HEALTH PROMOTION BOXES

P9-CFX-716

Gene Therapy, 57
The Percentage of Child Medication–Related Poisoning Deaths Is Increasing, 85
Air Pollution Reported as Largest Single Environmental Health Risk, 86
Low-Level Lead Exposure Harms Children: A Renewed Call for Primary Prevention, 88
Low-Risk Alcohol Drinking Guidelines, 92
Hyponatremia and Older Adults, 122
Potassium Intake: Hypertension and Stroke, 123
Tuberculosis and the Indigenous Population in Canada, 178
Risk of HIV Transmission Associated With Sexual Practices, 196
Glucocorticoids, Insulin, Inflammation, and Obesity, 222
Psychosocial Stress and Progression to Coronary Heart Disease, 223
Acute Emotional Stress and Adverse Heart Effects, 228
Partner's Survival and Spouse's Hospitalizations and/or Death, 228
Global Cancer Statistics and Risk Factors Associated With Causes of Cancer Death, 274
World Health Organization Cancer Prevention Strategies, 275
Increasing Use of Computed Tomography Scans and Associated Risks, 287
Rising Incidence of HPV-Associated Oropharyngeal Cancers, 293
Radiation Risks and Pediatric Computed Tomography: Data from the US National Cancer Institute, 306
Magnetic Fields and Development of Pediatric Cancer, 306
Bone Marrow Transplantation: Improving Outcomes for Canadian Children and Adolescent Cancer Patients, 307
Neuroplasticity, 313
Reducing Risk Factors Associated With Alzheimer's Disease, 376
Tourette Syndrome, 382
Prevention of Stroke in Women, 406
West Nile Virus, 414
Prevention of Fetal Alcohol Spectrum Disorders, 427
Growth Hormone Supplementation in Aging, 451
Vitamin D, 454
Type 1 Diabetes Mellitus, 479
Type 2 Diabetes Mellitus, 481
Sticky Platelets, 511
Prevention of Iron-Deficiency Anemia in Infants and Children, 561
B-type Natriuretic Peptide and Heart Failure, 598
Hypertension, 608
Obesity and Hypertension, 609
Recommendations for Managing Cholesterol, 619
Women and Microvascular Angina, 621
Canadian Heart Failure Statistics, 639
Sepsis Prevention: Central Line–Associated Bloodstream Infection, 651
The Surviving Sepsis Guidelines, 652
Endocarditis Risk, 666
Childhood Obesity in Canada, 676
Asthma, 706
Tips to Keep Lungs Healthy, 709
Ventilator-Associated Pneumonia, 712
Facts on Tobacco Use, 718
Lung Cancer, 720
Exercise-Induced Bronchoconstriction, 734
Cystic Fibrosis, 736
Vitamin D Supplementation, 752
Kidney Failure in Canada, 754
Urinary Tract Infection and Antibiotic Resistance, 766
Childhood Urinary Tract Infections, 789
Nutrition and Premenstrual Syndrome, 824
Nonsurgical Management of Vaginal Prolapse, 828
Screening With the Papanicolaou Test and with the Human Papillomavirus DNA Test, 834
Cervical Cancer Primary Prevention, 836
Breast Cancer Screening Mammography, 847
Acetaminophen and Acute Liver Failure, 915
Clostridium difficile and Diarrhea, 923
The Impact of Inflammatory Bowel Disease in Canada, 936
Promotion of Physical Activity in Canadian Schools, 940
Childhood Obesity and Fatty Liver Disease in Canada, 982
Tendon and Ligament Repair, 1007
Managing Tendinopathy, 1017
The Cost of Osteoporosis: Facts and Figures, 1022
Calcium, Vitamin D, and Bone Health, 1025
New Treatments for Osteoporosis, 1026
Musculo-skeletal Molecular Imaging, 1035
Psoriasis and Comorbidities, 1084
Melanoma in People With Darkly Pigmented Skin, 1094

evolve

ELSEVIER

YOU'VE JUST PURCHASED MORE THAN A TEXTBOOK!

Evolve Student Resources for *Huether: Understanding Pathophysiology, First Canadian Edition*, include the following:

- More than 100 **animations** help students visualize difficult material
- **Case studies** with questions and answers put content in real-life scenarios
- Printable **key points** put the "Did You Understand?" feature from the text into the hands of students for on-the-go review
- More than 585 **review questions** with answers provide a useful study tool

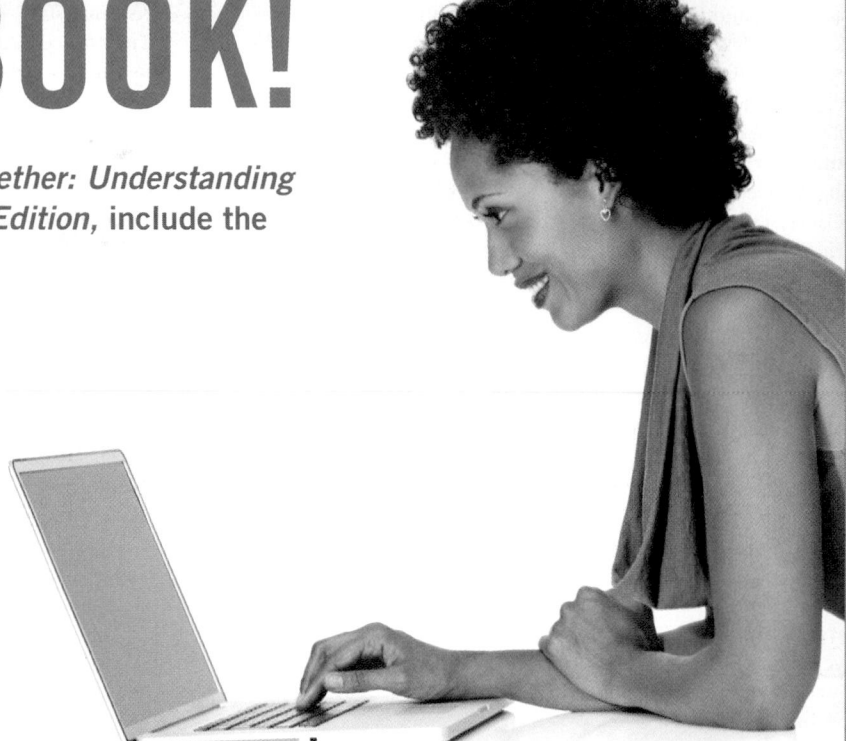

Activate the complete learning experience that comes with each textbook purchase by registering at

http://evolve.elsevier.com/Canada/Huether/pathophysiology

REGISTER TODAY!

You can now purchase Elsevier products on Evolve!
Go to evolve.elsevier.com/html/shop-promo.html to search and browse for products.

2015v1.0

First Canadian Edition

Understanding Pathophysiology

Mohamed Toufic El-Hussein, RN, PhD
Associate Professor, School of Nursing
Faculty of Health, Community & Education
Mount Royal University
Calgary, Alberta

Kelly Power-Kean, MHS, NP, RN
Center for Nursing Studies
Memorial University
St. John's, Newfoundland

Stephanie Zettel, BN, MN
Associate Professor
School of Nursing and Midwifery
Mount Royal University
Calgary, Alberta

U.S. AUTHORS

Sue E. Huether, MS, PhD
Professor Emeritus
College of Nursing
University of Utah
Salt Lake City, Utah

Kathryn L. McCance, MS, PhD
Professor Emeritus
College of Nursing
University of Utah
Salt Lake City, Utah

U.S. Section Editors

Valentina L. Brashers, MD
Professor of Nursing and Woodard Clinical Scholar
Attending Physician in Internal Medicine
University of Virginia Health System
Charlottesville, Virginia

Neal S. Rote, PhD
Academic Vice-Chair and Director of Research
Department of Obstetrics and Gynecology
University Hospitals Case Medical Center
William H. Weir, MD, Professor of Reproductive Biology and Pathology
Case Western Reserve University School of Medicine
Cleveland, Ohio

ELSEVIER

ELSEVIER

UNDERSTANDING PATHOPHYSIOLOGY, FIRST CANADIAN EDITION
ISBN: 978-1-77172-117-2
Copyright © 2018 Elsevier Canada, a division of Reed Elsevier Canada, Ltd.

This adaptation of *Understanding Pathophysiology*, Sixth Edition, by Sue E. Huether and Kathryn L. McCance is published by arrangement with Elsevier, Inc.

ISBN: 978-0-323-35409-7

Copyright © 2017, Elsevier Inc. All rights reserved.
Previous editions copyrighted 2012, 2008, 2004, 2000, 1996.

No part of this publication may be reproduced or transmitted in any form or by any means, electronic or mechanical, including photocopying, recording, or any information storage and retrieval system, without permission in writing from the publisher. Reproducing passages from this book without such written permission is an infringement of copyright law.

Requests for permission to make copies of any part of the work should be mailed to: College Licensing Officer, access ©, 1 Yonge Street, Suite 1900, Toronto, ON M5E 1E5. Fax: (416) 868-1621. All other inquiries should be directed to the publisher.

Every reasonable effort has been made to acquire permission for copyrighted material used in this edition and to acknowledge all such indebtedness accurately. Any errors and omissions called to the publisher's attention will be corrected in future printings.

Notices

Knowledge and best practice in this field are constantly changing. As new research and experience broaden our understanding, changes in research methods, professional practices, or medical treatment may become necessary.

Practitioners and researchers must always rely on their own experience and knowledge in evaluating and using any information, methods, compounds, or experiments described herein. In using such information or methods they should be mindful of their own safety and the safety of others, including parties for whom they have a professional responsibility.

With respect to any drug or pharmaceutical products identified, readers are advised to check the most current information provided (i) on procedures featured or (ii) by the manufacturer of each product to be administered, to verify the recommended dose or formula, the method and duration of administration, and contraindications. It is the responsibility of practitioners, relying on their own experience and knowledge of their patients, to make diagnoses, to determine dosages and the best treatment for each individual patient, and to take all appropriate safety precautions.

To the fullest extent of the law, neither the Publisher nor the authors, contributors, or editors assume any liability for any injury and/or damage to persons or property as a matter of products liability, negligence or otherwise, or from any use or operation of any methods, products, instructions, or ideas contained in the material herein.

Library and Archives Canada Cataloguing in Publication
Huether, Sue E., author
Understanding pathophysiology / Sue Huether, Kelly Power-Kean, Mohamed El-Hussein, Kathryn McCance, Stephanie Zettel. – First Canadian edition.
ISBN 978-1-77172-117-2 (softcover)
1. Physiology, Pathological–Textbooks. 2. Physiology, Pathological–Canada–Textbooks. I. Title.
RB113.H84 2018 616.07 C2017-903057-4

Cover Photo Credits
Outer left: Antibody and antigen – © Stefanie Winkler/Dreamstime.com
Inner left: Bacteria attacking the immune system – © Science Pics/Dreamstime.com
Inner right: Virus in blood – © Rangpl/Dreamstime.com
Outer right: T-cell – © Andreus/Dreamstime.com

VP Medical and Canadian Education: Madelene J. Hyde
Content Strategist (Acquisitions): Roberta A. Spinosa-Millman
Content Development Manager: Laurie Gower
Content Development Specialist: Martina van de Velde
Publishing Services Manager: Julie Eddy
Senior Project Manager: Richard Barber
Cover Designer: Brett J. Miller, BJM Graphic Design and Communications
Book Designer: Maggie Reid

Elsevier Canada
420 Main Street East, Suite 636, Milton, ON, Canada L9T 5G3
Phone: 416-644-7053

Printed in Canada

Last digit is the print number: 9 8 7 6 5 4 3 2 1

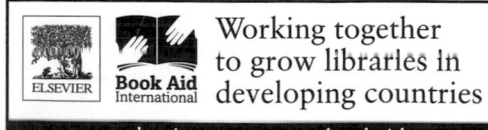

REVIEWERS

Colleen Battista, BScN, RN, MN
Nursing Faculty
Collaborative BScN Program
St. Lawrence College/Laurentian University
St. Lawrence College, Cornwall Campus
Cornwall, Ontario

Brenda Dafoe Enns, BA, RN, MN
Nursing Instructor
Baccalaureate Nursing Program
School of Health Sciences and Community Services
Red River College
Winnipeg, Manitoba

Daphne Gill, BA, PhD
Sessional Lecturer
Department of Biology
University of Prince Edward Island
Charlottetown, Prince Edward Island

Heather Helpard, BN, MN, PhD
Assistant Professor
School of Nursing
Dalhousie University
Halifax, Nova Scotia

Anne-Marie Kowatsch, BSc, MSc
Instructor
Baccalaureate Nursing Program
Red River College
Winnipeg, Manitoba

Tara Lyster, BScN, RN, MN
Sessional Lecturer
School of Nursing
Thompson Rivers University
Kamloops, British Columbia

Joan Mills, RN, MN, CCN(C)
Assistant Professor
Faculty of Nursing
MacEwan University
Edmonton, Alberta

Deborah Morrison, RN, BScN, MN
Nursing Chair—Interim
School of Health & Community Services
Durham College
Oshawa, Ontario

Maha Othman, MD, MSc, PhD
Professor
School of Baccalaureate Nursing
St. Lawrence College
Kingston, Ontario

Jennifer Perry, RN(EC), NP-PHC, PhD
Professor
School of Nursing
St. Lawrence College
Kingston, Ontario

Kara Sealock, BN, RN, MEd, CNCC(C)
Nursing Instructor
Faculty of Nursing
University of Calgary
Calgary, Alberta

CONTRIBUTORS

The editors would like to acknowledge the following contributors, whose work is the foundation on which the First Canadian Edition is based:

Barbara J. Boss, RN, PHD, CFNP, CANP
Retired Professor of Nursing
University of Mississippi Medical Center
Jackson, Mississippi

Kristen Lee Carroll, MD
Chief of Staff
Medical Staff/Orthopedics
Shriners Hospital for Children
Professor of Orthopedics
University of Utah
Salt Lake City, Utah

Margaret F. Clayton, PhD, APRN
Associate Professor and Assistant Dean for the PhD Program
College of Nursing
University of Utah
Salt Lake City, Utah

Christy L. Crowther-Radulewicz, RN, MS, CRNP
Nurse Practitioner
Orthopedic Surgery
Anne Arundel Orthopedic Surgeons
Annapolis, Maryland

Susanna G. Cunningham, BSN, MA, PhD, RN, FAHA, FAAN
Professor Emeritus
Department of Biobehavioral Nursing
School of Nursing
University of Washington
Seattle, Washington

Sara J. Fidanza, MS, RN, CNS-BC, CPNP-BC
Digestive Health Institute
Children's Hospital Colorado
Clinical Faculty
University of Colorado College of Nursing
Aurora, Colorado

Diane P. Genereux, PhD
Assistant Professor
Department of Biology
Westfield State
Westfield, Massachusetts

Todd Cameron Grey, MD
Chief Medical Examiner
Office of the Medical Examiner
State of Utah
Salt Lake City, Utah

Robert E. Jones, MD, FACP, FACE
Professor of Medicine
Endocrinology Division
University of Utah School of Medicine
Salt Lake City, Utah

Lynn B. Jorde, PhD
H.A. and Edna Benning Presidential Professor and Chair
Department of Human Genetics
University of Utah School of Medicine
Salt Lake City, Utah

Lynne M. Kerr, MD, PhD
Associate Professor
Department of Pediatrics, Division of Pediatric Neurology
University of Utah Medical Center
Salt Lake City, Utah

Nancy E. Kline,[†] PhD, RN, CPNP, FAAN
Director, Nursing Research, Medicine
Patient Services/Emergency Department
Boston Children's Hospital
Boston, Massachusetts

Lauri A. Linder, PhD, APRN, CPON
Assistant Professor
College of Nursing
University of Utah
Clinical Nurse Specialist
Cancer Transplant Center
Primary Children's Hospital
Salt Lake City, Utah

Sue Ann McCann, MSN, RN, DNC
Programmatic Nurse Specialist
Nursing
Clinical Research Coordinator
Dermatology
University of Pittsburgh Medical Center
Pittsburgh, Pennsylvania

Nancy L. McDaniel, MD
Associate Professor of Pediatrics
University of Virginia
Charlottesville, Virginia

Afsoon Moktar, PhD, EMBA, CT (ASCP)
Associate Professor
School of Physician Assistant Studies
Massachusetts College of Pharmacy and Health Sciences University
Boston, Massachusetts

Noreen Heer Nicol, PhD, RN, FNP, NEA-BC
Associate Professor
College of Nursing
University of Colorado
Denver, Colorado

Nancy Pike, PhD, RN, CPNP-AC, FAAN
Assistant Professor
UCLA School of Nursing
Pediatric Nurse Practitioner
Cardiothoracic Surgery
Children's Hospital Los Angeles
Los Angeles, California

Patricia Ring, RN, MSN, PNP, BC
Pediatric Nephrology
Children's Hospital of Wisconsin
Wauwatosa, Wisconsin

Anna E. Roche, MSN, RN, CPNP, CPON
Pediatric Nurse Practitioner
Dana Farber/Boston Children's Cancer and Blood Disorders Center
Boston, Massachusetts

George W. Rodway, PhD, APRN
Associate Clinical Professor
Betty Irene Moore School of Nursing at UC Davis
Sacramento, California

[†]Deceased.

Sharon Sables-Baus, PhD, MPA, RN, PCNS-BC
Associate Professor
University of Colorado
College of Nursing and School of Medicine
Department of Pediatrics
Pediatric Nurse Scientist
Children's Hospital Colorado
Aurora, Colorado

Anna Schwartz, PhD, FNP-C, FAAN
Associate Professor
School of Nursing
Northern Arizona University
Flagstaff, Arizona
Affiliate Associate Professor
Biobehavioral Nursing and Health Systems
University of Washington
Seattle, Washington

Joan Shea, MSN, RN, CPON
Staff Nurse III
Hematology/Oncology/Clinical Research
Boston Children's Hospital
Boston, Massachusetts

Lorey K. Takahashi, PhD
Professor of Psychology
Department of Psychology
University of Hawaii at Manoa
Honolulu, Hawaii

David M. Virshup, MD
Professor and Director
Program in Cancer and Stem Cell Biology
Duke-NUS Graduate Medical School
Singapore
Professor of Pediatrics
Duke University School of Medicine
Durham, North Carolina

PREFACE

Based on the sixth US edition of *Understanding Pathophysiology*, the first Canadian edition has been updated and revised with consideration of the rapid advances in molecular and cellular biology. Many sections have been rewritten or reorganized to provide a foundation for better understanding of the mechanisms of disease. Integrated throughout the text are concepts from the basic sciences, including genetics, epigenetics, gene–environment interaction, immunity, and inflammation. The text has been written to assist students with the translation of the concepts and processes of pathophysiology into clinical practice and to promote lifelong learning. All laboratory values were changed to measure results in SI units and to fit the Canadian context. Canadian statistics were also embedded, based on updated data from Health Canada, the Canadian Institute for Health Information, and other relevant governmental organizations. Furthermore, Indigenous perspectives were integrated and explored in relation to the epidemiology of pathophysiological conditions in Canada. Lastly, feedback from Canadian reviewers was addressed with a critical appreciation of relevant issues and application in current nursing practice.

Although the primary focus of the text is pathophysiology, we include discussions of the following interconnected topics to highlight their importance for clinical practice:

- A lifespan approach that includes special sections on aging and separate chapters on children
- Epidemiology and incidence rates showing regional and worldwide differences that reflect the importance of environmental and lifestyle factors on disease initiation and progression
- Sex differences that affect epidemiology and pathophysiology
- Molecular biology—mechanisms of normal cell function and how their alteration leads to disease
- Clinical manifestations, summaries of treatment, and health promotion/risk reduction

ORGANIZATION AND CONTENT

The book is organized into two parts: Part One, Basic Concepts of Pathophysiology, and Part Two, Body Systems and Diseases.

Part One: Basic Concepts of Pathophysiology

Part One introduces basic principles and processes that are important for a contemporary understanding of the pathophysiology of common diseases. The concepts include descriptions of cellular communication; forms of cell injury; genes and genetic disease; epigenetics; fluid and electrolytes and acid and base balance; immunity and inflammation; mechanisms of infection; stress, coping, and illness; and tumour biology. Chapter 3, *Epigenetics and Disease* explains the way heritable changes in gene expression—*phenotype* without a change in *genotype*—are influenced by several factors, including age, environment and lifestyle, and disease state.

The first Canadian edition includes significant revisions to Part One, incorporating new or updated information on the following topics:

- Updated content on cell membranes, cell junctions, intercellular communication, transport by vesicles, and stem cells (Chapter 1)
- Updated content on epigenetics and disease (Chapter 3)
- Updated content on cellular adaptations, oxidative stress, chemical injury, types of cell death, and aging, with a focus on Canadian epidemiology (Chapter 4)
- Updates regarding mechanisms of human defence—characteristics of innate and adaptive immunity (Chapters 6 and 7)
- Updated content on mechanisms of infection, antibiotic-resistant disease, and alterations in immune defence (Chapter 8)
- Updated content on stress, inflammation, hormones, and disease (Chapter 9)
- Updated chapter on tumour biology (after an extensive reorganization in the sixth US edition) (Chapter 10)
- Updated chapters on the epidemiology of cancer (after an extensive reorganization in the sixth US edition) (Chapters 11 and 12)

Part Two: Body Systems and Diseases

Part Two presents the pathophysiology of the most common alterations according to body system. To promote readability and comprehension, we have used a logical sequence and uniform approach in presenting the content of the units and chapters. Each unit focuses on a specific organ system and contains chapters related to anatomy and physiology, the pathophysiology of the most common diseases, and common alterations in children. The anatomy and physiology content is presented as a review to enhance the learner's understanding of the structural and functional changes inherent in pathophysiology. A brief summary of normal aging effects is included at the end of these review chapters. The general organization of each disease or disorder discussion includes an introductory paragraph on relevant risk factors and epidemiology, a significant focus on pathophysiology and clinical manifestations, and then a brief review of evaluation and treatment.

The information on reproductive pathophysiology is presented in two chapters, with a new chapter, *Alterations of the Male Reproductive System.* Other significant revisions to Part Two, which have been retained in the first Canadian edition, include new and/or updated information on the following topics:

- Mechanisms of pain transmission, pain syndromes, and categories of sleep disorders (Chapter 14)
- Alterations in levels of consciousness, seizure disorders, and delirium. Pathogenesis of degenerative brain diseases, the dementias, movement disorders, traumatic brain and spinal cord injury, stroke syndromes, headache, and infections and structural malformations of the central nervous system (Chapters 15, 16, 17)
- The pathogenesis of type 2 diabetes mellitus (Chapter 19)
- Platelet function and coagulation; anemias, alterations of leukocyte function and myeloid and lymphoid tumours (Chapters 20 and 21)
- Extensive chapter revisions of alterations of hematological function in children (Chapter 22)
- Extensive chapter revisions on structure and function of the cardiovascular and lymphatic systems (Chapter 23)
- Mechanisms of atherosclerosis, hypertension, coronary artery disease, heart failure, and shock (Chapter 24)
- Pediatric valvular disorders, heart failure, hypertension, obesity, and heart disease (Chapter 25)
- Pathophysiology of acute lung injury, asthma, pneumonia, lung cancer, respiratory distress in the newborn, and cystic fibrosis (Chapters 27 and 28)
- Mechanisms of kidney stone formation, immune processes of glomerulonephritis, and acute and chronic kidney injury (Chapters 30 and 31)
- Female and male reproductive disorders, female and male reproductive cancers, breast diseases and mechanisms of breast cancer, prostate cancer, male breast cancer, and sexually transmitted infections (Chapters 33 and 34)

- Gastroesophageal reflux, nonalcoholic liver disease, inflammatory bowel disease, viral hepatitis, obesity, gluten-sensitive enteropathy, and necrotizing enterocolitis (Chapters 36 and 37)
- Bone cells, bone remodelling, joint and tendon diseases, osteoporosis, rheumatoid arthritis, and osteoarthritis (Chapters 38 and 39)
- Congenital and acquired musculo-skeletal disorders, and muscular dystrophies in children (Chapter 40)
- Psoriasis, discoid lupus erythematosus, and atopic dermatitis (Chapters 41 and 42)
- Cancer of the various organ systems was updated for all chapters.

FEATURES TO PROMOTE LEARNING

A number of features are incorporated into this text that guide and support learning and understanding, including:

- *Chapter Outlines* including page numbers for easy reference
- *Quick Check* questions strategically placed throughout each chapter to help readers confirm their understanding of the material; answers are included on the textbook's Evolve website
- *Health Promotion* boxes with a strategic focus on evidence-informed health promotion and current health practices
- *Risk Factors* boxes for selected diseases
- End-of-chapter *Did You Understand?* summaries that condense the major concepts of each chapter into an easy-to-review list format; printable versions of these are available on the textbook's Evolve website
- *Key Terms* set in blue boldface in text and listed, with page numbers, at the end of each chapter
- Special boxes for *Aging* and *Pediatrics* content that highlight discussions of lifespan alterations

ART PROGRAM

All of the figures and photographs have been carefully reviewed, and some have been revised or updated. This edition features approximately 1 000 images. The figures are designed to help students visually understand sometimes difficult and complex material. Hundreds of high-quality photographs show clinical manifestations, pathological specimens, and clinical imaging techniques. Micrographs show normal and abnormal cellular structure. The combination of illustrations, algorithms, photographs, and use of colour for tables and boxes allows a more precise understanding of essential information.

TEACHING/LEARNING PACKAGE

For Students

The free electronic **Student Resources** on Evolve include review questions and answers, numerous animations, answers to the Quick Check questions in the book, printable key points, and bonus case studies with questions and answers. A comprehensive *Glossary* of pathophysiological conditions for the textbook of more than 600 terms helps students with the often difficult terminology related to pathophysiology; this is available both on Evolve and in the electronic version of the textbook. These electronic resources enhance learning options for students. Go to http://evolve.elsevier.com/Canada/Huether/pathophysiology.

For Instructors

The electronic **Instructor Resources** on Evolve are available free to instructors with qualified adoptions of the textbook and include the following: TEACH Lesson Plans with case studies to assist with clinical application; a Test Bank of more than 1 200 items; PowerPoint Presentations for each chapter, with integrated images, audience response questions, and case studies; and an Image Collection of approximately 1 000 key figures from the text. All of these teaching resources are also available to instructors on the book's Evolve website. Plus the Evolve Learning System provides a comprehensive suite of course communication and organization tools that allow you to upload your class calendar and syllabus, post scores and announcements, and more. Go to http://evolve.elsevier.com/Canada/Huether/pathophysiology.

The most exciting part of the learning support package is **Pathophysiology Online**, a complete set of online modules that provide thoroughly developed lessons on the most important and difficult topics in pathophysiology supplemented with illustrations, animations, interactive activities, interactive algorithms, self-assessment reviews, and exams. Instructors can use it to enhance traditional classroom lecture courses or for distance and online-only courses. Students can use it as a self-guided study tool.

ACKNOWLEDGMENTS

This book would not be possible without the knowledge and expertise of the contributors to the previous US editions. Their reviews and synthesis of the evidence and clear and concise presentation of information are strengths of this text, and facilitated the adaptation of this information for the Canadian context.

The reviewers for this edition provided excellent recommendations for focus of content and revisions, based on the Canadian context, with thoughtful consideration of Indigenous perspectives on health, wellness, and disease. We appreciate their insightful work.

We are thankful to Martina van de Velde, our Content Development Specialist, for overseeing this wonderful project, providing insights regarding formatting, and suggesting content to maintain a streamlined manuscript that flows seamlessly from one section to another. We are also thankful to Roberta A. Spinosa-Millman, Content Strategist, for recruiting such a great team! Collaborating with one another on this project has been a great learning experience, and one that would not have been possible without Roberta having brought us all together.

We have respected the contributions from US authors, Sue E. Huether and Kathryn L. McCance, in this first Canadian edition and recognize the innovation and clarity that these authors bring to pathophysiology.

Lastly, we would like to thank our families for their undying support. They are what makes this work possible!

Mohamed El-Hussein
Kelly Power-Kean
Stephanie Zettel

INTRODUCTION TO PATHOPHYSIOLOGY

The word root *"patho"* is derived from the Greek word *pathos*, which means suffering. The Greek word root *"logos"* means discourse or, more simply, system of formal study, and *"physio"* refers to functions of an organism. Altogether, pathophysiology is the study of the underlying changes in body physiology (molecular, cellular, and organ systems) that result from disease or injury. Important, however, is the inextricable component of suffering and the psychological, spiritual, social, cultural, and economic implications of disease.

The science of pathophysiology seeks to provide an understanding of the mechanisms of disease and to explain how and why alterations in body structure and function lead to the signs and symptoms of disease. Understanding pathophysiology guides health care providers in the planning, selection, and evaluation of therapies and treatments.

Knowledge of human anatomy and physiology and the interrelationship among the various cells and organ systems of the body is an essential foundation for the study of pathophysiology. Review of this subject matter enhances comprehension of pathophysiological events and processes. Understanding pathophysiology also entails the utilization of principles, concepts, and basic knowledge from other fields of study including pathology, genetics, epigenetics, immunology, and epidemiology. A number of terms are used to focus the discussion of pathophysiology; they may be used interchangeably at times, but that does not necessarily indicate that they have the same meaning. Those terms are reviewed here for the purpose of clarification.

Pathology is the investigation of structural alterations in cells, tissues, and organs, which can help identify the cause of a particular disease. Pathology differs from **pathogenesis**, which is the pattern of tissue changes associated with the *development* of disease. **Etiology** refers to the study of the *cause* of disease. Diseases may be caused by infection, heredity, gene–environment interactions, alterations in immunity, malignancy, malnutrition, degeneration, or trauma. Diseases that have no identifiable cause are termed **idiopathic**. Diseases that occur as a result of medical treatment are termed **iatrogenic** (e.g., some antibiotics can injure the kidney and cause kidney failure). Diseases that are acquired as a consequence of being in a hospital environment are called **health care–associated diseases**. An infection that develops as a result of a person's immune system being depressed after receiving cancer treatment during a hospital stay would be defined as a health care–associated infection.

Diagnosis is the naming or identification of a disease. A diagnosis is made from an evaluation of the evidence accumulated from the presenting signs and symptoms, health and medical history, physical examination, laboratory tests, and imaging. A **prognosis** is the expected outcome of a disease. **Acute disease** is the sudden appearance of signs and symptoms that last only a short time. **Chronic disease** develops more slowly, and the signs and symptoms last for a long time, perhaps for a lifetime. Chronic diseases may have a pattern of remission and exacerbation. **Remissions** are periods when symptoms disappear or diminish significantly. **Exacerbations** are periods when the symptoms become worse or more severe. A **complication** is the onset of a disease in a person who is already coping with another existing disease (e.g., a person who has undergone surgery to remove a diseased appendix may develop the complication of a wound infection or pneumonia). **Sequelae** are unwanted outcomes of having a disease or are the result of trauma, such as paralysis resulting from a stroke or severe scarring resulting from a burn.

Clinical manifestations are the signs and symptoms or *evidence* of disease. **Signs** are objective alterations that can be observed or measured by another person, measures of bodily functions such as pulse rate, blood pressure, body temperature, or white blood cell count. Some signs are **local**, such as redness or swelling, and other signs are **systemic**, such as fever. **Symptoms** are subjective experiences reported by the person with disease, such as pain, nausea, or shortness of breath; and they vary from person to person. The **prodromal period** of a disease is the time during which a person experiences vague symptoms such as fatigue or loss of appetite before the onset of specific signs and symptoms. The term **insidious symptoms** describes vague or nonspecific feelings and an awareness that there is a change within the body. Some diseases have a **latent period**, a time during which no symptoms are readily apparent in the affected person, but the disease is nevertheless present in the body; an example is the incubation phase of an infection or the early growth phase of a tumour. A **syndrome** is a group of symptoms that occur together and may be caused by several interrelated problems or a specific disease; severe acute respiratory syndrome (SARS), for example, presents with a set of symptoms that include headache, fever, body aches, an overall feeling of discomfort, and sometimes dry cough and difficulty breathing. A **disorder** is an abnormality of function; this term also can refer to an illness or a particular problem such as a bleeding disorder.

Epidemiology is the study of tracking patterns or disease occurrence and transmission among populations and by geographical areas. **Incidence** of a disease is the number of new cases occurring in a specific time period. **Prevalence** of a disease is the number of existing cases within a population during a specific time period.

Risk factors, also known as **predisposing factors**, increase the probability that disease will occur, but these factors are not the *cause* of disease. Risk factors include heredity, age, gender, race, environment, and lifestyle. A **precipitating factor** is a condition or event that *does* cause a pathological event or disorder. For example, asthma is precipitated by exposure to an allergen, or angina (pain) is precipitated by exertion.

Pathophysiology is an exciting field of study that is ever-changing as new discoveries are made. Understanding pathophysiology empowers health care providers with the knowledge of how and why disease develops and informs their decision making to ensure optimal health care outcomes. Embedded in the study of pathophysiology is understanding that suffering is a personal, individual experience and a major component of disease.

CONTENTS

PART ONE Basic Concepts of Pathophysiology

UNIT 1 The Cell

1 Cellular Biology, 1
Kathryn L. McCance and Stephanie Zettel
Prokaryotes and Eukaryotes, 1
Cellular Functions, 2
Structure and Function of Cellular Components, 2
Nucleus, 2
Cytoplasmic Organelles, 2
Plasma Membranes, 2
Cellular Receptors, 9
Cell-to-Cell Adhesions, 10
Extracellular Matrix, 10
Specialized Cell Junctions, 12
Cellular Communication and Signal Transduction, 12
Cellular Metabolism, 14
Role of Adenosine Triphosphate, 16
Food and Production of Cellular Energy, 16
Oxidative Phosphorylation, 16
Membrane Transport: Cellular Intake and Output, 17
Electrolytes as Solutes, 18
Transport by Vesicle Formation, 21
Movement of Electrical Impulses: Membrane Potentials, 24
Cellular Reproduction: The Cell Cycle, 25
Phases of Mitosis and Cytokinesis, 25
Rates of Cellular Division, 26
Growth Factors, 26
Tissues, 27
Tissue Formation, 27
Types of Tissues, 27

2 Genes and Genetic Diseases, 38
Lynn B. Jorde and Stephanie Zettel
DNA, RNA, and Proteins: Heredity at the Molecular Level, 38
Definitions, 38
From Genes to Proteins, 39
Chromosomes, 42
Chromosome Aberrations and Associated Diseases, 42
Elements of Formal Genetics, 49
Phenotype and Genotype, 49
Dominance and Recessiveness, 49
Transmission of Genetic Diseases, 50
Autosomal Dominant Inheritance, 50
Autosomal Recessive Inheritance, 52
X-Linked Inheritance, 54
Linkage Analysis and Gene Mapping, 56
Classic Pedigree Analysis, 56
Complete Human Gene Map: Prospects and Benefits, 57
Multifactorial Inheritance, 58

3 Epigenetics and Disease, 62
Diane P. Genereux, Lynn B. Jorde, and Stephanie Zettel
Epigenetic Mechanisms, 62
DNA Methylation, 62
Histone Modifications, 63
RNA-Based Mechanisms, 64
Epigenetics and Human Development, 64
Genomic Imprinting, 64
Prader-Willi and Angelman Syndromes, 64
Beckwith-Wiedemann Syndrome, 65
Russell-Silver Syndrome, 66
Inheritance of Epigenetic States, 66
Epigenetics and Nutrition, 66
Epigenetics and Maternal Care, 66
Epigenetics and Mental Illness, 67
Epigenetic Disease in the Context of Genetic Abnormalities, 67
Twin Studies Provide Insights on Epigenetic Modification, 68
Molecular Approaches to Understand Epigenetic Disease, 68
Epigenetics and Cancer, 68
DNA Methylation and Cancer, 68
microRNAs and Cancer, 69
Epigenetic Screening for Cancer, 69
Emerging Strategies for the Treatment of Epigenetic Disease, 69
Future Directions, 71

4 Altered Cellular and Tissue Biology, 74
Kathryn L. McCance, Todd Cameron Grey, and Stephanie Zettel
Cellular Adaptation, 75
Atrophy, 75
Hypertrophy, 76
Hyperplasia, 77
Dysplasia: Not a True Adaptive Change, 77
Metaplasia, 78
Cellular Injury, 78
General Mechanisms of Cellular Injury, 79
Hypoxic Injury, 80
Free Radicals and Reactive Oxygen Species Injury: Oxidative Stress, 82
Chemical or Toxic Injury, 83
Unintentional and Intentional Injuries, 93
Infectious Injury, 96
Immunological and Inflammatory Injury, 96
Manifestations of Cellular Injury: Accumulations, 96
Water, 97
Lipids and Carbohydrates, 97
Glycogen, 98
Proteins, 99
Pigments, 99
Calcium, 100
Urate, 100
Systemic Manifestations, 101

Cellular Death, 101
Necrosis, 101
Apoptosis, 105
Autophagy, 106
Aging and Altered Cellular and Tissue Biology, 107
Normal Lifespan, Life Expectancy, and Quality-Adjusted Life Year, 108
Degenerative Extracellular Changes, 108
Cellular Aging, 108
Tissue and Systemic Aging, 109
Frailty, 109
Somatic Death, 109

5 Fluids and Electrolytes, Acids and Bases, 115
Sue E. Huether and Stephanie Zettel
Distribution of Body Fluids and Electrolytes, 115
Water Movement Between Plasma and Interstitial Fluid, 115
Water Movement Between ICF and ECF, 116
Alterations in Water Movement, 116
Edema, 116
Sodium, Chloride, and Water Balance, 117
Alterations in Sodium, Chloride, and Water Balance, 120
Isotonic Alterations, 121
Hypertonic Alterations, 121
Hypotonic Alterations, 121
Alterations in Potassium and Other Electrolytes, 122
Potassium, 122
Other Electrolytes—Calcium, Phosphate, and Magnesium, 126
Acid-Base Balance, 126
Hydrogen Ion and pH, 126
Buffer Systems, 126
Acid-Base Imbalances, 128
PEDIATRIC CONSIDERATIONS: Distribution of Body Fluids, 132
GERIATRIC CONSIDERATIONS: Distribution of Body Fluids, 132

UNIT 2 Mechanisms of Self-Defence

6 Innate Immunity: Inflammation and Wound Healing, 135
Neal S. Rote and Stephanie Zettel
Human Defence Mechanisms, 135
First Line of Defence: Physical and Biochemical Barriers and the Human Microbiome, 135
Second Line of Defence: Inflammation, 138
Plasma Protein Systems and Inflammation, 140
Cellular Components of Inflammation, 142
Acute and Chronic Inflammation, 149
Local Manifestations of Acute Inflammation, 150
Systemic Manifestations of Acute Inflammation, 150
Chronic Inflammation, 150
Wound Healing, 152
Phase I: Inflammation, 153
Phase II: Proliferation and New Tissue Formation, 153
Phase III: Remodelling and Maturation, 154
Dysfunctional Wound Healing, 154
PEDIATRIC CONSIDERATIONS: Age-Related Factors Affecting Innate Immunity in the Newborn Child, 155
GERIATRIC CONSIDERATIONS: Age-Related Factors Affecting Innate Immunity in Older Adults, 155

7 Adaptive Immunity, 159
Neal S. Rote and Stephanie Zettel
Third Line of Defence: Adaptive Immunity, 159
Antigens and Immunogens, 161
Antibodies, 161
Classes of Immunoglobulins, 162
Antigen–Antibody Binding, 163
Function of Antibodies, 163
Immune Response: Collaboration of B Cells and T Cells, 165
Generation of Clonal Diversity, 165
Clonal Selection, 168
Cell-Mediated Immunity, 171
T-Lymphocyte Function, 171
PEDIATRIC CONSIDERATIONS: Age-Related Factors Affecting Mechanisms of Self-Defence in the Newborn Child, 174
GERIATRIC CONSIDERATIONS: Age-Related Factors Affecting Mechanisms of Self-Defence in Older Adults, 174

8 Infection and Defects in Mechanisms of Defence, 177
Neal S. Rote and Stephanie Zettel
Infection, 177
Microorganisms and Humans: A Dynamic Relationship, 177
Countermeasures Against Infectious Microorganisms, 188
Deficiencies in Immunity, 190
Initial Clinical Presentation, 190
Primary (Congenital) Immune Deficiencies, 191
Secondary (Acquired) Immune Deficiencies, 193
Evaluation and Care of Those With Immune Deficiency, 193
Replacement Therapies for Immune Deficiencies, 193
AIDS, 195
Hypersensitivity: Allergy, Autoimmunity, and Alloimmunity, 199
Mechanisms of Hypersensitivity, 202
Antigenic Targets of Hypersensitivity Reactions, 208

9 Stress and Disease, 216
Margaret F. Clayton, Kathryn L. McCance, Lorey K. Takahashi, and Stephanie Zettel
Historical Background and General Concepts, 216
Stress Overview: Allostasis, Multiple Mediators, and Systems, 219
The Stress Response, 220
Regulation of the Hypothalamic-Pituitary-Adrenal System, 220
Neuroendocrine Regulation: Autonomic Nervous System, 222

Histamine and Other Hormones, 224
Role of the Immune System, 227
Stress, Personality, Coping, and Illness, 227
Coping, 228
GERIATRIC CONSIDERATIONS: Aging and the Stress–Age Syndrome, 230

UNIT 3 Cellular Proliferation: Cancer

10 Biology of Cancer, 235
Neal S. Rote, David M. Virshup, and Stephanie Zettel
Cancer Terminology and Characteristics, 235
Tumour Classification and Nomenclature, 235
The Biology of Cancer Cells, 238
Sustained Proliferative Signalling, 240
Evading Growth Suppressors, 243
Genomic Instability, 244
Enabling Replicative Immortality, 247
Inducing Angiogenesis, 247
Reprogramming Energy Metabolism, 248
Resisting Apoptotic Cell Death, 249
Tumour-Promoting Inflammation, 250
Evading Immune Destruction, 252
Activating Invasion and Metastasis, 253
Clinical Manifestations of Cancer, 256
Paraneoplastic Syndromes, 256
Pain, 256
Fatigue, 256
Cachexia, 256
Anemia, 258
Leukopenia and Thrombocytopenia, 259
Infection, 259
Gastro-intestinal Tract, 260
Hair and Skin, 260
Diagnosis, Characterization, and Treatment of Cancer, 260
Diagnosis and Staging, 260
Classification of Tumours: Classic Histology and Modern Genetics, 261
Treatment, 262

11 Cancer Epidemiology, 268
Kathryn L. McCance and Stephanie Zettel
Genetics, Epigenetics, and Tissue, 268
Incidence and Mortality Trends, 274
In Utero and Early Life Conditions, 274
Environmental and Lifestyle Factors, 276
Tobacco Use, 276
Diet, 277
Nutrition, Obesity, Alcohol Consumption, and Physical Activity: Impacts on Cancer, 277
Ionizing Radiation, 285
Ultraviolet Radiation, 289
Electromagnetic Radiation, 291
Infection, and Sexual and Reproductive Behaviour, 292
Other Viruses and Microorganisms, 293
Air Pollution, 293
Chemical and Occupational Hazards as Carcinogens, 294

12 Cancer in Children and Adolescents, 303
Lauri A. Linder, Nancy E. Kline, and Stephanie Zettel
Incidence, Etiology, and Types of Childhood Cancer, 303
Etiology, 304
Genetic and Genomic Factors, 305
Environmental Factors, 305
Prognosis, 307

PART TWO Body Systems and Diseases

UNIT 4 The Neurological System

13 Structure and Function of the Neurological System, 309
Lynne M. Kerr, Sue E. Huether, Richard A. Sugerman, and Kelly Power-Kean
Overview and Organization of the Nervous System, 309
Cells of the Nervous System, 309
The Neuron, 310
Neuroglia and Schwann Cells, 310
Nerve Injury and Regeneration, 311
The Nerve Impulse, 313
Synapses, 313
Neurotransmitters, 313
The Central Nervous System, 313
The Brain, 313
The Spinal Cord, 320
Motor Pathways, 322
Sensory Pathways, 322
Protective Structures of the Central Nervous System, 323
Blood Supply of the Central Nervous System, 325
The Peripheral Nervous System, 327
The Autonomic Nervous System, 328
Anatomy of the Sympathetic Nervous System, 328
Anatomy of the Parasympathetic Nervous System, 331
Neurotransmitters and Neuroreceptors, 331
Functions of the Autonomic Nervous System, 331
GERIATRIC CONSIDERATIONS: Aging and the Nervous System, 335

14 Pain, Temperature, Sleep, and Sensory Function, 338
George W. Rodway, Sue E. Huether, Jan Belden, and Kelly Power-Kean
Pain, 338
Theories of Pain, 338
Neuroanatomy of Pain, 339
Pain Modulation, 340
Clinical Descriptions of Pain, 342
Temperature Regulation, 344
Control of Body Temperature, 344
Temperature Regulation in Infants and Older Adults, 345
Pathogenesis of Fever, 346
Benefits of Fever, 346
Disorders of Temperature Regulation, 346

Sleep, 347
Sleep Disorders, 348
The Special Senses, 349
Vision, 349
Hearing, 354
Olfaction and Taste, 356
Somatosensory Function, 356
Touch, 356
Proprioception, 356
GERIATRIC CONSIDERATIONS: Aging and Changes in Vision, 357
GERIATRIC CONSIDERATIONS: Aging and Changes in Hearing, 357
GERIATRIC CONSIDERATIONS: Aging and Changes in Olfaction and Taste, 357

15 **Alterations in Cognitive Systems, Cerebral Hemodynamics, and Motor Function,** 363
Barbara J. Boss, Sue E. Huether, and Kelly Power-Kean
Alterations in Cognitive Systems, 363
Alterations in Arousal, 363
Alterations in Awareness, 369
Data-Processing Deficits, 371
Seizure Disorders, 376
Types of Seizure, 376
Alterations in Cerebral Hemodynamics, 377
Increased Intracranial Pressure, 378
Cerebral Edema, 379
Hydrocephalus, 380
Alterations in Neuromotor Function, 380
Alterations in Muscle Tone, 380
Alterations in Muscle Movement, 381
Upper and Lower Motor Neuron Syndromes, 385
Motor Neuron Diseases, 387
Amyotrophic Lateral Sclerosis, 388
Alterations in Complex Motor Performance, 389
Disorders of Posture (Stance), 389
Disorders of Gait, 389
Disorders of Expression, 389
Extrapyramidal Motor Syndromes, 390

16 **Disorders of the Central and Peripheral Nervous Systems and Neuromuscular Junction,** 394
Barbara J. Boss, Sue E. Huether, and Kelly Power-Kean
Central Nervous System Disorders, 394
Traumatic Brain and Spinal Cord Injury, 394
Degenerative Disorders of the Spine, 402
Cerebrovascular Disorders, 406
Headache, 410
Infection and Inflammation of the Central Nervous System, 411
Demyelinating Disorders, 415
Peripheral Nervous System and Neuromuscular Junction Disorders, 416
Peripheral Nervous System Disorders, 416
Neuromuscular Junction Disorders, 417
Tumours of the Central Nervous System, 417
Brain Tumours, 417
Spinal Cord Tumours, 421

17 **Alterations of Neurological Function in Children,** 426
Lynne M. Kerr, Sue E. Huether, Vinodh Narayanan, and Kelly Power-Kean
Development of the Nervous System in Children, 426
Structural Malformations, 427
Defects of Neural Tube Closure, 427
Craniostenosis, 430
Malformations of Brain Development, 431
Alterations in Function: Encephalopathies, 433
Static Encephalopathies, 433
Inherited Metabolic Disorders of the Central Nervous System, 433
Acute Encephalopathies, 434
Infections of the Central Nervous System, 435
Cerebrovascular Disease in Children, 435
Perinatal Stroke, 435
Childhood Stroke, 435
Epilepsy and Seizure Disorders in Children, 436
Childhood Tumours, 436
Brain Tumours, 436
Embryonal Tumours, 438

UNIT 5 The Endocrine System

18 **Mechanisms of Hormonal Regulation,** 443
Valentina L. Brashers, Sue E. Huether, and Kelly Power-Kean
Mechanisms of Hormonal Regulation, 443
Regulation of Hormone Release, 443
Hormone Transport, 444
Mechanisms of Hormone Action, 444
Structure and Function of the Endocrine Glands, 447
Hypothalamic-Pituitary System, 447
Pineal Gland, 452
Thyroid and Parathyroid Glands, 452
Endocrine Pancreas, 455
Adrenal Glands, 457
GERIATRIC CONSIDERATIONS: Aging and Its Effects on Specific Endocrine Glands, 461

19 **Alterations of Hormonal Regulation,** 465
Valentina L. Brashers, Robert E. Jones, Sue E. Huether, and Kelly Power-Kean
Mechanisms of Hormonal Alterations, 465
Alterations of the Hypothalamic-Pituitary System, 466
Diseases of the Posterior Pituitary, 466
Diseases of the Anterior Pituitary, 468
Alterations of Thyroid Function, 471
Thyrotoxicosis/Hyperthyroidism, 471
Hypothyroidism, 473
Thyroid Carcinoma, 474
Alterations of Parathyroid Function, 474
Hyperparathyroidism, 474
Hypoparathyroidism, 475
Dysfunction of the Endocrine Pancreas: Diabetes Mellitus, 476
Types of Diabetes Mellitus, 476
Acute Complications of Diabetes Mellitus, 482
Chronic Complications of Diabetes Mellitus, 483
Alterations of Adrenal Function, 487
Disorders of the Adrenal Cortex, 487
Tumours of the Adrenal Medulla, 490

UNIT 6 The Hematological System

20 Structure and Function of the Hematological System, 496
Neal S. Rote, Kathryn L. McCance, and Kelly Power-Kean
Components of the Hematological System, 496
Composition of Blood, 496
Lymphoid Organs, 500
The Mononuclear Phagocyte System, 503
Development of Blood Cells, 503
Hematopoiesis, 503
Development of Erythrocytes, 506
Development of Leukocytes, 509
Development of Platelets, 509
Mechanisms of Hemostasis, 510
Function of Platelets and Blood Vessels, 510
Function of Clotting Factors, 512
Retraction and Lysis of Blood Clots, 513
PEDIATRIC CONSIDERATIONS: **Hematological Value Changes, 516**
GERIATRIC CONSIDERATIONS: Hematological Value Changes, 517

21 Alterations of Hematological Function, 520
Anna Schwartz, Kathryn L. McCance, Neal S. Rote, and Kelly Power-Kean
Alterations of Erythrocyte Function, 520
Classification of Anemias, 520
Macrocytic-Normochromic Anemias, 522
Microcytic-Hypochromic Anemias, 524
Normocytic-Normochromic Anemias, 526
Myeloproliferative Red Blood Cell Disorders, 526
Polycythemia Vera, 526
Iron Overload, 529
Alterations of Leukocyte Function, 529
Quantitative Alterations of Leukocytes, 529
Alterations of Lymphoid Function, 538
Lymphadenopathy, 538
Malignant Lymphomas, 538
Alterations of Splenic Function, 545
Hemorrhagic Disorders and Alterations of Platelets and Coagulation, 546
Disorders of Platelets, 546
Alterations of Platelet Function, 549
Disorders of Coagulation, 550

22 Alterations of Hematological Function in Children, 560
Joan Shea, Nancy E. Kline, Anna E. Roche, Kathryn L. McCance, and Kelly Power-Kean
Disorders of Erythrocytes, 560
Acquired Disorders, 560
Inherited Disorders, 564
Disorders of Coagulation and Platelets, 569
Inherited Hemorrhagic Disease, 569
Antibody-Mediated Hemorrhagic Disease, 569
Neoplastic Disorders, 570
Leukemia, 570
Lymphomas, 571

UNIT 7 The Cardiovascular and Lymphatic Systems

23 Structure and Function of the Cardiovascular and Lymphatic Systems, 575
Susanna G. Cunningham, Valentina L. Brashers, Kathryn L. McCance, and Mohamed El-Hussein
The Circulatory System, 575
The Heart, 575
Structures That Direct Circulation Through the Heart, 576
Structures That Support Cardiac Metabolism: The Coronary Vessels, 578
Structures That Control Heart Action, 580
Factors Affecting Cardiac Output, 587
The Systemic Circulation, 589
Structure of Blood Vessels, 589
Factors Affecting Blood Flow, 593
Regulation of Blood Pressure, 595
Regulation of the Coronary Circulation, 598
The Lymphatic System, 599

24 Alterations of Cardiovascular Function, 604
Valentina L. Brashers and Mohamed El-Hussein
Diseases of the Veins, 604
Varicose Veins and Chronic Venous Insufficiency, 604
Thrombus Formation in Veins, 605
Superior Vena Cava Syndrome, 605
Diseases of the Arteries, 606
Hypertension, 606
Orthostatic (Postural) Hypotension, 611
Aneurysm, 611
Thrombus Formation, 612
Embolism, 613
Peripheral Vascular Disease, 613
Atherosclerosis, 614
Peripheral Artery Disease, 617
Coronary Artery Disease, Myocardial Ischemia, and Acute Coronary Syndromes, 167
Disorders of the Heart Wall, 629
Disorders of the Pericardium, 629
Disorders of the Myocardium: The Cardiomyopathies, 630
Disorders of the Endocardium, 632
Cardiac Complications in AIDS, 638
Manifestations of Heart Disease, 638
Heart Failure, 638
Dysrhythmias, 643
Shock, 643
Impairment of Cellular Metabolism, 643
Clinical Manifestations of Shock, 648
Treatment for Shock, 648
Types of Shock, 648
Multiple Organ Dysfunction Syndrome, 653

25 Alterations of Cardiovascular Function in Children, 662
Nancy Pike, Nancy L. McDaniel, and Mohamed El-Hussein
Congenital Heart Disease, 662
Obstructive Defects, 664
Defects With Increased Pulmonary Blood Flow, 667

Defects With Decreased Pulmonary Blood Flow, 668
Mixing Defects, 670
Heart Failure, 672
Acquired Cardiovascular Disorders, 673
Kawasaki Disease, 673
Systemic Hypertension, 674

UNIT 8 The Pulmonary System

26 Structure and Function of the Pulmonary System, 679
Valentina L. Brashers and Mohamed El-Hussein
Structures of the Pulmonary System, 679
Conducting Airways, 679
Gas-Exchange Airways, 680
Pulmonary and Bronchial Circulation, 681
Control of the Pulmonary Circulation, 683
Chest Wall and Pleura, 683
Function of the Pulmonary System, 684
Ventilation, 684
Neurochemical Control of Ventilation, 684
Mechanics of Breathing, 686
Gas Transport, 688
GERIATRIC CONSIDERATIONS: **Aging and the Pulmonary System, 692**

27 Alterations of Pulmonary Function, 695
Valentina L. Brashers, Sue E. Huether, and Mohamed El-Hussein
Clinical Manifestations of Pulmonary Alterations, 695
Signs and Symptoms of Pulmonary Disease, 695
Conditions Caused by Pulmonary Disease or Injury, 697
Disorders of the Chest Wall and Pleura, 699
Chest Wall Restriction, 699
Pleural Abnormalities, 699
Pulmonary Disorders, 701
Restrictive Lung Diseases, 701
Obstructive Lung Diseases, 705
Respiratory Tract Infections, 711
Pulmonary Vascular Disease, 715
Malignancies of the Respiratory Tract, 717

28 Alterations of Pulmonary Function in Children, 725
Valentina L. Brashers, Sue E. Huether, and Mohamed El-Hussein
Disorders of the Upper Airways, 725
Infections of the Upper Airways, 725
Aspiration of Foreign Bodies, 727
Obstructive Sleep Apnea Syndrome, 727
Disorders of the Lower Airways, 728
Respiratory Distress Syndrome of the Newborn, 728
Bronchopulmonary Dysplasia, 730
Respiratory Tract Infections, 730
Aspiration Pneumonitis, 733
Bronchiolitis Obliterans, 733
Asthma, 733
Acute Lung Injury/Acute Respiratory Distress Syndrome, 735
Cystic Fibrosis, 735
Sudden Unexpected Infant Death, 737

UNIT 9 The Renal and Urological Systems

29 Structure and Function of the Renal and Urological Systems, 741
Sue E. Huether and Mohamed El-Hussein
Structures of the Renal System, 741
Structures of the Kidney, 741
Urinary Structures, 745
Renal Blood Flow, 746
Autoregulation of Intrarenal Blood Flow, 746
Neural Regulation of Renal Blood Flow, 747
Hormones and Other Factors Regulating Renal Blood Flow, 747
Kidney Function, 747
Nephron Function, 747
Hormones and Nephron Function, 752
Renal Hormones, 752
Tests of Renal Function, 753
Renal Clearance, 753
Plasma Creatinine Concentration, 754
Blood Urea Nitrogen, 754
PEDIATRIC CONSIDERATIONS: **Pediatrics and Renal Function, 756**
GERIATRIC CONSIDERATIONS: **Aging and Renal Function, 756**

30 Alterations of Renal and Urinary Tract Function, 759
Sue E. Huether and Mohamed El-Hussein
Urinary Tract Obstruction, 759
Upper Urinary Tract Obstruction, 759
Lower Urinary Tract Obstruction, 761
Tumours, 763
Urinary Tract Infection, 765
Causes of Urinary Tract Infection, 765
Types of Urinary Tract Infection, 765
Glomerular Disorders, 767
Glomerulonephritis, 767
Nephrotic and Nephritic Syndromes, 771
Acute Kidney Injury, 772
Classification of Kidney Dysfunction, 772
Classification of Acute Kidney Injury, 772
Chronic Kidney Disease, 775
Creatinine and Urea Clearance, 777
Fluid and Electrolyte Balance, 777
Calcium, Phosphate, and Bone, 778
Protein, Carbohydrate, and Fat Metabolism, 778
Cardiovascular System, 778
Pulmonary System, 779
Hematological System, 779
Immune System, 779
Neurological System, 779
Gastro-intestinal System, 779
Endocrine and Reproductive Systems, 779
Integumentary System, 779

31 Alterations of Renal and Urinary Tract Function in Children, 784
Patricia Ring, Sue E. Huether, and Mohamed El-Hussein
Structural Abnormalities, 784
Hypospadias, 784
Epispadias and Exstrophy of the Bladder, 785
Bladder Outlet Obstruction, 785

Ureteropelvic Junction Obstruction, 785
Hypoplastic or Dysplastic Kidneys, 786
Polycystic Kidney Disease, 786
Renal Agenesis, 786
Glomerular Disorders, 786
Glomerulonephritis, 786
Immunoglobulin A Nephropathy, 787
Nephrotic Syndrome, 787
Hemolytic Uremic Syndrome, 787
Nephroblastoma, 788
Bladder Disorders, 788
Urinary Tract Infections, 788
Vesicoureteral Reflux, 789
Urinary Incontinence, 790
Types of Incontinence, 790

UNIT 10 The Reproductive Systems

32 Structure and Function of the Reproductive Systems, 793
Afsoon Moktar, George W. Rodway, Sue E. Huether, and Kelly Power-Kean
Development of the Reproductive Systems, 793
Sexual Differentiation in Utero, 793
Puberty and Reproductive Maturation, 795
The Female Reproductive System, 796
External Genitalia, 796
Internal Genitalia, 798
Female Sex Hormones, 801
Menstrual Cycle, 802
Structure and Function of the Breast, 805
Female Breast, 805
Male Breast, 807
The Male Reproductive System, 807
External Genitalia, 807
Internal Genitalia, 809
Spermatogenesis, 810
Male Sex and Reproductive Hormones, 810
Aging and Reproductive Function, 811
Aging and the Female Reproductive System, 811
Aging and the Male Reproductive System, 812

33 Alterations of the Female Reproductive System, 816
Kathryn L. McCance, Afsoon Moktar, and Kelly Power-Kean
Abnormalities of the Female Reproductive Tract, 816
Alterations of Sexual Maturation, 817
Delayed or Absent Puberty, 818
Precocious Puberty, 818
Disorders of the Female Reproductive System, 819
Hormonal and Menstrual Alterations, 819
Infection and Inflammation, 823
Pelvic Organ Prolapse, 827
Benign Growths and Proliferative Conditions, 829
Cancer, 833
Sexual Dysfunction, 842
Impaired Fertility, 843
Disorders of the Female Breast, 843
Galactorrhea, 843
Benign Breast Disease and Conditions, 844
Breast Cancer, 845

34 Alterations of the Male Reproductive System, 868
George W. Rodway, Kathryn L. McCance, and Kelly Power-Kean
Alterations of Sexual Maturation, 868
Delayed or Absent Puberty, 868
Precocious Puberty, 868
Disorders of the Male Reproductive System, 869
Disorders of the Urethra, 869
Disorders of the Penis, 869
Disorders of the Scrotum, Testis, and Epididymis, 872
Disorders of the Prostate Gland, 876
Sexual Dysfunction, 888
Disorders of the Male Breast, 890
Gynecomastia, 890
Carcinoma, 891
Sexually Transmitted Infections, 891

UNIT 11 The Digestive System

35 Structure and Function of the Digestive System, 899
Sue E. Huether and Mohamed El-Hussein
The Gastro-Intestinal Tract, 899
Mouth and Esophagus, 899
Stomach, 902
Small Intestine, 905
Large Intestine, 909
Intestinal Microbiome, 910
Splanchnic Blood Flow, 910
Accessory Organs of Digestion, 910
Liver, 911
Gallbladder, 914
Exocrine Pancreas, 915
GERIATRIC CONSIDERATIONS: Aging and the Gastro-Intestinal System, 918

36 Alterations of Digestive Function, 921
Sue E. Huether and Mohamed El-Hussein
Disorders of the Gastro-Intestinal Tract, 921
Clinical Manifestations of Gastro-Intestinal Dysfunction, 921
Disorders of Motility, 925
Gastritis, 930
Peptic Ulcer Disease, 931
Malabsorption Syndromes, 935
Inflammatory Bowel Disease, 935
Diverticular Disease of the Colon, 938
Appendicitis, 939
Mesenteric Vascular Insufficiency, 939
Disorders of Nutrition, 940
Disorders of the Accessory Organs of Digestion, 943
Common Complications of Liver Disorders, 943
Disorders of the Liver, 947
Disorders of the Gallbladder, 951
Disorders of the Pancreas, 952
Cancer of the Digestive System, 953
Cancer of the Gastro-Intestinal Tract, 953
Cancer of the Accessory Organs of Digestion, 957

37 Alterations of Digestive Function in Children, 968
Sharon Sables-Baus, Sara J. Fidanza, and Mohamed El-Hussein
Disorders of the Gastro-Intestinal Tract, 968
Congenital Impairment of Motility, 968
Acquired Impairment of Motility, 972

Impairment of Digestion, Absorption, and Nutrition, 974
Diarrhea, 979
Disorders of the Liver, 979
Disorders of Biliary Metabolism and Transport, 979
Inflammatory Disorders, 980
Portal Hypertension, 981
Metabolic Disorders, 982
Gastro-Intestinal Malignancies in Children, 982
Hepatoblastoma, 982
Pancreatic Tumours, 982

UNIT 12 The Musculo-skeletal and Integumentary Systems

38 **Structure and Function of the Musculo-skeletal System,** 988
Christy L. Crowther-Radulewicz, Kathryn L. McCance, and Stephanie Zettel
Structure and Function of Bones, 988
Elements of Bone Tissue, 988
Types of Bone Tissue, 992
Characteristics of Bone, 994
Maintenance of Bone Integrity, 995
Structure and Function of Joints, 995
Fibrous Joints, 995
Cartilaginous Joints, 995
Synovial Joints, 998
Structure and Function of Skeletal Muscles, 998
Whole Muscle, 999
Components of Muscle Function, 1003
Tendons and Ligaments, 1006
Aging and the Musculo-skeletal System, 1006
Aging of Bones, 1006
Aging of Joints, 1007
Aging of Muscles, 1007

39 **Alterations of Musculo-skeletal Function,** 1011
Christy L. Crowther-Radulewicz, Kathryn L. McCance, and Stephanie Zettel
Musculo-skeletal Injuries, 1011
Skeletal Trauma, 1011
Support Structures, 1015
Disorders of Bones, 1020
Metabolic Bone Diseases, 1020
Infectious Bone Disease: Osteomyelitis, 1028
Disorders of Joints, 1029
Osteoarthritis, 1029
Classic Inflammatory Joint Disease, 1032
Disorders of Skeletal Muscle, 1041
Secondary Muscular Dysfunction, 1041
Fibromyalgia, 1041
Chronic Fatigue Syndrome, 1042
Muscle Membrane Abnormalities, 1043
Metabolic Muscle Diseases, 1043
Inflammatory Muscle Diseases: Myositis, 1044
Toxic Myopathies, 1046
Musculo-skeletal Tumours, 1047
Bone Tumours, 1047
Muscle Tumours, 1051

40 **Alterations of Musculo-skeletal Function in Children,** 1059
Kristen Lee Carroll, Lynne M. Kerr, Kathryn L. McCance, and Stephanie Zettel
Congenital Defects, 1059
Clubfoot, 1059
Developmental Dysplasia of the Hip, 1059
Osteogenesis Imperfecta, 1060
Bone Infection, 1062
Osteomyelitis, 1062
Septic Arthritis, 1063
Juvenile Idiopathic Arthritis, 1064
Osteochondroses, 1065
Legg-Calvé-Perthes Disease, 1065
Osgood-Schlatter Disease, 1065
Scoliosis, 1066
Muscular Dystrophy, 1067
Duchenne Muscular Dystrophy, 1067
Becker Muscular Dystrophy, 1068
Facioscapulohumeral Muscular Dystrophy, 1068
Myotonic Muscular Dystrophy, 1068
Musculo-skeletal Tumours, 1069
Benign Bone Tumours, 1069
Malignant Bone Tumours, 1069
Nonaccidental Trauma, 1071
Fractures in Nonaccidental Trauma, 1071

41 **Structure, Function, and Disorders of the Integument,** 1074
Sue Ann McCann, Noreen Heer Nicol, Sue E. Huether, and Stephanie Zettel
Structure and Function of the Skin, 1074
Layers of the Skin, 1074
Clinical Manifestations of Skin Dysfunction, 1076
Disorders of the Skin, 1081
Inflammatory Disorders, 1081
Papulosquamous Disorders, 1083
Vesiculobullous Diseases, 1085
Infections, 1087
Vascular Disorders, 1089
Benign Tumours, 1091
Skin Cancer, 1091
Burns, 1095
Cold Injury, 1099
Disorders of the Hair, 1101
Alopecia, 1101
Hirsutism, 1101
Disorders of the Nail, 1101
Paronychia, 1101
Onychomycosis, 1101
GERIATRIC CONSIDERATIONS: Aging and Changes in Skin Integrity, 1102

42 **Alterations of the Integument in Children,** 1107
Noreen Heer Nicol, Sue E. Huether, and Stephanie Zettel
Acne Vulgaris, 1107
Dermatitis, 1108
Atopic Dermatitis, 1108
Diaper Dermatitis, 1109

Infections of the Skin, 1109
Bacterial Infections, 1109
Fungal Infections, 1110
Viral Infections, 1111
Insect Bites and Parasites, 1113
Scabies, 1114
Pediculosis (Lice Infestation), 1114
Fleas, 1114
Bedbugs, 1114
Cutaneous Hemangiomas and Vascular Malformations, 1115
Cutaneous Hemangiomas, 1115
Cutaneous Vascular Malformations, 1116
Other Skin Disorders, 1116
Miliaria, 1116
Erythema Toxicum Neonatorum, 1116

Index, 1119

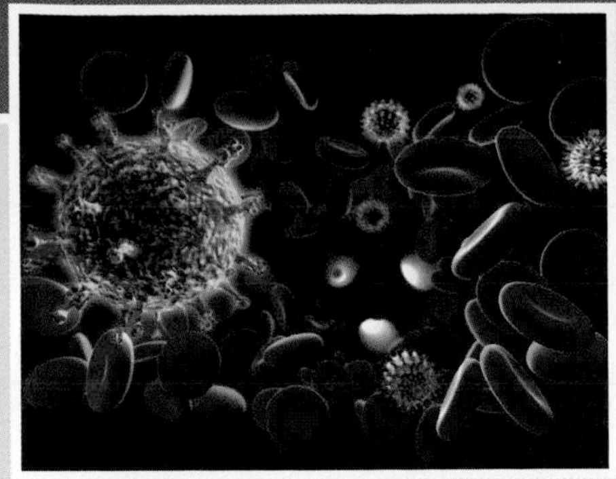

1

Cellular Biology

Kathryn L. McCance and Stephanie Zettel

EVOLVE WEBSITE

http://evolve.elsevier.com/Canada/Huether/pathophysiology
Student Review Questions
Key Points
Case Studies
Animations
Quick Check Answers

CHAPTER OUTLINE

Prokaryotes and Eukaryotes, 1
Cellular Functions, 2
Structure and Function of Cellular Components, 2
Nucleus, 2
Cytoplasmic Organelles, 2
Plasma Membranes, 2
Cellular Receptors, 9
Cell-to-Cell Adhesions, 10
Extracellular Matrix, 10
Specialized Cell Junctions, 12
Cellular Communication and Signal Transduction, 12
Cellular Metabolism, 14
Role of Adenosine Triphosphate, 16
Food and Production of Cellular Energy, 16
Oxidative Phosphorylation, 16
Membrane Transport: Cellular Intake and Output, 17
Electrolytes as Solutes, 18
Transport by Vesicle Formation, 21
Movement of Electrical Impulses: Membrane Potentials, 24
Cellular Reproduction: The Cell Cycle, 25
Phases of Mitosis and Cytokinesis, 25
Rates of Cellular Division, 26
Growth Factors, 26
Tissues, 27
Tissue Formation, 27
Types of Tissues, 27

All body functions depend on the integrity of cells. Therefore an understanding of cellular biology is increasingly necessary to comprehend disease processes. An overwhelming amount of information reveals how cells behave as a multicellular "social" organism. At the heart of it all is cellular communication (cellular "crosstalk")—how messages originate and are transmitted, received, interpreted, and used by the cell. Streamlined conversation between, among, and within cells maintains cellular function and specialization. Cells communicate with other cells in a way to promote the integrity of the entire organism (i.e., they are well differentiated), and cells that resemble each other interact with each other more effectively. For example, prokaryotic and eukaryotic cells are organized differently, which accounts for the difference in response to pharmacotherapy. Anti-infectives, such as penicillin, are only effective against bacteria. Pharmacotherapy against eukaryotic cells results in more severe adverse effects, because the cells that are being targeted with the therapy more closely resemble human cells. When cells become less differentiated (as a result of injury or mutation) or less like the surrounding cells, the conversation breaks down, and cells either adapt (sometimes altering function) or become vulnerable to isolation, injury, or diseases such as cancer.

PROKARYOTES AND EUKARYOTES

Living cells generally are divided into eukaryotes and prokaryotes. The cells of higher animals and plants are eukaryotes, as are the single-celled organisms, fungi, protozoa, and most algae. Prokaryotes include cyanobacteria (blue-green algae), bacteria, and rickettsiae. Prokaryotes traditionally were studied as core subjects of molecular biology. Today, emphasis is on the eukaryotic cell; much of its structure and function have no counterpart in bacterial cells.

Eukaryotes (*eu* = good; *karyon* = nucleus; also spelled *eucaryotes*) are larger and have more extensive intracellular anatomy and organization than prokaryotes. Eukaryotic cells have a characteristic set of membrane-bound intracellular compartments, called *organelles*, that includes a well-defined nucleus. The **prokaryotes** contain no organelles, and their nuclear material is not encased by a nuclear membrane. Prokaryotic cells are characterized by lack of a distinct nucleus.

Besides having structural differences, prokaryotic and eukaryotic cells differ in chemical composition and biochemical activity. The *nuclei* of prokaryotic cells carry genetic information in a single circular chromosome, and they lack a class of proteins called *histones*, which in eukaryotic cells bind with deoxyribonucleic acid (DNA) and are involved in the supercoiling of DNA. Eukaryotic cells have several or many chromosomes. Protein production, or synthesis, in the two classes of cells also differs because of major structural differences in ribonucleic acid (RNA)–protein complexes. Other distinctions include differences in mechanisms of transport across the outer cellular membrane and in enzyme content.

CELLULAR FUNCTIONS

Cells become specialized through the process of differentiation, or maturation, so that some cells eventually perform one kind of function and other cells perform other functions. Cells with a highly developed function, such as movement, often lack some other property, such as hormone production, which is more highly developed in other cells.

The eight chief cellular functions are as follows:

1. *Movement.* Muscle cells can generate forces that produce motion. Muscles that are attached to bones produce limb movements, whereas those muscles that enclose hollow tubes or cavities move or empty contents when they contract (e.g., the colon).
2. *Conductivity.* Conduction as a response to a stimulus is manifested by a wave of excitation, an electrical potential that passes along the surface of the cell to reach its other parts. Conductivity is the chief function of nerve cells.
3. *Metabolic absorption.* All cells can take in and use nutrients and other substances from their surroundings.
4. *Secretion.* Certain cells, such as mucous gland cells, can synthesize new substances from substances they absorb and then secrete the new substances to serve as needed elsewhere.
5. *Excretion.* All cells can rid themselves of waste products resulting from the metabolic breakdown of nutrients. Membrane-bound sacs (lysosomes) within cells contain enzymes that break down, or digest, large molecules, turning them into waste products that are released from the cell.
6. *Respiration.* Cells absorb oxygen, which is used to transform nutrients into energy in the form of adenosine triphosphate (ATP). Cellular respiration, or oxidation, occurs in organelles called *mitochondria.*
7. *Reproduction.* Tissue growth occurs as cells enlarge and reproduce themselves. Even without growth, tissue maintenance requires that new cells be produced to replace cells that are lost normally through cellular death. Not all cells are capable of continuous division (see Chapter 4).
8. *Communication.* Communication is vital for cells to survive as a society of cells. Appropriate communication allows the maintenance of a dynamic steady state.

STRUCTURE AND FUNCTION OF CELLULAR COMPONENTS

Figure 1-1, *A*, shows a "typical" eukaryotic cell, which consists of three components: an outer membrane called the plasma membrane, or plasmalemma; a fluid "filling" called cytoplasm (Figure 1-1, *B*); and the "organs" of the cell—the membrane-bound intracellular organelles, among them the nucleus.

Nucleus

The nucleus, which is surrounded by the cytoplasm and generally is located in the centre of the cell, is the largest membrane-bound organelle. Two pliable membranes compose the nuclear envelope (Figure 1-2, *A*). The nuclear envelope is pockmarked with pits, called nuclear pores, which allow chemical messages to exit and enter the nucleus (Figure 1-2, *B*). The outer membrane is continuous with membranes of the endoplasmic reticulum (see Figure 1-1). The nucleus contains the nucleolus (a small, dense structure composed largely of RNA), most of the cellular DNA, and the DNA-binding proteins (i.e., the histones) that regulate its activity. The DNA "chain" in eukaryotic cells is so long that it is easily broken. Therefore the histones that bind to DNA cause DNA to fold into chromosomes (Figure 1-2, *C*), which decreases the risk of breakage and is essential for cell division in eukaryotes.

The primary functions of the nucleus are cell division and control of genetic information. Other functions include the replication and repair of DNA and the transcription of the information stored in DNA. Genetic information is transcribed into RNA, which can be processed into messenger, transport, and ribosomal RNAs and introduced into the cytoplasm, where it directs cellular activities. Most of the processing of RNA occurs in the nucleolus. (The roles of DNA and RNA in protein synthesis are discussed in Chapter 2.)

Cytoplasmic Organelles

Cytoplasm is an aqueous solution (cytosol) that fills the cytoplasmic matrix—the space between the nuclear envelope and the plasma membrane. The cytosol represents about half the volume of a eukaryotic cell. It contains thousands of enzymes involved in intermediate metabolism and is *crowded* with ribosomes making proteins (see Figure 1-1, *B*). Newly synthesized proteins remain in the cytosol if they lack a signal for transport to a cell organelle.[1] The organelles suspended in the cytoplasm are enclosed in biological membranes, so they can simultaneously carry out functions requiring different biochemical environments. Many of these functions are directed by coded messages carried from the nucleus by RNA. The functions include synthesis of proteins and hormones and their transport out of the cell, isolation and elimination of waste products from the cell, performance of metabolic processes, breakdown and disposal of cellular debris and foreign proteins (antigens), and maintenance of cellular structure and motility. The cytosol is a storage unit for fat, carbohydrates, and secretory vesicles. Table 1-1 lists the principal cytoplasmic organelles.

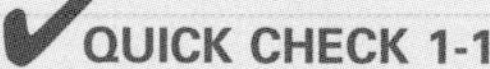

QUICK CHECK 1-1

1. Why is the process of differentiation essential to specialization? Give an example.
2. Describe at least two cellular functions.

Plasma Membranes

Every cell is contained within a membrane with gates, channels, and pumps. Membranes surround the cell or enclose an intracellular organelle and are exceedingly important to normal physiological function because they control the composition of the space, or compartment, they enclose. Membranes can allow or exclude various molecules and, because of selective transport systems, they can move molecules in or out of the space (Figure 1-3). By controlling the movement of substances from one compartment to another, membranes exert a powerful influence on metabolic pathways. Directional transport is facilitated by polarized domains, distinct apical and basolateral domains. Cell polarity, the direction of cellular transport, maintains normal cell and tissue structure for numerous functions (e.g., movement of nutrients in and out of the cell) and becomes altered with diseases (Figure 1-4). The plasma membrane also has an important role in cell-to-cell recognition. Other functions of the plasma membrane include cellular mobility and the maintenance of cellular shape (Table 1-2).

Membrane Composition

The basic structure of cell membranes is the lipid bilayer, composed of two apposing leaflets and proteins that span the bilayer or interact with the lipids on either side of the two leaflets (Figure 1-5). Lipid research is growing, and principles of membrane organization are being overhauled.[2] In short, the main constituents of cell membranes are lipids and proteins. Historically, the plasma membrane was described as a fluid lipid bilayer (fluid mosaic model) composed of a *uniform* lipid distribution with inserted moving proteins. It now appears that the lipid bilayer is a much more complex structure where lipids and

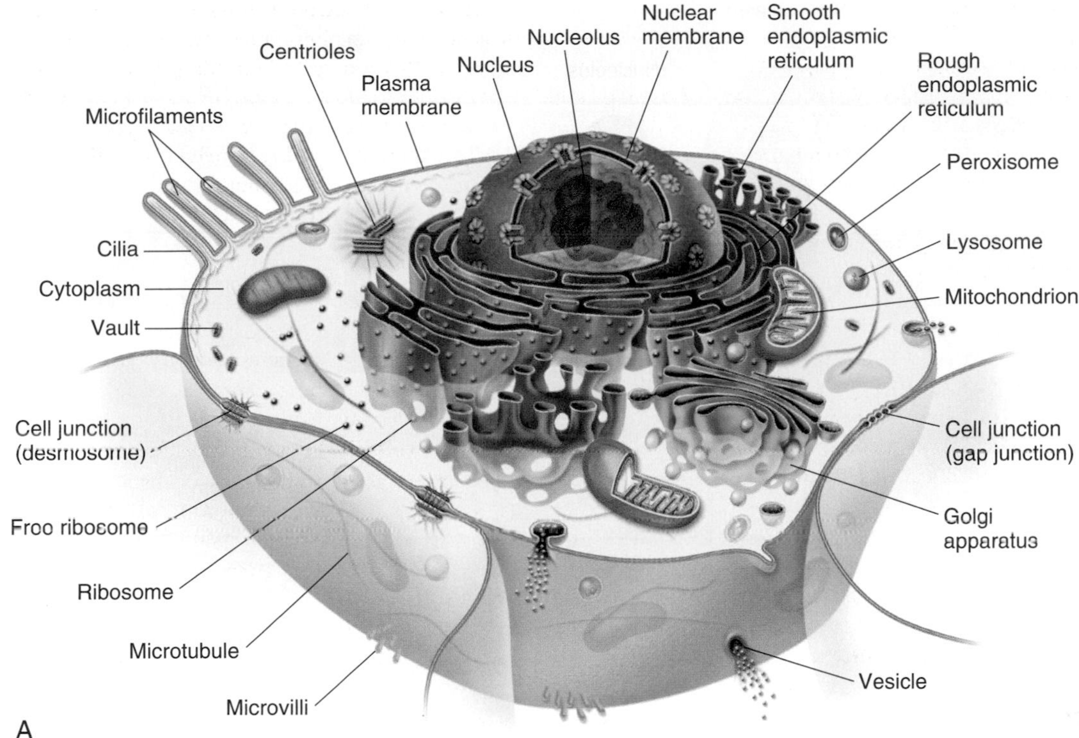

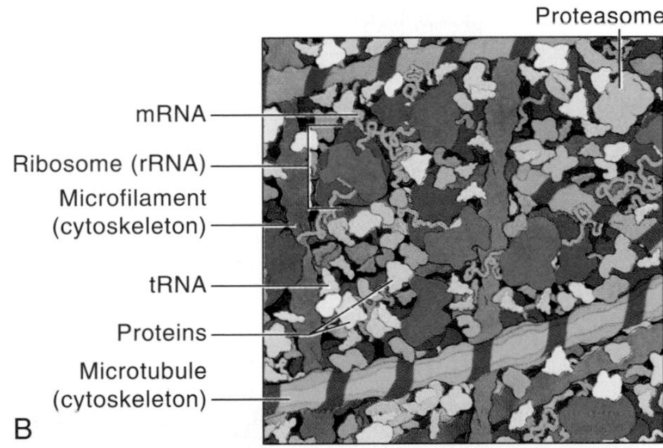

FIGURE 1-1 Typical Components of a Eukaryotic Cell and Structure of the Cytoplasm. **A,** Artist's interpretation of cell structure. Note the many mitochondria known as the "power plants of the cell." **B,** Colour-enhanced electron micrograph of a cell. The cell is crowded. Note, too, the innumerable dots bordering the endoplasmic reticulum. These are ribosomes, the cell's "protein factories." *mRNA,* messenger RNA; *tRNA,* transfer RNA. (**B,** from Patton, K.T., & Thibodeau, G.A. [2013]. *Anatomy & physiology* [8th ed.]. St. Louis: Mosby.)

proteins are not uniformly distributed but can separate into discrete units called *microdomains*, differing in their protein and lipid compositions.[3] Different membranes have varying percentages of lipids and proteins. Intracellular membranes may have a higher percentage of proteins than do plasma membranes, presumably because most enzymatic activity occurs within organelles. The membrane organization is achieved through noncovalent bonds that allow different physical states called *phases*. The lipid bilayer can be structured in three main phases: solid gel phase, fluid liquid-crystalline phase, and liquid-ordered phase (Figure 1-5, *B*). These phases can change under physiological factors such as temperature and pressure fluctuations. Carbohydrates are mainly associated with plasma membranes, in which they are chemically combined with lipids, forming **glycolipids**, and with proteins, forming **glycoproteins** (see Figure 1-5).

The outer surface of the plasma membrane in many types of cells, especially endothelial cells and adipocytes, is not smooth but dimpled with flask-shaped invaginations known as caveolae ("tiny caves"). Caveolae serve as a storage site for many receptors, provide a route for transport into the cell, and act as the initiator for relaying signals from several extracellular chemical messengers into the cell's interior (see p. 23).

Lipids. Each lipid molecule is said to be polar, or **amphipathic**, which means that one part is hydrophobic (uncharged, or "water hating") and another part is hydrophilic (charged, or "water loving") (Figure 1-6). The membrane spontaneously organizes itself into two layers because of these two incompatible solubilities. The hydrophobic region (hydrophobic tail) of each lipid molecule is protected from water, whereas the hydrophilic region (hydrophilic head) is immersed in it. The bilayer

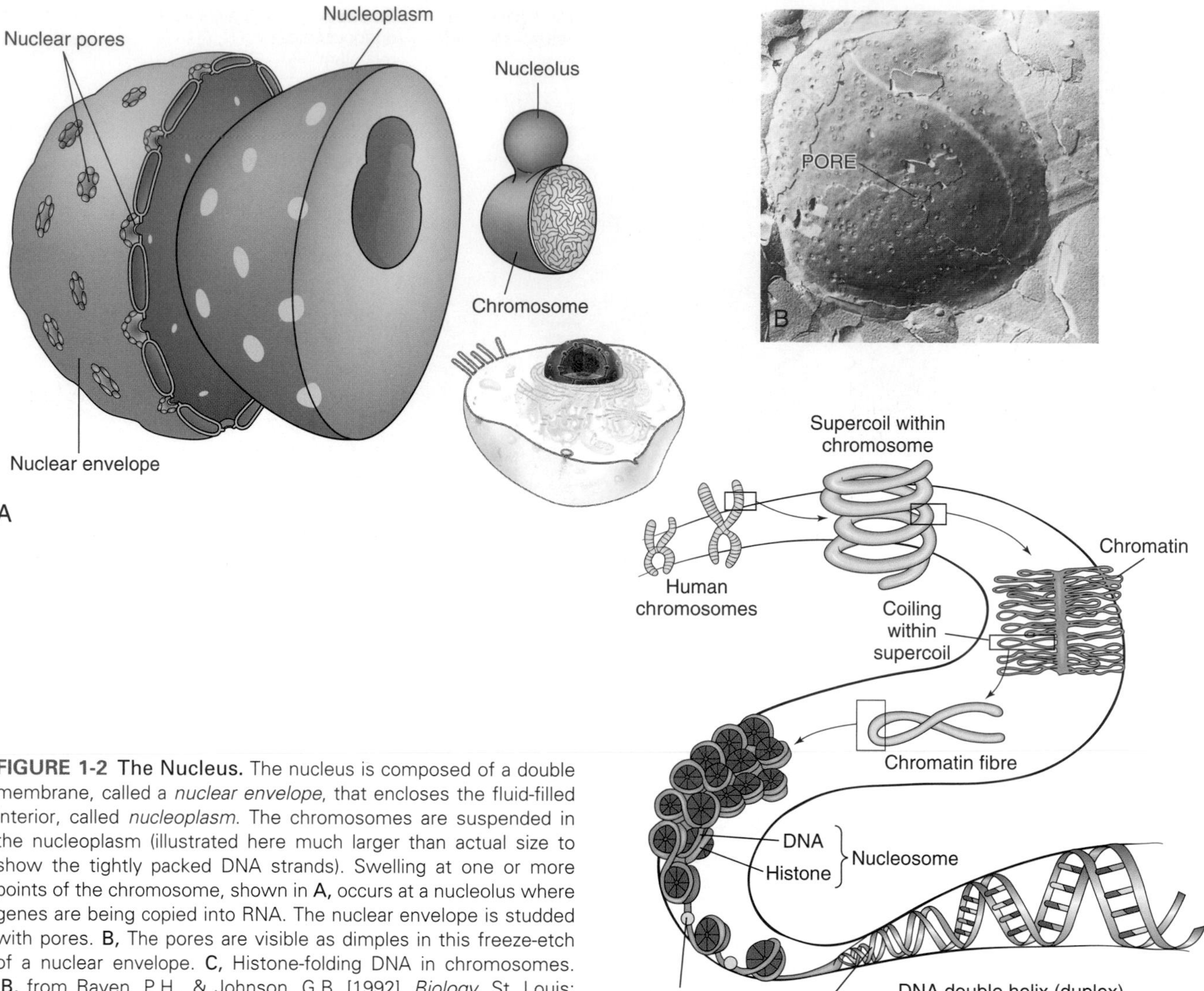

FIGURE 1-2 The Nucleus. The nucleus is composed of a double membrane, called a *nuclear envelope*, that encloses the fluid-filled interior, called *nucleoplasm*. The chromosomes are suspended in the nucleoplasm (illustrated here much larger than actual size to show the tightly packed DNA strands). Swelling at one or more points of the chromosome, shown in **A**, occurs at a nucleolus where genes are being copied into RNA. The nuclear envelope is studded with pores. **B**, The pores are visible as dimples in this freeze-etch of a nuclear envelope. **C**, Histone-folding DNA in chromosomes. (**B**, from Raven, P.H., & Johnson, G.B. [1992]. *Biology*. St. Louis: Mosby.)

TABLE 1-1 Principal Cytoplasmic Organelles

Organelle	Characteristics and Description
Ribosomes	RNA-protein complexes (nucleoproteins) synthesized in nucleolus and secreted into cytoplasm. They provide sites for cellular protein synthesis.
Endoplasmic reticulum	Network of tubular channels (cisternae) that extend throughout outer nuclear membrane. It specializes in synthesis and transport of protein and lipid components of most organelles.
Golgi complex	Network of smooth membranes and vesicles located near nucleus. It is responsible for processing and packaging proteins onto secretory vesicles that break away from the complex and migrate to various intracellular and extracellular destinations, including the plasma membrane. Best-known vesicles are those that have coats largely made of the protein *clathrin*. Proteins in the complex bind to the cytoskeleton, generating tension that helps organelle function and keep its stretched shape intact.
Lysosomes	Saclike structures that originate from the Golgi complex and contain enzymes for digesting most cellular substances to their basic form, such as amino acids, fatty acids, and carbohydrates (sugars). Cellular injury leads to release of lysosomal enzymes that cause cellular self-destruction.
Peroxisomes	Structures similar to lysosomes, but contain several oxidative enzymes (e.g., catalase, urate oxidase) that produce or use hydrogen peroxide; reactions detoxify various wastes.
Mitochondria	Structures that contain metabolic machinery needed for cellular energy metabolism. Enzymes of respiratory chain (electron-transport chain), found in the inner membrane of mitochondria, generate most of a cell's ATP (oxidative phosphorylation). They have a role in osmotic regulation, pH control, calcium homeostasis, and cell signalling.
Cytoskeleton	"Bone and muscle" of a cell. It is composed of a network of protein filaments, including microtubules and actin filaments (microfilaments); it forms cell extensions (microvilli, cilia, flagella).
Caveolae	Tiny indentations (caves) that can capture extracellular material and shuttle it inside the cell or across the cell.
Vaults	Cytoplasmic ribonucleoproteins shaped like octagonal barrels. They are thought to act as "trucks," shuttling molecules from the nucleus to elsewhere in the cell.

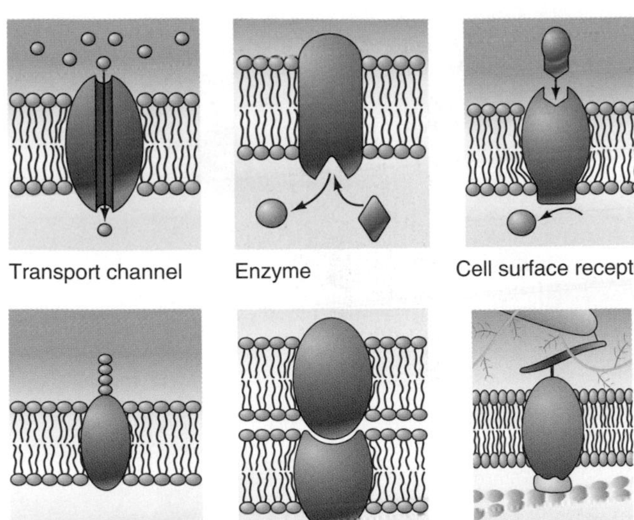

FIGURE 1-3 Functions of Plasma Membrane Proteins. The plasma membrane proteins illustrated here show a variety of functions performed by the different types of plasma membranes. (From Raven, P.H., & Johnson, G.B. [1995]. *Understanding biology* [3rd ed.]. Dubuque, IA: Brown.)

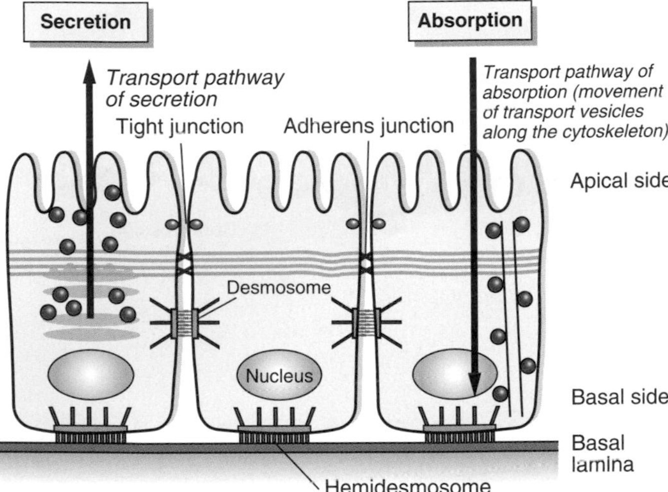

FIGURE 1-4 Cell Polarity of Epithelial Cells. Schematic of cell polarity (cell direction) of epithelial cells. Shown are the directions of the basal side and the apical side. Organelles and cytoskeleton are also arranged directionally to enable, for example, intestinal cell secretion and absorption. (Adapted from *Life science web textbook*, The University of Tokyo.)

serves as a barrier to the diffusion of water and hydrophilic substances, while allowing lipid-soluble molecules, such as oxygen (O_2) and carbon dioxide (CO_2), to diffuse through the membrane readily. The structure of the cell membrane also makes it more difficult for water-soluble medications and ionized medications to enter the cell.

A major component of the plasma membrane is a bilayer of lipid molecules—glycerophospholipids, sphingolipids, and sterols (e.g., cholesterol). The most abundant lipids are phospholipids. **Phospholipids** have a phosphate-containing hydrophilic head connected to a hydrophobic tail. Phospholipids and glycolipids form self-sealing lipid bilayers. Lipids along with protein assemblies act as "molecular glue" for the structural integrity of the membrane. Investigators are studying the concept of lipid rafts. **Membrane lipid rafts (MLRs)** appear to be

TABLE 1-2 Plasma Membrane Functions

Cellular Mechanism	Membrane Functions
Structure	Usually thicker than membranes of intracellular organelles Containment of cellular organelles Maintenance of relationship with cytoskeleton, endoplasmic reticulum, and other organelles Maintenance of fluid and electrolyte balance Outer surfaces of plasma membranes in many cells are not smooth but are dimpled with cavelike indentations called *caveolae*; they are also studded with cilia or even smaller cylindrical projections called *microvilli*; both are capable of movement
Protection	Barrier to toxic molecules and macromolecules (proteins, nucleic acids, polysaccharides) Barrier to foreign organisms and cells
Activation of cell	Hormones (regulation of cellular activity) Mitogens (cellular division; see Chapter 2) Antigens (antibody synthesis; see Chapter 6) Growth factors (proliferation and differentiation; see Chapter 10)
Storage	Storage site for many receptors Transport Diffusion and exchange diffusion Endocytosis (pinocytosis, phagocytosis) Exocytosis (secretion) Active transport
Cell-to-cell interaction	Communication and attachment at junctional complexes Symbiotic nutritive relationships Release of enzymes and antibodies to extracellular environment Relationships with extracellular matrix

Modified from King, D.W., Fenoglio, C.M., & Lefkowitch, J.H. (1983). *General pathology: Principles and dynamics*. Philadelphia: Lea & Febiger.

structurally and functionally distinct regions of the plasma membrane[4,5] and consist of cholesterol and sphingolipid-dependent microdomains that form a network of lipid–lipid, protein–protein, and protein–lipid interactions (Figures 1-5, *B*, and 1-7) Although discrepancies between experimental results exist, two main types of MLRs are hypothesized: those that contain the cholesterol-binding protein caveolin (see p. 24) and those that do not.[4] Researchers hypothesize that there are lipid rafts that have several functions, including (1) providing cellular polarity and organization of signalling trafficking; (2) acting as platforms for extracellular matrix (ECM) adhesion and intracellular cytoskeletal tethering to the plasma membrane through cell adhesion molecules (CAMs); (3) enabling signalling across the membrane, which can rearrange cytoskeletal architecture and regulate cell growth, migratio
and other functions; and (4) allowing entry of viruses, bacteria,
and nanoparticles.[4]

Proteins. A **protein** is made from a chain of amino
as **polypeptides**. There are 20 types of amino acids,
each type of protein has a unique sequence of a
are the major workhorses of the cell. After tra
protein from RNA, see Chapter 2) of a
modifications (PTMs) are the metho
numbers of proteins generated. Th
and functions of proteins and
standing diseases. Researchers

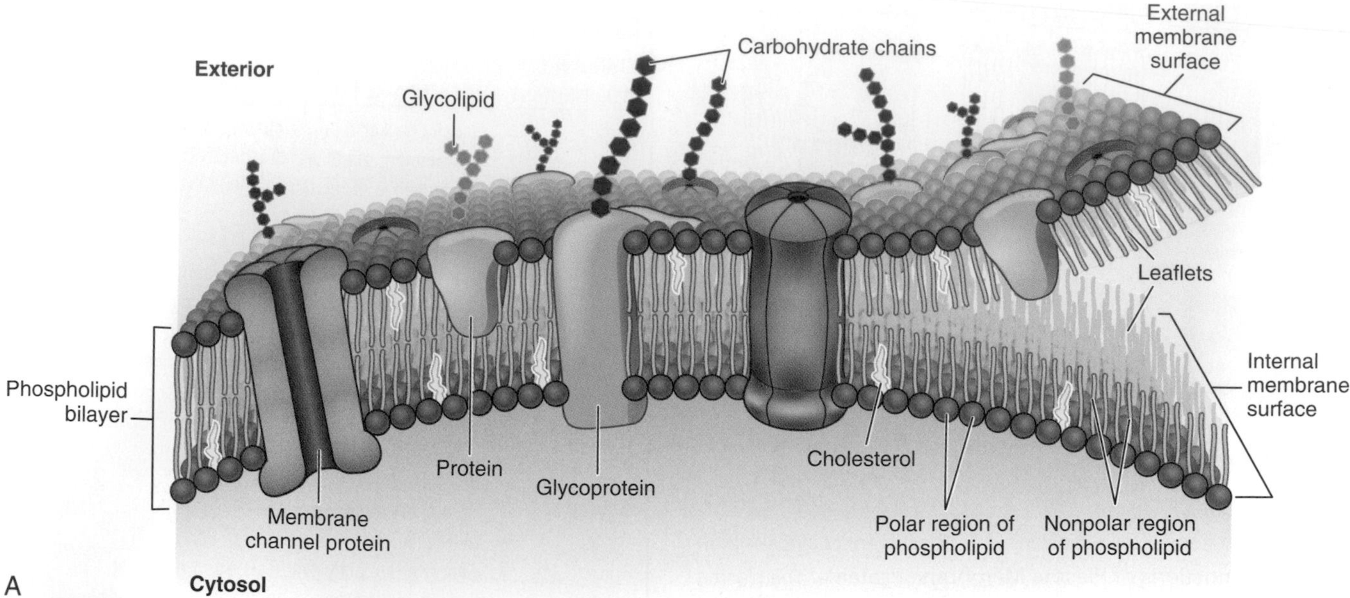

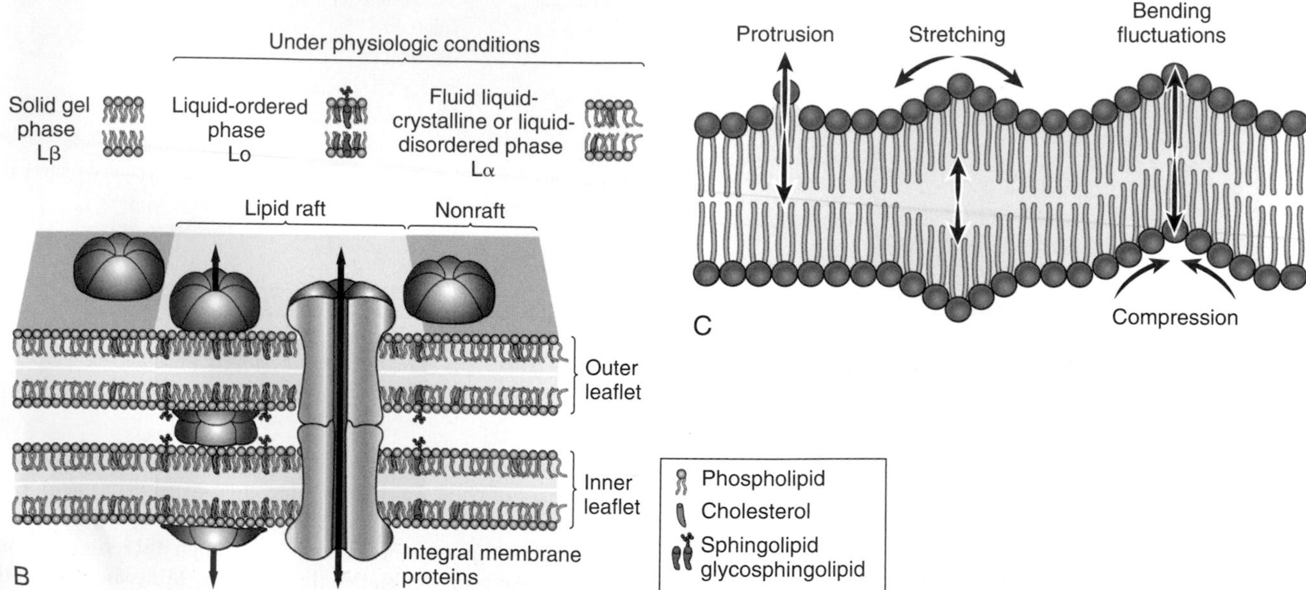

FIGURE 1-5 Lipid Bilayer Membranes. A, Concepts of biological membranes have markedly changed in the last two decades, from the classic fluid mosaic model to the current model that lipids and proteins are not evenly distributed but can isolate into microdomains, differing in their protein and lipid composition. **B,** An example of a microdomain is lipid rafts (*yellow*). Rafts are dynamic domain structures composed of cholesterol, sphingolipids, and membrane proteins important in different cellular processes. Various models exist to clarify the functions of domains. The three major phases of lipid bilayer organization include a solid gel phase (e.g., with low temperatures), a liquid-ordered phase (high temperatures), and a fluid liquid-crystalline (or liquid-disordered) phase. Some membrane-associated proteins are integrated into the lipid bilayer; other proteins are loosely attached to the outer and inner surfaces of the membrane. Transmembrane proteins protrude through the entire outer and inner surfaces of the membrane, and they can be attracted to microdomains through specific interactions with lipids. Interaction of the membrane proteins with distinct lipids depends on the hydrophobic thickness of the membrane, the lateral pressures of the membrane (mechanical force may shift protein channels from an open to closed state), the polarity or electrical charges at the lipid-protein interface, and the presence on the protein side of amino acid side chains. Important for pathophysiology is the proposal that protein-lipid interactions can be critical for correct insertion, folding, and orientation of membrane proteins. For example, diseases related to lipids that interfere with protein folding are becoming more prevalent. **C,** The cell membrane is not static but is always moving. Observed for the first time from measurements taken at the National Institute of Standards and Technology (NIST) and France's Institut Laue-Langevin (ILL). (Adapted from Bagatolli, L.A., Ipsen, J.H., Simonsen, A.C., et al. [2010]. *Prog Lipid Res,* [illegible] 378–389; Contreras, F.X., Ernst, A.M., Wieland, F., et al. [2011]. *Cold Spring Harb Perspect Biol, 3*[6], [illegible]4705; Cooper, G.M. [2000]. *The cell—a molecular approach* [2nd ed.]. Sunderland (MA): Sinauer [illegible]s; Defamie, N., & Mesnil, M. [2012]. *Biochim Biophys Acta, 1818*[8], 1866–1869; Woodka, A.C., [illegible] Porcar, L. et al. [2012]. *Phys Rev Lett, 109*[5], 058102.)

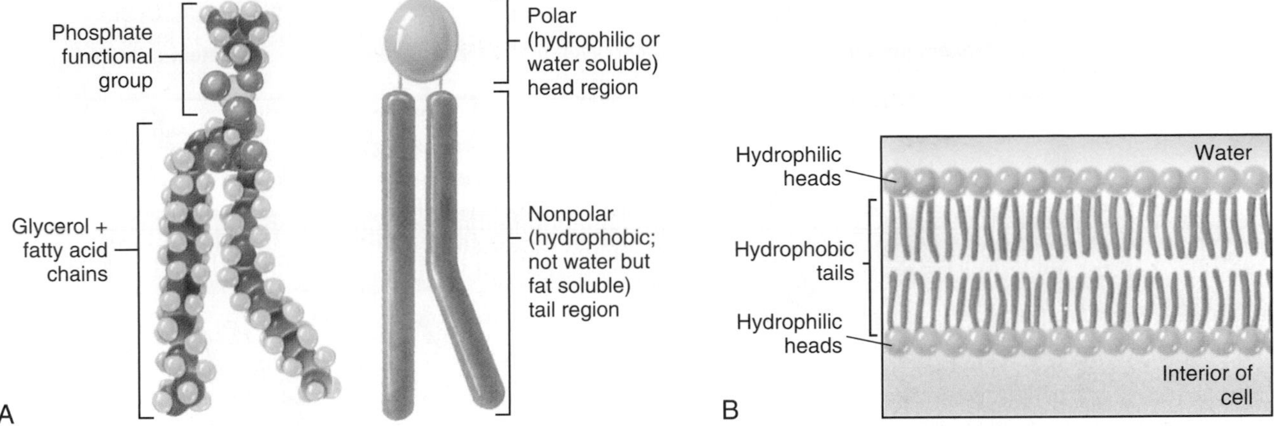

FIGURE 1-6 Structure of a Phospholipid Molecule. A, Each phospholipid molecule consists of a phosphate functional group and two fatty acid chains attached to a glycerol molecule. **B,** The fatty acid chains and glycerol form nonpolar, hydrophobic "tails," and the phosphate functional group forms the polar, hydrophilic "head" of the phospholipid molecule. When placed in water, the hydrophobic tails of the molecule face inward, away from the water, and the hydrophilic head faces outward, toward the water. (From Raven, P.H., & Johnson, G.B. [1995]. *Understanding biology* [3rd ed.]. Dubuque, IA: Brown.)

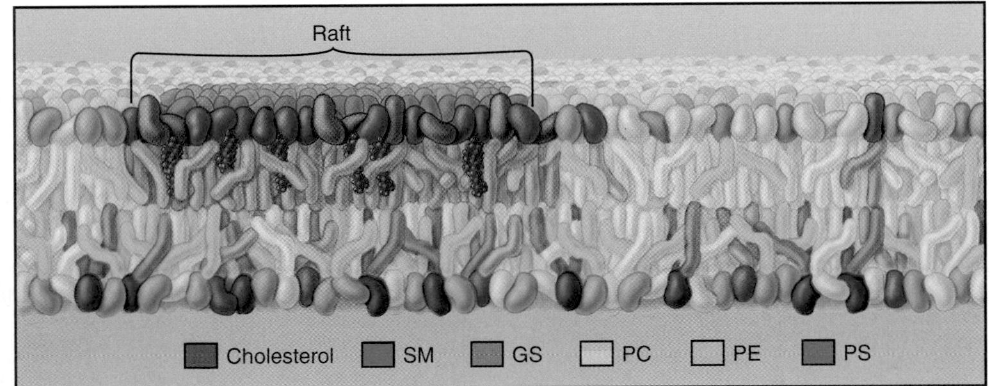

FIGURE 1-7 Lipid Rafts. The plasma membrane is composed of many lipids, including sphingomyelin (*SM*) and cholesterol, shown here as a small raft in the external leaflet. *GS*, glycosphingolipid; *PC*, phosphatidylcholine; *PE*, phosphatidylethanolamine; *PS*, phosphatidylserine. (From Pollard, T.D., & Ernshaw, W.C. [2004]. *Cell biology*. St. Louis: Saunders Elsevier.)

interfere with the host's PTMs.[6] New approaches are being used to understand changes in proteins—a field called **proteomics** is the study of the **proteome**, or entire set of proteins expressed by a genome from synthesis, translocation, and modification (e.g., folding), and the analysis of the roles of proteomes in a staggering number of diseases.

Membrane proteins associate with the lipid bilayer in different ways (Figure 1-8), including (1) **transmembrane proteins** that extend across the bilayer and are exposed to an aqueous environment on both sides of the membrane (Figure 1-8, *A*); (2) proteins located almost entirely in the cytosol and are associated with the cytosolic half of the lipid bilayer by an α helix exposed on the surface of the protein (Figure 1-8, *B*); (3) proteins that exist outside the bilayer, on one side or the other, and are attached to the membrane by one or more covalently attached lipid groups (Figure 1-8, *C*); and (4) proteins bound indirectly to one or the other bilayer membrane face and are held in place by their interactions with other proteins (Figure 1-8, *D*).[1]

Proteins directly attached to the membrane bilayer can be removed by dissolving the bilayer with detergents called **integral membrane proteins**. The remaining proteins that can be removed by gentler procedures that interfere with protein–protein interactions but do not dissolve the bilayer are known as **peripheral membrane proteins**.

Proteins exist in densely folded molecular configurations rather than straight chains; so most hydrophilic units are at the surface of the molecule, and most hydrophobic units are inside. Membrane proteins, like other proteins, are synthesized by the ribosome and then make their way, called *trafficking*, to different membrane locations of a cell.[7] Trafficking places unique demands on membrane proteins for folding, translocation, and stability.[7] Thus, much research is now being done to understand misfolded proteins (e.g., as a cause of disease; Box 1-1).

Although membrane structure is determined by the lipid bilayer, membrane functions are determined largely by proteins. Proteins act as (1) recognition and binding units (receptors) for substances moving into and out of the cell; (2) pores or transport channels for various electrically charged particles, called **ions** or *electrolytes*, and specific carriers for amino acids and monosaccharides; (3) specific enzymes that drive active pumps to promote concentration of certain ions, particularly potassium (K^+), within the cell while keeping concentrations of other ions (e.g., sodium, Na^+) less than concentrations found in the extracellular environment; (4) cell surface markers, such as glycoproteins (proteins attached to carbohydrates), that identify a cell to its neighbour; (5) **cell adhesion molecules (CAMs)**, or proteins that allow cells to hook together and form attachments of the cytoskeleton

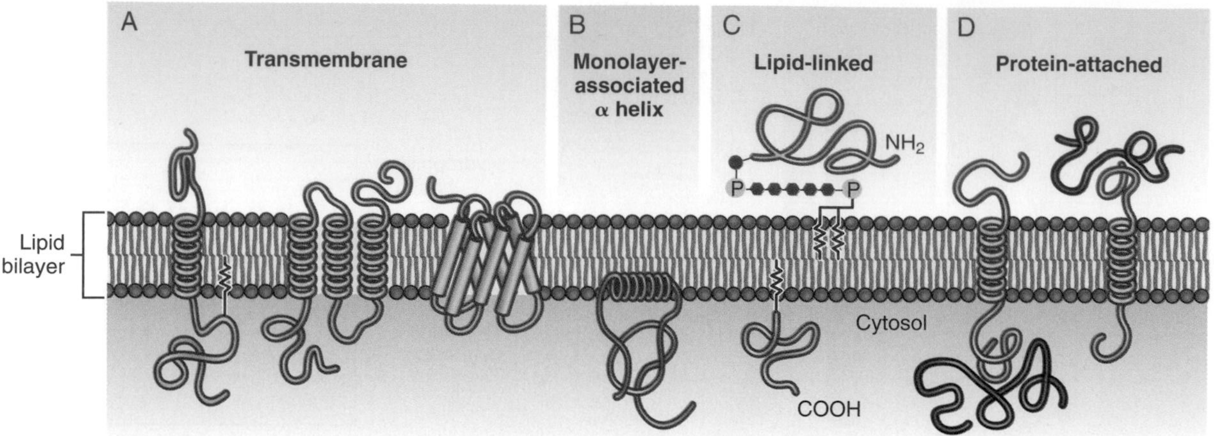

FIGURE 1-8 Proteins Attach to the Plasma Membrane in Different Ways. A, Transmembrane proteins extend through the membrane as a single α helix, as multiple α helices, or as a rolled-up barrel-like sheet called a β barrel. **B,** Some membrane proteins are anchored to the cytosolic side of the lipid bilayer by an amphipathic α helix. **C,** Some proteins are linked on either side of the membrane by a covalently attached lipid molecule. **D,** Proteins are attached by weak noncovalent interactions with other membrane proteins. *COOH,* carboxyl group; *NH_2,* amino group; *P,* protein. (**D,** adapted from Alberts, B. [2014]. *Essential cell biology* [4th ed.]. New York: Garland.)

BOX 1-1 Endoplasmic Reticulum, Protein Folding, and ER Stress

Protein folding in the endoplasmic reticulum (ER) is critical for us. As the biological workhorses, proteins perform vital functions in every cell. To do these tasks, proteins must fold into complex three-dimensional structures (see figure). Most secreted proteins *fold* and are modified in an error-free manner, but ER or cell stress, mutations, or random (stochastic) errors during protein synthesis can decrease the folding amount or the rate of folding. Pathophysiological processes, such as viral infections, environmental toxins, and mutant protein expression, can perturb the sensitive ER environment. Natural processes also can perturb the environment, such as the large protein-synthesizing load placed on the ER. These perturbations cause the accumulation of immature and abnormal proteins in cells, leading to **ER stress**. Fortunately, the ER is loaded with protective ways to help folding; for example, protein *chaperones* facilitate folding and prevent the formation of off-pathway types. Because specialized cells produce large amounts of secreted proteins, the movement or flux through the ER is tremendous. Therefore misfolded proteins not repaired in the ER are observed in some diseases and can initiate apoptosis or cell death. It has recently been shown that the endoplasmic reticulum mediates intracellular signalling pathways in response to the accumulation of unfolded or misfolded proteins; collectively, the pathways are known as the **unfolded-protein response (UPR)**. Investigators are studying UPR-associated inflammation and how the UPR is coupled to inflammation in health and disease. Specific diseases include Alzheimer's disease, Parkinson's disease, prion disease, amyotrophic lateral sclerosis, and diabetes mellitus. Additionally being studied is ER stress and how it may accelerate age-related dysfunction.

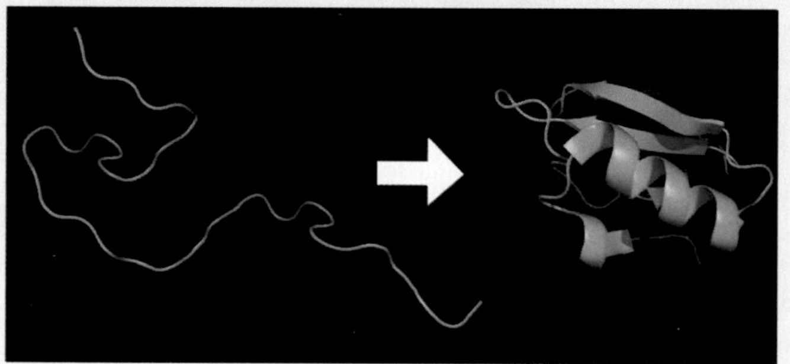

Protein Folding. Each protein exists as an unfolded polypeptide (*left*) or a random coil after the process of translation from a sequence of mRNA to a linear string of amino acids. From amino acids interacting with each other they produce a three-dimensional structure called the folded protein (*right*) that is its native state.

Data from Brodsky, J., & Skach, W.R. (2011). *Curr Opin Cell Biol, 23,* 464–475; Jäger, R., Bertrand, M.J.M., Gorman, A.M., et al. (2012). *Biol Cell, 104*(5), 259–270; Ron, D., & Walter, P. (2007). *Nat Rev Mol Cell Biol, 8,* 519–529.

for maintaining cellular shape; and (6) catalysts of chemical reactions (e.g., conversion of lactose to glucose; see Figure 1-3). Membrane proteins are key components of energy transduction, converting chemical energy into electrical energy, or electrical energy into either mechanical energy or synthesis of ATP.[7] Investigators are studying ATP enzymes and the changes in shape of biological membranes, particularly mitochondrial membranes, and their relationship to aging and disease.[8-10]

In animal cells, the plasma membrane is stabilized by a meshwork of proteins attached to the underside of the membrane called the cell cortex. Human red blood cells have a cell cortex that maintains their flattened biconcave shape.[1]

Protein regulation in a cell: protein homeostasis. The cellular protein pool is in constant change or flux. The number of copies of a protein in a cell depends on how quickly it is made and how long it survives or is broken down. This adaptable system of protein homeostasis is defined by the "proteostasis" network that comprises ribosomes (makers); chaperones (helpers); and two protein breakdown systems or proteolytic systems—lysosomes and the ubiquitin–proteasome system (UPS). These systems regulate protein homeostasis under a large variety

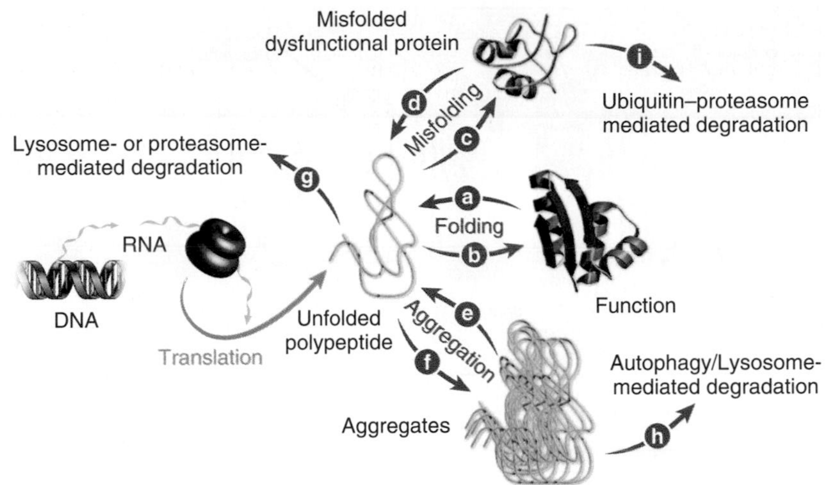

FIGURE 1-9 Protein Homeostasis System and Outcomes. A main role of the protein homeostasis network (*proteostasis*) is to minimize protein misfolding and protein aggregation. The network includes ribosome-mediated protein synthesis, chaperone- (folding helpers in the endoplasmic reticulum) and enzyme-mediated folding, breakdown systems of lysosome- and proteasome-mediated protein degradation, and vesicular trafficking. The network integrates biological pathways that balance folding, trafficking, and protein degradation depicted by arrows *b, d, e, f, g, h,* and *i*. (Adapted from Lindquist, S.L., & Kelly, J.W. [2011]. *Cold Spring Harb Perspect Biol, 3*[12], pii: a004507.)

of conditions, including variations in nutrient supply, the existence of oxidative stress or cellular differentiation, changes in temperature, and the presence of heavy metal ions and other sources of stress.[11] Malfunction or failure of the proteostasis network is associated with human disease[12] (Figure 1-9).

Carbohydrates. The short chains of sugars or carbohydrates (oligosaccharides) contained within the plasma membrane are generally bound to membrane proteins (glycoproteins) and lipids (glycolipids). Long polysaccharide chains attached to membrane proteins are called *proteoglycans*. All of the carbohydrate on the glycoproteins, proteoglycans, and glycolipids is located on the outside of the plasma membrane, and the carbohydrate coating is called the **glycocalyx**. The glycocalyx helps protect the cell from mechanical damage.[1] Additionally, the layer of carbohydrate gives the cell a slimy surface that assists the mobility of other cells, like leukocytes, to squeeze through the narrow spaces.[1] The functions of carbohydrates are more than protection and lubrication and include specific cell–cell recognition and adhesion. Intercellular recognition is an important function of membrane oligosaccharides; for example, the transmembrane proteins called *lectins*, which bind to a particular oligosaccharide, recognize neutrophils at the site of bacterial infection. This recognition allows the neutrophil to adhere to the blood vessel wall and migrate from the blood into the infected tissue to help eliminate the invading bacteria.[1]

Cellular Receptors

Cellular receptors are protein molecules on the plasma membrane, in the cytoplasm, or in the nucleus that can recognize and bind with specific smaller molecules called **ligands** (from the Latin *ligare*, "to bind") (Figure 1-10). The region of a protein that associates with a ligand is called its **binding site**. Hormones, for example, are ligands. Recognition and binding depend on the chemical configuration of the receptor and its smaller ligand, which must fit together somewhat like pieces of a jigsaw puzzle (see Chapter 18). Binding selectively to a protein receptor with high affinity to a ligand depends on formation of weak, noncovalent interactions—hydrogen bonds, electrostatic attractions, and van der Waals attractions—and favourable hydrophobic forces.[1] Numerous receptors are found in most cells, and ligand binding to receptors activates or inhibits the receptor's associated signalling or biochemical pathway.

Plasma membrane receptors protrude from or are exposed at the external surface of the membrane and are important for cellular uptake of ligands (see Figure 1-10). The ligands that bind with membrane receptors include hormones, neurotransmitters, antigens, complement components, lipoproteins, infectious agents, medications, and metabolites. Many new discoveries concerning the specific interactions of cellular receptors with their respective ligands have provided a basis for understanding disease.

Although the chemical nature of ligands and their receptors differs, receptors are classified based on their location and function. Cellular type determines overall cellular function, but plasma membrane receptors determine which ligands a cell will bind with and how the cell will respond to the binding. Specific processes also control intracellular mechanisms.

Receptors for different medications are found on the plasma membrane, in the cytoplasm, and in the nucleus. Membrane receptors have been found for certain anaesthetics, opiates, endorphins, enkephalins, antibiotics, cancer chemotherapeutic agents, digitalis, and other medications. Membrane receptors for endorphins, which are opiatelike peptides isolated from the pituitary gland, are found in large quantities in pain pathways of the nervous system (see Chapters 13 and 14). With binding to the receptor, the endorphins (or medications such as morphine) change the cell's permeability to ions, increase the concentration of molecules that regulate intracellular protein synthesis, and initiate molecular events that modulate pain perception.

Receptors for infectious microorganisms, or antigen receptors, bind bacteria, viruses, and parasites to the cell membrane. Antigen receptors on white blood cells (lymphocytes, monocytes, macrophages, granulocytes) recognize and bind with antigenic microorganisms and activate the immune and inflammatory responses (see Chapter 6).

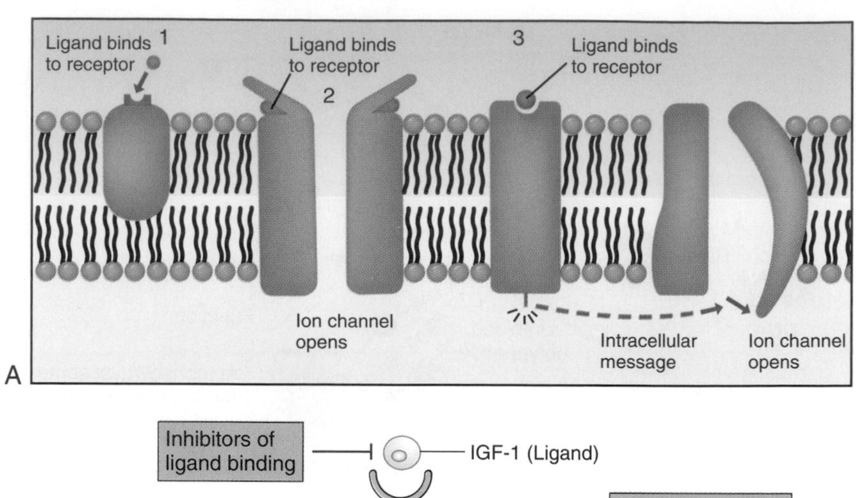

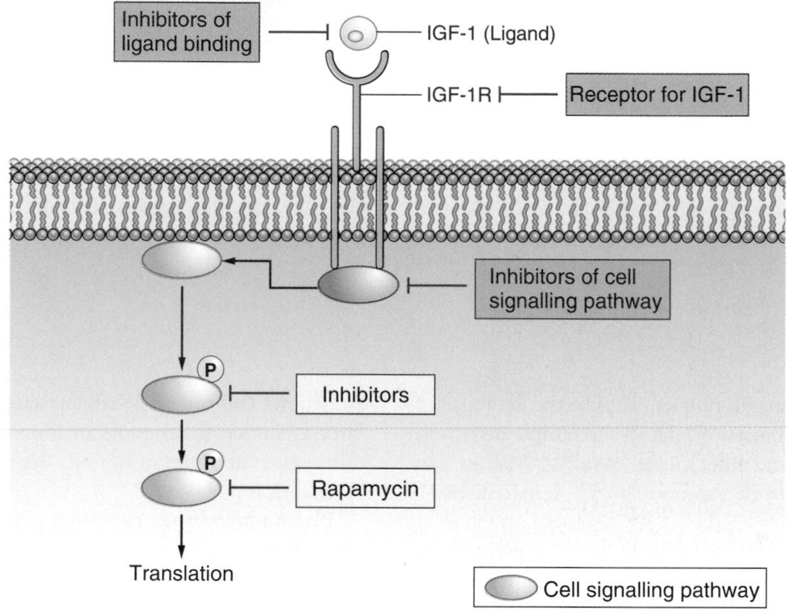

FIGURE 1-10 Cellular Receptors. **(A)** **1,** Plasma membrane receptor for a ligand (here, a hormone molecule) on the surface of an integral protein. A neurotransmitter can exert its effect on a postsynaptic cell by means of two fundamentally different types of receptor proteins: **2,** channel-linked receptors, and **3,** non–channel-linked receptors. Channel-linked receptors are also known as *ligand-gated channels.* **(B)** Example of ligand-receptor interaction. Insulinlike growth factor 1 (*IGF-1*) is a ligand and binds to the insulinlike growth factor 1 receptor (*IGF-1R*). With binding at the cell membrane the intracellular signalling pathway is activated, causing translation of new proteins (*P*) to act as intracellular communicators. This pathway is important for cancer growth. Researchers are developing pharmacological strategies to reduce signalling at and downstream of the IGF-1R, hoping this will lead to compounds useful in cancer treatment.

CELL-TO-CELL ADHESIONS

Cells are small and squishy, *not* like bricks. They are enclosed only by a flimsy membrane, yet the cell depends on the integrity of this membrane for its survival. How can cells be connected strongly, with their membranes intact, to form a muscle that can lift this textbook? Plasma membranes not only serve as the outer boundaries of all cells but also allow groups of cells to be held together robustly, in **cell-to-cell adhesions**, to form tissues and organs. Once arranged, cells are linked by three different means: (1) CAMs in the cell's plasma membrane, (2) the ECM, and (3) specialized cell junctions.

Extracellular Matrix

Cells can be united by attachment to one another or through the **extracellular matrix (ECM)** (including the **basement membrane**), which the cells secrete around themselves. The ECM is an intricate meshwork of fibrous proteins embedded in a watery, gel-like substance composed of complex carbohydrates (Figure 1-11). The matrix is similar to glue; however, it provides a pathway for diffusion of nutrients, wastes, and other water-soluble substances between the blood and tissue cells. Interwoven within the matrix are three groups of **macromolecules**: (1) fibrous structural proteins, including collagen and elastin; (2) adhesive glycoproteins, such as fibronectin; and (3) proteoglycans and hyaluronic acid.

- **Collagen** forms cablelike fibres or sheets that provide tensile strength or resistance to longitudinal stress. Collagen breakdown, such as occurs in osteoarthritis, destroys the fibrils that give cartilage its tensile strength.
- **Elastin** is a rubberlike protein fibre most abundant in tissues that must be capable of stretching and recoiling, such as tissues found in the lungs.
- **Fibronectin**, a large glycoprotein, promotes cell adhesion and cell anchorage. Reduced amounts have been found in certain types of cancerous cells; the reduced amount of this substance allows cancer

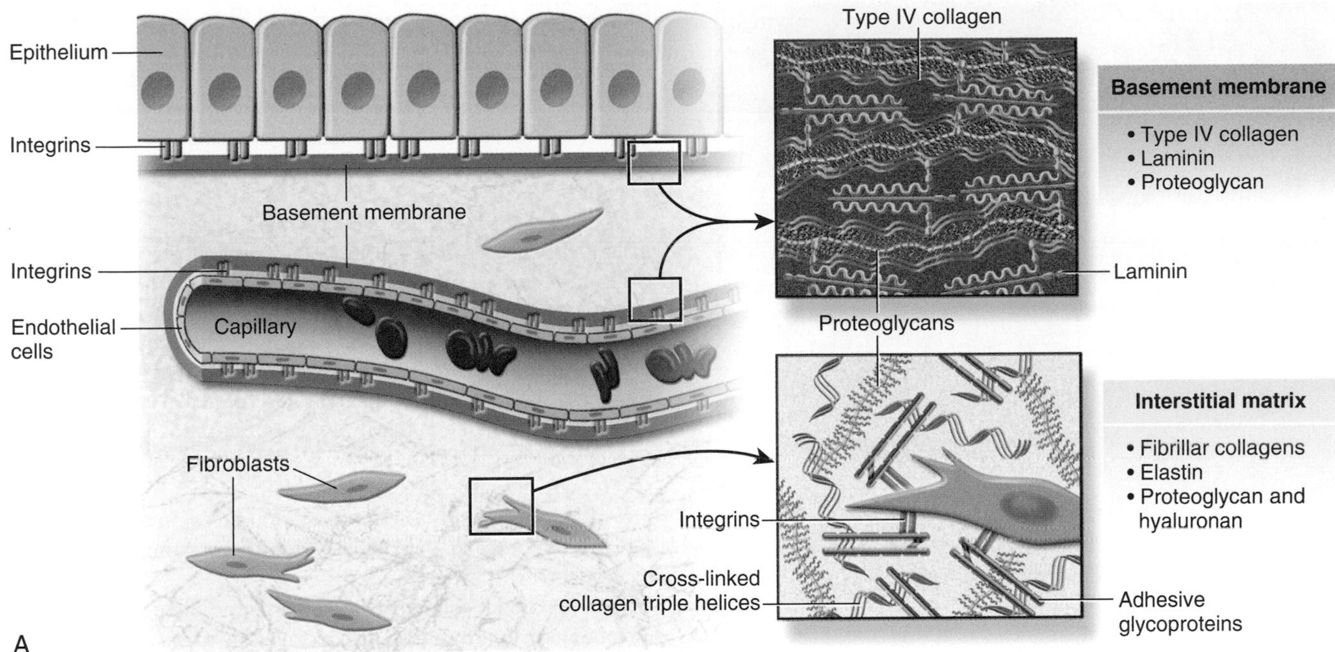

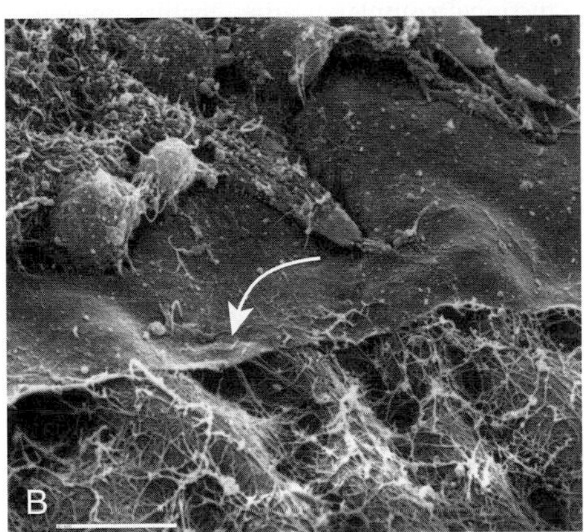

FIGURE 1-11 Extracellular Matrix. A, Tissues are not just cells but also extracellular space. The extracellular space is an intricate network of macromolecules called the *extracellular matrix* (*ECM*). The macromolecules that constitute the ECM are secreted locally (by mostly fibroblasts) and assembled into a meshwork in close association with the surface of the cell that produced them. Two main classes of macromolecules include proteoglycans, which are bound to polysaccharide chains called *glycosaminoglycans*, and fibrous proteins (e.g., collagen, elastin, fibronectin, and laminin), which have structural and adhesive properties. Together the proteoglycan molecules form a gel-like ground substance in which the fibrous proteins are embedded. The gel permits rapid diffusion of nutrients, metabolites, and hormones between the blood and the tissue cells. Matrix proteins modulate cell-matrix interactions, including normal tissue remodelling (which can become abnormal, e.g., with chronic inflammation). Disruptions of this balance result in serious diseases such as arthritis, tumour growth, and other pathological conditions. **B,** Scanning electron micrograph of a chick embryo where a portion of the epithelium has been removed, exposing the curtainlike ECM. (**A,** adapted from Kumar, V., Abbas, A.K., & Aster, J.C. [Eds.]. [2015]. *Robbins and Cotran pathologic basis of disease* [9th ed.]. Philadelphia: Saunders; **B,** © Robert L Trelstad; from Gartner, L.P., & Hiatt, J.L. [2006]. *Color textbook of histology* [3rd ed.]. St. Louis: Saunders/Elsevier.)

cells to travel, or metastasize, to other parts of the body. All of these macromolecules occur in intercellular junctions and cell surfaces and may assemble into two different components: interstitial matrix and basement membrane (see Figure 1-11).

The basement membrane is a thin, tough layer of ECM (connective tissue) underlying the epithelium of many organs and is also called the **basal lamina** (Figure 1-11, *B*).

The ECM is secreted by **fibroblasts** ("fibre formers") (Figure 1-12), local cells that are present in the matrix. The matrix and the cells within it are known collectively as **connective tissue** because they interconnect cells to form tissues and organs. Human connective tissues are enormously varied. They can be hard and dense, like bone; flexible, like tendons or the dermis of the skin; resilient and shock absorbing, like cartilage; or soft and transparent, similar to the jellylike substance that fills the eye.

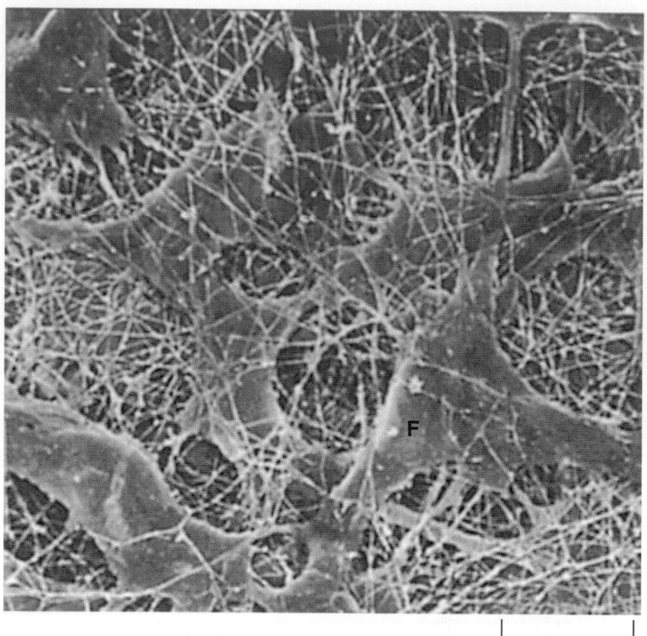

FIGURE 1-12 Fibroblasts in Connective Tissue. This micrograph shows tissue from the cornea of a rat. The extracellular matrix surrounds the fibroblasts (*F*). (From Nishida, T., Yasumoto, K., Otori, T., et al. [1988]. *Invest Ophthalmol Vis Sci, 29,* 1887–1890.)

In all these examples, the majority of the tissue is composed of ECM, and the cells that produce the matrix are scattered within it like raisins in a pudding (see Figure 1-12).

The matrix not only acts as passive scaffolding for cellular attachment but also helps regulate the function of the cells with which it interacts. The matrix helps regulate such important functions as cell growth and differentiation.

Specialized Cell Junctions

Cells in direct physical contact with neighbouring cells are often interconnected at specialized plasma membrane regions called **cell junctions**. Cell junctions are classified by their function: (1) some hold cells together and form a tight seal (tight junctions); (2) some provide strong mechanical attachments (adherens junctions, desmosomes, hemidesmosomes); (3) some provide a special type of chemical communication (e.g., inorganic ions and small water-soluble molecules to move from the cytosol of one cell to the cytosol of another cell), such as those causing an electrical wave (gap junctions); and (4) some maintain apicobasal polarity of individual epithelial cells (tight junctions) (Figure 1-13). Overall, cell junctions make the epithelium leak-proof and mediate mechanical attachment of one cell to another, allowing communicating tunnels and maintaining cell polarity.

Cell junctions can be classified as symmetrical and asymmetrical. Symmetrical junctions include tight junctions, the belt desmosome (zonula adherens), desmosomes (macula adherens), and gap junctions (also called *intercellular channels* or *communicating junctions*).[13] An asymmetrical junction is the hemidesmosome (see Figure 1-13). Together they form the **junctional complex**. **Desmosomes** unite cells either by forming continuous bands or belts of epithelial sheets or by developing buttonlike points of contact. Desmosomes also act as a system of braces to maintain structural stability. **Tight junctions** are barriers to diffusion, prevent the movement of substances through transport proteins in the plasma membrane, and prevent the leakage of small molecules between the plasma membranes of adjacent cells. **Gap junctions** are clusters of communicating tunnels or connexons that allow small ions and molecules to pass directly from the inside of one cell to the inside of another. **Connexons** are hemichannels that extend outward from each of the adjacent plasma membranes (Figure 1-13, *C*).

Multiple factors regulate gap junction intercellular communication, including voltage across the junction, intracellular pH, intracellular Ca^{++} concentration, and protein phosphorylation. The most abundant human connexin is connexin 43 (Cx43).[14] Investigators recently showed that loss of Cx43 expression in colorectal tumours is correlated with a shorter cancer-free survival rate.[15] This study is the first evidence that Cx43 acts as a tumour suppressor for colorectal cancer (enhances apoptosis) and therefore may be an important prognostic marker and target for therapy.[15] Investigators also recently reported that glycyrrhizic acid (GA), a glycoside of licorice root extracts, may be a strong chemopreventive agent against carcinogens; induced colon cancer in rats and Cx43 is one target.[16] Too much GA often in humans may lead to hypokalemia and hypertension.[17]

The junctional complex is a highly permeable part of the plasma membrane. Its permeability is controlled by a process called **gating**. Increased levels of cytoplasmic calcium cause decreased permeability at the junctional complex. Gating enables uninjured cells to protect themselves from injured neighbours. Calcium is released from injured cells.

CELLULAR COMMUNICATION AND SIGNAL TRANSDUCTION

Cells need to communicate with each other to maintain a stable internal environment, or **homeostasis**; to regulate their growth and division; to oversee their development and organization into tissues; and to coordinate their functions. Cells communicate by using hundreds of kinds of signal molecules, for example, insulin (Figure 1-10, *B*). Cells communicate in three main ways: (1) they display plasma membrane–bound signalling molecules (receptors) that affect the cell itself and other cells in direct physical contact (Figure 1-14, *A*); (2) they affect receptor proteins *inside* the target cell and the signal molecule has to enter the cell to bind to them (Figure 1-14, *B*); and (3) they form protein channels (gap junctions) that directly coordinate the activities of adjacent cells (Figure 1-14, *C*). Alterations in cellular communication affect disease onset and progression. In fact, if a cell cannot perform gap junctional intercellular communication, normal growth control and cell differentiation is compromised, thereby favouring cancerous tumour development (see Chapter 10). Secreted chemical signals involve communication locally and at a distance. Primary modes of intercellular signalling are contact-dependent, paracrine, hormonal, neurohormonal, and neurotransmitter. Autocrine stimulation occurs when the secreting cell targets itself (Figure 1-15).

Contact-dependent signalling requires cells to be in close membrane–membrane contact. In **paracrine signalling**, cells secrete local chemical mediators that are quickly taken up, destroyed, or immobilized. Paracrine signalling usually involves different cell types; however, cells also can produce signals to which they alone respond, called **autocrine signalling** (see Figure 1-15). For example, cancer cells use this form of signalling to stimulate their survival and proliferation. The mediators act only on nearby cells. **Hormonal signalling** involves specialized endocrine cells that secrete chemicals called *hormones*; hormones are released by one set of cells and travel through the bloodstream to produce a response in other sets of cells (see Chapter 18). In **neurohormonal signalling**, hormones are released into the blood by neurosecretory neurons. Like

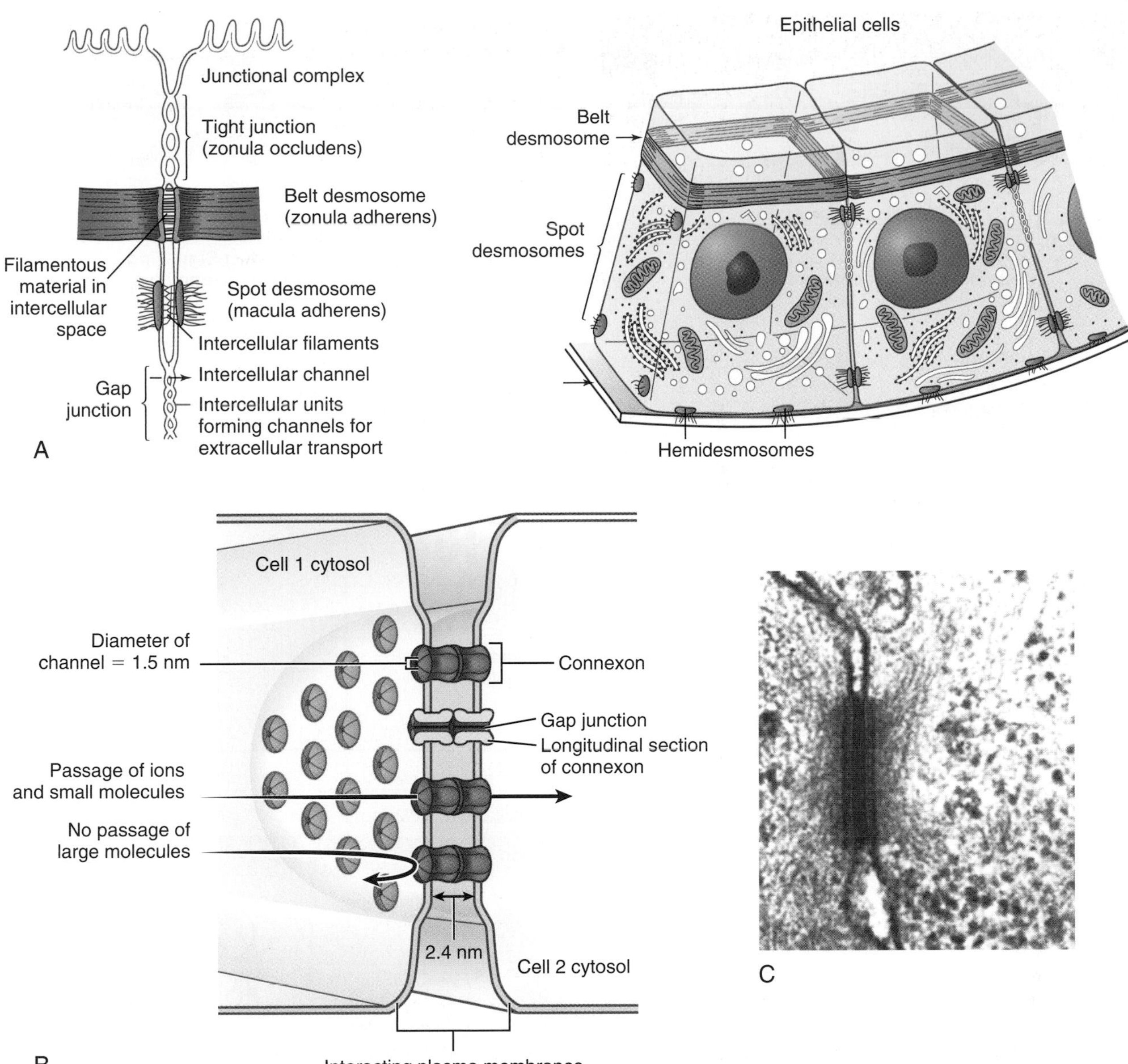

FIGURE 1-13 Junctional Complex. **A,** Schematic drawing of a belt desmosome between epithelial cells. This junction, also called the *zonula adherens*, encircles each of the interacting cells. The spot desmosomes and hemidesmosomes, like the belt desmosomes, are adhering junctions. This tight junction is an impermeable junction that holds cells together but seals them in such a way that molecules cannot leak between them. The gap junction, as a communicating junction, mediates the passage of small molecules from one interacting cell to the other. **B,** Connexons. The connexin gap junction proteins have four transmembrane domains and they play a vital role in maintaining cell and tissue function and homeostasis. Cells connected by gap junctions are considered ionically (electrically) and metabolically coupled. Gap junctions coordinate the activities of adjacent cells; for example, they are important for synchronizing contractions of heart muscle cells through ionic coupling and for permitting action potentials to spread rapidly from cell to cell in neural tissues. The reason gap junctions occur in tissues that are not electrically active is unknown. Although most gap junctions are associated with junctional complexes, they sometimes exist as independent structures. **C,** Electron micrograph of desmosomes. (**A** and **C,** from Raven, P.H., & Johnson, G.B. [1992]. *Biology*. St. Louis: Mosby; **B,** adapted from Gartner, L.P., & Hiatt, J.L. [2006]. *Color textbook of histology* [3rd ed.]. St. Louis: Saunders Elsevier; Sherwood, L. [2013]. *Learning* [8th ed.]. Belmont, CA: Brooks/Cole CENGAGE.)

endocrine cells, neurosecretory neurons release bloodborne chemical messengers, whereas ordinary neurons secrete short-range neurotransmitters into a small discrete space (i.e., synapse). Neurons communicate directly with the cells they innervate by releasing chemicals or **neurotransmitters** at specialized junctions called **chemical synapses**; the neurotransmitter diffuses across the synaptic cleft and acts on the postsynaptic target cell (see Figure 1-15). Many of these same signalling molecules are receptors used in hormonal, neurohormonal, and paracrine signalling. Important differences lie in the speed and selectivity with which the signals are delivered to their targets.[1]

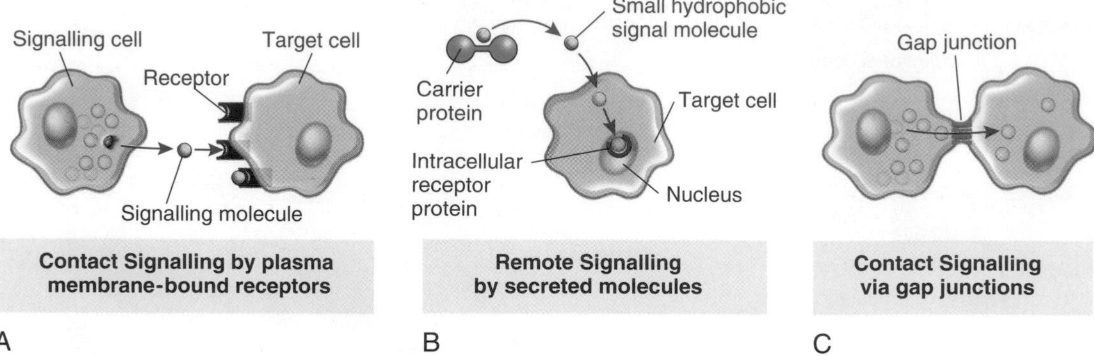

FIGURE 1-14 Cellular Communication. Three primary ways cells communicate with one another. (**B**, adapted from Alberts, B., Johnson, A., Lewis, J., et al. [2008]. *Molecular biology of the cell* [5th ed.]. New York: Garland.)

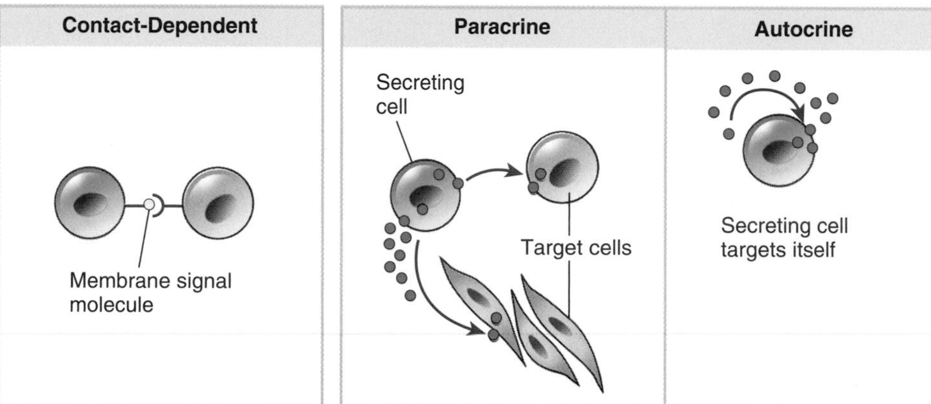

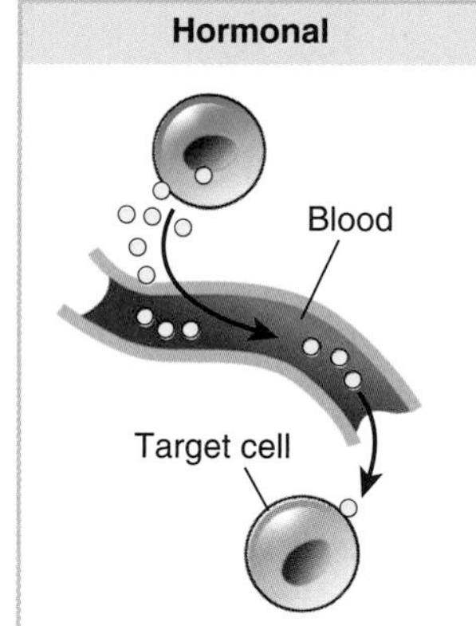

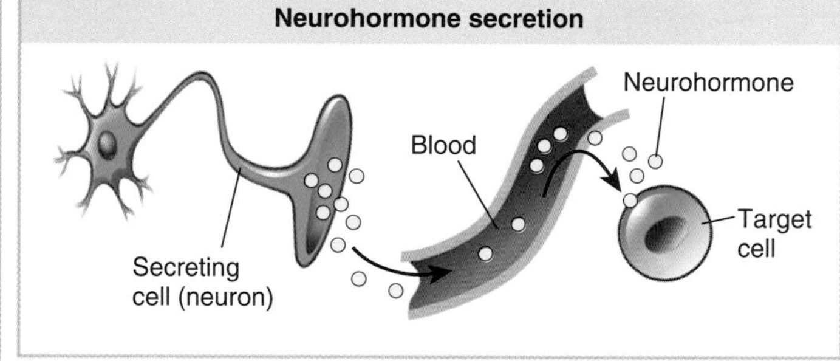

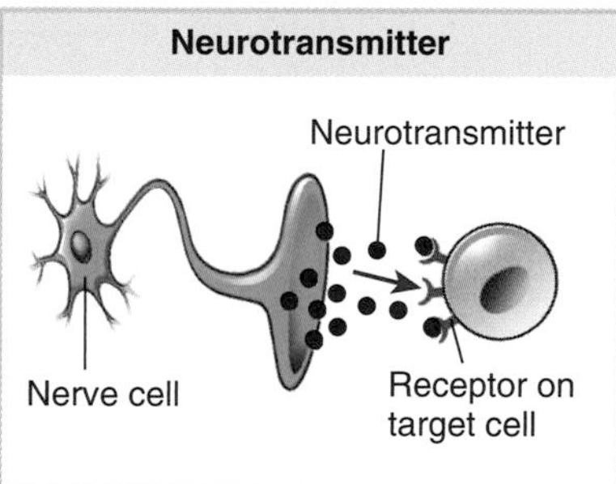

FIGURE 1-15 Primary Modes of Chemical Signalling. Five forms of signalling mediated by secreted molecules. Hormones, paracrines, neurotransmitters, and neurohormones are all intercellular messengers that accomplish communication between cells. Autocrines bind to receptors on the same cell. Not all neurotransmitters act in the strictly synaptic mode shown; some act in a contact-dependent mode as local chemical mediators that influence multiple target cells in the area.

Plasma membrane receptors belong to one of three classes that are defined by the signalling (transduction) mechanism used. Table 1-3 summarizes these classes of receptors. Cells respond to external stimuli by activating a variety of **signal transduction pathways**, which are communication pathways, or signalling cascades (Figure 1-16, *C*). Signals are passed between cells when a particular type of molecule is produced by one cell—the **signalling cell**—and received by another—the **target cell**—by means of a **receptor protein** that recognizes and responds specifically to the signal molecule (Figure 1-16, *A* and *B*). In turn, the signalling molecules activate a pathway of intracellular protein kinases that results in various responses, such as grow and reproduce, die, survive, or differentiate (Figure 1-16, *D*). If deprived of appropriate signals, most cells undergo a form of cell suicide known as *programmed cell death*, or *apoptosis* (see p. 105).

CELLULAR METABOLISM

All of the chemical tasks of maintaining essential cellular functions are referred to as **cellular metabolism**. The energy-using process of metabolism is called **anabolism** (*ana* = upward), and the energy-releasing process is known as **catabolism** (*kata* = downward). Metabolism provides the cell with the energy it needs to produce cellular structures.

TABLE 1-3 Classes of Plasma Membrane Receptors

Type of Receptor	Description
Ion channel coupled	Involve rapid synaptic signalling between electrically excitable cells; also called *transmitter-gated* ion channels. Channels open and close briefly in response to neurotransmitters, changing ion permeability of plasma membrane of postsynaptic cell.
Enzyme coupled	Once activated by ligands, function directly as enzymes or associate with enzymes.
G-protein coupled	Indirectly activate or inactivate plasma membrane enzyme or ion channel; interaction mediated by *GTP-binding regulatory protein (G-protein)*. May also interact with inositol phospholipids, which are significant in cell signalling, and with molecules involved in *inositol-phospholipid transduction pathway*.

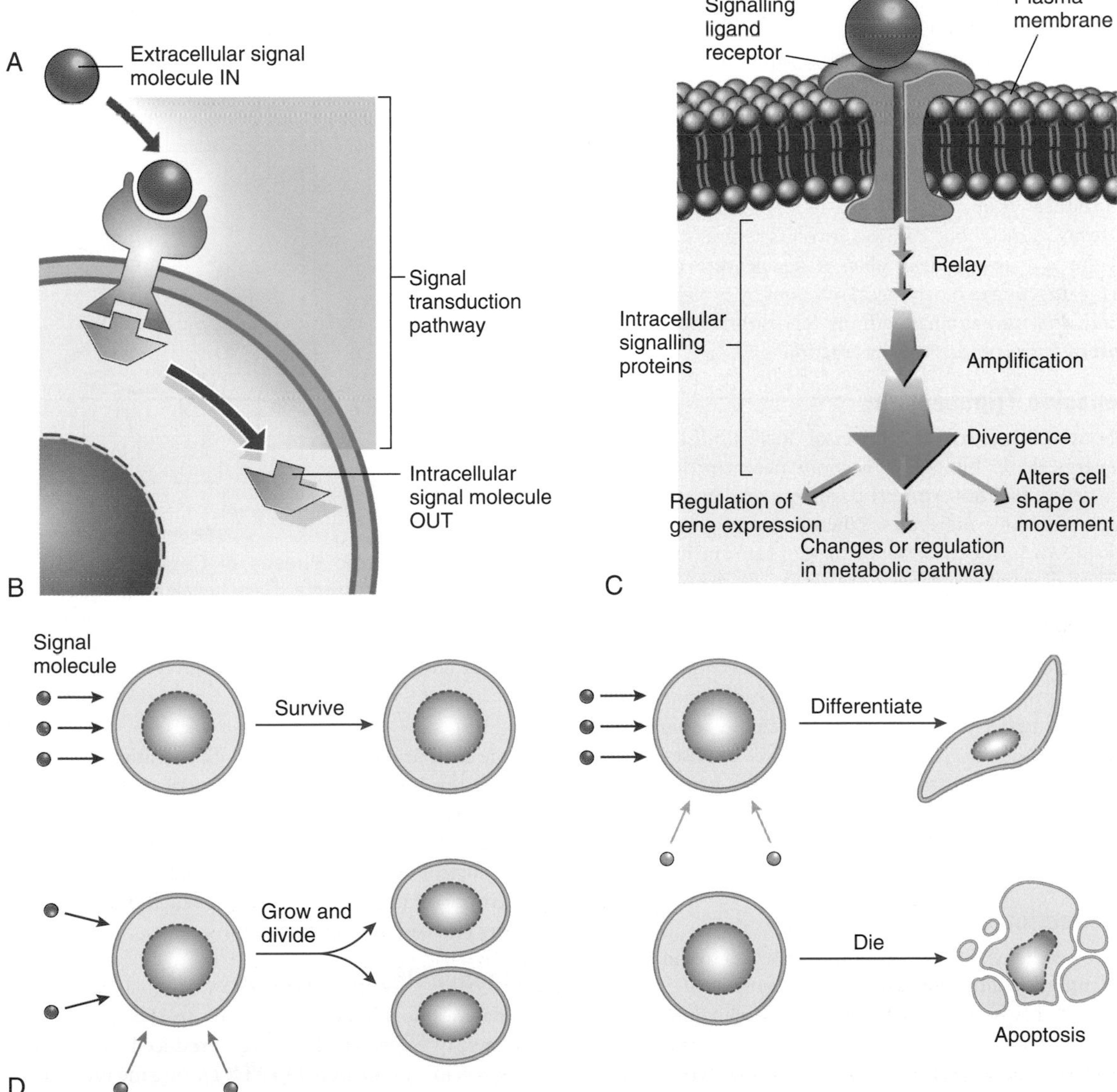

FIGURE 1-16 Schematic of a Signal Transduction Pathway. Like a telephone receiver that converts an electrical signal into a sound signal, a cell converts an extracellular signal, **A,** into an intracellular signal, **B. C,** An extracellular signal molecule (ligand) bonds to a receptor protein located on the plasma membrane, where it is transduced into an intracellular signal. This process initiates a signalling cascade that relays the signal into the cell interior, amplifying and distributing it during transit. Amplification is often achieved by stimulating enzymes. Steps in the cascade can be modulated by other events in the cell. **D,** Different cell behaviours rely on multiple extracellular signals.

BOX 1-2 Role of Adenosine Triphosphate Outside Cells

Emerging understandings are the role of adenosine triphosphate (ATP) *outside* cells—as a messenger. In animal studies, using the newly developed ATP probe, ATP has been measured in pericellular spaces. New research is clarifying the role of ATP as an extracellular messenger and its role in many physiological processes, including inflammation.

From Burnstock, G. (2007). *Physiol Rev, 87*(2), 659–797. doi:10.1152/physrev.00043.2006; Falzoni, S., Donvito, G., & Di Virgilio, F. (2013). *Interface Focus, 3*(3), 20120101. doi:10.1098/rsfs.2012.0101; Nurse, C.A., & Piskuric, N.A. (2012). *Semin Cell Dev Biol, 24*(1), 22–30. doi:10.1016/j.semcdb.2012.09.006.

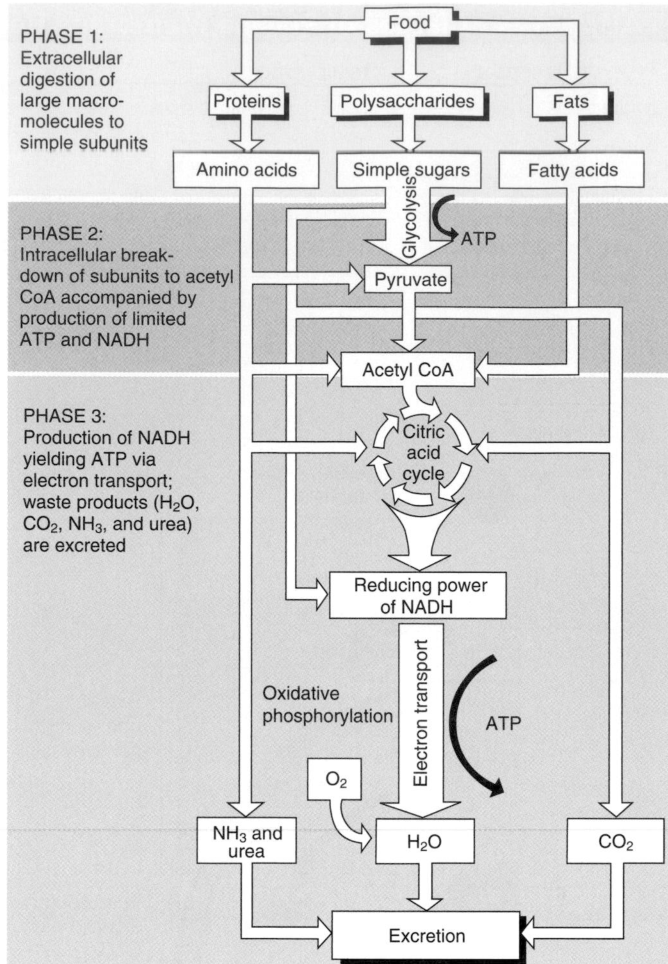

FIGURE 1-17 Three Phases of Catabolism, Which Lead from Food to Waste Products. These reactions produce adenosine triphosphate (*ATP*), which is used to power other processes in the cell. *CO_2*, carbon dioxide; *CoA*, coenzyme A; *H_2O*, water; *NADH*, reduced nicotinamide adenine dinucleotide; *NH_3*, ammonia; *O_2*, oxygen.

Dietary proteins, fats, and starches (i.e., carbohydrates) are hydrolyzed in the intestinal tract into amino acids, fatty acids, and glucose, respectively. These constituents are then absorbed, circulated, and incorporated into the cell, where they may be used for various vital cellular processes, including the production of ATP. The process by which ATP is produced is one example of a series of reactions called a **metabolic pathway**. A metabolic pathway involves several steps whose end products are not always detectable. A key feature of cellular metabolism is the directing of biochemical reactions by protein catalysts or enzymes. Each enzyme has a high affinity for a **substrate**, a specific substance converted to a product of the reaction.

Role of Adenosine Triphosphate

Best known about ATP is its role as a universal "fuel" *inside* living cells. This fuel or energy drives biological reactions necessary for cells to function. For a cell to function, it must be able to extract and use the chemical energy in organic molecules. When 1 mol of glucose metabolically breaks down in the presence of oxygen into carbon dioxide and water, 686 kcal of chemical energy are released. The chemical energy lost by one molecule is transferred to the chemical structure of another molecule by an energy-carrying or energy-transferring molecule, such as ATP. The energy stored in ATP can be used in various energy-requiring reactions and in the process is generally converted to adenosine diphosphate (ADP) and inorganic phosphate (Pi). The energy available as a result of this reaction is about 7 kcal/mol of ATP. The cell uses ATP for muscle contraction and active transport of molecules across cellular membranes. ATP not only stores energy but also *transfers* it from one molecule to another. Energy stored by carbohydrate, lipid, and protein is catabolized and transferred to ATP (Box 1-2).

Food and Production of Cellular Energy

Catabolism of the proteins, lipids, and polysaccharides found in food can be divided into the following three phases (Figure 1-17):

Phase 1: **Digestion**. Large molecules are broken down into smaller subunits: proteins into amino acids, polysaccharides into simple sugars (i.e., monosaccharides), and fats into fatty acids and glycerol. These processes occur outside the cell and are activated by secreted enzymes.

Phase 2: **Glycolysis** and **oxidation**. The most important part of phase 2 is glycolysis, the splitting of glucose. Glycolysis produces two molecules of ATP per glucose molecule through oxidation, or the removal and transfer of a pair of electrons. The total process is called *oxidative cellular metabolism* and involves 10 biochemical reactions (Figure 1-18).

Phase 3: **Citric acid cycle (Krebs cycle, tricarboxylic acid cycle)**. Most of the ATP is generated during this final phase, which begins with the citric acid cycle and ends with oxidative phosphorylation. About two thirds of the total oxidation of carbon compounds in most cells is accomplished during this phase. The major end products are CO_2 and two dinucleotides—reduced nicotinamide adenine dinucleotide (NADH) and the reduced form of flavin adenine dinucleotide ($FADH_2$)—both of which transfer their electrons into the electron-transport chain.

Oxidative Phosphorylation

Oxidative phosphorylation occurs in the mitochondria and is the mechanism by which the energy produced from carbohydrates, fats, and proteins is transferred to ATP. During the breakdown (catabolism) of foods, many reactions involve the removal of electrons from various intermediates. These reactions generally require a coenzyme (a nonprotein carrier molecule), such as nicotinamide adenine dinucleotide (NAD), to transfer the electrons and thus are called **transfer reactions**.

Molecules of NAD and flavin adenine dinucleotide (FAD) transfer electrons they have gained from the oxidation of substrates to molecular oxygen. The electrons from reduced NAD and FAD, NADH and $FADH_2$, respectively, are transferred to the **electron-transport chain** on the inner surfaces of the mitochondria with the release of hydrogen ions. Some carrier molecules are brightly coloured, iron-containing proteins

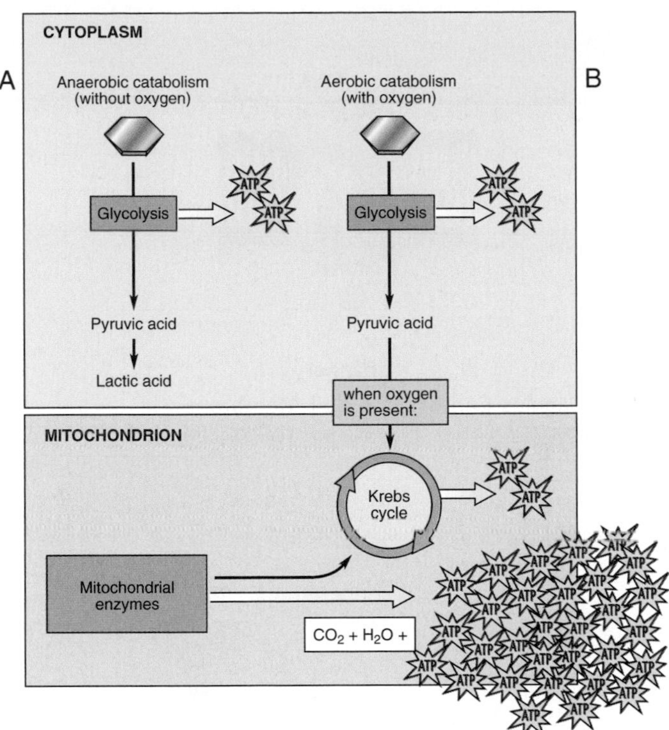

FIGURE 1-18 **Glycolysis.** Sugars are important for fuel or energy and they are oxidized in small steps to carbon dioxide (*CO_2*) and water (*H_2O*). Glycolysis is the process for oxidizing sugars or glucose. Breakdown of glucose. **A,** Anaerobic catabolism, to lactic acid and little adenosine triphosphate (*ATP*). **B,** Aerobic catabolism, to carbon dioxide, water, and lots of ATP. (From Herlihy, B. [2015]. *The human body in health and illness* [5th ed.]. St. Louis: Saunders.)

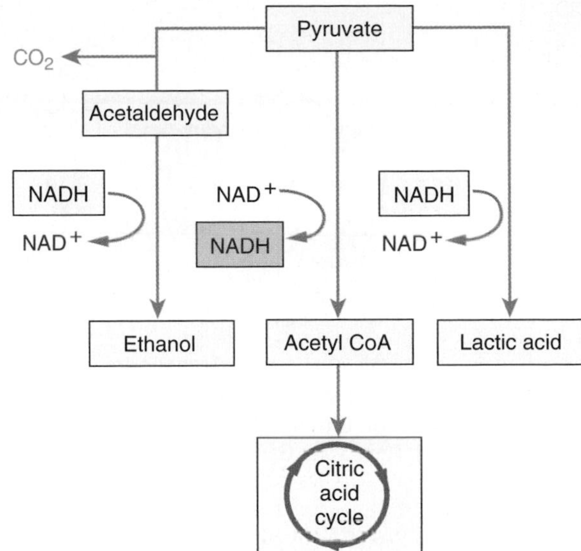

FIGURE 1-19 **What Happens to Pyruvate, the Product of Glycolysis?** In the presence of oxygen, pyruvate is oxidized to acetyl coenzyme A (*Acetyl CoA*) and enters the citric acid cycle. In the absence of oxygen, pyruvate instead is reduced, accepting the electrons extracted during glycolysis and carried by reduced nicotinamide adenine dinucleotide (*NADH*). When pyruvate is reduced directly, as it is in muscles, the product is lactic acid. When carbon dioxide (*CO_2*) is first removed from pyruvate and the remainder is reduced, as it is in yeasts, the resulting product is ethanol. *NAD^+*, oxidized nicotinamide adenine dinucleotide.

known as *cytochromes* that accept a pair of electrons. These electrons eventually combine with molecular oxygen.

If oxygen is not available to the electron-transport chain, ATP will not be formed by the mitochondria. Instead, an anaerobic (without oxygen) metabolic pathway synthesizes ATP. This process, called **substrate phosphorylation** or **anaerobic glycolysis**, is linked to the breakdown (glycolysis) of carbohydrate (see Figure 1-18). Because glycolysis occurs in the cytoplasm of the cell, it provides energy for cells that lack mitochondria. The reactions in anaerobic glycolysis involve the conversion of glucose to pyruvic acid (pyruvate) with the simultaneous production of ATP. With the glycolysis of one molecule of glucose, two ATP molecules and two molecules of pyruvate are liberated. If oxygen is present, the two molecules of pyruvate move into the mitochondria, where they enter the citric acid cycle (Figure 1-19).

If oxygen is absent, pyruvate is converted to lactic acid, which is released into the extracellular fluid. The conversion of pyruvic acid to lactic acid is reversible; therefore, once oxygen is restored, lactic acid is quickly converted back to either pyruvic acid or glucose. The anaerobic generation of ATP from glucose through glycolysis is not as efficient as the aerobic generation process. Adding an oxygen-requiring stage to the catabolic process (phase 3; see Figure 1-17) provides cells with a much more powerful method for extracting energy from food molecules.

MEMBRANE TRANSPORT: CELLULAR INTAKE AND OUTPUT

Cell survival and growth depend on the constant exchange of molecules with their environment. Cells continually import nutrients, fluids, and chemical messengers from the extracellular environment and expel metabolites, or the products of metabolism, and end products of lysosomal digestion. Cells also must regulate ions in their cytosol and organelles. Simple diffusion across the lipid bilayer of the plasma membrane occurs for such important molecules as O_2 and CO_2. However, the majority of molecular transfer depends on specialized **membrane transport proteins** that span the lipid bilayer and provide private conduits for select molecules.[1] Membrane transport proteins occur in many forms and are present in all cell membranes.[1] Transport by membrane transport proteins is sometimes called **mediated transport**. Most of these transport proteins allow selective passage (e.g., Na^+ but not K^+ or K^+ but not Na^+). Each type of cell membrane has its own transport proteins that determine which solute can pass into and out of the cell or organelle.[1] The two main classes of membrane transport proteins are *transporters* and *channels*. These transport proteins differ in the type of **solute**—small particles of dissolved substances—they transport. A **transporter** is specific, allowing only those ions that fit the unique binding sites on the protein (Figure 1-20, *A*). A transporter undergoes conformational changes to enable membrane transport. A **channel**, when open, forms a pore across the lipid bilayer that allows ions and selective polar organic molecules to diffuse across the membrane (Figure 1-20, *B*). Transport by a channel depends on the size and electrical charge of the molecule. Some channels are controlled by a gate mechanism that determines which solute can move into it. Ion channels are responsible for the electrical excitability of nerve and muscle cells and play a critical role in the membrane potential.

The mechanisms of membrane transport depend on the characteristics of the substance to be transported. In **passive transport**, water and small, electrically uncharged molecules move easily through pores in the plasma membrane's lipid bilayer (Figure 1-20). This process occurs naturally through any semipermeable barrier. Molecules will easily flow "downhill" from a region of high concentration to a region of low concentration; this movement is called *passive* because it does not require

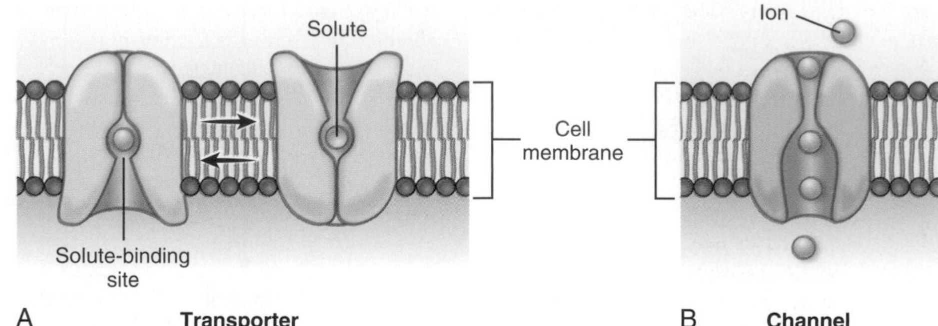

FIGURE 1-20 Inorganic Ions and Small, Polar Organic Molecules Can Cross a Cell Membrane Through Either a Transporter or a Channel. (Adapted from Alberts, B. [2014]. *Essential cell biology* [4th ed.]. New York: Garland.)

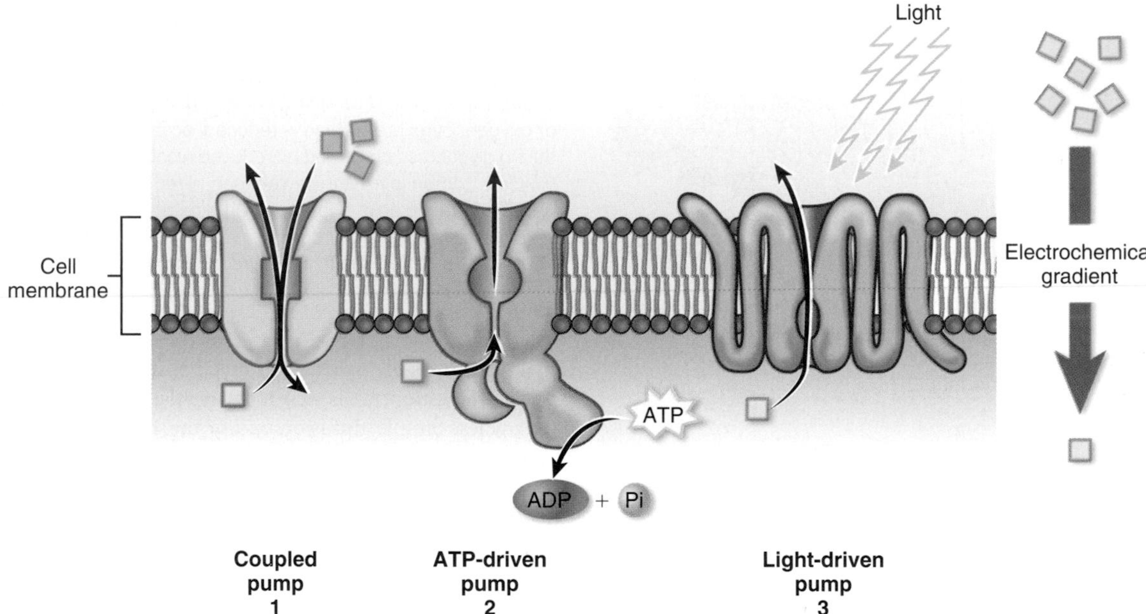

FIGURE 1-21 Pumps Carry Out Active Transport in Three Ways. **1,** *Coupled pumps* link the uphill transport of one solute to the downhill transport of another solute. **2,** *ATP-driven pumps* drive uphill transport from hydrolysis of ATP. **3,** *Light-driven pumps* are mostly found in bacteria and use energy from sunlight to drive uphill transport. *ADP*, adenosine diphosphate; *ATP*, adenosine triphosphate; *Pi*, inorganic phosphate. (Adapted from Alberts, B. [2014]. *Essential cell biology* [4th ed.]. New York: Garland.)

expenditure of energy or a driving force. It is driven by osmosis, hydrostatic pressure, and diffusion, all of which depend on the laws of physics and do not require life.

Other molecules are too large to pass through pores or are ligands bound to receptors on the cell's plasma membrane. Some of these molecules are moved into and out of the cell by **active transport**, which requires life, biological activity, and the cell's expenditure of metabolic energy (Figure 1-21). Unlike passive transport, active transport occurs across only living membranes that have to drive the flow "uphill" by coupling it to an energy source. Movement of a solute against its concentration gradient occurs by special types of transporters called *pumps* (see Figure 1-21). These transporter pumps must harness an energy source to power the transport process. Energy can come from ATP hydrolysis, a transmembrane ion gradient, or sunlight (see Figure 1-21). The best-known energy source is the Na^+–K^+-dependent adenosine triphosphatase (ATPase) pump (see Figure 1-26). It continuously regulates the cell's volume by controlling leaks through pores or protein channels and maintaining the ionic concentration gradients needed for cellular excitation and membrane conductivity. Large molecules (macromolecules), along with fluids, are transported by endocytosis (taking in) and exocytosis (expelling). Receptor-macromolecule complexes enter the cell by means of receptor-mediated endocytosis.

Mediated transport systems can move solute molecules singly or two at a time. Two molecules can be moved simultaneously in one direction (a process called **symport**; e.g., sodium-glucose in the digestive tract) or in opposite directions (called **antiport**; e.g., the sodium–potassium pump in all cells), or a single molecule can be moved in one direction (called **uniport**; e.g., glucose) (Figure 1-22).

Electrolytes as Solutes

Body fluids are composed of **electrolytes**, which are electrically charged and dissociate into constituent ions when placed in solution, and nonelectrolytes, such as glucose, urea, and creatinine, which do not dissociate. Electrolytes account for approximately 95% of the solute molecules in body water. Electrolytes exhibit **polarity** by orienting themselves toward the positive or negative pole. Ions with a positive charge are known as **cations** and migrate toward the negative pole, or cathode, if an electrical current is passed through the electrolyte solution. **Anions** carry a negative charge and migrate toward the positive pole, or anode, in the presence of electrical current. Anions and cations are located in both the intracellular fluid (ICF) and the extracellular fluid (ECF) compartments, although their concentration depends on their location. (Fluid and electrolyte balance between body compartments is discussed in Chapter 5.) For example, sodium (Na^+) is the predominant extracellular cation, and potassium (K^+) is the principal intracellular cation. The difference in ICF and ECF concentrations of these ions is important to the transmission of electrical impulses across the plasma membranes of nerve and muscle cells.

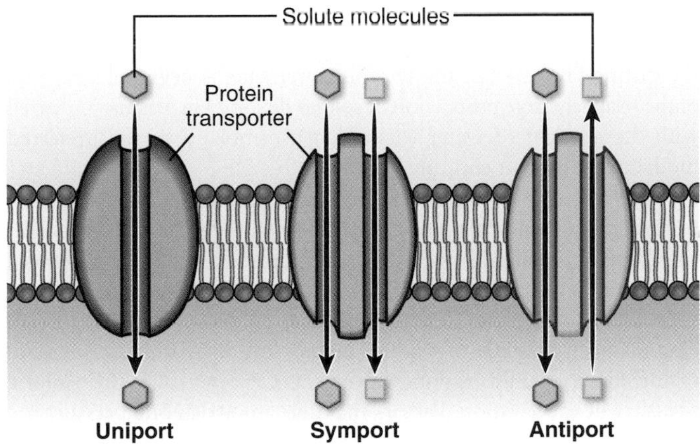

FIGURE 1-22 Mediated Transport. The illustration shows simultaneous movement of a single solute molecule in one direction (*Uniport*), of two different solute molecules in one direction (*Symport*), and of two different solute molecules in opposite directions (*Antiport*).

Electrolytes are measured in milliequivalents per litre (mEq/L) or millimoles per litre (mmol/L). The term *milliequivalent* indicates the chemical-combining activity of an ion, which depends on the electrical charge, or **valence**, of its ions. In abbreviations, valence is indicated by the number of plus or minus signs. One milliequivalent of any cation can combine chemically with 1 mEq of any anion: one monovalent anion will combine with one monovalent cation. Divalent ions combine more strongly than monovalent ions. To maintain electrochemical balance, one divalent ion will combine with two monovalent ions (e.g., $Ca^{++} + 2Cl^- \rightleftharpoons CaCl_2$).

Passive Transport: Diffusion, Filtration, and Osmosis

Diffusion. **Diffusion** is the movement of a solute molecule from an area of greater solute concentration to an area of lesser solute concentration. This difference in concentration is known as a **concentration gradient**. Although particles in a solution move randomly in any direction, if the concentration of particles in one part of the solution is greater than that in another part, the particles distribute themselves evenly throughout the solution. According to the same principle, if the concentration of particles is greater on one side of a permeable membrane than on the other side, the particles diffuse spontaneously from the area of greater concentration to the area of lesser concentration until equilibrium is reached. The higher the concentration on one side, the greater the diffusion rate.

The diffusion rate is influenced by differences of electrical potential across the membrane. Because the pores in the lipid bilayer are often lined with Ca^{++}, other cations (e.g., Na^+ and K^+) diffuse slowly because they are repelled by positive charges in the pores.

The rate of diffusion of a substance depends also on its size (diffusion coefficient) and its lipid solubility (Figure 1-23). Usually, the smaller the molecule and the more soluble it is in oil, the more hydrophobic or nonpolar it is and the more rapidly it will diffuse across the bilayer. Oxygen, carbon dioxide, and steroid hormones (e.g., androgens and estrogens) are all nonpolar molecules. Water-soluble substances, such as glucose and inorganic ions, diffuse very slowly, whereas uncharged lipophilic ("lipid-loving") molecules, such as fatty acids and steroids, diffuse rapidly. Ions and other polar molecules generally

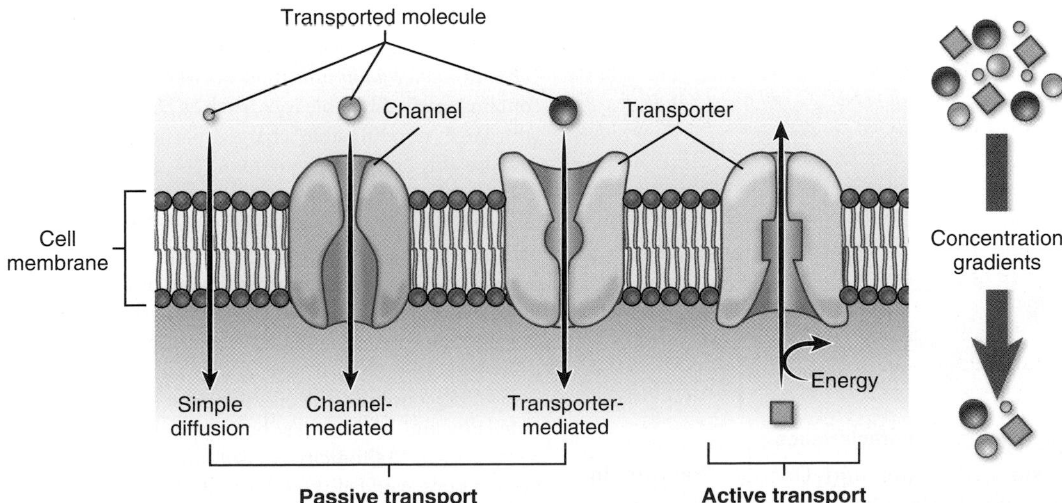

FIGURE 1-23 Passive Diffusion of Solute Molecules Across the Plasma Membrane. Oxygen, nitrogen, water, urea, glycerol, and carbon dioxide can diffuse readily down the concentration gradient. Macromolecules are too large to diffuse through pores in the plasma membrane. Ions may be repelled if the pores contain substances with identical charges. If the pores are lined with cations, for example, other cations will have difficulty diffusing because the positive charges will repel one another. Diffusion can still occur, but it occurs more slowly.

diffuse across cellular membranes more slowly than lipid-soluble substances.

Water readily diffuses through biological membranes because water molecules are small and uncharged. The dipolar structure of water allows it to rapidly cross the regions of the bilayer containing the lipid head groups. The lipid head groups constitute the two outer regions of the lipid bilayer.

Filtration: hydrostatic pressure. **Filtration** is the movement of water and solutes through a membrane because of a greater pushing pressure (force) on one side of the membrane than on the other side. **Hydrostatic pressure** is the mechanical force of water pushing against cellular membranes (Figure 1-24, *A*). In the vascular system, hydrostatic pressure is the blood pressure generated in vessels when the heart contracts. Blood reaching the capillary bed has a hydrostatic pressure of 25 to 30 mm Hg, which is sufficient force to push water across the thin capillary membranes into the interstitial space. Hydrostatic pressure is partially balanced by osmotic pressure, whereby water moving out of the capillaries is partially balanced by osmotic forces that tend to pull water into the capillaries (Figure 1-24, *B*). Water that is not osmotically attracted back into the capillaries moves into the lymph system (see the discussion of Starling forces in Chapter 5).

Osmosis. **Osmosis** is the movement of water "down" a concentration gradient—that is, across a semipermeable membrane from a region of higher water concentration to one of lower concentration. For osmosis to occur, (1) the membrane must be more permeable to water than to solutes, and (2) the concentration of solutes on one side of the membrane must be greater than that on the other side so that water moves more easily. Osmosis is directly related to both hydrostatic pressure and solute concentration but not to particle size or weight. For example, particles of the plasma protein albumin are small but are more concentrated in body fluids than the larger and heavier particles of globulin. Therefore albumin exerts a greater osmotic force than does globulin.

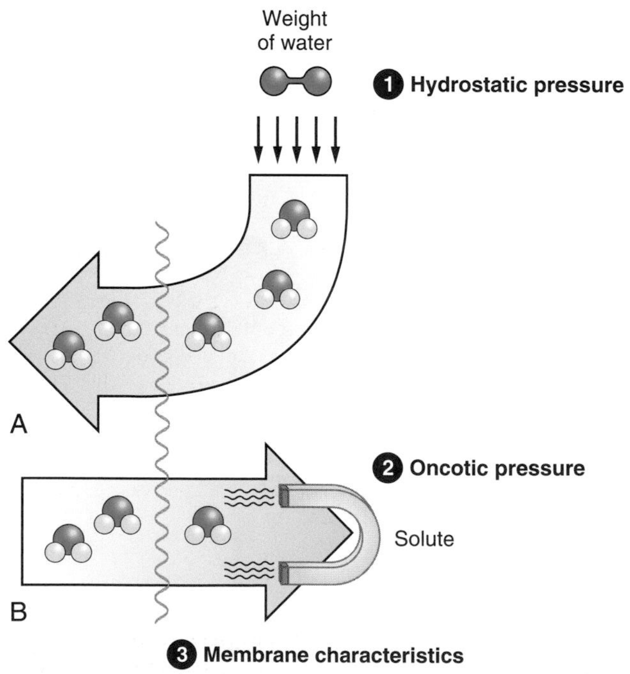

FIGURE 1-24 Hydrostatic Pressure and Oncotic Pressure in Plasma. 1, Hydrostatic pressure in plasma. **2,** Oncotic pressure exerted by proteins in the plasma usually tends to *pull* water into the circulatory system. The proteins are too big to cross the semipermeable membrane, and have a negative charge. **3,** Individuals with low protein levels (e.g., starvation) are unable to maintain a normal oncotic pressure; therefore water is not reabsorbed into the circulation and, instead, causes body edema.

Osmolality controls the distribution and movement of water between body compartments. The terms *osmolality* and *osmolarity* often are used interchangeably in reference to osmotic activity, but they define different measurements. **Osmolality** measures the number of milliosmoles per kilogram (mOsm/kg) of water, or the concentration of molecules per *weight* of water. **Osmolarity** measures the number of milliosmoles per litre of solution, or the concentration of molecules per *volume* of solution.

In solutions that contain only dissociable substances, such as sodium and chloride, the difference between the two measurements is negligible. When considering all the different solutes in plasma (e.g., proteins, glucose, lipids), however, the difference between osmolality and osmolarity becomes more significant. Osmolarity tends to be less than osmolality because it includes solute content as part of the solution volume. On the other hand, the osmolality of a solution is a measure of weight, and the solvent weight does not include any solutes. Though the distinction between the two measurements is negligible, because of the relatively large proportion of solutes dissolved in plasma compared with the amount of water (or solvent), osmolality is the preferred modality for human clinical assessment.

The normal osmolality of body fluids is 280 to 294 mOsm/kg. The osmolalities of intracellular and extracellular fluids tend to equalize, providing a measure of body fluid concentration and thus the body's hydration status. Hydration is affected also by hydrostatic pressure because the movement of water by osmosis can be opposed by an equal amount of hydrostatic pressure. The amount of hydrostatic pressure required to oppose the osmotic movement of water is called the **osmotic pressure** of the solution. Factors that determine osmotic pressure are the type and thickness of the plasma membrane, the size of the molecules, the concentration of molecules or the concentration gradient, and the solubility of molecules within the membrane.

Effective osmolality is sustained osmotic activity and depends on the concentration of solutes remaining on one side of a permeable membrane. If the solutes penetrate the membrane and equilibrate with the solution on the other side of the membrane, the osmotic effect will be diminished or lost.

Plasma proteins influence osmolality because they have a negative charge (see Figure 1-24, *B*). The principle involved is known as *Gibbs-Donnan equilibrium*; it occurs when the fluid in one compartment contains small, diffusible ions, such as Na^+ and chloride (Cl^-), together with large, nondiffusible, charged particles, such as plasma proteins. Because the body tends to maintain an electrical equilibrium, the nondiffusible protein molecules cause asymmetry in the distribution of small ions. Anions such as Cl^- are thus driven out of the cell or plasma, and cations such as Na^+ are attracted to the cell. The protein-containing compartment maintains a state of electroneutrality, but the osmolality is higher. The overall osmotic effect of colloids, such as plasma proteins, is called **oncotic pressure** or **colloid osmotic pressure**.

Tonicity describes the effective osmolality of a solution. (The terms *osmolality* and *tonicity* may be used interchangeably.) Solutions have relative degrees of tonicity. An isotonic solution (or isosmotic solution) has the same osmolality or concentration of particles (285 mOsm) as the ICF or ECF. A hypotonic solution has a lower concentration and is thus more dilute than body fluids (Figure 1-25). A hypertonic solution has a concentration of more than 285 to 294 mOsm/kg. The concept of tonicity is important when correcting water and solute imbalances by administering different types of replacement solutions (see Figure 1-25) (see Chapter 5).

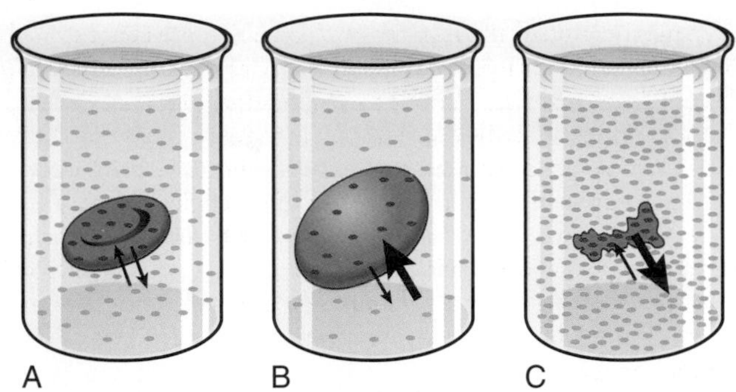

FIGURE 1-25 Tonicity. Tonicity is important, especially for red blood cell function. A, Isotonic solution. B, Hypotonic solution. C, Hypertonic solution. (From Waugh, A., & Grant, A. [2012]. *Ross and Wilson anatomy and physiology in health and illness* [12th ed.]. London: Churchill Livingstone.)

QUICK CHECK 1-2

1. What does glycolysis produce?
2. Define *membrane transport proteins.*
3. What are the differences between passive and active transport?
4. Why do water and small, electrically charged molecules move easily through pores in the plasma membrane?

Active Transport of Na^+ and K^+

The active transport system for Na^+ and K^+ is found in virtually all mammalian cells. The Na^+–K^+-antiport system (i.e., Na^+ moving out of the cell and K^+ moving into the cell) uses the direct energy of ATP to transport these cations. The transporter protein is ATPase, which requires Na^+, K^+, and magnesium (Mg^{++}) ions. The concentration of ATPase in plasma membranes is directly related to Na^+–K^+-transport activity. Approximately 60 to 70% of the ATP synthesized by cells, especially muscle and nerve cells, is used to maintain the Na^+–K^+-transport system. Excitable tissues have a high concentration of Na^+–K^+ ATPase, as do other tissues that transport significant amounts of Na^+. For every ATP molecule hydrolyzed, three molecules of Na^+ are transported out of the cell, whereas only two molecules of K^+ move into the cell. The process leads to an electrical potential and is called *electrogenic*, with the inside of the cell more negative than the outside. Although the exact mechanism for this transport is uncertain, it is possible that ATPase induces the transporter protein to undergo several conformational changes, causing Na^+ and K^+ to move short distances (Figure 1-26). The conformational change lowers the affinity for Na^+ and K^+ to the ATPase transporter, resulting in the release of the cations after transport.

Table 1-4 summarizes the major mechanisms of transport through pores and protein transporters in the plasma membranes. Many disease states are caused or manifested by loss of these membrane transport systems.

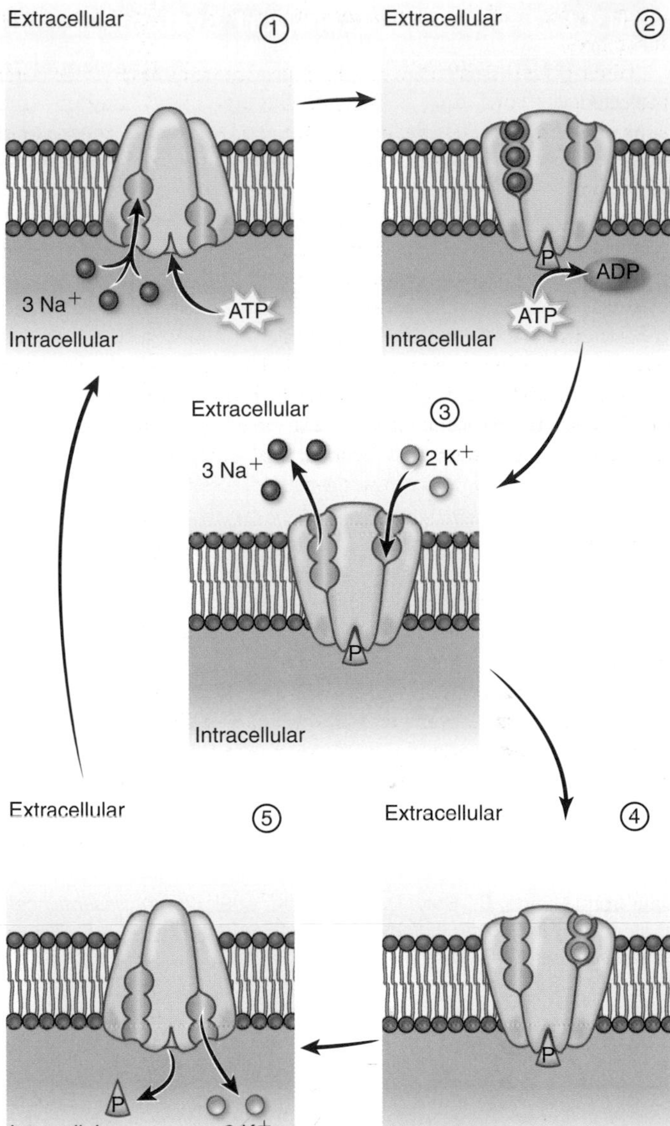

FIGURE 1-26 Active Transport and the Sodium–Potassium Pump. 1, Three sodium (Na^+) ions bind to sodium-binding sites on the carrier's inner face. 2, At the same time, an energy-containing adenosine triphosphate (*ATP*) molecule produced by the cell's mitochondria binds to the carrier. The ATP dissociates, transferring its stored energy to the carrier. 3 and 4, The carrier then changes shape, releases the three Na^+ ions to the outside of the cell, and attracts two potassium (K^+) ions to its potassium-binding sites. 5, The carrier then returns to its original shape, releasing the two K^+ ions and the remnant of the ATP molecule to the inside of the cell. The carrier is now ready for another pumping cycle. *ADP*, adenosine diphosphate; *P*, protein.

Transport by Vesicle Formation

Endocytosis and Exocytosis

The active transport mechanisms by which the cells move large proteins, polynucleotides, or polysaccharides (macromolecules) across the plasma membrane are very different from those that mediate small solute and ion transport. Transport of macromolecules involves the sequential formation and fusion of membrane-bound vesicles.

In **endocytosis**, a section of the plasma membrane enfolds substances from outside the cell, invaginates (folds inward), and separates from the plasma membrane, forming a vesicle that moves into the cell (Figure 1-27, *A*). Two types of endocytosis are designated based on the size of the vesicle formed. **Pinocytosis** (cell drinking) involves the ingestion of fluids, bits of the plasma membrane, and solute molecules through formation of small vesicles; and **phagocytosis** (cell eating) involves the ingestion of large particles, such as bacteria, through formation of large vesicles (vacuoles).

Because most cells continually ingest fluid and solutes by pinocytosis, the terms *pinocytosis* and *endocytosis* often are used interchangeably. In pinocytosis, the vesicle containing fluids, solutes, or both fuses with a

TABLE 1-4 Major Transport Systems in Mammalian Cells

Substance Transported	Mechanism of Transport[a]	Tissues
Carbohydrates		
Glucose	Passive: protein channel	Most tissues
	Active: symport with Na^+	
Fructose	Active: symport with Na^+	Small intestines and renal tubular cells
	Passive	Intestines and liver
Amino Acids		
Amino acid specific transporters	Coupled channels	Intestines, kidney, and liver
All amino acids except proline	Active: symport with Na^+	Liver
Specific amino acids	Active: group translocation	Small intestine
	Passive	
Other Organic Molecules		
Cholic acid, deoxycholic acid, and taurocholic acid	Active: symport with Na^+	Intestines
Organic anions (e.g., malate, α-ketoglutarate, glutamate)	Antiport with counter–organic anion	Mitochondria of liver cells
ATP–ADP	Antiport transport of nucleotides; can be active	Mitochondria of liver cells
Inorganic Ions		
Na^+	Passive	Distal renal tubular cells
Na^+/H^+	Active antiport, proton pump	Proximal renal tubular cells and small intestines
Na^+/K^+	Active: ATP driven, protein channel	Plasma membrane of most cells
Ca^{++}	Active: ATP driven, antiport with Na^+	All cells, antiporter in red cells
H^+/K^+	Active	Parietal cells of gastric cells secreting H^+
HCO_3^- (perhaps other anions)	Mediated: antiport (anion transporter–band 3 protein)	Erythrocytes and many other cells
Water	Osmosis passive	All tissues

[a]The known transport systems are listed here; others have been proposed. Most transport systems have been studied in only a few tissues and their sites of activity may be more limited than indicated.

ADP, adenosine diphosphate; *ATP*, adenosine triphosphate, Ca^{++}, calcium; Cl^-, chloride; H^+, hydrogen; HCO_3^-, bicarbonate; K^+, potassium; Na^+, sodium.

Data from Alberts, B., Bray, D., Hopkin, K., et al. (2014). *Essential cell biology* (4th ed.). New York: Garland; Alberts, B., Johnson, A., Lewis, J., et al. (2001). *Molecular biology of the cell* (4th ed.). New York: Wiley; Devlin, T.M. (Ed.). (1992). *Textbook of biochemistry: with clinical correlations* (3rd ed.). New York: Wiley; Raven, P.H., & Johnson, G.B. (1995). *Understanding biology* (3rd ed.). Dubuque, IA: Brown.

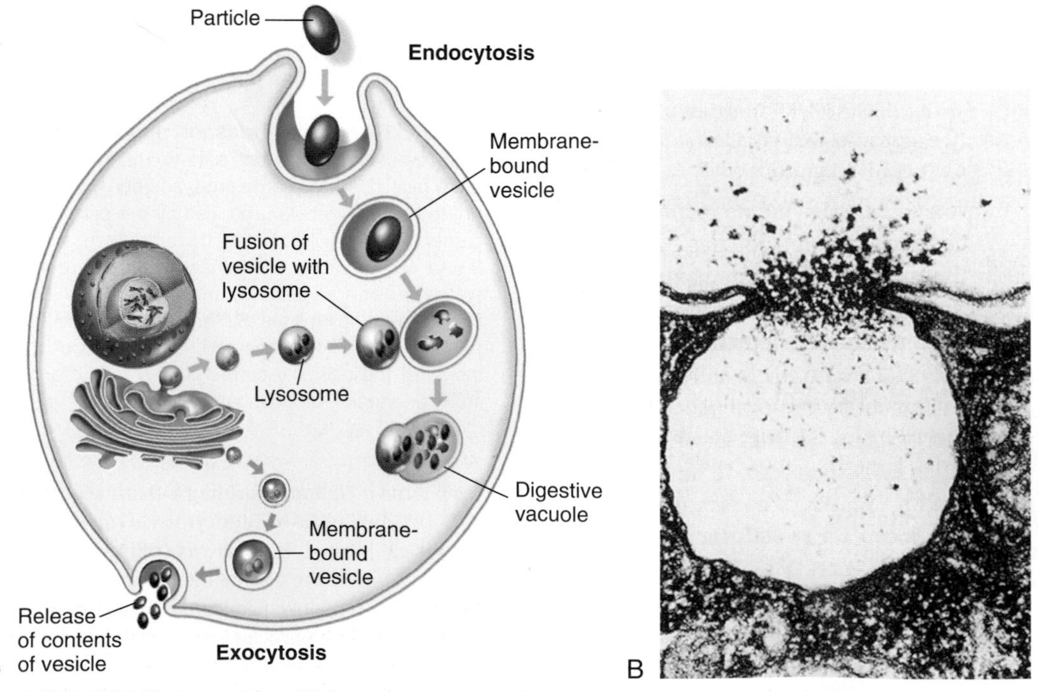

FIGURE 1-27 Endocytosis and Exocytosis. A, Endocytosis and fusion with lysosome and exocytosis. **B,** Electron micrograph of exocytosis. (**B,** from Raven, P.H., & Johnson, G.B. [1999]. *Biology* [5th ed.]. New York: McGraw-Hill.)

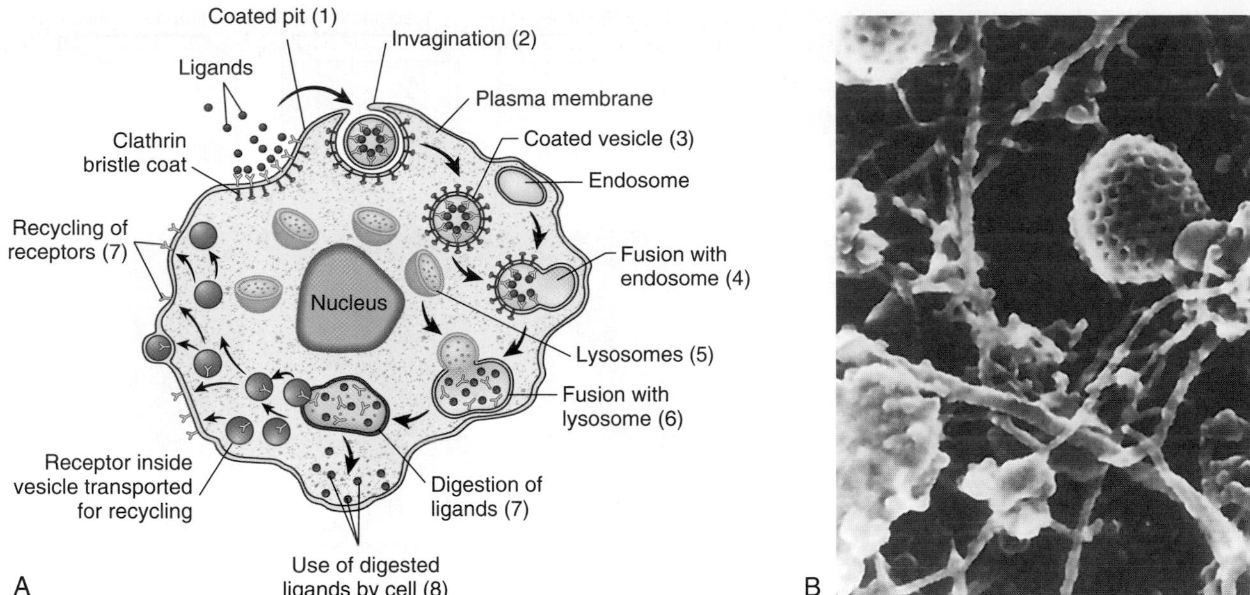

FIGURE 1-28 Ligand Internalization by Means of Receptor-Mediated Endocytosis. A, The ligand attaches to its surface receptor (through the bristle coat or clathrin coat) and, through receptor-mediated endocytosis, enters the cell. The ingested material fuses with a lysosome and is processed by hydrolytic lysosomal enzymes. Processed molecules can then be transferred to other cellular components. **B,** Electron micrograph of a coated pit showing different sizes of filaments of the cytoskeleton (×82 000) receptor-mediated endocytosis with coated pit and vesicle. (**B,** from Erlandsen, S.L., & Magney, J.E. [1992]. *Color atlas of histology*. St. Louis: Mosby.)

lysosome, and lysosomal enzymes digest the vesicle's contents for use by the cell. Vesicles that bud from membranes have a particular protein coat on their cytosolic surface and are called coated vesicles. The best studied are those that have an outer coat of bristlelike structures—the protein clathrin. Pinocytosis occurs mainly by the clathrin-coated pits and vesicles (Figure 1-28). After the coated pits pinch off from the plasma membrane, they quickly shed their coats and fuse with an endosome. An endosome is a vesicle pinched off from the plasma membrane from which its contents can be recycled to the plasma membrane or sent to lysosomes for digestion. In phagocytosis, the large molecular substances are engulfed by the plasma membrane and enter the cell so that they can be isolated and destroyed by lysosomal enzymes (see Chapter 6). Substances that are not degraded by lysosomes are isolated in residual bodies and released by exocytosis. Both pinocytosis and phagocytosis require metabolic energy and often involve binding of the substance with plasma membrane receptors before membrane invagination and fusion with lysosomes in the cell. New data are revealing that endocytosis has an even larger and more important role than previously known (Box 1-3).

In eukaryotic cells, secretion of macromolecules almost always occurs by exocytosis (Figure 1-27). Exocytosis has two main functions: (1) replacement of portions of the plasma membrane that have been removed by endocytosis and (2) release of molecules synthesized by the cells into the ECM.

Receptor-Mediated Endocytosis

The internalization process, called receptor-mediated endocytosis (ligand internalization), is rapid and enables the cell to ingest large amounts of receptor macromolecule complexes in clathrin-coated vesicles without ingesting large volumes of extracellular fluid (see Figure 1-28). The cellular uptake of cholesterol, for example, depends on receptor-mediated endocytosis. Additionally, many essential metabolites (e.g., vitamin B_{12} and iron) depend on receptor-mediated endocytosis, as does the influenza (flu) virus.

> **BOX 1-3 The New Endocytic Matrix**
>
> An explosion of new data is disclosing a much more involved role for endocytosis than just a simple way to internalize nutrients and membrane-associated molecules. These new data show that endocytosis not only is a master organizer of signalling pathways but also has a major role in managing signals in time and space. Endocytosis appears to control signalling; therefore, it determines the net output of biochemical pathways. The control of signalling occurs because endocytosis modulates the presence of receptors and their ligands as well as effectors at the plasma membrane or at intermediate stations of the endocytic route. The overall processes and anatomy of these new functions are sometimes called the *endocytic matrix*. All of these functions ultimately have a large impact on almost every cellular process, including the nucleus.

Caveolae

The outer surface of the plasma membrane is dimpled with tiny flask-shaped pits (cavelike) called caveolae. Caveolae are thought to form from membrane microdomains or lipid rafts. Caveolae are cholesterol- and glycosphingolipid-rich microdomains where the protein *caveolin* is thought to be involved in several processes, including clathrin-independent endocytosis, cellular cholesterol regulation and transport, and cellular communication. Many proteins, including a variety of receptors, cluster in these tiny chambers.

Caveolae are not only uptake vehicles but also important sites for signal transduction, a tedious process in which extracellular chemical messages or *signals* are communicated to the cell's interior for execution. For example, in vitro evidence now exists that plasma membrane estrogen

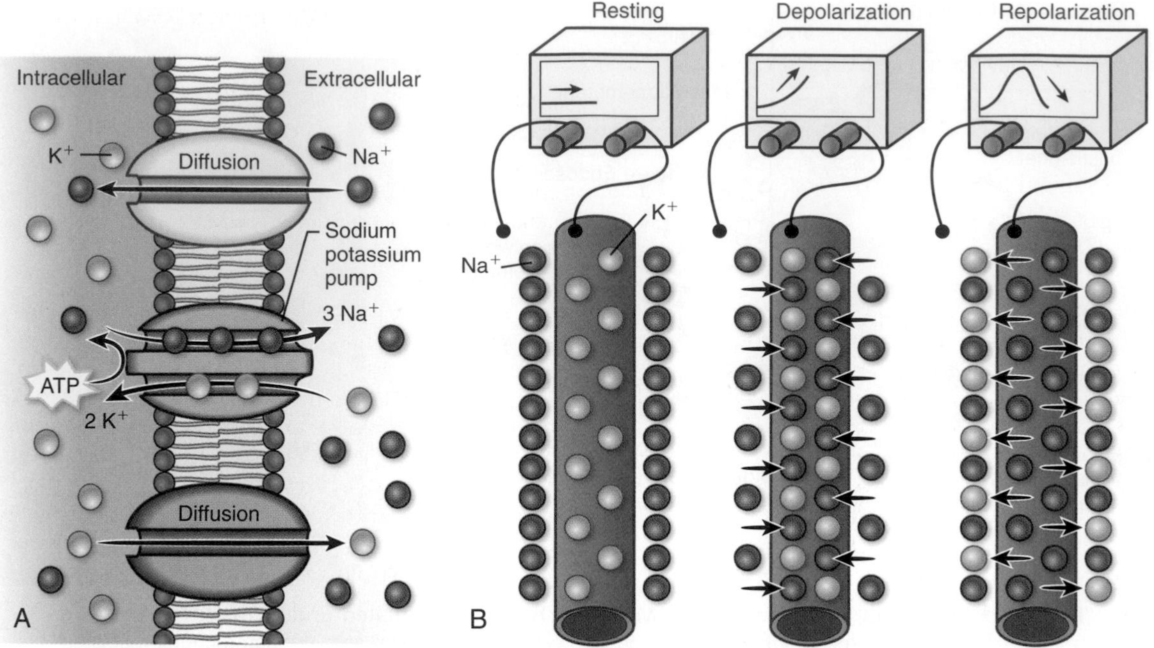

FIGURE 1-29 Sodium–Potassium Pump and Propagation of an Action Potential. A, Concentration difference of sodium (*Na*⁺) and potassium (*K*⁺) intracellularly and extracellularly. The direction of active transport by the sodium–potassium pump is also shown. **B,** The left diagram represents the polarized state of a neuronal membrane when at rest. The middle and right diagrams represent changes in sodium and potassium membrane permeabilities with depolarization and repolarization. *ATP,* adenosine triphosphate.

receptors can localize in caveolae, and crosstalk with estradiol facilitates several intracellular biological actions.[18]

Movement of Electrical Impulses: Membrane Potentials

All body cells are electrically polarized, with the inside of the cell more negatively charged than the outside. The difference in electrical charge, or voltage, is known as the **resting membrane potential** and is about −70 to −85 mV. The difference in voltage across the plasma membrane results from the differences in ionic composition of ICF and ECF. Sodium ions are more concentrated in the ECF, and potassium ions are more concentrated in the ICF. The concentration difference is maintained by the active transport of Na^+ and K^+ (the sodium–potassium pump), which transports sodium outward and potassium inward (Figure 1-29). Because the resting plasma membrane is more permeable to K^+ than to Na^+, K^+ diffuses easily from the ICF to the ECF. Because both Na^+ and K^+ are cations, the net result is an excess of anions inside the cell, resulting in the resting membrane potential.

Nerve and muscle cells are excitable and can change their resting membrane potential in response to electrochemical stimuli. Changes in resting membrane potential convey messages from cell to cell. When a nerve or muscle cell receives a stimulus that exceeds the membrane threshold value, a rapid change occurs in the resting membrane potential, known as the **action potential**. The action potential carries signals along the nerve or muscle cell and conveys information from one cell to another in a dominolike fashion. Nerve impulses are described in Chapter 13. When a resting cell is stimulated through voltage-regulated channels, the cell membranes become more permeable to sodium, so a net movement of sodium into the cell occurs and the membrane potential decreases, or moves forward, from a negative value (in millivolts) to zero. This decrease is known as **depolarization**. The depolarized cell is more positively charged, and its polarity is neutralized.

To generate an action potential and the resulting depolarization, the **threshold potential** must be reached. Generally this occurs when the cell has depolarized by 15 to 20 mV. When the threshold is reached, the cell will continue to depolarize with no further stimulation. The sodium gates open, and sodium rushes into the cell, causing the membrane potential to drop to zero and then become positive (depolarization). The rapid reversal in polarity results in the action potential.

During **repolarization**, the negative polarity of the resting membrane potential is re-established. As the voltage-gated sodium channels begin to close, voltage-gated potassium channels open. Membrane permeability to sodium decreases and potassium permeability increases, so potassium ions leave the cell. The sodium gates close, and with the loss of potassium the membrane potential becomes more negative. The Na^+–K^+ pump then returns the membrane to the resting potential by pumping potassium back into the cell and sodium out of the cell.

During most of the action potential, the plasma membrane cannot respond to an additional stimulus. This time is known as the **absolute refractory period** and is related to changes in permeability to sodium. During the latter phase of the action potential, when permeability to potassium increases, a stronger-than-normal stimulus can evoke an action potential; this time is known as the **relative refractory period**.

When the membrane potential is more negative than normal, the cell is in a **hyperpolarized state** (less excitable: decreased K^+ levels within the cell). A stronger-than-normal stimulus is then required to reach the threshold potential and generate an action potential. When the membrane potential is more positive than normal, the cell is in a **hypopolarized state** (more excitable than normal: increased K^+ levels within the cell) and a weaker-than-normal stimulus is required to reach the threshold potential. Changes in the intracellular and extracellular concentrations of ions or a change in membrane permeability can cause these alterations in membrane excitability.

QUICK CHECK 1-3

1. Identify examples of molecules transported in one direction (symport) and opposite directions (antiport).
2. If oxygen is no longer available to make ATP, what happens to the transport of Na^+?
3. Describe the differences between pinocytosis, phagocytosis, and receptor-mediated endocytosis.

CELLULAR REPRODUCTION: THE CELL CYCLE

Human cells are subject to wear and tear, and most do not last for the lifetime of the individual. In most tissues, new cells are created as fast as old cells die. Cellular reproduction is therefore necessary for the maintenance of life. Reproduction of gametes (sperm and egg cells) occurs through a process called *meiosis*, described in Chapter 2. The reproduction, or division, of other body cells (somatic cells) involves two sequential phases—**mitosis**, or nuclear division, and **cytokinesis**, or cytoplasmic division. Before a cell can divide, however, it must double its mass and duplicate all its contents. Separation for division occurs during the growth phase, called **interphase**. The alternation between mitosis and interphase in all tissues with cellular turnover is known as the **cell cycle**.

The four designated phases of the cell cycle (Figure 1-30) are (1) the **S phase** (S = synthesis), in which DNA is synthesized in the cell nucleus; (2) the **G_2 phase** (G = gap), in which RNA and protein synthesis occurs, namely, the period between the completion of DNA synthesis and the next phase (M); (3) the **M phase** (M = mitosis), which includes both nuclear and cytoplasmic division; and (4) the **G_1 phase**, which is the period between the M phase and the start of DNA synthesis. When cells are in the **G_0 phase**, they are neither dividing nor preparing to divide. Rather, they are continuing on with their regular function as part of the tissue or organ to which they belong. Understanding the cell cycle is important when considering the effectiveness of antineoplastic medications and the growth of cancer cells, which will be covered in Chapter 10.

Phases of Mitosis and Cytokinesis

Interphase (the G_1, S, and G_2 phases) is the longest phase of the cell cycle. During interphase, the **chromatin** (the substance that gives the nucleus its granular appearance) consists of very long, slender rods jumbled together in the nucleus. Late in interphase, strands of chromatin begin to coil, causing shortening and thickening.

The M phase of the cell cycle, mitosis and cytokinesis, begins with **prophase**, the first appearance of chromosomes. As the phase proceeds, each chromosome is seen as two identical halves called **chromatids**, which lie together and are attached by a spindle site called a **centromere**. (The two chromatids of each chromosome, which are genetically identical, are sometimes called *sister chromatids.*) The nuclear membrane, which surrounds the nucleus, disappears. **Spindle fibres** are microtubules formed in the cytoplasm. They radiate from two centrioles located at opposite poles of the cell and pull the chromosomes to opposite sides of the cell, beginning **metaphase**. Next, the centromeres become aligned in the middle of the spindle, which is called the **equatorial plate (or metaphase plate)** of the cell. In this stage, chromosomes are easiest to observe microscopically because they are highly condensed and arranged in a relatively organized fashion.

Anaphase begins when the centromeres split and the sister chromatids are pulled apart. The spindle fibres shorten, causing the sister chromatids to be pulled, centromere first, toward opposite sides of the cell. When the sister chromatids are separated, each is considered to be a chromosome. Thus the cell has 92 chromosomes during this stage. By the end of anaphase, there are 46 chromosomes lying at each side of the cell. Barring mitotic errors, each of the two groups of 46 chromosomes is identical to the original 46 chromosomes present at the start of the cell cycle.

During **telophase**, the final stage, a new nuclear membrane is formed around each group of 46 chromosomes, the spindle fibres disappear, and the chromosomes begin to uncoil. Cytokinesis causes the cytoplasm

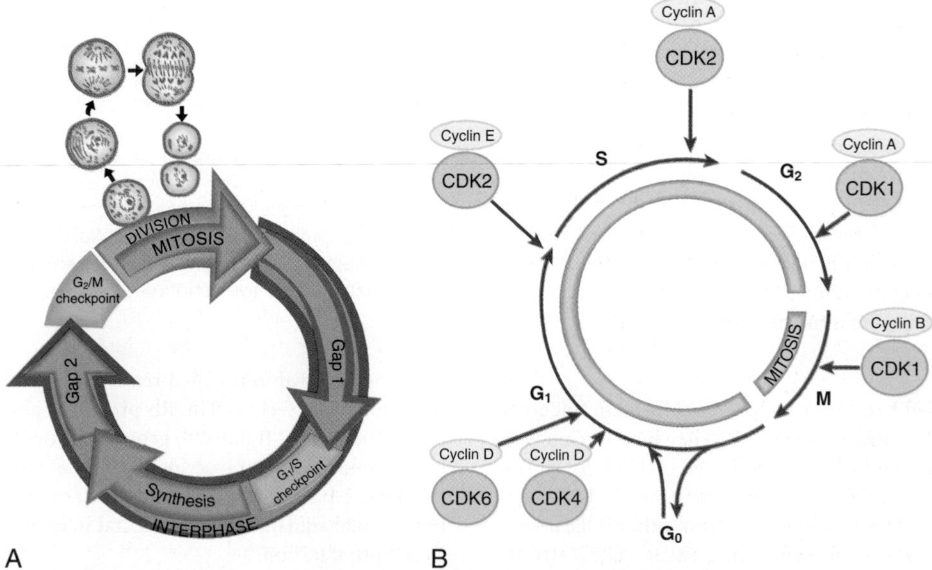

FIGURE 1-30 Interphase and the Phases of Mitosis. A, The G_1/S checkpoint is to "check" for cell size, nutrients, growth factors, and DNA damage. See text for resting phases. The G_2/M checkpoint checks for cell size and DNA replication. **B,** The orderly progression through the phases of the cell cycle is regulated by *cyclins* (so called because levels rise and fall) and cyclin-dependent protein kinases (*CDKs*) and their inhibitors. When cyclins are complexed with CDKs, cell cycle events are triggered.

TABLE 1-5 Examples of Growth Factors and Their Actions

Growth Factor	Physiological Actions
Platelet-derived growth factor (PDGF)	Stimulates proliferation of connective tissue cells and neuroglial cells
Epidermal growth factor (EGF)	Stimulates proliferation of epidermal cells and other cell types
Insulinlike growth factor 1 (IGF-1)	Collaborates with PDGF and EGF; stimulates proliferation of fat cells and connective tissue cells
Vascular endothelial growth factor (VEGF)	Mediates functions of endothelial cells; proliferation, migration, invasion, survival, and permeability
Insulinlike growth factor 2 (IGF-2)	Collaborates with PDGF and EGF; stimulates or inhibits response of most cells to other growth factors; regulates differentiation of some cell types (e.g., cartilage)
Transforming growth factor-beta (TGF-β; multiple subtypes)	Stimulates or inhibits response of most cells to other growth factors; regulates differentiation of some cell types (e.g., cartilage)
Fibroblast growth factor (FGF; multiple subtypes)	Stimulates proliferation of fibroblasts, endothelial cells, myoblasts, and other multiple subtypes
Interleukin-2 (IL-2)	Stimulates proliferation of T lymphocytes
Nerve growth factor (NGF)	Promotes axon growth and survival of sympathetic and some sensory and central nervous system neurons
Hematopoietic cell growth factors (IL-3, GM-CSF, G-CSF, erythropoietin)	Promote proliferation of blood cells

G-CSF, granulocyte colony-stimulating factor; *GM-CSF*, granulocyte-macrophage colony-stimulating factor.

to divide into almost equal parts during this phase. At the end of telophase, two identical diploid cells, called **daughter cells**, have been formed from the original cell.

Rates of Cellular Division

Although the complete cell cycle lasts 12 to 24 hours, about 1 hour is required for the four stages of mitosis and cytokinesis. All types of cells undergo mitosis during formation of the embryo, but many adult cells—such as nerve cells, lens cells of the eye, and muscle cells—lose their ability to replicate and divide. The cells of other tissues, particularly epithelial cells (e.g., cells of the intestine, lung, or skin), divide continuously and rapidly, completing the entire cell cycle in less than 10 hours.

The difference between cells that divide slowly and cells that divide rapidly is the length of time spent in the G_1 phase of the cell cycle. Once the S phase begins, however, progression through mitosis takes a relatively constant amount of time.

The mechanisms that control cell division depend on the integrity of genetic, epigenetic (heritable changes in genome function that occur without alterations in the DNA sequence; see Chapter 3), and protein growth factors. Protein growth factors govern the proliferation of different cell types. Individual cells are members of a complex cellular society in which survival of the entire organism is key—not survival or proliferation of just the individual cells. When a need arises for new cells, as in repair of injured cells, previously nondividing cells must be triggered rapidly to re-enter the cell cycle. With continual wear and tear, the cell birth rate and the cell death rate must be kept in balance.

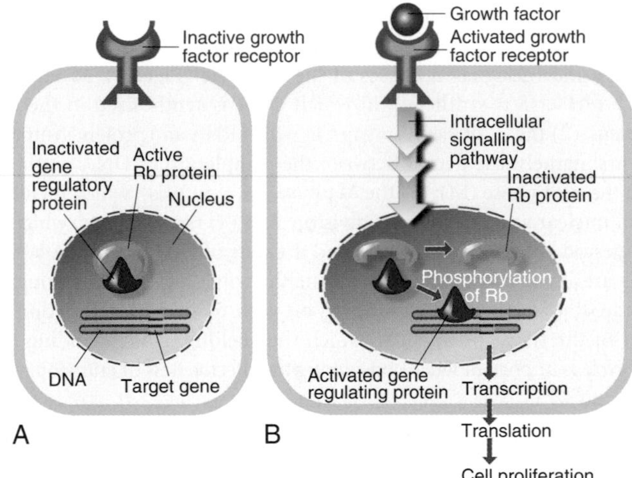

FIGURE 1-31 How Growth Factors Stimulate Cell Proliferation. **A,** Resting cell. With the absence of growth factors, the retinoblastoma (*Rb*) protein is not phosphorylated; thus it holds the gene regulatory proteins in an inactive state. The gene regulatory proteins are required to stimulate the transcription of genes needed for cell proliferation. **B,** Proliferating cell. Growth factors bind to the cell surface receptors and activate intracellular signalling pathways, leading to activation of intracellular proteins. These intracellular proteins phosphorylate and thereby inactivate the Rb protein. The gene regulatory proteins are now free to activate the transcription of genes, leading to cell proliferation.

Growth Factors

Growth factors, also called **cytokines**, are peptides (protein fractions) that transmit signals within and between cells. They have a major role in the regulation of tissue growth and development (Table 1-5). Having nutrients is not enough for a cell to proliferate; it must also receive stimulatory chemical signals (growth factors) from other cells, usually its neighbours or the surrounding supporting tissue called **stroma**. These signals act to overcome intracellular braking mechanisms that tend to restrain cell growth and block progress through the cell cycle (Figure 1-31).

An example of a brake that regulates cell proliferation is the **retinoblastoma (Rb) protein**, first identified through studies of a rare childhood eye tumour called *retinoblastoma*, in which the Rb protein is missing or defective. The Rb protein is abundant in the nucleus of all vertebrate cells. It binds to gene regulatory proteins, preventing them from stimulating the transcription of genes required for cell proliferation (see Figure 1-31). Extracellular signals, such as growth factors, activate intracellular signalling pathways that inactivate the Rb protein, leading to cell proliferation.

Different types of cells require different growth factors; for example, **platelet-derived growth factor (PDGF)** stimulates the production of connective tissue cells. Table 1-5 summarizes the most significant growth factors. Evidence shows that some growth factors also regulate other cellular processes, such as cellular differentiation. In addition to growth

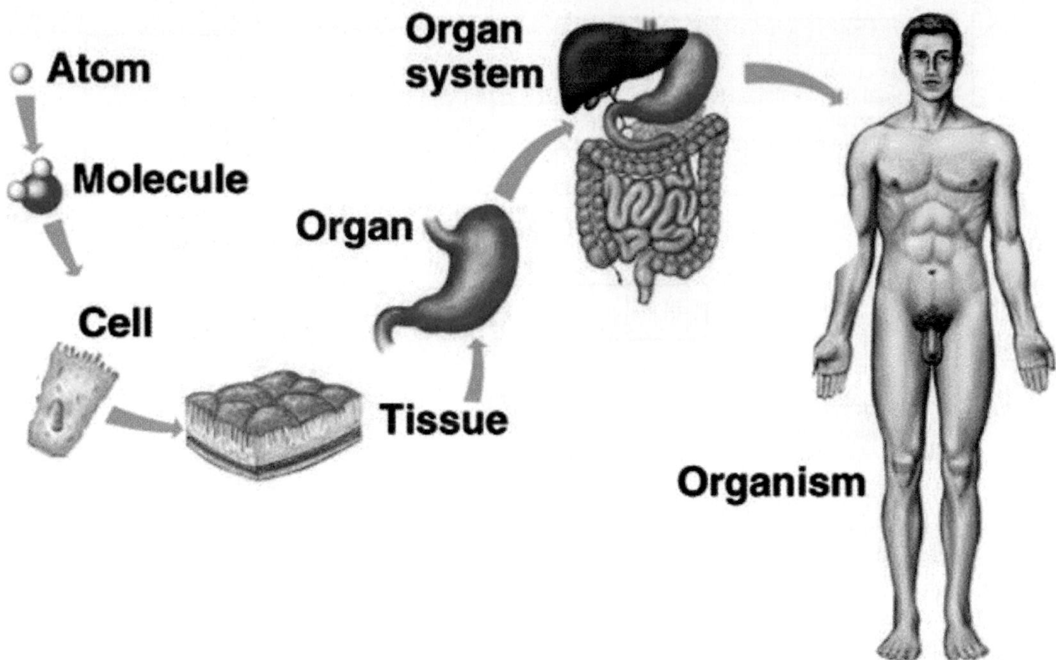

FIGURE 1-32 Cells, Tissues, Organs, and Organ Systems. The smallest level of organization shown in this diagram is the cell. Cells working together make up a tissue, which in turn is part of an organ. Organs working together form the different organ systems that make up a whole organism.

factors that stimulate cellular processes, there are factors that inhibit these processes; these factors are not well understood. Cells that are starved of growth factors come to a halt after mitosis and enter the **arrested (resting) (G_0) state** of the cell cycle (see p. 25 for cell cycle).[1]

TISSUES

Cells of one or more types are organized into tissues, and different types of tissues compose organs. Finally, organs are integrated to perform complex functions as tracts or systems (Figure 1-32).

All cells are in contact with a network of extracellular macromolecules known as the ECM (see p. 10). This matrix not only holds cells and tissues together but also provides an organized latticework within which cells can migrate and interact with one another.

Tissue Formation

To form tissues, cells must exhibit intercellular recognition and communication, adhesion, and memory. Specialized cells sense their environment through signals, such as growth factors, from other cells. This type of communication ensures that new cells are produced only when and where they are required. Different cell types have different adhesion molecules in their plasma membranes, sticking selectively to other cells of the same type. They can also adhere to ECM components. Because cells are tiny and squishy and enclosed by a flimsy membrane, it is remarkable that they form a strong human being. Strength can occur because of the ECM and the strength of the cytoskeleton with cell–cell adhesions to neighbouring cells. Cells have memory because of specialized patterns of gene expression evoked by signals that acted during embryonic development. Memory allows cells to autonomously preserve their distinctive character and pass it on to their progeny.[1]

Fully specialized or **terminally differentiated** cells that are lost are regenerated from proliferating *precursor cells*. These precursor cells have been derived from a smaller number of stem cells.[1] **Stem cells** are cells with the potential to develop into many different cell types during early development and growth. In many tissues, stem cells serve as an internal repair and maintenance system, dividing indefinitely. These cells can maintain themselves over very long periods of time, called **self-renewal**, and can generate all the differentiated cell types of the tissue or **multipotency**. This stem cell–driven tissue renewal is very evident in the epithelial lining of the intestine, stomach, blood cells, and skin, which is continuously exposed to environmental factors. A class of extracellular signalling proteins, known as **Wnt signals**, sustain tissue renewal and enable tissue to be continuously replenished and maintained over a lifetime.[19] When a stem cell divides, each daughter cell has a choice: it can remain as a stem cell or it can follow a pathway that results in terminal differentiation (Figure 1-33).

Types of Tissues

The four basic types of tissues are nerve, epithelial, connective, and muscle tissues. The structure and function of these four types underlie the structure and function of each organ system. Neural tissue is composed of highly specialized cells called *neurons*, which receive and transmit electrical impulses rapidly across junctions called *synapses* (see Figure 13-1). Different types of neurons have special characteristics that depend on their distribution and function within the nervous system. Epithelial, connective, and muscle tissues are summarized in Tables 1-6, 1-7, and 1-8, respectively.

QUICK CHECK 1-4
1. What is the cell cycle?
2. Describe the five types of intracellular communication.
3. Why is the extracellular matrix important for tissue cells?

Text continued on p. 34

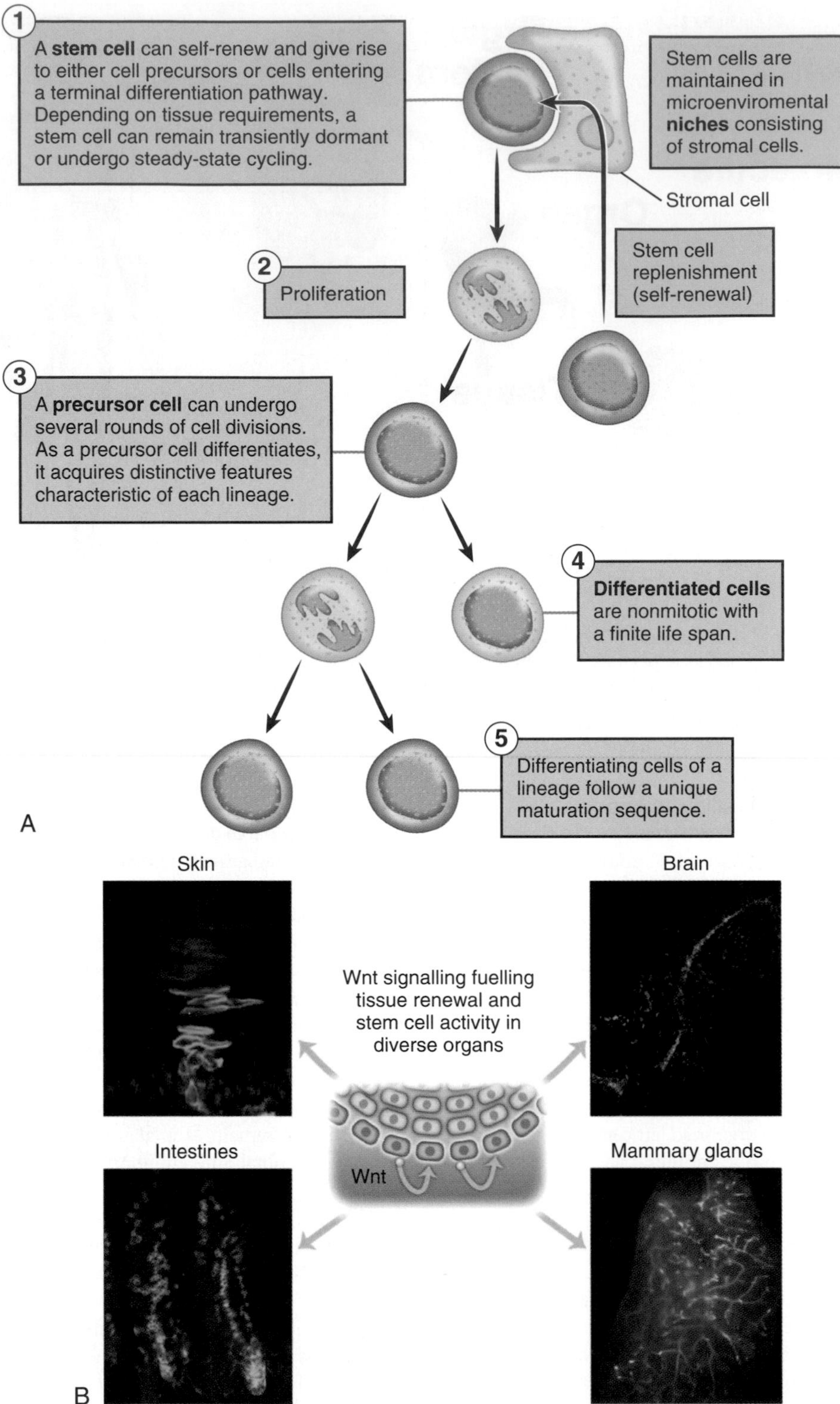
1
A stem cell can self-renew and give rise to either cell precursors or cells entering a terminal differentiation pathway. Depending on tissue requirements, a stem cell can remain transiently dormant or undergo steady-state cycling.
Stem cells are maintained in microenviromental niches consisting of stromal cells.
Stromal cell
2
Proliferation
Stem cell replenishment (self-renewal)
3
A precursor cell can undergo several rounds of cell divisions. As a precursor cell differentiates, it acquires distinctive features characteristic of each lineage.
4
Differentiated cells are nonmitotic with a finite life span.
5
Differentiating cells of a lineage follow a unique maturation sequence.
A
Skin
Brain
Wnt signalling fuelling tissue renewal and stem cell activity in diverse organs
Wnt
Intestines
Mammary glands
B

FIGURE 1-33 Properties of Stem Cell Systems. **A,** Stem cells have three characteristics: *self-renewal, proliferation,* and *differentiation* into mature cells. Stem cells are housed in *niches* consisting of *stromal cells* that provide factors for their maintenance. Stem cells of the embryo can give rise to cell precursors that generate all the tissues of the body. This property defines stem cells as *multipotent.* Stem cells are difficult to identify anatomically. Their identification is based on specific *cell surface markers* (cell surface antigens recognized by specific monoclonal antibodies) and on the lineage they generate following *transplantation.* **B,** Wnt signalling fuels tissue renewal. (**A,** from Kierszenbaum, A. [2012]. *Histology and cell biology: An introduction to pathology* [3rd ed.]. St. Louis: Elsevier. **B,** from Clevers, H., Loh, K.M., & Nusse, R. [2014]. *Science, 346*[6205], 54.)

TABLE 1-6 Characteristics of Epithelial Tissues

Simple Squamous Epithelium

Structure

Single layer of cells

Location and Function

Lining of blood vessels leads to diffusion and filtration

Lining of pulmonary alveoli (air sacs) leads to separation of blood from fluids in tissues

Bowman's capsule (kidney), where it filters substances from blood, forming urine

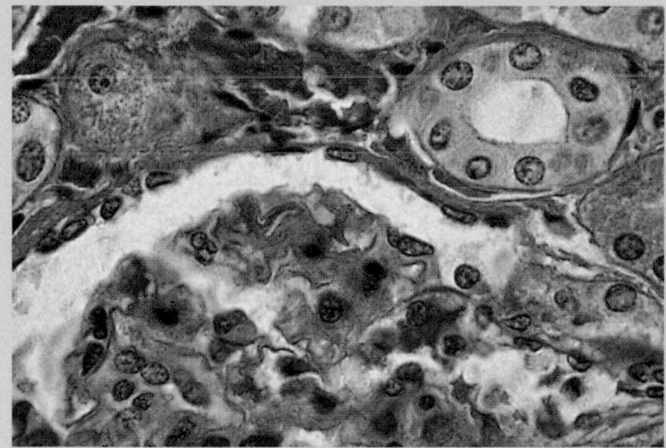

Simple Squamous Epithelial Cell. Photomicrograph of simple squamous epithelial cell in parietal wall of Bowman's capsule in kidney. (From Erlandsen, S.L., & Magney, J.E. [1992]. *Color atlas of histology.* St. Louis: Mosby.)

Stratified Squamous Epithelium

Structure

Two or more layers, depending on location, with cells closest to basement membrane tending to be cuboidal

Location and Function

Epidermis of skin and linings of mouth, pharynx, esophagus, and anus provide protection and secretion

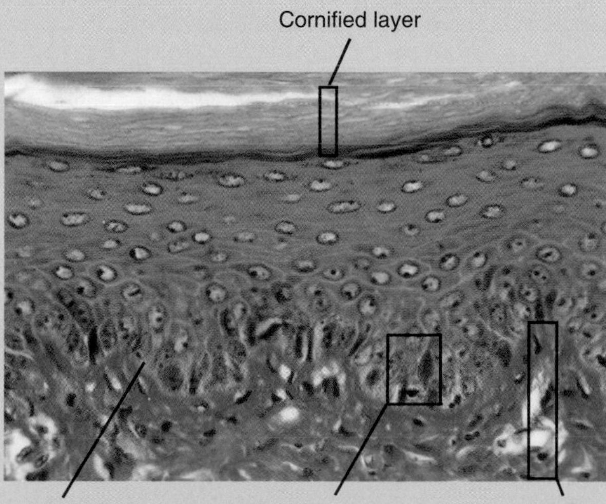

Cornified Stratified Squamous Epithelium. Diagram of stratified squamous epithelium of skin. (Copyright Ed Reschke. Used with permission.)

Transitional Epithelium

Structure

Vary in shape from cuboidal to squamous, depending on whether basal cells of bladder are columnar or are composed of many layers; when bladder is full and stretched, the cells flatten and stretch like squamous cells

Location and Function

Linings of urinary bladder and other hollow structures stretch, allowing expansion of the hollow organs

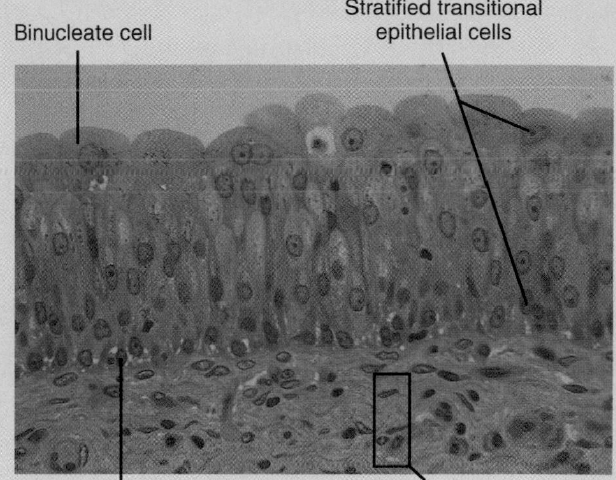

Stratified Squamous Transitional Epithelium. Photomicrograph of stratified squamous transitional epithelium of urinary bladder. (Copyright Ed Reschke. Used with permission.)

Simple Cuboidal Epithelium

Structure

Simple cuboidal cells; rarely stratified (layered)

Location and Function

Glands (e.g., thyroid, sweat, salivary) and parts of the kidney tubules and outer covering of ovary secrete fluids

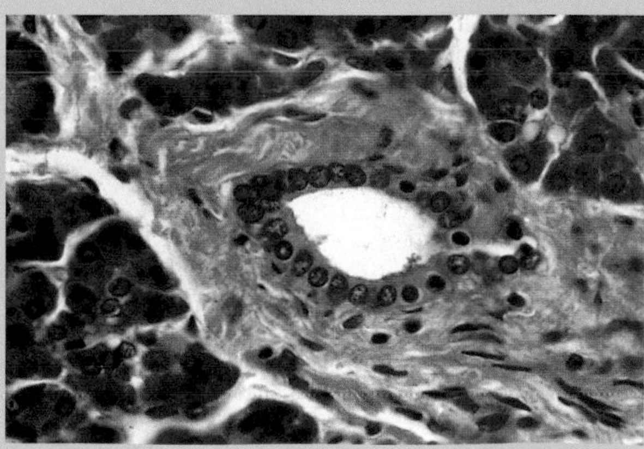

Simple Cuboidal Epithelium. Photomicrograph of simple cuboidal epithelium of pancreatic duct. (From Erlandsen, S.L., & Magney, J.E. [1992]. *Color atlas of histology.* St. Louis: Mosby.)

Continued

TABLE 1-6 Characteristics of Epithelial Tissues—cont'd

Simple Columnar Epithelium

Structure

Large amounts of cytoplasm and cellular organelles

Location and Function

Ducts of many glands and lining of digestive tract allow secretion and absorption from stomach to anus

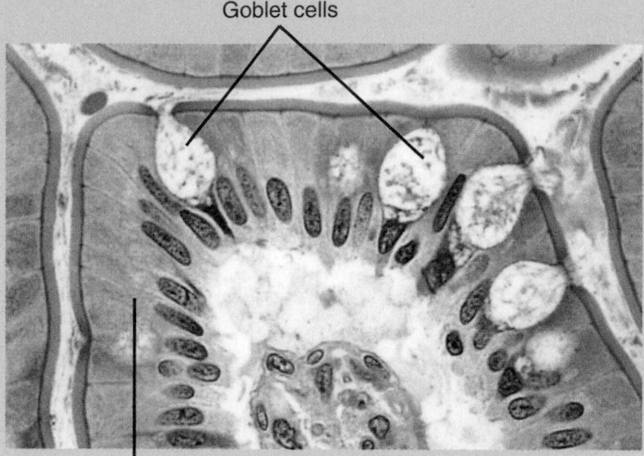

Simple Columnar Epithelium. Photomicrograph of simple columnar epithelium. (Copyright Ed Reschke. Used with permission.)

Ciliated Simple Columnar Epithelium

Structure

Same as simple columnar epithelium but ciliated

Location and Function

Linings of bronchi of lungs, nasal cavity, and oviducts allow secretion, absorption, and propulsion of fluids and particles

Stratified Columnar Epithelium

Structure

Small and rounded basement membrane (columnar cells do not touch basement membrane)

Location and Function

Linings of epiglottis, part of pharynx, anus, and male urethra provide protection

Pseudostratified Ciliated Columnar Epithelium

Structure

All cells in contact with basement membrane

Nuclei found at different levels within cell, giving stratified appearance

Free surface often ciliated

Location and Function

Linings of large ducts of some glands (parotid, salivary), male urethra, respiratory passages, and eustachian tubes of ears transport substances

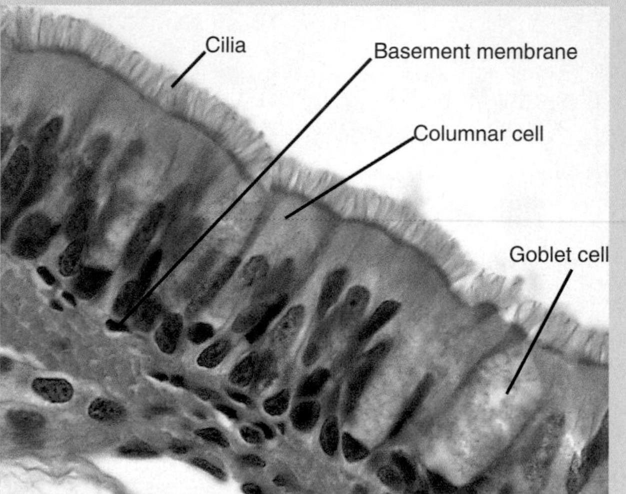

Pseudostratified Ciliated Columnar Epithelium. Photomicrograph of pseudostratified ciliated columnar epithelium of trachea. (Jose Luis Calvo/Shutterstock.com.)

TABLE 1-7 Connective Tissues

Loose or Areolar Tissue

Structure

Unorganized; spaces between fibres

Most fibres collagenous, some elastic and reticular

Includes many types of cells (fibroblasts and macrophages most common) and large amount of intercellular fluid

Location and Function

Attaches skin to underlying tissue; holds organs in place by filling spaces between them; supports blood vessels

Intercellular fluid transports nutrients and waste products

Fluid accumulation causes swelling (edema)

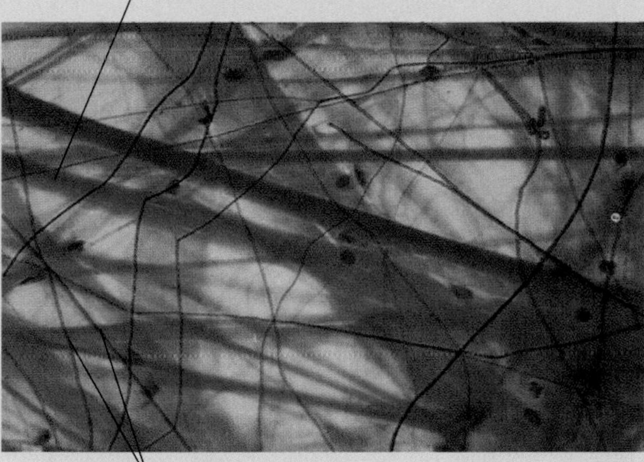

Loose Areolar Connective Tissue. (Copyright Ed Reschke. Used with permission.)

Dense Irregular Tissue

Structure

Dense, compact, and areolar tissue, with fewer cells and greater number of closely woven collagenous fibres than in loose tissue

Location and Function

Dermis layer of skin; acts as protective barrier

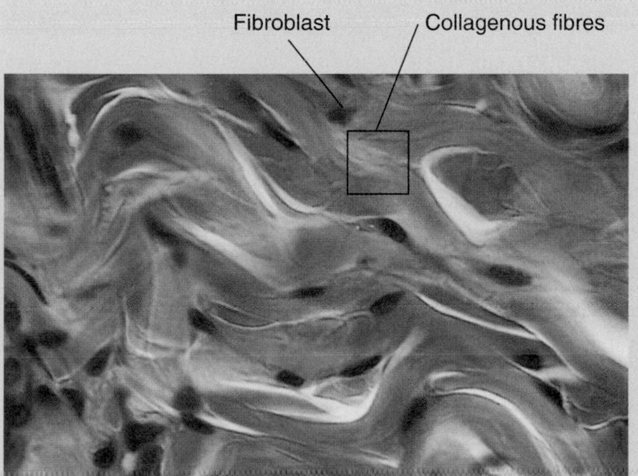

Dense, Irregular Connective Tissue. (Copyright Ed Reschke. Used with permission.)

Dense, Regular (White Fibrous) Tissue

Structure

Collagenous fibres and some elastic fibres, tightly packed into parallel bundles, with only fibroblast cells

Location and Function

Forms strong tendons of muscle, ligaments of joints, some fibrous membranes, and fascia that surrounds organs and muscles

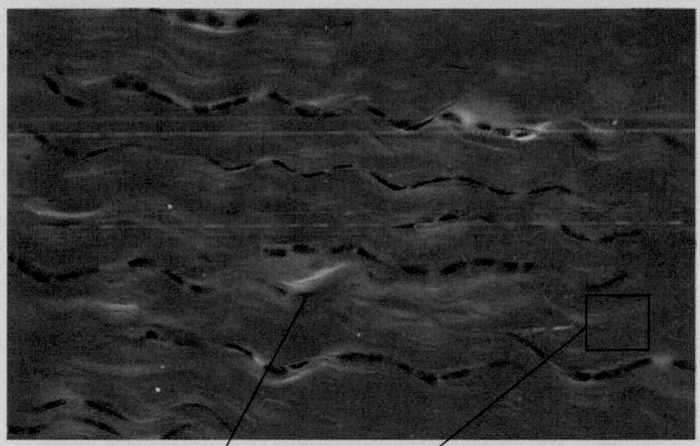

Dense, Regular (White Fibrous) Connective Tissue. (Copyright Ed Reschke. Used with permission.)

Elastic Tissue

Structure

Elastic fibres, some collagenous fibres, fibroblasts

Location and Function

Lends strength and elasticity to walls of arteries, trachea, vocal cords, and other structures

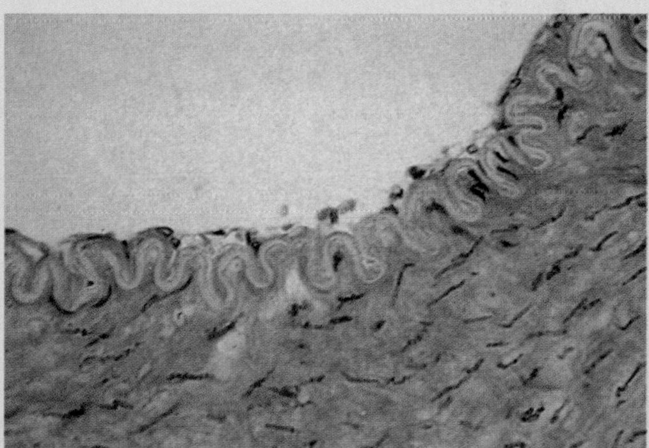

Elastic Connective Tissue. (From Erlandsen, S.L., & Magney, J.E. [1992]. *Color atlas of histology.* St. Louis: Mosby.)

Continued

TABLE 1-7 Connective Tissues—cont'd

Adipose Tissue

Structure

Fat cells dispersed in loose tissues; each cell containing a large droplet of fat flattens nucleus and forces cytoplasm into a ring around cell's periphery

Location and Function

Stores fat, which provides padding and protection

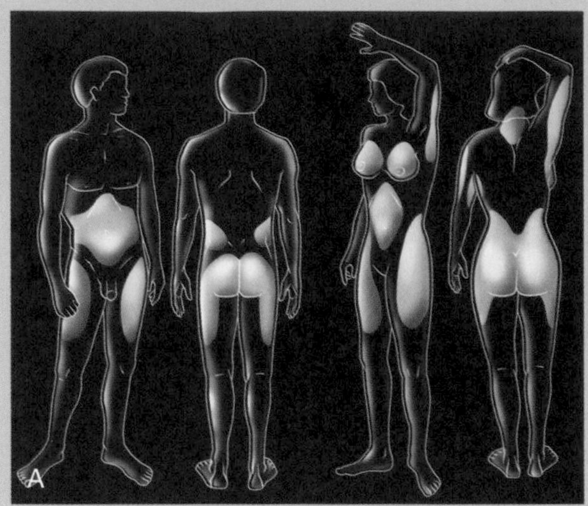

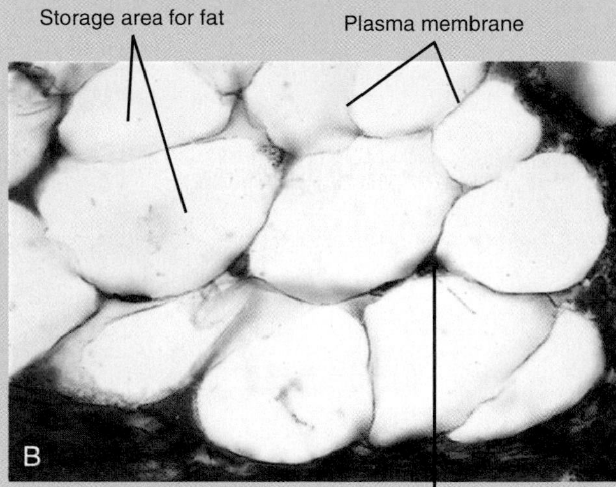

Adipose Tissue. **A,** Fat storage areas—distribution of fat in male and female bodies. **B,** Photomicrograph of adipose tissue. (**A,** from Thibodeau, G.A., & Patton, K.T. [2007]. *Anatomy & physiology* [6th ed.]. St. Louis: Mosby; **B,** copyright Ed Reschke. Used with permission.)

Cartilage (Hyaline, Elastic, Fibrous)

Structure

Collagenous fibres embedded in a firm matrix (chondrin); no blood supply

Location and Function

Gives form, support, and flexibility to joints, trachea, nose, ear, vertebral disks, embryonic skeleton, and many internal structures

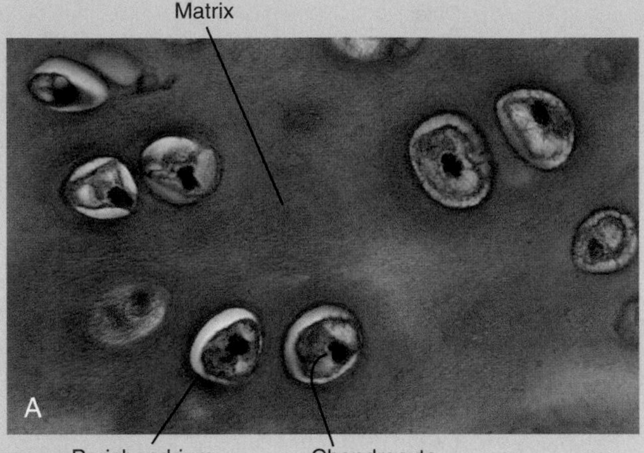

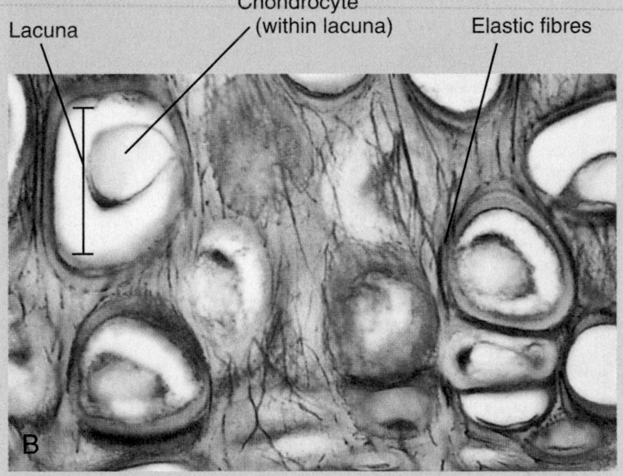

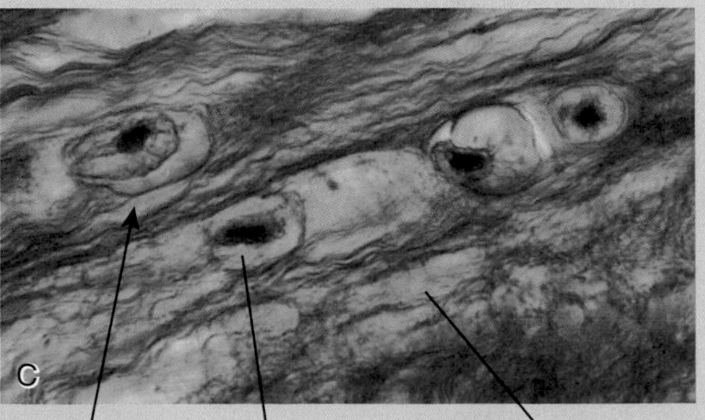

Cartilage. **A,** Hyaline cartilage. **B,** Elastic cartilage. **C,** Fibrous cartilage. (A, B, and C, copyright Ed Reschke. Used with permission.)

TABLE 1-7 Connective Tissues—cont'd

Bone
Structure
Rigid connective tissue consisting of cells, fibres, ground substances, and minerals

Location and Function
Lends skeleton rigidity and strength

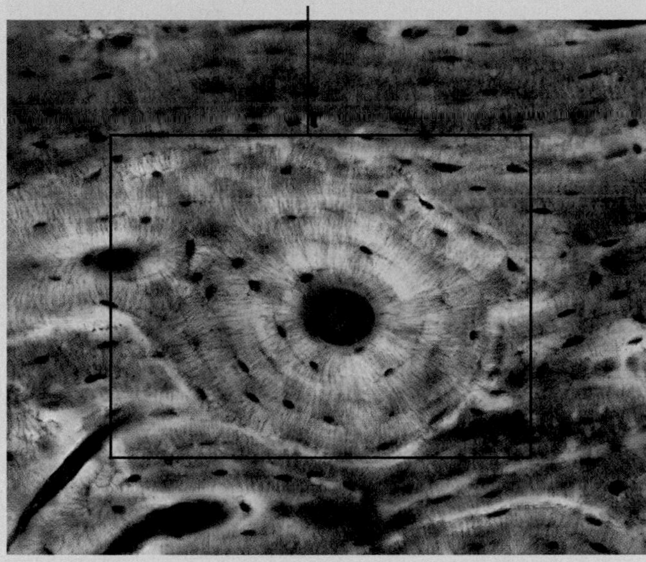

Bone. (Steve Gschmeissner/Science Source.)

Special Connective Tissues
Plasma
Structure
Fluid

Location and Function
Serves as matrix for blood cells

Macrophages in Tissue, Reticuloendothelial, or Macrophage System
Structure
Scattered macrophages (phagocytes) called Kupffer cells (in liver), alveolar macrophages (in lungs), microglia (in central nervous system)

Location and Function
Facilitate inflammatory response and carry out phagocytosis in loose connective, lymphatic, digestive, medullary (bone marrow), splenic, adrenal, and pituitary tissues

TABLE 1-8 Muscle Tissues

Skeletal (Striated) Muscle
Structure Characteristics of Cells
Long, cylindrical cells that extend throughout length of muscles
Striated myofibrils (proteins)
Many nuclei on periphery

Location and Function
Attached to bones directly or by tendons and provide voluntary movement of skeleton and maintenance of posture

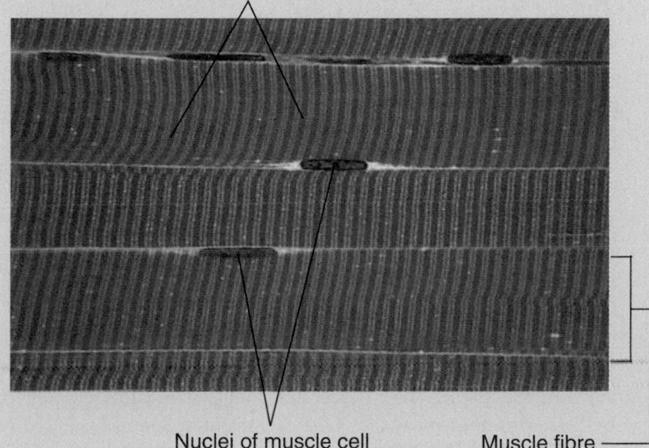

Skeletal (Striated) Muscle. (From Thibodeau, G.A., & Patton, K.T. [2007]. *Anatomy & physiology* [6th ed.]. St. Louis: Mosby.)

Cardiac Muscle
Structure Characteristics of Cells
Branching networks throughout muscle tissue
Striated myofibrils

Location and Function
Cells attached end-to-end at intercalated disks with tissue forming walls of heart (myocardium) to provide involuntary pumping action of heart

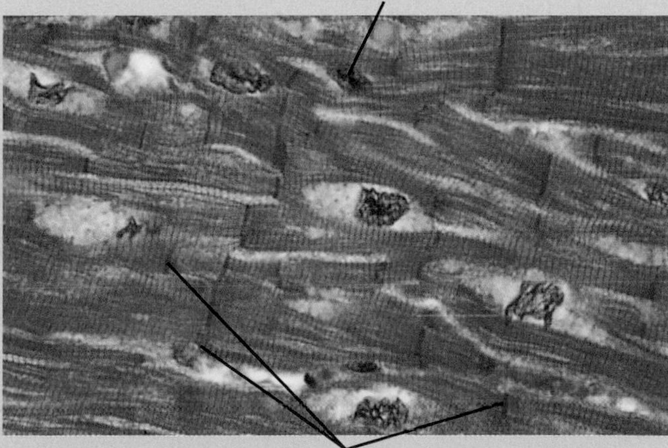

Cardiac Muscle. (Copyright Ed Reschke. Used with permission.)

Continued

TABLE 1-8 Muscle Tissues—cont'd

Smooth (Visceral) Muscle

Structure Characteristics of Cells

Long spindles that taper to a point
Absence of striated myofibrils

Location and Function

Walls of hollow internal structures, such as digestive tract and blood vessels (viscera), provide voluntary and involuntary contractions that move substances through hollow structures

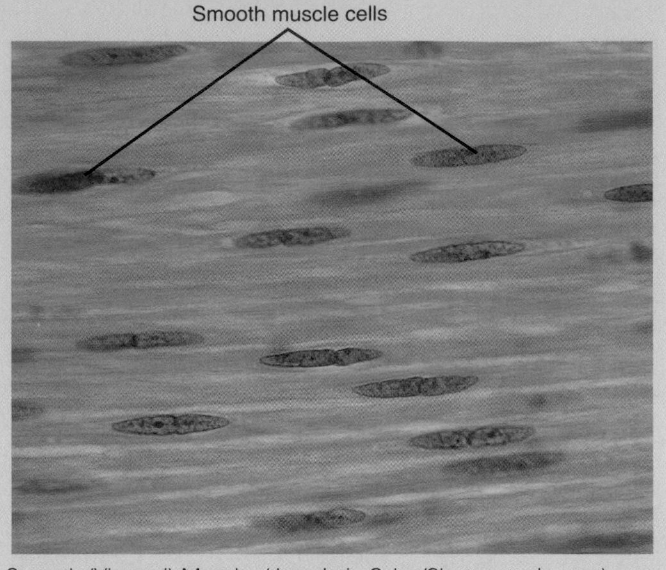

Smooth (Visceral) Muscle. (Jose Luis Calvo/Shutterstock.com.)

DID YOU UNDERSTAND?

Cellular Functions

1. Cells become specialized through the process of differentiation or maturation.
2. The eight specialized cellular functions are movement, conductivity, metabolic absorption, secretion, excretion, respiration, reproduction, and communication.

Structure and Function of Cellular Components

1. The eukaryotic cell consists of three general components: the plasma membrane, the cytoplasm, and the intracellular organelles.
2. The nucleus is the largest membrane-bound organelle and is found usually in the cell's centre. The chief functions of the nucleus are cell division and control of genetic information.
3. Cytoplasm is an aqueous solution (cytosol) that fills the cytoplasmic matrix—the space between the nuclear envelope and the plasma membrane.
4. The organelles are suspended in the cytoplasm and are enclosed in biological membranes.
5. The endoplasmic reticulum is a network of tubular channels (cisternae) that extend throughout the outer nuclear membrane. It specializes in the synthesis and transport of protein and lipid components of most of the organelles.
6. The Golgi complex is a network of smooth membranes and vesicles located near the nucleus. The Golgi complex is responsible for processing and packaging proteins into secretory vesicles that break away from the Golgi complex and migrate to a variety of intracellular and extracellular destinations, including the plasma membrane.
7. Lysosomes are saclike structures that originate from the Golgi complex and contain digestive enzymes. These enzymes are responsible for digesting most cellular substances to their basic form, such as amino acids, fatty acids, and carbohydrates (sugars).
8. Cellular injury leads to a release of the lysosomal enzymes, causing cellular self-digestion.
9. Peroxisomes are similar to lysosomes but contain several enzymes that either produce or use hydrogen peroxide.
10. Mitochondria contain the metabolic machinery necessary for cellular energy metabolism. The enzymes of the respiratory chain (electron-transport chain), found in the inner membrane of the mitochondria, generate most of the cell's ATP.
11. The cytoskeleton is the "bone and muscle" of the cell. The internal skeleton is composed of a network of protein filaments, including microtubules and actin filaments (microfilaments).
12. The plasma membrane encloses the cell and, by controlling the movement of substances across it, exerts a powerful influence on metabolic pathways. Principles of membrane structure are being overhauled.
13. Proteins are the major workhorses of the cell. Membrane proteins, like other proteins, are synthesized by the ribosome and then make their way, called *trafficking*, to different locations in the cell. Trafficking places unique demands on membrane proteins for folding, translocation, and stability. Misfolded proteins are emerging as an important cause of disease.
14. Protein regulation in a cell is called *protein homeostasis* and is defined by the proteostasis network. This network is composed of ribosomes (makers), chaperones (helpers), and protein breakdown or proteolytic systems. Malfunction of these systems is associated with disease.
15. Carbohydrates contained within the plasma membrane are generally bound to membrane proteins (glycoproteins) and lipids (glycolipids).
16. Protein receptors (recognition units) on the plasma membrane enable the cell to interact with other cells and with extracellular substances.
17. Membrane functions are determined largely by proteins. These functions include recognition by protein receptors and transport of substances into and out of the cell.

Cell-to-Cell Adhesions

1. Cell-to-cell adhesions are formed on plasma membranes, thereby allowing the formation of tissues and organs. Cells are held together by three different means: (a) the extracellular membrane, (b) cell adhesion molecules in the cell's plasma membrane, and (c) specialized cell junctions.

2. The extracellular matrix includes three groups of macromolecules: (a) fibrous structural proteins (e.g., collagen and elastin), (b) adhesive glycoproteins, and (c) proteoglycans and hyaluronic acid. The matrix helps regulate cell growth, movement, and differentiation.
3. The basement membrane is a tough layer of extracellular matrix underlying the epithelium of many organs; it is also called the *basal lamina*.
4. Cell junctions can be classified as symmetrical and asymmetrical. Symmetrical junctions include tight junctions, the belt desmosome, desmosomes, and gap junctions. An asymmetrical junction is the hemidesmosome.

Cellular Communication and Signal Transduction

1. Cells communicate in three main ways: (a) they form protein channels (gap junctions); (b) they display receptors that affect intracellular processes or other cells in direct physical contact; and (c) they use receptor proteins *inside* the target cell.
2. Primary modes of intercellular signalling include contact-dependent, paracrine, hormonal, neurohormonal, and neurotransmitter.
3. Signal transduction involves signals or instructions from extracellular chemical messengers that are conveyed to the cell's interior for execution. If deprived of appropriate signals, cells undergo a form of cell suicide known as programmed cell death, or apoptosis.

Cellular Metabolism

1. The chemical tasks of maintaining essential cellular functions are referred to as *cellular metabolism*. Anabolism is the energy-using process of metabolism, whereas catabolism is the energy-releasing process.
2. Adenosine triphosphate (ATP) functions as an energy-transferring molecule. It is fuel for cell survival. Energy is stored by molecules of carbohydrate, lipid, and protein, which, when catabolized, transfers energy to ATP.
3. Oxidative phosphorylation occurs in the mitochondria and is the mechanism by which the energy produced from carbohydrates, fats, and proteins is transferred to ATP.

Membrane Transport: Cellular Intake and Output

1. Cell survival and growth depends on the constant exchange of molecules with their environment. The two main classes of membrane transport proteins are transporters and channels. The majority of molecular transfer depends on specialized membrane transport proteins.
2. Water and small, electrically uncharged molecules move through pores in the plasma membrane's lipid bilayer in the process called *passive transport*.
3. Passive transport does not require the expenditure of energy; rather, it is driven by the physical effect of osmosis, hydrostatic pressure, and diffusion.
4. Larger molecules and molecular complexes are moved into the cell by active transport, which requires the cell to expend energy (by means of ATP).
5. The largest molecules (macromolecules) and fluids are transported by the processes of endocytosis (ingestion) and exocytosis (expulsion). Endocytosis, or vesicle formation, is when the substance to be transported is engulfed by a segment of the plasma membrane, forming a vesicle that moves into the cell.
6. Pinocytosis is a type of endocytosis in which fluids and solute molecules are ingested through formation of small vesicles.
7. Phagocytosis is a type of endocytosis in which large particles, such as bacteria, are ingested through formation of large vesicles, called *vacuoles*.
8. In receptor-mediated endocytosis, the plasma membrane receptors are clustered, along with bristlelike structures, in specialized areas called *coated pits*.
9. Endocytosis occurs when coated pits invaginate, internalizing ligand-receptor complexes in coated vesicles.
10. Inside the cell, lysosomal enzymes process and digest material ingested by endocytosis.
11. Two types of solutes exist in body fluids: electrolytes and nonelectrolytes. Electrolytes are electrically charged and dissociate into constituent ions when placed in solution. Nonelectrolytes do not dissociate when placed in solution.
12. Diffusion is the passive movement of a solute from an area of higher solute concentration to an area of lower solute concentration.
13. Filtration is the measurement of water and solutes through a membrane because of a greater pushing pressure.
14. Hydrostatic pressure is the mechanical force of water pushing against cellular membranes.
15. Osmosis is the movement of water across a semipermeable membrane from a region of lower solute concentration to a region of higher solute concentration.
16. The amount of hydrostatic pressure required to oppose the osmotic movement of water is called the *osmotic pressure* of the solution.
17. The overall osmotic effect of colloids, such as plasma proteins, is called the *oncotic pressure*, or *colloid osmotic pressure.*
18. All body cells are electrically polarized, with the inside of the cell more negatively charged than the outside. The difference in voltage across the plasma membrane is the resting membrane potential.
19. When an excitable (nerve or muscle) cell receives an electrochemical stimulus, cations enter the cell and cause a rapid change in the resting membrane potential, known as the *action potential.* The action potential "moves" along the cell's plasma membrane and is transmitted to an adjacent cell. This is how electrochemical signals convey information from cell to cell.

Cellular Reproduction: The Cell Cycle

1. Cellular reproduction in body tissues involves mitosis (nuclear division) and cytokinesis (cytoplasmic division).
2. Only mature cells are capable of division. Maturation occurs during a stage of cellular life called *interphase* (the growth phase).
3. The cell cycle is the reproductive process that begins after interphase in all tissues with cellular turnover. There are four phases of the cell cycle: (a) the S phase, during which DNA synthesis takes place in the cell nucleus; (b) the G_2 phase, the period between the completion of DNA synthesis and the next phase (M); (c) the M phase, which involves both nuclear (mitotic) and cytoplasmic (cytokinetic) division; and (d) the G_1 phase (growth phase), after which the cycle begins again.
4. The M phase (mitosis) involves four stages: prophase, metaphase, anaphase, and telophase.
5. The mechanisms that control cellular division depend on the integrity of genetic, epigenetic, and protein growth factors.

Tissues

1. Cells of one or more types are organized into tissues, and different types of tissues compose organs. Organs are organized to function as tracts or systems.
2. Three key factors that maintain the cellular organization of tissues are (a) recognition and cell communication, (b) selective cell-to-cell adhesion, and (c) memory.
3. Fully specialized or terminally differentiated cells that are lost are generated from proliferating *precursor cells* and they, in turn, have

been derived from a smaller number of stem cells. Stem cells are cells with the potential to develop into many different cell types during early development and growth. In many tissues, stem cells serve as an internal repair and maintenance system dividing indefinitely. These cells can maintain themselves over very long periods of time, called self-renewal, and can generate all the differentiated cell types of the tissue or multipotency.
4. Tissue cells are linked at cell junctions, which are specialized regions on their plasma membranes. Cell junctions attach adjacent cells and allow small molecules to pass between them.
5. The four basic types of tissues are epithelial, muscle, nerve, and connective tissues.
6. Neural tissue is composed of highly specialized cells called *neurons* that receive and transmit electrical impulses rapidly across junctions called *synapses*.
7. Epithelial tissue covers most internal and external surfaces of the body. The functions of epithelial tissue include protection, absorption, secretion, and excretion.
8. Connective tissue binds various tissues and organs together, supporting them in their locations and serving as storage sites for excess nutrients.
9. Muscle tissue is composed of long, thin, highly contractile cells or fibres called *myocytes*. Muscle tissue that is attached to bones enables voluntary movement. Muscle tissue in internal organs enables involuntary movement, such as the heartbeat.

KEY TERMS

Absolute refractory period, 24
Action potential, 24
Active transport, 18
Amphipathic, 3
Anabolism, 14
Anaphase, 25
Anion, 19
Antiport, 18
Arrested (resting) (G_0) state, 27
Autocrine signalling, 12
Basal lamina, 11
Basement membrane, 10
Binding site, 9
Catabolism, 14
Cation, 19
Caveolae, 23
Cell adhesion molecule (CAM), 7
Cell cortex, 8
Cell cycle, 25
Cell junction, 12
Cell polarity, 2
Cell-to-cell adhesion, 10
Cellular metabolism, 14
Cellular receptor, 9
Centromere, 25
Channel, 17
Chemical synapse, 13
Chromatid, 25
Chromatin, 25
Citric acid cycle (Krebs cycle, tricarboxylic acid cycle), 16
Clathrin, 23
Coated vesicle, 23
Collagen, 10
Concentration gradient, 19
Connective tissue, 11
Connexon, 12
Contact-dependent signalling, 12
Cytokinesis, 25
Cytoplasm, 2
Cytoplasmic matrix, 2
Cytosol, 2
Daughter cell, 26
Depolarization, 24
Desmosome, 12
Differentiation, 2
Diffusion, 19
Digestion, 16
Effective osmolality, 20
Elastin, 10
Electrolyte, 18
Electron-transport chain, 16
Endocytosis, 21
Endosome, 23
Equatorial plate (metaphase plate), 25
ER stress, 8
Eukaryote, 1
Exocytosis, 23
Extracellular matrix (ECM), 10
Fibroblast, 11
Fibronectin, 10
Filtration, 20
G_0 phase, 25
G_1 phase, 25
G_2 phase, 25
Gap junction, 12
Gating, 12
Glycocalyx, 9
Glycolipid, 3
Glycolysis, 16
Glycoprotein, 3
Growth factor (cytokine), 26
Homeostasis, 12
Hormonal signalling, 12
Hydrostatic pressure, 20
Hyperpolarized state, 24
Hypopolarized state, 24
Integral membrane protein, 7
Interphase, 25
Ions, 7
Junctional complex, 12
Ligand, 9
Lipid bilayer, 2
M phase, 25
Macromolecule, 10
Mediated transport, 17
Membrane lipid raft (MLR), 5
Membrane transport protein, 17
Metabolic pathway, 16
Metaphase, 25
Mitosis, 25
Multipotency, 27
Neurohormonal signalling, 12
Neurotransmitter, 13
Nuclear envelope, 2
Nuclear pores, 2
Nucleolus, 2
Nucleus, 2
Oncotic pressure (colloid osmotic pressure), 20
Organelle, 2
Osmolality, 20
Osmolarity, 20
Osmosis, 20
Osmotic pressure, 20
Oxidation, 16
Oxidative phosphorylation, 16
Paracrine signalling, 12
Passive transport, 17
Peripheral membrane protein, 7
Phagocytosis, 21
Phospholipid, 5
Pinocytosis, 21
Plasma membrane (plasmalemma), 2
Plasma membrane receptor, 9
Platelet-derived growth factor (PDGF), 26
Polarity, 19
Polypeptide, 5
Post-translational modification (PTM), 5
Prokaryote, 1
Prophase, 25
Protein, 5
Proteolytic, 8
Proteome, 7
Proteomic, 7
Receptor protein, 14
Receptor-mediated endocytosis (ligand internalization), 23
Relative refractory period, 24
Repolarization, 24
Resting membrane potential, 24
Retinoblastoma (Rb) protein, 26
Self-renewal, 27
Signalling cell, 14
Signal transduction pathway, 14
Solute, 17
S phase, 25
Spindle fibre, 25
Stem cell, 27
Stroma, 26
Substrate, 16
Substrate phosphorylation (anaerobic glycolysis), 17
Symport, 18
Target cell, 14
Telophase, 25
Terminally differentiated, 27
Threshold potential, 24
Tight junction, 12
Tonicity, 20
Transfer reaction, 16
Transmembrane protein, 7
Transporter, 17
Unfolded-protein response (UPR), 8
Uniport, 18
Valence, 19
Wnt signals, 27

REFERENCES

1. Alberts, B. (2014). *Essential cell biology* (4th ed.). New York: Garland.
2. Simons, K., & Sampaio, J. L. (2011). Membrane organization and lipid rafts. *Cold Spring Harbor Perspectives in Biology, 3*(10), a004697. doi:10.1101/cshperspect.a004697.
3. Contreras, F. X., Ernst, A. M., Wieland, F., et al. (2011). Specificity of intramembrane protein-lipid interactions. *Cold Spring Harbor Perspectives in Biology, 3*(6), pii: a004705. doi:10.1101/cshperspect.a004457.
4. Head, B. P., Patel, H. H., & Insel, P. A. (2014). Interaction of membrane/lipid rafts with the cytoskeleton: Impact on signaling and function: Membrane/lipid rafts, mediators of cytoskeletal arrangement and cell signaling. *Biochimica et Biophysica Acta, 1838*(2), 532–545. doi:10.1016/j.bbamem.2013.07.018.
5. Karnovsky, M. J., Kleinfeld, A. M., Hoover, R. L., et al. (1982). The concept of lipid domains in membranes. *Journal of Cell Biology, 94*(1), 1–6.
6. Ribert, D., & Cossart, P. (2010). Pathogen-mediated postranslational modification: A re-emerging field. *Cell, 143*, 694–702. doi:10.1016/j.cell.2010.11.019.
7. Vinothkumar, K. R., & Henderson, R. (2010). Structure of membrane proteins. *Quarterly Review of Biophysics, 43*(1), 65–158. doi:10.1017/S0033583510000041.
8. Cogliati, S., Frezza, C., Soriano, M. E., et al. (2013). Mitochondrial cristae shape determines respiratory chain supercomplexes assembly and respiratory efficiency. *Cell, 155*(1), 160–171. doi:10.1016/j.cell.2013.08.032.
9. Daum, B., Walter, A., Horst, A., et al. (2013). Age-dependent dissociation of ATP synthase dimers and loss of inner-membrane cristae in mitochondria. *Proceedings of the National Academy of Sciences of the United States of America, 110*(38), 15301–15306. doi:10.1073/pnas.1305462110.
10. Friedman, J. R., & Nunnari, J. (2014). Mitochondrial form and function. *Nature, 505*(7483), 335–343. doi:10.1038/nature12985.
11. Amm, I., Sommer, T., & Wolf, D. H. (2014). Protein quality control and elimination of protein waste: The role of the ubiquitin-proteosome system. *Biochimica et Biophysica Acta, 1843*(1), 182–196. doi:10.1016/j.bbamcr.2013.06.031.
12. Lindquist, S. L., & Kelly, J. W. (2011). Chemical and biological approaches for adapting proteostasis to ameliorate protein misfolding and aggregation diseases: Progress and prognosis. *Cold Spring Harbor Perspectives in Biology, 3*(12), pii: a004507. doi:10.1101/cshperspect.a004507.
13. Kierszenbaum, A. L., & Tres, L. T. (2011). *Histology and cell biology: An introduction to pathology* (3rd ed.). St. Louis: Elsevier.
14. Xu, Q., Kopp, R. F., Chen, Y., et al. (2012). Gating of connexin 43 gap junctions by a cytoplasmic loop calmodulin binding domain. *American Journal of Physiology. Cell Physiology, 302*(10), C1548–C1556. doi:10.1152/ajpcell.00319.2011.
15. Sirnes, S., Bruun, J., Kolberg, M., et al. (2012). Connexin43 acts as a colorectal tumor suppressor and predicts disease outcome. *International Journal of Cancer. Journal International du Cancer, 131*(3), 570–581. doi:10.1002/ijc.26392.
16. Khan, R., Khan, A. Q., Lateef, A., et al. (2013). Glycyrrhizic acid suppresses the development of precancerous lesions via regulating the hyperproliferation, inflammation, angiogenesis and apoptosis in the colon of Wistar rats. *PLoS ONE, 8*(2), e56020. doi:10.1371/journal.pone.0056020.
17. Zhang, M. Z., Xu, J., Yao, B., et al. (2009). Inhibition of 11β hydroxysteroid dehydrogenase type II selectively blocks the tumor COX-2 pathway and suppresses colon carcinogenesis in mice and humans. *Journal of Clinical Investigation, 119*(4), 876–885. doi:10.1172/JCI37398.
18. Chaudhri, R. A., Schwartz, N., Elbaradie, K., et al. (2014). Role of ERα36 in membrane-associated signaling by estrogen. *Steroids, 81*, 74–80. doi:10.1016/j.steroids.2013.10.020.
19. Clevers, H., Loh, K. M., & Nusse, R. (2014). Stem cell signaling. An integral program for tissue renewal and regeneration: Wnt signaling and stem cell control. *Science, 346*(6205), 1248012. doi:10.1126/science.1248012.

2

Genes and Genetic Diseases

Lynn B. Jorde and Stephanie Zettel

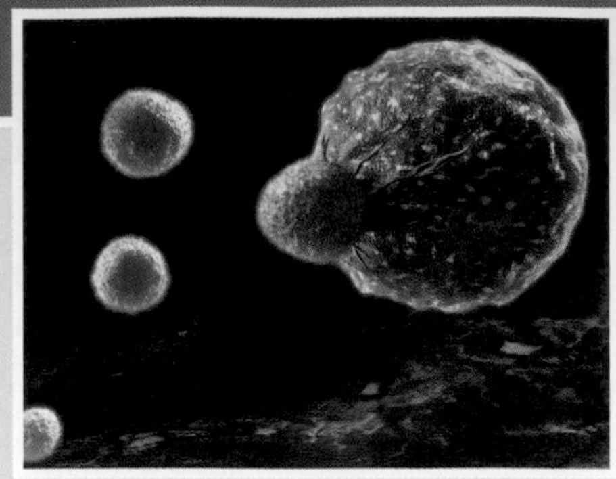

EVOLVE WEBSITE

http://evolve.elsevier.com/Canada/Huether/pathophysiology
Student Review Questions
Key Points
Case Studies
Animations
Quick Check Answers

CHAPTER OUTLINE

DNA, RNA, and Proteins: Heredity at the Molecular Level, 38
Definitions, 38
From Genes to Proteins, 39
Chromosomes, 42
Chromosome Aberrations and Associated Diseases, 42
Elements of Formal Genetics, 49
Phenotype and Genotype, 49
Dominance and Recessiveness, 49
Transmission of Genetic Diseases, 50
Autosomal Dominant Inheritance, 50
Autosomal Recessive Inheritance, 52
X-Linked Inheritance, 54
Linkage Analysis and Gene Mapping, 56
Classic Pedigree Analysis, 56
Complete Human Gene Map: Prospects and Benefits, 57
Multifactorial Inheritance, 58

Genetics occupies a central position in the entire study of biology. An understanding of genetics is essential to study human, animal, plant, or microbial life. Genetics is the study of biological inheritance. In the nineteenth century, microscopic studies of cells led scientists to suspect the nucleus of the cell contained the important mechanisms of inheritance. Scientists found that chromatin, the substance giving the nucleus a granular appearance, is observable in nondividing cells. Just before the cell divides, the chromatin condenses to form discrete, dark-staining organelles, which are called **chromosomes**. (Cell division is discussed in Chapter 1.) With the rediscovery of Gregor Mendel's important breeding experiments at the turn of the twentieth century, it soon became apparent the chromosomes contained **genes**, the basic units of inheritance (Figure 2-1).

The primary constituent of chromatin is **deoxyribonucleic acid (DNA)**. Genes are composed of sequences of DNA. By serving as the blueprints of proteins in the body, genes ultimately influence all aspects of body structure and function. Humans have approximately 20 000 protein-coding genes and an additional 9 000 to 10 000 genes that encode various types of RNA (see the following section) that are not translated into proteins. An error in one of these genes often leads to a recognizable genetic disease.

To date, more than 20000 genetic traits and diseases have been identified and catalogued. As infectious diseases continue to be more effectively controlled, the proportion of beds in pediatric hospitals occupied by children with genetic diseases has risen. In addition to children, many common diseases primarily affecting adults, such as hypertension, coronary heart disease, diabetes, and cancer, are now known to have important genetic components.

Great progress is being made in the diagnosis of genetic diseases and in the understanding of genetic mechanisms underlying them. With the huge strides being made in molecular genetics, "gene therapy"—the utilization of normal genes to correct genetic disease—has begun.

DNA, RNA, AND PROTEINS: HEREDITY AT THE MOLECULAR LEVEL

Definitions

Composition and Structure of DNA

Genes are composed of DNA, which has three basic components: the five-carbon monosaccharide deoxyribose; a phosphate molecule; and four types of nitrogenous bases. Two of the bases, **cytosine** and **thymine**, are single carbon-nitrogen rings called **pyrimidines**. The other two bases, **adenine** and **guanine**, are double carbon-nitrogen rings called **purines**. The four bases are commonly represented by their first letters: A (adenine), C (cytosine), T (thymine), and G (guanine).

Watson and Crick demonstrated how these molecules are physically assembled as DNA, proposing the **double-helix model**, in which DNA appears like a twisted ladder with chemical bonds as its rungs (Figure 2-2). The two sides of the ladder consist of deoxyribose and phosphate molecules, united by strong phosphodiester bonds. Projecting from each side of the ladder, at regular intervals, are the nitrogenous bases. The base projecting from one side is bound to the base projecting from the other by a weak hydrogen bond. Therefore the nitrogenous bases form the rungs of the ladder; adenine pairs with thymine, and guanine pairs with cytosine. Each DNA subunit—consisting of one

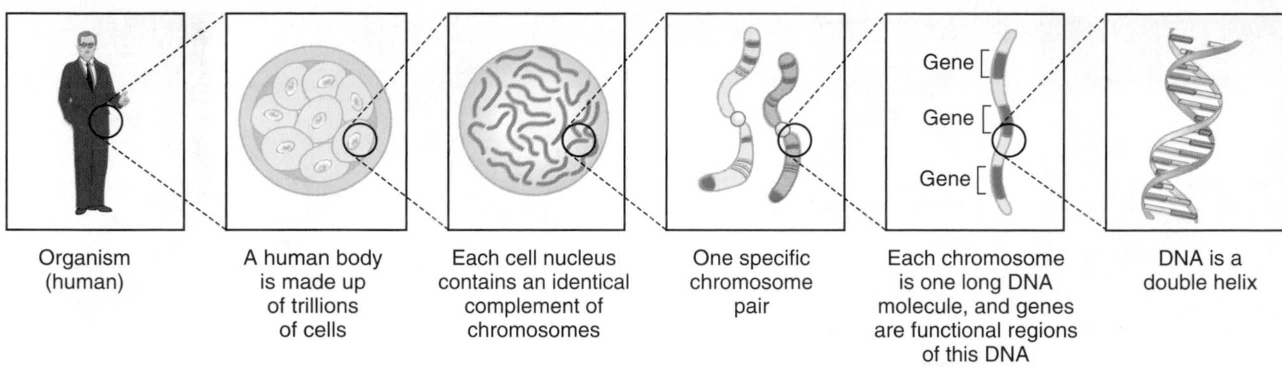

FIGURE 2-1 Successive Enlargements from a Human to the Genetic Material.

deoxyribose molecule, one phosphate group, and one base—is called a **nucleotide**.

DNA as the Genetic Code

DNA directs the synthesis of all the body's proteins. Proteins are composed of one or more **polypeptides** (intermediate protein compounds), which in turn consist of sequences of **amino acids**. The body contains 20 different types of amino acids; they are specified by the 4 nitrogenous bases. To specify (code for) 20 different amino acids with only 4 bases, different combinations of bases, occurring in groups of 3 (triplets), are used. These triplets of bases are known as **codons**. Each codon specifies a single amino acid in a corresponding protein. Because there are 64 (4 × 4 × 4) possible codons but only 20 amino acids, there are many cases in which several codons correspond to the same amino acid.

The genetic code is universal: *all* living organisms use precisely the same DNA codes to specify proteins except for mitochondria, the cytoplasmic organelles in which cellular respiration takes place (see Chapter 1)—they have their own extranuclear DNA. Several codons of mitochondrial DNA encode different amino acids, as compared with the same nuclear DNA codons.

Replication of DNA

DNA replication consists of breaking the weak hydrogen bonds between the bases, leaving a single strand with each base unpaired (Figure 2-3). The consistent pairing of adenine with thymine and of guanine with cytosine, known as **complementary base pairing**, is the key to accurate replication. The unpaired base attracts a free nucleotide only if the nucleotide has the proper complementary base. When replication is complete, a new double-stranded molecule identical to the original is formed. The single strand is said to be a **template**, or molecule on which a complementary molecule is built, and is the basis for synthesizing the new double strand.

Several different proteins are involved in DNA replication. The most important of these proteins is an enzyme known as **DNA polymerase**. This enzyme travels along the single DNA strand, adding the correct nucleotides to the free end of the new strand and checking to ensure that its base is actually complementary to the template base. This mechanism of DNA proofreading substantially enhances the accuracy of DNA replication.

Mutation

A **mutation** is any inherited alteration of genetic material. One type of mutation is the **base pair substitution**, in which one base pair replaces another. This replacement *can* result in a change in the amino acid sequence. However, because of the redundancy of the genetic code, many of these mutations do not change the amino acid sequence and thus have no consequence. Such mutations are called **silent mutations**. Base pair substitutions altering amino acids consist of two basic types: **missense** mutations, which produce a change (i.e., the "sense") in a single amino acid; and **nonsense** mutations, which produce one of the three stop codons (UAA, UAG, or UGA) in the messenger RNA (mRNA) (Figure 2-4). Missense mutations (Figure 2-4, *A*) produce a single amino acid change, whereas nonsense mutations (Figure 2-4, *B*) produce a premature stop codon in the mRNA. Stop codons terminate translation of the polypeptide.

The **frameshift mutation** involves the insertion or deletion of one or more base pairs of the DNA molecule. As Figure 2-5 shows, these mutations change the entire "reading frame" of the DNA sequence because the deletion or insertion is not a multiple of three base pairs (the number of base pairs in a codon). Frameshift mutations can thus greatly alter the amino acid sequence. (*In-frame* insertions or deletions, in which a multiple of three bases is inserted or lost, tend to have less severe disease consequences than do frameshift mutations.)

Agents known as **mutagens** increase the frequency of mutations. Examples include radiation and chemicals such as nitrogen mustard, vinyl chloride, alkylating agents, formaldehyde, and sodium nitrite.

Mutations are rare events. The rate of **spontaneous mutations** (those occurring in the absence of exposure to known mutagens) in humans is about 1.1×10^{-8} per gene per generation.[1] This rate varies from one gene to another. Some DNA sequences have particularly high mutation rates and are known as **mutational hot spots** (Box 2-1).[2]

> **BOX 2-1 Mutational Hot Spots and Antibiotic Resistance**
>
> Zhang and colleagues investigated mechanisms of antibiotic resistance (clofazimine [Lamprene]) in *Mycobacterium tuberculosis* and discovered two nucleotide sequences that accounted for more than 50% of the mutations resulting in resistance to clofazimine. The authors also discovered two new genes responsible for resistant organisms and concluded that this research will assist in more rapidly identifying those who are resistant to this antibiotic and enable the discovery of more effective treatments.
>
> From Zhang, S., Chen, J., Cui, P., et al. (2015). *J Antimicrob Chemother, 70*(9), 2507–2510. doi:10.1093/jac/dkv150.

From Genes to Proteins

DNA is formed and replicated in the cell nucleus, but protein synthesis takes place in the cytoplasm. The DNA code is transported from nucleus to cytoplasm, and subsequent protein is formed through two basic processes: transcription and translation. These processes are mediated by **ribonucleic acid (RNA)**, which is chemically similar to DNA except the sugar molecule is ribose rather than deoxyribose, and uracil rather

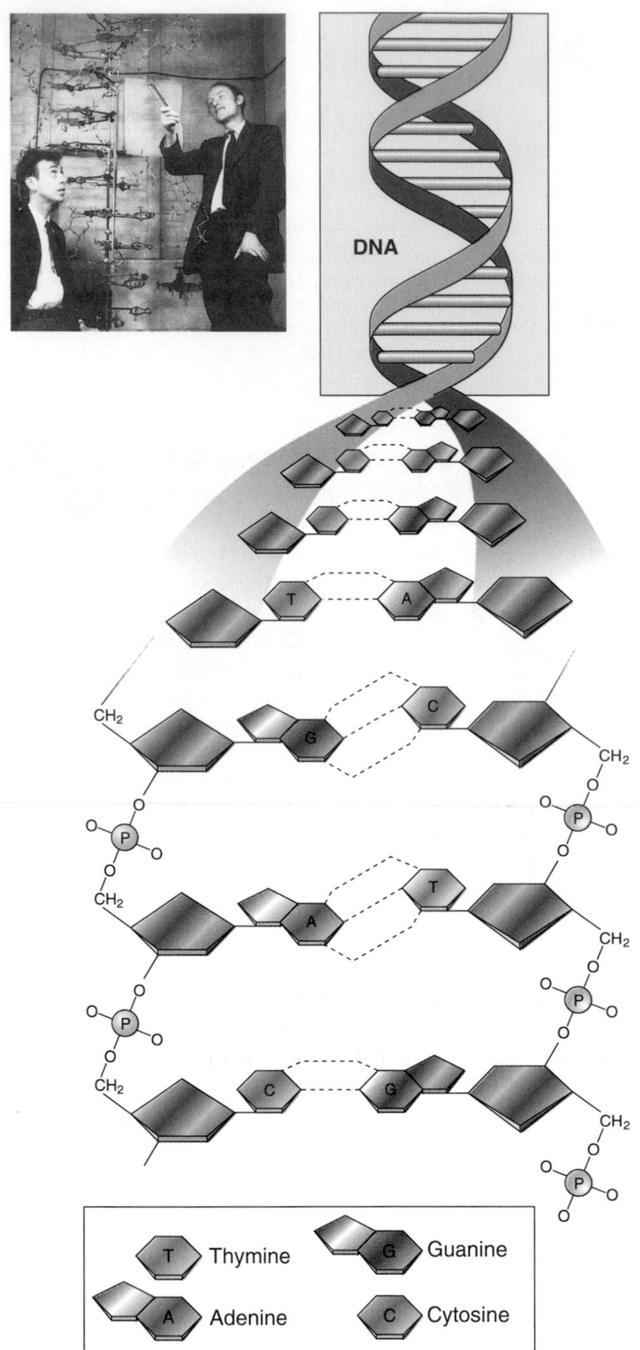

FIGURE 2-2 Watson–Crick Model of the DNA Molecule. The DNA structure illustrated here is based on that published by James Watson (*photograph, left*) and Francis Crick (*photograph, right*) in 1953. Note that each side of the DNA molecule consists of alternating sugar and phosphate groups. Each sugar group is bonded to the opposing sugar group by a pair of nitrogenous bases (adenine-thymine or cytosine-guanine). The sequence of these pairs constitutes a genetic code that determines the structure and function of a cell. (Illustration from Herlihy, B. [2015]. *The human body in health and illness* [5th ed.]. St. Louis: Saunders. Photo from Barrington Brown/Science Source.)

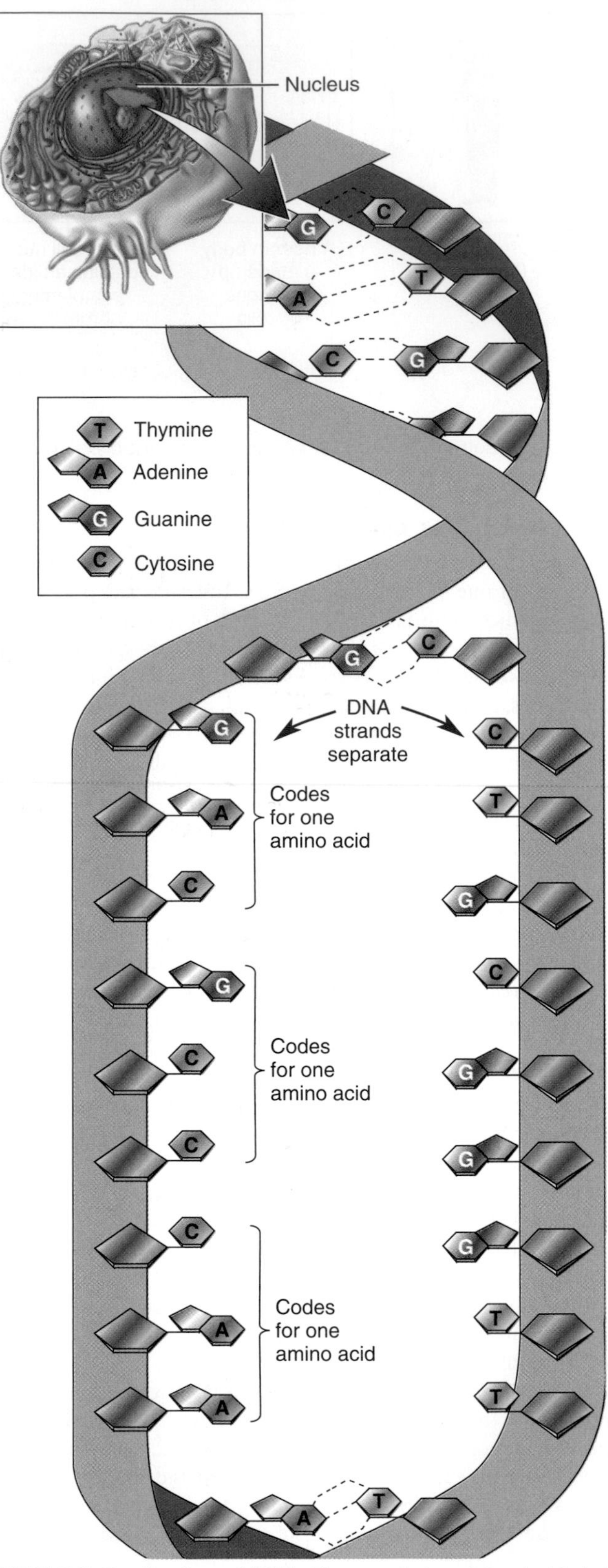

FIGURE 2-3 Replication of DNA. The two chains of the double helix separate and each chain serves as the template for a new complementary chain. (From Herlihy, B. [2015]. *The human body in health and illness* [5th ed.]. St. Louis: Saunders.)

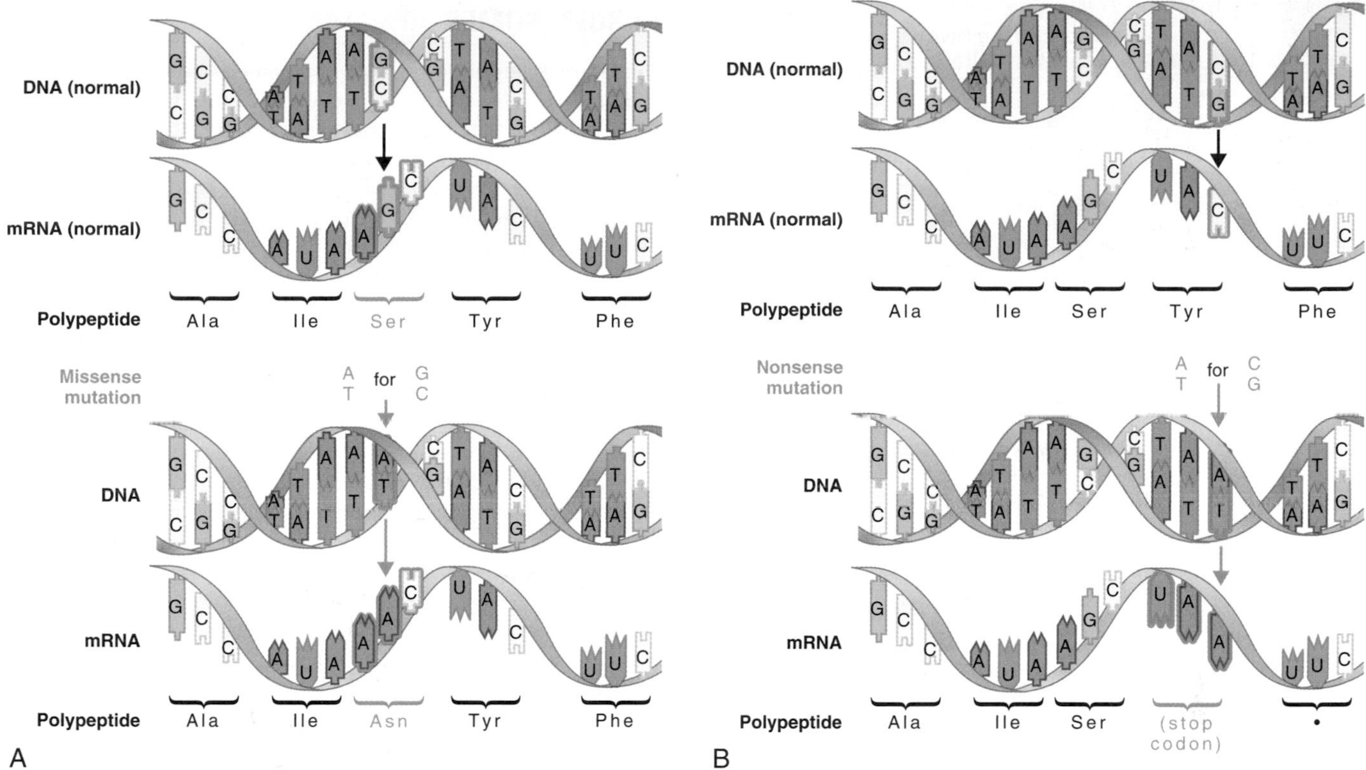

FIGURE 2-4 **Base Pair Substitution.** Missense mutations (**A**) produce a single amino acid change, whereas nonsense mutations (**B**) produce a stop codon in the messenger RNA (*mRNA*). Stop codons terminate translation of the polypeptide. (From *Science, 328*(5978), 636–639. doi:10.1126/science.1186802.)

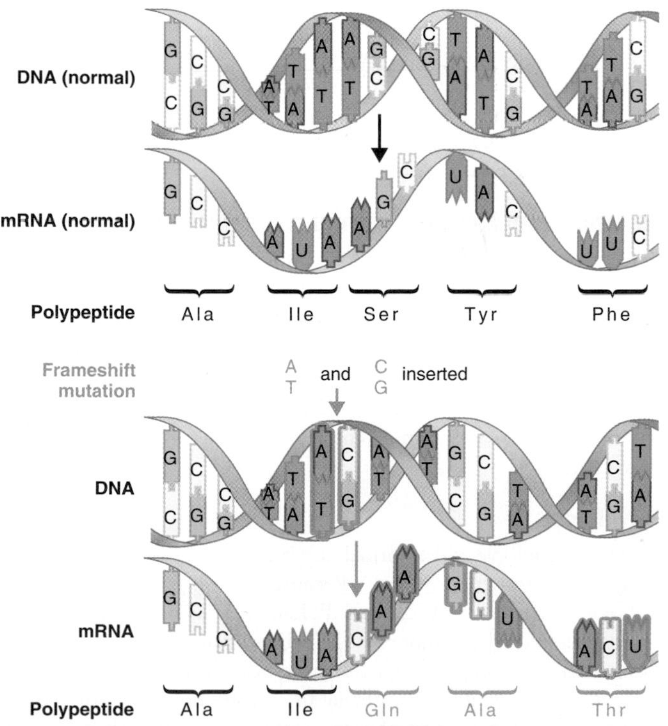

FIGURE 2-5 **Frameshift Mutations.** Frameshift mutations result from the addition or deletion of a number of bases that is not a multiple of 3. This mutation alters all of the codons downstream from the site of insertion or deletion. *mRNA*, messenger RNA. (From Jorde, L., L.B., Carey, J.C., & Bamshad, M.J. [2010]. *Medical genetics* [4th ed.]. St. Louis: Mosby.)

than thymine is one of the four nitrogenous bases. The other three bases of RNA, as in DNA, are adenine, cytosine, and guanine. Uracil is structurally similar to thymine, so it also can pair with adenine. Whereas DNA usually occurs as a double strand, RNA usually occurs as a single strand.

Transcription

In **transcription**, RNA is synthesized from a DNA template, forming **messenger RNA (mRNA)**. **RNA polymerase** binds to a **promoter site**, a sequence of DNA that specifies the beginning of a gene. RNA polymerase then separates a portion of the DNA, exposing unattached DNA bases. One DNA strand then provides the template for the sequence of mRNA nucleotides.

The sequence of bases in the mRNA is thus complementary to the template strand, and except for the presence of uracil instead of thymine, the mRNA sequence is identical to that of the other DNA strand. Transcription continues until a **termination sequence**, codons that act as signals for the termination of protein synthesis, is reached. Then the RNA polymerase detaches from the DNA, and the transcribed mRNA is freed to move out of the nucleus and into the cytoplasm (Figures 2-6 and 2-7).

Gene Splicing

When the mRNA is first transcribed from the DNA template, it reflects exactly the base sequence of the DNA. In eukaryotes, many RNA sequences are removed by nuclear enzymes, and the remaining sequences are spliced together to form the functional mRNA that migrates to the cytoplasm. The excised sequences are called **introns** (intervening sequences), and the sequences that are left to code for proteins are called **exons**.

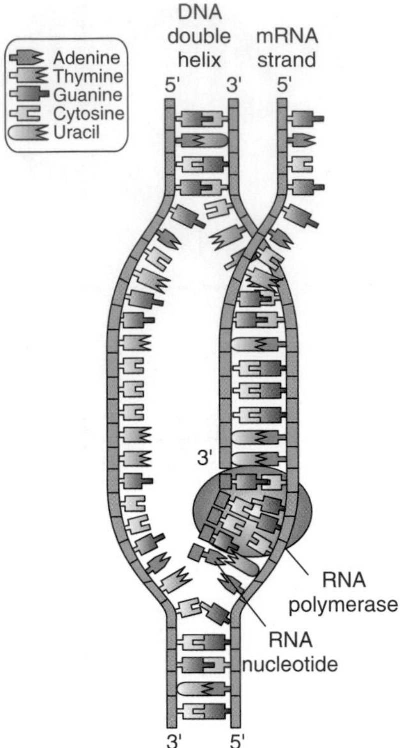

FIGURE 2-6 General Scheme of RNA Transcription. In transcription of messenger RNA (*mRNA*), a DNA molecule "unzips" in the region of the gene to be transcribed. RNA nucleotides already present in the nucleus temporarily attach themselves to exposed DNA bases along one strand of the unzipped DNA molecule according to the principle of complementary pairing. As the RNA nucleotides attach to the exposed DNA, they bind to each other and form a chainlike RNA strand called an *mRNA molecule.* Notice that the new mRNA strand is an exact copy of the base sequence on the opposite side of the DNA molecule. As in all metabolic processes, the formation of mRNA is controlled by an enzyme—in this case, the enzyme is called *RNA polymerase.* (From Ignatavicius, D.D., & Workman, L.D. [2010]. *Medical-surgical nursing* [6th ed.]. St. Louis: Saunders.)

Translation

In **translation**, RNA directs the synthesis of a polypeptide (see Figure 2-7), interacting with **transfer RNA (tRNA)**, a cloverleaf-shaped strand of about 80 nucleotides. The tRNA molecule has a site where an amino acid attaches. The three-nucleotide sequence at the opposite side of the cloverleaf is called the **anticodon**. It undergoes complementary base pairing with an appropriate codon in the mRNA, which specifies the sequence of amino acids through tRNA.

The site of actual protein synthesis is in the **ribosome**, which consists of approximately equal parts of protein and **ribosomal RNA (rRNA)**. During translation, the ribosome first binds to an initiation site on the mRNA sequence and then binds to its surface, so that base pairing can occur between tRNA and mRNA. The ribosome then moves along the mRNA sequence, processing each codon and translating an amino acid by way of the interaction of mRNA and tRNA.

The ribosome provides an enzyme that catalyzes the formation of covalent peptide bonds between the adjacent amino acids, resulting in a growing polypeptide. When the ribosome arrives at a termination signal on the mRNA sequence, translation and polypeptide formation cease; the mRNA, ribosome, and polypeptide separate from one another; and the polypeptide is released into the cytoplasm to perform its required function.

CHROMOSOMES

Human cells can be categorized into **gametes** (sperm and egg cells) and **somatic cells**, which include all cells other than gametes. Each somatic cell nucleus has 46 chromosomes in 23 pairs (Figure 2-8). These are **diploid cells**, and the individual's father and mother each donate one chromosome per pair. New somatic cells are formed through **mitosis** and **cytokinesis**. Gametes are **haploid cells**: they have only 1 member of each chromosome pair, for a total of 23 chromosomes. Haploid cells are formed from diploid cells by **meiosis** (Figure 2-9).

In 22 of the 23 chromosome pairs, the 2 members of each pair are virtually identical in microscopic appearance; thus they are **homologous** (Figure 2-10, *B*). These 22 chromosome pairs are homologous in both males and females and are termed **autosomes**. The remaining pair of chromosomes, the sex chromosomes, consists of two homologous X chromosomes in females and a nonhomologous pair, X and Y, in males.

Figure 2-10, *A*, illustrates a **metaphase spread**, which is a photograph of the chromosomes as they appear in the nucleus of a somatic cell during metaphase. (Chromosomes are easiest to visualize during this stage of mitosis.) In Figure 2-10, *A*, the chromosomes are arranged according to size, with the homologous chromosomes paired. The 22 autosomes are numbered according to length, with chromosome 1 being the longest and chromosome 22 the shortest. A **karyotype**, or **karyogram**, is an ordered display of chromosomes. Some natural variation in relative chromosome length can be expected from person to person, so it is not always possible to distinguish each chromosome by its length. Therefore the position of the centromere (region of DNA responsible for movement of the replicated chromosomes into the two daughter cells during mitosis and meiosis) also is used to classify chromosomes (see Figures 2-10, *B* and 2-11).

The chromosomes in Figure 2-10 were stained with Giemsa stain, resulting in distinctive **chromosome bands**. These bands form various patterns in the different chromosomes so that each chromosome can be distinguished easily. Using banding techniques, researchers can number chromosomes and study individual variations. Missing or duplicated portions of chromosomes, which often result in serious diseases, also are readily identified. More recently, techniques have been devised permitting each chromosome to be visualized with a different colour.

Chromosome Aberrations and Associated Diseases

Chromosome abnormalities are the leading known cause of intellectual disability and miscarriage. Estimates indicate that a major chromosome aberration occurs in at least 1 in 12 conceptions. Most of these fetuses do not survive to term; about 50% of all recovered first-trimester spontaneous abortuses have major chromosome aberrations.[3] The number of live births affected by these abnormalities is, however, significant; approximately 1 in 150 has a major diagnosable chromosome abnormality.[3]

Polyploidy

Cells with a multiple of the normal number of chromosomes are **euploid cells** (Greek *eu* = good or true). Because normal gametes are haploid and most normal somatic cells are diploid, they are both euploid forms. When a euploid cell has more than the diploid number of chromosomes, it is said to be a **polyploid cell**. Several types of body tissues, including some liver, bronchial, and epithelial tissues, are normally polyploid. A zygote that has three copies of each chromosome, rather than the usual two, has a form of polyploidy called **triploidy**. Nearly all triploid fetuses are spontaneously aborted or stillborn. The prevalence of triploidy among live births is approximately 1 in 10 000. **Tetraploidy**, a condition in which euploid cells have 92 chromosomes, has been found primarily in early abortuses, although occasionally affected infants have been

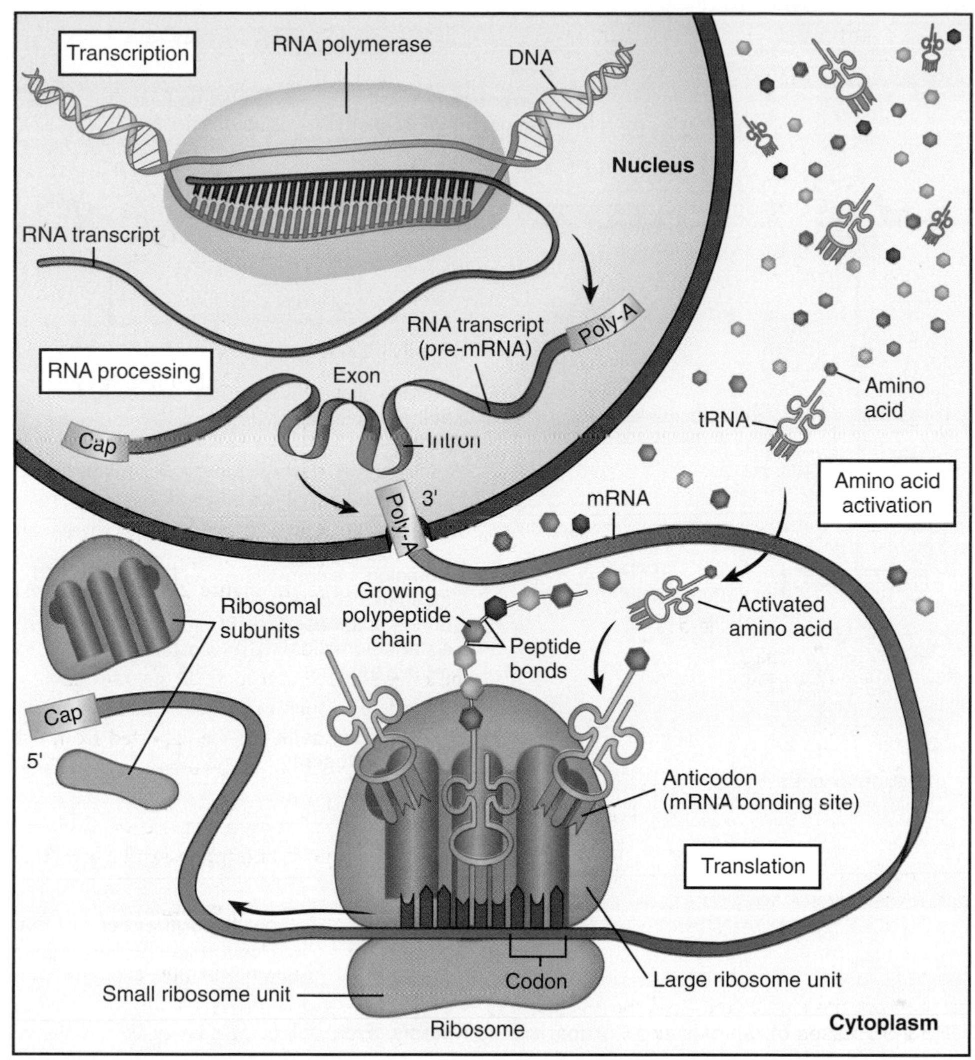

FIGURE 2-7 Protein Synthesis. The site of transcription is the nucleus and the site of translation is the cytoplasm. See the text for details. *mRNA,* messenger RNA; *tRNA,* transfer RNA.

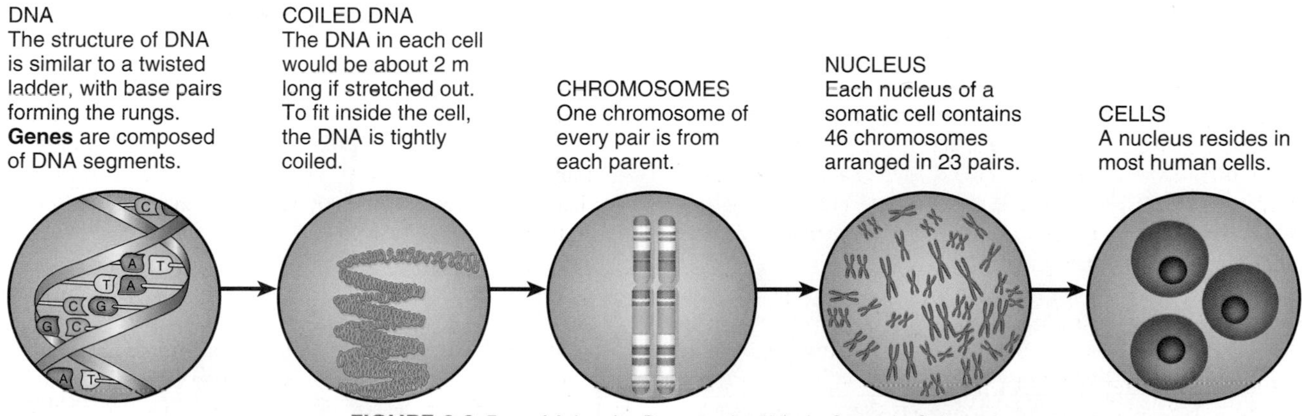

DNA
The structure of DNA is similar to a twisted ladder, with base pairs forming the rungs. **Genes** are composed of DNA segments.
COILED DNA
The DNA in each cell would be about 2 m long if stretched out. To fit inside the cell, the DNA is tightly coiled.
CHROMOSOMES
One chromosome of every pair is from each parent.
NUCLEUS
Each nucleus of a somatic cell contains 46 chromosomes arranged in 23 pairs.
CELLS
A nucleus resides in most human cells.

FIGURE 2-8 From Molecular Parts to the Whole Somatic Cell.

born alive. Like triploid infants, however, they do not survive. Triploidy and tetraploidy are relatively common conditions, accounting for approximately 10% of all known miscarriages.[4]

Aneuploidy

A cell that does not contain a multiple of 23 chromosomes is an **aneuploid cell**. A cell containing three copies of one chromosome is said to be trisomic (a condition termed **trisomy**) and is aneuploid. Monosomy, the presence of only one copy of a given chromosome in a diploid cell, is the other common form of aneuploidy. Among the autosomes, monosomy of any chromosome is lethal, but newborns with trisomy of chromosomes 13, 18, 21, or X can survive. This difference illustrates an important principle: *in general, loss of chromosome material has more serious consequences than duplication of chromosome material.*

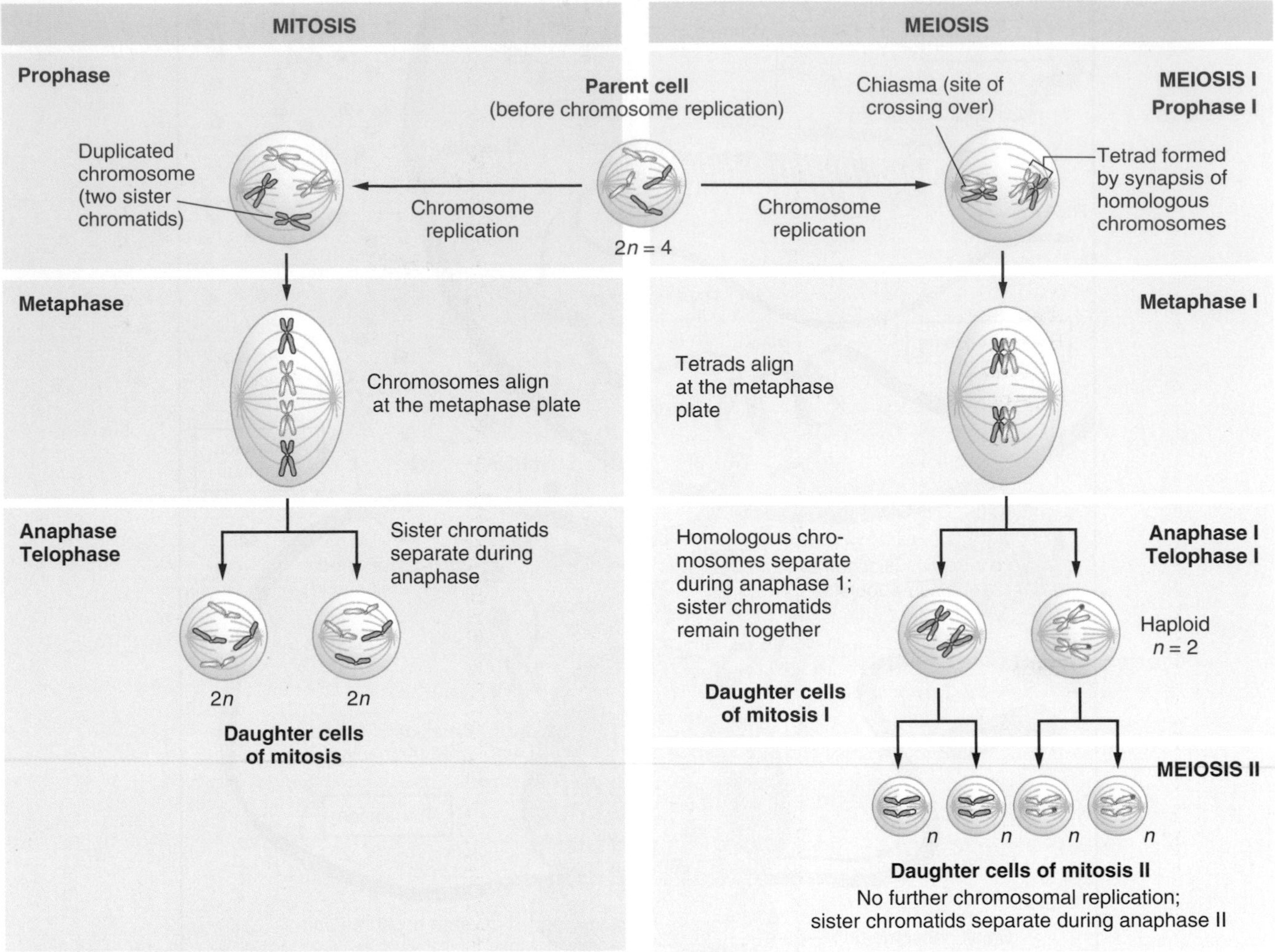

MITOSIS
MEIOSIS
Prophase
Parent cell
(before chromosome replication)
Chiasma (site of
crossing over)
MEIOSIS I
Prophase I
Duplicated
chromosome
(two sister
chromatids)
Chromosome
replication
Chromosome
replication
Tetrad formed
by synapsis of
homologous
chromosomes
2n = 4
Metaphase
Metaphase I
Chromosomes align
at the metaphase plate
Tetrads align
at the metaphase
plate
Anaphase
Telophase
Sister chromatids
separate during
anaphase
Homologous chro-
mosomes separate
during anaphase 1;
sister chromatids
remain together
Anaphase I
Telophase I
Haploid
n = 2
2n
2n
Daughter cells
of mitosis
Daughter cells
of mitosis I
MEIOSIS II
n
n
n
n
Daughter cells of mitosis II
No further chromosomal replication;
sister chromatids separate during anaphase II

FIGURE 2-9 Phases of Meiosis and Comparison to Mitosis. (From Jorde, L.B., Carey, J.C., & Bamshad, M.J. [2010]. *Medical genetics* [4th ed.]. St. Louis: Mosby.)

1
2
3
4
5
6
7
8
9
10
11
12
13
14
15
16
17
18
X
Y
19
20
21
22
A
9.2 μm
B
Homologous chromosomes
Homologous chromosomes
Kinetochore
Replication
Centromere
Cohesin
proteins
Kinetochores
Sister chromatids
Sister chromatids

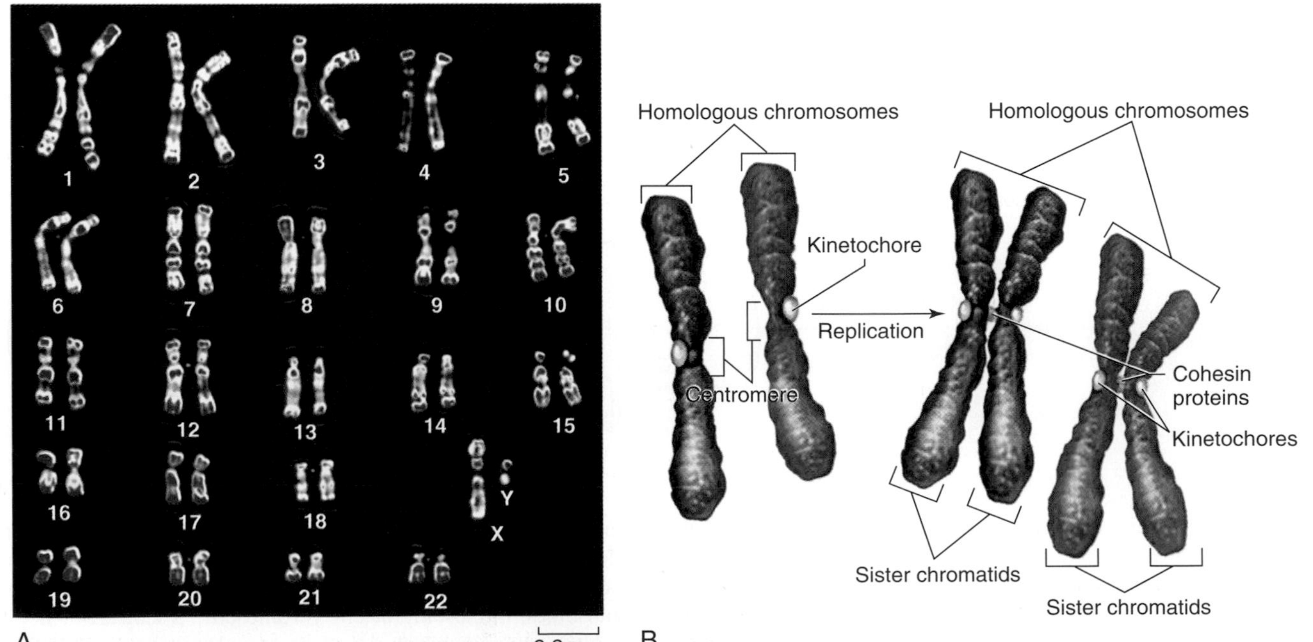

FIGURE 2-10 Karyotype of Chromosomes. **A,** Human karyotype. **B,** Homologous chromosomes and sister chromatids. (From Raven, P.H., Johnson, G., Mason, K., et al. [2008]. *Biology* [8th ed.]. New York: McGraw-Hill.)

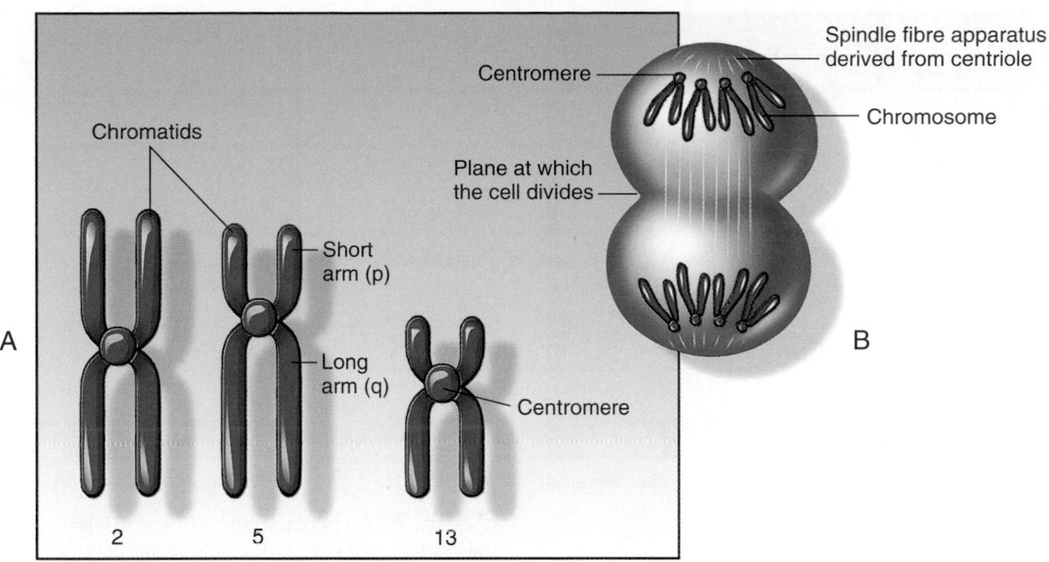

FIGURE 2-11 Structure of Chromosomes. A, Human chromosomes 2, 5, and 13. Each is replicated and consists of two chromatids. Chromosome 2 is a metacentric chromosome because the centromere is close to the middle; chromosome 5 is submetacentric because the centromere is set off from the middle; chromosome 13 is acrocentric because the centromere is at or very near the end. **B,** During mitosis, the centromere divides and the chromosomes move to opposite poles of the cell. At the time of centromere division, the chromatids are designated as chromosomes.

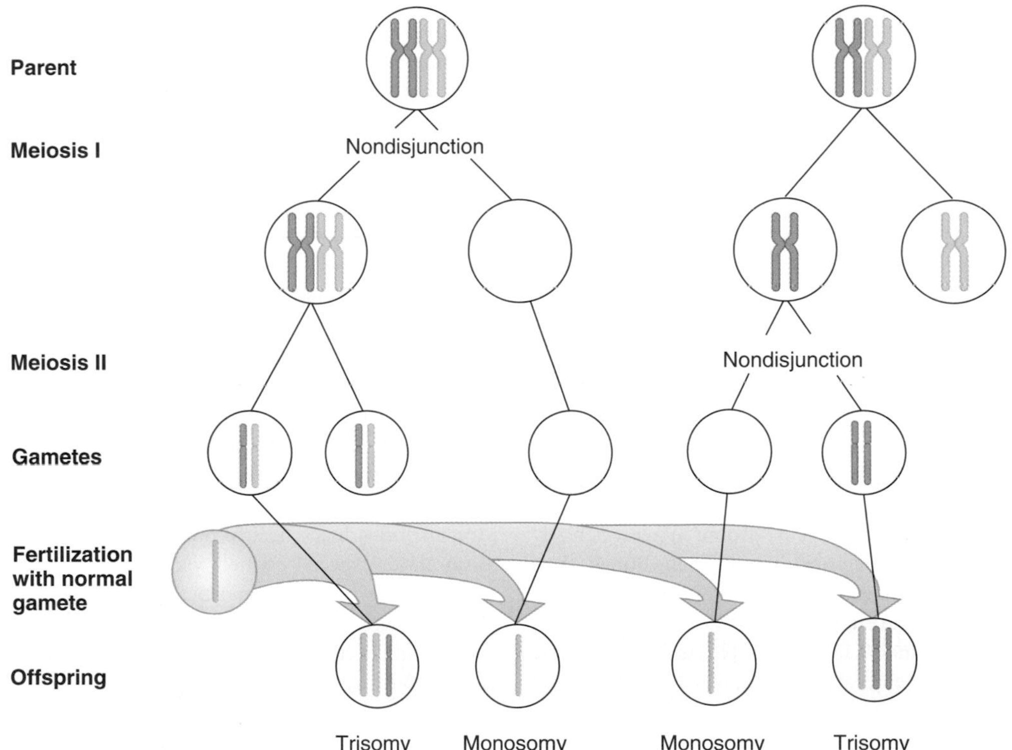

FIGURE 2-12 Nondisjunction. Nondisjunction causes aneuploidy when chromosomes or sister chromatids fail to divide properly. (From Jorde, L.B., Carey, J.C., & Bamshad, M.J. [2010]. *Medical genetics* [4th ed.]. St. Louis: Mosby.)

Aneuploidy of the sex chromosomes is less serious than that of the autosomes. Very little genetic material—only about 40 genes—is located on the Y chromosome. For the X chromosome, inactivation of extra chromosomes (see p. 54) largely diminishes their effect. A zygote bearing *no* X chromosome, however, will not survive.

Aneuploidy is usually the result of **nondisjunction**, an error in which homologous chromosomes or sister chromatids fail to separate normally during meiosis or mitosis (Figure 2-12). Nondisjunction produces some gametes that have two copies of a given chromosome and others that have no copies of the chromosome. When such gametes unite with

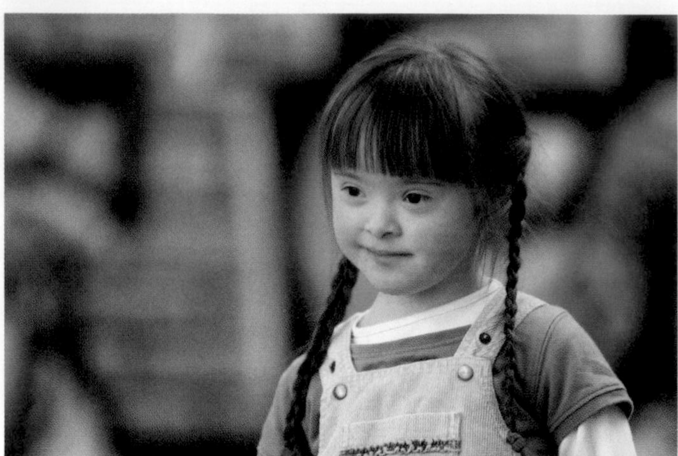

FIGURE 2-13 Child With Down Syndrome. (Dennis Kuvaev/ Shutterstock.com.)

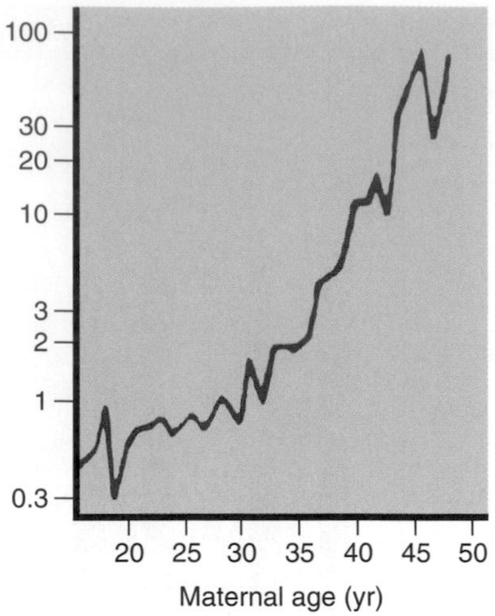

FIGURE 2-14 Down Syndrome Increases with Maternal Age. Rate is per 1 000 live births related to maternal age.

normal haploid gametes, the resulting zygote is monosomic or trisomic for that chromosome. Occasionally, a cell can be monosomic or trisomic for more than one chromosome.

Autosomal aneuploidy. Trisomy can occur for any chromosome, but fetuses with other trisomies of chromosomes (other than 13, 18, 21, or X) do not survive to term. Trisomy 16, for example, is the most common trisomy among abortuses, but it is not seen in live births.[5]

Partial trisomy, in which only an extra portion of a chromosome is present in each cell, can occur also. The consequences of partial trisomies are not as severe as those of complete trisomies. Trisomies may occur in only some cells of the body. Individuals thus affected are said to be chromosomal mosaics, meaning that the body has two or more different cell lines, each of which has a different karyotype. Mosaics are often formed by early mitotic nondisjunction occurring in one embryonic cell but not in others.

The best-known example of aneuploidy in an autosome is trisomy of chromosome 21, which causes Down syndrome (named after J. Langdon Down, who first described the syndrome in 1866). Down syndrome is seen in approximately 1 in 800 live births (from http://www.cdss.ca/positioning/positioning/down-syndrome-defined.html); its principal features are shown and outlined in Figure 2-13 and Table 2-1.

The risk of having a child with Down syndrome increases greatly with maternal age. As Figure 2-14 demonstrates, women younger than 30 years have a risk ranging from about 1 in 1 000 births to 1 in 2 000 births. The risk begins to rise substantially after 35 years of age, and reaches 3% to 5% for women older than 45 years. This dramatic increase in risk is caused by the age of maternal egg cells, which are held in an arrested state of prophase I from the time they are formed in the female embryo until they are shed in ovulation. Thus an egg cell formed by a 45-year-old woman is itself 45 years old. This long suspended state may allow defects to accumulate in the cellular proteins responsible for meiosis, leading to nondisjunction. The risk of Down syndrome, as well as other trisomies, does not increase with paternal age.[6]

Sex chromosome aneuploidy. The incidence of sex chromosome aneuploidies is fairly high. Among live births, about 1 in 500 males and 1 in 900 females have a form of sex chromosome aneuploidy.[7] Because these conditions are generally less severe than autosomal aneuploidies, all forms except complete absence of any X chromosome material allow at least some individuals to survive.

One of the most common sex chromosome aneuploidies, affecting about 1 in 1 000 newborn females, is trisomy X. Instead of two X chromosomes, these females have three X chromosomes in each cell. Most of these females have no overt physical abnormalities, although sterility, menstrual irregularity, or intellectual disability is sometimes seen. Some females have four X chromosomes, and they are more often intellectually disabled. Those with five or more X chromosomes generally are more severely intellectually disabled and have various physical defects.

A condition that leads to somewhat more serious problems is the presence of a single X chromosome and no homologous X or Y chromosome, so that the individual has a total of 45 chromosomes. The karyotype is usually designated 45,X, and it causes a set of symptoms known as Turner's syndrome (Figure 2-15; see Table 2-1). Individuals with at least two X chromosomes and one Y chromosome in each cell (47,XXY karyotype) have a disorder known as Klinefelter's syndrome (Figure 2-16; see Table 2-1).

Abnormalities of Chromosome Structure

In addition to the loss or gain of whole chromosomes, parts of chromosomes can be lost or duplicated as gametes are formed, and the arrangement of genes on chromosomes can be altered. Unlike aneuploidy and polyploidy, these changes sometimes have no serious consequences for an individual's health. Some of them can even remain entirely unnoticed, especially when very small pieces of chromosomes are involved. Nevertheless, abnormalities of chromosome structure can also produce serious disease in individuals or their offspring.

During meiosis and mitosis, chromosomes usually maintain their structural integrity, but chromosome breakage occasionally occurs. Mechanisms exist to "heal" these breaks and usually repair them perfectly with no damage to the daughter cell. However, some breaks remain or heal in a way that alters the chromosome's structure. The risk of chromosome breakage increases with exposure to harmful agents called clastogens (e.g., ionizing radiation, viral infections, and some types of chemicals).

Deletions. Broken chromosomes and lost DNA cause deletions (Figure 2-17). Usually, a gamete with a deletion unites with a normal gamete to form a zygote. The zygote thus has one chromosome with the normal complement of genes and one with some missing genes. Because many genes can be lost in a deletion, serious consequences result even though one normal chromosome is present. The most often

TABLE 2-1 **Characteristics of Various Chromosome Disorders**

Disease/Disorder	Features
Down Syndrome	
Trisomy of Chromosome 21	
IQ	It usually ranges from 20 to 70 (intellectual disability).
Male/female findings	Virtually all males are sterile; some females can reproduce.
Face	Distinctive features include low nasal bridge, epicanthal folds, protruding tongue, low-set ears.
Musculo-skeletal system	Features include poor muscle tone (hypotonia) and short stature.
Systemic disorders	Features include congenital heart disease (one third to half of cases), reduced ability to fight respiratory tract infections, and increased susceptibility to leukemia—overall reduced survival rate; by age 40 years usually develop symptoms similar to those of Alzheimer's disease.
Mortality	About 75% of fetuses with Down syndrome abort spontaneously or are stillborn; 20% of infants die before age 10 years; those who live beyond 10 years have life expectancy of about 60 years.
Causative factors	97% of cases are caused by nondisjunction during formation of one of parent's gametes or during early embryonic development; 3% result from translocations; in 95% of cases, nondisjunction occurs when mother's egg cell is formed; the remainder involve paternal nondisjunction; 1% are mosaics—these have a large number of normal cells, and effects of trisomic cells are attenuated and symptoms are generally less severe.
Turner's Syndrome	
(45,X) Monosomy of X Chromosome	
IQ	Individuals with this syndrome are not considered to be intellectually disabled, although the syndrome is associated with some impairment of spatial and mathematical reasoning ability.
Male/female findings	It is found only in females.
Musculo-skeletal system	Short stature is common; other features are characteristic webbing of neck, widely spaced nipples, and reduced carrying angle at elbow.
Systemic disorders	Features include coarctation (narrowing) of aorta, edema of feet in newborns; females are usually sterile and have gonadal streaks rather than ovaries; streaks are sometimes susceptible to cancer.
Mortality	About 15–20% of spontaneous abortions with chromosome abnormalities have this karyotype, most common single-chromosome aberration; highly lethal during gestation, only about 0.5% of these conceptions survive to term.
Causative factors	75% of cases inherit X chromosome from mother, thus caused by meiotic error in father; frequency is low compared with other sex chromosome aneuploidies (1 : 5000 newborn females); 50% have simple monosomy of X chromosome; the remainder have more complex abnormalities; combinations of 45,X cells with XX or XY cells common.
Klinefelter's Syndrome	
(47,XXY) XXY Condition	
IQ	A moderate degree of mental impairment may be present.
Male/female findings	Individuals have a male appearance but are usually sterile; 50% develop femalelike breasts (gynecomastia); occurs in 1 : 1000 male births.
Voice	Voice is somewhat high pitched.
Systemic disorders	Features include sparse body hair, sterility, and small testicles.
Causative factors	50% of cases are the result of nondisjunction of X chromosomes in mother, and frequency rises with increasing maternal age; also involves XXY and XXXY karyotypes with degree of physical and mental impairment increasing with each added X chromosome; mosaicism fairly common with most prevalent combination of XXY and XY cells.

cited example of a disease caused by a chromosomal deletion is the **cri du chat syndrome**. The term literally means "cry of the cat" and describes the characteristic cry of the affected child. Other symptoms include low birth weight, severe intellectual disability, microcephaly (smaller than normal head size), and heart defects. The disease is caused by a deletion of part of the short arm of chromosome 5.

Duplications. A deficiency of genetic material is more harmful than an excess, so **duplications** usually have less serious consequences than deletions. For example, a deletion of a region of chromosome 5 causes cri du chat syndrome, but a duplication of the same region causes intellectual disability but less serious physical defects.

Inversions. An **inversion** occurs when two breaks take place on a chromosome, followed by the reinsertion of the missing fragment at its original site but in inverted order. Therefore a chromosome symbolized as ABCDEFG might become ABEDCFG after an inversion.

Unlike deletions and duplications, no loss or gain of genetic material occurs, so inversions are "balanced" alterations of chromosome structure, and they often have no apparent physical effect. Some genes are influenced by neighbouring genes, however, and this **position effect**, a change in a gene's expression caused by its position, sometimes results in physical defects in these persons. Inversions can cause serious problems in the offspring of individuals carrying the inversion because the inversion can lead to duplications and deletions in the chromosomes transmitted to the offspring.

Translocations. The interchange of genetic material between nonhomologous chromosomes is called **translocation**. A **reciprocal translocation** occurs when breaks take place in two different chromosomes and the material is exchanged (Figure 2-18, *A*). As with inversions, the carrier of a reciprocal translocation is usually normal, but his or her offspring can have duplications and deletions.

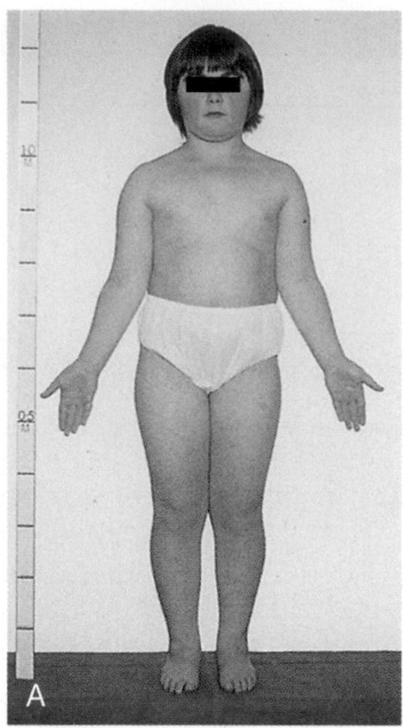

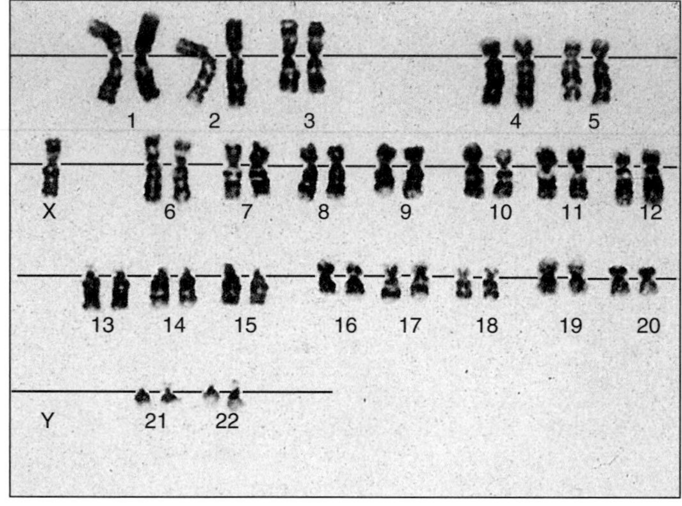

FIGURE 2-15 Turner's Syndrome. A, A sex chromosome is missing, and the person's chromosomes are 45,X. Characteristic signs are short stature, female genitalia, webbed neck, shieldlike chest with underdeveloped breasts and widely spaced nipples, and imperfectly developed ovaries. **B,** As this karyotype shows, Turner's syndrome results from monosomy of sex chromosomes (genotype XO). (From Patton, K.T., & Thibodeau, G.A. [2013]. *Anatomy & physiology* [8th ed.]. St. Louis: Mosby. Courtesy Nancy S. Wexler, PhD, Columbia University.)

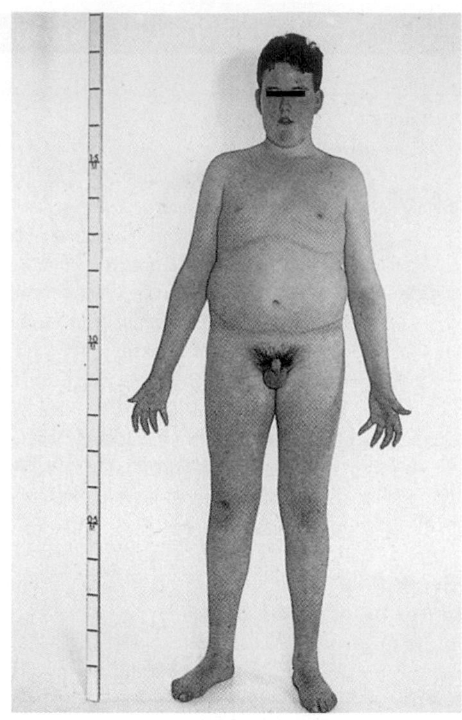

FIGURE 2-16 Klinefelter's Syndrome. This young man exhibits many characteristics of Klinefelter's syndrome: small testes, some development of the breasts, sparse body hair, and long limbs. This syndrome results from the presence of two or more X chromosomes with one Y chromosome (e.g., genotypes XXY or XXXY). (From Patton, K.T., & Thibodeau, G.A. [2016]. *Anatomy & physiology* [9th ed.]. St. Louis: Mosby. Courtesy Nancy S. Wexler, PhD, Columbia University.)

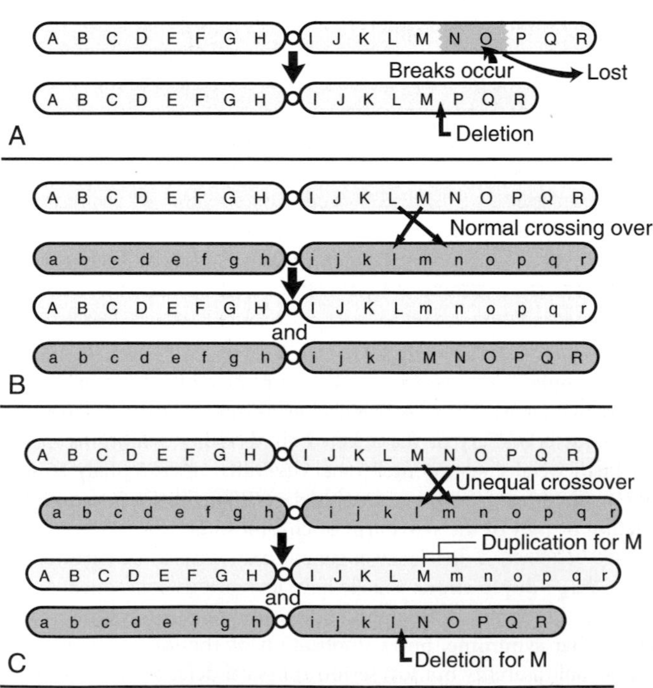

FIGURE 2-17 Abnormalities of Chromosome Structure. A, Deletion occurs when a chromosome segment is lost. **B,** Normal crossing over. **C,** The generation of duplication and deletion through unequal crossing over.

A second and clinically more important type of translocation is **Robertsonian translocation**. In this disorder, the long arms of two nonhomologous chromosomes fuse at the centromere, forming a single chromosome. Robertsonian translocations are confined to chromosomes 13, 14, 15, 21, and 22 because the short arms of these chromosomes are very small and contain no essential genetic material. The short arms are usually lost during subsequent cell divisions. Because the carriers of Robertsonian translocations lose no important genetic material, they are unaffected, although they have only 45 chromosomes in each cell. Their offspring, however, may have serious monosomies or trisomies.

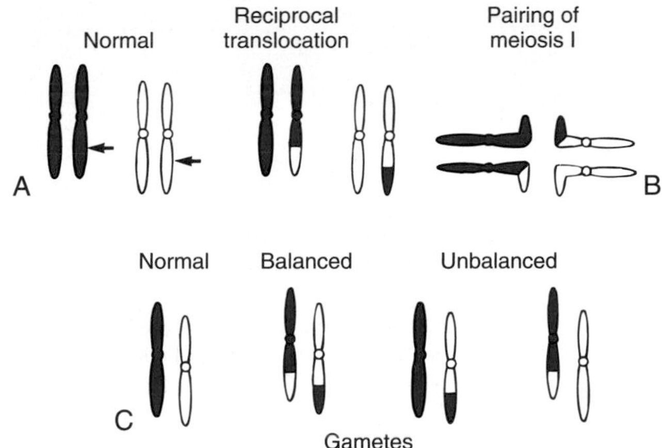

FIGURE 2-18 Normal and Abnormal Chromosome Translocation. **A,** Normal chromosomes and reciprocal translocation. **B,** Pairing at meiosis I. **C,** Consequences of translocation in gametes; unbalanced gametes result in zygotes that are partially trisomic and partially monosomic and consequently develop abnormally.

For example, a common Robertsonian translocation involves the fusion of the long arms of chromosomes 21 and 14. An offspring who inherits a gamete carrying the fused chromosome can receive an extra copy of the long arm of chromosome 21 and develop Down syndrome. Robertsonian translocations are responsible for approximately 3% to 5% of Down syndrome cases. Parents who carry a Robertsonian translocation involving chromosome 21 have an increased risk of producing multiple offspring with Down syndrome.

Fragile sites. A number of areas on chromosomes develop distinctive breaks and gaps (observable microscopically) when the cells are cultured. Most of these fragile sites do not appear to be related to disease. However, one fragile site, located on the long arm of the X chromosome, is associated with fragile X syndrome. The most important feature of this syndrome is intellectual disability. With a relatively high population prevalence (affecting approximately 1 in 4000 males and 1 in 8000 females), fragile X syndrome is the second most common genetic cause of intellectual disability (after Down syndrome).

In fragile X syndrome, females who inherit the mutation do not necessarily express the disease condition, but they can pass it on to descendants who do express it. Ordinarily, a male who inherits a disease gene on the X chromosome expresses the condition, because he has only one X chromosome. An uncommon feature of this disease is that about one third of carrier females are affected, although less severely than males. Unaffected transmitting males have been shown to have more than about 50 repeated DNA sequences near the beginning of the fragile X gene. These trinucleotide sequences, which consist of CGG sequences duplicated many times, cause fragile X syndrome when the number of copies exceeds 200.[8] The number of these repeats can increase from generation to generation. More than 20 other genetic diseases, including Huntington's disease and myotonic dystrophy, also are caused by this mechanism.[9]

QUICK CHECK 2-1

1. What is the major composition of DNA?
2. Define the terms *mutation, autosomes,* and *sex chromosomes.*
3. What is the significance of mRNA?
4. What is the significance of chromosomal translocation?

ELEMENTS OF FORMAL GENETICS

The mechanisms by which an individual's set of paired chromosomes produces traits are the principles of genetic inheritance. Mendel's work with garden peas first defined these principles. Later geneticists have refined Mendel's work to explain patterns of inheritance for traits and diseases that appear in families.

Analysis of traits that occur with defined, predictable patterns has helped geneticists to assemble the pieces of the human gene map. Current research focuses on determining the RNA or protein products of each gene and understanding the way they contribute to disease. Eventually, diseases and defects caused by single genes can be traced and therapies to prevent and treat such diseases can be developed. For example, researchers have identified a specific gene sequence which, when mutated, gives rise to sickle cell anemia. By identifying this gene sequence, they have been able to cut out the mutated gene and introduce the correct gene into hematopoietic stem cells, resulting in normal red blood cells.[10]

Traits caused by single genes are called *Mendelian traits* (after Gregor Mendel). Each gene occupies a position, or locus, on a chromosome. The genes at a particular locus can have different forms (i.e., they can be composed of different nucleotide sequences) called alleles. A locus that has two or more alleles that each occur with an appreciable frequency in a population is said to be polymorphic (or a polymorphism).

Because humans are diploid organisms, each chromosome is represented twice, with one member of the chromosome pair contributed by the father and one by the mother. At a given locus, an individual has one allele whose origin is paternal and one whose origin is maternal. When the two alleles are identical, the individual is homozygous at that locus. When the alleles are not identical, the individual is heterozygous at that locus.

Phenotype and Genotype

The composition of genes at a given locus is known as the genotype. The outward appearance of an individual, which is the result of both genotype and environment, is the phenotype. For example, an infant who is born with an inability to metabolize the amino acid phenylalanine has the single-gene disorder known as phenylketonuria (PKU) and thus has the PKU genotype. If the condition is left untreated, abnormal metabolites of phenylalanine will begin to accumulate in the infant's brain and irreversible intellectual disability will occur. Intellectual disability is thus one aspect of the PKU phenotype. By imposing dietary restrictions to exclude food that contains phenylalanine, however, intellectual disability can be prevented. Foods high in phenylalanine include proteins found in milk, dairy products, meat, fish, chicken, eggs, beans, and nuts. Although the child still has the PKU genotype, a modification of the environment (in this case, the child's diet) produces an outwardly normal phenotype.

Dominance and Recessiveness

In many loci, the effects of one allele mask those of another when the two are found together in a heterozygote. The allele whose effects are observable is said to be dominant. The allele whose effects are hidden is said to be recessive (from the Latin root for "hiding"). Traditionally, for loci having two alleles, the dominant allele is denoted by an uppercase letter and the recessive allele is denoted by a lowercase letter. When one allele is dominant over another, the heterozygote genotype *Aa* has the same phenotype as the dominant homozygote *AA*. For the recessive allele to be expressed, it must exist in the homozygote form, *aa*. When the heterozygote is distinguishable from both homozygotes, the locus is said to exhibit codominance.

A carrier is an individual who has a disease gene but is phenotypically normal. Many genes for a recessive disease occur in heterozygotes who carry one copy of the gene but do not express the disease. When recessive genes are lethal in the homozygous state, they are eliminated from the population when they occur in homozygotes. By "hiding" in carriers, however, recessive genes for diseases are passed on to the next generation.

TRANSMISSION OF GENETIC DISEASES

The pattern in which a genetic disease is inherited through generations is termed the **mode of inheritance**. Knowing the mode of inheritance can reveal much about the disease-causing gene itself, and members of families with the disease can be given reliable genetic counselling.

Mendel systematically studied modes of inheritance and formulated two basic laws of inheritance. His **principle of segregation** states that homologous genes separate from one another during reproduction and that each reproductive cell carries only one copy of a homologous gene. Mendel's second law, the **principle of independent assortment**, states that the hereditary transmission of one gene does not affect the transmission of another. Mendel discovered these laws in the mid-nineteenth century by performing breeding experiments with garden peas, even though he had no knowledge of chromosomes. Early twentieth-century geneticists found that chromosomal behaviour essentially corresponds to Mendel's laws, which now form the basis for the **chromosome theory of inheritance**.

The known single-gene diseases can be classified into four major modes of inheritance: autosomal dominant, autosomal recessive, X-linked dominant, and X-linked recessive. The first two types involve genes known to occur on the 22 pairs of autosomes. The last two types occur on the X chromosome; very few disease-causing genes occur on the Y chromosome.

The **pedigree** chart summarizes family relationships and shows which members of a family are affected by a genetic disease (Figure 2-19). Generally, the pedigree begins with one individual in the family, the **proband**. This individual is usually the first person in the family diagnosed or seen in a clinic.

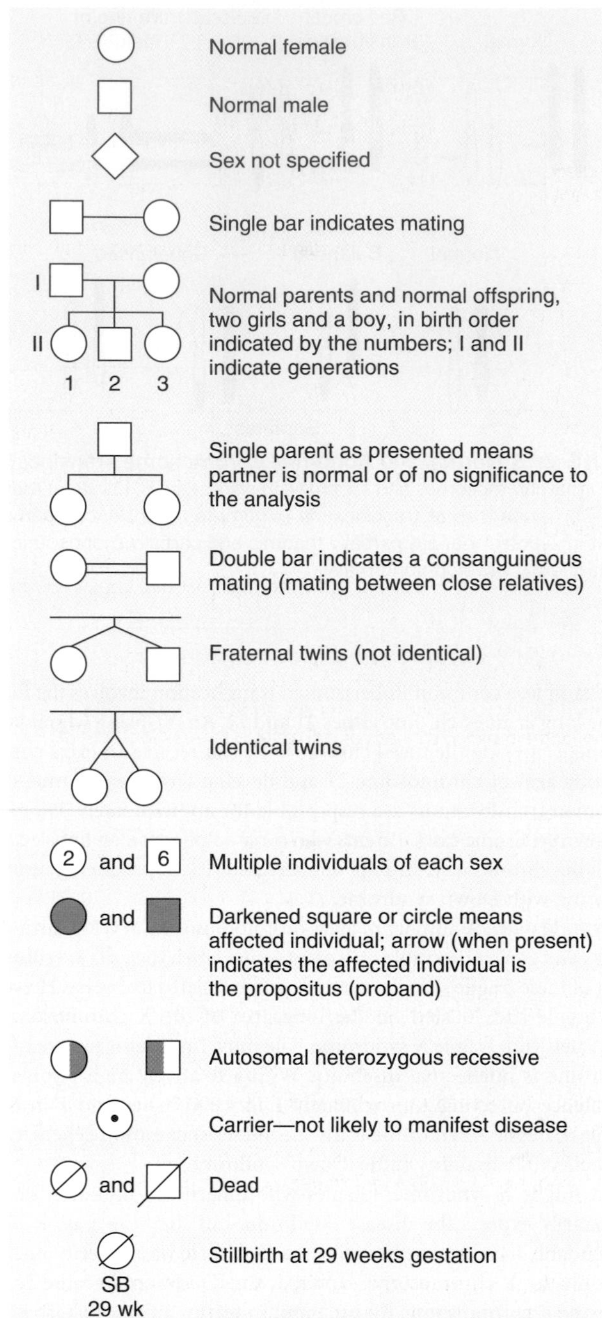

FIGURE 2-19 Symbols Commonly Used in Pedigrees. (From Jorde, L.B., Carey, J.C., & Bamshad, M.J. [2010]. *Medical genetics* [4th ed.]. St. Louis: Mosby.)

Autosomal Dominant Inheritance

Characteristics of Pedigrees

Diseases caused by autosomal dominant genes are rare, with the most common occurring in fewer than 1 in 500 individuals. Therefore it is uncommon for two individuals who are both affected by the same autosomal dominant disease to produce offspring together. Figure 2-20, *A*, illustrates this unusual pattern. Affected offspring are usually produced by the union of a normal parent with an affected heterozygous parent. The Punnett square in Figure 2-20, *B*, illustrates this mating. The affected parent can pass either a disease-causing allele or a normal allele to the next generation. On average, half the children will be heterozygous and will express the disease, and half will be normal.

The pedigree in Figure 2-21 shows the transmission of an autosomal dominant allele. Several important characteristics of this pedigree support the conclusion that the trait is caused by an autosomal dominant gene:

- The two sexes exhibit the trait in approximately equal proportions; males and females are equally likely to transmit the trait to their offspring.
- No generations are skipped. If an individual has the trait, one parent must also have it. If neither parent has the trait, none of the children have it (with the exception of new mutations, as discussed later).
- Affected heterozygous individuals transmit the trait to approximately half their children, and because gamete transmission is subject to chance fluctuations, all or none of the children of an affected parent may have the trait. When large numbers of matings of this type are studied, however, the proportion of affected children closely approaches one half. Skipped generations are not seen in classic autosomal dominant pedigrees.

Recurrence Risks

Parents at risk of producing children with a genetic disease nearly always ask the question, "What is the *chance* that our child will have this disease?" The probability that an individual will develop a genetic disease is termed the **recurrence risk**. When one parent is affected by an autosomal dominant disease (and is a heterozygote) and the other is unaffected, the recurrence risk for each child is one half.

An important principle is that each birth is an independent event, much like a coin toss. Thus, even though parents may have already had

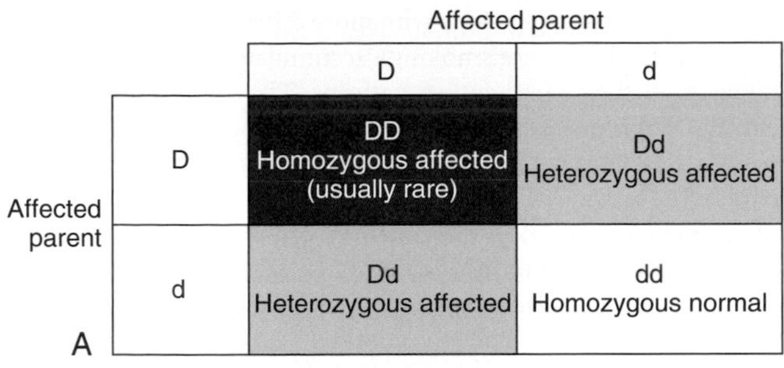

Affected parent
D
d
D
DD
Homozygous affected
(usually rare)
Dd
Heterozygous affected
Affected parent
d
Dd
Heterozygous affected
dd
Homozygous normal
A

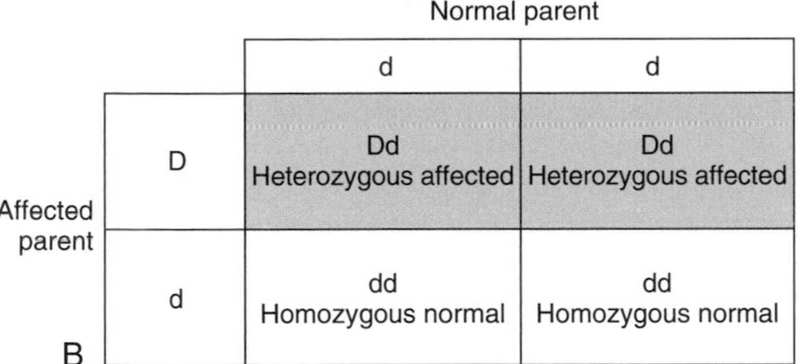

Normal parent
d
d
D
Dd
Heterozygous affected
Dd
Heterozygous affected
Affected parent
d
dd
Homozygous normal
dd
Homozygous normal
B

FIGURE 2-20 Punnett Square and Autosomal Dominant Traits. **A,** Punnett square for the mating of two individuals with an autosomal dominant gene. Here both parents are affected by the trait. **B,** Punnett square for the mating of a normal individual with a carrier for an autosomal dominant gene.

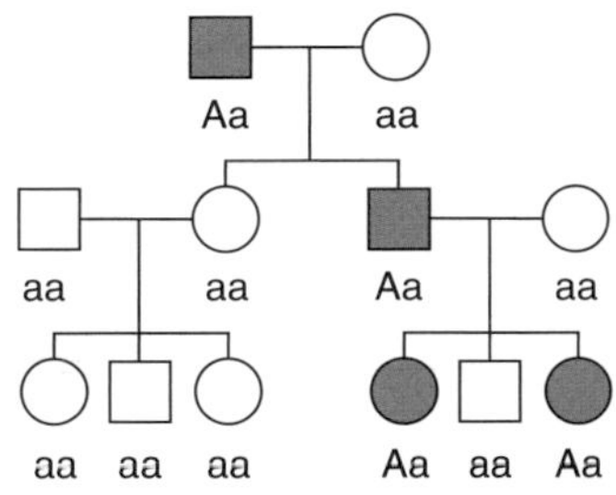

FIGURE 2-21 Pedigree Illustrating the Inheritance Pattern of Postaxial Polydactyly, an Autosomal Dominant Disorder. Affected individuals are represented by shading. (From Jorde, L.B., Carey, J.C., & Bamshad, M.J. [2010]. *Medical genetics* [4th ed.]. St. Louis: Mosby.)

a child with the disease, their recurrence risk remains one half. Even if they have produced several children, all affected (or all unaffected) by the disease, the law of independence dictates the probability their next child will have the disease is still one half. Parents' misunderstanding of this principle is a common problem encountered in genetic counselling.

If a child is born with an autosomal dominant disease and there is no history of the disease in the family, the child is probably the product of a new mutation. The gene transmitted by one of the parents has thus undergone a mutation from a normal to a disease-causing allele. The alleles at this locus in most of the parent's other germ cells are still normal. In this situation the recurrence risk for the parent's subsequent offspring is not greater than that of the general population. The offspring of the affected child, however, will have a recurrence risk of one half. Because these diseases often reduce the potential for reproduction, many autosomal dominant diseases result from new mutations.

Occasionally, two or more offspring have symptoms of an autosomal dominant disease when there is no family history of the disease. Because mutation is a rare event, it is unlikely that this disease would be a result of multiple mutations in the same family. The mechanism most likely

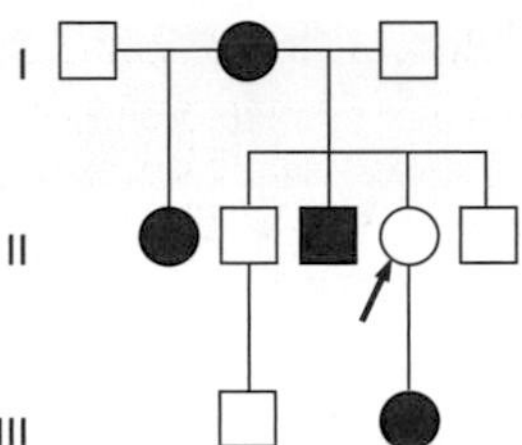

FIGURE 2-22 Pedigree for Retinoblastoma Showing Incomplete Penetrance. Female with marked arrow in line II must be heterozygous, but she does not express the trait.

responsible is termed **germline mosaicism**. During the embryonic development of one of the parents, a mutation occurred that affected all or part of the germline. Few or none of the somatic cells of the embryo were affected. Thus the parent carries the mutation in his or her germline but does not actually express the disease. As a result, the unaffected parent can transmit the mutation to multiple offspring. This phenomenon, although relatively rare, can have significant effects on recurrence risks.[11]

Delayed Age of Onset

One of the best-known autosomal dominant diseases is Huntington's disease, a neurological disorder whose main features are progressive dementia and increasingly uncontrollable limb movements (chorea; discussed further in Chapter 15). A key feature of this disease is its **delayed age of onset**: symptoms usually are not seen until 40 years of age or later. Thus those who develop the disease often have borne children before they are aware they have the disease-causing mutation. If the disease was present at birth, nearly all affected persons would die before reaching reproductive age and the occurrence of the disease-causing allele in the population would be much lower. An individual whose parent has the disease has a 50% chance of developing it during middle age. He or she is thus confronted with a torturous question: Should I have children, knowing that there is a fifty-fifty chance that I may have this disease-causing gene and will pass it to half of my children? A DNA test can now be used to determine whether an individual has inherited the trinucleotide repeat mutation that causes Huntington's disease.

Penetrance and Expressivity

The **penetrance** of a trait is the percentage of individuals with a specific genotype who also exhibit the expected phenotype. Incomplete penetrance means individuals who have the disease-causing genotype may not exhibit the disease phenotype at all, even though the genotype and the associated disease may be transmitted to the next generation. A pedigree illustrating the transmission of an autosomal dominant mutation with incomplete penetrance is provided in Figure 2-22. Retinoblastoma, the most common malignant eye tumour affecting children, typically exhibits incomplete penetrance. About 10% of the individuals who are **obligate carriers** of the disease-causing mutation (i.e., those who have an affected parent and affected children and therefore must themselves carry the mutation) do not have the disease. The penetrance of the disease-causing genotype is then said to be 90%.

The gene responsible for retinoblastoma is a **tumour-suppressor gene**: the normal function of its protein product is to regulate the cell cycle so cells do not divide uncontrollably. When the protein is altered because of a genetic mutation, its tumour-suppressing capacity is lost and a tumour can form[12] (see Chapters 10 and 17).

Expressivity is the extent of variation in phenotype associated with a particular genotype. If the expressivity of a disease is variable, penetrance may be complete but the severity of the disease can vary greatly. A good example of variable expressivity in an autosomal dominant

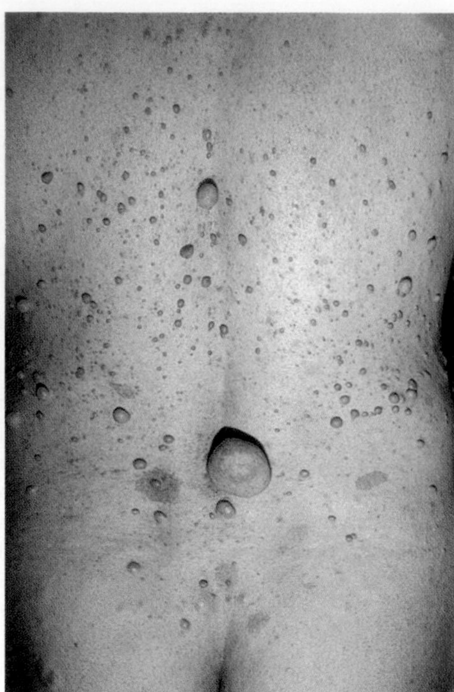

FIGURE 2-23 Neurofibromatosis. Tumours. The most common types are either sessile or pedunculated. Early tumours are soft, dome-shaped papules or nodules that have a distinctive violaceous hue. Most are benign. (From Habif, T.P., Campbell, J.L. Jr, Chapman, M.S., et al. [2005]. *Skin disease: Diagnosis and treatment* [2nd ed.]. St. Louis: Elsevier.)

disease is neurofibromatosis type 1, or von Recklinghausen disease. As in retinoblastoma, the mutations that cause neurofibromatosis type 1 occur in a tumour-suppressor gene.[13] The expression of this disease varies from a few harmless café-au-lait (light brown) spots on the skin to numerous neurofibromas, scoliosis, seizures, gliomas, neuromas, malignant peripheral nerve sheath tumours, hypertension, and learning disorders (Figure 2-23).

Several factors cause variable expressivity. Genes at other loci sometimes modify the expression of a disease-causing gene. Environmental factors also can influence expression of a disease-causing gene. Finally, different mutations at a locus can cause variation in severity. For example, a mutation that alters only one amino acid of the factor VIII gene usually produces a mild form of hemophilia A, whereas a "stop" codon (premature termination of translation) usually produces a more severe form of this blood coagulation disorder.

Epigenetics and Genomic Imprinting

Although this chapter focuses on DNA sequence variation and its consequence for disease, there is increasing evidence that the same DNA sequence can produce dramatically different phenotypes because of chemical modifications altering the *expression* of genes (these modifications are collectively termed **epigenetic**, Chapter 3). An important example of such a modification is **DNA methylation**, the attachment of a methyl group to a cytosine base followed by a guanine base in the DNA sequence (Figure 2-24). These sequences, which are common near many genes, are termed **CpG islands**. When the CpG islands located near a gene become heavily methylated, the gene is less likely to be transcribed into mRNA. In other words, the gene becomes transcriptionally inactive. One study showed that identical (monozygotic) twins accumulate different methylation patterns in the DNA sequences of their somatic cells as they age, causing increasing numbers of phenotypic differences.[14] Intriguingly, twins with more differences in their lifestyles (e.g., smoking versus nonsmoking) accumulated larger numbers of differences in their **methylation** patterns. The twins, despite having identical DNA sequences, become more and more different as a result of epigenetic changes, which in turn affect the expression of genes (see Figure 3-5).

Epigenetic alteration of gene activity can have important disease consequences. For example, a major cause of one form of inherited colon cancer (termed *hereditary nonpolyposis colorectal cancer [HNPCC]*) is the methylation of a gene whose protein product repairs damaged DNA. When this gene becomes inactive, damaged DNA accumulates, eventually resulting in colon tumours. Epigenetic changes are also discussed in Chapters 3, 10, and 11.

Approximately 100 human genes are thought to be methylated differently, depending on which parent transmits the gene. This epigenetic modification, characterized by methylation and other changes, is termed **genomic imprinting**. For each of these genes, one of the parents *imprints* the gene (inactivates it) when it is transmitted to the offspring. An example is the insulinlike growth factor 2 (*IGF-2*) gene on chromosome 11, which is transmitted by both parents, but the copy inherited from the mother is normally methylated and inactivated (imprinted). Thus only one copy of *IGF-2* is active in normal individuals. However, the maternal imprint is occasionally lost, resulting in two active copies of *IGF-2*. Having two active copies of *IGF-2* causes excess fetal growth and contributes to a condition known as *Beckwith-Weidemann syndrome* (see p. 65).

A second example of genomic imprinting is a deletion of part of the long arm of chromosome 15 (15q11-q13), which, when inherited from the father, causes the offspring to manifest a disease known as *Prader-Willi syndrome* (short stature, obesity, hypogonadism). When the same deletion is inherited from the mother, the offspring develop *Angelman syndrome* (intellectual disability, seizures, ataxic gait). The two different phenotypes reflect the fact that different genes are normally active in the maternally and paternally transmitted copies of this region of chromosome 15 (see pp. 64–65).

Autosomal Recessive Inheritance

Characteristics of Pedigrees

Like autosomal dominant diseases, diseases caused by autosomal recessive genes are rare in populations, although there can be numerous carriers. The most common lethal recessive disease in White children, cystic fibrosis, occurs in about 1 in 2 500 births. Approximately 1 in 25 White people carries a copy of a mutation that causes cystic fibrosis (see Chapter 28). Carriers are phenotypically unaffected. Some autosomal recessive diseases are characterized by delayed age of onset, incomplete penetrance, and variable expressivity.

Figure 2-25 shows a pedigree for cystic fibrosis. The gene responsible for cystic fibrosis encodes a chloride ion channel in some epithelial cells. Defective transport of chloride ions leads to a salt imbalance that results in secretions of abnormally thick, dehydrated mucus. Some digestive organs, particularly the pancreas, become obstructed, causing malnutrition, and the lungs become clogged with mucus, making them highly susceptible to bacterial infections. Death from lung disease or heart failure occurs before 40 years of age in about half of persons with cystic fibrosis.

The clustered regularly interspaced short palindromic repeats (CRISPR) system discovered in the bacterium *Streptococcus pyogenes* works as a mechanism to defend the bacteria against viruses and foreign DNA. This simple bacterial immune system has provided a revolutionary tool for targeted genome engineering (https://www.systembio.com/crispr-cas9/overview) and has future implications for correcting genetic abnormalities associated with cystic fibrosis.

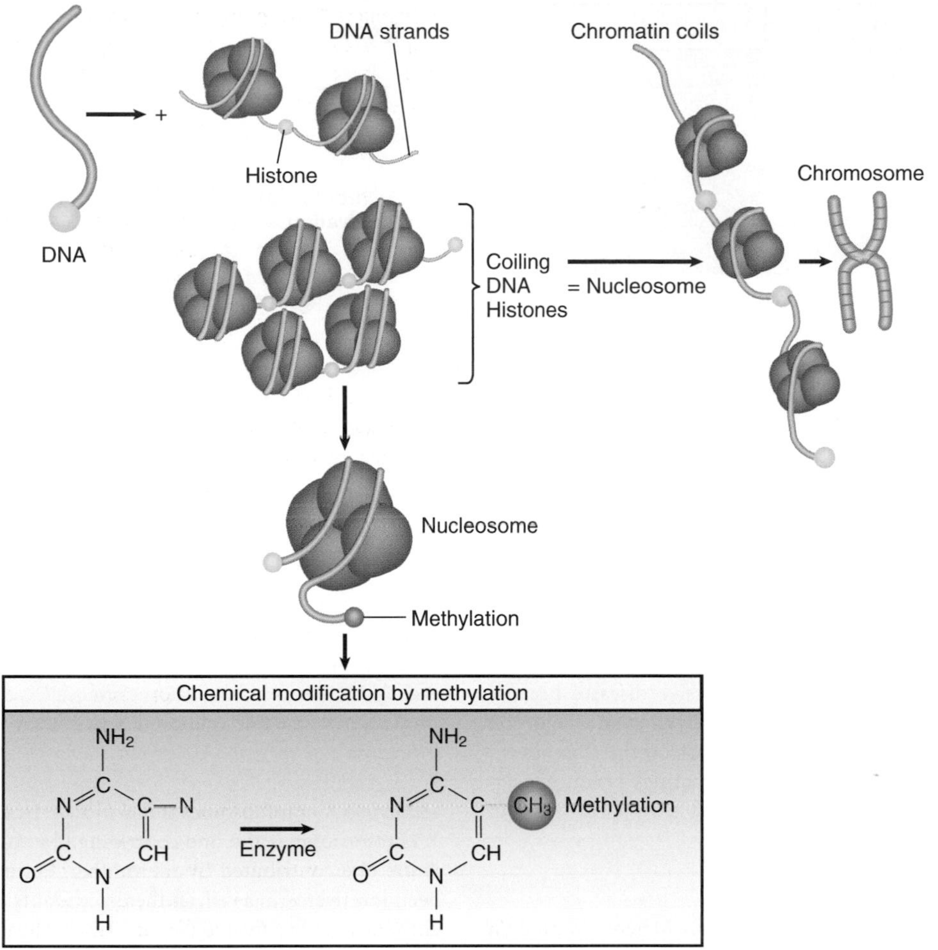

FIGURE 2-24 Epigenetic Modifications. Because DNA is a long molecule, it needs packaging to fit in the tiny nucleus. Packaging involves *coiling* of the DNA in a "left-handed" spiral around spools, made of four pairs of proteins individually known as histones and collectively termed the *histone octamer*. The entire spool is called a *nucleosome* (see also Figure 1-2). Nucleosomes are organized into chromatin, the repeating building blocks of a chromosome. Histone modifications are correlated with methylation, are reversible, and occur at multiple sites. Methylation occurs at the 5 position of cytosine and provides a "footprint" or signature as a unique epigenetic alteration (*red*). When genes are expressed, chromatin is open or active; however, when chromatin is condensed because of methylation and histone modification, genes are inactivated.

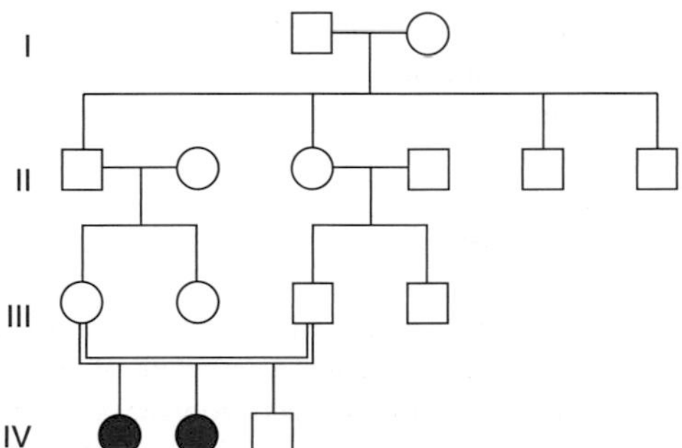

FIGURE 2-25 Pedigree for Cystic Fibrosis. Cystic fibrosis is an autosomal recessive disorder. The double bar denotes a consanguineous mating. Because cystic fibrosis is relatively common in European populations, most cases do not involve consanguinity.

Important criteria for discerning autosomal recessive inheritance include the following:

- Males and females are affected in equal proportions.
- Consanguinity (marriage between related individuals) is sometimes present, especially for rare recessive diseases.
- The disease may be seen in siblings of affected individuals but usually not in their parents.
- On average, one fourth of the offspring of carrier parents will be affected.

Recurrence Risks

In most cases of recessive disease, both of the parents of affected individuals are heterozygous carriers. On average, one fourth of their offspring will be normal homozygotes, half will be phenotypically normal carrier heterozygotes, and one fourth will be homozygotes with the disease (Figure 2-26). Thus the recurrence risk for the offspring of carrier parents is 25%. However, in any given family, there are chance fluctuations.

If two parents have a recessive disease, they each must be homozygous for the disease. Therefore all their children also must be affected. Homozygous genes for the disease distinguish recessive from dominant inheritance because two parents both affected by a dominant gene are nearly always both heterozygotes, resulting in only one fourth of their children being unaffected (i.e., having the recessive trait).

Because carrier parents usually are unaware that they both carry the same recessive allele, they often produce an affected child before

	D	d
D	DD Homozygous normal	Dd Heterozygous carrier
d	Dd Heterozygous carrier	dd Homozygous affected

FIGURE 2-26 Punnett Square for the Mating of Heterozygous Carriers Typical of Most Cases of Recessive Disease.

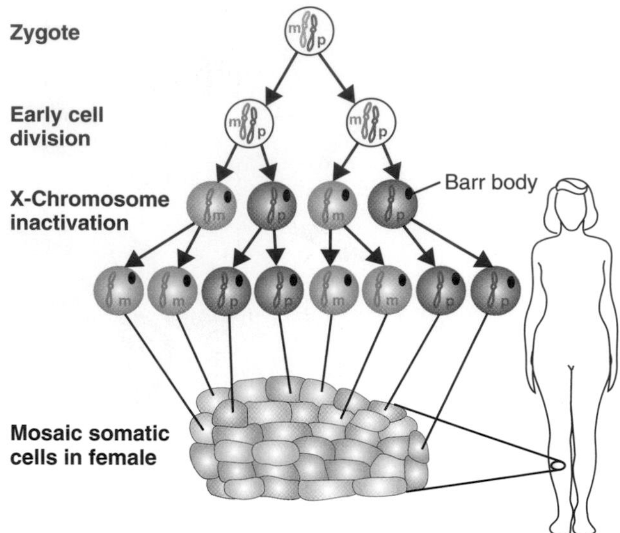

FIGURE 2-27 The X-Inactivation Process. The maternal (*m*) and paternal (*p*) X chromosomes are both active in the zygote and in early embryonic cells. X inactivation then takes place, resulting in cells having either an active paternal X or an active maternal X. Females are thus X chromosome mosaics, as shown in the tissue sample at the bottom of the figure. (From Jorde, L.B., Carey, J.C., & Bamshad, M.J. [2010]. *Medical genetics* [4th ed.]. St. Louis: Mosby.)

becoming aware of their condition. Carrier detection tests can identify heterozygotes by analyzing the DNA sequence to reveal a mutation. Some recessive diseases for which carrier detection tests are routinely used include phenylketonuria, sickle cell disease, cystic fibrosis, Tay-Sachs disease, hemochromatosis, and galactosemia.

Consanguinity

Consanguinity and inbreeding are related concepts. Consanguinity refers to the mating of two related individuals, and the offspring of such matings are said to be *inbred.* Consanguinity is sometimes an important characteristic of pedigrees for recessive diseases because relatives share a certain proportion of genes received from a common ancestor. The proportion of shared genes depends on the closeness of their biological relationship. Consanguineous matings produce a significant increase in recessive disorders and are seen most often in pedigrees for rare recessive disorders.

X-Linked Inheritance

Some genetic conditions are caused by mutations in genes located on the sex chromosomes, and this mode of inheritance is termed sex linked. Only a few diseases are known to be inherited as X-linked dominant or Y chromosome traits, so only the more common X-linked recessive diseases are discussed here.

Because females receive two X chromosomes, one from the father and one from the mother, they can be homozygous for a disease allele at a given locus, homozygous for the normal allele at the locus, or heterozygous. Males, having only one X chromosome, are hemizygous for genes on this chromosome. If a male inherits a recessive disease gene on the X chromosome, he will be affected by the disease because the Y chromosome does not carry a normal allele to counteract the effects of the disease gene. Because a single copy of an X-linked recessive gene will cause disease in a male, whereas two copies are required for disease expression in females, more males are affected by X-linked recessive diseases than are females.

X Inactivation

In the late 1950s Mary Lyon proposed that one X chromosome in the somatic cells of females is permanently inactivated, a process termed X inactivation.[15,16] This proposal, the Lyon hypothesis, explains why most gene products coded by the X chromosome are present in equal amounts in males and females, even though males have only one X chromosome and females have two X chromosomes. This phenomenon is called dosage compensation. The inactivated X chromosomes are observable in many interphase cells as highly condensed intranuclear chromatin bodies, termed Barr bodies (after Barr and Bertram, who discovered them in the late 1940s). Normal females have one Barr body in each somatic cell, whereas normal males have no Barr bodies.

X inactivation occurs very early in embryonic development—approximately 7 to 14 days after fertilization. In each somatic cell, one of the two X chromosomes is inactivated. In some cells, the inactivated X chromosome is the one contributed by the father; in other cells, it is the one contributed by the mother. Once the X chromosome has been inactivated in a cell, all the descendants of that cell have the same chromosome inactivated (Figure 2-27). Thus inactivation is said to be random but *fixed.*

Some individuals do not have the normal number of X chromosomes in their somatic cells. For example, males with Klinefelter's syndrome typically have two X chromosomes and one Y chromosome. These males do have one Barr body in each cell. Females whose cell nuclei have three X chromosomes have two Barr bodies in each cell, and females whose cell nuclei have four X chromosomes have three Barr bodies in each cell. Females with Turner's syndrome have only one X chromosome and no Barr bodies. Thus the number of Barr bodies is always one less than the number of X chromosomes in the cell. All but one X chromosome are always inactivated.

Persons with abnormal numbers of X chromosomes, such as those with Turner's syndrome or Klinefelter's syndrome, are not physically normal. This situation presents a puzzle because they presumably have only one active X chromosome, the same as individuals with normal numbers of chromosomes. The difference in the number of X chromosomes is probably because the distal tips of the short and long arms of the X chromosome, as well as several other regions on the chromosome arm, are not inactivated. Thus X inactivation is also known to be *incomplete.*

The inactivated X chromosome DNA is heavily methylated. Inactive X chromosomes can be at least partially reactivated in vitro by administering 5-azacytidine, a demethylating agent.

Sex Determination

The process of sexual differentiation, in which the embryonic gonads become either testes or ovaries, begins during the sixth week of gestation. A key principle of mammalian sex determination is that one copy of the Y chromosome is sufficient to initiate the process of gonadal differentiation that produces a male fetus. The number of X chromosomes

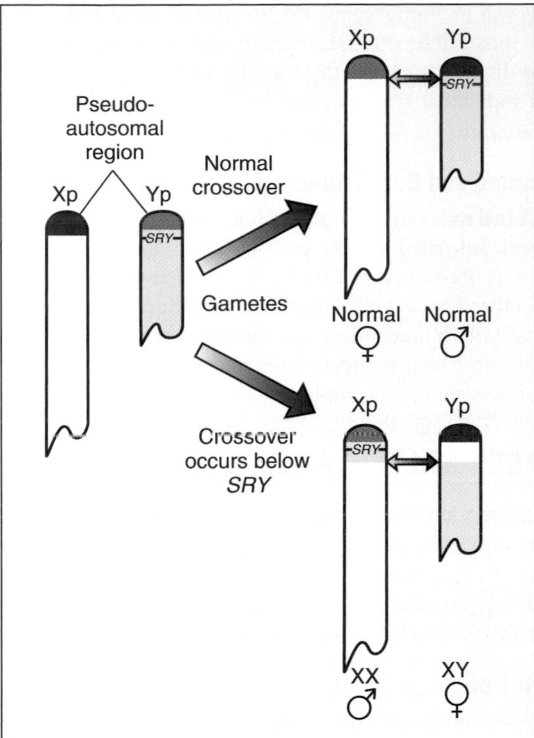

FIGURE 2-28 Distal Short Arms of the X and Y Chromosomes Exchange Material During Meiosis in the Male. The region of the Y chromosome in which this crossover occurs is called the *pseudoautosomal region.* The *SRY* gene, which triggers the process leading to male gonadal differentiation, is located just outside the pseudoautosomal region. Occasionally, the crossover occurs on the centromeric side of the *SRY* gene, causing it to lie on an X chromosome instead of a Y chromosome. An offspring receiving this X chromosome will be an XX male, and an offspring receiving the Y chromosome will be an XY female.

does not alter this process. For example, an individual with two X chromosomes and one Y chromosome in each cell is still phenotypically a male. Thus the Y chromosome contains a gene that begins the process of male gonadal development.

This gene, termed *SRY* (for "sex-determining region on the Y"), has been located on the short arm of the Y chromosome.[17] The *SRY* gene lies just outside the pseudoautosomal region (Figure 2-28), which pairs with the distal tip of the short arm of the X chromosome during meiosis and exchanges genetic material with it (crossover), just as autosomes do. The DNA sequences of these regions on the X and Y chromosomes are highly similar. The rest of the X and Y chromosomes, however, do not exchange material and are not similar in DNA sequence.

Other genes that contribute to male differentiation are located on other chromosomes. Thus *SRY* triggers the action of genes on other chromosomes. This concept is supported by the fact that the *SRY* protein product is similar to other proteins known to regulate gene expression.

Occasionally, the crossover between X and Y occurs closer to the centromere than it should, placing the *SRY* gene on the X chromosome after crossover. This variation can result in offspring with an apparently normal XX karyotype but a male phenotype. Such XX males are seen in about 1 in 20 000 live births and resemble males with Klinefelter's syndrome. Conversely, it is possible to inherit a Y chromosome that has lost the *SRY* gene (the result of either a crossover error or a deletion of the gene). This situation produces an XY female. Such females have gonadal streaks rather than ovaries and have poorly developed secondary sex characteristics.

QUICK CHECK 2-2

1. Why is the influence of environment significant to phenotype?
2. Describe the differences between a dominant and a recessive allele.
3. Why are the concepts of variable expressivity, incomplete penetrance, and delayed age of onset so important in relation to genetic diseases?
4. What is the recurrence risk for autosomal dominant inheritance and recessive inheritance?

Characteristics of Pedigrees

X-linked pedigrees show distinctive modes of inheritance. The most striking characteristic is that females seldom are affected. To express an X-linked recessive trait fully, a female must be homozygous: either both her parents are affected, or her father is affected and her mother is a carrier. Such matings are rare.

Four important principles of X-linked recessive inheritance are as follows:

1. The trait is seen much more often in males than in females.
2. Because a father can give a son only a Y chromosome, the trait is never transmitted from father to son.
3. The gene can be transmitted through a series of carrier females, causing the appearance of one or more "skipped generations."
4. The gene is passed from an affected father to all his daughters, who, as phenotypically normal carriers, transmit it to approximately half their sons, who are affected.

A relatively common X-linked recessive disorder is Duchenne muscular dystrophy (DMD), which affects approximately 1 in 3 500 males. As its name suggests, this disorder is characterized by progressive muscle degeneration. Affected individuals usually are unable to walk by age 10 or 12 years. The disease affects the heart and respiratory muscles, and death caused by respiratory or cardiac failure usually occurs before 20 years of age. Identification of the disease-causing gene (on the short arm of the X chromosome) has greatly increased our understanding of the disorder.[18] The *DMD* gene is the largest gene ever found in humans, spanning more than 2 million DNA bases. It encodes a previously undiscovered muscle protein, termed dystrophin. Extensive study of dystrophin indicates that it plays an essential role in maintaining the structural integrity of muscle cells: it may also help to regulate the activity of membrane proteins. When dystrophin is absent, as in DMD, the cell cannot survive, and muscle deterioration ensues. Most cases of DMD are caused by frameshift deletions of portions of the *DMD* gene and thus involve alterations of the amino acids encoded by the DNA following the deletion.

Recurrence Risks

The most common mating type involving X-linked recessive genes is the combination of a carrier female and a normal male (Figure 2-29, *A*). On average, the carrier mother will transmit the disease-causing allele to half her sons (who are affected) and half her daughters (who are carriers).

The other common mating type is an affected father and a normal mother (Figure 2-29, *B*). In this situation, all the sons will be normal because the father can transmit only his Y chromosome to them. Because all the daughters must receive the father's X chromosome, they will all be heterozygous carriers. Because the sons *must* receive the Y chromosome and the daughters *must* receive the X chromosome with the disease gene, these are precise outcomes and not probabilities. None of the children will be affected.

The final mating pattern, less common than the other two, involves an affected father and a carrier mother (Figure 2-29, *C*). With this pattern, on average, half the daughters will be heterozygous carriers,

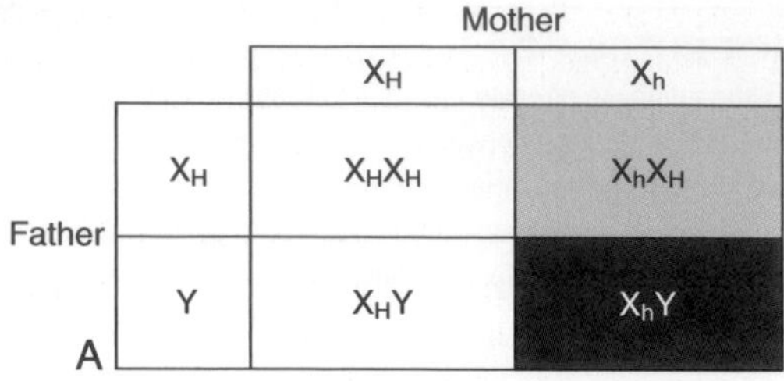

		Mother	
		X_H	X_H
Father	X_h	X_HX_h	X_HX_h
	Y	X_HY	X_HY

B

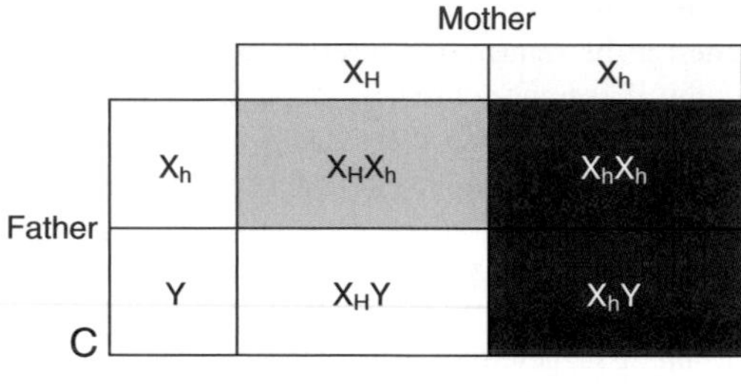

FIGURE 2-29 Punnett Square and X-Linked Recessive Traits. **A,** Punnett square for the mating of a normal male (X_HY) and a female carrier of an X-linked recessive gene (X_HX_h). **B,** Punnett square for the mating of a normal female (X_HX_H) with a male affected by an X-linked recessive disease (X_hY). **C,** Punnett square for the mating of a female who carries an X-linked recessive gene (X_HX_h) with a male who is affected with the disease caused by the gene (X_hY).

and half will be homozygous for the disease allele and thus affected. Half the sons will be normal, and half will be affected. Some X-linked recessive diseases, such as DMD, are fatal or incapacitating before the affected individual reaches reproductive age, and therefore affected fathers are rare.

Sex-Limited and Sex-Influenced Traits

A sex-limited trait can occur in only one sex, often because of anatomical differences. Inherited uterine and testicular defects are two obvious examples. A sex-influenced trait occurs much more often in one sex than the other. For example, male-pattern baldness occurs in both males and females but is much more common in males. Autosomal dominant breast cancer, which is much more commonly expressed in females than males, is another example of a sex-influenced trait.

LINKAGE ANALYSIS AND GENE MAPPING

Locating genes on specific regions of chromosomes has been one of the most important goals of human genetics. The location and identification of a gene can tell much about the function of the gene, the interaction of the gene with other genes, and the likelihood that certain individuals will develop a genetic disease.

Classic Pedigree Analysis

Mendel's second law, the principle of independent assortment, states that an individual's genes will be transmitted to the next generation independently of one another. This law is only partly true, however, because genes located close together on the same chromosome do tend to be transmitted together to the offspring. Thus Mendel's principle of independent assortment holds true for most pairs of genes but not those that occupy the same region of a chromosome. Such loci demonstrate linkage and are said to be linked.

During the first meiotic stage, the arms of homologous chromosome pairs intertwine and sometimes exchange portions of their DNA (Figure 2-30) in a process known as crossover. During crossover, new combinations of alleles can be formed. For example, two loci on a

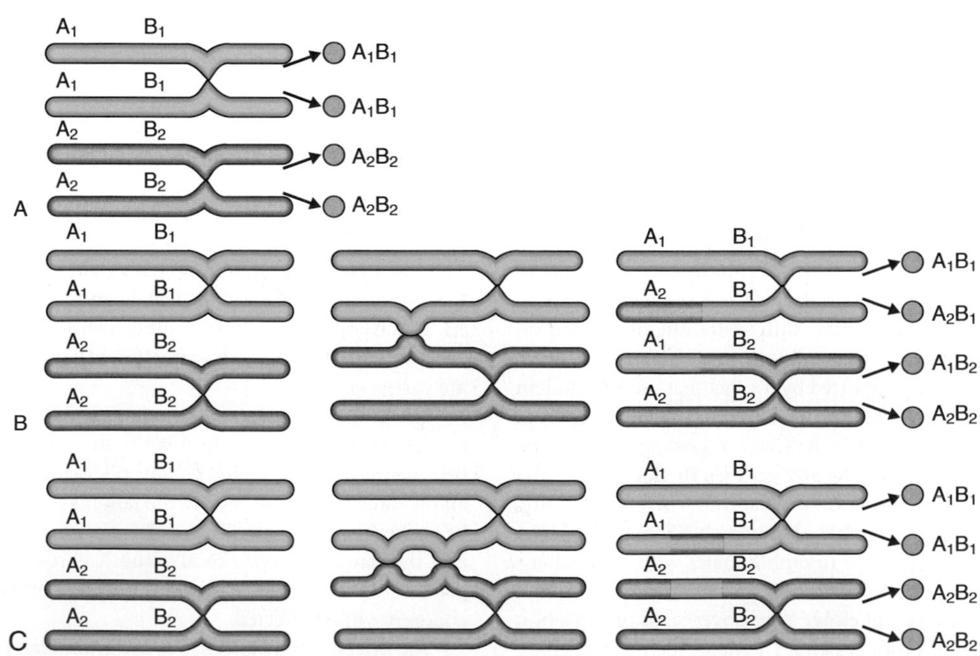

FIGURE 2-30 Genetic Results of Crossing Over. **A,** No crossing over. **B,** Crossing over with recombination. **C,** Double crossing over, resulting in no recombination.

chromosome have alleles A_1 and A_2 and alleles B_1 and B_2. Alleles A_1 and B_1 are located together on one member of a chromosome pair, and alleles A_2 and B_2 are located on the other member. The genotype of this individual is denoted as A_1B_1/A_2B_2.

As Figure 2-30, *A*, shows, the allele pairs A_1B_1 and A_2B_2 would be transmitted together when no crossover occurs. However, when crossover occurs (Figure 2-30, *B*), all four possible pairs of alleles can be transmitted to the offspring: A_1B_1, A_2B_1, A_1B_2, and A_2B_2. The process of forming such new arrangements of alleles is called **recombination**. Crossover does not necessarily lead to recombination, however, because double crossover between two loci can result in no actual recombination of the alleles at the loci (Figure 2-30, *C*).

Once a close linkage has been established between a disease-gene locus and a "marker" locus (a DNA sequence that varies among individuals) and once the alleles of the two loci that are inherited together within a family have been determined, reliable predictions can be made as to whether a member of a family will develop the disease. This type of analysis is called **linkage analysis**. Linkage has been established between several DNA polymorphisms and each of the two major genes that can cause autosomal dominant breast cancer (about 5% of breast cancer cases are caused by these autosomal dominant genes). Determining this kind of linkage means that it is possible for offspring of an individual with autosomal dominant breast cancer to know whether they also carry the gene and thus could pass it on to their own children. In most cases, specific disease-causing mutations can be identified, allowing direct detection and diagnosis. For some genetic diseases, prophylactic treatment is available if the condition can be diagnosed in time. An example of this is hemochromatosis, a recessive genetic disease in which excess iron is absorbed, causing degeneration of the heart, liver, brain, and other vital organs. Individuals at risk of developing the disease can be determined by testing for a mutation in the hemochromatosis gene and through clinical tests, and preventive therapy (periodic phlebotomy) can be initiated to deplete iron stores and ensure a normal lifespan.

Complete Human Gene Map: Prospects and Benefits

The major goals of the Human Genome Project were to find the locations of all human genes (the "gene map") and to determine the entire human DNA sequence. These goals have now been accomplished, and the genes responsible for more than 4 000 Mendelian conditions have been identified (Figure 2-31).[3,19,20] The project has greatly increased our understanding of the mechanisms that underlie many diseases, such as retinoblastoma, cystic fibrosis, neurofibromatosis, and Huntington's disease. The project also has led to more accurate diagnosis of these conditions and, in some cases, more effective treatment.

DNA sequencing has become much less expensive and more efficient in recent years. Consequently, many thousands of individuals have now been completely sequenced, leading in some cases to the identification of disease-causing genes (see *Health Promotion:* Gene Therapy).[21]

HEALTH PROMOTION: GENE THERAPY

Thousands of subjects are currently enrolled in more than 1 000 gene therapy protocols. Most of these protocols involve the genetic alteration of cells to combat various types of cancer. Others involve the treatment of inherited diseases, such as β-thalassemia, hemophilia B, severe combined immunodeficiency, and retinitis pigmentosa.

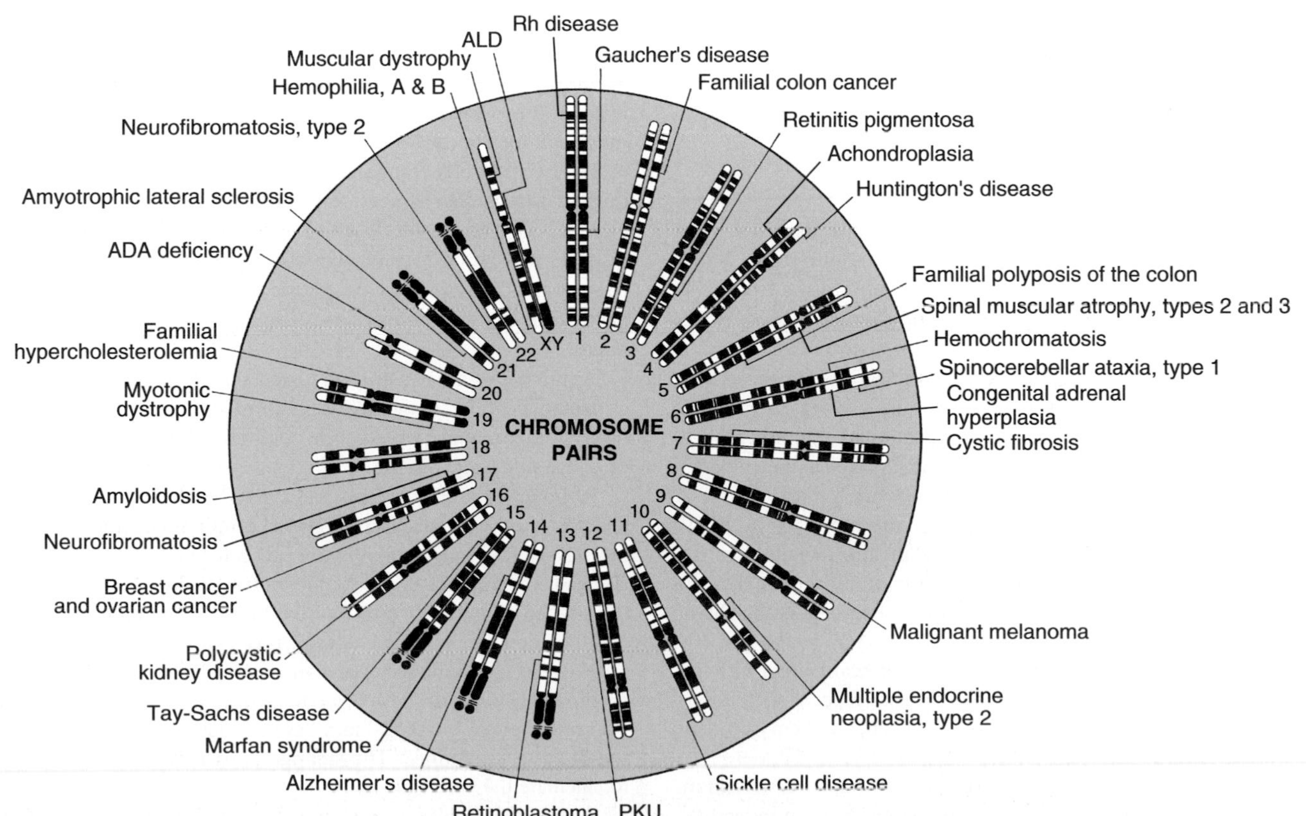

FIGURE 2-31 Example of Diseases: A Gene Map. *ADA*, adenosine deaminase; *ALD*, adrenoleukodystrophy; *PKU*, phenylketonuria.

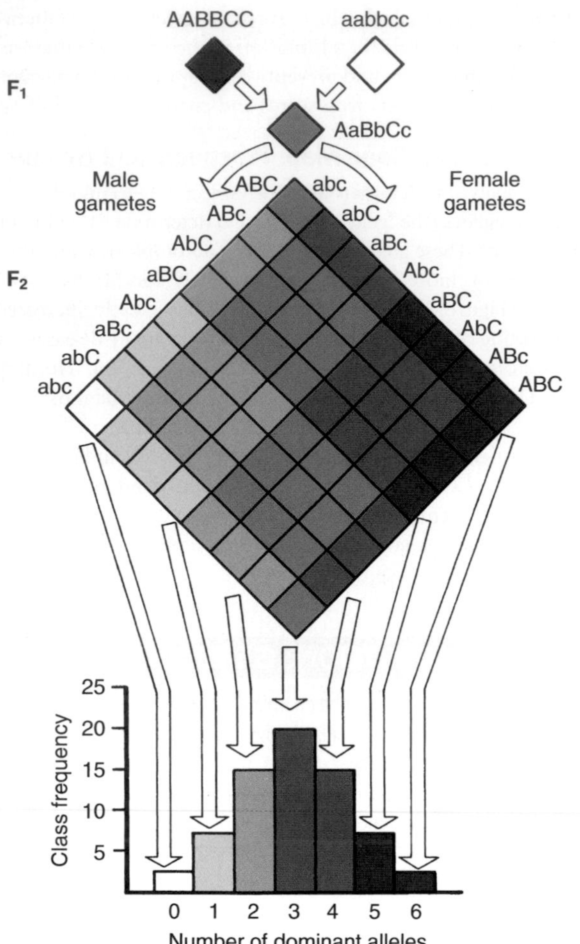

FIGURE 2-32 **Multifactorial Inheritance.** Analysis of mode of inheritance for grain colour in wheat. The trait is controlled by three independently assorted gene loci.

MULTIFACTORIAL INHERITANCE

Not all traits are produced by single genes; some traits result from several genes acting together. They are called **polygenic traits**. When environmental factors also influence the expression of the trait (as is usually the case), the term **multifactorial inheritance** is used. Many multifactorial and polygenic traits tend to follow a normal distribution in populations (the familiar bell-shaped curve). Figure 2-32 shows how three loci acting together can cause grain colour in wheat to vary in a gradual way from white to red, exemplifying multifactorial inheritance. If both alleles at each of the three loci are white alleles, the colour is pure white. If most alleles are white but a few are red, the colour is somewhat darker; if all are red, the colour is dark red.

Other examples of multifactorial traits include height and IQ. Although both height and IQ are determined in part by genes, they are influenced also by environment. For example, the average height of many human populations has increased by 5 to 10 cm in the past 100 years because of improvements in nutrition and health care. Also, IQ scores can be improved by exposing individuals (especially children) to enriched learning environments. Thus both genes and environment contribute to variation in these traits.

A number of diseases do not follow the bell-shaped distribution. Instead they appear to be either present in or absent from an individual. Yet they do not follow the patterns expected of single-gene diseases. Many of them are probably polygenic or multifactorial, but a certain

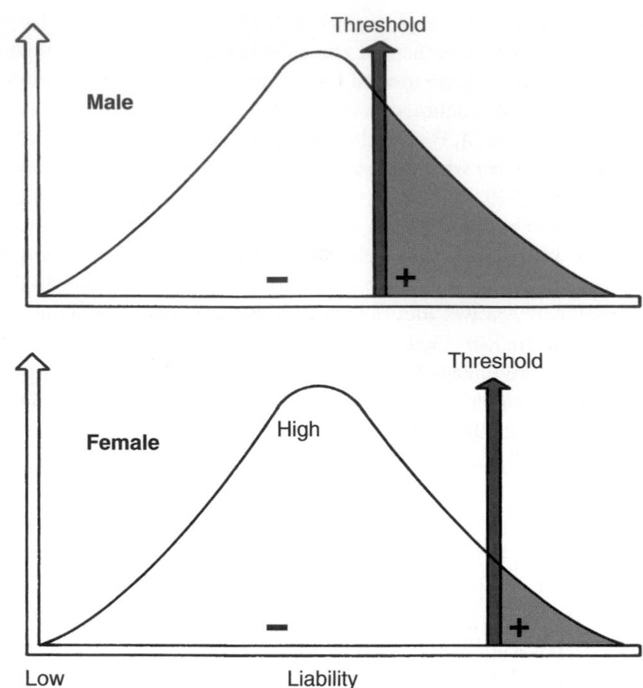

FIGURE 2-33 Threshold of Liability for Pyloric Stenosis in Males and Females.

threshold of liability must be crossed before the disease is expressed. Below the threshold, the individual appears normal; above it, the individual is affected by the disease (Figure 2-33).

A good example of such a threshold trait is pyloric stenosis, a disorder characterized by a narrowing or obstruction of the pylorus, the area between the stomach and small intestine. Chronic vomiting, constipation, weight loss, and electrolyte imbalance can result from the condition, but it is easily corrected by surgery. The prevalence of pyloric stenosis is about 3 in 1 000 live births in White people. This disorder is much more common in males than females, affecting 1 in 200 males and 1 in 1 000 females. The apparent reason for this difference is that the threshold of liability is much lower in males than females, as shown in Figure 2-33. Thus fewer defective alleles are required to generate the disorder in males. This situation also means the offspring of affected females are more likely to have pyloric stenosis because affected females necessarily carry more disease-causing alleles than do most affected males.

A number of other common diseases are thought to correspond to a threshold model. They include cleft lip and cleft palate, neural tube defects (anencephaly, spina bifida), clubfoot (talipes), and some forms of congenital heart disease.

Although recurrence risks can be given with confidence for single-gene diseases (e.g., 50% for autosomal dominants, 25% for autosomal recessives), it is considerably more difficult to do so for multifactorial diseases. The number of genes contributing to the disease is not known, the precise allelic constitution of the biological parents is not known, and the extent of environmental effects can vary from one population to another. For most multifactorial diseases, **empirical risks** (i.e., those based on direct observation) have been derived. To determine empirical risks, a large sample of biological families in which one child has developed the disease is examined. The siblings of each child are then surveyed to calculate the percentage who also develop the disease.

Another difficulty is distinguishing polygenic or multifactorial diseases from single-gene diseases having incomplete penetrance or variable expressivity. Large data sets and good epidemiological data

BOX 2-2 Criteria Used to Define Multifactorial Diseases

1. The recurrence risk becomes higher if more than one family member is affected. For example, the recurrence risk for neural tube defects in a British family increases to 10% if two siblings have been born with the disease. By contrast, the recurrence risk for single-gene diseases remains the same regardless of the number of siblings affected.
2. If the expression of the disease is more severe, the recurrence risk is higher. This finding is consistent with the liability model; a more severe expression indicates that the individual is at the extreme end of the liability distribution. Relatives of the affected individual are thus at a higher risk of inheriting disease genes. Cleft lip or cleft palate is a condition in which relatives are at a higher risk of inheriting disease genes.
3. Relatives of probands of the less commonly affected are more likely to develop the disease. As with pyloric stenosis, development of the disease occurs because an affected individual of the less susceptible sex is usually at a more extreme position on the liability distribution.
4. Generally, if the population frequency of the disease is *f*, the risk for offspring and siblings of probands is approximately $\sqrt{f}$. The same principle does not usually hold true for single-gene traits.
5. The recurrence risk for the disease decreases rapidly in more remotely related relatives. Although the recurrence risk for single-gene diseases decreases by 50% with each degree of relationship (e.g., an autosomal dominant disease has a 50% recurrence risk for siblings, 25% for uncle-nephew relationship, 12.5% for first cousins), the risk for multifactorial inheritance decreases much more quickly.

often are necessary to make the distinction. Box 2-2 lists criteria commonly used to define multifactorial diseases.

The genetics of common disorders such as hypertension, heart disease, and diabetes is complex and often confusing. Nevertheless, the public health impact of these diseases, together with the evidence for hereditary factors in their etiology, demands that genetic studies be pursued. Hundreds of genes contributing to susceptibility for these diseases have been discovered, and the next decade will undoubtedly witness substantial advancements in our understanding of these disorders.

✔ QUICK CHECK 2-3

1. Define linkage analysis; cite an example.
2. Why is "threshold of liability" an important consideration in multifactorial inheritance?
3. Describe the concept of multifactorial inheritance, and include two examples.

DID YOU UNDERSTAND?

DNA, RNA, and Proteins: Heredity at the Molecular Level

1. Genes, the basic units of inheritance, are composed of deoxyribonucleic acid (DNA) and are located on chromosomes.
2. DNA is composed of deoxyribose, a phosphate molecule, and four types of nitrogenous bases. The physical structure of DNA is a double helix.
3. The DNA bases code for amino acids, which in turn make up proteins. The amino acids are specified by triplet codons of nitrogenous bases.
4. DNA replication is based on complementary base pairing, in which a single strand of DNA serves as the template for attracting bases that form a new strand of DNA.
5. DNA polymerase is the primary enzyme involved in replication. It adds bases to the new DNA strand and performs "proofreading" functions.
6. A mutation is an inherited alteration of genetic material (i.e., DNA).
7. Substances that cause mutations are called *mutagens.*
8. The mutation rate in humans varies from locus to locus and is about 1.1×10^{-8} per gene per generation.
9. Transcription and translation, the two basic processes in which proteins are specified by DNA, both involve ribonucleic acid (RNA). RNA is chemically similar to DNA, but it is single stranded, has a ribose sugar molecule, and has uracil rather than thymine as one of its four nitrogenous bases.
10. Transcription is the process by which DNA specifies a sequence of messenger RNA (mRNA).
11. Much of the RNA sequence is spliced from the mRNA before the mRNA leaves the nucleus. The excised sequences are called *introns*, and those that remain to code for proteins are called *exons.*
12. Translation is the process by which RNA directs the synthesis of polypeptides. This process takes place in the ribosomes, which consist of proteins and ribosomal RNA (rRNA).
13. During translation, mRNA interacts with transfer RNA (tRNA), a molecule that has an attachment site for a specific amino acid.

Chromosomes

1. Human cells consist of diploid somatic cells (body cells) and haploid gametes (sperm and egg cells).
2. Humans have 23 pairs of chromosomes. Twenty-two of these pairs are autosomes. The remaining pair consists of the sex chromosomes. Females have two homologous X chromosomes as their sex chromosomes; males have an X and a Y chromosome.
3. A karyotype is an ordered display of chromosomes arranged according to length and the location of the centromere.
4. Various types of stains can be used to make chromosome bands more visible.
5. About 1 in 150 live births has a major diagnosable chromosome abnormality. Chromosome abnormalities are the leading known cause of intellectual disability and miscarriage.
6. Polyploidy is a condition in which a euploid cell has some multiple of the normal number of chromosomes. Humans have been observed to have triploidy (three copies of each chromosome) and tetraploidy (four copies of each chromosome); both conditions are lethal.
7. Somatic cells that do not have a multiple of 23 chromosomes are aneuploid. Aneuploidy is usually the result of nondisjunction.
8. Trisomy is a type of aneuploidy in which one chromosome is present in three copies in somatic cells. A partial trisomy is one in which only part of a chromosome is present in three copies.
9. Monosomy is a type of aneuploidy in which one chromosome is present in only one copy in somatic cells.
10. In general, monosomies cause more severe physical defects than do trisomies, illustrating the principle that the loss of chromosome material has more severe consequences than the duplication of chromosome material.

11. Down syndrome, a trisomy of chromosome 21, is the best-known disease caused by a chromosome aberration. It affects 1 in 800 live births and is much more likely to occur in the offspring of women older than 35 years.
12. Most aneuploidies of the sex chromosomes have less severe consequences than those of the autosomes.
13. The most commonly observed sex chromosome aneuploidies involve alterations in the number of X chromosomes, namely the 47,XXX karyotype, 45,X karyotype (Turner's syndrome), and 47,XXY karyotype (Klinefelter's syndrome).
14. Abnormalities of chromosome structure include deletions, duplications, inversions, and translocations.

Elements of Formal Genetics

1. Mendelian traits are caused by single genes, each of which occupies a position, or locus, on a chromosome.
2. Alleles are different forms of genes located at the same locus on a chromosome.
3. At any given locus in a somatic cell, an individual has two genes, one from each parent. An individual may be homozygous or heterozygous at a locus.
4. An individual's genotype is his or her genetic makeup, and the phenotype reflects the interaction of genotype and environment.
5. In a heterozygote, a dominant gene's effects mask those of a recessive gene. The recessive gene is expressed only when it is present in two copies.

Transmission of Genetic Diseases

1. Genetic diseases caused by single genes usually follow autosomal dominant, autosomal recessive, or X-linked recessive modes of inheritance.
2. Pedigree charts are important tools in the analysis of modes of inheritance.
3. Skipped generations are not seen in classic autosomal dominant pedigrees.
4. Recurrence risks specify the probability that future offspring will inherit a genetic disease. For single-gene diseases, recurrence risks remain the same for each offspring, regardless of the number of affected or unaffected offspring.
5. The recurrence risk for autosomal dominant diseases is usually 50%.
6. Germline mosaicism can alter recurrence risks for genetic diseases because unaffected parents can produce multiple affected offspring. This situation occurs because the germline of one parent is affected by a mutation but the parent's somatic cells are unaffected.
7. Males and females are equally likely to exhibit autosomal dominant diseases and to pass them on to their offspring.
8. Many genetic diseases have a delayed age of onset.
9. A gene that is not always expressed phenotypically is said to have incomplete penetrance.
10. Variable expressivity is a characteristic of many genetic diseases.
11. Genomic imprinting, which is associated with methylation, results in differing expression of a disease gene, depending on which parent transmitted the gene.
12. Epigenetics involves changes, such as the methylation of DNA bases, that do not alter the DNA sequence but can alter the expression of genes.
13. Most commonly, biological parents of children with autosomal recessive diseases are both heterozygous carriers of the disease gene.
14. The recurrence risk for autosomal recessive diseases is 25%.
15. Males and females are equally likely to be affected by autosomal recessive diseases.
16. Consanguinity is sometimes present in families with autosomal recessive diseases, and it becomes more prevalent with rarer recessive diseases.
17. Carrier detection tests for an increasing number of autosomal recessive diseases are available.
18. In each normal female somatic cell, one of the two X chromosomes is inactivated early in embryogenesis.
19. X inactivation is random, fixed, and incomplete (i.e., only part of the chromosome is actually inactivated). It may involve methylation.
20. Gender is determined embryonically by the presence of the *SRY* gene on the Y chromosome. Embryos that have a Y chromosome (and thus the *SRY* gene) become males, whereas those lacking the Y chromosome become females. When the Y chromosome lacks the *SRY* gene, an XY female can be produced. Similarly, an X chromosome that contains the *SRY* gene can produce an XX male.
21. X-linked genes are those that are located on the X chromosome. Nearly all known X-linked diseases are caused by X-linked recessive genes.
22. Males are hemizygous for genes on the X chromosome.
23. X-linked recessive diseases are seen much more often in males than in females because males need only one copy of the gene to express the disease.
24. Biological fathers cannot pass X-linked genes to their sons.
25. Skipped generations often are seen in X-linked recessive disease pedigrees because the gene can be transmitted through carrier females.
26. Recurrence risks for X-linked recessive diseases depend on the carrier and affected status of the mother and father.
27. A sex-limited trait is one that occurs only in one sex (gender).
28. A sex-influenced trait is one that occurs more often in one sex than the other.

Linkage Analysis and Gene Mapping

1. During meiosis I, crossover occurs and can cause recombinations of alleles located on the same chromosome.
2. The frequency of recombinations can be used to infer the map distance between loci on the same chromosome.
3. A marker locus, when closely linked to a disease-gene locus, can be used to predict whether an individual will develop a genetic disease.
4. The major goals of the Human Genome Project were to find the locations of all human genes (the "gene map") and to determine the entire human DNA sequence. These goals have now been accomplished, and the genes responsible for more than 4000 Mendelian conditions have been identified.

Multifactorial Inheritance

1. Traits that result from the combined effects of several loci are polygenic. When environmental factors also influence the expression of the trait, the term *multifactorial inheritance* is used.
2. Many multifactorial traits have a threshold of liability. Once the threshold of liability has been crossed, the disease may be expressed.
3. Empirical risks, based on direct observation of large numbers of families, are used to estimate recurrence risks for multifactorial diseases.
4. Recurrence risks for multifactorial diseases become higher if more than one biological family member is affected or if the expression of the disease in the proband is more severe.
5. Recurrence risks for multifactorial diseases decrease rapidly for more remote relatives.

KEY TERMS

Adenine, 38
Allele, 49
Amino acid, 39
Aneuploid cell, 43
Anticodon, 42
Autosome, 42
Barr body, 54
Base pair substitution, 39
Carrier, 49
Carrier detection test, 54
Chromosomal mosaic, 46
Chromosome, 38
Chromosome band, 42
Chromosome breakage, 46
Chromosome theory of inheritance, 50
Clastogen, 46
Codominance, 49
Codon, 39
Complementary base pairing, 39
Consanguinity, 54
CpG islands, 52
Cri du chat syndrome, 47
Crossover, 56
Cytokinesis, 42
Cytosine, 38
Delayed age of onset, 51
Deletion, 46
Deoxyribonucleic acid (DNA), 38
Diploid cell, 42
DNA methylation, 52
DNA polymerase, 39
Dominant, 49
Dosage compensation, 54
Double-helix model, 38
Down syndrome, 46
Duplication, 47
Dystrophin, 55
Empirical risk, 58
Epigenetic, 52
Euploid cell, 42
Exon, 41
Expressivity, 51
Fragile site, 49
Frameshift mutation, 39
Gamete, 42
Gene, 38
Genomic imprinting, 52
Genotype, 49
Germline mosaicism, 51
Guanine, 38
Haploid cell, 42
Hemizygous, 54
Heterozygote, 49
Heterozygous, 49
Homologous, 42
Homozygote, 49
Homozygous, 49
Inbreeding, 54
Intron, 41
Inversion, 47
Karyotype (karyogram), 42
Klinefelter's syndrome, 46
Linkage, 56
Linkage analysis, 57
Locus, 49
Meiosis, 42
Messenger RNA (mRNA), 41
Metaphase spread, 42
Methylation, 52
Missense, 39
Mitosis, 42
Mode of inheritance, 50
Multifactorial inheritance, 58
Mutagen, 39
Mutation, 39
Mutational hot spot, 39
Nondisjunction, 45
Nonsense, 39
Nucleotide, 39
Obligate carrier, 51
Partial trisomy, 46
Pedigree, 50
Penetrance, 51
Phenotype, 49
Polygenic trait, 58
Polymorphic (polymorphism), 49
Polypeptide, 39
Polyploid cell, 42
Position effect, 47
Principle of independent assortment, 50
Principle of segregation, 50
Proband, 50
Promoter site, 41
Pseudoautosomal, 55
Purine, 38
Pyrimidine, 38
Recessive, 49
Reciprocal translocation, 47
Recombination, 57
Recurrence risk, 50
Ribonucleic acid (RNA), 39
Ribosomal RNA (rRNA), 42
Ribosome, 42
RNA polymerase, 41
Robertsonian translocation, 48
Sex-influenced trait, 56
Sex-limited trait, 56
Sex linked (inheritance), 54
Silent mutation, 39
Somatic cell, 42
Spontaneous mutation, 39
Template, 39
Termination sequence, 41
Tetraploidy, 42
Threshold of liability, 58
Thymine, 38
Transcription, 41
Transfer RNA (tRNA), 42
Translation, 42
Translocation, 47
Triploidy, 42
Trisomy, 43
Tumour-suppressor gene, 51
Turner's syndrome, 46
X inactivation, 54

REFERENCES

1. Roach, J. C., Glusman, G., Smit, A. F., et al. (2010). Analysis of genetic inheritance in a family quartet by whole-genome sequencing. *Science, 328*(5978), 636–639. doi:10.1126/science.1186802.
2. Zhang, S., Chen, J., Cui, P., et al. (2015). Identification of novel mutations associated with clofazimine resistance in Mycobacterium tuberculosis. *Journal of Antimicrobial Chemotherapy, 70*(9), 2507–2510. doi:10.1093/jac/dkv150.
3. Jorde, L. B., Carey, J. C., & Bamshad, M. J. (2010). *Medical genetics* (4th ed.). St. Louis: Mosby.
4. Gardner, R. J. M., Sutherland, G. R., & Schaffer, L. G. (2012). *Chromosome abnormalities and genetic counseling*. Oxford: Oxford University Press.
5. Nagaoka, S. I., Hassold, T. J., & Hunt, P. A. (2012). Human aneuploidy: Mechanisms and new insights into an age-old problem. *Nature Reviews. Genetics, 13*(7), 493–504. doi:10.1038/nrg3245.
6. Antonarakis, S. E., & Epstein, C. J. (2006). The challenge of Down syndrome. *Trends in Molecular Medicine, 12*(10), 473–479. doi:10.1016/j.molmed.2006.08.005.
7. Gravholt, C. H. (2013). Sex chromosome abnormalities. In D. L. Rimoin, R. E. Pyeritz, & B. R. Korf (Eds.), *Emery and Rimoin's principles and practice of medical genetics* (6th ed.). Philadelphia: Elsevier.
8. Rooms, L., & Kooy, R. F. (2011). Advances in understanding fragile X syndrome and related disorders. *Current Opinion in Pediatrics, 23*(6), 601–606. doi:10.1097/MOP.0b013e32834c7f1a.
9. Nelson, D. L., Orr, H. T., & Warren, S. T. (2013). The unstable repeats—three evolving faces of neurological disease. *Neuron, 77*(5), 825–843. doi:10.1016/j.neuron.2013.02.022.
10. Hoban, M. D., Gregory, J. C., Mendel, M. C., et al. (2015). Correction of the sickle-cell disease mutation in human hematopoietic stem/progenitor cells. *Blood, 125*(17), 2597–2604. doi:10.1182/blood-2014-12-615948.
11. Biesecker, L. G., & Spinner, N. B. (2013). A genomic view of mosaicism and human disease. *Nature Reviews. Genetics, 14*(5), 307–320. doi:10.1038/nrg3424.
12. Tomlinson, I. (2015). The Mendelian colorectal cancer syndromes. *Annals of Clinical Biochemistry, 52*(6), 690–692. doi:10.1177/0004563215597944.
13. Pasmant, E., Vidaud, M., Vidaud, D., et al. (2012). Neurofibromatosis type 1: From genotype to phenotype. *Journal of Medical Genetics, 49*(8), 483–489. doi:10.1136/jmedgenet-2012-100978.
14. Livshits, G., Gao, F., Malkin, I., et al. (2016). Contribution of heritability and epigenetic factors to skeletal muscle mass variation in United Kingdom twins. *Journal of Clinical Endocrinology and Metabolism, 101*(6), 2450–2459. doi:10.1210/jc.2016-1219.
15. Lyon, M. F. (1999). X-chromosome inactivation. *Current Biology, 9*(7), R235–R237.
16. Lee, J. T., & Bartolomei, M. S. (2013). X-inactivation, imprinting, and long noncoding RNAs in health and disease. *Cell, 152*(6), 1308–1323. doi:10.1016/j.cell.2013.02.016.
17. Larney, C., Bailey, T. L., & Koopman, P. (2014). Switching on sex: Transcriptional regulation of the testis-determining gene *SRY*. *Development (Cambridge, England), 141*(11), 2195–2205. doi:10.1242/dev.107052.
18. Flanigan, K. M. (2012). The muscular dystrophies. *Seminars in Neurology, 32*(3), 255–263. doi:10.1055/s-0032-1329199.
19. Lander, E. S. (2011). Initial impact of the sequencing of the human genome. *Nature, 470*(7333), 187–197. doi:10.1038/nature09792.
20. Yang, Y., Muzny, D. M., Reid, J. G., et al. (2013). Clinical whole-exome sequencing for the diagnosis of Mendelian disorders. *The New England Journal of Medicine, 369*(16), 1502–1511. doi:10.1056/NEJMoa1306555.
21. Koboldt, D. C., Steinberg, K. M., Larson, D. E., et al. (2013). The next-generation sequencing revolution and its impact on genomics. *Cell, 155*(1), 27–38. doi:10.1016/j.cell.2013.09.006.

3

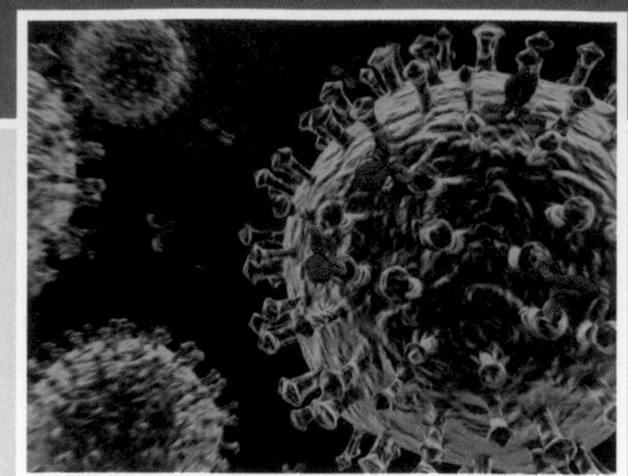

Epigenetics and Disease

Diane P. Genereux, Lynn B. Jorde, and Stephanie Zettel

EVOLVE WEBSITE

http://evolve.elsevier.com/Canada/Huether/pathophysiology
Student Review Questions
Key Points
Case Studies
Animations
Quick Check Answers

CHAPTER OUTLINE

Epigenetic Mechanisms, 62
DNA Methylation, 62
Histone Modifications, 63
RNA-Based Mechanisms, 64
Epigenetics and Human Development, 64
Genomic Imprinting, 64
Prader-Willi and Angelman Syndromes, 64
Beckwith-Wiedemann Syndrome, 65
Russell-Silver Syndrome, 66
Inheritance of Epigenetic States, 66
Epigenetics and Nutrition, 66
Epigenetics and Maternal Care, 66
Epigenetics and Mental Illness, 67
Epigenetic Disease in the Context of Genetic Abnormalities, 67
Twin Studies Provide Insights on Epigenetic Modification, 68
Molecular Approaches to Understand Epigenetic Disease, 68
Epigenetics and Cancer, 68
DNA Methylation and Cancer, 68
microRNAs and Cancer, 69
Epigenetic Screening for Cancer, 69
Emerging Strategies for the Treatment of Epigenetic Disease, 69
Future Directions, 71

Human beings exhibit an impressive diversity of physical and behavioural features. Some of this diversity is attributable to genetic variation. Another contributor to human diversity is epigenetic ("upon genetic") modification (a change in phenotype or gene expression that does not involve DNA mutation or changes in nucleotide sequence). Basically, epigenetics is the study of mechanisms that will switch genes "on," such that they are *expressed*, and "off," such that they are *silenced*. Epigenetic mechanisms include chemical modifications to DNA and associated histones, and the production of small RNA molecules. Gene regulation by epigenetic processes can occur at the level of either transcription or translation. Epigenetic modification is critical for fundamental processes of human development, including the differentiation of embryonic stem cells into specific cell types, and the inactivation of one of the two X chromosomes in each cell of a genetic female. Some genes are noted to be *imprinted*, a form of epigenetic regulation where the expression of a gene depends on whether it is inherited from the mother or the father.

EPIGENETIC MECHANISMS

A variety of diseases can result from abnormal epigenetic states. Metabolic disease can occur when there is aberrant expression of both copies of a locus that is typically imprinted. Environmental stressors can markedly increase the risk of aberrant epigenetic modification and are strongly associated with some cancers. It is because of their increasing clear role in a wide range of pathologies that abnormal epigenetic states are currently a focus of both preventive efforts and pharmaceutical intervention. Currently known epigenetic mechanisms include DNA methylation, histone modifications, and RNA-based mechanisms (Figure 3-1).

DNA Methylation

DNA methylation (see Figure 3-1) occurs through the attachment of a methyl group (CH_3) to a cytosine. Dense DNA methylation can be thought of as "insulation" that renders genes silent by blocking access by transcription factors. Dense methylation is typically coincident with hypoacetylation (decrease of the functional group acetyl) of the histone proteins around which the DNA is wound (see "Histone Modifications"). Together, DNA methylation and histone hypoacetylation can render a gene transcriptionally silent, preventing production of the encoded protein. Methylated cytosines have been found to occur principally at cytosines that are followed by a guanine base (sometimes known as cytosines in "CpG dinucleotides"). In human embryonic stem cells, methylation also can occur at cytosines outside of the CpG context (see Figure 2-24).

DNA methylation plays a prominent role in both human health and disease. For example, in each cell of a normal human female, one of the two X chromosomes is silenced by dense methylation and associated molecular marks, whereas the other X chromosome is transcriptionally active and largely devoid of methylation. During early embryonic development, there is epigenetic inactivation of one of the two X chromosomes in each cell of a human female—either the X chromosome inherited from her mother or the X chromosome inherited from her father. The determination of which chromosome is to be silenced occurs at random and independently in each of the cells present at this stage

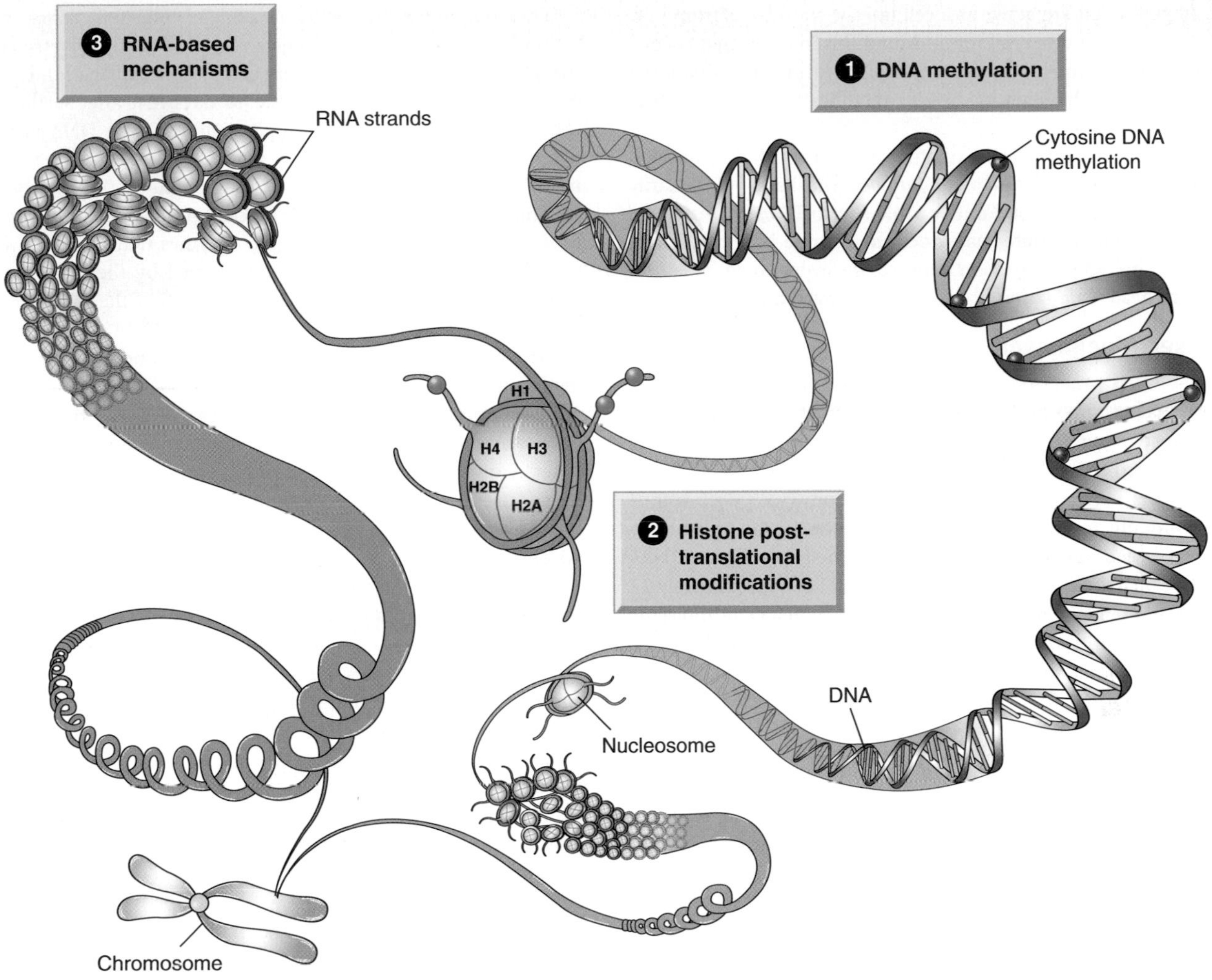

FIGURE 3-1 Three Types of Epigenetic Mechanisms. Investigators are studying three epigenetic mechanisms: **(1)** DNA methylation, **(2)** histone modifications, and **(3)** RNA-based mechanisms. See text for discussion.

of development; the silent state of that chromosome is inherited by all subsequent copies. If a woman's two X chromosomes carry different alleles at a given locus, random X inactivation can lead to somatic mosaicism, wherein the alleles active in two different cells can confer two very different traits. Striking examples include the patchy coloration of calico cats and anhidrotic ectodermal dysplasia, a condition characterized by patchy presence and absence of sweat glands in the skin of human females who have one X chromosome bearing a normal allele and one X chromosome bearing a mutant allele at the X-encoded locus. Because of the somatic mosaicism that arises through random inactivation of the X chromosome, females tend to have less severe phenotypes than do males for a variety of X-linked disorders, including colour blindness and fragile X syndrome.

Aberrant DNA methylation, either the presence of dense methylation where it is typically absent or the absence of methylation where it is typically present, can lead to misregulation of tumour-suppressor genes and oncogenes. Abnormal DNA methylation states are a common feature of several human cancers, including those of the colon[1-3] (see Figures 3-1 and 3-6 [p. 69]; see also Chapter 10).

Histone Modifications

Histone modifications (see Figure 3-1) include histone acetylation (adding an acetyl group) and deacetylation (deletion of an acetyl group) to the end of a histone protein. Like DNA methylation, these changes can alter the expression state of chromatin. Histones are proteins that facilitate compaction of genomic DNA into the nucleus of a cell, much as a spool helps to organize a long piece of thread for storage in a small space. When the DNA of the human genome is wound around histones, it is only ≈1/40 000 as long as it would be in its uncondensed state. Chemical modification of histones in a region of DNA can either upregulate or downregulate nearby gene expression by increasing or decreasing the tightness of the interaction between DNA and histones, thus modulating the extent to which DNA is accessible to transcription factors. DNA in association with histones is referred to as *chromatin*. At any given time, various regions of chromatin are typically in one of two forms: *euchromatin*, an open state in which most or all nearby genes are transcriptionally active; or *heterochromatin*, a closed state in which most or all nearby genes are transcriptionally inactive.

Chromatin structure plays a critical role in determining the developmental potential of a given cell lineage, and can undergo dramatic changes during organismal development. For example, chromatin states differ substantially between embryonic stem cells, which are poised to give rise to all of the different cell types that make up an individual, and terminally differentiated cells, which are committed to a specific developmental path. The fraction of DNA that is in the heterochromatic state increases as cells differentiate, consistent with the reduction in the number of genes that are active as a cell lineage transitions from pluripotency to terminal differentiation.[4] Mutations in genes that encode histone-modifying proteins have been implicated in congenital heart disease,[5] for example, highlighting histone modification states as critical for normal development.

In contrast to the vast majority of other cell types, including oocytes, sperm cells express not histones but *protamines*, which are evolutionarily derived from histones.[6] Protamines enable sperm DNA to wind into an even more compact state than does the histone-bound DNA in somatic cells. This tight compaction improves the hydrodynamic features of the sperm head, facilitating its movement toward the egg.

RNA-Based Mechanisms

Noncoding RNAs (ncRNAs) and other RNA-based mechanisms (see Figure 3-1) play an important role in regulating a wide variety of cellular processes, including RNA splicing and DNA replication. These ncRNAs have been likened to "sponges" in so far as they can "sop up" complementary RNAs, thus inhibiting their function (see, e.g., http://www.ncbi.nlm.nih.gov/pmc/articles/PMC2957044/). Of particular relevance to gene regulation are the hairpin-shaped microRNAs (miRNAs), which are encoded by DNA sequences of approximately 22 nucleotides, typically within the introns (a segment of a DNA molecule that does not code for proteins) of genes or in noncoding DNA located between genes (see Chapter 2). In contrast to DNA methylation and histone modification, both of which principally affect gene expression at the level of transcription, miRNAs typically modulate the stability and translational efficiency of existing messenger RNAs (mRNAs) encoded at other loci. Interaction between miRNAs and mRNAs target for degradation is typically mediated by regions of partial sequence complementarity. As a result, miRNAs can at once be specific enough so that they do not bind to *all* of the mRNAs in a cell and general enough to regulate a large number of different mRNA sequences. miRNAs also directly modulate translation by impairing ribosomal function. miRNAs regulate diverse signalling pathways; those that stimulate cancer development and progression are called *oncomirs*. For example, miRNAs have been linked to carcinogenesis because they alter the activity of oncogenes and tumour-suppressor genes (see Chapter 10).

EPIGENETICS AND HUMAN DEVELOPMENT

Each of the cells in the very early embryo has the potential to give rise to a somatic cell of any type. These embryonic stem cells are therefore said to be totipotent ("possessing all powers"). A key process in early development then is the differential epigenetic modification of specific DNA nucleotide sequences in these embryonic stem cells, ultimately leading to the differential gene-expression profiles that characterize the various differentiated somatic cell types. These early modifications ensure that specific genes are expressed only in the cells and tissue types in which their gene products typically function (e.g., factor VIII expression primarily in hepatocytes, or dopamine receptor expression in neurons).

Epigenetic modifications early in development also highlight a fundamental feature of genetics as compared with epigenetic information: all of the cells in a given individual contain almost exactly the same genetic information. It is the epigenetic information eventually placed on top of these sequences that enables them to achieve the diverse functions of differentiated somatic cells. A small percentage of genes, termed housekeeping genes, are necessary for the function and maintenance of all cells. These genes escape epigenetic silencing and remain transcriptionally active in all or nearly all cells. Housekeeping genes include encoding histones, DNA and RNA polymerases, and ribosomal RNA genes.

How do embryonic stem cells achieve epigenetic states typical of totipotency, whereby they can give rise to all of the diverse cell types that make up a fully developed organism? One explanation is that early embryogenesis (approximately the 10 days just after fertilization) is characterized by rapid fluctuation in genome-wide DNA methylation densities. Fertilization triggers a global loss of DNA methylation at most loci in both the oocyte-contributed and the sperm-contributed genomes. This loss of methylation is accomplished in part by suppression of the DNA methyltransferases, the enzymes that add methyl groups to DNA. Methylation is not directly copied by the DNA replication process. Instead, immediately following replication, the methyltransferases read the pattern of methylation on the parent DNA strand and use that information to determine which daughter-strand cytosines should be methylated. As embryonic cell division proceeds in the absence of DNA methyltransferases, cell division continues, eventually yielding cells that have nearly all of their loci in unmethylated, transcriptionally active states. Around the time of implantation in the uterus, the DNA methyltransferases become active again, permitting establishment of the cell-lineage–specific marks required for the establishment of organ systems.

GENOMIC IMPRINTING

A baby inherits two copies of each autosomal gene: one from its mother and one from its father. For a large subset of these genes, expression is biallelic, meaning that both the maternally and the paternally inherited copies contribute to offspring phenotype. For another, smaller subset of these genes, expression is stochastically monoallelic,[7] meaning that the maternal copy is randomly chosen for inactivation in some somatic cells and the paternal copy is randomly chosen for inactivation in other somatic cells. For a third and smaller subset of autosomes (about 1%) either the maternal copy or the paternal copy is imprinted, meaning that either the copy inherited through the sperm or the copy inherited through the egg is inactivated and remains in this inactive state in all of the somatic cells of the individual.

The subset of genes that are subject to imprinting is highly enriched for loci relevant to organismal growth. The *genetic conflict hypothesis*[7] was developed as a potential explanation for this pattern. Although both the mother and the father benefit genetically from the birth and survival of offspring, their interests are not entirely aligned. Because a mother makes a large physiological investment in each child, it is in her evolutionary best interest to limit the flow of energetic resources to any given offspring so as to maintain her physiological capacity to bear subsequent children. By contrast, except in cases of certain permanent and monogamous relationships, it is in the best interest of the father for his child to extract maximal resources from its mother, as his own future fecundity, or fertility, is not contingent on the sustained fecundity of the mother. In general, imprinting of maternally inherited genes tends to reduce offspring size; imprinting of paternally inherited genes tends to increase offspring size. One hallmark of imprinting-associated disease is that the phenotype of affected individuals is critically dependent on whether the mutation is inherited from the mother or from the father. Some examples are included in the following syndromes.

Prader-Willi and Angelman Syndromes

A well-known disease example of imprinting is associated with a deletion of about 4 million base pairs (Mb) of the long arm of chromosome 15. When this deletion is inherited from the father, the child manifests Prader-Willi syndrome, with features including short stature, hypotonia, small hands and feet, obesity, mild to moderate intellectual disability, and hypogonadism[8] (Figure 3-2, *A*). The same 4-Mb deletion, when

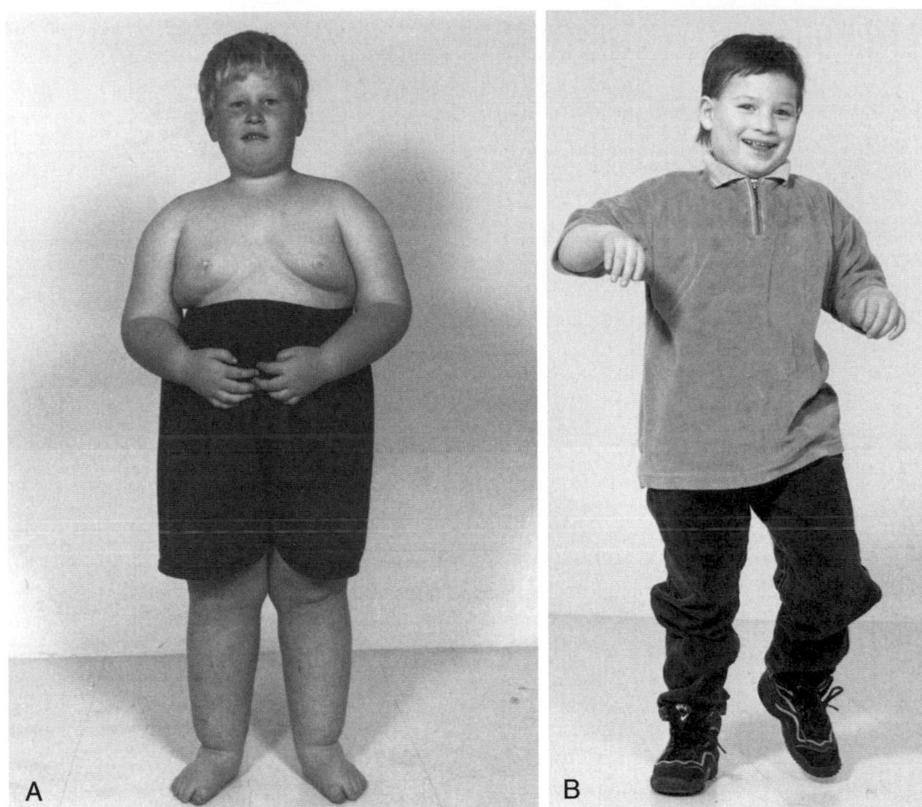

FIGURE 3-2 Prader-Willi and Angelman Syndromes. A, A child with Prader-Willi syndrome (truncal obesity, small hands and feet, inverted V-shaped upper lip). **B,** A child with Angelman syndrome (characteristic posture, ataxic gait, bouts of uncontrolled laughter). (From Jorde, L.B., Carey, J.C., & Bamshad, M.J. [2010]. *Medical genetics* [4th ed.]. Philadelphia: Mosby.)

inherited from the mother, causes Angelman syndrome, which is characterized by severe intellectual disability, seizures, and an ataxic gait (Figure 3-2, *B*).[9] These diseases are each observed in about 1 of every 15 000 live births; chromosome deletions are responsible for about 70% of cases of both diseases. The deletions that cause Prader-Willi and Angelman syndromes are indistinguishable at the DNA sequence level and affect the same group of genes.

For several decades, it was unclear how the same deletion could produce such disparate results in different individuals. Further analysis showed that the 4-Mb deletion (the *critical region*) contains several genes that are normally transcribed only on the copy of chromosome 15 that is inherited from the father.[10] These genes are transcriptionally inactive (imprinted) on the copy of chromosome 15 inherited from the mother. Similarly, other genes in the critical region are transcriptionally active only on the chromosome copy inherited from the mother and are inactive on the chromosome inherited from the father. Thus, several genes in this region are normally active on only one chromosome copy (Figure 3-3). If the single active copy of one of these genes is lost because of a chromosome deletion, then no gene product is produced, resulting in disease.

Molecular analysis has revealed much about genes in this critical region of chromosome 15.[10] The gene responsible for Angelman syndrome encodes a ligase involved in protein degradation during brain development (consistent with the intellectual disability and ataxia observed in this disorder). In brain tissue, this gene is active only on the chromosome copy inherited from the mother. Consequently, a maternally transmitted deletion removes the single active copy of this gene. Several genes in the critical region are associated with Prader-Willi syndrome, and they are transcribed only on the chromosome transmitted by the father. A paternally transmitted deletion removes the only active copies of these genes producing the features of Prader-Willi syndrome.

Beckwith-Wiedemann Syndrome

Another well-known example of imprinting is Beckwith-Wiedemann syndrome, an overgrowth condition accompanied by an increased predisposition to cancer. Beckwith-Wiedemann syndrome is usually identifiable at birth because of the presence of large size for gestational age, neonatal hypoglycemia, a large tongue, creases on the earlobe, and omphalocele (birth defect of infant intestines).[11] Children with Beckwith-Wiedemann syndrome have an increased risk of developing Wilms tumour or hepatoblastoma. Both of these tumours can be treated effectively if they are detected early; thus screening at regular intervals is an important part of management. Some children with Beckwith-Wiedemann syndrome also develop asymmetrical overgrowth of a limb or one side of the face or trunk (hemihyperplasia).

As with Angelman syndrome, a minority of Beckwith-Wiedemann syndrome cases (about 20 to 30%) are caused by the inheritance of two copies of a chromosome from the father and no copy of the chromosome from the mother (*uniparental disomy*, in this case affecting chromosome 11). Several genes on the short arm of chromosome 11 are imprinted on either the paternally or the maternally transmitted chromosome. These genes are found in two separate, differentially methylated regions (DMRs). In DMR1, the gene that encodes insulinlike growth factor 2 (IGF-2) is inactive on the maternally transmitted chromosome but active on the paternally transmitted chromosome. Thus, a normal individual has only one active copy of *IGF-2*. When two copies of the paternal chromosome are inherited (i.e., paternal uniparental disomy) or there is loss of imprinting on the maternal copy

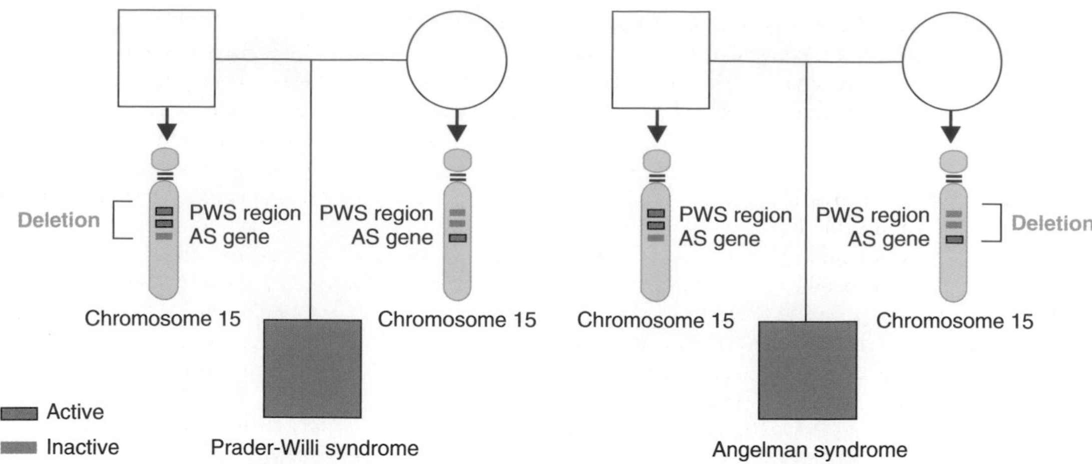

FIGURE 3-3 Prader-Willi Syndrome Pedigrees. These pedigrees illustrate the inheritance patterns of Prader-Willi syndrome (*PWS*), which can be caused by a deletion of about 4 million base pairs (Mb) of chromosome 15q when inherited from the father. In contrast, Angelman syndrome (*AS*) can be caused by the same deletion but only when it is inherited from the mother. The reason for this difference is that different genes in this region are normally imprinted (inactivated) in the copies of 15q transmitted by the mother and the father. (From Jorde, L.B., Carey, J.C., & Bamshad, M.J. [2010]. *Medical genetics* [4th ed.]. Philadelphia: Mosby.)

of *IGF-2*, an active *IGF-2* gene is present in double dose. These changes produce increased levels of IGF-2 during fetal development, contributing to the overgrowth features of Beckwith-Wiedemann syndrome. Note that, in contrast to Prader-Willi and Angelman syndromes, which are produced by a missing gene product, Beckwith-Wiedemann syndrome is caused, in part, by overexpression of a gene product.

Russell-Silver Syndrome

Russell-Silver syndrome is characterized by delayed growth, proportionate short stature, leg length discrepancy, and a small, triangular face. About one third of Russell-Silver syndrome cases are caused by imprinting abnormalities of chromosome 11p15.5 that lead to downregulation of *IGF-2* and therefore diminished growth. Another 10% of cases of Russell-Silver syndrome are caused by maternal uniparental disomy. Thus, whereas upregulation, or extra copies, of active *IGF-2* causes overgrowth in Beckwith-Wiedemann syndrome, downregulation of *IGF-2* causes the diminished growth seen in Russell-Silver syndrome.

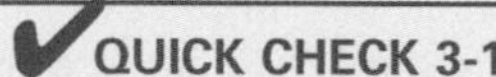

1. Define *epigenetics*.
2. What are the three types of epigenetic mechanisms?
3. What is meant by the genetic conflict hypothesis?
4. Compare and contrast the molecular and phenotypic features of Prader-Willi and Angelman syndromes.

INHERITANCE OF EPIGENETIC STATES

It is increasingly clear that imprinted genes are not the only loci for which epigenetic modifications persist over time. Conditions encountered in utero, during childhood, and even during adolescence or later can have long-term impacts on epigenetic states, sometimes with impacts that can be transmitted across generations.[12] A few such examples are discussed next.

Epigenetics and Nutrition

During the winter of 1943, millions of people in urban areas of the Netherlands suffered starvation conditions as a result of a Nazi blockade that prevented shipments of food from agricultural areas. When researchers sought to investigate how exposure to famine in utero had affected individuals born in a historically prosperous country, they found individuals who suffered nutritional deprivation in utero were more likely to suffer from obesity and diabetes as adults than individuals in the Netherlands who had not experienced nutritional deprivation during gestation. There also seemed to be a transgenerational impact, in that the children of individuals who were in utero during the Dutch Hunger Winter were found to be significantly smaller than the children of those not affected by the blockade. Other data sets reveal an elevated risk for cardiovascular and metabolic disease for offspring of individuals exposed during early development to fluctuations in agricultural yields.[13]

The specific molecular mechanisms that may mediate these apparent relationships between nutritional deprivation and disease risk on one or more generations are largely unknown. From some animal models, it seems that the *IGF-2* gene is a possible target of epigenetic modifications arising through nutritional deprivation. Exposure in utero and through lactation to some chemicals (including bisphenol A, a constituent of plastics sometimes used in food preparation and storage) seems to lead to epigenetic modifications similar to those that arise through nutritional deprivation in early life.[14]

Epigenetics and Maternal Care

It is increasingly clear that parenting style can affect epigenetic states, and that this information can be transmitted from one generation to the next. Mice and other rodents can exhibit two alternate styles of nursing behaviour: frequent arched-back nursing with a high level of licking and grooming behaviour, and an alternate style with infrequent arched-back nursing and much reduced licking and grooming behaviour. In one especially compelling study,[15] pups of mothers that engaged in frequent arched-backed nursing were found to have significantly lower methylation levels and higher transcription activity of a glucocorticoid receptor–encoding locus. Similarly, Anacker, O'Donnell, and Meaney investigated how parent–offspring interactions affect the epigenetic state and expression of genes, both in humans and nonhumans. Most of the products of these genes influence hypothalamic-pituitary-adrenal function.[16] Because the glucocorticoid receptor is involved in a pathway that intensifies fearfulness and response to stress, these findings suggest that alteration to methylation states could help explain the finding that exposure to stress early in life can modulate behaviour in adulthood. These findings also highlight the concept that epigenetic processes can help store information about the environment, and that the relevant epigenetic modifications can modulate behaviour later in life.

Epigenetics and Ethanol Exposure During Gestation

The impact of ethanol exposure in utero on skeletal and neural development was first reported in 1973[17] and led to broad awareness of fetal alcohol spectrum disorder. It was not until recently, however, that population-based and molecular-level studies began to clarify the epigenetic signals that mediate these impacts. At first, researchers found alcohol exposure in utero can affect the DNA methylation states of various genomic elements, but without specific emphasis on loci directly relevant to skeletal and neural development.[11] More recently, it was found that treating cultured neural stem cells with ethanol impairs their ability to differentiate to functional neurons; this impairment seems to be correlated with aberrant, dense methylation at loci that are active in normal neuronal tissue.[18] One possible explanation for these effects is that ethanol exposure in utero modulates fetal expression of the DNA methyltransferases.[19]

Epigenetics and Mental Illness

Researchers suggest that epigenetics also plays a role in psychiatric illness, resulting in many different phenotypes.[12] Schizophrenia, major depressive disorder, and bipolar disorder are just a few examples of how epigenetic influences can alter the course of an illness. These disorders are associated with alternating remissions and relapses, and the epigenetic changes that occur demonstrate how genetic activity is altered by the interactions of the organism with its environment. These epigenetic influences are reversible and can change over time. Further research in this area is considering how the environment impacts the expression of psychiatric conditions and the possibility of understanding the effect of environmental stimuli on the course of the illness with the intention to better treat and support individuals with these conditions.

Epigenetic Disease in the Context of Genetic Abnormalities

In some diseases, both genetic and epigenetic factors contribute to the origin of abnormal phenotypes. For example, several abnormal phenotypes can arise in individuals with mutations at the fragile X locus *FMR1* (Figure 3-4, *A*). Some of these phenotypes arise in individuals for

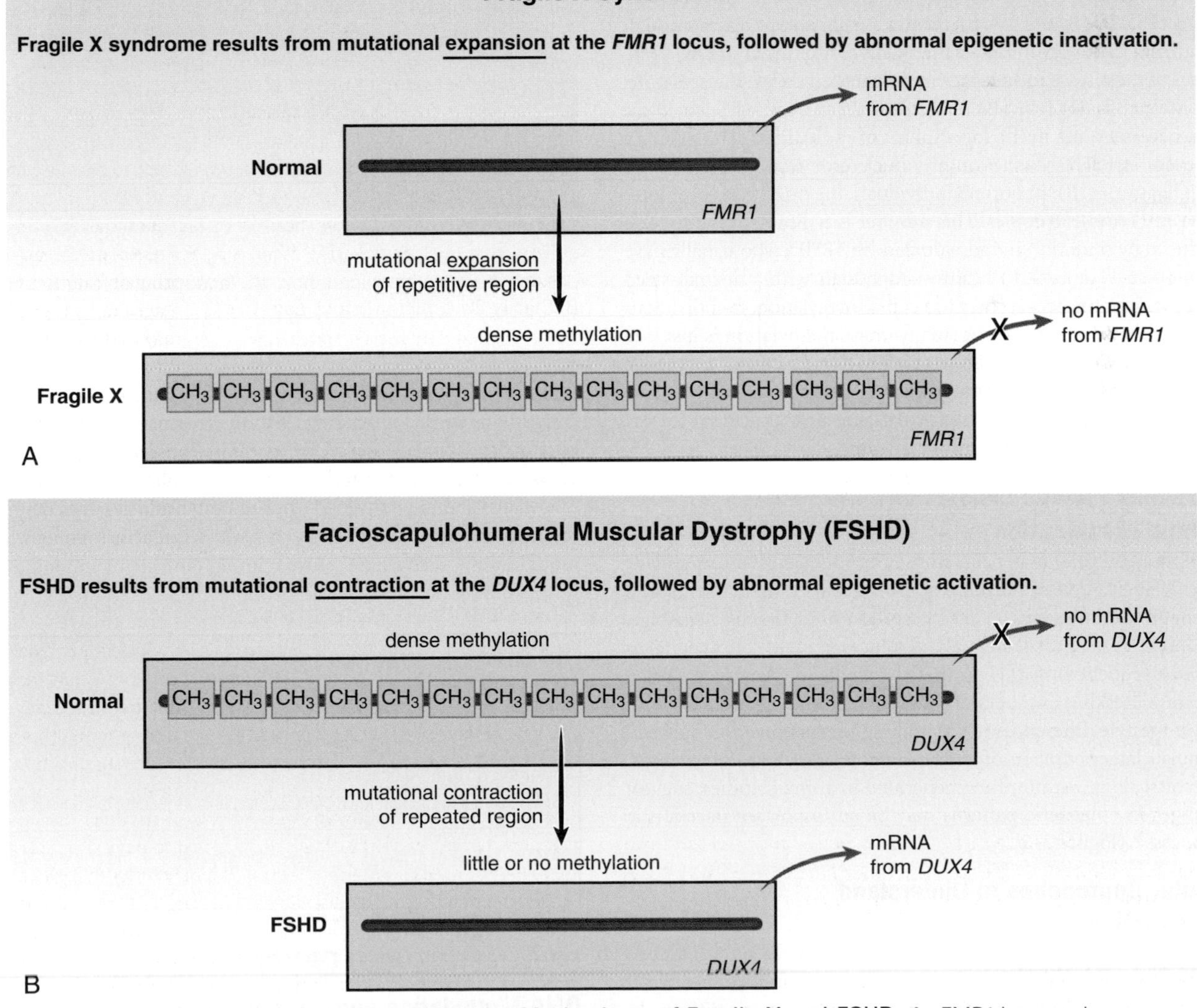

FIGURE 3-4 Comparing the Molecular Mechanisms of Fragile X and FSHD. **A,** *FMR1* in normal, expanded permutation, and full-mutation states. **B,** *DUX4* in normal and contracted states. *FSHD,* facioscapulohumeral muscular dystrophy; *mRNA,* messenger RNA.

whom epigenetic changes are coincident with genetic changes. The most common genetic abnormality at *FMR1* involves expansion in the number of cytosine-guanine (CG) dinucleotide repeats in the gene promoter. Females who have CG repeats in excess of the approximately 35 that are typical at this locus are at risk for fragile X–associated primary ovarian insufficiency, characterized by an elevated risk for early menopause.[20] Males with moderate expansions are at risk for fragile X tremor ataxia syndrome (FXTAS), characterized by a late-onset intention tremor.[21] Both of these conditions seem to arise through accumulation of excess levels of *FMR1* mRNAs in nuclear inclusion bodies.[20,22] Individuals with 200 repeats are at risk for fragile X syndrome, characterized by reduced IQ and a set of behavioural abnormalities. Remarkably, although possession of a large CG repeat in the *FMR1* promoter dramatically increases the probability that an individual will have fragile X syndrome, the disease can be present in males who have the large repeat but be absent in their brothers who have inherited an allele of very similar size.[23] This difference can be explained, at least in part, by the observation that acquisition of methylation-based silencing at *FMR1* is stochastic, meaning that the presence of a large repeat increases the probability of the dense promoter methylation that could lead to gene silencing, but does not guarantee it. It remains to be seen whether dietary or environmental features can modulate the probability that dense methylation at *FMR1* will accrue in individuals with the full-mutation allele.

In another genetic-epigenetic disease, **facioscapulohumeral muscular dystrophy (FSHD)** (Figure 3-4, *B*), the disease phenotype arises through loss of normal methylation rather than gain of abnormal methylation. Symptoms of the disease include adverse impacts on skeletal musculature. Though lifespan is not typically reduced by the disease, wheelchair use becomes necessary late in life for a subset of individuals. The primary genetic event in FSHD is deletion of a nucleotide repeat in the *DUX4* gene (see Figure 3-4, *B*). In normal individuals, the *D4Z4* gene promoter has between 11 and 150 copies. This number is typically found to have been reduced by mutation in individuals with FSHD, who usually have only 1 to 10 such repeats. In healthy individuals with a normal-sized allele, the *D4Z4* promoter typically has dense methylation. In individuals with reduced copy-counts, the normally dense methylation is lost (see Figure 3-4, *B*).[24] The disease allele typically also has fewer repressive histone marks than does the normal allele.[25] Together, fragile X syndrome and FSHD highlight that both abnormal gain and abnormal loss of epigenetic modifications can result in disease.

Twin Studies Provide Insights on Epigenetic Modification

Identical (monozygotic) twin pairs, whose DNA sequences are essentially the same, offer a unique opportunity to isolate and examine the impacts of epigenetic modifications. A recent study found that as twins age, they exhibit increasingly substantial differences in methylation patterns of the DNA sequences of their somatic cells; these changes are often reflected in increasing numbers of phenotypic differences. Twins with significant lifestyle differences (e.g., smoking versus nonsmoking) tend to accumulate larger numbers of differences in their methylation patterns. These results, along with findings generated in animal studies, suggest that changes in epigenetic patterns may be an important part of the aging process[26] (Figure 3-5).

Molecular Approaches to Understand Epigenetic Disease

Because epigenetic information is not encoded by DNA molecules but instead by chemical modifications to those molecules, conventional sequencing approaches are not sufficient to reveal epigenetic differences between normal individuals and those who have epigenetic modifications associated with disease. To collect information on DNA methylation states of individual nucleotides, DNA is typically subjected to bisulfite conversion before sequencing. Bisulfite treatment does not alter most nucleotides, including methylated cytosines, but deaminates unmethylated cytosines to uracil.[27] Because uracil complements adenine, not guanine, methylated and unmethylated cytosines can be distinguished in resulting sequence data, so long as the genetic sequence is known. Histone modification states can be assayed through the use of antibodies specific for histones with various modifications.[28]

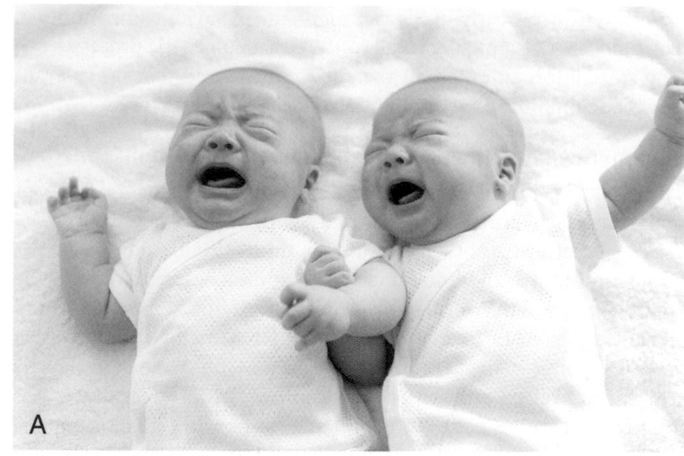

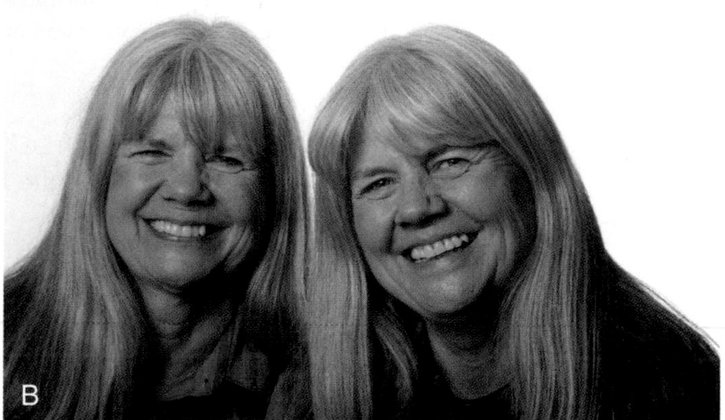

FIGURE 3-5 Twins and Aging. A, Twins as babies look very much alike but, **B,** as adults, twins have slight differences in appearance, possibly because of epigenetics. (**A,** leungchophan/Shutterstock.com. **B,** Stacey Bates/Shutterstock.com.)

QUICK CHECK 3-2

1. Evaluate the statement: "Epigenetic information is highly dynamic in early development."
2. How does the epigenetic regulation of imprinted genes compare with that of the rest of the genome?
3. Compare and contrast the molecular mechanisms leading to fragile X syndrome and to FSHD.
4. Why are pairs of identical twins especially useful in the study of epigenetic phenomena?

EPIGENETICS AND CANCER

DNA Methylation and Cancer

Some of the most extensive evidence for the role of epigenetic modification in human disease comes from studies of cancer (Figure 3-6).[29,30]

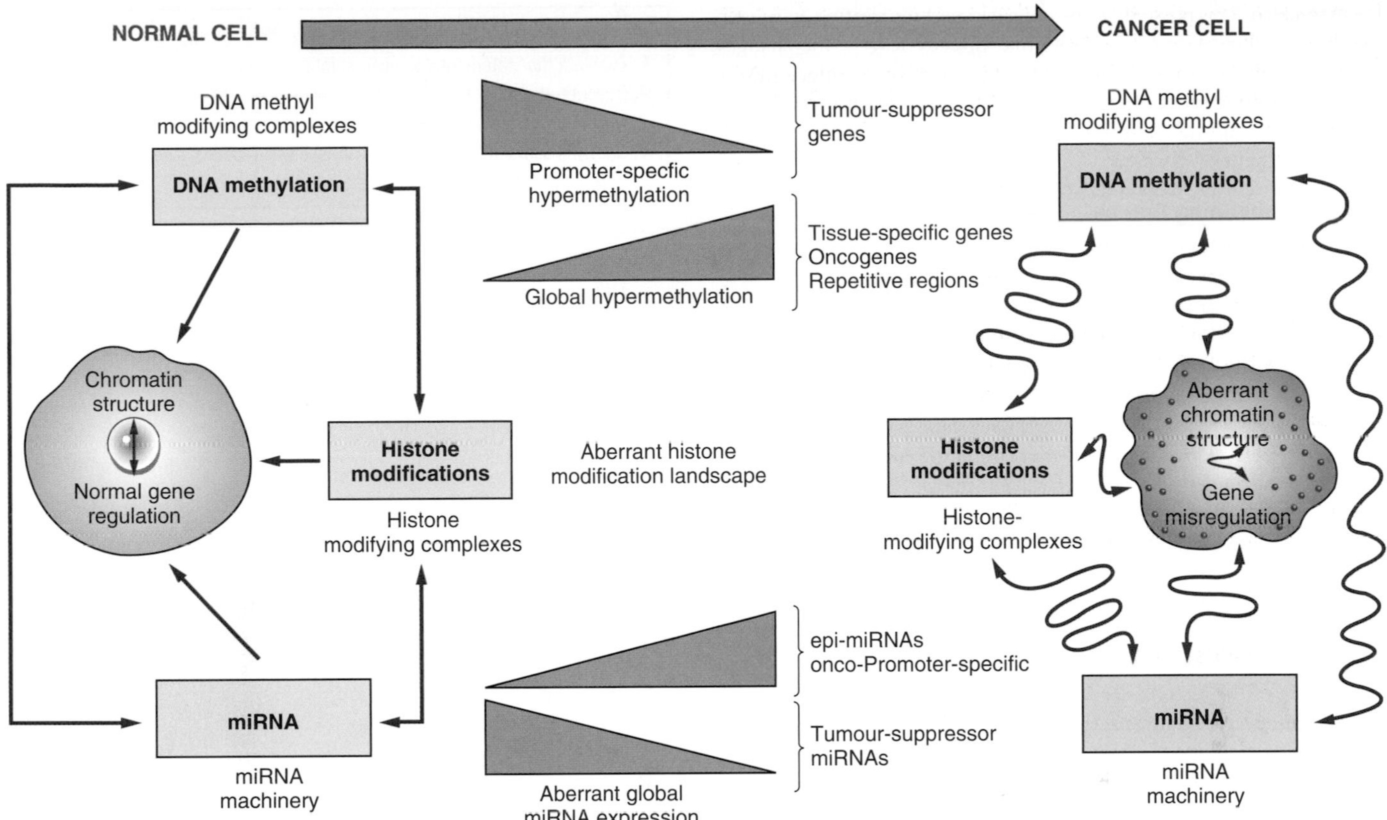

FIGURE 3-6 Global Epigenomic Alterations and Cancer. Oncogenesis often occurs through a combination of genetic mutations and epigenetic change. In cancer cells, the promoters of tumour-suppressor genes typically become hypermethylated, leading, in combination with histone modifications, to abnormal gene silencing. Because tumour-suppressor genes typically help to control cell division, their silencing can result in tumour progression. Global hypomethylation leads to chromosomal instability and fragility, and increases the risk of additional genetic mutations. As well, these modifications create abnormal messenger RNA and microRNA (*miRNA*) expression, which leads to activation of oncogenes and silencing of tumour-suppressor genes. (Reprinted from *Current Opinion in Genetics & Development,* 22(1), Sandoval, J., & Esteller, M., "Cancer epigenomics: beyond genomics," Pages 50–55, Copyright 2012, with permission from Elsevier.)

Tumour cells typically exhibit genome-wide hypomethylation (decreased methylation), which can increase the activity of oncogenes (see Chapter 10). Hypomethylation increases as tumours progress from benign neoplasms to malignancy. In addition, the promoter regions of tumour-suppressor genes are often hypermethylated, which decreases their rate of transcription and their ability to inhibit tumour formation. Hypermethylation of the promoter region of the *RB1* gene is often seen in retinoblastoma[31]; hypermethylation of the *BRCA1* gene is seen in some cases of inherited breast cancer (Chapter 33).[32]

A major cause of one form of inherited colon cancer (hereditary nonpolyposis colorectal cancer [HNPCC]) is the methylation of the promoter region of a gene, *MLH1*, whose protein product repairs damaged DNA. When *MLH1* becomes inactive, DNA damage accumulates, eventually resulting in colon tumours.[33,34] Abnormal methylation of tumour-suppressor genes also is common in the progression of Barrett esophagus, a condition in which the lining of the esophagus is replaced by cells that have features associated with the lower intestinal tract, and to adenocarcinoma possibly through upregulation of one of the enzymes that adds methyl groups to DNA.[35]

microRNAs and Cancer

Hypermethylation also is seen in miRNA genes, which encode small (22 base pair) RNA molecules that bind to the ends of mRNAs, degrading them and preventing their translation. More than 1 000 miRNA sequences have been identified in humans, and hypermethylation of specific subgroups of miRNAs is associated with tumourigenesis. When miRNA genes are methylated, their mRNA targets are overexpressed, and this overexpression has been associated with metastasis.[29]

Epigenetic Screening for Cancer

The common finding of epigenetic alteration in cancerous tissue raises the possibility that epigenetic screening approaches could complement or even replace existing early-detection methods. In some cases, epigenetic screening could be done using bodily fluids, such as urine or sputum, eliminating the need for the more invasive, costly, and risky strategies currently in place. Monitoring for misregulation of miRNAs has shown promise as a tool for early diagnosis of cancers of the colon,[36] breast,[37] and prostate.[38] Other epigenetics-based screening approaches have shown promise for detection of cancers of the bladder,[39] lung,[40] and prostate.[41]

Emerging Strategies for the Treatment of Epigenetic Disease

Epigenetic modifications are potentially reversible: DNA can be demethylated, histones can be modified to change the transcriptional state of nearby DNA, and miRNA-encoding loci can be upregulated or downregulated. This possibility raises the prospect for treating epigenetic disease with pharmaceutical agents that directly reverse the changes associated with the disease phenotype. In recent years, interventions involving all three types of epigenetic modulators (DNA methylation, histone modification, and miRNAs) have shown considerable promise for the treatment of disease.

DNA Demethylating Agents

5-Azacytidine has been used as a therapeutic drug in the treatment of leukemia and myelodysplastic syndrome (5-azacytosine, the active component of 5-azacytidine, is shown in Figure 3-7).[42] A cytosine analogue, **5-azacytidine**, is incorporated into DNA opposite its complementary nucleotide, guanine. 5-Azacytidine differs from cytosine in that it has a nitrogen, rather than a carbon, in the fifth position of its cytidine ring. As a result, the DNA methyltransferases cannot add methyl groups to 5-azacytidine, and DNA that contains 5-azacytidine declines in its methylation density over successive rounds of DNA replication.[43] Administration of 5-azacytidine is associated with various adverse effects, including digestive disturbance, but has shown promise in the treatment of diseases, including pancreatic cancer[44] and myelodysplastic syndromes.[45,46]

Histone Deacetylase Inhibitors

The activity of the histone deacetylases (HDACs) increases chromatin compaction, decreasing transcriptional activity (Figure 3-8). In many cases, excessive activity of HDACs results in transcriptional inactivation of tumour-suppressor genes, leading ultimately to the development of tumours. Treatment with HDAC inhibitors, either alone or in combination with other medications, has shown promise in the treatment of cancers of the breast[47] and prostate,[48] but only very limited success in the treatment of pancreatic cancer.[49]

microRNA Coding

A major challenge in developing medications that modify epigenetic alterations is to target only the genes responsible for a specific cancer. Therapeutic approaches that use miRNA offer a potential solution to this problem as treatment can be targeted to individual loci using sequence characteristics of relevant RNA molecules.

QUICK CHECK 3-3

1. Evaluate the statement: "Cancer is, in many cases, an epigenetic disease."
2. Describe the role of miRNAs in cancer.
3. Describe a potential strategy for the treatment of epigenetic disease.
4. Describe some of the challenges of developing pharmaceutical approaches to remedy abnormal epigenetic states.

A: Cytosine —DNMT1+*S*-Adenosylmethionine→ 5-Methylcytosine

B: 5-Azacytosine —DNMT1+*S*-Adenosylmethionine→ 5-Azacytosine

FIGURE 3-7 5-Azacytosine as Demethylating Agent. A, Unmethylated cytosines in DNA are typically subject to the addition of methyl groups by DNMT1, a DNA methyltransferase, using methyl groups supplied by the methyl donor *S*-adenosylmethionine. **B,** In 5-azacytosine, the 5′ carbon of cytosine is replaced with a nitrogen. This chemical difference is sufficient both to block the addition of a methyl group and to confer irreversible binding to DNMT1. Incorporation of 5-azacytosine into DNA is therefore sufficient to drive passive loss of methylation from replicating DNA, and thus to reactivate hypermethylated loci. 5-Azacytosine, bound to a sugar, can be integrated into DNA, and has been administered with some success in treating epigenetic diseases that arise through hypermethylation of individual loci.

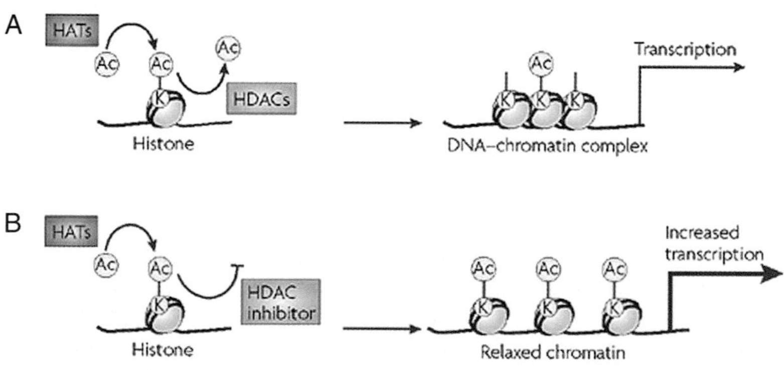

FIGURE 3-8 Effect of HDAC Inhibitors on Chromatin Remodelling and Transcription. A, Levels of histone acetylation at specific lysine (*K*) residues are determined by concurrent reactions of acetylation (*Ac*) and deacetylation, which are mediated by histone acetyltransferases (*HATs*) and histone deacetylases (*HDACs*). This histone acetylation is vital for establishing the conformational structure of DNA–chromatin complexes, and, subsequently, transcriptional gene expression. **B,** By blocking the deacetylation reaction, HDAC inhibitors change the equilibrium of histone acetylation levels, leading to increased acetylation, chromatin modification to relax conformation, and transcription upregulation. (Reprinted by permission from Macmillan Publishers Ltd: *Nature Reviews Drug Discovery* 7, 854–868 (2008).)

FUTURE DIRECTIONS

Robust experimental observations are clarifying the roles of epigenetic states in determining cell fates and disease phenotypes. The well-documented involvement of epigenetic abnormalities in carcinogenesis and the mounting evidence for these epigenetic changes in other common diseases (discussed in other chapters) will likely elucidate possibilities for reversing the epigenetic abnormalities and possibly preventing their establishment in utero.

DID YOU UNDERSTAND?

Epigenetic Mechanisms

1. Investigators are studying three major types of epigenetic mechanisms: (a) DNA methylation, which results from attachment of a methyl group to a cytosine; in the somatic cells, all or nearly all methylation occurs at cytosines that are followed by guanines ("CpG dinucleotides"); (b) histone modifications, through the addition of various chemical groups, including methyl and acetyl; and (c) noncoding RNAs (ncRNAs) or microRNAs (miRNAs), short nucleotides derived from introns of protein coding genes or transcribed as independent genes from regions of the genome whose functions, if any, remain poorly understood. miRNAs regulate diverse signalling pathways.
2. DNA methylation is, at present, the best-studied epigenetic process. When a gene becomes heavily methylated, the DNA is less likely to be transcribed into mRNA.
3. Methylation, along with histone hypoacetylation and condensation of chromatin, inhibits the binding of proteins that promote transcription, such that the gene becomes transcriptionally inactive.
4. Environmental factors, such as diet and exposure to certain chemicals, may cause epigenetic modification.
5. The heritable transmission to future generations of epigenetic modifications is called *transgenerational inheritance.*

Epigenetics and Human Development

1. Epigenetic modification alters gene expression without changes to DNA sequence.
2. Housekeeping genes are necessary for the function and maintenance of all cells, and they escape epigenetic silencing, remaining transcriptionally active in all (or nearly all) cells.
3. Fertilization triggers loss of DNA methylation and suppression of DNA methyltransferases (enzymes that add methyl groups to DNA), yielding cells that have nearly all of their loci in unmethylated and transcriptionally active states.
4. Implantation in the uterus activates the DNA methyltransferases and allows for cell-lineage–specific marks required for the development of organ systems.

Genomic Imprinting

1. Gregor Mendel's experiments with garden peas demonstrated that the phenotype is the same whether a given allele is inherited from the mother or the father. This principle, which has long been part of the central dogma of genetics, does not always hold. For some human genes, a given gene is transcriptionally active on only one copy of a chromosome (e.g., the copy inherited from the father). On the other copy of the chromosome (the one inherited from the mother) the gene is transcriptionally inactive. This process of gene silencing, in which genes are silenced depending on which parent transmits them, is known as *imprinting*; the transcriptionally silenced genes are said to be "imprinted."
2. When an allele is imprinted, it typically has heavy methylation. By contrast, the nonimprinted allele is typically not methylated.
3. A well-known disease example of imprinting is associated with a deletion of about 4 million base pairs (Mb) of the long arm of chromosome 15. When this deletion is inherited from the father, the child manifests Prader-Willi syndrome.
4. The same 4-Mb deletion, when inherited from the mother, causes Angelman syndrome.
5. Another well-known example of imprinting is Beckwith-Wiedemann syndrome, an overgrowth condition accompanied by an increased predisposition to cancer.
6. Whereas upregulation, or extra copies, of active *IGF-2* causes overgrowth in Beckwith-Wiedemann syndrome, downregulation of *IGF-2* causes the diminished growth seen in Russell-Silver syndrome.

Inheritance of Epigenetic States

1. Events encountered in utero, in childhood, and in adolescence can result in specific epigenetic changes that yield a wide range of phenotypic abnormalities, including metabolic syndromes.
2. Fetal alcohol spectrum disorder, which results from ethanol exposure in utero, may be mediated by the repressive impact of ethanol on the DNA methyltransferases.
3. Both abnormal gain of methylation, as in the case of fragile X syndrome, and abnormal loss of methylation, as in the case of facioscapulohumeral muscular dystrophy, can produce disease phenotypes.
4. As twins age, they demonstrate increasing differences in methylation patterns of their DNA sequences, causing increasing numbers of phenotypic differences.
5. In studies of twins with significant lifestyle differences (e.g., smoking versus nonsmoking) large numbers of differences in their methylation patterns are observed to accrue over time.

Epigenetics and Cancer

1. The best evidence for epigenetic effects on human disease risk comes from studies of cancer.
2. Methylation densities decline as tumours progress, which can increase the activity of oncogenes, causing tumours to progress from benign neoplasms to malignancy. Additionally, the promoter regions of tumour-suppressor genes are often hypermethylated. These elevated methylation levels decreases their rate of transcription at these critical genes, thus reducing the ability to inhibit tumour formation.
3. Hypermethylation also is seen in miRNA genes and is associated with tumourigenesis.
4. Unlike DNA sequence mutations, epigenetic modifications can be reversed through pharmaceutical intervention. For example, 5-azacytidine, a demethylating agent, has been used as a therapeutic drug in the treatment of leukemia and myelodysplastic syndrome.

Future Directions

1. Robust experimental observations are defining the roles of epigenetic states in shaping cell fates.
2. The well-documented involvement of epigenetic abnormalities in carcinogenesis and the mounting evidence for these epigenetic changes in other common diseases (discussed throughout the text) will likely elucidate new therapies with the possibilities of reversing the epigenetic abnormalities.

KEY TERMS

5-Azacytidine, 70
Angelman syndrome, 65
Beckwith-Wiedemann syndrome, 65
Biallelic, 64
DNA methylation, 62
Embryonic stem cell, 64
Epigenetics, 62
Facioscapulohumeral muscular dystrophy (FHMD), 68
Fragile X, 67
Histone, 63
Histone modification, 63
Housekeeping genes, 64
Imprinted, 64
MicroRNA (miRNA), 64
Monoallelic, 64
Noncoding RNA (ncRNA), 64
Prader-Willi syndrome, 64
Russell-Silver syndrome, 66

REFERENCES

1. King, W. D., Ashbury, J. E., Taylor, S. A., et al. (2014). A cross-sectional study of global DNA methylation and risk of colorectal adenoma. *BMC Cancer*, *14*(1), 488. doi:10.1186/1471-2407-14-488.
2. Dhimolea, E., Wadia, P. R., Murray, T. J., et al. (2014). Prenatal exposure to BPA alters the epigenome of the rat mammary gland and increases the propensity to neoplastic development. *PLoS ONE*, *9*(7), e99800. doi:10.1371/journal.pone.0099800.
3. Ashour, N., Angulo, J. C., Andrés, G., et al. (2014). A DNA hypermethylation profile reveals new potential biomarkers for prostate cancer diagnosis and prognosis. *Prostate*, *74*(12), 1171–1182. doi:10.1002/pros.22833.
4. Meshorer, E., & Misteli, T. (2006). Chromatin in pluripotent embryonic stem cells and differentiation. *Nature Reviews. Molecular Cell Biology*, *7*(7), 540–546. doi:10.1038/nrm1938.
5. Zaidi, S., Choi, M., Wakimoto, H., et al. (2013). De novo mutations in histone-modifying genes in congenital heart disease. *Nature*, *498*(7453), 220–223. doi:10.1038/nature12141.
6. Balhorn, R. (2007). The protamine family of sperm nuclear proteins. *Genome Biology*, *8*(9), 227. doi:10.1186/gb-2007-8-9-227.
7. Deng, Q., Ramsköld, D., Reinius, B., et al. (2014). Single-cell RNA-seq reveals dynamic, random monoallelic gene expression in mammalian cells. *Science*, *343*(6167), 193–196. doi:10.1126/science.1245316.
8. Cassidy, S. B., Schwartz, S., Miller, J. L., et al. (2012). Prader-Willi syndrome. *Genetics in Medicine*, *14*(1), 10–26. doi:10.1038/gim.0b013e31822bead0.
9. Williams, C. A., Beaudet, A. L., Clayton-Smith, J., et al. (2006). Angelman syndrome 2005: Updated consensus for diagnostic criteria. *American Journal of Medical Genetics. Part A*, *140*(5), 413–418. doi:10.1002/ajmg.a.31074.
10. Horsthemke, B., & Wagstaff, J. (2008). Mechanisms of imprinting of the Prader-Willi/Angelman region. *American Journal of Medical Genetics. Part A*, *146A*(16), 2041–2052. doi:10.1002/ajmg.a.32364.
11. Kaminen-Ahola, N., Ahola, A., Maga, M., et al. (2010). Maternal ethanol consumption alters the epigenotype and the phenotype of offspring in a mouse model. *PLoS Genetics*, *6*(1), e1000811. doi:10.1371/journal.pgen.1000811.
12. Stuffrein-Roberts, S., & Kennedy, J. (2008). Role of epigenetics in mental disorders. *Australian and New Zealand Journal of Psychiatry*, *42*(2), 97–107. doi:10.1080/00048670701787495.
13. Bygren, L. O., Tinghög, P., Carstensen, J., et al. (2014). Change in paternal grandmothers' early food supply influenced cardiovascular mortality of the female grandchildren. *BMC Genetics*, *15*, 12. doi:10.1186/1471-2156-15-12.
14. van Esterik, J. C., Dollé, M. E., Lamoree, M. H., et al. (2014). Programming of metabolic effects in C57BL/6JxFVB mice by exposure to bisphenol A during gestation and lactation. *Toxicology*, *321*, 40–52. doi:10.1016/j.tox.2014.04.001.
15. Weaver, I. C., Cervoni, N., Champagne, F. A., et al. (2004). Epigenetic programming by maternal behavior. *Nature Neuroscience*, *7*(8), 847–854. doi:10.1038/nn1276.
16. Anacker, C., O'Donnell, K. J., & Meaney, M. J. (2014). Early life adversity and the epigenetic programming of hypothalamic-pituitary-adrenal function. *Dialogues in Clinical Neuroscience*, *16*(3), 321–333.
17. Jones, K. L., Smith, D. W., Ulleland, C. N., et al. (1973). Pattern of malformation in offspring of chronic alcoholic mothers. *Lancet*, *1*(7815), 1267–1271.
18. Zhou, F. C., Balaraman, Y., Teng, M., et al. (2011). Alcohol alters DNA methylation patterns and inhibits neural stem cell differentiation. *Alcoholism, Clinical and Experimental Research*, *35*(4), 735–746. doi:10.1111/j.1530-0277.2010.01391.x.
19. Mukhopadhyay, P., Rezzoug, F., Kaikaus, J., et al. (2013). Alcohol modulates expression of DNA methyltransferases and methyl CpG-/CpG domain-binding proteins in murine embryonic fibroblasts. *Reproductive Toxicology*, *37*, 40–48. doi:10.1016/j.reprotox.2013.01.003.
20. Lu, C., Lin, L., Tan, H., et al. (2012). Fragile X premutation RNA is sufficient to cause primary ovarian insufficiency in mice. *Human Molecular Genetics*, *21*(23), 5039–5047. doi:10.1093/hmg/dds348.
21. Jacquemot, S. (2004). Penetrance of the fragile X–associated tremor/ataxia syndrome in a premutation carrier population. *JAMA: The Journal of the American Medical Association*, *291*(4), 460–469. doi:10.1001/jama.291.4.460.
22. Tassone, F., Hagerman, R. J., Garcia-Arocena, D., et al. (2004). Intranuclear inclusions in neural cells with premutation alleles in fragile X associated tremor/ataxia syndrome. *Journal of Medical Genetics*, *41*(4), e43.
23. Stöger, R., Kajimura, T. M., Brown, W. T., et al. (1997). Epigenetic variation illustrated by DNA methylation patterns of the fragile-X gene *FMR1*. *Human Molecular Genetics*, *6*(11), 1791–1801.
24. Cabianca, D. S., & Gabellini, D. (2010). The cell biology of disease: FSHD: Copy number variations on the theme of muscular dystrophy. *Journal of Cell Biology*, *191*(6), 1049–1060. doi:10.1083/jcb.201007028.
25. Bodega, B., Ramirez, G. D., Grasser, F., et al. (2009). Remodeling of the chromatin structure of the facioscapulohumeral muscular dystrophy (FSHD) locus and upregulation of FSHD-related gene 1 (*FRG1*) expression during human myogenic differentiation. *BMC Biology*, *7*, 41. doi:10.1186/1741-7007-7-41.
26. Fraga, M. F., Ballestar, E., Paz, M. F., et al. (2005). Epigenetic differences arise during the lifetime of monozygotic twins. *Proceedings of the National Academy of Sciences of the United States of America*, *102*(30), 10604–10609. doi:10.1073/pnas.0500398102.
27. Frommer, M., McDonald, L. E., Millar, D. S., et al. (1992). A genomic sequencing protocol that yields a positive display of 5-methylcytosine residues in individual DNA strands. *Proceedings of the National Academy of Sciences of the United States of America*, *89*(5), 1827–1831.
28. Peters, A. H., Kubicek, S., Mechtier, K., et al. (2003). Partitioning and plasticity of repressive histone methylation states in mammalian chromatin. *Molecular Cell*, *12*(6), 1577–1589.
29. Esteller, M. (2008). Epigenetics in cancer. *New England Journal of Medicine*, *358*(11), 1148–1159. doi:10.1056/NEJMra072067.
30. Sandoval, J., & Esteller, M. (2012). Cancer epigenomics: Beyond genomics. *Current Opinion in Genetics & Development*, *22*(1), 50–55. doi:10.1016/j.gde.2012.02.008.
31. Giacinti, C., & Giordano, A. (2006). RB and cell cycle progression. *Oncogene*, *25*(38), 5220–5227. doi:10.1038/sj.onc.1209615.
32. Hansmann, T., Pliushch, G., Leubner, M., et al. (2012). Constitutive promoter methylation of *BRCA1* and *RAD51C* in patients with familial ovarian cancer and early-onset sporadic breast cancer. *Human Molecular Genetics*, *21*(21), 4669–4679. doi:10.1093/hmg/dds308.
33. Lynch, H. T., & de la Chapelle, A. (2003). Hereditary colorectal cancer. *New England Journal of Medicine*, *348*(10), 919–932. doi:10.1056/NEJMra012242.
34. Pino, M. S., & Chung, D. C. (2011). Microsatellite instability in the management of colorectal cancer. *Expert Review of Gastroenterology & Hepatology*, *5*(3), 385–399. doi:10.1586/egh.11.25.
35. Hong, J., Li, D., Wands, J., et al. (2013). Role of NADPH oxidase NOX5-S, NF-κB, and DNMT1 in acid-induced p16 hypermethylation in Barrett's cells. *American Journal of Physiology. Cell Physiology*, *305*(10), C1069–C1079. doi:10.1152/ajpcell.00080.2013.
36. Tao, K., Yang, J., Guo, Z., et al. (2014). Prognostic value of miR-221-3p, miR-342-3p and miR-491-5p expression in colon cancer. *American Journal of Translational Research*, *6*(4), 391–401.
37. Ahmad, A., Sethi, S., Chen, W., et al. (2014). Up-regulation of microRNA-10b is associated with the development of breast cancer brain metastasis. *American Journal of Translational Research*, *6*(4), 384–390.
38. Ren, Q., Liang, J., Wei, J., et al. (2014). Epithelial and stromal expression of miRNAs during prostate cancer progression. *American Journal of Translational Research*, *6*(4), 329–339.
39. Dulaimi, E., Uzzo, R. G., Greenberg, R. E., et al. (2004). Detection of bladder cancer in urine by a tumor suppressor gene hypermethylation panel. *Clinical Cancer Research*, *10*(6), 1887–1893.
40. Guzmán, L., Depix, M. S., Salinas, A. M., et al. (2012). Analysis of aberrant methylation on promoter sequences of tumor suppressor genes and total DNA in sputum samples: A promising tool for early detection of COPD and lung cancer in smokers. *Diagnostic Pathology*, *7*, 87. doi:10.1186/1746-1596-7-87.
41. Henrique, R., & Jerónimo, C. (2004). Molecular detection of prostate cancer: A role for GSTP1 hypermethylation. *European Urology*, *46*(5), 660–669, discussion 669. doi:10.1016/j.eururo.2004.06.014.
42. Di Costanzo, A., Del Gaudio, N., Miglicaccio, A., et al. (2014). Epigenetic drugs against cancer: An evolving landscape. *Toxicology*, *88*(9), 1651–1668. doi:10.1007/s00204-014-1315-6.
43. Christman, J. K. (2002). 5-Azacytidine and 5-aza-2'-deoxycytidine as inhibitors of DNA methylation: Mechanistic studies and their implications for cancer therapy. *Oncogene*, *21*(35), 5483–5495. doi:10.1038/sj.onc.1205699.
44. Zhang, H., Zhou, W. C., Li, X., et al. (2014). 5-Azacytidine suppresses the proliferation of pancreatic cancer cells by inhibiting the Wnt/β-catenin signaling pathway. *Genetics and Molecular Research*, *13*(3), 5064–5072. doi:10.4238/2014.July.4.22.
45. Jabbour, E., & Garcia-Manero, G. (2015). Deacetylase inhibitors for the treatment of myelodysplastic syndromes. *Leukemia and Lymphoma*, *56*(5), 1205–1212. doi:10.3109/10428194.2014.946025.

46. Müller-Thomas, C., Rudelius, M., Rondak, I. C., et al. (2014). Response to azacitidine is independent of p53 expression in higher-risk myelodysplastic syndromes and secondary acute myeloid leukemia. *Haematologica*, *99*(10), e179–e181. doi:10.3324/haematol.2014.104760.
47. Tate, C. R., Rhodes, L. V., Segar, H. C., et al. (2012). Targeting triple-negative breast cancer cells with the histone deacetylase inhibitor panobinostat. *Breast Cancer Research: BCR*, *14*(3), R79. doi:10.1186/bcr3192.
48. Chen, C. S., Wang, Y. C., Yang, H. C., et al. (2007). Histone deacetylase inhibitors sensitize prostate cancer cells to agents that produce DNA double-strand breaks by targeting Ku70 acetylation. *Cancer Research*, *67*(11), 5318–5327. doi:10.1158/0008-5472.CAN-06-3996.
49. Koutsounas, I., Giagnis, C., & Theocharis, S. (2013). Histone deacetylase inhibitors and pancreatic cancer: Are there any promising clinical trials? *World Journal of Gastroenterology*, *19*(8), 1173–1181. doi:10.3748/wjg.v19.i8.1173.

4

Altered Cellular and Tissue Biology

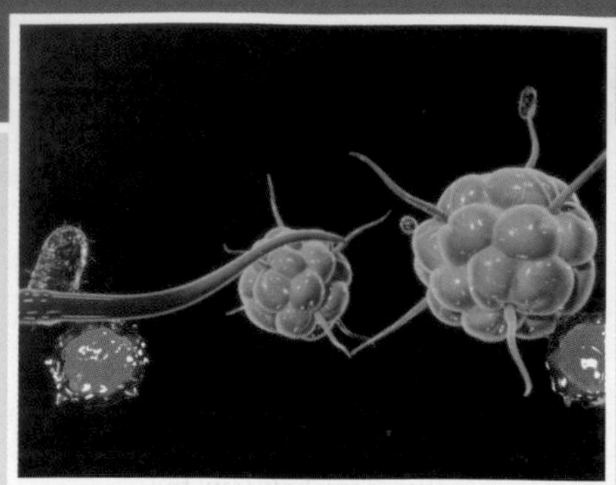

Kathryn L. McCance, Todd Cameron Grey, and Stephanie Zettel

EVOLVE WEBSITE

http://evolve.elsevier.com/Canada/Huether/pathophysiology
Student Review Questions
Key Points
Case Studies
Animations
Quick Check Answers

CHAPTER OUTLINE

Cellular Adaptation, 75
- Atrophy, 75
- Hypertrophy, 76
- Hyperplasia, 77
- Dysplasia: Not a True Adaptive Change, 77
- Metaplasia, 78

Cellular Injury, 78
- General Mechanisms of Cellular Injury, 79
- Hypoxic Injury, 80
- Free Radicals and Reactive Oxygen Species Injury: Oxidative Stress, 82
- Chemical or Toxic Injury, 83
- Unintentional and Intentional Injuries, 93
- Infectious Injury, 96
- Immunological and Inflammatory Injury, 96

Manifestations of Cellular Injury: Accumulations, 96
- Water, 97
- Lipids and Carbohydrates, 97
- Glycogen, 98
- Proteins, 99
- Pigments, 99
- Calcium, 100
- Urate, 100
- Systemic Manifestations, 101

Cellular Death, 101
- Necrosis, 101
- Apoptosis, 105
- Autophagy, 106

Aging and Altered Cellular and Tissue Biology, 107
- Normal Lifespan, Life Expectancy, and Quality-Adjusted Life Year, 108
- Degenerative Extracellular Changes, 108
- Cellular Aging, 108
- Tissue and Systemic Aging, 109
- Frailty, 109

Somatic Death, 109

The majority of diseases are caused by many factors acting together (i.e., *multifactorial*) or interacting with a genetically susceptible person. Injury to cells and their surrounding environment, called the *extracellular matrix* (ECM), leads to tissue and organ injury. Although the normal cell is restricted by a narrow range of structure and functions, including metabolism and specialization, it can *adapt* to physiological demands or stress to maintain a steady state called *homeostasis*. **Adaptation** is a reversible, structural, or functional response both to normal or physiological conditions and to adverse or pathological conditions. For example, the uterus adapts to pregnancy—a normal physiological state—by enlarging. Enlargement occurs because of an increase in the size and number of uterine cells. In an adverse condition, such as high blood pressure, myocardial cells are stimulated to enlarge by the increased work of pumping. Like most of the body's adaptive mechanisms, however, cellular adaptations to adverse conditions are usually only temporarily successful. Severe or long-term stressors overwhelm adaptive processes and cellular injury or death ensues. Altered cellular and tissue biology can result from adaptation, injury, neoplasia, accumulations, aging, or death. (Neoplasia is discussed in Chapters 10 and 11.)

Knowledge of the structural and functional reactions of cells and tissues to injurious agents, including genetic defects, is vital to understanding disease processes. Cellular injury can be caused by any factor that disrupts cellular structures or deprives the cell of oxygen and nutrients required for survival. Injury may be reversible (*sublethal*) or irreversible (*lethal*) and is classified broadly as chemical, hypoxic (lack of sufficient oxygen), free radical, intentional, unintentional, immunological, infection, and inflammatory. Cellular injuries from various causes have different clinical and pathophysiological manifestations. Stresses from metabolic derangements may be associated with intracellular *accumulations* and include carbohydrates, proteins, and lipids. Sites of cellular death can cause accumulations of calcium resulting in *pathological calcification*. Cellular death is confirmed by structural changes seen when cells are stained and examined under a microscope. The two main types of cellular death are *necrosis* and *apoptosis*, and nutrient deprivation can initiate *autophagy* that results in cellular death. All of these pathways of cellular death are discussed later in this chapter.

Cellular aging causes structural and functional changes that eventually may lead to cellular death or a decreased capacity to recover from injury.

Mechanisms explaining how and why cells age are not known, and distinguishing between pathological changes and physiological changes that occur with aging is often difficult. Aging clearly causes alterations in cellular structure and function, yet *senescence*, growing old, is both inevitable and normal.

CELLULAR ADAPTATION

Cells adapt to their environment to escape and protect themselves from injury. An adapted cell is neither normal nor injured—its condition lies somewhere between these two states. Adaptations are reversible changes in cell size, number, phenotype, metabolic activity, or functions of cells.[1] Adaptive responses have limits, however, and additional cell stresses can affect essential cell function leading to *cellular injury*. Cellular adaptations also can be a common and central part of many disease states. In the early stages of a successful adaptive response, cells may have enhanced function; thus, it is hard to distinguish a pathological response from an extreme adaptation to an excessive functional demand. The most significant adaptive changes in cells include atrophy (decrease in cell size), hypertrophy (increase in cell size), hyperplasia (increase in cell number), and metaplasia (reversible replacement of one mature cell type by another less mature cell type or a change in the phenotype). Dysplasia (deranged cellular growth) is not considered a true cellular adaptation but rather an atypical hyperplasia. These changes are shown in Figure 4-1.

Atrophy

Atrophy is a decrease or shrinkage in cellular size. If atrophy occurs in a sufficient number of an organ's cells, the entire organ shrinks or becomes atrophic. Atrophy can affect any organ, but it is most common in skeletal muscle, the heart, secondary sex organs, and the brain. Atrophy can be classified as *physiological* or *pathological*. **Physiological atrophy** occurs with early development. For example, the thymus gland undergoes physiological atrophy during childhood. **Pathological atrophy** occurs as a result of decreases in workload, pressure, use, blood supply, nutrition, hormonal stimulation, and nervous system stimulation (Figure 4-2). Individuals immobilized in bed for a prolonged period of time exhibit a type of skeletal muscle atrophy called **disuse atrophy**. Aging causes brain cells to become atrophic and endocrine-dependent organs, such as the gonads, to shrink as hormonal stimulation decreases. Whether atrophy is caused by normal physiological conditions or by pathological conditions, atrophic cells exhibit the same basic changes.

The atrophic muscle cell contains less endoplasmic reticulum (ER) and fewer mitochondria and myofilaments (part of the muscle fibre that controls contraction) than found in the normal cell. In muscular atrophy caused by nerve loss, oxygen consumption and amino acid uptake are immediately reduced. The mechanisms of atrophy include decreased protein synthesis, increased protein catabolism, or both. A new hypothesis includes ribosome function and its role as translation machinery or the conversion of messenger RNA (mRNA) into protein called *ribosome biogenesis*. Ribosome biogenesis has an important role in the regulation of skeletal muscle mass.[2] The primary pathway of protein catabolism is the **ubiquitin–proteasome pathway**, and catabolism involves **proteasomes** (protein-degrading complexes). Proteins degraded in this pathway are first conjugated to **ubiquitin** (another small protein) and then degraded by proteasomes. An increase in proteasome activity is characteristic of atrophic muscle changes. Deregulation of this pathway often leads to abnormal cell growth and is associated with cancer and other diseases (see Chapters 3 and 10).

Atrophy as a result of chronic malnutrition is often accompanied by a "self-eating" process called *autophagy* that creates **autophagic vacuoles** (see p. 75). These vacuoles are membrane-bound vesicles within the cell that contain cellular debris and hydrolytic enzymes, which function to break down substances to the simplest units of fat, carbohydrate, or protein. The levels of hydrolytic enzymes rise rapidly in atrophy. The enzymes are isolated in autophagic vacuoles to prevent

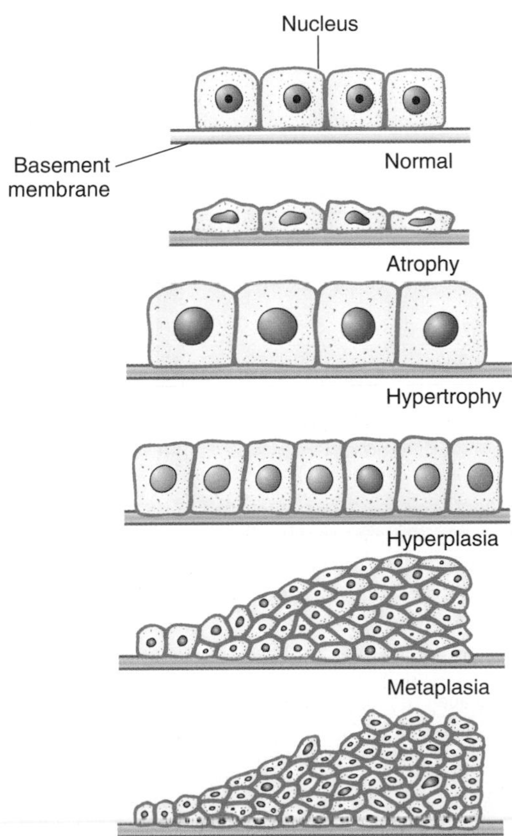

FIGURE 4-1 Adaptive and Dysplastic Alterations in Simple Cuboidal Epithelial Cells.

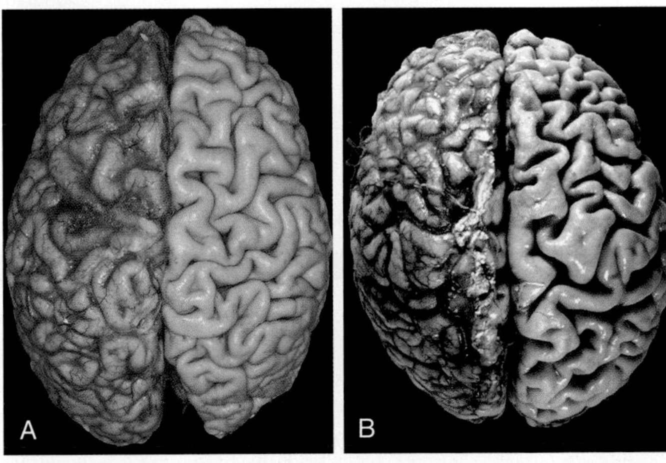

FIGURE 4-2 Atrophy. A, Normal brain of a young adult. **B,** Atrophy of the brain in an 82-year-old male with atherosclerotic cerebrovascular disease, resulting in reduced blood supply. Note that loss of brain substance narrows the gyri and widens the sulci. The meninges have been stripped from the right half of each specimen to reveal the surface of the brain. (From Kumar, V., Abbas, A.K., & Aster, J.C. [Eds.]. [2015]. *Robbins and Cotran pathologic basis of disease* [9th ed.]. Philadelphia: Saunders.)

uncontrolled cellular destruction. Thus the vacuoles form as needed to protect uninjured organelles from the injured organelles and are eventually engulfed and destroyed by lysosomes. Certain contents of the autophagic vacuole may resist destruction by lysosomal enzymes and persist in membrane-bound residual bodies. An example of granules that can persist and resist breakdown is granules containing **lipofuscin**, the yellow-brown age pigment. Lipofuscin accumulates primarily in liver cells, myocardial cells, and atrophic cells.

Hypertrophy

Hypertrophy is a compensatory increase in the size of cells in response to mechanical stimuli (also called *mechanical load* or *stress,* such as from repetitive stretching, chronic pressure, or volume overload) and consequently increases the size of the affected organ (Figures 4-3 and 4-4). The cells of the heart and kidneys are particularly prone to enlargement. Hypertrophy, as an adaptive response (muscular enlargement), occurs in the striated muscle cells of both the heart and skeletal

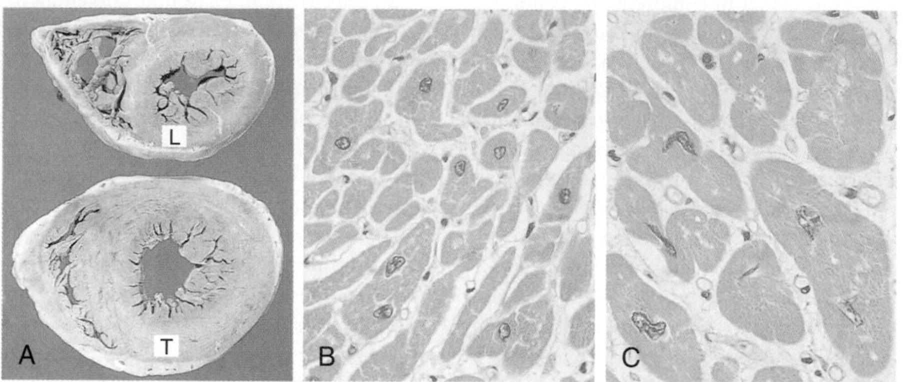

FIGURE 4-3 Hypertrophy of Cardiac Muscle in Response to Valve Disease. A, Transverse slices of a normal heart and a heart with hypertrophy of the left ventricle (*L*, normal thickness of left ventricular wall; *T*, thickened wall from heart in which severe narrowing of aortic valve caused resistance to systolic ventricular emptying). **B,** Histology of cardiac muscle from the normal heart. **C,** Histology of cardiac muscle from a hypertrophied heart. (From Stevens, A., & Lowe, J. [2000]. *Pathology: Illustrated review in color* [2nd ed.]. Edinburgh: Mosby.)

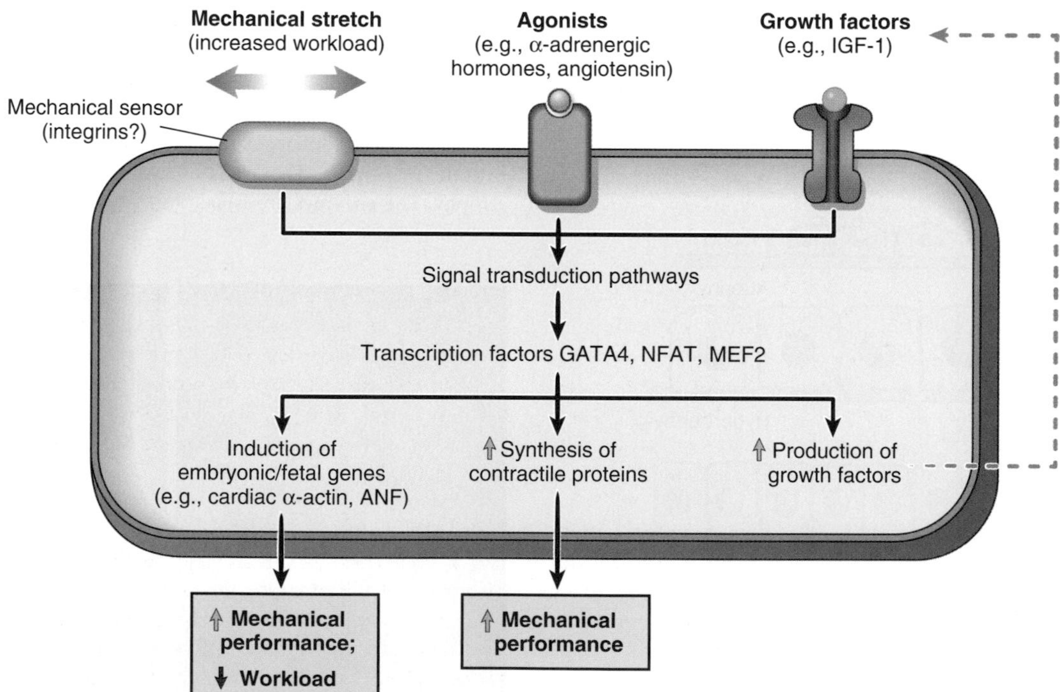

FIGURE 4-4 Mechanisms of Myocardial Hypertrophy. Mechanical sensors appear to be the main stimulators for physiological hypertrophy. Other stimuli possibly more important for pathological hypertrophy include agonists (initiators) and growth factors. These factors then signal transcription pathways whereby transcription factors then bind to DNA sequences, activating muscle proteins that are responsible for hypertrophy. These pathways include induction of embryonic/fetal genes, increased synthesis of contractile proteins, and production of growth factors. *ANF,* atrial natriuretic factor; *IGF-1,* insulinlike growth factor 1; *NFAT,* nuclear factor of activated T-cells; *MEF2,* myocyte enhancer factor-2. (Adapted from Kumar, V., Abbas, A.K., & Aster, J.C. [Eds.]. [2015]. *Robbins and Cotran pathologic basis of disease* [9th ed.]. Philadelphia: Saunders.)

muscles. Initial cardiac enlargement is caused by dilation of the cardiac chambers, is short lived, and is followed by increased synthesis of cardiac muscle proteins, allowing muscle fibres to do more work. The increase in cellular size is associated with an increased accumulation of protein in the cellular components (plasma membrane, ER, myofilaments, mitochondria) and *not* with an increase in cellular fluid. Yet, individual protein pools may expand or shrink.[3] Cardiac hypertrophy involves changes in signalling and transcription factor pathways resulting in increased protein synthesis, leading to left ventricular hypertrophy (LVH). Emerging evidence suggests that the ubiquitin–proteasome system (UPS) not only attends to damaged, misfolded, or mutant proteins by protein breakdown but also may attend to cell growth eventually leading to LVH.[4] With time, cardiac hypertrophy is characterized by ECM remodelling and increased growth of adult myocytes. The myocytes progressively increase in size and reach a limit beyond which no further hypertrophy can occur (see Chapter 24).[5,6]

Although hypertrophy can be classified as *physiological* or *pathological*, time may be the critical factor or determinant of the transition from physiological to pathological cardiac hypertrophy. With *physiological hypertrophy*, preservation of myocardial structure characterizes postnatal development, moderate endurance exercise training, pregnancy, and the early phases of increased pressure and volume loading on the adult human heart. This physiological response is temporary; however, aging, strenuous exercise, and sustained workload or stress lead to pathological hypertrophy with structural and functional manifestations. *Pathological hypertrophy* in the heart is secondary to hypertension, coronary heart disease, or problem valves and is presumably a key risk factor for heart failure. Additionally, it is associated with increased interstitial fibrosis, cellular death, and abnormal cardiac function (see Figure 4-3). Historically, the progression of pathological cardiac hypertrophy has been considered irreversible. However, emerging data from experimental studies and clinical observations show reversal of pathological cardiac hypertrophy in certain cases. Cardiac hypertrophy can be reversed when the increased wall stress is normalized, a process termed *regression*.[7] For example, unloading of hemodynamic stress by a left ventricular assist device (used in individuals with heart failure for bridging to heart transplantation) induces regression of cardiac hypertrophy and improvement of left ventricular function in those with end-stage heart failure.[8] Regression of cardiac hypertrophy is accompanied by activation of unique sets of genes, including fetal-type genes and those involved in protein degradation.[9,10] However, the signalling mechanisms mediating regression of cardiac hypertrophy have been poorly understood. Improvement in new blood vessel development (angiogenesis) in the hypertrophic heart can lead to regression of the hypertrophy and prevention of heart failure.[11,12] In mice, dietary supplementation of physiologically relevant levels of copper can reverse pathological cardiac hypertrophy.[12,13]

When a diseased kidney is removed, the remaining kidney adapts to the increased workload with an increase in both the size and the number of cells. The major contributing factor to this renal enlargement is hypertrophy. Another example of normal or physiological hypertrophy is the increased growth of the uterus and mammary glands in response to pregnancy.

Hyperplasia

Hyperplasia is an increase in the number of cells, resulting from an increased rate of cellular division. Hyperplasia, as a response to injury, occurs when the injury has been severe and prolonged enough to have caused cellular death. Loss of epithelial cells and cells of the liver and kidney triggers deoxyribonucleic acid (DNA) synthesis and mitotic division. Increased cell growth is a multistep process involving the production of growth factors, which stimulate the remaining cells to synthesize new cell components and, ultimately, to divide. Hyperplasia and hypertrophy often occur together, and both take place if the cells can synthesize DNA.

Two types of normal, or physiological, hyperplasia are compensatory hyperplasia and hormonal hyperplasia. **Compensatory hyperplasia** is an adaptive mechanism that enables certain organs to regenerate. For example, removal of part of the liver leads to hyperplasia of the remaining liver cells (hepatocytes) to compensate for the loss. Even with removal of 70% of the liver, regeneration is complete in about 2 weeks. Several growth factors and cytokines (chemical messengers) are induced and play critical roles in liver regeneration.

Not all types of mature cells have the same capacity for compensatory hyperplastic growth. Nondividing tissues contain cells that can no longer (i.e., postnatally) go through the cell cycle and undergo mitotic division. These highly specialized cells, for example, neurons and skeletal muscle cells, never divide again once they have differentiated—that is, they are *terminally differentiated*.[14] In human cells, cell growth and cell division depend on signals from other cells; but cell growth, unlike cell division, does not depend on the cell-cycle control system.[14] Nerve cells and most muscle cells do most of their growing after they have terminally differentiated and permanently ceased dividing.[14] Significant compensatory hyperplasia occurs in epidermal and intestinal epithelia, hepatocytes, bone marrow cells, and fibroblasts; and some hyperplasia is noted in bone, cartilage, and smooth muscle cells. Another example of compensatory hyperplasia is the callus, or thickening, of the skin as a result of hyperplasia of epidermal cells in response to a mechanical stimulus.

Hormonal hyperplasia occurs chiefly in estrogen-dependent organs, such as the uterus and breast. After ovulation, for example, estrogen stimulates the endometrium to grow and thicken in preparation for receiving the fertilized ovum. If pregnancy occurs, hormonal hyperplasia, as well as hypertrophy, enables the uterus to enlarge. (Hormone function is described in Chapters 19 and 33.)

Pathological hyperplasia is the abnormal proliferation of normal cells, usually in response to excessive hormonal stimulation or growth factors on target cells (Figure 4-5). The most common example is pathological hyperplasia of the endometrium (caused by an imbalance between estrogen and progesterone secretion, with oversecretion of estrogen) (see Chapter 33). Pathological endometrial hyperplasia, which causes excessive menstrual bleeding, is under the influence of regular growth-inhibition controls. If these controls fail, hyperplastic endometrial cells can undergo malignant transformation. Benign prostatic hyperplasia is another example of pathological hyperplasia and results from changes in hormone balance. In both of these examples, if the hormonal imbalance is corrected, hyperplasia regresses.[1]

Dysplasia: Not a True Adaptive Change

Dysplasia refers to abnormal changes in the size, shape, and organization of mature cells (Figure 4-6). Dysplasia is not considered a true adaptive process but is related to hyperplasia and is often called **atypical hyperplasia**. Dysplastic changes often are encountered in epithelial tissue of the cervix and respiratory tract, where they are strongly associated with common neoplastic growths and often are found adjacent to cancerous cells. Importantly, however, the term *dysplasia* does *not* indicate cancer and may not progress to cancer. Dysplasia is often classified as mild, moderate, or severe; yet, because this classification scheme is somewhat subjective, it has prompted some to recommend the use of either "low grade" or "high grade" instead. If the inciting stimulus is removed, dysplastic changes often are reversible. (Dysplasia is discussed further in Chapter 10.)

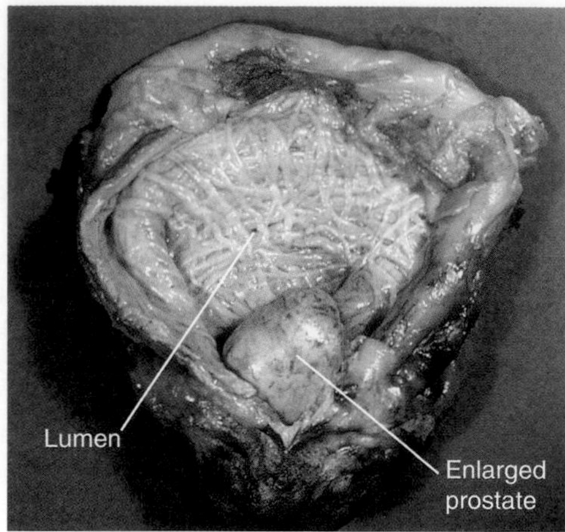

FIGURE 4-5 Hyperplasia of the Prostate with Secondary Thickening of the Obstructed Urinary Bladder (Bladder Cross-Section). The enlarged prostate is seen protruding into the lumen of the bladder, which appears trabeculated. These "trabeculae" result from hypertrophy and hyperplasia of smooth muscle cells that occur in response to increased intravesical pressure caused by urinary obstruction. (From Damjanov, I. [2012]. *Pathology for the health professions* [4th ed.]. St. Louis: Saunders.)

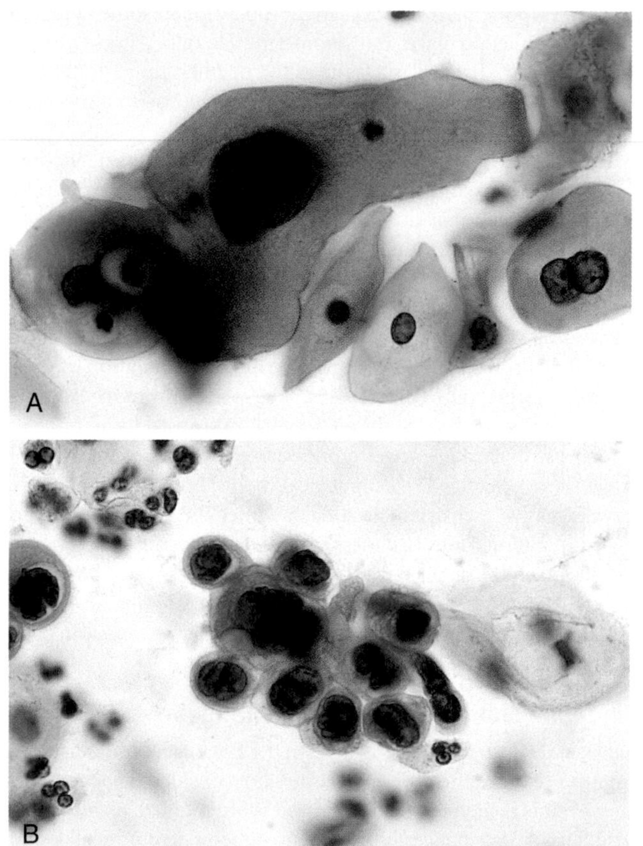

FIGURE 4-6 Dysplasia of the Uterine Cervix. A, Mild dysplasia. **B,** Severe dysplasia. (From Damjanov, I., & Linder, J. [1996]. *Anderson's pathology* [10th ed.]. St. Louis: Mosby.)

Metaplasia

Metaplasia is the reversible replacement of one mature cell type (epithelial or mesenchymal) by another, sometimes less differentiated, cell type. It is thought to develop (as an adaptive response better suited to withstand the adverse environment) from a reprogramming of stem cells that exist on most epithelia or of undifferentiated **mesenchymal (tissue from embryonic mesoderm) cells** present in connective tissue. These precursor cells mature along a new pathway because of signals generated by growth factors in the cell's environment. The best example of metaplasia is replacement of normal columnar ciliated epithelial cells of the bronchial (airway) lining by stratified squamous epithelial cells (Figure 4-7). The newly formed cells do not secrete mucus or have cilia, causing loss of a vital protective mechanism. Bronchial metaplasia can be reversed if the inducing stimulus, usually cigarette smoking, is removed. With prolonged exposure to the inducing stimulus, however, dysplasia and cancerous transformation can occur.

TABLE 4-1 Types of Progressive Cellular Injury and Responses

Type	Responses
Adaptation	Atrophy, hypertrophy, hyperplasia, metaplasia
Active cellular injury	Immediate response of "entire" cell
Reversible	Loss of ATP, cellular swelling, detachment of ribosomes, autophagy of lysosomes
Irreversible	"Point of no return" structurally when severe vacuolization of mitochondria occurs and Ca^{++} moves into cell
Necrosis	Common type of cellular death with severe cell swelling and breakdown of organelles
Apoptosis, or programmed cellular death	Cellular self-destruction for elimination of unwanted cell populations
Autophagy	Eating of self, cytoplasmic vesicles engulf cytoplasm and organelles, recycling factory
Chronic cellular injury (subcellular alterations)	Persistent stimuli response may involve only specific organelles or cytoskeleton (e.g., phagocytosis of bacteria)
Accumulations or infiltrations	Water, pigments, lipids, glycogen, proteins
Pathological calcification	Dystrophic and metastatic calcification

ATP, adenosine triphosphate; *Ca^{++}*, calcium.

CELLULAR INJURY

Injury to cells and to the ECM leads to injury of tissues and organs, ultimately determining the structural patterns of disease. Loss of function is derived from cell and ECM injury and cellular death. Cellular injury occurs if the cell is unable to maintain homeostasis—a normal or adaptive steady state—in the face of injurious stimuli or stress. Injured cells may recover (**reversible injury**) or die (**irreversible injury**). Injurious stimuli include chemical agents, lack of sufficient oxygen (hypoxia), free radicals, infectious agents, physical and mechanical factors, immunological reactions, genetic factors, and nutritional imbalances. Types of injuries and their responses are summarized in Table 4-1 and Figure 4-8.

The extent of cellular injury depends on the type, state (including level of cell differentiation and increased susceptibility to fully differentiated cells), and adaptive processes of the cell, as well as the type, severity, and duration of the injurious stimulus. Two individuals exposed to an identical stimulus may incur varying degrees of cellular injury. Modifying factors, such as nutritional status, can profoundly influence the extent of injury. The precise "point of no return" that leads to cellular death is a biochemical puzzle, but once changes to the nucleus

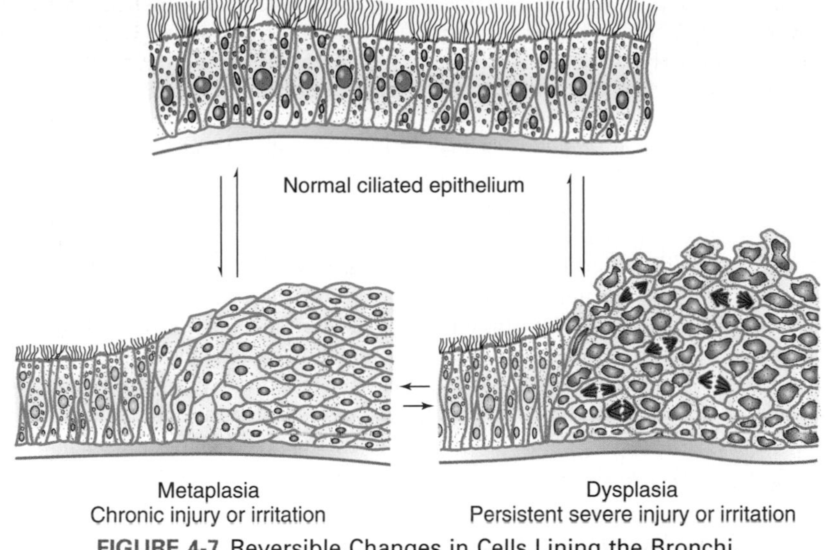

FIGURE 4-7 Reversible Changes in Cells Lining the Bronchi.

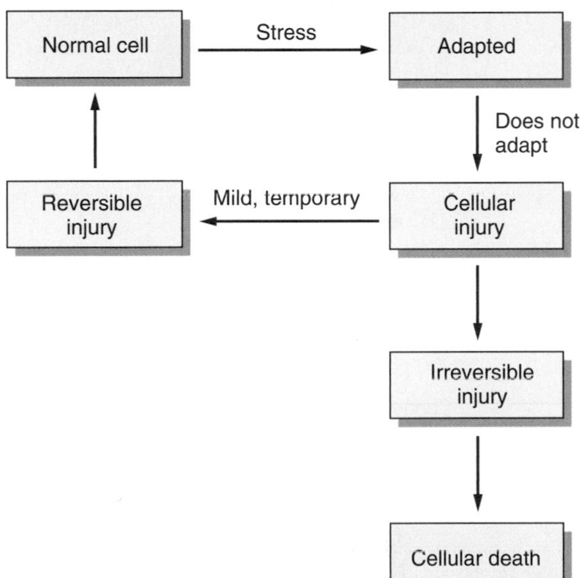

FIGURE 4-8 Stages of Cellular Adaptation, Injury, and Death. The normal cell responds to physiological and pathological stresses by adapting (atrophy, hypertrophy, hyperplasia, metaplasia). Cellular injury occurs if the adaptive responses are exceeded or compromised by injurious agents, stress, and mutations. The injury is reversible if it is mild or transient, but if the stimulus persists, the cell suffers irreversible injury and eventually death.

occur and cell membranes are disrupted, the cell moves to irreversible injury and death.

General Mechanisms of Cellular Injury

Common biochemical themes are important to understanding cellular injury and cellular death, regardless of the injuring agent. These include adenosine triphosphate (ATP) depletion, mitochondrial damage, oxygen and oxygen-derived free radical membrane damage (depletion of ATP), protein folding defects, DNA damage defects, and calcium-level alterations (Table 4-2). Examples of common forms of cellular injury are (1) hypoxic injury, (2) free radicals and reactive oxygen species injury, and (3) chemical injury.

TABLE 4-2 Common Themes in Cellular Injury and Cellular Death

Theme	Comments
ATP depletion	Loss of mitochondrial ATP and decreased ATP synthesis; results include cellular swelling, decreased protein synthesis, decreased membrane transport, and lipogenesis, all changes that contribute to loss of integrity of plasma membrane
Reactive oxygen species (↑ROS)	Lack of oxygen is key in progression of cellular injury in ischemia (reduced blood supply); activated oxygen species (ROS, $O_2^{\bar{\cdot}}$, H_2O_2, •OH) cause destruction of cell membranes and cell structure
Ca^{++} entry	Normally intracellular cytosolic calcium concentrations are very low; ischemia and certain chemicals cause an increase in cytosolic Ca^{++} concentrations; sustained levels of Ca^{++} continue to increase with damage to plasma membrane; Ca^{++} causes intracellular damage by activating a number of enzymes
Mitochondrial damage	Can be damaged by increases in cytosolic Ca^{++}, ROS; two outcomes of mitochondrial damage are loss of membrane potential, which causes depletion of ATP and eventual death or necrosis of cell, and activation of another type of cellular death (apoptosis) (see p. 105)
Membrane damage	Early loss of selective membrane permeability found in all forms of cellular injury, lysosomal membrane damage with release of enzymes causing cellular digestion
Protein misfolding, DNA damage	Proteins may misfold, triggering *unfolded protein response* that activates corrective responses; if overwhelmed, response activates cell suicide program or apoptosis; DNA damage (genotoxic stress) also can activate apoptosis (see p. 105)

ATP, adenosine triphosphate; *Ca^{++}*, calcium.

Hypoxic Injury

Hypoxia, or lack of sufficient oxygen within cells, is the single most common cause of cellular injury (Figure 4-9). Hypoxia can result from a reduced amount of oxygen in the air, loss of hemoglobin or decreased efficacy of hemoglobin, decreased production of red blood cells, diseases of the respiratory and cardiovascular systems, and poisoning of the oxidative enzymes (cytochromes) within the cells. Hypoxia plays a role in physiological processes including cell differentiation, angiogenesis, proliferation, erythropoiesis, and overall cell viability.[15] The main consumers of oxygen are mitochondria, and the cellular responses to hypoxia are reported to be mediated by the production of reactive oxygen species (ROS) at the mitochondrial complex III.[15] Investigators are studying the role of ROS as hypoxia signalling molecules. More commonly, hypoxia is associated with the pathophysiological conditions such as inflammation, ischemia, and cancer. Hypoxia can induce inflammation, and inflamed lesions can become hypoxic (Figure 4-10).[16] The cellular mechanisms involved in hypoxia and inflammation are emerging and include activation of immune responses and oxygen-sensing compounds called *prolyl hydroxylases* (PHDs) and hypoxia-inducible transcription factor (HIF). HIF is a family of transcription regulators that coordinate the expression of many genes in response to oxygen deprivation. Mammalian development occurs in a hypoxic environment.[17] Hypoxia-induced signalling involves complicated crosstalk between hypoxia and inflammation, linking hypoxia and inflammation to inflammatory bowel disease, certain cancers, and infections.[16] Research is ongoing to understand the mechanisms of how tumours adapt to low oxygen levels by inducing angiogenesis, increasing glucose consumption, and promoting the metabolic state of glycolysis (see Chapter 10).[18]

The most common cause of hypoxia is ischemia (reduced blood supply). Ischemic injury often is caused by the gradual narrowing of arteries (arteriosclerosis) or complete blockage by blood clots (thrombosis) or both. Progressive hypoxia caused by gradual arterial obstruction is better tolerated than the acute anoxia (total lack of oxygen) caused by a sudden obstruction, as with an embolus (a blood clot or other

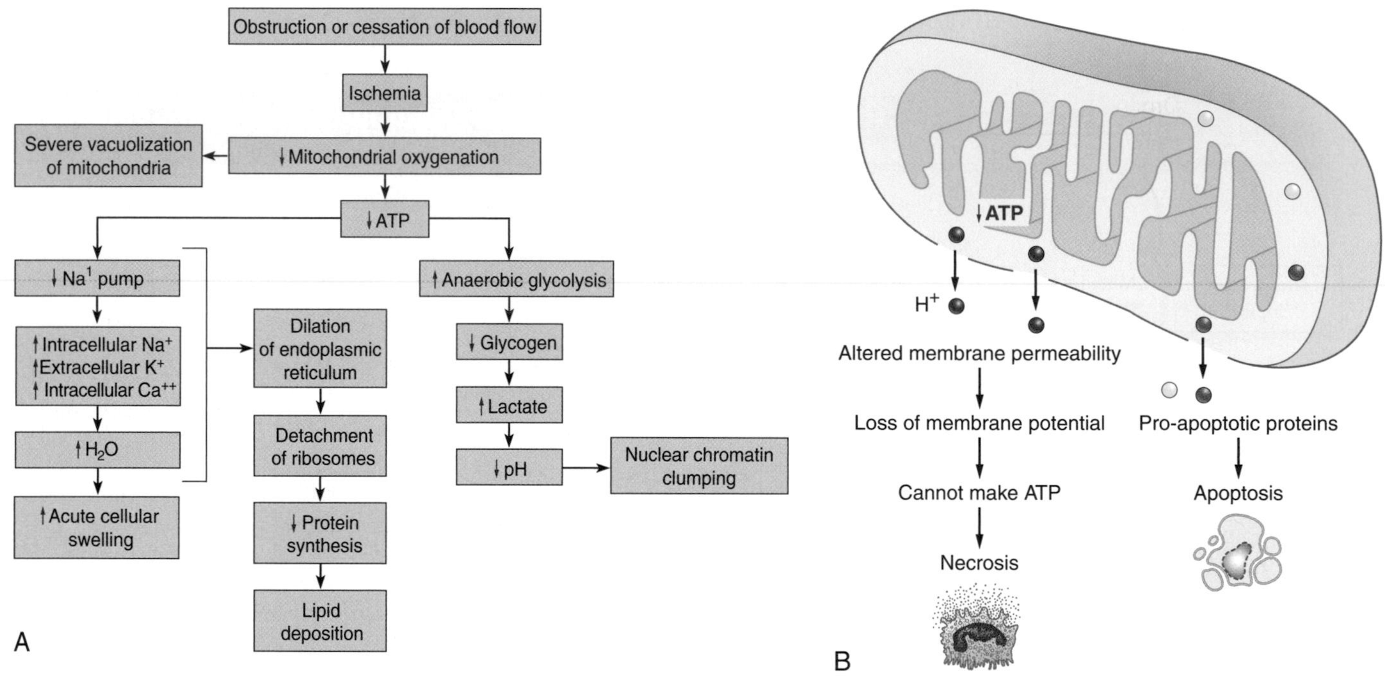

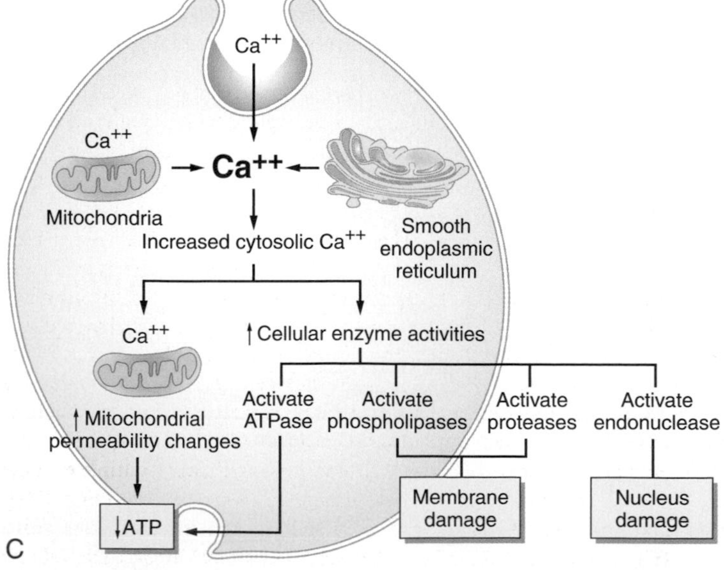

FIGURE 4-9 Hypoxic Injury Induced by Ischemia. A, Consequences of decreased oxygen delivery or ischemia with decreased adenosine triphosphate (*ATP*). The structural and physiological changes are reversible if oxygen (*H_2O*) is delivered quickly. Significant decreases in ATP result in cellular death, mostly by necrosis. **B,** Mitochondrial damage can result in changes in membrane permeability, loss of membrane potential, and decrease in ATP concentration. Between the outer and inner membranes of the mitochondria are proteins that can activate the cell's suicide pathways, called apoptosis. **C,** Calcium ions (*Ca^{++}*) are critical mediators of cellular injury. Ca^{++} are usually maintained at low concentrations in the cell's cytoplasm; thus ischemia and certain toxins can initially cause an increase in the release of Ca^{++} from intracellular stores and later an increased movement (influx) across the plasma membrane. (Adapted from Kumar, V., Abbas, A.K., & Aster, J.C. [Eds.]. [2015]. *Robbins and Cotran pathologic basis of disease* [9th ed.]. Philadelphia: Saunders.)

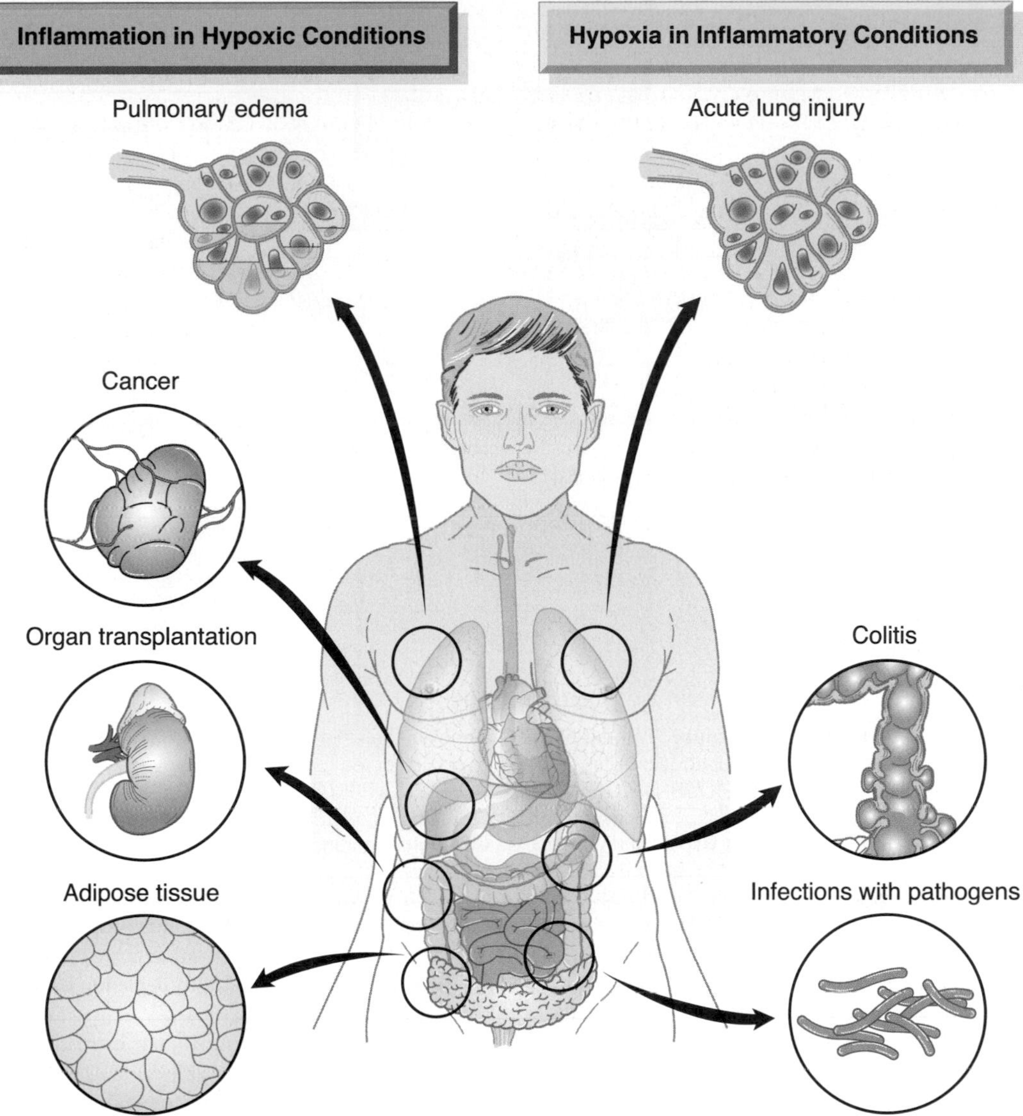

FIGURE 4-10 Hypoxia and Inflammation. Shown is a simplified drawing of clinical conditions characterized by tissue hypoxia that causes inflammatory changes (*left*) and inflammatory diseases that ultimately lead to hypoxia (*right*). These diseases and conditions are discussed in more detail in their respective chapters. (From *The New England Journal of Medicine,* Holger K. Eltzschig, Peter Carmeliet, "Hypoxia and Inflammation," 364:656–665. Copyright © 2011 Massachusetts Medical Society. Reprinted with permission from Massachusetts Medical Society.)

blockage in the circulation). An acute obstruction in a coronary artery can cause myocardial cellular death (infarction) within minutes if the blood supply is not restored, whereas the gradual onset of ischemia usually results in myocardial adaptation. Myocardial infarction and stroke, which are common causes of death in North America, generally result from atherosclerosis (a type of arteriosclerosis) and consequent ischemic injury. (Vascular obstruction is discussed in Chapter 24.)

Cellular responses to hypoxic injury caused by ischemia have been demonstrated in studies of the heart muscle. Within 1 minute after blood supply to the myocardium is interrupted, the heart becomes pale and has difficulty contracting normally. Within 3 to 5 minutes, the ischemic portion of the myocardium ceases to contract because of a rapid decrease in mitochondrial phosphorylation, causing insufficient ATP production. Lack of ATP leads to increased anaerobic metabolism, which generates ATP from glycogen when there is insufficient oxygen. When glycogen stores are depleted, even anaerobic metabolism ceases.

A reduction in ATP levels causes the plasma membrane's sodium–potassium (Na^+–K^+) pump and sodium–calcium exchange mechanism to fail, which leads to an intracellular accumulation of sodium and calcium and diffusion of potassium out of the cell. Sodium and water then can enter the cell freely, and cellular swelling, as well as early dilation of the ER, results. Dilation causes the ribosomes to detach from the rough ER, reducing protein synthesis. With continued hypoxia, the entire cell becomes markedly swollen, with increased concentrations of sodium, water, and chloride and decreased concentrations of potassium. These disruptions are reversible if oxygen is restored. If oxygen is not restored, however, vacuolation (formation of vacuoles) occurs within the cytoplasm, and swelling of lysosomes and marked mitochondrial swelling result from damage to the outer membrane. Continued hypoxic injury with accumulation of calcium subsequently activates multiple enzyme systems, resulting in membrane damage, cytoskeleton disruption, DNA and chromatin degradation, ATP depletion, and eventual cellular death (Figure 4-9, *C*). Structurally, with plasma membrane damage, extracellular

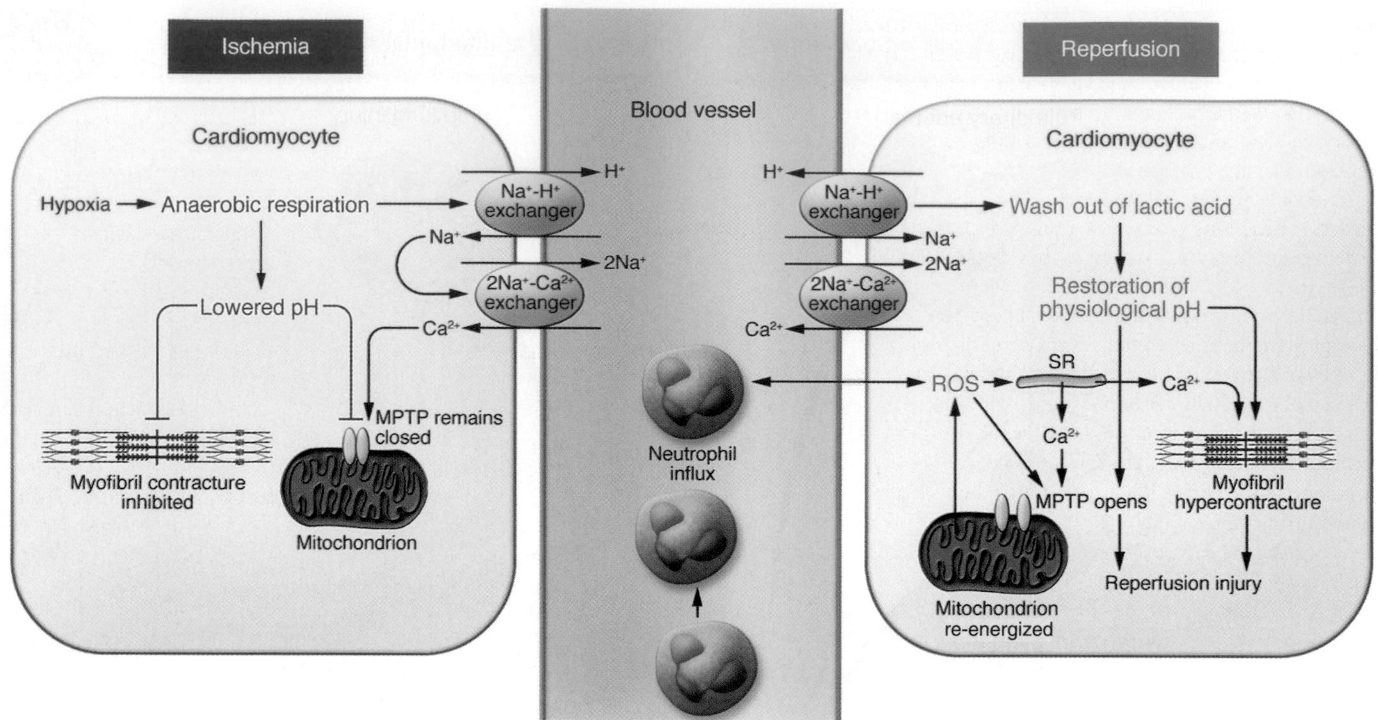

FIGURE 4-11 Reperfusion Injury. Without oxygen, or anoxia, the cells display hypoxic injury and become swollen. With reoxygenation, reperfusion injury increases because of the formation of reactive oxygen radicals that can cause cell necrosis. (JOURNAL OF CLINICAL INVESTIGATION. ONLINE by AMERICAN SOCIETY FOR CLINICAL INVESTIGATION. Reproduced with permission of AMERICAN SOCIETY FOR CLINICAL INVESTIGATION in the format Republish in a book via Copyright Clearance Center.)

calcium readily moves into the cell and intracellular calcium stores are released. Increased intracellular calcium levels activate cell enzymes (caspases) that promote cellular death by apoptosis. Persistent ischemia is associated with irreversible injury and necrosis. Irreversible injury is associated structurally with severe swelling of the mitochondria, severe damage to plasma membranes, and swelling of lysosomes. Overall, death is mainly by necrosis but apoptosis also contributes.[1]

Restoration of blood flow and oxygen, however, can cause additional injury called ischemia-reperfusion injury (Figure 4-11). Ischemia-reperfusion injury is very important clinically because it is associated with tissue damage during myocardial and cerebral infarction. Several mechanisms are now proposed for ischemia-reperfusion injury and include the following:

- *Oxidative stress*—Reoxygenation causes the increased generation of ROS and nitrogen species.[1] Highly reactive oxygen intermediates (oxidative stress) generated include hydroxyl radical (OH^-), superoxide radical ($O_2^{\bar{\cdot}}$), and hydrogen peroxide (H_2O_2). The nitrogen species include nitric oxide (NO) generated by endothelial cells, macrophages, neurons, and other cells. These radicals can all cause further membrane damage and mitochondrial calcium overload. The white blood cells (neutrophils) are especially affected with reperfusion injury, including neutrophil adhesion to the endothelium. Antioxidant treatment not only reverses neutrophil adhesion but also can reverse neutrophil-mediated heart injury. In one study of individuals undergoing elective percutaneous coronary intervention (PCI), pretreatment with vitamin C was associated with less myocardial injury.[19] The PREVEC Trial (prevention of reperfusion damage associated with percutaneous coronary angioplasty following acute myocardial infarction) seeks to evaluate whether vitamins C and E reduce infarct size in patients subjected to percutaneous coronary angioplasty after acute myocardial infarction.[20]
- *Increased intracellular calcium concentration*—Intracellular and mitochondrial calcium overload the cell; this process begins during acute ischemia. Reperfusion causes even more calcium influx because of cell membrane damage and ROS-induced injury to the sarcoplasmic reticulum. The increased calcium increases mitochondrial permeability, eventually leading to depletion of ATP and further cellular injury.
- *Inflammation*—Ischemic injury increases inflammation because danger signals (from cytokines) are released by resident immune cells when cells die and this signalling initiates inflammation.
- *Complement activation*—The activation of complement may increase the tissue damage from reperfusion-ischemia injury.[1]

QUICK CHECK 4-1
1. When does a cell become irreversibly injured?
2. Describe the pathogenesis of hypoxic injury.
3. What are the mechanisms of ischemia-reperfusion injury?

Free Radicals and Reactive Oxygen Species Injury: Oxidative Stress

An important mechanism of cellular injury is injury induced by free radicals, especially by ROS; this form of injury is called oxidative stress. Oxidative stress occurs when *excess* ROS overwhelm endogenous antioxidant systems. A free radical is an electrically uncharged atom or group of atoms that has an unpaired electron. Having one unpaired electron makes the molecule unstable; the molecule becomes stabilized by either donating or accepting an electron from another molecule. When the attacked molecule loses its electron, it becomes a free radical. Therefore it is capable of injurious chemical bond formation with proteins, lipids, and carbohydrates—key molecules in membranes and nucleic acids. Free radicals are difficult to control and initiate chain reactions. They are *highly* reactive because they have low chemical specificity, meaning that they can react with most molecules in their proximity. Oxidative stress can activate several intracellular signalling pathways because ROS can modulate enzymes and transcription factors. Oxidative stress is an important mechanism of cell damage in many conditions, including chemical and radiation injury, ischemia-reperfusion injury, cellular aging, and microbial killing by phagocytes, particularly neutrophils and macrophages.[1]

Free radicals may be generated within cells, first by the reduction–oxidation reactions (redox reactions) in normal metabolic processes such as respiration. Under normal physiological conditions, ROS serve as "redox messengers" in the regulation of intracellular signalling; however, excess ROS may produce irreversible damage to cellular components. All biological membranes contain redox systems, which also are important for cell defence (e.g., inflammation, iron uptake, growth and proliferation, and signal transduction). Second, absorption of extreme energy sources (e.g., ultraviolet light, radiation) produces free radicals. Third, enzymatic metabolism of exogenous chemicals or medications (e.g., $CCl_3^{\bullet}$, a product of carbon tetrachloride [CCl_4]) results in the formation of free radicals. Fourth, transition metals (i.e., iron and copper) donate or accept free electrons during intracellular reactions and activate the formation of free radicals such as in the Fenton reaction (i.e., when they react with H_2O_2 to create hydroxyl ions and water). Finally, NO is an important colourless gas that is an intermediate in many reactions generated by endothelial cells, neurons, macrophages, and other cell types. NO can act as a free radical and can be converted to highly reactive peroxynitrite anion ($ONOO^-$), nitrogen dioxide (NO_2), and nitrate (NO_3^-). Table 4-3 describes the most significant free radicals.

Free radicals cause several damaging effects by (1) **lipid peroxidation**, which is the destruction of polyunsaturated lipids (the same process by which fats become rancid), leading to membrane damage and increased permeability; (2) protein alterations, causing fragmentation of polypeptide chains that can lead to loss and protein misfolding; and (3) DNA damage, causing mutations (Figure 4-12). Because of the increased understanding of free radicals, a growing number of diseases and disorders have been linked either directly or indirectly to these reactive species (Box 4-1).

The body can eliminate free radicals. The oxygen free radical superoxide may spontaneously decay into oxygen and hydrogen peroxide. Table 4-4 summarizes other methods that contribute to inactivation or termination of free radicals. The toxicity of certain medications and chemicals can be attributed either to conversion of these chemicals to free radicals or to the formation of oxygen-derived metabolites (see the following discussion).

Mitochondrial Effects

Mitochondria are key players in cellular injury and cellular death because they produce ATP, or life-sustaining energy. Mitochondria can be damaged by ROS and by increases of cytosolic calcium ion (Ca^{++}) concentration (see Figure 4-9). Box 4-2 summarizes the three major types and consequences of mitochondrial damage. Currently, investigators are trying to identify the polypeptides (i.e., proteomes) directly involved in diseases associated with mitochondrial dysfunction. ROS not only damage proteins and mitochondria but also can promote damage in neighbouring cells. An important area of research emphasis is that protein aggregates can increase mitochondrial damage and damaged mitochondria can further induce protein damage, thus resulting in neuro-degeneration. An emerging area of research concerns mitochondrial DNA that escapes from autophagy, which may be a mechanism of tissue inflammation.[21]

Chemical or Toxic Injury

Mechanisms

Humans are constantly exposed to a variety of compounds termed **xenobiotics** (Greek *xenos*, "foreign"; *bios*, "life") that include toxic, mutagenic, and carcinogenic chemicals (Figure 4-13). Some of these chemicals are found in the human diet, for example, fungal mycotoxins such as aflatoxin B_1. Many xenobiotics are toxic to the liver (hepatotoxic). The liver is the initial site of contact for many ingested xenobiotics, medications, and alcohol, making this organ most susceptible to chemically induced injury. The toxicity of many chemicals results from absorption through the gastro-intestinal tract after oral ingestion. A main cause for withdrawing medications from the market is hepatotoxicity. Certain dietary supplements (e.g., chaparral and ma huang)

TABLE 4-3 Free Radicals as Contributors to Oxidative Stress

Name	Formula	Characteristics
Hyperoxide/ superoxide	$^{\bullet}O_2^-$	Highly unstable, signalling function, synaptic plasticity
Hydrogen peroxide	H_2O_2	Cell toxicity, signalling function, generation of other reactive oxygen species
Hydroxyl radical	$^{\bullet}OH$	Free radical, highly unstable, very reactive agent
Alkoxyl radical	$RO^{\bullet}$	Free radical, reaction product of lipids
Peroxyl radical	$ROO^{\bullet}$	Free radical, reaction product of lipids
Hypochlorite anion	OCl^-	Reactive oxygen species, reactive chlorine species, enzymatically generated by myeloperoxidase
Singlet oxygen	$^1O_2$	Induced/excited oxygen molecule, radical and nonradical form
Ozone	O_3	Environmental toxin
Nitric oxide	$^{\bullet}NO$	Environmental toxin, endogenous signal molecule
Peroxynitrite anion	$ONOO^-$	Highly reactive reaction intermediate of $^{\bullet}O_2$ and $^{\bullet}NO$
Nitrogen dioxide	$^{\bullet}NO_2$	Highly reactive radical, environmental toxin
Nitrogen oxides	NO_x	Environmental toxins, including NO and $^{\bullet}NO_2$, derived from the combustion process

From Domej, W., Oettl, K., & Renner, W. (2014). *Int J Chron Obstruct Pulmon Dis, 9*(1), 1207–1224, Table 1. *International Journal of Chronic Obstructive Pulmonary Disease* by DOVE Medical Press. Reproduced with permission of DOVE Medical Press in the format Republish in a book via Copyright Clearance Center.

BOX 4-1 Diseases and Disorders Linked to Oxygen-Derived Free Radicals

- Deterioration noted in aging
  - Atherosclerosis
  - Ischemic brain injury
  - Alzheimer's disease
- Neurotoxins
- Cancer
- Cardiac myopathy
- Chronic granulomatous disease
- Diabetes mellitus
- Eye disorders
  - Macular degeneration
  - Cataracts
- Inflammatory disorders
- Iron overload
- Lung disorders
  - Asbestosis
  - Oxygen toxicity
  - Emphysema
- Nutritional deficiencies
- Radiation injury
- Reperfusion injury
- Rheumatoid arthritis
- Skin disorders
- Toxic states
  - Xenobiotics (CCl_4, paraquat, cigarette smoke, etc.)
  - Metal irons (Ni, Cu, Fe, etc.)

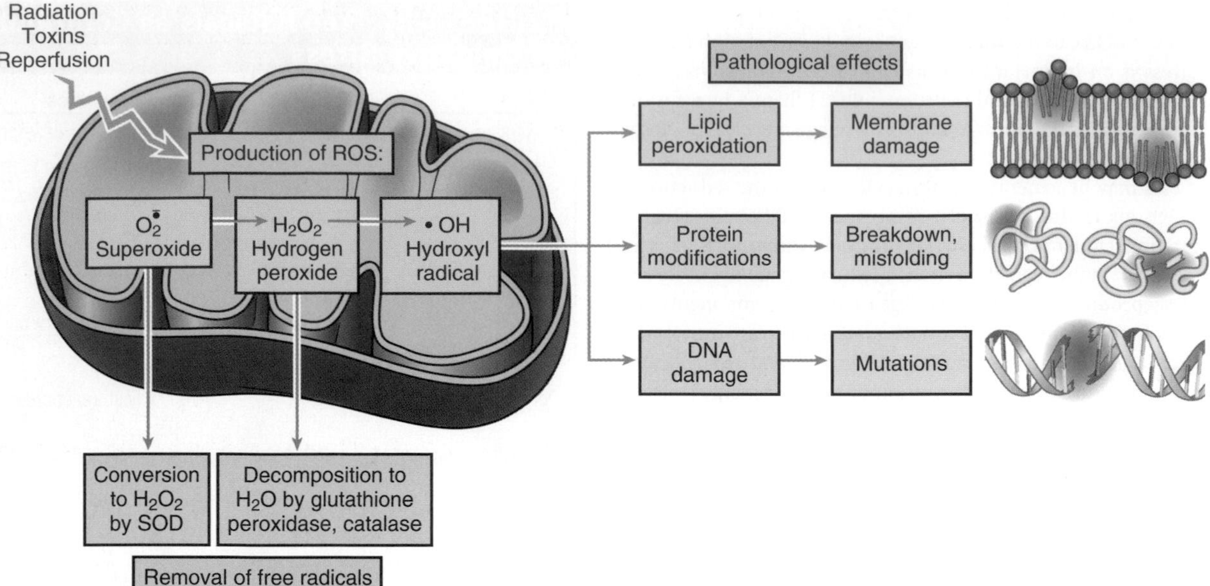

FIGURE 4-12 The Role of Reactive Oxygen Species in Cellular Injury. The production of reactive oxygen species (ROS) can be initiated by many cell stressors, such as radiation, toxins, and reperfusion of oxygen. Free radicals are removed by normal decay and enzymatic systems. ROS accumulates in cells because of insufficient removal or excess production leading to cellular injury, including lipid peroxidation, protein modifications, and DNA damage or mutations. *SOD,* superoxide dismutase. (Adapted from Kumar, V., Abbas, A.K., & Aster, J.C. [Eds.]. [2015]. *Robbins and Cotran pathologic basis of disease* [9th ed.]. Philadelphia: Saunders.)

TABLE 4-4 Methods Contributing to Inactivation or Termination of Free Radicals

Method	Process
Antioxidants	Endogenous or exogenous; either blocks synthesis or inactivates (e.g., scavenges) free radicals; includes vitamin E, vitamin C, cysteine, glutathione, albumin, ceruloplasmin, transferrin, γ-lipoacid, others
Enzymes	Superoxide dismutase,[a] which converts superoxide to hydrogen peroxide (H_2O_2); catalase[a] (in peroxisomes) decomposes H_2O_2; glutathione peroxidase[a] decomposes hydroxyl radical (OH^-) and H_2O_2

[a]These enzymes are important in modulating the cellular destructive effects of free radicals, also released in inflammation.

BOX 4-2 Three Major Types and Consequences of Mitochondrial Damage

1. Damage to the mitochondria results in the formation of the *mitochondrial permeability transition pore,* a high-conductance channel or pore. The opening of this channel results in the loss of mitochondrial membrane potential, causing failure of oxidative phosphorylation, depletion of adenosine triphosphate, and damage to mitochondrial DNA, leading to necrosis of the cell.
2. Altered oxidative phosphorylation leads to the formation of reactive oxygen species that can damage cellular components.
3. Because mitochondria store several proteins between their membranes, increased permeability of the outer membrane may result in leakage of pro-apoptotic proteins and cause cellular death by apoptosis.

Data from Kumar, V., Abbas, A.K., & Aster, J.C. (Eds.). (2015). *Robbins and Cotran pathologic basis of disease* (9th ed.). Philadelphia: Saunders.

are potent hepatotoxins.[22] Other common routes of exposure for xenobiotics are absorption through the skin and inhalation. The severity of chemically induced liver injury varies from minor liver injury to acute liver failure, cirrhosis, and liver cancer.[23]

The use of a systems biology approach includes delineation of toxicity pathways that may be defined as cellular response pathways, which when disturbed are expected to result in adverse health effects. Using this model of testing, investigators proposed screening and classifying compounds using a "cellular stress response pathway." Components or mechanisms of these pathways include oxidative stress, heat shock response, DNA damage response, hypoxia, ER stress (see Chapter 1), mental stress, inflammation, and osmotic stress. Many chemicals have already been classified under these mechanisms.

The liver as the principal site for xenobiotic metabolism, called *biotransformation,* converts the lipophilic xenobiotics to more hydrophilic forms for efficient excretion. Biotransformation, however, also can produce short-lived unstable highly reactive chemical intermediates that can lead to adverse effects.[24] These harmful intermediates, classified and catalogued, are called **toxicophores**. The intermediates include electrophiles, nucleophiles, free radicals, and redox-active reactants. **Electrophiles** (electron lovers) are atoms or molecules attracted to electrons and accept a pair of electrons to make a covalent bond. This process creates a partially or fully charged centre in electrophilic molecules.[24] A **nucleophile** is an atom or molecule that donates an electron pair to an electrophile to make a chemical bond. All chemical species with a free pair of electrons can act as nucleophiles. Nucleophiles are strongly attracted to positively charged regions in other chemicals and can be oxidized to free radicals and electrophiles.[24] In general, the majority of all *reactive* chemical species are electrophilic because the formation of nucleophiles is rare[24]. The generation of these excess reactive chemical species leads to molecular damage in liver cells. These reactive intermediates can interact with cellular macromolecules (such as proteins and DNA), can covalently bind to proteins and form **protein adducts**

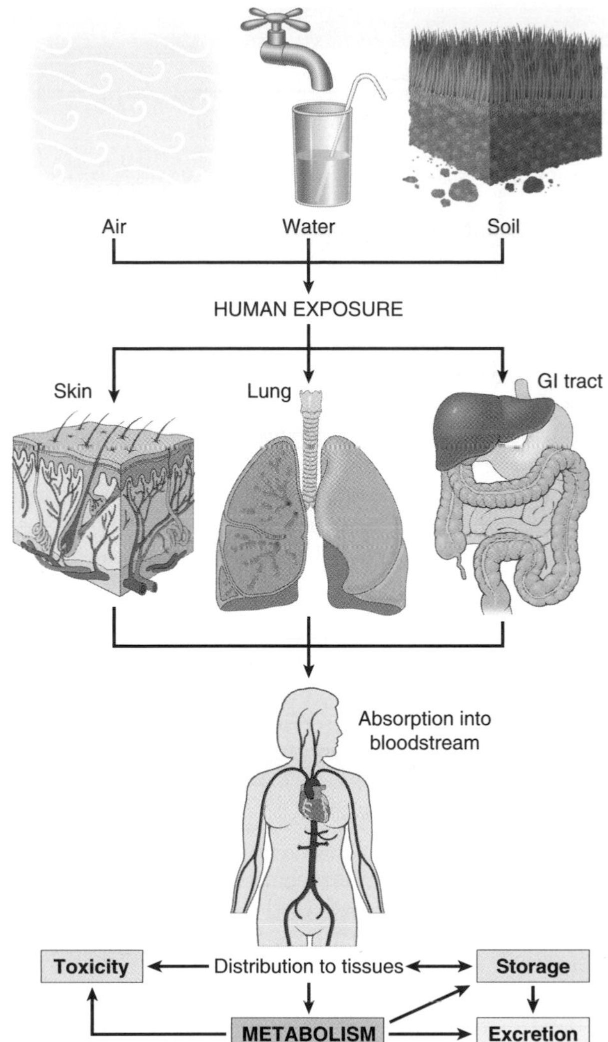

FIGURE 4-13 Human Exposure to Pollutants. Pollutants contained in air, water, and soil are absorbed through the lungs, gastro-intestinal (*GI*) tract, and skin. In the body, the pollutants may act at the site of absorption but are generally transported through the bloodstream to various organs where they can be stored or metabolized. Metabolism of xenobiotics may result in the formation of water-soluble compounds that are excreted, or a toxic metabolite may be created by activation of the agent. (From Kumar, V., Abbas, A.K., & Aster, J.C. [Eds.]. [2015]. *Robbins and Cotran pathologic basis of disease* [9th ed.]. Philadelphia: Saunders.)

(chemical bound to protein) and DNA adducts, or can react directly with cell structures to cause cell damage.[25] Adduct formation can lead to adverse conditions including disruption in protein function, excess formation of fibrous connective tissue (fibrogenesis), and activation of immune responses.[24] The identity of proteins modified by xenobiotics can be found in the resource known as the reactive metabolite target protein database.[26] The body has two major defence systems for counteracting these effects: (1) detoxification enzymes and their cofactors and (2) antioxidant systems. Phases of detoxification include phase I enzymes, such as cytochrome P-450 (CYP) oxidases, which are the most important oxidative reactions. Other phase I detoxification enzymes include those for reduction and hydrolysis. In phase II detoxification, conjugation enzymes, such as glutathione (GSH), detoxify reactive electrophiles and produce polar metabolites that cannot diffuse across membranes. Most conjugation enzymes are located in the cytosol. Phase III detoxification is often called the *efflux transporter system* because enzymes remove the parent medications, metabolites, and xenobiotics from cells. The liver has the highest supply of biotransformation enzymes of all organs and, therefore, has the key role in protection from chemical toxicity.[24] Figure 4-14 is a summary of chemically induced liver injury.

The consequence of self-propagating chain reactions of free radicals is lipid peroxidation. Free radicals react mainly with polyunsaturated fatty acids in membranes and can initiate lipid peroxidation. The breakdown of membrane lipids results in altered function of the mitochondria, ER, plasma membranes, and Golgi apparatus, and therefore has a role in acute liver cellular death (necrosis) and progression of liver injury (Figure 4-15).[24]

Chemical Agents, Including Medications

Numerous chemical agents cause cellular injury. Because chemical injury remains a constant problem in clinical settings, it is a major limitation to medication therapy. Over-the-counter and prescribed medications can cause cellular injury, sometimes leading to death. The leading cause of child poisoning is medications (see *Health Promotion:* The Percentage of Child Medication–Related Poisoning Deaths Is Increasing). The site of injury is frequently the liver, where many chemicals and medications are metabolized (see Figure 4-15). Long-term exposure to air pollutants, insecticides, and herbicides can cause cellular injury (see *Health Promotion:* Air Pollution Reported as Largest Single Environmental Health Risk).

HEALTH PROMOTION

The Percentage of Child Medication–Related Poisoning Deaths Is Increasing

Today, the second leading cause of childhood hospitalizations in Ontario is unintentional poisoning with prescription and over-the-counter medications. Children under 5 years of age account for 86% of all deaths and unintentional poisonings.

How can we increase the safety of children exposed to so many medications? Safe storage is the *most* important solution, and safe dosing from clinicians will reduce dosing errors. Medications should be locked away where children cannot reach them. Additionally, improvements are continuing through improved packaging and labelling of medications as well as education of parents and consumers on dosing information. See the following online resource for further information: https://members.oma.org/HEALTHPROMOTION/Pages/ChildPoisoning.aspx.

From Ontario Medical Association. (2016). *Preventing child poisoning.* Retrieved from https://www.oma.org/HEALTHPROMOTION/Pages/ChildPoisoning.aspx.

Another way to classify mechanisms by which medication actions, chemicals, and toxins produce injury includes (1) direct damage, also called *on-target toxicity*; (2) exaggerated response at the target, including overdose; (3) biological activation to toxic metabolites, including free radicals; (4) hypersensitivity and related immunological reactions; and (5) rare toxicities.[27] These mechanisms are not mutually exclusive; thus several may be operating concurrently.

Direct damage is when chemicals and medications injure cells by combining *directly* with critical molecular substances. For example, cyanide is highly toxic (e.g., poisonous) because it inhibits mitochondrial cytochrome oxidase and hence blocks electron transport. Many chemotherapeutic medications, known as antineoplastic agents, induce cell damage by direct cytotoxic effects. Exaggerated pharmacological responses at the target include tumours caused by industrial chemicals and the birth defects attributed to thalidomide.[27] Importantly, another

HEALTH PROMOTION

Air Pollution Reported as Largest Single Environmental Health Risk

The World Health Organization (WHO) reports that about 7 million people died in 2012 as a result of air pollution exposure. Improved measurements and better technology have enabled scientists to make more detailed analyses of health risks. These findings confirm that air pollution is now the world's largest single environmental health risk and reducing air pollution could save millions of lives. New data show a stronger link between indoor and outdoor air pollution exposure and cardiovascular diseases (e.g., strokes and ischemic heart disease) as well as the link between air pollution and cancer. These data are in addition to the role of air pollution and the development of respiratory diseases, including infections and chronic obstructive pulmonary diseases. Using these 2012 data for low- and middle-income countries, Southeast Asia and Western Pacific regions had the largest air pollution burden. Included in the analysis is a breakdown of deaths for adults and children attributed to specific diseases:

Outdoor Air Pollution–Caused Deaths—Breakdown by Disease:
- 40% ischemic heart disease
- 40% stroke
- 11% chronic obstructive pulmonary disease (COPD)
- 6% lung cancer
- 3% acute lower respiratory tract infections in children

Indoor Air Pollution–Caused Deaths—Breakdown by Disease:
- 34% stroke
- 26% ischemic heart disease
- 22% COPD
- 12% acute lower respiratory tract infections in children
- 6% lung cancer

WHO estimates that indoor air pollution was linked to 4.3 million deaths in 2012 from cooking over coal, wood, dung, and biomass stoves. Outdoor air pollution estimates were 3.7 million deaths in 2012 from urban and rural sources. WHO has suggested some recommendations for controlling air pollution in its *WHO Guideline for Indoor Air Quality: Household Fuel Combustion* (http://www.who.int/indoorair/guidelines/hhfc/en/).

Data from World Health Organization. (2014). *7 million premature deaths annually linked to air pollution* [Press release]. Retrieved from http://www.who.int/mediacentre/news/releases/2014/air-pollution/en/#.

TABLE 4-5 Common Drugs of Abuse

Class	Molecular Target	Example
Opioid narcotics	Mu opioid receptor (agonist)	Heroin, hydromorphone (Dilaudid)
		Oxycodone (Percodan, Percocet, OxyContin)
		Methadone (Metadol)
		Meperidine (Demerol)
Sedative-hypnotics	$GABA_A$ receptor (agonist)	Barbiturates
		Ethanol
		Methaqualone (Quaalude)
		Glutethimide (Doriden)
		Ethchlorvynol (Placidyl)
Psychomotor stimulants	Dopamine transporter (antagonist)	Cocaine
	Serotonin receptors (toxicity)	Amphetamines
		3,4-Methylenedioxymethamphetamine (MDMA, ecstasy)
Phencyclidinelike medications	NMDA glutamate receptor channel (antagonist)	Phencyclidine (PCP, angel dust)
		Ketamine
Cannabinoids	CB_1 cannabinoid receptors (agonist)	Marihuana
		Hashish
Hallucinogens	Serotonin 5-HT_2 receptors (agonist)	Lysergic acid diethylamide (LSD)
		Mescaline
		Psilocybin

5-HT_2, 5-hydroxytryptamine; *CB_1*, cannabinoid receptor type 1; *GABA*, gamma-aminobutyric acid; *NMDA*, *N*-methyl-D-aspartate.
From Hyman, S.E. (2001). *JAMA, 286*, 2586; Kumar, V., Abbas, A.K., & Aster, J.C. (2015). Cellular responses to stress and toxic insults: Adaptation, injury, and death. In V. Kumar, A.K. Abbas, & J.C. Aster (Eds.), *Robbins and Cotran pathologic basis of disease* (9th ed., 31–68). Philadelphia: Saunders.

example includes common drugs of abuse (Table 4-5). Drug abuse can involve mind-altering substances beyond therapeutic or social norms (Table 4-6). Drug addiction and overdose are serious public health issues.

Most toxic chemicals are not biologically active in their parent (native) form but must be converted to reactive metabolites, which then act on target molecules. This conversion is usually performed by the cytochrome P-450 oxidase enzymes in the smooth ER of the liver and other organs. These toxic metabolites cause membrane damage and cellular injury mostly from formation of *free radicals* and subsequent membrane damage from lipid peroxidation (see Figure 4-15). For example, acetaminophen (Paracetamol) is converted to a toxic metabolite in the liver, causing cellular injury (Figure 4-16). Acetaminophen is one of the most common causes of poisoning worldwide.[28] Many investigators are studying hepatoprotective strategies.[29]

Hypersensitivity reactions are a common medication toxicity and range from mild skin rashes to immune-mediated organ failure.[27] One type of hypersensitivity reaction is the delayed-onset reaction, which

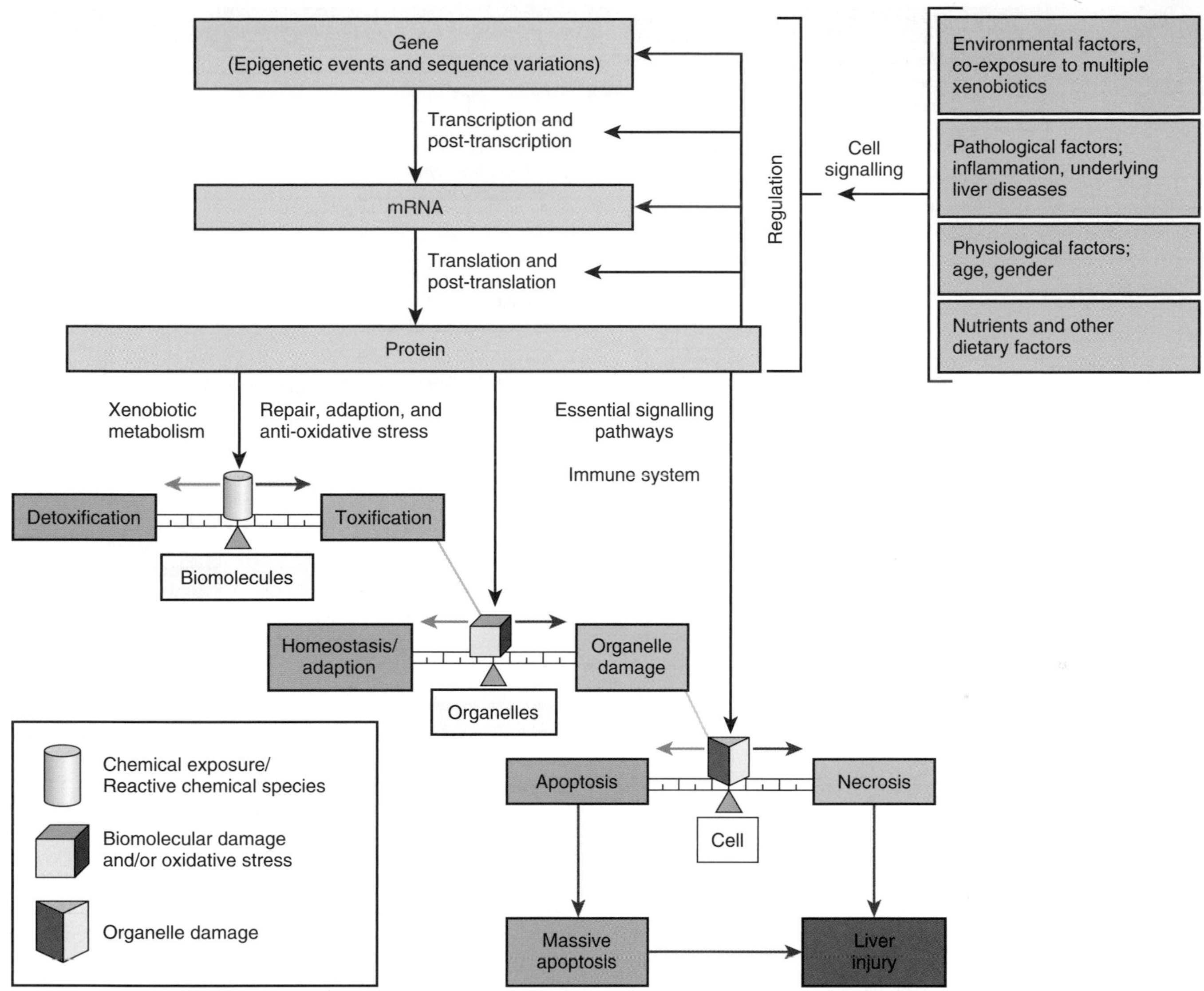

FIGURE 4-14 Chemical Liver Injury. Liver injury is a result of genetic, environmental, biological, and dietary factors. Certain chemicals can form toxic or chemically reactive metabolites. The risk of liver injury also can increase with increasing doses of a toxicant. Xenobiotic enzyme induction can lead to altered metabolism of chemicals, and medications can either inhibit or induce medication-metabolizing enzymes. These changes can lead to greater toxicity. The dose at the site of action is controlled by the Phase I to III xenobiotic metabolites, and metabolizing enzymes are encoded by numerous different genes. Therefore, the metabolism and toxicity outcomes can vary greatly among individuals. Additionally, all aspects of xenobiotic metabolism are regulated by certain transcription factors (cellular mediators of gene regulation). Overall, the extent of cell damage depends on the balance between reactive chemical species and protective responses aimed at decreasing oxidative stress, repairing macromolecular damage, or preserving cell health by inducing apoptosis or cellular death. Significant clinical outcomes of chemical-induced liver injury occur with necrosis and the immune response. Covalent binding of reactive metabolites to cellular proteins can produce new antigens (haptens) that initiate autoantibody production and T-cytotoxic cell responses. Necrosis, a form of cellular death, can result from extensive damage to the plasma membrane with altered ion transport, changes of membrane potential, cell swelling, and eventual dissolution. Altogether the pathogenesis of chemically induced liver injury is determined by genetics, environmental factors, and other underlying pathological conditions. Green arrows are pathways leading to cell recovery; red arrows indicate pathways to cell damage or death; black arrows are pathways leading to chemically induced liver injury. *mRNA*, messenger RNA. (Adapted from Gu, X., & Manautou, J.E. [2013]. *Exp Rev Mol Med, 14*, e4.)

occurs after multiple doses of a medication are administered. Some protein medications and large polypeptide medications (e.g., insulin) can directly stimulate antibody production (see Chapter 8). Most medications, however, act as haptens and bind covalently to serum or cell-bound proteins. The binding makes the protein immunogenic, stimulating antidrug antibody production, T-cell responses against the medication, or both. For example, penicillin itself is not antigenic but its metabolic degradation products can become antigenic and cause an allergic reaction. Rare toxicities simply mean infrequent occurrences as described previously by the other four mechanisms. These toxicities

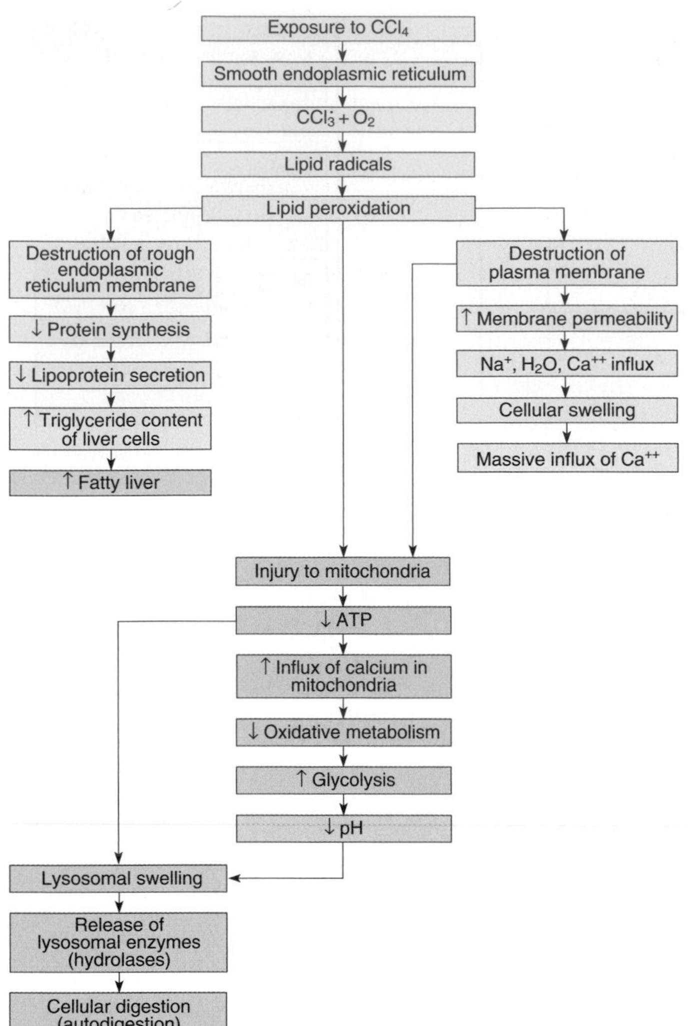

FIGURE 4-15 Chemical Injury of Liver Cells Induced by Carbon Tetrachloride Poisoning. Light blue boxes are mechanisms unique to chemical injury, purple boxes involve hypoxic injury, and green boxes are clinical manifestations. *CCl_4*, carbon tetrachloride; *$CCl_3^{\cdot}$*, trichloromethyl free radical; *O_2*, oxygen; *Na^+*, sodium, *H_2O*, water; *Ca^{++}*, calcium ion; *ATP*, adenosine triphosphate.

reflect individual genetic predispositions that affect medication or chemical metabolism, disposition, and immune responses.

Carbon monoxide, carbon tetrachloride, and social drugs, such as alcohol, can significantly alter cellular function and injure cellular structures. Accidental or suicidal poisonings by chemical agents cause numerous deaths. The injurious effects on cells of some agents—lead, carbon monoxide, ethyl alcohol, mercury—are common.

Lead. Lead (Pb) is a heavy toxic metal that persists in older homes, the environment, and the workplace. Lead may be found in hazardous concentrations in food, water, and air, and it is one of the most common overexposures found in industry.[30] Despite efforts to reduce exposure through government regulation, exposure still persists for many people, and toxicity is still a primary hazard for children[31] (see *Health Promotion:* Low-Level Lead Exposure Harms Children: A Renewed Call for Primary Prevention). Although Pb was removed from paint in Europe in 1922 and regulations to reduce the amount of Pb in paint were created in Canada in 2002, many homes in Canada still contain leaded paint, and chipped and peeling leaded paint constitutes a major source of current childhood exposure.[32-35] The chipped paint can disintegrate at friction surfaces to form Pb dust.[35] Another source of contamination is Pb dust dispersed along roadways from previous leaded gasoline

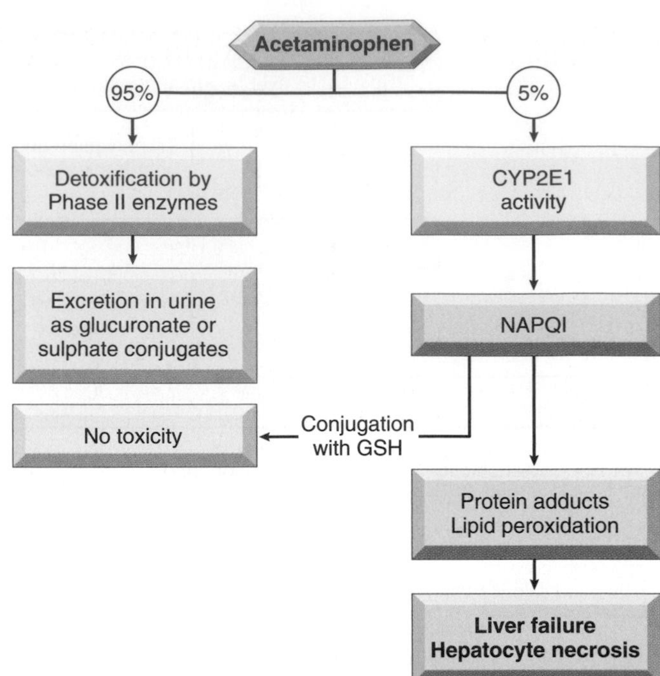

FIGURE 4-16 Acetaminophen Metabolism and Toxicity. *CYP2E1*, a cytochrome; *GSH*, glutathione; *NAPQI*, toxic byproduct.

HEALTH PROMOTION

Low-Level Lead Exposure Harms Children: A Renewed Call for Primary Prevention

Lead exposure is relatively low in Canada, and levels are often difficult to determine. Notable symptoms include headaches, irritability, abdominal pain, vomiting, anemia (general weakness, paleness), weight loss, poor attention span, noticeable learning difficulty, slowed speech development, and hyperactivity.

Low levels of lead exposure tend to create vague symptoms, and the cause often cannot be determined very easily. Exposure to lead is mainly through oral ingestion or absorption by the skin. Because children tend to touch everything and put things into their mouths, they are at greater risk of exposure, although blood lead levels of Canadian children are generally low (at less than 0.483 mcmol/L). Routine blood lead testing may be necessary in communities with a history of soil contamination (from nearby industrial activity). Further information on lead screening is available through Health Canada at http://www.hc-sc.gc.ca/ewh-semt/contaminants/lead-plomb/asked_questions-questions_posees-eng.php.

From Health Canada. (2009). *Lead information package—Some commonly asked questions about lead and human health.* Retrieved from http://www.hc-sc.gc.ca/ewh-semt/contaminants/lead-plomb/asked_questions-questions_posees-eng.php.

emissions.[35] When Pb was removed from gasoline, blood lead levels (BLLs) dropped significantly.[36-38] Previous emissions of leaded fuel created large dispersions of Pb dust in the environment. Particulate Pb (2 to 10 μm) does not degrade and persists in the environment, making it a notable source of human exposure.[39] Other airborne sources include smelters and piston-engine airplanes.[40] Drinking water exposed to Pb occurs from outdated fixtures, plumbing without corrosion control, and solders.[35] Well water may not be tested for Pb.[35] Although the average blood levels of Pb in children in Canada have dropped since the 1970s, there are at-risk populations with higher than average BLLs.[35] Children of lower social economic status or racial minority status are still at higher risk of Pb poisoning, and some regions in Canada have an increased

TABLE 4-6 Social or Street Drugs and Their Effects

Type of Drug	Description and Effects
Marihuana (pot)	*Active substance:* Δ9-tetrahydrocannabinol (THC), found in resin of *Cannabis sativa* plant With smoking (e.g., "joints"), about 5–10% is absorbed through lungs; with heavy use the following adverse effects have been reported: alterations of sensory perception; cognitive and psychomotor impairment (e.g., inability to judge time, speed, distance); an increase in heart rate and blood pressure; an increase in susceptibility to laryngitis, pharyngitis, bronchitis; coughing and hoarseness; possible contribution to lung cancer (different dosages need study; it contains large number of carcinogens); based on data from animal studies, reproductive changes, including reduced fertility, decreased sperm motility, and decreased levels of circulatory testosterone; fetal abnormalities, including low birth weight; increased frequency of infectious illness, which is thought to be result of depressed cell-mediated and humoral immunity; beneficial effects include decreased nausea secondary to cancer chemotherapy and decreased pain in certain chronic conditions
Methamphetamine (meth)	An amine derivation of amphetamine ($C_{10}H_{15}N$) used as crystalline hydrochloride CNS stimulant; in large doses causes irritability, aggressive (violent) behaviour, anxiety, excitement, auditory hallucinations, and paranoia (delusions and psychosis); mood changes are common and abuser can swiftly change from friendly to hostile; paranoiac swings can result in suspiciousness, hyperactive behaviour, and dramatic mood swings Appeals to abusers because body's metabolism is increased and produces euphoria, alertness, and perception of increased energy Stages: *Low intensity:* User is not psychologically addicted and uses methamphetamine by swallowing or snorting *Binge and high intensity:* User has psychological addiction and smokes or injects to achieve a faster, stronger high *Tweaking:* Most dangerous stage; user is continually under the influence, not sleeping for 3–15 days, extremely irritated, and paranoid
Cocaine and crack	Extracted from leaves of cocoa plant and sold as a water-soluble powder (cocaine hydrochloride) liberally diluted with talcum powder or other white powders; extraction of pure alkaloid from cocaine hydrochloride is "free-base" called *crack* because it "cracks" when heated Crack is more potent than cocaine; cocaine is widely used as an anaesthetic, usually in procedures involving oral cavity; it is a potent CNS stimulant, blocking reuptake of neurotransmitters norepinephrine, dopamine, and serotonin; also increases synthesis of norepinephrine and dopamine; dopamine induces sense of euphoria, and norepinephrine causes adrenergic potentiation, including hypertension, tachycardia, and vasoconstriction; cocaine can therefore cause severe coronary artery narrowing and ischemia; the reason cocaine increases thrombus formation is unclear; other cardiovascular effects include dysrhythmias, sudden death, dilated cardiomyopathy, rupture of descending aorta (i.e., secondary to hypertension); effects on fetus include premature labour, delayed fetal development, stillbirth, hyperirritability
Heroin	Opiate closely related to morphine, methadone, and codeine Highly addictive, and withdrawal causes intense fear ("I'll die without it"); sold "cut" with similar-looking white powder; dissolved in water it is often highly contaminated; feeling of tranquility and sedation lasts only a few hours and thus encourages repeated intravenous or subcutaneous injections; acts on the receptors enkephalins, endorphins, and dynorphins, which are widely distributed throughout body with high affinity to CNS; effects can include infectious complications, especially *Staphylococcus aureus*, granulomas of lung, septic embolism, and pulmonary edema—in addition, viral infections, including from HIV, from casual exchange of needles; sudden death is related to overdosage secondary to respiratory depression, decreased cardiac output, and severe pulmonary edema

CNS, central nervous system; *HIV*, human immunodeficiency virus.
Data from Kumar, V., Abbas, A.K., & Aster, J.C. (Eds.). (2015). *Robbins and Cotran pathologic basis of disease* (9th ed.). Philadelphia: Saunders; Nahas, G., Sutin, K., & Bennett, W.M. (2000). *N Engl J Med, 343*(7), 514–515.

prevalence of higher BLLs in children.[35] More importantly, the American Centers for Disease Control and Prevention (CDC) reports that "no safe blood lead level in children has been identified."[41] Common sources of Pb are included in Table 4-7.

Children are more susceptible to the effects of Pb than adults for several reasons, including (1) children have increased hand-to-mouth behaviour and exposure from the ingestion of Pb dust; (2) the blood–brain barrier in children is immature during fetal development, contributing to greater Pb accumulation in the developing brain; and (3) infant absorption of Pb is greater than that in adults, and bone turnover (in adults the body burden of Pb is found in bone) in children from skeletal growth results in continuous leaching of Pb into blood, causing constant body exposure.[35,41] If nutrition is compromised, especially if dietary intake of iron and calcium is insufficient, children are more likely to have elevated BLLs.[35] Particularly worrisome is Pb exposure during pregnancy because the developing fetal nervous system is especially vulnerable; Pb exposure can result in lower IQ, learning disorders, hyperactivity, and attention problems.[31]

The organ systems primarily affected by Pb ingestion include the nervous system, the hematopoietic system (tissues that produce blood cells), and the kidneys of the urological system. The neurological effect of Pb in exposed children is the driving factor for reducing Pb levels in the environment.[35] Elevated BLLs not only are linked to cognitive deficits but also are associated with behavioural changes including antisocial behaviour, acting out in school, and difficulty paying attention.[35] The cognitive and behavioural changes of Pb-exposed children persist after complete cessation of Pb exposure.[35] In 1991 the CDC lowered the definition of Pb intoxication to 0.483 mcmol/L BLL because several studies reported that children with BLLs of at least 10 μm/dL had impaired intellectual functioning[35] (Figure 4-17). Studies in animals have led to the hypothesis that Pb targets the learning and memory processes by inhibiting the *N*-methyl-D-aspartate receptor (NMDAR), which is necessary for hippocampus-mediated learning and memory.[35,42] Similar changes also have been found in cultured neuron systems.[35] Inhibition of either voltage-gated calcium channels or NMDARs by Pb results in reduction of Ca^{++} entry into the cell, thereby disrupting the

TABLE 4-7 Common Sources of Lead Exposure

Exposure	Source
Environmental	Lead paint, soil, or dust near roadways or lead-painted homes; plastic window blinds; plumbing materials (from pipes or solder); pottery glazes and ceramic ware; lead-core candle wicks; leaded gasoline; water (pipes)
Occupational	Lead mining and refining, plumbing and pipe fitting, auto repair, glass manufacturing, battery manufacturing and recycling, printing shop, construction work, plastic manufacturing, gas station attendant, firing-range attendant
Hobbies	Glazed pottery making, target shooting at firing ranges, lead soldering, preparing fishing sinkers, stained-glass making, painting, car or boat repair
Other	Gasoline sniffing, costume jewelry, cosmetics, contaminated herbal products

Data from Sanborn, M.D., Abelsohn, A., Campbell, M., et al. (2002). *CMAJ, 166*(10), 1287–1292.

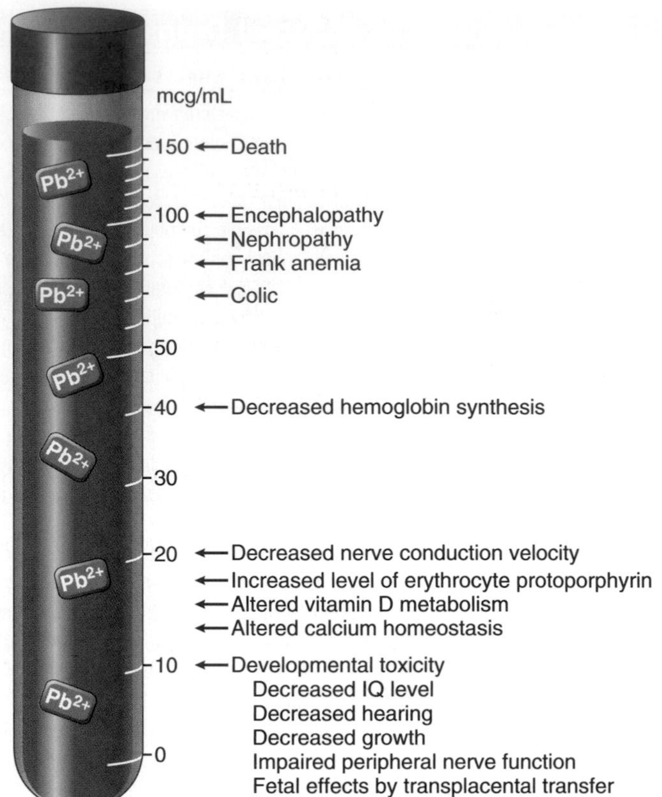

FIGURE 4-17 Lead Poisoning in Children Related to Blood Levels. (From Kumar, V., Abbas, A.K., & Aster, J.C. [Eds.]. [2015]. *Robbins and Cotran pathologic basis of disease* [9th ed.]. Philadelphia: Saunders.)

necessary Ca^{++} signalling for neurotransmission.[43,44] Pb induces cellular damage by increasing oxidative stress.[45] Lead toxicity involves the direct formation of ROS (singlet oxygen, hydrogen peroxides, hydroperoxides) and depletion of antioxidants.[45] Pb exposure leads to lowered levels of glutathione; and because glutathione is important for the metabolism of specific medications and other toxins, low Pb levels can increase their toxicity, as well as the levels of other metals.[45] From animal studies and human population studies, low-level Pb exposure may cause hypertension.[46] Pb interferes with the normal remodelling of cartilage and bone in children. From radiological studies of bone, "lead lines" are detectable and Pb also can be found in the gums as a result of hyperpigmentation. Pb inhibits several enzymes involved in hemoglobin synthesis and causes anemia (most obvious is a microcytic hypochromic anemia). Renal lesions can cause tubular dysfunction, resulting in glycosuria (glucose in the urine), aminoaciduria (amino acids in the urine), and hyperphosphaturia (excess phosphate in the urine). Gastro-intestinal symptoms are less severe and include nausea, loss of appetite, weight loss, and abdominal cramping.

Carbon monoxide. Gaseous substances can be classified according to their ability to asphyxiate (interrupt respiration) or irritate. Toxic asphyxiants, such as carbon monoxide, hydrogen cyanide, and hydrogen sulphide, directly interfere with cellular respiration.

Carbon monoxide (CO) is an odourless, colourless, nonirritating, and undetectable gas unless it is mixed with a visible or odorous pollutant. CO is produced by the incomplete combustion of fuels such as gasoline. Although CO is a chemical agent, the ultimate injury it produces is a hypoxic injury—namely, oxygen deprivation. As a systemic asphyxiant, CO causes death by inducing central nervous system (CNS) depression. Normally, oxygen molecules are carried to tissues bound to hemoglobin in red blood cells (see Chapter 27). Because CO's affinity for hemoglobin is 300 times greater than that of oxygen, CO quickly binds with the hemoglobin, preventing the oxygen molecules' ability to bind to the hemoglobin. Minute amounts of CO can produce a significant percentage of carboxyhemoglobin (carbon monoxide bound with hemoglobin). With increasing levels of carboxyhemoglobin, hypoxia occurs insidiously, evoking widespread ischemic changes in the CNS, and individuals are often unaware of their plight. The diagnosis is made from measurement of carboxyhemoglobin levels in the blood.

Symptoms related to CO poisoning include headache, giddiness, tinnitus (ringing in the ears), chest pain, confusion, nausea, weakness, and vomiting. CO is an *air pollutant* found in combustion fumes produced by cars and trucks, small gasoline engines, stoves, gas ranges, gas refrigerators, heating systems, lanterns, burning charcoal or wood, and cigarette smoke. Chronic exposure can occur in people working in confined spaces, such as underground garages and tunnels. Fumes can accumulate in enclosed or semienclosed spaces, and poisoning from breathing CO can occur in humans and animals. High levels of CO can cause loss of consciousness and death. Death can occur in individuals sleeping or intoxicated before experiencing any symptoms. Although all people and animals are at risk, those most susceptible to poisoning include unborn babies, infants, and people with chronic heart disease, respiratory problems, and anemia. For information on preventing CO poisoning from home appliances and on proper venting, see the following Government of Canada website: http://www.healthycanadians.gc.ca.

Ethanol. Alcohol (ethanol) is the most abused drug in Canada. In 2002, alcohol contributed to 2 000 deaths annually from alcoholic liver disease. A blood concentration of 17 mmol/L is the legal definition for drunk driving in Canada. This level of alcohol in an average person may be reached after consumption of three drinks (three 12-ounce bottles of beer, 15 ounces of wine, and 4 to 5 ounces of distilled liquor). The effects of alcohol vary by age, gender, and percentage of body fat; the rate of metabolism affects the blood alcohol level. Because alcohol is not only a psychoactive drug but also a food, it is considered part of the basic food supply in many societies.

A large intake of alcohol has enormous effects on nutritional status. Liver and nutritional disorders are the most serious consequences of alcohol abuse. Major nutritional deficiencies include magnesium, vitamin B_6, thiamine, and phosphorus. Folic acid deficiency is a common problem in chronic alcoholic populations. Ethanol alters folic acid (folate) homeostasis by decreasing intestinal absorption of folate, increasing

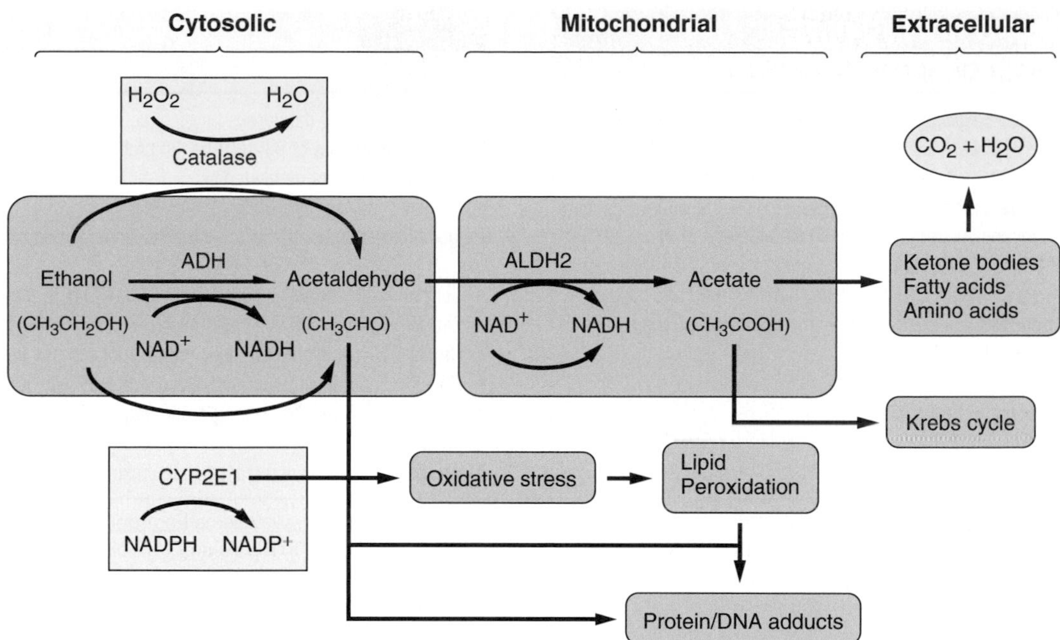

FIGURE 4-18 Ethanol Metabolism Pathway. Ethanol is metabolized into acetaldehyde through the cytosolic enzyme alcohol dehydrogenase (*ADH*), the microsomal enzyme cytochrome P-450 2E1 (*CYP2E1*), and the peroxisomal enzyme catalase. The ADH enzyme reaction is the main ethanol metabolic pathway involving an intermediate carrier of electrons, namely, nicotinamide adenine dinucleotide (*NAD*+), which is reduced by two electrons to form *NADH*. Acetaldehyde is metabolized mainly by aldehyde dehydrogenase 2 (*ALDH2*) in the mitochondria to acetate and NADH before being cleared into the systemic circulation. *CO_2*, carbon dioxide; *H_2O_2*, hydrogen peroxide; *H_2O*, water; *NADP*+, oxidized form of nicotinamide adenine dinucleotide phosphate; *NADPH*, dihydronicotinamide-adenine dinucleotide phosphate. (Reprinted from *Pharmacology & Therapeutics*, 132(1), Yingmei Zhang, Jun Ren, "ALDH2 in alcoholic heart diseases: Molecular mechanism and clinical implications," Pages 86–95, Copyright 2011, with permission from Elsevier.)

liver retention of folate, and increasing the loss of folate through urinary and fecal excretion.[47] Folic acid deficiency becomes especially serious in pregnant women who consume alcohol and may contribute to fetal alcohol spectrum disorder (see p. 92).

Most of the alcohol in blood is metabolized to *acetaldehyde* in the liver by three enzyme systems: alcohol dehydrogenase (ADH), the microsomal ethanol-oxidizing system (MEOS; CYP2E1), and catalase (Figure 4-18). The major pathway involves ADH, an enzyme located in the cytosol of hepatocytes. The MEOS depends on cytochrome P-450 (CYP2E1), an enzyme needed for cellular oxidation. Activation of CYP2E1 requires a high ethanol concentration and thus is thought to be important in the accelerated ethanol metabolism (i.e., tolerance) noted in persons with chronic alcoholism. Acetaldehyde has many toxic tissue effects and is responsible for some of the acute effects of alcohol and for development of head and neck cancer (HNC).[1] A recent and first study showed that HNC risk may be influenced by alcohol-metabolizing genes (*ADH1B* and *ALDH2*) and oral hygiene.[48]

The major effects of acute alcoholism involve the CNS. After alcohol is ingested, it is absorbed, unaltered, in the stomach and small intestine. Fatty foods and milk slow absorption. Alcohol then is distributed to all tissues and fluids of the body in direct proportion to the blood concentration. Individuals differ in their capability to metabolize alcohol. Genetic differences in the metabolism of liver alcohol, including levels of aldehyde dehydrogenases, have been identified.[49] These genetic polymorphisms may account for ethnic and gender differences in ethanol metabolism. Persons with chronic alcoholism develop tolerance because of production of enzymes, leading to an increased rate of metabolism (e.g., P-450).

Numerous studies have validated the so-called *J-* or *U-shaped* inverse association between alcohol and overall or cardiovascular mortality, such as from myocardial infarction and ischemic stroke. These studies have found that light to moderate (nonbinge) drinkers tend to have lower mortality than nondrinkers, and heavy drinkers have higher mortality.[50] (See *Health Promotion:* Low-Risk Alcohol Drinking Guidelines.) The suggested mechanisms for cardioprotection for light to moderate drinkers include increase in levels of high-density lipoprotein–cholesterol (HDL-C), decrease in levels of low-density lipoprotein (LDL), prevention of clot formation, reduction in platelet aggregation, decrease in blood pressure, increase in coronary vessel vasodilation, increase in coronary blood flow, decrease in coronary inflammation, decrease in atherosclerosis, limited ischemia-reperfusion injury (I/R injury), and a decrease in diabetic vessel pathology.[51] The Canadian Heart and Stroke Association recommends no more than 15 drinks per week for men and 10 drinks per week for women (one 341-mL beer, 118 mL of wine, 44 mL of 80-proof spirits, or 29 mL of 100-proof spirits). Drinking more alcohol can increase the risks of alcoholism, high blood pressure, obesity, stroke, breast cancer, suicide, and accidents.[52] Individuals who do not consume alcohol should not be encouraged to start drinking.[53]

Acute alcoholism (drunkenness) affects the CNS. Alcohol intoxication causes CNS depression. Depending on the amount consumed, CNS depression is associated with sedation, drowsiness, loss of motor coordination, delirium, altered behaviour, and loss of consciousness. Toxic amounts (65 to 86 mmol/L) result in a lethal coma or respiratory arrest because of medullary centre depression. Investigators studied the effects of snoring and multiple variables, including alcohol. They found that a low level of self-reported physical activity is a risk factor for future habitual snoring complaints in women independent of alcohol dependence, smoking, current weight, and weight gain. Furthermore, increased physical activity can modify the risk.[54]

HEALTH PROMOTION

Low-Risk Alcohol Drinking Guidelines

Canada's Low-Risk Alcohol Drinking Guidelines recommend no more than 10 drinks per week for women (15 drinks/week for men) with no more than 3 drinks at one time (4 drinks/one time for men). The annual national consumption of alcohol is 470 standard servings per person (or 9 servings/week) for individuals 15 years and over. Risky alcohol consumption is common in underage drinkers (30% at least monthly in 2010) and peaks between 19 and 24 years, with more than 50% of males and 45% of females drinking more than the recommended levels monthly, or more often. The guidelines recommend not drinking when you are:

- operating a motor vehicle
- using machinery or tools
- pregnant or planning to be pregnant
- responsible for the safety of others
- taking medicine or other drugs that interact with alcohol
- doing any kind of dangerous physical activity
- living with mental or physical health problems
- living with alcohol dependence
- making important decisions

The guidelines suggest the following safer drinking tips to prevent injury and illness:

- Set limits for yourself when you drink, and stick to them.
- Eat before and while you are drinking.
- Drink slowly: consume no more than 2 drinks in any 3 hours.
- Have one non-alcoholic drink for every drink of alcohol.
- Consider your age, body weight and health problems that might suggest lower limits.
- Do not start to drink or increase your drinking for perceived health benefits.

From Canadian Centre on Substance Abuse. (2013). *Drinking guidelines.* Retrieved from http://www.ccsa.ca/Eng/topics/alcohol/drinking-guidelines/Pages/default.aspx (accessed October 14, 2016); Statistics Canada. (2012). Table 183-0019: Volume of sales of alcoholic beverages in litres of absolute alcohol and per capita 15 years and over, fiscal years ended March 31, annual. Retrieved March 5, 2012, from http://www5.statcan.gc.ca/cansim/a26?lang=eng&retrLang=eng&id=1830019&paSer=&pattern=&stByVal=2&p1=-1&p2=-1&tabMode=dataTable&csid=; Canadian Centre on Substance Abuse. (2012). *Levels and Patterns of Alcohol Use in Canada. Alcohol Price Policy Series, Report 1 of 3.* Ottawa: CCSA. Retrieved from http://www.ccsa.ca/Resource%20Library/CCSA-Patterns-Alcohol-Use-Policy-Canada-2012-en.pdf.

Acute alcoholism may induce reversible hepatic and gastric changes.[1] Chronic and binge drinking causes alcoholic liver disease (ALD), with a spectrum from hepatic steatosis (fatty change) to steatohepatitis (fatty change and inflammation) and cirrhosis (see Chapter 36). These alterations can eventually lead to hepatocellular carcinoma. The pathogenesis of ALD is not fully characterized, and recent studies reveal a major role of mitochondria. Animal studies have shown that alcohol causes mitochondrial DNA damage, lipid accumulation, and oxidative stress. Acute alcoholism also contributes significantly to motor vehicle fatalities.

Chronic alcoholism causes structural alterations in practically all organs and tissues in the body because most tissues contain enzymes capable of ethanol oxidation or nonoxidative metabolism. The most significant activity, however, occurs in the liver. Alcohol is the leading cause of liver-related morbidity and mortality.[55] In general, hepatic changes, initiated by acetaldehyde, include inflammation, deposition of fat, enlargement of the liver, interruption of microtubular transport of proteins and their secretion, increase in intracellular water, depression of fatty acid oxidation in the mitochondria, increase in membrane rigidity, and acute liver cell necrosis (see Chapter 36). Specifically, chronic or binge alcohol consumption causes ALD with a spectrum ranging from simple fatty liver (steatosis), to steatohepatitis (fatty with inflammation), to cirrhosis (Figure 4-19) (see Chapter 36). Cirrhosis is associated with portal hypertension and an increased risk for hepatocellular carcinoma. Cellular damage is increased by ROS and oxidative stress. Activation of proinflammatory cytokines from neutrophils and lymphocytes mediates liver damage.[56] Oxidative stress is associated with cell membrane phospholipid depletion, which alters the fluidity and function of cell membranes as well as intercellular transport. Chronic alcoholism is related to several disorders, including injury to the myocardium (alcoholic cardiomyopathy); increased tendency to hypertension, acute gastritis, and acute and chronic pancreatitis; and regressive changes in skeletal muscle. Chronic alcohol consumption is associated with an increased incidence of cancer of the oral cavity, liver, esophagus, and breast.

Ethanol is implicated in the onset of a variety of immune defects, including effects on the production of cytokines involved in inflammatory responses. Alcohol can induce epigenetic variations in the developmental pathways of many types of immune cells (e.g., granulocytes, macrophages, and T lymphocytes) that promote increased inflammation.[57] Alcohol increases the development of serious medical conditions related to immune system dysfunction, including acute respiratory distress syndrome (ARDS) as well as liver cancer and ALD.[57] Binge and chronic drinking increases susceptibility to many infectious microorganisms and can enhance the progression of human immunodeficiency virus (HIV) by affecting innate and adaptive immunity.[57]

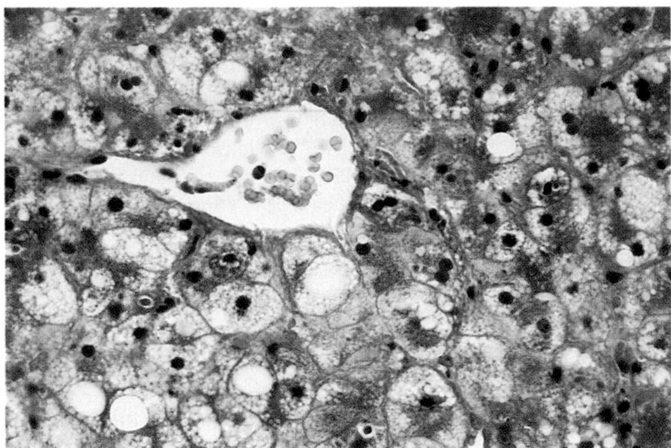

FIGURE 4-19 Alcoholic Hepatitis. Chicken-wire fibrosis extending between hepatocytes (Mallory trichrome stain). (From Damjanov, I., & Linder, J. [Eds.]. [1996]. *Anderson's pathology* [10th ed.]. St. Louis: Mosby.)

The deleterious effects of prenatal alcohol exposure can cause mental deficiency and neurobehavioural disorders, as well as fetal alcohol syndrome. **Fetal alcohol spectrum disorder** includes delayed growth, facial anomalies, cognitive impairment, and ocular malformations (Figure 4-20). It is among the common causes of mental deficiency.[58] Evidence of epigenetic alterations has led to the hypothesis that alcohol effects on fetal development may be caused not only by maternal alcohol consumption but also by the father's exposure as well.[58] Epigenetic alterations may be carried through the male germline for generations.[59] Alcohol crosses the placenta, reaching the fetus, and blood levels of the fetus may reach equivalent levels to maternal levels in 1 to 2 hours.[60] Research has demonstrated an unimpeded bidirectional movement of alcohol between the fetus and the mother. The fetus may completely

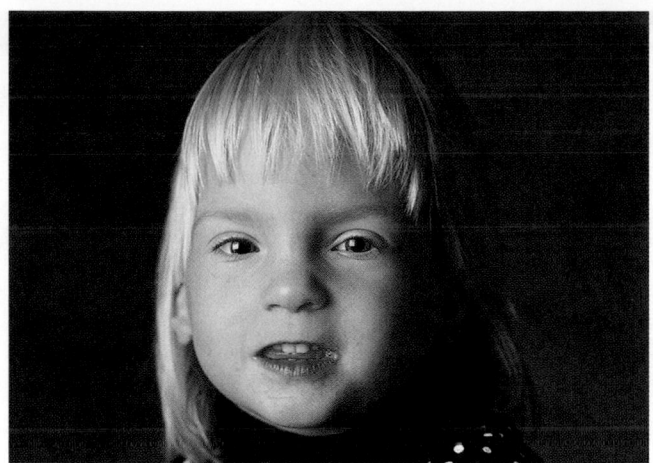

FIGURE 4-20 Fetal Alcohol Spectrum Disorder. When alcohol enters the fetal blood, the potential result can cause tragic congenital abnormalities, such as microcephaly ("small head"), low birth weight, and cardiovascular defects, as well as developmental disabilities, such as physical and intellectual disability, and even death. Note the small head, thinned upper lip, small eye openings (palpebral fissures), epicanthal folds, and receded upper jaw (retrognathia) typical of fetal alcohol spectrum disorder. (From Fortinash, K.M., & Holoday Worret, P.A. [2012]. *Psychiatric mental health nursing* [5th ed.]. St. Louis: Mosby.)

depend on maternal hepatic detoxification because the activity of alcohol dehydrogenase (ADH) in fetal liver is less than 10% of that in the adult liver.[60] Additionally, the amniotic fluid acts as a reservoir for alcohol, prolonging fetal exposure.[60] The specific mechanisms of injury are unknown; however, acetaldehyde can alter fetal development by disrupting differentiation and growth; DNA and protein synthesis; modification of carbohydrates, proteins, and fats; and flow of nutrients across the placenta; and neuro-circuitry dysfunction may be long-lasting.[58,60]

Mercury. Mercury is a global threat to human and environmental health. A recent report, *Global Mercury Assessment 2013*, presents an overview.[61] This report provides the most recent information on worldwide atmospheric mercury emissions, releases to the aquatic environment, and the fate of mercury in the global environment. Causes from human activity, called anthropogenic, are responsible for about 30% of annual emissions of mercury to air, another 10% arise from natural geological sources, and the remainder (60%) occurs from re-emissions or earlier released mercury that has increased over decades and centuries in surface soil and water.[61] The major sources of anthropogenic mercury emissions to air are artisanal and small-scale gold mining (ASGM) and coal burning. The next major sources are the production of ferrous and nonferrous metals, and cement production. Importantly, investigators report that emissions from industrial sectors have increased since 2005.[61] Types of aquatic releases of mercury include industrial sites (power plants, factories), old mines, landfills, and waste disposal locations. ASGM is a significant producer of aquatic mercury release. It is estimated that more than 90% of mercury in marine animals is from anthropogenic emissions.[61] Large amounts of inorganic mercury have accumulated in surface soils and in the oceans. Climate change, with thawing of enormous areas of frozen lands, may release even more long-stored mercury and organic matter into lakes, rivers, and oceans.[61]

Dental amalgams, or "silver fillings," are made of two almost equal parts of liquid mercury and a powder containing silver, tin, copper, zinc, and other metals.[40] When amalgams are placed or removed they can release a small amount of mercury vapour. Chewing can release a small amount of vapour, and people absorb the vapour by inhalation or ingestion.[40] Researchers are studying the effects of exposure to magnetic fields, such as from mobile phone use, and the release of mercury from amalgams.[62] Susceptibility to mercury toxicity varies in a dose-dependent fashion and, among individuals, based on multiple genes, not all of which have been identified.[63,64] Worldwide efforts are under way to phase down or eliminate the use of mercury dental amalgam.[64] Thimerosal, a mercury-containing preservative, was removed from all vaccines in 2001, with the exception of inactivated influenza vaccines.[65]

✔ QUICK CHECK 4-2

1. Why are children more susceptible to the toxic effects of lead exposure?
2. Describe the sources of lead exposure.
3. Describe the mechanisms of cellular injury related to chronic alcoholism.
4. What are the sources of mercury exposure?

Unintentional and Intentional Injuries

Unintentional and intentional injuries are an important health problem in Canada. Statistics on nonfatal injuries are harder to document accurately, but they are known to be a significant cause of morbidity and disability and to cost society billions of dollars annually. The more common terms used to describe and classify unintentional and intentional injuries and brief descriptions of important features of these injuries are discussed in Table 4-8.

Asphyxial Injuries

Asphyxial injuries are caused by a failure of cells to receive or use oxygen. Deprivation of oxygen may be partial (*hypoxia*) or total (*anoxia*). Asphyxial injuries can be grouped into four general categories: suffocation, strangulation, chemical asphyxiants, and drowning.

Suffocation. Suffocation, or oxygen failing to reach the blood, can result from a lack of oxygen in the environment (entrapment in an enclosed space or filling of the environment with a suffocating gas) or blockage of the external airways. Classic examples of these types of asphyxial injuries are a child who is trapped in an abandoned refrigerator or a person who commits suicide by putting a plastic bag over his or her head. A reduction in the ambient oxygen level to 16% (normal is 21%) is immediately dangerous. If the level is below 5%, death can ensue within a matter of minutes. The diagnosis of these types of asphyxial injuries depends on obtaining an accurate and thorough history because there will be no specific physical findings.

Diagnosis and treatment in choking asphyxiation (obstruction of the internal airways) depend on locating and removing the obstructing material. Injury or disease also may cause swelling of the soft tissues of the airway, leading to partial or complete obstruction and subsequent asphyxiation. Suffocation also may result from compression of the chest or abdomen (mechanical or compressional asphyxia), preventing normal respiratory movements. Usual signs and symptoms include florid facial congestion and petechiae (pinpoint hemorrhages) of the eyes and face.

Strangulation. Strangulation is caused by compression and closure of the blood vessels and air passages resulting from external pressure on the neck. Strangulation causes cerebral hypoxia or anoxia secondary to the alteration or cessation of blood flow to and from the brain. It is important to remember that the amount of force needed to close the jugular veins (2 kg) or carotid arteries (5 kg) is significantly less than that required to crush the trachea (15 kg). It is the alteration of cerebral blood flow in most types of strangulation that causes injury or death—not the lack of airflow. With complete blockage of the carotid arteries, unconsciousness can occur within 10 to 15 seconds.

A noose is placed around the neck, and the weight of the body is used to cause constriction of the noose and compression of the neck

TABLE 4-8 Unintentional and Intentional Injuries

Type of Injury	Description
BLUNT-FORCE INJURIES 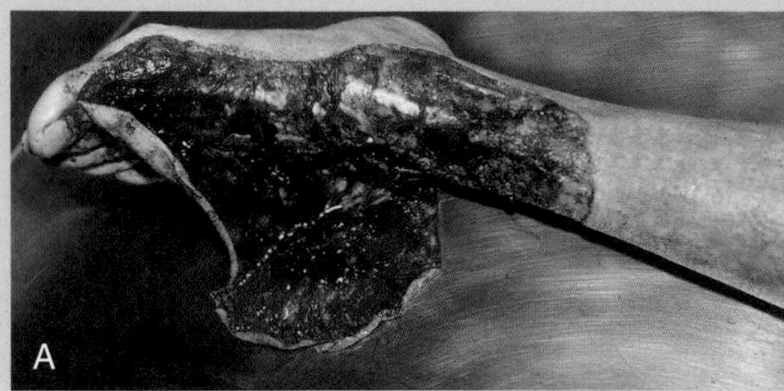	Mechanical injury to body resulting in tearing, shearing, or crushing; most common type of injury seen in health care settings; caused by blows or impacts; motor vehicle accidents and falls most common cause (see photo A) *Contusion* (*bruise*): Bleeding into skin or underlying tissues; initial colour will be red-purple, then blue-black, then yellow-brown or green (see Figure 4-24); duration of bruise depends on extent, location, and degree of vascularization; bruising of soft tissue may be confined to deeper structures; *hematoma* is collection of blood in soft tissue; *subdural hematoma* is blood between inner surface of dura mater and surface of brain; can result from blows, falls, or sudden acceleration/deceleration of head as occurs in *shaken baby syndrome; epidural hematoma* is collection of blood between inner surface of skull and dura; is most often associated with a skull fracture *Laceration:* Tear or rip resulting when tensile strength of skin or tissue is exceeded; is ragged and irregular with abraded edges; an extreme example is *avulsion,* where a wide area of tissue is pulled away; lacerations of internal organs are common in blunt-force injuries; lacerations of liver, spleen, kidneys, and bowel occur from blows to abdomen; thoracic aorta may be lacerated in sudden deceleration accidents; severe blows or impacts to chest may rupture heart with lacerations of atria or ventricles *Fracture:* Blunt-force blows or impacts can cause bone to break or shatter (see Chapter 39)
SHARP-FORCE INJURIES 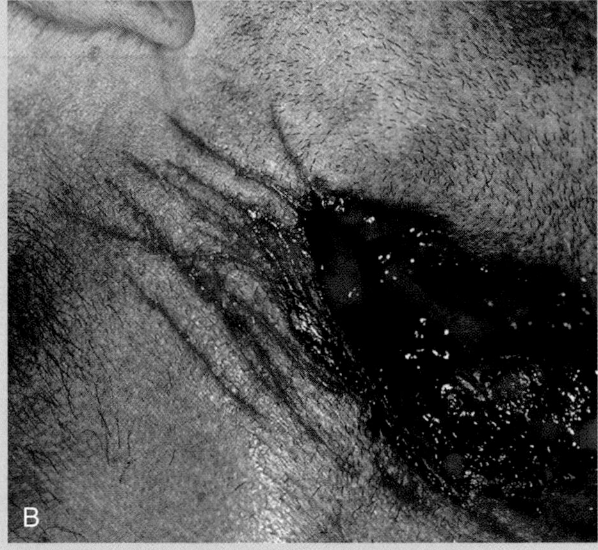	Sharp-force injuries are characterized by a relatively well-defined traumatic separation of tissues, occurring when a sharp-edged or pointed object comes into contact with the skin and underlying tissues. Three specific subtypes of sharp-force injuries exist, as follows: stab wounds, incised wounds, and chop wounds.[a] *Incised wound:* A wound that is *longer* than it is *deep;* wound can be straight or jagged with sharp, distinct edges without abrasion; usually produces significant external bleeding with little internal hemorrhage; these wounds are noted in sharp-force injury suicides; in addition to a deep, lethal cut, there will be superficial incisions in same area called *hesitation marks* (see photo B) *Stab wound:* A penetrating sharp-force injury that is *deeper* than it is *long;* if a sharp instrument is used, depths of wound are clean and distinct but can be abraded if object is inserted deeply and wider portion (e.g., hilt of a knife) impacts skin; depending on size and location of wound, external bleeding may be surprisingly small; after an initial spurt of blood, even if a major vessel or heart is struck, wound may be almost completely closed by tissue pressure, thus allowing only a trickle of visible blood despite copious internal bleeding *Puncture wound:* Instruments or objects with sharp points but without sharp edges produce puncture wounds; classic example is wound of foot after stepping on a nail; wounds are prone to infection, have abrasion of edges, and can be very deep *Chopping wound:* Heavy, edged instruments (axes, hatchets, propeller blades) produce wounds with a combination of sharp- and blunt-force characteristics
GUNSHOT WOUNDS 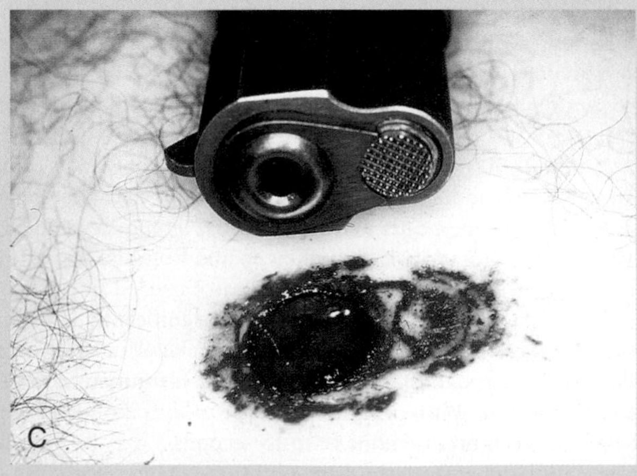	Gunshot wounds are either penetrating (bullet remains in body) or perforating (bullet exits body); bullet also can fragment; most important factors or appearances are whether it is an entrance or exit wound and range of fire *Entrance wound:* All wounds share some common features; overall appearance is most affected by range of fire *Contact range entrance wound:* Distinctive type of wound when gun is held so muzzle rests on or presses into skin surface; there is searing of edges of wound from flame and soot or smoke on edges of wound in addition to hole; hard contact wounds of head cause severe tearing and disruption of tissue (because of thin layer of skin and muscle overlying bone); wound is gaping and jagged, known as *blow back*; can produce a patterned abrasion that mirrors weapon used (see photo C)

TABLE 4-8 Unintentional and Intentional Injuries—cont'd

Type of Injury	Description
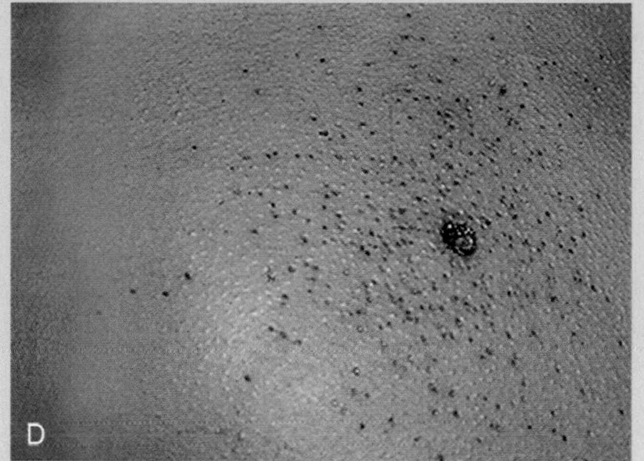	*Intermediate (distance) range entrance wound:* Surrounded by gunpowder tattooing or stippling; *tattooing* results from fragments of burning or unburned pieces of gunpowder exiting barrel and forcefully striking skin; *stippling* results when gunpowder abrades but does not penetrate skin (see photo D) *Indeterminate range entrance wound:* Occurs when flame, soot, or gunpowder does not reach skin surface but bullet does; *indeterminate* is used rather than *distant* because appearance may be same regardless of distance; for example, if an individual is shot at close range through multiple layers of clothing the wound may look the same as if the shooting occurred at a distance *Exit wound:* Has the same appearance regardless of range of fire; most important factors are speed of projectile and degree of deformation; size cannot be used to determine if hole is an exit or entrance wound; usually has clean edges that can often be re-approximated to cover defect; skin is one of toughest structures for a bullet to penetrate; thus it is not uncommon for a bullet to pass entirely through body but stopped just beneath skin on "exit" side *Wounding potential of bullets:* Most damage done by a bullet is a result of amount of energy transferred to tissue impacted; speed of bullet has much greater effect than increased size; some bullets are designed to expand or fragment when striking an object, for example, *hollow-point* ammunition; lethality of a wound depends on what structures are damaged; wounds of brain may not be lethal; however, they are usually immediately incapacitating and lead to significant long-term disability; a person with a "lethal" injury (wound of heart or aorta) also may not be immediately incapacitated

[a]From Prahlow, J.A. (2016). Forensic autopsy of sharp-force injuries. Retrieved from http://emedicine.medscape.com/article/1680082-overview.

in hanging strangulations. The body does not need to be completely suspended to produce severe injury or death. Depending on the type of ligature used, there usually is a distinct mark on the neck—an inverted V with the base of the V pointing toward the point of suspension. Internal injuries of the neck are actually quite rare in hangings, and only in judicial hangings, in which the body is weighted and dropped, is significant soft tissue or cervical spinal trauma seen. Petechiae of the eyes or face may be seen, but they are rare.

In ligature strangulation, the mark on the neck is horizontal without the inverted V pattern seen in hangings. Petechiae may be more common because intermittent opening and closure of the blood vessels may occur as a result of the victim's struggles. Internal injuries of the neck are rare.

Variable amounts of external trauma on the neck are found with contusions and abrasions in manual strangulation caused either by the assailant or by the victim clawing at his or her own neck in an attempt to remove the assailant's hands. Internal damage can be quite severe, with bruising of deep structures and even fractures of the hyoid bone and tracheal and cricoid cartilages. Petechiae are common.

Chemical asphyxiants. Chemical asphyxiants either prevent the delivery of oxygen to the tissues or block its utilization. Carbon monoxide is the most common chemical asphyxiant. Cyanide acts as an asphyxiant by combining with the ferric iron atom in cytochrome oxidase, thereby blocking the intracellular use of oxygen. A victim of cyanide poisoning will have the same cherry-red appearance as a carbon monoxide intoxication victim because cyanide blocks the use of circulating oxyhemoglobin. An odour of bitter almonds also may be detected. (The ability to smell cyanide is a genetic trait that is absent in a significant portion of the general population.) Hydrogen sulphide (sewer gas) is a chemical asphyxiant in which victims of hydrogen cyanide poisoning may have brown-tinged blood in addition to the nonspecific signs of asphyxiation.

Drowning. Drowning is an alteration of oxygen delivery to tissues resulting from the inhalation of fluid, usually water. In 2012 there were 495 drowning deaths in Canada.[66] Although research in the 1940s and 1950s indicated that changes in blood electrolyte levels and volume as a result of absorption of fluid from the lungs may be an important factor in some drownings, the major mechanism of injury is hypoxemia (low blood oxygen levels). Even in freshwater drownings, where large amounts of water can pass through the alveolar-capillary interface, there is no evidence that increases in blood volume cause significant electrolyte disturbances or hemolysis, or that the amount of fluid loading is beyond the compensatory capabilities of the kidneys and heart. Airway obstruction is the more important pathological abnormality, underscored by the fact that in as many as 15% of drownings little or no water enters the lungs because of vagal nerve–mediated laryngospasms. This phenomenon is called dry-lung drowning.

No matter what mechanism is involved, cerebral hypoxia leads to unconsciousness in a matter of minutes. Whether it progresses to death depends on a number of factors, including the age and the health of the individual. One of the most important factors is the temperature of the water. Irreversible injury develops much more rapidly in warm water than it does in cold water. Submersion times of up to 1 hour with subsequent survival have been reported in children who were submerged in very cold water. Complete submersion is not necessary for a person to drown. An incapacitated or helpless individual (epileptic, alcoholic, infant) may drown in water that is only a few centimetres deep.

It is important to remember that no specific or diagnostic findings *prove* that a person recovered from the water is actually a drowning victim. In cases where water has entered the lung, there may be large amounts of foam exiting the nose and mouth, although the same sign also can be seen in certain types of drug overdoses. A body recovered from water with signs of prolonged immersion could just as easily be a victim of some other type of injury with the immersion acting to obscure the actual cause of death. When working with a living victim recovered from water, it is essential to keep in mind that an underlying condition may have led to the person's becoming incapacitated and submerged—a condition that also may need to be treated or corrected while correcting hypoxemia and dealing with its sequelae.

> **QUICK CHECK 4-3**
> 1. Give examples of intentional and unintentional injury.
> 2. Describe unintentional injury as a form of injury in health care delivery in Canada.
> 3. What is the major mechanism of injury with drowning?

Infectious Injury

The pathogenicity (virulence) of microorganisms lies in their ability to survive and proliferate in the human body, where they injure cells and tissues. The disease-producing potential of a microorganism depends on its ability to (1) invade and destroy cells, (2) produce toxins, and (3) produce damaging hypersensitivity reactions. (See Chapter 8 for a description of infection and infectious organisms.)

Immunological and Inflammatory Injury

Cellular membranes are injured by direct contact with cellular and chemical components of the immune and inflammatory responses, such as phagocytic cells (lymphocytes, macrophages) and substances such as histamine, antibodies, lymphokines, complement, and proteases (see Chapter 6). Complement is responsible for many of the membrane alterations that occur during immunological injury.

Membrane alterations are associated with a rapid leakage of K^+ out of the cell and a rapid influx of water. Antibodies can interfere with membrane function by binding with and occupying receptor molecules on the plasma membrane. Antibodies also can block or destroy cellular junctions, interfering with intercellular communication. Other mechanisms of cellular injury are genetic and epigenetic factors, nutritional imbalances, and physical agents. These mechanisms are summarized in Table 4-9.

MANIFESTATIONS OF CELLULAR INJURY: ACCUMULATIONS

An important manifestation of cellular injury is the intracellular accumulation of abnormal amounts of various substances and the resultant metabolic disturbances. Cellular accumulations, also known as infiltrations, result not only from sublethal, sustained injury by cells but also from normal (but inefficient) cell function. Two categories of substances can produce accumulations: (1) *normal cellular substances* (such as excess water, proteins, lipids, and carbohydrates) and (2) *abnormal substances*, either endogenous (such as a product of abnormal metabolism or synthesis) or exogenous (such as infectious agents or a mineral). These products can accumulate transiently or permanently and can be toxic or harmless. Most accumulations are attributed to four types of mechanisms, all abnormal (Figure 4-21). Abnormal accumulations of these substances can occur in the cytoplasm (often in the lysosomes) or in the nucleus if (1) there is insufficient removal of the normal substance because of altered packaging and transport, for example, fatty change in the liver called *steatosis*; (2) an abnormal substance, often the result of a mutated gene, accumulates because of defects in protein folding, transport, or abnormal degradation; (3) an endogenous substance (normal or abnormal) is not effectively catabolized, usually because of lack of a vital lysosomal enzyme, called *storage diseases*; or (4) harmful exogenous materials, such as heavy metals, mineral dusts, or microorganisms, accumulate because of inhalation, ingestion, or infection.

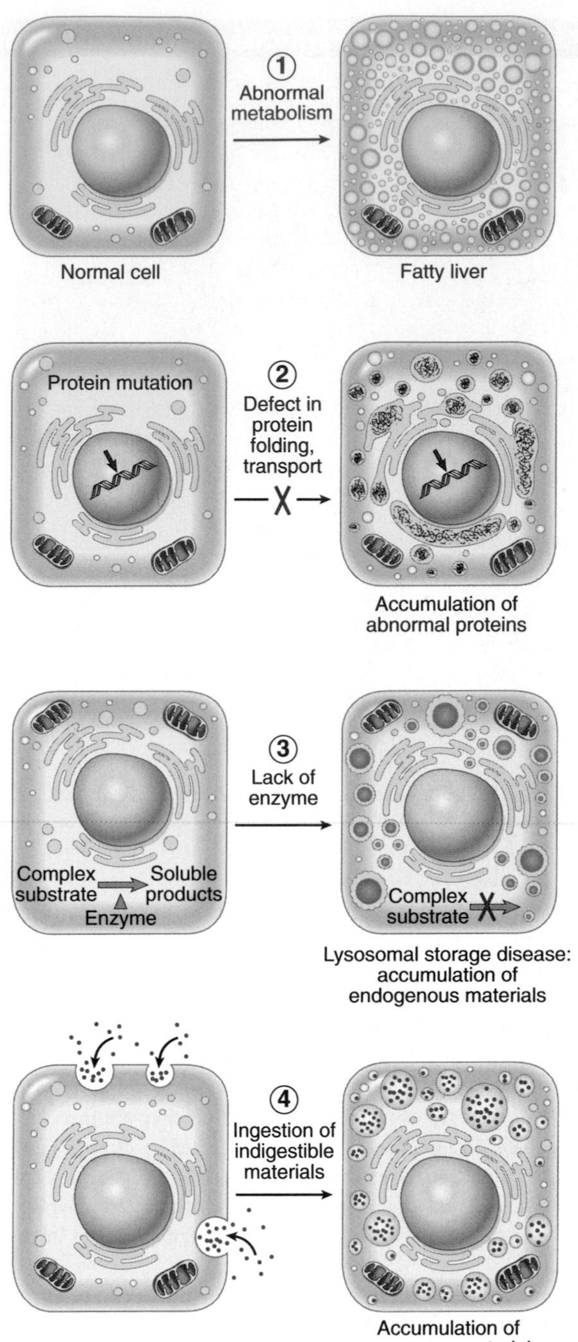

FIGURE 4-21 Mechanisms of Intracellular Accumulations. (From Kumar, V., Abbas, A.K., & Aster, J.C. [Eds.]. [2015]. *Robbins and Cotran pathologic basis of disease* [9th ed.]. Philadelphia: Saunders.)

In all storage diseases, the cells attempt to digest, or catabolize, the "stored" substances. As a result, excessive amounts of metabolites (products of catabolism) accumulate in the cells and are expelled into the ECM, where they are consumed by phagocytic cells called *macrophages* (see Chapter 6). Some of these scavenger cells circulate throughout the body, whereas others remain fixed in certain tissues, such as the liver or spleen. As more and more macrophages and other phagocytes migrate to tissues that are producing excessive metabolites, the affected tissues begin to swell. This mechanism causes enlargement of the liver

TABLE 4-9 **Mechanisms of Cellular Injury**

Mechanism	Characteristics	Examples
Genetic Factors	Alter cell's nucleus and plasma membrane's structure, shape, receptors, or transport mechanisms	Sickle cell anemia, Huntington's disease, muscular dystrophy, abetalipoproteinemia, familial hypercholesterolemia
Epigenetic Factors	Induction of mitotically heritable alterations in gene expression without changing DNA	Gene silencing in cancer
Nutritional Imbalances	Pathophysiological cellular effects develop when nutrients are not consumed in diet and transported to body's cells *or* when excessive amounts of nutrients are consumed and transported	Protein deficiency, protein-calorie malnutrition, glucose deficiency, lipid deficiency (hypolipidemia), dyslipidemia (increased lipoproteins in blood causing deposits of fat in heart, liver, and muscle), vitamin deficiencies
Physical Agents		
Temperature extremes	*Hypothermic injury* results from chilling or freezing of cells, creating high intracellular sodium concentrations; abrupt drops in temperature lead to vasoconstriction and increased viscosity of blood, causing ischemic injury, infarction, and necrosis; reactive oxygen species are important in this process	Frostbite
	Hyperthermic injury is caused by excessive heat and varies in severity according to nature, intensity, and extent of heat	Burns, burn blisters, heat cramps usually from vigorous exercise with water and salt loss; heat exhaustion with salt and water loss causes heme contraction; heat stroke is life-threatening with a clinical rectal temperature of 41°C (106°F)
	Tissue injury caused by compressive waves of air or fluid impinging on body, followed by sudden wave of decreased pressure; changes may collapse thorax, rupture internal solid organs, and cause widespread hemorrhage: carbon dioxide and nitrogen that are normally dissolved in blood precipitate from solution and form small bubbles (gas emboli), causing hypoxic injury and pain	Blast injury (air or immersion), decompression sickness (caisson disease or "the bends"); recently reported in a few individuals with subdural hematomas after riding high-speed roller coasters
Ionizing radiation	Refers to any form of radiation that can remove orbital electrons from atoms; source is usually environment and medical use; damage is to DNA molecule, causing chromosomal aberrations, chromosomal instability, and damage to membranes and enzymes; also induces growth factors and extracellular matrix remodelling; uncertainty exists regarding effects of low levels of radiation	X-rays, γ-rays, and α- and β-particles cause skin redness, skin damage, chromosomal damage, cancer
Illumination	Fluorescent lighting and halogen lamps create harmful oxidative stresses; ultraviolet light has been linked to skin cancer	Eyestrain, obscured vision, cataracts, headaches, melanoma
Mechanical stresses	Injury is caused by physical impact or irritation; they may be overt or cumulative	Faulty occupational biomechanics, leading to overexertion disorders
Noise	Can be caused by acute loud noise or cumulative effects of various intensities, frequencies, and duration of noise; considered a public health threat	Hearing impairment or loss; tinnitus, temporary threshold shift, or loss can occur as a complication of critical illness, from mechanical trauma, ototoxic medications, infections, vascular disorders, and noise

(hepatomegaly) or the spleen (splenomegaly) as a clinical manifestation of many storage diseases.

Water

Cellular swelling, the most common degenerative change, is caused by the shift of extracellular water into the cells. In hypoxic injury, movement of fluid and ions into the cell is associated with acute failure of metabolism and loss of ATP production. Normally, the pump that transports sodium ions (Na^+) out of the cell is maintained by the presence of ATP and adenosinetriphosphatase (ATPase), the active transport enzyme. In metabolic failure caused by hypoxia, reduced levels of ATP and ATPase permit sodium to accumulate in the cell while potassium (K^+) diffuses outward. The increased intracellular sodium concentration increases osmotic pressure, drawing more water into the cell. The cisternae of the ER become distended, rupture, and then unite to form large vacuoles that isolate the water from the cytoplasm, a process called *vacuolation.* Progressive vacuolation results in cytoplasmic swelling called **oncosis** (which has replaced the old term *hydropic [water] degeneration*) or **vacuolar degeneration** (Figure 4-22). If cellular swelling affects all the cells in an organ, the organ increases in weight and becomes distended and pale.

Cellular swelling is reversible and is considered sublethal. It is, in fact, an early manifestation of almost all types of cellular injury, including severe or lethal cellular injury. It is also associated with high fever, hypokalemia (abnormally low concentrations of potassium in the blood; see Chapter 5), and certain infections.

Lipids and Carbohydrates

Certain metabolic disorders result in the abnormal intracellular accumulation of carbohydrates and lipids. These substances may accumulate throughout the body but are found primarily in the spleen, liver, and CNS. Accumulations in cells of the CNS can cause neurological dysfunction

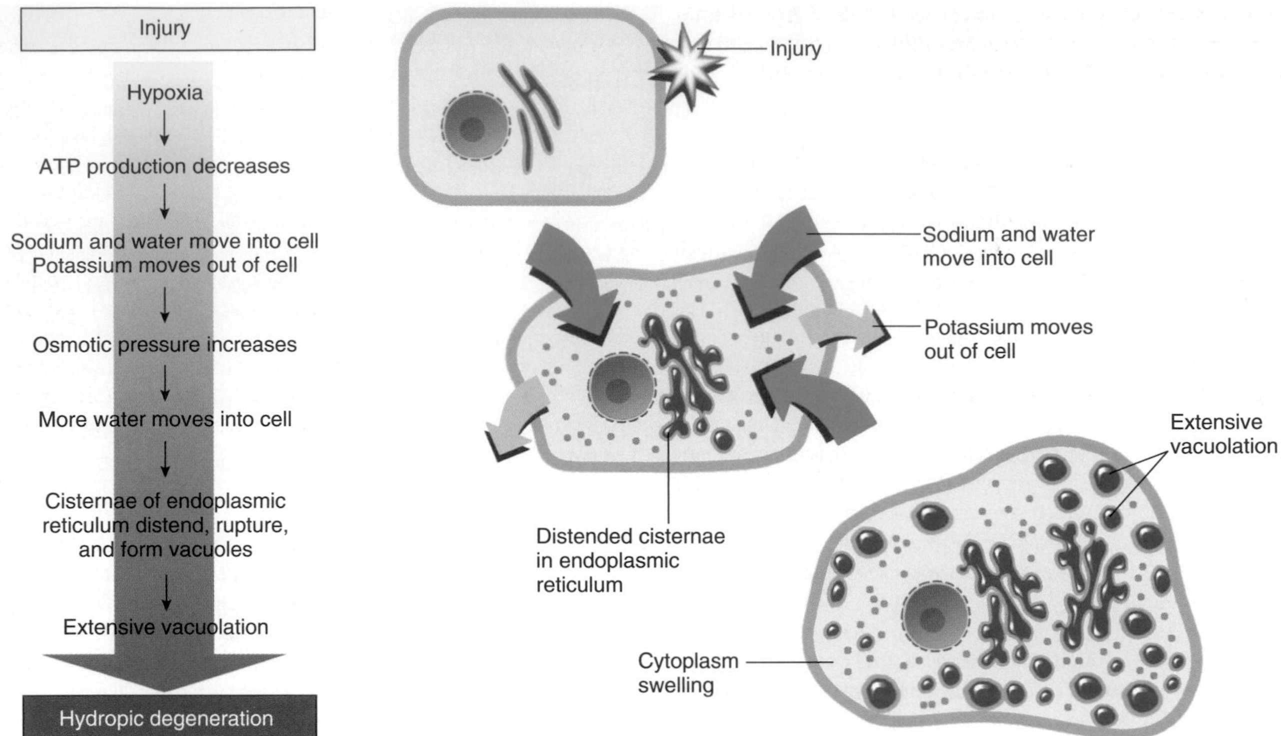

FIGURE 4-22 The Process of Oncosis (Formerly Referred to as "Hydropic Degeneration"). *ATP,* adenosine triphosphate.

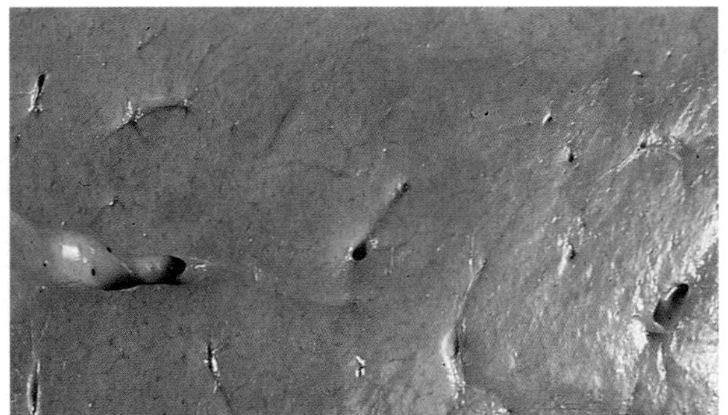

FIGURE 4-23 Fatty Liver. The liver appears yellow. (From Damjanov, I., & Linder, J. [2000]. *Pathology: A color atlas.* St. Louis: Mosby.)

and severe intellectual disability. Lipids accumulate in Tay-Sachs disease, Niemann-Pick disease, and Gaucher's disease; whereas in the diseases known as mucopolysaccharidoses, carbohydrates are in excess. The mucopolysaccharidoses are progressive disorders that usually involve multiple organs, including liver, spleen, heart, and blood vessels. The accumulated mucopolysaccharides are found in reticuloendothelial cells, endothelial cells, intimal smooth muscle cells, and fibroblasts throughout the body. These carbohydrate accumulations can cause clouding of the cornea, joint stiffness, and intellectual disability.

Although lipids sometimes accumulate in heart, muscle, and kidney cells, the most common site of intracellular lipid accumulation, or **fatty change (steatosis)**, is liver cells (Figure 4-23). Because hepatic metabolism and secretion of lipids are crucial to proper body function, imbalances and deficiencies in these processes lead to major pathological changes. In developed countries, the most common cause of fatty change in the liver is alcohol abuse. Other causes of fatty change include diabetes mellitus, protein malnutrition, toxins, anoxia, and obesity. As lipids fill the cells, vacuolation pushes the nucleus and other organelles aside. The liver's outward appearance is yellow and greasy. Alcohol abuse is one of the most common causes of fatty liver (see Chapter 36).

Lipid accumulation in liver cells occurs after cellular injury instigates one or more of the following mechanisms:

1. Increased movement of free fatty acids into the liver (starvation, e.g., increases the metabolism of triglycerides in adipose tissue, releasing fatty acids that subsequently enter liver cells)
2. Failure of the metabolic process that converts fatty acids to phospholipids, resulting in the preferential conversion of fatty acids to triglycerides
3. Increased synthesis of triglycerides from fatty acids (increased levels of the enzyme α-glycerophosphatase can accelerate triglyceride synthesis)
4. Decreased synthesis of apoproteins (lipid-acceptor proteins)
5. Failure of lipids to bind with apoproteins and form lipoproteins
6. Failure of mechanisms that transport lipoproteins out of the cell
7. Direct damage to the ER by free radicals released by alcohol's toxic effects

Many pathological states show accumulation of cholesterol and cholesterol esters. These states include atherosclerosis, in which atherosclerotic plaques, smooth muscle cells, and macrophages within the intimal layer of the aorta and large arteries are filled with lipid-rich vacuoles of cholesterol and cholesterol esters. Other states include cholesterol-rich deposits in the gallbladder and Niemann-Pick disease (type C), which involve genetic mutations of an enzyme affecting cholesterol transport.

Glycogen

Glycogen storage is important as a readily available energy source in the cytoplasm of normal cells. Intracellular accumulations of glycogen are seen in genetic disorders called *glycogen storage diseases* and in disorders of glucose and glycogen metabolism. As with water and lipid accumulation, glycogen accumulation results in excessive vacuolation of the cytoplasm. The most common cause of glycogen accumulation is the disorder of glucose metabolism (i.e., diabetes mellitus) (see Chapter 19).

Proteins

Proteins provide cellular structure and constitute most of the cell's dry weight. The proteins are synthesized on ribosomes in the cytoplasm from the essential amino acids lysine, threonine, leucine, isoleucine, methionine, tryptophan, valine, phenylalanine, and histidine. The accumulation of protein probably damages cells in two ways. First, metabolites, produced when the cell attempts to digest some proteins, are enzymes that when released from lysosomes can damage cellular organelles. Second, excessive amounts of protein in the cytoplasm push against cellular organelles, disrupting organelle function and intracellular communication.

Protein excess accumulates primarily in the epithelial cells of the renal convoluted tubules of the nephron unit and in the antibody-forming plasma cells (B lymphocytes) of the immune system. Several types of renal disorders cause excessive excretion of protein molecules in the urine (proteinuria). Normally, little or no protein is present in the urine, and its presence in significant amounts indicates cellular injury and altered cellular function.

Accumulations of protein in B lymphocytes can occur during active synthesis of antibodies during the immune response. The excess aggregates of protein are called *Russell bodies* (see Chapter 6). Russell bodies have been identified in multiple myeloma (plasma cell tumour) (see Chapter 21).

Mutations in protein can slow protein folding, resulting in the accumulation of partially folded intermediates. An example is α_1-antitrypsin deficiency, which can cause emphysema. Certain types of cellular injury are associated with the accumulation of cytoskeleton proteins. For example, the *neurofibrillary tangle* found in the brain in Alzheimer's disease contains these types of proteins.

Pigments

Pigment accumulations may be normal or abnormal, endogenous (produced within the body) or exogenous (produced outside the body). Endogenous pigments are derived, for example, from amino acids (e.g., tyrosine, tryptophan). They include melanin and the blood proteins porphyrins, hemoglobin, and hemosiderin. Lipid-rich pigments, such as lipofuscin (the aging pigment), give a yellow-brown colour to cells undergoing slow, regressive, and often atrophic changes. The most common exogenous pigment is carbon (coal dust), a pervasive air pollutant in urban areas. Inhaled carbon interacts with lung macrophages and is transported by lymphatic vessels to regional lymph nodes. This accumulation blackens lung tissues and involved lymph nodes. Other exogenous pigments include mineral dusts containing silica and iron particles, lead, silver salts, and dyes for tattoos.

Melanin

Melanin accumulates in epithelial cells (keratinocytes) of the skin and retina. It is an extremely important pigment because it protects the skin against long exposure to sunlight and is considered an essential factor in the prevention of skin cancer (see Chapters 11 and 41). Ultraviolet light (e.g., sunlight) stimulates the synthesis of melanin, which probably absorbs ultraviolet rays during subsequent exposure. Melanin also may protect the skin by trapping the injurious free radicals produced by the action of ultraviolet light on skin.

Melanin is a brown-black pigment derived from the amino acid *tyrosine*. It is synthesized by epidermal cells called *melanocytes* and is stored in membrane-bound cytoplasmic vesicles called *melanosomes.*

Melanin also can accumulate in melanophores (melanin-containing pigment cells), macrophages, or other phagocytic cells in the dermis. Presumably these cells acquire the melanin from nearby melanocytes or from pigment that has been extruded from dying epidermal cells. This mechanism causes freckles. Melanin also occurs in the benign form of pigmented moles called *nevi* (see Chapter 41). Malignant melanoma is a cancerous skin tumour that contains melanin.

A decrease in melanin production occurs in the inherited disorder of melanin metabolism called *albinism.* Albinism is often diffuse, involving all the skin, the eyes, and the hair. Albinism is also related to phenylalanine metabolism. In classic types, the person with albinism is unable to convert tyrosine to 3,4-dihydroxyphenylalanine (DOPA), an intermediate in melanin biosynthesis. Melanocytes are present in normal numbers, but they are unable to make melanin. Individuals with albinism are very sensitive to sunlight and quickly become sunburned. They are also at high risk for skin cancer.

Hemoproteins

Hemoproteins are among the most essential of the normal endogenous pigments. They include hemoglobin and the oxidative enzymes, the cytochromes. Central to an understanding of disorders involving these pigments is knowledge of iron uptake, metabolism, excretion, and storage (see Chapter 20). Hemoprotein accumulations in cells are caused by excessive storage of iron, which is transferred to the cells from the bloodstream. Iron enters the blood from three primary sources: (1) tissue stores, (2) the intestinal mucosa, and (3) macrophages that remove and destroy dead or defective red blood cells. The amount of iron in blood plasma depends also on the metabolism of the major iron transport protein, *transferrin.*

Iron is stored in tissue cells in two forms: as ferritin and, when increased levels of iron are present, as hemosiderin. Hemosiderin is a yellow-brown pigment derived from hemoglobin. With pathological states, excesses of iron cause hemosiderin to accumulate within cells, often in areas of bruising and hemorrhage and in the lungs and spleen after congestion caused by heart failure. With local hemorrhage, the skin first appears red-blue and then lysis of the escaped red blood cells occurs, causing the hemoglobin to be transformed to hemosiderin. The colour changes noted in bruising reflect this transformation (Figure 4-24).

Hemosiderosis is a condition in which excess iron is stored as hemosiderin in the cells of many organs and tissues. This condition is common in individuals who have received repeated blood transfusions or prolonged parenteral administration of iron. Hemosiderosis is associated also with increased absorption of dietary iron, conditions in which iron storage and transport are impaired, and hemolytic anemia. Excessive alcohol (e.g., wine) ingestion also can lead to hemosiderosis. Normally, absorption of excessive dietary iron is prevented by an iron absorption process in the intestines. Failure of this process can lead to total body iron accumulations in the range of 60 to 80 g, compared with normal iron stores of 4.5 to 5 g. Excessive accumulations of iron, such as occur in hemochromatosis (a genetic disorder of iron metabolism and the most severe example of iron overload), are associated with liver and pancreatic cell damage.

Bilirubin is a normal, yellow-to-green pigment of bile derived from the porphyrin structure of hemoglobin. Excess bilirubin within cells and tissues causes jaundice (icterus), or yellowing of the skin. Jaundice occurs when the bilirubin level exceeds 25 to 34 mmol/L of plasma, compared with the normal values of 6.8 to 17.1 mmol/L. Hyperbilirubinemia occurs with (1) destruction of red blood cells (erythrocytes), such as in hemolytic jaundice; (2) diseases affecting the metabolism and excretion of bilirubin in the liver; and (3) diseases that cause obstruction of the common bile duct, such as gallstones or pancreatic tumours. Certain medications (specifically chlorpromazine [Largactil]

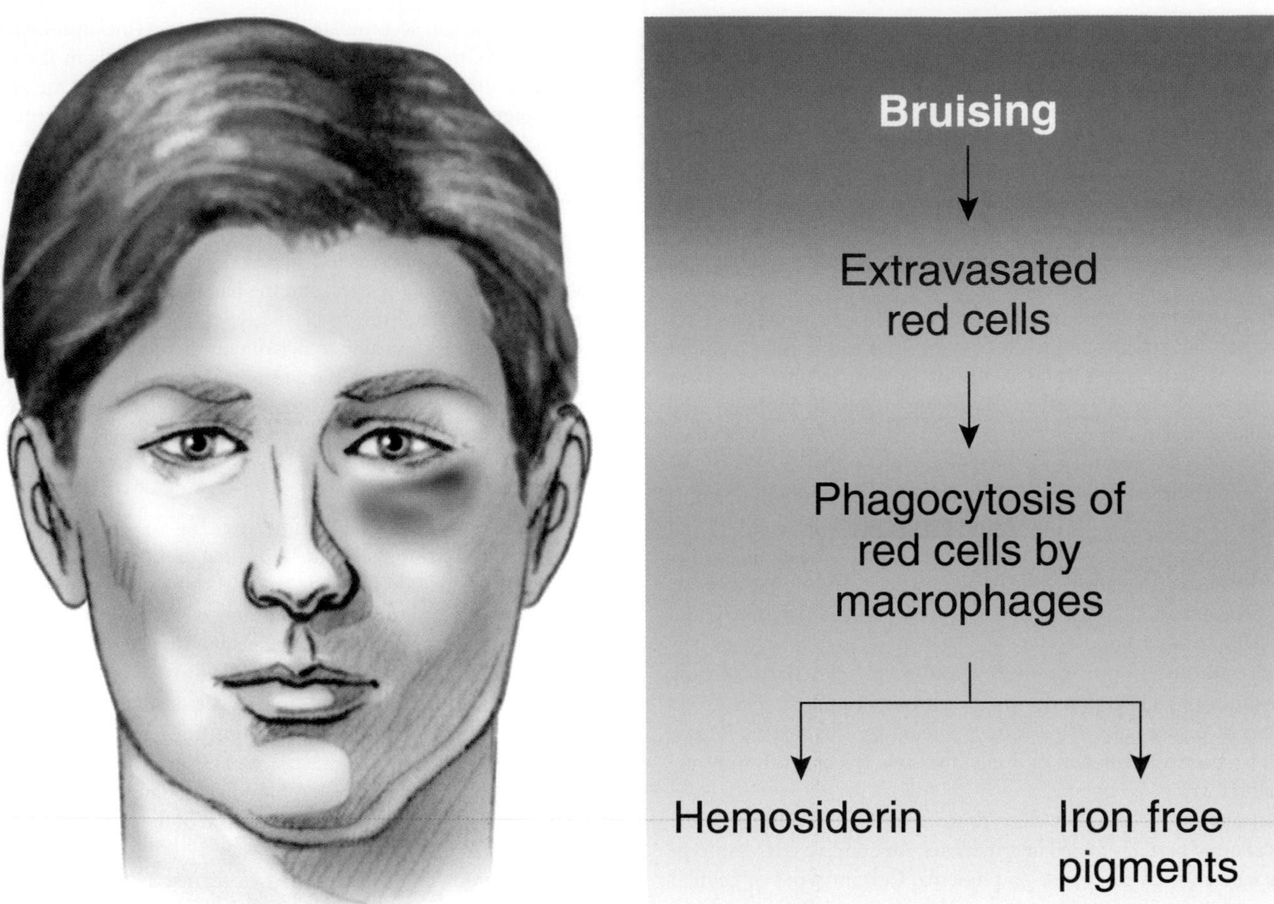

FIGURE 4-24 Hemosiderin Accumulation Is Noted as the Colour Changes in a "Black Eye."

and other phenothiazine derivatives), estrogenic hormones, and halothane (Fluothane) (an anaesthetic) can cause the obstruction of normal bile flow through the liver.

Because unconjugated bilirubin is lipid soluble, it can injure the lipid components of the plasma membrane. Albumin, a plasma protein, provides significant protection by binding unconjugated bilirubin in plasma. Unconjugated bilirubin causes two cellular outcomes: uncoupling of oxidative phosphorylation and a loss of cellular proteins. These two changes could cause structural injury to the various membranes of the cell.

Calcium

Calcium salts accumulate in both injured and dead tissues (Figure 4-25). An important mechanism of cellular calcification is the influx of extracellular calcium in injured mitochondria. Another mechanism that causes calcium accumulation in alveoli (gas-exchange airways of the lungs), gastric epithelium, and renal tubules is the excretion of acid at these sites, leading to the local production of hydroxyl ions. Hydroxyl ions result in precipitation of calcium hydroxide, $Ca(OH)_2$, and hydroxyapatite, $Ca_5(PO_4)_3OH$, a mixed salt. Damage occurs when calcium salts cluster and harden, interfering with normal cellular structure and function.

Pathological calcification can be dystrophic or metastatic. **Dystrophic calcification** occurs in dying and dead tissues in areas of necrosis (see also the types of necrosis: coagulative, liquefactive, caseous, and fatty). It is present in chronic tuberculosis of the lungs and lymph nodes, advanced atherosclerosis (narrowing of the arteries as a result of plaque accumulation), and heart valve injury (Figure 4-26). Calcification of the heart valves interferes with their opening and closing, causing heart murmurs (see Chapter 24). Calcification of the coronary arteries predisposes them to severe narrowing and thrombosis, which can lead to myocardial infarction. Another site of dystrophic calcification is the centre of tumours. Over time, the centre is deprived of its oxygen supply, dies, and becomes calcified. The calcium salts appear as gritty, clumped granules that can become hard as stone. When several layers clump together, they resemble grains of sand and are called **psammoma bodies**.

Metastatic calcification consists of mineral deposits that occur in undamaged normal tissues as the result of hypercalcemia (excess calcium in the blood; see Chapter 5). Conditions that cause hypercalcemia include hyperparathyroidism, toxic levels of vitamin D, hyperthyroidism, idiopathic hypercalcemia of infancy, Addison's disease (adrenocortical insufficiency), systemic sarcoidosis, milk-alkali syndrome, and the increased bone demineralization that results from bone tumours, leukemia, and disseminated cancers. Hypercalcemia also may occur in advanced renal failure with phosphate retention. As phosphate levels increase, the activity of the parathyroid gland increases, causing higher levels of circulating calcium.

Urate

In humans, uric acid (**urate**) is the major end product of purine catabolism because of the absence of the enzyme urate oxidase. Serum urate concentration is, in general, stable: approximately 297.4 mcmol/L in postpubertal males and 243.9 mcmol/L in postpubertal females. Disturbances in maintaining serum urate levels result in hyperuricemia

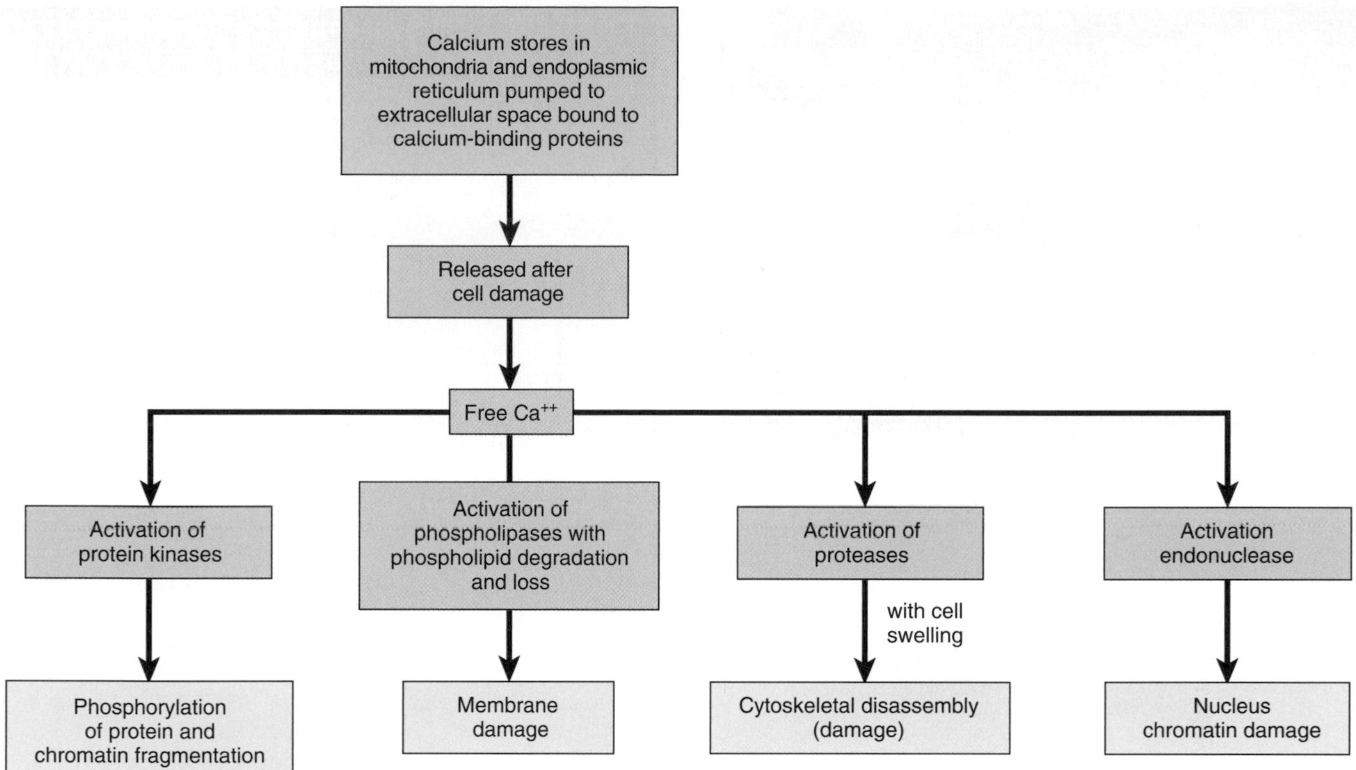

FIGURE 4-25 Free Cytosolic Calcium: A Destructive Agent. Normally, calcium (*Ca*$^{++}$) is removed from the cytosol by adenosine triphosphate (ATP)–dependent calcium pumps. In normal cells, calcium is bound to buffering proteins, such as calbindin or parvalbumin, and is contained in the endoplasmic reticulum and the mitochondria. If there is abnormal permeability of calcium-ion channels, direct damage to membranes, or depletion of ATP (i.e., hypoxic injury), calcium increases in the cytosol. If the free calcium cannot be buffered or pumped out of cells, uncontrolled enzyme activation takes place, causing further damage. Uncontrolled entry of calcium into the cytosol is an important final common pathway in many causes of cellular death.

and the deposition of sodium urate crystals in the tissues, leading to painful disorders collectively called *gout.* These disorders include acute arthritis, chronic gouty arthritis, tophi (firm, nodular, subcutaneous deposits of urate crystals surrounded by fibrosis), and nephritis (inflammation of the nephron). Chronic hyperuricemia results in the deposition of urate in tissues, cellular injury, and inflammation. Because urate crystals are not degraded by lysosomal enzymes, they persist in dead cells.

Systemic Manifestations

Systemic manifestations of cellular injury include a general sense of fatigue and malaise, a loss of well-being, and altered appetite. Fever is often present because of biochemicals produced during the inflammatory response. Table 4-10 summarizes the most significant systemic manifestations of cellular injury.

CELLULAR DEATH

In response to significant external stimuli, cellular injury becomes irreversible and cells are forced to die. Cellular death has historically been classified as necrosis and apoptosis. Necrosis is characterized by rapid loss of the plasma membrane structure, swelling of organelles, dysfunction of the mitochondria, and lack of typical features of apoptosis.[67] Apoptosis is known as a regulated or programmed cell process characterized by the "dropping off" of cellular fragments called *apoptotic bodies.* Too little or too much apoptosis is linked to many disorders, including neuro-degenerative diseases, ischemic damage, autoimmune disorders, and cancers. Yet, apoptosis can have normal functions, and unlike necrosis it is not always linked with a pathological process. Until recently, necrosis was only considered passive or accidental cellular death occurring after severe and sudden injury. It is the main outcome in several common injuries including ischemia, toxin exposure, certain infections, and trauma. It has now been proposed that under certain conditions, such as activation of death proteases, necrosis may be *regulated* or *programmed* in a well-orchestrated way as a backup for apoptosis (apoptosis may progress to necrosis)[68]—hence the new term **programmed necrosis**, or **necroptosis**. Necroptosis shares traits with both necrosis and apoptosis. Although the identification of the signalling mechanisms for necroptosis is incomplete, necroptosis is recognized in both normal physiological conditions and pathological conditions, including bone growth plate disorders, cellular death in fatty liver disease, acute pancreatitis, reperfusion injury, and certain neuro-degenerative disorders, such as Parkinson's disease.[1]

Historically, programmed cellular death only referred to apoptosis. Figure 4-27 illustrates the structural changes in cellular injury resulting in necrosis or apoptosis. Table 4-11 compares the unique features of necrosis and apoptosis. Other forms of cell loss include autophagy (self-eating) (see p. 105).

Necrosis

Cellular death eventually leads to cellular dissolution, or necrosis. **Necrosis** is the sum of cellular changes after local cellular death and

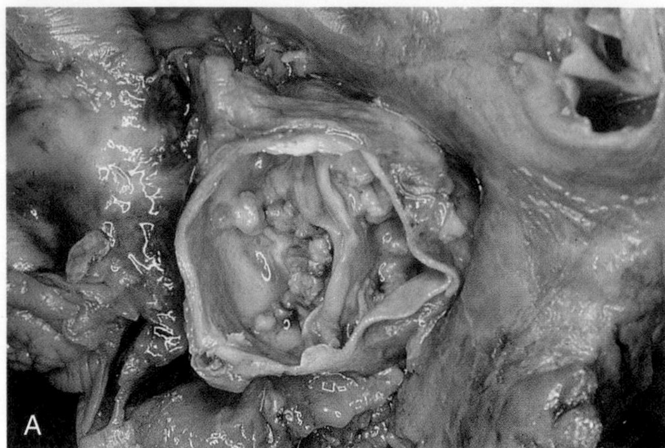

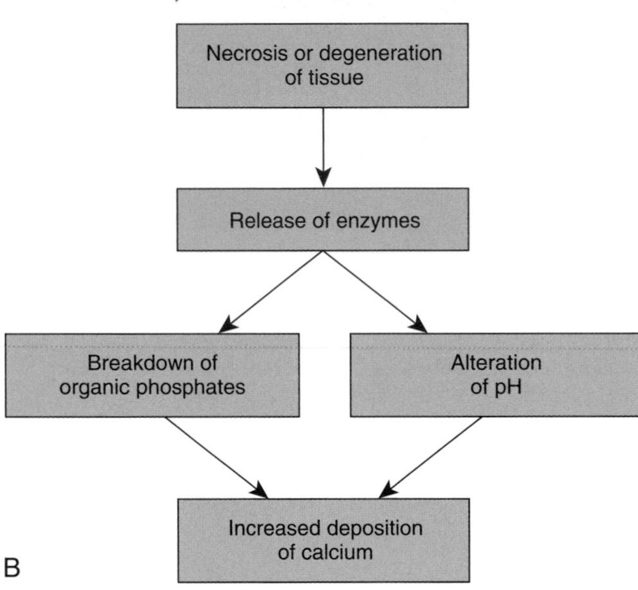

FIGURE 4-26 Aortic Valve Calcification. **A,** This calcified aortic valve is an example of dystrophic calcification. **B,** This algorithm shows the dystrophic mechanism of calcification. (**A,** from Damjanov, I. [2012]. *Pathology for the health professions* [4th ed.]. St. Louis: Saunders.)

the process of cellular self-digestion, known as autodigestion or autolysis (see Figure 4-27). Cells die long before any necrotic changes are noted by light microscopy. The structural signs that indicate irreversible injury and progression to necrosis are dense clumping and progressive disruption both of genetic material and of plasma and organelle membranes. Because membrane integrity is lost, necrotic cell contents leak out and may cause the signalling of inflammation in surrounding tissue. In later stages of necrosis, most organelles are disrupted, and karyolysis (nuclear dissolution and lysis of chromatin from the action of hydrolytic enzymes) is under way. In some cells the nucleus shrinks and becomes a small, dense mass of genetic material (pyknosis). The pyknotic nucleus eventually dissolves (by karyolysis) as a result of the action of hydrolytic lysosomal enzymes on DNA. Karyorrhexis means fragmentation of the nucleus into smaller particles, or "nuclear dust."

Although necrosis still refers to death induced by nonspecific trauma or injury (e.g., cell stress or the heat shock response), with the very recent identification of molecular mechanisms regulating the process of necrosis, the study of necrosis has experienced a new twist. Unlike apoptosis, necrosis has been viewed as passive with cellular death occurring in a disorganized and unregulated manner. Some molecular regulators governing programmed necrosis have been identified and

TABLE 4-10 Systemic Manifestations of Cellular Injury

Manifestation	Cause
Fever	Release of endogenous pyrogens (interleukin-1, tumour necrosis factor-alpha, prostaglandins) from bacteria or macrophages; acute inflammatory response
Increased heart rate	Increase in oxidative metabolic processes resulting from fever
Increase in leukocytes (leukocytosis)	Increase in total number of white blood cells because of infection; normal is 5 000–9 000/mm^3 (increase is directly related to severity of infection)
Pain	Various mechanisms, such as release of bradykinins, obstruction, pressure
Presence of cellular enzymes	Release of enzymes from cells of tissue[a] in extracellular fluid
Lactate dehydrogenase (LDH) (LDH isoenzymes)	Release from red blood cells, liver, kidney, skeletal muscle
Creatine kinase (CK) (CK isoenzymes)	Release from skeletal muscle, brain, heart
Aspartate aminotransferase (AST/SGOT)	Release from heart, liver, skeletal muscle, kidney, pancreas
Alanine aminotransferase (ALT/SGPT)	Release from liver, kidney, heart
Alkaline phosphatase (ALP)	Release from liver, bone
Amylase	Release from pancreas
Aldolase	Release from skeletal muscle, heart

[a]The rapidity of enzyme transfer is a function of the weight of the enzyme and the concentration gradient across the cellular membrane. The specific metabolic and excretory rates of the enzymes determine how long levels of enzymes remain elevated.

TABLE 4-11 Features of Necrosis and Apoptosis

Feature	Necrosis	Apoptosis
Cell size	Enlarged (swelling)	Reduced (shrinkage)
Nucleus	Pyknosis → karyorrhexis → karyolysis	Fragmentation into nucleosome-size fragments
Plasma membrane	Disrupted	Intact; altered structure, especially orientation of lipids
Cellular contents	Enzymatic digestion; may leak out of cell	Intact; may be released in apoptotic bodies
Adjacent inflammation	Frequent	No
Physiological or pathological role	Invariably pathological (culmination of irreversible cellular injury)	Often physiological, means of eliminating unwanted cells; may be pathological after some forms of cellular injury, especially DNA damage

From Kumar, V., Abbas, A.K., & Aster, J.C. (2015). Cellular responses to stress and toxic insults: Adaptation, injury, and death. In V. Kumar, A.K. Abbas, & J.C. Aster (Eds.), *Robbins and Cotran pathologic basis of disease* (9th ed., pp. 31–68). Philadelphia: Saunders.

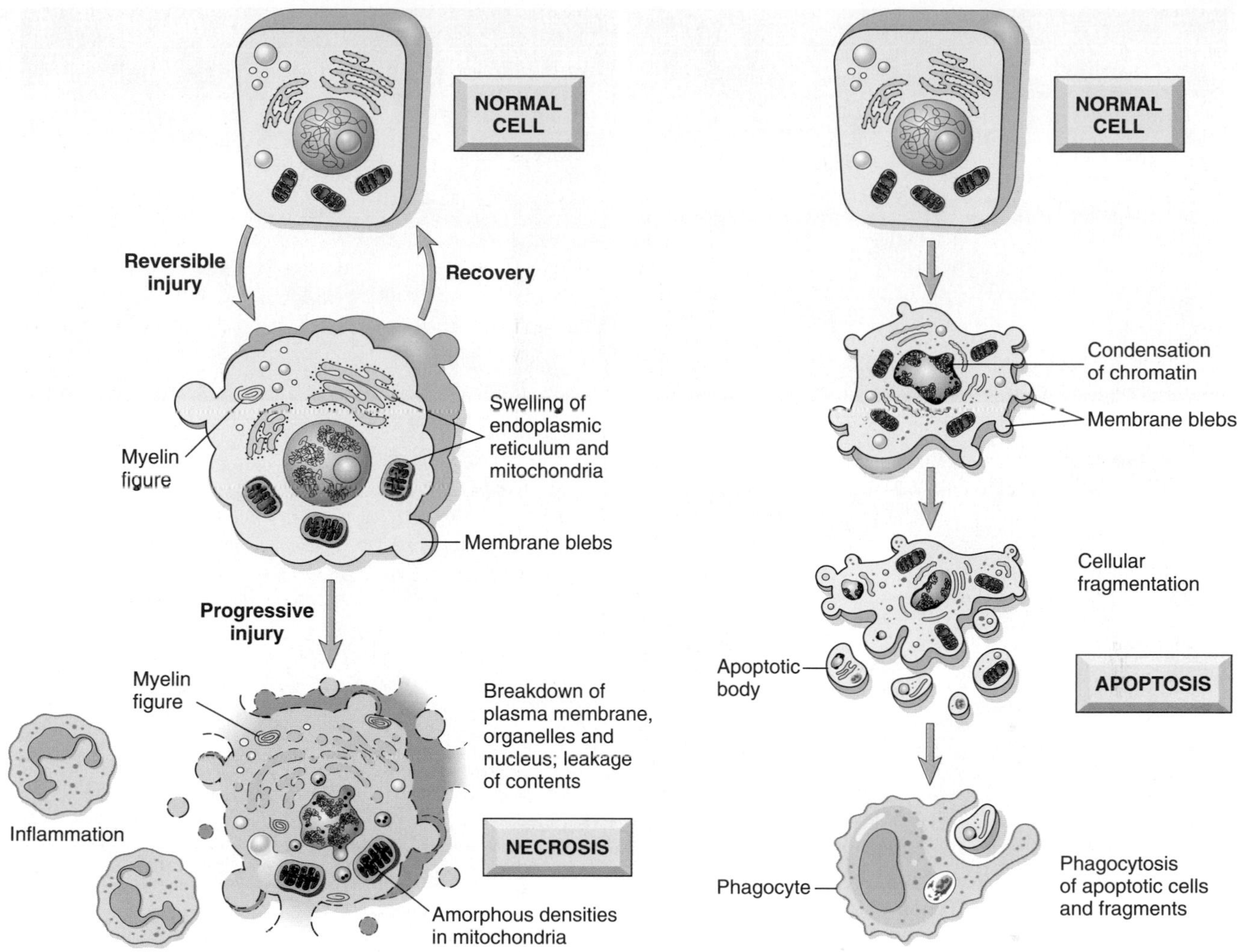

FIGURE 4-27 Schematic Illustration of the Morphological Changes in Cellular Injury Culminating in Necrosis or Apoptosis. Myelin figures come from degenerating cellular membranes and are noted within the cytoplasm or extracellularly. (From Kumar, V., Abbas, A.K., & Aster, J.C. [Eds.]. [2015]. *Robbins and Cotran pathologic basis of disease* [9th ed.]. Philadelphia: Saunders.)

demonstrated to be interconnected by a large network of signalling pathways.[69] Emerging evidence shows that programmed necrosis is associated with pathological diseases and provides innate immune response to viral infection.[69]

Different types of necrosis tend to occur in different organs or tissues and sometimes can indicate the mechanism or cause of cellular injury. The four major types of necrosis are coagulative, liquefactive, caseous, and fatty. Another type, gangrenous necrosis, is *not* a distinctive type of cellular death but refers instead to larger areas of tissue death. These necroses are summarized as follows:

1. **Coagulative necrosis**. It occurs primarily in the kidneys, heart, and adrenal glands; it commonly results from hypoxia caused by severe ischemia or hypoxia caused by chemical injury, especially ingestion of mercuric chloride. Coagulation is a result of protein denaturation, which causes the protein albumin to change from a gelatinous, transparent state to a firm, opaque state (Figure 4-28, *A*). The area of coagulative necrosis is called an **infarct**.
2. **Liquefactive necrosis**. It commonly results from ischemic injury to neurons and glial cells in the brain (Figure 4-28, *B*). Dead brain tissue is readily affected by liquefactive necrosis because brain cells are rich in digestive hydrolytic enzymes and lipids, and the brain contains little connective tissue. Cells are digested by their own hydrolases, so the tissue becomes soft, liquefies, and segregates from healthy tissue, forming cysts. This process can be caused by bacterial infection, especially *Staphylococci*, *Streptococci*, and *Escherichia coli*.
3. **Caseous necrosis**. It usually results from tuberculous pulmonary infection, especially by *Mycobacterium tuberculosis* (Figure 4-28, *C*). It is a combination of coagulative and liquefactive necroses. The dead cells disintegrate, but the debris is not completely digested by the hydrolases. Tissues resemble clumped cheese in that they are soft and granular. A granulomatous inflammatory wall encloses areas of caseous necrosis.
4. **Fatty necrosis**. Fat necrosis is cellular dissolution caused by powerful enzymes, called *lipases*, that occur in the breast, pancreas, and other abdominal structures (Figure 4-28, *D*). Lipases break down triglycerides, releasing free fatty acids that then combine with calcium, magnesium, and sodium ions, creating soaps (saponification). The necrotic tissue appears opaque and chalk-white.
5. **Gangrenous necrosis**. Although it refers to death of tissue, this type of gangrene is not a specific pattern of cellular death. It results from severe hypoxic injury, which commonly occurs because of arteriosclerosis, or blockage, of major arteries, particularly those in the lower leg (Figure 4-29). With hypoxia and subsequent bacterial invasion, the tissues can undergo necrosis. *Dry gangrene* is usually

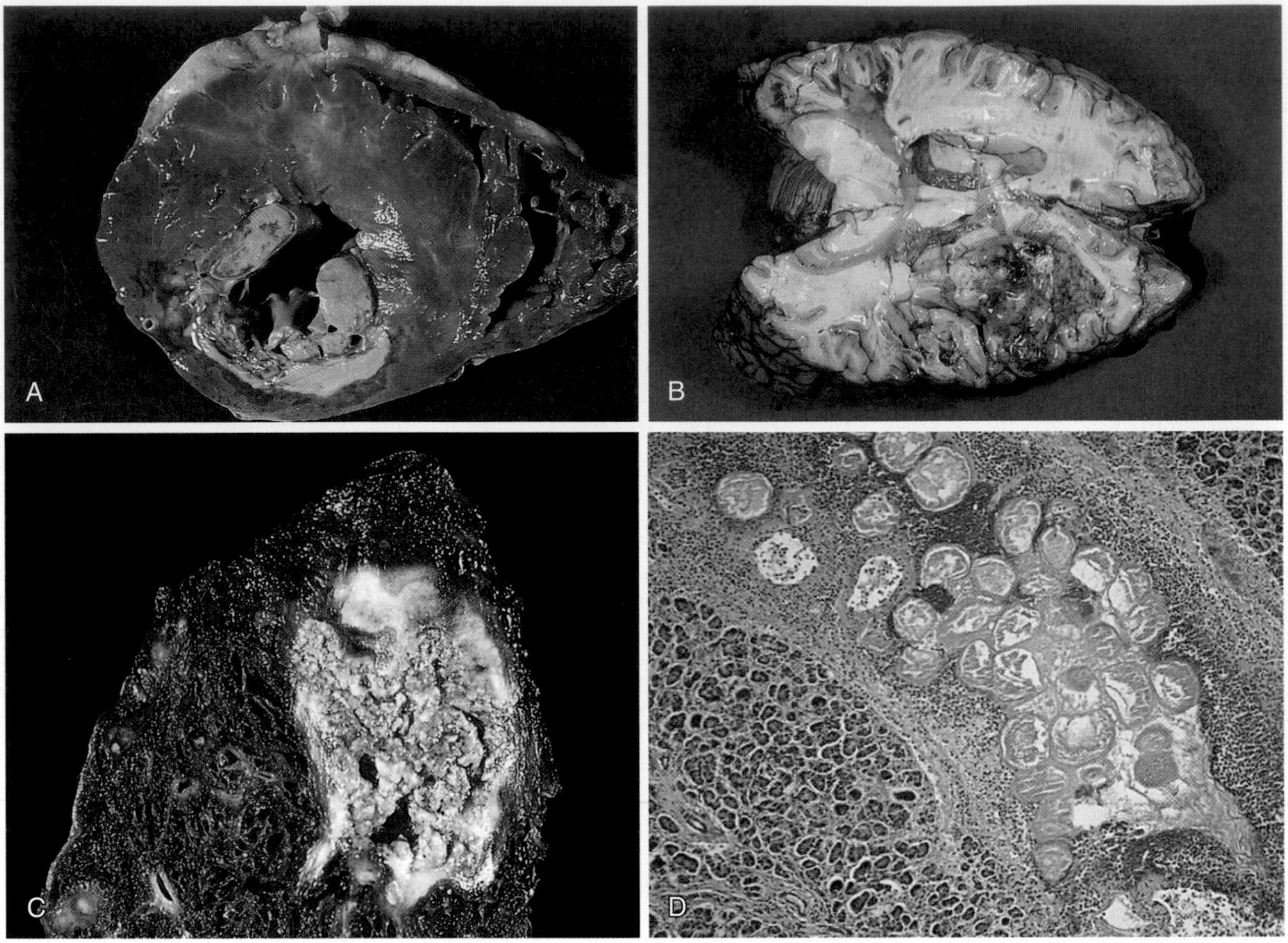

FIGURE 4-28 Types of Necrosis. A, Coagulative necrosis. A wedge-shaped kidney infarct (*yellow*). **B,** Liquefactive necrosis of the brain. The area of infarction is softened as a result of liquefaction necrosis. **C,** Caseous necrosis. Tuberculosis of the lung, with a large area of caseous necrosis containing yellow-white and cheesy debris. **D,** Fat necrosis of pancreas. Interlobular adipocytes are necrotic; acute inflammatory cells surround these. (**A** and **C,** from Kumar, V., Abbas, A.K., & Aster, J.C. [Eds.]. [2015]. *Robbins and Cotran pathologic basis of disease* [9th ed.]. Philadelphia: Saunders. **B,** from Damjanov, I. [2012]. *Pathology for the health professions* [4th ed.]. St. Louis: Saunders. **D,** from Damjanov, I., & Linder, J. [Eds.]. [1996]. *Anderson's pathology* [10th ed.]. St. Louis: Mosby.)

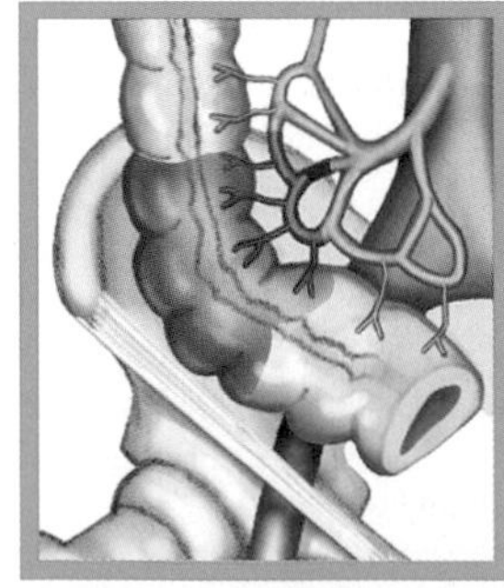

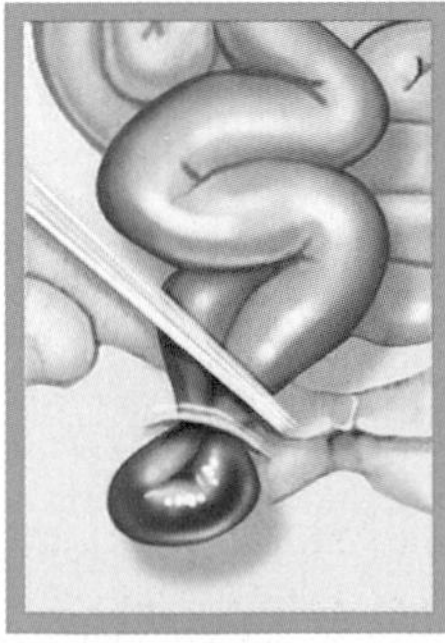

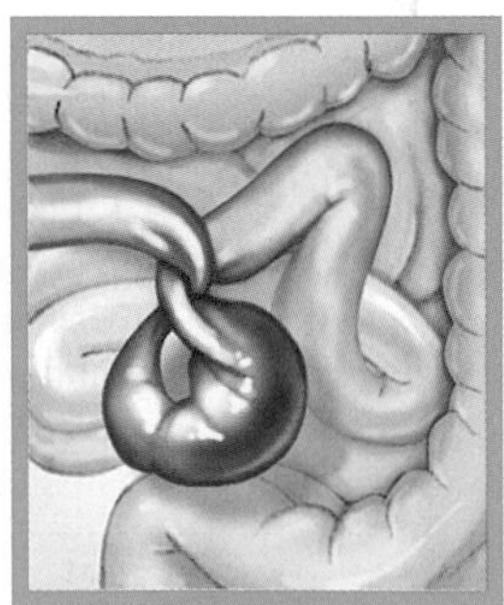

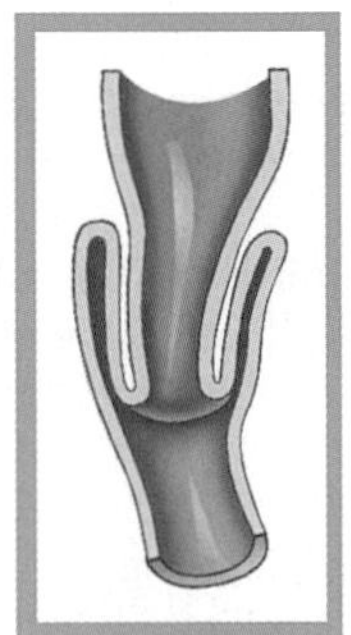

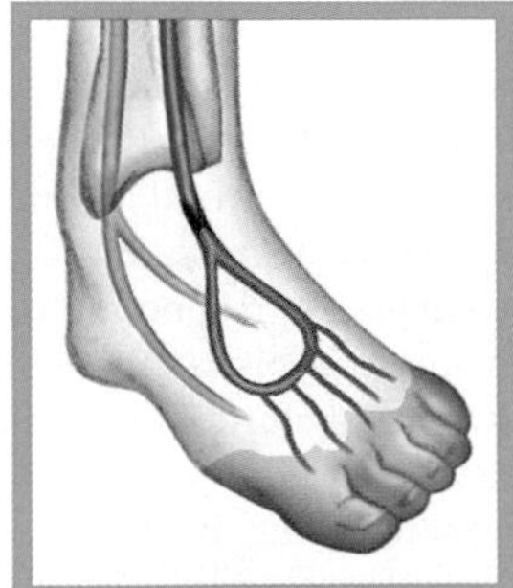

FIGURE 4-29 Gangrene, a Complication of Necrosis. In certain circumstances, necrotic tissue will be invaded by putrefactive organisms that are both saccharolytic and proteolytic. Foul-smelling gases are produced, and the tissue becomes green or black as a result of breakdown of hemoglobin. Obstruction of the blood supply to the bowel almost inevitably is followed by gangrene.

the result of coagulative necrosis. The skin becomes very dry and shrinks, resulting in wrinkles, and its colour changes to dark brown or black. *Wet gangrene* develops when neutrophils invade the site, causing liquefactive necrosis. Wet gangrene also usually occurs in internal organs, causing the site to become cold, swollen, and black. A foul odour is present, and if systemic symptoms become severe, death can ensue.

6. **Gas gangrene**. This type of gangrene is caused by infection of injured tissue by one of many species of *Clostridium*. These anaerobic bacteria produce hydrolytic enzymes and toxins that destroy connective tissue and cellular membranes and cause bubbles of gas to form in muscle cells. Gas gangrene can be fatal if enzymes lyse the membranes of red blood cells, destroying their oxygen-carrying capacity. Death is caused by shock.

Apoptosis

Apoptosis ("dropping off") is an important distinct type of cellular death that differs from necrosis in several ways (see Figure 4-27 and Table 4-11). Apoptosis is an active process of cellular self-destruction called *programmed cellular death* and is implicated in both normal and pathological tissue changes. Cells need to die; otherwise, endless proliferation would lead to gigantic bodies. The average adult may create 10 billion new cells every day—and destroy the same number.[70] Death by apoptosis causes loss of cells in many pathological states, including the following:

- *Severe cellular injury.* When cellular injury exceeds repair mechanisms, the cell triggers apoptosis. *DNA damage* can result either directly or indirectly from production of free radicals.
- *Accumulation of misfolded proteins.* This state may result from genetic mutations or free radicals. Excessive accumulation of misfolded proteins in the ER leads to a condition known as **ER stress** (see Chapter 1). ER stress results in apoptotic cellular death. This mechanism has been linked to several degenerative diseases of the CNS and other organs (Figure 4-30).
- *Infections* (*particularly viral*). Apoptosis may be the result of the virus directly or indirectly by the host immune response. Cytotoxic T lymphocytes respond to viral infections by inducing apoptosis and, therefore, eliminating the infectious cells. This process can cause tissue damage, and it is the same for cellular death in tumours and rejection of tissue transplants.
- *Obstruction in tissue ducts.* In organs with duct obstruction, including the pancreas, kidney, and parotid gland, apoptosis causes pathological atrophy.

Excessive or insufficient apoptosis is known as *dysregulated apoptosis.* A low rate of apoptosis can permit the survival of abnormal cells, for example, mutated cells that can increase cancer risk. Defective apoptosis may not eliminate lymphocytes that react against host tissue (self-antigens), leading to autoimmune disorders. Excessive apoptosis is known to occur in several neuro-degenerative diseases, from ischemic injury (such as myocardial infarction and stroke), and from death of virus-infected cells (such as seen in many viral infections).

Apoptosis depends on a tightly regulated cellular program for its initiation and execution.[70] This death program involves enzymes that divide other proteins—proteases, which are activated by proteolytic activity in response to signals that induce apoptosis. These proteases are called **caspases**, a family of aspartic acid–specific proteases. The

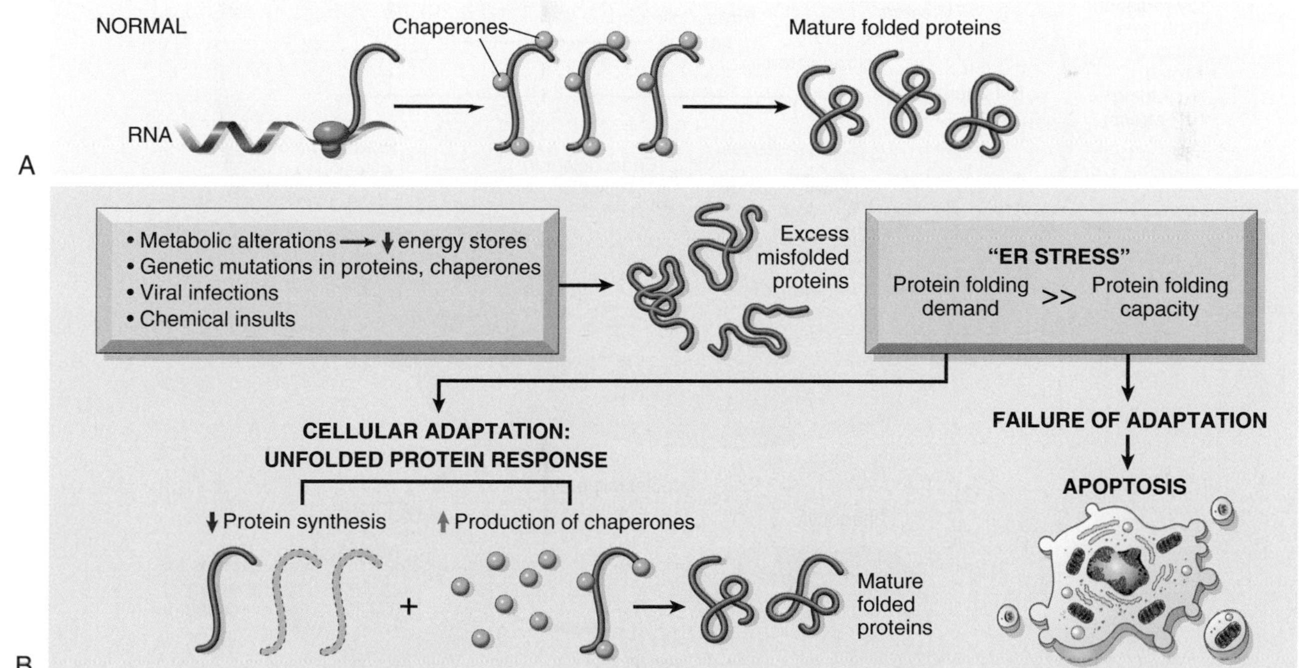

FIGURE 4-30 The Unfolded Protein Response, Endoplasmic Stress, and Apoptosis. A, In normal or healthy cells the newly made proteins are folded with help from chaperones and then incorporated into the cell or secreted. **B,** Various stressors can cause endoplasmic reticulum (ER) stress whereby the cell is challenged to cope with the increased load of misfolded proteins. The accumulation of the protein load initiates the *unfolded protein response* in the ER; if restoration of the protein fails, the cell dies by apoptosis. An example of a disease caused by misfolding of proteins is Alzheimer's disease. (From Kumar, V., Abbas, A.K., & Aster, J.C. [Eds.]. [2015]. *Robbins and Cotran pathologic basis of disease* [9th ed.]. Philadelphia: Saunders.)

activated suicide caspases cleave and, thereby, activate other members of the family, resulting in an amplifying "suicide" cascade. The activated caspases then cleave other key proteins in the cell, killing the cell quickly and neatly. The two different pathways that converge on caspase activation are called the *mitochondrial* (*intrinsic*) *pathway* and the *death receptor* (*extrinsic*) *pathway* (Figure 4-31). Cells that die by apoptosis release chemical factors that recruit phagocytes that quickly engulf the remains of the dead cell, thus reducing chances of inflammation. With necrosis, cellular death is not tidy because cells that die as a result of acute injury swell, burst, and spill their contents all over their neighbours, causing a likely damaging inflammatory response.

Autophagy

The Greek term **autophagy** means "eating of self." Autophagy, as a "recycling factory," is a self-destructive process and a survival mechanism. Basically, autophagy involves the delivery of cytoplasmic contents to the lysosome for degradation. Box 4-3 contains the terms used to describe autophagy.

When cells are starved or nutrient deprived, the autophagic process institutes cannibalization and recycles the digested contents.[1,71] Autophagy can maintain cellular metabolism under starvation conditions and remove damaged organelles under stress conditions, improving the survival of cells. With the central role of autophagy in cell homeostasis, autophagy has been implicated in cancer, heart disease, neuro-degenerative

BOX 4-3 The Major Forms of Autophagy

Macroautophagy, the most common term to refer to autophagy, involves the sequestration and transportation of parts (cargo) of the cytosol in an autophagic vacuole (autophagosome).

Microautophagy is the inward invagination of the lysosomal membrane for cargo delivery.

Chaperone-mediated autophagy is the chaperone-dependent proteins that direct cargo across the lysosomal membrane.

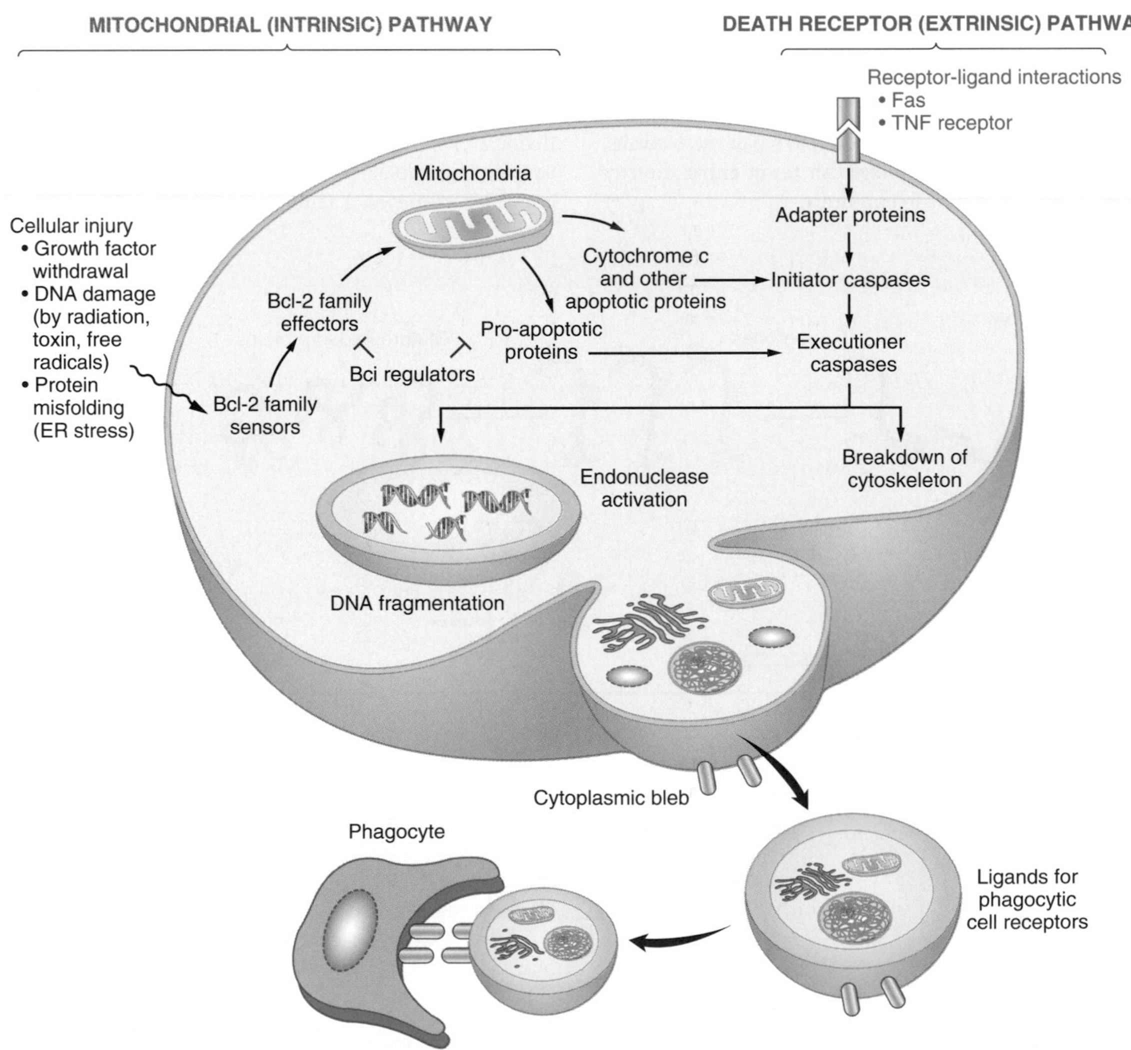

FIGURE 4-31 Mechanisms of Apoptosis. The two pathways of apoptosis differ in their induction and regulation, and both culminate in the activation of "executioner" caspases. The induction of apoptosis by the mitochondrial pathway involves the Bcl-2 family, which causes leakage of mitochondrial proteins. The regulators of the death receptor pathway involve the proteases, called *caspases. TNF*, tumour necrosis factor. (Adapted from Kumar, V., Abbas, A.K., & Aster, J.C. [Eds.]. [2015]. *Robbins and Cotran pathologic basis of disease* [9th ed.]. Philadelphia: Saunders.)

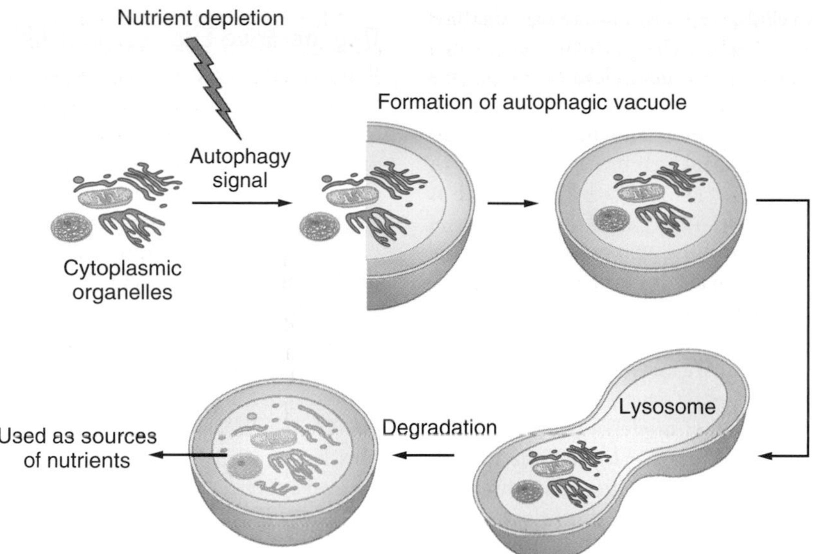

FIGURE 4-32 Autophagy. Cellular stresses, such as nutrient deprivation, activate autophagy genes that create vacuoles in which cellular organelles are sequestered and then degraded following fusion of the vesicles with lysosomes. The digested materials are recycled to provide nutrients for the cell.

diseases, inflammation, and infection.[72] Autophagy begins with a membrane, also known as a *phagophore* (although controversial) (Figure 4-32).[73] This cup-shaped, curved phagophore expands and engulfs intracellular cargo—organelles, ribosomes, proteins—forming a double membrane *autophagosome.* The cargo-laden autophagosome fuses with the lysosome, now called an *autophagolysosome*, which promotes the degradation of the autophagosome by lysosomal acid proteases. The phagophore membrane is highly curved along the rim of the open cup, suggesting that mechanisms responsible for its formation and growth may depend on membrane curvature–dependent events.[74] Lysosomal transporters export amino acids and other byproducts of degradation out of the cytoplasm where they can be reused for the synthesis of macromolecules and for metabolism.[75,76] ATP is generated and cellular damage is reduced during autophagy that removes nonfunctional proteins and organelles.[71]

Investigators are excited about the utilization of autophagy for therapeutic strategies. Autophagy is a critical garbage collecting and recycling process in healthy cells, and this process becomes less efficient and less discriminating as the cell ages. Consequently, harmful agents accumulate in cells, damaging cells and leading to aging: for example, failure to clear protein products in neurons of the CNS can cause dementia; failure to clear ROS-producing mitochondria can lead to nuclear DNA mutations and cancer. Thus these processes may even partially define aging. Therefore normal autophagy may potentially rejuvenate an organism and prevent cancer development as well as other degenerative diseases.[77] In addition, autophagy may be the last immune defence against infectious microorganisms that penetrate intracellularly.[78]

QUICK CHECK 4-4

1. Why is an increase in the concentration of intracellular calcium injurious?
2. Compare and contrast necrosis and apoptosis.
3. Why is apoptosis significant?
4. Define *autophagy.*

AGING AND ALTERED CELLULAR AND TISSUE BIOLOGY

The terms *aging* and *lifespan* tend to be used synonymously; however, they are not equivalent. **Aging** is usually defined as a normal physiological process that is universal and inevitable, whereas **lifespan** is the time from birth to death and has been used to study the aging process.[79] Aging is associated with a gradual loss of homeostatic mechanisms whose underlying cause is perplexing,[80] and is a complex process because of a multiplicity of factors. Investigators are focused on genetic, epigenetic, inflammatory, oxidative stress, and metabolic origins of aging, including the study of genetic signatures in humans with exceptional longevity; the identification and recent discovery of epigenetic mechanisms that modulate gene expression; the role of intrauterine environment and lifelong patterns of health; the effects of personality, behaviour, and social support; the influence of insulin/insulinlike growth factor 1 (IGF-1) signalling; and the contributions of cellular dysfunction and senescence to an inflammatory microenvironment that leads to chronic disease, frailty, and decreased lifespan. To focus more simply, the factors that may be most important for aging include increased damage to the cell, reduced capacity to divide (replicative senescence), reduced ability to repair damaged DNA, and increased likelihood of defective protein balance or homeostasis.[1] A major challenge of aging research has been to separate the causes of cell and tissue aging from the vast changes that accompany it.[80] Public health issues related to healthy aging require understanding of the nature of aging and the factors that predict healthy aging and delayed transition to increasing vulnerability and frailty.

Traditionally, aging has not been considered a disease because it is "normal"; disease is usually considered "abnormal." Conceptually, this distinction seems clear until the concept of "injury" or "damage" is introduced; disease has been defined by some pathologists as the result of injury. *Chronological aging* has been defined as the time-dependent loss of structure and function that proceeds very slowly and in such small increments that it appears to be the result of the accumulation of small, imperceptible injuries—a gradual result of wear and tear. One of the hallmarks of aging is the accumulation of damaged macromolecules. DNA damage can lead to cellular dysfunction both directly and indirectly as a consequence of cellular responses to damage that can lead to altered gene expression.[81,82] Age-related changes to macromolecules for long-lived cells, such as neurons and myofibres, lead to gradual loss of structure and function.

Replicative aging or *senescence* is the accumulation of cellular damage in continuously dividing cells, for example, epithelia of the skin or gastro-intestinal tract. One mechanism of replicative senescence is the progressive shortening of telomeres—the repeated sequences of DNA at the ends of chromosomes. Replicative aging and chronological aging are particularly important for adult stem cells because they divide throughout life.[83] As mutations increase with age, cell fates include apoptosis, malignant transformation, cell-cycle arrest, or senescence.[84]

Despite the fact that aging and death are inevitable, lifespan, on the other hand, can be experimentally changed.[81] Genetic and environmental interventions have extended the lifespan of model organisms, such as the nematode worm *Caenorhabditis elegans* (*C. elegans*), the fruit fly *Drosophilia melanogaster*, and mice.[85,86] Extending lifespan, however, is not equivalent to delaying aging![80] For example, treatment of an acute infection can prevent death but the fundamental *rate* of aging continues. Yet, investigators will study and try to isolate, manipulate, and reset so-called longevity genes to slow the rate of aging.

Recent advances in stem cell biology have begun to reveal the molecular mechanisms behind reprogramming events that occur during fertilization and when the nucleus of a mature somatic cell is transferred to an enucleated oocyte. Called *somatic cell nuclear transfer* (SCNT), this process gave rise to the first cloned mammal, Dolly the sheep, and led to the explosion of research in cloning.[80] SCNT is important in terms of demonstrating the ability of the oocyte cytoplasm to reprogram the donor nucleus. These reprogramming events have led to the process to create induced pluripotent stem cells (iPSCs).[87] The major emphasis of reprogramming research is the reversal of the differentiated program and attainment of a pluripotent state (differentiated cells in all three germ layers of the embryo) and not the reversal of aging.[80,88] Nevertheless, each of these processes is discussed in the context of resetting the aging clock.

Restoration of youthfulness to aged cells and tissues has created so-called rejuvenating interventions. Experiments to test whether cells and tissues from an old animal can be restored to a younger self include the approach called *heterochronic* (i.e., young-to-old or old-to-young) *transplantations* and *heterochronic parabiosis*, when the systemic circulations of two animals are joined. The systemic environment may become more youthful with restoration of protein components in the blood and tissues, especially chemokines and cytokines.[89] For example, investigators found a protein, GDF-11, may reverse age-associated cardiac hypertrophy when injected into old animals.[90]

Administration of the medication rapamycin (Sirolimus), an mTOR inhibitor, can extend the lifespan of mice.[91] These and future studies may not just change differentiation programs of cells and tissue but also possibly alter the aging clock. Observations in *C. elegans* suggest strongly that the causes of aging may be largely epigenetic.[80,92,93]

Normal Lifespan, Life Expectancy, and Quality-Adjusted Life Year

The **maximal lifespan** of humans is between 80 and 100 years and does not vary significantly among populations. **Life expectancy** is the *average* number of years of life remaining at a given age, however, it does not include quality of life. The **quality-adjusted life year (QALY)** is a measure of disease burden including quality and not just quantity of live lived. Statistics Canada reported in 2009 that the life expectancy at birth was 79 years and 83 years for males and females, respectively. The lowest life expectancy was in Newfoundland/Labrador at 77 years for males and 81 years for males, and the highest was in British Columbia (80 years for males; 84 years for females).[94]

Degenerative Extracellular Changes

Extracellular factors that affect the aging process include the binding of collagen; the increase in the effects of free radicals on cells; the structural alterations of fascia, tendons, ligaments, bones, and joints; and the development of peripheral vascular disease, particularly arteriosclerosis (see Chapter 24).

Aging affects the ECM with increased cross-linking (e.g., aging collagen becomes more insoluble, chemically stable but rigid, resulting in decreased cell permeability), decreased synthesis, and increased degradation of collagen. The ECM determines the tissue's physical properties.[95] These changes, together with the disappearance of elastin and changes in proteoglycans and plasma proteins, cause disorders of the ground substance that result in dehydration and wrinkling of the skin (see Chapter 41). Other age-related defects in the ECM include skeletal muscle alterations (e.g., atrophy, decreased tone, loss of contractility), cataracts, diverticula, hernias, and rupture of intervertebral discs.

Free radicals of oxygen that result from oxidative cellular metabolism, *oxidative stress* (e.g., respiratory chain, phagocytosis, prostaglandin synthesis), damage tissues during the aging process. The oxygen radicals produced include superoxide radical, hydroxyl radical, and hydrogen peroxide. These oxygen products are extremely reactive and can damage nucleic acids, destroy polysaccharides, oxidize proteins, peroxidize unsaturated fatty acids, and kill and lyse cells. Oxidant effects on target cells can lead to malignant transformation, presumably through DNA damage. That progressive and cumulative damage from oxygen radicals may lead to harmful alterations in cellular function is consistent with those alterations of aging. This hypothesis is founded on the wear-and-tear theory of aging, which states that damages accumulate with time, decreasing the organism's ability to maintain a steady state. Because these oxygen-reactive species not only can permanently damage cells but also may lead to cellular death, there is new support for their role in the aging process.

Of much interest is the relationship between aging and the disappearance or alteration of extracellular substances important for vessel integrity. With aging, lipid, calcium, and plasma proteins are deposited in vessel walls. These depositions cause serious basement membrane thickening and alterations in smooth muscle functioning, resulting in arteriosclerosis (a progressive disease that causes such problems as stroke, myocardial infarction, renal disease, and peripheral vascular disease).

Cellular Aging

Cellular changes characteristic of aging include atrophy, decreased function, and loss of cells, possibly caused by apoptosis (Figure 4-33). Loss of cellular function from any of these causes initiates the compensatory mechanisms of hypertrophy and hyperplasia of the remaining cells, which can lead to metaplasia, dysplasia, and neoplasia. All of these changes can alter receptor placement and function, nutrient pathways, secretion of cellular products, and neuroendocrine control mechanisms. In the aged cell, DNA, RNA, cellular proteins, and membranes are most susceptible to injurious stimuli. DNA is particularly vulnerable to such injuries as breaks, deletions, and additions. Lack of DNA repair increases the cell's susceptibility to mutations that may be lethal or may promote the development of neoplasia (see Chapter 10).

Mitochondria are the organelles responsible for the generation of most of the energy used by eukaryotic cells. **Mitochondrial DNA (mtDNA)** encodes some of the proteins of the electron-transfer chain, the system necessary for the conversion of ADP to ATP. Mutations in mtDNA can deprive the cell of ATP, and mutations are correlated with the aging process. The accumulation of mutations could be caused by errors in replication or by unrepaired damage.[96,97]

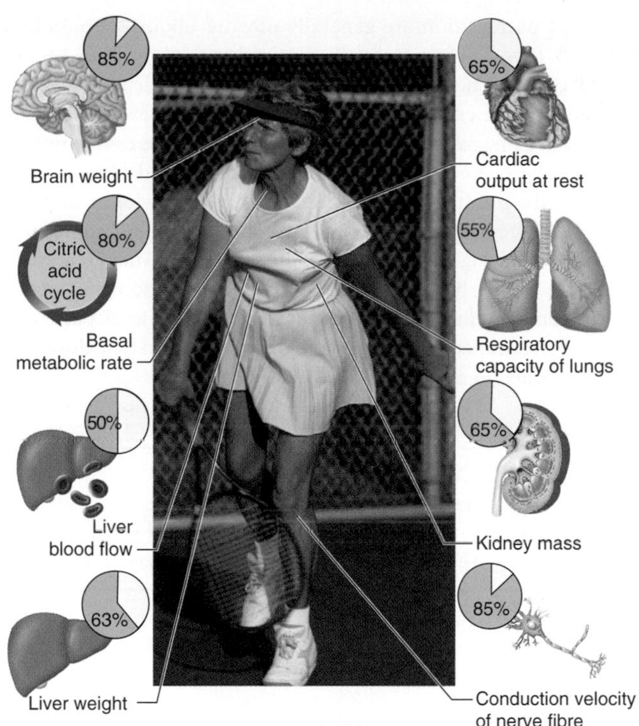

FIGURE 4-33 Some Biological Changes Associated with Aging. Insets show the proportion of remaining functions in the organs of a person in late adulthood compared with those of a 20-year-old.

The most common age-related mtDNA mutation in humans is a large rearrangement called the *4977 deletion*, or *common deletion*, and is found in humans older than 40 years. It is a deletion that removes all or part of 7 of the 13 protein-encoding mtDNA genes and 5 of the 22 transfer RNA genes. Individual cells containing this deletion have a condition known as *heteroplasmy*. Heteroplasmy levels rise with aging. Cumulative damage of mtDNA is implicated in the progression of such common diseases as diabetes, cancer, heart failure, and neuro-degenerative disorders.

Tissue and Systemic Aging

It is probably safe to say that every physiological process functions less efficiently with increasing age. The most characteristic tissue change with age is a progressive stiffness or rigidity that affects many systems, including the arterial, pulmonary, and musculo-skeletal systems. A consequence of blood vessel and organ stiffness is a progressive increase in peripheral resistance to blood flow. The movement of intracellular and extracellular substances also decreases with age, as does the diffusion capacity of the lung. Blood flow through organs also decreases.

Changes in the endocrine and immune systems include thymus atrophy. Although this occurs at puberty, causing a decreased immune response to T-dependent antigens (foreign proteins), increased formation of autoantibodies and immune complexes (antibodies that are bound to antigens), and an overall decrease in the immunological tolerance for the host's own cells further diminish the effectiveness of the immune system later in life. In women the reproductive system loses ova, and in men spermatogenesis decreases. Responsiveness to hormones decreases in the breast and endometrium.

The stomach experiences decreases in the rate of emptying and secretion of hormones and hydrochloric acid. Muscular atrophy diminishes mobility by decreasing motor tone and contractility. **Sarcopenia**, loss of muscle mass and strength, can occur into old age. The skin of the aged individual is affected by atrophy and wrinkling of the epidermis and by alterations in the underlying dermis, fat, and muscle.

Total body changes include a decrease in height; a reduction in circumference of the neck, thighs, and arms; widening of the pelvis; and lengthening of the nose and ears. Several of these changes are the result of tissue atrophy and of decreased bone mass caused by osteoporosis and osteoarthritis. Some body composition changes include an increase in body weight, which begins in middle age (men gain until 50 years of age and women until 70 years), and an increase in fat mass followed by a decrease in stature, weight, fat-free mass, and body cell mass at older ages. **Fat-free mass (FFM)** includes all minerals, proteins, and water plus all other constituents except lipids. As the amount of fat increases, the percentage of total body water decreases. Increased body fat and centralized fat distribution (abdominal area) are associated with non–insulin-dependent diabetes and heart disease. Total body potassium concentration also decreases because of decreased cellular mass. An increased sodium–potassium ratio suggests that the decreased cellular mass is accompanied by an increased extracellular compartment.

Although some of these alterations are probably inherent in aging, others represent consequences of the process. Advanced age increases susceptibility to disease, and death occurs after an injury or insult because of diminished cellular, tissue, and organ function.

Frailty

Frailty is a common clinical syndrome in older adults, leaving a person vulnerable to falls, functional decline, disability, disease, and death. With an increasing aged population worldwide, efforts to promote independence and decrease frailty are challenging and needed. Sarcopenia and cachexia are a common consequence of aging and many acute and chronic illnesses.[98] Investigators are grappling with a common nomenclature to develop consensus for definitions of sarcopenia and cachexia. One proposal has been to define each condition simply as "muscle wasting disease," which can be applied in both acute and chronic settings.[98] An acceptable vocabulary and classification system is yet to be developed.

The determinants of sarcopenia include environmental and genetic factors, which presently are poorly understood.[99] Common themes of mechanisms for sarcopenia include the following: (1) decrease in the number of skeletal muscle fibres, mainly type II fibres; (2) decline in muscle protein synthesis with age; (3) decline in muscle fractions, such as myofibrillar and mitochondrial, with age; (4) reduction in protein turnover adversely affecting muscle function by inducing protein loss and protein accumulation; (5) loss of alpha motor neurons in the spinal column; (6) dysregulation of anabolic hormones; (7) cytokine productions and inflammation; (8) inadequate nutrition; and (9) sedentary history.[99,100] For research and clinical purposes, the criteria indicating compromised energetics include low grip strength, slowed walking speed, low physical activity, and unintentional weight loss.[101] The syndrome is complex and involves other alterations such as osteopenia, cognitive impairment, and anemia, as well as gender differences.

SOMATIC DEATH

Somatic death is death of the entire person. Unlike the changes that follow cellular death in a live body, **postmortem change** is diffuse and does not involve components of the inflammatory response. Within minutes after death, postmortem changes appear, eliminating any difficulty in determining that death has occurred. The most notable manifestations are complete cessation of respiration and circulation. The surface of the skin usually becomes pale and yellowish; however, the lifelike colour of the cheeks and lips may persist after death caused by carbon monoxide poisoning, drowning, or chloroform poisoning.[102]

Body temperature falls gradually immediately after death and then more rapidly (approximately 1°C/hr [33.8°F/hr]) until, after 24 hours, body temperature equals that of the environment.[103] After death caused by certain infective diseases, body temperature may continue to rise for a short time. Postmortem reduction of body temperature is called **algor mortis**.

Blood pressure within the retinal vessels decreases, causing muscle tension to decrease and the pupils to dilate. The face, nose, and chin become sharp or peaked-looking as blood and fluids drain from these areas.[104] Gravity causes blood to settle in the most dependent, or lowest, tissues, which develop a purple discoloration called **livor mortis**. Incisions made at this time usually fail to cause bleeding. The skin loses its elasticity and transparency.

Within 6 hours after death, acidic compounds accumulate within the muscles because of the breakdown of carbohydrates and the depletion of ATP. This increased acidity interferes with ATP-dependent detachment of myosin from actin (contractile proteins), and muscle stiffening, or **rigor mortis**, develops. The smaller muscles are usually affected first, particularly the muscles of the jaw. Within 12 to 14 hours, rigor mortis usually affects the entire body.

Signs of putrefaction are generally obvious about 24 to 48 hours after death. Rigor mortis gradually diminishes, and the body becomes flaccid at 36 to 62 hours. Putrefactive changes vary depending on the temperature of the environment. The most visible is greenish discoloration of the skin, particularly on the abdomen. The discoloration is thought to be related to the diffusion of hemolyzed blood into the tissues and the production of sulfhemoglobin, choleglobin, and other denatured hemoglobin derivatives.[103,104] Slippage or loosening of the skin from underlying tissues occurs at the same time. After this, swelling or bloating of the body and liquefactive changes occur, sometimes causing opening of the body cavities. At a microscopic level, putrefactive changes are associated with the release of enzymes and lytic dissolution called **postmortem autolysis**.

✔QUICK CHECK 4-5

1. Aging is a complex process. Describe the multitude of mechanisms of aging.
2. What are the body composition changes that occur with aging?
3. Define *frailty* and possible endocrine–immune system involvement.

DID YOU UNDERSTAND?

Cellular Adaptation

1. Cellular adaptation is a reversible, structural, or functional response both to normal or physiological conditions and to adverse or pathological conditions. Cells can adapt to physiological demands or stress to maintain a steady state called *homeostasis*.
2. The most significant adaptive changes in cells include atrophy, hypertrophy, hyperplasia, and metaplasia.
3. Atrophy is a decrease in cellular size caused by aging, disuse, or reduced/absent blood supply, hormonal stimulation, or neural stimulation. The amounts of endoplasmic reticulum (ER), mitochondria, and microfilaments decrease. The mechanisms of atrophy probably include decreased protein synthesis, increased protein catabolism, or both. A new hypothesis called ribosome biogenesis involves the role of messenger RNA (mRNA) and protein translation.
4. Hypertrophy is an increase in the size of cells in response to mechanical stimuli and consequently increases the size of the affected organ. The amounts of protein in the plasma membrane, ER, microfilaments, and mitochondria increase. Hypertrophy can be classified as physiological or pathological.
5. Hyperplasia is an increase in the number of cells caused by an increased rate of cellular division. Hyperplasia is classified as physiological (compensatory and hormonal) and pathological.
6. Dysplasia, or *atypical hyperplasia*, is an abnormal change in the size, shape, and organization of mature tissue cells. It is considered atypical rather than a true adaptational change.
7. Metaplasia is the reversible replacement of one mature cell type by another less mature cell type.

Cellular Injury

1. Injury to cells and to the extracellular matrix (ECM) lead to injury of tissues and organs, ultimately determining the structural patterns of disease. Cellular injury occurs if the cell is unable to maintain homeostasis—a normal or adaptive steady state—in the face of injurious stimuli or stress. Injured cells may recover (reversible injury) or die (irreversible injury).
2. Four biochemical themes are important to cellular injury: (a) adenosine triphosphate (ATP) depletion, resulting in mitochondrial damage; (b) accumulation of oxygen and oxygen-derived free radicals, causing membrane damage; (c) protein folding defects; and (d) increased intracellular calcium concentration and loss of calcium steady state.
3. Injury is caused by lack of oxygen (hypoxia), free radicals, caustic or toxic chemicals, infectious agents, inflammatory and immune responses, genetic factors, insufficient nutrients, or physical and mechanical trauma from many causes.
4. The sequence of events leading to cellular death is commonly decreased ATP production, failure of active transport mechanisms (the sodium–potassium pump), cellular swelling, detachment of ribosomes from the ER, cessation of protein synthesis, mitochondrial swelling as a result of calcium accumulation, vacuolation, leakage of digestive enzymes from lysosomes, autodigestion of intracellular structures, lysis of the plasma membrane, and death.
5. The initial insult in hypoxic injury is usually ischemia (the cessation of blood flow into vessels that supply the cell with oxygen and nutrients).
6. Free radicals cause cellular injury because they have an unpaired electron that makes the molecule unstable. To stabilize itself, the molecule either donates or accepts an electron from another molecule. Therefore it forms injurious chemical bonds with proteins, lipids, and carbohydrates—key molecules in membranes and nucleic acids.
7. The damaging effects of free radicals, especially activated oxygen species such as superoxide radical ($O_2^{\bar{\cdot}}$), hydroxyl radical (OH^-), and hydrogen peroxide (H_2O_2), called oxidative stress, include (a) peroxidation of lipids, (b) alteration of ion pumps and transport mechanisms, (c) fragmentation of DNA, and (d) damage to mitochondria, releasing calcium into the cytosol.
8. Restoration of oxygen, however, can cause additional injury, called reperfusion injury. The mechanisms discussed for reperfusion injury include oxidative stress, increased intracellular calcium concentration, inflammation, and complement activation.

9. Humans are exposed to thousands of chemicals that have inadequate toxicological data. A systems biology approach is now being used to investigate toxicity pathways that include oxidative stress, heat shock proteins, DNA damage response, hypoxia, ER stress, mental stress, inflammation, and osmotic stress.
10. Unintentional and intentional injuries are an important health problem in Canada. Death as a result of these injuries is more common for men than women.
11. Injuries by blunt force are the result of the application of mechanical energy to the body, resulting in tearing, shearing, or crushing of tissues. The most common types of blunt-force injuries include motor vehicle accidents and falls.
12. A contusion is bleeding into the skin or underlying tissues as a consequence of a blow. A collection of blood in soft tissues or an enclosed space may be referred to as a *hematoma*.
13. An abrasion (scrape) results from removal of the superficial layers of the skin caused by friction between the skin and injuring object. Abrasions and contusions may have a patterned appearance that mirrors the shape and features of the injuring object.
14. A laceration is a tear or rip resulting when the tensile strength of the skin or tissue is exceeded.
15. An incised wound is a cut that is longer than it is deep. A stab wound is a penetrating sharp-force injury that is deeper than it is long.
16. Gunshot wounds may be either penetrating (bullet retained in the body) or perforating (bullet exits the body). The most important factors determining the appearance of a gunshot injury are whether it is an entrance or an exit wound and the range of fire.
17. Asphyxial injuries are caused by a failure of cells to receive or use oxygen. These injuries can be grouped into four general categories: suffocation, strangulation, chemical asphyxiants, and drowning.
18. Activation of inflammation and immunity, which occurs after cellular injury or infection, involves powerful biochemicals and proteins capable of damaging normal (uninjured and uninfected) cells.
19. Genetic disorders injure cells by altering the nucleus and the plasma membrane's structure, shape, receptors, or transport mechanisms.
20. Deprivation of essential nutrients (proteins, carbohydrates, lipids, vitamins) can cause cellular injury by altering cellular structure and function, particularly of transport mechanisms, chromosomes, the nucleus, and DNA.
21. Injurious physical agents include temperature extremes, changes in atmospheric pressure, ionizing radiation, illumination, mechanical stresses, and noise.
22. Errors in health care are a leading cause of injury or death in Canada. Errors involve medicines, surgery, diagnosis, equipment, and laboratory reports. They can occur anywhere in the health care system, including hospitals, clinics, outpatient surgery centres, physicians' and nurse practitioners' offices, pharmacies, and the individual's home.

Manifestations of Cellular Injury: Accumulations

1. An important manifestation of cellular injury is the resultant metabolic disturbances of intracellular accumulation (infiltration) of abnormal amounts of various substances. Two categories of accumulations are (a) normal cellular substances (e.g., excess water, proteins, lipids, and carbohydrates) and (b) abnormal substances, either endogenous (e.g., a product of abnormal metabolism or synthesis) or exogenous (e.g., a virus).
2. Most accumulations are attributed to four types of mechanisms, all abnormal: (a) an endogenous substance is produced in excess or at an increased rate; (b) an abnormal substance, often the result of a mutated gene, accumulates; (c) an endogenous substance is not effectively catabolized; and (d) a harmful exogenous substance accumulates because of inhalation, ingestion, or infection.
3. Accumulations harm cells by "crowding" the organelles and by causing excessive (and sometimes harmful) metabolites to be produced during their catabolism. The metabolites are released into the cytoplasm or expelled into the ECM.
4. Cellular swelling, the accumulation of excessive water in the cell, is caused by the failure of transport mechanisms and is a sign of many types of cellular injury. Oncosis is a type of cellular death resulting from cellular swelling.
5. Accumulations of organic substances—lipids, carbohydrates, glycogen, proteins, pigments—are caused by disorders in which (a) cellular uptake of the substance exceeds the cell's capacity to catabolize (digest) or use it or (b) cellular anabolism (synthesis) of the substance exceeds the cell's capacity to use or secrete it.
6. Dystrophic calcification (accumulation of calcium salts) is always a sign of pathological change because it occurs only in injured or dead cells. Metastatic calcification, however, can occur in uninjured cells in individuals with hypercalcemia.
7. Disturbances in urate metabolism can result in hyperuricemia and deposition of sodium urate crystals in tissue—leading to a painful disorder called gout.
8. Systemic manifestations of cellular injury include fever, leukocytosis, increased heart rate, pain, and serum elevations of enzymes in the plasma.

Cellular Death

1. Cellular death has historically been classified as necrosis and apoptosis. Necrosis is characterized by rapid loss of the plasma membrane structure, organelle swelling, mitochondrial dysfunction, and the lack of features of apoptosis. Apoptosis is known as regulated or programmed cellular death and is characterized by "dropping off" of cellular fragments, called apoptotic bodies. It is now understood that under certain conditions necrosis is regulated or programmed, hence the new term *programmed necrosis*, or necroptosis.
2. The four major types of necrosis are coagulative, liquefactive, caseous, and fatty. Different types of necrosis occur in different tissues.
3. Structural signs that indicate irreversible injury and progression to necrosis are the dense clumping and disruption of genetic material and the disruption of the plasma and organelle membranes.
4. Apoptosis, a distinct type of sublethal injury, is a process of selective cellular self-destruction that occurs in both normal and pathological tissue changes.
5. Death by apoptosis causes loss of cells in many pathological states, including (a) severe cellular injury, (b) accumulation of misfolded proteins, (c) infections, and (d) obstruction in tissue ducts.
6. Excessive accumulation of misfolded proteins in the ER leads to a condition known as *ER stress*. ER stress results in apoptotic cellular death, and this mechanism has been linked to several degenerative diseases of the central nervous system and other organs.
7. Excessive or insufficient apoptosis is known as *dysregulated apoptosis*.
8. *Autophagy* means "eating of self," and as a recycling factory it is a self-destructive process and a survival mechanism. When cells are starved or nutrient deprived, the autophagic process institutes cannibalization and recycles the digested contents. Autophagy can maintain cellular metabolism under starvation conditions and remove damaged organelles under stress conditions, improving the survival of cells. Autophagy declines and becomes less efficient as the cell ages, thus contributing to the aging process.
9. Gangrenous necrosis, or gangrene, is tissue necrosis caused by hypoxia and the subsequent bacterial invasion.

Aging and Altered Cellular and Tissue Biology

1. It is difficult to determine the physiological (normal) from the pathological changes of aging. Investigators are focused on genetic, epigenetic, inflammatory, oxidative stress, and metabolic origins of aging.
2. Important factors in aging include increased damage to the cell, reduced capacity to divide, reduced ability to repair damaged DNA, and increased likelihood of defective protein balance or homeostasis.
3. Frailty is a common clinical syndrome in older adults, leaving a person vulnerable to falls, functional decline, disability, disease, and death. Sarcopenia and cachexia are a common consequence of aging.

Somatic Death

1. Somatic death is death of the entire person. Postmortem change is diffuse and does not involve components of the inflammatory response.
2. Manifestations of somatic death include cessation of respiration and circulation, gradual lowering of body temperature, dilation of the pupils, loss of elasticity and transparency in the skin, stiffening of the muscles (rigor mortis), and discoloration of the skin (livor mortis). Signs of putrefaction are obvious about 24 to 48 hours after death.

KEY TERMS

Adaptation, 74
Aging, 107
Algor mortis, 110
Anoxia, 80
Anthropogenic, 93
Apoptosis, 105
Asphyxial injury, 93
Atrophy, 75
Autolysis, 102
Autophagic vacuole, 75
Autophagy, 106
Bilirubin, 99
Carbon monoxide (CO), 90
Carboxyhemoglobin, 90
Caseous necrosis, 103
Caspase, 105
Cellular accumulations (infiltrations), 96
Cellular swelling, 97
Chemical asphyxiant, 95
Choking asphyxiation, 93
Coagulative necrosis, 103
Compensatory hyperplasia, 77
Cyanide, 95
Cytochrome, 99
Disuse atrophy, 75
Drowning, 95
Dry-lung drowning, 95
Dysplasia (atypical hyperplasia), 77
Dystrophic calcification, 100
Electrophile, 84
ER stress, 105
Ethanol, 90
Fat-free mass (FFM), 109
Fatty change (steatosis), 98
Fatty necrosis, 103
Fetal alcohol spectrum disorder, 92
Frailty, 109
Free radical, 82
Gangrenous necrosis, 103
Gas gangrene, 105
Hanging strangulation, 95
Hemoprotein, 99
Hemosiderin, 99
Hemosiderosis, 99
Hormonal hyperplasia, 77
Hydrogen sulphide, 95
Hyperplasia, 77
Hypertrophy, 76
Hypoxia, 80
Hypoxia-inducible transcription factor (HIF), 80
Infarct, 103
Irreversible injury, 78
Ischemia, 80
Ischemia-reperfusion injury, 82
Karyolysis, 102
Karyorrhexis, 102
Lead (Pb), 88
Life expectancy, 108
Lifespan, 107
Ligature strangulation, 95
Lipid peroxidation, 83
Lipofuscin, 76
Liquefactive necrosis, 103
Livor mortis, 110
Manual strangulation, 95
Maximal lifespan, 108
Melanin, 99
Mesenchymal (tissue from embryonic mesoderm) cell, 78
Metaplasia, 78
Metastatic calcification, 100
Mitochondrial DNA (mtDNA), 108
Necrosis, 101
Nucleophile, 84
Oncosis (vacuolar degeneration), 97
Oxidative stress, 82
Pathological atrophy, 75
Pathological hyperplasia, 77
Physiological atrophy, 75
Postmortem autolysis, 110
Postmortem change, 109
Programmed necrosis (necroptosis), 101
Proteasome, 75
Protein adduct, 84
Psammoma body, 100
Pyknosis, 102
Quality-adjusted life year (QALY), 108
Reperfusion injury, 82
Reversible injury, 78
Rigor mortis, 110
Sarcopenia, 109
Somatic death, 109
Strangulation, 93
Suffocation, 93
Toxicophore, 84
Ubiquitin, 75
Ubiquitin–proteasome pathway, 75
Urate, 100
Vacuolation, 81
Xenobiotic, 83

REFERENCES

1. Kumar, V., Abbas, A. K., & Aster, J. C. (Eds.), (2015). *Robbins and Cotran pathologic basis of disease* (9th ed.). Philadelphia: Saunders.
2. Chaillou, T., Kirby, T. J., & McCarthy, J. J. (2014). Ribosome biogenesis: Emerging evidence for a central role in the regulation of skeletal muscle mass. *Journal of Cellular Physiology*, *229*(11), 1584–1594. doi:10.1002/jcp.24604.
3. Lam, M. P. Y., Wang, D., Lau, E., et al. (2014). Protein kinetic signatures of the remodeling heart following isoproterenol stimulation. *Journal of Clinical Investigation*, *124*(4), 1734–1744. doi:10.1172/JCI73787.
4. Cacciapuoti, F. (2014). Role of ubiquitin–proteasome system (UPS) in left ventricular hypertrophy (LVH). *American J Cardiovascular Disease*, *4*(1), 1–5.
5. Hill, J. A., & Olson, E. N. (2008). Cardiac plasticity. *New England Journal of Medicine*, *358*(13), 1370–1380. doi:10.1056/NEJMra072139.
6. Leri, A., Kajstura, P. A., Dimmeler, S., et al. (2011). Role of cardiac stem cells in cardiac pathophysiology: A paradigm shift in human myocardial biology. *Circulation Research*, *109*, 941–961. doi:10.1161/CIRCRESAHA.111.243154.
7. Hariharan, N., Ikeda, Y., Hong, C., et al. (2013). Autophagy plays an essential role in mediating regression of hypertrophy during unloading of the heart. *PLoS ONE*, *8*(1), e51632. doi:10.1371/journal.pone.0051632.
8. Zafeiridis, A., Jeevandandam, V., Houser, S. R., et al. (1998). Regression of cellular hypertrophy after left ventricular assist device support. *Circulation*, *98*, 656d–662d. doi:10.1161/01.CIR.98.7.656.
9. Depre, C., Shipley, G. L., Chen, W., et al. (1998). Unloaded heart in vivo replicates fetal gene expression of cardiac hypertrophy. *Nature Medicine*, *4*, 1269–1275. doi:10.1038/3253.
10. Friddle, C. J., Koga, T., Rubin, E. M., et al. (2000). Expression profiling reveals distinct sets of genes altered during induction and regression of cardiac hypertrophy. *Proceedings of the National Academy of Sciences of the United States of America*, *97*, 6745–6750. doi:10.1073/pnas.100127897.
11. Jiang, Y., Reynolds, C., Xiao, C., et al. (2007). Dietary copper supplementation reverses hypertrophic cardiomyopathy induced by chronic pressure overload in mice. *Journal of Experimental Medicine*, *204*, 657–666. doi:10.1084/jem.20061943.
12. Zhou, Y., Jiang, Y., & Kang, Y. J. (2008). Copper reverses cardiomyocyte hypertrophy through vascular endothelial growth factor-mediated reduction in the cell size. *Journal of Molecular and Cellular Cardiology*, *45*, 106–117. doi:10.1016/j.yjmcc.2008.03.022.
13. Zhou, Y., Bourcey, K., & Kang, Y. J. (2009). Copper-induced regression of cardiomyocyte hypertrophy is associated with enhanced vascular endothelial growth factor receptor-1 signalling

pathway. *Cardiovascular Research, 84*, 54–63. doi:10.1093/cvr/cvp178.
14. Alberts, B., Bray, D., Hopkin, K., et al. (2014). *Essential cell biology* (4th ed.). New York: Garland Press.
15. Hamanaka, R. B., & Chandel, N. S. (2009). Mitochondrial reactive oxygen species regulate hypoxic signaling. *Current Opinion in Cell Biology, 21*(6), 894–899. doi:10.1016/j.ceb.2009.08.005.
16. Eltzschig, H. K., & Carmeliet, P. (2011). Hypoxia and inflammation. *New England Journal of Medicine, 364*(7), 656–665. doi:10.1056/NEJMra0910283.
17. Choi, H. J., Sanders, T. A., Tormos, K. V., et al. (2013). ECM-dependent HIF induction directs trophoblast stem cell fate via LIMK1-mediated cytoskeletal rearrangement. *PLoS ONE, 8*(2), e56949. doi:10.1371/journal.pone.0056949.
18. Choksi, S., Lin, Y., Pobezinskaya, Y., et al. (2011). A HIF-1, ATIA, protects cells from apoptosis by modulating the mitochondrial thioredoxin, TRX2. *Molecular Cell, 42*(5), 597–609. doi:10.1016/j.molcel.2011.03.030.
19. Wang, Z. J., Hu, W. K., Liu, Y. Y., et al. (2014). The effect of intravenous vitamin C infusion on periprocedural myocardial injury for patients undergoing elective percutaneous coronary intervention. *Canadian Journal of Cardiology, 30*(1), 96–101. doi:10.1016/j.cjca.2013.08.018.
20. Rodrigo, R., Hasson, D., Prieto, J. C., et al. (2014). The effectiveness of antioxidant vitamins C and E in reducing myocardial infarct size in patients subjected to percutaneous coronary angioplasty (PREVEC Trial): Study protocol for a pilot randomized double-blind controlled trial. *Trials, 15*, 192. doi:10.1186/1745-6215-15-192.
21. Oka, T., Hikoso, S., Yamaguchi, O., et al. (2012). Mitochondrial DNA that escapes from autophagy causes inflammation and heart failure. *Nature, 485*(7397), 251–255. doi:10.1038/nature10992.
22. Seeff, L. B. (2007). Herbal hepatotoxicity. *Clinics in Liver Disease, 11*, 577–596. doi:10.1016/j.cld.2007.06.005.
23. Carithers, R. L., Jr., & McClain, C. J. (2010). Alcoholic liver disease. In M. Feldman, L. S. Friedman, & L. J. Brandt (Eds.), *Sleisenger and Fordtran's gastrointestinal and liver disease: Pathophysiology, diagnosis, management* (9th ed., pp. 1383–1400). Philadelphia: Saunders/Elsevier.
24. Gu, X., & Manautou, J. E. (2013). Molecular mechanisms underlying chemical liver injury. *Expert Reviews in Molecular Medicine, 14*, e4. doi:10.1017/S1462399411002110.
25. Jones, D. P., & Delong, M. J. (2000). Detoxification and protective functions of nutrients. In M. Stipanuk (Ed.), *Biochemical and physiological aspects of nutrition*. Philadelphia: Saunders.
26. Hanzlik, R. P., Koen, Y. M., Theertham, B., et al. (2007). The reactive metabolite target protein database (TPDB)—a web-accessible resource. *BMC Bioinformatics, 8*, 95. doi:10.1186/1471-2105-8-95.
27. Liebler, D. C., & Guengerich, F. P. (2005). Elucidating mechanisms of drug-induced toxicity. *Nature, 4*, 410–420. doi:10.1038/nrd1720.
28. Gunnell, D., Murray, V., & Hawton, K. (2000). Use of Paracetamol (acetaminophen) for suicide and nonfatal poisoning: Worldwide patterns of use and misuse. *Suicide and Life-Threatening Behavior, 30*, 313–326.
29. Grespan, R., Agular, R. P., Giubilei, F. N., et al. (2014). Hepatoprotective effect of pretreatment with thymus vulgaris essential oil in experimental model of acetaminophen-induced injury. *Evidence-based Complementary and Alternative Medicine, 2014*, 954136. doi:10.1155/2014/954136.
30. Occupational Safety and Health Administration. (2012). *Lead*. Washington, DC: U.S. Department of Labor.
31. Murata, K., Iwata, T., Dakeishi, M., et al. (2009). Lead toxicity: Does the critical level of lead resulting in adverse effects differ between adults and children? *Journal of Occupational Health, 51*(1), 1–12.
32. Gibson, J. L. (2005). A plea for painted railings and painted walls of rooms as the source of lead poisoning amongst Queensland children, 1904. *Public Health Reports, 120*, 301.
33. Gilbert, S. G., & Weiss, B. (2006). A rationale for lowering the blood lead action level from 10 to 2 microg/dL. *Neurotoxicology, 27*, 693. doi:10.1016/j.neuro.2006.06.008.
34. Jacobs, D. E., Clickner, R. P., Zhou, J. Y., et al. (2002). The prevalence of lead-based paint hazards in U.S. housing. *Environmental Health Perspectives, 110*, 599.
35. Neal, A. P., & Guilarte, T. R. (2013). Mechanisms of lead and manganese neurotoxicity. *Toxicological Research, 2*, 99–114. doi:10.1039/C2TX20064C.
36. Nichani, V., Li, W. I., Smith, M. A., et al. (2006). Blood lead levels in children after phase-out of leaded gasoline in Bombay, India. *Science of the Total Environment, 363*, 95. doi:10.1016/j.scitotenv.2005.06.033.
37. Pirkle, L., Kaufmann, R. B., Brody, D. J., et al. (1997). Exposure of the U.S. population to lead, 1991–1994. *Environmental Health Perspectives, 106*, 745.
38. Strömberg, U., Lundh, T., & Skerfving, S. (2008). Yearly measurements of blood lead in Swedish children since 1978: The declining trend continues in the petrol-lead-free period 1995–2007. *Environmental Research, 107*, 332. doi:10.1016/j.envres.2008.03.007.
39. Luo, X. S., Yu, S., & Li, X. D. (2011). Distribution, availability, and sources of trace metals in different particle size fractions of urban soils in Hong Kong: Implications for assessing the risk to human health. *Environmental Pollution (Barking, Essex: 1987), 159*, 1317. doi:10.1016/j.envpol.2011.01.013.
40. United States Environmental Protection Agency. (2008). *Fact sheet: Final revisions to the national quality air standards for lead*. Washington, DC: Author. Retrieved from https://www.epa.gov/sites/production/files/2016-03/documents/final_rule_20081015_pb_factsheet.pdf.
41. Centers for Disease Control and Prevention. (2013). *Blood lead levels in children aged 1–5 years—United States, 1999–2010*. Atlanta, GA: Author.
42. Morris, R. G., Anderson, E., Lynch, G. S., et al. (1986). Selective impairment of learning and blockade of long-term potentiation by an *N*-methyl-D-aspartate receptor antagonist, AP5. *Nature, 319*(6056), 774–776. doi:10.1038/319774a0.
43. Konur, S., & Ghosh, A. (2005). Calcium signaling and the control of dendritic development. *Neuron, 46*, 401–405. doi:10.1016/j.neuron.2005.04.022.
44. Waites, C. L., & Garner, C. C. (2011). Presynaptic function in health and disease. *Trends in Neurosciences, 34*, 326–337. doi:10.1016/j.tins.2011.03.004.
45. Jomova, K., & Valko, M. (2011). Advances in metal-induced oxidative stress and human disease. *Toxicology, 283*, 65–87. doi:10.1016/j.tox.2011.03.001.
46. Abadin, H., Ashizawa, A., Stevens, Y. W., et al. (2007). *Toxicological profile for lead*. Atlanta, GA: Agency for Toxic Substances and Disease Registry (US).
47. Romanoff, R., Ross, D. M., & McMartin, K. E. (2007). Acute ethanol exposure inhibits renal folate transport, but repeated exposure upregulates folate transport proteins in rats and human cells. *Journal of Nutrition, 137*, 1260–1265.
48. Tsai, S. T., Wong, T. Y., Ou, C. Y., et al. (2014). The interplay between alcohol consumption, oral hygiene, ALDH2, and ADH1B in the risk of head and neck cancer. *International Journal of Cancer. Journal International du Cancer, 135*(10), 2424–2436. doi:10.1002/ijc.28885.
49. Hines, L. M., Ray, L., Hutchison, K., et al. (2005). Alcoholism: The dissection for endophenotypes. *Dialogues in Clinical Neuroscience, 7*(2), 153–163.
50. Rostron, B. (2012). Epidemiology alcohol consumption and mortality risks in the USA. *Alcohol and Alcoholism (Oxford, Oxfordshire), 47*(3), 334–339. doi:10.1093/alcalc/agr171.
51. Krenz, M., & Korthius, R. J. (2013). Moderate ethanol ingestion and cardiovascular protection: From epidemiologic associations to cellular mechanisms. *Journal of Molecular and Cellular Cardiology, 52*(1), 93–104. doi:10.1016/j.yjmcc.2011.10.011.
52. Canadian Heart and Stroke Association. (2016). *Lifestyle risk factors*. Ottawa: Author. Retrieved from http://www.heartandstroke.ca/heart/risk-and-prevention/lifestyle-risk-factors.
53. Costanzo, S., Di Castelnuovo, A., Donati, M. B., et al. (2010). Cardiovascular and overall mortality risk in relation to alcohol consumption in patients with cardiovascular disease. *Circulation, 121*, 1951–1959. doi:10.1161/CIRCULATIONAHA.109.865840.
54. Spörndly-Nees, S., Asenlöf, P., Theorell-Haglöw, J., et al. (2014). Leisure-time physical activity predicts complaints of snoring in women: A prospective cohort study over 10 years. *Sleep Medicine, 15*, 415–421. doi:10.1016/j.sleep.2013.09.020.
55. Nassir, F., & Ibdah, J. A. (2014). Role of mitochondria in alcoholic liver disease. *World Journal of Gastroenterology, 20*(9), 2136–2142. doi:10.3748/wjg.v20.i9.2136.
56. Leiber, C. S. (2005). Metabolism of alcohol. *Clinics in Liver Disease, 9*(1), 1–35. doi:10.1016/j.cld.2004.10.005.
57. Curtis, B. J., Zahs, A., & Kovacs, E. J. (2013). Epigenetic targets for reversing immune defects caused by alcohol exposure. *Alcohol Res, 35*(1), 97–113.
58. Sadrian, B., Wilson, D. A., & Saito, M. (2013). Long-lasting circuit dysfunction following developmental ethanol exposure. *Brain Sci, 3*(2), 704–727. doi:10.3390/brainsci3020704.
59. Govorko, D., Bekdash, R. A., Zhang, C., et al. (2012). Male germline transmits fetal alcohol adverse effect on hypothalamic proopiomelanocortin gene across generations. *Biological Psychiatry, 72*, 378–388. doi:10.1016/j.biopsych.2012.04.006.
60. Burd, L., Blair, J., & Dropps, K. (2012). Prenatal alcohol exposure, blood alcohol concentrations and alcohol elimination rates for the mother, fetus and newborn. *Journal of Perinatology, 32*(9), 652–659. doi:10.1038/jp.2012.57.
61. UNEP. (2013). *Global mercury assessment 2013: sources, emissions, releases and environmental transport*. Geneva: UNEP Chemicals Branch.
62. Mortazavi, S. M., Neghab, M., Anoosheh, S. M., et al. (2014). High-field MRI and mercury release from dental amalgam fillings. *International Journal of Occupational Medicine, 5*(2), 101–105.
63. Geier, D. A., Carmody, T., Kern, J. K., et al. (2012). A dose-dependent relationship between mercury exposure from dental amalgams and urinary mercury levels: A further assessment of the Casa Pia Children's Dental Amalgam Trial. *Human and Experimental Toxicology, 31*(1), 11–17. doi:10.1177/0960327111417264.
64. Homme, K. G., Kern, J. K., Haley, B. E., et al. (2014). New science challenges old notion that mercury dental amalgam is safe. *Biometals: An International Journal on the Role of Metal Ions in Biology, Biochemistry, and Medicine, 27*(1), 19–24. doi:10.1007/s10534-013-9700-9.
65. Schecter, R., & Grether, J. K. (2008). Continuing increases in autism reported to California's developmental services system, mercury in retrograde. *Archives of General Psychiatry, 65*(1), 19–24. doi:10.1001/archgenpsychiatry.2007.1.
66. Drowning Prevention Research Centre Canada.. (2015). *Canadian Drowning Report, 2015 Edition*. Retrieved from http://www.lifesavingsociety.ns.ca.
67. Hitomi, J., Christofferson, D. E., Ng, A., et al. (2008). Identification of a molecular signaling network that regulates a cellular necrotic cell death pathway by a genome wide siRNA screen. *Cell, 135*(7), 1311–1323. doi:10.1016/j.cell.2008.10.044.
68. Feokstova, M., & Leverkus, M. (2015). Programmed necrosis and necroptosis signaling. *FEBS Journal, 282*(1), 19–31. doi:10.1111/febs.13120.
69. Wang, Z., Jiang, H., Chen, S., et al. (2012). The mitochondrial phosphatase PGAM5 functions at the convergence point of multiple necrotic death pathways. *Cell, 148*, 228–243. doi:10.1016/j.cell.2011.11.030.

70. Raloff, J. (2001). Coming to terms with death: Accurate descriptions of a cell's demise may offer clues to diseases and treatments. *Science News, 159*, 378–380. doi:10.2307/3981880.
71. Glick, D., Barth, S., & Macleod, K. F. (2010). Autophagy: Cellular and molecular mechanisms. *Journal of Pathology, 221*(1), 3–12. doi:10.1002/path.2697.
72. Ge, L., Baskaran, S., Schekman, R., et al. (2014). The protein-vesicle network of autophagy. *Current Opinion in Cell Biology, 29*, 18–24. doi:10.1016/j.ceb.2014.02.005.
73. Cuda, C., Pope, R., & Perlman, H. (2016). The inflammatory role of phagocyte apoptotic pathways in rheumatic diseases. *Nature Reviews. Rheumatology, 12*(9), 543–558. doi:10.1038/nrrheum.2016.132.
74. Dancourt, J., & Melia, T. J. (2014). Lipidation of the autophagy proteins LC3 and GABARAP is a membrane-curvature dependent process. *Autophagy, 10*(8), 1470–1471. doi:10.4161/auto.29468.
75. Mizushima, N. (2007). Autophagy: Process and function. *Genes & Development, 21*(22), 2861–2873, review. doi:10.1101/gad.1599207.
76. Shen, H. M., & Mizushima, N. (2014). At the end of the autophagic road: An emerging understanding of lysosomal functions in autophagy. *Trends in Biochemical Sciences, 39*(2), 61–71. doi:10.1016/j.tibs.2013.12.001.
77. Butow, R. A., & Avadhani, N. G. (2004). Mitochondrial signaling: The retrograde response. *Molecular Cell, 14*(1), 1–15.
78. Levine, B., Mizushima, N., & Virgin, H. W. (2011). Autophagy in immunity and inflammation. *Nature, 469*, 323–335. doi:10.1038/nature09782.
79. Tissenbaum, H. A. (2012). Genetics, life span, health span, and the aging process in *Caenorhabditis elegans. Journals of Gerontology. Series A, Biological Sciences and Medical Sciences, 67A*(5), 503–510. doi:10.1093/gerona/gls088.
80. Rando, T. A., & Chang, H. Y. (2012). Aging rejuvenation, and epigenetic reprogramming: Resetting the aging clock. *Cell, 148*, 46–57. doi:10.1016/j.cell.2012.01.003.
81. Campisi, J., & Vijg, J. (2009). Does damage to DNA and other macromolecules play a role in aging? If so, how? *Journals of Gerontology. Series A, Biological Sciences and Medical Sciences, 64*, 175–178. doi:10.1093/gerona/gln065.
82. Seviour, E. G., & Lin, S. Y. (2010). The DNA damage response: Balancing the scale between cancer and ageing. *Aging (Albany, NY), 2*, 900–907. doi:10.18632/aging.100248.
83. Charville, G. W., & Rando, T. A. (2011). Stem cell ageing and non-random chromosome segregation. *Philosophical Transactions of the Royal Society of London. Series B, Biological Sciences, 366*, 85–93. doi:10.1098/rstb.2010.0279.
84. Kuilman, T., Michaloglou, C., Mooi, W. J., et al. (2010). The essence of senescence. *Genes & Development, 24*, 2463–2479. doi:10.1101/gad.1971610.
85. Fontana, L., Partridge, L., & Longo, V. D. (2010). Extending healthy life span—from yeast to humans. *Science, 328*, 321–326. doi:10.1126/science.1172539.
86. Kenyon, C. J. (2010). The genetics of ageing. *Nature, 464*, 504–512. doi:10.1038/nature08980.
87. Takahashi, K., & Yamanaka, S. (2006). Induction of pluripotent stem cells from mouse embryonic and adult fibroblast cultures by defined factors. *Cell, 126*, 663–676. doi:10.1016/j.cell.2006.07.024.
88. Hanna, J. H., Saha, K., & Jaenisch, R. (2010). Pluripotency and cellular reprogramming: Facts, hypotheses, unresolved issues. *Cell, 143*, 508–525. doi:10.1016/j.cell.2010.10.008.
89. Villeda, S. A., Luo, J., Mosher, K. I., et al. (2011). The ageing systemic milieu negatively regulates neurogenesis and cognitive function. *Nature, 477*, 90–94. doi:10.1038/nature10357.
90. Loffredo, F. S., Steinhauser, M. L., Jay, S. M., et al. (2013). Growth differentiation factor 11 is a circulating factor that reverses age-related cardiac hypertrophy. *Cell, 153*, 828–839. doi:10.1016/j.cell.2013.04.015.
91. Harrison, D. E., Strong, R., Sharp, Z. D., et al. (2009). Rapamycin fed late in life extends lifespan in genetically heterogeneous mice. *Nature, 460*, 392–395. doi:10.1038/nature08221.
92. Armstrong, L., Al-Aama, J., Stojkovic, M., et al. (2014). Concise review: The epigenetic contribution to stem cell ageing—can we rejuvenate our older cells? *Stem Cells, 32*(9), 2291–2298. doi:10.1002/stem.1720.
93. Greer, E. L., Maures, T. J., Ucar, D., et al. (2011). Transgenerational epigenetic inheritance of longevity in *Caenorhabditis elegans. Nature, 479*, 365–371. doi:10.1038/nature10572.
94. Statistics Canada. (2013). *Life Tables, Canada, Provinces and Territories, 2009 to 2011*. Ottawa: Minister of Industry.
95. Fausto, A., Campbell, J. S., & Riehle, K. J. (2006). Liver regeneration. *Hepatology (Baltimore, Md.), 43*, S45–S53. doi:10.1002/hep.20969.
96. Itsara, L. S., Kennedy, S. R., Fox, E. J., et al. (2014). Oxidative stress is not a major contributor to somatic mitochondrial DNA mutations. *PLoS Genetics, 10*(2), e1003974. doi:10.1371/journal.pgen.1003974.
97. Sevini, F., Giuliani, C., Vianello, D., et al. (2014). mtDNA mutations in human aging and longevity: Controversies and new perspectives opened by high-throughput technologies. *Experimental Gerontology, 56*, 234–244. doi:10.1016/j.exger.2014.03.022. Retrieved from http://dx.doi.org/10.1016/j.exger.2014.03.022.
98. Anker, S. D., Coats, A. J., Morley, J. E., et al. (2014). Muscle wasting disease: A proposal for a new disease classification. *Journal of Cachexia, Sarcopenia and Muscle, 5*(1), 1–3. doi:10.1007/s13539-014-0135-0.
99. Walrand, S., Guillet, C., Salles, J., et al. (2011). Physiopathological mechanism of sarcopenia. *Clinics in Geriatric Medicine, 27*, 365–385. doi:10.1016/j.cger.2011.03.005.
100. Ali, S., & Garcia, J. M. (2011). Sarcopenia, cachexia and aging: Diagnosis, mechanism and therapeutic options—a mini-review. *Gerontology, 60*(4), 294–305. doi:10.1159/000356760.
101. Walston, J. D. (2011). Frailty. Preface. *Clinics in Geriatric Medicine, 27*(1), xi. doi:10.1016/j.cger.2010.09.001.
102. Shennan, T. (1935). *Postmortems and morbid anatomy* (3rd ed.). Baltimore: William Wood.
103. Riley, M. W. (1990). Foreword: the gender paradox. In M. G. Ory & H. R. Warner (Eds.), *Gender, health, and longevity: multidisciplinary perspectives*. New York: Springer.
104. Katsumata, Y., Sato, K., & Yada, S. (1985). Green pigments in epidermal blisters of decomposed cadavers. *Forensic Science International, 28*(3–4), 167–174.

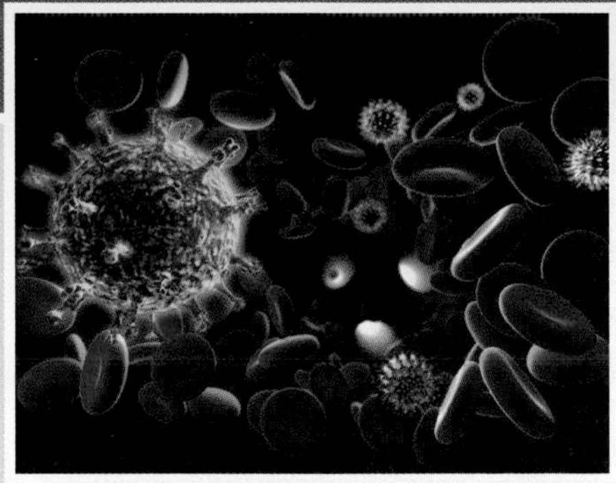

5

Fluids and Electrolytes, Acids and Bases

Sue E. Huether and Stephanie Zettel

EVOLVE WEBSITE

http://evolve.elsevier.com/Canada/Huether/pathophysiology
Student Review Questions
Key Points
Case Studies
Animations
Quick Check Answers

CHAPTER OUTLINE

Distribution of Body Fluids and Electrolytes, 115
- Water Movement Between Plasma and Interstitial Fluid, 115
- Water Movement Between ICF and ECF, 116

Alterations in Water Movement, 116
- Edema, 116

Sodium, Chloride, and Water Balance, 117

Alterations in Sodium, Chloride, and Water Balance, 120
- Isotonic Alterations, 121
- Hypertonic Alterations, 121
- Hypotonic Alterations, 121

Alterations in Potassium and Other Electrolytes, 122
- Potassium, 122
- Other Electrolytes—Calcium, Phosphate, and Magnesium, 126

Acid-Base Balance, 126
- Hydrogen Ion and pH, 126
- Buffer Systems, 126
- Acid-Base Imbalances, 128

PEDIATRIC CONSIDERATIONS: **Distribution of Body Fluids, 132**

GERIATRIC CONSIDERATIONS: **Distribution of Body Fluids, 132**

The cells of the body live in a fluid environment with electrolyte and acid-base concentrations maintained within a narrow range. Changes in electrolyte concentration affect the electrical activity of nerve and muscle cells and cause shifts of fluid from one compartment to another. Alterations in acid-base balance disrupt cellular functions. Fluid fluctuations also affect blood volume and cellular function. Disturbances in these functions are common and can be life-threatening. Understanding how alterations occur and how the body compensates or corrects the disturbance is important for comprehending many pathophysiological conditions.

DISTRIBUTION OF BODY FLUIDS AND ELECTROLYTES

The sum of fluids within all body compartments constitutes **total body water (TBW)**—about 60% of body weight in adults (Table 5-1). The volume of TBW is usually expressed as a percentage of body weight in kilograms. One litre of water weighs 1 kg. The rest of the body weight is composed of fat and fat-free solids, particularly bone.

Body fluids are distributed among functional compartments, or spaces, and provide a transport medium for cellular and tissue function. **Intracellular fluid (ICF)** comprises all the fluid within cells, about two thirds of TBW. **Extracellular fluid (ECF)** is all the fluid outside the cells (about one third of TBW) and includes **interstitial fluid** (the space between cells and outside the blood vessels) and **intravascular fluid** (blood plasma) (Table 5-2). The total volume of body water for a 70-kg person is about 42 litres. Other ECF compartments include lymph and transcellular fluids, such as synovial, intestinal, and cerebrospinal fluid; sweat; urine; and pleural, peritoneal, pericardial, and intraocular fluids.

Electrolytes and other solutes are distributed throughout the intracellular and extracellular fluid (Table 5-3). Note that ECF contains a large amount of *sodium* and *chloride* and a small amount of *potassium*, whereas the opposite is true of ICF. The concentrations of *phosphates* and *magnesium* are greater in ICF, and the concentration of *calcium* is greater in ECF. These differences are important for the maintenance of electroneutrality between the extracellular and intracellular compartments, the transmission of electrical impulses, and the movement of water among body compartments (see Chapter 1).

Although the amount of fluid within the various compartments is relatively constant, solutes (e.g., salts) and water are exchanged between compartments to maintain their unique compositions. The percentage of TBW varies with the amount of body fat and age. Because fat is water repelling (hydrophobic), very little water is contained in adipose (fat) cells. Individuals with more body fat have proportionately less TBW and tend to be more susceptible to dehydration.

The distribution and the amount of TBW change with age (see the *Pediatric Considerations* and *Geriatric Considerations* boxes later in this chapter), and although daily fluid intake may fluctuate widely, the body regulates water volume within a relatively narrow range. Water obtained by drinking, water ingested in food, and water derived from oxidative metabolism are the primary sources of body water. Normally, the largest amounts of water are lost through renal excretion, with lesser amounts lost through the stool and vaporization from the skin and lungs (insensible water loss) (Table 5-4).

Water Movement Between Plasma and Interstitial Fluid

The distribution of water and the movement of nutrients and waste products between the capillary and interstitial spaces occur as a result

TABLE 5-1 Total Body Water (%) in Relation to Body Weight

Body Build	Adult Male	Adult Female	Child (1–10 yr)	Infant (1 mo–1 yr)	Newborn (Up to 1 mo)
Normal	60	50	65	70	70–80
Lean	70	60	50-60	80	
Obese	50	42	50	60	

NOTE: Total body water is a percentage of body weight.
mo, month; *yr*, year.

TABLE 5-2 Distribution of Body Water (70-kg Man)

Fluid Compartment	% of Body Weight	Volume (L)
Intracellular fluid (ICF)	40	28
Extracellular fluid (ECF)	20	14
Interstitial	15	11
Intravascular	5	3
Total body water (TBW)	60	42

TABLE 5-3 Representative Distribution of Electrolytes in Body Compartments

Electrolytes	ECF (mmol/L)	ICF (mmol/L)
Cations		
Sodium	142	12
Potassium	4.2	150
Calcium	2.5	0
Magnesium	1	12
TOTAL	149.7	174
Anions		
Bicarbonate	24	12
Chloride	103	4
Phosphate	2	100
Proteins	16	65
Other anions	8	6
TOTAL	153	187

ECF, extracellular fluid; *ICF*, intracellular fluid.

TABLE 5-4 Normal Water Gains and Losses (70-kg Man)

	Daily Intake (mL)		Daily Output (mL)
Drinking	1 400–1 800	Urine	1 400–1 800
Water in food	700–1 000	Stool	100
Water of oxidation	300–400	Skin	300–500
		Lungs	600–800
TOTAL	2 400–3 200	**TOTAL**	2 400–3 200

of changes in hydrostatic pressure (pushes water) and osmotic or oncotic pressure (pulls water) at the arterial and venous ends of the capillary (see Figure 1-24). Water, sodium, and glucose readily move across the capillary membrane. The plasma proteins normally do not cross the capillary membrane and maintain effective osmolality by generating plasma oncotic pressure (particularly albumin).

As plasma flows from the arterial to the venous end of the capillary, four forces determine whether fluid moves out of the capillary and into the interstitial space (filtration) or whether fluid moves back into the capillary from the interstitial space (reabsorption). These four forces acting together are described as **net filtration** or **Starling forces**:

1. **Capillary hydrostatic pressure (blood pressure)** facilitates the outward movement of water from the capillary to the interstitial space.
2. **Capillary (plasma) oncotic pressure** osmotically attracts water from the interstitial space back into the capillary.
3. **Interstitial hydrostatic pressure** facilitates the inward movement of water from the interstitial space into the capillary.
4. **Interstitial oncotic pressure** osmotically attracts water from the capillary into the interstitial space.

The forces moving fluid back and forth across the capillary wall are summarized as follows:

Net filtration = (Forces favouring filtration) − (Forces opposing filtration)

Forces favouring filtration = Capillary hydrostatic pressure and interstitial oncotic pressure

Forces opposing filtration = Capillary oncotic pressure and interstitial hydrostatic pressure

At the arterial end of the capillary, hydrostatic pressure exceeds capillary oncotic pressure and fluid moves into the interstitial space (filtration). At the venous end of the capillary, capillary oncotic pressure exceeds capillary hydrostatic pressure and fluids are attracted back into the circulation (reabsorption). Interstitial hydrostatic pressure promotes the movement of about 10% of the interstitial fluid along with small amounts of protein into the lymphatics, which then returns to the circulation. Because albumin does not normally cross the capillary membrane, interstitial oncotic pressure is normally minimal. Figure 5-1 illustrates net filtration.

Water Movement Between ICF and ECF

Water moves between ICF and ECF compartments primarily as a function of osmotic forces. Water moves freely by diffusion through the lipid bilayer cell membrane and through **aquaporins**, a family of water channel proteins that provide permeability to water.[1] Sodium is responsible for the ECF osmotic balance, and potassium maintains the ICF osmotic balance. The osmotic force of ICF proteins and other nondiffusible substances is balanced by the active transport of ions out of the cell. Water crosses cell membranes freely, so the osmolality of TBW is normally at equilibrium. Normally ICF is not subject to rapid changes in osmolality, but when ECF osmolality changes, water moves from one compartment to another until osmotic equilibrium is re-established (see "Isotonic Alterations," p. 121).

ALTERATIONS IN WATER MOVEMENT

Edema

Edema is excessive accumulation of fluid within the interstitial spaces. The forces favouring fluid movement from the capillaries or lymphatic channels into the tissues are increased capillary hydrostatic pressure, decreased plasma oncotic pressure, increased capillary membrane permeability, and lymphatic channel obstruction[2] (Figure 5-2).

PATHOPHYSIOLOGY Capillary hydrostatic pressure increases as a result of venous obstruction or salt and water retention. Venous obstruction causes hydrostatic pressure to increase behind the obstruction,

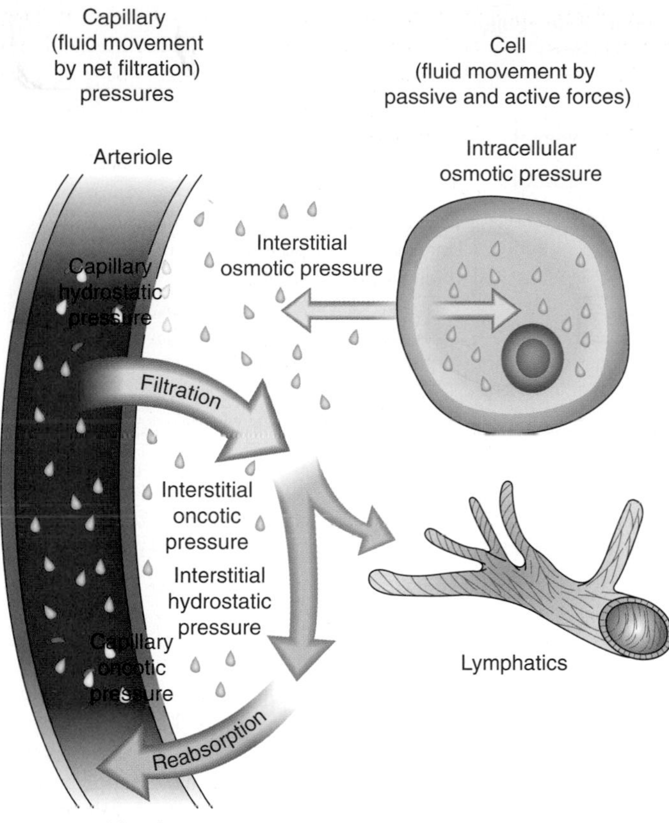

FIGURE 5-1 Net Filtration—Fluid Movement Between Plasma and Interstitial Space. The movement of fluid between the vascular, interstitial spaces and the lymphatics is the result of net filtration of fluid across the semipermeable capillary membrane. Capillary hydrostatic pressure is the primary force for fluid movement out of the arteriolar end of the capillary and into the interstitial space. At the venous end, capillary oncotic pressure (from plasma proteins) attracts water back into the vascular space. Interstitial hydrostatic pressure promotes the movement of fluid and proteins into the lymphatics. Osmotic pressure accounts for the movement of fluid between the interstitial space and the intracellular space. Normally, intracellular and extracellular fluid osmotic pressures are equal (280 to 294 mOsm) and water is equally distributed between the interstitial and intracellular compartments.

pushing fluid from the capillaries into the interstitial spaces. Thrombophlebitis (inflammation of veins), hepatic obstruction, tight clothing around the extremities, and prolonged standing are common causes of venous obstruction. Heart failure, renal failure, and cirrhosis of the liver are associated with excessive salt and water retention, which cause plasma volume overload, increased capillary hydrostatic pressure, and edema.

Since plasma albumin acts like a magnet to attract water, loss or diminished production (e.g., from liver disease or protein malnutrition) contributes to decreased plasma oncotic pressure. Plasma proteins are lost in glomerular diseases of the kidney, serous drainage from open wounds, hemorrhage, burns, and cirrhosis of the liver. The decreased oncotic attraction of fluid within the capillary causes filtered capillary fluid to remain in the interstitial space, resulting in edema.

Capillaries become more permeable with inflammation and immune responses, especially with trauma such as burns or crushing injuries, neoplastic disease, and allergic reactions. Proteins escape from the vascular space and produce edema through decreased capillary oncotic pressure and interstitial fluid protein accumulation.

The lymphatic system normally absorbs interstitial fluid and a small amount of proteins. When lymphatic channels are blocked or surgically removed, proteins and fluid accumulate in the interstitial space, causing **lymphedema**.[3] For example, lymphedema of the arm or leg occurs after surgical removal of axillary or femoral lymph nodes, respectively, for treatment of carcinoma. Inflammation or tumours may cause lymphatic obstruction, leading to edema of the involved tissues.

CLINICAL MANIFESTATIONS Edema may be localized or generalized. *Localized edema* is usually limited to a site of trauma, as in a sprained finger. Another kind of localized edema occurs within particular organ systems and includes cerebral, pulmonary, and laryngeal edema; pleural effusion (fluid accumulation in the pleural space); pericardial effusion (fluid accumulation within the membrane around the heart); and ascites (accumulation of fluid in the peritoneal space). Edema of specific organs, such as the brain, lung, or larynx, can be life-threatening. *Generalized edema* is manifested by a more uniform distribution of fluid in interstitial spaces. Dependent edema, in which fluid accumulates in gravity-dependent areas of the body, might signal more generalized edema. Dependent edema appears in the feet and legs when standing and in the sacral area and buttocks when supine (lying on back). It can be identified by pressing on tissues overlying bony prominences. A pit left in the skin indicates edema (hence the term *pitting edema*) (Figure 5-3).

Edema usually is associated with weight gain, swelling and puffiness, tight-fitting clothes and shoes, limited movement of affected joints, and symptoms associated with the underlying pathological condition. Fluid accumulations increase the distance required for nutrients and waste products to move between capillaries and tissues. Blood flow may be impaired also. Therefore wounds heal more slowly, and with prolonged edema the risks of infection and pressure sores over bony prominences increase. As edematous fluid accumulates, it is trapped in a "third space" (i.e., the interstitial space, pleural space, pericardial space) and is unavailable for metabolic processes or perfusion. Dehydration can develop as a result of this sequestering. Such sequestration occurs with severe burns, where large amounts of vascular fluid are lost to the interstitial spaces, reducing plasma volume and causing shock (see Chapter 24).

EVALUATION AND TREATMENT Specific conditions causing edema require diagnosis. Edema may be treated symptomatically until the underlying disorder is corrected. Supportive measures include elevating edematous limbs, using compression stockings, avoiding prolonged standing, restricting salt intake, and taking diuretics. Administration of intravenous (IV) albumin can be required in severe cases.

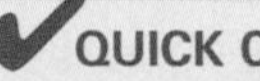
QUICK CHECK 5-1

1. How does an increase in capillary hydrostatic pressure cause edema?
2. How does a decrease in capillary oncotic pressure cause edema?

SODIUM, CHLORIDE, AND WATER BALANCE

The kidneys and hormones have a central role in maintaining sodium and water balance. Because water follows the osmotic gradients established by changes in salt concentration, sodium concentration and water balance are intimately related. Sodium concentration is regulated by renal effects of aldosterone (see Figure 18-18). Water balance is regulated primarily by **antidiuretic hormone (ADH**; also known as *vasopressin*).

Sodium (Na^+) accounts for 90% of the ECF cations (positively charged ions) (see Table 5-3). Along with its constituent anions (negatively

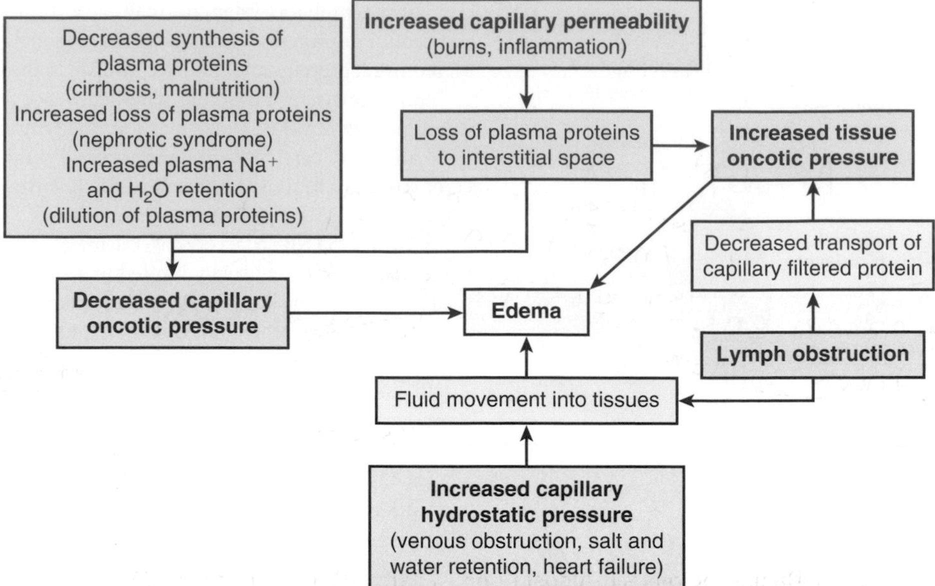

FIGURE 5-2 Mechanisms of Edema Formation. *H_2O*, water; *Na^+*, sodium.

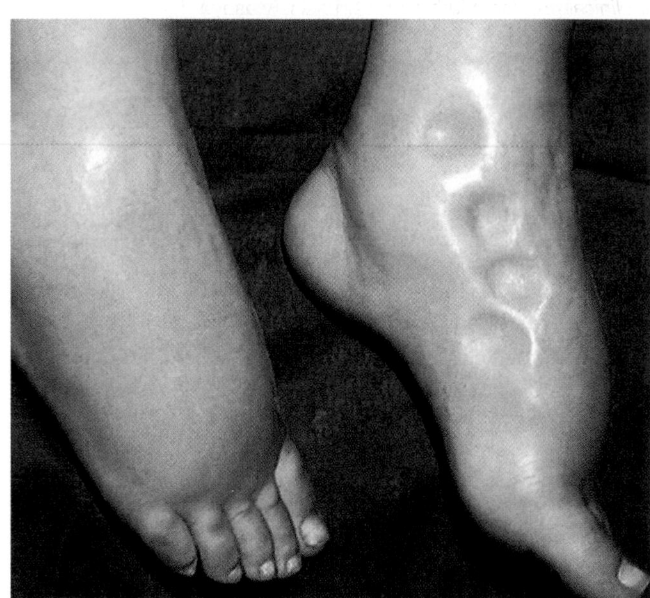

FIGURE 5-3 Pitting Edema. (From Bloom, A., & Ireland, J. [1992]. *Color atlas of diabetes* [2nd ed.]. St. Louis: Mosby.)

charged ions) chloride and bicarbonate, sodium regulates extracellular osmotic forces and therefore regulates water balance. Sodium is important in other functions, including maintenance of neuromuscular irritability for conduction of nerve impulses (in conjunction with potassium and calcium; see Figure 1-29), regulation of acid-base balance (using sodium bicarbonate and sodium phosphate), participation in cellular chemical reactions, and transport of substances across the cellular membrane.

The kidney, in conjunction with neural and hormonal mediators, maintains normal serum sodium concentration within a narrow range (136 to 145 mmol/L) primarily through renal tubular reabsorption. Hormonal regulation of sodium (and potassium) balance is mediated by **aldosterone**, a mineralocorticoid synthesized and secreted from the adrenal cortex as a component of the **renin-angiotensin-aldosterone system**. Aldosterone secretion is influenced by circulating blood volume, blood pressure, and plasma concentrations of sodium and potassium. When circulating blood volume or blood pressure is reduced, sodium levels are depressed, or potassium levels are increased, **renin**, an enzyme secreted by the juxtaglomerular cells of the kidney, is released. Renin stimulates the formation of **angiotensin I**, an inactive polypeptide. Angiotensin-converting enzyme (ACE) in pulmonary vessels converts angiotensin I to **angiotensin II**, which stimulates the secretion of aldosterone and ADH and also causes vasoconstriction. The aldosterone promotes renal sodium and water reabsorption and excretion of potassium, increasing blood volume (Figure 5-4; see also Figure 29-9). Vasoconstriction elevates the systemic blood pressure and restores renal perfusion (blood flow). This restoration inhibits the further release of renin.

Natriuretic peptides are hormones primarily produced by the myocardium. Atrial natriuretic hormone (ANH) is produced by the atria. B-type natriuretic peptide (BNP) is produced by the ventricles. Urodilatin (an ANP analogue) is synthesized within the kidney. Natriuretic peptides are released when there is an increase in transmural atrial pressure (increased volume), which may occur with heart failure or when there is an increase in mean arterial pressure[4] (Figure 5-5). They are natural antagonists to the renin-angiotensin-aldosterone system. Natriuretic peptides cause vasodilation and increase sodium and water excretion, decreasing blood pressure. Natriuretic peptides are sometimes called a "third factor" in sodium regulation. (Increased glomerular filtration rate is thus the first factor and aldosterone the second factor.)

Chloride (Cl^-) is the major anion in ECF and provides electroneutrality, particularly in relation to sodium. Chloride transport is generally passive and follows the active transport of sodium so that increases or decreases in chloride concentration are proportional to changes in sodium concentration. Chloride concentration tends to vary inversely with changes in the concentration of bicarbonate (HCO_3^-), the other major anion.

Water balance is regulated by the secretion of ADH. ADH is secreted when plasma osmolality increases or circulating blood volume decreases and blood pressure drops (Figure 5-6). Increased plasma osmolality occurs with water deficit or sodium excess in relation to TBW. The increased osmolality stimulates hypothalamic **osmoreceptors**. In addition to causing thirst, these osmoreceptors signal the posterior pituitary gland to release ADH. Thirst stimulates water drinking and

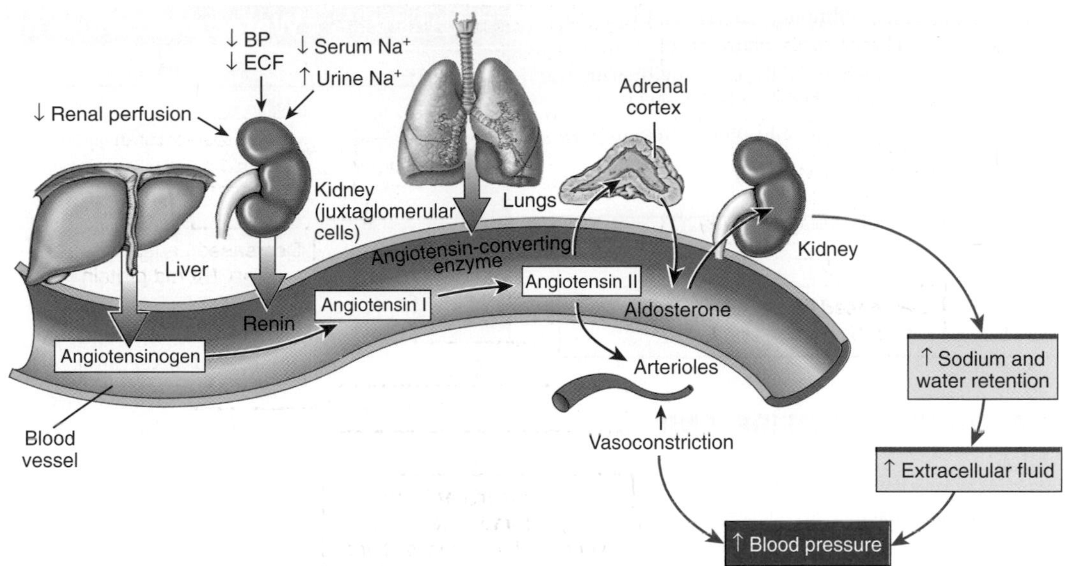

FIGURE 5-4 The Renin-Angiotensin-Aldosterone System. *BP*, blood pressure; *ECF*, extracellular fluid; *Na+*, sodium. (Modified from Herlihy, B., & Maebius, N. [2011]. *The human body in health and disease* [4th ed.]. Philadelphia: Saunders. Borrowed from Lewis, S.L., Bucher, L., Heitkemper, M.M., et al. [2014]. *Medical-surgical nursing: Assessment and management of clinical problems* [9th ed.]. St. Louis: Mosby.)

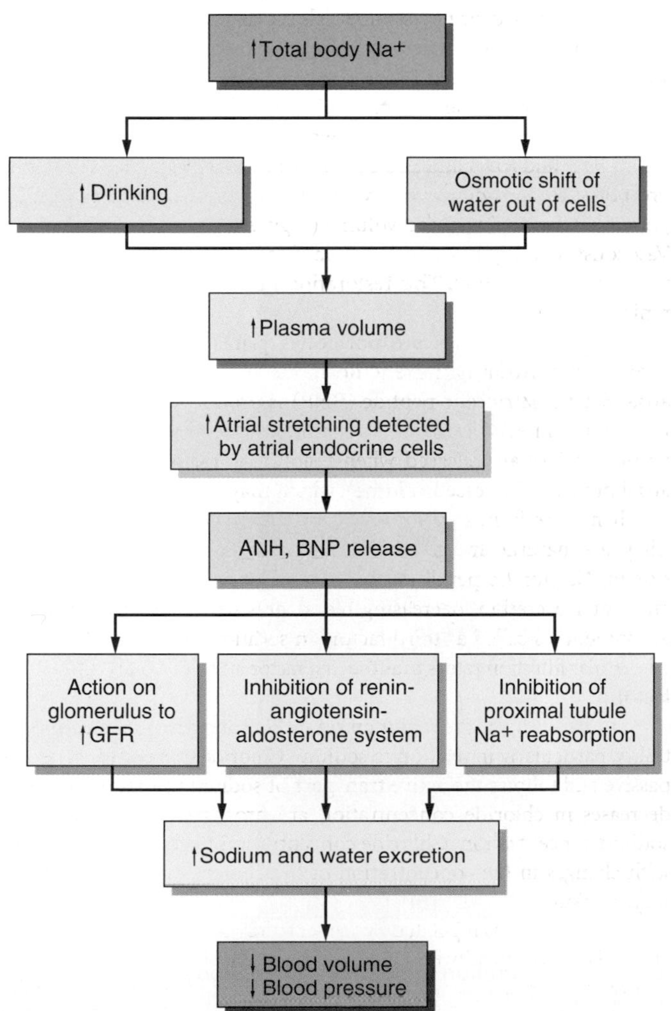

FIGURE 5-5 The Natriuretic Peptide System. *ANH*, atrial natriuretic hormone; *BNP*, brain natriuretic peptide; *GFR*, glomerular filtration rate; *Na+*, sodium

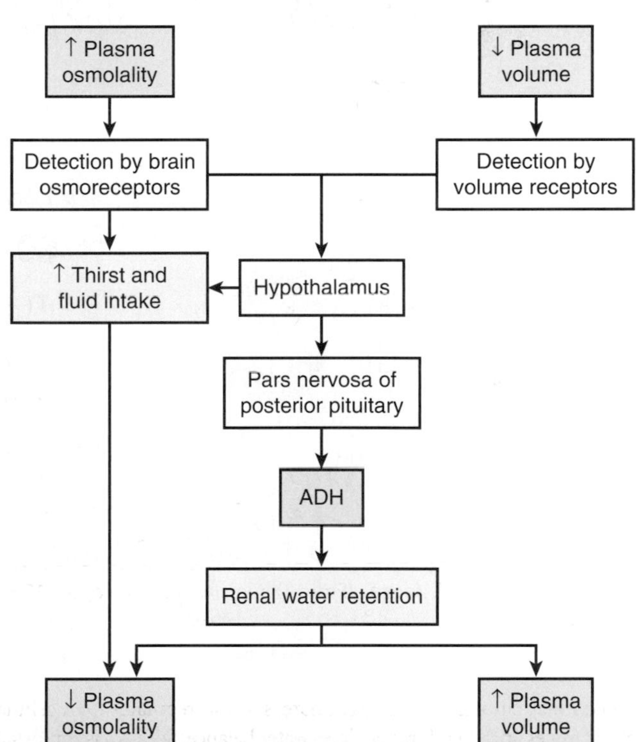

FIGURE 5-6 The Antidiuretic Hormone System. *ADH*, antidiuretic hormone.

ADH increases water reabsorption into the plasma from the distal tubules and collecting ducts of the kidney (see Chapter 29). The reabsorbed water decreases plasma osmolality, returning it toward normal, and urine concentration increases.

With fluid loss (dehydration) from vomiting, diarrhea, or excessive sweating, a decrease in blood volume and blood pressure often occurs. **Volume-sensitive receptors** and **baroreceptors** (nerve endings that are sensitive to changes in volume and pressure) also stimulate the release of ADH from the pituitary gland and stimulate thirst. The volume receptors are located in the right and left atria and thoracic vessels;

baroreceptors are found in the aorta, pulmonary arteries, and carotid sinus. ADH secretion also occurs when atrial pressure drops, as occurs with decreased blood volume and with the release of angiotensin II (see Figure 29-9). The reabsorption of water mediated by ADH then promotes the restoration of plasma volume and blood pressure (see Figure 5-6).

QUICK CHECK 5-2

1. What forces promote net filtration?
2. How do hormones regulate salt and water balance?
3. What are aquaporins?

ALTERATIONS IN SODIUM, CHLORIDE, AND WATER BALANCE

Alterations in sodium and water balance are closely related. Sodium imbalances occur with gains or losses of body water. Water imbalances develop with gains or losses of salt. In general, these alterations can be classified as changes in tonicity, the change in the concentration of solutes in relation to water: isotonic, hypertonic, or hypotonic (Table 5-5 and Figure 5-7; see also Figure 1-25). Changes in tonicity also alter the volume of water in the intracellular and extracellular compartments, resulting in isovolemia, hypervolemia, or hypovolemia.

TABLE 5-5 Water and Solute Imbalances

Tonicity	Mechanism
Isotonic (iso-osmolar) imbalance Serum osmolality = 280–294 mOsm/kg	Gain or loss of ECF resulting in concentration equivalent to 0.9% sodium chloride solution (normal saline); no shrinking or swelling of cells
Hypertonic (hyperosmolar) imbalance Serum osmolality >294 mOsm/kg	Imbalances that result in ECF concentration >0.9% salt solution (i.e., water loss or solute gain); cells shrink in hypertonic fluid
Hypotonic (hypo-osmolar) imbalance Serum osmolality <280 mOsm/kg	Imbalance that results in ECF <0.9% salt solution (i.e., water gain or solute loss); cells swell in hypotonic fluid
Formula for calculating serum osmolarity	(2 × [Na] + [Glu])/18 + BUN/2.8

BUN, blood serum urea nitrogen level (mmol/L); *ECF*, extracellular fluid; *[Glu]*, serum glucose concentration (mmol/L); *[Na]*, serum sodium concentration (mmol/L).

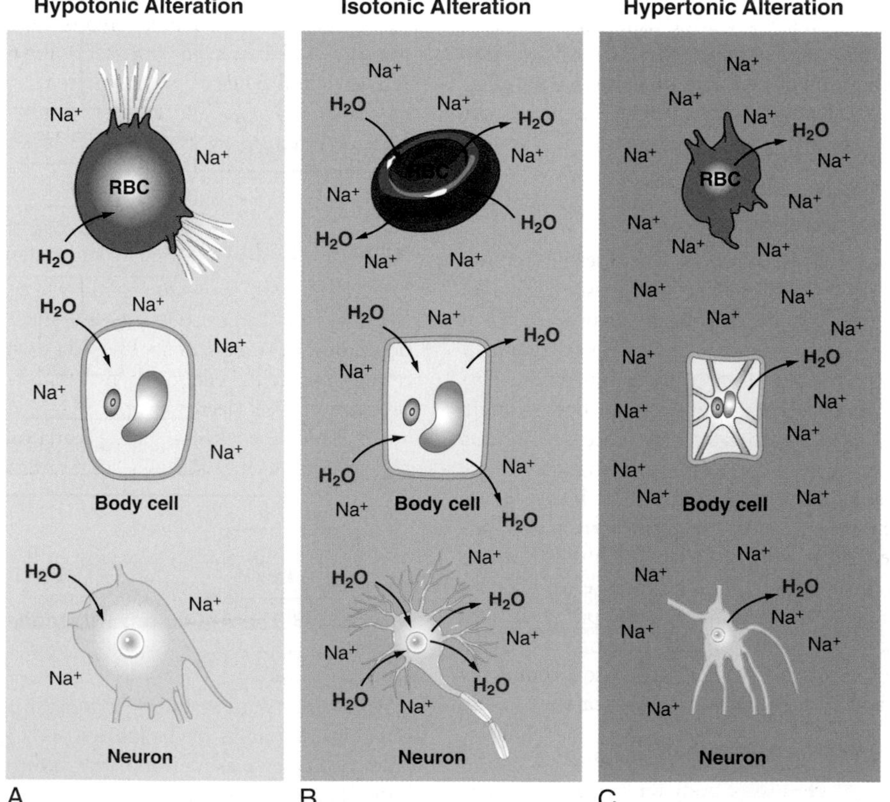

FIGURE 5-7 Effects of Alterations in Extracellular Sodium Concentration in Red Blood Cell, Body Cell, and Neuron. A, Hypotonic alteration: Decrease in extracellular fluid (ECF) sodium (*Na^+*) concentration (hyponatremia) results in intracellular fluid osmotic attraction of water (*H_2O*) with swelling and potential bursting of cells. **B,** Isotonic alteration: Normal concentration of sodium in ECF and no change in shifts of fluid in or out of cells. **C,** Hypertonic alteration: An increase in ECF sodium concentration (hypernatremia) results in osmotic attraction of water out of cells with cell shrinkage. *RBC*, red blood cell.

Isotonic Alterations

Isotonic alterations are the most common kinds of alterations, and they occur when TBW changes are accompanied by proportional changes in the concentrations of electrolytes (see Figure 5-7). Isotonic fluid loss causes dehydration and hypovolemia. For example, if an individual loses pure plasma or ECF, fluid volume is depleted but the concentration and type of electrolytes and the osmolality remain in the normal range (280 to 294 milliosmoles [mOsm]). Causes include hemorrhage, severe wound drainage, excessive diaphoresis (sweating), and inadequate fluid intake. There is loss of ECF volume with weight loss, dryness of skin and mucous membranes, decreased urine output, and symptoms of hypovolemia. Indicators of hypovolemia include a rapid heart rate, flattened neck veins, and normal or decreased blood pressure. In severe states, hypovolemic shock can occur (see Chapter 24). Isotonic fluids containing electrolytes and glucose are given orally, intravenously (i.e., 0.9% saline solution or 5% dextrose in 0.225% saline solution), or, in some cases, subcutaneously (hypodermoclysis).

Isotonic fluid excess causes hypervolemia. Common causes include excessive administration of IV fluids, hypersecretion of aldosterone, or the effects of medications such as cortisone (which causes renal reabsorption of sodium and water). As plasma volume expands, hypervolemia develops with weight gain. The diluting effect of excess plasma volume leads to decreased hematocrit and decreased plasma protein concentration. The neck veins may distend, and the blood pressure increases. Increased capillary hydrostatic pressure leads to edema formation. Ultimately, pulmonary edema and heart failure may develop. Diuretics are commonly used for treatment.

Hypertonic Alterations

Hypertonic fluid alterations develop when the osmolality of ECF is elevated above normal (greater than 294 mOsm). The most common causes are increased concentration of ECF sodium (hypernatremia) or deficit of ECF water, or both. In both instances, ECF hypertonicity attracts water from the intracellular space, causing ICF dehydration (see Figure 5-7).

Hypernatremia

PATHOPHYSIOLOGY Hypernatremia occurs when serum sodium levels exceed 145 mmol/L. Increased levels of serum sodium cause hypertonicity. Hypernatremia can be isovolemic, hypovolemic, or hypervolemic, depending on the accompanying ECF water volume.

Isovolemic hypernatremia is the most common type and occurs when there is a *loss of free water* with a near-normal body sodium concentration. Causes include inadequate water intake; excessive sweating (sweat is hypotonic), fever, or respiratory tract infections, which increase the respiratory rate and enhance water loss from the lungs; burns; vomiting; diarrhea; and central or nephrogenic diabetes insipidus (lack of ADH or inadequate renal response to ADH). Infants with severe diarrhea are vulnerable and have increased risk because they cannot communicate thirst. Insufficient water intake occurs particularly in individuals who are comatose, confused, or immobilized or are receiving gastric feedings. Dehydration refers to water deficit but also is commonly used to indicate both sodium and water loss (isotonic or iso-osmolar dehydration).[5]

Hypovolemic hypernatremia occurs where there is loss of sodium accompanied by a relatively greater loss of body water. Causes include use of loop diuretics, osmotic diuresis (i.e., from hyperglycemia related to uncontrolled diabetes mellitus or use of mannitol), or failure of the kidneys to concentrate urine.

Hypervolemic hypernatremia is rare and occurs when there is increased TBW and a greater increase in total body sodium level, resulting in hypervolemia. Causes include infusion of hypertonic saline solutions (e.g., as sodium replacement for treatment of salt depletion, which can occur with renal impairment, heart failure, or gastro-intestinal losses); oversecretion of adrenocorticotropic hormone (ACTH) or aldosterone (e.g., Cushing's syndrome, adrenal hyperplasia); and near salt water drowning.[6] High amounts of dietary sodium rarely cause hypernatremia in a healthy individual because the sodium is eliminated by the kidneys.

Because chloride follows sodium, hyperchloremia (elevation of serum chloride concentration greater than 106 mmol/L) often accompanies hypernatremia, as well as plasma bicarbonate deficits (such as in metabolic acidosis)[7]. There are no specific symptoms or treatment for chloride excess.

CLINICAL MANIFESTATIONS When there is excessive sodium intake or decreased sodium loss in relation to water, water is osmotically redistributed to the hypertonic extracellular space, resulting in hypervolemia, and intracellular dehydration ensues. Clinical manifestations include thirst, weight gain, bounding pulse, and increased blood pressure. Central nervous system signs are the most serious and are related to alterations in membrane potentials and shrinking of brain cells (sodium cannot cross brain capillaries because of their tight endothelial junctions). Signs include muscle twitching and hyper-reflexia (hyperactive reflexes), confusion, coma, convulsions, and cerebral hemorrhage from stretching of veins. Hypernatremia with marked water deficit is manifested by signs and symptoms of intracellular and extracellular dehydration with volume depletion (Box 5-1).

EVALUATION AND TREATMENT Serum sodium levels are greater than 147 mmol/L and urine specific gravity will be greater than 1.030. The history and physical examination provide information about underlying disorders and events. The treatment of hypernatremia and water deficit is to give oral fluids or isotonic salt-free fluid (5% dextrose in water) until the serum sodium level returns to normal. Fluid replacement must be given slowly to prevent cerebral edema. Serum sodium levels need to be monitored. Hypervolemia or hypovolemia requires treatment of the underlying clinical condition.

Hypotonic Alterations

Hypotonic fluid imbalances occur when the osmolality of ECF is less than 280 mmol (see Figure 5-7). The most common causes are sodium deficit or water excess. Either leads to *intracellular overhydration* (cellular edema) and cell swelling. When there is a sodium deficit, the osmotic pressure of ECF decreases and water moves into the cell where the osmotic pressure is greater. The plasma volume then decreases, leading to symptoms of hypovolemia. With water excess, increases in both ICF

BOX 5-1 Signs and Symptoms of Dehydration

Increased serum sodium concentration	Soft eyeballs
Thirst	Sunken fontanels in infants
Headache	Prolonged capillary refill time
Weight loss	Tachycardia
Oliguria and concentrated urine	Weak pulses
Hard stools	Low blood pressure
Decreased skin turgor	Postural hypotension
Dry mucous membranes	Hypovolemic shock
Decreased sweating and tears	Confusion
Elevated temperature	Coma

and ECF volume occur, causing symptoms of hypervolemia and water intoxication with cerebral and pulmonary edema.

Hyponatremia

PATHOPHYSIOLOGY Hyponatremia develops when the serum sodium concentration falls below 135 mmol/L. Hyponatremia occurs when there is loss of sodium, inadequate intake of sodium, or dilution of sodium by water excess.[8] Sodium depletion usually causes hypo-osmolality with movement of water into cells and rupture of cell membranes.

Isovolemic hyponatremia occurs when there is loss of sodium without a significant loss of water (pure sodium deficit). Causes can include syndrome of inappropriate antidiuretic hormone[9] (SIADH [see Chapter 19], which enhances water retention), hypothyroidism, pneumonia, and glucocorticoid deficiency. Inadequate intake of dietary sodium is rare but possible in individuals on low-sodium diets, particularly with use of diuretics.

Hypervolemic hyponatremia occurs when total body sodium level increases. The increased sodium leads to an increase in TBW and dilution of sodium in the extracellular space. Causes include heart failure, cirrhosis of the liver, and nephrotic syndrome. Edema is present.

Hypovolemic hyponatremia occurs with a loss of TBW, but there is a greater loss of body sodium. The extracelluar volume is decreased. Causes include prolonged vomiting, severe diarrhea, inadequate secretion of aldosterone (e.g., adrenal insufficiency), and renal losses from diuretics.

Dilutional hyponatremia (water intoxication) occurs when there is intake of large amounts of free water or replacement of fluid loss with IV 5% dextrose in water, which dilutes sodium. The glucose is metabolized to carbon dioxide and water, leaving a hypotonic solution with a diluting effect. Excessive sweating stimulates thirst and intake of large amounts of free water (as can occur in endurance athletes), which dilutes sodium. Some individuals with psychogenic disorders develop water intoxication from compulsive water drinking. Other causes can include tap water enemas, near fresh water drowning, and use of selective serotonin reuptake inhibitors (SSRIs). When the body is functioning normally, it is almost impossible to produce an excess of TBW because water balance is regulated by the kidneys.

Hypochloremia, a low level of serum chloride (less than 98 mmol/L), usually occurs with hyponatremia or an elevated bicarbonate concentration, as in metabolic alkalosis. Sodium deficit related to restricted intake, use of diuretics, vomiting, or nasogastric suction is accompanied by chloride deficiency. Cystic fibrosis is characterized by hypochloremia (see Chapter 28). Treatment of the underlying cause is required.

CLINICAL MANIFESTATIONS The serum sodium concentration will be less than 136 mmol/L. Sodium depletion usually causes hypo-osmolality with movement of water into cells. The hematocrit is reduced from the dilutional effect of water excess in dilutional hyponatremia. The high amount of intracellular solutes compared with the low amount of extracellular solutes as a result of the hyponatremia causes an intracellular osmotic shift of water, resulting in cell swelling. The most life-threatening consequence is cerebral edema and increased intracranial pressure. Neurological changes include lethargy, confusion, apprehension, seizures, and coma. A decrease in sodium concentration changes the cell's ability to depolarize and repolarize normally, altering the action potential in neurons and muscle (see Chapter 1). Muscle twitching, depressed reflexes, and weakness are common. Nausea and vomiting are more common with less severe hyponatremia (i.e., decreases between 120 and 130 mmol/L). Hypovolemic hyponatremia has signs of hypotension, tachycardia, and decreased urine output. Hypervolemic hyponatremia is accompanied by weight gain, edema, ascites, and jugular vein distension. Hyponatremia is a major cause of morbidity and mortality in critical care units and in older adults (see *Health Promotion:* Hyponatremia and Older Adults).

HEALTH PROMOTION

Hyponatremia and Older Adults

Hyponatremia is the most common of the electrolyte disorders, and prevalence is highest among older hospitalized individuals. Isovolemic hyponatremia caused by SIADH is thought to be the most common cause and can occur with central nervous system injury, pulmonary disease, malignancies, nausea, pain, and aging changes. Other contributing factors include use of thiazide diuretics, proton pump inhibitors, age-related decrease in thirst with dehydration, and diminished urine concentrating ability. Hyponatremia contributes to cognitive deficits, gait disturbances, falls, fractures, long-term hospitalization, the need for long-term care, and death. Older adults need to be assessed for risk, implementation of preventive strategies, and early intervention.

SIADH, syndrome of inappropriate antidiuretic hormone.
From Ayus, J.C., Negri, A.L., Kalantar-Zadeh, K., et al. (2012). *Nephrol Dial Transplant, 27*(10), 3725–3731; Berl, T. (2013). *Clin J Am Soc Nephrol, 8*(3), 469–475; Cowen, L.E., Hodak, S.P., & Verbalis, J.G. (2013). *Endocrinol Metab Clin North Am, 42*(2), 349–370; Cumming, K., Hoyle, G.E., Hutchison, J.D., et al. (2014). *PLoS One, 9*(2), e88272; Mannesse, C.K., Vondeling, A.M., van Marum, R.J., et al. (2013). *Ageing Res Rev, 12*(1), 165–173; Schrier, R.W., Sharma, S., & Shchekochikhin, D. (2013). *Nat Rev Nephrol, 9*(1), 37–50 (Erratum in [2013]. *Nat Rev Nephrol* 9[3], 124).

EVALUATION AND TREATMENT The cause of hyponatremia must be determined and treatment planned accordingly. Small amounts of IV hypertonic sodium chloride (i.e., 3% sodium chloride) can be given when neurological manifestations are severe, but they must be given slowly to prevent osmotic demyelination syndrome in the brain.[9] Restriction of water intake is required in most cases of dilutional hyponatremia because body sodium levels may be normal or increased even though serum sodium levels are low. Arginine vasopressin (ADH) receptor antagonists (vaptans) are a class of medications used for the treatment of hypervolemic and euvolemic hyponatremia.[10] Serum sodium concentration must be monitored.[8]

✔ QUICK CHECK 5-3

1. What causes isotonic imbalance?
2. What are some causes of hypernatremia?
3. What is the most severe complication of hyponatremia?

ALTERATIONS IN POTASSIUM AND OTHER ELECTROLYTES

Potassium

Potassium (K^+) is the major intracellular electrolyte and is essential for normal cellular functions. Total body potassium content is about 4000 mmol, with most of it (98%) located in the cells. The ICF concentration of potassium is 150 to 160 mmol/L; the ECF potassium concentration is 3.5 to 5.0 mmol/L. The difference in concentration is maintained by a sodium–potassium adenosinetriphosphatase active transport system (Na^+–K^+ ATPase pump) (see Figure 1-26).

As the predominant ICF ion, potassium exerts a major influence on the regulation of ICF osmolality and fluid balance as well as on intracellular electrical neutrality in relation to hydrogen (H^+) and sodium.

Potassium is required for glycogen and glucose deposition in liver and skeletal muscle cells. It also maintains the resting membrane potential, as reflected in the transmission and conduction of nerve impulses (see Figure 1-29), the maintenance of normal cardiac rhythms, and the contraction of skeletal muscle and smooth muscle.

Dietary potassium moves rapidly into cells after ingestion. However, the distribution of potassium between intracellular and extracellular fluids is influenced by several factors. Insulin, aldosterone, epinephrine, and alkalosis facilitate the shift of potassium into cells. Insulin deficiency, aldosterone deficiency, acidosis, cell lysis, and strenuous exercise facilitate the shift of potassium out of cells. Glucagon blocks entry of potassium into cells, and glucocorticoids promote potassium excretion. Potassium also will move out of cells along with water when there is increased ECF osmolarity.

Although potassium is found in most body fluids, the kidney is the most efficient regulator of potassium balance. Potassium is freely filtered by the renal glomerulus, and 90% is reabsorbed by the proximal tubule and loop of Henle. In the distal tubules, principal cells secrete potassium and intercalated cells reabsorb potassium. These cells determine the amount of potassium excreted from the body. The gut may also sense the amount of K^+ ingested and stimulate renal K^+ excretion independent of aldosterone.[11]

The potassium concentration in the distal tubular cells is determined primarily by the plasma concentration in the peritubular capillaries. When plasma potassium concentration increases from increased dietary intake or shifts of potassium from ICF to ECF occur, potassium is secreted into the urine by the distal tubules. Decreased levels of plasma potassium result in decreased distal tubular secretion, although approximately 5 to 15 mmol/day will continue to be lost. Changes in the rate of filtrate (urine) flow through the distal tubule also influence the concentration gradient for potassium secretion. When the urine flow rate is high, as with the use of diuretics, potassium concentration in the distal tubular urine is lower, leading to the secretion of potassium into the urine.

Changes in pH and thus in hydrogen ion concentration also affect potassium balance. During acute acidosis, hydrogen ions accumulate in the ICF and potassium shifts out of the cell to the ECF to maintain a balance of cations across the cell membrane. This response occurs in part because of a decrease in Na^+–K^+ ATPase pump activity. Decreased ICF potassium results in decreased secretion of potassium by the distal tubular cells, contributing to hyperkalemia. In acute alkalosis, intracellular fluid levels of hydrogen diminish and potassium shifts into the cell; in addition, the distal tubular cells increase their secretion of potassium, further contributing to hypokalemia.[12]

Besides conserving sodium, *aldosterone* also regulates potassium concentration. Elevated plasma potassium concentration causes the release of renin by renal juxtaglomerular cells and the adrenal secretion of aldosterone through the renin-angiotensin-aldosterone system. Aldosterone then stimulates the release of potassium into the urine by the distal renal tubules. Aldosterone also increases the secretion of potassium from sweat glands.

Insulin helps regulate plasma potassium levels by stimulating the Na^+–K^+ ATPase pump, thus promoting the movement of potassium into liver and muscle cells, particularly after eating. Insulin can also be used to treat hyperkalemia. Dangerously low levels of plasma potassium can result when insulin is given while potassium levels are depressed. Potassium balance is especially significant in the treatment of conditions requiring insulin administration, such as insulin-dependent diabetes mellitus.

Potassium adaptation is the ability of the body to adapt to increased levels of potassium intake over time. A sudden increase in potassium may be fatal, but if the intake of potassium is slowly increased by amounts of more than 120 mmol/day, the kidney can increase the urinary excretion of potassium and maintain potassium balance.

Hypokalemia

PATHOPHYSIOLOGY Potassium deficiency, or **hypokalemia**, develops when the serum potassium concentration falls to less than 3.5 mmol/L. Because cellular and total body stores of potassium are difficult to measure, changes in potassium balance are described, although not always accurately, by the plasma concentration. Generally, lowered serum potassium level indicates loss of total body potassium. With potassium loss from ECF, the concentration gradient change favours movement of potassium from the cell to the ECF. The ICF/ECF concentration ratio is maintained, but the amount of total body potassium is depleted.

Factors contributing to the development of hypokalemia include reduced intake of potassium, increased entry of potassium into cells, and increased loss of body potassium. Dietary deficiency of potassium is more common in older adults with both low protein intake and inadequate intake of fruits and vegetables and in individuals with alcoholism or anorexia nervosa (see *Health Promotion:* Potassium Intake: Hypertension and Stroke). Reduced potassium intake generally becomes a problem when combined with other causes of potassium depletion.

HEALTH PROMOTION

Potassium Intake: Hypertension and Stroke

Enriched dietary intake of potassium is associated with lower risk of hypertension and stroke. The Canadian diet often exceeds recommendations for sodium intake and has a deficiency in potassium intake. There is increased risk of high blood pressure, cardiovascular disease, and mortality when the plasma ratio of sodium concentration to potassium concentration is high. Potassium attenuates the effects of high dietary salt with reduction in blood pressure, stroke rates, and cardiovascular disease risk. The exact mechanism of how potassium affects blood pressure is unknown, but it is thought to be related to renal handling of sodium, endothelial cell function, decreased vascular resistance, and reduced oxidative stress. A large prospective study of older women showed that a lower risk of ischemic but not hemorrhagic stroke was associated with higher intakes of potassium, especially in women without hypertension. Lower risk of mortality was found in all women with higher intakes of potassium. Increased dietary intake of potassium is recommended for most individuals without impaired renal handling of potassium.

Data from Aaron, K.J., & Sanders, P.W. (2013). *Mayo Clin Proc, 88*(9), 987–995; Arjun, S., Mossavar-Rahmani, Y., Kamensky, V., et al. (2014). *Stroke, 45*(10), 2874–2880. doi:10.1161/STROKEAHA.114.006046; Castro, H., & Raij, L. (2013). *Semin Nephrol, 33*(3), 277–289; Whelton, P.K., & He, J. (2014). *Curr Opin Lipidol, 25*(1), 75–79.

ECF hypokalemia can develop without losses of total body potassium. For example, potassium shifts from the ECF to the ICF in exchange for hydrogen to maintain plasma acid-base balance during respiratory or metabolic alkalosis. Insulin promotes cellular uptake of potassium and insulin administration may cause an ECF potassium deficit.

Potassium shifts from the ICF to the ECF in conditions such as diabetic ketoacidosis, in which the increased hydrogen ion concentration in the ECF causes H^+ to shift into the cell in exchange for potassium. A normal level of potassium is maintained in the plasma, but potassium continues to be lost in the urine, causing a deficit in the amount of total body potassium. Severe, even fatal, hypokalemia may occur if insulin is administered without also providing potassium supplements. Thus total body potassium depletion becomes evident when insulin treatment and rehydration therapy are initiated. Potassium replacement is instituted cautiously to prevent hyperkalemia.

Losses of potassium from body stores are usually caused by gastro-intestinal and renal disorders. Diarrhea, intestinal drainage tubes or fistulae, and laxative abuse also result in hypokalemia. Normally, only 5 to 10 mmol of potassium and 100 to 150 mL of water are excreted in the stool each day. With diarrhea, fluid and electrolyte losses can be voluminous, with several litres of fluid and 100 to 200 mmol of potassium lost per day. Vomiting or continuous nasogastric suctioning often is associated with potassium depletion, partly because of the potassium lost from the gastric fluid but principally because of renal compensation for volume depletion and the metabolic alkalosis (elevated bicarbonate levels) that occurs from sodium, chloride, and hydrogen ion losses. The loss of fluid and sodium stimulates the secretion of aldosterone, which in turn causes renal losses of potassium.

Renal potassium losses occur with increased secretion of potassium by the distal tubule. Use of potassium-wasting diuretics, excessive aldosterone secretion, increased distal tubular flow rate, and low plasma magnesium concentration all may contribute to urinary losses of potassium. The elevated flow of bicarbonate at the distal tubule during alkalosis also contributes to renal excretion of potassium because the increased tubular lumen electronegativity attracts potassium. Many diuretics inhibit the reabsorption of sodium chloride, causing the diuretic effect. The distal tubular flow rate then increases, promoting potassium excretion. If sodium loss is severe, the compensating aldosterone secretion may further deplete potassium stores. Primary hyperaldosteronism with excessive secretion of aldosterone from an adrenal adenoma (tumour) also causes potassium wasting. Many kidney diseases reduce the ability to conserve sodium. The disordered sodium reabsorption produces a diuretic effect, and the increased distal tubule flow rate favours the secretion of potassium. Magnesium deficits increase renal potassium secretion and promote hypokalemia. Certain antibiotics (i.e., carbenicillin disodium [Geocillin] and amphotericin B [Fungizone]) are known to cause hypokalemia by increasing the rate of potassium excretion. Rare hereditary defects in renal potassium transport (e.g., Bartter and Gitelman syndromes) also can cause hypokalemia.

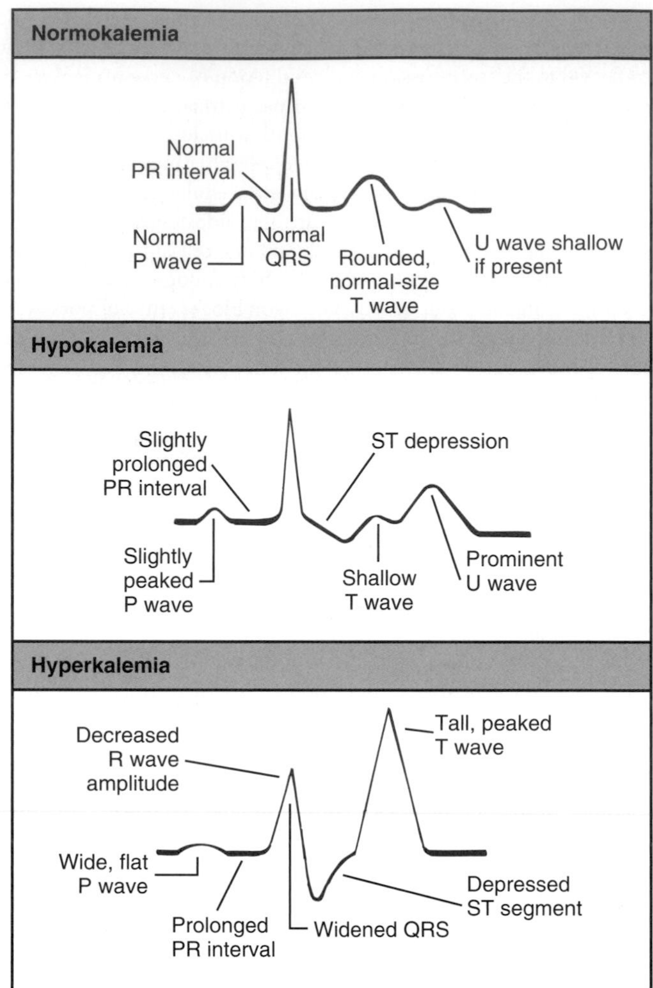

FIGURE 5-8 Electrocardiogram Changes with Potassium Imbalance.

CLINICAL MANIFESTATIONS Mild losses of potassium are usually asymptomatic. Severe loss of potassium results in neuromuscular and cardiac manifestations. Neuromuscular excitability decreases, causing skeletal muscle weakness, smooth muscle atony, cardiac dysrhythmias, glucose intolerance, and impaired urinary concentrating ability.[13]

Symptoms occur in relation to the rate of potassium depletion. Because the body can accommodate slow losses of potassium, the decrease in ECF concentration may allow potassium to shift from the intracellular space, restoring the potassium concentration gradient toward normal, with less severe neuromuscular changes. With acute and severe losses of potassium, changes in neuromuscular excitability are more profound. Skeletal muscle weakness occurs initially in the larger muscles of the legs and arms and ultimately affects the diaphragm and depresses ventilation. Paralysis and respiratory arrest can occur with severe losses. Loss of smooth muscle tone is manifested by constipation, intestinal distension, anorexia, nausea, vomiting, and paralytic ileus (paralysis of the intestinal muscles).

The cardiac effects of hypokalemia are related also to changes in membrane excitability. As ECF potassium concentration decreases, the resting membrane potential becomes more negative (i.e., from −90 to −100 mV [hypopolarization]). Because potassium contributes to the repolarization phase of the action potential, hypokalemia delays ventricular repolarization. Various dysrhythmias may occur, including sinus bradycardia, atrioventricular block, and paroxysmal atrial tachycardia. The characteristic changes in the electrocardiogram (ECG) reflect *delayed repolarization*. For example, the amplitude of the T wave decreases, the amplitude of the U wave increases, and the ST segment is depressed (Figure 5-8). In severe states of hypokalemia, P waves peak, the QT interval is prolonged, and T wave inversions may be seen. Hypokalemia enhances the therapeutic effect of digitalis and increases the risk of digitalis toxicity.

A wide range of metabolic dysfunctions may result from potassium deficiency (Table 5-6). Carbohydrate metabolism is affected because hypokalemia depresses insulin secretion and alters hepatic and skeletal muscle glycogen synthesis. Renal function is impaired, with a decreased ability to concentrate urine. Polyuria (increased urine) and polydipsia (increased thirst) are associated with decreased responsiveness to ADH. Long-term potassium deficits lasting more than 1 month may damage renal tissue, with interstitial fibrosis and tubular atrophy.

EVALUATION AND TREATMENT The diagnosis of hypokalemia is significantly related to the medical history and the identification of disorders associated with potassium loss or shifts of extracellular potassium to the intracellular space. Treatment involves an estimation of total body potassium losses and correction of acid-base imbalances. Further losses of potassium should be prevented and the individual should be encouraged to eat foods rich in potassium. The maximal rate of oral replacement is 40 to 80 mmol/day if renal function is normal. A maximal safe rate of IV replacement is 20 mmol/hr. Because potassium

TABLE 5-6 Clinical Manifestations of Potassium Level Alterations

Organ System	Hypokalemia	Hyperkalemia
Cardiovascular	Dysrhythmias ECG changes (flattened T waves, U waves, ST depression, peaked P wave, prolonged QT interval) Cardiac arrest Weak, irregular pulse rate Postural hypotension	Dysrhythmias ECG changes (peaked T waves, prolonged PR interval, absent P wave with widened QRS complex) Bradycardia Heart block Cardiac arrest
Nervous	Lethargy Fatigue Confusion Paresthesias	Anxiety Tingling Numbness
Gastro-intestinal	Nausea and vomiting Decreased motility Distension Decreased bowel sounds Ileus	Nausea and vomiting Diarrhea Colicky pain
Kidney	Water loss Thirst Inability to concentrate urine Increased tubular production of ammonia and ammonium Kidney damage	Oliguria Kidney damage
Skeletal and smooth muscle	Weakness Flaccid paralysis Respiratory arrest Constipation Bladder dysfunction	Early: hyperactive muscles Late: weakness and flaccid paralysis

is irritating to blood vessels, a maximal concentration of 40 mmol/L should be used. Serum potassium values are monitored until normokalemia is achieved.

Hyperkalemia

PATHOPHYSIOLOGY Elevation of ECF potassium concentration greater than 5.0 mmol/L constitutes **hyperkalemia**.[14] Because of efficient renal excretion, increases in total body potassium level are relatively rare. Acute increases in serum potassium level are handled quickly through increased cellular uptake and renal excretion of body potassium excesses.

Hyperkalemia may be caused by increased intake of potassium, a shift of potassium from cells to ECF, decreased renal excretion, or medications that decrease renal potassium excretion (i.e., ACE inhibitors, angiotensin receptor blockers, and aldosterone antagonists). If renal function is normal, slow, long-term increases in potassium intake are usually well tolerated through potassium adaptation, although short-term potassium loading can exceed renal excretion rates. Dietary excesses of potassium are uncommon, but accidental ingestion of potassium salt substitutes can cause toxicity. Use of stored whole blood and IV boluses of potassium penicillin G or replacement potassium can precipitate hyperkalemia, particularly with impaired renal function. Potassium moves from ICF to ECF with cell trauma or a change in cell membrane permeability, acidosis, insulin deficiency, or cell hypoxia. Burns, massive crushing injuries, and extensive surgeries can cause release of potassium to ECF as a result of cell trauma. If renal function is sustained, potassium is excreted. As cell repair begins, hypokalemia develops without an adequate replacement of potassium.

In acidosis, ECF hydrogen ions shift into cells in exchange for ICF potassium and sodium; hyperkalemia and acidosis therefore often occur simultaneously. Because insulin promotes cellular entry of potassium, insulin deficits, which occur with such conditions as diabetic ketoacidosis, are accompanied by hyperkalemia. Hypoxia can lead to hyperkalemia by diminishing the efficiency of cell membrane active transport, resulting in the escape of potassium to ECF. Digitalis overdose (toxicity) may cause hyperkalemia by inhibiting the Na^+–K^+ ATPase pump, and thus allowing potassium to remain outside the cell.

Decreased renal excretion of potassium commonly is associated with hyperkalemia. Renal failure that results in oliguria (urine output of 30 mL/hr or less) is accompanied by elevations of serum potassium level. The severity of hyperkalemia is related to the amount of potassium intake, the degree of acidosis, and the rate of renal cell damage. Decreases in the secretion or renal effects of aldosterone also can cause decreases in the urinary excretion of potassium. For example, Addison's disease (a disease of adrenal cortical insufficiency) results in decreased production and secretion of aldosterone (and other steroids) and thus contributes to hyperkalemia.

CLINICAL MANIFESTATIONS Symptoms vary with the severity of hyperkalemia. During mild attacks, increased neuromuscular irritability may be manifested as restlessness, intestinal cramping, and diarrhea. Severe hyperkalemia decreases the resting membrane potential (i.e., from −90 to −70 mV [hyperpolarization]) and causes muscle weakness, loss of muscle tone, and paralysis. In mild states of hyperkalemia, there is more rapid repolarization, reflected in the ECG as narrow and taller T waves with a shortened QT interval. Severe hyperkalemia causes delayed cardiac conduction and prevents repolarization of the heart muscle. Severe hyperkalemia depresses the ST segment, prolongs the PR interval, and widens the QRS complex because of decreased conduction velocity from inactivated sodium channels (see Figure 5-8). Bradydysrhythmias and delayed conduction are common in hyperkalemia; severe hyperkalemia can cause ventricular fibrillation or cardiac arrest.[15]

As with hypokalemia, changes in the ratio of intracellular to extracellular potassium concentration contribute to the symptoms of hyperkalemia (see Table 5-6). The neuromuscular effects of hyperkalemia are related to the increase in rate of repolarization and the presence of other contributing factors, such as acidosis and calcium balance. Long-term increases in ECF potassium concentration result in shifts of potassium into the cell, because the tendency is to maintain a normal ratio of ICF to ECF potassium concentrations. Acute elevations of extracellular potassium concentration affect neuromuscular irritability because this ratio is disrupted. Increases in ECF calcium concentration can override the neuromuscular effects of hyperkalemia because calcium is also a cation and affects the threshold potential (see Chapter 1).

EVALUATION AND TREATMENT Hyperkalemia should be investigated when there is a history of renal disease, massive trauma, insulin deficiency, Addison's disease, use of potassium salt substitutes, or metabolic acidosis. The acuity of the onset of symptoms may be related to the underlying cause.

Management of hyperkalemia includes treating the contributing causes and correcting the potassium excess. When serum potassium levels are dangerously high, calcium gluconate can be administered to restore normal neuromuscular irritability and to stabilize the resting cardiac membrane potential by making the threshold potential less negative. Administration of glucose (which readily stimulates insulin secretion) or administration of both glucose and insulin for diabetic individuals facilitates cellular entry of potassium. Sodium bicarbonate corrects metabolic acidosis and lowers serum potassium concentration. Oral or rectal administration of cation exchange resins, which exchange sodium for potassium in the intestine, can be effective. Dialysis effectively removes potassium when renal failure has occurred.

QUICK CHECK 5-4

1. What role does potassium play in the body? What metabolic dysfunctions occur in potassium deficiency? In potassium excess?
2. Explain how a person can have normal total body potassium levels but still exhibit hypokalemia.
3. What is the most prominent ECG change associated with hyperkalemia? With hypokalemia?

Other Electrolytes—Calcium, Phosphate, and Magnesium

The specifics of balance for the other body electrolytes—calcium (Ca^{++}), phosphate (PO_4^{3+}), and magnesium (Mg^{++})—are summarized in Table 5-7. Parathyroid hormone and vitamin D are important for the regulation of these minerals[16] (see Chapter 18).

ACID-BASE BALANCE

Acid-base balance must be regulated within a narrow range for the body to function normally. Slight changes in amounts of hydrogen and changes in pH can significantly alter biological processes in cells and tissues.[17] Hydrogen ion is needed to maintain membrane integrity and the speed of metabolic enzyme reactions. Most pathological conditions disturb acid-base balance, producing circumstances possibly more harmful than the disease process itself.

Hydrogen Ion and pH

The concentration of hydrogen ions in body fluids is very small—approximately 0.000 000 1 mg/L. This number, which may be expressed as 10^{-7} mg/L, is indicated as pH 7.0. The symbol *pH* represents the acidity or alkalinity of a solution. As the pH changes 1 unit (e.g., from pH 7.0 to pH 6.0), the $[H^+]$ ($[H^+]$ = hydrogen ion concentration) changes tenfold. The greater the $[H^+]$, the more acidic the solution and the lower the pH. The lower the $[H^+]$, the more alkaline or basic the solution and the higher the pH. In biological fluids, a pH of less than 7.4 is defined as acidic and a pH greater than 7.4 is defined as alkaline, or basic (Table 5-8).

Body acids are formed as end products of protein, carbohydrate, and fat metabolism, and acids can release hydrogen ion. Acids must be balanced by the amount of basic substances in the body to maintain normal pH. The lungs, kidneys, and bones are the major organs involved in regulating acid-base balance. The systems work together to regulate short- and long-term changes in acid-base status.

Body acids exist in two forms: **volatile** (can be eliminated as carbon dioxide [CO_2] gas) and **nonvolatile** (can be eliminated by the kidney). The volatile acid is carbonic acid (H_2CO_3), a *weak acid* (i.e., it does not release its hydrogen easily). In the presence of the enzyme carbonic anhydrase, it readily dissociates into CO_2 and water (H_2O). The carbon dioxide is then eliminated by pulmonary ventilation.

Nonvolatile acids are sulphuric, phosphoric, and other organic acids. They are *strong acids* (readily release their hydrogens). Nonvolatile acids are secreted into the urine by the renal tubules in amounts of about 60 to 100 mmol of hydrogen per day or about 1 mmol per kilogram of body weight.

Buffer Systems

Buffering occurs in response to changes in acid-base status. **Buffers** can absorb excessive hydrogen ion (H^+) (acid) or hydroxyl ion (OH^-) (base) and prevent a significant change in pH. The buffer systems are located in both the ICF and the ECF compartments, and they function at different rates (Table 5-9). The most important plasma buffer systems are carbonic acid–bicarbonate and the protein hemoglobin (Figure 5-9). Phosphate and protein are the most important intracellular buffers and provide a first line of defence. Ammonia and phosphate can attach hydrogen ions and are important renal buffers.

Carbonic Acid–Bicarbonate Buffering

The **carbonic acid–bicarbonate buffer** pair *operates in both the lung and the kidney* and is a major extracellular buffer. The lungs are a second line of defence and can relatively quickly (within seconds to minutes) decrease the amount of carbonic acid by blowing off carbon dioxide and leaving water. The kidneys are a third line of defence (hours to days) and can reabsorb bicarbonate (a type of base) or regenerate new bicarbonate from carbon dioxide and water. The relationship between bicarbonate (HCO_3^-) and carbonic acid (H_2CO_3) is usually expressed as a ratio. Normal bicarbonate level is about 24 mmol/L, and normal carbonic acid level is about 1.2 mmol/L (when the partial pressure of carbon dioxide in arterial blood [$PaCO_2$] is 40 mm Hg), producing a 20:1 (24/1.2) ratio and the normal pH of 7.4 (Figure 5-10). These two systems are very effective together because the lungs can adjust acid concentration rapidly by ventilation, and bicarbonate is easily reabsorbed or regenerated by the kidney tubules, although more slowly.

Renal and respiratory adjustments to primary changes in pH are known as **compensation**. The respiratory system compensates for changes in pH by increasing or decreasing the concentration of carbon dioxide (carbonic acid) by changing ventilation. The renal system compensates by producing more acidic or more alkaline urine. The values for $PaCO_2$ and bicarbonate will vary from normal levels in an attempt to maintain a ratio of 20:1. **Correction** occurs when the values for both components of the buffer pair (carbonic acid and bicarbonate) return to normal levels.

Protein Buffering

Both intracellular and extracellular proteins have negative charges and can serve as buffers for hydrogen, but because most proteins are inside cells, they are primarily an intracellular buffer system. Hemoglobin (Hb) is an excellent intracellular blood buffer because it can bind with hydrogen ion (H^+) (forming HHb) and carbon dioxide (forming $HHbCO_2$). Hemoglobin bound to hydrogen ion becomes a weak acid. Hemoglobin not saturated with oxygen (venous blood) is a better buffer than hemoglobin saturated with oxygen (arterial blood). The pH control mechanism is illustrated in Figure 5-9.

Renal Buffering

The distal tubule of the kidney regulates acid-base balance by secreting hydrogen into the urine and reabsorbing bicarbonate into the plasma. Dibasic phosphate ($HPO_4^=$) and ammonia (NH_3) are two important renal buffers because they can attach hydrogen ions and be secreted into the urine. The renal buffering of hydrogen ions requires the use of carbon dioxide (CO_2) and water (H_2O) to form carbonic acid (H_2CO_3). The enzyme carbonic anhydrase catalyzes the reaction. The hydrogen in the carbonic acid is then secreted from the tubular cell and buffered in the lumen by phosphate and ammonia (i.e., forms $H_2PO_4^-$ and NH_4^+). The remaining bicarbonate is reabsorbed. The end effect is the addition of new bicarbonate to the plasma, which contributes to the alkalinity

TABLE 5-7 **Alterations in Calcium, Phosphate, and Magnesium**

Parameter	Calcium	Phosphate	Magnesium
Normal values	Serum: 2.1–2.6 mmol/L (total, adult), 1.9–2.6 mmol/L) total, less than 10 days), 1.05–1.30 mmol/L (ionized, adult); 99% in bone as hydroxyapatite; remainder in plasma and body cells with 50% bound to plasma proteins; 40% free or ionized; ionized form most important physiologically	Serum: 0.8–1.5 mmol/L (adult), 1.45–2.10 mmol/L in infants and young children; mainly in bone with some in ICF and ECF; exists as phospholipids, phosphate esters, and inorganic phosphate (ionized form)	Serum: 0.75–0.95 mmol/L (adult); 40–60% stored in bone, 33% bound to plasma proteins; primary intracellular divalent cation
Function	Needed for fundamental metabolic processes; major cation for structure of bone and teeth; enzymatic cofactor for blood clotting; required for hormone secretion and function of cell receptors; directly related to plasma membrane stability and permeability, transmission of nerve impulses, and contraction of muscles; parathyroid hormone, vitamin D_3, and calcitonin act together to control calcium absorption and excretion (see Chapter 18)	Intracellular and extracellular anion buffer in regulation of acid-base balance; provides energy for muscle contraction (as ATP); parathyroid hormone, vitamin D_3, and calcitonin act together to control phosphate absorption and excretion (see Chapter 18)	Cofactor in intracellular enzymatic reactions and causes neuromuscular excitability; often interacts with calcium and potassium in reactions at cellular level and has important role in smooth muscle contraction and relaxation; magnesium is absorbed in the intestine and eliminated by the kidney
Excess	**Hypercalcemia** (serum concentrations >2.6 mmol/L)	**Hyperphosphatemia** (serum concentrations >1.5 mmol/L)	**Hypermagnesemia** (serum concentrations >1.25 mmol/L)
Causes	Hyperparathyroidism; bone metastases with calcium resorption from breast, prostate, renal, and cervical cancer; sarcoidosis; excess vitamin D; many tumours that produce PTH	Acute or chronic renal failure with significant loss of glomerular filtration; treatment of metastatic tumours with chemotherapy that releases large amounts of phosphate into serum; long-term use of laxatives or enemas containing phosphates; hypoparathyroidism	Usually renal insufficiency or failure; also excessive intake of magnesium-containing antacids, adrenal insufficiency
Effects	Many nonspecific; fatigue, weakness, lethargy, anorexia, nausea, constipation; impaired renal function, kidney stones; dysrhythmias, bradycardia, cardiac arrest; bone pain, osteoporosis	Symptoms primarily related to low serum calcium levels (caused by high phosphate levels) similar to results of hypocalcemia; when prolonged, calcification of soft tissues in lungs, kidneys, joints	Skeletal smooth muscle contraction; excess nerve function; loss of deep tendon reflexes; nausea and vomiting; muscle weakness; hypotension; bradycardia; respiratory distress
Deficit	**Hypocalcemia** (serum calcium concentration <2.1 mmol/L)	**Hypophosphatemia** (serum phosphate concentration <0.4 mmol/L—critical value)	**Hypomagnesemia** (serum magnesium concentration <0.75 mmol/L)
Causes	Related to inadequate intestinal absorption, deposition of ionized calcium into bone or soft tissue, blood administration, or decreases in PTH and vitamin D; nutritional deficiencies occur with inadequate sources of dairy products or green leafy vegetables	Most commonly by intestinal malabsorption related to vitamin D deficiency, use of magnesium- and aluminum-containing antacids, long-term alcohol abuse, and malabsorption syndromes; respiratory alkalosis; increased renal excretion of phosphate associated with hyperparathyroidism	Malnutrition, malabsorption syndromes, alcoholism, urinary losses (renal tubular dysfunction, loop diuretics)
Effects	Increased neuromuscular excitability; tingling, muscle spasm (particularly in hands, feet, and facial muscles), intestinal cramping, hyperactive bowel sounds; severe cases show convulsions and tetany; prolonged QT interval, cardiac arrest	Conditions related to reduced capacity for oxygen transport by red blood cells and disturbed energy metabolism; leukocyte and platelet dysfunction; deranged nerve and muscle function; in severe cases, irritability, confusion, numbness, coma, convulsions; possibly respiratory failure (because of muscle weakness), cardiomyopathies, bone resorption (leading to rickets or osteomalacia)	Behavioural changes, irritability, increased reflexes, muscle cramps, ataxia, nystagmus, tetany, convulsions, tachycardia, hypotension

ATP, adenosine triphosphate; *PTH*, parathyroid hormone.

of the plasma because the hydrogen ion is excreted from the body (Figure 5-11).

Acid-Base Imbalances

Pathophysiological changes in the concentration of hydrogen ion in the blood lead to acid-base imbalances.[18,19] In acidemia the pH of arterial blood is less than 7.4. A systemic increase in hydrogen ion concentration or a loss of base is termed acidosis. In alkalemia the pH of arterial blood is greater than 7.4. A systemic decrease in hydrogen ion concentration or an excess of base is termed alkalosis (Figure 5-12). These changes may be caused by metabolic or respiratory processes. Figure 5-10 summarizes the relationship among pH, the partial pressure of carbon dioxide (respiratory regulation), and the concentration of bicarbonate (renal regulation) during alkalosis and acidosis. Acid-base imbalances are assessed using measurement of arterial blood gases, which includes the reporting of pH, $PaCO_2$, and HCO_3^-. The medical history and clinical symptoms are important in determining the cause of the disorder. Figure 5-13 summarizes the relationships among pH, $PaCO_2$, and bicarbonate during different acid-base alterations.

Metabolic Acidosis

In metabolic acidosis the concentrations of non–carbonic acids increase or bicarbonate is lost from ECF or cannot be regenerated by the kidney (Table 5-10). Metabolic acidosis can occur either quickly, as in lactic acidosis caused by poor perfusion or hypoxemia, or slowly over an extended time, as in renal failure, diabetic ketoacidosis, or starvation (anion gap acidosis).[20] There is a decrease in the 20:1 ratio of HCO_3^- to H_2CO_3.

The buffering systems normally compensate for excess acid and maintain arterial pH within normal range. When acidosis is severe, buffers become depleted and cannot compensate, and the ratio of the concentrations of bicarbonate to carbonic acid decreases to less than 20:1 (see Figure 5-10). An increase in the plasma concentration of chloride out of proportion of sodium causes hyperchloremic acidosis (nonanion gap acidosis). The specific type of acidosis can be determined by examining the serum anion gap (see Table 5-10).

Metabolic acidosis is manifested by changes in the function of the neurological, respiratory, gastro-intestinal, and cardiovascular systems. Early symptoms include headache and lethargy, which progress to confusion and coma in severe acidosis. The respiratory system's efforts to compensate for the increase in metabolic acids result in what are termed *Kussmaul respirations* (a form of hyperventilation), which are deep and rapid. This response represents the body's attempt to increase pH by expelling carbon dioxide, which decreases carbonic acid concentration. Other symptoms include anorexia, nausea, vomiting, diarrhea, and abdominal discomfort. Death can result in the most severe and prolonged cases preceded by dysrhythmias and hypotension. The underlying condition must be diagnosed to establish effective treatment.

Metabolic Alkalosis

When excessive loss of metabolic acids occurs, bicarbonate concentration increases, causing metabolic alkalosis[21] (see Figure 5-13). When acid loss is caused by vomiting, renal compensation is not very effective because loss of chloride (an anion) in hydrochloric acid (HCl) stimulates renal retention of bicarbonate (an anion). The result is known as hypochloremic metabolic alkalosis.[21] Hyperaldosteronism also can lead to alkalosis as a result of sodium bicarbonate retention and loss of hydrogen and potassium. Diuretics may produce a mild alkalosis because they promote greater excretion of sodium, potassium, and chloride than of bicarbonate.

Some common signs and symptoms of metabolic alkalosis are weakness, muscle cramps, hyperactive reflexes, tetany, confusion, convulsions, and atrial tachycardia. Respirations may be shallow, and slow ventilation may manifest as the lungs attempt to compensate by increasing carbon dioxide retention. The manifestations vary with the cause and severity of the alkalosis. The symptoms of hyperactive reflexes and tetany occur because alkalosis increases binding of Ca^{++} to plasma proteins, thus decreasing ionized calcium concentration. The decreased

TABLE 5-8 pH of Body Fluids

Body Fluid	pH	Factors Affecting pH
Gastric juices	1.0–3.0	Hydrochloric acid production
Urine	5.0–6.0	Hydrogen ion excretion from waste products
Arterial blood	7.35–7.45	pH is slightly higher because there is less carbonic acid
Venous blood	7.37	pH is slightly lower because there is more carbonic acid
Cerebrospinal fluid	7.32	Decreased bicarbonate and higher carbon dioxide content decrease pH
Pancreatic fluid	7.8–8.0	Contains bicarbonate produced by exocrine cells
Bile	7.0–8.0	Contains bicarbonate
Small intestine fluid	6.5–7.5	Contains alkaline fluid from pancreas, liver, and gallbladder

TABLE 5-9 Buffer Systems

Buffer Pairs	Buffer System	Chemical Reaction	Rate
HCO_3^-/H_2CO_3	Bicarbonate	$H^+ + HCO_3^- \gtrless H_2O + CO_2$	Instantaneously
Hb^-/HHb	Hemoglobin	$HHb \rightleftharpoons H^+ + Hb^-$	Instantaneously
$HPO_4^=/H_2PO_4^-$	Phosphate	$H_2PO_4^- + H^+ + HPO_4^=$	Instantaneously
Pr^-/HPr	Plasma proteins	$HPr \rightleftharpoons H^+ + Pr^-$	Instantaneously
Organs	**Physiological Mechanism**		**Rate**
Lung ventilation	Regulates retention or elimination of CO_2 and therefore H_2CO_3 concentration		Minutes to hours
Ionic shifts	Exchange of intracellular potassium and sodium for hydrogen		2–4 hours
Kidney tubules	Bicarbonate reabsorption and regeneration, ammonia formation, phosphate buffering		Hours to days
Bone	Exchanges of calcium and phosphate and release of carbonate		Hours to days

CO_2, Carbon dioxide; *H^+*, hydrogen; *Hb^-*, hemoglobin; *HCO_3^-*, bicarbonate; *H_2CO_3*, carbonic acid; *HHb*, hydrogenated hemoglobin; *H_2O*, water; *$HPO_4^=$*, dibasic phosphate; *$H_2PO_4^-$*, monobasic phosphate; *HPr*, hydrogenated protein; *Pr^-*, protein.

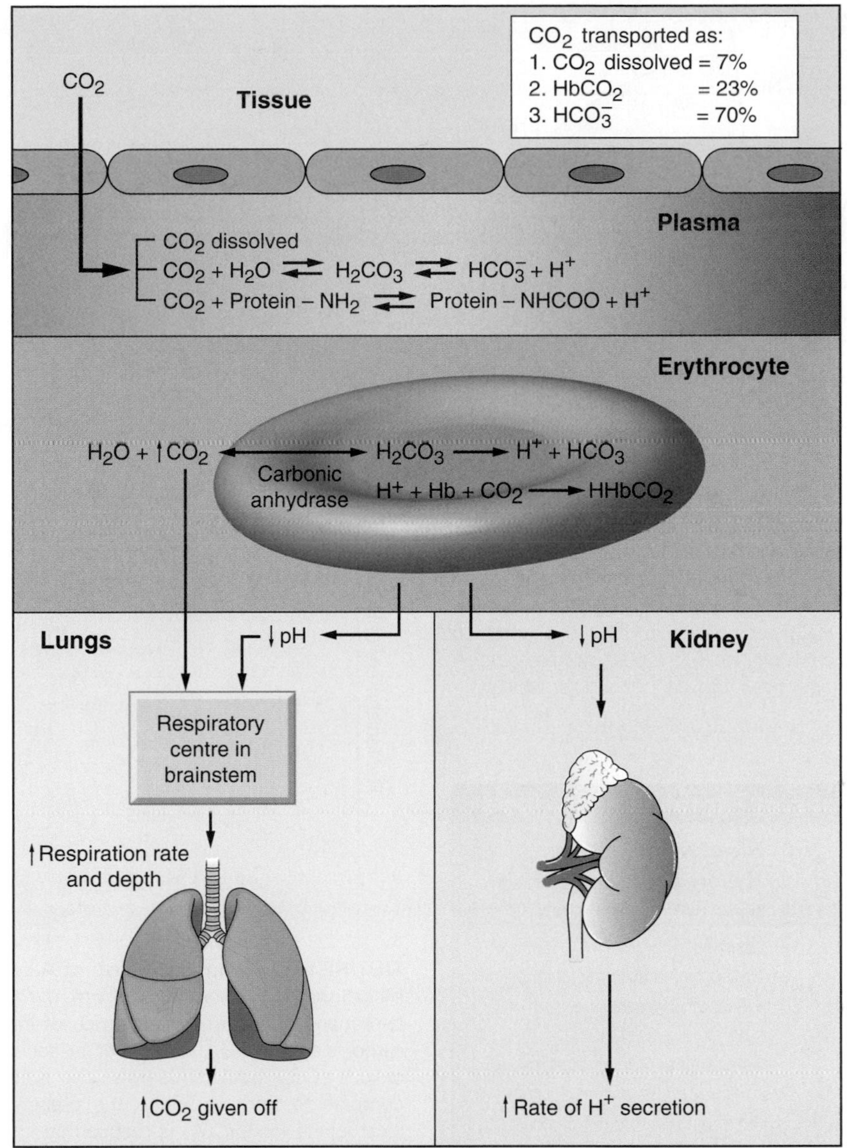

FIGURE 5-9 Integration of pH Control Mechanisms (Example for Acidosis). Carbon dioxide (*CO_2*) is produced in tissue cells and diffuses to plasma, where it is transported as dissolved CO_2, or it combines with water (*H_2O*) to form carbonic acid (*H_2CO_3*), or it combines with protein from which hydrogen has been released. Most of the CO_2 diffuses into the red blood cells and combines with water to form H_2CO_3. The H_2CO_3 dissociates to form hydrogen ion (*H^+*) and bicarbonate (*HCO_3^-*). Hydrogen combines with hemoglobin (*Hb*) that has released its oxygen to form HHb, which buffers the hydrogen and makes venous blood slightly more acidic than arterial blood. The increase in H^+ coupled with elevated CO_2 levels results in $HhbCO_2$ and an increase in the respiratory rate and secretion of H^+ by the kidneys. *$HhbCO_2$*, carbaminohemoglobin; *NH_2*, amiodogen; *NHCOO*, carbamate.

ionized calcium concentration causes excitable cells to become hypopolarized, initiating an action potential more easily and causing muscle contraction.

Treatments are related to the underlying cause of the condition. With hypochloremic alkalosis or contraction alkalosis with volume depletion, a sodium chloride solution is required for correction because chloride must be replaced before bicarbonate can be excreted by the kidney.

Respiratory Acidosis

Respiratory acidosis occurs when there is alveolar hypoventilation, resulting in an excess of carbon dioxide in the blood (hypercapnia). The arterial carbon dioxide tension (or pressure) ($PaCO_2$) is greater than 45 mm Hg and the pH is less than 7.35 (see Figure 5-13). A decrease in alveolar ventilation in relation to the metabolic production of carbon dioxide produces respiratory acidosis by an increase in the concentration of carbonic acid. Respiratory acidosis can be acute or chronic.[22] Common causes include depression of the respiratory centre (e.g., from medications or head injury), paralysis of the respiratory muscles, disorders of the chest wall (e.g., kyphoscoliosis or broken ribs), and disorders of the lung parenchyma (e.g., pneumonia, pulmonary edema, emphysema, asthma, bronchitis). Renal compensation occurs by elimination of hydrogen ion and retention of bicarbonate.

The signs and symptoms seen often include headache, blurred vision, breathlessness, restlessness, and apprehension followed by lethargy, disorientation, muscle twitching, tremors, convulsions, and coma.

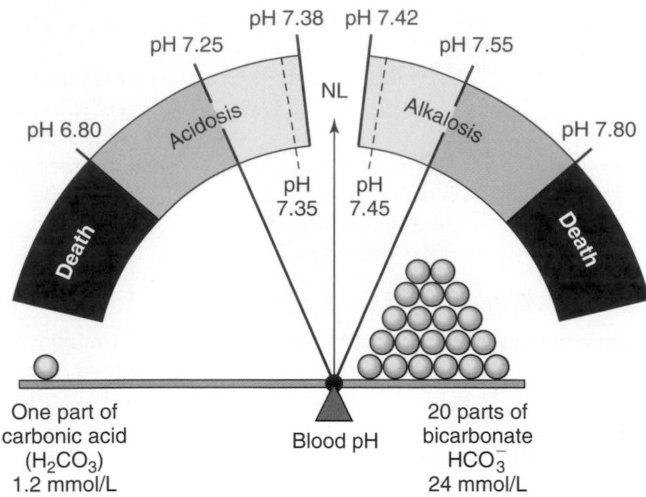

FIGURE 5-10 **Ratio of Carbonic Acid and Bicarbonate Concentration in Maintaining pH Within Normal Limits.** An increase in carbonic acid (*H_2CO_3*) or decrease in bicarbonate (*HCO_3^-*) concentration causes acidosis. A decrease in H_2CO_3 or increase in HCO_3^- concentration causes alkalosis. *NL*, normal. (From Monahan, F.D. [2007]. *Medical-surgical nursing: Health and illness perspectives* [8th ed.]. St. Louis: Mosby.)

TABLE 5-10 Causes of Metabolic Acidosis

Increased Non–Carbonic Acids (Elevated Anion Gap[a])	Bicarbonate Loss or Hyperchloremic Acidosis (Normal Anion Gap)
Increased H^+ load	Diarrhea
Ketoacidosis (e.g., diabetes mellitus, starvation)	Ureterosigmoidoscopy (chloride absorbed in excess of sodium in small intestine)
Lactic acidosis (e.g., shock, hypoxemia)	Renal failure (loss of bicarbonate)
Ingestion (e.g., ammonium chloride, ethylene glycol, methanol, salicylates, paraldehyde)	Proximal renal tubular acidosis (loss of more renal sodium in relation to chloride)
Decreased renal H^+ excretion	
Uremia	
Distal renal tubule acidosis	

[a]***Anion gap*** refers to anions not usually measured in laboratory reports (e.g., sulphate, phosphate, and lactate). The anions usually measured are chloride (Cl^-) and bicarbonate (HCO_3^-). When the sum of the concentrations of measured anions (e.g., chloride and bicarbonate) is subtracted from the sum of the concentrations of measured cations (e.g., sodium and potassium), there is a "gap" of approximately 10–12 mmol/L; this is the normal anion gap. An elevated anion gap provides clues to the cause of the acidosis (i.e., to the addition of endogenously or exogenously generated acids). In a normal anion gap acidosis, chloride is retained to replace lost bicarbonate.

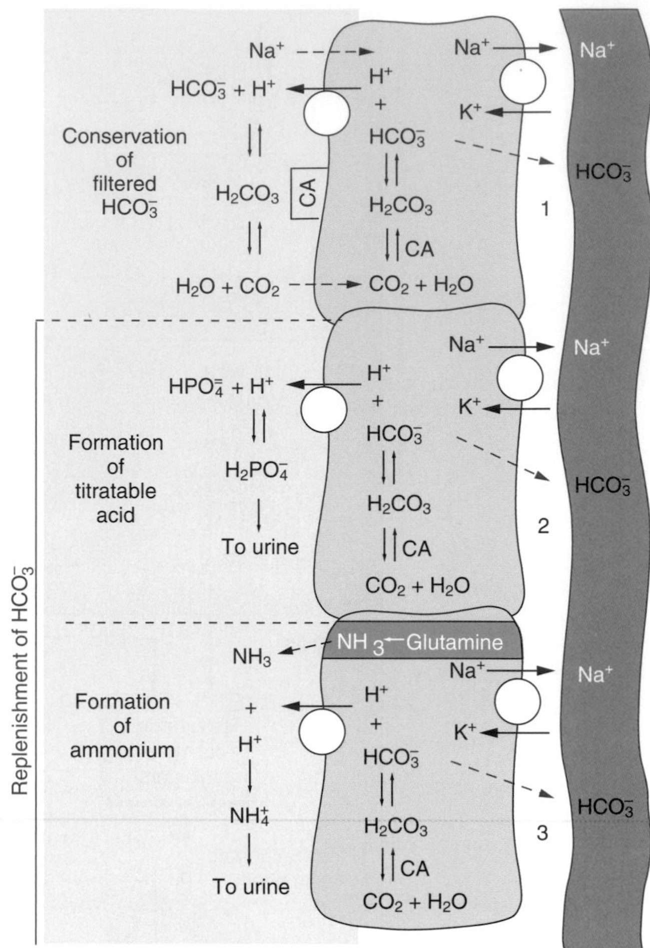

FIGURE 5-11 **Renal Excretion of Acid. 1, Conservation of filtered bicarbonate.** Filtered bicarbonate (*HCO_3^-*) combines with secreted hydrogen ion (*H^+*) in the presence of carbon anhydrase (*CA*) to form carbonic acid (*H_2CO_3*), which then dissociates to water (*H_2O*) and carbon dioxide (*CO_2*); both diffuse into the epithelial cell. The CO_2 and H_2O combine to form H_2CO_3 in the presence of CA, and the resulting bicarbonate ion (*HCO_3^-*) is reabsorbed into the capillary. **2, Formation of titratable acid.** Hydrogen ion is secreted and combines with dibasic phosphate (*$HPO_4^=$*) to form monobasic phosphate (*$H_2PO_4^-$*). The secreted H^+ is formed from the dissociation of H_2CO_3, and the remaining HCO_3^- is reabsorbed into the capillary. **3, Formation of ammonium.** Ammonia (NH_3) is produced from glutamine in the epithelial cell and diffuses to the tubular lumen, where it combines with H^+ to form ammonium ion (NH_4^+). Once NH_4^+ has been formed, it cannot return to the epithelial cell (diffusional trapping), and the bicarbonate remaining in the epithelial cell is reabsorbed into the capillary. *K^+*, potassium; *NA^+*, sodium.

Respiratory rate is rapid at first and gradually becomes depressed as the respiratory centre adapts to increasing levels of carbon dioxide. The skin may be warm and flushed because the elevated carbon dioxide concentration causes vasodilation. The restoration of adequate alveolar ventilation is necessary to remove the excess CO_2 (and decrease H_2CO_3).

Respiratory Alkalosis

Respiratory alkalosis occurs when there is alveolar hyperventilation (deep, rapid respirations). Excessive reduction in plasma carbon dioxide levels **(hypocapnia)** decreases carbonic acid concentration.[23,24] The $PaCO_2$ is less than 35 mm Hg and the pH is greater than normal (see Figure 5-13). Respiratory alkalosis can be chronic or acute. Hypoxemia (caused by pulmonary disease, heart failure, or high altitudes), hypermetabolic states (e.g., fever, anemia, thyrotoxicosis), early salicylate intoxication, hysteria, cirrhosis, and Gram-negative sepsis stimulate hyperventilation. Improper use of mechanical ventilators also can cause iatrogenic (treatment-related) respiratory alkalosis, and secondary alkalosis may develop as a result of hyperventilation stimulated by

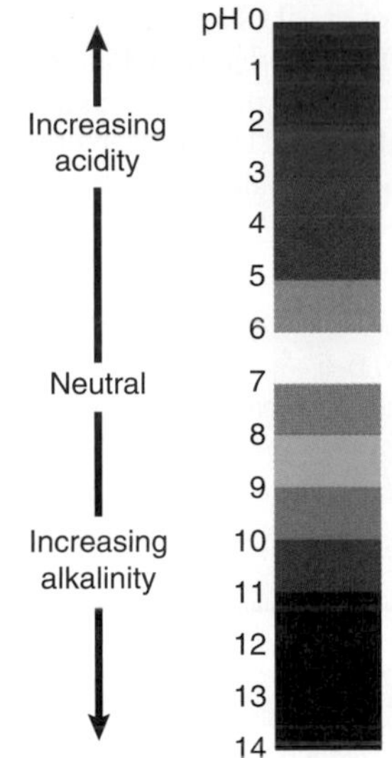

FIGURE 5-12 Acid-Base Imbalances.

metabolic or respiratory acidosis. The kidneys compensate by decreasing hydrogen excretion and bicarbonate reabsorption.

The central and peripheral nervous systems are stimulated by respiratory alkalosis, causing dizziness, confusion, tingling of extremities (paresthesias), convulsions, and coma. Cerebral vasoconstriction reduces cerebral blood flow. Carpopedal spasm (spasm of muscles in the fingers and toes), tetany, and other symptoms of hypocalcemia (see Table 5-7) are similar to those of metabolic alkalosis. The underlying disturbance must be treated, particularly hypoxemia.

Arterial Blood Gas Analysis

Interpreting arterial blood gases (ABGs) is an essential component to understanding acid-base balance and the compensatory mechanisms involved with restoring (or attempting to restore) acid-base balance. The *6 Easy Steps to ABG Analysis* is a useful resource for nurses to use for this process.[25] The six steps to ABG analysis are as follows:

1. Is the pH normal?
2. Is the CO_2 normal?
3. Is the HCO_3^- normal?

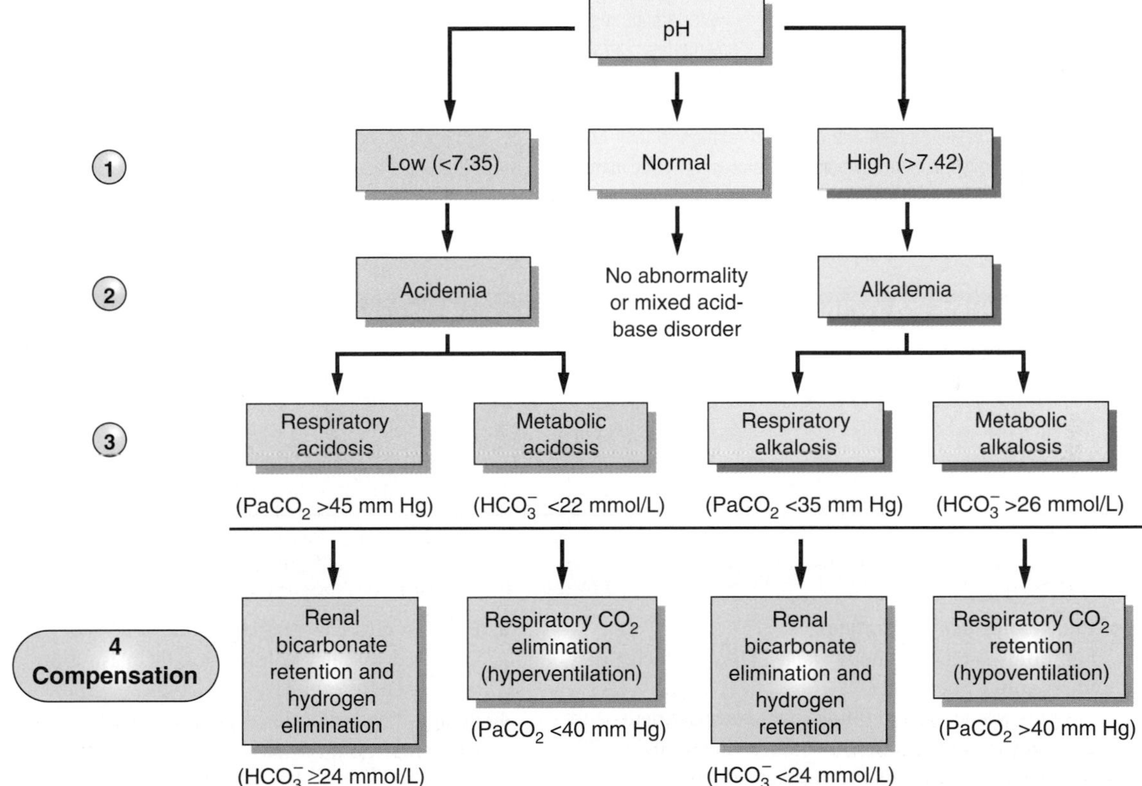

FIGURE 5-13 Primary and Compensatory Acid-Base Changes. A systematic approach can be used to interpret the cause of an acid-base imbalance. **1,** Is the pH low or high? **2,** If the pH is low (acidemia), is the cause respiratory (high $PaCO_2$) or metabolic (low HCO_3^-)? **3,** If the pH is high (alkalemia), is the cause respiratory (low $PaCO_2$) or metabolic (high HCO_3^-)? **4,** Is there compensation for the primary acid-base disorder? (a) HCO_3^- will be ≥24 mmol/L if there is renal compensation for a primary respiratory acidosis; (b) $PaCO_2$ will be <40 mm Hg if there is respiratory compensation of a primary metabolic acidosis; (c) HCO_3^- will be <24 mmol/L if there is renal compensation for primary respiratory alkalosis; (d) $PaCO_2$ will be >40 mm Hg if there is respiratory compensation for primary metabolic alkalosis. NOTE: Examine the pH first to determine whether there is acidemia or alkalemia. Then examine the changes in HCO_3^- and $PaCO_2$. **1,** HCO_3^- will be elevated when there is primary metabolic alkalosis or renal compensation for primary respiratory acidosis. **2,** HCO_3^- will be decreased when there is primary metabolic acidosis or renal compensation for primary respiratory alkalosis. **3,** $PaCO_2$ will be elevated when there is primary respiratory acidosis or respiratory compensation for primary metabolic alkalosis. **4,** $PaCO_2$ will be decreased when there is primary respiratory alkalosis or respiratory compensation for metabolic acidosis. *HCO_3^-*, bicarbonate; *$PaCO_2$*, partial pressure of carbon dioxide in arterial blood.

4. Match the CO_2 or the HCO_3^- with the pH.
5. Does the CO_2 or the HCO_3^- go the opposite direction of the pH?
6. Are the partial pressure of oxygen in arterial blood (PaO_2) and the oxygen (O_2) saturation normal?

First, determine whether the pH is normal (7.35 to 7.45), acidic (less than 7.35), or alkaline (greater than 7.45). Then, look at the CO_2 level (normal is 35 to 45 mmol/L). Less than 35 mmol/L is considered alkalotic, whereas greater than 45 mmol/L is considered acidotic. Next, look at the HCO_3^- level (normal is 22 to 26 mmol/L). An HCO_3^- level that is less than 22 mmol/L is acidotic, and a level that is greater than 26 mmol/L is alkalotic. The next step is to match the CO_2 or the HCO_3^- level with the pH to determine the type of disorder—respiratory or metabolic. For example, an acidic CO_2 level of 50 mmol/L with a pH of 7.30 would indicate respiratory acidosis. To determine whether there is compensation, note whether the CO_2 level or the HCO_3^- level is in the opposite direction of the pH. For example, if the HCO_3^- is 27 mmol/L (alkalotic) and the pH is 7.30, that would indicate some compensation by the metabolic system (i.e., the kidneys; see Chapter 29) and other buffering systems in the body. The last step of the process is to look at PaO_2 and O_2 saturation. Low values of each are evidence of hypoxemia (see Chapter 27).

QUICK CHECK 5-5

1. What is the difference between compensation and correction of acid-base disturbances?
2. What two chemicals are altered in metabolic acid-base disturbances?
3. How do alterations in carbon dioxide concentration influence acid-base status?

PEDIATRIC CONSIDERATIONS

Distribution of Body Fluids

Newborn Infants

At birth TBW represents about 75 to 80% of body weight and decreases to about 67% during the first year of life. Physiological loss of body water amounting to 5% of body weight occurs as an infant adjusts to a new environment. Infants are particularly susceptible to significant changes in TBW because of a high metabolic rate and greater body surface area, as compared with adults. Consequently, they have a greater fluid intake and output in relation to their body size. Renal mechanisms of fluid and electrolyte conservation may not be mature enough to counter abnormal losses related to vomiting or diarrhea, thereby allowing dehydration to occur. Symptoms of dehydration include increased thirst, decreased urine output, decreased body weight, decreased skin elasticity, sunken fontanels, absent tears, dry mucous membranes, increased heart rate, and irritability.

Children and Adolescents

TBW slowly decreases to 60 to 65% of body weight. At adolescence the percentage of TBW approaches adult levels and differences according to gender appear. Males have a greater percentage of body water because of increased muscle mass, and females have more body fat because of the influence of estrogen and thus less water.

GERIATRIC CONSIDERATIONS

Distribution of Body Fluids

The further decline in the percentage of TBW in older adults is in part the result of a decreased free fat mass and decreased muscle mass, as well as a reduced ability to regulate sodium and water balance. Kidneys are less efficient in producing either a concentrated or a diluted urine, and sodium-conserving responses are sluggish. Thirst perception also may decline, and loss of cognitive function can influence access to beverages. Healthy older adults can adequately maintain their hydration status. When disease is present, a decrease in TBW, dehydration, and hypernatremia can become life-threatening.

DID YOU UNDERSTAND?

Distribution of Body Fluids and Electrolytes

1. The sum of all fluids is the total body water (TBW), which varies with age and amount of body fat.
2. Body fluids are distributed among functional compartments and are classified as intracellular fluid (ICF) and extracellular fluid (ECF).
3. Water moves between ICF and ECF compartments principally by osmosis.
4. Water moves between plasma and interstitial fluid by osmosis (pulling of water) and hydrostatic pressure (pushing of water), which occur across the capillary membrane.
5. Movement across the capillary wall is called *net filtration* and is described according to Starling forces (the balance between hydrostatic and osmotic forces).

Alterations in Water Movement

1. Edema is a problem of fluid distribution that results in accumulation of fluid within the interstitial spaces.
2. The pathophysiological process that leads to edema is related to an increase in forces favouring fluid filtration from the capillaries or lymphatic channels into the tissues.
3. Edema is caused by arterial dilation, venous or lymphatic obstruction, increased vascular volume, loss of plasma proteins, or increased capillary permeability.
4. Edema may be localized or generalized and usually is associated with weight gain, swelling and puffiness, tighter-fitting clothes and shoes, and limited movement of the affected area.

Sodium, Chloride, and Water Balance

1. There is an intimate relationship between the balance of sodium and water levels; chloride levels are generally proportional to changes in sodium levels.
2. Water balance is regulated by the sensation of thirst and by antidiuretic hormone (ADH), which is secreted in response to an increase in plasma osmolality or a decrease in circulating blood volume.
3. Sodium balance is regulated by aldosterone, which increases reabsorption of sodium from the urine into the blood by the distal tubules of the kidney.
4. Renin and angiotensin are enzymes that promote secretion of aldosterone and thus regulate sodium and water balance.

5. Natriuretic peptides are involved in decreasing tubular reabsorption and promoting urinary excretion of sodium.

Alterations in Sodium, Chloride, and Water Balance

1. Alterations in sodium and water balance may be classified as isotonic, hypertonic, or hypotonic.
2. Isotonic alterations occur when changes in TBW are accompanied by proportional changes in electrolytes.
3. Hypertonic alterations develop when the osmolality of ECF is elevated above normal, usually because of an increased concentration of ECF sodium or a deficit of ECF water.
4. Hypernatremia (sodium levels of more than 145 mmol/L) may be caused by an acute increase in sodium level or a loss of water.
5. Hypernatremia can be isovolemic, hypovolemic, or hypervolemic, depending on accompanying changes in the level of body water.
6. Hypernatremia with marked water deficit is manifested by hypovolemia and dehydration.
7. Hyperchloremia is caused by an excess of sodium or a deficit of plasma bicarbonate.
8. Hypotonic alterations occur when the osmolality of ECF is less than normal.
9. Hyponatremia (serum sodium concentration less than 135 mmol/L) usually causes movement of water into cells.
10. Hyponatremia may be caused by sodium loss, inadequate sodium intake, or dilution of the body's sodium level with excess water.
11. Hyponatremia can be isovolemic, hypervolemic, hypovolemic, or dilutional, depending on accompanying changes in the amount of body water.
12. Hypochloremia usually is the result of hyponatremia or elevated bicarbonate concentrations.

Alterations in Potassium and Other Electrolytes

1. Potassium is the predominant ICF ion; it regulates ICF osmolality, maintains the resting membrane potential, and is required for deposition of glycogen in liver and skeletal muscle cells.
2. Potassium balance is regulated by the kidney, by aldosterone and insulin secretion, and by changes in pH.
3. Potassium adaptation allows the body to accommodate slowly to increased levels of potassium intake.
4. Hypokalemia (serum potassium concentration of less than 3.5 mmol/L) indicates loss of total body potassium, although ECF hypokalemia can develop without losses of total body potassium, and plasma potassium levels may be normal or elevated when total body potassium is depleted.
5. Hypokalemia may be caused by reduced potassium intake, a shift of potassium from ECF to ICF, increased aldosterone secretion, increased renal excretion, and alkalosis.
6. Hyperkalemia (potassium levels that are greater than 5.0 mmol/L) may be caused by increased potassium intake, a shift of potassium from ICF to ECF, or decreased renal excretion.
7. Calcium is an ion necessary for bone and teeth formation, blood coagulation, hormone secretion and cell receptor function, and membrane stability.
8. Phosphate acts as a buffer in acid-base regulation and provides energy for muscle contraction.
9. Calcium and phosphate concentrations are rigidly controlled by parathyroid hormone (PTH), vitamin D, and calcitonin.
10. Hypocalcemia (serum calcium concentration less than 2.1 mmol/L) is related to inadequate intestinal absorption, deposition of calcium into bone or soft tissue, blood administration, or decreased PTH and vitamin D levels.
11. Hypercalcemia (serum calcium concentration greater than 2.6 mmol/L) can be caused by a number of diseases, including hyperparathyroidism, bone metastases, sarcoidosis, and excess vitamin D.
12. Hypophosphatemia is usually caused by intestinal malabsorption and increased renal excretion of phosphate.
13. Hyperphosphatemia develops with acute or chronic renal failure when there is significant loss of glomerular filtration.
14. Magnesium is a major intracellular cation and is regulated principally by PTH.
15. Magnesium functions in enzymatic reactions and often interacts with calcium at the cellular level.
16. Hypomagnesemia (serum magnesium concentration less than 0.75 mmol/L) may be caused by malabsorption syndromes.
17. Hypermagnesemia (serum magnesium concentration greater than 1.25 mmol/L) is rare and usually is caused by renal insufficiency or failure.

Acid-Base Balance

1. Hydrogen ions, which maintain membrane integrity and the speed of enzymatic reactions, must be concentrated within a narrow range if the body is to function normally.
2. Hydrogen ion concentration, $[H^+]$, is expressed as pH, which represents the negative logarithm (i.e., 10^{-7}) of hydrogen ions in solution (i.e., 0.000 000 1 mg/L).
3. Different body fluids have different pH values; values less than 7.4 are defined as acidic and values greater than 7.4 are defined as alkaline, or basic.
4. The renal and respiratory systems, together with the body's buffer systems, are the principal regulators of acid-base balance.
5. Buffers are substances that can absorb excessive acid or base without a significant change in pH.
6. Buffers exist as acid-base pairs; the principal plasma buffers are carbonic acid (H_2CO_3), bicarbonate (HCO_3^-), protein (hemoglobin), and phosphate.
7. The lungs and kidneys act to compensate for primary changes in pH by increasing or decreasing ventilation and by producing more acidic or more alkaline urine.
8. Correction is a process different from compensation; correction occurs when the values for both components of the buffer pair return to normal as the primary disorder is treated or resolves.
9. Acid-base imbalances are caused by changes in the concentration of hydrogen ion in the blood; an increase causes acidosis, and a decrease causes alkalosis.
10. An abnormal increase or decrease in bicarbonate concentration causes metabolic alkalosis or metabolic acidosis; changes in the rate of alveolar ventilation and removal of carbon dioxide produce respiratory acidosis or respiratory alkalosis.
11. Metabolic acidosis is caused by an increase in the levels of non–carbonic acids or by the loss of bicarbonate from ECF.
12. Metabolic alkalosis occurs with an increase in bicarbonate concentration, which is usually caused by loss of metabolic acids from conditions such as vomiting or gastro-intestinal suctioning or by excessive bicarbonate intake, hyperaldosteronism, and diuretic therapy.
13. Respiratory acidosis occurs with decreased alveolar ventilation, which in turn causes hypercapnia (an increase in carbon dioxide concentration in the blood) and increased carbonic acid concentration.
14. Respiratory alkalosis occurs with alveolar hyperventilation and excessive reduction of carbon dioxide level, or hypocapnia with decreases in carbonic acid concentration.

KEY TERMS

Acidemia, 128
Acidosis, 128
Aldosterone, 118
Alkalemia, 128
Alkalosis, 128
Angiotensin I, 118
Angiotensin II, 118
Anion gap, 128
Antidiuretic hormone (ADH), 117
Aquaporin, 116
Baroreceptor, 119
Buffer, 126
Buffering, 126
Capillary hydrostatic pressure (blood pressure), 116
Capillary (plasma) oncotic pressure, 116
Carbonic acid–bicarbonate buffer, 126
Chloride (Cl^-), 118
Compensation, 126
Correction, 126
Dehydration, 121
Dilutional hyponatremia (water intoxication), 122
Edema, 116
Extracellular fluid (ECF), 115
Hypercapnia, 129
Hyperchloremia, 121
Hyperkalemia, 125
Hypernatremia, 121
Hypertonic fluid alterations, 121
Hypervolemic hypernatremia, 121
Hypervolemic hyponatremia, 122
Hypocapnia, 130
Hypochloremia, 122
Hypochloremic metabolic alkalosis, 128
Hypokalemia, 123
Hyponatremia, 122
Hypotonic fluid imbalance, 121
Hypovolemic hypernatremia, 121
Hypovolemic hyponatremia, 122
Interstitial fluid, 115
Interstitial hydrostatic pressure, 116
Interstitial oncotic pressure, 116
Intracellular fluid (ICF), 115
Intravascular fluid, 115
Isotonic alteration, 121
Isotonic fluid excess, 121
Isotonic fluid loss, 121
Isovolemic hypernatremia, 121
Isovolemic hyponatremia, 122
Lymphedema, 117
Metabolic acidosis, 128
Metabolic alkalosis, 128
Natriuretic peptide, 118
Net filtration, 116
Nonvolatile, 126
Nonvolatile acids, 126
Osmoreceptor, 118
Potassium (K^+), 122
Potassium adaptation, 123
Renin, 118
Renin-angiotensin-aldosterone system, 118
Respiratory acidosis, 129
Respiratory alkalosis, 130
Sodium (Na^+), 117
Starling forces, 116
Total body water (TBW), 115
Volatile, 126
Volume-sensitive receptor, 119
Water balance, 118

REFERENCES

1. Day, R. E., Kitchen, P., Owen, D. S., et al. (2014). Human aquaporins: Regulators of transcellular water flow. *Biochimica Biophysica Acta, 1840*(5), 1492–1506. doi:10.1016/j.bbagen.2013.09.033.
2. Trayes, K. P., Studdiford, J. S., Pickle, S., et al. (2013). Edema: Diagnosis and management. *American Family Physician, 88*(2), 102–110.
3. Ridner, S. H. (2013). Pathophysiology of lymphedema. *Seminars in Oncology Nursing, 29*(1), 4–11. doi:10.1016/j.soncn.2012.11.002.
4. Motiwala, S. R., & Januzzi, J. L., Jr. (2013). The role of natriuretic peptides as biomarkers for guiding the management of chronic heart failure. *Clinical Pharmacology and Therapeutics, 93*(1), 57–67. doi:10.1038/clpt.2012.187.
5. Cheuvront, S. N., Kenefick, R. W., Charkoudian, N., et al. (2013). Physiologic basis for understanding quantitative dehydration assessment. *American Journal of Clinical Nutrition, 97*(3), 455–462. doi:10.3945/ajcn.112.044172.
6. Sam, R., & Feizi, I. (2012). Understanding hypernatremia. *American Journal of Nephrology, 36*(1), 97–104. doi:10.1159/000339625.
7. Berend, K., van Hulsteijn, L. H., & Gans, R. O. (2012). Chloride: The queen of electrolytes? *European Journal of Internal Medicine, 23*(3), 203–211. doi:10.1016/j.ejim.2011.11.013.
8. Sterns, R. H. (2015). Disorders of plasma sodium—Causes, consequences, and correction. *New England Journal of Medicine, 372*(1), 55–65. doi:10.1056/NEJMra1404489.
9. Gross, P. (2012). Clinical management of SIADH. *Therapeutic Advances in Endocrinology and Metabolism, 3*(2), 61–73. doi:10.1177/2042018812437561.
10. Lehrich, R. W., Ortiz-Melo, D. I., Patel, M. B., et al. (2013). Role of vaptans in the management of hyponatremia. *American Journal of Kidney Diseases, 62*(2), 364–376. doi:10.1053/j.ajkd.2013.01.034.
11. Youn, J. H. (2013). Gut sensing of potassium intake and its role in potassium homeostasis. *Seminars in Nephrology, 33*(3), 248–256. doi:10.1016/j.semnephrol.2013.04.005.
12. Lee Hamm, L., Hering-Smith, K. S., & Nakhoul, N. L. (2013). Acid-base and potassium homeostasis. *Seminars in Nephrology, 33*(3), 257–264. doi:10.1016/j.semnephrol.2013.04.006.
13. Pepin, J., & Shields, C. (2012). Advances in diagnosis and management of hypokalemic and hyperkalemic emergencies. *Emergency Medicine Practice, 14*(2), 1–17.
14. Lim, S. (2007). Approach to hyperkalemia. *Acta Medica Indonesiana, 39*(2), 99–103.
15. Maxwell, A. P., Linden, K., O'Donnell, S., et al. (2013). Management of hyperkalaemia. *Journal of the Royal College of Physicians of Edinburgh, 43*(3), 246–251. doi:10.4997/JRCPE.2013.312.
16. Moe, S. M. (2008). Disorders involving calcium, phosphorus and magnesium. *Primary Care, 35*(2), 215–237. doi:10.1016/j.pop.2008.01.007.
17. Adeva-Andany, M. M., Carneiro-Freire, N., Donapetry-García, C., et al. (2014). The importance of the ionic product for water to understand the physiology of the acid-base balance in humans. *BioMed Research International*, 695281. doi:10.1155/2014/695281.
18. Berend, K., de Vries, A. P., & Gans, R. O. (2014). Physiological approach to assessment of acid-base disturbances. *New England Journal of Medicine, 371*(15), 1434–1445. doi:10.1056/NEJMra1003327. Erratum in (2014). *N Engl J Med, 371*(20), 1948.
19. Carmody, J. B., & Norwood, V. F. (2012). A clinical approach to paediatric acid-base disorders. *Postgraduate Medical Journal, 88*(1037), 143–151. doi:10.1136/postgradmedj-2011-130191.
20. Kraut, J. A., & Madias, N. E. (2012). Differential diagnosis of nongap metabolic acidosis: Value of a systematic approach. *Clinical Journal of the American Society of Nephrology: CJASN, 7*(4), 671–679. doi:10.2215/CJN.09450911.
21. Soifer, J. T., & Kim, H. T. (2014). Approach to metabolic alkalosis. *Emergency Medicine Clinics of North America, 32*(2), 453–463. doi:10.1016/j.emc.2014.01.005.
22. Bruno, C. M., & Valenti, M. (2012). Acid-base disorders in patients with chronic obstructive pulmonary disease: A pathophysiological review. *Journal of Biomedicine & Biotechnology, 2012*, 915150. doi:10.1155/2012/915150.
23. Palmer, B. F. (2012). Evaluation and treatment of respiratory alkalosis. *American Journal of Kidney Diseases, 60*(5), 834–838. doi:10.1053/j.ajkd.2012.03.025.
24. Madias, N. E. (2010). Renal acidification responses to respiratory acid base disorders. *Journal of Nephrology, 16*(Suppl. 16), S85–S91.
25. Woodruff, D. (2006). *6 Easy steps to ABG analysis.* Macedonia, OH: Ed4Nurses. Retrieved from https://herzing.blackboard.com/bbcswebdav/pid-5299257-dt-content-rid-11795236_1/courses/06-2132-A-PN108-1/ABGebook.pdf.

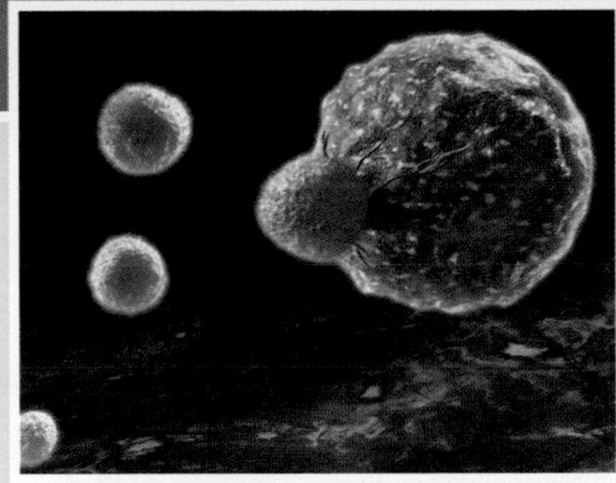

6

Innate Immunity: Inflammation and Wound Healing

Neal S. Rote and Stephanie Zettel

EVOLVE WEBSITE

http://evolve.elsevier.com/Canada/Huether/pathophysiology
Student Review Questions
Key Points
Case Studies
Animations
Quick Check Answers

CHAPTER OUTLINE

Human Defence Mechanisms, 135
First Line of Defence: Physical and Biochemical Barriers and the Human Microbiome, 135
Second Line of Defence: Inflammation, 138
Plasma Protein Systems and Inflammation, 140
Cellular Components of Inflammation, 142
Acute and Chronic Inflammation, 149
Local Manifestations of Acute Inflammation, 150
Systemic Manifestations of Acute Inflammation, 150
Chronic Inflammation, 150
Wound Healing, 152
Phase I: Inflammation, 153
Phase II: Proliferation and New Tissue Formation, 153
Phase III: Remodelling and Maturation, 154
Dysfunctional Wound Healing, 154
PEDIATRIC CONSIDERATIONS: **Age-Related Factors Affecting Innate Immunity in the Newborn Child, 155**
GERIATRIC CONSIDERATIONS: **Age-Related Factors Affecting Innate Immunity in Older Adults, 155**

The human body is continually exposed to a large variety of conditions that result in damage, such as sunlight, pollutants, agents that can cause physical trauma, and infectious agents (viruses, bacteria, fungi, parasites). Damage can also arise from within, such as cancers. The damage may be at the level of a single cell, which can be easily repaired, or may be at the level of multiple cells or tissues or organs, which can result in disease and potentially the death of the individual. To protect us from these conditions, the body has developed a highly sophisticated, multilevel system of interactive defence mechanisms.

HUMAN DEFENCE MECHANISMS

The human body has developed several means of protecting itself from injury and infection. **Innate immunity**, also known as natural or native immunity, includes natural barriers (physical and biochemical) and inflammation. Physical and biochemical barriers form the first line of defence at the body's surfaces and are in place at birth to prevent damage by substances in the environment and thwart infection by pathogenic microorganisms. Surface barriers may also harbour a group of micro-organisms known as the "normal flora" that can protect us from pathogens. If the surface barriers are breached, the second line of defence, the **inflammatory response**, is activated to protect the body from further injury, prevent infection of the injured tissue, and promote healing. The inflammatory response is a rapid activation of biochemical and cellular mechanisms that are relatively nonspecific, with similar responses being initiated against a wide variety of causes of tissue damage. The third line of defence, **adaptive (acquired) immunity** (also known as *specific immunity*), is induced in a relatively slower and more specific process and targets particular invading microorganisms for the purpose of eradicating them. Adaptive immunity also involves "memory," which results in a more rapid response during future exposure to the same microorganism. Comparisons among defence mechanisms are described in Table 6-1. The information presented in this chapter introduces the components and processes of innate immunity and sets the stage for Chapter 7, which presents an overview of adaptive immunity, and Chapter 8, which discusses processes of infection and alterations in immune defences. Innate immunity in the newborn and changes associated with aging are reviewed in the *Pediatric* and *Geriatric Considerations* boxes.

First Line of Defence: Physical and Biochemical Barriers and the Human Microbiome

Physical Barriers

The physical barriers that cover the external parts of the human body offer considerable protection from damage and infection. These barriers are composed of tightly associated epithelial cells of the skin and of the linings of the gastro-intestinal, genitourinary, and respiratory tracts (Figure 6-1). When pathogens attempt to penetrate this physical barrier, they may be removed by mechanical means—sloughed off with dead skin cells as they are routinely replaced, expelled by coughing or sneezing, vomited from the stomach, or flushed from the urinary tract by urine. Epithelial cells of the upper respiratory tract also produce mucus and have hairlike cilia that trap and move pathogens upward to be expelled by coughing or sneezing. Additionally, the low temperature (such as on the skin) and the low pH (such as of the skin and stomach) generally inhibit microorganisms, most of which routinely require temperatures near 37°C (98.6°F) and pH near neutral for efficient growth.

TABLE 6-1 Overview of Human Defences

Characteristics	Barriers	Innate Immunity	Adaptive (Acquired) Immunity
Level of defence	First line of defence against infection and tissue injury	Second line of defence; occurs as response to tissue injury or infection (inflammatory response)	Third line of defence; initiated when innate immune system signals cells of adaptive immunity
Timing of defence	Constant	Immediate response	Delay between primary exposure to antigen and maximal response; immediate against secondary exposure to antigen
Specificity	Broadly specific	Broadly specific	Response is very specific toward "antigen"
Cells	Epithelial cells Microbiome	Mast cells, granulocytes (neutrophils, eosinophils, basophils), monocytes/ macrophages, natural killer (NK) cells, platelets, endothelial cells	T cells, B cells, macrophages, dendritic cells
Memory	No memory involved	No memory involved	Specific immunological memory by T and B cells
Active molecules	Defensins, cathelicidins, collectins, lactoferrin, bacterial toxins	Complement, clotting factors, kinins, cytokines	Antibodies, complement, cytokines
Protection	Protection includes anatomical barriers (i.e., skin and mucous membranes), cells and secretory molecules (e.g., lysozymes, low pH of stomach and urine), and ciliary activity	Protection includes vascular responses, cellular components (e.g., mast cells, neutrophils, macrophages), secretory molecules or cytokines, and activation of plasma protein systems	Protection includes activated T and B cells, cytokines, and antibodies

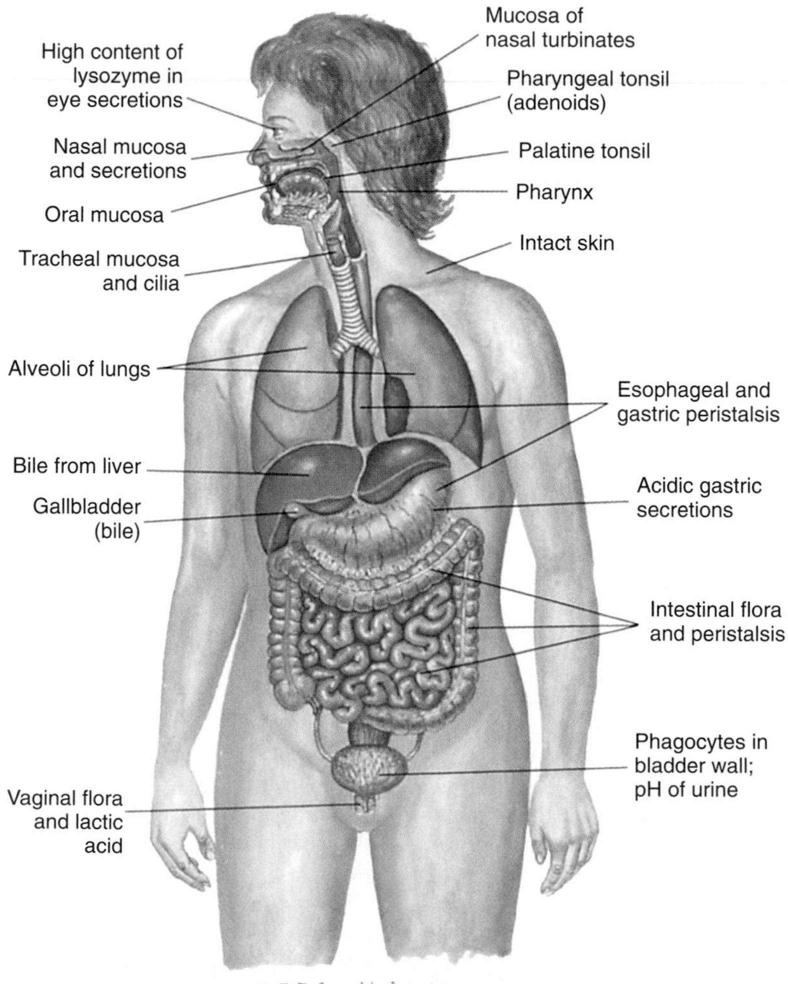

FIGURE 6-1 The Closed Barrier. The digestive, respiratory, and genitourinary tracts and skin form closed barriers between the internal organs and the environment. (From Grimes, D.E. [1991]. *Infectious diseases.* St. Louis: Mosby.)

Epithelial Cell–Derived Chemicals

Epithelial cells secrete an array of substances that protect against infection, including mucus, perspiration (or sweat), saliva, tears, and earwax. These can trap potential invaders and contain substances that will kill microorganisms. Perspiration, tears, and saliva contain an enzyme (**lysozyme**) that attacks the cell walls of Gram-positive bacteria. Sebaceous glands in the skin also secrete fatty acids and lactic acid that kill bacteria and fungi. These glandular secretions create an acidic (pH 3 to 5) and inhospitable environment for most bacteria.

Epithelial cell secretions also contain small-molecular-weight **antimicrobial peptides** that kill or inhibit the growth of disease-causing bacteria, fungi, and viruses.[1] These antimicrobial peptides are generally positively charged polypeptides of approximately 15 to 95 amino acids. More than a thousand antimicrobial peptides have been found, but the best studied are **cathelicidins** and **defensins**.

Several cathelicidins have been discovered in other species, but only one is currently known to function in humans. Bacteria have cholesterol-free cell membranes into which cathelicidin can insert and disrupt the membrane, killing the bacteria. Cathelicidin is produced by epithelial cells of the skin, gut, urinary tract, and respiratory tract, and is stored in neutrophils, mast cells, and monocytes and can be released during inflammation.

In contrast, many different human defensins have been identified. Defensin molecules can be further subdivided into α types (at least six identified in humans) and β types (at least six identified, but perhaps up to 40 different molecules). The α-defensins often require activation by proteolytic enzymes, whereas the β-defensins are synthesized in active forms. Given the similarity in their chemical charges, defensins may kill bacteria in the same way as cathelicidin. The α-defensins are particularly rich in the granules of neutrophils and may contribute to the killing of bacteria by those cells. They are also found in Paneth cells lining the small intestine, where they protect against a variety of disease-causing microorganisms. The β-defensins are found in epithelial cells lining the respiratory, urinary, and intestinal tracts, as well as in the skin. In addition to antibacterial properties, β-defensins may also help protect epithelial surfaces from infection with adenovirus (one of the causes of the common cold) and human immunodeficiency virus (HIV). Both classes of antimicrobial peptides also can activate cells of the next levels of defence: innate and acquired immunity.

The lung also produces and secretes a family of glycoproteins, **collectins**, which includes surfactant proteins A through D and mannose-binding lectin. Collectins react with carbohydrates on the surface of a wide array of pathogenic microorganisms and help cells of the innate immune system (macrophages) to recognize and kill the microorganism. **Mannose-binding lectin (MBL)** recognizes a sugar commonly found on the surface of microbes and is a powerful activator of a plasma protein system (complement), resulting in damage to bacteria or increased recognition by macrophages.

The Normal Microbiome

The body's surfaces are colonized with an array of microorganisms, the **normal microbiome** (previously known as **normal flora**). Each surface (the skin and the mucous membranes of the eyes, upper and lower gastro-intestinal [GI] tracts, upper respiratory tract, urethra, and vagina) is colonized by a combination of bacteria and fungi that is unique to the particular location and individual[2] (Table 6-2). The microorganisms in the microbiome do not normally cause disease, and although their relationship with humans has been referred to as *commensal* (to the benefit of one organism without affecting the other), the relationship may be more *mutualistic* (to the benefit of both organisms). Using the colon for an example, at birth the lower gut is relatively sterile but colonization with bacteria begins quickly, with the number, diversity, and concentration increasing progressively during the first year of life.

The normal microbiome benefits us in many ways; bacteria in the GI tract produce (1) enzymes that facilitate the digestion and utilization of many molecules in the human diet, such as fatty acids and large polysaccharides; (2) usable metabolites (e.g., vitamin K, B vitamins); and (3) antibacterial factors that prevent colonization by pathogenic

TABLE 6-2 The Human Microbiome

Location	Microorganisms
Skin	Predominantly Gram-positive cocci and rods; *Staphylococcus epidermidis*, corynebacteria, mycobacteria, and streptococci are primary inhabitants; *Staphylococcus aureus* in some people; also yeasts (*Candida*, *Pityrosporum*) in some areas of skin
	Numerous transient microorganisms may become temporary residents
	In moist areas, Gram-negative bacteria
	Around sebaceous glands, *Propionibacterium* and *Brevibacterium*
	Mite *Demodex folliculorum* lives in hair follicles and sebaceous glands around face
Nose	Predominantly Gram-positive cocci and rods, especially *S. epidermidis*
	Some people are nasal carriers of pathogenic bacteria, including *S. aureus*, β-hemolytic streptococci, and *Corynebacterium diphtheria*
Mouth	Complex of bacteria that includes several species of streptococci, *Actinomyces*, lactobacilli, and *Haemophilus*
	Anaerobic bacteria and spirochetes colonize gingival crevices
Pharynx	Similar to flora in mouth plus staphylococci, *Neisseria*, and diphtheroids
	Some asymptomatic persons also harbour pathogens: pneumococcus, *Haemophilus influenzae*, *Neisseria meningitidis*, and *C. diphtheria*
Distal small intestine	Enterobacteria, streptococci, lactobacilli, anaerobic bacteria, and *C. albicans*
Colon	Bacteroides, lactobacilli, clostridia, *Salmonella*, *Shigella*, *Klebsiella*, *Proteus*, *Pseudomonas*, *enterococci*, and other streptococci, bacilli, and *Escherichia coli*
Distal urethra	Typical bacteria found on skin, especially *S. epidermidis* and diphtheroids; also lactobacilli and nonpathogenic streptococci
Vagina	Birth to 1 month: similar to adult
	1 month to puberty: *S. epidermidis*, diphtheroids, *E. coli*, and streptococci
	Puberty to menopause: *Lactobacillus acidophilus*, diphtheroids, staphylococci, streptococci, and variety of anaerobes
	Postmenopause: similar to prepubescence

Adapted from Bennett, J.E., Dolin, R., & Blaser, M.J. (Eds.). (2015). *Mandell, Douglas, and Bennett's principles and practice of infectious diseases* (8th ed.). Philadelphia: Saunders.

microorganisms (see Chapter 8). For example, members of the normal microbiome in the colon produce chemicals (ammonia, phenols, indoles, and other toxic materials) and proteins (*bacteriocins*) that are toxic to more pathogenic microorganisms. They also compete with pathogens for nutrients and block attachment to the epithelium, which is an obligatory first step in the infectious process by most pathogens. Additionally, the normal microbiome of the gut helps train the adaptive immune system by inducing growth of gut-associated lymphoid tissue (where most cells of the adaptive immune system reside) and the development of both local and systemic adaptive immunity. Bidirectional communication between the brain and GI tract (brain–gut axis) is influenced by GI bacteria with importance for cognitive function, behaviour, pain modulation, and stress responses.[3]

Prolonged treatment with broad-spectrum antibiotics can alter the normal microbiome, decreasing its protective activity, and lead to an overgrowth of pathogenic microorganisms. In the intestine, overgrowth of the yeast *Candida albicans* or the bacteria *Clostridium difficile* (a cause of pseudomembranous colitis, an infection of the colon) may occur. The bacterium *Lactobacillus* is a major constituent of the normal GI and vaginal microbiome in healthy women.[4] This microorganism produces a variety of chemicals (e.g., hydrogen peroxide, lactic acid, bacteriocins) that help prevent infections of the vagina and urinary tract by other bacteria and yeast. Prolonged antibiotic treatment can diminish colonization with *Lactobacillus* and increase the risk for urological or vaginal infections, such as vaginosis.

The mutualistic relationship with the microbiome is maintained through the physical integrity of the skin and mucosal epithelium and other mechanisms that protect the microbiome from the immune and inflammatory systems. Some members of the normal bacterial microbiome are opportunistic; **opportunistic microorganisms** can cause disease if the individual's defences are compromised. These microorganisms are normally controlled by the innate and adaptive immune systems and contribute to our defences. For example, *Pseudomonas aeruginosa* is a member of the normal microbiome of the skin and produces a toxin that protects against infections with staphylococcal and other bacteria. However, severe burns compromise the integrity of the skin and may lead to life-threatening systemic infections with *Pseudomonas*.

QUICK CHECK 6-1

1. How do physical barriers contribute to defence mechanisms?
2. What are antimicrobial peptides?
3. What two types of defensins contribute to the biochemical barrier?
4. What is the normal microbiome? What is its role in defence?
5. What are opportunistic microorganisms?

Second Line of Defence: Inflammation

Whereas the physical and biochemical barriers of the innate immune system are relatively static, **inflammation** is programmed to respond to cellular or tissue damage, whether the damaged tissue is septic or sterile. The response is a rapid initiation of an interactive system of humoral (soluble in the blood) and cellular systems designed to limit the extent of tissue damage, destroy contaminating infectious microorganisms, initiate the adaptive immune response, and begin the healing process.

The inflammatory response (1) occurs in tissues with a blood supply (vascularized); (2) is activated *rapidly* (within seconds) after damage occurs; (3) depends on the activity of both *cellular and chemical components*; and (4) is *nonspecific*, meaning that it takes place in approximately the same way, regardless of the type of stimulus or whether exposure to the same stimulus has occurred in the past.

Inflammation will be activated by virtually any injury to vascularized tissues, including infection or tissue necrosis (e.g., ischemia, trauma, physical or chemical injury, foreign bodies, immune reactions). The classic or cardinal signs of acute inflammation were described in the first century by a Roman named Celsus and included rubor (redness), calor (heat), tumour (swelling), and dolor (pain). A fifth sign, functio laesa (loss of function), was added later. Microscopic inflammatory changes occur within seconds in the microcirculation (arterioles, capillaries, and venules) near the site of an injury and include the following processes (Figure 6-2):

1. Vasodilation (increased size of the blood vessels), which causes slower blood velocity and increases blood flow to the injured site
2. Increased vascular permeability (the blood vessels become porous from contraction of endothelial cells) and leakage of fluid out of

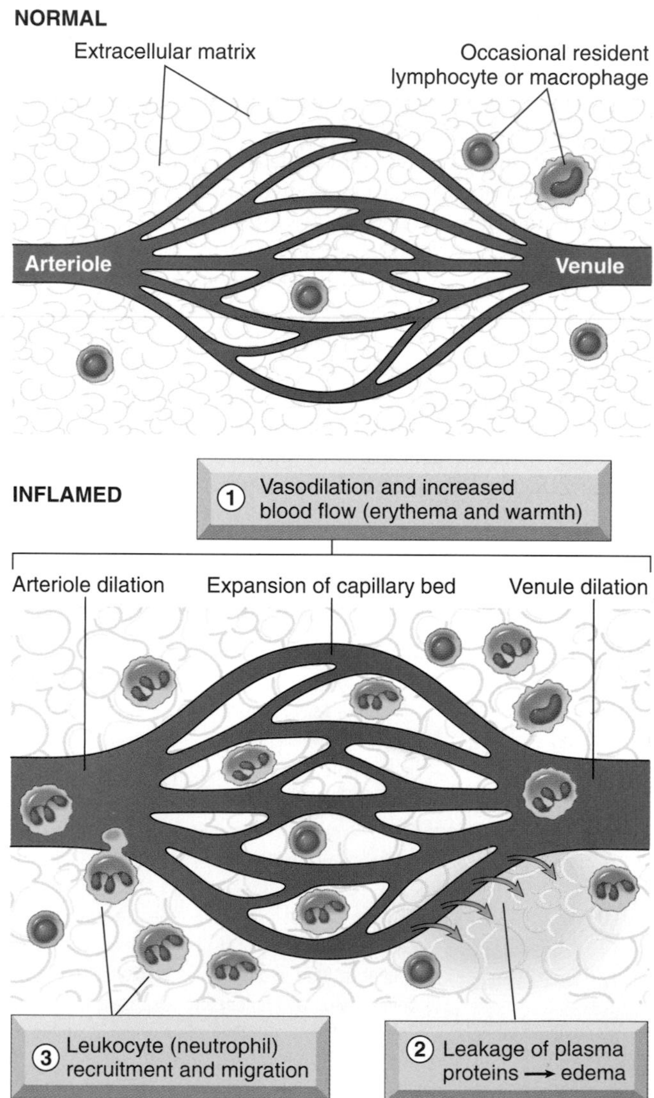

FIGURE 6-2 The Major Local Changes in the Process of Inflammation. Compared with normal circulation, inflammation is characterized by **(1)** dilation of the blood vessels and increased blood flow, leading to erythema and warmth; **(2)** increased vascular permeability with leakage of plasma from the vessels, leading to edema; and **(3)** movement of leukocytes from the vessels into the site of injury. (From Kumar, V., Abbas, A.K., Aster, J.C., et al. [Eds.] [2010]. *Robbins and Cotran pathologic basis of disease* [8th ed.]. Philadelphia: Saunders.)

the vessel (exudation), causing swelling (edema) at the site of injury; as plasma moves outward, blood in the microcirculation becomes more viscous and flows more slowly, and the increased blood flow and increasing concentration of red cells at the site of inflammation cause locally increased redness (erythema) and warmth

3. White blood cell adherence to the inner walls of vessels and their migration through enlarged junctions between the endothelial cells lining the vessels into the surrounding tissue

Each of the characteristic changes associated with inflammation is the direct result of the activation and interactions of a host of chemicals and cellular components found in the blood and tissues. The vascular changes deliver leukocytes (particularly neutrophils), plasma proteins, and other biochemical mediators to the site of injury, where they act in concert. Some of these chemical mediators activate pain fibres. The tissue injury, pain, and swelling contribute to loss of function. Figure 6-3 summarizes the process of acute inflammation. The lymphatic vessels drain the extravascular fluid to the lymph nodes and may, themselves, become secondarily inflamed: lymphangitis of the lymph vessels and lymphadenitis of the nodes, which become hyperplastic, enlarged, and frequently painful.

There are several benefits of inflammation, including the following:

- It prevents infection and further damage by invading microorganisms. The inflammatory exudate dilutes toxins produced by bacteria and released from dying cells. The activation of plasma protein systems (e.g., complement and clotting systems) helps contain and destroy bacteria. The influx of phagocytes (e.g., neutrophils, macrophages) destroys cellular debris and microorganisms.
- It limits and controls the inflammatory process. The influx of plasma protein systems (e.g., clotting system), plasma enzymes, and cells (e.g., eosinophils) prevents the inflammatory response from spreading to areas of healthy tissue.
- It interacts with components of the adaptive immune system to elicit a more specific response to contaminating pathogen(s) through the influx of macrophages and lymphocytes that destroy pathogens.
- It prepares the area of injury for healing and repair through removal of bacterial products, dead cells, and other products of inflammation (e.g., by way of channels through the epithelium or drainage by lymphatic vessels).

Fluid and debris that accumulate at an inflamed site are drained by lymphatic vessels. This process also facilitates the development of acquired immunity because microbial antigens in lymphatic fluid pass through the lymph nodes, where they encounter lymphocytes.

QUICK CHECK 6-2

1. Why are innate immunity and inflammation described as "nonspecific"?
2. How are the five classic superficial symptoms of inflammation related to the process of inflammation?
3. Describe the basic steps in acute inflammation.
4. What are the benefits of inflammation?

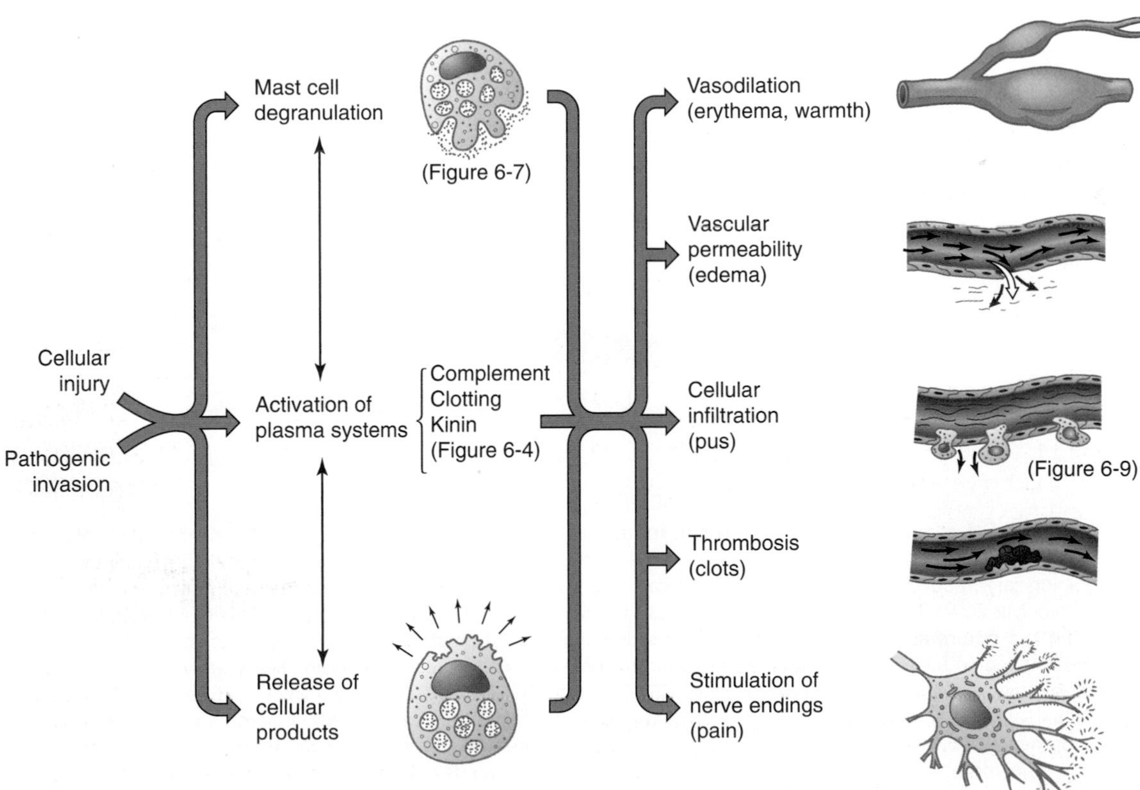

FIGURE 6-3 Acute Inflammatory Response. Inflammation is usually initiated by cellular injury and may be complicated by infection. Mast cell degranulation, the activation of three plasma systems, and the release of subcellular components from the damaged cells occur as a consequence. These systems are interdependent, so that induction of one (e.g., mast cell degranulation) can result in the induction of the other two. The result is the development of the characteristic microscopic and clinical hallmarks of inflammation. The figure numbers refer to additional figures in which more detailed information may be found on that portion of the response.

Plasma Protein Systems and Inflammation

Three key **plasma protein systems** are essential to an effective inflammatory response: the complement system, the clotting system, and the kinin system (Figure 6-4). Although each system has a unique role in inflammation, they have many similarities. Each system consists of multiple proteins found in the blood, usually in inactive forms; several are enzymes that circulate as proenzymes. Each system contains a few proteins that can be activated early in inflammation. Activation of the first components results in sequential activation of other components of the system, leading to a biological function that helps protect the individual. This sequential activation is referred to as a *cascade*. Thus, we occasionally refer to the complement cascade, the clotting cascade, or the kinin cascade. In some cases, activation of a particular protein in the system may require that it be enzymatically cut into two pieces of different size. Usually the larger fragment continues the cascade by activating the next component, and the smaller fragment frequently has potent proinflammatory activities.

Complement System

The **complement system** consists of a large number of proteins (sometimes called *complement factors*) that together constitute about 10% of the total circulating serum protein. Activation of the complement system produces several factors that can destroy pathogens directly or can activate or increase the activity of many other components of the

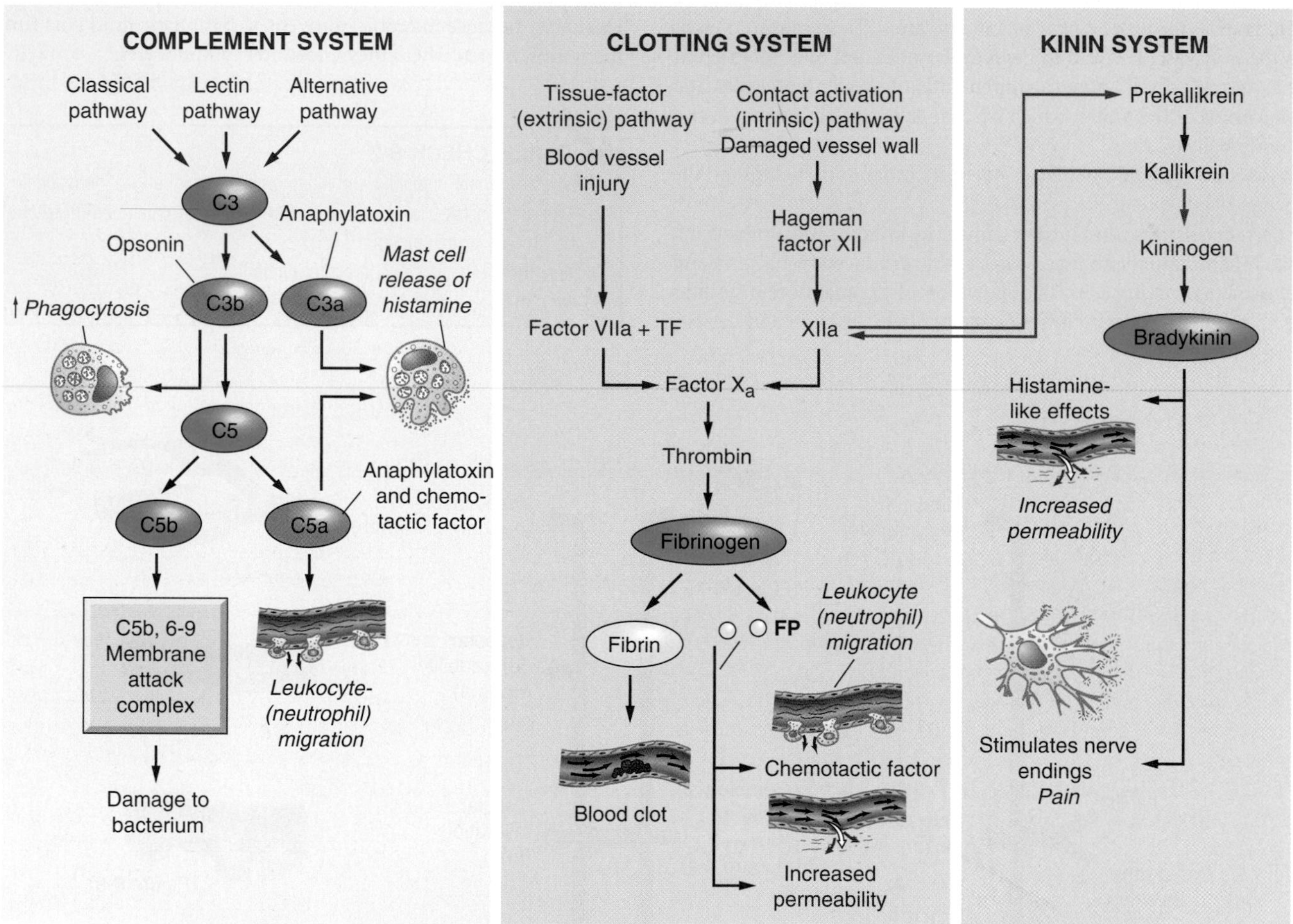

FIGURE 6-4 Plasma Protein Systems in Inflammation: Complement, Clotting, and Kinin Systems. Each plasma protein system consists of a family of proteins that are activated in sequence to create potent biological effects. The complement system can be activated by three mechanisms, each of which results in proteolytic activation of C3. The fragments of C3 activation, C3a and C3b, are major components of inflammation. C3a is a potent anaphylatoxin, which induces degranulation of mast cells. C3b can bind to the surface or cells, such as bacteria, and either serve as an opsonin for phagocytosis or proteolytically activate the next component of the complement cascade, C5. The smaller fragment of C5 activation is C5a, a powerful anaphylatoxin, and is also chemotactic for neutrophils, attracting them to the site of inflammation. The larger fragment, C5b, activates the components of the membrane attack complex (C5–C9), which damage the bacterial membrane and kill the bacteria. The clotting system can be activated by the tissue factor (extrinsic) pathway and the contact activation (intrinsic) pathway. All routes of clotting initiation lead to activation of factor X and thrombin. Thrombin is an enzyme that proteolytically activates fibrinogen to form fibrin and small fibrinopeptides (FPs). Fibrin polymerizes to form a clot, and the FPs are highly active as chemotactic factors and cause increased vascular permeability. The XIIa produced by the clotting system can also be activated by kallikrein of the kinin system (*red arrow*). Prekallikrein is enzymatically converted to kininogen, which activates bradykinin. Bradykinin functions similarly to histamine and increases vascular permeability. Bradykinin can also stimulate nerve endings to cause pain. *FP*, fibrinopeptide; *TF*, tissue factor.

inflammatory and adaptive immune response. Factors produced during activation of the complement system are among the body's most potent defenders, particularly against bacterial infection.

The most important function of the complement cascade is activation of C3 and C5, which results in a variety of molecules that are (1) opsonins, (2) chemotactic factors, or (3) anaphylatoxins.[5] **Opsonins** coat the surface of bacteria and increase their susceptibility to being phagocytized (eaten) and killed by inflammatory cells, such as neutrophils and macrophages. **Chemotactic factors** diffuse from a site of inflammation and attract phagocytic cells to that site. **Anaphylatoxins** induce rapid degranulation of mast cells (i.e., release of histamine that induces vasodilation and increased capillary permeability), a major cellular component of inflammation. The most potent complement products are C3b (opsonin), C3a (anaphylatoxin), and C5a (anaphylatoxin, chemotactic factor). Activation of terminal complement components C5b through C9 (membrane attack complex, or MAC) results in a complex that creates pores in the outer membranes of cells or bacteria. The pores disrupt the cell's membrane and permit water to enter, causing the death of the cell.

Three major pathways control the activation of complement (see Figure 6-4). The **classical pathway** is primarily activated by antibodies, which are proteins of the acquired immune system. Antibodies must first bind to their targets, called *antigens*, which can be proteins or carbohydrates from bacteria or other infectious agents. Antibodies activate the first component of complement, C1, which leads to activation of other complement components, leading to activation of C3 and C5. Thus, antibodies of the acquired immune response can use the complement system to kill bacteria and activate inflammation.

The **alternative pathway** is activated by several substances found on the surface of infectious organisms (e.g., lipopolysaccharides [endotoxin] on the bacterial surface or yeast cell wall carbohydrates [zymosan]). This pathway uses unique proteins (factor B, factor D, and properdin) to form a complex that activates C3. C3 activation leads to C5 activation and convergence with the classical pathway. Thus, the complement system can be directly activated by certain infectious organisms without antibody being present.

The **lectin pathway** is similar to the classical pathway but is independent of antibody. It is activated by several plasma proteins, particularly MBL. MBL binds to bacterial polysaccharides containing the carbohydrate mannose and activates complement through two proteins that are similar to C1—mannose-binding lectin-associated serine protease 1 (MASP-1) and MASP-2.[6] Thus, infectious agents that do not activate the alternative pathway may be susceptible to complement through the lectin pathway.

In summary, the complement cascade can be activated by at least three different means, and its products have four functions: (1) opsonization (C3b); (2) anaphylatoxic activity resulting in mast cell degranulation (C3a, C5a); (3) leukocyte chemotaxis (C5a); and (4) cell lysis (C5b–C9 [MAC]).

Clotting System

The **clotting (coagulation) system** is a group of plasma proteins that, when activated sequentially, form a blood clot. A **blood clot** is a meshwork of protein (fibrin) strands that contains platelets (the primary cellular initiator of clotting) and traps other cells, such as erythrocytes, phagocytes, and microorganisms. Clots (1) plug damaged vessels and stop bleeding, (2) trap microorganisms and prevent their spread to adjacent tissues, and (3) provide a framework for future repair and healing. Specific details and illustrations of the clotting system are presented in Chapter 20 (see also Figure 20-18), and only the relationship between clotting and inflammation is presented here.

The clotting system can be activated by many substances that are released during tissue injury and infection, including collagen, proteinases, kallikrein, and plasmin, as well as by bacterial products such as endotoxins. Like the complement cascade, the coagulation cascade can be activated through different pathways that converge and result in the formation of a clot (see Figure 6-4). The **tissue factor (extrinsic) pathway** is activated by **tissue factor (TF)** (also called **tissue thromboplastin**) that is released by damaged endothelial cells in blood vessels and reacts with activated factor VII (VIIa). The **contact activation (intrinsic) pathway** is activated when the vessel wall is damaged and **Hageman factor (factor XII)** in plasma contacts negatively charged subendothelial substances. The pathways converge at factor X. Activation of factor X begins a common pathway leading to activation of fibrin that polymerizes to form a fibrin clot.

As with the complement system, activation of the clotting system produces protein fragments known as fibrinopeptides (FPs) A and B that enhance the inflammatory response. Fibrinopeptides are released from fibrinogen when fibrin is produced. Both FPs (especially fibrinopeptide B) are chemotactic for neutrophils and increase vascular permeability by enhancing the effects of bradykinin (formed from the kinin system) on endothelial cells.

Kinin System

The third plasma protein system, the **kinin system** (see Figure 6-4), interacts closely with the coagulation system. Both the clotting and kinin systems can be initiated through activation of Hageman factor (factor XII) to factor XIIa. Another name for factor XIIa is *prekallikrein* activator because it enzymatically activates the first component of the kinin system, prekallikrein. The final product of the kinin system is a small-molecular-weight molecule, **bradykinin**, which is produced from a larger precursor molecule, kininogen. Bradykinin causes dilation of blood vessels, acts with prostaglandins to induce pain, causes smooth muscle cell contraction, and increases vascular permeability.

Control and Interaction of Plasma Protein Systems

The three plasma protein systems are highly interactive so that activation of one results in production of a large number of very potent, biologically active substances that further activate the other systems. Very tight regulation of these processes is essential for the following two reasons:

1. The inflammatory process is critical for an individual's survival; thus, efficient activation must be guaranteed regardless of the cause of tissue injury. Interaction among the plasma systems may result in activation of the entire inflammatory response, regardless of which system is activated initially.
2. The biochemical mediators generated during these processes are potent and potentially detrimental to the individual, and their actions must be strictly confined to injured or infected tissues.

Therefore, multiple mechanisms are available to either activate or inactivate (regulate) these plasma protein systems. For example, the plasma that enters the tissues during inflammation (edema) contains enzymes that destroy mediators of inflammation. **Carboxypeptidase** inactivates the anaphylatoxic activities of C3a and C5a, and kininases degrade kinins. **Histaminase** degrades histamine and kallikrein and downregulates the inflammatory response.

The formation of clots also activates a **fibrinolytic system** that is designed to limit the size of the clot and remove the clot after bleeding has ceased. Thrombin of the clotting system activates **plasminogen** in the blood to form the enzyme plasmin. The primary activity of **plasmin** is to degrade fibrin polymers in clots. However, plasmin can also activate the complement cascade through components C1, C3, and C5 and the kinin cascade by activating factor XII and producing prekallikrein activator.

Another example of a common regulator is **C1 esterase inhibitor (C1 INH)**. C1 INH inhibits complement activation through C1 (classical pathway), MASP-2 (lectin pathway), and C3b (alternative pathway). It is also a major inhibitor of the clotting and kinin pathway components (e.g., kallikrein, factor XIIa). A genetic defect in C1 INH (C1 INH deficiency) results in hereditary angioedema, which is a self-limiting edema of cutaneous and mucosal layers resulting from stress, illness, or a relatively minor or unapparent trauma. The disease is characterized by hyperactivation of all three plasma protein systems, although excessive production of bradykinin appears to be the principal cause of increased vascular permeability.

Many cells are protected from inadvertent complement system damage by factors linked to the external surface of the plasma membrane. Two examples are decay accelerating factor (DAF) and CD59; DAF prevents activation of C3, and CD59 inhibits the membrane attack complex.

QUICK CHECK 6-3

1. What are the three most important products of the complement system?
2. How is the coagulation cascade activated? How is it related to the plasma kinin cascade?
3. What factors control the plasma protein systems of inflammation?

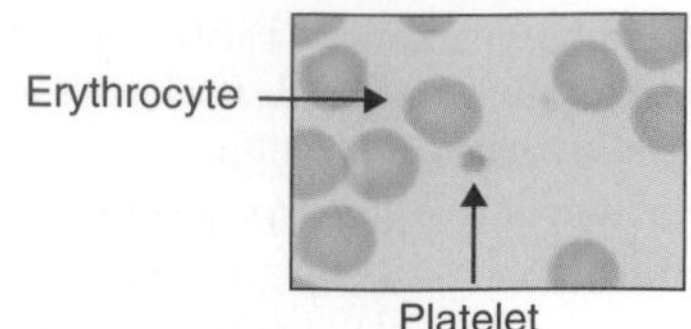

LEUKOCYTES

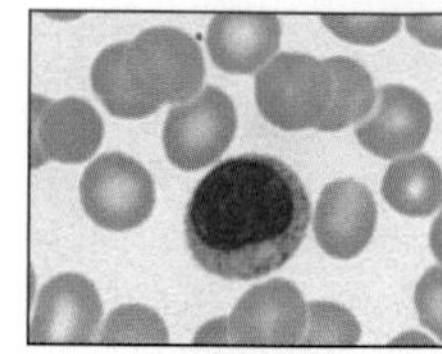

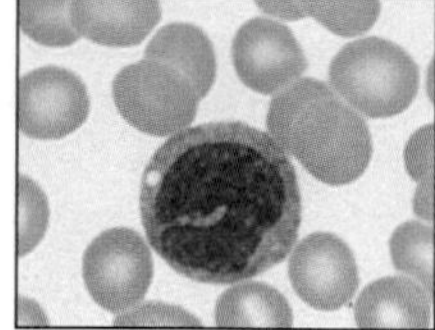

Granulocytes

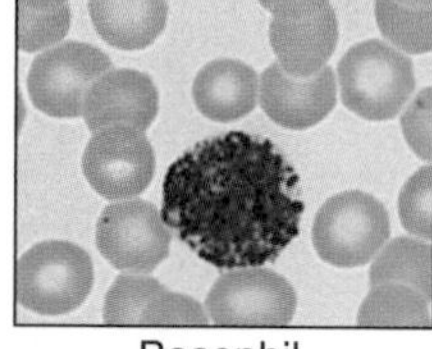

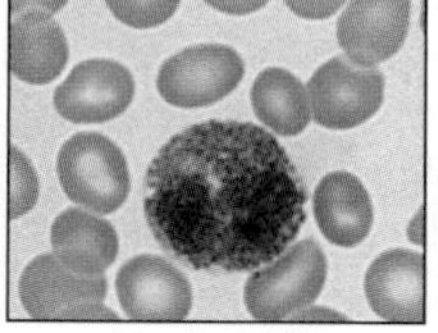

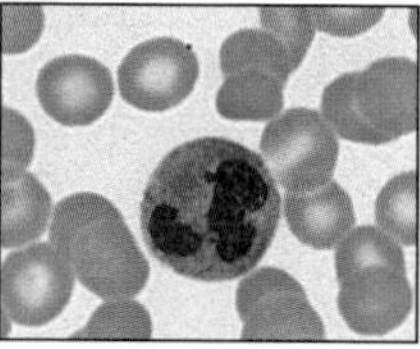

FIGURE 6-5 Cellular Components of the Blood. Cells in the blood can be classified as red blood cells (erythrocytes), cellular fragments (platelets), or white blood cells (leukocytes). Leukocytes consist of lymphocytes, monocytes, and granulocytes (neutrophils, eosinophils, basophils). (Erythrocyte plate from Goldman, L., & Schafer, A.I. [Eds.]. [2012]. *Goldman's Cecil medicine* [24th ed.]. Philadelphia: Saunders; rest of plates from McPherson, R.A. [Ed.]. [2012]. *Henry's clinical diagnosis and management by laboratory methods* [22nd ed.]. Philadelphia: Saunders.)

Cellular Components of Inflammation

Inflammation is a process in vascular tissue; thus, the cellular components can be found in the blood or in tissue surrounding the blood vessels. The blood vessels are lined with endothelial cells, which under normal conditions actively maintain blood flow. During inflammation the vascular endothelium becomes a principal coordinator of blood clotting and the passage of cells and fluid into the tissue. The tissues close to the vessels contain mast cells, which are probably the most important activators of inflammation, and dendritic cells, which connect the innate and acquired immune responses. The blood contains a complex mixture of cells (Figure 6-5 and see also Chapter 20). Blood cells are divided into erythrocytes (red blood cells), platelets, and leukocytes (white blood cells). Erythrocytes carry oxygen to the tissues, and platelets are small cell fragments involved in blood clotting. Leukocytes are subdivided into granulocytes (containing many enzyme-filled cytoplasmic granules), monocytes, and lymphocytes. Granulocytes are the most common leukocytes and are classified by the type of stains needed to visualize enzyme-containing granules in their cytoplasm (basophils, eosinophils, and neutrophils). Monocytes are precursors of macrophages that are found in the tissue. Various forms of lymphocytes participate in the innate immune response (e.g., natural killer [NK] cells) and the acquired immune response (B and T cells).

Cells of both innate and acquired immune systems respond to molecules produced at a site of cellular damage and are recruited to that site to augment the protective response. These molecules originate from destroyed or damaged cells, contaminating microbes, activation of the plasma protein systems, or secretions by other cells of the innate or acquired immune systems. Each cell has a set of cell surface receptors that specifically bind these molecules, resulting in activation of intracellular signalling pathways and activation of the cell itself. Activation may result in the cell gaining a function critical to the inflammatory response or the induction of the release of additional cellular products that increase inflammation, or both. Most of these inflammatory cells and protein systems, along with the substances they produce, act at the site of tissue injury to confine the extent of damage; kill microorganisms; remove the cellular debris; and activate healing, tissue regeneration (a process known as *resolution*), or repair.

Cellular Receptors

As will be discussed in Chapter 7, B and T lymphocytes of the adaptive immune system have evolved surface receptors (i.e., the T-cell antigen receptor, or TCR, and the B-cell antigen receptor, or BCR) that bind a large spectrum of antigens. Cells involved in innate resistance have evolved a different set of receptors that recognize a much more limited array of specific molecules (ligands). These receptors are referred to as pattern recognition receptors (PRRs). PRRs recognize two types of molecular *patterns*: molecules that are expressed by infectious agents, either found on their surface or released as soluble molecules (pathogen-associated molecular patterns, or PAMPs); or products of cellular damage (damage-associated molecular patterns, or DAMPs). Thus, cells of the innate immune system can respond to both sterile (through DAMPs) and septic (through PAMPs and DAMPs) tissue damage. It is estimated that at least 100 different PRRs are expressed that recognize more than 1 000 different molecules.

PRRs are generally expressed on cells in tissues near the body's surface (i.e., skin, respiratory tract, GI tract, genitourinary tract) where they monitor the environment for products of cellular damage and potentially infectious microorganisms. Classes of cellular PRRs primarily differ in the specificity of ligands they bind. PRRs can be found as cell surface receptors that bind extracellular ligands, in endosomes in contact with ingested microbes and other materials, in the cytosol where they bind intracellular materials resulting from cellular damage, or secreted into the extracellular environment. An example of a secreted PRR is MBL of the lectin pathway of complement activation.

Toll-like receptors (TLRs) primarily recognize a large variety of PAMPs located on the microorganism's cell wall or surface (e.g., bacterial lipopolysaccharide [LPS], peptidoglycans, lipoproteins, yeast zymosan,

TABLE 6-3 Cellular Source and Microbial Target for Each Toll-Like Receptor

Receptor	Cellular Expression Pattern	PAMP Recognition
TLR1	Cell surface (ubiquitous): neutrophils, monocytes/macrophages, dendritic cells, T cells, B cells, natural killer (NK) cells	Fungal, bacterial, viral; forms heterodimer with TLR2 (see TLR2 recognition)
TLR2	Cell surface: neutrophils, monocytes/macrophages, dendritic cells	Fungal (yeast zymosan), bacterial (Gram-positive bacterial peptidoglycan, lipoproteins), viral (lipoproteins)
TLR3	Intracellular: monocytes/macrophages, dendritic cells, T cells, NK cells, epithelial cells	Double-stranded RNA produced by many viruses
TLR4	Cell surface: granulocytes, monocytes/macrophages, dendritic cells, T cells, B cells, epithelial cells	Bacterial (primarily Gram-negative bacterial LPS, lipoteichoic acids), viral (RSV F protein, hepatitis C)
TLR5	Cell surface: granulocytes, monocytes/macrophages, dendritic cells, NK cells, epithelial cells	Bacterial (flagellin); forms heterodimer with TLR4
TLR6	Cell surface: monocytes/macrophages, dendritic cells, B cells, NK cells	Fungal, bacterial, viral; forms heterodimer with TLR2 (see TLR2 recognition)
TLR7	Intracellular: monocytes/macrophages, dendritic cells, B cells	Natural ligand uncertain; may bind viral single-strand RNA
TLR8	Cell surface: monocytes/macrophages, dendritic cells, NK cells	Natural ligand uncertain; may bind fungal PAMPs or viral single-stranded RNA
TLR9	Intracellular: monocytes/macrophages, dendritic cells, B cells	Bacterial (unmethylated DNA [CpG dinucleotides])
TLR10	Cell surface: monocytes/macrophages, dendritic cells, B cells	Natural ligand uncertain; may form heterodimers with TLR2
TLR11	*TLR11* gene does not code a full-length protein in humans	No known immune response

PAMP, pathogen-associated molecular pattern; *RSV*, respiratory syncytial virus; *TLR*, toll-like receptor.

viral coat proteins), other surface structures (e.g., bacterial flagellin), or microbial nucleic acid (e.g., bacterial DNA, viral double-stranded RNA).[7] Eleven different TLRs have been described in humans (Table 6-3). They are expressed on the surface of many cells that have direct and early contact with potential pathogenic microorganisms, including mucosal epithelial cells, mast cells, neutrophils, macrophages, dendritic cells, and some subpopulations of lymphocytes. TLRs are linked to pathways that produce two groups of transcription factors: *NF-κB*, which controls synthesis and release of cytokines; and *interferon regulatory factors* (*IRFs*), which control the production of antiviral type I interferons.[8]

Complement receptors are found on many cells of the innate and acquired immune responses (e.g., granulocytes, monocytes/macrophages, lymphocytes, mast cells, erythrocytes, platelets), as well as some epithelial cells. They recognize several fragments produced through activation of the complement system, particularly C3a, C5a, and C3b.

Scavenger receptors are primarily expressed on macrophages and facilitate recognition and phagocytosis of bacterial pathogens, as well as damaged cells and altered soluble lipoproteins associated with vascular damage (e.g., high-density lipoprotein [HDL], acetylated low-density lipoprotein [LDL], oxidized LDL).[9] More than eight receptors have been identified. Some scavenger receptors (e.g., SR-PSOX) recognize the cell membrane phospholipid phosphatidylserine (PS). PS is normally sequestered on the cytoplasmic surface of the cell membrane, but it is externalized under a very limited variety of conditions, including erythrocyte senescence and cellular apoptosis. Thus macrophages, through this receptor, can identify and remove old red blood cells and cells undergoing apoptosis.

NOD-like receptors (NLRs) are cytoplasmic receptors that recognize products of microbes and damaged cells. At least 22 NLRs have been identified in humans. NOD-1 and NOD-2 are cytoplasmic and recognize fragments of peptidoglycans from intracellular bacteria and initiate production of proinflammatory mediators, such as tumour necrosis factor (TNF) and interleukin-6 (IL-6).[10] Other NLRs associate with intracellular multiprotein complexes called **inflammasomes**. Inflammasomes primarily bind cellular stress-related molecules, a type of DAMP, and control the production of the inflammatory cytokines interleukin-1β (IL-1β) and IL-18.[11]

Cellular Products

To elicit an effective inflammatory (or adaptive immune) response, intercellular communication and cooperation are necessary. **Cytokines** constitute a large family of small-molecular-weight soluble intercellular-signalling molecules that are secreted, bind to specific cell membrane receptors, and regulate innate or adaptive immunity (Figure 6-6). Cytokines may be either *proinflammatory* or *anti-inflammatory* in nature, depending on whether they tend to induce or inhibit the inflammatory response. These molecules usually diffuse over short distances, but some effects occur over long distances, such as the systemic induction of fever by some cytokines (i.e., endogenous pyrogens) that are produced at an inflammatory site. Binding of cytokines to a target cell often induces synthesis of additional cellular products. For example, binding of the cytokine **tumour necrosis factor-alpha (TNF-α)** to a cell may result in synthesis and release of interleukin-1.

A large number of cytokines have been described and are classified into several families.[12] The terms *lymphokines* and *monokines* refer respectively to cytokines secreted from lymphocytes or monocytes, although cytokines are secreted by many different types of cells. **Chemokines** are members of a special family of cytokines that are chemotactic and primarily attract leukocytes to sites of inflammation.[13] Chemokines are synthesized by many cell types, including macrophages, fibroblasts, and endothelial cells, in response to proinflammatory cytokines, such as TNF-α. To date, more than 50 different human chemokines have been described. Examples include those that primarily attract macrophages (e.g., monocyte/macrophage chemotactic proteins [MCP-1, MCP-2, and MCP-3]), macrophage inflammatory proteins (MIP-α and MIP-1β), or neutrophils (e.g., interleukin-8 [IL-8]).

Interleukins (ILs) are produced predominantly by macrophages and lymphocytes in response to stimulation of PRRs or by other cytokines.[14] More than 30 ILs have been identified. Their effects include the following:

- Alteration of adhesion molecule expression on many types of cells
- Attraction of leukocytes to a site of inflammation (chemotaxis)
- Induction of proliferation and maturation of leukocytes in the bone marrow
- General enhancement or suppression of inflammation
- Development of the acquired immune response

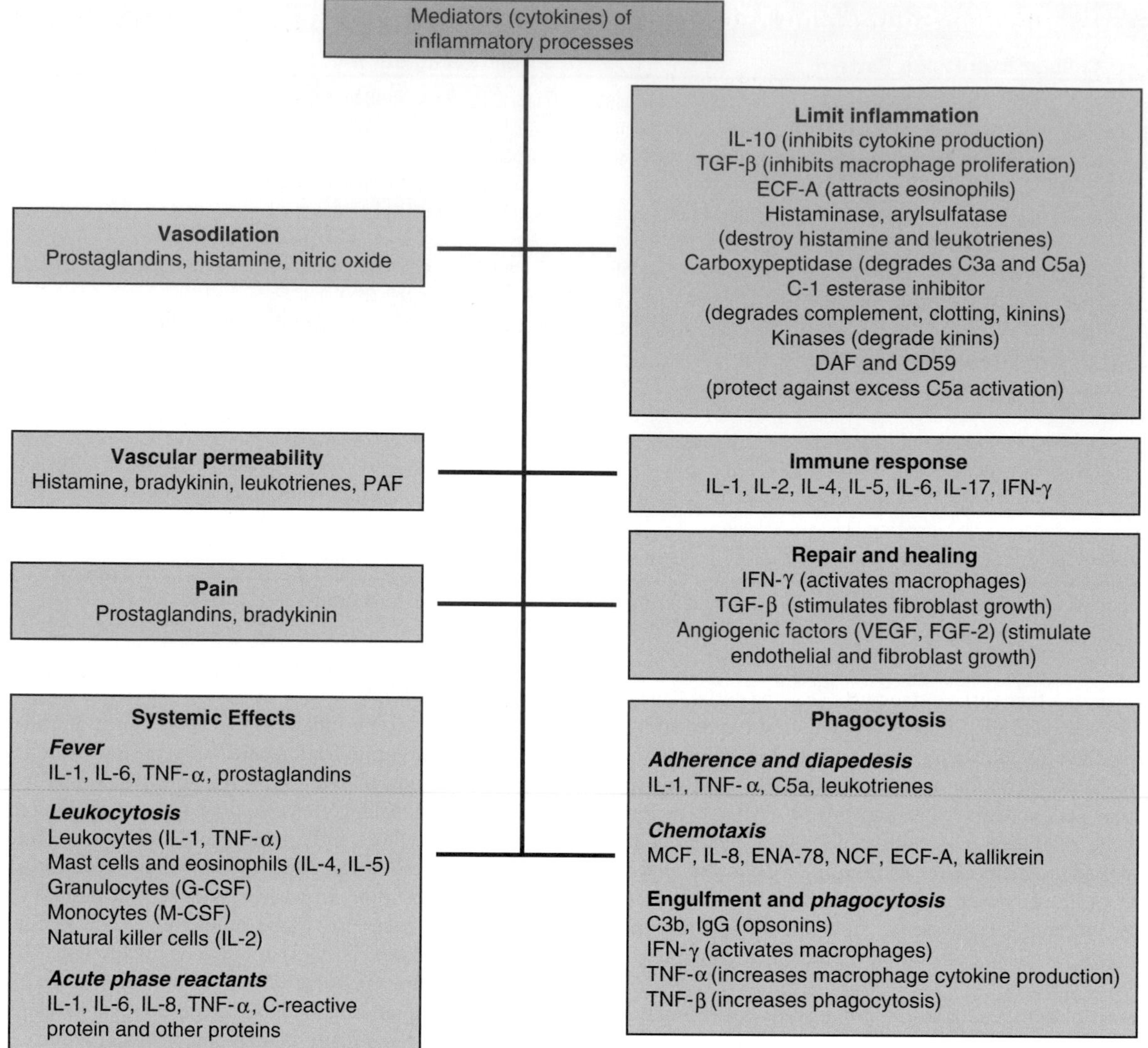

FIGURE 6-6 Principal Mediators of Inflammatory Processes. *C3b,* large fragment produced from complement component C3; *C5a,* small fragment produced from complement component C5; *DAF,* decay accelerating factor; *ECF-A,* eosinophil chemotactic factor of anaphylaxis; *ENA-78,* epithelial neutrophil activating peptide-78; *FGF,* fibroblast growth factor; *G-CSF,* granulocyte colony-stimulating factor; *IFN,* interferon; *IgG,* immunoglobulin G (predominant class of antibody in the blood); *IL,* interleukin; *MCF,* monocyte chemotactic factor; *M-CSF,* macrophage colony-stimulating factor; *NCF,* neutrophil chemotactic factor; *PAF,* platelet-activating factor; *TGF,* T-cell growth factor; *TNF,* tumour necrosis factor; *VEGF,* vascular endothelial growth factor.

Two major proinflammatory ILs are interleukin-1 and interleukin-6, which cooperate closely with another cytokine, TNF-α. **Interleukin-1 (IL-1)** is produced in two forms, IL-1α and IL-1β, mainly by macrophages.[15] IL-1 activates monocytes, other macrophages, and lymphocytes, thereby enhancing both innate and acquired immunity, and acts as a growth factor for many cells. It has several effects on neutrophils, including induction of proliferation (resulting in an increase in the number of circulating neutrophils), attraction to an inflammatory site (chemotaxis), and increased cellular respiration and lysosomal enzyme activity (both effects resulting in increased cellular killing of bacteria). IL-1 is an endogenous pyrogen (i.e., fever-causing cytokine) that reacts with receptors on cells of the hypothalamus and affects the body's thermostat, resulting in fever.

Interleukin-6 (IL-6) is produced by macrophages, lymphocytes, fibroblasts, and other cells. IL-6 directly induces hepatocytes (liver cells) to produce many of the proteins needed in inflammation (acute-phase reactants, discussed later in this chapter). IL-6 also stimulates growth and differentiation of blood cells in the bone marrow and the growth of fibroblasts (required for wound healing).

Although not classified as an interleukin, TNF-α is secreted by macrophages and other cells (e.g., mast cells) in response to stimulation of TLRs. TNF-α induces a multitude of proinflammatory effects, particularly on the vascular endothelium and macrophages. When secreted in large amounts, TNF-α has systemic effects that include the following:

- Inducing fever by acting as an endogenous pyrogen
- Causing increased synthesis of inflammation-related serum proteins by the liver
- Causing muscle wasting (cachexia) and intravascular thrombosis in cases of severe infection and cancer

Very high levels of TNF-α can be lethal and are probably responsible for fatalities from shock caused by Gram-negative bacterial infections.

Some cytokines are anti-inflammatory and diminish the inflammatory response. The most important are interleukin-10 and transforming growth factor-beta. **Interleukin-10 (IL-10)** is primarily produced by lymphocytes and suppresses the growth of other lymphocytes and the production of proinflammatory cytokines by macrophages, leading to downregulation of both inflammatory and acquired immune responses. **Transforming growth factors**, including **transforming growth factor-beta (TGF-β)**, are produced by many cells in response to inflammation and induce cell division and differentiation of other cell types, such as immature blood cells.

Interferons (IFNs) are members of a family of cytokines that protect against viral infections and modulate the inflammatory response. (Mechanisms of viral infection are described in Chapter 8.) Type I interferons (primarily IFN-α, IFN-β) are produced and released by virally infected cells in response to viral double-stranded RNA and other viral PAMPs. These IFNs do not kill viruses directly but instead are secreted and induce antiviral proteins and protection in neighbouring healthy cells. Type II interferon (IFN-γ) is produced primarily by lymphocytes; it activates macrophages, resulting in increased capacity to kill infectious agents (including viruses and bacteria), and enhances the development of acquired immune responses against viruses.

Mast Cells and Basophils

The mast cell is probably the most important cellular activator of the inflammatory response. **Mast cells** are filled with granules and located in the loose connective tissues close to blood vessels near the body's outer surfaces (i.e., in the skin and lining the GI and respiratory tracts). **Basophils** are found in the blood and probably function in the same way as tissue mast cells.[16] A great number of stimuli activate mast cells to release potent soluble inducers of inflammation. These inducers are released by (1) **degranulation** (the release of the contents of mast cell granules) and (2) *synthesis* (the new production and release of mediators in response to a stimulus) (Figure 6-7).

Degranulation. In response to a stimulus, biochemical mediators in the mast cell granules, including histamine, chemotactic factors, and cytokines (e.g., TNF-α, IL-4), are released within seconds and exert their effects immediately. **Histamine** is a small-molecular-weight molecule with potent effects on many other cells, particularly those that control the circulation. Histamine, along with serotonin (found in many cells, but not human mast cells), is called a *vasoactive amine*. These molecules cause temporary, rapid constriction of smooth muscle and dilation of the postcapillary venules, which results in increased blood flow into the microcirculation. Histamine also causes increased vascular permeability resulting from retraction of endothelial cells lining the capillaries and increased adherence of leukocytes to the endothelium. Histamine affects cells by binding to histamine H1 and H2 receptors on the target cell surface (Figure 6-8). Antihistamines are medications that block the binding of histamine to its receptors, resulting in decreased inflammation.

Binding of histamine to the *H1 receptor* is essentially proinflammatory; that is, it promotes inflammation. On the other hand, binding to the *H2 receptor* is generally anti-inflammatory because it results in suppression of leukocyte function. The H1 receptor is present on smooth muscle cells, especially those of the bronchi, and causes bronchial smooth muscle to contract (bronchoconstriction) when stimulated. Both types of receptors are distributed among many different cells and are often present on the same cells and may act in an antagonistic fashion. For example, stimulation of H1 receptors on neutrophils results in augmentation of neutrophil chemotaxis, whereas H2 receptor stimulation results in its inhibition. The H2 receptor is especially abundant on parietal cells of the stomach mucosa and induces the secretion of gastric acid as part of the normal physiology of the stomach.

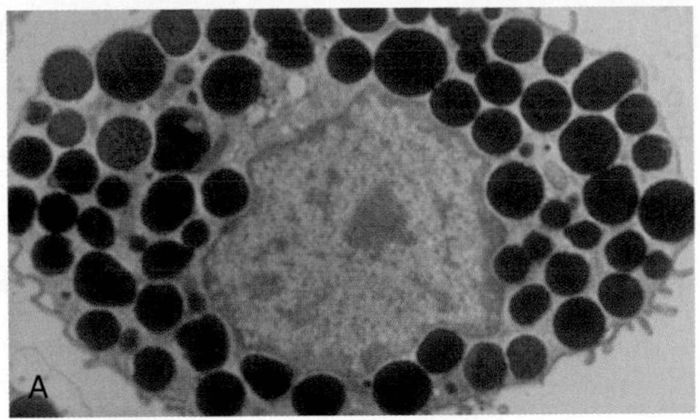

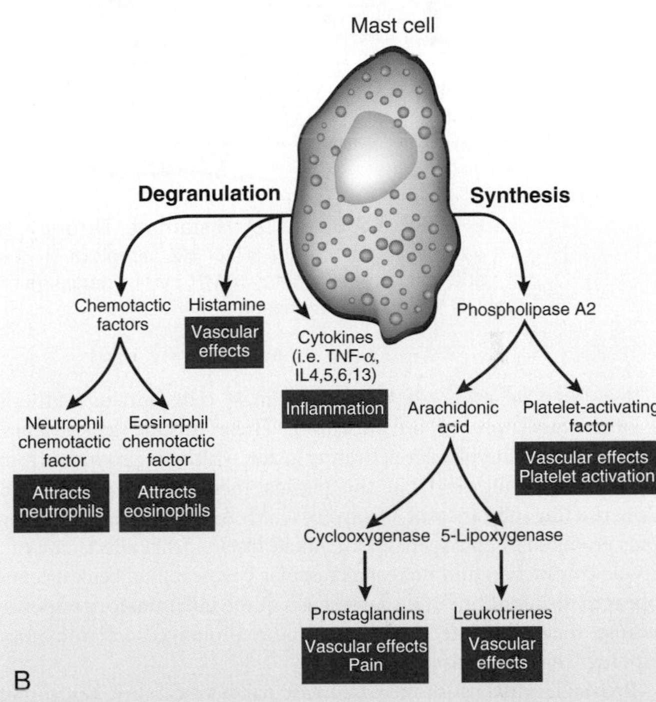

FIGURE 6-7 Mast Cell and Mast Cell Degranulation and Synthesis of Biological Mediators During Inflammation. A, Colourized photomicrograph of mast cell; dense red granules contain histamine and other biologically active substances. Among these are histamine, which is a major initiator of vascular changes, and a variety of chemotactic factors. **B,** Mast cell degranulation (*left*) and synthesis (*right*). Histamine and other biologically active substances are released immediately after stimulation of mast cells. Different pharmacological compounds block the synthesis or action of biological mediators during inflammation in specific ways: corticosteroids work by inhibiting phospholipases; non-steroidal anti-inflammatory drugs inhibit cyclo-oxygenase from producing prostaglandins; and acetaminophen blocks a variant of cyclo-oxygenase (i.e., it has no anti-inflammatory effect). *IL,* interleukin; *TNF-α,* tumour necrosis factor-alpha. (**A,** from Roitt, I.M., Broistoff, J., & Male, D.K. [1993]. *Immunology* [3rd ed.]. St. Louis: Mosby.)

The role of histamine receptors and hypersensitivity is discussed in Chapter 8.

Mast cell granules also contain chemotactic factors, two of which are **neutrophil chemotactic factor (NCF)** and **eosinophil chemotactic factor of anaphylaxis (ECF-A)**. **Chemotaxis** is directional movement of cells along a chemical gradient formed by a chemotactic factor. Neutrophils are the predominant cell needed to kill bacteria in the early stages of inflammation. Eosinophils help regulate the inflammatory response. Both cells are discussed in more detail later in this chapter.

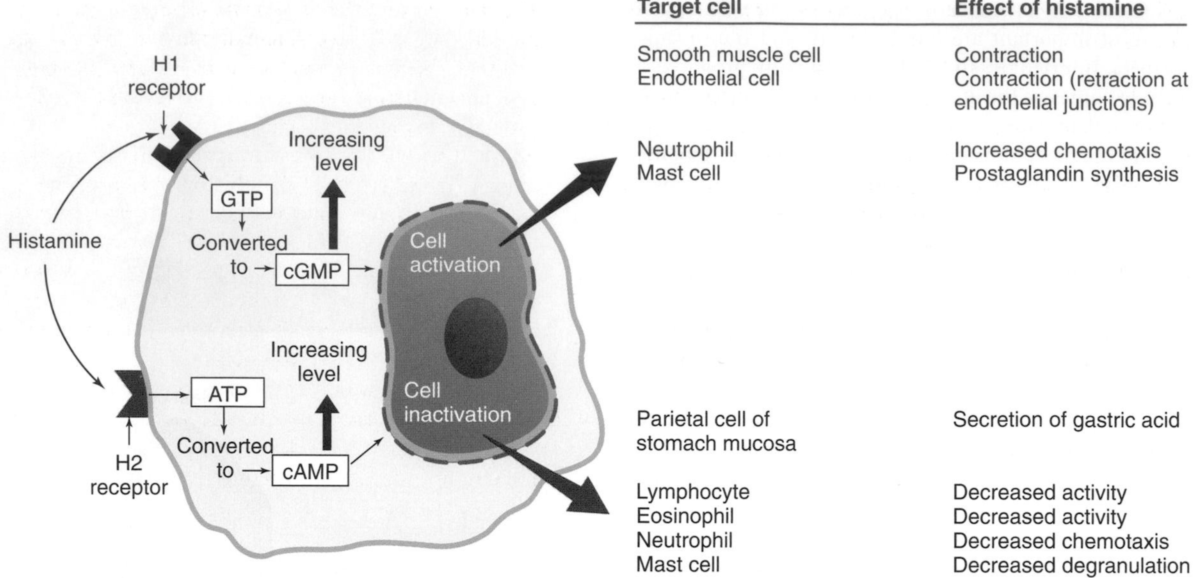

FIGURE 6-8 Effects of Histamine Through H1 and H2 Receptors. The effects depend on (1) the density and affinity of H1 or H2 receptors on the target cell and (2) the identity of the target cell. *ATP*, adenosine triphosphate; *cAMP*, cyclic adenosine monophosphate; *cGMP*, cyclic guanosine monophosphate; *GTP*, guanosine triphosphate.

Synthesis of mediators. Activated mast cells initiate synthesis of other mediators of inflammation. These include leukotrienes, prostaglandins, and platelet-activating factor, which are produced from lipids (arachidonic acid) in the plasma membrane. Leukotrienes (slow-reacting substances of anaphylaxis [SRS-A]) are sulphur-containing lipids produced by lipoxygenase that initiate histaminelike effects: smooth muscle contraction and increased vascular permeability. Leukotrienes appear to be important in the later stages of the inflammatory response because they stimulate slower and more prolonged inflammatory responses than does histamine.

Prostaglandins cause increased vascular permeability, neutrophil chemotaxis, and pain by direct effects on nerves. They are long-chain, unsaturated fatty acids produced by the action of the enzyme cyclo-oxygenase (COX) on arachidonic acid; prostaglandins are classified into groups (E, D, A, F, and B) according to their structure with numeral subscripts designating the number of double bonds. Prostaglandins E_1 and E_2 cause increased vascular permeability and smooth muscle contraction. COX exists in two different forms: COX-1 is found in most tissues and COX-2 is associated with inflammation. Acetylsalicylic acid (Aspirin) and other nonsteroidal anti-inflammatory drugs (NSAIDs) inhibit both COX-1 and COX-2, but inhibition of COX-1 causes complications, such as GI toxicity. Selective COX-2 inhibitors are now available.

Platelet-activating factor (PAF) is produced by removal of a fatty acid from the plasma membrane phospholipids by phospholipase A_2. Although mast cells are a major source of PAF, this molecule also can be produced by neutrophils, monocytes, endothelial cells, and platelets. The biological activity of PAF is virtually identical to that of leukotrienes, namely, PAF causes endothelial cell retraction to increase vascular permeability, leukocyte adhesion to endothelial cells, and platelet activation.

Endothelium

The lining of blood vessels consists of a layer of endothelial cells that adhere to an underlying matrix of connective tissue that contains a variety of proteins, including collagen, fibronectin, and laminins. Endothelial cells regulate circulating components of the inflammatory system and maintain normal blood flow by preventing spontaneous activation of platelets and members of the clotting system. Nitric oxide (NO) produced from arginine and prostacyclin (PGI_2) from arachidonic acid maintain blood flow and pressure and inhibit platelet activation. PGI_2 and NO are synergistic. NO is released continually to relax vascular smooth muscle and suppress the effects of low levels of cytokines, thus maintaining vascular tone. PGI_2 production varies a great deal and is increased when additional regulation is needed.

Damage to the endothelial cell lining of the vessel exposes the subendothelial connective tissue matrix, which is prothrombogenic and initiates platelet activation and formation of clots (the contact activation [intrinsic] clotting pathway). Proinflammatory mediators (e.g., histamine, prostacyclin, and many others) affect the endothelium, resulting in adherence of leukocytes to the vessel surface, invasion of leukocytes into the tissue, and efflux of plasma from the vessel.

Platelets

Platelets are anucleate cytoplasmic fragments formed from *megakaryocytes*. They circulate in the bloodstream until vascular injury occurs, resulting in platelet activation by many products of tissue destruction and inflammation, including collagen, thrombin, and PAF. Activated platelets (1) interact with components of the coagulation cascade to stop bleeding; (2) degranulate, releasing biochemical mediators such as serotonin, which has vascular effects similar to those of histamine; and (3) synthesize thromboxane A_2 (TXA_2) from prostaglandin H_2. TXA_2 is a potent vasoconstrictor and inducer of platelet aggregation. Prolonged use of low-dose Aspirin preferentially suppresses production of TXA_2 without interfering with the production of anti-inflammatory PGI_2 by the endothelium. Platelets also release growth factors that promote wound healing. (Platelet function is described in detail in Chapter 20.)

Phagocytes

The primary role of most granulocytes (neutrophils, eosinophils, basophils) and monocytes/macrophages is phagocytosis—the process by which a cell ingests and disposes of damaged cells and foreign material, including microorganisms.

Neutrophils. The **neutrophil**, or **polymorphonuclear neutrophil (PMN)**, is a member of the granulocytic series of white blood cells and is named for the characteristic staining pattern of its granules as well as its multilobed nucleus. Neutrophils are the predominant phagocytes in the early inflammatory site, arriving within 6 to 12 hours after the initial injury. Several inflammatory mediators (e.g., some bacterial proteins, complement fragments C3a and C5a, and mast cell NCF) specifically and rapidly attract neutrophils from the circulation and activate them.[17]

Because the neutrophil is a mature cell that is incapable of division and sensitive to acidic environments, it is short lived at the inflammatory site and becomes a component of the purulent exudate, or pus, which is removed from the body through the epithelium or drained from the infected site via the lymphatic system. (The lymphatic system is described in Chapter 23.) The primary roles of the neutrophil are removal of debris and dead cells in sterile lesions, such as burns, and destruction of bacteria in nonsterile lesions.

Eosinophils. Another population of granulocytes is the **eosinophil**. Although eosinophils are only mildly phagocytic, they have two specific functions: (1) they serve as the body's primary defence against parasites, and (2) they help regulate vascular mediators released from mast cells. The role of eosinophils in resistance to parasites occurs in collaboration with specific antibodies produced by the acquired immune system (discussed in Chapter 7).[18]

Regulation of mast cell–derived inflammatory mediators is critical to control inflammation. The acute inflammatory response is needed only in a circumscribed area and for a limited time. Therefore, control mechanisms are necessary to prevent biochemical mediators from evoking more inflammation than necessary. Mast cell eosinophil chemotactic factor of anaphylaxis (ECF-A) attracts eosinophils to the site of inflammation. Eosinophil lysosomal granules contain enzymes that degrade vasoactive molecules, thereby controlling the vascular effects of inflammation. Histaminase degrades histamine, and arylsulfatase B degrades leukotrienes.

Basophils. The basophil is the least prevalent granulocyte in the blood. It is very similar to mast cells in the content of its granules. In addition, it is an important source of the cytokine IL-4, which is a key regulator of the adaptive immune response. Although often associated with allergies and asthma, its primary role is yet unknown.

Monocytes and macrophages. **Monocytes** are the largest normal blood cells (14 to 20 μm in diameter). Monocytes are produced in the bone marrow, enter the circulation, and migrate to the inflammatory site where they develop into macrophages. Monocytes also appear to be the precursors of macrophages that are found in tissues (tissue macrophages) including Kupffer cells in the liver, alveolar macrophages in the lungs, and microglia in the brain. **Macrophages** are generally larger (20 to 40 μm) and are more active as phagocytes than their monocytic precursors. Macrophages, particularly those residing in the tissues, are often important cellular initiators of the inflammatory response.

Monocyte-derived macrophages from the circulation may appear at the inflammatory site as soon as 24 hours after the initial neutrophil infiltration, but usually arrive 3 to 7 days later. Neutrophils and monocytes/macrophages differ chiefly in the following ways:

- *Speed:* Neutrophils arrive at the injury site first, whereas macrophages move more sluggishly.
- *Active lifespan:* Macrophages survive and divide in the acidic inflammatory site, whereas neutrophils cannot.
- *Chemotactic factors:* Neutrophils and macrophages are not attracted by the same factors, such as macrophage chemotactic factor, which is released by neutrophils.
- *Enzymatic content of their lysosomes, or digestive vacuoles:* Neutrophils have a more active nicotinamide adenine dinucleotide phosphate (NADPH) oxidase and produce more hydrogen peroxide; macrophage phagolysosomes are more acidic, favouring the activity of acidic proteases and other enzymes.
- *Role in the immune response:* Macrophages, but not neutrophils, are involved in activation of the adaptive immune system.
- *Role in wound repair:* Macrophages are the primary cells that infiltrate tissue in wounds, remove cells and cellular debris, promote angiogenesis, and produce cytokines and growth factors that suppress further inflammation and initiate healing by promoting epithelial cell division, activating fibroblasts, and promoting synthesis of extracellular matrix and collagen.

The bactericidal activity of macrophages can increase markedly with the help of inflammatory cytokines produced by cells of the acquired immune system (subsets of T lymphocytes) or cells activated through TLRs. Macrophage activation results in two subpopulations of cells.[19] M1 macrophages are activated through TLRs by substances found in sites of inflammation and have greater bacterial killing capacity. M2 macrophages are activated by lymphocyte-produced cytokines and are primarily involved in healing and repair.[20]

Several bacteria are resistant to killing by granulocytes and can even survive inside macrophages. Microorganisms, such as *Mycobacterium tuberculosis* (tuberculosis), *Mycobacterium leprae* (leprosy), *Salmonella typhi* (typhoid fever), *Brucella abortus* (brucellosis), and *Listeria monocytogenes* (listeriosis), can remain dormant or multiply inside the phagolysosomes of macrophages.

Dendritic cells. **Dendritic cells** provide one of the major links between the innate and acquired immune responses. They are the primary phagocytic cells located in the peripheral organs and skin, where molecules released from infectious agents are encountered, recognized through PRRs, and internalized through phagocytosis. Dendritic cells then migrate through the lymphatic vessels to lymphoid tissue, such as lymph nodes, and interact with **T lymphocytes (T cells)** to generate an acquired immune response.[21] Through the production of a family of cytokines, they guide development of a subset of T cells (T-helper cells) that coordinate the development of functional B and T cells (discussed in Chapter 7).

Phagocytosis. The two most important phagocytes are neutrophils and macrophages. Both cells are circulating in the blood and must first leave the circulation and migrate to the site of inflammation before initiating phagocytosis (Figure 6-9). Many products of inflammation affect expression of surface molecules involved in cell-to-cell adherence. Both leukocytes and endothelial cells begin expressing molecules (selectins and integrins) that increase adhesion, or stickiness, causing the leukocytes to adhere more avidly to the endothelial cells in the walls of the capillaries and venules in a process called **margination**, or **pavementing**. Leukocyte-endothelial interactions lead to **diapedesis**, or emigration of the cells through the interendothelial junctions that have loosened in response to inflammatory mediators.[22]

Once inside the tissue, leukocytes undergo a process of directed migration (chemotaxis) by which they are attracted to the inflammatory site by chemotactic factors.[23] The primary chemotactic factors include many bacterial products, NCF produced by mast cells, the chemokine IL-8, complement fragments C3a and C5a, and products of the clotting and kinin systems. Red blood cells cannot repair themselves and are phagocytized by macrophages at the end of their lifespan (Figure 6-10).

At the inflammatory site, the process of phagocytosis involves five steps: (1) recognition and adherence of the phagocyte to its target, (2) engulfment (ingestion or endocytosis), (3) formation of a phagosome, (4) fusion of the phagosome with lysosomal granules within the

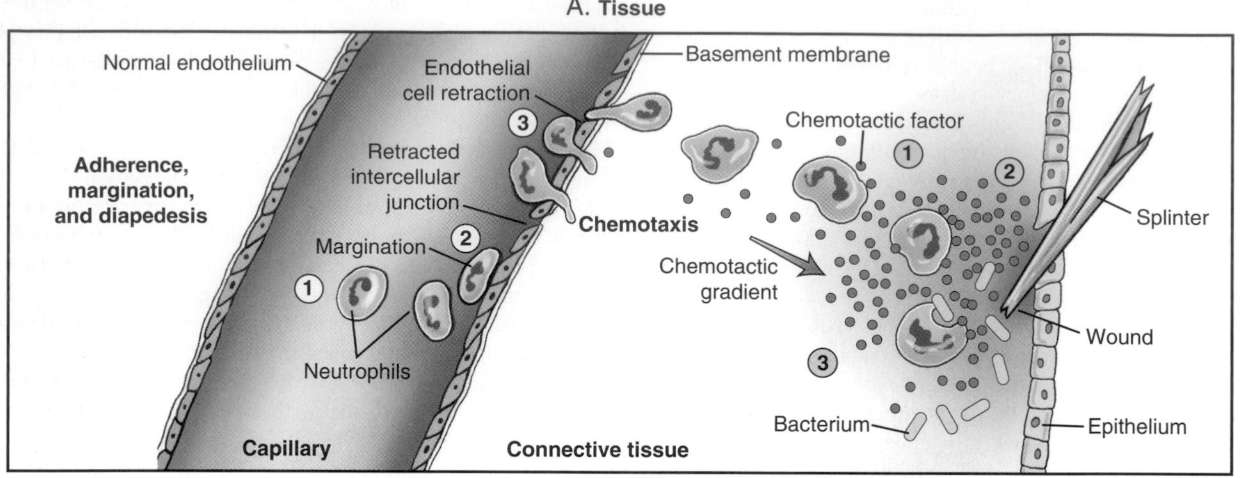

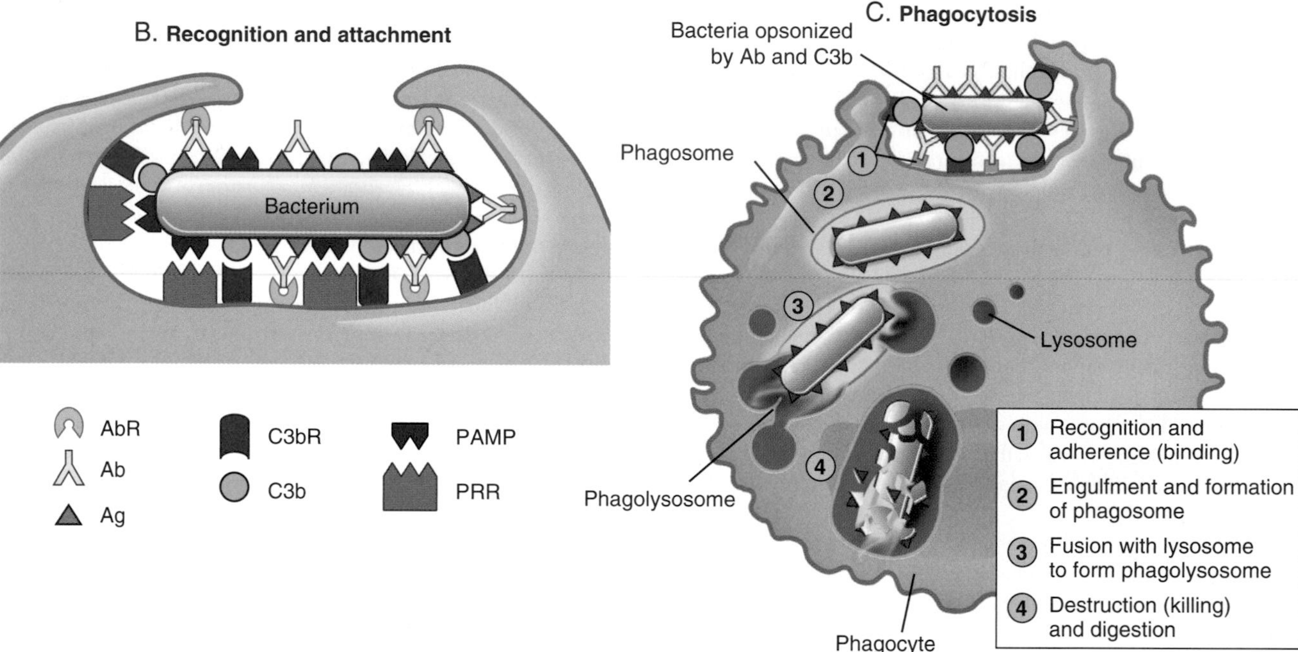

FIGURE 6-9 Process of Phagocytosis. The process that results in phagocytosis is characterized by three interrelated steps: adherence and diapedesis, tissue invasion by chemotaxis, and phagocytosis. **A,** *Adherence, margination, diapedesis, and chemotaxis:* The primary phagocyte in the blood is the neutrophil, which usually moves freely within the vessel **(1)**. At sites of inflammation, the neutrophil progressively develops increased adherence to the endothelium, leading to accumulation along the vessel wall (margination, or pavementing) **(2)**. At sites of endothelial cell retraction, the neutrophil exits the blood by means of diapedesis **(3)**. *Chemotaxis:* In the tissues, the neutrophil detects chemotactic factor gradients through surface receptors **(1)** and migrates toward higher concentrations of the factors **(2)**. The high concentration of chemotactic factors at the site of inflammation immobilizes the neutrophil **(3)**. **B,** *Specific receptors for recognition and attachment.* **C,** *Phagocytosis*: Opsonized microorganisms bind to the surface of a phagocyte through specific receptors **(1)**. The microorganism is ingested into a phagocytic vacuole, or phagosome **(2)**. Lysosomes fuse with the phagosome, resulting in the formation of a phagolysosome **(3)**. During this process the microorganism is exposed to products of the lysosomes, including a variety of enzymes and products of the hexose-monophosphate shunt (e.g., hydrogen peroxide [H_2O_2], superoxide [O_2^-]). The microorganism is killed and digested **(4)**. *Ab,* antibody; *AbR,* antibody receptor; *Ag,* antigen; *C3b,* complement component C3b; *C3bR,* complement C3b receptor; *PAMP,* pathogen-associated molecular pattern; *PRR,* pattern recognition receptor.

phagocyte, and (5) destruction of the target. Throughout the process, both the target and the digestive enzymes are isolated within membrane-bound vesicles. Isolation protects the phagocyte itself from the harmful effects of the target microorganisms, as well as its own enzymes.

Most phagocytes can trap and engulf bacteria using PRRs, although the process is relatively slow. **Opsonization** greatly enhances adherence by acting as a glue to tighten the affinity of adherence between the phagocyte and the target cell. The most efficient opsonins are antibodies and C3b produced by the complement system. Antibodies are made

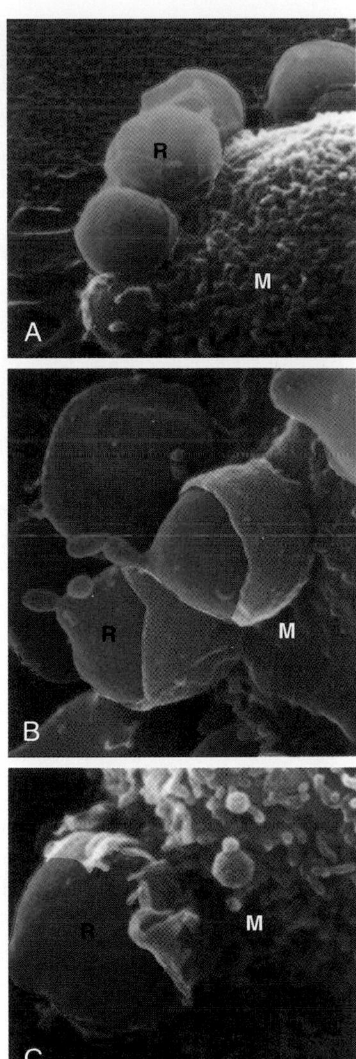

FIGURE 6-10 Phagocytosis of Red Blood Cell. This scanning electron micrograph shows the progressive steps in phagocytosis. **A,** Red blood cells (*R*) attach to the surface of a macrophage (*M*). **B,** Part of the macrophage (*M*) membrane starts to enclose the red blood cell (*R*). **C,** The red blood cells are almost totally engulfed by the macrophage. (Modified from King, D.W., Fenoglio, C.M., & Lefkowitch, J.H. [1983]. *General pathology: Principles and dynamics.* Philadelphia: Lea & Febiger.)

against antigens on the surface of bacteria and are highly specific to that particular microorganism. Certain bacterial and fungal polysaccharide coatings activate the alternative and lectin pathways of complement activation, which deposits C3b on the bacterial surface and increases phagocytosis. The surface of phagocytes contains a variety of specific receptors that will strongly bind to opsonins. These receptors include complement receptors that bind to C3b and Fc receptors that bind to a site on antibody molecules.

Engulfment (endocytosis) is carried out by small pseudopods that extend from the plasma membrane and surround the adherent microorganism, forming an intracellular phagocytic vacuole, or phagosome (see Figures 6-9 and 6-10). After the formation of the phagosome, lysosomes converge, fuse with the phagosome, and discharge their contents, creating a phagolysosome. Destruction of the bacterium takes place within the phagolysosome and is accomplished by both oxygen-dependent and oxygen-independent mechanisms.

Oxygen-dependent killing mechanisms result from the production of toxic oxygen species. Phagocytosis is accompanied by a burst of oxygen uptake by the phagocyte; this process is termed the *respiratory burst* and results from a shift in much of the cell's glucose metabolism to the hexose-monophosphate shunt, which produces NADPH. A membrane-associated enzyme, NADPH oxidase, uses NADPH to generate superoxide (O_2^-), hydrogen peroxide (H_2O_2), and other reactive oxygen species that can be highly damaging to bacteria. Hydrogen peroxide also can collaborate with the lysosomal enzyme *myeloperoxidase* and halide anions (chloride [Cl^-] and bromide [Br^-]) to form acids that kill bacteria and fungi.

Oxygen-independent mechanisms of microbial killing include (1) the acidic pH (3.5 to 4.0) of the phagolysosome, (2) cationic proteins that bind to and damage target cell membranes, (3) enzymatic attack of the microorganism's cell wall by lysozyme and other enzymes, and (4) inhibition of bacterial growth by lactoferrin binding of iron.

When a phagocyte dies at an inflammatory site, it frequently lyses (breaks open) and releases its cytoplasmic contents into the tissue. For example, contents of neutrophil primary granules (lysozyme, hydrolases, neutral proteases) and secondary granules (lysozyme, collagenase, gelatinase) can digest the connective tissue matrix, causing much of the tissue destruction associated with inflammation.[24] The destructive effects of many enzymes and reactive oxygen molecules released by dying phagocytes are minimized by natural inhibitors found in the blood, such as superoxide dismutase (breaks down O_2^-), catalase (breaks down H_2O_2), and the antiproteinases α1-antitrypsin and α_2-macroglobulin (both produced by the liver). An inherited deficiency of α_1-antitrypsin often leads to chronic lung damage and emphysema as a result of inflammation. (The pulmonary effects of α_1-antitrypsin deficiency are described in Chapter 27.)

Natural Killer Cells and Lymphocytes

The main function of natural killer (NK) cells is recognition and elimination of cells infected with viruses, although they also are somewhat effective at elimination of other abnormal cells, specifically cancer cells.[25] NK cells seem to be more efficient in this role when they encounter an infected cell within the circulatory system as opposed to within tissues. NK cells have inhibitory and activating receptors that allow differentiation between infected or tumour cells and normal cells. If the NK cell binds to a target cell through activating receptors, it produces several cytokines and toxic molecules that can kill the target.[26] NK cells and lymphocytes, which are the principal cells of the adaptive immune response, will be discussed in much more detail in Chapter 7.

QUICK CHECK 6-4

1. What are pattern recognition receptors?
2. What are cytokines? How do cytokines promote inflammation?
3. What products do the mast cells release during inflammation, and what are their effects?
4. What phagocytic cell types are involved in the acute inflammatory response? What is the role of each?
5. What are the five steps in the process of phagocytosis?

ACUTE AND CHRONIC INFLAMMATION

Inflammation can be divided into phases of acute and chronic inflammation. The acute inflammatory response is self-limiting—that is, it continues only until the threat to the host is eliminated. This usually takes 8 to 10 days from onset to healing. If the acute inflammatory response proves inadequate, a chronic inflammation may develop and persist for weeks or months. If healing has not been initiated, inflammation may progress to a granulomatous response that is designed to contain the cause of tissue damage so it no longer poses any harm to the individual. The characteristics of the early (i.e., acute) inflammatory response differ from those of the later (i.e., chronic) response, and each phase involves different biochemical mediators and cells that function together. Depending on the successful containment of tissue damage and infection, the acute and chronic phases may lead to healing without progression to the next phase.

Local Manifestations of Acute Inflammation

The cells and plasma protein systems of the inflammatory response interact to produce all the characteristics of inflammation, whether local or systemic (discussed in the next section), as well as determine the duration of inflammation, either acute or chronic. All the local characteristics of **acute inflammation** (i.e., swelling, pain, heat, and redness [erythema]) result from vascular changes and the subsequent leakage of circulating components into the tissue.

The **exudate** of inflammation results from increased vascular permeability and varies in composition, depending on the stage of the inflammatory response and, to some extent, the injurious stimulus. In early or mild inflammation, the exudate may be watery (**serous exudate**) with very few plasma proteins or leukocytes, such as the fluid in a blister. In more severe or advanced inflammation, the exudate may be thick and clotted (**fibrinous exudate**), such as in the lungs of individuals with pneumonia. If a large number of leukocytes accumulate, as in persistent bacterial infections, the exudate consists of pus and is called a **purulent (suppurative) exudate**. Purulent exudate is characteristic of walled-off lesions (**cysts** or **abscesses**). If bleeding occurs, the exudate is filled with erythrocytes and is described as a **hemorrhagic exudate**.

Systemic Manifestations of Acute Inflammation

The three primary systemic changes associated with the acute inflammatory response are fever, leukocytosis (a transient increase in the levels of circulating leukocytes), and increased levels of circulating plasma proteins.

Fever

Fever is partially induced by specific cytokines (e.g., IL-1, released from neutrophils and macrophages). These cytokines are known as **endogenous pyrogens** to differentiate them from pathogen-produced *exogenous pyrogens.* **Pyrogens** act directly on the hypothalamus, the portion of the brain that controls the body's thermostat. (Mechanisms of temperature regulation and fever are discussed in Chapter 14.) A fever can be beneficial because some microorganisms (e.g., those that cause syphilis or gonococcal urethritis) are highly sensitive to small increases in body temperature. On the other hand, fever may have harmful adverse effects because it may enhance the host's susceptibility to the effects of endotoxins associated with Gram-negative bacterial infections (bacterial toxins are described in Chapter 8).

Leukocytosis

Leukocytosis is an increase in the number of circulating white blood cells (greater than 11 000/mL^3 in adults). During many infections, leukocytosis may be accompanied by a *left shift* in the ratio of immature to mature neutrophils, so that the more immature forms of neutrophils, such as band cells, metamyelocytes, and occasionally myelocytes, are present in relatively greater than normal proportions. (Chapter 20 contains a more complete discussion of the development and maturation of blood cells.) Production of immature leukocytes increases primarily from proliferation and release of granulocyte and monocyte precursors in the bone marrow, which is stimulated by several products of inflammation.

TABLE 6-4 Circulating Levels of Acute-Phase Reactants During Inflammation

Function	Increased	Decreased
Coagulation components	Fibrinogen Prothrombin Factor VIII Plasminogen	None
Protease inhibitors	α_1-Antitrypsin α_1-Antichymotrypsin	Inter-α1-antitrypsin
Transport proteins	Haptoglobin Hemopexin Ceruloplasmin Ferritin	Transferrin
Complement components	C1s, C2, C3, C4, C5, C9, factor B, C1 inhibitor	Properdin
Miscellaneous proteins	α_1-Acid glycoprotein Fibronectin Serum amyloid A (SAA) C-reactive protein (CRP)	Albumin Prealbumin α_1-Lipoprotein β-Lipoprotein

Plasma Protein Synthesis

The synthesis of many plasma proteins, mostly products of the liver, is increased during inflammation. These proteins, which can be either proinflammatory or anti-inflammatory in nature, are referred to as **acute-phase reactants** (Table 6-4). Acute-phase reactants reach maximal circulating levels within 10 to 40 hours after the start of inflammation. IL-1 is indirectly responsible for the synthesis of acute-phase reactants through the induction of IL-6, which directly stimulates liver cells to synthesize most of these proteins.

Common laboratory tests for inflammation measure levels of acute-phase reactants. For example, an increase in blood levels of acute-phase reactants, primarily fibrinogen, is associated with an increased adhesion among erythrocytes and a corresponding increase in the sedimentation rate. The erythrocyte sedimentation rate is a measurement of the rate at which red blood cells sediment in a tube over a prescribed time span (usually an hour). Although increased erythrocyte sedimentation is a nonspecific reaction, it is considered a good indicator of an acute inflammatory response.

Chronic Inflammation

Superficially, the difference between acute and chronic inflammation is duration; **chronic inflammation** lasts 2 weeks or longer, regardless of cause. Chronic inflammation is sometimes preceded by an unsuccessful acute inflammatory response (Figure 6-11). For example, if bacterial contamination or foreign objects (e.g., dirt, wood splinter, silica, and glass) persist in a wound, an acute response may be prolonged beyond 2 weeks. Pus formation, suppuration (purulent discharge), and incomplete wound healing may characterize this type of chronic inflammation.

Chronic inflammation can occur also as a distinct process without previous acute inflammation. Some microorganisms (e.g., mycobacteria that cause tuberculosis) have cell walls with a very high lipid and wax content, making them relatively insensitive to breakdown by phagocytes. Other microorganisms (e.g., those that cause leprosy, syphilis, and brucellosis) can survive within the macrophage and avoid removal by the acute inflammatory response. Other microorganisms produce toxins that damage tissue and cause persistent inflammation even after the

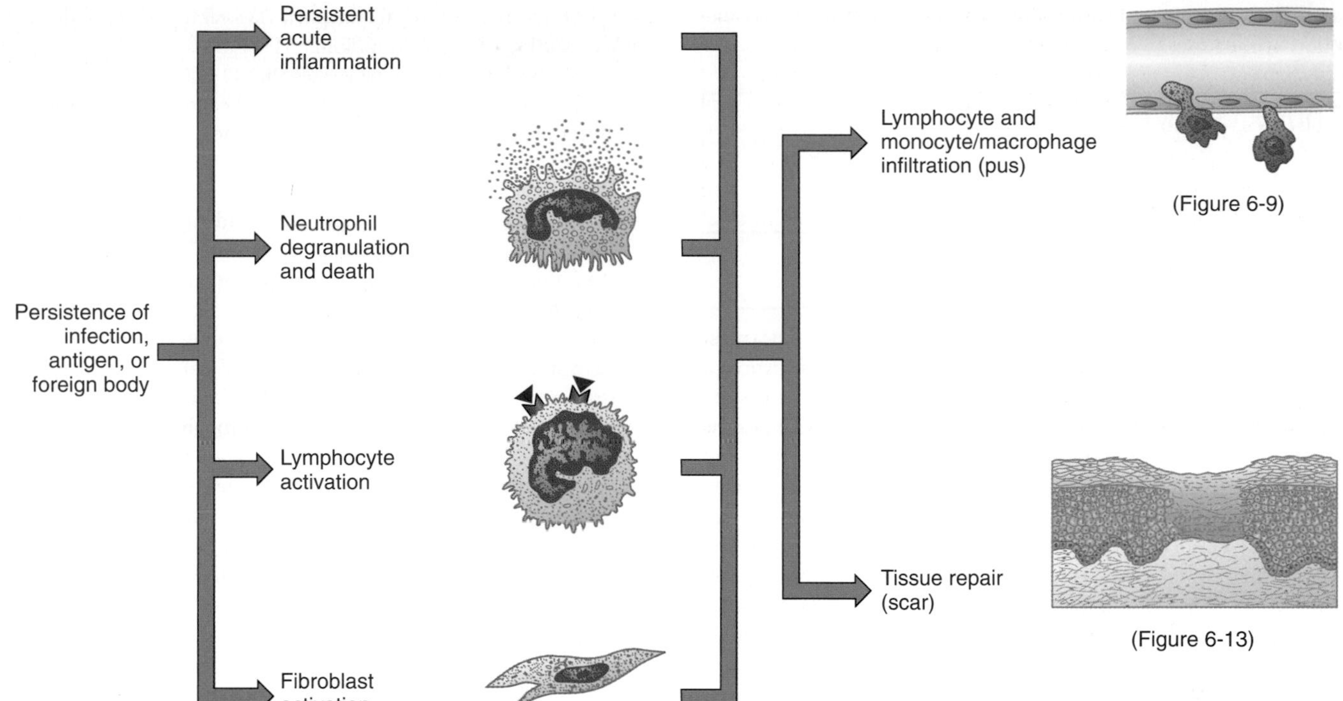

FIGURE 6-11 The Chronic Inflammatory Response. Inflammation usually becomes chronic because of the persistence of an infection, an antigen, or a foreign body in the wound. Chronic inflammation is characterized by the persistence of many of the processes of acute inflammation. In addition, large amounts of neutrophil degranulation and death, the activation of lymphocytes, and the concurrent activation of fibroblasts result in the release of mediators that induce the infiltration of more lymphocytes and monocytes/macrophages and the beginning of wound healing and tissue repair. For more detailed information on each portion of the response, see the figures referenced in this illustration.

organism is killed. Finally, chemicals, particulate matter, or physical irritants (e.g., inhaled dusts, wood splinters, and suture material) can cause a prolonged inflammatory response.

Chronic inflammation is characterized by a dense infiltration of lymphocytes and macrophages. If macrophages are unable to protect the host from tissue damage, the body attempts to wall off and isolate the infected area, thus forming a **granuloma** (Figure 6-12). For example, infections caused by some bacteria (listeriosis, brucellosis), fungi (histoplasmosis, coccidioidomycosis), and parasites (leishmaniasis, schistosomiasis, toxoplasmosis) can result in granuloma formation. TNF-α primarily drives granuloma formation.[27] Some macrophages differentiate into large **epithelioid cells**, which specialize in taking up debris and other small particles. Other macrophages fuse into multinucleated **giant cells**, which are active phagocytes that can engulf very large particles—larger than those that can be engulfed by a single macrophage. These two types of specialized cells form the centre of the granuloma, which is surrounded by a wall of lymphocytes. The granuloma itself is often encapsulated by fibrous deposits of collagen and may become cartilaginous or possibly calcified by deposits of calcium carbonate and calcium phosphate.

The classic granuloma associated with tuberculosis is characterized by a wall of epithelioid cells surrounding a cheeselike proteinaceous centre derived from dead and decaying tissue (caseous necrosis) and mycobacteria.[28] Decay of cells within the granuloma results in the release of acids and the enzymatic contents of lysosomes from dead phagocytes. In this inhospitable environment, the cellular debris is broken down into its basic constituents, and a clear fluid may remain (liquefactive necrosis). Eventually, this fluid diffuses out and leaves a hollow,

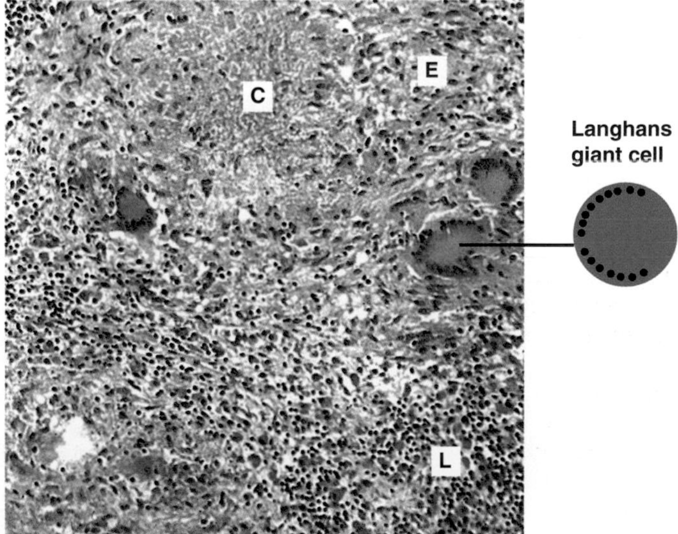

FIGURE 6-12 Tuberculous Granuloma. A central area of amorphous caseous necrosis (*C*) is surrounded by a zone of lymphocytes (*L*) and enlarged epithelioid cells (*E*). Activated macrophages frequently fuse to form multinucleated cells (Langhans giant cells). In tuberculoid granulomas the nuclei of the giant cells move to the cellular margins in a horseshoelike formation.

thick-walled structure that has replaced normal tissue and reduced the function of the lung.

> **✔QUICK CHECK 6-5**
> 1. Describe how acute inflammation differs from chronic inflammation. What characteristics do they share?
> 2. List the types of exudate produced in inflammation.

WOUND HEALING

The conclusion of inflammation is healing and repair. The most favourable outcome is a return to normal structure and function if damage is minor, no complications occur, and destroyed tissues are capable of **regeneration** (replacement of damaged tissue with healthy tissue, such as occurs in the epithelia of the skin and intestines and in some organs, such as the liver) (Figure 6-13). This restoration is called **resolution** and may take up to 2 years, and local production of IL-10 appears to play a critical role.[29] Resolution may not be possible if extensive damage is present, the tissue is not capable of regeneration, infection results in abscess or granuloma formation, or fibrin persists in the lesion. In those cases, repair takes place instead of resolution. **Repair** is the replacement of destroyed tissue with scar tissue. **Scar tissue** is composed primarily of collagen that fills in the lesion and restores strength but cannot carry out the physiological functions of destroyed tissue, resulting in loss of function.

Wound healing involves processes that (1) fill in, (2) seal, and (3) shrink the wound. These characteristics of healing vary in importance and duration among different types of wounds. A clean incision, such as a paper cut or a sutured surgical wound, heals primarily through the process of collagen synthesis. Because this type of wound has minimal tissue loss and close apposition of the wound edges, very little sealing **(epithelialization)** and shrinkage **(contraction)** are required. Wounds that heal under conditions of minimal tissue loss are said to heal by **primary intention** (see Figure 6-13).

Other wounds do not heal as easily. Healing of an open wound, such as a stage IV pressure ulcer (decubitus ulcer), requires a great deal of tissue replacement so that epithelialization, scar formation, and contraction take longer and healing occurs through **secondary intention** (see Figure 6-13). Healing by either primary or secondary intention may occur at different rates for different types of tissue injury.

Epidermal wounds that heal by secondary intention and unsutured internal lesions are not completely restored by healing. At best, repaired tissue regains 80% of its original tensile strength. Only epithelial, hepatic (liver), and bone marrow cells are capable of the complete mitotic regeneration of the normal tissue known as *compensatory hyperplasia*. In fibrous connective tissue, such as joints and ligaments, normal healing results in replacement of the original tissue with new tissue that does

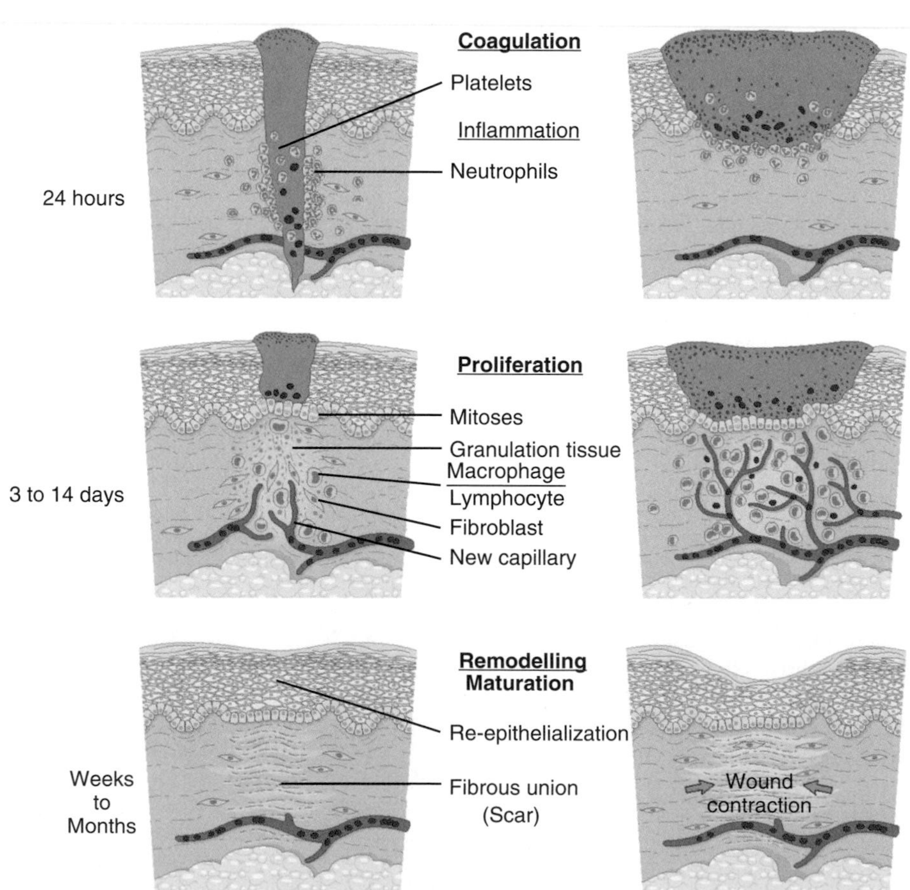

FIGURE 6-13 Wound Healing by Primary and Secondary Intention, and Phases of Wound Healing. Phases of wound healing (coagulation, inflammation, proliferation, remodelling, and maturation) and steps in wound healing by primary intention (*left*) and secondary intention (*right*). Note large amounts of granulation tissue and wound contraction in healing by secondary intention. (From Roberts, J.R., & Custalow, C.B. [2013]. *Roberts and Hedges' clinical procedures in emergency medicine* [6th ed.]. Philadelphia: Saunders.)

not have exactly the same structure or function as that of the original. Some tissues heal without replacement of cells. For example, damage resulting from myocardial infarction heals with a scar composed of fibrous tissue rather than with cardiac muscle.

Wound healing occurs in three overlapping phases: inflammation, proliferation and new tissue formation, and remodelling and maturation.

Phase I: Inflammation

The early phase of wound healing, the transition from acute inflammation to healing, begins almost immediately. The **inflammatory phase** includes coagulation or hemostasis and the infiltration of cells that participate in wound healing, including platelets, neutrophils, and macrophages (Figure 6-14). The fibrin mesh of the blood clot acts as a scaffold for cells that participate in healing. Platelets contribute to clot formation and, as they degranulate, release growth factors that initiate proliferation of undamaged cells. Neutrophils clear the wound of debris and bacteria and are later replaced by macrophages. Macrophages are essential to wound healing because they clear debris, release wound healing mediators and growth factors, recruit fibroblasts, and help promote formation of a new blood supply **(angiogenesis)** during the proliferative phase of wound healing.

Phase II: Proliferation and New Tissue Formation

The proliferative phase begins 3 to 4 days after the injury and continues for as long as 2 weeks. The wound is sealed and the fibrin clot is replaced by normal tissue or scar tissue during this phase. The **proliferative phase** is characterized by macrophage invasion of the dissolving clot and recruitment and proliferation of fibroblasts (connective tissue cells), followed by fibroblast collagen synthesis, epithelialization, contraction of the wound, and cellular differentiation. Macrophages secrete a variety of biochemical mediators that promote healing, including:

- TGF-β stimulates fibroblasts entering the lesion to synthesize and secrete the collagen precursor procollagen.
- **Angiogenesis factors**, such as vascular endothelial growth factor (VEGF) and fibroblast growth factor-2 (FGF-2), stimulate vascular endothelial cells to form capillary buds that grow into the lesion; decreased pH and decreased wound oxygen tension also promote angiogenesis.[30]
- **Matrix metalloproteinases (MMPs)** degrade and remodel extracellular matrix proteins (e.g., collagen and fibrin) at the site of injury.[31]

Granulation tissue grows into the wound from surrounding healthy connective tissue and consists of invasive cells, new lymphatic vessels, and new capillaries derived from capillaries in the surrounding tissue, giving the granulation tissue a red, granular appearance. During this process the healing wound must be protected. Epithelialization is the process by which epithelial cells grow into the wound from surrounding healthy tissue.[32] Epithelial cells migrate under the clot or scab using MMPs to unravel collagen. Migrating epithelial cells contact similar cells from all sides of the wound and seal it. The epithelial cells remain active, undergoing differentiation to give rise to the various epidermal layers (see Chapter 41). Epithelialization of a skin wound can be hastened if the wound is kept moist, preventing the fibrin clot from becoming a scab.

Fibroblasts are important cells during healing because they secrete collagen and other connective tissue proteins. Fibroblasts are stimulated by macrophage-derived TGF-β to proliferate, enter the lesion, and deposit connective tissue proteins in débrided areas about 6 days after the fibroblasts have entered the lesion. **Collagen** is the most abundant protein in the body.[33] It contains high concentrations of the amino acids glycine, proline, and lysine, many of which are enzymatically modified. Modification of proline and lysine requires several cofactors that are absolutely necessary for proper collagen polymerization and function. These include iron, ascorbic acid (vitamin C), and molecular oxygen (O_2); absence

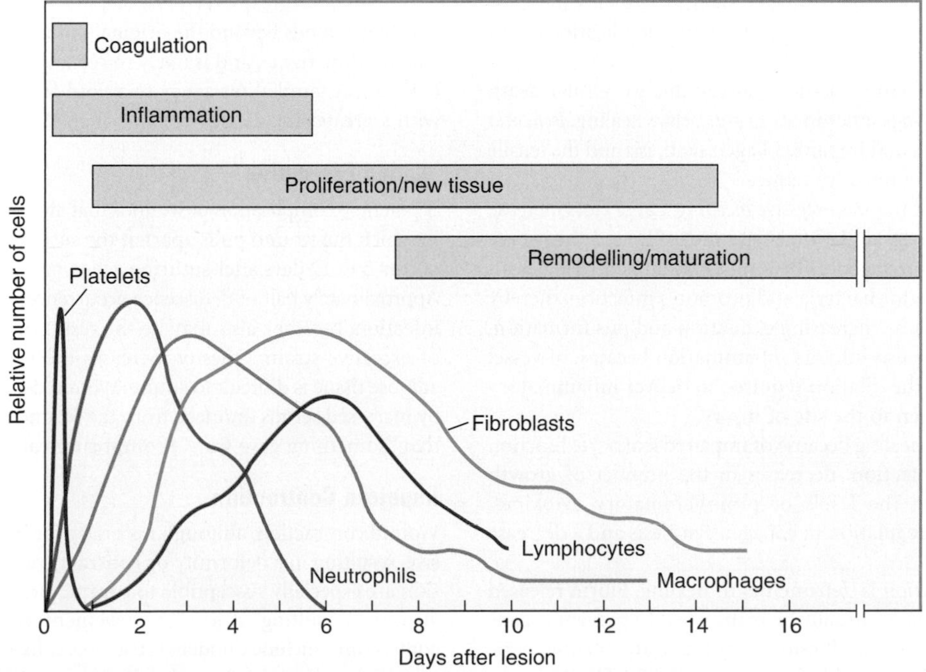

FIGURE 6-14 Time Course of Cells Infiltrating a Wound. Neutrophils and macrophages are the predominant cells that infiltrate a wound during inflammation. Lymphocytes appear later and peak at day 7. Fibroblasts are the predominant cells during the proliferative and remodelling phases of the healing process. (Adapted from Townsend, C.M., Beauchamp, D.R., Evers, B.M., et al. [Eds.]. [2012]. *Sabiston textbook of surgery* [19th ed.]. St. Louis: Elsevier.)

of any of these results in impaired wound healing. As healing progresses, collagen molecules are cross-linked by intermolecular covalent bonds to form collagen fibrils that are further cross-linked to form collagen fibres. The complete process takes several months.

In granulation tissue, TGF-β induces some fibroblasts to transition into **myofibroblasts**, specialized cells responsible for wound contraction.[34] Myofibroblasts have features of both smooth muscle cells and fibroblasts. They appear microscopically similar to fibroblasts but differ in that their cytoplasm contains bundles of parallel fibres similar to those found in smooth muscle cells. **Wound contraction** occurs as extensions from the plasma membrane of myofibroblasts establish connections between neighbouring cells, contract their fibres, and exert tension on the neighbouring cells while anchoring themselves to the wound bed. Wound contraction is necessary for closure of all wounds, especially those that heal by secondary intention. Contraction is noticeable 6 to 12 days after injury.

Phase III: Remodelling and Maturation

Tissue remodelling and maturation begins several weeks after injury and is normally complete within 2 years. During this phase, there is continuation of cellular differentiation, scar formation, and scar remodelling. The fibroblast is the major cell of tissue remodelling with the deposition of collagen into an organized matrix. Tissue regeneration and wound contraction continue in the remodelling and maturation phase—a phase for recovering normal tissue structure that can persist for years. For wounds that heal by scarring, scar tissue is remodelled and capillaries disappear, leaving the scar avascular. Within 2 to 3 weeks after maturation has begun, the scar tissue has gained about two thirds of its eventual maximal strength.

Dysfunctional Wound Healing

Dysfunctional wound healing and impaired epithelialization may occur during any phase of the healing process. The cause of dysfunctional wound healing includes ischemia, excessive bleeding, obesity, excessive fibrin deposition, a predisposing disorder such as diabetes mellitus, wound infection, inadequate nutrients, numerous medications, and tobacco smoke.[35]

Oxygen-deprived (ischemic) tissue is susceptible to cellular death and infection, which prolongs inflammation and delays healing. *Ischemia* reduces energy production and impairs collagen synthesis and the tensile strength of regenerating connective tissue.

Healing is prolonged if there is *excessive bleeding*. Large clots increase the amount of space that granulation tissue must fill, and they serve as mechanical barriers to oxygen diffusion. Accumulated blood is an excellent culture medium for bacteria and promotes infection, thereby prolonging inflammation by increasing exudation and pus formation. Decreased blood volume also inhibits inflammation because of vessel constriction rather than the dilation required to deliver inflammatory cells, nutrients, and oxygen to the site of injury.

Obesity delays wound healing because of impaired leukocyte function and predisposition to infection, decreases in the number of growth factors, and increases in the levels of proinflammatory cytokines. Additionally, there is dysregulation in collagen synthesis and a decrease in angiogenesis.[36]

Excessive fibrin deposition is detrimental to healing. Fibrin released in response to injury must eventually be reabsorbed to prevent organization into fibrous adhesions. Adhesions formed in the pleural, pericardial, or abdominal cavities can bind organs together by fibrous bands and distort or strangulate the affected organ.

Persons with *diabetes* are at risk for prolonged wound healing. Wounds are often ischemic because of the potential for small-vessel diseases that impair the microcirculation and alter (glycosylated) hemoglobin, which has an increased affinity for oxygen and thus does not readily release oxygen in tissues. Consequences of hyperglycemia also include suppression of macrophages and increased risk for wound infection.

Wound infection is caused by the infiltration of pathogens. Pathogens damage cells, stimulate the continued release of inflammatory mediators, consume nutrients, and delay wound healing.

Optimal *nutrition* is important during all phases of healing because metabolic needs increase. Leukocytes need glucose to produce adenosine 5′-triphosphate (5′-adenosine triphosphate [ATP]) necessary for chemotaxis, phagocytosis, intercellular killing, and initiation of healing; therefore the wounds of persons with diabetes who receive insufficient insulin heal poorly. Hypoproteinemia impairs fibroblast proliferation and collagen synthesis. Prolonged lack of vitamins A and C results in poorly formed connective tissue and greatly impaired healing because they are cofactors required for collagen synthesis.[37] Other nutrients, including iron, zinc, manganese, and copper, are also required as cofactors for collagen synthesis. Malnutrition increases risk for wound infection, delays healing, and reduces wound tensile strength.

Medications, including antineoplastic (anticancer) agents, NSAIDs, and steroids, delay wound healing. Antineoplastic agents slow cell division and inhibit angiogenesis. Although NSAIDs inhibit prostaglandin production and suppress acute inflammation and relieve pain, they also can delay wound healing, particularly bone formation, and may contribute to the formation of excessive scarring. Steroids prevent macrophages from migrating to the site of injury and inhibit release of collagenase and plasminogen activator. Steroids also inhibit fibroblast migration into the wound during the proliferative phase and delay epithelialization. Toxic agents in *tobacco smoke* (i.e., nicotine, carbon monoxide, and hydrogen cyanide) delay wound healing and increase the risk for wound infection.

Dysfunctional collagen synthesis may involve excessive production of collagen, leading to a hypertrophic scar or keloid.[38] A **hypertrophic scar** is raised but remains within the original boundaries of the wound and tends to regress over time (Figure 6-15, *A*). A **keloid** is a raised scar that extends beyond the original boundaries of the wound, invades surrounding tissue, and is likely to recur after surgical removal (Figure 6-15, *B*). A familial tendency to keloid formation has been observed, with a greater incidence in Blacks than IN Whites.

Wound Disruption

A potential complication of wounds that are sutured closed is **dehiscence**, in which the wound pulls apart at the suture line. Dehiscence generally occurs 5 to 12 days after suturing, when collagen synthesis is at its peak. Approximately half of dehiscence occurrences are associated with wound infection, but they also may be the result of sutures breaking because of excessive strain. Obesity increases the risk for dehiscence because adipose tissue is difficult to suture. Wound dehiscence usually is heralded by increased serous drainage from the wound and a patient's perception that "something gave way." Prompt surgical attention is required.

Impaired Contraction

Wound contraction, although necessary for healing, may become excessive, resulting in a deformity or **contracture of scar tissue**. Burns of the skin are especially susceptible to contracture development, particularly at joints, resulting in loss of movement around the joints. Internal contractures include duodenal strictures caused by dysfunctional healing of a peptic ulcer; esophageal strictures caused by chemical burns, such as lye ingestion; or abdominal adhesions caused by surgery, infection, or radiation. Contracture may occur in cirrhosis of the liver, constricting vascular flow and contributing to the development of portal hypertension and esophageal varices. Proper positioning, range-of-motion

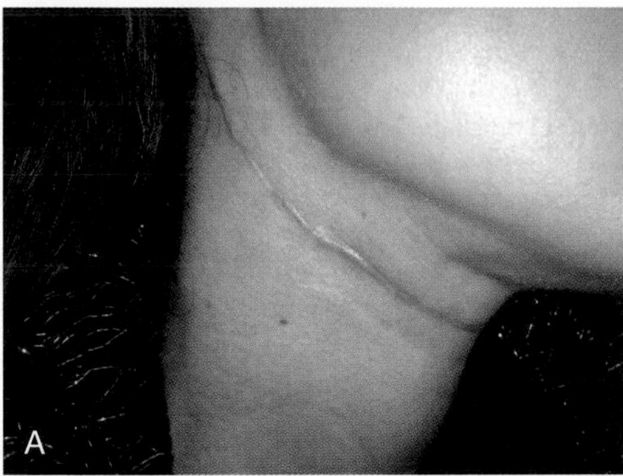

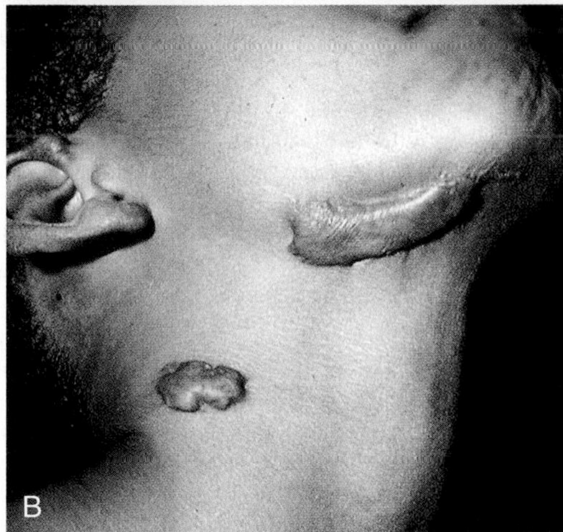

FIGURE 6-15 Hypertrophic Scar and Keloid Scar Formation. Hypertrophic scar (**A**) and keloid scar (**B**) caused by excessive synthesis of collagen at suture sites. (**A,** from Flint, P.W., Haughey, B.H., Lund, V.J., et al. [2015]. *Cummings otolaryngology: Head & neck surgery* [6th ed.]. Philadelphia: Mosby; **B,** from Damjanov, I., & Linder, J. [1996]. *Anderson's pathology* [10th ed.]. St. Louis: Mosby.)

exercises, and surgery are among the physical means used to overcome excessive skin contractures. Surgery is performed to release internal contractures.

QUICK CHECK 6-6

1. How does regeneration of tissue differ from repair of tissue?
2. What does it mean to heal by primary intention?
3. What is the role of fibroblasts in wound healing?
4. Describe various ways in which wound healing may be dysfunctional.

PEDIATRIC CONSIDERATIONS

Age-Related Factors Affecting Innate Immunity in the Newborn Child

- Newborn physiological immunity is acquired from the mother through the placenta and breast milk.
- Newborns have transiently depressed inflammatory responses.
- Neutrophils are incapable of chemotaxis, lacking fluidity in the plasma membrane.
- Complement levels are diminished, especially components of the alternative pathways (e.g., factor B), particularly in premature newborns.
- Monocyte/macrophage numbers are normal, but chemotaxis of monocytes is delayed.
- There is a tendency for infections associated with chemotactic defects, for example, cutaneous abscesses caused by staphylococci and cutaneous candidiasis.
- There are diminished oxidative and bacterial responses in those stressed by in utero infection or respiratory insufficiency.
- There is a tendency to develop severe overwhelming sepsis and meningitis when infected by bacteria against which no maternal antibodies are present.
- The establishment of the gut microbiome is facilitated by breast milk.
- Caesarean-delivered newborns have reduced gut microbial diversity.

GERIATRIC CONSIDERATIONS

Age-Related Factors Affecting Innate Immunity in Older Adults

- Older adults have normal numbers of cells of innate immunity, but the cells may have diminished function (e.g., decreased phagocytic activity, decreased antibody production, and altered cytokine synthesis).
- The incidence of chronic inflammation is higher, possibly related to an increased production of proinflammatory mediators.
- Older adults are at risk for impaired healing and infection associated with chronic illness (e.g., diabetes mellitus, peripheral vascular disease, or cardiovascular disease) and decreased phagocytosis.
- The use of medications may interfere with healing (e.g., anti-inflammatory steroids).
- A loss of subcutaneous fat diminishes layers of protection against injury.
- Atrophied epidermis, including underlying capillaries, decreases perfusion and increases the risk of hypoxia in the wound bed.
- The aging of the immune system can diminish the effectiveness of vaccines.

DID YOU UNDERSTAND?

Human Defence Mechanisms

1. The three lines of human defence from injury and infection are innate immunity (which includes natural barriers), inflammatory response, and adaptive (acquired) immunity.
2. Physical barriers are the first lines of defence that prevent damage to the individual and prevent invasion by pathogens; these include the skin and mucous membranes.
3. Antibacterial peptides (cathelicidins, defensins, collectins, and mannose-binding lectin) in mucous secretions, perspiration, saliva, tears, and other secretions provide a biochemical barrier against pathogenic microorganisms.
4. The skin and mucous membranes are colonized by commensal or mutualistic microorganisms that provide protection by releasing chemicals that facilitate immune responses, prevent colonization by pathogens, and facilitate digestion in the gastro-intestinal tract.
5. The second line of defence is the inflammatory response (inflammation), a rapid and nonspecific protective response to cellular injury from any cause. It can occur only in vascularized tissue.

6. The macroscopic hallmarks of inflammation are redness, swelling, heat, pain, and loss of function of the inflamed tissues.
7. The microscopic hallmarks of inflammation are vasodilation, increased capillary permeability, and an accumulation of fluid and cells at the inflammatory site.
8. Inflammation is mediated by three key plasma protein systems: the complement system, the clotting system, and the kinin system. The components of all three systems are a series of inactive proteins that are activated sequentially.
9. The complement system can be activated by antigen-antibody reactions (through the classical pathway) or by other products, especially bacterial polysaccharides (through the lectin pathway or the alternative pathway), resulting in the production of biologically active fragments that recruit phagocytes, activate mast cells, and destroy pathogens.
10. The most biologically potent products of the complement system are C3b (opsonin), C3a (anaphylatoxin), and C5a (anaphylatoxin, chemotactic factor).
11. The clotting system stops bleeding, localizes microorganisms, and provides a meshwork for repair and healing.
12. Bradykinin is the most important product of the kinin system and causes vascular permeability, smooth muscle contraction, and pain.
13. Control of inflammation regulates inflammatory cells and enzymes and localizes the inflammatory response to the area of injury or infection.
14. Carboxypeptidase, histaminase, and C1 esterase inhibitor are inactivating enzymes, and the fibrinolytic system and plasmin facilitate clot degradation after bleeding is stopped.
15. Many different types of cells are involved in the inflammatory process, including mast cells, endothelial cells, platelets, phagocytes (neutrophils, eosinophils, monocytes/macrophages, dendritic cells), natural killer cells, and lymphocytes.
16. Most cells express plasma membrane pattern recognition receptors that recognize molecules produced by infectious microorganisms (pathogen-associated molecular patterns, or PAMPs), or products of cellular damage (damage-associated molecular patterns, or DAMPs). Toll-like receptors and NOD-like receptors are expressed on many inflammatory cells, recognize PAMPs and DAMPs, and promote release of cytokines and inflammatory mediators that eliminate damaged cells and protect against invasion by microbes.
17. The cells of the innate immune system secrete many biochemical mediators (cytokines) that are responsible for activating other cells and regulating the inflammatory response; these cytokines include chemokines, interleukins, interferons, and other molecules.
18. Chemokines induce chemotaxis of leukocytes, fibroblasts, and other cells to promote phagocytosis and wound healing.
19. Interleukins are produced primarily by lymphocytes and macrophages and promote or inhibit inflammation by activating growth and differentiation of leukocytes and lymphocytes.
20. The most important proinflammatory interleukins are interleukin-1 (IL-1), interleukin-6 (IL-6), and tumour necrosis factor-alpha. IL-6 and interleukin-10 downregulate the inflammatory response.
21. Interferons are produced by cells that are infected by viruses. Once released from infected cells, interferons can stimulate neighbouring healthy cells to produce substances that prevent viral infection.
22. The most important activator of the inflammatory response is the mast cell, which is located in connective tissue near capillaries and initiates inflammation by releasing biochemical mediators (histamine, chemotactic factors) from preformed cytoplasmic granules and synthesizing other mediators (prostaglandins, leukotrienes, and platelet-activating factor) in response to a stimulus. Basophils are found in the blood and probably function in the same way as tissue mast cells.
23. Histamine is the major vasoactive amine released from mast cells. It causes dilation of capillaries and retraction of endothelial cells lining the capillaries, which increases vascular permeability.
24. The endothelial cells lining the circulatory system (vascular endothelium) normally regulate circulating components of the inflammatory system and maintain normal blood flow by preventing spontaneous activation of platelets and members of the clotting system.
25. Platelets interact with the coagulation cascade to stop bleeding and release a number of mediators that promote and control inflammation.
26. During inflammation the endothelium expresses receptors that help leukocytes leave the vessel and retract to allow fluid to pass into the tissues.
27. The polymorphonuclear neutrophil, the predominant phagocytic cell in the early inflammatory response, exits the circulation by diapedesis through the retracted endothelial cell junctions and moves to the inflammatory site by chemotaxis.
28. Eosinophils release products that control the inflammatory response and are the principal cell that kills parasitic organisms.
29. The macrophage, the predominant phagocytic cell in the late inflammatory response, is highly phagocytic, is responsive to cytokines, and promotes wound healing.
30. Dendritic cells connect the innate and acquired immune systems by collecting antigens at the site of inflammation and transporting them to sites, such as the lymph nodes, where immunocompetent B and T cells reside and are transformed into functional cells.
31. Phagocytosis is a multistep cellular process for the elimination of pathogens and foreign debris. The steps are (a) recognition and attachment, (b) engulfment, (c) formation of a phagosome, (d) fusion of the phagosome with lysosomal granules within the phagocyte, and (e) destruction of the target. Phagocytic cells engulf microorganisms and enclose them in phagocytic vacuoles (phagolysosomes), within which toxic products (especially metabolites of oxygen) and degradative lysosomal enzymes kill and digest the microorganisms.
32. Opsonins, such as antibody and complement component C3b, coat microorganisms and make them more susceptible to phagocytosis by binding them more tightly to the phagocyte.

Acute and Chronic Inflammation

1. Acute inflammation is self-limiting and usually resolves within 8 to 10 days.
2. Local manifestations of inflammation are the result of the vascular changes associated with the inflammatory process, including vasodilation and increased capillary permeability. The symptoms include redness, heat, swelling, and pain.
3. The principal systemic effects of inflammation are fever and increases in levels of circulating leukocytes (leukocytosis) and plasma proteins (acute-phase reactants [i.e., IL-1 and IL-6]).
4. Chronic inflammation can be a continuation of acute inflammation that lasts 2 weeks or longer. It also can occur as a distinct process without much preceding acute inflammation.
5. Chronic inflammation is characterized by a dense infiltration of lymphocytes and macrophages. The body may wall off and isolate the infection to protect against tissue damage by formation of a granuloma.

Wound Healing

1. Resolution and regeneration refer to the return of tissue to nearly normal structure and function. Repair refers to healing by scar tissue formation.
2. Damaged tissue proceeds to resolution (restoration of the original tissue structure and function) if little tissue has been lost or if injured tissue is capable of regeneration. Wounds that heal under conditions of minimal tissue loss are said to heal by primary intention.
3. Tissues that sustained extensive damage or those incapable of regeneration heal by the process of repair resulting in the formation of a scar. This process is called healing by secondary intention.
4. Resolution and repair occur in two separate phases: the reconstructive phase in which the wound begins to heal and the maturation phase in which the healed wound is remodelled.
5. Dysfunctional wound healing can be related to ischemia, excessive bleeding, obesity, excessive fibrin deposition, a predisposing disorder such as diabetes mellitus, wound infection, inadequate nutrients, numerous medications, and tobacco smoke.
6. Dehiscence is a disruption in which the wound pulls apart at the suture line.
7. A contracture of scar tissue is a deformity caused by the excessive shortening of collagen in scar tissue.

Pediatric Considerations: Age-Related Factors Affecting Innate Immunity in the Newborn Child

1. Newborns have transiently depressed inflammatory function, particularly neutrophil chemotaxis and alternative complement pathway activity.

Geriatric Considerations: Age-Related Factors Affecting Innate Immunity in Older Adults

1. Older adults are at risk for impaired wound healing, usually because of chronic illnesses.

KEY TERMS

Abscess, 150
Acute inflammation, 150
Acute-phase reactant, 150
Adaptive (acquired) immunity, 135
α_1-Antitrypsin, 149
Alternative pathway, 141
Anaphylatoxin, 141
Angiogenesis, 153
Angiogenesis factor, 153
Antimicrobial peptide, 137
Basophil, 145
Blood clot, 141
Bradykinin, 141
C1 esterase inhibitor (C1 INH), 141
C1 INH deficiency, 142
Carboxypeptidase, 141
Cathelicidin, 137
Chemokine, 143
Chemotactic factor, 141
Chemotaxis, 145
Chronic inflammation, 150
Classical pathway, 141
Clotting (coagulation) system, 141
Collagen, 153
Collectin, 137
Complement receptor, 143
Complement system, 140
Contact activation (intrinsic) pathway, 141
Contraction, 152
Contracture of scar tissue, 154
Cyst, 150
Cytokine, 143
Damage-associated molecular pattern (DAMP), 142
Defensin, 137
Degranulation, 145
Dehiscence, 154
Dendritic cell, 147
Diapedesis, 147
Endogenous pyrogen, 150
Endothelial cell, 146
Eosinophil, 147
Eosinophil chemotactic factor of anaphylaxis (ECF-A), 145
Epithelialization, 152
Epithelioid cell, 151
Exudate, 150
Fc receptor, 149
Fever, 150
Fibrinolytic system, 141
Fibrinous exudate, 150
Fibroblast, 153
Giant cell, 151
Granulation tissue, 153
Granuloma, 151
Hageman factor (factor XII), 141
Hemorrhagic exudate, 150
Hereditary angioedema, 142
Hexose-monophosphate shunt, 149
Histaminase, 141
Histamine, 145
Hypertrophic scar, 154
Inflammasomes, 143
Inflammation, 138
Inflammatory phase, 153
Inflammatory response, 135
Innate immunity, 135
Interferon (IFN), 145
Interleukin (IL), 143
Interleukin-1 (IL-1), 144
Interleukin-6 (IL-6), 144
Interleukin-10 (IL-10), 145
Keloid, 154
Kinin system, 141
Lectin pathway, 141
Leukocytosis, 150
Leukotriene (slow-reacting substance of anaphylaxis [SRS-A]), 146
Lymphocyte, 142
Lysozyme, 137
Macrophage, 147
Mannose-binding lectin (MBL), 137
Margination (pavementing), 147
Mast cell, 145
Matrix metalloproteinase (MMP), 153
Monocyte, 147
Myofibroblast, 154
Natural killer (NK) cell, 149
Neutrophil (polymorphonuclear neutrophil [PMN]), 147
Neutrophil chemotactic factor (NCF), 145
Nitric oxide (NO), 146
NOD-like receptors (NLRs), 143
Normal flora, 137
Normal microbiome, 137
Opportunistic microorganism, 138
Opsonin, 141
Opsonization, 148
Pathogen-associated molecular pattern (PAMP), 142
Pattern recognition receptor (PRR), 142
Phagocyte, 139
Phagocytosis, 146
Phagolysosome, 149
Phagosome, 149
Plasma protein system, 140
Plasmin, 141
Plasminogen, 141
Platelet, 146
Platelet-activating factor (PAF), 146
Primary intention, 152
Proliferative phase, 153
Prostacyclin (PGI_2), 146
Prostaglandin, 146
Purulent (suppurative) exudate, 150
Pyrogen, 150
Regeneration, 152
Repair, 152
Resolution, 152
Scar tissue, 152
Scavenger receptors, 143
Secondary intention, 152
Serous exudate, 150
T lymphocyte (T cell), 147
Tissue factor (extrinsic) pathway, 141
Tissue factor (TF; tissue thromboplastin), 141
Toll-like receptor (TLR), 142
Transforming growth factor, 145
Transforming growth factor-beta (TGF-β), 145
Tumour necrosis factor-alpha (TNF-α), 143
Wound contraction, 154

REFERENCES

1. Peterson, L. W., & Artis, D. (2014). Intestinal epithelial cells: Regulators of barrier function and immune homeostasis. *Nature Reviews. Immunology*, *14*(3), 141–153. doi:10.1038/nri3608.
2. Human Microbiome Project Consortium. (2012). Structure, function and diversity of the healthy human microbiome. *Nature*, *486*(7402), 207–214. doi:10.1038/nature11234.
3. Mayer, E. A., Tillisch, K., & Gupta, A. (2015). Gut/brain axis and the microbiota. *Journal of Clinical Investigation*, *125*(3), 926–938. doi:10.1172/JCI76304.
4. Liévin-Le Moal, V., & Servin, A. L. (2014). Anti-infective activities of *Lactobacillus* strains in the human intestinal microbiota: From probiotics to gastrointestinal anti-infectious biotherapeutic agents. *Clinical Microbiology Reviews*, *27*(2), 167–199. doi:10.1128/CMR.00080-13.
5. Ricklin, D., & Lambris, J. D. (2013). Complement in immune and inflammatory disorders: Therapeutic interventions. *Journal of Immunology*, *190*(8), 3839–3847. doi:10.4049/jimmunol.1203200.
6. Sekine, H., Takahashi, M., Iwaki, D., et al. (2013). The role of MASP-1/3 in complement activation. *Advances in Experimental Medicine and Biology*, *735*, 41–53.
7. O'Neil, L. A., Golenbock, D., & Bowie, A. G. (2013). The history of Toll-like receptors—redefining innate immunity. *Nature Reviews. Immunology*, *13*(6), 453–460. doi:10.1038/nri3446.
8. Qian, C., & Cao, X. (2013). Regulation of Toll-like receptor signaling pathways in innate immune responses. *Annals of the New York Academy of Sciences*, *1283*, 67–74. doi:10.1111/j.1749-6632.2012.06786.x.
9. Canton, J., Neculai, D., & Grinstein, S. (2013). Scavenger receptors in homeostasis and immunity. *Nature Reviews. Immunology*, *13*(9), 621–634. doi:10.1038/nri3515.
10. Philpott, D. J., Sorbara, M. T., Robertson, S. J., et al. (2014). NOD proteins: Regulators of inflammation in health and disease. *Nature Reviews. Immunology*, *14*(1), 9–23. doi:10.1038/nri3565.
11. Saxena, M., & Yeretssian, G. (2014). NOD-like receptors: Master regulators of inflammation and cancer. *Frontiers in Immunology*, *5*, 327. doi:10.3389/fimmu.2014.00327.
12. Schett, G., Elewaut, D., McInnes, I. B., et al. (2013). Toward a cytokine-based disease taxonomy. *Nature Medicine*, *19*(7), 822–824. doi:10.1038/nm.3260.
13. Martins-Green, M., Petreaca, M., & Wang, L. (2013). Chemokines and their receptors are key players in the orchestra that regulates wound healing. *Advances in Wound Care*, *2*(7), 327–347. doi:10.1089/wound.2012.0380.
14. Akdis, M., Burgler, S., Crameri, R., et al. (2011). Interleukins, from 1 to 37 and interferon-γ: Receptors, functions, and roles in diseases. *Journal of Allergy and Clinical Immunology*, *127*(3), 701–721. doi:10.1016/j.jaci.2010.11.050.
15. Ivashkiv, L. B., & Donlin, L. T. (2014). Regulation of type I interferon responses. *Nature Reviews. Immunology*, *14*(1), 36–49. doi:10.1038/nri3581.
16. Cromheecke, J. L., Nguyen, K. T., & Huston, D. P. (2014). Emerging role of human basophil biology in health and disease. *Current Allergy and Asthma Reports*, *14*(1), 408. doi:10.1007/s11882-013-0408-2.
17. Kolaczkowska, E., & Kubes, P. (2013). Neutrophil recruitment and function in health and inflammation. *Nature Reviews. Immunology*, *13*(3), 159–175. doi:10.1038/nri3399.
18. Melo, R. C., Liu, L., Xenakis, J. J., et al. (2013). Eosinophil-derived cytokines in health and disease: Unraveling novel mechanisms of selective secretion. *Allergy*, *68*(3), 274–284. doi:10.1111/all.12103.
19. Wynn, T. A., Chawla, A., & Pollard, J. W. (2013). Macrophage biology in development, homeostasis and disease. *Nature*, *496*(7446), 445–455. doi:10.1038/nature12034.
20. Van Dyken, S. J., & Locksley, R. M. (2013). Interleukin-4- and interleukin-13-mediated alternatively activated macrophages: Roles in homeostasis and disease. *Annual Review of Immunology*, *31*(2013), 317–343. doi:10.1146/annurev-immunol-032712-095906.
21. Platt, A. M., & Randolph, G. J. (2013). Dendritic cell migration through the lymphatic vasculature to lymph nodes. *Advances in Immunology*, *120*, 51–68. doi:10.1016/B978-0-12-417028-5.00002-8.
22. Herter, J., & Zarbock, A. (2013). Integrin regulation during leukocyte recruitment. *Journal of Immunology*, *190*(9), 4451–4457. doi:10.4049/jimmunol.1203179.
23. Weninger, W., Biro, M., & Jain, R. (2014). Leukocyte migration in the interstitial space of non-lymphoid organs. *Nature Reviews. Immunology*, *14*(4), 232–248. doi:10.1038/nri3641.
24. Wilgus, T. A., Roy, S., & McDaniel, J. C. (2013). Neutrophils and wound repair: Positive actions and negative reactions. *Advances in Wound Care*, *2*(7), 379–388. doi:10.1089/wound.2012.0383.
25. Campbell, K. S., & Hasegawa, J. (2013). Natural killer cell biology: An update and future directions. *Journal of Allergy and Clinical Immunology*, *132*(3), 536–544. doi:10.1016/j.jaci.2013.07.006.
26. Long, E. O., Kim, H. S., Liu, D., et al. (2013). Controlling natural killer cell responses: Integration of signals for activation and inhibition. *Annual Review of Immunology*, *31*, 227–258. doi:10.1146/annurev-immunol-020711-075005.
27. Dorhoi, A., & Kaufmann, S. H. (2014). Tumor necrosis factor alpha in mycobacterial infection. *Seminars in Immunology*, *26*(3), 203–209. doi:10.1016/j.smim.2014.04.003.
28. O'Garra, A., Redford, P. S., McNab, F. W., et al. (2013). The immune response to tuberculosis. *Annual Review of Immunology*, *31*, 475–527. doi:10.1146/annurev-immunol-032712-095939.
29. King, A., Balaji, S., Le, L. D., et al. (2014). Regenerative wound healing: The role of interleukin-10. *Advances in Wound Care*, *3*(4), 315–323. doi:10.1089/wound.2013.0461.
30. Raju, R., Palapetta, S. M., Sandhya, V. K., et al. (2014). A network map of EGF-1/FGFR signaling system. *Journal of Signal Transduction*, *2014*, 962962. doi:10.1155/2014/962962.
31. Khokha, R., Murthy, A., & Weiss, A. (2013). Metalloproteinases and their natural inhibitors in inflammation and immunity. *Nature Reviews. Immunology*, *13*(9), 649–665. doi:10.1038/nri3499.
32. Longmate, W. M., & Dipersio, C. M. (2014). Integrin regulation of epidermal function in wounds. *Advances in Wound Care*, *3*(3), 229–246. doi:10.1089/wound.2013.0516.
33. Mienaltowski, M. J., & Birk, D. E. (2014). Structure, physiology, and biochemistry of collagens. *Advances in Experimental Medicine and Biology*, *802*(2014), 5–29. doi:10.1007/978-94-007-7893-1_2.
34. Yang, X., Chen, B., Liu, T., et al. (2014). Reversal of myofibroblast differentiation: A review. *European Journal of Pharmacology*, *734*, 83–90. doi:10.1016/j.ejphar.2014.04.007.
35. Pierpont, Y. N., Dinh, T. P., Salas, R. E., et al. (2014). Obesity and surgical wound healing: A current review. *ISRN Obesity*, *2014*, 638936. doi:10.1155/2014/638936.
36. Pence, B. D., & Woods, J. A. (2014). Exercise, obesity, and cutaneous wound healing: Evidence from rodent and human studies. *Advances in Wound Care*, *3*(1), 71–79. doi:10.1089/wound.2012.0377.
37. Moores, J. (2013). Vitamin C: A wound healing perspective. *British Journal of Community Nursing Supplement*, *S6*, S8–S11.
38. Monstrey, S., Middelkoop, E., Vranckx, J. J., et al. (2014). Updated scar management practical guidelines: Non-invasive and invasive measures. *Journal of Plastic, Reconstructive and Aesthetic Surgery*, *67*(8), 1017–1025. doi:10.1016/j.bjps.2014.04.011.

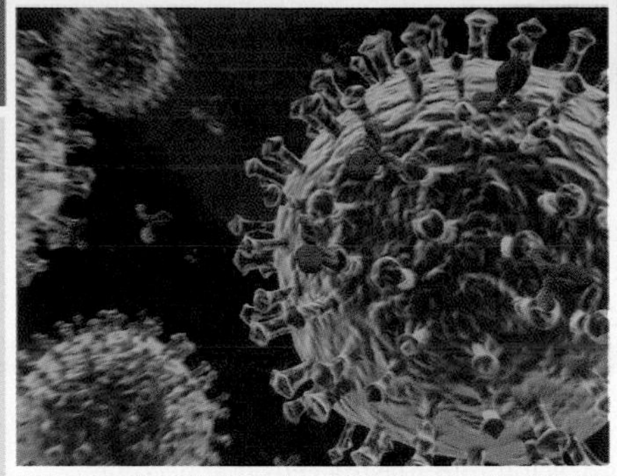

7

Adaptive Immunity

Neal S. Rote and Stephanie Zettel

EVOLVE WEBSITE

http://evolve.elsevier.com/Canada/Huether/pathophysiology
Student Review Questions
Key Points
Case Studies
Animations
Quick Check Answers

CHAPTER OUTLINE

Third Line of Defence: Adaptive Immunity, 159
Antigens and Immunogens, 161
Antibodies, 161
Classes of Immunoglobulins, 162
Antigen–Antibody Binding, 163
Function of Antibodies, 163
Immune Response: Collaboration of B Cells and T Cells, 165
Generation of Clonal Diversity, 165
Clonal Selection, 168
Cell-Mediated Immunity, 171
T-Lymphocyte Function, 171
PEDIATRIC CONSIDERATIONS: **Age-Related Factors Affecting Mechanisms of Self-Defence in the Newborn Child, 174**
GERIATRIC CONSIDERATIONS: **Age-Related Factors Affecting Mechanisms of Self-Defence in Older Adults, 174**

The third line of defence in the human body is **adaptive (acquired) immunity**, often called the **immune response** or **immunity**, and consists of **lymphocytes** (Figure 7-1) and serum proteins called *antibodies*. Once external barriers have been compromised and inflammation (innate immunity, see Chapter 6) has been activated, the adaptive immune response is called into action. Inflammation is the "first responder" that contains the initial injury and slows the spread of infection, whereas adaptive immunity slowly augments the initial defences against infection and provides long-term security against re-infection.

THIRD LINE OF DEFENCE: ADAPTIVE IMMUNITY

Inflammation and adaptive immunity differ in several key ways. First, the components of inflammation are activated immediately after tissue damage. Adaptive immunity is *inducible*; the effectors of the immune response, lymphocytes and antibodies, do not pre-exist but must be produced in response to infection. Thus, adaptive immunity develops more slowly than inflammation. Second, the inflammatory response is similar regardless of differences in the cause of tissue damage or whether the inflammatory site is sterile or contaminated with infectious microorganisms. The immune response is exquisitely *specific*. The lymphocytes and antibodies induced in response to infection are extremely specific to the infecting microbe. Third, the residual mediators of inflammation must be removed quickly to limit damage to surrounding healthy tissue and allow healing. The effectors of the immune response are *long-lived* and systemic, providing long-term protection against specific infections. Finally, the inflammatory response to both recurrent tissue damage and infection is identical. The immune response has *memory*. If re-infected with the same microbe, protective lymphocytes and antibody are produced immediately, thus providing permanent long-term protection against infection.

Despite the differences, the innate and adaptive immune systems are highly interactive and complementary. Many components of innate resistance are necessary for the development of the adaptive immune response. Conversely, products of the adaptive immune response activate components of innate resistance. Thus, both systems are essential for complete protection against infectious disease.

The mechanisms underlying the immune response will be discussed in this chapter. As with Chapter 6, a complete description of all the important components and processes of an effective immune response would require far more space than available. Therefore, this chapter will focus on the basic concepts and the most important, or well-studied, mediators of the immune response.

The adaptive immune response has its own vocabulary (Figure 7-2). **Antigens** are the molecular targets of antibodies and lymphocytes. Antigens are generally small molecules, usually within proteins, carbohydrates, or lipids, found on the surface of microbes or infected cells, although this definition will be expanded as we discuss immunological diseases in Chapter 8. In the fetus, well before being exposed to any infectious microorganisms, lymphocytes have undergone extensive differentiation. Some lymphoid stem cells enter the thymus and differentiate into **T lymphocytes (T cells,** *T* indicates thymus derived), whereas others enter specific regions of the bone marrow and differentiate into **B lymphocytes (B cells,** *B* indicates bone-marrow–derived). Each type of cell develops origin-specific cell surface proteins that identify them as T or B cells. Both B and T cells also develop cell surface antigen receptors. The receptors are remarkable because an individual lymphocyte is programmed to recognize only one specific antigen before having encountered that antigen. It is estimated that before birth each individual has produced a population of B and T cells capable of recognizing at least 10^8 different antigens. This process is called generation of **clonal diversity** and refers to the process by which the extensive diversity of antigen receptors on B and T cells is established (see Figure 7-2).

Lymphocytes leave the primary lymphoid organs (bone marrow and thymus) as immunocompetent, but naive, B and T cells. The cells are **immunocompetent** in that they have the capacity to respond to antigens, but they are *naive* in that they have not yet encountered antigen. These cells enter the blood and lymphatic vessels and migrate to the **secondary lymphoid organs** (e.g., lymph nodes, spleen) of the systemic immune system (Figure 7-3). Some take up residence in B-cell and T-cell–rich areas of those organs, and others re-enter the circulation. Approximately 60 to 70% of circulating lymphocytes are immunocompetent T cells, and 10 to 20% are immunocompetent B cells.

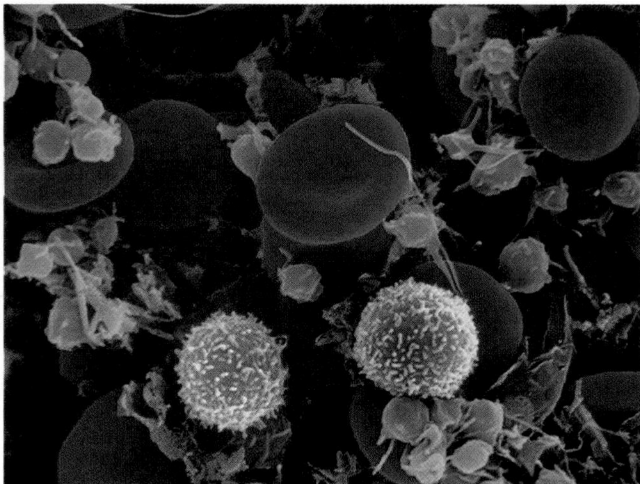

FIGURE 7-1 Lymphocytes. A scanning electron micrograph showing lymphocytes (yellow, like cotton candy), red blood cells, and platelets. (Dennis Kunkel Microscopy / Science Source).

A second process, *clonal selection*, is initiated when an infection occurs. This process requires the cooperation among a variety of cells in the secondary lymphoid organs; antigen needs to be *processed* by phagocytic cells, primarily dendritic cells, which also express the processed antigen on their surfaces and *present* the antigen to lymphocytes. Thus begins a symphony of cellular interactions, referred to as **clonal selection**, involving several subsets of B and T cells, intercellular adhesion through antigen receptors and specific intercellular adhesion molecules, the production and response to multiple cytokines, and eventual differentiation of immunocompetent B and T cells into highly specialized effector cells. B cells develop into **plasma cells** that become factories for the production of antibody. T cells develop into several subsets that can identify and kill a target cell (**T-cytotoxic cells, Tc cells**), regulate the immune response by helping the clonal selection process (**T-helper cells, Th cells**), or suppress inappropriate immune responses (**T-regulatory cells, Treg cells**). Both B and T cells also differentiate into very long-lived **memory cells** that exist for decades or, in some cases, for the life of the individual. Memory cells are rapidly activated if a second infection occurs with the same microbe.

Antibodies circulate in the blood and defend against extracellular microbes and microbial toxins. This response is referred to as the *humoral immune response*, or **humoral immunity**. Effector T cells are found in the blood and tissues and defend against intracellular pathogens (e.g., viruses) and cancer cells. This response is referred to as the *cellular immune response*, or **cellular immunity** (also cell-mediated immunity).

The preceding overview describes what is termed **active immunity (active acquired immunity)**, which develops in response to antigens. In certain clinical situations, preformed antibody or lymphocytes may be administered to an individual, termed **passive immunity (passive acquired immunity)**. Examples include individuals exposed to an infectious agent without having a pre-existing vaccine-induced immunity (e.g., hepatitis A virus or rabies virus) (Table 7-1). Passive immunization with specific T cells has been used to treat several forms of cancer. Whereas active acquired immunity is long lived, passive immunity is only temporary because the donor's antibodies or T cells are eventually destroyed.

TABLE 7-1 Clinical Use of Antigen or Antibody

	USE OF ANTIGEN OR ANTIBODY			
Antigen Source	**Protection: Combat Active Disease**	**Protection: Vaccination**	**Diagnosis**	**Therapy**
Infectious agents	Neutralize or destroy pathogenic microorganisms (e.g., antibody response against viral infections)	Induce safe and protective immune response (e.g., recommended childhood vaccines)	Measure circulating antigen from infectious agent or antibody (e.g., diagnosis of hepatitis B infection)	Passive treatment with antibody to treat or prevent infection (e.g., administration of antibody against hepatitis A)
Cancers	Prevent tumour growth or spread (e.g., immune surveillance to prevent early cancers)	Prevent cancer growth or spread (e.g., vaccination with cancer antigens)	Measure circulating antigen (e.g., circulating PSA for diagnosis of prostate cancer)	Immunotherapy (e.g., treatment of cancer with antibodies against cancer antigens)
Environmental substances	Prevent entrance into body (e.g., secretory IgA limits systemic exposure to potential allergens)	No clear example	Measure circulating antigen or antibody (e.g., diagnosis of allergy by measuring circulating IgE)	Immunotherapy (e.g., administration of antigen for desensitization of individuals with severe allergies)
Self-antigens	Immune system tolerance to self-antigens, which can be altered by an infectious agent leading to autoimmune disease (see Chapter 8)	Some cases of vaccination alter tolerance to self-antigens, leading to autoimmune disease	Measure circulating antibody against self-antigen for diagnosis of autoimmune disease (see Chapter 8)	Oral administration of self-antigens to diminish production of autoimmune disease–associated autoantibodies

PSA, prostate-specific antigen.

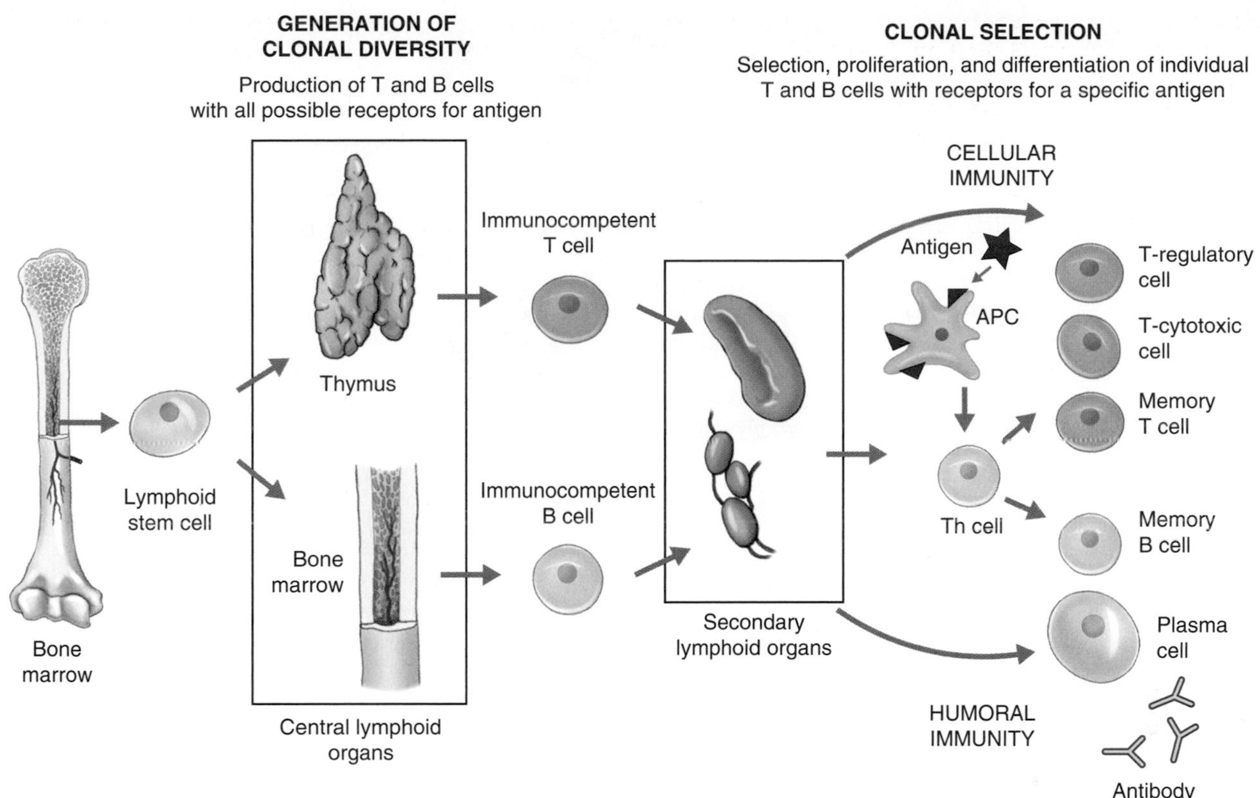

FIGURE 7-2 Overview of the Immune Response. The immune response can be separated into two phases: the *generation of clonal diversity* and *clonal selection.* During the generation of clonal diversity, lymphoid stem cells from the bone marrow migrate to the central lymphoid organs (the thymus or regions of the bone marrow), where they undergo a series of cellular division and differentiation stages resulting in either immunocompetent T cells from the thymus or immunocompetent B cells from the bone marrow. These cells are still naive in that they have never encountered foreign antigen. The immunocompetent cells enter the circulation and migrate to the secondary lymphoid organs (e.g., spleen and lymph nodes), where they establish residence in B- and T-cell–rich areas. The clonal selection phase is initiated by exposure to foreign antigen. The antigen is usually processed by antigen-presenting cells (*APCs*) for presentation to T-helper cells (*Th cells*). The intercellular cooperation among APCs, Th cells, and immunocompetent T and B cells results in a second stage of cellular proliferation and differentiation. Because the antigen has "selected" those T and B cells with compatible antigen receptors, only a small population of T and B cells undergo this process at one time. The result is an active cellular immunity or humoral immunity, or both. Cellular immunity is mediated by a population of effector T cells that can kill targets (T-cytotoxic cells) or regulate the immune response (T-regulatory cells), as well as a population of memory cells (memory T cells) that can respond more quickly to a second challenge with the same antigen. Humoral immunity is mediated by a population of soluble proteins (antibodies) produced by plasma cells and by a population of memory B cells that can produce more antibody rapidly to a second challenge with the same antigen.

ANTIGENS AND IMMUNOGENS

We need to initially understand the molecules against which an immune response is directed. Although the terms *antigen* and *immunogen* are commonly used as synonyms, there are clinically important differences between the two. *Antigen* is commonly used to describe a molecule that can *bind with* antibodies or antigen receptors on B and T cells. A molecule that will *induce* an immune response is an **immunogen**. Thus all immunogens are antigens but not all antigens are immunogens. For example, immunogenicity is frequently related to the size of the antigen. In general, large molecules (those greater than 10 000 daltons), such as proteins and polysaccharides, are most immunogenic. Many low-molecular-weight molecules can function as **haptens**; they are too small to be immunogens by themselves but become immunogenic after combining with larger molecules that function as carriers for the hapten. Poison ivy contains an oily sap called *urushiol* (molecular weight approximately 1 500 daltons), which upon contact with the skin is chemically altered, binds to large proteins in the skin, and becomes immunogenic, resulting in a T-cell response and onset of a classic poison ivy rash. Similar conditions will be discussed in Chapter 8.

> **QUICK CHECK 7-1**
> 1. Define *acquired immunity.*
> 2. Distinguish between innate immunity and acquired immunity.
> 3. Distinguish between humoral immunity and cell-mediated immunity.
> 4. What are the differences among antigens, immunogens, and haptens?

ANTIBODIES

A basic understanding of antibodies and how they react with antigens provides a foundation for more complex topics, such as the B cell and

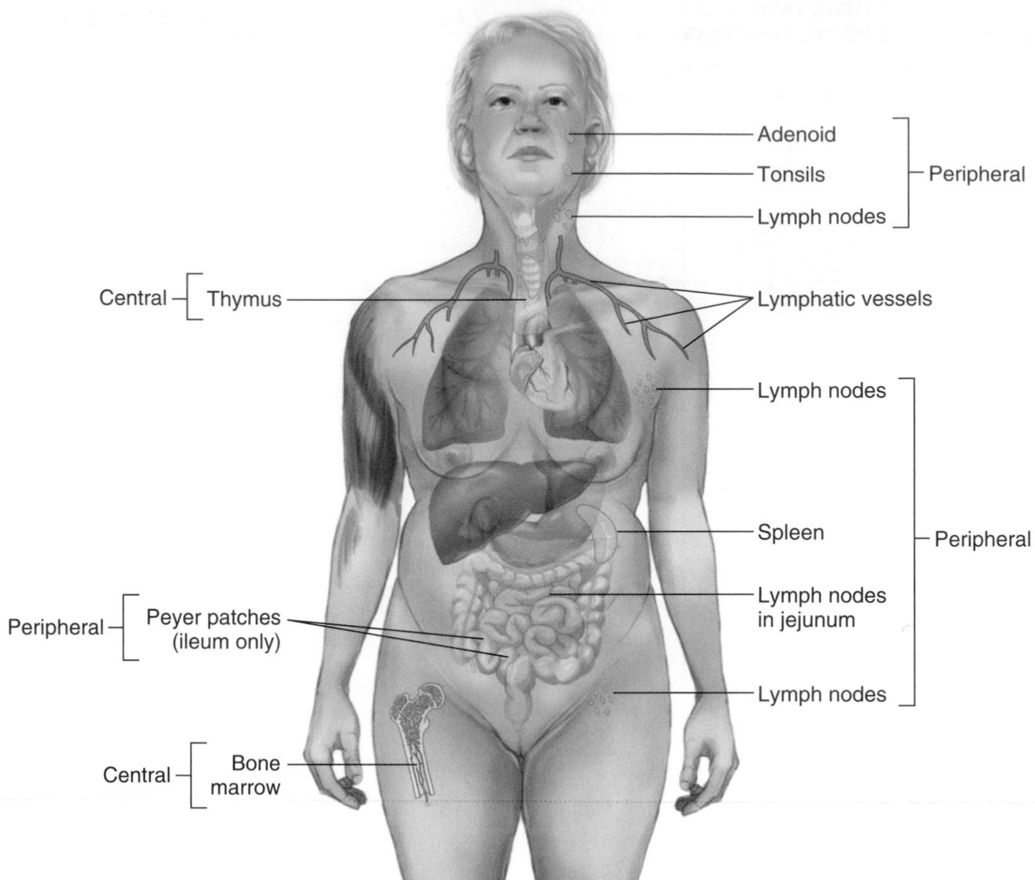

FIGURE 7-3 Lymphoid Tissues: Sites of B-Cell and T-Cell Differentiation. Immature lymphocytes migrate through central (primary) lymphoid tissues: the bone marrow (central lymphoid tissue for B lymphocytes) and the thymus (central lymphoid tissue for T lymphocytes). Mature lymphocytes later reside in the T- and B-lymphocyte–rich areas of the peripheral (secondary) lymphoid tissues.

T cell antigen receptors, the generation of clonal diversity, and intercellular collaborations during clonal selection, which are discussed later in this chapter. The terms **antibody** and **immunoglobulin (Ig)** are frequently used interchangeably. In general, *immunoglobulin* is frequently used as a generic description of a general group of antibodies, whereas *antibody* commonly denotes one particular set of immunoglobulins known to have specificity for a particular antigen.

Classes of Immunoglobulins

There are five classes of immunoglobulins (IgG, IgA, IgM, IgE, and IgD), which are characterized by differences in structure and function (Figure 7-4). Both IgG and IgA have subclasses (Table 7-2).

IgG is the most abundant class of immunoglobulins, constituting 80 to 85% of the immunoglobulins in the blood and accounting for most of the protective activity against infections. During pregnancy, maternal IgG is transported across the placenta and protects the newborn child during the first 6 months of life.

IgA is found in the blood and in bodily secretions as secretory IgA (subclass IgA2). Secretory IgA is a *dimer* consisting of two IgA2 molecules held together through a J chain and secretory piece. The secretory piece is attached to dimeric IgA during transportation through mucosal epithelial cells to protect against degradation by enzymes also found in secretions.

IgM is the largest immunoglobulin and usually exists as a pentamer (a molecule consisting of five identical smaller molecules) that is stabilized by a J chain. It is the first antibody produced during the initial, or primary, response to antigens. IgM is usually synthesized early in neonatal life, but may be increased as a response to infection in utero.

IgE is normally at low concentrations in the circulation. It has very specialized functions as a mediator of many common allergic responses (see Chapter 8) and in the defence against parasitic infections.[1]

IgD is found in low concentrations in the blood. Its primary function is as an antigen receptor on the surface of early B cells.

Molecular Structure

There are three parts to an antibody molecule (Figure 7-5). Two identical fragments have the ability to bind antigen and are termed **antigen-binding fragments (Fabs)**. The third fragment is termed the **crystallizable fragment (Fc)**. The Fab portions contain the recognition sites (receptors) for antigens and confer the molecule's specificity toward a particular antigen. The Fc portion is responsible for most of the biological functions of antibodies.[2]

An immunoglobulin molecule consists of four polypeptide chains: two identical light (L) chains and two identical heavy (H) chains. The class of antibody is determined by different amino acid sequences in the heavy chains. The light and heavy chains are held together by noncovalent bonds and covalent disulphide linkages. A set of disulphide bridges between the heavy chains occurs in the hinge region and, in some instances, lends a degree of flexibility at that site.

Each L and H chain is further subdivided structurally into constant (C) and variable (V) regions. The constant regions have relatively stable amino acid sequences within a particular immunoglobulin class.

TABLE 7-2 Properties of Immunoglobulins

Class	Subclass	Adult Serum Levels (mcmol/L)	Present in Secretions	Complement Activation	Opsonin	Agglutinin	Mast Cell Activation	Placental Transfer
IgG	IgG1	—53-60	+	++	++	+	–	+++
	IgG2	—18-20	+	+	–	+	–	+
	IgG3	—6-6.8	+	+++	++	+	–	+++
	IgG4	3.3	–	–	–	+	+	++
IgM		—1.2-1.5	+	++++	–	++++	–	–
IgA	IgA1	—17.5-18.8	+	–	–	+	–	–
	IgA2	3.1	+	–	–	+	–	–
	sIgA	0.3	++++	–	–	+	–	–
IgD		3[a]	–	–	–	–	–	–
IgE		0.03[a]	+	–	–	–	+++	–

[a]Unit of measurement is mg/dL.

sIgA, secretory immunoglobulin A; – indicates lack of activity; + to ++++ indicate relative activity or concentration.

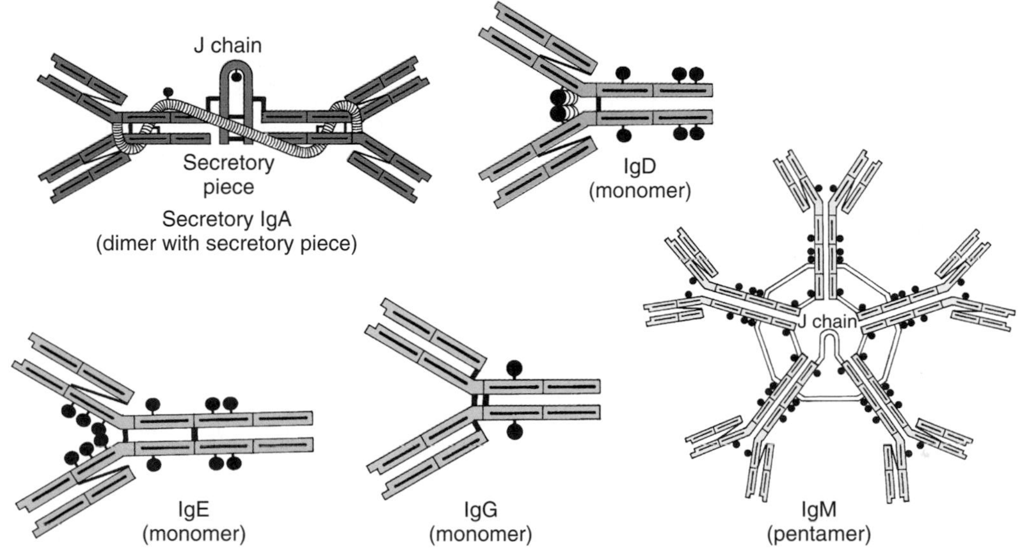

FIGURE 7-4 Structures of Different Immunoglobulins. Secretory IgA, IgD, IgE, IgG, and IgM. The black circles attached to each molecule represent carbohydrate residues.

Conversely, among different antibodies, the sequences of the variable regions have a large number of amino acid differences, and these variable regions are called **complementarity determining regions (CDRs)**. They determine the specificity of an antibody for a particular antigen. The regions between CDRs are called *framework regions* (FRs), and they have more stable amino acid sequences (see Figure 7-5).

Antigen–Antibody Binding

Because antigens are relatively small, a large molecule (e.g., protein, polysaccharide, nucleic acid) usually contains multiple and diverse antigens. The precise area of the antigen that is recognized by an antibody is called its **antigenic determinant**, or **epitope**. The matching portion on the antibody is sometimes referred to as the **antigen-binding site**, or **paratope**. The antigen fits into the antigen-binding site of the antibody with the specificity of a key into a lock and is held there by noncovalent chemical interactions.

Function of Antibodies

The chief function of antibodies is to protect against infection. The mechanism can be either *direct*—through the action of antibody alone—or *indirect*—requiring activation of other components of the innate immune response (Figure 7-6). Directly, antibodies can affect infectious agents or their toxic products by **neutralization** (inactivating or blocking the binding of antigens to receptors), **agglutination** (clumping insoluble particles that are in suspension), or **precipitation** (making a soluble antigen into an insoluble precipitate). For example, many pathogens initiate infection by attaching to specific receptors on cells. Viruses that cause the common cold or the influenza virus must attach to specific receptors on respiratory tract epithelial cells. Some bacteria, such as *Neisseria gonorrhoeae* that causes gonorrhea, must attach to specific sites on urogenital epithelial cells. Antibodies may protect the host by covering sites on the microorganism that are needed for attachment, thereby preventing infection. Many viral infections can be prevented by vaccination with inactivated or attenuated (weakened) viruses designed to induce neutralizing antibody production at the site of the entrance of the virus into the body. Vaccination against influenza using an inhaled vaccine particularly induces protective IgA in the respiratory tract.

Some bacteria secrete toxins that harm individuals. For example, specific bacterial toxins cause the symptoms of tetanus or diphtheria. Most toxins are proteins that bind to surface molecules on cells and damage those cells. Protective antibodies produced against the toxin

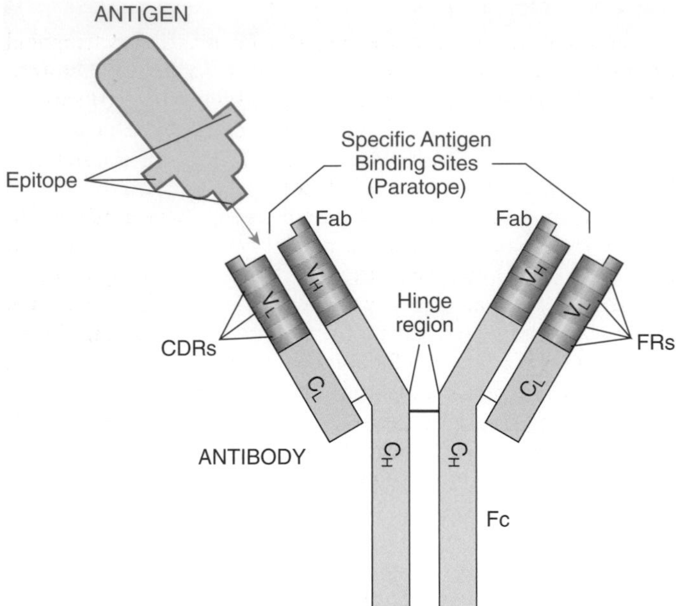

FIGURE 7-5 Antigen–Antibody Binding. *CDRs*, complementarity determining regions; C_H, constant region heavy chain; C_L, constant region light chain; *Fab*, antigen-binding fragment; *Fc*, crystallizable fragment; *FRs*, framework regions; V_H, variable region heavy chain; V_L, variable region light chain; red lines are disulphide linkages.

(referred to as *antitoxins*) can bind to the toxins, prevent their interaction with host cells, and neutralize their biological effects (see Chapter 8).

Indirectly, through the Fc portion, antibodies activate components of innate resistance, including complement and phagocytes (Figure 7-7). Through the classical pathway, complement component C1 will be activated by binding simultaneously to the Fc regions of two adjacent antibodies bound to a microbe, resulting in activation of the entire cascade. Phagocytic cells express receptors that bind the Fc portion of antibody; thus antibody is an opsonin that facilitates phagocytosis of bacteria.[3] IgM is the best complement-activating antibody, and IgG is the best opsonin. Some antibodies are more protective than others. It is now a common procedure to clone the "best" antibodies (monoclonal antibodies) for use in diagnostic tests and for therapy (Box 7-1).

Immunoglobulin E

IgE is a special class of antibody that protects the individual from infection with large parasitic worms (helminths).[4] However, when IgE is produced against relatively innocuous environmental antigens, it is also the primary cause of common allergies (e.g., hay fever, dust allergies, bee stings). The role of IgE in allergies is discussed in Chapter 8.

Large multicellular parasites usually invade mucosal tissues. Many antigens from the parasites induce IgE, as well as other antibody classes. IgG, IgM, and IgA bind to the surface of parasites, activate complement, generate chemotactic factors for neutrophils and macrophages, and serve as opsonins for those phagocytic cells. This response, however, does not greatly damage parasites. The only inflammatory cell that can

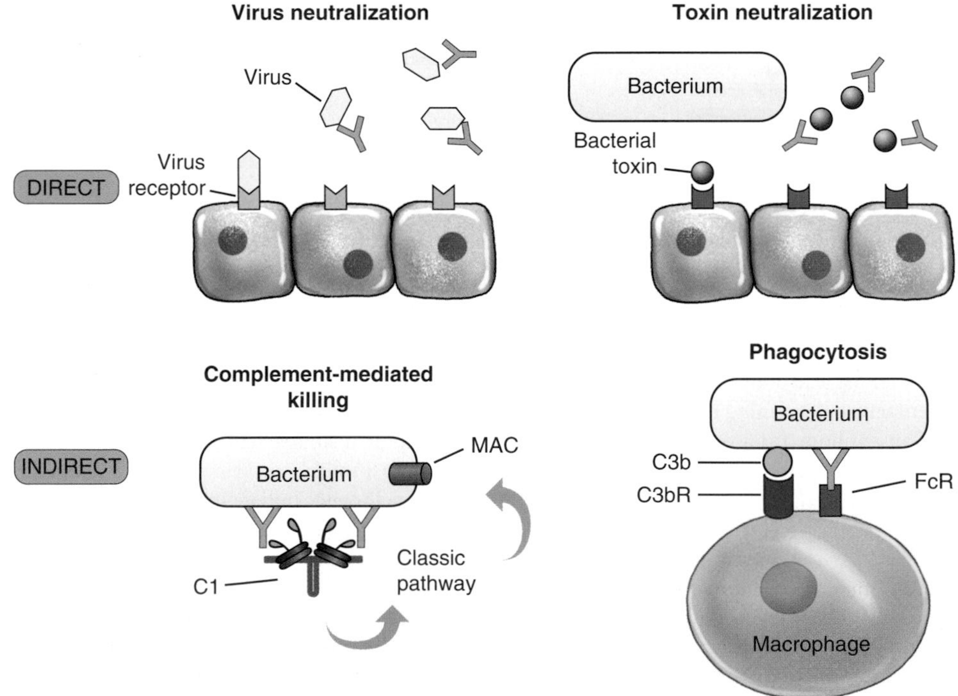

FIGURE 7-6 Direct and Indirect Functions of Antibodies. Protective activities of antibodies can be direct (through the action of antibodies alone) or indirect requiring activation of other components of the innate immune response, usually through the crystallizable fragment (Fc) region. *Direct* means include neutralization of viruses or bacterial toxins before they bind to receptors on the surface of the host's cells. *Indirect* means include activation of the classical complement pathway through C1, resulting in formation of the membrane attack complex (*MAC*), or increased phagocytosis of bacteria opsonized with antibody and complement components bound to appropriate surface receptors (*FcR* and *C3bR*). *C3b*, large fragment produced from complement component C3; *C3bR*, complement C3b receptor; *FcR*, crystallizable fragment receptor.

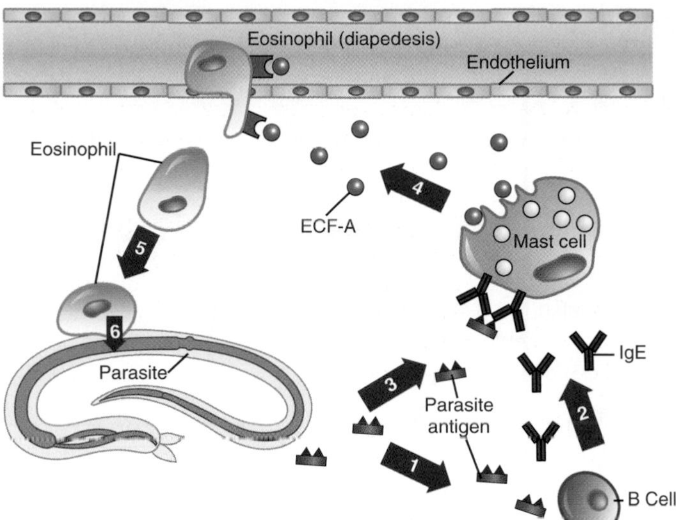

FIGURE 7-7 IgE Function. 1, Soluble antigens from a parasitic infection cause production of IgE antibody by B cells. **2,** Secreted IgE binds to IgE-specific receptors on the mast cell. **3,** Additional soluble parasite antigen cross-links the IgE on the mast cell surface, **4,** leading to mast cell degranulation and release of many proinflammatory products, including eosinophil chemotactic factor of anaphylaxis (*ECF-A*). **5,** ECF-A attracts eosinophils from the circulation. **6,** The eosinophil attaches to the surface of the parasite and releases potent lysosomal enzymes that damage microorganisms.

BOX 7-1 Monoclonal Antibodies

Most humoral immune responses are polyclonal—that is, a mixture of antibodies produced from multiple B cells. Most antigenic molecules have multiple antigenic determinants, each of which induces a different group of antibodies. Thus, a polyclonal response is a mixture of antibody classes, specificities, and function, some of which are more protective than others.

A monoclonal antibody is produced in the laboratory from one B cell that has been cloned; thus the entire antibody is of the same class, specificity, and function. The advantages of monoclonal antibodies are that (1) a single antibody of known antigenic specificity is generated rather than a mixture of different antibodies; (2) monoclonal antibodies have a single, constant binding affinity; (3) monoclonal antibodies can be diluted to a constant titre (concentration in fluid) because the actual antibody concentration is known; and (4) the antibody can be easily purified. Thus, a highly concentrated antibody with optimal function has been used to develop extremely specific and sensitive laboratory tests (e.g., home and laboratory pregnancy tests) and therapies (e.g., for certain infectious diseases or several experimental therapies for cancer).

adequately damage a parasite is the eosinophil because of the special contents of its granules, including major basic protein, eosinophil cationic protein, eosinophil peroxidase, and eosinophil neurotoxin, each of which can damage infectious worms. Thus, IgE is designed to specifically initiate an inflammatory reaction that preferentially attracts eosinophils to the site of parasitic infection.

Mast cells in the tissues have Fc receptors that specifically and with high affinity bind IgE. IgE antibodies against antigens of the parasite are rapidly bound to the mast cell surface. Soluble parasite molecules with multiple antigenic determinants diffuse to neighbouring mast cells and simultaneously bind to multiple IgE molecules. This reaction initiates a cascade of effects that can ultimately kill the parasite. The steps of the cascade are presented in Figure 7-7.

Secretory Immune System

Immunocompetent lymphocytes migrate among secondary lymphoid organs and tissue as part of the **systemic immune system**. Another, partially independent, immune system protects the external surfaces of the body through lacrimal and salivary glands and a network of lymphoid tissues residing in the breasts, bronchi, intestines, and genitourinary tract. This system is called the **secretory (mucosal) immune system** (Figure 7-8). Plasma cells in those sites secrete antibodies in bodily secretions such as tears, sweat, saliva, mucus, and breast milk to prevent pathogenic microorganisms from infecting the body's surfaces and possibly penetrating to cause systemic disease.[5] Alternatively, the microorganisms may reside in the membranes without causing disease, be shed, and cause infection for other individuals. Thus, an individual may become a carrier for a particular infectious organism. For example, in the 1950s two vaccines were developed to prevent infection with poliovirus, which enters through the gastro-intestinal tract. The Sabin vaccine was administered orally as an attenuated (i.e., inactivated so as to render relatively harmless) live virus. This route caused a transient, limited infection and induced effective systemic and secretory immunity that prevented both the disease and the establishment of a carrier state. The Salk vaccine, on the other hand, consisted of killed viruses administered by injection in the skin. It induced adequate systemic protection but did not generally prevent an intestinal carrier state. Thus, recipients of the Salk vaccine were protected from disease but could still shed the virus and infect others.

IgA is the dominant **secretory immunoglobulin**, although IgM and IgG also are present in secretions. The primary role of IgA is to prevent the attachment and invasion of pathogens through mucosal membranes, such as those of the gastro-intestinal, pulmonary, and genitourinary tracts. Dimeric IgA antibodies containing the J chain are produced by plasma cells of the mucosa. Mucosal epithelium expresses a cell surface immunoglobulin receptor that binds and internalizes IgA. The IgA, along with the epithelial receptor (secretory piece), is secreted as secretory IgA (sIgA).

The lymphoid tissues of the secretory immune system are connected; thus many foreign antigens in a mother's gastro-intestinal tract (e.g., poliovirus) induce secretion of specific antibodies into the breast milk. Colostral antibodies (i.e., those found in the colostrum of breast milk) may protect the nursing newborn against infectious disease agents that enter through the gastro-intestinal tract. Although colostral antibodies provide the newborn with passive immunity against gastro-intestinal infections, they do not provide systemic immunity because transport across the newborn's gut into the bloodstream is discontinued after the first 24 hours of life. Maternal antibodies that pass across the placenta into the fetus before birth provide passive systemic immunity.

IMMUNE RESPONSE: COLLABORATION OF B CELLS AND T CELLS

Generation of Clonal Diversity

The immune response occurs in two phases: generation of clonal diversity and clonal selection (Table 7-3, and see Figure 7-2). *Clonal diversity* is the production of a large population of B cells and T cells before birth that have the capacity to recognize almost any foreign antigen found in the environment. This process mostly occurs in specialized lymphoid organs (the **primary [central] lymphoid organs**): the bone marrow for B cells and the thymus for T cells.[6] The result is the differentiation of **lymphoid stem cells** into B and T cells with the ability to react against almost any antigen that will be encountered throughout life. It is estimated that B and T cells can collectively recognize more than 10^8 different antigenic determinants. Lymphocytes are released from these organs into the circulation as immunocompetent cells that have the

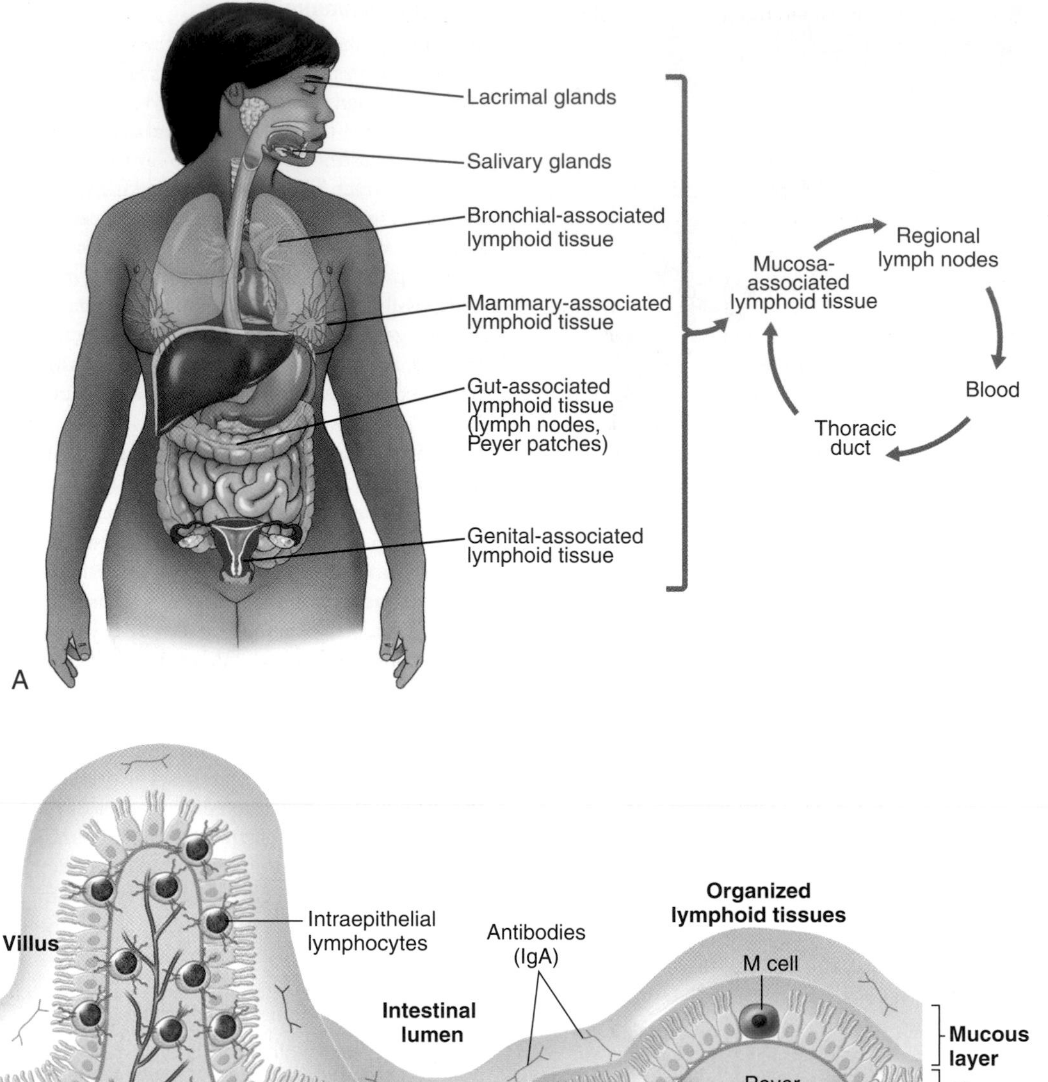

FIGURE 7-8 Secretory Immune System. **A**, Lymphocytes from the mucosal-associated lymphoid tissues circulate throughout the body in a pattern separate from other lymphocytes. For example, lymphocytes from the gut-associated lymphoid tissue circulate through the regional lymph nodes, the thoracic duct, and the blood and return to other mucosal-associated lymphoid tissues rather than to lymphoid tissue of the systemic immune system. **B**, Lymphoid tissue associated with mucous membranes is called *mucosa-associated lymphoid tissue* (MALT). *M cell*, microfold cell.

capacity to react with antigens and migrate to the circulation and other (secondary) lymphoid organs in the body.

Development of B Lymphocytes

Lymphocytes destined to become B cells circulate through the specialized regions of the bone marrow, where they are exposed to hormones and cytokines that induce proliferation and differentiation into B cells (see Figure 7-2). Lymphoid stem cells in the bone marrow interact with stromal cells through a variety of intercellular adhesion molecules. As the stem cell begins to mature, it progressively develops a variety of necessary surface markers important for the further differentiation and proliferation of the B cell.[7] The next stage in development is formation of the B cell antigen receptor (BCR).

The **B cell antigen receptor (BCR)** is a complex of antibodies bound to the cell surface and other molecules involved in intracellular signalling (Figure 7-9). Its role is to recognize an antigen and communicate that information to the cell's nucleus. The BCRs in immunocompetent cells are membrane-associated IgM (mIgM) and IgD (mIgD) immunoglobulins that have identical specificities for antigen. The mIgM is a monomer rather than the pentamer primarily found in the blood.

As described previously, the variable regions of antibodies, as well as the BCR, contain CDR areas. The diversity of these CDRs is responsible for the variety of antigens that can be recognized by immunocompetent B cells.[8] The enormous repertoire of specificities is made possible by rearrangement of existing DNA during B-cell development in the primary lymphoid organs, a process known as **somatic recombination**. Multiple loci in the DNA that encode for the variable regions of immunoglobulins are recombined to generate receptors that collectively can recognize and bind to any possible antigen.[8] To create the variable region of a light chain, different regions are rearranged using enzymes encoded by *recombination activating genes* (*RAG-1*, *RAG-2*). The DNA is cut and spliced (repaired) so that after this manipulation, the progeny of a single lymphocyte will synthesize immunoglobulins with identical variable regions. Those variable regions, however, are cut and spliced differently from those of another lymphocyte, making each cell unique and therefore able to react with different antigens. The gene for the H chain undergoes similar rearrangement.

Somatic rearrangement of the variable regions will frequently result in a BCR that recognizes the individual's own antigens, which may result in an inadvertent attack on "self" antigens expressed on various

TABLE 7-3 Generation of Clonal Diversity Versus Clonal Selection

	Generation of Clonal Diversity	Clonal Selection
Purpose?	To produce large numbers of T and B cells with maximum diversity of antigen receptors	To select, expand, and differentiate clones of T and B cells against specific antigens
When does it occur?	Primarily in fetus	Primarily after birth and throughout life
Where does it occur?	Central lymphoid organs: thymus for T cells, bone marrow for B cells	Peripheral lymphoid organs, including lymph nodes, spleen, and other lymphoid tissues
Is foreign antigen involved?	No	Yes, the antigen determines which clones of cells will be selected
What hormones or cytokines are involved?	Thymic hormones, IL-7, others	Many cytokines produced by Th cells and APCs
Final product?	Immunocompetent T and B cells that can react with the antigen, but have not seen the antigen, and migrate to secondary lymphoid organs	Plasma cells that produce antibodies, effector T cells that help (Th cells), kill targets (Tc cells), or regulate immune responses (Treg cells); memory B and T cells

APCs, antigen-presenting cells; *IL-7*, interleukin-7; *Tc cells*, T-cytotoxic cells; *Th cells*, T-helper cells; *Treg cells*, T-regulatory cells.

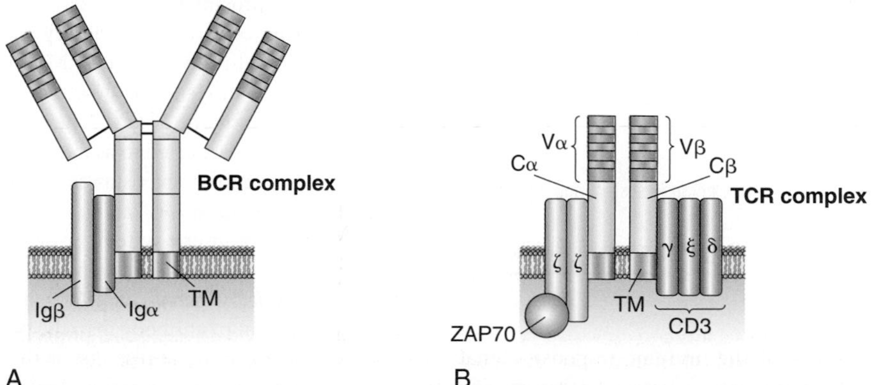

FIGURE 7-9 B Cell Antigen Receptor and T Cell Antigen Receptor. A, The antigen receptor on the surface of B cells (B cell antigen receptor *[BCR] complex*) is a monomeric (single) antibody with a structure similar to that of circulating antibody, with an additional transmembrane region (*TM*) that anchors the molecule to the cell surface. The active BCR complex contains molecules (*Igα* and *Igβ*) that are responsible for intracellular signalling after the receptor has bound antigen. **B,** The T-cell receptor (*TCR*) consists of an α- and a β-chain joined by a disulphide bond. Each chain consists of a constant region (*Cα* and *Cβ*) and a variable region (*Vα* and *Vβ*). Each variable region contains complementarity determining regions and framework regions in a structure similar to that of an antibody. The active TCR is associated with several molecules that are responsible for intracellular signalling after antigen binding. These include the CD3, which is a complex of gamma (*γ*), *epsilon* (*ξ*), and delta (*δ*) subunits and a complex of two zeta (*ζ*) molecules. The ζ molecules are attached to a cytoplasmic protein kinase (*ZAP70*) that is critical to intracellular signalling.

tissues and organs, thereby causing autoimmune disease or hypersensitivities. Many of these "autoreactive" B cells are eliminated in the bone marrow. It is estimated that more than 90% of developing B cells are induced to undergo apoptosis. This process is referred to as **central tolerance**, so that resultant immunocompetent B cells are against foreign antigens and "tolerant" to *self-antigens*. The process of peripheral tolerance is discussed on p. 173.

B-cell differentiation also is characterized by the development of a variety of important surface molecules that are markers for B cells. These include CD21 (a complement receptor) and CD40 (adhesion molecule required for later interactions with T cells).

Development of T Lymphocytes

The process of T-cell proliferation and differentiation is similar to that for B cells (see Figure 7-2). The primary lymphoid organ for T-cell development is the thymus.[9] Lymphoid stem cells journey through the thymus, where, under influence of thymic hormones and the cytokine interleukin-7 (IL-7), they are driven to undergo cell division and simultaneously produce receptors (**T cell antigen receptors [TCRs]**) against the diversity of antigens the individual will encounter throughout life. They exit the thymus through the blood vessels and lymphatics as mature (immunocompetent) T cells with antigen-specific receptors on the cell surface and establish residence in secondary lymphoid organs.

Production of the TCR proceeds in a manner very similar to that described earlier for B cells. The most common TCR resembles an antibody Fab region and consists of two protein chains, α- and β-chains, each of which has a variable region and a constant region (see Figure 7-9). The variable regions also undergo somatic recombination. As with the BCR, a set of intracellular signalling molecules co-assemble in the membrane with the TCR. The complex of these signalling molecules is called **CD3**.[10] Thus, all immunocompetent T cells can be identified by the presence of CD3 on the surface.

Differentiation of T cells in the thymus also results in expression in a variety of other important surface molecules. Initially, proteins called **CD4** and **CD8** are concurrently expressed on the developing cells. Th cells express the CD4 surface protein, whereas Tc cells express the CD8 surface protein. Approximately 60% of immunocompetent T cells in the circulation express CD4 and 40% express CD8.

Central tolerance also occurs in the thymus, where more than 95% of developing T cells are deleted. Like B cells, T cells can also become autoreactive.

✔ QUICK CHECK 7-2

1. What are the major functions of antibodies?
2. What is the difference between the secretory immune system and systemic immune system?
3. What are the different types of T cells, and what function does each have?

Clonal Selection

Antigens initiate the second phase of the immune response, clonal selection. *Clonal selection* is the processing of antigen for a specific immune response. This process involves a complex interaction among cells in the secondary lymphoid organs (see Figure 7-2). To initiate an effective immune response, most antigens must be *processed* because they cannot react directly with most cells of the immune system and must be shown or *presented* to the immune cells in a specific manner. This is the job of **antigen-processing (antigen-presenting) cells (APCs)** (usually **dendritic cells**, macrophages, or similar cells). The interaction among APCs, subpopulations of T cells that facilitate immune responses (Th cells), and immunocompetent B or T cells results in differentiation of B cells into active antibody-producing cells (plasma cells) and T cells into effector cells, such as Tc cells. Both lines also develop into memory cells that respond even faster when that antigen enters the body again. Thus, activation of the immune system produces a long-lasting protection against specific antigens (see Figure 7-2). Defects in any aspect of cellular collaboration will lead to defects in cell-mediated immunity, humoral immunity, or both and, depending on the particular defect, potentially the individual's death from infection (see Chapter 8).

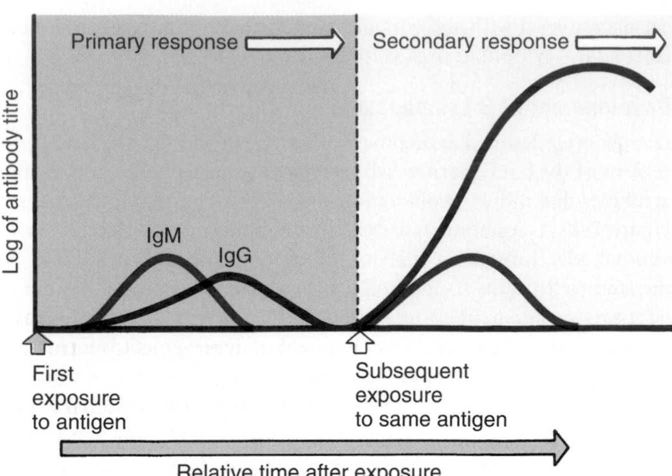

FIGURE 7-10 Primary and Secondary Immune Responses. The initial administration of antigen induces a primary response during which IgM is initially produced, followed by IgG. Another administration of the antigen induces the secondary response in which IgM is transiently produced and larger amounts of IgG are produced over a longer period of time.

Primary and Secondary Immune Responses

The immune response to an antigen has classically been divided into two phases—the primary and secondary responses—that are most easily demonstrated by measuring concentrations of circulating antibodies over time (Figure 7-10). After a single initial exposure to most antigens, there is a latent period, or lag phase, during which clonal selection occurs. After approximately 5 to 7 days, IgM antibody is detected in the circulation. This response is the **primary immune response**, characterized typically by initial production of IgM followed by production of IgG against the same antigen. The quantity of IgG may be about equal to or less than the amount of IgM. The amount of antibody in a serum sample is frequently referred to as the **titre**; a higher titre indicates more antibodies. If no further exposure to the antigen occurs, the circulating antibody is catabolized (broken down) and measurable quantities fall. The individual's immune system, however, has been primed.

A second challenge by the same antigen results in the **secondary immune response**, which is characterized by the more rapid production of a larger amount of antibody than the primary response. The rapidity of the secondary immune response is the result of memory cells that require less further differentiation. IgM may be transiently produced in the secondary response, but IgG production is increased considerably, making it the predominant antibody class. Natural infection (e.g., rubella) may result in measurable levels of protective IgG for the life of the individual. Some vaccines (e.g., polio) also may produce extremely long-lived protection, although most vaccines require boosters at specified intervals.

Antigen Processing and Presentation

For most antigens, the first step in clonal selection is processing and presentation by APCs. Antigens are usually expressed on large molecules found on microbes, which undergo phagocytosis and destruction by dendritic cells and macrophages. These antigens are referred to as *exogenous antigens*. Other antigens, *endogenous antigens*, originate within a cell that has been infected by a virus or has become cancerous.

Processing results in the release of small antigenic determinants, which are presented on the surface of APCs by specialized molecules, molecules of the **major histocompatibility complex (MHC)**. MHC molecules in humans also are called **human leukocyte antigens (HLAs)** (discussed in more detail in Chapter 8) and are related to their role in transplantation. MHC molecules are glycoproteins found on the surface of all human cells except red blood cells. They are divided into two general classes, class I and class II, based on their molecular structure, distribution among cell populations, and function in antigen presentation. MHC class I molecules are composed of a large alpha (α) chain along with a smaller chain called β_2-microglobulin. MHC class II molecules are composed of α- and β-chains that differ from the ones used for MHC class I. The α- and β-chains of the MHC molecules are encoded from different genetic loci located as a large complex of genes on human chromosome 6 (Figure 7-11). MHC genes are probably the most polymorphic of any human genes; therefore no two individuals, except identical twins, will have a complete set of identical MHC molecules.

MHC class I molecules present endogenous antigens, which are primarily recognized by Tc cells. Because MHC class I molecules are expressed on all cells, except red blood cells, any change in that cell caused by viral infection or malignancy may result in foreign antigens being presented. MHC class II molecules present exogenous antigens (Figure 7-12). Antigen presented by MHC class II molecules is preferentially recognized by Th cells. Thus, antigen presentation to Tc cells is *MHC class I restricted* and presentation to Th cells *is MHC class II restricted*. MHC class II molecules are co-expressed with MHC class I molecules on a limited number of cells that have APC function, including macrophages, dendritic cells, and B cells.

Thus, the term **antigen processing** relates to the process by which large exogenous and endogenous antigens are cut up by enzymes into small antigenic fragments that are linked with the appropriate MHC molecules and inserted into the membrane of the APC.[11] Lipid antigens are frequently presented by a molecule unrelated to the MHC, CD1, which is not discussed here.

Coded on Chromosome 6
HLA Molecules

Class I MHC Molecules (HLA-A, HLA-B, HLA-C)	Class II MHC Molecules (HLA-DR, HLA-DP, HLA-DQ)
Expressed on all nucleated cells and platelets	Expressed only on antigen-presenting cells (APCs): Macrophages, Dendritic cells, B cells
Presents endogenous antigen	Presents exogenous antigen
Recruits CD8+ Tc-Cells	Recruits CD4+ Th-Cells

T cells recognize antigenic fragments complexed to HLA-encoded molecules as "non-self."

FIGURE 7-11 Antigen-Presenting Molecules. *HLA*, human leukocyte antigen; *MHC*, major histocompatibility complex; *Tc cells*, T-cytotoxic cells; *Th cells*, T-helper cells.

Cellular Interactions in the Immune Response

The second step in clonal selection is a finely tuned set of intercellular collaborations that result in the production of effector cells (plasma cells, Th cells, Tc cells) and memory cells.[12] Each collaboration requires three complementary intracellular signalling events: antigen-specific recognition through the TCR complex, activation of intercellular adhesion molecules, and the response to specific groups of cytokines. Without each signalling event, a protective immune response will not be produced.

T-helper lymphocytes. Regardless of whether an antigen primarily induces a cellular or humoral immune response, APCs usually must present antigens to Th cells. The APC presents antigen held by the polymorphic regions ($\alpha 1$ and $\beta 1$) of the α- and β-chains of MHC class II molecules.[13] The antigen also binds to the TCR on the Th cell (see Figure 7-9). The strength of the intercellular antigen binding is increased by CD4 on the Th cell, which binds to a nonpolymorphic region of the $\beta 2$ region of the MHC class II molecule. The cytoplasmic portions of CD3 and CD4 interact to activate intracellular signalling pathways. A second co-stimulatory signal results from the interaction of a variety of adhesion molecules; the most critical is B7 on the APC and CD28 on the Th cell.

The third signal occurs through Th-cell cytokine receptors. In the early stages of Th-cell differentiation, IL-1 secreted by the APC provides this signal through the IL-1 receptor on the Th cell (Figure 7-13). The initial differentiation response by the Th cell includes the production of the cytokine IL-2 and upregulation of IL-2 receptors. IL-2 is secreted and acts in an autocrine (self-stimulating) fashion to induce further maturation and proliferation of the Th cell. Without IL-2 production, the Th cell cannot efficiently mature into a functional helper cell.

At this point and depending on the predominant cytokines in the immediate environment, Th cells undergo differentiation into one of several subsets: Th1, Th2, Th17, or Treg cells.[14] These subsets have different functions: **Th1 cells** preferentially provide help in developing Tc cells (cell-mediated immunity); **Th2 cells** provide more help for developing B cells (humoral immunity); **Th17 cells** are lymphokine-secreting cells that activate macrophages; and Treg cells limit the immune response (Treg cells are discussed later in this chapter).[15] The Th subsets differ considerably in the spectrum of cytokines they produce. Additionally, Th1 and Th2 cells may suppress each other so that the immune response may favour either antibody formation, with suppression of a cell-mediated response, or the opposite. For example, antigens derived from viral or bacterial pathogens and those derived from cancer cells seem to induce a greater number of Th1 cells relative to Th2 cells, whereas antigens derived from multicellular parasites and allergens may result in production of more Th2 cells. Many antigens (e.g., tetanus vaccine), however, will produce excellent humoral and cell-mediated responses simultaneously. Th cells are necessary for development of most humoral and cellular immune responses; therefore the virus that causes acquired immune deficiency syndrome (AIDS) results in life-threatening infections because it specifically infects and destroys Th cells (see Chapter 8).

Superantigens. Several pathogenic microorganisms, particularly viruses and bacteria, manipulate the normal interaction between APCs and Th cells to the detriment of the individual and the benefit of the microbe. A group of microbial molecules are called **superantigens (SAGs)**. SAGs bind to the portion of the TCR outside of its normal antigen-specific binding site, as well as to MHC class II molecules outside of their antigen presentation sites (Figure 7-14). Some SAGs also react with CD28 on the Th cells and provide a co-stimulatory signal. Thus, SAGs are not processed by an APC to be presented to an immune cell. This binding, which is independent of antigen recognition, provides a signal for Th-cell activation, proliferation, and cytokine production.

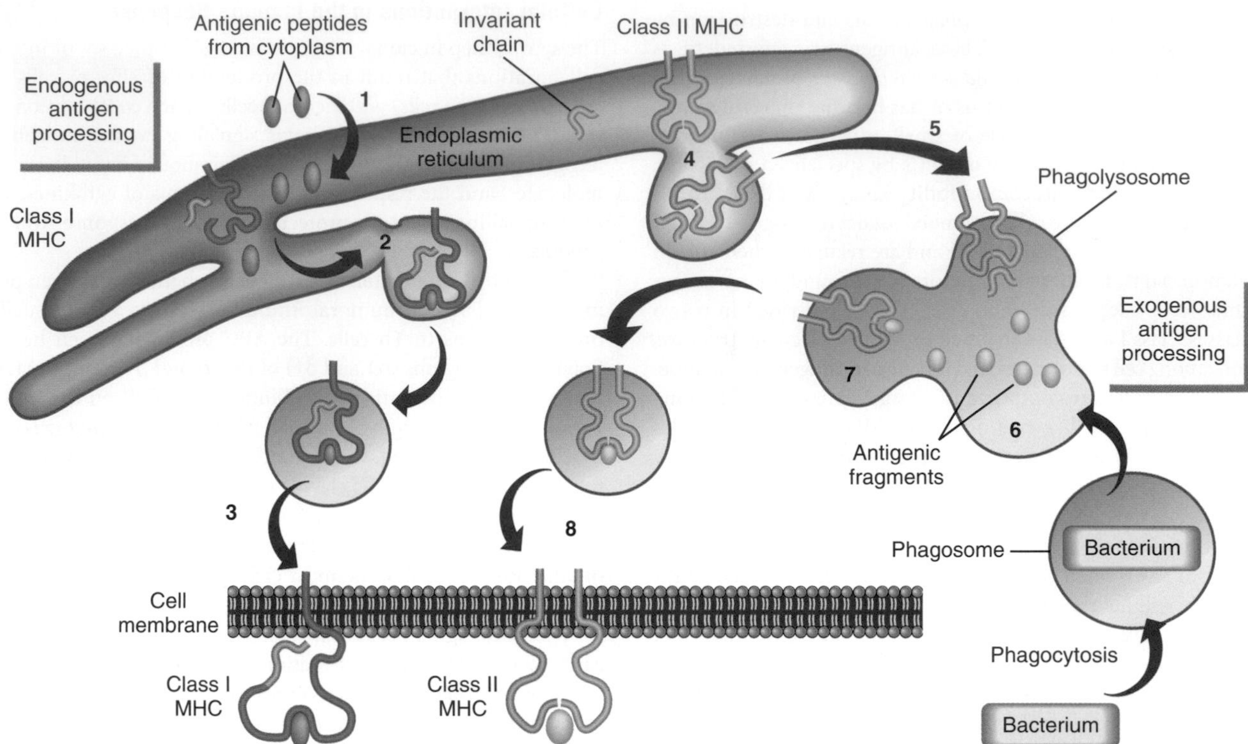

FIGURE 7-12 Antigen Processing. Antigen processing and presentation are required for initiation of most immune responses. Foreign antigens may be either endogenous (cytoplasmic protein) or exogenous (e.g., bacterium). Endogenous antigenic peptides are transported into the endoplasmic reticulum (ER) **(1)**, where the major histocompatibility complex (*MHC*) molecules are being assembled. In the ER, antigenic peptides bind to the α-chains of the MHC class I molecule **(2)**, and the complex is transported to the cell surface **(3)**. The α- and β-chains of the MHC class II molecules are also being assembled in the ER **(4)**, but the antigen-binding site is blocked by a small molecule (invariant chain) to prevent interactions with endogenous antigenic peptides. The MHC class II–invariant chain complex is transported to phagolysosomes **(5)**, where exogenous antigenic fragments have been produced as a result of phagocytosis **(6)**. In the phagolysosomes, the invariant chain is digested and replaced by exogenous antigenic peptides **(7)**, after which the MHC class II–antigen complex is inserted into the cell membrane **(8)**.

The normal antigen-specific recognition between Th cells and APCs results in activation of relatively few cells—only those cells with specific TCRs against that antigen. SAGs activate a large population of Th cells, regardless of antigen specificity, and induce excessive production of cytokines, including IL-2, interferon gamma (IFN-γ), and tumour necrosis factor-alpha (TNF-α). The overproduction of inflammatory cytokines results in symptoms of a systemic inflammatory reaction, including fever, low blood pressure, and, potentially, fatal shock. Some examples of SAGs are the bacterial toxins produced by *Staphylococcus aureus* and *Streptococcus pyogenes* (SAGs that cause toxic shock syndrome and food poisoning).[16]

T-cytotoxic lymphocytes. The differentiation of immunocompetent T cells into effector Tc cells requires similar intercellular communications as described for Th cells, with some very important differences. Rather than interacting with an APC, the immunocompetent Tc cell recognizes antigen presented by MHC class I molecules on the surface of a virus-infected cell or cancerous cell (Figure 7-15). The Tc cell expresses CD8, rather than CD4. CD8 binds to the MHC class I molecule and, as with Th-cell differentiation, the proximity of the CD3 and CD8 cytoplasmic portions activates intercellular signalling pathways. Cytokine signals, especially IL-2, are produced by Th1 cells and activate cytokine receptors on the Tc cells.

B-cell clonal selection. A further sequence of cellular interactions is required to produce an effective antibody response. The immunocompetent B cell is also an APC and expresses surface mIgM and mIgD BCRs (Figure 7-16). Unlike the TCR that can only *see* processed and presented antigens, the BCR can react with soluble antigens that have not been processed. B cells also express surface CD21, which is a receptor for opsonins produced by complement activation. Antigen binding through the BCR and CD21 activates the B cell, resulting in internalization, processing, and presentation of antigen fragments by MHC class II molecules.[17] The antigen presented on the B-cell surface is recognized by a Th2 cell through the TCR and CD4. The intercellular bridges created through antigen and other intercellular adhesion molecules induce the Th2 cell to secrete cytokines (particularly IL-4) that initiate B-cell proliferation and maturation into plasma cells.[18]

A major component of B-cell maturation is **class switch**, the process that results in the change in antibody production from one class to another (e.g., IgM to IgG during the primary immune response). Before exposure to antigens and Th2 cells, the B cell produces IgM and IgD, which are used as cell membrane receptors. During the clonal selection process, a B cell proliferates and develops into antibody-secreting plasma cells, and each B cell has the option of becoming a secretor of IgM or changing the class of antibody to a secreted form of IgG, IgA, or IgE. Class switch occurs by another round of somatic recombination with the variable region of the antibody heavy chain being combined with a different constant region of the heavy chain. Because the variable region is conserved and the light chain remains unchanged, the antigenic

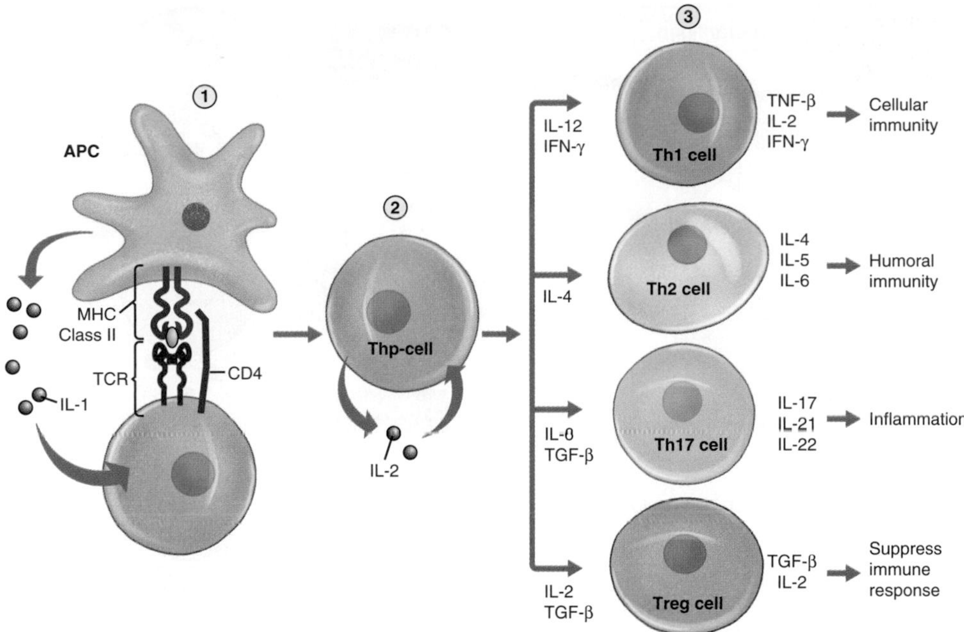

FIGURE 7-13 Development of T-Cell Subsets. The most important step in clonal selection is the production of populations of T-helper cells (*Th1, Th2,* and *Th17 cells*) and T-regulatory cells (*Treg cells*) that are necessary for the development of cellular and humoral immune responses. In this model, antigen-presenting cells (*APCs*) **(1)** (probably multiple populations) may influence whether a precursor Th cell (*Thp cell*) **(2)** will differentiate into a Th1, Th2, Th17, or Treg cell **(3)**. Differentiation of the Thp cell is initiated by three signalling events. The antigen signal is produced by the interaction of the T-cell receptor (*TCR*) and CD4 with antigen presented by major histocompatibility complex (*MHC*) class II molecules. A set of co-stimulatory signals is produced from interactions between adhesion molecules (not shown). A third signal is produced by the interactions of cytokines (particularly interleukin-1 [*IL-1*]) with appropriate cytokine receptors on the Thp cell. The Thp cell upregulates IL-2 production and expression of the IL-2 receptor, which acts in an autocrine fashion to accelerate Thp cell differentiation and proliferation. Commitment to a particular phenotype results from the relative concentrations of other cytokines. IL-12 and interferon gamma (*IFN-γ*) produced by some populations of APCs favour differentiation into the Th1 cell phenotype; IL-4, which is produced by a variety of cells, favours differentiation into the Th2 cell phenotype; IL-6 and transforming growth factor-beta (*TGF-β*) facilitate differentiation into Th17 cells; IL-2 and TGF-β induce differentiation into Treg cells. The Th1 cell is characterized by the production of cytokines that assist in the differentiation of T-cytotoxic cells, leading to cellular immunity, whereas the Th2 cell produces cytokines that favour B-cell differentiation and humoral immunity. Th1 and Th2 cells affect each other through the production of inhibitory cytokines: IFN-γ will inhibit the development of Th2 cells, and IL-4 will inhibit the development of Th1 cells. Th17 cells produce cytokines that affect phagocytes and increase inflammation. Treg cells produce immunosuppressive cytokines that prevent the immune response from being excessive. *TNF-β,* tumour necrosis factor-beta.

specificity of the antibody also remains unchanged. The particular constant region chosen by each cell during class switch appears to be, at least partially, under the control of specific Th2 cytokines. For example, IL-4 and IL-13 appear to preferentially stimulate switch to IgE secretion, and transforming growth factor-beta (TGF-β) and IL-5 appear to play major roles in class switch to IgA secretion. Thus, during clonal selection, a B cell may produce a population of plasma cells that are capable of producing many different classes of antibodies against the same antigen.

Although most antigens require B cells to interact with Th cells, a few antigens can bypass the need for cellular interactions and can directly stimulate B-cell maturation and proliferation. These antigens are called *T-cell–independent antigens* (Figure 7-17). They are mostly bacterial products that are large and are likely to have repeating identical antigenic determinants that bind and cross-link several BCRs. The accumulated intracellular signal is adequate to induce differentiation into a plasma cell but is not adequate to induce a change in the class of antibody that will be produced. Therefore, T-cell–independent antigens usually induce relatively pure IgM primary and secondary immune responses.

Memory cells. During the clonal selection process, both B cells and T cells differentiate and proliferate into an extremely large population of long-lived memory cells.[19] Memory cells remain inactive until subsequent exposure to the same antigen. Upon re-exposure, these memory cells do not require much further differentiation and will therefore rapidly become new plasma cells or effector T cells without the cellular interactions described previously.

CELL-MEDIATED IMMUNITY

The rather straightforward function of antibodies has been discussed earlier in this chapter. The function of effector T cells is more complex and utilizes the principles of intercellular recognition necessary for clonal selection.

T-Lymphocyte Function

The clonal selection process produces several subsets of effector T cells. Th cells and T memory cells have already been discussed. Other effector

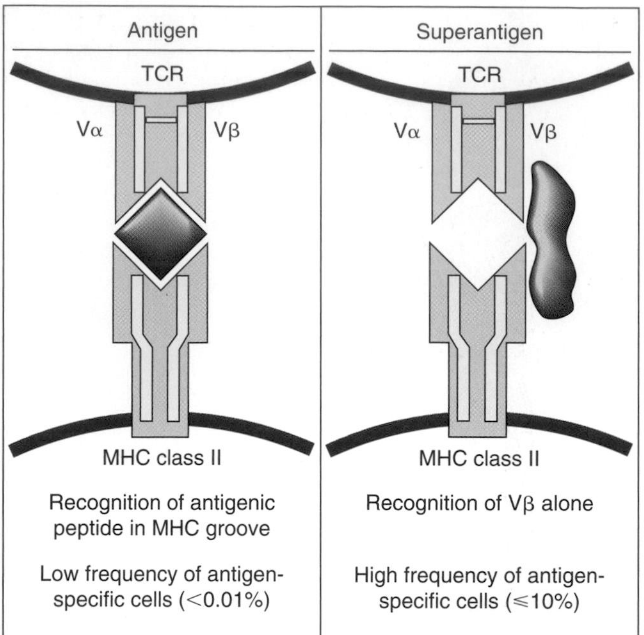

FIGURE 7-14 Superantigens. The T cell antigen receptor (*TCR*) and major histocompatibility complex (*MHC*) class II molecule are normally held together by processed antigen. Superantigens, such as some bacterial exotoxins, bind directly to the variable region of the TCRβ-chain and the MHC class II molecule. Each superantigen activates sets of Vβ chains independently of the antigen specificity of the TCR. *Vα* and *Vβ*, variable regions.

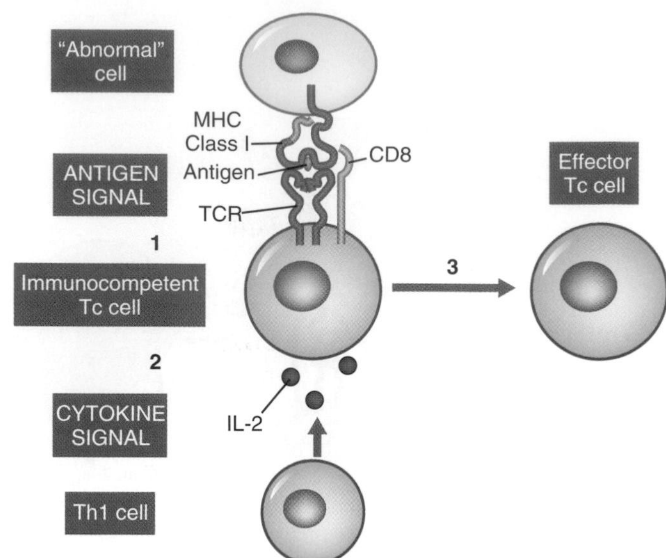

FIGURE 7-15 T-Cytotoxic Cell Clonal Selection. The immunocompetent T-cytotoxic cell (*Tc cell*) can react with the antigen but cannot yet kill target cells. During clonal selection, this cell reacts with the antigen presented by major histocompatibility complex (*MHC*) class I molecules on the surface of a virally infected or cancerous *abnormal* cell. **1,** The antigen–MHC class I complex is recognized simultaneously by the T cell antigen receptor (*TCR*), which binds to the antigen, and CD8, which binds to the MHC class I molecule. **2,** A separate signal is provided by cytokines, particularly interleukin-2 (*IL-2*) from T-helper (*Th1*) cells. **3,** In response to these signals, the Tc cell develops into an effector Tc cell with the ability to kill abnormal cells.

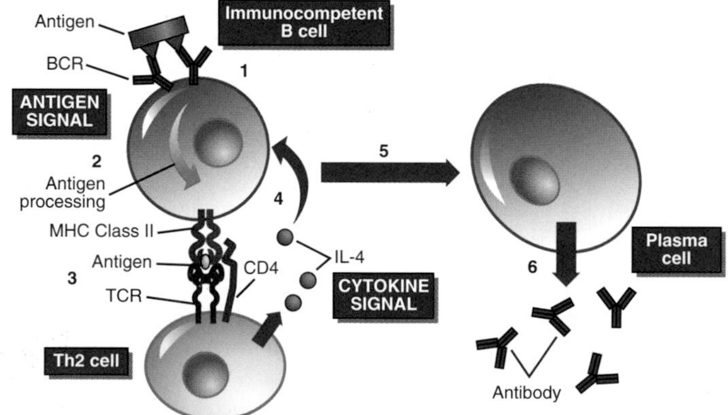

FIGURE 7-16 B-Cell Clonal Selection. Immunocompetent B cells undergo proliferation and differentiation into antibody-secreting plasma cells. Multiple signals are necessary **(1)**. The B cell itself can directly bind soluble antigen through the B cell antigen receptor (*BCR*) and act as an antigen-processing cell. The antigen is internalized, processed **(2)**, and presented **(3)** to the T cell antigen receptor (*TCR*) on a T-helper (*Th2*) cell by major histocompatibility complex (*MHC*) class II molecules **(4)**. A cytokine signal is provided by the Th2 cell cytokines (e.g., interleukin-4 [*IL-4*]) that react with the B cell **(5)**. The B cell differentiates into plasma cells that secrete the antibody **(6)**.

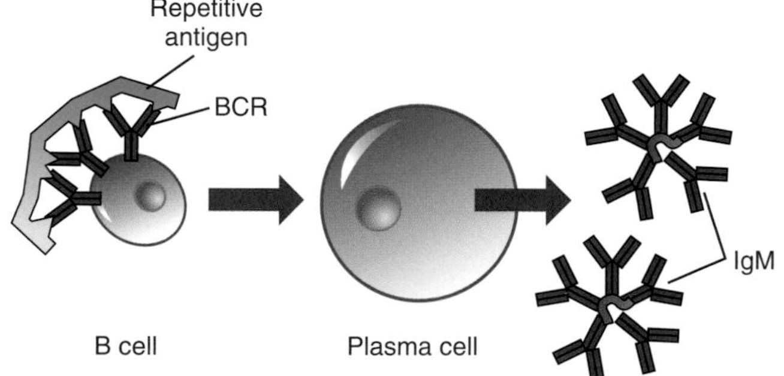

FIGURE 7-17 Activation of a B Cell by a T-Cell–Independent Antigen. Molecules containing repeating identical antigenic determinants may interact simultaneously with several receptors on the surface of the B cell and induce the proliferation and production of immunoglobulins. Because T-helper cells do not participate, class switch does not occur and the resultant antibody response is IgM. *BCR*, B cell antigen receptor.

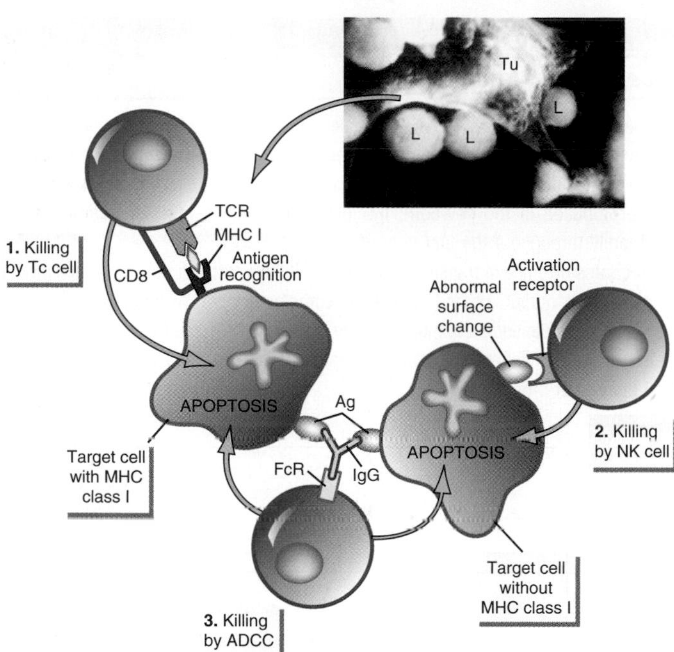

FIGURE 7-18 Cellular Killing Mechanisms. Several cells have the capacity to kill abnormal (e.g., virally infected, cancerous) target cells. **1,** T-cytotoxic cells (Tc cells) recognize endogenous antigen presented by major histocompatibility complex (*MHC*) class I molecules. The *Tc cell* mobilizes multiple killing mechanisms that induce apoptosis of the target cell. **2,** Natural killer (*NK*) cells identify and kill target cells through receptors that recognize abnormal surface changes. NK cells specifically kill targets that do not express surface MHC class I molecules. **3,** Several cells, including macrophages and NK cells, can kill by antibody-dependent cell-mediated cytotoxicity (*ADCC*). IgG antibodies bind to the foreign antigen (*Ag*) on the target cell, and cells involved in ADCC bind IgG through crystallizable fragment receptors (*FcR*) and initiate killing. The insert is a scanning electron microscopic view of Tc cells (*L*) attacking a much larger tumour cell (*Tu*). (Insert from Abbas, A., & Lichtman, A. [2003]. *Cellular and molecular immunology* [5th ed.]. Philadelphia: Saunders.)

T cells include Tc cells that attack and destroy cells expressing antigens from intracellular (endogenous) origins, Treg cells that limit (suppress) the immune response, and lymphokine-secreting T cells that secrete cytokines and activate other cells.

T-Cytotoxic Lymphocytes

Tc cells are responsible for the cell-mediated destruction of tumour cells or cells infected with viruses. In a fashion similar to intercellular recognition during the clonal selection process, the Tc cell must directly adhere to the target cell through antigen presented by MHC class I molecules and CD8 (Figure 7-18). Because of the broad cellular distribution of MHC class I molecules, Tc cells can recognize antigens on the surface of almost any type of cell that has been infected by a virus or has become cancerous. Unlike clonal selection, the roles of co-stimulatory signals through adhesion molecules and cytokines are of less importance here. Attachment to a target cell activates multiple killing mechanisms through which the Tc cell induces the target cell to undergo apoptosis.

Various other cells kill targets in a fashion similar to Tc cells. Prominent among these cells are natural killer cells. **Natural killer (NK) cells** are a special group of lymphoid cells that are similar to T cells but lack antigen-specific receptors. Instead, they express a variety of cell surface activation receptors (similar to pattern recognition receptors, see Chapter 6) that identify protein changes on the surface of cells infected with viruses or that have become cancerous. After attachment, the NK cell kills its target in a manner similar to that of Tc cells. NK cells also have receptors for MHC class I molecules. However, NK cells lack CD8; therefore, binding to MHC class I molecules results in inactivation of the NK cell. Thus, NK cells complement the effects of Tc cells. In some instances, a virus-infected or cancerous cell will "protect" itself by downregulating MHC class I molecule expression. Without surface MHC class I molecules, a cell becomes resistant to Tc-cell recognition and killing. NK cells primarily kill target cells that have suppressed the expression of MHC class I molecules.

NK cells, as well as some macrophages, can specifically kill targets through use of antibodies. NK cells express Fc receptors for IgG. If antigens on the infected or cancerous cell bind IgG, the NK cell can attach through Fc receptors and activate its normal killing mechanisms. This is referred to as **antibody-dependent cell-mediated cytotoxicity (ADCC)**.

Lymphokine-Secreting T Cells

Two subsets of Th cells amplify inflammation. Th1 cells, in addition to assisting Tc-cell clonal selection, secrete cytokines that activate M1 macrophages to increase phagocytic and microbial killing functions (described in Chapter 6). The most important cytokine for macrophage activation is IFN-γ. Th2 cells, in addition to assisting B-cell clonal selection, secrete cytokines (e.g., IL-4, IL-13) that activate M2 macrophages for healing and repair of damaged tissue (described in Chapter 6). Th17 cells secrete a set of cytokines (e.g., IL-17, IL-22, chemokines) that recruit phagocytic cells to a site of inflammation.[20] Th17-cell cytokines also may activate cells, particularly epithelial cells, to produce antimicrobial proteins in defence against certain bacterial and fungal pathogens.

T-Regulatory Lymphocytes

Treg cells are a diverse group of T cells that control the immune response, usually suppressing the response and maintaining tolerance against self-antigens.[21] This process occurs in the secondary lymphoid organs and other tissues, known as **peripheral tolerance**, in contrast to the process of central tolerance described earlier. This population of Treg cells that differentiate from the Th-cell population expresses CD4 and binds to antigens presented by MHC class II molecules. Unlike other Th cells, however, Treg cells express consistently high levels of CD25 (the IL-2 receptor). Differentiation from the Th precursor cell is controlled, primarily by TGF-β and IL-2. Treg cells produce very high levels of immunosuppressive cytokines TGF-β and IL-10, which generally decrease Th1 and Th2 activity by suppressing antigen recognition and Th-cell proliferation.

✔ QUICK CHECK 7-3

1. What are antigen-presenting cells?
2. Describe B cell antigen receptors and T cell antigen receptors.
3. What is the role of T-helper cells?
4. Why are cytokines important to the immune response?
5. What is the difference between central tolerance and peripheral tolerance?

Age-related mechanisms of self-defence in the newborn child and in older adults are listed in the *Pediatric Considerations* and *Geriatric Considerations* boxes.

PEDIATRIC CONSIDERATIONS

Age-Related Factors Affecting Mechanisms of Self-Defence in the Newborn Child

- Maternal IgG antibodies are transported across the placenta into the fetal blood and protect the neonate for the first 6 months, after which they are replaced by the child's own antibodies.
- Maternal antibodies provide protection within the newborn's circulation (see the figure in this box).
- Deficits in specific maternal transplacental antibody may lead to a tendency to develop severe, overwhelming sepsis and meningitis in the newborn.
- Normal human newborns are immunologically immature; they have deficient antibody production, phagocytic activity, and complement activity, especially components of alternative pathways (e.g., factor B).
- The newborn cannot produce all classes of antibody; IgM is produced by the newborn (develops in the last trimester) to in utero infections (e.g., cytomegalovirus, rubella virus, and *Toxoplasma gondii*); only limited amounts of IgA are produced in the newborn; IgG production begins after birth and rises steadily throughout the first year of life.
- Neonates often have transiently depressed inflammatory function, particularly neutrophil chemotaxis and alternative complement pathway activity.
- The T-cell–independent immune response is adequate in the fetus and neonate, but the T-cell–dependent immune response develops slowly during the first 6 months of life.

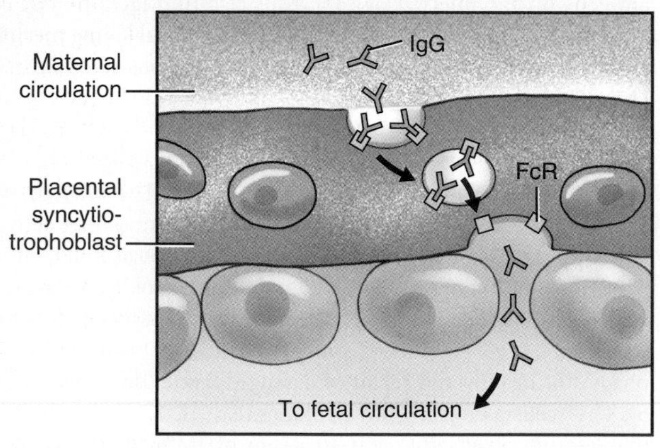

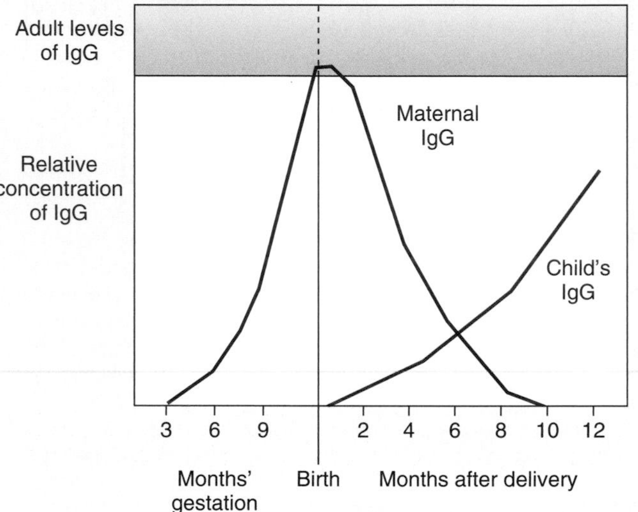

Antibody Levels in Umbilical Cord Blood and in Neonatal Circulation. Early in gestation, maternal IgG begins active transport across the placenta and enters the fetal circulation. At birth, the fetal circulation may contain nearly adult levels of IgG, which is almost exclusively from the maternal source. The fetal immune system has the capacity to produce IgM and small amounts of IgA before birth (not shown). After delivery, maternal IgG is rapidly destroyed and neonatal IgG production increases. *FcR*, crystallizable fragment receptor.

GERIATRIC CONSIDERATIONS

Age-Related Factors Affecting Mechanisms of Self-Defence in Older Adults

- Immune function decreases with age; diminished T-cell function and reduced antibody responses to antigenic challenges occur with age.
- The thymus reaches maximum size at sexual maturity and then undergoes involution until it is a vestigial remnant by middle age; by 45 to 50 years of age, the thymus is only 15% of its maximum size.
- With age there is a decrease in thymic hormone production and the organ's ability to mediate T-cell differentiation.
- T-cell function and antibody production are somewhat deficient in older adults. Older adults also tend to have increased levels of circulating autoantibodies (antibodies against self-antigens).
- Older adults are at risk for impaired wound healing, usually because of chronic illnesses.

DID YOU UNDERSTAND?

Third Line of Defence: Adaptive Immunity

1. Adaptive immunity is a state of protection, primarily against infectious agents, that differs from inflammation by being slower to develop, being more specific, and having memory that makes it much longer lived.
2. The adaptive immune response is most often initiated by cells of the innate system. These cells process and present portions of invading pathogens (i.e., antigens) to lymphocytes in peripheral lymphoid tissue.
3. The adaptive immune response is mediated by two different types of lymphocytes—B cells and T cells. Each has distinct functions. B cells are responsible for humoral immunity that is mediated by circulating antibodies (immunoglobulins), whereas T cells are responsible for cell-mediated immunity, in which

they kill targets directly or stimulate the activity of other leukocytes.
4. Adaptive immunity can be either active or passive depending on whether immune response components originated in the host or came from a donor.
5. The humoral immune response consists of molecules (antibodies) produced by B cells.
6. The induction of an immune response, or clonal selection, begins when antigen enters the individual's body.

Antigens and Immunogens

1. Antigens are molecules that bind and react with components of the immune response, such as antibodies and antigen receptors on B and T cells. Most antigens can induce an immune response, and these antigens are called *immunogens*.
2. All immunogens are antigens but not all antigens are immunogens.
3. Large molecules, such as proteins, polysaccharides, and nucleic acids, are most immunogenic. Thus molecular size is an important factor for antigen immunogenicity.
4. Haptens are antigens too small to be immunogens by themselves but become immunogenic after combining with larger molecules.

Antibodies

1. Antibodies are plasma glycoproteins that can be classified by chemical structure and biological activity as IgG, IgM, IgA, IgE, or IgD.
2. A typical antibody molecule is constructed of two identical heavy (H) chains and two identical light (L) chains and has two antigen-binding fragment portions that bind antigen and a crystalline fragment portion that interacts with complement or receptors on cells.
3. The antigenic determinant, or epitope, is the precise chemical structure with which an antibody or B cell or T cell antigen receptor reacts.
4. The protective effects of antibodies may be *direct* through the action of antibody alone or *indirect* requiring activation of other components of the innate immune response.
5. IgE is a special class of antibody produced against environmental antigens that are the primary cause of common allergies. It also protects the individual from infection caused by large parasitic worms (helminths).
6. The secretory immune system protects the external surfaces of the body by secreting antibodies in bodily secretions, such as tears, sweat, saliva, mucus, and breast milk. IgA is the dominant secretory immunoglobulin.

Immune Response: Collaboration of B Cells and T Cells

1. The generation of clonal diversity results in production of B and T cells with receptors against millions of antigens that possibly will be encountered in an individual's lifetime occurs in the fetus in the primary lymphoid organs: the thymus for T cells and portions of the bone marrow for B cells.
2. The generation of clonal diversity concludes when immunocompetent T and B cells migrate from the primary lymphoid organs into the circulation and secondary lymphoid organs to await antigen.
3. Lymphoid stem cells interact with stromal cells through a variety of adhesion factors. As the stem cell matures, it develops a variety of surface markers or receptors, one of the earliest being interleukin-7 (IL-7) receptor. IL-7, produced by stromal cells, is critical for driving differentiation and proliferation of the B cell.
4. The role of the B cell antigen receptor (BCR) is to recognize an antigen and communicate that information to the cell's nucleus.
5. The variable regions of antibodies, as well as the BCR, contain complementarity determining regions (CDRs). The diversity of these CDRs is responsible for the variety of antigens recognized by immunocompetent B cells. The enormous repertoire of antibody specificities is made possible by rearrangement of existing DNA during B-cell development in the primary lymphoid organs, a process called *somatic recombination*.
6. Somatic rearrangement of the antibody variable regions will frequently result in a BCR that recognizes the individual's own antigens, which may result in attack on "self" antigens expressed on various tissue and organs. Many of these "autoreactive" B cells are eliminated in the bone marrow. Most of the developing B cells undergo apoptosis. This entire process is referred to as *central tolerance*.
7. The process of T-cell proliferation and differentiation is similar to that for B cells. The primary lymphoid organ for T-cell development is the thymus. Lymphoid stem cells travel through the thymus, where thymic hormones and the cytokine IL-7 promote lymphoid stem cell division and the production of receptors. They exit the thymus as mature immunocompetent T cells with antigen-specific receptors on the cell surface.
8. The T cell antigen receptor (TCR) proceeds in a manner similar to the BCR. Initially proteins called CD4 and CD8 are expressed on the developing cells. Eventually CD4 cells develop into T-helper cells (Th cells) and CD 8 cells become T-cytotoxic cells (Tc cells). Other mature T cells include T-regulatory cells (Treg cells) and memory cells.
9. Most antigens must first interact with antigen-presenting cells (APCs) (e.g., macrophages). Dendritic cells present in the skin, mucosa, and lymphoid tissues also present antigens.
10. The response to antigens can be divided into two phases: primary immune response and secondary immune response. The primary immune response of humoral immunity is usually dominated by IgM, with lesser amounts of IgG. The secondary immune response has a more rapid production of a larger amount of antibodies, predominantly IgG.
11. Antigens are processed in APCs and presented on the cell surface by molecules of the major histocompatibility complex (MHC). The particular MHC molecule (class I or class II) that presents the antigen determines which cell will respond to that antigen. Th cells require that the antigen be presented in a complex with MHC class II molecules. Tc cells require that the antigen be presented by MHC class I molecules.
12. Th cells consist of Th1 cells, which help Tc cells respond to antigens; Th2 cells, which help B cells develop into plasma cells; and Th17 cells, which help activate macrophages.
13. Tc cells bind to and kill cellular targets such as cells infected with viruses or cancer cells.
14. The T cell sees the presented antigen through the TCR and accessory molecules (CD4 or CD8). CD4 is found on Th cells and reacts specifically with MHC class II molecules. CD8 is found on Tc cells and reacts specifically with MHC class I molecules.
15. The natural killer (NK) cell has some characteristics of the Tc cells and is important for killing target cells in which viral infection or malignancy has resulted in the loss of cellular MHC molecules.
16. Self-antigens are antigens on an individual's own cells. The individual's immune system does not normally recognize self-antigens as immunogenic, and this condition is known as peripheral tolerance.

KEY TERMS

Active immunity (active acquired immunity), 160
Adaptive (acquired) immunity, 159
Agglutination, 163
Antibody, 162
Antibody-dependent cell-mediated cytotoxicity (ADCC), 173
Antigen, 159
Antigen-binding fragment (Fab), 162
Antigen-binding site (paratope), 163
Antigenic determinant (epitope), 163
Antigen processing, 169
Antigen-processing (antigen-presenting) cell (APC), 168
B cell antigen receptor (BCR), 167
B lymphocyte (B cell), 159
CD3, 168
CD4, 168
CD8, 168
Cellular immunity, 160
Central tolerance, 168
Class switch, 170
Clonal diversity, 160
Clonal selection, 160
Complementarity determining region (CDR), 163
Crystallizable fragment (Fc), 162
Dendritic cell, 168
Hapten, 161
Human leukocyte antigen (HLA), 169
Humoral immunity, 160
Immune response, 159
Immunity, 159
Immunocompetent, 160
Immunogen, 161
Immunoglobulin (Ig), 162
Lymphocyte, 159
Lymphoid stem cell, 165
Major histocompatibility complex (MHC), 169
Memory cell, 160
Natural killer (NK) cell, 173
Neutralization, 163
Passive immunity (passive acquired immunity), 160
Peripheral tolerance, 173
Plasma cell, 160
Precipitation, 163
Primary (central) lymphoid organ, 165
Primary immune response, 168
Secondary immune response, 168
Secondary lymphoid organ, 160
Secretory immunoglobulin, 165
Secretory (mucosal) immune system, 165
Somatic recombination, 167
Superantigen (SAG), 169
Systemic immune system, 165
T cell antigen receptor (TCR), 168
T lymphocyte (T cell), 159
T-cytotoxic cell (Tc cell), 160
Th1 cell, 169
Th2 cell, 169
Th17 cell, 169
T-helper cell (Th cell), 160
Titre, 168
T-regulatory cell (Treg cell), 160

REFERENCES

1. Wu, L. C., & Zarrin, A. A. (2014). The production and regulation of IgE by the immune system. *Nature Reviews. Immunology, 14*(4), 247–259. doi:10.1038/nri3632.
2. Sela-Culang, I., Kunik, V., & Ofran, Y. (2013). The structural basis of antibody-antigen recognition. *Frontiers in Immunology, 4*, 302. doi:10.3389/fimmu.2013.00302.
3. Guilliams, M., Bruhns, P., Saeys, Y., et al. (2014). The function of Fcγ receptors in dendritic cells and macrophages. *Nature Reviews. Immunology, 14*(2), 94–108. doi:10.1038/nri3582.
4. Fitzsimmons, C. M., Falcone, F. H., & Dunne, D. W. (2014). Helminth allergens, parasite-specific IgE, and its protective role in human immunity. *Frontiers in Immunology, 5*, 61. doi:10.3389/fimmu.2014.00061.
5. Rescigno, M. (2013). Mucosal immunology and bacterial handling in the intestine. *Best Practice & Research. Clinical Gastroenterology, 27*(1), 17–24. doi:10.1016/j.bpg.2013.03.004.
6. Miyazaki, K., Miyazaki, M., & Murre, C. (2014). The establishment of B versus T cell identity. *Trends in Immunology, 35*(5), 205–210. doi:10.1016/j.it.2014.02.009.
7. Clark, M. R., Mandal, M., Ochiai, K., et al. (2014). Orchestrating B cell lymphopoiesis through interplay of IL-7 receptor and pre-B cell receptor signalling. *Nature Reviews. Immunology, 14*(2), 69–89. doi:10.1038/nri3570.
8. Shih, H.-Y., & Krangel, M. S. (2013). Chromatin architecture, CCCTC-binding factor, and V(D)J recombination: Managing long-distance relationships at antigen receptor loci. *Journal of Immunology, 190*(10), 4915–4921. doi:10.4049/jimmunol.1300218.
9. Boehm, T., & Swann, J. B. (2013). Thymus involution and regeneration: Two sides of the same coin? *Nature Reviews. Immunology, 13*(11), 831–838. doi:10.1038/nri3534.
10. Brownlie, R. J., & Zamoyska, R. (2013). T cell receptor signalling networks: Branching, diversified and bounded. *Nature Reviews. Immunology, 13*(4), 257–269. doi:10.1038/nri3403.
11. Blum, J. S., Wearsch, P. A., & Cresswell, P. (2013). Pathways of antigen processing. *Annual Review of Immunology, 31*(2013), 443–473. doi:10.1146/annurev-immunol-032712-095910.
12. Batista, F. D., & Dustin, M. L. (2013). Cell:cell interactions in the immune system. *Immunological Reviews, 251*(1), 7–12. doi:10.1111/imr.12025.
13. Fooksman, D. R. (2014). Organizing MHC class II presentation. *Frontiers in Immunology, 5*, 158. doi:10.3389/fimmu.2014.00158.
14. Yamane, H., & Paul, W. E. (2013). Early signaling events that underlie fate decisions of naïve CD4⁺ T cells toward distinct T-helper cell subsets. *Immunological Reviews, 252*(1), 12–23. doi:10.1111/imr.12032.
15. Jiang, S., & Dong, C. (2013). A complex issue on $CD4^+$ T-cell subsets. *Immunological Reviews, 252*(1), 5–11. doi:10.1111/imr.12041.
16. Ramachandran, G. (2014). Gram-positive and gram-negative bacterial toxins in sepsis: A brief review. *Virulence, 5*(1), 213–218. doi:10.4161/viru.27024.
17. Avalos, A. M., & Ploegh, H. L. (2014). Early BCR events and antigen capture, processing, and loading on MHC class II on B cells. *Frontiers in Immunology, 5*, 92. doi:10.3389/fimmu.2014.00092.
18. Njau, M. N., & Jacob, J. (2013). The CD28/B7 pathway: A novel regulator of plasma cell function. *Advances in Experimental Medicine and Biology, 785*(2013), 67–75. doi:10.1007/978-1-4614-6217-0_8.
19. Farber, D. L., Yudanin, N. A., & Restifo, N. P. (2014). Human memory T cells: Generation, compartmentalization and homeostasis. *Nature Reviews. Immunology, 14*(1), 24–35. doi:10.1038/nri3567.
20. Annunziato, F., Cosmi, L., Liotta, F., et al. (2013). Main features of human T helper 17 cells. *Annals of the New York Academy of Sciences, 1284*(2013), 66–70. doi:10.1111/nyas.12075.
21. Singer, B. D., King, L. S., & D'Alessio, F. R. (2014). Regulatory T cells as immunotherapy. *Frontiers in Immunology, 5*, 46. doi:10.3389/fimmu.2014.00046.

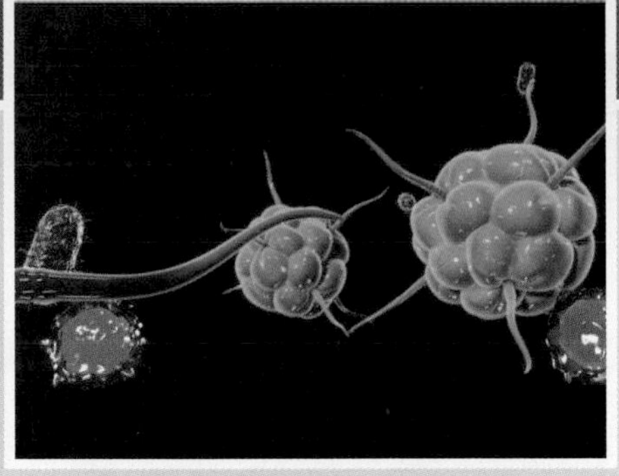

8

Infection and Defects in Mechanisms of Defence

Neal S. Rote and Stephanie Zettel

EVOLVE WEBSITE

http://evolve.elsevier.com/Canada/Huether/pathophysiology
Student Review Questions
Key Points
Case Studies
Animations
Quick Check Answers

CHAPTER OUTLINE

Infection, 177
Microorganisms and Humans: A Dynamic Relationship, 177
Countermeasures Against Infectious Microorganisms, 188
Deficiencies in Immunity, 190
Initial Clinical Presentation, 190
Primary (Congenital) Immune Deficiencies, 191
Secondary (Acquired) Immune Deficiencies, 193
Evaluation and Care of Those With Immune Deficiency, 193
Replacement Therapies for Immune Deficiencies, 193
AIDS, 195
Hypersensitivity: Allergy, Autoimmunity, and Alloimmunity, 199
Mechanisms of Hypersensitivity, 202
Antigenic Targets of Hypersensitivity Reactions, 208

The defensive system protecting the body from infection is a finely tuned network, but it is not perfect. Sometimes infectious agents can inhibit or escape defence mechanisms or the system may break down, leading to inadequate protection or inappropriate activation. An inadequate response (commonly called an *immune deficiency*) may range from relatively mild defects to life-threatening severity. Inappropriate responses (hypersensitivity reactions) may be (1) exaggerated against noninfectious environmental substances (allergy); (2) misdirected against the body's own cells (autoimmunity); or (3) directed against beneficial foreign tissues, such as transfusions or transplants (alloimmunity). Several of these inappropriate responses can be serious or life-threatening. This chapter provides an overview of conditions under which our protective systems have failed.

INFECTION

Modern health care has shown great progress in preventing and treating infectious diseases. In Canada, heart disease and malignancies greatly surpass infectious disease as major causes of death.[1] However, since the severe acute respiratory syndrome (SARS) epidemic that took place in 2003, the challenge in treating **infectious diseases** has become a key issue. Hospitals have implemented measures geared toward controlling health care–associated infections.[2] Most deaths related to infections occur in individuals whose protective systems are compromised (children, older adults, and those with chronic disease).

Infectious disease remains a significant threat to life in many parts of the world, including India, Africa, and Southeast Asia.[3] Sanitary living conditions, clean water, uncontaminated food, vaccinations, and antimicrobial medications have improved the health of many; but inefficient health care systems, endemic poverty, political unrest, and other factors have slowed progress in some regions. As a result of initiatives to prevent and treat infectious diseases, smallpox has been eradicated from the globe (the last reported case was in 1975 in Somalia). Worldwide, polio has declined by more than 99% and been eradicated from the Western hemisphere. Measles was decreased by 78% and was nearly eliminated in the Western hemisphere. Although vaccines and antimicrobials have diminished the frequency of some infectious diseases, new diseases have emerged, such as West Nile virus, SARS, Middle East respiratory syndrome coronavirus (MERS-CoV), and *Hantavirus*. Some diseases have spread uncontrollably, such as Ebola virus disease, into new regions of Africa. As well, many multiple medication–resistant microorganisms continue to develop. All of these examples reflect the ongoing intense challenges in the struggle to prevent and control infectious diseases.

In Canada, First Nations people and the Inuit have higher rates of contagious disease, resulting in shorter life expectancies. Human immunodeficiency virus (HIV)/acquired immunodeficiency syndrome (AIDS), influenza, West Nile virus, and tuberculosis (TB) are just a few of the common conditions found in the Indigenous population[4] (see *Health Promotion:* Tuberculosis and the Indigenous Population in Canada).

Microorganisms and Humans: A Dynamic Relationship

The increase in antibiotic resistance, in particular, places more importance on maintenance of an intact inflammatory and immune system. Individuals with immune deficiencies become easily infected with opportunistic microorganisms—those that normally would not cause disease but seize the opportunity provided by the person's decreased immune or inflammatory responses.

Unlike opportunistic infections, true pathogens have devised means to circumvent the normal controls provided by the innate and adaptive

HEALTH PROMOTION

Tuberculosis and the Indigenous Population in Canada

Indigenous people have one of the highest rates of tuberculosis (TB) in Canada. In 2012, Indigenous people in Canada accounted for 4% of the population, but 23% of the active cases of TB. TB incidence in the Inuit population was 400 times higher than TB incidence in the Canadian-born non-Indigenous population, and the incidence rate for First Nations people was 32 times higher. The rate of TB incidence in the Indigenous population can be explained partly by the living conditions on reserves. For example, many homes on reserves are overcrowded and poorly ventilated. A lack of proper nutrition can further increase the risk for those with latent TB infection to progress to an active disease state. Many individuals in First Nations communities also have pre-existing co-morbidities such as diabetes and HIV that further contribute to this risk. Moreover, many of these communities are remote and isolated, which results in decreased access to health care services.

In 2014, the federal government developed a framework for action to lower the incidence of TB in Canada. The key areas of focus for this framework are as follows:

1. Optimizing and enhancing current efforts to prevent and control active TB disease
2. Facilitating the identification and treatment of latent TB infection for those at high risk for developing active TB disease
3. Championing collaborative action to address the underlying risk factors for TB

The report *Tuberculosis Prevention and Control in Canada: A Federal Framework for Action* presents the federal government's framework for action and associated initiatives in relation to addressing TB in Canada.

© All rights reserved. *Tuberculosis Prevention and Control in Canada: A Federal Framework for Action.* Public Health Agency of Canada, 2014. Adapted and reproduced with permission from the Minister of Health, 2017. Retrieved from http://www.phac-aspc.gc.ca/tbpc-latb/pubs/tpc-pct/assets/pdf/tpc-pcta-eng.pdf.

TABLE 8-1 Classes of Microorganisms Infectious to Humans

Class	Size	Site of Reproduction	Example
Virus	20–300 nm	Intracellular	Poliomyelitis
Chlamydiae	200–1 000 nm	Intracellular	Urethritis
Rickettsiae	300–1 200 nm	Intracellular	Rocky Mountain spotted fever
Mycoplasma	125–350 nm	Extracellular	Atypical pneumonia
Bacteria	0.8–15 mcg	Skin	Staphylococcal wound infection
		Mucous membranes	Cholera
		Extracellular	Streptococcal pneumonia
		Intracellular	Tuberculosis
Fungi	2–200 mcg	Skin	Tinea pedis (athlete's foot)
		Mucous membranes	Candidiasis (e.g., thrush)
		Extracellular	Sporotrichosis
		Intracellular	Histoplasmosis
Protozoa	1–50 mm	Mucosal	Giardiasis
		Extracellular	Sleeping sickness
Helminths	3 mm to 10 m	Intracellular	Trichinosis
		Extracellular	Filariasis

immune systems. Several factors influence the capacity of a pathogen to cause disease:

- **Communicability**: The ability to spread from one individual to others (e.g., measles and pertussis spread very easily; HIV is of lower communicability)
- **Infectivity**: The ability of the pathogen to invade and multiply in the host (e.g., herpes simplex virus can survive for long periods in a latent stage)
- **Virulence**: The capacity of a pathogen to cause severe disease (e.g., measles virus is of low virulence; rabies and Ebola viruses are highly virulent)
- **Pathogenicity**: The ability of an agent to produce disease—success depends on communicability, infectivity, extent of tissue damage, and virulence (e.g., HIV can kill T lymphocytes [T cells])
- **Portal of entry**: The route by which a pathogenic microorganism infects the host (e.g., direct contact, inhalation, ingestion, or bites of an animal or insect)
- **Toxigenicity**: The ability to produce soluble toxins or endotoxins, factors that greatly influence the pathogen's degree of virulence

Infectivity is facilitated by the ability of pathogens to attach to cell surfaces, release enzymes that dissolve protective barriers, multiply rapidly, escape the action of phagocytes, or resist the effect of low pH. After penetrating protective barriers (invasion), pathogens then multiply and spread through the lymph and blood to tissues and organs, where they continue multiplying and cause disease. In humans the route of entrance of many pathogenic microorganisms also becomes the site of shedding of new infectious agents to other individuals, completing a cycle of infection.

Infectious disease can be caused by microorganisms that range in size from 20 nm (poliovirus) to 10 m (tapeworm). Classes of pathogenic microorganisms and their characteristics are summarized in Table 8-1. Some mechanisms of tissue damage caused by microorganisms are summarized in Table 8-2. The multiple layers of defence against infection are described in Chapters 6 and 7. Table 8-3 contains examples of microorganisms that defeat our protective systems.

Bacterial Disease

Bacteria are prokaryotes (lacking a discrete nucleus) and are relatively small. They can be aerobic or anaerobic and motile or immotile. Spherical bacteria are called *cocci*, rodlike forms are called *bacilli*, and spiral forms are termed *spirochetes*. Gram stain differentiates the microorganisms as Gram-positive or Gram-negative bacteria. Examples of human diseases caused by specific bacteria are listed in Table 8-4. The general structure of bacteria is reviewed in Figure 8-1.

Bacterial survival and growth depend on the effectiveness of the body's defence mechanisms and on the bacterium's ability to resist these defences. A vast amount of information has been published about bacterial pathogenesis. The main aspects of how bacteria cause disease may be illustrated in how one particular microorganism, *Staphylococcus aureus*, has adapted to become a life-threatening pathogen.

S. aureus has become a major cause of hospital-acquired (health care–associated) infections and is now spreading throughout communities. This microorganism is a common commensal inhabitant of normal skin and nasal passages (estimates indicate that from 30 to 80% of individuals may be nasal carriers) and can be transmitted by direct skin-to-skin contact or by contact with shared items or surfaces that have become contaminated by another person (e.g., towels, used bandages).[5]

TABLE 8-2 Examples of Microorganisms That Cause Tissue Damage

Pathogens That Directly Cause Tissue Damage	
Produce Exotoxin	
Streptococcus pyogenes	Tonsillitis, scarlet fever
Staphylococcus aureus	Boils, toxic shock syndrome, food poisoning
Corynebacterium diphtheria	Diphtheria
Clostridium tetani	Tetanus
Vibrio cholerae	Cholera
Produce Endotoxin	
Escherichia coli	Gram-negative sepsis
Haemophilus influenzae	Meningitis, pneumonia
Salmonella typhi	Typhoid
Shigella	Bacillary dysentery
Pseudomonas aeruginosa	Wound infection
Yersinia pestis	Plague
Cause Direct Damage With Invasion	
Variola	Smallpox
Varicella-zoster	Chickenpox, shingles
Hepatitis B virus	Hepatitis
Poliovirus	Poliomyelitis
Measles virus	Measles, subacute sclerosing panencephalitis
Influenza virus	Influenza
Herpes simplex virus	Cold sores
Pathogens That Indirectly Cause Tissue Damage	
Produce Immune Complexes	
Hepatitis B virus	Kidney disease
S. pyogenes	Glomerulonephritis
Treponema pallidum	Kidney damage in secondary syphilis
Most acute infections	Transient renal deposits
Cause Cell-Mediated Immunity	
Mycobacterium tuberculosis	Tuberculosis
Mycobacterium leprae	Tuberculoid leprosy
Lymphocytic choriomeningitis virus	Aseptic meningitis
Borrelia burgdorferi	Lyme arthritis
Herpes simplex virus	Herpes stromal keratitis

Data modified from Janeway, C.A., Travers, P., Walport, M., et al. (2001). *Immunobiology: The system in health and disease* (5th ed.). New York: Garland.

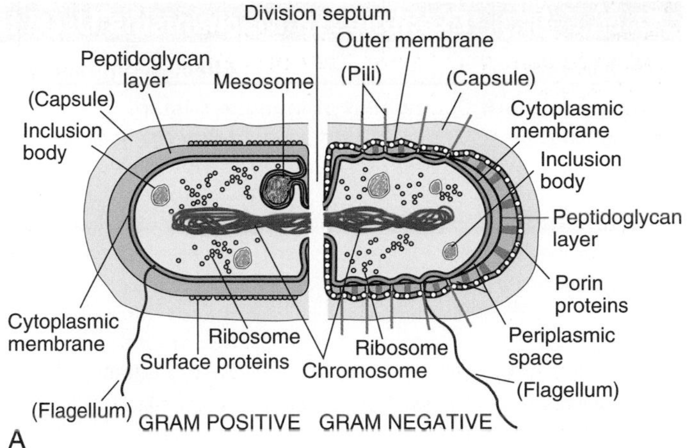

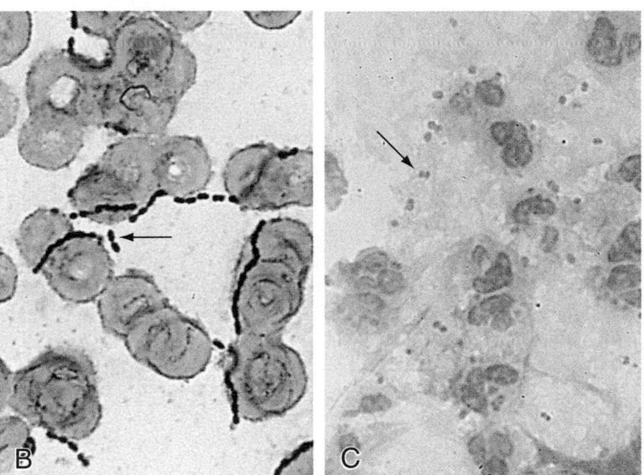

FIGURE 8-1 General Structure of Bacteria. A, The structure of the bacterial cell wall determines its staining characteristics with Gram stain. A Gram-positive bacterium has a thick layer of peptidoglycan (*left*). A Gram-negative bacterium has a thick peptidoglycan layer and an outer membrane (*right*). **B,** Example of a Gram-positive (darkly stained microorganisms, *arrow*) group A *Streptococcus*. This microorganism consists of cocci that frequently form chains. **C,** Example of a Gram-negative (pink microorganisms, *arrow*) *Neisseria meningitides* in cerebrospinal fluid. *Neisseria* form complexes of two cocci (diplococci). (**A,** from Murray, P.R., Rosenthal, K.S., & Pfaller, M.A. [2013]. *Medical microbiology* [7th ed.]. Philadelphia: Saunders; **B, C,** from Murray, P.R., Rosenthal, K.S., Kobayashi, G.S., et al. [2002]. *Medical microbiology* [4th ed.]. St. Louis: Mosby.)

Although a relatively benign commensal microorganism under normal conditions, *S. aureus* is well equipped to act as a life-threatening pathogen when the opportunity arises; thus it is an opportunistic microorganism. Skin infections may occur at sites of trauma, such as cuts and abrasions, and at areas of the body covered by hair (e.g., back of neck, groin, buttock, armpit, beard area of men). Most infections are relatively mild and localized, appearing as red and swollen pustules on the skin, containing pus or other drainage. They can develop into abscesses, boils, carbuncles, cellulitis, or furunculosis. Invasive disease may originate from wound infections (e.g., trauma, surgical wounds, indwelling medical devices, prosthetic joints) and lead to fatal septicemia and abscesses in internal organs (e.g., lungs, kidney, bones, skeletal muscle, meninges, or heart) (Figure 8-2).

Microscopically, staphylococci are Gram-positive cocci that generally grow in grapelike clusters. However, this microorganism possesses a myriad of potential virulence factors that determine the severity, location, and clinical features of infection. It should be noted that individual strains of this opportunistic pathogen utilize only some of the entire array of virulence factors.

Microorganisms frequently exist as part of complex multicellular masses called *biofilms*. **Biofilms** consist of mixed species of microorganisms, including bacteria, fungi, and viruses. Growth of bacteria in biofilms offers survival advantage by protection from the host's responses and exposure to antibiotics. These structures are associated with otitis media; urinary tract infections secondary to indwelling catheters; foot ulcers in diabetic persons; infected burn wounds; vaginitis; osteomyelitis; pneumonia secondary to cystic fibrosis; and diseases of

TABLE 8-3 Examples of Mechanisms Used by Pathogens to Resist the Immune System

Mechanisms	Effect on Immunity	Example of Specific Microorganisms
Destroy or Block Component of Immune System		
Produce toxins	Kills phagocyte or interferes with chemotaxis	*Staphylococcus*
	Prevents phagocytosis by inhibiting fusion between phagosome and lysosomal granules	*Streptococcus* *Mycobacterium tuberculosis*
Produce antioxidants (e.g., catalase, superoxide dismutase)	Prevents killing by oxygen-dependent mechanisms Promotes bacterial attachment	*Mycobacterium* sp. *Salmonella typhi*
Produce protease to digest IgA		*Neisseria gonorrhoeae* (urinary tract infection), *Haemophilus influenzae*, and *Streptococcus pneumoniae* (pneumonia)
Produce surface molecules that mimic crystallizable fragment (Fc) receptors and bind antibodies	Prevents activation of complement system Prevents antibody functioning as opsonin	*Staphylococcus* Herpes simplex virus
Mimic Self-Antigens		
Produce surface antigens (e.g., M protein, red blood cell antigens) that are similar to self-antigens	Resembles individual's own tissue; in some individuals, antibodies can be formed against self-antigen, leading to hypersensitivity disease (e.g., antibody to M protein also reacts with cardiac tissue, causing rheumatic heart disease; antibody to red blood cell antigens can cause anemia)	Group A *Streptococcus* (M protein) *Mycoplasma pneumoniae* (red cell antigens)
Change Antigenic Profile		
Undergo mutation of antigens or activate genes that change surface molecules	Delays immune response because of failure to recognize new antigen	Influenza HIV Some parasites

TABLE 8-4 Examples of Common Bacterial Infections

Microorganism	Gram Stain	Respiratory Pathway	Intracellular or Extracellular
Respiratory Tract Infections			
Upper Respiratory Tract Infections			
Corynebacterium diphtheriae (diphtheria)	Gram +	Facultative anaerobic	Extracellular
Haemophilus influenzae	Gram –	Facultative anaerobic	Extracellular
Streptococcus pyogenes (group A)	Gram +	Facultative anaerobic	Extracellular
Otitis Media			
Haemophilus influenzae	Gram –	Facultative anaerobic	Extracellular
Streptococcus pneumoniae	Gram +	Facultative anaerobic	Extracellular
Lower Respiratory Tract Infections			
Bacillus anthracis (pulmonary anthrax)	Gram +	Facultative anaerobic	Extracellular
Bordetella pertussis (whooping cough)	Gram –	Aerobic	Extracellular
Chlamydia pneumonia	Not stainable	Aerobic	Obligate intracellular
Escherichia coli	Gram –	Facultative anaerobic	Extracellular
Haemophilus influenzae	Gram –	Facultative anaerobic	Extracellular
Legionella pneumophila	Gram –	Aerobic	Facultative intracellular
Mycobacterium tuberculosis	Gram + (weakly)	Aerobic	Extracellular
Mycoplasma pneumoniae	Not stainable	Aerobic	Extracellular
Neisseria meningitidis (develops into meningitis)	Gram –	Aerobic	Extracellular
Pseudomonas aeruginosa	Gram –	Aerobic	Extracellular
Streptococcus agalactiae (group B; develops into meningitis)	Gram +	Facultative anaerobic	Extracellular
Streptococcus pneumoniae	Gram +	Facultative anaerobic	Extracellular
Yersinia pestis (plague)	Gram –	Facultative anaerobic	Extracellular

TABLE 8-4 Examples of Common Bacterial Infections—cont'd

Microorganism	Gram Stain	Respiratory Pathway	Intracellular or Extracellular
Gastro-intestinal Infections			
Inflammatory Gastro-intestinal Infections			
Bacillus anthracis (gastro-intestinal anthrax)	Gram +	Facultative anaerobic	Extracellular
Clostridium difficile	Gram +	Anaerobic	Extracellular
Escherichia coli O157:H7	Gram –	Facultative anaerobic	Extracellular
Vibrio cholerae	Gram –	Facultative anaerobic	Extracellular
Invasive Gastro-intestinal Infections			
Brucella abortus (brucellosis, undulant fever, leading to sepsis, heart infection)	Gram –	Aerobic	Intracellular
Helicobacter pylori (gastritis and peptic ulcers)	Gram –	Microaerophilic	Extracellular
Listeria monocytogenes (leading to sepsis and meningitis)	Gram +	Aerobic	Intracellular
Salmonella typhi (typhoid fever)	Gram –	Anaerobic	Extracellular
Shigella sonnei	Gram –	Facultative anaerobic	Extracellular
Food Poisoning			
Bacillus cereus	Gram +	Facultative anaerobic	Extracellular
Clostridium botulinum	Gram +	Anaerobic	Extracellular
Clostridium perfringens	Gram +	Anaerobic	Extracellular
Staphylococcus aureus	Gram +	Facultative anaerobic	Extracellular
Sexually Transmitted Infections			
Chlamydia trachomatis (pelvic inflammatory disease)	Not stainable	Aerobic	Intracellular
Neisseria gonorrhoeae (urethritis)	Gram –	Aerobic	Facultative intracellular
Treponema pallidum (spirochete; syphilis)	Gram –	Aerobic	Extracellular
Skin and Wound Infections			
Bacillus anthracis (cutaneous anthrax)	Gram +	Facultative anaerobic	Extracellular
Borrelia burgdorferi (Lyme disease; spirochete)	Gram –	Aerobic	Extracellular
Clostridium tetani (tetanus)	Gram +	Anaerobic	Extracellular
Clostridium perfringens (gas gangrene)	Gram +	Anaerobic	Extracellular
Mycobacterium leprae (leprosy)	Gram + (weakly)	Aerobic	Extracellular
Pseudomonas aeruginosa	Gram –	Aerobic	Extracellular
Rickettsia prowazekii (rickettsia; typhus)	Gram –	Aerobic	Obligate intracellular
Staphylococcus aureus	Gram +	Facultative anaerobic	Extracellular
Streptococcus pyogenes (group A)	Gram +	Facultative anaerobic	Extracellular
Eye Infections			
Chlamydia trachomatis (conjunctivitis)	Not stainable	Aerobic	Obligate intracellular
Haemophilus aegyptius (pink eye)	Gram –	Facultative anaerobic	Extracellular
Zoonotic Infections			
Bacillus anthracis (anthrax)	Gram +	Facultative anaerobic	Extracellular
Brucella abortus (brucellosis, also called undulant fever)	Gram –	Aerobic	Intracellular
Borrelia burgdorferi (spirochete; Lyme disease)	Gram –	Aerobic	Extracellular
Listeria monocytogenes	Gram +	Aerobic	Intracellular
Rickettsia rickettsii (rickettsia; Rocky Mountain spotted fever)	Gram –	Aerobic	Obligate intracellular
Rickettsia prowazekii (rickettsia; typhus)	Gram –	Aerobic	Obligate intracellular
Yersinia pestis (plague)	Gram –	Facultative anaerobic	Extracellular
Health Care–Associated Infections			
Enterococcus faecalis	Gram +	Facultative anaerobic	Extracellular
Enterococcus faecium	Gram +	Facultative anaerobic	Extracellular
Escherichia coli (cystitis)	Gram –	Facultative anaerobic	Extracellular
Pseudomonas aeruginosa	Gram –	Obligate anaerobic	Extracellular
Staphylococcus aureus	Gram +	Facultative anaerobic	Extracellular
Staphylococcus epidermidis	Gram +	Facultative anaerobic	Extracellular

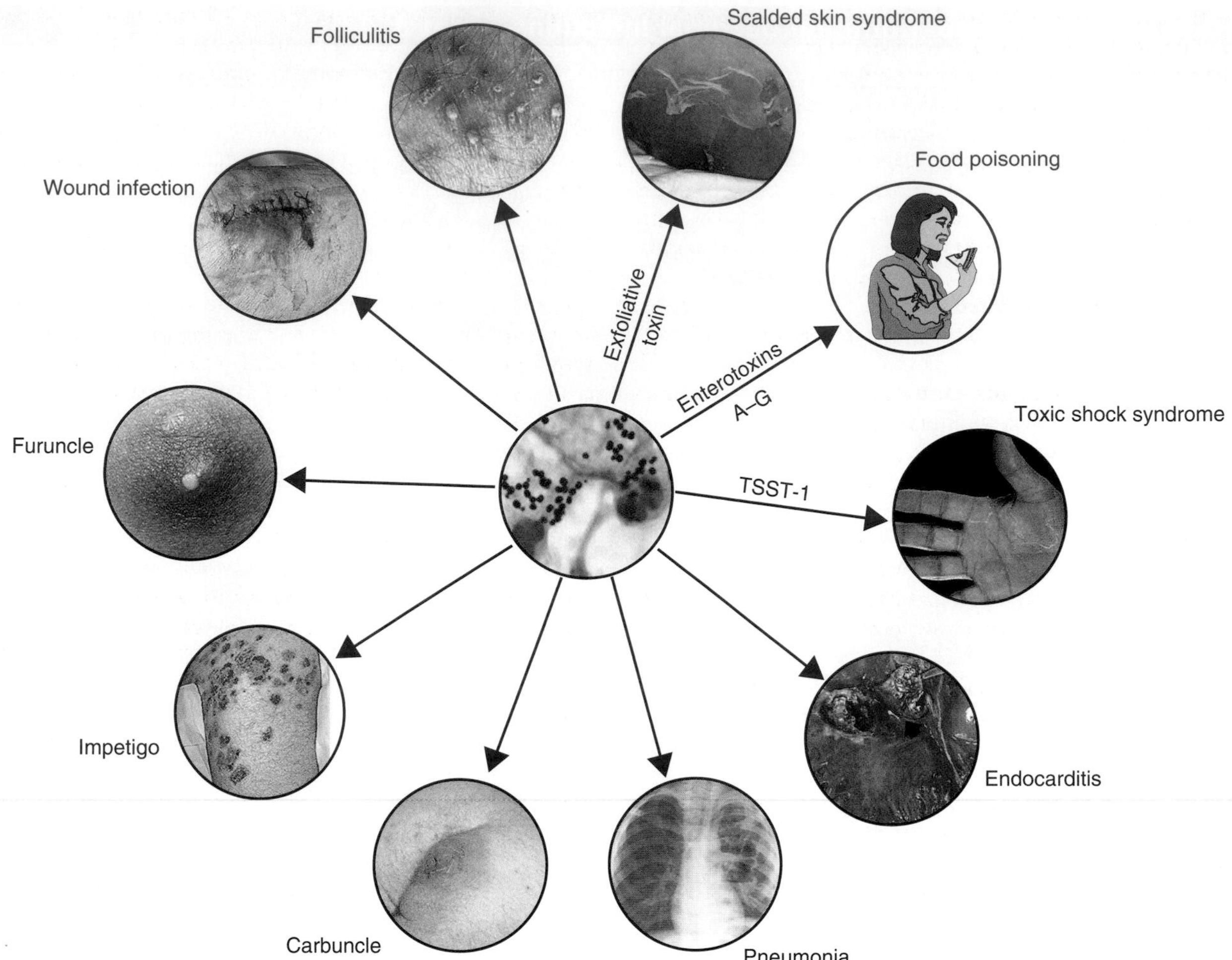

FIGURE 8-2 ***Staphylococcus aureus*** **Infections.** Different strains of *Staphylococcus aureus* (Gram-positive cocci in sputum from an individual with pneumonia [*centre photograph*]) cause a variety of infections. The particular infection may depend on the toxin produced: exfoliative toxin (scalded skin syndrome), enterotoxins A–G (food poisoning), or toxic shock syndrome toxin-1 (*TSST-1*). (Toxic shock syndrome, carbuncle, impetigo, and wound infection photos from Cohen, J., & Powderly, W.G. [2010]. *Infectious diseases* [3rd ed.]. St. Louis: Mosby; folliculitis photo from Goldman, L., & Ausiello, D. [2012]. *Cecil medicine* [24th ed.]. Philadelphia: Saunders; centre photo and photos of food poisoning and endocarditis from Kumar, V., Abbas, A.K., Fausto, N., et al. [Eds.] [2010]. *Robbins and Cotran pathologic basis of disease* [8th ed.]. Philadelphia: Saunders; furuncle photo from Long, S.S., Pickering, L.K., & Prober, C.G. [2012]. *Principles and practice of pediatric infectious diseases* [4th ed.]. Philadelphia: Saunders; scalded skin syndrome and pneumonia photos from Mandell, G., Bennett, J., & Dolin, R. [2010]. *Principles and practice of infectious diseases* [7th ed.]. Philadelphia: Churchill Livingstone.)

the oral cavity related to dental plaque, such as dental caries and periodontitis. *S. aureus* biofilms are associated with persistent nasopharyngeal colonization and colonization of implanted devices.[6]

A variety of surface proteins mediate adherence among microorganisms in biofilms and to connective tissue (laminin, fibrin, fibronectin) and endothelium. Attachment to collagen occurs in strains causing osteomyelitis and septic arthritis. The capsular polysaccharide mediates attachment to prosthetic devices and also protects against phagocytosis. One surface protein, protein A, binds immunoglobulin G (IgG) by the crystallizable fragment (Fc) portion so that the antigen-binding fragment (Fab) regions are facing outward.

Thus, the bacteria appear coated with a self-protein, and, with the Fc bound directly to protein A, the IgG cannot activate complement or act as an opsonin.[7] Staphylococcal protein A and a protein called *staphylococcal binder of immunoglobulin* are secreted; they both bind and neutralize IgG. *Staphylococcus* produces proteins that inhibit complement activity, including activation of C3 and C5, preventing production of C3b, C3a, and C5a.[8] A coagulase that induces fibrin clotting on the bacterial surface also masks bacterial antigens under a surface of self-proteins.

Some strains of *S. aureus* are also programmed to avoid innate immunity. They can produce inhibitors of antimicrobial peptides and avoid recognition by Toll-like receptors.[9] Even when engulfed by a phagocyte, *S. aureus* may resist intracellular oxidative killing by inactivating hydrogen peroxide and other reactive oxygen species. They also resist lysozyme by changing the chemistry of the cell wall.[10]

Many bacteria use toxins as virulence factors, including exotoxins and endotoxins. Exotoxins are secreted molecules and are immunogenic, eliciting production of antibodies known as **antitoxins** (important for vaccine development, see page 189). The most poisonous yet discovered is botulinum neurotoxin produced by *Clostridium botulinum*; less than 1 ng/kg is toxic to humans. Strains of *S. aureus* are capable of producing a wide array of secreted toxic molecules, or exotoxins. They include those that damage the cell membrane (α-toxin, which forms pores in membranes; hemolysin, which destroys erythrocytes; β-toxin, which is a sphingomyelinase; δ-toxin, a detergentlike toxin; and leukocidin, which lyses phagocytes). Other toxins include coagulase, which causes blood clots; staphylokinase, which breaks down clots; exfoliative toxins, which cause separation of the epidermis resulting in scalded skin syndrome; lipase, which degrades lipids on the skin surface and facilitates abscess formation; enterotoxins, which cause food poisoning; and superantigens (discussed in Chapter 7).[11] Each infectious strain of *S. aureus* may produce a few of these toxins so that strains differ in their capacities to cause particular diseases; thus, different strains may cause purulent dermal infections, food poisoning, or toxic shock syndrome.

Antibiotic resistance has become a major problem with *S. aureus*. For several decades pathogenic strains have commonly produced β-lactamase, an enzyme that destroys penicillin. More recently, staphylococci have developed resistance to broad-spectrum antibiotics, including methicillinlike antibiotics (methicillin-resistant *Staphylococcus aureus* [MRSA]), which were widely used to treat penicillin-resistant microorganisms.

It is clear that *S. aureus* succeeds as an opportunistic pathogen because of a wide array of virulence factors that neutralize important components of the innate and adaptive immune systems, destroy tissue, and resist much of our repertoire of antibiotics. The major remaining option is the development of an effective vaccine, a task that is sometimes difficult.[12] As mentioned in the beginning of this section, *S. aureus* is only one of many bacteria that have developed similar characteristics.

Gram-negative microbes produce an endotoxin (lipopolysaccharide [LPS]) that is a structural portion of the cell wall and is released during growth, lysis, or destruction of the bacteria or during treatment with antibiotics. Therefore, antibiotics cannot prevent the toxic effects of the endotoxin. Bacteria that produce endotoxins are called *pyrogenic bacteria* because they activate the inflammatory process and produce fever. The innermost part of the lipopolysaccharide, lipid A, consists of polysaccharide and fatty acids and is responsible for the substance's toxic effects.

Bacteremia occurs when bacteria are present in the blood. Gram-negative sepsis (sepsis or septicemia) occurs when bacteria are growing in the blood and release large amounts of endotoxin, which can cause endotoxic shock with up to 50% mortality.[13] Released endotoxin, as well as other bacterial products, reacts with pattern recognition receptors (PRRs) and induces the overproduction of proinflammatory cytokines, particularly tumour necrosis factor-alpha (TNF-α), interleukin-1 (IL-1), and interleukin-6 (IL-6), which may secondarily be immunosuppressive.[14] Endotoxin also is a potent activator of the complement and clotting systems, leading to a degree of capillary permeability sufficient to permit escape of large volumes of plasma into surrounding tissue, contributing to hypotension and, in severe cases, cardiovascular shock (see Chapter 24). Activation of the coagulation cascade leads to the syndrome of disseminated (or diffuse) intravascular coagulation (see Chapter 21).

Viral Disease

Viral diseases are the most common afflictions of humans and range from the common cold (caused by many viruses) to the "cold sore" of herpes simplex virus to cancers to AIDS. Examples of human diseases caused by specific viruses are listed in Table 8-5. Viruses are very simple microorganisms consisting of nucleic acid protected from the environment by a layer or layers of proteins (capsid). The viral genome can be double-stranded DNA (dsDNA), single-stranded DNA (ssDNA), double-stranded RNA (dsRNA), or single-stranded RNA (ssRNA). A select group of viruses (e.g., HIV, herpesviruses, influenza virus) bud from the surface of an infected cell, retaining a portion of the cell's plasma membrane (envelope) as added protection. Viral replication depends totally on their ability to infect a permissive host cell—a cell that cannot resist viral invasion and replication. Thus, viruses are obligatory intracellular microbes. Transmission is usually from one infected individual to an uninfected individual by aerosols of respiratory tract fluids, contact with infected blood, sexual contact, or transmission from an animal reservoir (zoonotic infection) usually through a vector, such as mosquitoes.[15]

To understand the basic concepts of viral pathogenicity, it may be best to look closely at a single virus. Influenza is an ssRNA virus with a segmented genome (eight pieces of ssRNA). It is transmitted through aerosols or body fluids and is highly infectious. Symptoms begin 1 to 4 days after infection and may include chills, fever, sore throat, muscle aches, severe headaches, coughing, weakness, generalized discomfort, nausea, and vomiting and may lead to pneumonia. It can be fatal, particularly in young children and older adults.[16] The normal rate of infectivity is about 5 to 15%, with a mortality of about 0.1%, and in most cases recovery occurs in 1 to 2 weeks. Yearly seasonal influenza outbreaks result in about 250 000 to 500 000 deaths worldwide.

The life cycle of every virus is completely intracellular and involves several steps, the first being *attachment* to a receptor on the target cell (Figure 8-3). The influenza virion expresses two surface proteins that are essential to virulence. The hemagglutinin (HA) protein is a glycoprotein that is necessary for entrance into cells by binding to glycan receptors on the surface of respiratory tract epithelium. The viral surface neuraminidase (NA) is an enzyme that is necessary for release of new virions from infected cells by cleaving cellular sialic acids (a common component of mammalian cell membranes). The specificity of this virus–receptor interaction (tropism) dictates the range of host cells that a particular virus will infect and, therefore, the clinical symptoms that reflect the alteration of the function of the infected cells. Other viruses also use specific receptors; for example, HIV attaches to CD4 on T-helper cells, Epstein-Barr virus (EBV, a cause of mononucleosis and Burkitt lymphoma) attaches to complement receptor 2 (CR2) on B lymphocytes (B cells), and Rhinovirus (a group of viruses that cause the common cold) attaches to intracellular adhesion molecule-1 (ICAM-1) on respiratory tract epithelium.

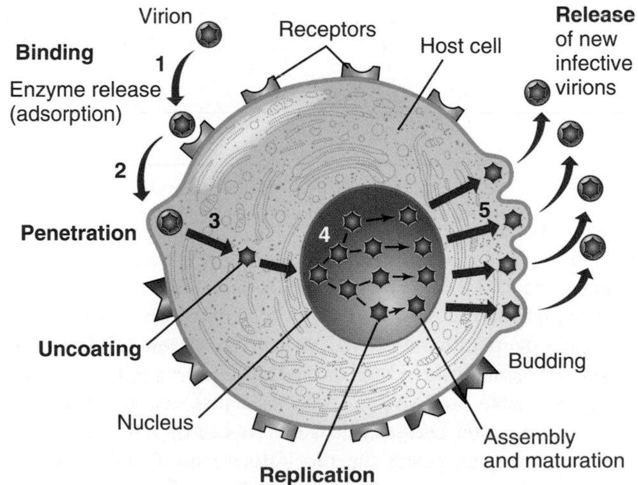

FIGURE 8-3 Stages of Viral Infection of a Host Cell. The virion (1) becomes attached to the cell's plasma membrane by absorption; (2) releases enzymes that weaken the membrane and allow it to penetrate the cell; (3) uncoats itself; (4) replicates; and (5) matures and escapes from the cell by budding from the plasma membrane. The infection then can spread to other host cells.

TABLE 8-5 Examples of Human Diseases Caused by Specific Viruses

Baltimore Classification	Family	Virus	Envelope	Main Route of Transmission	Disease
dsDNA	Adenoviruses	Adenovirus	No	Droplet contact	Acute febrile pharyngitis
	Herpesviruses	Herpes simplex type 1 (HSV-1)	Yes	Direct contact with saliva or lesions	Lesions in mouth, pharynx, conjunctivitis
		Herpes simplex type 2 (HSV-2)	Yes	Sexually, contact with lesions during birth	Sores on labia, meningitis in children
		Herpes simplex type 8 (HSV-8)	Yes	Sexually?, body fluids	Kaposi sarcoma
		Epstein-Barr virus (EBV)	Yes	Saliva	Mononucleosis, Burkitt lymphoma
		Cytomegalovirus (CMV)	Yes	Body fluids, mother's milk, transplacental	Mononucleosis, congenital infection
		Varicella-zoster virus (VZV)	Yes	Droplet contact	Chickenpox, shingles
ssDNA	Papovaviruses	Papillomavirus	No	Direct contact	Warts, cervical carcinoma
dsRNA	Reoviruses	Rotavirus	No	Fecal-oral	Severe diarrhea
ssRNA+	Picornaviruses	Coxsackievirus	No	Fecal-oral, droplet contact	Nonspecific febrile illness, conjunctivitis, meningitis
		Hepatitis A virus	No	Fecal-oral	Acute hepatitis
		Poliovirus	No	Fecal-oral	Poliomyelitis
		Rhinovirus	No	Droplet contact	Common cold
	Flaviviruses	Hepatitis C virus	Yes	Blood, sexually	Acute or chronic hepatitis, hepatocellular carcinoma
		Yellow fever virus	Yes	Mosquito vector	Yellow fever
		Dengue virus	Yes	Mosquito vector	Dengue fever
		West Nile virus	Yes	Mosquito vector	Meningitis, encephalitis
	Togaviruses	Rubella virus	Yes	Droplet contact, transplacental	Acute or congenital rubella
	Coronaviruses	SARS	Yes	Droplets in aerosol or direct contact	Severe respiratory tract disease
	Caliciviruses	Norovirus	No	Fecal-oral	Gastroenteritis
ssRNA–	Orthomyxoviruses	Influenza virus	Yes	Droplet contact	Influenza
	Paramyxoviruses	Measles virus	Yes	Droplet contact	Measles
		Mumps virus	Yes	Droplet contact	Mumps
		Parainfluenza virus	Yes	Droplet contact	Croup, pneumonia, common cold
		Respiratory syncytial virus (RSV)	Yes	Droplet contact, hand-to-mouth	Pneumonia, influenzalike syndrome
	Rhabdoviruses	Rabies virus	Yes	Animal bite, droplet contact	Rabies
	Bunyaviruses	Hantavirus	Yes	Aerosolized animal fecal material	Viral hemorrhagic fever
	Filoviruses	Ebola virus	Yes	Direct contact with body fluids	Viral hemorrhagic fever
		Marburg virus	Yes	Direct contact with body fluids	Viral hemorrhagic fever
	Arenavirus	Lassa virus	Yes	Aerosolized animal fecal material	Viral hemorrhagic fever
ssRNA+ with RT	Retroviruses	HIV	Yes	Sexually, blood products	AIDS
dsDNA with RT	Hepadnaviruses	Hepatitis B virus	Yes	All body fluids	Acute or chronic hepatitis, hepatocellular carcinoma

dsDNA, double-stranded DNA; *dsRNA*, double-stranded RNA; *RT*, reverse transcriptase; ssDNA, single-stranded DNA; ssRNA+, positive-sense single-stranded RNA; ssRNA–, negative-sense single-stranded RNA.

Attachment is followed by *penetration* (entrance into the cell by endocytosis or membrane fusion), *uncoating* (release of viral nucleic acid from the viral capsid by viral or host enzymes), *replication* (synthesis of messenger RNA [mRNA] and viral proteins), *assembly* (formation of new virions), and *release* (exit from the cell by lysis or budding). The influenza virus enters the respiratory tract epithelial cells by endocytosis. Low pH leads to intermembrane fusion between the endosome and viral envelop and uncoating.[17] The viral ssRNA is transported to the nucleus where transcription and replication occur using the viral RNA-dependent RNA polymerase.[18] Viral proteins assemble in the cytoplasm to form the matrix around the viral genome, and the virion buds from the cell surface. Infected cells usually die as a direct effect of the virus. The severity of clinical symptoms is usually secondary to the level of cytokines produced by the infected cells or in response to death of the cells.

The effects of a virus on the infected cell vary greatly. Some viruses, such as herpesviruses, will initiate a latency phase during which the host cell is transformed (i.e., herpes simplex viruses 1 and 2 establish latency in neurons). During this phase, the viral DNA may be integrated into the DNA of the host cell and become a permanent passenger in that cell and its progeny. In response to stimuli, such as stress, hormonal changes, or disease, the virus may exit latency and enter a productive cycle. Herpesviruses 1 and 2 are released from the neurons and infect skin epithelium, where lesions in the skin are a result of the immune response against the infected epithelium.

Cytopathic effects caused by other viruses include the following:

- Cessation of DNA, RNA, and protein synthesis (e.g., herpesvirus)
- Disruption of lysosomal membranes, resulting in release of digestive lysosomal enzymes that can kill the cell (e.g., herpesvirus)
- Fusion of host cells, producing multinucleated giant cells (e.g., respiratory syncytial virus)
- Alteration of the antigenic properties, or identity, of the infected cell, causing the individual's immune system to attack the cell as if it were foreign (e.g., hepatitis B virus)
- Transformation of host cells into cancerous cells, resulting in uninhibited and unregulated growth (e.g., human papillomavirus)
- Promotion of secondary bacterial infection in tissues damaged by viruses

The principal method by which influenza virus eludes the immune system is by changing viral surface antigens, a process known as **antigenic variation**. Antibodies against the HA and NA antigens are responsible for protection against influenza infection. Infections are seasonal and protection gained from the previous year's infection does not totally protect against influenza in the following year because the HA and NA antigens undergo yearly change. Usually antigenic variation is relatively minor (**antigenic drift**) and results from mutations. Individuals frequently have partial protection resulting from the previous year's infection, which lessens the clinical effects of the disease. Two groups of influenza virus—influenza A and influenza B—infect humans, and the yearly vaccine against influenza is a trivalent mixture of inactivated proteins from two influenza A subtypes and one influenza B subtype. Influenza B almost exclusively infects humans and mutates at a much lower rate than influenza A. Influenza A has antigenically distinct subtypes based on HA (17 forms) and NA (10 forms) antigens. Currently, subtypes H1N1, H1N2, and H3N2 are the primary causes of influenza worldwide.

Influenza A periodically undergoes major antigenic changes (**antigenic shifts**) (Figure 8-4). Influenza A can infect birds and mammals, and shifts occur in animals co-infected by a human and an avian strain of influenza. The genome is segmented and the segments can undergo recombination, during which the human virus obtains a new HA or NA antigen. Without a shift occurring, clinical influenza is usually considered epidemic (the number of new infections exceeds the number usually observed at other times of the year). When major antigenic changes occur, previous protection may not exist, resulting in a major pandemic (an epidemic that spreads over a large area, such as a continent or worldwide) and much more severe disease.

The concern with zoonotic influenza is that a lethal influenza virus that infects birds or other animals may suddenly develop the capacity to infect humans.[15] These infections are monitored closely by agencies such as the Centers for Disease Control and Prevention (CDC) in the United States, and by the Public Health Agency of Canada (PHAC) (http://www.phac-aspc.gc.ca). The PHAC is currently monitoring human cases of several zoonotic influenza outbreaks, including swine influenza virus (H1N1), a pathogenic H5N1 avian influenza virus, and a new strain of avian influenza (H7N9).

Viral pathogens bypass many defence mechanisms by hiding within cells and away from normal inflammatory or immune responses. Some viruses spread from cell to cell through the bloodstream (e.g., influenza,

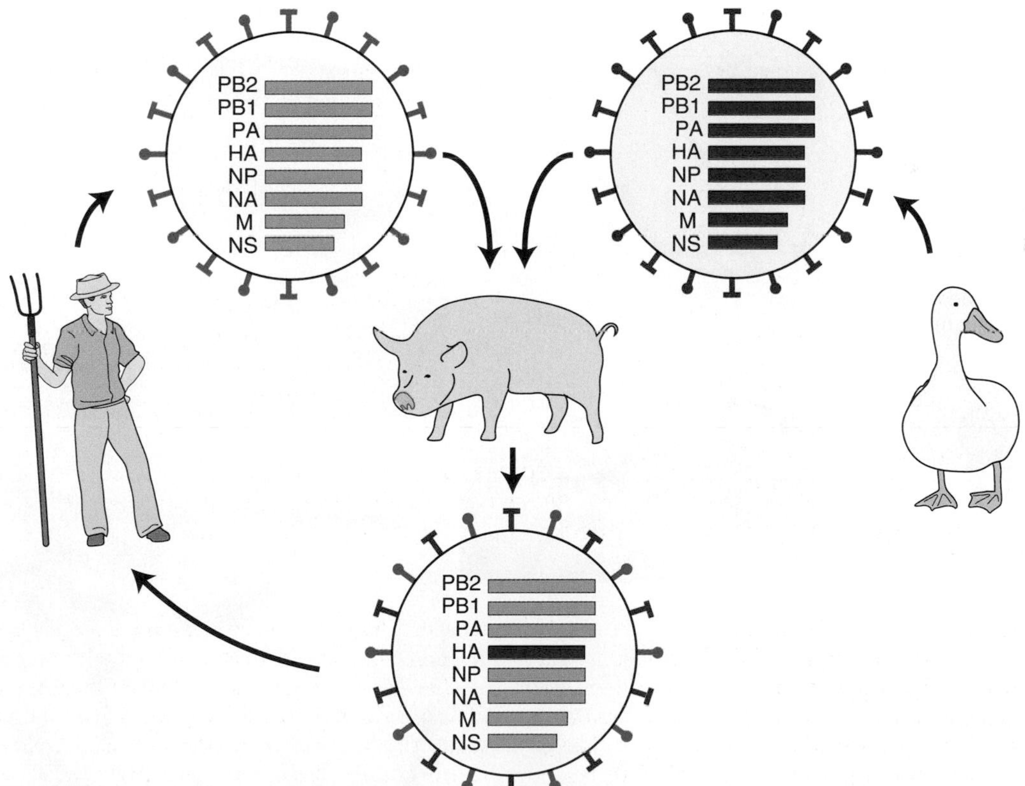

FIGURE 8-4 Antigenic Shifts in Influenza Virus. One theory proposes that antigenic shifts occur when a human influenza virus (*blue*) and an avian influenza virus (*red*) co-infect a species that is permissive for both. The eight single-stranded RNA strands are co-expressed in the same infected cell, resulting in mixing of the strands so that a hybrid virus can be produced. The hybrid virus indicated here contains all the genetic information of the original virus that infected humans but contains a new hemagglutinin (*HA*)-containing stand from the avian virus. This virus expresses a new HA antigen and will be less susceptible to residual immunity that normally provides partial protection against yearly influenza infections.

rubella) and are highly sensitive to neutralizing antibodies that block viral spread and eventually cure the infection; therefore, the disease is described as self-limiting. Other viruses (e.g., measles, herpes) are inaccessible to antibodies after initial infection because they remain inside infected cells, spreading by direct cell-to-cell contact. Most viruses have developed additional defence mechanisms. For example, influenza virus produces NS1 protein (viral nonstructural protein-1) that blocks the antiviral effects of type I interferon.

Fungal Disease

Fungi are relatively large eukaryotic microorganisms with thick walls that have two basic structures: single-celled yeasts (spheres) or multicellular moulds (filaments or hyphae) (Figure 8-5). Some fungi can exist in either form and are called **dimorphic fungi**. The cell walls of fungi are rigid and multilayered and composed of polysaccharides different from the peptidoglycans of bacteria. The lack of peptidoglycans allows fungi to resist the action of bacterial cell wall inhibitors such as penicillin and cephalosporin. Moulds are aerobic, and yeasts are facultative anaerobes, which adapt to, but do not require, anaerobic conditions. They usually reproduce by simple division or budding.

Diseases caused by fungi are called **mycoses**. Mycoses can be superficial, deep, or opportunistic. Superficial mycoses occur on or near skin or mucous membranes and usually produce mild and superficial disease. Fungi that invade the skin, hair, or nails are known as **dermatophytes**. The diseases they produce are called *tineas* (ringworm)—for example, tinea capitis (scalp), tinea pedis (feet), and tinea cruris (groin). Chapter 41 discusses the various skin disorders caused by fungi.

Pathological fungi cause disease by adapting to the host environment. Fungi that colonize the skin can digest keratin. Other fungi can grow with wide temperature variations in lower oxygen environments. Still other fungi have the capacity to suppress host immune defences. Phagocytes and T cells are important in controlling fungi. Low white blood cell counts promote fungal infection, and infection control is particularly important for individuals who are immunosuppressed. Common pathological fungi are summarized in Table 8-6.

Candida albicans is the most common cause of fungal infections in humans. It is an opportunistic yeast that is a commensal inhabitant in the normal microbiome of many healthy individuals, residing in the skin, gastro-intestinal tract, mouth (30 to 55% of healthy individuals), and vagina (20% of healthy women). *C. albicans* is normally under the control of local defence mechanisms, including members of the bacterial microbiome that produce antifungal agents. In healthy individuals antibiotic therapy can diminish the microbiome (e.g., diminished levels of *Lactobacillus* in the gastro-intestinal or vaginal microbiome). *Candida* overgrowth may occur, resulting in localized infection such as vaginitis or oropharyngeal infection (thrush).

In immunocompromised individuals, particularly those with diminished levels of neutrophils (neutropenia), disseminated infection may occur. *Candida* is the most common fungal infection in people with cancer (particularly acute leukemia and other hematological cancers), transplantation (bone marrow and solid organ), and HIV/AIDS. Invasive candidiasis also may be secondary to indwelling catheters, intravenous lines, or peritoneal dialysis, which provides direct entrance into the bloodstream.

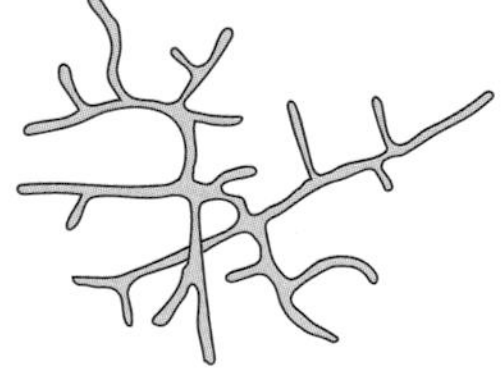

MOULDS
Filamentous fungi grow as multinucleate, branching hyphae, forming a mycelium (i.e., ringworm)

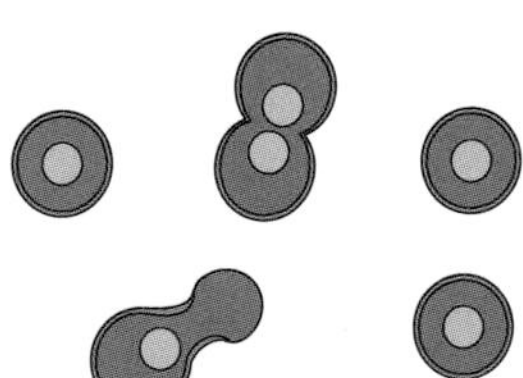

YEASTS
Yeasts grow as ovoid or spherical; single cells multiply by budding and division (i.e., *Histoplasma*)
A

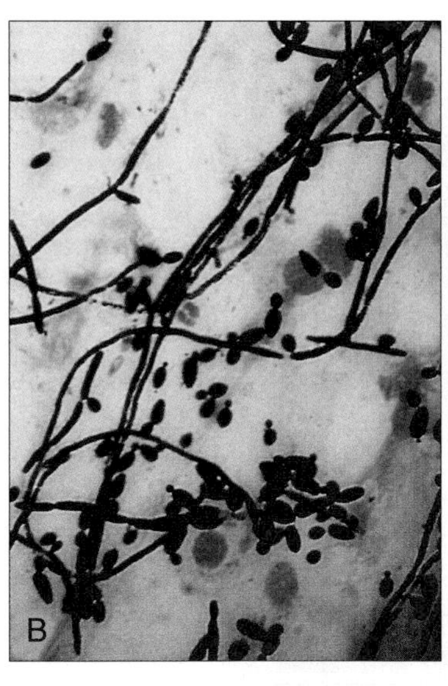

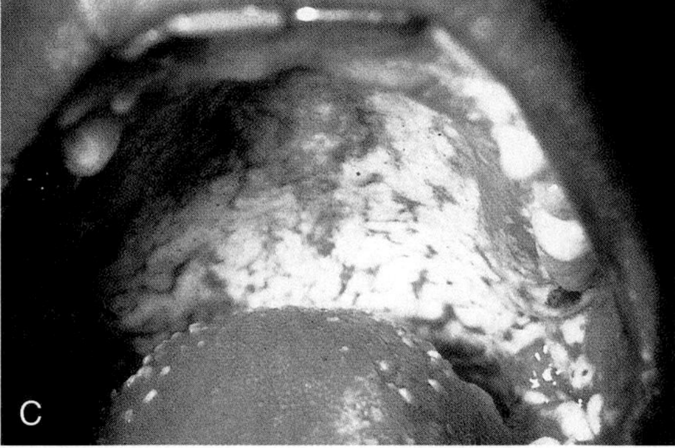

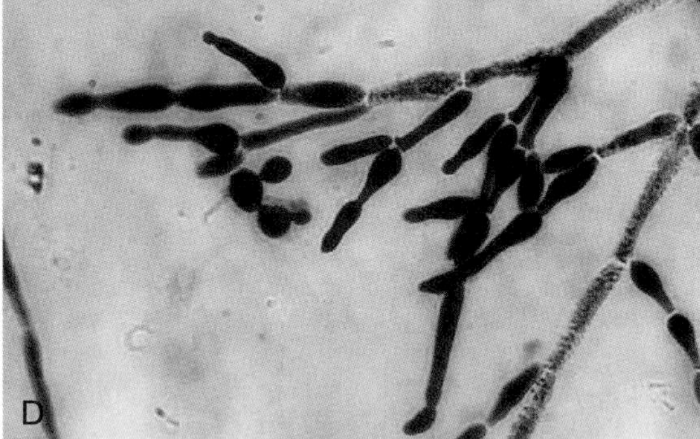

FIGURE 8-5 Morphology of Fungi. **(A)** Fungi may be either mould or yeast forms, or dimorphic. **(B)** Photograph showing *Candida albicans* with both the mycelial and the yeast forms. **(C)** Oral infection with *C. albicans* (candidiasis, i.e., thrush). **(D)** Gram stain of sputum showing that clinical isolates of *C. albicans* present as chains of elongated budding yeasts (× 1 000). (**A, B,** from Goering, R., Dockrell, H., Zuckerman, M., et al. [2013]. *Mims' medical microbiology* [5th ed.]. London: Saunders. **C,** from McPherson, R., & Pincus, M. [2012]. *Henry's clinical diagnosis and management by laboratory methods* [22nd ed.]. Philadelphia: Saunders; **D,** courtesy Dr. Stephen Raffanti.)

TABLE 8-6 Common Pathogenic Fungi

Primary Site of Infection	Fungus	Disease (Primary)	Symptoms
Superficial (no tissue invasion, little inflammation)	*Malassezia furfur*	Tinea versicolour, seborrheic dermatitis, dandruff	Red rash on body
Cutaneous (no tissue invasion, inflammatory response)	Dermatophytes	Tinea pedis (athlete's foot)	Scaling, fissures, pruritus
	Trichophyton mentagrophytes	Tinea cruris (jock itch)	Rash, pruritus
	Trichophyton rubrum	Tinea corporis (ringworm)	Lesion, raised border, scaling
	Microsporum canis		
	Candida albicans	Cutaneous candidiasis	Lesions in most areas of skin, mucous membranes, thrush, vaginal infection
Subcutaneous (tissue invasion)	*Sporothrix schenckii*	Sporotrichosis	Ulcers or abscesses on skin and other organ systems
Systemic (dimorphic; causes disease in healthy individuals)	*Stachybotrys chartarum*, or "black mould"	Black mould disease	Rash, headaches, nausea, pain
	Coccidioides immitis	Coccidioidomycosis	Valley fever, flulike symptoms
	Histoplasma capsulatum	Histoplasmosis	Lung, flulike symptoms, disseminates to multiple organs, eye
	Blastomyces dermatitidis	Blastomycosis	Flulike symptoms, chest pains
Systemic (opportunistic)	*Aspergillus fumigatus*, *Aspergillus flavus*	Aspergillosis	Invasive to lungs and other organs
	Pneumocystis jiroveci	Pneumocystis pneumonia (PCP)	Pneumonia
	Cryptococcus neoformans	Cryptococcosis	Pneumonialike illness, skin lesions, disseminates to brain, meningitis
	C. albicans	Systemic candidiasis	Sepsis, endocarditis, meningitis

TABLE 8-7 Examples of Parasites That Are Important in Humans

Category	Subgroup	Species	Disease	Organs Affected/Symptoms
Protozoa	Ameboid	*Entamoeba histolytica*	Amebiasis	Dysentery, liver abscess
	Flagellate	*Giardia lamblia*	Giardiasis[a]	Diarrhea
		Trichomonas vaginalis	Trichomoniasis	Inflammation of reproductive organs
		Trypanosoma cruzi, T. brucei	Chagas disease: African sleeping sickness	Generalized, blood and lymph nodes, progressing to cardiac and central nervous system (CNS)
	Ciliate	*Balantidium coli*	Balantidiasis	Small intestines, invasion of colon, diarrhea
	Sporozoa (nonmotile)	*Cryptosporidium parvum, C. hominis*	Cryptosporidiosis[a]	Intestine, diarrhea
		Plasmodium spp.	Malaria	Blood, liver
		Toxoplasma gondii	Toxoplasmosis[a]	Intestine, eyes, blood, heart, liver
Helminths	Flukes (trematodes)	*Fasciola hepatica*	Fasciolosis	Liver destruction
		Schistosoma mansoni	Schistosomiasis	Blood, diarrhea, bladder, generalized symptoms
	Tapeworms (cestodes)	*Taenia solium*	Pork tapeworm	Encysts in muscle, brain, liver
	Roundworms (nematodes)	*Ascaris lumbricoides*	Ascariasis	Intestinal obstruction, bile duct obstruction
		Necator americanus (hookworm)	Hookworm disease	Intestinal parasite
		Trichinella spiralis	Trichinosis[a]	Intestine, diarrhea, muscle, CNS, death
		Wuchereria bancrofti	Filariasis, elephantiasis	Lymphatics
		Enterobius vermicularis (pinworm)	Pinworm infection	Intestines
		Onchocerca volvulus	Onchocerciasis	Blindness, dermatitis

[a]Most common in the United States and Canada.

Disseminated candidiasis may involve deep infections of several internal organs, including abscesses in the kidney, brain, liver, and heart, and is characterized by persistent or recurrent fever, Gram-negative shocklike symptoms (hypotension, tachycardia), and disseminated intravascular coagulation (DIC). The death rates of septic or disseminated candidiasis are in the range of 30 to 40%.

Parasitic Disease

Parasitic microorganisms establish a relationship in which the parasite benefits at the expense of the other species. Parasites range from unicellular protozoa to large worms. Parasitic worms (helminths) include intestinal and tissue nematodes (e.g., hookworm, roundworm), flukes (e.g., liver fluke, lung fluke), and tapeworms. A protozoan is a eukaryotic, unicellular microorganism with a nucleus and cytoplasm. Pathogenic protozoa include malaria (*Plasmodium*), amoebae (e.g., *Entamoeba histolytica*, which causes amoebic dysentery), and flagellates (e.g., *Giardia lamblia*, which causes diarrhea; *Trypanosoma*, which causes sleeping sickness). Although less common in Canada, parasites and protozoa are common causes of infections worldwide, with a significant effect on the mortality and morbidity of individuals in developing countries. Important parasites of humans are listed in Table 8-7.

Malaria is one of the most common infections worldwide. In 2012, the World Health Organization (WHO) estimated that there were 207 million cases of malaria with an estimated 627 000 deaths; 90% were in Africa, where 82% of the deaths were children younger than age 5 years.[19] Malaria is caused by *Plasmodium falciparum*, a protozoan (unicellular) parasite.

Many protozoan parasites are transmitted through vectors or ingested. Vectors include the tsetse fly (*Trypanosoma cruzi*, which causes Chagas disease in South America; *Trypanosoma brucei*, which causes sleeping sickness in Africa) and sand fleas (leishmaniasis). Water and food can be contaminated with protozoal parasites (e.g., *E. histolytica*, *G. lamblia*). Transmission of *Plasmodium* is through the bite of an infected female *Anopheles* mosquito, where the parasite grows in the salivary gland.

The initial attachment to cells depends on the presence of the microorganism in the bloodstream or gastro-intestinal tract. Microorganisms in the bloodstream have surface proteins that allow them to attach to various receptors to infect macrophages, red blood cells, or organ cells such as the liver. For example, multiplication of *Plasmodium* occurs in erythrocytes and results in the release of additional parasites that infect other erythrocytes. Periodic (48 to 72 hours) lysis of the erythrocytes results in anemia and induction of cytokines (e.g., TNF-α, gamma interferon [IFN-γ], IL-1) that provoke fever, chills, sweating, headache, muscle pains, and vomiting. Severe symptoms include anemia, pulmonary edema, and other complications causing death. Neurological complications may result from infected red blood cells adhering to endothelium in capillaries of the brain.

TABLE 8-8 Reduction in Vaccine-Preventable Diseases in the United States, 2011

Disease	Baseline 20th-Century Annual Cases[a]	2011[b] Cases	% Reduction
Diphtheria	175 885	0	100.0
Measles	503 282	212	99.9
Mumps	152 209	370	99.4
Pertussis	147 271	15 216	90.8
Smallpox	48 164	0	100.0
Polio	16 316	0	100.0
Rubella	47 745	4	99.9
Tetanus	1 314	9	99.9
Haemophilus influenzae type b, invasive	20 000	1 170	94.2

[a]Average number of reported cases over multiple years before initiation of vaccine.
[b]Data from provisional cases of selected notifiable diseases, United States.
From Centers for Disease Control and Prevention. (2012). *MMWR Morb Mortal Wkly Rep, 60*(51), 1762–1775. Retrieved from https://www.cdc.gov/mmwr/preview/mmwrhtml/mm6052md.htm?s_cid=mm6052md_w.

Countermeasures Against Infectious Microorganisms

The body's innate and adaptive responses against microorganisms are numerous and involve an interaction between the immune and inflammatory systems. Pathogenic microorganisms, however, have developed means of circumventing the individual's protective defences. Therefore, prophylactic or interventive procedures have been developed either to prevent the pathogen from initiating disease (vaccines, public health measures) or to destroy the pathogen once the disease process has started (antimicrobials). Most vaccine development has focused on preventing the most severe and common infections (Table 8-8). With the initial success of antibiotic therapy, there was no perceived need for vaccination against many common and non–life-threatening infections. The increasing problem of antibiotic-resistant pathogens, however, has forced a reappraisal of that strategy, and a greater emphasis now is being placed on the development of new vaccines.

Infection Control Measures

Although effective means of safeguarding populations from exposure to infectious disease are well-known, lack of implementation or breakdowns in application of these initiatives has led to the re-emergence of some infectious diseases, particularly in less developed countries. The following are some examples of environmental infection control measures:

- Hand hygiene
- Sanitary disposal of sewage, garbage, and animal waste
- Provision of water treatment and prevention of water contamination
- Maintenance of sanitation practices for the transport, preparation, and serving of food
- Control of insect vectors by draining standing water and implementation of mosquito eradication programs
- Support of research to develop safe agents for insecticide-resistant insect vectors

Antimicrobials

Since initiation of the widespread use of penicillin during World War II, antibiotics have significantly prevented the spread of infections.

TABLE 8-9 Chemicals or Antimicrobials Identified That Prevent Growth of or Destroy Microorganisms

Mechanism of Action	Agents
Inhibits synthesis of cell wall	Penicillins, cephalosporins, monobactams, carbapenems, vancomycin, bacitracin, cycloserine, fosfomycin
Inhibits cell membrane function	Amphotericin, ketoconazole, polymycin
Damages cytoplasmic membrane	Polymyxins, polyene antifungals, imidazoles
Alters metabolism of nucleic acid	Quinolones, rifampin, nitrofurans, nitroimidazoles
Inhibits protein synthesis	Aminoglycosides, tetracyclines, chloramphenicol, macrolides, clindamycin, spectinomycin
Inhibits folic acid synthesis (needed for protein synthesis)	Sulfonamides, trimethoprim
Alters energy metabolism	Trimethoprim, dapsone, isoniazid

Adapted from Brenner, G.M., & Stevens, C.W. (2013). *Pharmacology* (4th ed.). Philadelphia: Saunders.

Antibiotics are natural products of fungi, bacteria, and related microorganisms that affect the growth of other microorganisms. Some antibacterial antibiotics are *bactericidal* (kill the microorganism), whereas others are *bacteriostatic* (inhibit growth until the microorganism is destroyed by the individual's own protective mechanisms). The mechanisms of action of most antibiotics include inhibition of the function or production of the cell wall or membrane; inhibition of protein synthesis; blockage of DNA replication; and interference with folic acid metabolism. See Table 8-9 for a list of mechanisms of action against a variety of pathogens. Because viruses use the enzymes of the host's cells, there has been far less success in developing antiviral antibiotics.

Immediately after antibiotics became widely used, antibiotic-resistant microorganisms were observed. By 1944 an adequate supply of penicillin allowed its widespread use to treat infections. In 1946 a hospital in Britain reported that 14% of all *S. aureus* infections were penicillin resistant, producing β-lactamase, an enzyme that destroys penicillin. The same hospital reported an increase to 59% by 1950 and to greater than 89% in the 1990s.

More than 2 million individuals develop antibiotic-resistant infections yearly, resulting in more than 23 000 deaths. Antibiotic resistance to a single antibiotic has rapidly progressed to **multiple-antibiotic resistance**. The CDC released a lengthy report on the matter—*Antibiotic Resistance Threats in the United States, 2013*—in which 18 pathogens were sorted into "Urgent Threats," "Serious Threats," and "Concerning Threats."[20] The most urgent threats are *Clostridium difficile*, carbapenem (an "antibiotic of last resort" against penicillin-resistant organisms) resistant Enterobacteriaceae species (i.e., *Klebsiella* and *E. coli*), and medication-resistant *Neisseria gonorrhoeae.*

Similarly, the *Chief Public Health Officer's Report on the State of Public Health in Canada, 2013* addresses the following concerns: immunization and vaccine-preventable diseases (and how to improve programs across Canada), health care–associated infections (and some of the more common ones, such as *C. difficile*, MRSA, and vancomycin-resistant enterocci), antimicrobial resistance (including methods of spread and ways to minimize the impact on the population), the resurgence of TB (particularly in vulnerable populations), foodborne and waterborne infections, and sexually transmitted infections.[21]

Many other infections considered routine and easily treatable are now resistant to almost all currently available antibiotics, including MRSA and *Streptococcus pneumoniae*, which causes pneumonia, meningitis, and acute otitis media (middle ear infection), which were once routinely susceptible to penicillin. Additionally, there are major increases in resistant *Salmonella typhi* (typhoid fever), *Shigella* (bloody diarrhea), *Acinetobacter* (pneumonia), *Campylobacter* (bloody diarrhea), *Enterococcus* (sepsis, wound infection, urinary tract infection), *Pseudomonas aeruginosa* (burn infection, sepsis), and *Mycobacterium tuberculosis* (tuberculosis).[22] Antibiotic-resistant fungi (e.g., fluconazole-resistant *C. albicans*) have evolved, and malarial parasites have recently developed broad medication resistance, including to chloroquine—the previous mainstay of the preventive and therapeutic arsenal of antimalarial medications.

Antibiotic resistance is usually a result of *genetic mutations* that can be transmitted directly to neighbouring microorganisms by plasmid exchange or incorporation of free DNA. Some microorganisms can *inactivate antibiotics*, penicillin resistance being the classic example. Other forms of resistance result from *modification of the target molecule.* Azidothymidine (AZT) is a family of antivirals that suppresses the enzymatic activity of reverse transcriptase, a viral-specific enzyme responsible for the replication of viral RNA and the production of a DNA copy. HIV frequently mutates and produces an AZT-resistant reverse transcriptase. Multidrug transporters in the microorganism's membrane mediate a third mechanism of resistance. These transporters affect the rate of intracellular accumulation of the antimicrobial *by preventing entrance* or, more commonly, *by increasing active efflux of the antibiotic.* Antibiotic-resistant strains of *M. tuberculosis* are protected from aminoglycosides and tetracycline by a multidrug pump that increases efflux.

Why have multiple-antibiotic–resistant microorganisms appeared? Lack of adherence in completing the therapeutic regimen with antibiotics allows the selective resurgence of microorganisms that are more relatively resistant to the antibiotic. Overuse of antibiotics can lead to the destruction of the normal microbiome, allowing the selective overgrowth of antibiotic-resistant strains or pathogens that had previously been controlled. There also is concern that overuse of antibiotics to promote growth in cattle results in ingestion of antibiotic-containing meat.[23]

Active Immunization

Recovery from an infection generally results in the strongest resistance to a future infection with the same microbe. **Vaccines** are biological preparations of antigens that when administered stimulate production of protective antibodies or cellular immunity against a specific pathogen without causing potentially life-threatening disease. The purpose of **vaccination** is to induce long-lasting protective immune responses under safe conditions. The primary immune response from vaccination is generally short lived; therefore, booster injections are used to push the immune response through multiple secondary responses that result in large numbers of memory cells and sustained protective levels of antibody or T cells, or both.

Mass vaccination programs have been tremendously successful and have led to major changes in the health of the world's population.[24] In the early 1950s an estimated 50 million cases of smallpox occurred each year, with about 15 million deaths. The WHO conducted an aggressive immunization campaign from 1967 to 1977 that resulted in the global eradication of smallpox by 1979. The Government of Canada publishes vaccine schedules at its website: https://www.canada.ca/en/public-health/services/provincial-territorial-immunization-information/provincial-territorial-routine-vaccination-programs-infants-children.html.

Development of a successful vaccine is costly and depends on several factors. They include identification of the protective immune response and the appropriate antigen to induce that response. For example, individuals with ongoing HIV infection produce a great deal of antibody against several HIV antigens. However, for development of a successful vaccine, it is important to first understand which antibody, if any, will protect against an initial infection.

Once a good candidate antigen is identified, it must be developed into an effective, cost-efficient, stable, and safe vaccine. Most vaccines against viral infection (measles, mumps, rubella, varicella [chickenpox]) contain live viruses that are weakened (**attenuated virus**) so they continue to express appropriate antigens but establish only a limited and easily controlled infection. Limited replication of the virus appears to afford better long-term protection than using viral antigen. Current exceptions are the hepatitis B vaccine, which uses a recombinant viral protein, and the hepatitis A vaccine, which is an inactivated (killed) virus and normally should not cause an infection.

Even attenuated viruses can establish life-threatening infections in individuals whose immune systems are deficient or suppressed. The risk of infection by the vaccine strain of a virus is extremely small, but it may affect the choice of recommended vaccines. For example, the Sabin vaccine for polio was an attenuated virus that was administered orally. It provided systemic protection and induced a secretory immune response to prevent growth of the poliovirus in the intestinal tract. Being a live virus, the vaccine could cause polio in some children who had unsuspected immune deficiencies (about 1 case in 2.4 million doses). The Salk vaccine was a completely inactivated virus administered by injection. It induced protective systemic immunity but did not provide adequate secretory immunity. Therefore, even if the individual was protected from systemic infection by poliovirus, the virus could establish a limited infection in the individual's intestinal mucosa, be shed, and infect others. When polio was epidemic, the oral vaccine was preferred. However, the live attenuated vaccine itself caused about eight cases of paralytic polio per year in the United States in individuals with inadequate immune systems. As a result, the current recommendation of the CDC is vaccination with the killed virus. The Sabin vaccine, or trivalent vaccine, is also no longer recommended or available in Canada, because most cases of paralytic polio from 1980 to 1995 were associated with this vaccine.[25]

Some common bacterial vaccines are killed microorganisms or extracts of bacterial antigens. The vaccine against pneumococcal pneumonia consists of a mixture of capsular polysaccharides from 23 strains of *S. pneumoniae*. Of the more than 90 known strains of this microorganism, these 23 cause the most severe illnesses. However, the capsular vaccine is not very immunogenic in young children. A *conjugated* vaccine is available that contains capsular polysaccharides from 13 strains conjugated to carrier proteins to increase **immunogenicity**. A similar vaccine is available for *Haemophilus influenzae* type b (Hib).

Some bacterial pathogens are not invasive, but colonize mucosal membranes or wounds and release potent exotoxins that act locally or systemically. Vaccination against systemic exotoxins (e.g., diphtheria, tetanus, pertussis) has been achieved using **toxoids**—purified exotoxins that have been chemically detoxified without loss of immunogenicity. Pertussis (whooping cough) vaccine has been changed from a killed whole-cell vaccine to cellular extract (acellular) vaccine that contains the pertussis toxoid and additional bacterial antigens. This change has dramatically reduced adverse effects (fever, local inflammatory reactions, and others) of vaccination.

With so many recommended vaccines, there has been an effort to combine vaccines to minimize the number of required injections. One of the first licensed vaccine mixtures was DPT, which now usually contains diphtheria (D) and tetanus (T) toxoids and acellular pertussis vaccine (aP). More recent mixtures include DTaP with inactivated poliovirus, either with Hib conjugate to tetanus toxoid or with hepatitis B antigen.

Common problems confronting vaccination programs include access to the programs in less developed countries or lack of adherence of the susceptible population even when vaccination programs are available. A certain percentage of the population will be genetically unresponsive or less responsive to a particular vaccine and therefore will not produce a protective immune response. As many as 10% of the population may not respond adequately to the recommended series of injections. With most vaccines, the percentage of unresponsive individuals is low, and they will benefit from successful immunization of the rest of the population. Depending on the microorganism, a certain percentage of the population (usually about 85%) should be immunized to achieve protection of the total population. This form of immunity is referred to as **herd immunity**. If this level of immunization is not achieved, outbreaks of infection can occur. In 2013, 89% of children in Canada received the measles, mumps, and rubella (MMR) vaccine by the age of 2. This percentage is still lower than the suggested 95% for herd immunity against this virus, and there have been several recent outbreaks of both the mumps and measles in various regions across Canada.[26] In several European countries, antivaccine groups have disrupted immunization programs. As a result, the incidence of pertussis (whooping cough) increased by 10 to 100 times in those countries compared with neighbouring countries that maintained a high incidence of immunization. Immunizations should be complete before children start school.

The reluctance to vaccinate has generally been based on potential vaccine dangers.[27] As with any medicine, complications can arise. In the case of vaccines, these complications include pain and redness at the injection site, fever, allergic reactions to vaccine ingredients, and infection associated with attenuated viruses in immune-deficient individuals. More severe dangers do exist, although they are extremely rare. More commonly the reluctance to vaccination is based on inadequate information.[28] A common fear relates to the presence of the preservative thimerosal in vaccines. Thimerosal is a mercury-containing compound that had been used as a preservative since the 1930s. Although no cases of mercury toxicity have been reported secondary to vaccination, thimerosal was removed from all vaccines in 2001, with the exception of some inactivated influenza vaccines. In 2003 groups in northern Nigeria claimed that the oral vaccine was unsafe and was tainted with antifertility medications (estradiol), HIV, and cancer-causing agents.[29] The reasoning appeared to be secondary to mounting distrust of Western nations because of conflicts in the Middle East. The effect was suspension of polio immunization for almost 1 year in two Nigerian states and reduction of immunization in three other states. The incidence of polio rose dramatically, and more than 27 000 cases of paralysis resulted. The goal of the WHO is to eradicate polio worldwide by 2022. As of November 2014, the total global number of wild polio (naturally occurring) cases was 291; the highest number of cases was in Pakistan (246).[30]

Passive Immunotherapy

Passive immunotherapy is a form of countermeasure against pathogens in which preformed antibodies are given to the individual. Passive immunotherapy with human immunoglobulin has been approved for several infections, including hepatitis A and hepatitis B. Treatment of potential rabies infection after a bite combines passive and active immunization. The rabies virus proliferates very slowly.[31] Individuals who have been bitten receive a onetime injection with human rabies immunoglobulin, or, more recently, with monoclonal antibody to slow further viral proliferation, followed by multiple injections with a killed viral vaccine to induce greater protective immunity. More specific therapy with monoclonal antibodies is being evaluated for other infectious diseases. A monoclonal antibody against respiratory syncytial virus has been approved for therapy, and recently, an experimental monoclonal antibody preparation seems to have neutralized the Ebola virus.

In the past, vaccines and therapeutic antibodies were developed only for the most deadly pathogens. With the increase in antibiotic-resistant microorganisms, the development and widespread use of new vaccines and antibodies against these microorganisms must be considered.[32]

> **✔ QUICK CHECK 8-1**
> 1. How do antigenic changes in viral pathogens promote disease?
> 2. What are three mechanisms pathogens use to block the immune system?
> 3. What is the difference between an endotoxin and an exotoxin?
> 4. How do bacteria develop antibiotic resistance?

DEFICIENCIES IN IMMUNITY

An **immune deficiency** (also called *immunodeficiency*) is the failure of the immune or inflammatory response to function normally, resulting in increased susceptibility to infections. **Primary (congenital) immune deficiency** is caused by a genetic defect, whereas **secondary (acquired) immune deficiency** is caused by another condition, such as cancer, infection, or normal physiological changes, such as aging. Acquired forms of immune deficiency are far more common than the congenital forms.

Initial Clinical Presentation

The clinical hallmark of immune deficiency is a tendency to develop unusual or recurrent, severe infections. The most severe primary immune deficiencies develop in young children, 2 years old and younger. Preschool and school-age children normally may have 6 to 12 infections per year, and adults may have 2 to 4 infections per year. Most of these are not severe and are limited to viral infections of the upper respiratory tract, recurrent streptococcal pharyngitis, or mild otitis media (middle ear infection).

Potential immune deficiencies should be considered if the individual has experienced severe, documented bouts of pneumonia, otitis media, sinusitis (sinus infection), bronchitis, septicemia (blood infection), or meningitis or infections with rare opportunistic microorganisms (e.g., *Pneumocystis carinii*).[33] Infections are generally recurrent with only short intervals of relative health, and multiple simultaneous infections are common. Individuals with immune deficiencies often have eight or more purulent ear infections, two or more serious sinus infections, and two or more pneumonias, recurrent abscesses, or persistent fungal infections (particularly thrush) within a year. Invasive fungal infections are rare in healthy individuals and strongly indicate a defective immune system. Recurrent internal infections, such as meningitis, osteomyelitis, or sepsis, are common. Prolonged antibiotic use is commonly ineffective by oral or injected routes and may necessitate intravenous administration. Children frequently present with failure to thrive because of chronic diarrhea and other chronic symptoms. A familial history of immune deficiency may be found in some types of primary deficiency.

Routine care of individuals with immune deficiencies must be tempered with the knowledge that the immune system may be totally ineffective. It is unsafe to administer conventional immunizing agents or blood products to many of these individuals because of the risk of causing an uncontrolled infection. Infection is a particular problem when attenuated vaccines that contain live but weakened microorganisms are used (e.g., live polio vaccine; vaccines against measles, mumps, and rubella).

The type of recurrent infections may indicate the type of immune defect. Deficiencies in T-cell immune responses are associated with recurrent infections caused by certain viruses (e.g., varicella herpes, cytomegalovirus), fungi, and yeasts (e.g., *Candida*, *Histoplasma*), or atypical microorganisms (e.g., *P. carinii*). B-cell deficiencies and phagocyte deficiencies, however, are suggested if the individual has documented, recurrent infections with microorganisms that require opsonization (e.g., encapsulated bacteria) or with viruses against which humoral immunity is normally effective (e.g., rubella). Some complement deficiencies resemble defects in antibody or phagocyte function, but others are associated with disseminated infections with bacteria of the genus *Neisseria* (*Neisseria meningitides* and *Neisseria gonorrhoeae*).

Primary (Congenital) Immune Deficiencies

Most primary immune deficiencies are the result of *single gene defects* (Table 8-10). Generally, the mutations are sporadic and not inherited: a family history exists in only about 25% of individuals. The sporadic mutations occur before birth, but the onset of symptoms may be early or later, depending on the particular syndrome. In some instances, symptoms of immune deficiency appear within the first 2 years of life. Other immune deficiencies are progressive, with the onset of symptoms appearing in the second or third decade of life.

Individually, primary immune deficiencies are rare. In Canada, about 2 000 people were diagnosed with primary immune deficiencies in 2009, but the number of actual cases is thought to be much greater because the condition is highly undiagnosed.[34] Many such conditions are subtle with minor deficiencies, but several result from major defects and lead to recurrent life-threatening infections. The distribution between genders is about even, although some specific diseases have a male or female predominance. The three most commonly diagnosed deficiencies are common variable immune deficiency (a deficiency in IgG, IgM, and IgA affecting 34% of individuals with primary immune deficiencies), selective immunoglobulin A (IgA) deficiency (24%), and IgG subclass deficiency (17%).

Primary immune deficiencies have recently been reclassified into nine groups, based on the principal component of the immune or inflammatory systems that is defective.[35] The major groups include combined with or without nonimmune defects (both B and T cells are deficient, although this group contains some diseases previously classified as T-cell defects), predominantly antibody deficiencies, immune dysregulation (defects in control of lymphocyte proliferation, T-regulatory cells defects), phagocytic defects (inadequate numbers or function), **defects in innate immunity**, and complement defects. To provide a better understanding of the diversity and severity of primary immune deficiencies, a few select examples will be discussed.

Combined Deficiencies

Combined deficiencies include the most life-threatening disorders and result from defects that directly affect the development of both T and B cells. However, the severity depends on the degree to which B and T cells are affected.[36] The most severe disorders are called **severe combined immunodeficiencies (SCIDs)**. Most individuals with SCIDs have few detectable lymphocytes in the circulation and secondary lymphoid organs (spleen, lymph nodes). The thymus usually is underdeveloped because of the absence of T cells. Immunoglobulin levels, especially IgM and IgA, are absent or greatly reduced. Several forms of SCID are caused by autosomal recessive enzymatic defects that result in the accumulation of toxic metabolites, and rapidly dividing cells, such as lymphocytes, are especially sensitive. For example, **adenosine deaminase deficiency (ADA deficiency)** results in the accumulation of toxic purines. **X-linked SCID** results from a common defect in most of the important IL receptors needed for lymphocyte maturation (e.g., IL-2, IL-4, IL-7).

Even if nearly adequate numbers of B and T cells are produced, their cooperation may be defective. The **bare lymphocyte syndrome** is an immune deficiency characterized by an inability of lymphocytes and macrophages to produce **major histocompatibility complex (MHC)** class I or class II molecules. Without MHC molecules, antigen presentation and intercellular cooperation cannot occur effectively. Children with this deficiency develop serious, life-threatening infections and usually die before the age of 5 years.

Some combined immune deficiencies result in depressed development of a small portion of the immune system. For example, an individual can be unable to produce a certain class of antibody, as in **Wiskott-Aldrich syndrome (WAS**, an X-linked recessive disorder), where IgM antibody production is greatly depressed. Antibody responses against antigens that elicit primarily an IgM response, such as polysaccharide antigens from bacterial cell walls (e.g., *P. aeruginosa*, *S. pneumoniae*, *H. influenzae*, and other microorganisms with polysaccharide outer capsules), are deficient.

Many combined immune deficiencies also are associated with other characteristic defects, some of which appear to be unrelated to the immune system yet may be life-threatening by themselves. These associated symptoms can be useful diagnostically and can clarify the pathophysiology of the disease. WAS results from a mutation in the *WAS* gene that affects the actin cytoskeleton, which is important for platelet function. Thus, WAS has an associated major defect in platelet function and is classified as a combined deficiency with nonimmune defects. Clinical manifestations include bleeding secondary to thrombocytopenia (low platelet counts), eczema, and recurrent infections (e.g., otitis media, pneumonia, herpes simplex, cytomegalovirus).

DiGeorge syndrome (congenital thymic aplasia or hypoplasia and diminished parathyroid gland development) is caused by the lack or partial lack of the thymus, resulting in greatly decreased T-cell numbers and function. Defective development of the third and fourth pharyngeal pouches during embryonic development results in the thymic defects

TABLE 8-10 Examples of Primary Immune Deficiencies

Classification	Example	Immune Deficiency	Outcome
Combined Immune Deficiencies: Without Nonimmune Defects			
Defective development of both B cells and T cells	Severe combined immunodeficiencies (SCIDs)	Lack of both T and B cells, little or no antibody production or cellular immunity	Recurrent, life-threatening infections with variety of microorganisms
	X-linked SCID	Defective interleukin receptors needed for lymphocyte maturation	Recurrent, life-threatening infections with variety of microorganisms
Defects in cooperation among B cells, T cells, and antigen-presenting cells	Bare lymphocyte syndrome	No antigen presentation because of lack of major histocompatibility complex (MHC) class I or MHC class II molecules on cell surface	Recurrent, life-threatening infections with variety of microorganisms
Combined Immune Deficiencies: With Nonimmune Defects			
Defect in actin cytoskeleton	Wiskott-Aldrich syndrome	Decreased IgM antibody	Recurrent infections with encapsulated bacteria; thrombocytopenia; eczema
Defective development of T cells in central lymphoid organ (thymus)	DiGeorge syndrome	Lack of T cells	Recurrent, life-threatening fungal and viral infections; defective parathyroid gland; abnormal facial development
Predominantly Antibody Deficiencies			
Defect in class-switch to IgA	Selective IgA deficiency	Diminished or absent IgA	Asymptomatic or recurrent mild sinus, pulmonary, and gastro-intestinal infections
Defect in development of B cells in the bone marrow	Bruton agammaglobulinemia	Few B cells	Recurrent bacterial infections
Phagocytic Defects			
Defects in production of neutrophils	Severe congenital neutropenia	Lack of neutrophils	Recurrent, life-threatening bacterial infections
Defects in bacterial killing	Chronic granulomatous disease	Lack of production of oxygen products (e.g., hydrogen peroxide)	Recurrent infections with bacteria that are sensitive to killing by oxygen-dependent mechanisms
Defects in Innate Immunity			
Defect in development of cellular immunity against specific antigen	Chronic mucocutaneous candidiasis	Lack of T-cell response to *Candida*	Recurrent and disseminated infections with fungus *Candida albicans*
Complement Deficiencies			
Defective production of C3	C3 deficiency	Little or no C3 produced	Recurrent, life-threatening bacterial infections
Defective production of component of membrane attack complex	C6, C7, C8, or C9 deficiency	Little or no C6, C7, C8, or C9 produced	Recurrent disseminated infections with *Neisseria gonorrhoeae* or *Neisseria meningitides*
Defective production of component of lectin pathway	Mannose-binding lectin deficiency	Little or no activation of lectin pathway	Recurrent infections with bacteria and yeast with mannose-containing capsules

and the lack of the parathyroid gland (causing an inability to regulate calcium concentration). Low blood calcium levels cause the development of tetany or involuntary rigid muscular contraction. DiGeorge syndrome is frequently associated with abnormal development of facial features that are controlled by the same embryonic pouches; these include low-set ears, fish-shaped mouth, and other altered features (Figure 8-6). Other examples of combined immune deficiencies include defects in CD3 resulting in the loss of T cell antigen receptor intracellular signalling, defective somatic gene rearrangement of variable region genes or constant region genes, IL-2 receptor defects, and defects in DNA repair.

Predominantly Antibody Deficiencies

Predominantly antibody deficiencies result from defects in B-cell maturation or function and are the most common of immune deficiencies.[37] T-cell immune responses are not affected in pure B-cell deficiencies. The results are lower levels of circulating immunoglobulins (**hypogammaglobulinemia**) or occasionally totally or nearly absent immunoglobulins (**agammaglobulinemia**).

Some defects may involve a particular class of antibody, such as **selective IgA deficiency**, in which only IgA is suppressed. This deficiency may result from a failure to class-switch to IgA and mature into IgA-producing plasma cells. Many individuals are asymptomatic, although others have a history of recurring sinus, pulmonary, and gastro-intestinal infections. Individuals with IgA deficiency often have chronic intestinal candidiasis (infection with *C. albicans*). Complications of IgA deficiency include severe allergic disease and autoimmune diseases. Secretory IgA normally may prevent the uptake of allergens from the environment; therefore, IgA deficiency may lead to a more intense challenge to the immune system by environmental antigens.

Bruton agammaglobulinemia is caused by blocked development of mature B cells in the bone marrow. There are few or no circulating B cells, although T-cell number and function are normal, resulting in

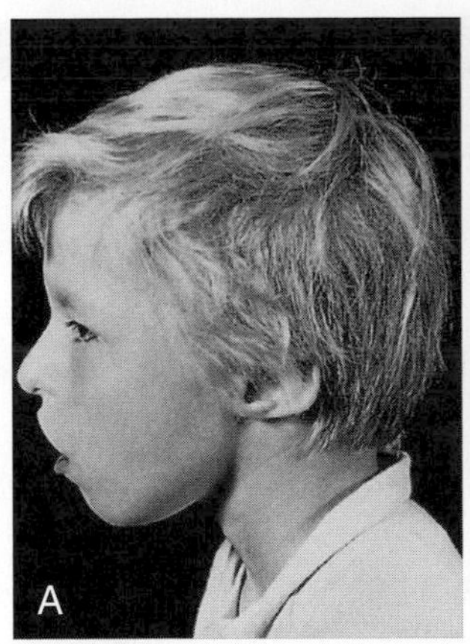
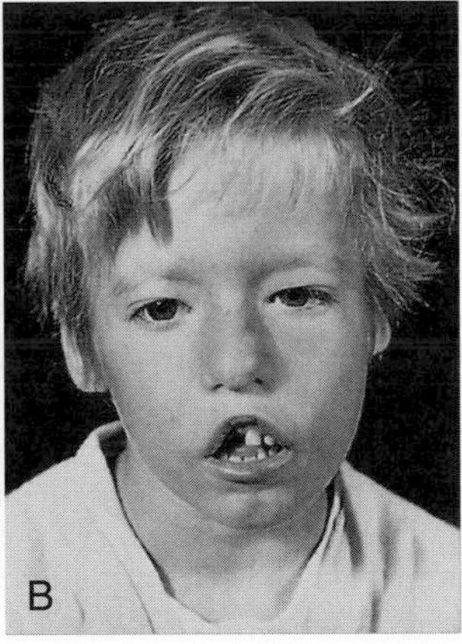

FIGURE 8-6 Facial Anomalies Associated With DiGeorge Syndrome. Note the wide-set eyes, low-set ears, and shortened structure of the upper lip. (From Male, D., Brostoff, J., Roth, D., et al. [2013]. *Immunology* [8th ed.]. Philadelphia: Mosby.)

repeated bacterial infections, such as otitis media, streptococcal sore throat, and conjunctivitis, and more serious conditions, such as septicemia.

Other predominantly antibody deficiencies include severe reduction in particular classes or subclasses of antibody; defects in B-cell surface receptors, such as CD21 and CD40; and defects in class-switch, which may result in a hyper-IgM syndrome.

Phagocyte Defects

Phagocyte defects range from inadequate numbers of phagocytes (e.g., severe congenital neutropenia) to defects in phagocyte function that can result in recurrent infections with the same group of microorganisms (encapsulated bacteria) associated with antibody, and complement deficiencies. Chronic granulomatous disease (CGD) is a severe defect in the myeloperoxidase–hydrogen peroxide system—a major means of bacterial destruction using the enzyme myeloperoxidase, halides (e.g., chloride ion), and hydrogen peroxide.[38] As a result of phagocytosis, neutrophils and other phagocytes switch much of their glucose metabolism to the hexose-monophosphate shunt. A byproduct of this pathway is the conversion of molecular oxygen by nicotinamide adenine dinucleotide phosphate (NADPH) oxidase into highly reactive oxygen derivatives, including hydrogen peroxide. Mutations in NADPH oxidase result in deficient production of hydrogen peroxide and other oxygen products needed for phagocytic killing. Thus, affected individuals have adequate myeloperoxidase and halide but lack the necessary hydrogen peroxide. A lack of hydrogen peroxide (and other highly reactive oxygen species) results in recurrent severe pneumonias; tumourlike granulomata in lungs, skin, and bones; and other infections with some opportunistic microorganisms, such as *S. aureus*, *Serratia marcescens*, and *Aspergillus* species. Other phagocytic deficiencies include defects in various leukocyte adhesion molecules, defects in the phagocytosis process or bacterial killing, and defects in cytokine receptors.

Defects in Innate Immunity

Some immune deficiencies are characterized by a defect in the capacity to produce an immune response against a particular antigen. In chronic mucocutaneous candidiasis, interaction between the Th17 lymphocytes and macrophages is ineffective related to a specific infectious agent, *C. albicans*. Thus the macrophage cannot be activated, and individuals with this immune deficiency usually have mild to extremely severe recurrent *Candida* infections involving the mucous membranes and skin. Other defects in innate immunity include defects in Toll-like receptors and natural killer (NK) cells.

Complement Deficiencies

Many complement deficiencies have been described. C3 deficiency is the most severe defect because of its central role in the complement cascade. Loss of C3b and C3a production and the inability to activate C5 result in recurrent life-threatening infections with encapsulated bacteria (e.g., *H. influenzae* and *S. pneumoniae*) at an early age. Deficiencies of any of the terminal components of the complement cascade (C5, C6, C7, C8, or C9 deficiencies) are associated with increased infections with only one group of bacteria—those of the genus *Neisseria* (*N. meningitides* or *N. gonorrhoeae*). *Neisseria* bacteria usually cause localized infections (meningitis or gonorrhea), but terminal pathway defects result in an 8 000-fold increased risk for systemic infections with atypical strains of these microorganisms.

Mannose-binding lectin (MBL) deficiency is the primary defect of the lectin pathway of complement activation. This defect, as well as defects in the alternative pathway, results in increased risk of infection with microorganisms that have polysaccharide capsules rich in mannose, particularly the yeast *Saccharomyces cerevisiae* and encapsulated bacteria such as *N. meningitidis* and *S. pneumoniae*. Other complement deficiencies include defects in components C1, C4, C2, C5, C1 inhibitor, factor B, factor D, properdin, complement control factors, MBL-associated serine protease, or complement receptors.

Secondary (Acquired) Immune Deficiencies

Secondary, or acquired, immune deficiencies are far more common than primary deficiencies. These deficiencies are complications of other physiological, psychological, or pathophysiological conditions. Some conditions that are known to be associated with acquired immune deficiencies are summarized in Box 8-1.

Although secondary deficiencies are common, many are not clinically relevant. In many cases, the degree of the immune deficiency is relatively minor and without any apparent increased susceptibility to infection. Alternatively, the immune system may be substantially suppressed, but only for a short duration, thus minimizing the incidence of clinically relevant infections. Some secondary immune deficiencies (e.g., AIDS or immunosuppression by cancer), however, are extremely severe and may result in recurrent life-threatening infections.

Evaluation and Care of Those With Immune Deficiency

A review of clinical characteristics can help select the appropriate tests. A basic screening test is a complete blood count (CBC) with a differential. The CBC provides information on the numbers of red blood cells, white blood cells, and platelets, and the differential indicates the quantities of lymphocytes, granulocytes, and monocytes in the blood. Quantitative determination of immunoglobulins (IgG, IgM, IgA) is a screening test for antibody production, and an assay for total complement (total hemolytic complement, CH_{50}) is useful if a complement defect is suspected. Further testing is described in Table 8-11.

Replacement Therapies for Immune Deficiencies

Many immune deficiencies can be successfully treated by replacing the missing component of the immune system. Individuals with B-cell deficiencies that cause hypogammaglobulinemia or agammaglobulinemia usually are treated by administration of intravenous immune globulin (IVIg), antibody-rich fractions prepared from plasma pooled from large numbers of donors.[39] Administration of IVIg replaces the individual's antibodies temporarily; these antibodies have a half-life of 3 to 4 weeks. Thus individuals must be treated repeatedly to maintain a protective level of antibodies in the blood.

BOX 8-1 Some Conditions Known to Be Associated With Acquired Immunodeficiencies

Normal Physiological Conditions
Pregnancy
Infancy
Aging

Psychological Stress
Emotional trauma
Eating disorders

Dietary Insufficiencies
Malnutrition caused by insufficient intake of large categories of nutrients, such as protein or calories
Insufficient intake of specific nutrients, such as vitamins, iron, or zinc

Infections
Congenital infections, such as rubella, cytomegalovirus, hepatitis B
Acquired infections, such as AIDS

Malignancies
Malignancies of lymphoid tissues, such as Hodgkin's disease, acute or chronic leukemia, or myeloma
Malignancies of nonlymphoid tissues, such as sarcomas and carcinomas

Physical Trauma
Burns

Medical Treatments
Stress caused by surgery
Anaesthesia
Immunosuppressive treatment with corticosteroids or antilymphocyte antibodies
Splenectomy
Cancer treatment with cytotoxic medications or ionizing radiation

Other Diseases or Genetic Syndromes
Diabetes
Alcoholic cirrhosis
Sickle cell disease
Systemic lupus erythematosus
Chromosome abnormalities, such as trisomy 21

TABLE 8-11 Laboratory Evaluation of Immune Deficiencies

Function Tested	Laboratory Test	Significance of Test
Tests of Humoral Immune Function		
Antibody production	Total immunoglobulin levels, including IgG, IgM, and IgA	Decrease or absence of total antibody production or of specific classes of antibody, which is associated with many B-cell and combined deficiencies
	Levels of isohemagglutinins	Production of specific IgM antibodies, which is decreased in some combined deficiencies; not useful with persons who are blood type AB and do not have naturally occurring isohemagglutinins
	Levels of antibodies against vaccines—especially diphtheria and tetanus toxoids	Production of specific IgG antibodies, which is decreased when B cells are deficient or class-switch is blocked
B-cell numbers	Numbers of lymphocytes with surface immunoglobulin	Production of circulating B cells, which is decreased in many severe B-cell or combined deficiencies
Antibody subclasses	Level-specific subclasses, particularly IgG1, IgG2, and IgG3	Decrease or absence of a particular subclass, which is characteristic of several immune deficiencies
Tests of Cellular Immune Function		
Delayed hypersensitivity skin test	Skin test reaction against previously encountered antigens, especially *Candida albicans* or tetanus toxoid	Defects in antigen-responsive T cells and skin test cellular interactions (e.g., lymphokine activity and macrophage function)
T-cell numbers	Numbers of T cells expressing characteristic membrane antigens (CD3 or CD11)	Defects in production of circulating T cells
T-cell proliferation in vitro	Proliferative response to nonspecific mitogens (e.g., phytohemagglutinin)	General T-cell defects in response to nonspecific stimulation (mitogens)
	Proliferative response to antigens (e.g., tetanus toxoid)	Defects in response of T cells to specific antigens
T-cell subpopulations	Quantify percentage of T cells with specific markers for total T cells (CD3), T-helper cells (CD4), T-cytotoxic cells (CD8)	Decrease in numbers of CD4 cells, which is related to AIDS progression

Defects in lymphoid cell development in the primary lymphoid organs (e.g., SCID, WAS) can sometimes be treated by replacement of stem cells through transplantation of bone marrow, umbilical cord cells, or other cell populations that are rich in stem cells. Thymic defects (e.g., DiGeorge syndrome, chronic mucocutaneous candidiasis) may be treated by transplantation of fetal thymus tissue or thymic epithelial cells (the cells that produce thymic hormones). However, in most cases improvement is only temporary.

Enzymatic defects that cause SCID (e.g., ADA deficiency) have been treated successfully with transfusions of glycerol frozen-packed erythrocytes. The donor erythrocytes contain the needed enzyme and can, at least temporarily, provide sufficient enzyme for normal lymphocyte function.

Bone marrow transplants containing hematopoietic stem cells are routinely used to treat SCID. However, as discussed later in this chapter, the donor and recipient should be matched as closely as possible for **human leukocyte antigens (HLAs)**. Individuals with SCID are at risk for **graft-versus-host disease (GVHD)**. GVHD occurs if T cells in a transplanted graft (e.g., transfused blood, bone marrow transplants) are mature and therefore capable of cell-mediated immunity against the recipient's HLA. The primary targets for GVHD are the skin (e.g., rash, loss or increase of pigment, thickening of skin), liver (e.g., damage to bile duct, hepatomegaly), mouth (e.g., dry mouth, ulcers, infections), eyes (e.g., burning, irritation, dryness), and gastro-intestinal tract (e.g., severe diarrhea), and the disease may lead to death from infections. The risk of GVHD can be diminished by removing mature T cells from tissue used to treat individuals with immune deficiencies.[40]

Injection of **mesenchymal stem cells (MSCs)** may be useful in these individuals. Stem cells are relatively undifferentiated cells and can be obtained from a variety of sources (e.g., embryos, bone marrow, adult tissues). MSCs are present in all adult tissues. These particular stem cells undergo differentiation into other cell types and, more importantly, have potent immunosuppressive properties.[41] Several clinical trials have demonstrated complete suppression of GVHD in a large number of recipients of MSCs.[42]

The first successful therapeutic replacement of defective genes was performed in two girls with SCID caused by an ADA deficiency.[43] The normal gene for ADA was cloned and inserted into a retroviral vector.[44] The gene for ADA replaced some retroviral genes, resulting in a virus that carried the normal human gene but did not cause disease. The virus was used to infect bone marrow stem cells from these children. The retrovirus inserted the normal *ADA* gene into the individuals' genetic material. The genetically altered stem cells were infused into the children, resulting in reconstitution of their immune systems. Gene therapy trials have verified immune reconstitution in individuals with ADA deficiency, X-linked SCID, CGD, and WAS.[45] However, the treatment trials have not been without some major complications, such as leukemia, that raise questions concerning the use of retroviral vectors for the insertion of new genes.

AIDS

Acquired immunodeficiency syndrome (AIDS) is a secondary immune deficiency that develops in response to viral infection. The **human immunodeficiency virus (HIV)** infects and destroys the CD4-positive ($CD4^+$) T-helper cells (Th cells), which are necessary for the development of both plasma cells and T-cytotoxic cells (Tc cells). Therefore, HIV suppresses the immune response against itself and secondarily creates a generalized immune deficiency by suppressing the development of immune responses against other pathogens and opportunistic micro-organisms, leading to the development of AIDS. New developments in the management of HIV infection have made it more of a chronic illness when the condition is well managed (with immune modifiers and effective antiviral agents). Many people live with HIV infection for long periods without progressing to AIDS.

Despite major efforts by health care agencies around the world, the number of cases and deaths from HIV infection and AIDS (HIV/AIDS) remains a major health concern. The WHO estimated that at the end of 2013, 35.3 million people were living with HIV/AIDS worldwide and more than 2.5 million were newly infected.[46] Approximately 3 million deaths occur each year from AIDS. Since 1980 it is estimated that more than 36 million individuals have died from AIDS worldwide. The majority of cases are in sub-Saharan Africa, where about 1 in 20 adults is living with HIV, but the epidemic is worldwide and the number of new cases is increasing rapidly, particularly in Asia.

In Canada, the spread of HIV/AIDS remains somewhat stable. The PHAC reported that 71 300 people were living with HIV/AIDS in Canada in 2011, and 25% of them were unaware that they were infected. Heterosexual transmission of HIV/AIDS is increasing, and people are living longer with the condition. There were 3 175 new cases of HIV in Canada in 2011, and the disease is being diagnosed at a younger age.[47] Before the implementation of massive public health campaigns and the use of antiviral medications, the progression from HIV infection to AIDS and death was unrelenting. In 1995 AIDS became the number one killer of individuals between the ages of 25 and 44 years in the United States and remains the eighth most common cause of death in that age group. With the advent of effective therapy to stabilize progression of the disease in the mid-1990s, HIV infection has become a chronic disease in Canada and the United States, with many fewer deaths.

Epidemiology of AIDS

HIV is a bloodborne pathogen with the following routes of transmission: blood or blood products, intravenous medication abuse, both heterosexual and homosexual activity, and maternal–child transmission before or during birth. Although the disease first gained attention in the United States related to sexual transmission between males, the most common route worldwide is through heterosexual activity (see *Health Promotion:* Risk of HIV Transmission Associated With Sexual Practices). Worldwide, women constitute more than half of those living with HIV/AIDS. In Canada, as in the rest of the world, the predominant means of transmission to women is through heterosexual contact. Hundreds of thousands of cases of HIV/AIDS have been reported in children who contracted the virus from their mothers across the placenta, through contact with infected blood during delivery, or through the milk during breastfeeding.

Pathogenesis of AIDS

HIV is a member of a family of viruses called *retroviruses*, which carry genetic information in the form of RNA rather than DNA (Figure 8-7). Retroviruses use a viral enzyme, **reverse transcriptase**, to convert RNA into dsDNA. Using a second viral enzyme, **HIV integrase**, the new DNA is inserted into the infected cell's genetic material, where it may remain dormant. If the cell is activated, translation of the viral information may be initiated, resulting in the formation of new virions, lysis and death of the infected cell, and shedding of infectious HIV particles. During that process, **HIV protease** is essential in processing proteins needed from the viral internal structure (capsid). If, however, the cell remains relatively dormant, the viral genetic material may remain latent for years and is probably present for the life of the individual.

The primary surface receptor on HIV is the envelope protein gp120, which binds to the molecule CD4 on the surface of Th cells. Several other necessary co-receptors, particularly the chemokine receptor CCR5, have been identified on target cells. Thus the major immunological finding in AIDS is the striking decrease in the number of $CD4^+$ Th cells (Figure 8-8).

Clinical Manifestations of AIDS

Depletion of $CD4^+$ Th cells has a profound effect on the immune system, causing a severely diminished response to a wide array of infectious pathogens and cancers (Box 8-2). At the time of diagnosis, the individual may present with one of several different conditions: serologically negative (no detectable antibody), serologically positive (positive for antibody

HEALTH PROMOTION

Risk of HIV Transmission Associated With Sexual Practices

High Risk (in descending order of risk)
Receptive anal intercourse with ejaculation (no condom)
Receptive vaginal intercourse with ejaculation (no condom)
Insertive anal intercourse (no condom)
Insertive vaginal intercourse (no condom)
Receptive anal intercourse with withdrawal before ejaculation
Insertive anal intercourse with withdrawal before ejaculation
Receptive vaginal intercourse (with spermicidal foam but no condom)
Insertive vaginal intercourse (with spermicidal foam but no condom)
Receptive anal or vaginal intercourse (with a condom)
Insertive anal or vaginal intercourse (with a condom)

Some Risk (in descending order of risk)
Oral sex with men with ejaculation
Oral sex with women
Oral sex with men with pre-ejaculation fluid (precum)
Oral sex with men, no ejaculation or precum
Oral sex with men (with a condom)

Some Risk (depending on situation, intactness of mucous membranes, etc.)
Mutual masturbation with external or internal touching
Sharing sex toys
Anal or vaginal fisting

No Risk
Masturbating with another person without touching one another
Hugging/massage/dry kissing
Frottage (rubbing genitals while remaining clothed)
Masturbating alone
Abstinence

Unresolved Issues
The role of precum in transmission
The protection offered by covering female genitals with a dental dam during oral sex on the women
The risk of transmission from wet kissing

From Public Health Agency of Canada. (2012). *HIV transmission risk: A summary of the evidence.* Ottawa: Her Majesty the Queen in Right of Canada, pp. 2–10. Retrieved from http://www.catie.ca/sites/default/files/HIV-TRANSMISSION-RISK-EN.pdf.

against HIV proteins) but asymptomatic, early stages of HIV disease, or AIDS (Figure 8-9).

The presence of circulating antibody against the HIV protein p24 followed by more complex tests for antibodies against additional HIV proteins (e.g., Western blot analysis) or for HIV DNA (e.g., polymerase chain reaction) indicates infection by the virus, although many of these individuals are asymptomatic. Antibody appears rather rapidly after infection through blood products, usually within 4 to 7 weeks, although some individuals have been seronegative for longer periods. The period between infection and the appearance of antibody is referred to as the *window period*. Although a person does not have antibody against HIV, he or she may have the virus growing, have the virus in the blood and body fluids, and be infectious to others.

Those with the early stages of HIV disease (early-stage disease) usually initially present with relatively mild and nonspecific symptoms resembling influenza, such as headaches, fever, or fatigue. These symptoms disappear after 1 to 6 weeks, and although individuals appear to be in clinical latency, the virus is actively proliferating in lymph nodes.

BOX 8-2 AIDS-Defining Opportunistic Infections and Neoplasms Found in Individuals With HIV Infection

Infections

Protozoal and Helminthic Infections
Cryptosporidiosis or isosporiasis (enteritis)
Pneumocystosis (pneumonia or disseminated infection)
Toxoplasmosis (pneumonia or central nervous system [CNS] infection)

Fungal Infections
Candidiasis (esophageal, tracheal, or pulmonary)
Coccidioidomycosis (disseminated)
Cryptococcosis (CNS infection)
Histoplasmosis (disseminated)

Bacterial Infections
Mycobacteriosis ("atypical," e.g., *Mycobacterium avium-intracellulare*, disseminated or extrapulmonary
Mycobacterium tuberculosis, disseminated or extrapulmonary)
Nocardiosis (pneumonia, meningitis, disseminated)
Salmonella infections (septicemia, recurrent)

Viral Infections
Cytomegalovirus (pulmonary, intestinal, retinitis, or CNS)
Herpes simplex virus (localized or disseminated)
Progressive multifocal leukoencephalopathy
Varicella-zoster virus (localized or disseminated)

Neoplasms
Invasive cancer of the uterine cervix
Kaposi sarcoma
Non-Hodgkin's lymphomas (Burkitt, immunoblastic)
Primary lymphoma of brain

From Kumar, V., Abbas, A.K., & Aster, J.C. (Eds.). (2015). *Robbins and Cotran pathologic basis of disease* (9th ed.). Philadelphia: Saunders.

The currently accepted definition of AIDS relies on both laboratory tests and clinical symptoms. If the individual is positive for antibodies against HIV, the diagnosis of AIDS is made in association with various clinical symptoms (Figure 8-10; see also Box 8-2). The symptoms include atypical or opportunistic infections and cancers, as well as indications of debilitating chronic disease (e.g., wasting syndrome, recurrent fevers). Most commonly, new cases of AIDS are diagnosed initially by decreased $CD4^+$ Th cell numbers. Individuals who are not HIV infected typically have 800 to 1 000 $CD4^+$ Th cells per cubic millimetre of blood, with a range from 600 to 1 200/mm^3. A diagnosis of AIDS can be made if the $CD4^+$ Th cell numbers decrease to less than 200/mm^3. Without treatment, the average time from infection to development of AIDS is just over 10 years. Some estimates are that approximately 99% of untreated HIV-infected individuals would eventually progress to AIDS.

Treatment and Prevention of AIDS

Approved AIDS medications are classified by mechanism of action: nucleoside and non-nucleoside inhibitors of reverse transcriptase (**reverse transcriptase inhibitors**), inhibitors of the viral protease (**HIV protease inhibitors**), inhibitors of the viral integrase (**HIV integrase inhibitors**), inhibitors of viral entrance into the target cell (**HIV fusion inhibitors**),

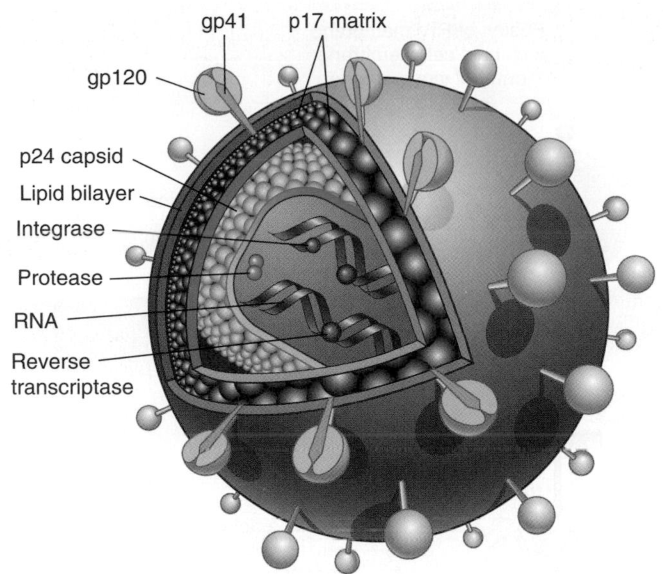

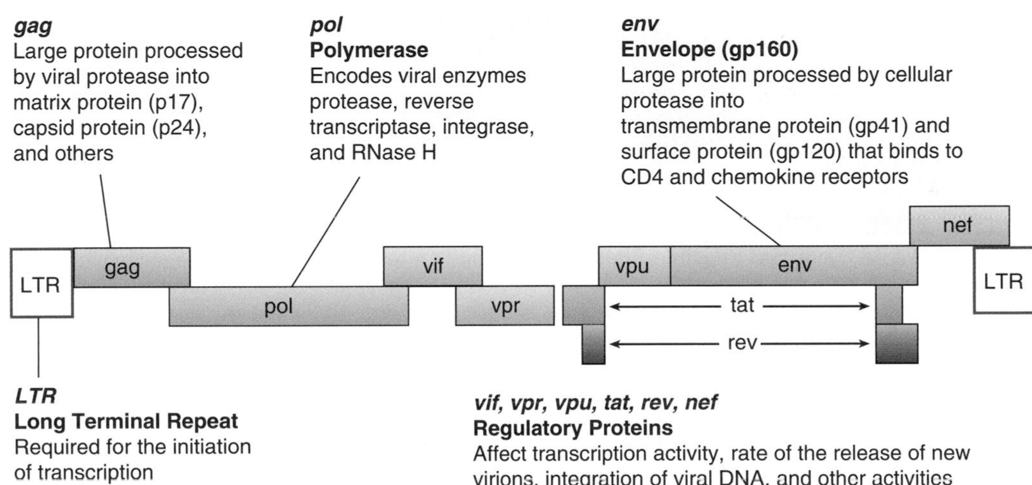

FIGURE 8-7 The Structure and Genetic Map of HIV-1. The human immunodeficiency virus type 1 (HIV-1) virion consists of a core of two identical strands of viral RNA molecules of viral enzymes (reverse transcriptase, protease, integrase) encoated in a core capsid structure consisting primarily of the structural viral protein p24. The capsid is further encased in a matrix consisting primarily of viral protein p17. The outer surface is an envelope consisting of the plasma membrane of the cell from which the virus budded (lipid bilayer) and two viral glycoproteins: a transmembrane glycoprotein, gp41, and a noncovalently attached surface protein, gp120. The HIV-1 genome contains regions that encode the structural proteins (*gag*), the viral enzymes (*pol*), and the envelope proteins (*env*). The genome of complex retroviruses, such as HIV-1, often contains a variety of small regions that regulate expression of the virus. (Modified from Kumar, V., Abbas, A.K., & Aster, J.C. [Eds.]. [2015]. *Robbins and Cotran pathologic basis of disease* [9th ed.]. Philadelphia: Saunders.)

and a **CCR5 antagonist** (inhibitor of viral attachment) (see Figure 8-8). The current regimen for treatment of HIV infection is a combination of medications, termed **antiretroviral therapy (ART)**. ART protocols require a combination of synergist medications from different classes, and specific regimens (e.g., timing of medication administration, doses, medication combinations) are adapted on the basis of age of the individual, secondary clinical symptoms (renal or hepatic insufficiency), CD4+ Th cell levels, viral load, specific co-infections, pre-existing cardiac risk factors, past history of treatment failure, suspected medication resistance, and other parameters.[48,49] The clinical benefits of ART are profound. Death from AIDS-related diseases has been reduced significantly since the introduction of ART. However, resistant variants to these medications have been identified. Medication therapy for AIDS is not curative because HIV incorporates into the genetic material of the host, particularly $CD4^+$ T memory cells, and may never be removed by antimicrobial therapy.[50] Therefore, medication administration to control the virus may have to continue for the lifetime of the individual. Additionally, HIV may persist in regions where the antiviral medications are not as effective, such as the central nervous system (CNS).

The chronic nature of HIV/AIDS resulting from successful ART has led to additional concerns. Long-term toxicity of ART medications has resulted in increased risk for cardiovascular disease, metabolic disorders, and organ failure. Treated individuals frequently fail to reconstitute their immune system and develop chronic immune activation characterized by activation of monocytes and T cells, production of proinflammatory cytokines (e.g., IFN-γ, IL-6), and depletion of Th17 cells.[51]

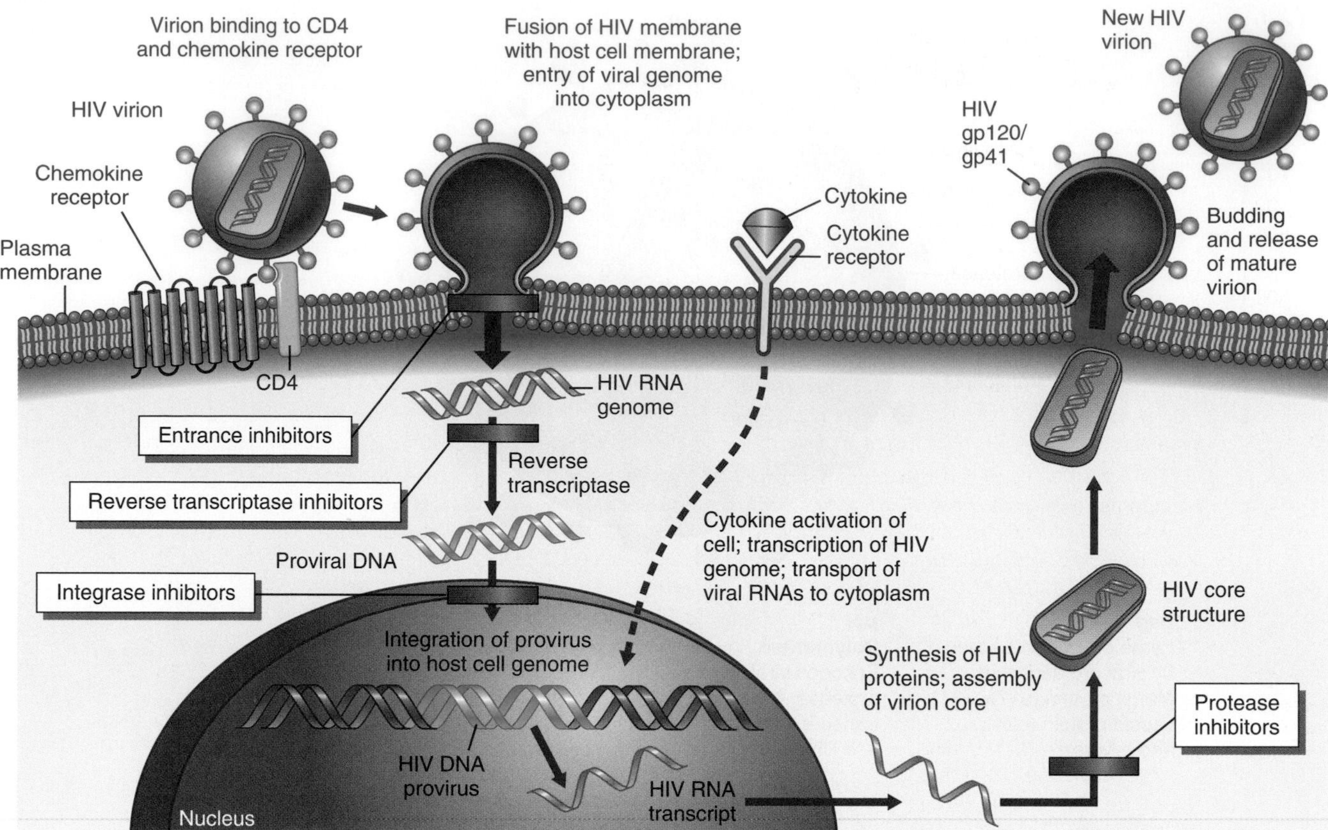

FIGURE 8-8 Life Cycle and Possible Sites of Therapeutic Intervention of HIV. The human immunodeficiency virus (*HIV*) virion consists of a core of two identical strands of viral RNA encoated in a protein structure with viral proteins gp41 and gp120 on its surface (envelope). HIV infection begins when a virion binds to CD4 and chemokine co-receptors on a susceptible cell and follows the process described here. The provirus may remain latent in the cell's DNA until it is activated (e.g., by cytokines). The HIV life cycle is susceptible to blockage at several sites (see the text for further information), including entrance inhibitors, reverse transcriptase inhibitors, integrase inhibitors, and protease inhibitors. (Modified from Kumar, V., Abbas, A.K., & Aster, J.C. [Eds.]. [2015]. *Robbins and Cotran pathologic basis of disease* [9th ed.]. Philadelphia: Saunders.)

Chronic immune activation tends to exacerbate clinical disease in adults and neonates.[52]

Vaccine development should be the most effective means of preventing HIV infection and may be useful in treating pre-existing infection. Most of the common viral vaccines (e.g., rubella, mumps, influenza) induce protective antibodies that block the initial infection. Only one vaccine (rabies) is used after the infection has occurred. The rabies vaccine is successful because the rabies virus proliferates and spreads very slowly. However, the ability of an HIV vaccine to either successfully prevent or treat HIV infection is questionable for several reasons.[53] First, the AIDS virus is genetically and antigenically variable, like the influenza virus, so that a vaccine created against one variant may not provide protection against another variant. Second, although individuals with HIV/AIDS have high levels of circulating antibodies against the virus, these antibodies do not appear to be protective. Therefore, even if a circulating antibody response can be induced by vaccination, that response might not be effective. A vaccine may have to induce both circulating and secretory (to prevent initial infection of the mucosal T cell) antibody and Tc cells.

Pediatric AIDS and Central Nervous System Involvement

HIV can be transmitted from mother to child during pregnancy, at the time of delivery, or through breastfeeding, although the risk of mother-to-child transmission has dropped precipitously since the use of antiretroviral medications in pregnant women. The clinical diagnosis of HIV infection in young children born of HIV-infected mothers is very often a difficult task because the presence of maternal antibodies may result in a misleading false-positive test for antibodies against HIV for as long as 18 months after birth. Testing for antibody against HIV can be performed recurrently from birth until 18 months; if the test results become negative and remain so after 12 months, the child can be considered uninfected.

The report *WHO Recommendations on the Diagnosis of HIV Infection in Infant and Children* suggests that in children younger than 18 months, testing for HIV or viral components should occur in two separate specimens, not including cord blood.[54] Testing involves detection of HIV nucleic acid or p24 antigen, or direct isolation of HIV in viral cultures.

HIV infection of babies is generally more aggressive than in adults; on average, an untreated child will die by his or her second birthday. Neurological involvement occurs more commonly in children than in adults and results from CNS involvement, rather than effects on peripheral portions of the nervous system. HIV encephalopathy occurs with varying degrees of severity and is a clinical component in the diagnosis of AIDS in children. Most HIV-infected newborns appear normal but may progressively develop signs of CNS involvement. These

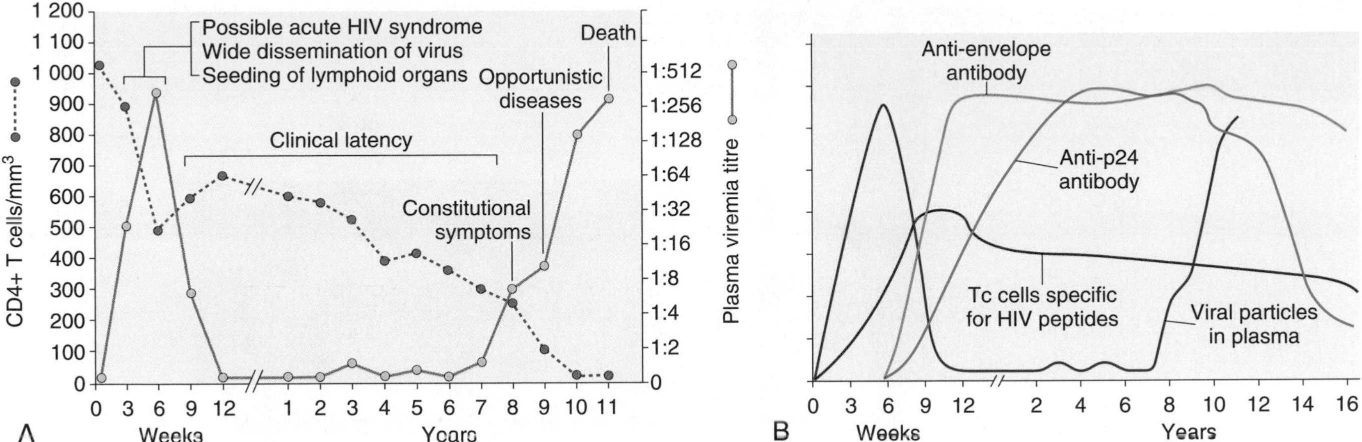

FIGURE 8-9 Typical Progression From HIV Infection to AIDS in Untreated Persons. A, Clinical progression begins within weeks after infection; the person may experience symptoms of acute human immunodeficiency virus (HIV) syndrome. During this early period, the virus progressively infects T cells and other cells and spreads to the lymphoid organs, with a sharp decrease in the number of circulating CD4+ Th cells. During a period of clinical latency, the virus replicates and T-cell destruction continues, although the person is generally asymptomatic. The individual may develop HIV-related disease (constitutional symptoms)—a variety of symptoms of acute viral infection that do not involve opportunistic infections or malignancies. When the number of CD4+ Th cells is critically suppressed, the individual becomes susceptible to a variety of opportunistic infections and cancers with a diagnosis of acquired immunodeficiency syndrome (AIDS). The length of time for progression from HIV infection to AIDS may vary considerably from person to person. **B,** Laboratory tests are changing throughout infection. Antibody and Tc cell (T-cytotoxic cells [*Tc cells*]) levels change during the progression to AIDS. During the initial phase antibodies against HIV-1 are not yet detectable (window period), but viral products, including proteins and RNA, and infectious virus may be detectable in the blood a few weeks after infection. Most antibodies against HIV are not detectable in the early phase. During the latent phase of infection antibody levels against p24 and other viral proteins, as well as HIV-specific Tc cells, increase, and then remain constant until the development of AIDS. (**A,** redrawn from Fauci, A.S., & Lane, H.C. [1997]. Human immunodeficiency virus disease: AIDS and related conditions. In A.S. Fauci, E. Braunwald, K.J. Isselbacher, et al. [Eds.], *Harrison's principles of internal medicine* [14th ed.]. New York: McGraw-Hill; **B,** from Kumar, V., Abbas, A.K., & Aster, J.C. [Eds.]. [2015]. *Robbins and Cotran pathologic basis of disease* [9th ed.]. Philadelphia: Saunders.)

signs usually appear as failure to attain (or loss of) developmental milestones or loss of intellectual ability, verified by standard developmental scale or neuropsychological tests; acquired symmetrical motor deficits, seen in children older than age 1 month; impaired brain growth or acquired microcephaly, demonstrated by head circumference measurements; or brain atrophy, demonstrated by computed tomography (CT) or magnetic resonance imaging (MRI) (serial imaging is required in children younger than 2 years of age).

It may be difficult to completely differentiate the effect of HIV infection on the CNS from other risk factors, including prenatal medication exposure, prematurity, chronic illness, and a chaotic social atmosphere. The pathogenesis of HIV encephalopathy in children is poorly understood, but the presence of inflammatory mediators may be a contributing factor.

Because HIV infection in infants progresses very rapidly, treatment must begin at the diagnosis of infection. In older children the criteria for treatment are similar to those used in adults. A growing number of investigational protocols are available for treatment of children with HIV. In general, treatment is focused on the preservation and maintenance of the immune system, aggressive response to opportunistic infections, support and relief of symptomatic occurrences, and administration of ART.

QUICK CHECK 8-2

1. Why is the development of recurrent or unusual infections the clinical hallmark of immunodeficiency?
2. Compare and contrast the most common infections in individuals with defects in cell-mediated immune response and those with defects in humoral immune response.
3. What are the new treatments for HIV?

HYPERSENSITIVITY: ALLERGY, AUTOIMMUNITY, AND ALLOIMMUNITY

Allergy, autoimmunity, and alloimmunity are classified as *hypersensitivity reactions.* **Hypersensitivity** is an altered immunological response to an antigen that results in disease or damage to the individual. Allergy, autoimmunity, and alloimmunity (also termed *isoimmunity*) can be most easily understood in relationship to the source of the antigen against which the hypersensitivity response is directed (Table 8-12). **Allergy** refers to a hypersensitivity to environmental antigens. These can include medicines, natural products (e.g., pollens, bee stings),

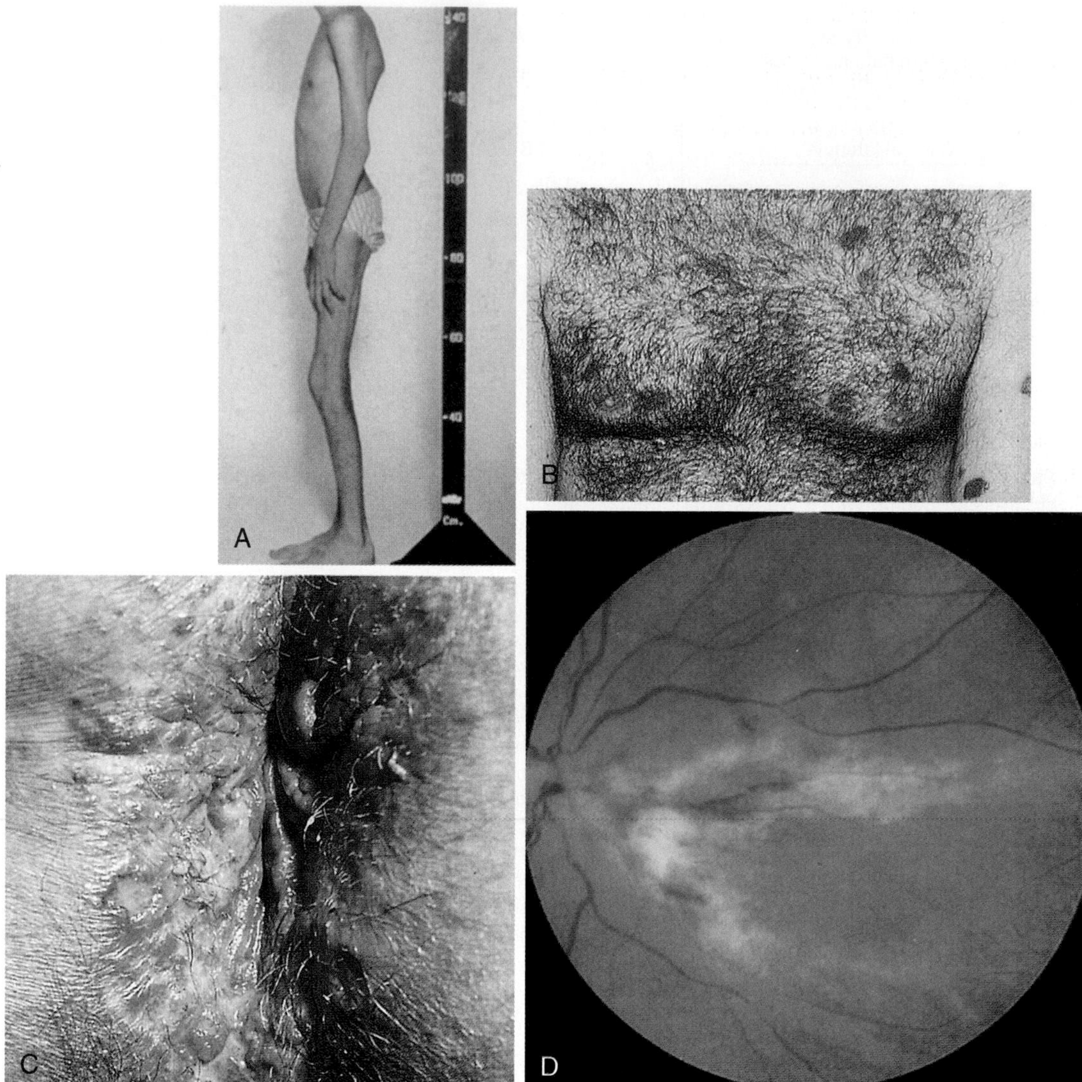

FIGURE 8-10 Clinical Symptoms of AIDS. **A,** Severe weight loss and anorexia. **B,** Kaposi sarcoma lesions. **C,** Perianal lesions of herpes simplex infection. **D,** Deterioration of vision from cytomegalovirus retinitis leading to areas of infection, which can lead to blindness. (**A** and **D,** from Taylor, P.K. [1995]. *Diagnostic picture tests in sexually transmitted diseases.* London: Mosby; **B** and **C,** from Morse, S.A., Holmes, K.K., & Balllard, R.C. [Eds.]. [2011]. *Atlas of sexually transmitted diseases and AIDS* [4th ed.]. London: Saunders.)

TABLE 8-12 Relative Incidence and Examples of Hypersensitivity Diseases[a]

	MECHANISM			
	Type I (IgE Mediated)	**Type II (Tissue Specific)**	**Type III (Immune Complex Mediated)**	**Type IV (Cell Mediated)**
Allergy Target antigens: environmental antigens	++++ Hay fever	+ Hemolysis in medication allergies	+ Gluten (wheat) allergy	++ Poison ivy allergy
Autoimmunity Target antigens: self-antigens	+ May contribute to some type III reactions	++ Autoimmune thrombocytopenia	+++ Systemic lupus erythematosus	++ Hashimoto thyroiditis
Alloimmunity Target antigens: another person's antigens	+ May contribute to some type III reactions	++ Hemolytic disease of the newborn	+ Individuals who do not make their own IgA may have an anaphylactic response against IgA in human immune globulin	++ Graft rejection

[a]The frequency of each reaction is indicated in a range from rare (+) to very common (++++). An example of each reaction is given.

infectious agents, and any other antigen that is not naturally found in the individual.

Autoimmunity is a disturbance in the immunological tolerance of self-antigens. The immune system normally does not strongly recognize the individual's own antigens. Healthy individuals of all ages, but particularly older adults, may produce low quantities of antibodies against their own antigens (*autoantibodies*) without developing overt autoimmune disease. Therefore, the presence of low quantities of autoantibodies does not necessarily indicate a disease state. Autoimmune diseases occur when the immune system reacts against self-antigens to such a degree that autoantibodies or autoreactive T cells damage the individual's tissues. Many clinical disorders are associated with autoimmunity and are generally referred to as **autoimmune diseases** (Table 8-13). Autoimmune diseases are more prevalent in women and the overall prevalence is rising.[55]

Alloimmune diseases occur when the immune system of one individual produces an immunological reaction against tissues of another individual. **Alloimmunity** can be observed during immunological reactions against transfusions, transplanted tissue, or the fetus during pregnancy.

The mechanism that initiates the onset of hypersensitivity, whether allergy, autoimmunity, or alloimmunity, is not completely understood. It is generally accepted that genetic, infectious, and possibly environmental factors contribute to the development of hypersensitivity reactions.

TABLE 8-13 Examples of Autoimmune Disorders

System Disease	Organ or Tissue	Probable Self-Antigen
Endocrine System		
Hyperthyroidism (Graves' disease)	Thyroid gland	Receptors for thyroid-stimulating hormone on plasma membrane of thyroid cells
Hashimoto's disease	Thyroid gland	Thyroid cell surface antigens, thyroglobulin
Insulin-dependent diabetes	Pancreas	Islet cells, insulin, insulin receptors on pancreatic cells
Addison's disease	Adrenal gland	Surface antigens on steroid-producing cells; microsomal antigens
Male infertility	Testis	Surface antigens on spermatozoa
Skin		
Pemphigus vulgaris	Skin	Intercellular substances in stratified squamous epithelium
Bullous pemphigoid	Skin	Basement membrane
Vitiligo	Skin	Surface antigens on melanocytes (melanin-producing cells)
Neuromuscular Tissue		
Multiple sclerosis	Neural tissue	Surface antigens of nerve cells
Myasthenia gravis	Neuromuscular junction	Acetylcholine receptors; striations of skeletal and cardiac muscle
Rheumatic fever	Heart	Cardiac tissue antigens that cross-react with group A streptococcal antigen
Cardiomyopathy	Heart	Cardiac muscle
Gastro-intestinal System		
Ulcerative colitis	Colon	Mucosal cells
Pernicious anemia	Stomach	Surface antigens of parietal cells; intrinsic factor
Primary biliary cirrhosis	Liver	Cells of bile duct
Chronic active hepatitis	Liver	Surface antigens of hepatocytes, nuclei, microsomes, smooth muscle
Eye		
Sjögren's syndrome	Lacrimal gland	Antigens of lacrimal gland, salivary gland, thyroid, and nuclei of cells
Connective Tissue		
Ankylosing spondylitis	Joints	Sacroiliac and spinal apophyseal joint
Rheumatoid arthritis	Joints	Collagen, IgG
Systemic lupus erythematosus	Multiple sites	Numerous antigens in nuclei, organelles, and extracellular matrix
Renal System		
Immune complex glomerulonephritis	Kidney	Numerous immune complexes
Goodpasture's syndrome	Kidney	Glomerular basement membrane
Hematological System		
Idiopathic neutropenia	Neutrophil	Surface antigens on polymorphonuclear neutrophils
Idiopathic lymphopenia	Lymphocytes	Surface antigens on lymphocytes
Autoimmune hemolytic anemia	Erythrocytes	Surface antigens on erythrocytes
Autoimmune thrombocytopenic purpura	Platelets	Surface antigens on platelets
Respiratory System		
Goodpasture's syndrome	Lung	Septal membrane of alveolus

TABLE 8-14 Immunological Mechanisms of Tissue Destruction

Type	Name	Rate of Development	Class of Antibody Involved	Principal Effector Cells Involved	Participation of Complement	Examples of Disorders
I	IgE-mediated reaction	Immediate	IgE	Mast cells	No	Seasonal allergic rhinitis Asthma
II	Tissue-specific reaction	Immediate	IgG IgM	Macrophages in tissues	Frequently	Autoimmune thrombocytopenic purpura, Graves' disease, autoimmune hemolytic anemia
III	Immune complex–mediated reaction	Immediate	IgG IgM	Neutrophils	Yes	Systemic lupus erythematosus
IV	Cell-mediated reaction	Delayed	None	Lymphocytes Macrophages	No	Contact sensitivity to poison ivy, metals (jewelry), and latex

Mechanisms of Hypersensitivity

Hypersensitivity reactions can be characterized also by the particular immune mechanism that results in the disease (Table 8-14). These mechanisms are apparent in most hypersensitivity reactions and have been divided into four distinct types: *type I* (IgE-mediated reactions), *type II* (tissue-specific reactions), *type III* (immune complex–mediated reactions), and *type IV* (cell-mediated reactions). This classification is artificial and seldom is a particular disease associated with only a single mechanism. The four mechanisms are interrelated, and in most hypersensitivity reactions several mechanisms can be functioning simultaneously or sequentially.

As with all immune responses, hypersensitivity reactions require sensitization against a particular antigen that results in a primary immune response. Disease symptoms appear after an adequate secondary immune response occurs. Hypersensitivity reactions are immediate or delayed, depending on the time required to elicit clinical symptoms after re-exposure to the antigen. Reactions that occur within minutes to a few hours after exposure to an antigen are termed **immediate hypersensitivity reactions**. **Delayed hypersensitivity reactions** may take several hours to appear and are at maximal severity days after re-exposure to the antigen. Generally, immediate reactions are caused by antibody, whereas delayed reactions are caused by cells (e.g., T cells, NK cells, macrophages).

The most rapid and severe immediate hypersensitivity reaction is **anaphylaxis**. Anaphylaxis occurs within minutes of re-exposure to the antigen and can be either systemic (generalized) or cutaneous (localized). Symptoms of systemic anaphylaxis include pruritus, erythema, vomiting, abdominal cramps, diarrhea, and breathing difficulties, and the most severe reactions may include contraction of bronchial smooth muscle, edema of the throat, and decreased blood pressure that can lead to shock and death.[56] Examples of systemic anaphylaxis are allergic reactions to bee stings, peanuts, shellfish, or eggs. Cutaneous anaphylaxis results in local symptoms, such as pain, swelling, and redness, which occur at the site of exposure to an antigen (e.g., a painful local reaction to an injected vaccine or medication).

Type I: IgE-Mediated Hypersensitivity Reactions

Type I hypersensitivity reactions are mediated by antigen-specific IgE and the products of tissue mast cells (Figure 8-11). Most common allergic reactions are type I reactions. In addition, most type I reactions occur against environmental antigens and are therefore allergic. Because of this strong association, many health care providers use the term *allergy* to indicate only IgE-mediated reactions. However, IgE can contribute to some autoimmune and alloimmune diseases, and many common allergies (e.g., poison ivy) are not mediated by IgE.

IgE has a relatively short lifespan in the blood because it rapidly binds to Fc receptors on mast cells.[57] Unlike Fc receptors on phagocytes, which bind IgG that has previously reacted with an antigen, the Fc receptors on mast cells specifically bind IgE that has not previously interacted with antigen. After a large amount of IgE has bound to the mast cells, an individual is considered *sensitized*. Further exposure of a sensitized individual to the allergen results in degranulation of the mast cell and the release of mast cell products (see Chapter 6).

Mechanisms of IgE-mediated hypersensitivity. The most potent mediator of IgE-mediated hypersensitivity is histamine, which affects several key target cells. Acting through H1 receptors, histamine contracts bronchial smooth muscles (bronchial constriction), increases vascular permeability (edema), and causes vasodilation (increased blood flow) (see Chapter 6). The interaction of histamine with H2 receptors results in increased gastric acid secretion. Blocking histamine receptors with antihistamines can control some type I responses.

Clinical manifestations of IgE-mediated hypersensitivity. The clinical manifestations of type I reactions are attributable mostly to the biological effects of histamine. The tissues most commonly affected by type I responses contain large numbers of mast cells and are sensitive to the effects of histamine released from them. These tissues are found in the gastro-intestinal tract, the skin, and the respiratory tract (Figure 8-12 and Table 8-15).

Gastro-intestinal allergy is caused by allergens that enter through the mouth—usually foods or medicines. Symptoms include vomiting, diarrhea, or abdominal pain. Foods most often implicated in gastro-intestinal allergies are milk, chocolate, citrus fruits, eggs, wheat, nuts, peanut butter, and fish.[58] The most common food allergy in adults is a reaction to shellfish, which may initiate an anaphylactic response and death.[59] When food is the source of an allergen, the active immunogen may be an unidentifiable product of how the food is processed during manufacture or broken down by digestive enzymes.[60] Sometimes the allergen is a medication, an additive, or a preservative in the food. For example, cows treated for mastitis with penicillin yield milk containing trace amounts of this antibiotic. Thus hypersensitivity apparently caused by milk proteins may instead be the result of an allergy to penicillin.

Urticaria, or hives, is a dermal (skin) manifestation of allergic reactions (see Figure 8-12). The underlying mechanism is the localized release of histamine and increased vascular permeability, resulting in limited areas of edema. Urticaria is characterized by white fluid-filled blisters (wheals) surrounded by areas of redness (flares). This **wheal and flare reaction** is usually accompanied by pruritus. Not all urticarial symptoms are caused by immunological reactions. Some, termed *nonimmunological urticaria*, result from exposure to cold temperatures,

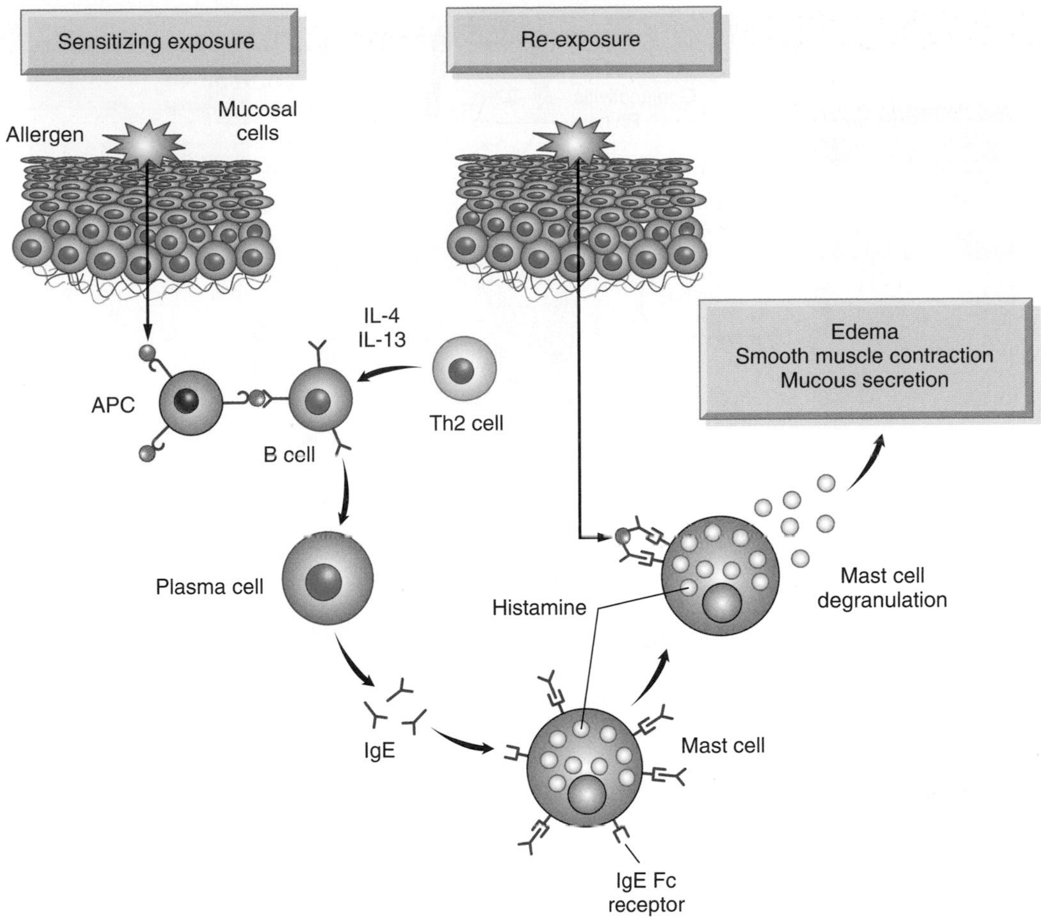

FIGURE 8-11 Mechanism of Type I, IgE-Mediated Reactions. First exposure to an allergen leads to antigen processing and presentation of antigen by an antigen-presenting cell (*APC*) to B cells, which is under the direction of T-helper 2 cells (*Th2 cells*). Th2 cells produce specific cytokines (e.g., interleukin-4 [*IL-4*], *IL-13*, and others) that favour maturation of the B cells into plasma cells that secrete IgE. The IgE is adsorbed to the surface of the mast cell by binding with IgE-specific crystallizable fragment (*Fc*) receptors. When an adequate amount of IgE is bound, the mast cell is sensitized. During re-exposure, the allergen cross-links the surface-bound IgE and causes degranulation of the mast cell. Contents of the mast cell granules, primarily histamine, induce local edema, smooth muscle contraction, mucous secretion, and other characteristics of an acute inflammatory reaction. (See Chapter 6 for more details on the role of mast cells in inflammation.)

emotional stress, medications, systemic diseases, or malignancies (e.g., lymphomas).

Effects of allergens on the mucosa of the eyes, nose, and respiratory tract include conjunctivitis (inflammation of the membranes lining the eyelids) (see Figure 8-12), rhinitis (inflammation of the mucous membranes of the nose), and asthma (constriction of the bronchi). Symptoms are caused by vasodilation, hypersecretion of mucus, edema, and swelling of the respiratory mucosa. Because the mucous membranes lining the respiratory tract are continuous, they are all adversely affected. The degree to which each is affected determines the symptoms of the disease; most anaphylactic reactions are type I hypersensitivities.

The central problem in allergic diseases of the lung is obstruction of the large and small airways (bronchi) of the lower respiratory tract by bronchospasm (constriction of smooth muscle in airway walls), edema, and thick secretions. This obstruction leads to ventilatory insufficiency, wheezing, and difficult or laboured breathing (see Chapter 27).

Certain individuals are genetically predisposed to develop allergies and are called **atopic**. In families in which one parent has an allergy, allergies develop in about 40% of the offspring. If both parents have allergies, the incidence may be as high as 80%. Atopic individuals tend to produce higher quantities of IgE and have more Fc receptors for IgE on their mast cells. The airways and the skin of atopic individuals have increased responsiveness to a wide variety of both specific and nonspecific stimuli.

Evaluation and treatment of IgE hypersensitivity. Allergic reactions can be life-threatening; therefore, it is essential that severely allergic individuals be informed of the specific allergen against which they are sensitized and instructed to avoid contact with that material. Several tests are available to evaluate allergic individuals. These include food challenges, skin tests with allergens, and laboratory tests for total IgE and allergen-specific IgE.

Type II: Tissue-Specific Hypersensitivity Reactions

Type II hypersensitivities are generally reactions against a specific cell or tissue. Cells express a variety of antigens on their surfaces, some of which are called **tissue-specific antigens** because they are expressed on the plasma membranes of only certain cells. Platelets, for example, have groups of antigens that are found on no other cells of the body. The symptoms of many type II diseases are determined by which tissue or

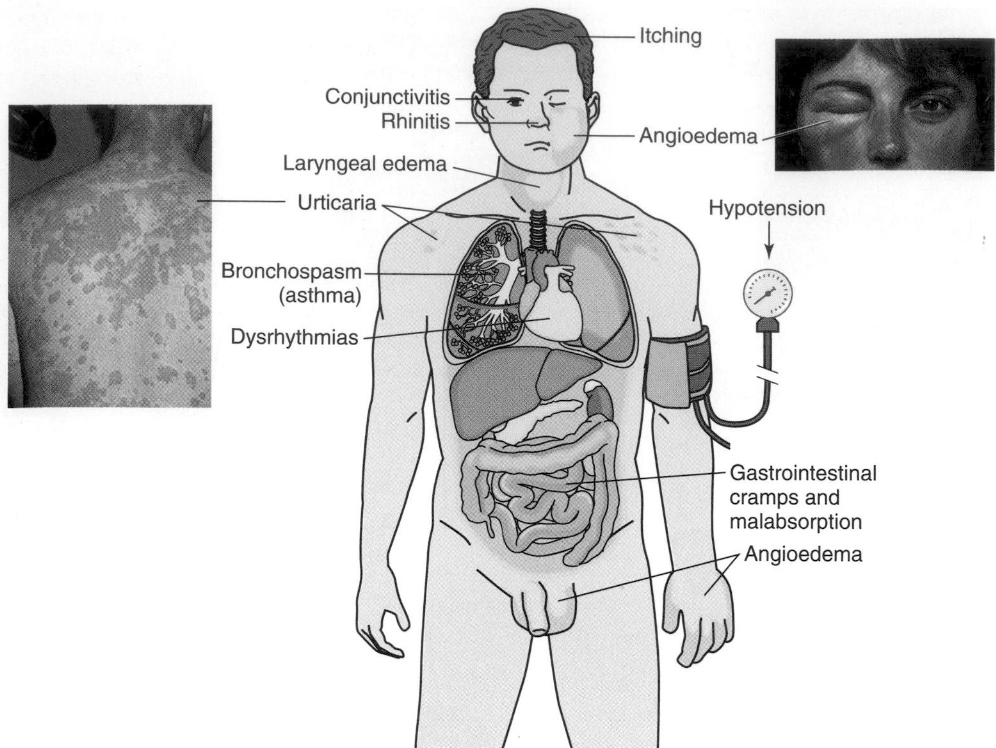

FIGURE 8-12 Type I, IgE-Mediated Hypersensitivity Reactions. Manifestations of allergic reactions as a result of type I hypersensitivity include pruritus, angioedema (swelling caused by exudation), edema of the larynx, urticaria (hives), bronchospasm (constriction of airways in the lungs), hypotension (low blood pressure), and dysrhythmias (irregular heartbeat) because of anaphylactic shock, and gastro-intestinal cramping caused by inflammation of the gastro-intestinal mucosa. Photographic inserts show a diffuse allergiclike eye and skin reaction on an individual. The skin lesions have raised edges and develop within minutes or hours, with resolution occurring after about 12 hours. (Inserts from Male, D., Brostoff, J., Roth, D., et al. [2013]. *Immunology* [8th ed.]. Philadelphia: Mosby.)

organ expresses the particular antigen. Environmental antigens (e.g., medications or their metabolites) may bind to the plasma membranes of specific cells (especially erythrocytes and platelets) and function as targets of type II reactions. The five general mechanisms by which type II hypersensitivity reactions can affect cells are shown in Figure 8-13. Each mechanism begins with antibody binding to tissue-specific antigens or antigens that have attached to particular tissues.

The cell may be destroyed by antibodies and complement (Figure 8-13, *A*). IgM or IgG reacts with an antigen on the surface of the cell, causing activation of the complement cascade through the classical pathway. Formation of the membrane attack complex (C5-9) damages the membrane and may result in lysis of the cell. For example, erythrocytes are destroyed by complement-mediated lysis in individuals with autoimmune hemolytic anemia (see Chapters 21 and 22) or as a result of an alloimmune reaction to mismatched transfused blood cells.

Antibody may cause cell destruction through phagocytosis by macrophages (Figure 8-13, *B*). The antibody may additionally activate complement, resulting in the deposition of C3b on the cell surface. Receptors on the macrophage recognize and bind opsonins (e.g., antibody or C3b) and increase phagocytosis of the target cell. For example, antibodies against platelet-specific antigens or against red blood cell antigens of the Rh system cause their removal by phagocytosis in the spleen.

Tissue damage may be caused by toxic products produced by neutrophils (Figure 8-13, *C*). Soluble antigens such as medications, molecules released from infectious agents, or molecules released from an individual's own cells may enter the circulation. In some instances, the antigens are deposited on the surface of tissues, where they bind antibody. The antibody may activate complement, resulting in the release of C3a and C5a, which are chemotactic for neutrophils, and the deposition of complement component C3b. Neutrophils are attracted, bind to the tissues through receptors for the Fc portion of antibody (Fc receptor) or for C3b, and release their granules onto the healthy tissue. The components of neutrophil granules, as well as the toxic oxygen products produced by these cells, will damage the tissue.

Antibody-dependent cell-mediated cytotoxicity (ADCC) *involves NK cells* (Figure 8-13, *D*). Antibody on the target cell is recognized by Fc receptors on the NK cells, which release toxic substances that destroy the target cell.

The last mechanism does not destroy the target cell but causes the cell to malfunction (Figure 8-13, *E*). The antibody is usually directed against antigenic determinants associated with specific cell surface receptors. The antibody changes the function of the receptor by preventing interactions with their normal ligands, replacing the ligand and inappropriately stimulating the receptor, or destroying the receptor. For example, in the hyperthyroidism (excessive thyroid activity) of Graves' disease, the autoantibody binds to and activates receptors for thyroid-stimulating hormone (TSH) (a pituitary hormone that controls the production of the hormone thyroxine by the thyroid). In this way, the antibody stimulates the thyroid cells to produce thyroxine. Under normal conditions, the increasing levels of thyroxine in the blood would signal the pituitary to decrease TSH production, which would result in less stimulation of the TSH receptor in the thyroid and a concomitant decrease in thyroxine production. Increasing amounts of thyroxine in

TABLE 8-15 Causes of Clinical Allergic Reactions

Typical Allergen	Mechanism of Hypersensitivity	Clinical Manifestation
Ingestants		
Foods	Type I	Gastro-intestinal allergy
Drugs	Types I, II, III	Urticaria, immediate medication reaction, hemolytic anemia, serum sickness
Inhalants		
Pollens, dust, moulds	Type I	Allergic rhinitis, bronchial asthma
Aspergillus fumigatus	Types I, III	Allergic bronchopulmonary aspergillosis
Thermophilic actinomycetes[a]	Types III, IV	Extrinsic allergic alveolitis
Injectants		
Drugs	Types I, II, III	Immediate medication reaction, hemolytic anemia, serum sickness
Bee venom	Type I	Anaphylaxis
Vaccines	Type III	Localized Arthus reaction
Serum	Types I, III	Anaphylaxis, serum sickness
Contactants		
Poison ivy, metals	Type IV	Contact dermatitis
Latex	Types I, IV	Contact dermatitis, anaphylaxis

[a]An order of fungi that grows best at high temperatures (between 45 and 80°C [113 and 176°F]).

Modified from Bellanti, J.A. (1985). *Immunology III*. Philadelphia: Saunders.

the blood have no effect on anti-TSH receptor antibodies, which continue to stimulate despite decreasing amounts of TSH (see Chapter 19).

Type III: Immune Complex–Mediated Hypersensitivity Reactions

Mechanisms of type III hypersensitivity. Most type III hypersensitivity disease reactions are caused by antigen–antibody (immune) complexes that are formed in the circulation and deposited later in vessel walls or other tissues (Figure 8-14). The primary difference between type II and type III mechanisms is that in type II hypersensitivity antibody binds to an antigen on the cell surface, whereas in type III antibody binds to soluble antigen that was released into the blood or body fluids, and the complex is then deposited in the tissues. Type III reactions are not organ specific, and symptoms are mostly unrelated to the particular antigenic target of the antibody. The harmful effects of immune complex deposition are caused by complement activation, particularly through the generation of chemotactic factors for neutrophils. The neutrophils bind to antibody and C3b contained in the complexes and attempt to ingest the immune complexes. They are often unsuccessful because the complexes are bound to large areas of tissue. During the attempted phagocytosis, large quantities of lysosomal enzymes are released into the inflammatory site instead of into phagolysosomes. The attraction of neutrophils and the subsequent release of lysosomal enzymes cause most of the resulting tissue damage.

Immune complex disease. Two prototypic models of type III hypersensitivity help explain the variety of diseases in this category. Serum sickness is a model of systemic type III hypersensitivities, and the Arthus reaction is a model of localized or cutaneous reactions.

Serum sickness–type reactions are caused by the formation of immune complexes in the blood and their subsequent generalized deposition in target tissues. Typically affected tissues are the blood vessels, joints, and kidneys. Symptoms include fever, enlarged lymph nodes, rash, and pain at sites of inflammation. Serum sickness was initially described as a complication of therapeutic administration of horse serum that contained antibody against tetanus toxin. Foreign serum is not administered to individuals today, although serum sickness reactions can be caused by the repeated intravenous administration of other antigens, such as medications, and the characteristics of serum sickness are observed in systemic type III autoimmune diseases.

A form of serum sickness is Raynaud phenomenon, a condition caused by the temperature-dependent deposition of immune complexes in the capillary beds of the peripheral circulation. Certain immune complexes precipitate at temperatures below normal body temperature, particularly in the tips of the fingers, toes, and nose, and are called cryoglobulins. The precipitates block the circulation and cause localized pallor and numbness, followed by cyanosis (a bluish tinge resulting from oxygen deprivation) and eventually gangrene if the circulation is not restored.

An Arthus reaction is caused by repeated local exposure to an antigen that reacts with preformed antibody and forms immune complexes in the walls of the local blood vessels. Symptoms of an Arthus reaction begin within 1 hour of exposure and peak 6 to 12 hours later. The lesions are characterized by a typical inflammatory reaction, with increased vascular permeability, an accumulation of neutrophils, edema, hemorrhage, clotting, and tissue damage.

Arthus reactions may be observed after injection, ingestion, or inhalation of allergens. Skin reactions can follow subcutaneous or intradermal inoculation with medications, fungal extracts, or antigens used in skin tests. Gastro-intestinal reactions, such as gluten-sensitive enteropathy (celiac disease), follow ingestion of an antigen, usually gluten from wheat products (see Chapter 37). Allergic alveolitis (farmer lung, pigeon breeder disease) is an Arthus-like acute hemorrhagic inflammation of the air sacs (alveoli) of the lungs resulting from inhalation of fungal antigens, usually particles from mouldy hay or pigeon feces (see Chapter 27).

Type IV: Cell-Mediated Hypersensitivity Reactions

Whereas types I, II, and III hypersensitivity reactions are mediated by antibody, type IV hypersensitivity reactions are mediated by T cells and do not involve antibody (Figure 8-15). Type IV mechanisms occur through either Tc cells or lymphokine-producing Th1 and Th17 cells. Tc cells attack and destroy cellular targets directly. Th1 and Th17 cells produce cytokines that recruit and activate phagocytic cells, especially macrophages. Destruction of the tissue is usually caused by direct killing by Tc cells or the release of soluble factors, such as lysosomal enzymes and toxic reactive oxygen species, from activated macrophages.

Clinical examples of type IV hypersensitivity reactions include graft rejection, the skin test for TB, and allergic reactions resulting from contact with such substances as poison ivy and metals. A type IV component also may be present in many autoimmune diseases. For example, T cells against type II collagen (a protein present in joint tissues) contribute to the destruction of joints in rheumatoid arthritis; T cells against a thyroid cell–surface antigen contribute to the destruction of the thyroid in autoimmune thyroiditis (Hashimoto's disease); and T cells against an antigen on the surface of pancreatic beta cells (the

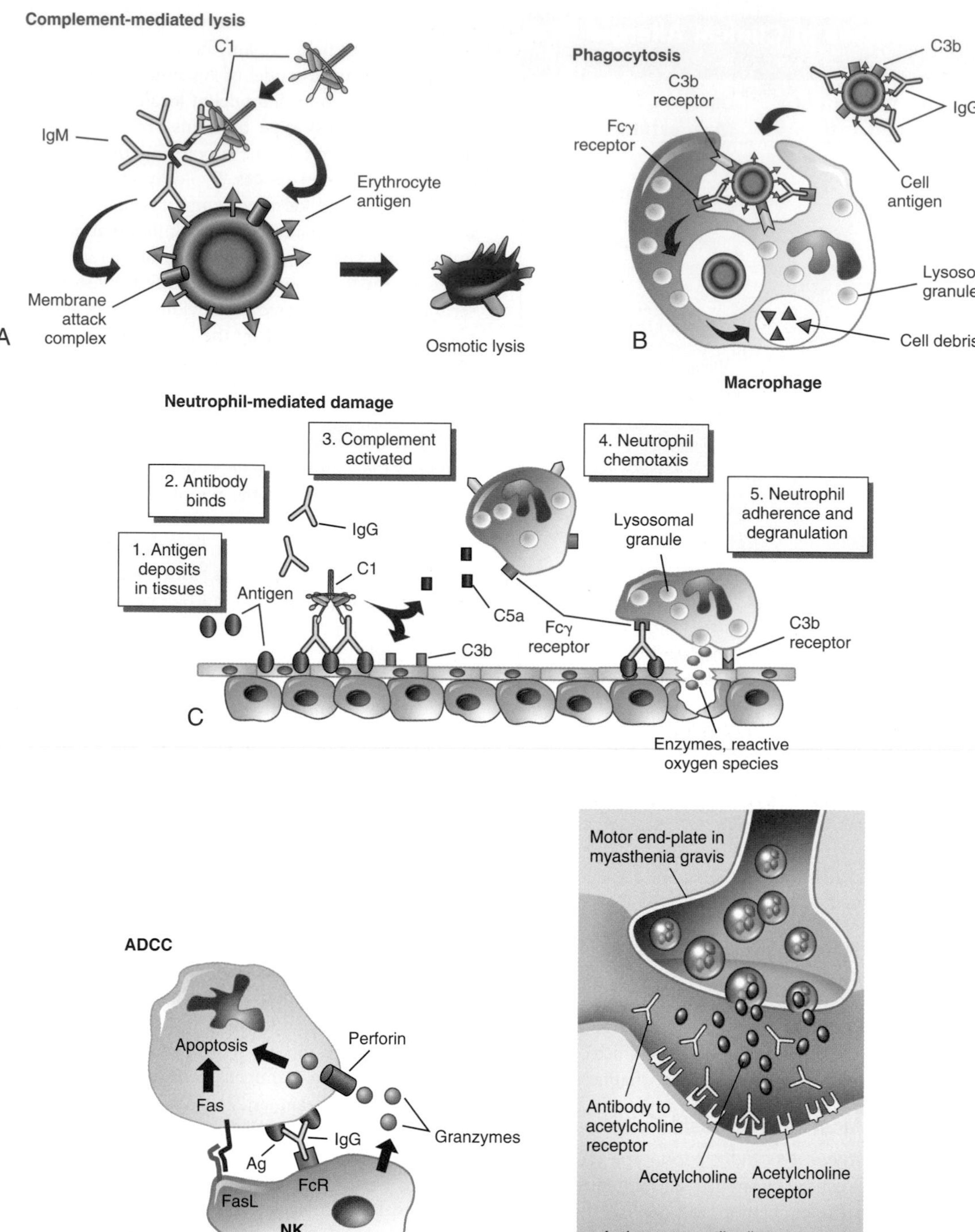

FIGURE 8-13 Mechanisms of Type II, Tissue-Specific Hypersensitivity Reactions. Antigens on the target cell bind with antibody and are destroyed or prevented from functioning by one of the following mechanisms: **(A)** complement-mediated lysis (an erythrocyte target is illustrated here); **(B)** clearance (phagocytosis) by macrophages in the tissue; **(C)** neutrophil-mediated damage; **(D)** antibody-dependent cell-mediated cytotoxicity (*ADCC*) (apoptosis of target cells is induced by natural killer [*NK*] cells by two mechanisms: by the release of granzymes and perforin, which is a molecule that creates pores in the plasma membrane, and enzymes [granzymes] that enter the target through the perforin pores; by the interactions of Fas ligand [*FasL*; a molecule similar to tumour necrosis factor-alpha] on the surface of NK cells with *Fas* [the receptor for FasL] on the surface of target cells); or **(E)** modulation or blocking of the normal function of receptors by antireceptor antibody. This example of mechanism **(E)** depicts myasthenia gravis in which acetylcholine receptor antibodies block acetylcholine from attaching to its receptors on the motor end-plates of skeletal muscle, thereby impairing neuromuscular transmission and causing muscle weakness. *Ag*, antigen; *C1*, complement component C1; *C3b*, complement fragment produced from C3, which acts as an opsonin; *C5a*, complement fragment produced from C5, which acts as a chemotactic factor for neutrophils; *Fcγ receptor*, cellular receptor for the crystallizable fragment (Fc) portion of IgG; *FcR*, Fc receptor.

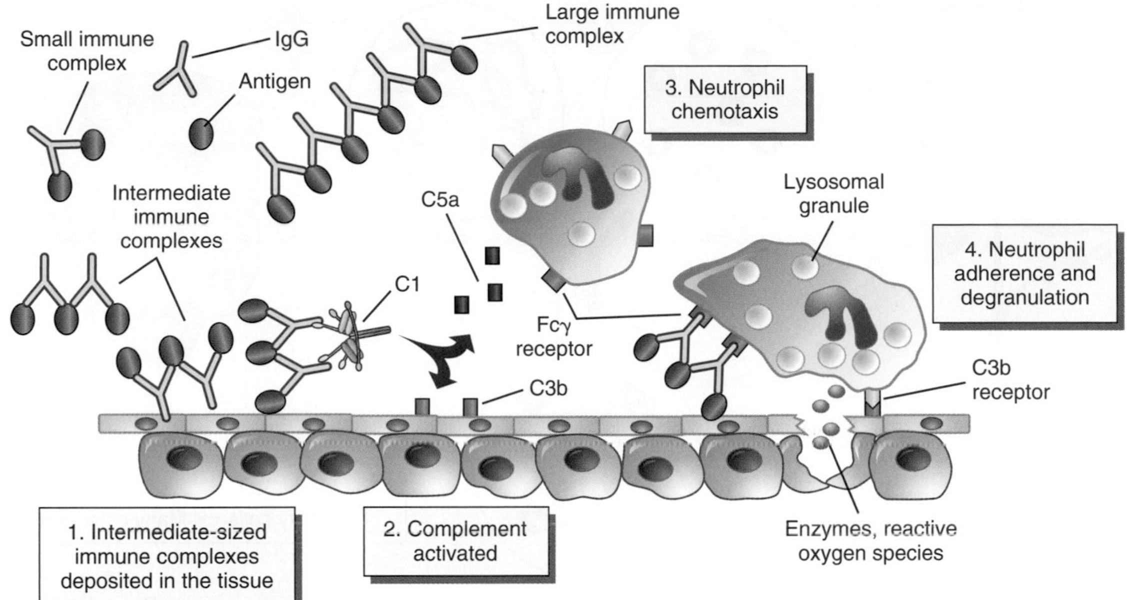

FIGURE 8-14 Mechanisms of Type III, Immune Complex–Mediated Hypersensitivity Reactions. Immune complexes form in the blood from circulating antigen and antibody. Both small and large immune complexes are removed successfully from the circulation and do not cause tissue damage. Intermediate-sized complexes are deposited in certain target tissues in which the circulation is slow or filtration of the blood occurs. The complexes activate the complement cascade through C1 and generate fragments including C5a and C3b. C5a is chemotactic for neutrophils, which migrate into the inflamed area and attach to the IgG and C3b in the immune complexes. The neutrophils attempt unsuccessfully to phagocytose the tissue and in the process release a variety of degradative enzymes that destroy the healthy tissues. *C1*, complement component C1; *C3b*, complement fragment produced from C3, which acts as an opsonin; *C5a*, complement fragment produced from C5, which acts as a chemotactic factor for neutrophils; *Fcγ receptor*, cellular receptor for the crystallizable fragment (Fc) portion of IgG.

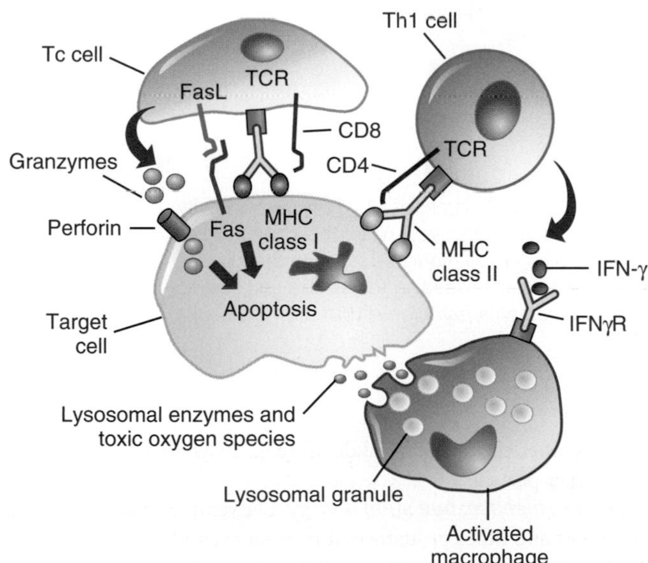

FIGURE 8-15 Mechanisms of Type IV, Cell-Mediated Hypersensitivity Reactions. Antigens from target cells stimulate T cells to differentiate into T-cytotoxic cells (*Tc cells*), which have direct cytotoxic activity, and T-helper cells (*Th1 cells*) involved in delayed hypersensitivity. The Th1 cells produce lymphokines (especially interferon-γ [*IFN-γ*]) that activate the macrophage through specific receptors (e.g., IFN-γ receptor [*IFNγR*]). The macrophages can attach to targets and release enzymes and reactive oxygen species that are responsible for most of the tissue destruction. *FasL*, a molecule similar to tumour necrosis factor-alpha; *MHC*, major histocompatibility complex; *TCR*, T cell antigen receptor.

cell that normally produces insulin) are responsible for beta-cell destruction in insulin-dependent (type 1) diabetes mellitus.

In 1891 Paul Ehrlich was the first to thoroughly describe a type IV hypersensitivity reaction in the skin, leading to the development of a diagnostic skin test for TB. The reaction follows an intradermal injection of tuberculin antigen into a suitably sensitized individual and is called a **delayed hypersensitivity skin test** because of its slow onset—24 to 72 hours to reach maximal intensity. The reaction site is infiltrated with T cells and macrophages, resulting in a clear hard centre **(induration)** and a reddish surrounding area **(erythema)**.

Allergic type IV reactions are elicited by some environmental antigens that are haptens (Chapter 7) and become immunogenic after binding to larger (carrier) proteins in the individual. In allergic **contact dermatitis**, the carrier protein is in the skin. The best-known example is poison ivy (Figure 8-16). The antigen is a plant catechol, urushiol, which reacts with normal skin proteins and evokes a cell-mediated immune response. Skin reactions to industrial chemicals, cosmetics, detergents, clothing, food, metals, and topical medicines (such as penicillin) are elicited by the same mechanism. Contact dermatitis consists of lesions only at the site of contact with the allergen, such as a metal allergy to jewelry.

QUICK CHECK 8-3

1. Distinguish among the four types of hypersensitivity mechanisms.
2. What is the mechanism of anaphylaxis?
3. What are some clinical examples of type IV hypersensitivity?

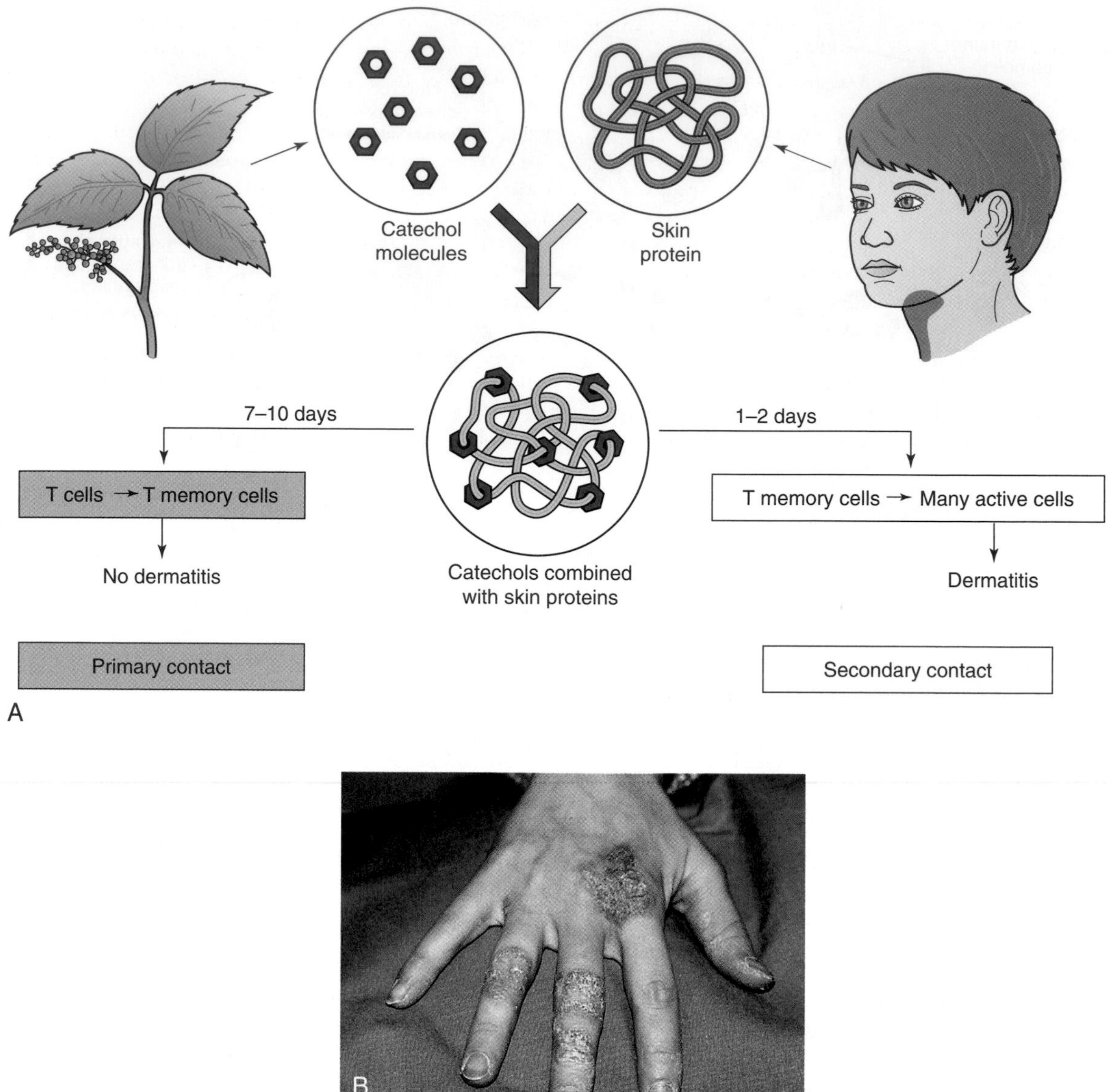

FIGURE 8-16 Development of Allergic Contact Dermatitis. A, The development of type IV hypersensitivity to poison ivy. The first (primary) contact with allergen sensitizes (produces reactive T cells) the individual but does not produce a rash (dermatitis). Secondary contact activates a type IV cell-mediated reaction that causes dermatitis. **B,** Contact dermatitis caused by a delayed hypersensitivity reaction leading to vesicles and scaling at the sites of contact. (From Damjanov, I., & Linder, J. [1996]. *Anderson's pathology* [10th ed.]. St. Louis: Mosby.)

Antigenic Targets of Hypersensitivity Reactions

Allergy

Allergens. Allergies are the most common hypersensitivity reactions. The majority of allergies are type I reactions that lead to annoying symptoms, including rhinitis, sneezing, and other relatively mild reactions. In some individuals, however, these reactions can be excessive and life-threatening (anaphylaxis). Antigens that cause allergic responses are called **allergens**. It is not known why some antigens are allergens and others are not. Typical allergens include pollens (e.g., ragweed), moulds and fungi (e.g., *Penicillium chrysogenum*), foods (e.g., milk, eggs, fish), animals (e.g., cat dander, dog dander), cigarette smoke, and components of house dust (e.g., fecal pellets of house mites). Often the allergen is contained within a particle that is too large to be phagocytosed or is surrounded by a protective nonallergenic coat. The actual allergen is released after enzymatic breakdown (e.g., by lysozyme in secretions) of the larger particle.

Allergic disease: bee sting allergy. Bee venoms contain a mixture of enzymes and other proteins that may serve as allergens and cause a type I hypersensitivity reaction. About 1% of children may have an anaphylactic reaction to bee venom.[61] Within minutes they may develop excessive swelling (edema) at the bee sting site, followed by generalized hives, pruritus, and swelling in areas distal from the sting (e.g., eyes, lips), and other systemic symptoms including flushing, sweating, dizziness, and headache. The most severe symptoms may include gastro-intestinal (e.g., stomach cramps, vomiting), respiratory (e.g., tightness in the throat, wheezing, difficulty breathing), and vascular (e.g., low blood pressure, shock) reactions. Severe respiratory tract and vascular reactions may lead to death.

For an individual with known bee sting hypersensitivity, lifestyle changes include avoidance of stinging or biting insects. If a child has experienced a previous anaphylactic reaction, the chance of having another is about 60%. The primary life-threatening symptoms result from contraction of respiratory tract smooth muscle. Autonomic nervous system mediators, such as epinephrine, bind to specific receptors on smooth muscle and reverse the effects of histamine, resulting in muscle relaxation. Thus most individuals with bee sting allergies carry self-injectable epinephrine. The administration of antihistamines has little effect because histamine has already bound H1 receptors and initiated severe bronchial smooth muscle contraction.

Clinical **desensitization** to allergens can be achieved in some individuals. Minute quantities of the allergen are injected in increasing doses over a prolonged period. The procedure may reduce the severity of the allergic reaction in the treated individual. However, this form of therapy may trigger systemic anaphylaxis, which can be severe and life-threatening. This approach works best for routine respiratory tract allergens and biting insect allergies (80 to 90% rate of desensitization over 5 years of treatment).[62] Food allergies have been very difficult to suppress, but some promising trials are under way to evaluate desensitization by oral or sublingual administration of increasing amounts of allergen.

Autoimmunity

Autoimmune diseases originate from an initiating event in a genetically predisposed individual. Current models of factors related to autoimmune diseases include genetic factors, environmental factors, and random or stochastic changes.[63] Some autoimmune diseases can be familial and attributed to the presence of a very small number of susceptibility genes; affected family members may not all develop the same disease, but have different disorders characterized by a variety of hypersensitivity reactions, including autoimmune and allergic. For example, the HLA antigen B27 is a risk factor for developing **ankylosing spondylitis (AS)**, an autoimmune inflammatory disease of the spine; 95% of individuals diagnosed with AS express HLA-B27, whereas only 4 to 8% of the general population expresses this antigen.[64] (HLA is discussed further under "Alloimmune Disease: Transplant Rejection," p. 211.) Although most autoimmune diseases appear as isolated events without a positive family history, susceptibility for developing such diseases appears to be linked to a combination of multiple genes.

Breakdown of tolerance. An individual is usually tolerant to his or her own antigens. **Tolerance** is a state of immunological control so that the individual does not make a detrimental immune response against his or her own cells and tissues. Autoimmune disease results from a breakdown of this tolerance.

The initiating event that breaks tolerance is unclear for most autoimmune diseases. It is also unclear as to the bodily site initially involved to cause autoimmunity.[63] Potential infectious initiators of autoimmune disease are being investigated,[65] but only one example is known: acute rheumatic fever. In a small number of individuals with group A streptococcal sore throats, the M proteins in the bacterial capsule mimic (*antigenic mimicry*) normal heart antigens and induce antibodies that also react with proteins in the heart valve, damaging the valve.[66] Thus acute rheumatic fever is a type II autoimmune hypersensitivity. Additionally, some streptococcal skin or throat infections release bacterial antigens into the blood that form circulating immune complexes. The complexes may deposit in the kidneys and initiate an immune complex–mediated glomerulonephritis (inflammation of the kidney).[67] Thus streptococcal antigens (an environmental antigen) may also cause a type III allergic hypersensitivity (poststreptococcal glomerulonephritis).

Autoimmune disease: systemic lupus erythematosus. **Systemic lupus erythematosus (SLE)** is the most common, complex, and serious of the autoimmune disorders. SLE is characterized by the production of a large variety of antibodies (autoantibodies) against self-antigens, including nucleic acids, erythrocytes, coagulation proteins, phospholipids, lymphocytes, platelets, and many other self-components. The most characteristic autoantibodies are against nucleic acids (e.g., ssDNA, dsDNA), histones, ribonucleoproteins, and other nuclear materials. Approximately 98% of persons with SLE have detectable antibodies against nuclear antigens. The blood normally contains many of these products of cellular turnover and breakdown so that autoantibodies react with the circulating antigen and form circulating immune complexes. The deposition of circulating DNA/anti-DNA complexes in the kidneys can cause severe kidney inflammation. Similar reactions can occur in the brain, heart, spleen, lung, gastro-intestinal tract, peritoneum, and skin. Thus some of the symptoms of SLE result from a type III hypersensitivity reaction. Other symptoms, such as destruction of red blood cells (anemia), lymphocytes (lymphopenia), and other cells, may be type II hypersensitivity reactions.

SLE, like most autoimmune diseases, occurs more often in women (approximately a 9 : 1 predominance of females), especially in the 20- to 40-year-old age group.[68] Blacks are affected more often than Whites (about an eightfold increased risk). A genetic predisposition for the disease has been implicated on the basis of increased incidence in twins and the existence of autoimmune disease in the families of individuals with SLE.

As with many autoimmune diseases, clinical manifestations of SLE may wax and wane; the individual may go through periods of remission and be relatively disease free until the onset of a *flare* (exacerbated disease activity). Symptoms include arthralgias or arthritis (90% of individuals), vasculitis and rash (70 to 80% of individuals), renal disease (40 to 50% of individuals), hematological abnormalities (50% of individuals, with anemia being the most common complication), and cardiovascular diseases (30 to 50% of individuals) (see "Discoid (Cutaneous) Lupus Erythematosus" in Chapter 41). Because the signs and symptoms affect almost every body system and tend to vacillate, SLE is extremely difficult to diagnose. As a result, a list of 11 common clinical findings,[69] which has been modified slightly to increase sensitivity of the diagnosis,[70] has been developed. The serial or simultaneous presence of at least four of these findings indicates that the individual has SLE. The findings are as follows:

1. Facial rash confined to the cheeks (malar rash)
2. Discoid rash (raised patches, scaling)
3. Photosensitivity (development of skin rash as a result of exposure to sunlight)
4. Oral or nasopharyngeal ulcers
5. Nonerosive arthritis of at least two peripheral joints
6. Serositis (inflammation of membranes of lung [pleurisy] or heart [pericarditis])
7. Renal disorder (persistent proteinuria of greater than 0.5 g/day or greater than 3 by dipstick, or cellular casts)
8. Neurological disorders (seizures or psychosis in the absence of known causes)
9. Hematological disorders (hemolytic anemia, leukopenia, lymphopenia, or thrombocytopenia)
10. Immunological disorders (anti-dsDNA, anti–Smith [Sm] antigen, false-positive serological test for syphilis, or antiphospholipid antibodies [anticardiolipin antibody or lupus anticoagulant])
11. Presence of antinuclear antibody (ANA)

Laboratory diagnosis is usually based on a positive ANA screening test; about 98% of individuals with SLE are positive, but a substantial number of false-positives occur in healthy individuals and those with other diseases. Because SLE is a progressive and slowly developing disease, some laboratory tests, including the ANA, may be positive years before the onset of clinical symptoms.[65] Detection of a positive ANA is usually followed by one or more specific tests (e.g., antibodies against Sm, dsDNA) that are complicated by low sensitivity (only a portion of individuals with SLE will be positive, although the number of false-positives is low).

There is no cure for SLE or most other autoimmune diseases. Fatalities resulting from SLE are usually related to infection, organ failure, or cardiovascular disease. The goals of treatment are to control symptoms and prevent further damage by suppressing the autoimmune response. Nonsteroidal anti-inflammatory drugs, such as acetylsalicylic acid (Aspirin), ibuprofen (Advil), or naproxen (Apo-Naproxren), reduce inflammation and relieve pain. Corticosteroids are often prescribed for more serious active disease. Immunosuppressive medications (e.g., methotrexate [Apo-Methotrexate], azathioprine [Nu-azathioprine], or cyclophosphamide [Procytox]) are used to treat severe symptoms involving internal organs. Antimalarial medications (e.g., hydroxychloroquine [Plaquenil]) are preferred treatments for individuals with stable disease.[65] Ultraviolet light may initiate flares, and protection from sun exposure is helpful. Prolonged use of certain medications can cause transient SLE-like symptoms, and the medication history is important for differential diagnosis.

Alloimmunity

Alloantigens. Genetic diversity is the norm in humans. Diversity also is observed among self-antigens, so that two individuals may have different antigens on their tissues and, therefore, make an immune response against each other's tissues. Some self-antigens, such as the ABO blood group, have limited diversity with very few different antigens being expressed in the population, whereas others, such as the HLA system, have tremendous diversity.

Alloimmune disease: transfusion reactions. Red blood cells (erythrocytes) express several important surface antigens, which are known collectively as the **blood group antigens** and can be targets of alloimmune reactions. More than 80 different red cell antigens are grouped into several dozen blood group systems. The most important of these, because they provoke the strongest humoral alloimmune response, are the ABO and Rh systems.

The **ABO blood group** consists of two major carbohydrate antigens, labelled A and B (Figure 8-17), that are expressed on virtually all cells. These are codominant, so both A and B can be simultaneously expressed, resulting in an individual having any one of four different blood types. The erythrocytes of blood type A express the type A carbohydrate antigen, those with blood type B express the B antigen, those with blood type AB express both A and B antigens on the same cell, and those of blood type O express neither the A nor the B antigen. A person with type A blood also has circulating antibodies to the B carbohydrate antigen. If this person receives blood from a type AB or B individual, a severe transfusion reaction occurs, and the transfused erythrocytes are destroyed by agglutination or complement-mediated lysis. Similarly, a type B individual (whose blood contains anti-A antibodies) cannot receive blood from a type A or AB donor. Type O individuals, who have neither antigen but have both anti-A and anti-B antibodies, cannot accept blood from any of the other three types. These naturally occurring antibodies, called **isohemagglutinins**, are IgM immunoglobulins and are induced early in life against similar antigens expressed on naturally occurring bacteria in the intestinal tract.

Because individuals with type O blood lack both types of antigens, they are considered **universal donors**, meaning that anyone can accept their red blood cells. Similarly, type AB individuals are considered **universal recipients** because they lack both anti-A and anti-B antibodies

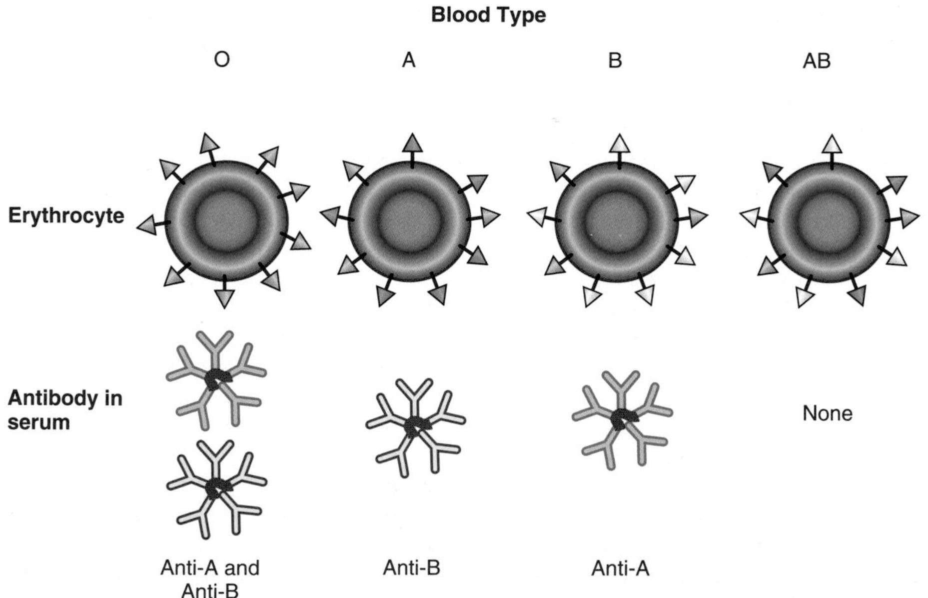

FIGURE 8-17 ABO Blood Types. This figure shows the relationship of antigens and antibodies associated with the ABO blood groups. The surfaces of erythrocytes of individuals with blood group O have a core carbohydrate that is present on cells of all ABO blood groups (H antigen). The sera of blood group O individuals contain IgM antibodies against both A and B carbohydrates. In individuals of the blood group A, some of the H antigens have been modified into A antigens. The sera of these individuals have IgM antibodies against the B antigen. In individuals with blood group B, some of the H antigens have been modified into B antigens. These individuals have IgM antibodies against the A antigen in their sera. In individuals of the blood group AB, some of the H antigens have been modified into both the A and B antigens. These individuals do not have antibodies to either A or B antigens.

and can be transfused with any ABO blood type. Harmful transfusion reactions can be prevented only by complete and careful ABO matching between donor and recipient.

The **Rh blood group** is a group of antigens expressed only on red blood cells. This blood group has the most diverse group of red cell antigens, consisting of at least 45 separate antigens, although only 1 is considered of major importance: the D antigen. Individuals who express the D antigen on their red cells are Rh-positive, whereas individuals who do not express the D antigen are Rh-negative. When discussing the gene for the Rh antigen, the letter *d* is used to indicate lack of D. Rh-positive individuals can have either a *DD* or *Dd* genotype, whereas Rh-negative individuals have the *dd* genotype. About 85% of North Americans are Rh-positive. Rh-negative individuals can make an IgG antibody to the D antigen (anti-D) if exposed to Rh-positive erythrocytes.

A disease called *hemolytic disease of the newborn* was most commonly caused by IgG anti-D alloantibody produced by Rh-negative mothers against erythrocytes of their Rh-positive fetuses (see Chapter 22). The mother's antibody crossed the placenta and destroyed the red blood cells of the fetus. The occurrence of this particular form of the disease has decreased dramatically because of the use of prophylactic anti-D immunoglobulin (i.e., WinRho). By mechanisms that are still not completely understood, administration of anti-D antibody within a few days of exposure to RhD-positive erythrocytes completely prevents sensitization against the D antigen. Because hemolytic disease of the newborn related to the D antigen has been controlled, alloantibodies against the other Rh antigens have become more important. In general, these alloantibodies are associated with a less severe hemolytic disease.

Alloimmune disease: transplant rejection. Molecules of the MHC were discussed in Chapter 7 as antigen-presenting molecules. MHC molecules are also a major target of transplant rejection. As a result of studies of transplantation, the human MHC molecules are also referred to as *human leukocyte antigens (HLAs)* and the different MHC genetic loci are commonly called *HLA-A, HLA-B, HLA-C, HLA-DR, HLA-DQ,* and *HLA-DP* (Figure 8-18). Additional genes for complement components (e.g., C4, factor B) are also contained in the MHC region and are referred to as class III loci. The class I (HLA-A, HLA-B, and HLA-C) and class II MHC loci (HLA-DR, HLA-DQ, and HLA-DP) are the most genetically diverse (polymorphic) of any human genetic loci. Within the human population, the number of possible different alleles (i.e., forms of the gene) expressed by each locus is astounding. For example, more than 300 different HLA-A molecules are expressed in the population. These numbers are based on the polymorphism of observed DNA sequences and may not reflect differences in function.

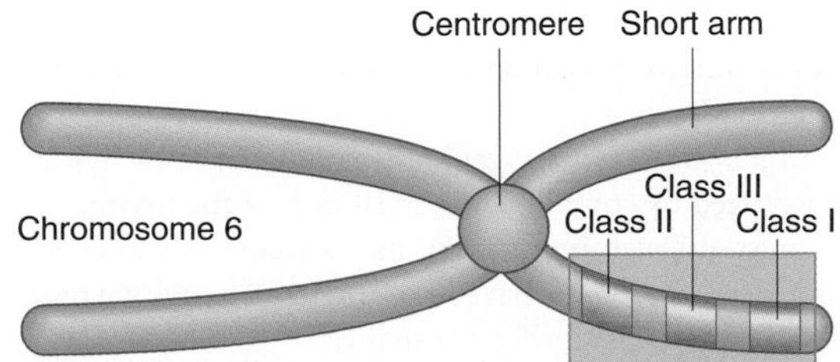

FIGURE 8-18 Human Leukocyte Antigens. The major histocompatibility complex is located on the short arm of chromosome 6 and contains genes that code for class I antigens, class II antigens, and class III proteins (i.e., complement proteins and cytokines). (From Peakman, M., & Vergani, D. [2009]. *Basic and clinical immunology* [2nd ed.]. London: Churchill Livingstone.)

Clearly, not every allele is expressed in the same individual. Humans have two copies of each MHC locus (one inherited from each parent) that are codominant so that molecules encoded by each parent's genes are expressed on the surface of every cell, except erythrocytes. Within an individual, each locus will express only one allele. For example, each person will have at most two different HLA-A proteins (one from each parent). However, with the tremendous number of possible alleles that can be expressed throughout the population, it is likely that any two unrelated individuals will have different MHC antigens.

The diversity of MHC molecules becomes clinically relevant during organ transplantation. The recipient of a transplant can mount an immune response against the foreign HLA antigens on the donor tissue, resulting in rejection. To minimize the chance of tissue rejection, the donor and recipient are often tissue-typed beforehand to identify differences in HLA antigens. Because of the large number of different alleles, it is highly unlikely that a perfect match can be found between someone who needs a transplant and a potential donor from the general population. The more similar two individuals are in their HLA tissue type, the more likely a transplant from one to the other will be successful. Clearly, the most successful transplants would be between identical twins because they are identical genetically.

The specific combination of alleles at the six major HLA loci on one chromosome (A, B, C, DR, DQ, and DP) is termed a *haplotype*. Each individual has two HLA haplotypes, one from the paternal chromosome 6 and another from the maternal chromosome (Figure 8-19). Each parent passes on one set of HLA antigens to each of his or her offspring, meaning that children usually share half their HLA antigens with each parent. Odds dictate that children will share one haplotype with half their siblings and either no haplotypes or both haplotypes with a quarter of their siblings. Thus the chance of finding a match among siblings is much higher (25%) than the general population.

Transplant rejection may be classified as hyperacute, acute, or chronic, depending on the amount of time that elapses between transplantation and rejection. **Hyperacute rejection** is immediate and rare. When the circulation is re-established to the grafted area, the graft may immediately turn white (the so-called white graft) instead of a normal pink colour. Hyperacute rejection usually occurs because of pre-existing antibody (type II reaction) to HLA antigens on the vascular endothelial cells in the grafted tissue.

Acute rejection is a cell-mediated immune response that occurs within days to months after transplantation. This type of rejection occurs when the recipient develops an immune response against unmatched HLA antigens after transplantation. A biopsy of the rejected organ usually shows an infiltration of lymphocytes and macrophages characteristic of a type IV reaction.

Chronic rejection may occur after a period of months or years of normal function. It is characterized by slow, progressive organ failure. Chronic rejection usually results from a weak cell-mediated (type IV) reaction against minor histocompatibility antigens on the grafted tissue. However, antibodies against HLA and other antigens also may cause chronic rejection through activation of complement or ADCC with NK cells.

QUICK CHECK 8-4

1. Why do certain medications become immunogenic to the host?
2. Why is systemic lupus erythematosus considered an autoimmune disease?
3. Define the different types of graft rejection.

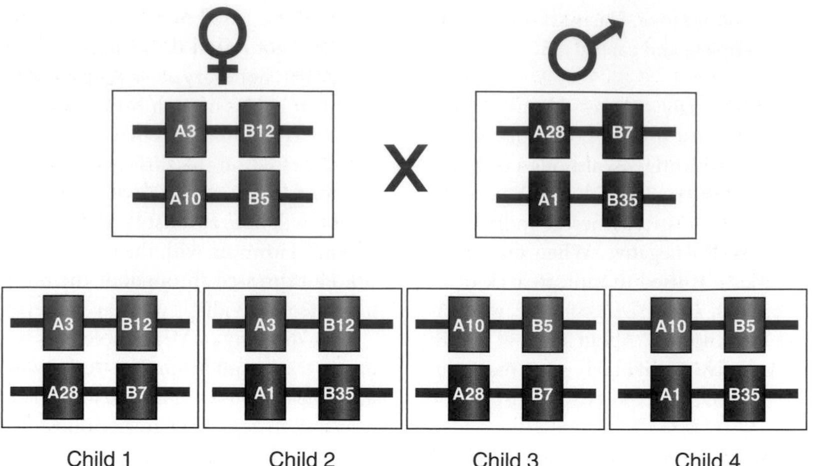

FIGURE 8-19 Inheritance of Human Leukocyte Antigens. Human leukocyte antigen (HLA) alleles are inherited in a codominant fashion; both maternal and paternal antigens are expressed. Specific HLA alleles are commonly given numbers to indicate different antigens. In this example, the mother has linked genes for HLA-A3 and HLA-B12 on one chromosome 6 and genes for HLA-A10 and HLA-B5 on the second chromosome 6. The father has HLA-A28 and HLA-B7 on one chromosome and HLA-A1 and HLA-B35 on the second chromosome. The children from this pairing may have one of four possible combinations of maternal and paternal HLA.

DID YOU UNDERSTAND?

Infection

1. Infectious disease is a significant cause of morbidity and mortality worldwide.
2. Pathogens have unique characteristics that influence their ability to cause disease.
3. Bacteria injure cells by producing exotoxins or endotoxins. Exotoxins are enzymes that can damage the plasma membranes of host cells or can inactivate enzymes critical to protein synthesis, and endotoxins activate the inflammatory response and produce fever.
4. Septicemia is the proliferation of bacteria in the blood. Endotoxins released by bloodborne bacteria cause the release of vasoactive enzymes that increase the permeability of blood vessels. Leakage from vessels causes hypotension that can result in endotoxic shock.
5. Viruses enter host cells and use the metabolic processes of host cells to proliferate and cause disease.
6. Viruses that have invaded host cells may decrease protein synthesis, disrupt lysosomal membranes, form inclusion bodies where synthesis of viral nucleic acids is occurring, fuse with host cells to produce giant cells, alter antigenic properties of the host cell, transform host cells into cancerous cells, and promote bacterial infection.
7. Diseases caused by fungi are called *mycoses*, and they occur in two forms: yeasts (spheres) and multicellular moulds (filaments or hyphae).
8. Dermatophytes are fungi that infect skin, hair, and nails with diseases such as ringworm and athlete's foot.
9. Fungi release toxins and enzymes that are damaging to tissue. *Candida albicans* is the most common cause of fungal infections in humans.
10. Parasitic microorganisms range from unicellular protozoa to large worms. Although less common in Canada and the United States, parasites and protozoa are common causes of infection worldwide.
11. Parasitic and protozoal infections are rarely transmitted from human to human. Infection mainly spreads through vectors (e.g., by mosquito bites) or through contaminated water or food (i.e., malaria, Chagas disease, sleeping sickness, and leishmaniasis).
12. Infection control measures include implementation of clean food and water, management of sewage and waste, control of insects that transmit disease, vaccination, appropriate use of antimicrobials, and passive immunotherapy.

Deficiencies in Immunity

1. An immune deficiency is the failure of mechanisms of self-defence to function in their normal capacity.
2. Immunodeficiencies are either congenital (primary) or acquired (secondary). Congenital immunodeficiencies are caused by genetic defects that disrupt lymphocyte development, whereas acquired immunodeficiencies are secondary to disease or other physiological alterations.
3. The clinical hallmark of immunodeficiency is a propensity to unusual or recurrent severe infections. The type of infection usually reflects the immune system defect.
4. The most common infections in individuals with defects of cell-mediated immune response are fungal and viral, whereas infections in individuals with defects of the humoral immune response or complement function are primarily bacterial.
5. Severe combined immunodeficiency (SCID) is a total lack of T-cell function and a severe (either partial or total) lack of B-cell function.
6. Wiskott-Aldrich syndrome is caused by decreased production of IgM antibody.
7. DiGeorge syndrome (congenital thymic aplasia or hypoplasia) is characterized by complete or partial lack of the thymus (resulting in depressed T-cell immunity) and is frequently associated with diminished or absent parathyroid gland activity (resulting in hypocalcemia) and cardiac anomalies.
8. Antibody deficiencies result from defects in B-cell maturation or function, the lymphoid organs required for B-cell maturation (as in Bruton agammaglobulinemia), to deficiencies in a single class of immunoglobulins (e.g., selective IgA deficiency).
9. Phagocyte defects include inadequate numbers or alteration in function, such as inadequate adhesion to bacteria or ineffective killing.

10. Complement and mannose-binding lectin deficiencies also are rare causes of increased risk for infection.
11. Acquired immunodeficiencies are caused by superimposed conditions, such as malnutrition, medical therapies, physical trauma, psychological stress, or infections.
12. Immunodeficiency syndromes usually are treated by replacement therapy. Deficient antibody production is treated by replacement of missing immunoglobulins with commercial gamma-globulin preparations. Lymphocyte deficiencies are treated by the replacement of host lymphocytes with transplants of bone marrow, fetal liver, or fetal thymus from a donor. Gene therapy trials are ongoing.
13. AIDS is an acquired dysfunction of the immune system caused by a retrovirus (HIV) that infects and destroys $CD4^+$ Th cells.

Hypersensitivity: Allergy, Autoimmunity, and Alloimmunity

1. Hypersensitivity is an immune response misdirected against the host's own tissues (autoimmunity) or directed against beneficial foreign tissues, such as transfusions or transplants (alloimmunity); or it can be exaggerated responses against environmental antigens (allergy).
2. Mechanisms of hypersensitivity are classified as type I (IgE-mediated reactions), type II (tissue-specific reactions), type III (immune complex–mediated reactions), and type IV (cell-mediated reactions).
3. Hypersensitivity reactions can be immediate (developing within seconds or hours) or delayed (developing within hours or days).
4. Anaphylaxis, the most rapid immediate hypersensitivity reaction, is an explosive reaction that occurs within minutes of re-exposure to the antigen and can lead to shock and death.
5. Type I (IgE-mediated) hypersensitivity reactions occur after antigen reacts with IgE on tissue mast cells, leading to mast cell degranulation and the release of histamine and other inflammatory substances.
6. Type II (tissue-specific) hypersensitivity reactions are caused by five possible mechanisms: complement-mediated lysis, phagocytosis by macrophages, neutrophil-mediated damage, antibody-dependent cell-mediated cytotoxicity, and modulation of cellular function.
7. Type III (immune complex–mediated) hypersensitivity reactions are caused by the formation of immune complexes that are deposited in target tissues, where they activate the complement cascade, generating chemotactic fragments that attract neutrophils into the inflammatory site.
8. Immune complex disease can be a systemic reaction, such as serum sickness (e.g., Raynaud phenomenon), or localized, such as the Arthus reaction.
9. Type IV (cell-mediated) hypersensitivity reactions are caused by specifically sensitized lymphocytes, which either kill target cells directly or release lymphokines that activate other cells, such as macrophages.
10. Allergens are antigens that cause allergic responses, usually a type I hypersensitivity response.
11. Autoimmune disease is loss of tolerance to self-antigens. There can be a genetic predisposition, and the diseases can be a type II or type III hypersensitivity reaction.
12. Alloimmunity is the immune system's reaction against antigens on the tissues of other members of the same species.
13. Alloimmune disorders include hemolytic disease of the newborn, in which the maternal immune system becomes sensitized against antigens expressed by the fetus; and transplant rejection and transfusion reactions, in which the immune system of the recipient of an organ transplant or blood transfusion reacts against foreign antigens on the donor's cells.

KEY TERMS

ABO blood group, 210
Acquired immunodeficiency syndrome (AIDS), 195
Acute rejection, 211
Adenosine deaminase deficiency (ADA deficiency), 191
Agammaglobulinemia, 192
Allergen, 208
Allergy, 199
Alloimmune disease, 201
Alloimmunity, 201
Anaphylaxis, 202
Ankylosing spondylitis (AS), 209
Antibiotic resistance, 183
Antibody-dependent cell-mediated cytotoxicity (ADCC), 204
Antigenic drift, 185
Antigenic shift, 185
Antigenic variation, 185
Antiretroviral therapy (ART), 197
Antitoxin, 182
Arthus reaction, 205
Atopic, 203
Attenuated virus, 189
Autoimmune disease, 201
Autoimmunity, 201
Bacteremia, 183
Bare lymphocyte syndrome, 191
β-Lactamase, 183
Biofilms, 179
Blood group antigen, 210
Bruton agammaglobulinemia, 192
C3 deficiency, 193
CCR5 antagonist, 197
Chronic granulomatous disease (CGD), 193
Chronic mucocutaneous candidiasis, 193
Chronic rejection, 211
Combined deficiencies, 191
Communicability, 178
Complement deficiency, 193
Contact dermatitis, 207
Cryoglobulins, 205
Defects in innate immunity, 191
Delayed hypersensitivity reaction, 202
Delayed hypersensitivity skin test, 207
Dermatophyte, 186
Desensitization, 209
DiGeorge syndrome, 191
Dimorphic fungus (*pl.*, fungi), 186
Endotoxic shock, 183
Endotoxin (lipopolysaccharide [LPS]), 183
Erythema, 207
Exotoxin, 183
Graft-versus-host disease (GVHD), 195
Herd immunity, 190
HIV fusion inhibitor, 196
HIV integrase, 195
HIV integrase inhibitor, 196
HIV protease, 195
HIV protease inhibitor, 196
Human immunodeficiency virus (HIV), 195
Human leukocyte antigen (HLA), 195
Hyperacute rejection, 211
Hypersensitivity, 199
Hypogammaglobulinemia, 192
Immediate hypersensitivity reaction, 202
Immune deficiency, 190
Immunogenicity, 190
Induration, 207
Infectious diseases, 177
Infectivity, 178
Influenza, 183
Isohemagglutinin, 210
Major histocompatibility complex (MHC), 191
Mannose-binding lectin (MBL) deficiency, 193
Mesenchymal stem cell (MSC), 195
Methicillin-resistant *Staphylococcus aureus* (MRSA), 183
Multiple-antibiotic resistance, 189
Mycosis (*pl.*, mycoses), 186
Parasitic microorganisms, 187
Passive immunotherapy, 190
Pathogenicity, 178
Phagocytic defects, 193
Portal of entry, 178
Predominantly antibody deficiency, 192
Primary (congenital) immune deficiency, 190
Raynaud phenomenon, 205

Reverse transcriptase, 195
Reverse transcriptase inhibitor, 196
Rh blood group, 211
Secondary (acquired) immune deficiency, 190
Selective IgA deficiency, 192
Sepsis, 183
Septicemia, 183
Serum sickness, 205
Severe combined immunodeficiency (SCID), 191
Severe congenital neutropenia, 193
Systemic lupus erythematosus (SLE), 209
Tissue-specific antigen, 203
Tolerance, 209
Toxigenicity, 178
Toxoid, 190
Tropism, 183
Type I hypersensitivity, 202
Type II hypersensitivity, 203
Type III hypersensitivity, 205
Type IV hypersensitivity, 205
Universal donor, 210
Universal recipient, 210
Urticaria (hives), 202
Vaccination, 189
Vaccine, 189
Virulence, 178
Wheal and flare reaction, 202
Wiskott-Aldrich syndrome (WAS), 191
X-linked SCID, 191
Zoonotic infection, 183

REFERENCES

1. Canadian Cancer Society, & Government of Canada. (2015). *Canadian cancer statistics, 2015*. Toronto: Author. Retrieved from https://www.cancer.ca/~/media/cancer.ca/CW/cancer%20information/cancer%20101/Canadian%20cancer%20statistics/Canadian-Cancer-Statistics-2015-EN.pdf.
2. Musau, J., Baumann, A., Kolotylo, C., et al. (2015). Infectious disease outbreaks and increased complexity of care. *International Nursing Review, 62*(3), 404–411. doi:10.1111/inr.12188.
3. Murthy, S., Keystone, J., & Kissoon, N. (2013). Infections of the developing world. *Critical Care Clinics, 29*(3), 485–507. doi:10.1016/j.ccc.2013.03.005.
4. Health Canada. (2016). *First Nations and Inuit health: Disease and health conditions*. Ottawa: Author. Retrieved from http://www.hc-sc.gc.ca/fniah-spnia/diseases-maladies/index-eng.php.
5. Brown, A. F., Leech, J. M., Rogers, T. R., et al. (2014). *Staphylococcus aureus* colonization: Modulation of host immune response and impact on human vaccine design. *Frontiers in Immunology, 4*, 507. doi:10.3389/fimmu.2013.00507.
6. Scherr, T. D., Heim, C. E., Morrison, J. M., et al. (2014). Hiding in plain sight: Interplay between staphylococcal biofilms and host immunity. *Frontiers in Immunology, 5*, 37. doi:10.3389/fimmu.2014.00037.
7. Foster, T. J., Geoghegan, J. A., Ganesh, V. K., et al. (2014). Adhesion, invasion and evasion: The many functions of the surface proteins of *Staphylococcus aureus*. *Nature Reviews. Microbiology, 12*(1), 49–62. doi:10.1038/nrmicro3161.
8. Zecconi, A., & Scali, F. (2013). *Staphylococcus aureus* virulence factors in evasion from innate immune defenses in human and animal diseases. *Immunology Letters, 150*, 12–22. doi:10.1016/j.imlet.2013.01.00.
9. Monack, D. M., & Hultgren, S. J. (2013). The complex interactions of bacterial pathogens and host defenses. *Current Opinion in Microbiology, 16*(1), 1–3. doi:10.1016/j.mib.2013.03.001.
10. Baxt, L. A., Garza-Mayers, A. C., & Goldberg, M. B. (2013). Bacterial subversion of host innate immune pathways. *Science, 340*(6133), 697–701. doi:10.1126/science.1235771.
11. Alonzo, F., 3rd, & Torres, V. J. (2014). The bicomponent pore-forming leucocidins of *Staphylococcus aureus*. *Microbiology and Molecular Biology Reviews : MMBR, 78*(2), 199–230. doi:10.1128/MMBR.00055-13.
12. Scully, I. L., Liberator, P. A., Jansen, K. U., et al. (2014). Covering all the bases: Preclinical development of an effective *Staphylococcus aureus* vaccine. *Frontiers in Immunology, 5*, 109. doi:10.3389/fimmu.2014.00109.
13. Huet, O., & Chin-Dusting, J. P. F. (2014). Septic shock: Desperately seeking treatment. *Clinical Science, 126*(1), 31–39. doi:10.1042/CS20120668.
14. Hotchkiss, R. S., Monneret, G., & Payen, D. (2013). Sepsis-induced immunosuppression: From cellular dysfunctions to immunotherapy. *Nature Reviews. Immunology, 13*(12), 862–874. doi:10.1038/nri3552.
15. Bean, A. G., Baker, M. L., Stewart, C. R., et al. (2013). Studying immunity to zoonotic diseases in the natural host—Keeping it real. *Nature Reviews. Immunology, 13*(12), 851–861. doi:10.1038/nri3551.
16. Ramsey, C. D., & Kumar, A. (2013). Influenza and endemic viral pneumonia. *Critical Care Clinics, 29*, 1069–1086. doi:10.1016/j.ccc.2013.06.003.
17. Sun, X., & Whittaker, G. R. (2013). Entry of influenza virus. *Advances in Experimental Medicine and Biology, 790*, 72–82. doi:10.1007/978-1-4614-7651-1_4.
18. Schrauwen, E. J. A., de Graaf, M., Herfst, S., et al. (2014). Determinants of virulence of influenza A virus. *European Journal of Clinical Microbiology & Infectious Diseases, 33*(4), 479–490. doi:10.1007/s10096-013-1984-8.
19. World Health Organization. (2015). *Malaria fact sheet no 94*. Retrieved from http://www.who.int/mediacentre/factsheets/fs094/en/.
20. Centers for Disease Control and Prevention. (2013). *Antibiotic resistance threats in the United States, 2013*. Retrieved from http://www.cdc.gov/drugresistance/threat-report-2013/pdf/ar-threats-2013-508.pdf.
21. Public Health Agency of Canada. (2013). *The Chief Public Health Officer's report on the state of public health in Canada, 2013: Infectious disease—The never-ending threat*. Ottawa: Author. Retrieved from http://www.phac-aspc.gc.ca/cphorsphc-respcacsp/2013/assets/pdf/2013-eng.pdf.
22. Rubinstein, E., & Keynan, Y. (2013). Vancomycin-resistant enterococci. *Critical Care Clinics, 29*, 841–852. doi:10.1016/j.ccc.2013.06.006.
23. Kennedy, D. (2013). Time to deal with antibiotics. *Science, 342*(6160), 776–777.
24. Rappuoli, R., Pizza, M., Del Giudice, G., et al. (2014). Vaccines, new opportunities for a new society. *Proceedings of the National Academy of Sciences of the United States of America, 111*(34), 12288–12293. doi:10.1073/pnas.1402981111.
25. Hampton, L. M., Farrell, M., Ramirez-Gonzalez, A., et al. (2016). Cessation of use of trivalent oral polio vaccine and introduction of inactivated poliovirus vaccine worldwide, 2016. *Weekly Epidemiological Record, 36*(37), 421–427. Retrieved from http://apps.who.int/iris/bitstream/10665/254485/1/WER9136_37_421-427.pdf.
26. Iorfida, C. (2015, July 21). *Measles vaccinations of toddlers at 89%, below "herd immunity level*. CBC News. Retrieved from http://www.cbc.ca/news/health/measles-vaccinations-of-toddlers-at-89-below-herd-immunity-level-1.3161617.
27. Larson, H. J., Smith, D. M., Paterson, P., et al. (2013). Measuring vaccine confidence: Analysis of data obtained by a media surveillance system used to analyse public concerns about vaccines. *Lancet Infectious Diseases, 13*(7), 606–613. doi:10.1016/S1473-3099(13)70108-7.
28. Smith, J. C., Appleton, M., & MacDonald, N. E. (2013). Building confidence in vaccines. *Advances in Experimental Medicine and Biology, 764*, 81–98.
29. Centers for Disease Control and Prevention. (2010). Progress toward poliomyelitis eradication—Nigeria, January 2009–June 2010. *MMWR. Morbidity and Mortality Weekly Report, 59*(26), 802–807.
30. Global Polio Eradication Initiative. (2014). *Data and monitoring*, November 19. Retrieved from http://polioeradication.org/Dataandmonitoring/Poliothisweek.aspx.
31. Hemachudha, T., Ugolini, G., Wacharapluesadee, S., et al. (2013). Human rabies: Neuropathogenesis, diagnosis, and management. *Lancet. Neurology, 12*(5), 498–513. doi:10.1016/S1474-4422(13)70038-3.
32. Graham, B. S. (2013). Advances in antiviral vaccine development. *Immunological Reviews, 255*(1), 230–242. doi:10.1111/imr.12098.
33. Cant, A., & Battersby, A. (2013). When to think of immunodeficiency. *Advances in Experimental Medicine and Biology, 764*, 167–177.
34. CSL Behring Canada. (n.d.) *Primary immune deficiency fact sheet*. Retrieved from http://www.cslbehring.ca/docs/483/664/Primary%20Immune%20Deficiency_Fact%20Sheet_24nov09,0.pdf.
35. Al-Herz, W., Bousifha, A., Casanova, J. L., et al. (2014). Primary immunodeficiency diseases: An update on the classification from the International Union of Immunological Societies Expert Committee for Primary Immunodeficiency. *Frontiers in Immunology, 5*, 162. doi:10.3389/fimmu.2014.00162.
36. van der Burg, M., & van Zelm, M. C. (2014). Clinical spectrum of SCID: The key is the thymus? *Frontiers in Immunology, 5*, 111. doi:10.3389/fimmu.2014.00111.
37. Durandy, A., Kracker, S., & Fischer, A. (2013). Primary antibody deficiencies. *Nature Reviews. Immunology, 13*(7), 510–533.
38. Holland, S. M. (2013). Chronic granulomatous disease. *Hematology/Oncology Clinics of North America, 27*, 89–99, viii. doi:10.1016/j.hoc.2012.11.002.
39. Schwab, I., & Nimmerjahn, F. (2014). Intravenous immunoglobulin therapy: How does IgG modulate the immune system? *Nature Reviews. Immunology, 13*(3), 176–189. doi:10.1038/nri3401.
40. Horn, B., & Cowan, M. J. (2013). Unresolved issues in hematopoietic stem cell transplantation for severe combined immunodeficiency: Need for safer conditioning and reduced late effects. *Journal of Allergy and Clinical Immunology, 131*(5), 1306–1311. doi:10.1016/j.jaci.2013.03.014.
41. Eggenhofer, E., Luk, F., Dahlke, M., et al. (2014). The life and fate of mesenchymal stem cells. *Frontiers in Immunology, 5*, 148. doi:10.3389/fimmu.2014.00148.
42. Toubai, T., Paczesny, S., Shono, Y., et al. (2009). Mesenchymal stem cells for treatment and prevention of graft-versus-host disease after allogeneic hematopoietic cell transplantation. *Current Stem Cell Research & Therapy, 4*(4), 252–259. doi:10.2174/157488809789649269.
43. Blaese, R. M. (1993). Development of gene therapy for immunodeficiency: Adenosine deaminase deficiency. *Pediatric Research, 33*(1 Suppl.), S49–S53. doi:10.1203/00006450-199305001-00278.
44. Onodera, M., Nelson, D. M., Sakiyama, Y., et al. (1999). Gene therapy for severe combined immunodeficiency caused by adenosine deaminase deficiency: Improved retroviral vectors for clinical trials. *Acta Haematologica, 101*(2), 89–96.
45. Mukherjee, S., & Thrasher, A. J. (2013). Gene therapy for PIDs: Progress, pitfalls, and prospects. *Gene, 525*, 174–181. doi:10.1016/j.gene.2013.03.098.
46. World Health Organization (WHO). (2009). *Towards universal access: Scaling up priority HIV/AIDS*

interventions in the health sector: Progress report 2009. Geneva: Author.

47. Public Health Agency of Canada. (2014). *HIV and AIDS in Canada: Surveillance report to December 31, 2013*. Ottawa: Public Health Agency of Canada. Retrieved from http://www.phac-aspc.gc.ca/aids-sida/publication/survreport/2013/dec/assets/pdf/hiv-aids-surveillence-eng.pdf70.
48. World Health Organization. (2012). *Patient evaluation and antiretroviral treatment for adults and adolescents clinical protocol for the WHO European Region 2012*, revision. Geneva: Author.
49. National Institutes of Health. (2014). *Guidelines for the use of antiretroviral agents in HIV-1-infected adults and adolescents*. Retrieved from https://aidsinfo.nih.gov/contentfiles/lvguidelines/adultandadolescentgl.pdf.
50. Archin, N. M., & Margolis, D. M. (2014). Emerging strategies to deplete the HIV reservoir. *Current Opinion in Infectious Diseases, 27*(1), 29–35. doi:10.1097/QCO.0000000000000026.
51. Smith, P. L., Tanner, H., & Dalgleish, A. (2014). Developments in HIV-1 immunotherapy and therapeutic vaccination. *F1000prime Reports, 6*, 43. doi:10.12703/P6-43.
52. Roff, S. R., Noon-Song, E. N., & Yamamoto, J. K. (2014). The significance of interferon-γ in HIV-1 pathogenesis, therapy, and prophylaxis. *Frontiers in Immunology, 4*, 498. doi:10.3389/fimmu.2013.00498.
53. Chiodi, F., & Weiss, R. A. (2014). Human immunodeficiency virus antibodies and the vaccine problem. *Journal of Internal Medicine, 275*(5), 444–455. doi:10.1111/joim.12225.
54. World Health Organization. (2010). *WHO recommendations on the diagnosis of HIV in infants and children*. Geneva: Author. Retrieved from http://www.who.int/hiv/pub/paediatric/diagnosis/en/.
55. Ngo, S. T., Steyn, F. J., & McCombe, P. A. (2014). Gender differences in autoimmune disease. *Frontiers in Endocrinology, 35*(3), 347–369. doi:10.1016/j.yfrne.2014.04.004.
56. Brown, S. G. A., Stone, S. F., Fatovich, D. M., et al. (2013). Anaphylaxis: Clinical patterns, mediator release, and severity. *Journal of Allergy and Clinical Immunology, 132*(11), 1141–1149. doi:10.1016/j.jaci.2013.06.015.
57. Eckl-Dorna, J., & Niederberger, V. (2013). What is the source of serum allergen-specific IgE? *Current Allergy and Asthma Reports, 13*(3), 281–287. doi:10.1007/s11882-013-0348-x.
58. Longo, G., Berti, I., Burks, A. W., et al. (2013). IgE-mediated food allergy in children. *Lancet, 382*(9905), 1656–1664. doi:10.1016/S0140-6736(13)60309-8.
59. Lopata, A. L., & Jeebhay, M. F. (2013). Airborne seafood allergens as a cause of occupational allergy and asthma. *Current Allergy and Asthma Reports, 13*(3), 288–297. doi:10.1007/s11882-013-0347-y.
60. Mueller, G. A., Maleki, S. J., & Pedersen, L. C. (2014). The molecular basis of peanut allergy. *Current Allergy and Asthma Reports, 14*(5), 429–438. doi:10.1007/s11882-014-0429-5.
61. Golden, D. B. K. (2013). Advances in diagnosis and management of insect sting allergy. *Annals of Allergy, Asthma and Immunology, 111*(4), 84–89. doi:10.1016/j.anai.2013.05.026.
62. Burks, A. W., Calderon, M. A., Casale, T., et al. (2013). Update on allergy immunotherapy: American Academy of Allergy, Asthma & Immunology/European Academy of Allergy and Clinical Immunology/PRACTALL consensus report. *Journal of Allergy and Clinical Immunology, 131*(5), 1288–1296. doi:10.1016/j.jaci.2013.01.049.
63. Deane, K. D., & El-Gabalawy, H. (2014). Pathogenesis and prevention of rheumatic disease: Focus on preclinical RA and SLE. *Nature Reviews. Rheumatology, 10*(4), 212–228. doi:10.1038/nrrheum.2014.6.
64. Sorrentino, R., Böckmann, R. A., & Florillo, M. T. (2014). HLA-B27 and antigen presentation: At the crossroads between immune defense and autoimmunity. *Molecular Immunology, 57*(1), 22–27. doi:10.1016/j.molimm.2013.06.017.
65. Root-Bernstein, R., & Fairweather, D. (2014). Complexities in the relationship between infection and autoimmunity. *Current Allergy and Asthma Reports, 14*(1), 407–414. doi:10.1007/s11882-013-0407-3.
66. Alam, J., Kim, Y. C., & Choi, Y. (2014). Potential role of bacterial infection in autoimmune diseases: A new aspect of molecular mimicry. *Immune Network, 14*(1), 7–13. doi:10.4110/in.2014.14.1.7.
67. Kurts, C., Panzer, U., Anders, H. J., et al. (2013). The immune system and kidney disease: Basic concepts and clinical implications. *Nature Reviews. Immunology, 13*(10), 738–753. doi:10.1038/nri3523.
68. Kiriakidou, M., Cotton, D., Taichman, D., et al. (2013). Systemic lupus erythematosus. *Annals of Internal Medicine, 159*(1), ITC4-1–ITC4-16. doi:10.7326/0003-4819-159-7-201310010-01004.
69. Hochberg, M. C. (1997). Updating the American College of Rheumatology revised criteria for the classification of systemic lupus erythematosus. *Arthritis and Rheumatism, 40*(9), 1725. doi:10.1002/1529-0131(199709)40:9<1725::AID-ART29>3.0.CO;2-Y.
70. Petri, M., Orbai, A. M., Alarcón, G. S., et al. (2012). Derivation and validation of the Systemic Lupus International Collaborating Clinics classification for systemic lupus erythematosus. *Arthritis and Rheumatism, 64*(8), 2677–2686. doi:10.1002/art.34473.

9

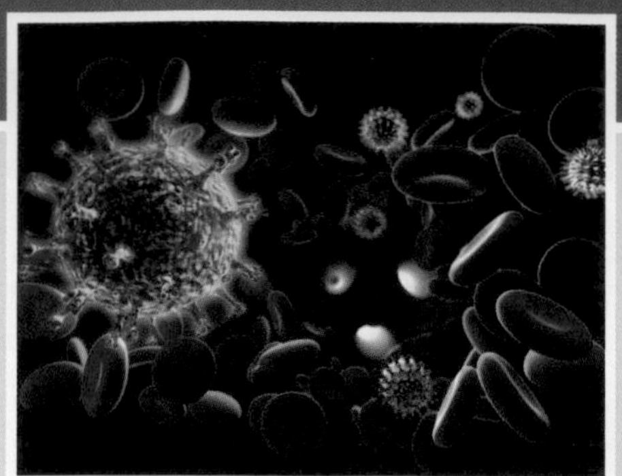

Stress and Disease

Margaret F. Clayton, Kathryn L. McCance, Lorey K. Takahashi, and Stephanie Zettel

EVOLVE WEBSITE

http://evolve.elsevier.com/Canada/Huether/pathophysiology
Student Review Questions
Key Points
Case Studies
Animations
Quick Check Answers

CHAPTER OUTLINE

Historical Background and General Concepts, 216
Stress Overview: Allostasis, Multiple Mediators, and Systems, 219
The Stress Response, 220
Regulation of the Hypothalamic-Pituitary-Adrenal System, 220
Neuroendocrine Regulation: Autonomic Nervous System, 222
Histamine and Other Hormones, 224
Role of the Immune System, 227
Stress, Personality, Coping, and Illness, 227
Coping, 228
GERIATRIC CONSIDERATIONS: **Aging and the Stress–Age Syndrome, 230**

Stress is broadly defined as a perceived or anticipated threat that disrupts a person's well-being or **homeostasis**. Stress involves a complex interaction between the body and brain in the face of random and constant external and internal challenges called **stressors**.[1,2] A stressor may stem from psychological/emotional (fear, social rejection), physical (dramatic temperature changes, abuse), or physiological (infection, inflammation) stimuli that trigger the **stress response**. Many physical and physiological stressors also are discussed in various chapters. This chapter highlights the effects of psychological and emotional stressors on modulating the onset of human diseases.

Exposure to acute stress activates defensive neural, autonomic, and immune systems to facilitate adaptation and survival.[3-5] However, unremitting or toxic stress induces adverse effects by promoting pathophysiology in the very systems that function to meet the challenges of acute stress. For example, whereas acute stress enhances the immune system to protect the individual, adverse situations that cannot be resolved and are accompanied by prolonged activation of the body's stress systems may lead to immunosuppression that impairs the body's ability to fight diseases.[6]

Although modern society offers many positive opportunities, events perceived as especially stressful and uncontrollable, such as loss of a family member, loss of a job, cancer diagnosis, physical abuse, social neglect, or financial hardships, may induce unhealthy coping strategies (e.g., smoking, drinking alcohol, drug abuse) and poor decisions, such as foregoing sleep, eating high-calorie comfort foods, and withdrawing from physical activity. Continued engagement in these behavioural activities is linked to a number of serious illnesses, such as hypertension, depression, diabetes, and obesity (Figure 9-1).[4,7,8] Thus, information should be made widely available to inform people of the positive benefits of coping behaviour (e.g., mindfulness, yoga, exercise) or to seek social support from others and health care providers to maintain a healthy behavioural and physiological profile.

HISTORICAL BACKGROUND AND GENERAL CONCEPTS

Walter B. Cannon used the term *stress* in both a physiological and a psychological sense as early as 1914, and coined the term "fight-or-flight response" to describe the body's preparation to deal with threat.[9] He applied the engineering concepts of stress and strain in a physiological context and believed that emotional stimuli also were capable of causing stress. The physiological reactions to stress included increased heart rate and blood supply of oxygen and glucose to muscles and the brain, elevated respiration, dilation of pupils, and inhibition of gastric secretions.

In 1946, Hans Selye further popularized and advanced the concept of stress in terms of a chemical or physical change (i.e., physiological stress, in response either to the external environment or within the body itself). His work showed that **physiological stress** involved (1) enlargement of the adrenal gland, (2) decreased lymphocyte levels in the blood from damage to lymphatic structures of the immune system, and (3) development of bleeding ulcers in the stomach and duodenal lining. Selye concluded that physiological stress will impair the ability of the organism to resist future stressors and represented the hallmark pattern of a nonspecific stress response that was labelled **general adaptation syndrome (GAS)**.[10]

GAS involved three successive stages: (1) the alarm stage, (2) the resistance or adaptation stage, and (3) the exhaustion stage. The **alarm stage** is the emergency reaction that prepares the body to fight or flee from threat. This stage involves the secretion of hormones and catecholamines to support physiological and metabolic activity (Figures 9-2 and 9-3) and boosts the immune system to thwart infection and disease. The ensuing **resistance or adaptation stage** requires continued mobilization of the body's resources to cope and overcome a sustained challenge. The **exhaustion stage** (currently described as *allostatic overload*)

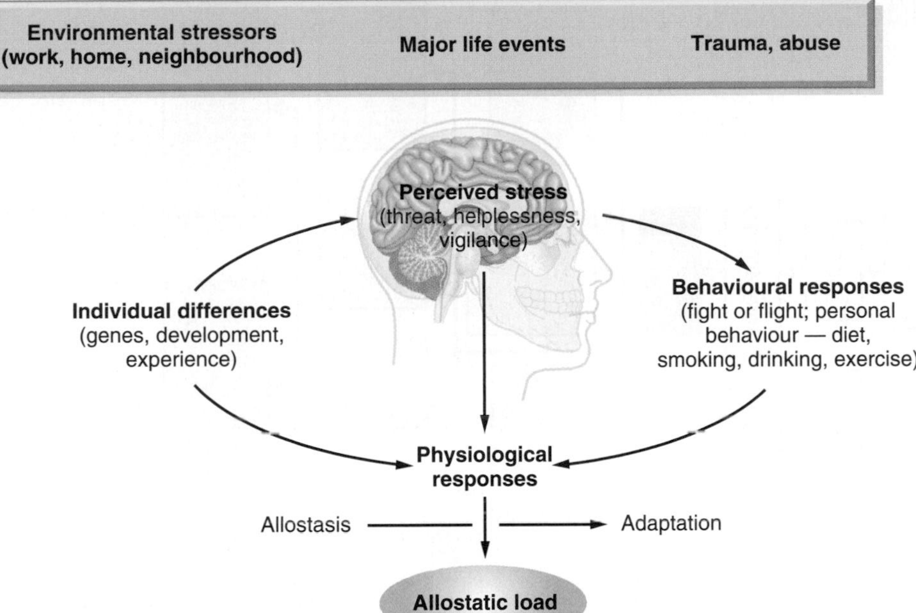

FIGURE 9-1 Physiological and Behavioural Stress Responses. Stress processes arise from bidirectional communication patterns between the brain and other physiological systems (autonomic, immune, neural, and endocrine). Importantly, these bidirectional mechanisms are protective, promoting short-term adaptation (allostasis). Chronic stress mechanisms, however, can lead to long-term dysregulation and promote behavioural responses and physiological responses that lead to stress-induced disorders/diseases (allostatic load), compromising health. (Reprinted from *European Journal of Pharmacology*, 583[2–3], McEwen, B.S., "Central effects of stress hormones in health and disease: understanding the protective and damaging effects of stress and stress mediators," Pages 174–185, Copyright 2008, with permission from Elsevier.)

occurs when the body's physiological and immune systems no longer effectively cope with the stressor and marks the onset of diseases (**diseases of adaptation**). That is, when stress continues unabated and adaptation is not successful, body organs that are weak, such as the heart and kidney, may no longer function and lead to death.

Although GAS is considered a cornerstone of stress research, the concept that stress is entirely the result of a physical disturbance is an oversimplification. In the mid-1950s, studies emerged demonstrating that psychological stressors were highly effective in activating adrenal hormone secretion. For example, stress hormone levels increased when monkeys were re-exposed to a clicking sound previously paired with electric shock.[11] Similarly, stress hormone secretion in humans increased when exposed to psychological stressors,[12] such as a stressful interview.[13] According to Mason a number of psychological factors, such as degree of comfort, unpleasantness, or suddenness of an unanticipated stimulus, could modulate the magnitude of the stress response.[14]

Research from the 1970s has demonstrated a remarkable sensitivity of the central nervous system (CNS) and endocrine system to emotional, psychological, and social influences. Psychological stressors can elicit a reactive or anticipatory stress response. For example, an examination with no physical stressor may elicit a **reactive response** involving physiological changes, such as increased heart rate and dry mouth. **Anticipatory responses** occur when physiological responses develop in anticipation of psychological stress or threat. Anticipatory responses can be generated by the fear of a potential encounter with a dangerous, unconditioned stimulus (such as a predator) or in conditioned situations when a person learns that a specific event was associated with an aversive situation.[15] Anticipation of re-exposure to these unwanted events produces a physiological stress response. For example, a child with a history of parental abuse may experience a physiological stress response in anticipation of further abuse when that parent enters the room. Another well-known example of a conditioned emotional response is the development of post-traumatic stress disorder (PTSD) in some military veterans and survivors of natural disasters.

Psychoneuroimmunology (PNI) is the study of how consciousness (*psycho*), mediated by the CNS (*neuro*), interacts with the immune system (*immunology*) to defend the body against infection. Psychoneuroimmunology assumes that immune-mediated diseases result from

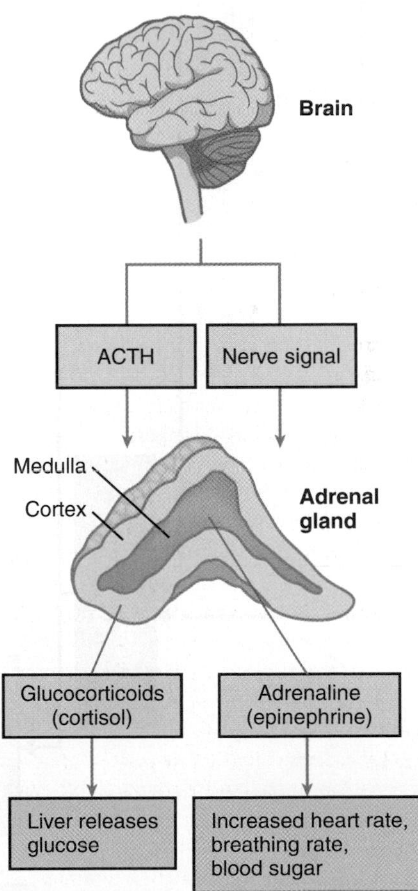

FIGURE 9-2 The Alarm Reaction. The alarm reaction includes increased secretion of glucocorticoids (cortisol) by the adrenal cortex and increased secretion of epinephrine and small amounts of norepinephrine from the adrenal medulla. The response to the release of cortisol and sympathetic nerve activation is summarized in Figure 9-3. *ACTH*, adrenocorticotropic hormone. (Adapted from Thibodeau, G.A., & Patton, K.T. [2016]. *Anatomy & physiology* [9th ed.]. St. Louis: Mosby.)

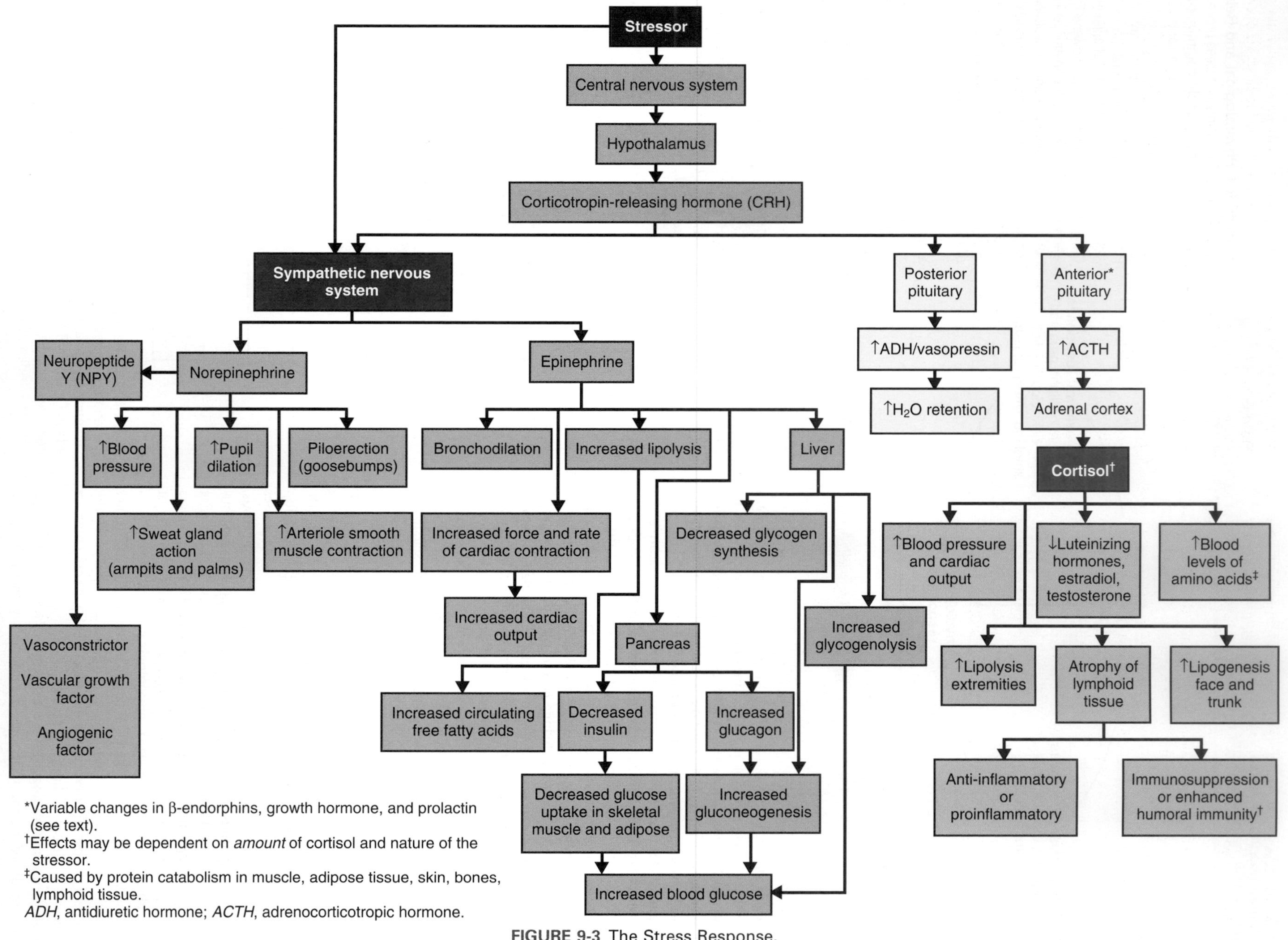

*Variable changes in β-endorphins, growth hormone, and prolactin (see text).
†Effects may be dependent on *amount* of cortisol and nature of the stressor.
‡Caused by protein catabolism in muscle, adipose tissue, skin, bones, lymphoid tissue.
ADH, antidiuretic hormone; *ACTH*, adrenocorticotropic hormone.

FIGURE 9-3 The Stress Response.

complex interrelationships among psychosocial, emotional, genetic, neurological, endocrine, immunological, and behavioural factors.[16-18] The immune system is integrated with other physiological processes and sensitive to changes in CNS and endocrine functioning linked to psychological states. Stressors include a broad range of physical and emotional sources—for example, infection, noise, decreased oxygen supply, pain, malnutrition, heat, cold, trauma, prolonged exertion, radiation, responses to life events (including anxiety, depression, anger, fear, loss, and excitement), obesity, advanced age, medications, disease, surgery, and medical treatment.

The study of PNI has generated broad scientific debate, especially with respect to the causal role of personality and emotional factors in cancer mortality and morbidity. For example, mouse models suggest a strong link between stress and breast cancer progression, but this effect is not consistently found in humans.[19,20] What is becoming increasingly clear is that secretion of stress hormones influences many metabolic systems and physiological events in both adults and children.[21] Furthermore, studies now point to a strong association between modulation of the immune system by psychosocial stressors and health outcomes.[22] With increased understanding of the relationship between stress and human diseases, new strategies are emerging to treat stress-related disorders.

Stress Overview: Allostasis, Multiple Mediators, and Systems

Increased knowledge of the link between stress and disease is supported by the concept of **allostasis**, introduced by Sterling and Eyer,[23] and refers to "stability through change." This concept differs from the "fixed homeostasis model" in which physiological regulation revolves around an unchanging set point. For example, after exposure to a challenging stressor, heighted physiological secretion of stress hormones (e.g., cortisol) must return to basal levels. By contrast, allostasis involves a dynamic strategy with the brain continuously monitoring many parameters to anticipate what is required from the neuroendocrine and autonomic systems to meet the challenges of future events.[3,24,25] Hence, return to initial basal hormone levels may not be the most adaptive strategy to cope with anticipated stress encounters. However, when chronic activation of regulatory systems taxes the body and brain, diseases and disorders may emerge. **Allostatic overload** is the term used to describe overactivation of adaptive regulatory physiological systems that may lead to clinical pathophysiology and increase susceptibility of disease.

Research suggests that allostasis and allostatic overload are highly individualized; that is, an event or situation that is considered normal in one person may be stressful to another.[26,27] When we experience allostatic overload, this load exacts a "wear and tear" toll on our bodies. Because the brain is a key player in perceiving stress, it is influential in determining when we have reached allostatic overload. Thus, psychological stress is increasingly recognized both as a precipitating factor for some diseases and as a contributor that worsens symptoms and negative outcomes in anxiety, persistent pain and fatigue syndromes, ulcers, asthma, obesity, metabolic syndrome, essential hypertension, and type 2 diabetes. In addition, stress disrupts the biological process of sleep and growth and reproductive functions.[28-32] Some of these disorders are the leading causes of death in both the United States and Canada (Table 9-1).

In response to acute and chronic stress, brain regions, including the hippocampus, amygdala, and prefrontal cortex, may respond by undergoing structural remodelling that alters behavioural and physiological responses to increase the risk of developing cognitive impairments and depression.[1,25] Key physiological systems involved in allostatic overload include exaggerated secretion of cortisol, catecholamines of the sympathetic nervous system, and proinflammatory cytokines, as well as a decline in parasympathetic activity. A prevalent example is sleep deprivation from being "stressed out." Sleep deprivation and disturbances, such as sleep apnea, short sleep duration, and insomnia, have significant associations with allostatic load, leading to damaging effects including elevated evening cortisol concentration; elevated insulin and blood glucose levels; increased blood pressure; reduced parasympathetic activity; increased levels of proinflammatory cytokines; and increased secretion of the hormone ghrelin (primarily by cells of the stomach and pancreas), which increases appetite.[33,34] Overall, the dynamic and damaging effects of allostatic overload can induce sleep deprivation, which then facilitates increased caloric intake, depressed mood, cognitive deficits, and a host of other unhealthy responses.

TABLE 9-1 Examples of Stress-Related Diseases and Conditions

Target Organ or System	Disease or Condition	Target Organ or System	Disease or Condition
Cardiovascular system	Coronary artery disease Hypertension Stroke Disturbances of heart rhythm	Gastro-intestinal system	Ulcer Irritable bowel syndrome Diarrhea Nausea and vomiting Ulcerative colitis
Muscle	Tension headaches Muscle contraction backache	Genitourinary system	Diuresis Impotence Frigidity
Connective tissues	Rheumatoid arthritis (autoimmune disease) Related inflammatory diseases of connective tissue	Skin	Eczema Neurodermatitis Acne
Pulmonary system	Asthma (hypersensitivity reaction) Hay fever (hypersensitivity reactions)	Endocrine system	Type 2 diabetes mellitus Amenorrhea
Immune system	Immunosuppression or deficiency Autoimmune diseases	Central nervous system	Fatigue and lethargy Type A behaviour Overeating Depression Insomnia

✔QUICK CHECK 9-1

1. How is stress related to unhealthy coping behaviours?
2. Briefly describe the three stages of the general adaptation syndrome.
3. Define *allostatic load* and *allostatic overload.*

THE STRESS RESPONSE

Because evidence points to the important role that stress plays in many disease processes, research has begun to focus on physiological mechanisms underlying mind–body interactions to understand and prevent stress-related diseases (see also the *Geriatric Considerations:* Aging and the Stress–Age Syndrome box). Using a multidisciplinary approach involving molecular biology, immunology, neurology, endocrinology, and behavioural science, researchers are investigating how stressful life events occurring over a prolonged period of time impair immune functions. Knowledge emerging from the various disciplines offers a holistic and complex model of the biochemical relationships among the CNS, autonomic nervous system (ANS), endocrine system, and immune system.

Regulation of the Hypothalamic-Pituitary-Adrenal System

A key stress hormone relationship is the regulation of the **hypothalamic-pituitary-adrenal (HPA) system** (Figure 9-4). In sequence, the perception of stress activates the hypothalamus to secrete **corticotropin-releasing hormone (CRH)**, which binds to specific receptors on anterior pituitary cells that, in turn, produce **adrenocorticotropic hormone (ACTH)**. ACTH is then transported through the blood to the adrenal glands located on the top of the kidneys. After binding to specific receptors on the cortex of the adrenal glands, glucocorticoid hormones (primarily cortisol) are released.

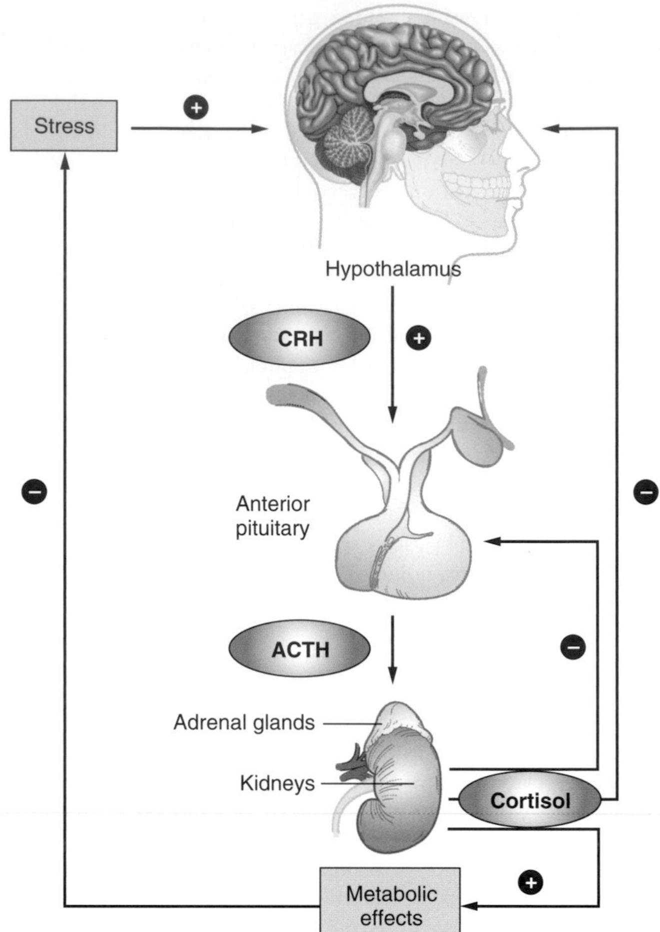

FIGURE 9-4 Hypothalamic-Pituitary-Adrenal Axis. The response to stress begins in the brain. The hypothalamus is the control centre in the brain for many hormones, including corticotropin-releasing hormone. *ACTH*, adrenocorticotropic hormone; *CRH*, corticotropin-releasing hormone.

Physiological Effects of Cortisol

During stress, the secretion of glucocorticoid hormones, primarily **cortisol** (cortisol is known outside the body as *hydrocortisone*), reaches all tissues, including the brain, easily penetrates cell membranes, and reacts with numerous intracellular glucocorticoid receptors (see Figure 9-3). Because they spare almost no tissue or organ and influence a large proportion of the human genome, glucocorticoids exert significant diverse biological actions.[28] They regulate many functions of the CNS, including arousal, cognition, mood, sleep, metabolism, maintenance of cardiovascular tone, the immune and inflammatory reaction, and growth and reproduction.

Cortisol mobilizes substances needed for cellular metabolism and stimulates gluconeogenesis or the formation of glucose from noncarbohydrate sources, such as amino acids or free fatty acids in the liver. In addition, cortisol enhances the elevation of blood glucose levels that is promoted by other hormones, such as epinephrine, glucagon, and growth hormone. Cortisol also inhibits the uptake and oxidation of glucose by many body cells. Overall, cortisol's actions on carbohydrate metabolism result in increased blood glucose levels, thereby energizing the body to combat the stressor. The effects of cortisol are summarized in Table 9-2.

Cortisol also affects protein metabolism. It has an anabolic effect by increasing the rate of protein synthesis and RNA in the liver. This effect is countered by its catabolic effect on protein stores in other tissues. Protein catabolism acts to increase levels of circulating amino acids; therefore, chronic exposure to excess cortisol can severely deplete protein stores in muscle, bone, connective tissue, and skin.

Another important adaptive function of cortisol is to enhance immunity during acute stress.[35] Cortisol exerts beneficial effects by inhibiting initial inflammatory effects, for example, vasodilation and increased capillary permeability. Cortisol also promotes resolution and repair. These actions are mainly accomplished by facilitating the effects of glucocorticoid receptor, namely, the transcription of genetic material (through DNA binding) within leukocytes.[36]

Pathophysiological Effects of Cortisol

Chronic dysregulation of the HPA axis, especially abnormal elevated levels of cortisol, has been linked to a wide variety of disorders, including obesity, sleep deprivation, lipid abnormalities, hypertension, diabetes, atherosclerosis, and loss of bone density.[3,27,28,37] In the brain, chronic glucocorticoid secretion may reduce hippocampal volume, enlarge the ventricles, and modulate reversible cortical atrophy.[1,28] These CNS changes may contribute to cognitive impairments and emotional disorders.

In the periphery, heightened stress-induced cortisol levels promote gastric secretion in the parietal cells of the stomach. This increased acid secretion along with *Helicobacter pylori* infection, which effectively erodes the protective mucosal layer of the stomach, may account for the gastro-intestinal ulceration observed by Selye in his experiments. Furthermore, glucocorticoids contribute to the development of metabolic syndrome and the pathogenesis of obesity (see *Health Promotion:* Glucocorticoids, Insulin, Inflammation, and Obesity) by directly causing

TABLE 9-2 **Physiological Effects of Cortisol**

Functions Affected	Physiological Effects
Carbohydrate and lipid metabolism	It diminishes peripheral uptake and utilization of glucose; promotes gluconeogenesis in liver metabolism cells; and enhances gluconeogenic response to other hormones. It promotes lipolysis in adipose tissue.
Protein metabolism	It increases protein synthesis in liver and decreases protein synthesis (including immunoglobulin synthesis) in muscle, lymphoid tissue, adipose tissue, skin, and bone. It increases plasma level of amino acids; stimulates deamination in liver.
Anti-inflammatory effects (systemic effects)	High levels of cortisol used in medication therapy suppress inflammatory response and inhibit proinflammatory activity of many growth factors and cytokines; however, over time, some individuals may develop tolerance to glucocorticoids, causing an increased susceptibility to both inflammatory and autoimmune diseases.
Proinflammatory effects (possible local effects)	Cortisol levels released during stress response may increase proinflammatory effects.
Lipid metabolism	Lipolysis takes place in extremities, and lipogenesis takes place in the face and trunk.
Immune effects	*Treatment* levels of glucocorticoids are immunosuppressive; thus they are valuable agents used in numerous diseases/conditions. T-cell or innate immune system is particularly affected by these larger doses of glucocorticoids, with suppression of Th1 function or innate immunity. *Stress* can cause a different pattern of immune response. These nontherapeutic levels can suppress innate (Th1) and increase adaptive (Th2) immunity—the so-called Th2 shift. Several factors influence this complex physiology and include long-term adaptations, reproductive hormones (i.e., overall, androgens suppress and estrogens stimulate immune responses), defects of the hypothalamic-pituitary-adrenal axis, histamine-generated responses, and acute versus chronic stress. Thus stress seems to cause a Th2 shift *systemically*, whereas *locally*, under certain conditions, it can induce proinflammatory activities and by these mechanisms may influence onset or course of infections, autoimmune/inflammatory, allergic, and neoplastic diseases.
Digestive function	It promotes gastric secretion.
Urinary function	It enhances excretion of calcium.
Connective tissue function	It decreases proliferation of fibroblasts in connective tissue (thus delaying healing).
Muscle function	It maintains normal contractility and maximal work output for skeletal and cardiac muscle.
Bone function	It decreases bone formation.
Vascular system/myocardial function	It maintains normal blood pressure; permits increased responsiveness of arterioles to constrictive action of adrenergic stimulation; and optimizes myocardial performance.
Central nervous system function	It somehow modulates perceptual and emotional functioning. It is essential for normal arousal and initiation of daytime activity.
Possible synergism with estrogen in pregnancy?	It may suppress the maternal immune system to prevent rejection of the fetus.

insulin resistance and influencing genetic variations that predispose to obesity.[38-40]

The impact of cortisol on fetal development and subsequent risk for future disease also has been investigated. Reynolds has offered convincing data associating high maternal cortisol levels during pregnancy with low birth weight.[41] The consequences of cortisol-induced low birth weight now extend to disease risk in later life, for example, obesity; cardiovascular conditions, such as hypertension; and behavioural disorders attributed to altered brain structure.[41-43] Thus, glucocorticoids dramatically affect human pathophysiology and, consequently, longevity.[3,28,37]

The feedback mechanisms of the HPA axis sense and determine the circulating glucocorticoid levels, whereas other tissues passively accept the actions of circulating glucocorticoids.[28] Thus, discrepancy in the glucocorticoid sensing network between the HPA axis and peripheral tissues could possibly produce peripheral tissue hypercortisolism or hypocortisolism. For example, both high HPA axis reactivity to stress and increased peripheral tissue sensitivity to glucocorticoids are associated with the severity of coronary artery disease (see *Health Promotion:* Psychosocial Stress and Progression to Coronary Heart Disease).[44,45]

Cortisol secretion during stress exerts beneficial effects by inhibiting initial inflammatory effects, for example, vasodilation and increased capillary permeability.[36] Cortisol also promotes resolution and repair. These actions are mainly accomplished by facilitating the effects of glucocorticoid receptor, namely, the transcription of genetic material (through DNA binding) within leukocytes.[36] Because glucocorticoids are so widely expressed, they influence virtually all immune cells. The adaptiveness or destructiveness of cortisol-induced effects may depend on the intensity, type, and duration of the stressor; the tissue involved; and the subsequent concentration and length of cortisol exposure. Finally, glucocorticoids have been shown to induce T lymphocyte (T-cell) apoptosis.[36,46]

Effects of Exogenous Glucocorticoids

Stress hormones, especially glucocorticoids (cortisol), are used therapeutically as powerful anti-inflammatory/immunosuppressive agents. The synthetic forms of glucocorticoid hormones (exogenous types of anti-inflammatory glucocorticoids administered for a pharmaceutical reaction) are poorly metabolized when compared with endogenous glucocorticoids, leading to a longer half-life and no circadian rhythm for these compounds. Moreover, these synthetic compounds bind with different targets, so each has a unique effect.[47]

Elevated levels of glucocorticoids and catecholamines (epinephrine and norepinephrine), both endogenous and exogenously administered, may decrease innate immunity and increase autoimmune responses. In addition, prolonged effects of cortisol may accentuate inflammation and potentially increase neuronal death (e.g., in stroke victims)[47] and induce T-cell apoptosis.[36,46]

Initially, immune responses are regulated by cells of innate immunity called antigen-presenting cells (APCs), such as monocytes/macrophages (see Chapter 7), dendritic cells, and other phagocytic cells, and by Th1

HEALTH PROMOTION

Glucocorticoids, Insulin, Inflammation, and Obesity

The signs and symptoms of Cushing's syndrome (e.g., excess glucocorticoids) include truncal obesity, relatively thin extremities, a "moon face," and a "buffalo [neck] hump." In such individuals, the possibility of associated hypertension is high, and the risk of infection and metabolic syndrome or frank type 2 diabetes is increased. In addition, the likelihood of an elevated ratio of intra-abdominal subcutaneous fat mass to nonabdominal fat mass is high because the glucocorticoids mediate the redistribution of stored calories into the abdominal region. The specific increase in abdominal fat stores is a consequence of elevated levels of glucocorticoids combined with increased insulin action. However, the increased levels of glucocorticoids need not be present in the circulation; instead, they can be generated locally in fat by conversion of inactive cortisone to active cortisol through the action of the isoenzyme 11β-hydroxysteroid dehydrogenase (11β-HSD) type 1. This conversion is referred to as "pre-receptor" metabolism of cortisol. The active steroid is secreted directly to the liver through the portal vein. In vitro insulin synthesis and secretion from the pancreas are inhibited by the glucocorticoids. However, increasing levels of glucocorticoids in vivo are associated with increasing insulin secretion, possibly because of an anti-insulin effect on the liver, which appears to be vulnerable to the negative effects of glucocorticoids on insulin action. Hepatic insulin resistance is strongly associated with abdominal obesity.

Recent data reveal that the plasma concentration of inflammatory mediators, such as tumour necrosis factor-alpha (TNF-α) and interleukin-6 (IL-6), is increased in the insulin-resistant states of obesity and type 2 diabetes. Two mechanisms might be involved in the pathogenesis of inflammation: (1) glucose and macronutrient intake (i.e., which can be mediated through chronic stress) causes oxidative stress; and (2) the increased concentrations of TNF-α and IL-6 associated with obesity and type 2 diabetes might interfere with insulin signal transduction. This interference might promote inflammation. Chronic overnutrition (obesity) might thus be a proinflammatory state with oxidative stress.

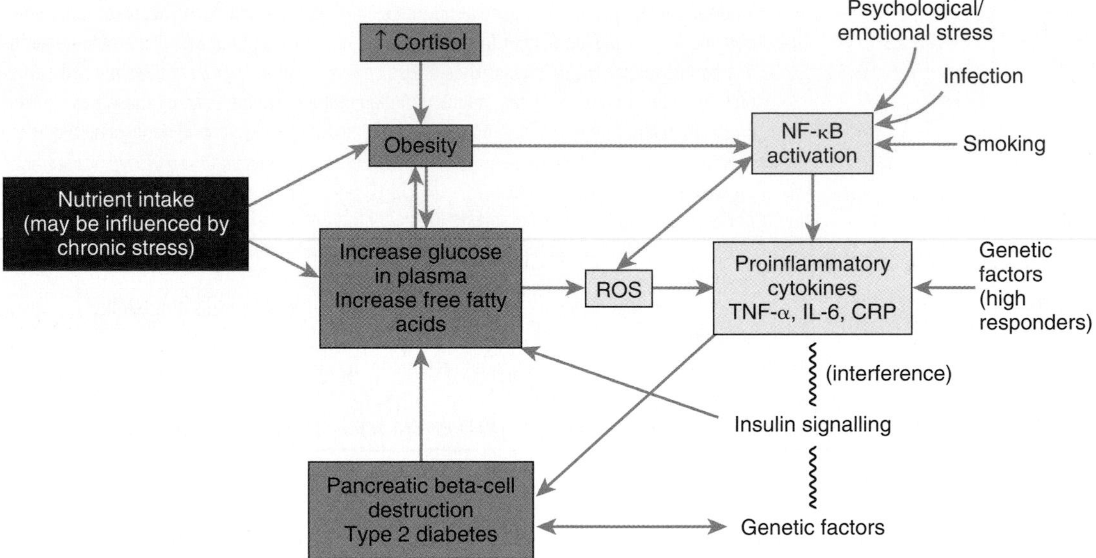

Stress, Inflammation, Obesity, and Type 2 Diabetes. The induction of reactive oxygen species (*ROS*) generation and inflammation through the proinflammatory transcription factor NF-κB activates most proinflammatory genes. Macronutrient intake, obesity, free fatty acids, infection, smoking, psychological stress, and genetic factors increase the production of ROS. Interference with insulin signalling (insulin resistance) leads to hyperglycemia and proinflammatory changes. Proinflammatory changes increase levels of TNF-α and IL-6, and also lead to the inhibition of insulin signalling and insulin resistance. Inflammation in pancreatic beta cells leads to beta-cell dysfunction, which in combination with insulin resistance leads to type 2 diabetes. *CRP*, C-reactive protein; *IL-6*, interleukin-6; *TNF-α*, tumour necrosis factor-alpha.

Data from Dallman, M.F., la Fleur, S.E., Pecoraro, N.C., et al. (2004). *Endocrinology, 145*(6), 2633–2638; Dandona, P., Aljada, A., & Bandyopadhyay, A. (2004). *Trends Immunol, 25*(1), 4–7; Khadir, A., Tiss, A., Kavalakatt, S., et al. (2015). *Mediators Inflamm, 2015,* 512603; Kim, S.P., Ellmerer, M., Van Citters, G.W., et al. (2003). *Diabetes, 52,* 2453–2460; Masuzaki, H., Paterson, J., Sinyama, H., et al. (2001). *Science, 294,* 2166–2170; Padgett, D.A., & Glaser, R. (2003). *Trends Immunol, 24*(8), 444–448; Shimanoe, C., Hara, M., Nishida, Y., et al. (2015). *PLoS One, 10*(2), e0118105; Spencer, S.J., & Tilbrook, A. (2011). *Stress, 14*(3), 233–246; Strack, A.M., Sebastian, R.J., Schwartz, M.W., et al. (1995). *Am J Physiol, 268,* R142–R149; Wagen Knecht, L.E., Langefeld, C.D., Scherzinger, A.L., et al. (2003). *Diabetes, 52*(10), 2490–2496.

and Th2 lymphocytes (T-helper cells involved in adaptive immunity; see Chapter 7). These cells secrete cytokines, the chemical messengers that regulate innate and adaptive immune responses. APCs also release cytokines that induce T cells to differentiate into Th1 cells. Th1 cells and APC cytokines work together to stimulate the activity of T-cytotoxic cells (Tc cells), natural killer (NK) cells, and activated macrophages—the major components of innate immunity (see Chapter 6).

Cytokines secreted by Th2 cells also act to inhibit Th1 cells and can promote adaptive immunity by stimulating growth and activating mast cells and eosinophils, as well as the differentiation of B lymphocyte (B-cell) immunoglobulins. Thus, these cytokines are considered to be the major anti-inflammatory cytokines (Figure 9-5).[48] The decrease in Th1 activity and increase in Th2 activity is sometimes called a **Th1 to Th2 shift.**

Neuroendocrine Regulation: Autonomic Nervous System

Sympathetic Nervous System

The sympathetic nervous system is aroused, simultaneously with the HPA system during stress, to release norepinephrine (adrenergic

HEALTH PROMOTION

Psychosocial Stress and Progression to Coronary Heart Disease

The link between stress and coronary heart disease was proposed as early as the 1970s; however, it was only recently that conclusive evidence and proposed mechanisms for development of the disease were identified. Much work continues to focus on elucidating the interaction between stress and cardiovascular disease.

One of the primary risk factors for coronary heart disease is hypertension. A new designation of prehypertension was recently created and found to be a good predictor for future cardiovascular events. Prehypertension is defined as a systolic blood pressure of 120 to 139 mm Hg or a diastolic blood pressure of 80 to 90 mm Hg. Individuals with prehypertension are much more likely to develop frank hypertension and, eventually, coronary heart disease.

Studies show that persons with a highly reactive personality type who experience high levels of anxiety with stress are much more likely to progress from prehypertension to hypertension and then to develop cardiac disease, specifically coronary heart disease, than those who have better coping abilities. Further long-term psychological stress, such as that experienced in a strained marriage or an unhappy work environment, not only was shown to accelerate the progression of hypertension and coronary heart disease but also is correlated with higher mortality rates from coronary heart disease.

Trait anger, defined as a stable personality trait characterized by frequency, intensity, and duration of anger, also was shown to be a factor in the development of coronary heart disease at higher rates than in the general population. Individuals with trait anger also experienced more strokes. Hostile individuals with advanced cardiovascular disease may be particularly susceptible to stress-induced increases in sympathetic activity and inflammation.

One popular mechanism for the interaction between psychosocial stress and cardiovascular disease suggests that stress triggers an inflammatory response that, over time, increases the chances of developing coronary heart disease. The primary mechanisms proposed are chronically elevated cortisol levels and dysregulation of the circadian rhythm for cortisol release. Further, chronic stress alters HPA function, resulting in an abnormal stress response pattern. This alteration in HPA activity was found in persons with coronary heart disease along with increased inflammatory markers. A newer and emerging mechanism is the involvement of T-regulatory cells (Treg cells). Treg cells play an important role in maintaining peripheral tolerance of tissue antigens, preventing autoimmune diseases, and decreasing chronic inflammatory diseases. Studies have shown that naturally occurring CD4+CD25+ Treg cells are downregulated in individuals with acute coronary syndrome (ACS). Additionally, the sympathetic nervous system plays an important role in immune homeostasis by maintaining the number of Treg cells in the periphery and this may be affected by psychological stress. The Treg-cell lineage, however, is heterogeneous.

Because coronary heart disease is one of the major causes of death in industrialized countries, development of successful interventional programs is of high priority. Programs in which dietary changes, exercise, stress management, and positive support systems are implemented continue to show positive results for slowing the progression of heart disease and decreasing the risk factors for disease development. Further, individuals in these programs report decreased levels of depression and stress as well as overall improvement in mental health.

Data from Bhowmick, S., Anurag, S., Flavell, R.A., et al. (2009). *J Leukoc Biol, 86*(6), 1275–1283; Brydon, L., Strike, P.C., Bhattacharyya, M.R., et al. (2010). *J Psychosom Res, 68*(2), 109–116; Cheng, X., Yu, X, Ding, Y.J., et al. (2008). *Clin Immunol, 127*, 89–97; Davidson, K.W. (2008). *Cleve Clin J Med, 75*(Suppl. 2), S15–S19; Miyara, M., & Sakaguchi, S. (2007). *Trends Mol Med, 13*, 108–116; Mor, A., Luboshits, G., Planer, D., et al. (2006). *Eur Heart J, 27*, 2530–2537; Nijm, J., Kristenson, M., Olsson, A.G., et al. (2007). *J Int Med, 262*(3), 375–384; Sakaguchi, S., Yamaguchi, T., Nomura, T., et al. (2008). *Cell, 133*, 775–787; Sardella, G., De Luca, L., Francavilla, V., et al. (2007). *Thromb Res, 120*, 631–634; Sawant, D.V., & Vignali, D.A. (2014). *Immunol Rev, 259*(1), 173–191; Shamaei-Tousi, A., Steptoe, A., O'Donnell, K., et al. (2007). *Cell Stress Chaperones, 12*(4), 384–392; Shevach, E.M. (2000). *Annu Rev Immunol, 18*, 423–449; Steptoe, A., & Brydon, L. (2009). *Neurosci Biobehav Rev, 33*, 63–70; Vignali, D.A., Collison, L.W., & Workman, C.J. (2008). *Nat Rev Immunol, 8*, 523–532; Vizza, J., Neatrour, D.M., Felton, P.M., et al. (2007). *J Cardiopulm Rehabil Prev, 27*(6), 376–383; Zhu, Z., Meng, K., Zhong, Y.-C., et al. (2014). *PLoS One, 9*(2), e88775.

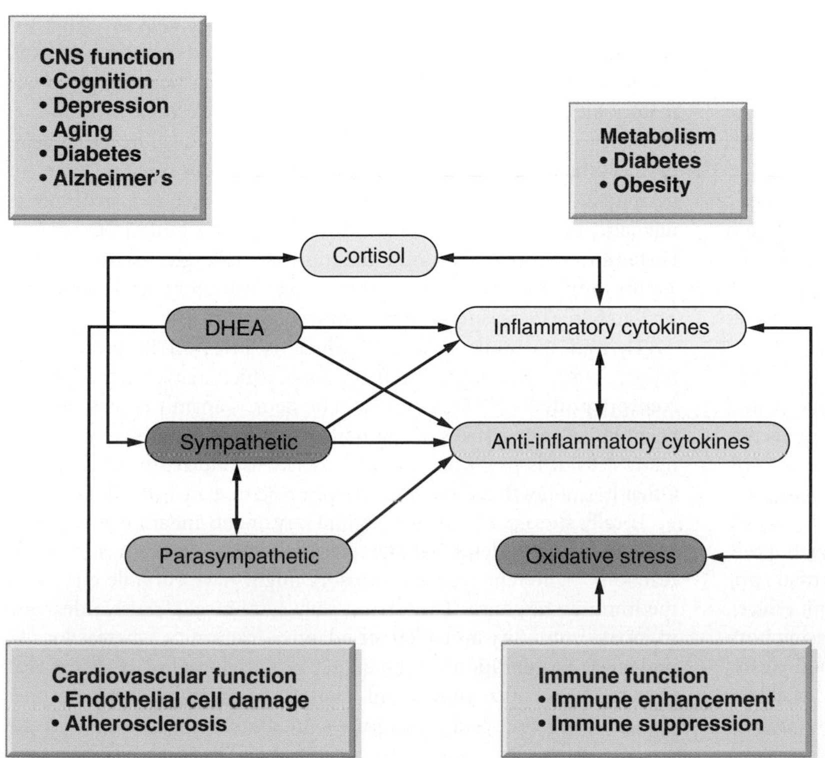

FIGURE 9-5 Stress Interactions Are Nonlinear and Complex. Nonlinearity means that when one mediator is increased or decreased, the subsequent compensatory changes in other mediators depend on time and level of change, causing multiple interacting variables. The inevitable consequences from adapting to daily life over time include changes in behavioural responses. For example, these changes include sleeping patterns, smoking, alcohol consumption, physical activity, and social interactions. These behavioural patterns are a part of the allostatic overload with chronic elevations in cortisol level, sympathetic activity, and levels of proinflammatory cytokines, and a decrease in parasympathetic activity. *CNS*, central nervous system; *DHEA*, dehydroepiandrosterone. (Reprinted from *European Journal of Pharmacology*, 583[2–3], McEwen, B.S., "Central effects of stress hormones in health and disease: understanding the protective and damaging effects of stress and stress mediators," Pages 174–185, Copyright 2008, with permission from Elsevier.)

TABLE 9-3 Physiological Effects of Catecholamines[a]

Organ/Tissue	Process or Result
Brain	Increased blood flow; increased glucose metabolism
Cardiovascular system	Increased rate and force of contraction Peripheral vasoconstriction
Pulmonary system	Bronchodilation
Skeletal muscle	Increased glycogenolysis Increased contraction Increased dilation of muscle vasculature Decreased glucose uptake and utilization (decreases insulin release)
Liver	Increased glucose production Increased glycogenolysis
Adipose tissue	Increased lipolysis Decreased glucose uptake
Skin	Decreased blood flow
Gastro-intestinal and genitourinary tracts	Decreased protein synthesis Decreased smooth muscle contraction Increased renin release Increased gastro-intestinal sphincter tone
Lymphoid tissue	Acute and chronic stress inhibits several components of innate immunity, particularly decreasing natural killer cells
Macrophages	Inhibited and stimulated macrophage activity Depends on availability of type 1/proinflammatory cytokines, presence or absence of antigenic stressors, and peripheral corticotropin-releasing hormone (CRH)

[a]Some of these responses require glucocorticoids (e.g., cortisol) for maximal activity (see text for explanation).

Data from Elenkov, I.J., & Chrousos, G.P. (2002). *Ann N Y Acad Sci, 966*, 290–303; Granner, D.K. (2000). Hormones of the adrenal medulla. In R.K. Murray, P.A. Mayes, D.K. Granner, et al. (Eds.), *Harper's biochemistry* (25th ed.). New York: McGraw-Hill.

stimulation) and stimulate the medulla of the adrenal gland to release catecholamines (80% epinephrine and 20% norepinephrine) into the bloodstream. Sympathetic nerves also contain nonadrenergic mediators that amplify or antagonize the effects of adrenal catecholamines.

Circulating catecholamines essentially mimic direct sympathetic stimulation. Catecholamines cannot cross the blood–brain barrier and are synthesized locally in the brain. The physiological effects of the catecholamines on organs and tissues are summarized in Table 9-3. Norepinephrine regulates blood pressure, promotes arousal, and increases vigilance, anxiety, and other protective emotional responses.

The catecholamines stimulate two major classes of receptors: α-adrenergic receptors (α_1 and α_2) and β-adrenergic receptors (β_1 and β_2). Table 13-7 summarizes the actions of the two subclasses of adrenergic receptors. (A discussion of receptors can be found in Chapters 1, 18, and 23.) Epinephrine binds with and activates both α and β receptors, whereas norepinephrine binds primarily with α receptors.

Epinephrine in the liver and skeletal muscles is rapidly metabolized. Epinephrine influences cardiac action by enhancing myocardial contractility (inotropic effect), increasing heart rate (chronotropic effect), and increasing venous return to the heart, ultimately increasing both cardiac output and blood pressure. Epinephrine dilates blood vessels supplying skeletal muscles, allowing for greater oxygenation. Metabolically, it causes transient hyperglycemia (high blood sugar), reduces glucose uptake in the muscles and other organs, and decreases insulin release from the pancreas, thus preventing glucose uptake by peripheral tissue and preserving it for the CNS. Epinephrine also mobilizes free fatty acids and cholesterol.

Catecholamine secretion also increases proinflammatory cytokine production, which elevates heart rate and blood pressure and impairs wound healing.[49] Recent research further indicates that chronic stress-induced increases in norepinephrine levels ultimately result in increased production of inflammatory leukocytes that adhere to vessel walls and promote the development of plaque.[45,50] Proteases released from these inflammatory leukocytes further promote risk of myocardial infarction and stroke by weakening the fibrous cap of the plaque, which can promote plaque rupture.[45] In addition to a stress-induced increased risk of cardiovascular disease, the effects of stress on inflammatory cytokine secretion also influence depression, autoimmune disorders, and virally mediated cancers,[51,52] and may be important in functional decline that leads to frailty, disability, and untimely death.[30,53] Finally, stress-induced excessive levels of inflammatory cytokines during infection or inflammatory illness may activate a collection of nonspecific symptoms called the "sickness syndrome."

Parasympathetic Nervous System

The parasympathetic system balances the sympathetic nervous system and thus also influences adaptation or maladaptation to stressful events. The parasympathetic system generally opposes the sympathetic system; for example, the parasympathetic nervous system slows the heart rate. The parasympathetic system also has anti-inflammatory effects.[47] Under conditions of allostatic overload, the parasympathetic system may decrease its containment of the sympathetic system, resulting in increased or prolonged inflammatory responses.[3] Researchers evaluate the relative balance of the parasympathetic and sympathetic nervous systems using a technique known as heart rate variability (the measurement of R wave variability from heartbeat to heartbeat).

Histamine and Other Hormones

The immune system is integrated with other physiological processes and is sensitive to changes in CNS and endocrine functioning, such as those that accompany psychological states.[54,55] Stressors can elicit the stress response through the action of the nervous and endocrine systems, specifically CRH from the hypothalamus and from peripheral inflammatory sites (called *peripheral [immune] CRH*).[56,57] **Peripheral (immune) CRH** is proinflammatory, causing an increase in vasodilation and vascular permeability. Therefore, it appears that mast cells are the target of peripheral CRH. Mast cells release histamine, which is a well-known mediator of acute inflammation and allergic reactions (Figure 9-6). Histamine induces acute inflammation and allergic reactions while suppressing Th1 activity (decreasing innate immunity) and promoting Th2 activity (increasing adaptive immunity).[58-61]

Thyroid hormone synthesis, which is involved in growth and reproduction, is suppressed during stress, which may conserve energy. **Neuropeptide Y (NPY)**, a sympathetic neurotransmitter, has recently been shown to be a stress mediator. Because NPY is a growth factor for many cells, it is implicated in atherosclerosis and tissue remodelling. Other hormones that influence the stress response are listed in Table 9-4.

Locally, stress can exert proinflammatory or anti-inflammatory effects. Moreover, some evidence indicates that stress is not a uniform, nonspecific reaction.[62] Different types of stressors might have variable effects on the immune response. Thus, stress may systemically cause a decrease in innate immunity and enhance adaptive immunity, whereas locally, under certain conditions, it can induce proinflammatory activities that may influence the onset and cause of infection, autoimmune/inflammatory, and allergic responses. In summary, stress can activate

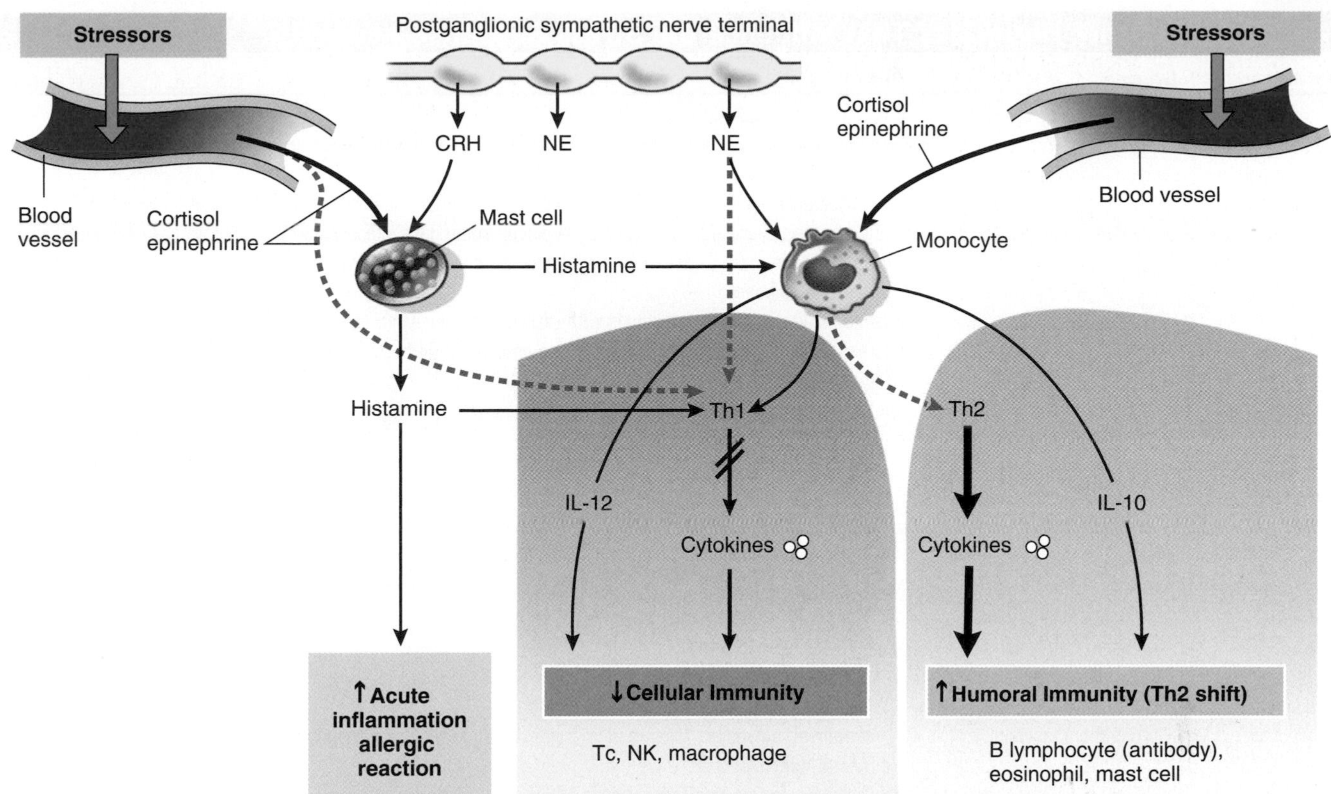

FIGURE 9-6 Effect of Corticotropin-Releasing Hormone–Mast Cell–Histamine Axis, Cortisol, and Catecholamines on the Th1/Th2 Balance—Innate and Adaptive Immunity. Adaptive immunity provides protection against multicellular parasites, extracellular bacteria, some viruses, soluble toxins, and allergens. Innate immunity provides protection against intracellular bacteria, fungi, protozoa, and several viruses. Type 1 cytokines or proinflammatory cytokines include IL-12, IFN-γ, and TNF-α. Type 2 cytokines or anti-inflammatory cytokines include IL-10 and IL-4. Solid lines (*black*) represent stimulation, whereas dashed lines (*blue*) represent inhibition (i.e., Th1 and Th2 are mutually inhibitory, IL-12 and IFN-γ inhibit Th2, and vice versa; IL-4 and IL-10 inhibit Th1 responses). Stress and CRH modulate inflammatory/immune and allergic responses by stimulating cortisol (glucocorticoid), catecholamines, and peripheral (immune) CRH secretion and by changing the production of regulatory cytokines and histamines. *CRH* (peripheral, immune), corticotropin-releasing hormone; *IFN-γ*, interferon-gamma; *IL*, interleukin; *NE*, norepinephrine; *NK*, natural killer cell; *Tc*, T-cytotoxic cell; *Th*, T-helper cell; *TNF-α*, tumour necrosis factor-alpha; *dashed lines*, decreased (inhibited); *solid lines*, increased (stimulation). (Reprinted from *Trends in Endocrinology & Metabolism,* 10(9), Elenkov, I.J., & Chrousos, G.P., "Stress hormones, Th1/Th2 patterns, pro/anti-inflammatory cytokines and susceptibility to disease," Pages 359–368, Copyright 1999, with permission from Elsevier.)

TABLE 9-4 Other Hormones That Influence the Stress Response

Hormone	Source	Action
β-Endorphins (endogenous opiates)	Pituitary and hypothalamus	They activate endorphin (opiate) receptors on peripheral sensory nerves, leading to pain relief or analgesia. Hemorrhage increases levels to inhibit blood pressure or delay compensatory changes that would increase blood pressure.[a]
Growth hormone (somatotropin)	Anterior pituitary gland	It affects protein, lipid, and carbohydrate metabolism. It counters the effects of insulin. It is involved in tissue repair. It may participate in growth and function of immune system.[b] Levels increase after a variety of stressful stimuli (cardiac catheterization, electroshock therapy, gastroscopy, surgery, fever, physical exercise). Increased levels are associated with psychological stimuli (taking examinations, viewing violent or sexually arousing films, participating in certain psychological performance tests). Prolonged stress (chronic stress) suppresses growth hormone.
Prolactin	Anterior pituitary gland; numerous extrapituitary tissue sites[c]	It increases in response to many stressful stimuli (including procedures such as gastroscopy, proctoscopy, pelvic examination, and surgery).[d] It is increased for in situ breast cancer.[e] It requires more intense stimuli than those leading to increases in catecholamine or cortisol levels. Levels show little change after exercise.

Continued

TABLE 9-4 Other Hormones That Influence the Stress Response—cont'd

Hormone	Source	Action
Oxytocin	Hypothalamus	It promotes bonding and social attachment.[f] In animals, it is associated with reduced hypothalamic-pituitary-adrenal activation levels and reduced anxiety.[f]
Testosterone	Leydig cells in testes	It regulates male secondary sex characteristics and libido. Levels decrease after stressful stimuli (anaesthesia, surgery, marathon running, mountain climbing).[g] It is decreased by psychological stimuli; however, some data indicate that psychological stress associated with competition (e.g., pistol shooting) increases both testosterone and cortisol levels, especially in athletes older than 45 years.[h] It is markedly reduced in individuals with respiratory failure, burns, and heart failure.[i] Decreased levels occur during aging and are associated with lowered cortisol responsiveness to stress-induced inflammation.[j]
Estrogen	Ovaries	It works in concert with oxytocin, exerting calming effect during stressful situations.[k]
Melatonin	Produced by pineal gland	It increases during stress response. Release is suppressed by light and increased in dark. Receptors have been identified on lymphoid cells, possibly higher density of receptors on T cells than on B cells. Suppression of lymphocyte function by trauma was reversed by melatonin.[l]
Somatostatin (SOM)	Produced by sensory nerve terminals found in and released from lymphoid cells and hypothalamus	Natural killer function and immunoglobulin synthesis are decreased by SOM. Growth hormone secretion is decreased by SOM.
Vasoactive intestinal peptide (VIP)	Found in neurons of CNS and in peripheral nerves	VIP increases during stress. VIP-containing nerves are located in both primary and secondary lymphoid tissues, around blood vessels, and in gastro-intestinal tract. VIP receptors are on both T and B cells; VIP may influence lymphocyte maturation. Cytokine production by T cells is modified by VIP; and B-cell and antibody production is influenced by VIP.
Calcitonin gene–related peptide (CGRP)	Found in spinal cord motor neurons and in sensory neurons near dendritic cells of skin and in primary and secondary lymphoid tissues	CGRP receptors are present on T and B lymphocytes (T cells and B cells); thus it is likely that CGRP can modulate immune function. CGRP may enhance acute inflammatory response because it is a vasodilator. Maturation of immune B cells is inhibited by CGRP; and IL-1 is inhibited by CGRP, which is important for activation of T cells. It has been shown to interfere with lymphocyte activation.
Neuropeptide Y (NPY)	Present in neurons of CNS and in neurons throughout body; colocalized in nerve terminals in lymphatic tissues with norepinephrine	Lymphocytes have receptors for NPY and thus may modulate their function.[m] Several lines of evidence suggest that NPY is a neurotransmitter and neurohormone involved in stress response. Increased levels of NPY occur in plasma in response to severe or prolonged stress; may be responsible for stress-induced regional vasoconstriction (splanchnic, coronary, and cerebral); and may also increase platelet aggregation.[b] It may be important in preventing depression.
Substance P (SP)	Produced by neuropeptide classified as tachykinin (increases heart rate subsequent to lowering blood pressure) found in brain, as well as nerves innervating secondary lymphoid tissues	SP increases in response to stress. Receptors for SP are found on membranes of both T and B cells, mononuclear phagocytic cells, and mast cells. Proinflammatory activity induces release of histamine from mast cells during stress response. It causes smooth muscle contraction, causes macrophages and T cells to release cytokines, and increases antibody production.

[a]Amico, J.A., Mantella, R.C., Vollmer, R.R., et al. (2004). *J Neuroendocrinol, 16*(4), 319–324.
[b]Rabin, B.S. (1999). The nervous system—immune system connection. In *Stress, immune function, and health: The connection.* New York: Wiley-Liss.
[c]Cacioppo, J.T., Berntson, G.G., Malarkey, W.B., et al. (1998). *Ann N Y Acad Sci, 840*, 664–673.
[d]Rohleder, N., Kudielka, B.M., Hellhammer, D.H., et al. (2002). *J Neuroimmunol, 126*(1–2), 69–77.
[e]Tikk, K., Sookthai, D., Fortner, R.T., et al. (2015). *Breast Cancer Research, 17*(1), 49.
[f]Lieberwirth, C., & Wang, Z. (2014). *Front Neurosci, 8*, 171.
[g]Chesnokova, V., & Melmed, S. (2002). *Endocrinology, 143*(5), 1571–1574.
[h]Guezennec, C.Y., Lafarge, J.P., Bricout, V.A., et al. (1995). *Int J Sports Med, 16*(6), 368–372.
[i]Volterrani, M., Rosano, G., & Iallamo, F. (2012). *Endocrine, 42*(2), 272–277.
[j]Bauer-Wu, S.M. (2002). *Clin J Oncol Nurs, 6*(4), 243–246.
[k]Kudwa, A.E., McGivern, R.F., & Handa, R.J. (2014). *Physiol Behav, 129*, 287–296.
[l]Maestroni, G.J. (1999). *Adv Exp Med Biol, 460*, 396.
[m]Petitto, J.M., Huang, Z., & McCarthy, D.B. (1994). *J Neuroimmunol, 54*, 81–86.

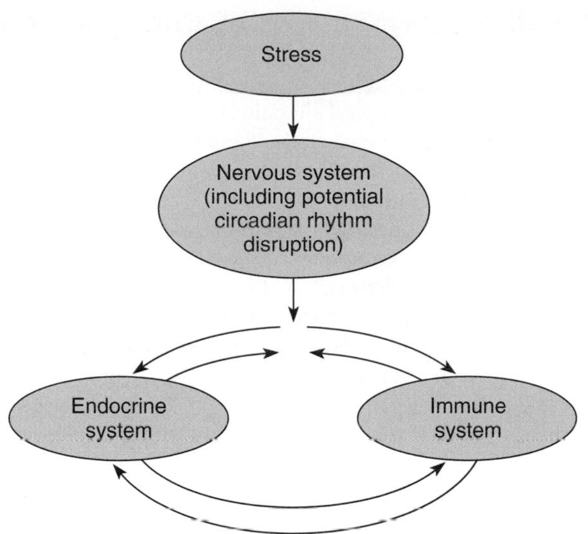

FIGURE 9-7 Nervous System/Endocrine System/Immune System Interactions. Interconnections or pathways of communication among the immune, nervous, and endocrine systems.

an excessive immune response and, through cortisol and the catecholamines, suppress Th1 responses while enhancing Th2 responses.

Role of the Immune System

The immune, nervous, and endocrine systems communicate through similar (and highly complex) pathways using hormones, neurotransmitters, neuropeptides, and immune cell products.[36] Various components of immune system responses are affected by neuroendocrine-produced factors involved in the stress reaction. Conversely, immune cell–derived cytokines and other products affect neurocrine and endocrine cells.[54,63,64] Several pathways regulate communication among these systems (Figure 9-7).

Stress-induced secretion of HPA hormones and catecholamines of the ANS sympathetic branch directly influences the immune system. Immune cells have receptors for ACTH, CRH, endorphins, norepinephrine, growth hormone, steroids, and other products of the stress response.[55] In addition, cholinergic, adrenergic, and peptidergic nerves innervate lymphoid organs, such as the thymus, spleen, lymph nodes, and bone marrow.[63] Exposure to stress increases endogenous opiate secretion to enhance or suppress immune cell functions in a concentration-dependent manner (see Table 9-4).[63,65-68]

Lymphocytes also produce ACTH and endorphins in small amounts that influence the immune response in an autocrine (same cell stimulation) or paracrine (cell to cell) manner in ongoing immune and memory cytotoxic responses.[63,69,70] The T-cell growth factor interleukin-2 (IL-2) can upregulate pituitary ACTH. Immune-derived cytokines have direct and indirect effects on HPA and adrenal cell functions. Thus, the immune system has an adaptive role as a signal organ to alert other systems of internally threatening stimuli (e.g., infection, tissue damage, tumour cells). The release of immune inflammatory mediators (IL-6, tumour necrosis factor-beta [TNF-β], interferon) is triggered by bacterial or viral infections, cancer, tissue injury, and other stressors that in turn initiate a stress response through the HPA pathway. Enhanced systemic production of these cytokines also induces other CNS and behaviour changes during an acute infectious episode.[71-74]

Although acute stress activates HPA hormone secretion and immune system products, such as interleukin-1 (IL-1), continued stress-induced secretion of glucocorticoids inhibits production of IL-1 by activated macrophages and monocytes.[63,75] Prolonged severe stress may lead to enlargement of the adrenal gland with simultaneous involution of the thymus and lymph nodes. Increased secretion of glucocorticoids may be an important mechanism underlying stress-related immune structure alterations and suppression of the immune response.[54]

In addition to the HPA and sympathetic nervous system, the pineal gland regulates the immune response and mediates the effects of circadian rhythm on immunity. When melatonin production by the pineal gland is blocked (by continuous light or by pharmacological means), the immune response is suppressed, whereas administration of melatonin reverses these effects.[76] This immunomodulation pathway may effect immune changes found with sleep disturbance and dysregulated circadian rhythm,[77] which are common among acutely ill, stressed persons.

In summary, neuropeptides and hormones have significant effects on the immune system. Whether this impact on immune system functions is suppressive or potentiating depends on the type of factor secreted (some factors enhance, some suppress, and some both enhance and suppress), the concentration and length of exposure, and the target cell.[74] Neuropeptides and neuroendocrine hormones may directly control biochemical events affecting cell proliferation, differentiation, and function or may indirectly control immune cell behaviour by affecting the production or activity of cytokines.[63,64] Chronic stress affects many immune cell functions, including decreased NK-cell and T-cell cytotoxicity and impaired B-cell function.[31,70] Importantly, these impairments in the immune system may have negative health consequences for stressed individuals, such as increased risk of infection and some types of cancer.[78,79] Common pathophysiological origins relating to chronic inflammatory processes include cardiovascular disease, osteoporosis, arthritis, type 2 diabetes mellitus, chronic obstructive pulmonary disease, other diseases associated with aging, and some cancers; all are characterized by the prolonged presence of proinflammatory cytokines.[15,80]

It is important to note that although inflammation is a normal response and considered beneficial, excessive inflammation can damage tissue. Stress and negative emotions are associated directly with the production of increased levels of proinflammatory cytokines, providing a link between stress, immune function, and disease.[81-83]

STRESS, PERSONALITY, COPING, AND ILLNESS

Extreme physiological stressors, such as severe burn injury, represent a predictable stimulus for stress responses. A less severe and defined event or situation, however, can be a stressor for one person and not for another. As discussed previously, stress itself is not an independent entity but a system of interdependent processes moderated by the nature, intensity, and duration of the stressor and the perception, appraisal, and coping efficacy of the affected individual, all of which in turn mediate the psychological and physiological response to stress. Further, adjustment to repetitive stressors is known to be individualized, based on a person's appraisal of a situation.[26] Illustrating the influence of an individualized stress appraisal on physiological processes, a meta-analysis of the relationship between stressors and immunity found that a higher perception of stress was associated with reduced Tc-cell cytotoxicity, although not with levels of circulating Th cells or Tc cells.

Psychosocial distress may be predictive of psychological, social, and physical health outcomes (see *Health Promotion:* Acute Emotional Stress and Adverse Heart Effects). A psychologically distressed individual may experience a general stress-induced state of unpleasant arousal that manifests as physiological, emotional, cognitive, and behaviour changes.[84] Periods of depression and emotional upheaval associated with adverse life events may place the affected individual at increased risk for immunological deficits accompanied by ill health.[54] For example, studies showed a relationship between depression and reduction in lymphocyte proliferation and NK-cell activity.[85] Multiple moderating factors may be important in immune modulation in depressed individuals, including alcoholism and other lifestyle factors, such as social support. Examples of triggering circumstances include bereavement, academic pressures, and marital conflict. Aging also may increase psychosocial distress and is associated with immune changes (see *Health Promotion:* Partner's Survival and Spouse's Hospitalizations and/or Death).[80,81]

HEALTH PROMOTION

Acute Emotional Stress and Adverse Heart Effects

Myocardial Ischemia

- Individuals with coronary heart disease may develop myocardial ischemia during mental or acute emotional stress even though their exercise or chemical nuclear test results are negative.
- Systemic vascular resistance increases during periods of mental or acute emotional stress with concomitant increased myocardial oxygen demand.

Left Ventricular Dysfunction

- More evidence for left ventricular dysfunction exists in older women.
- After acute emotional stress or trauma, there is an increase in sudden chest pain and shortness of breath.
- Left ventricular dysfunction is more common in the cardiac apex.
- Alterations are possibly a result of increased levels of catecholamines.

Ventricular Dysrhythmias

- Intense or unusual acute stress precipitates about 20% of serious ventricular dysrhythmias or sudden cardiac death.
- Altered brain activity may lead to changes in ventricular repolarization and electrical instability of the cardiac muscle.

Data from Pimple, P., Shah, A., Rooks, C., et al. (2015). *Am Heart J, 169*(1), 115–121; Ramadan, R., Sheps, D., Esteves, F., et al. (2013). *J Am Heart Assoc, 2*(5), e000321; Wei, J., Rooks, C., Ramadan, R., et al. (2014). *Am J Cardiol, 114*(2), 187–192; Wittstein, I.S., Thiemann, D.R., Lima, J.A.C., et al. (2005). *N Engl J Med, 352*(6), 539–548; Ziegelstein, R.C. (2007). *JAMA, 298*(3), 324–329.

HEALTH PROMOTION

Partner's Survival and Spouse's Hospitalizations and/or Death

A Harvard study shows that a spouse's chances of dying increase not only when the partner dies but also when that partner becomes seriously ill. The 9-year follow-up study consisted of 518 240 older adult couples. Mortality after the partner's hospitalization varied according to the spouse's diagnosis. For older adults whose spouse had been hospitalized, the short-term risk of dying approached that of an older adult after his or her spouse's death. A wife's hospitalization increased her husband's chances of dying within 1 month by 35%; a husband's hospitalization increased his wife's chances of dying by 44%. Likewise, a wife's death increased her partner's 1-month mortality risk by 53%, and a husband's death raised his partner's risk by 61%. The researchers commented that a spouse's illness or death can increase a partner's mortality by causing severe stress and removing a primary source of emotional, psychological, practical, and financial support.

Data from Carey, F.M., Shah, S.M., DeWilde, S., et al. (2014). *JAMA Int Med, 174*(4), 598–605; Christakis, N.A., & Allison, P.D. (2006). *N Engl J Med, 354*(7), 719–730.

Personality characteristics are associated with differences in appraisal and response to stressors. Specific personality characteristics, such as academic achievement, motivation, optimism, and aggression, are correlated with immunological alterations. For example, aggression is positively associated with changes in T- and B-cell numbers in male military personnel. In addition, optimism, perceived stress, and anxiety enhance responses to influenza vaccinations after age 50.[68,86]

Stressful life events and mood are important factors that exacerbate symptoms in acquired immunodeficiency syndrome (AIDS) infection, diabetes, and multiple sclerosis.[64,87,88] In addition, the interaction with health care providers in a clinical setting, the diagnosis of a major illness, and the process of undergoing various clinical procedures (e.g., blood sampling, injections, examinations, surgical procedures) may represent significant negative life events to many individuals (Figure 9-8). These additional stresses may interfere with the efficacy of the medical intervention. Identifying and reducing stress in the clinical setting have particular applicability for both preventing disease and managing illness.

Many studies have linked severe psychosocial stress resulting from negative life events to chronic disorders with mental and physical consequences. A life-threatening event may lead to the development of PTSD.[89-92] Early research with breast cancer survivors demonstrated a link between sympathetic activity and HPA-axis activation, noting that some women reported symptoms of PTSD (heart palpitations, panic, shakiness, nausea) when they thought about cancer recurrence or when they found themselves near the hospital where treatment began.[93] Furthermore, the threat of cancer recurrence (using a simulated mammography event as a stressor to elicit thoughts of cancer recurrence) elicited greater alterations in heart rate variability when compared with another simulated controlled stressor.[94] These studies show a connection between re-exposure to mammography, which occurred repeatedly throughout breast cancer survivorship, and activation of the ANS.

These uncontrolled stressful events may negatively affect the course of illness and interfere with the efficacy of the medical intervention. Identifying and reducing stress in the clinical setting have particular applicability in both disease prevention and illness management. In addition to medical procedures, patient–provider communication provides an important area for future research. Recent studies of cancer communication and patient–provider interaction indicate a link between communication events and emotional outcomes, such as uncertainty and mood state in breast cancer survivors.[95,96]

Coping

Coping is the process of managing stressful challenges that tax the individual's resources.[67] Coping responses may be adaptive or maladaptive, and the extent to which an individual responds to distress, using effective positive coping strategies, determines the degree of successful moderation of the stress challenge. For example, studies are beginning to support a role for stress reduction in slowing human immunodeficiency virus (HIV) progression.[41,45,51,97] Other investigations are under way to determine the benefits offered by exercise and mindfulness, as well as others, such as inclusion of green space in urban environments.[30] Studies also are focusing on mediating factors that influence stress susceptibility or resilience, such as age, socioeconomic status, gender, social support, religious or spiritual factors, personality, self-esteem, genetics, past experiences, and current health status (Figure 9-9).[98]

Coping strategies are especially beneficial when they are problem-focused and individuals seek social support.[67,76] Evidence suggests that effective interventions may result in greater stress resilience and improved psychological and physiological outcomes.[99] For example, women with

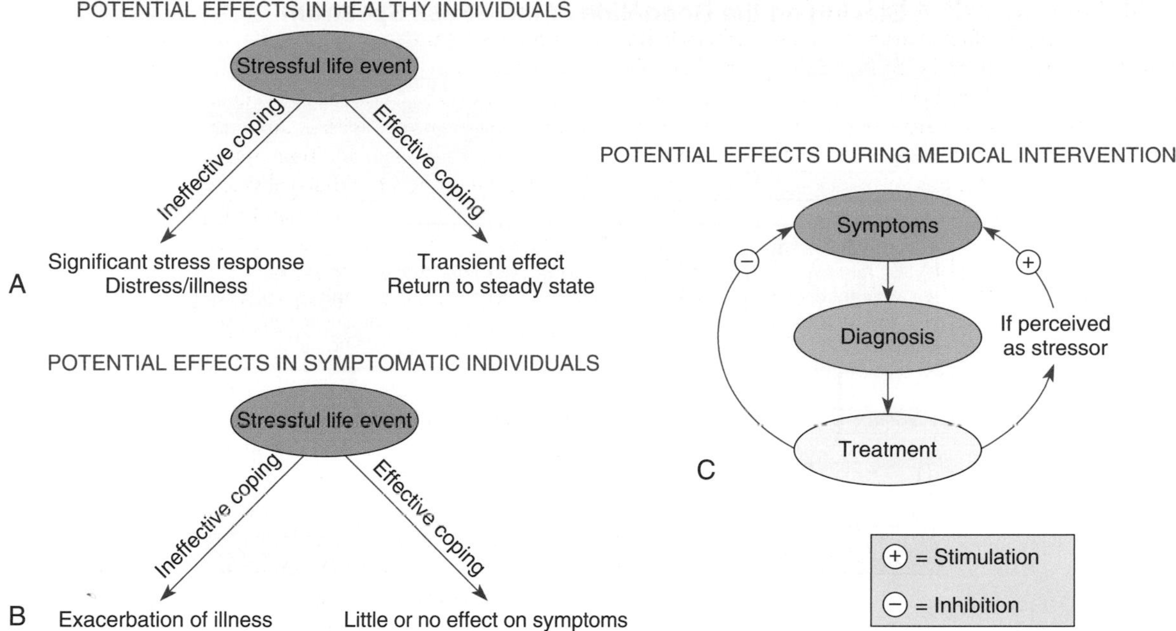

FIGURE 9-8 Health Outcome Determination in Stressful Life Situations Is Moderated by Numerous Factors. Whether a life-challenged individual experiences distress or illness depends on the person's appraisal of the event and the coping strategies used during the stressful period. Models **(A)** and **(B)** reflect possible outcomes in stressed healthy and symptomatic individuals. Model **(C)** illustrates the dynamic clinical setting in which the diagnosis of a serious illness and subsequent medical interventions may be perceived as stressful challenges and have potentially detrimental influences on physical outcome.

recurrent metastatic breast cancer and provided weekly group counselling in conjunction with routine medical treatment lived an average of 19 months longer than control subjects, suggesting a positive influence of group support for these women.[74,76]

Maladaptive coping can result in a change in behaviour contributing to potentially adverse health effects (e.g., increased smoking, change in eating habits). Serious disturbances of the sleep–wake cycle observed in many stressed people and in experimental and many clinical settings[33,100] may exacerbate the pathophysiological status of some individuals.[101-103] Sleep deprivation and circadian disruption, even in young, otherwise healthy individuals, have detrimental influences on respiratory and immune system function. Even partial sleep deprivation was associated with reduced NK-cell activity in healthy subjects, and only recently have seriously ill individuals been assessed for adequacy and structure of sleep during recovery.[101]

Behavioural styles, such as overcommitment to employment-related tasks, repression, denial, escape–avoidance, and concealment, are associated with altered immune functions.[55,104] Repression is associated with lower monocyte counts, higher eosinophil counts, higher serum glucose levels, and more self-reported medication reactions in medical outpatients,[77] and with higher Epstein-Barr virus antibody titres in students.[75] A prospective long-term study also found increased markers of accelerated HIV infection in gay men who concealed their homosexual identity.[64] Schoolteachers who devoted long hours without reward and who were unable to disengage from work-related tasks were found to have lowered innate immune responses.[104]

The importance of social support for seriously ill individuals also needs to be considered in the health of caregivers. Significant stress manifested as depression, anxiety, and fatigue has been noted in family caregivers of those with cancer, Alzheimer's disease, and burn trauma.[105] Enhanced social support of caregivers improves measures of immune function.[65,66,76,106,107]

Interventions to potentially prevent or manage stress-related psychological or physical problems include both short- and long-term education on evaluating and adopting effective coping strategies. Approaches may be used or investigated on an individual or group basis. Incorporation of effective stress management approaches into clinical education facilitates their use in the clinical arena. Future research could focus on the efficacy of such approaches with different populations because it is clear one size does not fit all (coping of cancer survivors may be vastly different from coping of combat veterans).

In summary, the mind and body are connected through a multitude of complex physical and emotional interactions.[108] Understanding the complexity of these interactions is a challenge for researchers. Areas of promise include investigating relationships between the effects of stress on illness, as well as developing effective stress management techniques and approaches that improve health outcomes.

QUICK CHECK 9-2

1. Define the *hypothalamic-pituitary-adrenal axis.*
2. Define *psychoneuroimmunology.*
3. How does the immune system participate in stress-related diseases?
4. Why do stress-related diseases occur?
5. What intervention or prevention activities reduce stress-related diseases?

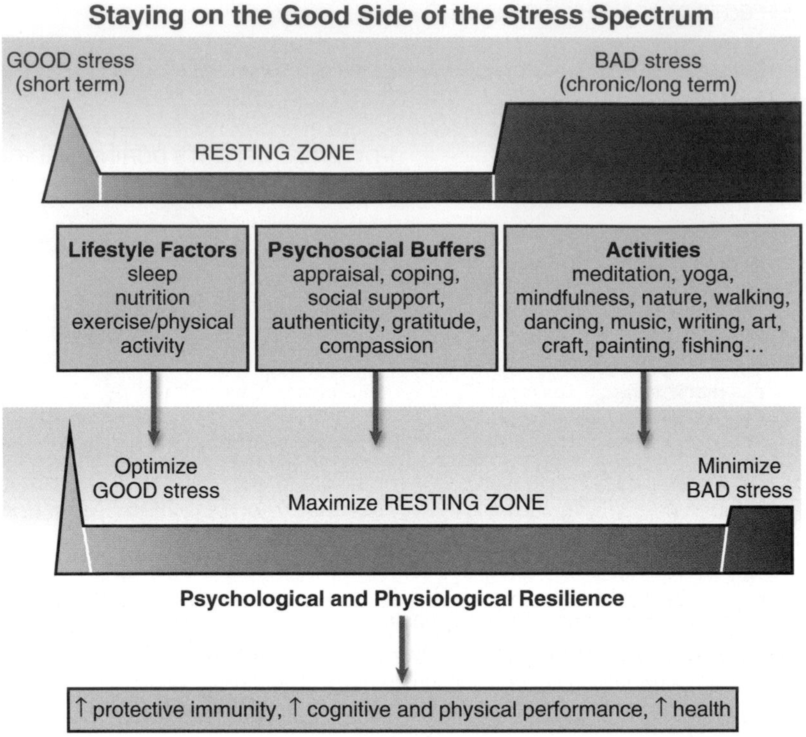

Staying on the Good Side of the Stress Spectrum

GOOD stress (short term) | RESTING ZONE | BAD stress (chronic/long term)

Lifestyle Factors	**Psychosocial Buffers**	**Activities**
sleep nutrition exercise/physical activity	appraisal, coping, social support, authenticity, gratitude, compassion	meditation, yoga, mindfulness, nature, walking, dancing, music, writing, art, craft, painting, fishing...

Optimize GOOD stress | Maximize RESTING ZONE | Minimize BAD stress

Psychological and Physiological Resilience

↑ protective immunity, ↑ cognitive and physical performance, ↑ health

FIGURE 9-9 Staying on the Good Side of the Stress Spectrum. GOOD stress is shown on the left of the spectrum and involves a rapid biological response to the stressor, followed by a rapid shutdown of the response upon cessation of the stressor. These responses support physiological conditions that are likely to enhance protective immunity, cognitive and physical performance, and overall health. BAD stress, represented on the right of the spectrum, involves exposure to chronic or long-term biological changes that are likely to result in dysregulation or suppression of immune function, a decrease in cognitive and physical performance, and an increased likelihood of disease. Short-term stress or long-term stress (or both) is generally superimposed on a psychophysiological RESTING ZONE of low/no stress that also represents a state of health maintenance/restoration. To maintain health, one needs to optimize GOOD stress, maximize the RESTING ZONE, and minimize BAD stress. Achieving psychological and physiological resilience involves a multipronged approach. Sleep of a quality and duration that helps one feel rested in the morning, a moderate and healthy diet, and consistent and moderate exercise or physical activity are three LIFESTYLE FACTORS that are likely to enable one to stay on the "good" side of the stress spectrum. Effective appraisal and coping mechanisms, genuine gratitude, social support, and compassion toward others and oneself are likely to provide PSYCHOSOCIAL BUFFERS against bad stress and enable one to stay on the "good" side of the stress spectrum. Additionally, depending on individual preferences, ACTIVITIES, such as, meditation, yoga, being in nature, exercise/physical activity, music, art, craft, dance, fishing, painting, also may reduce BAD stress, extend the RESTING ZONE, and optimize GOOD stress. Such personal activities are likely to involve different strokes for different folks and need not always be meditative or reflective in nature. (Adapted from Dhabhar, F.S., & McEwen, B.S. [2007]. Bidirectional effects of stress on immune function: Possible explanations for salubrious as well as harmful effects. In R. Ader [Ed.], *Psychoneuroimmunology IV*. San Diego: Elsevier.)

GERIATRIC CONSIDERATIONS

Aging and the Stress–Age Syndrome

With aging, sometimes a set of neurohormonal and immune alterations, as well as tissue and cellular changes, develop. These changes have been defined as stress–age syndrome and include the following:

- Alterations in the excitability of structures of the limbic system and hypothalamus
- Increase of the blood concentrations of catecholamines, ADH, ACTH, and cortisol
- Decrease of the concentrations of testosterone, thyroxine, and others
- Alterations of opioid peptides
- Immunodepression and pattern of chronic inflammation
- Alterations in lipoproteins
- Hypercoagulation of the blood
- Free radical damage of cells

Some of the alterations are adaptational, whereas others are potentially damaging. These stress-related alterations of aging can influence the course of developing stress reactions and lower adaptive reserve and coping capacity.

ACTH, adrenocorticotropic hormone; *ADH*, antidiuretic hormone.
Data from Frolkis, V.V. (1998). *Mech Ageing Dev, 69*(1–2), 93–107.

DID YOU UNDERSTAND?

Overview

1. Stress is broadly defined as a threat that is perceived or anticipated, resulting in interactions between the body and the brain (the stress response).

Historical Background and General Concepts

1. Cannon used the term *stress* in both a physiological and a psychological sense in 1914. The idea that stressful events could cause physiological responses was further developed by Selye in 1946. Selye's work demonstrated that internal or external stressors could result in adrenal gland enlargement, immune alterations (increased leukocytes), and gastro-intestinal manifestations (ulcers). These global physiological responses were labelled the general adaptation syndrome (GAS).
2. GAS occurs in three stages: the alarm stage, the resistance or adaptation stage, and the exhaustion stage (now referred to as *allostatic overload*). Diseases of adaptation develop if the resistance or adaptation stage does not restore homeostasis. Although important, the concept that stress is entirely the result of a physical disturbance is greatly oversimplified.
3. Continuing the evolution of this research, adrenal gland hormone responses to stressors were suggested in the 1950s and central nervous system (CNS) and endocrine responses were proposed in the 1970s.
4. Psychological stressors can be anticipatory and triggered by expectations of an upcoming stressor or can be reactive to a stressor. Both of these psychological stressors are capable of eliciting a physiological stress response.
5. The study of the body's response to stressors continues to evolve and has become known by the term *psychoneuroimmunology* (PNI).
6. The concepts of allostasis (stability through change; monitoring the environment for adaptive response) and homeostasis (return to base levels reflecting an unchanging set point) both indicate physiological responses. Allostatic overload can occur when there is overactivation of adaptive responses that may in turn increase susceptibility to disease.
7. The stress response is initiated when a stressor is present in the body or perceived by the mind. Psychological stress may cause or worsen several diseases or disorders, including anxiety, depression, insomnia, persistent pain and fatigue syndromes, obesity, metabolic syndrome, essential hypertension, type 2 diabetes, atherosclerosis and its cardiovascular consequences, osteoporosis, and autoimmune inflammatory and allergic disorders. A classic example of stress and allostatic overload is sleep alteration and the associated damaging effects of elevated evening cortisol, insulin, and glucose.

The Stress Response

1. The stress response involves the nervous system (sympathetic branch of the autonomic nervous system), the endocrine system (pituitary and adrenal glands), and the immune system. More simply, these relationships are often cited together as the hypothalamic-pituitary-adrenal (HPA) axis.
2. The physiology of managing stressful events is complex, involving mechanisms of both protection and injury. The two major stress regulation systems are the autonomic nervous system (ANS) and the HPA system.
3. Activation of the ANS consists of sympathetic stimulation of the adrenal medulla and nerve endings to rapidly secrete catecholamines (norepinephrine, epinephrine, neuropeptide Y).
4. Activation of the HPA system involves sequential secretion of corticotropin-releasing hormone from the hypothalamus, which stimulates receptors in the anterior pituitary to secrete adrenocorticotropic hormone (ACTH) that, in turn, stimulates the adrenal cortex to secrete glucocorticoids, particularly cortisol.
5. Glucocorticoids reach all tissues, including the brain, easily penetrate cell membranes, and react with numerous intracellular glucocorticoid receptors. Because they spare almost no tissue or organ and influence a large proportion of the human genome, they broadly exert diverse biological actions. For example, glucocorticoids have an important modulatory role in the CNS. These hormones regulate memory, cognition, mood, and sleep and influence many other body systems.
6. In general, catecholamines of the sympathetic system prepare the body to act; for example, cortisol mobilizes glucose (for energy) and other substances.
7. Cortisol is the primary glucocorticoid produced during stress.
8. Cortisol's chief effects involve metabolic processes. By inhibiting the use of metabolic substances while promoting their formation, cortisol mobilizes glucose, amino acids, lipids, and fatty acids and delivers them to the bloodstream. As an example, anabolic effects of cortisol increase the rate of protein synthesis in the liver, whereas the catabolic effects of cortisol increase levels of amino acids, ultimately depleting protein stores in muscle, bone, skin, and connective tissue.
9. Cortisol contributes to elevated blood glucose and inhibits glucose uptake by body cells providing energy to combat perceived or anticipated stressors.
10. Chronic dysregulation of the HPA axis, especially abnormal elevated levels of cortisol, has been linked to a wide variety of disorders, including obesity, sleep deprivation, lipid abnormalities, hypertension, diabetes, atherosclerosis, and loss of bone density.
11. Glucocorticoids contribute to the development of metabolic syndrome and the pathogenesis of obesity. They can directly cause insulin resistance and influence genetic variations that predispose to obesity.
12. The impact of cortisol on fetal development and subsequent risk of future disease is being considered.
13. Elevated levels of glucocorticoids and catecholamines (epinephrine and norepinephrine), both endogenous and exogenous (synthetic pharmaceuticals), may decrease innate immunity and increase autoimmune responses. However, prolonged effects of cortisol may accentuate inflammation. Overall, stress activates an excessive immune response and, through cortisol and the catecholamines, suppresses Th1 responses while enhancing Th2 responses.
14. Glucocorticoids from the adrenal cortex, in response to ACTH from the pituitary gland, comprise the major stress hormones along with the catecholamines epinephrine and norepinephrine.
15. Norepinephrine's chief effects complement those of epinephrine. Norepinephrine constricts blood vessels of the viscera and skin; this has the effect of shifting blood flow to the vessels dilated by epinephrine. Norepinephrine also increases mental alertness.
16. Epinephrine exerts its chief effects on the cardiovascular system. Epinephrine increases cardiac output and increases blood flow to the heart, brain, and skeletal muscles by dilating vessels that supply these organs. It also dilates the airways, thereby increasing delivery of oxygen to the bloodstream.
17. The parasympathetic system balances or restrains the sympathetic system, resulting in slowed heart rates, and anti-inflammatory effects. During prolonged stress (allostatic overload) the parasympathetic system is less effective in opposing the sympathetic system.

18. Other hormones, including β-endorphins, growth hormone, prolactin, oxytocin, the steroid sex hormones, and antidiuretic hormone, influence the stress response by their diverse actions.

Stress, Personality, Coping, and Illness

1. Stress is a system of interdependent processes that are moderated by the nature, intensity, and duration of the stressor and the coping efficacy of the affected individual, all of which in turn mediate the psychological and physiological response to stress.
2. Personality characteristics are associated with individual differences in appraisal and response to stressors. Further, the appraisal of events as distressful may be predictive of psychological, social, and physical health outcomes (maladaptive coping, depression, post-traumatic stress disorder, heart disease, altered immunity).
3. Coping styles associated with altered immunity include repression, denial, escape–avoidance, and concealment. Coping strategies are more beneficial when they are problem-focused and may result in improved resilience and better psychological and physiological outcomes.

Geriatric Considerations: Aging and the Stress–Age Syndrome

1. With aging, often a set of neurohormonal and immune alterations, including tissue and cellular changes, occur. These changes are collectively called *stress–age syndrome*.
2. The changes are numerous, with some being adaptive whereas others are potentially damaging.
3. Coping techniques for managing stress may mitigate the effects of stress on maladaptive behaviours such as excessive alcohol ingestion and smoking, and, by extension, impact the effects of existing chronic illness.

KEY TERMS

Adrenocorticotropic hormone (ACTH), 220
Alarm stage (in GAS), 000
Allostasis, 219
Allostatic overload, 219
Anticipatory response, 217
Coping, 228
Corticotropin-releasing hormone (CRH), 220
Cortisol, 220
Diseases of adaptation, 217
Exhaustion stage (in GAS), 216
General adaptation syndrome (GAS), 216
Homeostasis, 216
Hypothalamic-pituitary-adrenal (HPA) system, 220
Neuropeptide Y (NPY), 224
Peripheral (immune) CRH, 224
Physiological stress, 216
Psychoneuroimmunology (PNI), 217
Reactive response, 217
Resistance or adaptation stage (in GAS), 216
Stressor, 216
Stress response, 216
Th1 to Th2 shift, 222

REFERENCES

1. McEwen, B. S. (2012). Brain on stress: How the social environment gets under the skin. *Proceedings of the National Academy of Sciences of the United States of America*, *109*, 17180–17185. doi:10.1073/pnas.1121254109.
2. Nicolaides, N. C., Charmandari, E., Chrousos, G. P., et al. (2014). Circadian endocrine rhythms: The hypothalamic-pituitary-adrenal axis and its actions. *Annals of the New York Academy of Sciences*, *1318*, 71–80. doi:10.1111/nyas.12464.
3. McEwen, B. S. (2008). Central effects of stress hormones in health and disease: Understanding the protective and damaging effects of stress and stress mediators. *European Journal of Pharmacology*, *583*(2–3), 174–185. doi:10.1016/j.ejphar.2007.11.071.
4. Dhabhar, F. S., Malarkey, W. B., Neri, E., et al. (2012). Stress induced redistribution of immune cells—From barracks to boulevards to battlefields: A tale of three hormones. *Psychoneuroendocrinology*, *37*, 1345–1368. doi:10.1016/j.psyneuen.2012.05.008.
5. Ulrich-Lai, Y. M., & Herman, J. P. (2009). Neural regulation of endocrine and autonomic stress responses. *Nature Reviews. Neuroscience*, *10*, 397–409. doi:10.1038/nrn2647.
6. Dhabhar, F. S., & McEwen, B. S. (1999). Enhancing versus suppressive effects of stress hormones on skin immune function. *Proceedings of the National Academy of Sciences of the United States of America*, *96*(3), 1059–1064.
7. Compare, A., Zarbo, C., Shonin, E., et al. (2014). Emotional regulation and depression: A potential mediator between heart and mind. *Cardiovascular Psychiatry and Neurology*, *2014*, 324374. doi:10.1155/2014/324374.
8. Peskind, E. R., Li, G., Shofer, J. B., et al. (2014). Influence of lifestyle modifications on age-related free radical injury to brain. *JAMA Neurology*, *71*(9), 150–154. doi:10.1001/jamaneurol.2014.1428.
9. Cannon, W. B., Binger, C. A. L., & Fitz, R. (1914). Experimental hyperthyroidism. *American Journal of Physiology*, *36*, 363.
10. Selye, H. (1946). The general adaptation syndrome and the diseases of adaptation. *Journal of Clinical Endocrinology*, *6*, 117–230.
11. Mason, J. W., & Brady, J. V. (1956). Plasma 17-hydroxycorticosteroid changes related to reserpine effects on emotional behaviors. *Science*, *124*, 983.
12. Hill, S. R., Goetz, F. C., Fox, H. M., et al. (1956). Studies on adrenocortical and psychological responses to stress in man. *Archives of Internal Medicine*, *97*, 269. doi:10.1001/archinte.1956.00250210015002.
13. Hetzel, B. S., Schottstaedt, W. W., Grace, W. J., et al. (1955). Changes in urinary 17-hydroxycorticosteroid excretion during stressful life experiences in man. *Journal of Clinical Endocrinology and Metabolism*, *15*(9), 1057–1068.
14. Mason, J. W. (1972). Organization of psychoendocrine mechanisms: A review and reconsideration of research. In N. S. Greenfield & R. A. Steinbach (Eds.), *Handbook of psychophysiology*. New York: Holt, Rinehart, & Winston.
15. Herman, J. P., Figueredo, H., Mueller, N. K., et al. (2003). Central mechanisms of stress integration: Hierarchical circuitry controlling hypothalamo-pituitary-adrenocortical responsiveness. *Frontiers in Neuroendocrinology*, *24*(3), 151–158.
16. Bauer-Wu, S. M. (2002). Psychoneuroimmunology. Part I: Physiology. *Clinical Journal of Oncology Nursing*, *6*(3), 167–170. doi:10.1188/02.CJON.167-170.
17. Bauer-Wu, S. M. (2002). Psychoneuroimmunology. Part II: Mind-body interventions. *Clinical Journal of Oncology Nursing*, *6*(4), 243–246. doi:10.1188/02.CJON.243-246.
18. Irwin, M. R. (2008). Human psychoneuroimmunology: 20 years of discovery. *Brain, Behavior, and Immunity*, *22*(2), 129–139. doi:10.1016/j.bbi.2007.07.013.
19. Ranchor, A. V., Sanderman, R., & Coyne, J. C. (2010). Invited commentary: Personality as a causal factor in cancer risk and mortality—Time to retire a hypothesis? *American Journal of Epidemiology*, *172*(4), 386–388. doi:10.1093/aje/kwq210.
20. Sloan, E. K., Priceman, S. J., Cox, B. F., et al. (2010). The sympathetic nervous system induces a metastatic switch in primary breast cancer. *Cancer Research*, *70*(18), 7042–7052. doi:10.1158/0008-5472.CAN-10-0522.
21. McVicar, A., Ravalier, J. M., & Greenwood, C. (2013). Biology of stress revisited: Intracellular mechanisms and the conceptualization of stress. *Stress Health*, *30*(4), 272–279. doi:10.1002/smi.2508.
22. Finnerty, C. C., Mabvuure, N. T., Ali, A., et al. (2013). The surgically induced stress response. *JPEN. Journal of Parenteral and Enteral Nutrition*, *37*(Suppl. 1), 21S–29S. doi:10.1177/0148607113496117.
23. Sterling, P., & Eyer, J. (1988). Allostasis: A new paradigm to explain arousal pathology. In S. Fisher & J. Reason (Eds.), *Handbook of life stress, cognition, and health* (pp. 629–649). New York: John Wiley and Sons.
24. Sterling, P. (2012). Allostasis: A model of predictive regulation. *Physiology and Behavior*, *106*, 5–15. doi:10.1016/j.physbeh.2011.06.004.
25. Schulkin, J. (2011). Social allostasis: Anticipatory regulation of the internal milieu. *Frontiers in Evolutionary Neuroscience*, *2*, e111. doi:10.3389/fnevo.2010.00111.
26. Dich, N., Doan, S. N., Kivimäki, M., et al. (2014). A non-linear association between self-reported negative emotional response to stress and subsequent allostatic load: Prospective results from the Whitehall II cohort study. *Psychoneuroendocrinology*, *49C*, 54–61. doi:10.1016/j.psyneuen.2014.07.001.
27. Seeman, T., Epel, E., Gruenewald, T., et al. (2010). Socio-economic differentials in peripheral biology: Cumulative allostatic load. *Annals of the New York Academy of Sciences*, *1186*, 223–239. doi:10.1111/j.1749-6632.2009.05341.x.
28. Chrousos, G. P., & Kino, T. (2009). Glucocorticoid signaling in the cell: Expanding clinical complications to complex human behavioral and

somatic disorders. *Annals of the New York Academy of Sciences, 1179*, 153–166. doi:10.1111/j.1749-6632.2009.04988.x.
29. Everson-Rose, S. A., Roetker, N. S., Lutsey, P. L., et al. (2014). Chronic stress, depressive symptoms, anger, hostility, and risk of stroke and transient ischemic attack in the multi-ethnic study of atherosclerosis. *Stroke; a Journal of Cerebral Circulation, 45*(8), 2318–2323. doi:10.1161/STROKEAHA.114.004815.
30. Jonker, M. F., van Lenthe, F. J., Donkers, B., et al. (2014). The effect of urban green on small-area (healthy) life expectancy. *Journal of Epidemiology and Community Health, 68*(10), 999–1002. doi:10.1136/jech-2014-203847.
31. Kiecolt-Glaser, J. K., McGuire, L., Robles, T. F., et al. (2002). Psychoneuroimmunology: Psychological influences on immune function and health. *Journal of Consulting and Clinical Psychology, 70*(3), 537–547.
32. Liu, L. Y., Coe, C. L., Swenson, C. A., et al. (2002). School examinations enhance airway inflammation to antigen challenge. *American Journal of Respiratory and Critical Care Medicine, 165*(8), 1062–1067. doi:10.1164/ajrccm.165.8.2109065.
33. Chen, X., Redline, S., Shields, A. E., et al. (2014). Associations of allostatic load with sleep apnea, insomnia, short sleep duration, and other sleep disturbances: Findings from the National Health and Nutrition Examination Survey 2005 to 2008. *Annals of Epidemiology, 24*(8), 612–619. doi:10.1016/j.annepidem.2014.05.014.
34. McEwen, B. S. (2006). Sleep deprivation as neurobiologic and physiologic stressor, allostasis and allostatic load. *Metabolism: Clinical and Experimental, 55*(10, Suppl. 2), S20–S23. doi:10.1016/j.metabol.2006.07.008.
35. Dhabhar, F. S. (2014). Effects of stress on immune function: The good, the bad, and the beautiful. *Immunologic Research, 58*, 193–210. doi:10.1007/s12026-014-8517-0.
36. Coutinho, A. E., & Chapman, K. E. (2011). The anti-inflammatory and immunosuppressive effects of glucocorticoids, recent developments and mechanistic insights. *Molecular and Cellular Endocrinology, 335*(1), 2–13. doi:10.1016/j.mce.2010.04.005.
37. Monaghan, P. (2014). Organismal stress, telomeres and life histories. *Journal of Experimental Biology, 217*(Pt. 1), 57–66. doi:10.1242/jeb.090043.
38. Martinac, M., Pehar, D., Karlovic, D., et al. (2014). Metabolic syndrome, activity of the hypothalamic-pituitary-adrenal axis and inflammatory mediators in depressive disorder. *Acta Clinica Croatica, 53*(1), 55–71.
39. Nakamura, A. (2015). Genotypes of the renin-angiotensin system and glucocorticoid complications. *Pediatrics International, 57*(1), 72–78. doi:10.1111/ped.12434.
40. Paredes, S., & Ribiero, L. (2014). Cortisol: The villain in metabolic syndrome? *Revista Da Associacao Medica Brasileira, 60*(1), 84–92.
41. Reynolds, R. M. (2013). Glucocorticoid excess and the developmental origins of disease: Two decades of testing the hypothesis—2012 Curt Richter award winner. *Psychoneuroendocrinology, 38*(1), 1–11. doi:10.1016/j.psyneuen.2012.08.012.
42. Kajantie, E., Feldt, K., Räikkönnen, K., et al. (2007). Body size at birth predicts hypothalamic-pituitary-adrenal axis response to psychosocial stress at 60 to 70 years. *Journal of Clinical Endocrinology and Metabolism, 92*(11), 4094–4100. doi:10.1210/jc.2007-1539.
43. Painter, R. C., Roseboom, T. J., & de Rooij, S. R. (2012). Long-term effects of prenatal stress and glucocorticoid exposure. *Birth Defects Research. Part C, Embryo Today: Reviews, 96*(4), 315–324. doi:10.1002/bdrc.21021.
44. Alevizaki, M., Cimponeriu, A., Lekakis, J., et al. (2007). High anticipatory stress plasma cortisol levels and sensitivity to glucocorticoids predict severity of coronary artery disease in subjects undergoing coronary angiography. *Metabolism: Clinical and Experimental, 56*(2), 222–226. doi:10.1016/j.metabol.2006.09.017.
45. Hanna, R. N., & Hedrick, C. C. (2014). Stressing out stem cells: Linking stress and hematopoiesis in cardiovascular disease. *Nature Medicine, 20*(7), 707–708. doi:10.1038/nm.3631.
46. Liddicoat, D. R., Kyparissoudis, K., Berzins, S. P., et al. (2014). The glucocorticoid receptor 1A3 promoter correlates with high sensitivity to glucocorticoid-induced apoptosis in human lymphocytes. *Immunology and Cell Biology, 92*(10), 825–836. doi:10.1038/icb.2014.57.
47. Sorrells, S. F., Caso, J. R., Munhoz, C. D., et al. (2009). The stressed CNS: When glucocorticoids aggravate inflammation (review). *Neuron, 64*(1), 33–39. doi:10.1016/j.neuron.2009.09.032.
48. Elenkov, I. J., Iezzoni, D. G., Daly, A., et al. (2005). Cytokine dysregulation, inflammation, and well-being. *Neuroimmunomodulation, 12*(5), 255–269. doi:10.1159/000087104.
49. Kim, M. H., Gorouhi, F., Ramirez, S., et al. (2014). Catecholamine stress alters neutrophil trafficking and impairs wound healing by β2-adrenergic receptor-mediated upregulation of IL-6. *Journal of Investigative Dermatology, 134*(3), 809–817. doi:10.1038/jid.2013.415.
50. Heidt, T., Sager, H. B., Courties, G., et al. (2014). Chronic variable stress activates hematopoietic stem cells. *Nature Medicine, 20*(7), 754–758. doi:10.1038/nm.3589.
51. Chhatre, S., Metzger, D. S., Frank, I., et al. (2013). Effects of behavioral stress reduction transcendental meditation intervention in persons with HIV. *AIDS Care, 25*(10), 1291–1297. doi:10.1080/09540121.2013.764396.
52. Heinzelmann-Schwarz, V. A., Kind, A. B., & Jacob, F. (2014). Management of human papillomavirus-related gynecological malignancies. *Current Problems in Dermatology, 45*, 216–224. doi:10.1159/000358408.
53. Brüünsgard, H., & Pedersen, B. K. (2003). Age-related inflammatory cytokines and disease. *Immunology and Allergy Clinics of North America, 23*(1), 15–39.
54. Shelby, J., Ku, W. W., & Nelson, H. C. (1996). Neurohormone and neuropeptide regulation of the post-traumatic immune response. In E. Faist (Ed.), *Host defense alterations of trauma, shock, and sepsis: Multi-organ failure/immunotherapy of sepsis*. Berlin: Pabst.
55. Sundar, S. K., Cierpial, M. A., Kilts, C., et al. (1990). Brain IL-1–induced immunosuppression occurs through activation of both pituitary-adrenal axis and sympathetic nervous system by corticotropin-releasing factor. *Journal of Neuroscience, 10*(11), 3701–3706.
56. Calcagni, E., & Elenkov, I. (2006). Stress system activity, innate and T helper cytokines, and susceptibility to immune-related diseases (review). *Annals of the New York Academy of Sciences, 1069*, 62–76. doi:10.1196/annals.1351.006.
57. Lagier, B., Lebel, B., Bousquet, J., et al. (1997). Different modulation by histamine of IL-4 and interferon-gamma (IFN-gamma) release according to the phenotype of human Th0, Th1, and Th2 clones. *Clinical and Experimental Immunology, 108*(3), 545–551.
58. Jochem, J., Josko, J., & Gwozdz, B. (2001). Endogenous opioid peptides system in haemorrhagic shock—Central cardiovascular regulation. *Medical Science Monitor, 7*(3), 545–549.
59. Molina, P. E. (2001). Opiate modulation of hemodynamic, hormonal, and cytokine responses to hemorrhage. *Shock (Augusta, Ga.), 15*(6), 471–478.
60. Molina, P. E. (2002). Stress-specific opioid modulation of haemodynamic counter-regulation. *Clinical and Experimental Pharmacology and Physiology, 29*(3), 248–253.
61. Rocklin, R. E. (Ed.), (1990). *Histamine and H2 antagonists in inflammation and immunodeficiency*. New York: Marcel Dekker.
62. Burguera, B., Muruais, C., Peñalva, A., et al. (1990). Dual and selective actions of glucocorticoid upon basal and stimulated growth hormone release in man. *Neuroendocrinology, 51*(1), 51–58.
63. Reiche, E. M. V., Nunes, S. O., & Morimoti, H. K. (2004). Stress, depression, the immune system, and cancer (review). *Lancet Oncology, 5*(10), 617–625. doi:10.1016/S1470-2045(04)01597-9.
64. Coyle, P. K. (1996). The neuroimmunology of multiple sclerosis. *Advances in Neuroimmunology, 6*(2), 143–154.
65. Baron, R. S., Cutrona, C. E., Hicklin, D., et al. (1990). Social support and immune function among spouses of cancer patients. *Journal of Personality and Social Psychology, 59*(2), 344–352.
66. Fawzy, F. I., Fawzy, N. W., Hyun, C. S., et al. (1993). Malignant melanoma: Effects of an early structured psychiatric intervention, coping, and affective state on recurrence and survival 6 years later. *Archives of General Psychiatry, 50*(9), 681–689.
67. Folkman, S., & Lazarus, R. S. (1988). The relationship between coping and emotion: Implications for theory and research. *Social Science and Medicine, 26*(3), 309–317.
68. Granger, D. A., Booth, A., & Johnson, D. R. (2000). Human aggression and enumerative measures of immunity. *Psychosomatic Medicine, 62*(4), 583–590.
69. Cole, S. W., Kemeny, M. E., Taylor, S. E., et al. (1996). Accelerated course of human immunodeficiency virus infection in gay men who conceal their homosexual identity. *Psychosomatic Medicine, 58*(3), 219–231.
70. Johnson, E. W., Hughes, T. K., Jr., & Smith, E. M. (2005). ACTH enhancement of T-lymphocyte cytotoxic responses. *Cellular and Molecular Neurobiology, 25*(3–4), 743–757. doi:10.1007/s10571-005-3972-8.
71. Busbridge, N. J., & Grossman, A. B. (1991). Stress and the single cytokine: Interleukin modulation of the pituitary-adrenal axis. *Molecular and Cellular Endocrinology, 82*(2–3), C209–C214.
72. Hori, T., Nakashima, T., Take, S., et al. (1991). Immune cytokines and regulation of body temperature, food intake, and cellular immunity. *Brain Research Bulletin, 27*(3–4), 309–313.
73. Navarra, P., Tsagarakis, S., Faris, M. S., et al. (1991). Interleukins-1 and -6 stimulate the release of corticotropin-releasing hormone-41 from rat hypothalamus in vitro via the eicosanoid cyclooxygenase pathway. *Endocrinology, 128*(1), 37–44. doi:10.1210/endo-128-1-37.
74. Spiegel, D. (1997). Psychosocial aspects of breast cancer treatment. *Seminars in Oncology, 24*(1 Suppl. 1), S1–S47.
75. Esterling, B., Antoni, M. H., Kumar, M., et al. (1990). Emotional repression, stress disclosure responses, and Epstein-Barr viral capsid antigen titers. *Psychosomatic Medicine, 52*(4), 397–410.
76. Spiegel, D., Sephton, S. E., Terr, A. I., et al. (1998). Effects of psychosocial treatment in prolonging cancer survival may be mediated by neuroimmune pathways. *Annals of the New York Academy of Sciences, 840*, 674–683.
77. Jamner, L. D., Schwartz, G. E., & Leigh, H. (1988). The relationship between repressive and defensive coping styles and monocyte, eosinophil, and serum glucose levels: Support for the opioid peptide hypothesis of regression. *Psychosomatic Medicine, 50*(6), 567–575.
78. Imai, K., Matsuyama, S., Miyake, S., et al. (2000). Natural cytotoxic activity of peripheral-blood lymphocytes and cancer incidence: An 11-year follow-up study of a general population. *Lancet, 356*(9244), 1795–1799. doi:10.1016/S0140-6736(00)03231-1.
79. Teicher, M. H., Andersen, S. L., Polcari, A., et al. (2002). Developmental neurobiology of childhood stress and trauma. *Psychiatric Clinics of North America, 25*(2), 297–426.
80. Frolkis, V. V. (1993). Stress-age syndrome. *Mechanisms of Ageing and Development, 69*(1–2), 93–107.
81. Hirokawa, K. (1997). Reversing and restoring immune functions. *Mechanisms of Ageing and Development, 93*(1–3), 119–124.
82. Kopnisky, K. L., Stoff, D. M., & Rausch, D. M. (2004). Workshop report: The effects of psychological variables on the progression of HIV-1

disease. *Brain, Behavior, and Immunity, 18*(3), 246–261. doi:10.1016/j.bbi.2003.08.003.
83. Wellen, K. E., & Hotamisligil, G. S. (2005). Inflammation, stress, and diabetes. *Journal of Clinical Investigation, 115*(5), 1111–1119. doi:10.1172/JCI25102.
84. Thoits, P. A. (1983). Dimensions of life events that influence psychological distress: An evaluation and synthesis of the literature. In H. B. Kaplan (Ed.), *Psychosocial stress: Trends in theory and research.* Orlando: Academic Press.
85. Irwin, M. (1999). Immune correlates of depression. *Advances in Experimental Medicine and Biology, 461*, 1–24. doi:10.1007/978-0-585-37970-8_1.
86. Hayney, M. S., Coe, C. L., Muller, D., et al. (2014). Age and psychological influences on immune responses to trivalent inactivated influenza vaccine in the Meditation or Exercise for Preventing Acute Respiratory Infection (MEPARI) trial. *Human Vaccines & Immunotherapeutics, 10*(1), 83–91. doi:10.4161/hv.26661.
87. Solomon, G. F., Kemeny, M. E., & Temoshok, L. (1991). Psychoneuroimmunologic aspects of human immunodeficiency virus infection. In R. Ader, D. L. Felten, & N. Cohen (Eds.), *Psychoneuroimmunology* (2nd ed., pp. 1081–1113). New York: Academic Press.
88. Surwit, R. S., & Schneider, M. S. (1993). Role of stress in the etiology and treatment of diabetes mellitus. *Psychosomatic Medicine, 55*(4), 380–393.
89. Bremner, J. D., Narayan, M., Staib, L. H., et al. (1999). Neural correlates of memories of childhood sexual abuse in women with and without posttraumatic stress disorder. *American Journal of Psychiatry, 156*(11), 1787–1795. doi:10.1176/ajp.156.11.1787.
90. Busso, D. S., McLaughlin, K. A., & Sheridan, M. A. (2014). Media exposure and sympathetic nervous system reactivity predict PTSD symptoms after the Boston marathon bombings. *Depression and Anxiety, 31*(7), 551–558. doi:10.1002/da.22282.
91. Clohessy, S., & Ehlers, A. (1999). PTSD symptoms, response to intrusive memories and coping in ambulance service workers. *British Journal of Clinical Psychology, 38*(Pt. 3), 251–265.
92. Donnelly, C. L., Amaya-Jackson, L., & March, J. S. (1999). Psychopharmacology of pediatric posttraumatic stress disorder. *Journal of Child and Adolescent Psychopharmacology, 9*(3), 203–220. doi:10.1089/cap.1999.9.203.
93. Cordova, M. J., Andrykowski, M. A., Kenady, D. E., et al. (1995). Frequency and correlates of posttraumatic-stress-disorder-like symptoms after treatment for breast cancer. *Journal of Consulting and Clinical Psychology, 63*(6), 981–986.
94. Ma, Z., Faber, A., & Dubé, L. (2007). Exploring women's psychoneuroendocrine responses to cancer threat, insights from a computer-based guided imagery task. *Canadian Journal of Nursing Research, 39*(1), 98–115.
95. Clayton, M. F., Dudley, W. N., & Musters, A. (2008). Communication with breast cancer survivors. *Health Communication, 23*(3), 207–221. doi:10.1080/10410230701808376.
96. Porter, L. S., Mishel, M., Neelon, V., et al. (2003). Cortisol levels and responses to mammography screening in breast cancer survivors: A pilot study. *Psychosomatic Medicine, 65*(5), 842–848.
97. Vedhara, K., & Irwin, M. (Eds.), (2005). *Human psychoimmunology*. Oxford: Oxford University Press.
98. Hunsche, C., Hernandez, O., & de la Fuente, M. (2016). Impaired immune response in old mice suffering from obesity and premature immunosenescence in adulthood. *Journals of Gerontology. Series A, Biological Sciences and Medical Sciences, 71*(8), 983–991. doi:10.1093/gerona/glv082.
99. Lazar, J. S. (1996). Mind-body medicine in primary care. Implications and applications. *Primary Care, 23*(1), 169–182.
100. Jiang, Y., & Zhu, J. (2015). Effects of sleep deprivation on behaviors and abnormal hippocampal BDNF/miR-10B expression in rats with chronic stress depression. *International Journal of Clinical and Experimental Pathology, 8*(1), 586–593.
101. Irwin, M., Mascovich, A., Gillin, J. C., et al. (1994). Partial sleep deprivation reduces natural killer cell activity in humans. *Psychosomatic Medicine, 56*(6), 493–498.
102. Pollmächer, T., Mullington, J., Korth, C., et al. (1995). Influence of host defense activation on sleep in humans. *Advances in Neuroimmunology, 5*(2), 155–169.
103. White, D. P., Douglas, N. J., Pickett, C. K., et al. (1983). Sleep deprivation and the control of ventilation. *American Review of Respiratory Disease, 128*(6), 984–986. doi:10.1164/arrd.1983.128.6.984.
104. Bellingrath, S., Rohleder, N., & Kudielka, B. M. (2010). Healthy working school teachers with high effort-reward-imbalance and overcommitment show increased pro-inflammatory immune activity and a dampened innate immune defence. *Brain, Behavior, and Immunity, 24*(8), 1332–1339. doi:10.1016/j.bbi.2010.06.011.
105. Pinquart, M., & Sörensen, S. (2003). Differences between caregivers and noncaregivers in psychological health and physical health: A meta-analysis. *Psychology and Aging, 18*(2), 250–267.
106. Kiecolt-Glaser, J., Glaser, R., Shuttleworth, E. C., et al. (1987). Chronic stress and immunity in family caregivers of Alzheimer's disease victims. *Psychosomatic Medicine, 49*(5), 523–535.
107. Shelby, J., Sullivan, J., Groussman, M., et al. (1992). Severe burn injury: Effects on psychologic and immunologic function in noninjured close relatives. *Journal of Burn Care and Rehabilitation, 13*(1), 58–63.
108. Epel, E. S., & Lithgow, G. J. (2014). Stress biology and ageing mechanisms: Toward understanding the deep connection between adaptation to stress and longevity. *Journals of Gerontology. Series A, Biological Sciences and Medical Sciences, 69*(S1), S10–S16. doi:10.1093/gerona/glu055.

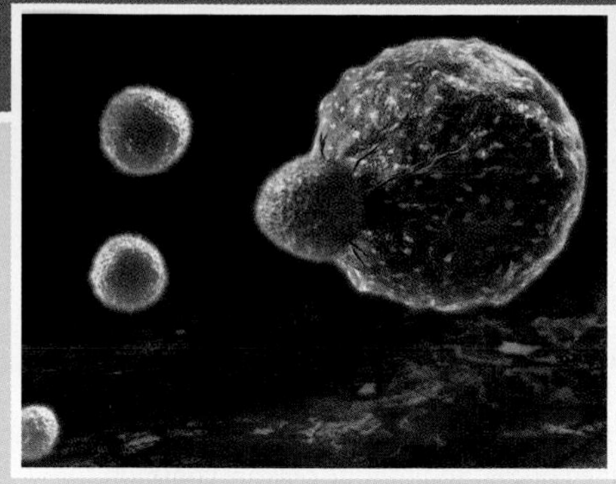

Biology of Cancer

Neal S. Rote, David M. Virshup, and Stephanie Zettel

EVOLVE WEBSITE

http://evolve.elsevier.com/Canada/Huether/pathophysiology
Student Review Questions
Key Points
Case Studies
Animations
Quick Check Answers

CHAPTER OUTLINE

Cancer Terminology and Characteristics, 235
Tumour Classification and Nomenclature, 235
The Biology of Cancer Cells, 238
Sustained Proliferative Signalling, 240
Evading Growth Suppressors, 243
Genomic Instability, 244
Enabling Replicative Immortality, 247
Inducing Angiogenesis, 247
Reprogramming Energy Metabolism, 248
Resisting Apoptotic Cell Death, 249
Tumour-Promoting Inflammation, 250
Evading Immune Destruction, 252
Activating Invasion and Metastasis, 253
Clinical Manifestations of Cancer, 256
Paraneoplastic Syndromes, 256
Pain, 256
Fatigue, 256
Cachexia, 256
Anemia, 258
Leukopenia and Thrombocytopenia, 259
Infection, 259
Gastro-intestinal Tract, 260
Hair and Skin, 260
Diagnosis, Characterization, and Treatment of Cancer, 260
Diagnosis and Staging, 260
Classification of Tumours: Classic Histology and Modern Genetics, 261
Treatment, 262

Cancer is a leading cause of suffering and death in the developed world. Over the past 35 years, intensive research has led to a significantly enhanced understanding of this complex and frightening disease. We now understand that cancer is a collection of more than 100 different diseases, each caused by a specific and often unique age-related accumulation of genetic and epigenetic alterations. Environment, heredity, and behaviour interact to modify the risk of developing cancer and the response to treatment. Improvements in treatment strategies and supportive care, coupled with new, often individualized therapies based on advances in our fundamental understanding of the basic pathophysiology of malignancy, have contributed to an increasing number of effective options for these diverse, often lethal, disorders collectively called cancer.

CANCER TERMINOLOGY AND CHARACTERISTICS

Any discussion of cancer must start with a definition of what it is and what it is not. Although most readers may have an intuitive understanding of this disorder, composing an exact definition that encompasses this broad category is more challenging. The US National Cancer Institute (NCI) of the National Institutes of Health (NIH) defines *cancer* as "diseases in which abnormal cells divide without control and are able to invade other tissues."[1]

The term **cancer** comes from the Latin translation of the Greek word for crab, *karkinoma*, which the physician Hippocrates used to describe the appendagelike projections extending from tumours into adjacent tissue. The word **tumour** originally referred to any swelling that is caused by inflammation but is now generally reserved for describing a new growth, or **neoplasm**.

Tumour Classification and Nomenclature

The careful evaluation of each cancer is important for many reasons. Different cancers will have different causes, different rates and patterns of progression, and different responses to treatment. The classification starts with knowing the tissue and organ of origin, the extent of distribution to other sites, and the microscopic appearance of the lesion. Increasingly, it also includes a detailed description of the critical genetic changes in the cancer. (See Figure 10-1 for a flow chart showing how cancer begins and spreads.)

Benign and Malignant

Not all tumours or neoplasms, however, are cancer; they can be benign or malignant (cancerous). **Benign tumours** are usually encapsulated with connective tissue and contain fairly well-differentiated cells and well-organized **stroma** (Figure 10-2). They retain recognizable normal tissue structure and do not invade beyond their capsule, nor do they spread to regional lymph nodes or distant locations. Mitotic cells are very rarely present during microscopic analysis. Benign tumours are generally named according to the tissues from which they arise with the suffix "-oma," which indicates a tumour or mass. For example, a benign tumour of the smooth muscle of the uterus is a *leiomyoma*, and a benign tumour of fat cells is a *lipoma*. It is important to understand that benign tumours can become extremely large and, depending on their location in the body, can cause morbidity or be life-threatening. For example, a benign meningioma at the base of the skull may cause symptoms by compressing adjacent normal brain tissue.

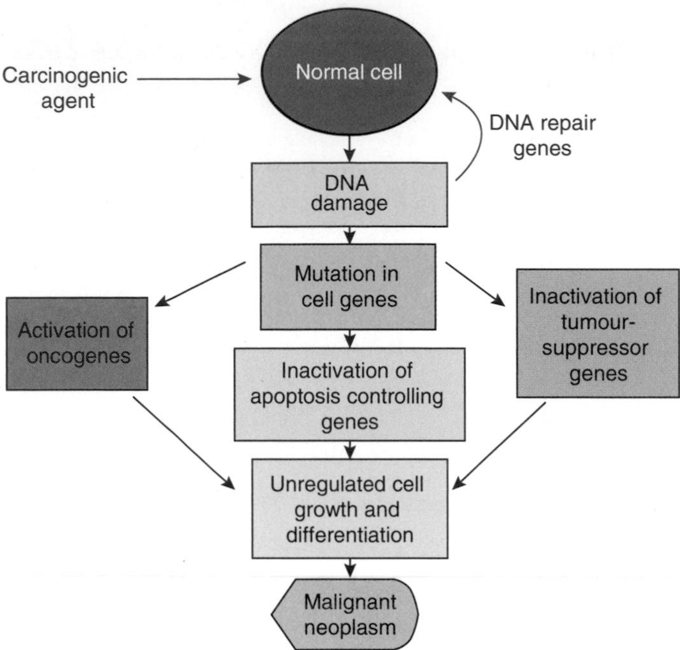

FIGURE 10-1 The Carcinogenic Process.

Some tumours initially described as benign can progress to cancer and then are referred to as **malignant tumours**, which are distinguished from benign tumours by more rapid growth rates and specific microscopic alterations, including loss of differentiation and absence of normal tissue organization (Figure 10-3). One of the microscopic hallmarks of cancer cells is **anaplasia**, the loss of cellular differentiation. Malignant cells are also **pleomorphic**, with marked variability of size and shape. They often have large darkly stained nuclei, and mitotic cells are common. Malignant tumours may have a substantial amount of stroma, but it is disorganized, with loss of normal tissue structure. Malignant tumours lack a capsule and grow to invade nearby blood vessels, lymphatics, and surrounding structures. The most important and most deadly characteristic of malignant tumours is their ability to spread far beyond the tissue of origin, a process known as *metastasis*.

Unlike benign tumours, which are named related to the tissue of origin, cancers generally are named according to the cell type from which they originate. Cancers arising in epithelial tissue are called **carcinomas**, and if they arise from or form ductal or glandular structures are named **adenocarcinomas**. Hence, a malignant tumour arising from breast glandular tissue is a mammary adenocarcinoma, whereas an example of a benign breast tumour is a fibroadenoma. Cancers arising from mesenchymal tissue (including connective tissue, muscle, and bone) usually have the suffix **sarcoma**. For example, malignant cancers of skeletal muscle are known as rhabdomyosarcomas. Cancers of lymphatic tissue are called **lymphomas**, whereas cancers of blood-forming cells are called **leukemias**. However, many cancers, such as Hodgkin's disease and Ewing sarcoma, are named for historical reasons that do not follow this nomenclature convention.

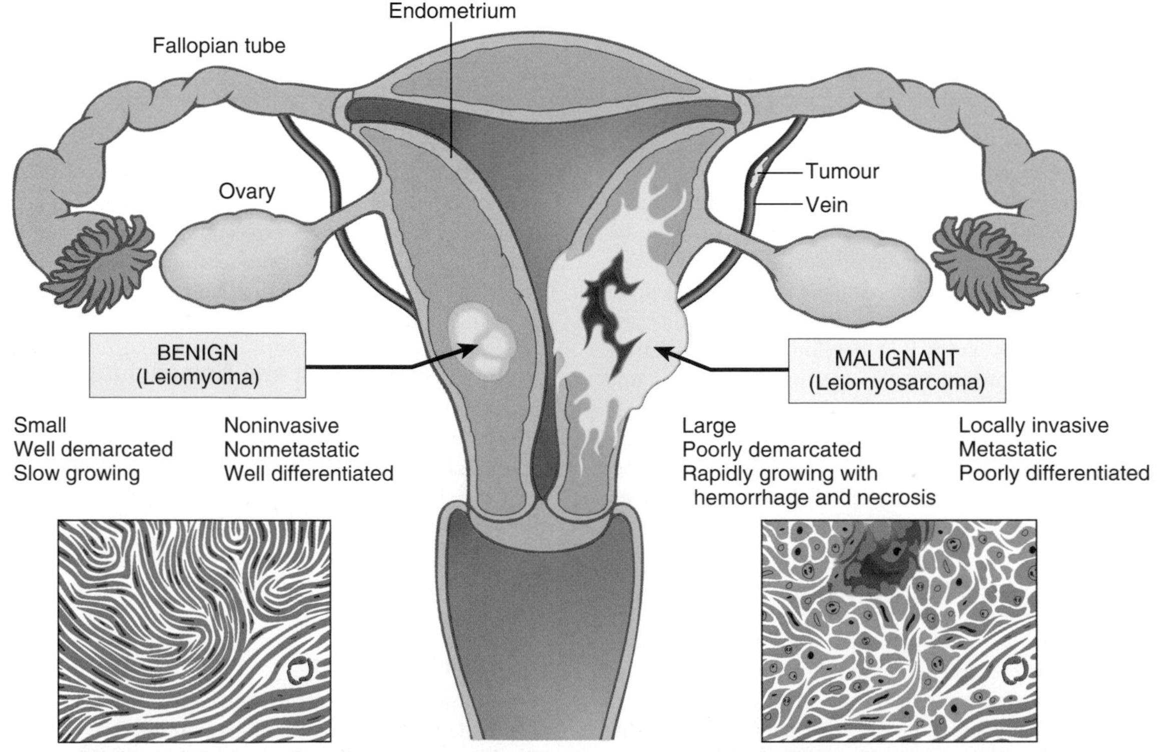

FIGURE 10-2 Comparison Between a Benign Tumour and a Malignant Tumour of the Same Origin. (From Kumar, V., Abbas, A.K., & Aster, J.C. [Eds.]. [2015]. *Robbins and Cotran pathologic basis of disease* [9th ed.]. Philadelphia: Saunders.)

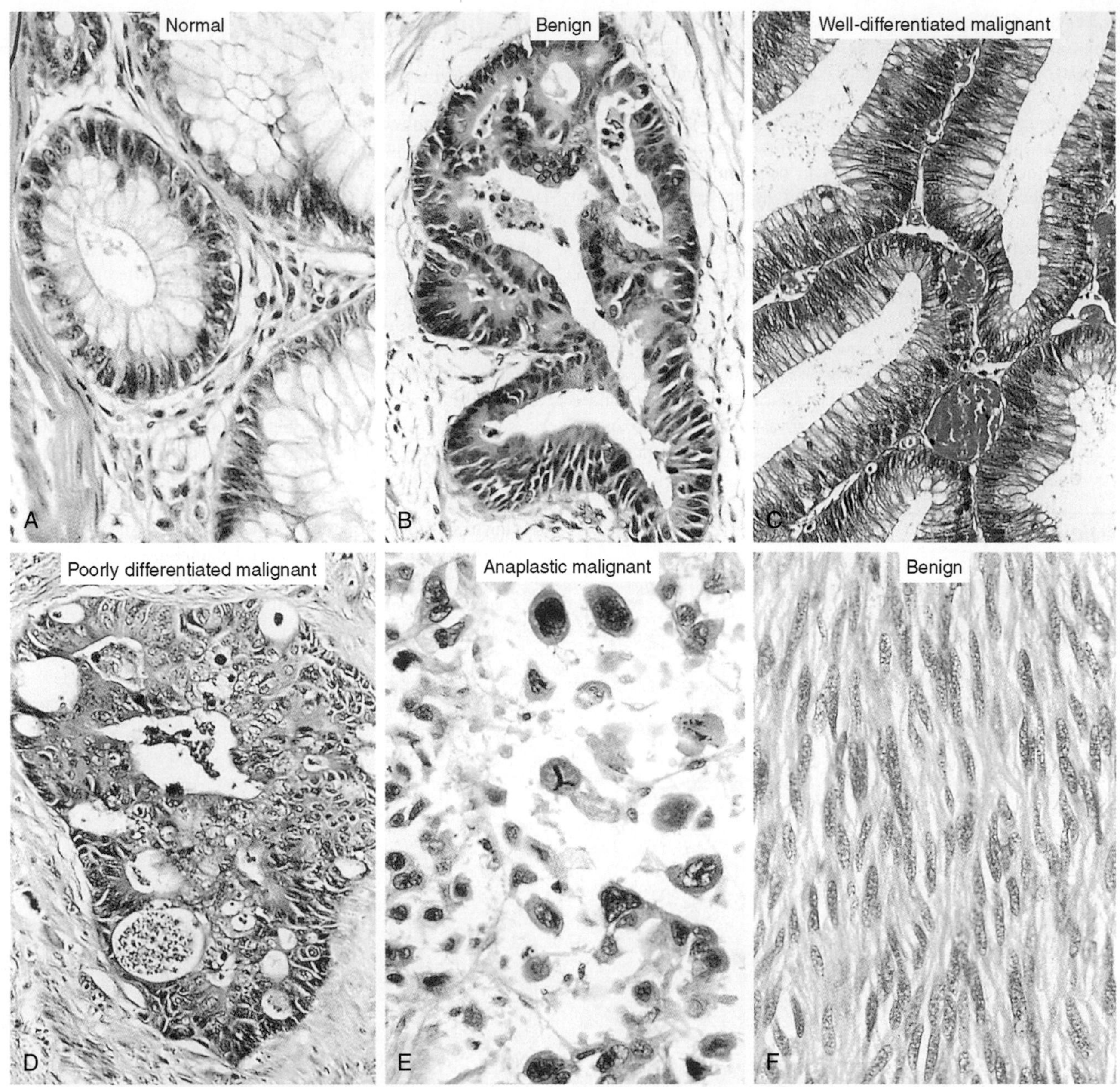

FIGURE 10-3 Loss of Cellular and Tissue Differentiation During the Development of Cancer. The cells of a benign neoplasm **(B)** resemble those of the normal colonic epithelium **(A)**, in that they are columnar and have an orderly arrangement. Loss of some degree of differentiation is evident in that the neoplastic cells do not show much mucin vacuolization (large, clear cytoplasmic vacuoles in **A**). Cells of the well-differentiated malignant neoplasm **(C)** of the colon have a haphazard arrangement, and although gland lumina are formed they are architecturally abnormal and irregular. Nuclei vary in shape and size, especially when compared with those illustrated in **(A)**. Cells in the poorly differentiated malignant neoplasm **(D)** have an even more haphazard arrangement, with very poor formation of gland lumina. Nuclei show greater variation in shape and size compared with the well-differentiated malignant neoplasm **(C)**. Cells in anaplastic malignant neoplasms **(E)** bear no relation to the normal epithelium, with no recognizable gland formation. Tremendous variation is found in the size of cells and their nuclei, with very intense staining (hyperchromatic nuclei). Not knowing the site of origin makes it impossible to classify this tumour by microscopic appearance alone. Well-differentiated tumours often resemble their cell of origin, as shown in the example of a benign tumour of smooth muscles **(F)**. (From Stevens, A., & Lowe, J. [2000]. *Pathology* [2nd ed.]. London: Mosby.)

Carcinoma in Situ

Carcinoma in situ (often abbreviated CIS) refers to preinvasive epithelial tumours of glandular or squamous cell origin. Cancers develop incrementally, as they accumulate specific genetic lesions. Careful surveillance for cancer often detects abnormal growths in epithelial tissues that have atypical cells and increased proliferation rate compared with normal surrounding tissues. These early-stage cancers are localized to the epithelium and have not penetrated the local basement membrane or invaded the surrounding stroma. Based on these characteristics, they are not malignant. CIS occurs in a number of sites, including the cervix, skin, oral cavity, esophagus, and bronchus. In glandular epithelium, in situ lesions occur in the stomach, endometrium, breast, and large bowel. In the breast, ductal carcinoma in situ (DCIS) fills the mammary ducts but has not progressed to local tissue invasion.[2] DCIS lesions are readily treatable, although the optimal therapeutic approach is controversial. CIS lesions can have one of the following three fates: (1) they can remain stable for a long time, (2) they can progress to invasive and metastatic cancers, or (3) they can regress and disappear. CIS can vary from low-grade to high-grade dysplasia, with the high-grade lesions having the highest likelihood of becoming invasive cancers. The time that such preinvasive lesions remain in situ before becoming invasive is unknown. Some carcinomas of the cervix appear as preinvasive lesions in situ for several years before they progress to invasive carcinoma and metastatic tumours (Figure 10-4). Knowing how to best treat low-grade CIS lesions is challenging, because the proportion that progress to cancer versus the proportion that will never cause clinical problems is usually not known. Although most persons prefer removal of any CIS as opposed to "watchful waiting," this topic continues to be a source of great debate.

QUICK CHECK 10-1

1. What is cancer?
2. Identify the major differences between benign and malignant tumours.
3. What is carcinoma in situ?

THE BIOLOGY OF CANCER CELLS

In two seminal publications, Drs. Douglas Hanahan and Robert Weinberg[3,4] described what they considered the hallmarks of cancer. Both articles stimulated considerable discussion and, especially, debate. The original publication contained six hallmarks, but with time and new research findings, increased to eight hallmarks and two traits that enable cancer progression. Their analysis remains the leading overview of why a cell is malignant. The following discussion is organized in the context of those 10 hallmarks/enablers (Figure 10-5). Two fundamental concepts are the foundation for understanding the biology of cancer. Cancer is a complex genetic disease, and the microenvironment of a tumour is a heterogeneous mixture of cells, both cancerous and benign. These concepts affect every stage of cancer development and evolve during that development. **Tumour initiation**, the process that produces the initial cancer cells, is dependent on specific mutations and characteristics of the microenvironment. **Tumour promotion**, the process during which the population of cancer cells expands with diversity of cancer cell phenotypes, is dependent on additional mutations and a changing tumour microenvironment. **Tumour progression**, the process leading to spread of the tumour to adjacent and distal sites (metastasis), is governed by further mutations and changing microenvironments at the primary tumour and at sites of metastasis.

Cancer is a disease of cumulative genetic changes during aging. The fraction of individuals who develop cancer increases dramatically with

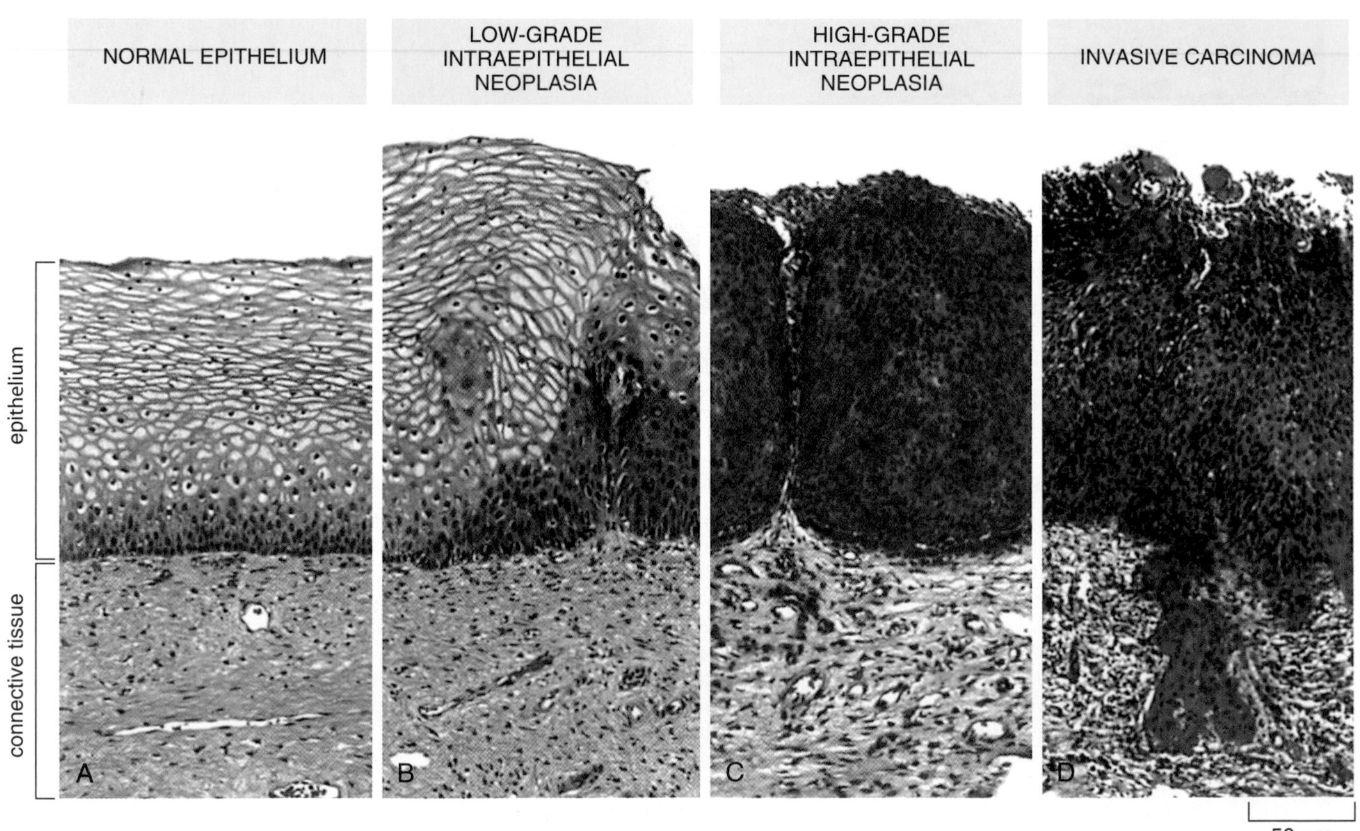

FIGURE 10-4 Progression From Normal to Neoplasm in the Uterine Cervix. A sequence of cellular and tissue changes progressing from low-grade to high-grade intraepithelial neoplasms (also called *carcinoma in situ*) and then to invasive cancer is seen often in the development of cancer. In this example of the early stages of cervical neoplastic changes, the presence of anaplastic cells and loss of normal tissue architecture signify the development of cancer. The high rate of cell division and the presence of local mutagens and inflammatory mediators all contribute to the accumulation of genetic abnormalities that lead to cancer. (Courtesy of Andrew J. Connolly. From Alberts, B., Johnson, A., Lewis, J., et al. [2008]. *Molecular biology of the cell* [5th ed.]. New York: Garland.)

age. Genetic changes may occur by both mutational and epigenetic mechanisms. Mutation generally means an alteration in the DNA sequence affecting expression or function of a gene (Figure 10-6). Mutations include small-scale changes in DNA, such as **point mutations**; the alteration of one or a few nucleotide base pairs (see Chapter 2). This type of mutation can have profound effects on the activity of resultant proteins. **Chromosome translocations** are large changes in chromosome structure in which a piece of one chromosome is translocated to another chromosome. **Gene amplification** is the result of repeated duplication of a region of a chromosome, so that instead of the normal two copies of a gene, tens or even hundreds of copies are present. Gene expression also may be altered indirectly by epigenetic effects including **DNA methylation**, histone acetylation, or altered expression of **noncoding RNA (ncRNA)** (see Chapter 3). Some mutations, referred to as *driver mutations*, "drive" the progression of cancer. There may be as many as 140 different driver mutations, although some are more critical than others, and each cancer only has a relatively small number of these.[5] Not all mutations in cancer contribute to the malignant phenotype. Some are just random events and are referred to as *passenger mutations*; they are just along for the ride. After a critical number of driver mutations have occurred, the cell becomes cancerous. The cancer cell has a selective advantage over its neighbours; its progeny can accumulate faster than its nonmutant neighbours. This selective advantage is referred to as **clonal proliferation** or **clonal expansion** (Figure 10-7). As a clone with mutations proliferates, it may become an early-stage tumour, for example, a carcinoma in situ or a benign colonic polyp. The increasingly rapid cell division and impaired DNA repair mechanisms of cancer cells result in a continuing accumulation of mutations throughout the progression to the most aggressive metastatic lesion. Thus, **transformation**, the process by which a normal cell becomes a cancer cell, is directed by progressive accumulation of genetic changes that alter the basic nature of the cell and drive it to malignancy. The process of tumour development is a form of Darwinian evolution; cells with a heritable change that confers a survival advantage out-compete their neighbours. Each cancer cell may develop its own set of mutations

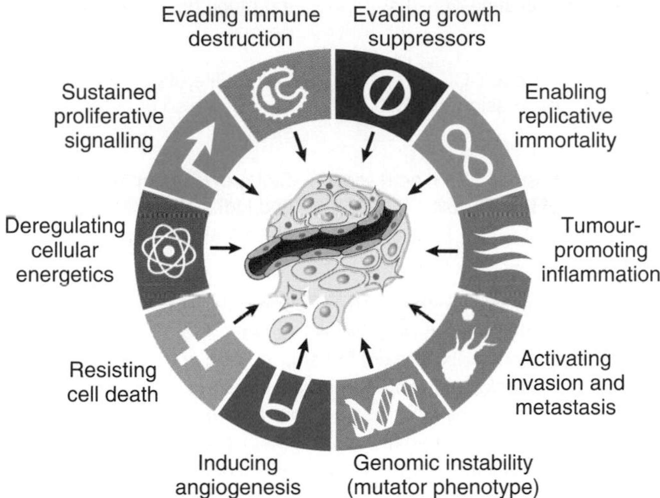

FIGURE 10-5 Hallmarks of Cancer. (Adapted from *Cell*, 144(5), Hanahan, D. & Weinberg, R.A., "Hallmarks of Cancer: The Next Generation," Pages 646–674, Copyright 2011, with permission from Elsevier. Found in Kumar, V., Abbas, A.K., & Aster, J.C. [Eds.]. [2015], *Robbins and Cotran pathologic basis of disease* [9th ed.]. Philadelphia: Saunders.)

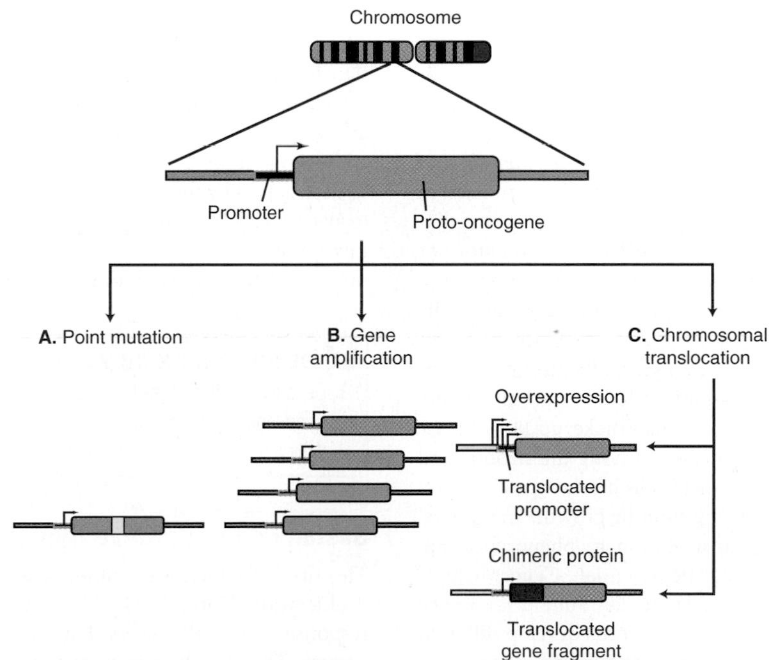

FIGURE 10-6 Oncogene Activation Mechanisms. Cellular genes may become cancerous oncogenes as a result of **(A)** point mutations that alter one or a few nucleotide base pairs, causing the production of a protein that is activated as a result of the altered sequence (e.g., RAS); **(B)** amplification of the cellular gene, resulting in higher levels of protein expression (e.g., MYCN [v-myc avian myelocytomatosis viral oncogene neuroblastoma derived homologue] in neuroblastoma); or **(C)** chromosomal translocations that either (1) lead to the juxtaposition of a strong promoter, causing increased protein expression (myelocytomatosis viral oncogene homologue in Burkitt lymphoma), or (2) produce a novel fusion protein that is derived from gene fragments normally present on different chromosomes (BCR-ABL in chronic myeloid leukemia). (From Haber, D.A. [2004]. Molecular genetics of cancer. In *ACP medicine*. Danbury, CT: WebMD.)

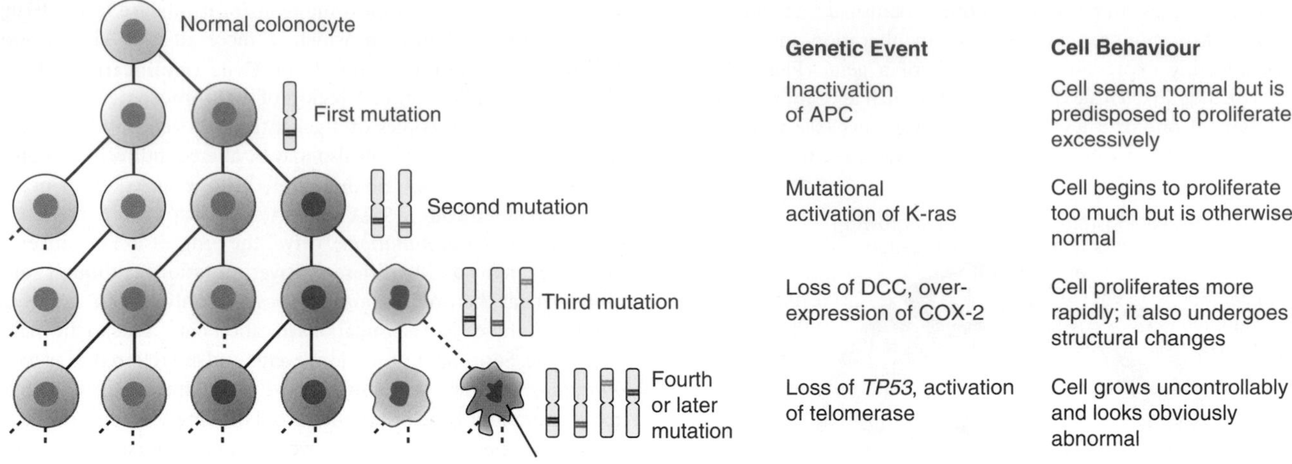

Normal colonocyte
First mutation
Second mutation
Third mutation
Fourth or later mutation
Malignant cell
Genetic Event
Cell Behaviour
Inactivation of APC
Cell seems normal but is predisposed to proliferate excessively
Mutational activation of K-ras
Cell begins to proliferate too much but is otherwise normal
Loss of DCC, over-expression of COX-2
Cell proliferates more rapidly; it also undergoes structural changes
Loss of TP53, activation of telomerase
Cell grows uncontrollably and looks obviously abnormal

FIGURE 10-7 Clonal Proliferation Model of Neoplastic Progression in the Colon. During clonal proliferation, progressively altered populations of colon cells (colonocytes) arise over time. As genetic and epigenetic changes occur, different subclones (indicated by different colour cells) coexist for a time. Clones that grow the fastest out-compete other clones, producing even more malignant, and abnormal-appearing, growths. The sequential accumulation of mutations has been well studied in the progression from a normal colon cell to a benign intestinal polyp to a malignant colon cancer. One of the earliest mutations in colon cancer is loss of the tumour-suppressor gene *APC*. Additional mutations (often in the oncogene *RAS*), activation of COX-2, and loss of the tumour suppressors *DCC* and *TP53* occur as the lesion progresses from a benign polyp to an invasive carcinoma. *APC*, adenomatous polyposis coli; *COX-2*, cyclo-oxygenase-2; *DCC*, deleted in colon cancer; *TP53*, tumour protein p53 gene. (Modified from Kumar, V., Cotran, R.S., & Robbins, S.L. [1997]. *Basic pathology* [6th ed.]. Philadelphia: Saunders; and Mendelsohn, I., Howley, P., Israel, M.A., et al. [2001]. *The molecular basis of cancer* [2nd ed.]. Philadelphia: Saunders.)

resulting in a genomically heterogeneous mixture of cells with subsets that have accumulated more and more mutations that increase the cell's malignant potential.[6] Thus many cancer cells that do not accumulate a critical set of mutations lose the competition and die during this process.

The processes occurring during the development of cancer are, in many ways, analogous to wound healing. The initial proliferation of cancer cells and enlargement of the tumour elicit the synthesis of proinflammatory mediators by the cancer cells and adjacent nonmalignant cells. As with wound healing, mediators recruit inflammatory or immune cells (primarily T lymphocytes [T cells] and macrophages, but also B lymphocytes [B cells] and neutrophils) and cells normally associated with tissue repair (fibroblasts, adipocytes, mesenchymal stem cells, endothelial cells, and pericytes). These cells form the stroma (tumour microenvironment) that surrounds and infiltrates the tumour (Figure 10-8).[7] In some conditions, stromal cells may make up 90% of the tumour mass.[8] Extensive paracrine signalling among the stromal and cancer cells affects both populations; cancer cells increase proliferation and become more heterogeneous during tumour growth, and several populations of stromal cells undergo evolution to phenotypes that promote cancer progression and metastatic potential.[9] Cancer heterogeneity arises from ongoing proliferation and mutation. Tumour-associated endothelial cells, fibroblasts, and inflammatory cells develop different and distinct gene expression profiles with unique cell surface molecules and patterns of secreted molecules. During this process there is generally a great deal of cancer cell death, but the surviving cells are more aggressive and many take on a metastatic phenotype. Because continuing somatic mutations may be random, cancer cells in different regions of the tumour may be genetically diverse. Additionally, a population of cancer stem cells may arise, the origin of which is still unclear. Many of the hallmarks of cancer are consequences of cancer-stromal interactions (discussed later in this chapter).

Several of the hallmarks or enablers are primarily genomic alterations that initiate and maintain development of cancer. These genomic alterations will be discussed first and include sustained proliferative signalling, evading growth suppressors, genomic instability, and enabling replicative immortality (see Figure 10-5). Other hallmarks or enablers are secondary to genomic change and include inducing angiogenesis and reprogramming energy metabolism. A third group, tumour resistance to destruction by the host's protective mechanisms, includes resistance to apoptotic cell death, tumour-promoting inflammation, and evading immune destruction. The last hallmark is the culmination of the previous nine: activating invasion and metastasis.

QUICK CHECK 10-2

1. Describe the differences between point mutations, chromosomal translocations, and gene amplification in the process of cancer.
2. Why is the tumour microenvironment important to cancer progression?

Sustained Proliferative Signalling

The first and foremost hallmark of cancer is uncontrolled cellular proliferation. Normal cells generally only enter proliferative phases in response to growth factors that bind to specific receptors on the cell surface. The cytoplasmic components of the receptors are associated with signalling molecules that undergo activation and in turn activate intracellular signalling pathways leading to induction or activation of regulatory factors affecting DNA synthesis, entrance into the cell cycle, and changes in expression of other genes related to cell metabolism for optimal growth (Figure 10-9). One example is initiation of proliferation by epidermal growth factor (EGF). EGF binds and cross-links two EGF receptors on the cell surface. The cytoplasmic portions of the receptors are tyrosine kinases that attach phosphorus to tyrosine in neighbouring

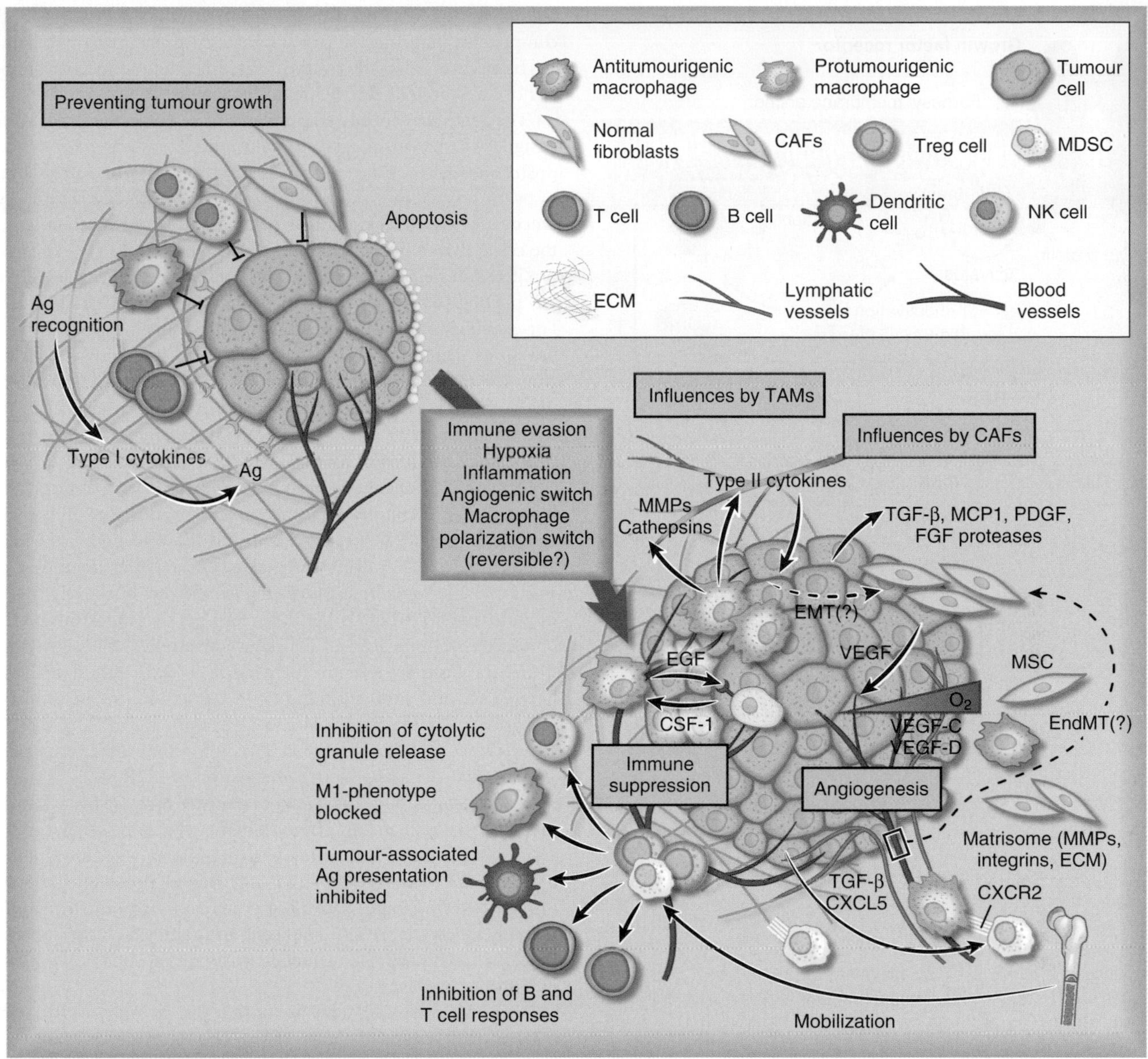

FIGURE 10-8 Cancers Live in a Complex Microenvironment. Cancer cells express tumour-specific antigens that ideally can be recognized by cells of the immune system and inflammatory systems (natural killer cells [*NK cells*], antitumourigenic M1 macrophages, T-cytotoxic cells) and destroyed by apoptosis or undergo growth suppression by type I cytokines. However, successful cancers produce a variety of cytokines and chemokines that are chemoattractants for stromal cells that infiltrate the tumour and undergo change to protumourigenic phenotypes. The affected cells include tumour-associated M2 macrophages, cancer-associated fibroblasts (*CAFs*), mesenchymal stem cells (*MSCs*), and immune suppressor cells of T-cell origin (T-regulatory cells [*Treg cells*]) and myeloid origin (myeloid-derived suppressor cells [*MDSC*]). Through multiple receptor-mediated interactions between other stromal cells and the cancer cells, the stromal cells, as well as the cancer cells, collectively produce a battery of additional cytokines (e.g., TGF-β, type II cytokines), chemokines (e.g., CXCL5), growth factors (e.g., VEGF, EGF, CSF-1, FGF, PDGF), and proteases (e.g., MMPs) and secrete components of the extracellular matrix [*ECM*]. The stromal reaction promotes tumour progression, including new blood vessel growth (angiogenesis), tumour cell proliferation and differentiation, suppression of immune rejection and tumour cell apoptosis, invasion, and commitment to metastasis. *Ag*, antigen; *CSF-1*, colony-stimulating factor-1; *CXCL5*, C-X-C motif chemokine 5; *CXCR2*, C-X-C chemokine receptor type 2; *EGF*, epidermal growth factor; *EMT*, epithelial-mesenchymal transition; *FGF*, fibroblast growth factor; *MCP-1*, macrophage chemotactic protein-1; *MMPs*, matrix metalloproteinases; O_2, oxygen; *PDGF*, platelet-derived growth factor; *TAM*, tumour-associated macrophage; *TGF-β*, transforming growth factor-beta; *VEGF*, vascular endothelial growth factor. (Modified from Quail, D.F., & Joyce, J.A. [2013]. *Nat Med, 19*[11], 1423–1437.)

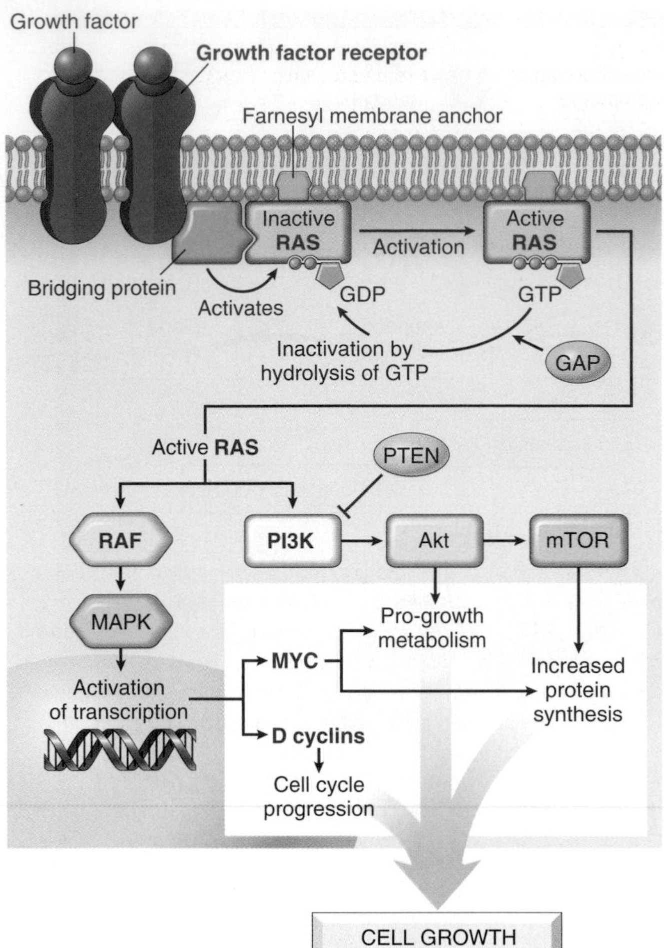

FIGURE 10-9 Growth Factor Signalling Pathways in Cancer. Growth factor receptors, RAS, PI3K, MYC, and D cyclins are oncoproteins that are activated by mutations in various cancers. GAPs apply brakes to *RAS* activation, and PTEN serves the same function for *PI3K*. *Akt*, protein kinase B; *GAP*, GTPase-activating protein; *GDP*, guanosine diphosphate; *GTP*, guanosine triphosphate; *MAPK*, mitogen-activated protein kinase; *mTOR*, mammalian target of rapamycin; *MYC*, myelocytomatosis viral oncogene homologue; *PI3K*, phosphoinositidyl-3-kinase; *PTEN*, phosphatase and tensin homologue; *RAF*, rapidly accelerated fibrosarcoma. (From Kumar, V., Abbas, A.K., & Aster, J.C. [Eds.]. [2015]. *Robbins and Cotran pathologic basis of disease* [9th ed.]. Philadelphia: Saunders.)

proteins, including each other (autophosphorylation). Phosphorylation allows the receptor to attach to bridging protein, which links the EGF receptors to plasma membrane–associated inactive RAS. **RAS** is an acronym for "rat sarcoma," where it was found originally. Inactive RAS is associated with guanine diphosphate (GDP). Association between the EGF receptor and inactive RAS modifies the binding of GDP, which is replaced with guanosine triphosphate (GTP). GTP activates RAS, which is a GTPase that converts GTP to GDP, during which it can activate signalling pathways such as the mitogen-activated protein kinase (MAPK) pathway and the phosphatidylinositol-3-kinase (PI3K) pathway. These signalling pathways phosphorylate other cytoplasmic proteins and affect activity and nuclear localization of transcription factors, such as myelocytomatosis viral oncogene homologue (MYC), that govern the transcription of cell cycle regulators (i.e. G_1 phase of the cell cycle), such as cyclins, and entrance into cellular proliferation. Proliferation can be discontinued through this pathway by decreased levels of growth factors in the environment or inactivation of signalling pathway components. Targeting these cyclins that effectively "turn on" cell division has been a promising area for the development of monoclonal antibodies in novel research of the treatment of cancer.

The genes that encode components of receptor-mediated pathways designed to regulate normal cellular proliferation are collectively called **proto-oncogenes**. Cancerous cells characteristically express mutated or overexpressed proto-oncogenes, which are referred to as **oncogenes**. Oncogenes are independent of normal regulatory mechanisms; thus the cell is driven into a state of unregulated constitutive expression of proliferation signals and uncontrolled cell growth. Oncogenes can affect any portion of the growth factor pathways, such as described for EGF. For example, most growth factors originate from neighbouring cells, but some cancers acquire the ability to secrete growth factors that stimulate their own growth, a process known as **autocrine stimulation**. As described later in this chapter, noncancerous stromal cells within a tumour are frequently modified to benefit the cancer. In some instances, stromal cells produce excessive growth factors that drive the proliferation of cancer cells. Other cancers increase the expression of growth factor receptors; for example, in breast cancer production of the human epidermal growth factor receptor 2 (HER2, also known as the EGF receptor gene [*ERBB-2*]) is upregulated and is hyper responsive to low levels of EGF. Some breast and lung cancers are effectively treated by inhibitors of HER2 and other EGF receptors that block this pathway.[10]

Oncogenes may lead to constant activation of the signal cascade from the cell surface receptor to the nucleus. Up to a third of all cancers have an activating mutation in the *RAS* gene resulting in a continuous cell growth signal even when growth factors are missing (see Figure 10-9). Other mutations in the EGF receptor pathway include excessive proliferation signalling by hyperactivation of PI3K.

Several types of genetic events can activate oncogenes. A point mutation that is frequently observed in lung cancer results in continuous activation of the EGF **receptor tyrosine kinase**. A point mutation in the *RAS* gene converts it from a regulated proto-oncogene to an unregulated oncogene. Activating point mutations in *RAS* are found in many cancers, especially pancreatic and colorectal cancer. Specialized tests, such as direct DNA sequencing, can detect such point mutations in clinical samples.

Translocations can activate oncogenes in one of two distinct mechanisms (Figure 10-10). First, a translocation can cause excess and inappropriate production of a proliferation factor. One of the best examples is the t(8;14) translocation found in many Burkitt lymphomas; t(8;14) designates a chromosome that has a piece of chromosome 8 fused to a piece of chromosome 14 (see Chapter 21).[11] Burkitt lymphoma is an aggressive cancer of B lymphocytes. The *MYC* proto-oncogene found on chromosome 8 is normally activated at low levels in proliferating lymphocytes and is inactivated in mature lymphocytes. If the t(8;14) translocation occurs, the *MYC* gene is aberrantly placed under the control of a B-cell immunoglobulin gene (*IG*) present on chromosome 14. The *IG* gene is very active in maturing B cells. The t(8;14) translocation alters the control of *MYC*; its normal low-level expression is switched to high levels, as directed by an *IG* gene promoter. Hyperproduction of MYC protein drives proliferation and blocks differentiation.

Second, chromosome translocations can lead to the production of novel proteins with growth-promoting properties. In chronic myeloid (or *myelogenous*) leukemia (CML) a specific chromosome translocation is almost always present (see Figure 10-10). This translocation, t(9;22), was first identified in association with CML in Philadelphia in 1960 and is often referred to as the *Philadelphia chromosome*.[12] Translocation fuses two chromosomes in the middle of two different genes: *BCR* (breakpoint cluster region gene) on chromosome 9 and *ABL* (Abelson gene) on chromosome 22. The result is production of a BCR-ABL fusion protein containing the first half of BCR and the second half of ABL (a nonreceptor tyrosine kinase). BCR-ABL is an unregulated protein tyrosine kinase that promotes growth of myeloid cells. Imatinib (Gleevec), a medication that specifically targets this tyrosine kinase, represents the first successful chemotherapy targeted against the product of a specific oncogenic mutation. Imatinib and related tyrosine kinase inhibitors (TKIs) are highly effective in the treatment of CML and, because of their specificity, lack the toxic adverse effects noted with nonspecific anticancer medications. However, imatinib is not effective in cancers that do not have the t(9;22) translocation or related mutations. In modern personalized cancer therapy, knowledge of the specific genetic alteration can dictate the optimal medications for the individual.

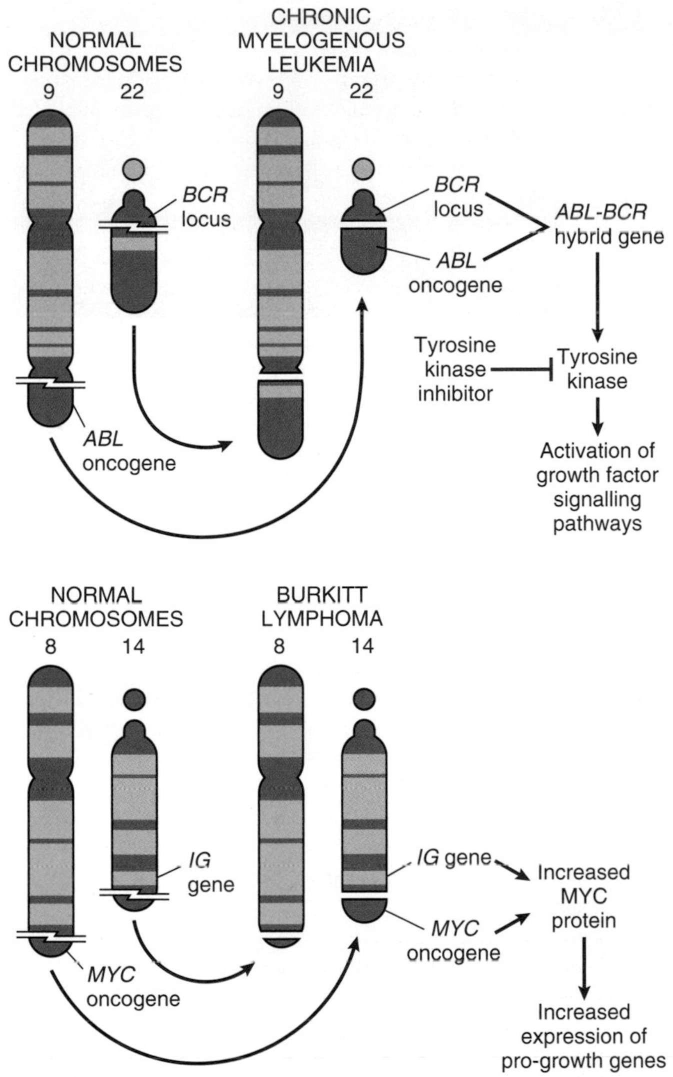

Oncogenes also may be activated by gene amplification (Figure 10-11). Gene amplification results in increased expression of an oncogene, or in some cases medication-resistance genes. The N-*MYC* oncogene, a member of the *MYC* family, is amplified in 25% of childhood neuroblastoma and confers a poor prognosis. The HER2 gene (*ERBB2*) is amplified in 20% of breast cancers.

FIGURE 10-10 Examples of Chromosomal Translocations and Associated Oncogenes. See text for further explanation. *ABL*, Abelson gene; *BCR*, breakpoint cluster region gene; *IG*, immunoglobulin gene; *MYC*, myelocytomatosis viral oncogene homologue. (From Kumar, V., Abbas, A.K., & Aster, J.C. [Eds.]. [2015]. *Robbins and Cotran pathologic basis of disease* [9th ed.]. Philadelphia: Saunders.)

Evading Growth Suppressors

Uncontrolled cancer cell proliferation also is related to inactivation of tumour-suppressor genes. **Tumour-suppressor genes** normally regulate the cell cycle, inhibit proliferation resulting from growth signals, stop cell division when cells are damaged, and prevent mutations. Hence, they also have been referred to as *antioncogenes.* Whereas oncogenes are *activated* in cancers, tumour suppressors must be *inactivated* to allow cancer to occur (Table 10-1 and Figure 10-12). A single genetic event can activate an oncogene because it can act in a dominant manner in the cell. However, we have two copies of each tumour-suppressor gene, one from each parent. Both copies must be inactivated; therefore, two mutations are necessary.

A prototypical tumour-suppressor gene is the **retinoblastoma (*RB*) gene**. Normal cells receive diverse "antigrowth" signals from their normal environment. Contact with other cells, with basement membranes, and with some soluble factors normally signal cells to stop proliferating. Tumour-suppressor genes, such as *RB*, monitor antigrowth cellular signals and block activation of the growth and division phase in the cell cycle; thus mutations in *RB* lead to persistent cell growth. Antiproliferative activity of *RB* depends on the degree of protein phosphorylation.[13] Low levels of phosphorylation (hypophosphorylation) result in *RB* binding to and inhibiting transcription factors that regulate genes controlling passage through the cell cycle. Growth factor–regulated kinases increase phosphorylation (hyperphosphorylation) and inactivation of *RB*. A variety of genetic mutations in cancers also inactivate *RB*, resulting in unregulated and continuous cellular proliferation. *RB* is mutated in childhood retinoblastoma, and in many lung, breast, and bone cancers as well. The *RB* gene resides on chromosome 13, in a region referred to as q14 (13q14). Most individuals with *RB* mutations have a subtle mutation, such as a point mutation, in one allele. The *RB* gene in the other chromosome may be inactivated through loss of the 13q14 region or epigenetic mechanisms.

Another classic tumour-suppressor gene is **tumour protein p53 (*TP53*)**. The protein p53 has been called the *guardian of the genome.*

TABLE 10-1 Comparison of Cancer Gene Types

Gene Type	Normal Function	Mutation Effect
Caretaker genes	Maintain DNA and chromosome stability	Chromosome instability leads to increased rates of mutation
Dominant oncogenes[a]	Encode proteins that promote growth (e.g., growth factors)	Overexpression or amplification causes gain of function
Tumour suppressors (recessive oncogenes)	Encode proteins that inhibit proliferation and prevent or repair mutations	Loss of function of both alleles increases cancer risk

[a]Nonmutant state referred to as proto-oncogene.

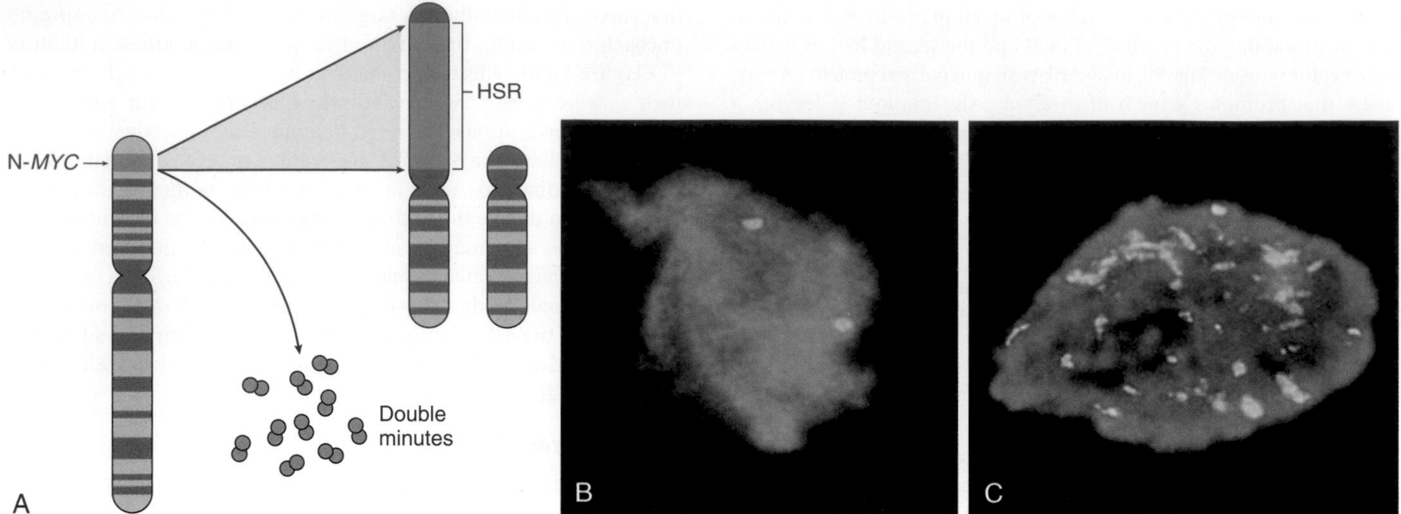

FIGURE 10-11 N-*MYC* **Gene Amplification in Neuroblastoma. A,** The N-*MYC* gene is present on chromosome 2, becomes amplified, and is seen either as extra chromosomal double minutes or as a chromosomal homologous staining region (*HSR*). The N-*MYC* gene is detected in human neuroblastoma cells using a technique called FISH (fluorescent in situ hybridization). **B,** A single pair of N-*MYC* genes is detected in normal cells and in low-grade neuroblastoma. **C,** Multiple, amplified copies of the N-*MYC* gene are detected in some cases of neuroblastoma. Amplification of the N-*MYC* gene is strongly associated with a poor prognosis in childhood neuroblastoma. (**A,** from Kumar, V., Abbas, A.K., & Aster, J.C. [Eds.]. [2015]. *Robbins and Cotran pathologic basis of disease* [9th ed.]. Philadelphia: Saunders. **B, C,** Courtesy Arthur R. Brothman, PhD, FACMG, University of Utah School of Medicine, Salt Lake City, UT.)

TP53 monitors intracellular signals related to stress and activates caretaker genes—genes that are responsible for the maintenance of genomic integrity (Figure 10-13). Many types of cellular stress (e.g., anoxia, oncogene expression, nuclear damage) produce intracellular signals (e.g., levels of nucleotides and glucose, degree of oxygenation, DNA damage, and other indicators of cellular abnormalities) detectable by p53. Normally p53 is in an inactive complex with inhibitor molecules. Stress activates kinases that phosphorylate p53 into an active suppressor of cell division and activator of caretaker genes. Caretaker genes encode proteins that are involved in repairing damaged DNA, such as occurs with errors in DNA replication, mutations caused by ultraviolet or ionizing radiation, and mutations caused by chemicals and medications. The p53 protein also controls initiation of cellular senescence or apoptosis, and suppresses cell division until DNA repair is complete or other effects of stress are corrected. If not corrected, the cell enters senescence or apoptosis, thus preventing further DNA damage and mutations. Loss of function of *TP53* or caretaker genes leads to increased mutation rates and cancer.[14]

Because inactivation of tumour-suppressor genes requires at least two mutations (one in each allele), a single germ cell mutation (sperm or egg) results in the transmission of cancer-causing genes from one generation to the next, producing families with a high risk for specific cancers. These inherited mutations that predispose to cancer are almost invariably in tumour-suppressor genes because only a single additional mutation in any other cell (somatic cell mutation) is needed to inactivate completely the tumour-suppressor gene (Table 10-2).[15]

An example of increased risk for cancer that can be inherited is the familial form of retinoblastoma. A mutation in one *RB* allele is inherited so that only one additional mutation in the normal allele will lead to cancer (see Table 10-2). Approximately half of children with retinoblastoma have the inheritable form, and most will develop tumours in both eyes (bilateral retinoblastoma). Also, Li-Fraumeni syndrome is a very rare inheritable loss-of-function mutation in *TP53* in one allele resulting in a 25-fold increase of developing malignancy at early age (less than 50 years of age). These malignancies may include breast cancer, brain tumours, acute leukemia, soft tissue sarcomas, bone sarcoma, and adrenal cortical carcinoma. Other familial cancers with inheritable mutations in tumour-suppressor genes include Wilms tumour, a childhood cancer of the kidney (*WT1* gene); neurofibromatosis (*NF1* gene); and familial polyposis coli or adenomas of the colon (*APC* gene). Characterization of cancer-causing genes and other genetic factors helps identify individuals prone to developing cancer and contributes to our understanding of sporadic cancers. Individuals known to carry mutations in tumour-suppressor genes are offered targeted cancer screening to facilitate early cancer detection and therapy.

TABLE 10-2 Some Familial Cancer Syndromes Caused by Tumour-Suppressor Gene Function Loss

Syndrome	Gene
Retinoblastoma	*RB1*
Li-Fraumeni syndrome	*p53 (TP53)*
Familial melanoma	*p16$^{NK\alpha}$ (CDKN2A)*
Neurofibromatosis	*Neurofibromin (NF1)*
Familial adenomatous polyps	*APC*
Breast cancer	*BRCA1*

Genomic Instability

Genomic instability refers to an increased tendency of alterations—mutability—in the genome during the life cycle of cells. Inherited and acquired mutations in caretaker genes that protect the integrity of the genome and DNA repair increase the level of genomic instability and risk for developing cancer. In other words, these mutations cause

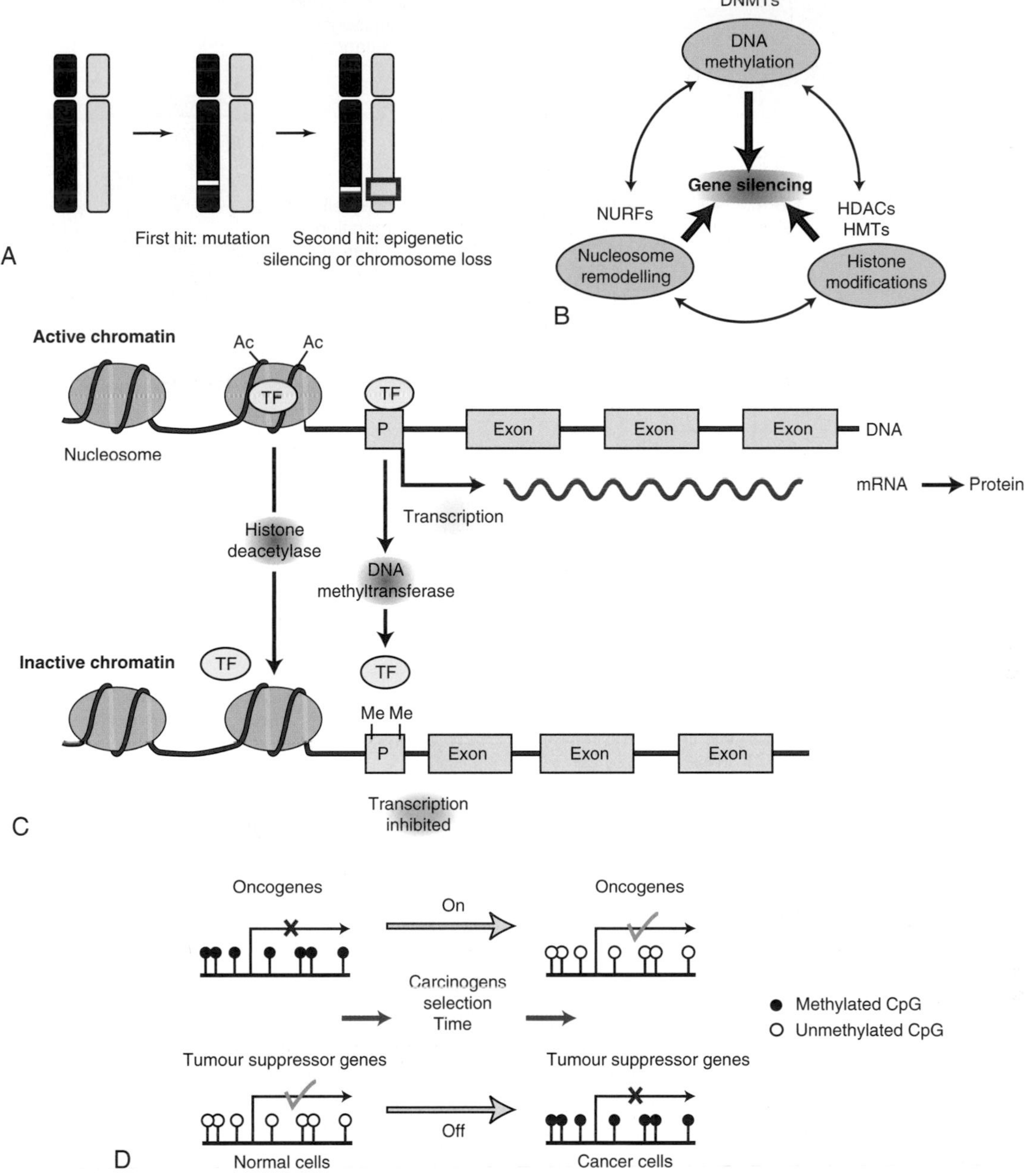

FIGURE 10-12 Silencing Tumour-Suppressor Genes. Tumour-suppressor genes can be deactivated by a variety of mechanisms. **A,** In this example, the first hit is a point mutation in a tumour-suppressor gene (*white box*), followed by either epigenetic silencing or chromosome loss of the second allele (*red box*). **B,** Genes can normally be silenced by a variety of interacting processes, including DNA methylation, histone modification, nucleosomal remodelling, and microRNA changes (not shown). A number of cellular enzymes contribute to these modifications, including DNA methyltransferases (*DNMTs*), histone deacetylases (*HDACs*), histone methyltransferases (*HMTs*), and complex nucleosomal remodelling factors (*NURFs*). Gene silencing is essential for normal development and differentiation. **C,** Histone modification and promoter methylation (*Me*) regulate gene expression (exons code for resultant messenger [*mRNA*] after the introns are spliced out). Genes are transcribed when chromatin is modified by addition of acetyl (*Ac*) groups to specific lysine groups in histones. Gene expression can be turned off when specific acetyl groups are removed (by HDACs) or when the CpG-rich promoter regions of genes are modified by direct DNA methylation (by DNA methyltransferase). In addition, small endogenous RNA molecules (microRNAs) can bind to mRNA and reduce gene expression. **D,** Changes in promoter methylation turn cancer genes off and on. Oncogenes can be turned on by promoter hypomethylation, and tumour-suppressor genes can be turned off by promoter hypermethylation. Each of these changes can produce selective growth and survival advantages for the cancer cell. *P,* promoter region; *TF,* transcription factor. (**B,** Reprinted from *Cell,* 128(4), Jones, P.A., & Baylin, S.B., "The epigenomics of cancer," Pages 683–692, Copyright 2007, with permission from Elsevier. **C,** From *The New England Journal of Medicine,* Peter D. Gluckman, Mark A. Hanson, Cyrus Cooper, et al, "Effect of In Utero and Early Life Conditions on Adult Health and Disease," 359:61–73. Copyright © 2008 Massachusetts Medical Society. Reprinted with permission from Massachusetts Medical Society. **D,** from Shames, D.S., Minna, J.D., & Gazdar, A.F. [2007]. *Curr Mol Med,* 7[1], 85–102.)

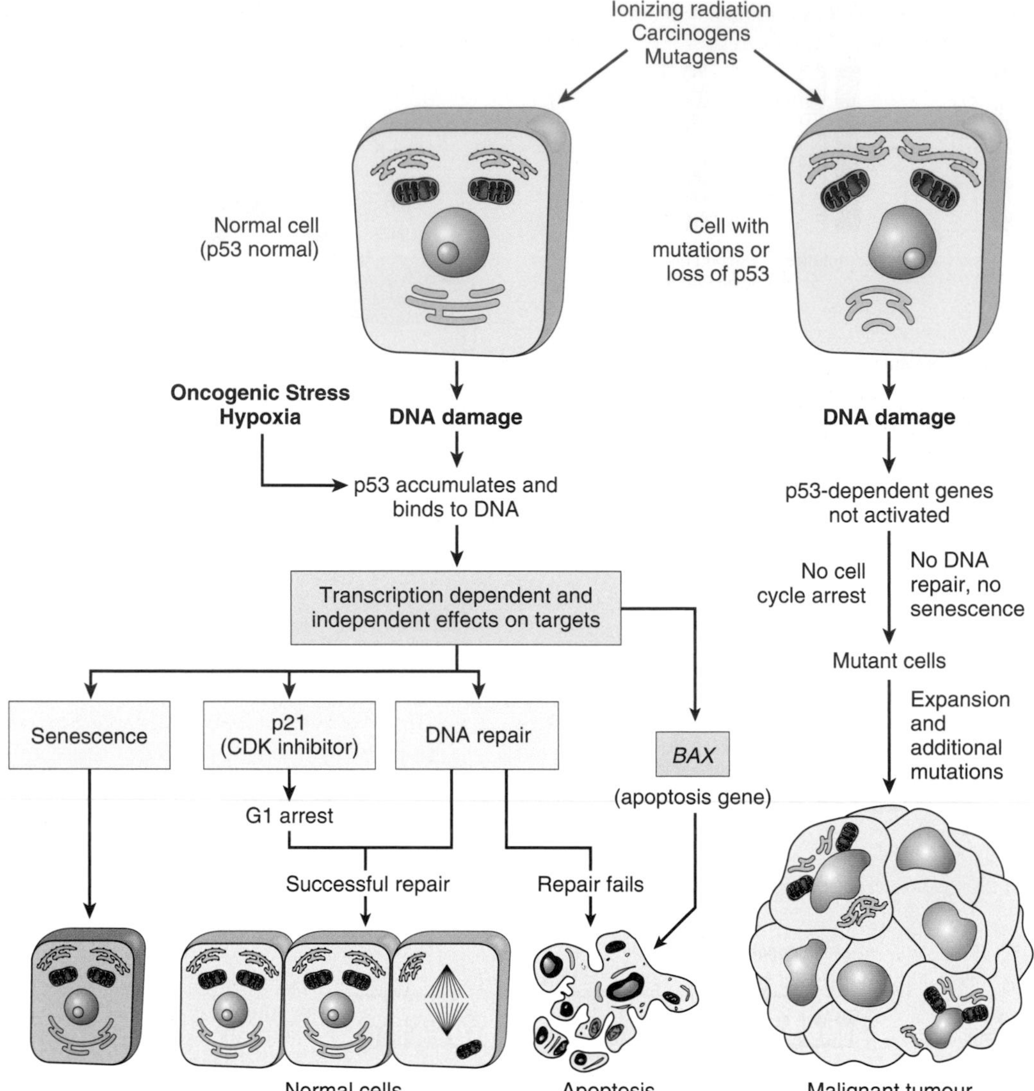

FIGURE 10-13 The Role of p53 in Maintaining the Integrity of the Genome. Activation of normal p53 by DNA-damaging agents or by hypoxia leads to cell cycle arrest in G_1 by upregulation of the cell cycle inhibitor p21 and induction of DNA repair transcriptional upregulation of the cyclin-dependent kinase inhibitor *CDKN1A* (encoding the cyclin-dependent kinase inhibitor p21) and the *GADD45* genes. Successful repair of DNA allows cells to proceed with the cell cycle. If DNA repair fails, p53 triggers either apoptosis or senescence. In cells with loss or mutation of the *p53* gene, DNA damage does not induce cell cycle arrest or DNA repair, and genetically damaged cells proliferate, giving rise eventually to malignant neoplasms. *BAX*, Bcl-2–associated X protein gene; *CDK*, cyclin-dependent kinase. (From Kumar, V., Abbas, A.K., & Aster, J.C. [Eds.]. [2015]. *Robbins and Cotran pathologic basis of disease* [9th ed.]. Philadelphia: Saunders.)

stable cells to become more labile. Acquired mutations in "guardians of the genome," such as *TP53*, that detect DNA damage and activate repair mechanisms result in an increasing accumulation of mutations. Xeroderma pigmentosum is a defect in the repair of DNA pyrimidine dimers created by ultraviolet (UV) light that increases the risk for skin cancers. Hereditary nonpolyposis colorectal cancer results from an inherited defect in repairing DNA base pair mismatches that occur occasionally during DNA replication. Affected individuals have an increased rate of small insertions and deletions in DNA (and more labile cells), leading to a high rate of colon and other cancers. Some inherited mutations threaten the integrity of entire chromosomes. Bloom's syndrome, caused by mutations in a DNA helicase, presents with an increased risk of several forms of cancer, and those with Fanconi aplastic anemia, caused by loss of function for repairing DNA double-strand breaks, have a particularly increased risk of acute myelogenous leukemia. These examples are autosomal recessive disorders in which affected individuals demonstrate marked chromosomal instability.

Genomic instability also may result from increased epigenetic silencing or modulation of gene function (Chapter 3). Many cancers have increased methylation of DNA in the promoter region of tumour-suppressor genes. They also have associated changes in the modification of histones in the chromatin, often correlated with methylation of DNA. These changes alter the promoter regions of genes, leading to their silencing or altered gene expression.

Changes in gene regulation can affect not just single genes but also entire intracellular signalling networks. Gene expression networks can be regulated by changes in microRNAs (miRNAs, or *miRs*) and other ncRNAs.[16] miRNAs regulate diverse signalling pathways; the miRNAs that stimulate cancer development and progression are termed oncomirs.[17] miRNAs decrease the stability and expression of other genes by pairing with mRNA.

Mutations in *BRCA1* and *BRCA2* (breast cancer 1 and 2, early-onset genes) are currently of clinical importance. Both are tumour suppressors and caretaker genes that repair double-stranded DNA breaks. Inherited mutations in either gene greatly increase the risk for a variety of tumours, especially breast cancer in both women and men, and ovarian or prostate cancers. Approximately 12% of women generally will develop breast cancer within their lifetime, whereas about 60% of women with a high-risk *BRCA1* mutation and 45% with a *BRCA2* mutation will develop cancer by age 70.[18] Ovarian cancer occurs in approximately 1.4% of the general population, but about 39% of women with an inherited mutation in *BRCA1* and about 15% with a mutation in *BRCA2* will develop ovarian cancer by age 70. At-risk women are currently offered prophylactic surgery to reduce the risk of cancer.

In addition to specific gene mutations and abnormal epigenetic silencing, chromosome instability also appears to be increased in malignant cells, resulting in a high rate of chromosome loss, as well as loss of heterozygosity and chromosome amplification. The underlying mechanism of this instability is not clear but may be caused by malfunctions in the cellular machinery that regulates chromosome segregation at mitosis.

Enabling Replicative Immortality

A hallmark of cancer cells is their immortality, in that they seem to have an unlimited lifespan and will continue to divide for years under appropriate laboratory conditions. One of the most commonly used laboratory cell lines, HeLa cells, was derived from a cervical cancer specimen obtained in 1951 that continues to grow and divide in laboratories around the world.[19] Most normal cells are not immortal and can divide only a limited number of times (known as the Hayflick limit) before they either enter senescence (cease dividing) or enter crisis (apoptosis) and die. One major block to unlimited cell division (i.e., immortality) is the size of a specialized structure called the *telomere*. Telomeres are protective ends, or caps, of repeating hexanucleotides (six nucleotide units) on each chromosome and are placed and maintained by a specialized enzyme called telomerase (Figure 10-14).[20] As one might expect, telomerase is usually active only in germ cells (in ovaries and testes) and in stem cells. All other cells of the body lack telomerase activity. Therefore, when nongerm cells begin to proliferate abnormally their telomere caps shorten with each cell division. Short telomeres normally signal the cell to cease cell division. If the telomeres become critically small, the chromosomes become unstable and fragment, and the cells die.

Cancer cells are very heterogeneous, and many cells die as the cancer develops. When they reach a critical age, most cancer cells activate telomerase to restore and maintain their telomeres, thereby allowing continuous division.[21] The trigger for re-expression of telomerase activity remains unclear, but it seems to require expression of specific oncogenes, such as *RAS* or *MYC*, and loss of function of certain tumour-suppressor genes, such as *p53* and *RB*. Telomerase activity is restored in about 90% of cancers. The remaining cancers appear to recruit or originate from stem cells, becoming cancer stem cells that maintain levels of telomerase activity characteristically found in somatic stem cells.[22] Because telomerase is specifically activated in cancer cells, and potentially in cancer stem cells, it is an attractive therapeutic target.

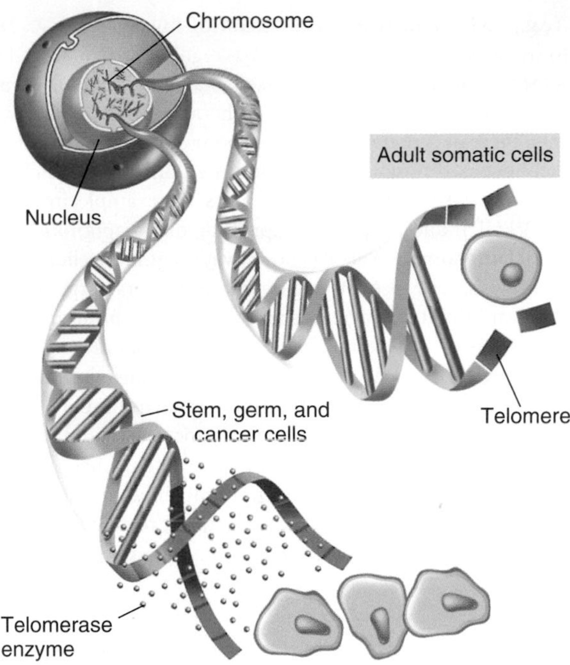

FIGURE 10-14 Control of Immortality: Telomeres and Telomerase. Normal adult somatic cells cannot divide indefinitely because the ends of their chromosomes are capped by telomeres. In the absence of the telomerase enzyme, telomeres become progressively shorter with each division until, when they are critically short, they signal to the cell to stop dividing. In germ cells, adult stem cells, and cancer cells the telomerase gene is "switched on," producing an enzyme that rebuilds the telomeres. Thus, like germ cells, the cancer cell becomes immortal and able to divide indefinitely without losing its telomeres.

QUICK CHECK 10-3

1. What are the heritable changes in cells that contribute to cancer development?
2. Define *oncogene*, *proto-oncogene*, and *tumour-suppressor gene*.
3. Biologically, why do tumour-suppressor genes have to be inactivated to cause cancer?
4. Define *epigenetics* and *epigenetic silencing*.
5. Distinguish between mutations in somatic cells versus in germ cells.
6. Define *telomeres*, *telomerase*, and *senescence*, and describe their effects on cancer.

Inducing Angiogenesis

A major component of wound healing is the process of establishing new blood vessels within the tissue undergoing repair (called neovascularization or angiogenesis). Access to a blood supply also is obligatory to the growth and spread of cancer. Without a blood supply to deliver oxygen and nutrients, growth of a tumour is limited to about a millimetre in diameter.

Angiogenic factors and angiogenic inhibitors normally control development of new vessels. In cancerous tumours several mechanisms increase and maintain secretion of angiogenic factors by the cancer cells, as well as prevent release of angiogenic inhibitors. Hypoxia-inducible factor-1 alpha (HIF-1α), an oxygen-sensitive transcription factor, is a major regulator of angiogenesis in normal tissue; HIF-1α is stabilized under hypoxic conditions and induces expression of proangiogenic factors, such as vascular endothelial growth factor (VEGF) and basic fibroblast growth factor (bFGF). Inactivation of tumour-suppressor genes (e.g., *p53*) or increased expression of oncogenes (e.g., *HER2*) leads to increased expression of HIF-1α–regulated angiogenic factors and increased vascularization. Increased expression of HIF-1α also is related to increased resistance to chemotherapy, increased tumour cell glycolysis, increased metastasis, and a poor prognosis. These effects may likely occur through an autocrine mechanism by which VEGF activates tumour-associated VEGF receptors. For example, in soft tissue sarcomas VEGF induces increased expression of antiapoptotic proteins (e.g., B-cell lymphoma 2 [Bcl-2]) and activation of intracellular survival signal pathways. The use of angiogenic inhibitors targeting VEGF signalling can inhibit angiogenesis and diminish tumour growth.

Other routes of angiogenic factor induction include mutations in cancer oncogenes (e.g., *RAS*, *MYC*) that increase transcription of VEGF by cancer cells. Most cells in the tumour microenvironment also secrete VEGF, including tumour-infiltrating monocytes, endothelial cells, adipocytes, and cancer-associated fibroblasts. Angiogenesis inhibitors, such as **thrombospondin-1 (TSP-1)**, normally bind to cellular surface receptors on inflammatory cells and negatively regulate angiogenesis in wound healing and tissue remodelling. The expression of angiogenesis inhibitors is under the control of *p53*, which is suppressed in cancer cells, thus diminishing the control of stromal inflammatory cell secretion of angiogenic factors.

Cancer cells and stromal cells may increase production of **matrix metalloproteinases (MMPs**; e.g., MMP-9) (Figure 10-15). MMPs are zinc-dependent proteases that digest the surrounding extracellular matrix (ECM). The ECM contains stored latent (inactive) forms of some angiogenic factors (e.g., bFGF, transforming growth factor-beta [TGF-β]). MMPs activate the stored forms into functional angiogenic factors.

The vessels formed within tumours differ from those in healthy tissue. They originate from endothelial sprouting from existing capillaries and irregular branching, rather than regular branching seen in healthy tissue. The interendothelial cell contact is less tight so the vessels are more porous and prone to hemorrhage, as well as allowing passage of tumour cells into the vascular system.

Reprogramming Energy Metabolism

Cancer cells live in a distinct environment from normal cells and have different nutritional requirements from nonproliferating cells. The

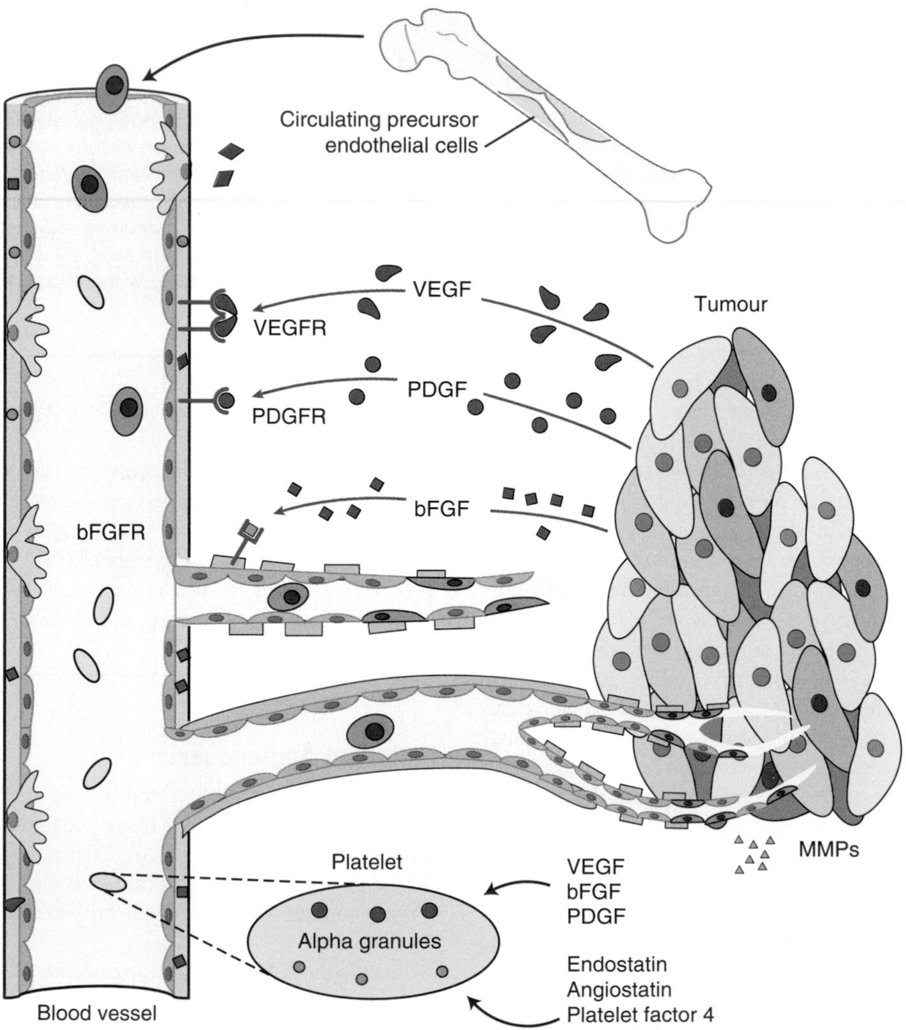

FIGURE 10-15 Tumour-Induced Angiogenesis. Malignant tumours secrete angiogenic factors and tissue-remodelling matrix metalloproteinases (*MMPs*) that actively induce formation of new blood vessels. New blood vessels are formed from both local endothelial cells and circulating precursor cells recruited from the bone marrow. Circulating platelets can also release regulatory proteins into the tumour. *bFGF* and *bFGFR*, basic fibroblast growth factor and its receptor, respectively; *PDGF* and *PDGFR*, platelet-derived growth factor and its receptor, respectively; *VEGF* and *VEGFR*, vascular endothelial growth factor and its receptor, respectively. (Reprinted by permission from Macmillan Publishers Ltd: NATURE REVIEWS DRUG DISCOVERY, Folkman, J., "Angiogenesis: an organizing principle for drug discovery?," 6[4]: 273–286, copyright 2007.)

successful cancer cell divides rapidly, with the consequent requirement for the building blocks to construct new cells. Nonmalignant cells in the presence of adequate oxygen normally generate adenosine triphosphate (ATP) by mitochondrial oxidative phosphorylation (OXPHOS), generating 36 ATP molecules from each glucose molecule that is broken down to water and carbon dioxide. In the absence of sufficient oxygen (hypoxia) normal cells perform glycolysis (anaerobic glycolysis), generating only two ATP molecules per molecule of glucose, with lactic acid and pyruvate as byproducts.

Even in the presence of adequate oxygen, cancer cells may not use OXPHOS, but are reprogrammed to glycolysis (Warburg effect) (Figure 10-16). Thus, the Warburg effect is the use of glycolysis under normal oxygen conditions, hence the name **aerobic glycolysis**. Although aerobic glycolysis was postulated to arise from cancer-specific mitochondrial dysfunction, it is now apparent that this is instead a highly regulated and beneficial adaptation for cancer cells.[23] The shift from OXPHOS to glycolysis allows lactate and other products of glycolysis to be used for the more efficient production of lipids, nucleosides, amino acids, and other molecular building blocks needed for rapid cell growth.

A new model, the **reverse Warburg effect**, may play a role in certain cancers. Cancer cells may continue using the OXPHOS to generate large amounts of ATP. However, they also may manipulate the cancer-associated fibroblasts (CAFs), perhaps by inducing oxidative stress, to undergo aerobic glycolysis and secrete metabolites (e.g., lactate, pyruvate) that the cancer cells can use in the citric acid cycle (Krebs cycle) to feed OXPHOS and produce ATP.[24] A secondary consequence would be induction of autophagy in the CAFs, resulting in consumption of the CAFs and release of materials needed by the cancer cell in the synthesis of new organelles.

Promoters of aerobic glycolysis are activated by oncogenes and mutated tumour-suppressor molecules. Upregulation of glucose transporter 1 (GLUT1) under the control of oncogenes (e.g., *RAS*, *MYC*) and mutant tumour suppressors (e.g., *TP53*) increases transport of glucose into the cytoplasm. These and other oncogenes or mutant tumour-suppressor genes inhibit OXPHOS and promote the aerobic glycolytic pathway and related metabolic pathways that support the rapid growth of cancers.[25]

Clinically the high glucose utilization of a cancer can be exploited for its detection.[26] ^{18}F-fluorodeoxyglucose (FDG) is incorporated into cells in the same way as glucose, with two key differences. Because it is missing a key hydroxyl group it cannot be broken down by glycolysis and, thus, FDG accumulates in cells. Because it is tagged with ^{18}F, it can be imaged by a positron emission tomography (PET) scan. Small metastatic tumour masses that are consuming huge amounts of glucose can readily be detected with this imaging method (Figure 10-17).

Resisting Apoptotic Cell Death

Programmed cell death (**apoptosis**) is a mechanism by which individual cells can self-destruct under conditions of tissue remodelling or as a protection against aberrant cell growth that may lead to malignancy. Two pathways may trigger apoptosis (Figure 10-18). The intrinsic pathway (mitochondrial pathway) monitors cellular stress. Cellular stress may include DNA damage, genomic instability, aberrant proliferation, loss of adhesion to ECM or to adjacent cells, and other causes and characteristics of abnormal cellular physiology. The extrinsic pathway is activated through a plasma membrane receptor complex linked to intracellular activators of apoptosis (known as the *death receptor*).

The balance between proapoptotic (e.g., Bcl-2–associated X protein [BAX] and Bcl-2–homologous antagonist/killer [BAK]) and antiapoptotic (e.g., Bcl-2) members of the Bcl-2 family regulates apoptosis. Both groups regulate mitochondrial release of proapoptotic molecules (e.g., cytochrome *c*). As mentioned previously, expression of the tumour-suppressor gene *p53* is affected by intracellular stress, particularly DNA damage. If DNA damage is irreparable, *p53* is activated by phosphorylation and induces transcription of proapoptotic factors.

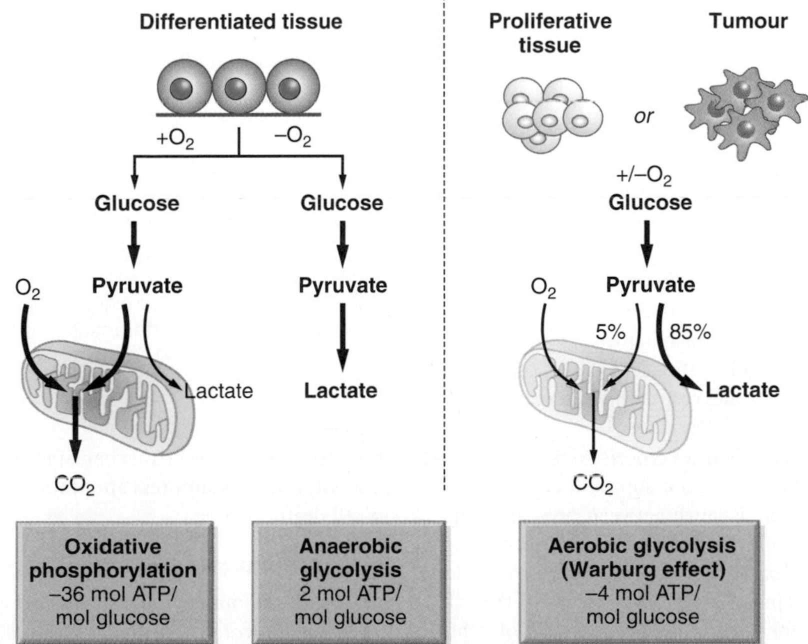

FIGURE 10-16 Cancers Have Altered Metabolism. Normal tissues use oxidative phosphorylation (OXPHOS) to turn glucose into carbon dioxide (CO_2) and energy (in the form of adenosine triphosphate [*ATP*]). Cancers take a different approach; even in the presence of oxygen (O_2), they do not use OXPHOS. Instead, they consume large quantities of glucose to make cellular building blocks, supporting rapid proliferation. (From Vander Heiden, M.G., Cantley, L.C., & Thompson, C.B. [2009]. *Science, 324*, 1029–1033.)

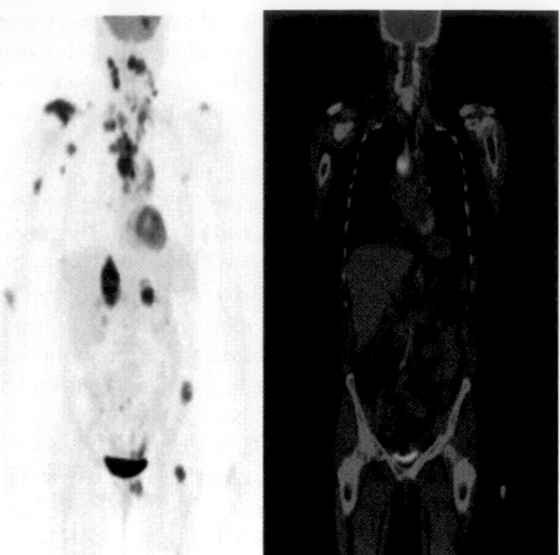

FIGURE 10-17 The Intense Glucose Requirement of Cancer Aids in Diagnosis. This 54-year-old woman had a non–small cell lung carcinoma (NSCLC) surgically removed. Five years later, these images were obtained. The positron emission tomography (PET) scan using ^{18}F-deoxyglucose shows metastatic lesions in the brain, right shoulder, and mediastinal and cervical lymph nodes as well as the liver, left pelvis, and proximal femur. *Left,* PET whole-body image. *Right,* Representative coronal image from the whole-body FDG-PET/CT–fused image of the same patient. The fused image consists of the computed tomography [CT] image with the metabolic information superimposed in colour. The pattern of distribution is most likely from the primary tumour to the large mediastinal lymph nodes, followed by lymphatic spread to cervical lymph nodes. Bloodborne dissemination produced the bone, brain, and liver metastases. Normally, only the heart, brain, and bladder show a strong signal on PET scan. *FDG,* fluorodeoxyglucose. (Images courtesy John Hoffman, MD, Huntsman Cancer Institute, Salt Lake City, UT.)

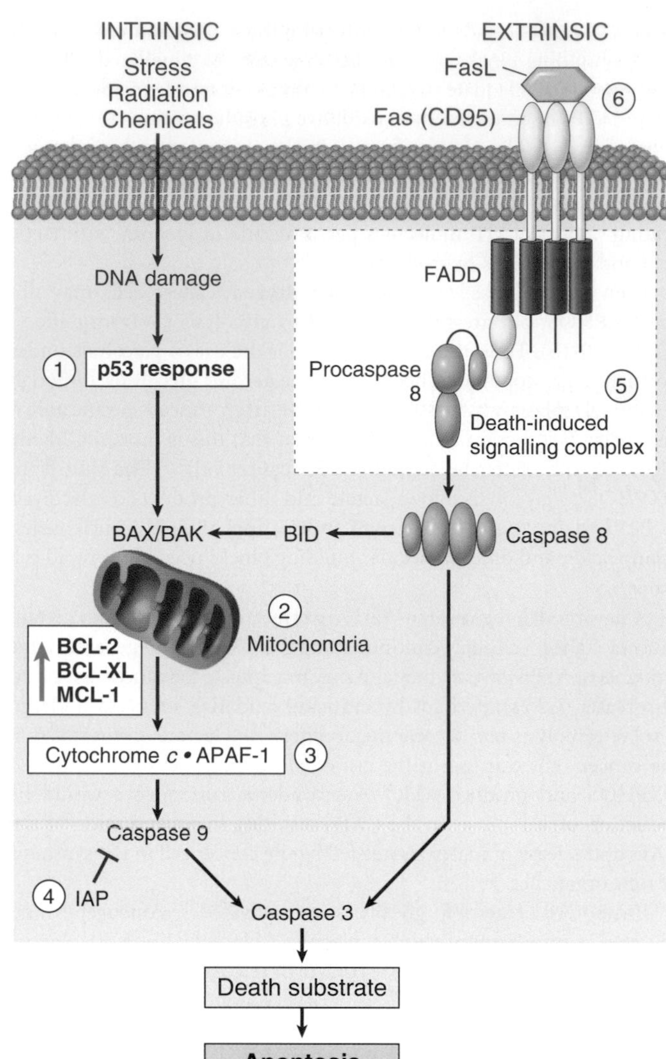

FIGURE 10-18 Extrinsic and Intrinsic Pathways of Apoptosis and Mechanisms Used by Tumour Cells to Evade Cell Death. (1) Loss of p53 leading to reduced function of proapoptotic factors, such as BAX. **(2)** Reduced egress of cytochrome *c* from mitochondria as a result of upregulation of antiapoptotic factors, such as Bcl-2. **(3)** Loss of apoptotic peptidase-activating factor 1 (*APAF1*). **(4)** Upregulation of inhibitors of apoptosis (*IAP*). **(5)** Reduced CD95 levels. **(6)** Inactivation of death domain signalling complex (Fas-associated death domain [*FADD*]). *BAK,* Bcl-2–homologous antagonist or killer; *Bcl-2,* B-cell lymphoma 2; *Bcl-XL,* B-cell lymphoma-extra large; *BID,* BH3 interacting-domain death agonist (related to Bcl-2); *Fas,* apoptosis antigen 1 receptor; *FasL,* Fas ligand; *MCL-1,* myeloid leukemia cell differentiation protein. (From Kumar, V., Abbas, A.K., & Aster, J.C. [Eds.]. [2015]. *Robbins and Cotran pathologic basis of disease* [9th ed.]. Philadelphia: Saunders.)

The extrinsic pathway is relatively dormant until the death receptor is activated. The principal apoptotic receptor is called Fas/CD95 (the CD95 nomenclature is an alternative for Fas) (see Figure 10-18). Fas is a receptor for Fas ligand (FasL) and similar molecules, such as tumour necrosis factor (TNF). T-cytotoxic lymphocytes (Tc cells) and natural killer (NK) cells express surface and soluble FasL and can produce TNF, thus inducing apoptosis in target cells. The Fas receptor is linked to a complex of intracellular proteins (the Fas-associated death domain [FADD] signalling complex) that triggers apoptosis.

Both pathways activate a series of intracellular effector enzymatic molecules (caspases). Proapoptotic molecules released by mitochondria in the intrinsic pathway activate caspase 9, which in turn activates caspase 3. Caspase 3 cuts DNA and other substrates, leading to cell death. Activation of the extrinsic pathway activates caspase 8, which can directly activate caspase 3.

Apoptotic pathways are dysregulated in most cancers. Most commonly, loss-of-function mutations to the *TP53* gene suppress activation of apoptosis during DNA damage. The balance between pro- and antiapoptotic molecules also can be affected by overexpression of antiapoptotic molecules or diminished expression of antiapoptotic molecules resulting from mutations. Overexpression of Bcl-2 occurs in the vast majority of follicular B-cell lymphomas. Excess expression of other antiapoptotic members of the Bcl-2 family also may provide increased resistance to chemotherapeutic medications, many of which act through induction of apoptosis. Other mechanisms of providing resistance to apoptosis include downregulation of caspases or production of caspase inhibitors. By whatever mechanism, or combination of mechanisms, successful cancers suppress apoptotic pathways and increase resistance to cell death.

Tumour-Promoting Inflammation

Historically, an immune/inflammatory response to cancer was considered a detrimental condition that successful tumours evolved methods of evading. We now realize that the relationship between a cancer and the inflammatory system is much more complex.[27] The inflammatory response may contribute to the onset of cancer and be manipulated throughout the process to benefit tumour progression and spread.[28]

Chronic inflammation has been recognized for close to 150 years as being an important factor in the development of cancer.[29] Chronic inflammations may result from many causes, for example, solar irradiation, asbestos exposure (mesothelioma), pancreatitis, and infection (Table 10-3). Additionally, some organs appear to be more susceptible to the oncogenic effects of chronic inflammation (e.g., the gastro-intestinal [GI] tract, prostate, thyroid gland). Individuals who have suffered with ulcerative colitis for 10 years or more have up to a 30-fold increase in the risk of developing colon cancer.[30] Chronic viral hepatitis caused by hepatitis B virus (HBV) or hepatitis C virus (HCV) infection markedly increases the risk of liver cancer.

TABLE 10-3 Chronic Inflammatory Conditions and Infectious Agents Associated With Neoplasms

Inflammatory Condition	Associated Neoplasm(s)
Asbestosis, silicosis	Mesothelioma, lung carcinoma
Bronchitis	Lung carcinoma
Cystitis, bladder inflammation	Bladder carcinoma
Gingivitis, lichen planus	Oral squamous cell carcinoma
Inflammatory bowel disease, Crohn's disease, chronic ulcerative colitis	Colorectal carcinoma
Lichen sclerosus	Vulvar squamous cell carcinoma
Chronic pancreatitis, hereditary pancreatitis	Pancreatic carcinoma
Reflux esophagitis, Barrett esophagus	Esophageal carcinoma
Sialadenitis	Salivary gland carcinoma
Sjögren syndrome, Hashimoto thyroiditis	Mucosa-associated lymphoid tissue (MALT) lymphoma
Skin inflammation	Melanoma
Infectious Agent (Nonviral)	**Associated Neoplasm(s)**
Helicobacter pylori	Gastric adenocarcinoma, MALT lymphoma
Chronic bacterial cholecystitis	Gallbladder cancer
Schistosomiasis	Bladder, liver, rectal carcinoma; follicular lymphoma of spleen
Liver flukes	Cholangiocarcinoma
Infectious Agent (Viral)	**Associated Neoplasm(s)**
Human immunodeficiency virus type 1 (HIV-1)	Non-Hodgkin's lymphoma, squamous cell carcinomas, Kaposi sarcoma
Hepatitis B (HBV) and hepatitis C (HCV)	Hepatocellular carcinoma
Epstein-Barr virus (EBV)	B-cell non-Hodgkin's lymphoma, Burkitt lymphoma, nasopharyngeal carcinoma
Kaposi sarcoma herpesvirus (KSHV)/human herpesvirus 8 (HHV8) and immunodeficiency	Kaposi sarcoma
Human papillomavirus (HPV)-16, -18, -31, others	Cervical, anogenital
Human T-cell lymphotropic virus type 1 (HTLV-1)	Adult T-cell leukemia/lymphoma

From Kuper, H., Adami. H.O., & Trichopoulos, D. (2000). *J Intern Med, 248*(3), 171–183.

A specific example is the association between gastric inflammation induced by infection with the bacterium *Helicobacter pylori* and the risk for gastric cancer. *H. pylori* is a bacterium that infects more than half of the world's population. Chronic infection with *H. pylori* is an important cause of peptic ulcer disease and is strongly associated with gastric carcinoma, a leading cause of cancer deaths worldwide. It also is associated with a less common cancer, gastric mucosa-associated lymphoid tissue (MALT) lymphomas.[31] *H. pylori* infection is often acquired in childhood and disproportionately affects lower socioeconomic classes. Although most infections are asymptomatic, prolonged chronic inflammation can lead to increased gastric acid secretion, atrophic gastritis, and duodenal ulcers, or benign cellular proliferation that can, in a small fraction of individuals, progress to dysplastic changes and, finally, gastric adenocarcinoma. *H. pylori* infection can both directly and indirectly produce genetic and epigenetic changes in cells of infected stomachs, including mutations in *TP53* and alterations in the methylation of specific genes. Eradication of *H. pylori* from infected individuals before the development of dysplasia may prevent the development of cancer. However, there is no expert consensus on the value of population screening and treatment strategies. The MALT lymphomas associated with chronic *H. pylori* infections may depend on chronic inflammation and antigenic stimulation associated with infections, and therefore, treatment with antibiotics may be useful even in cases of early lymphoma.

Once cells with malignant phenotypes have developed, additional complex interactions occur between the tumour and the surrounding stroma and cells of the immune and inflammatory systems. Cancers disrupt the environment, initiate or enhance inflammation, and, in turn, recruit local and distant cells (macrophages, lymphocytes, and other cellular components of inflammation). The acute inflammatory response is initially designed to eliminate infection, but evolves to initiate and direct the healing process (see Chapter 6). Successful tumours appear capable of manipulating cells of the inflammatory response from a rejection response toward the phenotypes associated with wound healing and tissue regeneration; this process includes induction in the damaged tissue of cellular proliferation, neovascularization, and local immune suppression.[32] These activities benefit cancer progression, as well as increase resistance to chemotherapeutic agents.

One of the key cells that promote tumour survival is the **tumour-associated macrophage (TAM)**. Tumours commonly produce cytokines and chemokines that are chemotactic factors for monocytes/macrophages (e.g., colony-stimulating factor-1 [CSF-1; also known as *macrophage colony-stimulating factor*, or M-CSF], the chemokine ligand 2 [CCL2; also known as *macrophage chemotactic protein-1*, or MCP-1]). Levels of CCL2 in human breast cancer and cancers of the esophagus are related to the degree of macrophage infiltration and progression of the tumour. Most tumours have large numbers of TAMs, whose presence frequently correlates with a worse prognosis. Thus, monocytes are attracted from the blood and into the tumour, where they mature into macrophages. Monocytes have the capacity to differentiate into several macrophage phenotypes, depending upon the conditions in the micro-environment. The classic proinflammatory macrophage (M1) is the primary macrophage in the acute inflammatory response and is responsible for removal and destruction of infectious agents. During healing, however, a different phenotype (M2) produces anti-inflammatory mediators to suppress ongoing inflammation and induce cellular proliferation, angiogenesis, and wound healing.[33] TAMs appear to phenotypically mimic the M2 phenotype.

TAMs have diminished cytotoxic response and develop the capacity to block Tc-cell and NK-cell functions and produce cytokines that are advantageous for tumour growth and spread. TAMs secrete cellular growth factors (e.g., TGF-β and fibroblast growth factor-2 [FGF-2]) that favour tumour cell proliferation, angiogenesis, and tissue remodelling, similar to their activities in wound healing. They also secrete angiogenesis factors (e.g., VEGF) that induce neovascularization and MMPs that degrade intercellular matrix. The overall effect is increased tumour growth, invasion of the blood vessels, increased oxygen to the tumour, and invasion through the degraded matrix into the local tissue.

Cancer-associated fibroblasts (CAFs) synthesize the ECM that surrounds and permeates the tumour.[34] Cytokines and growth factors stored in the matrix as well as growth factors, metalloproteases, proteoglycans, and other molecules secreted by CAFs contribute greatly to cancer progression, local spread, and metastasis.

Evading Immune Destruction

Many cancers express cell surface antigens that are not generally found on normal cells from the same tissue. Tumour-associated antigens include products of oncogenes, antigens from oncogenic viruses, oncofetal antigens (expressed in embryonic tissues and tumours), and altered glycoproteins and glycolipids.[35] Viral and tumour antigens are processed by the tumour cell and presented on the cell surface by major histocompatibility complex (MHC) class I molecules and are targets of CD8+ Tc cells (see Chapter 7). NK cells recognize altered cell surface glycoproteins and glycolipids. Thus, cancer cells should be recognized as foreign and destroyed by the immune system. In the laboratory, T cells and NK cells recognize and kill cancer cells. This observation gave rise to two hypotheses—immune surveillance and immunotherapy. The immune surveillance hypothesis predicts that most developing malignancies are suppressed by an efficient immune response against tumour-associated antigens. The immunotherapy hypothesis predicts that the immune system could be used to target tumour-associated antigens and destroy tumours clinically. Immunotherapy could be either active, by immunization with tumour antigens to elicit or enhance the immune response against a particular cancer, or passive, by injecting the cancer patient with antibodies or lymphocytes directed against the tumour antigens. However, the interactions between cancer and the immune system are more complex than originally envisioned, and both hypotheses remain controversial.

What is the role of the immune system in protecting against cancer? The most clearly documented effective immune response is prophylactic and directed against oncogenic viruses. Several viruses have been associated with human cancer; human papillomavirus (HPV), Epstein-Barr virus (EBV; also known as *HHV4*), Kaposi sarcoma herpesvirus (KSHV; also known as HHV8), and hepatitis B and C viruses (HBV, HCV) are associated with about 15% of all human cancers worldwide (see Table 10-3).[36] Cancer of the cervix and hepatocellular carcinoma account for approximately 80% of virus-linked cancer cases.

Virtually all cervical cancer is caused by infection with specific types of HPV, which infects basal skin cells and commonly causes warts. There are more than 120 HPV types, but only about 40 can infect human mucosal tissue, and only a few (HPV-16, -18, -31, and -45) are associated with the highest risk of developing cervical, anogenital, and penile cancer. Most HPV infection is handled effectively and rapidly by the immune system and does not cause cancer. Cancer is more common in people with prolonged infection with HPV (a decade or more), during which the viral DNA becomes integrated into the genomic DNA of the infected basal cell of the cervix and directs the persistent production of viral oncogenes. Early oncogenic HPV infection is readily detected by the Papanicolaou (Pap) test, an examination of cervical epithelial scrapings. Early detection of atypical cells in a Pap test alerts health care providers to the possibility of cervical carcinoma in situ, which can be effectively treated. The Pap test is probably the most effective cancer-screening test developed to date. For women age 30 to 65 years old, additional testing for HPV infection of cervical cells (HPV test) should be added.[37] Vaccines protecting against the common oncogenic HPV types (HPV-16 and HPV-18 [types that cause 70% of cervical cancers] and HPV-6 and HPV-11 [types that cause 90% of genital warts]) were approved for clinical use beginning in 2006; if these vaccines are administered to young women and men before an initial HPV infection, this is likely to prevent many cases of cervical cancer.

Chronic hepatitis B infections are common in parts of Asia and Sub-Saharan Africa and confer up to a 200-fold increased risk of developing liver cancer. Chronic hepatitis C infections have become increasingly recognized in Western countries. Up to 80% of liver cancer cases worldwide are associated with chronic hepatitis caused either by HBV or by HCV. The initial infection with HBV or HCV is not associated with cancer; instead, it is acquisition of a chronic viral hepatitis that markedly increases cancer risk. In both cases, it appears that a lifetime of chronic liver inflammation predisposes to the development of hepatocellular carcinoma. Widespread use of the HBV vaccine is expected to significantly decrease the incidence of chronic hepatitis B and hence hepatocellular carcinoma. Unfortunately, a vaccine for HCV is not yet available.

For most other human tumour viruses, immunoprophylaxis is not yet available. EBV and HHV8 are members of the Herpesviridae family. More than 90% of adults have been infected with EBV, usually as children and without symptoms. EBV infection during adolescence may cause infectious mononucleosis. The virus infects B cells and stimulates their limited proliferation and usually becomes latent throughout the individual's life. If the individual is immunosuppressed because of HIV infection or because of medications given for an organ transplant, persistent EBV infection can lead to the development of B-cell lymphomas. EBV infection also is associated with Burkitt lymphoma in areas of endemic malaria and with nasopharyngeal carcinoma, a cancer endemic in Chinese populations in Southeast Asia. HHV8 is linked to the development of Kaposi sarcoma, a cancer that was once seen primarily in older men but now occurs in a markedly more virulent form in immunosuppressed individuals, especially those with acquired immunodeficiency syndrome (AIDS). HHV8 also has been linked to several rare lymphomas. **Human T-cell lymphotropic virus type 1 (HTLV-1)** is an oncogenic retrovirus linked to the development of adult T-cell leukemia and lymphoma (ATLL). HTLV-1 is transmitted vertically (i.e., inherited by children from infected parents) and horizontally (e.g., by breastfeeding, sexual intercourse, blood transfusions, and exposure to infected needles). Infection with HTLV-1 may be asymptomatic, and only a small fraction of infected individuals develop ATLL, often many years after acquiring the virus.

Thus immunization has proven beneficial in preventing viral-induced cancers. The immune surveillance hypothesis, however, would predict that components of the immune system, especially T cells, monitor the body and destroy most nascent tumours, even those not caused by viruses. If the immune surveillance hypothesis is correct, compromise of the immune system by immunosuppressive medications or development of genetic or acquired immune deficiencies would result in increased incidences of all types of cancer.[38] However, defective immune responses generally only increase the risk for lymphoid cancers, many of which are associated with viral infections. For example, individuals taking chronic powerful immunosuppressive medications, such as those given for kidney, heart, or liver transplant, have a much higher risk of developing viral-associated cancers, with a 10-fold increased risk of non-Hodgkin's lymphoma (caused by EBV) and up to a 1 000-fold increased risk of Kaposi sarcoma (caused by HHV8). The same immunosuppressed individuals, however, have only a slight increase in the risk of common cancers such as lung and colon cancer (and this could well be because of increased inflammation at those sites), and no increase in the risk of breast or prostate cancer.

However, many tumours have an abundance of tumour-infiltrating lymphocytes (TILs). Although the immune cells frequently found in tumours were once thought to be futile attempts at an antitumour response, instead it appears that cancers actively recruit an immune and stromal response to assist in the remodelling of tissues, formation of new blood vessels, and promotion of metastasis.[39] NK cells are generally in low amounts in tumours. The predominant TILs are T-regulatory (Treg) cells. Treg cells are CD4+ cells that differentiate under the control of specific cytokines, primarily TGF-β. The role of Treg cells during wound healing is to control or limit the immune response to protect the host's own tissues against autoimmune reactions. Their role in tumours is manipulated to prevent a destructive antitumour immune response and provide cytokines that facilitate tumour cell proliferation and spread. Treg cells and TAMs, as well as other stromal cells, produce very high levels of TGF-β and interleukin-10 (IL-10). IL-10 is an immunosuppressive cytokine, which generally decreases T-helper cell 1 (Th1) and Th2 activity, suppresses antigen recognition and cell proliferation by Th cells, and suppresses the capacity of CD8+ Tc cells to recognize, proliferate, and kill tumour cells.[40] The goal of current immunotherapy regimens is to reverse this relationship and facilitate T-cell–mediated cancer cell death (discussed later in this chapter).

The release of immunosuppressive factors into the tumour microenvironment also increases resistance of the tumour to chemotherapy and radiotherapy. Increased levels of Treg cells in blood and lymph nodes and infiltrating the tumour correlate with poor outcomes in breast and GI tumours. In advanced non–small cell lung cancer, an elevated ratio of Treg to Tc cells is related to a poor response to platinum-based chemotherapy. Immunosuppressive cytokines additionally lower the cancer cell's sensitivity to immune-mediated death (Figure 10-19). With increasing heterogeneity of cells within the tumour, subpopulations of antigen-negative cancer cell variants may selectively outgrow more immune-sensitive cells.[41] Variants may suppress the production of particular antigens or suppress levels of antigen-presenting MHC class I molecules. Other cytokines appear to increase the cancer cells' resistance to apoptosis. For example, the Th2 cytokine IL-4 increases the resistance of thyroid cancer to chemotherapy; IL-6 produced by Th cells, adipocytes, and fibroblasts activates survival pathways in breast cancer, leading to resistance to radiotherapy; and adipocytes enhance the transcription of the antiapoptotic factor Bcl-2 in leukemia cells.

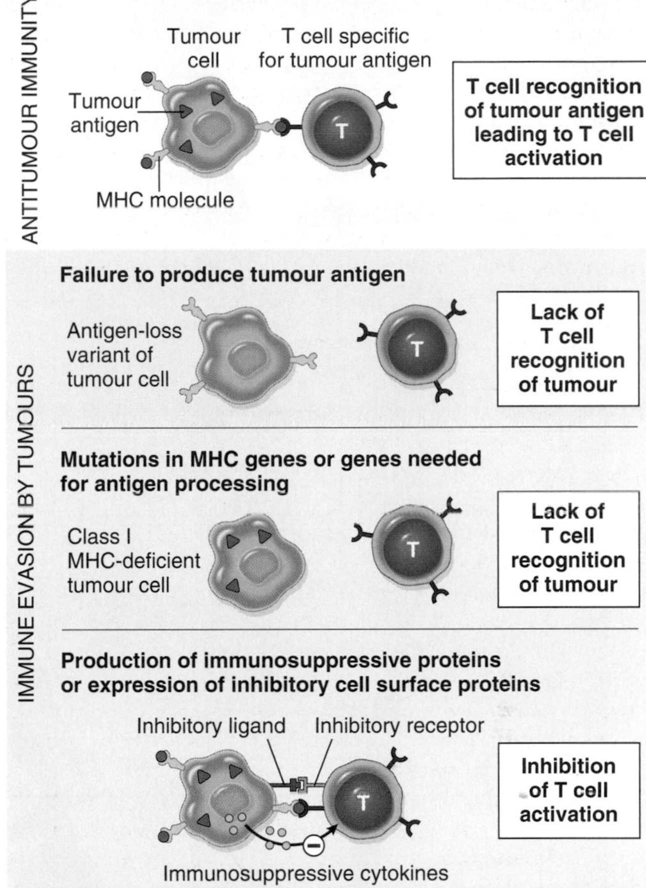

FIGURE 10-19 Mechanisms by Which Tumour Cells Evade the Immune System. Tumours may evade the immune response by losing expression of antigens or major histocompatibility complex (*MHC*) molecules or by producing immunosuppressive cytokines or ligands for inhibitory receptors on T cells. (From Kumar, V., Abbas, A.K., & Aster, J.C. [Eds.]. [2015]. *Robbins and Cotran pathologic basis of disease* [9th ed.]. Philadelphia: Saunders.)

Activating Invasion and Metastasis

Metastasis is the spread of cancer cells from the site of the original tumour to distant tissues and organs through the body. Metastasis is a defining characteristic of cancer and is the major cause of death from cancer. Cancer that has not metastasized can often be cured by a combination of surgery, chemotherapy, and radiation. These same therapies are frequently ineffective against cancer that has metastasized. For example, in appropriately treated women with localized low-stage breast cancer, the 5-year survival rate is often greater than 90%. Tragically, less than 30% of women with metastatic breast cancer are still alive 5 years after diagnosis. A growing body of basic and clinical research is defining the biological principles of metastasis, with the hope that this improved understanding will lead to novel diagnostic approaches and better therapies to prevent and treat metastatic cancers.

How do cancer cells develop the ability to metastasize? Metastasis is a highly inefficient process. Cancer cells must surmount multiple physical and physiological barriers to spread, survive, and proliferate in distant locations, and the destination must be receptive to the growth of the cancer. Changes in the tumour microenvironment initiate the metastatic process and may include stromal cell adaptation to increase tumour mass and intratumour hypoxia.[42] As this diversity increases within the changing tumour microenvironment, some cancer cells evolve with multiple new abilities that can facilitate metastasis. The model for transition to metastatic cancer cells is called epithelial-mesenchymal transition (EMT).[43]

Epithelial-mesenchymal transition (EMT) has been most extensively described for carcinomas, which originate from highly differentiated and polarized epithelial cells that form structured sheets stabilized by multiple adherences to neighbouring cells and to a basement membrane (an extracellular meshwork of collagens and other connective tissue proteins) along the cell's basal surface. Although the degree of malignant transformation resulting in a primary carcinoma may be adequate for local expansion of the tumour, neoplastic cells usually retain some epithelial-like characteristics that prevent dissociation from the ECM and preclude successful metastasis to distal sites. A greater degree of cellular "dedifferentiation" is necessary to produce the phenotype that can separate from the primary tumour and flourish in a potentially hostile secondary site. This results from a programmed transition of the still partially epithelial-like carcinoma to a more undifferentiated mesenchymal-like phenotype (Figure 10-20). A similar process occurs with tumours of endothelial origin (endothelial-mesenchymal transition).

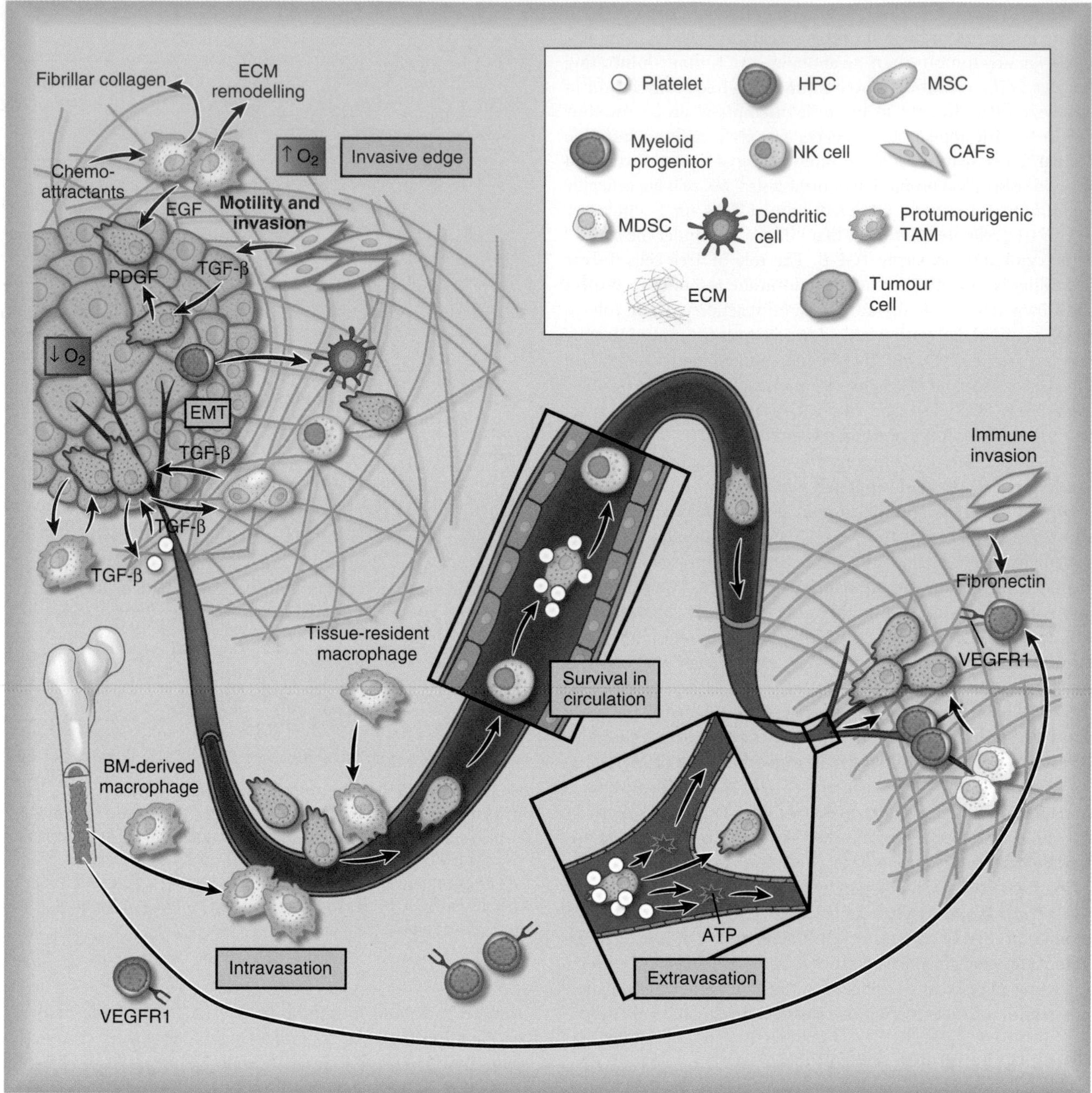

FIGURE 10-20 Epithelial-Mesenchymal Transition and Metastasis. The microenvironment supports metastatic dissemination and colonization at secondary sites. Stromal cells (e.g., mesenchymal stem cells [*MSC*]), possibly facilitated by a relative decrease in oxygen (O_2) levels in the tumour, contribute to the epithelial-mesenchymal transition (*EMT*) through which tumour cells develop a metastatic phenotype characterized by suppression of adhesion molecules and reduced adherence to adjacent cells and extracellular matrix (*ECM*), increased local invasion, and access to the blood and lymphatic circulations. One major mediator of this process is transforming growth factor-beta (*TGF-β*), which is secreted by the tumour stroma. Intravascularization of tumour cells into the circulation is facilitated by protumourigenic tumour-associated macrophage (*TAMs*), and cancer-associated fibroblasts (*CAFs*) tend to cluster at the leading edge of the invading cancer cells and secrete matrix metalloproteinases that promote digestion and remodelling of the surrounding ECM. Survival in the circulation is promoted by association with platelets and clotting factors that shield the cancer cells from cytotoxic immune cells (T-cytotoxic cells and natural killer cells [*NK cells*]) that also are suppressed by myeloid-derived suppressor cells (*MDSC*). Potential metastatic sites are prepared by induction of fibronectin, which provides a site for the influx of hematopoietic progenitor cells (*HPC*) that have receptors for vascular endothelial cell growth factor. HPC appear essential for establishment of a metastatic site. At a metastatic site, cancer cells will adhere to local vascular endothelium, undergo extravascularization facilitated by the effects of adenosine triphosphate (*ATP*) on the endothelium, and undergo mesenchymal-to-epithelial transition. The premetastatic niche may have been prepared by molecular signalling from the cancer and initiation of a favourable microenvironment. *BM*, bone marrow; *EGF*, epidermal growth factor; *PDGF*, platelet-derived growth factor; *VEGFR1*, vascular endothelial cell growth factor receptor 1. (Reprinted by permission from Macmillan Publishers Ltd: NATURE MEDICINE, Quail, D.F., & Joyce, J.A., "Microenvironmental regulation of tumor progression and metastasis," 19[11]: 1423–1437, copyright 2013.)

EMT is a process that occurs normally in embryonic development, as well as wound healing and tissue repair. Generally, cells that have transitioned into a mesenchymal-like phenotype have suppressed expression of adhesion molecules with a loss of polarity, increased migratory capacity, elevated resistance to apoptosis, and demonstrated the potential to redifferentiate into other cell types.[44] The transition to a mesenchymal-like phenotype is, in most cases, driven by cytokines and chemokines produced within the tumour microenvironment.[45] IL-8 is an effective driver of carcinoma cells into EMT.

Invasion, or local spread, is a prerequisite for metastasis. In its earliest stages local invasion may occur by direct tumour extension. Eventually, however, cells migrate away from the primary tumour and invade the surrounding tissues (see Figure 10-20). Invasion is a multistep process within EMT that includes diminished cell-to-cell adhesion, digestion of the surrounding ECM, and increased motility of individual cancer cells. TGF-β induces changes in expression of E-cadherin (an integral component of tight junctions) and of β_4-integrin in mammary gland tumour cells. The loss of E-cadherin in particular allows cells to detach from the ECM and migrate more readily.

Recruitment of TAMs and other cell types is critical for invasion. Cells are normally attached to the ECM. TAMs and other stromal cells secrete proteases and protease activators, such as the MMPs and plasminogen activators, which promote digestion of connective tissue capsules and other structural barriers. Degradation of the surrounding ECM creates pathways through which cells can move, while releasing bioactive peptides as digestion products that further stimulate tumour growth and mobility.

Normal cells, when separated from their ECM, undergo *anoikis*, a form of apoptosis. Tumour cells adapted to a hypoxic environment have already been selected for resistance to apoptosis, often by loss of normal cell death pathways. The process of EMT frequently increases resistance to apoptosis. For example, neuroblastomas with loss of the proapoptotic caspase 8 genes are able to avoid apoptosis after loss of integrins and are more able to metastasize than the same cells with normal levels of caspase 8. Accordingly, individuals whose neuroblastomas have low levels of caspase 8 have a poor prognosis.

To transition from local to distant metastasis, the cancer cells must also be able to invade local blood and lymphatic vessels, a task facilitated by stimulation of neoangiogenesis and lymphangiogenesis by factors such as VEGF. After release from the ECM and digestion of basement membranes, mobile cancer cells gain access to the circulation, perhaps facilitated by the leaky newly made vessels and attraction of the cells because of chemoattractants coming from these new vessels. Once in the circulation, metastatic cells must be able to withstand the physiological stresses of travel in the blood and lymphatic circulation, including high shear rates and exposure to immune cells. One mechanism is for tumour cells to bind to blood platelets, giving them a protective coat of non-malignant blood cells that both shields the tumour cells and creates a small tumour embolus, or cancer clot, that can promote cancer cell survival in distant locations (see Figure 10-20).

Cancer cells spread through vascular and lymphatic pathways. The neovascularization of a cancer offers malignant cells direct access into the venous blood and draining lymphatic vessels. The venous and lymphatic drainage networks associated with the primary tumour frequently determine the pattern of metastasis. Single cells, clumps, and even tumour fragments can disseminate by these routes. Anatomical patterns of lymphatic and venous blood flow help determine how colon cancers spread to the liver, liver cancers spread through the portal vein to the lungs, lung cancers spread through the systemic circulation to the brain, and breast cancer spreads through the lymphatics to axillary lymph nodes. Cancers often spread first to regional lymph nodes through the lymphatics and then to distant organs through the bloodstream.

There also is a major yet poorly understood selectivity of different cancers for different sites. Metastatic breast cancer often spreads through the bloodstream to bones but rarely to kidney or spleen, whereas lymphomas often spread to the spleen but uncommonly spread to bone. In a key study, different types of cancer cells were injected into the carotid artery of mice.[46] In spite of identical blood flow–mediated distribution of the cancer cells, each cell type produced cancers in very different parts of the brain. This tissue selectivity is likely caused by specific interactions between the cancer cells and specific receptors on the small blood vessels in different organs. Experimental metastasis studies in mice are beginning to reveal additional molecular reasons for this tissue specificity. Examples include interaction between $\alpha3\beta1$ integrins binding to laminin-5 receptors in the lung, and the chemokine receptor CXCR4 on breast cancer cells promoting homing to lung tissues expressing the ligand CXCL12.[47]

A cancer's ability to establish a metastatic lesion in a new location requires that the cancer survive in the specific environment and be capable of forming complex and heterogeneous tumours. In some cases, these tumour-initiating cells are very rare. Human cancers transplanted into special immune-deficient mice will grow and can metastasize. Experiments have been performed to determine how few cancer cells are capable of establishing a tumour; only 1 in 10 000 human colon cancer cells are able to re-form a complex and heterogeneous colon cancer in mice; however, in human melanomas 1 in 4 cells can initiate a complex tumour in the appropriate mouse model. Thus, the number of potentially metastatic cells may vary greatly with the particular cancer.

The degree of dedifferentiation may be variable, but most cells undergoing EMT acquire stem cell traits that facilitate initial growth in a new microenvironment.[48] The EMT is not a stable transition; after taking residence in the metastatic site, the tumour tends to regain some characteristics of the primary tumour, thus reverting to some extent to its epithelial origins. Because metastasis requires successful completion of each and every step, there may be many opportunities to interrupt this potentially lethal pathway.

However, metastasis does not universally result in proliferation at a new site. Some cancer cells survive at a new site but do not proliferate to form a clinically relevant metastatic site. These cancer cells appear to exist in a state of *dormancy*. **Dormancy** is cellular quiescence—a stable, nonproliferative state that is reversible. Cells may remain quiescent for years before initiating proliferation. About two thirds of breast cancer deaths occur after a 5-year disease-free interval. In other conditions, solitary tumour cells can be detected in the blood years after a complete clinical remission in individuals, and many people with detectable micrometastases will not develop clinically obvious metastases. Cancer cell dormancy may be extremely common, even without a history of clinical cancer. Studies of deceased individuals without any history of cancer suggest that most of us have dormant cancer cells that never adjusted to form a malignant tumour.[49]

The causes of dormancy and, more importantly, escape from dormancy and development of a malignant cancer are unknown. Dormancy may result from features of the cell or the environmental niche, or both. Individuals with clinical cancers may shed disseminated tumour cells very early from premetastatic lesions.[50] These early cells may have developed inadequately to a metastatic phenotype and thus cannot recruit cells into a supportive stroma or initiated angiogenesis. Another consideration is the niche itself. It is not clear whether a developing cancer secretes factors that enter the bloodstream and prepare potential metastatic niches.[51] If so, early disseminated cancer cells may encounter nonsupportive niches that foster dormancy. A clear understanding of dormancy is needed because existing cancer therapies do not address this condition.

QUICK CHECK 10-4

1. Why is the stroma important for cancer growth and invasion?
2. Identify cancers that are the result of chronic inflammation.
3. Why does inflammation fuel cancer development or invasion?
4. Identify common viruses that can cause cancer.
5. How do cancers protect themselves from cell death?
6. Why is angiogenesis important to cancer development?

CLINICAL MANIFESTATIONS OF CANCER

The clinical manifestations of cancer are numerous and depend on the localization and type of tumour, and some are apparent before actual diagnosis of a malignancy. Generally, the variety and intensity of symptoms will increase as the malignancy progresses.

Paraneoplastic Syndromes

Paraneoplastic syndromes are symptom complexes that are triggered by a cancer but are not caused by direct local effects of the tumour mass. They are most commonly caused by biological substances released from the tumour (e.g., hormones, cytokines) or by an immune response triggered by the tumour. For example, a small fraction of carcinoid tumours release substances, including serotonin, into the bloodstream that cause flushing, diarrhea, wheezing, and rapid heartbeat. A number of cancers trigger an antibody response that attacks the nervous system, causing a variety of neurological disorders that can precede other symptoms of cancer by months.

Although infrequent, paraneoplastic syndromes are significant because they may be the earliest symptom of an unknown cancer and, in affected individuals, can be serious, often irreversible, and sometimes life-threatening. Table 10-4 presents the classifications of paraneoplastic syndromes.

Pain

Pain is one of the most feared complications of advanced cancer. Although pain can be one of the presenting symptoms of cancer, most commonly there is little or no pain during the early stages of malignant disease. Significant pain, however, occurs in a large fraction of those individuals who are terminally ill with cancer. Pain is strongly influenced by fear, anxiety, sleep loss, fatigue, and overall physical deterioration. It occurs through an interaction among physiological, cultural, and psychological components. (The neurophysiology of pain is discussed in Chapter 14.)

Cancer-associated pain can arise from a variety of direct and indirect mechanisms. Direct pressure, obstruction, invasion of a sensitive structure, stretching of visceral surfaces, tissue destruction, infection, and inflammation all can cause pain. Pain can occur at the site of the primary tumour or can result from a distant metastatic lesion. Furthermore, pain may be referred away from the involved site and manifest, for example, as back pain.

Specific sites are more prone to cancer-associated pain. Bone metastases, common in advanced breast and prostate cancer, can cause significant pain because of periosteal irritation, medullary pressure, vertebral collapse, and pathological fractures. Brain tumours (primary or metastatic) can, depending on the location, cause headache, seizures, or neurological deficits. Pain in the abdomen may be caused by bowel obstruction, or inflammation and infection. Hepatic malignancies can stretch the liver, resulting in a dull pain or a feeling of fullness over the right upper abdominal quadrant. Mucosal surfaces can develop painful ulcerative lesions from the cancer, chemotherapy, and radiation or leukopenia (or both).

The diagnosis and treatment of pain is one of the primary responsibilities of the medical team. The individual's perception and, hence, reporting of pain can vary widely and be affected by such factors as age and cultural background. The first priority of treatment is to control pain rapidly and completely as judged by the individual. The second priority is to prevent recurrence of pain. Objective measurements of pain are increasingly being included along with the reporting of more traditional vital signs. Many institutions are using specialized pain management teams that are trained to recognize different types of acute and persistent pain, as well as the individual's response to that pain. Many modalities are available to treat pain, ranging from combinations of nonsteroidal anti-inflammatory drugs (NSAIDs) and narcotics to palliative surgery and radiation therapy. Individual-controlled analgesia provides many benefits, not the least of which is regaining some control over one's own body. Although cancer pain is a complex problem arising from multiple sources, individuals should be assured that suffering is not inevitable and that relief is attainable.

Fatigue

Fatigue is the most frequently reported symptom of cancer and cancer treatment. The exact mechanisms that produce fatigue are poorly understood. Suggested causes include sleep disturbances, various biochemical changes secondary to disease and treatment, numerous psychosocial factors, and environmental and physical factors.

The physiological understanding of fatigue probably includes mechanisms for decreased muscle contractility. Overall, studies of muscle function suggest that some individuals with cancer may lose portions of muscle function needed to perform normal physical activities. Other areas of research include muscle function consequences from metabolic products of cancer treatment and associated muscle loss from circulating cytokines (e.g., TNF and IL-1). Similar to pain, fatigue is a subjective clinical manifestation. Individuals with cancer describe fatigue in many ways (e.g., weakness, lack of energy, depression). Some of these symptoms have been termed "chemo brain," or mild cognitive impairment. The changes in cognitive function can be caused by the cancer itself or by the stress associated with the diagnosis of cancer, because symptoms similar to "chemo brain" also occur in individuals who have not received chemotherapy.

Cachexia

The multiorgan syndrome of cachexia includes a constellation of clinical manifestations, including anorexia; wasting; thermogenesis; altered heart and liver function; gut malabsorption; early satiety (filling); taste alterations; and altered protein, lipid, and carbohydrate metabolism (Figure 10-21).

Although several definitions of *cachexia* exist, two factors are significant: weight loss and inflammation. Severe weight loss is primarily from loss of skeletal muscle and body fat.[52] The wasting that occurs in muscle may be dependent on alterations in other organs or tissues including white adipose tissue.[52] Important is that cachexia is multifactorial, involving changes in many metabolic pathways. The cachetic syndrome involves abnormalities in heart function, alterations in liver protein synthesis, changes in hypothalamic mediators, and activation of brown adipose tissue and GI function.[52] All of these changes result in a major decrease in quality of life and indirectly result in death in some individuals. The incidence of the syndrome among individuals with cancer is very high and varies by tumour type.[52]

Molecular Basis of Cachexia

Cachexia has been discussed as a type of energy balance disorder where energy intake is decreased and energy expenditure is increased.[52] Energy intake and expenditure depends on the tumour type and its growth

TABLE 10-4 **Paraneoplastic Syndromes**

Clinical Syndromes	Major Forms of Underlying Cancer	Causal Mechanism
Endocrinopathies		
Cushing's syndrome	Small cell lung carcinoma Pancreatic carcinoma Neural tumours	ACTH or ACTH-like substance
Syndrome of inappropriate antidiuretic hormone (SIADH) secretion	Small cell lung carcinoma; intracranial neoplasms	Antidiuretic hormone or atrial natriuretic hormones
Hypercalcemia	Squamous cell carcinoma of lung Breast carcinoma Renal carcinoma Adult T-cell leukemia or lymphoma Ovarian carcinoma	PTHRP, TGF-α, TNF, IL-1
Hypoglycemia	Fibrosarcoma Other mesenchymal sarcomas Hepatocellular carcinoma	Insulin or insulinlike substance
Carcinoid syndrome	Bronchial adenoma (carcinoid) Pancreatic carcinoma Gastric carcinoma	Serotonin, bradykinin
Polycythemia	Renal carcinoma Cerebellar hemangioma Hepatocellular carcinoma	Erythropoietin
Nerve and Muscle Syndromes		
Myasthenia	Bronchogenic carcinoma	Immunological
Disorders of central and peripheral nervous systems	Breast carcinoma	Unknown
Dermatological Disorders		
Acanthosis nigricans	Gastric carcinoma Lung carcinoma Uterine carcinoma	Immunological; secretion of epidermal growth factor
Dermatomyositis	Bronchogenic, breast carcinoma	Immunological
Osseous, Articular, and Soft Tissue Changes		
Hypertrophic osteoarthropathy and clubbing of fingers	Bronchogenic carcinoma	Unknown
Vascular and Hematological Changes		
Venous thrombosis (Trousseau phenomenon)	Pancreatic carcinoma Bronchogenic carcinoma Other cancers	Tumour products (mucins that activate clotting)
Nonbacterial thrombotic endocarditis	Advanced cancers	Hypercoagulability
Anemia	Thymic neoplasms	Unknown
Others		
Nephrotic syndrome	Various cancers	Tumour antigens, immune complexes

From Kumar, V., Abbas, A.K., & Fausto, N. (Eds.). (2005). *Pathologic basis of disease* (7th ed.). Philadelphia: Saunders.
ACTH, adrenocorticotropic hormone; *IL*, interleukin; *PTHRP*, parathyroid hormone–related protein; *TGF-α*, transforming growth factor-alpha; *TNF*, tumour necrosis factor.

phase. Because individuals who are being administered total parenteral nutrition still lose weight, increased resting energy expenditure may be the cause of the wasting syndrome.[52] Investigators are studying the role of both mitochondria and sarcoplasmic reticulum (SR) in muscle function and its relationship to cachexia. Hypotheses related to these functions include increased production of peroxisome-proliferator–activated receptor-γ coactivator-1 alpha (PGC1α), which can activate a mitochondrial protein (mitofusin-2 [MFN2]) that interacts with muscle SR and controls interorganelle calcium (Ca^{2+}) signalling. Therefore, one hypothesis is the overexpression of PGC1α can activate MFN2 expression, leading to Ca^{2+} deregulation, which is closely associated with muscle wasting.[52] Muscle weakness and fatigue is related to loss of myofibrillar proteins in muscle cells. Abnormalities in protein and amino acid metabolism are noted in cachetic muscle (Figure 10-22).

Contributing further to muscle wasting is an increase in apoptosis and an impaired capacity for regeneration.[52] Many signalling pathways are involved in protein turnover leading to the wasting process and are activated by inflammatory mediators including cytokines, myostatin, and tumour-derived factors. In addition to muscle wasting, miRNAs may be involved in stimulating the breakdown of adipose tissue.[53,54] In cancer cachexia, skeletal muscle loss includes major loss of white adipose tissue (WAT). The WAT loss is thought to be caused by (1) increased lipolysis, (2) decreased activity of lipoprotein lipase (LPL), and (3) decreased new or de novo lipogenesis in adipose tissue.[52]

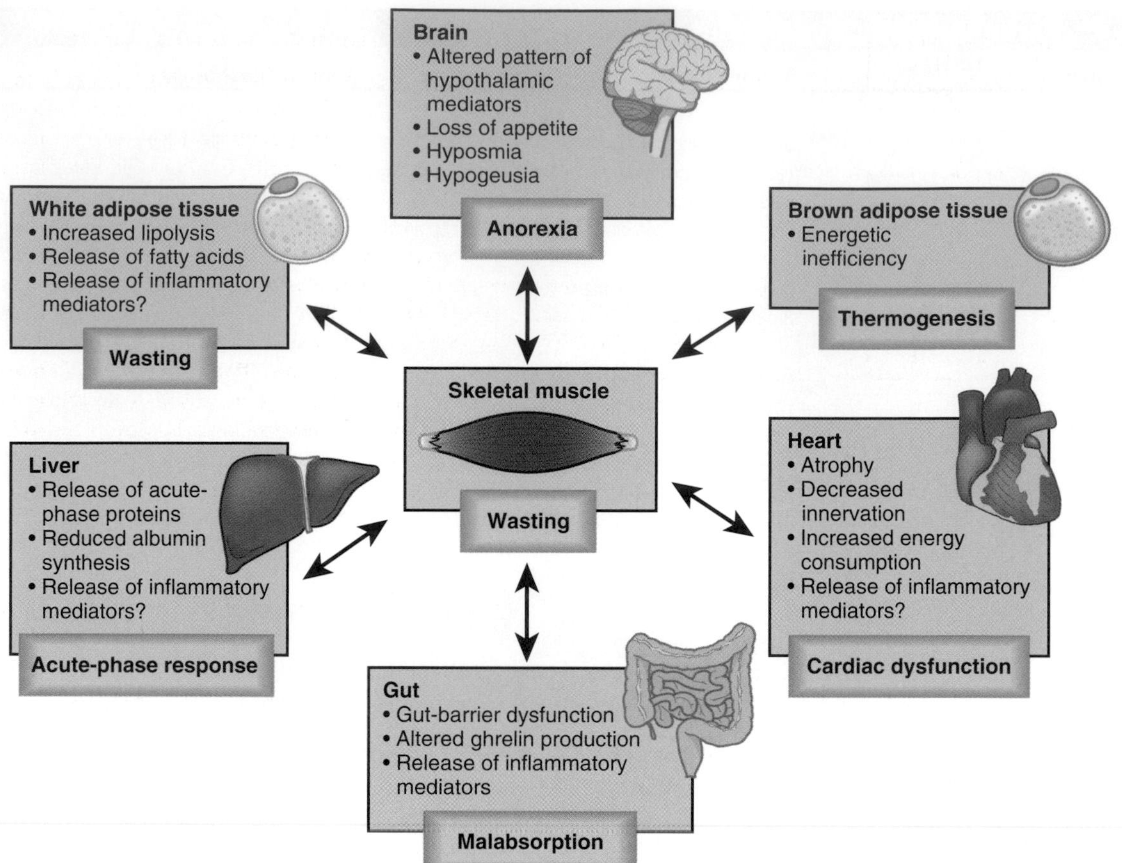

FIGURE 10-21 Cachexia: A Multiorgan Syndrome. Loss of skeletal muscle and of adipose tissue are major contributors to cachexia. But many other organs have a role in the cachexia syndrome, and the wasting that takes place in muscle may be dependent on alterations in these other organs or tissues. Changes in hypothalamic function and activation of brown adipose tissue, as well as alterations in liver and heart function, also are involved in the syndrome. Recent studies support a role for gut microbiota in cancer cachexia and the possibility of a gut-microbiota-skeletal muscle relationship. Recent data suggest that the conversion of white adipose tissue to brown adipose tissue is triggered by both humoral inflammatory mediators (such as interleukin-6) and tumour-derived compounds (such as parathyroid-hormone–related protein). (From Bindels, L.B., Beck, R., Schakman, O., et al. [2012]. *PLoS One, 7*[6], e37971; Bindels, L.B., & Delzenne, N.M. [2013]. *Int J Biochem Cell Biol, 45*, 2186–2190.)

New data show that WAT cells undergo a "browning" process during cancer cachexia where they change to beige cells called *BAT-like cells*.[55,56] Browning is associated with increased thermogenesis. Tumour-derived compounds, such as IL-6 (which also may be released by immune cells) and parathyroid-hormone–related protein (PTHRP), may be the drivers of thermogenesis.[55]

An unusual and frustrating component of cancer care is the person's early satiety, or a sense of being full after only a few mouthfuls of food. Brain mediators are involved in the regulation of food intake and include appetite, satiation, taste, and smell of food. Therefore, the brain is an important organ in anorexia and consequently altered energy balance. Profoundly altered are both *orexigenic* (appetite-stimulating) and *anorexigenic* (appetite-suppressing) brain pathways.[57] (Cytokines are discussed in detail in Chapters 6 and 7.)

Anemia

Anemia is commonly associated with malignancy; 20% of persons diagnosed with cancer have hemoglobin concentrations of less than 14 g/L (normal value = 23 g/L). Mechanisms that cause anemia include chronic bleeding (resulting in iron deficiency), severe malnutrition, cytotoxic chemotherapy, and malignancy in blood-forming organs. Chronic bleeding and iron deficiency can accompany colorectal or genitourinary malignancy. Iron also is malabsorbed in persons with gastric, pancreatic, or upper-intestinal cancer. Often there is a defect in the reutilization of iron because of lack of transfer of iron from the storage pool to blood cell precursors. This defect may be caused by increased secretion of IL-6 and hepcidin (a hormone secreted by the liver that regulates the body's iron distribution) (see Chapter 20). Defects in erythropoietin production and shortened duration of red cell survival also have been documented. In addition, anorexia can cause both iron and folate deficiency. Megaloblastic (large red cell) anemias also may develop after methotrexate treatment.

Administration of erythropoietin, which stimulates production of erythrocytes, has been effective in correcting anemia in persons with cancer; fewer red blood cell transfusions were required in most of the studied subjects. In addition, anemias occurring after chemotherapy or radiotherapy have been treated successfully with erythropoietin. However, recent studies have shown that aggressive use of erythropoietin increases the risk of blood clots and can decrease cancer survival.

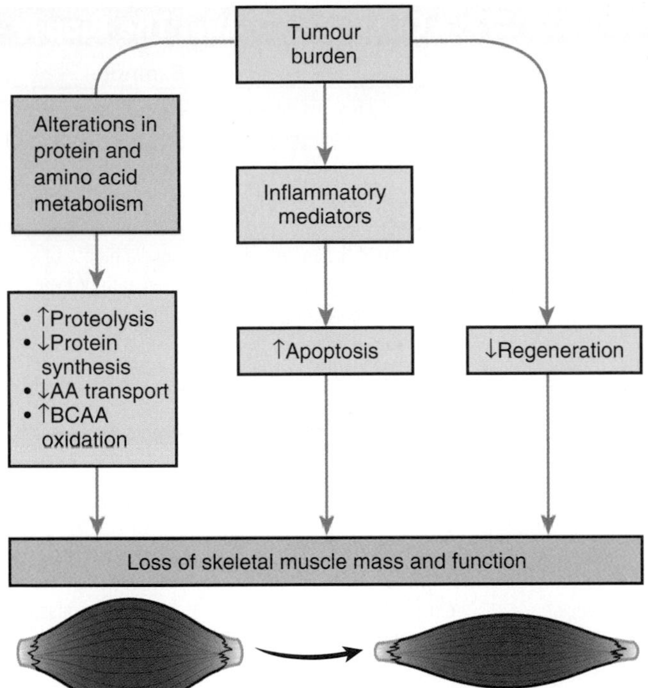

FIGURE 10-22 Wasting of Skeletal Muscle. Inflammation plays a major role in muscle wasting and is linked to alterations in protein and amino acid metabolism, activation of muscle cell apoptosis, and decreased regeneration. *AA,* amino acid; *BCAA,* branched-chain amino acid. (Reprinted by permission from Macmillan Publishers Ltd: NATURE REVIEWS CANCER, Josep M. Argilés, Sílvia Busquets, Britta Stemmler, Francisco J. López-Soriano, "Cancer cachexia: understanding the molecular basis," 14, 754–762, copyright 2014.)

Leukopenia and Thrombocytopenia

Direct tumour invasion of the bone marrow causes both leukopenia (a decreased total white blood cell count) and thrombocytopenia (a decreased number of platelets). More commonly, many chemotherapeutic medications, which primarily affect rapidly dividing cells, are toxic to the bone marrow, often causing granulocytopenia and thrombocytopenia. Granulocytopenia also can result from radiation therapy if it encompasses significant areas of the bone marrow. The duration of granulocytopenia and hence the risk of serious infection can be lessened by treatment with recombinant human granulocyte colony-stimulating factor (rhG-CSF, filgrastim). rhG-CSF stimulates white blood cell precursors in the marrow to proliferate and differentiate rapidly. Thrombocytopenia is a major cause of hemorrhage in persons with cancer and is often treated with platelet transfusions. Thrombocytopenia also is an accompanying disorder of disseminated intravascular coagulation that occurs in persons with acute promyelocytic leukemia (see Chapter 21) and severe infections.

Infection

Infection is the most significant cause of complications and death in persons with malignant disease. Advanced malignancies are highly immunosuppressive, as are the radiotherapy and chemotherapy used to treat it. (Factors that predispose persons with cancer to infection are summarized in Table 10-5.) When the absolute granulocyte count falls below 500 cells per microlitre, the risk of serious microbial (bacterial and fungal) infection increases. Surgery also can lower resistance to infection because removal of large quantities of tissue, together with hemorrhage, dead spaces, and poor tissue perfusion, can create favourable sites for infection. Hospital-related (health care–associated) infections increase because of indwelling medical devices, inadequate wound care, and the introduction of microorganisms from visitors and other individuals.

TABLE 10-5 Factors Predisposing Individuals With Cancer to Infection

Factor	Basis
Age	Many common malignancies occur mostly in older age. Immunological functions decline with age. General debility reduces immunocompetence. Immobility predisposes to infection. Far-advanced cancer often results in immobility and general debility that worsen with age. Older adults are predisposed to nutritional inadequacies. Malnutrition impairs immunocompetence.
Tumour	Nutritional derangements can result. Sites and circumstances favourable to growth of microorganisms (obstruction, serous or blood effusion, ulceration) can be created. Far-advanced disease predisposes individuals to debility and immobility. Humoral or cellular immune defects may result. Metastasis to bone marrow may cause leukopenia or other defects in immunity.
Leukemias	Inadequate granulocyte production (impaired phagocytosis) results. Thrombocytopenia (bleeding) can occur. Late effect: chronic lung disease from *Pneumocystis carinii* pneumonia can develop during therapy.
Lymphomas and other mononuclear phagocyte malignancies	Humoral and cellular immune defects (anergy, altered immunoglobulin production) result. Late effect: splenectomy in children can cause increased susceptibility to infection.
Surgical treatment	Invasive procedure interrupts first lines of defence. Radical nature of surgery (removal of large blocks of tissue in lengthy procedures) causes hemorrhage, decreased tissue perfusion, creation of dead spaces, devitalization of tissues. Procedure may be "dirty" surgery (bowel, infected or contaminated areas). Surgery patients are often older and at poor risk. Long preoperative hospitalization often precedes surgery. Patients may have received previous adrenocorticosteroid therapy. Patients may have infections at sites remote from operative area. Nutritional derangements (especially important in head and neck surgery) may result. Lymph node dissection may predispose patient to local infection and impair containment to area. Gynecological surgery may result in fistulae. Lung surgery may cause bronchopleural fistulae. Debility and immobility may result.

Data from Donovan, M.I., & Girton, S.F. (1984). *Cancer care nursing* (2nd ed.). New York: Appleton-Century-Crofts; Murphy, G.P., Lawrence, W., & Lenhard, R.E. (Eds.). (1995). *Clinical oncology* (2nd ed.). Atlanta: American Cancer Society.

Gastro-intestinal Tract

The entire GI tract relies on rapidly growing cells to produce an effective barrier to trauma and infection and to provide an absorptive surface for nutrients. Both chemotherapy and radiation therapy may cause a decreased cell turnover, thereby leading to oral ulcers (stomatitis), malabsorption, and diarrhea. The disruption of barrier defences also increases the risk for infection, especially invasion by a person's own GI microbiome.

Therapy-induced nausea, thought to be caused by an agent's direct action upon the central nervous system's vomiting centres, historically has been a major obstacle for continuing therapy. Aggressive anti-nausea (antiemetic) therapy, including the centrally acting serotonin 5-hydroxytryptamine (5-HT3) antagonists (such as ondansetron [Zofran] or dolasetron [Anzemet]), has allowed better tolerance of highly emetogenic protocols. Other popular antiemetics include steroids and phenothiazines. Synthetic cannabinoids, the active ingredients in marihuana, increase appetite in addition to having antinausea properties. Analgesia often includes opiate agents, vital in treating severe cases of mucosal lesions. Supplemental nutrition through enteral or parenteral routes may be needed to combat malnutrition. Good oral hygiene may help prevent complications arising from mucosal membrane breakdown.

Hair and Skin

Alopecia (hair loss) results from chemotherapy effects on hair follicles. Alopecia is usually temporary, although hair may regrow with a different texture initially. Not all chemotherapeutic agents cause alopecia. Decreased renewal rates of the epidermal layers in the skin may lead to skin breakdown and dryness, altering the normal barrier protection against infection. Radiation therapy may cause skin erythema (redness) and contribute to breakdown.

TABLE 10-6 Obtaining Tissue: The Biopsy

Procedure	Purpose	Example
Excisional biopsy	The complete removal of area of interest, usually with a margin of normal tissue	Full resection (e.g., mastectomy, partial colectomy)
Incisional biopsy	The removal of a portion of a lesion	Lymph node biopsy, muscle mass biopsy
Core needle biopsy	The removal of tissue with a needle; often performed with direct vision, or guided with ultrasound or CT; provides an intact core tissue sample	Needle biopsy of prostate or liver mass
Fine needle aspirate	The removal of dissociated cells with a small-gauge needle for cytological study; does not preserve tissue structure	Thyroid, breast mass
Exfoliative cytology	The removal of cells shed from surface (e.g., from cervix, sputum [lung], or urine)	Brushings from lung or colon endoscopy

CT, computed tomography.

DIAGNOSIS, CHARACTERIZATION, AND TREATMENT OF CANCER

The diagnosis of cancer has a profound effect on individuals and their families. Responses range from depression to resigned fatalism to an aggressive no-holds-barred pursuit of therapy. The choice of therapy should be based on full consideration by the individual, the family, and the medical team of the individual's diagnosis, prognosis, and therapeutic options. Many types of cancer can be effectively treated with chemotherapy, radiotherapy, surgery, and combinations of these modalities. Caregivers must recognize that many individuals seek additional non–science-based explanations and therapies and often use these therapies, either concurrently or sequentially.

Diagnosis and Staging

Histological Staging

Cancer can be discovered in many ways: after screening tests, from routine examinations, and after investigation of symptoms. The symptoms a cancer produces are as diverse as the types of cancer. The location of the cancer can determine symptoms by physical pressure, obstruction, and loss of normal function, or a cancer can cause problems far away from its source by pressing on nerves or secreting bioactive compounds. Whatever the initial complaint, once the diagnosis is suspected and a tumour has been identified, it is essential that tumour tissue be obtained to establish a definitive diagnosis and correctly classify the disease. Various methods of obtaining tissue are described in Table 10-6.

Once tissue is obtained, it is examined microscopically by the pathologist for the histological hallmarks of cancer detailed in the beginning of this chapter. The classification of the cancer can be further facilitated by a variety of clinically available tests, including immunohistochemical stains, flow cytometry, electron microscopy, chromosome analysis, and genetic studies.

If the diagnosis of cancer is established, it is critical to determine whether the cancer has spread, known as the **stage of cancer**. Staging initially involves determining the size of the tumour, the degree to which it has locally invaded, and the extent to which it has spread (metastasized) (Figure 10-23). Specific molecular tests are increasingly used in staging as well. Diverse schemes are used for staging different tumours. In general, a four-stage system is used, with carcinoma in situ regarded as a special case. Cancer confined to the organ of origin is stage 1; cancer that is locally invasive is stage 2; cancer that has spread to regional structures, such as lymph nodes, is stage 3; and cancer that has spread to distant sites, such as a liver cancer spreading to lung or a prostate cancer spreading to bone, is stage 4. One common scheme for standardizing staging is the World Health Organization's TNM system: *T* indicates tumour spread, *N* indicates node involvement, and *M* indicates the presence of distant metastasis (see Figure 10-23). The prognosis generally worsens with increasing tumour size, lymph node involvement, and metastasis. Staging also may alter the choice of therapy, with more aggressive therapy being delivered to more invasive disease.

Tumour Markers

During surveillance or diagnosis of cancer as well as following therapy, specific biochemical markers of tumours have proven to be helpful. These **tumour markers** are substances produced by both benign and malignant cells that are either present in or on tumour cells or found in blood, spinal fluid, or urine. Some tumour markers have been known for many decades. Tumour markers include hormones, enzymes, genes, antigens, and antibodies (Table 10-7). If the tumour marker itself has biological activity, then it can cause symptoms, such as those described in Table 10-7. For example, the adrenal medulla normally secretes the catecholamine epinephrine (adrenaline). Benign tumours of the adrenal medulla (pheochromocytoma) can produce catecholamines (e.g., adrenaline) in vast excess, leading to rapid pulse rate, high blood pressure, diaphoresis (i.e., sweating), and tremors. Detection of elevated blood

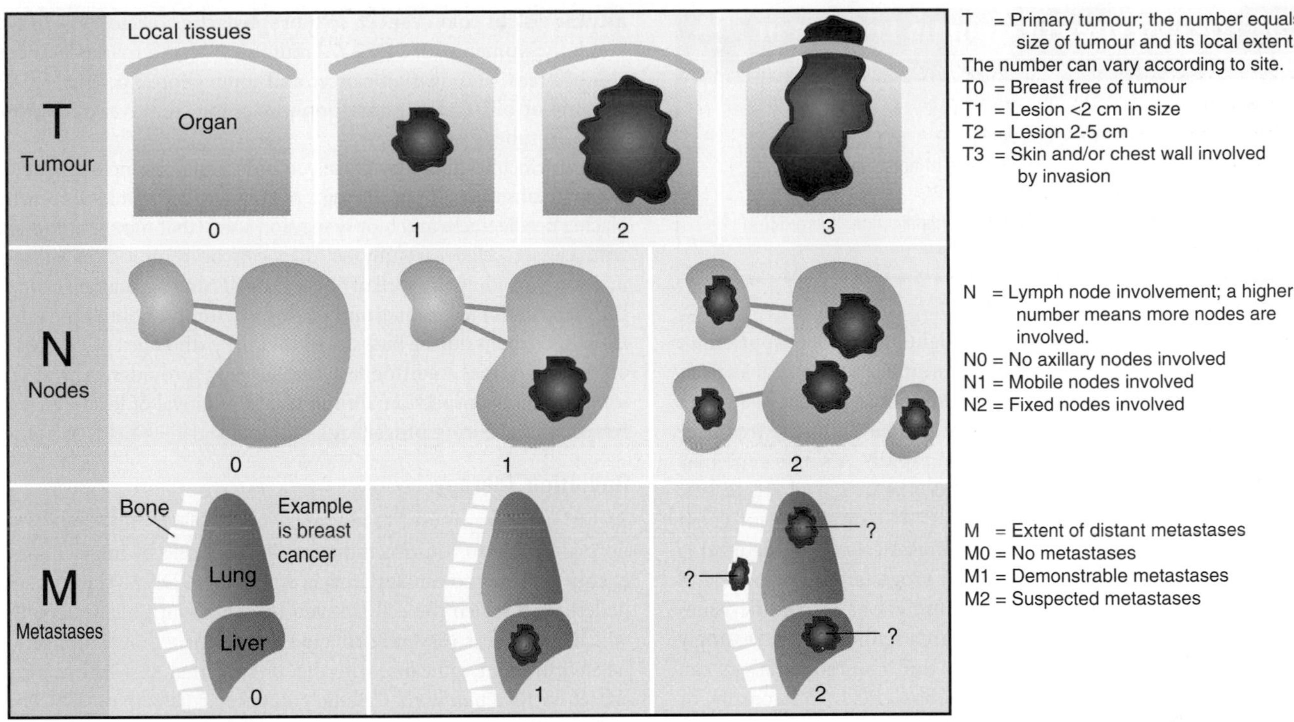

FIGURE 10-23 **Tumour Staging by the TNM System.** Example of staging for breast cancer. (See figure for explanation of the abbreviations.)

TABLE 10-7 Examples of Tumour Markers

Marker Name	Nature	Type of Tumour
Adrenocorticotropic hormone (ACTH)	Peptide hormone	Pituitary adenomas
Alpha fetoprotein (AFP)	70-kDa protein	Hepatic, germ cell
Beta-human chorionic gonadotropin (β-HCG)	Glycopeptide hormone	Germ cell
Cancer agent (CA)15-3/ CA27.29	Protein antigen	Breast
CA-125	Glycoprotein antigen	Ovary
Carcinoembryonic antigen (CEA)	200-kDa glycoprotein	Gastro-intestinal, pancreas, lung, breast, etc.
Catecholamines	Epinephrine and precursors	Pheochromocytoma (adrenal medulla)
Estrogen receptor (ER)/ progesterone receptor (PR)	Extracted receptor	Breast
Homovanillic acid/ vanillylmandelic acid (HVA/VMA)	Catecholamine metabolites	Neuroblastoma
Prostate-specific antigen (PSA)	33-kDa glycoprotein	Prostate
Urinary Bence Jones protein	Immunoglobulin light chain	Multiple myeloma

or urine levels of catecholamines helps to confirm the diagnosis, and treatment of the disease relieves the symptoms. Tumour markers can be used in three ways: (1) to screen and identify individuals at high risk for cancer; (2) to help diagnose the specific type of tumour in individuals with clinical manifestations relating to their tumour, as in adrenal tumours or enlarged liver or prostate; and (3) to follow the clinical course of a tumour.

To date, no tumour marker has proven satisfactory to screen populations of healthy individuals for cancer.[58] Testing large populations will always detect a few normal individuals with test results at the high end of the normal distribution ("false positives"), which can lead to expensive and invasive additional tests, and unnecessary concern. Similarly, some individuals with disease will have test results in the normal range ("false negatives"). More importantly, some nonmalignant conditions also can produce tumour markers. The presence of an elevated tumour marker therefore may suggest a specific diagnosis, but it is not used alone as a definitive diagnostic test. For example, prostate tumours secrete prostate-specific antigen (PSA) into the blood. But, enthusiasm has waned for routine testing for PSA levels. Most men (approximately 75%) with elevated levels of PSA do not have cancer upon biopsy.[59] A taskforce to study the use of PSA detection concluded that for every 1 000 men (ages 55 to 69) screened repeatedly, only zero to one prostate cancer–related death would be avoided, 100 to 120 men would undergo unnecessary biopsies with some complications, and 110 men would be diagnosed with prostate cancer (frequently slow growing and not life-threatening) and 50 of these would have major complications related to treatment.[60] However, falling levels of PSA after radiation or surgical therapy may indicate successful treatment for prostate cancer, and a later rise may indicate a recurrence. Identification of ideal sensitive and specific tumour markers that are elevated early in the course of common cancers remains a high priority because the early detection of cancer often improves the treatment outcome.

Classification of Tumours: Classic Histology and Modern Genetics

Because our knowledge about the cellular and molecular alterations in individual cancers can influence the choices of therapy, it becomes increasingly important for clinicians to accurately classify each cancer (Box 10-1). The classification, and hence the treatment decisions, of

BOX 10-1 Types of Genetic Lesions in Cancer

1. Point mutations
2. Subtle alterations (insertions, deletions)
3. Chromosome changes (aneuploidy and loss of heterozygosity)
4. Amplifications
5. Gene silencing (DNA methylation, histone modification, microRNAs)
6. Exogenous sequences (tumour viruses)

cancers was originally based on gross and light microscopic appearance and is now commonly accompanied by immunohistochemical analysis of protein expression. Increasingly, this immunohistochemical analysis is supplemented by a more extensive genetic analysis of the tumours. The range of genetic analysis is expanding rapidly. A single gene may be examined (e.g., to determine whether there is a characteristic chromosomal translocation diagnostic of CML), or a panel of genes and proteins may be examined (e.g., in breast cancer) to determine if the tumour expresses estrogen receptor, progesterone receptor, and the EGF receptor HER2, or if there are mutations in specific genes that modify response to therapy. In a research setting and increasingly in clinical settings, global gene expression and mutation analysis can be measured using polymerase chain reaction (PCR), microarray, or advanced DNA sequencing technology. These analyses can be used to classify tumours more precisely and may predict the most effective therapy. This detailed analysis of each tumour is a form of **personalized medicine** that offers therapy based on a very detailed knowledge of the characteristics of each individual's specific cancer.[61] This enhanced molecular characterization subdivides cancers into therapeutically and prognostically relevant smaller groups. As an example, breast cancers can now be subclassified into over four types (luminal A, luminal B, basal-like, and others) based on their expression of specific markers, such as estrogen receptor, HER2/neu (a type of receptor tyrosine kinase), and other specific genes and proteins. Each subtype has a different response to therapy and a different prognosis.

Treatment

Until late in the last century the mainstays of cancer therapy have been surgery, chemotherapy, and radiation therapy. These approaches have been highly successful for certain types of cancer but have many limitations. Immunotherapy has been the Holy Grail of cancer therapists, but successes have been few. Cancer therapy is now in a process of rapid evolution. Armed with a more clear understanding that cancer is, in fact, multiple diseases that share general hallmarks and enablers, and that the specific mechanisms underlying each hallmark may vary considerably among cancers (e.g., the large variety of oncogenes that may be used to differentiate cancers), modern cancer therapy is reaching a stage where complete genetic analysis of an individual cancer may determine the appropriate combination of therapies. Thus, effective therapy may include a combination of reagents targeting several hallmarks and under constant modification to target the evolving cancer cells.

Surgery

Surgery plays many roles in the care of individuals with cancer. The multiple approaches to obtaining tissue for diagnosis have been discussed. Surgery is often the definitive treatment of cancers that do not spread beyond the limits of surgical excision. It also is indicated for the relief of symptoms, for example, those caused by tumour mass obstruction. In selected high-risk diseases, surgery plays a role in the prevention of cancer. For example, individuals with familial adenomatous polyposis because of germline mutations of the *APC* gene have close to a 100% lifetime risk of colon cancer, so a prophylactic colectomy is indicated. Similarly, women with *BRCA1/2* mutations have a markedly increased risk of breast and ovarian cancer and often choose prophylactic mastectomy or bilateral salpingo-oophorectomy (removal of ovaries and fallopian tubes), or both.

Key principles apply specifically to cancer surgery, including obtaining adequate surgical margins during a resection to prevent local recurrences, placing needle tracks and biopsy incision scars (that may be contaminated with cancer cells) carefully so they can be removed in subsequent incisions, avoiding the spread of cancer cells during surgical procedures through careful technique, and paying attention to obtaining adequate tissue specimens during biopsies so that the pathologist can be confident of the diagnosis. Additionally, the surgeon provides critical staging information by inspection, sampling, and removal of local and regional lymph nodes during procedures.

Radiation Therapy

Radiation therapy is used to kill cancer cells while minimizing damage to normal structures. Ionizing radiation damages cells by imparting enough energy to cause molecular damage, especially to DNA. The damage may be lethal, in which the cell is killed by radiation; potentially lethal, in which the cell is so severely affected by radiation that modifications in its environment will cause it to die; or sublethal, in which the cell can subsequently repair itself. Cellular compartments with rapidly renewing cells are, in general, more radiosensitive. Effective cell killing by radiation also requires good local delivery of oxygen, something not always present in large cancers. Radiation produces slow changes in most cancers and irreversible changes in normal tissues as well. Because of these irreversible changes, each tissue has a maximum lifetime dose of radiation it can tolerate. Radiation is well suited to treat localized disease in areas that are hard to reach surgically, for example, in the brain and pelvis. A number of radiation delivery methods are available, with external beam being the most common. Radiation sources, such as small ^{125}I-labelled capsules (also called *seeds*), can also be temporarily placed into body cavities, a delivery method termed **brachytherapy**. Brachytherapy is useful in the treatment of cervical, prostate, and head and neck cancers.

Chemotherapy

The era of modern chemotherapy began with the observation in World War II that mustard gas exposure caused suppression of the bone marrow. Related compounds, such as nitrogen mustard and cyclophosphamide (Procytox), were then tested and produced clinical responses in hematological malignancies, including lymphomas. Also in the late 1940s, based on the remarkable clinical observation that the vitamin folic acid could *increase* leukemia growth, antifolate medications were developed (leading ultimately to methotrexate [Apo-Methotrexate]) that produced remissions in previously untreatable leukemia.

All chemotherapeutic agents take advantage of specific vulnerabilities in target cancer cells. Antimetabolites, such as methotrexate and L-asparaginase (Elspar), block normal growth pathways in all cells, but leukemia and other cancer cells are exquisitely sensitive to folic acid and asparagine deprivation, whereas nonmalignant cells are far less sensitive. Similarly, some cancer cells are highly sensitive to DNA-damaging agents, such as cyclophosphamide and anthracyclines, because of the oncogenic mutations that accelerate the cell cycle and DNA synthesis. Cellular checkpoints prevent normal cells treated with microtubule-directed medications, such as vincristine (Oncovin) and the taxanes, from undergoing mitosis, whereas cancer cells treated with these agents lack normal checkpoints, continue through mitosis, and undergo mitotic catastrophe (see Chapter 1).

Single chemotherapeutic agents often shrink cancers, but these medications given alone rarely, if ever, provide a cure. Hence, chemotherapy medications are usually given in combinations designed to attack a cancer from many different weaknesses at the same time and to limit the dose and therefore the toxicity of any single agent. Cancers contain a very large number of cells, and commonly a small fraction of those cells may be resistant to a particular medication. However, those cells are likely to be sensitive to the second or third medication in a chemotherapy cocktail. Scheduling of medication administration is also very important, with many studies showing cancers are more likely to develop medication resistance if there are significant delays between planned courses of chemotherapy.

Chemotherapy can be used for several distinct purposes. **Induction chemotherapy** seeks to cause shrinkage or disappearance of tumours. In Hodgkin's disease, for example, chemotherapy alone can be used in some cases to cure the disease. In other settings, chemotherapy may shrink the tumour and improve symptoms without ultimately providing a cure. **Adjuvant chemotherapy** is given after surgical excision of a cancer with the goal of eliminating micrometastases. **Neoadjuvant chemotherapy** is given before localized (surgical or radiation) treatment of a cancer. As with induction chemotherapy, the effectiveness, or lack thereof, of neoadjuvant therapy can be measured (e.g., with follow-up scans). Neoadjuvant therapy can shrink a cancer so that surgery may spare more normal tissue. For example, in the bone cancer osteogenic sarcoma, neoadjuvant therapy often converts a large tumour mass into a much smaller mass, allowing the surgeon to perform a limb-sparing excision rather than an amputation.

Immunotherapy

The expression of unique antigens on cancer cells that can be targeted by T cells has driven the quest for effective therapies to initiate an immune response, boost a currently inadequate immune response, or convert a tumour-protective immune response to a destructive one. Since the 1950s this quest has been characterized by promises and frustrations.

Vaccines have been extremely effective in protecting us against infective agents. Although they generally induce a prophylactic immune response, at least one vaccine (against rabies) is administered after the infection. Vaccines against oncogenic viruses provide protection and prevent the onset of viral-induced tumours. For approximately 50 years, numerous potential therapeutic vaccines have been tested with little success. Initially, whole tumour cell vaccines prepared from an individual's own cancer (autologous) or from cancers from other individuals (allogeneic) were used, with or without adjuvants that induced inflammatory responses (e.g., bacille Calmette-Guérin [BCG]) or augmented the vaccine's immunogenicity. Several allogeneic cancer cell vaccines continue to be tested. So far, none has been shown to be effective enough to be licensed. Other approaches have included immunization with the following:

- Protein extracts from cancers
- Peptides that represented the epitope from these proteins
- Dendritic cells that have processed and present cancer antigens
- DNA containing the genetic sequence for cancer antigens that transfects the recipient's cells and expresses that antigen
- Viral vectors that contain the genetic information for cancer antigens[62]

Sipuleucel-T (Provenge) is one such drug that has been approved for the treatment of metastatic prostate cancer that is resistant to conventional therapy and has been available in Canada since February 2015. Dendritic cells are obtained from an individual with prostate cancer and incubated with a protein resulting from the fusion of prostatic acid phosphatase, a cancer antigen found in 95% of prostate cancers, and granulocyte-macrophage colony-stimulating factor, an immune cell stimulating cytokine. The dendritic cells process and present the antigen and are infused back into the patient. In clinical trials, treatment with sipuleucel-T extended the lives of patients by 4.1 months. These results may not seem spectacular, but they were meaningful in this group of patients with very advanced and terminal disease. The medication is extremely costly, at over $100 000 per treatment. Other vaccine approaches against B-cell lymphoma and melanoma have shown promising results.[63]

Passive immunotherapy using lymphocytes against cancer cell antigens has been attempted, with limited success, since the early 1970s. In recent years, passive administration of tumour-targeting lymphocytes (adoptive cell therapy [ACT]) has developed more promise as a result of various pretreatment ex vivo techniques that improve treatment efficacy. A major source of patient's lymphocytes is those that have infiltrated the tumour.[64] The efficacy of these cells is increased by depleting the Treg cells within the population or by engineering the T-cell receptor for greater specificity against the tumour.[65]

A family of monoclonal antibodies, called *checkpoint inhibitors*, is under investigation. These antibodies are directed against co-stimulatory molecules involved in repressing T-cell immune responses (see Chapter 7). By blocking inhibitory signals, Tc cells may retain tumour-killing capacity.

Targeted Disruption of Cancer

As discussed previously, cancers appear to share a variety of hallmarks that contribute to the malignant phenotype. Recent molecular and genetic analyses of groups of cancer can classify an individual's cancer by the spectrum of mutations underlying the cancer phenotype.[66] However, each of the therapeutic approaches described previously generally treats specific vulnerabilities of the cancer rather than a variety of contributing factors. That approach is not successful in most invasive cancers because some cancer cells may undergo further mutation, leading to therapeutic resistance.

Exceptions include targeted medications, used in combination with conventional chemotherapy, against very specific characteristics of selected cancers. For example, imatinib is a competitive inhibitor of tyrosine kinases, primarily the BCR-ABL tyrosine kinase (Table 10-8). It is highly effective in treating CML but ineffective in virtually all other

TABLE 10-8 Examples of Molecular-Era Anticancer Medications

Medication (Trade Name)	Type of Medication	Molecular Target	Disease
Imatinib (Gleevec)	Small molecule TKI	BCR-ABL tyrosine kinase, FGF receptor tyrosine kinase	Chronic myeloid leukemia, gastro-intestinal stromal tumour
Erlotinib (Tarceva)	Small molecule TKI	EGF receptor tyrosine kinase	Subset of lung cancer
Trastuzumab (Herceptin)	Monoclonal antibody	HER2 receptor tyrosine kinase	HER2-positive breast cancer
Bevacizumab (Avastin)	Monoclonal antibody	VEGFR	Advanced colorectal cancer
Rituximab (Rituxan)	Monoclonal antibody	CD20 antigen on B lymphocytes	B-cell malignancies

EGF, epidermal growth factor; *FGF*, fibroblast growth factor; *HER2*, human epidermal growth factor receptor 2; *TKI*, tyrosine kinase inhibitor; *VEGFR*, vascular endothelial growth factor receptor.

cancers. Monoclonal antibodies against the CD20 antigen expressed on some B-cell lymphomas, the EGF receptor on colon cancers and head and neck cancers, and the EGF receptor HER2 on breast cancer are relatively successful.[67] These medications are so tightly targeted they have much less toxicity than conventional chemotherapies that have targets in virtually all cells.

Tumour growth and progression is dependent on a variety of mutations leading to expression of oncogenes, inactivation of tumour-suppressor molecules, and interactions with inflammatory cells in the tumour microenvironment that foster angiogenesis, resistance to apoptosis and immune-mediated cancer cell death, altered tumour cell metabolism, and metastasis. A more efficacious therapeutic approach, therefore, may be a combination of medications highly targeted to cancer hallmarks.[68]

The NCI lists more than 25 medications as cancer-targeting agents that inactivate oncogenes, block angiogenesis, and affect cancer cell metabolism.[69] Monoclonal antibodies are available that induce apoptosis in tumour-infiltrating cells such as TAM, Treg cells, and tumour endothelium.[70] Additionally, specific antagonists may neutralize the effects of cytokines, chemokines, and other tumour-enhancing mediators produced in the tumour microenvironment.[71] These antagonists are usually in the form of monoclonal antibodies, which are available against TNF-α, VEGF, HER-2, and other ligands and their receptors. Such highly specific targeting would minimize secondary toxic effects.

✔QUICK CHECK 10-5

1. Describe the major clinical manifestations of cancer.
2. How is cancer diagnosed?
3. What are the most common treatments of cancer?

DID YOU UNDERSTAND?

Cancer Terminology and Characteristics

1. Benign tumours are usually encapsulated and well differentiated and do not spread to distant locations.
2. Malignant tumours, compared with benign tumours, have more rapid growth rates, specific microscopic alterations (anaplasia, loss of differentiation), absence of normal tissue organization, and no capsule. They invade blood vessels and lymphatics and have distant metastases.
3. Carcinomas arise from epithelial tissue, and leukemias are cancers of blood-forming cells. Carcinoma in situ (CIS) refers to noninvasive epithelial tumours of glandular or squamous cell origin.

The Biology of Cancer Cells

1. Genetic changes are the basis of cancer. These changes include small and large DNA mutations that alter genes, chromosomes, and noncoding RNAs, as well as epigenetic changes because of altered chemical modifications of DNA and histones.
2. The incidence of cancer increases with age as the individual acquires genetic hits or mutations with time. Mutations activate growth-promotion pathways, block antigrowth signals, prevent apoptosis, stimulate telomerase and new blood vessel growth, and allow tissue invasion and distant metastasis.
3. Some mutations are more important for cancer progression. These mutations can be called *driver mutations*. *Passenger mutations* are random mutations that presumably do not contribute to cancer progression.
4. Key genetic mechanisms have a role in human carcinogenesis: (a) mutations of proto-oncogenes, resulting in hyperactivity of growth-related gene products (such genes are called *oncogenes*); (b) mutation of genes, resulting in loss or inactivity of gene products that normally would inhibit growth (such genes are called *tumour-suppressor genes*); and (c) mutation of caretaker genes that normally prevent mutations.
5. Oncogenes are independent of normal regulatory mechanisms and signal uncontrolled proliferation.
6. Some oncogenes, such as *RAS*, result from point mutations.
7. Oncogenes can result from genetic translocations. The Philadelphia chromosome in chronic myeloid leukemia (CML) results from a translocation that creates a novel protein fusion of the *BCR* and *ABL* genes and expression of an unregulated promoter of cell growth.
8. Tumour-suppressor genes must be inactivated in cancer cells by mutations to each allele, one from each parent.
9. A common mutation in cancer cells is inactivation of the tumour-suppressor gene tumour protein p53 (*TP53*), which controls expression of many genes that repair DNA damage, suppression of cellular proliferation during genomic repair, and initiation of apoptosis. Inactivation of p53 results in increased mutation rates and cancer.
10. Caretaker genes are responsible for maintaining genomic integrity. Inherited mutations can disrupt caretaker genes and cause chromosome instability.
11. Abnormal gene silencing is emerging as a major factor in cancer progression. Gene expression can be regulated in a heritable manner (i.e., passed from a parent to a child or from a single cell to its progeny) by an "epigenetic" mechanism called *silencing*.
12. In rare families, an initial inheritable mutation in a tumour-suppressor gene, such as *TP53*, the retinoblastoma gene (*RB*), or the breast cancer genes (*BRCA1* and *BRCA2*), may lead to a greatly increased risk of developing particular cancers.
13. Changes in gene regulation can affect not just single genes but entire networks of signalling. Gene expression networks can be regulated by changes in microRNAs (miRNAs or miRs) and other ncRNAs.
14. Cancer cells are immortal.
15. When they reach a critical age, cancer cells activate telomerase to restore and maintain their telomeres, thereby allowing cancer cells to divide repeatedly or become immortal.
16. Like many normal adult tissues, cancers can contain rare stem cells that provide a source of immortal cells. To fully eradicate a cancer, it may be necessary to target the cancer stem cell.
17. Access to the vascular system is essential for tumour growth.
18. Stromal cells and cancer cells can secrete multiple factors, such as vascular endothelial growth factor (VEGF), that stimulate new blood vessel growth (called *neovascularization* or *angiogenesis*).
19. The successful cancer cell divides rapidly, with the consequent requirement for the building blocks of new cells; cancer cell division often occurs in a hypoxic and acidic environment. Many cancer genes also encourage aerobic glycolysis and promote high glucose utilization of a cancer.
20. In cancer, defects in the intrinsic or extrinsic pathways, or both, provide resistance to apoptotic cell death.

21. Overexpression of B-cell lymphoma 2 (Bcl-2) blocks apoptosis in most follicular B-cell lymphomas.
22. Some conditions of chronic inflammation increase the risk of developing cancer. A prime example is the association between gastric cancer and infection with *Helicobacter pylori.*
23. Cells recruited to the tumour microenvironment are essential to the growth and spread of cancer and are active participants in induction of cellular proliferation, angiogenesis, degradation of extracellular matrix (ECM), suppression of infiltrating immune cells, and the development and spread of metastatic cells.
24. Unique antigens and other markers on tumour cells can be recognized by T lymphocytes and natural killer cells of the immune system, leading to destruction of the tumour cell.
25. Cancer cells can evade rejection by the immune system by production of immunosuppressive factors, induction of immunosuppressive T-regulatory cells, evolution of tumour–antigen-negative variants, or suppressed expression of antigen-presenting MHC class I molecules.
26. Antibodies induced by vaccines against oncogenic viruses, such as human papillomavirus (HPV) and hepatitis B virus (HBV), protect against initial infection and development of cervical and liver tumours, respectively.
27. Defects in the immune system increase the risk of viral-associated cancers but have a minimal effect on the risk of other cancers.
28. Metastasis is the major cause of death from cancer.
29. Metastasis is a complex process that requires cells to have many new abilities, including the ability to invade, survive, and proliferate in a new environment.
30. Carcinomas undergo a process of epithelial-mesenchymal transition (EMT) during which many epithelial-like characteristics are lost (e.g., polarity, adhesion to basement membrane), resulting in increased migratory capacity, increased resistance to apoptosis, and a dedifferentiated stem cell–like state that favours growth in foreign microenvironments and establishment of metastatic disease.
31. Invasion consists of loss of cell-to-cell contact, degradation of the ECM, and migration of tumour cells to the vascular or lymphatic systems. Stromal cells, particularly tumour-associated macrophages (TAMs), are essential to this process.
32. Some cancers appear to selectively home to particular metastatic sites, which may be a result of expression of particular receptors for ligands expressed by cells at the site.

Clinical Manifestations of Cancer

1. Paraneoplastic syndromes are rare symptom complexes, often caused by biologically active substances released from a tumour or by an immune response triggered by a tumour, that manifest as symptoms not directly caused by the local effects of the cancer.
2. Clinical manifestations of cancer include pain, fatigue, cachexia, anemia, leukopenia, thrombocytopenia, and infection.
3. Pain is generally associated with the late stages of cancer. It can be caused by pressure, obstruction, invasion of a structure sensitive to pain, stretching, tissue destruction, and inflammation.
4. Fatigue is the most frequently reported symptom of cancer and cancer treatment.
5. Cachexia is a multiorgan syndrome with many clinical manifestations including anorexia; muscle wasting; thermogenesis; altered heart and liver function; gut malabsorption; early satiety; taste alterations; and altered protein, lipid, and carbohydrate metabolism. Two factors are most significant: muscle loss and inflammation. Muscle wasting involves many protein signalling pathways and inflammatory mediators. Profoundly altered are both appetite-stimulating and appetite-suppressing brain pathways.
6. Anemia associated with cancer usually occurs because of malnutrition, chronic bleeding and resultant iron deficiency, chemotherapy, radiation, and malignancies in the blood-forming organs.
7. Leukopenia is usually a result of chemotherapy (which is toxic to bone marrow) or radiation (which kills circulating leukocytes).
8. Thrombocytopenia is usually the result of chemotherapy or malignancy in the bone marrow.
9. Infection may be caused by leukopenia, immunosuppression, or debility associated with advanced disease. It is the most significant cause of complications and death.
10. The gastro-intestinal tract relies on rapidly growing cells to provide an absorptive surface for nutrients. Both chemotherapy and radiation therapy may cause decreased cell turnover, thereby leading to oral ulcers (stomatitis), malabsorption, and diarrhea.
11. Alopecia (hair loss) results from chemotherapy effects on hair follicles. Alopecia is usually temporary, although hair may initially regrow with a different texture. Not all chemotherapeutic agents cause alopecia. Decreased renewal rates of the epidermal layers in the skin may lead to skin breakdown and dryness, altering the normal barrier protection against infection.

Diagnosis, Characterization, and Treatment of Cancer

1. The diagnosis of cancer requires a biopsy and examination of tumour tissue by a pathologist. Cancer classification is established by a variety of tests.
2. Tumour staging involves the size of the tumour, the degree to which it has locally invaded, and the extent to which it has spread. A standard scheme for staging is the T (tumour spread), N (node involvement), and M (metastasis) system.
3. The classification, and hence the treatment decisions, of cancers was originally based on gross and light microscopic appearance and is now commonly accompanied by immunohistochemical analysis of protein expression. Increasingly, staging is supplemented by a more extensive molecular analysis of the tumours.
4. Tumour markers are substances (i.e., hormones, enzymes, genes, antigens, antibodies) found in cancer cells and in blood, spinal fluid, or urine. They are used to screen and identify individuals at high risk for cancer, to help diagnose specific types of tumours, and to follow the clinical course of cancer.
5. Cancer is treated routinely with surgery, radiation therapy, chemotherapy, and combinations of these modalities.
6. Surgical therapy is used for nonmetastatic disease (in which cure is possible by removing the tumour) and as a palliative measure to alleviate symptoms.
7. Ionizing radiation causes cell damage; therefore, the goal of radiation therapy is to damage the tumour without causing excessive toxicity or damage to nondiseased structures.
8. The theoretical basis of chemotherapy is the vulnerability of tumour cells in various stages of the cell cycle.
9. Modern chemotherapy uses combinations of medications with different targets and different toxicities.
10. Immunotherapy attempts to modify the immune system from a cancer-protective state to a destructive condition.
11. Future treatment of tumours will, most likely, use a careful histological and genetic analysis of individual cancers that prescribes a combination of tumour-targeting medications to simultaneously disrupt multiple hallmarks of that particular cancer.

KEY TERMS

Adenocarcinoma, 236
Adjuvant chemotherapy, 263
Aerobic glycolysis, 249
Anaplasia, 236
Angiogenesis, 247
Angiogenic factor, 247
Apoptosis, 249
Autocrine stimulation, 242
Benign tumour, 235
Brachytherapy, 262
Cachexia, 256
Cancer, 235
Cancer-associated fibroblasts (CAFs), 252
Carcinoma, 236
Carcinoma in situ (CIS), 237
Caretaker gene, 244
Chromosome instability, 247
Chromosome translocation, 239
Clonal expansion, 239
Clonal proliferation, 239
DNA methylation, 239
Dormancy, 255
Epigenetic silencing, 246
Epithelial-mesenchymal transition (EMT), 253
Gene amplification, 239
Germ cell mutation, 244
Human T-cell lymphotropic virus type 1 (HTLV-1), 252
Hypoxia-inducible factor-1 alpha (HIF-1α), 247
Induction chemotherapy, 263
Leukemia, 236
Lymphoma, 236
Malignant tumour, 236
Matrix metalloproteinase (MMP), 248
Metastasis, 253
MicroRNA (miRNA), 247
Neoadjuvant chemotherapy, 263
Neoplasm, 235
Neovascularization, 247
Noncoding RNA (ncRNA), 239
Oncogene, 242
Oncomir, 247
Paraneoplastic syndrome, 256
Personalized medicine, 262
Pleomorphic, 236
Point mutation, 239
Proto-oncogene, 242
RAS, 242
Receptor tyrosine kinase, 242
Retinoblastoma (*RB*) gene, 243
Reverse Warburg effect, 249
Sarcoma, 236
Silencing, 246
Somatic cell mutation, 244
Stage of cancer, 260
Stroma, 235
Telomerase, 247
Telomere, 247
Thrombospondin-1 (TSP-1), 248
Transformation, 239
Tumour, 235
Tumour-associated macrophage (TAM), 251
Tumour initiation, 238
Tumour marker, 260
Tumour progression, 238
Tumour promotion, 238
Tumour protein p53 (*TP53*), 243
Tumour-suppressor gene, 243

REFERENCES

1. National Cancer Institute. (2014). *What is cancer?* Retrieved from http://www.cancer.gov/cancertopics/cancerlibrary/what-is-cancer.
2. Pieri, A., Harvey, J., & Bundred, N. (2014). Pleomorphic lobular carcinoma in situ of the breast: Can the evidence guide practice? *World Journal of Clinical Oncology, 5*(3), 546–553. doi:10.5306/wjco.v5.i3.546.
3. Hanahan, D., & Weinberg, R. A. (2000). Hallmarks of cancer. *Cell, 100*(1), 57–70.
4. Hanahan, D., & Weinberg, R. A. (2011). Hallmarks of cancer: The next generation. *Cell, 144*(5), 646–674. doi:10.1016/j.cell.2011.02.013.
5. Vogelstein, B., Papadopoulos, N., Velculescu, V. E., et al. (2013). Cancer genome landscapes. *Science, 339*(6127), 1546–1558. doi:10.1126/science.1235122.
6. Alexandrov, L. B., & Stratton, M. R. (2014). Mutational signatures: The patterns of somatic mutations hidden in cancer genomes. *Current Opinion in Genetics & Development, 24*, 52–60. doi:10.1016/j.gde.2013.11.014.
7. Hanahan, D., & Coussens, L. M. (2012). Accessories to the crime: Functions of cells recruited to the tumor microenvironment. *Cancer Cell, 21*(3), 309–322. doi:10.1016/j.ccr.2012.02.022.
8. Berns, A., & Pandolfi, P. P. (2014). Tumor microenvironment revisited. *EMBO Reports, 15*(5), 458–459. doi:10.1002/embr.201438794.
9. Quail, D. F., & Joyce, J. A. (2013). Microenvironmental regulation of tumor progression and metastasis. *Nature Medicine, 19*(11), 1423–1437. doi:10.1038/nm.3394.
10. Perez, E. A., Cortés, J., Gonzalez-Angulo, A. M., et al. (2014). HER2 testing: Current status and future directions. *Cancer Treatment Reviews, 40*(2), 276–281. doi:10.1016/j.ctrv.2013.09.001.
11. Ott, G., Rosenwald, A., & Campo, E. (2013). Understanding MYC-driven aggressive B-cell lymphomas: Pathogenesis and classification. *Hematology / The Education Program of the American Society of Hematology, 2013*, 575–583. doi:10.1182/asheducation-2013.
12. Jabbour, E., & Kantarjian, H. (2014). Chronic myeloid leukemia: 2014 update on diagnosis, monitoring, and management. *American Journal of Hematology, 89*(5), 547–556. doi:10.1002/ajh.23691.
13. Rubin, S. M. (2013). Deciphering the retinoblastoma protein phosphorylation code. *Trends in Biochemical Sciences, 38*(1), 12–19. doi:10.1016/j.tibs.2012.10.007.
14. Muller, P. A. J., & Vousden, K. H. (2014). Mutant p53 in cancer: New functions and therapeutic opportunities. *Cancer Cell, 25*(3), 304–317. doi:10.1016/j.ccr.2014.01.021.
15. Rahman, N. (2014). Realizing the promise of cancer predisposition genes. *Nature, 505*(7483), 302–308. doi:10.1038/nature12981.
16. Kim, E.-W., Kim, E. Y., Jeon, D., et al. (2014). Differential microRNA expression signatures and cell type-specific association with Taxol resistance in ovarian cancer cells. *Drug Design, Development and Therapy, 8*, 293–314. doi:10.2147/DDDT.S51969.
17. Jerónimo, C., & Henrique, R. (2014). Epigenetic biomarkers in urological tumors: A systemic review. *Cancer Letters, 342*(2), 264–274. doi:10.1016/j.canlet.2011.12.026.
18. National Cancer Institute. (2014). *BRCA1 and BRCA2: Cancer risk and genetic testing*. Retrieved from http://www.cancer.gov/cancertopics/factsheet/Risk/BRCA.
19. Lucey, B. P., Nelson-Rees, W. A., & Hutchins, G. M. (2009). HeLa cells, and cell culture contamination. *Archives of Pathology & Laboratory Medicine, 133*(9), 1463–1467. doi:10.1043/1543-2165-133.9.1463.
20. Azzalin, C. M., & Lingner, J. (2014). Telomere functions grounding on TERRA firma. *Trends in Cell Biology, 25*(1), 29–36. doi:10.1016/j.tcb.2014.08.007.
21. Shay, J. W., & Wright, W. E. (2011). Role of telomeres and telomerase in cancer. *Seminars in Cancer Biology, 21*(6), 349–353. doi:10.1016/j.semcancer.2011.10.001.
22. Beck, B., & Blanpain, C. (2013). Unravelling cancer stem cell potential. *Nature Reviews. Cancer, 13*(10), 727–738. doi:10.1038/nrc3597.
23. Xie, J., Wu, H., Dai, C., et al. (2014). Beyond Warburg effect—Dual metabolic nature of cancer cells. *Scientific Reports, 4*, 4927. doi:10.1038/srep04927.
24. Morandi, A., & Chiarugi, P. (2014). Metabolic implication of tumor: Stroma crosstalk in breast cancer. *Journal of Molecular Medicine, 92*(2), 117–126. doi:10.1007/s00109-014-1124-7.
25. Zhao, Y., Butler, E. G., & Tan, M. (2013). Targeting cellular metabolism to improve cancer therapeutics. *Cell Death & Disease, 4*, e532. doi:10.1038/cddis.2013.60.
26. Parks, S. K., Chiche, J., & Pouysségur, J. (2013). Disrupting proton dynamics and energy metabolism for cancer therapy. *Nature Reviews. Cancer, 13*(9), 611–623. doi:10.1038/nrc3579.
27. Okada, F. (2014). Inflammation-related carcinogenesis: Current findings in epidemiological trends, causes and mechanisms. *Yonago Acta Medica, 57*(2), 65–72.
28. Coffelt, S. B., & De Visser, K. E. (2014). Cancer: Inflammation lights the way to metastasis. *Nature, 507*(7490), 48–49. doi:10.1038/nature13062.
29. Elinav, E., Nowarski, R., Thaiss, C. A., et al. (2013). Inflammation-induced cancer: Crosstalk between tumours, immune cells and microorganisms. *Nature Reviews. Cancer, 13*(11), 759–771. doi:10.1038/nrc3611.
30. Rogler, G. (2014). Chronic ulcerative colitis and colorectal cancer. *Cancer Letters, 345*(2), 235–241. doi:10.1016/j.canlet.2013.07.032.
31. Pasechnikov, V., Chukov, S., Federov, E., et al. (2014). Gastric cancer: Prevention, screening and early diagnosis. *World Journal of Gastroenterology, 20*(38), 13842–13862. doi:10.3748/wjg.v20.i38.13842.
32. Goubran, H., Kotb, R. R., Stakiw, J., et al. (2014). Regulation of tumor growth and metastasis: The role of tumor microenvironment. *Cancer Growth and Metastasis, 7*, 9–18. doi:10.4137/CGM.S11285.
33. Van Overmeire, E., Laoui, D., Kerisse, J., et al. (2014). Mechanisms driving macrophage diversity and specialization in distinct tumor microenvironments and parallelisms with other tissues. *Frontiers in Immunology, 5*, 127. doi:10.3389/fimmu.2014.00127.
34. Miles, F. L., & Sikes, R. A. (2014). Insidious changes in stromal matrix fuel cancer progression. *Molecular Cancer Research, 12*(3), 297–312. doi:10.1158/1541-7786.MCR-13-0535.
35. Coulie, P. G., Van den Eynde, B. J., van der Bruggen, P., et al. (2014). Tumour antigens recognized by T lymphocytes: At the core of cancer immunotherapy. *Nature Reviews. Cancer, 14*(2), 135–146. doi:10.1038/nrc3670.
36. Mesri, E. A., Feitelson, M. A., & Munger, K. (2014). Human viral oncogenesis: A cancer hallmarks analysis. *Cell Host & Microbe, 15*(3), 266–282. doi:10.1016/j.chom.2014.02.011.
37. Volerman, A., & Cifu, A. S. (2014). Cervical cancer screening. *JAMA: The Journal of the American Medical Association, 312*(21), 2279–2280. doi:10.1001/jama.2014.14992.
38. Corthay, A. (2014). Does the immune system naturally protect against cancer? *Frontiers in Immunology, 5*, 197. doi:10.3389/fimmu.2014.00197.
39. Stockmann, C., Schadendorf, D., Klose, R., et al. (2014). The impact of the immune system on tumor: Angiogenesis and vascular remodeling.

Frontiers in Oncology, 4, 69. doi:10.3389/fonc.2014.00069.
40. Talmadge, J. E., & Gabrilovich, D. I. (2013). History of myeloid-derived suppressor cells. *Nature Reviews. Cancer, 13*(10), 739–752. doi:10.1038/nrc3581.
41. Jamal-Hanjani, M., Thanopoulou, E., Peggs, K. S., et al. (2013). Tumour heterogeneity and immune-modulation. *Current Opinion in Pharmacology, 13*(4), 497–503. doi:10.1016/j.coph.2013.04.006.
42. Gilkes, D. M., Semenza, G. L., & Wirtz, D. (2014). Hypoxia and the extracellular matrix: Drivers of tumour metastasis. *Nature Reviews. Cancer, 14*(6), 430–439. doi:10.1038/nrc3726.
43. Kothari, A. N., Mi, Z., Zapf, M., et al. (2014). Novel clinical therapeutics targeting the epithelial to mesenchymal transition. *Clinical and Translational Medicine, 3*(35), 1–14. doi:10.1186/s40169-014-0035-0.
44. De Craene, B., & Berx, G. (2013). Regulatory networks defining EMT during cancer initiation and progression. *Nature Reviews. Cancer, 13*(2), 97–110. doi:10.1038/nrc3447.
45. Smith, H. A., & Kang, Y. (2013). The metastasis-promoting roles of tumor-associated immune cells. *Journal of Molecular Medicine, 91*(4), 411–429. doi:10.1007/s00109-013-1021-5.
46. Fidler, I. J., Schackert, G., Zhang, R. D., et al. (1999). The biology of melanoma brain metastasis. *Cancer Metastasis Reviews, 18*(3), 387–400.
47. Domanska, U. M., Kruizinga, R. C., Nagengast, W. B., et al. (2013). A review on CXCR4/CXCL12 axis in oncology: No place to hide. *European Journal of Cancer, 49*(1), 219–230. doi:10.1016/j.ejca.2012.05.005.
48. Barcellos-de-Souza, P., Gori, V., Bambi, F., et al. (2013). Tumor microenvironment: Bone marrow-mesenchymal stem cells as key players. *Biochimica et Biophysica Acta, 1836*(2), 321–335. doi:10.1016/j.bbcan.2013.10.004.
49. Benzekry, S., Gandolfi, A., & Hahnfeldt, P. (2014). Global dormancy of metastases due to systemic inhibition of angiogenesis. *PLoS ONE, 9*(1), e84249. doi:10.1371/journal.pone.0084249.
50. Sosa, M. S., Bragado, P., & Aguirre-Ghiso, J. A. (2014). Mechanisms of disseminated cancer dormancy: An awakening field. *Nature Reviews. Cancer, 14*(9), 611–622. doi:10.1038/nrc3793.
51. Klein-Goldberg, A., Maman, S., & Witz, I. P. (2014). The role played by the microenvironment in site-specific metastasis. *Cancer Letters, 352*(1), 54–58. doi:10.1016/j.canlet.2013.08.029.
52. Argilés, J. M., Busquets, S., Stemmler, B., et al. (2014). Cancer cachexia: Understanding the molecular basis. *Nature Reviews. Cancer, 14*(11), 754–762. doi:10.1038/nrc3829.
53. He, W. A., Calore, F., Londhe, P., et al. (2014). Microvesicles containing miRNAs promote muscle cell death in cancer cachexia via TLR7. *Proceedings of the National Academy of Sciences of the United States of America, 111*(12), 4525–4529. doi:10.1073/pnas.1402714111.
54. Hitachi, K., & Tsuchida, K. (2013). Role of microRNAs in skeletal muscle hypertrophy. *Frontiers in Physiology, 4*, 408. doi:10.3389/fphys.2013.00408.
55. Kir, S., White, J. P., Kleiner, S., et al. (2014). Tumour-derived PTH-related protein triggers tissue browning and cancer cachexia. *Nature, 513*(7516), 100–104. doi:10.1038/nature13528.
56. Petruzzelli, M., Schweiger, M., Schreiber, R., et al. (2014). A switch from white to brown fat increases energy expenditure in cancer-associated cachexia. *Cell Metabolism, 20*(3), 433–447. doi:10.1016/j.cmet.2014.06.011.
57. Ramos, E. J., Suzuki, S., Marks, D., et al. (2004). Cancer anorexia-cachexia syndrome: Cytokines and neuropeptides. *Current Opinion in Clinical Nutrition and Metabolic Care, 7*(4), 427–434.
58. American Cancer Society. (2014). *Tumor markers*. Retrieved from https://www.cancer.gov/about-cancer/diagnosis-staging/diagnosis/tumor-markers-fact-sheet.
59. National Cancer Institute. (2014). *Prostate-specific antigen (PSA) test*. Retrieved from http://www.cancer.gov/cancertopics/factsheet/detection/PSA.
60. Moyer, V. A., & U.S. Preventive Services Task Force. (2012). Screening for prostate cancer: U.S. Preventive Services Task Force recommendation statement. *Annals of Internal Medicine, 157*(2), 120–134. doi:10.7326/0003-4819-157-2-201207170-00459.
61. Shames, D. S., & Wistuba, I. I. (2014). The evolving genomic classification of lung cancer. *Journal of Pathology, 232*(2), 121–133. doi:10.1002/path.4275.
62. National Cancer Institute. (2014). *Immunotherapy: Using the immune system to treat cancer*. Retrieved from http://www.cancer.gov/researchandfunding/progress/immunotherapy-using-immune-system-to-treat-cancer.
63. Gao, J., Bernatchez, C., Sharma, P., et al. (2013). Advances in the development of cancer immunotherapies. *Trends in Immunology, 34*(2), 90–98. doi:10.1016/j.it.2012.08.004.
64. Hinrichs, C. S., & Rosenberg, S. A. (2014). Exploiting the curative potential of adoptive T-cell therapy for cancer. *Immunological Reviews, 257*(1), 56–71. doi:10.1111/imr.12132.
65. Phan, G. Q., & Rosenberg, S. A. (2013). The potential and promise of cancer immunotherapy. *Cancer Control, 20*(4), 289–297.
66. Hoadley, K. A., Yau, C., Wolf, D. M., et al. (2014). Multiplatform analysis of 12 cancer types reveals molecular classification within and across tissues of origin. *Cell, 158*(4), 929–944. doi:10.1016/j.cell.2014.06.049.
67. Sliwkowski, M. X., & Mellman, I. (2013). Antibody therapeutics in cancer. *Science, 341*(6151), 1192–1198. doi:10.1126/science.1241145.
68. Hanahan, D. (2014). Rethinking the war on cancer. *Lancet, 383*(9916), 558–563. doi:10.1016/S0140-6736(13)62226-6.
69. Nero, T. L., Moton, C. J., Holien, J. K., et al. (2014). Oncogenic protein interfaces: Small molecules, big challenges. *Nature Reviews. Cancer, 14*(4), 248–262. doi:10.1038/nrc3690.
70. Tan, J. (2014). Waging war on cancer with the sword of immunity. *Cell, 158*, 233–234.
71. O'Shea, J. J., Kanno, Y., & Chan, A. C. (2014). In search of magic bullets: The golden age of immunotherapeutics. *Cell, 157*(1), 227–240. doi:10.1016/j.cell.2014.03.010.

11

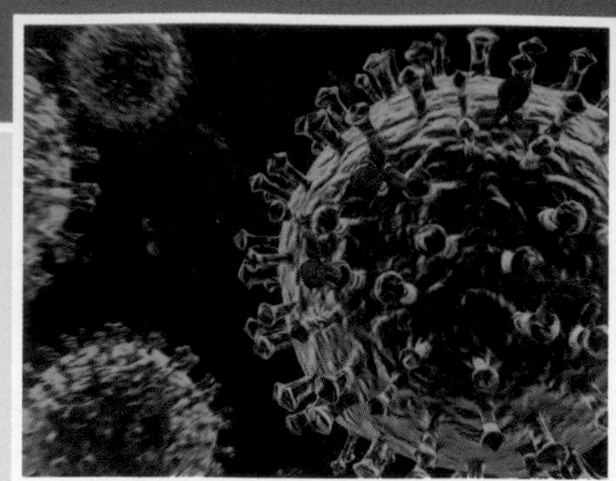

Cancer Epidemiology

Kathryn L. McCance and Stephanie Zettel

EVOLVE WEBSITE

http://evolve.elsevier.com/Canada/Huether/pathophysiology
Student Review Questions
Key Points
Case Studies
Animations
Quick Check Answers

CHAPTER OUTLINE

Genetics, Epigenetics, and Tissue, 268
Incidence and Mortality Trends, 274
In Utero and Early Life Conditions, 274
Environmental and Lifestyle Factors, 276
Tobacco Use, 276
Diet, 277
Nutrition, Obesity, Alcohol Consumption, and Physical Activity: Impacts on Cancer, 277
Ionizing Radiation, 285
Ultraviolet Radiation, 289
Electromagnetic Radiation, 291
Infection, and Sexual and Reproductive Behaviour, 292
Other Viruses and Microorganisms, 293
Air Pollution, 293
Chemical and Occupational Hazards as Carcinogens, 294

Although cancer arises from a complicated and an interacting web of multiple etiologies, avoiding high-risk behaviours and exposure to **individual carcinogens**, or cancer-causing substances, will prevent many types of cancer (Figure 11-1). Research has shown that lifestyle behaviours, dietary and environmental factors, and occupational exposure contribute to the number of cancer cases and deaths.[1-3] In this context, any of the following factors can contribute to the development of cancer[4-6]:

- Lifestyle choices, such as smoking, alcohol use, and nutritional intake
- Lack of physical exercise; overweight, obesity
- Infections, sexual practices
- Environmental conditions, including exposure to sunlight, natural and medical radiation, workplace exposures, and involuntary or unknown exposures
- Prescribed and illicit medications
- Socioeconomic factors that affect exposures and susceptibility
- Carcinogenic substances present in air, water, and soil

Estimates of environmental factors and their attributable risk for cancer vary. The International Agency for Research on Cancer (IARC) completed a review of the more than 100 chemicals, occupations, physical agents, biological agents, and other agents classified as carcinogenic to humans.[4] Simplified tables with a list of classifications by cancer sites with sufficient or limited evidence in humans are contained in Table 11-1.

GENETICS, EPIGENETICS, AND TISSUE

Cancers are caused by environmental and lifestyle factors, and by genetic and epigenetic factors (Figure 11-2). *Patterns* of cancer incidence around the world are environmental in origin—and not primarily genetic. At the level of the cell, cancer is *driven* by genetic alterations and epigenetic abnormalities with included variations in detoxifying enzymes or DNA repair genes. Interacting factors causing cancer risk are a weaker immune system and differences in hormone levels and metabolic factors (see Chapter 10). These interacting factors are influenced by the greater external environment and the cell's immediate environment. The biological environment surrounding cells includes metabolic and hormonal factors, for example, excess estrogen production, inflammation, and disordered glucose and lipid metabolism. Thus, the biological environment is modified by metabolic requirements, physical activity, infections, nutrition, occupational carcinogens, air pollution, and many other environmental factors. Investigators are challenged to connect the complex web between genotype, phenotype, and the environment to understand a person's chances of developing cancer.

Cancer development and progression involve the tissue microenvironment, or stroma. Emerging in importance is the microenvironment's interaction with environmental factors, because stromal tissue has various immune cells that can promote inflammation. Chronic inflammation is at the interface of environmental factors and genetics. Inflammation caused by environmental factors includes, for example, inhaled tobacco smoke, asbestos fibres, or fine particles in the air from diesel engine exhaust and other industrial sources. These sources are major factors in lung and other respiratory tract cancers.[7,8] Once malignant phenotypes have developed, complex interactions occur between the tumour, the surrounding stroma, and the cells of the immune and inflammatory systems (see Chapter 10).

Text continued on p. 274

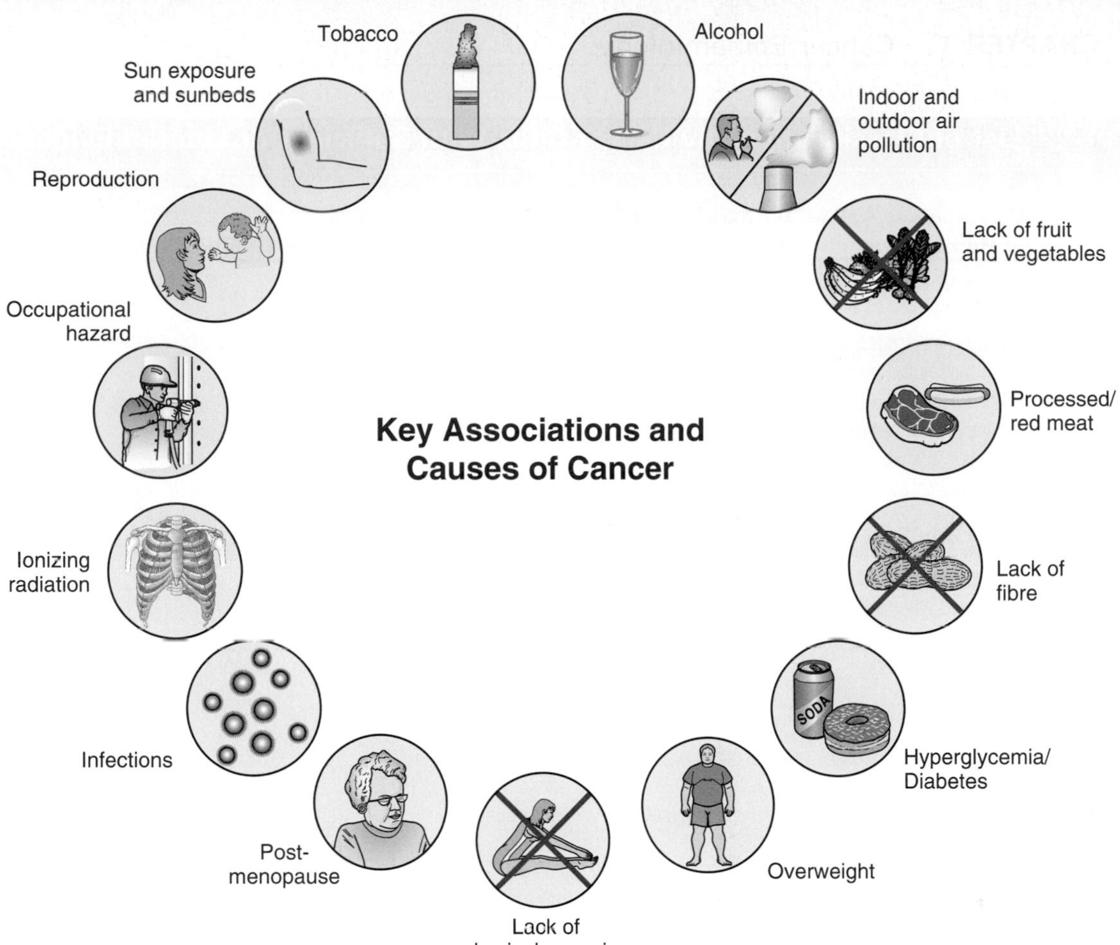

FIGURE 11-1 Key Associations and Causes of Cancer. Tobacco, diet, alcohol, obesity, lack of physical activity, hormones, infections, ionizing radiation, occupational hazards, reproductive factors, and ultraviolet light are key factors for cancer. Although diet is key and known to affect cancer risk, identifying specific dietary factors that elevate risk has been very difficult.

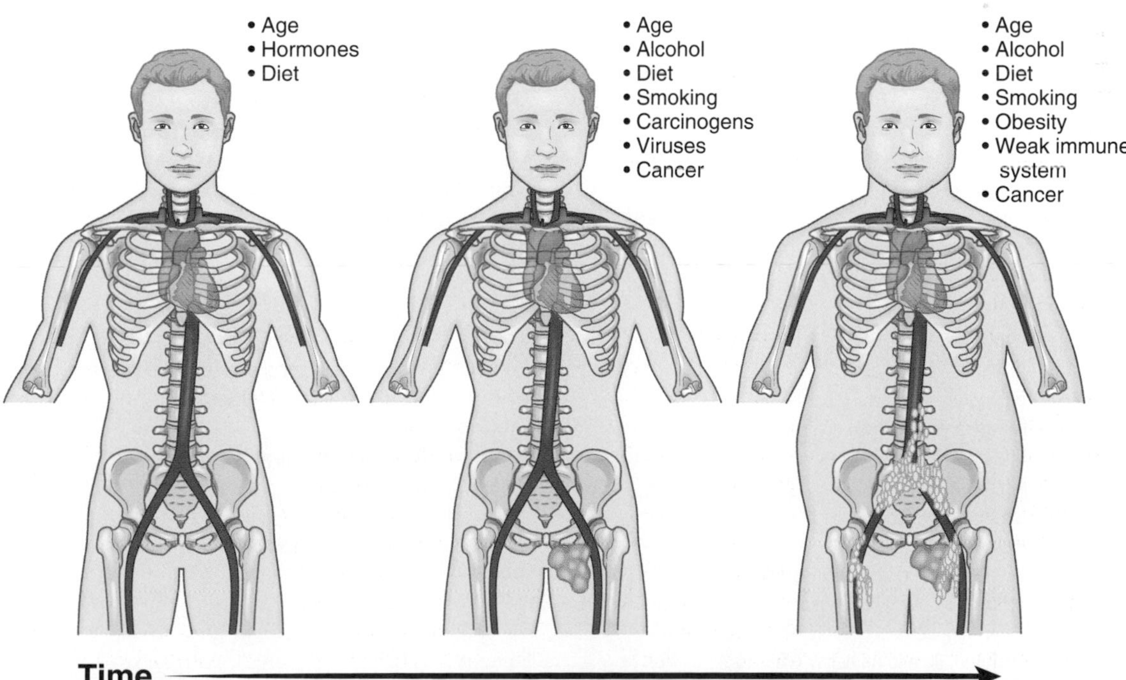

FIGURE 11-2 Environmental Factors and Genetic, Epigenetic, and Other Host Factors. Over time a person's internal genetic makeup persistently interacts with external or environmental factors. Environmental factors (e.g., diet, smoking, alcohol use, hormones, certain viruses, chemical carcinogens) collectively interact with internal epigenetic factors and genetic mutations to destabilize normal biological factors including immune factors for balancing growth and maturation. (Adapted from National Cancer Institute. [2007]. *Understanding cancer series: Cancer: Inside and outside factors.* Washington, DC: National Cancer Institute, National Institutes of Health.)

TABLE 11-1 List of Classifications by Cancer Sites With Sufficient or Limited Evidence in Humans

Cancer Site	Carcinogenic Agents With Sufficient Evidence in Humans	Agents With Limited Evidence in Humans
Lip, Oral Cavity, and Pharynx		
Lip		Solar radiation
Oral cavity	Alcoholic beverages	
	Betel quid with tobacco	
	Betel quid without tobacco	
	Human papillomavirus (HPV) type 16	
	Tobacco, smokeless	
	Tobacco smoking	
Salivary gland	X-radiation, γ-radiation	Radioiodines, including iodine-131
Tonsil	HPV-16	
Pharynx	Alcoholic beverages	Asbestos (all forms)
	Betel quid with tobacco	Mate drinking, hot
	HPV-16	Printing presses
	Tobacco smoking	Tobacco smoke, secondhand
Nasopharynx	Epstein-Barr virus (EBV)	
	Formaldehyde	
	Salted fish, Chinese style	
	Wood dust	
Digestive tract, upper	Acetaldehyde associated with consumption of alcoholic beverages	
Digestive Organs		
Esophagus	Acetaldehyde associated with consumption of alcoholic beverages	Dry cleaning
	Alcoholic beverages	Mate drinking, hot
	Betel quid with tobacco	Pickled vegetables (traditional Asian)
	Betel quid without tobacco	Rubber production industry
	Tobacco, smokeless	Tetrachloroethylene
	Tobacco smoking	
	X-radiation, γ-radiation	
Stomach	*Helicobacter pylori*	Asbestos (all forms)
	Rubber production industry	EBV
	Tobacco smoking	Lead compounds, inorganic
	X-radiation, γ-radiation	Nitrate or nitrite (ingested) under conditions that result in endogenous nitrosation
		Pickled vegetables (traditional Asian)
		Salted fish (Chinese style)
Colon and rectum	Alcoholic beverages	Asbestos (all forms)
	Tobacco smoking	*Schistosoma japonicum*
	X-radiation, γ-radiation	
Anus	Human immunodeficiency virus type 1 (HIV-1)	HPV-18, HPV-33
	HPV-16	
Liver and bile duct	Aflatoxins	Androgenic (anabolic) steroids
	Alcoholic beverages	Arsenic and inorganic arsenic compounds
	Clonorchis sinensis	Betel quid without tobacco
	Estrogen-progestogen contraceptives	HIV-1
	Hepatitis B virus (HBV)	Polychlorinated biphenyls
	Hepatitis C virus (HCV)	*S. japonicum*
	Opisthorchis viverrini	Trichloroethylene
	Plutonium	X-radiation, γ-radiation
	Thorium-232 and its decay products	
	Tobacco smoking (in smokers and in smokers' children)	
	Vinyl chloride	
Gallbladder	Thorium-232 and its decay products	
Pancreas	Tobacco, smokeless	Alcoholic beverages
	Tobacco smoking	Thorium-232 and its decay products
		X-radiation, γ-radiation
Digestive tract, unspecified		Radioiodines, including iodine-131

TABLE 11-1 List of Classifications by Cancer Sites With Sufficient or Limited Evidence in Humans—cont'd

Cancer Site	Carcinogenic Agents With Sufficient Evidence in Humans	Agents With Limited Evidence in Humans
Respiratory Organs		
Nasal cavity and paranasal sinus	Isopropyl alcohol production	Carpentry and joinery
	Leather dust	Chromium (VI) compounds
	Nickel compounds	Formaldehyde
	Radium-226 and its decay products	Textile manufacturing
	Radium-228 and its decay products	
	Tobacco smoking	
	Wood dust	
Larynx	Acid mists, strong inorganic	HPV-16
	Alcoholic beverages	Mate drinking, hot
	Asbestos (all forms)	Rubber production industry
	Tobacco smoking	Sulphur mustard
		Tobacco smoke, secondhand
Lung	Aluminum production	Acid mists, strong inorganic
	Arsenic and inorganic arsenic compounds	Art glass, glass containers, and pressed ware (manufacture of)
	Beryllium and beryllium products	Biomass fuel (primarily wood), indoor emissions from household combustion of
	Bis(chloromethyl) ether; chloromethyl methyl ether (technical grade)	Bitumens, oxidized, and their emissions during roofing
	Cadmium and cadmium compounds	Bitumens, hard, and their emissions during mastic asphalt work
	Chromium (VI) compounds	Carbon electrode manufacture
	Coal, indoor emissions from household combustion	α-Chlorinated toluenes and benzyl chloride (combined exposure)
	Coal gasification	Cobalt metal with tungsten carbide
	Coal-tar pitch	Creosotes
	Coke production	Engine exhaust, diesel
	Hematite mining (underground)	Frying, emissions from high-temperature
	Iron and steel founding	Insecticides, nonarsenical (occupational exposures in spraying and application)
	MOPP (vincristine-prednisone-nitrogen mustard-procarbazine mixture)	Printing processes
	Nickel compounds	2,3,7,8-Tetrachlorodibenzo-*para*-dioxin
	Painting	Welding fumes
	Plutonium	
	Radon-222 and its decay products	
	Rubber production industry	
	Silica dust, crystalline	
	Soot	
	Sulphur mustard	
	Tobacco smoke, secondhand	
	Tobacco smoking	
	X-radiation, γ-radiation	
Bone, Skin, Mesothelium, Endothelium, and Soft Tissue		
Bone	Plutonium	Radioiodines, including iodine-131
	Radium-224 and its decay products	
	Radium-226 and its decay products	
	Radium-228 and its decay products	
	X-radiation, γ-radiation	
Skin (melanoma)	Solar radiation	
	Ultraviolet-emitting tanning devices	
Skin (other malignant neoplasms)	Arsenic and inorganic arsenic compounds	Creosotes
	Azathioprine	HIV-1
	Coal-tar distillation	HPV-5 and HPV-8 (in individuals with epidermodysplasia verruciformis)
	Coal-tar pitch	Nitrogen mustard
	Cyclosporine	Petroleum refining (occupational exposures)
	Methoxypsoralen plus ultraviolet A	Ultraviolet-emitting tanning devices
	Mineral oils, untreated or mildly treated	Merkel cell polyomavirus (MCPyV)
	Shale oils	
	Solar radiation	
	Soot	
	X-radiation, γ-radiation	

Continued

TABLE 11-1 List of Classifications by Cancer Sites With Sufficient or Limited Evidence in Humans—cont'd

Cancer Site	Carcinogenic Agents With Sufficient Evidence in Humans	Agents With Limited Evidence in Humans
Mesothelium (pleura and peritoneum)	Asbestos (all forms) Erionite Painting	
Endothelium (Kaposi sarcoma)	HIV-1 Kaposi sarcoma herpesvirus	
Soft tissue		Polychlorophenols or their sodium salts (combined exposures) Radioiodines, including iodine-131 2,3,7,8-Tetrachlorodibenzo-*p*-dioxin
Breast and Female Genital Organs		
Breast	Alcoholic beverages Diethylstilbestrol Estrogen-progestogen contraceptives Estrogen-progestogen menopausal therapy X-radiation, γ-radiation	Estrogen menopausal therapy Ethylene oxide Shiftwork that involves circadian disruption Tobacco smoking
Vulva	HPV-16	HIV-1
Vagina	Diethylstilbestrol (exposure in utero) HPV-16	HIV-1
Uterine cervix	Diethylstilbestrol (exposure in utero) Estrogen-progestogen contraceptives HIV-1 HPV-16, 18, 31, 33, 35, 39, 45, 51, 52, 56, 58, 59 Tobacco smoking	HPV-26, 53, 66, 67, 68, 70, 73, 82 Tetrachloroethylene
Endometrium	Estrogen menopausal therapy Estrogen-progestogen menopausal therapy Tamoxifen	Diethylstilbestrol
Ovary	Asbestos (all forms) Estrogen menopausal therapy Tobacco smoking	Talc-based body powder (perineal use) X-radiation, γ-radiation
Male Genital Organs		
Penis	HPV-16	HIV-1 HPV-18
Prostate		Androgenic (anabolic) steroids Arsenic and inorganic arsenic compounds Cadmium and cadmium compounds Rubber production industry Thorium-232 and its decay products X-radiation, γ-radiation
Testis		Diethylstilbestrol exposure in utero
Urinary Tract		
Kidney	Tobacco smoking X-radiation, γ-radiation	Arsenic and inorganic arsenic compounds Cadmium and cadmium compounds Printing processes
Renal pelvis and ureter	Aristolochic acids, plants containing phenacetin Phenacetin, analgesic mixtures containing Tobacco smoking	Aristolochic acids
Urinary bladder	Aluminum production 4-Aminobiphenyl Arsenic and inorganic arsenic compounds Auramine production Benzidine Chlornaphazine Cyclophosphamide Magenta production 2-Naphthylamine	4-Chloro-*ortho*-toluidine Coal-tar pitch Coffee Dry cleaning Engine exhaust, diesel Hairdressers and barbers (occupational exposure) Printing processes Soot Textile manufacturing

TABLE 11-1 List of Classifications by Cancer Sites With Sufficient or Limited Evidence in Humans—cont'd

Cancer Site	Carcinogenic Agents With Sufficient Evidence in Humans	Agents With Limited Evidence in Humans
	Painting Rubber production industry *Schistosoma haematobium* Tobacco smoking *ortho*-Toluidine X-radiation, γ-radiation	
Eye, Brain, and Central Nervous System		
Eye	HIV-1 Ultraviolet-emitting tanning devices Welding	Solar radiation
Brain and central nervous system	X-radiation, γ-radiation	Radiofrequency electromagnetic fields (including from wireless phones)
Endocrine Glands		
Thyroid	Radioiodines, including iodine-131 X-radiation, γ-radiation	
Lymphoid, Hematopoietic, and Related Tissue		
Leukemia and lymphoma, or both	Azathioprine Benzene Busulfan 1,3-Butadiene Chlorambucil Cyclophosphamide Cyclosporine EBV Etoposide with cisplatin and bleomycin Fission products, including strontium-90 Formaldehyde *H. pylori* HCV HIV-1 Human T-cell lymphotropic virus type 1 Kaposi sarcoma herpesvirus Melphalan MOPP (vincristine-prednisone-nitrogen mustard-procarbazine mixture) Phosphorus-32 Rubber production industry Semustine (methyl-CCNU) Thiotepa Thorium-23 and its decay products Tobacco smoking Treosulfan X-radiation, γ-radiation	Bis(chloroethyl)nitrosourea Chloramphenicol Ethylene oxide Etoposide HBV Magnetic fields, extremely low frequency (childhood leukemia) Mitoxantrone Nitrogen mustard Painting (childhood leukemia from maternal exposure) Petroleum refining (occupational exposures) Polychlorophenols or their sodium salts (combined exposures) Radioiodines, including iodine-131 Radon-222 and its decay products Styrene Teniposide Tetrachloroethylene Trichloroethylene 2,3,7,8-Tetrachlorodibenzo-*para*-dioxin Tobacco smoking (childhood leukemia in smokers' children) Malaria (caused by infection with *Plasmodium falciparum* in holoendemic areas)
Multiple or Unspecific Sites		
Multiple sites (unspecified)	Cyclosporine Fission products, including strontium-90 X-radiation, γ-radiation (exposure in utero)	Chlorophenoxy herbicides Plutonium
All cancer sites (combined)	2,3,7,8-Tetrachlorodibenzo-*para*-dioxin	

NOTE: This table does not include factors not covered in the IARC monographs, notably genetic traits, reproductive status, and some nutritional factors.

Adapted from Cogliano, V.J., Baan, R., Straif, K., et al. (2011). *J Natl Cancer Inst, 103*, 1–13. Retrieved from http://jnci.oxfordjournals.org/content/early/2011/12/11/jnci.djr483.short?rss=1.

QUICK CHECK 11-1

1. Describe what is meant by the statement "environment is the main cause of cancer."
2. What is the role of the microenvironment in cancer development and progression?

INCIDENCE AND MORTALITY TRENDS

Cancer is predicted to become a major cause of morbidity and mortality in the coming decades in all regions of the world[9] (see *Health Promotion:* Global Cancer Statistics and Risk Factors Associated With Causes of Cancer Death). According to GLOBACAN, in 2012 worldwide, there were 14.1 million new cancer cases and 8.2 million cancer deaths, and 32.6 million people were living with cancer (diagnosed in the past 5 years).[10] The global cancer burden is shifting from the more developed countries to economically disadvantaged countries.[11] Canadian cancer statistics are compiled annually by the Government of Canada (see http://www.cancer.ca).[12] Approximately 2 in 5 Canadians will develop cancer within their lifetime, and about 1 in 4 Canadians will die of cancer. In 2015, it was estimated that 196 900 Canadians would develop cancer, and 78 000 would die of it. Most of the new cancer cases (51%) were predicted to be lung, breast, colorectal, and prostate cancer. Lung cancer is the leading cause of cancer death in Canada, and it accounts for more cancer deaths among Canadians than the other three major cancer types combined. The lung cancer death rate has actually dropped (especially for men) over the past 25 years. This drop is possibly related to changes in lifestyle habits (i.e., smoking cessation), which have resulted in a decline in the cancer death rate since the early 1990s overall. The prevalence of cancer is higher in men than in women in Canada, and most (89%) Canadians who develop cancer are older (over the age of 50). The survival rate for people diagnosed with cancer is 63%, but this number varies according to the cancer. For example, thyroid cancer has a very high 5-year relative survival rate (98%), whereas the survival rate for pancreatic cancer is very low (8%).[12] Measuring the cancer burden in Canada is very important because it informs both research priorities and the allocation of appropriate resources for the effective treatment and management of its various forms. The World Health Organization (WHO) has suggested that prevention is the most effective long-term strategy for preventing cancer (see *Health Promotion:* World Health Organization Cancer Prevention Strategies).

IN UTERO AND EARLY LIFE CONDITIONS

From studies of the etiology of certain cancers, it is widely accepted that a long latency period precedes the onset of adult cancers. Accumulating data suggest that early life events influence later susceptibility to certain chronic diseases (Figure 11-3).[13] **Developmental plasticity** is the degree to which an organism's development is contingent (external cues) on its environment. Specifically, the developmental origins' hypothesis postulates that nutrition and other environmental factors affect cellular pathways during gestation, enabling a single genotype to produce a broad range of adult phenotypes.[14] *Plasticity* refers to the ability of genes to organize physiologically or structurally in response to environmental conditions during fetal development. The hypothesis also postulates that persistent epigenetic adaptations that occur early in development in response to maternal nutrition and the environment are associated with increased susceptibility to cancer and other adult-onset chronic diseases.[15] Throughout in utero development, the placenta plays

HEALTH PROMOTION

Global Cancer Statistics and Risk Factors Associated With Causes of Cancer Death

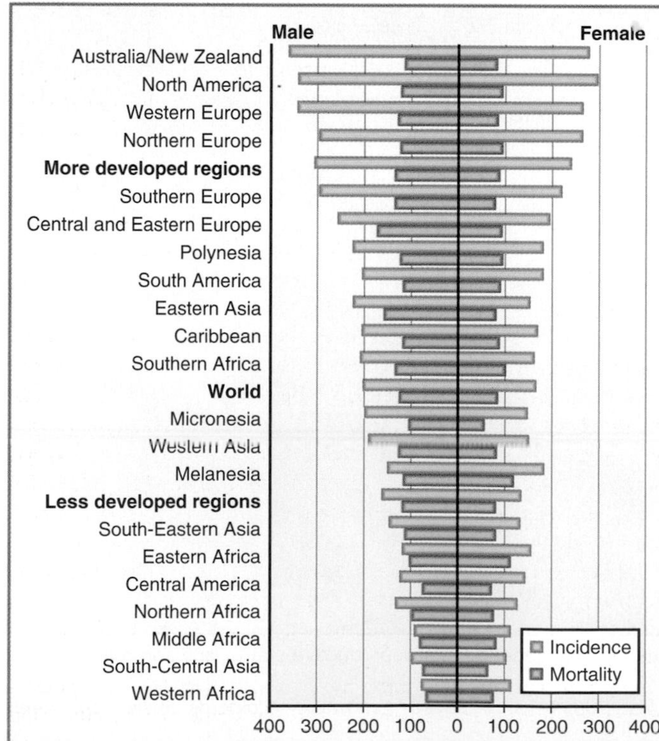

The growth of an aging population and increasing prevalence of established risk factors—smoking, overweight, physical inactivity, changing reproductive patterns associated with urbanization, and economic development—are increasing the occurrence of cancer. According to GLOBOCAN, in 2012 worldwide, there were 14.1 million new cancer cases and 8.2 million cancer deaths. Lung cancer is the leading cause of cancer death among males in both developed and developing countries, and lung cancer has surpassed breast cancer as the leading cause of cancer death among females in more developed countries. Breast cancer is the leading cause of cancer death among females in less developed countries. In developed countries, other leading causes of cancer death include colorectal cancer among males and females and prostate cancer among males. In less developed countries, the leading causes of cancer death are liver and stomach cancer among males and cervical cancer among females. Of concern is that cancer incidence rates for all cancers combined are nearly twice as high in more developed countries in both genders as compared with developing countries, but mortality rates are only 8 to 15% higher in more developed countries. This disparity reflects many factors, including geographical regional differences in the mix of types of cancer, which is affected by risk factors, detection practices, and availability of treatment. Risk factors associated with leading causes of cancer death include tobacco use (lung, colorectal, stomach, and liver cancer), overweight and obesity and physical inactivity (breast and colorectal cancer), and infection (liver, stomach, and cervical cancer). Effective application of tobacco control, vaccination, and use of early detection tests could prevent a substantial portion of cancer cases and deaths.

Data from Torre, L.A., Bray, F., Siegel, R.L., et al. (2015). *Cancer J Clin, 65*(2), 87–108.

HEALTH PROMOTION

World Health Organization Cancer Prevention Strategies

The World Health Organization suggests that prevention offers the most cost-effective, long-term strategy for controlling cancer and other noncommunicable diseases. Reducing the risk of developing cancer can be achieved through the following approaches, among other measures:

- *Avoid smoking*—Tobacco is responsible for nearly one-quarter of cancer deaths worldwide, making it the single greatest avoidable risk factor for cancer.
- *Follow a healthy lifestyle*—Eating a diet high in vegetables, fruit, and fibre, and low in red and processed meat, maintaining a healthy body weight, and being physically active can prevent about one-third of the 12 major cancers worldwide, according to the American Institute for Cancer Research and the World Cancer Research Fund.
- *Reduce alcohol consumption*—Reducing alcohol can be a factor for many different types of cancer, and the risk for cancer increases with the amount of alcohol consumed.
- *Avoid overexposure to sunlight and not using tanning beds or sun lamps*—Limiting time in mid-day sun, wearing protective clothing, seeking shade, and using sunscreen can help reduce the risk for skin cancer, while still allowing people to receive the health benefits of sun exposure. Indoor tanning does not provide a safe alternative to the sun and should be avoided.
- *Avoid infections*—Certain vaccines can help reduce the risk for some infections associated with cancer (e.g., human papillomavirus, and hepatitis B and C).
- *Avoid environmental and occupational carcinogens*—Testing and awareness can help reduce the risk for some environmental causes of cancer (e.g., radon), and occupational carcinogens (e.g., industrial chemicals).

Data from World Health Organization. (2017). *Cancer prevention*. Retrieved from http://www.who.int/cancer/prevention/en/.

a major role in controlling growth and development.[16] Because the placenta is a regulator of the intrauterine environment and can be influenced by exposures throughout pregnancy,[16] much research is being done with DNA methylation linking environmental cues to placental pathologies and adult life. The Dutch Famine Birth Cohort is a well-known study of the effects of prenatal undernutrition in humans. Undernutrition was linked to increased heart disease, metabolic disorders, and a possible link with breast cancer decades later.[17] Early versus late undernutrition in pregnancy indicated that the first trimester of pregnancy is particularly vulnerable to disease outcome in adulthood.[18] Much research is needed to understand nutrition in pregnancy and child vulnerabilities later in life. Recently, a striking experiment in mice demonstrated how extra vitamin doses during pregnancy in the mother's diet changed the fur colour of pups.[19] This was the first study to show maternal nutrition and subsequent phenotype changes. The nutrients (B_{12}, folic acid, choline, and betaine) silenced the gene that rendered mice fat and yellow but did not alter its DNA sequence. Silencing, or switching the gene off, linked prenatal diet to such diseases as diabetes, obesity, and cancer. These concepts, called the *developmental basis of health and disease*, are defining the hypothesis of disease onset. Subsequently, the focus of disease prevention and intervention needs to include the decades before onset—that is, in utero and neonatal periods. It is hoped that emerging studies on epigenetic mechanisms in dietary-associated transgenerational human disease will lead to beneficial health outcomes in the next generation.[18]

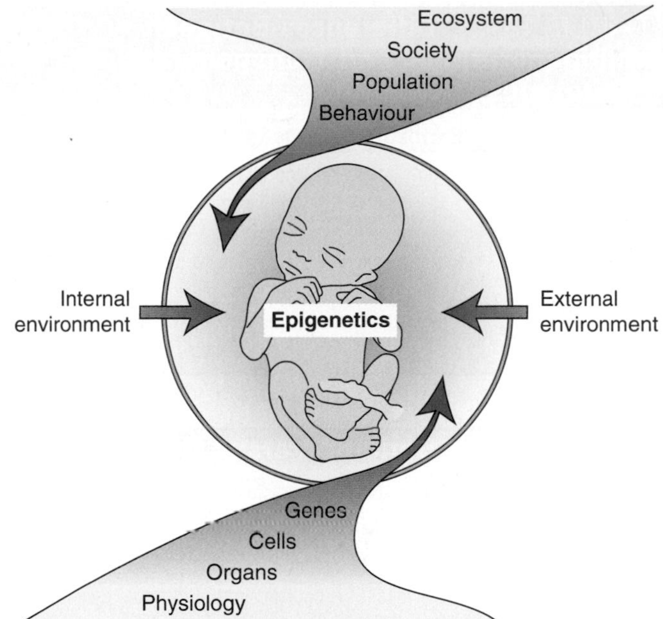

FIGURE 11-3 Fetal Vulnerability to External and Internal Environments. The fetus is particularly vulnerable to changes in the external and internal environments, which can have immediate and lifelong consequences. Such environmentally induced changes can occur at multiple levels, including molecular and behavioural. Ultimately these alterations may be epigenetic, inducing mitotically heritable alterations in gene expression without changing the DNA. (Adapted from Crews, E., & McLachlan, J.A. [2006]. *Endocrinology, 147*[6 Suppl.], S4–S10.)

Perhaps one of the best examples of early life events and future cancer is the chemical exposure to diethylstilbestrol (DES), a synthetic nonsteroidal estrogen. This medication was prescribed between 1938 and 1971 in an attempt to prevent multiple pregnancy-related problems, such as miscarriage, premature birth, and abnormal bleeding.[20] By the 1950s it became clear that DES interfered with the *development* of the reproductive system in the fetus and did not prevent miscarriage. Data suggest that a DES-associated increase in cancer of the female genital tract is elevated throughout a woman's reproductive years.[21,22] More recent studies have revealed that daughters of women who took DES during pregnancy may have a slightly increased risk for breast cancer before age 40 (i.e., 1.9 times the risk compared with unexposed women at age 40).[23] For every 1 000 DES-exposed women ages 45 to 49, it is estimated that 4 will be diagnosed with breast cancer.

Research from animal studies has demonstrated a relationship between DES exposure and an increased rate of a rare type of testicular cancer (rete testis) and prostate cancer.[24] Whether DES-exposed sons have increased risks of testicular cancer and prostate cancer is unclear, and more evidence is needed as the cohort of men ages.[22] Meta-analysis provides evidence that testicular cancer, hypospadias, and cryptorchidism are all positively associated with prenatal exposure to DES.[25] DES inhibits the hypothalamic-pituitary-gonadal axis, thereby blocking testicular synthesis of testosterone, lowering plasma testosterone levels, and inducing a chemical castration.[22] Testicular cancer is becoming more common in low- and middle-income countries where optimal treatment may not exist.[26]

In summary, fetal programming defines, in part, the developmental origins of health and disease.[27,28] The evidence for specific DNA methylation marks, in utero environments, and future phenotypes is growing. Increasing the complexity of our understanding of in utero

TABLE 11-2 Differences Between Multigenerational and Transgenerational Phenotypes

Phenotype	Exposure	Definition
Multigenerational	Direct	Simultaneous exposure of multiple generations to an environmental factor
Transgenerational	Initial germline exposure (ancestral)	Transgenerational phenotype that is transmitted to future generations via germline inheritance

TABLE 11-3 Somatic Versus Germ Cell Inheritance

Cell Type	Biological Response
Somatic cells	It is critical for adult-onset disease in an exposed individual; it is not transmitted to future generations as transgenerational effect.
Germ cells	It allows transmission between generations; it promotes transgenerational phenotype.

and early life conditions is the recent report that genotype and gene–environmental interactions explain substantial proportions of interindividual variation in the **methylome** (set of nucleic acid methylation modifications in the genome or cell) at birth.[29] A 2013 report suggests the possible importance in both fixed genetic variation and environmental factors in understanding epigenetic variation. In addition, epigenetic effects may help explain transgenerational effects[30] (Tables 11-2 and 11-3). For example, Newbold and colleagues[31] demonstrated that DES-related reproductive cancers in mice also occurred in the grandsons and granddaughters of mothers treated with DES.

QUICK CHECK 11-2

1. Describe briefly the incidence rates and death rates of common cancers in developing and developed countries.
2. Define *developmental plasticity.*
3. Describe how epigenetic processes can be modified by environmental factors.
4. Define the *developmental basis of health and disease.*

ENVIRONMENTAL AND LIFESTYLE FACTORS

Tobacco Use

Cigarette smoking is carcinogenic and remains the most important cause of cancer. Tobacco smoking causes cancer in more than 15 organ sites, and exposure to secondhand smoke and parental smoking causes cancer in daughters and sons and in other nonsmokers.[32,33] The largest preventable cause for cancer is tobacco use. More than 20 million premature deaths are attributable to smoking and exposure to secondhand smoke.[34] The risk is greatest in those who begin to smoke when young and continue throughout life, but tobacco smoking is pandemic, affecting more than 1 billion people of all ages.[32] Importantly, the eradication of tobacco use can only be achieved by preventing children and adolescents from starting tobacco use. Globally, tobacco use is greatest in developing countries, where 84% of 1.3 billion current smokers live.[35] Asia is now considered the largest tobacco producer and consumer in the world.[36] The WHO reports that tobacco use causes more than 6 million deaths per year from cancer, chronic lung disease, cardiovascular disease, and stroke.[37] On average, smokers die 13 to 14 years earlier than nonsmokers[38]; about 25% will die prematurely during middle age (35 to 69 years).[39]

Cigarette smoking is a leading cause of death in Canada.[40] In 2013, 14.6% of all Canadian adults smoked cigarettes. Estimates of cigarette smoking by age were as follows: 10.7%, ages 15 to 19 (4.6% of 15- to 16-year-olds and 18.5% of 19-year-olds were smokers); 17.9%, ages 20 to 24; 18.5%, ages 25 to 34; 16.7%, ages 35 to 44; 16.3%, ages 45 to 544; and 10.8%, ages 55 and older (Figure 11-4 shows a downward trend in smoking rates in Canada between 1965 and 2013).[40] Cigarette smoking is more common among men (16%) than women (13.3%), and there is a negative correlation between mental health and smoking rates, especially among youth. Smoking rates tend to also be higher with lower socioeconomic conditions. Average consumption of cigarettes has decreased by three cigarettes per day since 1999. The quit ratio for smoking in 2013 was the highest it has ever been; 64% of people who have ever been smokers had quit.[40]

Smoking affects nearly every organ of the body[41] (Figure 11-5). Nonsmokers are also affected by secondhand smoke. Every year in Canada, secondhand smoke causes 800 deaths from lung cancer and heart disease in nonsmokers.[42] In Canada in 2013, 59.1% of respondents to a survey on tobacco use had been exposed within the last month, and 12.9% were exposed to secondhand smoke on a daily basis.[40] Secondhand smoke, also called **environmental tobacco smoke (ETS)**, is the combination of sidestream smoke (burning end of a cigarette, cigar, or pipe) and mainstream smoke (exhaled by the smoker). More than 7000 chemicals have been identified in mainstream tobacco smoke. Nonsmokers who live with smokers are at greatest risk for lung cancer as well as numerous noncancerous conditions.[43] Additionally, secondhand smoke results in infant deaths due to sudden unexpected infant death (SUID) or complications from low birth weight or other conditions as a result of parental smoking, particularly by the mother.

Smoking tobacco is linked to cancers of the lung, upper aerodigestive tract (oral cavity, pharynx, larynx, nasal cavity, paranasal sinuses, esophagus, and stomach), lower urinary tract (renal pelvis, penis, and bladder), kidney, pancreas, cervix, and uterus, as well as acute myeloid leukemia (see Figure 11-5). The new list of disease risks includes liver cancer and colorectal cancer. Secondhand smoke is a cause of stroke; increases the risk of death in people with cancer and cancer survivors, as well as those with age-related macular degeneration, tuberculosis, ectopic pregnancy, and diabetes mellitus; increases inflammation; impairs immunity; and is a cause of rheumatoid arthritis. Smoking causes even more deaths from vascular, respiratory, and other diseases than from cancer. The epidemic of smoking ranks among the greatest health catastrophes of the century and has caused an enormous avoidable public health tragedy.[34]

Cigar or pipe smoking, or both, is strongly and causally related to cancers of the oral cavity, oropharynx, hypopharynx, larynx, esophagus, and lung. Cigar smokers who inhale deeply may be at increased risk of developing coronary heart disease and chronic obstructive pulmonary disease.[44] Pipe smokers have an increased risk of dying from cancers of the lung, lip, throat, esophagus, larynx, pancreas, colon, and rectum.[45] Consumption of loose tobacco (i.e., roll-your-own cigarette tobacco and pipe tobacco) changed substantially from 2000 to 2011.[46] Roll-your-own cigarette equivalent consumption decreased by 56.3%, whereas pipe tobacco consumption increased by 482.1%. Changes also were observed with cigars, whereby consumption of small cigars decreased 65% and consumption of large cigars increased 233.1%. Bidi smoking, a small amount of tobacco wrapped in the leaf of another plant (used in South Asia), delivers higher amounts of nicotine per gram of tobacco

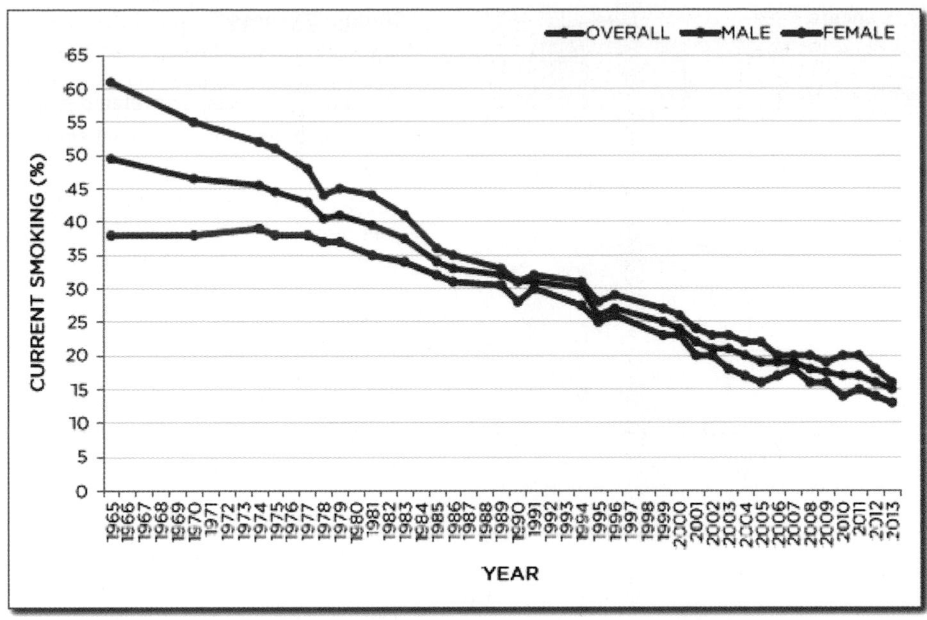

FIGURE 11-4 Smoking Prevalence in Canada, Adults Aged 15+, 1965–2013. NOTE: Includes daily and nondaily smokers. (From Reid JL, Harnmond D, Rynard VL, Burkhalter R. *Tobacco Use in Canada: Patterns and Trends, 2017 Edition*. Waterloo, ON: Propel Centre for Population Health Impact, University of Waterloo. Retrieved from https://uwaterloo.ca/tobacco-use-canada/.)

and comparable or greater amounts of tar compared with cigarettes.[47] Case-controlled studies indicate bidi smoking can cause cancers of the respiratory and digestive sites. A recent study in India showed that esophageal cancer is associated with smoking (including bidi) and alcohol.[48] The IARC reports *sufficient evidence* in humans that smokeless tobacco is associated with oral cavity, esophageal, and pancreatic cancers.[4]

The Tobacco Control Liasion Committee (created in 2000 by the federal, provincial, and territorial Advisory Committee on Population Health and Health Security [ACPHHS] to enable collaboration around implementation of the New Directions for Tobacco Control in Canada—A National Strategy) and the WHO Framework Convention on Tobacco Control (WHO FCTC) are national and global tobacco control initiatives for reducing both the demand for and supply of tobacco products. Control policies enforce bans on tobacco advertising, promotion, and sponsorship and provide evidence that calls for dramatic action.

Diet

Understanding dietary factors that increase the risk for cancer is most important but can be difficult. The ways in which diet affects one's likelihood of developing cancer are complicated by the variety of foods consumed, the many constituents of foods, the metabolic consequences of eating, and the temporal changes in the patterns of food use. Cancer risks in older adults may depend as much on diet in early life as on current eating practices.[49] In addition, studies in humans targeting diet and disease associations face a variety of challenges, including measurements of specific nutrients, food types, and dietary patterns.

Dietary sources of carcinogenic substances include compounds produced in the cooking of fat, meat, or protein and naturally occurring carcinogens associated with plant food substances, such as alkaloids or mould byproducts.[50] Figure 11-6 is a summary of convincing and probable judgements related to food and physical activity risk factors and the prevention of cancer.[50] Dietary components can act directly as mutagens or interfere with mutagen elimination. Abundant evidence exists that nutritional factors in many metabolic processes are related to cancer development (Figure 11-7).

Research is ongoing to understand the complexity of genomics, epigenomics, transcription factors (transcriptomics), proteomics, and metabolic factors (metabolomics) and the way that modifying any one or more of these factors influences cancer risk. **Nutrigenomics** is the study of the effects of nutrition on the phenotypic variability of individuals based on genomic differences (see Figure 11-7). Investigators are focusing on the sequence and functions of genes, single nucleotide polymorphisms (SNPs), and amplifications and deletions within the DNA sequences as modifiers of the response to foods and drinks and their components.[50]

Nutrition, Obesity, Alcohol Consumption, and Physical Activity: Impacts on Cancer

What we eat, how much we weigh, and how much we move influence our risks of developing cancer. Mounting evidence is clear—everyday *choices* impact our chances of getting or preventing cancer. Ongoing tedious and comprehensive investigative work is linking diet, body weight, and exercise to risk for specific cancers.

Nutrition

The implementation of dietary patterns (e.g., Mediterranean dietary pattern) and the promotion of specific dietary recommendations (e.g., dietary approaches to lower blood pressure) are becoming more widespread for fostering lifelong health.[51] The results of decades of research activity on the association of *specific* nutrients and foods and many forms of cancer have been controversial. Although so much in the cancer literature regarding nutrition is argued, it is difficult to ignore the data showing changes in cancer risk among individuals in low-risk countries compared with those in high-risk countries. For example, much of the geological variation in incidence across the world for

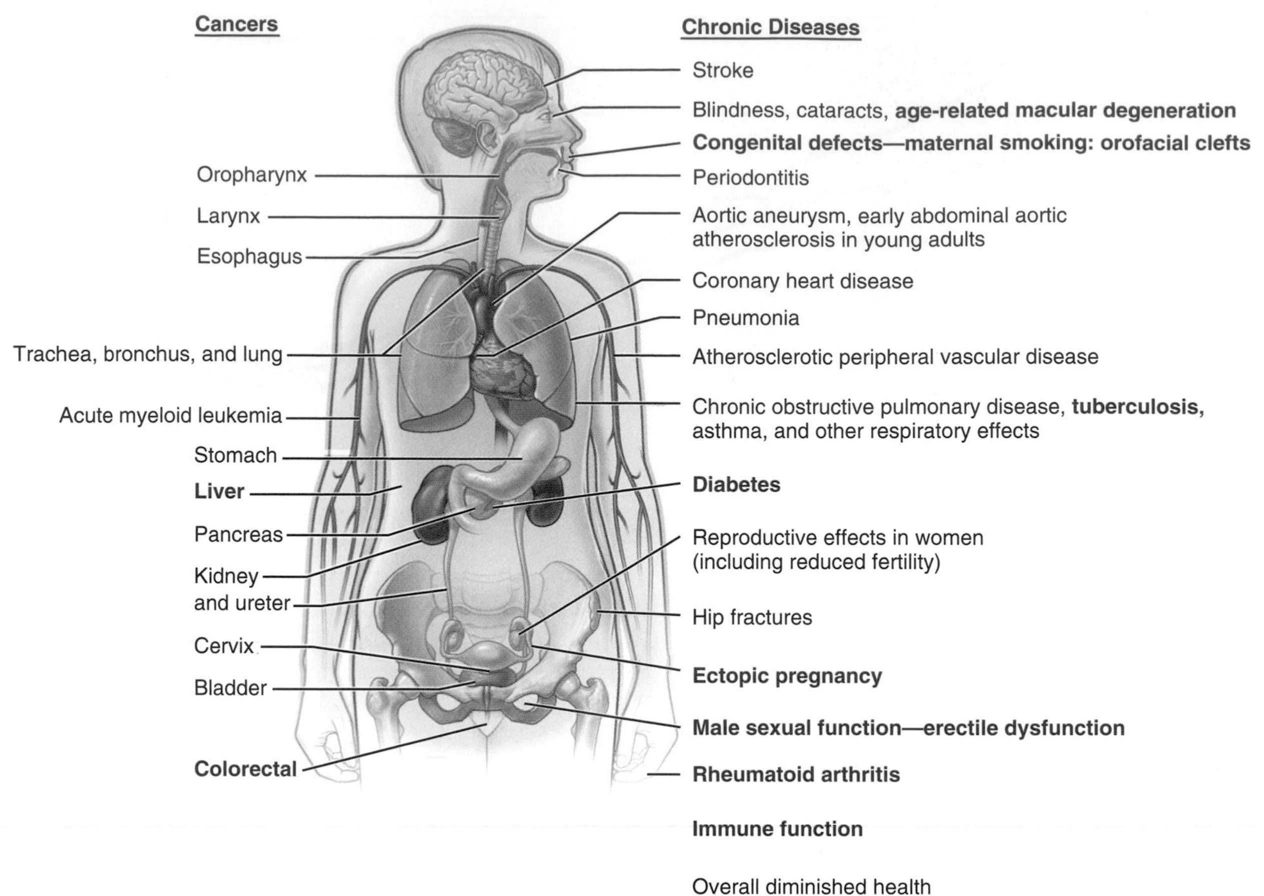

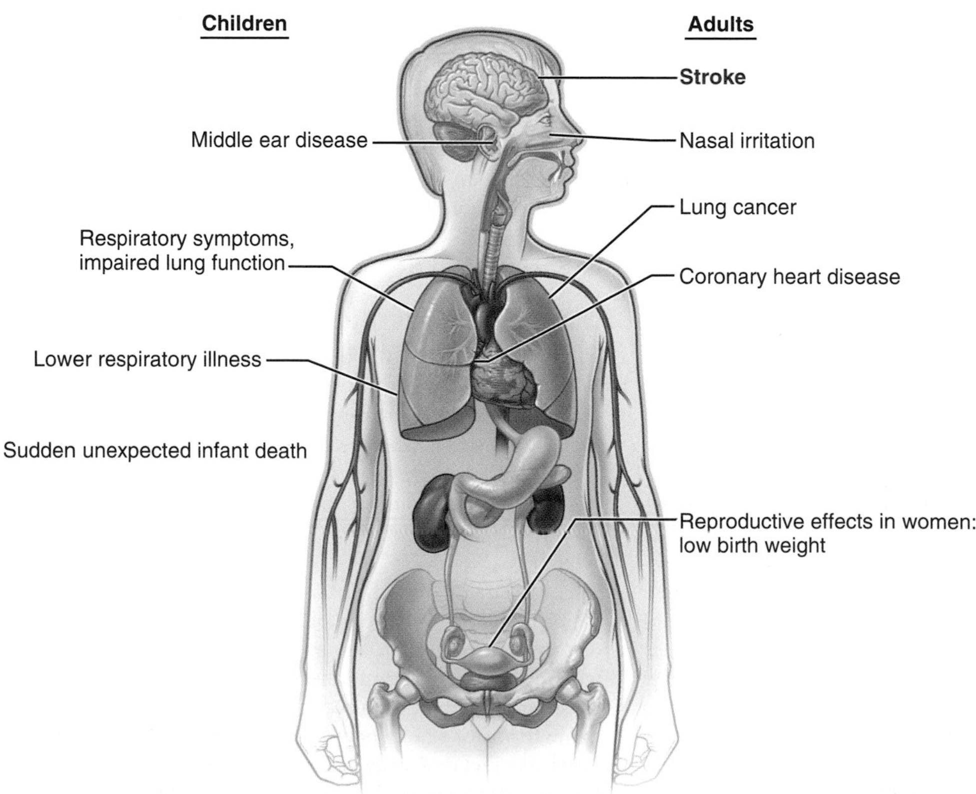

FIGURE 11-5 The Health Consequences Linked to Smoking. NOTE: The conditions in red are new diseases that have causally been linked to smoking. See text for discussion.

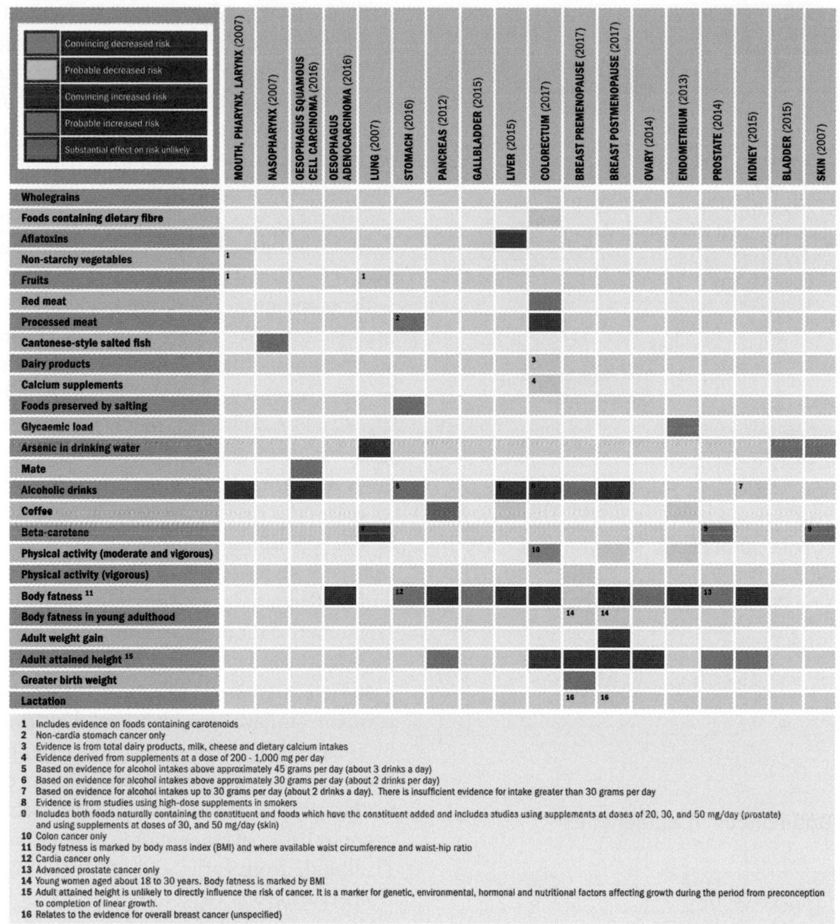

FIGURE 11-6 Summary of Convincing and Probable Judgements. (This material has been adapted from the WCRF/AICR Continuous Update Project: Diet, Nutrition, Physical Activity and the Prevention of Cancer. Summary of Strong Evidence. Available at: wcrf.org/cupmatrix accessed on 03-11-2017.)

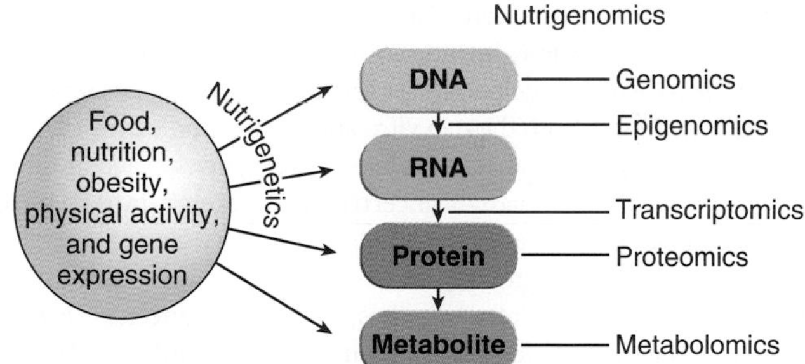

FIGURE 11-7 Basis for the Study of Food, Nutrition, Obesity, Physical Activity, and the Cancer Process. The genetic message in the DNA code is translated to RNA, and then into protein synthesis, and so determines metabolic processes. Research methods, called "-omics," address these different stages. (This material has been adapted from the 2007 WCRF/AICR Report Food, Nutrition, Physical Activity and the Prevention of Cancer: a Global Perspective.)

colorectal cancer has been attributed to differences in diet, particularly the consumption of red and processed meat, fibre, and alcohol, as well as body weight and physical activity.[52,53] With migration, these changes in risk are rapid, and the most plausible determinants of such changes are the adoption of the so-called "Western" diet. Japan has seen a rapid increase in the incidence of colorectal cancer with westernization of their diet.[54] It seems clear that focusing on dietary patterns, as well as meaningful biomarkers reflecting specific nutritional factors relevant to carcinogenesis, may be a more successful approach. The following important cellular processes are affected by nutrition (see a complete list in Figure 11-8):

- The cell cycle
- The balance between cell proliferation and cell death (e.g., apoptosis)
- Cell differentiation
- Genes, including oncogenes and tumour-suppressor genes
- Cell signalling
- Gene expression
- Cellular microenvironment that influences gene expression
- Epigenetic regulation
- Hormonal regulation
- DNA damage and repair
- Carcinogen metabolism
- Inflammation and immunity

Gene expression is influenced by epigenetic processes such as DNA methylation or acetylation (addition of an acetyl group) (see Chapters 3 and 10). Dietary sources of methyl groups, including folate, methionine, betaine, serine, and choline, are primary potential donors as modulators of DNA methylation[55] (Figure 11-9). A recent study by the European Prospective Investigation into Cancer and Nutrition (EPIC) found that

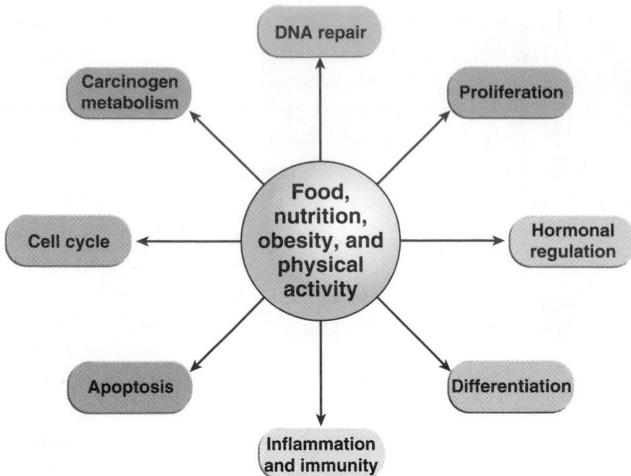

FIGURE 11-8 Food, Nutrition, Obesity, Physical Activity, and Cellular Processes Linked to Cancer. Food, nutrition, and physical activity can influence fundamental processes shown here, which may promote or inhibit cancer development and progression. (This material has been adapted from the 2007 WCRF/AICR Report Food, Nutrition, Physical Activity and the Prevention of Cancer: a Global Perspective.)

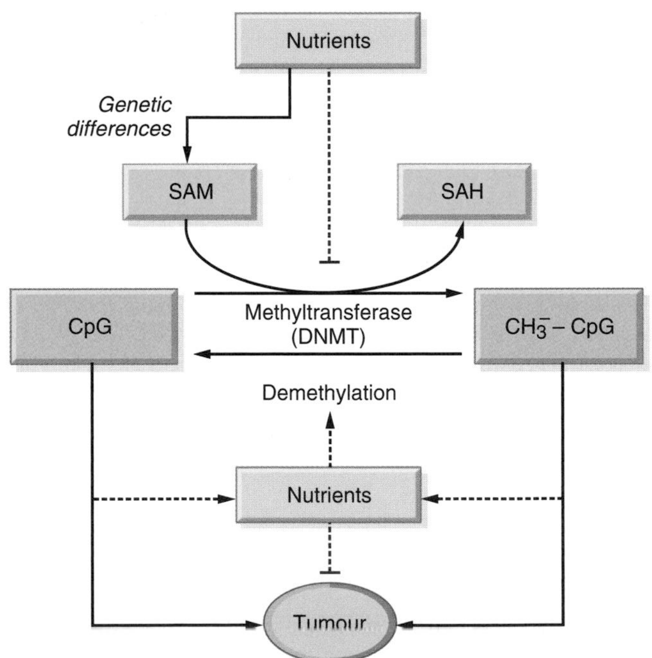

FIGURE 11-9 Dietary Factors, DNA Methylation, and Cancer. Certain dietary factors (see Table 11-5) may supply methyl groups (+CH_3) that can be donated through *S*-adenosylmethionine (*SAM*) to many acceptors in the cell (DNA, proteins, lipids, and metabolites). Donation and removal (demethylation) are affected by numerous enzymes, including DNA methyltransferase (*DNMT*). Increased DNMT activity occurs in many tumour cells. Hypermethylation can inhibit or silence tumour-suppressor genes (see Chapter 10), and DNA methylation inhibitors as anticancer agents can block DNMT, thus reactivating tumour-suppressor genes. DNA hypomethylation can reactivate and mutate genes, including cancer-causing oncogenes. *SAH*, *S*-adenosylhomocysteine.

individuals with high plasma concentrations of methionine, choline, and betaine may be at reduced risk for colorectal cancer.[56]

B vitamins, coenzymes in one-carbon metabolism (vitamins B_2, B_6, B_{12}), also are modulators of DNA methylation.[57] To date, there are limited human studies of the effects of methyl donor supply on methylation of specific genomic sequences.[55] However, a study[58] found that periconceptional maternal supplementation with 400 mcg of folic acid per day was associated with increased methylation in offspring aged 17 months. In experimental animals, maternal diet during the periconceptional period established DNA methylation in the offspring with permanent phenotypic changes.[59] In the Waterland study,[60] methylation effects were found to be similar in all tissues examined, suggesting that the mechanism may alter markings in stem cells early in embryogenesis before tissue differentiation and persist into adult life. Choline deficiency in pregnancy results in hypermethylation of genomic DNA and of the insulinlike growth factor 2 (*IGF-2*) gene.[61] Several studies have reported that severe folate deficiency (which increases the risk for hepatocellular cancer) induces hypomethylation of the *p53* tumour-suppressor gene.[62-64] In vitro studies have shown that several bioactive food components, including tea polyphenols and bioflavonoids, inhibit DNA methyltransferase (DNMT)-mediated DNA methylation in a dose-dependent manner[65] (see Figure 11-9). Acetylation and deacetylation are mediated by enzyme histones, histone acetyl transferase (HAT), and histone deacetylase (HDAC). Dietary components have been identified that act as regulators of gene expression by epigenetic mechanisms.[66,67] For example, there is strong evidence for the epigenetic effects of organosulphur compounds from garlic and of isothiocyanates from cruciferous vegetables.[66] Butyrate produced in the colon by bacterial fermentation of nonstarch polysaccharide (fibre), diallyl disulphide from garlic and other allium vegetables, and sulforaphane from cruciferous vegetables can act as HDAC inhibitors to maintain DNA stability or modify transcription.[50] A recent laboratory study found sulforaphane to inhibit modulators of inflammation in human mammary epithelial cells.[68]

Studies involving cultured cancer cells and animal models have illustrated the potential protective role of dietary polyphenols, such as curcumin, resveratrol, genistein, epigallocatechin-3-gallate, and indole-3-carbinol and its derivative 3,3′-diindolylmethane. The effects of these dietary agents may include antiproliferation and pro-apoptosis through the epigenetic regulation of microRNAs (miRNAs).[69] Because of the promising results from these in vitro and in vivo studies, the efficacies of these natural agents in cancer therapies are being investigated in clinical trials (see http://www.canadiancancertrials.ca). Interest in resveratrol, a polyphenolic compound with anti-inflammatory, antioxidant, and anticancer activities, is growing because of its demonstrable role in possibly delaying age-related diseases, including cancers.[70] Feeding mice a diet supplemented with human equivalent doses of 105 and 210 mg of resveratrol daily resulted in inhibition of colorectal tumours through an epigenetic mechanism (miR-96, an miRNA).[70] Yet, a recent prospective cohort study in community-dwelling older adults found total urinary resveratrol metabolite concentration was not associated with inflammatory markers, cardiovascular disease, or cancer, or predictive of all-cause mortality.[71] More research needs to be done with resveratrol.

MiRNA expression in response to diet may be involved in several cancers.[50] Several dietary factors, including macronutrients (fat, protein, and alcohol) and micronutrients (folate and vitamin E, curcumin), alter the expression of many miRNAs in animals and humans[55,72] (see Chapter 10). Curcumin analogues (compared with just curcumin) with increased anticancer activity and solubility, such as EF24 (3,5-bis[2-fluorobenzylidene]piperidin-4-one), show enhanced expression of potential tumour-suppressor miRNAs.[73]

Bioactive components have a profound effect on differentiation, and a major area of investigation is on the differentiation of cancer stem cells. Cancer stem cells have been isolated and identified in hematopoietic and epithelial cancers, including cancers of the brain, breast, ovary, prostate, colon, and stomach.[50,74] Stem cells are found among most adult tissues, where they maintain and regenerate tissues. Stem cells can remodel organs in response to physiological triggers—*adaptive resizing*.[75] Cancer stem cells utilize several developmental mechanisms for self-renewal and these mechanisms appear to be fundamental to the initiation and recurrence of tumours. Even if chemotherapy or radiation eliminates cancer cells, it is only when the cancer stem cells are destroyed that a full recovery is achievable.[74] Repopulation with radioresistant or chemoresistant stem cells may significantly contribute to therapy resistance. Evidence from both medication and bioactive food constituents shows modifications in cancer stem cell self-renewal capabilities; for example, retinoic acid may promote differentiation of breast cancer stem cells.[76] Adequate consumption of specific food compounds, including vitamins A and D, genistein, green tea, epigallocatechin gallate (EGCG), sulforaphane, theanine, curcumin, choline, and possibly many others, may suppress cancer stem renewal.[74] An uncontrolled self-renewal process may be initiated by abnormal developmental signals that come from the extracellular microenvironment known as "niches." The loss of regulation in self-renewal signals, including Wnt, Notch, and hedgehog pathways, is a characteristic of cancer stem cells.[74] Various food bioactive components can modulate the signalling pathway.

A variety of food constituents may influence DNA repair[50,77] (Figure 11-10). Observational studies suggest that malnutrition can reduce DNA repair from damage.[78] In vivo studies have demonstrated that healthy adults consuming kiwi fruits, cooked carrots, or supplemental coenzyme Q_{10} improved their DNA repair.[50] Consumption of lycopene-rich vegetable juice was associated with significantly decreased damage to the DNA of lung epithelial cells in healthy adults.[79]

Humans are constantly exposed to a variety of compounds termed **xenobiotics** (the Greek word *xenos* means "foreign"; *bios* means "life") that include toxic, mutagenic, and carcinogenic chemicals. Many of these chemicals are found in the human diet. Most xenobiotics are transported in the blood by lipoproteins and penetrate lipid membranes (see Chapter 4). The body has two main defence systems for counteracting these effects: (1) detoxification enzymes and (2) antioxidant systems (see Chapter 4). Enzymes that activate xenobiotics are called **phase I activation enzymes**. **Phase II detoxification enzymes** then protect further against a large array of reactive intermediates and nonactivated xenobiotics.[50] These enzymes are located predominantly in the liver and provide clearance of compounds through the portal circulation, thereby preventing the potentially carcinogenic agent(s) from entering the body through the gastro-intestinal tract and portal circulation. They also occur in the skin epithelia and can be induced in other extrahepatic tissue, such as the lung. They represent a potential target to influence carcinogen metabolism. Isothiocyanates from cruciferous vegetables induce the expression of phase II detoxification enzymes. Food and nutrition modify carcinogen metabolism and may modify carcinogenesis.

Glutathione-*S*-transferases (GSTs) are enzyme housekeepers involved in the metabolism of environmental carcinogens and reactive oxygen species (ROS). Individuals who lack these enzymes may be at higher risk for cancers because of decreased capacity to dispose of activated carcinogens. For example, the fungi that produce aflatoxins can grow on certain crops such as peanuts and some cereals (e.g., grains). Aflatoxins are carcinogens triggered by phase I activation enzymes in the liver that

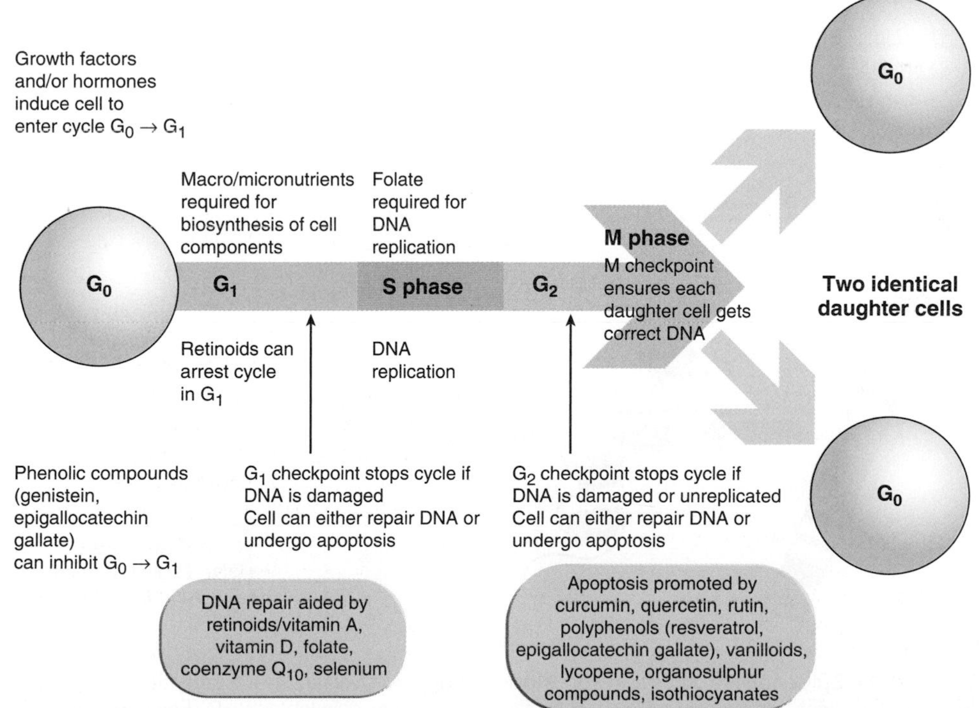

FIGURE 11-10 Cell Cycle and Nutrition Regulation. Nutrition may influence the regulation of the normal cell cycle, which ensures correct DNA replication. *G_0* represents the resting phase; *G_1*, the growth and preparation of the chromosome for replication; *S phase*, the synthesis of DNA; *G_2*, the preparation of the cell for division; and *M phase*, mitosis. (Adapted from World Cancer Research Fund/American Institute for Cancer Research. [2007]. *Food, nutrition, physical activity, and the prevention of cancer: A global perspective.* Washington, DC: American Institute for Cancer Research.)

can produce DNA adducts. Individuals lacking these enzymes are at a higher risk for colon cancer. Diets high in isothiocyanates (from cruciferous vegetables) may decrease this risk.[80] Individuals who consume diets high in red meat and processed meat and who carry certain genetic polymorphisms have an increased risk of developing colorectal cancer.[50,81-83] Processed meats include those treated by preservatives or by smoking, curing, or salting. The EPIC study, which included 478 040 people from 10 countries, reported that the most convincing data are from meats, including sausages, bratwursts, frankfurters, and hot dogs, all of which have nitrites, nitrates, or other preservatives. These *N*-nitroso compounds can increase nitrogenous residues in the colon and cause DNA damage.[50] Dietary components either can be activated into potential carcinogens through metabolic processes or can be inactivated and prevent DNA damage.[50] High intake of red meat may result in the synthesis of higher levels of heme iron; iron can activate oxidative stress and inflammation in the colon. Meat may have certain thermoresistant oncogenic bovine viruses (e.g., polyoma or papilloma virus) or possible single-stranded DNA viruses.[84] Certain SNPs in the *N*-acetyltransferase gene alter the activity of the enzyme involved in the activation of heterocyclic amines from cooking meat at high temperatures and may increase the risk for colon cancer.[50]

Red cabbage leads to changes in meat-derived mutagens in urine.[50] Flavonoids found in plants may alter carcinogen metabolism, and dietary indole-3-carbinol has been found to inhibit spontaneous occurrence of endometrial adenocarcinomas in rats.[50]

Chronic inflammation and immune function may help explain patterns of cancer around the world. People who are undernourished or live in poverty may have impaired immune status, which can be a factor in cancers caused by infectious agents, for example, cancers of the liver and cervix.[50]

Diet affects many pathways to cancer (see p. 277), and many of these processes are likely influenced, if not regulated, by DNA methylation, an epigenetic mechanism that affects gene function (see also Chapter 3). As illustrated in Figure 11-11, it is possible that many environmental factors interact with the genome to produce altered epigenetic markers that change the expression of cancer-causing genes, tumour-suppressor genes, and oncogenes. Future research is needed to define robust biomarkers of cancer risk.

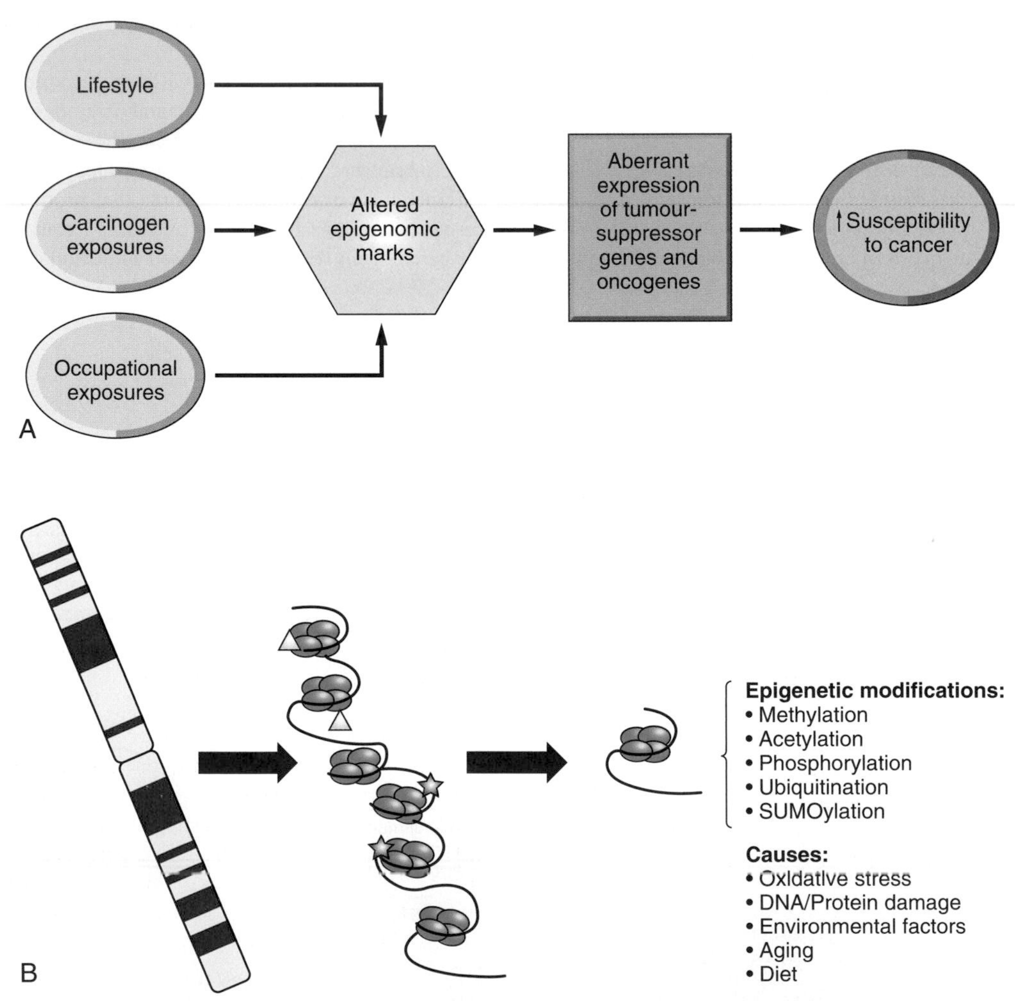

FIGURE 11-11 Epigenetic Modulation and Modifications. **A,** Overview of the potential role of epigenetic modulation by dietary and other environmental factors in cancer development. **B,** Epigenetic modulation model according to current knowledge. The different types of chemical modifications, such as methylation or acetylation, of promoter regions and/or other regulatory DNA sequences outside the gene can have a severe impact on gene transcription and translation and a resultant high modulation of gene expression and product (protein) functionality. (**B,** Reprinted from *Cancer Letters,* 342(2), Nowsheen, S., Aziz, K., Tran, P. T., Gorgoulis, V. G., Yang, E. S., & Georgakilas, A. G., "Epigenetic inactivation of DNA repair in breast cancer," Pages 213–222, Copyright 2014, with permission from Elsevier.)

Obesity

Obesity in most developed countries (and in urban areas of many developing countries) has been increasing rapidly over the past 20 years. Obesity in Canada is an epidemic and constitutes a startling setback to major improvements in other areas of health.[85] One in four adult Canadians and 1 in 10 children suffer from clinical obesity, which means that there are 6 million Canadians living with obesity who may require immediate support in managing and controlling their weight. As a leading cause of type 2 diabetes, high blood pressure, heart disease, stroke, arthritis, and cancer, the condition impacts the entire community.[85]

Numerous health conditions are linked to obesity and physical inactivity. The substantial suffering and long-term human and societal costs of obesity underlie the urgency to accelerate progress in obesity prevention.[86] Studies have significantly improved the understanding of the relationship between overweight or obesity, energy balance and cancer risk, cancer recurrence, and survival.[50,87,88] Consensus now exists that obesity is a risk factor for cancers of the endometrium, colorectum, kidney, esophagus, breast (postmenopausal), and pancreas. Evidence is evolving of the association between obesity and cancers of the thyroid, gallbladder, liver, and ovary, as well as aggressive types of prostate cancer and non-Hodgkin's lymphoma.[50,87] Importantly, obesity is recognized as a poor prognostic factor for several cancers.[89-91]

The only globally accepted criteria for overweight and obesity are based on the body mass index (BMI). Widely accepted standards based on BMI criteria for overweight and obesity are recommended by the WHO[50] (Table 11-4) and supported by other panels and federal agencies. According to the WHO, worldwide obesity has doubled since 1980, and more than 1.9 billion adults, 18 years of age and older, were overweight in 2014. Of these, more than 600 million were obese. Worldwide, 41 million children younger than age 5 were overweight or obese in 2014.[92]

The mechanisms of obesity-associated cancer risks are unclear and may vary by type of tumour and distribution of body fat. Emerging, however, are three main factors related to obesity and cancer: (1) the insulin–insulinlike growth factor 1 (IGF-1) axis, (2) sex hormones, and (3) adipokines or adipocyte-derived cytokines.[93] These three factors are linked to metabolic dysregulation of adipose tissue and endocrine and paracrine altered signalling of adipose tissue in obesity.[93,94] Metabolic changes in adipose tissue from obesity result in several alterations and include insulin resistance, hyperglycemia, dyslipidemia, hypoxia, and chronic inflammation.[93,95] Because tumour growth is regulated by interactions between tumour cells and their tissue microenvironment or stromal compartments that are rich in adipose tissue, adipocytes function as endocrine cells and critically shape the tumour microenvironment. Dysfunctional adipose tissue can create altered signalling pathways that involve proinflammatory mediators, macrophages, and cancer-associated fibroblasts. All of these cells are tumour-promoting cell types and, with insulin resistance and hypoxia, can trigger compensatory angiogenesis and an energy reservoir for the embedded cancer cells.[93] The cancer-associated adipocytes (CAAs) undergo both structural and functional alterations during cancer progression that altogether create an environment toward increased cancer invasiveness and aggression[93] (Figure 11-12).

TABLE 11-4 World Health Organization Classification of Body Mass Index

BMI (kg/m²)[a]	WHO Classification	Other Descriptions
<18.5	Underweight	Thin
18.5–24.9	Normal range	"Healthy," "normal," or "acceptable" weight
25.0–29.9	Preobese	Overweight
30.0–34.9	Obese class I	Obesity
35.0–39.9	Obese class II	—[a]
>40.0	Obese class III	Morbidly overweight

[a]The cutoffs are somewhat arbitrary, although they are derived from epidemiological studies of BMI and overall mortality. It is important to understand that within each category of BMI there can be substantial individual variation in total and visceral adiposity and in related metabolic factors. These variations are also true for the normal range BMI.

BMI, body mass index; *WHO*, World Health Organization.

Data available at World Health Organization. (n.d.). *Body mass index (BMI)*. Retrieved from http://www.euro.who.int/en/health-topics/disease-prevention/nutrition/a-healthy-lifestyle/body-mass-index-bmi.

Alcohol Consumption

Alcohol is classified by the IARC as a human carcinogen. Excessive alcohol plays a contributory role in several common cancers.[50] Overall, there are strong data linking alcohol with cancers of the mouth, pharynx, larynx, esophagus, liver, colorectum, and breast[4,50,55,96] (Table 11-5). The evidence does not show any "safe limit" of alcohol intake, and the health effect is from ethanol, regardless of the type of drink.[50]

Mechanisms involved in alcohol-related carcinogenesis include the effect of acetaldehyde, the first metabolite of ethanol oxidation; the induction of cytochrome P-450 2E1 (genetic variant CYP2E1), leading to the generation of ROS; increased procarcinogen activation (e.g., nitrosamines); modulation of cellular regeneration (cell cycle); nutritional deficiencies (retinol, retinyl esters, folic acid, other vitamins) that may predispose to altered mucosal integrity and enzyme and metabolic dysfunction; and other structural abnormalities. Inherited factors also put some individuals at increased risk in DNA repair ability, carcinogen metabolism, and cell cycle control.[84] Recent investigation is concerned with epigenetic mechanisms and alcohol metabolism.[97,98] Figure 11-13 summarizes some of these epigenetic mechanisms and the effects of alcohol metabolism that may be important for cancer pathogenesis.

Physical Activity

Physical activity reduces the risk for breast and colon cancers and may reduce the risk for other cancers, including endometrial, lung, and prostate cancers.[99] Several biological mechanisms causing this effect have been proposed and include decreasing insulin and IGF levels; decreasing obesity; increasing free radical scavenger systems; altering inflammatory mediators; decreasing levels of circulating sex hormones and metabolic hormones; improving immune function; enhancing cytochrome P-450, thus modifying carcinogen activation; and increasing gut motility.[100-102] For colon cancer, physical activity increases gut motility, which reduces the length of time (transit time) that the bowel lining is exposed to potential mutagens.[103] For breast cancer, vigorous physical activity may decrease exposure of breast tissue to ovarian hormones, insulin, and IGF. A randomized trial found that after 12 months of moderate-intensity exercise, postmenopausal women had significantly decreased levels of serum estrogens.[104] Physical activity also helps prevent type 2 diabetes, which has been associated with risk for cancer of the colon and pancreas.[103,105]

Many questions are unanswered regarding frequency, intensity, and duration of exercise. Much of the literature suggests that between 3.5 and 4 hours of vigorous activity per week are necessary to optimize protection for colon cancer.[102] There is likely a dose–response relationship for colon cancer and breast cancer, and 30 to 60 minutes per day of moderate to vigorous intensity activity is proposed to decrease breast cancer risk.[106] The Canadian Physical Activity Guidelines and Canadian Sedentary

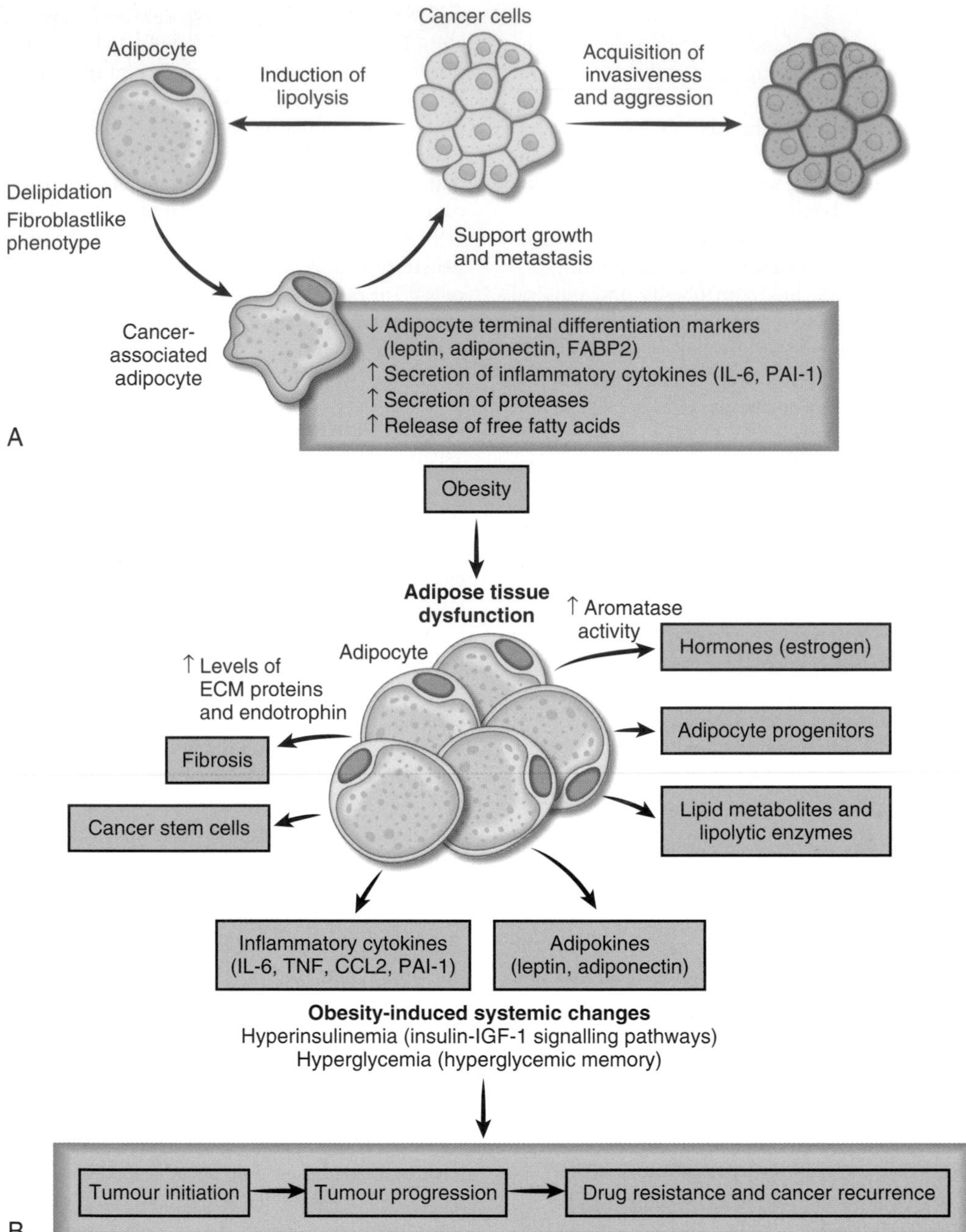

FIGURE 11-12 Structural and Functional Changes in Adipocytes and Interaction With the Microenvironment Contribute to Cancer Progression and Metastases: A Working Model. A, Signalling interactions occur between cancer cells and cancer-associated adipocytes. This interaction within the tumour microenvironment creates a place, or *niche*, permissive for cancer growth. Cancer cells stimulate the breakdown of lipids in adipocytes, leading to *delipidation* and the emergence of a fibroblastlike phenotype in adipocytes. The continuing alterations are associated with functional changes in the cells and include increased secretion of inflammatory mediators (cytokines) and proteases, and increased release of free fatty acids. All of these changes can support tumour growth and invasiveness. **B,** Obesity leads to excessive levels of proinflammatory cytokines, sex hormones, lipid metabolites, and altered adipokines. The altered adipose tissue becomes a source of various extracellular matrix proteins, cancer stem cells, and cancer-associated adipokines. Collectively these alterations contribute to tumour initiation, growth, and recurrence. The systemic metabolic changes of obesity—hyperinsulinemia and hyperglycemia—can further contribute to a tumour-permissive environment. *CCL2,* chemokine ligand 2; *ECM,* extracellular matrix; *FABP2,* fatty acid binding protein 2; *IGF-1,* insulinlike growth factor 1; *IL-6,* interleukin-6; *PAI-1,* plasminogen activator inhibitor-1; *TNF,* tumour necrosis factor. (Reprinted by permission from Macmillan Publishers Ltd: NAT REV ENDOCRINOL, 10[8], Park, J., et al, "Obesity and cancer—mechanisms underlying tumour progression and recurrence," pages 455–465, copyright 2014.)

TABLE 11-5 Alcoholic Drinks and Risk for Cancer[a]

	DECREASES RISK		INCREASES RISK	
	Exposure	Cancer Site	Exposure	Cancer Site
Convincing			Alcoholic drinks	Mouth, pharynx and larynx, esophagus Colorectum (men)[b] Breast (pre- and postmenopause)
Probable			Alcoholic drinks	Liver[c] Colorectum (women)[b]
Limited—suggestive				
Substantial effect on risk unlikely	Alcoholic drinks (adverse effect): kidney[d]			

[a]In the judgement of the panel (World Cancer Research Fund/American Institute for Cancer Research), the factors listed modify the risk for cancer. Judgements are graded according to the strength of the evidence.
[b]The judgements for men and women are different because there are fewer data for women. Increased risk is only apparent above a threshold of 30 g/day of ethanol for both genders.
[c]Cirrhosis is an essential precursor of liver cancer caused by alcohol. The International Agency for Research on Cancer has graded alcohol as a class 1 carcinogen for liver cancer. Alcohol alone only causes cirrhosis in the presence of other factors.
[d]The evidence was sufficient to judge that alcoholic drinks are unlikely to have an adverse effect on the risk for kidney cancer; it was inadequate to draw a conclusion regarding the protective effect.
Adapted from World Cancer Research Fund/American Institute for Cancer Research. (2007). *Food, nutrition, physical activity, and the prevention of cancer: A global perspective.* Washington, DC: American Institute for Cancer Research.

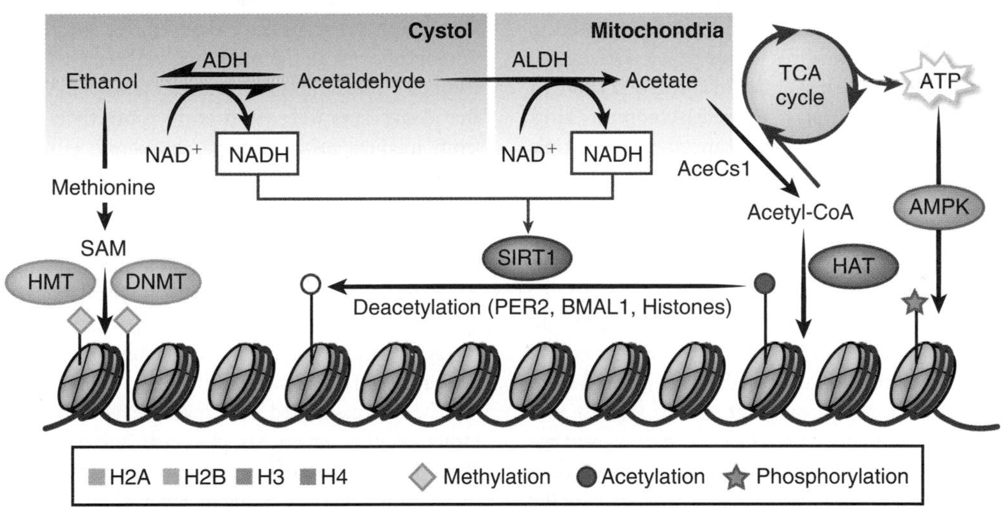

FIGURE 11-13 Alcohol Metabolism and Epigenetics. Chronic alcohol intake leads to decreased methylation called *hypomethylation* by decreasing *S*-adenosylmethionine (*SAM*) that is used by DNA enzymes called methyltransferases (*DNMTs*) and histone enzymes called methyltransferases (*HMTs*) to methylate DNA and histones. Additionally, alcohol metabolism increases the ratio of the coenzyme reduced nicotinamide adenine dinucleotide (*NADH*) to the oxidized nicotinamide adenine dinucleotide (*NAD*+); this step inhibits the sirtuin enzyme SIRT1, which interferes with normal histone acetylation patterns. *AceCs1*, acetyl-coenzyme A synthetase 1; *Acetyl-CoA*, acetyl-coenzyme A; *ADH*, alcohol dehydrogenase; *ALDH*, aldehyde dehydrogenase; *AMPK*, adenosine monophosphate–activated protein kinase; *ATP*, adenosine triphosphate; *BMAL1*, brain and muscle-like aryl hydrocarbon receptor nuclear translocator-like protein 1; *HAT*, histone acetyltransferase; *PER2*, period 2; *TCA*, tricarboxylic acid. (Adapted from Zakhari, S. [2013]. *Alcohol Res, 35*[1], 6–16.)

Behaviour Guidelines (http://www.csep.ca/view.asp?ccid=508) suggest that being active for at least 150 minutes per week can help reduce the risk for many conditions, including certain types of cancer. Physical activity can also result in improved fitness, strength, and mental health.[107]

A Cochrane review found that aerobic exercise was beneficial for adults with cancer-related fatigue during and after cancer treatment.[108] Another Cochrane review found that exercise in children with cancer was associated with improved body composition, flexibility, and cardiorespiratory fitness.[109] More research on exercise for adults and children for prevention of cancer, postcancer treatment, and survivors of cancer is needed.

Ionizing Radiation

Much of the knowledge of the effects of ionizing radiation (IR) on human cancer has stemmed from observations of the Hiroshima and Nagasaki atomic bomb exposures, particularly data from the Life Span Study. These data provide the best estimate of human cancer risk over the dose range from 20 to 250 cGy for low linear energy transfer (LET)

TABLE 11-6 Cancer Associated With Exposure to Ionizing Radiation

Cancer Type	AB	AS	PM	TC	TH	RP	UM	RD
Leukemia	x	x			x			x
Thyroid	x			x				
Breast	x		x					
Lung	x	x			x		x	
Bone						x		
Stomach	x	x						
Esophagus	x	x						
Lymphoma	x	x						x
Brain			x				x	
Liver				x				
Skin				x			x	x

AB, atomic bomb survivors; *AS*, ankylosing spondylitis patients; *PM*, postpartum mastitis patients; *RD*, radiologists; *RP*, radium dial painters; *TC*, tinea capitis patients; *TH*, individuals receiving Thorotrast; *UM*, underground miners.

Data from Jones, J.A., Casey, R.C., & Karouia, F. (2010). Ionizing radiation as a carcinogen. In C.A. McQueen (Ed.), *Comprehensive toxicology* (2nd ed.). St. Louis: Elsevier.

radiation, such as X-rays or γ-rays. Other evidence is derived from groups exposed for medical reasons, underground miners exposed to radon gas, and other occupational exposures (Table 11-6). The atomic bomb exposures in Japan caused acute leukemias in adults and children and increased frequencies of thyroid and breast carcinomas. Lung, stomach, colon, esophageal, and urinary tract cancers and multiple myeloma have been added to the list. At Nagasaki and Hiroshima, leukemia incidence in individuals 15 years or younger reached its peak 6 to 7 years after the explosions and has steadily declined since 1952. People 45 years and older at the time of exposure had a latent period of 20 years before developing acute leukemia.

Recently, standard models and evaluations of age of exposure to radiation and radiation-induced cancer risks have been questioned.[110-112] Epidemiological data from Japanese atomic bomb survivors and from children exposed to radiation for medical intervention suggest that excess relative risks (ERRs) for radiation-induced cancers at a given age are exceptionally higher for individuals exposed during childhood than for those exposed at older ages.[113] These data also are published by the International Commission on Radiological Protection (ICRP) and the National Academy of Sciences's Committee on the Biological Effects of Ionizing Radiation (BEIR Committee).[114] What is at question is the ERRs of radiation exposure in *adulthood* and radiation-induced cancer risk. Recent analyses of Japanese bomb survivors suggest that the ERR for cancer induction decreases with increasing age at exposure only until exposure ages of 30 to 40 years; with radiation exposure at older ages, the ERR does not decrease further, and for many individual cancer sites (liver, colon, lung, stomach, and bladder) the ERR may actually increase in all solid cancers combined.[110,112,115] These new data present a challenge to the conceptual understanding of the mechanisms of cancer induction.[112] Biological models of cancer development all predict that ERRs should decrease continuously with increasing age of radiation exposure. However, recent models of radiation carcinogenesis show IR acts not only as an *initiator* of premalignant cell clones but also as a *promoter* of pre-existing premalignant cell alterations.[110,112,115] Promotion is used here to mean the process by which an initiated cell clonally expands. Therefore, promotional processes from radiation can result in increasing excess lifetime cancer risks with increasing age at exposure. From these new data investigators propose that radiation-induced cancer risks after exposure in middle age may be almost twice as high as previously estimated.[112]

Human exposure to IR includes emissions from the environment (e.g., radon), X-rays, computed tomography (CT) scans, radioisotopes, and other radioactive sources. Health risks involve not only neoplastic diseases but also cardiovascular disease and stroke following high doses in therapeutic medicine and lower doses in A-bomb survivors (BEIR VII report).[114,116] Late effects of radiation in A-bomb survivors show persistent elevations of inflammatory markers, implying immunological damage may be the cause of later cardiovascular effects.[117] For the first time, investigators using a model of umbilical vein endothelial cells have shown that low doses (0.05 Gy) of X-rays induce DNA damage and apoptosis in endothelial cells. These findings will need continued research.[118] Cardiac and blood vessel damage may manifest years after completion of radiation therapy.[119] Other risks include somatic mutations that may contribute to other diseases (e.g., birth defects and eye maladies) and, from animal studies, inherited mutations that may affect the incidence of diseases in future generations. Exposure to diagnostic radiography in utero has been associated with childhood cancer, particularly leukemia.[120-122] The link or association between in utero irradiation and childhood cancer is, however, controversial and varies with study methodology.[123] Heritable mutations are of particular concern for women because the number of oocytes is presumably fixed at birth and mutations, if not repaired, are cumulative.[124] An important summary point in BEIR VII[114] is the concern from high-dose medical exposure, for example, CT scans (see *Health Promotion:* Increasing Use of Computed Tomography Scans and Associated Risks). In 2009 the US National Council on Radiation Protection and Measurements (NCRP)[125] reported that Americans were exposed to more than seven times as much IR from medical procedures as compared with that in the 1980s. The increased exposure is mostly because of the rapid increase in the use of CT imaging.[126] The increase in imaging is likely driven by several factors, including improvements in the technology, that have led to increased clinical applications, patient demand, physician demand, defensive medical practices, and medical uncertainty.[127] Similarly, in Canada, the Canadian Nuclear Safety Commission has reported that medical procedures account for roughly 40% of the total annual radiation dose received by Canadians.[128]

The risks associated with low-dose radiation are being debated among radiobiologists, geneticists, physicists, and others because of the potential effect on the health of current and future generations.[129] The expression of radiation-induced damage depends not only on dose, fractionation, and protraction but also on repair mechanisms; bystander effects; radioprotective substances, such as antioxidants; and the mechanism of radiation delivery.[124]

Radiation-Induced Cancer

Ionizing radiation is a mutagen and carcinogen and can penetrate cells and tissues and deposit energy in tissues at random in the form of ionizations (e.g., excitation or removal of an electron from the target atom). These ionizations can lead to irreversible or indirect damage from formation and attack by water-based free radicals (radiolysis).[129] The *general* characteristics of IR-induced carcinogenesis are well established.[130] The past two decades have focused on *specific* cellular and molecular mechanisms that relate to the induction of cancer, including dose–response relationships for chromosome aberrations, cell transformation, gene expression (genetic and epigenetic), alternative targets, mutagenesis in somatic cells, the biological effects that occur in nonirradiated cells (i.e., nontargeted effects), and effects on the microenvironment.[131] IR is a potent DNA-damaging agent causing cross-linking, nucleotide base damage, and single-strand breaks (SSBs) and double-strand breaks (DSBs)[132] to DNA, and disrupted cellular

HEALTH PROMOTION

Increasing Use of Computed Tomography Scans and Associated Risks

A review article in the *New England Journal of Medicine* on computed tomography (CT) and radiation exposure has received much media attention. The article was written by radiology researchers at Columbia University. In short, the numbers of CT scans have greatly increased in the United States (and in Canada). This increase has occurred both as a diagnostic treatment for individuals with symptoms and as a diagnostic modality for individuals without symptoms (heart, lung, colon, and whole-body screening). Faster scanning times are partly responsible for increased CT use in pediatric populations. Typical doses are larger from CT scans than for a conventional examination (e.g., 50 times more radiation to stomach than an X-ray), and the organs of the body differ in their sensitivity to radiation dose (see the figure that follows). Based on data correlations from Japanese survivors of atomic bombs, the authors estimated that 1.5 to 2.0% of cancers in the United States might be attributable to CT radiation. The authors noted that CT scans are sometimes ordered excessively and repeated unnecessarily because of defensive medicine. They also include three ways to reduce radiation exposure from CT: (1) reduce radiation doses in individual studies (i.e., use modern scanners), (2) substitute ultrasonography with magnetic resonance imaging (MRI) for CT whenever possible, and (3) order CT scans only when absolutely necessary.

Relative Tissue/Organ Sensitivity to Ionizing Radiation (adapted from ICRP 2007 recommendations, Annex B, p. 261)

Organ/Tissue	Number of Tissues	*Tissue Weighting Factor, w_t	Total Contribution
Lungs, stomach, colon, bone marrow, breast, remainder**	6	0.12	0.72
⁺Gonads	1	0.08	0.08
Thyroid, esophagus, bladder, liver	4	0.04	0.16
Bone surface, skin, brain, salivary glands	4	0.01	0.04

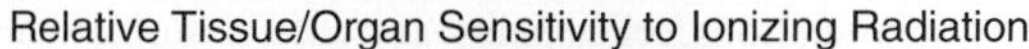

*Tissue weighting factor is a measurement of relative risk of exposure and varies, depending on the tissue.

**Remainder tissues are adrenals, extrathoracic tissue, heart, gall bladder, kidneys, lymph nodes, muscle, oral mucosa, pancreas, prostate (males), small intestine, spleen, thymus, and uterus/cervix (females).

⁺The tissue weighting factor for gonads is applied to the mean doses to testes and ovaries.

Relative Tissue/Organ Sensitivity to Ionizing Radiation

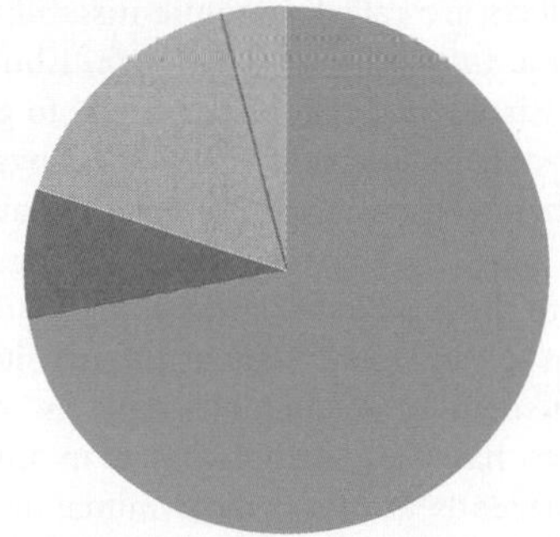

- Lung, stomach, colon, bone marrow, breast, remainder
- Gonads
- Thyroid, esophagus, bladder, liver
- Bone surface, skin, brain, salivary glands

Data retrieved from the International Commission on Radiological Protection (ICRP), 2007 (Annex B, p. 261).

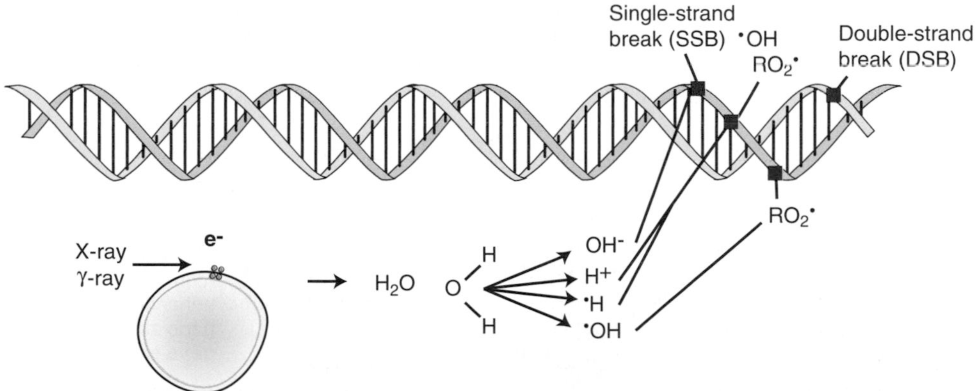

FIGURE 11-14 Free Radicals. Free radicals formed by water nearby and around DNA cause indirect effects. These effects have a short life of single free radicals. Oxygen can modify the reaction, enabling longer lifetimes of oxidative free radicals. *H*, hydrogen; *H*$^+$, hydrogen ion; *•H*, hydrogen free radical; H_2O, water; *O*, oxygen; *OH*$^-$, hydroxyl ion; *•OH*, hydroxyl free radical; $RO_2^{\bullet}$, reactive oxygen species.

regulation processes can lead to carcinogenesis.[132] The DSB (Figure 11-14) is considered the characteristic lesion observed for the effects of IR. In certain experimental systems, one DSB may lead to cell cycle arrest and possible further repair. Yet many DSBs appear to result from clustered damage, a consequence of the pattern of distribution of ionizations with DNA. These patterns of clustered damage may be more difficult to accurately repair.[133] Importantly, DSBs are mostly repaired by the nonhomologous end joining (NHEJ) pathway. This pathway is efficient for joining the DNA broken ends; however, errors can occur and repair may decline with age.[134] Irradiated human cells unable to execute the NHEJ pathway are supersensitive to the introduction of large-scale mutations and chromosomal aberrations.[129]

Although evidence suggests that interindividual differences in radiation responses may be attributed to certain genes, IR can activate oncogenes, resulting in uncontrolled cell growth[131,135] (see Chapter 10). Tumour-suppressor genes also are sensitive to IR. Several tumour-suppressor genes have been identified that are deactivated by IR that promotes carcinogenesis.[131,135] Recent research has shown that cells can detect and respond epigenetically, altering gene expression after low doses of radiation.[131] Gene expression can change as a function of radiation dose and radiation type.[131]

Nontargeted Effects

A long-held assumption is that cellular alterations—mutations and malignant transformation—occur only in cells directly radiated. It is now known that cells not directly exposed to radiation, but instead the progeny of cells that were irradiated many cell divisions previously, may express a high level of gene mutations, cell lethality, and chromosomal aberration. Altogether these effects are called **genomic instability**. Investigators are studying genomic instability as it may contribute to secondary cancers. The directly irradiated cells also can lead to genetic effects in so-called bystander cells or innocent cells (called **bystander effects**), even though they themselves received no direct radiation exposure.[129] For example, using an in vivo mouse model, investigators found that localized radiation to the head led to induced bystander effects in the lead-shielded distant spleen tissue.[136] These radiosensitive mice showed unexpected enhancement of medulloblastoma in their cerebellum. The bystander effect has been demonstrated in three-dimensional human tissues and recently in other whole animal organisms.[101] Both DSBs and apoptotic cell death were induced by bystander effects, supporting the role of signalling between the irradiated cells (the targeted cells) and unirradiated cells (the nontargeted, or bystander, cells) (Figure 11-15). Such communication is thought to occur from direct physical connection between cells or gap junctions, called gap junctional intercellular communication (see p. 12), and from signalling pathways. Numerous intercellular and intracellular signalling pathways are implicated in the bystander response, and these effects have been shown to be transmitted to their descendants. These various effects demonstrated in vivo may reflect an ongoing inflammatory response (oxidative stress response) to the initial radiation-induced injury[137] (Box 11-1). One hypothesis is the stress response is due to elevated ROS affecting genomic instability. Importantly, therapeutic interference with specific signalling pathways (e.g., p38MAPK) may result in genome stabilization.[138] Both the bystander and the genomic instability effects have been termed **nontargeted effects**.

Acute, Latent, and Microenvironmental Effects

IR causes acute and persistent short- and long-term effects.[102-104] Acute exposure to IR can cause damage to several organ systems, especially those with highly proliferative cells such as the hematopoietic system,

BOX 11-1 A Paradigm Shift? Responses to Ionizing Radiation Mediated by Inflammatory Mechanisms

Many observations have not been supportive of the conventional paradigm of biological responses to ionizing radiation (IR). The conventional paradigm is that the consequences of exposure to IR have been attributed solely to mutational DNA damage or cell death induced in irradiated cells at the time of exposure. The challenges to this paradigm come from three types of published data: (1) **abscopal**, or "out-of field," effects, where radiation treatment to one local area of the body results in an antitumour effect distant to the radiation site; (2) detection of plasma factors in vivo (clastogenic [or capable of chromosome damage] factors) that can affect the survival and function of irradiated cells; and (3) effects in nonirradiated cells that are in the vicinity of irradiated cells (bystander effects) or in the descendants of irradiated cells several generations after the initial radiation exposure (genomic instability). These nontargeted effects are different than the targeted effects that arise in cells upon immediate deposition of energy at the time of radiation exposure. The nontargeted effects arise as a result of intracellular signalling and appear to represent a genotype-dependent balance (and various epigenetic influences) of toxic factors and cellular responses that may involve both oxidative stress and inflammatory type processes (see Figure 11-15).

Data from El Azzam, Jay-Gerin, J.P., & Pain, D. (2012). *Cancer Lett, 327*(1–2), 48–60; Mukherjee, D., Coates, P.J., Lorimore, S.A., et al. (2014). *J Pathol, 232*(3), 289–299.

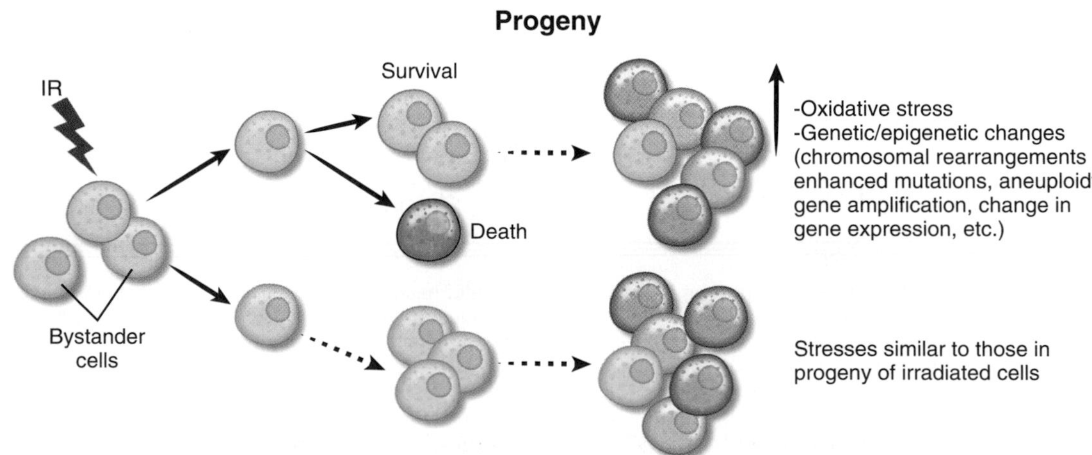

FIGURE 11-15 Radiation: Targeted and Nontargeted or Bystander Effects. Signalling from cells exposed to irradiation causes stressful effects, including oxidative stress, to those cells not directly radiated called bystander cells and their progeny. These induced effects may be similar to those reported in the progeny of irradiated cells. *IR*, ionizing radiation. (Reprinted from *Cancer Lett,* 327(1–2), El Azzam, Jay-Gerin, J.P., & Pain, D., "Ionizing radiation-induced metabolic oxidative stress and prolonged cell injury," Pages 48–60, Copyright 2012, with permission from Elsevier.)

the skin, and the gastro-intestinal system[105] (see Chapter 4). Investigators have postulated that radiation's carcinogenic potential persists because of nontargeted radiation effects that alter cell and tissue signalling and change the microenvironment.[106,139] Investigators report the brain's innate immune system is very vulnerable to cranial irradiation, altering the microenvironment and causing the recruitment and infiltration of macrophages.[140] With improvement in cancer survival, the long-term risks for a second cancer developing from treatment become more important.[141]

Radiation-induced cancer in humans has latent periods, usually 5 to 10 years, but can be decades.[131] British investigators reported the following results: for solid cancers, radiation-related excess risk starts to appear about 5 years after exposure in therapeutically irradiated groups; and for leukemia, it starts to appear within 5 years of exposure.[141] In the United States, using Surveillance Epidemiology and End Results (SEER) data, the estimated excess of second cancers that could be related to radiotherapy was found to be about 8%; data from the United Kingdom, which included diagnostic procedures and excluded therapeutic irradiation, yielded an estimation of 15%.[141,142]

Low Dose and Dose Rate

Recent events, including the 2011 Fukushima nuclear accident in Japan, terrorist attacks, and exposure to radiation from medical procedures, have increased the need to understand the human health effects of exposure to low-level IR.[143] Risk estimates for human exposure at low-dose, low-LET ionizing radiation (0 to 100 mSv, or less than 0.1 Gy) are constantly debated. Although investigators have reported that accurate measurements of risks from low doses of radiation are statistically difficult because they require such large populations, researchers have developed an in silico simulation model of a population-based cohort study for conducting future epidemiological studies of excess cancer risks in CT-exposed individuals.[144] Simulation models may provide reasonable approximations, and theoretical models are still used to estimate response curves (Box 11-2).

Ultraviolet Radiation

Ultraviolet radiation (**UV radiation**), comes from sunlight. Other sources of UV radiation include electric lights, black lights, and tanning lamps.[145] UV radiation is divided into three major wavelengths: UVA, UVB, and UVC radiation. Most of the UV radiation received on earth is UVA and some UVB.[145] UVA radiation is weaker than UVB, but UVA penetrates deeper into the skin and is more constant throughout the year despite the weather.[145] UVB affects the outer layer of the skin, and UVC radiation does not increase health risks as much as UVB.[145] UV radiation also can be important to health and produces vitamin D that helps in the absorption of calcium and phosphorus from food, which are all important for bone development. The WHO recommends 5 to 15 minutes of sun exposure two to three times a week; however, overexposure can result in acute and chronic health effects on the skin, eyes, and immune system.[146]

BOX 11-2 Theoretical Models to Understand Low-Dose Ionizing Radiation

Several models estimate the risk of low-dose ionizing radiation. They include the linear no-threshold (LNT) model, which assumes that any dose, including very low doses, has the potential to cause mutations (see **A**). Another model, the linear-quadratic dose–response model, illustrates a relationship between dose and biological response that is curved (i.e., response = dose^2) and implies that the rate of change in response is different at different doses; the response may change slowly at low doses, for example, but rapidly at high doses, (see **B**). The threshold model proposes a threshold dose below which radiation may not cause cancer in humans (see **C**). Proponents of this model argue that such thresholds are derived, for example, from the ability to repair damage caused by lower doses of radiation. There is some evidence that low doses may actually produce a higher level of risk per unit of dose, which is called the supralinear hypothesis (see **D**). The stochastic (or random probability) model (see **E**) is a major model for understanding low-dose radiation. Currently, the shape of the response curve for the low-dose region is really unknown.

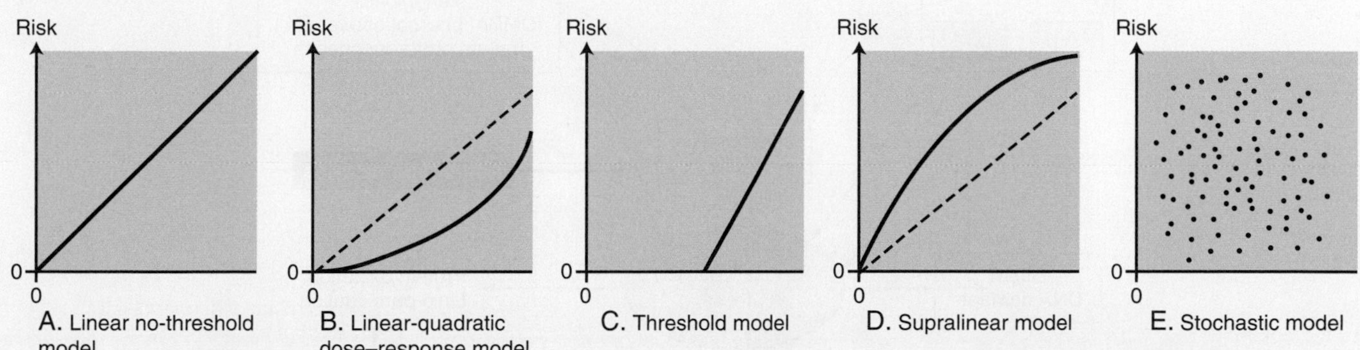

Theoretical Models for Estimating the Risk of Low-Dose Ionizing Radiation. Collective population dose is expressed as a person-rem (roentgen equivalent, man). Estimating a collective dose then enables an application of a "constant risk factor" to obtain a statistical estimate of the number of additional cancers (above background radiation) from that exposure. These computations apply to low doses–low-dose rates only. Many propose the best fit is the LNT model (**A**). The most common alternative to the LNT model is the linear-quadratic model (**B**). The quadratic term is the square of the dose. The linear term is equal to zero. The threshold model (**C**) is a threshold below which there is *no* increase in cancer risk. Proponents of this model argue that because some toxic chemicals and materials exhibit such thresholds, radiation must also have a threshold. Their arguments are related to repair of the radiation damage caused by lower doses of radiation. Some evidence exists that low levels of radiation produce a higher level of risk per unit dose, which is called the *supralinear model* (**D**). The stochastic model (**E**) describes effects that are random and proposes that events cannot be predicted. (Adapted from Makhijani, A., Smith, B., & Thorne, M.C. [2006]. *Science for the vulnerable: Setting radiation and multiple exposure environmental health standards to protect those at most risk.* Takoma Park, MD: Institute for Energy and Environmental Research.)

There are three main types of skin cancer: cancer that forms in melanocytes (pigment cells) called **melanoma**, cancer in the lower part of the epidermis or outer layer of the skin called **basal cell carcinoma (BCC)**, and cancer in the flat cells that form the surface of the skin called **squamous cell carcinoma (SCC)** (see Chapter 41). Melanoma, the most lethal form of skin cancer, can occur on any skin surface; however, in men it is often found on the skin on the head, the neck, between the shoulders, and the hips. In women it is more commonly found on the skin on the lower legs, between the shoulders, and the hips. Although rare in people with dark skin, melanoma is usually found under the fingernails, under the toenails, on the palms of the hands, or on the soles of the feet.[147] BCC commonly occurs on the head and neck. SCC is found more commonly in men who work outdoors, but can occur in anyone. SCC occurs on sun-exposed areas of the skin, including the nose, ears, lower lip, and dorsa of the hand. SCCs are composed of keratinizing cells and are more aggressive then BCC, but the development into invasive SCC is low.[148] For a more complete discussion about these skin cancers, see Chapter 41.

The incidence of BCC and SCC is strongly correlated with lifetime sunlight exposure (i.e., photocarcinogenesis). Specific patterns of sunlight exposure, intermittent or chronic, confer different host effects, acute or cumulative. Intense intermittent recreational sun exposure has been associated with melanoma and BCC. Chronic occupational sun exposure has been associated with SCC. Tanning bed use also has been associated with an increased risk for BCC. The risk was higher in females and with higher use of indoor tanning facilities.[149] For other occupational factors linked to skin cancers, see Chapter 41. Depending on the time of day and a person's skin type, acute sun exposure may result in sunburn.[147] From epidemiological studies, a sunburn is defined as a burn or pain and possible blistering that lasts for 2 or more days.[147] Cumulative sun exposure is the additive effects of intermittent sun exposure, chronic sun exposure, or both. Other skin cancer risk factors include IR, chronic arsenic ingestion, immunosuppression, and genetic factors. These skin cancers have a higher incidence among people with a light or fair skin tone, but they can occur in anyone and in those who do not burn from sunlight.[150]

UV radiation is known to cause specific gene mutations; for example, SCC involves mutation in the tumour protein p53 (*TP53*) gene, BCC in the patched 1 tumour-suppressor gene (*PTCH1*), and melanoma in the *p16* gene.[151] The patched or hedgehog intracellular signalling pathway plays a central role in both sporadic BCCs and nevoid basal cell carcinoma syndrome (Gorlin syndrome) tumour growth.[152] Investigators are identifying aberrant DNA methylation and histone modifications in tumour tissues and cell lines for skin cancers.[153-155] In addition, UV light induces the release of tumour necrosis factor-alpha (TNF-α) in the epidermis, which may reduce immune surveillance against skin cancer.[156] The identification of transcription factors and chemokine receptors suggests a critical role of inflammation in skin carcinogenesis.[157]

Skin exposure to UV radiation and IR, as well as chemical (xenobiotic) agents or medications, produces ROS in large quantities.[158] Uncontrolled release of ROS is an important contributor to skin carcinogenesis.[158] Imbalances in ROS and antioxidants can lead to oxidative stress, tissue injury, and direct DNA damage (Figure 11-16). ROS can induce a number of transcription factors (e.g., activator protein-1 [AP-1] and NF-κB)[159] and increase regulating genes that induce inflammation.[158,160] Inflammation is a critical component of tumour progression.

The incidence of melanoma has been increasing annually at rates of 2 to 7% in White populations since the 1980s.[161] Incidence is increasing worldwide, and in Canada incidence increased by 2.3% for men and 2.9% for women between 2001 and 2010.[162] Although pediatric melanoma is rare, most studies have indicated that its incidence has been rising.[163] However, a recent study found that the incidence of new cases of pediatric melanoma in the United States actually decreased from 2004 to 2010, but only in those children with good prognostic indicators.[163] Therefore, health programs need to continue to encourage sun protective behaviour (protective clothing, sunscreen use, decreased time spent outside, decreased indoor tanning) to reduce melanoma incidence. Because death rates from melanoma have not risen as rapidly as incidence rates,

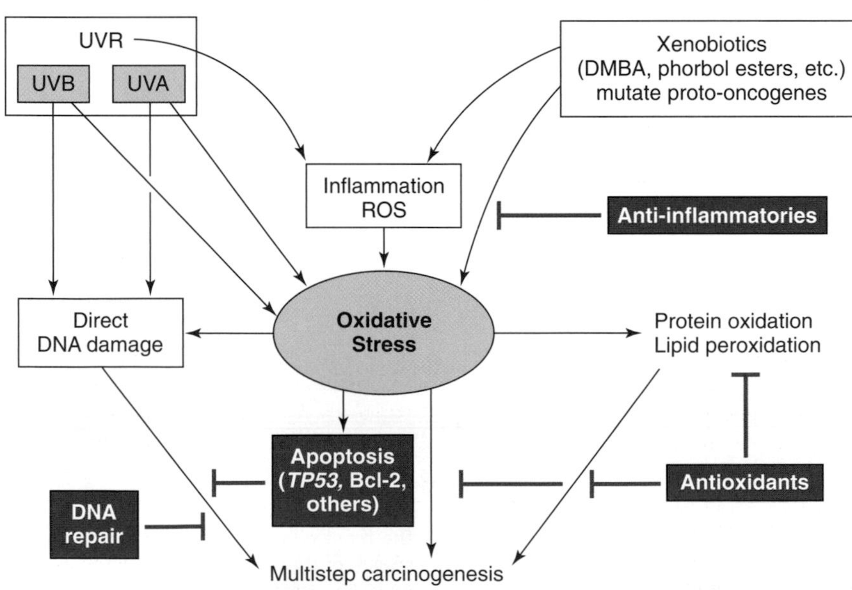

FIGURE 11-16 Theoretical Scheme of Multistep Skin Carcinogenesis. Ultraviolet radiation (*UVR*), inflammation, and xenobiotics lead to oxidative stress, resulting in direct DNA damage, protein oxidation, lipid peroxidation, and apoptosis. The protective mechanisms shown in *red* include apoptosis, DNA repair, and antioxidants. *Bcl-2,* B-cell lymphoma 2; *DMBA,* 7,12-dimethylbenz[a]anthracene; *ROS,* reactive oxygen species; *TP53,* tumour protein p53 gene; *UVA,* ultraviolet A; *UVB,* ultraviolet B. (Adapted from Sander, C.D., et al. [2004]. Role of oxidative stress and the antioxidant network in cutaneous carcinogenesis. *Int J Dermatol,* 43[5]: 326–335. Copyright © 2004, John Wiley and Sons.)

controversy still exists about whether some of the incidence is a result of overdiagnosis.[164,165] Melanomas can appear suddenly and without warning, and can arise from or near a mole (melanocytic nevus) and freckles.[166] Complex interactions between UV exposure profiles and genotype combinations determine nevus numbers and size, as well as facial freckling.[166] When detected in the early stages, melanoma is highly curable.[167] Early-stage melanoma is classified as radial growth phase (RGP). Later-stage melanoma, called vertical growth phase (VGP), is characterized by invasion into the dermal layer and is frequently metastatic.[168] Much research is ongoing to understand the mechanisms that promote progression from less invasive RGP melanoma to aggressive VGP melanoma. Recent progress in understanding the molecular alterations in melanoma will likely advance its diagnosis, prognosis, and treatment.

The pathogenesis of melanoma is very complex, involving genetic and environmental factors. The genetic factors can be inherited, for example, in high-susceptibility genes (i.e., *cyclin-dependent kinase inhibitor 2A [CDKN2A]*) or in low-susceptibility genes (i.e., *melanocortin-1*). About 10 to 15% of melanomas are inherited as an autosomal dominant trait with variable penetrance.[169] The majority of melanomas are sporadic and seem to involve UV radiation damage.[169] UV radiation is correlated with DNA damage. Epidemiological and case-control studies suggest that UV radiation exposure is the most significant factor for the development of melanoma (episodes of intense, intermittent exposure [measured as history of sunburn]). Other evidence, however, reports that rates of melanoma are uncommon in persons with outdoor occupations. Furthermore, because melanomas sometimes occur in dark-skinned individuals, other environmental factors may be important. Recent analyses in Iceland and Italy and a previous large prospective study in Norway and Sweden suggest sunbed use as a reason for increased melanoma, especially in women.[170-172] Indoor tanning (sunbed use) is a risk factor for melanoma[173] (i.e., frequent indoor tanning increases melanoma risk). Certain skin conditions also are treated with UVA and UVB light therapy. Family history (i.e., genetic factors), skin type, and the density of moles are important in determining the risk of developing melanoma. Traits associated with a high risk for melanoma are light-coloured hair, eyes, and skin; an inability to tan; and a tendency to freckle, sunburn, and develop nevi.

The emerging molecular changes associated with melanoma emphasize that melanoma, like many other cancers, is not a single disease but a diverse group of disorders. The most frequent driver mutations in melanoma involve cell cycle control, progrowth pathways, and telomerase.[169] Although other genes may be involved, melanoma progression is often associated with a mutation in the *BRAF* oncogene.[168] The most common mutation in *BRAF*^{V600E} promotes the progression of melanoma through activation of the mitogen-activated protein kinase (MAPK) signalling cascade.[168] Investigators report disease progression may involve factors secreted by the melanoma cells that activate extracellular matrix enzymes (matrix metalloproteinase-1 [MMP-1]) and adjacent stromal fibroblasts in the tumour microenvironment.[168]

Although avoiding sunlight by keeping in the shade and covering up is very important for protection, more data are needed to understand whether sunscreen prevents melanoma. A significant benefit from regular sunscreen use has not yet demonstrated primary prevention for BCC and melanoma.[174] Increased knowledge of the intricate cellular interactions in melanoma will increase understanding of melanoma etiology and pathogenesis. This knowledge is essential for early detection and treatment.

Electromagnetic Radiation

Health risks associated with **radiofrequency electromagnetic radiation (RF-EMR)** are very controversial. RF-EMR is in the frequency range of 30 kHz to 300 GHz. Electromagnetic fields (EMFs) generated by RF sources couple with the body and result in induced electric and magnetic fields with associated currents inside tissue.[175] Exposure to electric and magnetic fields is widespread. Microwaves, radar, mobile phones (e.g., cellphones and smartphones), cordless phones, cellphone towers (base stations), power frequency radiation associated with electricity and radio waves, fluorescent lights, computers, and other electric equipment create EMRs of varying strength. Despite the breadth of literature on microwaves (MW), the impact of EMR on human health has not been fully assessed. Scientific evidence is accumulating, although it has been hampered by the scarcity of methods to accurately measure exposure, the lack of a clear dose–response relationship, and the difficulty in reproducing effects. In addition, with competing priorities such as convenience, financial interest, and health necessity, a consensus on the risk–benefit ratio of EMR exposure may be difficult to achieve, and safety standards vary significantly, up to 1 000 times among countries.[176,177] The National Institute of Environmental Health Sciences Electric and Magnetic Fields Working Group[178] in the United States recommended that low-frequency EMFs be classified as possible carcinogens. Overall, there is limited evidence that magnetic fields cause childhood leukemia and insufficient evidence for other cancers in children.[179-182] A recent large census-cohort study from Switzerland did not suggest an association between predicted RF-EMF exposure from broadcast transmitters and childhood leukemia.[183] Studies of magnetic field exposure from power lines and electric blankets in adults reveal little evidence of an association with leukemia, brain tumours, or breast cancer.[179]

The most extensively studied exposure is from the use of wireless telephones (mobile and cordless phones); other exposures include occupational settings and sources from the general environment.[175] One cohort study and five case-control studies did not show an increased rate of brain tumours after the increase in mobile phone use. However, these studies had limitations because most of the analyses examined trends only in the early 2000s.[175] The INTERPHONE study,[184] a multicentre case-control study, is the largest study so far that studies the relationship between mobile phone use and brain tumours (i.e., glioma, acoustic neuroma, and meningioma). Results for cordless phones are lacking in the INTERPHONE study.[185] The pooled analyses included 2 708 glioma cases and 2 972 controls. The odds ratios (ORs) in terms of time spent on the phone showed that the highest time spent on the phone (greater than 1 640 hours of use) was related to glioma risk (OR 1.40; 95% confidence interval [CI] 1.03 to 1.89). There was a suggestion of increased risk for tumours on the same side of the head as the phone use (ipsilateral exposure) in the temporal lobe, where RF-EMF exposure is highest.[175] The OR for glioma increased with an increasing RF dose for exposures 7 years or more before diagnosis, but there was no association with estimated dose for exposures less than 7 years before diagnosis.[175] A Swedish investigative group performed a pooled analysis of two similar studies between the relationship of glioma, acoustic neuroma, and meningioma manifestation and mobile and cordless phone use.[186] Study participants who used a mobile phone for more than 1 year had an OR for glioma of 1.3 (95% CI 1.1 to 1.6). The OR increased with increasing time since first use and with total call time, attaining 3.2 (2.0 to 5.1) for more than 2 000 hours of use.[175] Ipsilateral use of the phone was associated with higher risk.[175] Similar findings were reported for cordless phones.[175] Although the INTERPHONE and Swedish studies were judged susceptible to bias, the WHO IARC Monograph Working Group concluded that the findings could not be dismissed because of bias alone and a causal relationship between mobile phones and glioma is possible.[175] The WHO Working Group concluded that there is "limited evidence in humans" for the carcinogenicity of RF-EMF based on associations between glioma and acoustic neuroma and exposure to RF-EMF from wireless phones.[175]

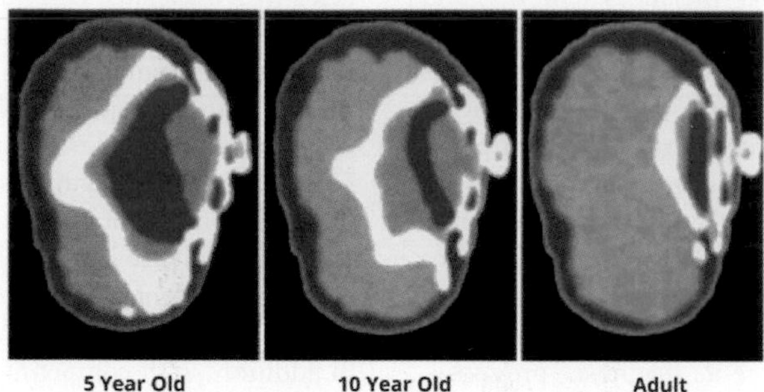

FIGURE 11-17 Electromagnetic Radiation From a Cellphone Can Penetrate the Skull. Electromagnetic radiation from a cellphone can penetrate the skull and deposit energy 4 to 6 cm into the brain. A 50-minute cellphone exposure was associated with increased brain glucose metabolism in the region closest to the antenna. This finding is of unknown clinical significance. (From Volkow, N.D., Tomasi, D., Wang, G.-J., et al. [2011]. *JAMA, 305*[8], 808–813.)

The WHO Working Group reviewed numerous mechanisms of carcinogenicity from RF-EMF.[175] The mechanisms included genotoxicity, effects on immune function, gene and protein expression, cell signalling, oxidative stress, apoptosis, and the blood–brain barrier. Other suggested mechanisms may include altered DNA repair mechanisms and epigenetic changes to DNA.[185] The WHO Working Group classified RF-EMF as "possibly carcinogenic to humans" (a Group 2B carcinogen, per IARC classification).

EMR from a cellphone can penetrate the skull and deposit energy 4 to 6 cm into the brain (Figure 11-17).[187] Investigators found that a 50-minute cellphone exposure was associated with increased brain glucose metabolism in the region closest to the antenna.[188] Children have a smaller head and thinner skull bone than adults, and investigators have reported higher conductivity and higher absorption from RF-EMF than for adults.[189-191] Concern is for children in whom the effects may be compounded because of increased vulnerability to radiation and their longer use of cellphones into adulthood. Advice about reducing exposures through simple precautions is increasing; for example, individuals should not hold a cellphone directly to their head, pregnant women should keep cellphones away from their abdomen, and children should not be allowed to play with or use a cellphone. Mobile phone manufacturers themselves are issuing advice on reducing exposure.[192] Ongoing unbiased research is desperately needed. Absolute proof of causation may be hindered because of the ethical questions associated with exposing individuals to potentially harmful interventions.

QUICK CHECK 11-3

1. What are the cancers associated with cigarette smoking?
2. How are dietary components related to cancer?
3. What are the possible pathophysiological mechanisms of obesity-associated cancer risk?
4. How does ionizing radiation contribute to carcinogenesis? Ultraviolet radiation?
5. Discuss the difficulty in determining cancer risks with electromagnetic radiation.

Infection, and Sexual and Reproductive Behaviour

Infection is an important contributor to cancer worldwide. In developed countries, 7% of all cancers are thought to be due to infections.[193] The prevalence of cancer cases attributable to infections varies widely by region. In 2008, de Martel and colleagues estimated that 7.4% of cases occurred in more developed regions, and 22.9% occurred in less developed regions.[194] The highest prevalence occurred in sub-Saharan Africa, at 32.7%.[194] De Martel and colleagues used cancer-causing agents classified by the IARC to determine the prevalence of cancers attributable to infections because the strength of published evidence is controversial. According to investigators, these prevalence rates are probably conservative and underestimate the true burden of infection-associated cancers.[194] The top four notable infections associated with new cancer cases are human papillomavirus (HPV), *Helicobacter pylori* (*H. pylori*), hepatitis B virus (HBV), and hepatitis C virus (HCV) (Table 11-7). Hepatitis B and hepatitis C can infect the liver and together account for the large majority of liver cancer cases (see Chapter 36). It has been estimated that *H. pylori* accounted for about 75% of all stomach cancers[195]; however, updated estimates using both enzyme-linked immunosorbent assay (ELISA) and Western blot for detection of anti–*H. pylori* antibodies include an additional 120 000 cases of gastric cancer for a total percentage of 89%.[196] Additional sources of cancer include the Epstein-Barr virus (EBV), which is linked to cancers of the nasopharynx, Hodgkin's disease, and non-Hodgkin's lymphoma; the human herpes virus type 8, which is linked to Kaposi sarcoma; and human T-cell lymphotropic virus type 1, which is linked to leukemia and lymphoma. The following discussion will concern HPV.

At least 50% of sexually active people will have genital HPV at some time in their lives.[197] HPVs are a group of more than 150 related viruses. More than 40 of these viruses can easily spread from direct skin contact or through vaginal, rectal, or oral sex.[198] *Low-risk HPVs* do not cause cancer but can cause skin warts, called *condylomata acuminata*. *High-risk HPVs*, or oncogenic HPVs, can cause cancer. Even though about a dozen HPVs have been identified, HPV types 16 and 18 are responsible for the majority of cancers.[198] However, most high-risk HPV infections may cause cytological abnormalities or abnormal cell changes that disappear unexpectedly. According to the US National Cancer Institute, most infections will be suppressed by the immune system.[199] Persistence of infection with high-risk HPV is a prerequisite for the development of cervical intraepithelial neoplasia (CIN) lesions (see Figure 33-16) and invasive cervical cancers.[12,199] HPV infection has been identified as a definite carcinogen for six types of cancer: cervix, penis, vulva, anus, and some oropharynx (including the base of the tongue and tonsils).[199,200] The incidence of HPV-associated oropharyngeal cancer has increased

TABLE 11-7 **Number of New Cancer Cases[a] in 2008 Attributable to Infection, by Infectious Agent, and Development Status[b]**

	Less Developed Regions	More Developed Regions	World
Hepatitis B and C viruses	520 000 (32.0%)	80 000 (19.4%)	600 000 (29.5%)
Human papillomavirus	490 000 (30.2%)	120 000 (29.2%)	610 000 (30.0%)
Helicobacter pylori	470 000 (28.9%)	190 000 (46.2%)	660 000 (32.4%)
Epstein-Barr virus	96 000 (5.9%)	16 000 (3.9%)	110 000 (5.5%)
Human herpesvirus type 8	39 000 (2.4%)	4 100 (1.0%)	43 000 (2.1%)
Human T-cell lymphotropic virus type 1	660 (0.0%)	1 500 (0.4%)	2 100 (0.1%)
Opisthorchis viverrini and *Clonorchis sinensis*	2 000 (0.1%)	0 (0.0%)	2 000 (0.1%)
Schistosoma haematobium	6 000 (0.4%)	0 (0.0%)	6 000 (0.3%)
Total	**1 623 660 (100.0%)**	**411 600 (100.0%)**	**2 035 260 (100.0%)**

[a]Numbers are rounded to two significant digits.

[b]Data are the number of new cancer cases attributed to a particular infectious agent (proportion of the total number of new cases attributed to infection that is due to a specific agent).

Data from de Martel, C., Ferlay, J., Franceschi, S., et al. (2012). *Lancet Oncol, 13*(6), 607-615.

during the past 20 years, especially among men. Factors that may increase the risk of developing cancer following a high-risk HPV infection include smoking, decreased immunity, having many children (increased risk for cervical cancer), long-term oral contraceptive use (increased risk for cervical cancer), poor oral hygiene (increased risk for oropharyngeal cancer), and chronic inflammation.[201] Although the main mode of HPV transmission occurs through genital contact (oral, touching, or sexual intercourse), HPV has been found in virginal women before first intercourse.[202] Consensus is that newborn babies can be exposed to cervical HPV infection from the mother.[202] The possible modes of transmission in children, however, are controversial.[203] The *Health Promotion:* Rising Incidence of HPV-Associated Oropharyngeal Cancers contains information on the rising incidence of HPV-associated oropharyngeal cancers.

The Society of Obstetricians and Gynaecologists of Canada (SOGC) current guidelines (2007) recommend that women should have a Papanicolaou smear (Pap test) every 2 to 3 years up to the age of 70, depending on the province, beginning once they have become sexually active.[205] Women with certain risk factors may need more frequent screening or to continue screening beyond age 65. Women who have received the HPV vaccine still need regular cervical screening[199,204] (see Chapter 33 for a discussion on the HPV vaccine). HPV vaccines protect males and females against diseases, including cancers, when given to the recommended age groups. HPV vaccines are given in three shots over 6 months.[206]

Other Viruses and Microorganisms

A discussion of the relationship between viruses, bacteria, and cancer appears in Chapter 10 and appropriate chapters in Unit II. Other microorganisms involved in carcinogenesis include parasites such as *Opisthorchis viverrini* (bile duct cancer) and *Schistosoma haematobium* (bladder cancer). Their specific roles in carcinogenesis are reported to be related to cofactors or carcinogens, or both.

Air Pollution

Outdoor air pollution is a complex mixture of many known carcinogens, and its relationship to lung cancer has been studied for more than 50 years.[207] Past reviews of outdoor and household air pollution indicated that both were associated with increased rates of lung cancer, most particularly with exposures to increased levels of particles called **particulate matter (PM)**. Particulate matter, also known as *particle pollution*, is a mixture of extremely small particles and liquid droplets. PM consists of a complex mix of acids (such as nitrates and sulphates), organic chemicals, metals, and soil or dust particles. The IARC recently concluded that exposure to outdoor air pollution and to PM in outdoor air is "carcinogenic to humans" (IARC Group 1 carcinogen) and causes lung cancer.[208,209] The IARC's evaluation came from long-term epidemiological studies of residential exposure to air pollution. Specifically, focused

HEALTH PROMOTION

Rising Incidence of HPV-Associated Oropharyngeal Cancers

The incidence of head and neck cancers has fallen with a decrease in smoking in both the United States and Canada; however, the incidence of human papillomavirus (HPV)-associated oropharyngeal cancers (tonsil and tongue base) appears to be rising—especially in young White men. The two classes of oropharyngeal squamous cell carcinoma seem to have different causes: HPV-positive oral cancers are possibly associated with sex-related risk factors, whereas HPV-negative cancers are associated with tobacco and alcohol consumption. Epidemiological studies support little interaction between the two sets of risk factors, suggesting that HPV-positive cancer and HPV-negative cancer have *distinct* pathogenesis. Tobacco use and alcohol use are known etiological factors in head and neck cancers; it is surprising that most cases of oropharyngeal cancers in nonsmokers are HPV-related. Not yet known is whether this increase is attributed to changes in sexual norms (from past generations), with more oral sex partners or oral sex at an earlier age. Smoking, however, has an adverse effect on both HPV-positive and HPV-negative oral cancers. In Sweden the incidence of oropharyngeal cancers caused by HPV increased from 23% in the 1970s to 57% in the 1990s to 93% in 2007. Emerging data indicate that HPV is now the primary cause of tonsillar cancer in North America and Europe. The mechanism of HPV-oropharyngeal cancer is different than that related to tobacco use: *P53* degradation occurs (i.e., *P53* helps direct genetic repair and cell death [see Chapter 10]), the *RB* pathway is inactivated (cell signalling pathway), and the risk for HPV-16 (i.e., *P16*) is increased. Tobacco-related oropharyngeal cancers are characterized by *TP53* mutation and a decrease in the *CDKN2A* mutation (cell cycle gene), and thus a decrease in *P16*. Individuals with *P16*-positive tumours have a better prognosis than those with *P16*-negative tumours.

CDKN2A, cyclin-dependent kinase inhibitor 2A gene; *RB*, retinoblastoma gene; *TP53*, tumour protein p53 gene.

Data from Chaturvedi, A.K., Engels, E.A., Pfeiffer, R.M., et al. (2011). *J Clin Oncol, 29*(32), 4294–4301; Lowy, D.R., & Munger, K. (2010). *N Engl J Med, 363*(1), 82–84; Marur, S., D'Souza, G., Westra, W.H., et al. (2010). *Lancet Oncol, 11*(8), 781–789; Nasman, A., Attner, P., Hammarstedt, L., et al. (2009). *Int J Cancer, 125*(2), 362–366.

reviews of lung cancer risk are with prominent components of PM in outdoor air ($PM_{2.5}$ particles with aerodynamic diameter equal to or less than 2.5 μm, or fine particles and PM_{10} [equal to or less than 10 μm, or inhalable particles]) (Figure 11-18).

$PM_{2.5}$ includes a higher proportion of mutagenic agents.[210] Importantly, analyses by continent of study (including North America, Europe, and others) yielded consistent, positive associations between $PM_{2.5}$ and lung cancer.[207] *Primary particles* are emitted directly from a source, for example, construction sites, unpaved roads, fields, smokestacks, or fires. *Secondary particles* are emitted from power plants, industries, and automobiles. These particles are a complex of chemicals including sulphur dioxide and nitrogen oxides and make up most of the fine particle pollution in Canada.[211] Fine or ultrafine particles are easily absorbed by the lungs and phagocytosed by macrophages and neutrophils that release tissue-damaging inflammatory mediators. Acute exposure to diesel exhaust that contains fine particles is linked to lung, throat, and eye irritations; asthma attacks; and myocardial ischemia (Figure 11-19).[212] Importantly, according to the WHO, diesel exhaust is carcinogenic and causes lung cancer.[213] The central hypothesis, based on

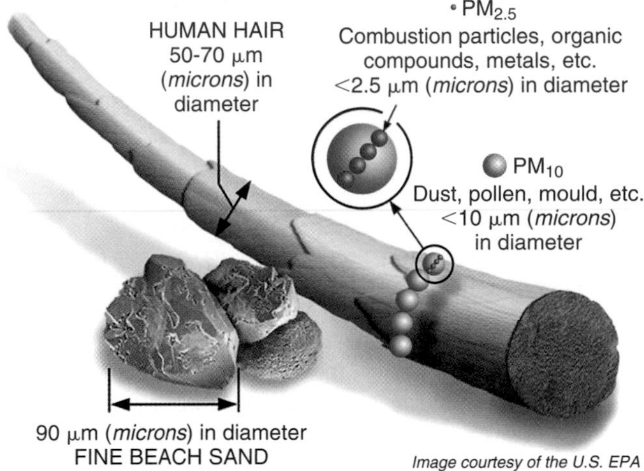

FIGURE 11-18 Particle Sizes and Pollution. *PM,* particulate matter. (From Environmental Protection Agency. [2013]. *Particulate matter updated March 18, 2013.* Washington, DC: Author.)

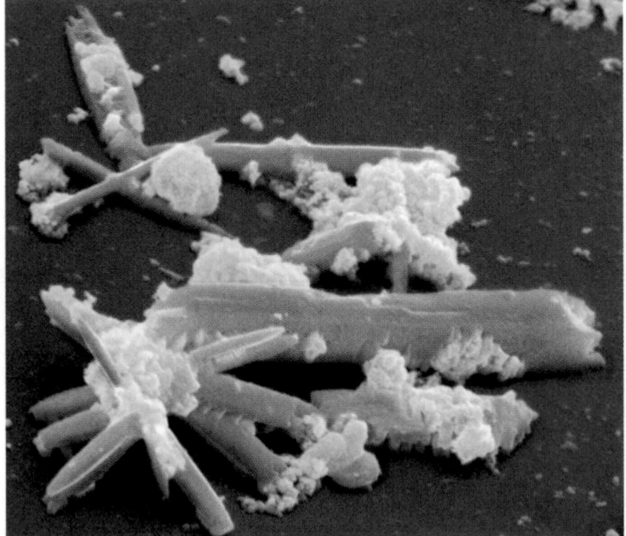

FIGURE 11-19 Exhaust Particulate Matter. Diesel exhaust is carcinogenic and causes lung cancer. (Thomas Deerinck, NCMIR/Science Source.)

rat studies, for the mechanisms related to particle-induced lung carcinogenesis is that insoluble particles cause pulmonary inflammation (e.g., cytokine release, ROS), which leads to oxidative stress and oxidation of DNA, proliferative response, and tissue remodelling that progresses toward fibrosis and tumour development.

The Global Burden of Disease collaboration estimated that approximately 3.22 million deaths were caused by exposure to air pollution in 2010, an increase from 2.91 million deaths attributed to air pollution in 1990.[214] From data in 2010, cancers of the trachea, bronchus, or lung represent about 7% of total mortality attributable to $PM_{2.5}$.[214] So far, data have not been conclusive about the relationship between air pollution and lung cancer risk for former heavy smokers and light smokers.[207]

Living close to certain industries is a recognized cancer risk factor.[215] Overall, fine particle pollution also is linked to other health problems and includes (1) premature death in people with heart or lung disease; (2) nonfatal heart attacks; (3) irregular heartbeat; (4) aggravated asthma; (5) decreased lung function; and (6) respiratory symptoms, including irritation of the airways, coughing, and shortness of breath.[211] In addition, other effects of particle pollution include reduced visibility (haze); environmental damage in lakes and streams, coastal waters, and river basins; depletion of nutrients in soil; and damage to forests and food crops.[211]

Indoor air pollution is generally considered worse than outdoor air pollution, partly because of cigarette smoke. ETS (secondhand smoke) can cause the formation of reactive oxygen free radicals and thus DNA damage. The IARC has classified ETS as a human carcinogen. Another significant indoor air pollutant is radon gas. **Radon** is a natural radioactive gas derived from the radioactive decay of uranium that is ubiquitous in rock and soil; it can become trapped in houses and form radioactive decay products known to be carcinogenic to humans. The most hazardous houses can be identified by testing and then be modified to prevent further radon contamination. Exposure levels are greater from underground mines than from houses. Most of the lung cancers associated with radon are bronchogenic; however, small cell carcinoma does occur with greater frequency in underground miners. Radon increases the risk for lung cancer in underground miners in spite of their smoking status.

In China, some regions report very high levels of lung cancer in women who spend much of their time indoors. Exposures from heating and cooking combustion sources (e.g., oil vapours) and asbestos are identified as risk factors for lung cancer.[216] In addition, domestic coal use and ETS increase the risk for lung cancer in women and men.[217,218]

Chemical and Occupational Hazards as Carcinogens

An estimated 100 000 synthetic chemicals are used in North America.[219] Of those, only about 7% have been tested for their health effects[220]; another 1 000 chemicals are added each year.[219] Exposure to chemicals occurs every day—chemicals are present in air, soil, food, water, household products, toys, personal care products, workplaces, and homes. The number of known carcinogens in experimental animals is large. It is suspected that most of these chemical carcinogens are potentially carcinogenic in humans, but documentation is lacking. Table 11-1 (pp. 270–273) provides a summary of the chemicals according to sufficient or limited evidence in humans by cancer site. Known and probable carcinogenic agents are updated by the IARC.

Chemical carcinogenesis involves the classic genotoxic mechanisms, and exposure to genotoxic carcinogens also might involve a variety of nongenotoxic effects in cells.[221] A number of studies reported that the carcinogenic effects induced by several chemicals, including 2-acetylaminofluorene, tamoxifen, trichloroethylene, aflatoxin B_1, ochratoxin, nickel, and chromium, do not follow a classic genotoxic carcinogenesis model, but rather involve a spectrum of cellular alterations encompassing epigenetic alterations.[222] These epigenetically reprogrammed cells show an epigenetic profile similar to that frequently observed in cancer cells, including altered histone patterns, hypomethylation of DNA repetitive elements, alterations in proto-oncogenes, and hypermethylation of tumour-suppressor genes. Altered epigenetic status confers genome instability and loss of controlled growth signals, typically observed in cancer cells.[223] According to the director of the US National Institute of Environmental Health Sciences, "exposure to gene-altering substances, particularly in the womb and shortly after birth can lead to increased susceptibility to disease. There is a huge potential impact from these exposures, partly because the changes may be inherited across generations."[224]

A substantial percentage of cancers of the upper respiratory passages, lung, bladder, and peritoneum are attributed to occupational factors; however, fewer studies of nonsmokers exist.[225] One notable occupational factor is asbestos-silicate mineral woven into fabrics, used in fire-resistant, insulating materials, and many other industrial sources. Chrysotile asbestos, more than any other type, accounts for a majority of asbestos in buildings in North America. Asbestos increases the risk for mesothelioma and lung cancer and possibly other cancers. Benign conditions of asbestos exposures include pleural plaques, diffuse pleural thickening, and pulmonary fibrosis. The asbestos-related disorders (ARDs) are currently of significant occupational and public health concern.[226] Asbestos was used in homes and buildings built before the 1970s to insulate ceiling tiles, flooring, and pipe covers. In Western Europe, the epidemic of mesothelioma in building workers and other workers born after 1940 did not become apparent until the 1990s because of long latency. Asbestos usage has been banned in most developed countries, but it is still used in many developing countries and the incidence of cases of ARDs is rising.[226] No exposure to asbestos is without risk.

Inorganic arsenic, found principally in underground water (at levels ranging from 1 000 to 4 000 mcg/L), is found in many regions of the world. According to the IARC, strong evidence indicates an increased risk for bladder, skin, and lung cancers following consumption of water with high levels of arsenic (generally greater than 200 mcg/L).[227] Evidence for cancers of the liver, colon, and kidney is weaker. Other sources of inorganic arsenic are related to occupational exposures (see Table 11-1).

Carcinoma of the bladder has been linked with the manufacture of dyes, rubber, paint, and aromatic amines, especially β-naphthylamine and benzidine. Benzol inhalation is linked to leukemia in shoemakers and in workers in the rubber cement, explosives, and dyeing industries. Other notable occupational hazards include heavy metals (e.g., high-nickel alloy, chromium VI compounds, inorganic arsenic), silica, polycyclic aromatic hydrocarbons, sulphuric acid, and chloromethyl ether. Data from the Nurse's Health Study in the United States showed an increased risk of lung cancer associated with PM air pollution exposure.[228] Data from the European Study of Cohorts for Air Pollution Effects indicated that PM contributes to lung cancer incidence in Europe.[229] Studies of occupational exposure to diesel exhaust found an increased risk for lung cancer.[230] Other important exposures are included in Table 11-1 (pp. 270–273). Disentangling data related to lung cancer, air pollution, and occupational risks is complex, especially in combination with active and passive smoking and the interplay of environmental factors and genetic polymorphisms at multiple loci.

QUICK CHECK 11-4

1. Identify the high-risk types of HPV that are carcinogenic.
2. What components of air pollution are considered most important for carcinogenesis?
3. Why do certain chemicals present a notable challenge to the environment and cancer?

DID YOU UNDERSTAND?

Overview

1. Cancer arises from a complicated and interacting web of multiple etiologies. Avoiding high-risk behaviours and exposure to individual carcinogens will prevent development of many types of cancers.
2. Lifestyle behaviours, dietary and environmental factors, and occupational exposure contribute to the number of cancer cases and deaths.

Genetics, Epigenetics, and Tissue

1. Cancers are caused by environmental and lifestyle factors, and genetic and epigenetic factors. Driven by genetic alterations and epigenetic abnormalities, biological processes also include variations in detoxifying enzymes or DNA repair genes. Interacting factors are weaker immune systems, differences in hormone levels, and metabolic factors. These factors are influenced by the surrounding microenvironment, or stroma.
2. Altogether, the biological environment is modified by metabolic and hormonal factors, inflammation, and disordered glucose and lipid metabolism. Once malignant phenotypes have developed, complex interactions occur between the tumour, the surrounding stroma, and the cells of the immune and inflammatory systems.

Incidence and Mortality Trends

1. Cancer is predicted to become a major cause of morbidity and mortality in the coming decades in all regions of the world.
2. The global cancer burden is shifting from the more developed countries to economically disadvantaged countries.
3. Overall, cancer death rates have been declining since the early 1990s for both men and women.

In Utero and Early Life Conditions

1. Emerging data suggest that early life events influence later susceptibility to chronic diseases.
2. Developmental plasticity is the degree to which an organism's development is contingent on its environment. Plasticity refers to the ability of genes to organize physiologically or structurally in response to environmental conditions during fetal development.
3. Studies of early versus late undernutrition in pregnancy indicate that the first trimester of pregnancy is particularly vulnerable to disease outcome in adulthood.
4. Research on DNA methylation marks, in utero environments, and future phenotypes is growing.

Environmental and Lifestyle Factors

Tobacco Use

1. Cigarette smoking is carcinogenic and the most important cause of cancer. Tobacco smoking causes cancer in more than 15 organ sites, and exposure to secondhand smoke and parental smoking causes cancer in daughters and sons and in other nonsmokers. The risk is

greatest in those who begin to smoke when young and continue smoking throughout life. However, smoking is pandemic, affecting all ages.

2. Smoking tobacco is linked to cancers of the lung, upper aerodigestive tract, lower urinary tract, kidney, pancreas, cervix, uterus, and myeloid leukemia. Recently added to the list are liver cancer and colorectal cancer.
3. Secondhand smoke is a cause of stroke, and 800 people in Canada die of lung cancer and heart disease related to secondhand smoke every year. Secondhand smoke increases the risk of death in people with cancer and cancer survivors as well as those with age-related macular degeneration, tuberculosis, ectopic pregnancy, and diabetes mellitus. Smoking increases inflammation, impairs immunity, and is a cause of rheumatoid arthritis. Smoking causes even more deaths from vascular and respiratory diseases.
4. Cigar or pipe smoking is causally related to cancers of the oral cavity, oropharynx, hypopharynx, larynx, esophagus, and lung. Pipe smokers have an increased risk of dying from cancers of lung, lip, throat, esophagus, larynx, pancreas, colon, and rectum.
5. Bidi smoking can cause cancers of the respiratory and digestive sites.

Diet

1. Understanding diet as a factor for increasing the risk for cancer is difficult yet essential. The complexity is due to the variety of foods consumed, the many constituents of foods, the metabolic consequences of eating, and the temporal changes in the patterns of food use.
2. Carcinogenic substances from diet can develop from the cooking of fat, meat, or protein (e.g., heterocyclic aromatic amines), and from naturally occurring compounds associated with plant foods.
3. Nutrigenomics is the study of the effects of nutrition on the phenotypic variability of individuals based on genomic differences. Investigators are focused on genes, single nucleotide polymorphisms, amplifications, and deletions within the DNA sequences as modifiers of the response to foods and drinks.

Nutrition, Obesity, Alcohol Consumption, and Physical Activity: Impacts on Cancer

1. Results from decades of research on specific nutrients and foods and cancers have been controversial. Less controversial are the implementation of dietary patterns, for example, the Mediterranean dietary pattern, and the promoting of specific dietary recommendations, for example, approaches to lower blood pressure.
2. The importance of diet has been illustrated by data showing changes in cancer risk among individuals in low-risk countries compared with those in high-risk countries. With migration, these changes (low risk becomes high risk) are rapid, and a plausible determinant of such changes is the adoption of the "Western" diet.
3. Most relevant to carcinogenesis, because many cellular functions are affected by nutrition (i.e., cell cycle, cell differentiation, proliferation, microRNA expression, self-renewal, DNA repair, hormonal axes), is focusing on dietary patterns and meaningful biomarkers specific to nutritional factors.
4. Nutrition may directly influence epigenetic factors that silence genes that should be active or activate genes that should be silent.
5. Dietary components can act directly as mutagens or interfere with their elimination.
6. Obesity has been increasing in developed countries and in urban areas of developing countries. Obesity in Canada is an epidemic. Studies have significantly improved the understanding of the relationship between overweight or obesity, energy balance and cancer risk, cancer recurrence, and survival.
7. Obesity is a risk factor for cancers of the endometrium, colorectum, kidney, esophagus, breast (postmenopausal), and pancreas. Evidence is evolving for other cancers.
8. The mechanisms of obesity-associated cancer risks are unclear and vary by type of tumour and distribution of body fat. Emerging are three main factors related to obesity and cancer: (a) insulin–insulinlike growth factor (IGF) 1 axis, (b) sex hormones, and (c) adipokines or adipocyte-derived cytokines.
9. Metabolic changes in adipose tissue from obesity result in several alterations and include insulin resistance, hyperglycemia, dyslipidemia, hypoxia, and chronic inflammation. Tumour growth is regulated by interactions between tumour cells and stromal compartments that are rich in adipose tissue; adipocytes function as endocrine cells and shape the tumour microenvironment.
10. Alcohol plays a contributory role in several common cancers. Strong data link alcohol with cancers of the mouth, pharynx, larynx, esophagus, liver, colorectum, and breast. The evidence does not show any "safe limit" of alcohol intake, and the health effect is from ethanol, regardless of the type of drink.
11. Alcohol-related carcinogenesis involves acetaldehyde; reactive oxygen species; increased procarcinogen activation; modulation of cellular regeneration; nutritional deficiencies that may predispose to altered mucosal integrity, and enzyme and metabolic dysfunction; and other structural abnormalities. Under investigation are epigenetic alterations and the effects of alcohol metabolism.
12. Physical activity reduces the risk for breast and colon cancers and may reduce the risk for other cancers.
13. Biological mechanisms for the protective effects of physical activity include decreasing insulin and IGF levels, decreasing obesity, increasing free radical scavenger systems, altering inflammatory mediators, decreasing levels of circulating sex hormones and metabolic hormones, improving immune function, enhancing cytochrome P-450 activity (thus modifying carcinogen activation), and increasing gut motility.
14. Physical activity helps prevent type 2 diabetes, which has been associated with risk for cancer of the colon and pancreas.
15. Many unanswered questions remain regarding frequency, intensity, and duration of exercise and its protective effects.
16. The Canadian Physical Activity Guidelines and Canadian Sedentary Behaviour Guidelines suggest that being active for at least 150 minutes per week can help reduce the risk for many conditions, including certain types of cancer.
17. Exercise in children with cancer was associated with improved body composition, flexibility, and cardiorespiratory fitness.

Ionizing Radiation

1. Much of the knowledge of the effects of ionizing radiation (IR) on human cancer has come from Hiroshima and Nagasaki atomic bomb exposures, particularly data from the Life Span Study. Other evidence is from exposure to radiation for medical reasons, underground miners, and other occupational exposures. Human exposure includes emissions from the environment, X-rays, computed tomography (CT) scans, radioisotopes, and other radioactive sources.
2. From the atomic bomb exposures in Japan, increased frequencies of cancers occurred in thyroid and breast tissue, and lung, stomach, colon, esophageal, and urinary tract cancers increased, as did multiple myeloma.
3. Excess relative risks (ERRs) for radiation-induced cancers at a given age are much higher for individuals exposed during childhood. What is in question now is the ERRs of radiation exposure in adulthood.
4. New models of carcinogenesis identify IR not only as an initiator of premalignant cell clones but also as a promoter of pre-existing premalignant damage.

5. Other health risks from radiation include cardiovascular effects and somatic mutations that may contribute to other diseases. These effects may manifest years after completion of radiation therapy.
6. An important summary point from BEIR VII is the concern about the increased IR exposure from medical procedures, particularly CT scans and nuclear medicine procedures.
7. The risks from low-dose radiation are being debated among radiobiologists, geneticists, physicists, and others because of the potential effect on the health of current and future generations.
8. IR is a mutagen and carcinogen; it can penetrate cells and tissues and deposit energy in tissues at random in the form of ionizations.
9. IR affects many cellular processes, including gene expression, mitochondrial function, nucleotide base damage, and single-strand breaks and double-strand breaks to DNA. These changes can lead to carcinogenesis.
10. It is now known that radiation may induce a type of genomic instability to the progeny of the directly irradiated cells over many generations of cell divisions and can affect so-called bystander cells. Investigators are studying genomic instability as it may contribute to secondary cancers.
11. Epigenetic events after radiation include alterations in pathways affecting cell adhesion, extracellular matrix interactions, and cell-to-cell communication.

Ultraviolet Radiation

1. Ultraviolet (UV) radiation comes from sunlight. Other sources of UV radiation include electric lights, black lights, and tanning lamps. Most of the UV radiation received on earth is UVA and some UVB. UVA radiation is weaker than UVB, but UVA penetrates deeper into the skin and is more constant throughout the year despite the weather.
2. The incidence of basal cell carcinoma (BCC) and squamous cell carcinoma (SCC) is strongly correlated with lifetime sunlight exposure. Intense intermittent recreational sun exposure has been associated with melanoma and BCC. Tanning bed use has been associated with an increased risk for BCC and data suggest sunbed use as a reason for increased melanoma, especially in women. Chronic occupational sun exposure has been associated with SCC.
3. Cumulative sun exposure is the additive effects of intermittent sun exposure, chronic sun exposure, or both.
4. UV radiation is known to cause specific gene mutations: for example, SCC involves mutation in the *TP53* gene, BCC in the patched 1 tumour-suppressor gene (*PTCH1*), and melanoma in the *p16* gene. Investigators are identifying epigenetic alterations in tumour tissues and cell lines for skin cancers.
5. Skin exposure to UV radiation produces ROS in large quantities that can overwhelm tissue antioxidants and other oxygen-degrading pathways. Imbalances in ROS can lead to oxidative stress, tissue injury, and direct DNA damage.
6. UV radiation can activate the transcription factor NF-κB and other free radicals important in regulating genes that induce inflammation. Inflammation is a critical component of tumour progression.
7. Melanoma is the most lethal skin cancer and the incidence of melanoma has been increasing worldwide. The pathogenesis of melanoma is complex, including genetic and environmental factors.

Electromagnetic Radiation

1. Radiofrequency electromagnetic radiation (RF-EMR) is a type of nonionizing and low-frequency radiation. Health risks associated with RF-EMR are controversial. Exposure to electric and magnetic fields is widespread.
2. RF-EMR sources include microwaves, radar, mobile phones, cordless phones, cellphone towers (base stations), power frequency radiation associated with electricity and radio waves, fluorescent lights, computers, and other electric equipment.
3. Data regarding the effects of RF-EMR have been slow to emerge because of lack of methods to accurately measure exposure, lack of clear dose–response relationships, reproducing effects, financial interests, and other priorities, such as convenience.
4. Overall, there is limited evidence that magnetic fields cause childhood leukemia and insufficient evidence for other cancers in children.
5. The WHO International Agency for Research on Cancer (IARC) Monograph Working Group classified RF-EMF as "possibly carcinogenic to humans" (a Group 2B carcinogen, per IARC classification).

Infection, and Sexual and Reproductive Behaviour

1. Infection is an important contributor to cancer worldwide. The top four notable infections associated with new cancer cases are human papillomavirus (HPV), *Helicobacter pylori*, hepatitis B virus (HBV), and hepatitis C virus (HCV).
2. Although about a dozen HPVs have been identified, HPV types 16 and 18 are responsible for the majority of cancers. Persistence of infection with high-risk HPV is a prerequisite for the development of cervical intraepithelial neoplasia (CIN) lesions and invasive cancer.
3. HPV infection has been identified as a definite carcinogen for six types of cancer: cervix, penis, vulva, anus, and some oropharynx (including the base of the tongue and tonsils).
4. The incidence of HPV-associated oropharyngeal cancer has increased during the past 20 years, especially among men.
5. Biological factors that may interact with HPV infection to increase cancer risk include long-term oral contraceptive use, smoking, decreased immunity, having many children, poor oral hygiene (increased risk for oropharyngeal cancer), and chronic inflammation.
6. HPV may be transmitted by genital contact (oral, touching, or sexual intercourse). The possible modes of transmission in children are controversial; newborn babies can be exposed to cervical HPV infection from the mother.

Air Pollution

1. Indoor and outdoor air pollution are both associated with increased rates of lung cancer. The IARC concluded that exposure to outdoor air pollution and to particulate matter (PM) in outdoor air is carcinogenic to humans.
2. $PM_{2.5}$ includes a higher proportion of mutagenic agents. Primary particles are emitted directly from a source, for example, construction sites, unpaved roads, or smokestacks. Secondary particles are emitted from power plants, industries, and automobiles. Diesel exhaust is carcinogenic and causes lung cancer.
3. Acute exposure to diesel exhaust that contains fine particles is linked to lung, throat, and eye irritations; asthma attacks; and myocardial ischemia.
4. The hypothesis for the mechanisms related to particle-induced lung carcinogenesis is that insoluble particles cause pulmonary inflammation, which leads to oxidative stress and oxidation of DNA, proliferative response, tissue remodelling that progresses toward fibrosis, and tumour development.
5. Fine particle pollution also is linked to premature death in people with heart or lung disease, nonfatal heart attacks, irregular heartbeat, and decreased lung function.
6. Indoor air pollution is generally considered worse than outdoor air pollution. Sources of indoor air pollution include secondhand smoke, heating and cooking combustion sources, radon, and coal use.

Chemicals and Occupational Hazards as Carcinogens

1. An estimated 100 000 synthetic chemicals are used in North America; only about 7% have been tested for their health effects.
2. Exposure to chemicals occurs from air, soil, food, water, household products, toys, personal care products, medications, workplaces, and homes.
3. The IARC has classified carcinogenic agents as known and probable.
4. Chemical carcinogenesis involves genotoxic and epigenetic alterations. Other mechanisms include hormonal disruption, interference with cell signalling mechanisms, and other unknown effects.
5. Exposure to gene-altering substances, particularly in the womb and shortly after birth, can lead to increased susceptibility to disease.
6. A substantial percentage of cancers of the upper respiratory passages, lung, bladder, and peritoneum are attributed to occupational factors.
7. Asbestos is linked to an epidemic of mesothelioma in Western Europe. Asbestos usage has been banned in most developed countries, but it is still used in many developing countries.

KEY TERMS

Abscopal, 288
Asbestos-silicate mineral, 295
Basal cell carcinoma (BCC), 290
Bystander effect, 288
Developmental plasticity, 274
Environmental tobacco smoke (ETS), 276
Genomic instability, 288
Individual carcinogen, 268
Melanoma, 290
Methylome, 276
Nontargeted effect, 288
Nutrigenomics, 277
Particulate matter (PM), 293
Phase I activation enzymes, 281
Phase II detoxification enzymes, 281
Radiofrequency electromagnetic radiation (RF-EMR), 291
Radon, 294
Squamous cell carcinoma (SCC), 290
UV radiation, 289
Xenobiotic, 281

REFERENCES

1. Clapp, R. W., Howe, G. K., & Jacobs, M. M. (2007). Environmental and occupational causes of cancer: A call to act on what we know. *Biomedicine & Pharmacotherapy, 61*(10), 631–639. doi:10.1016/j.biopha.2007.08.001.
2. Clapp, R. W., Jacobs, M. M., & Loechler, E. L. (2008). Environmental and occupational causes of cancer; New evidence 2005–2007. *Reviews on Environmental Health, 23*(1), 1–37.
3. World Health Organization. (2014). *World cancer report 2014*. Geneva: WHO Agency for Research on Cancer.
4. Cogliano, V. J., Baan, R., Straif, K., et al. (2011). Preventable exposures associated with human cancers. *Journal of the National Cancer Institute, 103*(24), 1827–1839. doi:10.1093/jnci/djr483.
5. Institute of Medicine. (2001). *Rebuilding the unity of health and the environment: A new vision of environmental health for the 21st century [workshop summary]*. Washington, DC: National Academy Press.
6. National Toxicology Program. (2011). *Report on carcinogens* (12th ed.). Washington, DC: U.S. Department of Health and Human Services.
7. International Agency for Research on Cancer. (2012). *Special report: Policy—A review of human carcinogens—Part C: Metals, arsenic, dusts, and fibres*. Retrieved from http://monographs.iarc.fr/ENG/Monographs/vol100C/index.php.
8. Straif, K., Benbrahim-Tallaa, L., Baan, R., et al. (2009). A review of human carcinogens—Part C: Metals, arsenic, dusts, and fibres. *Lancet Oncology, 10*(5), 453–454.
9. Bray, F., Jemal, M., Grey, N., et al. (2012). Global cancer transitions according to the Human Development Index (2008–2030): A population-based study. *Lancet Oncology, 13*(8), 790–801. doi:10.1016/S1470-2045(12)70211-5.
10. Ferlay, J., Soerjomataram, I., Dikshit, R., et al. (2015). Cancer incidence and mortality worldwide: Sources, methods, and major patterns in GLOBOCAN 2012. *International Journal of Cancer, 136*(5), E359–E386. doi:10.1002/ijc.29210.
11. National Cancer Institute. (2014). *Epidemiology and genomics research global health and cancer epidemiology*. Bethesda, MD: Author.
12. Canadian Cancer Society. (2016). *Canadian cancer statistics*. Retrieved from http://www.cancer.ca/en/cancer-information/cancer-101/cancer-statistics-at-a-glance/?region=on.
13. Gluckman, P. D., Hanson, M. A., & Mitchell, M. D. (2010). Developmental origins of health and disease: Reducing the burden of chronic disease in the next generation. *Genome Medicine, 2*(2), 14. doi:10.1186/gm135.
14. Bateson, P., Barker, D., Clutton-Brock, T., et al. (2004). Developmental plasticity and human health. *Nature, 430*(6998), 419–421. doi:10.1038/nature02725.
15. Waterland, R. A., & Jirtle, R. J. (2004). Early nutrition, epigenetic changes at transposons and imprinted genes, and enhanced susceptibility to adult chronic disease. *Nutrition, 20*, 63–68.
16. Koukoura, O., Sifakis, S., & Spandidos, D. A. (2012). DNA methylation in the human placenta and fetal growth. *Molecular Medicine Reports, 5*, 883–889. doi:10.3892/mmr.2012.763.
17. Painter, R. C., de Rooij, S. R., Bossuyt, P. M., et al. (2006). Early onset of coronary artery disease after prenatal exposure to the Dutch famine. *American Journal of Clinical Nutrition, 84*, 322–327.
18. Jang, H., & Serra, C. (2014). Nutrition, epigenetics, and diseases. *Clinical Nutrition Research, 3*(1), 1–8. doi:10.7762/cnr.2014.3.1.1.
19. Waterland, R. A. (2009). Early environmental effects on epigenetic regulation in humans. *Epigenetics, 4*(8), 523–525.
20. Rubin, M. M. (2007). Antenatal exposure to DES: Lessons learned … future concerns. *Obstetrical and Gynecological Survey, 62*(8), 548–555. doi:10.1097/01.ogx.0000271138.31234.d7.
21. Park, S. K., Kang, D., McGlynn, K. A., et al. (2008). Intrauterine environments and breast cancer risk: Meta-analysis and systematic review. *Breast Cancer Research, 10*(1), R8. doi:10.1186/bcr1850.
22. National Cancer Institute. (2011). *Diethylstibestrol (DES) and cancer*. Washington, DC: National Institutes of Health.
23. Palmer, J. R., Wise, L. A., Hatch, E. E., et al. (2006). Prenatal diethylstilbestrol exposure and risk of breast cancer. *Cancer Epidemiology, Biomarkers and Prevention, 15*(8), 1509–1514. doi:10.1158/1055-9965.EPI-06-0109.
24. Newbold, R. R. (2008). Prenatal exposure to diethylstilbestrol (DES). *Fertility and Sterility, 89*(2 Suppl.), e55–e56. doi:10.1016/j.fertnstert.2008.01.062.
25. Martin, O., Shialis, T., Lester, J., et al. (2008). Testicular dysgenesis syndrome and the estrogen hypothesis: A quantitative meta-analysis. *Ciên Saúde Colet, 13*(5), 1601–1618. Retrieved from http://www.scielo.br/scielo.php?script=sci_arttext&pid=S1413-81232008000500024&lng=en&nrm=iso.
26. Znaor, A., Lortet-Tieulent, J., Jemal, A., et al. (2014). International variations and trends in testicular cancer incidence and mortality. *European Urology, 65*(6), 1095–1106. doi:10.1016/j.eururo.2013.11.004.
27. Gluckman, P. D., Hanson, M. A., Cooper, C., et al. (2008). Effect of in utero and early-life conditions on adult health and disease. *New England Journal of Medicine, 359*(1), 61–73. doi:10.1056/NEJMra0708473.
28. Gluckman, P. D., Hanson, M. A., Buklijas, T., et al. (2009). Epigenetic mechanisms that underpin metabolic and cardiovascular diseases. *Nature Reviews. Endocrinology, 5*(7), 401–408. doi:10.1038/nrendo.2009.102.
29. Teh, A. L., Pan, H., Chen, L., et al. (2014). The effect of genotype and in utero environment on inter-individual variation in neonate DNA methylomes. *Genome Research, 24*(7), 1064–1074. doi:10.1101/gr.171439.113.
30. Luteijn, M. J., & Ketting, R. F. (2013). PIWI-interacting RNAs: From generation to transgenerational epigenetics. *Nature Reviews. Genetics, 14*(8), 523–534. doi:10.1038/nrg3495.
31. Newbold, R. R., Padilla-Banks, E., & Jefferson, W. N. (2006). Adverse effects of the model environmental estrogen diethylstilbestrol are transmitted to subsequent generations. *Endocrinology, 147*(6 Suppl.), S11–S17. doi:10.1210/en.2005-1164.
32. International Agency for Research on Cancer. (2011). *IARC handbooks of cancer prevention. Tobacco control: Effectiveness of tax and price policies for tobacco*. Geneva: Author.
33. Secretan, B., Straif, K., Baan, R., et al. (2009). A review of human carcinogens—Part E: Tobacco, areca nut, alcohol, coal smoke, and salted fish. *Lancet Oncology, 10*(11), 1033–1034.
34. Office of the Surgeon General. (2014). *The health consequences of smoking—50 years of progress. A report of the Surgeon General executive summary*. Rockville, MD: U.S. Department of Health and Human Services.
35. Centers for Disease Control and Prevention. (2008). Global youth tobacco surveillance, 2000–2007. *MMWR. Morbidity and Mortality Weekly Report, 57*(5501), 1–21.
36. Zheng, W., McLerran, D. F., Rolland, B. A., et al. (2014). Burden of total and cause-specific mortality related to tobacco smoking among adults aged ≥45 years in Asia: A pooled analysis of 21 cohorts. *PLoS*

Medicine, 11(4), e1001631. doi:10.1371/journal.pmed.1001631.
37. World Health Organization. (2011). *WHO report on the global tobacco epidemic, 2011. Warning about the dangers of tobacco, executive summary*. Geneva: Author.
38. Centers for Disease Control and Prevention. (2002). Annual smoking-attributable mortality, years of potential life lost, and productivity losses—United States, 1995–1999. *MMWR. Morbidity and Mortality Weekly Report, 51*(14), 300–303.
39. World Health Organization. (2008). *World cancer report: Global cancer rates could increase by 50% to 15 million by 2020*. Retrieved from http://www.WHO.int/mediacentre/news/release/2003/pr27/en/.
40. Propel Centre for Population Health Impact. (2015). *Tobacco use in Canada: Patterns and trends: 2015 edition*. Waterloo, ON: University of Waterloo. Retrieved from https://uwaterloo.ca/tobacco-use-canada/sites/ca.tobacco-use-canada/files/uploads/files/tobaccouseincanada_2015_accessible_final-s.pdf.
41. Lushniak, B. D. (2014). A historic moment: The 50th anniversary of the first Surgeon General's Report on smoking and health. *Public Health Reports, 129*(1), 5–6.
42. Government of Canada. (2015). *Dangers of secondhand smoke*. Retrieved from http://healthycanadians.gc.ca/healthy-living-vie-saine/tobacco-tabac/avoid-second-hand-smoke-eviter-fumee-secondaire/second-hand-smoke-fumee-secondaire/dangers-eng.php.
43. Centers for Disease Control and Prevention. (2010). *Smoking and secondhand smoke*. Retrieved from http://www.cdc.gov/cancer/lung.
44. Centers for Disease Control and Prevention. (2010). *Cigar smoking and cancer*. Retrieved from http://www.cancer.gov/cancertopics/factsheet/Tobacco/cigars.
45. American Cancer Society. (2014). *What are the health risks of smoking pipes or cigars?* Atlanta, GA: Author.
46. Centers for Disease Control and Prevention. (2012). Consumption of cigarettes and combustible tobacco—United States, 2000–2011. *MMWR. Morbidity and Mortality Weekly Report, 61*(30).
47. Taioli, E. (2008). Gene-environment interaction in tobacco-related cancers. *Carcinogenesis, 29*(8), 1467–1474. doi:10.1093/carcin/bgn062.
48. Giri, P. A., Singh, K. K., & Phalke, D. B. (2014). Study of socio-demographic determinants of esophageal cancer at a tertiary care teaching hospital of Western Maharashtra, India. *South Asian Journal of Cancer, 3*(1), 54–56. doi:10.4103/2278-330X.126526.
49. Farvid, M. S., Cho, E., Eliassen, A. H., et al. (2014). Dietary protein sources in early adulthood and breast cancer incidence: Prospective cohort study. *British Medical Journal, 348*, g3437. doi:10.1136/bmj.g3437.
50. World Cancer Research Fund/American Institute for Cancer Research. (2007). *Food, nutrition, physical activity, and the prevention of cancer: A global perspective*. Washington, DC: American Institute for Cancer Research.
51. Kiefte-de Jong, J. C., Mathers, J. C., & Franco, O. H. (2014). Nutrition and healthy aging: The key ingredients. *Proceedings of the Nutrition Society, 73*(2), 249–259. doi:10.1017/S0029665113003881.
52. Cancer Research UK. (2013). *Bowel cancer incidence statistics*. London: Registered Charity in England, Wales, Scotland, and the Isle of Man.
53. Hjartaker, A., Aagnes, B., Robsahm, T. E., et al. (2014). Subsite-specific dietary risk factors for colorectal cancer: A review of cohort studies. *Journal of Oncology*, 703854. doi:10.1155/2013/703854.
54. Center, M. M., Jemal, A., & Ward, E. (2009). International trends in colorectal cancer incidence rates. *Cancer Epidemiology, Biomarkers and Prevention, 18*(6), 1688–1694. doi:10.1158/1055-9965.EPI-09-0090.
55. Mathers, J. C., Strathdee, G., & Relton, C. L. (2010). Induction of epigenetic alterations by dietary and other environmental factors. *Advances in Genetics, 71*, 3–39. doi:10.1016/B978-0-12-380864-6.00001-8.
56. Nitter, M., Norgard, B., de Vogel, S., et al. (2014). Plasma methionine, choline, betaine, and dimethylglycine, in relation to colorectal cancer risk in the European Prospective Investigation into Cancer and Nutrition (EPIC). *Annals of Oncology, 25*(8), 1609–1615. doi:10.1093/annonc/mdu185.
57. Choi, S.-W., Corrocher, R., & Friso, S. (2009). Nutrients and DNA methylation. In S.-W. Choi & S. Friso (Eds.), *Nutrients and epigenetics* (pp. 105–126). Boca Raton, FL: CRC Press Taylor & Francis Group.
58. Steegers-Theunissen, R. P., Obermann-Borst, S. A., Kremer, D., et al. (2009). Periconceptional maternal folic acid use of 400 mcg per day is related to increased methylation of the *IGF2* gene in the very young child. *PLoS ONE, 4*(11), e7845.
59. Dominguez-Salas, P., Moore, S. E., Baker, M. S., et al. (2014). Maternal nutrition at conception modulates DNA methylation of human metastable epialleles. *Nature Communications, 5*, 3746. doi:10.1038/ncomms4746.
60. Waterland, R. A., & Jirtle, R. L. (2003). Transposable elements: Targets for early nutritional effects on epigenetic gene regulation. *Molecular and Cellular Biology, 23*(15), 5293–5300.
61. Kovacheva, V. P., Mellott, T. J., Davison, J. M., et al. (2007). Gestational choline deficiency causes global and Igf2 gene DNA hypermethylation by up-regulation of Dnmt1 expression. *Journal of Biological Chemistry, 282*(43), 31777–31788. doi:10.1074/jbc.M705539200.
62. Kim, Y. I., Pgribny, I. P., Basnakian, A. G., et al. (1997). Folate deficiency in rats induces DNA strand breaks and hypomethylation within the p53 tumor suppressor gene. *American Journal of Clinical Nutrition, 65*(1), 46–52.
63. Persson, E. C., Schwartz, L. M., Park, Y., et al. (2013). Alcohol consumption, folate intake, hepatocellular carcinoma, and liver disease mortality. *Cancer Epidemiology, Biomarkers and Prevention, 22*(3), 415–421. doi:10.1158/1055-9965.EPI-12-1169.
64. Wu, M. Y., Kuo, C. S., Lin, C. Y., et al. (2009). Lymphocytic mitochondrial DNA deletions, biochemical folate status and hepatocellular carcinoma susceptibility in a case-control study. *British Journal of Nutrition, 102*(5), 715–721.
65. Lee, W. J., Shim, J. Y., & Zhu, B. T. (2005). Mechanisms for the inhibition of DNA methyltransferases by tea catechins and bioflavonoids. *Molecular Pharmacology, 68*(4), 1018–1030.
66. Delage, B., & Dashwood, R. H. (2008). Dietary manipulation of histone structure and function. *Annual Review of Nutrition, 28*, 347–366.
67. Miozzo, M., Vaira, V., & Sirchia, S. M. (2015). Epigenetic alterations in cancer and personalized cancer treatment. *Future Oncology (London, England), 11*(2), 333–348.
68. Kim, H. N., Kim, D.-H., Kim, E.-H., et al. (2014). Sulforaphane inhibits phorbol ester-stimulated IKK-NK-$_{\kappa}$B signaling and COX-2 expression in human mammary epithelial cells by targeting NF-κB activating kinase and ERK. *Cancer Letters, 351*(1), 41–49.
69. Phuah, N. H., & Nagoor, N. H. (2014). Regulation of microRNAs by natural agents: New strategies in cancer therapies. *BioMed Research International, 2014*, 804510.
70. Saud, S. M., Li, W., Morris, N. L., et al. (2014). Resveratrol prevents tumorigenesis in mouse model of Kras activated colorectal cancer by suppressing oncogenic Kras expression. *Carcinogenesis, 35*(12), 2778–2786.
71. Semba, R. D., Ferrucci, L., Bartali, B., et al. (2014). Resveratrol levels and all-cause mortality in older community-dwelling adults. *JAMA Internal Medicine, 174*(7), 1077–1084.
72. Dahmke, I. N., Backes, C., Rudsitis-Auth, J., et al. (2013). Curcumin intake affects miRNA signature in murine melanoma with mmu-miR-205-5p most significantly altered. *PLoS ONE, 8*(12), e81122.
73. Yang, C. H., Yue, J., Sims, M., et al. (2013). The curcumin analog EF24 targets NF-κB and miRNA-21, and has potent anticancer activity in vitro and in vivo. *PLoS ONE, 8*(8), e71130.
74. Kim, Y. S., Farrar, W., Colburn, N. H., et al. (2012). Cancer stem cells: Potential target for bioactive food components. *Journal of Nutritional Biochemistry, 23*, 691–698.
75. O'Brien, L. E., Solimna, S. S., Li, X., et al. (2011). Altered modes of stem cell division drive adaptive intestinal growth. *Cell, 147*, 603–614.
76. Ginestier, C., Wicinski, J., Cervera, N., et al. (2009). Retinoid signaling regulates breast cancer stem cell differentiation. *Cell Cycle (Georgetown, Tex.), 8*, 3297–3302.
77. Slyskova, J., Lorenzo, Y., Karlsen, A., et al. (2014). Both genetic and dietary factors underlie individual differences in DNA damage levels and DNA repair capacity. *DNA Repair, 16*, 66–73.
78. González, C., Nájera, O., Cortés, E., et al. (2002). Hydrogen peroxide-induced DNA damage and DNA repair in lymphocytes from malnourished children? *Environmental and Molecular Mutagenesis, 39*, 33–42.
79. Arab, L., Steck-Scott, S., & Fleishauer, A. T. (2002). Lycopene and the lung. *Experimental Biology and Medicine (Maywood, N.J.), 227*, 894–899.
80. Yang, G., Gao, Y.-T., Shu, X.-O., et al. (2010). Isothiocyanate exposure, glutathione S-transferase polymorphisms, and colon cancer risk. *American Journal of Nutrition, 91*(3), 704–711.
81. Corpet, D. E. (2014). Epidemiological evidence for the association between red and processed meat intake and colorectal cancer. *Science, 98*, 115.
82. Eichholzer, M., Rohrmann, S., Barbir, A., et al. (2012). Polymorphisms in heterocyclic aromatic amines metabolism-related genes are associated with colorectal adenoma risk. *International Journal of Molecular Epidemiology and Genetics, 3*(2), 96–106.
83. World Cancer Research Fund/American Institute for Cancer Research. (2011). *WCRF/AICR systematic literature review continuous update project report, 2011*. Retrieved from http://www.wcrf.org/sites/default/files/SLR_pancreatic_cancer_2011.pdf.
84. zur Hausen, H. (2012). Red meat consumption and cancer: Reasons to suspect involvement of bovine infectious factors in colorectal cancer. *International Journal of Cancer, 130*(11), 2475–2483.
85. Canadian Obesity Network. (2016). *Understanding obesity*. Retrieved from http://www.obesitynetwork.ca/understanding-obesity.
86. Glickman, D., Greenwood, M. R. C., Purcell, W., III, et al. (2012). *Accelerating progress in obesity prevention: Solving the weight of the nation*. Washington, DC: The National Academies Press.
87. Demark-Wahnefried, W., Platz, E. A., Ligibel, J. A., et al. (2012). The role of obesity in cancer survival and recurrence. *Cancer Epidemiology, Biomarkers and Prevention, 21*(8), 1244–1259.
88. Haslam, D. (2007). Obesity: A medical history. *Obesity Reviews, 8*(Suppl. 1), 31–36.
89. Cao, Y., & Ma, J. (2011). Body mass index, prostate cancer-specific mortality, and biochemical recurrence: A systematic review and meta-analysis. *Cancer Prevention Research, 4*, 486–501.
90. Ewertz, M., Jensen, M.-B., Gunnarsdóttir, K. A., et al. (2011). Effect of obesity on prognosis after early-stage breast cancer. *Journal of Clinical Oncology, 29*, 25–31.
91. Sinicrope, F. A., Foster, N. R., Sargent, D. J., et al. (2010). Obesity is an independent prognostic variable in colon cancer survivors. *Clinical Cancer Research, 16*, 1884–1893.
92. World Health Organization. (2016). *Obesity and overweight*. Retrieved from http://www.who.int/mediacentre/factsheets/fs311/en/.
93. Park, J., Morley, T. S., Kim, M., et al. (2014). Obesity and cancer—Mechanisms underlying tumor progression and recurrence. *Nature Reviews. Endocrinology, 10*(8), 455–465.
94. Park, J., Euhus, D. M., & Scherer, P. E. (2011). Paracrine and endocrine effects of adipose tissue on cancer development and progression. *Endocrine Reviews, 32*(4), 550–570.

95. Pérez-Hernández, A. I., Catalán, V., Gómez-Ambrosi, J., et al. (2014). Mechanisms linking excess adiposity and carcinogenesis promotion. *Frontiers in Endocrinology (Lausanne)*, *5*, 65.
96. American Cancer Society. (2012). *Cancer treatment and survivorship facts & figures 2012–2013*. Atlanta, GA: Author.
97. Mandrekar, P. (2011). Epigenetic regulation in alcoholic liver disease. *World Journal of Gastroenterology*, *17*(20), 2456–2464.
98. Zakhari, S. (2013). Alcohol metabolism and epigenetic changes. *Alcohol Research*, *35*(1), 6–16.
99. National Cancer Institute. (2009). *Physical activity and cancer*. Washington, DC: National Institutes of Health. Retrieved from http://www.cancer.gov/cancertopics/factsheet/prevention/physicalactivity.
100. Soria, G., Polo, S. E., & Almouzni, G. (2012). Prime, repair, restore: The active role of chromatin in the DNA response. *Molecular Cell*, *46*(6), 722–734.
101. Bertucci, A., Pocock, R. D. J., Randers-Pehrson, G., et al. (2009). Microbeam irradiation of the *C. elegans* nematode. *Journal of Radiation Research*, *50*, A49–A54.
102. Mancuso, M., Pasquali, E., Leonardi, S., et al. (2008). Oncogenic bystander radiation effects in patched heterozygous mouse cerebellum. *Proceedings of the National Academy of Sciences of the United States of America*, *105*(34), 12445–12450.
103. Nguyen, D. H., Oketch-Rabah, H. A., Illa-Bochaca, I., et al. (2011). Radiation acts on the microenvironment to affect breast carcinogenesis by distinct mechanisms that decrease cancer latency and affect tumor type. *Cancer Cell*, *19*, 640–651.
104. Ojima, M., Fururtani, A., Ban, N., et al. (2011). Persistence of DNA double-strand breaks in normal human cells induced by radiation-induced bystander effect. *Radiation Research*, *175*, 90–96.
105. Chute, J. P. (2012). To survive radiation injury, remember you're APCs. *Nature Medicine*, *18*(7), 1013–1014.
106. Barcellos-Hoff, M. H., & Nguyen, D. H. (2009). Radiation carcinogenesis in context: How do irradiated tissues become tumors? *Health Physics*, *97*(5), 446–457.
107. Canadian Society for Exercise Physiology. (2012). *Canadian physical activity, and sedentary behaviour guidelines*. Ottawa: Author. Retrieved from http://www.csep.ca/cmfiles/guidelines/csep_guidelines_handbook.pdf.
108. Cramp, F., & Byron-Daniel, J. (2012). Exercise for the management of cancer-related fatigue in adults. *Cochrane Database of Systematic Reviews*, (11), CD006145.
109. Braam, K. I., van der Torre, P., Takken, T., et al. (2013). Physical exercise training interventions for children and young adults during and after treatment for childhood cancer. *Cochrane Database of Systematic Reviews*, (4), CD008796.
110. Little, M. P. (2009). Heterogeneity of variation of relative risk by age at exposure in the Japanese atomic bomb survivors. *Radiation and Environmental Biophysics*, *48*(3), 253–262.
111. Shuryak, I., Hahnfeldt, P., Hlatky, L., et al. (2009). A new view of radiation-induced cancer: Integrating short- and long-processes. Part l: Approach. *Radiation and Environmental Biophysics*, *48*(3), 263–274.
112. Shuryak, I., Sachs, R. K., & Brenner, D. J. (2010). Cancer risks after radiation exposure in middle age. *Journal of the National Cancer Institute*, *102*(21), 1606–1609.
113. Preston, D. L., Ron, E., Tokuoka, S., et al. (2007). Solid cancer incidence in atomic bomb survivors: 1958–1998. *Radiation Research*, *168*(1), 1–64.
114. Committee on the Biological Effects of Ionizing Radiation. (2006). *Health risks from exposure to low levels of ionizing radiation, BEIR VII Phase 2*. Washington, DC: National Academies Press.
115. Walsh, L. (2009). Heterogeneity of variation of relative risk by age at exposure in Japanese atomic bomb survivors. *Radiation and Environmental Biophysics*, *48*(3), 345–347.
116. Preston, D. L., Shimizu, Y., Pierce, D. A., et al. (2003). Studies of mortality of atomic bomb survivors. Report 13: Solid cancer and noncancer disease mortality: 1950–1997. *Radiation Research*, *160*, 381–407.
117. Hoel, D. G. (2006). Ionizing radiation and cardiovascular disease. *Annals of the New York Academy of Sciences*, *1076*, 309–317.
118. Rombouts, C., Aerts, A., Beck, M., et al. (2013). Differential response to acute low dose radiation in primary and immortalized endothelial cells. *International Journal of Radiation Biology*, *89*(10), 841–850.
119. Yusuf, S. W., Sami, S., & Daher, I. N. (2011). Radiation-induced heart disease: A clinical update. *Cardiology Research and Practice*, *317659*, 2011.
120. Linet, M. S., Kim, K. P., & Rajaraman, P. (2009). Children's exposure to diagnostic medical radiation and cancer risk: Epidemiologic and dosimetric considerations. *Pediatric Radiology*, *39*(Suppl. 1), S4–S26.
121. Schulze-Rath, R., Hammer, G. P., & Blettner, M. (2008). Are pre- or postnatal diagnostic X-rays a risk factor for childhood cancer? A systematic review. *Radiation and Environmental Biophysics*, *47*, 301–312.
122. Wakeford, R. (2008). Childhood leukaemia following medical diagnostic exposure to ionizing radiation in utero or after birth. *Radiation Protection Dosimetry*, *132*, 166–174.
123. Harbron, R. W. (2012). Cancer risks from low dose exposure to ionising radiation—Is the linear no-threshold model still relevant? *Radiography*, *18*, 28–33.
124. Prasad, K. N., Cole, W. C., & Hasse, G. M. (2004). Health risks of low dose ionizing radiation in humans: A review. *Experimental Biology and Medicine*, *229*(5), 378–382.
125. National Council on Radiation Protection and Measurement. (2009). *1929–2009 medical radiation exposure of the U.S. population greatly increased since the early 1980s*. Retrieved from http://NCRPonline.org.
126. Brenner, D. J., & Hall, E. J. (2007). Computed tomography—An increasing source of radiation exposure. *New England Journal of Medicine*, *357*(22), 2277–2284.
127. Smith-Bendman, R., Miglioretti, D. L., Johnson, E., et al. (2012). Use of diagnostic imaging studies and associated radiation exposure for patients enrolled in large integrated health care system, 1996–2010. *JAMA: Journal of the American Medical Association*, *307*(22), 2400–2409.
128. Canadian Nuclear Safety Commission. (2015). *Radiation doses*. Retrieved from http://nuclearsafety.gc.ca/eng/resources/radiation/introduction-to-radiation/radiation-doses.cfm.
129. Little, J. B. (2006). Cellular radiation effects and the bystander response. *Mutation Research*, *597*, 113–118.
130. Little, J. B. (2000). Radiation carcinogenesis. *Carcinogenesis*, *21*(3), 397–404.
131. Jones, J. A., Casey, R. C., & Karouia, F. (2010). Ionizing radiation as a carcinogen. In C. A. McQueen (Ed.), *Comprehensive toxicology* (2nd ed., pp. 181–228). St. Louis: Elsevier.
132. Kovalchuk, O., & Baulch, J. E. (2008). Epigenetic changes and nontargeted radiation effects—Is there a link? *Environmental and Molecular Mutagenesis*, *49*(1), 16–25.
133. Cunniffe, S., O'Neill, P., Greenberg, M. M., et al. (2014). Reduced repair capacity of a DNA clustered damage site comprised of 8-oxo-7,8-dihydro-2′-deoxyguanosine and 2-deoxyribonolactone results in an increased mutagenic potential of these lesions. *Mutation Research—Fundamental and Molecular Mechanisms of Mutagenesis*, *762*, 32–39.
134. Vaidya, A., Mao, Z., Tian, X., et al. (2014). Knock-in reporter mice demonstrate that DNA repair by non-homologous end joining declines with age. *PLoS Genetics*, *10*(7), e1004511.
135. Nag, S., Qin, J., Srivenugopal, K. S., et al. (2013). The MDM2-p53 pathway revisited. *Journal of Biomedical Research*, *27*(4), 254–271.
136. Koturbash, I., Loree, J., Kutanzi, K., et al. (2008). In vivo bystander effects: Cranial X-irradiation leads to elevated DNA damage, altered cellular proliferation and apoptosis, and increased p53 levels in shielded spleen. *International Journal of Radiation Oncology, Biology, Physics*, *70*(2), 554–562.
137. Mukherjee, D., Coates, P. J., Lorimore, S. A., et al. (2014). Responses to ionizing radiation mediated by inflammatory mechanisms. *Journal of Pathology*, *232*(3), 289–299.
138. Werner, E., Wang, H., & Doetsch, P. W. (2014). Opposite roles for p38MAPK-driven responses and reactive oxygen species in the persistence and resolution of radiation-induced genomic instability. *PLoS ONE*, *9*(10), e108234.
139. Wright, E. G. (2010). Manifestations and mechanisms of non-targeted effects of ionizing radiation. *Mutation Research*, *687*(1–2), 28–33.
140. Morganti, J. M., Jopson, T. D., Liu, S., et al. (2014). Cranial irradiation alters the brain's microenvironment and permits CCR2+ macrophage infiltration. *PLoS ONE*, *9*(4), e93650.
141. Barrington de Gonzalez, A., Curtis, R. E., Kry, S. F., et al. (2011). Proportion of second cancers attributable to radiotherapy treatment in adults: A prospective cohort study in the US SEER cancer registries. *Lancet Oncology*, *12*(4), 353–360.
142. Parkin, D. M., & Darby, S. C. (2011). Cancers in 2010 attributable to ionising radiation exposure in the UK. *British Journal of Cancer*, *105*, S57–S65.
143. Institute of Medicine. (2014). *Findings from research on health effects of low-level ionizing radiation exposure: Opportunities for the Armed Forces Radiobiology Research Institute*. Washington DC: Author.
144. Shuryak, I., Lubin, J. H., & Brenner, D. J. (2014). Potential for adult-based epidemiological studies to characterize overall cancer risks associated with a lifetime of CT scans. *Radiation Research*, *181*(6), 584–591.
145. Centers for Disease Control and Prevention. (2014). *Radiation and your health*. Atlanta, GA: Author. Retrieved from http://www.cdc.gov/nceh/radiation/.
146. World Health Organization. (2014). *Ultraviolet radiation and the INTERSUN*. Geneva: Author.
147. National Cancer Institute. (2011). *Types of skin cancer*. Washington, DC: National Institutes of Health. Retrieved from http://www.cancer.gov/cancertopics/wyntk/skin/page4.
148. National Cancer Institute. (2013). *Cellular classification of skin cancer*. Washington, DC: National Institutes of Health.
149. National Cancer Institute. (2014). *Genetics of skin cancer*. Washington, DC: National Institutes of Health.
150. National Cancer Institute. (2011). *Anyone can get skin cancer*. Washington, DC: National Institutes of Health.
151. Cleaver, J. E., & Crowley, E. (2002). UV damage, DNA repair, and skin carcinogenesis. *Frontiers in Bioscience*, *7*, d1024–d1043.
152. Atwood, S. X., Whitson, R. J., & Oro, A. E. (2014). Advanced treatment for basal cell carcinomas. *Cold Spring Harbor Perspectives in Medicine*, *4*(7), a013581.
153. Besaratinia, A., & Tommasi, S. (2014). Epigenetics of human melanoma: Promises and challenges. *Journal of Molecular Cell Biology*, *6*(5), 356–367.
154. Stamatelli, A., Vlachou, C., Aroni, K., et al. (2014). Epigenetic alterations in sporadic basal cell carcinomas. *Archives of Dermatological Research*, *306*(6), 561–569.
155. Wu, J., Zhang, J. R., & Qin, J. (2014). Clinical significance of methylation of E-cadherin and p14ARF gene promoters in skin squamous cell carcinoma tissues. *International Journal of Clinical and Experimental Medicine*, *7*(7), 1808–1812.
156. Streilein, J. W., Taylor, J. R., Vincek, V., et al. (1994). Immune surveillance and sunlight-induced skin cancer. *Immunology Today*, *15*(4), 174–179.
157. Maru, G. B., Gandhi, K., Ramchandani, A., et al. (2014). The role of inflammation in skin cancer. *Advances in Experimental Medicine and Biology*, *816*, 437–469.
158. Bickers, D. R., & Ather, M. (2006). Oxidative stress in the pathogenesis of skin disease. *The Journal of Investigative Dermatology*, *126*, 2562–2575.

159. Dhar, A., Young, M. R., & Colburn, N. H. (2002). The role of AP-1, NF-kappaB, and ROS/NOS in skin carcinogenesis: The JB6 model is predictive. *Molecular and Cellular Biochemistry, 234*(1–2), 185–193.
160. Sander, C. D., Chang, H., Hamm, F., et al. (2004). Role of oxidative stress and the antioxidant network in cutaneous carcinogenesis. *International Journal of Dermatology, 43*(5), 326–335.
161. Lin, J., Hocker, T. L., Singh, M., et al. (2008). Genetics of melanoma. *British Journal of Dermatology, 159*(2), 286–291.
162. Canadian Cancer Society's Advisory Committee on Cancer Statistics. (2016). *Canadian cancer statistics 2015.* Toronto: Canadian Cancer Society. Retrieved from https://www.cancer.ca/~/media/cancer.ca/CW/cancer%20information/cancer%20101/Canadian%20cancer%20statistics/Canadian-Cancer-Statistics-2015-EN.pdf.
163. Campbell, L. B., Kreicher, K. L., Gittleman, H. R., et al. (2015). Melanoma incidence in children and adolescents: Decreasing trends in the United States. *Journal of Pediatrics, 166*(6), 1505–1513. doi:10.1016/j.jpeds.2015.02.050.
164. Frangos, J. E., Duncan, L. M., Piris, A., et al. (2012). Increased diagnosis of thin superficial spreading melanomas: A 20-year study. *Journal of the American Academy of Dermatology, 67*(3), 387–394. doi:10.1016/j.jaad.2011.10.026.
165. Welch, H. G., & Black, W. C. (2010). Overdiagnosis in cancer. *Journal of the National Cancer Institute, 102*(9), 605–613. doi:10.1093/jnci/djq099.
166. Barón, A. E., Asdigian, N. L., Gonzalez, V., et al. (2014). Interactions between ultraviolet light and MC1R and OCA2 variants are determinants of childhood nevus and freckle phenotypes. *Cancer Epidemiology, Biomarkers and Prevention, 23*(12), 2829–2839. doi:10.1158/1055-9965.EPI-14-0633.
167. Heymann, W. R. (2007). Screening for melanoma. *Journal of the American Academy of Dermatology, 56*(1), 144–145. doi:10.1016/j.jaad.2006.08.046.
168. Whipple, C. A., & Brinkerhoff, C. E. (2014). BRAF(v600E) melanoma cells secrete factors that activate stromal fibroblasts and enhance tumorigenicity. *British Journal of Cancer, 111*(8), 1625–1633. doi:10.1038/bjc.2014.452.
169. Kumar, V., Abbas, A. K., & Aster, J. C. (Eds.), (2015). *Robbins and Cotran pathologic basis of disease* (9th ed.). Philadelphia: Saunders.
170. Doré, J. F., & Chignol, M. C. (2012). Tanning salons and skin cancer. *Photochemistry and Photobiology, 11*(1), 30–37. doi:10.1039/c1pp05186e.
171. Gandini, S., Stanganelli, I., Magi, S., et al. (2014). Melanoma attributable to sunbed use and tan seeking behaviours: An Italian survey. *European Journal of Dermatology, 24*(1), 35–40. doi:10.1684/ejd.2013.2214.
172. Héry, C., Tryggvadóttir, L., Sigurdsson, T., et al. (2010). A melanoma epidemic in Iceland: Possible influence of sunbed use. *American Journal of Epidemiology, 172*(7), 762–767. doi:10.1093/aje/kwq238.
173. Lazovich, D., Vogel, R. I., Berwick, M., et al. (2010). Indoor tanning and risk of melanoma: A case-control study in a highly exposed population. *Cancer Epidemiology, Biomarkers and Prevention, 19*(60), 1557–1568. doi:10.1158/1055-9965.EPI-09-1249.
174. Bens, G. (2014). Sunscreens. *Advances in Experimental Medicine and Biology, 810*, 429–463.
175. Baan, R., Grosse, Y., Lauby-Secretan, B., et al. (2011). Carcinogenicity of radiofrequency electromagnetic fields. *Lancet Oncology, 12*(7), 624–626.
176. Genuis, S. J. (2008). Fielding a current idea: Exploring the public health impact of electromagnetic radiation. *Public Health, 122*(2), 113–124. doi:10.1016/j.puhe.2007.04.008.
177. Belyaev, I. Y. (2010). Dependence of non-thermal biological effects of microwaves on physical and biological variables: Implications for reproducibility and safety standards. *European Journal of Oncology Library, 5*, 187–219.
178. National Institute of Environmental Health Sciences Working Group Report. (1998). *Assessment of health effects from exposure to power-line frequency electric and magnetic fields.* Washington, DC: U.S. Government Printing Office.
179. National Cancer Institute. (2005). *Electromagnetic fields and cancer.* Retrieved from http://www.cancer.gov/cancertopics/factsheet/Risk/magnetic-fields.
180. UK Childhood Cancer Study Investigators. (1999). Exposure to power-frequency magnetic fields and the risk of childhood cancer. *Lancet, 354*(9194), 1925–1931.
181. UK Childhood Cancer Study Investigators. (2000). Childhood cancer and residential proximity to power lines. *British Journal of Cancer, 83*(11), 1573–1580. doi:10.1054/bjoc.2000.1550.
182. Bunch, K. J., Keegan, T. J., Swanson, J., et al. (2014). Residential distance at birth from overhead high-voltage powerlines: Childhood cancer risk in Britain 1962–2008. *British Journal of Cancer, 110*(5), 1402–1408. doi:10.1038/bjc.2014.15.
183. Hauri, D. D., Spycher, B., Huss, A., et al. (2014). Exposure to radio-frequency electromagnetic fields from broadcast transmitters and risk of childhood cancer: A census-based cohort study. *American Journal of Epidemiology, 179*(7), 843–851. doi:10.1093/aje/kwt442.
184. INTERPHONE Study Group. (2010). Brain tumour risk in relation to mobile telephone use: Results of the INTERPHONE International Case-control Study. *International Journal of Epidemiology, 39*(3), 675–694. doi:10.1093/ije/dyq079.
185. Hardell, L., Carlberg, M., & Hansson Mild, K. (2013). Use of mobile phones and cordless phones is associated with increased risk for glioma and acoustic neuroma. *Pathophysiology, 20*(2), 85–110. doi:10.1016/j.pathophys.2012.11.001.
186. Hardell, L., Carlberg, M., & Hansson Mild, K. (2011). Pooled analysis of case-control studies on malignant brain tumours and the use of mobile and cordless phones including living and deceased subjects. *International Journal of Oncology, 38*(5), 1465–1474. doi:10.3892/ijo.2011.947.
187. Christensen, H. C., Schüz, J., Kosteljanetz, M., et al. (2004). Cellular telephone use and risk of acoustic neuroma. *American Journal of Epidemiology, 159*(3), 277–283.
188. Volkow, N. D., Tomasi, D., Wang, G. J., et al. (2011). Effects of cell phone radiofrequency signal exposure on brain glucose metabolism. *JAMA: The Journal of the American Medical Association, 305*(8), 808–813. doi:10.1001/jama.2011.186.
189. Cardis, E., Deltour, I., Mann, S., et al. (2008). Distribution of RF energy emitted by mobile phones in anatomical structures of the brain. *Physics in Medicine and Biology, 53*(11), 2771–2783. doi:10.1088/0031-9155/53/11/001.
190. Christ, A., Gosselin, M. C., Christopoulou, M., et al. (2010). Age-dependent tissue-specific exposure of cell phone users. *Physics in Medicine and Biology, 55*(7), 1767–1783. doi:10.1088/0031-9155/55/7/001.
191. Gandhi, O. P., Morgan, L. L., de Salles, A. A., et al. (2012). Exposure limits: The underestimation of absorbed cell phone radiation, especially in children. *Electromagnetic Biology and Medicine, 31*(1), 34–51. doi:10.3109/15368378.2011.622827.
192. Davis, D. L., Kesari, S., Soskolne, C. L., et al. (2013). Swedish review strengthens grounds for concluding that radiation from cellular and cordless phones is a probable human carcinogen. *Pathophysiology, 20*(2), 123–129. doi:10.1016/j.pathophys.2013.03.001.
193. Canadian Cancer Society. (2016). *Viruses and bacteria.* Retrieved from http://www.cancer.ca/en/prevention-and-screening/be-aware/viruses-and-bacteria/?region=sk.
194. de Martel, C., Ferlay, J., Franceschi, S., et al. (2012). Global burden of cancers attributable to infections in 2008: A review and synthetic analysis. *Lancet Oncology, 13*(6), 607–615. doi:10.1016/S1470-2045(12)70137-7.
195. Dart, H., Wolin, K. Y., & Colditz, G. A. (2012). Commentary: Eight ways to prevent cancer: A framework for effective prevention messages for the public. *Cancer Causes and Control, 23*(4), 601–608. doi:10.1007/s10552-012-9924-y.
196. Plummer, M., Franceschi, S., Vignat, J., et al. (2014). Global burden of gastric cancer attributable to *Helicobacter pylori. International Journal of Cancer, 136*(2), 487–490. doi:10.1002/ijc.28999.
197. Centers for Disease Control and Prevention. (2012). *Human papillomavirus (HPV).* Atlanta, GA: Author.
198. National Cancer Institute. (2012). *HPV and cancer.* Washington, DC: Author.
199. National Cancer Institute. (2014). *Pap and HPV testing.* Retrieved from http://www.cancer.gov/cancertopics/factsheet/detection/Pap-HPV-testing.
200. International Agency for Research on Cancer. (2012). *IARC monographs on the evaluation of carcinogenic risks to humans, Biological agents 100B: A review of human carcinogens.* Lyon, France: Author. Retrieved from http://monographs.iarc.fr/ENG/Monographs/vol100B/index.php.
201. Schiffman, M., Castle, P. E., Jeronimo, J., et al. (2007). Human papillomavirus and cervical cancer. *Lancet, 370*(9590), 890–907. doi:10.1016/S0140-6736(07)61416-0.
202. Smith, E. M., Parker, M. A., Rubenstein, L. M., et al. (2010). Evidence for vertical transmission of HPV from mothers to infants. *Infectious Diseases in Obstetrics and Gynecology, 2010*, 326369. doi:10.1155/2010/326369. Retrieved from http://dx.doi.org/10.1155/2010/326369.
203. Syrjänen, S., & Puranen, M. (2000). Human papillomavirus infections in children: The potential role of maternal transmission. *Critical Reviews in Oral Biology & Medicine, 11*(2), 259–274.
204. Moyer, V. A., & U.S. Preventive Services Task Force. (2012). Screening for cervical cancer: U.S. Preventive Services Task Force recommendation statement. *Annals of Internal Medicine, 156*(12), 880–891. doi:10.7326/0003-4819-156-12-201206190-00424.
205. Murphy, K. J., & Howlett, R. (2007). Screening for cervical cancer (Chapter 5 in Canadian consensus on human papillomavirus). *Journal of Obstetrics and Gynaecology, 29*(8), s27–s36.
206. Centers for Disease Control and Prevention. (2015). *Genital HPV infection—CDC fact sheet.* Atlanta GA: Author.
207. Hamra, G. B., Guha, N., Cohen, A., et al. (2014). Outdoor particulate matter exposure and lung cancer: A systematic review and meta-analysis. *Environmental Health Perspectives, 122*(9), 906–911. doi:10.1289/ehp.1408092.
208. International Agency for Research on Cancer. (2016). *IARC monographs on the evaluation of carcinogenic risks to humans: Outdoor air pollution* (Vol. 109). Lyon, France: Author.
209. Loomis, D., Grosse, Y., Lauby-Secretan, B., et al. (2013). The carcinogenicity of outdoor air pollution. *Lancet Oncology, 14*, 1262–1263.
210. Buschini, A., Cassoni, F., Anceschi, E., et al. (2001). Urban airborne particulate: Genotoxicity evaluation of different size fractions by mutagenesis tests on microorganisms and comet assay. *Chemosphere, 44*(8), 1723–1736.
211. Government of Canada. (2016). *Ambient levels of fine particulate matter.* Retrieved from https://www.ec.gc.ca/indicateurs-indicators/default.asp?lang=en&n=029BB000-.
212. Puett, R. C., Hart, J. E., Yanosky, J. D., et al. (2009). Chronic fine and course particulate exposure, mortality, and coronary heart disease in the Nurses' Health Study. *Environmental Health Perspectives, 117*(11), 1697–1701.
213. Gulland, A. (2012). Diesel engine exhaust causes lung cancer, says WHO. *British Medical Journal, 344*, e4174. doi:10.1136/bmj.e4174.
214. Lim, S. S., Vos, T., Flaxman, A. D., et al. (2012). A comparative risk assessment of burden of disease and injury attributable to 67 risk factors and risk factor clusters in 21 regions, 1990–2010: A systematic analysis for the Global Burden of Disease Study 2010. *Lancet, 380*, 2224–2260. doi:10.1016/S0140-6736(12)61766-8.
215. Boffetta, P., Soutar, A., Cherrie, J. W., et al. (2004). Mortality among workers employed in the titanium dioxide production industry in Europe. *Cancer Causes and Control, 15*(7), 697–706. doi:10.1023/B:CACO.0000036188.23970.22.

216. Hecht, S. S., Seow, A., Wang, M., et al. (2010). Elevated levels of volatile organic carcinogen and toxicant biomarkers in Chinese women who regularly cook at home. *Cancer Epidemiology, Biomarkers and Prevention, 19*(5), 1185–1192. doi:10.1158/1055-9965.EPI-09-1291.
217. Barone-Adesi, F., Chapman, R. S., Silverman, D. T., et al. (2012). Risk of lung cancer associated with domestic use of coal in Xuanwei, China: Retrospective cohort study. *British Medical Journal, 345*, e5414. doi:10.1136/bmj.e5414.
218. Zhao, Y., Wang, S., Aunan, K., et al. (2006). Air pollution and lung cancer risks in China—Meta-analysis. *Science of the Total Environment, 366*(2–3), 500–513. doi:10.1016/j.scitotenv.2005.10.010.
219. Agency for Toxic Substances and Disease Registry. (2014). *Chemicals, cancer, and you*. Atlanta, GA: Author. Retrieved from https://www.atsdr.cdc.gov/emes/public/docs/Chemicals,%20Cancer,%20and%20You%20FS.pdf.
220. Gray, J. (2008). *State of the evidence 2008: The connection between breast cancer and the environment*. San Francisco: Breast Cancer Fund.
221. Tryndyak, V. P., Muskhelishvili, L., Kovalchuk, O., et al. (2006). Effect of long-term tamoxifen exposure on genotoxic and epigenetic changes in rat liver: Implications for tamoxifen-induced hepatocarcinogenesis. *Carcinogenesis, 27*(8), 1713–1720. doi:10.1093/carcin/bgl050.
222. Karpinets, T. V., & Foy, B. D. (2005). Tumorigenesis: The adaptation of mammalian cells to sustained stress environment by epigenetic alterations and succeeding matched mutations. *Carcinogenesis, 26*(8), 1323–1334. doi:10.1093/carcin/bgi079.
223. Tabish, A. M., Poels, K., Hoet, P., et al. (2012). Epigenetic factors in cancer risk: Effect of chemical carcinogens on global DNA methylation pattern in human TK6 cells. *PLoS ONE, 7*(4), e34674.
224. Hileman, B. (2009). Chemicals can turn genes on and off; new tests needed, scientists say. In *Environmental health news*. Charlottesville, VA: National Institute of Environmental Health Sciences.
225. Neuberger, J. S., & Field, R. W. (2003). Occupation and lung cancer in nonsmokers. *Reviews on Environmental Health, 18*(4), 251–267.
226. Prazakova, S., Thomas, P. S., Sandrini, A., et al. (2014). Asbestos and the lung in the 21st century: An update. *Clinical Respiratory Journal, 8*(1), 1–10. doi:10.1111/crj.12028.
227. Borm, P. J., Schins, R. P., & Albrecht, C. (2004). Inhaled particles and lung cancer, part B: Paradigms and risk assessment. *International Journal of Cancer, 110*(1), 3–14. doi:10.1002/ijc.20064.
228. Puett, R. C., Hart, J. E., Yanosky, J. D., et al. (2014). Particulate matter air pollution exposure, distance to road, and incident lung cancer in the Nurses' Health Study cohort. *Environmental Health Perspectives, 122*(9), 926–932. doi:10.1289/ehp.1307490.
229. Raaschou-Nielsen, O., Andersen, Z. J., Beelen, R., et al. (2013). Air pollution and lung cancer incidence in 17 European cohorts: Prospective analyses from the European Study of Cohorts for Air Pollution Effects (ESCAPE). *Lancet Oncology, 14*(9), 813–822. doi:10.1016/S1470-2045(13)70279-1.
230. Vineis, P., Forastiere, F., Hoek, G., et al. (2004). Outdoor air pollution and lung cancer: Recent epidemiologic evidence. *International Journal of Cancer, 111*(5), 647–652. doi:10.1002/ijc.20292.

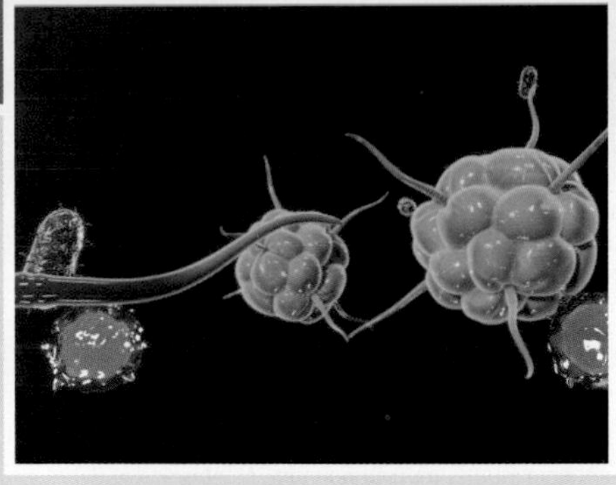

Cancer in Children and Adolescents

Lauri A. Linder, Nancy E. Kline, and Stephanie Zettel

EVOLVE WEBSITE

http://evolve.elsevier.com/Canada/Huether/pathophysiology
Student Review Questions
Key Points
Case Studies
Animations
Quick Check Answers

CHAPTER OUTLINE

Incidence, Etiology, and Types of Childhood Cancer, 303
Etiology, 304
Genetic and Genomic Factors, 305
Environmental Factors, 305
Prognosis, 307

Cancer can occur at any age, but its impact at a younger age can be particularly devastating. While cancer in children and adolescents is rare, according to Statistics Canada, in 2011, cancer was the leading cause of disease-related death in children under the age of 15 years.[1] Survival rates among children and adolescents with cancer have dramatically improved since the 1960s. Among the factors leading to improved cure rates include the use of combination chemotherapy, the incorporation of research data obtained from clinical trials, and the utilization of multimodal treatment for solid tumours.

INCIDENCE, ETIOLOGY, AND TYPES OF CHILDHOOD CANCER

Between 2009 and 2013, there were 4715 new cases of cancer in children from birth to 14 years of age in Canada, an average of 943 cases per year. Between 2008 and 2012, there were 595 cancer deaths in children from birth to 14 years of age in Canada, an average of 119 deaths per year.[2] Childhood cancer accounts for less than 1% of all new cancer cases in Canada, and the three types of cancer that account for most of the cases between birth and 14 years of age are leukemia (32%), brain and central nervous system cancers (19%), and lymphoma (11%). Similarly, most cancer deaths in children from birth to 14 years of age are related to brain and central nervous system cancers (34%), leukemia (26%), and neuroblastoma and other peripheral nervous cell tumours (11%). Between 2006 and 2010, the most common types of cancer found in adolescents and young adults (15 to 29 years of age)[2] were as follows:

- Thyroid—16%
- Testicular—13%
- Hodgkin's lymphoma—12%
- Melanoma—8%

Young men are more likely to die from cancer than young women.

The types of malignancies that occur in children are vastly different from those that affect adults. The most common types of cancer among adults include prostate, breast, lung, and colon cancer. In contrast, children tend to develop leukemias, brain tumours, and sarcomas. Although many adult cancers have associated environmental and lifestyle factors that could theoretically be avoided, such as sun exposure and smoking, very few such factors have been linked to pediatric malignancies. More data are emerging that the developing child may be affected by epigenetic modifications resulting from parental exposures before conception, exposures in utero, and nutrition during early life.[3,4]

Most childhood cancers originate from the **mesodermal germ layer**, which develops into connective tissue, bone, cartilage, muscle, blood, blood vessels, gonads, kidney, and the lymphatic system (Figure 12-1). Thus the more common childhood cancers are leukemias, sarcomas, and embryonic tumours.

Leukemias are circulating tumours that primarily involve the blood and bone marrow, whereas lymphoma tends to localize to lymph tissue. Common manifestations of these disorders are related to myelosuppression or organ dysfunction secondary to the infiltration of white blood cells. These malignancies also tend to present with nonspecific symptoms such as malaise, weakness, unexplained fever, night sweats, and recurrent infections (those affected will often have large, nontender lymph nodes). Classification of hematological neoplasms is based on the cell type of the neoplasm, rather than its location in the body. Myeloid cancers involve cells from the myeloid lineage (e.g., erythrocytes, granulocytes, platelets, and monocytes), and lymphoid cancers are derived from B lymphocytes, T lymphocytes, and natural killer cells. Hodgkin's lymphoma is another example of a lymphoid cancer.[5]

Embryonic tumours originate during intrauterine life and contain abnormal cells that appear to be immature embryonic tissue unable to mature or differentiate into fully developed functional cells. Embryonic tumours are most often diagnosed early in life (usually by 5 years of age) and are rare in older children, adolescents, and adults. The names of these tumours often include the root term *blast* (e.g., neuroblastoma, retinoblastoma), which indicates the embryonic stage of development.

Sarcomas, leukemias, and lymphomas are cancers observed in childhood and also may occur in adults. Most adult cancers, however,

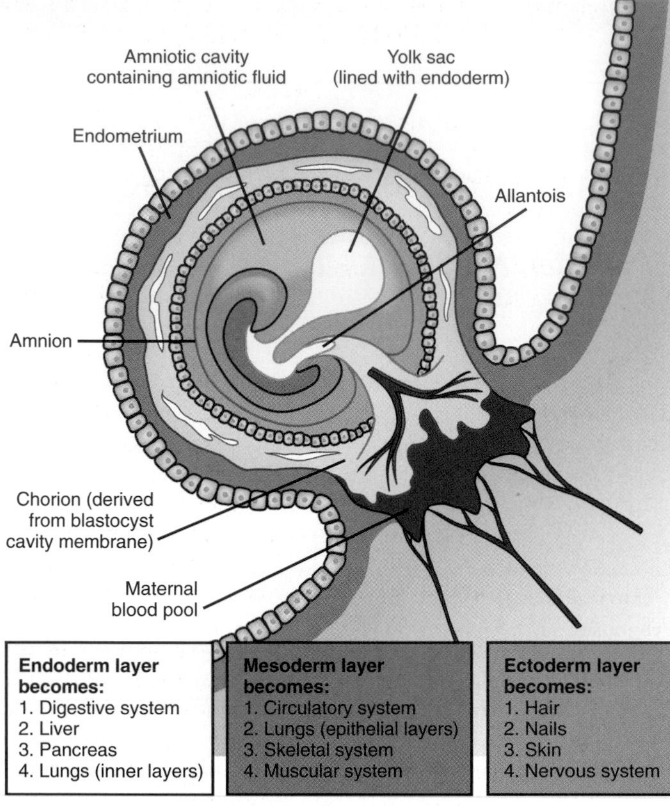

FIGURE 12-1 Mesodermal Germ Layer.

involve epithelial tissue and are, therefore, carcinomas. Carcinomas rarely occur in children because these cancers most commonly result from environmental carcinogens and require a long period from exposure to the appearance of the carcinoma. Carcinomas begin to increase in incidence between the ages of 15 and 19 years, becoming the most common cancer tissue type observed after adolescence.[6]

Childhood cancers are often diagnosed during peak times of physical growth and maturation, accounting for the bimodal distribution in their incidence. In general, they are extremely fast-growing cancers, resulting in a relatively short latency period—that is, the time from the initial exposure to the onset of symptoms. The distribution of cancer types also changes during childhood and adolescence. Leukemias and embryonal tumours have a peak incidence before the child is 5 years of age. Brain tumours, the second leading type of childhood cancer overall, have a peak incidence among children less than 15 years of age. The incidence of specific subtypes of brain tumours does, however, vary across childhood and adolescence. Lymphomas, both Hodgkin's and non-Hodgkin's, represent the third most common type of childhood cancer. Lymphoma is rare in children less than 5 years of age and occurs with increasing frequency in children and adolescents 10 years of age and older. Rhabdomyosarcoma is the most common soft tissue sarcoma of childhood. Rhabdomyosarcoma has a bimodal age distribution with two thirds of cases occurring in children less than 6 years of age and one third occurring in children and adolescents 10 years of age and older. The two most common types of bone tumours are osteosarcoma and Ewing sarcoma. These cancers are more likely to occur in adolescents ages 15 and older.

Etiology

The causes of cancer in children are largely unknown. A few environmental factors are known to predispose a child to cancer, but causal factors have not been established for most childhood cancers. A number of host factors, many of which are genetic risk factors or congenital conditions, have been implicated in the development of childhood cancer (Table 12-1).

Because of their relatively short latency period, most childhood cancers do not lend themselves to early cancer warning signs. Certainly

TABLE 12-1 Congenital Factors Associated With Childhood Cancer

Syndrome	Associated Childhood Cancer
Chromosome Alterations	
Down syndrome	Acute leukemia
13q syndrome	Retinoblastoma
Chromosome Instability	
Ataxia-telangiectasia	Lymphoma
Bloom's syndrome	Acute leukemia, lymphoma, Wilms tumour
Fanconi anemia	Acute myelogenous leukemia, myelodysplastic syndrome, hepatic tumours
Hereditary Syndromes	
Beckwith-Wiedemann syndrome	Wilms tumour, sarcoma, brain tumours, neuroblastoma, hepatoblastoma
Neurofibromatosis type I	Brain tumour, sarcomas, neuroblastomas, Wilms tumour, nonlymphocytic leukemia
Neurofibromatosis type II	Meningioma (malignant or benign), acoustic neuroma or schwannoma, gliomas, ependymomas
Tuberous sclerosis	Glial tumours
Li-Fraumeni syndrome	Sarcoma, adrenocortical carcinoma
Von Hippel-Lindau disease	Cerebellar hemangioblastoma, retinal angioma, renal cell carcinoma, pheochromocytomas
Ataxia-telangiectasia	Leukemia, lymphoma, brain tumours
Gorlin syndrome	Medulloblastoma, skin tumours
Immunodeficiency Disorders	
Congenital	
Agammaglobulinemia	Lymphoma, leukemia, brain tumours
Immunoglobulin A (IgA) deficiency	Lymphoma, leukemia, brain tumours
Wiskott-Aldrich syndrome	Leukemia, lymphoma
Acquired	
Aplastic anemia	Leukemia
HIV/AIDS	
Organ transplantation	Leukemia, lymphoma
Congenital Malformation Syndromes	
Aniridia, hemihypertrophy, hamartoma, genitourinary anomalies	Wilms tumour
Cryptorchidism	Testicular tumour
Gonadal dysgenesis	Gonadoblastoma
Family Susceptibility	
Twin or sibling with leukemia	Leukemia

HIV/AIDS, human immunodeficiency virus/acquired immunodeficiency syndrome.

the American Cancer Society's seven warning signs of cancer (which have been adopted in Canada and many other countries) do not apply because they describe adult, environmentally caused carcinomas. Likewise, efforts to establish early screening strategies for childhood cancers have not been effective. Although host factors are important in identifying populations of children at risk for cancer, most children who are diagnosed with cancer do not have known predisposing environmental or host factors.

Multiple causation theory provides a useful framework for interpreting the results of epidemiological studies. For example, laboratory and epidemiological studies may indicate that exposure to a certain chemical can cause leukemia, but not all children exposed to that chemical will develop leukemia. Additional studies will be needed to determine what other host and environmental factors must interact with chemical exposure to cause the disease.

Genetic and Genomic Factors

Acquired or inherited mutations in individual genes may contribute to the development of cancer in children and adolescents. Mutations in more than 150 oncogenes and tumour-suppressor genes have been associated with the subsequent development of both childhood and adult cancers (Table 12-2). Fanconi anemia and Bloom's syndrome are two autosomal recessive conditions that result in impaired DNA repair and are risk factors for the development of acute leukemia.[7] Retinoblastoma, a malignant embryonic tumour of the eye, occurs either as an inherited defect in the *RB1* gene or as an acquired mutation (see Chapter 17).

Although leukemia is not inherited as a genetic condition, siblings of children with leukemia have a two to four times increased risk for the development of leukemia relative to that of siblings of healthy children. The occurrence of leukemia in monozygous twins is estimated to be as high as 25%.

Li-Fraumeni syndrome (LFS) is an autosomal dominant disorder involving the *TP53* tumour-suppressor gene. For individuals with a mutation in the *TP53* gene, the risk of developing cancer as a child or adult is significantly higher than the risk in the unaffected population. Children and adults in families affected by LFS are at risk for soft tissue sarcoma, breast cancer, leukemia, osteosarcoma, melanoma, and cancer of the colon, pancreas, adrenal cortex, and brain. Individuals with LFS also are at increased risk of developing multiple primary cancers.[8]

Chromosomal abnormalities also may contribute to the development of childhood cancer. Chromosomal abnormalities include aneuploidy, deletions, amplifications, translocations, and fragility (see Chapter 2). These abnormalities may occur within the affected cancer cells as a consequence of malignant transformation or may be present as the consequence of a congenital syndrome.

A chromosomal translocation results from the rearrangement of two nonhomologous chromosomes. Translocations may result in the creation of a fusion gene in which the two previously separate gene regions unite. Two fusion genes associated with acute lymphocytic leukemia (ALL) in children are the *BCR-ABL* gene, resulting from a translocation between chromosomes 9 and 22, and the *TEL-AML1* gene, resulting from a translocation between chromosomes 12 and 21.[9,10]

Several syndromes associated with specific congenital malformations are linked to a higher incidence of cancer development. In some cases, these children may be carefully followed and screened for tumour development. One of the more recognized syndromes is trisomy 21 (Down syndrome), which has an increased susceptibility to acute leukemia. The risk of developing leukemia is 10 to 20 times greater among children with Down syndrome than in children without Down syndrome. The age distribution for developing ALL among children with Down syndrome is similar to that of children without Down syndrome.[11,12]

Wilms tumour, a malignant tumour of the kidney, is particularly recognized for its association with a number of congenital anomalies, including genitourinary anomalies, aniridia (congenital absence of the iris), hemihypertrophy (muscular overgrowth of half of the body or face), and intellectual disabilities. Identifiable malformations and congenital predisposition syndromes are present in approximately 17% of children diagnosed with Wilms tumour.[13]

TABLE 12-2 Selected Oncogenes and Tumour-Suppressor Genes Associated With Childhood Cancer

Gene	Associated Pediatric Tumour
Oncogenes	
ABL	Acute lymphoblastic leukemia
MYCN	Neuroblastoma
MYB	Neural tumours, leukemia, lymphoma, rhabdomyosarcoma, Wilms tumour, neuroblastoma
erbB	Glioblastomas
NRAS	Neuroblastoma, leukemia
HRAS/KRAS	Neuroblastoma, rhabdomyosarcoma, leukemia
ATM	Lymphoma, leukemia
Tumour-Suppressor Genes	
RB1	Retinoblastoma, sarcoma
WT1, WT2	Wilms tumour, leukemia
NF-1	Sarcoma, primitive neuroectodermal tumour, juvenile chronic myelocytic leukemia
NF-2	Brain tumours, melanoma, meningiomas
p16	Brain tumours, leukemia
TP53	Sarcoma, leukemia, brain tumours, lymphoma
DCC	Ewing sarcoma, rhabdomyosarcoma
CDKN2A	Glioblastoma, acute lymphoblastic leukemia
CDC2L1	Non-Hodgkin's lymphoma, neuroblastoma

Data from Beamer, L.C., Linder, L., Wu, B., et al. (2013). *Nurs Clin North Am, 48*(4), 585–626; Esparza, S.D., Sakamoto, K.M., Milton, B.A., et al. (2016). *Childhood cancer genetics*. Retrieved from http://emedicine.medscape.com/article/989983-overview#a1.

Environmental Factors

Finding the cause of any disease is typically a long, slow process. Epidemiological studies require many years to determine whether a risk factor is possibly related to the development of childhood cancer. No single factor determines whether an individual will develop cancer, even if a specific environmental exposure explains a high proportion of the occurrence of a specific cancer (Box 12-1).

Prenatal Exposure

Prenatal exposure to some medications and to ionizing radiation has been linked to childhood cancers. The most well-described medication is diethylstilbestrol (DES), which was prescribed by physicians to prevent spontaneous miscarriage (in women with previous miscarriage). In 1971 DES was identified as a transplacental chemical carcinogen because a small percentage of the daughters of women who took DES developed adenocarcinomas of the vagina. Since then, other studies have attempted to identify other medications taken by pregnant women that may cause cancer in their offspring, but no other medications have been found

BOX 12-1 Factors That May Contribute to the Development of Childhood and Adolescent Cancer

- Genetic and epigenetic factors
- Diet
- Immune function
- Occupational exposure
- Ionizing radiation
- Hormonal variations
- Viral illnesses
- Individual characteristics, such as the biological, social, and physical environment

TABLE 12-3 Medications That May Increase Risk for Childhood Cancer

Medication Class	Uses	Cancer Risk
Anabolic androgenic steroids	To stimulate bone growth and appetite; induce puberty; increase muscle mass and physical strength	Hepatocellular carcinoma
Epipodophyllotoxin and anthracycline chemotherapy agents	To treat cancer	Leukemia
Immunosuppressive agents	To prevent organ rejection following transplantation surgery	Lymphoma

to have this effect. Current evidence suggests that an increased risk for childhood leukemia is associated with low levels of exposure to antenatal X-rays.[14] An association between antenatal X-ray exposure and childhood brain tumours has not been identified.[15] Other current areas of research include exploring epigenetic modifications resulting from prenatal exposures and their role in future cancer development.[7]

Childhood Exposure

Childhood exposure to ionizing radiation, medications, electromagnetic fields, or viruses has been associated with the risk of developing cancer. Retrospective research has shown a significant correlation between radiation-induced malignancies and either radiotherapy (cancer treatment) or radiation exposure from diagnostic imaging[16] (see *Health Promotion:* Radiation Risks and Pediatric Computed Tomography: Data From the US National Cancer Institute). In addition to the medication and environmental agents that are known to cause cancer in adults and, therefore, also are risks for exposure during childhood, a few medications may particularly increase cancer risk during childhood (Table 12-3).

The relationship between childhood cancer and other environmental factors (e.g., electromagnetic fields, small appliances, radon) has been the focus of many epidemiological studies. Although associations between some environmental exposures and acute leukemia have been demonstrated, no conclusive causal evidence has been reported[17-19]

HEALTH PROMOTION

Radiation Risks and Pediatric Computed Tomography: Data From the US National Cancer Institute

The use of pediatric computed tomography (CT) has been increasing rapidly. As a result, radiation risks for children have become a growing concern. Children are more sensitive to radiation than adults, as demonstrated in epidemiological studies. Children have a longer life expectancy than adults, increasing the window of opportunity to express radiation damage, and children may receive a higher radiation dose than necessary if CT is not adjusted for their smaller size. Although CT scans comprise up to about 12% of diagnostic radiological procedures in large US hospitals, it is estimated that they account for approximately 49% of the US population's collective radiation dose from all medical X-ray examinations. CT is the largest contributor to medical radiation exposure among the US population. It is important to stress that the absolute cancer risks associated with CT scans are small. The lifetime risks of cancer because of CT scans, which have been estimated in the literature using projection models based on atomic bomb survivors, are about 1 case of cancer for every 1 000 people who are scanned, with a maximal incidence of about 1 case of cancer for every 500 people who are scanned. The benefits of properly performed and clinically justified CT examinations should always outweigh the risks for an individual child; unnecessary exposure is associated with unnecessary risk. Minimizing radiation exposure from pediatric CT, whenever possible, will reduce the projected number of CT-related cancers.

Data from National Cancer Institute, National Institutes of Health. (2012). *NCI radiation risks and pediatric computed tomography (CT): A guide for health care workers.* Bethesda, MD: National Cancer Institute.

HEALTH PROMOTION

Magnetic Fields and Development of Pediatric Cancer

Several recent reports have suggested an association between environmental sources and the development of cancer in children. The presence of low-frequency magnetic fields has been a concern for many years as causing leukemia in children. The World Health Organization (WHO) research agenda identified the importance of such an analysis as a high research priority in 2007. A recent meta-analysis evaluated nine case-control studies, representing eight different countries, conducted between 1997 and 2013 and involving 11 699 cases of children with leukemia and 13 194 controls. This meta-analysis identified an increased risk for childhood leukemia associated with high levels of magnetic field exposure (greater than or equal to 0.4 μT). For additional perspective, the WHO estimates that only about 1 to 4% of children worldwide live in conditions that exceed this level of exposure. Ongoing research needs to be done in this area because environmental factors may require many years of exposure to cause disease. Additionally, an association between an environmental factor and childhood cancer does not establish causality. Ongoing research is needed to better understand the relationships between environmental factors and other factors associated with childhood cancer, as well as potential underlying mechanisms by which environmental factors may contribute to the development of childhood cancer.

Data from World Health Organization. (2015). *Electromagnetic fields and public health: Exposure to extremely low frequency fields.* Retrieved from http://www.who.int/peh-emf/publications/facts/fs322/en/; Zhao, L., Liu, X., Wang, C., et al. (2014). *Leuk Res, 38*(3), 269–274.

(see *Health Promotion:* Magnetic Fields and Development of Pediatric Cancer).

The strongest association between viruses and the development of cancer in children has been the Epstein-Barr virus (EBV), which is linked to Burkitt lymphoma, nasopharyngeal carcinoma, and Hodgkin's disease.[20] Children with acquired immunodeficiency syndrome (AIDS), caused by human immunodeficiency virus (HIV), have an increased risk of developing non-Hodgkin's lymphoma and Kaposi sarcoma. However, with the use of highly active antiretroviral therapy in the developed world, the incidence of AIDS-related malignancies has declined dramatically.[21]

PROGNOSIS

More than 70% of children diagnosed with cancer are cured. Some of the factors leading to improved cure rates in pediatric oncology include the use of combination chemotherapy or multimodal treatment for solid childhood tumours and improvements in nursing and supportive care. The development of research centres for comprehensive childhood cancer treatment and cooperative study groups also have facilitated refinements in treatment protocols and data sharing, leading to improved survival rates.

The management of hematological malignancies in children and adolescents focuses on the use of combination chemotherapy to kill the malignant cells, followed by a stem cell transplant to rescue and restore bone marrow function[5] (see *Health Promotion:* Bone Marrow Transplantation: Improving Outcomes for Canadian Children and Adolescent Cancer Patients). Induction chemotherapy is used to try to remove as many of the neoplastic cells as possible. It is followed by the consolidation phase, which has the aim of eliminating nondetectable cells. Maintenance chemotherapy is often administered to prolong remission of the cancer. Chemotherapy is often administered into the cerebrospinal fluid intrathecally because malignant blood and lymph cells can migrate across the blood–brain barrier to the central nervous system. The donor and host cells must be extensively cross-matched to ensure the transplantation is successful. There is a possibility of the transplanted donor cells mounting an immune attack on the host's tissues, resulting in *graft-versus-host disease*, which can be life-threatening.

Survival rates for children younger than 15 years of age who have been diagnosed with cancer have increased at a rate of 1.5% per year in the United States, which is similar to increases in survival for adults older than 50 years of age. Adolescents and young adults between 15 and 24 years of age, however, have experienced increases in survival of less than 0.5% per year.[6] Survival rates in Canada have been similar.[2] A partial explanation for the relative lack of progress in curing the adolescent population at the same rate as that realized in the younger pediatric population is the lack of clinical trials. At the time of writing, only 18 out of 818 Canadian cancer trials were recruiting adolescents; this number stands in contrast to the 17 cancer trials for infants and 249 cancer trials for children.[22] In the United States, the National Cancer Institute (NCI) and pediatric and adult cooperative groups sponsored by the NCI have launched a national initiative to increase the number of adolescents and young adults in clinical trials.[23]

Survivors of childhood cancer are at increased risk of developing a second malignancy during their lifetime. This risk may be associated with a variety of factors, including previous chemotherapy or radiotherapy, genetic factors, and type of primary cancer (e.g., soft tissue sarcoma, neuroblastoma).

Because childhood cancer should be viewed as a chronic disease instead of a fatal illness, treatment includes attention to quality of life and symptom management. Even those cancers that cannot be cured generally can be treated, resulting in significantly improved quality of life. Children and adolescents whose cancers are regarded as cured still face residual and late effects of their treatment. These late effects are more significant in children than in adults because treatment given during childhood occurs in a physically immature, growing individual. Late effects that need further study include physical impairments, reproductive dysfunction, soft tissue and bone atrophy, learning disabilities, secondary cancers, and psychological sequelae. More must be learned about the genetic factors associated with childhood malignancies and about the genetic consequences of treatment. A referral to genetic services is appropriate for families of children whose cancer is known to be transmitted genetically (e.g., retinoblastoma, LFS).

HEALTH PROMOTION

Bone Marrow Transplantation: Improving Outcomes for Canadian Children and Adolescent Cancer Patients

Allogeneic bone marrow transplantation (BMT) provides the chance of a cure to patients with potentially fatal leukemias and lymphomas. Allogeneic transplants involve the donation of bone marrow from an otherwise healthy donor and have dramatically improved patient outcomes in a number of ways. However, there are risks and side effects associated with BMT. Treatments include antimicrobials with greater specificity for bacterial and fungal infections that result from prolonged neutropenia, as well as the use of growth factors such as granulocyte colony-stimulating factors in the supportive care of patients with infections associated with transplantation.

While research continues into mechanisms that explain why some BMTs fail (i.e., due to graft-versus-host disease), efforts to identify the best possible marrow donors in Canada also have the potential to dramatically improve transplant outcomes. Extensive human leukocyte antigen (HLA) typing is essential for the "best" match and the "best" outcomes. Signing up to be a marrow donor is easy, and it is voluntary. Increasing the number of donors in the registry and the specificity of HLA typing ensures the usefulness of this registry for both recipients and donors in years to come.

Based on Cancer Advocacy Coalition of Canada. (2011). *Report card on cancer in Canada, 2010–11.* Toronto: Author, pp. 33–37. Retrieved from http://www.canceradvocacy.ca/reportcard/2010/2010-2011%20REPORT%20CARD%20ON%20CANCER%20IN%20CANADA.pdf.

QUICK CHECK 12-1

1. What are the most common childhood cancers, and how do they differ from adult cancers?
2. Why are children less likely to develop carcinomas?
3. Compare and contrast different etiological factors associated with the development of childhood cancer.

DID YOU UNDERSTAND?

Overview

1. Childhood cancer is a rare disease, but it remains the leading cause of death that is attributable to disease in children.

Incidence, Etiology, and Types of Childhood Cancer

1. The most common type of childhood cancer is leukemia, and the second most common type is cancer involving the brain or central nervous system.
2. Although many adult cancers are associated with environmental and lifestyle factors, very few such factors have been linked to pediatric malignancies because children have not lived long enough to be affected by them.
3. Children with immunodeficiencies are at increased risk of developing cancer because of an ineffective immune system.
4. Children with Down syndrome are at increased risk of developing leukemia.
5. Risk factors that may be associated with the development of childhood cancer include inherited and acquired genetic and epigenetic factors, diet, immune function, occupational exposure, ionizing radiation, hormonal variations, viral illnesses, and other individual characteristics (e.g., the biological, social, or physical environment).

Prognosis

1. Survivors of childhood cancer are at increased risk of developing a second malignancy during their lifetime, compared with the general population.

KEY TERMS

Embryonic tumour, 303
Li-Fraumeni syndrome (LFS), 305
Mesodermal germ layer, 303
Multiple causation, 305
Wilms tumour, 305

REFERENCES

1. Statistics Canada. (2015). *Childhood cancer incidence and mortality in Canada*. Retrieved from http://www.statcan.gc.ca/pub/82-624-x/2015001/article/14213-eng.htm.
2. Canadian Cancer Society. (2016). *Childhood cancer statistics*. Retrieved from http://www.cancer.ca/en/cancer-information/cancer-101/childhood-cancer-statistics/?region=on.
3. Burdge, G. C., Lillycrop, K. A., & Jackson, A. A. (2009). Nutrition in early life, and risk of cancer and metabolic disease: Alternative endings in an epigenetic tale? *British Journal of Nutrition*, *101*(5), 619–630. doi:10.1017/S0007114508145883.
4. Kaur, P., Shorey, L. E., Ho, E., et al. (2013). The epigenome as a potential mediator of cancer prevention by dietary phytochemicals: The fetus as a target. *Nutrition Reviews*, *71*(7), 441–457. doi:10.1111/nure.12030.
5. Kotter, M., & Banasik, J. (2013). Malignant disorders of white blood cells. In L. Copstead & J. Banasik (Eds.), *Pathophysiology* (5th ed.). St. Louis: Elsevier.
6. Howlader, N., Noone, A. M., Krapcho, M., et al. (Eds.). (2013). *SEER cancer statistics review, 1975–2011*. Bethesda, MD: National Cancer Institute. Retrieved from http://seer.cancer.gov/csr/1975_2011/.
7. Seif, A. E. (2011). Pediatric leukemia predisposition syndromes: Clues to understanding leukemogenesis. *Cancer Genetics*, *204*(5), 227–244. doi:10.1016/j.cancergen.2011.04.005.
8. McBride, K. A., Ballinger, M. L., Killick, E., et al. (2014). Li-Fraumeni syndrome: Cancer risk assessment and clinical management. *Nature Reviews. Clinical Oncology*, *11*(5), 260–271. doi:10.1038/nrclinonc.2014.41.
9. Izraeli, S. (2014). Beyond Philadelphia: "pH-like" B cell precursor acute lymphoblastic leukemia–Diagnostic challenges and therapeutic promises. *Current Opinion in Hematology*, *21*(4), 289–296. doi:10.1097/MOH.0000000000000050.
10. Linka, Y., Ginzel, S., Krüger, M., et al. (2013). The impact of TEL-AML1 (ETV6-RUNX1) expression in precursor B cells and implications for leukaemia using three different genome-wide screening methods. *Blood Cancer Journal*, *3*, e151. doi:10.1038/bcj.2013.48.
11. Maloney, K. W. (2011). Acute lymphoblastic leukaemia in children with Down syndrome: An updated review. *British Journal of Haematology*, *155*(4), 420–425. doi:10.1111/j.1365-2141.2011.08846.x.
12. Whitlock, J. A., Sather, H. N., Gaynon, P., et al. (2005). Clinical characteristics and outcome of children with Down syndrome and acute lymphoblastic leukemia: A Children's Cancer Group study. *Blood*, *106*(13), 4043–4049. doi:10.1182/blood-2003-10-3446.
13. Dumoucel, S., Gauthier-Villars, M., Stoppa-Lyonnet, D., et al. (2014). Malformations, genetic abnormalities, and Wilms tumor. *Pediatric Blood & Cancer*, *61*(1), 140–144. doi:10.1002/pbc.24709.
14. Wakeford, R. (2013). The risk of childhood leukaemia following exposure to ionising radiation. *Journal of Radiological Protection*, *33*(1), 1–25. doi:10.1088/0952-4746/33/1/1.
15. Milne, E., Greenop, K. R., Fritschi, L., et al. (2014). Childhood and parental diagnostic radiological procedures and risk of childhood brain tumors. *Cancer Causes and Control*, *25*(3), 375–383. doi:10.1007/s10552-014-0338-x.
16. Miglioretti, D. L., Johnson, E., Williams, A., et al. (2013). Pediatric computed tomography and associated radiation exposure and estimated cancer risk. *JAMA Pediatrics*, *167*(8), 700–707. doi:10.1001/jamapediatrics.2013.311.
17. Heck, J. E., Park, A. S., Qiu, J., et al. (2014). Risk of leukemia in relation to exposure to ambient air toxins in pregnancy and early childhood. *International Journal of Hygiene and Environmental Health*, *217*(6), 662–668. doi:10.1016/j.ijheh.2013.12.003.
18. Sermage-Faure, C., Demoury, C., Rudant, J., et al. (2013). Childhood leukemia close to high-voltage power lines—The Geocap study, 2002–2007. *British Journal of Cancer*, *108*(9), 1899–1906. doi:10.1038/bjc.2013.128.
19. Zhao, L., Liu, X., Wang, C., et al. (2014). Magnetic fields exposure and childhood leukemia risk: A meta-analysis based on 11,699 cases and 13,194 controls. *Leukemia Research*, *38*(3), 269–274. doi:10.1016/j.leukres.2013.12.008.
20. Houldcroft, C. J., & Kellam, P. (2015). Host genetics of Epstein-Barr virus infection, latency and disease. *Reviews in Medical Virology*, *25*(2), 71–84. doi:10.1002/rmv.1816.
21. Simard, E. P., Pfeiffer, R. M., & Engels, E. A. (2012). Mortality due to cancer among people with AIDS: A novel approach using registry-linkage data and population attributable risk methods. *AIDS (London, England)*, *26*(10), 1311–1318. doi:10.1097/QAD.0b013e328353f38e.
22. Canadian Partnership Against Cancer Corporation. (2017). *Canadian cancer trials*. Retrieved from http://www.canadiancancertrials.ca.
23. Adolescent and Young Adult Oncology Press Review Group, LiveStrong Young Adult Alliance. (2006). *Closing the gap: Research and care imperatives for adolescents and young adults with cancer*. Bethesda, MD: National Cancer Institute. Retrieved from http://planning.cancer.gov/library/AYAO_PRG_Report_2006_FINAL.pdf.

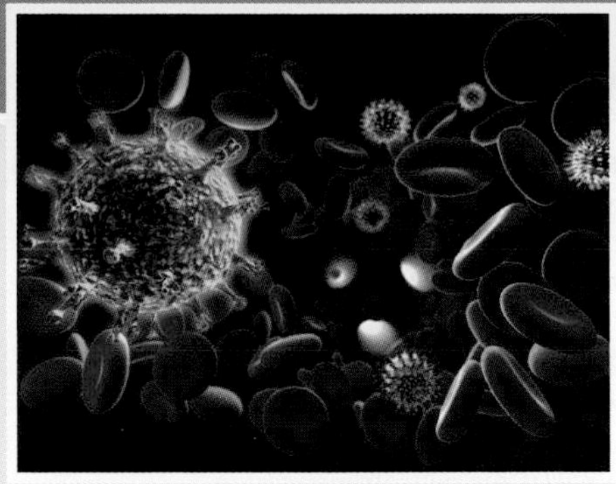

13

Structure and Function of the Neurological System

Lynne M. Kerr, Sue E. Huether, Richard A. Sugerman, and Kelly Power-Kean*

EVOLVE WEBSITE

http://evolve.elsevier.com/Canada/Huether/pathophysiology
Student Review Questions
Key Points
Case Studies
Animations
Quick Check Answers

CHAPTER OUTLINE

Overview and Organization of the Nervous System, 309
Cells of the Nervous System, 309
The Neuron, 310
Neuroglia and Schwann Cells, 310
Nerve Injury and Regeneration, 311
The Nerve Impulse, 313
Synapses, 313
Neurotransmitters, 313
The Central Nervous System, 313
The Brain, 313
The Spinal Cord, 320
Motor Pathways, 322
Sensory Pathways, 322
Protective Structures of the Central Nervous System, 323
Blood Supply of the Central Nervous System, 325
The Peripheral Nervous System, 327
The Autonomic Nervous System, 328
Anatomy of the Sympathetic Nervous System, 328
Anatomy of the Parasympathetic Nervous System, 331
Neurotransmitters and Neuroreceptors, 331
Functions of the Autonomic Nervous System, 331
***GERIATRIC CONSIDERATIONS:* Aging and the Nervous System, 335**

The human nervous system is a remarkable structure responsible for decision making, for the body's ability to interact with the environment, and for the regulation and control of activities involving our internal organs. It is a network composed of complex structures that transmit electrical and chemical signals between the brain and the body's many organs and tissues. Aging changes occur throughout life and vary among individuals (see the *Geriatric Considerations:* Aging and the Nervous System box). This chapter provides a basic overview of the structure and function of the nervous system and supports the understanding of nervous system pathophysiology in the following chapters.

OVERVIEW AND ORGANIZATION OF THE NERVOUS SYSTEM

Although the nervous system functions as a unified whole, structures and functions have been divided here to facilitate understanding. Structurally, the nervous system is divided into the central nervous system and the peripheral nervous system. The **central nervous system (CNS)** consists of the brain and spinal cord, enclosed within the protective cranial vault and vertebrae, respectively. The **peripheral nervous system (PNS)** is composed of the **cranial nerves** and the spinal nerves and their ganglia. Peripheral nerve pathways are differentiated into **afferent pathways (ascending pathways)**, which carry sensory impulses toward the CNS, and **efferent pathways (descending pathways)**, which innervate skeletal muscle or effector organs by transmitting motor impulses away from the CNS.

Functionally, the PNS can be divided into the somatic nervous system and the autonomic nervous system. The **somatic nervous system** consists of pathways that regulate voluntary motor control (e.g., skeletal muscle). The **autonomic nervous system (ANS)** is involved with regulation of the body's internal environment (viscera) through involuntary control of organ systems. The ANS is further divided into sympathetic and parasympathetic divisions. Organs innervated by specific components of the nervous system are called **effector organs**.

CELLS OF THE NERVOUS SYSTEM

Two basic types of cells constitute nervous tissue: neurons and supporting non-neuronal cells. The **neuron** is the primary cell of the nervous system. It is an electrically excitable cell and transmits information. Cells, such as **neuroglial cells** (astrocytes, microglia, and oligodendrocytes in the CNS) and **Schwann (neurilemma) cells** and **satellite cells** (in the PNS), provide structural support, protection, and nutrition for the neurons.

*Dr. Richard A. Sugerman contributed to this chapter in the US 5th edition.

The Neuron

Working alone or in units, neurons detect environmental changes and initiate body responses to maintain a dynamic steady state. Neuronal size and structure vary markedly, so that each neuron is adapted to perform specialized functions. The fuel source for the neuron is predominantly glucose. Insulin, however, is not required for cellular glucose uptake in the CNS. The cellular constituents of neurons include microtubules (which transport substances within the cell), neurofibrils (very thin supportive fibres that extend throughout the neuron), microfilaments (thought to be involved in transport of cellular products), and Nissl substances (endoplasmic reticulum and ribosomes; involved in protein synthesis).

A neuron (Figure 13-1) has three components: a cell body (soma), the dendrites (thin branching fibres of the cell), and the axons. Most cell bodies are located within the CNS; those in the PNS usually are found in groups called ganglia (or plexuses—a group of relay nerves). The dendrites are extensions that carry nerve impulses toward the cell body. Axons are long, conductive projections that carry nerve impulses away from the cell body. The axon hillock is the cone-shaped process where the axon leaves the cell body. The first part of the axon hillock has the lowest threshold for stimulation, so action potentials begin there. A typical neuron has only one axon, which may be wrapped with a segmented layer of lipid material called myelin, an insulating substance that speeds impulse propagation. This entire membrane is referred to as the myelin sheath (Figures 13-2 and 13-25, *B*). The myelin sheaths are interrupted at regular intervals by the nodes of Ranvier. Axons can branch at the nodes of Ranvier. In the CNS, myelin is produced by oligodendrocytes. In the PNS, myelin is produced by Schwann cells. Telodendria form presynaptic vesicles for neurotransmission.

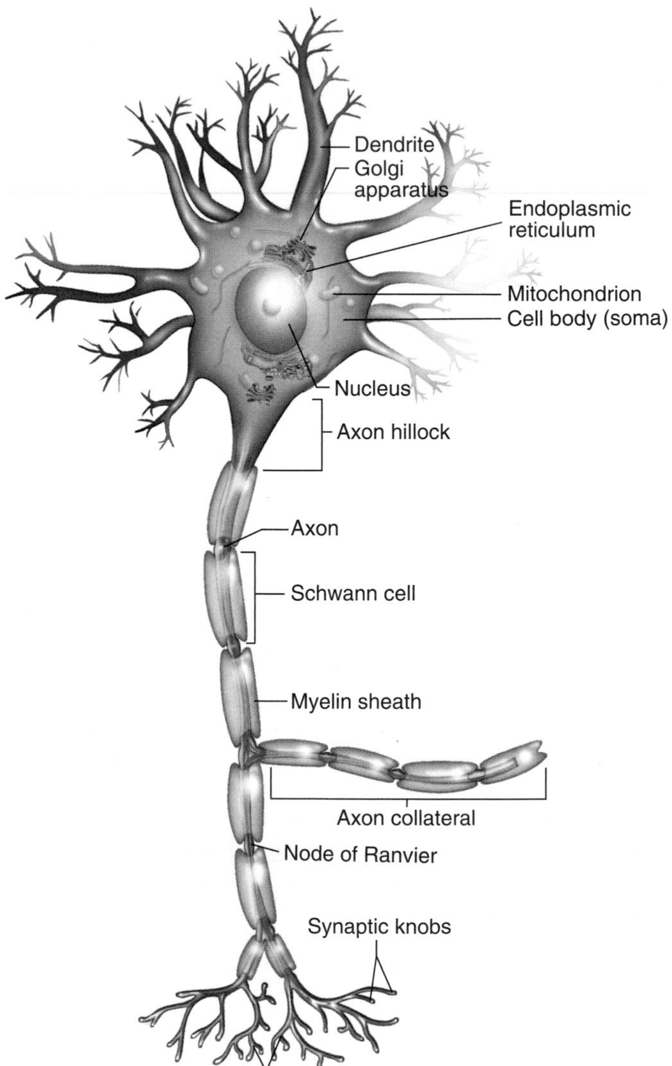

FIGURE 13-1 Neuron With Composite Parts. Multipolar neuron: PNS neuron with multiple extensions from the cell body. *PNS*, peripheral nervous system. (Modified from Patton, K.T., Thibodeau, G.A., & Douglas, M.M. [2012]. *Essentials of anatomy & physiology.* St. Louis: Mosby.)

The principle of *divergence* refers to the ability of axonal branches to influence many different neurons. *Convergence* applies when branches of various numbers of neurons "converge" on and influence a single neuron. Nutrient exchange is not possible through the myelin sheath, although it can occur at the nodes of Ranvier where the axon is not insulated. Where there is myelin, the velocity of nerve impulses increases. Myelin acts as an insulator that allows an action potential to leap between segments rather than flow along the entire length of the membrane, yielding the increased velocity. This mechanism is referred to as saltatory conduction. Disorders of the myelin sheath (demyelinating diseases), such as multiple sclerosis and Guillain-Barré syndrome, demonstrate the important role myelin plays in nerve conduction (see Chapter 16). Conduction velocities depend not only on the myelin coating but also on the diameter of the axon. Larger axons transmit impulses at a faster rate.

Neurons are structurally classified on the basis of the number of processes (projections) extending from the cell body. There are four basic types of cell configuration: (1) unipolar, (2) pseudounipolar, (3) bipolar, and (4) multipolar. Unipolar neurons have one process that branches shortly after leaving the cell body. One example is found in the retina. Pseudounipolar neurons (some authors call them *unipolar*) also have one process; the dendritic portion of each of these neurons extends away from the CNS, and the axon portion projects into the CNS (see Figure 13-2). This configuration is typical of sensory neurons in both cranial and spinal nerves. Bipolar neurons have two distinct processes arising from the cell body. This type of neuron connects the rod and cone cells of the retina. Multipolar neurons are the most common and have multiple processes capable of extensive branching. A motor neuron is typically multipolar (see Figure 13-2).

Functionally, there are three types of neurons (their direction of transmission and typical configuration are noted in parentheses): (1) sensory (afferent, mostly pseudounipolar), (2) associational (interneurons, multipolar), and (3) motor (efferent, multipolar). Sensory neurons carry impulses from peripheral sensory receptors to the CNS. Associational neurons (interneurons) transmit impulses from neuron to neuron—that is, from sensory to motor neurons. They are located solely within the CNS. Motor neurons transmit impulses away from the CNS to an effector (i.e., skeletal muscle or organs). In skeletal muscle the end processes form a neuromuscular (myoneural) junction (see Figure 13-15).

Neuroglia and Schwann Cells

Neuroglia ("nerve glue") are the general classification of non-neuronal cells that support the neurons of the CNS. They comprise approximately half of the total brain and spinal cord volume and are 5 to 10 times more numerous than neurons. Different types of neuroglia serve different functions. Astrocytes, for example, surround blood vessels, fill the spaces between neurons, and contribute to synaptic function in the CNS.[1] Oligodendroglia (oligodendrocytes) form myelin sheaths within the CNS. Ependymal cells line the cerebrospinal fluid (CSF)–filled cavities of the CNS. Microglia remove debris (phagocytosis) in the CNS. Schwann

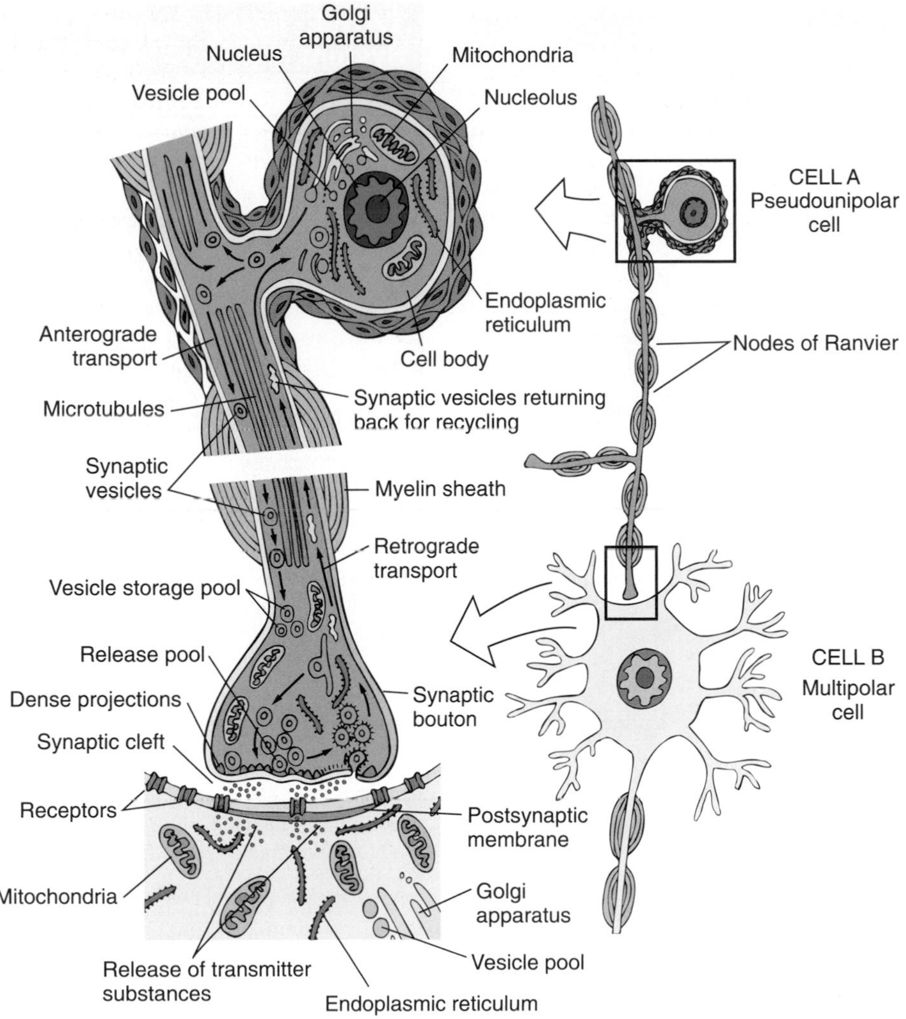

FIGURE 13-2 Neuronal Transmission and Synaptic Cleft. Electrical impulse travels along axon of first neuron (presynaptic cell) to synapse. Chemical transmitter is secreted into synaptic space to depolarize membrane (dendrite or cell body) of next neuron (postsynaptic cell) in pathway. *Cell A* represents pseudounipolar cell; *cell B* represents multipolar cell.

cells form the myelin sheath around axons and direct axonal regrowth and functional recovery in the PNS.[2] **Nonmyelinating Schwann cells** provide metabolic support. (Characteristics of neuroglia and Schwann cells are summarized in Figure 13-3 and Table 13-1.)

Nerve Injury and Regeneration

Mature nerve cells do not divide, and injury can cause permanent loss of function. When an axon is severed, **Wallerian degeneration** occurs in the distal axon: (1) a characteristic swelling appears within the portion of the axon distal to the cut; (2) the neurofilaments hypertrophy; (3) the myelin sheath shrinks and disintegrates; and (4) the axon degenerates and disappears. The myelin sheaths re-form into Schwann cells that align in a column between the severed part of the axon and the effector organ.

At the proximal end of the injured axon, similar changes occur but only back to the next node of Ranvier. The cell body responds to trauma by swelling and dying by chromatolysis (dispersing the Nissl substance) or apoptosis. During the repair process, the cell increases protein synthesis and mitochondrial activity. Approximately 7 to 14 days after the injury, new terminal sprouts project from the proximal segment and may enter the remaining Schwann cell pathway. (Figure 13-4 contains a more detailed representation of these events.) This process, however, is limited to myelinated fibres and generally occurs only in the PNS. The regeneration of axonal constituents in the CNS is limited by an increased incidence of scar formation and the different nature of myelin formed by the oligodendrocyte.

Nerve regeneration depends on many factors, such as location of the injury, the type of injury, the presence of inflammatory responses, and the process of scarring. The closer to the cell body of the nerve, the greater the chances that the nerve cell will die and not regenerate. A crushing injury allows recovery more fully than does a cut injury. Crushed nerves sometimes recover fully, whereas cut nerves form connective tissue scars that block or slow regenerating axonal branches. Peripheral nerves injured close to the spinal cord recover poorly and slowly because of the long distance between the cell body and the peripheral termination of the axon.[3]

QUICK CHECK 13-1

1. How do the functions of the somatic and autonomic nervous systems differ?
2. What are the three components of a neuron?
3. How does myelin affect nerve impulses?
4. Name the process through which injured axons are repaired, and describe the process.

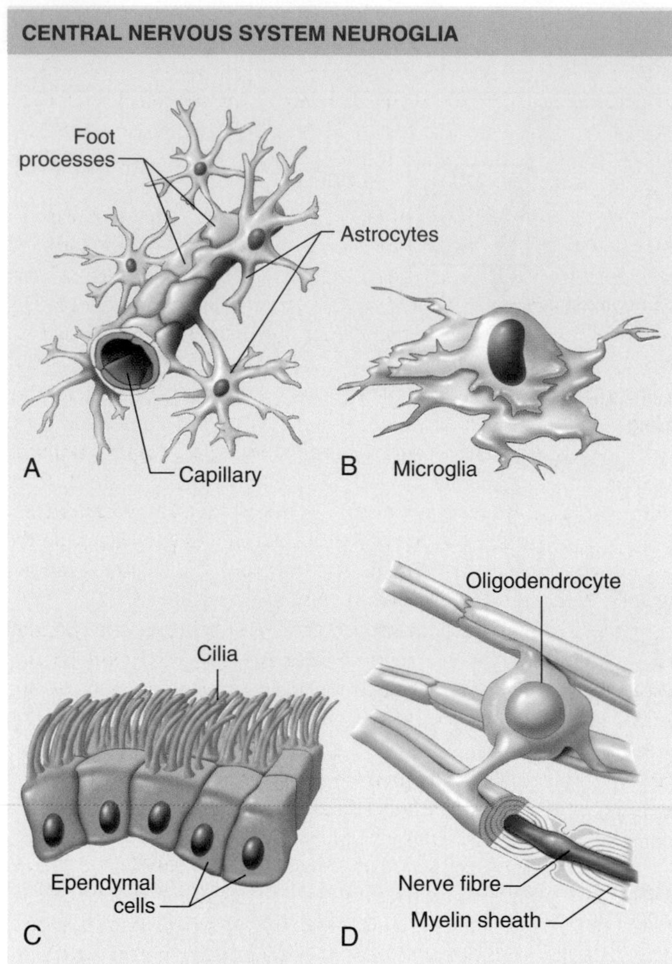

FIGURE 13-3 Types of Neuroglial Cells. Central nervous system (CNS) neuroglia: **A,** Astrocytes attached to the outside of a capillary blood vessel in the brain. **B,** A phagocytic microglial cell. **C,** Ciliated ependymal cells forming a sheet that usually lines fluid cavities in the brain. **D,** An oligodendrocyte with processes that wrap around nerve fibres in the CNS to form myelin sheaths. Peripheral nervous system (PNS) neuroglia: **E,** A Schwann cell supporting a bundle of nerve fibres in the PNS. **F,** Another type of Schwann cell encircling a peripheral nerve fibre to form a thick myelin sheath. (From Patton, K.T., Thibodeau, G.A., & Douglas, M.M. [2012]. *Essentials of anatomy & physiology*. St. Louis: Mosby.)

TABLE 13-1 Support Cells of the Nervous System

Cell Type	Primary Functions
Astrocytes	Form specialized contacts between neuronal surfaces and blood vessels Provide rapid transport for nutrients and metabolites Are thought to form an essential component of blood–brain barrier Appear to be scar-forming cells of CNS, which may be foci for seizures Appear to work with neurons in processing information and memory storage
Oligodendroglia (oligodendrocytes)	Form the myelin sheath in CNS
Schwann cells	Form the myelin sheath in PNS
Nonmyelinating Schwann cells	Provide neuronal metabolic support and regeneration in PNS
Microglia	Are responsible for clearing cellular debris (phagocytic properties)
Ependymal cells	Serve as a lining for ventricles and choroid plexuses involved in production of cerebrospinal fluid

CNS, central nervous system; *PNS*, peripheral nervous system.
Data from Martinez Banaclocha, M.A. (2005). *Int J Neurosci, 115*(3), 329–337; Sofroniew, M.V., & Vinters, H.V. (2010). *Acta Neuropathol, 119*(1), 7–35; Vanderah, T., & Gould, D. (2015). *Nolte's The human brain: An introduction to its functional anatomy* (7th ed.). St. Louis: Mosby.

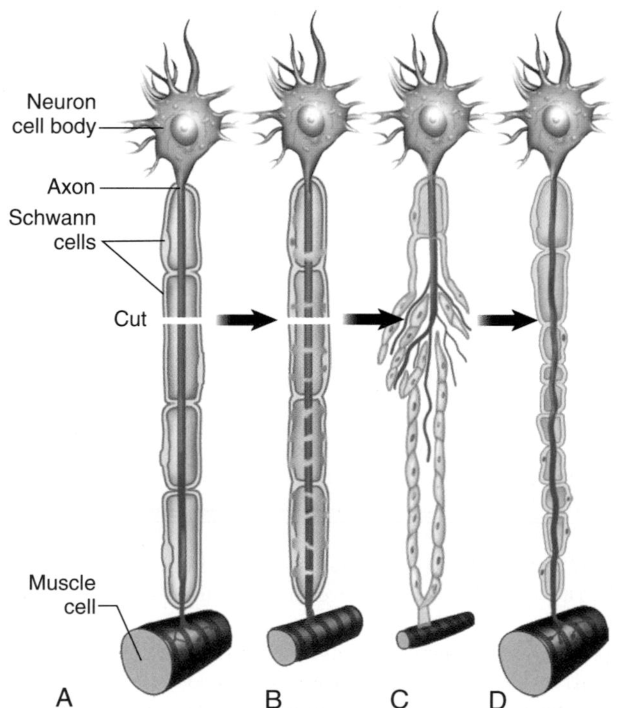

FIGURE 13-4 Repair of a Peripheral Nerve Fibre. When cut, a damaged motor axon can regrow to its distal connection only if the Schwann cells remain intact (to form a guiding tunnel) and if scar tissue does not block its way. (From Patton, K.T., & Thibodeau, G.A. [2013]. *Anatomy & physiology* [8th ed.]. St. Louis: Mosby.)

THE NERVE IMPULSE

Neurons generate and conduct electrical and chemical impulses by selectively changing the electrical potential of the plasma membrane and influencing other nearby neurons by releasing chemicals (**neurotransmitters**). An unexcited neuron maintains a resting membrane potential. When the membrane potential is sufficiently raised, an action potential is generated and the nerve impulse then flows to all parts of the neuron. The action potential response occurs only when the stimulus is strong enough; if it is too weak, the membrane remains unexcited. This property is termed the *all-or-none response* (see Chapter 1 for a discussion of electrical impulse conduction).

Synapses

Neurons are not physically continuous with one another. The region between adjacent neurons is called a **synapse** (see Figure 13-2). Impulses are transmitted across the synapse by chemical and electrical conduction (see Figure 13-2); only chemical conduction is discussed here. Chapter 1 contains information on electrical conduction (see Figure 1-29). The neurons that conduct a nerve impulse are named according to whether they relay impulses toward (**presynaptic neurons**) or away from (**postsynaptic neurons**) the synapse. When an impulse originates in a presynaptic neuron, the impulse reaches the vesicles, where chemicals (neurotransmitters) are stored in the **synaptic bouton**. Once released from the vesicles, the neurotransmitters diffuse across the **synaptic cleft** (the space between the neurons) and bind to specific neurotransmitter (protein) receptor sites on the plasma membrane of the postsynaptic neuron, relaying the impulse (see Figure 13-2). Brain synapses can change in strength and number throughout life, and this ability is known as synaptic plasticity, or **neuroplasticity** (see *Health Promotion:* Neuroplasticity).

HEALTH PROMOTION

Neuroplasticity

Scientists investigating neuroplasticity ask how to encourage this process of brain reorganization. Research provides important information for the improvement of health related to diseases of aging. Researchers have discovered that the adult brain continues to form novel neural connections and grow new neurons in response to learning or training as we age.

Recent research suggests that physical activity can have a major impact on brain function. It has been shown that sustained, consistent, aerobic exercise has produced major improvements in cognitive processes and brain growth. It promotes **neurogenesis** by increasing the production of **neurotrophic factors** and is also associated with improvements in spatial memory. New research aims to develop lifestyle behaviours that could improve normal brain development as well as repair damaged brains.

Although the benefits of aerobic exercise have yet to be fully investigated, substantial data support the utility of exercise for promoting brain plasticity and improving CNS function in many conditions, including normal aging and dementia. Behaviour, environmental factors, thought, and emotions may also contribute to neoplastic change, which has significant implications for healthy development, learning, memory, and recovery from brain injury.

Based on Cramer, S.A., Sur, M., Dobkin, B.H., et al. (2011). *Brain, 134*(6), 1591–1609. doi:10.1093/brain/awr039; Liou, S. (2010, June 26). *Neurobiology* [Blog post]. Retrieved from http://web.stanford.edu/group/hopes/cgi-bin/hopes_test/neuroplasticity/.

Neurotransmitters

Neurotransmitters are chemicals synthesized in the neuron and localized in the presynaptic terminal (synaptic bouton). Neurotransmitters are then released into the synaptic cleft and bind to a receptor site (binding site) on the postsynaptic membrane of another neuron or effector, where they affect ion channels (see Figure 13-2). Each neurotransmitter is removed by a specific mechanism from its site of action. Many substances are neurotransmitters, including norepinephrine, acetylcholine, dopamine, histamine, and serotonin. Many of these transmitters have more than one function.[4] Neurotransmitter and neuromodulator substances are summarized in Table 13-2.

Because the neurotransmitter is normally stored on one side of the synaptic cleft and the receptor sites are on the other side, chemical synapses operate in one direction. Therefore, action potentials are transmitted along a multineuronal pathway in one direction. The binding of the neurotransmitter at the receptor site changes the permeability of the postsynaptic neuron and, consequently, its membrane potential. Two possible scenarios can then follow: (1) the postsynaptic neuron may be excited (depolarized; **excitatory postsynaptic potentials [EPSPs]**) or (2) the postsynaptic neuron's plasma membrane may be inhibited (hyperpolarized; **inhibitory postsynaptic potentials [IPSPs]**). Cannabinoid transmitters have been discovered that are released from postsynaptic neurons and modulate neurotransmitter release from the presynaptic neurons (retrograde transmission).[5,6] (Chapter 1 reviews electrical impulses and membrane potentials.)

Usually, a single EPSP cannot induce a neuron's action potential and the propagation of the nerve impulse. Whether this response occurs depends on the number and frequency of potentials the postsynaptic neuron receives—a concept known as **summation. Temporal summation** (time relationship) refers to the effects of successive, rapid impulses received from a single neuron at the same synapse. **Spatial summation** (spacing effect) is the combined effects of impulses from a number of neurons onto a single neuron at the same time. **Facilitation** refers to the effect of EPSP on the plasma membrane potential. The plasma membrane is facilitated when summation brings the membrane closer to the threshold potential and decreases the stimulus required to induce an action potential. The effect that a chemical neurotransmitter has on the plasma membrane potential depends on the balance of these effects. The mechanisms of **convergence** (many neurons firing and converging on one neuron), **divergence** (one neuron firing and diverging on many neurons), summation, and facilitation allow for the integrative processes of the nervous system.

QUICK CHECK 13-2

1. Explain the process of the chemical conduction of impulses.
2. What are neurotransmitters? Give two examples.
3. Compare summation and facilitation.

THE CENTRAL NERVOUS SYSTEM

The Brain

The brain is a functionally integrated circuit of millions of neurons with different genomes, structures, molecular composition, networks, and connections. It weighs approximately 3 pounds and receives 15 to 20% of the total cardiac output. The brain enables a person to reason, function intellectually, express personality and mood, and perceive and interact with the environment.

The three major structural divisions of the brain are (1) the forebrain (prosencephalon), which includes the telencephalon and diencephalon; (2) the midbrain (mesencephalon), which connects the pons to the diencephalon; and (3) the hindbrain (rhombencephalon), which includes the **cerebellum**, pons, and medulla (Table 13-3 and Figure 13-5). The midbrain, medulla, and pons comprise the **brainstem**, which connects the hemispheres of the brain, cerebellum, and spinal cord. A collection of nerve cell bodies (nuclei) within the brainstem makes up the **reticular**

TABLE 13-2 Substances That Are Neurotransmitters or Neuromodulators

Substance	Location	Effect	Clinical Example
Acetylcholine	Many parts of brain, spinal cord, neuromuscular junction of skeletal muscle, and many ANS synapses	Excitatory or inhibitory	Alzheimer's disease (a type of dementia) is associated with a decrease in acetylcholine-secreting neurons. Myasthenia gravis (weakness of skeletal muscles) results from a reduction in acetylcholine receptors.
Monoamines			
Norepinephrine	Many areas of brain and spinal cord; also in some ANS synapses	Excitatory or inhibitory	Cocaine and amphetamines[a] result in overstimulation of postsynaptic neurons.
Serotonin	Many areas of brain and spinal cord	Generally inhibitory	It is involved with mood, anxiety, and sleep induction. Levels of serotonin are elevated in schizophrenia (delusions, hallucinations, withdrawal).
Dopamine	Some areas of brain and ANS synapses	Generally excitatory	Parkinson's disease (depression of voluntary motor control) results from the destruction of dopamine-secreting neurons. Medications used to increase dopamine production induce vomiting and schizophrenia.
Histamine	Posterior hypothalamus	Excitatory (H1 and H2 receptors) and inhibitory (H3 receptors)	No clear indication exists of histamine-associated pathological conditions. Histamine is involved with arousal and attention and links to other brain transmitter systems.
Amino Acids			
Gamma-aminobutyric acid (GABA)	Most neurons of CNS have GABA receptors	Majority of postsynaptic inhibition in brain	Medications that increase GABA function have been used to treat epilepsy by inhibiting excessive discharge of neurons.
Glycine	Spinal cord	Most postsynaptic inhibition in spinal cord	Glycine receptors are inhibited by strychnine.
Glutamate and aspartate	Widespread in brain and spinal cord	Excitatory	Medications that block glutamate or aspartate, such as riluzole, are used to treat amyotrophic lateral sclerosis. These medications might prevent overexcitation from seizures and neural degeneration.
Neuropeptides			
Endorphins and enkephalins	Widely distributed in CNS and PNS	Generally inhibitory	Morphine and heroin bind to endorphin and enkephalin receptors on presynaptic neurons and reduce pain by blocking the release of neurotransmitter.
Substance P	Spinal cord, brain, and sensory neurons associated with pain, gastro-intestinal tract	Generally excitatory	Substance P is a neurotransmitter in pain transmission pathways. Blocking release of substance P by morphine reduces pain.

[a]They increase the release and block the reuptake of norepinephrine.
ANS, autonomic nervous system; *CNS*, central nervous system; *PNS*, peripheral nervous system.
From Daroff, R.B., Fenichel, G.M., Jankovic, J., et al. (2012). *Bradley's neurology in clinical practice* (6th ed.). Philadelphia: Saunders.

formation (Figure 13-6). The reticular formation is a large network of diffuse nuclei that connect the brainstem to the cortex and control vital reflexes, such as cardiovascular function and respiration. It is essential for maintaining wakefulness and attention and, therefore, is referred to as the reticular activating system (RAS) (see Figure 13-6). Some nuclei within the reticular formation cause specific motor movements, such as balance and posture.[4]

Divisions of the brain are associated with different functions, but attributing specific functions to definite regions of the brain is not entirely accurate. However, for clinical considerations functional specificity is very useful for localizing pathological conditions in various nervous system regions. Dr. Brodmann, a neuropsychiatrist, is credited with postulating that various activities are correlated to many regions of the cerebral cortex.[7] (Figure 13-7, *C* illustrates these regions and describes some of the areas.) The mapping of brain networks is also helpful in discovering how varying parts of the brain are interconnected when performing a specific function[8,9] (Box 13-1).

Forebrain

Telencephalon. The telencephalon (cerebral hemispheres) consists of the cerebral cortex (the largest portion of the brain) and the basal ganglia (composed of several *nuclei*). The surface of the cerebral cortex is covered with convolutions called *gyri* (see Figure 13-7), which greatly increase the cortical surface area and the number of neurons. Grooves between adjacent gyrus are termed sulci; deeper grooves are termed *fissures*. The cerebral cortex contains an outer layer of cell bodies of neurons (grey matter). White matter lies beneath the cerebral cortex and is composed of myelinated nerve fibres.

TABLE 13-3 Divisions of the Central Nervous System

Primary Brain Vesicles	Secondary Vesicles	Structures in Secondary Vesicles
Forebrain (prosencephalon)	Telencephalon	Cerebral hemispheres Cerebral cortex Basal ganglia
	Diencephalon	Epithalamus Thalamus Hypothalamus Subthalamus
Midbrain (mesencephalon)	Mesencephalon	Corpora quadrigemina (tectum–superior and inferior colliculi) Cerebral peduncles
Hindbrain (rhombencephalon)	Metencephalon	Cerebellum Pons
	Myelencephalon	Medulla oblongata
Spinal cord	Spinal cord	Spinal cord

BOX 13-1 Brain Networks

The architecture and integrated function of neural nodes, networks, and interconnected pathways within the brain are being mapped in the advancing field of human connectomics. Imaging techniques include positron emission tomography (PET; it measures pairs of gamma rays emitted by an introduced positron-emitting radionuclide), tracer diffusion tensor magnetic resonance imaging (MRI; it measures diffusion of water in tissue), functional MRI (it measures changes in blood flow), magnetoencephalography (MEG; it measures magnetic fields produced by electric currents generated by neurons), and electroencephalography (EEG, it measures voltage changes in brain neurons), which are combined with mathematical and computational models.

The figure that follows provides an illustration of brain connectivity showing interconnecting cortical pathways using diffusion tensor imaging tracking technology. Such mapping of the brain contributes to an understanding of the commonalities and individual differences of the normally functioning brain and changes associated with aging and disease (i.e., degenerative brain disease, epilepsy, schizophrenia, and brain tumours).

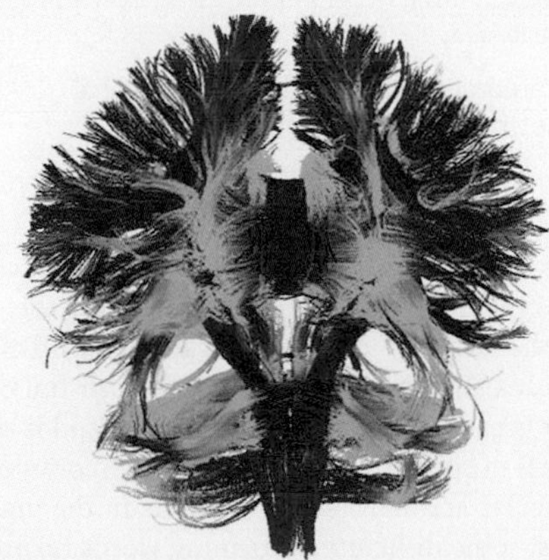

(Reprinted from *The Lancet Neurology*, 12[12], Filippi, M., "Assessment of system dysfunction in the brain through MRI-based connectomics," Pages 1189–1199, Copyright 2013, with permission from Elsevier.)

From Park, H.J., & Friston, K. (2013). *Science, 342*(6158), 1238411; Pollock, J.D., Wu, D.-Y., & Satterlee, J. (2014). *Trends Neurosci, 37*(2), 106–123; Sporns, O. (2013). *Neuroimage, 80*, 53–61; see also the Human Connectome Project at http://humanconnectome.org/about/project/.

FIGURE 13-5 Structural Divisions of the Brain. (From Standring, S., [Ed.]. [2008]. *Gray's anatomy: The anatomical basis of clinical practice* [40th ed.]. Edinburgh: Churchill Livingstone.)

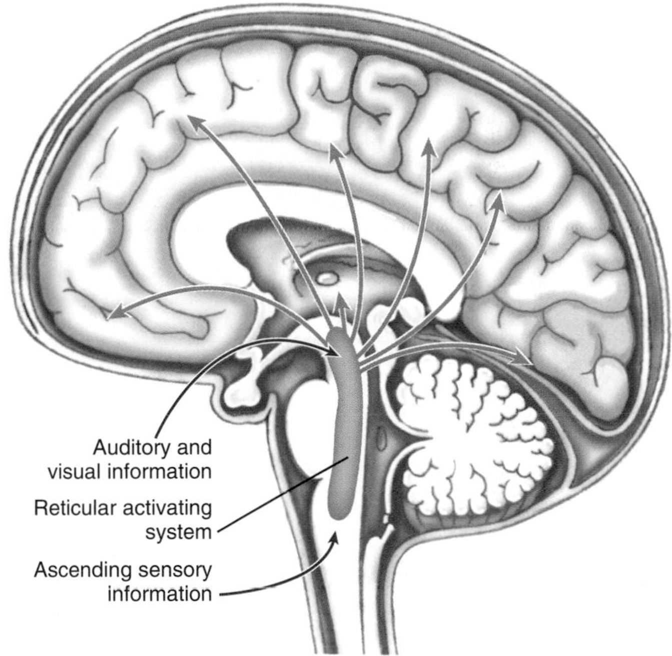

FIGURE 13-6 Reticular Activating System. The reticular activating system (RAS) consists of nuclei in the brainstem reticular formation plus fibres that conduct sensory information to the nuclei and fibres that conduct from the nuclei to widespread areas of the cerebral cortex. Functioning of the RAS is essential for consciousness.

The two cerebral hemispheres are separated by a deep groove known as the **longitudinal fissure**. The surface of each hemisphere is divided into lobes named after the region of the skull under which each lobe lies. The posterior margin of the **frontal lobe** is on the **central sulcus (fissure of Rolando)**, and it borders inferiorly on the **lateral sulcus (sylvian fissure, lateral fissure)** (see Figure 13-7). The **prefrontal area** is responsible for goal-oriented behaviour (e.g., the ability to concentrate), short-term or recall memory, the elaboration of thought, and inhibition of the limbic areas of the CNS. The **premotor area (Brodmann area 6)** (see Figure 13-7, *C*) is involved in programming motor movements. This area contains the cell bodies that form part of the **basal ganglia system (extrapyramidal system**—efferent pathways outside the pyramids of the medulla oblongata). The frontal eye fields (the lower portion of

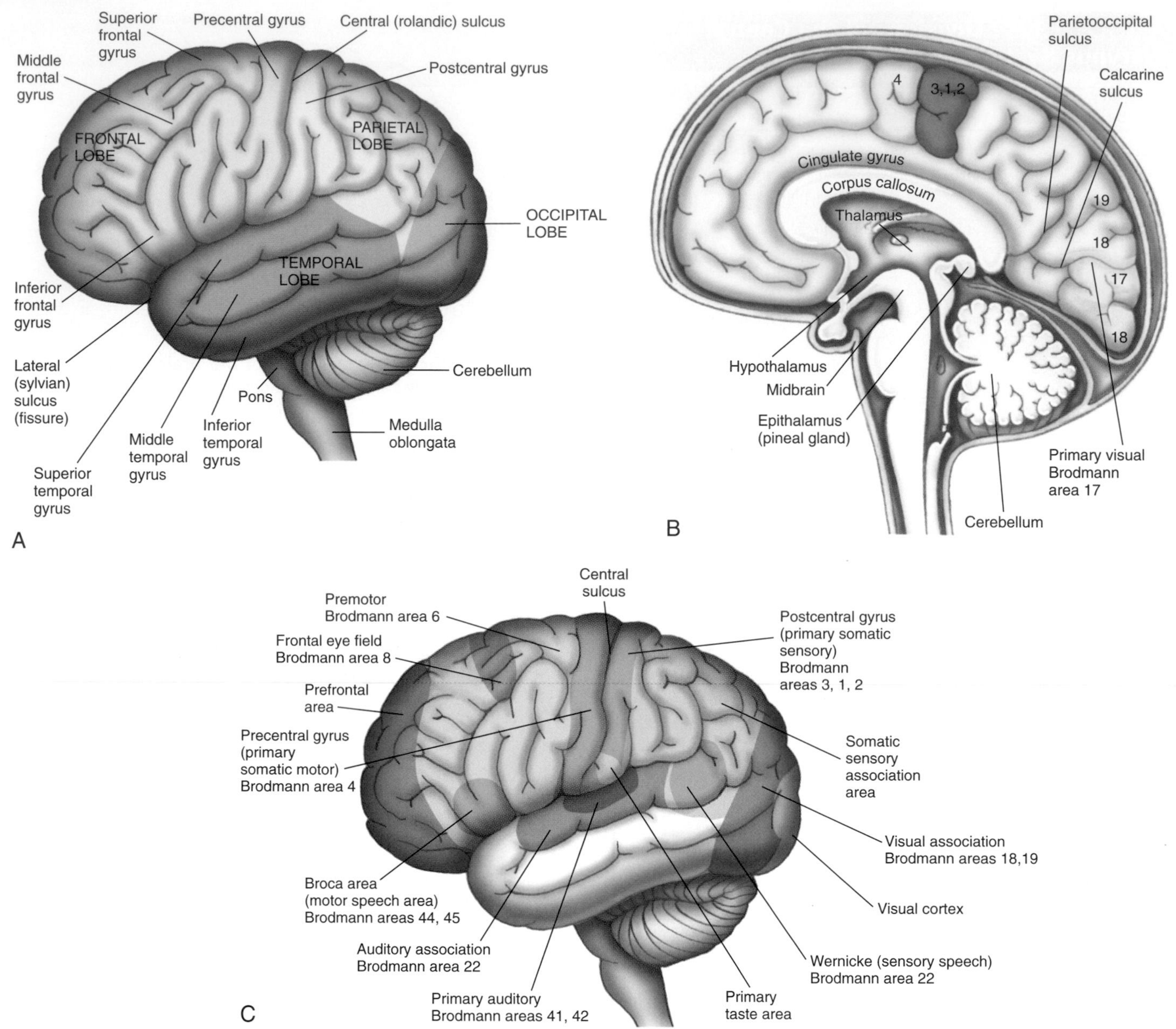

FIGURE 13-7 The Cerebral Hemispheres. **A,** Left hemisphere of cerebrum, lateral view. **B,** Functional areas of the cerebral cortex, midsagittal view. **C,** Functional areas of the cerebral cortex, lateral view.

Brodmann area 8), which are involved in controlling eye movements, are located on the middle frontal gyrus.

The **primary motor area (Brodmann area 4)** is located along the **precentral gyrus** forming the **primary voluntary motor area**, which has a somatotopic organization that is often referred to as a *homunculus* (little human) (Figure 13-8). Electrical stimulation of specific areas of this cortex causes specific muscles of the body to move. For example, stimulation of Brodmann area 4 in the medial longitudinal fissure affects the lower limb and foot, whereas stimulation of the superior lateral surface of the precentral gyrus affects the torso and arm, the middle third of the hand, and the lower third of the face and the mouth and throat. The axons travelling from the cell bodies in and on either side of this gyrus project fibres (axons) that form the **pyramidal system**. This system includes the **corticobulbar tract** that synapses in the brainstem and provides voluntary control of muscles in the head and neck, and the **corticospinal tracts (pyramidal system)** that descend into the spinal cord and provide voluntary control of muscles throughout the body. Cerebral impulses control function on the opposite side of the body, a phenomenon called **contralateral control** (Figure 13-9, *A*). The **Broca area (Brodmann areas 44, 45)** is rostral on the inferior frontal gyrus. It is usually on the left hemisphere and is responsible for the motor aspects of speech. Damage to this area, commonly as a result of a cerebrovascular accident (stroke), results in the inability to form words or at least some difficulty in forming words (expressive aphasia or dysphasia) (see Chapter 15).

The **parietal lobe** lies within the borders of the central, parietooccipital, and lateral sulci. This lobe contains the major area for somatic sensory input, located primarily along the **postcentral gyrus** (Brodmann areas 3, 1, 2) (see Figure 13-7), which is adjacent to the primary motor area. Communication between the motor and sensory areas (and among other regions in the cortex) is provided by **association fibres**. Much of this region is involved in sensory association (storage, analysis, and

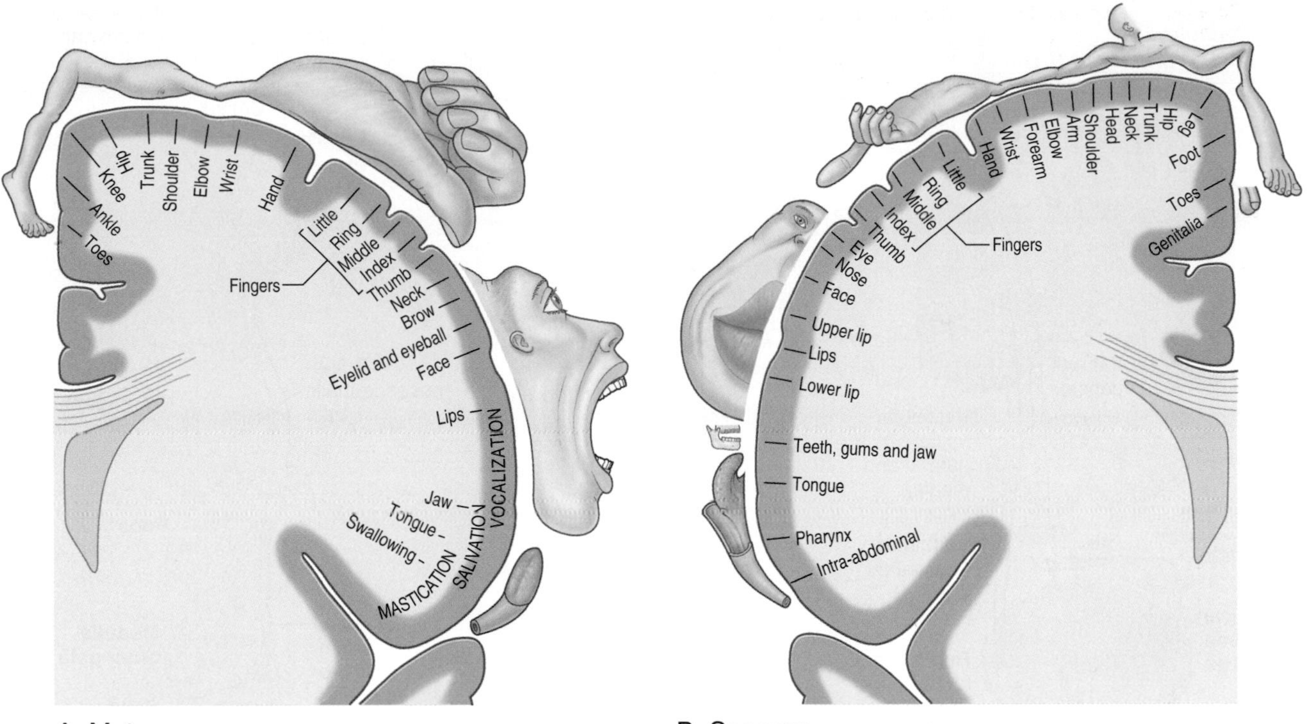

FIGURE 13-8 Primary Somatic Motor and Sensory Areas of the Cortex. A, The motor homunculus shows proportional somatotopical representation in the main motor area. **B,** The sensory homunculus shows proportional somatotopical representation in the somaesthetic cortex. (From Standring, S. [Ed.]. [2008]. *Gray's Anatomy: The anatomical basis of clinical practice* [40th ed.]. Edinburgh: Churchill Livingstone.)

interpretation of stimuli). (Figure 13-8 shows the distribution of functions associated with both the primary motor area and the primary sensory area of the cerebral cortex.)

The **occipital lobe** lies caudal to the parietooccipital sulcus and is superior to the cerebellum. The primary visual cortex (Brodmann area 17) is located in this region and receives input from the retinas. Much of the remainder of this lobe is involved in visual association (Brodmann areas 18, 19). The **temporal lobe** lies inferior to the lateral fissure and is composed of the superior, middle, and inferior temporal gyri. The primary auditory cortex (Brodmann area 41) and its related association area (Brodmann area 42) lie deep within the lateral sulcus on the superior temporal gyrus. The **Wernicke area**, along with adjacent portions of the parietal lobe, constitutes a *sensory speech area*. This area is responsible for reception and interpretation of speech, and dysfunction may result in receptive aphasia or dysphasia. The temporal lobe also is involved in memory consolidation and smell.

Another lobe, the **insula (insular lobe)**, lies hidden from view in the lateral sulci between the temporal and frontal lobes of each hemisphere. The insula processes sensory and emotional information and routes the information to other areas of the brain. Lying directly beneath the longitudinal fissure is a mass of white matter pathways called the **corpus callosum (transverse or commissural fibres)**. This structure connects the two cerebral hemispheres through sensory and motor contralateral projection of axons and is essential in coordinating activities between hemispheres (see Figure 13-7).

Inside the cerebrum are numerous tracts (white matter) and nuclei (grey matter). The major **cerebral nuclei** are called the **basal ganglia (basal nuclei)** system. The basal ganglia system is a group of nuclei that includes the **caudate nucleus**, **putamen**, and **globus pallidus**. The putamen and globus pallidus together are called the **lentiform nucleus**. The caudate nucleus and putamen together are called the **striatum**[7] (Figure 13-10). Other structures in the basal ganglia include the *substantia nigra*, the *nucleus accumbens*, and the *subthalamic nucleus*. The nuclei of the basal ganglia are important for voluntary movement and cognitive and emotional functions.

The **internal capsule** is a thick layer of white matter in which axons of afferent (sensory) and efferent (motor) pathways pass to and from the cerebral cortex through the centre of the cerebral hemispheres and between the caudate and lentiform nuclei (Figure 13-10, *B*).

The basal ganglia plus their direct and indirect interconnections with the thalamus, premotor cortex, red nucleus, reticular formation, and spinal cord have been considered part of the extrapyramidal system. The **extrapyramidal system** is a part of the motor control system that causes involuntary reflexes and movement and has a stabilizing effect on motor control. Parkinson's disease (substantia nigra) and Huntington's disease (striatum) are characterized by various involuntary or exaggerated motor movements (see Chapter 15).

The **limbic system** is a group of interconnected structures located between the telencephalon and diencephalon and surrounding the corpus callosum. It is composed of the amygdala, hippocampus, fornix, hypothalamus, and related autonomic nuclei (see Figure 13-10). It is an extension or modification of the olfactory system and influences the autonomic and endocrine systems. The limbic system mediates emotion and long-term memory through connections in the prefrontal cortex (limbic cortex). Its principal effects are involved in primitive behavioural responses, visceral reaction to emotion, motivation, mood, feeding behaviours, biological rhythms, and the sense of smell.

Diencephalon. The **diencephalon (interbrain)**, surrounded by the cerebrum and sitting on top of the brainstem, has four divisions: **epithalamus**, **thalamus**, **hypothalamus**, and **subthalamus** (see Table 13-3 and Figure 13-7). The epithalamus forms the roof of the third ventricle (a brain cavity) and composes the most superior portion of

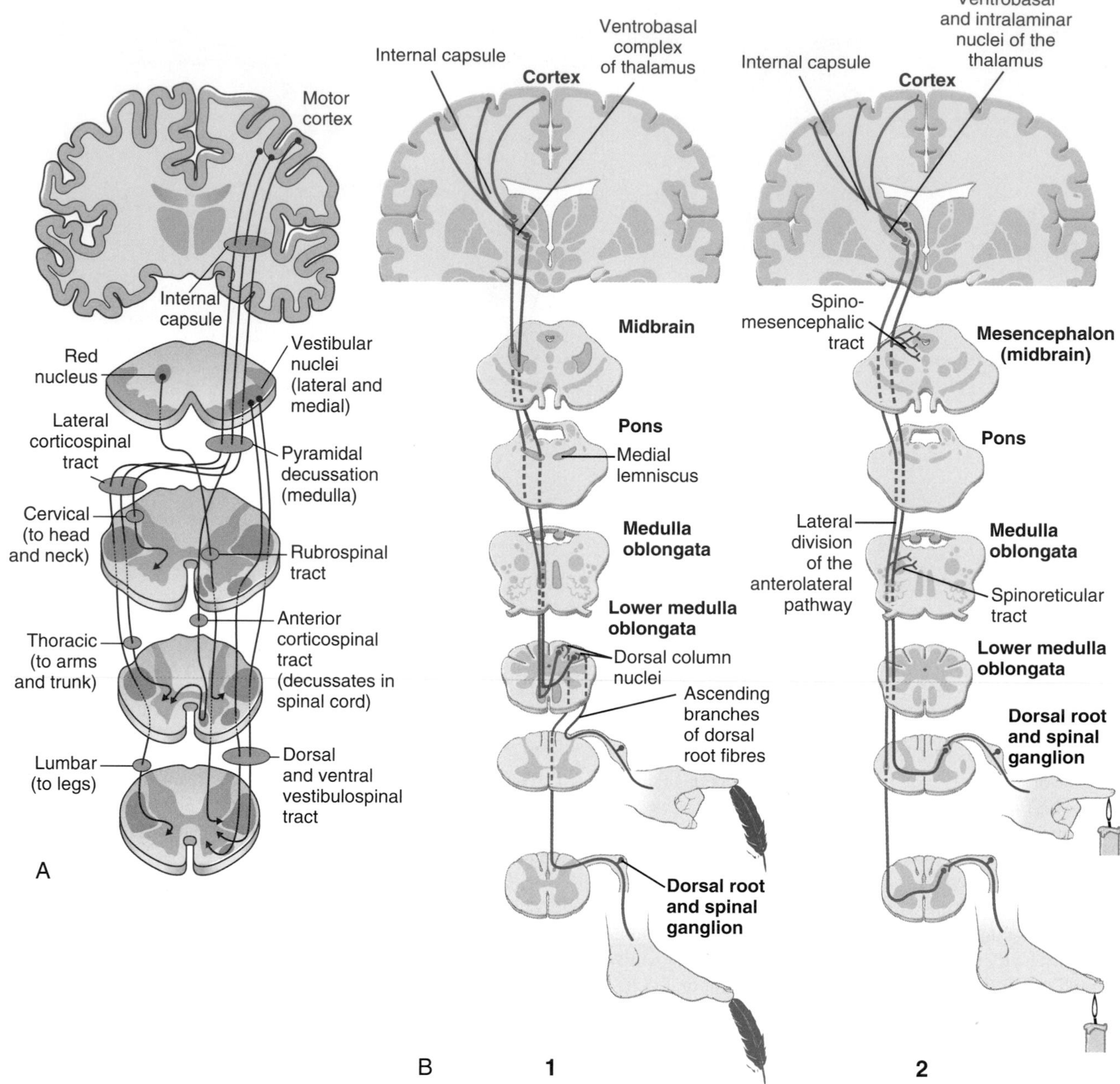

FIGURE 13-9 Examples of Somatic Motor and Sensory Pathways. A, Motor tracts. The pyramidal pathway through the lateral corticospinal tract and the extrapyramidal pathways through the rubrospinal, reticulospinal, and vestibulospinal tracts. **B,** Sensory tracts. **1,** The dorsal column-medial lemniscal pathway for transmitting critical types of tactile signals: touch and proprioception. Note the lateral corticospinal tract decussation is in the lower medulla. **2,** Anterior and lateral divisions of the anterolateral sensory pathway: pain and temperature. Note the decussation is in the spinal cord. (**A,** from Compston, A., McDonald, I., Noseworthy, J., et al. [2006]. *McAlpine's multiple sclerosis* [4th ed.]. London: Churchill Livingstone. **B,** from Hall, J.E. [2016]. *Guyton and Hall textbook of medical physiology* [13th ed.]. Philadelphia: Saunders.)

the diencephalon. The diencephalon controls vital functions and visceral activities and is closely associated with those of the limbic system.

The thalamus borders and surrounds the third ventricle. It is a major integrating centre for afferent impulses to the cerebral cortex. Various sensations are perceived at this level, but cortical processing is required for interpretation. The thalamus serves also as a relay centre for information from the basal ganglia and cerebellum to the appropriate motor area.

The hypothalamus forms the base of the diencephalon. The hypothalamus functions to (1) maintain a constant internal environment and (2) implement behavioural patterns. Integrative centres control ANS function, regulate body temperature and endocrine function, and adjust emotional expression. The hypothalamus exerts its influence through the endocrine system, as well as through neural pathways (Box 13-2). The subthalamus flanks the hypothalamus laterally. It serves as an important basal ganglia centre for motor activities.

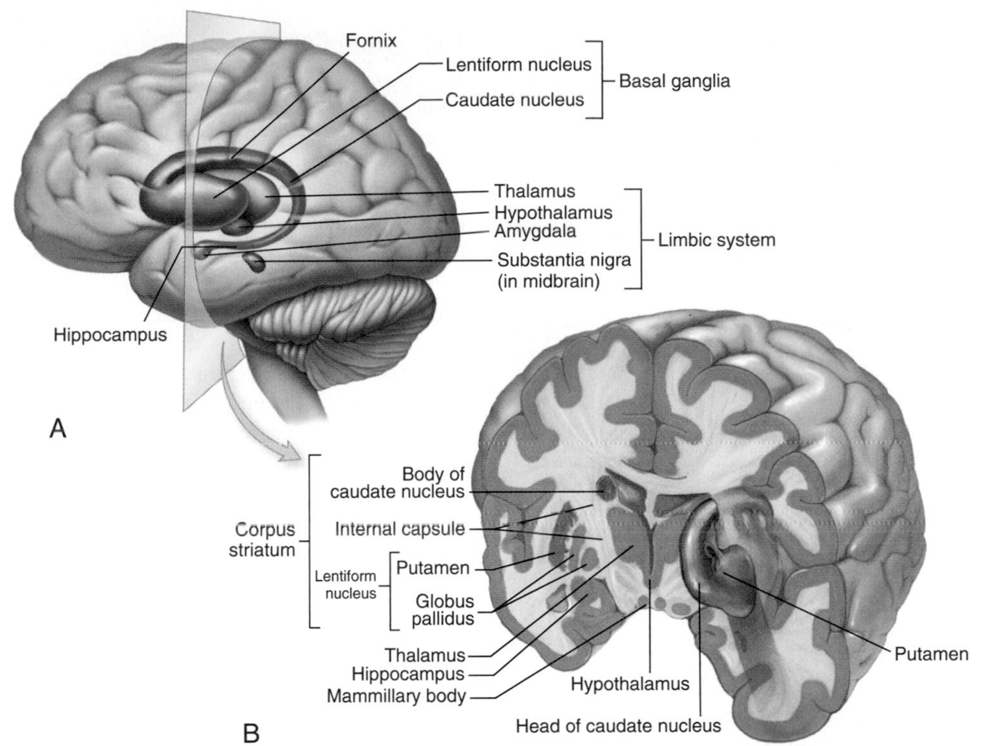

FIGURE 13-10 Basal Ganglia. A, The basal ganglia seen through the cortex of the left cerebral hemisphere. B, The basal ganglia seen in a frontal (coronal) section of the brain. (From Patton, K.T., & Thibodeau, G.A. [2016]. *Anatomy & physiology* [9th ed.]. St. Louis: Mosby.)

BOX 13-2 Functions of the Hypothalamus

- Visceral and somatic responses
- Affectual responses
- Hormone synthesis
- Sympathetic and parasympathetic activity
- Temperature regulation
- Fluid balance
- Appetite and feeding responses
- Physical expression of emotions
- Sexual behaviour
- Pleasure–punishment centres
- Level of arousal or wakefulness

Midbrain

Mesencephalon. The midbrain (mesencephalon) is composed of three structures: the corpora quadrigemina (located on the tectum, the ceiling of the midbrain), which is composed of the two pairs of superior colliculi and two pairs of inferior colliculi; the tegmentum (the floor of the midbrain), which is composed of the red nucleus, substantia nigra, and the basis pedunculi. The tegmentum and basis pedunculi are collectively called the cerebral peduncles.

The superior colliculi are involved with voluntary and involuntary visual motor movements (e.g., the ability of the eyes to track moving objects in the visual field). The inferior colliculi accomplish similar motor activities but involve movements affecting the auditory system (e.g., positioning the head to improve hearing). The red nucleus receives ascending sensory information from the cerebellum and projects a minor motor pathway, the rubrospinal tract, to the cervical spinal cord. The last portion of the basal ganglia is the substantia nigra, which synthesizes dopamine, a neurotransmitter and precursor of norepinephrine. Its dysfunction is associated with Parkinson's disease and schizophrenia. The basis pedunculi are made up of efferent fibres of the corticospinal, corticobulbar, and corticopontocerebellar tracts.

Other notable structures of this region are the nuclei of the third and fourth cranial nerves. The cerebral aqueduct (aqueduct of Sylvius), which carries CSF, also traverses this structure. Obstruction of this aqueduct is often the cause of hydrocephalus.

Hindbrain

Metencephalon. The major structures of the metencephalon are the cerebellum and the pons. The cerebellum (see Figure 13-7) is composed of grey and white matter, and its cortical surface is convoluted like the surface of the cerebrum. It also is divided by a central fissure into two lobes connected by the vermis.

The cerebellum is responsible for reflexive, involuntary fine-tuning of motor control and for maintaining balance and posture through extensive neural connections with the medulla (through the inferior cerebellar peduncle) and with the midbrain (through the superior cerebellar peduncle). The two hemispheres are connected to the pons by the middle cerebellar peduncles. These connections allow extensive sampling of visual, vestibular, and proprioceptive data from other regions of the CNS and periphery.

The pons (bridge) is easily recognized by its bulging appearance below the midbrain and above the medulla. Primarily it transmits information from the cerebellum to the brainstem and between the two cerebellar hemispheres. The nuclei of cranial nerves V through VIII are located in this structure.

Myelencephalon. The myelencephalon (usually called the medulla oblongata) forms the lowest portion of the brainstem. Reflex activities—such as heart rate, respiration, blood pressure, coughing, sneezing, swallowing, and vomiting—are controlled in this area. The nuclei of cranial nerves IX through XII are located in this region.

A major portion of the descending motor pathways (i.e., corticospinal tracts) cross to the other side, or decussate, at the medulla (see Figure 13-9). These pathways, together with other areas of decussation in the CNS, are the basis for the phenomenon of *contralateral control.* Sleep–wake rhythms also are processed by neural influences from lower brain centres and are associated with a complex group of diffuse structures and functions (see Chapter 14), including the RAS (cells that receive collateral signals from the afferent sensory pathways and project the signals to the higher brain centres, thus controlling CNS activity) (see Figure 13-6).

QUICK CHECK 13-3

1. Name the three major divisions of the brain and their component parts.
2. Describe the limbic system's functions.
3. What are the two major functions of the hypothalamus?

The Spinal Cord

The **spinal cord** is the portion of the CNS that lies within the vertebral canal and is surrounded and protected by the **vertebral column**. The spinal cord has many functions, which include a long nerve cable that connects the brain and body, somatic and autonomic reflexes, motor pattern control centres, and sensory and motor modulation. It originates in the medulla oblongata and ends at the level of the first or second lumbar vertebra in adults (Figure 13-11). The end of the spinal cord, the **conus medullaris**, is cone shaped. Spinal nerves continue from the end of the spinal cord and form a nerve bundle called the **cauda equina**. The filament anchor from the conus medullaris to the coccyx is the **filum terminale** (see Figure 13-11). The coverings of the spinal cord are illustrated in Figure 13-12.

Grossly, the spinal cord is divided into vertebral sections (8 cervical, 12 thoracic, 5 lumbar, 5 sacral, and 1 coccygeal) that correspond to

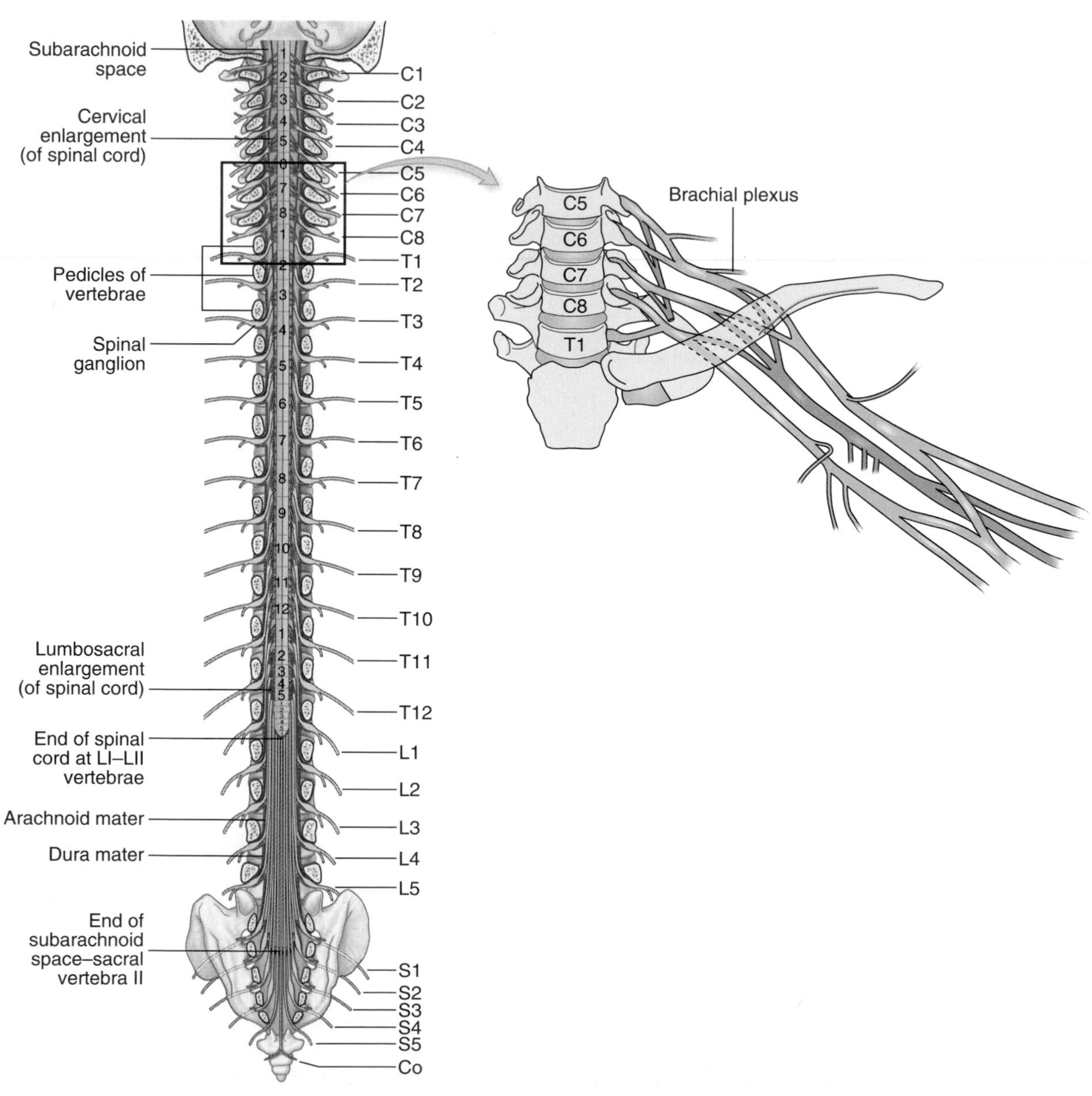

FIGURE 13-11 Vertebral Canal, Spinal Cord, and Spinal Nerves. Enlarged schematic of the brachial plexus is shown. (From Drake, R., Vogl, A.W., & Mitchell, A.W.M. [2015]. *Gray's anatomy for students* [3rd ed.]. London: Churchill Livingstone. **Inset,** from Chung, K.C., Yang, L. J.-S., & McGillicuddy, J.E. [Eds.]. [2012]. *Practical management of pediatric and adult brachial plexus palsies.* London: Saunders.)

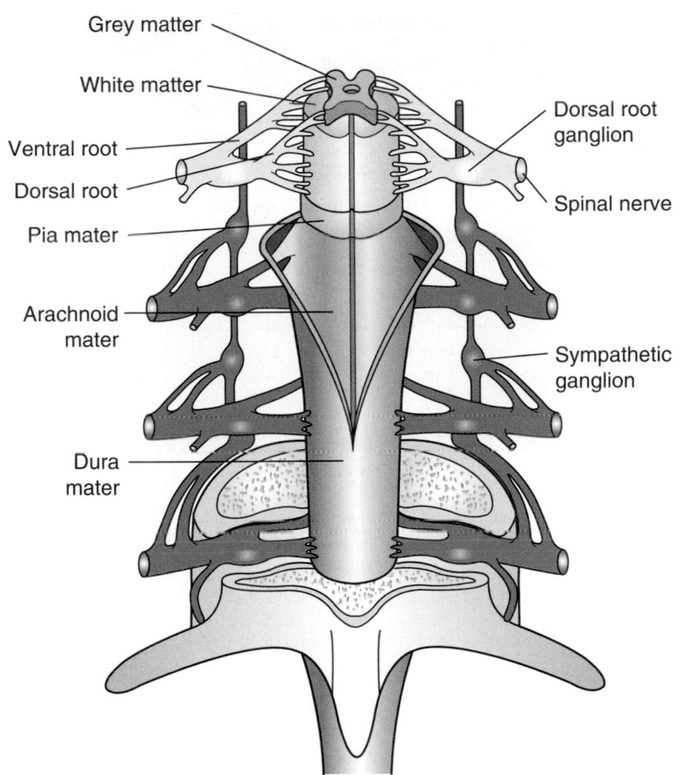

FIGURE 13-12 Coverings of the Spinal Cord. The dura mater is shown in natural colour. Note how it extends to cover the spinal nerve roots and nerves. The arachnoid is highlighted in purple and the pia mater in pink. (From Patton, K.T., & Thibodeau, G.A. [2016]. *Structure and function of the body* [15th ed.]. St. Louis: Mosby.)

paired nerves (see Figure 13-11). A cross-section of the spinal cord (Figure 13-13) is characterized by a butterfly-shaped inner core of grey matter (containing nerve cell bodies). The **central canal** lies in the centre of this region and extends through the spinal cord from its origin in the fourth ventricle. The grey matter of the spinal cord is divided into three regions and displays specific functional characteristics. These regions include the **posterior horn**, or **dorsal horn** (composed primarily of interneurons and axons from sensory neurons whose cell bodies lie in the **dorsal root ganglion**). At the tip of the posterior horn is the **substantia gelatinosa**, a structure involved in pain transmission (see Chapter 14). The **lateral horn** contains cell bodies involved with the ANS. The **anterior horn (ventral horn)** contains the nerve cell bodies for efferent pathways that leave the spinal cord by way of spinal nerves.

Surrounding the grey matter is white matter that forms ascending and descending pathways called **spinal tracts**. Spinal tracts are named to denote their beginning and ending points. For example, the **spinothalamic tract** (see Figure 13-13) carries nerve impulses from the spinal cord to the thalamus in the diencephalon. Numerous spinal tracts are grouped into columns according to their location within the white matter. These columns include the **anterior columns**, **lateral columns**, and posterior (dorsal) columns (see Figure 13-13).

Neural circuits in the spinal cord, when activated, display specific sets of motor responses. **Reflex arcs** form basic units that respond to stimuli and provide protective circuitry for motor output. Structures needed for a reflex arc are a receptor, an **afferent (sensory) neuron**, an **efferent (motor) neuron**, and an effector muscle or gland. A simple reflex arc may contain only two neurons (Figure 13-14). Interneurons are usually present and provide a link between sensory and motor neurons. The motor effects of reflex arcs generally occur before the

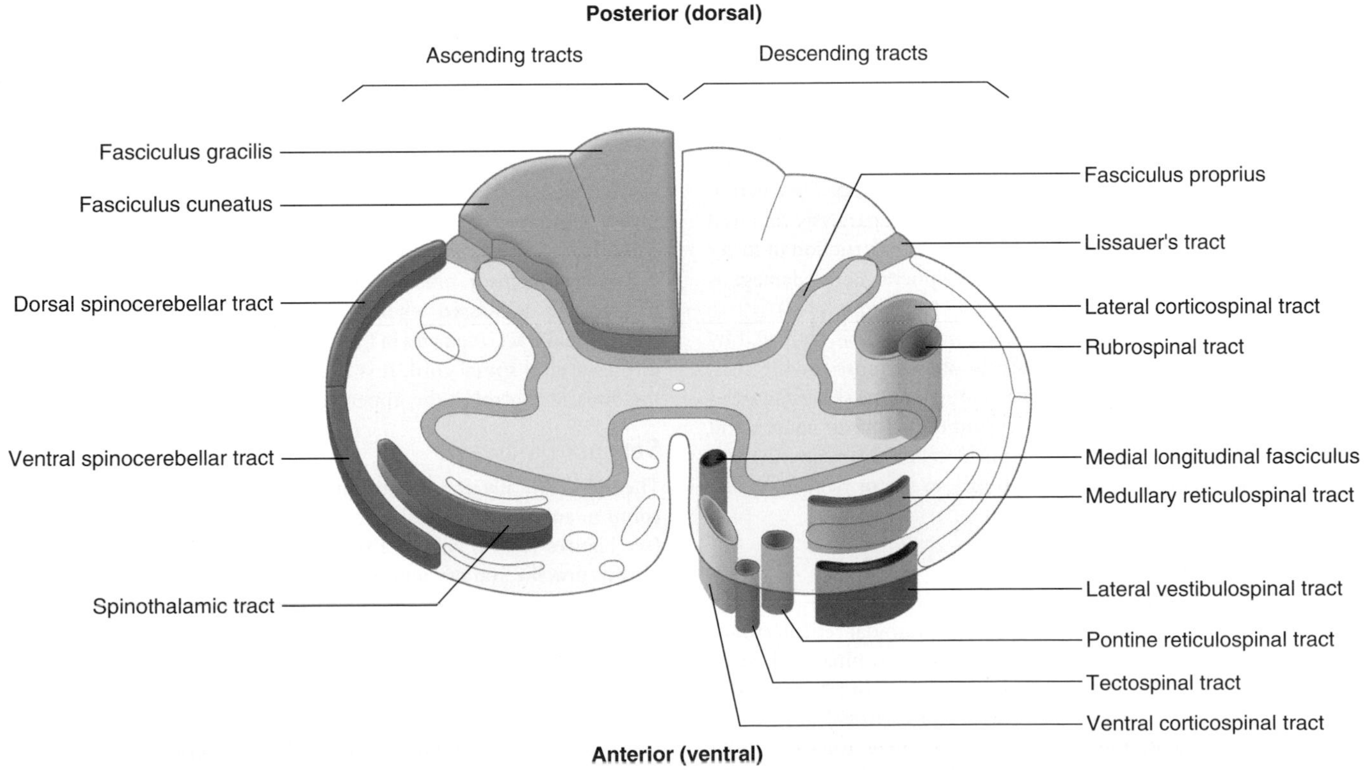

FIGURE 13-13 Ascending and Descending Tracts of the Spinal Cord. All ascending (*sensory*) and descending (*motor*) tracts are present bilaterally. In this figure, ascending tracts are emphasized on the left side and descending tracts are emphasized on the right side. The location of Lissauer's tract and the fasciculus proprius (which contain both ascending and descending fibres) are also shown. (From Crossman, A.R., & Neary, D. [2015]. *Neuroanatomy: An illustrated colour text* [4th ed.]. London: Churchill Livingstone.)

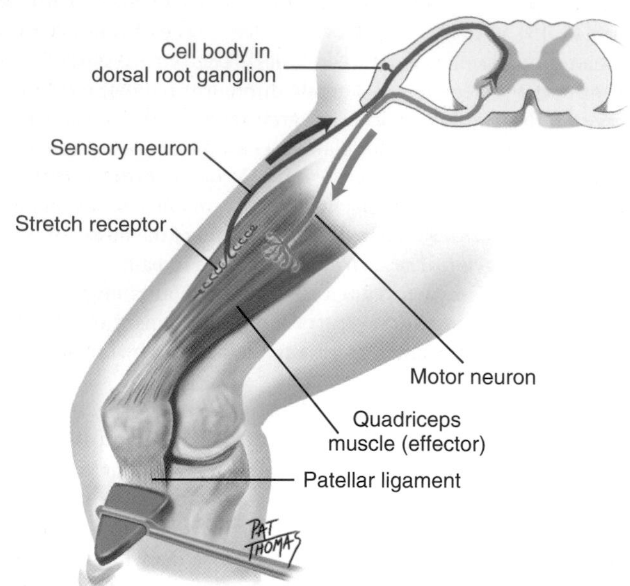

FIGURE 13-14 Cross Section of Spinal Cord Showing Simple Reflex Arc. (From Jarvis, C. [2016]. *Physical examination & health assessment* [7th ed.]. St. Louis: Saunders.)

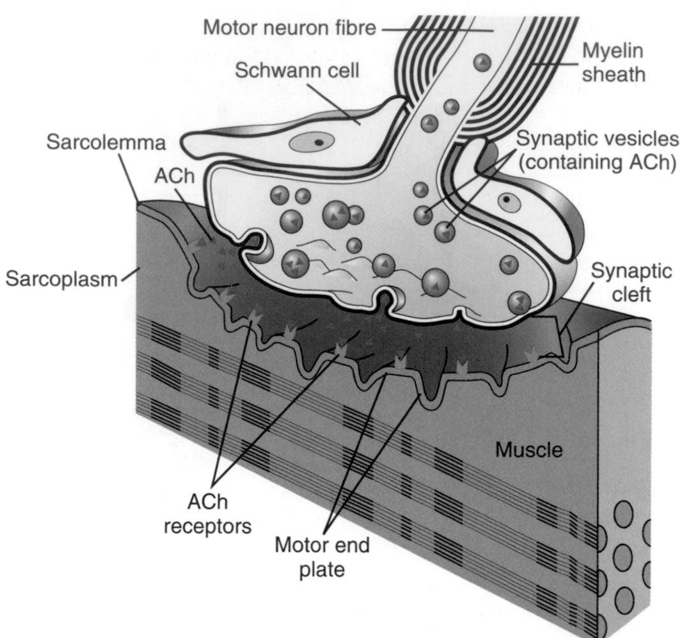

FIGURE 13-15 Normal Neuromuscular Junction This figure shows how the distal end of a motor neuron fibre forms a synapse, or "chemical junction," with an adjacent muscle fibre. Neurotransmitters (specifically, acetylcholine [*ACh*]) are released from the neuron's synaptic vesicles and diffuse across the synaptic cleft. There, they stimulate receptors in the motor end-plate region of the sarcolemma. (From Damjanov, I. [2012]. *Pathology for the health professions* [4th ed.]. St. Louis: Saunders.)

event is perceived in the brain's higher centres. Much internal environmental regulation is mediated by reflex activity involving the ANS.

Afferent pathways transmit information from peripheral receptors, and eventually it terminates in the cerebral or cerebellar cortex, or both. Efferent pathways primarily relay information from the cerebrum to the brainstem or spinal cord. **Upper motor neurons** are completely contained within the CNS. Their primary roles are controlling fine motor movement and influencing or modifying spinal reflex arcs and circuits. Generally, upper motor neurons form synapses with interneurons, which then form synapses with lower motor neurons that project into the periphery. **Lower motor neurons** directly influence muscles. Their cell bodies lie in the grey matter of the brainstem and spinal cord, but their processes extend out of the CNS and into the PNS. Destruction of upper motor neurons usually results in initial paralysis followed within days or weeks by partial recovery, whereas destruction of lower motor neurons leads to paralysis unless peripheral nerve damage is followed by nerve regeneration and recovery (see Figure 13-4).

Muscle activity (i.e., stimulation and contraction) is regulated by nerve impulses. Motor neurons innervate one or more muscle cells, forming **motor units**, which consist of a neuron and the skeletal muscles it stimulates. The junction between the axon of the motor neuron and the plasma membrane of the muscle cell is called the *neuromuscular (myoneural) junction* (Figure 13-15). (Injury to motor neurons is discussed in Chapter 16.)

Motor Pathways

Clinically relevant motor pathways are the lateral corticospinal and corticobulbar pyramidal tracts; and the extrapyramidal reticulospinal, vestibulospinal, and rubrospinal tracts. The corticospinal and corticobulbar pathways are essentially the same tract and consist of a two-neuron chain. The cell bodies (upper motor neurons) originate in and around the precentral gyrus; pass through the corona radiata of the cerebrum, the internal capsule, middle three fifths of the cerebral pedunculus, pons, and pyramid; and decussate (cross contralaterally) in the medulla oblongata and form the lateral corticospinal tract of the spinal cord (see Figures 13-9, *A* and 13-13) and thus control the opposite side of the body. The **corticobulbar tract axons** synapse on motor cranial nuclei within the brainstem that control muscles of the face, head, and neck. The lateral corticospinal tract axons leave the tract to go to specific interneurons or motor neurons in the anterior horn. The **lateral corticospinal tract** has the same somatotopic organization as the body (see Figure 13-8). These lower motor neurons project through nerves to specific muscles. These tracts are involved in precise motor movements. The **reticulospinal tract** (see Figure 13-13) modulates motor movement by inhibiting and exciting spinal activity. The **vestibulospinal tract** arises from a vestibular nucleus in the pons and causes the extensor muscles of the body to rapidly contract, most dramatically witnessed when a person starts to fall backward. The **rubrospinal tract** originates in the red nucleus, decussates, and terminates in the cervical spinal cord. It is important for muscle movement and fine muscle control in the upper extremities.

Sensory Pathways

The three clinically important spinal afferent pathways are the posterior column, anterior spinothalamic tract, and lateral spinothalamic tract (see Figures 13-9, *B* and 13-13). The **posterior (dorsal) column (fasciculus gracilis** and **fasciculus cuneatus)** carries fine-touch sensation, two-point discrimination, and proprioceptive information (i.e., **epicritic information**). The posterior column is formed by a three-neuron chain. The first neuron of the chain is the primary afferent neuron. It also is the sensory neuron of the reflex arc. After entering the spinal cord, it sends its axon ipsilaterally up the spinal cord to a specific part of the posterior column and synapses in the three posterior column nuclei in the medulla oblongata. A basketball playing centre has primary afferent neurons that could be more than 2 m long, running from the great toe up to the medulla oblongata. The axon of the second-order neuron crosses contralaterally at the medial lemniscus and ascends and synapses with a specific nucleus of the thalamus. The third-order neuron, originating in the thalamus, continues the tract into the internal capsule, corona radiata, and postcentral gyrus (Brodmann areas 3, 1, 2) (see Figures 13-7, and 13-9, *B*).

The **anterior** and **lateral spinothalamic tracts** are responsible for vague touch sensation and for pain and temperature perception, respectively (see Figure 13-9, *B*). These modalities are referred to as **protopathic**. These tracts also form a three-neuron chain. However, their primary afferent neurons synapse in the posterior horn of the spinal cord, not just at the level they enter the intervertebral foramen but in a number of spinal segments above and below their point of entry. This action is an example of divergence. The axons of the second-order neurons in the posterior horn cross to the contralateral side in the spinal cord in the lateral column, ascend to the same thalamic nucleus as the posterior column pathway, and continue with the posterior column pathway to the postcentral gyrus.

Protective Structures of the Central Nervous System

Cranium

The cranium is composed of eight bones. The cranial vault encloses and protects the brain and its associated structures. The soft tissue that encapsulates the cranium is called the *scalp*, which consists of five layers: skin, connective tissue, epicranial aponeurosis, loose areolar tissue, and pericranium. The **galea aponeurotica**, which is a component of the epicranial aponeurosis, is a thick, fibrous band of tissue overlying the cranium between the frontal and occipital muscles that affords added protection to the skull. The subgaleal space has venous connections with the dural sinuses, and with increased intracranial pressure, blood can be shunted to the space, thus reducing pressure in the intracranial cavity. The subgaleal space is also a common site for wound drains after intracranial surgery.

The floor of the cranial vault is irregular and contains many foramina (openings) for cranial nerves, blood vessels, and the spinal cord to exit. The cranial floor is divided into three fossae (depressions). The frontal lobes lie in the **anterior fossa**, the temporal lobes and base of the diencephalon lie in the **middle fossa (temporal fossa)**, and the cerebellum lies in the **posterior fossa**. These terms are commonly used anatomical landmarks to describe the location of intracranial lesions.

Meninges

Surrounding the brain and spinal cord are three protective membranes: the dura mater, the arachnoid, and the pia mater. Collectively they are called the **meninges** (Figure 13-16, *C*). The **dura mater** (meaning literally "hard mother") is composed of two layers, with the venous sinuses formed between them. The outermost layer forms the **periosteum (endosteal layer)** of the skull. The **inner dura (meningeal layer)** is responsible for forming rigid membranes that support and separate various brain structures.

One of these membranes, the **falx cerebri**, dips between the two cerebral hemispheres along the longitudinal fissure. The falx cerebri is anchored anteriorly to the base of the brain at the crista galli of the ethmoid bone. The **tentorium cerebelli**, a common landmark, is a membrane that separates the cerebellum below from the cerebral structures above. Internal to the dura mater is the location of the **arachnoid**, a spongy, weblike structure that loosely follows the contours of the cerebral structures.

The **subdural space** lies between the dura and arachnoid. Many small bridging veins that have little support traverse the subdural space. Their disruption results in a subdural hematoma (see Chapter 16). The **subarachnoid space** lies between the arachnoid and the **pia mater** and contains CSF (Figure 13-16, *A* and *C*). Unlike the dura mater and arachnoid, the delicate pia mater adheres to the contours of the brain and spinal cord. It provides support for blood vessels serving brain tissue. The **choroid plexuses**, structures that produce CSF, arise from the pial membrane (Figure 13-16, *B*). The spinal cord is anchored to the vertebrae by extension of the meninges. The meninges continue beyond the end of the spinal cord (at vertebrae levels L1 and L2) to the lower portion of the sacrum. CSF contained within the subarachnoid space also circulates inferiorly to about the second sacral vertebra.

The meninges form potential and real spaces important to understanding functional and pathological mechanisms. For example, between the dura mater and skull lies a potential space termed the **extradural space** (see Figure 13-16, *C*). The arterial supply to the meninges consists of blood vessels that lie within grooves in the skull. A skull fracture can sever one of these vessels and produce an epidural hematoma.

Cerebrospinal Fluid and the Ventricular System

Cerebrospinal fluid (CSF) is a clear, colourless fluid similar to blood plasma and interstitial fluid. The intracranial and spinal cord structures float in CSF and are thereby partially protected from jolts and blows. The buoyant properties of the CSF also prevent the brain from tugging on meninges, nerve roots, and blood vessels. (Constituents of CSF are listed in Table 13-4.) Between 125 and 150 mL of CSF is circulating within the **ventricles** (small cavities) and subarachnoid space at any given time. Approximately 600 mL of CSF is produced daily.

The choroid plexuses in the lateral, third, and fourth ventricles produce the major portion of CSF. (Ventricles are illustrated in Figure 13-16.) These plexuses are characterized by a rich network of blood vessels, supplied by the pia mater, that lie close to the ependymal cells of the ventricles. The tight junctions of the choroid blood vessel provide a limiting barrier between the CSF and blood that functions similarly to the blood–brain barrier (see Figures 13-16, *B* and 13-16, *C*).

The CSF exerts pressure within the brain and spinal cord. When a person is supine, CSF pressure is about 80 to 180 mm of water pressure, or approximately 5 to 14 mm of mercury pressure, but doubles when the person moves to an upright position. CSF flow results from the pressure gradient between the arterial system and the CSF-filled cavities. Beginning in the lateral ventricles, the CSF flows through the **interventricular foramen (foramen of Monro)** into the third ventricle and then passes through the cerebral aqueduct (aqueduct of Sylvius) into

TABLE 13-4 Composition of Cerebrospinal Fluid

Constituent	Normal Value
Na^+	135–150 mmol/L of CSF
K^+	2.7–3.9 mmol/L of CSF
Cl^-	116–127 mmol/L of CSF
HCO_3^-	22.9 mmol/L of CSF
Glucose (fasting)	2.8–4.2 mmol/L of CSF (60–70% of blood glucose)
pH	7.28–7.32
Protein	0.15–0.45 g/L of CSF to 0.7 g/L
Albumin	56–76%
Globulin	6–19%
Cells	
White (lymphocyte)	0–5 × 10^6 WBCs/L (0–10 cells/μL)
Red	0

Cl^-, chloride; *CSF*, cerebrospinal fluid; *HCO_3^-*, bicarbonate; *K^+*, potassium; *Na^+*, sodium; *WBC*, white blood cell.
Sofronescu, A., & Wheeler, T. (2015). *Cerebrospinal fluid analysis*. Retrieved from http://emedicine.medscape.com/article/2093316-overview.

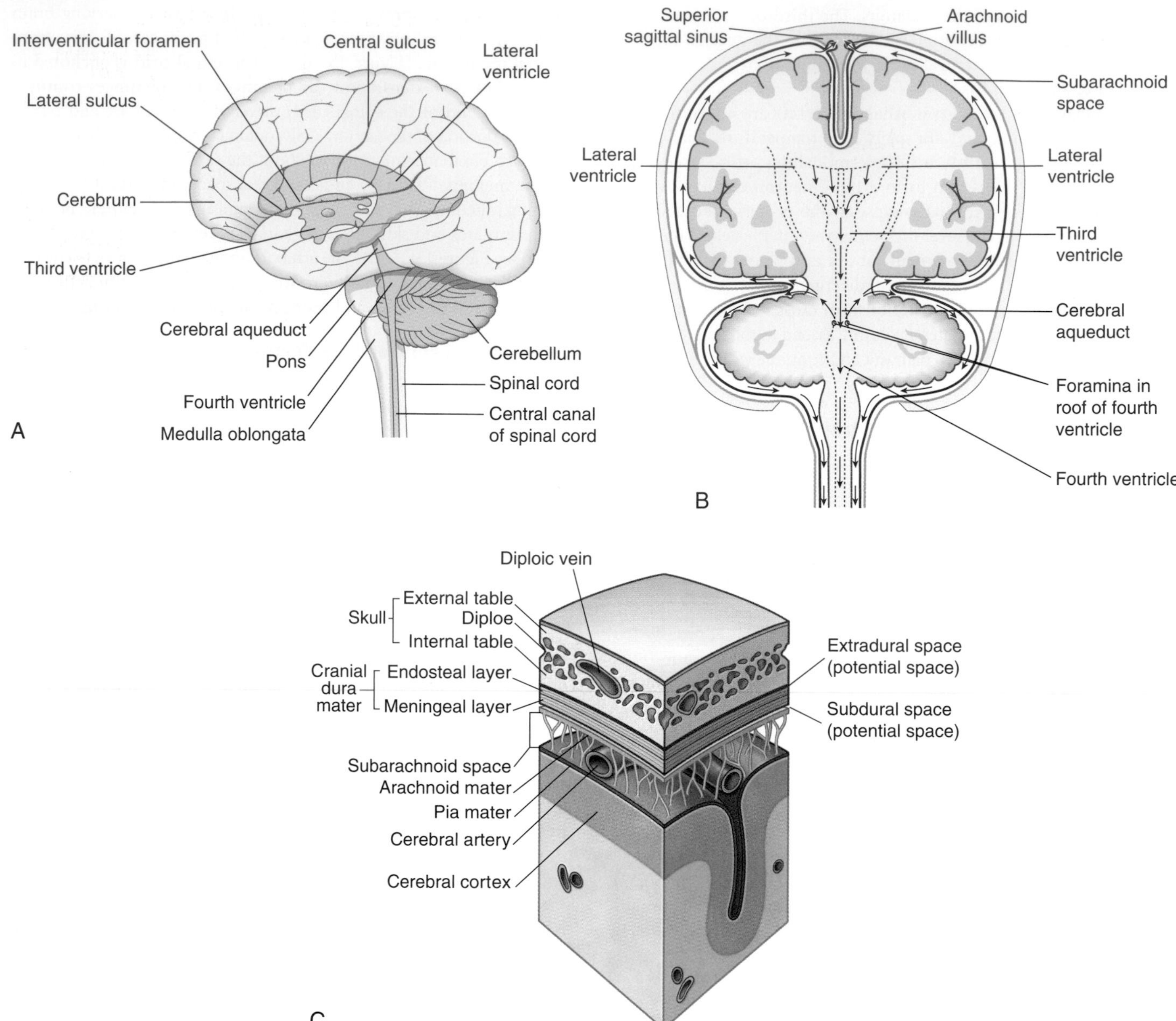

FIGURE 13-16 Flow of Cerebrospinal Fluid and Meninges of the Brain. **A,** Ventricles highlighted in blue within a translucent brain in a left lateral view. **B,** Flow of cerebrospinal fluid (CSF). The fluid produced by filtration of blood by the choroid plexus of each ventricle flows inferiorly through the lateral ventricles, interventricular foramen, third ventricle, cerebral aqueduct, fourth ventricle, and subarachnoid space to the blood. **C,** Meninges of the brain in relation to CSF and venous blood flow. (**A, B,** from Waugh, A., & Grant, A. [2012]. *Ross and Wilson anatomy and physiology in health and illness* [12th ed.]. London: Churchill Livingstone. **C,** from Drake, R., Vogl, A.W., & Mitchell, A.W.M. [2015]. *Gray's anatomy for students* [3rd ed.]. London: Churchill Livingstone.)

the fourth ventricle. From the fourth ventricle the CSF may pass through either the paired **lateral apertures (foramen of Luschka)** or the **median aperture (foramen of Magendie)** before communicating with the subarachnoid spaces of the brain and spinal cord. The CSF does not, however, accumulate. Instead, it is reabsorbed into the venous circulation through the arachnoid villi. The **arachnoid villi** protrude from the arachnoid space, through the dura mater, and lie within the blood flow of the venous sinuses (see Figure 13-16, *B*). CSF is reabsorbed through a pressure gradient between the arachnoid villi and the cerebral venous sinuses. The villi function as one-way valves directing CSF outflow into the blood but preventing blood flow into the subarachnoid space. Thus CSF is formed from the blood, and after circulating throughout the CNS, it returns to the blood.

Vertebral Column

The vertebral column (Figure 13-17) is composed of 33 vertebrae: 7 cervical, 12 thoracic, 5 lumbar, 5 fused sacral, and 4 fused coccygeal. Between each interspace (except for the fused sacral and coccygeal vertebrae) is an **intervertebral disc** (Figure 13-18). At the centre of the intervertebral disc is the **nucleus pulposus**, a pulpy mass of elastic fibres. The intervertebral disc absorbs shocks, preventing damage to the vertebrae. The intervertebral disc is also a common source of back

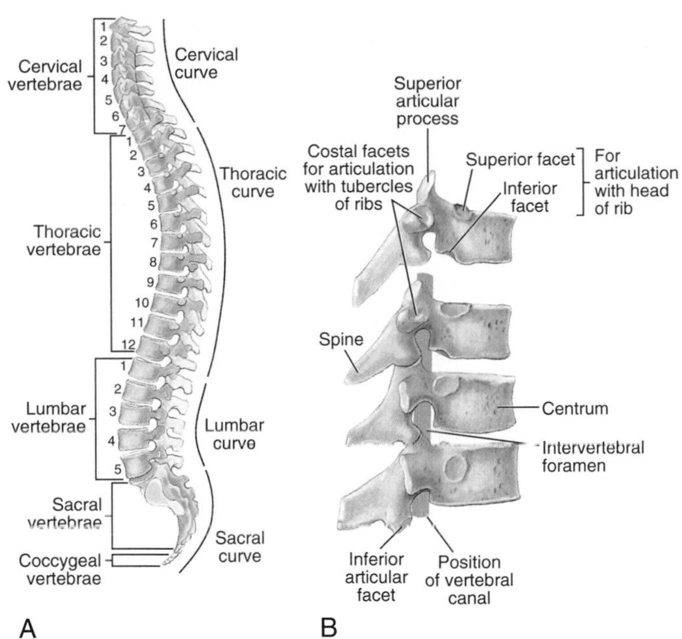

FIGURE 13-17 Vertebral Column. A, The normal curves and regions of the vertebral column. The vertebrae in each region are numbered. **B,** Lateral view of several vertebrae showing how they articulate. (From Solomon, E. [2016]. *Introduction to human anatomy and physiology* [4th ed.]. St. Louis: Saunders.)

problems. If too much stress is applied to the vertebral column, the disc contents may rupture and protrude into the spinal canal, causing compression of the spinal cord or nerve roots.

QUICK CHECK 13-4
1. What information is conveyed in the ascending and descending spinal tracts?
2. Contrast the functions of upper and lower motor neurons.
3. Name the protective structures of the central nervous system, and briefly describe each.

Blood Supply of the Central Nervous System

Blood Supply to the Brain

The brain receives approximately 20% of the cardiac output, or 800 to 1000 mL of blood flow per minute. Carbon dioxide is a primary regulator for blood flow within the CNS. It is a potent vasodilator, and its effects ensure an adequate blood supply.

The brain derives its arterial supply from two systems: the **internal carotid arteries** and the **vertebral arteries** (Figure 13-19). The internal carotid arteries supply a proportionately greater amount of blood flow. They originate at the common carotid arteries, enter the cranium through the base of the skull, and pass through the **cavernous sinus**. After forming some small branches, these arteries divide into the anterior and middle cerebral arteries. The vertebral arteries originate at the subclavian arteries and pass through the transverse foramina of the cervical vertebrae, entering the cranium through the foramen magnum. They join at the junction of the pons and medulla to form the **basilar artery** (Figure 13-20). The basilar artery divides at the level of the midbrain to form paired posterior cerebral arteries.

The **circle of Willis** (see Figure 13-20) provides an alternative route for blood flow when one of the contributing arteries is obstructed (collateral blood flow). The circle of Willis is formed by the posterior cerebral arteries, posterior communicating arteries, internal carotid arteries, anterior cerebral arteries, and anterior communicating artery. The anterior cerebral, middle cerebral, and posterior cerebral arteries leave the circle of Willis and extend to various brain structures. The border zone is the area between the major arterial territories. (Table 13-5 and Figure 13-21 identify the structures served, functional

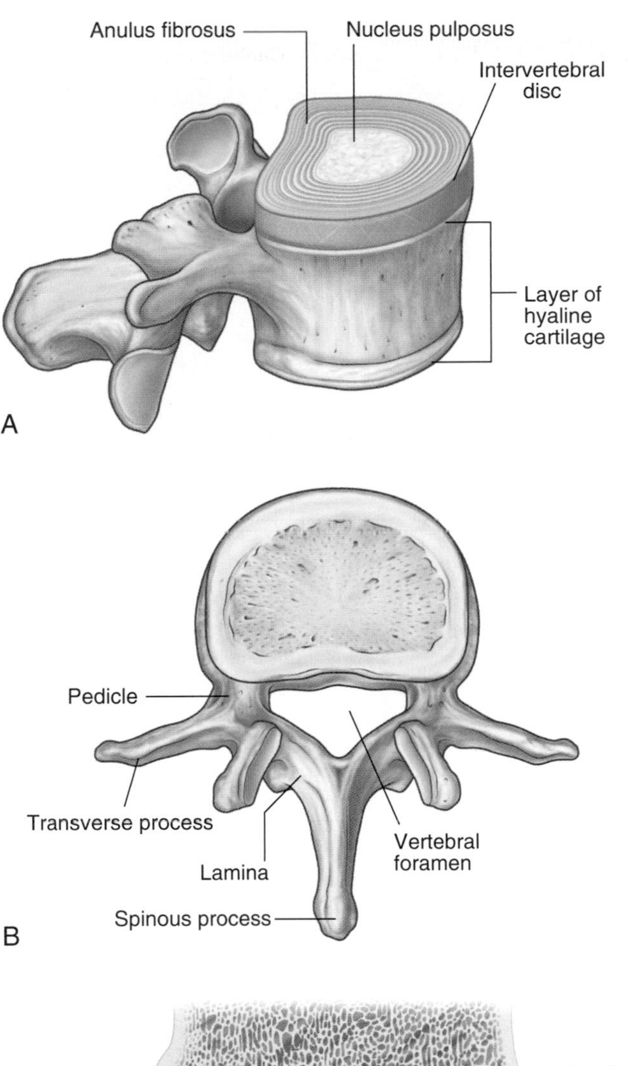

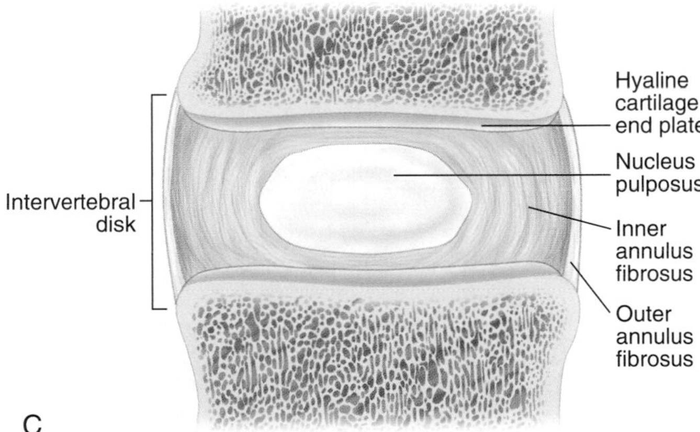

FIGURE 13-18 Intervertebral Disc. A, Sagittal illustration. **B,** Superior view of the structures of a typical vertebra. **C,** Magnified illustration. (**A** and **B,** from Drake, R., Vogl, A.W., & Mitchell, A.W.M. [2015]. *Gray's anatomy for students* [3rd ed.]. London: Churchill Livingstone. **C,** from Lawry, G.V., Kreder, H., Hawker, G., et al. [2010]. *Fam's musculoskeletal examination and joint injection techniques* [2nd ed.]. Philadelphia: Mosby.)

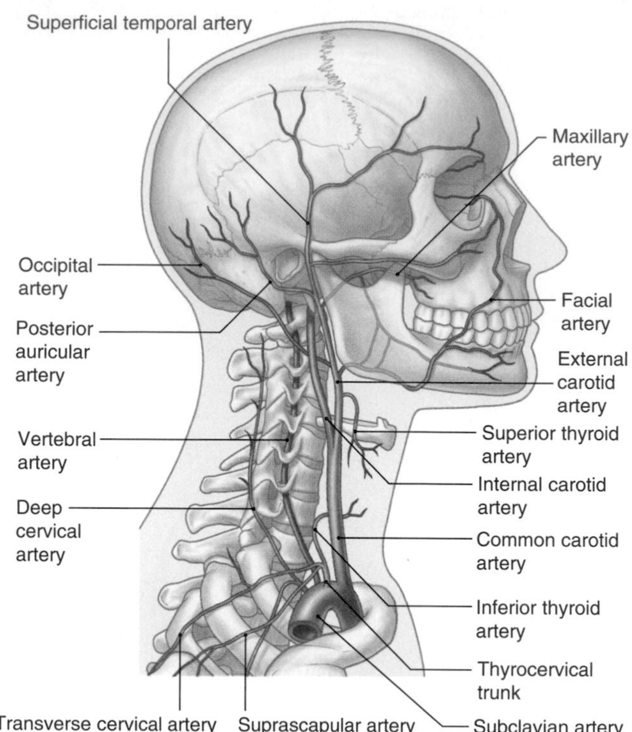

FIGURE 13-19 Major Arteries of the Head and Neck. (From Moses, K.P., Nava, P., Banks, J., et al. [2013]. *Atlas of clinical gross anatomy* [2nd ed.]. Philadelphia: Saunders.)

relationships, and pathological considerations related to occlusion of cerebral arteries.)

Cerebral venous drainage does not parallel its arterial supply, whereas the venous drainage of the brainstem and cerebellum does parallel the arterial supply of these structures. The cerebral veins are classified as superficial veins and deep veins. The veins drain into venous plexuses and dural sinuses (formed between the dural layers) and eventually join the internal jugular veins at the base of the skull (Figure 13-22). Adequacy of venous outflow can significantly affect intracranial pressure. For example, head-injured individuals who turn or let their heads fall to the side partially occlude venous return, and the intracranial pressure can increase then because of decreased flow through the jugular veins.

Blood–Brain Barrier

The **blood–brain barrier (BBB)** describes cellular structures that selectively inhibit certain potentially harmful substances in the blood from entering the interstitial spaces of the brain or CSF, allowing neurons to function normally. Endothelial cells in brain capillaries with their intracellular tight junctions are the site of the BBB. Supporting cells include astrocytes, pericytes, and microglia[10] (Figure 13-23, and see Chapter 1). The exact nature of this mechanism is debated, but it appears that certain metabolites, electrolytes, and chemicals can cross into and out of the brain to varying degrees. This exchange has substantial implications for medication therapy because certain types of antibiotics and chemotherapeutic medications show a greater propensity than others for crossing this barrier. Breakdown of the BBB can contribute to neuro-inflammation and neuro-degeneration.

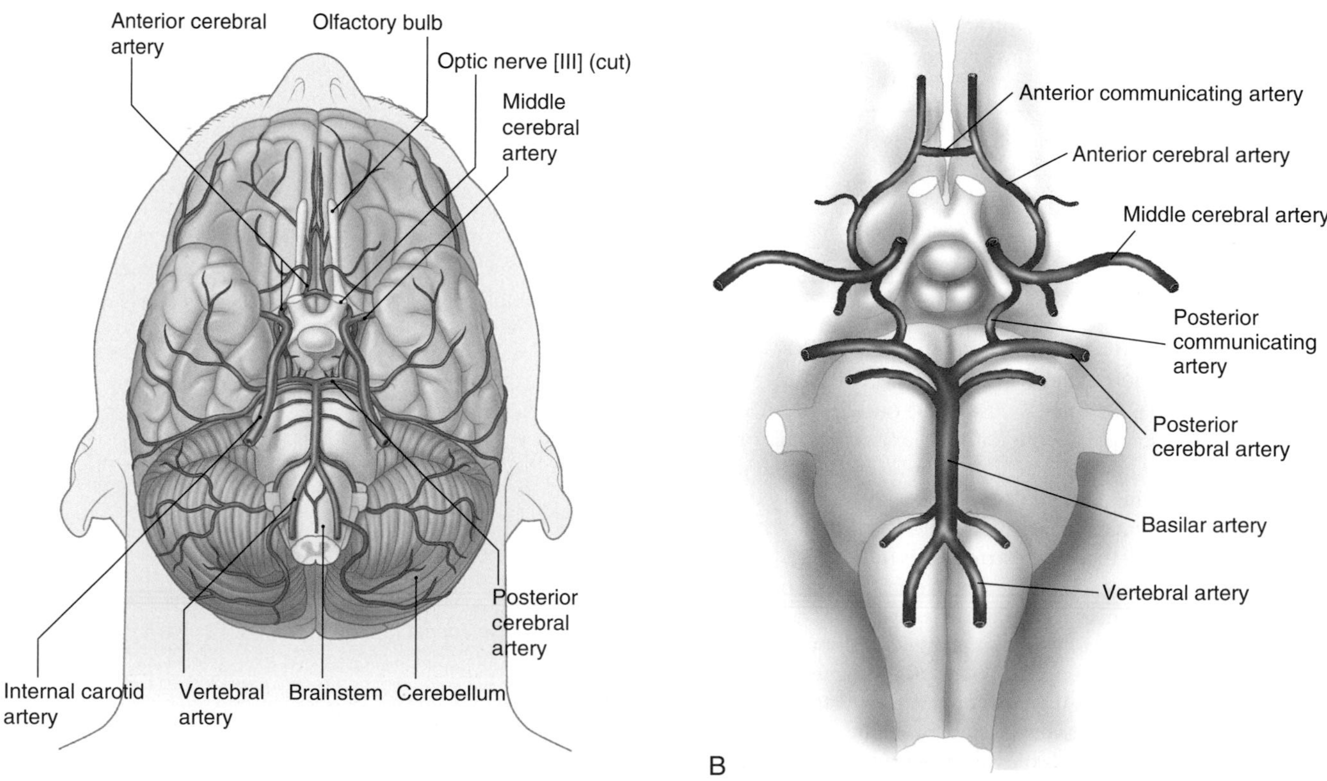

FIGURE 13-20 Arteries at the Base of the Brain. The arteries that compose the circle of Willis are the two anterior cerebral arteries, joined to each other by the anterior communicating artery and two short segments of the internal carotids, off of which the posterior communicating arteries connect to the posterior cerebral arteries. (**A,** from Moses, K.P., Nava, P., Banks, J., et al. [2013]. *Atlas of clinical gross anatomy* [2nd ed.]. Philadelphia: Saunders. **B,** from Hagen-Ansert, S. [2012]. *Textbook of diagnostic sonography* [7th ed.]. St. Louis: Mosby.)

TABLE 13-5 Arterial Systems Supplying the Brain

Arterial Origin	Structures Served	Conditions Caused by Occlusion
Anterior cerebral artery	Basal ganglia; corpus callosum; medial surface of cerebral hemispheres; superior surface of frontal and parietal lobes	Hemiplegia on contralateral side of body, greater in lower than in upper extremities
Middle cerebral artery	Frontal lobe; parietal lobe; temporal lobe (primarily cortical surfaces)	Aphasia in dominant hemisphere and contralateral hemiplegia (see Chapter 15)
Posterior cerebral artery	Part of diencephalon (thalamus, hypothalamus) and temporal lobe; occipital lobe	Visual loss; sensory loss; contralateral hemiplegia if cerebral peduncle affected

From Pike-MacDonald, S.A. (2013). *Mosby's Canadian manual of diagnostic and laboratory tests* (Cdn. ed.). Toronto: Elsevier.

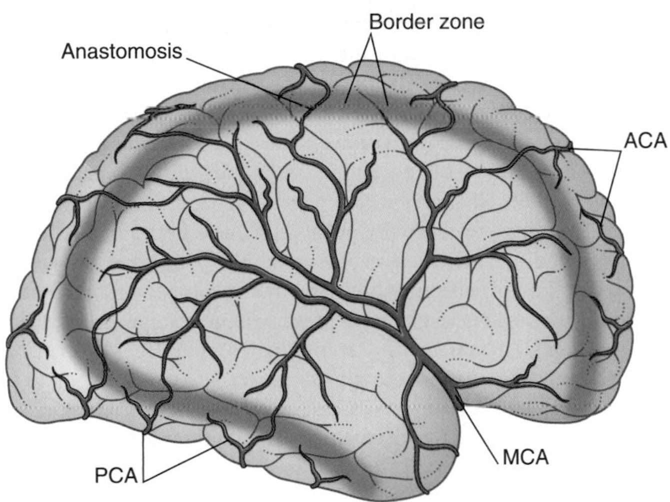

FIGURE 13-21 Areas of the Brain Affected by Occlusion of the Anterior, Middle, and Posterior Cerebral Artery Branches. *ACA*, grey area affected by occlusion of branches of anterior cerebral artery; *MCA*, pink area affected by occlusion of branches of middle cerebral artery; *PCA*, orange area affected by occlusion of branches of posterior cerebral artery. Occlusions can occur in the cortical or deep areas of the border zone. (From Fitzgerald, M.J.T., Gruener, G., & Mtui, E. [2012]. *Clinical neuroanatomy and neuroscience* [6th ed.]. Philadelphia: Saunders.)

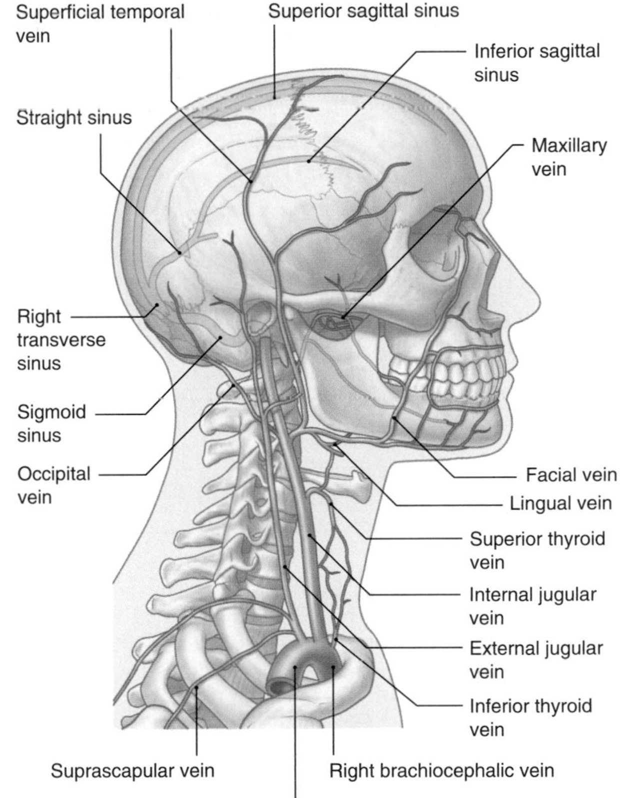

FIGURE 13-22 Veins of the Head and Neck. Deep veins and dural sinuses are projected on the skull. Note two superficial veins in the face are tributaries that send blood through emissary veins in the skull foramen into deep veins inside the skull terminating in the internal jugular vein. (From Moses, K.P., Nava, P., Banks, J., et al. [2013]. *Atlas of clinical gross anatomy* [2nd ed.]. Philadelphia: Saunders.)

Blood Supply to the Spinal Cord

The spinal cord derives its blood supply from branches off the vertebral arteries and from branches from various regions of the aorta (Figure 13-24). The **anterior spinal artery** and the paired **posterior spinal arteries** branch from the vertebral artery at the base of the cranium and descend alongside the spinal cord. Arterial branches from vessels exterior to the spinal cord follow the spinal nerve through the intervertebral foramina, pass through the dura, and divide into the anterior and posterior radicular arteries.

The radicular arteries eventually connect to the spinal arteries. Branches from the radicular and spinal arteries form plexuses whose branches penetrate the spinal cord, supplying the deeper tissues. Venous drainage parallels the arterial supply closely and drains into venous sinuses located between the dura and periosteum of the vertebrae.

THE PERIPHERAL NERVOUS SYSTEM

The cranial and spinal nerves, including their branches and ganglia, constitute the peripheral nervous system (PNS). A peripheral nerve (cranial or spinal) is composed of individual axons wrapped in a myelin sheath. These individual fibres are arranged in bundles called **fascicles** (Figure 13-25, *B*).

The 31 pairs of spinal nerves derive their names from the vertebral level from which they exit. There are 8 cervical, 12 thoracic, 5 lumbar, and 5 sacral pairs, and 1 coccygeal pair. The first cervical nerve exits above the first cervical vertebra, and the rest of the spinal nerves exit below their corresponding vertebrae. From the thoracic region (and inferiorly), nerves correspond to the vertebral level above their exit.

Spinal nerves contain both sensory and motor neurons and are called **mixed nerves**. They arise as rootlets lateral to anterior and posterior horns of the spinal cord. These two spinal nerve roots converge in the

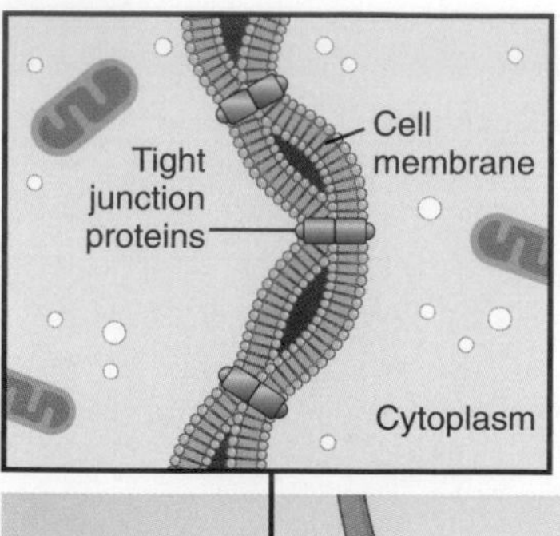

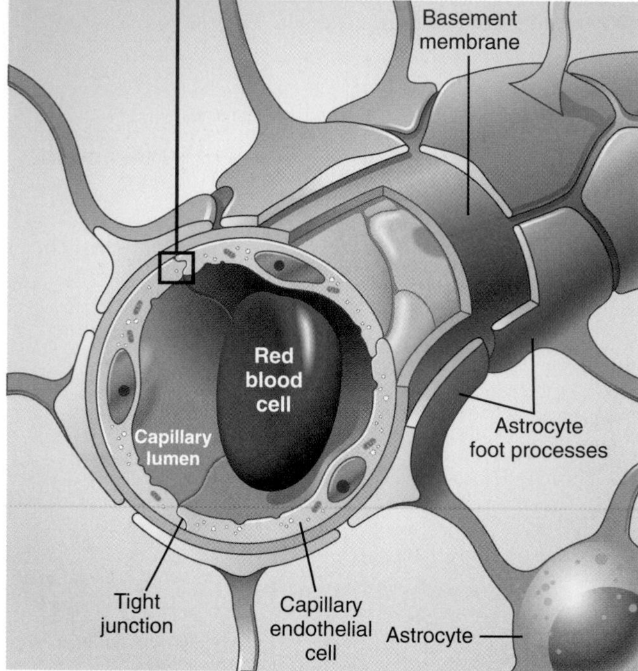

FIGURE 13-23 Blood–Brain Barrier. Cell membranes with tight junctions create a physical barrier between capillary blood and the cytoplasm of astrocytes. (From Bradley, W.G. [Ed.]. [2007]. *Neurology in clinical practice* [5th ed.]. London: Butterworth-Heinemann.)

region of the intervertebral foramen to form the spinal nerve trunk. Shortly after converging, the spinal nerve divides into anterior and posterior rami (branches). The anterior rami (except the thoracic) initially form plexuses (networks of nerve fibres), which then branch into the peripheral nerves. Instead of forming plexuses, the thoracic nerves pass through the intercostal spaces and innervate regions of the thorax.

The main spinal nerve plexuses innervate the skin and the underlying muscles of the limbs. The brachial plexus, for example, is formed by the last four cervical nerves (C5 to C8) and the first thoracic nerve (T1) (see Figure 13-11). The brachial plexus innervates the nerves of the arm, wrist, and hand. The lumbar plexus (L1 to L4) and sacral plexus (L5 to S5) contain nerves that innervate the anterior and posterior portions of the lower body, respectively.

The posterior rami of each spinal nerve, with their many processes, are distributed to a specific area in the body. Sensory signals thus arise from specific sites associated with a specific spinal cord segment. Specific areas of cutaneous innervation at these spinal cord segments are called dermatomes (Figure 13-25, *C*).

Like spinal nerves, cranial nerves are categorized as peripheral nerves. Most cranial nerves are mixed nerves (like the spinal nerves), although some are purely sensory or purely motor. Cranial nerves (Figure 13-25, *A*) connect to nuclei in the brain and brainstem. Table 13-6 describes structural and functional characteristics of the cranial nerves.

QUICK CHECK 13-5

1. Describe the circle of Willis and explain its role in supplying blood to the brain.
2. What is the source of the spinal cord's blood supply?
3. Describe the anatomy and function of the peripheral nervous system (PNS).
4. What are the plexuses? Give two examples in the PNS.
5. What are the cranial nerves? Give three examples.

THE AUTONOMIC NERVOUS SYSTEM

The structure and function of the autonomic nervous system (ANS) are complex and still not well understood. Components of the ANS are located in both the CNS and the PNS; however, the ANS is considered to be part of the efferent division of the PNS, even though visceral afferent neurons are certainly an important part of this system. Many neurons of the ANS travel in the spinal nerves and certain cranial nerves. The widespread activity of this system indicates that its components are distributed all over the body. The peripheral autonomic nerves carry mainly efferent fibres. The motor component of the ANS is a two-neuron system consisting of preganglionic neurons (myelinated) and postganglionic neurons (unmyelinated) (Figure 13-26). This arrangement contrasts with the somatic nervous system, where a single motor neuron travels from the CNS to the innervated structure. Visceral afferent neurons have their cell bodies in some sensory and cranial ganglia and their fibre processes travelling in peripheral nerves.

The CNS has autonomic areas in the intermediolateral horns of the spinal cord, the cardiovascular and respiratory centres in the reticular formation, and both sympathetic and parasympathetic areas in the hypothalamus. CNS pathways interconnect all these areas.

The ANS coordinates and maintains a steady state among visceral (internal) organs, such as regulation of cardiac muscle, smooth muscle, and the glands of the body. This system is considered an involuntary system because one generally cannot *will* these functions to happen. The ANS is separated both structurally and functionally into two divisions: (1) the sympathetic nervous system and (2) the parasympathetic nervous system (Figure 13-27).

Anatomy of the Sympathetic Nervous System

The sympathetic nervous system mobilizes energy stores in times of need (e.g., in the "fight-or-flight response" or acute stress response) (see Figure 9-3; see also Chapter 9). The sympathetic division is innervated by cell bodies located from the first thoracic (T1) through the second lumbar (L2) regions of the spinal cord and therefore is called the thoracolumbar division. The preganglionic axons of the sympathetic division form synapses shortly after leaving the spinal cord in the sympathetic (paravertebral) ganglia. These preganglionic axons travel several different ways: (1) directly synapsing with postganglionic neurons in the sympathetic chain ganglion at their level; (2) up or down the sympathetic chain ganglion before forming synapses with a higher or lower postganglionic neuron; or (3) through the sympathetic chain ganglion, postganglionic neurons within collateral ganglia (see Figure 13-27). Some preganglionic axons form pathways called splanchnic nerves, which lead to collateral ganglia on the front of the aorta. The collateral ganglia are named according to the branches of the aorta nearest them, namely, the celiac, superior mesenteric, and inferior mesenteric. The preganglionic neurons synapse with postganglionic neurons within the collateral ganglia. These postganglionic neurons

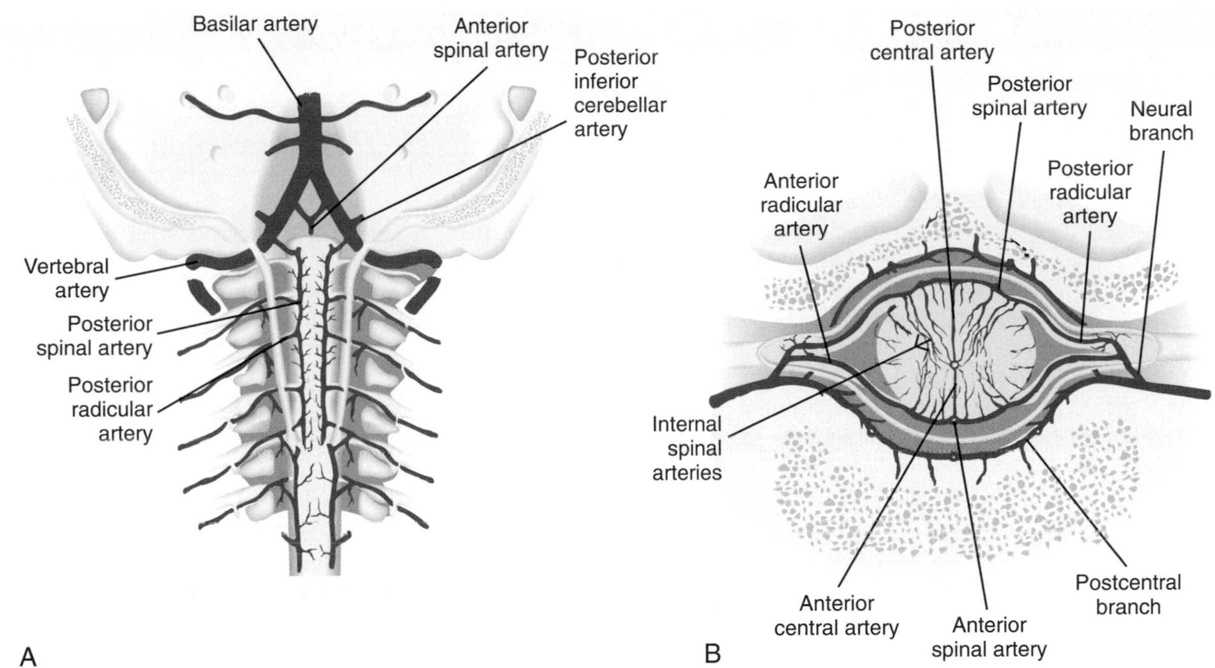

FIGURE 13-24 Arteries of the Spinal Cord. A, Arteries of cervical cord exposed from the rear. **B,** Arteries of spinal cord diagrammatically shown in horizontal section. (Redrawn from Rudy, E.B. [Ed.]. [1984]. *Advanced neurological and neurosurgical nursing.* St. Louis: Mosby.)

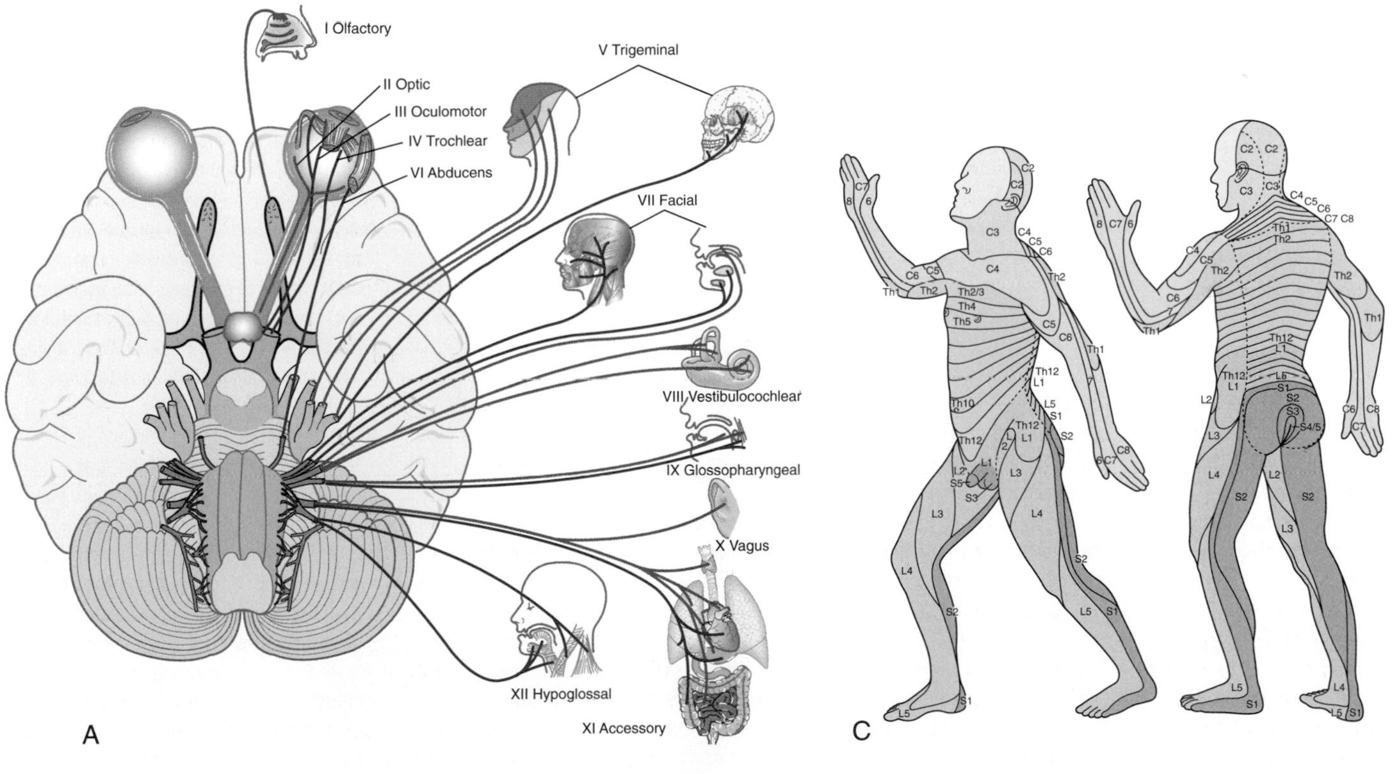

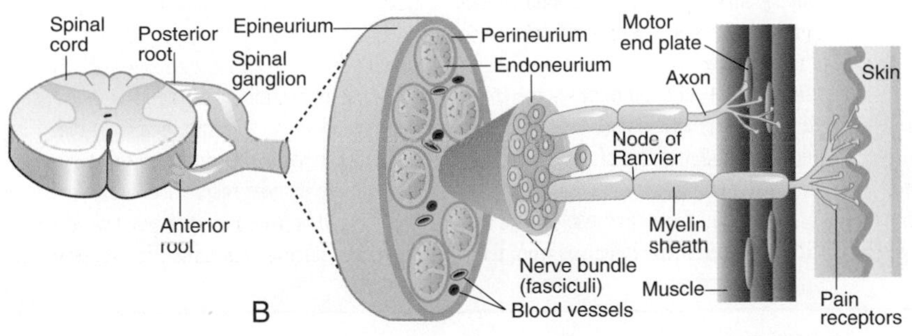

FIGURE 13-25 Cranial and Peripheral Nerves and Skin Dermatomes. A, Ventral surface of the brain showing attachment of the cranial nerves. The red lines indicate motor function, and the blue lines indicate sensory function. **B,** Peripheral nerve trunk and coverings. **C,** Dermatome map, anterolateral view (*left*) and posterolateral view (*right*). (**A,** from Applegate, E. [2011]. *The anatomy and physiology learning system* [4th ed.]. St. Louis: Saunders. **C,** from Salvo, S.G. [2014]. *Mosby's pathology for massage therapists* [3rd ed.]. St. Louis: Mosby.)

TABLE 13-6 The Cranial Nerves

Number and Name	Origin and Course	Function	How Tested
I. Olfactory	Fibres arise from nasal olfactory epithelium and form synapses with olfactory bulbs, which transmit impulses to temporal lobe.	It is purely sensory; it carries impulses for sense of smell.	Person is asked to sniff aromatic substances, such as oil of cloves and vanilla, and to identify them.
II. Optic	Fibres arise from retina of eye to form the optic nerve, which passes through sphenoid bone; two optic nerves then form optic chiasma (with partial crossover of fibres) and eventually end in the occipital cortex.	It is purely sensory; it carries impulses for vision.	Vision and visual field are tested with an eye chart and by testing the point at which the person first sees an object (finger) moving into the visual field; inside of eye is viewed with ophthalmoscope to observe blood vessels of eye interior.
III. Oculomotor	Fibres emerge from the midbrain and exit from the skull to run to the eye.	It contains motor fibres to the inferior oblique and to superior, inferior, and medial rectus extraocular muscles that direct the eyeball; levator muscles of the eyelid; smooth muscles of iris and ciliary body; and proprioception (sensory) to the brain from extraocular muscles.	Pupils are examined for size, shape, and equality; pupillary reflex is tested with a penlight (pupils should constrict when illuminated); and the ability to follow moving objects is tested.
IV. Trochlear	Fibres emerge from the posterior midbrain and exit from the skull to run to the eye.	Proprioceptor and motor fibres for superior oblique muscle of eye (extraocular muscle).	It is tested in common with cranial nerve III relative to the ability to follow moving objects.
V. Trigeminal	Fibres emerge from the pons and form three divisions that exit from the skull and run to the face and cranial dura mater.	It provides both motor and sensory impulses for the face; it conducts sensory impulses from the mouth, nose, surface of eye, and dura mater; it also contains motor fibres that stimulate chewing muscles.	Sensations of pain, touch, and temperature are tested with a safety pin and hot and cold objects; corneal reflex is tested with a wisp of cotton; motor branch is tested by asking subject to clench teeth, open mouth against resistance, and move jaw from side to side.
VI. Abducens	Fibres leave the inferior pons and exit from the skull to run to the eye.	It contains motor fibres to lateral rectus muscle and proprioceptor fibres from the same muscle to the brain.	It is tested in common with cranial nerve III relative to the ability to move each eye laterally.
VII. Facial	Fibres leave the pons and travel through temporal bone to reach face.	Mixed: (1) it supplies motor fibres to muscles of facial expression and to lacrimal and salivary glands, and (2) it carries sensory fibres from taste buds of anterior part of tongue	Anterior two thirds of the tongue are tested for the ability to taste sweet (sugar), salty, sour (vinegar), and bitter (quinine) substances; symmetry of face is checked; the subject is asked to close eyes, smile, whistle, and so on; tearing is tested with ammonia fumes.
VIII. Vestibulocochlear (acoustic)	Fibres run from the inner ear (hearing and equilibrium receptors in temporal bone) to enter brainstem just below the pons.	It is purely sensory; the vestibular branch transmits impulses for sense of equilibrium; cochlear branch transmits impulses for sense of hearing.	Hearing is checked by air and bone conduction by use of a tuning fork; vestibular tests: Bárány and caloric tests.
IX. Glossopharyngeal	Fibres emerge from the medulla and leave the skull to run to the throat.	Mixed: (1) motor fibres serve pharynx (throat) and salivary glands, and (2) sensory fibres carry impulses from pharynx, posterior tongue (taste buds), and pressure receptors of carotid artery.	Gag and swallow reflexes are checked; the subject is asked to speak and cough; the posterior one third of tongue may be tested for taste.
X. Vagus	Fibres emerge from the medulla, pass through the skull, and descend through the neck region into the thorax and abdominal region.	Fibres carry sensory and motor impulses for pharynx; a large part of this nerve is parasympathetic motor fibres, which supply smooth muscles of abdominal organs; it receives sensory impulses from viscera.	The test is the same as for cranial nerve IX (IX and X are tested in common) because they both serve muscles of the throat.
XI. Spinal accessory	Fibres arise from the medulla and superior spinal cord and travel to muscles of neck and back.	It provides sensory and motor fibres for sternocleidomastoid and trapezius muscles, and muscles of soft palate, pharynx, and larynx.	Sternocleidomastoid and trapezius muscles are checked for strength by asking the subject to rotate head and shrug shoulders against resistance.
XII. Hypoglossal	Fibres arise from the medulla and exit from the skull to travel to the tongue.	It carries motor fibres to muscles of the tongue and sensory impulses from the tongue to the brain.	The subject is asked to stick out tongue, and any position abnormalities are noted.

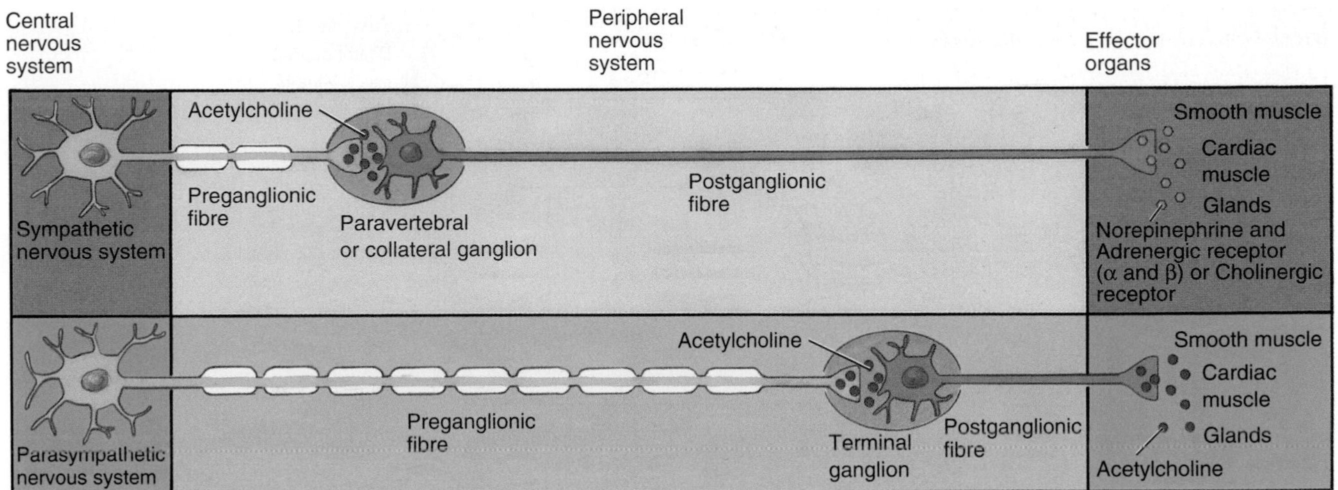

FIGURE 13-26 Preganglionic and Postganglionic Fibres of the Autonomic Nervous System. (From Applegate, E. [2011]. *The anatomy and physiology learning system* [4th ed.]. St. Louis: Saunders.)

leave the collateral ganglia and innervate the viscera below the diaphragm.

Preganglionic sympathetic neurons that innervate the adrenal medulla also travel in the splanchnic nerves and *do not* synapse before reaching the gland. The secretory cells in the adrenal medulla are considered modified postganglionic neurons. Because preganglionic sympathetic fibres are all myelinated, travel to the adrenal medulla is quick, and innervation causes the rapid release of epinephrine and norepinephrine. Epinephrine and norepinephrine are mediators of the fight-or-flight response (see Chapter 9).

Anatomy of the Parasympathetic Nervous System

The parasympathetic nervous system conserves and restores energy. The nerve cell bodies of this division are located in the cranial nerve nuclei and in the sacral region of the spinal cord and therefore constitute the **craniosacral division**. Unlike the sympathetic branch, the preganglionic fibres in the parasympathetic division travel close to the organs they innervate before forming synapses with the relatively short postganglionic neurons (see Figure 13-27). Parasympathetic nerves arising from nuclei in the brainstem travel to the viscera of the head, thorax, and abdomen within cranial nerves—including the oculomotor (III), facial (VII), glossopharyngeal (IX), and vagus (X) nerves.

Preganglionic parasympathetic nerves that originate from the sacral region of the spinal cord run either separately or together with some spinal nerves. The preganglionic axons unite to form the **pelvic nerve**, which innervates the viscera of the pelvic cavity. These preganglionic axons synapse with postganglionic neurons in terminal ganglia located close to the organs they innervate.

Neurotransmitters and Neuroreceptors

Sympathetic preganglionic fibres and parasympathetic preganglionic and postganglionic fibres release **acetylcholine**—the same neurotransmitter released by somatic efferent neurons (see Figure 13-26). These fibres are characterized by **cholinergic transmission**. Most postganglionic sympathetic fibres release **norepinephrine** (adrenaline) and thus are considered to function by **adrenergic transmission**. A few postganglionic sympathetic fibres, such as those that innervate the sweat glands, release acetylcholine.

The action of catecholamines varies with the type of neuroreceptor stimulated. It should be remembered that catecholamines also are released by the adrenal medulla gland that physiologically and biochemically resembles the sympathetic nervous system. Two types of adrenergic receptors exist, α and β. Cells of the effector organs may have only one or both types of adrenergic receptors. The **α-adrenergic receptors** have been further subdivided according to the action produced. α_1-Adrenergic activity is associated mostly with excitation or stimulation; α_2-adrenergic activity is associated with relaxation or inhibition. Most of the α-adrenergic receptors on effector organs belong to the α_1 class. The **β-adrenergic receptors** are classified as β_1-adrenergic receptors (which facilitate increased heart rate and contractility and cause the release of renin from the kidney) and β_2-adrenergic receptors (which facilitate all remaining effects attributed to β receptors).[11] Norepinephrine stimulates all α_1 and β_1 receptors and only certain β_2 receptors. The primary response from norepinephrine, however, is stimulation of the α_1-adrenergic receptors that cause vasoconstriction. Epinephrine strongly stimulates all four types of receptors and induces general vasodilation because of the predominance of β receptors in muscle vasculatures. (Table 13-7 summarizes the effects of neuroreceptors on their effector organs.)

Functions of the Autonomic Nervous System

Many body organs are innervated by both the sympathetic and parasympathetic nervous systems. The two divisions often cause opposite responses; for example, sympathetic stimulation of the stomach causes decreased peristalsis, whereas parasympathetic stimulation of the intestine increases peristalsis. In general, sympathetic stimulation promotes responses for the protection of the individual. For example, sympathetic activity increases blood glucose levels and temperature and raises the blood pressure. In emergency situations, a generalized and widespread discharge of the sympathetic system occurs, the fight-or-flight response, or acute stress response (see Chapter 9). This response is accomplished by an increased firing frequency of sympathetic fibres and by activation of sympathetic fibres normally silent and at rest (fibres to the sweat glands, pilomotor muscles, and the adrenal medulla, as well as vasodilator fibres to muscle). Regulation of vasomotor tone is considered the single most important function of the sympathetic nervous system. (Figure 13-28 illustrates some of the most important functions of the sympathetic nervous system.)

Increased parasympathetic activity promotes rest and tranquility and is characterized by reduced heart rate and enhanced visceral functions

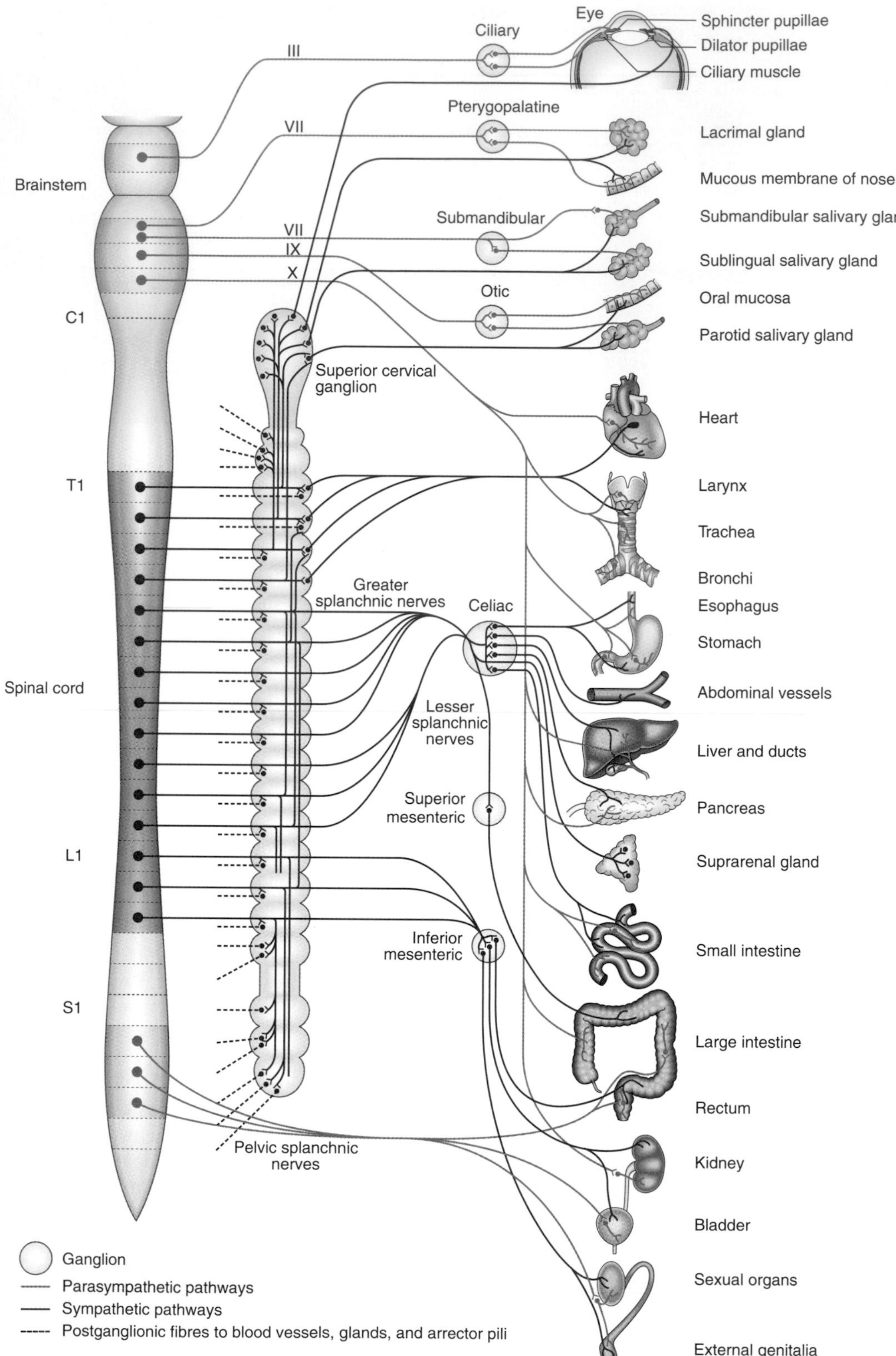

FIGURE 13-27 Sympathetic and Parasympathetic Divisions of the Autonomic Nervous System. Preganglionic neuron cell bodies are located in the brainstem and sacral cord segments (parasympathetic or "cranio-sacral" division) and thoracic and upper lumbar cord segments (sympathetic or "thoraco-lumbar" division). The axons of these neurons synapse with postganglionic neurons, which innervate smooth muscle, cardiac muscle, and glands of the body. The postganglionic neuron cell bodies may be located in distinct autonomic ganglia (represented with circles), or in or very near the wall of the innervated visceral organ. Note that sympathetic fibres provide the only innervation to peripheral effectors (sweat glands, arrector pili muscles, adipose tissue, and blood vessels). (From Cramer, D., & Darby, S. [2005]. *Basic and clinical anatomy of the spine, spinal cord, and ANS* [2nd ed.]. St. Louis: Elsevier Mosby.)

TABLE 13-7 Actions of Autonomic Nervous System Neuroreceptors

Effector Organ or Tissue	Adrenergic Receptors	Adrenergic Effects	Cholinergic Effects (Nicotine and Muscarinic[a] Receptors)
Eye, iris			
Radial muscle	α_1	Dilation	—
Sphincter muscle	—	—	Constriction
Eye, ciliary muscle	β_2	Relaxation for far vision	Contraction for near vision
Lacrimal glands	α_1	Secretion	Secretion
Nasopharyngeal glands	—	—	Secretion
Salivary glands	α_1	Secretion of potassium and water	Secretion of potassium and water
	β	Secretion of amylase	—
Heart			
Sinoatrial (SA) node	β_1, β_2	Increase heart rate	Decrease heart rate; vagus arrest
Atrial	β_1, β_2	Increase contractility and conduction velocity	Decrease contractility; shorten action potential duration
Atrioventricular (AV) junction	β_1, β_2	Increase automaticity and propagation velocity	Decrease automaticity and propagation velocity
Purkinje system	β_1, β_2	Increase automaticity and propagation velocity	—
Ventricles	β_1, β_2	Increase contractility	Slight decrease in contraction
Arterioles			
Coronary	α_1, α_2, β_2	Constriction, dilation	Dilation
Skin and mucosa	α_1, α_2	Constriction	Dilation
Skeletal muscle	α, β_2	Dilation, constriction	Dilation
Cerebral	α_1	Constriction (slight)	Dilation
Pulmonary	α_1, β_2	Constriction, dilation	Dilation
Mesenteric	α_1	Constriction	Dilation
Renal	α_1, β_1, β_2	Constriction, dilation	Dilation
Salivary glands	α_1, α_2	Constriction	Dilation
Veins, systemic	α_1, α_2, β_2	Constriction, dilation	—
Lung			
Bronchial muscle	α_2	Relaxation	Contraction
Bronchial glands	α_1, β_2	Decrease secretion; increase secretion	Stimulation
Stomach			
Motility	α_1, α_2, β_1, β_2	Decrease (usually)	Increase
Sphincters	α_1	Contraction (usually)	Relaxation (usually)
Secretion	α_2	Inhibition	Stimulation
Liver	α_1, β_2	Glycogenolysis and gluconeogenesis	—
Gallbladder and ducts	β_2	Relaxation	Contraction
Pancreas			
Acini	α	Decrease secretion	Secretion
Islet cells	α_2, β_2	Decrease secretion; increase secretion	—
Intestine			
Motility and tone	α_1, α_2, β_1, β_2	Decrease	Increase
Sphincters	α_1	Contraction	Relaxation (usually)
Secretion	α_2	Inhibition	Stimulation
Adrenal medulla	—	Secretion of epinephrine and norepinephrine (nicotinic effect)	
Kidney			
Renin secretion	α_1, β_1	Decrease; increase	—
Ureter			
Motility and tone	β_1	Increase	Increase (?)
Urinary bladder			
Detrusor	β_2	Relaxation	Contraction
Trigone and sphincter	α_1	Contraction	Relaxation
Sex organs, male	α_1	Ejaculation	Erection
Skin			
Pilomotor muscles	α_1	Contraction	—
Sweat glands	α_1	Localized secretion	—
Fat cells	α_2, β_1, β_2, β_3	Inhibition of lipolysis; stimulation of lipolysis	—
Pineal gland	β	Melatonin synthesis	—

[a]Muscarinic receptors respond to circulating muscarinic antagonists.

Modified from Brunton, L.L., Chabner, B.A., & Knollmann, B.C. (Eds.). (2011). *Goodman & Gilman's The pharmacological basis of therapeutics* (12th ed.). New York: McGraw-Hill; Yagiela, J.A., Dowd, F., Johnson, B., et al. (2011). *Pharmacology and therapeutics for dentistry* [6th ed.]. St. Louis: Mosby.

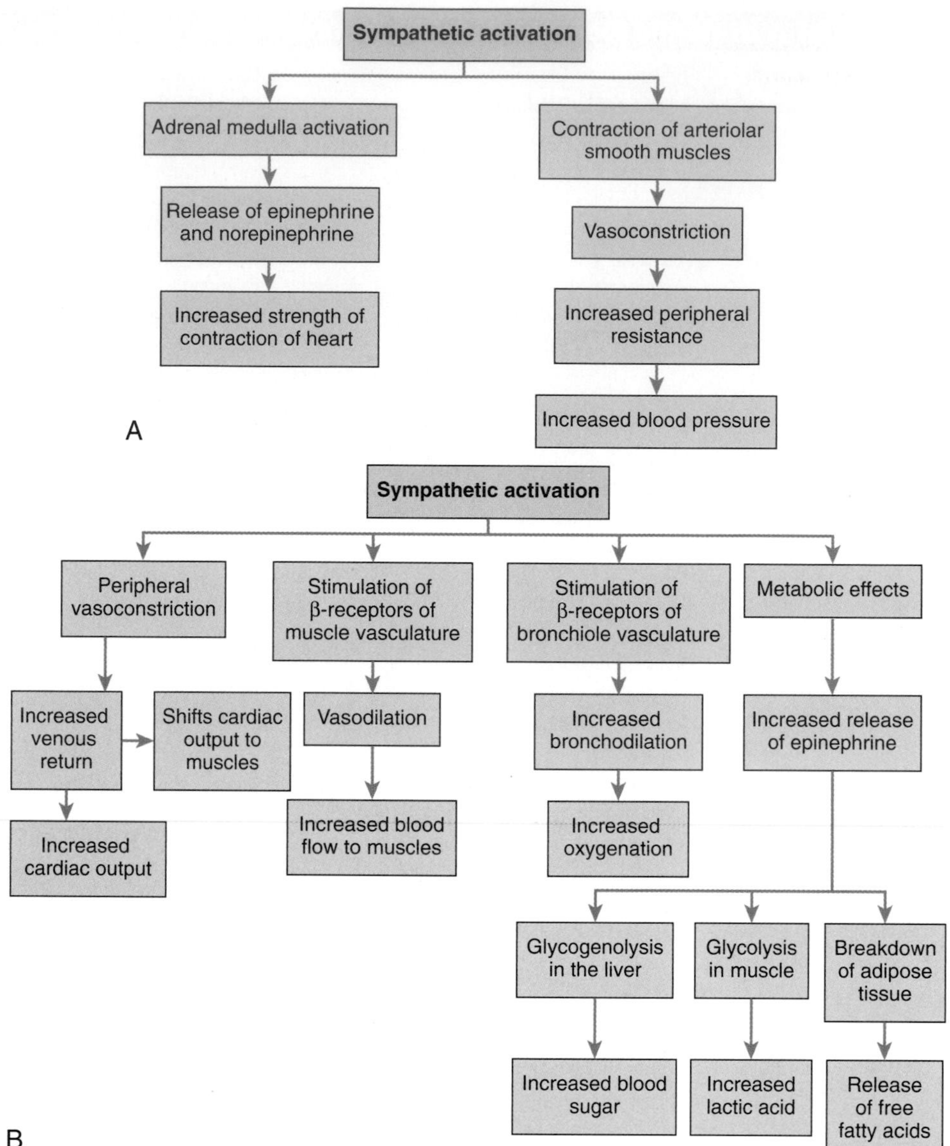

FIGURE 13-28 Examples of Important Functions of the Sympathetic Nervous System. A, Regulation of vasomotor tone. **B,** Regulation of strenuous muscular exercise ("fight-or-flight response," or acute stress response). (See also Chapter 9 and Figure 9.3 for more details on the stress response.)

concerned with digestion. Stimulation of the vagus nerve (cranial nerve X) in the gastro-intestinal tract increases peristalsis and secretion, as well as the relaxation of sphincters. Activation of parasympathetic fibres in the head, provided by cranial nerves III, VII, and IX, causes constriction of the pupil, tear secretion, and increased salivary secretion. Stimulation of the sacral division of the parasympathetic system contracts the urinary bladder and facilitates the process of genital erection.

The parasympathetic system lacks the generalized and widespread response of the sympathetic system. Specific parasympathetic fibres are activated to regulate particular functions. Although the actions of the parasympathetic and sympathetic systems are usually antagonistic, there are exceptions. Peripheral vascular resistance, for example, is increased dramatically by sympathetic activation but is not altered appreciably by activity of the parasympathetic system. Most blood vessels involved in the control of blood pressure are innervated by sympathetic nerves. To decrease blood pressure, therefore, it is more important to block or paralyze the continuous (tonic) discharge of the sympathetic system than to promote parasympathetic activity.

QUICK CHECK 13-6

1. What are the structural and functional divisions of the autonomic nervous system?
2. Compare cholinergic and adrenergic transmission.
3. What are the functions of the autonomic nervous system?

GERIATRIC CONSIDERATIONS

Aging and the Nervous System

Structural Changes With Aging
- Decrease in brain weight and size, particularly frontal regions
- Increase in ventricular volume
- Fibrosis and thickening of the meninges
- Narrowing of gyri and widening of sulci
- Increase in size of ventricles

Cellular Changes With Aging
- Decrease in number of neurons not consistently related to changes in mental function
- Decrease in myelin
- Lipofuscin deposition (a pigment resulting from cellular autodigestion)
- Decrease in number of dendritic processes and synaptic connections
- Intracellular neurofibrillary tangles; significant accumulation in cortex associated with Alzheimer's dementia
- Imbalance in amount and distribution of neurotransmitters
- Decrease in glucose metabolism

Cerebrovascular Changes With Aging
- Arterial atherosclerosis (may cause infarcts and scars)
- Increase in permeability of blood–brain barrier
- Decrease in vascular density

Functional Changes With Aging*
- Decrease in tendon reflexes
- Progressive deficit in taste and smell
- Decrease in vibratory sense
- Decrease in accommodation and colour vision
- Decrease in neuromuscular control with change in gait and posture
- Sleep disturbances
- Memory impairments
- Cognitive alterations associated with chronic disease

*Functional changes and nervous system aging have significant individual variation.

Data from Chételat, G., Landeau, B., Salmon, E., et al. (2013). *Neuroimage, 76*, 167–177; Fjell, A.M., McEvoy, L., Holland, D., et al. (2014). *Prog Neurobiol, 117*, 20–40; Fjell, A.M., & Walhovd, K.B. (2010). *Rev Neurosci, 21*(3), 187–221; Xekardaki, A., Kövari, E., Gold, G., et al. (2015). *Adv Exp Med Biol, 821*, 11–17.

DID YOU UNDERSTAND?

Overview and Organization of the Nervous System

1. The divisions of the nervous system have been categorized as either structural (central nervous system [CNS] and peripheral nervous system [PNS]) or functional (somatic nervous system and autonomic nervous system [ANS]).
2. The CNS consists of the brain and spinal cord.
3. The PNS is composed of the cranial and spinal nerves, which carry impulses toward the CNS (afferent—sensory) and away from the CNS (efferent—motor) to and from target organs or skeletal muscle.

Cells of the Nervous System

1. The neuron and neuroglial cells (non-nerve cells) constitute nervous tissue. The neuron is specialized in transmitting and receiving electrical and chemical impulses, whereas the neuroglial cell provides supportive and maintenance functions.
2. The neuron is composed of a cell body, dendrite(s), and an axon. A myelin sheath around selected axons forms insulation that allows faster nerve impulse conduction.
3. The neuron is further divided into unipolar, pseudounipolar, bipolar, and multipolar categories, according to its structure and particular mechanics of impulse transmission.

The Nerve Impulse

1. The region between the neurons is the synapse, and the region between the neuron and muscle is the myoneural junction.
2. Neurotransmitters are responsible for chemical conduction across the synapse, and the myoneural junction nerve impulse is regulated predominantly by a balance of inhibitory postsynaptic potentials (IPSPs) and excitatory postsynaptic potentials (EPSPs), temporal and spatial summation, and convergence and divergence.

The Central Nervous System

1. The brain is contained within the cranial vault and is divided into three distinct regions: (a) forebrain, (b) midbrain, and (c) hindbrain.
2. The forebrain comprises the two cerebral hemispheres and allows conscious perception of internal and external stimuli, thought and memory processes, and voluntary control of skeletal muscles. The deep portion of the forebrain is termed the *diencephalon* and processes incoming sensory data. The centre for voluntary control of skeletal muscle movements is located along the precentral gyrus in the frontal lobe, whereas the centre for perception is along the postcentral gyrus in the parietal lobe. The Broca area (inferior frontal gyrus) and the Wernicke area (superior temporal gyrus) are major speech centres.
3. The midbrain is primarily a relay centre for motor and sensory tracts, as well as a centre for auditory and visual reflexes.
4. The hindbrain allows sampling and comparison of sensory data, which are received from the periphery and motor impulses of the cerebral hemispheres, for the purpose of coordination and refinement of skeletal muscle movement.
5. The spinal cord contains most of the nerve fibres that connect the brain with the periphery. The corticospinal tracts are descending pyramidal (motor) pathways from the motor cortex. The rubrospinal and reticulospinal tracts are descending extrapyramidal tracts that coordinate movement. The posterior column, anterior spinothalamic tract, and lateral spinothalamic tract carry sensory information to the brainstem and thalamus, where information is relayed to the sensory cortex. Reflex arcs are sensory and motor circuits completed in the spinal cord and influenced by the higher centres in the brain.
6. The CNS is protected by the scalp, bony cranium, meninges (dura mater, arachnoid, and pia mater), cerebrospinal fluid (CSF), and the vertebral column. CSF is formed from blood components in the choroid plexuses of the ventricles and is reabsorbed in the arachnoid villi (located in the dural venous sinuses) after circulating through the brain and subarachnoid space.
7. The paired carotid and vertebral arteries supply blood to the brain and connect to form the circle of Willis. The major branches projecting from the circle of Willis are the anterior, middle, and posterior

cerebral arteries. Drainage of blood from the brain is accomplished through the venous sinuses and jugular veins.
8. The blood–brain barrier is provided by tight junctions between the cells of brain capillary endothelial cells and surrounding supporting cells.
9. Blood supply to the spinal cord originates from the vertebral arteries and branches arising from the aorta.

The Peripheral Nervous System

1. The cranial and spinal nerves constitute the PNS. The PNS relays information from the CNS to muscle and effector organs through cranial and spinal nerve tracts arranged in fascicles (multiple fascicles bound together form the peripheral nerve).

The Autonomic Nervous System

1. The ANS is responsible for maintaining a steady state in the internal environment. Two opposing systems make up the ANS: (a) the sympathetic nervous system (thoracolumbar division) responds to stress by mobilizing energy stores and prepares the body to defend itself, and (b) the parasympathetic nervous system (craniosacral division) conserves energy and the body's resources. Both systems function, more or less, at the same time.

KEY TERMS

Acetylcholine, 331
Adrenergic transmission, 331
Afferent pathway (ascending pathway), 309
Afferent (sensory) neuron, 321
α-Adrenergic receptor, 331
Anterior column, 321
Anterior fossa, 323
Anterior horn (ventral horn), 321
Anterior spinal artery, 327
Anterior spinothalamic tract, 323
Arachnoid, 323
Arachnoid villi, 324
Association fibre, 316
Associational neuron (interneuron), 310
Astrocyte, 310
Autonomic nervous system (ANS), 309
Axon, 310
Axon hillock, 310
Basal ganglia (basal nuclei), 317
Basal ganglia system (extrapyramidal system), 315
Basilar artery, 325
Basis pedunculi, 319
β-Adrenergic receptor, 331
Bipolar neuron, 310
Blood–brain barrier (BBB), 326
Brachial plexus, 328
Brain network, 314
Brainstem, 313
Broca area (Brodmann areas 44, 45), 316
Cauda equina, 320
Caudate nucleus, 317
Cavernous sinus, 325
Celiac, 328
Central canal, 321
Central nervous system (CNS), 309
Central sulcus (fissure of Rolando), 315
Cerebellum, 313
Cerebral aqueduct (aqueduct of Sylvius), 319
Cerebral cortex, 314
Cerebral nuclei, 317
Cerebral peduncle, 319
Cerebrospinal fluid (CSF), 323
Cholinergic transmission, 331
Choroid plexus, 323
Circle of Willis, 325
Collateral ganglia, 328
Contralateral control, 316
Conus medullaris, 320
Convergence, 313
Corpora quadrigemina, 319
Corpus callosum (transverse or commissural fibres), 317
Corticobulbar tract, 316
Corticobulbar tract axon, 322
Corticospinal tract (pyramidal system), 316
Cranial nerve, 309
Craniosacral division, 331
Dendrite, 310
Dermatome, 328
Diencephalon (interbrain), 317
Divergence, 313
Dopamine, 319
Dorsal root ganglion, 321
Dura mater, 323
Efferent (motor) neuron, 321
Effector organ, 309
Efferent pathway (descending pathway), 309
Ependymal cell, 310
Epicritic information, 322
Epithalamus, 317
Excitatory postsynaptic potential (EPSP), 313
Extradural space, 323
Extrapyramidal system, 317
Facilitation, 313
Falx cerebri, 323
Fascicle, 327
Filum terminale, 320
Frontal lobe, 315
Galea aponeurotica, 323
Ganglia (plexus), 310
Globus pallidus, 317
Grey matter, 314
Hypothalamus, 317
Inferior colliculi, 319
Inferior mesenteric, 328
Inhibitory postsynaptic potential (IPSP), 313
Inner dura (meningeal layer), 323
Insula (insular lobe), 317
Internal capsule, 317
Internal carotid artery, 325
Interventricular foramen (foramen of Monro), 323
Intervertebral disc, 324
Lateral aperture (foramen of Luschka), 324
Lateral column, 321
Lateral corticospinal tract, 322
Lateral horn, 321
Lateral spinothalamic tract, 323
Lateral sulcus (sylvian fissure, lateral fissure), 315
Lentiform nucleus, 317
Limbic system, 317
Longitudinal fissure, 315
Lower motor neuron, 322
Lumbar plexus, 328
Median aperture (foramen of Magendie), 324
Meninges, 323
Metencephalon, 319
Microfilament, 310
Microglia, 310
Microtubule, 310
Midbrain (mesencephalon), 319
Middle fossa (temporal fossa), 323
Mixed nerves, 327
Motor unit, 322
Multipolar neuron, 310
Myelencephalon (medulla oblongata), 319
Myelin, 310
Myelin sheath, 310
Neurofibril, 310
Neurogenesis, 313
Neuroglia, 310
Neuroglial cell, 309
Neuromuscular (myoneural) junction, 310
Neuron, 309
Neuroplasticity, 313
Neurotransmitter, 313
Neurotrophic factors, 313
Nissl substance, 310
Nodes of Ranvier, 310
Nonmyelinating Schwann cell, 311
Norepinephrine, 331
Nucleus pulposus, 324
Occipital lobe, 317
Oligodendroglia (oligodendrocyte), 310
Parasympathetic nervous system, 328
Parietal lobe, 316
Pelvic nerve, 331
Periosteum (endosteal layer), 323
Peripheral nervous system (PNS), 309
Pia mater, 323
Plexus, 328
Pons, 319
Postcentral gyrus, 316
Posterior (dorsal) column (fasciculus gracilis, fasciculus cuneatus), 322
Posterior fossa, 323
Posterior horn (dorsal horn), 321
Posterior spinal artery, 327
Postganglionic neuron, 328
Postsynaptic neuron, 313
Precentral gyrus, 316
Prefrontal area, 315
Preganglionic neuron, 328
Premotor area (Brodmann area 6), 315
Presynaptic neuron, 313
Primary motor area (Brodmann area 4), 316
Primary voluntary motor area, 316
Protopathic, 323
Pseudounipolar neuron, 310
Putamen, 317

Pyramidal system, 316
Red nucleus, 319
Reflex arc, 321
Reticular activating system (RAS), 314
Reticular formation, 313
Reticulospinal tract, 322
Rubrospinal tract, 322
Sacral plexus, 328
Saltatory conduction, 310
Satellite cell, 309
Schwann (neurilemma) cell, 309
Sensory neuron, 310
Somatic nervous system, 309
Spatial summation, 313
Spinal cord, 320
Spinal tract, 321
Spinothalamic tract, 321
Splanchnic nerve, 328
Striatum, 317
Subarachnoid space, 323
Subdural space, 323
Substantia gelatinosa, 321
Substantia nigra, 319
Subthalamus, 317
Sulci, 314
Summation, 313
Superior colliculi, 319
Superior mesenteric, 328
Sympathetic nervous system, 328
Sympathetic (paravertebral) ganglia, 328
Synapse, 313
Synaptic bouton, 313
Synaptic cleft, 313
Tegmentum, 319
Telencephalon (cerebral hemisphere), 314
Temporal lobe, 317
Temporal summation, 313
Tentorium cerebelli, 323
Thalamus, 317
Thoracolumbar division, 328
Unipolar neuron, 310
Upper motor neuron, 322
Ventricle, 323
Vermis, 319
Vertebral artery, 325
Vertebral column, 320
Vestibulospinal tract, 322
Wallerian degeneration, 311
Wernicke area, 317
White matter, 314

REFERENCES

1. Bernardinelli, Y., Muller, D., & Nikonenko, I. (2014). Astrocyte-synapse structural plasticity. *Neural Plasticity, 2014*, 232105. doi:10.1155/2014/232105.
2. Kim, H. A., Mindos, T., & Parkinson, D. B. (2013). Plastic fantastic: Schwann cells and repair of the peripheral nervous system. *Stem Cells Translational Medicine, 2*(8), 553–557. doi:10.5966/sctm.2013-0011.
3. Sulaiman, W., & Gordon, T. (2013). Neurobiology of peripheral nerve injury, regeneration, and functional recovery: From bench top research to bedside application. *The Ochsner Journal, 13*(1), 100–108.
4. Kolb, B., Whishaw, I. Q., & Teskey, G. C. (2016). *An introduction to brain and behavior* (5th ed.). New York: Worth.
5. Elphick, M. R. (2012). The evolution and comparative neurobiology of endocannabinoid signalling. *Philosophical Transactions of the Royal Society of London. Series B, Biological Sciences, 367*(1607), 3201–3215. doi:10.1098/rstb.2011.0394.
6. Castillo, P. E., Younts, T. J., Chávez, A. E., et al. (2012). Endocannabinoid signaling and synaptic function. *Neuron, 76*(1), 70–81. doi:10.1016/j.neuron.2012.09.020.
7. Vanderah, T., & Gould, D. (2015). *Nolte's The human brain: An introduction to its functional anatomy* (7th ed.). St. Louis: Mosby.
8. Meehan, T. P., & Bressler, S. L. (2012). Neurocognitive networks: Findings, models, and theory. *Neuroscience and Biobehavioral Reviews, 36*(10), 2232–2247. doi:10.1016/j.neubiorev.2012.08.002.
9. Stam, C. J., & van Straaten, E. C. (2012). The organization of physiological brain networks. *Clinical Neurophysiology, 123*(6), 1067–1087. doi:10.1016/j.clinph.2012.01.011.
10. Obermeier, B., Daneman, R., & Ransohoff, R. M. (2013). Development, maintenance and distribution of the blood-brain barrier. *Nature Medicine, 19*, 1584–1596. doi:10.1038/nm.3407.
11. Brady, S. T., Siegel, G. J., Albers, R. W., et al. (2012). *Basic neurochemistry: Principles of molecular, cellular, and medical neurobiology* (8th ed.). Waltham, MA: Academic Press.

14

Pain, Temperature, Sleep, and Sensory Function

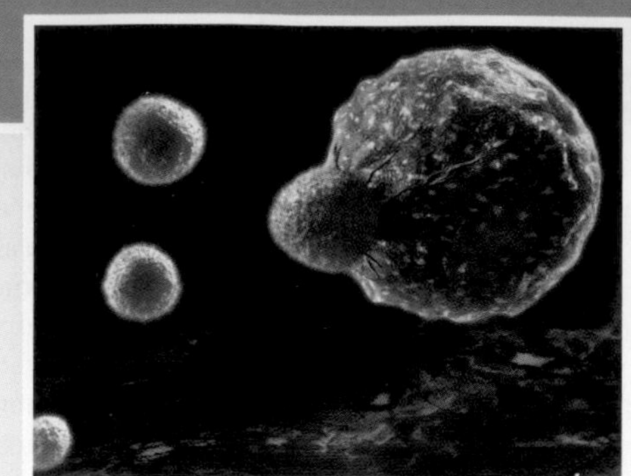

George W. Rodway, Sue E. Huether, Jan Belden, and Kelly Power-Kean*

EVOLVE WEBSITE

http://evolve.elsevier.com/Canada/Huether/pathophysiology

Student Review Questions
Key Points
Case Studies
Animations
Quick Check Answers

CHAPTER OUTLINE

Pain, 338
Theories of Pain, 338
Neuroanatomy of Pain, 339
Pain Modulation, 340
Clinical Descriptions of Pain, 342
Temperature Regulation, 344
Control of Body Temperature, 344
Temperature Regulation in Infants and Older Adults, 345
Pathogenesis of Fever, 346
Benefits of Fever, 346
Disorders of Temperature Regulation, 346
Sleep, 347
Sleep Disorders, 348
The Special Senses, 349
Vision, 349
Hearing, 354
Olfaction and Taste, 356
Somatosensory Function, 356
Touch, 356
Proprioception, 356
GERIATRIC CONSIDERATIONS: **Aging and Changes in Vision, 357**
GERIATRIC CONSIDERATIONS: **Aging and Changes in Hearing, 357**
GERIATRIC CONSIDERATIONS: **Aging and Changes in Olfaction and Taste, 357**

Alterations in sensory function may involve dysfunctions of the general or the special senses. Dysfunctions of the general senses include persistent pain (also referred to as *chronic pain*), abnormal temperature regulation, and tactile or proprioceptive dysfunction. Pain is an unpleasant but protective phenomenon that is uniquely experienced by each individual, and it cannot be adequately defined, identified, or measured by an observer. Like pain, variations in temperature can signal disease. Fever is a common manifestation of dysfunction and is often the first symptom observed in an infectious or inflammatory condition.

Sleep is a normal cyclic process that restores the body's energy and maintains normal functioning. Sleep is so essential to both physiological and psychological functions that sleep deprivation causes a wide range of clinical manifestations.

The special senses of vision, hearing, touch, smell, and taste are the means by which individuals perceive stimuli that are essential in interacting with the environment. Dysfunctions of the special senses include visual, auditory, vestibular, olfactory, and gustatory (taste) disorders.

*Jan Belden contributed to this chapter in the US 5th edition.

PAIN

Pain is a complex experience. It involves dynamic interactions between physical, cognitive, spiritual, emotional, and environmental factors and cannot be characterized as only a response to injury. McCaffery defined *pain* as "whatever the experiencing person says it is, existing whenever he says it does."[1] The Canadian Pain Coalition concurs with the International Association for the Study of Pain definition of *pain*, which is "an unpleasant sensory and emotional experience associated with actual or potential tissue damage or described in terms of such damage."[2] Acute pain is protective and promotes withdrawal from painful stimuli, allows the injured part to heal, and teaches avoidance of painful stimuli.

Theories of Pain

The theories of pain include the specificity theory, pattern theory, gate control theory, and neuromatrix theory.

Specificity theory proposes that injury activates specific pain receptors and fibres that project to the brain. *Intensity of pain* is directly related to the amount of associated tissue injury (i.e., pricking one's finger with a needle would cause minimal pain, whereas cutting one's hand with a knife would produce more pain). The theory is useful when applied to specific injuries and the acute pain associated with them. It does not account for persistent pain or cognitive and emotional elements that contribute to more complex types of pain.[3]

Pattern theory describes the role of impulse intensity and the repatterning of the central nervous system (CNS) in activating the perception of pain. Pattern theory is limited because it does not account for all types of pain experiences.[3]

Gate control theory integrates and builds upon features of the other theories to explain the complex multidimensional aspects of pain perception and pain modulation.[3] Pain transmission is modulated by a balance of impulses conducted to the spinal cord where cells in the substantia gelatinosa function as a "gate." The spinal gate regulates pain transmission to higher centres in the CNS. Largely myelinated **A delta (Aδ) fibres** and small unmyelinated **C fibres** respond to a broad range of painful stimuli (mechanical, thermal, and chemical). These fibres terminate on interneurons in the substantia gelatinosa (laminae in the dorsal horn of the spinal cord). **Nociceptive transmissions** on these fibres "open" the spinal gate and increase the perception of pain. Closure or partial closure of the spinal gates can occur from **non-nociceptive stimulation** (i.e., from touch sensors in the skin). These signals are carried on non-nociceptive larger **A beta (Aβ) fibres** (large myelinated fibres that transmit touch and vibration sensations) and decrease pain perception. The closure or partial closure of spinal gates through non-nociceptive stimulation (e.g., rubbing a painful area) explains why some of the pain or discomfort may be alleviated. Other efferent CNS pathways descend to the spinal cord and may close, partially close, or open the gate modulation of the pain experience. Gate control theory, bolstered by progress in understanding neuronal pathways in the peripheral and central nervous systems, has greatly advanced our understanding of pain. As good as the gate control theory has been, however, there are observations about pain in paraplegics that "do not fit the theory."

Neuromatrix theory proposes that the brain produces patterns of nerve impulses drawn from various inputs, including genetic, psychological, and cognitive experiences.[3] The qualities we normally feel from the body, including pain, also can be felt in the absence of inputs from the body (as noted with phantom limb pain). In other words, stimuli may trigger the patterns but do not produce them. Neuromatrix patterns are normally activated by sensory inputs from the periphery, but may originate independently in the brain with no external input.[3] The neuromatrix theory illustrates the plasticity (adaptable change in structure and function) of the brain. It does not supplant our understanding of gate control theory, and what we know about peripheral inflammation, spinal modulation, and midbrain descending control of pain. Neuromatrix theory builds upon gate control theory by explaining an integrated body–self, thus providing a holistic and dynamic consideration of pain. However, there are many different kinds of pain, and no single theory is adequate to explain the complex dynamics of the pain experience. Continuing research is advancing our understanding of the neural mechanisms of pain.[3]

Neuroanatomy of Pain

Three portions of the nervous system are responsible for the sensation of, perception of, and response to pain:

1. The *afferent pathways*, which begin in the peripheral nervous system (PNS), travel to the spinal gate in the dorsal horn and then ascend to higher centres in the CNS
2. The *interpretive centres* located in the brainstem, midbrain, diencephalon, and cerebral cortex
3. The *efferent pathways* that descend from the CNS back to the dorsal horn of the spinal cord

The processing of potentially harmful (noxious) stimuli through a normally functioning nervous system is called **nociception**.[2] **Nociceptors**, or pain receptors, are free nerve endings in the afferent PNS. When they are stimulated, they cause **nociceptive pain**. The cell bodies of nociceptors are located in the dorsal root ganglia for the body and in the trigeminal ganglion for the face. Nociceptors have a peripheral and central axonal branch that innervates their target organ and the spinal cord, respectively. Nociceptors are unevenly distributed throughout the body, so the relative sensitivity to pain differs according to their location (Table 14-1). Nociceptors respond to different types of noxious stimuli: mechanical (pressure or mechanical distortion), thermal (extreme temperatures), or chemical (acids or chemicals of inflammation such as bradykinin, histamine, leukotrienes, or prostaglandins). Nociception involves four phases: transduction, transmission, perception, and modulation.[4,5]

TABLE 14-1 Stimuli That Activate Nociceptors (Pain Receptors)

Location of Receptor	Provoking Stimuli
Skin	Pricking, cutting, crushing, burning, freezing
Gastro-intestinal tract	Engorged or inflamed mucosa, distension or spasm of smooth muscle, traction on mesenteric attachment
Skeletal muscle	Ischemia, injuries of connective tissue sheaths, necrosis, hemorrhage, prolonged contraction, injection of irritating solutions
Joints	Synovial membrane inflammation
Arteries	Piercing, inflammation
Head	Traction, inflammation, or displacement of arteries, meningeal structures, and sinuses; prolonged muscle contraction
Heart	Ischemia and inflammation
Bone	Periosteal injury: fractures, tumour, inflammation

Pain transduction begins when nociceptors are activated by a noxious stimulus, causing ion channels (sodium, potassium, calcium) on nociceptors to open, creating electrical impulses that travel through axons of two primary types of nociceptors that are transmitted to the spinal cord, brainstem, thalamus, and cortex (see Figure 13-9).[6] There are two primary types of nociceptors: Aδ fibres and C fibres. Aδ fibres are larger myelinated fibres that rapidly transmit sharp, well-localized "fast" pain sensations, such as a burn or pinprick to the skin. Activation of these fibres causes a spinal reflex withdrawal of the affected body part from the stimulus before a pain sensation is perceived.[7] C fibres are the most numerous, are smaller and unmyelinated, and are located in muscle, tendons, body organs, and in the skin. They slowly transmit dull, aching, or burning sensations that are poorly localized and often constant.[4,7,8]

Pain transmission is the conduction of pain impulses along the Aδ and C fibres (primary order neurons) into the dorsal horn of the spinal cord (Figure 14-1). Here they form synapses with excitatory or inhibitory interneurons (second-order neurons) in the substantia gelatinosa of the dorsal horn. The impulses then synapse with projection neurons (third-order neurons), cross the midline of the spinal cord, and ascend to the brain through two lateral spinothalamic tracts. The neospinothalamic tract (anterior spinal thalamic tract) carries fast impulses for acute sharp pain. The paleospinothalamic tract (lateral spinothalamic tract) carries slow impulses for dull or persistent pain. The fast sharp pain is perceived first, followed by dull, throbbing pain. These tracts connect to the reticular formation, hypothalamus, thalamus (the major relay station of sensory information), and the limbic system. The impulses

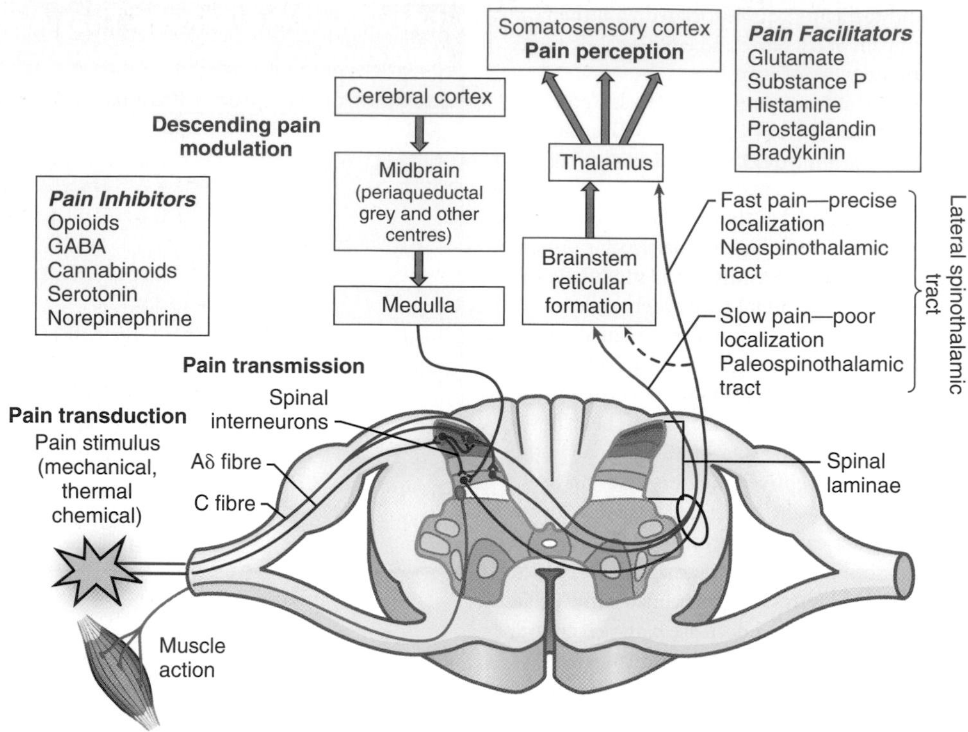

FIGURE 14-1 Transmission of Pain Sensations. The Aδ and C fibres synapse in the laminae of the dorsal horn, cross over to the contralateral spinothalamic tract, and then ascend to synapse in the midbrain through the neospinothalamic and paleospinothalamic tracts. Impulses are then conducted to the sensory cortex. Descending pain inhibition is initiated in the cerebral cortex or from the midbrain and medulla. *GABA*, gamma-aminobutyric acid.

are then projected to the somatosensory cortex for interpretation of location and intensity of pain (see Figure 14-1), and to other areas of the brain for an integrated response to pain.

Pain perception is the conscious awareness of pain, which occurs primarily in the reticular and limbic systems and the cerebral cortex. Interpretation of pain is influenced by many factors including genetics, cultural influences, gender roles, and life experience, including past pain experiences and level of health.[9] Three systems interact to produce the perception of pain.[10] The **sensory-discriminative system** is mediated by the somatosensory cortex and is responsible for identifying the presence, character, location, and intensity of pain. The **affective-motivational system** determines an individual's conditioned avoidance behaviours and emotional responses to pain. It is mediated through the reticular formation, limbic system, and brainstem. The **cognitive-evaluative system** overlies the individual's learned behaviour concerning the experience of pain and therefore can modulate perception of pain. It is mediated through the cerebral cortex. The integration of these three systems is referred to as the "pain matrix."[11]

Pain threshold and tolerance are subjective phenomena that influence an individual's perception of pain. They can be influenced by genetics, gender, cultural perceptions, expectations, role socialization, physical and mental health, and age[12,13] (Table 14-2). Clinicians often find it helpful to use pain scales to assess their patients' pain. Various pain scales are available for use with neonates, infants, children, adolescents, adults, older adults, and persons who have impaired communication skills.

Pain threshold is defined as the lowest intensity of pain that a person can recognize.[2] Intense pain at one location may increase the threshold in another location. For example, a person with severe pain in one knee is more likely to experience less intense persistent back pain (called **perceptual dominance**). Because of perceptual dominance, pain at one site may mask other painful areas. Stress, excessive physical exertion, acupuncture, sexual activity, and other factors can increase the levels of circulating neuromodulators, thereby raising the pain threshold.

Pain tolerance is defined as the greatest intensity of pain that a person can endure.[2] It varies greatly among people and in the same person over time because of the body's ability to respond differently to noxious stimuli (see Table 14-2). Pain tolerance generally *decreases* with repeated exposure to pain, fatigue, anger, boredom, apprehension, and sleep deprivation and may *increase* with alcohol consumption, persistent use of opioid medications, hypnosis, distracting activities, and strong beliefs or faith.

Pain Modulation

Pain modulation involves many different mechanisms that increase or decrease the transmission of pain signals throughout the nervous system. Depending on the mechanism, modulation can occur before, during, or after pain is perceived.[8]

Neurotransmitters of Pain Modulation

A wide variety of neurotransmitters act to modulate control over transmission of pain impulses in the periphery, spinal cord, and brain.[14,15] The peripheral triggering mechanisms that initiate release of **excitatory neurotransmitters** include tissue injury (prostaglandins, histamine, bradykinin) and chronic inflammatory lesions (lymphokines). Glutamate, aspartate, substance P, and calcitonin are common excitatory neurotransmitters in the brain and spinal cord. These substances sensitize nociceptors by reducing the activation threshold, leading to increased responsiveness of nociceptors.[16]

TABLE 14-2 Pain Perception in Infants, Children, and Older Adults

	Infants	Children	Older Adults
Pain threshold	Painful neonatal experiences increase pain sensitivity (lower threshold); pain may be increased with future procedures	Lower or same as adults	Individual responses, which vary, but pain threshold may be lower
Physiological symptoms	Increased heart rate, blood pressure, and respiratory rate; flushing or pallor, sweating, and decreased oxygen saturation	Same as infants; nausea and vomiting	Same as infants and children; nausea and vomiting; may be decreased in individuals with cognitive impairment
Behavioural responses	Changes in facial expression, crying, and body movements, with lowered brows drawn together; vertical bulge and furrows in forehead between brows; broadened nasal root; tightly closed eyes; angular, square-shaped mouth, chin quiver; withdrawal of affected limbs, rigidity, flailing	Individual responses, which vary	Individual responses, which vary, and may be influenced by presence of painful chronic diseases and decline in renal, intestinal, hepatic, cardiovascular, and neurological function; individuals with cognitive impairment may demonstrate changes in behaviour (e.g., combative or withdrawn, increased confusion)

Data from Maxwell, L.G., Malavolta, C.P., & Fraga, M.V. (2013). *Clin Perinatol, 40*(3), 457–469; Molton, I.R., & Terrill, A.L. (2014). *Am Psychol, 69*(2), 197–207; Tracy, B., & Sean Morrison, R. (2013). *Clin Ther, 35*(11), 1659–1668; Walker, S.M. (2014). *Paediatr Anaesth, 24*(1), 39–48.

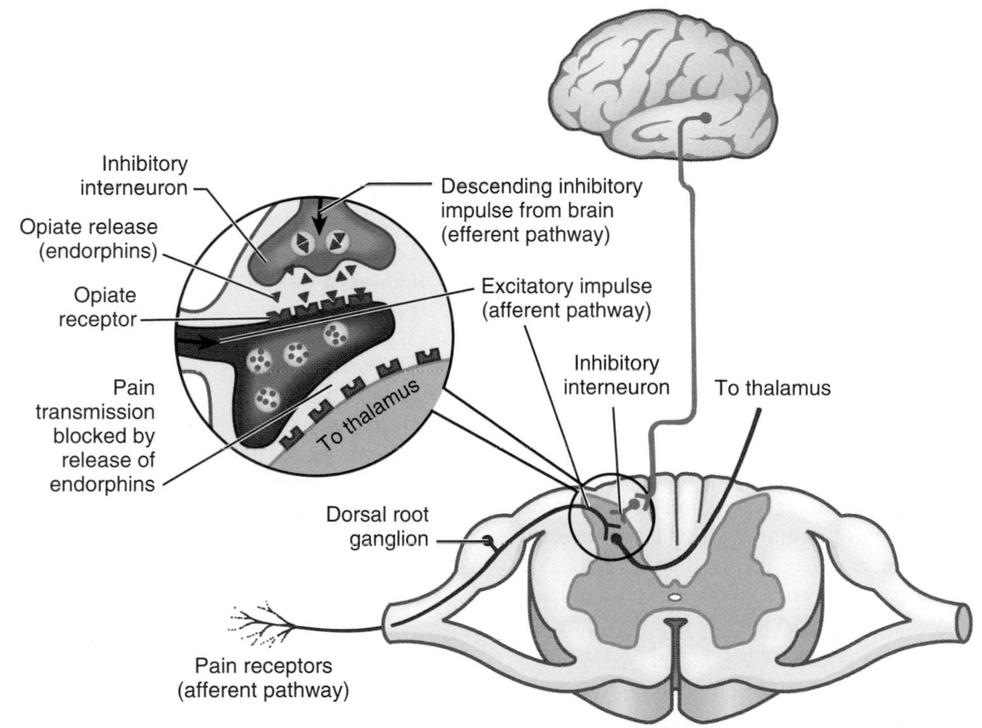

FIGURE 14-2 Descending Pathway and Endorphin Response. In this figure, a descending inhibitory impulse is transmitted from the brain to an inhibitory interneuron in the dorsal horn stimulating the release of endorphin. The endorphin activates a μ opioid receptor and results in inhibition of pain transmission to ascending pathways.

Inhibitory neurotransmitters in the spinal cord include gamma-aminobutyric acid (GABA) and glycine. Norepinephrine and 5-hydroxytryptamine (serotonin) contribute to pain inhibition in the medulla and pons, but can excite peripheral nerves.[5]

Endogenous opioids are a family of morphinelike neuropeptides that inhibit transmission of pain impulses in the periphery, spinal cord, and brain by binding with specific opioid receptors (mu [μ], kappa [κ], and delta [δ]) on neurons. They inhibit ion channels, preventing the release of excitatory neurotransmitters, such as substance P and glutamate, in the dorsal horn. In the midbrain they influence descending inhibitory pathways[17] (Figure 14-2). In peripheral inflamed tissue, opioids are produced and released from immune cells and activate opioid receptors on sensory nerve terminals.[18] Opioid receptors are widely distributed throughout the body and are responsible for general sensations of well-being and modulation of many physiological processes, including control of respiratory and cardiovascular functions, stress and immune responses, gastro-intestinal function, reproduction, and neuroendocrine control.[19,20]

Enkephalins are the most prevalent of the natural opioids and bind to δ opioid receptors. **Endorphins** (endogenous morphine) are produced in the brain. The best-studied endorphin is β-endorphin, which binds to μ receptors and is purported to produce the greatest sense of exhilaration as well as substantial natural pain relief. Dynorphins are the most potent of the endogenous opioids, binding strongly with κ receptors to impede pain signals. Paradoxically, they play a role in neuropathic pain and in mood disorders and medication addiction.[21] Endomorphins bind with μ receptors and have potent analgesic effects.[22] Nociceptin/orphanin FQ is an opioid that *induces* pain or hyperalgesia but does not interact with opioid receptors. The nociceptin receptor is widely distributed throughout the PNS and CNS and is also associated with inflammation, immune regulation, mood, and emotion.[23]

Synthetic and natural opiates have pharmacological actions similar to morphine and bind as direct agonists to the opioid receptors. Morphine has a 50 times higher affinity for μ receptors in comparison with other opioids. Naloxone (Narcan) is the only clinically used opioid receptor antagonist, with a higher affinity for the μ receptors than for the other receptors.[24]

Endocannabinoids are synthesized from phospholipids and are classified as eicosanoids. They activate cannabinoid CB_1 (primarily in the CNS) and CB_2 receptors (primarily in immune tissue [e.g., the spleen]) to modulate pain and other functions including memory, appetite, immune function, sleep, stress response, thermoregulation, and addiction. CB_1 receptors decrease pain transmission by inhibiting release of excitatory neurotransmitters in the spinal dorsal horn, periaqueductal grey, thalamus, rostral ventromedial medulla (RVM), and amygdala. Cannabis (marihuana) produces a resin containing cannabinoids. Cannabinoids are analgesic in humans, but their use is limited by their psychoactive and addictive properties. Work is in progress to develop cannabinoid receptor agonists that do not have addictive side effects.[25-27]

Pathways of Modulation

Descending inhibitory pathways, descending facilitatory pathways, and nuclei inhibit or facilitate pain. Afferent stimulation of the ventromedial medulla and periaqueductal grey (PAG) (grey matter surrounding the cerebral aqueduct), in particular, in the midbrain stimulates efferent pathways, which inhibit afferent pain signals at the dorsal horn.[28] The RVM stimulates efferent pathways that facilitate or inhibit pain in the dorsal horn.[29] Inhibitory pathways can activate opioid receptors and inhibit release of excitatory neurotransmitters, facilitate release of inhibitory neurotransmitters, or stimulate inhibitory interneurons.

Segmental pain inhibition occurs when Aβ fibres are stimulated and the impulses arrive at the same spinal level as impulses from Aδ or C fibres. They stimulate an inhibitory interneuron and decrease pain transmission. An example is rubbing an area that has been injured to relieve pain.[8]

Diffuse noxious inhibitory control (DNIC) is an inhibitory pain system that involves a spinal-medullary-spinal pathway. Pain is relieved when two noxious stimuli occur at the same time from different sites (pain inhibiting pain). This system also is known as heterosegmental pain inhibition and is the basis for pain relief with acupuncture, deep massage, or intense cold or heat.[30]

Expectancy-related cortical activation (placebo effect [beneficial expectations] or nocibo effect [adverse expectations]) can exert control over analgesic systems to attenuate or intensify pain.[31] In other words, cognitive expectations can cause real, measurable physiological effects that share some of the same descending pain pathways as the pain modulatory systems.

Clinical Descriptions of Pain

Pain can be described in a variety of ways. Because of the complex nature of pain, however, many terms overlap and more than one description is often used. The broad categories of pain are summarized in Box 14-1. Some of the most common clinical pain presentations are summarized next.

BOX 14-1 Categories of Pain

I. Neurophysiological Pain
- A. **Nociceptive pain**
  1. Somatic (e.g., skin, muscle, bone)
  2. Visceral (e.g., intestine, liver, stomach)
  3. Referred
- B. **Neuropathic (non-nociceptive)**
  1. Central pain (lesion in brain or spinal cord)
  2. Peripheral pain (lesion in peripheral nervous system)

II. Neurogenic Pain
- A. **Neuralgia (pain in the distribution of a nerve)**
- B. **Constant**
  1. Sympathetically independent
  2. Sympathetically dependent

III. Temporal Pain (time related, duration)
- A. **Acute pain**
  1. Somatic (e.g., pain resulting from skin laceration)
  2. Visceral (e.g., pain resulting from inflammation associated with appendicitis)
  3. Referred (e.g., shoulder pain referred from inflammation of the gallbladder)
- B. **Persistent pain**

IV. Pain Location
- A. **Abdominal pain**
- B. **Chest pain**
- C. **Headache**
- D. **Low back pain**
- E. **Orofacial pain**
- F. **Pelvic pain**

V. Etiological Pain
- A. **Cancer pain**
- B. **Dental pain**
- C. **Inflammatory pain**
- D. **Ischemic pain**
- E. **Vascular pain**

Adapted from Mersky, H. (2014). Taxonomy and classification of chronic pain syndromes. In H.T. Benzon, J.P. Rathmell, C.L. Wu, et al. (Eds.), *Practical management of pain* (5th ed., pp. 13–18). St. Louis: Mosby.

Acute pain (nociceptive pain) is a normal protective mechanism that alerts the individual to a condition or experience that is immediately harmful to the body and mobilizes the individual to take prompt action to relieve it. Acute pain is transient, usually lasting minutes to several weeks.[32] It begins suddenly and is relieved after the chemical mediators that stimulate pain receptors are removed.[33] Stimulation of the autonomic nervous system results in physical manifestations including increased heart rate, hypertension, diaphoresis, and dilated pupils. Anxiety related to the pain experience, including its cause, treatment, and prognosis, is common, as is the hope of recovery and expectation of limited duration.[9]

Acute pain arises from cutaneous, deep somatic, or visceral structures and can be classified as (1) somatic, (2) visceral, or (3) referred. Somatic pain arises from the skin, joints, and muscles. It is either sharp and

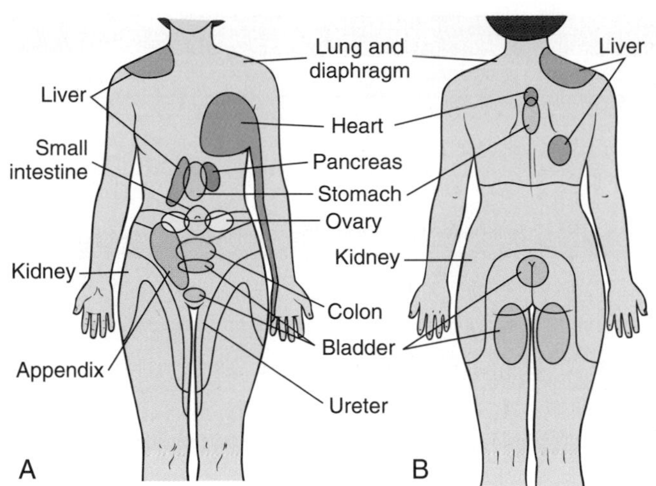

FIGURE 14-3 Sites of Referred Pain. **A**, Anterior view. **B**, Posterior view.

well localized (especially fast pain carried by Aδ fibres) or dull, aching, throbbing, and poorly localized as seen in polymodal C fibre transmissions. **Visceral pain** is transmitted by C fibres and refers to pain in internal organs and the lining of body cavities; it tends to be poorly localized with an aching, gnawing, throbbing, or intermittent cramping quality. It is carried by sympathetic fibres and is associated with nausea and vomiting, hypotension, and, in some cases, shock. Visceral pain often radiates (spreads away from the actual site of the pain) or is referred. **Referred pain** is felt in an area removed or distant from its point of origin—the area of referred pain is supplied by the same spinal segment as the actual site of pain. Impulses from many cutaneous and visceral neurons converge on the same ascending neuron, and the brain cannot distinguish between the different sources of pain. Because the skin has more receptors, the painful sensation is experienced at the referred site instead of at the site of origin.[34] Referred pain can be acute or persistent. Figure 14-3 illustrates common areas of referred pain and their associated sites of origin. (Figure 13-25 illustrates cranial and peripheral nerves and skin dermatomes; see also Box 14-1.)

Persistent pain (intractable pain) has been defined as lasting for more than 3 to 6 months and is pain lasting well beyond the expected normal healing time. It varies with type of injury.[35] Persistent pain serves no purpose and is poorly understood and causes suffering. It often appears to be out of proportion to any observable tissue injury. It may be ongoing (e.g., low back pain) or intermittent (e.g., migraine headaches). Changes in the PNS and CNS that cause dysregulation of nociception and pain modulation processes (peripheral and central sensitization) are thought to lead to persistent pain[36,37] (see the discussion of neuropathic pain, described later in this section).

Neuroimaging studies have demonstrated brain changes in individuals with persistent pain, which may lead to cognitive deficits and decreased ability to cope with pain.[38] These negative manifestations of persistent pain are thought to be due, in part, to the stress of coping with continuous pain and may be reversible when pain is controlled.[39-41] Because it is not yet possible to predict when acute pain will develop into persistent pain, early treatment of acute pain is encouraged.[42]

Physiological responses to intermittent persistent pain are similar to those for acute pain. Persistent pain, however, allows for physiological adaptation, producing normal heart rate and blood pressure. This normalization may lead many to mistakenly conclude that people with persistent pain are malingering because they do not appear to be in pain. As persistent pain progresses, certain behavioural and psychological changes often emerge, including depression, difficulty eating and sleeping, preoccupation with the pain, and avoidance of pain-provoking stimuli.[43] The desire to relieve pain and the need to hide it become conflicting drives for those with persistent pain, who fear being labelled as complainers.[44] Persistent pain is perceived as meaningless and is often associated with a sense of hopelessness as more time elapses and no cure seems possible. A few persistent pain syndromes are listed in Table 14-3. Comparison of acute and persistent pain is summarized in Table 14-4. Persistent pain associated with specific organ systems is discussed in later chapters.

Neuropathic pain is persistent pain initiated or caused by a primary lesion or dysfunction in the nervous system and leads to long-term changes in pain pathway structures (neuroplasticity) and abnormal processing of sensory information.[45] There is amplification of pain without stimulation by injury or inflammation. Neuropathic pain is often described as burning, shooting, shocklike, or tingling. It is characterized by increased sensitivity to painful or nonpainful stimuli with hyperalgesia, **allodynia** (the induction of pain by normally nonpainful stimuli), and the development of spontaneous pain.[46] Neuropathic pain is classified as either peripheral or central and is associated with central and peripheral sensitization.[47] **Peripheral neuropathic pain** is caused by peripheral nerve lesions and an increase in the sensitivity and excitability of primary sensory neurons and cells in the dorsal root ganglion (**peripheral sensitization**). Examples include nerve entrapment, diabetic neuropathy, or chronic pancreatitis.

Central neuropathic pain is caused by a lesion or dysfunction in the brain or spinal cord. A progressive repeated stimulation of group C neurons (wind-up) in the dorsal horn leads to increased sensitivity of central pain signalling neurons (**central sensitization**). This central sensitization results in pathological changes in the CNS that cause persistent pain.[48] Examples include brain or spinal cord trauma, tumours, vascular lesions, multiple sclerosis, Parkinson's disease, postherpetic neuralgia, and phantom limb pain.[36,37]

The following mechanisms have been implicated in the cause of neuropathic pain[46,49,50]:

- Changes in sensitivity of neurons—lower threshold with peripheral and central sensitization
- Spontaneous impulses from regenerating peripheral nerves
- Alterations in the dorsal root ganglion and spinothalamic tract in response to peripheral nerve injury (i.e., deafferentation pain—loss of pain-related afferent information to the brain)
- Loss of pain inhibition and stimulation of pain facilitation by excitatory neurotransmitters in the dorsal horn (e.g., release of glutamate by stimulation of *N*-methyl-D-aspartate [NMDA] receptors)
- Loss of descending inhibitory pain modulation
- Hyperexcitable spinal interneurons stimulated by Aβ fibres (nonpainful stimulation of pain)
- Release of nociceptive inflammatory cytokines, chemokines, and growth factors by activated glial cells
- Structural and functional alterations in brain processing neural networks

Because of the complexity of the causes of neuropathic pain syndromes, they are difficult to treat. Multimodal therapy is often needed, including nonmedication treatment.[51]

QUICK CHECK 14-1

1. What is the difference between Aδ and C fibres?
2. Give two examples of pain excitatory and inhibitory neurotransmitters.
3. How do Aβ fibres inhibit pain and cause pain?
4. What are two differences between nociceptive pain and neuropathic pain?

TABLE 14-3 Persistent Pain Syndromes

Condition	Description
Persistent low back pain	It is the most common persistent pain condition. It results from poor muscle tone, inactivity, muscle strain, or sudden, vigorous exercise.
Myofascial pain syndromes	Pain results from muscle spasm, tenderness, stiffness, or injury to muscle and fascia with peripheral and central sensitization. Examples include myositis, fibrositis, myalgia, fibromyalgia, and muscle strain. It involves trigger points—small hypersensitive regions in muscle or connective tissues that, when stimulated, produce pain in a specific area. As the disorder progresses, pain becomes increasingly generalized.
Chronic postoperative pain	It involves persistent pain that can occur with disruption or cutting of sensory nerves. Examples include post-thoracotomy, postmastectomy. Risk factors may include pre-existing pain and genetic susceptibility.
Cancer pain	It is attributed to the advance of disease, treatment, or coexisting disease entities.
Deafferentation pain	This pain is due to the loss of sensory input into the central nervous system (CNS) caused by lesion in peripheral nerves (e.g., brachial plexus injury) or pathology of the CNS (e.g., complex regional pain syndrome). It is described as a constant, vicelike ache with paroxysms of burning or shocklike sensations. Common types include severe burning pain triggered by various stimuli, such as cold, light touch, or sound, and complex regional pain syndromes (occur after peripheral nerve injury and are characterized by continuous, severe, burning pain associated with vasomotor changes and muscle wasting).
Hyperalgesia	It is an increased sensitivity to pain and a decreased pain threshold to tactile and painful stimuli. Pain is diffuse, modified by fatigue and emotion, and mixed with other sensations. It may result from chronic irritation of CNS areas.
Hemiagnosia	It is the loss of ability to identify a source of pain on one side of the body. Painful stimuli on that side produce discomfort, anxiety, moaning, agitation, and distress, but no attempt to withdraw from stimulus. It is associated with stroke.
Phantom limb pain	It is pain experienced in an amputated limb after the stump has completely healed. It may be immediate or occur months later. It is associated with preamputation pain and acute postoperative pain. The exact cause is unknown, thought to originate in the brain. It can be influenced by emotions or sympathetic stimulation.

From c.p.van.wilgen@sport.umcg.nl.

TABLE 14-4 Comparison of Acute and Persistent Pain

Characteristic	Acute Pain	Persistent Pain
Experience	An event	A situation; state of existence
Source	External agent or internal disease, injury, or inflammation	Unknown; if known, treatment is prolonged or ineffective
Onset	Usually sudden	May be sudden or develop insidiously
Duration	Transient (up to 3 months); usually of short duration Resolves with treatment and healing	Prolonged (months to years); lasts beyond expected normal healing time
Pain identification	Painful and nonpainful areas generally well identified	Painful and nonpainful areas less easily differentiated; change in sensations becomes more difficult to evaluate
Clinical signs	Typical response pattern with more visible signs Anxiety and emotional distress common	Response patterns vary; fewer overt signs (adaptation) Pain can interfere with sleep, productivity, and quality of life
Significance	Significant (informs person something is wrong); protective	Person looks for significance and meaning; serves no useful purpose
Pattern	Self-limiting or readily corrected	Continuous or intermittent; intensity may vary or remain constant
Course	Suffering usually decreases over time	Suffering usually increases over time
Actions	Leads to actions to relieve pain	Leads to actions to modify pain experience
Prognosis	Likelihood of eventual complete relief	Complete relief usually not possible

TEMPERATURE REGULATION

Human temperature regulation (**thermoregulation**) is achieved through precise balancing of heat production, heat conservation, and heat loss. The normal range of body temperature is considered to be 36.2° to 37.7°C (96.2° to 99.4°F) overall, but a person's individual body parts will vary in temperature. Body temperature rarely exceeds 41°C. The extremities are generally cooler than the trunk and the temperature at the core of the body (as measured by rectal temperature) is generally 0.5°C higher than the surface temperature (as measured by oral temperature). Internal temperature varies in response to activity, environmental temperature, and daily fluctuation (circadian rhythm). Oral temperatures fluctuate within 0.2° to 0.5°C during a 24-hour period. Women tend to have wider fluctuations that follow the menstrual cycle, with a sharp rise in temperature just before ovulation. The daily fluctuating temperature in both genders peaks around 6 p.m. and is at its lowest during sleep. Maintenance of body temperature within the normal range is necessary for life.

Control of Body Temperature

Thermoregulation is mediated primarily by the hypothalamus and endocrine system. Peripheral thermoreceptors in the skin and abdominal

TABLE 14-5 Mechanisms of Heat Production and Heat Loss

Condition	Description
Heat Production	
Chemical reactions of metabolism	Reactions occur during ingestion and metabolism of food and while maintaining body at rest (basal metabolism); occur in body core (e.g., liver)
Skeletal muscle contraction	Gradual increase in muscle tone or rapid muscle oscillations (shivering)
Chemical thermogenesis	Epinephrine is released and produces rapid, transient increase in heat production by raising basal metabolic rate; quick, brief effect that counters heat lost through conduction and convection; involves brown adipose tissue, which decreases markedly in older adults; thyroid hormone increases metabolism
Heat Loss	
Radiation	Heat loss through electromagnetic waves emanating from surfaces with temperature higher than surrounding air
Conduction	Heat loss by direct molecule-to-molecule transfer from one surface to another, so that warmer surface loses heat to cooler surface
Convection	Transfer of heat through currents of gases or liquids; exchanges warmer air at body's surface with cooler air in surrounding space
Vasodilation	Diversion of core-warmed blood to surface of body, with heat transferred by conduction to skin surface and from there to surrounding environment; occurs in response to autonomic stimulation under control of hypothalamus
Evaporation	Body water evaporates from surface of skin and linings of mucous membranes; major source of heat reduction connected with increased sweating in warmer surroundings
Decreased muscle tone	Exhausted feeling caused by moderately reduced muscle tone and curtailed voluntary muscle activity
Increased respiration	Air is exchanged with environment through normal process; minimal effect
Voluntary mechanisms	"Stretching out" and "slowing down" in response to high body temperatures; increasing body surface area available for heat loss; dressing in light-coloured, loose-fitting garments
Adaptation to warmer climates	Gradual process beginning with lassitude, weakness, and faintness; proceeding through increased sweating, lowered sodium content, decreased heart rate, and increased stroke volume and extracellular fluid volume; and terminating in improved warm weather functioning and decreased symptoms of heat intolerance (work output, endurance, and coordination increase; subjective feelings of discomfort decrease)

organs (unmyelinated C fibres and thinly myelinated Aδ fibres) and central thermoreceptors in the hypothalamus, spinal cord, and other central locations provide the hypothalamus with information about skin and core temperatures. If these temperatures are low or high, the hypothalamus triggers heat production and heat conservation or heat loss mechanisms.

Body heat is produced by the chemical reactions of metabolism and skeletal muscle tone and contraction. The heat-producing mechanism (chemical or nonshivering thermogenesis) begins with hypothalamic thyrotropin-stimulating hormone-releasing hormone (TSH-RH); it stimulates the anterior pituitary to release thyroid-stimulating hormone (TSH), which acts on the thyroid gland and stimulates the release of thyroxine. Thyroxine then acts on the adrenal medulla, causing the release of epinephrine into the bloodstream. Epinephrine causes vasoconstriction, stimulates glycolysis, and increases metabolic rate, thus increasing body heat. Norepinephrine and thyroxine activate brown fat thermogenesis where energy is released as heat instead of as adenosine triphosphate (ATP). Heat is distributed by the circulatory system.[52]

The hypothalamus also triggers heat conservation by stimulating the sympathetic nervous system, which stimulates the adrenal cortex and results in increased skeletal muscle tone, initiating the shivering response and producing vasoconstriction. By constricting peripheral blood vessels, centrally warmed blood is shunted away from the periphery to the core of the body where heat can be retained. This involuntary mechanism takes advantage of the insulating layers of the skin and subcutaneous fat to protect core temperature. The hypothalamus relays information to the cerebral cortex about cold, and voluntary responses result. Individuals typically bundle up, keep moving, or curl up in a ball. These types of voluntary physical activities respectively provide insulation, increase skeletal muscle activity, and decrease the amount of skin surface available for heat loss through radiation, convection, and conduction.[53]

The hypothalamus responds to warmer core and peripheral temperatures by reversing the same mechanisms, resulting in heat loss. Heat loss is achieved through (1) radiation, (2) conduction, (3) convection, (4) vasodilation, (5) evaporation of sweat, (6) decreased muscle tone, (7) increased respiration, (8) voluntary measures, and (9) adaptation to warmer climates (i.e., increasing or decreasing the volume of sweat). Table 14-5 summarizes further information about mechanisms of heat production and heat loss.

Temperature Regulation in Infants and Older Adults

Infants (particularly low-birth-weight infants) and older adults require special attention to maintenance of body temperature. Term infants produce sufficient body heat, primarily through metabolism of brown fat, but cannot conserve heat produced because of their small body size, greater ratio of body surface to body weight, and inability to shiver. Infants also have little subcutaneous fat and thus are not as well insulated as adults.[54] Children also have a greater ratio of body surface to body weight, lower sweating rate, higher peripheral blood flow in the heat, and a greater extent of vasoconstriction in the cold than adults. They can acclimatize to changes in environmental temperatures, but do so at a lower rate than adults.[55]

Older adults respond poorly to environmental temperature extremes because of their slowed blood circulation, structural and functional skin changes, overall decreased heat-producing activities, and the presence of disease (i.e., heart failure, chronic lung disease, diabetes mellitus, or peripheral vascular disease). Cold stress in older adults also decreases coronary perfusion.[56] In addition, older adults have a decreased shivering response (delayed onset and decreased effectiveness), slowed metabolic rate, decreased vasoconstrictor response, diminished or absent ability to sweat, decreased peripheral sensation, desynchronized circadian rhythm, decreased perception of heat and cold, decreased thirst, decreased nutritional reserves, and decreased brown adipose tissue.[57]

Pathogenesis of Fever

Fever (febrile response) is a temporary resetting of the hypothalamic thermostat to a higher level in response to exogenous or endogenous pyrogens. Exogenous pyrogens (endotoxins produced by pathogens; see Chapter 8) stimulate the release of endogenous pyrogens from phagocytic cells, including tumour necrosis factor-alpha (TNF-α), interleukin-1 (IL-1), interleukin-6 (IL-6), and interferon (IFN). These pyrogens raise the thermal set point by inducing the hypothalamic synthesis of prostaglandin E_2 (PGE_2). The release of PGE_2 produces an integrated response that raises body temperature through an increase in heat production and conservation (Figure 14-4). The individual feels colder, dresses more warmly, decreases body surface area by curling up, and may go to bed in an effort to get warm. Body temperature is maintained at the new level until the fever "breaks," when the set point begins to return to normal with decreased heat production and increased heat reduction mechanisms. The individual feels very warm, dons cooler clothes, throws off the covers, and stretches out. Once the body has returned to a normal temperature, the individual feels more comfortable and the hypothalamus adjusts thermoregulatory mechanisms to maintain the new temperature.

Fever of unknown origin (FUO) is a body temperature greater than 38.3°C [101°F]) for longer than 3 weeks' duration that remains undiagnosed after 3 days of hospital investigation, 3 outpatient visits, or 1 week of ambulatory investigation. The clinical categories of FUO include infectious, rheumatic or inflammatory, neoplastic, human immunodeficiency virus (HIV)-associated, and miscellaneous disorders.[58]

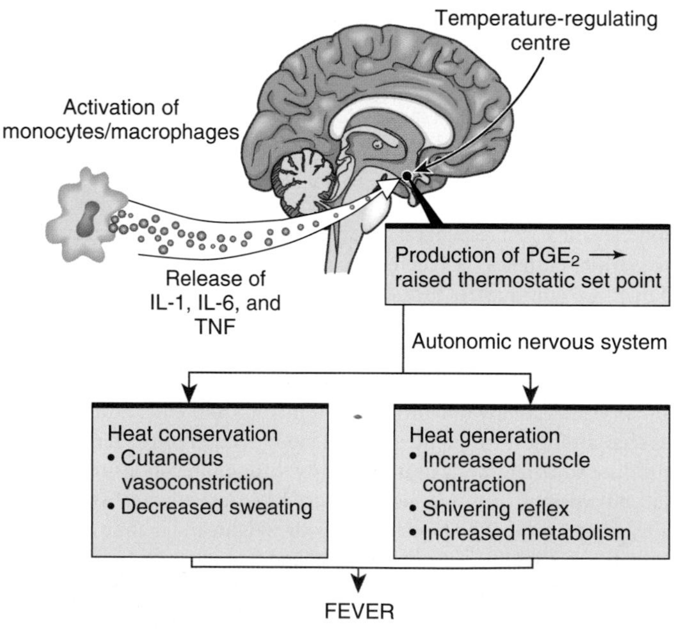

FIGURE 14-4 Production of Fever. When monocytes or macrophages are activated, they secrete cytokines such as interleukin-1 (*IL-1*), interleukin-6 (*IL-6*), and tumour necrosis factor (*TNF*), which reach the hypothalamic temperature-regulating centre. These cytokines promote the synthesis and secretion of prostaglandin E_2 (*PGE_2*) in the anterior hypothalamus. PGE_2 increases the thermostatic set point, and the autonomic nervous system is stimulated, resulting in shivering, muscle contraction, peripheral vasoconstriction, and increased metabolism mediated by thyroid hormone. (From Lewis, S.M., Bucher, L., Heitkemper, M.M., et al. [2014]. *Medical-surgical nursing: Assessment and management of clinical problems* [9th ed.]. St. Louis: Mosby.)

Benefits of Fever

Moderate fever helps the body respond to infectious processes through several mechanisms[59,60]:

- Raising of the body temperature kills many microorganisms and adversely affects their growth and replication.
- Higher body temperatures decrease serum levels of iron, zinc, and copper—minerals needed for bacterial replication.
- Increased temperature causes lysosomal breakdown and autodestruction of cells, preventing viral replication in infected cells.
- Heat increases lymphocytic transformation and motility of polymorphonuclear neutrophils, facilitating the immune response.
- Phagocytosis is enhanced, and the production of antiviral interferon is augmented.

Suppression of fever with antipyrogenic medications can be effective but should be used with caution.[61,62] Infection and fever responses in older adults and children may vary. Box 14-2 lists the principal features associated with fever at the extremes of age.[63]

Disorders of Temperature Regulation

Hyperthermia

Hyperthermia is elevation of the body temperature without an increase in the hypothalamic set point. Hyperthermia can produce nerve damage, coagulation of cell proteins, and death. At 41°C (105.8°F), nerve damage produces convulsions in the adult. Death results at 43°C (109.4°F). Hyperthermia may be therapeutic, accidental, or associated with stroke or head trauma. Prevention of hyperthermia in stroke and head trauma assists in limiting brain injury.[64]

Therapeutic hyperthermia is a form of local, regional, or whole-body hyperthermia used to destroy pathological microorganisms or tumour cells by facilitating the host's natural immune process or tumour blood flow.[65]

The forms of accidental hyperthermia are summarized as follows[66]:

- Heat cramps are severe, spasmodic cramps in the abdomen and extremities that follow prolonged sweating and associated sodium loss. They usually occur in those not accustomed to heat or those performing strenuous work in very warm climates. Fever, rapid pulse rate, and increased blood pressure accompany the cramps.
- Heat exhaustion results from prolonged high core or environmental temperatures, which cause profound vasodilation and profuse sweating, leading to dehydration, decreased plasma volumes, hypotension, decreased cardiac output, and tachycardia. Symptoms include weakness, dizziness, confusion, nausea, and fainting.
- Heat stroke is a potentially lethal result of an overstressed thermoregulatory centre. Heat stroke can be caused by exertion, by

BOX 14-2 Effects of Fever at the Extremes of Age

Older Adults

They show decreased or no fever response to infection; therefore, benefits of fever are reduced.

High morbidity and mortality result from lack of beneficial aspects.

Children

They develop higher temperatures than adults do for relatively minor infections.

Febrile seizures before age 5 years are not uncommon.

overexposure to environmental heat, or from impaired physiological mechanisms for heat loss. With very high core temperatures (greater than 40°C [104°F]), the regulatory centre ceases to function and the body's heat loss mechanisms fail. Symptoms include high core temperature, absence of sweating, rapid pulse rate, confusion, agitation, and coma. Complications include cerebral edema, degeneration of the CNS, swollen dendrites, renal tubular necrosis, and hepatic failure with delirium, coma, and eventually death if treatment is not undertaken.[67]

- **Malignant hyperthermia** is a potentially lethal hypermetabolic complication of a rare inherited muscle disorder that may be triggered by inhaled anaesthetics and depolarizing muscle relaxants.[68] The syndrome involves altered calcium function in muscle cells with hypermetabolism, uncoordinated muscle contractions, increased muscle work, increased oxygen consumption, and a raised level of lactic acid production. Acidosis develops, and body temperature rises, with resulting tachycardia and cardiac dysrhythmias, hypotension, decreased cardiac output, and cardiac arrest. Signs resemble those of coma—unconsciousness, absent reflexes, fixed pupils, apnea, and occasionally a flat electroencephalogram (EEG). Oliguria and anuria are common. It is most common in children and adolescents.

Hypothermia

Hypothermia (core body temperature less than 35°C [95°F]) produces depression of the CNS and the respiratory system, vasoconstriction, alterations in microcirculation and coagulation, and ischemic tissue damage. Hypothermia may be accidental or therapeutic (Box 14-3). Most tissues can tolerate low temperatures in controlled situations, such as surgery. However, in severe hypothermia, ice crystals form on the inside of the cell, causing cells to rupture and die. Tissue hypothermia slows cell metabolism, increases the blood viscosity, slows microcirculatory blood flow, facilitates blood coagulation, and stimulates profound vasoconstriction (see also the discussion of frostbite in Chapter 41).

Trauma and Temperature

Major body trauma can affect temperature regulation through various mechanisms. Damage to the CNS, inflammation, increased intracranial pressure, or intracranial bleeding typically produces a body temperature of greater than 39°C (102.2°F). This sustained noninfectious fever, often referred to as a "**central fever**," appears with or without bradycardia. A central fever does not induce sweating and is very resistant to antipyretic therapy.[69] Other traumatic mechanisms that produce temperature alterations include accidental injuries, hemorrhagic shock, major surgery, and thermal burns. The severity and type of alteration (hyperthermia or hypothermia) vary with the severity of the cause and the body system affected.

QUICK CHECK 14-2

1. Why is temperature regulation important?
2. What are the principal heat production methods? Heat loss methods?
3. How does the hypothalamus alter its set point to change body temperature?
4. Compare and contrast hyperthermia and hypothermia and their effects on the body.

BOX 14-3 Defining Characteristics of Hypothermia

Accidental Hypothermia

The unintentional decrease in core temperature to less than 35°C (95°F) results from sudden immersion in cold water, prolonged exposure to cold environments, diseases that diminish the ability to generate heat, or altered thermoregulatory mechanisms. It is most common among young people and older adults.

Factors That Increase Risk

1. Hypothyroidism
2. Hypopituitarism
3. Malnutrition
4. Parkinson's disease
5. Rheumatoid arthritis
6. Chronic increased vasodilation
7. Failure of thermoregulatory control resulting from cerebral injury, ketoacidosis, uremia, sepsis, and drug overdose

Response Mechanisms

1. Peripheral vasoconstriction—shunts blood away from cooler skin to core to decrease heat loss and produces peripheral tissue ischemia
2. Intermittent reperfusion of extremities (Lewis phenomenon) helps preserve peripheral oxygenation until core temperature drops dramatically
3. Hypothalamic centre induces shivering; thinking becomes sluggish, and coordination is depressed
4. Stupor; heart rate and respiratory rate decline; cardiac output diminishes; metabolic rate falls; acidosis; eventual ventricular fibrillation and asystole occur at 30°C (86°F) and lower

Treatment

1. Most changes are reversible with rewarming
2. Core temperature greater than 30°C (86°F)—active rewarming (external)
3. Core temperature less than 30°C (86°F) or with severe cardiovascular problems—active core rewarming (internal)

Therapeutic Hypothermia

It is used to slow metabolism and preserve ischemic tissue during surgery (e.g., limb re-implantation), postcardiac arrest management of patients presenting with ventricular fibrillation or ventricular tachycardia, or following neurological injury.

Effects and Cautions

1. It stresses the heart, leading to ventricular fibrillation and cardiac arrest (may be the desired outcome in open heart surgery when the heart must be stopped).
2. It exhausts liver glycogen stores by prolonged shivering.
3. Surface cooling may cause burns, frostbite, and fat necrosis.
4. It may lead to immunosuppression with increased infection risk.
5. It slows drug metabolism.

From Corneli, H.M. (2012). *Pediatr Emerg Care, 28*(5), 475–480; Frink, M., Flohé, S., van Griensven, M., et al. (2012). *Mediators Inflamm, 2012*, 762840; Lantry, J., Dezman, Z., & Hirshon, J.M. (2012). *Br J Hosp Med (Lond), 73*(1), 31–37.

SLEEP

Sleep is an active multiphase process that provides restorative functions and promotes memory consolidation. Complex neural circuits, interacting hormones, and neurotransmitters involving the hypothalamus, thalamus, brainstem, and cortex control the timing of the sleep–wake cycle and coordinate this cycle with circadian rhythms (24-hour rhythm cycles).[70] Normal sleep has two phases that can be documented by EEG: **rapid eye movement (REM) sleep** (20 to 25% of sleep time) and slow-wave (non-REM) sleep. Non-REM sleep is further divided into three stages (N1, N2, N3) from light to deep sleep followed by REM sleep. Four to six cycles of REM and non-REM sleep occur each night in an adult.[71]

The hypothalamus is a major sleep centre and the hypocretins (orexins), acetylcholine, and glutamate are neuropeptides secreted by the hypothalamus that promote wakefulness. Prostaglandin D_2, adenosine, melatonin, serotonin, l-tryptophan, GABA, and growth factors promote sleep. The pontine reticular formation is primarily responsible for generating REM sleep, and projections from the thalamocortical network produce non-REM sleep.[72]

REM sleep is initiated by *REM-on* and *REM-off* neurons in the pons and mesencephalon. REM sleep occurs about every 90 minutes beginning 1 to 2 hours after non-REM sleep begins. This sleep is known as *paradoxical sleep* because the EEG pattern is similar to that of the normal awake pattern and the brain is very active with dreaming. REM and non-REM sleep alternate throughout the night, with lengthening intervals of REM sleep and fewer intervals of deeper stages of non-REM sleep toward morning. The changes associated with REM sleep include increased parasympathetic activity and variable sympathetic activity associated with rapid eye movement; muscle relaxation; loss of temperature regulation; altered heart rate, blood pressure, and respiration; penile erection in men and clitoral engorgement in women; release of steroids; and many memorable dreams. Respiratory control appears largely independent of metabolic requirements and oxygen variation. Loss of normal voluntary muscle control in the tongue and upper pharynx may produce some respiratory obstruction. Cerebral blood flow increases.

Non–rapid eye movement (NREM) sleep accounts for 75 to 80% of sleep time in adults and is initiated when inhibitory signals are released from the hypothalamus. Sympathetic tone is decreased and parasympathetic activity is increased during NREM sleep, creating a state of reduced activity. The basal metabolic rate falls by 10 to 15%; temperature decreases 0.5° to 1.0°C (0.9° to 1.8°F); heart rate, respiration, blood pressure, and muscle tone decrease; and knee jerk reflexes are absent. Pupils are constricted. During the various stages, cerebral blood flow to the brain decreases and growth hormone is released, with corticosteroid and catecholamine levels depressed. Box 14-4 summarizes the sleep characteristics of infants and older adults.

BOX 14-4 Sleep Characteristics of Infants and Older Adults

Infants

- Infants sleep 10 to 16 hours per day: 50% REM (active) sleep, 25% non-REM (inactive) sleep.
- Infant sleep cycles are 50 to 60 minutes in length; 10 to 45 minutes of REM sleep accompanied by movement of the arms, legs, and facial muscles followed by about 20 minutes of non-REM sleep.
- At 1 year, REM and non-REM sleep cycles are about equal in length and infants sleep through the night with about two naps per day.

Older Adults

- Total sleep time is decreased with a longer time to fall asleep and poorer quality sleep.
- Total time in slow-wave and final phase of non-REM sleep decreases by 15 to 30%.
- Increases occur in stage 1 and 2 non-REM sleep, attributable to an increased number of spontaneous arousals.
- Older adults tend to go to sleep earlier in the evening and wake earlier in the morning because of a phase advance in their normal circadian sleep cycle.
- Alterations in sleep patterns occur about 10 years later in women than in men.
- Sleep disorders are more likely in older adults and increase the risk for morbidity and mortality.

REM, rapid eye movement.
From Edwards, B.A., O'Driscoll, D.M., Asad, A., et al. (2010). *Semin Respir Crit Care Med, 31*(5), 618–633; Galland, B.C., Taylor, B.J., Elder, D.E., et al. (2012). *Sleep Med Rev, 16*(3), 213–222; Neikrug, A.B., & Ancoli-Israel, S. (2010). *Gerontology, 56*(2), 181–189; Ng, D.K., & Chan, C.H. (2013). *Pediatr Neonatol, 54*(2), 82–87.

Sleep Disorders

Because classification of sleep disorders is complex, the International Classification of Sleep Disorders III (ISCD-3) has been established by the American Academy of Sleep Medicine and includes six classifications: (1) insomnia, (2) sleep-related breathing disorders, (3) central disorders of hypersomnolence, (4) circadian rhythm sleep–wake disorders, (5) parasomnias, and (6) sleep-related movement disorders.[73] The most common disorders are summarized here.

Common Dyssomnias

Insomnia is the inability to fall or stay asleep; it is accompanied by fatigue during wakefulness and may be mild, moderate, or severe. It may be transient, lasting a few days or months (primary insomnia), and related to travel across time zones or caused by acute stress.[74] Chronic insomnia can be idiopathic, start at an early age, and be associated with drug or alcohol abuse, persistent pain disorders, chronic depression, the use of certain medications, obesity, aging, genetics, and environmental factors that result in hyperarousal.[75]

Obstructive sleep apnea syndrome (OSAS) is the most commonly diagnosed sleep disorder. The Public Health Agency of Canada states that 3% of Canadians over the age of 18 years reported being diagnosed with sleep apnea. In addition, more than one in four Canadian adults (26%) were at high risk developing OSAS, based on the presence of identified risk factors. Major risk factors include obesity, male gender, and older age.[76] A lack of daytime sleepiness often lessens awareness of a potential sleep disorder, and many persons are never properly diagnosed and treated.[77] OSAS results from partial or total upper airway collapse with obstruction to airflow recurring during sleep with excessive loud snoring, gasping, and multiple apneic episodes that last 10 seconds or longer. The periodic breathing eventually produces arousal, which interrupts the sleep cycle, reducing total sleep time and producing sleep and REM deprivation. Associated conditions include decreased sensitivity to carbon dioxide and oxygen tensions, upper airway obstruction, a small airway, and decreased airway dilator muscle activation. **Obesity hypoventilation syndrome** may be related to leptin resistance because leptin also is a respiratory stimulant. Sleep apnea produces hypercapnia and low oxygen saturation and eventually leads to polycythemia, pulmonary hypertension, systemic hypertension, stroke, right-sided heart failure, dysrhythmias, liver congestion, cyanosis, and peripheral edema.[78] **Hypersomnia** (excessive daytime sleepiness) is associated with OSAS. Individuals may fall asleep while driving a car, working, or even while conversing, with consequent significant safety concerns.[79] Sleep deprivation also can result in impaired mood and cognitive function characterized by impairments of attention, episodic memory, working memory, and executive functions.[80]

Polysomnography is needed to diagnose OSAS, in addition to the history and physical examination. Treatments include use of nasal continuous positive airway pressure and dental devices, surgery of the upper airway and jaw in selected individuals, and management of obesity.[81] Adenotonsillar hypertrophy is the major cause of OSAS in children, and obesity increases the risk. Adenotonsillectomy is the treatment of choice.[82,83]

Narcolepsy is a primary hypersomnia characterized by hallucinations, sleep paralysis, and, rarely, cataplexy (brief spells of muscle weakness).

Narcolepsy is usually sporadic or can occur in families. Narcolepsy without cataplexy is associated with immune-mediated destruction of hypocretin (orexin)-secreting cells in the hypothalamus. Orexins stimulate wakefulness.[84]

Circadian rhythm sleep disorders are common disorders of the 24-hour sleep–wake schedule (circadian rhythm sleep disorders). They can result from having rapid time-zone changes (or jet-lag syndrome), alternating the sleep schedule (rotating work shifts) involving 3 hours or more in sleep time, or changing the total sleep time from day to day. They can also result from being diagnosed either with advanced sleep phase disorder (early morning waking–early evening sleeping), which results in sleep loss if social requirements lead to later bedtime, or with delayed sleep phase disorder (late morning waking–late night to early morning sleeping), which results in sleep loss because of required early morning rising (common in adolescents). These changes desynchronize the circadian rhythm, which can depress the degree of vigilance, performance of psychomotor tasks, and arousal.[85,86] A circadian rhythm sleep disorder known as **shift work sleep disorder** affects many shift workers who rotate or swing long shifts (such as nurses), particularly between the hours of 2200 (10:00 p.m.) and 0600 (6:00 a.m.).[87,88] Our sleep–wake cycle is driven by circadian rhythms, and the disruption of this circadian influence may cause problems in the short term, such as cognitive deficits and difficulty concentrating. However, long-term health consequences of shift work sleep disorder may be quite serious and include depression or anxiety, increased risk for cardiovascular disease, and increased all-cause mortality.[85] Sleep cycle phenotype also has a genetic basis and influences the timing and cycles of sleep and can affect advances or delays in sleep–wake times.[89,90]

Common Parasomnias

Parasomnias are unusual behaviours occurring during NREM stage 3 (slow-wave) sleep.[91] These behaviours include sleepwalking, having night terrors, rearranging furniture, eating food, exhibiting sleep sex or violent behaviour, and having restless legs syndrome. REM sleep behaviour disorder is manifested by loss of REM paralysis, leading to potentially injurious dream enactment.[92,93]

Two dysfunctions of sleep (somnambulism and night terrors) are common in children and may be related to CNS immaturity. **Somnambulism (sleepwalking)** is a disorder primarily of childhood and appears to resolve within a few years. Sleepwalking is therefore not associated with dreaming, and the child has no memory of the event on awakening. Sleepwalking in adults is often associated with sleep-disordered breathing. **Night terrors** are characterized by sudden apparent arousals in which the child expresses intense fear or emotion. However, the child is not awake and can be difficult to arouse. Once awakened, the child has no memory of the night terror event. Night terrors are not associated with dreams. Although this problem occurs most often in children, adults also may experience it with corresponding daytime anxiety.

Restless Legs Syndrome

Restless legs syndrome (RLS), or **Willis-Ekbom disease**, is a common sensorimotor disorder associated with unpleasant sensations (prickling, tingling, crawling) and nonvolitional periodic leg movements that occurs at rest and is worse in the evening or at night. There is a compelling urge to move the legs for relief with a significant effect on sleep and quality of life. The disorder is more common in women, during pregnancy, older adults, and individuals with iron deficiency. RLS has a familial tendency and is associated with a circadian fluctuation of dopamine in the substantia nigra. Iron is a cofactor in dopamine production, and some individuals respond to iron administration as well as dopamine agonists.[94] Diagnostic and treatment guidelines have been established to assist with disease management.[95]

> **QUICK CHECK 14-3**
> 1. Describe REM and non-REM sleep.
> 2. What is the major difference between the dyssomnias and parasomnias?

THE SPECIAL SENSES

Vision

The eyes are complex sense organs responsible for vision. Within a protective casing, each eye has receptors, a lens system for focusing light on the receptors, and a system of nerves for conducting impulses from the receptors to the brain. Visual dysfunction may be caused by abnormal ocular movements or alterations in visual acuity, refraction, colour vision, or accommodation. Visual dysfunction also may be the secondary effect of another neurological disorder.

The Eye

The wall of the eye consists of three layers: (1) sclera, (2) choroid, and (3) retina (Figure 14-5). The **sclera** is the thick, white, outermost layer. It becomes transparent at the **cornea**—the portion of the sclera in the central anterior region that allows light to enter the eye. The **choroid** is the deeply pigmented middle layer that prevents light from scattering inside the eye. The **iris**, part of the choroid, has a round opening, the **pupil**, through which light passes. Smooth muscle fibres control the size of the pupil so that it adjusts to bright light or dim light and to close or distant vision.

The **retina** is the innermost layer of the eye, and contains millions of rods and cones—special photoreceptors that convert light energy into nerve impulses. **Rods** mediate peripheral and dim light vision and are densest at the periphery. **Cones**, densest in the centre of the retina, are colour and detail receptors. There are no photoreceptors where the optic nerve leaves the eyeball; this point of entry creates the **optic disc**, or blind spot. Lateral to each optic disc is the **macula lutea**, the area of most distinct vision, and in the centre is the **fovea centralis**, a tiny area that contains only cones and provides the greatest visual acuity (see Figure 14-5).

As shown in Figure 14-11, nerve impulses pass through the **optic nerves** (second cranial nerve) to the **optic chiasm**. The nerves from

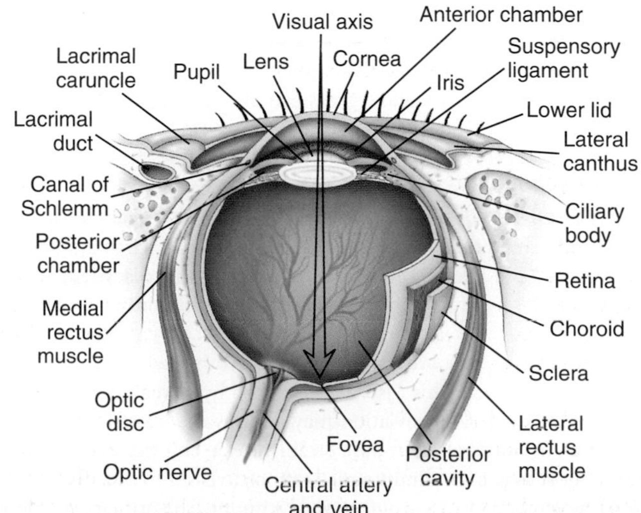

FIGURE 14-5 Internal Anatomy of the Eye. (Adapted from Patton, K.T., & Thibodeau, G.A. [2008]. *Structure & function of the human body* [13th ed.]. St. Louis: Mosby.)

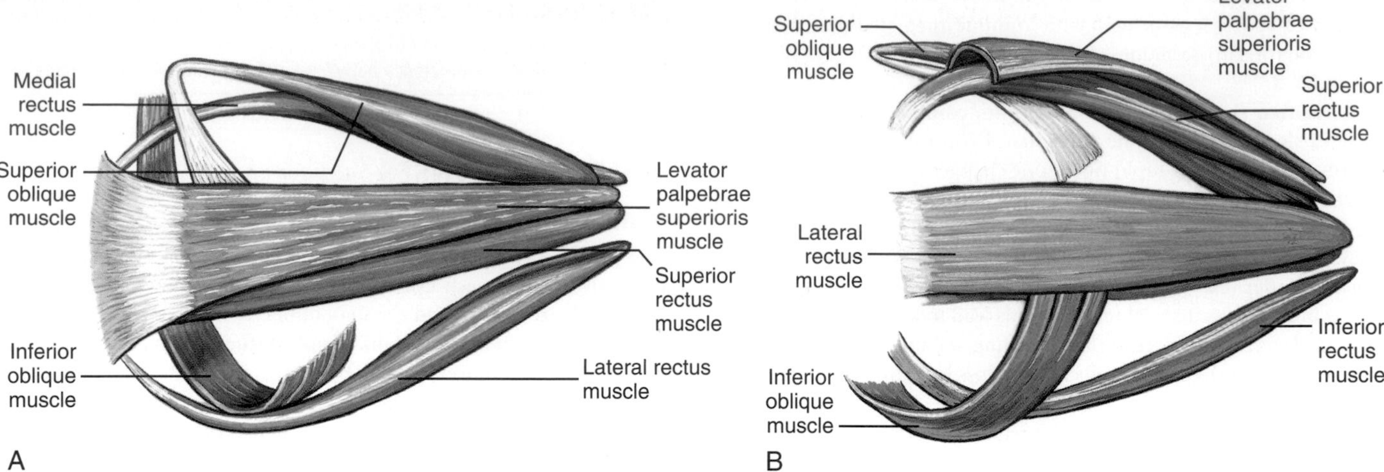

FIGURE 14-6 Extrinsic Muscles of the Right Eye. A, Superior view. **B,** Lateral view. (From Dutton, J.J. [2011]. *Atlas of clinical and surgical orbital anatomy* [2nd ed.]. Philadelphia: Saunders.)

the inner (nasal) halves of the retinas cross to the opposite side and join fibres from the outer (temporal) halves of the retinas to form the optic tracts. The fibres of the optic tracts synapse in the dorsal lateral geniculate nucleus and pass by way of the optic radiation (or geniculocalcarine tract) to the primary visual cortex in the occipital lobe of the brain. Some fibres terminate in the **suprachiasmatic nucleus (SCN)** (located above the optic chiasm) and are involved in regulating the sleep–wake cycle. Light entering the eye is focused on the retina by the **lens**—a flexible, biconvex, crystal-like structure. The flexibility of the lens allows a change in curvature with contraction of the ciliary muscles, called **accommodation**, and allows the eye to focus on objects at different distances. The lens divides the anterior chamber into (1) the aqueous chamber and (2) the vitreous chamber. **Aqueous humor** fills the aqueous chamber and helps maintain pressure inside the eye, as well as provide nutrients to the lens and cornea. Aqueous humor is secreted by the ciliary processes and reabsorbed into the canal of Schlemm. If drainage is blocked, intraocular pressure increases (causing glaucoma). The vitreous chamber is filled with a gel-like substance called **vitreous humor**. Vitreous humor helps to prevent the eyeball from collapsing inward.

The central retinal artery provides blood to the inner retinal surface, and the choroid supplies nutrients to the outer surface of the retina. Six extrinsic eye muscles allow gross eye movements and permit eyes to follow a moving object (Figure 14-6).

Visual Dysfunction

Alterations in ocular movements. Abnormal ocular movements result from oculomotor, trochlear, or abducens cranial nerve dysfunction (see Table 13-6). The three types of eye movement disorders are (1) strabismus, (2) nystagmus, and (3) paralysis of individual extraocular muscles.

In **strabismus**, one eye deviates from the other when the person is looking at an object. This disorder is caused by a weak or hypertonic muscle in one eye. The deviation may be upward, downward, inward (entropia), or outward (extropia). Strabismus in children requires early intervention to prevent **amblyopia** (reduced vision in the affected eye caused by cerebral blockage of the visual stimuli). The primary symptom of strabismus is **diplopia** (double vision). Causes include neuromuscular disorders of the eye muscle, diseases involving the cerebral hemispheres, or thyroid disease.

Nystagmus is an involuntary unilateral or bilateral rhythmic movement of the eyes. It may be present at rest or when the eye moves. **Pendular nystagmus** is characterized by a regular back-and-forth movement of the eyes. In **jerk nystagmus**, one phase of the eye movement is faster than the other. Nystagmus may be caused by imbalanced reflex activity of the inner ear, vestibular nuclei, cerebellum, medial longitudinal fascicle, or nuclei of the oculomotor, trochlear, and abducens cranial nerves (see Table 13-6 and Figure 13-25). Drugs, retinal disease, and diseases involving the cervical cord also may produce nystagmus.

Paralysis of specific extraocular muscles may cause limited abduction, abnormal closure of the eyelid, ptosis (drooping of the eyelid), or diplopia (double vision) as a result of unopposed muscle activity. Trauma or pressure in the area of the cranial nerves or diseases such as diabetes mellitus and myasthenia gravis also paralyze specific extraocular muscles.

Alterations in visual acuity. Visual acuity is the ability to see objects in sharp detail. With advancing age, the lens of the eye becomes less flexible and adjusts slowly, and there is altered refraction of light by the cornea and lens. Thus, visual acuity declines with age. Table 14-6 contains a summary of changes in the eye caused by aging. Specific causes of visual acuity changes are (1) amblyopia, (2) scotoma, (3) cataracts, (4) papilledema, (5) dark adaptation, (6) glaucoma, (7) retinal detachment (Figure 14-7), and (8) macular degeneration (Table 14-7).

A **cataract** is a cloudy or opaque area in the ocular lens and leads to visual loss when located on the visual axis. It is the leading cause of blindness in the world. The incidence of cataracts increases with age as the lens enlarges. Cataracts develop because of alterations of metabolism and transport of nutrients within the lens. Although the most common form of cataract is degenerative, cataracts also may occur congenitally or as a result of infection, radiation, trauma, medications, or diabetes mellitus. Cataracts cause decreased visual acuity, blurred vision, glare, and decreased colour perception. Cataracts are treated by removal of the entire lens and replacement with an intraocular artificial lens.[96]

Glaucomas are the second leading cause of blindness and are characterized by intraocular pressures greater than 12 to 20 mm Hg with death of retinal ganglion cells and their axons.[97]

There are three primary types of glaucoma (Figure 14-8).[98]

1. *Open angle.* This type of glaucoma is characterized by outflow obstruction of aqueous humor at the trabecular meshwork or canal of Schlemm even though there is adequate space for drainage; often

TABLE 14-6 Changes in the Eye Caused by Aging

Structure	Change	Consequence
Cornea	Thicker and less curved	Increase in astigmatism
Formation of grey ring at edge of cornea (arcus senilis)	Not detrimental to vision	
Anterior chamber	Decrease in size and volume caused by thickening of lens	Occasionally exerts pressure on Schlemm canal and may lead to increased intraocular pressure and glaucoma
Lens	Increase in opacity	Decrease in refraction with increased light scattering (blurring) and decreased colour vision (green and blue); can lead to cataracts
Ciliary muscles	Reduction in pupil diameter, atrophy of radial dilation muscles	Persistent constriction (senile miosis); decrease in critical flicker frequency[a]
Retina	Reduction in number of rods at periphery, loss of rods and associated nerve cells	Increase in minimum amount of light necessary to see an object

[a]The rate at which consecutive visual stimuli can be presented and still be perceived as separate.

TABLE 14-7 Causes of Visual Acuity Changes

Disorder	Description
Amblyopia	Reduced or dimmed vision; cause unknown Associated with strabismus Accompanies such diseases as diabetes mellitus, renal failure, and malaria and use of drugs such as alcohol and tobacco
Scotoma	Circumscribed defect of central field of vision Often associated with retrobulbar neuritis and multiple sclerosis, compression of optic nerve by tumour, inflammation of optic nerve, pernicious anemia, methyl alcohol poisoning, and use of tobacco
Cataracts	Cloudy or opaque area in ocular lens Incidence increases with age because most commonly a result of degeneration; other causes are congenital
Papilledema	Edema and inflammation of optic nerve where it enters eyeball Caused by obstruction of venous return from retina by one of three main sources: increased intracranial pressure, retrobulbar neuritis, or changes in retinal blood vessels
Dark adaptation	With age, eye does not adapt as readily to dark Also, changes in quantity and quality of rhodopsin are causative; vitamin A deficiencies can produce this at any age
Glaucoma	Increased intraocular pressures (>12–20 mm Hg) Loss of acuity results from pressure on optic nerve, which blocks flow of nutrients to optic nerve fibres, leading to their death; sixth leading cause of blindness
Retinal detachment	Tear or break in retina with accumulation of fluid and separation from underlying tissue; seen as floaters, flashes of light, or a curtain over visual field; risks include extreme myopia, diabetic retinopathy, sickle cell disease

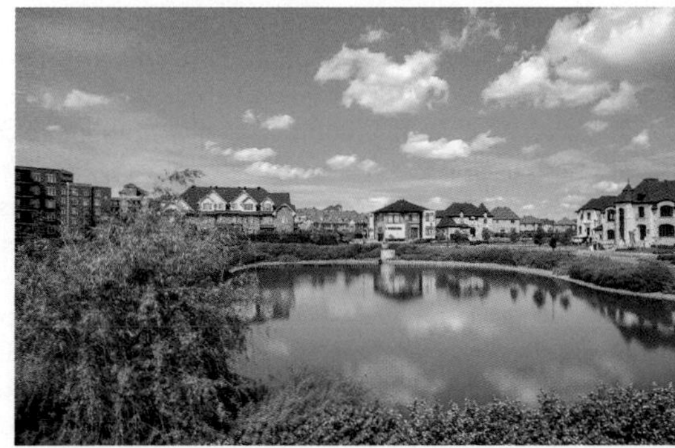
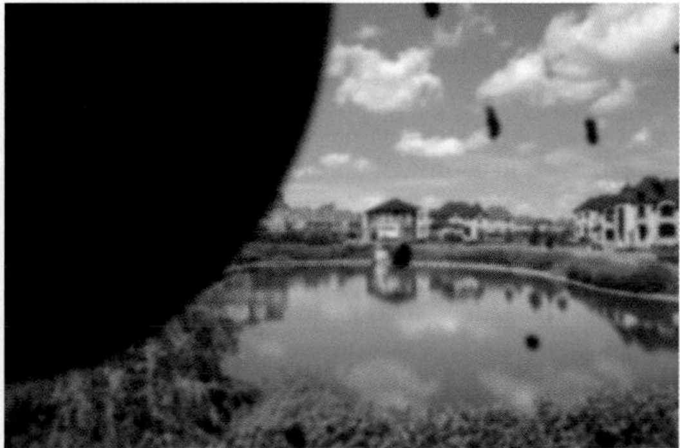

FIGURE 14-7 Perceived Visual Field of an Individual With a Retinal Detachment. (BakerJarvis / Shutterstock.com.)

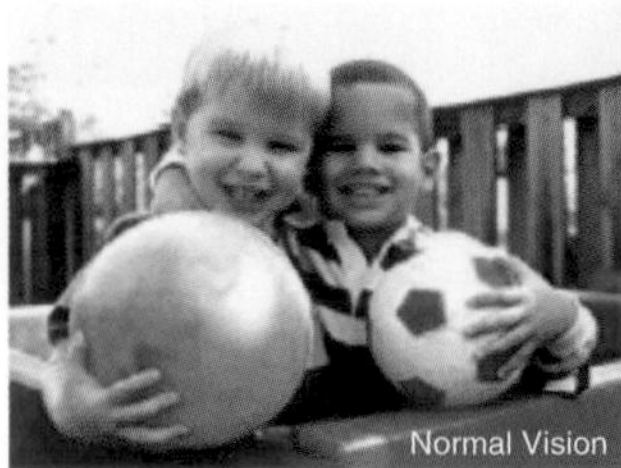

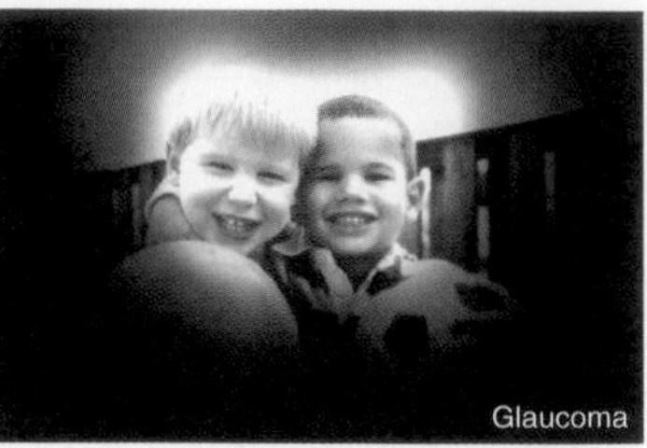

FIGURE 14-8 Glaucoma Vision. (From National Eye Institute, https://www.flickr.com/photos/nationaleyeinstitute/7544734516/in/album-72157646474384400/.)

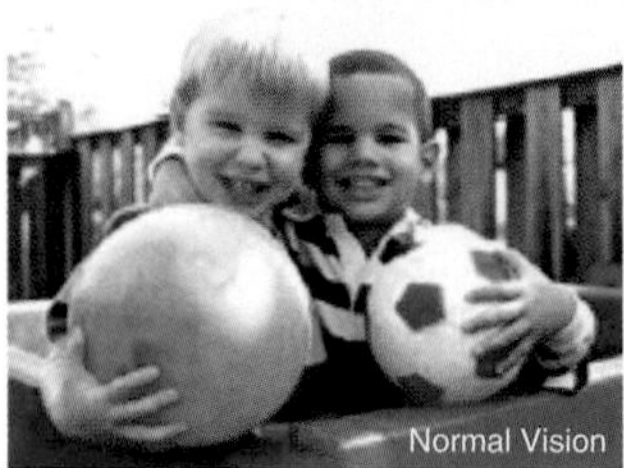

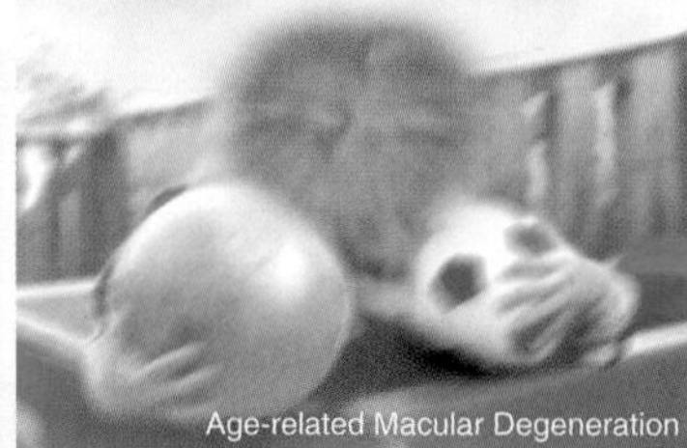

FIGURE 14-9 Age-Related Macular Degeneration. (From National Eye Institute, https://www.flickr.com/photos/nationaleyeinstitute/7544733860/sizes/l/.)

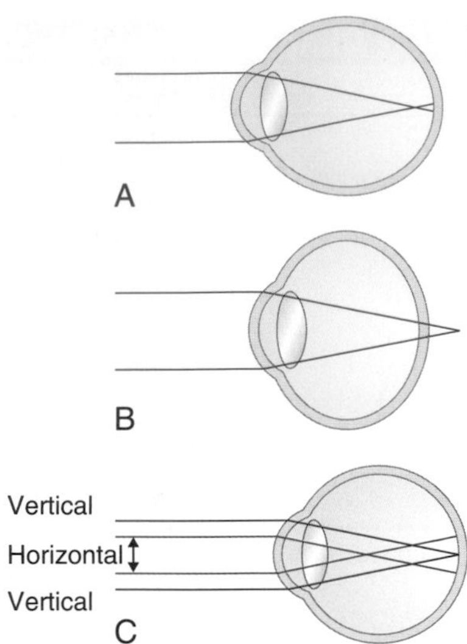

FIGURE 14-10 Alterations in Refraction. A, Myopic eye. Parallel rays of light are brought to a focus in front of the retina. **B,** Hyperopic eye. Parallel rays of light come to a focus behind the retina in the unaccommodative eye. **C,** Simple myopic astigmatism. The vertical bundle of rays is focused on the retina; the horizontal rays are focused in front of the retina. (From Stein, H.A., Stein, R.M., & Freeman, M.I. [2013]. *The ophthalmic assistant: A text for allied and associated ophthalmic personnel* [9th ed.]. Philadelphia: Saunders.)

this is an inherited disease and is a leading cause of blindness with few preliminary symptoms.

2. *Angle closure.* In this type of glaucoma there is displacement of the iris toward the cornea with obstruction of the trabecular meshwork and obstruction of outflow of aqueous humor from the anterior chamber; it may occur acutely with a sudden rise in intraocular pressure, causing pain and visual disturbances.
3. *Congenital closure.* This is a rare disease associated with congenital malformations and other genetic anomalies.

Glaucoma is often asymptomatic and diagnosis may not occur until a late stage of disease. Both medical and surgical therapies are available.[99]

Age-related macular degeneration (AMD) (Figure 14-9) is a severe and irreversible loss of vision and a major cause of blindness in older adults. Hypertension, cigarette smoking, diabetes mellitus, and family history of AMD are risk factors. The degeneration usually occurs after the age of 60 years. There are two forms: atrophic (dry, nonexudative) and neovascular (wet, exudative). The atrophic form is more common and is slowly progressive, with inflammation and accumulation of lipofuscin (a lysosomal pigmented residue) and drusen (waste products from photoreceptors) in the retina and may include limited night vision and difficulty reading. The neovascular form includes accumulation of drusen and lipofuscin, abnormal choroidal blood vessel growth, leakage of blood or serum, retinal detachment, fibrovascular scarring, loss of photoreceptors, and more severe and rapid loss of central vision. Treatment includes antivascular endothelial growth factor (anti-VEGF) injection for wet macular degeneration and antioxidant vitamins for dry macular degeneration.[100] Two carotenoids, lutein and zeaxanthin, are antioxidants that selectively accumulate in the retina and may protect the eye from AMD.[101]

Alterations in accommodation. *Accommodation* refers to changes in the thickness of the lens. Accommodation is needed for clear vision and is mediated through the oculomotor nerve. Pressure, inflammation, age, and disease of the oculomotor nerve may alter accommodation, causing diplopia, blurred vision, and headache.

Loss of accommodation with advancing age is termed **presbyopia**, a condition in which the ocular lens becomes larger, firmer, and less elastic. The major symptom is reduced near vision, causing the individual to hold reading material at arm's length. Treatment includes corrective forward, contact, and intraocular lenses or laser refractive surgery for monovision.[102,103]

Alterations in refraction. Alterations in refraction are the most common visual problem. Causes include irregularities of the corneal curvature, the focusing power of the lens, and the length of the eye. The major symptoms of refraction alterations are blurred vision and headache. The three most common types of refraction are as follows (Figure 14-10):

1. **Myopia** (nearsightedness). Light rays are focused in front of the retina when the person is looking at a distant object.
2. **Hyperopia** (farsightedness). Light rays are focused behind the retina when a person is looking at a near object.
3. **Astigmatism** (unequal curvature of the cornea). Light rays are bent unevenly and do not come to a single focus on the retina. Astigmatism may coexist with myopia, hyperopia, or presbyopia.

Alterations in colour vision. Normal sensitivity to colour diminishes with age because of the progressive yellowing of the lens that occurs with aging. All colours become less intense, although colour discrimination for blue and green is greatly affected. (See the *Geriatric Considerations:* Aging and Changes in Vision box.) Colour vision deteriorates more rapidly for individuals with diabetes mellitus than for the general population.

Abnormal colour vision also may be caused by **colour blindness** and is an X-linked genetic trait. Colour blindness affects 6 to 8% of the male population and about 0.5% of the female population. Although many forms of colour blindness exist, most commonly the affected individual cannot distinguish red from green.[104] In the most severe form individuals see only shades of grey, black, and white.

Neurological disorders causing visual dysfunction. Vision may be disrupted at many points along the visual pathway, causing various defects in the visual field. Visual changes may cause defects or blindness

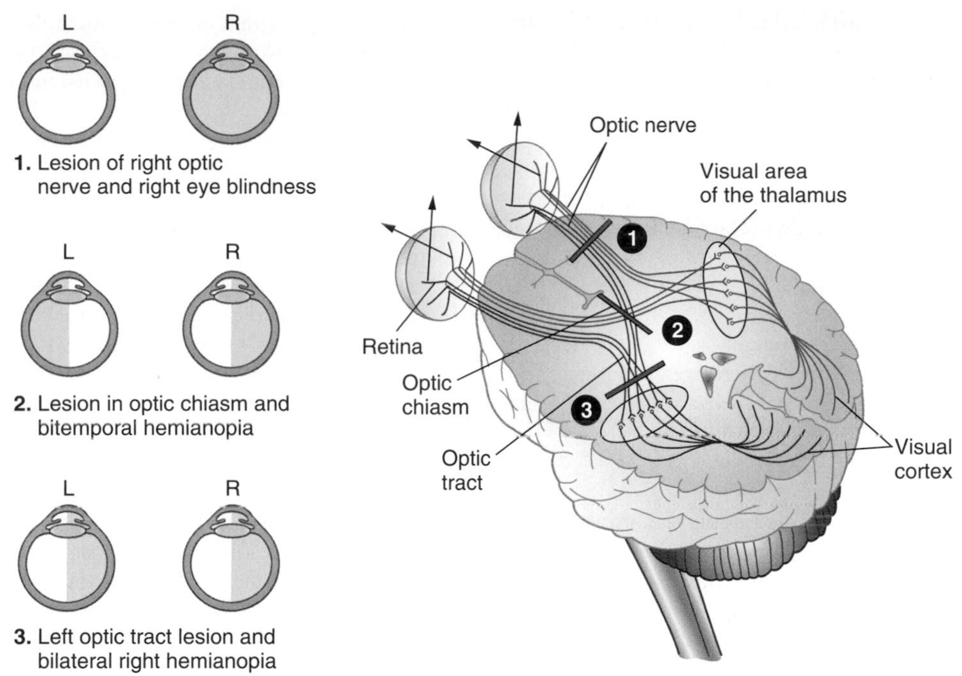

FIGURE 14-11 Visual Pathways and Defects. (Modified from Thompson, J.M., McFarland, G.K., Hirsch, J.E., et al. [2002]. *Mosby's clinical nursing* [5th ed.]. St. Louis: Mosby.)

in the entire visual field or in half of a visual field (hemianopia). (Figure 14-11 illustrates the many areas along the visual pathway that may be damaged and the associated visual changes.) Injury to the optic nerve causes same-side blindness. Injury to the optic chiasm (the X-shaped crossing of the optic nerves) can cause various defects, depending on the location of the injury. Possible causes of optic tract damage include stroke, congenital defects, tumours, infection, and surgery.

External Eye Structure and Disorders

Protective external eye structures include the eyelids (palpebrae), conjunctivae, and lacrimal apparatus. The eyelids control the amount of light reaching the eyes, and the conjunctiva lines the eyelids. Tears released from the lacrimal apparatus bathe the surface of the eye and prevent friction, maintain hydration, and wash out foreign bodies and other irritants (Figure 14-12).

Infection and inflammatory responses are the most common conditions affecting the supporting structures of the eyes. **Blepharitis** is an inflammation of the eyelids caused by *Staphylococcus* or seborrheic dermatitis. A **hordeolum (stye)** is an infection (usually staphylococcal) of the sebaceous glands of the eyelids usually centered near an eyelash. A **chalazion** is a noninfectious lipogranuloma of the meibomian (oil-secreting) gland that often occurs in association with a hordeolum and appears as a deep nodule within the eyelid. These conditions present with redness, swelling, and tenderness and are treated symptomatically. **Entropion** is a common eyelid malposition in which the lid margin turns inward against the eyeball. There are both surgical and nonsurgical treatments to reposition the lid margin.

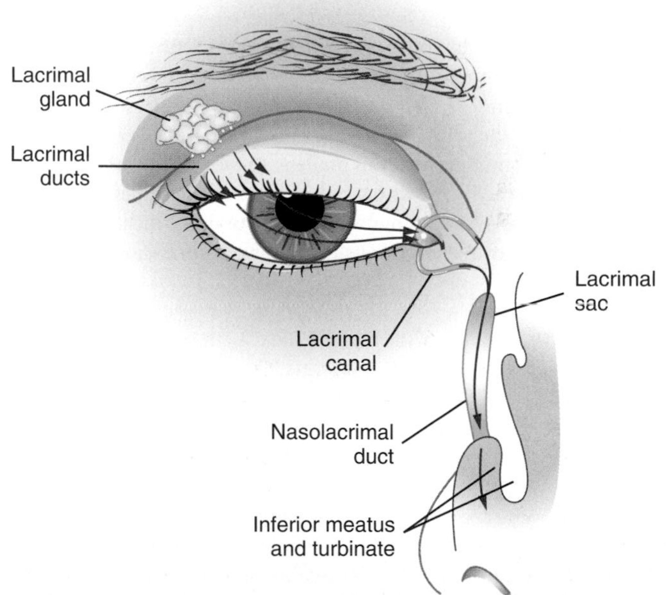

FIGURE 14-12 Lacrimal Apparatus. Fluid produced by lacrimal glands (tears) streams across the eye surface, enters the canals, and then passes through the nasolacrimal duct to enter the nose. (From Applegate, E. [2011]. *The anatomy and physiology learning system* [4th ed.]. St. Louis: Saunders.)

Conjunctivitis is an inflammation of the conjunctiva (mucous membrane covering the front part of the eyeball) caused by viruses (most common), bacteria, allergies, or chemical irritants.[105] **Acute bacterial conjunctivitis (pinkeye)** is highly contagious and often caused by *Staphylococcus, Haemophilus, Streptococcus pneumoniae,* and *Moraxella catarrhalis,* although other bacteria may be involved. In children younger than 6 years, *Haemophilus* infection often leads to otitis media (conjunctivitis–otitis syndrome). Preventing the spread of the microorganism with meticulous handwashing and use of separate towels is important. The disease also is treated with antibiotics.

Viral conjunctivitis is caused by an adenovirus. Again, it is contagious, with symptoms of watering, redness, and photophobia. **Allergic conjunctivitis** is associated with a variety of antigens, including pollens. **Chronic conjunctivitis** results from any persistent conjunctivitis.

Trachoma (chlamydial conjunctivitis) is caused by *Chlamydia trachomatis* and often is associated with poor sanitary conditions. It is the leading cause of preventable blindness in the world.

Keratitis is an infection of the cornea caused by bacteria or viruses. Bacterial infections can cause corneal ulceration, and type 1 herpes simplex virus can involve both the cornea and the conjunctiva. *Acanthamoeba* keratitis can occur from contact lens wear because of poor hygiene. Severe ulcerations with residual scarring require corneal transplantation.

Hearing

Age-related hearing loss usually occurs gradually as we grow older. The loss of hearing usually arises from inner ear changes, but it may also involve the middle ear or changes in neural pathways between the ear and the brain.

The Normal Ear

The ear is divided into three areas: (1) the external ear, involved only with hearing; (2) the middle ear, involved only with hearing; and (3) the inner ear, involved with both hearing and equilibrium.

The external ear is composed of the pinna (auricle), which is the visible portion of the ear, and the external auditory canal, a tube that leads to the middle ear (Figure 14-13). The external auditory canal is surrounded by the bones of the cranium. The opening (meatus) of the canal is just above the mastoid process. The air-filled sinuses, called mastoid air cells, of the mastoid process promote conductivity of sound between the external and the middle ear. The tympanic membrane separates the external ear from the middle ear. Sound waves entering the external auditory canal hit the tympanic membrane (eardrum) and cause it to vibrate.

The middle ear is composed of the tympanic cavity, a small chamber in the temporal bone. Three ossicles (small bones known as the malleus [hammer], incus [anvil], and stapes [stirrup]) transmit the vibration of the tympanic membrane to the inner ear. When the tympanic membrane moves, the malleus moves with it and transfers the vibration to the incus, which passes it on to the stapes. The stapes presses against the oval window, a small membrane of the inner ear. The movement of the oval window sets the fluids of the inner ear in motion (Figure 14-14).

The eustachian (pharyngotympanic) tube connects the middle ear with the pharynx. Normally flat and closed, the eustachian tube opens briefly when a person swallows or yawns, and it equalizes the pressure in the middle ear with atmospheric pressure. Equalized pressure permits the tympanic membrane to vibrate freely. Through the eustachian tube the mucosa of the middle ear is continuous with the mucosal lining of the throat.

The inner ear is a system of osseous labyrinths (bony, mazelike chambers) filled with perilymph. The bony labyrinth is divided into the cochlea, the vestibule, and the semicircular canals (see Figure 14-13). Suspended in the perilymph is the endolymph-filled membranous labyrinth that basically follows the shape of the bony labyrinth.

Within the cochlea is the organ of Corti, which contains hair cells (hearing receptors). Sound waves that reach the cochlea through vibrations of the tympanic membrane, ossicles, and oval window set the cochlear fluids into motion. Receptor cells on the basilar membrane are stimulated when their hairs are bent or pulled by fluid movement. Once stimulated, hair cells transmit impulses along the cochlear nerve (a division of the vestibulocochlear nerve) to the auditory cortex of the temporal lobe in the brain (see Figure 14-14 and view an animation at https://www.youtube.com/watch?v=46aNGGNPm7s). The auditory cortex of the temporal lobe is where interpretation of the sound occurs.

The semicircular canals and vestibule of the inner ear contain equilibrium receptors. In the semicircular canals, the dynamic equilibrium receptors respond to changes in direction of movement. Within each semicircular canal is the crista ampullaris, a receptor region composed of a tuft of hair cells covered by a gelatinous cupula. When the head is rotated, the endolymph in the canal lags behind and moves in the direction opposite to the head's movement. The hair cells are stimulated, and impulses are transmitted through the vestibular nerve (a division of the vestibulocochlear nerve) to the cerebellum.

The vestibule in the inner ear contains maculae—receptors essential to the body's sense of static equilibrium. As the head moves, otoliths (small pieces of calcium salts) move in a gel-like material in response to changes in the pull of gravity. The otoliths pull on the gel, which in turn pulls on the hair cells in the maculae. Nerve impulses in the hair cells are triggered and transmitted to the brain (see Figure 14-14). Thus the ear not only permits the hearing of a large range of sounds but also assists with maintaining balance through the sensitive equilibrium

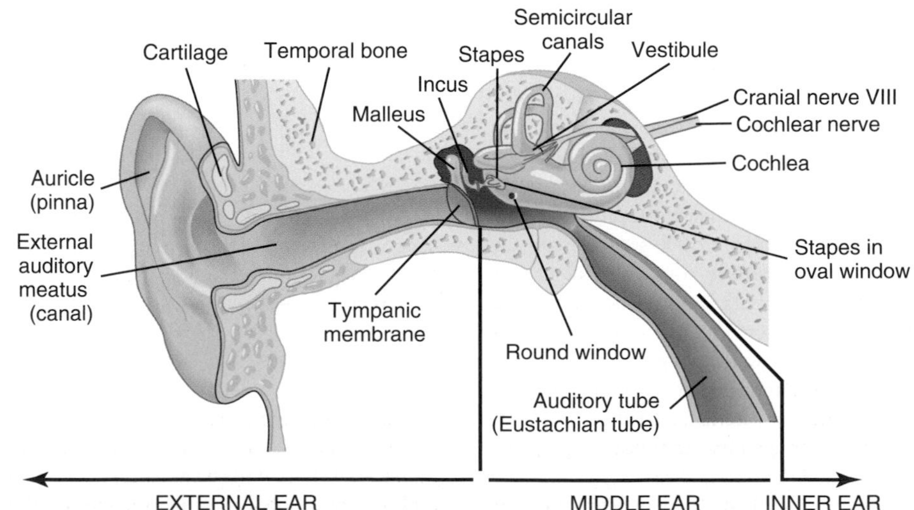

FIGURE 14-13 The Ear. External, middle, and inner ears. (Anatomical structures are not drawn to scale.) (From Applegate, E. [2011]. *The anatomy and physiology learning system* [4th ed.]. St. Louis: Saunders.)

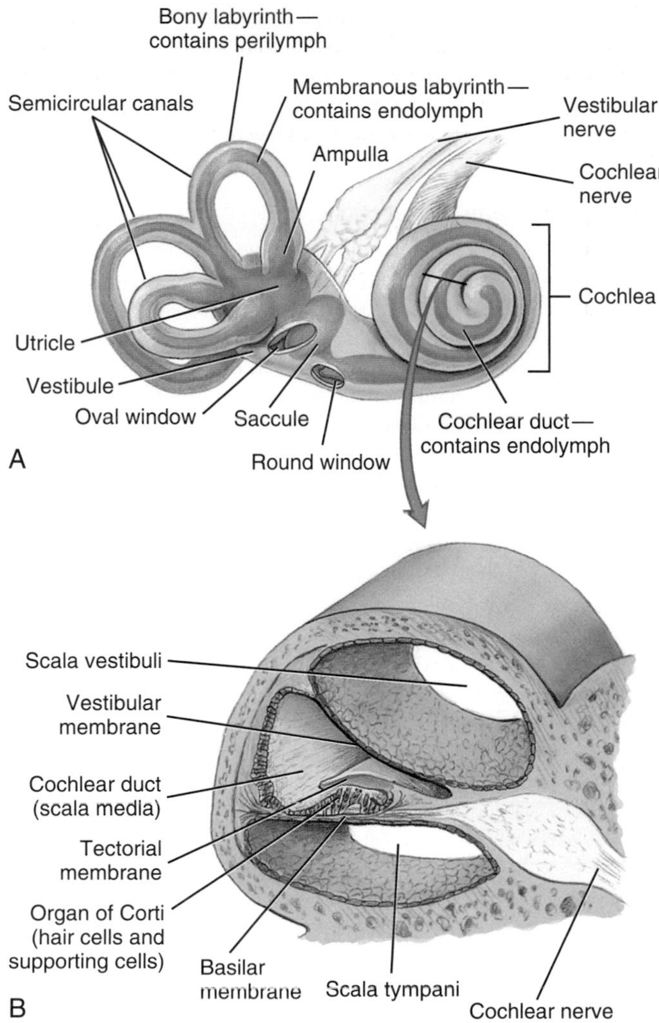

FIGURE 14-14 The Inner Ear. A, The bony labyrinth (*tan*) is the hard outer wall of the entire inner ear and includes the semicircular canals, vestibule, and cochlea. Within the bony labyrinth is the membranous labyrinth (*purple*), which is surrounded by perilymph and filled with endolymph. Each ampulla in the vestibule contains a crista ampullaris that detects changes in head position and sends sensory impulses through the vestibular nerve to the brain. **B,** Section of the membranous cochlea. Hair cells in the organ of Corti detect sound and send the information through the cochlear nerve. The vestibular and cochlear nerves join to form the eighth cranial nerve. (From Applegate, E. [2011]. *The anatomy and physiology learning system* [4th ed.]. St. Louis: Saunders.)

receptors (see an animation at https://www.youtube.com/watch?v=YMIMvBa8XGs).

Auditory Dysfunction

Between 5 and 10% of the general population have impaired hearing, and it is the most common sensory defect. The major categories of auditory dysfunction are conductive hearing loss, sensorineural hearing loss, mixed hearing loss, and functional hearing loss. Hearing loss may range from mild to profound. Auditory changes caused by aging are common and incremental (see the *Geriatric Considerations:* Aging and Changes in Hearing box).

Conductive hearing loss. A conductive hearing loss occurs when a change in the outer or middle ear impairs conduction of sound from the outer to the inner ear. Conditions that commonly cause a conductive hearing loss include impacted cerumen, foreign bodies lodged in the ear canal, benign tumours of the middle ear, carcinoma of the external auditory canal or middle ear, eustachian tube dysfunction, otitis media, acute viral otitis media, chronic suppurative otitis media, cholesteatoma (accumulation of keratinized epithelium), and otosclerosis.

Symptoms of conductive hearing loss include diminished hearing and soft speaking voice. The voice is soft because often the individual hears his or her voice, conducted by bone, as loud.

Sensorineural hearing loss. A sensorineural hearing loss is caused by impairment of the organ of Corti or its central connections. The loss may occur gradually or suddenly. Conditions causing sensorineural loss include congenital and hereditary factors, noise exposure, aging, Ménière's disease, ototoxicity, systemic disease (syphilis, Paget's disease, collagen diseases, diabetes mellitus), neoplasms, and autoimmune processes.[106] Congenital and neonatal sensorineural hearing loss may be caused by maternal rubella, ototoxic medications, prematurity, traumatic delivery, erythroblastosis fetalis, bacterial meningitis, and congenital hereditary malfunction. Diagnosis often is made when delayed speech development is noted. Sudden-onset bilateral sensorineural hearing loss is a medical emergency.[107]

Presbycusis is the most common form of sensorineural hearing loss in older adults. Its cause may be atrophy of the basal end of the organ of Corti, loss of auditory receptors, changes in vascularity, or stiffening of the basilar membranes. Ototoxic components (substances that cause destruction of auditory function) have been observed after exposure to various medications and chemicals—for example, antibiotics such as streptomycin, neomycin, gentamicin, and vancomycin; diuretics such as ethacrynic acid (Edecrin) and furosemide (Apo-Furosemide); and chemicals such as salicylate, quinine, carbon monoxide, nitrogen mustard, arsenic, mercury, gold, tobacco, and alcohol. In most instances, the medications and chemicals listed initially cause tinnitus (ringing in the ear), followed by a progressive high-tone sensorineural hearing loss that is permanent.

Mixed and functional hearing loss. A mixed hearing loss is caused by a combination of conductive and sensorineural losses. With functional hearing loss, which is rare, the individual does not respond to voice and appears not to hear. It is thought to be caused by emotional or psychological factors.

Ménière's disease. Ménière's disease (endolymphatic hydrops) is an episodic disorder of the middle ear with an unknown etiology that can be unilateral or bilateral. There is excessive endolymph and pressure in the membranous labyrinth that disrupts both vestibular and hearing functions. There are four symptoms: recurring episodes of vertigo (often accompanied by severe nausea and vomiting), hearing loss, ringing in the ears (tinnitus), and a feeling of fullness in the ear. Treatment is symptomatic with medical management or surgical management when medications fail.[108]

Ear Infections

Otitis externa. Otitis externa is the most common inflammation of the outer ear and may be acute or persistent, infectious or noninfectious. The most common origins of acute infections are bacterial microorganisms including *Pseudomonas*, *Staphylococcus aureus*, and, less commonly, *Escherichia coli*. Fungal infections are less common. Infection usually follows prolonged exposure to moisture (swimmer's ear). The earliest symptoms are inflammation with pruritus, swelling, and clear drainage progressing to purulent drainage with obstruction of the canal. Tenderness and pain with earlobe retraction accompany inflammation. Acidifying solutions are used for early treatment and topical antimicrobials usually provide effective treatment for later stages of disease.[109] Chronic infections are more often related to allergy or skin disorders.

Otitis media. Otitis media is a common infection of infants and children. Most children have one episode by 3 years of age. The most common pathogens are *S. pneumoniae*, *Haemophilus influenzae*, and *M. catarrhalis*. Predisposing factors include allergy, sinusitis, submucosal cleft palate, adenoidal hypertrophy, eustachian tube dysfunction, and immune deficiency. Breastfeeding is a protective factor. Recurrent acute otitis media may be genetically determined.[110]

Acute otitis media (AOM) is associated with ear pain, fever, irritability, inflamed tympanic membrane, and fluid in the middle ear. The appearance of the tympanic membrane progresses from erythema to opaqueness with bulging as fluid accumulates. There is an increasing prevalence of AOM caused by penicillin-resistant microorganisms. Otitis media with effusion (OME) is the presence of fluid in the middle ear without symptoms of acute infection.

Treatment includes symptom management, particularly of pain, with watchful waiting, antimicrobial therapy for severe illness, and placement of tympanostomy tubes when there is persistent bilateral effusion and significant hearing loss. Complications include mastoiditis, brain abscess, meningitis, and chronic otitis media with hearing loss. Persistent middle ear effusions may affect speech, language, and cognitive abilities. Multivalent vaccines for prevention of otitis media are effective for reducing disease incidence.[111,112]

Olfaction and Taste

Olfaction (smell) is a function of cranial nerve I and part of cranial nerve V. Taste (gustation) is a function of multiple nerves in the tongue, soft palate, uvula, pharynx, and upper esophagus innervated by cranial nerves VII and IX. Both of these cranial nerves are influenced by hormones within the sensory cells. Dysfunctions of smell and taste may occur separately or jointly. The strong relationship between smell and taste creates the sensation of flavour. If either sensation is impaired, the perception of flavour is altered. Olfactory structures are illustrated in Figure 14-15.

Olfactory cells, located in the olfactory epithelium, are the receptor cells for smell. Seven different primary classes of olfactory stimulants have been identified: (1) camphoraceous, (2) musky, (3) floral, (4) peppermint, (5) ethereal, (6) pungent, and (7) putrid. The primary sensations of taste are (1) sour, (2) salty, (3) sweet, (4) bitter, and (5) umami (savouriness). Taste buds (fungiform, foliate, and circumvallate) sensitive to each of the primary sensations are located in specific areas of the tongue.[113]

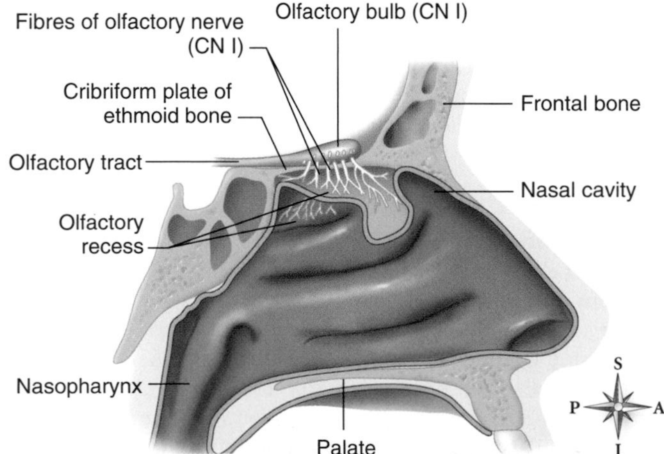

FIGURE 14-15 Olfaction. Midsagittal section of the nasal area shows the location of major olfactory sensory structures. (From Patton, K.T., Thibodeau, G.A., & Douglas, M.M. [2012]. *Essentials of anatomy & physiology*. St. Louis: Mosby.)

Sensitivity to odours declines steadily with aging. See the *Geriatric Considerations:* Aging and Changes in Olfaction and Taste box for a summary of changes in olfaction and taste with aging.

Olfactory and Taste Dysfunctions

Olfactory dysfunctions include the following:

- Hyposmia—impaired sense of smell
- Anosmia—complete loss of sense of smell
- Olfactory hallucinations—smelling odours that are not really present
- Parosmia—abnormal or perverted sense of smell

The sense of taste can be impaired by injury. Altered taste may be attributed to impaired smell associated with injury near the hippocampus.

Hypogeusia is a decrease in taste sensation, whereas ageusia is an absence of the sense of taste. These disorders result from cranial nerve injuries and can be specific to the area of the tongue innervated. Dysgeusia is a perversion of taste in which substances possess an unpleasant flavour (i.e., metallic). Alterations in taste may compromise adequate nutrition or cause anorexia.[114]

QUICK CHECK 14-4

1. List the major structures of the eye.
2. Visual disorders fall into several categories; name them.
3. How does fluid accumulate in the middle ear during otitis media?
4. What factors are involved in the sensation of flavour?

SOMATOSENSORY FUNCTION

Touch

The sensation of touch involves four afferent fibre types that mediate tactile sensation, and there may be an additional sensory nerve that transmits pleasurable touch.[115] Receptors sensitive to touch are present in the skin with high densities in the fingers and lips. Meissner corpuscles and pacinian corpuscles are fast-adapting receptors and sense movement across the skin and vibration, respectively. The slowly adapting Merkel discs sense sustained light touch, and Ruffini endings respond to deep sustained pressure, stretch, and joint position. Specific sensory input is carried to the higher levels of the CNS by the dorsal column of the spinal cord and the anterior spinothalamic tract.

The cutaneous senses develop before birth, but structural growth continues into early adulthood. Then a gradual decline occurs, with loss in tactile discrimination with advancing age.[116] Abnormal tactile perception may be caused by alterations at any level of the nervous system, from the receptor to the cerebral cortex. Factors that interrupt or impair reception, transmission, perception, or interpretation of touch—including trauma, tumour, infection, metabolic changes, vascular changes, and degenerative diseases—may cause tactile dysfunction. In addition, most tactile sensations evoke affective responses that determine whether the sensation is unpleasant, pleasant, or neutral.

Proprioception

Proprioception is the awareness of the position of the body and its parts. It depends on impulses from the inner ear and from receptors in joints and ligaments. Sensory data are transmitted to higher centres, primarily through the dorsal columns and the spinocerebellar tracts, with some data passing through the medial lemnisci and thalamic radiations to the cortex. These stimuli are necessary for the coordination of movements, the grading of muscular contraction, and the maintenance of equilibrium.

A progressive loss of proprioception has been reported in older adults and is associated with an increased risk for falls and injury.[117] As with tactile dysfunction, any factor that interrupts or impairs the reception, transmission, perception, or interpretation of proprioceptive stimuli also alters proprioception and increases risk for falls and injury. Two common causes of alterations in proprioception are vestibular dysfunction and neuropathy.

Specific vestibular dysfunctions are vestibular nystagmus and vertigo. **Vestibular nystagmus** is the constant, involuntary movement of the eyeball and develops when the semicircular canal system is overstimulated. **Vertigo** is the sensation of spinning that occurs with inflammation of the semicircular canals in the ear. The individual may feel either that he or she is moving in space or that the world is revolving. Vertigo often causes loss of balance, and nystagmus may occur. Ménière's disease can cause loss of proprioception during an acute attack, so that standing or walking is impossible.

Peripheral neuropathies also can cause proprioceptive dysfunction. They may be caused by several conditions and commonly are associated with renal disease and diabetes mellitus. Although the exact sequence of events is unknown, neuropathies cause a diminished or absent sense of body position or position of body parts. Gait changes often occur.

QUICK CHECK 14-5

1. How are different touch receptors distributed over the body?
2. What are two common causes of alterations in proprioception?

GERIATRIC CONSIDERATIONS

Aging and Changes in Vision

- The incidence of cataracts increases with age.
- Age-related macular degeneration (AMD) is a major cause of blindness in older adults. It is a severe and irreversible loss of vision.
- Presbyopia is the loss of visual accommodation associated with advancing age.
- Colour discrimination diminishes with age, with blue and green affected most.
- See Tables 14-6 and 14-7 for additional information.

GERIATRIC CONSIDERATIONS

Aging and Changes in Hearing[a]

Changes in Structure	Changes in Function
Cochlear hair cell degeneration	Inability to hear high-frequency sounds (presbycusis, sensorineural loss); interferes with understanding speech; hearing may be lost in both ears at different times
Loss of auditory neurons in spiral ganglia of organ of Corti	Inability to hear high-frequency sounds (presbycusis, sensorineural loss); interferes with understanding speech; hearing may be lost in both ears at different times
Degeneration of basilar (cochlear) conductive membrane of cochlea	Inability to hear at all frequencies but more pronounced at higher frequencies (cochlear conductive loss)
Decreased vascularity of cochlea	Equal loss of hearing at all frequencies (strial loss); inability to disseminate localization of sound
Loss of cortical auditory neurons	Equal loss of hearing at all frequencies (strial loss); inability to disseminate localization of sound

[a]Hearing loss affects about 33% of older adults.
Data from Frisina, R.D. (2009). *Ann N Y Acad Sci, 1170*, 708–717; Roth, T.N. (2015). *Handb Clin Neurol, 129*, 357–373.

GERIATRIC CONSIDERATIONS

Aging and Changes in Olfaction and Taste

- Decline in sensitivity to odours, usually after age 80, occurs.
- Loss of olfaction may diminish appetite, taste, and food selection and may affect nutrition.
- Inability to smell toxic fumes or gases can pose a safety hazard.
- Decline in taste sensitivity is more gradual than decline in sense of smell.
- Higher concentrations of flavours are required to stimulate taste.
- Taste may be influenced by decreased salivary secretion.

DID YOU UNDERSTAND?

Pain

1. Pain (nociception) is a complex, unpleasant sensory experience that involves dynamic interactions between physical, cognitive, spiritual, emotional, and environmental factors. Pain is protective.
2. Three portions of the nervous system are responsible for sensation, perception, and response to pain: (a) the afferent pathways, (b) the interpretive centres of the central nervous system, and (c) the efferent pathways.
3. Nociception involves four phases: transduction, transmission, perception, and modulation.
4. There are two primary types of nociceptors: Aδ fibres and C fibres. Myelinated Aδ fibres transmit sharp, well-localized "fast" pain. Smaller, unmyelinated C fibres more slowly transmit dull, aching, or burning sensations that are less localized.
5. The somatosensory cortex mediates localization and intensity of pain. The reticular formation, limbic system, and brainstem control emotional and affective responses to pain. The cortex coordinates the meaning an experience of pain.
6. Pain threshold is the lowest intensity of pain that a person can recognize. Pain tolerance is the greatest intensity of pain that an individual can endure. Both are subjective and influenced by many factors.
7. Neuromodulators of pain include substances that (a) stimulate pain nociceptors (e.g., prostaglandins, bradykinins, lymphokines, substance P, glutamate) and (b) suppress pain (e.g., GABA, endogenous opioids, endocannabinoids). Some substances excite peripheral nerves but inhibit central nerves (e.g., serotonin, norepinephrine).
8. Endogenous opioids inhibit pain transmission and include enkephalins, endorphins, dynorphins, and endomorphins. They are produced in the central nervous system.
9. Descending inhibitory and facilitatory pathways and nuclei inhibit or facilitate pain. Efferent pathways from the ventromedial medulla and periaqueductal grey inhibit pain impulses at the dorsal horn. The rostroventromedial medulla stimulates efferent pathways that facilitate or inhibit pain in the dorsal horn.
10. Segmental pain inhibition occurs when impulses from Aβ fibres (touch and vibration sensations) arrive at the same spinal level as impulses from Aδ or C fibres.
11. Diffuse noxious inhibitory control occurs when pain signals from two different sites are transmitted simultaneously and inhibit pain through a spinal-medullary-spinal pathway.
12. Classifications of pain include nociceptive pain (with a known physiological cause), non-nociceptive pain (neuropathic pain), acute pain (signal to the person of a harmful stimulus), and persistent pain (persistence of pain of unknown cause or unusual response to therapy).
13. Acute pain may be (a) somatic (superficial), (b) visceral (internal), or (c) referred (present in an area distant from its origin). The area of referred pain is supplied by the same spinal segment as the actual site of pain.
14. Persistent pain is pain lasting well beyond the expected normal healing time and may be intermittent (e.g., low back pain) or persistent (e.g., migraine headaches).
15. Psychological, behavioural, and physiological responses to persistent pain include depression, sleep disorders, preoccupation with pain, lifestyle changes, and physiological adaptation.
16. Neuropathic pain is increased sensitivity to painful stimuli and results from abnormal processing of pain information in the peripheral or central nervous system.

Temperature Regulation

1. Temperature regulation is achieved through precise balancing of heat production, heat conservation, and heat loss. The normal range of body temperature is considered to be 36.2° to 37.7°C (96.2° to 99.4°F) overall.
2. Temperature regulation is mediated by the hypothalamus through central thermoreceptors in the skin, hypothalamus, spinal cord, abdominal organs, and other central locations.
3. Body heat is produced through chemical reactions of metabolism and skeletal muscle tone and contraction.
4. Heat is conserved through vasoconstriction and voluntary mechanisms.
5. Body heat is lost through radiation, conduction, convection, vasodilation, evaporation of sweat, decreased muscle tone, increased respiration, voluntary measures, and adaptation to warmer climates.
6. Infants do not conserve heat well because of their greater body surface to body weight and low amount of subcutaneous fat. Older adults have poor responses to environmental temperature extremes as a result of slowed blood circulation, structural and functional changes in the skin, and overall decreased heat-producing activities.
7. Fever is triggered by the release of exogenous pyrogens from bacteria or the release of endogenous pyrogens (cytokines) from phagocytic cells. Fever is both a normal immunological mechanism and a symptom of disease.
8. Fever involves the "resetting of the hypothalamic thermostat" to a higher level. When the fever breaks, the set point returns to normal.
9. Fever of unknown origin is a body temperature greater than 38.3°C (101°F) for longer than 3 weeks' duration that remains undiagnosed after 3 days of hospital investigation, 3 outpatient visits, or 1 week of ambulatory investigation.
10. Fever production aids responses to infectious processes. Higher temperatures kill many microorganisms, promote immune responses, and decrease serum levels of iron, zinc, and copper, which are needed for bacterial replication.
11. Hyperthermia (marked warming of core temperature) can produce nerve damage, coagulation of cell proteins, and death. Forms of accidental hyperthermia include heat cramps, heat exhaustion, heat stroke, and malignant hyperthermia. Heat stroke and malignant hyperthermia are potentially lethal.
12. Hypothermia (marked cooling of core temperature) slows the rate of chemical reaction (tissue metabolism), increases the viscosity of the blood, slows blood flow through the microcirculation, facilitates blood coagulation, and stimulates profound vasoconstriction. Hypothermia may be accidental or therapeutic.

Sleep

1. Sleep is an active multiphase process divided into rapid eye movement (REM) and non–rapid eye movement (non-REM) sleep, each of which has its own series of stages. While asleep, an individual progresses through REM and non-REM (slow wave) sleep in a predictable cycle.
2. REM sleep is controlled by mechanisms in the pons and mesencephalon. Non-REM sleep is controlled by release of inhibitory signals from the hypothalamus and accounts for 75 to 80% of sleep time.
3. The sleep patterns of infants, young children, and older adults vary in total sleep time, cycle length, and percentage of time spent in each sleep cycle. Older adults experience a decrease in total sleep time.

4. Sleep disorders include (a) dyssomnias (disorders of initiating sleep [i.e., insomnia, sleep-disordered breathing, hypersomnia, or disorders of the sleep–wake schedule]) and (b) parasomnias (i.e., sleepwalking or night terrors and restless legs syndrome).
5. The restorative, reparative, and growth processes occur during slow-wave (non-REM) sleep. Sleep deprivation can cause profound changes in personality and functioning.

The Special Senses

1. The wall of the eye has three layers: sclera, choroid, and retina. The retina contains millions of baroreceptors known as rods and cones that receive light through the lens and then convey signals to the optic nerve and subsequently to the visual cortex of the brain.
2. The eye is filled with vitreous and aqueous humor which prevent it from collapsing.
3. The major alterations in ocular movement include strabismus, nystagmus, and paralysis of specific extraocular muscles.
4. Structural eye changes caused by aging result in decreased visual acuity.
5. Alterations in visual acuity can be caused by amblyopia, scotoma, cataracts, papilledema, glaucoma, and macular degeneration.
6. A cataract is a cloudy or opaque area in the ocular lens and leads to visual loss when located on the visual axis.
7. Glaucomas are characterized by intraocular pressures greater than 12 to 20 mm Hg with death of retinal ganglion cells and their axons.
8. Age-related macular degeneration is irreversible loss of vision with dry or wet forms.
9. Alterations in accommodation develop with increased intraocular pressure, inflammation, and disease of the oculomotor nerve. Presbyopia is loss of accommodation caused by loss of elasticity of the lens with aging.
10. Alterations in refraction, including myopia, hyperopia, and astigmatism, are the most common visual disorders.
11. Alterations in colour vision can be related to yellowing of the lens with aging and colour blindness, an inherited trait.
12. The eyelids, conjunctivae, and lacrimal apparatus protect the eye. Infections are the most common conditions affecting the supporting structures of the eyes; they include blepharitis, conjunctivitis, chalazion, and hordeolum.
13. Trauma or disease of the optic nerve pathways, or optic radiations, can cause blindness in the visual fields.
14. Blepharitis is an inflammation of the eyelid; a hordeolum (stye) is an infection of the eyelid's sebaceous gland; and a chalazion is an infection of the eyelid's meibomian gland.
15. Conjunctivitis can be acute or chronic, bacterial, viral, or allergic. Redness, edema, pain, and lacrimation are common symptoms. Chlamydial conjunctivitis is the leading cause of blindness in the world and is associated with poor sanitary conditions.
16. Keratitis is a bacterial or viral infection of the cornea that can lead to corneal ulceration. Photophobia, pain, and tearing are common symptoms.
17. The ear is composed of the external ear, middle ear, and inner ear. The external structures are the pinna, auditory canal, and tympanic membrane. The tympanic cavity (containing three bones: the malleus, the incus, and the stapes), oval window, eustachian tube, and fluid compose the middle ear and transmit sound vibrations to the inner ear.
18. The inner ear includes the bony and membranous labyrinths that transmit sound waves through the cochlea to the acoustic division of the eighth cranial nerve. The semicircular canals and vestibule help maintain balance through the equilibrium receptors.
19. Hearing loss can be classified as conductive, sensorineural, mixed, or functional.
20. Conductive hearing loss occurs when sound waves cannot be conducted through the middle ear.
21. Sensorineural hearing loss develops with impairment of the organ of Corti or its central connections. Presbycusis is the most common form of sensorineural hearing loss in older adults.
22. A combination of conductive and sensorineural loss is a mixed hearing loss.
23. Loss of hearing with no known organic cause is a functional hearing loss.
24. Ménière's disease is a disorder of the middle ear that affects hearing and balance.
25. Otitis externa is an infection of the outer ear associated with prolonged exposure to moisture.
26. Otitis media is an infection of the middle ear that is common in children. Accumulation of fluid (effusion) behind the tympanic membrane is a common finding.
27. The perception of flavour is altered if olfaction or taste dysfunctions occur. Sensitivity to odour and taste decreases with aging.
28. Hyposmia is a decrease in the sense of smell, and anosmia is the complete loss of the sense of smell. Inflammation of the nasal mucosa and trauma or tumours of the olfactory nerve lead to a diminished sense of smell.
29. Hypogeusia is a decrease in taste sensation, and ageusia is the absence of the sense of taste. Loss of taste buds or trauma to the facial or glossopharyngeal nerves decreases taste sensation.

Somatosensory Function

1. Tactile sensation is a function of receptors present in the skin (pacinian corpuscles), and the sensory response is conducted to the brain through the dorsal column and anterior spinothalamic tract.
2. Alterations in touch can result from disruption of skin receptors, sensory transmission, or central nervous system perception.
3. Proprioception is the awareness of the position and location of the body and its parts. Proprioceptors are located in the inner ear, joints, and ligaments. Proprioceptive stimuli are necessary for balance, coordinated movement, and grading of muscular contraction.
4. Disorders of proprioception can occur at any level of the nervous system and result in impaired balance and lack of coordinated movement.

Geriatric Considerations: Aging and Changes in Hearing

1. Approximately one third of older adults have hearing loss.

KEY TERMS

A beta (Aβ) fibres, 339
A delta (Aδ) fibres, 339
Accidental hyperthermia, 346
Accommodation, 350
Acute bacterial conjunctivitis (pinkeye), 353
Acute otitis media (AOM), 356
Acute pain, 342
Affective-motivational system, 340
Age-related macular degeneration (AMD), 352
Ageusia, 356

Allergic conjunctivitis, 353
Allodynia, 343
Amblyopia, 350
Anosmia, 356
Aqueous humor, 350
Astigmatism, 352
Blepharitis, 353
Cannabinoid, 342
Cannabis, 342
Cataract, 350
Central fever, 347
Central neuropathic pain, 343
Central sensitization, 343
C fibres, 339
Chalazion, 353
Choroid, 349
Chronic conjunctivitis, 353
Circadian rhythm sleep disorder, 349
Cochlea, 354
Cognitive-evaluative system, 340
Colour blindness, 352
Conductive hearing loss, 355
Cone, 349
Conjunctivitis, 353
Cornea, 349
Crista ampullaris, 354
Descending facilitatory pathway, 342
Descending inhibitory pathway, 342
Diffuse noxious inhibitory control (DNIC), 342
Diplopia, 350
Dynorphin, 342
Dysgeusia, 356
Endocannabinoid, 342
Endogenous opioid, 341
Endogenous pyrogen, 346
Endomorphin, 342
Endorphin, 341
Enkephalin, 341
Entropion, 353
Equilibrium receptor, 354
Eustachian (pharyngotympanic) tube, 354
Excitatory neurotransmitter, 340
Exogenous pyrogen, 346
Expectancy-related cortical activation, 342
External auditory canal, 354
Fever, 346
Fever of unknown origin (FUO), 346
Fovea centralis, 349
Functional hearing loss, 355
Gate control theory, 339
Glaucoma, 350
Hair cell, 354
Heat cramp, 346
Heat exhaustion, 346
Heat stroke, 346
Heterosegmental pain inhibition, 342
Hordeolum (stye), 353
Hyperopia, 352
Hypersomnia, 348
Hyperthermia, 346
Hypogeusia, 356
Hyposmia, 356
Hypothermia, 347
Incus (anvil), 354
Inhibitory neurotransmitter, 341
Insomnia, 348
Intractable pain, 343
Iris, 349
Jerk nystagmus, 350
Keratitis, 354
Lens, 350
Macula lutea, 349
Maculae, 354
Malignant hyperthermia, 347
Malleus (hammer), 354
Mastoid air cell, 354
Mastoid process, 354
Meissner corpuscle, 356
Ménière's disease, 355
Merkel disc, 356
Mixed hearing loss, 355
Myopia, 352
Narcolepsy, 348
Neuromatrix theory, 339
Neuropathic pain, 343
Night terrors, 349
Nociceptin/orphanin FQ, 342
Nociception, 339
Nociceptive pain, 339
Nociceptive transmissions, 339
Nociceptor, 339
Non-nociceptive stimulation, 339
Non–rapid eye movement (NREM) sleep, 348
Nystagmus, 350
Obesity hypoventilation syndrome, 348
Obstructive sleep apnea syndrome (OSAS), 348
Olfaction, 356
Olfactory hallucination, 356
Optic chiasm, 349
Optic disc, 349
Optic nerve, 349
Organ of Corti, 354
Otitis externa, 355
Otitis media, 356
Otitis media with effusion (OME), 356
Otolith, 354
Oval window, 354
Pacinian corpuscle, 356
Pain modulation, 340
Pain perception, 340
Pain threshold, 340
Pain tolerance, 340
Pain transduction, 339
Pain transmission, 339
Parasomnia, 349
Parosmia, 356
Pattern theory, 339
Pendular nystagmus, 350
Perceptual dominance, 340
Perilymph, 354
Peripheral neuropathic pain, 343
Peripheral sensitization, 343
Persistent pain, 343
Pinna, 354
Presbycusis, 355
Presbyopia, 352
Proprioception, 356
Pupil, 349
Rapid eye movement (REM) sleep, 347
Referred pain, 343
Restless legs syndrome (RLS), 349
Retina, 349
Rod, 349
Ruffini ending, 356
Sclera, 349
Segmental pain inhibition, 342
Semicircular canal, 354
Sensorineural hearing loss, 355
Sensory-discriminative system, 340
Shift work sleep disorder, 349
Sleep, 347
Somatic pain, 342
Somnambulism (sleepwalking), 349
Specificity theory, 338
Stapes (stirrup), 354
Strabismus, 350
Suprachiasmatic nucleus (SCN), 350
Taste, 356
Therapeutic hyperthermia, 346
Thermoregulation, 344
Tinnitus, 355
Touch, 356
Trachoma, 354
Tympanic cavity, 354
Tympanic membrane, 354
Vertigo, 357
Vestibular nystagmus, 357
Vestibule, 354
Viral conjunctivitis, 353
Visceral pain, 343
Vitreous humor, 350
Willis-Ekbom disease, 349

REFERENCES

1. McCaffery, M. (1968). *Nursing practice theories related to cognition, bodily pain and nonenvironment interactions.* Los Angeles: University of California at Los Angeles Students' Store.
2. International Association for the Study of Pain. (2014). *IASP taxonomy.* Retrieved from http://www.iasp-pain.org/Taxonomy?navItemNumber=576.
3. McCance, K. L., & Huether, S. E. (2015). *Pathophysiology: The biologic basis for disease in adults and children* (7th ed., p. 485). St. Louis: Mosby.
4. Arnstein, P. (2010). *Clinical coach for effective pain management.* Philadelphia: FA Davis.
5. Pasero, C., & McCaffery, M. (2011). *Pain assessment and pharmacologic management.* St. Louis: Mosby.
6. Basbaum, A. I., Bautista, D. M., Scherrer, G., et al. (2009). Cellular and molecular mechanisms of pain. *Cell, 139*(2), 267–284.
7. Helms, J. E., & Barone, C. P. (2008). Physiology and treatment of pain. *Critical Care Nurse, 28*(6), 38–40.
8. Marchand, S. (2008). The physiology of pain mechanisms: From the periphery to the brain. *Rheumatic Diseases Clinics of North America, 34*(2), 285–309. doi:10.1016/j.rdc.2008.04.003.
9. Argoff, C. E., Albrecht, P., Irving, G., et al. (2009). Multimodal analgesia for chronic pain: Rationale and future directions. *Pain Medicine (Malden, Mass.), 10*(S2), S53–S66. doi:10.1111/j.1526-4637.2009.00669.x.
10. Casey, K. L. (1999). Forebrain mechanisms of nociception and pain: Analysis through imaging. *Proceedings of the National Academy of Sciences of the United States of America, 96*(14), 7668–7674.
11. Garcia-Larrea, L., & Peyron, R. (2013). Pain matrices and neuropathic pain matrices: A review. *Pain, 154*(Suppl. 1), S29–S43. doi:10.1016/j.pain.2013.09.001.
12. Wandner, L. D., Scipio, C. D., Hirsch, A. T., et al. (2013). The perception of pain in others: How gender, race, and age influence pain expectations. *Journal of Pain, 13*(3), 220–227. doi:10.1016/j.jpain.2011.10.014.
13. Bartley, E. J., & Fillingim, R. B. (2013). Sex differences in pain: A brief review of clinical and experimental findings. *British Journal of Anaesthesia, 111*(1), 52–58. doi:10.1093/bja/aet127.
14. Ossipov, M. H., Dussor, G. O., & Porreca, F. (2010). Central modulation of pain. *Journal of Clinical Investigation, 120*(11), 3779–3787. doi:10.1172/JCI43766.
15. Fields, H. L., Basbaum, A. I., & Heinricher, M. M. (2005). Central nervous system mechanism of pain modulation. In S. McMahon & M. Koltzenburg (Eds.), *Wall and Melzack's textbook of pain* (5th ed., pp. 125–142). Edinburgh: Churchill Livingstone.

16. Gangadharan, V., & Kuner, R. (2013). Pain hypersensitivity mechanisms at a glance. *Disease Models & Mechanisms, 6*(4), 889–895. doi:10.1242/dmm.011502.
17. Lau, B. K., & Vaughan, C. W. (2014). Descending modulation of pain: The GABA disinhibition hypothesis of analgesia. *Current Opinion in Neurobiology, 29C*, 159–164. doi:10.1016/j.conb.2014.07.010.
18. Ninkovic, J., & Roy, S. (2013). Role of the mu-opioid receptor in opioid modulation of immune function. *Amino Acids, 45*(1), 9–24. doi:10.1007/s00726-011-1163-0.
19. Bodnar, R. J. (2010). Endogenous opiates and behavior: 2009. *Peptides, 31*(12), 2325–2359. doi:10.1016/j.peptides.2010.09.016.
20. Busch-Dienstfertig, M., & Stein, C. (2010). Opioid receptors and opioid peptide-producing leukocytes in inflammatory pain—Basic and therapeutic aspects. *Brain, Behavior, and Immunity, 24*(5), 683–694. doi:10.1016/j.bbi.2009.10.013.
21. Lutz, P. E., & Kieffer, B. L. (2013). The multiple facets of opioid receptor function: Implications for addiction. *Current Opinion in Neurobiology, 23*(4), 473–479. doi:10.1016/j.conb.2013.02.005.
22. Perlikowska, R., & Janecka, A. (2014). Bioavailability of endomorphins and the blood–brain barrier—A review. *Medicinal Chemistry (Shariqah, United Arab Emirates), 10*(1), 2–17.
23. Tariq, S., Nurulain, S. M., Tekes, K., et al. (2013). Deciphering intracellular localization and physiological role of nociceptin and nocistatin. *Peptides, 43*, 174–183. doi:10.1016/j.peptides.2013.02.010.
24. Koob, G. F., Arends, M. A., & Le Moal, M. (Eds.), (2014). *Drugs, addiction and the brain* (pp. 133–171). Amsterdam: Academic Press.
25. Davis, M. P. (2014). Cannabinoids in pain management: CB1, CB2 and non-classic receptor ligands. *Expert Opinion on Investigational Drugs, 23*(8), 1123–1140. doi:10.1517/13543784.2014.918603.
26. Guindon, J., & Hohmann, A. G. (2009). The endocannabinoid system and pain. *CNS and Neurological Disorders Drug Targets, 8*(6), 403–421.
27. Ulugöl, A. (2014). The endocannabinoid system as a potential therapeutic target for pain modulation. *Balkan Medical Journal, 31*(2), 115–120. doi:10.5152/balkanmedj.2014.13103.
28. Mason, P. (2005). Deconstructing endogenous pain modulations. *Journal of Neurophysiology, 94*(3), 1659–1663. doi:10.1152/jn.00249.2005.
29. Dogrul, A., Ossipov, M. H., & Porreca, F. (2009). Differential mediation of descending pain facilitation and inhibition by spinal 5HT-3 and 5HT-7 receptors. *Brain Research, 1280*, 52–59. doi:10.1016/j.brainres.2009.05.001.
30. van Wijk, G., & Veldhuijzen, D. S. (2010). Perspective on diffuse noxious inhibitory controls as a model of endogenous pain modulation in clinical pain syndromes. *Journal of Pain, 11*(5), 408–419. doi:10.1016/j.jpain.2009.10.009.
31. Colloca, L., & Grillon, C. (2014). Understanding placebo and nocebo responses for pain management. *Current Pain and Headache Reports, 18*(6), 419. doi:10.1007/s11916-014-0419-2.
32. Canadian Pain Coalition Pain Resource Centre. (2016). *About pain*. Retrieved from http://prc.canadianpaincoalition.ca/en/about_pain.html.
33. Costigan, M., Scholz, J., & Woolf, C. J. (2009). Neuropathic pain: A maladaptive response of the nervous system to damage. *Annual Review of Neuroscience, 32*, 1–32. doi:10.1146/annurev.neuro.051508.135531.
34. Thibodeau, G. A., & Patton, K. T. (2003). *Anatomy & physiology* (5th ed.). St. Louis: Mosby.
35. Apkarian, A. V., Baliki, M. N., & Geha, P. Y. (2009). Towards a theory of chronic pain. *Progress in Neurobiology, 87*(2), 8197. doi:10.1016/j.pneurobio.2008.09.018.
36. Mifflin, K. A., & Kerr, B. J. (2014). The transition from acute to chronic pain: Understanding how different biological systems interact. *Canadian Journal of Anaesthesia, 61*(2), 112–122. doi:10.1007/s12630-013-0087-4.
37. Fornasari, D. (2012). Pain mechanisms in patients with chronic pain. *Clinical Drug Investigation, 32*(Suppl. 1), 45–52. doi:10.2165/11630070-000000000-00000.
38. Attal, N., Masselin-Dubois, A., Martinez, V., et al. (2014). Does cognitive functioning predict chronic pain? Results from a prospective surgical cohort. *Brain: A Journal of Neurology, 137*(Pt. 3), 904–917. doi:10.1093/brain/awt354.
39. May, A. (2008). Chronic pain may change the structure of the brain. *Pain, 137*(1), 7–15. doi:10.1016/j.pain.2008.02.034.
40. Rodriquez-Raecke, R., Niemeier, A., Ihle, K., et al. (2009). Brain gray matter decrease in chronic pain is the consequence and not the cause of pain. *Journal of Neuroscience, 29*(44), 12746–12750. doi:10.1523/JNEUROSCI.3687-09.2009.
41. Tracey, I., & Bushnell, M. C. (2009). How neuroimaging studies have challenged us to rethink: Is chronic pain a disease? *Journal of Pain, 10*(11), 1113–1120. doi:10.1016/j.jpain.2009.09.001.
42. McGreevy, K., Bottros, M. M., & Raja, S. N. (2011). Preventing chronic pain following acute pain: Risk factors, preventive strategies, and their efficacy. *European Journal of Pain Supplement, 5*(2), 365–372. doi:10.1016/j.eujps.2011.08.013.
43. Garland, E. L. (2012). Pain processing in the human nervous system: A selective review of nociceptive and biobehavioral pathways. *Primary Care, 39*(3), 561–571. doi:10.1016/j.pop.2012.06.013.
44. Miles, A., Curran, H. V., Pearce, S., et al. (2005). Managing constraint: The experience of people with chronic pain. *Social Science and Medicine, 61*(2), 431–441. doi:10.1016/j.socscimed.2004.11.065.
45. Nickel, F. T., Seifert, F., Lanz, S., et al. (2012). Mechanisms of neuropathic pain. *European Neuropsychopharmacology, 22*(2), 81–91. doi:10.1016/j.euroneuro.2011.05.005.
46. Jensen, T. S., & Finnerup, N. B. (2014). Allodynia and hyperalgesia in neuropathic pain: Clinical manifestations and mechanisms. *Lancet Neurology, 13*(9), 924–935. doi:10.1016/S1474-4422(14)70102-4.
47. Smith, H. S., & Meek, P. D. (2011). Pain responsiveness to opioids: Central versus peripheral neuropathic pain. *Journal of Opioid Management, 7*(5), 391–400.
48. Woolf, C. J. (2011). Central sensitization: Implications for the diagnosis and treatment of pain. *Pain, 152*(3 Suppl.), S2–S15. doi:10.1016/j.pain.2010.09.030.
49. Cohen, S. P., & Mao, J. (2014). Neuropathic pain: Mechanisms and their clinical implications. *British Medical Journal, 348*, f7656. doi:10.1136/bmj.f7656.
50. Gold, M. S., & Miroslay, M. B. (2015). Pain: from neurobiology to disease. In M. J. Zigmond, L. P. Rowland, & J. T. Coyle (Eds.), *Neurobiology of brain disorders: Biological basis of neurological and psychiatric disorders* (pp. 674–692). London: Academic Press.
51. Vranken, J. H. (2012). Elucidation of pathophysiology and treatment of neuropathic pain. *Central Nervous System Agents in Medicinal Chemistry, 12*(4), 304–314.
52. Clapham, J. C. (2012). Central control of thermogenesis. *Neuropharmacology, 63*(1), 111–123. doi:10.1016/j.neuropharm.2011.10.014.
53. Rothwell, N. J. (1994). CNS regulation of thermogenesis. *Critical Reviews in Neurobiology, 8*(1–2), 1–10.
54. Baumgart, S. (2008). Iatrogenic hyperthermia and hypothermia in the neonate. *Clinics in Perinatology, 35*(1), 183–197, ix–x. doi:10.1016/j.clp.2007.11.002.
55. Falk, B., & Dotan, R. (2011). Temperature regulation and elite young athletes. *Medicine and Sport Science, 56*, 126–149. doi:10.1159/000320645.
56. Gao, Z., Wilson, T. E., Drew, R. C., et al. (2012). Altered coronary vascular control during cold stress in healthy older adults. *American Journal of Physiology, Heart and Circulatory Physiology, 302*(1), H312–H318. doi:10.1152/ajpheart.00297.2011.
57. Saely, C. H., Geiger, K., & Drexel, H. (2012). Brown versus white adipose tissue. A mini-review. *Gerontology, 58*(1), 15–23. doi:10.1159/000321319.
58. Kaya, A., Ergul, N., Kaya, S. Y., et al. (2013). The management and the diagnosis of fever of unknown origin. *Expert Review of Anti-infective Therapy, 11*(8), 805–815. doi:10.1586/14787210.2013.814436.
59. Barone, J. E. (2009). Fever: Fact and fiction. *The Journal of Trauma, 67*(2), 406–409. doi:10.1097/TA.0b013e3181a5f335.
60. Cannon, J. G. (2013). Perspective on fever: The basic science and conventional medicine. *Complementary Therapies in Medicine, 21*(Suppl. 1), S54–S60. doi:10.1016/j.ctim.2011.08.002.
61. Purssell, E., & While, A. E. (2013). Does the use of antipyretics in children who have acute infections prolong febrile illness? A systematic review and meta-analysis. *Journal of Pediatrics, 163*(3), 822–827. doi:10.1016/j.jpeds.2013.03.069.
62. Wing, R., Dor, M. R., & McQuilkin, P. A. (2013). Fever in the pediatric patient. *Emergency Medicine Clinics of North America, 31*(4), 1073–1096. doi:10.1016/j.emc.2013.07.006.
63. Roghmann, M. C., Warner, J., & Mackowiak, P. A. (2001). The relationship between age and fever magnitude. *American Journal of the Medical Sciences, 322*(2), 68–70.
64. Wang, H., Wang, B., Normoyle, K. P., et al. (2014). Brain temperature and its fundamental properties: A review for clinical neuroscientists. *Frontiers in Neuroscience, 8*, 307. doi:10.3389/fnins.2014.00307.
65. Ahmed, K., & Zaidi, S. F. (2013). Treating cancer with heat: Hyperthermia as promising strategy to enhance apoptosis. *Journal of the Pakistan Medical Association, 63*(4), 504–508.
66. Gomez, C. R. (2014). Disorders of body temperature. *Handbook of Clinical Neurology, 120*, 947–957. doi:10.1016/B978-0-7020-4087-0.00062-0.
67. Atha, W. F. (2013). Heat-related illness. *Emergency Medicine Clinics of North America, 31*(4), 1097–1108. doi:10.1016/j.emc.2013.07.012.
68. Bandschapp, O., & Girard, T. (2012). Malignant hyperthermia. *Swiss Medical Weekly, 142*, w13652. doi:10.4414/smw.2012.13652.
69. Hocker, S. E., Tian, L., Li, G., et al. (2013). Indicators of central fever in the neurologic intensive care unit. *JAMA Neurology, 70*(12), 1499–1504. doi:10.1001/jamaneurol.2013.4354.
70. Albrecht, U. (2012). Timing to perfection: The biology of central and peripheral circadian clocks. *Neuron, 74*(2), 246–260. doi:10.1016/j.neuron.2012.04.006.
71. Iber, C., Ancoli-Israel, S., Chesson, A., et al. (2007). *The AASM manual for the scoring of sleep and associated events*. Westchester IL: American Academy of Sleep Medicine.
72. España, R. A., & Scammell, T. E. (2011). Sleep neurobiology from a clinical perspective. *Sleep, 34*(7), 845–858. doi:10.5665/SLEEP.1112.
73. American Academy of Sleep Medicine (2014). *International classification of sleep disorders: Diagnostic and coding manual* (3rd ed.). Westchester, IL: Author.
74. Ellis, J. G., Gehrman, P., Espie, C. A., et al. (2012). Acute insomnia: Current conceptualizations and future directions. *Sleep Medicine Reviews, 16*(1), 5–14. doi:10.1016/j.smrv.2011.02.002.
75. Buysse, D. J. (2013). Insomnia. *JAMA: The Journal of the American Medical Association, 309*(7), 706–716. doi:10.1001/jama.2013.193.
76. Public Health Agency of Canada. (2009). *What is the impact of sleep apnea on Canadians?* Retrieved from http://www.phac-aspc.gc.ca/cd-mc/sleepapnea-apneesommeil/ff-rr-2009-eng.php.
77. Berry, R. B. (2012). *Fundamentals of sleep medicine*. Philadelphia: Elsevier.
78. Ayas, N. T., Hirsch, A. A., Laher, I., et al. (2014). New frontiers in obstructive sleep apnoea. *Clinical Science, 127*(4), 209–216. doi:10.1042/CS20140070.
79. De Backer, W. (2013). Obstructive sleep apnea/hypopnea syndrome. *Panminerva Medica, 55*(2), 191–195.
80. Gagnon, K., Baril, A. A., Gagnon, J. F., et al. (2014). Cognitive impairment in obstructive sleep apnea. *Pathologie-Biologie, 62*(5), 233–240. doi:10.1016/j.patbio.2014.05.015.

81. Freedman, N. (2014). Improvements in current treatments and emerging therapies for adult obstructive sleep apnea. *F1000prime Reports*, *6*, 36. doi:10.12703/P6-36.
82. Carter, K. A., Hathaway, N. E., & Lettieri, C. F. (2014). Common sleep disorders in children. *American Family Physician*, *89*(5), 368–377.
83. Mannarino, M. R., Di Filippo, F., & Pirro, M. (2012). Obstructive sleep apnea syndrome. *European Journal of Internal Medicine*, *23*(7), 586–593. doi:10.1016/j.ejim.2012.05.013.
84. Mignot, E. J. (2012). A practical guide to the therapy of narcolepsy and hypersomnia syndromes. *Neurotherapeutics*, *9*(4), 739–752. doi:10.1007/s13311-012-0150-9.
85. Baron, K. G., & Reid, K. J. (2014). Circadian misalignment and health. *International Review of Psychiatry (Abingdon, England)*, *26*(2), 139–154. doi:10.3109/09540261.2014.911149.
86. Nesbitt, A. D., & Dijk, D. J. (2014). Out of synch with society: An update on delayed sleep phase disorder. *Current Opinion in Pulmonary Medicine*, *20*(6), 581–587. doi:10.1097/MCP.0000000000000095.
87. Morrissette, D. A. (2013). Twisting the night away: A review of the neurobiology, genetics, diagnosis, and treatment of shift work disorder. *CNS Spectrums*, *18*(Suppl. 1), 45–53. doi:10.1017/S109285291300076X.
88. Thorpy, M. (2011). Understanding and diagnosing shift work disorder. *Postgraduate Medicine*, *123*(5), 96–105. doi:10.3810/pgm.2011.09.2464.
89. Hida, A., Kitamura, S., & Mishima, K. (2012). Pathophysiology and pathogenesis of circadian rhythm sleep disorders. *Journal of Physiological Anthropology*, *31*, 7. doi:10.1186/1880-6805-31-7.
90. Jones, C. R., Huang, A. L., Ptáček, L. J., et al. (2013). Genetic basis of human circadian rhythm disorders. *Experimental Neurology*, *243*, 28–33. doi:10.1016/j.expneurol.2012.07.012.
91. Matwiyoff, G., & Lee-Chiong, T. (2010). Parasomnias: An overview. *Indian Journal of Medical Research*, *131*, 333–337.
92. Howell, M. J. (2012). Parasomnias: An updated review. *Neurotherapeutics*, *9*(4), 753–775. doi:10.1007/s13311-012-0143-8.
93. Zadra, A., & Pilon, M. (2011). NREM parasomnias. *Handbook of Clinical Neurology*, *99*, 851–868. doi:10.1016/B978-0-444-52007-4.00011-4.
94. Wijemanne, S., & Jankovic, J. (2015). Restless legs syndrome: Clinical presentation diagnosis and treatment. *Sleep Medicine*, *16*(6), 678–690. doi:10.1016/j.sleep.2015.03.002.
95. Allen, R. P. (2014). Restless legs syndrome/Willis-Ekbom disease: Evaluation and treatment. *International Review of Psychiatry (Abingdon, England)*, *26*(2), 248–262. doi:10.3109/09540261.2014.904279.
96. Voleti, V. B., & Hubschman, J. P. (2013). Age-related eye disease. *Maturitas*, *75*(1), 29–33. doi:10.1016/j.maturitas.2013.01.018.
97. Casson, R. J., Chidlow, G., Wood, J. P., et al. (2012). Definition of glaucoma: Clinical and experimental concepts. *Clinical & Experimental Ophthalmology*, *40*(4), 341–349. doi:10.1111/j.1442-9071.2012.02773.x.
98. Agarwal, R., Gupta, S. K., Agarwal, P., et al. (2009). Current concepts in the pathophysiology of glaucoma. *Indian Journal of Ophthalmology*, *57*(4), 257–266. doi:10.4103/0301-4738.53049.
99. Weinreb, R. N., Aung, T., & Medeiros, F. A. (2014). The pathophysiology and treatment of glaucoma: A review. *JAMA: The Journal of the American Medical Association*, *311*(18), 1901–1911. doi:10.1001/jama.2014.3192.
100. Khan, M., Agarwal, K., Loutfi, M., et al. (2014). Present and possible therapies for age-related macular degeneration. *ISRN Ophthalmology*, *2014*, 608390. doi:10.1155/2014/608390.
101. Hampton, B. M., Kovach, J. L., & Schwartz, S. G. (2015). Pharmacogenetics and nutritional supplementation in age-related macular degeneration. *Clinical Ophthalmology*, *9*, 873–876. doi:10.2147/OPTH.S84155.
102. Liu, H. H., Hu, Y., & Cui, H. P. (2015). Femtosecond laser in refractive and cataract surgeries. *International Journal of Ophthalmology*, *8*(2), 419–426. doi:10.3980/j.issn.2222-3959.2015.02.36.
103. Lichtinger, A., & Rootman, D. S. (2012). Intraocular lenses for presbyopia correction: Past, present, and future. *Current Opinion in Ophthalmology*, *23*(1), 40–46. doi:10.1097/ICU.0b013e32834cd5be.
104. Neitz, J., & Neitz, M. (2011). The genetics of normal and defective color vision. *Vision Research*, *51*(7), 633–651. doi:10.1016/j.visres.2010.12.002.
105. Azari, A. A., & Barney, N. P. (2013). Conjunctivitis: A systematic review of diagnosis and treatment. *JAMA: The Journal of the American Medical Association*, *310*(16), 1721–1729. doi:10.1001/jama.2013.280318.
106. Kozak, A. T., & Grundfast, K. M. (2009). Hearing loss. *Otolaryngologic Clinics of North America*, *42*(1), 79–85. doi:10.1016/j.otc.2008.09.008.
107. Sara, S. A., Teh, B. M., & Friedland, P. (2014). Bilateral sudden sensorineural hearing loss: Review. *Journal of Laryngology and Otology*, *128*(Suppl. 1), S8–S15. doi:10.1017/S002221511300306X.
108. Foster, C. A., & Breeze, R. E. (2013). The Ménière attack: An ischemia/reperfusion disorder of inner ear sensory tissues. *Medical Hypotheses*, *81*(6), 1108–1115. doi:10.1016/j.mehy.2013.10.015.
109. Wipperman, J. (2014). Otitis externa. *Primary Care*, *41*(1), 1–9. doi:10.1016/j.pop.2013.10.001.
110. Rye, M. S., Blackwell, J. M., & Jamieson, S. E. (2012). Genetic susceptibility to otitis media in childhood. *Laryngoscope*, *122*(3), 665–675. doi:10.1002/lary.22506.
111. Pichichero, M. E. (2013). Otitis media. *Pediatric Clinics of North America*, *60*(2), 391–407. doi:10.1016/j.pcl.2012.12.007.
112. Principi, N., Baggi, E., & Esposito, S. (2012). Prevention of acute otitis media using currently available vaccines. *Future Microbiology*, *7*(4), 457–465. doi:10.2217/fmb.12.23.
113. Roper, S. D. (2013). Taste buds as peripheral chemosensory processors. *Seminars in Cell and Developmental Biology*, *24*(1), 71–79. doi:10.1016/j.semcdb.2012.12.002.
114. Visvanathan, R., & Chapman, I. M. (2009). Undernutrition and anorexia in the older person. *Gastroenterology Clinics of North America*, *38*(3), 393–409. doi:10.1016/j.gtc.2009.06.009.
115. McGlone, F., & Reilly, D. (2010). The cutaneous sensory system. *Neuroscience and Biobehavioral Reviews*, *34*(2), 148–159. doi:10.1016/j.neubiorev.2009.08.004.
116. Norman, J. F., Kappers, A. M., Cheeseman, J. R., et al. (2013). Aging and curvature discrimination from static and dynamic touch. *PLoS ONE*, *8*(7), e68577. doi:10.1371/journal.pone.0068577.
117. Proske, U., & Gandevia, S. C. (2012). The proprioceptive senses: Their roles in signaling body shape, body position and movement, and muscle force. *Physiological Reviews*, *92*(4), 1651–1697. doi:10.1152/physrev.00048.2011.

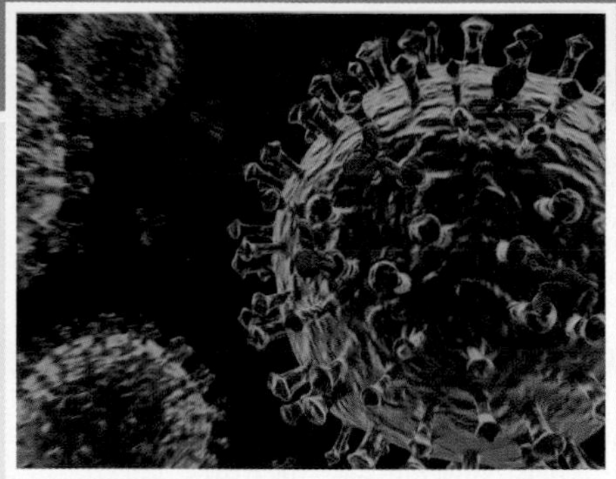

15

Alterations in Cognitive Systems, Cerebral Hemodynamics, and Motor Function

Barbara J. Boss, Sue E. Huether, and Kelly Power-Kean

EVOLVE WEBSITE

http://evolve.elsevier.com/Canada/Huether/pathophysiology

Student Review Questions

Key Points

Case Studies

Animations

Quick Check Answers

CHAPTER OUTLINE

Alterations in Cognitive Systems, 363
- Alterations in Arousal, 363
- Alterations in Awareness, 369
- Data-Processing Deficits, 371
- Seizure Disorders, 376
- Types of Seizure, 376

Alterations in Cerebral Hemodynamics, 377
- Increased Intracranial Pressure, 378
- Cerebral Edema, 379
- Hydrocephalus, 380

Alterations in Neuromotor Function, 380
- Alterations in Muscle Tone, 380
- Alterations in Muscle Movement, 381
- Upper and Lower Motor Neuron Syndromes, 385
- Motor Neuron Diseases, 387
- Amyotrophic Lateral Sclerosis, 388

Alterations in Complex Motor Performance, 389
- Disorders of Posture (Stance), 389
- Disorders of Gait, 389
- Disorders of Expression, 389

Extrapyramidal Motor Syndromes, 390

A person achieves cognitive and behavioural functional competence by integrated processes of cognitive systems, sensory systems, and motor systems. The purpose of this chapter is to present the concepts and processes of alterations in these systems as an approach to understanding the manifestations of neurological dysfunction and disease.

The neural systems that are essential to cognitive function are (1) attentional systems that provide arousal and maintenance of attention over time; (2) memory and language systems by which information is communicated; and (3) affective or emotive systems that mediate mood, emotion, and intention. These core systems are fundamental to the processes of abstract thinking and reasoning. The products of abstraction and reasoning are organized and made operational through the executive attentional networks. The normal functioning of these networks manifests through the motor network in a behavioural array viewed by others as appropriate to human activity and successful living.

ALTERATIONS IN COGNITIVE SYSTEMS

Full **consciousness** is a state of awareness both of oneself and of the environment, and a set of responses to that environment. The fully conscious individual initiates spontaneous, purposeful activity independently to a perceived stimulus. Any decrease in this state of awareness and varied responses is a decrease in consciousness.

Consciousness has two distinct components: arousal (state of awakeness) and awareness (content of thought). **Arousal** is mediated by the reticular activating system, which regulates aspects of attention and information processing and maintains consciousness. Awareness encompasses all cognitive functions and is mediated by attentional systems, memory systems, language systems, and executive systems.

Alterations in Arousal

Alterations in level of arousal may be caused by structural, metabolic, or psychogenic (functional) disorders.

PATHOPHYSIOLOGY **Structural alterations in arousal** are divided according to the original location of the pathological condition. Causes include infection, vascular alterations, neoplasms, traumatic injury, congenital alterations, degenerative changes, polygenic traits, and metabolic disorders.

Supratentorial disorders (above the tentorium cerebelli) produce changes in arousal by either diffuse or localized dysfunction. The **tentorium cerebelli** is an extension of the dura mater that separates the cerebellum from the inferior portion of the occipital lobes. Diffuse dysfunction may be caused by disease processes affecting the cerebral cortex or the underlying subcortical white matter (e.g., encephalitis). Disorders outside the brain but within the cranial vault (extracerebral) can produce diffuse dysfunction, including neoplasms, closed-head trauma with subsequent subdural bleeding, and accumulation of pus in the subdural space. Disorders within the brain substance (intracerebral)—bleeding, infarcts, emboli, and tumours—function primarily as masses. Such localized destructive processes directly impair function of the thalamic or hypothalamic activating systems or secondarily compress these structures in a process of herniation.

Infratentorial disorders (below the tentorium cerebelli) produce a decline in arousal by (1) direct destruction or compression of the reticular activating system and its pathways (e.g., accumulations of blood or pus, neoplasms, and demyelinating disorders) or (2) destruction of the brainstem (midbrain, pons, medulla) either by direct invasion or by indirect impairment of its blood supply.

Metabolic disorders produce a decline in arousal by alterations in delivery of energy substrates as occurs with hypoxia, electrolyte disturbances, or hypoglycemia. Metabolic disorders caused by liver or renal failure cause alterations in neuronal excitability because of failure to metabolize or eliminate medications and toxins. All the systemic diseases that eventually produce nervous system dysfunction are part of this metabolic category.

Psychogenic alterations in arousal (unresponsiveness), although uncommon, may signal general psychiatric disorders. Despite apparent unconsciousness, the person actually is physiologically awake and the neurological examination reflects normal responses.

CLINICAL MANIFESTATIONS AND EVALUATION Five patterns of neurological function are critical to the evaluation process: (1) level of consciousness, (2) pattern of breathing, (3) pupillary reaction, (4) oculomotor responses, and (5) motor responses. Patterns of clinical manifestations help in determining the extent of brain dysfunction and serve as indexes for identifying increasing or decreasing central nervous system (CNS) function. Distinctions are made between metabolically induced and structurally induced manifestations (Table 15-1). The types of manifestations suggest the cause of the altered arousal state (Table 15-2).

Level of consciousness is the most critical clinical index of nervous system function, with changes indicating either improvement or deterioration of the individual's condition. A person who is alert and oriented to self, others, place, and time is considered to be functioning at the highest level of consciousness, which implies full use of all the person's cognitive capacities. From this normal alert state, levels of consciousness diminish in stages from confusion and disorientation (which can occur simultaneously) to coma, each of which is clinically defined (Table 15-3).

Patterns of breathing help evaluate the level of brain dysfunction and coma (Figure 15-1). Rate, rhythm, and pattern should be evaluated. Breathing patterns can be categorized as hemispheric or brainstem patterns (Table 15-4).

With normal breathing, a neural centre in the forebrain (cerebrum) produces a rhythmic pattern. When consciousness decreases, lower brainstem centres regulate the breathing pattern by responding only to changes in partial pressure of carbon dioxide in arterial blood ($PaCO_2$) levels; this breathing pattern is called *posthyperventilation apnea*. *Cheyne-Stokes respiration* is an abnormal rhythm of ventilation with alternating periods of tachypnea and apnea (crescendo–decrescendo pattern). Increases in $PaCO_2$ levels lead to tachypnea. The $PaCO_2$ level then decreases to below normal and breathing stops (apnea) until the carbon dioxide reaccumulates and again stimulates tachypnea (see Figure 15-1). In cases of opiate or sedative medication overdose, the respiratory centre is depressed so the rate of breathing gradually decreases until respiratory failure occurs.

Pupillary changes indicate the presence and level of brainstem dysfunction because brainstem areas that control arousal are adjacent to areas that control the pupils (Figure 15-2). For example, severe ischemia and hypoxia usually produce dilated, fixed pupils. Hypothermia may cause fixed pupils.

Some drugs affect pupils and must be considered in evaluating individuals in comatose states. Large doses of atropine and scopolamine fully dilate and fix pupils. Doses of sedatives (e.g., benzodiazepines) in sufficient amounts to produce coma, and taken in combination with other CNS-depressant agents (e.g., alcohol or barbiturates), cause the pupils to become midposition or moderately dilated, unequal, and commonly fixed to light. Opiates cause pinpoint pupils. Severe barbiturate intoxication may produce fixed pupils.

Oculomotor responses (resting, spontaneous, and reflexive eye movements) change at various levels of brain dysfunction in comatose individuals. Persons with metabolically induced coma, except with barbiturate-hypnotic and phenytoin poisoning, generally retain ocular

TABLE 15-1 Clinical Manifestations of Metabolic and Structural Causes of Altered Arousal

Manifestations	Metabolically Induced	Structurally Induced
Blink to threat (cranial nerves II, VII)	Equal	Asymmetrical
Optic discs (cranial nerve II)	Flat, good pulsation	Papilledema
Extraocular movement (cranial nerves III, IV, VI)	Roving eye movements; normal oculocephalic reflex (Doll's eyes phenomenon) and oculovestibular reflex (caloric ice water test)	Gaze paresis, nerve palsy
Pupils (cranial nerves II, III)	Equal and reactive; may be dilated (e.g., atropine), pinpoint (e.g., opiates), or midposition and fixed (e.g., benzodiazepines combined with other central nervous system–depressant agents)	Asymmetrical or nonreactive; may be midposition (midbrain injury), pinpoint (pons injury), large (tectal injury)
Corneal reflex (cranial nerves V, VII)	Symmetrical response	Asymmetrical response
Grimace to pain (cranial nerve VII)	Symmetrical response	Asymmetrical response
Motor function movement	Symmetrical	Asymmetrical
Muscle tone	Symmetrical	Paratonic (rigid), spastic, flaccid, especially if asymmetrical
Posture	Symmetrical	Decorticate, especially if symmetrical; decerebrate, especially if asymmetrical (see Figure 15-6)
Deep tendon reflexes	Symmetrical	Asymmetrical
Babinski sign	Absent or symmetrical response	Present
Sensation	Symmetrical	Asymmetrical

TABLE 15-2 Differential Characteristics of States Causing Altered Arousal

Mechanism	Manifestations
Supratentorial mass lesions compressing or displacing diencephalon or brainstem	Initiating signs usually of focal cerebral dysfunction: vomiting, headache, hemiparesis, ocular signs, seizures, coma Signs of dysfunction progress rostral to caudal Neurological signs at any given time point to one anatomical area (e.g., diencephalon, mesencephalon, medulla) Motor signs often asymmetrical
Infratentorial mass of destruction causing coma	History of preceding brainstem dysfunction or sudden onset of coma Localizing brainstem signs precede or accompany onset of coma and always include oculovestibular abnormality Cranial nerve palsies usually manifest "bizarre" respiratory patterns that appear at onset
Metabolic coma Exogenous toxins (medications) Endogenous toxins (organ system failure)	Confusion and stupor commonly precede motor signs Motor signs usually are symmetrical Pupillary reactions usually are preserved Asterixis, myoclonus, tremor, and seizures are common Acid–base imbalance with hyperventilation or hypoventilation is common
Psychiatric unresponsiveness	Lids close actively; pupils reactive or dilated (cycloplegics) Oculocephalic reflexes are unpredictable; oculovestibular reflexes are physiological (nystagmus is present) Motor tone is inconsistent or normal Eupnea or hyperventilation is usual No pathological reflexes are present Electroencephalogram (EEG) is normal

TABLE 15-3 Levels of Altered Consciousness

State	Definition
Confusion	Loss of ability to think rapidly and clearly; impaired judgement and decision making
Disorientation	The person may exhibit restlessness, anxiety, and irritation; disorientation to time occurs first, followed by disorientation to place and familiar others (family members) and impaired memory; recognition of self is lost last
Lethargy	Limited spontaneous movement or speech; easy arousal with normal speech or touch; may or may not be oriented to time, place, or person
Obtundation	Mild to moderate reduction in arousal (awakeness) with limited response to environment; falls asleep unless stimulated verbally or tactilely; answers questions with minimal response
Stupor	Condition of deep sleep or unresponsiveness from which person may be aroused or caused to open eyes only by vigorous and repeated stimulation; response is often withdrawal or grabbing at stimulus
Light coma	Associated with purposeful movement on stimulation
Coma	Associated with nonpurposeful movement only on stimulation
Deep coma	Associated with unresponsiveness or no response to any stimulus

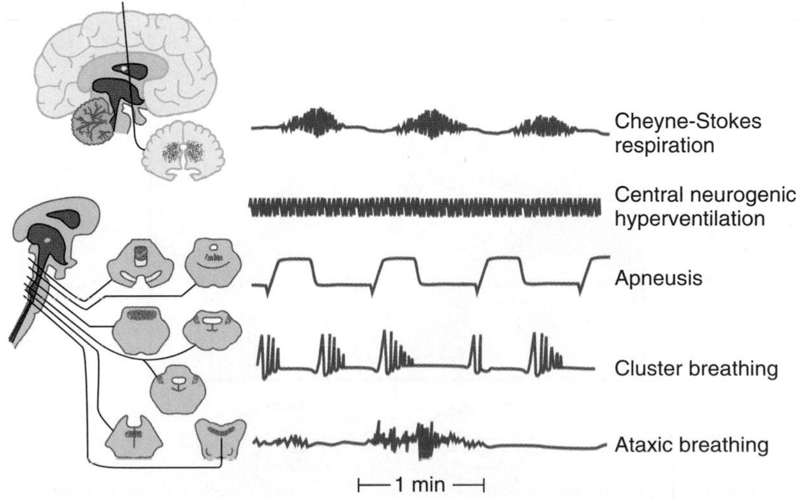

FIGURE 15-1 Abnormal Respiratory Patterns With Corresponding Level of Central Nervous System Activity. (From Urden, L.D., Stacy, K.M., & Lough, M.E. [2010]. *Critical care nursing: Diagnosis and management* [6th ed.]. St. Louis: Mosby.)

TABLE 15-4 Patterns of Breathing

Breathing Pattern	Description	Location of Injury
Hemispheric Breathing Patterns		
Normal	After a period of hyperventilation that lowers partial pressure of carbon dioxide in arterial blood ($PaCO_2$), the individual continues to breathe regularly but with reduced depth.	Response of nervous system to an external stressor—not associated with injury to central nervous system (CNS)
Posthyperventilation apnea	Respirations stop after hyperventilation has lowered partial pressure of carbon dioxide (PCO_2) level below normal. Rhythmic breathing returns when PCO_2 level returns to normal.	Associated with diffuse bilateral metabolic or structural disease of cerebrum
Cheyne-Stokes respirations	Breathing pattern has a smooth increase (crescendo) in rate and depth of breathing (hyperpnea), which peaks and is followed by a gradual smooth decrease (decrescendo) in rate and depth of breathing to the point of apnea, when the cycle repeats itself. The hyperpneic phase lasts longer than the apneic phase.	Bilateral dysfunction of deep cerebral or diencephalic structures; seen with supratentorial injury and metabolically induced coma states
Brainstem Breathing Patterns		
Central neurogenic hyperventilation	A sustained, deep, rapid, but regular pattern (hyperpnea) occurs, with a decreased $PaCO_2$ and a corresponding increase in pH and PO_2.	May result from CNS damage or disease that involves midbrain and upper pons; seen after increased intracranial pressure and blunt head trauma
Apneusis	A prolonged inspiratory cramp (a pause at full inspiration) occurs; a common variant of this is a brief end-inspiratory pause of 2 or 3 seconds, often alternating with an end-expiratory pause.	Indicates damage to respiratory control mechanism located at pontine level; most commonly associated with pontine infarction but documented with hypoglycemia, anoxia, and meningitis
Cluster breathing	A cluster of breaths has a disordered sequence with irregular pauses between breaths.	Dysfunction in lower pontine and high medullary areas
Ataxic breathing	Completely irregular breathing occurs, with random shallow and deep breaths and irregular pauses. The rate is often slow.	Originates from a primary dysfunction of medullary neurons controlling breathing
Gasping breathing pattern (agonal gasps)	A pattern of deep "all-or-none" breaths is accompanied by a slow respiratory rate.	Indicative of a failing medullary respiratory centre

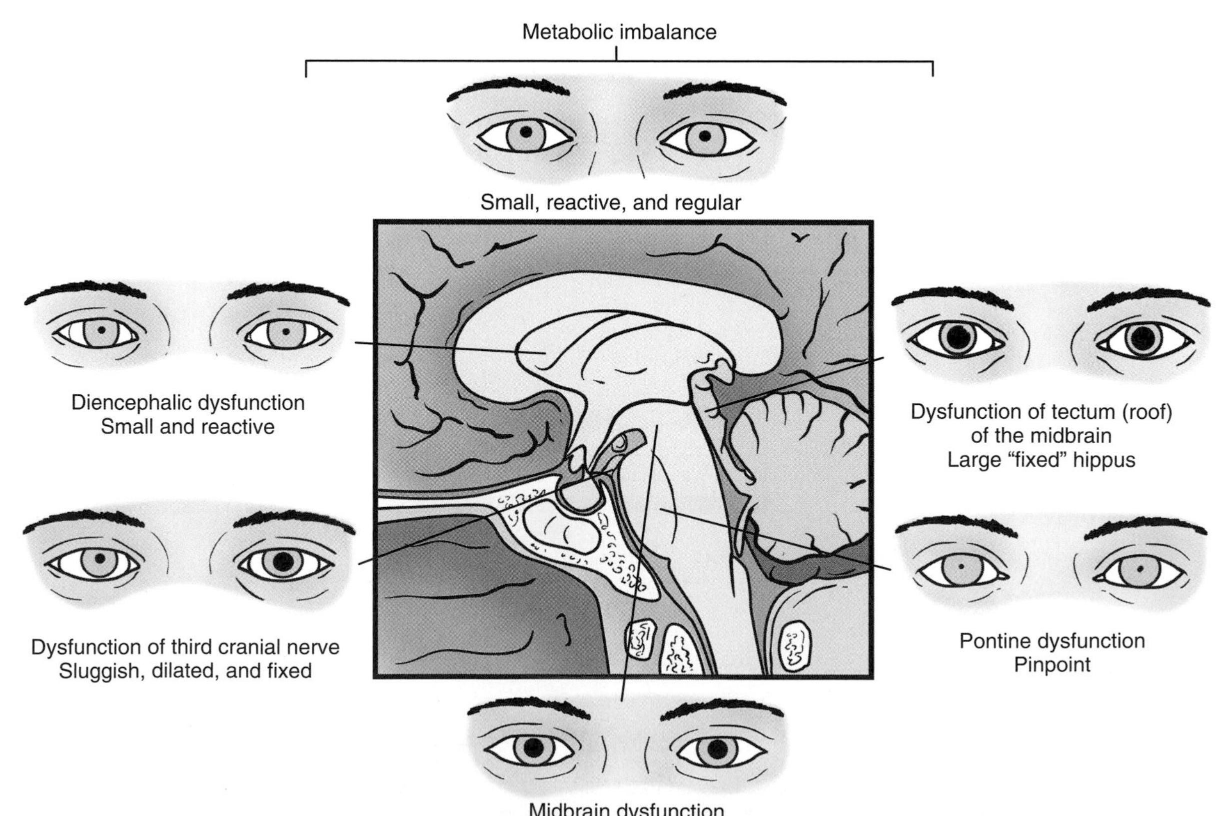

FIGURE 15-2 Appearance of Pupils at Different Levels of Consciousness.

reflexes even when other signs of brainstem damage are present. Destructive or compressive injury to the brainstem causes specific abnormalities of the oculocephalic and oculovestibular reflexes (Figures 15-3 and 15-4). Injuries that involve an oculomotor nucleus or nerve cause the involved eye to deviate outward, producing a resting dysconjugate lateral position of the eye.

FIGURE 15-3 Test for Oculocephalic Reflex Response (Doll's Eyes Phenomenon). **A,** Normal response—eyes turn together to side opposite from turn of head. **B,** Abnormal response—eyes do not turn in conjugate manner. **C,** Absent response—eyes move in direction of head movement (brainstem injury). (From Rudy, E.B. [1984]. *Advanced neurological and neurosurgical nursing*. St. Louis: Mosby.)

Assessment of **motor responses** helps to evaluate the level of brain dysfunction and determine the most severely damaged side of the brain. The pattern of response noted may be (1) purposeful; (2) inappropriate, generalized motor movement; or (3) not present. Motor signs indicating loss of cortical inhibition that are commonly associated with decreased consciousness include primitive reflexes and rigidity **(paratonia)** (Figure 15-5). Primitive reflexes include grasping, reflex sucking, snout reflex, and palmomental reflex, all of which are normal in the newborn but disappear in infancy. Abnormal flexor and extensor responses in the upper and lower extremities are defined in Table 15-5 and illustrated in Figure 15-6.

Vomiting, **yawning**, and **hiccups** are complex reflexlike motor responses that are integrated by neural mechanisms in the lower brainstem. These responses may be produced by compression or diseases involving tissues of the medulla oblongata (e.g., infection, neoplasm, infarction) but also occur relative to other more benign stimuli to the vagal nerve. Most CNS disorders produce nausea and vomiting. Vomiting without nausea indicates direct involvement of the central neural mechanism (or pyloric obstruction; see Chapters 36 and 37). Vomiting often accompanies CNS injuries that (1) involve the vestibular nuclei or its immediate projections, particularly when double vision (diplopia) also is present; (2) impinge directly on the floor of the fourth ventricle; or (3) produce brainstem compression secondary to an increase in intracranial pressure.

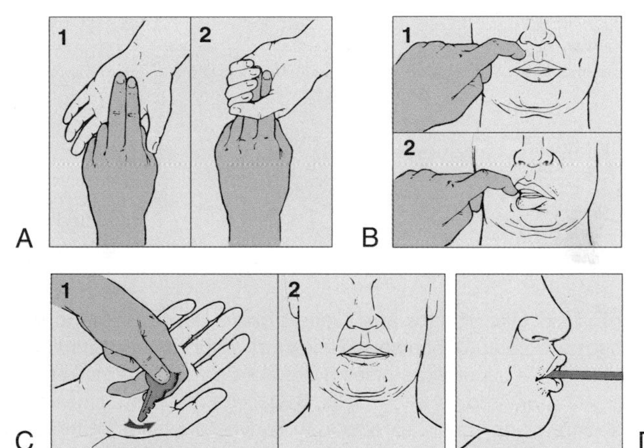

FIGURE 15-5 Pathological Reflexes. **A,** Grasp reflex. **B,** Snout reflex. **C,** Palmomental reflex. **D,** Suck reflex.

A 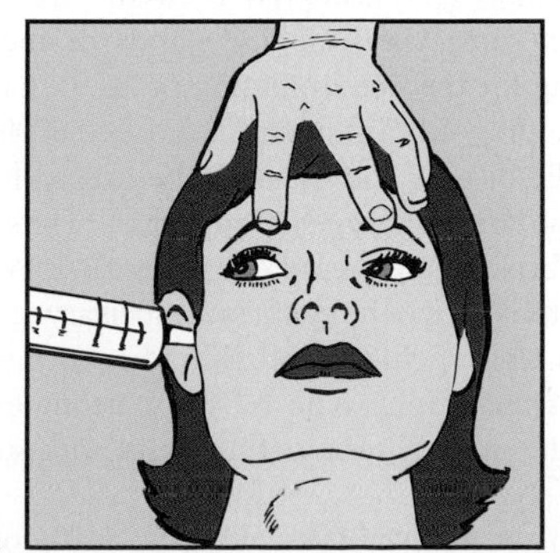 B 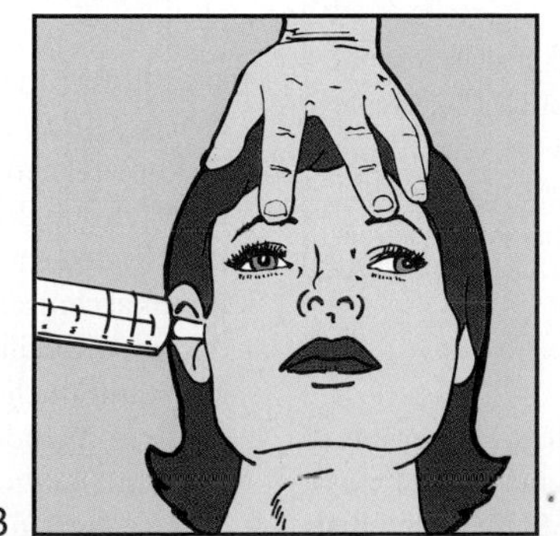 C 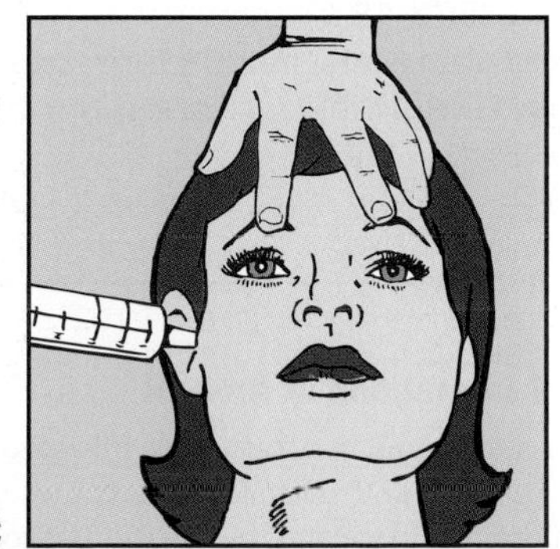

FIGURE 15-4 Test for Oculovestibular Reflex (Caloric Ice Water Test). **A,** Ice water is injected into the ear canal. Normal response—conjugate eye movements. **B,** Abnormal response—dysconjugate or asymmetrical eye movements. **C,** Absent response—no eye movements.

TABLE 15-5 Abnormal Motor Responses With Decreased Responsiveness

Motor Response	Description	Location of Injury
Decorticate posturing/rigidity: upper extremity flexion, lower extremity extension	Slowly developing flexion of arm, wrist, and fingers with adduction in the upper extremity and extension, internal rotation, and plantar flexion of lower extremity	Hemispheric damage above midbrain releasing medullary and pontine reticulospinal systems
Decerebrate posturing/rigidity: upper and lower extremity extensor responses	Opisthotonos (hyperextension of vertebral column) with clenching of teeth; extension, abduction, and hyperpronation of arms; and extension of lower extremities	Associated with severe damage involving midbrain or upper pons
	In acute brain injury, shivering and hyperpnea may accompany unelicited recurrent decerebrate spasms	Acute brain injury often causes limb extension regardless of location
Extensor responses in upper extremities accompanied by flexion in lower extremities		Pons
Flaccid state with little or no motor response to stimuli		Lower pons and upper medulla

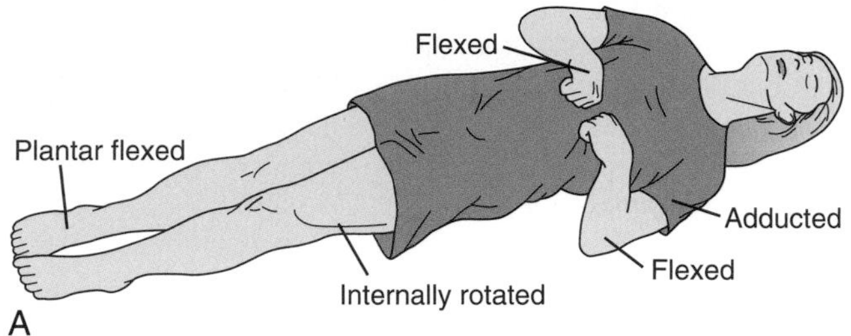

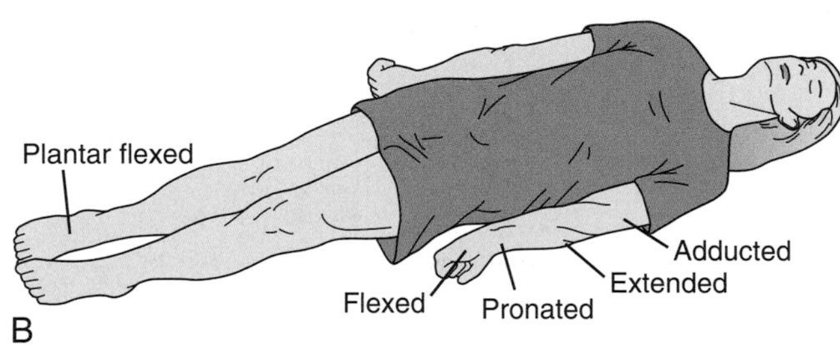

FIGURE 15-6 Decorticate and Decerebrate Posture/Responses. **A,** Decorticate posture/response. Flexion of arms, wrists, and fingers with adduction in upper extremities Bilateral extension, internal rotation, and plantar flexion in lower extremities. **B,** Decerebrate posture/response. All four extremities in rigid extension with hyperpronation of forearms and plantar extension of feet. (From deWit, S.C., & Kumagai, C.K. [2013]. *Medical-surgical nursing* [2nd ed.]. St. Louis: Saunders.)

✔ QUICK CHECK 15-1

1. Why are structural as well as metabolic factors capable of producing coma?
2. Why is level of consciousness the most critical index of central nervous system function?
3. Why does Cheyne-Stokes respiration appear in a comatose individual?
4. Why are oculomotor changes associated with levels of brain injury?

Outcomes of Alterations in Arousal

Outcomes of alterations in arousal fall into two categories: *extent of disability* (*morbidity*) and *mortality*. Outcomes depend on the cause and extent of brain damage and the duration of coma. Some individuals may recover consciousness and an original level of function, some may have permanent disability, and some may never regain consciousness and experience neurological death. Two forms of neurological death—brain death and cerebral death—result from severe pathological conditions and are associated with irreversible coma. Other possible outcomes are a vegetative state, a minimally conscious state, or locked-in syndrome. The extent of disability has four subcategories: recovery of consciousness, residual cognitive function, psychological function, and vocational function.

BOX 15-1 Canadian Minimal Criteria for Neurological Determination of Death

1. Established etiology capable of causing neurological death in the absence of reversible conditions capable of mimicking neurological death
2. Unresponsive coma with bilateral absence of motor responses, excluding spinal reflexes
3. No spontaneous respiration (apnea)
4. No brainstem functions, defined by absent gag and cough reflexes and the bilateral absence of corneal responses, pupillary responses to light, with pupils at mid-size or greater, and ocular responses to head turning or caloric stimulation (see Figures 15-3 and 15-4)
5. Absent confounding factors

From Shemie, S.D., Doig, C., Dickens, B., et al. (2006). *CMAJ, 174*(6), S1–S12. doi:10.1503/cmaj.045142. Copied under licence from Access Copyright. Further reproduction, distribution or transmission is prohibited except as otherwise permitted by law.

Brain death (total brain death) occurs when the brain is damaged so completely that it can never recover (irreversible) and cannot maintain the body's internal homeostasis. Canadian guidelines define *brain death*, or *neurological determination of death* (NDD), as the irreversible cessation of all brainstem functions. Clear medical standards, including criteria and minimal testing for the determination of NDD, have been established. The abnormality of brain function must result from structural or known metabolic disease and must *not* be caused by a depressant medication, alcohol poisoning, or hypothermia.[1] The clinical criteria used to determine brain death are noted in Box 15-1. When any of the minimal clinical criteria cannot be confirmed, ancillary tests are required. Accepted ancillary tests include cerebral radiocontrast angiography and radionuclide angiography. The NDD in neonates, infants, and children includes the same criteria as for adults, with some additional recommendations.[2]

Cerebral death, or **irreversible coma**, is death of the cerebral hemispheres exclusive of the brainstem and cerebellum. Brain damage is permanent, and the individual is forever unable to respond behaviourally in any significant way to the environment. The brainstem may continue to maintain internal homeostasis (i.e., body temperature, cardiovascular functions, respirations, and metabolic functions). The survivor of cerebral death may remain in a coma or emerge into a persistent vegetative state or a minimally conscious state. In coma, the eyes are usually closed with no eye opening. The person does not follow commands, speak, or have voluntary movement.[3]

A **persistent vegetative state (VS)** is complete unawareness of the self or surrounding environment and complete loss of cognitive function. The individual does not speak any comprehensible words or follow commands. Sleep–wake cycles are present, eyes open spontaneously, and blood pressure and breathing are maintained without support. Brainstem reflexes (pupillary, oculocephalic, chewing, swallowing) are intact but cerebral function is lost. There is bowel and bladder incontinence. Recovery is unlikely if the state persists for 12 months. In a **minimally conscious state (MCS)** individuals may follow simple commands, manipulate objects, gesture or give yes/no responses, have intelligible speech, and have movements such as blinking or smiling.[4]

With **locked-in syndrome** there is complete paralysis of voluntary muscles with the exception of eye movement. Content of thought and level of arousal are intact, but the efferent pathways are disrupted (injury at the base of the pons with the reticular formation intact, often caused by basilar artery occlusion).[5] Thus, the individual cannot communicate through speech or body movement but is fully conscious, with intact cognitive function. Vertical eye movement and blinking are a means of communication.

Alterations in Awareness

Awareness (content of thought) encompasses all cognitive functions, including awareness of self, environment, and affective states (i.e., moods). Awareness is mediated by all of the core networks under the guidance of executive attention networks including selective attention and memory. Executive attention networks involve abstract reasoning, planning, decision making, judgement, error correction, and self-control. Each attentional function is a network of interconnected brain areas and not localized to a single brain area.

Selective attention (orienting) refers to the ability to select specific information to be processed from available, competing environmental and internal stimuli, and to focus on that stimulus (i.e., to concentrate on a specific task without being distracted).[6] *Selective visual attention* is the ability to select objects from multiple visual stimuli and process them to complete a task. *Selective auditory* or *hearing attention* is the ability to select or filter specific sounds and process them to complete a task. Multiple areas of the brain are involved in selective attention including cortical areas, thalamic nuclei, and the limbic system. **Selective attention deficits** can be temporary, permanent, or progressive. Disorders associated with selective attention deficits include seizure activity, parietal lobe contusions, subdural hematomas, stroke, gliomas or metastatic tumour, late Alzheimer's dementia, frontotemporal dementia, and psychotic disorders.

Memory is the recording, retention, and retrieval of information. **Amnesia** is the loss of memory and can be mild or severe. Two types of amnesia are retrograde amnesia and anterograde amnesia. The person experiencing **retrograde amnesia** has difficulty retrieving past personal history memories or past factual memories. **Anterograde amnesia** is the inability to form new personal or factual memories but memories of the distant past are retained and retrieved. **Image processing** is a higher level of memory function and includes the ability to use sensory data and language to form concepts, assign meaning, and make abstractions. Alterations in image processing include an inability to form concepts and generalizations or to reason. Thinking is very concrete. These **memory disorders** may be temporary (e.g., after a seizure) or permanent (e.g., after severe head injury or in Alzheimer's disease).

BOX 15-2 Attention-Deficit/Hyperactivity Disorder

Initially attention-deficit/hyperactivity disorder (ADHD) was viewed as a neurodevelopmental disorder of childhood. It is now recognized that 50 to 75% of persons diagnosed in childhood have continuing symptoms into adulthood. Often the diagnosis is first made in adolescence or young adulthood when behavioural control and self-organization are expected of the person. The ability to function at work, at home, and in social situations is often impaired because of inattentiveness, hyperactivity, impulsivity, and problems with executive function. Continued treatment including medications for symptomatic adults is supported; substance abuse, which is more common in persons with ADHD, is reduced with continued treatment. The multifactorial patterns of inheritance and gene–environment interactions are under investigation, as are the pathogenesis and pathophysiology of this complex disorder. Findings from structural and functional neuroimaging suggest the involvement of developmentally abnormal brain networks related to cognition, attention, emotion, and sensorimotor functions. It is hoped that new findings will lead to improved prevention, diagnosis, treatment options, and functional outcomes.

Data from Baroni, A., & Castellanos, F.X. (2015). *Curr Opin Neurobiol, 30*, 1–8; Harstad, E., & Levy, S. (2014). *Pediatrics, 134*(1), e293–e301; Matthews, M., Nigg, J.T., & Fair, D.A. (2014). *Curr Top Behav Neurosci, 16*, 235–266; Sharma, A., & Couture, J. (2014). *Ann Pharmacother, 48*(2), 209–225.

There may be only the memory disorder, or the memory disorder may be associated with other cognitive disorders.

Executive attention deficits include the inability to maintain sustained attention and a working memory deficit. Sustained attention deficit is an inability to set goals and recognize when an object meets a goal. A working memory deficit is an inability to remember instructions and information needed to guide behaviour. Executive attention deficits may be temporary, progressive, or permanent. Attention-deficit/hyperactivity disorder (ADHD) is a common disorder of childhood that can continue through adulthood (Box 15-2). Table 15-6 summarizes alterations in attention and memory.

PATHOPHYSIOLOGY Very generally, the primary pathophysiological mechanisms that operate in disorders of awareness are (1) direct destruction caused by ischemia and hypoxia or indirect destruction resulting from compression and (2) the effects of toxins and chemicals or metabolic disorders. Disorders of selective attention, at least as they relate to visual orienting behaviour, are produced by disease that involves portions of the midbrain. Disease affecting the superior colliculi manifests as a slowness in orienting attention. Parietal lobe disease may produce *unilateral neglect syndrome* or lack of awareness of one side of the body or lack of response to stimuli on one side of the body and can occur after a stroke. An individual may groom or dress on only one side or eat food from only one side of the plate. **Sensory inattentiveness** is a form of neglect. The person is able to recognize individual sensory input from the dysfunctional side when asked, but ignores the sensory input from the dysfunctional side when stimulated from both sides **(extinction)**. The entire complex of denial of dysfunction, loss of recognition of one's own body parts, and extinction sometimes is referred to as hemineglect or **neglect syndrome**. A disorder in vigilance may be produced by disease in the prefrontal areas. Dysfunction in the right anterior cingulate gyrus and basal ganglia may cause detection problems, whereas problems with working memory may be produced with left lateral frontal injury. Anterograde amnesia originates from pathological conditions in the hippocampus and related temporal lobe structures; the diencephalic region including the thalamus; and the basal forebrain.

TABLE 15-6 Clinical Manifestations of Alterations in Attention and Memory

Deficit	Clinical Signs	Symptoms
Attention		
Selective attention (orienting)	Inability to focus attention; decreased eye, head, and body movements associated with focusing on stimuli; decreased search and scanning; faulty orientation to stimuli, causing safety problems	Person reports inability to focus attention, failure to perceive objects and other stimuli (history of injuries, falls, safety problems); can exhibit neglect syndrome (i.e., unilateral neglect with failure to groom or recognize one side of the body)
Memory		
Antegrade amnesia (inability to form new memories)	*Left hemisphere:* disorientation to time, situation, place, name, person (verbal identification); impaired language memory (e.g., names of objects); impaired semantic memory	Person reports disorientation, confusion, "not listening," "not remembering"; reports by others of person being disoriented, not able to remember, not able to learn new information
	Right hemisphere: disorientation to self, person (visual), place (visual); impaired episodic memory (personal history); impaired emotional memory	
	Either or both hemispheres: confusion; behavioural change	
Retrograde amnesia (loss of past memories)	*Left hemisphere:* inability to retrieve personal history, past medical history; unaware of recent current events	Person reports remote memory problems; others report that person cannot recall formerly known information
	Right hemisphere: inability to recognize persons, places, objects, music, and so on from past	
Image processing	Inability to categorize (identify similarities and differences) or sort; inability to form concepts; inability to analyze relationships; misinterpretations; inability to interpret proverbs	Reports by others of frequent misinterpretation of data, failure to conceptualize or generalize information
	Inability to perform deductive reasoning (convergent reasoning); inability to perform inductive reasoning (divergent reasoning); inability to abstract; concrete reasoning demonstrated; delusions	Reports by others of predominantly concrete thinking; lack of understanding of everyday situations, health care regimens, and such; delusional thinking
Executive Attention Deficits		
Vigilance	Failure to stay alert and orient to stimuli	Person reports decreased alertness or ability to orient
Detection	Lack of initiative (anergy); lack of ambition; lack of motivation; flat affect; no awareness of feelings; appears depressed, apathetic, and emotionless; fails to appreciate deficit; disinterested in appearance; lacks concern about childish or crude behaviour	Reports by others of laziness or apathy, flat affect, or lack of emotional expression; failure to exhibit or be aware of feelings
Mild	Responds to immediate environment but no new ideas; grooming and social graces are lacking	Reports by others of lack of ambition, motivation, or initiative; failure to carry out adult tasks; lack of social graces and new ideas
Severe	Motionless; lack of response to even internal cues; does not respond to physical needs; does not interact with surroundings	Reports by others of failure to groom or toilet self, unawareness of surroundings and own physical needs
	Inability to use feedback regarding behaviour; failure to recognize omissions and errors in self-care, speech, writing, and arithmetic; impaired cue utilization; overestimation of performance	Reports by others of not changing behaviour when requested; unawareness of limitations; does not recognize and correct errors in dressing, grooming, toileting, eating, and such; fails to recognize speech and arithmetic errors; careless speech
	Failure to shift response set; failure to change behaviour when conditions change; cue utilization may be impaired	Reports by others of failure to use feedback; inability to incorporate feedback (does not correct when feedback is given)
Working memory (recent or short-term memory)	Inability to set goals or form goals; indecisiveness	Reports by others of failure to set goals, indecisiveness
	Failure to make plans; inability to produce a complete line of reasoning; inability to make up a story; appears impulsive	Reports by others of failure to plan, impulsiveness, "does not think things through"
	Failure to initiate behaviour; failure to maintain behaviour; failure to discontinue behaviour; slowness to alternate response for the next step; motor perseveration	Reports by others of not knowing where to begin, inability to carry out sequential acts (maintain a behaviour), inability to cease a behaviour

Retrograde amnesia and higher-level memory deficits originate from pathological conditions in the widely distributed association areas of the cerebral cortex (Figure 13-7, *C*). Executive attention deficits are associated with alterations in the frontal and prefrontal cortex including the anterior cingulate gyrus, supplementary motor area, and portions of the basal ganglia.

CLINICAL MANIFESTATIONS Clinical manifestations of selective attention deficits, memory deficits, and executive attention function deficits are presented in Table 15-6.

EVALUATION AND TREATMENT Immediate medical management is directed at diagnosing the cause and treating reversible factors. Rehabilitative measures generally focus on compensatory or restorative activities and recently have been greatly facilitated by computer technology and other electronic devices.

QUICK CHECK 15-2

1. Why is irreversible coma different from brain death?
2. What is the difference between anterograde and retrograde amnesia?
3. What is an example of neglect syndrome?

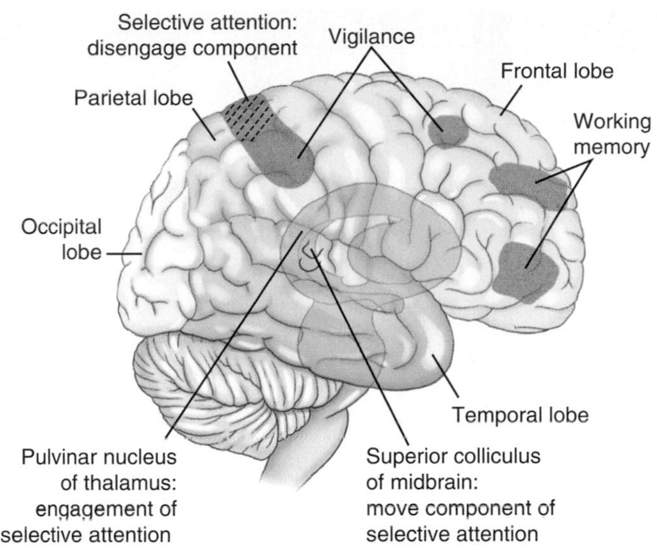

FIGURE 15-7 Right Cortical, Subcortical, and Brainstem Areas of the Brain Mediating Cognitive Function. (From Boss, G.J., & Wilkerson, R. [2008]. Communication: Language and pragmatics. In S.P. Hoeman [Ed.], *Rehabilitation nursing: Prevention, intervention & outcomes* [4th ed., p. 508]. St. Louis: Mosby.)

Data-Processing Deficits

Data-processing deficits are problems associated with recognizing and processing sensory information and include agnosia, dysphasia, and acute confusional states and delirium.

Agnosia

Agnosia is a defect of pattern recognition—a failure to recognize the form and nature of objects. Agnosia can be tactile, visual, or auditory, but generally only one sense is affected. For example, an individual may be unable to identify a safety pin by touching it with a hand but is able to name it when looking at it. Agnosia may be as minimal as a finger agnosia (failure to identify by name the fingers of one's hand) or more extensive, such as a colour agnosia. Although agnosia is associated most commonly with cerebrovascular accidents, it may arise from any pathological process that injures specific areas of the brain.

Dysphasia

Dysphasia is impairment of comprehension or production of language with impaired communication. Comprehension or use of symbols, in either written or verbal language, is disturbed or lost. **Aphasia** is a more severe form of dysphasia and an inability to communicate using language. Often the terms *dysphasia* and *aphasia* are used interchangeably. The term *dysphasia* is used here. Dysphasia results from dysfunction in the left cerebral hemisphere (i.e., Broca area [inferior frontal gyrus] and Wernicke area [superior temporal gyrus]) and the subcortical and cortical connecting networks (Figure 15-7 and see Figure 13-7). Dysphasias usually are associated with a cerebrovascular accident involving the middle cerebral artery or one of its many branches. Language disorders, however, may arise from a variety of injuries and diseases including vascular, neoplastic, traumatic, degenerative, metabolic, or infectious causes. Most language disorders result from acute processes or a chronic residual deficit of the acute process.

Dysphasias have been classified anatomically (i.e., Wernicke or Broca area dysphasias) or functionally as disorders of fluency (quality and content of speech). *Expressive dysphasia* (also known as Broca, motor, or nonfluent dysphasia) involves loss of ability to produce spoken or written language, with slow or difficult speech. Verbal comprehension is usually present. Expressive dysphasia is differentiated from *dysarthria,* in which words cannot be articulated clearly as a result of cranial nerve damage or muscle impairment. *Receptive dysphasia* (also known as Wernicke, sensory, or fluent dysphasia) involves an inability to understand written or spoken language. Speech is fluent, flowing at a normal rate, but words and phrases have no meaning. *Anomic aphasia* is a sensory aphasia distinguished by difficulty finding words and naming a person or object. Circumlocution, or describing an object as a way of trying to name something, is common in anomic aphasia. Auditory comprehension is present in *conductive dysphasia,* but there is impaired verbatim repetition. Naming also can be impaired. The person recognizes the errors and tries to correct them. Speech is fluent but words and sounds may be transposed. Damage is in the left hemisphere to networks that connect Broca and Wernicke areas. *Transcortical dysphasias* are rare and can be motor, sensory, or mixed. They involve areas of the brain that connect into the language centres. *Global dysphasia* is the most severe dysphasia and involves both expressive and receptive dysphasia. The individual is nonfluent or mute; cannot read or write; and has impaired comprehension, naming, reading, and writing. Global dysphasia is usually associated with a cerebrovascular accident involving the middle cerebral artery. Table 15-7 compares types of dysphasias, and Table 15-8 illustrates some of the language disturbances. Pure dysphasias are rare and are often mixed, making diagnosis difficult. All types of dysphasia usually improve with speech rehabilitation.

Acute Confusional States and Delirium

Acute confusional states (also may be known as *acute organic brain syndromes*) are transient disorders of awareness and may have either a sudden or a gradual onset. Delirium can be considered as a type of acute confusional state, but for this discussion acute confusional states and delirium are considered to be synonymous. There are many medical conditions associated with delirium, and they are summarized in Box 15-3.

PATHOPHYSIOLOGY Acute confusional states arise from disruption of a widely distributed neural network involving the reticular activating system of the upper brainstem and its projections into the thalamus, basal ganglion, and specific association areas of the cortex and

TABLE 15-7 Major Types of Dysphasia

Type	Expression	Verbal Comprehension	Repetition	Reading Comprehension	Writing	Location of Lesion	Cause of Lesion
Expressive							
Broca, nonfluent or motor aphasia	Cannot find words, difficulty writing	Relatively intact	Impaired	Variable	Impaired	Left posteroinferior frontal lobe (Broca area)	Occlusion of one or several branches of left middle cerebral artery supplying inferior frontal gyrus
Transcortical motor, nonfluent dysphasia	Halting speech	Intact	Intact	Impaired	Impaired	Anterior superior frontal lobe	Occlusion at the border zone between two arterial territories
Receptive							
Wernicke, receptive fluent or sensory dysphasia	Meaningless verbal language, inappropriate words or unable to monitor language for correctness so errors are not recognized Intonation, accent, cadence, rhythm, and articulation normal	Impaired; disturbance in understanding all language	Impaired	Impaired	Impaired	Left posterosuperior temporal lobe (Wernicke area)	Occlusion of inferior division of left middle cerebral artery
Conductive dysphasia	Difficulty repeating words, phrases spoken to them; naming is impaired	Intact	Severely impaired	Variable	Variable	Inferior and posterior temporal lobe; parietotemporal junction	Occlusion in distributions of left middle cerebral artery
Anomic dysphasia	Hesitancy, difficulty recalling names, objects, or numbers	Intact	Impaired	Variable	Intact except for anomia	Left temporoparietal zones; arcuate fasciculus	Diffuse left hemisphere brain disease
Transcortical sensory, fluent dysphasia	Repeats words and phrases spoken to them	Poor	Intact	Impaired	Impaired	Posterior temporal lobe	Occlusion at the border zone between two cerebral arterial territories
Other							
Transcortical mixed motor and sensory, nonfluent	Repeats words and phrases spoken to them	Impaired	Intact	Impaired	Impaired	Left cerebral hemisphere; spares the perisylvian cortex	Occlusion at the border zone between two cerebral arterial territories
Global or nonfluent; summation of motor and sensory aphasia	Mute	Impaired	Impaired	Impaired	Impaired	Large areas of the left cortex and subcortical regions	Occlusion of left middle cerebral artery of left internal carotid artery, tumours, other mass lesions, hemorrhage, embolic occlusion of ascending parietal or posterior temporal branch of middle cerebral artery

TABLE 15-8 Examples of Dysphasia

Disorder	Example
Receptive Dysphasia	
Wernicke/Fluent/Sensory Dysphasia	
Verbal paraphasia	*Question:* What did the car do?
	Patient: The car would spit sweetly down the road. (The car sped swiftly down the road.)
Conductive	*Request:* Say, "Persistence is essential to success."
	Patient: Mesastence is instans to success.
Neologism	*Question:* What do you call this? (Pointing to a plant.)
Anomic aphasia (circumlocution example)	*Patient:* It's a logper.
	Question: What do you call this? (Pointing to a plant.)
	Patient: Something that grows.
	Patient: It's ...
	Or
	Question: What did you do this morning?
	Patient: Reading.
	Question: Were you reading a book or newspaper?
	Patient: One of those.
Expressive Dysphasia	
Nonfluent/Broca/Motor Dysphasia	
Telegraphic style	*Question:* Where is your daughter?
	Patient: Calgary ... home ... Monday.

From Boss, B.J. (1984). *J Neurosurg Nurs, 16*(3), 151–160.

BOX 15-3 Conditions Causing Acute Confusional States or Delirium

Drug intoxication
Alcohol or drug withdrawal
Metabolic disorders (e.g., hypoglycemia, thyroid storm)
Brain trauma or surgery
Postanaesthesia
Febrile illnesses or heat stroke
Electrolyte imbalance, dehydration
Heart, kidney, or liver failure

limbic areas. **Delirium (hyperactive confusional state)** is associated with autonomic nervous system overactivity and typically develops over 2 to 3 days. It most commonly occurs in Critical Care Units, following surgery, or during withdrawal from CNS depressants (i.e., alcohol or narcotic agents). Delirium is associated with right-upper middle-temporal gyrus or left temporal-occipital junction disruption, and several neurotransmitters (i.e., acetylcholine and dopamine) are involved.[7] **Excited delirium syndrome (ExDS)**, also known as *agitated delirium*, is a type of hyperkinetic delirium that can lead to sudden death. Its symptoms include altered mental status, combativeness, aggressiveness, tolerance to significant pain, rapid breathing, sweating, severe agitation, elevated temperature, noncompliance or poor awareness in following direction from police or medical personnel, inability to become fatigued, unusual or superhuman strength, and inappropriate clothing for the current environment. **Hypoactive delirium (hypoactive confusional state)** is more likely to be associated with right-sided frontal-basal ganglion disruption.

Most metabolic disturbances (i.e., hypoglycemia, thyroid disorders, liver or kidney disease) that produce delirium interfere with neuronal metabolism or synaptic transmission. Many drugs and toxins also interfere with neurotransmission function at the synapse.

CLINICAL MANIFESTATIONS Delirium initially manifests as difficulty in concentrating, restlessness, irritability, insomnia, tremulousness, and poor appetite. Some persons experience seizures. Unpleasant, even terrifying, dreams or hallucinations may occur. In a fully developed delirium state, the individual is completely inattentive and perceptions are grossly altered, with extensive misperception and misinterpretation. The person appears distressed and often perplexed; conversation is incoherent. Frank tremor and high levels of restless movement are common. Violent behaviour may be present. The individual cannot sleep, is flushed, and has dilated pupils, a rapid pulse rate (tachycardia), elevated temperature, and profuse sweating (diaphoresis). Delirium typically abates suddenly or gradually in 2 to 3 days, although occasionally delirium states persist for weeks.

Hypoactive delirium is associated with underactivity and may occur in individuals who have fevers or metabolic disorders (i.e., chronic liver or kidney failure) or who are under the influence of CNS depressants. The individual exhibits decreases in mental function, specifically alertness, attention span, accurate perception, interpretation of the environment, and reaction to the environment. Forgetfulness and apathy are prominent, speech may be slow, and the individual dozes frequently.

EVALUATION AND TREATMENT The initial goals are to (1) establish that the individual is confused and (2) determine the cause of the confusion (organic or functional) (Table 15-9). The next step is to differentiate whether the confusion is delirium or an underlying dementia. Individuals with dementia are at increased risk of developing delirium. A complete history, physical examination, and laboratory tests (electrocardiogram and blood, urine, cerebrospinal fluid [CSF], and radiological studies) are needed. Several assessment scales are available to guide evaluation (such as Clinical Assessment of Confusion A and B, Confusion Assessment Method for the Intensive Care Unit [CAM-ICU], and Intensive Care Delirium Screening Checklist).[8-11] Once the cause is established, treatment is directed at controlling the primary disorder with supportive measures used as appropriate. Delirium is preventable in some individuals.[12] Table 15-10 contains a comparison of the features differentiating delirium and dementia.

QUICK CHECK 15-3

1. What are two types of dysphasia?
2. How does dysphasia differ from dysarthria?
3. What are some causes of delirium?

Dementia

Dementia is an acquired deterioration and a progressive failure of many cerebral functions that includes impairment of intellectual processes with a decrease in orienting, memory, language, judgement, and decision making. Because of declining intellectual ability, the individual may exhibit alterations in behaviour, for example, agitation, wandering, and aggression.

PATHOPHYSIOLOGY Mechanisms leading to dementia include neuron degeneration, compression of brain tissue, atherosclerosis of cerebral vessels, and brain trauma. Genetic predisposition is associated with the neuro-degenerative diseases, including Alzheimer's, Huntington's, and Parkinson's diseases. CNS infections, including the human

TABLE 15-9 Differences Between Organic and Functional Confusion

Factor	Organic Confusion	Functional Confusion
Memory impairment	Recent more impaired than remote	No consistent difference between recent and remote
Disorientation		
Time	Within own lifetime or reasonably near future	May not be related to person's lifetime
Place	Familiar place or one where person might easily be found	Bizarre or unfamiliar places
Person	Sense of identity usually preserved Misidentification of others as familiar	Sense of identity diminished Misidentification of others based on delusion system
Hallucinations	Visual, vivid Animals and insects common	Auditory more frequent Bizarre and symbolic
Illusions	Common	Not prominent
Delusions	Concern everyday occurrences and people	Bizarre and symbolic
Confused	Spotty confusion Clear intervals mixed with confused episodes Worse at night	More consistent No tendency to become worse at night

From Morris, M., & Rhodes, M. (1972). *Am J Nurs, 72*(9), 1632.

TABLE 15-10 Comparison of Delirium and Dementia

Feature	Delirium	Dementia
Age	Usually older	Usually older
Onset	Acute—common during hospitalization	Usually insidious; acute in some cases of strokes/trauma
Associated conditions	Urinary tract infection, thyroid disorders, hypoxia, hypoglycemia, toxicity, fluid-electrolyte imbalance, renal insufficiency, trauma, postsurgical anaesthesia	May have no other conditions Brain trauma
Course	Fluctuating/reversible with treatment	Chronic slow decline
Duration	Hours to weeks	Months to years
Attention	Impaired	Intact early; often impaired late
Sleep–wake cycle	Disrupted	Usually normal
Alertness	Impaired	Normal
Orientation	Impaired	Intact early; impaired late
Behaviour	Agitated, withdrawn or depressed	Intact early
Speech	Incoherent, rapid or slowed	Word-finding problems
Thoughts	Disorganized, delusions	Impoverished
Perceptions	Hallucinations/illusions	Usually intact early

Adapted from Caplan, J.P., & Rabinowitz, T. (2010). *Med Clin North Am, 94*(6), 1103–1116, ix.

immunodeficiency virus (HIV) and slow-growing viruses associated with Creutzfeldt-Jakob disease, also lead to nerve cell degeneration and brain atrophy.

CLINICAL MANIFESTATIONS Clinical manifestations of the major dementias are presented in Table 15-11.

EVALUATION AND TREATMENT Establishing the cause for dementia may be complicated, but individuals with clinical manifestations of dementia should be evaluated with laboratory and neuropsychological testing to identify underlying conditions that may be treatable. Unfortunately, no specific cure exists for most progressive dementias. Therapy is directed at maintaining and maximizing use of the remaining capacities, restoring functions if possible, and accommodating to lost abilities. Helping the family to understand the process and to learn ways to assist the individual is essential.

Alzheimer's Disease

Alzheimer's disease (AD) (dementia of Alzheimer's type [DAT], senile disease complex) is the leading cause of severe cognitive dysfunction in older adults. The three forms of AD are nonhereditary sporadic or late-onset AD (70 to 90%), early-onset familial AD (FAD), and early-onset AD (very rare). More than 747 000 Canadians have AD or another form of dementia, and the numbers are expected to increase to 1.4 million by 2031.[13]

PATHOPHYSIOLOGY The exact cause of AD is unknown. Early-onset FAD has been linked to three genes with mutations on chromosome 21 (abnormal amyloid precursor protein 14 [*APP14*], abnormal presenilin 1 [*PSEN1*], and abnormal presenilin 2 [*PSEN2*]). Late-onset AD may be related to the involvement of chromosome 19 with the apolipoprotein E gene-allele 4 (*APOE4*). Studies are ongoing to classify the genetic variations of AD.[14] DNA methylation is an epigenetic marker for AD.[15] Sporadic late-onset AD is the most common form and does not have a specific genetic association; however, the cellular pathology is the same as that for gene-associated early- and late-onset AD.[16] Pathological alterations in the brain include accumulation of extracellular **neuritic plaques** containing a core of amyloid beta protein, intraneuronal neurofibrillary tangles, and degeneration of basal forebrain cholinergic neurons with loss of acetylcholine. Failure to process and clear amyloid precursor protein results in the accumulation of toxic fragments of amyloid beta protein that leads to formation of diffuse neuritic plaques,

TABLE 15-11 **Clinical Manifestations of the Major Degenerative Dementias**

Disease	First Symptom	Mental Status	Neurobehaviour	Neurological Examination
Alzheimer's disease	Memory loss; impaired learning	Episodic memory loss	Initially normal, progressive cognitive impairment	Initially normal
Creutzfeldt-Jakob disease	Dementia, mood, anxiety, movement disorders	Variable, frontal/executive, focal cortical, memory	Depression, anxiety	Myoclonus, rigidity, parkinsonism
Dementia with Lewy body	Visual hallucinations; delusions that family members/friends are someone else; REM sleep disorder; delirium; parkinsonism	Drawing and frontal/ executive; spares memory; delirium prone	Visual hallucinations, depression, sleep disorder, delusions	Parkinsonism
Frontotemporal dementia	Apathy; poor judgement/reasoning, speech/language	Frontal/executive, language; spares drawing	Apathy, decline in person or social conduct, euphoria, depression	Due to PSP/CBD overlap; vertical gaze palsy, axial rigidity, dystonia, alien hand
Vascular dementia	Often but not always sudden, usually within 3 months of a stroke; variable: apathy, falls, focal weakness	Frontal/executive, cognitive slowing; memory can be intact	Apathy, delusions, anxiety	Usually motor slowing; can be normal

CBD, cortical basal degeneration; *PSP*, progressive supranuclear palsy; *REM*, rapid eye movement.
Adapted from Bird, T.D., & Miller, B.L. (2008). Dementia. In A.S. Fauci, E. Braunwald, D.L. Kasper, et al. (Eds.), *Harrison's principles of internal medicine* (17th ed., p. 2538). New York: McGraw-Hill.

disruption of nerve impulse transmission, and death of neurons. The tau protein, a microtubule-binding protein, in neurons detaches and forms an insoluble filament called a **neurofibrillary tangle**, contributing to neuronal death (Figure 15-8). Neuritic plaques and neurofibrillary tangles are more concentrated in the cerebral cortex and hippocampus. The loss of neurons results in brain atrophy with widening of sulci and shrinkage of gyri (see Figure 15-8). Loss of synapses, acetylcholine, and other neurotransmitters contributes to the decline of memory and attention and the loss of other cognitive functions associated with AD.[17]

CLINICAL MANIFESTATIONS AD has a long preclinical and prodromal course, and pathophysiological changes can occur decades before the appearance of the clinical dementia syndrome. The disease progresses from mild short-term memory deficits culminating in total loss of cognitive and executive functions. Initial clinical manifestations are insidious and often are attributed to forgetfulness, emotional upset, or other illness. The individual becomes progressively more forgetful over time, particularly in relation to recent events. Memory loss increases as the disorder advances, and the person becomes disoriented and confused and loses the ability to concentrate. Abstraction, problem solving, and judgement gradually deteriorate with failure in mathematical calculation ability, language, and visuospatial orientation. **Dyspraxia** may appear. The mental status changes induce behavioural changes, including irritability, agitation, and restlessness. Mood changes also result from the deterioration in cognition. The person may become anxious, depressed, hostile, emotionally labile, and prone to mood swings. Motor changes may occur if the posterior frontal lobes are involved, causing rigidity and flexion posturing. Weight loss can be significant. Great variability in age of onset, intensity and sequence of symptoms, and location and extent of brain abnormalities is common. Stages for the progression of AD are summarized in Table 15-12.

EVALUATION AND TREATMENT The diagnosis of AD is made by ruling out other causes. Clinical criteria have been developed to assist diagnosis.[18] The clinical history, including mental status examinations (Mini–Mental Status Examination, clock drawing, and Geriatric Depression Scale), laboratory tests, brain imaging of structure, blood flow and metabolism, and the course of the illness (which may span 5 years or more), is used to assess progression of the disease. Efforts are in progress to identify imaging and biochemical markers for risk assessment and early diagnosis

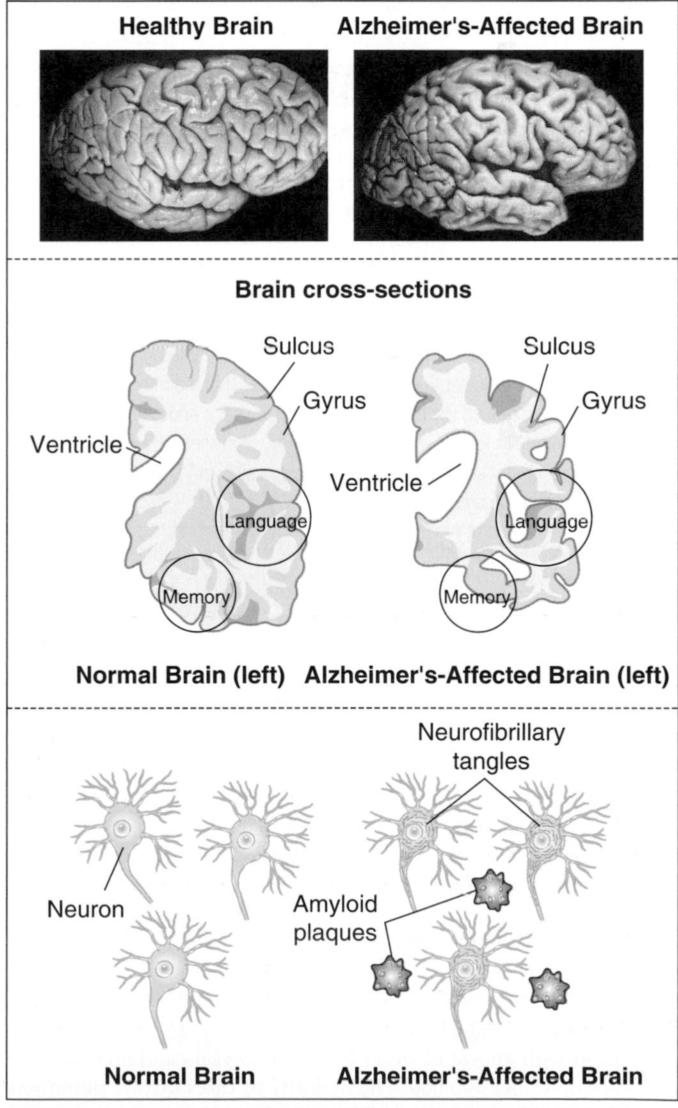

FIGURE 15-8 Common Pathological Findings in Alzheimer's Disease. The middle panel represents coronal slices through the left brain (facing anterior).

TABLE 15-12 Progression of Alzheimer's Disease

Stage	Mild Cognitive Impairment	Early Stage	Middle Stage	Late Stage	End Stage
Cognitive	Mild memory loss	Measurable short-term memory loss; difficulty with word finding; other cognition problems compared with previous behaviour	Moderate to severe cognitive problems: impaired reasoning, judgement, and problem solving; disorientation to time, place, and person; difficulty planning and organizing; progressive memory loss	Little cognitive ability; language not clear	No significant cognitive function; loss of orientation to self
Functional	Possibly depression (versus apathy); mild anxiety	Mild IADL problems	IADL-dependent; some ADL problems	ADL-dependent; incontinent	Nonambulatory/bedbound; unable to eat related to failure to sense hunger or thirst, difficulty swallowing

ADL, (basic) activities of daily living; *IADL*, instrumental activities of daily living.
Adapted from National Conference of Gerontological Nurse Practitioners and the National Gerontological Nursing Association. (2008). *Counseling Points, 1*(1), 6; Peña-Casanova, J., Sánchez-Benavides, G., de Sola-Llopis, S., et al. (2012). *Arch Med Res, 43*(8), 686–693.

and progression of Alzheimer's type and other neuro-degenerative causes of dementia.[19] See *Health Promotion:* Reducing Risk Factors Associated With Alzheimer's Disease.

HEALTH PROMOTION

Reducing Risk Factors Associated With Alzheimer's Disease

When considering risk factors and the likelihood of becoming affected by a certain disease, four main characteristics are considered: (1) the characteristics of the person, (2) lifestyle, (3) environment, and (4) genetic background. When considering Alzheimer's disease, risk factors do not cause the disease but rather increase the chance of being affected by the disease. Nonmodifiable risk factors include age and genetic makeup; however, some risk factors can be modified. The Alzheimer Society of Canada states that maintaining a healthy lifestyle can help reduce the risk for Alzheimer's disease and other dementias. Seven key modifiable risk factors have been identified: (1) diabetes, (2) hypertension, (3) obesity, (4) smoking, (5) depression, (6) cognitive inactivity or low education, (7) and physical inactivity.

Data from Alzheimer Society Canada. (2014). *Risk factors.* Retrieved from http://www.alzheimer.ca/en/About-dementia/Alzheimer-s-disease/Risk-factors.

Treatment is directed at using devices to compensate for the impaired cognitive function, such as memory aids; maintaining unimpaired cognitive functions; and maintaining or improving the general state of hygiene, nutrition, and health. Cholinesterase inhibitors have shown a modest effect on cognitive function in mild to moderate AD. An *N*-methyl-D-aspartate (NMDA) receptor antagonist blocks glutamate activity and may slow progression of disease in moderate to severe AD. Treatments, beginning in the preclinical stage, are being developed to prevent, modify, or halt disease pathology.[20]

Frontotemporal Dementia

Frontotemporal dementia (FTD), previously known as **Pick disease**, is the second most common form of dementia and is a degenerative disease of the frontal and anterior frontal lobes. There is a familial association with an age of onset less than 60 years and an estimated incidence of 15 per 100 000. The majority of cases involve mutations of genes encoding tau protein. Three distinct clinical syndromes are presented in frontotemporal degeneration, depending on the site of atrophy: (1) behavioural variant of FTD, (2) progressive nonfluent aphasia, and (3) semantic dementia. Differentiating pathological and clinical diagnostic criteria are in development.[21] There is no specific treatment.

Seizure Disorders

Seizure disorders represent a manifestation of disease and not a specific disease entity. A **seizure** is a sudden, transient disruption in brain electrical function caused by abnormal excessive discharges of cortical neurons. **Epilepsy** is the recurrence of seizures and a type of seizure disorder for which no underlying, correctable cause for the seizure can be found. The term **convulsion** is sometimes applied to seizures and refers to the tonic–clonic (jerky, contract–relax) movement associated with some seizures. Seizures in children are presented in Chapter 17.

Conditions Associated With Seizure Disorders

Any disorder that alters the neuronal environment may cause seizure activity. Conditions that may produce a seizure are metabolic disorders, congenital malformations, genetic predisposition, perinatal injury, postnatal trauma, myoclonic syndromes, infection, brain tumour, vascular disease, and medication or alcohol abuse. The onset of seizures also may indicate the presence of an ongoing primary neurological disease. Structural and metabolic causes of recurrent seizures in adults are summarized in Table 15-13. The cause of seizures is often unknown.

The threshold for seizures may be lowered by hypoglycemia, fatigue or lack of sleep, emotional or physical stress, fever, large amounts of water ingestion, constipation, use of antipsychotic medications (i.e., chlorpromazine [Largactil] and clozapine [Clozaril]) especially when combined with alcohol, withdrawal from depressant medications (including alcohol), or hyperventilation (respiratory alkalosis). Some environmental stimuli, such as blinking lights, a poorly adjusted television screen, loud noises, certain music, certain odours, or merely being startled, have been known to initiate a seizure. Women may have increased seizure activity immediately before or during menses.

Types of Seizure

Seizures are classified in different ways: by clinical manifestations, site of origin, electroencephalogram (EEG) correlates, or response to therapy. Types of seizures and clinical manifestations are presented in Chapter 17 (see Table 17-6). Terms used to describe seizure activity are defined in Table 15-14.

Epilepsy now is considered to be the result of the interaction of complex genetic mutations with environmental effects that cause

TABLE 15-13 Structural and Metabolic Causes of Recurrent Seizures in Adults

Age at Onset	Probable Cause
Young adults (18 to 35 years)	Alcohol or drug withdrawal (e.g., barbiturates, benzodiazepines) Brain tumour Idiopathic Illicit drug use (e.g., cocaine, amphetamine) Posttraumatic brain injury Perinatal insults
Older adults (>35 years)	Alcohol or drug withdrawal (e.g., barbiturates, benzodiazepines) Brain tumour Cerebrovascular disease (e.g., stroke, aneurysm, arteriovenous malformations, infection) Central nervous system degenerative diseases (e.g., Alzheimer's disease, multiple sclerosis) Idiopathic Metabolic disorders (e.g., uremia, hepatic failure, electrolyte abnormalities, hypoglycemia) Posttraumatic brain injury

Data from Daroff, R.B., Fenichel, G.M., Jankovic, J., et al. (2012). *Bradley's neurology in clinical practice* (6th ed.). Philadelphia: Saunders.

TABLE 15-14 Terminology Applied to a Seizure Disorder

Term	Definition
Preictal Phase	
Prodroma	Early clinical manifestation (such as malaise, headache, or sense of depression) that may occur a few days to hours before onset of a seizure
Aura	A partial seizure experienced as a peculiar sensation preceding onset of generalized seizure that may take the form of gustatory, visual, or auditory experience or a feeling of dizziness, numbness, or just "a funny feeling"
Ictal Phase	The event of the seizure
Tonic phase	A state of muscle contraction in which there is excessive muscle tone
Clonic phase	A state of alternating contraction and relaxation of muscles
Postictal Phase	Time period immediately following cessation of seizure activity

abnormalities in synaptic transmission, an imbalance in the brain's neurotransmitters, or the development of abnormal nerve connections after injury.[22] A group of neurons may exhibit a paroxysmal depolarization shift and function as an **epileptogenic focus**. These neurons are hypersensitive and are more easily activated by hyperthermia, hypoxia, hypoglycemia, hyponatremia, repeated sensory stimulation, and certain sleep phases. Epileptogenic neurons fire more frequently and with greater amplitude. When the intensity reaches a threshold point, cortical excitation spreads. Excitation of the subcortical, thalamic, and brainstem areas corresponds to the **tonic phase** (muscle contraction with increased muscle tone) and is associated with loss of consciousness. The **clonic phase** (alternating contraction and relaxation of muscles) begins when inhibitory neurons in the cortex, anterior thalamus, and basal ganglia react to the cortical excitation. The seizure discharge is interrupted, producing intermittent muscle contractions that gradually decrease and finally cease. The epileptogenic neurons are exhausted.

During seizure activity, oxygen is consumed at a high rate—about 60% greater than normal. Although **cerebral blood flow (CBF)** also increases, oxygen is rapidly depleted, along with glucose, and lactate accumulates in brain tissue. Continued, severe seizure activity has the potential for progressive brain injury and irreversible damage. In addition, if a seizure focus in the brain is active for a prolonged period, a **mirror focus** may develop in contralateral normal tissue and cause seizure activity.

CLINICAL MANIFESTATIONS The clinical manifestations associated with seizure depend on its type (see Table 17 6). Two types of symptoms signal the **preictal phase** of a generalized tonic–clonic seizure: **prodroma**, early manifestations occurring hours to days before a seizure and that may include anxiety, depression, or inability to think clearly; and a partial seizure that immediately precedes the onset of a generalized tonic–clonic seizure. Both may become familiar to the person experiencing recurrent generalized seizures and may enable the person to prevent injuries during the seizure. The **ictus** is the episode of the epileptic seizure with tonic–clonic activity. Relaxation of urinary and bowel sphincters may occur, leading to bladder and bowel incontinence. Airway maintenance needs to be ensured. **Status epilepticus** in adults is a state of continuous seizures lasting more than 5 minutes, or rapidly recurring seizures before the person has fully regained consciousness from the preceding seizure, or a single seizure lasting more than 30 minutes. The **postictal phase** follows an epileptic seizure and can include signs of headache, confusion, dysphasia, memory loss, and paralysis that may last hours or a day or two. Deep sleep also is common.[23]

EVALUATION AND TREATMENT The health history, physical examination, and laboratory tests of blood and urine (concentrations of blood glucose, serum calcium, blood urea nitrogen, and urine sodium; and creatinine clearance time) can identify systemic diseases known to promote seizures. Brain imaging and CSF examination help identify neurological diseases associated with seizures. The EEG is used to assess the type of seizure and determine its focus in brain tissue.

Treatment for a seizure disorder is to first correct or control its cause, if possible. If this treatment is not possible, the major means of management is the judicious administration of antiseizure medications. Dietary treatments (e.g., ketogenic and Atkins diet) are effective for some individuals. Surgical interventions can improve seizure control and quality of life in people with medication-resistant epilepsy.[24,25]

✔ QUICK CHECK 15-4

1. What is an epileptogenic focus?
2. Why can so many conditions precipitate seizures?
3. Why is continued seizing dangerous?

ALTERATIONS IN CEREBRAL HEMODYNAMICS

An injured brain reacts with structural, chemical, and pathophysiological changes. Primary brain injury is the original trauma and secondary brain injury is a consequence of alterations in CBF, **intracranial pressure (ICP)**, and oxygen delivery (Box 15-4 and see Chapter 16).

Alterations in CBF may be related to three injury states: (1) inadequate cerebral perfusion, (2) normal cerebral perfusion but with an elevated ICP, and (3) excessive **cerebral blood volume (CBV)**. Treatments for these injury states are directed at improving or maintaining cerebral perfusion pressure (CPP), as well as controlling ICP.

Increased Intracranial Pressure

Increased intracranial pressure (increased ICP) may result from an increase in intracranial content (as occurs with tumour growth), edema, excess CSF, or hemorrhage. It necessitates an equal reduction in volume of the other cranial contents. The most readily displaced content is CSF. If ICP remains high after CSF displacement out of the cranial vault, CBV and blood flow are altered.

In *stage 1 of intracranial hypertension*, vasoconstriction and external compression of the venous system occur in an attempt to further decrease the ICP. Thus, during the first stage of intracranial hypertension, ICP may not change because of the effective compensatory mechanisms, and there may no detectable symptoms (Figure 15-9). Small increases in volume, however, cause an increase in pressure, and the pressure may take longer to return to baseline. This pressure change can be detected with ICP monitoring.

BOX 15-4 Cerebral Hemodynamics

Cerebral blood flow to the brain is normally maintained at a rate that matches local metabolic needs of the brain.

Cerebral perfusion pressure (70 to 90 mm Hg) is the pressure required to perfuse the cells of the brain.

Cerebral blood volume is the amount of blood in the intracranial vault at a given time.

Cerebral blood oxygenation is measured by oxygen saturation in the internal jugular vein.

Intracranial pressure normally is 1 to 15 mm Hg, or 60 to 180 cm H_2O.

In *stage 2 of intracranial hypertension*, there is continued expansion of intracranial contents. The resulting increase in ICP may exceed the ability of the brain's compensatory mechanisms to adjust. The pressure begins to compromise neuronal oxygenation, and systemic arterial vasoconstriction occurs in an attempt to elevate the systemic blood pressure sufficiently to overcome the increased ICP. Clinical manifestations at this stage usually are subtle and transient, including episodes of confusion, restlessness, drowsiness, and slight pupillary and breathing changes (see Figure 15-9). Interventions at this stage reduce ICP and promote better clinical outcomes.

In *stage 3 of intracranial hypertension*, ICP begins to approach arterial pressure, the brain tissues begin to experience hypoxia and hypercapnia, and the individual's condition rapidly deteriorates. Clinical manifestations include decreasing levels of arousal or central neurogenic hyperventilation, widened pulse pressure, bradycardia, and small, sluggish pupils (see Figure 15-9).

Dramatic sustained rises in ICP are not seen until all compensatory mechanisms have been exhausted. Then dramatic rises in ICP occur over a very short period. Autoregulation, the compensatory alteration in the diameter of the intracranial blood vessels designed to maintain a constant blood flow during changes in CPP, is lost with progressively increased ICP. Accumulating carbon dioxide may still cause vasodilation locally, but without autoregulation this vasodilation causes the blood pressure in the vessels to drop and the blood volume to increase. The brain volume is thus further increased and ICP continues to rise. Small increases in volume cause dramatic increases in ICP, and the pressure takes much longer to return to baseline. As the ICP begins to approach systemic blood pressure, CPP falls and cerebral perfusion slows dramatically. The brain tissues experience severe hypoxia, hypercapnia, and acidosis.

In *stage 4 of intracranial hypertension*, brain tissue shifts (herniates) from the compartment of greater pressure to a compartment of lesser

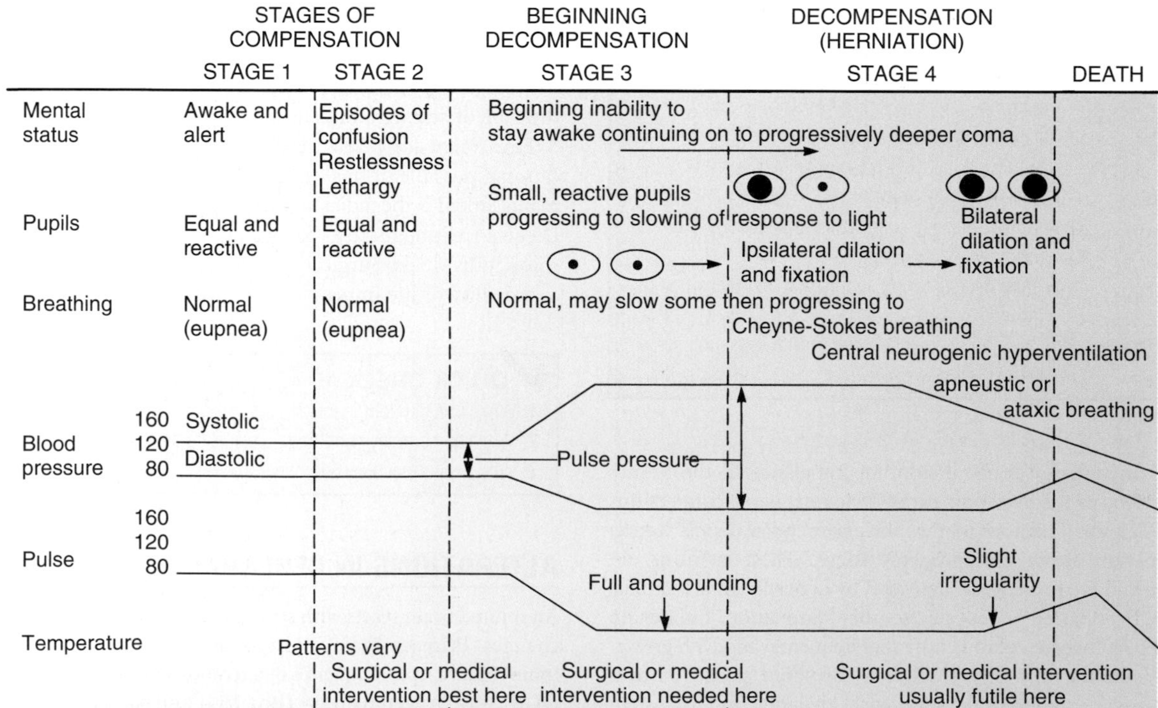

FIGURE 15-9 Clinical Correlates of Compensated and Uncompensated Stages of Intracranial Hypertension. (From Beare, P.G., & Myers, J.L. [1998]. *Principles and practice of adult health nursing* [3rd ed.]. St. Louis: Mosby.)

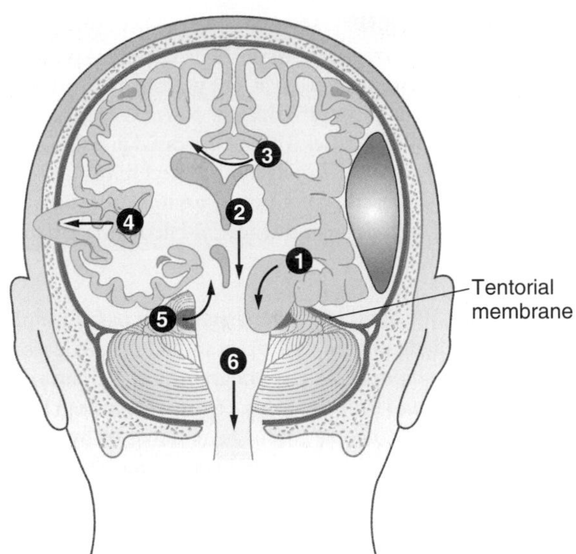

FIGURE 15-10 Brain Herniation Syndromes. Herniations can occur both above and below the tentorial membrane. Supratentorial: **1,** uncal (transtentorial); **2,** central; **3,** cingulate; **4,** transcalvarial (external herniation through an opening in the skull). Infratentorial: **5,** upward herniation of cerebellum; **6,** cerebellar tonsillar move down through foramen magnum.

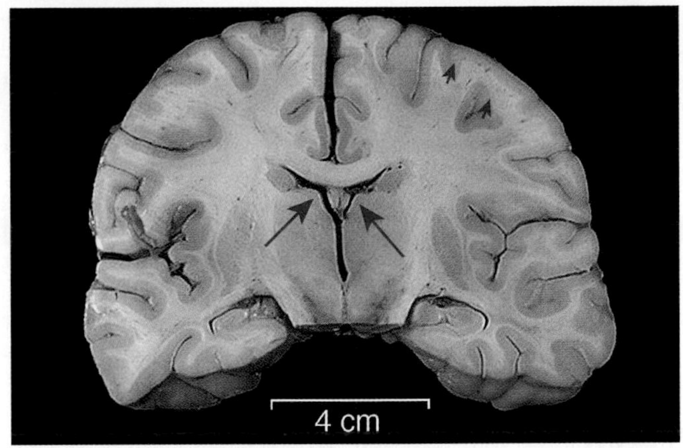

FIGURE 15-11 Brain Edema. This coronal section of the cerebrum demonstrates marked compression in the lateral ventricles (*long arrows*) and flattening of gyri (*short arrows*) from extensive bilateral cerebral edema. Edema increases intracranial pressure, leading to herniation. (From Klatt, E.C. [2010]. *Robbins and Cotran atlas of pathology* [2nd ed.]. Philadelphia: Saunders.)

pressure and increased ICP in one compartment of the cranial vault is not evenly distributed throughout the other vault compartments (see Figures 15-9 and 15-10). With this shift in brain tissue, the herniating brain tissue's blood supply is compromised, causing further ischemia and hypoxia in the herniating tissues. The volume of content within the lower pressure compartment increases, exerting pressure on the brain tissue that normally occupies that compartment, and thus impairs its blood supply. For example, herniation into the brainstem impairs the vital cardiovascular and respiratory regulatory centres and can cause death. The herniation process markedly and rapidly increases ICP. Mean systolic arterial pressure soon equals ICP, and CBF ceases at this point. The types of brain herniation syndromes are outlined in Box 15-5.

Cerebral Edema

Cerebral edema is an increase in the fluid content of brain tissue (Figure 15-11). The result is increased extracellular or intracellular tissue volume. It occurs after brain insult from trauma, infection, hemorrhage, tumour, ischemia, infarction, or hypoxia. The harmful effects of cerebral edema are caused by distortion of blood vessels, displacement of brain tissues, increase in ICP, and eventual herniation of brain tissue to a different brain compartment.

Three types of cerebral edema are (1) vasogenic edema, (2) cytotoxic (metabolic) edema, and (3) interstitial edema. **Vasogenic edema** is clinically the most important type and is caused by the increased permeability of the capillary endothelium of the brain after injury to the vascular structure. The selective permeability of capillaries that comprise the blood–brain barrier is disrupted. Plasma proteins leak into the extracellular spaces, drawing water to them and increasing the water content of the brain parenchyma. Vasogenic edema begins in the area of injury and spreads, with fluid accumulating in the white matter of the ipsilateral side because the parallel myelinated fibres separate more easily. Edema promotes more edema because of ischemia from the increasing ICP.

Clinical manifestations of vasogenic edema include focal neurological deficits, disturbances of consciousness, and a severe increase in ICP. Vasogenic edema resolves by slow diffusion.

BOX 15-5 Brain Herniation Syndromes

Supratentorial Herniation

1. *Uncal herniation.* It occurs when the uncus or hippocampal gyrus, or both, shifts from the middle fossa through the tentorial notch into the posterior fossa, compressing the ipsilateral third cranial nerve, the contralateral third cranial nerve, and the mesencephalon. Uncal herniation generally is caused by an expanding mass in the lateral region of the middle fossa. The classic manifestations of uncal herniation are a decreasing level of consciousness, pupils that become sluggish before fixing and dilating (first the ipsilateral, then the contralateral pupil), Cheyne-Stokes respirations (which later shift to central neurogenic hyperventilation), and the appearance of decorticate and then decerebrate posturing.
2. *Central herniation.* It occurs when there is a straight downward shift of the diencephalon through the tentorial notch. It may be caused by injuries or masses located around the outer perimeter of the frontal, parietal, or occipital lobes; extracerebral injuries around the central apex (top) of the cranium; bilaterally positioned injuries or masses; and unilateral cingulate gyrus herniation. The individual rapidly becomes unconscious; moves from Cheyne-Stokes respirations to apnea; develops small, reactive pupils and then dilated, fixed pupils; and passes from decortication to decerebration.
3. *Cingulate gyrus herniation.* It occurs when the cingulate gyrus shifts under the falx cerebri. Little is known about its clinical manifestations.
4. *Transcalvarial.* The brain shifts through a skull fracture or a surgical opening in the skull. This type of external herniation may occur during a craniectomy—surgery in which a flap of skull is removed. This type of herniation prevents the piece of skull from being replaced.

Infratentorial Herniation

1. The most common syndrome is *cerebellar tonsillar.* The cerebellar tonsil shifts through the foramen magnum because of increased pressure within the posterior fossa. The clinical manifestations are an arched stiff neck, paresthesias in the shoulder area, decreased consciousness, respiratory abnormalities, and pulse rate variations. Occasionally the force produces an *upward transtentorial* herniation of a cerebellar tonsil or the lower brainstem. There is increased intracranial pressure but no specific set of clinical manifestations associated with infratentorial herniation (see Figure 15-10).

In **cytotoxic (metabolic) edema**, toxic factors directly affect the cellular elements of the brain parenchyma (neuronal, glial, and endothelial cells), causing failure of the active transport systems. The cells lose their potassium and gain larger amounts of sodium. Water follows by osmosis into the cells, so that the cells swell. Cytotoxic edema occurs principally in the grey matter and may increase vasogenic edema.

Interstitial edema is seen most often with noncommunicating hydrocephalus. The edema is caused by transependymal movement of CSF from the ventricles into the extracellular spaces of the brain tissues. The brain fluid volume increases predominantly around the ventricles, with increased hydrostatic pressure within the white matter. The size of the white matter is reduced because of the rapid disappearance of myelin lipids.

Hydrocephalus

The term **hydrocephalus** refers to various conditions characterized by excess fluid in the cerebral ventricles, subarachnoid space, or both. Hydrocephalus occurs because of interference with CSF flow caused by increased fluid production, obstruction within the ventricular system, or defective reabsorption of the fluid. A tumour of the choroid plexus may, in rare instances, cause overproduction of CSF. The types of hydrocephalus are reviewed in Table 15-15.

Hydrocephalus may develop from infancy through adulthood. **Communicating hydrocephalus** is defective resorption of CSF from the cerebral subarachnoid space and is found more often in adults. **Noncommunicating hydrocephalus (internal hydrocephalus, intraventricular hydrocephalus)** is obstruction within the ventricular system and is seen more often in children (see Figure 17-6). Congenital hydrocephalus is ventricular enlargement before birth and is rare.

PATHOPHYSIOLOGY The obstruction of CSF flow associated with hydrocephalus produces increased pressure and dilation of the ventricles proximal to the obstruction. The increased pressure and dilation cause atrophy of the cerebral cortex and degeneration of the white matter tracts. Selective preservation of grey matter occurs. When excess CSF fills a defect caused by atrophy, a degenerative disorder, or a surgical excision, this fluid is not under pressure; therefore, atrophy and degenerative changes do not occur.

TABLE 15-15 Types of Hydrocephalus

Type	Mechanism	Cause
Noncommunicating	Obstruction of CSF flow between ventricles Aqueduct stenosis Arnold-Chiari malformation (brain extension through foramen magnum) Compression by tumour	Congenital abnormality
Communicating	Impaired absorption of CSF within subarachnoid space Compression of subarachnoid space by a tumour High venous pressure in sagittal sinus Head injury Congenital malformation	Infection with inflammatory adhesions
	Increased CSF secretion by choroid plexus	Secreting tumour

CSF, cerebrospinal fluid.

CLINICAL MANIFESTATIONS Most cases of hydrocephalus develop gradually and insidiously over time. **Acute hydrocephalus** presents with signs of rapidly developing increased ICP. The person quickly deteriorates into a deep coma if not promptly treated. **Normal-pressure hydrocephalus** (dilation of the ventricles without increased pressure) develops slowly, with the individual or family noting declining memory and cognitive function. The triad symptoms of an unsteady, broad-based gait with a history of falling; incontinence; and dementia are common and may be treated surgically.[26]

EVALUATION AND TREATMENT The diagnosis is based on physical examination, computed tomography (CT) scan, and magnetic resonance imaging (MRI). A radioisotopic cisternogram may be performed to diagnose normal-pressure hydrocephalus. Hydrocephalus can be treated by surgery to resect cysts, neoplasms, or hematomas or by ventricular bypass into the normal intracranial channel or into an extracranial compartment using a shunting procedure, one of the three most common neurosurgical procedures. Excision or coagulation of the choroid plexus occasionally is needed when a papilloma is present. In normal-pressure hydrocephalus, reduction in CSF is achieved through diuresis or placement of a ventriculoperitoneal shunt.[27]

✔ QUICK CHECK 15-5

1. What are the four stages of increased intracranial pressure?
2. How does supratentorial herniation differ from infratentorial herniation?
3. What are the different types of cerebral edema?
4. How is communicating hydrocephalus different from noncommunicating hydrocephalus?

ALTERATIONS IN NEUROMOTOR FUNCTION

Movements are complex patterns of activity controlled by the cerebral cortex, the pyramidal system, the extrapyramidal system, and the motor units. Dysfunction in any of these areas can cause motor dysfunction. General neuromotor dysfunctions are associated with changes in muscle tone, movement, and complex motor performance.

Alterations in Muscle Tone

Normal muscle tone involves a slight resistance to passive movement. Throughout the range of motion, the resistance is smooth, constant, and even. The alterations of muscle tone and their characteristics and causes are presented in Table 15-16.

Hypotonia

In **hypotonia** (decreased muscle tone), passive movement of a muscle occurs with little or no resistance. Causes include cerebellar damage and pure pyramidal tract damage (a rare occurrence). The hypotonia contributes to the ataxia and intention tremor in cerebellar damage and manifests with minimal weakness and normal or slightly exaggerated reflexes. A pure pyramidal tract injury produces hypotonia and weakness. Hypotonia also occurs when the nerve impulses needed for muscle tone are lost, such as in spinal cord injury or cerebrovascular accident.

Individuals with hypotonia tire easily or are weak. They may have difficulty rising from a sitting position, sitting down without using arm support, and walking up and down stairs, as well as an inability to stand on their toes. Because of their weakness, accidents during ambulatory and self-care activities are common. The joints become hyperflexible, so persons with hypotonia may be able to assume positions that require extreme joint mobility. The joints may appear loose. The muscle mass

TABLE 15-16 **Alterations in Muscle Tone**

Alterations	Characteristics	Cause
Hypotonia	Passive movement of a muscle mass with little or no resistance	Thought to be caused by decreased muscle spindle activity as a result of decreased excitability of neurons (e.g., muscular dystrophy, cerebral palsy)
	Muscles may be moved rapidly without resistance	
Flaccidity	Associated with limp, atrophied muscles, and paralysis	Occurs typically when nerve impulses necessary for muscle tone are lost
Hypertonia	Increased muscle resistance to passive movement May be associated with paralysis	Results when lower motor unit reflex arc continues to function but is not mediated or regulated by higher centres (e.g., stroke, brain tumours, multiple sclerosis)
	May be accompanied by muscle hypertrophy	
Spasticity	A gradual increase in tone causing increased resistance until tone suddenly diminishes, which results in clasp-knife phenomenon; increased deep tendon reflexes (hyperreflexia); clonus (spread of reflexes)	Exact mechanism unclear; appears to arise from an increased excitability of alpha motor neurons to any input because of absence of descending inhibition of pyramidal systems (e.g., multiple sclerosis, brain trauma, cerebral palsy)
Paratonia (gegenhalten)	Resistance to passive movement, which varies in direct proportion to force applied	Exact mechanism unclear; associated with frontal lobe injury (e.g., progressive Alzheimer's dementia)
Dystonia	Sustained involuntary muscle contraction with twisting movement	Produced by slow muscular contraction; lack of reciprocal inhibition of muscle (e.g., neuroleptic medication adverse effects, meningitis)
Rigidity	Muscle resistance to passive movement of a rigid limb that is uniform in both flexion and extension throughout the motion	Occurs as a result of constant, involuntary contraction of muscle—usually involves extrapyramidal tracts (e.g., Parkinson's disease)
Plastic or lead-pipe rigidity	Increased muscular tone relatively independent of degree of force used in passive movement; does not vary throughout the passive movement	Associated with basal ganglion damage (e.g., Parkinson's disease)
Cogwheel rigidity	Uniform resistance may be interrupted by a series of brief jerks, resulting in movements much like a ratchet, cogwheel phenomenon	Associated with basal ganglion damage
Gamma rigidity	Characterized by extensor posturing (decerebrate rigidity)	Loss of excitation of extensor inhibitory areas by cerebral cortex decreasing inhibition of alpha and gamma motor neurons
Alpha rigidity	Impaired relaxation characterized by extensor rigidity of skeletal muscle after contraction	Loss of cerebellum input to lateral vestibular nuclei

atrophies because of decreased input entering the motor unit, and muscles appear flabby and flat. Muscle cells are gradually replaced by connective tissue and fat. Fasciculations may be present in some cases.

Hypertonia

In **hypertonia** (increased muscle tone), passive movement of a muscle occurs with resistance to stretch and is caused by upper motor neuron damage (see p. 381). The four types of hypertonia are **spasticity** (usually corticospinal in origin) (Figures 15-12 and 15-13), **paratonia (gegenhalten)**, dystonia (Figure 15-14), and **rigidity** (usually extrapyramidal in origin). Four types of rigidity are described: plastic or lead-pipe, cogwheel, gamma (independent of stretch reflex pathways), and alpha (dependent on stretch reflex pathways) (see Table 15-16).

Individuals with hypertonia tire easily or are weak. Passive movement and active movement are affected equally, except in paratonia, in which more active than passive movement is possible. As a result of hypertonia and weakness, accidents occur during ambulatory and self-care activities.

The muscles may atrophy because of decreased use. However, hypertrophy occasionally occurs as a result of the overstimulation of muscle fibres. Overstimulation occurs when the motor unit reflex arc remains intact and functioning but is not inhibited by higher centres. This lack of higher-centre inhibition causes continual muscle contraction, resulting in enlargement of the muscle mass and the development of firm muscles.

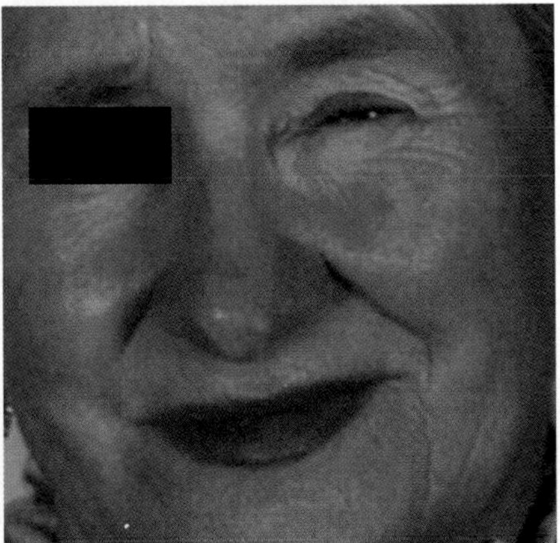

FIGURE 15-12 Paroxysm of Left-Sided Hemifacial Spasm. (From Perkin, G.D. [2002]. *Mosby's color atlas and text of neurology* [2nd ed.]. London: Mosby.)

Alterations in Muscle Movement

Movement requires a change in the contractile state of muscles. Abnormal movements occur when CNS dysfunction alters muscle innervation. The neurotransmitter *dopamine* has a role in several movement disorders. Some movement disorders (e.g., the akinesias) result from too little

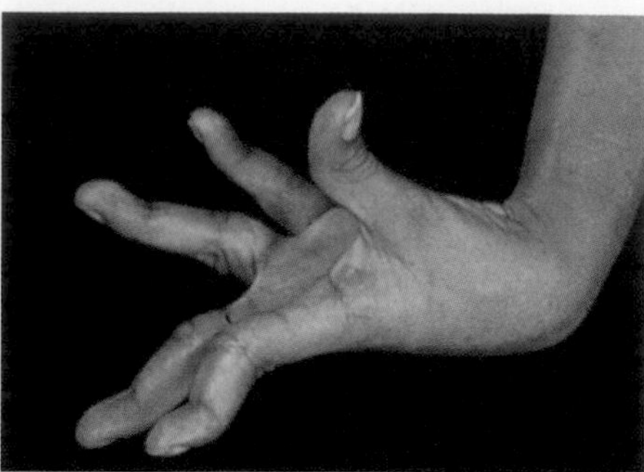

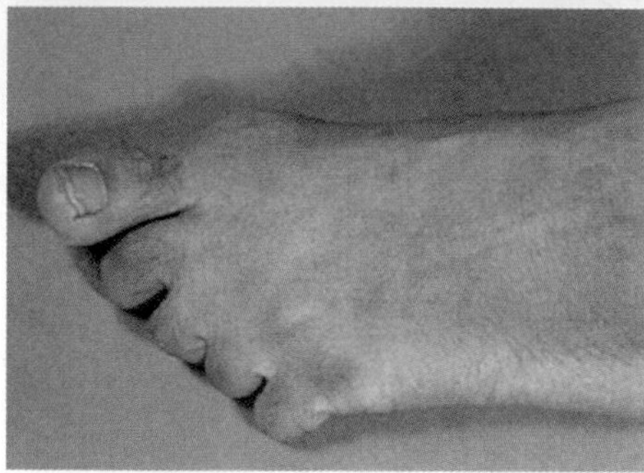

FIGURE 15-13 Dystonic Posturing of the Hand and Foot. (From Perkin, G.D. [2002]. *Mosby's color atlas and text of neurology* [2nd ed.]. London: Mosby.)

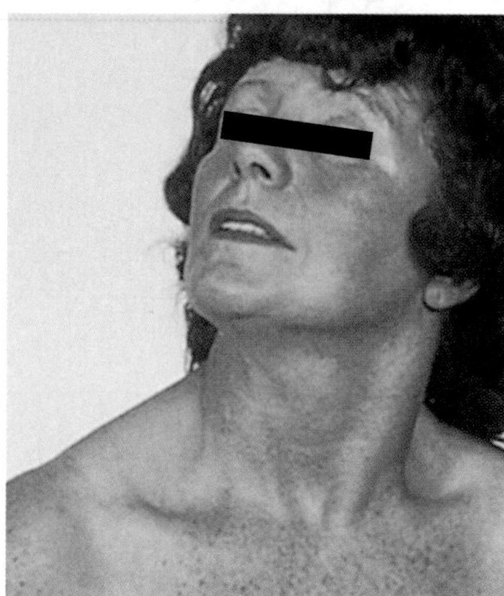

FIGURE 15-14 Spasmodic Torticollis. A characteristic head posture related to spasticity. (From Perkin, G.D. [2002]. *Mosby's color atlas and text of neurology* [2nd ed.]. London: Mosby.)

dopaminergic activity, whereas others (e.g., chorea, ballism, tardive dyskinesia) result from too much dopaminergic activity. Still others are not primarily related to dopamine function. Movement disorders are not necessarily associated with muscle mass, strength, or tone but are neurological dysfunctions resulting in insufficient or excessive movement or involuntary movement.

Hyperkinesia is excessive, purposeless movement and represents the second broad category of abnormal movements. Within this category are a number of specific dysfunctions including tremors (Table 15-17). Also included under the general category of hyperkinesias are *dyskinesias* and abnormal involuntary movements. Huntington's disease symptoms are the hallmark of hyperkinesia.

Paroxysmal dyskinesias are abnormal, involuntary movements that occur as spasms. The type of dyskinesia varies depending on the specific disorder.

Tardive dyskinesia is the involuntary movement of the face, lip, tongue, trunk, and extremities. Although the condition occurs occasionally in individuals with Parkinson's disease, it usually occurs as a adverse effect of prolonged antipsychotic medication therapy. The most common symptom of tardive dyskinesia is rapid, repetitive, stereotypical movements, such as continual chewing with intermittent protrusions of the tongue, lip smacking, and facial grimacing. The symptoms also are called *extrapyramidal symptoms* because the extrapyramidal system controls involuntary reflexes and coordination of movement and posture (see Table 15-19).

Other movement disorders in this category are (1) complex repetitive movements, including automatism (unconscious behaviour), stereotypy (ritualistic behaviour such as rocking), complex tics such as Tourette syndrome (see *Health Promotion:* Tourette Syndrome), compulsions, perseverations, and mannerisms; (2) excessive reactions to certain stimuli; and (3) paroxysmal excessive activity, including cataplexy and excessive startle reaction.

HEALTH PROMOTION

Tourette Syndrome

There is growing evidence that Tourette syndrome (TS) occurs worldwide and has common features across all races and cultures. The hallmark of TS is the presence of motor tics (sudden, rapid, repetitive nonrhythmic movements) and vocal tics. The tics may be either simple, involving only an individual muscle group (e.g., eye blinking or grunting), or complex, requiring coordinated movement of muscle groups (e.g., head banging or repeating of another person's words). The syndrome has a complex multifactorial etiology with undetermined genetic, environmental, immune, and hormonal factors. Recent research has indicated that exposure to certain environmental factors during the prenatal, perinatal, and postnatal periods may impact the onset and progression of TS. The pregnancy-related exposures include maternal smoking and prenatal life stressors. Other factors that may cause a worsening of TS-related tics include low birth weight and forceps use during delivery. Further studies have also indicated that exposure to certain pathogens may be linked to the disease. Additional studies exploring these relationships may hold promise for the improvement of the course of TS related to these modifiable risk factors.

Data from Hoekstra, P.J., Dietrich, A., Edwards, M.J., et al. (2013). *Neurosci Biobehav Rev, 37*(6), 1040–1049.

Hypokinesia is decreased amplitude of movement, bradykinesia is decreased speed of movement, and akinesia is absence of voluntary movement. All of these terms represent a deficit of voluntary movement. Parkinson's disease symptoms are the hallmark of a lack of voluntary movement.

Huntington's Disease

Huntington's disease (HD), also known as *chorea*, is a relatively rare, hereditary, degenerative hyperkinetic movement disorder diffusely involving the basal ganglia and cerebral cortex. The onset of HD is usually between 25 and 45 years of age, when the trait may already have been passed to the person's children. The disorder has a prevalence rate of approximately 5 to 10 per 100 000 persons and occurs in all races.[28]

PATHOPHYSIOLOGY HD is inherited from one or both parents who have the autosomal dominant trait with high penetrance. The genetic

TABLE 15-17 Types of Hyperkinesia and Tremor

Type	Characteristics	Causes
Hyperkinesia		
Chorea[a]	Nonrepetitive muscular contractions, usually of extremities of face; random pattern of irregular, involuntary rapid contractions of groups of muscles; disappears with sleep, decreases with resting; increases with emotional stress and attempted voluntary movement	Associated with excess concentration of or supersensitivity to dopamine within basal ganglia
Athetosis[a]	Disorder of distal muscle postural fixation; slow, sinuous, irregular movements most obvious in distal extremities, more rhythmic than choreiform movements and always much slower; movements accompany characteristic hand posture; slowly fluctuating grimaces	Occurs most commonly as result of injury to putamen of basal ganglion; exact pathophysiological mechanism is not known
Ballism	Disorder of proximal muscle postural fixation with wild flinging movement of limbs; movement is severe and stereotyped, usually lateral; does not lessen with sleep; ballism is most common on one side of body, a condition termed *hemiballism*	Results from injury to subthalamic nucleus (one of nuclei that comprise basal ganglia); thought to be caused by reduced inhibitory influence in nucleus, a release phenomenon; hemiballism results from injury to contralateral subthalamic nucleus
Hyperactivity	State of prolonged, generalized, increased activity that is largely involuntary but may be subject to some voluntary control; not highly stereotyped but rather manifests as continuous changes in total body posture or in excessive performance of some simple activity, such as pacing under inappropriate circumstances	May be caused by frontal and reticular activating system injury
Wandering	Tendency to wander without regard for environment	"Release phenomenon" associated with bilateral injury to globus pallidus or putamen
Akathisia	Special type of hyperactivity; mild compulsion to move (usually more localized to legs); severe, frenzied motion possible; movements are partly voluntary and may be transiently suppressed; carrying out movement brings sense of relief; frequent complication of antipsychotic medications	Dopaminergic transmission may be involved
Tremor at Rest	Rhythmic, oscillating movement affecting one or more body parts	Caused by regular contraction of opposing groups of muscles
Parkinsonian tremor	Regular, rhythmic, slower flexion-extension contraction; involves principally metacarpophalangeal and wrist joints; alternating movements between thumb and index finger described as "pill rolling"; disappears during voluntary movement	Loss of inhibitory influence of dopamine in the basal ganglia, causing instability of basal ganglial feedback circuit within cerebral cortex
Postural Tremor		
Asterixis (tremor of hepatic encephalopathy)	Irregular flapping movement of hands accentuated by outstretching arms	Exact mechanisms responsible unknown; thought to be related to accumulation of products normally detoxified by liver (e.g., ammonia)
Metabolic	Rapid, rhythmic tremor affecting fingers, lips, and tongue; accentuated by extending body part; enhanced physiological tremor	Occurs in conditions associated with disturbed metabolism or toxicity, as in thyrotoxicosis (hyperthyroidism), alcoholism, and chronic use of barbiturates, amphetamines, lithium, or amitriptyline (Elavil); exact mechanism responsible unknown
Essential (familial)	Tremor of fingers, hands, and feet; absent at rest but accentuated by extension of body part, prolonged muscular activity, and stress	Not associated with any other neurological abnormalities; cause unknown
Intention Tremor		
Cerebellar	Tremor initiated by movement, maximal toward end of movement	Occurs in disease of dentate nucleus (one of deep cerebellar nuclei responsible for efferent output) and superior cerebellar peduncle (stalklike structure connected to pons); caused by errors in feedback from periphery and errors in preprogramming goal-directed movement
Rubral	Rhythmic tremor of limbs that originates proximally by movement	Results from lesions involving dentatorubrothalamic tract (a spinothalamic tract connecting red nucleus in reticular formation and dentate nucleus in cerebellum)
Myoclonus	Series of shocklike, nonpatterned contractions of portion of a muscle, entire muscle, or group of muscles that cause throwing movements of a limb; usually appear at random but frequently triggered by sudden startle; do not disappear during sleep	Associated with an irritable nervous system and spontaneous discharge of neurons; structures associated with myoclonus include cerebral cortex, cerebellum, reticular formation, and spinal cord

[a]Choreoathetosis involves both chorea and athetosis; precise pathophysiology is unknown.

defect of HD is on the short arm of chromosome 4. There is an abnormally long polyglutamine tract in the huntingtin (htt) protein that is toxic to neurons caused by a cytosine-adenine-guanine (CAG) trinucleotide repeat expansion (40 to 70 repeats instead of 9 to 34) with abnormal protein folding. Age of symptom onset is related to the length of the repeat sequences and mechanisms of toxicity. Repeat lengths greater than 60 cause the juvenile form of the disease.[29] Fathers, but not mothers, with high normal alleles do not develop HD but are at risk of transmitting potentially penetrant HD alleles (greater than or equal to 36) to their offspring, who can develop HD.[30]

The principal pathological feature of HD is severe degeneration of the basal ganglia, particularly the caudate nucleus. Tangles of protein (htt protein) collect in the brain cells and chains of glutamine on the abnormal molecules stick to each other and contribute to neuronal loss. Basal ganglia and nigral depletion of gamma-aminobutyric acid (GABA), an inhibitory neurotransmitter, is the principal biochemical alteration in HD. It alters the integration of motor and mental function.[31]

CLINICAL MANIFESTATIONS Symptoms of HD progress slowly and include involuntary fragmentary movements, such as chorea, athetosis, and ballism (see Table 15-17). Chorea, the most common type of abnormal movement, begins in the face and arms, eventually affecting the entire body. There is emotional lability and progressive dysfunction of intellectual and thought processes (dementia). Any one of these features may mark the onset of the disease. Cognitive deficits include loss of working memory and reduced capacity to plan, organize, and sequence. Thinking is slow, and apathy is present. Restlessness, disinhibition, and irritability are common. Euphoria or depression may be present.

EVALUATION AND TREATMENT The diagnosis of HD is based on family history and clinical presentation of the disorder. Neuroradiological abnormalities can be demonstrated up to 15 years before clinical symptoms. No known treatment is effective in halting the degeneration or progression of symptoms, and the disease is fatal. Symptomatic medication therapies are available.[32]

Hypokinesia

Hypokinesia (decreased movement) is loss of voluntary movement despite preserved consciousness and normal peripheral nerve and muscle function. Types of hypokinesia include akinesia, bradykinesia, and loss of associated movement.

Akinesia and bradykinesia. Akinesia is a decrease in voluntary and associated movements. It is related to dysfunction of the extrapyramidal system and caused by either a deficiency of dopamine or a defect of the postsynaptic dopamine receptors, which occurs in parkinsonism. Bradykinesia is slowness of voluntary movements. All voluntary movements become slow, laboured, and deliberate, with difficulty in (1) initiating movements, (2) continuing movements smoothly, and (3) performing synchronous (at the same time) and consecutive tasks. Both akinesia and bradykinesia involve a delay in the time it takes to start to perform a movement.

Loss of associated movement. In hypokinesia, the normal, habitually associated movements that provide skill, grace, and balance to voluntary movements are lost. Decreased associated movements accompanying emotional expression cause an expressionless face, a statuelike posture, absence of speech inflection, and absence of spontaneous gestures. Decreased associated movements accompanying locomotion cause reduction in arm and shoulder movements, hip swinging, and rotary motion of the cervical spine.

Parkinson's Disease

Parkinson's disease (PD) is a complex motor disorder accompanied by systemic nonmotor and neurological symptoms. Etiological classification of parkinsonism includes primary parkinsonism and secondary parkinsonism. Primary PD begins after the age of 40 years, with the incidence increasing after age 60 years. It is more prevalent in males and a leading cause of neurological disability in individuals older than 60 years. In 2010–11, an estimated 55 000 Canadians aged 18 or older reported that they had been diagnosed with PD.[33] The familial form represents about 10% of PD; however, the majority of cases are sporadic or idiopathic. Secondary parkinsonism is parkinsonism caused by disorders other than PD (i.e., head trauma, infection, neoplasm, atherosclerosis, toxins, medication intoxication). Medication-induced parkinsonism, caused by neuroleptics, antiemetics, and antihypertensives, is the most common secondary form and usually is reversible.

PATHOPHYSIOLOGY The pathogenesis of primary PD is unknown. Several gene mutations have been identified that influence nerve function in PD. Gene–environment interactions are probable causes of neuro-degeneration in PD. The primary pathology is degeneration of the basal ganglia (see Figure 13-10) with dysfunctional or misfolded α-synuclein protein and loss of dopamine-producing neurons in the substantia nigra and dorsal striatum. The resulting depletion of dopamine, an inhibitory neurotransmitter, and relative excess of cholinergic (excitatory) activity in the feedback circuit are manifested by hypertonia (tremor and rigidity) and akinesia, producing a syndrome of abnormal movement called parkinsonism (Parkinson's syndrome, parkinsonian syndrome, paralysis agitans) (Figure 15-15). Neuroimaging shows degeneration of dopaminergic neurons preceding the onset of motor symptoms by as long as 3 to 6 years.[34] Dementia may develop over decades with infiltration of Lewy bodies (accumulation of abnormal protein in nerve cells) and plaque formation similar to AD.[35] Loss of cholinergic subcortical input into the cortex is associated with nonmotor symptoms of PD.[36]

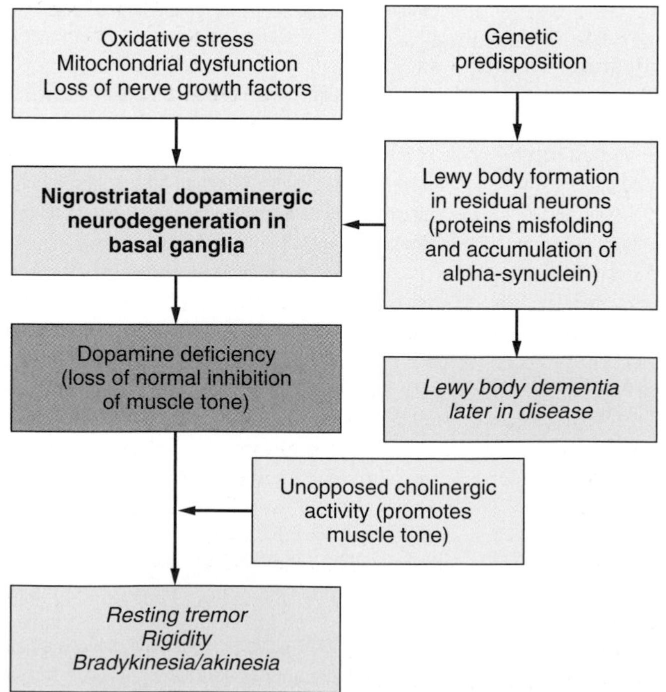

FIGURE 15-15 Pathophysiology of Parkinson's Disease.

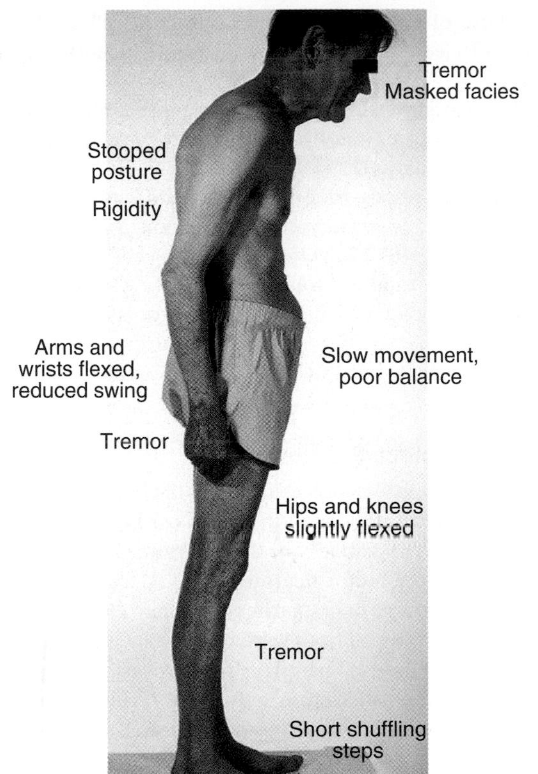

FIGURE 15-16 Stooped Posture of Parkinson's Disease. (From Perkin, D.G. [2002]. *Mosby's color atlas and text of neurology* [2nd ed.]. London: Mosby.)

CLINICAL MANIFESTATIONS The classic manifestations of PD are resting tremor, rigidity, bradykinesia or akinesia, postural disturbance, dysarthria, and dysphagia. They may develop alone or in combination, but as the disease progresses, all are usually present. There is no true paralysis. The symptoms are always bilateral but usually involve one side early in the illness. Because the onset is insidious, the beginning of symptoms is difficult to document. Early in the disease, reflex status, sensory status, and mental status usually are normal. Loss of smell can be an early nonmotor symptom. Postural abnormalities (flexed, forward leaning), difficulty walking, and weakness develop as neuro-degeneration progresses (Figure 15-16). Speech may be slurred.

Disorders of equilibrium result from postural abnormalities. The person with PD cannot make the appropriate postural adjustment to tilting or falling and falls like a post when starting to tilt. The festinating gait (short, accelerating steps) of the individual with PD is an attempt to maintain an upright position while walking. Individuals are also unable to right themselves when changing from a reclining or crouching position to a standing position and when rolling over from a supine to a lateral or prone position. Sleep disorders and excessive daytime sleepiness are commonly experienced. Sensory disturbances (pain and impaired smell and vision), urinary urgency, difficulty concentrating, depression, and hallucinations are some of the nonmotor symptoms of PD.[37,38] Autonomic–neuroendocrine changes also contribute to nonmotor symptoms and include inappropriate diaphoresis, orthostatic hypotension, drooling, gastric retention, constipation, and urinary retention.

Progressive dementia is more common in persons older than 70 years. Mental status may be further compromised by the adverse effects of the medication taken to control symptoms.

TABLE 15-18 Upper and Lower Motor Neuron Syndromes Signs and Symptoms

Upper Motor Neuron (Pyramidal Cells—Motor Cortex)	Lower Motor Neuron (Cranial Nerve Nuclei—Brainstem; Ventral Horn—Spinal Cord)
Muscle groups are affected	Individual muscles may be affected
Mild weakness	Mild weakness
Minimal disuse muscle atrophy	Marked muscle atrophy
No fasciculations	Fasciculations
Increased muscle stretch reflexes (clasp-knife spasticity; resistance to passive flexion that releases abruptly to allow easy flexion)	Decreased muscle stretch reflexes
Clonus may be present	Clonus not present
Hypertonia, spasticity	Hypotonia, flaccidity Hyporeflexia
Pathological reflexes (Babinski and Hoffmann signs, loss of abdominal reflexes)	No Babinski sign
Often initial impairment of only skilled movements	Asymmetrical and may involve one limb only in beginning to become generalized as disease progresses

EVALUATION AND TREATMENT The diagnosis of PD is based on the history and the clinical features of the disease. Causes of secondary parkinsonism are first excluded. Specific gene panels and imaging studies are evolving for early diagnosis.[39] Treatment of PD is symptomatic with medication therapy to decrease akinesia. Because of troublesome adverse effects and loss of effectiveness, however, medication therapy may not be started until the symptoms become incapacitating. Deep brain stimulation (i.e., subthalamic neurostimulation) is replacing surgery to treat persons unresponsive to medication therapy. Implants of stem cells and fetal cells, as well as gene therapy, are strategies for future treatments.[40] Dysphagia and general immobility are special problems of the individual with PD requiring interdisciplinary efforts to improve functional status.[41]

Upper and Lower Motor Neuron Syndromes

Paresis and paralysis are symptoms of upper and lower motor neuron syndromes (Table 15-18). **Paresis** (weakness) is partial paralysis with incomplete loss of muscle power. **Paralysis** is loss of motor function so that a muscle group is unable to overcome gravity.

Upper Motor Neuron Syndromes

Upper motor neuron syndromes are the result of damage to descending motor pathways at cortical, brainstem, or spinal cord levels. **Upper motor neuron paresis or paralysis** is known also as *spastic paresis/paralysis*, and different terms are used to describe the specific disorders (Box 15-6).

Upper motor neuron paresis or paralysis is associated with a **pyramidal motor syndrome**, which involves a series of motor dysfunctions resulting from interruption of the pyramidal system (Figures 15-17 and 15-18). The injury may be in the cerebral cortex, the subcortical white matter, the internal capsule, the brainstem, or the spinal cord. The clinical manifestations reflect muscle overactivity and include excessive movements, such as clonus and spasms, occurring regularly as a result of loss of higher motor centre control. There is great variation, depending on the suddenness of onset and the age of the individual.

Spinal shock is the temporary loss of all spinal cord functions below the lesion (below the level of the pons). It is characterized by complete flaccid paralysis, absence of reflexes, and marked disturbances of bowel and bladder function. Hypotension can occur from loss of sympathetic tone at higher levels of spinal cord injury. A major factor in spinal shock is the sudden destruction of the efferent pathways. If destruction occurs more slowly, spinal shock may not develop (see Chapter 16).

If the pyramidal system is interrupted above the level of the pons, the hand and arm muscles are greatly affected. Paralysis rarely involves all the muscles on one side of the body, even when the hemiplegia results from complete damage to the internal capsule. Bilateral movements, such as those of the eye, jaw, and larynx, as well as those of the trunk, are affected only slightly, if at all. Predominantly the limbs are influenced.

Paralysis associated with a pyramidal motor syndrome rarely remains flaccid for a prolonged time. After a few days or weeks, a gradual return of spinal reflexes marks the end of spinal shock. Reflexes then become hyperactive, and muscle tone increases significantly, particularly in antigravity muscles. *Spasticity* is common, although rigidity occasionally occurs (see Table 15-16). Most often, passive range-of-motion movements cause "clasp-knife" rigidity, probably by activating the stretch receptors in the muscle spindles and the Golgi tendon organ. (Muscle function is discussed in Chapter 38.) With pyramidal motor syndrome, predominantly the flexors of the arms and the extensors of the legs are affected.

BOX 15-6 Upper Motor Neuron Paresis or Paralysis

Hemiparesis/hemiplegia is paresis/paralysis of the upper and lower extremities on one side.

Diplegia is paralysis of corresponding parts of both sides of the body as a result of cerebral hemisphere injuries.

Paraparesis/paraplegia is weakness/paralysis of the lower extremities as a result of lower spinal cord injury.

Quadriparesis/quadriplegia is paresis/paralysis of all four extremities as a result of upper spinal cord injury (spinal cord injury is discussed in Chapter 16).

Lower Motor Neuron Syndromes

Lower (primary, alpha) motor neurons are the large motor neurons in the anterior (or ventral) horn of the spinal cord and the motor nuclei of the brainstem. The axons from these nerve cell bodies bring nerve impulses from upper motor neurons to the skeletal muscles through the anterior spinal roots or cranial nerves (Figure 15-19). Lower motor neuron syndromes impair both voluntary and involuntary movement. The degree of paralysis or paresis is proportional to the number of lower motor neurons affected. If only some of the motor units that supply a muscle are affected, only partial paralysis (or paresis) results.

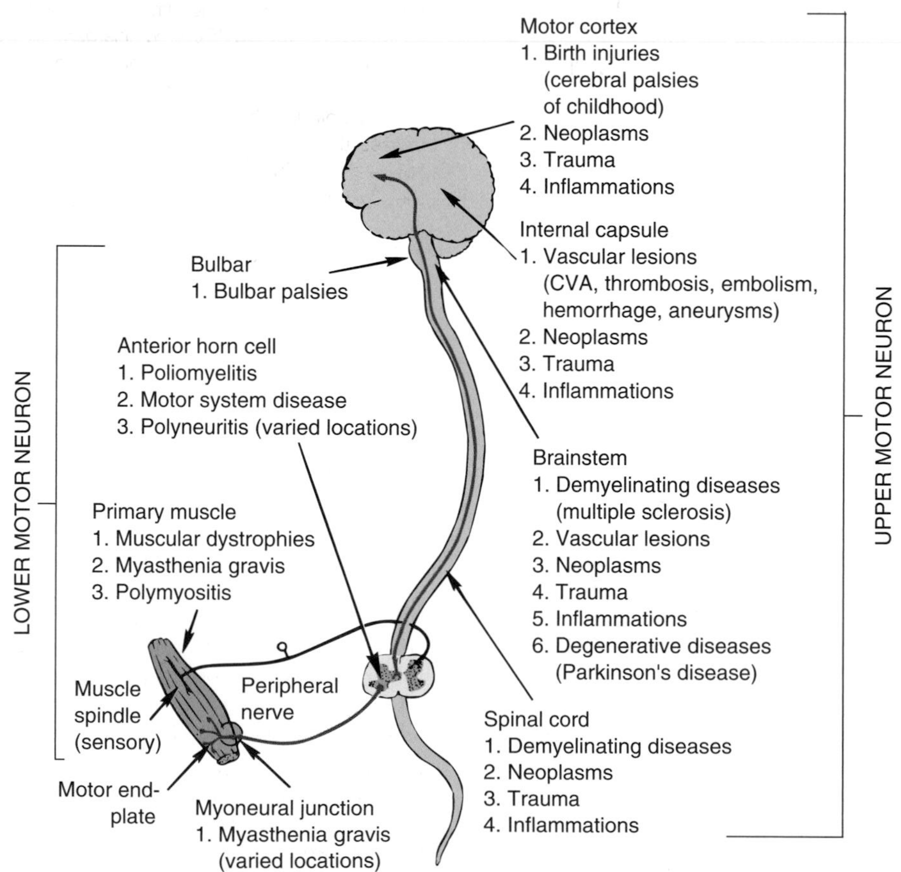

FIGURE 15-17 Motor Function Syndromes. Disturbances in motor function are classified pathologically along upper and lower motor neuron structures. It should be noted that the same pathological condition occurs at more than one site in an upper motor neuron (*top right*). A few pathological conditions involve both upper and lower motor neuron structures, as in amyotrophic lateral sclerosis, for example. Other lesion sites include myoneural junction and primary muscle, making it possible to classify conditions as neuromuscular and muscular, respectively.

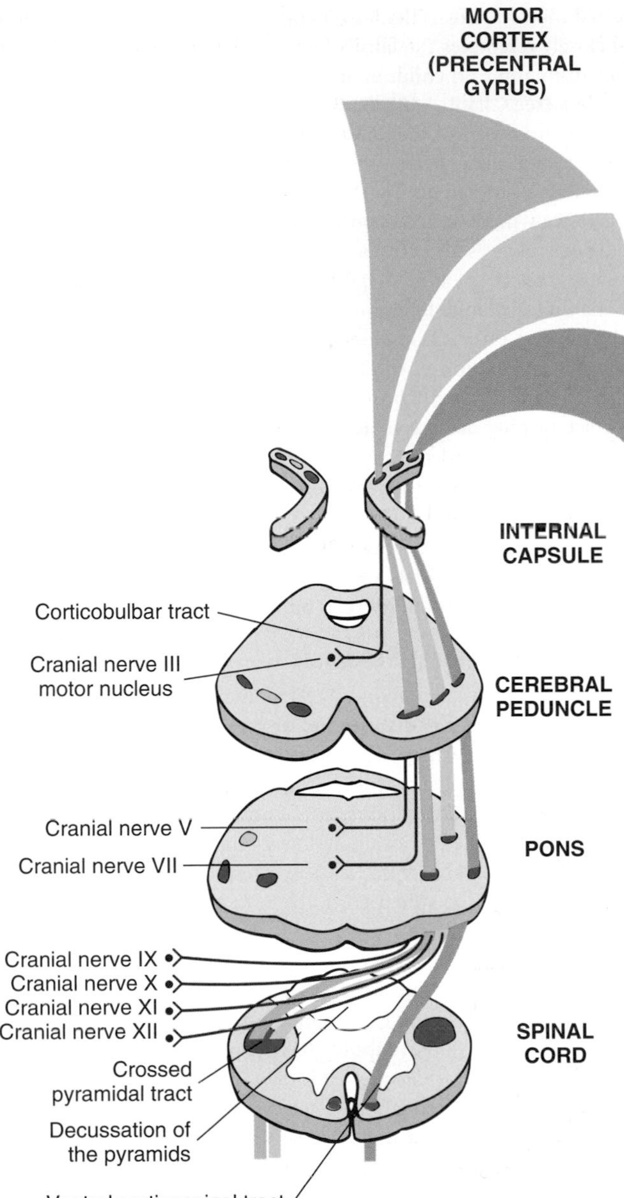

FIGURE 15-18 Structures of the Upper Motor Neuron, or Pyramidal, System. Pyramidal system fibres are shown to originate primarily in cells in the precentral gyrus of the motor cortex; to converge at the internal capsule; to descend to form the central third of the cerebral peduncle; to descend further through the pons, where small fibres supply cranial nerve motor nuclei along the way; to form pyramids at the medulla, where most of the fibres decussate; and then to continue to descend in the lateral column of white matter of the spinal cord. A few fibres descend without crossing at the level of the medulla (i.e., the ventral [anterior] corticospinal tract).

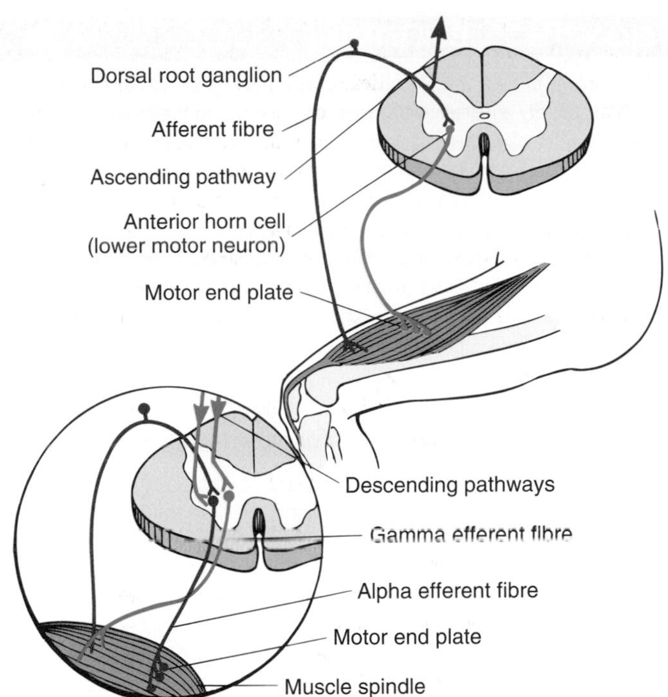

FIGURE 15-19 Structures Composing Lower Motor Neuron, Including Motor (Efferent) and Sensory (Afferent) Elements. (*Top*) Anterior horn cell (in anterior grey column of spinal cord and its axon), terminating in motor end plate as it innervates extrafusal muscle fibres in quadriceps muscle. (*Detailed enlargement*) Sensory and motor elements of gamma loop system. Gamma efferent fibres shown innervating the muscle spindle (sensory receptor of skeletal muscle). Contraction of muscle spindle fibres stretches the central portion of the spindle and causes the gamma afferent spindle fibre to transmit impulse centrally to the cord. Muscle spindle gamma afferent fibres in turn synapse on the anterior horn cell, and impulses are transmitted by way of alpha efferent fibres to skeletal (extrafusal) muscle, causing it to contract. Muscle spindle discharge is interrupted by active contraction of skeletal muscle fibres.

If all motor units are affected, complete paralysis results. Other clinical manifestations also are proportional to the degree of dysfunction, but the precise manifestations depend on the location of the dysfunction in the motor unit and in the CNS.

Small motor (gamma) neurons, which maintain muscle tone and protect the muscle from injury, are needed for normal motor movement. They depend on input from the muscle spindle (arriving through an afferent limb rising to the cord). Dysfunction in this motor system (the gamma loop) impairs tone and reduces tendon reflexes, causing hyporeflexia. The muscles become susceptible to damage from hyperextensibility.

Generally, the large and small motor neuron systems are equally affected. Therefore, the muscle has reduced or absent tone and is accompanied by hyporeflexia or **areflexia** (loss of tendon reflexes) and **flaccid paresis/paralysis**.

Denervated muscles (i.e., muscles that have lost their nervous system input) atrophy over weeks to months, mostly from disuse, and demonstrate **fasciculations** (muscle rippling or quivering under the skin). Occasionally, denervated muscles cramp. **Fibrillation** is isolated contraction of a single muscle fibre because of metabolic changes in denervated muscle and is not clinically visible.

Motor Neuron Diseases

Motor neuron diseases result from progressive degeneration of upper or lower motor neurons in the spinal cord, brainstem, or cortex. Amyotrophic lateral sclerosis and paralytic poliomyelitis (see Chapter 8) are examples of these diseases.

Several pathological processes may give rise to motor neuron diseases that can be sporadic or inherited. A virally induced or postinfectious or postvaccination inflammatory process may injure or destroy anterior horn cells or cranial nerve cell bodies. Most of these inflammatory processes are mild and are followed by rapid cellular recovery (Box 15-7).

BOX 15-7 Bell's Palsy

The etiology of Bell's palsy (unilateral facial nerve palsy) remains unknown. There is usually an inflammatory reaction compressing the facial nerve, particularly in the narrowest segment, followed by demyelinating neural change. The most distressing signs are unilateral facial weakness and the inability to smile or whistle. Bell's palsy may be caused by reactivation of herpes viruses in cranial nerve VII (facial), geniculate ganglia, or an autoimmune response. The signs usually have an acute onset (within 72 hours). Herpes simplex type 1 has been detected in up to 78% of cases, and herpes zoster has been detected in 30% of cases. Severe pain with facial palsy and a vesicular rash in the ear or mouth suggest herpes zoster infection. Ramsay Hunt syndrome (herpes zoster oticus) is rare, but complete recovery is less than 50%. Recovery from Bell's palsy is usually complete. Both disorders may be treated with combination antivirals and oral steroids. Treatment should be individualized according to severity of symptoms.

Data from Baugh, R.F., Basura, G.J., Ishii, L.E., et al. (2013). *Otolaryngol Head Neck Surg, 149*(3 Suppl.), S1–S27. Retrieved from http://oto.sagepub.com/content/149/3_suppl/S1.full); De Ru, J.A., & Van Benthem, P.P. (2014). *Evid Based Med, 19*(1), 15; Glass, G.E., & Tzafetta, K. (2014). *Fam Pract, 31*(6), 631–642; Greco, A., Gallo, A., Fusconi, M., et al. (2012). *Autoimmun Rev, 12*(2), 323–328.

In motor neuron disease, muscle strength, muscle tone, and muscle bulk are affected in the muscles innervated by the involved motor neurons. The paresis and paralysis associated with anterior horn cell injury are segmental, but because each muscle is supplied by two or more roots, the segmental character of the weakness may be difficult to recognize. When cranial nerve motor nuclei are affected (they lack nerve roots and have only small rootlets near the point of exit from the brainstem), the distribution of the motor weakness follows that of the peripheral nerve. The weakness may involve distal muscles, proximal muscles, and the muscles of midline structures. Hypotonia and hyporeflexia or areflexia are present.

The atrophy associated with motor neuron disease is segmental when the anterior horn cells of the spinal cord are involved and follows the distribution of the peripheral nerve when the motor nuclei of the cranial nerves are affected. The atrophy may be in distal, proximal, or midline muscles. Fasciculations are particularly associated with primary motor neuron injury, and muscle cramps are common. Mild fatigue is a common complaint. If the pathological process is limited to the primary motor neuron, no sensory changes are evident.

Because degenerative disorders can cause loss of nerve cells in the anterior horn or motor nuclei, the surviving cells are small, shrunken, and filled with lipofuscin. Lost neurons are replaced by astrocytes. The roots or rootlets are thin, and the muscles show denervation and atrophy.

Several brainstem syndromes involve damage to one or more of the cranial nerve nuclei. These syndromes are called *cranial nerve palsy* and may be caused by vascular occlusion, tumour, aneurysm, tuberculosis, or hemorrhage.

The anterior horn cells and the motor nuclei of the cranial nerves may be affected secondarily in many severe pathological processes that primarily involve the peripheral nerves. The condition may extend proximally to affect the nerve roots or rootlets and the motor neurons themselves, a process commonly seen, for example, in **Guillain-Barré syndrome** (see Chapter 16). If sufficient numbers of motor neurons are destroyed, permanent loss of motor function results because regeneration of the damaged axons requires a living neuronal cell body.

A group of degenerative disorders principally cause progressive motor cell atrophy. One of these disorders is **progressive spinal muscular atrophy**, in which the anterior horn cells of the spinal cord are the affected motor neurons that degenerate. This disorder occurs in adults and closely resembles the familial progressive muscular atrophies that occur in infants and children and are considered inherited metabolic disorders (see Chapter 40). If the motor nuclei of the cranial nerves are affected instead of the anterior horn cells, the disorder is labelled **progressive bulbar palsy**, so named because the myelencephalon originally was called the *bulb* and a degenerative process causes a progressively more serious condition. When any lower motor neuron syndrome involves the cranial nerves that arise from the bulb (i.e., cranial nerves IX, X, and XII), the dysfunction is called a **bulbar palsy**.

The clinical manifestations of bulbar palsy include paresis or paralysis of the jaw, face, pharynx, and tongue musculature. Articulation is affected, especially articulation of the lingual (*r*, *n*, *l*), labial (*b*, *m*, *p*, *f*), dental (*d*, *t*), and palatal (*k*, *g*) consonants. Modulation is impaired, making the voice rasping or nasal. Pharyngeal reflexes are diminished or lost. Palate and vocal cord movement during phonation is impaired, and chewing and swallowing are affected. The facial muscles are weak, and the face appears to droop. The jaw jerk is decreased. Atrophy eventually becomes apparent, as do fasciculations. All of these manifestations become progressively worse, leading to aspiration, malnutrition, possible dehydration, and an inability to communicate verbally.

Amyotrophic Lateral Sclerosis

Amyotrophic lateral sclerosis (ALS; sporadic motor neuron disease, sporadic motor system disease, motor neuron disease [MND], Lou Gehrig's disease) is a worldwide neuro-degenerative disorder that diffusely involves lower and upper motor neurons, resulting in progressive muscle weakness. *Amyotrophic* (without muscle nutrition or progressive muscle wasting) refers to the predominant lower motor neuron component of the syndrome. *Lateral sclerosis*, scarring of the corticospinal tract in the lateral column of the spinal cord, refers to the upper motor neuron component of the syndrome.

ALS occurs in young adults or older adults, but it is most commonly diagnosed in middle to late adulthood. It affects both men and women with about 2 cases per 100 000 population in Canada.[42] Most cases of ALS are sporadic. A subset (about 10%) of persons has a familial form with genetic mutations in superoxide dismutase (SOD) that contribute to the neurotoxicity affecting motor neurons. Mutated TAR RNA-binding protein 43 (TDP-43) is a major constituent of the neuronal protein inclusions in ALS. Gene and environmental interactions are being evaluated as a cause of ALS.[43]

PATHOPHYSIOLOGY The cause of ALS is unknown. Oxidative stress, mitochondrial dysfunction, defects in axonal transport, excitotoxicity and glutamate transport, neuronal cytoplasmic inclusions (i.e., TDP-43 protein), and neuro-inflammation as causes of neuron degeneration are under investigation.[44]

The principal pathological feature of ALS is degeneration of lower and upper motor neurons. There is a decrease in large motor neurons in the spinal cord, brainstem, and cerebral cortex (premotor and motor areas), with ongoing degeneration in the remaining motor neurons. Death of the motor neuron results in axonal degeneration and secondary demyelination with glial proliferation and sclerosis (scarring). Widespread neural degeneration of nonmotor neurons in the spinal cord and motor cortices, as well as in the premotor, sensory, and temporal cortices, has been found.

Lower motor neuron degeneration denervates motor units. Adjacent, still viable lower motor neurons attempt to compensate by distal intramuscular sprouting, reinnervation, and enlargement of motor units.

CLINICAL MANIFESTATIONS The initial symptoms of the disease are heterogeneous and may be related to lower or upper motor neuron dysfunction or both. About 60% of individuals have a spinal form of the disease with focal muscle weakness beginning in the arms and legs and progressing to muscle atrophy, spasticity, and loss of manual dexterity and gait. No associated mental, sensory, or autonomic symptoms are present. ALS with progressive bulbar palsy presents with difficulty speaking and swallowing, and peripheral muscle weakness and atrophy usually occur within 1 to 2 years. These individuals have a poorer response to treatment with mechanical ventilation.[45] FTD may occur concurrently.[46]

EVALUATION AND TREATMENT Diagnosis of ALS is based predominantly on the history and physical examination with no evidence of other neuromuscular disorders. Electromyography and muscle biopsy results verify lower motor neuron degeneration and denervation. Imaging studies and CSF biomarkers can assist in making the diagnosis. Little treatment is available to alter the overall course of the ALS syndrome. The medication riluzole (Rilutek), an antiglutamate, has extended the length of time patients do not require ventilatory assistance. Supportive and rehabilitative management are directed toward preventing complications of immobility. Psychological support of the affected individual and the family is extremely important.[47] ALS is fatal from respiratory failure usually within 3 years of diagnosis. A small percentage of individuals live 5 to 10 years or longer.[48]

ALTERATIONS IN COMPLEX MOTOR PERFORMANCE

Alterations in complex motor performance include disorders of posture (stance), disorders of gait, and disorders of expression.

Disorders of Posture (Stance)

An inequality of tone in muscle groups, because of a loss of normal postural reflexes, results in a posturing of limbs. Equilibrium and balance are disrupted. Many reflex systems govern tone and posture, but the most important factor in posture control is the stretch reflex, in which extensor (antigravity) muscle stretching causes increased extensor tone and inhibited flexor tone. Four types of disorders of posture are (1) dystonic posture, (2) decorticate posture/response, (3) decerebrate posture/response, and (4) basal ganglion posture.

Dystonia is the maintenance of an abnormal posture through muscular contractions. When muscular contractions are sustained for several seconds, they are called **dystonic movements**; when contractions last for longer periods, they are called **dystonic postures**. Dystonic postures may last for weeks, causing permanent, fixed contractures. Dystonia has been associated with basal ganglia abnormality, but the exact pathophysiological mechanisms are unknown. One dystonic posture is decorticate posture/response (striatal posture or upper motor neuron dysfunction posture), which may be unilateral or bilateral.

Decorticate posture/response (also referred to as **antigravity posture** or **hemiplegic posture**) is characterized by upper extremities flexed at the elbows and held close to the body and by lower extremities that are externally rotated and extended (see Figure 15-6). Decorticate posture/response is thought to occur when the brainstem is not inhibited by the cerebral cortex motor area. Upper motor neuron posture is more commonly described as the arm flexed at the elbow with a wrist drop, the leg inadequately bent at the knee, the hip excessively circumabducted, and the presence of footdrop.

Decerebrate posture/response refers to increased tone in extensor muscles and trunk muscles, with active tonic neck reflexes. When the head is in a neutral position, all four limbs are rigidly extended (see Figure 15-6). The decerebrate posture is caused by severe injury to the brain and brainstem, resulting in overstimulation of the postural righting and vestibular reflexes.

Basal ganglion posture refers to a stooped, hyperflexed posture with a narrow-based, short-stepped gait. This posture abnormality results from the loss of normal postural reflexes and not from defects in proprioceptive, labyrinthine, or visual function. Dysfunctional equilibrium results when the individual loses stability and cannot make the appropriate postural adjustment to tilting or loss of balance, falling instead. Dysfunctional righting is the inability to right oneself when changing from a lying or crouching to a standing position or when rolling from the supine to the lateral or prone position. Dysfunctional postural fixation is the involuntary flexion of the head and neck, causing the person difficulty in maintaining an upright trunk position while standing or walking. Basal ganglion dysfunction accounts for this posture.

Disorders of Gait

Four predominant types of gait associated with neurological disorders are (1) upper motor neuron dysfunction gait, (2) cerebellar (ataxic) gait, (3) basal ganglion gait, and (4) frontal lobe ataxic gait. As with posture, equilibrium and balance are affected with gait disturbances.[49]

Several types of **upper motor neuron gait** exist. With mild forms, the individual may have footdrop with fatigue and hip and leg pain. A spastic gait, which is associated with unilateral injury, manifests by a shuffling gait with the leg extended and held stiff, causing a scraping over the floor surface. The leg swings improperly around the body rather than being appropriately lifted and placed. The foot may drag on the ground, and the person tends to fall to the affected side. A scissors gait is associated with bilateral injury and spasticity. The legs are adducted so they touch each other. As the person walks, the legs are swung around the body but then cross in front of each other because of adduction. Injury to the pyramidal system accounts for these gaits (e.g., stroke, cerebral palsy, multiple sclerosis, spinal cord tumour).

A **cerebellar (ataxic) gait** is wide-based, with the feet apart and often turned outward or inward for greater stability. The pelvis is held stiff, and the individual staggers when walking. Cerebellar dysfunction with loss of coordination accounts for this particular gait.

A **basal ganglion gait** is a broad-based gait in which the person walks with small steps and a decreased arm swing. The head and body are flexed and the arms semiflexed and abducted, whereas the legs are flexed and rigid in more advanced states. Basal ganglion dysfunction accounts for this gait and is associated with PD.

A **frontal lobe ataxic gait** is wide-based with increased body sway and falls, loss of control of truncal motion, gait ignition failure, start hesitation, shuffling, and freezing. The gait is associated with frontal lobe damage or degeneration. The pattern may change as the frontal disease progresses. The slowness of walking, lack of heel–shin or upper limb ataxia, dysarthria, or nystagmus distinguishes the wide stance from cerebellar ataxic gait.[50]

Gait disorders are often accompanied by balance, coordination, and sensory dysfunction that further alter mobility and increase risk for falls. Assessment and intervention strategies are important for prevention of injury.

Disorders of Expression

Disorders of expression involve the motor aspects of communication and include (1) hypermimesis, (2) hypomimesis, and (3) apraxia or dyspraxia. **Hypermimesis** commonly manifests as pathological laughter or crying. Pathological laughter is associated with right hemisphere injury, and pathological crying is associated with left hemisphere injury. The exact pathophysiology is not known. **Hypomimesis** manifests as *aprosody*—the loss of emotional language. *Receptive aprosody* involves an inability to understand emotion in speech and facial expression.

TABLE 15-19 Pyramidal Versus Extrapyramidal Motor Syndrome

Manifestations	Pyramidal Motor Syndrome	Extrapyramidal Motor Syndrome
Unilateral movement	Paralysis of voluntary movement	Little or no paralysis of voluntary movement
Tendon reflexes	Increased tendon reflexes	Normal or slightly increased tendon reflexes
Babinski sign	Present	Absent
Involuntary movements	Absence of involuntary movements	Presence of tremor, chorea, athetosis, or dystonia
Muscle tone	Spasticity in muscles (e.g., clasp-knife phenomenon)	Plastic rigidity (equal throughout movement) or intermittent—cogwheel rigidity (generalized but predominantly in flexors of limbs and trunk)
	Hypertonia present in flexors of arms and extensors of legs	Hypotonia, weakness and gait disturbances in cerebellar disease

Expressive aprosody involves the inability to express emotion in speech and facial expression. Aprosody is associated with right hemisphere damage.

Apraxia or dyspraxia is a disorder of learned skilled movements with difficulty planning and executing coordinated motor movements. The term is often used interchangeably with *dyspraxia*. It can be developmental, beginning at birth (developmental apraxia), or associated with vascular disorders (common in stroke), trauma, tumours, degenerative disorders, infections, or metabolic disorders. People with apraxia have difficulty performing tasks requiring motor skills, including speaking, writing, using tools or utensils, playing sports, following instructions, and focusing.[51]

True apraxias occur when the connecting pathways between the left and right cortical areas are interrupted. Apraxias may result from any pathological process that disrupts the cortical areas necessary for the conceptualization and execution of a complex motor act or the communication pathways within the left hemisphere or between the hemispheres.[51,52]

EXTRAPYRAMIDAL MOTOR SYNDROMES

Because the extrapyramidal system encompasses all the motor pathways except the pyramidal system, two types of motor dysfunction make up the **extrapyramidal motor syndromes**: (1) basal ganglia motor syndromes and (2) cerebellar motor syndromes. Unlike pyramidal motor syndromes, both extrapyramidal motor syndromes result in movement or posture disturbance without significant paralysis, along with other distinctive symptoms (Table 15-19).

Basal ganglia motor syndromes are caused by an imbalance of dopaminergic and cholinergic activity in the corpus striatum. A relative excess of cholinergic activity produces akinesia and hypertonia. A relative excess of dopaminergic activity produces hyperkinesia and hypotonia. Symptoms associated with Parkinson's and Huntington's diseases are exemplary of disorders of the basal ganglia. **Cerebellar motor syndromes** are associated with ataxia and other symptoms affecting coordinated movement. Cerebellar motor syndromes primarily influence the same side of the body; for example, damage to the right cerebellum generally causes symptoms on the right side of the body.

Medication-induced extrapyramidal effects may also be encountered with short- or long-term use of certain medications. The medications involved, including the antipsychotic haloperidol (Haldol) and the antiemetic metoclopramide (Metoclopramide), antagonize the dopamine D2 receptors, resulting in extrapyramidal adverse effects.

✔ QUICK CHECK 15-6

1. Why are there so many causes of hypertonia?
2. How is chorea different from athetosis?
3. Why is paresis/paralysis a type of hypokinesia?
4. What structures are involved in alterations of complex motor performance?

DID YOU UNDERSTAND?

Alterations in Cognitive Systems

1. Full consciousness is an awareness of oneself and the environment with an ability to respond to external stimuli with a wide variety of responses.
2. Consciousness has two components: arousal (level of awakeness) and awareness (content of thought).
3. An altered level of arousal occurs by diffuse bilateral cortical dysfunction, bilateral subcortical (reticular formation, brainstem) dysfunction, localized hemispheric dysfunction, and metabolic disorders.
4. An alteration in breathing pattern and the level of consciousness reflect the level of brain dysfunction.
5. Pupillary changes reflect changes in level of brainstem function, medication action, and response to hypoxia and ischemia.
6. Abnormal eye movements, including nystagmus, reflect alterations in brainstem function.
7. Level of brain function manifests by changes in generalized motor responses or no responses.
8. Loss of cortical inhibition associated with decreased consciousness produces abnormal flexor and extensor movements.
9. Brain death results from irreversible brain damage, with an inability to maintain internal homeostasis.
10. Cerebral death, or irreversible coma, represents permanent brain damage, with an ability to maintain cardiac, respiratory, and other vital functions.
11. Arousal returns in vegetative states, but awareness is absent.
12. Alterations in awareness include alterations in executive attention (abstract reasoning, planning, decision making, judgement, error correction, and self-control) and memory.
13. With a deficit in selective attention, mediated by midbrain, thalamus, and parietal lobe structures, the individual cannot focus on selective stimuli and thus neglects those stimuli.
14. In retrograde amnesia, some past memories are lost; and in anterograde amnesia, new memories cannot be formed.
15. Frontal areas mediate vigilance, detection, and working (short-term) memory.

16. With vigilance deficits, the person cannot maintain sustained concentration.
17. With detection deficits, the person is unmotivated and may be perceived by others as lazy or apathetic, demonstrated by the inability to set goals and plan.
18. Data-processing deficits include agnosias, dysphasias, acute confusional states, and dementias.
19. Agnosias are defects of recognition and may be tactile, visual, or auditory. They are caused by dysfunction in the primary sensory area or the interpretive areas of the cerebral cortex.
20. Dysphasia (aphasia) is an impairment of comprehension or production of language. Most dysphasias are expressive or receptive.
21. Acute confusional states are characterized chiefly by a loss of detection and, in the case of delirium, intense autonomic nervous system hyperactivity.
22. Alzheimer's disease is a chronic irreversible dementia that is related to altered production or failure to clear amyloid from the brain with plaque formation, formation of neurofibrillary tangles, and loss of basal forebrain cholinergic neurons.
23. Frontotemporal dementias are rare early-onset degenerative diseases similar to Alzheimer's disease.
24. Seizures represent a sudden, chaotic discharge of cerebral neurons with transient alterations in brain function. Seizures may be generalized or focal and can result from cerebral lesions, biochemical disorders, trauma, or epilepsy.

Alterations in Cerebral Hemodynamics

1. Alterations in cerebral blood flow are related to changes in cerebral perfusion pressure, changes in cerebral blood volume, and cerebral blood oxygenation.
2. Increased intracranial pressure (increased ICP) may result from edema, excess cerebrospinal fluid (CSF), hemorrhage, or tumour growth. When ICP approaches arterial pressure, hypoxia and hypercapnia produce brain damage.
3. Cerebral edema is an increase in the fluid content of the brain resulting from infection, hemorrhage, tumour, ischemia, infarction, or hypoxia. Cerebral edema can cause increased ICP.
4. The shifting or herniation of brain tissue from one compartment to another disrupts the blood flow of both compartments and damages brain tissue.
5. Supratentorial herniation involves the temporal lobe and hippocampal gyrus shifting from the middle fossa to posterior fossa; transtentorial herniation involves a downward shift of the diencephalon through the tentorial notch; and shifting of the cingulate gyrus can occur under the falx cerebri.
6. The most common infratentorial herniation is a shift of the cerebellar tonsils through the foramen magnum.
7. Hydrocephalus comprises a variety of disorders characterized by an excess of fluid within the ventricles, subarachnoid space, or both. Hydrocephalus occurs because of interference with CSF flow caused by increased fluid production or obstruction within the ventricular system or by defective reabsorption of the fluid.

Alterations in Neuromotor Function

1. General neuromotor dysfunctions are associated with changes in muscle tone, movement, and complex motor performance.
2. Hypotonia and hypertonia are the main categories of altered tone.
3. Hypotonia is associated with pyramidal tract or cerebellar injury. Muscles are flaccid and weak with atrophy.
4. The four types of hypertonia are spasticity, paratonia (gegenhalten), dystonia, and rigidity.
5. Hyperkinesia, hypokinesia, paresis, and paralysis are the main categories of alterations in muscle movement.
6. Included in the category of hyperkinesia are chorea, athetosis, ballism, akathisia, tremor, and myoclonus.
7. Huntington's disease (chorea) is a rare hereditary disease involving the basal ganglia and cerebral cortex that commonly manifests between 25 and 45 years of age.
8. The major pathological feature of Huntington's disease is severe degeneration of the basal ganglia and the cerebral cortex with an excess of dopaminergic activity that causes involuntary, fragmentary hyperkinetic movements.
9. Types of hypokinesia include akinesia, bradykinesia, and loss of associated movement.
10. Parkinson's disease is a commonly occurring degenerative disorder of the basal ganglia (corpus striatum) involving degeneration of the dopamine-secreting nigrostriatal pathway.
11. Dopamine depletion in the basal ganglia and excess cholinergic activity in the cortex, basal ganglia, and thalamus cause tremor and rigidity in Parkinson's disease. Progressive dementia may be associated with an advanced stage of the disease.
12. An upper motor neuron syndrome is characterized by paresis or paralysis, hypertonia, and hyperreflexia.
13. Two subtypes of paresis or paralysis are upper motor neuron spastic paresis/paralysis and lower motor neuron flaccid paresis/paralysis.
14. Upper motor neuron syndromes are the result of damage to descending motor pathways at cortical, brainstem, or spinal cord levels and result in spastic paralysis.
15. Spinal shock is temporary loss of all spinal cord function below the lesion (below the level of the pons). It is characterized by complete flaccid paralysis, absence of reflexes, and marked disturbances of bowel and bladder function.
16. Lower motor neuron syndromes manifest by impaired voluntary and involuntary movements and flaccid paralysis.
17. Partial paralysis occurs with only partial loss of alpha motor neurons, and total paralysis is complete loss of alpha motor neurons. Loss of gamma motor neurons impairs muscle tone and decreases tendon reflexes.
18. Lower (primary, alpha) motor neuron syndromes involve the large motor neurons in the anterior (or ventral) horn of the spinal cord and the motor nuclei of the brainstem and cause flaccid paralysis.
19. Amyotrophic lateral sclerosis involves degeneration of both upper and lower motor neurons with progressive muscle weakness and atrophy.

Alterations in Complex Motor Performance

1. Alterations in complex motor performance include disorders of posture (stance), disorders of gait, and disorders of expression.
2. Disorders of posture include dystonic posture, decerebrate posture/response, basal ganglion posture, and senile posture.
3. Disorders of gait include upper motor neuron gait, cerebellar (ataxic) gait, basal ganglion gait, and frontal lobe ataxic gait.
4. Disorders of expression include hypermimesis, hypomimesis, and apraxia (dyspraxia).
5. Apraxia is an impairment of the conceptualization or execution of a complex motor act.

Extrapyramidal Motor Syndromes

1. Extrapyramidal motor syndromes include basal ganglia and cerebellar motor syndromes.
2. Basal ganglia motor syndromes manifest by alterations in muscle tone and posture, including rigidity, involuntary movements, and loss of postural reflexes.
3. Cerebellar motor syndromes result in loss of muscle tone, difficulty with coordination, and disorders of equilibrium and gait.

KEY TERMS

Acute confusional state, 371
Acute hydrocephalus, 380
Agnosia, 371
Akinesia, 384
Alzheimer's disease (AD) (dementia of Alzheimer's type [DAT], senile disease complex), 374
Amnesia, 369
Amyotrophic lateral sclerosis, 388
Anterograde amnesia, 369
Aphasia, 371
Apraxia or dyspraxia, 390
Areflexia, 387
Arousal, 363
Autoregulation, 378
Awareness, 369
Basal ganglia motor syndrome, 390
Basal ganglion gait, 389
Basal ganglion posture, 389
Bradykinesia, 384
Brain death (total brain death), 368
Bulbar palsy, 388
Cerebellar (ataxic) gait, 389
Cerebellar motor syndrome, 390
Cerebral blood flow (CBF), 377
Cerebral blood oxygenation, 378
Cerebral blood volume (CBV), 377
Cerebral death (irreversible coma), 368
Cerebral edema, 379
Cerebral perfusion pressure (CPP), 378
Clonic phase, 377
Communicating hydrocephalus, 380
Consciousness, 363
Convulsion, 376
Cytotoxic (metabolic) edema, 380
Decerebrate posture/response, 389
Decorticate posture/response (antigravity posture, hemiplegic posture), 389
Delirium (hyperactive confusional state), 373
Dementia, 373
Diplegia, 386
Dysphasia, 371
Dyspraxia, 375
Dystonia, 389
Dystonic movement, 389
Dystonic posture, 389
Epilepsy, 376
Epileptogenic focus, 377
Excited delirium syndrome (ExDS), 373
Executive attention deficit, 369
Extinction, 369
Extrapyramidal motor syndrome, 390
Fasciculation, 387
Fibrillation, 387
Flaccid paresis/paralysis, 387
Frontal lobe ataxic gait, 389
Frontotemporal dementia (FTD) (Pick disease), 376
Guillain-Barré syndrome, 388
Hemiparesis, 386
Hemiplegia, 386
Hiccup, 367
Huntington's disease (HD), 382
Hydrocephalus, 380
Hyperkinesia, 382
Hypermimesis, 389
Hypertonia, 381
Hypoactive delirium (hypoactive confusional state), 373
Hypokinesia, 384
Hypomimesis, 389
Hypotonia, 380
Ictus, 377
Image processing, 369
Increased intracranial pressure (increased ICP), 378
Interstitial edema, 380
Intracranial pressure (ICP), 377
Level of consciousness, 364
Locked-in syndrome, 369
Lower motor neuron syndromes, 386
Memory, 369
Memory disorder, 369
Minimally conscious state (MCS), 369
Mirror focus, 377
Motor response, 367
Neglect syndrome, 369
Neuritic plaques, 374
Neurofibrillary tangle, 375
Noncommunicating hydrocephalus (internal hydrocephalus, intraventricular hydrocephalus), 380
Normal-pressure hydrocephalus, 380
Oculomotor response, 364
Paralysis, 385
Paraparesis, 386
Paraplegia, 386
Paratonia (gegenhalten), 381
Paresis, 385
Parkinsonism (Parkinson's syndrome, parkinsonian syndrome, paralysis agitans), 384
Parkinson's disease (PD), 384
Paroxysmal dyskinesia, 382
Patterns of breathing, 364
Persistent vegetative state (VS), 369
Postictal phase, 377
Preictal phase, 377
Prodroma, 377
Progressive bulbar palsy, 388
Progressive spinal muscular atrophy, 388
Psychogenic alterations in arousal (unresponsiveness), 364
Pupillary change, 364
Pyramidal motor syndrome, 385
Quadriparesis, 386
Quadriplegia, 386
Retrograde amnesia, 369
Rigidity, 381
Secondary parkinsonism, 384
Seizure, 376
Selective attention, 369
Selective attention deficit, 369
Sensory inattentiveness, 369
Spasticity, 381
Spinal shock, 386
Status epilepticus, 377
Structural alterations in arousal, 363
Tardive dyskinesia, 382
Tentorium cerebelli, 363
Tonic phase, 377
Tourette syndrome, 382
Upper motor neuron gait, 389
Upper motor neuron paresis or paralysis, 385
Vasogenic edema, 379
Vomiting, 367
Yawning, 367

REFERENCES

1. Shemie, S. D., Doig, C., Dickens, B., et al. (2006). Severe brain injury to neurological determination of death: Canadian forum recommendations. *CMAJ : Canadian Medical Association Journal, 174*(6), S1–S12. doi:10.1503/cmaj.045142.
2. Shemie, S. D., Doig, C., Dickens, B., et al. (2006). Brain arrest: The neurological determination of death and organ donor management in Canada. *CMAJ : Canadian Medical Association Journal, 174*(6), S1–S30. doi:10.1503/cmaj.045142.
3. Overgaard, M. (2009). How can we know if patients in coma, vegetative state or minimally conscious state are conscious? *Progress in Brain Research, 177*, 11–19. doi:10.1016/S0079-6123(09)17702-6.
4. Hirschberg, R., & Giacino, J. T. (2011). The vegetative and minimally conscious states: Diagnosis, prognosis and treatment. *Neurologic Clinics, 29*(4), 773–786. doi:10.1016/j.ncl.2011.07.009.
5. Lacroix, G., Couret, D., Combaz, X., et al. (2012). Transient locked-in syndrome and basilar artery vasospasm. *Neurocritical Care, 16*(1), 145–147. doi:10.1007/s12028-011-9655-z.
6. Carrasco, M. (2011). Visual attention: The past 25 years. *Vision Research, 51*(13), 1484–1525. doi:10.1016/j.visres.2011.04.012.
7. Zaal, I. J., & Slooter, A. J. (2012). Delirium in critically ill patients: Epidemiology, pathophysiology, diagnosis and management. *Drugs, 72*(11), 1457–1471. doi:10.2165/11635520-000000000-00000.
8. Barr, J., Fraser, G. L., Puntillo, K., et al. (2013). Clinical practice guidelines for the management of pain, agitation, and delirium in adult patients in the intensive care unit. *Critical Care Medicine, 41*(1), 263–306. doi:10.1097/CCM.0b013e3182783b72. Retrieved from http://www.learnicu.org/pages/guidelines.aspx.
9. Devlin, J. W., Brummel, M. E., & Al-Qadheeb, N. S. (2012). Optimising the recognition of delirium in the intensive care unit. *Best Practice and Research. Clinical Anaesthesiology, 26*(3), 385–393. doi:10.1016/j.bpa.2012.08.002.
10. Grover, S., & Kate, N. (2012). Assessment scales for delirium: A review. *World Journal of Psychiatry, 2*(4), 58–70. doi:10.5498/wjp.v2.i4.58.
11. Morandi, A., McCurley, J., Vasilevskis, E. E., et al. (2012). Tools to detect delirium superimposed on dementia: A systematic review. *Journal of the American Geriatrics Society, 60*(11), 2005–2013. doi: 10.1111/j.1532-5415.2012.04199.x. Erratum in *J Am Geriatr Soc, 61*(1), 174, 2013.
12. Zhang, H., Lu, Y., Liu, M., et al. (2013). Strategies for prevention of postoperative delirium: A systematic review and meta-analysis of randomized trials. *Critical Care, 17*(2), R47. doi:10.1186/cc12566.
13. Alzheimer Society Canada. (2016). *Dementia numbers in Canada*. Retrieved from http://www.alzheimer.ca/en/About-dementia/What-is-dementia/Dementia-numbers.

14. Reitz, C., & Mayeux, R. (2014). Alzheimer disease: Epidemiology, diagnostic criteria, risk factors and biomarkers. *Biochemical Pharmacology, 88*(4), 640–651. doi:10.1016/j.bcp.2013.12.024.
15. Coppieters, N., Dieriks, B. V., Lill, C., et al. (2014). Global changes in DNA methylation and hydroxymethylation in Alzheimer's disease human brain. *Neurobiology of Aging, 35*(6), 1334–1344. doi:10.1016/j.neurobiolaging.2013.11.031.
16. Loy, C. T., Schofield, P. R., Turner, A. M., et al. (2014). Genetics of dementia. *Lancet, 383*(9919), 828–840. doi:10.1016/S0140-6736(13)60630-3.
17. Bloom, G. S. (2014). Amyloid-β and tau: The trigger and bullet in Alzheimer disease pathogenesis. *JAMA Neurology, 71*(4), 505–508. doi:10.1001/jamaneurol.2013.5847.
18. Cummings, J. L., Dubois, B., Molinuevo, J. L., et al. (2013). International Work Group criteria for the diagnosis of Alzheimer disease. *Medical Clinics of North America, 97*(3), 363–368. doi:10.1016/j.mcna.2013.01.001.
19. Wurtman, R. (2015). Biomarkers in the diagnosis and management of Alzheimer's disease. *Metabolism: Clinical and Experimental, 64*(3 Suppl. 1), S47–S50. doi:10.1016/j.metabol.2014.10.034.
20. Kumar, A., Singh, A., & Ekavali. (2015). A review on Alzheimer's disease pathophysiology and its management: An update. *Pharmacological Reports, 67*(2), 195–203. doi:10.1016/j.pharep.2014.09.004.
21. Rohan, Z., & Matej, R. (2014). Current concepts in the classification and diagnosis of frontotemporal lobar degenerations: A practical approach. *Archives of Pathology & Laboratory Medicine, 138*(1), 132–138. doi:10.5858/arpa.2012-0510-RS.
22. Casillas-Espinosa, P. M., Powell, K. L., & O'Brien, T. J. (2012). Regulators of synaptic transmission: Roles in the pathogenesis and treatment of epilepsy. *Epilepsia, 53*(Suppl. 9), 41–58. doi:10.1111/epi.12034.
23. Rémi, J., & Noachtar, S. (2010). Clinical features of the postictal state: Correlation with seizure variables. *Epilepsy and Behavior, 19*(2), 114–117. doi:10.1016/j.yebeh.2010.06.039.
24. Kumar, A., Valentín, A., Humayon, D., et al. (2013). Preoperative estimation of seizure control after resective surgery for the treatment of epilepsy. *Seizure, 22*(10), 818–826. doi:10.1016/j.seizure.2013.06.010.
25. Payne, N. E., Cross, J. H., Sander, J. W., et al. (2011). The ketogenic and related diets in adolescents and adults—A review. *Epilepsia, 52*(11), 1941–1948. doi:10.1111/j.1528-1167.2011.03287.x.
26. Kiefer, M., & Unterberg, A. (2012). The differential diagnosis and treatment of normal-pressure hydrocephalus. *Deutsches Ärzteblatt International, 109*(1–2), 15–25. doi:10.3238/arztebl.2012.0015.
27. Ziebell, M., Wetterslev, J., Tisell, M., et al. (2013). Flow-regulated versus differential pressure-regulated shunt valves for adult patients with normal pressure hydrocephalus. *Cochrane Database of Systematic Reviews*, (5), CD009706, doi:10.1002/14651858.CD009706.pub2.
28. Agostinho, L. A., Dos Santos, S. R., Alvarenga, R. M., et al. (2013). A systematic review of the intergenerational aspects and the diverse genetic profiles of Huntington's disease. *Genetics and Molecular Research, 12*(2), 1974–1981. doi:10.4238/2013.June.13.6.
29. Labbadia, J., & Morimoto, R. I. (2013). Huntington's disease: Underlying molecular mechanisms and emerging concepts. *Trends in Biochemical Sciences, 38*(8), 378–385. doi:10.1016/j.tibs.2013.05.003.
30. Ross, C. A., & Tabrizi, S. J. (2011). Huntington's disease: From molecular pathogenesis to clinical treatment. *Lancet. Neurology, 10*(1), 83–98. doi:10.1016/S1474-4422(10)70245-3.
31. Kumar, P., Kalonia, H., & Kumar, A. (2010). Huntington's disease: Pathogenesis to animal models. *Pharmacological Reports, 62*(1), 1–14.
32. Dayalu, P., & Albin, R. L. (2015). Huntington disease: Pathogenesis and treatment. *Neurologic Clinics, 33*(1), 101–114. doi:10.1016/j.ncl.2014.09.003.
33. Statistics Canada. (2015). *Parkinson's disease: Prevalence, diagnosis and impact.* Retrieved from http://www.statcan.gc.ca/pub/82-003-x/2014011/article/14112-eng.htm.
34. Gaig, C., & Tolosa, E. (2009). When does Parkinson's disease begin? *Movement Disorders, 24*(Suppl. 2), S656–S664. doi:10.1002/mds.22672.
35. Hirsch, E. C., Jenner, P., & Przedborski, S. (2013). Pathogenesis of Parkinson's disease. *Movement Disorders, 28*(1), 24–30. doi:10.1002/mds.25032.
36. Yarnall, A., Rochester, L., & Burn, D. J. (2011). The interplay of cholinergic function, attention, and falls in Parkinson's disease. *Movement Disorders, 26*(14), 2496–2503. doi:10.1002/mds.23932.
37. Chaudhuri, K. R., & Odin, P. (2010). The challenge of non-motor symptoms in Parkinson's disease. *Progress in Brain Research, 184*, 325–341. doi:10.1016/S0079-6123(10)84017-8.
38. Sprenger, F., & Poewe, W. (2013). Management of motor and non-motor symptoms in Parkinson's disease. *CNS Drugs, 27*(4), 259–272. doi:10.1007/s40263-013-0053-2.
39. Miller, D. B., & O'Callaghan, J. P. (2015). Biomarkers of Parkinson's disease: Present and future. *Metabolism: Clinical and Experimental, 64*(3 Suppl. 1), S40–S46. doi:10.1016/j.metabol.2014.10.030.
40. Buttery, P. C., & Barker, R. A. (2014). Treating Parkinson's disease in the 21st century: Can stem cell transplantation compete? *Journal of Comparative Neurology, 522*(12), 2802–2816. doi:10.1002/cne.23577.
41. Giugni, J. C., & Okun, M. S. (2014). Treatment of advanced Parkinson's disease. *Current Opinion in Neurology, 27*(4), 450–460. doi:10.1097/WCO.0000000000000118.
42. Amyotrophic Lateral Sclerosis Society of Canada. (2015). *ALS quick facts.* Retrieved from https://www.als.ca/sites/default/files/files/ALS_Quick_Facts%282%29.pdf.
43. Al-Chalabi, A., & Hardiman, O. (2013). The epidemiology of ALS: A conspiracy of genes, environment and time. *Nature Reviews. Neurology, 9*(11), 617–628. doi:10.1038/nrneurol.2013.203.
44. Turner, M. R., Bowser, R., Bruijn, L., et al. (2013). Mechanisms, models and biomarkers in amyotrophic lateral sclerosis. *Amyotrophic Lateral Sclerosis and Frontotemporal Degeneration, 14*(Suppl. 1), 19–32. doi:10.3109/21678421.2013.778554.
45. Radunovic, A., Annane, D., Jewitt, K., et al. (2013). Mechanical ventilation for amyotrophic lateral sclerosis/motor neuron disease. *Cochrane Database of Systematic Reviews*, (3), CD004427, doi:10.1002/14651858.CD004427.pub3.
46. Bennion Callister, J., & Pickering-Brown, S. M. (2014). Pathogenesis/genetics of frontotemporal dementia and how it relates to ALS. *Experimental Neurology, 262*(Pt. B), 84–90. doi:10.1016/j.expneurol.2014.06.001.
47. Gordon, P. H. (2013). Amyotrophic lateral sclerosis: An update for 2013 Clinical Features, Pathophysiology, Management and Therapeutic Trials. *Aging and Disease, 4*(5), 295–310. doi:10.14336/AD.2013.0400295.
48. Wijesekera, L. C., & Leigh, P. N. (2009). Amyotrophic lateral sclerosis. *Orphanet Journal of Rare Diseases, 4*, 3. doi:10.1186/1750-1172-4-3.
49. Snijders, A. H., van de Warrenburg, B. P., Giladi, N., et al. (2007). Neurological gait disorders in elderly people: Clinical approach and classification. *Lancet. Neurology, 6*(1), 63–74. doi:10.1016/S1474-4422(06)70678-0.
50. Thompson, P. D. (2012). Frontal lobe ataxia. *Handbook of Clinical Neurology, 103*, 619–622. doi:10.1016/B978-0-444-51892-7.00044-9.
51. Foundas, A. L. (2013). Apraxia: Neural mechanisms and functional recovery. *Handbook of Clinical Neurology, 110*, 335–345. doi:10.1016/B978-0-444-52901-5.00028-9.
52. Zadikoff, C., & Lang, A. E. (2005). Apraxia in movement disorders. *Brain, 128*(Pt. 7), 1480–1497. doi:10.1093/brain/awh560.

16

Disorders of the Central and Peripheral Nervous Systems and Neuromuscular Junction

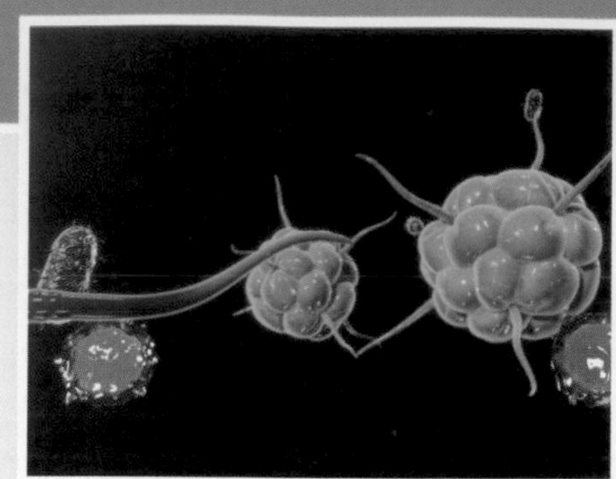

Barbara J. Boss, Sue E. Huether, and Kelly Power-Kean

EVOLVE WEBSITE

http://evolve.elsevier.com/Canada/Huether/pathophysiology
Student Review Questions
Key Points
Case Studies
Animations
Quick Check Answers

CHAPTER OUTLINE

Central Nervous System Disorders, 394
Traumatic Brain and Spinal Cord Injury, 394
Degenerative Disorders of the Spine, 402
Cerebrovascular Disorders, 406
Headache, 410
Infection and Inflammation of the Central Nervous System, 411
Demyelinating Disorders, 415
Peripheral Nervous System and Neuromuscular Junction Disorders, 416
Peripheral Nervous System Disorders, 416
Neuromuscular Junction Disorders, 417
Tumours of the Central Nervous System, 417
Brain Tumours, 417
Spinal Cord Tumours, 421

Alterations in central nervous system (CNS) function are caused by traumatic injury, vascular disorders, tumour growth, infectious and inflammatory processes, and metabolic derangements (including those arising from nutritional deficiencies and medications or chemicals). Alterations in peripheral nervous system function involve the nerve roots, a nerve plexus or the nerves themselves, or the neuromuscular junction.

CENTRAL NERVOUS SYSTEM DISORDERS

Traumatic Brain and Spinal Cord Injury

Traumatic Brain Injury

Traumatic brain injury (TBI) is an alteration in brain function or other evidence of brain pathology caused by an external force. In Canada, TBI is the primary cause of death and disability in individuals under the age of 40, occurring at a rate of 500 out of 100 000 individuals annually. TBI has an annual incidence rate greater than all combined cases of multiple sclerosis, spinal cord injury, human immunodeficiency virus (HIV)/acquired immune deficiency syndrome (AIDS), and breast cancer. It is reported that 30% of all TBIs are sustained by children and youth, many of them while participating in sports and recreational-related activities. The incidence of TBI among First Nations people is estimated to be four to five times the rate of the general population.[1]

In recent years, individuals with TBI have shown improved survival outcomes. Advancements have been made in enhanced safety measures (e.g., passive seat restraints, air bags, protective head gear), reduced transport time to hospitals or trauma centres, improved on-scene medical management, and prevention and management of secondary brain injury.

TBI can be classified as primary or secondary. Primary brain injury is caused by direct impact and can be focal, affecting one area of the brain, or diffuse (diffuse axonal injury [DAI]), involving more than one area of the brain.[2] Focal brain injury and DAI each account for half of all injuries. Focal brain injury accounts for more than two thirds of head injury deaths. DAI accounts for less than one third of deaths. More severely disabled survivors, including those surviving in an unresponsive state or reduced level of consciousness, have DAI. Secondary injury is an indirect consequence of the primary injury and includes systemic responses and a cascade of cellular and molecular cerebral events. TBI can be mild, moderate, or severe. The Glasgow Coma Scale is used to grade severity of injury (Table 16-1). Most TBIs are mild. The hallmark of a severe TBI is loss of consciousness for 6 hours or more.[3] Review Chapter 15 for information about increased intracranial pressure (ICP).

Primary brain injury

Focal brain injury. Focal brain injury can be caused by closed (blunt) trauma or open (penetrating) trauma. Closed injury is more common and involves either the head striking a hard surface or a rapidly moving object striking the head, or by blast waves. The dura remains intact, and brain tissues are not exposed to the environment. Blunt trauma may result in both focal brain injuries and diffuse axonal injuries, and they can occur at the same time (Table 16-2). Open injury occurs with penetrating trauma or skull fracture. A break in the dura results in exposure of the cranial contents to the environment.[3]

Closed brain injuries are specific, grossly observable brain lesions that occur in a precise location; 75 to 90% of blunt trauma injuries are mild. Injury to the vault, vessels, and supporting structures can produce more severe damage, including contusions and epidural, subdural, and intracerebral hematomas. The injury may be a **coup injury** (at the site of impact) or **contrecoup injury** (from brain rebounding and hitting opposite side of skull) (Figure 16-1). Compression of the skull at the point of impact produces **contusions** or brain bruising from blood leaking from an injured vessel. The severity of contusion varies with the amount of energy transmitted by the skull to underlying brain tissue. The smaller the area of impact, the more severe the injury because of the concentration of force. Brain edema forms around and in damaged neural tissues, contributing to increasing ICP (see Chapter 15). Multiple hemorrhages, edema, infarction, and necrosis can occur within the contused areas. The tissue has a pulpy quality. The maximal effects of these injuries peak 18 to 36 hours after severe head injury.

Contusions are found most commonly in the frontal lobes, particularly at the poles and along the inferior orbital surfaces; in the temporal lobes, especially at the anterior poles and along the inferior surface; and at the frontotemporal junction. They cause changes in attention, memory, executive attention functions (see Chapter 15), affect, emotion, and behaviour. Less commonly, contusions occur in the parietal and occipital lobes. Focal cerebral contusions are usually superficial, involving just the gyri. Hemorrhagic contusions may coalesce into a large confluent intracranial hematoma.

A contusion may be evidenced by immediate loss of consciousness (generally accepted to last no longer than 5 minutes), loss of reflexes (individual falls to the ground), transient cessation of respiration, brief period of bradycardia, and decrease in blood pressure (lasting 30 seconds to a few minutes). Increased cerebrospinal fluid (CSF) pressure and electrocardiogram (ECG) and electroencephalogram (EEG) changes occur on impact. Vital signs may stabilize to normal values in a few seconds; reflexes then return and the person regains consciousness over minutes to days. Residual deficits may persist, and some persons never regain a full level of consciousness.

Evaluation is based on results of the health history, level of consciousness according to the Glasgow Coma Scale (see Table 16-1), outcomes of imaging studies (e.g., computed tomography [CT], magnetic resonance imaging [MRI], and positron emission tomography [PET] scans), and assessment of vital parameters (e.g., ICP and EEG). Large contusions and lacerations with hemorrhage may be surgically excised. Treatment is otherwise directed at controlling ICP and managing symptoms.

Epidural (extradural) hematomas (bleeding between the dura mater and the skull) represent 1 to 2% of major head injuries and occur in all age groups, but most commonly in those 20 to 40 years old. An artery is the source of bleeding in 85% of epidural hematomas, usually accompanied by a skull fracture; 15% of these injuries result from injury to the meningeal vein or dural sinus (Figure 16-2). The

TABLE 16-1 Glasgow Coma Scale[a]

Score[b]	Best Eye Response Score (4)	Best Verbal Response Score (5)	Best Motor Response Score (6)
1	No eye opening	No verbal response	No motor response
2	Eye opening to pain	Incomprehensible sounds	Extension to pain
3	Eye opening to verbal command	Inappropriate words	Flexion to pain
4	Eyes open spontaneously	Confused	Withdrawal from pain
5	NA	Oriented	Localizing pain
6	NA	NA	Obeys commands

[a]The Glasgow Coma Scale (GCS) is scored between 3 and 15, with 3 being the worst and 15 the best. It is composed of the sum of three parameters: Best Eye Response, Best Verbal Response, and Best Motor Response. Mild Brain Injury = 13 or higher; Moderate Brain Injury = 9 to 12; Severe Brain Injury = 8 or less.

[b]It is important to break the scoring report into its components, for example, E3V3M5 = GCS 11. A total score is meaningless without this information. Age affects the GCS. Older adults with traumatic brain injury (TBI) have better GCS scores than younger individuals with TBI with similar TBI severity (i.e., older adults have higher GCS scores than those of younger individuals with TBI with similar anatomical TBI severity).

Data from Salottolo, K., Levy, A.S., Slone, D.S., et al. (2014). *JAMA Surg, 149*(7), 727–734; Teasdale, G., & Jennett, B. (1974). *Lancet, 2*, 81–84.

TABLE 16-2 Classification of Brain Injuries

Type of Injury	Mechanism
Primary Brain Injury	
Focal Brain Injury	Localized injury from impact
Closed injury	Blunt trauma
Coup	Injury is directly below site of forceful impact
Contrecoup	Injury is on opposite side of brain from site of forceful impact
Epidural (extradural) hematoma	Vehicular accidents, minor falls, sporting accidents
Subdural hematoma	Forceful impact: vehicular accidents or falls, especially in older adults or persons with chronic alcohol misuse
Subarachnoid hemorrhage	Bleeding caused by forceful impact, usually vehicular accidents or long-distance falls
Open injury	Penetrating trauma: missiles (bullets) or sharp projectiles (knives, ice picks, axes, screwdrivers)
Compound fracture	Objects strike head with great force or head strikes object forcefully; temporal blows, occipital blows, upward impact of cervical vertebrae (basilar skull fracture)
Diffuse Axonal Injury (can occur with focal injury)	Traumatic shearing forces; tearing of axons from twisting and rotational forces with injury over widespread brain areas; moving head strikes hard, unyielding surface or moving object strikes stationary head; torsional head motion without impact
Secondary Brain Injury	
Secondary brain injury	Decrease in CBF caused by edema, hemorrhage, increased ICP; neuro-inflammation
Cell death	Release of excitatory neurotransmitters (glutamate); failure of cell ion pumps, mitochondrial failure

CBF, cerebral blood flow; *ICP*, intracranial pressure.

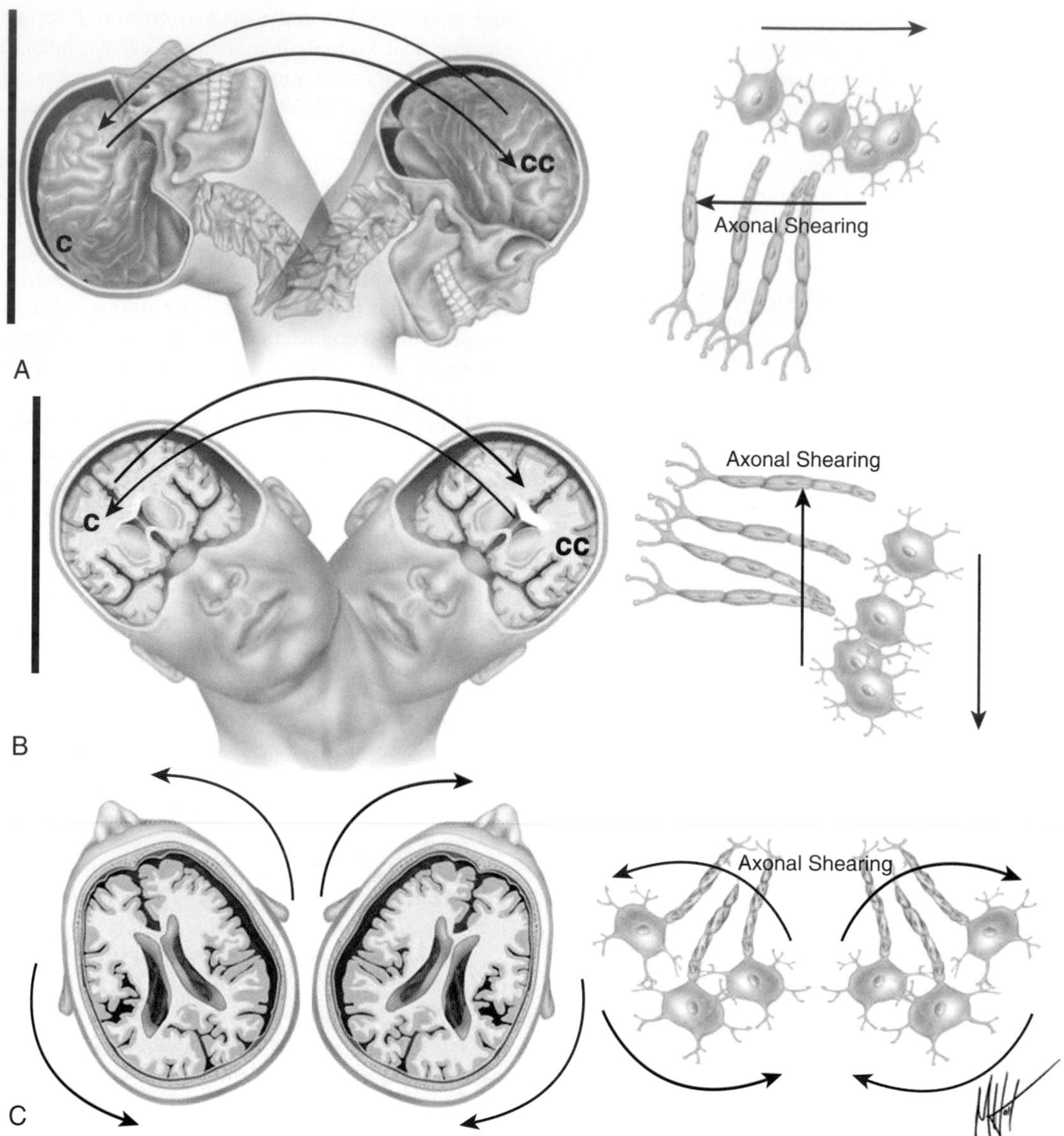

FIGURE 16-1 **Coup and Contrecoup Focal Injury With Acceleration/Deceleration Axonal Shearing.** **A,** Sagittal force causing coup (*c*) and contrecoup injury (*cc*). **B,** Lateral force causing coup (*c*) and contrecoup (*cc*) injury. **C,** Axial or rotational injury with shearing of axons, particularly at base of brain. Acceleration/deceleration axonal shearing injury occurs throughout the brain (red and blue directional arrows in all three images). (Borrowed from Pascual, J.M., & Preito, R. [2012]. Chapter 133: Surgical management of severe closed head injury in adults. In A. Quinones-Hinojosa [Ed.], *Schmidek and Sweet operative neurosurgical techniques* [6th ed., Vol. 2, pp. 1513–1538]. Philadelphia: Saunders. Originally redrawn from Adams, J.H. [1990]. Brain damage in fatal nonmissile head injury in man. In R. Braakman [Ed.], *Handbook of clinical neurology, head injury* [Vol. 13, pp. 43–63]. Amsterdam: Elsevier Science Publishers BV; Gennarelli, T.A., Thibault, L.E., Adams, J.H., et al. [1982]. *Ann Neurol, 12,* 564–574.)

temporal fossa is the most common site of epidural hematoma caused by injury to the middle meningeal artery or vein. The temporal lobe shifts medially, precipitating uncal and hippocampal gyrus herniation through the tentorial notch. Epidural hemorrhages are found occasionally in the subfrontal area, especially in the young and older adult populations, caused by injury to the anterior meningeal artery or a venous sinus; and in the occipital-suboccipital area, resulting in herniation of the posterior fossa contents through the foramen magnum (see Figure 15-10).

Individuals with temporal epidural hematomas lose consciousness at injury; one third of those affected then become lucid for a few minutes to a few days (if a vein is bleeding). As the hematoma accumulates, a headache of increasing severity, vomiting, drowsiness, confusion, seizure, and hemiparesis may develop. Because temporal lobe herniation occurs, the level of consciousness is rapidly lost, with ipsilateral pupillary dilation and contralateral hemiparesis. A CT scan or MRI usually is needed to diagnose epidural hematoma. The prognosis is good if intervention is initiated before bilateral dilation of the pupils occurs. Epidural hematomas are almost always medical emergencies requiring monitoring and evaluation or surgical evacuation of the hematoma.[4]

Subdural hematomas (bleeding between the dura mater and the brain) arise in 10 to 20% of persons with TBI. *Acute subdural hematomas* develop rapidly, commonly within hours, and usually are located at the top of the skull (the cerebral convexities). Bilateral hematomas occur

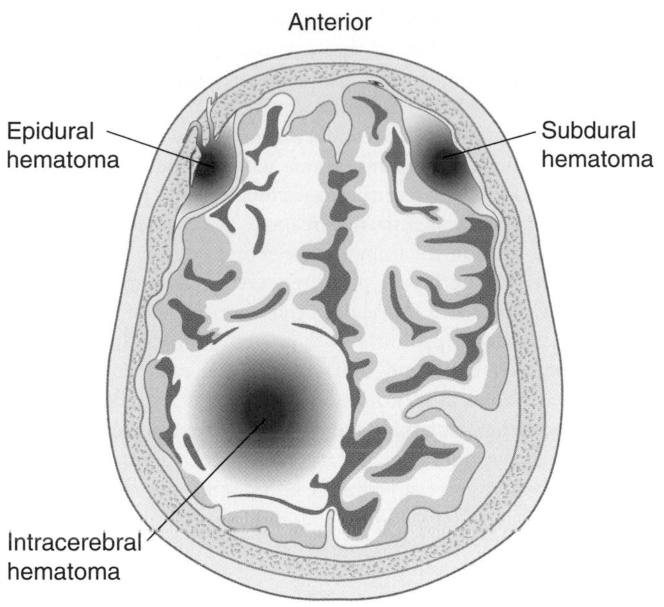

FIGURE 16-2 Brain Hematomas.

in 15 to 20% of persons. Subacute subdural hematomas develop more slowly, often over 48 hours to 2 weeks. *Chronic subdural hematomas* (commonly found in older adults and persons who abuse alcohol and have some degree of brain atrophy with a subsequent increase in extradural space) develop over weeks to months. Bridging veins tear, causing both rapidly and subacutely developing subdural hematomas, although torn cortical veins or venous sinuses and contused tissue also may be the source. These subdural hematomas act like expanding masses, increasing ICP that eventually compresses the bleeding vessels (see Figure 16-2). Brain herniation can result. With a chronic subdural hematoma, the existing subdural space gradually fills with blood. A vascular membrane forms around the hematoma in approximately 2 weeks. Further enlargement may take place.

In acute, rapidly developing subdural hematomas, the expanding clots directly compress the brain. As ICP rises, bleeding veins are compressed. Thus, bleeding is self-limiting, although cerebral compression and displacement of brain tissue can cause temporal lobe herniation.

An acute subdural hematoma classically begins with headache, drowsiness, restlessness or agitation, slowed cognition, and confusion. These symptoms worsen over time and progress to loss of consciousness, respiratory pattern changes, and pupillary dilation (i.e., the symptoms of temporal lobe herniation). Homonymous hemianopia (defective vision in either the right or the left field [see Figure 14-11]), dysconjugate gaze, and gaze palsies also may occur.

Of those individuals affected by chronic subdural hematomas, 80% have chronic headaches and tenderness over the hematoma on palpation. Most persons appear to have a progressive dementia with generalized rigidity (paratonia). Chronic subdural hematomas require a craniotomy to evacuate the gelatinous blood. Percutaneous drainage for chronic subdural hematomas has proven successful. However, reaccumulation often occurs unless the surrounding membrane is removed.

Intracerebral hematomas (bleeding within the brain) occur in 2 to 3% of persons with head injuries, may be single or multiple, and are associated with contusions. Although most commonly located in the frontal and temporal lobes, they may occur in the hemispheric deep white matter. Penetrating injury or shearing forces traumatize small blood vessels. The intracerebral hematoma then acts as an expanding mass, increasing ICP, compressing brain tissues, and causing edema (see Figure 16-2). Delayed intracerebral hematomas may appear 3 to 10 days after the head injury. Intracerebral hematomas also can occur with nontraumatic brain injury, such as hemorrhagic stroke (see p. 408).

Intracerebral hematomas cause a decreasing level of consciousness. Coma or a confusional state from other injuries, however, can make the cause of this increasing unresponsiveness difficult to detect. Contralateral hemiplegia also may occur and, as ICP rises, temporal lobe herniation may appear. In delayed intracerebral hematoma, the presentation is similar to that of a hypertensive brain hemorrhage—sudden, rapidly progressive decreased level of consciousness with pupillary dilation, breathing pattern changes, hemiplegia, and bilateral positive Babinski reflexes.

History and physical examination help to establish the diagnosis, and CT scan, MRI, and cerebral angiography confirm it. Evacuation of a singular intracerebral hematoma has only occasionally been helpful, mostly for subcortical white matter hematomas. Otherwise, treatment is directed at reducing the ICP and allowing the hematoma to reabsorb slowly.

Open brain injury (trauma that penetrates the dura mater) produces both focal and diffuse injuries and includes compound skull fractures and missile injuries (e.g., bullets, rocks, shell fragments, knives, and blunt instruments). A **compound skull fracture** opens a communication between the cranial contents and the environment and should be investigated whenever lacerations of the scalp, tympanic membrane, sinuses, eye, or mucous membranes are present. Such fractures may involve the cranial vault or the base of the skull (basilar skull fracture). Cranial nerve damage and spinal fluid leak may occur with a basilar skull fracture.

The mechanisms of open brain trauma are crush injury (laceration and crushing of whatever the missile touches) and stretch injury (blood vessels and nerves damaged without direct contact as a result of stretching). The tangential injury is to the coverings and the brain (scalp and brain lacerations) and may also include skull fractures and meningeal or cerebral lacerations from projectiles and debris driven into the brain substance.

Most persons lose consciousness with open brain injury. The depth and duration of the coma are related to the location of injury, extent of damage, and amount of bleeding. Open brain injury often requires debridement of the traumatized tissues to prevent infection and to remove blood clots, thereby reducing ICP. Intracranial pressure also is managed with steroids, dehydrating agents, osmotic diuretics, or a combination of these medications. Broad-spectrum antibiotics are administered to prevent infection.

A compound fracture may be diagnosed through physical examination, skull X-ray films, or both. Basilar skull fracture is determined on the basis of clinical findings, such as spinal fluid leaking from the ear or nose. Skull X-rays often do not demonstrate the fracture, although intracranial air or air in the sinuses on X-ray film, CT scan, or MRI is indirect evidence of a basilar skull fracture. Bed rest and close observation for meningitis and other complications are prescribed for a basilar skull fracture.

Diffuse brain injury. **Diffuse brain injury (diffuse axonal injury [DAI])** involves widespread areas of the brain. Mechanical effects from high levels of acceleration and deceleration, such as whiplash, or rotational forces cause shearing of delicate axonal fibres and white matter tracts that project to the cerebral cortex (see Figure 16-1). The most severe axonal injuries are located more peripheral to the brainstem, causing extensive cognitive and affective impairments, as seen in survivors of TBI from motor vehicle crashes. Axonal damage reduces the speed of information processing and responding and disrupts the individual's attention span.[5]

Pathophysiologically, axonal damage can be seen only with an electron microscope and involves numerous axons, either alone or in conjunction with actual tissue tears. Advanced imaging techniques assist in defining areas of injury. Areas where axons and small blood vessels are torn appear as small hemorrhages, particularly in the corpus callosum and dorsolateral quadrant of the rostral brainstem at the superior cerebellar peduncle. More damaged axons are visible 12 hours to several days after the initial injury. The severity of diffuse injury correlates with how much shearing force was applied to the brainstem. DAI is not associated with intracranial hypertension immediately after injury; however, acute brain swelling caused by increased intravascular blood flow within the brain, vasodilation, and increased cerebral blood volume is seen often and can result in death.

Several categories of diffuse brain injury exist: mild concussion, classic cerebral concussion, mild DAI, moderate DAI, and severe DAI.

Mild concussion (mild traumatic brain injury) is characterized by immediate but transitory clinical manifestations. CSF pressure rises, and ECG and EEG changes occur without loss of consciousness.[6] Approximately 75 to 90% of blunt trauma injuries cause mild concussion. The Glasgow Coma Scale score for mild concussion is 13 to 15. The initial confusional state lasts for 1 to several minutes, possibly with amnesia for events preceding the trauma (retrograde amnesia). Anterograde amnesia (lack of memories) may also exist transiently. Persons may experience headache and complain of nervousness and "not being themselves" for up to a few days.

Classic cerebral concussion is any loss of consciousness lasting less than 6 hours accompanied by retrograde and anterograde amnesia with a confusional state lasting for hours to days. Transient cessation of respiration can occur with brief periods of bradycardia and a decrease in blood pressure lasting 30 seconds or less. Vital signs stabilize within a few seconds to within normal limits. Reflexes fail and are regained as responsiveness returns.

DAI is a severe brain injury and produces coma lasting more than 6 hours because of axonal disruption. Three forms of DAI exist: mild, moderate, and severe. In mild diffuse axonal injury, coma lasts 6 to 24 hours with 30% of persons displaying decerebrate or decorticate posturing (see Figure 15-6). They may experience prolonged periods of stupor or restlessness.

In moderate diffuse axonal injury, the score on the Glasgow Coma Scale is 4 to 8 initially and 6 to 8 by 24 hours; 35% of victims have transitory decerebration or decortication, with unconsciousness lasting days or weeks. On awakening, the person is confused and suffers a long period of post-traumatic anterograde and retrograde amnesia. There is often permanent deficit in memory, attention, abstraction, reasoning, problem solving, executive functions, vision or perception, and language. Mood and affect changes range from mild to severe.

In severe diffuse axonal injury, injury involves both hemispheres and the brainstem. Coma may last days to months. The person experiences immediate autonomic dysfunction (hypertension, tachycardia, tachypnea, extensor posturing) that disappears in a few weeks. increased ICP appears 4 to 6 days after injury. Pulmonary complications occur often. Profound sensorimotor and cognitive system deficits are present, including spastic paralysis, dysarthria, dysphagia, memory loss, inability to learn and reason, and failure to modulate behaviour. Irreversible coma and death can occur.

High-resolution CT scan and MRI assist in the diagnosis of focal and diffuse injuries. Medical management must address endocrine and metabolic derangements. The goal of treatment is to maintain cerebral perfusion and oxygenation, and promote neuroprotection. Implementation of TBI guidelines decreases death and improves neurological outcome. The Corticosteroid Randomization After Significant Head Injury (CRASH) trial showed that corticosteroids increase mortality with acute TBI; consequently, these medications are no longer used.[3,7] Guidelines are available to direct treatment.[8]

Secondary brain injury. Secondary brain injury is an indirect result of primary brain injury, including trauma and stroke syndromes. Systemic and cerebral processes are contributing factors. Systemic processes include hypotension, hypoxia, anemia, hypercapnia, and hypocapnia. Cerebral contributions include inflammation, cerebral edema, increased ICP, decreased cerebral perfusion pressure, cerebral ischemia, and brain herniation. Cellular and molecular brain damage from the effects of primary injury develops hours to days later. Astrocyte swelling and proliferation alter the blood–brain barrier and cause increased ICP. Ischemia contributes to excitotoxicity with release of excitatory neurotransmitters, such as glutamate and aspartate. They cause cellular influx of calcium, damage mitochondria, and cause neuronal hyperexcitability. A hypermetabolic state, poor perfusion, influx of inflammatory mediators, fluctuations in cellular sodium and potassium ion channels, and mitochondrial failure all contribute to cytotoxic edema, axonal swelling, and neuronal death.[2]

The management of secondary brain injury is related to prevention and includes removal of hematomas and management of hypotension, hypoxemia, anemia, ICP, fluid and electrolyte balance, body temperature, and ventilation. Thyrotropin-releasing hormone, statins, and other agents are under investigation and may be neuroprotective by decreasing excitotoxicity, neuro-inflammation, and other mechanisms of secondary injury.[2,9] Progress is difficult because of the lack of predictive biomarkers and medications that can cross the blood–brain barrier. Fluid and nutrition management has emerged as critically important in the care of individuals with severe brain injury.[10] Long-term recovery can be influenced by systemic complications, such as pneumonia, fever, infections, and immobility that contribute to further brain injury, and delays in repair and recovery.

Complications of Traumatic Brain Injury

Many complications are associated with TBI and are related to the severity of injury and the parts of the brain that are affected. Altered states of consciousness can range from confusion to deep coma (see Table 15-3). Cognitive deficits; hydrocephalus; sensory-motor disorders, including pain, paresis, and paralysis; and loss of coordination may be present. Three of the most common post-traumatic brain syndromes are summarized next.

Postconcussion syndrome, including headache, dizziness, fatigue, nervousness or anxiety, irritability, insomnia, depression, inability to concentrate, and forgetfulness, may last for weeks to months after a concussion. Treatment entails reassurance and symptomatic relief in addition to 24 hours of close observation after the concussion in the event bleeding or swelling in the brain occurs. Symptoms requiring further evaluation and treatment include drowsiness or confusion, nausea or vomiting, severe headache, memory deficit, seizures, drainage of CSF from the ear or nose, weakness or loss of feeling in the extremities, asymmetry of the pupils, and double vision. Guidelines for the management of pediatric and adult concussion are available.[11-13] Guidelines have been published for the management of sports-related concussion.[14]

Post-traumatic seizures occur in about 2 to 16% of TBIs, with the highest risk among open brain injuries. Seizures can occur early, within days, and up to 2 to 5 years or longer after the trauma. Causal mechanisms are poorly understood, and cellular and molecular changes in the brain associated with injury and repair, such as sprouting of new neurons with hyperexcitability and decreases in GABAergic inhibition, may cause the hyperexcitable state that leads to epileptogenesis. Seizure prevention using medications, such as phenytoin (Dilantin), is initiated for moderate to severe TBI at the time of injury. Clinical trials are ongoing to test medications that prevent the development of post-traumatic seizures.[15]

Chronic traumatic encephalopathy (CTE) (previously called *dementia pugilistica*) is a progressive dementing disease that develops with repeated brain injury associated with sporting events, blast injuries in soldiers, or work-related head trauma. Tau neurofibrillary tangles are present in the brain, and research is in progress to discover the mechanistic link between neurotrauma and CTE. It is diagnosed from history and clinical evaluation, and at autopsy.[16,17]

QUICK CHECK 16-1

1. How is a concussion different from a contusion?
2. Why do epidural, subdural, and intracerebral hematomas act like expanding masses?
3. Why is head motion the principal causative mechanism of diffuse brain injury?

Spinal Cord and Vertebral Injury

Each year, approximately 4 259 persons in Canada experience serious spinal cord injury. Male gender and ages 20 to 39 years are strong risk factors for experiencing a traumatic spinal cord injury. Motor vehicle accidents, sports activities, and violence are the leading cause of injury in this age group. A significant number of injuries also occurs in persons aged 70 years and older, mainly as a result of falls.[18] Older adults are particularly at risk for trauma that results in serious spinal cord injury because of pre-existing degenerative vertebral disorders.

PATHOPHYSIOLOGY **Primary spinal cord injury** occurs with the initial mechanical trauma and immediate tissue destruction. Injuries to the cord are summarized in Table 16-3. Primary spinal cord injury occurs if an injured spine is not adequately immobilized immediately following injury. Primary spinal cord injury also may occur in the absence of vertebral fracture or dislocation from longitudinal stretching of the cord with or without flexion or extension of the vertebral column, or both. The stretching causes altered axon transport, edema, myelin degeneration, and retrograde or Wallerian degeneration (see Chapter 13).

Secondary spinal cord injury is a pathophysiological cascade of vascular, cellular, and biochemical events that begins within a few minutes after injury and continues for weeks. Edema, ischemia, excitotoxicity (excessive stimulation by excitatory neurotransmitters such as glutamate), inflammation, oxidative damage, and activation of necrotic and apoptotic cell death signal events similar to those previously described for TBI.[19]

With secondary spinal cord injury, microscopic hemorrhages appear in the central grey matter and pia-arachnoid, increasing in size until the entire grey matter is hemorrhagic and necrotic. Edema in the white matter occurs, impairing the microcirculation of the cord. Hemorrhages and edema are followed by reduced vascular perfusion and development of ischemic areas, which are maximal at the level of injury and two cord segments above and below it. Cellular and subcellular alterations and tissue necrosis occur. Cord swelling increases the individual's degree of dysfunction, making it difficult to distinguish functions permanently lost from those temporarily impaired. In the cervical region, cord swelling may be life-threatening. Diaphragm function may be impaired because phrenic nerves exit at C3 to C5. Cardiovascular and respiratory functions mediated by the medulla oblongata can be lost.

Circulation in the white matter tracts of the spinal cord returns to normal in about 24 hours, but grey matter circulation remains altered. Phagocytes appear 36 to 48 hours after injury, and microglia proliferate with altered astrocytes. Red blood cells then begin to disintegrate, and resorption of hemorrhages and edema begins. Degenerating axons are engulfed by macrophages in the first 10 days after injury. The traumatized cord is replaced by acellular collagenous tissue, usually in 3 to 4 weeks. Meninges thicken as part of the scarring process.

Vertebral injuries result from acceleration, deceleration, or deformation forces occurring at impact. These forces cause vertebral fractures, dislocations, and bone fragments that can cause compression to the tissues, pull or exert traction (tension) on the tissues, or cause shearing of tissues so they slide into one another (Figures 16-3 to 16-6). Vertebral injuries can be classified as (1) simple fracture—a single break usually affecting transverse or spinous processes; (2) compressed (wedged) vertebral fracture—vertebral body compressed anteriorly; (3) comminuted (burst) fracture—vertebral body shattered into several fragments; and (4) dislocation.

The vertebrae fracture readily with both direct and indirect trauma. When the supporting ligaments are torn, the vertebrae move out of alignment and dislocations occur. A horizontal force moves the vertebrae

TABLE 16-3 Spinal Cord Injuries

Injury	Description
Cord concussion	Results in temporary disruption of cord-mediated functions
Cord contusion	Bruising of neural tissue causes swelling and temporary loss of cord-mediated functions
Cord compression	Pressure on cord causes ischemia to tissues; must be relieved (decompressed) to prevent permanent damage to spinal cord
Laceration	Tearing of neural tissues of spinal cord; may be reversible if only slight damage sustained by neural tissues; may result in permanent loss of cord-mediated functions if spinal tracts are disrupted
Transection	Severing of spinal cord causes permanent loss of function
Complete	All tracts in spinal cord are completely disrupted; all cord-mediated functions below transection are completely and permanently lost
Incomplete	Some tracts in spinal cord remain intact, together with functions mediated by these tracts; has potential for recovery although function is temporarily lost
Preserved sensation only	Some demonstrable sensation below level of injury
Preserved motor nonfunctional	Preserved motor function without useful purpose; sensory function may or may not be preserved
Preserved motor functional	Preserved voluntary motor function that is functionally useful
Hemorrhage	Bleeding into neural tissue as a result of blood vessel damage; usually no major loss of function
Damage or obstruction of spinal blood supply	Causes local ischemia

straight forward; if the individual is in a flexed position at the time of injury, the vertebrae are then angulated. Flexion and extension injuries may result in dislocations. (Bone, ligament, and joint injuries are presented in Table 16-4.)

Vertebral injuries in adults occur most often at vertebrae C1 to C2 (cervical), C4 to C7, and T10 (thoracic) to L2 (lumbar) (see Figure 13-11), the most mobile portions of the vertebral column. The spinal cord occupies most of the vertebral canal in the cervical and lumbar regions, so it can be easily injured in these locations.

CLINICAL MANIFESTATIONS Spinal shock develops immediately after injury because of loss of continuous tonic discharge from the brain or brainstem and inhibition of suprasegmental impulses caused by cord hemorrhage, edema, or anatomical transection. Normal activity of spinal cord cells at and below the level of injury ceases with complete loss of reflex function, flaccid paralysis, absence of sensation, loss of bladder and rectal control, transient drop in blood pressure, and poor venous circulation. The condition also results in disturbed thermal control because the sympathetic nervous system is damaged. The hypothalamus cannot regulate body heat through vasoconstriction and increased metabolism; therefore, the individual assumes the temperature of the air (poikilothermia). Spinal shock generally lasts 7 to 20 days, with a range of a few days to 3 months. It terminates with the reappearance of reflex activity, hyper-reflexia, spasticity, and reflex emptying of the bladder. Table 16-5 summarizes the clinical manifestations of spinal cord injury.

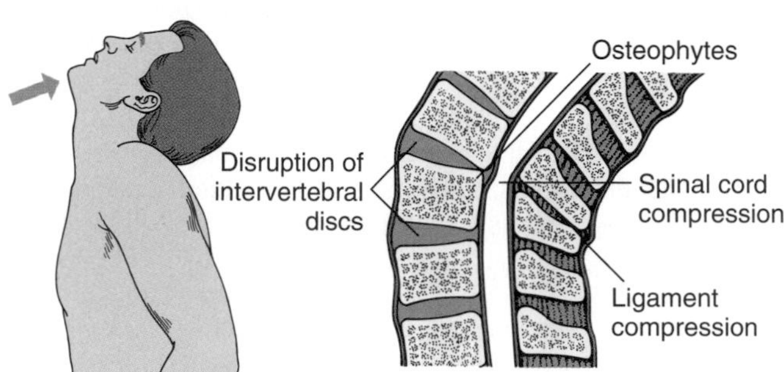

FIGURE 16-3 Hyperextension Injuries of the Spine. Hyperextension injuries of the spine can result in fracture or nonfracture injuries with spinal cord damage.

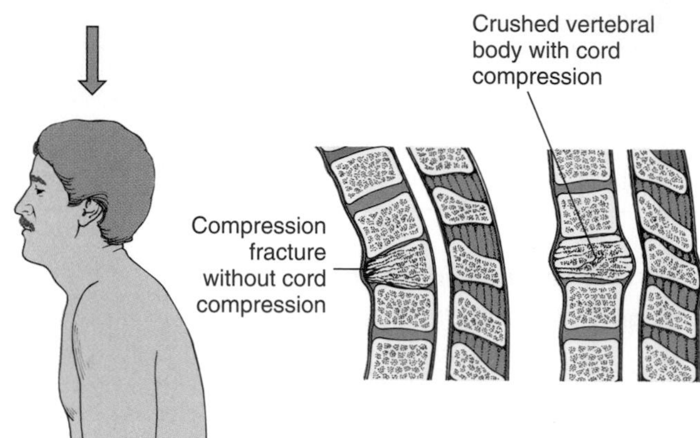

FIGURE 16-5 Axial Compression Injuries of the Spine. In axial compression injuries of the spine, the spinal cord is contused directly by retropulsion of bone or disc material into the spinal canal.

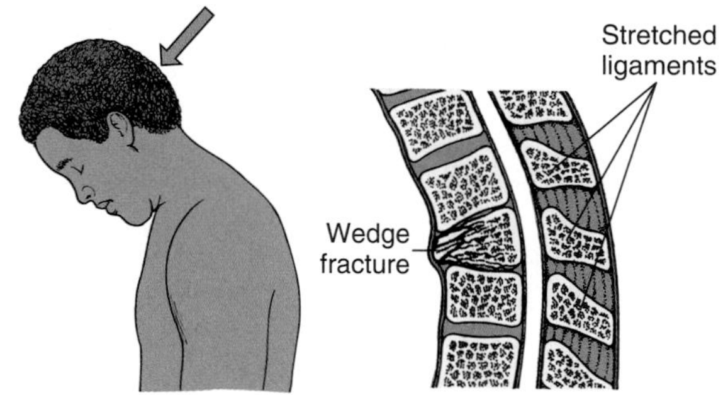

FIGURE 16-4 Flexion Injury of the Spine. Hyperflexion produces translation (subluxation) of vertebrae that compromises the central canal and compresses spinal cord parenchyma or vascular structures.

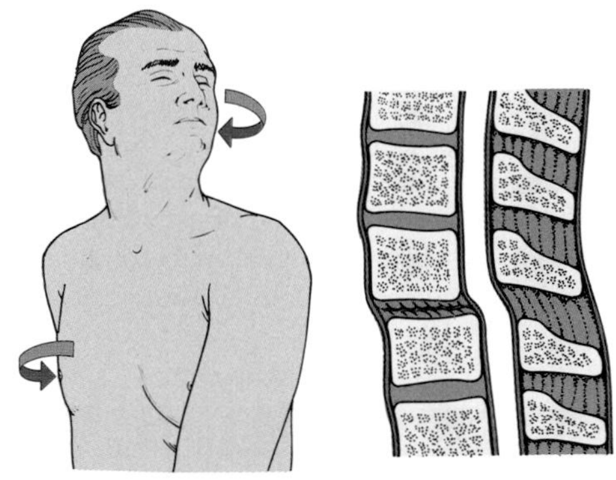

FIGURE 16-6 Flexion-Rotation Injuries of the Spine.

TABLE 16-4 Mechanisms of Vertebral Injury Involving Bone, Ligaments, and Joints

Mechanism of Injury	Location of Vertebral Injury	Forces of Injury	Location of Injury
Hyperextension	Fracture and dislocation of posterior elements, such as spinous processes, transverse processes, laminae, pedicles, or posterior ligaments	Results from forces of acceleration–deceleration and sudden reduction in anteroposterior diameter of spinal cord	Cervical area
Hyperflexion	Fracture or dislocation of vertebral bodies, discs, or ligaments	Results from sudden and excessive force that propels neck forward or causes an exaggerated lateral movement of neck to one side	Cervical area
Vertical compression (axial loading)	Shattering fractures	Results from a force applied along an axis from top of cranium through vertebral bodies	T12 to L2
Rotational forces (flexion-rotation)	Rupture support ligaments in addition to producing fractures	Add shearing force to acceleration forces	Cervical area

TABLE 16-5 Clinical Manifestations of Spinal Cord Injury

Stage	Clinical Manifestations
Spinal Shock Stage	
Complete spinal cord transection	Loss of motor function 1. Quadriplegia with injuries of cervical spinal cord 2. Paraplegia with injuries of thoracic spinal cord Muscle flaccidity Loss of all reflexes below level of injury Loss of pain, temperature, touch, pressure, and proprioception below level of injury Pain at site of injury caused by zone of hyperesthesia above injury Atonic bladder and bowel Paralytic ileus with distension Loss of vasomotor tone in lower body parts; low and unstable blood pressure Loss of perspiration below level of injury Loss or extreme depression of genital reflexes such as penile erection and bulbocavernous reflex Dry and pale skin; possible ulceration over bony prominences Respiratory impairment
Partial spinal cord transection	Asymmetrical flaccid motor paralysis below level of injury Asymmetrical reflex loss Preservation of some sensation below level of injury Vasomotor instability less severe than that seen with complete cord transection Bowel and bladder impairment less severe than that seen with complete cord transection Preservation of ability to perspire in some portions of body below level of injury *Brown-Séquard's syndrome* (associated with penetrating injuries, hyperextension and flexion, locked facets, and compression fractures) 1. Ipsilateral paralysis or paresis below level of injury 2. Ipsilateral loss of touch, pressure, vibration, and position sense below level of injury 3. Contralateral loss of pain and temperature sensations below level of injury *Central cervical cord syndrome* (acute cord compression between bony bars or spurs anteriorly and thickened ligamentum flavum posteriorly associated with hyperextension) 1. Motor deficits in upper extremities, especially hands, more dense than in lower extremities 2. Varying degrees of bladder dysfunction *Burning hand syndrome* (variant of central cord syndrome; in 50% of cases an underlying spine fracture/dislocation is present) 1. Severe burning paresthesias and dysesthesias in the hands or feet *Anterior cord syndrome* (compromise of anterior spinal artery by occlusion or pressure effect of disc) 1. Loss of motor function below level of injury 2. Loss of pain and temperature sensations below level of injury 3. Touch, pressure, position, and vibration senses intact *Posterior cord syndrome* (associated with hyperextension injuries with fractures of vertebral arch) 1. Impaired light touch and proprioception *Conus medullaris syndrome* (compression injury at T12 from disc herniation or burst fracture of body of T12) 1. Flaccid paralysis of legs 2. Flaccid paralysis of anal sphincter 3. Variable sensory deficits *Cauda equina syndrome* (compression of nerve roots below L1 caused by fracture and dislocation of spine or large posterocentral intervertebral disc herniation) 1. Lower extremity motor deficits 2. Variable sensorimotor dysfunction 3. Variable reflex dysfunction 4. Variable bladder, bowel, and sexual dysfunction *Syndrome of neuropraxia* (postathletic injury, associated with congenital spinal stenosis) 1. Dramatic but transient neurological deficits, including quadriplegia *Horner's syndrome* (injury to preganglionic sympathetic trunk or postganglionic sympathetic neurons of superior cervical ganglion) 1. Ipsilateral pupil smaller than contralateral pupil 2. Sunken ipsilateral eyeball 3. Ptosis of affected eyeball 4. Lack of perspiration on ipsilateral side of face

Continued

TABLE 16-5 Clinical Manifestations of Spinal Cord Injury—cont'd

Stage	Clinical Manifestations
Heightened Reflex Activity Stage	Emergence of Babinski reflexes, possibly progressing to a triple reflex; possible development of still later flexor spasms Reappearance of ankle and knee reflexes, which become hyperactive Contraction of reflex detrusor muscle leading to urinary incontinence Appearance of reflex defecation Mass reflex with flexion spasms, profuse sweating, piloerection, and bladder and occasional bowel emptying may be evoked by autonomic stimulation of skin or from full bladder Episodes of hypertension Defective heat-induced sweating Eventual development of extensor reflexes, first in muscles of hip and thigh, later in leg Possible paresthesias below level of transection: dull, burning pain in lower back, abdomen, buttocks, and perineum

Neurogenic shock, also called *vasogenic shock*, occurs with cervical or upper thoracic cord injury above T5 and may be seen in addition to spinal shock. Neurogenic shock is caused by the absence of sympathetic activity through loss of supraspinal control and unopposed parasympathetic tone mediated by the intact vagus nerve. Symptoms include vasodilation, hypotension, bradycardia, and failure of body temperature regulation. Neurogenic shock may be complicated by hypovolemic or cardiogenic shock if there is concurrent heart failure or blood loss (see Chapter 24).

Autonomic hyper-reflexia (dysreflexia) is a syndrome of sudden, massive reflex sympathetic discharge associated with spinal cord injury at level T6 or above where descending inhibition is blocked (Figure 16-7). It may occur after spinal shock resolves and be a recurrent complication. Characteristics involve changes in the body's autonomic functions, including paroxysmal hypertension (up to 300 mm Hg, systolic), a pounding headache, blurred vision, sweating above the level of the lesion with flushing of the skin, nasal congestion, nausea, piloerection caused by pilomotor spasm, bradycardia (30 to 40 beats/min), and automatic bladder emptying. The symptoms may develop singly or in combination. The condition can cause serious complications (stroke, seizures, myocardial ischemia, and death) and requires immediate treatment.

In autonomic hyper-reflexia, sensory receptors below the level of the cord lesion are stimulated. The intact autonomic nervous system reflexively responds with an arteriolar spasm that increases blood pressure. Baroreceptors in the cerebral vessels, the carotid sinus, and the aorta sense the hypertension and stimulate the parasympathetic system. The heart rate decreases, but the visceral and peripheral vessels do not dilate because efferent impulses cannot pass through the cord.

The most common cause is a distended bladder or rectum; however, any sensory stimulation (i.e., skin or pain receptors) can elicit autonomic hyper-reflexia. Intravenous fluids may be required to maintain blood pressure. Medication therapy may be required to lower blood pressure and reduce complications. Bladder, bowel, and skin care management are important preventive strategies. Education of the individual and family regarding triggers and acute management are important, as is wearing a medic alert tag.[20]

EVALUATION AND TREATMENT Diagnosis of spinal cord injury is based on physical examination and imaging studies. Neurogenic shock must be differentiated from other kinds of shock (i.e., hypovolemic shock). For a suspected or confirmed vertebral fracture or dislocation, regardless of the presence or absence of spinal cord injury, the immediate intervention is immobilization of the spine to prevent further injury. Decompression and surgical fixation may be necessary. Corticosteroids may be given at the time of injury to decrease secondary cord injury from inflammation and thereafter for several days.[21] Therapeutic hypothermia has shown some encouraging evidence for improved outcomes, particularly for cervical cord injuries; however, more research is needed.[22] Clinical trials are in progress to treat acute spinal cord injury, including cell-based therapies, immune modulators, vasculature selective treatments, and functional electrical stimulation.[23] Nutrition; lung function; skin integrity; prevention of pressure ulcers, in particular; and bladder and bowel management must be addressed. Plans for rehabilitation need early consideration.

Degenerative Disorders of the Spine

Low Back Pain

Low back pain (LBP) affects the area between the lower rib cage and gluteal muscles and often radiates into the thighs. The incidence rate of LBP in Canada is estimated to be 18.6%, with a higher percentage among older adults.[24] LBP is the primary cause of disability worldwide.[25] The burdens of disability include psychological, financial, occupational, and social effects on the person and family members.

Risk factors include occupations that require repetitious lifting in the forward bent-and-twisted position; exposure to vibrations caused by vehicles or industrial machinery; obesity; and cigarette smoking. Some people have a genetic predisposition for LBP.

PATHOGENESIS Most cases of LBP are idiopathic or nonspecific, and no precise diagnosis is possible. *Acute* LBP is often associated with muscle or ligament strain and is more common in individuals younger than 50 years of age without a history of cancer. Common causes of *chronic* LBP include degenerative disc disease, spondylolysis, spondylolisthesis (vertebra slides forward or slips in relation to a vertebra below), spinal osteochondrosis, spinal stenosis, and lumbar disc herniation. Other causes include tension caused by tumours or disc prolapse, bursitis, synovitis, rising venous and tissue pressures (found in degenerative joint disease), abnormal bone pressures, spinal immobility, inflammation caused by infection (as in osteomyelitis), and pain referred from viscera or the posterior peritoneum. Systemic causes of LBP include bone diseases, such as osteoporosis or osteomalacia, and hyperparathyroidism. Anatomically, LBP must originate from innervated structures, but deep pain is widely referred and varies. The nucleus pulposus has no intrinsic innervation, but when extruded or herniated through a prolapsed disc, it irritates the spinal nerve dural membranes and causes pain referred to the segmental area[26] (Figure 16-8).

The interspinous bursae can be a source of pain between L3, L4, L5, and S1 but also may affect L1, L2, and L3 spinous processes. The anterior and posterior longitudinal ligaments of the spine and the interspinous and supraspinous ligaments are abundantly supplied with pain receptors, as is the ligamentum flavum. All of these ligaments are vulnerable to traumatic tears (sprains) and fracture. Discogenic pain also may be related to inflammation and nerve sprouting within the disc.[27]

CLINICAL MANIFESTATIONS About 1% of individuals with acute LBP have pain along the distribution of a lumbar nerve root (radicular pain), most commonly involving the sciatic nerve (sciatica). Sciatica is often accompanied by sensorineural and motor deficits, such as tingling, numbness, and weakness in various parts of the leg and foot. Major or progressive motor or sensory deficit, **cauda equina syndrome** (new-onset bowel or bladder incontinence or urinary retention, loss of anal sphincter tone, and saddle anaesthesia), history of cancer metastasis to bone, and suspected spinal infection can be associated with chronic LBP.

EVALUATION AND TREATMENT Diagnosis of LBP is based on the history and physical examination. Imaging and nerve conduction studies are obtained with severe neurological deficit or serious underlying disease. Diagnosis and treatment guidelines are available to plan therapy.[28] Most individuals with acute LBP benefit from a nonspecific short-term treatment regimen of analgesic medications, exercises, physiotherapy, and education. Individuals should be advised to stay active and continue their usual activity, including work, within the limits permitted by pain. Surgical treatments, specifically discectomy and spinal fusions, are used for individuals not responding to medical management or for emergency management of cauda equina syndrome. Individuals with chronic LBP may benefit from anti-inflammatory and muscle relaxant medications, exercise programs, massage, topical heat, spinal manipulation, acupuncture, cognitive-behavioural therapies, and interdisciplinary care.[29] There is scant evidence for efficacy of opioids for chronic LBP, but a high risk for addiction.[30] The complexity of causes contributes to the difficulty in defining pathogenesis and clearly defining the most effective therapies.

Degenerative Joint Disease

Degenerative disc disease. **Degenerative disc disease (DDD)** is common in individuals 30 years of age and older. It is, in part, a process of normal aging as a response to continuous vertical compression of the spine (axial loading). DDD includes a genetic component, involving genes that code the cartilage intermediate layer protein (CILP). The combination of environmental interactions and genetic predisposition increases susceptibility to lumbar disc disease by disrupting normal building and maintenance of cartilage.[27] Causes include biochemical (e.g., inflammatory mediators) and biomechanical alterations (e.g., mechanical loading and compression) of the intervertebral disc tissue. For example, loss of disc proteoglycans and collagen with disc dehydration and loss of hydrostatic pressure alters disc structure and function. The annulus can tear and the disc can herniate, pinching nerves or placing strain on the spine. The pathological findings in DDD include disc

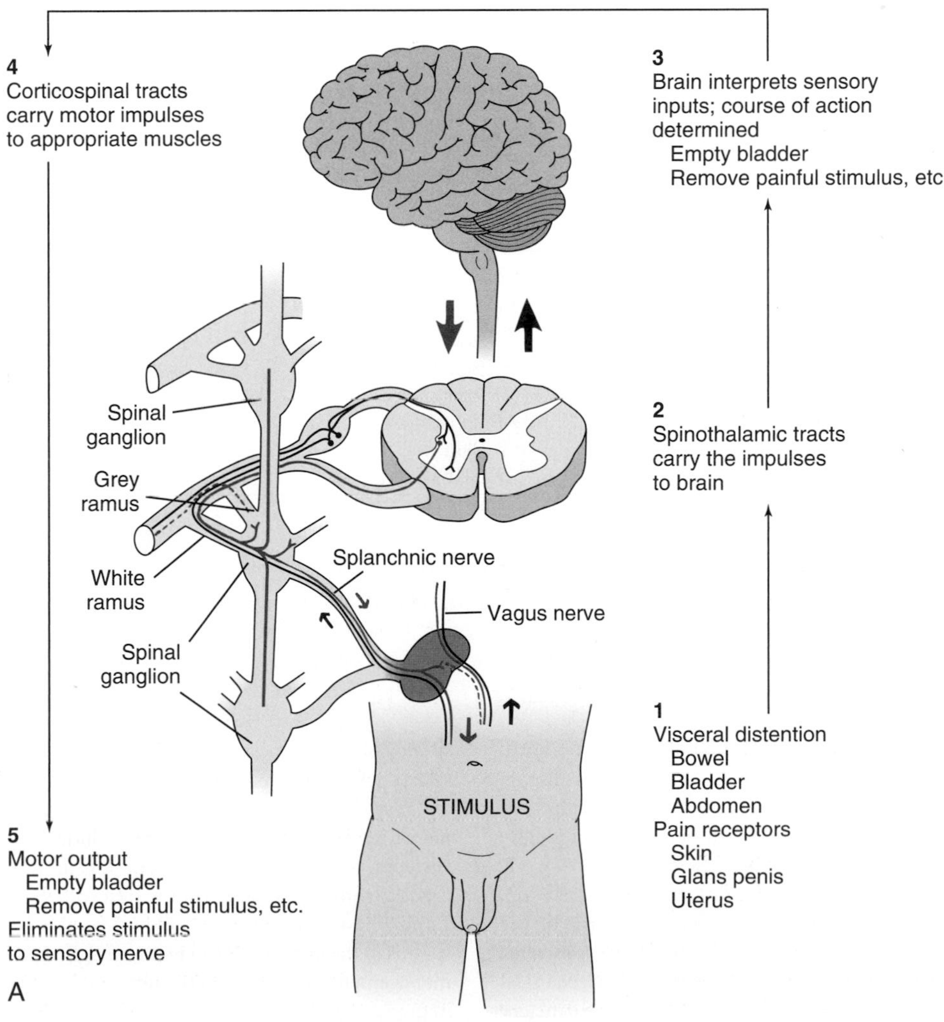

FIGURE 16-7 Autonomic Hyper-Reflexia. A, Normal response pathway. *Continued*

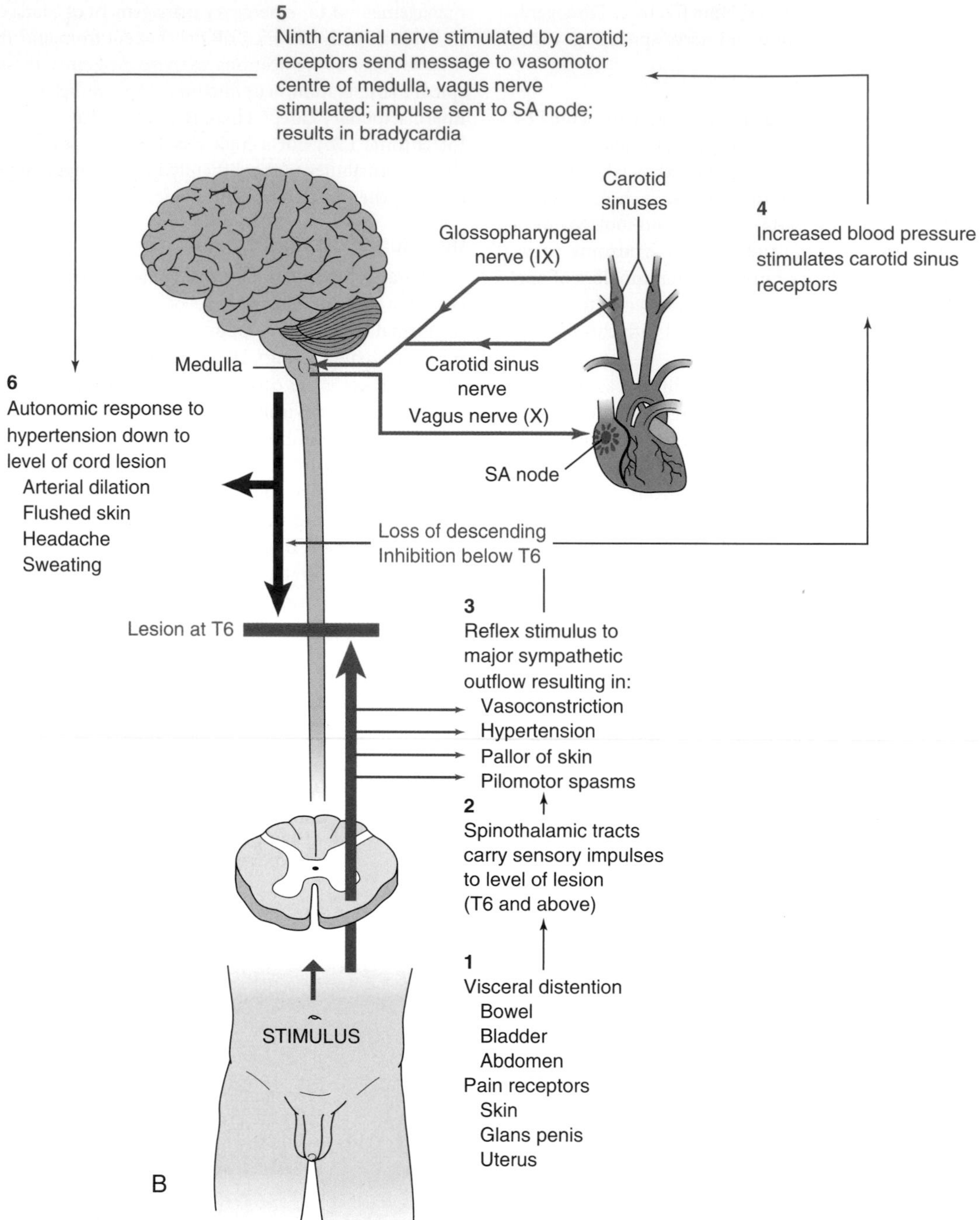
5
Ninth cranial nerve stimulated by carotid; receptors send message to vasomotor centre of medulla, vagus nerve stimulated; impulse sent to SA node; results in bradycardia
Carotid sinuses
4
Increased blood pressure stimulates carotid sinus receptors
Glossopharyngeal nerve (IX)
Medulla
Carotid sinus nerve
Vagus nerve (X)
6
Autonomic response to hypertension down to level of cord lesion
Arterial dilation
Flushed skin
Headache
Sweating
SA node
Loss of descending Inhibition below T6
Lesion at T6
3
Reflex stimulus to major sympathetic outflow resulting in:
Vasoconstriction
Hypertension
Pallor of skin
Pilomotor spasms
2
Spinothalamic tracts carry sensory impulses to level of lesion (T6 and above)
1
Visceral distention
Bowel
Bladder
Abdomen
Pain receptors
Skin
Glans penis
Uterus
STIMULUS
B

FIGURE 16-7, cont'd B, Autonomic dysreflexia pathway. *SA*, sinoatrial. (Modified from Rudy, E.B. [1984]. *Advanced neurological and neurosurgical nursing.* St. Louis: Mosby.)

protrusion; spondylolysis, subluxation (spondylolisthesis), or both; degeneration of vertebrae; and spinal stenosis. Lumbar disc disease causes one third of all back pain that affects 70 to 90% of adults at some point in their lives. However, only a small percentage of people with DDD have any functional incapacity because of pain.

Spondylolysis. Spondylolysis is a structural defect (degeneration, fracture, or developmental defect) in the pars interarticularis of the vertebral arch (the joining of the vertebral body to the posterior structures). The lumbar spine at L5 is affected most often. Mechanical pressure may cause an anterior or posterior displacement of the deficient vertebra (spondylolisthesis). Heredity plays a significant role, and spondylolysis is associated with an increased incidence of other congenital spinal defects. Symptoms include lower back and lower limb pain.

Spondylolisthesis. Spondylolisthesis, an osseous defect of the pars interarticularis, allows a vertebra to slide anteriorly in relation to the vertebra below, commonly occurring at L5-S1. Spondylolisthesis is graded from 1 to 4 based on the percentage of slip that occurs. Grades 1 and 2 have symptoms of pain in the lower back and buttocks, muscle spasms in the lower back and legs, and tightened hamstrings. Conservative management includes exercise, rest, and back bracing. Vertebral slippage in grades 3 and 4 usually requires surgical decompression, stabilization, or both.

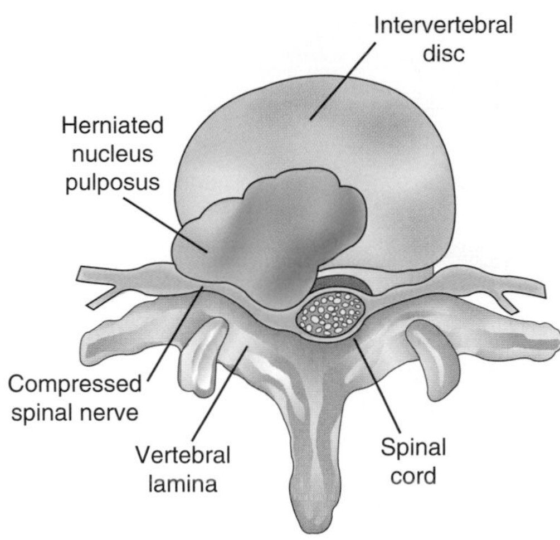

FIGURE 16-8 Herniated Nucleus Pulposus.

Spinal stenosis. Spinal stenosis is a narrowing of the spinal canal that causes pressure on the spinal nerves or cord and can be congenital or acquired (more common) and associated with trauma or arthritis. It is categorized by the area of the spine affected: cervical, thoracic, or lumbar. Acquired conditions include a bulging disc, facet hypertrophy, or a thick ossified posterior longitudinal ligament. Symptoms are related to the area of the spine affected and can produce pain; numbness; and tingling in the neck, hands, arms, or legs with weakness and difficulty walking. Surgical decompression is recommended for those with chronic symptoms and those who do not respond to medical management.

Herniated Intervertebral Disc

Herniation of an intervertebral disc is a displacement of the nucleus pulposus or annulus fibrosus beyond the intervertebral disc space (see Figure 16-8). Rupture of an intervertebral disc usually is caused by trauma, DDD, or both. Risk factors are weight-bearing sports, light weight lifting, and certain work activities, such as repeated lifting. Men are affected more often than women, with the highest incidence in the 30- to 50-year age group. Most commonly affected are the lumbosacral discs L4-L5 and L5-S1. Herniation is typically at higher vertebrae in older adults. Disc herniation occasionally occurs in the cervical area, usually at C5-C6 and C6-C7. Herniations at the thoracic level are extremely rare. The herniation may occur immediately, within a few hours, or months to years after injury.

PATHOPHYSIOLOGY In a herniated disc, the ligament and posterior capsule of the disc are usually torn, allowing the nucleus pulposus to extrude and compress the nerve root. The vascular supply may be compromised and cause inflammatory changes in the nerve root (radiculitis). Occasionally, the injury tears the entire disc loose, causing the disc capsule and nucleus pulposus to protrude onto the nerve root or compress the spinal cord. Multiple nerve root compression may be found at the L5-S1 level, where the cauda equina may be compressed, causing cauda equina syndrome (see Table 16-5).

CLINICAL MANIFESTATIONS The location and size of the herniation into the spinal canal, together with the amount of space in the canal, determine the clinical manifestations associated with the injury (Figure 16-9). Compression or inflammation, or both, of a spinal nerve resulting from disc herniation follows a dermatomal distribution called radiculopathy (Figure 16-10). A herniated disc in the lumbosacral area is associated with pain that radiates along the sciatic nerve course over the buttock and into the calf or ankle. The pain occurs with straining,

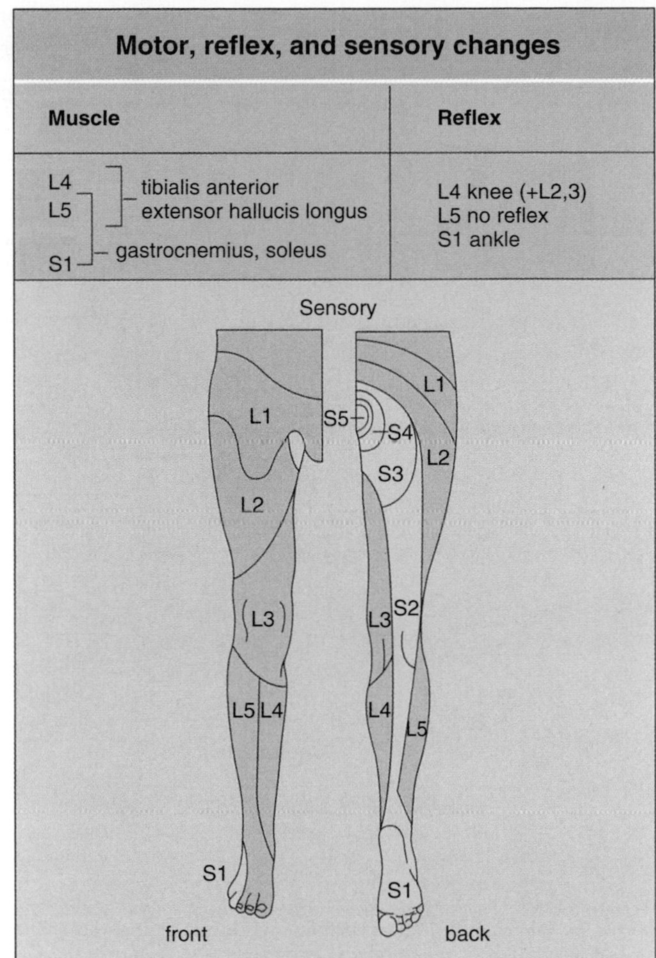

FIGURE 16-9 Clinical Features of a Herniated Nucleus Pulposus.

including coughing and sneezing, and usually on straight leg raising. Other clinical manifestations include limited range of motion of the lumbar spine; tenderness on palpation in the sciatic notch and along the sciatic nerve; impaired pain, temperature, and touch sensations in the L4-L5 or L5-S1 dermatomes of the leg and foot; decreased or absent ankle jerk reflex; and mild weakness of the foot. More rarely, there is development of cauda equina syndrome.

With the herniation of a lower cervical disc, paresthesias and pain are present in the upper arm, forearm, and hand along the affected nerve root distribution. Neck motion and straining, including coughing and sneezing, may increase neck and nerve root pain. Neck range of motion is diminished. Slight weakness and atrophy of biceps or triceps muscles may occur; the biceps or triceps reflex may decrease. Occasionally, signs of corticospinal and sensory tract impairments appear, including motor weakness of the lower extremities, sensory disturbances in the lower extremities, and presence of a Babinski reflex.

EVALUATION AND TREATMENT Diagnosis of a herniated intervertebral disc is made through the history and physical examination, spinal X-ray films, electromyelography, CT scan, MRI, myelography, discography, and nerve conduction studies. Evidence-based practice guidelines have been published to guide treatment options.[31] Most herniated discs heal spontaneously over time and do not require surgery. A surgical approach is indicated if there is evidence of severe compression (weakness or decreased deep tendon, bladder, or bowel reflexes) or if a conservative

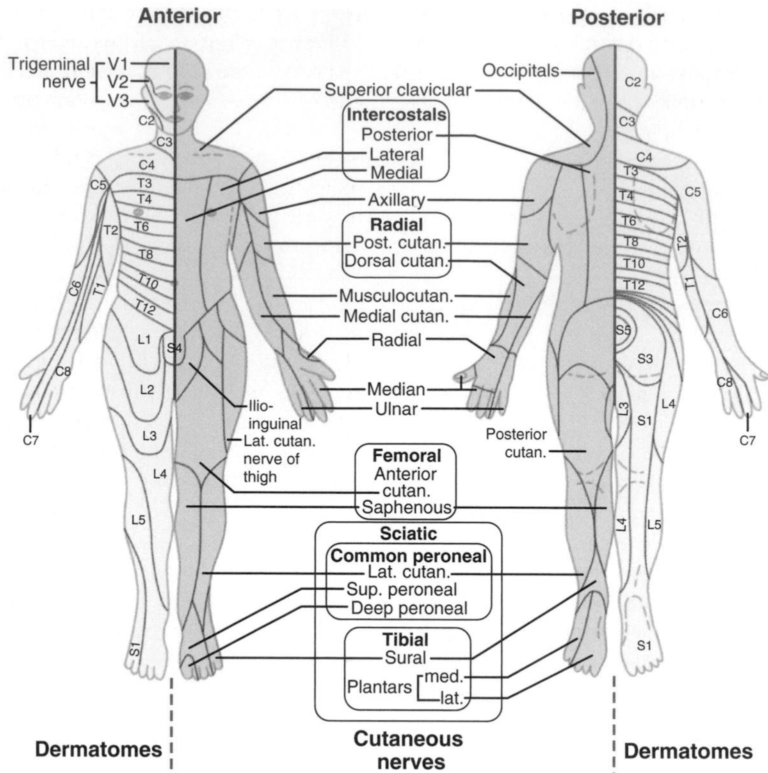

FIGURE 16-10 Sensory Nerve Distribution of Skin Dermatomes. (Redrawn from Patton, H.D., Sundsten, J.W., Crill, W.E., et al. [Eds.]. [1976]. *Introduction to basic neurology*. Philadelphia: Saunders. Borrowed from Canale, S.T., & Beaty, J.H. [2013]. *Campbell's operative orthopaedics* [12th ed.]. St. Louis: Mosby.)

approach is unsuccessful.[32] Cauda equina syndrome requires emergency surgical evaluation.[33]

Cerebrovascular Disorders

Cerebrovascular disease is the most frequently occurring neurological disorder, accounting for more than 50% of the persons admitted to general hospitals with neurological problems. Any abnormality of the brain caused by a pathological process in the blood vessels is referred to as a *cerebrovascular disease*. Included in this category are lesions of the vessel wall, occlusion of the vessel lumen by thrombus or embolus, rupture of the vessel, and alteration in blood quality such as increased blood viscosity.

The brain abnormalities induced by cerebrovascular disease are either (1) ischemia with or without infarction (death of brain tissues) or (2) hemorrhage. The common clinical manifestation of cerebrovascular disease is a **cerebrovascular accident (CVA)** or stroke. The symptoms occur suddenly and are focal (i.e., slurred speech, difficulty swallowing, limb weakness, or paralysis). In its mildest form, a CVA is so minimal that it is almost unnoticed. In its most severe form, hemiplegia, coma, and death result.

Cerebrovascular Accidents (Stroke Syndromes)

CVAs are the leading cause of disability and the third leading cause of death in Canada, with over 13 000 persons dying from CVAs annually. It is estimated that about 80% of all CVAs can be prevented[34] (see *Health Promotion:* Prevention of Stroke in Women). Persons with both hypertension and type 2 diabetes mellitus have a fourfold increase of CVA incidence and an eightfold increase in stroke mortality.[35] Research has shown that First Nations people, Inuit, and Métis are more likely to be diagnosed with hypertension and type 2 diabetes, which puts them at a higher risk for CVAs than the general population.[36]

HEALTH PROMOTION

Prevention of Stroke in Women

Stroke is a leading cause of death in Canadian women. The number of women with stroke will increasingly outnumber men in the future. The Heart and Stroke Foundation of Canada recommends a number of ways women can reduce the risk for stroke. A summary of these recommendations is as follows:

- Become and remain smoke-free
- Achieve and maintain a healthy body weight
- Be physically active for at least 150 minutes of moderate to vigorous-intensity aerobic physical activity per week
- Maintain a healthy blood pressure through lifestyle changes (such as increased physical activity) and, when needed, through medication
- Eat a healthy diet that is lower in fat and higher in fibre, and includes foods from each of the four food groups in Canada's Food Guide
- Use medications to reduce the risk for stroke as prescribed by your health care provider; for example, medications for hypertension, dyslipidemia, and diabetes, or other medications such as acetylsalicylic acid (Aspirin)
- Identify causes of excess stress and employ strategies to reduce them
- Be aware of a possible increased risk for stroke related to your family background
- Be aware of stroke risk factors (e.g., obesity, hypertension, and diabetes) at an early age
- Be aware that hormone therapy (conjugated equine estrogen) with or without medroxyprogesterone (Provera) should not be used for primary or secondary prevention of stroke in postmenopausal women

From Heart and Stroke Foundation of Canada. (2017). Women's unique risk factors. Retrieved from http://www.heartandstroke.ca/heart/risk-and-prevention/womens-unique-risk-factors.

The mortality rate of stroke has decreased by more than 75% over the past 60 years, and is associated with improved control of hypertension, diabetes, and dyslipidemia, as well as smoking cessation.[37]

CVAs (stroke syndromes) are classified pathophysiologically as ischemic, hemorrhagic, or associated with hypoperfusion. Risk factors for stroke include the following:

- Poorly or uncontrolled arterial hypertension
- Smoking, which increases the risk for stroke by 50%
- Insulin resistance and diabetes mellitus
- Polycythemia and thrombocythemia
- High total cholesterol or low high-density lipoprotein (HDL) cholesterol, elevated lipoprotein-a
- Congestive heart disease and peripheral vascular disease
- Hyperhomocysteinemia
- Atrial fibrillation
- *Chlamydia pneumoniae* infection

Ischemic stroke. Ischemic stroke occurs when there is obstruction to arterial blood flow to the brain from thrombus formation, an embolus, or hypoperfusion related to decreased blood volume or heart failure. The inadequate blood supply results in ischemia (inadequate cellular oxygen) and can progress to infarction (death of tissue).

Transient ischemic attacks (TIAs) are episodes of neurological dysfunction lasting no more than 1 hour and resulting from focal cerebral ischemia. The clinical manifestations of a TIA may include weakness, numbness, sudden confusion, loss of balance, or a sudden severe headache. The use of brain imaging modalities often reveals a brain infarction. About 3 to 17% of individuals who experience a TIA will have a stroke within 90 days.[38]

Thrombotic strokes (cerebral thromboses) arise from arterial occlusions caused by thrombi formation in arteries supplying the brain or intracranial vessels. Conditions causing increased coagulation or inadequate cerebral perfusion (e.g., dehydration, hypotension, prolonged vasoconstriction from malignant hypertension) increase the risk for thrombosis. Cerebral thrombosis develops most often from atherosclerosis and inflammatory disease processes that damage arterial walls. It may take as long as 20 to 30 years for obstruction to develop at the branches and curvature found in the cerebral circulation (see Chapter 24 for a discussion of atherogenesis). The smooth stenotic area can degenerate, forming an ulcerated area of the vessel wall. Platelets and fibrin adhere to the damaged wall, and a clot forms, gradually occluding the artery. The clot may enlarge both distally and proximally. Thrombotic strokes also occur when parts of a clot detach, travel upstream, and obstruct blood flow, causing acute ischemia.

Embolic stroke involves fragments that break from a thrombus formed outside the brain, usually in the heart, aorta, or common carotid artery. Other sources of embolism include fat, air, tumour, bacterial clumps, and foreign bodies. The embolus usually involves small brain vessels and obstructs at a bifurcation or other point of narrowing, thus causing ischemia. An embolus may plug the lumen entirely and remain in place or shatter into fragments and become part of the vessel's blood flow. Risk factors for an embolic stroke include atrial fibrillation, left ventricular aneurysm or thrombus, left atrial thrombus, recent myocardial infarction, endocarditis, rheumatic valve disease, mechanical valvular prostheses, atrioseptal defects, patent foramen ovale, and primary cardiac tumours. In persons who experience an embolic stroke, a second stroke usually follows because the source of emboli continues to exist. Embolization is usually in the distribution of the middle cerebral artery (the largest cerebral artery). Ischemic strokes in children are associated with congenital heart disease, cerebral arteriovenous malformations, and sickle cell disease (see Chapter 17).

Lacunar strokes (lacunar infarcts or small vessel disease) are usually caused by occlusion of a single, deep perforating artery that supplies small penetrating subcortical vessels, causing ischemic lesions (0.5 to 15 mm, or lacunes) predominantly in the basal ganglia, internal capsules, and pons. These strokes are rare and, because of the location and small area of infarction, they may have pure motor or sensory deficits.[39]

Hypoperfusion, or hemodynamic stroke, is associated with *systemic* hypoperfusion caused by cardiac failure, pulmonary embolism, or bleeding that results in inadequate blood supply to the brain. Stroke may occur more readily if there is carotid artery occlusion. Symptoms are usually bilateral and diffuse.[40]

PATHOPHYSIOLOGY Cerebral infarction results when an area of the brain loses its blood supply because of vascular occlusion. Causes include (1) abrupt vascular occlusion (e.g., embolus or thrombi), (2) gradual vessel occlusion (e.g., atheroma), and (3) partial occlusion of stenotic vessels. Cerebral thrombi and cerebral emboli most commonly produce occlusion, but atherosclerosis and hypertension are the dominant underlying processes.

There is a central core of irreversible ischemia and necrosis with cerebral infarction. The central core is surrounded by a zone of borderline ischemic tissue, the ischemic penumbra. Ischemia in the penumbra is not severe enough to result in structural damage. Prompt restoration of perfusion in the penumbra by injection of thrombolytic agents promotes perfusion and may prevent necrosis and loss of neurological function. The window of opportunity for protecting the penumbra is about 3 hours.

Cerebral infarctions are ischemic or hemorrhagic. In *ischemic infarcts*, the affected area becomes pale and softens 6 to 12 hours after the occlusion. Necrosis, swelling around the insult, and mushy disintegration appear by 48 to 72 hours after infarction. There is infiltration of macrophages and phagocytosis of necrotic tissue. The necrosis resolves by about the second week, ultimately leaving a cavity surrounded by glial scarring.

In *hemorrhagic infarcts*, bleeding occurs into the infarcted area through leaking vessels when the embolic fragments resolve and reperfusion begins to occur. Hemorrhagic transformation of ischemic stroke may be exacerbated by thrombolytic therapy.[41]

CLINICAL MANIFESTATIONS Clinical manifestations of thrombotic and embolic stroke vary, depending on the artery obstructed. Different sites of obstruction create different occlusion syndromes (e.g., carotid artery, dysphasia and contralateral motor [i.e., paresis] sensory [i.e., numbness] deficits, conjugate ipsilateral eye deviation), middle cerebral artery syndromes (dysphasia and contralateral motor and sensory deficits), or vertebrobasilar system syndromes (dizziness and ataxia, can progress to quadriplegia and coma).[42] Contralateral motor and sensory manifestations occur on the opposite side of the body from the location of the brain lesion because motor tracts originate in the cortex and most cross over in the medulla. Sensory tracts originate in the periphery and cross over in the spinal cord. Ipsilateral manifestations occur on the same side as the brain lesion. See Figure 16-11 for the Heart and Stroke Foundation of Canada's simple assessment tool for persons presenting with signs and symptoms of stroke.

EVALUATION AND TREATMENT Imaging is used to diagnose stroke. Treatment of ischemic stroke is focused on (1) restoring brain perfusion in a time frame that does not contribute to reperfusion injury, (2) counteracting the ischemic cascade pathways, (3) lowering cerebral metabolic demand so that the susceptible brain tissue is protected against impaired perfusion, (4) preventing recurrent ischemic events, and (5) promoting tissue restoration. Thrombolysis, using tissue-type plasminogen activator (tPA), is given within 3 and up to 4.5 hours of onset of symptoms. Endovascular intra-arterial thrombolysis may be used to

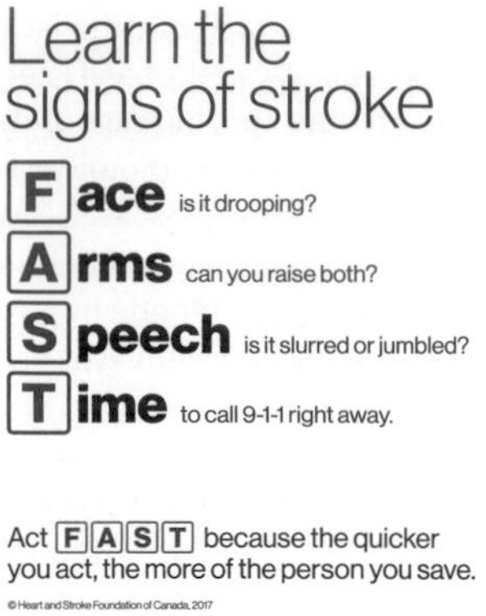

Learn the signs of stroke

Face is it drooping?

Arms can you raise both?

Speech is it slurred or jumbled?

Time to call 9-1-1 right away.

Act FAST because the quicker you act, the more of the person you save.

© Heart and Stroke Foundation of Canada, 2017

FIGURE 16-11 Signs of Stroke. (From Heart and Stroke Foundation of Canada. [2017]. *Signs of stroke.* Retrieved from http://www.heartandstroke.ca/stroke/signs-of-stroke.)

treat those who cannot receive tPA.[43] Supportive management is given to control cerebral edema and increased ICP and to provide neuroprotection. Arresting the disease process by control of risk factors is critical, and antiplatelet therapy may be instituted. A template and guidelines are available for the assessment and management of acute ischemic stroke.[44,45]

In embolic strokes, treatment is directed at preventing further embolization by instituting anticoagulation therapy and correcting the primary problem. Rehabilitation is indicated for ischemic strokes, and recovery of function is often possible.

Hemorrhagic stroke. Hemorrhagic stroke (intracranial hemorrhage) is the third most common cause of CVA. A hemorrhagic stroke can occur within the brain tissue (intraparenchymal) or in the subarachnoid or subdural spaces. The primary cause of intraparenchymal hemorrhagic stroke is hypertension with other causes including tumours, coagulation disorders, trauma, or illicit drug use, particularly cocaine. Prevention or control of hypertension reduces the incidence of hemorrhagic stroke.

Subarachnoid hemorrhage is associated with ruptured aneurysms or arteriovenous malformations (see p. 409) or brain trauma. Subdural hemorrhage (hematoma) is usually associated with brain trauma (see p. 394). Hypertensive causes of hemorrhagic stroke involve primarily smaller arteries and arterioles, resulting in thickening of the vessel walls and increased cellularity of the vessels. Necrosis may be present. Microaneurysms in these smaller vessels or arteriolar necrosis may precipitate the bleeding.

PATHOPHYSIOLOGY A mass of blood is formed as bleeding continues into the brain tissue. Adjacent brain tissue is deformed, compressed, and displaced, producing ischemia, edema, increased ICP, and necrosis. Rupture or seepage of blood into the ventricular system often occurs and is associated with higher mortality. Hemorrhages are described as massive, small, slit, or petechial. Massive hemorrhages are several centimetres in diameter, small hemorrhages are 1 to 2 cm in diameter, a slit hemorrhage lies in the subcortical area, and a petechial hemorrhage is the size of a pinhead bleed. The most common sites for hypertensive hemorrhages are in the putamen of the basal ganglia, the thalamus, the cortex and subcortex, the pons, the caudate nucleus, and the cerebellar hemispheres. Because neurons surrounding the ischemic or infarcted areas undergo changes that disrupt plasma membranes, cellular edema results, causing further compression of capillaries. Maximal cerebral edema develops in approximately 72 hours and takes about 2 weeks to subside. Most persons survive an initial hemispheric ischemic stroke unless there is massive cerebral edema, which is nearly always fatal. The cerebral hemorrhage resolves through reabsorption. Macrophages and astrocytes clear blood from the area. A cavity forms, surrounded by a dense gliosis (glial scar) after removal of the blood.

CLINICAL MANIFESTATIONS The clinical manifestations of hemorrhagic stroke are similar to those for embolic and thrombotic stroke and depend on the location and size of the bleed. Symptoms can occur suddenly and with activity. Once a deep unresponsive state occurs, the person rarely survives. The immediate prognosis is grave; however, if the person survives, recovery of function is often possible.

It is difficult to differentiate ischemic from hemorrhagic stroke based on symptoms. Individuals experiencing intracranial hemorrhage from a ruptured or leaking aneurysm have one of three sets of symptoms: (1) onset of an excruciating generalized headache with an almost immediate lapse into an unresponsive state, (2) headache but with consciousness maintained, and (3) sudden lapse into unconsciousness. If the hemorrhage is confined to the subarachnoid space, there may be no local signs. If bleeding spreads into the brain tissue, hemiparesis or paralysis, dysphasia, or homonymous hemianopia may be present. Warning signs of an impending aneurysm rupture include headache, transient unilateral weakness, transient numbness and tingling, and transient speech disturbance. However, such warning signs are often absent.

EVALUATION AND TREATMENT Treatment of an intracranial bleed, regardless of cause, focuses on stopping or reducing the bleeding, controlling the increased ICP, preventing a rebleed, and preventing vasospasm. There are some attempts to drain blood in a cerebral bleed, but the benefit is not documented in studies. Microsurgical interventions are under investigation.[46] Surgical treatments are options for ruptured aneurysms, vascular malformations, and subarachnoid hemorrhage.

Intracranial aneurysm. Intracranial aneurysms may result from arteriosclerosis, congenital abnormality, cocaine use, trauma, inflammation, and vascular sheer wall stress. The size may vary from 2 mm to 2 or 3 cm. Most aneurysms are located at bifurcations in or near the circle of Willis, in the vertebrobasilar arteries, or within the carotid system where there is higher wall sheer stress and flow turbulence (see Figures 13-19 and 13-20). Aneurysms may be single, but in 20 to 25% of the cases, more than one is present. In these instances, the aneurysms may be unilateral or bilateral. Peak incidence of rupture occurs in persons 50 to 59 years of age, with the incidence in postmenopausal women slightly higher than that in men.

PATHOPHYSIOLOGY No single pathological mechanism exists. Aneurysms may be classified on the basis of shape and form. Saccular aneurysms (berry aneurysms) occur frequently (in approximately 2% of the population) and likely result from congenital abnormalities in the tunica media of the arterial wall and hemodynamic and molecular changes.[47] The sac gradually grows over time. A saccular aneurysm may be (1) round with a narrow stalk connecting it to the parent artery, (2) broad-based without a stalk, or (3) cylindrical (Figure 16-12). Saccular aneurysms are rare in childhood; their highest incidence of rupturing or bleeding (subarachnoid hemorrhage) is among persons 20 to 50 years of age.

Fusiform aneurysms (giant aneurysms) are less common, occur as a result of diffuse arteriosclerotic changes, and are found most commonly in the basilar arteries or terminal portions of the internal carotid arteries. They act as space-occupying lesions.

Aneurysms rupture through thin areas often at bifurcation sites, causing hemorrhage into the subarachnoid space that spreads rapidly, producing localized changes in the cerebral cortex and focal irritation of nerves and arteries (see the discussion of Laplace law in Chapter

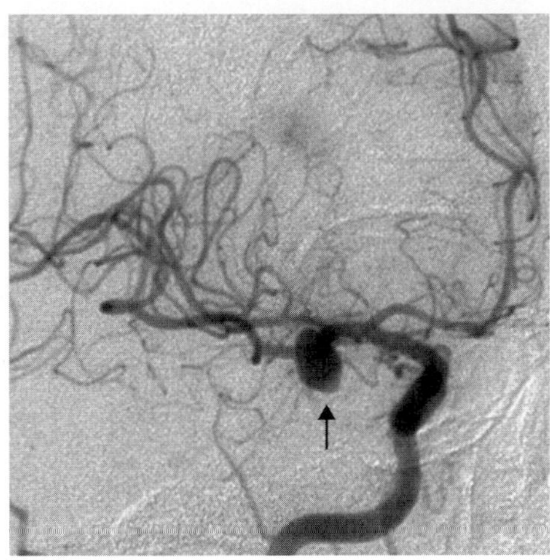

FIGURE 16-12 Berry Aneurysm, Angiogram. In this lateral view, with contrast filling a portion of the cerebral arterial circulation, a berry aneurysm (*arrow*) involving the middle cerebral artery of the circle of Willis at the base of the brain is shown. (From Klatt, E.C. [2015]. *Robbins and Cotran atlas of pathology* [3rd ed.]. Philadelphia: Saunders.)

23). Bleeding ceases when a fibrin-platelet plug forms at the point of rupture and as a result of compression. Blood undergoes reabsorption through arachnoid villi within 3 weeks.

CLINICAL MANIFESTATIONS Aneurysms often are asymptomatic. Of all persons undergoing routine autopsy, 5% are found to have one or more intracranial aneurysms. Clinical manifestations include dizziness or headache and cranial nerve compression, but the signs vary depending on the location and size of the aneurysm. Cranial nerves III, IV, V, and VI (see Table 13-6) are affected most often. Unfortunately, the most common first indication of the presence of an aneurysm is an acute subarachnoid hemorrhage, intracerebral hemorrhage, or combined subarachnoid-intracerebral hemorrhage (see "Hemorrhagic Stroke," p. 408).

EVALUATION AND TREATMENT Diagnosis before a bleeding episode is made through arteriography. After a subarachnoid or intracerebral hemorrhage, a tentative diagnosis of an aneurysm is based on clinical manifestations, history, and imaging. Treatments for intracranial aneurysm are both medical (i.e., control of hypertension) and surgical (i.e., microvascular clipping or placement of endovascular coils).[48]

Vascular malformation. Vascular malformations are rare congenital vascular lesions. An **arteriovenous malformation (AVM)** is a mass of dilated vessels between the arterial and venous systems (arteriovenous fistula) without an intervening capillary bed, may occur in any part of the brain, and vary in size from a few millimetres to large malformations extending from the cortex to the ventricle. AVMs occur equally in males and females and occasionally occur in families. Although AVMs are usually present at birth, symptoms exhibit a delayed age of onset and commonly occur before 30 years of age.

PATHOPHYSIOLOGY AVMs have abnormal blood vessel structure, are abnormally thin, and have complex growth and remodelling patterns.[49] There is direct shunting of arterial blood into the venous vasculature without the dissipation of the arterial blood pressure with increased risk for rupture. One or several arteries may feed the AVM and, over time, they become tortuous and dilated. With moderate to large AVMs, sufficient blood is shunted into the malformation to deprive surrounding tissue of adequate blood perfusion.

CLINICAL MANIFESTATIONS Twenty percent of persons with an AVM have a characteristic chronic, nondescript headache, although some experience migraine. Fifty percent of persons experience seizures. The other 50% experience an intracerebral, subarachnoid, or subdural hemorrhage with progressive neurological deficits. Bleeding from an AVM into the subarachnoid space causes symptoms identical to those associated with a ruptured aneurysm. If bleeding is into the brain tissue, focal signs that develop resemble a stroke that is progressing in severity. Ten percent of persons experience hemiparesis or other focal signs. At times, noncommunicating hydrocephalus (see Chapter 15) develops with a large AVM that extends into the ventricular lining.

EVALUATION AND TREATMENT A systolic bruit over the carotid artery in the neck or the mastoid process (or the eyeball in a young person), representing audible turbulent blood flow, is almost always diagnostic of an AVM. Confirming diagnosis is made by CT and MRI, followed by magnetic resonance angiography (MRA). Treatment options include direct surgical excision, endovascular embolization, or radiotherapy.[50]

Subarachnoid hemorrhage. **Subarachnoid hemorrhage (SAH)** is the escape of blood from a defective or injured vessel into the subarachnoid space. Individuals at risk for a subarachnoid hemorrhage are those with intracranial aneurysm, intracranial AVM, hypertension, or a family history of SAH, and those who have sustained head injuries. Subarachnoid hemorrhages often recur, especially from a ruptured intracranial aneurysm.

PATHOPHYSIOLOGY When a vessel is leaking, blood oozes into the subarachnoid space. When a vessel tears, blood under pressure is pumped into the subarachnoid space. The blood increases the intracranial volume, and it is also extremely irritating to the neural tissues and produces an inflammatory reaction. In addition, the blood coats nerve roots, clogs arachnoid granulations (impairing CSF reabsorption), and obstructs foramina within the ventricular system (impairing CSF circulation). Intracranial pressure immediately increases to almost diastolic levels but returns to near baseline in about 10 minutes. Cerebral blood flow and cerebral perfusion pressure decrease. Autoregulation of blood flow is impaired, and there is a compensatory increase in systolic blood pressure.[51] The expanding hematoma acts like a space-occupying lesion, compressing and displacing brain tissue with increased ICP, decreased cerebral blood flow, blood–brain barrier breakdown, brain edema, inflammation, and cell death. Secondary brain injury can occur as described for TBI. Granulation tissue is formed, and meningeal scarring with impairment of CSF reabsorption and secondary hydrocephalus often results. Mortality in subarachnoid hemorrhage is 50% at 1 month.

Delayed cerebral ischemia, a syndrome of progressive neurological deterioration, is associated with *cerebral artery vasospasm*. From 40 to 60% of persons with an SAH experience vasospasms in adjacent and, occasionally, in nonadjacent vessels. Vasospasm may occur because of leukocyte–endothelial cell interactions or the effects of vasoactive substances (e.g., calcium, prostaglandins, serotonin, catecholamines) on the arteries of the subarachnoid space. Edema, medial necrosis, and proliferation of the tunica intima in cerebral arterioles have been found. Vasospasm causes decreased cerebral blood flow, ischemia, and possibly infarct and can lead to delayed ischemic injury and death 3 to 14 days after the initial hemorrhage.[52]

CLINICAL MANIFESTATIONS Early manifestations associated with leaking vessels are episodic and include headache, changes in mental status or level of consciousness, nausea or vomiting, and focal neurological defects. A ruptured vessel causes a sudden, throbbing, "explosive" headache, accompanied by nausea and vomiting, visual disturbances, motor deficits, and loss of consciousness related to a dramatic rise in ICP. Meningeal irritation and inflammation often occur, causing neck stiffness (nuchal rigidity), photophobia, blurred vision, irritability, restlessness, and low-grade fever. A positive Kernig sign (straightening the knee with the hip and knee in a flexed position produces pain in the back and neck regions) and a positive Brudzinski sign (passive flexion of the neck produces neck pain and increased rigidity) may appear. No localizing signs are present if the bleed is confined completely to the subarachnoid space.

The Hunt and Hess SAH grading system is based on description of the clinical manifestations (Table 16-6).[53] Rebleeding is a significant risk with a high mortality (up to 70%). The period of greatest risk is during the first 72 hours and up to 2 weeks after the initial bleed. Rebleeding is manifested by a sudden increase in blood pressure and ICP, along with a deteriorating neurological status.[54]

Seizures occur in 25% of persons with an SAH, and hydrocephalus after a bleed occurs in 20% of cases. Hypothalamic dysfunction, manifested by salt wasting, hyponatremia, and ECG changes, is common.

EVALUATION AND TREATMENT The diagnosis of an SAH is based on the clinical presentation, imaging, and CSF evaluation. Treatment is directed at controlling ICP, improving cerebral perfusion pressure, preventing ischemia and hypoxia of neural tissues, and avoiding rebleeding episodes. Surgical intervention is common. Treatment guidelines are available to direct therapy.[48]

TABLE 16-6 Subarachnoid Hemorrhage Classification Scale

Category	Description
Grade I	Neurological status intact; mild headache, slight nuchal rigidity
Grade II	Neurological deficit evidenced by cranial nerve involvement; moderate to severe headache with more pronounced meningeal signs (e.g., photophobia, nuchal rigidity)
Grade III	Drowsiness and confusion with or without focal neurological deficits; pronounced meningeal signs
Grade IV	Stuporous with pronounced neurological deficits (e.g., hemiparesis, dysphasia); nuchal rigidity
Grade V	Deep coma state with decerebrate posturing and other brainstem functioning

From Tateshima, S., & Duckwiler, G. (2012). Vascular diseases of the nervous system. In R.B. Daroff, G.M. Fenichel, J. Jankovic, et al. (Eds.), *Bradley's neurology in clinical practice*. Philadelphia: Saunders.

✔ QUICK CHECK 16-2

1. Why is atherosclerosis a risk factor for thrombotic stroke?
2. Why do the signs and symptoms of a TIA resolve completely?
3. Why do lacunar strokes involve small infarcts?
4. How is an arteriovenous malformation different from an aneurysm?

Headache

Headache is a common neurological disorder and is usually a benign symptom. However, it can be associated with serious disease such as brain tumour, meningitis, or cerebrovascular disease (e.g., giant cell arteritis, cerebral aneurysm, or cerebral bleeds). The headache syndromes discussed here are the chronic, recurring type not associated with structural abnormalities or systemic disease and include migraine, cluster, and tension-type headaches. Characteristics of the major types of headache syndromes are summarized in Table 16-7.

Migraine

Migraine is an episodic neurological disorder characterized by a headache lasting 4 to 72 hours. It is diagnosed when any two of the following features occur: unilateral head pain, throbbing pain, pain worsens with activity, moderate or severe pain intensity; *and* at least one of the following: nausea and/or vomiting, or photophobia and phonophobia.[55] Migraine is broadly classified as (1) *migraine with aura* with visual, sensory, or motor symptoms; and, more commonly, (2) *migraine without aura.*

Migraine occurs in 11.8% of women and 4.7% of men in Canada, and can occur in children. It is more common in those who are in their 30s and 40s. There often is a family history of migraine. In susceptible women, migraine occurs most frequently before and during menstruation and is decreased during pregnancy and menopause. The cyclic withdrawal of estrogen and progesterone may trigger attacks of migraine.[56,57]

Migraine is caused by a combination of multiple genetic and environmental factors. Persons with migraine have an increased risk for epilepsy, depression, anxiety disorders, cardiovascular disease, and stroke. Migraine may be precipitated by triggers. Individuals with migraine are likely to have a genetically determined reduced threshold for triggers. Triggers can include becoming tired or oversleeping, missed meals, overexertion, weather change, stress or relaxation from stress,

TABLE 16-7 Characteristics of Common Headaches

	MIGRAINE		Cluster Headache/	
	Without Aura	With Aura (25–30%)	Proximal Hemicrania	Tension-Type Headache
Age of onset	Childhood, adolescence, or young adulthood	Childhood, adolescence, or young adulthood	Young adulthood, middle age	Young adulthood, middle age
Gender	Higher in females	Higher in females	Male	Not gender specific
Family history of headaches	Yes	Yes	No	Yes
Onset and evolution	Slow to rapid	Slow to rapid	Rapid	Slow to rapid
Time course	Episodic	Episodic	Clusters in time	Episodic, may become constant
Quality	Usually throbbing	Usually throbbing	Steady	Steady
Location	Variable, unilateral to bilateral	Variable, unilateral to bilateral	Orbit, temple, cheek	Variable
Associated features	Prodrome, vomiting	Aura: visual, sensory, language, and motor disturbance Prodrome, vomiting	Lacrimation, rhinorrhea, Horner syndrome	None

hormonal changes (menstrual periods), excess afferent stimulation (bright lights, strong smells), and chemicals (alcohol or nitrates).

The pathophysiological basis for migraine is complex and not clearly established. There is no identifiable pathology, but there are associated changes in brain metabolism and blood flow. Current theories includes neurological, vascular, hormonal, and neurotransmitter components. Migraine aura is associated with cortical spreading depression (CSD). CSD is a spontaneous self-propagating wave of glial and neuronal depolarization resulting in hyperactivity that starts in the occipital region and spreads across the cortex.[58] CSD initiates the release of neurotransmitters that activate the trigeminal vascular system (afferent projections from cranial nerve V), stimulating vasodilation of dural blood vessels, activation of inflammation, peripheral and central sensitization of pain receptors (hypersensitivity to pain), and activation of areas of the brainstem and forebrain that modulate pain. Release of inflammatory mediators with sterile meningeal inflammation and edema of blood vessels may be an important component of migraine pain. Vasodilation of blood vessels is not sufficient to account for the pain of migraine. Calcitonin gene-related peptide (CGRP) release by the trigeminal vascular system is related to migraine pain. The mechanism is not clear, but CGRP antagonists stop the headache. Glutamate (an excitatory neurotransmitter) concentration is increased and 5-hydroxytryptamine (5-HT, serotonin) concentration is decreased. 5-HT causes vasoconstriction and antagonizes CGRP. Consequently, 5-HT(1B/1D) receptor agonists (i.e., triptans) and CGRP receptor and glutamate receptor antagonists have been used for the acute treatment of migraine.[59-61]

The clinical phases of a migraine attack are as follows:

1. *Premonitory phase:* Up to one third of persons have premonitory symptoms hours to days before onset of aura or headache. These symptoms may include tiredness, irritability, loss of concentration, stiff neck, and food cravings.
2. *Migraine aura:* Up to one third of persons have aura symptoms at least some of the time that may last up to 1 hour. Symptoms can be visual, sensory, or motor.
3. *Headache phase:* Throbbing pain usually begins on one side and spreads to include the entire head. Headache may be accompanied by fatigue, nausea, and vomiting or dizziness. There may be hypersensitivity to anything touching the head. Symptoms may last from 4 to 72 hours (usually about a day).
4. *Recovery phase:* Irritability, fatigue, or depression may take hours or days to resolve.

Differentiation of types of migraine headache is summarized in Table 16-7. The diagnosis of migraine is made from medical history and physical examination. Differential diagnosis is confirmed by imaging and EEG. Functional neuroimaging and genetic studies are advancing the understanding of the mechanisms involved in migraine attacks and individual variants involved with disease susceptibility.[62] The management of migraine includes avoidance of triggers (e.g., darkening the room, applying ice). Sleeping can provide some relief with the onset of acute migraine. Pharmacological management for the treatment and prevention of migraine is available.[63,64] A transcutaneous electrical stimulation device providing trigeminal neurostimulation has been approved by Health Canada for the prevention of migraine.[65]

Chronic migraines usually begin as episodic migraines that increase in frequency over time. Chronic migraine occurs at least 15 days in a month (can occur daily or on a near-daily basis) for more than 3 months. Chronic migraines are associated with overuse of analgesic migraine medications (sometimes called *rebound headaches*), obesity, and caffeine overuse. Treatment is similar to that for episodic migraine. Individuals with chronic migraine unresponsive to medical treatment should be evaluated for intracranial hypertension without papilledema and the possibility of sinus venous stenosis.[66]

Cluster Headache

Cluster headaches are one of a group of disorders referred to as *trigeminal autonomic cephalagias* (headaches involving the autonomic division of the trigeminal nerve).[67] They occur in one side of the head, primarily in men between 20 and 50 years of age. The pain may alternate sides with each headache episode and is severe, stabbing, and throbbing. These uncommon headaches occur in clusters (up to 8 attacks per day) and last for minutes to hours for a period of days, followed by a long period of spontaneous remission. Cluster headache has an episodic and a chronic form with extreme pain intensity and short duration. If the cluster of attacks occurs more frequently without sustained spontaneous remission, they are classified as *chronic cluster headaches* (10 to 20% of cases) (see Table 16-7). Triggers are similar to those that cause migraine headache.

Trigeminal activation occurs but the mechanism is unclear. Functional imaging indicates a role for concomitant posterior hypothalamic and pain neuromatrix activation with opioid system involvement.[68] The pathogenic mechanism for pain is related to the release of vasoactive substances and the formation of neurogenic inflammation. Autonomic dysfunction is characterized by sympathetic underactivity and parasympathetic activation. There is unilateral trigeminal distribution of severe pain with ipsilateral autonomic manifestations, including tearing on affected side, ptosis of the ipsilateral eye, and congestion of the nasal mucosa. Prophylactic medications are used to treat cluster headache, as well as avoidance of triggers. Acute attacks are managed with oxygen inhalation, sumatriptan (Imitrex) or inhaled ergotamine tartrate (Medihaler Ergotamine) administration, and nerve stimulation.[69] New medications are under investigation.

Tension-Type Headache

Tension-type headache (TTH) is the most common type of headache. The average age of onset is during the second decade of life. It is a mild to moderate bilateral headache with a sensation of a tight band or pressure around the head with gradual onset of pain. The headache occurs in episodes and may last for several hours or several days. It is not aggravated by physical activity. Chronic tension-type headache (CTTH) evolves from episodic TTH and represents headache that occurs at least 15 days per month for at least 3 months.

Both central and peripheral mechanisms operate in causing tension headaches. The central pain mechanism is associated with CTTH, and a peripheral mechanism is associated with episodic TTH. The central pain mechanism probably involves hypersensitivity of pain fibres from the trigeminal nerve that leads to central sensitization. The peripheral sensitization of myofascial sensory nerves may contribute to muscular hypersensitivity and the development of CTTH. Headache sufferers have more localized pain and tenderness of pericranial muscles. Many individuals have both TTHs and migraines.

Mild TTHs are treated with ice, and more severe forms are treated with Aspirin or nonsteroidal anti-inflammatory medications. CTTHs are best managed with a tricyclic antidepressant and behavioural and relaxation therapy. Some individuals benefit from injection of botulinum toxin A. Long-term use of analgesics or other medications, such as muscle relaxants, antihistamines, tranquilizers, caffeine, and ergot alkaloids, should be avoided.[70]

Infection and Inflammation of the Central Nervous System

The CNS may be infected by bacteria, viruses, fungi, parasites, and mycobacteria. The invading organisms enter the nervous system either by spreading through arterial blood vessels (Figure 16-13) or by directly invading the nervous tissue from another site of infection. Neurological

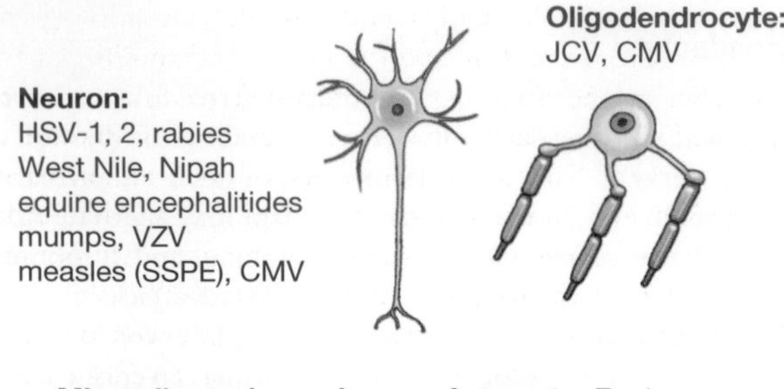

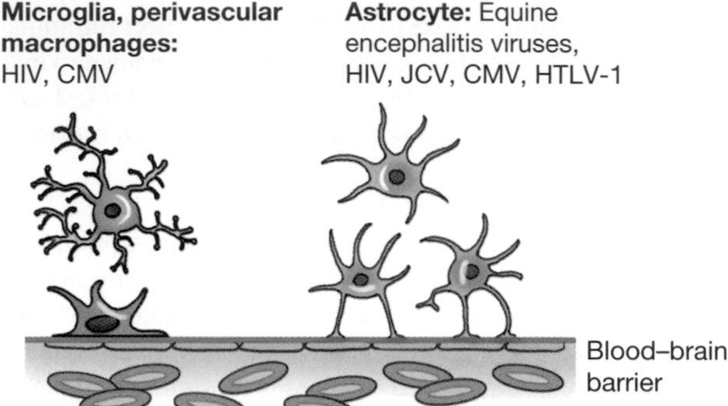

FIGURE 16-13 Viral Infection in the Central Nervous System. Viruses infect specific cell types within the central nervous system, depending on the particular properties of the virus together with individual cell membrane proteins expressed on permissive cell types. Normally the brain is protected from circulating pathogens and toxins by the blood–brain barrier. *CMV,* cytomegalovirus; *HIV,* human immunodeficiency virus; *HSV,* herpes simplex virus; *HTLV-1,* human T-cell lymphotropic virus type 1 (causes T-cell leukemia); *JCV,* John Cunningham virus (a polyomavirus causing progressive multifocal leukoencephalopathy); *SSPE,* subacute sclerosing panencephalitis; *VZV,* varicella-zoster virus. (Adapted from Power, C., & Noorbakhsh, G. [2007]. Central nervous system viral infections: Clinical aspects and pathogenic mechanisms. In S. Gilman [Ed.], *Neurobiology of disease* [p. 488]. Burlington, MA: Elsevier.)

infections produce disease by several mechanisms: direct neuronal or glial infection, mass lesion formation, inflammation with subsequent edema, interruption of CSF pathways, neuronal or vascular damage, and secretion of neurotoxins. An immune process may initiate an inflammatory reaction.

Meningitis

Meningitis is inflammation of the brain or spinal cord. Infectious meningitis may be caused by bacteria, viruses, fungi, parasites, or toxins. The infection may be acute, subacute, or chronic with the pathophysiology, clinical manifestations, and treatment differing for each type of microorganism.

Fungal meningitis is a chronic, much less common condition than bacterial or viral meningitis. The infection most often occurs in persons with impaired immune responses or alterations in normal body flora. It develops insidiously, usually over days or weeks. Fungi in the nervous system usually produce a granulomatous reaction, forming granulomata or gelatinous masses in the meninges at the base of the brain. Fungi also may extend along the perivascular sites in the subarachnoid space and into the brain tissue, producing arteritis with thrombosis, infarction, and communicating hydrocephalus. Meningeal fibrosis develops later in the inflammatory process. Cranial nerve dysfunction, caused by compression, often results from the granulomata and fibrosis. The first manifestations are often those of dementia (see Chapter 15) or communicating hydrocephalus (see Chapter 15). The individual is characteristically afebrile.

Viral meningitis (aseptic or nonpurulent meningitis) is thought to be limited to the meninges. An identifiable bacterium cannot be found in the CSF. The most common viruses are enteroviral viruses (echovirus, coxsackievirus, and nonparalytic poliomyelitis), arboviruses, and herpes simplex type 2. Viruses enter the nervous system by crossing the blood–brain barrier, by direct spread along peripheral nerves, or through the choroid plexus epithelium. Recognition of viral antigens by immune cells activates the inflammatory response. The clinical manifestations of viral meningitis are similar to those of bacterial meningitis, but milder. Viral meningitis is managed pharmacologically with antiviral medications and steroids.

Bacterial meningitis is primarily an infection of the pia mater and arachnoid, the subarachnoid space, the ventricular system, and the CSF. Meningococci (*Neisseria meningitidis*) and pneumococci (*Streptococcus pneumoniae*) are the most common pathogens. An increase of medication-resistant strains of *S. pneumoniae* is an emerging problem worldwide. About 1 in 100 000 persons are affected by bacterial meningitis annually.[71] Meningococcus has been identified worldwide, and there are six serogroups: A, B, C, W-135, X, and Y. Most cases are sporadic and occur predominantly in children younger than 1 year of age and adolescents. Local outbreaks may occur in student residences, military bases, or sub-Saharan Africa. With pneumococcal meningitis, young persons and those more than 40 years of age are mostly affected. Predisposing conditions are otitis or sinusitis (25%), immunocompromised status (16%), and pneumonia (12%). The disease is spread by respiratory droplets and contact with contaminated saliva or respiratory tract secretions (kissing, coughing, sneezing, or sharing utensils, food, and drink).[72] Carriers of the meningococcal bacteria do not develop meningitis but may pass it on to others.

PATHOPHYSIOLOGY Meningococci and pneumococci are inhaled and attach to epithelial cells in the nasopharynx where they cross the mucosal barrier, enter the bloodstream, travel to cerebral blood vessels, cross the blood–brain barrier, and infect the meninges. With bacterial infection, large numbers of neutrophils are recruited to the subarachnoid space. Release of cytotoxic inflammatory agents and bacterial toxins alter the blood–brain barrier, cause cerebral edema, and damage brain tissue. The inflammatory exudate thickens the CSF and interferes with normal CSF flow around the brain and spinal cord, possibly obstructing arachnoid villi and producing hydrocephalus. Meningeal cells become edematous, and the combined exudate and edematous cells increase ICP. Engorged blood vessels and thrombi can disrupt blood flow, causing further injury.[73] Acute infectious **purpura fulminans** is a rare rapidly progressive syndrome of hemorrhagic infarction of the skin and disseminated intravascular coagulation that can lead to multiple organ failure, ischemic necrosis of digits and limbs with amputation required, and death. It is caused by bacterial endotoxin and inflammatory cytokines.

CLINICAL MANIFESTATIONS The clinical manifestations of bacterial meningitis can be grouped into infectious signs, meningeal signs, and neurological signs. The clinical manifestations of systemic infection include fever, tachycardia, and chills. The clinical manifestations of meningeal irritation are a severe throbbing headache, severe photophobia, nuchal rigidity, and positive Kernig and Brudzinski signs. The neurological signs include a decrease in consciousness, cranial nerve palsies, focal neurological deficits (such as hemiparesis or hemiplegia and ataxia), and seizures. Often there is projectile vomiting. As ICP increases, papilledema develops and delirium may progress to unconsciousness and death.

With meningococcal meningitis, a petechial or purpuric rash covers the skin and mucous membranes.

EVALUATION AND TREATMENT Rapid diagnosis, antibiotic administration, and supportive treatment are important to prevent morbidity and mortality from bacterial meningitis. Diagnosis is based on physical examination, blood cultures, and the results of nasopharyngeal smear and antigen tests. CSF analysis and cultures are required for differential diagnosis.[73,74] Serious complications, including septic shock, disseminated intravascular coagulation, purpura fulminans, limb damage, and multiple organ failure, require intensive multidisciplinary care.

Vaccinations are available to prevent meningococcal, pneumococcal, and *Haemophilus influenzae* meningitis.[75] Meningococcal vaccine promotes antibody protection within 7 to 14 days.[76] Vaccination of children ages 11 or 12 years is recommended, with a booster to be given between ages 16 and 18 years or older, particularly postsecondary students living in student residences.

Brain or Spinal Cord Abscess

Abscesses, localized collections of pus, may form within the parenchyma of the brain or spinal cord but are rare.

Brain abscesses are classified as epidural, subdural, or intracerebral. *Epidural brain abscesses (empyemas)* are associated with osteomyelitis in a cranial bone. *Subdural brain abscesses (empyemas)* arise from a sinus infection or a vascular source. *Intracerebral brain abscesses* arise from a vascular source. Spinal cord abscesses are classified as epidural or intramedullary. Epidural spinal abscesses usually originate as osteomyelitis in a vertebra; the infection then spreads into the epidural space. (Osteomyelitis is discussed in Chapter 39.)

PATHOPHYSIOLOGY Microorganisms gain entrance to the CNS by direct extension or distribution along the wall of a vein. Infective emboli carry organisms from distant sites. Users of illicit drugs who share needles are at risk, as are immunosuppressed persons. For example: *Toxoplasma gondii* is producing an ever-increasing number of CNS abscesses in persons with AIDS.[77] Streptococci, staphylococci, and *Bacteroides*, often combined with anaerobes, are the most common bacteria that cause abscesses; however, yeast and fungi also may be involved.[78]

Brain abscesses progress from localized inflammation to a necrotic core with the formation of a connective tissue capsule, usually within 14 days or longer.[79] Existing abscesses also tend to spread and form daughter abscesses.

CLINICAL MANIFESTATIONS Early manifestations include low-grade fever, headache (most common symptom), nausea and vomiting, neck pain and stiffness, confusion, drowsiness, sensory deficits, and communication deficits. Later manifestations are associated with an expanding mass and include decreased attention span, memory deficits, decreased visual acuity and narrowed visual fields, papilledema, ocular palsy, ataxia, dementia, and seizures. The development of symptoms may be very insidious, often making an abscess difficult to diagnose.[80]

Extradural brain abscesses are associated with localized pain, purulent drainage from the nasal passages or auditory canal, fever, localized tenderness, and neck stiffness. Clinical manifestations of spinal cord abscesses have four stages: (1) spinal aching; (2) severe root pain, accompanied by spasms of the back muscles and limited vertebral movement; (3) weakness caused by progressive cord compression; and (4) paralysis.

EVALUATION AND TREATMENT The diagnosis is suggested by clinical features and confirmed by imaging studies. Antibiotics and surgical aspiration or excision is usually indicated. Intracranial pressure may have to be managed. Spinal cord abscesses are treated with surgical decompression or aspiration, antibiotic therapy, and supportive therapy.

Encephalitis

Encephalitis is an acute febrile illness, usually of viral origin, with nervous system involvement. The most common forms are caused by bites of mosquitoes, ticks, or flies. Herpes simplex type 1 is the most common sporadic cause of encephalitis. Viruses infect specific cell types in the CNS, as shown in Figure 16-13. Referred to as *infectious viral encephalitides*, encephalitis may occur as a complication of systemic viral diseases such as poliomyelitis, rabies, or mononucleosis, or it may arise after recovery from viral infections such as rubella, varicella, rubeola, or yellow fever. Encephalitis also may follow vaccination with a live attenuated virus vaccine if the vaccine has an encephalitis component, for example, measles, mumps, and rubella. Typhus, trichinosis, malaria, and schistosomiasis also are associated with encephalitis. Toxoplasmosis may acutely reactivate in immunosuppressed persons when the once-dormant parasite in cyst form disseminates in brain tissues.[81]

With the exception of the California viral encephalitis, which is endemic, the arthropodborne encephalitides occur in epidemics, varying in geographic and seasonal incidence (Table 16-8 and *Health Promotion*: West Nile Virus). Eastern equine encephalitis is the most serious but least common of the encephalitides.

TABLE 16-8 Common Arboviruses of North America

Virus	Distribution	Insect Vector	Immediate Vertebrate Host
West Nile	United States, Canada, Mexico	Mosquito (*Culex* sp)	Passiform birds (jays, blackbirds, crows, finches, sparrows)
St. Louis encephalitis	United States, Canada, Mexico	Mosquito (*Culex* sp)	Passerine birds (sparrows, house finches)
Eastern equine encephalitis	Atlantic and Gulf Coast states, upper New York, Michigan, Eastern Canada	Mosquito (*Culex* sp)	Fresh water swamp birds
Western equine encephalitis	Western United States, Canada	Mosquito (*Culex* sp)	Passerine birds, jackrabbit
Venezuelan encephalitis	Mexico, Florida, Texas	Mosquito (*Culex* and *Aedes* sp)	Rodents, aquatic birds
Powassan encephalitis	Northern United States, Canada	Ixodes ticks	Squirrels, mice, ground hogs, voles
La Crosse or Jamestown encephalitis	North central and northeast United States	Mosquito (*Aedes triseriatus*)	Chipmunks, squirrels
Colorado tick fever	Rocky Mountain states, Canada	Tick (*Dermacentor andersoni*)	Chipmunks, squirrels, small mammals
Dengue	Mexico and Florida	Mosquito (*Aedes* sp)	Humans and nonhuman primates

From Davis, L.E., Beckham, J.D., & Tyler, K.L. (2008). *Neurol Clin, 26*(3), 727–757 (Table 2). doi:10.1016/j.ncl.2008.03.012

HEALTH PROMOTION

West Nile Virus

West Nile virus (WNV), a *Flavivirus* transmitted predominantly by the *Culex* mosquito, emerged in New York State in 1999. It is the most common cause of epidemic meningoencephalitis and the leading cause of arboviral encephalitis in North America. The first human case of WNV infection in Canada was reported in 2002. Humans and horses, as well as other mammals, are incidental hosts. Birds and mosquitoes are life cycle hosts. In most parts of Canada, the risk of becoming infected with WNV starts mid-April and ends after the first hard frost. Besides mosquito transmission, WNV can be transmitted through blood transfusions and organ transplants. Health experts think that transmission from mother to unborn child and through breast milk is possible.

The most effective way to avoid infection with WNV is to prevent mosquito bites. Since mosquitoes are most active at dawn and dusk, avoiding outdoor activities during those times reduces the risk of bites. It is recommended during outdoor activities to wear long pants and long-sleeved loose shirts, socks, and a hat, and light-coloured clothing. In addition, the use of an insect repellant that contains DEET or icaridin is recommended. Since mosquitoes lay their eggs in standing water, eliminating any areas of standing water around the home is suggested. The use of window and door screens also assists in preventing mosquitoes from entering the home.

Data from Government of Canada. (2016). *Prevention of West Nile virus.* Retrieved from http://healthycanadians.gc.ca/diseases-conditions-maladies-affections/disease-maladie/west-nile-nil-occidental/prevention-eng.php; Petersen, L.R., Brault, A.C., & Nasci, R.S. (2013). *JAMA, 310*(3), 308–315; Reisen, W.K. (2013). *Viruses, 5*(9), 2079–2105.

PATHOPHYSIOLOGY Viruses gain access to the CNS through the bloodstream, olfactory bulb, or choroid plexus, or through an intraneuronal route from peripheral nerves. Meningeal involvement is present in all encephalitides. The various encephalitides may cause widespread nerve cell degeneration. Edema, necrosis with or without hemorrhage, and increased ICP develop.

CLINICAL MANIFESTATIONS Encephalitis ranges from a mild infectious disease to a life-threatening disorder. Mild symptoms include malaise, headache, body aches, nausea, and vomiting. Dramatic clinical manifestations include fever, delirium, or confusion progressing to unconsciousness, difficulty with word finding, seizure activity, cranial nerve palsies, paresis and paralysis, involuntary movement, and abnormal reflexes. Signs of marked ICP may be present.

EVALUATION AND TREATMENT Diagnosis is made by history and clinical presentation aided by CSF examination and culture, serological studies, white blood cell count, CT scan, or MRI. Empirical treatment is specific to the type of virus and may include antiviral agents, antibiotics, and steroids. Herpes encephalitis is treated with antiviral agents, such as acyclovir (Zovirax). Measures to control ICP are paramount.[82]

Neurological Complications of AIDS

From 40 to 60% of all persons with AIDS (see Chapter 8) have neurological complications. The most common neurological disorder is HIV-associated neurocognitive disorder. Others are peripheral neuropathies, vacuolar (spongy softening) myelopathy, opportunistic infections of the CNS, neoplasms, and, less commonly, stroke syndromes.[83]

HIV-associated neurocognitive disorder. A variety of names are used for HIV-associated neurocognitive disorder (HAND), including *HIV-associated cognitive dysfunction*, *HIV encephalopathy*, *subacute encephalitis*, *HIV-associated dementia complex*, *HIV cognitive motor complex*, *AIDS encephalopathy*, *AIDS dementia complex*, and *AIDS-related dementia*. Both adults and children may be affected by progressive cognitive dysfunction with motor and behavioural alterations. The syndrome typically develops later in the disease but may be an early or singular manifestation in some persons. The syndrome is more prevalent in drug users with HIV. Highly active antiretroviral therapy (HAART) with more efficient CNS medication penetration has reduced the prevalence and improved survival for severe HAND, but milder forms of the disease may persist because of longer life.

The neurological syndromes develop from properties of the virus, genetic characteristics of the host, and interactions with the environment (including treatment). At the time of primary HIV infection, HIV infects the perivascular macrophages, microglial cells, and astrocytes, particularly the basal ganglia and deep white matter. Affected macrophages, macrophage-derived multinucleated cells, and microglia cause an immune-mediated demyelination process in white matter. Focal and diffuse demyelination of white matter and spongy changes of the spinal cord are present.

HAND is insidious in onset and unpredictable in its course. Most persons experience a steady progression of mental decline characterized by abrupt accelerations of signs over several months to more than 1 year. The triad of clinical manifestations are neurocognitive impairment, behavioural disturbance, and motor abnormalities. Specific manifestations can include an organic psychosis with agitation, inappropriate behaviour, and hallucinosis. Motor signs include difficulty speaking; progressive loss of balance; gait ataxia; spastic paraparesis or paralysis; and generalized hyper-reflexia sometimes accompanied by decreased writing ability, tremor, myoclonus, and seizure.

Diagnosis is difficult, especially in early stages, and CSF analysis, CT scan, and MRI data help establish the diagnosis. HIV antiretroviral treatment is continued. Although CNS medication penetration is reduced, there is decreased prevalence and improved survival for individuals with severe HAND.[84]

HIV myelopathy. HIV myelopathy involves diffuse degeneration of the spinal cord in persons with HIV. *Vacuolar myelopathy* is thought to be a direct consequence of HIV. The lateral and posterior columns of the lumbar spinal cord are affected. Progressive spastic paraparesis with ataxia is the predominant clinical manifestation. Leg weakness, upper motor neuron signs, incontinence, and posterior column sensory loss may be present. Diagnosis is made on the basis of history, physical findings, and supporting data from diagnostic procedures. Treatment is supportive.

HIV-associated peripheral neuropathy. HIV may directly infect nerves and cause HIV distal symmetric polyneuropathy, most commonly sensory neuropathy.[85] Persons experience neuropathic pain, including pain burning sensations and numbness commonly in the extremities. Weakness and decreased or absent distal reflexes may be present. Diagnosis is established through the history and physical findings, laboratory data, and nerve conduction and electromyogram (EMG) studies.

Viral meningitis and HIV. Some persons develop acute viral meningitis at approximately the time of seroconversion. The presentation of acute viral meningitis may represent the initial infection of the nervous system by the virus. Symptoms include headache, fever, and meningismus (headache, photophobia, nuchal rigidity). Cranial nerve involvement, especially V and VII, may appear, but the disease is self-limiting and requires only symptomatic treatment.

Opportunistic infections and HIV. Opportunistic infections may be bacterial, fungal, or viral in origin and may produce neurological disease. Typically, bacterial infections are caused by unusual microorganisms. Cryptococcal infection is the most common fungal disorder and the third leading cause of neurological disease in persons with AIDS.

The symptoms are vague, such as fever, headache, malaise, and meningismus. Herpes encephalitis and herpes varicella-zoster radiculitis may develop. Papovavirus may produce a demyelinating disorder. Cytomegalovirus encephalitis, toxoplasmosis (a protozoal infection), and tuberculosis meningitis have a high incidence in African countries.[86,87]

Central nervous system neoplasms and HIV. The incidence of HIV-associated CNS neoplasms has declined significantly with HAART, particularly primary CNS lymphoma. Other neoplasms associated with HIV include systemic non-Hodgkin's lymphoma and metastatic Kaposi sarcoma. Primary CNS lymphoma is a large-cell tumour that presents as rapidly developing and expanding multicentric intracranial mass lesions. The meninges and, possibly, the cranial nerves and spinal cord are invaded in systemic non-Hodgkin's lymphoma. Metastasis of a Kaposi sarcoma to the CNS is uncommon.[88]

Demyelinating Disorders

Demyelinating disorders result from damage to the myelin nerve sheath and affect neural transmission. They can occur in either the central (i.e., multiple sclerosis) or the peripheral (i.e., Guillain-Barré syndrome) nervous system. Contributing factors include genetics, infections, autoimmune reactions, environmental toxins, and unknown factors.

Multiple Sclerosis

Multiple sclerosis (MS) is a chronic inflammatory disease involving degeneration of CNS myelin, scarring (sclerosis or plaque formation), and loss of axons. Canada has the highest rate of MS in the world, with an estimated 100 000 Canadians living with the disease.[89] MS is caused by an autoimmune response to self or microbial antigens in genetically susceptible individuals. The onset of MS is usually between 20 and 40 years of age and is more common in women. Men may have a more severe progressive course. The prevalence rate is higher in northern latitudes. Risk factors that may be involved include smoking, vitamin D deficiency, and Epstein-Barr virus infection.[90] The etiology of MS is unknown.

PATHOPHYSIOLOGY MS is a diffuse and progressive disease with patches of damage that can occur throughout the brain and spinal cord. Autoreactive T lymphocytes (T cells) and B lymphocytes (B cells) cross the blood–brain barrier and recognize myelin and oligodendrocyte autoantigens, triggering inflammation and loss of oligodendrocytes (myelin-producing cells). Activation of microglia cells (brain macrophages) contributes to inflammation and injury with plaque formation and axonal degeneration. Loss of myelin disrupts nerve conduction with subsequent death of neurons and brain atrophy. Normal-appearing white matter can be microscopically very abnormal, and grey matter lesions and atrophy have been documented during later stages of the disease process.[91] These degenerative processes begin before symptom onset and progress throughout a person's life (Figure 16-14).[92] Myelin degeneration also can present as *optic neuritis* or involve the spinal cord. *Spinal MS* can occur concurrently or independently of brain lesions. The multifocal, multistaged features of MS lesions in established disease produce symptoms that are multiple and variable.

CLINICAL MANIFESTATIONS The most common initial symptoms of MS are paresthesias of the face, trunk, or limbs; weakness; impaired gait; visual disturbances; or urinary incontinence, indicating diffuse CNS involvement. Cerebellar and corticospinal involvement presents as nystagmus, ataxia, and weakness with all four limbs involved. Intention tremor and slurred speech may also occur.

The onset, duration, and severity of symptoms are different for each person. Disease exacerbations (also known as relapses or flares) are the temporary occurrence or worsening of symptoms. The symptoms may be mild or serious, may last for several days or weeks, and may be followed by progressive symptoms, including paresthesias, difficulty speaking, ataxia, or visual changes. The mechanism of these exacerbations is related to delayed or blocked conduction caused by inflammation and demyelination. Various events can occur immediately before the exacerbation of symptoms and are regarded as precipitating factors or triggers, including trauma, emotional stress, and pregnancy. Painful sensory events, spastic paralysis, and bowel and bladder incontinence are common with spinal involvement.[93] Recovery from symptoms during remissions is caused by downregulation of inflammation and the restoration of axonal function, either by remyelination, the resolution of inflammation, or the restoration of conduction to demyelinated axons.

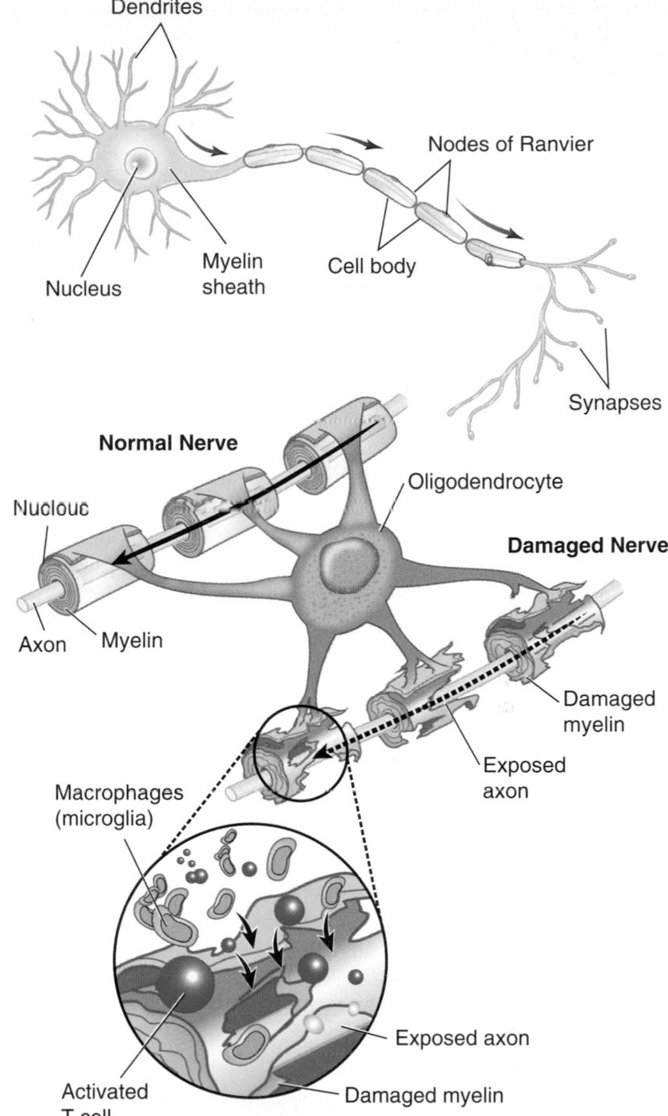

FIGURE 16-14 Pathogenesis of Multiple Sclerosis.

The subtypes of MS are based on the clinical course: (1) *remitting-relapsing*, initial onset of symptoms followed by remission and exacerbations; (2) *primary progressive*, a steady decline from onset; (3) *secondary-progressive*, initial remitting and relapsing symptoms with a steady decline in function; and (4) *progressive-relapsing*, a progressive course from onset with superimposed relapses. Initially, 85 to 90% of persons present with a remitting-relapsing course and without treatment transition to the progressive types with insidious neurological decline. Early cognitive changes are common and may include poor judgement, apathy, emotional lability, and depression.

EVALUATION AND TREATMENT There is no single test available to diagnose or rule out MS. Diagnostic criteria include the history and clinical examination in combination with MRI (most sensitive test), CSF findings, and evoked potentials.[94] Persistently elevated levels of CSF immunoglobulin G (IgG) are found in about two thirds of individuals with MS, and oligoclonal IgG bands on electrophoresis are found in more than 90% of MS patients. Evoked potential studies aid diagnosis by detecting decreased conduction velocity in visual, auditory, and somatosensory pathways. MRI is the most sensitive available method of detecting demyelinated plaques and monitoring disease.

The treatment goal in MS is prevention of exacerbations, prevention of permanent neurological damage, and control of symptoms. Disease-modifying medications are initiated with diagnosis and include corticosteroids, immunosuppressants, and immune system modulators. Continuous monitoring is important because of the increased risk for infection when taking these medications. Plasma exchange may be used in persons who do not respond to steroids. Medications are also available for symptom control. The long-term benefit of these medications is under investigation.[95] Supportive care includes participation in a regular exercise program; cessation of smoking; and avoidance of overwork, extreme fatigue, and heat exposure. The administration of vitamin D to prevent disease progression is being evaluated.[96] Stem cell therapy is under investigation.[97]

A recent theory has emerged associating chronic cerebrospinal venous insufficiency (CCSVI) with the symptoms of MS. It has been suggested that the presence of a blockage or narrowing of the veins in the head and neck does not allow for efficient removal of blood from the CNS, causing these symptoms. The proposed treatment for CCSVI, referred to as "liberation therapy," is an angioplasty procedure, which involves opening blocked or narrowed veins to allow for improved blood flow and drainage of blood from the brain. Global clinical studies have been conducted on this treatment with conflicting results. The procedure is not approved for treatment of MS in Canada.[98]

Guillain-Barré Syndrome

Guillain-Barré syndrome is a rare demyelinating disorder caused by a humoral and cell-mediated immunological reaction directed at the peripheral nerves. It usually occurs after a respiratory tract or gastro-intestinal infection. The clinical manifestations can vary from paresis of the legs to complete quadriplegia, respiratory insufficiency, and autonomic nervous system instability. Intravenous immunoglobulin or plasmapheresis is used during the acute phase and followed by aggressive rehabilitation.[99] Recovery occurs within weeks to months or up to 2 years. About 30% of individuals have residual weakness.

✔ QUICK CHECK 16-3

1. What are two differences between the symptoms of migraine and cluster headaches?
2. How can bacterial meningitis lead to an amputation?
3. What are the autoimmune mechanisms that cause multiple sclerosis lesions?

PERIPHERAL NERVOUS SYSTEM AND NEUROMUSCULAR JUNCTION DISORDERS

Peripheral Nervous System Disorders

Disease processes may injure the axons travelling to and from the brainstem and spinal cord neuronal cell bodies. The injury may affect a distinct anatomical area on the axon, or the spinal nerves may be injured at the roots, at the plexus (**plexus injuries**) before peripheral nerve formation, or at the nerves themselves. The cranial nerves do not have roots or plexuses and are affected only within themselves. Autonomic nerve fibres may be injured as they travel in certain cranial nerves and emerge through the ventral root and plexuses to pass through the peripheral nerves of the body. Peripheral nervous system disorders are summarized in Table 16-9.

TABLE 16-9 Peripheral Nervous System Disorders

Disorder	Pathology	Clinical Manifestations
Radiculopathies	Involves injury to spinal roots as they exit or enter vertebral canal; caused by compression, inflammation, direct trauma	Strength, tone, and bulk of muscles innervated by involved roots affected; pattern is similar to that seen in amyotrophies, with tone and deep tendon reflexes decreased, rarely absent; fasciculations; mild fatigue; sensory alterations, pain
Plexus injuries	Involve nerve plexus distal to spinal roots but proximal to formation of peripheral nerves; caused by trauma, compression, infiltration, or iatrogenic (positioning or intramuscular injection)	Motor weakness, muscle atrophy, sensory loss in affected areas; paralysis common
Neuropathies	Called *sensorimotor* if sensory, motor, and reflex effects; pure sensory caused by leprosy, industrial solvents, chloramphenicol, and hereditary mechanisms; motor caused by Guillain-Barré syndrome, infectious mononucleosis, viral hepatitis, acute porphyria, or lead, mercury, and triorthocresylphosphate (TCP) poisoning	Muscle strength, tone, and bulk affected; whole muscles or groups may be paretic or paralyzed; muscles of feet and legs first, then hands and arms; tone and deep tendon reflexes generally decreased with atrophy and fasciculation; mild fatigue; some specific symptoms of paresthesia and dysesthesia; altered reflexes; autonomic disturbances; deformities; metabolic changes
Guillain-Barré syndrome (several antibody subtypes have been identified)	Involves acute onset of motor, sensory, or autonomic symptoms caused by autoimmune inflammatory response, resulting in axonal demyelination; most commonly manifests as ascending motor paralysis; often preceded by respiratory tract or gastro-intestinal viral infection	Clinical manifestations are related to antibody subtypes; manifestations can include paresis of legs to complete quadriplegia, paralysis of eye muscles, respiratory insufficiency, autonomic nervous system instability; sensory symptoms (pain, numbness, paresthesias); may progress to respiratory arrest or cardiovascular collapse

From Vucic, S., Kiernan, M.C., & Cornblath, D.R. (2009). *J Clin Neurosci, 16*(6), 733–741.

Neuromuscular Junction Disorders

Transmission of the nerve impulse at the neuromuscular junction requires the release of adequate amounts of neurotransmitter from the presynaptic terminals of the axon and effective binding of the released transmitter to the receptors on the membranes of muscle cells (see Figure 13-15). Myasthenia gravis is the most prevalent of the neuromuscular junction disorders and is presented next.

Myasthenia Gravis

Myasthenia gravis is an acquired chronic autoimmune disease mediated by antibodies against the acetylcholine receptor (AChR) at the post-synaptic membrane of the neuromuscular junction. The Canadian incidence of this disease is about 5.3 per million population,[100] and it is more common in women. Thymic tumours, pathological changes in the thymus, and other autoimmune diseases are associated with the disorder. (Autoimmune mechanisms are discussed in Chapter 8.) **Ocular myasthenia**, more common in males, involves weakness of the eye muscles and eyelids, and may include swallowing difficulties and slurred speech.

PATHOPHYSIOLOGY Myasthenia gravis results from a defect in nerve impulse transmission at the neuromuscular junction. The postsynaptic AChRs on the muscle cell's plasma membrane are no longer recognized as "self" and elicit T-cell–dependent formation of IgG autoantibodies. The autoantibodies fix onto AChR sites, blocking the binding of acetylcholine. Eventually the antibody action destroys receptor sites. This loss of AChR sites causes diminished transmission of the nerve impulse across the neuromuscular junction and decreased muscle depolarization. Symptomatic individuals without anti-AChR antibodies may have antibodies against muscle-specific kinase (MuSK) with similar symptoms. Why this autosensitization occurs is unknown.

CLINICAL MANIFESTATIONS Myasthenia gravis has an insidious onset. The variable distribution of AChR sites or the number of and different isoforms of antibodies may determine when and which muscle groups are affected first. The muscles of the eyes, face, mouth, throat, and neck usually are affected first. There can be drooling and difficulty chewing and swallowing food. These problems can affect nutrition and put the person at risk for respiratory aspiration. The muscles of the neck, shoulder girdle, and hip flexors are less frequently affected, but muscle fatigue is common after exercise and there can be progressive weakness. The respiratory muscles of the diaphragm and chest wall can become weak with impaired ventilation. Clinical manifestations may first appear during pregnancy, during the postpartum period, or in conjunction with the administration of certain anaesthetic agents. The progression of myasthenia gravis varies, appearing first as a mild case that spontaneously remits, with a series of relapses and symptom-free intervals ranging from weeks to months. Over time, the disease can progress. **Myasthenic crisis** can develop as the disease progresses and occurs when severe muscle weakness causes extreme quadriparesis or quadriplegia, respiratory insufficiency with shortness of breath, and extreme difficulty in swallowing. The individual in myasthenic crisis is in danger of respiratory arrest.

Cholinergic crisis may arise from anticholinesterase medication toxicity with increased intestinal motility, episodes of diarrhea and complaints of intestinal cramping, bradycardia, pupillary constriction, increased salivation, and diaphoresis. These symptoms are caused by the smooth muscle hyperactivity secondary to excessive accumulation of acetylcholine at the neuromuscular junctions and excessive parasympatheticlike activity. As in myasthenic crisis, the individual is in danger of respiratory arrest.

EVALUATION AND TREATMENT The diagnosis of myasthenia gravis is made on the basis of a response to edrophonium chloride (Tensilon), results of EMG studies, and detection of anti-AChR or MuSK antibodies. With the intravenous administration of the medication, immediate demonstrable improvement in muscle strength usually persists for several minutes. Mediastinal tomography and MRI help determine whether a thymoma is present. Current treatments for myasthenia gravis have improved prognosis, including in those who have ocular myasthenia.

Anticholinesterase medications, steroids, and immunosuppressant medications (e.g., azathioprine [Imuran] and cyclosporine [Sandimmune] are used to treat myasthenia gravis and prevent myasthenic crisis. For individuals with cholinergic crisis, anticholinergic medications are withheld until blood levels are nontoxic; in addition, ventilatory support is provided and respiratory complications are prevented. Plasmapheresis may be lifesaving. Thymectomy is the treatment of choice in individuals with a thymoma and those with anti-AChR antibodies because this terminates the production of self-reactive T cells and B cells that produce the antibodies.[101,102]

QUICK CHECK 16-4

1. Where in the peripheral nervous system can disease occur?
2. Why do antibodies contribute to the symptoms of myasthenia gravis?
3. How do myasthenic crisis and cholinergic crisis differ in terms of cause and treatment?

TUMOURS OF THE CENTRAL NERVOUS SYSTEM

CNS tumours include both brain and spinal cord tumours. In 2012, the estimated number of new cases of primary brain tumours in Canada was 2 800, and the estimated number of deaths was 1 850.[103] The incidence of cancer increases with age, with 69% of new cases and 62% of cancer deaths occurring among those 50 to 79 years of age. CNS tumours are the second most common type of cancer occurring in children, second to leukemia.[104] Approximately 70 to 75% of all intracranial tumours in children are located infratentorially (see Chapter 17), and in adults 70% are located supratentorially. Peripheral nerve tumours are rare in children and common in adults. Carcinogenesis is discussed in Chapter 10, pituitary tumours are discussed in Chapter 19, and cerebral tumours in children are discussed in Chapter 17.

Brain Tumours

Tumours within the cranium can be either primary or metastatic. *Primary brain tumours* originate from brain substance, including neuroglia, neurons, cells of blood vessels, and connective tissue. *Extracerebral tumours* originate outside substances of the brain and include meningiomas, acoustic nerve tumours, and tumours of pituitary and pineal glands. *Metastatic (secondary) brain tumours* arise in organ systems outside the brain and spread to the brain. Common sites of intracranial tumours are illustrated in Figure 16-15.

Local effects of cranial tumours are caused by the destructive action of the tumour itself on a particular site in the brain and by compression causing decreased cerebral blood flow. Generalized effects result from increased ICP caused by growth of the tumour, obstruction of the ventricular system, hemorrhages in and around the tumour, or cerebral edema (Figure 16-16). Manifestations include seizures, visual disturbances, unstable gait, and cranial nerve dysfunction.

Intracranial brain tumours do not metastasize as readily as tumours in other organs because there are no lymphatic channels within the brain substance. If metastasis does occur, it is usually through seeding

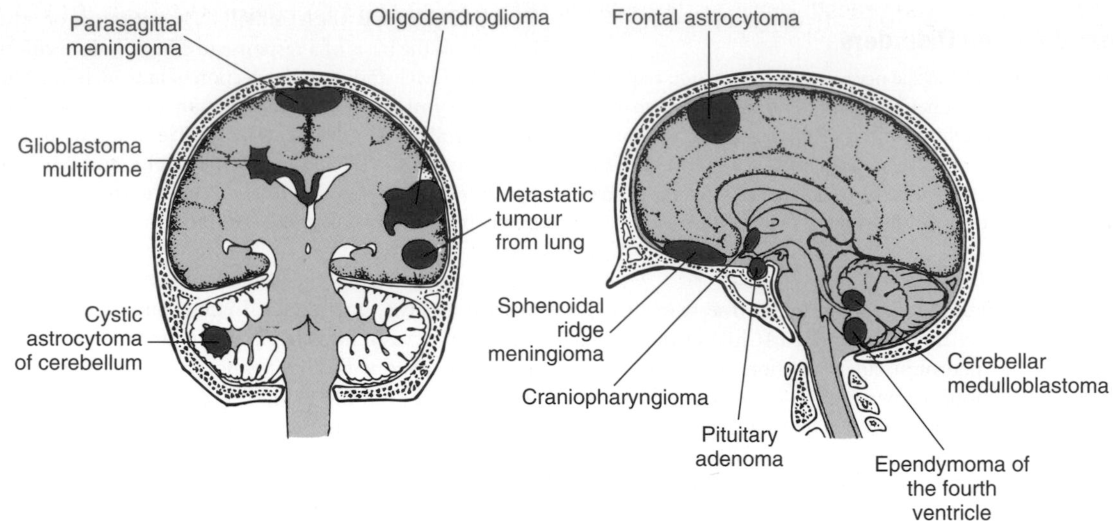

FIGURE 16-15 Common Sites of Intracranial Tumours.

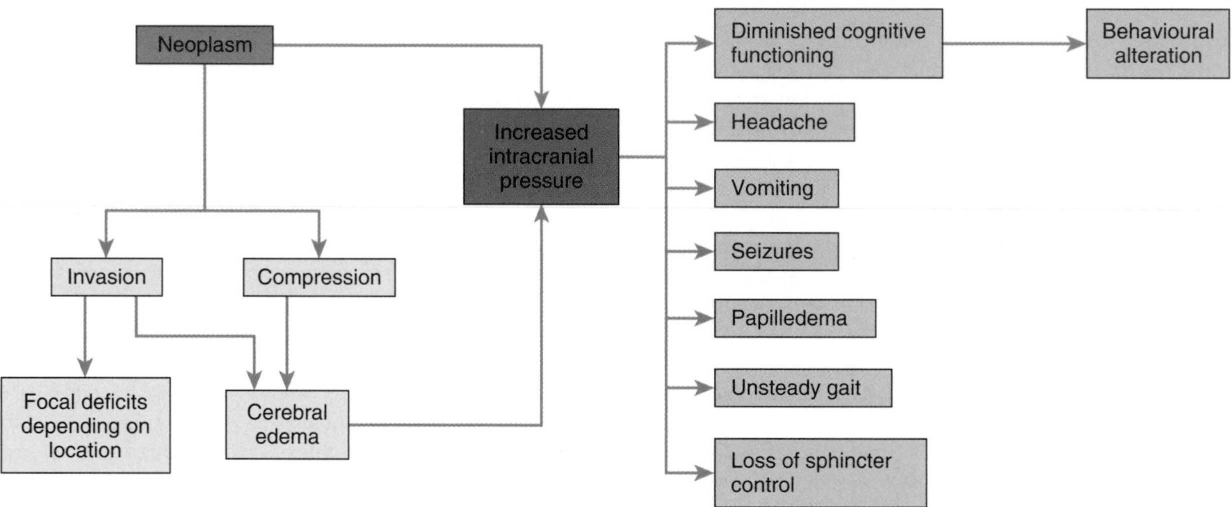

FIGURE 16-16 Origin of Clinical Manifestations Associated With an Intracranial Neoplasm.

of cerebral blood or CSF during cranial surgery or through artificial shunts.

Primary Brain (Intracerebral) Tumours

Primary brain (intracerebral) tumours, also called gliomas, include astrocytomas, oligodendrogliomas, and ependymomas. They make up 50 to 60% of all adult brain tumours and about 2% of all cancers in Canada (Table 16-10). The World Health Organization (WHO) divides gliomas into four grades based on histopathological features, cellular density, atypia, mitotic activity, microvascular proliferation, and necrosis (Table 16-11). Grades I and II are generally benign or slow growing. Grades III and IV are malignant tumours. Etiology for primary brain tumours is not clearly known. Ionizing radiation is the only known environmental risk factor. There may be an association between mobile phone use and gliomas and acoustic neuromas.[105,106]

Surgical or radiosurgical excision, surgical decompression, chemotherapy, radiotherapy, and hyperthermia are treatment options for these tumours. Supportive treatment is directed at reducing edema. New treatment options are emerging. (Cancer treatment is discussed in Chapter 10.)

Astrocytoma. Astrocytomas are the most common glioma (about 35 to 50% of all tumours of the brain and spinal cord)[104] and are classified by grade and type (see Table 16-11). These tumour cells are thought to have lost normal growth restraint and thus proliferate uncontrollably. Astrocytomas are graded I through IV, with grades I and II being slow-growing tumours that are most common in children. Grade I and II astrocytomas commonly progress to a higher grade, faster growing tumour. They may occur anywhere in the brain or spinal cord, and are generally located in the cerebrum, hypothalamus, or pons. Low-grade astrocytomas tend to be located laterally or supratentorially in adults and in a midline or near-midline position in children.

Headache and subtle neurobehavioural changes may be early signs, with other neurological symptoms evolving slowly and increased ICP occurring late in the tumour's course. Onset of a focal seizure disorder between the second and sixth decade of life suggests an astrocytoma. Low-grade astrocytomas are treated with surgery or by external radiation, and at least 50% of persons survive 5 years when surgery is followed by radiation therapy.[104,107]

Grades III and IV astrocytomas are found predominantly in the frontal lobes and cerebral hemispheres, although they may occur in the brainstem, cerebellum, and spinal cord. Men are twice as likely to have astrocytomas as women; in the 15- to 34-year-old age group they are the third most common brain cancer, whereas in the 35- to 54-year-old age group they are the fourth most common.

TABLE 16-10 **Brain and Spinal Cord Tumours**

Neoplasm	Location	Characteristics	Cell of Origin
Gliomas			
Astrocytoma	Anywhere in brain or spinal cord	Slow growing, invasive	Astrocytes
Glioblastoma multiforme	Predominantly in cerebral hemispheres	Highly invasive and malignant	Thought to arise from mature astrocytes
Oligodendrocytoma	Most commonly in frontal lobes deep in white matter; may arise in brainstem, cerebellum, and spinal cord	Relatively avascular; tends to be encapsulated; more malignant form called *oligodendroblastoma*	Oligodendrites
Ependymoma	Intramedullary: wall of ventricles; may arise in caudal tail of spinal cord	More common in children, variable growth rates; more malignant, invasive form is called *ependymoblastoma*; may extend into ventricle or invade brain tissue	Ependymal cells
Neuronal Cell			
Medulloblastoma	Posterior cerebellar vermis, roof of fourth ventricle	Well demarcated but infiltrating, rapid growing; fills fourth ventricle	Embryonic cells
Mesodermal Tissue			
Meningioma	Intradural, extramedullary: sylvian fissure region, superior parasagittal surface of frontal and parietal lobes, olfactory groove, wing of sphenoid bone, superior surface of cerebellum, cerebellopontine angle, spinal cord	Slow growing, circumscribed, encapsulated, sharply demarcated from normal tissues, compressive in nature	Arachnoid cells; may be from fibroblasts
Choroid Plexus			
Papillomas	Choroid plexus of ventricular system, lateral ventricle in children, fourth ventricle in adults	Usually benign; slow expansion inducing hemorrhage and hydrocephalus; malignant tumour is rare	Epithelial cells
Cranial Nerves and Spinal Nerve Roots			
Neurilemmoma	Cranial nerves (most commonly vestibular division of cranial nerve VIII)	Slow growing	Schwann cells
Neurofibroma	Extramedullary—spinal cord	Slow growing	Neurilemma, Schwann cells
Pituitary Tumours			
	Pituitary gland; may extend to or invade floor of third ventricle	Age linked, several types, slow growing, macroadenomas and microadenomas	Pituitary cells, pituitary chromophobes, basophils, eosinophils
Germ Cell Tumours			
	Neurohypophysis, hypothalamus, pineal region Primarily in adolescents More common in males than females Variable prognosis	Rare, 0.5% of all primary brain tumours	Several types—germinoma, embryonal carcinoma, yolk sac tumour, choriocarcinoma, teratoma, mixed germ cell tumour—with different cell origins
Pineal region	Pineal region; pineal parenchyma	Several types (germinoma, pineocytoma, teratoma)	Several types with different cell origins
Blood Vessel Tumours			
Angioma	Predominantly in posterior cerebral hemispheres	Slow growing	Arising from congenitally malformed arteriovenous connections
Hemangioblastomas	Predominantly in cerebellum	Slow growing	Embryonic vascular tissue

Grade IV astrocytoma, **glioblastoma multiforme**, is the most lethal and common type of primary brain tumour. This type is highly vascular and extensively irregular and infiltrative, making it difficult to remove surgically. Fifty percent of glioblastomas are bilateral or at least occupy more than one lobe at the time of death. The typical clinical presentation for a glioblastoma multiforme is that of diffuse, nonspecific clinical signs, such as headache, irritability, and "personality changes" that progress to more clear-cut manifestations of increased ICP, including headache on position change, papilledema, vomiting, or seizure activity. Symptoms may progress to include definite focal

TABLE 16-11 Grades of Astrocytomas

Grade[a]	Type	Description	Characteristics
I	Pilocytic astrocytoma	Common in children and young adults and people with neurofibromatosis type 1; common in cerebellum	Least malignant, well differentiated; grows slowly; near-normal microscopic appearance, noninfiltrating
II	Diffuse, low-grade astrocytoma (fibrillary, gemistocytic, protoplasmic) Oligodendroglioma	Common in young adults; more common in cerebrum but can occur in any part of brain	Abnormal microscopic appearance; grows slowly; infiltrates to adjacent tissue; may recur at higher grade
III	Anaplastic (malignant) astrocytoma Anaplastic oligodendroglioma	Common in young adults	Malignant; many cells undergoing mitosis; infiltrates adjacent tissue; frequently recurs at higher grade
IV	Glioblastoma (glioblastoma multiforme)	Common in older adults, particularly men Predominant in cerebral hemispheres	Poorly differentiated; increased number of cells undergoing mitosis; bizarre microscopic appearance; widely infiltrates; neovascularization; central necrosis

[a]World Health Organization Grading of Central Nervous System Tumours.
Data from American Brain Tumor Association. (2010). *Brain tumor primer* (9th ed.). Chicago: Author. Retrieved from http://neurosurgery.mgh.harvard.edu/abta/; Louis, D.N., Ohgaki, H., Wiestler, O.D., et al. (2007). *Acta Neuropathol, 114*(2), 97–109.

signs, such as hemiparesis, dysphasia, dyspraxia, cranial nerve palsies, and visual field deficits.

Higher grade astrocytomas are treated surgically and with radiotherapy and chemotherapy. Recurrence is common, and survival time is less than 5 years.[108]

Oligodendroglioma. Oligodendrogliomas constitute about 2% of all brain tumours and 10 to 15% of all gliomas. They are typically slow-growing tumours, and most oligodendrogliomas are macroscopically indistinguishable from other gliomas and may be a mixed type of oligodendroglioma and astrocytoma. Most are found in the frontal and temporal lobes, often in the deep white matter, but they are found also in other parts of the brain and spinal cord. Many are found in young adults with a history of temporal lobe epilepsy. Malignant degeneration occurs in approximately one third of persons with oligodendrogliomas, and the tumours are then referred to as *oligodendroblastomas*.

More than 50% of individuals experience a focal or generalized seizure as the first clinical manifestation. Only half of those with an oligodendroglioma have increased ICP at the time of diagnosis and surgery, and only one third develop focal manifestations. Treatment includes surgery, radiotherapy, and chemotherapy.

Ependymoma. Ependymomas are nonencapsulated gliomas that arise from ependymal cells; they are rare in adults, usually occurring in the spinal cord.[109] However, in children ependymomas are typically located in the brain. They constitute about 6% of all primary brain tumours in adults and 10% in children and adolescents. Approximately 70% of these tumours occur in the fourth ventricle, with others found in the third and lateral ventricles and caudal portion of the spinal cord. Approximately 40% of infratentorial ependymomas occur in children younger than 10 years. Cerebral (supratentorial) ependymomas occur at all ages.

Fourth ventricle ependymomas present with difficulty in balance, unsteady gait, uncoordinated muscle movement, and difficulty with fine motor movement. The clinical manifestations of a lateral and third ventricle ependymoma that involves the cerebral hemispheres are seizures, visual changes, and hemiparesis. Blockage of the CSF pathway produces hydrocephalus and presents with headache, nausea, and vomiting.

The interval between first manifestations and surgery may be as short as 4 weeks or as long as 7 or 8 years. Ependymomas are treated with radiotherapy, radiosurgery, and chemotherapy. About 20 to 50% of persons survive 5 years. Some persons benefit from a shunting procedure when the ependymoma has caused a noncommunicating hydrocephalus.

Primary Extracerebral Tumours

Meningioma. Meningiomas constitute about 34% of all intracranial tumours. These tumours usually originate from the arachnoidal (meningeal) cap cells in the dura mater and rarely from arachnoid cells of the choroid plexus of the ventricles. Meningiomas are located most commonly in the olfactory grooves, on the wings of the sphenoid bone (at the base of the skull), in the tuberculum sellae (next to the sella turcica), on the superior surface of the cerebellum, and in the cerebellopontine angle and spinal cord. Rarely, they can involve the optic nerve sheath with loss of visual acuity.[110] The cause of meningiomas is unknown.

A meningioma is sharply circumscribed and adapts to the shape it occupies. It may extend to the dural surface and erode the cranial bones or produce an osteoblastic reaction. A few meningiomas exhibit malignant, invasive qualities.

Meningiomas are slow growing, and clinical manifestations occur when they reach a certain size and begin to indent the brain parenchyma. Focal seizures are often the first manifestation, and increased ICP is less common than with gliomas.

There is a 20% recurrence rate even with complete surgical excision. If only partial resection is possible, the tumour recurs. Radiation therapies also are used to slow growth.

Nerve sheath tumours. Neurofibromas (benign nerve sheath tumours) are a group of autosomal dominant disorders of the nervous system. They include neurofibromatosis type 1 (NF1) (previously known as von Recklinghausen's disease) and neurofibromatosis type 2 (NF2); NF1 and NF2 are also known as *peripheral neurofibromatosis* and *central neurofibromatosis*, respectively.

NF1 is the most prevalent type of nerve sheath tumour, with an incidence of about 1 in 3 500 people, and causes multiple cutaneous neurofibromas, cutaneous macular lesions (café-au-lait spots and freckles), and less commonly bone and soft tissue tumours. Inactivation of the *NF1* gene results in loss of function of neurofibromin in Schwann cells and promotes tumourigenesis (neurofibromas). Learning disabilities are present in about 50% of affected individuals.[111]

NF2 is rare and occurs in about 1 in 60 000 people. The *NF2* gene product is neurofibromin 2 (merlin), a tumour-suppressor protein, and mutations promote development of CNS tumours, particularly schwannomas, although other tumour types can occur (meningiomas, ependymomas, astrocytomas, and neurofibromas). Schwannomas of the vestibular nerves present with hearing loss and deafness. Other symptoms may include loss of balance and dizziness. Schwannomas also may develop in other cranial, spinal, and peripheral nerves, and cutaneous signs are less prominent.

Genetic testing is available for the management of families susceptible to NF, and prenatal diagnosis is possible. Diagnosis is based on clinical manifestations and neuroimaging studies, and diagnostic criteria have been established for NF1.[112,113] Surgery is the major treatment. Individuals with NF2 have extensive morbidity and reduced life expectancy, particularly with early age of onset. Genetically tailored medications are likely to provide personalized therapy for both of these devastating conditions.

Metastatic brain tumours. Metastatic brain tumours from systemic cancers are 10 times more common than primary brain tumours, and 20 to 40% of persons with cancer have metastasis to the brain.[114] Common primary sites include lung, breast, and skin (e.g., melanomas), as well as kidney, colorectal, and other types of cancer. Metastasis to the brain is thought to be through vascular channels (see Chapter 10).

Metastatic brain tumours produce signs resembling those of glioblastomas, although several unusual syndromes do exist. Carcinomatous (metastatic cancer) encephalopathy causes headache, nervousness, depression, trembling, confusion, forgetfulness, and gait disorder. In carcinomatosis of the cerebellum, headache, dizziness, and ataxia are found. Carcinomatosis of the craniospinal meninges (also called *carcinomatous meningitis*) manifests with headache, confusion, and symptoms of cranial or spinal nerve root dysfunction. Metastatic brain tumours carry a poor prognosis. Treatment is guided by the pathology of the original tumour; number, size and location of the brain metastasis; and prior cancer treatments. With the development of new medications that cross the blood–brain barrier, chemotherapy is increasingly recommended.[115] Survival is about 1 year.

Spinal Cord Tumours

Primary spinal cord tumours are rare and represent about 2% of CNS tumours. They may be extramedullary extradural, intradural extramedullary, or intradural intramedullary. Intramedullary tumours originate within the neural tissues of the spinal cord. Extramedullary tumours originate from tissues outside the spinal cord. Intramedullary tumours are primarily gliomas (astrocytomas and ependymomas). Gliomas are difficult to resect completely, and radiotherapy is required. Spinal ependymomas may be completely resected and are more common in adults. Extramedullary tumours are either peripheral nerve sheath tumours (neurofibromas or schwannomas) or meningiomas. Neurofibromas are generally found in the thoracic and lumbar region, whereas meningiomas are more evenly distributed through the spine. Complete resection of these tumours can be curative. Other extramedullary tumours are sarcomas, vascular tumours, chordomas, and epidermoid tumours. Intramedullary tumours include ependymoma, astrocytoma, and hemangioblastoma.

Metastatic spinal cord tumours are usually carcinomas (i.e., from breast, lung, or prostate cancer), lymphomas, or myelomas. Their location is often extradural, having proliferated to the spine through direct extension from tumours of the vertebral structures or from extraspinal sources extending through the interventricular foramen or bloodstream.

PATHOPHYSIOLOGY Intramedullary spinal cord tumours produce dysfunction by both invasion and compression. Extramedullary spinal cord tumours produce dysfunction by compressing adjacent tissue, not by direct invasion. Metastases from spinal cord tumours occur from direct extension or seeding through the CSF or bloodstream.

CLINICAL MANIFESTATIONS An acute onset of clinical manifestations suggests a vascular occlusion of vessels supplying the spinal cord, whereas gradual and progressive symptoms suggest compression. The compressive syndrome (sensorimotor syndrome) involves both the anterior and the posterior spinal tracts, and motor function and sensory function are affected as the tumour grows. Pain is usually a presenting symptom.

The irritative syndrome (radicular syndrome) combines the clinical manifestations of a cord compression with radicular pain that occurs in the sensory root distribution and indicates root irritation. The segmental manifestations include segmental sensory changes, such as paresthesias and impaired pain and touch perception; motor disturbances, including cramps, atrophy, fasciculations, and decreased or absent deep tendon reflexes; and continuous spinal pain.

EVALUATION AND TREATMENT The diagnosis of a spinal cord tumour is made through bone scan, PET, CT-guided needle biopsy, or open biopsy. Involvement of specific cord segments is established. Any metastases also are identified. Treatment varies depending on the nature of the tumour and the person's clinical status, but surgery is essential for all spinal cord tumours.[116]

QUICK CHECK 16-5

1. How is an encapsulated central nervous system (CNS) tumour different from a nonencapsulated CNS tumour?
2. What are three types of spinal cord tumours?
3. What are some common signs and symptoms of compressive and irritative spinal cord tumour syndromes?

DID YOU UNDERSTAND?

Central Nervous System Disorders

1. Thirty percent of all traumatic brain injuries are sustained by children and youth, many of them while participating in sports and recreational-related activities.
2. Primary brain injury is caused by direct impact and involves neural injury, primary glial injury, and vascular responses.
3. Primary brain injuries can be focal or diffuse.
4. Focal brain injury can be caused by closed (blunt) trauma or open (penetrating) trauma. Closed injury is more common. Open injury involves a skull fracture with exposure of the cranial vault to the environment.
5. Focal brain injury includes contusion, laceration, epidural (extradural) hematoma, subdural hematoma, intracerebral hematoma, and open brain injury.
6. Diffuse brain injury (diffuse axonal injury [DAI]) results from shearing forces that result in axonal damage ranging from mild concussion to severe DAI.
7. Secondary brain injury develops from systemic and intracranial responses to primary brain trauma that result in further brain injury and neuronal death.
8. Spinal cord injury involves damage to neural tissues by compressing tissue, pulling or exerting tension on tissue, or shearing tissues so that they slide into one another. Vertebral fracture occurs with direct or indirect trauma.
9. Spinal cord injury may cause spinal shock with cessation of all motor, sensory, reflex, and autonomic functions below the transected area. Loss of motor and sensory function depends on the level of injury.

10. Neurogenic shock occurs with cervical or upper thoracic cord injury (above T5) and can occur concurrently with spinal shock.
11. Autonomic hyper-reflexia (dysreflexia) is a syndrome of sudden, massive reflex sympathetic discharge associated with spinal cord injury at level T6 or above. Flexor spasms are accompanied by profuse sweating, piloerection, and automatic bladder emptying.
12. Complete spinal cord transection results in paralysis. Paralysis of the lower half of the body with both legs involved is called *paraplegia*. Paralysis involving all four extremities is called *quadriplegia*.
13. Return of spinal neuron excitability occurs slowly. Reflex activity can return in 1 to 2 weeks in most persons with acute spinal cord injury. A pattern of flexion reflexes emerges, involving first the toes, then the feet and the legs. Eventually, reflex voiding and bowel elimination appear.
14. Low back pain is pain between the lower rib cage and gluteal muscles and often radiates into the thighs.
15. Most causes of low back pain are unknown; however, some secondary causes are disc prolapse, tumours, bursitis, synovitis, degenerative joint disease, osteoporosis, fracture, inflammation, and sprain.
16. Degenerative disc disease is an alteration in intervertebral disc tissue and can be related to normal aging.
17. Spondylolysis is a structural defect of the spine with displacement of the deficient vertebra.
18. Spondylolisthesis involves forward slippage of a vertebra and can include a crack or fracture of the pars interarticularis, usually at the L5-S1 vertebrae.
19. Herniation of an intervertebral disc is a displacement of the nucleus pulposus or annulus fibrosus beyond the intervertebral disc space. Herniation most commonly affects the lumbosacral discs L5-S1 and L4-5. The extruded pulposus compresses the nerve root, causing pain that radiates along the sciatic nerve course.
20. Cerebrovascular disease is the most frequently occurring neurological disorder. Any abnormality of the blood vessels of the brain is referred to as a *cerebrovascular disease*.
21. Cerebrovascular disease is associated with two types of brain abnormalities: (a) ischemia with or without infarction and (b) hemorrhage.
22. Transient ischemic attacks are episodes of neurological dysfunction lasting no more than 1 hour and resulting from focal cerebral ischemia.
23. Cerebrovascular accidents (stroke syndromes) are classified pathophysiologically as ischemic (thrombotic or embolic), hemorrhagic (intracranial hemorrhage), or associated with hypoperfusion.
24. Intracranial aneurysms result from defects in the vascular wall and are classified on the basis of form and shape. They are often asymptomatic, but the signs vary depending on the location and size of the aneurysm.
25. An arteriovenous malformation is a mass of dilated blood vessels. Although usually present at birth, symptoms are delayed and usually occur before age 30.
26. A subarachnoid hemorrhage occurs when blood escapes from defective or injured vasculature into the subarachnoid space. When a vessel tears, blood under pressure is pumped into the subarachnoid space. The blood produces an inflammatory reaction in these tissues and increased intracranial pressure results.
27. Migraine is an episodic headache that can be associated with triggers, and it may have an aura associated with a cortical spreading depression that alters cortical blood flow. Pain is related to overactivity in the trigeminal vascular system.
28. Cluster headaches are a group of disorders known as *trigeminal autonomic cephalalgias* and occur primarily in men. They occur in clusters over a period of days with extreme pain intensity and short duration, and are associated with trigeminal activation.
29. Tension-type headache is the most common headache. Episodic-type headaches involve a peripheral pain mechanism, and the chronic type involves a central pain mechanism and may be related to hypersensitivity to pain in craniocervical muscles.
30. Infection and inflammation of the central nervous system (CNS) can be caused by bacteria, viruses, fungi, protozoa, and rickettsiae. Bacterial infections are pyogenic or pus producing.
31. Meningitis (infection of the meninges) is classified as bacterial (i.e., meningococci), aseptic (viral or nonpurulent), or fungal. Bacterial meningitis primarily is an infection of the pia mater, the arachnoid, and the fluid of the subarachnoid space. Aseptic meningitis is thought to be limited to the meninges. Fungal meningitis is a chronic, less common type of meningitis.
32. Brain abscesses often originate from infections outside the CNS. Organisms gain access to the CNS from adjacent sites or spread along the wall of a vein. A localized inflammatory process develops with formation of exudate. After a few days, the infection becomes delimited with a centre of pus and a wall of granular tissue.
33. Encephalitis is an acute febrile illness of viral origin with nervous system involvement. The most common encephalitides are caused by bites of mosquitoes, ticks, or flies; viruses; and herpes simplex type 1. Meningeal involvement appears in all encephalitides.
34. Herpes encephalitis is treated with antiviral agents. No definitive treatment exists for the other encephalitides.
35. The common neurological complications of AIDS are HIV-associated neurocognitive disorder, HIV myelopathy, opportunistic infections, cytomegalovirus encephalitis, parasitic infection, and neoplasms. Pathologically, there may be diffuse CNS involvement, focal pathological changes, and obstructive hydrocephalus.
36. Multiple sclerosis is a chronic inflammatory demyelinating disorder with scarring (sclerosis) and loss of axons. Although the pathogenesis is unknown, the demyelination is thought to result from an immunogenetic-viral cause in genetically susceptible individuals.
37. Guillain-Barré syndrome is a demyelinating disorder caused by a humoral and cell-mediated immunological reaction directed at the peripheral nerves.

Peripheral Nervous System and Neuromuscular Junction Disorders

1. With disorders of the roots of spinal cord nerves, the roots may be compressed, inflamed, or torn. Clinical manifestations include local pain or paresthesias in the sensory root distribution. Treatment may involve surgery, antibiotics, steroids, radiation therapy, and chemotherapy.
2. Plexus injuries involve the plexus distal to the spinal roots. Paralysis can occur with complete plexus involvement.
3. When peripheral nerves are affected, axon and myelin degeneration may be present. These syndromes are classified as sensorimotor, sensory, or motor and are characterized by varying degrees of sensory disturbance, paresis, and paralysis. Secondary atrophy may be present.
4. Myasthenia gravis is a disorder of voluntary muscles characterized by muscle weakness and fatigability. It is considered an autoimmune disease and is associated with an increased incidence of other autoimmune diseases.
5. Myasthenia gravis results from a defect in nerve impulse transmission at the postsynaptic membrane of the neuromuscular junction. Immunoglobulin G antibody is secreted against the "self" acetylcholine receptors and blocks the binding of acetylcholine. The antibody action destroys the receptor sites, causing decreased transmission of the nerve impulse across the neuromuscular junction.

Tumours of the Central Nervous System

1. Two main types of tumours occur within the cranium: primary and metastatic. Primary tumours are classified as intracerebral tumours (astrocytomas, oligodendrogliomas, and ependymomas) or extracerebral tumours (meningioma or nerve sheath tumours). Metastatic tumours can be found inside or outside the brain substance.
2. CNS tumours cause local and generalized manifestations. The effects are varied, and local manifestations include seizures, visual disturbances, unstable gait, and cranial nerve dysfunction.
3. Spinal cord tumours are classified as intramedullary tumours (within the neural tissues) or extramedullary tumours (outside the spinal cord). Metastatic spinal cord tumours are usually carcinomas, lymphomas, or myelomas.
4. Extramedullary spinal cord tumours produce dysfunction by compression of adjacent tissue, not by direct invasion. Intramedullary spinal cord tumours produce dysfunction by both invasion and compression.

KEY TERMS

Arteriovenous malformation (AVM), 409
Astrocytomas, 418
Autonomic hyper-reflexia (dysreflexia), 402
Bacterial meningitis, 412
Brain abscess, 413
Brudzinski sign, 410
Cauda equina syndrome, 403
Cerebral infarction, 407
Cerebrovascular accident (CVA), 406
Cholinergic crisis, 417
Chronic traumatic encephalopathy (CTE), 399
Classic cerebral concussion, 398
Closed brain injuries, 394
Cluster headache, 411
Compound skull fracture, 397
Compressive syndrome (sensorimotor syndrome), 421
Contrecoup injury, 395
Contusion, 395
Coup injury, 395
Degenerative disc disease (DDD), 403
Diffuse brain injury (diffuse axonal injury [DAI]), 397
Embolic stroke, 407
Encephalitis, 413
Ependymoma, 420
Epidural (extradural) hematoma, 395
Focal brain injury, 394
Fungal meningitis, 412
Fusiform aneurysm (giant aneurysm), 408
Glioblastoma multiforme, 419
Glioma, 418
Guillain-Barré syndrome, 416
Headache, 410
Hemorrhagic stroke (intracranial hemorrhage), 408
HIV-associated neurocognitive disorder (HAND), 414
HIV distal symmetric polyneuropathy, 414
HIV myelopathy, 414
Hypoperfusion, or hemodynamic stroke, 407
Intracerebral hematoma, 397
Intracranial aneurysm, 408
Irritative syndrome (radicular syndrome), 421
Ischemic penumbra, 407
Ischemic stroke, 407
Kernig sign, 410
Lacunar stroke (lacunar infarct or small vessel disease), 407
Low back pain (LBP), 402
Meningioma, 420
Meningitis, 412
Metastatic brain tumours, 421
Migraine, 410
Mild concussion, 398
Mild diffuse axonal injury, 398
Moderate diffuse axonal injury, 398
Multiple sclerosis (MS), 415
Myasthenia gravis, 417
Myasthenic crisis, 417
Neurofibroma (benign nerve sheath tumour), 420
Neurofibromatosis type 1 (NF1), 420
Neurofibromatosis type 2 (NF2), 420
Neurogenic shock, 402
Ocular myasthenia, 417
Oligodendroglioma, 420
Open brain injury, 397
Open (penetrating) trauma, 394
Plexus injury, 416
Postconcussion syndrome, 398
Post-traumatic seizure, 398
Primary brain (intracerebral) tumour, 418
Primary spinal cord injury, 399
Purpura fulminans, 412
Radiculopathy, 405
Saccular aneurysm (berry aneurysm), 408
Secondary brain injury, 398
Secondary spinal cord injury, 399
Severe diffuse axonal injury, 398
Spinal cord abscess, 413
Spinal cord tumours, 421
Spinal shock, 400
Spinal stenosis, 405
Spondylolisthesis, 404
Spondylolysis, 404
Subarachnoid hemorrhage (SAH), 409
Subdural hematoma, 396
Tension-type headache (TTH), 411
Thrombotic stroke (cerebral thrombosis), 407
Transient ischemic attack (TIA), 407
Traumatic brain injury (TBI), 394
Viral meningitis (aseptic or nonpurulent meningitis), 412
West Nile virus (WNV), 414

REFERENCES

1. Northern Brain Injury Association. (2014). *Brain injury statistics, 2014*. Retrieved from http://nbia.ca/brain-injury-statistics/.
2. Perry, E. C., 3rd, Ahmed, H. M., & Origitano, T. C. (2014). Neurotraumatology. *Handbook of Clinical Neurology, 121*, 1751–1772. doi:10.1016/B978-0-7020-4088-7.00113-9.
3. Edwards, P., Arango, M., Balica, L., et al. (2005). Final results of MRC CRASH, a randomised placebo-controlled trial of intravenous corticosteroid in adults with head injury—Outcomes at 6 months. *Lancet, 365*(9475), 1957–1959. doi:10.1016/S0140-6736(05)66552-X.
4. Zakaria, Z., Kaliaperumal, C., Kaar, G., et al. (2013). Extradural haematoma—To evacuate or not? Revisiting treatment guidelines. *Clinical Neurology and Neurosurgery, 115*(8), 1201–1205. doi:10.1016/j.clineuro.2013.05.012.
5. Johnson, V. E., Stewart, W., & Smith, D. H. (2013). Axonal pathology in traumatic brain injury. *Experimental Neurology, 246*, 35–43. doi:10.1016/j.expneurol.2012.01.013.
6. Jagoda, A. S. (2010). Mild traumatic brain injury: Key decisions in acute management. *Psychiatric Clinics of North America, 33*(4), 797–806. doi:10.1016/j.psc.2010.09.004.
7. Sauerlaud, S., & Maegele, M. A. (2004). CRASH landing in severe head injury. *Lancet, 364*(9442), 729–782. doi:10.1016/S0140-6736(04)17202-4.
8. Marshall, S., Bayley, M., McCullagh, S., et al. (2012). Clinical practice guidelines for mild traumatic brain injury and persistent symptoms. *Canadian Family Physician, 58*(3), 257–267. Retrieved from http://www.cfp.ca/content/58/3/257.
9. Kabadi, S. V., & Faden, A. I. (2014). Neuroprotective strategies for traumatic brain injury: Improving clinical translation. *International Journal of Molecular Sciences, 15*(1), 1216–1236. doi:10.3390/ijms15011216.
10. Wang, X., Dong, Y., Han, X., et al. (2013). Nutritional support for patients sustaining traumatic brain injury: A systematic review and meta-analysis of prospective studies. *PLoS ONE, 8*(3), e58838. doi:10.1371/journal.pone.0058838.
11. Farrell, C. A., & Canadian Paediatric Society & Acute Care Committee. (2013). Management of the paediatric patient with acute head trauma. *Paediatrics and Child Health, 18*(5), 253–258. Retrieved from http://www.cps.ca/en/documents/position/paediatric-patient-with-acut e-head-trauma.
12. Kochanek, P. M., Carney, N., Adelson, P. D., et al. (2012). Guidelines for the acute medical management of severe traumatic brain injury in infants, children, and adolescents—Second edition. *Pediatric Critical Care Medicine, 13*(Suppl. 1), S1–S82. doi:10.1097/PCC.0b013e31823f435c.
13. Ontario Neurotrauma Foundation. (2014). *Guidelines for diagnosing and managing pediatric concussion*. Toronto: Author. Retrieved from http://onf.org/documents/guidelines-diagnosing-and-managing-pediatric-concussion.
14. Purcell, L. K., & Canadian Paediatric Society & Healthy Active Living and Sports Medicine Committee. (2014). Sport-related concussion: Evaluation and management. *Paediatrics and Child Health, 19*(3), 152–158. Retrieved from http://

www.cps.ca/documents/position/sport-related-concussion-evaluation-management.
15. Szaflarski, J. P., Nazzal, Y., Dreer, L. E., et al. (2014). Post-traumatic epilepsy: Current and emerging treatment options. *Neuropsychiatric Disease and Treatment, 10*, 1469–1477. doi:10.2147/NDT.S50421.
16. Lucke-Wold, B. P., Turner, R. C., Logsdon, A. F., et al. (2014). Linking traumatic brain injury to chronic traumatic encephalopathy: Identification of potential mechanisms leading to neurofibrillary tangle development. *Journal of Neurotrauma, 31*(13), 1129–1138. doi:10.1089/neu.2013.3303.
17. Rabinowitz, A. R., & Levin, H. S. (2014). Cognitive sequelae of traumatic brain injury. *Psychiatric Clinics of North America, 37*(1), 1–11. doi:10.1016/j.psc.2013.11.004.
18. Urban Futures (2010). *The incidence and prevalence of spinal cord injury in Canada: Overview and estimates based on current evidence*. Vancouver: Rick Hansen Institute and Urban Features. Retrieved from http://fecst.inesss.qc.ca/fileadmin/documents/photos/LincidenceetlaprevalencedestraumamedullaireauCanada.pdf.
19. Oyinbo, C. A. (2011). Secondary injury mechanisms in traumatic spinal cord injury: A nugget of this multiply cascade. *Acta Neurobiologiae Experimentalis, 71*(2), 281–299.
20. Milligan, J., Lee, J., McMillan, C., et al. (2012). Autonomic dysreflexia: Recognizing a common serious condition in patients with spinal cord injury. *Canadian Family Physician, 58*(8), 831–835.
21. Priestley, J. V., Michael-Titus, A. T., & Tetzkaff, W. (2012). Limiting spinal cord injury by pharmacological intervention. *Handbook of Clinical Neurology, 109*, 463–484. doi:10.1016/B978-0-444-52137-8.00029-2.
22. Hansebout, R. R., & Hansebout, C. R. (2014). Local cooling for traumatic spinal cord injury: Outcomes in 20 patients and review of the literature. *Journal of Neurosurgery. Spine, 20*(5), 550–561. doi:10.3171/2014.2.SPINE13318.
23. Rabchevsky, A. G., Patel, S. P., & Springer, J. E. (2011). Pharmacological interventions for spinal cord injury: Where do we stand? How might we step forward? *Pharmacology & Therapeutics, 132*(1), 15–29. doi:10.1016/j.pharmthera.2011.05.001.
24. Cassidy, J. D., Côté, P., Carroll, L. J., et al. (2005). Incidence and course of lower back pain episodes in the general population. *Spine (Phila Pa 1976), 30*(24), 2813–2823.
25. Hoy, D., March, L., Brooks, P., et al. (2014). The global burden of low back pain: Estimates from the Global Burden of Disease 2010 study. *Annals of the Rheumatic Diseases, 73*(6), 968–974. doi:10.1136/annrheumdis-2013-204428.
26. Golob, A. L., & Wipf, J. E. (2014). Low back pain. *Medical Clinics of North America, 98*(3), 405–428. doi:10.1016/j.mcna.2014.01.003.
27. Ito, K., & Creemers, L. (2013). Mechanisms of intervertebral disk degeneration/injury and pain: A review. *Global Spine Journal, 3*(3), 145–152. doi:10.1055/s-0033-1347300.
28. Towards Optimized Practice (TOP) Low Back Pain Working Group (2015). *Evidence-informed primary care management of lower back pain: Clinical practice guideline*. Edmonton: Author. Retrieved from http://www.topalbertadoctors.org/download/1885/LBPguideline.pdf?_20160225091721.
29. Koes, B. W., van Tulder, M., Lin, C. W., et al. (2010). An updated overview of clinical guidelines for the management of non-specific low back pain in primary care. *European Spine Journal, 19*(12), 2075–2094. doi:10.1007/s00586-010-1502-y.
30. Deyo, R. A., Von Korff, M., & Duhrkoop, D. (2015). Opioids for low back pain. *British Medical Journal, 350*, g6380. doi:10.1136/bmj.g6380.
31. Kreiner, D. S., Hwang, S. W., Easa, J. E., et al. (2014). An evidence-based clinical guideline for the diagnosis and treatment of lumbar disc herniation with radiculopathy. *The Spine Journal, 14*(1), 180–191. doi:10.1016/j.spinee.2013.08.003.
32. Jacobs, W. C., Rubinstein, S. M., Koes, B., et al. (2013). Evidence for surgery in degenerative lumbar spine disorders. *Best Practice and Research. Clinical Rheumatology, 27*(5), 673–684. doi:10.1016/j.berh.2013.09.009.
33. Bruggeman, A. J., & Decker, R. C. (2011). Surgical treatment and outcomes of lumbar radiculopathy. *Physical Medicine and Rehabilitation Clinics of North America, 22*(1), 161–177. doi:10.1016/j.pmr.2010.10.002.
34. Heart and Stroke Foundation. (2016). *About us*. Retrieved from http://www.heartandstroke.com/site/c.ikIQLcMWJtE/b.3479075/k.C8B0/About_Us.htm.
35. Bradley, W. G., Daroff, R. B., Fenichel, G. M., et al. (2008). *Neurology in clinical practice* (5th ed., pp. 1165–1169). Philadelphia: Butterworth-Heinemann.
36. Heart and Stroke Foundation of Canada. (2016). *Indigenous peoples resources*. Retrieved from http://www.heartandstroke.mb.ca/site/c.lgLSIVOyGpF/b.3660995/k.1B8/First_Nations_Inuit__M233tis_Resources.htm.
37. Heart and Stroke Foundation. (2016). *Statistics*. Retrieved from http://www.heartandstroke.com/site/c.ikIQLcMWJtE/b.3483991/k.34A8/Statistics.htm.
38. Gupta, H. V., Farrell, A. M., & Mittal, M. K. (2014). Transient ischemic attacks: Predictability of future ischemic stroke or transient ischemic attack events. *Therapeutics and Clinical Risk Management, 10*, 27–35. doi:10.2147/TCRM.S54810.
39. Wardlaw, J. M., Doubal, F., Armitage, P., et al. (2009). Lacunar stroke is associated with diffuse blood-brain barrier dysfunction. *Annals of Neurology, 65*(2), 194–202. doi:10.1002/ana.21549.
40. Klijn, C. J., & Kappelle, L. J. (2010). Haemodynamic stroke: Clinical features, prognosis, and management. *Lancet. Neurology, 9*(10), 1008–1017. doi:10.1016/S1474-4422(10)70185-X.
41. Jickling, G. C., Liu, D., Stamova, B., et al. (2014). Hemorrhagic transformation after ischemic stroke in animals and humans. *Journal of Cerebral Blood Flow and Metabolism, 34*(2), 185–199. doi:10.1038/jcbfm.2013.203.
42. Pare, J. R., & Kahn, J. H. (2012). Basic neuroanatomy and stroke syndromes. *Emergency Medicine Clinics of North America, 30*(3), 601–615. doi:10.1016/j.emc.2012.05.004.
43. Kelley, R. E., & Martin-Schild, S. (2012). Ischemic stroke: Emergencies and management. *Neurologic Clinics, 30*(1), 187–210, ix. doi:10.1016/j.ncl.2011.09.014.
44. Heart and Stroke Foundation of Canada. (2015). *Emergency department evaluation of acute stroke and TIA order and documentation template*. Retrieved from http://www.strokebestpractices.ca/wp-content/uploads/2016/03/CSBPR-Order-and-Documentation-Template_ED-evaluation-of-Acute-Stroke-and-TIA_2016March1.pdf.
45. Casaubon, L. K., Boulanger, J.-M., Blacquiere, D., et al. (2015). *Canadian stroke best practice recommendations: Hyperacute stroke care guidelines, update 2015*. Retrieved from http://www.sasksurgery.ca/pdf/Hyperacute-Guidelines-Canadian-Stroke-Best-Practices-Update2015.pdf.
46. Gomes, J. A., & Manno, E. (2013). New developments in the treatment of intracerebral hemorrhage. *Neurologic Clinics, 31*(3), 721–735. doi:10.1016/j.ncl.2013.03.002.
47. Francis, S. E., Tu, J., Qian, Y., et al. (2013). A combination of genetic, molecular and haemodynamic risk factors contributes to the formation, enlargement and rupture of brain aneurysms. *Journal of Clinical Neuroscience, 20*(7), 912–918. doi:10.1016/j.jocn.2012.12.003.
48. Connolly, E. S., Jr., Rabinstein, A. A., Carhuapoma, J. R., et al. (2012). Guidelines for the management of aneurysmal subarachnoid hemorrhage: A guideline for healthcare professionals from the American Heart Association/American Stroke Association. *Stroke, 43*(6), 1711–1737. doi:10.1161/STR.0b013e3182587839.
49. Novakovic, R. L., Lazzarro, M. A., Castonguay, A. C., et al. (2013). The diagnosis and management of brain arteriovenous malformations. *Neurologic Clinics, 31*(3), 749–763. doi:10.1016/j.ncl.2013.03.003.
50. Gross, B. A., & Du, R. (2014). Diagnosis and treatment of vascular malformations of the brain. *Current Treatment Options in Neurology, 16*(1), 279. doi:10.1007/s11940-013-0279-9.
51. Budohoski, K. P., Czosnyka, M., Kirkpatrick, P. J., et al. (2013). Clinical relevance of cerebral autoregulation following subarachnoid haemorrhage. *Nature Reviews. Neurology, 9*(3), 152–163. doi:10.1038/nrneurol.2013.11.
52. Ciurea, A. V., Palade, C., Voinescu, D., et al. (2013). Subarachnoid hemorrhage and cerebral vasospasm—literature review. *Journal of Medicine and Life, 6*(2), 120–125.
53. Cavanaugh, S. J., & Gordon, V. L. (2002). Grading scales used in the management of aneurismal subarachnoid hemorrhage: A critical review. *Journal of Neuroscience Nursing, 34*(6), 288–295.
54. Guo, L. M., Zhou, H. Y., Xu, J. W., et al. (2011). Risk factors related to aneurysmal rebleeding. *World Neurosurgery, 76*(3–4), 292–298, discussion 253–254. doi:10.1016/j.wneu.2011.03.025.
55. International Headache Society. (2005). *IHS classification ICHD-II 1. Migraine*. Retrieved from http://ihs-classification.org/en/02_klassifikation/02_teil1/01.00.00_migraine.html.
56. Ramage-Morin, P. L., & Gilmour, H. (2014). Prevalence of migraine in the Canadian household population. *Statistics Canada Health Reports, 25*(6), 10–16. Retrieved from http://www.statcan.gc.ca/pub/82-003-x/2014006/article/14033-eng.pdf.
57. Sacco, S., Ricci, S., Degan, D., et al. (2012). Migraine in women: The role of hormones and their impact on vascular diseases. *Journal of Headache and Pain, 13*(3), 177–189. doi:10.1007/s10194-012-0424-y.
58. Ferrari, M. D., Kiever, R. R., Terwindt, G. M., et al. (2015). Migraine pathophysiology: Lessons from mouse models and human genetics. *Lancet. Neurology, 14*(1), 65–80. doi:10.1016/S1474-4422(14)70220-0.
59. Akerman, S., & Goadsby, P. J. (2014). Pathophysiology of migraine. In M. J. Aminoff & R. B. Daroff (Eds.), *Encyclopedia of the neurological sciences* (2nd ed., pp. 67–71). London: Academic Press.
60. Edvinsson, L., Villalón, C. M., & Maassen Van Den Brink, A. (2012). Basic mechanisms of migraine and its acute treatment. *Pharmacology & Therapeutics, 136*(3), 319–333. doi:10.1016/j.pharmthera.2012.08.011.
61. Pietrobon, D., & Moskowitz, M. A. (2013). Pathophysiology of migraine. *Annual Review of Physiology, 75*, 365–391. doi:10.1146/annurev-physiol-030212-183717.
62. Cutrer, F. M., & Smith, J. H. (2013). Human studies in the pathophysiology of migraine: Genetics and functional neuroimaging. *Headache, 53*(2), 401–412. doi:10.1111/head.12024.
63. Reddy, D. S. (2013). The pathophysiological and pharmacological basis of current drug treatment of migraine headache. *Expert Review of Clinical Pharmacology, 6*(3), 271–288. doi:10.1586/ecp.13.14.
64. Armstrong, C., & American Academy of Neurology, & American Headache Society. (2013). AAN/AHS update recommendations for migraine prevention in adults. *American Family Physician, 87*(8), 584–585. Retrieved from http://www.aafp.org/afp/2013/0415/p584.html.
65. Health Canada. (2012). *Medical devices: Active licence listing*. Retrieved from http://www.hc-sc.gc.ca/dhp-mps/md-im/index-eng.php.
66. De Simone, R., Ranieri, A., Montella, S., et al. (2014). Intracranial pressure in unresponsive chronic migraine. *Journal of Neurology, 261*(7), 1365–1373. doi:10.1007/s00415-014-7355-2.
67. Benoliel, R., & Eliav, E. (2013). Primary headache disorders. *Dental Clinics of North America, 57*(3), 513–539. doi:10.1016/j.cden.2013.04.005.
68. Iacovelli, E., Coppola, G., Tinelli, E., et al. (2012). Neuroimaging in cluster headache and other trigeminal autonomic cephalalgias. *Journal of*

Headache and Pain, *13*(1), 11–20. doi:10.1007/s10194-011-0403-8.
69. Weaver-Agostoni, J. (2013). Cluster headache. *American Family Physician*, *88*(2), 122–128.
70. Freitag, F. (2013). Managing and treating tension-type headache. *Medical Clinics of North America*, *97*(2), 281–292. doi:10.1016/j.mcna.2012.12.003.
71. Thigpen, M. C., Whitney, C. G., Messonnier, N. E., et al. (2011). Bacterial meningitis in the United States, 1998–2007. *New England Journal of Medicine*, *364*(21), 2016–2025. doi:10.1056/NEJMoa1005384.
72. Coureuil, M., Join-Lambert, O., Lécuyer, H., et al. (2013). Pathogenesis of meningococcemia. *Cold Spring Harbor Perspectives in Medicine*, *3*(6), doi:10.1101/cshperspect.a012393. pii, a012393.
73. Heckenberg, S. G., Brouwer, M. C., & van de Beek, D. (2014). Bacterial meningitis. *Handbook of Clinical Neurology*, *121*, 1361–1375. doi:10.1016/B978-0-7020-4088-7.00093-6.
74. Putz, K., Hayani, K., & Zar, F. A. (2013). Meningitis. *Primary Care*, *40*(3), 707–726. doi:10.1016/j.pop.2013.06.001.
75. Centers for Disease Control and Prevention. (2015). *Vaccines and vaccination; Meningococcal vaccination*. Retrieved from http://www.cdc.gov/meningococcal/vaccine-info.html.
76. Campsall, P. A., Laupland, K. B., & Niven, D. J. (2013). Severe meningococcal infection: A review of epidemiology, diagnosis, and management. *Critical Care Clinics*, *29*(3), 393–409. doi:10.1016/j.ccc.2013.03.001.
77. Yan, J., Huang, B., Liu, G., et al. (2013). Meta-analysis of prevention and treatment of toxoplasmic encephalitis in HIV-infected patients. *Acta Tropica*, *127*(3), 236–244. doi:10.1016/j.actatropica.2013.05.006.
78. Brouwer, M. C., Coutinho, J. M., & van de Beek, D. (2014). Clinical characteristics and outcome of brain abscess: Systematic review and meta-analysis. *Neurology*, *82*(9), 806–813. doi:10.1212/WNL.0000000000000172.
79. Alvis Miranda, H., Castellar-Leones, S. M., Elzain, M. A., et al. (2013). Brain abscess: Current management. *Journal of Neurosciences in Rural Practice*, *4*(Suppl. 1), S67–S81. doi:10.4103/0976-3147.116472.
80. Muzumdar, D., Jhawar, S., & Goel, A. (2011). Brain abscess: An overview. *International Journal of Surgery*, *9*(2), 136–144. doi:10.1016/j.ijsu.2010.11.005.
81. Rust, R. S. (2012). Human arboviral encephalitis. *Seminars in Pediatric Neurology*, *19*(3), 130–151. doi:10.1016/j.spen.2012.03.002.
82. Roos, K. L. (2014). Encephalitis. *Handbook of Clinical Neurology*, *121*, 1377–1381. doi:10.1016/B978-0-7020-4088-7.00094-8.
83. Sen, S., Rabinstein, A. A., Elkind, M. S., et al. (2012). Recent developments regarding human immunodeficiency virus infection and stroke. *Cerebrovascular Diseases*, *33*(3), 209–218. doi:10.1159/000335300.
84. Spudich, S. (2013). HIV and neurocognitive dysfunction. *Current HIV/AIDS Reports*, *10*(3), 235–243. doi:10.1007/s11904-013-0171-y.
85. Centner, C. M., Bateman, K. J., & Heckmann, J. M. (2013). Manifestations of HIV infection in the peripheral nervous system. *Lancet. Neurology*, *12*(3), 295–309. doi:10.1016/S1474-4422(13)70002-4.
86. Alkali, N. H., Bwala, S. A., Nyandaiti, Y. W., et al. (2013). NeuroAIDS in sub-Saharan Africa: A clinical review. *Annals of African Medicine*, *12*(1), 1–10. doi:10.4103/1596-3519.108242.
87. Chang, C. C., Crane, M., Zhou, J., et al. (2013). HIV and co-infections. *Immunological Reviews*, *254*(1), 114–142. doi:10.1111/imr.12063.
88. Malfitano, A., Barbaro, G., Perretti, A., et al. (2012). Human immunodeficiency virus-associated malignancies: A therapeutic update. *Current HIV Research*, *10*(2), 123–132.
89. Multiple Sclerosis Society of Canada. (2016). *What is MS?* Retrieved from https://mssociety.ca/about-ms/what-is-ms.
90. O'Gorman, C., Lucas, R., & Taylor, B. (2012). Environmental risk factors for multiple sclerosis: A review with a focus on molecular mechanisms. *International Journal of Molecular Sciences*, *13*(9), 11718–11752. doi:10.3390/ijms130911718.
91. Klaver, R., De Vries, H. E., Schenk, G. J., et al. (2013). Grey matter damage in multiple sclerosis: A pathology perspective. *Prion*, *7*(1), 66–75. doi:10.4161/pri.23499.
92. Kakalacheva, K., Münz, C., & Lünemann, J. D. (2011). Viral triggers of multiple sclerosis. *Biochimica et Biophysica Acta*, *1812*(2), 132–140. doi:10.1016/j.bbadis.2010.06.012.
93. Courtney, A. M. (2009). Multiple sclerosis. *Medical Clinics of North America*, *93*(2), 451–476, ix–x. doi:10.1016/j.mcna.2008.09.014.
94. Milo, R., & Miller, A. (2014). Revised diagnostic criteria of multiple sclerosis. *Autoimmunity Reviews*, *13*(4–5), 518–524. doi:10.1016/j.autrev.2014.01.012.
95. Wingerchuk, D. M., & Carter, J. L. (2014). Multiple sclerosis: Current and emerging disease-modifying therapies and treatment strategies. *Mayo Clinic Proceedings*, *89*(2), 225–240. doi:10.1016/j.mayocp.2013.11.002.
96. Hewer, S., Lucas, R., van der Mei, I., et al. (2013). Vitamin D and multiple sclerosis. *Journal of Clinical Neuroscience*, *20*(5), 634–641. doi:10.1016/j.jocn.2012.10.005.
97. National Institutes of Health, Northwestern University. (2006). *Stem cell therapy for patients with multiple sclerosis failing alternate approved therapy—A randomized study [verified June 2016]*. Retrieved from http://clinicaltrials.gov/ct2/show/NCT00273364.
98. Multiple Sclerosis Society of Canada. (2016). *Chronic cerebrospinal venous insufficiency (CCSVI)*. Retrieved from https://mssociety.ca/hot-topics/chronic-cerebrospinal-venous-insufficiency-ccsvi.
99. Winer, J. B. (2014). An update in Guillain-Barré syndrome. *Autoimmune Diseases*, *2014*, 793024. doi:10.1155/2014/793024.
100. Carr, A. S., Cardwell, C. R., McCarron, P. O., et al. (2010). A systematic review of population based epidemiological studies in myasthenia gravis. *BMC Neurology*, *10*(46), doi:10.1186/1471-2377-10-46.
101. Mehndiratta, M. M., Pandey, S., & Kuntzer, T. (2011). Acetylcholinesterase inhibitor treatment for myasthenia gravis. *Cochrane Database of Systematic Reviews*, (2), CD006986, doi:10.1002/14651858.CD006986.pub2.
102. Zieliński, M. (2011). Management of myasthenic patients with thymoma. *Thoracic Surgery Clinics*, *21*(1), 47–57, vi. doi:10.1016/j.thorsurg.2010.08.009.
103. Canadian Cancer Society's Steering Committee on Cancer Statistics (2012). *Canadian cancer statistics 2012*. Toronto: Author. Retrieved from http://www.cancer.ca/~/media/cancer.ca/CW/cancer%20information/cancer%20101/Canadian%20cancer%20statistics/Canadian-Cancer-Statistics-2012-EN.pdf.
104. American Cancer Society (2015). *Cancer facts & figures 2015*. Atlanta: Author. Retrieved from http://www.cancer.org/acs/groups/content/@editorial/documents/document/acspc-044552.pdf.
105. Hardell, L., & Carlberg, M. (2013). Using the Hill viewpoints from 1965 for evaluating strengths of evidence of the risk for brain tumors associated with use of mobile and cordless phones. *Reviews on Environmental Health*, *28*(2–3), 97–106. doi:10.1515/reveh-2013-0006.
106. Hardell, L., Carlberg, M., Söderqvist, F., et al. (2013). Case-control study of the association between malignant brain tumours diagnosed between 2007 and 2009 and mobile and cordless phone use. *International Journal of Oncology*, *43*(6), 1833–1845. doi:10.3892/ijo.2013.2111.
107. Grier, J. T., & Batchelor, T. (2006). Low grade gliomas in adults. *The Oncologist*, *11*, 681–693. doi:10.1634/theoncologist.11-6-681.
108. Venur, V. A., Peereboom, D. M., & Ahluwalia, M. S. (2015). Current medical treatment of glioblastoma. *Cancer Treatment and Research*, *163*, 103–115. doi:10.1007/978-3-319-12048-5_7.
109. Oh, M. C., Kim, J. M., Kaur, G., et al. (2013). Prognosis by tumor location in adults with spinal ependymomas. *Journal of Neurosurgery. Spine*, *18*(3), 226–235. doi:10.3171/2012.12.SPINE12591.
110. Ashpole, N. M., Sanders, J. E., Hodges, G. L., et al. (2015). Growth hormone, insulin-like growth factor-1 and the aging brain. *Experimental Gerontology*, *68*, 76–81. doi:10.1016/j.exger.2014.10.002.
111. Ferner, R. E., & Gutmann, D. H. (2013). Neurofibromatosis type 1 (NF1): Diagnosis and management. *Handbook of Clinical Neurology*, *115*, 939–955. doi:10.1016/B978-0-444-52902-2.00053-9.
112. Lloyd, S. K., & Evans, D. G. (2013). Neurofibromatosis type 2 (NF2): Diagnosis and management. *Handbook of Clinical Neurology*, *115*, 957–967. doi:10.1016/B978-0-444-52902-2.00054-0.
113. DeBella, K., Szudek, J., & Friedman, J. M. (2000). Use of the National Institutes of Health criteria for diagnosis of neurofibromatosis 1 in children. *Pediatrics*, *105*(3 Pt. 1), 608–614.
114. Walbert, T., & Gilbert, M. R. (2009). The role of chemotherapy in the treatment of patients with brain metastases from solid tumors. *International Journal of Clinical Oncology*, *14*(4), 299–306. doi:10.1007/s10147-009-0916-1.
115. Gállego Pérez-Larraya, J., & Hildebrand, J. (2014). Brain metastases. *Handbook of Clinical Neurology*, *121*, 1143–1157. doi:10.1016/B978-0-7020-4088-7.00077-8.
116. Tredway, T. L. (2014). Minimally invasive approaches for the treatment of intramedullary spinal tumors. *Neurosurgery Clinics of North America*, *25*(2), 327–336. doi:10.1016/j.nec.2013.12.010.

17

Alterations of Neurological Function in Children

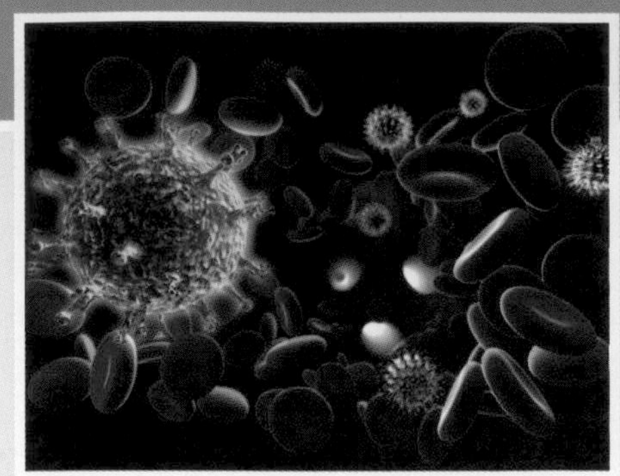

Lynne M. Kerr, Sue E. Huether, Vinodh Narayanan, and Kelly Power-Kean*

EVOLVE WEBSITE

http://evolve.elsevier.com/Canada/Huether/pathophysiology

Student Review Questions
Key Points
Case Studies
Animations
Quick Check Answers

CHAPTER OUTLINE

Development of the Nervous System in Children, 426
Structural Malformations, 427
Defects of Neural Tube Closure, 427
Craniostenosis, 430
Malformations of Brain Development, 431
Alterations in Function: Encephalopathies, 433
Static Encephalopathies, 433
Inherited Metabolic Disorders of the Central Nervous System, 433
Acute Encephalopathies, 434
Infections of the Central Nervous System, 435
Cerebrovascular Disease in Children, 435
Perinatal Stroke, 435
Childhood Stroke, 435
Epilepsy and Seizure Disorders in Children, 436
Childhood Tumours, 436
Brain Tumours, 436
Embryonal Tumours, 438

Neurological disorders in children can occur from infancy through adolescence and include congenital malformations, genetic defects in metabolism, brain injuries, infection, tumours, and other disorders that affect neurological function.

DEVELOPMENT OF THE NERVOUS SYSTEM IN CHILDREN

The nervous system develops from the embryonic ectoderm through a complex, sequential process that can be arbitrarily divided into stages. These include (1) formation of the neural tube (3 to 4 weeks' gestation), (2) development of the forebrain from the neural tube (2 to 3 months' gestation), (3) neuronal proliferation and migration (3 to 5 months' gestation), (4) formation of network connections and synapses (5 months' gestation to many years postnatally), and (5) myelination (birth to many years postnatally). Many different events happen simultaneously, and critical periods must pass uninterrupted if the vulnerable fetus is to develop normally. Genetic and environmental factors (e.g., nutrition, hormones, oxygen levels, toxins, alcohol, medications, drugs, maternal infections, maternal disease) can have a significant effect on neural development[1,2] (see *Health Promotion:* Prevention of Fetal Alcohol Spectrum Disorders).

The growth and development of the brain occurs most rapidly from the third month of gestation through the first year of life, reflecting the proliferation of neurons and glial cells. Although basically all of the neurons that an individual will ever have are present at birth, development of skills, such as walking, talking, and thinking, depends on these cells making correct connections with other cells and on myelination of the axons making those connections. The head is the fastest-growing body part during infancy. One half of postnatal brain growth is achieved by the first year and is 90% complete by age 6 years. The cortex thickens with maturation, and the sulci deepen as a result of rapid expansion of the surface area of the brain. Cerebral blood flow and oxygen consumption during these years are about twice those of the adult brain.

The bones of the infant's skull are separated at the suture lines, forming two **fontanelles**, or "soft spots": one diamond-shaped anterior fontanelle and one triangular-shaped posterior fontanelle. The sutures allow for expansion of the rapidly growing brain. The posterior fontanelle may be open until 2 to 3 months of age; the anterior fontanelle normally does not fully close until 18 months of age (Figure 17-1). Head growth almost always reflects brain growth. Monitoring the fontanelles and careful measurement and plotting of the head circumference on standardized growth charts are essential elements of the pediatric examination. A common cause of accelerating head growth and macrocephaly is hydrocephalus, a condition in which the cerebrospinal fluid (CSF) compartment (ventricles) is enlarged. Increased intracranial pressure (ICP), with distension or bulging of the fontanelles, and separation of the sutures are key signs of hydrocephalus. Microcephaly (head circumference below the second percentile for age) can be the result of prenatal infection, toxin exposure, or malnutrition, or have a primary genetic etiology (see p. 427).

Because of the immaturity of much of the human forebrain at birth, neurological examination of the infant detects mostly reflex responses

*Vinodh Narayanan contributed to this chapter in the US 5th edition.

HEALTH PROMOTION

Prevention of Fetal Alcohol Spectrum Disorders

The term *fetal alcohol spectrum disorder* (FASD) is used to describe the full range of damage that prenatal alcohol exposure can cause in the unborn child. Alcohol crosses the placenta and the blood–brain barrier and exerts teratogenic effects on the developing brain throughout fetal development. Damage can vary from mild to severe physical defects and cognitive, behavioural, emotional, and adaptive functioning deficits. FASD includes diagnoses of fetal alcohol syndrome (FAS), partial FAS, alcohol-related neurodevelopmental disorder (ARND), and alcohol-related birth defects (ARBD).[1,2] ARND has long-lasting neurobehavioural and cognitive deficiencies. It is among the most common causes of mental deficits that persist throughout adulthood. ARND is 100% preventable. Rates of alcohol consumption by women during pregnancy range from 5 to 15%.[2-5] Studies indicate that the incidence of FAS in Canada is higher among Indigenous people.[6] As there is no known amount of alcohol that is safe to consume while pregnant, the Canadian Paediatric Society has made the following recommendations related to screening, education, and prevention programs to promote alcohol-free pregnancies:

- Address the effects of FAS through classroom or community education programs.
- Encourage women to avoid consuming alcohol before conception and throughout pregnancy.
- Identify women who are drinking while pregnant and promote reduction in their consumption.
- Recommend abstinence from alcohol during the first prenatal visit.[6]
- Promptly refer pregnant individuals who are unable to stop drinking alcohol for alcohol treatment.[4-5]

References

1. Interagency Coordinating Committee on Fetal Alcohol Spectrum Disorders. (2011). *Consensus statement on recognizing alcohol-related neurodevelopmental disorder (ARND) in primary health care of children.* Retrieved from https://niaaa.nih.gov/sites/default/files/ARNDConferenceConsensusStatementBooklet_Complete.pdf.
2. Roussotte, F. F., Sulik, K. K., Mattson, S. N., et al. (2012). *Human Brain Mapping, 33*(4), 920–937.
3. Centers for Disease Control and Prevention. (2012). *MMWR Morbidity and Mortality Weekly Report, 61*(28), 534–538.
4. May, P. A., Blankenship, J., Marais, A. S., et al. (2013). *Drug and Alcohol Dependence, 133*(2), 502–512.
5. Zelner, I., & Koren, G. (2013). *Journal of Population Therapeutics and Clinical Pharmacology, 20*(2), e201–e206.
6. Canadian Paediatric Society. (2002). *Position statement: Fetal alcohol syndrome* [Reaffirmed February 1, 2016]. Retrieved from http://www.cps.ca/en/documents/position/fetal-alcohol-syndrome.

that require an intact spinal cord and brainstem. Some of these reflex patterns are inhibited as cerebral cortical function matures, and these patterns disappear at predictable times during infancy (Table 17-1).

Absence of expected reflex responses at the appropriate age indicates general depression of central or peripheral motor functions. Asymmetrical responses may indicate lesions in the motor cortex or peripheral nerves, or may occur with fractures of bones after traumatic delivery or postnatal injury. As the infant matures, the neonatal reflexes disappear in a predictable order as voluntary motor functions supersede them. Abnormal persistence of these reflexes is seen in infants with developmental delays or with central motor lesions.

QUICK CHECK 17-1

1. When does development of neuronal myelination occur?
2. What is a major function of the fontanelles?
3. Why do many of the reflexes of infancy disappear by 1 year of age?

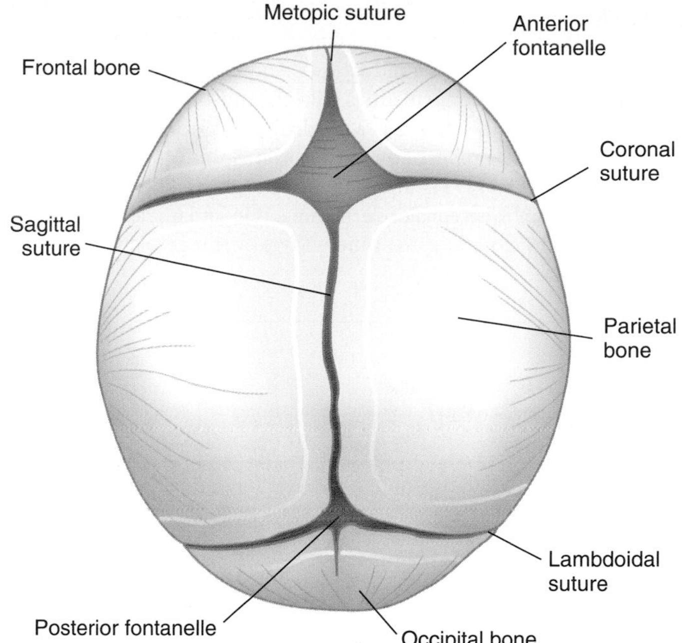

FIGURE 17-1 Cranial Sutures and Fontanelles in Infancy. Fibrous union of suture lines and interlocking of serrated edges (occurs by 6 months; solid union requires approximately 12 years). (Head growth charts are available from the Centers for Disease Control and Prevention at http://www.cdc.gov/nchs/data/series/sr_11/sr11_246.pdf.)

TABLE 17-1 Reflexes of Infancy

Reflex	Age of Appearance of Reflex	Age at Which Reflex Should No Longer Be Obtainable
Moro	Birth	3 months
Stepping	Birth	6 weeks
Sucking	Birth	4 months awake 7 months asleep
Rooting	Birth	4 months awake 7 months asleep
Palmar grasp	Birth	6 months
Plantar grasp	Birth	10 months
Tonic neck	2 months	5 months
Neck righting	4 to 6 months	24 months
Landau	3 months	24 months
Parachute reaction	9 months	Persists indefinitely

STRUCTURAL MALFORMATIONS

Central nervous system (CNS) malformations are responsible for 75% of fetal deaths and 40% of deaths during the first year of life. CNS malformations account for 33% of all apparent congenital malformations, and 90% of CNS malformations are defects of neural tube closure.

Defects of Neural Tube Closure

Neural tube defects (NTDs) are caused by an arrest of the normal development of the brain and spinal cord during the first month of embryonic development. This disorder is relatively common, with a prevalence rate of approximately 4.1 per 10 000 births in Canada (although there are significant provincial prevalence variations).[3] Fetal death often occurs in the more severe forms, thereby reducing the actual prevalence of neural defects at birth.[4] Defects of neural tube closure are divided into two categories: (1) anterior midline defects (ventral induction) and (2) posterior defects (dorsal induction). Anterior midline defects may cause brain and face abnormalities with the most extreme form being **cyclopia**, in which the child has a single midline orbit and eye with a protruding noselike proboscis above the orbit. **Spina bifida (split spine)** is the most common NTD and includes anencephaly (*an*, "without"; *enkephalos*, "brain"), encephalocele, meningocele, and myelomeningocele. Vertebrae fail to close in spina bifida. Myelomeningocele is a form of spina bifida with incomplete development of the spine and protrusion of both the spinal cord and the meninges through the skin. Meningocele is a form of spina bifida in which there is protrusion of the meninges, but the spinal cord remains in the spinal canal. Disorders of embryonic neural development are summarized in Figure 17-2.

The cause of NTDs is believed to be multifactorial (a combination of genes and environment). No single gene has been found to cause NTDs, but there can be associated mutations in folate-responsive or folate-dependent pathways.[5] Folic acid deficiency during preconception

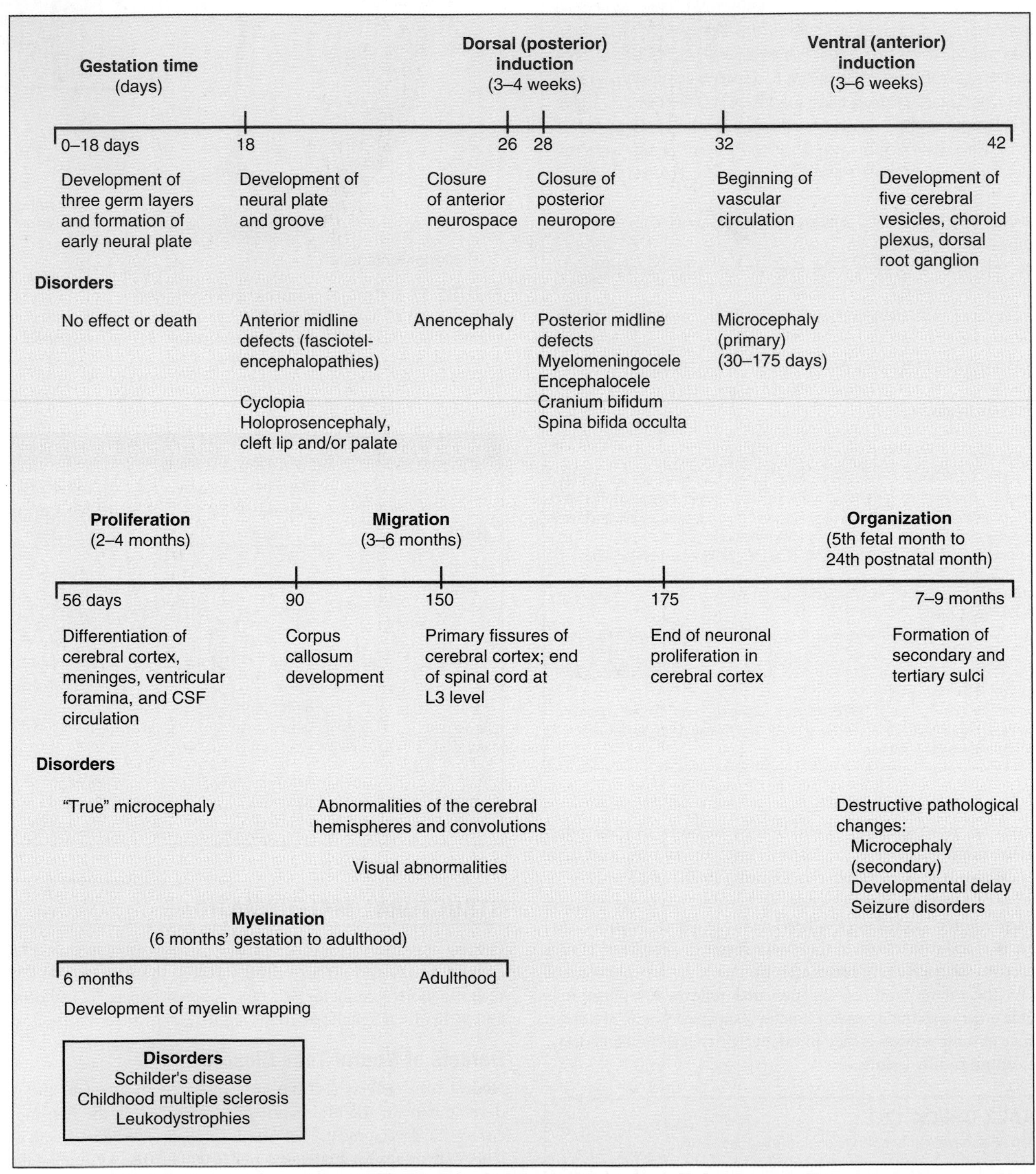

FIGURE 17-2 Disorders Associated With Specific Stages of Embryonic Development. *CSF,* cerebrospinal fluid.

and early stages of pregnancy increases the risk for NTDs, and supplementation (400 mcg of folic acid per day) ensures adequate folate status.[6] Results have shown that the introduction of the mandatory fortification of flour with folic acid in Canada has resulted in a significant reduction in the incidence of NTDs. Other considerations include the increasing use of folic acid supplements and increased prenatal screening and diagnosis leading to pregnancy termination.[3] Other risk factors include a previous NTD pregnancy, maternal diabetes or obesity, use of anticonvulsant medications (particularly valproic acid [Valproate Sodium]), and maternal hyperthermia.[7,8]

Anencephaly is an anomaly in which the soft, bony component of the skull and part of the brain are missing.[9] There is a prevalence rate of 0.8 per 10 000 births in Canada each year.[3] These infants are stillborn or die within a few days after birth. The pathological mechanism is unknown. Diagnosis is often made prenatally by using ultrasound or evaluating maternal serum alpha fetoprotein (AFP).

Encephalocele refers to a herniation or protrusion of the brain and meninges through a defect in the skull, resulting in a saclike structure.[10] There is a prevalence rate of 0.6 per 10 000 births in Canada each year.[3]

Meningocele is a saclike cyst of meninges filled with spinal fluid and is a mild form of spina bifida (Figure 17-3). It develops during the first 4 weeks of pregnancy when the neural tube fails to close completely. The cystic dilation of meninges protrudes through the vertebral defect but does not involve the spinal cord or nerve roots and may produce no neurological deficit or symptoms. Meningoceles occur with equal frequency in the cervical, thoracic, and lumbar spine areas.

Myelomeningocele (meningomyelocele; spina bifida cystica) is a hernial protrusion of a saclike cyst (containing meninges, spinal fluid, and a portion of the spinal cord with its nerves) through a defect in the posterior arch of a vertebra. Eighty percent of myelomeningoceles are located in the lumbar and lumbosacral regions, the last regions of the neural tube to close. Myelomeningocele is one of the most common developmental anomalies of the nervous system, affecting 1 out of every 1 200 children born in Canada.[11]

Meningocele and myelomeningoceles are evident at birth as a pronounced skin defect on the infant's back (see Figure 17-3). The bony prominences of the unfused neural arches can be palpated at the lateral border of the defect. The defect usually is covered by a transparent membrane that may have neural tissue attached to its inner surface. This membrane may be intact at birth or may leak CSF, thereby increasing the risks of infection and neuronal damage.

The spinal cord and nerve roots are malformed below the level of the lesion, resulting in loss of motor, sensory, reflex, and autonomic functions. A brief neurological examination concentrating on motor function in the legs, reflexes, and sphincter tone is usually sufficient to determine the level above which spinal cord and nerve root function is preserved (Table 17-2). This examination is useful to predict whether the child will ambulate, require bladder catheterization, or be at high risk of developing scoliosis (see Chapter 40).

Hydrocephalus occurs in 85% of infants with myelomeningocele.[12] Seizures also occur in 30% of those with myelodysplasia. Visual and perceptual problems, including ocular palsies, astigmatism, and visuoperceptual deficits, are common. Motor and sensory functions below the level of the lesions are altered. Often these problems worsen as the child grows and the cord ascends within the vertebral canal, pulling primary scar tissue and tethering the cord.[13] Several musculo-skeletal deformities are related to this diagnosis, as are spinal deformities.

Myelomeningoceles are almost always associated with the **Chiari II malformation (Arnold-Chiari malformation)**.[12] This structural defect is a complex malformation of the brainstem and cerebellum in which the cerebellar tonsils are displaced downward into the cervical spinal

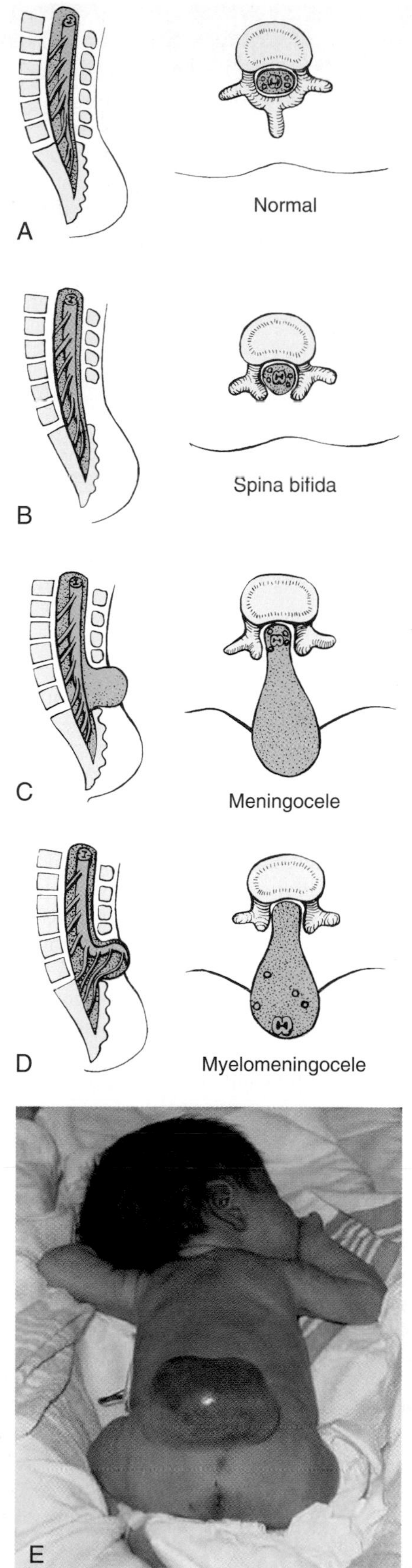

FIGURE 17-3 Normal Spine, Spina Bifida, Meningocele, and Myelomeningocele. (From Hockenberry, M.J., & Wilson, D. [2015]. *Wong's nursing care of infants and children* [10th ed.]. St. Louis: Mosby.)

TABLE 17-2 Functional Alterations in Myelodysplasia Related to Level of Lesion

Level of Lesion	Functional Implications
Thoracic	Flaccid paralysis of lower extremities; variable weakness in abdominal trunk musculature; high thoracic level may mean respiratory compromise; absence of bowel and bladder control
High lumbar	Voluntary hip flexion and adduction; flaccid paralysis of knees, ankles, and feet; may walk with extensive braces and crutches; absence of bowel and bladder control
Mid lumbar	Strong hip flexion and adduction; fair knee extension; flaccid paralysis of ankles and feet; absence of bowel and bladder control
Low lumbar	Strong hip flexion, extension, and adduction and knee extension; weak ankle and toe mobility; may have limited bowel and bladder function
Sacral	Normal function of lower extremities; normal bowel and bladder function

Modified from Sandler, A.D. (2010). *Pediatr Clin North Am, 57*(4), 879–892.

canal; the upper medulla and lower pons are elongated and thin; and the medulla is also displaced downward and sometimes has a "kink" (Figure 17-4). The Chiari II malformation is associated with hydrocephalus from pressure that blocks the flow of CSF; syringomyelia, an abnormality causing cysts at multiple levels within the spinal cord; and cognitive and motor deficits.[14]

Other types of Chiari malformations are not associated with spina bifida. Type I Chiari malformation does not involve the brainstem and may be asymptomatic. In type III, the brainstem or cerebellum extends into a high cervical myelomeningocele. Type IV is characterized by lack of cerebellar development.

Most cases of meningocele and myelomeningocele are diagnosed prenatally by a combination of maternal serological testing (AFP) and prenatal ultrasound. In these cases, the fetus is usually delivered by elective Caesarean section to minimize trauma during labour. Surgical repair is critical and can be performed by in utero fetal surgery or during the first 72 hours of life.[15,16]

It is possible for a defect to occur without any visible exposure of meninges or neural tissue, and the term **spina bifida occulta** is then used. The defect is common and occurs to some degree in 10 to 25% of infants. Spina bifida occulta usually causes no neurological dysfunction because the spinal cord and spinal nerves are normal. **Tethered cord syndrome** may develop after surgical correction for myelomeningocele. The cord becomes abnormally attached or tethered as a result of scar tissue as the cord transcends the vertebral canal with growth.[17]

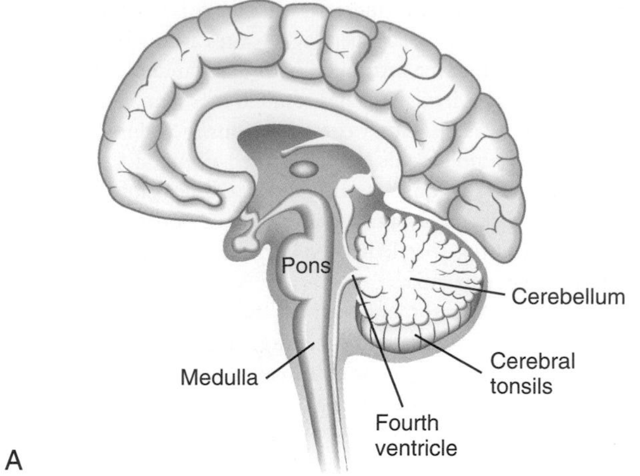

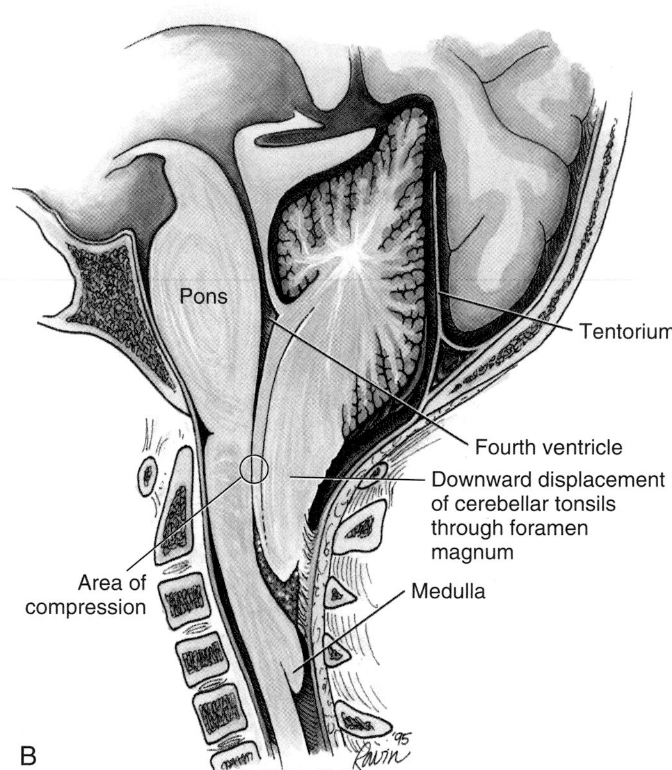

FIGURE 17-4 Normal Brain and Chiari II Malformation. **A,** Diagram of normal brain. **B,** Diagram of Chiari II malformation with downward displacement of cerebellar tonsils and medulla through foramen magnum causing compression and obstruction to flow of cerebrospinal fluid. (**B,** Used with permission from Barrow Neurological Institute, Phoenix, Arizona.)

Craniostenosis

Skull malformations range from minor, insignificant defects to major defects that are incompatible with life. **Craniostenosis** (also termed *craniosynostosis*) is the premature closure of one or more of the cranial sutures (sagittal, coronal, lambdoid, metopic) during the first 18 to 20 months of the infant's life. The incidence of craniostenosis is 1 per 1 800 to 2 500 live births.[18] Males are affected twice as often as females. Fusion of a cranial suture prevents growth of the skull perpendicular to the suture line, resulting in an asymmetrical shape of the skull. The general term *plagiocephaly*, meaning "misshapen skull," is used to describe deformities that result from craniostenosis or from asymmetrical head posture (positional). When a single coronal suture fuses prematurely, the head is flattened on that side in front. When the sagittal suture fuses prematurely, the head is elongated in the anteroposterior direction (scaphocephaly).[19] Single suture craniostenosis is usually only a cosmetic issue. Rarely, when multiple sutures fuse prematurely, brain growth may be restricted, and surgical repair may prevent neurological dysfunction (Figure 17-5). Syndromic craniostenosis involves deformities in other systems (i.e., the heart, limbs, and CNS).

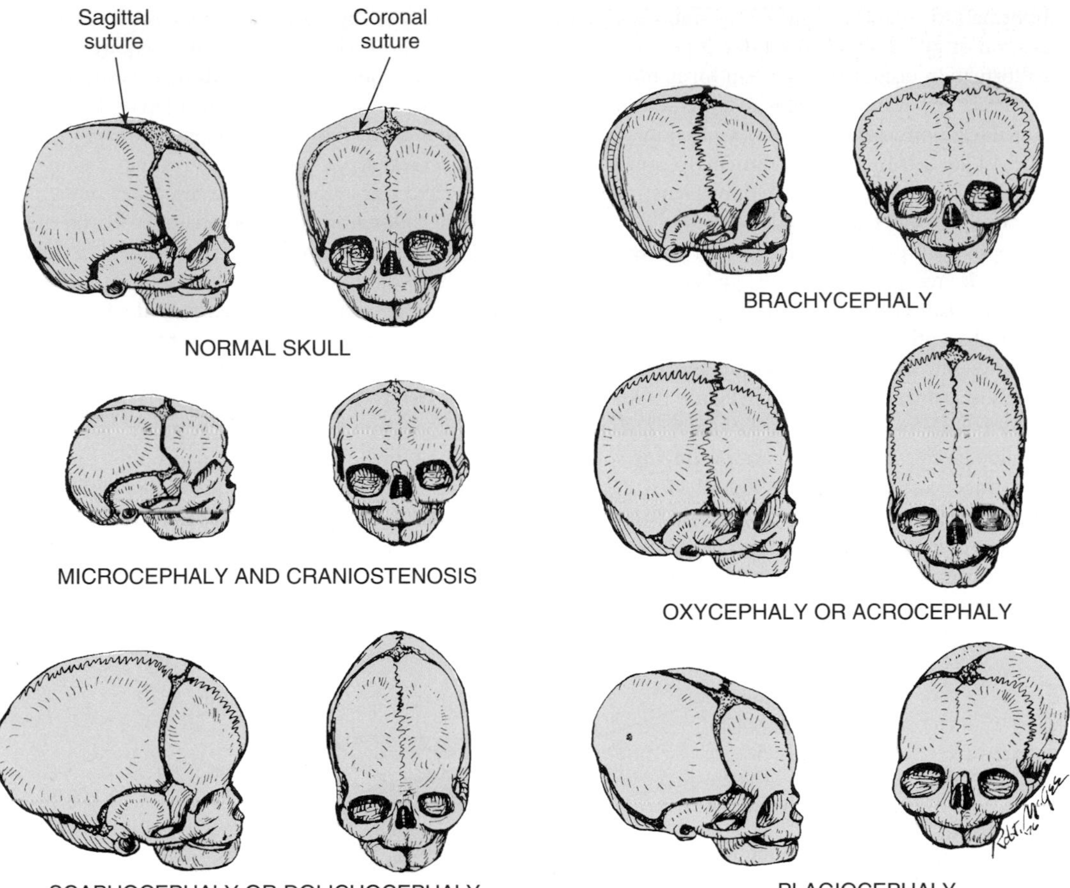

FIGURE 17-5 Normal and Abnormal Head Configurations. *Normal skull:* Bones separated by membranous seams until sutures gradually close. *Microcephaly and craniostenosis:* Microcephaly is head circumference more than 2 standard deviations below the mean for age, gender, race, and gestation and reflects a small brain; craniostenosis is premature closure of sutures. *Scaphocephaly or dolichocephaly* (frequency 56%): Premature closure of sagittal suture, resulting in restricted lateral growth. *Brachycephaly:* Premature closure of coronal suture, resulting in excessive lateral growth. *Oxycephaly or acrocephaly* (frequency 5.8 to 12%): Premature closure of all coronal and sagittal sutures, resulting in accelerated upward growth and small head circumference. *Plagiocephaly* (frequency 13%): Unilateral premature closure of coronal suture, resulting in asymmetrical growth. (From Hockenberry, M.J., & Wilson, D. [2015]. *Wong's nursing care of infants and children* [10th ed.]. St. Louis: Mosby.)

Malformations of Brain Development

Reduced proliferation or accelerated apoptosis causes congenital microcephaly (microencephaly—small brain) and increased proliferation causes megalencephaly (abnormally large brain).

Microcephaly is a defect in brain growth as a whole (see Figure 17-5). Cranial size is significantly below average for the infant's age, gender, race, and gestation. The small size of the skull reflects a small brain (microencephaly), which is caused by reduced proliferation or accelerated apoptosis (Table 17-3). *True (primary) microcephaly* is usually caused by an autosomal recessive genetic or chromosomal defect. *Secondary (acquired) microcephaly* is associated with various causes including infection, trauma, metabolic disorders, maternal anorexia experienced during the third trimester of pregnancy, and the presence of other genetic syndromes. Children with microcephaly are usually developmentally delayed.

TABLE 17-3 Causes of Microcephaly

Defects in Brain Development	Intrauterine Infections	Perinatal and Postnatal Disorders
Hereditary (recessive) microcephaly	Congenital rubella	Intrauterine or neonatal anoxia
Down syndrome and other trisomy syndromes	Cytomegalovirus infection	Severe malnutrition in early infancy
Fetal ionizing radiation exposure	Congenital toxoplasmosis	Neonatal herpesvirus infection
Maternal phenylketonuria	Zika virus infection	
Cornelia de Lange's syndrome		
Rubinstein-Taybi syndrome		
Smith-Lemli-Opitz syndrome		
Fetal alcohol spectrum disorder		
Angelman syndrome		
Seckel's syndrome		

Cortical dysplasias are a heterogeneous group of disorders caused by defects in brain development. These disorders may range from a small area of abnormal tissue (e.g., heterotopia, which are pieces of grey matter that did not migrate to their normal position in the cortex of the brain; and focal cortical dysplasias, where brain organization in one small area is abnormal) to an entire brain that is smooth without the normal configuration of gyri and sulci of a developed brain (lissencephaly). The malformation occurs during brain formation. There is a specific genetic defect for some of these disorders; others are multifactorial or acquired (e.g., intrauterine trauma or infection). Cortical dysplasias increase the risk for seizures that are difficult to control, and cause developmental delay and motor dysfunction. Genetic testing assesses risk in other family members and guides therapy.[20]

Congenital hydrocephalus is present at birth and characterized by increased CSF pressure. It may be caused by blockage within the ventricular system where the CSF flows, an imbalance in the production of CSF, or a reduced reabsorption of CSF.[21] The increased pressure within the ventricular system dilates the ventricles and pushes and compresses the brain tissue against the skull cavity (Figure 17-6). When hydrocephalus develops before fusion of the cranial sutures, the skull can expand to accommodate this additional space-occupying volume and preserve neuronal function (see photo in Figure 17-6, *C*). The overall incidence of hydrocephalus is approximately 1 to 3 per 1 000 live births.[22] The incidence of hydrocephalus that is not associated with myelomeningocele is approximately 0.5 to 1 per 1 000 live births.[22] (Types of hydrocephalus are discussed in Chapter 15.)

Congenital hydrocephalus may cause fetal death in utero, or the increased head circumference may require Caesarean delivery of the infant. Symptoms depend directly on the cause and rate of hydrocephalus development. When there is separation of the cranial sutures, a resonant note sounds when the skull is tapped, a manifestation termed **Macewen sign ("cracked pot" sign)**. The eyes may assume a staring expression, with sclera visible above the cornea, called *sunsetting*. Cognitive impairment in children with hydrocephalus is often related to associated brain malformations, or episodes of shunt failure or infection. Approximately 30 to 40% of children with uncomplicated congenital hydrocephalus complete schooling and are employed when treated successfully with shunting or endoscopic third ventriculostomy and choroid plexus cauterization.[23-25]

The **Dandy-Walker malformation (DWM)** is a congenital defect of the cerebellum characterized by a large posterior fossa cyst that communicates with the fourth ventricle and an atrophic, upwardly rotated cerebellar vermis.[26] DWM is commonly associated with hydrocephalus caused by compression of the aqueduct of Sylvius. Other causes of obstructions within the ventricular system that can result in hydrocephalus include brain tumours, cysts, trauma, arteriovenous malformations, blood clots, infections, and the Chiari malformations (see p. 429).

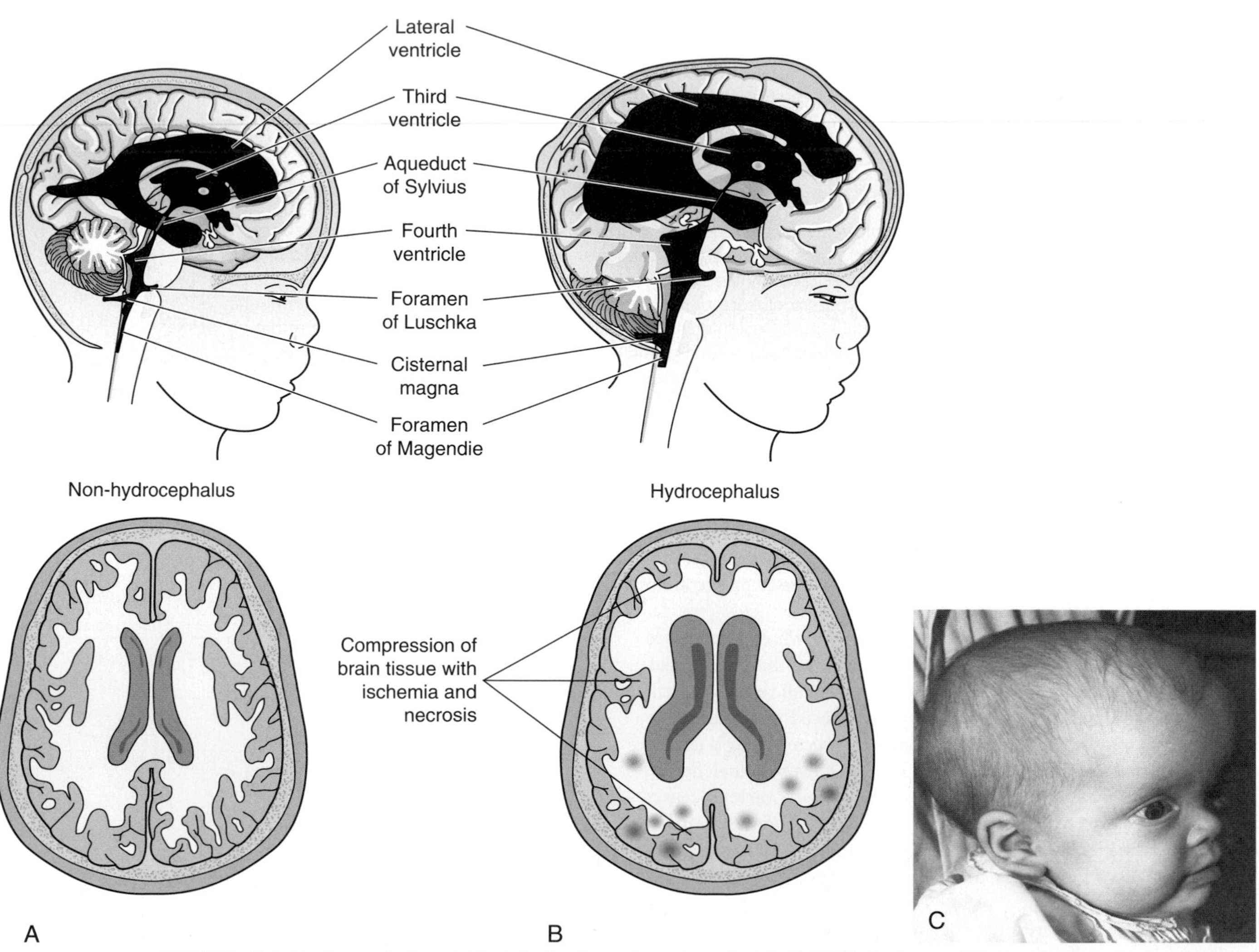

FIGURE 17-6 Hydrocephalus. A block in the flow of cerebrospinal fluid (CSF). **A,** Patent CSF circulation. **B,** Enlarged lateral and third ventricles caused by obstruction of circulation (e.g., stenosis of aqueduct of Sylvius). **C,** Infant born with hydrocephalus. (**C,** from McCance, K.L., & Huether, S.E. [2014]. *Pathophysiology: The biological basis for disease in adults and children* [7th ed.]. St. Louis: Elsevier, p. 668.)

QUICK CHECK 17-2

1. List two defects of neural tube closure.
2. Why do motor and sensory functions worsen with growth in a child with a neural tube defect?
3. What food source or dietary supplement helps to prevent neural tube defects?

ALTERATIONS IN FUNCTION: ENCEPHALOPATHIES

Encephalopathy, which means brain pathology, is a general category that includes a number of syndromes and diseases (see Chapter 16). These disorders may be acute or chronic, as well as static or progressive.

Static Encephalopathies

Static or nonprogressive encephalopathy describes a neurological condition caused by a fixed lesion without active and ongoing disease. Causes include brain malformations (disorders of neuronal migration) or brain injury that may occur during gestation or birth, or at any time during childhood. The degree of neurological impairment is directly related to the extent of the injury or malformation. Anoxia, trauma, and infections are the most common factors that cause injury to the nervous system in the perinatal period. Infections, metabolic disturbances (acquired or genetic), trauma, toxins, and vascular disease may injure the nervous system in the postnatal period.[27]

Cerebral palsy is a disorder of movement, muscle tone, or posture that is caused by injury or abnormal development in the immature brain before, during, or after birth up to 1 year of age. Cerebral palsy is one of the most common crippling disorders of childhood, affecting nearly 50 000 children in Canada alone. Although the exact incidence is unknown, studies suggest that the prevalence is approximately 1 in 500, and 1 in 1 000 newborns in Canada.[28]

Risk factors include prenatal or perinatal cerebral hypoxia, hemorrhage, infection, genetic abnormalities, or low birth weight. Cerebral palsy can be classified on the basis of neurological signs and motor symptoms, with the major types involving spasticity, dystonia, ataxia, or a combination of these symptoms (mixed). Diplegia, hemiplegia, or tetraplegia may be present.

Pyramidal/spastic cerebral palsy results from damage to corticospinal pathways (upper motor neurons) and is associated with increased muscle tone, persistent primitive reflexes, hyperactive deep tendon reflexes, clonus, rigidity of the extremities, scoliosis, and contractures. This form of cerebral palsy accounts for approximately 70 to 80% of cases. Extrapyramidal/nonspastic cerebral palsy is caused by damage to cells in the basal ganglia, thalamus, or cerebellum and includes two subtypes: dystonic and ataxic. Dystonic cerebral palsy is associated with extreme difficulty in fine motor coordination and purposeful movements. Movements are stiff, uncontrolled, and abrupt, resulting from injury to the basal ganglia or extrapyramidal tracts. This form of cerebral palsy accounts for approximately 10 to 20% of cases. Ataxic cerebral palsy is caused by damage to the cerebellum with alterations in coordination and movement. There is a broad based gait in an attempt to maintain balance and tremor is common with intentional movements. This form of cerebral palsy accounts for approximately 5 to 10% of cases. A child may have symptoms of each of these cerebral palsy types, which leads to a mixed disorder accounting for approximately 13% of cases.[29]

Children with cerebral palsy often have associated neurological disorders, such as seizures (about 50%), and intellectual impairment ranging from mild to severe (about 67%). Other complications include visual impairment, communication disorders, respiratory problems, bowel and bladder problems, and orthopedic disabilities.[30]

Inherited Metabolic Disorders of the Central Nervous System

A large number of inherited metabolic disorders have been identified, typically leading to diffuse brain dysfunction. Early diagnosis and treatment is vital if these infants are to survive without severe neurological problems. Newborn screening in Canada for specific metabolic conditions varies by province or territory and has led to children at risk of developing metabolic conditions being identified before symptoms develop. Table 17-4 lists some of these inherited metabolic disorders. Inborn errors of metabolism are present at birth, and most cause disturbances of the nervous system, although they may not manifest until childhood or even adulthood. Defects in amino acid and lipid metabolism are among the most common.

Defects in Amino Acid Metabolism

Biochemical defects in amino acid metabolism include (1) those in which the transport of an amino acid is impaired, (2) those involving an enzyme or cofactor deficiency, and (3) those encompassing certain chemical components, such as branched-chain or sulphur-containing amino acids. Most of these disorders are caused by genetic defects resulting in lack of a normal protein and absence of enzymatic activity.

Phenylketonuria. Phenylketonuria (PKU) is an example of an inborn error of metabolism characterized by phenylalanine hydroxylase

TABLE 17-4 Inherited Metabolic Disorders of the Central Nervous System

Age of Onset	Disorder
Neonatal period	Pyridoxine dependency, galactosemia, urea cycle defects, maple syrup urine disease and its variant, phenylketonuria (PKU), Menkes' kinky hair syndrome
Early infancy	Tay-Sachs disease and its variants, infantile Gaucher's disease, infantile Niemann-Pick disease, Krabbe disease (leukodystrophy), Farber lipogranulomatosis, Pelizaeus-Merzbacher disease and other sudanophilic leukodystrophies, spongy degeneration of central nervous system (Canavan disease), Alexander's disease, Alpers disease, Leigh disease (subacute necrotizing encephalomyelopathy), congenital lactic acidosis, Zellweger encephalopathy, Lowe disease (oculocerebrorenal disease)
Late infancy and early childhood	Disorders of amino acid metabolism, metachromatic leukodystrophy, adrenoleukodystrophy, late infantile GM_1 gangliosidosis, late infantile Gaucher's and Niemann-Pick diseases, neuroaxonal dystrophy, mucopolysaccharidosis, mucolipidosis, fucosidosis, mannosidosis, aspartylglycosaminuria, neuronal ceroid lipofuscinoses (Jansky-Bielschowsky disease, Batten's disease, Vogt-Spielmeyer disease, neuronal ceroid lipofuscinosis), Cockayne's syndrome, ataxia telangiectasia
Later childhood and adolescence	Progressive cerebellar ataxias of childhood and adolescence, hepatolenticular degeneration (Wilson's disease), Hallervorden-Spatz disease, Lesch-Nyhan syndrome, Aicardi-Goutieres syndrome, progressive myoclonus epilepsies, homocystinuria, Fabry's disease

Data from Volpe, J.J. (2008). *Neurology of the newborn* (5th ed.). Philadelphia: Saunders. For information regarding screening and parent education, see Medical Home Portal at http://www.medicalhomeportal.org.

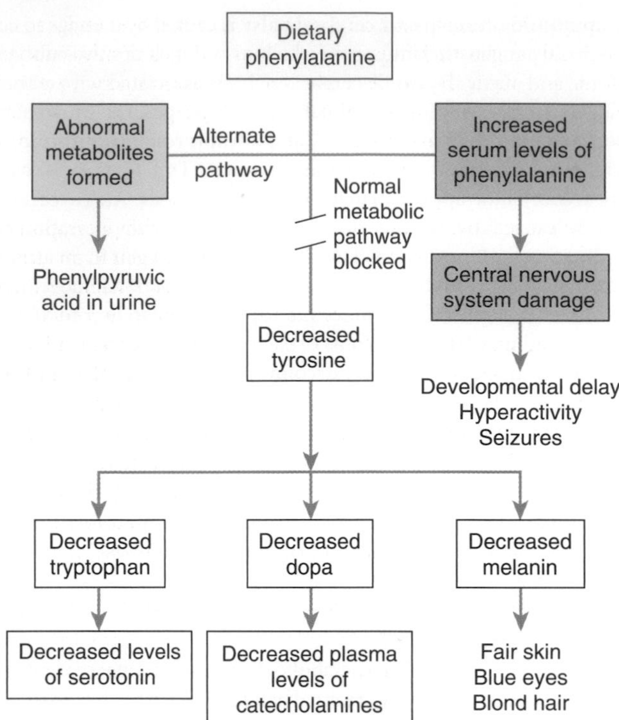

FIGURE 17-7 Metabolic Error and Consequences in Phenylketonuria. (From Hockenberry, M.J., & Wilson, D. [2015]. *Wong's nursing care of infants and children* [10th ed.]. St. Louis: Mosby.)

deficiency and the inability of the body to convert the essential amino acid phenylalanine to tyrosine (Figure 17-7). PKU is an autosomal recessive inborn error of metabolism characterized by mutations of the phenylalanine hydroxylase (*PAH*) gene. PKU has an incidence of 1 per 12 000 live births in North America.[31,32]

Most natural food proteins contain about 15% phenylalanine, an essential amino acid. Phenylalanine hydroxylase controls the conversion of this essential amino acid to tyrosine in the liver. The body uses tyrosine in the biosynthesis of proteins, melanin, thyroxine, and the catecholamines in the brain and adrenal medulla. Phenylalanine hydroxylase deficiency causes an accumulation of phenylalanine in the serum. Elevated phenylalanine levels result in developmental abnormalities of the cerebral cortical layers, defective myelination, and cystic degeneration of the grey and white matter. Unfortunately, brain damage occurs before the metabolites can be detected in the urine, and damage continues as long as phenylalanine levels remain high. Nonselective newborn screening is used to detect PKU in Canada and in more than 30 other countries. Treatment, consisting of reduction of dietary phenylalanine (PKU diet), is effective and allows for normal development. Supplementation with other essential amino acids and nutrients is required to promote adequate growth and development. Mutations in the *PAH* gene are by far the most common cause of PKU, although there are other types of PKU as well. In one such variation, there is impaired synthesis of cofactors (e.g., tetrahydrobiopterin [BH_4]), which contributes to elevated levels of phenylalanine. Individuals with impaired synthesis of BH_4 have a positive response when sapropterin (Kuvan), a synthetic form of tetrahydrobiopterin, is included in their treatment.[33]

Storage Diseases

Disorders of lipid metabolism are termed **lysosomal storage diseases** because each disorder in this group can be traced to a missing lysosomal enzyme. Lysosomal storage disorders are rare and include more than

TABLE 17-5 Common Poisons

Pharmacological Agents	Heavy Metals	Miscellaneous Agents
Acetaminophen	Lead	Botulinum toxin
Amphetamines	Acute exposure	Alcohols
Anticonvulsants	Chronic exposure	Ethyl
Antidepressants	Mercury	Isopropyl
Antihistamines	Thallium	Methyl
Atropine	Arsenic	Pesticides
Barbiturates	Iron supplements	Organophosphates
Methadone		Chlorinated hydrocarbons
Phencyclidine		Mushrooms
Salicylates		Venoms
Tranquilizers		Snakebite
		Tick paralysis
		Ethylene glycol
		Furniture polish
		Paint solvents

Data from Shannon, M.W., Borron, S.W., & Burns, M. (2007). *Haddad and Winchester's clinical management of poisoning and drug overdose* (4th ed.). Philadelphia: Saunders; Swaiman, K.F., Ashwal, S., Ferriero, D.M., et al. (2012). *Pediatric neurology: Principles and practice* (5th ed., Vol 2). St. Louis: Mosby.

50 known genetic disorders. The prevalence of lysosomal storage disorders ranges from 1:50 000 births to 1:4 000 000 births.[1,34] These disorders cause an excessive accumulation of a particular cell product, occurring in the brain, liver, spleen, bone, and lung, and thus involving several organ systems. Generally, these disorders are not included in newborn screening. Some of these disorders may be treated with enzyme replacement therapy.[35] Perhaps the best known of the lysosomal storage disorders is **Tay-Sachs disease (GM_2 gangliosidosis)**, an autosomal recessive disorder (*HexA* gene on chromosome 15) caused by deficiency of the lysosomal enzyme hexosaminidase A (HexA), an enzyme that degrades GM_2 gangliosides (fatty acids) within nerve cell lysosomes. Approximately 80% of individuals diagnosed are of Jewish ancestry, although sporadic cases appear in the non-Jewish population. Onset of this disease usually occurs when the infant is 4 to 6 months old. Symptoms of Tay-Sachs include an exaggerated startle response to loud noise, seizures, developmental regression, dementia, and blindness. Death from this disease is almost universal and occurs by 5 years of age. Screening for carriers of the gene defect concomitant with counselling to prevent disease transmission is possible.[36]

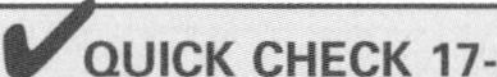

QUICK CHECK 17-3

1. List three types of cerebral palsy.
2. Why does failure to metabolize phenylalanine produce such widespread and devastating effects on development?

Acute Encephalopathies

Intoxications of the Central Nervous System

Medication-induced encephalopathies must always be considered a possibility in the child with unexplained neurological changes. Such encephalopathies may result from accidental ingestion, therapeutic overdose, intentional overdose, or ingestion of environmental toxins (the most commonly ingested poisons are listed in Table 17-5). Approximately 900 children are hospitalized, and approximately 3 children die annually in Canada as a result of unintentional poisoning.[37,38]

Lead poisoning results in high blood levels of lead. If lead poisoning is untreated, lead encephalopathy results and is responsible for serious and irreversible neurological damage. Those at greatest risk are children ages 2 to 3 years and children prone to the practice of pica—the habitual, purposeful, and compulsive ingestion of non-food substances, such as clay, soil, and paint chips or paint dust. Lead intoxication also may occur from chronic exposure to lead in cosmetics, inhalation of gasoline vapors, and ingestion of airborne lead.[39]

National statistics on current blood lead levels in Canadian children are not available. However, in the United States, an estimated 535 000 children 1 to 5 years of age (2.2% of children 1 month to 5 years of age) have excessive amounts of lead in their blood.[40,41] Data from one Canadian study revealed that Indigenous infants had greater prenatal exposure to lead.[41] The *Canadian Family Physician* has published recommendations for the treatment of lead poisoning, depending on blood lead levels.[42] Fetal neurotoxicity occurs with maternal lead exposure, particularly during the first trimester.[43]

Infections of the Central Nervous System

Meningitis is an infection of the meninges and subarachnoid space of the brain and spinal cord, whereas the word encephalitis reflects inflammation within the brain. In many infections of the meninges, encephalitis also is present and the term *meningoencephalitis* is used. The origin of such inflammation and acute encephalopathy can be caused by bacteria, viruses, or other microorganisms. Aseptic meningitis has no evidence of bacterial infection but may be associated with viral infection, systemic disease, or medications.

Bacterial Meningitis

Acute bacterial meningitis is one of the most serious infections to which infants and children are susceptible. Between 2006 and 2011, approximately 196 cases of bacterial meningitis was reported annually in Canada, with an incidence of 0.58 cases per 100 000 population and a fatality ratio of 8.1%. The highest incidence rates were among infants aged less than 1 year.[44] The introduction of conjugate vaccines against *Haemophilus influenzae* type B, *Streptococcus pneumoniae*, and *Neisseria meningitidis* (meningococcus) has decreased the incidence of bacterial meningitis.[45] A vaccine for serogroup B *N. meningitidis* has been newly licensed in Canada but is not recommended for routine immunization programs for infants, children, adolescents, or adults.[46]

Group B *Streptococcus* causes lethal meningitis and sepsis in neonates and is transmitted to the child from the mother's birth canal. *S. pneumoniae* is the most common microorganism in children 1 to 23 months of age. Staphylococcal or streptococcal meningitis can occur in children of any age but shows a predilection for children who have had neurosurgery, skull fracture, or a complication of systemic bacterial infection. Infections that originate in the middle ear, sinuses, or mastoid cells also may lead to *S. pneumoniae* infection in children. Children with sickle cell disease or who have had a splenectomy are particularly at high risk for infection.[47]

Escherichia coli and group B beta-hemolytic streptococci are the most common causes of meningitis in the newborn period. The second most common microorganism causing bacterial meningitis, particularly in children younger than 4 years, is *Neisseria meningitidis* (meningococcus) and it has the potential to occur in epidemics. Approximately 2 to 5% of healthy children are carriers of *N. meningitidis*. As the incidence of *N. meningitidis* infection increases in adolescence and with crowded environments, such as in student residences and among military personnel, it is recommended that all individuals 11 to 18 years of age receive two immunizations against this pathogen.[48]

Pathogens enter the nervous system by direct extension from a contiguous source (e.g., paranasal sinuses or mastoid cells) or, more commonly, by hematogenous spread (e.g., infective endocarditis, pneumonia, neurosurgical procedures, severe burns). Pathogens then cross the blood–brain barrier, enter the CSF, and multiply. Bacterial toxins increase cerebrovascular permeability, causing alterations in blood flow and edema. Increased cranial pressure may intensify further by obstruction to the CSF circulation. Herniation of the brainstem causes death.

Acute bacterial meningitis often is preceded by an upper respiratory tract or a gastro-intestinal infection. Inflammation leads to the general symptoms of fever, headache, vomiting, and irritability and the CNS symptoms of photophobia, nuchal and spinal rigidity, decreased level of consciousness, and seizures. Irritation of the meninges and spinal roots causes pain and resistance to neck flexion (nuchal rigidity), a positive Kernig sign (resistance to knee extension in the supine position with the hips and knees flexed against the body), and a positive Brudzinski sign (flexion of the knees and hips when the neck is flexed forward rapidly). With severe meningeal irritation, the child may demonstrate opisthotonic posturing (rigid arching of the back with the head extended). Infants may have bulging fontanelles. Meningococcal meningitis can produce a characteristic petechial rash.

Viral meningitis (aseptic or nonpurulent meningitis) may result from a direct infection of a virus, or it may be secondary to disease, such as measles, mumps, herpes, or leukemia. The hallmark of viral meningitis is a mononuclear response in the CSF and the presence of normal glucose levels as well. The clinical manifestations are similar to those in bacterial meningitis, although usually milder.

Viral encephalitis in children is similar to viral encephalitis in adults (see Chapter 16, Figure 16-13) and can be difficult to distinguish from viral meningitis. Viruses can directly invade the brain, causing inflammation; or postinfectious encephalitis can develop as a result of an autoimmune response.[49] Encephalopathy resulting from human immunodeficiency virus (HIV) is discussed in Chapter 8 and Chapter 16.

CEREBROVASCULAR DISEASE IN CHILDREN

Perinatal Stroke

Perinatal arterial ischemic stroke is estimated at 1 in 4 000 live births and is a leading cause of perinatal brain injury, cerebral palsy, and lifelong disability. Although a cause for perinatal stroke is usually not found, clotting abnormalities may make the child prone to further vascular events.

Childhood Stroke

Childhood stroke occurs in 1.3 to 1.6 per 100 000 children per year and may be divided into two categories: ischemic and hemorrhagic.[50,51]

Ischemic (occlusive) stroke is rare in children and may result from embolism, sinovenous thrombosis, or congenital or iatrogenic narrowing of vessels leading to decreased flow of blood and oxygen to areas of the brain. Children with arterial ischemic stroke do not have the typical adult risk factors of atherosclerosis and hypertension. Risk factors include cardiac diseases, hematological and vascular disorders, and infection. Approximately 40% of children with acute ischemic stroke have no identifiable risk factors.[52] Sickle cell disease, cerebral arteriopathies, and cardiac anomalies are the common disorders associated with arterial ischemic stroke.[53]

Hemorrhagic stroke (intracranial hemorrhage) is most commonly caused by bleeding from congenital cerebral arteriovenous malformations and is rare in children younger than 19 years. Intraventricular hemorrhage associated with premature birth is related to immature blood vessels and unstable blood pressure. There is a high risk of developing post-hemorrhagic hydrocephalus.[54]

Moyamoya disease is a rare, chronic, progressive vascular stenosis of the circle of Willis. There is obstruction of arterial flow to the brain and the development of basal arterial collateral vessels that vascularize hypoperfused brain distal to the occluded vessels.[55] *Moyamoya* means a "puff of smoke" in Japanese. The disease is idiopathic or associated with other disorders (moyamoya syndrome).

Clinical presentation varies according to the vessels involved, the cause of the disease, and the age of the individual. Symptoms include hemiplegia, weakness, seizures, headaches, high fever, nuchal rigidity, hemianopia, sensory changes, facial palsy, and temporary aphasia. Obtaining a thorough history of evolving symptoms and risk factors is important for diagnosis. Laboratory studies may be indicated. Neuroimaging studies assist in determining the cause of the disease. Surgery is an option for treatment, and anticoagulants and antithrombotics may be used in selected cases.

Epilepsy and Seizure Disorders in Children

The incidence of epilepsy varies greatly with age, geographical location, and study design. In Canada, 44% of children diagnosed with epilepsy are under the age of 5 years, 55% are under the age of 10 years, and 75 to 85% are under the age of 18 years. Approximately 15 500 people in Canada are newly diagnosed each year.[56]

Seizures are the abnormal discharge of electrical activity within the brain. When a sufficient number of neurons become overexcited, they discharge abnormally, which sometimes results in clinical manifestations (seizures) with alterations in motor function, sensation, autonomic function, behaviour, and consciousness. The manifestations depend on the site and spread of abnormal electrical activity. If a child has more than one unprovoked seizure, that child is said to have **epilepsy**, although there are a few exceptions—one example being febrile seizures. Seizures may result from diseases that are primarily neurological (CNS) or are systemic and affect CNS function secondarily (such as diabetes). Seizures can be caused by structural abnormalities of the brain, hypoxia, intracranial hemorrhage, CNS infection, traumatic injury, electrolyte imbalance, or inborn metabolic disturbances. Febrile seizures occur in about 2 to 5% of children between ages 6 months and 5 years; they are benign and the most common type of childhood seizure. Seizures are sometimes clearly familial. Often the cause of epilepsy is unknown and presumed to have a genetic basis. Table 17-6 summarizes the major types of seizure disorders found in children (see also Chapter 15 and Table 15-14).

CHILDHOOD TUMOURS

Brain Tumours

Brain tumours are the most common solid tumour and second most common primary neoplasm in children. In Canada, CNS tumours account for nearly 20% of all childhood cancers under the age of 15 years, with approximately 94% of CNS cancers occurring in the brain. About 3% are malignancies of the cerebral meninges, and the remainder occur in the spinal cord or cranial nerves.[57] Five-year survival for childhood brain tumours is about 73%, varying significantly by tumour type, although there is often significant morbidity.

TABLE 17-6 Major Types of Seizure Disorders Found in Children

Disorder	Manifestations
Generalized Seizure	First clinical manifestations indicate that seizure activity starts in or involves both cerebral hemispheres; consciousness may be impaired; bilateral manifestations; may be preceded by an aura
Tonic-clonic	Musculature stiffens, then intense jerking as trunk and extremities undergo rhythmic contraction and relaxation
Atonic	Sudden, momentary loss of muscle tone; drop attacks
Myoclonic	Sudden, brief contractures of a muscle or group of muscles
Absence seizure	Brief loss of consciousness with minimal or no loss of muscle tone; may experience 20 or more episodes a day lasting approximately 5 to 10 sec each; may have minor movement, such as lip smacking, twitching of eyelids
Partial (Focal) Seizure	Seizure activity that begins with and usually is limited to one part of left or right hemisphere; an aura is common
Simple	Seizure activity that occurs without loss of consciousness
Complex	Seizure activity that occurs with impairment of consciousness
Epilepsy Syndromes	Seizure disorders that display a group of signs and symptoms that occur collectively and characterize or indicate a particular condition
Infantile spasms (West's syndrome)	Form of epilepsy with episodes of sudden flexion or extension involving neck, trunk, and extremities; clinical manifestations range from subtle head nods to violent body contractions (jackknife seizures); onset between 3 and 12 months of age; may be idiopathic, genetic, result of metabolic disease, or in response to central nervous system insult; spasms occur in clusters of 5 to 150 times per day; EEG shows large-amplitude, chaotic, and disorganized pattern called *hypsarrhythmia*
Lennox-Gastaut syndrome	Epileptic syndrome with onset in early childhood, 1 to 5 years of age; includes various generalized seizures—tonic-clonic, atonic (drop attacks), akinetic, absence, and myoclonic; EEG has characteristic "slow spike and wave" pattern; results in intellectual disability and delayed psychomotor developments
Juvenile myoclonic epilepsy	Onset in adolescence; multifocal myoclonus; seizures often occur early in morning, aggravated by lack of sleep or after excessive alcohol intake; occasional generalized convulsions; require long-term medication treatment
Benign rolandic epilepsy	Epileptic syndrome typically occurring in the preadolescent age (6 to 12 years); strong association with sleep (seizures typically occur a few hours after sleep onset or just before waking in morning); complex partial seizures with orofacial signs (drooling, distortion of facial muscles); characteristic EEG with centrotemporal (Rolandic fissure) spikes
Status Epilepticus	Continuing or recurring seizure activity in which recovery from seizure activity is incomplete; unrelenting seizure activity can last 30 min or more; medical emergency that requires immediate intervention
Febrile Seizure	Seizure activity associated with a high body temperature but without any serious underlying health issue occurring most commonly in children between the ages of 6 months and 5 years

EEG, electroencephalogram.

Primary brain tumours arise from brain tissue and do not metastasize outside the brain. The cause of brain tumours is unknown, although genetic, environmental, and immune factors have been investigated. Exposure to radiation therapy has been the only environmental factor consistently related to the development of brain tumours.[58]

Brain tumours can arise from any CNS cell, and tumours are classified by cell type. The types and characteristics of childhood brain tumours are summarized in Table 17-7. Medulloblastoma, ependymoma, astrocytoma, brainstem glioma, craniopharyngioma, and optic nerve glioma constitute approximately 75 to 80% of all pediatric brain tumours. Germ cell tumours are rare. Two thirds of all pediatric brain tumours in children are located in the posterior fossa (Figure 17-8). Treatment strategies and prognoses vary, depending on diagnosis.

Signs and symptoms of brain tumours in children vary from generalized and vague to localized and related specifically to an anatomical area. Signs of increased ICP may occur, including headache, vomiting, lethargy, and irritability. If a young child complains of repeated and worsening headache, a thorough investigation should take place because headache is an uncommon complaint in young children. Headache caused by increased ICP usually is worse in the morning and gradually improves during the day when the child is upright and venous drainage is enhanced. The frequency of headache and other symptoms increases as the tumour grows. Irritability or possible apathy and increased somnolence also may result. Like headache, vomiting occurs more commonly in the morning. Often it is *not* preceded by nausea and may become projectile, differing from a gastro-intestinal disturbance in that the child may be ready to eat immediately after vomiting. Other signs and symptoms include increased head circumference with bulging fontanelles in the child younger than 2 years, cranial nerve palsies, and papilledema (Box 17-1).

Localized findings relate to the degree of disturbance in physiological functioning in the area where the tumour is located. Children with infratentorial tumours exhibit localized signs of impaired coordination and balance, including ataxia, gait difficulties, truncal ataxia, and loss of balance. **Medulloblastoma** occurs as an invasive malignant tumour that develops in the vermis of the cerebellum and may extend into the fourth ventricle. **Ependymoma** develops in the fourth ventricle and arises from the ependymal cells that line the ventricular system. Because both tumours are located in the posterior fossa region along the midline,

TABLE 17-7 Brain Tumours in Children

Type	Characteristics
Astrocytoma	Arises from astrocytes, often in cerebellum or lateral hemisphere Slow growing, solid or cystic Often very large before diagnosed Varies in degree of malignancy
Optic nerve glioma	Arises from optic chiasm or optic nerve (association with neurofibromatosis type 1) Slow-growing, low-grade astrocytoma
Medulloblastoma (infiltrating glioma)	Often located in cerebellum, extending into fourth ventricle and spinal fluid pathway Rapidly growing malignant tumour Can extend outside central nervous system
Brainstem glioma	Arises from pons Numerous cell types Compresses cranial nerves V through X
Ependymoma	Arises from ependymal cells lining ventricles Circumscribed, solid, nodular tumours
Craniopharyngioma	Arises near pituitary gland, optic chiasm, and hypothalamus Cystic and solid tumours that affect vision, pituitary, and hypothalamic functions
Germ cell tumour	Arises from germ cells and is most common in pineal and suprasellar region, usually occurring during adolescence

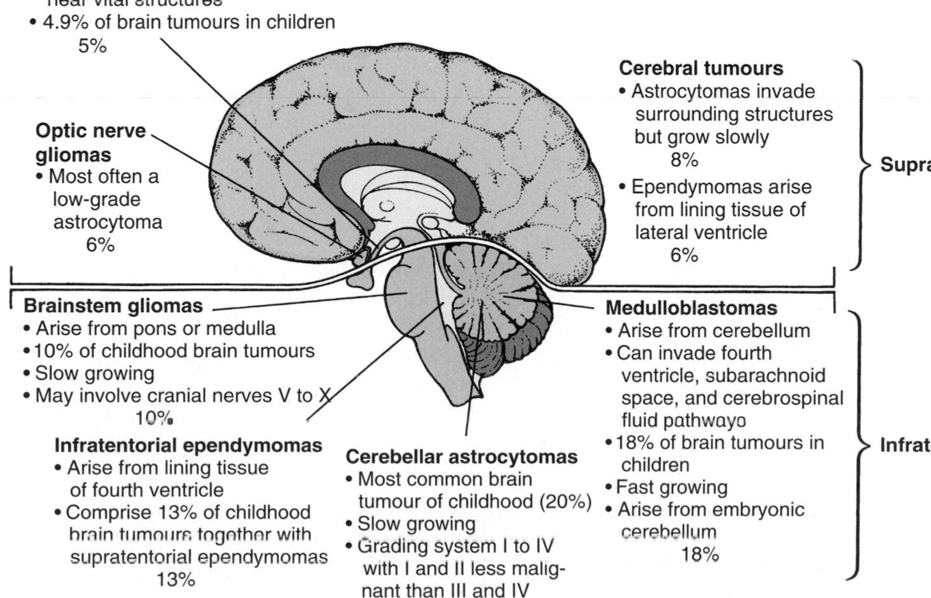
Craniopharyngiomas
• Located adjacent to the sella turcica (structure containing the pituitary gland), often considered to lie supratentorial
• Considered to have benign properties but is life threatening because of its location near vital structures
• 4.9% of brain tumours in children
5%
Optic nerve gliomas
• Most often a low-grade astrocytoma
6%
Cerebral tumours
• Astrocytomas invade surrounding structures but grow slowly
8%
• Ependymomas arise from lining tissue of lateral ventricle
6%
Supratentorial
Brainstem gliomas
• Arise from pons or medulla
• 10% of childhood brain tumours
• Slow growing
• May involve cranial nerves V to X
10%
Infratentorial ependymomas
• Arise from lining tissue of fourth ventricle
• Comprise 13% of childhood brain tumours together with supratentorial ependymomas
13%
Cerebellar astrocytomas
• Most common brain tumour of childhood (20%)
• Slow growing
• Grading system I to IV with I and II less malignant than III and IV
20%
Medulloblastomas
• Arise from cerebellum
• Can invade fourth ventricle, subarachnoid space, and cerebrospinal fluid pathways
• 18% of brain tumours in children
• Fast growing
• Arise from embryonic cerebellum
18%
Infratentorial
FIGURE 17-8 Location of Brain Tumours in Children.

BOX 17-1 Clinical Manifestations of Brain Tumours

Headache
Recurrent and progressive
In frontal or occipital area
Worse on arising; pain lessens during the day
Intensified by lowering head and straining, such as when defecating, coughing, sneezing

Vomiting
With or without nausea or feeding
Progressively more projectile
More severe in morning
Relieved by moving and changing position

Neuromuscular Changes
Uncoordination or clumsiness
Loss of balance (use of wide-based stance, falling, tripping, banging into object)
Poor fine motor control
Weakness
Hyporeflexia or hyper-reflexia
Positive Babinski sign
Spasticity
Paralysis

Behavioural Changes
Irritability
Decreased appetite
Failure to thrive
Fatigue (frequent naps)
Lethargy
Coma
Bizarre behaviour (staring, automatic movements)

Cranial Nerve Neuropathy
Cranial nerve involvement varies according to tumour location
Most common signs:
Head tilt
Visual defects (nystagmus, diplopia, strabismus, episodic "greying out" of vision, and visual field defects)

Vital Sign Disturbances
Decreased pulse and respiratory rates
Increased blood pressure
Decreased pulse pressure
Hypothermia or hyperthermia

Other Signs
Seizures
Cranial enlargement*
Tense, bulging fontanelle at rest*
Separating suture*
Nuchal rigidity
Papilledema (edema of optic nerve)

*Present only in infants and young children.
From Hockenberry, M.N. (2007). *Wong's essentials of pediatric nursing* (7th ed.). St. Louis: Mosby.

presenting signs and symptoms are similar and are usually related to hydrocephalus and increased ICP. In contrast, **cerebellar astrocytomas** are located on the surface of the right or left cerebellar hemisphere and cause unilateral symptoms (occurring on the same side as the tumour), such as head tilt, limb ataxia, and nystagmus.

Brainstem gliomas often cause a combination of cranial nerve involvement (facial weakness, limitation of horizontal eye movement), cerebellar signs of ataxia, and corticospinal tract dysfunction. Increased ICP generally does not occur.

The area of the sella turcica, the structure containing the pituitary gland, is the site of several childhood brain tumours; most common of this group is the **craniopharyngioma**. This tumour originates from the pituitary gland or hypothalamus. Usually slow growing, it may be quite large by the time of diagnosis. Symptoms include headache, seizures, diabetes insipidus, early onset of puberty, and growth delay. Other tumours located in this region of the brain include **optic gliomas**. Optic nerve gliomas are associated with neurofibromatosis type 1, a neurocutaneous condition characterized by café-au-lait macules on the skin and benign tumours of the skin. Tumours that involve the optic tract may cause complete unilateral blindness and hemianopia of the other eye. Optic atrophy is another common finding. Supratentorial tumours of the cerebral hemispheres are more common in neonates and adolescents.[59]

Embryonal Tumours

Neuroblastoma

Neuroblastoma is an embryonal tumour originating outside the CNS in the developing sympathetic nervous system (sympathetic ganglia and the adrenal medulla). Because neuroblastoma involves a defect of embryonic tissue and is the most common cancer in infants less than 1 year of age, 75% of neuroblastomas are found before the child is 5 years old and is rare after 10 years of age. Occasionally, these tumours have been diagnosed at birth with metastasis apparent in the placenta. Approximately 50 to 70 new cases of neuroblastoma are diagnosed every year in Canada. Although it accounts for only about 6% of pediatric malignancies, neuroblastoma causes about 15% of cancer deaths in children.[60,61]

Neuroblastoma is the most common and immature form of the sympathetic nervous system tumours. Areas of necrosis and calcification often are present in the tumour. More than with any other cancer, neuroblastoma has been associated with spontaneous remission, commonly in infants. Prognosis is worse for children older than 2 years of age with disseminated disease.[62]

Although familial tendency has been noted in individual cases, a nonfamilial or sporadic pattern is found in most children with neuroblastoma. Familial cases of neuroblastoma are considered to have an autosomal dominant pattern of inheritance (mechanisms of inheritance are discussed in Chapter 2).

The most common location of neuroblastoma is in the retroperitoneal region (65% of cases), most often the adrenal medulla. The tumour is evident as an abdominal mass and may cause anorexia, bowel and bladder alteration, and sometimes spinal cord compression. The second most common location of neuroblastoma is the mediastinum (15% of cases), where the tumour may cause dyspnea or infection related to airway obstruction. Less commonly, neuroblastoma may arise from the cervical sympathetic ganglion (3 to 4% of cases). Cervical neuroblastoma often causes Horner's syndrome, which consists of miosis (pupil contraction), ptosis (drooping eyelid), enophthalmos (backward displacement of the eyeball), and anhidrosis (sweat deficiency). Neuroblastoma rarely presents with a cerebellar neurological syndrome called opsoclonus-myoclonus syndrome.[63] Children develop conjugate chaotic eye movements, jerky movements of the limbs, and ataxia.

A number of systemic signs and symptoms are characteristic of neuroblastoma, including weight loss, irritability, fatigue, and fever. Intractable diarrhea occurs in 7 to 9% of children and is caused by tumour secretion of a hormone called *vasoactive intestinal polypeptide.*

More than 90% of children with neuroblastoma have increased amounts of catecholamines and associated metabolites in their urine. High levels of urinary catecholamines and serum ferritin are associated with a poor prognosis.

Retinoblastoma

Retinoblastoma is a rare congenital eye tumour of young children that originates in the retina of one or both eyes (Figure 17-9). Two forms of retinoblastoma are exhibited: inherited and acquired. The inherited form of the disease generally is diagnosed during the first year of life. The acquired disease most commonly is diagnosed in children 2 to 3 years of age and involves unilateral disease.[64]

Approximately 40% of retinoblastomas are inherited as an autosomal dominant trait with incomplete penetrance (see Figure 2-22). The remaining 60% are acquired. In the early 1970s, Knudson proposed the "two-hit" hypothesis to explain the occurrence of both hereditary and acquired forms of the disease.[65] This hypothesis predicts that two separate transforming events or "hits" must occur in a normal retinoblast cell to cause the cancer. Further, it proposes that in the inherited form, the first hit or mutation occurs in the germ cell (inherited from either parent), and the mutation is contained in every cell of the child's body. Only a second, random mutation in a retinoblast cell is needed to transform that cell into cancer. Multiple tumours are observed in the inherited form because these second mutations are likely to occur in several of the approximately 1 to 2 million retinoblast cells. In contrast, the acquired form of retinoblastoma requires two independent hits or mutations to occur in the same somatic cell (after the egg is fertilized) for the transformation to cancer. As a result, the acquired form of retinoblastoma is much less likely to occur. Figure 17-10 illustrates the two-mutation model for these two patterns of mutation.

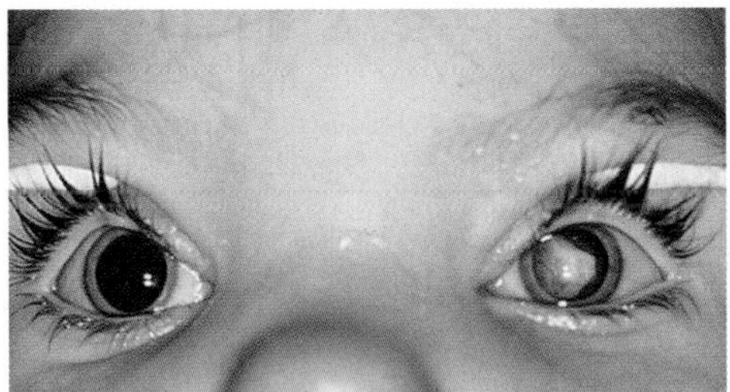

FIGURE 17-9 Retinoblastoma. The tumour occupies a large portion of the inside of the eye globe. (From Damjanov, I. [2006]. *Pathology for the health professions* [3rd ed.]. St. Louis: Saunders. Courtesy Dr. Walter Richardson and Dr. Jamsheed Khan, Kansas City, KS.)

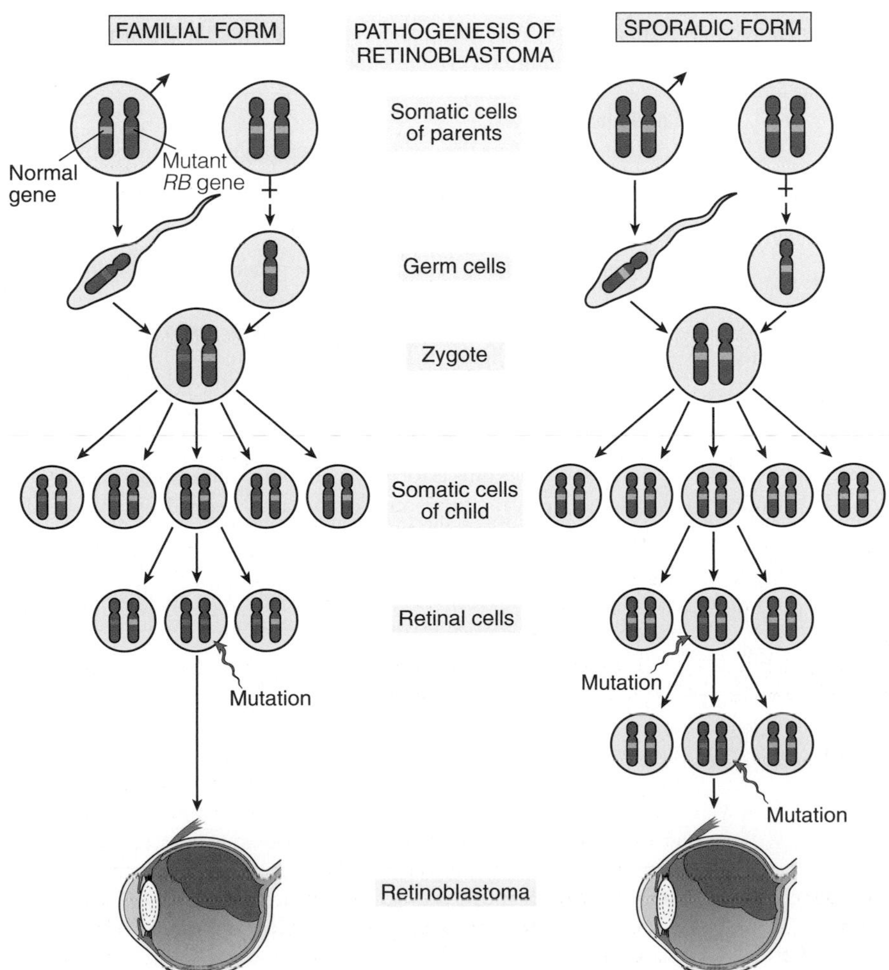

FIGURE 17-10 The Two-Mutation Model of Retinoblastoma Development. In inherited retinoblastoma, the first mutation is transmitted through the germline of an affected parent. The second mutation occurs somatically in a retinal cell, leading to development of the tumour. In sporadic retinoblastoma, development of a tumour requires two somatic mutations.

The primary sign of retinoblastoma is leukocoria, a white pupillary reflex (white reflex) also called *cat's eye reflex*, which is caused by the mass behind the lens (see Figure 17-9). This easy-to-identify sign can be missed. Other signs and symptoms include strabismus; a red, painful eye; and limited vision.

Because retinoblastoma is a treatable tumour, dual priorities are saving the child's life and restoring useful vision. The prognosis for most children with retinoblastoma is excellent, with a greater than 90% long-term survival.

QUICK CHECK 17-4

1. Why are the principal symptoms of brain tumours in children related to brainstem function?

DID YOU UNDERSTAND?

Development of the Nervous System in Children

1. The growth and development of the brain occur most rapidly from the third month of gestation through the first year of life.
2. The bones of the skull are separated at the suture lines; and the wide, membranous junctions of the suture lines (known as *fontanelles*) allow for brain growth and close by 18 months of age.

Structural Malformations

1. Spina bifida (split spine) is the most common disorder of neural tube closure and includes anencephaly (absence of part of the skull and brain), encephalocele (herniation of the meninges and brain through a skull defect), meningocele (a saclike meningeal cyst that protrudes through a vertebral defect), and myelomeningocele.
2. Premature closure of one or more of the cranial sutures causes craniostenosis and prevents normal skull expansion, resulting in compression of growing brain tissue.
3. Microcephaly is lack of brain growth with delayed mental and motor development.
4. Congenital hydrocephalus results from overproduction, impaired absorption, or blockage of circulation of cerebrospinal fluid. Dandy-Walker malformation is caused by cystic dilation of the fourth ventricle and aqueductal compression.

Alterations in Function: Encephalopathies

1. Static encephalopathies are nonprogressive disorders of the brain that can occur during gestation, birth, or at any time during childhood and can be caused by endogenous or exogenous factors.
2. Cerebral palsy can be caused by prenatal cerebral hypoxia or perinatal trauma. Symptoms may include motor dysfunction (including increased muscle tone, increased reflexes, and loss of fine motor coordination), intellectual disability, seizure disorders, or developmental delays.
3. Inherited metabolic disorders that damage the nervous system include defects in amino acid metabolism (phenylketonuria) and lipid metabolism (Tay-Sachs disease) and result in abnormal behaviour, seizures, and deficient psychomotor development.
4. Accidental poisonings from a variety of toxins can cause serious neurological damage.
5. Bacterial meningitis is commonly caused by *Neisseria meningitidis* or *Streptococcus pneumoniae* and may result from respiratory tract or gastro-intestinal infections; symptoms include fever, headaches, photophobia, seizures, rigidity, and stupor.
6. Viral meningitis may result from direct infection or be secondary to a systemic viral infection (e.g., measles, mumps, herpes, or leukemia).

Cerebrovascular Disease in Children

1. Ischemic (occlusive) stroke is rare in children but can occur from embolism, sickle cell disease, cerebral arteriopathies, and cardiac anomalies.
2. Hemorrhagic stroke can occur in association with immature blood vessels associated with prematurity or congenital cerebral arteriovenous malformations.
3. Moyamoya disease is a rare, chronic, progressive vascular stenosis of the circle of Willis that obstructs arterial blood flow to the brain.
4. Seizure disorders involve abnormal discharges of electrical activity within the brain. They are associated with numerous nervous system disorders and more often are a generalized rather than a partial type of seizure.
5. Generalized seizures include tonic-clonic, atonic, myoclonic, and absence seizures.
6. Partial seizures suggest more localized brain dysfunction.
7. Febrile seizures are provoked and usually limited to children between the ages of 6 months and 5 years. They are benign in nature and the most common type of childhood seizure.

Childhood Tumours

1. Brain tumours are the most common tumours of the nervous system and the second most common type of childhood cancer.
2. Tumours in children most often are located below the tentorial plate (infratentorial tumours).
3. Symptoms of brain tumours may be generalized or localized. The most common general symptoms are the result of increased intracranial pressure and include headache, irritability, vomiting, somnolence, and bulging of fontanelles.
4. Localized signs of infratentorial tumours in the cerebellum include impaired coordination and balance. Cranial nerve signs occur with tumours in or near the brainstem.
5. Signs and symptoms associated with brain tumours and the degree of physiological functioning disturbance depend on the specific location of the tumour.
6. Neuroblastoma is an embryonal tumour of the sympathetic nervous system and can be located anywhere there is sympathetic nervous tissue. Symptoms are related to tumour location and size of metastasis.
7. Retinoblastoma is a congenital eye tumour that has two forms: inherited and acquired.

KEY TERMS

Acute bacterial meningitis, 435
Anencephaly, 429
Aseptic meningitis, 435
Ataxic cerebral palsy, 433
Brainstem glioma, 438
Cerebellar astrocytoma, 438
Cerebral palsy, 433
Chiari II malformation (Arnold-Chiari malformation), 429
Congenital hydrocephalus, 432
Cortical dysplasia, 431
Craniopharyngioma, 438
Craniostenosis, 430
Cyclopia, 428

Dandy-Walker malformation (DWM), 432
Dystonic cerebral palsy, 433
Encephalitis, 435
Encephalocele, 429
Encephalopathy, 433
Ependymoma, 437
Epilepsy, 436
Extrapyramidal/nonspastic cerebral palsy, 433
Fontanelle, 426
Hemorrhagic stroke (intracranial hemorrhage), 435
Ischemic (occlusive) stroke, 435
Lead poisoning, 435
Lysosomal storage disease, 434
Macewen sign ("cracked pot" sign), 432
Medulloblastoma, 437
Meningitis, 435
Meningocele, 429
Microcephaly, 431
Moyamoya disease, 436
Myelomeningocele, 429
Neural tube defect (NTD), 427
Neuroblastoma, 438
Optic glioma, 438
Phenylketonuria (PKU), 433
Pica, 435
Pyramidal/spastic cerebral palsy, 433
Retinoblastoma, 439
Spina bifida (split spine), 428
Spina bifida occulta, 430
Tay-Sachs disease (GM_2 gangliosidosis), 434
Tethered cord syndrome, 430
Viral encephalitis, 435
Viral meningitis (aseptic or nonpurulent meningitis), 435

REFERENCES

1. Beard, J. L. (2008). Why iron deficiency is important in infant development. *Journal of Nutrition, 138*(12), 2534–2536.
2. Todorich, B., Pasquini, J. M., Garcia, C. I., et al. (2009). Oligodendrocytes and myelination: The role of iron. *Glia, 57*(5), 467–478. doi:10.1002/glia.20784.
3. Public Health Agency of Canada (2013). *Congenital anomalies in Canada 2013: A perinatal health surveillance report.* Ottawa: Author. Retrieved from http://publications.gc.ca/collections/collection_2014/aspc-phac/HP35-40-2013-eng.pdf.
4. Kaufman, B. (2004). Neural tube defects. *Pediatric Clinics of North America, 51*(2), 389–419. doi:10.1016/S0031-3955(03)00207-4.
5. Copp, A. J., Stanier, P., & Greene, N. D. (2013). Neural tube defects: Recent advances, unsolved questions, and controversies. *Lancet. Neurology, 12*(8), 799–810. doi:10.1016/S1474-4422(13)70110-8.
6. Khodr, Z. G., Lupo, P. J., Agopian, A. J., et al. (2014). Preconceptional folic acid-containing supplement use in the national birth defects prevention study. *Birth Defects Research. Part A, Clinical and Molecular Teratology, 100*(6), 472–482. doi:10.1002/bdra.23238.
7. Centers for Disease Control and Prevention. (2010). CDC grand rounds: Additional opportunities to prevent neural tube defects with folic acid fortification. *MMWR. Morbidity and Mortality Weekly Report, 59*(31), 980–984.
8. Meador, K. J. (2013). Comment: Valproate dose effects differ across congenital malformations. *Neurology, 81*(11), 1002. doi:10.1212/WNL.0b013e3182a43eb7.
9. Centers for Disease Control and Prevention. (2015). *Facts about anencephaly.* Retrieved from http://www.cdc.gov/ncbddd/birthdefects/Anencephaly.html.
10. Centers for Disease Control and Prevention. (2014). *Facts about encephalocele.* Retrieved from http://www.cdc.gov/ncbddd/birthdefects/Encephalocele.html.
11. Spina Bifida and Hydrocephalus Association of Canada. (2016). *About spina bifida.* Retrieved from http://sbhac.ca/about-spina-bifida/.
12. Tamburrini, G., Frassanito, P., Iakovaki, K., et al. (2013). Myelomeningocele: The management of the associated hydrocephalus. *Child's Nervous System, 29*(9), 1569–1579. doi:10.1007/s00381-013-2179-4.
13. Adzick, N. S. (2009). Fetal myelomeningocele: Natural history, pathophysiology, and in-utero intervention. *Seminars in Fetal and Neonatal Medicine, 15*(1), 9–14. doi:10.1016/j.siny.2009.05.002.
14. Salman, M. S. (2011). Posterior fossa decompression and the cerebellum in Chiari type II malformation: A preliminary MRI study. *Child's Nervous System, 27*(3), 457–462. doi:10.1007/s00381-010-1359-8.
15. Adzick, N. S., Thom, E. A., Spong, C. Y., et al. (2011). MOMS investigators: A randomized trial of prenatal versus postnatal repair of myelomeningocele. *New England Journal of Medicine, 364*(11), 993–1004. doi:10.1056/NEJMoa1014379.
16. Adzick, N. S. (2013). Fetal surgery for spina bifida: Past, present, future. *Seminars in Pediatric Surgery, 22*(1), 10–17. doi:10.1053/j.sempedsurg.2012.10.003.
17. Moldenhauer, J. S. (2014). In utero repair of spina bifida. *American Journal of Perinatology, 31*(7), 595–604. doi:10.1055/s-0034-1372429.
18. The Hospital for Sick Children. (2014). *Craniosynostosis: What is craniosynostosis?* Retrieved from http://www.sickkids.ca/Craniofacial/What we do/Craniofacial Conditions/Craniosynostosis/.
19. Ciurea, A. V., Toader, C., & Mihalache, C. (2011). Actual concepts in scaphocephaly: (An experience of 98 cases). *Journal of Medicine and Life, 4*(4), 424–431.
20. Barkovich, J. A., Guerrini, R., Kuzniecky, R. I., et al. (2012). A developmental and genetic classification for malformations of cortical development: Update 2012. *Brain, 135*(Pt. 5), 1348–1369. doi:10.1093/brain/aws019.
21. McAllister, J. P., Jr. (2012). Pathophysiology of congenital and neonatal hydrocephalus. *Seminars in Fetal and Neonatal Medicine, 17*(5), 285–294. doi:10.1016/j.siny.2012.06.004.
22. Garton, H. J., & Piatt, J. H., Jr. (2004). Hydrocephalus. *Pediatric Clinics of North America, 51*(2), 305–325. doi:10.1016/j.pcl.2003.12.002.
23. Constantini, S., Sgouros, S., & Kulmarni, A. (2013). Neuroendoscopy in the youngest age group. *World Neurosurgery, 79*(2 Suppl.), S23.e1–S23.e11. doi:10.1016/j.wneu.2012.02.003.
24. Vinchon, M., Baroncini, M., & Delestret, I. (2012). Adult outcome of pediatric hydrocephalus. *Child's Nervous System, 28*(6), 847–854. doi:10.1007/s00381-012-1723-y.
25. Warf, B. C. (2013). Congenital idiopathic hydrocephalus of infancy: The results of treatment by endoscopic third ventriculostomy with or without choroid plexus cauterization and suggestions for how it works. *Child's Nervous System, 29*(6), 935–940. doi:10.1007/s00381-013-2072-1.
26. Gandolfi Colleoni, G., Contro, E., Carletti, A., et al. (2012). Prenatal diagnosis and outcome of fetal posterior fossa fluid collections. *Ultrasound in Obstetrics and Gynecology, 39*(6), 625–631. doi:10.1002/uog.11071.
27. Marret, S., Vanhullle, C., & Laquerriere, A. (2013). Pathophysiology of cerebral palsy. *Handbook of Clinical Neurology, 111*, 169–176. doi:10.1016/B978-0-444-52891-9.00016-6.
28. MediResource Inc. (2016). *Cerebral palsy: The facts.* Retrieved from http://bodyandhealth.canada.com/condition/getcondition/Cerebral-Palsy.
29. Krigger, K. W. (2006). Cerebral palsy: An overview. *American Family Physician, 73*(1), 91–100.
30. Pruitt, D. W., & Tsai, T. (2009). Common medical comorbidities associated with cerebral palsy. *Physical Medicine and Rehabilitation Clinics of North America, 20*(3), 453–467. doi:10.1016/j.pmr.2009.06.002.
31. Blau, N., van Spronsen, F. J., & Levy, H. L. (2010). Phenylketonuria. *Lancet, 376*(9750), 1417–1427. doi:10.1016/S0140-6736(10)60961-0.
32. CanPKU.org. (2016). *About PKU.* Retrieved from http://canpku.org/about-pku-2.
33. Burton, B. K., Nowacka, M., Hennermann, J. B., et al. (2011). Safety of extended treatment with sapropterin dihydrochloride in patients with phenylketonuria: Results of a phase 3b study. *Molecular Genetics and Metabolism, 103*(4), 315–322. doi:10.1016/j.ymgme.2011.03.020.
34. Meikle, P. J., Ranieri, E., Simonsen, H., et al. (2013). Newborn screening for lysosomal storage disorders: Clinical evaluation of a two-tier strategy. *Pediatrics, 114*(4), 909–916. doi:10.1542/peds.2004 0583.
35. Parenti, G., Pignata, C., Vajro, P., et al. (2013). New strategies for the treatment of lysosomal storage diseases (review). *International Journal of Molecular Medicine, 31*(1), 11–20. doi:10.3892/ijmm.2012.1187.
36. Patterson, M. C. (2013). Gangliosidoses. *Handbook of Clinical Neurology, 113*, 1707–1708. doi:10.1016/B978-0-444-59565-2.00039-3.
37. Bronstein, A. C., Spyker, D. A., Cantilena, L. R., Jr., et al. (2010). 2009 annual report of the American Association of Poison Control Centers' National Poison Data System (NPDS): 27th annual report. *Clinical Toxicology (Philadelphia, Pa.), 48*(10), 979–1178. doi:10.3109/15563650.2010.543906. Retrieved from http://www.aapcc.org/dnn/Portals/0/correctedannualreport.pdf.
38. Mowry, J. B., Spyker, D. A., Cantilena, L. R., Jr., et al. (2013). 2012 annual report of the American Association of Poison Control Centers' National Poison Data System (NPDS): 30th annual report. *Clinical Toxicology (Philadelphia, Pa.), 51*(10), 949–1229. doi:10.3109/15563650.2013.863906.
39. Advisory Committee on Childhood Lead Poisoning Prevention. (2007). Interpreting and managing blood lead levels <10 μg/dL in children and reducing childhood exposures to lead: Recommendations of CDC's Advisory Committee on Childhood Lead Poisoning Prevention. *MMWR Recommendations and Reports, 56*(RR–8), 1–14. Retrieved from http://www.cdc.gov/mmwr/preview/mmwrhtml/rr5608a1.htm.
40. Centers for Disease Control and Prevention. (2013). Blood lead levels in children aged 1–5 years—United States, 1999–2010. *MMWR. Morbidity and Mortality Weekly Report, 62*(13), 245–248.
41. Tsekrekos, S. N., & Buka, I. (2005). Lead levels in Canadian children: Do we have to review the standard? *Paediatrics and Child Health, 10*(4), 215–220.
42. Abelsohn, A. R., & Sanborn, M. (2010). Lead in children: Clinical management for family physicians. *Canadian Family Physician, 56*(6), 531–535.
43. Liu, J., Gao, D., Chen, Y., et al. (2014). Lead exposure at each stage of pregnancy and neurobehavioral development of neonates. *Neurotoxicology, 44*, 1–7. doi:10.1016/j.neuro.2014.03.003.
44. Public Health Agency of Canada. (2015). *Invasive meningococcal disease.* Retrieved from http://www.phac-aspc.gc.ca/im/vpd-mev/meningococcal/professionals-professionnels-eng.php.
45. Kim, K. S. (2010). Acute bacterial meningitis in infants and children. *Lancet Infectious Diseases, 10*(1), 32–42. doi:10.1016/S1473-3099(09)70306-8.
46. Public Health Agency of Canada. (2014). *The recommended use of the multicomponent Meningococcal B (4CMenB) vaccine in Canada.* Retrieved from http://www.phac-aspc.gc.ca/naci-ccni/mening-4cmenb-exec-resum-eng.php.
47. Ramakrishnan, M., Moïsi, J. C., Klugman, K. P., et al. (2010). Increased risk of invasive bacterial infections in African people with sickle-cell disease: A systematic review and meta-analysis. *Lancet*

Infectious Diseases, 10(5), 329–337. doi:10.1016/S1473-3099(10)70055-4.

48. Centers for Disease Control and Prevention. (2014). *Vaccines and preventable diseases: Meningococcal: Who needs to be vaccinated*? Retrieved from http://www.cdc.gov/vaccines/vpd-vac/mening/who-vaccinate.htm.
49. Weingarten, L., Enarson, P., & Klassen, T. (2013). Encephalitis. *Pediatric Emergency Care, 29*(2), 235–241. doi:10.1097/PEC.0b013e318280d7f3.
50. Kirton, A., & deVeber, G. (2015). Paediatric stroke: Pressing issues and promising directions. *Lancet. Neurology, 14*(1), 92–102. doi:10.1016/S1474-4422(14)70227-3.
51. Mallick, A. A., & O'Callaghan, F. J. (2010). The epidemiology of childhood stroke. *European Journal of Paediatric Neurology, 14*(3), 197–205. doi:10.1016/j.ejpn.2009.09.006.
52. Lopez-Vicente, M., Ortega-Gutierrez, S., Amlie-Lefond, C., et al. (2010). Diagnosis and management of pediatric arterial ischemic stroke. *Journal of Stroke and Cerebrovascular Diseases, 19*(3), 175–183. doi:10.1016/j.jstrokecerebrovasdis.2009.03.013.
53. Numis, A. L., & Fox, C. K. (2014). Arterial ischemic stroke in children: Risk factors and etiologies. *Current Neurology and Neuroscience Reports, 14*(1), 422. doi:10.1007/s11910-013-0422-8.
54. Tsitouras, V., & Sgouros, S. (2011). Infantile posthemorrhagic hydrocephalus. *Child's Nervous System, 27*(10), 1595–1608. doi:10.1007/s00381-011-1521-y.
55. Kronenburg, A., Braun, K. P., van der Zwan, A., et al. (2014). Recent advances in moyamoya disease: Pathophysiology and treatment. *Current Neurology and Neuroscience Reports, 14*(1), 423. doi:10.1007/s11910-013-0423-7.
56. Epilepsy Canada. (2016). *Epilepsy facts*. Retrieved from http://www.epilepsy.ca/epilepsy-facts.html.
57. Public Health Agency of Canada. (2014). *Cancer in Canada: An epidemiological overview*. Retrieved from http://www.phac-aspc.gc.ca/cd-mc/cancer/cic_eo-cac_ae-eng.php#s4r.
58. American Cancer Society. (2014). *What are the risk factors for brain and spinal cord tumours in children?* Retrieved from http://www.cancer.org/cancer/braincnstumorsinchildren/detailedguide/brain-and-spinal-cord-tumors-in-children-risk-factors.
59. Jacques, G., & Cormac, O. (2013). Central nervous system tumors. *Handbook of Clinical Neurology, 112*, 931–958. doi:10.1016/B978-0-444-52910-7.00015-5.
60. American Cancer Society. (2015). *What are the key statistics about neuroblastoma*? Retrieved from http://www.cancer.org/cancer/neuroblastoma/detailedguide/neuroblastoma-key-statistics.
61. Neuroblastoma Canada. (2015). *Neuroblastoma statistics*. Retrieved from http://neuroblastoma.ca/neuroblastoma/statistics/.
62. National Cancer Institute. (2014). *General information about neuroblastoma*. Retrieved from http://www.cancer.gov/cancertopics/pdq/treatment/neuroblastoma/HealthProfessional/page1.
63. Singhi, P., Sahu, J. K., Sarkar, J., et al. (2014). Clinical profile and outcome of children with opsoclonus-myoclonus syndrome. *Journal of Child Neurology, 29*(1), 58–61. doi:10.1177/0883073812471433.
64. Rodriguez-Galindo, C., Orbach, D. B., & VanderVeen, D. (2015). Retinoblastoma. *Pediatric Clinics of North America, 62*(1), 201–223. doi:10.1016/j.pcl.2014.09.014.
65. Knudson, A. G., Jr. (1971). Mutation and cancer: A statistical study of retinoblastoma. *Proceedings of the National Academy of Sciences of the United States of America, 68*(4), 820–823.

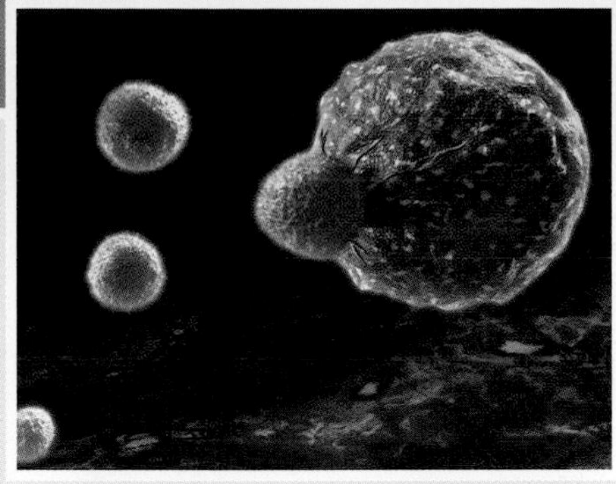

18

Mechanisms of Hormonal Regulation

Valentina L. Brashers, Sue E. Huether, and Kelly Power-Kean

EVOLVE WEBSITE

http://evolve.elsevier.com/Canada/Huether/pathophysiology
Student Review Questions
Key Points
Case Studies
Animations
Quick Check Answers

CHAPTER OUTLINE

Mechanisms of Hormonal Regulation, 443
Regulation of Hormone Release, 443
Hormone Transport, 444
Mechanisms of Hormone Action, 444
Structure and Function of the Endocrine Glands, 447
Hypothalamic-Pituitary System, 447
Pineal Gland, 452
Thyroid and Parathyroid Glands, 452
Endocrine Pancreas, 455
Adrenal Glands, 457
***GERIATRIC CONSIDERATIONS:* Aging and Its Effects on Specific Endocrine Glands, 461**

The endocrine system is composed of various glands located throughout the body (Figure 18-1). These glands can synthesize and release special chemical messengers called *hormones*. The endocrine system has five general functions: (1) differentiation of the reproductive and central nervous systems in the developing fetus; (2) stimulation of sequential growth and development during childhood and adolescence; (3) coordination of the male and female reproductive systems, which makes sexual reproduction possible; (4) maintenance of an optimal internal environment throughout life; and (5) initiation of corrective and adaptive responses when emergency demands occur. The endocrine, nervous, and immune systems work together to regulate responses to the internal and external environments. Hormones convey specific regulatory information among cells and organs and are integrated with the nervous system to maintain communication and control. The mechanisms of communication and control occur within a cell (*autocrine*), between local cells (*paracrine*), and between cells located remotely from each other (*endocrine*). Changes in the structure and function of the endocrine glands occur with aging and are summarized in the *Geriatric Considerations* box.

MECHANISMS OF HORMONAL REGULATION

Endocrine glands respond to specific signals by synthesizing and releasing **hormones** into the circulation, which then trigger intracellular responses. All hormones share certain general characteristics:

1. Hormones have specific rates and rhythms of secretion. Three basic patterns of secretion are (a) diurnal patterns, (b) pulsatile and cyclic patterns, and (c) patterns that depend on levels of circulating substrates (e.g., calcium, sodium, potassium, or the hormones themselves).
2. Hormones operate within feedback systems, either negative or positive, to maintain an optimal internal environment.
3. Hormones affect only target cells with specific receptors for the hormone and then act on these cells to initiate specific cell functions or activities.
4. Steroid hormones are either excreted directly by the kidneys or metabolized by the liver, which inactivates them and renders the hormone more water soluble for renal excretion. Peptide hormones are catabolized by circulating enzymes and eliminated in the feces or urine.

Hormones may be classified according to structure, gland of origin, effects, or chemical composition. (Table 18-1 categorizes known hormones based on structure.) The secretion and mechanisms of action of hormones represent an extremely complex system of integrated responses. The endocrine and nervous systems work together to regulate responses to the internal and external environments.

Regulation of Hormone Release

Hormones are released either to respond to an altered cellular environment or to maintain the level of another hormone or substance. One or more of the following mechanisms regulates hormone release: (1) chemical factors (such as blood glucose or calcium levels), (2) endocrine factors (a hormone from one endocrine gland controlling another endocrine gland), and (3) neural control. For example, insulin is secreted by the chemical stimulation of increased plasma glucose levels, cortisol from the adrenal cortex is an endocrine factor that regulates and stimulates insulin secretion, and direct stimulation of the insulin-secreting cells of the pancreas by the autonomic nervous system is a form of neural control.

Feedback systems provide precise monitoring and control of the cellular environment. Both negative- and positive-feedback systems are important for maintaining hormone levels within physiological ranges. **Negative feedback** is the most common and occurs when a changing chemical, neural, or endocrine response to a stimulus decreases the

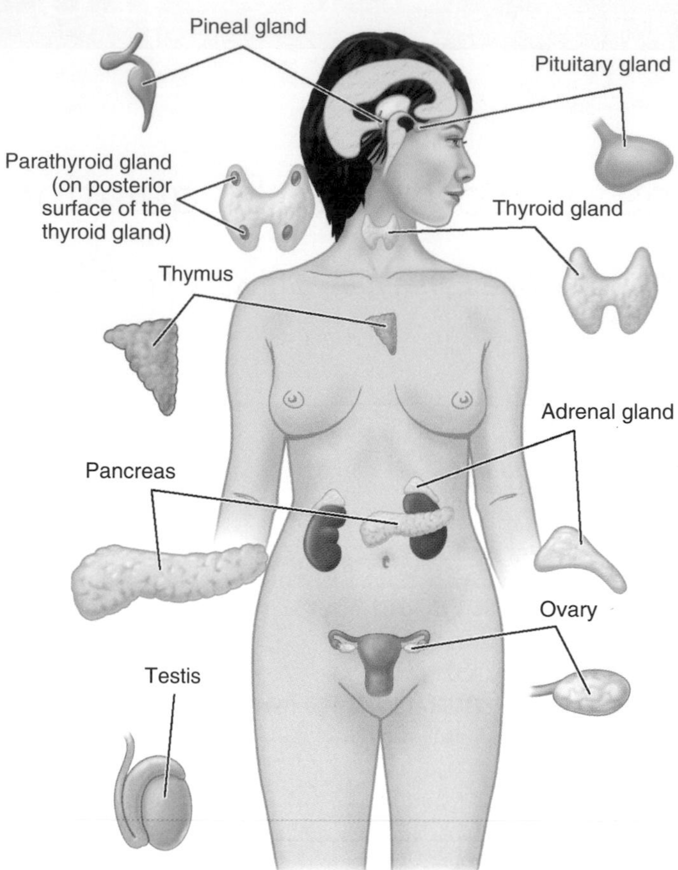

FIGURE 18-1 Major Endocrine Glands. (From Applegate, E. [2011]. *The anatomy and physiology learning system* [4th ed.]. St. Louis: Saunders.)

TABLE 18-1 Structural Categories of Hormones

Structural Category	Examples
Water Soluble	
Peptides	Growth hormone Insulin Leptin Parathyroid hormone Prolactin
Glycoproteins	Follicle-stimulating hormone Luteinizing hormone Thyroid-stimulating hormone
Polypeptides	Adrenocorticotropic hormone Antidiuretic hormone Calcitonin Endorphins Glucagon Hypothalamic hormones Lipotropins Melanocyte-stimulating hormone Oxytocin Somatostatin Thymosin Thyrotropin-releasing hormone
Amines	Epinephrine Norepinephrine
Lipid Soluble	
Thyroxine (an amine, but lipid soluble)	Both thyroxine and triiodothyronine
Steroids (cholesterol is a precursor for all steroids)	Estrogens Glucocorticoids (cortisol) Mineralocorticoids (aldosterone) Progestins (progesterone) Testosterone
Derivatives of arachidonic acid (autocrine or paracrine action)	Leukotrienes Prostacyclins Prostaglandins Thromboxanes

synthesis and secretion of a hormone. **Positive feedback** occurs when a neural, chemical, or endocrine response increases the synthesis and secretion of a hormone. For example, Figure 18-2, *A*, illustrates negative feedback within the hypothalamic-pituitary axis and the thyroid gland. Decreased serum levels of the thyroid hormones thyroxine (T_4) and triiodothyronine (T_3) stimulate secretion of **thyrotropin-releasing hormone (TRH)** from the hypothalamus, which stimulates the secretion of **thyroid-stimulating hormone (TSH)**. Secretion of TSH stimulates the synthesis and secretion of T_3 and T_4. Increasing levels of T_4 and T_3 then generate negative feedback on the pituitary and hypothalamus to inhibit TSH and TRH synthesis and decrease the synthesis and production of thyroid hormones. The lack of negative-feedback inhibition on hormonal release often results in pathological excessive hormone production (see Chapter 19).

An example of positive feedback is found in the female reproductive cycle. The cyclic rise of estradiol levels provides positive feedback on the anterior pituitary and hypothalamus, causing a subsequent increase in gonadotropin-releasing hormone and follicle-stimulating hormone. These changes result in ovulation (see Chapter 32).

Hormone Transport

Once hormones are released into the circulatory system, they are distributed throughout the body. The protein (peptide) hormones (see Table 18-1) are water soluble and generally circulate in free (unbound) forms. Water-soluble hormones generally have a half-life of seconds to minutes because they are catabolized by circulating enzymes. For example, insulin has a half-life of 3 to 5 minutes and is catabolized by insulinases. Lipid-soluble hormones (see Table 18-1), such as cortisol and adrenal androgens, are transported bound to a water-soluble carrier or transport protein and can remain in the blood for hours to days. Only free hormones (those not bound to a carrier protein) can signal a target cell. Because there is equilibrium between the concentrations of free hormones and hormones bound to plasma proteins, a significant change in the concentration of binding proteins can affect the concentration of free hormones in the plasma (Table 18-2). (Mechanisms of hormone binding are discussed in Chapter 1.)

Mechanisms of Hormone Action

Although a hormone is distributed throughout the body, only those cells with appropriate receptors, termed **target cells**, for that hormone are affected. *Hormone receptors* of the target cell have two main functions: (1) to recognize and bind specifically and with high affinity to their particular hormones and (2) to initiate a signal to appropriate intracellular effectors.

The sensitivity of the target cell to a particular hormone is related to the total number of receptors per cell or the affinity (binding) for

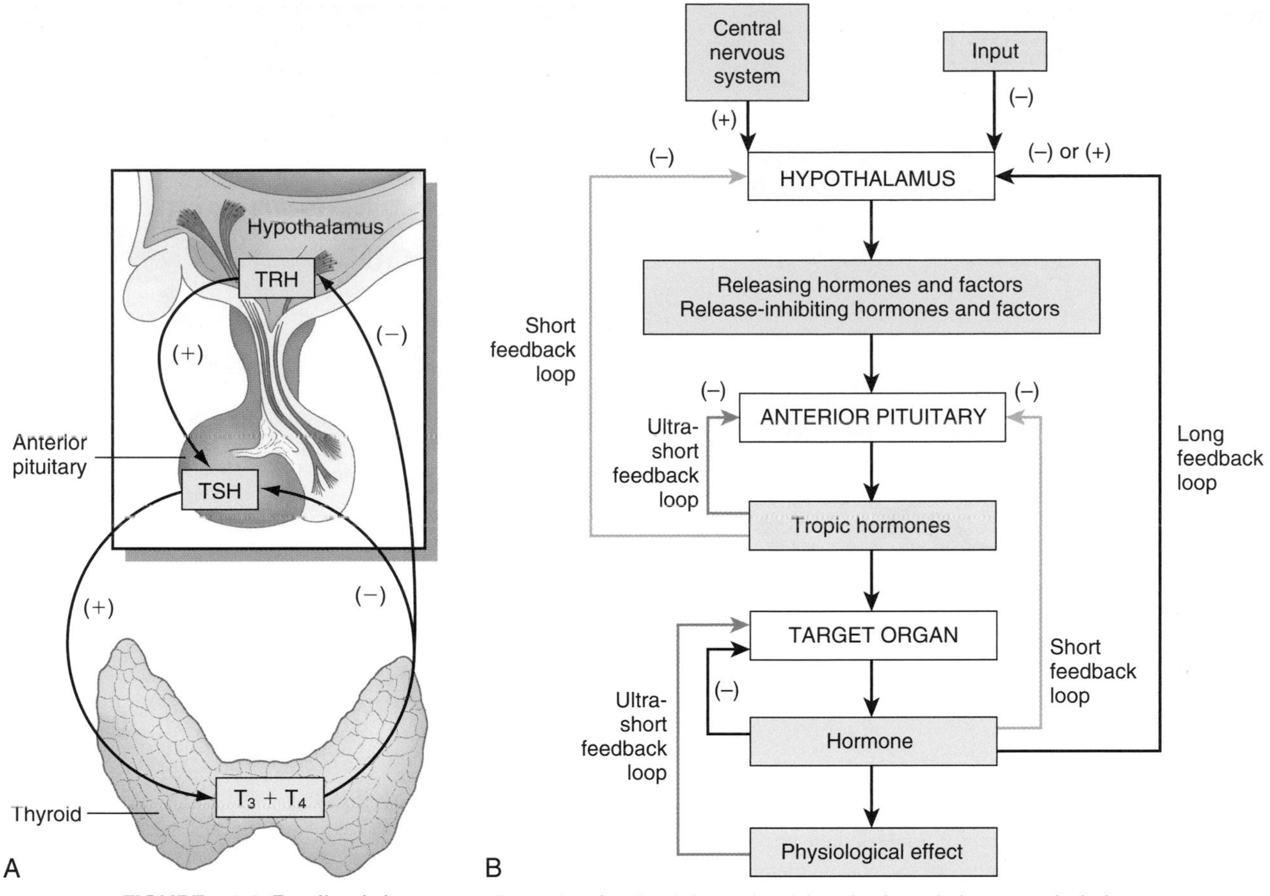

FIGURE 18-2 Feedback Loops. A, Endocrine feedback loops involving the hypothalamus and pituitary gland, and end organs; in this example, the thyroid gland is illustrated (endocrine regulation). **B,** General model for control and negative feedback to hypothalamic-pituitary target organ systems. Negative-feedback regulation is possible at three levels: target organ (ultra-short feedback), anterior pituitary (short feedback), and hypothalamus (long feedback). *T_3*, triiodothyronine *T_4*, thyroxine (tetraiodothyronine); *TRH*, thyroid-releasing hormone; *TSH*, thyroid-stimulating hormone.

TABLE 18-2 Binding Proteins, Their Hormones, and Variables That Affect Their Circulating Levels

Binding Protein	Hormone	Factors That Increase Binding Protein Levels	Factors That Decrease Binding Protein Levels
Corticosteroid-binding globulin	Cortisol	Estrogen	Liver disease
	Progesterone		
Sex hormone–binding globulin	Dihydrotestosterone	—	Androgens
	Testosterone	Hypothyroidism	
	Estradiol	Liver disease	
Thyroid-binding globulin	Thyroxine	Estrogen	Testosterone
	Triiodothyronine	Hyperthyroidism	Glucocorticoids
			Liver disease
Albumin	All lipid-soluble hormones	Estrogen	Liver disease
			Malnutrition
			Renal disease

the receptors to the hormone: the more receptors or the higher the affinity of the receptors, the more sensitive the cell to the stimulating effects of the hormone. Low concentrations of hormone increase the number or affinity of receptors per cell; this is called **upregulation**. High concentrations of hormone decrease the number or affinity of receptors; this is called **downregulation** (Figure 18-3). Thus the cell can adjust its sensitivity to the concentration of the signalling hormone. The receptors on the plasma membrane are continuously synthesized and degraded, so that changes in receptor concentration or affinity may occur within hours. The regulation of hormone receptors is of particular importance in type 2 diabetes, in which there is a decrease in insulin receptor sensitivity and hyperglycemia (see Chapter 19). Various

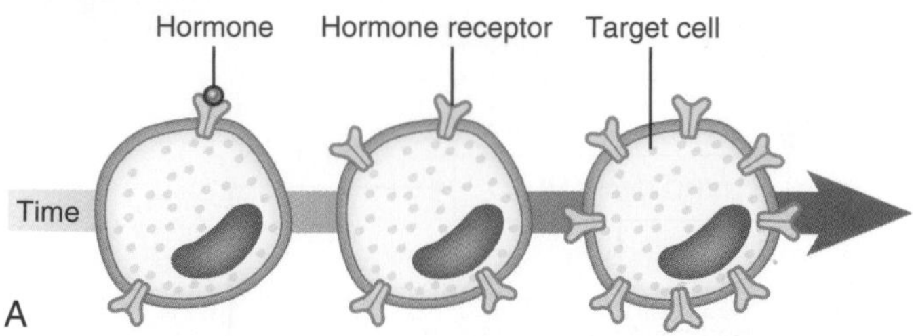

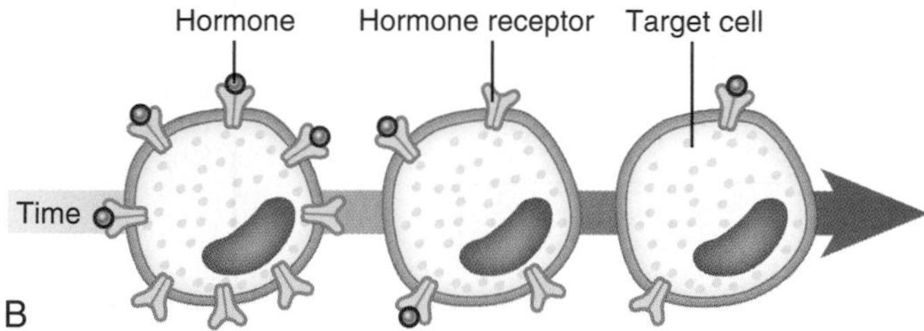

FIGURE 18-3 Regulation of Target Cell Sensitivity. **A,** Low hormone level and upregulation, or an increase in the number of receptors. **B,** High hormone level and downregulation, or a decrease in the number of receptors.

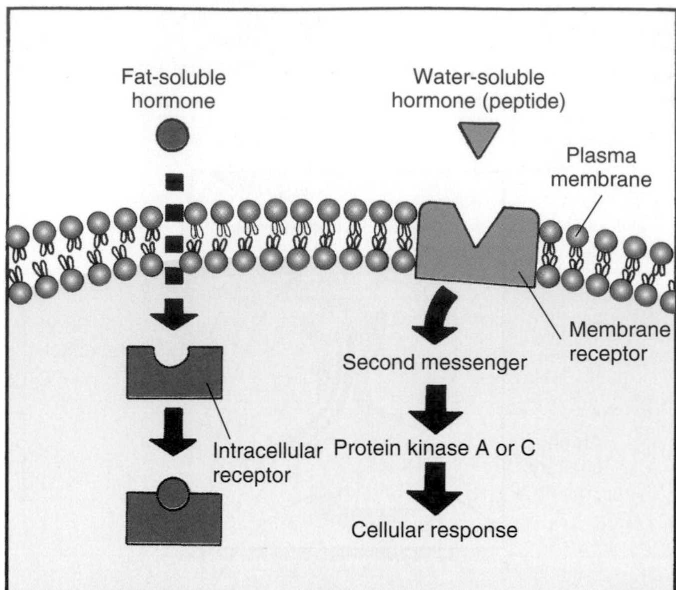

FIGURE 18-4 Hormone Binding at Target Cell.

physiochemical conditions can affect both the receptor number and the affinity of the hormone for its receptor. Some of these physiochemical conditions are the fluidity and structure of the plasma membrane, pH, temperature, ion concentration, diet, and the presence of other chemicals (e.g., medications).

Hormones affect target cells directly or permissively. **Direct effects** are the obvious changes in cell function that result specifically from stimulation by a particular hormone. **Permissive effects** are less obvious hormone-induced changes that facilitate the maximal response or functioning of a cell. For example, insulin via insulin receptors has a direct effect on skeletal muscle cells, causing increased glucose transport into these cells. Insulin also has a permissive effect on mammary cells, facilitating the response of these cells to the direct effects of prolactin.

Some hormones have biphasic effects that are dependent on the concentration or secretion pattern of the hormone. For example, in primary hyperparathyroidism, continuous hypersecretion of parathyroid hormone (PTH) leads to bone destruction by osteoclasts. Conversely, bone formation is stimulated when recombinant PTH is given in low doses at intermittent intervals, as a treatment for osteoporosis with high risk for fracture[1] (see Chapter 39). Methods of hormone measurement are summarized in Box 18-1.

Hormone Receptors

Hormone receptors may be located in the plasma membrane or in the intracellular compartment of the target cell (Figure 18-4). Water-soluble (peptide) hormones, which include the protein hormones and the catecholamines, have a high molecular weight and cannot diffuse across the cell membrane. They interact or bind with receptors located in or on the cell membrane. Fat-soluble steroids, vitamin D, retinoic acid, and thyroid hormones diffuse freely across the plasma and nuclear membranes and bind with cytosolic or nuclear receptors. The hormone-receptor complex binds to a specific region in the DNA and stimulates the expression of a specific gene. Some fat-soluble hormones (e.g., estrogen [see Chapter 32]) may also bind with plasma membrane receptors and can have rapid cellular effects.[2-4]

BOX 18-1 Methods of Hormone Measurement

Radioimmunoassay (RIA)

In this immunological technique, known amounts of antibody and radio-labelled hormone are placed in an assay tube with the unlabelled hormone. The radio-labelled hormone competes chemically with the unlabelled hormone molecules for binding sites on the antibodies. When increasing amounts of unlabelled hormones are added to the assay, the limited binding sites of the antibody can bind less of the radio-labelled hormone. Therefore, the higher the concentration of unlabelled hormone, the fewer the number of radioactive *counts*, or labelled hormone, that bind with the fixed concentration of antibody. A quantitative value is established by use of standard reference curves.

Enzyme-Linked Immunosorbent Assay (ELISA)

This assay is used to determine circulating hormone levels. The method is similar to that of RIA but is less expensive and easier to conduct. Instead of radio-labelled hormones, an enzyme-labelled hormone is used. The enzyme activity in either the bound or the unbound fraction is determined and related to the concentration of the unlabelled hormone.

Bioassay

This assay uses graded doses of hormone in a reference preparation and then compares the results with an unknown sample. Bioassays are used more commonly in investigative endocrinology than in clinical laboratories.

First and Second Messengers

All water-soluble hormones and some steroid hormones have hormone-specific receptors located in the plasma membranes of cells. Hormone binding with the plasma membrane receptor initiates a complex cascade of intracellular effects. In this cascade, the hormone is termed the **first messenger**. The hormone–receptor interaction initiates a signal that generates a small molecule inside the cell, called the **second messenger**. Second messengers include cyclic adenosine monophosphate (cAMP), cyclic guanosine monophosphate (cGMP), calcium, inositol triphosphate, and the tyrosine kinase system (Table 18-3). The second messenger conveys the signal from the receptor to the cytoplasm and

TABLE 18-3 Second Messengers Identified for Specific Hormones

Second Messenger	Associated Hormones
Cyclic adenosine monophosphate (cAMP)	Adrenocorticotropic hormone (ACTH) Luteinizing hormone (LH) Human chorionic gonadotropin (hCG) Follicle-stimulating hormone (FSH) Thyroid-stimulating hormone (TSH) Antidiuretic hormone (ADH) Thyrotropin-releasing hormone (TRH) Parathyroid hormone (PTH) Glucagon
Cyclic guanosine monophosphate (cGMP)	Atrial natriuretic peptide
Calcium (Ca^{++}) and inositol triphosphate (IP_3)	Angiotensin II Gonadotropin-releasing hormone (GnRH) Antidiuretic hormone (ADH) Luteinizing hormone–releasing hormone (LHRH)
Tyrosine kinases	Insulin Growth hormone (GH) Leptin Prolactin

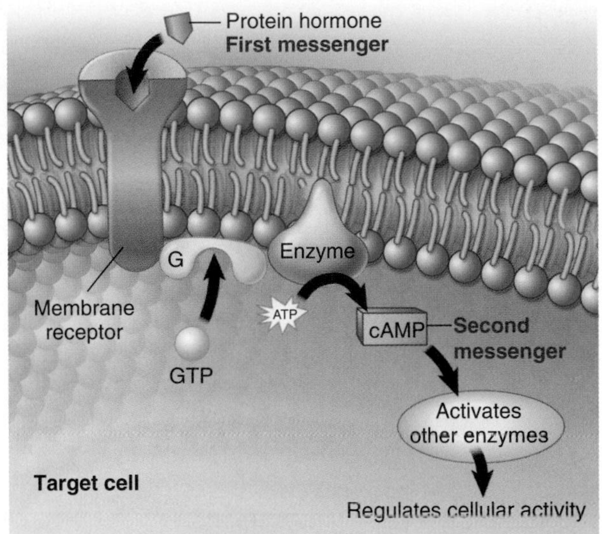

FIGURE 18-5 Mechanism of First and Second Messenger Action. The hormone acts as a "first messenger," delivering its message via the bloodstream to a membrane receptor in the target cell much like a key fits into a lock. The "second messenger" causes the cell to respond and perform its specialized function. *ATP,* adenosine triphosphate; *cAMP,* cyclic adenosine monophosphate; *G,* G protein; *GTP,* guanosine triphosphate. (From Patton, K.T., & Thibodeau, G.A. [2016]. *Structure & function of the body* [15th ed.]. St. Louis: Mosby.)

nucleus of the cell and mediates the effect of the hormone on the target cell (e.g., membrane permeability alterations, protein synthesis, inhibition of specific metabolic pathways, enzyme activation, or cellular growth).

When first messengers from the anterior pituitary gland, adrenocorticotropic hormone (ACTH) and TSH, bind to a cell membrane receptor, intracellular levels of cAMP increase. Second-messenger cAMP activates protein kinases, leading to phosphorylation of cellular proteins. This either activates or deactivates intracellular enzymes, thus directing the actions or products of specific cells (Figure 18-5).

cGMP functions as a second messenger following receptor binding of first messengers (e.g., atrial natriuretic peptide and nitric oxide). These hormones play crucial roles in cardiovascular and pulmonary health and disease. Medications such as phosphodiesterase inhibitors that target cGMP are being explored for treatment of various diseases.[5,6]

Hormone-receptor binding of first-messenger angiotensin II and antidiuretic hormone (ADH) results in generation of the second messenger, inositol triphosphate. Inositol triphosphate triggers a release of intracellular calcium, another second messenger. Increased intracellular calcium levels can lead to the formation of the calcium–calmodulin complex, which mediates the effects of calcium on intracellular activities that are crucial for cell metabolism and growth. For example, calmodulin-dependent protein kinases control intracellular contractile components (myosin and actin, which cause muscle contraction), alter plasma membrane permeability to calcium, and regulate the intracellular enzyme activity that promotes hormone secretion.

Some hormone first messengers, such as insulin, growth hormone (GH), and prolactin, bind to surface receptors that directly activate second messengers of the tyrosine kinase family. These tyrosine kinases include the Janus family of tyrosine kinases (JAK) and signal transducers and activators of transcription (STAT). They regulate a wide range of intracellular processes that contribute to cellular metabolism and growth, and are being targeted in emerging treatments for diabetes and cancer.[7-9]

Lipid-Soluble (Steroid) Hormone-Receptor Binding

With the exception of thyroid hormones, the lipid-soluble hormones are synthesized from cholesterol (giving rise to the term *steroid*). These include androgens, estrogens, progestins, glucocorticoids, mineralocorticoids, vitamin D, and retinoid. Because these are relatively small, lipophilic, hydrophobic molecules, lipid-soluble hormones can cross the lipid plasma membrane by simple diffusion (see Chapter 1). Receptors for lipid-soluble hormones are in the cytosol and nucleus and direct gene expression (Figure 18-6). Modulation of gene expression can take hours to days. Studies also reveal that receptors for lipid-soluble hormones are in the plasma membrane and are associated with rapid responses (seconds to minutes) as shown in Figure 18-6.[10,11]

✔ QUICK CHECK 18-1
1. What are hormones? By what mechanisms do they function?
2. What is meant by negative-feedback regulation of hormone release?
3. How do first messengers differ from second messengers?
4. Where are the receptors located for lipid-soluble hormones?

STRUCTURE AND FUNCTION OF THE ENDOCRINE GLANDS

Hypothalamic-Pituitary System

The hypothalamic-pituitary axis forms the structural and functional basis for central integration of the neurological and endocrine systems, creating what is called the neuroendocrine system. The hypothalamic-pituitary axis produces several hormones that affect a number of diverse body functions (Figure 18-7), including thyroid, adrenal, and reproductive functions.

The **hypothalamus** is located at the base of the brain. It is connected to the pituitary gland by the pituitary stalk (Figure 18-8). The hypothalamus

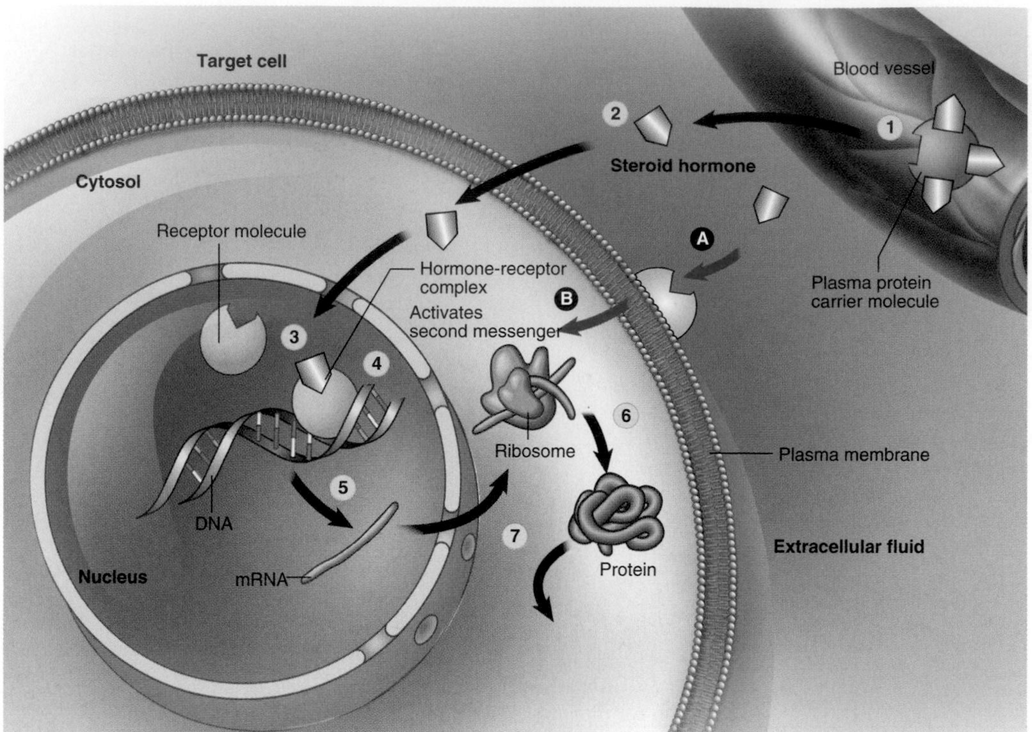

FIGURE 18-6 Steroid Hormone Mechanism. Lipid-soluble steroid hormone molecules detach from the carrier protein **(1)** and pass through the plasma membrane **(2)**. Hormone molecules then diffuse into the nucleus, where they bind to a receptor to form a hormone-receptor complex **(3)**. This complex then binds to a specific site on a DNA molecule **(4)**, triggering transcription of the genetic information encoded there **(5)**. The resulting messenger RNA (*mRNA*) molecule moves to the cytosol, where it associates with a ribosome, initiating synthesis of a new protein **(6)**. This new protein—usually an enzyme or channel protein—produces specific effects on the target cell **(7)**. The classic genomic action is typically slow (*red arrows*). Steroids also may exact rapid effects (*green arrows*) by binding to receptors on the plasma membrane **(A)** and activating an intercellular second messenger **(B)**. (From Patton, K.T., & Thibodeau, G.A. [2016]. *Anatomy & physiology* [9th ed.]. St. Louis: Mosby.)

is connected to the anterior pituitary through hypophysial portal blood vessels (Figure 18-9) and to the posterior pituitary via a nerve tract referred to as the *hypothalamohypophysial tract* (Figure 18-10). These connections are vital to the functioning of the hypothalamic-pituitary system. The hypothalamus contains special neurosecretory cells that are like other neurons in that they have similar electrical properties, organelles, membranes, and synapses. Hypothalamic neurosecretory cells, however, can synthesize and secrete the hypothalamic-releasing hormones that regulate the release of hormones from the anterior pituitary. In addition, these cells synthesize the hormones **antidiuretic hormone (ADH)** and **oxytocin** that are released from the posterior pituitary gland. These hormones are summarized in Table 18-4.

The **pituitary gland** is located in the sella turcica (a saddle-shaped depression of the sphenoid bone at the base of the skull). It weighs approximately 0.5 g, except during pregnancy when its weight increases by about 30%. It is composed of two distinctly different lobes: (1) the anterior pituitary, or adenohypophysis, and (2) the posterior pituitary, or neurohypophysis (see Figure 18-8). These two lobes differ in their embryonic origins, cell types, and functional relationship to the hypothalamus.

The Anterior Pituitary

The **anterior pituitary** (adenohypophysis) accounts for 75% of the total weight of the pituitary gland. It is composed of three regions: (1) the pars distalis, (2) the pars tuberalis, and (3) the pars intermedia. The **pars distalis** is the major component of the anterior pituitary and is the source of the anterior pituitary hormones. The **pars tuberalis** is a thin layer of cells on the anterior and lateral portions of the pituitary stalk. The **pars intermedia** lies between the two and secretes **melanocyte-stimulating hormone (MSH)** in the fetus. In the adult, the distinct pars intermedia disappears and the individual cells are distributed diffusely throughout the pars distalis and pars nervosa (neural lobe) of the posterior pituitary.

The anterior pituitary is composed of two main cell types: (1) the **chromophobes**, which appear to be nonsecretory, and (2) the **chromophils**, which are considered the secretory cells of the adenohypophysis. The chromophils are subdivided into seven secretory cell types, and each cell type secretes a specific hormone or hormones. In general, the anterior pituitary hormones are regulated by (1) secretion of hypothalamic peptide hormones or releasing factors, (2) feedback effects of the hormones secreted by target glands, and (3) direct effects of other mediating neurotransmitters. (Feedback loops are summarized in Figure 18-2.)

The anterior pituitary secretes **tropic hormones** that affect the physiological function of specific target organs (see Figure 18-7 and Table 18-5). MSH promotes the pituitary secretion of melanin, which darkens skin colour. The glycoprotein hormones **follicle-stimulating hormone (FSH)** and **luteinizing hormone (LH)** influence reproductive function and are discussed in Chapter 32. **Adrenocorticotropic hormone (ACTH)** regulates the release of cortisol from the adrenal cortex.

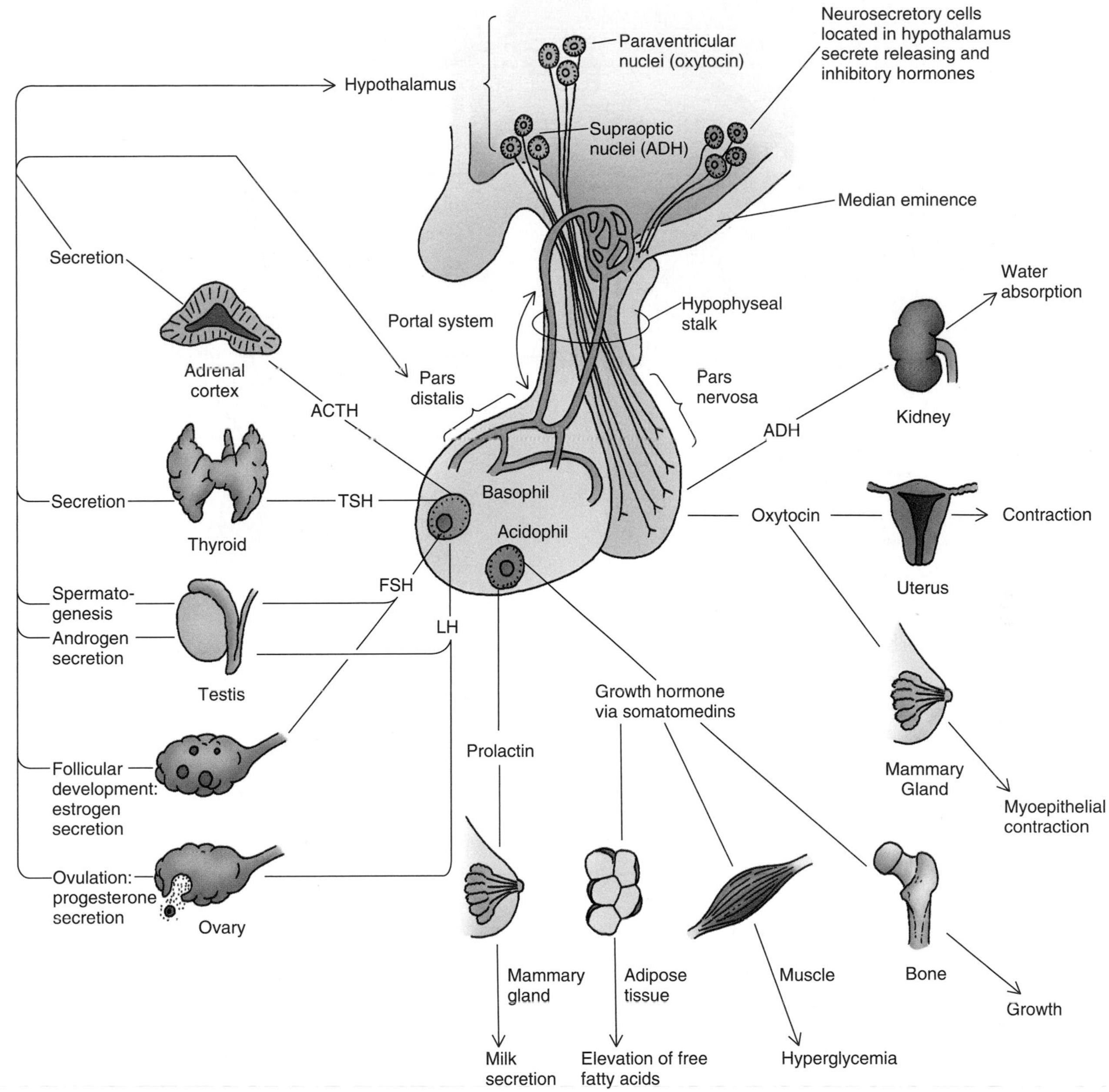

FIGURE 18-7 Pituitary Gland and Its Target Organs. *ACTH*, adrenocorticotropic hormone; *ADH*, antidiuretic hormone; *FSH*, follicle-stimulating hormone; *LH*, luteinizing hormone; *TSH*, thyroid-stimulating hormone. (From Gartner, L.P., & Hiatt, J.L. [2007]. *Color textbook of histology* [3rd ed.]. Philadelphia: Saunders.)

TABLE 18-4 Hypothalamic Hormones (Hypophysiotropic Hormones)

Hormone	Target Tissue	Action
Thyrotropin-releasing hormone (TRH)	Anterior pituitary	Stimulates release of thyroid-stimulating hormone (TSH); modulates prolactin secretion
Gonadotropin-releasing hormone (GnRH)	Anterior pituitary	Stimulates release of follicle-stimulating hormone (FSH) and luteinizing hormone (LH)
Somatostatin	Anterior pituitary	Inhibits release of growth hormone (GH) and TSH
Growth hormone–releasing hormone (GHRH)	Anterior pituitary	Stimulates release of GH
Corticotropin-releasing hormone (CRH)	Anterior pituitary	Stimulates release of adrenocorticotropic hormone (ACTH) and β-endorphin
Substance P	Anterior pituitary	Inhibits synthesis and release of ACTH; stimulates secretion of GH, FSH, LH, and prolactin
Prolactin-inhibiting factor (PIF, dopamine)	Anterior pituitary	Inhibits synthesis and secretion of prolactin
Prolactin-releasing factor (PRF)	Anterior pituitary	Stimulates secretion of prolactin

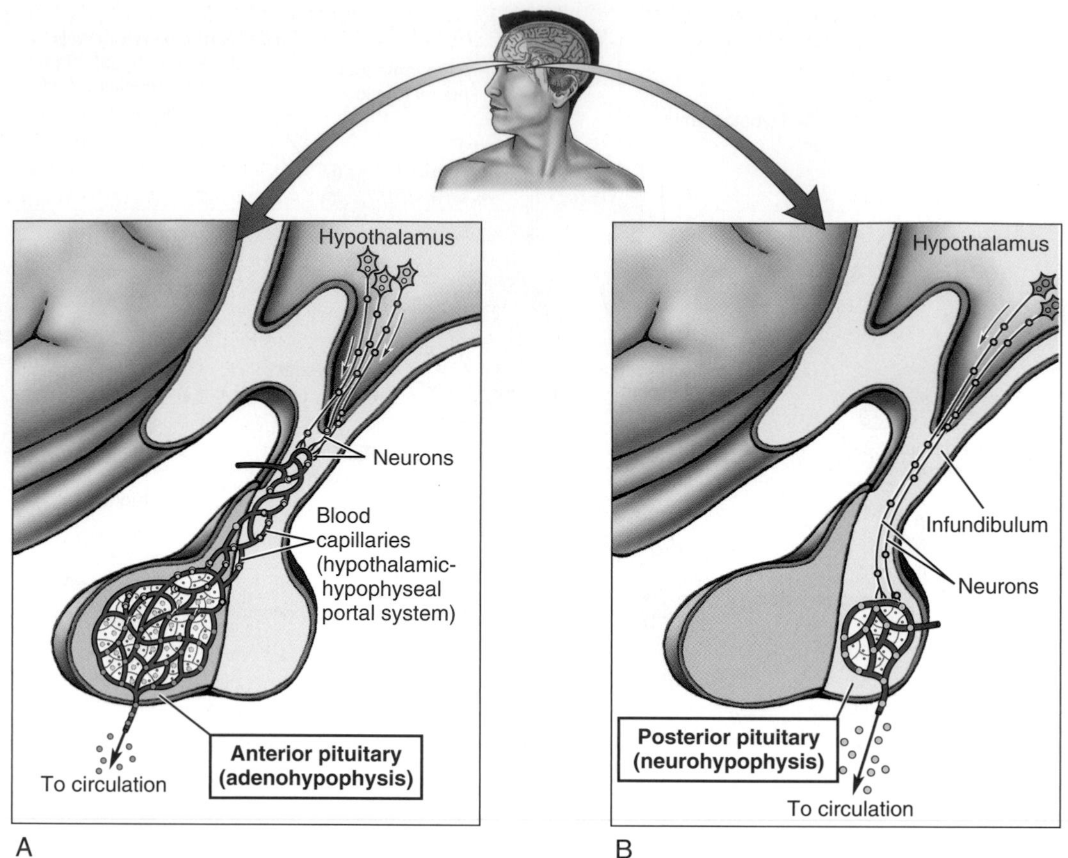

FIGURE 18-8 Pituitary Gland. The pituitary gland sits within the sella turcica of the sphenoid bone of the skull. **A,** Relationship of the hypothalamus to the anterior pituitary gland. **B,** Relationship of the hypothalamus to the posterior pituitary gland. (From Herlihy, B. [2015]. *The human body in health and illness* [5th ed.]. St. Louis: Saunders.)

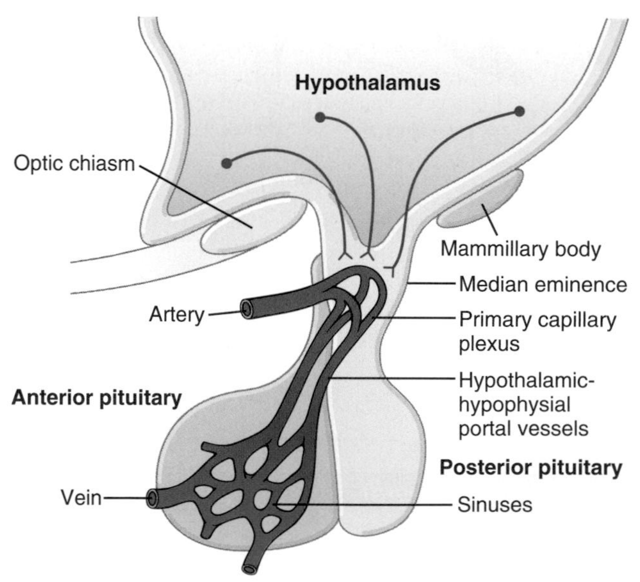

FIGURE 18-9 Hypophysial Portal System. (From Hall, J.E. [2016]. *Guyton and Hall textbook of medical physiology* [13th ed.]. Philadelphia: Saunders.)

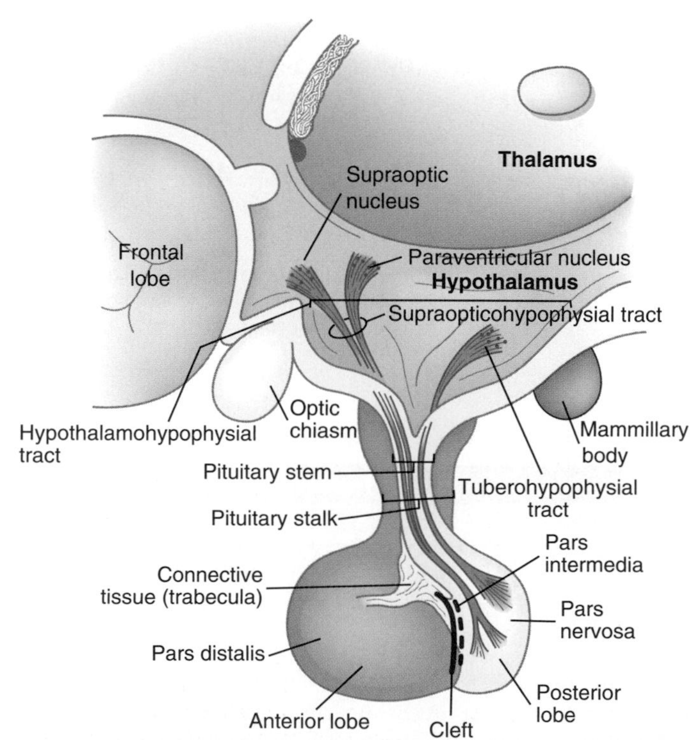

FIGURE 18-10 Nerve Tracts From Hypothalamus to Posterior Lobe of Pituitary Gland.

TABLE 18-5 Tropic Hormones of the Anterior Pituitary and Their Functions

Hormone	Secretory Cell Type	Target Organs	Functions
Adrenocorticotropic hormone (ACTH)	Corticotropic	Adrenal gland (cortex)	Increases steroidogenesis (cortisol and androgenic hormones); synthesis of adrenal proteins contributing to maintenance of adrenal gland
Melanocyte-stimulating hormone (MSH)	Melanotropic	Anterior pituitary	Promotes secretion of melanin and lipotropin by anterior pituitary; makes skin darker
Somatotropic Hormones			
Growth hormone (GH)	Somatotropic	Muscle, bone, liver	Regulates metabolic processes related to growth and adaptation to physical and emotional stressors, muscle growth, increased protein synthesis, increased liver glycogenolysis, increased fat mobilization
		Liver	Induces formation of somatomedins, or insulinlike growth factors (IGFs) that have actions similar to insulin
Prolactin	Lactotropic	Breast	Induces milk production
Glycoprotein Hormones			
Thyroid-stimulating hormone (TSH)	Thyrotropic	Thyroid gland	Increases production and secretion of thyroid hormone Increases iodide uptake; promotes hypertrophy and hyperplasia of thymocytes
Luteinizing hormone (LH)	Gonadotropic	In women: granulosa cells In men: Leydig cells	Stimulates ovulation, progesterone production Stimulates testicular growth, testosterone production
Follicle-stimulating hormone (FSH)	Gonadotropic	In women: granulosa cells In men: Sertoli cells	Stimulates follicle maturation, estrogen production Stimulates spermatogenesis
β-Lipotropin	Corticotropic	Adipose cells	Promotes fat breakdown and release of fatty acids
β-Endorphins	Corticotropic	Adipose cells; brain opioid receptors	Produces analgesia; may regulate body temperature, food and water intake

TSH regulates the activity of the thyroid gland. The roles of ACTH and TSH are discussed later in this chapter. **Growth hormone (GH)** and **prolactin** are called the *somatotropic hormones* and have diverse effects on body tissues. GH secretion is controlled by two hormones from the hypothalamus: growth hormone–releasing hormone (GHRH), which increases GH secretion; and somatostatin, which inhibits GH secretion. GH is essential to normal tissue growth and maturation and also impacts aging, sleep, nutritional status, stress, and reproductive hormones. Many of the anabolic functions of GH are mediated, at least in part, by the insulinlike growth factors (IGFs), which are also known as the *somatomedins*.[12]

There are two primary forms of IGF: IGF-1 and IGF-2, of which IGF-1 is the most biologically active. They both circulate bound to a group of IGF-binding proteins (IGFBPs) modulating their availability. IGF-1 binds to IGF-1 receptors mediating the anabolic effects of GH. IGF-1 also binds to insulin receptors, providing an insulinlike effect on skeletal muscle. IGF-2 has important effects on fetal growth, but suppresses GH in the adult. Because of the anabolic effects of GH and IGF-1, they can be used to treat growth disorders, increase muscle mass, and potentially slow the aging process, but their use has also been linked to increased rates of cancer[13,14] (see *Health Promotion:* Growth Hormone Supplementation in Aging).

HEALTH PROMOTION

Growth Hormone Supplementation in Aging

Aging is a multifactorial process that is influenced by genetic and environmental factors. The aging process is associated with many hormonal and metabolic changes. The amounts of growth hormone (GH) and insulinlike growth factor (IGF) decline with aging, a process that has been called the "somatopause." Clinical findings related to somatotropic hormone changes with aging include increased visceral fat, decreased lean body mass, decreased bone density, and changes in reproductive and cognitive function. The underlying mechanisms of aging and its relationship to GH and IGF are complex. For example, GH and IGF promote bone and muscle growth, and a recent study suggests that the brain receptor for IGF-1 (an IGF ligand) may be a significant factor in determining overall lifespan and ability to respond to physiological stress. GH and IGF effects on inflammation and immunity also are important in the aging process. Unfortunately, there remains much confusion and controversy over the role of these hormones. Even so, thousands of Canadians self-medicate with a synthetic formulation of GH as an antiaging remedy, with the goal of improving strength, energy, and immunity, as well as use for treatment of heart disease, cancer, impotence, and Alzheimer's disease.

Despite enthusiasm for the use of therapeutic doses of recombinant human growth hormone (rhGH) as a way to slow the aging process, studies have not been consistently positive. Evidence shows that rhGH supplementation can be harmful, and that lower lifetime levels of these hormones may confer longevity by providing protection from cancer and other age-related diseases. Health Canada warns consumers not to self-medicate with human growth hormone GHR-15 due to risks associated with unsubstantiated health claims and its other potential harmful effects.

Data from Anisimov, V.N., & Bartke, A. (2013). *Crit Rev Oncol Hematol, 87*(3), 201–223; Ashpole, N.M., Sanders, J.E., Hodges, E.L., et al. (2015). *Exp Gerontol, 68*, 76–81; Government of Canada. (2005). *Healthy Canadians: Health Canada warns consumers not to use human growth hormone drug called GHR-15.* Retrieved from http://www.healthycanadians.gc.ca/recall-alert-rappel-avis/hc-sc/2005/13695a-eng.php; Haber, D. (2016). *Health promotion and aging: Practical application for health professionals* (7th ed.). New York: Springer; Junnila, R.K., List, E.O., Berryman, D.E., et al. (2013). *Nat Rev Endocrinol, 9*(6), 366–376; Nass, R. (2013). *Endocrinol Metab Clin North Am, 42*(2), 187–199; Sattler, F.R. (2013). *Best Pract Res Clin Endocrinol Metab, 27*(4), 541–555.

Prolactin primarily functions to induce milk production during pregnancy and lactation. It has immune stimulatory effects and modulates immune and inflammatory responses with both physiological and pathological reactions.[15] Its synthesis is stimulated by vasoactive intestinal polypeptide, serotonin, and growth factors. Release of prolactin is inhibited by dopamine.

The Posterior Pituitary

The embryonic **posterior pituitary** (neurohypophysis) is derived from the hypothalamus and is composed of three parts: (1) the median eminence, located at the base of the hypothalamus; (2) the pituitary stalk; and (3) the infundibular process, also known as the *pars nervosa* or *neural lobe*. The **median eminence** is composed largely of the nerve endings of axons from the ventral hypothalamus. It is often designated as part of the posterior pituitary but contains at least 10 biologically active hypothalamic-releasing hormones, as well as the neurotransmitters dopamine, norepinephrine, serotonin, acetylcholine, and histamine. The **pituitary stalk** contains the axons of neurons that originate in the supraoptic and paraventricular nuclei of the hypothalamus and connects the pituitary gland to the brain. Axons originating in the hypothalamus terminate in the **pars nervosa**, which secretes the hormones of the posterior pituitary (see Figure 18-10).

The posterior pituitary secretes two polypeptide hormones: (1) ADH, also called *arginine vasopressin*, and (2) oxytocin. These hormones differ by only two amino acids. They are synthesized—along with their binding proteins, the neurophysins—in the supraoptic and paraventricular nuclei of the hypothalamus (see Figure 18-10). They are packaged in secretory vesicles and are moved down the axons of the pituitary stalk to the pars nervosa for storage. The posterior pituitary thus can be seen as a storage and releasing site for hormones synthesized in the hypothalamus. The release of ADH and oxytocin is mediated by cholinergic and adrenergic neurotransmitters. The major stimulus to both ADH and oxytocin release is glutamate, whereas the major inhibitory input is through gamma-aminobutyric acid (GABA).[16] Before release into the circulatory system, ADH and oxytocin are split from the neurophysins and are secreted in unbound form.

Antidiuretic hormone. The major homeostatic function of the posterior pituitary is the control of plasma osmolality as regulated by ADH (see Chapter 5). At physiological levels, ADH increases the permeability of the distal renal tubules and collecting ducts (see Chapter 29). This increased permeability leads to increased water reabsorption into the blood, thus concentrating the urine and reducing serum osmolality. Hypercalcemia, prostaglandin E, and hypokalemia can inhibit this water reabsorption.

The secretion of ADH is regulated primarily by the osmoreceptors of the hypothalamus, located near or in the supraoptic nuclei. As plasma osmolality increases these osmoreceptors are stimulated, the rate of ADH secretion increases, more water is reabsorbed by the kidney, and the plasma is diluted back to its set-point osmolality. ADH has no direct effect on electrolyte levels, but by increasing water reabsorption, serum electrolyte concentrations may decrease because of a dilutional effect.

ADH secretion also is increased by changes in intravascular volume, as monitored by baroreceptors in the left atrium, in the carotid arteries, and in the aortic arches. A volume loss of 7 to 25% acts on these receptors to stimulate ADH secretion. Stress, trauma, pain, exercise, nausea, nicotine, exposure to heat, and medications such as morphine also increase ADH secretion. ADH secretion decreases with decreased plasma osmolality, increased intravascular volume, hypertension, alcohol ingestion, and an increase in estrogen, progesterone, or angiotensin II levels.

Physiological levels of ADH do not significantly impact vessel tone. However, ADH was originally named *vasopressin* because, in extremely high levels, it causes vasoconstriction and a resulting increase in arterial blood pressure. For example, high doses of ADH (given as the medication vasopressin [Pitressin]) may be administered to achieve hemostasis during hemorrhage and to raise blood pressure in shock states.[17,18]

Oxytocin. Oxytocin is responsible for contraction of the uterus and milk ejection in lactating women and may affect sperm motility in men. In both genders, oxytocin has an antidiuretic effect similar to that of ADH. In women, oxytocin is secreted in response to suckling and mechanical distension of the female reproductive tract. Oxytocin binds to its receptors on myoepithelial cells in the mammary tissues and causes contraction of those cells, which increases intramammary pressure and milk expression ("let-down" reflex). Oxytocin also acts on the uterus to stimulate contractions. Oxytocin functions near the end of labour to enhance the effectiveness of contractions, promote delivery of the placenta, and stimulate postpartum uterine contractions, thereby preventing excessive bleeding. The function of this hormone is discussed in detail in Chapter 32.

QUICK CHECK 18-2

1. What is the relationship between the hypothalamus and the pituitary?
2. What is the action of antidiuretic hormone?

Pineal Gland

The pineal gland is located near the centre of the brain and is composed of photoreceptive cells that secrete **melatonin**. It is innervated by noradrenergic sympathetic nerve terminals controlled by pathways within the hypothalamus. Melatonin release is stimulated by exposure to dark and inhibited by light exposure. It is synthesized from tryptophan, which is first converted to serotonin and then to melatonin. Melatonin regulates circadian rhythms and reproductive systems, including the secretion of the gonadotropin-releasing hormones and the onset of puberty. It also plays an important role in immune regulation and is postulated to impact the aging process. Further effects of melatonin include increasing nitric oxide release from blood vessels, removing toxic oxygen free radicals, and decreasing insulin secretion.[19] Melatonin has been used therapeutically in humans to help with sleep disturbances, jet lag, and psychological and inflammatory disorders. Its utility for numerous other disorders is being explored.[20]

Thyroid and Parathyroid Glands

The thyroid gland, located in the neck just below the larynx, produces hormones that control the rates of metabolic processes throughout the body. The four parathyroid glands are near the posterior side of the thyroid and function to control serum calcium levels (Figure 18-11).

Thyroid Gland

Two lobes of the **thyroid gland** lie on either side of the trachea, inferior to the thyroid cartilage and joined by a small band of tissue termed the **isthmus**. The pyramidal lobe is superior to the isthmus (see Figure 18-11). The normal thyroid gland is not visible on inspection, but it may be palpated on swallowing, which causes it to be displaced upward.

The thyroid gland consists of **follicles** that contain follicular cells surrounding a viscous substance called *colloid* (Figure 18-12). The follicular cells synthesize and secrete the thyroid hormones. Neurons terminate on blood vessels within the thyroid gland and on the follicular cells themselves, so neurotransmitters (acetylcholine, catecholamines) may directly affect the secretory activity of follicular cells and thyroid blood flow. Approximately a 2-month supply of thyroid hormones is stored in the gland.

Also found in the thyroid are parafollicular cells, or C cells (see Figure 18-12). **C cells** secrete various polypeptides, including calcitonin. At high levels, **calcitonin**, also called *thyrocalcitonin*, lowers serum calcium levels by inhibiting bone-resorbing osteoclasts (Table 18-6) (bone resorption is explained in Chapter 38). However, in humans the metabolic consequences of calcitonin deficiency or excess do not appear to be significant. Calcitonin can be used therapeutically to treat a number of bone disorders, including osteogenesis imperfecta, osteoporosis, and Paget's disease, among others. Parafollicular cells can give rise to medullary thyroid carcinoma.

Regulation of thyroid hormone secretion. Thyroid hormone (TH) is regulated through a negative-feedback loop involving the hypothalamus, the anterior pituitary, and the thyroid gland (see Figure 18-2). This loop is initiated by TRH, which is synthesized and stored within the hypothalamus. TRH is released into the hypothalamic-pituitary portal system and circulates to the anterior pituitary, where it stimulates the release of TSH. The levels of TRH increase with exposure to cold or stress and from decreased levels of thyroxine.

TSH is a glycoprotein synthesized and stored within the anterior pituitary. When TSH is secreted by the anterior pituitary, it circulates to bind with receptors on the plasma membrane of the thyroid follicular cells.

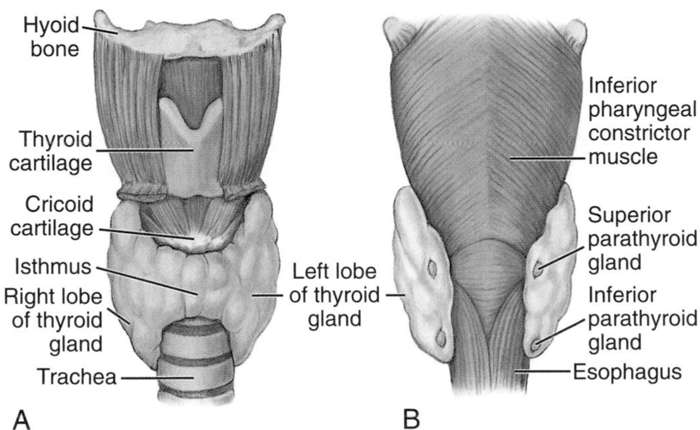
Hyoid bone
Thyroid cartilage
Cricoid cartilage
Isthmus
Right lobe of thyroid gland
Trachea
Left lobe of thyroid gland
Inferior pharyngeal constrictor muscle
Superior parathyroid gland
Inferior parathyroid gland
Esophagus
A
B

FIGURE 18-11 Thyroid and Parathyroid Glands. **A,** Anterior view. **B,** Posterior view. (From Fehrenbach, M.J., & Herring, S.W. [2012]. *Illustrated anatomy of the head and neck* [4th ed.]. St. Louis: Saunders.)

The primary effect of TSH on the thyroid gland is to cause an immediate release of stored TH and an increase in TH synthesis. TSH also increases growth of the thyroid gland by stimulating thymocyte hyperplasia and hypertrophy. As TH levels rise, there is a negative-feedback effect on the hypothalamic-pituitary axis to inhibit TRH and TSH release, which then results in decreased TH synthesis and secretion. TH synthesis is also controlled by serum iodide levels and by circulating selenium-dependent enzymes, called deiodinases, which inactivate the precursor molecule thyroxine.[21] Thyroid gland hormones and their regulation and function are summarized in Table 18-6.

Synthesis of thyroid hormone. TH synthesis is summarized in the following steps:

1. Uniodinated thyroglobulin (a large glycoprotein) is produced by the endoplasmic reticulum of the thyroid follicular cells.
2. Tyrosine is incorporated into the thyroglobulin as it is synthesized.
3. Iodide (the inorganic form of iodine) is actively transferred (pumped) from the blood into the colloid by carrier proteins located in the outer membrane of the follicular cells. This active transport system is called the iodide trap and is very efficient at accumulating the trace amounts of iodide from the blood.
4. Iodide is oxidized and quickly attaches to tyrosine within the thyroglobulin molecule.
5. Coupling of iodinated tyrosine forms thyroid hormones. Triiodothyronine (T_3) is formed from coupling of monoiodotyrosine (one iodine atom and tyrosine) and diiodotyrosine (two iodine atoms and tyrosine). Tetraiodothyronine, commonly known as thyroxine (T_4), is formed from coupling of two diiodotyrosines.
6. Thyroid hormones are stored attached to thyroglobulin within the colloid until they are released into the circulation.

The thyroid gland normally produces 90% T_4 and 10% T_3. Once released into the circulation, T_3 and T_4 are primarily transported bound to **thyroxine-binding globulin**, though some TH is transported by thyroxine-binding prealbumin (transthyretin), albumin, or lipoproteins. The bound form serves as a reservoir, while the unbound form is active. In the body tissues, most of the T_4 is converted to T_3, which acts on the target cell.[22]

Actions of thyroid hormone. TH has a significant effect on the growth, maturation, and function of cells and tissues throughout the body. TH is essential for normal growth and neurological development in the fetus and infant and affects metabolic, neurological, cardiovascular,

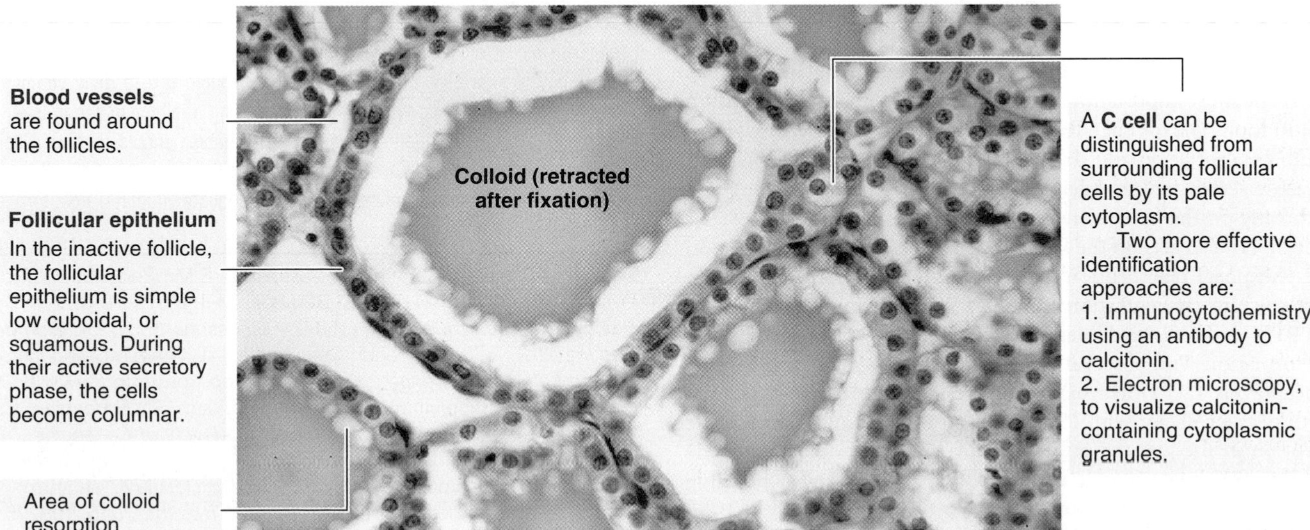
Blood vessels are found around the follicles.
Follicular epithelium
In the inactive follicle, the follicular epithelium is simple low cuboidal, or squamous. During their active secretory phase, the cells become columnar.
Area of colloid resorption
Colloid (retracted after fixation)
A **C cell** can be distinguished from surrounding follicular cells by its pale cytoplasm.
Two more effective identification approaches are:
1. Immunocytochemistry, using an antibody to calcitonin.
2. Electron microscopy, to visualize calcitonin-containing cytoplasmic granules.

FIGURE 18-12 Thyroid Follicle Cells.

TABLE 18-6 Thyroid Gland Hormones and Their Regulation and Functions

Hormone	Regulation	Functions
Thyroxine (T_4) and triiodothyronine (T_3)	T_4 and T_3 levels are controlled by thyroid-stimulating hormone; released in response to metabolic demand Influences on amount secreted: Gender Pregnancy Gonadal- and adrenocortical-increased steroids = ↑ levels Exposure to extreme cold = ↑ levels Nutritional state Chemicals Growth hormone–inhibiting hormone = ↓ levels Dopamine = ↓ levels Catecholamines = ↑ levels	Regulate protein, fat, and carbohydrate catabolism in all cells Regulate metabolic rate of all cells Regulate body heat production Serve as insulin antagonists Maintain growth hormone secretion, skeletal maturation Affect central nervous system development Are necessary for muscle tone and vigour Maintain cardiac rate, force, and output Maintain secretion of gastro-intestinal (GI) tract Affect respiratory rate and oxygen utilization Maintain calcium mobilization Affect red blood cell production Stimulate lipid turnover, free fatty acid release, and cholesterol synthesis
Calcitonin	Elevated serum calcium level—major stimulant for calcitonin Other stimulants: Gastrin Calcium-rich foods (regardless of serum calcium levels) Pregnancy Lowered serum calcium level—suppresses calcitonin release	Lowers serum calcium level by opposing bone-resorbing effects of parathyroid hormone, prostaglandins, and calciferols by inhibiting osteoclastic activity Lowers serum phosphate levels Decreases calcium and phosphorous absorption in GI tract

From Monahan, F.D., Sands, J., Neighbors, M., et al. (2007). *Phipps' medical-surgical nursing: Health and illness perspectives* (8th ed.). St. Louis: Mosby.

and respiratory functioning across the lifespan. In addition, TH is required for the metabolism and function of blood cells as well as normal muscle functioning and the integrity of skin, nails, and hair. Similar to some steroid hormones, TH binds to intracellular receptor complexes and then influences the genetic expression of specific proteins. TH also affects cell metabolism by altering protein, fat, and glucose metabolism and, as a result, increasing heat production and oxygen consumption. Additionally, TH has permissive effects throughout the body by optimizing the actions of other hormones and neurotransmitters (see Table 18-6). Use of TH and its analogues is being explored for the therapy of many metabolic disorders, such as obesity and type 2 diabetes mellitus.[23]

Parathyroid Glands

Normally two pairs of small parathyroid glands are present behind the upper and lower poles of the thyroid gland (see Figure 18-11). However, their number may range from two to six.

The parathyroid glands produce parathyroid hormone (PTH), which is the single most important factor in the regulation of serum calcium concentration. The overall effect of PTH secretion is to increase serum calcium concentration and decrease the level of serum phosphate. A decrease in serum-ionized calcium level stimulates PTH secretion. PTH acts directly on the bone to release calcium by stimulating osteoclast activity. PTH also acts on the kidney to increase calcium reabsorption while phosphate reabsorption is decreased. The resultant increase in serum calcium concentration inhibits PTH secretion. Paradoxically, when PTH is administered intermittently and at a low dose, it stimulates bone formation. This observation led to the use of PTH for treatment of osteoporosis. 1,25-Dihydroxy-vitamin D_3 (the active form of vitamin D) works as a cofactor with PTH to promote calcium and phosphate absorption in the gut and enhance bone mineralization. Vitamin D also plays an important role in metabolic processes and controlling inflammation. It has been reported that approximately one third (32%) of Canadians had concentrations of vitamin D below the recommended level[24] (see *Health Promotion:* Vitamin D).

HEALTH PROMOTION

Vitamin D

Vitamin D is essential for bone health and is widely used for the prevention and treatment of postmenopausal osteoporosis and renal osteodystrophy. Vitamin D deficiency affects 32% of all Canadians; 59% of those affected are between the ages of 20 and 39 years. Inadequate serum levels of vitamin D have been linked to infections, cancer, heart disease, dementia, diabetes, persistent pain syndromes, and autoimmune disorders. Controversies continue as to whether these associations indicate a direct cause and effect between low levels of vitamin D and the pathophysiology of these diseases, and whether vitamin D supplementation reduces risk or improves outcomes. However, many health organizations recommend increased intake of vitamin D–containing foods (fatty fish, egg yolks, vitamin D–fortified juices, and milk products), increased exposure to sunlight, and supplementation with vitamin D. Health Canada currently recommends that all Canadians over the age of 2, including pregnant and lactating women, consume 500 mL of milk or fortified soy beverages every day. Adults over the age of 50 years should take a daily vitamin D supplement of 400 units with a goal of achieving a minimum serum level of 50 nmol/L. Lastly, all healthy breastfed term babies should receive a daily vitamin D supplement of 400 units starting at birth and continuing until 1 year of age. Infants who are formula fed receive adequate vitamin D from fortified formula.

Data from Balvers, M.G., Brouwer-Brolsma, E.M., Endenburg, S., et al. (2015). *J Nutr Sci, 4*, e23; Berridge, M.J. (2015). *Biochem Biophys Res Commun, 460*(1), 53–71; Guessous, I. (2015). *Biomed Res Int, 2015*, 563403; Health Canada. (2012). *Vitamin D and calcium: Updated dietary reference intakes.* Retrieved from http://www.hc-sc.gc.ca/fn-an/nutrition/vitamin/vita-d-eng.php; Janz, T., & Pearson, C. (2015). *Health at a glance: Vitamin D blood levels of Canadians* (Statistics Canada Catalogue no. 82-624-X). Retrieved from http://www.statcan.gc.ca/pub/82-624-x/2013001/article/11727-eng.htm; Mozos, I., & Marginean, O. (2015). *Biomed Res Int, 2015*, 109275; Schöttker, B., & Brenner, H. (2015). *Nutrients, 7*(5), 3264–3278.

Phosphate and magnesium concentrations also affect PTH secretion. An increase in serum phosphate level decreases serum calcium level by causing calcium-phosphate precipitation into soft tissue and bone, which indirectly stimulates PTH secretion. Hypomagnesemia in persons with normal calcium levels acts as a mild stimulant to PTH secretion; however, in persons with hypocalcemia, hypomagnesemia decreases PTH secretion.[25]

QUICK CHECK 18-3

1. How does the anterior pituitary regulate the thyroid gland?
2. What form of thyroid hormone is biologically active?
3. What two organs are the sites of action of parathyroid hormone?

Endocrine Pancreas

The pancreas is both an endocrine gland that produces hormones and an exocrine gland that produces digestive enzymes. (The exocrine function of the pancreas is discussed in Chapter 35.) The pancreas is located behind the stomach, between the spleen and the duodenum, and houses the islets of Langerhans. The islets of Langerhans have four types of hormone-secreting cells: alpha cells, which secrete glucagon; beta cells, which secrete insulin and amylin; delta cells, which secrete gastrin and somatostatin; and F (or PP) cells, which secrete pancreatic polypeptide. These hormones regulate carbohydrate, fat, and protein metabolism. (The pancreas is illustrated in Figure 18-13.) Nerves from both the sympathetic and the parasympathetic divisions of the autonomic nervous system innervate the pancreatic islets.

Insulin

The beta cells of the pancreas synthesize insulin from the precursor proinsulin, which is formed from a larger precursor molecule, preproinsulin. Proinsulin is composed of A peptide and B peptide connected by a C peptide and two disulphide bonds. C peptide is cleaved by proteolytic enzymes, leaving the bonded A and B peptides as the insulin molecule. Insulin circulates freely in the plasma and is not bound to a carrier. C peptide level can be measured in the blood and used as an indirect measurement of serum insulin synthesis.

Secretion of insulin is regulated by chemical, hormonal, and neural control. Insulin secretion is pulsatile, increasing when the beta cells are stimulated by the parasympathetic nervous system, usually before eating a meal. Other factors stimulating insulin secretion include increased blood levels of glucose, amino acids (leucine, arginine, and lysine), and gastro-intestinal hormones (glucagon, gastrin, cholecystokinin, and secretin). Insulin secretion diminishes in response to low blood levels of glucose (hypoglycemia), high levels of insulin (through negative feedback to the beta cells), and sympathetic stimulation of the beta cells in the islets. Prostaglandins also inhibit insulin secretion.

At the target cell, insulin signalling is initiated when insulin binds and activates its cell surface receptor. These receptors are found on cells throughout the body. Insulin promotes cellular glucose uptake through glucose transporters (GLUTs). An intracellular cascade of phosphorylation events, protein–protein interactions, and second-messenger generation then occurs, resulting in diverse metabolic events throughout the body[26] (see details in Figure 18-14).

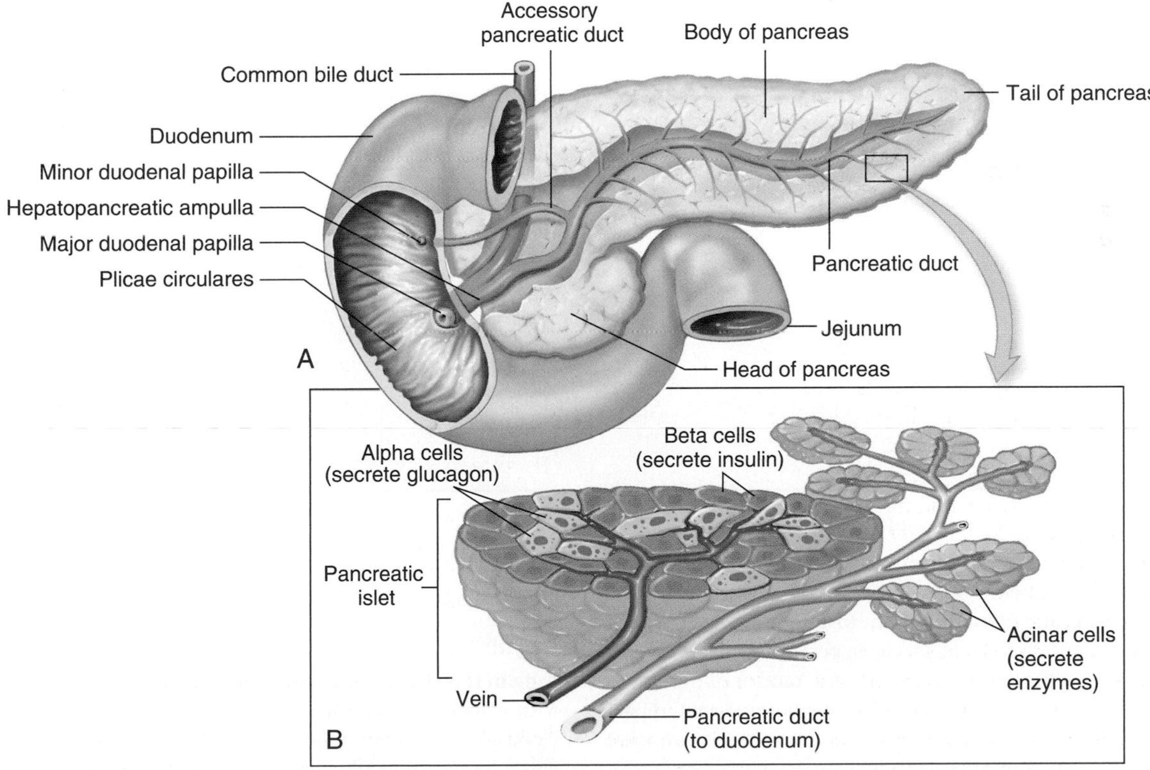

FIGURE 18-13 The Pancreas. A, Pancreas dissected to show main and accessory ducts. The main duct may join the common bile duct, as shown here, to enter the duodenum by a single opening at the major duodenal papilla, or the two ducts may have separate openings. The accessory pancreatic duct is usually present and has a separate opening into the duodenum. **B,** Exocrine glandular cells (around small pancreatic ducts) and endocrine glandular cells of the pancreatic islets (adjacent to blood capillaries). Exocrine pancreatic cells secrete pancreatic juice, alpha endocrine cells secrete glucagon, and beta cells secrete insulin and amylin. (From Patton, K.T., & Thibodeau, G.A. [2016]. *Structure & function of the body* [15th ed.]. St. Louis: Mosby.)

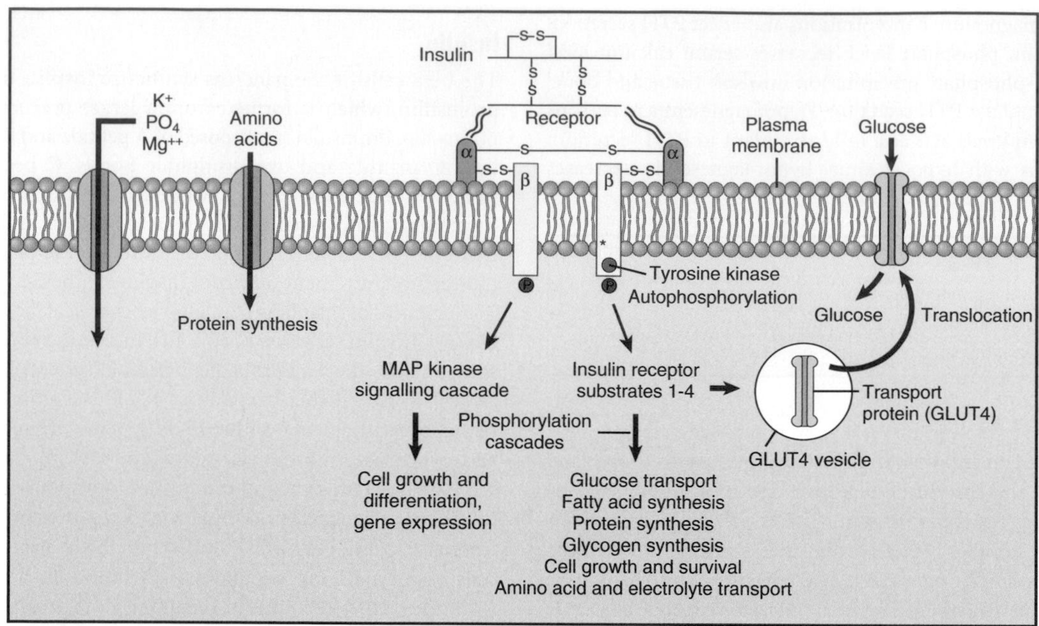

FIGURE 18-14 Insulin Action on Cells. Binding of insulin to its receptor causes autophosphorylation of the receptor, which then itself acts as a tyrosine kinase that phosphorylates insulin receptor substrates 1-4. Numerous target enzymes, such as protein kinase B and mitogen-activated protein (*MAP*) kinase, are activated and these enzymes have a multitude of effects on cell function. The glucose transporter (*GLUT4*) is recruited to the plasma membrane, where it facilitates glucose entry into the cell. The transport of amino acids, potassium (*K*+), magnesium (*Mg*++), and phosphate (*PO*4) into the cell is also facilitated. The synthesis of various enzymes is induced or suppressed, and cell growth is regulated by signal molecules that modulate gene expression. (Redrawn from Levy, M.N., Koeppen, B.M., & Stanton, B.A. [Eds.]. [2006]. *Berne & Levy principles of physiology* [4th ed.]. St. Louis: Mosby.)

TABLE 18-7 Insulin Actions

	SITES OF INSULIN ACTION		
Actions	**Liver Cells**	**Muscle Cells**	**Adipose Cells**
Glucose uptake	Increased	Increased	Increased
Glucose use	—	—	Increased glycerol phosphate
Glycogenesis	Increased	Increased	—
Glycogenolysis	Decreased	Decreased	—
Glycolysis	Increased	Increased	Increased
Gluconeogenesis	Increased	—	—
Other	Increased fatty acid synthesis Decreased ketogenesis Decreased urea cycle activity	Increased amino acid uptake Increased protein synthesis Decreased proteolysis	Increased fat esterification Decreased lipolysis Increased fat storage

The sensitivity of the insulin receptor is a key component in maintaining normal cellular function. Insulin sensitivity is affected by age, weight, abdominal fat, and physical activity. Insulin resistance has been implicated in numerous diseases, including hypertension, heart disease, and type 2 diabetes mellitus. Adipocytes release a number of hormones and cytokines that are altered in obesity and have an important impact on insulin sensitivity. The most effective measures shown to improve insulin sensitivity in humans are weight loss and exercise.[27]

Insulin is an anabolic hormone that promotes glucose uptake primarily in liver, muscle, and adipose tissue. It also increases the synthesis of proteins, carbohydrates, lipids, and nucleic acids. It functions mainly in the liver, muscle, and adipose tissue. Table 18-7 summarizes the actions of insulin. The net effect of insulin in these tissues is to stimulate protein and fat synthesis and decrease blood glucose level. The brain, red blood cells, kidney, and lens of the eye do not require insulin for glucose transport. Insulin also facilitates the intracellular transport of potassium, phosphate, and magnesium.

Amylin

Amylin (or islet amyloid polypeptide) is a peptide hormone cosecreted with insulin by beta cells in response to nutrient stimuli. It regulates blood glucose concentration by delaying gastric emptying and suppressing glucagon secretion after meals. Amylin also has a satiety effect, which reduces food intake. Through these mechanisms, amylin has an antihyperglycemic effect.[28]

Glucagon

Glucagon is produced by the alpha cells of the pancreas and by cells lining the gastro-intestinal tract. Glucagon acts primarily in the liver and increases blood glucose concentration by stimulating glycogenolysis and gluconeogenesis in muscle and lipolysis in adipose tissue. Amino acids, such as alanine, glycine, and asparagine, stimulate glucagon secretion. Glucagon release is inhibited by high glucose levels and stimulated by low glucose levels and sympathetic stimulation; thus it is antagonistic to insulin.[29]

Pancreatic Somatostatin

Somatostatin is produced by delta cells of the pancreas in response to food intake and is essential in carbohydrate, fat, and protein metabolism. It is different from hypothalamic somatostatin, which inhibits the release of GH and TSH. Pancreatic somatostatin is involved in regulating alpha-cell and beta-cell function within the islets by inhibiting secretion of insulin, glucagon, and pancreatic polypeptide.[30]

Gastrin, Ghrelin, and Pancreatic Polypeptide

Pancreatic gastrin stimulates the secretion of gastric acid. It is postulated that fetal pancreatic gastrin secretion is necessary for adequate islet cell development. Ghrelin stimulates GH secretion, controls appetite, and plays a role in obesity and the regulation of insulin sensitivity. Pancreatic polypeptide is released by F cells in response to hypoglycemia and protein-rich meals. It inhibits gallbladder contraction and exocrine pancreas secretion and is frequently increased in individuals with pancreatic tumours or diabetes mellitus.[31]

Adrenal Glands

The adrenal glands are paired, pyramid-shaped organs behind the peritoneum and close to the upper pole of each kidney. Each gland is surrounded by a capsule, embedded in fat, and well supplied with blood from the aorta and phrenic and renal arteries. Venous return from the left adrenal gland is to the renal vein and from the right adrenal gland is to the inferior vena cava.

Each adrenal gland consists of two separate portions: an outer cortex and an inner medulla. These two portions have different embryonic origins, structures, and hormonal functions. The adrenal cortex and medulla function like two separate but interrelated glands (Figure 18-15).

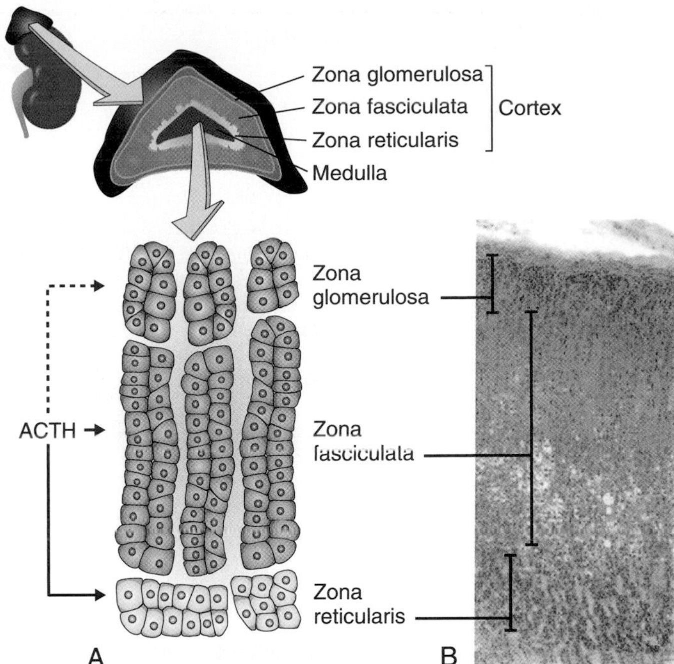

FIGURE 18-15 Structure of the Adrenal Glands Showing Cell Layers (Zonae) of the Cortex. A, Adrenal glands. Each gland consists of cortex and medulla. The cortex has three layers: zona glomerulosa, zona fasciculata, and zona reticularis. **B,** A portion of the medulla is visible at the lower right in the photomicrograph (× 35) and at the bottom of the drawing. (**A,** from Damjanov, I. [2008]. *Pathophysiology*. Philadelphia: Saunders; **B,** from Kierszenbaum, A. [2002]. *Histology and cell biology*. St. Louis: Mosby.)

Adrenal Cortex

The adrenal cortex accounts for 80% of the weight of the adult gland. The cortex is histologically subdivided into the following three zones[32]:

1. The zona glomerulosa, the outer layer, constitutes about 15% of the cortex and primarily produces the mineralocorticoid aldosterone.
2. The zona fasciculata, the middle layer, constitutes 78% of the cortex and secretes the glucocorticoids cortisol, cortisone, and corticosterone.
3. The zona reticularis, the inner layer, constitutes 7% of the cortex and secretes mineralocorticoids (aldosterone), adrenal androgens and estrogens, and glucocorticoids.

The cells of the adrenal cortex are stimulated by ACTH from the pituitary gland. All hormones of the adrenal cortex are synthesized from cholesterol. The best known pathway of steroidogenesis involves the conversion of cholesterol to pregnenolone, which is then converted to the major corticosteroids.

Glucocorticoids

Functions of the glucocorticoids. The glucocorticoids are steroid hormones that have metabolic, neurological, anti-inflammatory, and growth-suppressing effects. These functions (Figure 18-16) have direct effects on carbohydrate metabolism. These hormones increase blood glucose concentration by promoting gluconeogenesis in the liver and by decreasing uptake of glucose into muscle cells, adipose cells, and lymphatic cells. In extrahepatic tissues, the glucocorticoids stimulate protein catabolism and inhibit amino acid uptake and protein synthesis. The ultimate effect on the body is protein catabolism.

The glucocorticoids act at several sites to suppress immune and inflammatory reactions. One major immunosuppressant effect is the glucocorticoid-mediated decrease in the proliferation of T lymphocytes (T cells), primarily T-helper cells (Th cells). There is a greater effect on T-helper 1 (Th1) cytokine production (including antiviral interferons) than there is on T-helper 2 (Th2) cytokine production, and therefore greater depression of cellular immunity than humoral immunity (see Chapter 7). Glucocorticoids affect innate immunity through several pathways, including decreasing the activity of pattern receptors on the surface of macrophages (see Chapter 6). Anti-inflammatory effects of glucocorticoids also include decreased function of natural killer cells, suppression of inflammatory cytokines, and stabilization of lysosomal membranes, which decreases the release of proteolytic enzymes. The pro-inflammatory effects of glucocorticoids are not clearly understood.[32] Psychological and physiological stress increases glucocorticoid production, which provides a pathway for the well-described decrease in immunity seen in both acute and chronic stress conditions (see Chapter 9). Use of glucocorticoids for the treatment of disease also leads to suppression of innate and adaptive immunity and the challenging complications of infection and poor wound healing (see Chapter 8).

Other effects of glucocorticoids include inhibition of bone formation, inhibition of ADH secretion, and stimulation of gastric acid secretion. Glucocorticoids appear to potentiate the effects of catecholamines, including sensitizing the arterioles to the vasoconstrictive effects of norepinephrine. TH and GH effects on adipose tissue are also potentiated by glucocorticoids. A metabolite of cortisol may act like a barbiturate and depress nerve cell function in the brain, accounting for the noted effects on mood, such as anxiety and depression, associated with steroid level fluctuation in disease or stress.

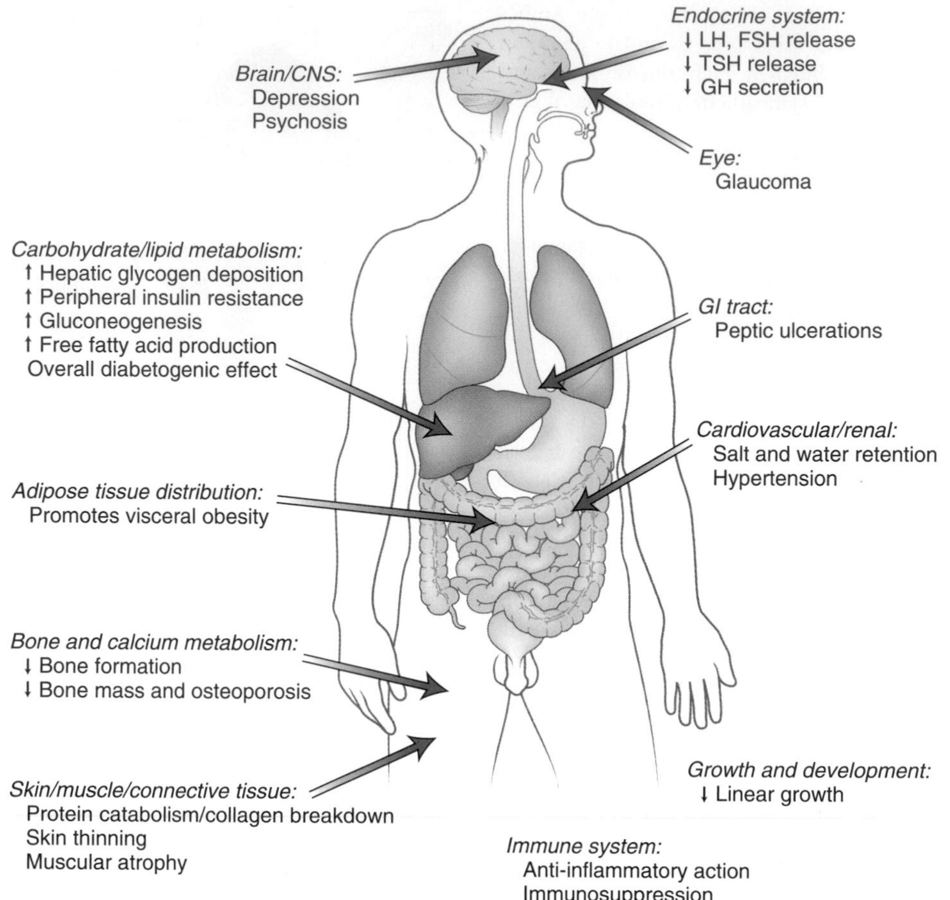

FIGURE 18-16 Effects of Glucocorticoids on the Body. *CNS*, central nervous system; *FSH*, follicle-stimulating hormone; *GH*, growth hormone; *GI*, gastro-intestinal; *LH*, luteinizing hormone; *TSH*, thyroid-stimulating hormone. (From Stewart, P.M., & Krone, N.P. [2011]. The adrenal cortex. In S. Melmed, K.S. Polonsky, P.R. Larsen, et al. [Eds.], *Williams textbook of endocrinology* [12th ed.]. Philadelphia: Saunders.)

Pathologically high levels of glucocorticoids increase the number of circulating erythrocytes (leading to polycythemia), increase the appetite, promote fat deposition in the face and cervical areas, increase uric acid excretion, decrease serum calcium levels (possibly by inhibiting gastro-intestinal absorption of calcium), suppress the secretion and synthesis of ACTH, and interfere with the action of GH so that somatic growth is inhibited (see Chapter 19).

Cortisol. The most potent naturally occurring glucocorticoid is **cortisol**. It is the main secretory product of the adrenal cortex and is needed to maintain life and protect the body from stress (see Figure 9-2). The liver is primarily responsible for the deactivation of cortisol.

Cortisol secretion is regulated primarily by the hypothalamus and the anterior pituitary gland (Figure 18-17). **Corticotropin-releasing hormone (CRH)** is produced by several nuclei in the hypothalamus and stored in the median eminence. Once released, CRH travels through the portal vessels to stimulate the production of ACTH, β-lipotropin, γ-lipotropin, endorphins, and enkephalins by the anterior pituitary. ACTH is the main regulator of cortisol secretion and adrenocortical growth.

ACTH is synthesized as part of a precursor called proopiomelanocortin (POMC). Three factors appear to be primarily involved in regulating the secretion of ACTH: (1) negative-feedback effects of high circulating levels of cortisol and synthetic glucocorticoids suppress both CRH and ACTH, whereas low cortisol levels stimulate their secretion; (2) diurnal rhythms affect ACTH and cortisol levels (in persons with regular sleep–wake patterns, ACTH peaks 3 to 5 hours after sleep begins and declines throughout the day, and cortisol levels follow a similar pattern); and (3) psychological and physiological (e.g., hypoxia, hypoglycemia, hyperthermia, exercise) stress increases ACTH secretion, leading to increased cortisol levels. (Neurological mechanisms regulating sleep are discussed in Chapter 14.) A form of immunoreactive ACTH (irACTH) is produced by the cells of the immune system and may account, in part, for integration of the immune and endocrine systems.

Once ACTH is secreted, it binds to specific plasma membrane receptors on the cells of the adrenal cortex and on other extra-adrenal tissues. Because both adrenal and extra-adrenal tissues have ACTH receptors, a number of effects result from stimulation by ACTH. In addition to increasing adrenocortical secretion of cortisol, ACTH maintains the size and synthetic functions of the adrenal cortex through activation of crucial enzymes and storage of cholesterol for metabolism into steroid hormones. Extra-adrenal effects of ACTH include stimulation of melanocytes and activation of tissue lipase.

Once ACTH stimulates the cells of the adrenal cortex, cortisol synthesis and secretion immediately occur. In the healthy person, the secretory patterns of ACTH and cortisol are nearly identical. After secretion, some cortisol circulates in bound form attached to albumin

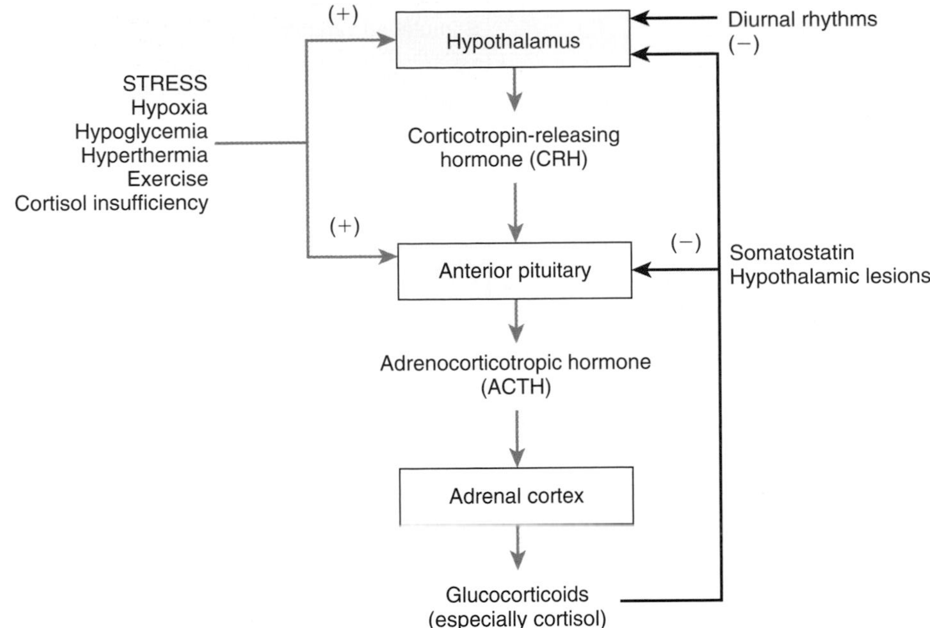

FIGURE 18-17 Feedback Control of Glucocorticoid Synthesis and Secretion.

but primarily it is bound to the plasma protein transcortin. A smaller amount circulates in the free form and diffuses into cells with specific intracellular receptors for cortisol. ACTH is rapidly inactivated in the circulation, and the liver and kidneys remove the deactivated hormone.

Mineralocorticoids: aldosterone. Mineralocorticoid steroids directly affect ion transport by renal tubular epithelial cells, causing sodium retention and potassium and hydrogen loss. Aldosterone is the most potent naturally occurring mineralocorticoid and conserves sodium by increasing the activity of the sodium–potassium pump of epithelial cells. (The sodium–potassium pump is described in Chapter 1.)

The initial stages of aldosterone synthesis occur in the zona fasciculata and zona reticularis. The final conversion of corticosterone to aldosterone is confined to the zona glomerulosa. Aldosterone synthesis and secretion is regulated primarily by the renin-angiotensin-aldosterone system (described in Chapter 29). The renin-angiotensin-aldosterone system is activated by sodium and water depletion, increased potassium levels, and a diminished effective blood volume (Figure 18-18). Angiotensin II is the primary stimulant of aldosterone synthesis and secretion; however, sodium and potassium levels also may directly affect aldosterone secretion. ACTH may transiently stimulate aldosterone synthesis but does not appear to be a major regulator of secretion.

When sodium and potassium levels are within normal limits, approximately 50 to 250 mg of aldosterone is secreted daily. Of the secreted aldosterone, 50 to 75% binds to plasma proteins. The large proportion of unbound aldosterone contributes to its rapid metabolic turnover in the liver, its low plasma concentration, and its short half-life (about 15 minutes). Aldosterone is degraded in the liver and is excreted by the kidney.

Aldosterone maintains extracellular volume by acting on distal nephron epithelial cells to increase reabsorption of sodium and excretion of potassium and hydrogen. This renal effect takes 90 minutes to 6 hours. Fluid and electrolyte regulation is addressed in more detail in Chapter 5. Other effects of aldosterone include enhancement of cardiac muscle contraction, stimulation of ectopic ventricular activity through secondary cardiac pacemakers in the ventricles, stiffening of blood vessels with increased vascular resistance, and decrease in fibrinolysis. Pathologically elevated levels of aldosterone have been implicated in the myocardial changes associated with heart failure, resistant hypertension, insulin resistance, and systemic inflammation.[33]

Adrenal estrogens and androgens. The healthy adrenal cortex secretes minimal amounts of estrogen and androgens. ACTH appears to be the major regulator. Some of the weakly androgenic substances secreted by the cortex (dehydroepiandrosterone [DHEA], androstenedione) are converted by peripheral tissues to stronger androgens, such as testosterone, thus accounting for some androgenic effects initiated by the adrenal cortex. Peripheral conversion of adrenal androgens to estrogens is enhanced in aging or obese persons as well as in those with liver disease or hyperthyroidism.[34] The biological effects and metabolism of the adrenal sex steroids do not vary from those produced by the gonads (see Chapter 32).

Adrenal Medulla

The chromaffin cells (pheochromocytes) of the adrenal medulla secrete and store the catecholamines epinephrine (adrenaline) and norepinephrine (noradrenaline). Both are synthesized from the amino acid phenylalanine (Figure 18-19). The adrenal medulla, together with the sympathetic division of the autonomic nervous system, is embryonically derived from neural crest cells. Only 30% of circulating epinephrine comes from the adrenal medulla; the other 70% is released from nerve terminals. The medulla is only a minor source of norepinephrine. The adrenal medulla functions as a sympathetic ganglion without postganglionic processes. Sympathetic cholinergic preganglion fibres terminate on the chromaffin cells and secrete catecholamines directly into the bloodstream. The catecholamines acting in the blood are therefore hormones and not neurotransmitters.

Physiological stress to the body (e.g., traumatic injury, hypoxia, hypoglycemia, and many others) triggers release of adrenal catecholamines through acetylcholine (from the preganglionic sympathetic fibres), which depolarizes the chromaffin cells (see Chapter 9). Depolarization causes exocytosis of the storage granules from the chromaffin cells with release of epinephrine and norepinephrine into the bloodstream.

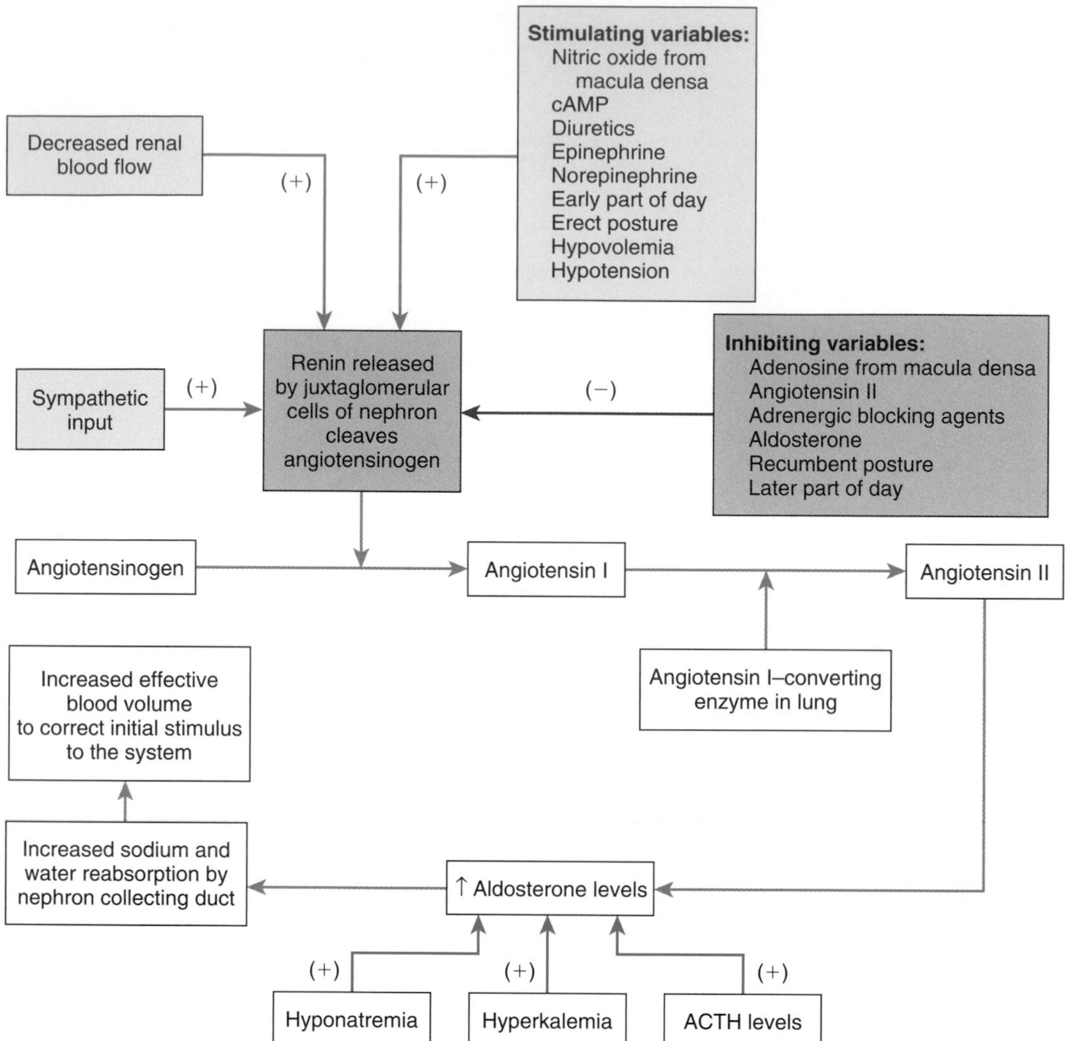

FIGURE 18-18 **The Feedback Mechanisms Regulating Aldosterone Secretion.** *ACTH*, adrenocorticotropic hormone; *cAMP*, cyclic adenosine monophosphate.

Secretion of adrenal catecholamines also is increased by ACTH and the glucocorticoids.[35]

Once released, the catecholamines remain in the plasma for only seconds to minutes. The catecholamines exert their biological effects after binding to plasma membrane receptors (α_1, α_2, β_1, β_2, and β_3) in target cells. This binding activates the adenylyl cyclase system. Catecholamines are rapidly removed from the plasma by being absorbed by neurons for storage in new cytoplasmic granules, or they may be metabolically inactivated and excreted in the urine. The catecholamines directly inhibit their own secretion by decreasing the formation of the enzyme tyrosine hydroxylase (the rate-limiting step).

Catecholamines have diverse effects on the entire body. Their release and the body's response have been characterized as the "fight-or-flight response" (stress response) (see Figures 9-2 and 9-3 and Tables 9-3 and 9-4). Metabolic effects of catecholamines promote hyperglycemia through a variety of mechanisms including interference with the usual glucose regulatory feedback mechanisms.

QUICK CHECK 18-4

1. What are the islets of Langerhans? Where are they located?
2. Compare and contrast the actions of alpha, beta, delta, and F cells.
3. What is the most potent naturally occurring glucocorticoid, and how is its secretion related to that of adrenocorticotropic hormone?
4. How does aldosterone influence fluid and electrolyte balance?
5. What are catecholamines?

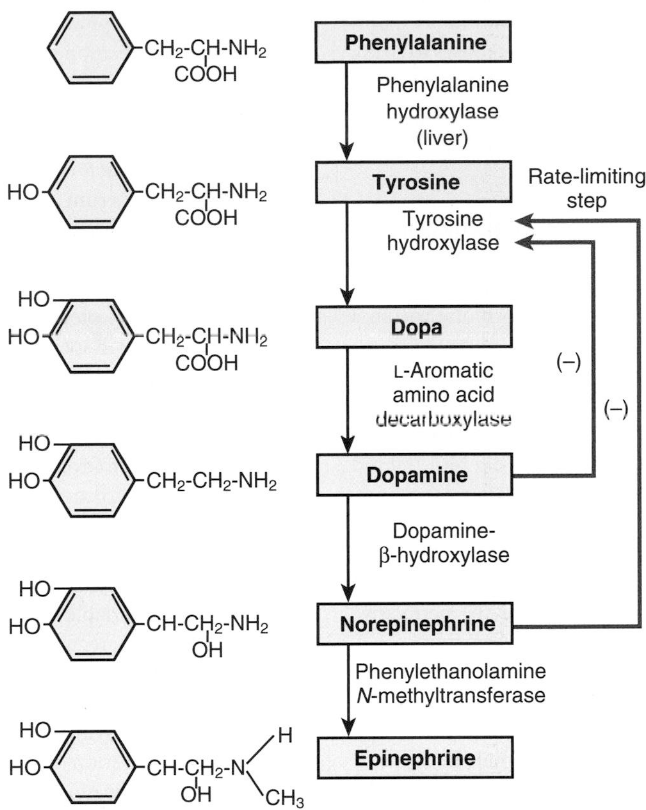

FIGURE 18-19 Synthesis of Catecholamines.

GERIATRIC CONSIDERATIONS

Aging and Its Effects on Specific Endocrine Glands

General Endocrine Changes With Aging

Aging has many effects on the neuroendocrine system. There are complex changes within the hypothalamic-pituitary axis; and altered biological activity of hormones, altered circulating levels of hormones, altered secretory response of the endocrine glands, altered metabolism of hormones, and loss of circadian control of hormone secretion are among the findings.

Pituitary

Posterior: Decrease in size; reduced antidiuretic hormone secretion.

Anterior: Increased fibrosis and moderate increase in size of gland; decline in growth hormone (GH) release.

Thyroid

Glandular atrophy, fibrosis, nodularity, and increased inflammatory infiltrates; decreased thyroxine secretion and turnover, decline in triiodothyronine (especially in men), diminished thyroid-stimulating hormone (TSH) secretion; reduced response of plasma TSH concentration to thyroid-releasing hormone (TRH) administration (especially in men).

Growth Hormone and Insulinlike Growth Factors

The amounts of GH and insulinlike growth factor decline with aging, which contributes to decreases in muscle size and function, reduced fat and bone mass, and changes in reproductive and cognitive function. Increased visceral fat, decreased lean body mass, and decreased bone density are common in older adults.

Pancreas

It is common for older adults to have glucose intolerance or diabetes, and these disorders frequently are undiagnosed in aging adults. Mechanisms include decreased insulin receptor activity and decreased beta-cell secretion of insulin.

Adrenal

Decreased dehydroepiandrosterone levels lead to decreased synthesis of androgen-derived estrogen and testosterone; decreased metabolic clearance of glucocorticoids and cortisol causes decreased cortisol secretion; there also are decreased levels of aldosterone. Circadian patterns of adrenocorticotropic hormone and cortisol secretion may change with aging.

Gonads

Postmenopausal women have decreased estrogen and progesterone, increased follicle-stimulating hormone, and relative increases in androgen levels; these changes have numerous physiological and pathophysiological consequences (see Chapter 32); in men there is a gradual decrease in serum testosterone levels, leading to decreased sexual activity, decreased muscle strength, and decreased bone mineralization.

DID YOU UNDERSTAND?

Overview

1. The endocrine system has diverse functions, including sexual differentiation, growth and development, and continuous maintenance of the body's internal environment and responses to stress.
2. Hormones are chemical messengers synthesized by endocrine glands and when released have intracrine, autocrine, paracrine, and endocrine effects.

Mechanisms of Hormonal Regulation

1. Hormones have specific negative- and positive-feedback mechanisms. Most hormone levels are regulated by negative feedback, in which hormone secretion raises the level of a specific hormone, ultimately causing secretion to subside, maintaining the hormone within a normal physiological range.
2. Endocrine feedback is described in terms of short, long, and ultra-short feedback loops.
3. Water-soluble hormones circulate throughout the body in unbound form, whereas lipid-soluble hormones (e.g., steroid and thyroid hormones) circulate throughout the body bound to carrier proteins.
4. Hormones affect only target cells with appropriate receptors and then act on these cells to initiate specific cell functions or activities.
5. Hormones have two general types of effects on cells: (a) direct effects, or obvious changes in cell function, and (b) permissive effects, or less obvious changes that facilitate cell function.
6. Receptors for hormones may be located on the plasma membrane or in the intracellular compartment of the target cell.
7. Water-soluble hormones act as first messengers, binding to receptors in the cell's plasma membrane. The signals initiated by hormone-receptor binding are then transmitted into the cell by the action of second messengers (i.e., cyclic adenosine monophosphate, cyclic guanosine monophosphate, or tyrosine kinase) and mediate the action of the hormone on the target cell (i.e., protein synthesis or cellular growth).
8. Lipid-soluble hormones (including steroid and thyroid hormones) cross the plasma membrane by diffusion. These hormones diffuse directly into the cell nucleus and bind to nuclear receptors. Rapid responses of steroid hormones may be mediated by plasma membrane receptors.

Structure and Function of the Endocrine Glands

1. The pituitary gland, consisting of anterior and posterior portions, is connected to the central nervous system through the hypothalamus.
2. The hypothalamus regulates anterior pituitary function by secreting releasing or inhibiting hormones and factors into the portal circulation.
3. Hypothalamic hormones include prolactin-releasing factor, which stimulates secretion of prolactin; prolactin-inhibiting factor (dopamine), which inhibits prolactin secretion; thyrotropin-releasing hormone, which affects release of thyroid hormones; growth hormone–releasing hormone, which stimulates the release of growth hormone (GH); somatostatin, which inhibits the release of GH; gonadotropin-releasing hormone, which facilitates the release of follicle-stimulating hormone (FSH) and luteinizing hormone (LH); corticotropin-releasing hormone (CRH), which facilitates the release of adrenocorticotropic hormone (ACTH) and endorphins; and substance P, which inhibits ACTH release and stimulates the release of a variety of other hormones.
4. Hormones of the anterior pituitary are regulated by (a) secretion of hypothalamic peptide hormones or releasing factors, (b) feedback effects of the hormones secreted by target glands, and (c) direct effects of other mediating neurotransmitters.
5. Hormones of the anterior pituitary include ACTH, melanocyte-stimulating hormone, somatotropic hormones (GH, prolactin), and glycoprotein hormones (FSH, LH, and thyroid-stimulating hormone [TSH]).
6. The posterior pituitary secretes antidiuretic hormone (ADH), which also is called *vasopressin*, and oxytocin.
7. ADH controls serum osmolality, increases permeability of the renal tubules to water, and causes vasoconstriction when administered pharmacologically in high doses. ADH also may regulate some central nervous system functions.
8. Oxytocin causes uterine contraction and lactation in women and may have a role in sperm motility in men. In both men and women, oxytocin has an antidiuretic effect similar to that of ADH.
9. Melatonin is secreted by the pineal gland and regulates circadian rhythms and reproduction.
10. The two-lobed thyroid gland contains follicles, which secrete some of the thyroid hormones, and C cells, which secrete calcitonin and somatostatin.
11. Regulation of thyroid hormone (TH) levels is complex and involves the hypothalamus, anterior pituitary, thyroid gland, and numerous biochemical variables.
12. TH secretion is regulated by thyroid-releasing hormone through a negative-feedback loop that involves the anterior pituitary and hypothalamus.
13. TSH, which is synthesized and stored in the anterior pituitary, stimulates secretion of TH by activating intracellular processes, including uptake of iodine necessary for the synthesis of TH in the thyroid gland.
14. Once secreted, TH acts on the thyroid gland, the anterior pituitary, and the median eminence to regulate further TH production.
15. Synthesis of TH depends on the glycoprotein thyroglobulin, which contains a precursor of TH, tyrosine. Tyrosine then combines with iodine to form precursor molecules of the thyroid hormones thyroxine (T_4) and triiodothyronine (T_3). These hormones are then stored within thyroid colloid until released into the circulation.
16. When released into the circulation, T_3 and T_4 are bound by carrier proteins in the plasma, which store these hormones and provide a buffer for rapid changes in hormone levels. The free form is the active form.
17. Thyroid hormones alter protein synthesis and have a wide range of metabolic effects on proteins, carbohydrates, lipids, vitamins, and other hormones and neurotransmitters. Thyroid hormones also affect heat production and cardiac function.
18. The paired parathyroid glands normally are located behind the upper and lower poles of the thyroid. These glands secrete parathyroid hormone (PTH), an important regulator of serum calcium and phosphate levels.
19. PTH secretion increases levels of ionized calcium and decreases levels of phosphate in the plasma.
20. In bone, PTH causes bone breakdown and resorption. At low doses it can promote bone formation. In the kidney, PTH increases reabsorption of calcium and decreases reabsorption of phosphorus and bicarbonate.
21. The endocrine pancreas contains the islets of Langerhans, which secrete hormones responsible for much of the carbohydrate metabolism in the body.

22. The islets of Langerhans consist of alpha cells, beta cells, delta cells, and F cells, which release hormones that regulate protein, fat, and carbohydrate metabolism.
23. Alpha cells produce glucagon, which is secreted inversely to blood glucose concentrations.
24. Beta cells secrete insulin and amylin, which suppresses glucagon secretion and has a satiety effect.
25. Delta cells secrete gastrin and somatostatin (which inhibits glucagon and insulin secretion).
26. F cells secrete pancreatic polypeptide, which inhibits gallbladder contraction and exocrine pancreatic secretion.
27. Insulin is a hormone that regulates blood glucose concentrations and overall body metabolism of fat, protein, and carbohydrates.
28. The paired adrenal glands are situated above the kidneys. Each gland consists of an adrenal medulla, which secretes catecholamines, and an adrenal cortex, which secretes steroid hormones.
29. The steroid hormones secreted by the adrenal cortex are synthesized from cholesterol. These hormones include glucocorticoids, mineralocorticoids, and adrenal androgens and estrogens.
30. Glucocorticoids directly affect carbohydrate metabolism by increasing blood glucose concentration through gluconeogenesis in the liver and by decreasing use of glucose. Glucocorticoids also inhibit immune and inflammatory responses, suppress growth, and promote protein catabolism.
31. The most potent naturally occurring glucocorticoid is cortisol, which is necessary for the maintenance of life and for protection from stress. Secretion of cortisol is regulated by the hypothalamus and anterior pituitary.
32. Cortisol secretion is related to secretion of ACTH, which is stimulated by CRH. ACTH binds with receptors of the adrenal cortex, which activates intracellular mechanisms (specifically cyclic adenosine monophosphate) and leads to cortisol release.
33. Mineralocorticoids are steroid hormones that directly affect ion transport by renal tubular epithelial cells, causing sodium retention and potassium and hydrogen loss.
34. Aldosterone is the most potent naturally occurring mineralocorticoid. Its primary role is renal reabsorption of sodium and excretion of potassium and hydrogen.
35. Aldosterone secretion is regulated primarily by the renin-angiotensin-aldosterone system, which is activated by sodium and water depletion, increased potassium levels, and a decreased blood volume..
36. Aldosterone acts by binding to a site on the cell nucleus and altering protein production within the cell. Its principal site of action is the kidney, where it causes sodium reabsorption and potassium and hydrogen excretion.
37. Androgens and estrogens secreted by the adrenal cortex act in the same way as those secreted by the gonads.
38. The adrenal medulla secretes the catecholamines epinephrine and norepinephrine. Their release is stimulated by sympathetic nervous system stimulation, ACTH, and glucocorticoids.
39. Catecholamines bind with various target cells and are taken up by neurons or excreted in the urine. They cause a range of metabolic effects characterized as the "fight-or-flight response" and include hyperglycemia and immunosuppression.

KEY TERMS

Adrenal cortex, 457
Adrenal gland, 457
Adrenal medulla, 459
Adrenocorticotropic hormone (ACTH), 448
Aldosterone, 459
Alpha cell, 455
Amylin, 456
Anterior pituitary, 448
Antidiuretic hormone (ADH), 448
Beta cell, 455
C cell, 453
Calcitonin, 453
Chromophil, 448
Chromophobe, 448
Corticotropin-releasing hormone (CRH), 458
Cortisol, 458
Delta cell, 455
Direct effect, 446
Downregulation, 445
F (or PP) cell, 455
First messenger, 446
Follicle, 452
Follicle-stimulating hormone (FSH), 448
Gastrin, 457
Ghrelin, 457
Glucagon, 456
Glucocorticoid, 457
Growth hormone (GH), 451
Hormone, 443
Hormone receptor, 446
Hypothalamus, 447
Insulin, 455
Islet of Langerhans, 455
Isthmus, 452
Luteinizing hormone (LH), 448
Median eminence, 452
Melanocyte-stimulating hormone (MSH), 448
Melatonin, 452
Mineralocorticoid, 459
Negative feedback, 443
1,25-Dihydroxy-vitamin D_3, 454
Oxytocin, 448
Pancreas, 455
Pancreatic polypeptide, 457
Parathyroid hormone (PTH), 454
Pars distalis, 448
Pars intermedia, 448
Pars nervosa, 452
Pars tuberalis, 448
Permissive effect, 446
Pituitary gland, 448
Pituitary stalk, 452
Positive feedback, 444
Posterior pituitary, 452
Prolactin, 451
Second messenger, 446
Somatostatin, 457
Target cell, 444
Thyroid gland, 452
Thyroid hormone (TH), 453
Thyroid-stimulating hormone (TSH), 444
Thyrotropin-releasing hormone (TRH), 444
Thyroxine-binding globulin, 453
Tropic hormone, 448
Upregulation, 445
Zona fasciculata, 457
Zona glomerulosa, 457
Zona reticularis, 457

REFERENCES

1. Fujita, T., Fukunaga, M., Itabashi, A., et al. (2014). Once-weekly injection of low-dose teriparatide (28.2 μg) reduced the risk of vertebral fracture in patients with primary osteoporosis. *Calcified Tissue International, 94*(2), 170–175. doi:10.1007/s00223-013-9777-8.
2. Bellavance, M. A., & Rivest, S. (2014). The HPA-immune axis and the immunomodulatory actions of glucocorticoids in the brain. *Frontiers in Immunology, 31*(5), 136. doi:10.3389/fimmu.2014.00136.
3. Levin, E. R. (2015). Extranuclear steroid receptors are essential for steroid hormone actions. *Annual Review of Medicine, 66*, 271–280. doi:10.1146/annurev-med-050913-021703.
4. Spiegel, A., Carter-Su, C., Taylor, S. I., et al. (2011). Mechanisms of action of hormones that act at the cell surface. In S. Melmed, K. S. Polonsky, P. R. Larsen, et al. (Eds.), *Williams textbook of endocrinology* (12th ed.). Philadelphia: Saunders.
5. Das, A., Durrant, D., Salloum, F. N., et al. (2015). PDE5 inhibitors as therapeutics for heart disease, diabetes and cancer. *Pharmacology & Therapeutics, 147*, 12–21. doi:10.1016/j.pharmthera.2014.10.003.
6. Bubb, K. J., Trinder, S. L., Baliga, R. S., et al. (2014). Inhibition of phosphodiesterase 2 augments cGMP and cAMP signaling to ameliorate pulmonary

hypertension. *Circulation, 130*(6), 496–507. doi:10.1161/CIRCULATIONAHA.114.009751.
7. Salisbury, T. B., & Tomblin, J. K. (2015). Insulin/Insulin-like growth factors in cancer: New roles for the aryl hydrocarbon receptor, tumor resistance mechanisms, and new blocking strategies. *Frontiers in Endocrinology (Lausanne), 2*(6), 12. doi:10.3389/fendo.2015.00012.
8. Miklossy, G., Hilliard, T. S., & Turkson, J. (2013). Therapeutic modulators of STAT signaling for human diseases. *Nature Reviews Drug Discovery, 12*(8), 611–629. doi:10.1038/nrd4088.
9. Prada, P. O., & Saad, M. J. (2013). Tyrosine kinase inhibitors as novel drugs for the treatment of diabetes. *Expert Opinion on Investigational Drugs, 22*(6), 751–763. doi:10.1517/13543784.2013.802768.
10. Wang, C., Liu, Y., & Cao, J. M. (2014). G protein-coupled receptors: Extranuclear mediators for the non-genomic actions of steroids. *International Journal of Molecular Sciences, 15*(9), 15412–15425. doi:10.3390/ijms150915412.
11. Lazar, M. A. (2011). Mechanism of action of hormones that act on nuclear receptors. In S. Melmed, K. S. Polonsky, P. R. Larsen, et al. (Eds.), *Williams textbook of endocrinology* (12th ed.). Philadelphia: Saunders.
12. Annunziata, M., Granata, R., & Ghigo, E. (2011). The IGF system. *Acta Diabetologica, 48*(1), 1–9. doi:10.1007/s00592-010-0227-z.
13. Baxter, R. C. (2014). IGF binding proteins in cancer: Mechanistic and clinical insights. *Nature Reviews. Cancer, 14*(5), 329–341. doi:10.1038/nrc3720.
14. Reed, M. L., Merriam, G. R., & Kargi, A. Y. (2013). Adult growth hormone deficiency—Benefits, side effects, and risks of growth hormone replacement. *Frontiers in Endocrinology, 4*, 64. doi:10.3389/fendo.2013.00064.
15. Pereira Suarez, A. L., López-Rincón, G., Martínez Neri, P. A., et al. (2015). Prolactin in inflammatory response. *Advances in Experimental Medicine and Biology, 846*, 243–264. doi:10.1007/978-3-319-12114-7_11.
16. Robinson, A. G., & Verbalis, J. (2011). Posterior pituitary. In S. Melmed, K. S. Polonsky, P. R. Larsen, et al. (Eds.), *Williams textbook of endocrinology* (12th ed.). Philadelphia: Saunders.
17. Oba, Y., & Lone, N. A. (2014). Mortality benefit of vasopressor and inotropic agents in septic shock: A Bayesian network meta-analysis of randomized controlled trials. *Journal of Critical Care, 29*(5), 706–710. doi:10.1016/j.jcrc.2014.04.011.
18. Russell, J. A. (2011). Bench-to-bedside review: Vasopressin in the management of septic shock. *Critical Care, 15*(4), 226–245. doi:10.1186/cc8224.
19. Lochner, A., Huisman, B., & Nduhirabandi, F. (2013). Cardioprotective effect of melatonin against ischaemia/reperfusion damage. *Frontiers in Bioscience (Elite Edition), 5*, 305–315.
20. Anderson, G., & Maes, M. (2014). Local melatonin regulates inflammation resolution: A common factor in neurodegenerative, psychiatric and systemic inflammatory disorders. *CNS and Neurological Disorders Drug Targets, 13*(5), 817–827. doi:10.2174/1871527313666140711091400.
21. Verloop, H., Dekkers, O. M., Peeters, R. P., et al. (2014). Genetics in endocrinology: Genetic variation in deiodinases: A systematic review of potential clinical effects in humans. *European Journal of Endocrinology, 171*(3), R123–R135. doi:10.1530/EJE-14-0302.
22. Salvatore, D., Davies, T. F., Schlumberger, M. J., et al. (2011). Thyroid physiology and diagnostic evaluation of patients with thyroid disorders. In S. Melmed, K. S. Polonsky, P. R. Larsen, et al. (Eds.), *Williams textbook of endocrinology* (12th ed.). Philadelphia: Saunders.
23. Shoemaker, T. J., Kono, T., Mariash, C. N., et al. (2012). Thyroid hormone analogues for the treatment of metabolic disorders: New potential for unmet clinical needs? *Endocrine Practice, 18*(6), 954–964. doi:10.4158/EP12086.RA.
24. Janz, T., & Pearson, C. (2015). *Health at a glance: Vitamin D blood levels of Canadians* (Statistics Canada Catalogue no. 82-624-X). Retrieved from http://www.statcan.gc.ca/pub/82-624-x/2013001/article/11727-eng.htm.
25. Castiglioni, S., Cazzaniga, A., Albisetti, W., et al. (2013). Magnesium and osteoporosis: Current state of knowledge and future research directions. *Nutrients, 5*(8), 3022–3033. doi:10.3390/nu5083022.
26. Buse, J. B., Polonsky, K. S., & Burant, C. F. (2011). Type II diabetes mellitus. In S. Melmed, K. S. Polonsky, P. R. Larsen, et al. (Eds.), *Williams textbook of endocrinology* (12th ed.). Philadelphia: Saunders.
27. Conn, V. S., Koopman, R. J., Ruppar, T. M., et al. (2014). Insulin sensitivity following exercise interventions: Systematic review and meta-analysis of outcomes among healthy adults. *Journal of Primary Care & Community Health, 5*(3), 211–222. doi:10.1177/2150131913520328.
28. Yang, F. (2014). Amylin in vasodilation, energy expenditure and inflammation. *Frontiers in Bioscience (Landmark Edition), 19*, 936–944. doi:10.2741/4258.
29. Gylfe, E., & Gilon, P. (2014). Glucose regulation of glucagon secretion. *Diabetes Research and Clinical Practice, 103*(1), 1–10. doi:10.1016/j.diabres.2013.11.019.
30. Vella, A., & Drucker, D. J. (2011). Gastrointestinal hormones and gut endocrine tumors. In S. Melmed, K. S. Polonsky, P. R. Larsen, et al. (Eds.), *Williams textbook of endocrinology* (12th ed.). Philadelphia: Saunders.
31. Stores, R. D., & Cone, J. K. (2011). Neuroendocrine control of energy stores. In S. Melmed, K. S. Polonsky, P. R. Larsen, et al. (Eds.), *Williams textbook of endocrinology* (12th ed.). Philadelphia: Saunders.
32. Stewart, P. M., & Krone, N. P. (2011). The adrenal cortex. In S. Melmed, K. S. Polonsky, P. R. Larsen, et al. (Eds.), *Williams textbook of endocrinology* (12th ed.). Philadelphia: Saunders.
33. Bollag, W. B. (2014). Regulation of aldosterone synthesis and secretion. *Comprehensive Physiology, 4*(3), 1017–1055. doi:10.1002/cphy.c130037.
34. Lamberts, S. W. (2011). Endocrinology of aging. In S. Melmed, K. S. Polonsky, P. R. Larsen, et al. (Eds.), *Williams textbook of endocrinology* (12th ed.). Philadelphia: Saunders.
35. Young, W. F. (2011). Endocrine hypertension. In S. Melmed, K. S. Polonsky, P. R. Larsen, et al. (Eds.), *Williams textbook of endocrinology* (12th ed.). Philadelphia: Saunders.

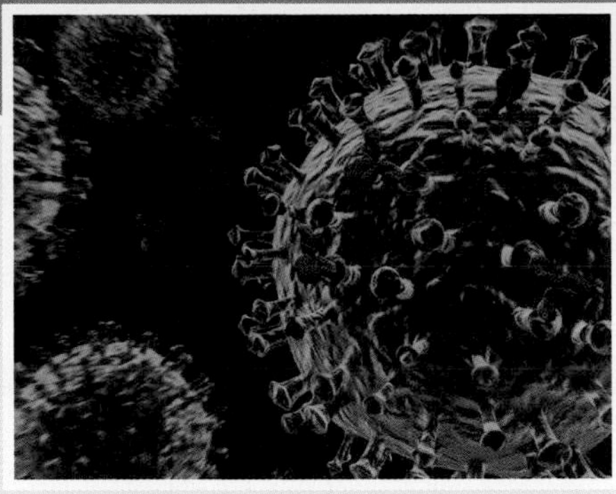

19

Alterations of Hormonal Regulation

Valentina L. Brashers, Robert E. Jones, Sue E. Huether, and Kelly Power-Kean

EVOLVE WEBSITE

http://evolve.elsevier.com/Canada/Huether/pathophysiology
Student Review Questions
Key Points
Case Studies
Animations
Quick Check Answers

CHAPTER OUTLINE

Mechanisms of Hormonal Alterations, 465
Alterations of the Hypothalamic-Pituitary System, 466
Diseases of the Posterior Pituitary, 466
Diseases of the Anterior Pituitary, 468
Alterations of Thyroid Function, 471
Thyrotoxicosis/Hyperthyroidism, 471
Hypothyroidism, 473
Thyroid Carcinoma, 474
Alterations of Parathyroid Function, 474
Hyperparathyroidism, 474
Hypoparathyroidism, 475
Dysfunction of the Endocrine Pancreas: Diabetes Mellitus, 476
Types of Diabetes Mellitus, 476
Acute Complications of Diabetes Mellitus, 482
Chronic Complications of Diabetes Mellitus, 483
Alterations of Adrenal Function, 487
Disorders of the Adrenal Cortex, 487
Tumours of the Adrenal Medulla, 490

Functions of the endocrine system involve complex interactions between hormones and most body systems that maintain dynamic steady states and influence tissue growth and reproductive capabilities. Endocrine system dysfunction is usually caused by hypersecretion or hyposecretion of the various hormones, leading to abnormal hormone concentrations in the blood. Dysfunction also may result from abnormal cell receptor function or from altered intracellular response to the hormone-receptor complex.

MECHANISMS OF HORMONAL ALTERATIONS

Significantly elevated or significantly depressed hormone levels may result from various causes (Table 19-1). Dysfunction of an endocrine gland may involve its failure to produce adequate amounts of biologically free or active hormone (hyposecretion), or a gland may synthesize or release too much hormone (hypersecretion). Feedback systems that recognize the need for a particular hormone may fail to function properly or may respond to inappropriate signals. Once hormones are released into the circulation, they may be degraded at an altered rate or be inactivated before reaching the target cell by antibodies that function as circulating hormone inhibitors (e.g., thyroid disease). Other causes of decreased hormone delivery to the target cell include an inadequate blood supply to the gland or target tissues or an insufficient amount of the appropriate carrier proteins in the serum. Ectopic sources of hormones (hormones produced by nonendocrine tissues) may cause abnormally elevated hormone levels without the benefit of the normal feedback system for hormone control (e.g., hormone-producing tumours); in this case, the ectopic hormone production is said to be autonomous.

Target cells may not respond appropriately to hormonal stimulation for a number of reasons. The following are the two general types of target cell insensitivity to hormones:

1. *Cell surface receptor–associated disorders.* These disorders have been identified primarily in water-soluble hormones, such as insulin. They may involve a decrease in the number of receptors, leading to decreased or defective hormone-receptor binding; impairment of receptor function, resulting in insensitivity to the hormone; presence of antibodies against specific receptors that either reduce available binding sites or mimic hormone action, suppressing or exaggerating, respectively, the target cell response; or unusual expression of receptor function, as occurs in some tumour cells.
2. *Intracellular disorders.* These disorders involve acquired defects in postreceptor signalling cascades or inadequate synthesis of a second messenger, such as cyclic adenosine monophosphate (cAMP), needed to transduce the hormonal signal into intracellular events. The target cell for water-soluble hormones may have a faulty response to hormone-receptor binding and thus fail to generate the required second messenger, or the cell may respond abnormally to the second messenger if levels of intracellular enzymes or proteins are altered. (Second messengers for various hormones are listed in Table 18-3.) As a result, the target cell fails to express the usual hormonal effect (e.g., pseudohypoparathyroidism, see p. 475).

TABLE 19-1 Mechanisms of Hormone Alterations

Inappropriate Amounts of Hormone Delivered to Target Cell	Inappropriate Response by Target Cell
Inadequate Hormone Synthesis	**Cell Surface Receptor–Associated Disorders**
1. Inadequate quantity of hormone precursors	1. Decrease in the number of receptors
2. Secretory cell unable to convert precursors to active hormone	2. Impaired receptor function (altered affinity for hormones)
Failure of Feedback Systems	3. Presence of antibodies against specific receptors
1. Do not recognize positive feedback, leading to inadequate hormone synthesis	4. Unusual expression of receptor function
2. Do not recognize negative feedback, leading to excessive hormone synthesis	
Inactive Hormones	**Intracellular Disorders**
1. Inadequate biologically free hormone	1. Acquired defects in postreceptor signalling cascades
2. Hormone degraded at an altered rate	2. Inadequate synthesis of a second messenger
3. Circulating hormone inhibitors	3. Intracellular enzymes or proteins are altered
Dysfunctional Delivery System	
1. Inadequate blood supply	4. Alterations in nuclear co-regulators
2. Inadequate carrier proteins	
3. Ectopic production of hormones	5. Altered protein synthesis

Pathogenic mechanisms affecting target cell response for lipid-soluble hormones are recognized less often than those affecting water-soluble hormones. When they do occur, the mechanisms are similar to those for water-soluble hormones, including changes in the number and binding affinity of intracellular receptors or altered generation of new messenger RNA (mRNA) and substrates for new protein synthesis. In other cases, hormone responsiveness may be linked to alterations in nuclear co-regulators, which are proteins (such as cAMP response element–binding protein) that facilitate or inhibit the transcription of the target gene.[1]

ALTERATIONS OF THE HYPOTHALAMIC-PITUITARY SYSTEM

Perhaps the most common cause of apparent hypothalamic dysfunction is interruption of the pituitary stalk caused by destructive lesions, rupture after head injury, surgical transection, or tumour. In these cases, interruption of the physical connections between the hypothalamus and the pituitary gland causes apparent pituitary disease. For example, without hypothalamic hormones (Figure 19-1), women cease to menstruate and men experience hypogonadism and impaired spermatogenesis. Adrenocorticotropic hormone (ACTH) response to low serum cortisol levels is decreased because of the absence of corticotropin-releasing hormone (CRH). Hypothalamic hypothyroidism is caused by the absence of thyrotropin-releasing hormone (TRH). Low levels of growth hormone–releasing hormone (GHRH) result in growth hormone (GH) deficiency and growth failure in children. Hyperprolactinemia is caused by an absence of the usual inhibitory control of prolactin secretion (dopamine).

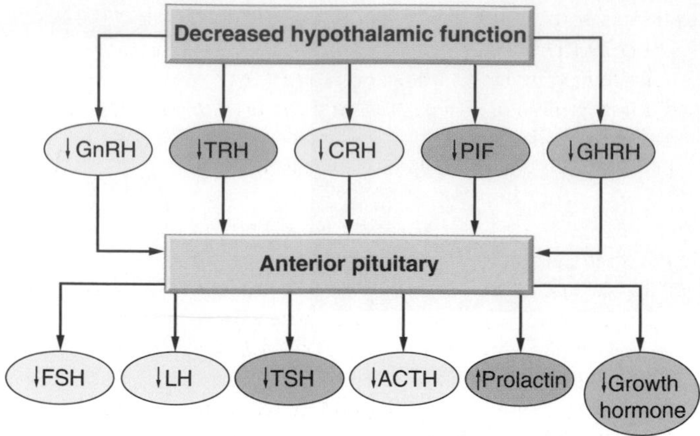

FIGURE 19-1 Loss of Hypothalamic Hormones. *ACTH*, adrenocorticotropic hormone; *CRH*, corticotropin-releasing hormone; *FSH*, follicle-stimulating hormone; *GHRH*, growth hormone–releasing hormone; *GnRH*, gonadotropin-releasing hormone; *LH*, luteinizing hormone; *PIF*, prolactin-inhibiting factor (probably dopamine); *TRH*, thyrotropin-releasing hormone; *TSH*, thyroid-stimulating hormone.

Diseases of the Posterior Pituitary

Diseases of the posterior pituitary cause abnormal secretion of antidiuretic hormone (ADH, also called *arginine vasopressin*). An excess amount of this hormone results in water retention and a hypo-osmolar state, whereas deficiencies in the amount or response to ADH result in serum hyperosmolarity (see Chapter 5). These complex pathophysiological states not only have significant clinical effects on the modulation of body fluids and electrolytes but also affect cognitive and emotional responses to stress.

Syndrome of Inappropriate Antidiuretic Hormone

The **syndrome of inappropriate antidiuretic hormone (SIADH)** is characterized by high levels of ADH in the absence of normal physiological stimuli for its release. A common cause of SIADH is the ectopic production of ADH by tumours, such as small cell carcinoma of the duodenum, stomach, and pancreas; cancers of the bladder, prostate, and endometrium; lymphomas; and sarcomas. Pulmonary disorders associated with SIADH include bronchogenic carcinoma, pneumonia (e.g., tuberculosis), asthma, cystic fibrosis, and respiratory failure requiring mechanical ventilation. Central nervous system disorders that may cause SIADH include encephalitis, meningitis, intracranial hemorrhage, tumours, and trauma.

Another important cause of SIADH is surgery. Any surgery can result in increased ADH secretion for as long as 5 to 7 days after surgery. The precise mechanism is uncertain but is likely related to fluid and volume changes following surgery, the amount and type of intravenous fluids given, and the use of opioid analgesics. Transient SIADH also may follow pituitary surgery because stored ADH is released in an unregulated fashion.[2]

Medications are an important cause of SIADH, especially in older adults. These include hypoglycemic medications (e.g., glyburide [Glycron]), opioids, general anaesthetics, antidepressants, antipsychotics, chemotherapeutic agents, nonsteroidal anti-inflammatory medications, and synthetic ADH analogues.[3]

PATHOPHYSIOLOGY The cardinal features of SIADH are the result of enhanced renal water retention. ADH increases renal collecting duct permeability to water by inducing the insertion of aquaporin-2, a water channel protein, into the tubular luminal membrane, which increases water reabsorption by the kidneys.[4] (Renal function is discussed in Chapter 29.) This water reabsorption results in an expansion of extracellular fluid volume that leads to dilutional hyponatremia (low serum sodium concentration), hypo-osmolarity, and urine that is inappropriately concentrated with respect to serum osmolarity because water is reabsorbed that normally would be excreted.

CLINICAL MANIFESTATIONS The symptoms of SIADH result from hyponatremia (see Chapter 5) and are determined by its severity and rapidity of onset. Thirst, impaired taste, anorexia, dyspnea on exertion, fatigue, and dulled sensorium occur when the serum sodium level decreases rapidly from 140 to 130 mmol/L. Peripheral edema is absent. Gastro-intestinal (GI) symptoms, including vomiting and abdominal cramps, occur with a drop in sodium concentration from 130 to 120 mmol/L. There is weight gain from water retention, even with nausea and vomiting. Even if hyponatremia develops slowly, serum sodium levels below 110 to 115 mmol/L cause confusion, lethargy, muscle twitching, and convulsions; severe and sometimes irreversible neurological damage may occur. Symptoms usually resolve with correction of hyponatremia (see Chapter 5).

EVALUATION AND TREATMENT A diagnosis of SIADH requires the following manifestations: (1) serum hypo-osmolality and hyponatremia; (2) urine hyperosmolarity (i.e., urine osmolality is greater than expected for the concomitant serum osmolality); (3) urine sodium excretion that matches sodium intake (i.e., sodium excretion is normal in spite of excessive water reabsorption); (4) normal adrenal and thyroid function; and (5) absence of conditions that can alter volume status (e.g., heart failure, hypovolemia from any cause, or renal insufficiency).

The treatment of SIADH involves the correction of any underlying causal problems and fluid restriction with careful monitoring of sodium status and neurological symptoms. In severe SIADH, emergency correction of severe hyponatremia by careful administration of hypertonic saline may be required. Resolution usually occurs within 3 days, with a 2- to 3-kg weight loss and correction of hyponatremia and salt wasting. If hyponatremia is corrected too rapidly, a severe neurological syndrome called *central pontine myelinolysis* can ensue. Demeclocycline (Declomycin), which causes the renal tubules to develop resistance to ADH, may be used to treat resistant or chronic SIADH. Vasopressin (ADH) receptor antagonists, known as *vaptans*, have recently been shown to be effective in treating SIADH.[5]

Diabetes Insipidus

Diabetes insipidus (DI) is an insufficiency of ADH activity, leading to polyuria (frequent urination) and polydipsia (frequent drinking). The two forms of DI are as follows:

1. *Neurogenic or central DI.* Caused by the insufficient secretion of ADH, it occurs when any organic lesion of the hypothalamus, pituitary stalk, or posterior pituitary interferes with ADH synthesis, transport, or release. Causative lesions include primary brain tumours, hypophysectomy, aneurysms, thrombosis, infections, and immunological disorders. Central DI is a well-recognized complication of traumatic brain injury. It can also be caused by hereditary disorders that affect ADH genes or result in structural changes in the pituitary gland.
2. *Nephrogenic DI.* Caused by inadequate response of the renal tubules to ADH, nephrogenic DI is usually acquired or may be genetic. Acquired nephrogenic DI is generally related to disorders and medications that damage the renal tubules or inhibit the generation of cAMP in the tubules. These disorders include pyelonephritis, amyloidosis, destructive uropathies, and polycystic kidney disease, all of which lead to irreversible DI. Medications that may induce a reversible form of nephrogenic DI include lithium carbonate, colchicines, amphotericin B, loop diuretics, general anaesthetics (such as methoxyflurane [Penthrane]), and demeclocycline (Declomycin). Several genetic causes of nephrogenic DI have been identified. One of the best described is a mutation in the gene that codes for aquaporin-2, which is one of the four water transport channels in the renal tubule.[6]

There is a rare form of DI associated with pregnancy. In gestational DI, the level of the vasopressin-degrading enzyme vasopressinase is increased. Clinical manifestations are usually mild and do not require treatment.[4,7]

Dipsogenic or *primary polydipsia* may be confused with DI. It is caused by the chronic ingestion of extremely large quantities of fluid that wash out the renal medullary concentration gradient, which results in a partial resistance to ADH. This condition resolves with decreased fluid ingestion. Psychogenic causes of polydipsia must be differentiated from true DI because administering an ADH analogue to an individual with psychogenic DI will result in severe hypo-osmolality.

PATHOPHYSIOLOGY Individuals with DI have a partial to total inability to concentrate urine. Insufficient ADH activity causes excretion of large volumes of dilute urine, leading to increased plasma osmolality. In conscious individuals, the thirst mechanism is stimulated and induces polydipsia—usually a craving for cold drinks. Dehydration develops rapidly without ongoing fluid replacement. If the individual with DI cannot conserve as much water as is lost in the urine, serum hypernatremia and hyperosmolality occur. Concentrations of other serum electrolytes generally are not affected.

CLINICAL MANIFESTATIONS The clinical manifestations of DI include polyuria, nocturia, continuous thirst, and polydipsia. The urine output is varied but can increase from the normal output of 1 to 2 L/day to as much as 8 to 12 L/day and can be higher than daily fluid intake. Individuals with longstanding DI develop a large bladder capacity and hydronephrosis (see Chapter 30). Neurogenic DI usually has an abrupt onset, and many individuals can specifically recall the date of onset of their symptoms. Nephrogenic DI usually has a more gradual onset. Table 19-2 compares the signs and symptoms of DI and SIADH.

TABLE 19-2 Signs and Symptoms of Diabetes Insipidus and Syndrome of Inappropriate Antidiuretic Hormone

Signs and Symptoms	Diabetes Inspidus	Syndrome of Inappropriate Antidiuretic Hormone
Urine output	High	Low (no hypovolemia)
Urine osmolality	Low (<100–200 mmol/kg H_2O)	High (>800 mmol/kg H_2O)
Urine specific gravity	Low (<1.010)	High (>1.020)
Serum sodium	Hypernatremia (>145 mmol/L)	Hyponatremia (<135 mmol/L)
Serum osmolality	Hyperosmolar (>300 mmol/kg)	Hypo-osmolar (<285 mmol/kg)
Symptoms	Polyuria, thirst, high urine output, signs of dehydration	Water retention, low urine output, nausea, vomiting, mental changes

EVALUATION AND TREATMENT DI must be distinguished from other polyuric states, including diabetes mellitus, osmotically induced diuresis, and psychogenic polydipsia. The criteria for the diagnosis of DI include low urine specific gravity, low urine osmolality, hypernatremia, high serum osmolality, and continued diuresis despite a serum sodium concentration of 145 mmol/L or greater. The diagnosis of DI is generally confirmed through water deprivation testing. Psychogenic polydipsia can be differentiated from nephrogenic DI based on plasma ADH levels. ADH levels are low in psychogenic polydipsia and normal or high in nephrogenic DI.

Treatment of neurogenic DI is based on the extent of the ADH deficiency and on the patient's age, endocrine and cardiovascular status, and lifestyle. Some individuals require ADH replacement, but fluid replacement using oral or intravenous routes is usually adequate. ADH replacement therapy for symptomatic central or neurogenic DI includes intravascular or, more commonly, oral or intranasal administration of the synthetic vasopressin analogue desmopressin (DDAVP).[8] Management of nephrogenic DI requires treatment of any reversible underlying disorders, discontinuation of etiological medications, and correction of associated electrolyte disorders. Surprisingly, thiazide diuretics may improve renal tubular salt and water retention in individuals with moderate nephrogenic DI. New treatments aimed at reversing aquaporin-2 dysfunction are being developed.[6] Medications that potentiate the action of otherwise insufficient amounts of endogenous ADH, such as chlorpropamide, carbamazepine (Tegretol), and clofibrate (Atromid), may be used in individuals with incomplete ADH deficiency.

Diseases of the Anterior Pituitary

Hypopituitarism

Hypopituitarism can be characterized by the absence of one or more anterior pituitary hormones or the complete failure of all anterior pituitary hormone functions. Hypopituitarism results from either an inadequate supply of hypothalamic-releasing hormones, because of damage to the pituitary stalk, or an inability of the gland to produce hormones. The most common causes of hypopituitarism are pituitary infarction or space-occupying lesions, such as pituitary adenomas or aneurysms. Pituitary infarction may occur in women during the postpartum period (Sheehan's syndrome) because of blood loss and hypovolemic shock.[9] Traumatic brain injury is increasingly recognized as an important cause of hypopituitarism and can have a significant impact on acute and long-term recovery.[10] Other causes of hypopituitarism include removal or destruction of the gland, infections (e.g., meningitis, syphilis, tuberculosis), autoimmune hypophysitis, certain medications (e.g., bexarotene [Targretin], carbamazepine, ipilimumab [Yervoy]), or mutation of the prophet of pituitary transcription factor (*PROP-1*) gene involved in early embryonic pituitary development.[11]

PATHOPHYSIOLOGY The pituitary gland is highly vascular and relies heavily upon portal blood flow from the hypothalamus. It is, therefore, vulnerable to ischemia and infarction. Infarction results in tissue necrosis and edema with swelling of the gland. Expansion of the pituitary within the fixed compartment of the sella turcica further impedes blood supply to the pituitary. Over time, fibrosis of pituitary tissue occurs and the symptoms of hypopituitarism develop. Adenomas and aneurysms may compress otherwise normal secreting pituitary cells and lead to compromised hormonal output.

CLINICAL MANIFESTATIONS The signs and symptoms of hypofunction of the anterior pituitary are variable and depend on which hormones are affected. In **panhypopituitarism**, all hormones are deficient and the individual suffers from multiple complications, including cortisol deficiency from lack of ACTH, thyroid deficiency from lack of thyroid-stimulating hormone (TSH), and loss of secondary sex characteristics because of the lack of follicle-stimulating hormone (FSH) and luteinizing hormone (LH). Low levels of GH and insulinlike growth factor 1 (IGF-1) affect growth in children and can cause physiological and psychological symptoms in adults. Finally, postpartum women cannot lactate because of decreased or absent prolactin.

ACTH deficiency with associated loss of cortisol is a potentially life-threatening disorder. ACTH deficiency usually is encountered with generalized pituitary hypofunction; it rarely occurs as an isolated event. Within 2 weeks of the complete absence of ACTH, symptoms of cortisol insufficiency develop, including nausea, vomiting, anorexia, fatigue, and weakness. Hypoglycemia results from increased insulin sensitivity, decreased glycogen reserves, and decreased gluconeogenesis associated with hypocortisolism. ACTH deficiency also limits maximal aldosterone secretion, although the renin-angiotensin system can stimulate some aldosterone secretion. The glomerular filtration rate decreases, causing decreased urine output.

TSH deficiency is rarely seen in isolation but often occurs with other pituitary hormone deficiencies. Symptoms develop 4 to 8 weeks after hypothyrotropinemia occurs and include cold intolerance, skin dryness, mild myxedema, lethargy, and decreased metabolic rate. The symptoms usually are less severe than those of primary hypothyroidism.

The onset of FSH and LH deficiencies in women of reproductive age is associated with amenorrhea and atrophy of the vagina, uterus, and breasts. In postpubertal males, the testicles atrophy and facial hair growth is diminished. Both men and women experience decreased body hair and diminished libido.

GH deficiency occurs in both children and adults. Several genetic defects have been identified in the GH axis in children, including a recessive mutation in the GH gene, resulting in a failure of GH secretion. Mutations also may involve the GH receptor, IGF-1 biosynthesis, IGF-1 receptors, or defects in GH signal transduction.[12] In adults, GH deficiency is most often caused by structural or functional abnormalities of the pituitary. In both children and adults, acute GH and IGF-1 deficiency has been implicated in significant metabolic perturbations seen with critical illness.

GH deficiency in children is manifested by growth failure and a condition known as hypopituitary dwarfism (Figure 19-2); however, not all children with short stature have GH deficiency. Symptoms of chronic adult GH deficiency syndrome include increased body fat, decreased strength and lean body mass, osteoporosis, reduced sweating, dry skin, and psychological problems, including depression, social withdrawal, fatigue, loss of motivation, and a diminished feeling of well-being. Without adequate GH replacement, increased mortality can occur as a result of myocardial infarction and stroke associated with dyslipidemias and atherosclerosis.[13]

EVALUATION AND TREATMENT The diagnostic evaluation of suspected pituitary disease is often challenging and must be carefully interpreted together with the individual's signs and symptoms. Simultaneous measurements of the levels of tropic hormones from the pituitary and target endocrine glands are crucial, and the more complicated dynamic testing of insulin, TRH, and gonadotropin-releasing hormone (GnRH) may be indicated. Imaging of the pituitary (magnetic resonance imaging [MRI] or computed tomography [CT] scans) is critical to assess for anatomical lesions, such as tumours.

Management of hypopituitarism requires correction of the underlying disorder as quickly as possible. Replacement of target gland hormones that are deficient because of lack of tropic anterior pituitary hormones is essential (such as cortisol, thyroid hormone, GH, and gender-specific steroid hormones).[14] In cases of circulatory collapse, immediate therapy with glucocorticoids and intravenous fluids is critical.

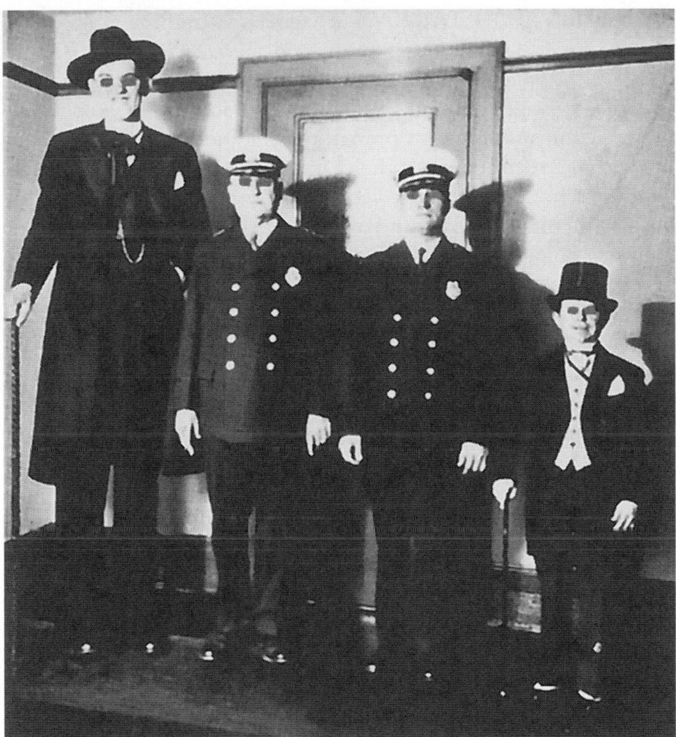

FIGURE 19-2 Hypopituitary Dwarfism and Pituitary Giantism. A pituitary giant and dwarf contrasted with normal-size men. Excessive secretion of growth hormone by the anterior lobe of the pituitary gland during the early years of life produces giants of this type, whereas deficient secretion of this substance produces well-formed dwarfs. (From Patton, K.T., & Thibodeau, G.A. [2013]. *Anatomy & physiology* [8th ed.]. St. Louis: Mosby.)

Hyperpituitarism: Primary Adenoma

Pituitary adenomas usually are benign, slow-growing tumours that arise from cells of the anterior pituitary. The cause of pituitary adenomas is not known and most occur sporadically. Altered gene expression is commonly detected and familial pituitary adenomas occur as part of syndromes affecting other organs, such as multiple endocrine neoplasia.[15] Most are microscopic (microadenomas) and are found only on post-mortem examinations or incidentally discovered on MRI examinations. The majority of pituitary microadenomas are hormonally silent and do not pose significant hazards to the individual. Larger adenomas (macroadenomas) are associated with morbidity and mortality attributable to alterations in hormone secretion or to invasion or impingement of surrounding structures.

PATHOPHYSIOLOGY Local expansion of the adenoma may impinge on the optic chiasma and cause various visual disturbances, depending on the portion of the nerve compressed. If the tumour is locally aggressive, invasion of the cavernous sinuses may occur, resulting in compromise of the oculomotor, trochlear, abducens, and trigeminal nerves with attending symptoms (see Table 13-6 for review of cranial nerves). Extension to the hypothalamus disturbs control of wakefulness, thirst, appetite, and temperature.

Hormonal effects of adenomas include hypersecretion from the adenoma itself and hyposecretion from surrounding pituitary cells. The adenomatous tissue secretes the hormone of the cell type from which it arose, without regard to the needs of the body and without benefit of regulatory feedback mechanisms (autonomous function). Because of the pressure exerted by the tumour in the unexpandable bony sella turcica, hyposecretion from those cells that are most sensitive to pressure is common (GH-, FSH-, and LH-secreting cells).[16]

CLINICAL MANIFESTATIONS The clinical manifestations of pituitary adenomas are related to tumour growth and hormone hypersecretion or hyposecretion. Increased tumour size causes headache, fatigue, neck pain or stiffness, and seizures. Visual changes include visual field impairments (often beginning in one eye and progressing to the other) and temporary blindness. If the tumour infiltrates other cranial nerves, neuromuscular function is affected.

Pituitary adenomas are most often associated with increased secretion of GH and prolactin (see "Hypersecretion of Growth Hormone: Acromegaly" and "Prolactinoma"). Gonadotropic hyposecretion results in menstrual irregularity in women, decreased libido, and receding secondary sex characteristics in both men and women. If the tumour exerts sufficient pressure, thyroid and adrenal hypofunction may occur because of lack of TSH and ACTH, resulting in the symptoms of hypothyroidism and hypocortisolism, respectively.

EVALUATION AND TREATMENT Diagnosis of pituitary adenoma involves physical and laboratory evaluations, including pertinent hormone assays and radiographic examination of the skull (MRI [preferred] or contrast-enhanced CT). The goal of treatment is to protect the individual from the effects of tumour growth and to control hormone hypersecretion while minimizing damage to appropriately secreting portions of the pituitary. Depending on tumour size and type, individuals may be treated by administration of specific medications to suppress tumour growth, trans-sphenoidal tumour resection, or radiation therapy including stereotactic treatments.[16]

QUICK CHECK 19-1

1. What is the mechanism of cell surface receptor–associated disorders?
2. Why do individuals with the syndrome of inappropriate antidiuretic hormone (SIADH) secrete concentrated urine?
3. Why may individuals with a pituitary adenoma develop visual disturbances?

Hypersecretion of Growth Hormone: Acromegaly

Acromegaly results from continuous exposure to high levels of GH and IGF-1; it almost always is caused by a GH-secreting pituitary adenoma (it rarely results from the ectopic production of GHRH).[17]

Acromegaly usually occurs in adults in the 40- to 59-year-old age group, although it is often present for years before diagnosis. It is a slowly progressive disease and, if untreated, is associated with a decreased life expectancy. Deaths from acromegaly are caused by heart disease secondary to hypertension and coronary artery disease, stroke, diabetes mellitus, or malignancy (colon or lung cancers).

PATHOPHYSIOLOGY With a GH-secreting adenoma, the usual GH baseline secretion pattern and sleep-related GH peaks are lost, and a totally unpredictable secretory pattern ensues. However, GH levels in acromegalics are never completely suppressed. Only slight elevations of GH and IGF-1 can stimulate growth. In children and adolescents whose epiphyseal plates have not yet closed, the effect of increased GH levels is termed **giantism** (see Figure 19-2). Skeletal growth is excessive, with some individuals becoming 2.4 or 2.7 metres tall. In the adult, epiphyseal closure has occurred, and increased amounts of GH and IGF-1 cause connective tissue proliferation and increased cytoplasmic matrix, as well as bony proliferation that results in the characteristic appearance of acromegaly (Figure 19-3).

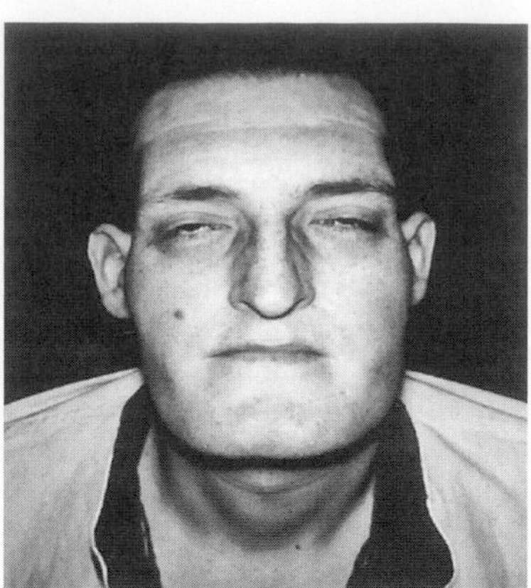

FIGURE 19-3 Acromegaly. (From McCance, K.L., & Huether, S.E. [2015]. *Pathophysiology: The biological basis for disease in adults and children* [7th ed.]. St. Louis: Elsevier, Figure 22-5.)

GH also has significant effects on glucose, lipid, and protein metabolism. Hyperglycemia results from adipocyte inflammation and GH inhibition of peripheral glucose uptake and increased hepatic glucose production, followed by compensatory hyperinsulinism and, finally, insulin resistance.[18] Diabetes mellitus occurs when the pancreas cannot secrete enough insulin to offset the effects of GH. Excessive levels of GH and IGF-1 also affect the cardiovascular system. Although the associated pathophysiological mechanism is not clearly understood at present, hypertension and left ventricular heart failure are seen in one-third to one-half of individuals with acromegaly. Cardiomyopathy associated with progressive and unrestrained myocardial growth is a significant factor.[19] GH also acts on the renal tubules to increase phosphate reabsorption, leading to mild hyperphosphatemia. Because the adenoma becomes increasingly a space-occupying lesion, hypopituitarism may occur because of compression of surrounding hormone-secreting cells. Hyperprolactinemia can occur in 30 to 40% of individuals with acromegaly.[17]

CLINICAL MANIFESTATIONS With connective tissue proliferation, individuals with acromegaly have an enlarged tongue, interstitial edema, enlarged and overactive sebaceous and sweat glands (leading to increased body odour), and coarse skin and body hair. Bony proliferation involves periosteal vertebral growth and enlargement of the bones of the face (see Figure 19-3), hands, and feet. The lower jaw and forehead also protrude. Skeletal abnormalities are irreversible.

Increased IGF-1 levels cause ribs to elongate at the bone-cartilage junction, leading to a barrel-chested appearance, and increased proliferation of cartilage in joints, which causes backache and arthralgias. With bony and soft tissue overgrowth, nerve entrapment occurs, leading to peripheral nerve damage manifested by weakness, muscular atrophy, footdrop, and sensory changes in the hands.

Symptoms of diabetes mellitus, such as polyuria and polydipsia, may occur because of decreased insulin sensitivity. Acromegaly-associated hypertension is usually asymptomatic until heart failure symptoms develop. Increased tumour size results in central nervous system symptoms of headache, seizure activity, visual disturbances, and papilledema. If compression hypopituitarism occurs, gonadotropin secretion may be affected, causing amenorrhea in women and sexual dysfunction in men. Approximately 20% of GH-secreting tumours also secrete prolactin, resulting in hypogonadism. Cardiovascular, metabolic, and tumour compression symptoms often improve with treatment.

EVALUATION AND TREATMENT Diagnosis is confirmed by clinical features of the disease, MRI scans, and elevated levels of IGF-1.[20] GH level is typically elevated and not suppressed with oral glucose tolerance testing. The goals of treatment are to normalize or reduce GH secretion and relieve or prevent complications related to tumour expansion. The treatment of choice in acromegaly is trans-sphenoidal surgical removal of the GH-secreting adenoma. Radiation therapy may be effective when rapid control of GH levels is not essential, when the individual is not a good surgical candidate, or when hyperfunction persists after subtotal resection. Somatostatin analogues, such as octreotide (SandoSTATIN), octreotide LAR (SandoSTATIN LAR), and lanreotide (Somatuline), normalize IGF-1 levels and lower GH levels. Pegvisomant (Somavert) can be used to supplement somatostatin analogues and is an effective medication that induces tissue insensitivity to GH by blocking the GH receptor.[17] Dopaminergic agonists, such as cabergoline (Dostinex), also may be helpful, especially if the tumour also secretes prolactin.

Prolactinoma

Pituitary tumours that secrete prolactin, **prolactinomas**, are the most common hormonally active pituitary tumours. Other conditions or medications can elevate prolactin levels in the absence of a pituitary pathological condition. For example, renal failure, polycystic ovarian disease, primary hypothyroidism, breast stimulation, or even the stress of venipuncture can increase prolactin levels. Prolactin is under tonic inhibitory hypothalamic control through the secretion of dopamine. Thus medications that block the effects of dopamine can increase prolactin level and stimulate proliferation of prolactin-secreting cells (lactotrophs). These include antipsychotics (risperidone [Risperdal], chlorpromazine [Largactil]), metoclopramide (Reglan), tricyclic antidepressants, and methyldopa (Aldomet). Estrogens increase prolactin concentration by stimulating hyperplasia of prolactin-secreting cells. Any process that interferes with the delivery of dopamine from the hypothalamus to the lactotrophs (pituitary stalk tumour, pituitary stalk transection, or compressive pituitary tumour) also results in hyperprolactinemia. Because TRH stimulates prolactin secretion, in addition to enhancing TSH release, prolactin concentration may be elevated in individuals with primary hypothyroidism.

PATHOPHYSIOLOGY The hallmark of a prolactinoma is sustained increases in the levels of serum prolactin. The physiological actions of prolactin include breast development during pregnancy, postpartum milk production, and suppression of ovarian function in nursing women. Pathological elevation of prolactin levels in women results in amenorrhea, nonpuerperal milk production (galactorrhea), hirsutism, and osteopenia or osteoporosis resulting from estrogen deficiency. Hyperprolactinemia in men causes hypogonadism and erectile dysfunction.

Because the adenoma becomes an increasingly space-occupying lesion, hypopituitarism may occur because of the compression of surrounding hormone-secreting cells. Central nervous system symptoms may develop because of growth and pressure of the adenoma within the sella turcica. These complications are especially common with what are called macro (greater than 1 cm in diameter) or giant (greater than 4 cm in diameter) prolactinomas and are often more difficult to treat.[21]

CLINICAL MANIFESTATIONS Women with hyperprolactinemia generally present with galactorrhea (nonpuerperal milk production) and menstrual disturbances including amenorrhea. In susceptible women, hirsutism develops because of estrogen deficiency. If not detected until after many years, this estrogen deficiency also may result in osteopenia or osteoporosis. Men often develop hypogonadism, gynecomastia, and erectile dysfunction, but may present late when symptoms related to the increasing size of the adenoma occur (i.e., headache or visual impairment).

EVALUATION AND TREATMENT The diagnostic evaluation of hyperprolactinemia includes a careful history to exclude medications that may cause elevations in prolactin concentration. Symptoms of hypothyroidism should be elicited, and screening with a serum TSH level is mandatory. MRI scanning of the pituitary is indicated to determine the size and location of an adenoma. If serum prolactin level is less than 50 mcg/L, a careful search for a nonpituitary cause should be pursued.

Dopaminergic agonists (cabergoline) are the treatment of choice for prolactinomas. Restoration of fertility in previously anovulatory women is common. In individuals resistant or intolerant to these medications, trans-sphenoidal surgery and radiotherapy are options.[22] New chemotherapeutic and targeted molecular therapies are being explored in selected cases.[23]

ALTERATIONS OF THYROID FUNCTION

Disorders of thyroid function develop as a result of primary dysfunction or disease of the thyroid gland or, secondarily, as a result of pituitary or hypothalamic alterations. **Primary thyroid disorders** result in alterations of thyroid hormone (TH) levels with secondary feedback effects on pituitary TSH. For example, when there are primary elevations in TH level, TSH level will secondarily decrease because of negative feedback. When TH level is decreased because of a condition affecting the thyroid gland, TSH level will be elevated. Thyroid disease also can present with minimal or no symptoms but with abnormal laboratory values, known as **subclinical thyroid disease**. **Central (secondary) thyroid disorders** are related to disorders of pituitary gland TSH production. When there is excessive TSH production, TH level is elevated secondary to the primary elevation of TSH concentration. The reverse is true with inadequate TSH production.

Thyrotoxicosis/Hyperthyroidism

PATHOPHYSIOLOGY **Thyrotoxicosis** is a condition that results from any cause of increased TH levels. **Hyperthyroidism** is a form of thyrotoxicosis in which excess amounts of TH are secreted from the thyroid gland (Figure 19-4). The terms *thyrotoxicosis* and *hyperthyroidism* are often used interchangeably. Common diseases that cause primary hyperthyroidism include Graves' disease, toxic multinodular goitre, and solitary toxic adenoma. *Central (secondary) hyperthyroidism* is less common and is caused by TSH-secreting pituitary adenomas. Thyrotoxicosis not associated with hyperthyroidism includes ectopic thyroid tissue and ingestion of excessive TH. Each condition is associated with a specific pathophysiology and manifestations; however, all forms of thyrotoxicosis share some common characteristics.

CLINICAL MANIFESTATIONS The clinical features of thyrotoxicosis are attributable to the metabolic effects of increased circulating levels of thyroid hormones. This usually results in an increased metabolic rate with heat intolerance and increased tissue sensitivity to stimulation by the sympathetic nervous system. The major manifestations are summarized in Figure 19-5. Enlargement of the thyroid gland (goitre) is common in hyperthyroid conditions caused by stimulation of TSH receptors.

Elevated serum thyroxine (T_4) and triiodothyronine (T_3) levels and suppressed serum TSH levels are diagnostic for primary hyperthyroidism. By contrast, central (secondary) hyperthyroidism caused by TSH-secreting pituitary tumours is characterized by normal to increased TSH levels

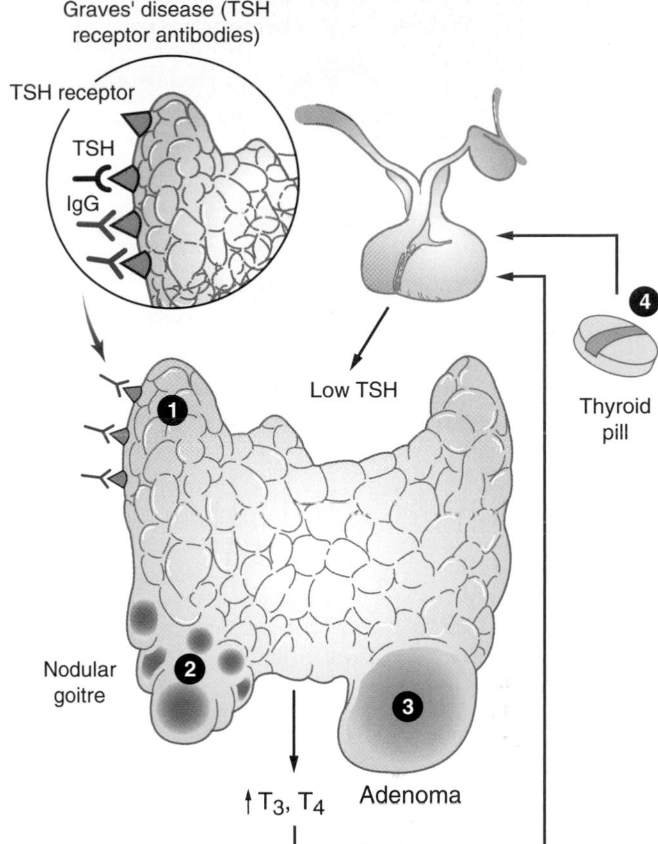

FIGURE 19-4 Common Causes of Hyperthyroidism. Hyperthyroidism may have several causes, among them: **1**, Graves' disease; **2**, toxic multinodular goitre; **3**, follicular adenoma; **4**, thyroid medication. *IgG*, immunoglobulin G; *TSH*, thyroid-stimulating hormone; T_4, thyroxine; T_3, triiodothyronine. (Adapted from Damjanov, I. [2012]. *Pathology for the health professions* [4th ed.]. St. Louis: Saunders.)

despite elevated TH concentrations. Radioactive iodine is used to test for increased uptake in primary hyperthyroidism (Figure 19-6). Treatment is directed at controlling excessive TH production, secretion, or action and employs antithyroid medication therapy, radioactive iodine therapy (absorbed only by thyroid tissue, causing death of cells), and surgery.[24] A major complication of all forms of treatment for hyperthyroidism is excessive ablation of the gland leading to hypothyroidism.

Graves' Disease

Graves' disease is the underlying cause of 50 to 80% of cases of hyperthyroidism with a prevalence of approximately 1% in the Canadian population. It occurs more commonly in women. Although the exact cause of Graves' disease is not known, genetic factors interacting with environmental triggers play an important role in the pathogenesis. Graves' disease is classified as an autoimmune disease and results from a form of type II hypersensitivity (see Chapter 8) in which there is stimulation of the thyroid by autoantibodies directed against the TSH receptor. These autoantibodies, called thyroid-stimulating immunoglobulins (TSIs), override the normal regulatory mechanisms. The TSI stimulation of TSH receptors in the gland results in hyperplasia of the gland (goitre) and increased synthesis of TH, especially of T_3. Increased levels of TH result in the classic signs and symptoms of hyperthyroidism illustrated in Figure 19-5. TSH production by the pituitary is inhibited through the usual negative feedback loop.[24,25]

TSI also contributes to the two major distinguishing clinical manifestations of Graves' disease (ophthalmopathy and dermopathy [pretibial

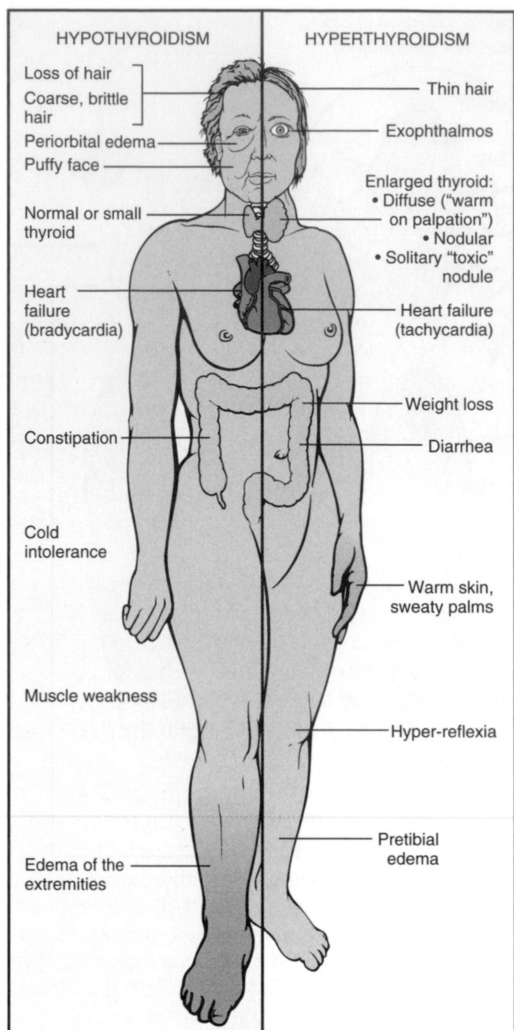

FIGURE 19-5 Clinical Manifestations of Hyperthyroidism and Hypothyroidism. (From Damjanov, I. [2012]. *Pathology for the health professions* [4th ed.]. St. Louis: Saunders.)

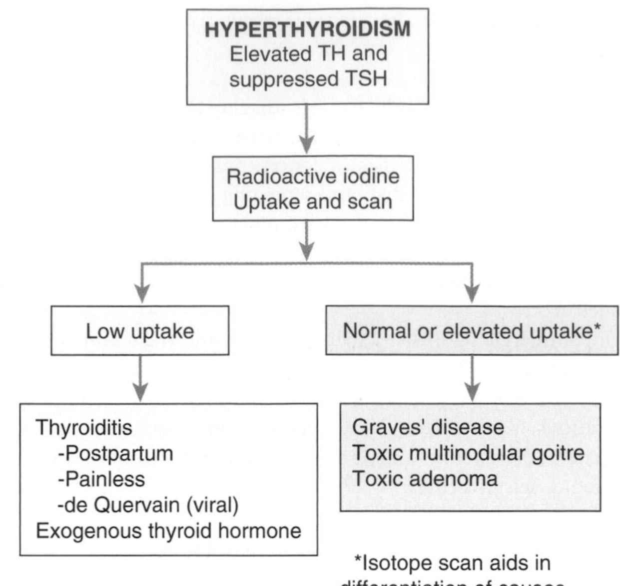

FIGURE 19-6 Evaluation of Hyperthyroidism. Radioactive iodine is used in the differential diagnosis of hyperthyroidism. *TH*, thyroid hormone; *TSH*, thyroid-stimulating hormone.

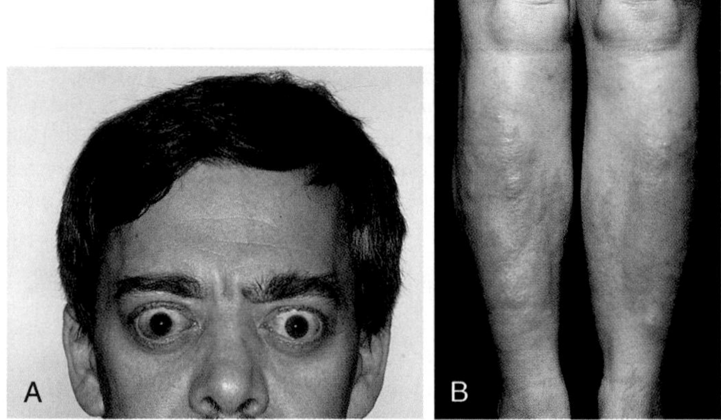

FIGURE 19-7 Thyrotoxicosis (Graves' Disease). A, Exophthalmos (large and protruding eyeballs often in association with a large goitre). **B,** Pretibial myxedema associated with Graves' disease; note lumpy and swollen appearance from accumulation of connective tissue and pinkish purple discoloration. (**A,** from Belchetz, P., & Hammond, P. [2003]. *Mosby's color atlas and text of diabetes and endocrinology*. Edinburgh: Mosby; **B,** from Habif, T. [2009]. *Clinical dermatology* [5th ed.]. St. Louis: Mosby.)

myxedema]). Two categories of ophthalmopathy associated with Graves' disease (Figure 19-7) are (1) functional abnormalities resulting from hyperactivity of the sympathetic division of the autonomic nervous system (lag of the globe on upward gaze and of the upper lid on downward gaze) and (2) infiltrative changes involving the orbital contents with enlargement of the ocular muscles. These changes affect more than half of individuals with Graves' disease. Orbital connective tissue accumulation, inflammation, and edema of the orbital contents result in exophthalmos (protrusion of the eyeball), periorbital edema, and extraocular muscle weakness, leading to diplopia (double vision).[26] The individual may experience irritation, pain, lacrimation, photophobia, blurred vision, decreased visual acuity, papilledema, visual field impairment, exposure keratosis, and corneal ulceration.

A small number of individuals with Graves' disease and very high levels of TSI experience **pretibial myxedema (Graves' dermopathy)**, characterized by subcutaneous swelling on the anterior portions of the legs and by indurated and erythematous skin. Graves' dermopathy is associated with thyrotropin receptor antigens on fibroblasts and recruited T lymphocytes (T cells) that stimulate excessive amounts of hyaluronic acid production in the dermis and subcutaneous tissue.[27] These manifestations occasionally appear on the hands, giving the appearance of clubbing of the fingers (thyroid acropachy).

Hyperthyroidism resulting from nodular thyroid disease. The thyroid gland normally enlarges in response to the increased demand for TH that occurs in puberty, pregnancy, and iodine-deficient states as well as in individuals with immunological, viral, or genetic disorders. When the condition resulting in increased TH resolves, TSH secretion normally subsides and the thyroid gland returns to its original size.

Irreversible changes can occur in some follicular cells so these cells function autonomously and produce excessive amounts of TH. On the other hand, some follicular cells may cease to function. The balance between the amount of TH produced by hyperfunctioning nodules and that produced by the remainder of the gland determines whether an individual develops hyperthyroidism. **Toxic multinodular goitre** occurs when there are several hyperfunctioning nodules leading to hyperthyroidism.

Unlike Graves' disease, there is absence of an autoimmune stimulus. If only one nodule is hyperfunctioning, it is termed toxic adenoma. The classic clinical manifestations of hyperthyroidism (see Figure 19-5) usually develop slowly, and exophthalmos and pretibial myxedema do not occur. Nodules may be palpable on physical examination and there is increased uptake of radioactive iodine. The incidence of malignancy in toxic nodular goitre is estimated to be as high as 9%, so most individuals should undergo a fine needle aspiration biopsy of suspicious nodules before treatment. Treatment consists of a combination of radioactive iodine, surgery, and antithyroid medications.[28]

Thyrotoxic crisis. Thyrotoxic crisis (thyroid storm) is a rare but dangerous worsening of the thyrotoxic state in which death can occur within 48 hours without treatment. The condition may develop spontaneously, but it usually occurs in individuals who have undiagnosed or partially treated Graves' disease and are subjected to excessive stress, such as infection, pulmonary or cardiovascular disorders, trauma, seizures, surgery (especially thyroid surgery), obstetrical complications, emotional distress, or dialysis. The symptoms of thyroid crisis are caused by the increased action of T_4 and T_3 exceeding metabolic demands.[29]

The systemic symptoms of thyrotoxic crisis include hyperthermia; tachycardia, especially atrial tachydysrhythmias; high-output heart failure; agitation or delirium; and nausea, vomiting, or diarrhea contributing to fluid volume depletion. Treatment includes (1) the use of medications that block TH synthesis (i.e., propylthiouracil or methimazole), (2) the use of beta-blockers for control of cardiovascular symptoms, the administration of (3) steroids or (4) iodine (e.g., saturated solution of potassium iodide [SSKI]), and (5) supportive care.

Hypothyroidism

Hypothyroidism results from deficient production of TH by the thyroid gland. Hypothyroidism is the most common disorder of thyroid function, affects 2% of the Canadian population, and occurs more commonly in women. It may be primary or central. Primary hypothyroidism accounts for 99% of all cases. Central (secondary) hypothyroidism is less common and is related to either pituitary or hypothalamic failure.

The most common cause of primary hypothyroidism in Canada is autoimmune thyroiditis (Hashimoto's disease, chronic lymphocytic thyroiditis), which results in gradual inflammatory destruction of thyroid tissue by infiltration of autoreactive T cells and circulating thyroid autoantibodies (antithyroid peroxidase and antithyroglobulin antibodies). This disorder is linked with several genetic risk factors and is commonly associated with other autoimmune conditions. Infiltration of thyroid autoantibodies, autoreactive T cells, natural killer cells, and inflammatory cytokines and induction of apoptosis are involved in the tissue destruction seen in Hashimoto's thyroiditis.[30] Radioactive iodine uptake is normal or elevated.

Spontaneous recovery of thyroid function is seen in three conditions: subacute thyroiditis, painless thyroiditis, and postpartum thyroiditis. Subacute thyroiditis (de Quervain's thyroiditis) is a rare nonbacterial inflammation of the thyroid gland often preceded by a viral infection. It is accompanied by fever, tenderness, and enlargement of the thyroid gland. The inflammatory process initially results in elevated levels of TH through the release of stored thyroglobulin, which then is associated with transient hypothyroidism before the gland recovers normal activity. Thyroid antibodies are not present in the blood. Symptoms may last for 2 to 4 months, and nonsteroidal anti-inflammatory medications or corticosteroids usually resolve symptoms. Painless (silent) thyroiditis has a course similar to that of subacute thyroiditis but is pathologically identical to Hashimoto's disease. Postpartum thyroiditis is pathologically related to Hashimoto's disease and generally occurs up to 6 months after delivery with a course similar to that seen in subacute thyroiditis. Thus a hyperthyroid phase (with a low thyroid radioiodine uptake) precedes the hypothyroid phase in typical cases of subacute, painless, or postpartum thyroiditis. Spontaneous recovery occurs in 95% of these conditions.

Congenital Hypothyroidism

Hypothyroidism in infants occurs when thyroid tissue is absent (thyroid dysgenesis) or with hereditary defects in TH synthesis. Thyroid dysgenesis occurs more often in female infants, with permanent abnormalities in 1 of every 4000 live births. Because TH is essential for embryonic growth, particularly of brain tissue, the infant will be cognitively disabled if there is no T_4 during fetal life.[31] The fetus is dependent on maternal T_4 for the first 20 weeks of gestation.[32] Hypothyroidism may not be evident at birth. Symptoms may include high birth weight, hypothermia, delay in passing meconium, and neonatal jaundice. Cord blood can be examined in the first days of life for measurement of T_4 and TSH levels. The probability of normal growth and intellectual function is high if treatment with levothyroxine is started before the child is 3 or 4 months old. The earlier TH replacement is initiated, the better the child's outcome.[33]

Without early screening, hypothyroidism may not be evident until after 4 months of age. Symptoms include difficulty eating, hoarse cry, and protruding tongue caused by myxedema of oral tissues and vocal cords; hypotonic muscles of the abdomen with constipation, abdominal protrusion, and umbilical hernia; subnormal temperature; lethargy; excessive sleeping; slow pulse rate; and cold, mottled skin. Skeletal growth is stunted because of impaired protein synthesis, poor absorption of nutrients, and lack of bone mineralization. The child will be dwarfed with short limbs, if not treated. Dentition is often delayed. Cognitive disability varies with the severity of hypothyroidism and the length of delay before treatment is initiated.

PATHOPHYSIOLOGY In *primary hypothyroidism*, loss of thyroid function leads to decreased production of TH and increased secretion of TSH and TRH (Figure 19-8). The most common causes of primary hypothyroidism in adults include autoimmune thyroiditis (Hashimoto's disease), iatrogenic loss of thyroid tissue after surgical or radioactive treatment for hyperthyroidism or after head and neck radiation therapy, medications (e.g., lithium and amiodarone [Cordarone]), and endemic iodine deficiency. Infants and children may present with hypothyroidism because of congenital defects. *Central (secondary) hypothyroidism* is

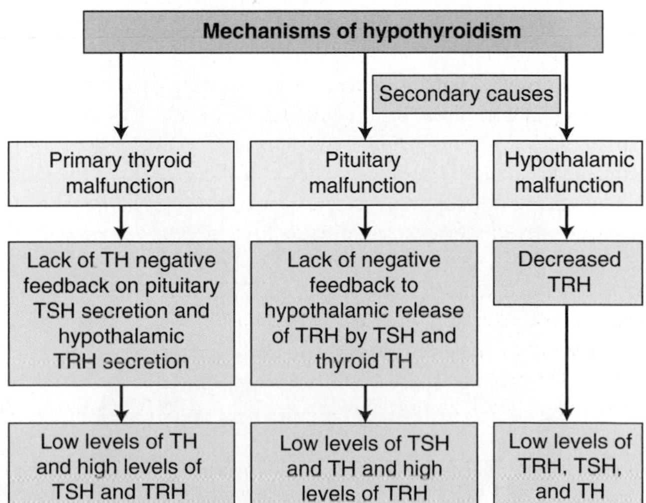

FIGURE 19-8 Mechanisms of Primary and Secondary Hypothyroidism. *TH,* thyroid hormone; *TRH,* thyrotropin-releasing hormone; *TSH,* thyroid-stimulating hormone.

caused by the pituitary's failure to synthesize adequate amounts of TSH or a lack of TRH. Pituitary tumours that compress surrounding pituitary cells or the consequences of their treatment are the most common causes of central hypothyroidism. Other causes include traumatic brain injury, subarachnoid hemorrhage, or pituitary infarction. Hypothalamic dysfunction results in low levels of TH, TSH, and TRH.[34] **Subclinical hypothyroidism** is a mild thyroid failure estimated to occur in 4 to 8% of adults. It is defined as an elevation in TSH levels with normal levels of circulating TH.[35]

CLINICAL MANIFESTATIONS Hypothyroidism generally affects all body systems and occurs insidiously over months or years. The decrease in TH level lowers energy metabolism and heat production. The individual develops a low basal metabolic rate, cold intolerance, lethargy, and slightly lowered basal body temperature (see Figure 19-5). The decrease in the level of TH can lead to excessive TSH production, which stimulates thyroid tissue and causes goitre.

The characteristic sign of severe or longstanding hypothyroidism is **myxedema**, which results from the altered composition of the dermis and other tissues. The connective tissue fibres are separated by large amounts of protein and mucopolysaccharide. This complex binds water, producing nonpitting, boggy edema, especially around the eyes, hands, and feet and in the supraclavicular fossae (Figure 19-9). The tongue and laryngeal and pharyngeal mucous membranes thicken, producing thick, slurred speech and hoarseness. **Myxedema coma**, a medical emergency, is a diminished level of consciousness associated with severe hypothyroidism. Signs and symptoms include hypothermia without shivering, hypoventilation, hypotension, hypoglycemia, and lactic acidosis. Older adults with comorbid conditions, such as pulmonary or urinary infections, heart failure, or cerebrovascular accident, and with moderate or untreated hypothyroidism are particularly at risk of developing myxedema coma. It also may occur after overuse of opioids or sedatives or after an acute illness in hypothyroid individuals. Symptoms of hypothyroidism in older adults should not be attributed to normal aging changes.[29]

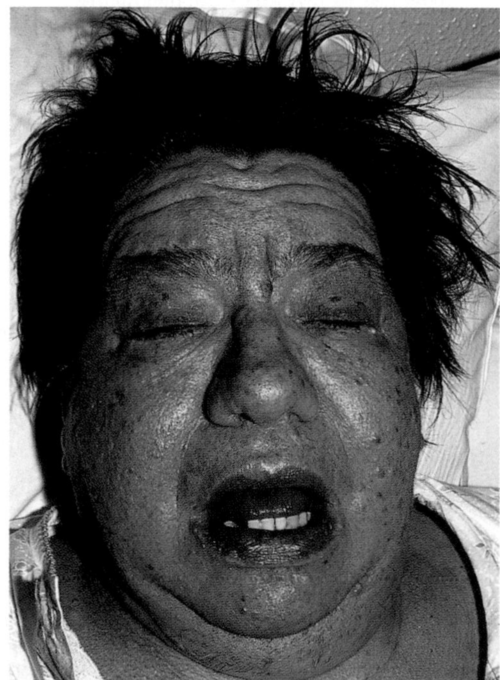

FIGURE 19-9 Myxedema. Note edema around eyes and facial puffiness. The hair is dry. (From Bolognia, J.L., Jorizzo, J., & Schaffer, J. [2012]. *Dermatology* [3rd ed.]. St. Louis: Mosby.)

EVALUATION AND TREATMENT The diagnosis of primary hypothyroidism is made by documentation of the clinical symptoms of hypothyroidism, and measurement of increased levels of TSH and decreased levels of TH (total T_3 and both total and free T_4). When hypothyroidism is caused by pituitary deficiencies, serum TSH levels and basal metabolic rate (BMR) decrease. Hormone replacement therapy with the hormone levothyroxine (Synthroid) is the treatment of choice. The restoration of normal TH levels should be timed appropriately; a regimen of hormonal therapy depends on the individual's age, the duration and severity of the hypothyroidism, and the presence of other disorders, particularly cardiovascular disorders.[36] Pregnant women need to be evaluated for thyroid function.[37]

Thyroid Carcinoma

Thyroid carcinoma is the seventh most common cancer in Canada, with approximately 5 700 persons diagnosed in 2011. The incidence rates of thyroid cancer have been increasing significantly worldwide, but the reasons for this phenomenon are unclear. Researchers at the Canadian Cancer Society are examining the role of suspected lifestyle and reproductive factors related to this increased incidence.[38] Exposure to ionizing radiation, especially during childhood, is the most consistent causal factor. Papillary and follicular thyroid carcinomas are the most common types, and medullary and anaplastic thyroid carcinomas are less common. Most tumours are well differentiated.

Most individuals with thyroid carcinoma have normal T_3 and T_4 levels and are therefore euthyroid. The cancer is typically discovered as a small thyroid nodule or metastatic tumour in the lungs, brain, or bone. Changes in voice and swallowing and difficulty breathing are related to tumour growth impinging on the trachea or esophagus. Ultrasonographic characteristics may be suggestive of malignancy, but are neither sensitive nor specific.[39] The diagnosis of thyroid cancer is generally made by fine needle aspiration of a thyroid nodule.

Treatment may include partial or total thyroidectomy, TSH suppression therapy (levothyroxine), radioactive iodine therapy (in iodine-concentrating tumours), postoperative radiation therapy, and chemotherapy (especially in anaplastic carcinoma). New insights into the molecular pathogenesis of thyroid carcinoma are leading to new therapies.[40]

QUICK CHECK 19-2

1. Compare the clinical manifestations of hyperthyroidism and hypothyroidism.
2. What is Graves' disease?
3. What is myxedema?
4. What is the most common cause of thyroid carcinoma?

ALTERATIONS OF PARATHYROID FUNCTION

Hyperparathyroidism

Hyperparathyroidism is characterized by greater than normal secretion of parathyroid hormone (PTH) and hypercalcemia. Hyperparathyroidism is classified as primary, secondary, or tertiary.[41]

PATHOPHYSIOLOGY **Primary hyperparathyroidism** is characterized by inappropriate excess secretion of PTH by one or more of the parathyroid glands. It is one of the most common endocrine disorders. Approximately 80 to 85% of cases are caused by parathyroid adenomas, another 10 to 15% result from parathyroid hyperplasia, and approximately 1% of cases are caused by parathyroid carcinoma. In addition, primary hyperparathyroidism may be caused by a variety of genetic causes, especially the genes that cause multiple endocrine neoplasia.[42]

In primary hyperparathyroidism, PTH secretion is increased and is not under the usual feedback control mechanisms. The calcium level in the blood increases because of increased bone resorption and GI absorption of calcium, but fails to inhibit PTH secretion by the parathyroid gland.

Secondary hyperparathyroidism is a compensatory response of the parathyroid glands to chronic hypocalcemia, which can be associated with decreased renal activation of vitamin D (renal failure) (see Chapter 30). Secretion of PTH is elevated, but PTH cannot achieve normal calcium levels because of insufficient levels of activated vitamin D. Other causes of secondary hyperparathyroidism include dietary deficiency in vitamin D or calcium; decreased intestinal absorption of vitamin D or calcium; and ingestion of medications, such as phenytoin (Dilantin), phenobarbital, and laxatives, which either accelerate the metabolism of vitamin D or decrease intestinal absorption of calcium.

Tertiary hyperparathyroidism is excessive secretion of PTH and hypercalcemia that occurs after longstanding secondary hyperparathyroidism. The etiology is unknown but represents autonomous secretion of PTH from persistent parathyroid stimulation even after withdrawal of calcium and calcitriol therapy.[43] Treatment is surgical removal of one of the parathyroid glands.

CLINICAL MANIFESTATIONS Hypercalcemia and hypophosphatemia are the hallmarks of primary hyperparathyroidism and may be discovered incidentally. Hypercalcemia and hypophosphatemia may be asymptomatic or affected individuals may present with symptoms related to the muscular, nervous, and GI systems, including fatigue, headache, depression, anorexia, and nausea and vomiting. Excessive osteoclastic and osteocytic activity resulting in bone resorption may cause pathological fractures, kyphosis of the dorsal spine, and compression fractures of the vertebral bodies. (Bone resorption is discussed in Chapter 39.)

The increased renal filtration load of calcium leads to hypercalciuria. Hypercalcemia also affects proximal renal tubular function, causing metabolic acidosis and production of an abnormally alkaline urine.[44] PTH hypersecretion enhances renal phosphate excretion and results in hypophosphatemia (see Chapter 5) and hyperphosphaturia. The combination of these three variables—hypercalciuria, alkaline urine, and hyperphosphaturia—predisposes the individual to the formation of calcium stones, particularly in the renal pelvis or renal collecting ducts. These may be associated with infections. Both kidney stones and renal infection can lead to impaired renal function. Hypercalcemia also impairs the concentrating ability of the renal tubule by decreasing its response to ADH. Chronic hypercalcemia of hyperparathyroidism is associated with mild insulin resistance, necessitating increased insulin secretion to maintain normal glucose levels.

Secondary hyperparathyroidism caused by renal disease presents clinically not only with bone resorption but also with the symptoms of hypocalcemia and hyperphosphatemia. Hypocalcemia can cause many significant clinical problems (see Chapter 5), and hyperphosphatemia can cause deleterious effects on the cardiovascular system.

EVALUATION AND TREATMENT The concurrent findings of increased ionized calcium concentration despite elevated PTH concentration are suggestive of primary hyperparathyroidism. PTH levels also may be inappropriately within the normal range because hypercalcemia should completely suppress PTH production. Imaging procedures are used to localize adenomas before surgery. Observation of asymptomatic individuals with mild hypercalcemia is recommended; these individuals are advised to avoid dehydration and limit dietary calcium intake. Definitive treatment of severe primary hyperparathyroidism involves surgical removal of the solitary adenoma or, in the case of hyperplasia, complete removal of three and partial removal of the fourth hyperplastic parathyroid glands. In those individuals for whom surgery is not an option, other treatments such as bisphosphonates and calcimimetics (e.g., cinacalcet [Sensipar]) may be considered.

If serum calcium concentration is low but PTH level is elevated, secondary hyperparathyroidism is likely. Evaluation for renal function may indicate chronic renal disease. Treatment for secondary hyperparathyroidism in chronic renal disease requires calcium replacement, dietary phosphate restriction and phosphate binders, and vitamin D replacement. Treatment also may include calcimimetics, which work to increase parathyroid calcium receptor sensitivity, thus lowering PTH levels.[45,46]

Hypoparathyroidism

Hypoparathyroidism (abnormally low PTH levels) is most commonly caused by damage to the parathyroid glands during thyroid surgery. This occurs because of the anatomical proximity of the parathyroid glands to the thyroid (see Figure 18-11). Hypoparathyroidism also is associated with genetic syndromes, including familial hypoparathyroidism and DiGeorge syndrome (see Chapter 8). Hypomagnesemia also can cause a decrease in both PTH secretion and PTH function. An idiopathic or autoimmune form of hypoparathyroidism also is recognized.[47] There is an inherited condition associated with hypocalcemia but with normal to elevated levels of PTH called *pseudohypoparathyroidism*; it is caused by a postreceptor defect in PTH action.

PATHOPHYSIOLOGY A lack of circulating PTH causes depressed serum calcium levels and increased serum phosphate levels. In the absence of PTH, resorption of calcium from bone and regulation of calcium reabsorption from the renal tubules are impaired. Phosphate reabsorption by the renal tubules is therefore increased, causing decreased renal phosphate excretion and hyperphosphatemia.

Hypomagnesemia inhibits PTH secretion. When serum magnesium levels return to normal, however, PTH secretion returns to normal, as does the responsiveness of peripheral tissues to PTH. Hypomagnesemia may be related to chronic alcoholism, malnutrition, malabsorption, increased renal clearance of magnesium caused by the use of aminoglycoside antibiotics or certain chemotherapeutic agents, or prolonged magnesium-deficient parenteral nutritional therapy.

CLINICAL MANIFESTATIONS Symptoms associated with hypoparathyroidism are primarily those of hypocalcemia (see Table 5-7). Hypocalcemia causes a lowered threshold for nerve and muscle excitation so that a nerve impulse may be initiated by a slight stimulus anywhere along the length of a nerve or muscle fibre. This creates tetany, a condition characterized by muscle spasms, hyper-reflexia, clonic-tonic convulsions, laryngeal spasms, and, in severe cases, death by asphyxiation. Chvostek's and Trousseau's signs may be used to evaluate for neuromuscular irritability. Chvostek's sign is elicited by tapping the cheek, resulting in twitching of the upper lip. Trousseau's sign is elicited by sustained inflation of a sphygmomanometer placed on the upper arm to a level above the systolic blood pressure with resultant painful carpal spasm. Other symptoms of hypocalcemia include dry skin, loss of body and scalp hair, hypoplasia of developing teeth, horizontal ridges on the nails, cataracts, basal ganglia calcifications (which may be associated with a parkinsonian syndrome), and bone deformities, including brachydactyly and bowing of the long bones.

Phosphate retention caused by increased renal reabsorption of phosphate is also associated with hypoparathyroidism. Hyperphosphatemia results from PTH deficiency and, in turn, hyperphosphatemia further lowers calcium concentration by inhibiting the activation of vitamin D, thereby lowering the GI absorption of calcium.

EVALUATION AND TREATMENT A low serum calcium concentration and a high phosphorous level in the absence of renal failure, intestinal disorders, or nutritional deficiencies suggest hypoparathyroidism. PTH levels are low in hypoparathyroidism and measurement of serum magnesium level and urinary calcium excretion also can help in diagnosis. Treatment is directed toward alleviation of the hypocalcemia. In acute states, this treatment involves parenteral administration of calcium, which corrects serum calcium concentration within minutes. Maintenance of serum calcium level is achieved with pharmacological doses of cholecalciferol (vitamin D_3) and oral calcium.[48] Hypoplastic dentition, cataracts, bone deformities, and basal ganglia calcifications do not respond to the correction of hypocalcemia, but the other symptoms of hypocalcemia are reversible.

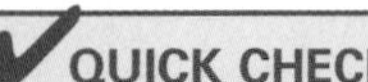

QUICK CHECK 19-3

1. How does excessive parathyroid hormone (PTH) affect bones?
2. What are the results of a lack of circulating PTH?

DYSFUNCTION OF THE ENDOCRINE PANCREAS: DIABETES MELLITUS

Diabetes mellitus is a group of metabolic diseases characterized by hyperglycemia resulting from defects in insulin secretion, insulin action, or both. In 2009, Canada had a 6.8% prevalence rate of diabetes. It is estimated that by 2019, 3.7 million Canadians will be diagnosed with the disease.[49] The Canadian Diabetes Association classifies four categories of diabetes mellitus[49] (Table 19-3), as follows:

1. Type 1 (beta-cell destruction, usually leading to absolute insulin deficiency)
2. Type 2 (ranging from predominantly insulin resistance with relative insulin deficiency to predominantly an insulin secretory defect with insulin resistance)
3. Other specific types
4. Gestational diabetes

The diagnosis of diabetes mellitus is based on **glycosylated hemoglobin (A_{1C})** levels; fasting plasma glucose (FPG) levels; 2-hour plasma glucose levels during oral glucose tolerance testing (OGTT) using a 75-g oral glucose load; or random glucose levels in an individual with symptoms (Box 19-1).[49] Glycosylated hemoglobin refers to the permanent attachment of glucose to hemoglobin molecules and reflects the average plasma glucose exposure over the life of a red blood cell (approximately 120 days). It provides a more accurate measure for monitoring long-term control of blood glucose levels. This test is critically dependent on the method of measurement and must be related to established standards.

The Canadian Diabetes Association classification "prediabetes" describes nondiabetic elevations of A_{1C}, FPG, or 2-hour plasma glucose value during OGTT (see Box 19-1).[49] The Canadian Diabetes Association estimates that the Canadian prevalence of prediabetes in 2015 was 22.1%, and by 2025 will increase to 23.2%.[50] This classification includes impaired glucose tolerance (IGT), which results from diminished insulin secretion, and impaired fasting glucose (IFG), which is caused by enhanced hepatic glucose output. Individuals with IGT and IFG are at increased risk for cardiovascular disease and premature death and carry a 15 to 50%, 5-year risk of developing diabetes, particularly type 2 diabetes.[51] Thus, prevention of diabetes with lifestyle interventions is essential.[51]

BOX 19-1 Diagnostic Criteria for Diabetes Mellitus

1. A_{1C} ≥6.5% in adults using a standardized, validated assay in the absence of factors that affect the accuracy of the A_{1C} and not for suspected type 1 diabetes
   OR
2. FPG 7.0 mmol/L (fasting is defined as no caloric intake for at least 8 hours)*
   OR
3. 2-hr PG in a 75 g OGTT ≥11.1 mmol/L*
   OR
4. Random PG ≥11.1 mmol/L

Diagnosis of Prediabetes

1. FPG 6.1–6.9 mmol/L
   OR
2. 2-hr PG in a 75 g OGTT 7.8–11.1 mmol/L
   OR
3. A_{1C} 6.0–6.4%

*In the absence of symptomatic hyperglycemia, if a single laboratory test result is in the diabetes range, a repeat confirmatory laboratory test (FPG, A_{1C}, 2-hr PG in a 75 g OGTT) must be done on another day. It is preferable that the same test be repeated (in a timely fashion) for confirmation, but a random PG in the diabetes range in an asymptomatic individual should be confirmed with an alternate test. In the case of symptomatic hyperglycemia, the diagnosis has been made and a confirmatory test is not required before treatment is initiated. In individuals in whom type 1 diabetes is likely (younger or lean or symptomatic hyperglycemia, especially with ketonuria or ketonemia), confirmatory testing should not delay initiation of treatment to avoid rapid deterioration. If results of two different tests are available and both are above the diagnostic cutpoints, the diagnosis of diabetes is confirmed.

A_{1C}, hemoglobin A_{1C} or glycosylated hemoglobin; *FPG*, fasting plasma glucose; *OGTT*, oral glucose tolerance testing; *PG*, plasma glucose.

Data from Canadian Diabetes Association Clinical Practice Guidelines Expert Committee. (2013). *Can J Diabetes, 37*(Suppl. 1), S1–S212. Retrieved from http://guidelines.diabetes.ca/app_themes/cdacpg/resources/cpg_2013_full_en.pdf.

Types of Diabetes Mellitus

Type 1 Diabetes Mellitus

Type 1 diabetes mellitus is the most common pediatric chronic disease, with approximately 5 to 10% of Canadians having this form of diabetes. The Canadian prevalence rate of diabetes in children aged 19 years and under is 0.3%, and the incidence is increasing.[51] Between 10 and 13% of individuals with newly diagnosed type 1 diabetes have a first-degree relative (parent or sibling) with type 1 diabetes. There is a 50% concordance rate in twins. Diagnosis is rare during the first 9 months of life and peaks at 12 years of age. Two distinct types of type 1 diabetes have been identified: idiopathic and autoimmune.

PATHOPHYSIOLOGY Idiopathic type 1 diabetes is far less common than autoimmune diabetes, has a strong genetic component, and occurs mostly in people of Asian or African descent. Affected individuals have varying degrees of insulin deficiency.

Autoimmune type 1 diabetes mellitus is a slowly progressive autoimmune T-cell–mediated disease that destroys beta cells of the pancreas. There is a deficient immune tolerance linked to abnormalities in immune cells and changes in beta-cell antigens. Destruction of beta cells is related to genetic susceptibility and environmental factors. The strongest genetic association is with human leukocyte antigen (HLA) class II alleles

TABLE 19-3 Epidemiology and Etiology of Diabetes Mellitus in Canada

	Type 1 Diabetes: Primary Beta-Cell Defect or Failure	Type 2 Diabetes: Insulin Resistance With Inadequate Insulin Secretion
Incidence		
Frequency	5–10% of all cases of diabetes mellitus Incidence of 15–35 per 100 000 population of all cases of diabetes mellitus	Accounts for most cases (≈85–90%) Incidence rate for all diabetes in adults over the age of 20 is 6.3 per 100 000 population Estimated prevalence of diabetes was 4.2% in 2000 and 7.6% in 2010; and it is 10.8% for 2020
Change in incidences	Rates among children and youth have been increasing globally. Canada was found to have one of the highest incidence rates of type 1 diabetes for children under 14 years of age	Estimated prevalence increase in diabetes was 103% from 2000–10; and it is 57% from 2010–20 and 220% from 2000–20 Currently, one in four Canadians lives with diabetes, undiagnosed diabetes, or prediabetes; this rate is expected to rise to one in three by 2020 if current trends continue
Characteristics		
Age at onset	Peak onset at age 11–13 years (slightly earlier for girls than for boys); rare in children younger than 1 year and adults older than 30 years	Risk of developing diabetes increases after age 40 years Incidence is increasing among youth
Gender	Similar in males and females	More males than females
Racial distribution	Rate for White people is 1.5–2 times higher than for visible minorities	Diabetes diagnosed among Indigenous people is described as an epidemic, with a prevalence three times or higher than that of the general population. In addition, people of South and Southeast Asian, African, and Latin American descent have higher rates of childhood type 2 diabetes, gestational diabetes mellitus, and type 2 diabetes
Obesity	Generally normal or underweight	Frequent contributing factor to precipitate type 2 diabetes among those susceptible
Etiology		
Common theory	*Autoimmune:* genetic and environmental factors, resulting in gradual process of autoimmune destruction in genetically susceptible individuals *Nonautoimmune:* Unknown	Genetic susceptibility (polygenic) combined with environmental determinants; defects in beta-cell function combined with insulin resistance Associated with long-duration obesity
Presence of antibody	Autoantibodies to insulin and to glutamic acid decarboxylase (GAD_{65})	Autoantibodies not present
Insulin resistance	Insulin resistance at diagnosis is unusual, but may occur as individual ages and gains weight	Insulin resistance is virtually universal and multifactorial in origin
Insulin secretion	Severe insulin deficiency or no insulin secretion at all	Typically increased at time of diagnosis, but progressively declines over course of illness

Data from Canadian Diabetes Association. (n.d.). *Diabetes: Canada at the tipping point: Charting a new path.* Retrieved from https://www.diabetes.ca/CDA/media/documents/publications-and-newsletters/advocacy-reports/canada-at-the-tipping-point-english.pdf; Centers for Disease Control. (2015). *National diabetes statistics report, 2014.* Retrieved from http://www.cdc.gov/diabetes/pubs/statsreport14/national-diabetes-report-web.pdf; Public Health Agency of Canada. (2011). *Diabetes in Canada: Facts and figures from a public health perspective.* Retrieved from http://www.phac-aspc.gc.ca/cd-mc/publications/diabetes-diabete/facts-figures-faits-chiffres-2011/index-eng.php.

HLA-DQ and *HLA-DR*. The *HLA-DR* marker is associated with other autoimmune disorders, such as celiac, Graves', Hashimoto's, and Addison's diseases. Environmental factors that have been implicated include exposure to certain medications, foods, and viruses. These gene–environment interactions result in the formation of autoantigens that are expressed on the surface of pancreatic beta cells and circulate in the bloodstream and lymphatics (Figure 19-10). Cellular immunity (T-cytotoxic cells and macrophages) and humoral immunity (autoantibodies) are stimulated, resulting in beta-cell destruction and apoptosis. The destruction of beta cells results from lymphocyte and macrophage infiltration of the islets, resulting in release of inflammatory cytokines, activation of T-helper and T-cytotoxic lymphocytes, and death of islet beta cells. Beta-cell destruction also is mediated by the production of autoantibodies against islet cells, insulin, glutamic acid decarboxylase (GAD), and other cytoplasmic proteins.[52] Insulin synthesis declines and hyperglycemia develops over time.

For insulin synthesis to decline enough such that hyperglycemia occurs, 80 to 90% of the insulin-secreting beta cells of the islets of Langerhans must be destroyed. Insulin normally suppresses secretion of glucagon and, thus, hypoinsulinemia leads to a marked increase in glucagon secretion. **Glucagon**, a hormone produced by the alpha cells of the islets, acts in the liver to increase blood glucose level by stimulating glycogenolysis and gluconeogenesis. In addition to the decline in insulin secretion, there is decreased secretion of **amylin**, another beta-cell hormone. One of the critical actions of amylin is to suppress glucagon release from the alpha cells. Thus both alpha-cell and beta-cell functions are abnormal, and both a lack of insulin and a relative excess of glucagon contribute to hyperglycemia in type 1 diabetes.

CLINICAL MANIFESTATIONS Historically, type 1 diabetes was thought to have an abrupt onset. It is now known, however, that the natural history involves a long preclinical period with gradual destruction of beta cells, eventually leading to insulin deficiency and hyperglycemia. In general, this latent period is longer in adults with onset of type 1 diabetes and often results in misclassification of those affected as having type 2 diabetes.

Type 1 diabetes affects the metabolism of fat, protein, and carbohydrates. Glucose accumulates in the blood and appears in the urine as the renal threshold for glucose is exceeded, producing an osmotic diuresis and symptoms of polyuria and thirst (Table 19-4). Wide fluctuations in blood glucose levels occur. In addition, protein and fat breakdown occurs because of the lack of insulin, resulting in weight loss. Increased metabolism of fats and proteins leads to high levels of circulating ketones, causing a condition known as **diabetic ketoacidosis (DKA)**.

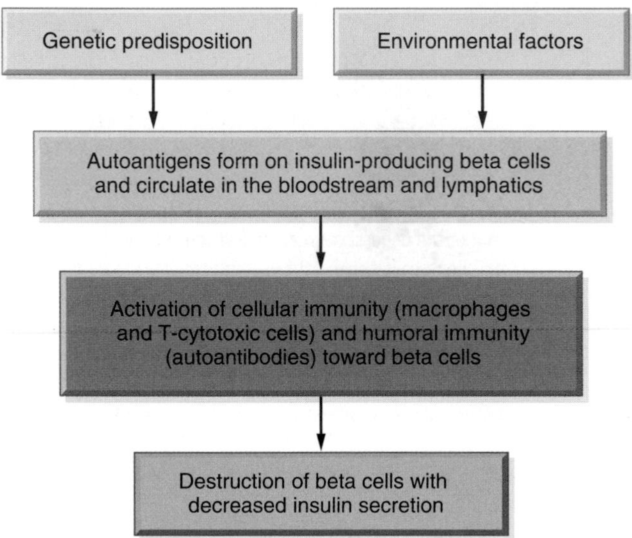

FIGURE 19-10 Pathophysiology of Type 1 Diabetes Mellitus.

Currently half of individuals with type 1 diabetes are obese, and an increasing number of individuals have both type 1 diabetes and the clinical manifestations of metabolic syndrome, including obesity, dyslipidemia, and hypertension.[53] (see Box 19-1). These individuals are at high risk for chronic complications of diabetes, including heart disease and stroke.

EVALUATION AND TREATMENT The criteria for diagnosis of type 1 diabetes are the same as those for type 2 diabetes.[51] (See Box 19-1.) Many children are first diagnosed when they present with the signs and symptoms of DKA. In DKA, acetone (a volatile form of ketones) is exhaled by hyperventilation and gives the breath a sweet or "fruity" odour. Occasionally, diabetic coma is the initial symptom of the disease. The diagnosis of diabetes is not difficult when the symptoms of polydipsia, polyuria, polyphagia, weight loss, and hyperglycemia are present in fasting and postprandial states. C-peptide, a component of proinsulin released during insulin production, can be measured in the serum as a surrogate for insulin levels and is indicative of residual beta-cell mass and function. The zinc transporter 8 autoantibody (ZnT8Ab) test has been approved for diagnosis of type 1 diabetes. Other important aspects of evaluation include looking for evidence of the chronic complications of type 1 diabetes, including renal, nervous system, cardiac, peripheral vascular, retinal, and bony tissue damage.

Currently, treatment regimens are designed to achieve optimal glucose level control (as measured by the A_{1C} value) without causing episodes of significant hypoglycemia.[51] Management requires individual planning according to type of disease, age, and activity level, but all individuals require some combination of insulin therapy, meal planning, and exercise regimen. Several different types of insulin preparations are available, and there are new technologies for more physiological insulin delivery systems (e.g., insulin pump therapy).[54] Many different kinds of therapies are being tested to prevent the autoimmune destruction of beta cells, including immunosuppression with antirejection medications (see *Health Promotion:* Type 1 Diabetes Mellitus). Finally, islet cell, stem cell,

TABLE 19-4 Clinical Manifestations and Mechanisms for Type 1 Diabetes Mellitus

Manifestation	Rationale
Polydipsia	Because of elevated blood glucose levels, water is osmotically attracted from body cells, resulting in intracellular dehydration and stimulation of thirst in hypothalamus
Polyuria	Hyperglycemia acts as an osmotic diuretic; the amount of glucose filtered by glomeruli of kidney exceeds that which can be reabsorbed by renal tubules; glycosuria results, accompanied by large amounts of water lost in urine
Polyphagia	Depletion of cellular stores of carbohydrates, fats, and protein results in cellular starvation and a corresponding increase in hunger
Weight loss	Weight loss occurs because of fluid loss in osmotic diuresis and loss of body tissue as fats and proteins are used for energy
Fatigue	Metabolic changes result in poor use of food products, contributing to lethargy and fatigue
Recurrent infections (e.g., boils, carbuncles, and bladder infection)	Growth of microorganisms is stimulated by increased glucose levels, and diabetes is associated with some immunocompromised individuals
Prolonged wound healing	Impaired blood supply hinders healing
Genital pruritus	Hyperglycemia and glycosuria favour fungal growth; candidal infections, resulting in pruritus, are a common presenting symptom in women
Visual changes	Blurred vision occurs as water balance in eye fluctuates because of elevated blood glucose levels; diabetic retinopathy may ensue
Paresthesias	Paresthesias are common manifestations of diabetic neuropathies
Cardiovascular symptoms (e.g., chest pain, extremity pain, and neurological deficits)	Diabetes contributes to formation of atherosclerotic plaques that involve coronary, peripheral, and cerebrovascular circulations and alterations in microvessels

HEALTH PROMOTION

Type 1 Diabetes Mellitus

The exact causes of type 1 diabetes mellitus are not fully understood. It is believed that behavioural patterns, coupled with environmental factors, often accelerate the disease in genetically disposed people. Studies have shown that the interaction between genetic and environmental factors varies among populations and ethnic groups. Type 1 diabetes is most frequently associated with the White population, particularly those of northern European descent.

Unfortunately, preventive measures for type 1 diabetes remain undefined. Genetic and environmental risk factors have been identified related to type 1 diabetes. By targeting environmental risk factors, increasing awareness of diabetes, and identifying people at risk, people may be able to reduce or delay the development of type 1 diabetes.

A person who has a first-degree relative with type 1 diabetes has a 10% chance of developing the disease. Researchers have identified several genes they suspect are linked with type 1 diabetes, but have been unable to find a specific gene that can accurately predict the development of diabetes.

Viral infections, in particular enteroviruses and dietary microbial toxins, are also suspected as factors that may precipitate the development of type 1 diabetes. Studies have also revealed possible risk factors, which may include exposure to autoantibodies and cow's milk protein in infancy. When considering the global increased incidence of type 1 diabetes, additional studies have shown a possible association related to changes in early feeding patterns, early growth in the first year of life, and hygiene practices such as the use of antibacterial disinfectants.

When considering the prevention of type 1 diabetes, studies have identified factors that may reduce the risk of developing the disease. These factors include breastfeeding and ensuring optimal vitamin D levels. Breastfeeding is felt to have a protective effect from developing type 1 diabetes; however, a short duration of breastfeeding has been identified as a predisposing factor, especially for those at an increase genetic risk. It has also been suggested that obesity may promote the development of insulin resistance, which in turn triggers an autoimmune response resulting in the destruction of pancreatic beta cells.

Data from Public Health Agency of Canada. (2011). *Diabetes in Canada: Facts and figures from a public health perspective.* Retrieved from http://www.phac-aspc.gc.ca/cd-mc/publications/diabetes-diabete/facts-figures-faits-chiffres-2011/index-eng.php.

and whole pancreas transplantation has been successful in selected individuals.[52,55]

Type 2 Diabetes Mellitus

Type 2 diabetes mellitus accounts for 90% of all diabetes in Canada.[56] There is an increased prevalence among Indigenous people, as well as people of South and Southeast Asian, African, and Latin American descent. There also is an increased prevalence of type 2 diabetes in children, especially in obese children (see Table 19-3).

A genetic and environmental interaction appears to be responsible for type 2 diabetes.[57] The most well-recognized risk factors are age, obesity, hypertension, physical inactivity, and family history. More than 60 genes have been identified that are associated with type 2 diabetes, including those that code for beta-cell mass, beta-cell function (ability to sense blood glucose levels, insulin synthesis, and insulin secretion), proinsulin and insulin molecular structures, insulin receptors, hepatic synthesis of glucose, glucagon synthesis, and cellular responsiveness to insulin stimulation.[58] These genetic abnormalities, combined with environmental influences such as obesity, result in the basic pathophysiological mechanisms of type 2 diabetes, which are insulin resistance and decreased insulin secretion by beta cells (Figure 19-11).

There is increasing evidence that diet, including diet during pregnancy, influences the long-term risk of developing type 2 diabetes in children and adults.[59] **Metabolic syndrome** is a constellation of disorders (central obesity, dyslipidemia, prehypertension, and an elevated fasting blood glucose level) that together confer a high risk of developing type 2 diabetes and associated cardiovascular complications (Box 19-2). It is estimated that 21% of Canadian adults aged 18 to 79 have metabolic syndrome.[60] Metabolic syndrome often develops during childhood and is prevalent among overweight children and adolescents. Metabolic syndrome is characterized by many of the same genetic and environmental risks as type 2 diabetes, and individuals should be screened on a regular basis (see Box 19-2). Early recognition and treatment, including vigorous lifestyle changes, are critical to reducing cardiovascular events and improving clinical outcomes for individuals with prediabetes and metabolic syndrome.[61]

PATHOPHYSIOLOGY Many organs contribute to insulin resistance, chronic hyperglycemia, and the consequences of type 2 diabetes (Figure 19-12). **Insulin resistance** is defined as a suboptimal response of insulin-sensitive tissues (especially liver, muscle, and adipose tissue) to insulin and is associated with obesity. Several mechanisms are involved

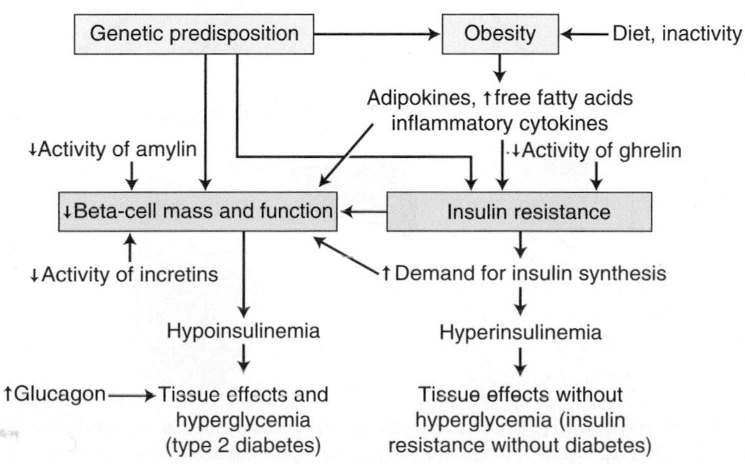

FIGURE 19-11 Pathophysiology of Type 2 Diabetes Mellitus.

BOX 19-2 Criteria for the Diagnosis of Metabolic Syndrome

Three or more of the following five traits:

1. Increased waist circumference (≥102 centimetres in men; ≥88 centimetres in women) for those of North American descent—these measurements are adjusted for certain ethnic groups
2. Plasma triglycerides ≥1.7 mmol/L
3. Plasma high-density lipoprotein (HDL) cholesterol <1.0 mmol/L (men) or <1.3 mmol/L (women)
4. Blood pressure systolic ≥130 mm Hg and/or diastolic ≥ 85 mm Hg
5. Fasting plasma glucose ≥5.6 mmol/L

Data from Canadian Diabetes Association Clinical Practice Guidelines Expert Committee. (2013). *Can J Diabetes, 37*(Suppl. 1), S1–S212. Retrieved from http://guidelines.diabetes.ca/app_themes/cdacpg/resources/cpg_2013_full_en.pdf.

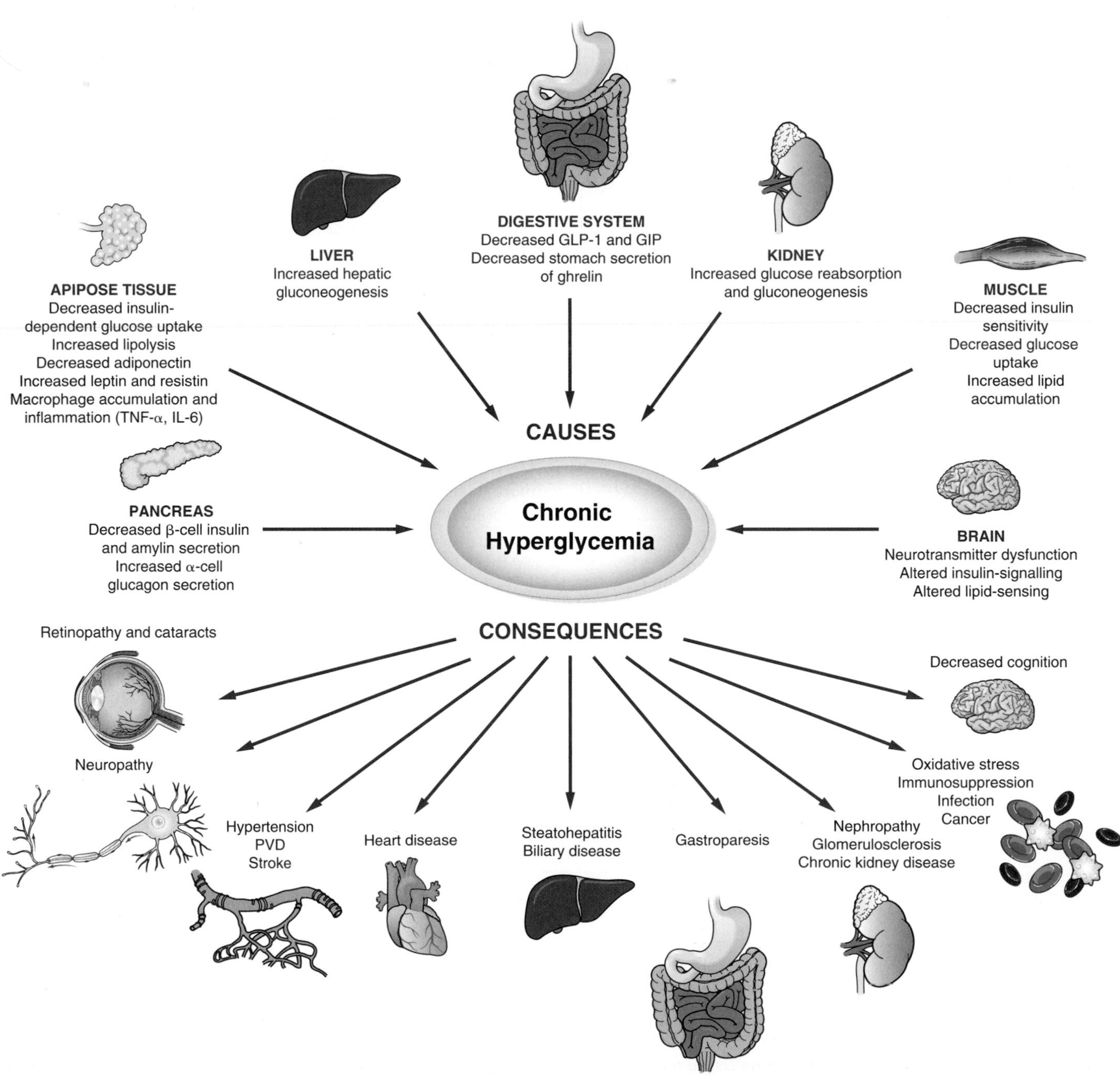

FIGURE 19-12 Multiorgan Causes and Common Consequences of Chronic Hyperglycemia in Type 2 Diabetes Mellitus. *GIP*, gastric inhibitory polypeptide; *GLP-1*, glucagonlike peptide 1; *IL-6*, interleukin-6; *PVD*, peripheral vascular disease; *TNF-α*, tumour necrosis factor-alpha.

in abnormalities of the insulin signalling pathway and contribute to insulin resistance. These mechanisms include an abnormality of the insulin molecule, high amounts of insulin antagonists, downregulation of the insulin receptor, and alteration of glucose transporter (GLUT) proteins.

Obesity is one of the most important contributors to insulin resistance and diabetes and acts through several important mechanisms:

1. Adipokines (leptin and adiponectin) are hormones produced in adipose tissue. Obesity results in increased serum levels of leptin and decreased levels of adiponectin. These changes are associated with inflammation and decreased insulin sensitivity.[62]
2. Elevated levels of serum free fatty acids (FFAs) and intracellular deposits of triglycerides and cholesterol are also found in obese individuals. These changes interfere with intracellular insulin signalling, decrease tissue responses to insulin, alter incretin actions, and promote inflammation.
3. Inflammatory cytokines are released from intra-abdominal adipocytes or adipocyte-associated mononuclear cells and induce insulin resistance and are cytotoxic to beta cells.[63]
4. Obesity is correlated with hyperinsulinemia and decreased insulin receptor density.

Compensatory hyperinsulinemia prevents the clinical appearance of diabetes for many years. Eventually, however, **beta-cell dysfunction** develops and leads to a relative deficiency of insulin activity.[57] The islet dysfunction is caused by a combination of a decrease in beta-cell mass and a reduction in normal beta-cell function.[64] A progressive decrease in the weight and number of beta cells occurs and many of the remaining cells develop "exhaustion" from increased demand for insulin biosynthesis.

Glucagon concentration is increased in type 2 diabetes because pancreatic alpha cells become less responsive to glucose inhibition, resulting in an increase in glucagon secretion. These abnormally high levels of glucagon increase blood glucose level by stimulating glycogenolysis and gluconeogenesis. As was discussed under type 1 diabetes, type 2 diabetes also is associated with a deficiency in amylin, further increasing glucagon levels.

Amylin (islet amyloid polypeptide) is another beta-cell hormone that is decreased in both type 1 and type 2 diabetes. Amylin increases satiety and suppresses glucagon release from the alpha cells. It also contributes to islet cell destruction through the deposition of abnormal (misfolded) amyloid polypeptide in the pancreas.[65] Pramlintide, a synthetic analogue of amylin, is used for treatment in type 2 diabetes in the United States, but has not been approved for use in Canada.

Hormones released from the GI tract play a role in insulin resistance, beta-cell function, and diabetes. **Ghrelin** is a peptide produced in the stomach and pancreatic islets that regulates food intake, energy balance, and hormonal secretion.[66] Decreased levels of circulating ghrelin have been associated with insulin resistance and increased fasting insulin levels. The **incretins** are a class of peptides that are released from the GI tract in response to food intake and function to increase the secretion of insulin and have many other positive effects on metabolism. The most studied incretin is called glucagonlike peptide 1 (GLP-1), and studies have demonstrated that beta-cell responsiveness to GLP-1 is reduced both in prediabetes and in type 2 diabetes.[67]

The kidneys also influence the pathophysiology of type 2 diabetes. Renal reabsorption of glucose through the sodium-glucose cotransporter 2 (SGLT2) is an important controller of serum glucose levels, and new medications aimed at blocking it have resulted in decreased measurements for blood glucose level, weight, and blood pressure.[68]

CLINICAL MANIFESTATIONS The clinical manifestations of type 2 diabetes are nonspecific. The affected individual is often overweight, dyslipidemic, hyperinsulinemic, and hypertensive. The individual with type 2 diabetes may show some classic symptoms of diabetes, such as polyuria and polydipsia, but more often will have nonspecific symptoms such as fatigue, recurrent infections, visual changes, or symptoms of neuropathy (paresthesias or weakness). In those whose diabetes has progressed without treatment, symptoms related to coronary artery, peripheral artery, and cerebrovascular disease may develop.

EVALUATION AND TREATMENT The diagnostic criteria for type 2 diabetes are the same as those for type 1 (see Box 19-1). Prevention of type 2 diabetes, especially in those individuals with prediabetes, hinges on diet and exercise, although there is increasing support for the use of some diabetes medications in high-risk individuals. (See *Health Promotion:* Type 2 Diabetes Mellitus.)

HEALTH PROMOTION

Type 2 Diabetes Mellitus

The incidence of diabetes is increasing worldwide, with an estimated 285 million adults affected. Approximately 85 to 95% of those affected have type 2 diabetes mellitus. Despite advances in treatment options, 49% of Canadians with type 2 diabetes have failed to achieve the glycosylated hemoglobin (A_{1c}) target levels recommended by the Canadian Diabetes Association.

Health promotion interventions play an important role in the prevention and management of type 2 diabetes. The Canadian Diabetes Association has suggested three strategies to use as the best prevention for diabetes and its complications:

1. Changing risk factors and conditions by promoting healthy eating, physical activity, and emotional well-being
2. Early identification and effective management of the disease
3. Rehabilitation

Although **modifying** lifestyle factors (e.g., increasing physical activity, eating healthy, and achieving and maintaining a healthy weight) can decrease the occurrence of diabetes, successfully accomplishing these modifications can be a challenging endeavour. Therefore, it is essential that a comprehensive approach to preventing type 2 diabetes incorporate both population-based and high-risk individual strategies. Health promotion strategies also require leadership from government, local communities, nongovernmental organizations, the business sector, and committed individuals.

Data from Ontario Ministry of Health. (1999). *Diabetes: Strategies for prevention.* Retrieved from http://health.gov.on.ca/en/common/ministry/publications/reports/diabetes/diabetes.aspx#identify.

As with type 1 diabetes, the goal of treatment for individuals with type 2 diabetes is the restoration of near-euglycemia (a normal blood glucose level) and correction of related metabolic disorders. The first approach to treatment of the individual with type 2 diabetes is maintaining an appropriate diet and exercise program.[69] Diet should match activity levels and include more complex carbohydrates (rather than simple sugars), foods low in fats, adequate protein, and fibre. Weight loss results in improved glucose tolerance. Bariatric surgery improves glycemic control, decreases the risk for cardiovascular disease, and promotes weight loss in those morbidly obese. For individuals who require further intervention, oral hypoglycemic agents are indicated. Currently, metformin (Glucophage) is considered the primary pharmacological choice for the treatment of type 2 diabetes and a second oral agent, a GLP-1 receptor agonist, or basal insulin is added if the A_{1C} target is not maintained over 3 months. An increasing number of persons are being treated with incretins. A combination of medications may be required. Insulin therapy may be needed in the later stage of type 2 diabetes because of loss of beta-cell function, which is progressive over time.

Other Specific Types of Diabetes Mellitus and Gestational Diabetes Mellitus

The Canadian Diabetes Association's classification of diabetes mellitus includes not only the most common forms of diabetes (type 1 and type 2) (see Table 19-3) but also "other specific types" of diabetes mellitus and "gestational diabetes mellitus." Other specific types of diabetes include genetic defects in beta-cell function, genetic defects in insulin action, diseases of the exocrine pancreas, endocrinopathies, medication- or chemical-induced beta-cell dysfunction, infections, and other uncommon autoimmune and inherited disorders that are associated with diabetes. **Maturity-onset diabetes of youth (MODY)** is the best described of these other specific types of diabetes. MODY includes six specific autosomal dominant mutations that affect critical enzymes involved in beta-cell function or insulin action. It is estimated that only 1% of cases of diabetes are monogenic and, therefore, are classified as MODY.[70] Diagnosis and management are similar to those techniques used for type 2 diabetes.

Gestational diabetes mellitus (GDM) has been defined as any degree of glucose intolerance with onset or first recognition during pregnancy. However, this definition meant that many women with previously undiagnosed type 1 or type 2 diabetes were diagnosed with GDM, and many of them had progressive disease after delivery. Therefore, the Canadian Diabetes Association recommends that women found to have diabetes at their initial prenatal visit receive a 75 g OGTT between 6 weeks and 6 months postpartum. GDM complicates approximately 7% of all pregnancies. Screening for GDM is recommended in asymptomatic, pregnant women between 24 and 28 weeks of gestation.[71] The Canadian Diabetes Association's preferred approach for diagnosis of GDM includes sequential screening with a 50 g glucose change test (GCT), followed by a 75 g OGTT using the glucose thresholds of fasting 5.3 mmol/L (1 hour: 10.6 mmol/L, and 2 hours: 9.0 mmol/L).[49] Women diagnosed with GDM requiring medication for glycemic control should be managed with insulin therapy. Women with type 2 diabetes who are planning a pregnancy should switch from noninsulin antihyperglycemic agents to insulin for glycemic control.[49] Tight glucose control prenatally, during pregnancy, and after delivery is essential to the short- and long-term health of both mother and baby. Women who have GDM have a greatly increased subsequent diabetes risk, making consistent follow-up important.

Acute Complications of Diabetes Mellitus

The major acute complications of diabetes mellitus are hypoglycemia, DKA, and **hyperosmolar hyperglycemic syndrome (HHS)** (see comparison in Table 19-5). The **Somogyi effect** (low blood glucose level during night that may lead to morning rise in blood glucose level) and **dawn phenomenon** (early morning rise in blood glucose level related to release of GH, cortisol, and catecholamines without preceding hypoglycemia) also may be seen.

Hypoglycemia in diabetes is sometimes called *insulin shock* or *insulin reaction*. Individuals with type 2 diabetes are at less risk for hypoglycemia than those with type 1 diabetes because they retain relatively intact glucose counter-regulatory mechanisms. However, hypoglycemia does occur in type 2 diabetes when treatment involves insulin secretogogues (e.g., sulfonylureas) or exogenous insulin. Symptoms include pallor, tremor, anxiety, tachycardia, palpitations, diaphoresis, headache, dizziness, irritability, fatigue, poor judgement, confusion, visual disturbances, hunger, seizures, and coma. Treatment requires immediate replacement of glucose either orally or intravenously. Glucagon for home use can be prescribed for individuals who are at high risk. Prevention is achieved with individualized management of medications and diet, monitoring of blood glucose levels, and education.

DKA is a serious complication related to a deficiency of insulin and an increase in the levels of insulin counter-regulatory hormones (catecholamines, cortisol, glucagon, GH) (Figure 19-13). DKA occurs in approximately 30% of children with type 1 diabetes, and 5% of children with type 2 diabetes.[72] DKA is much more common in type 1 diabetes because insulin is more deficient (see Table 19-5). It is characterized by hyperglycemia, acidosis, and ketonuria. Insulin normally stimulates lipogenesis and inhibits lipolysis, thus preventing fat

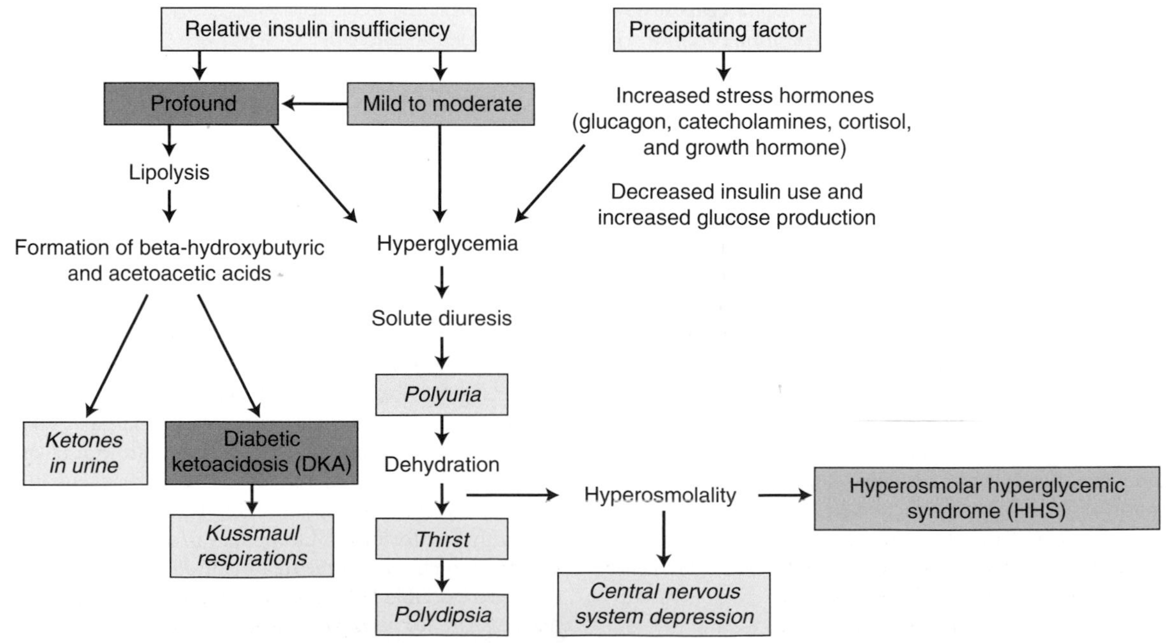

FIGURE 19-13 Pathophysiology of Diabetic Ketoacidosis and Hyperosmolar Hyperglycemia Syndrome in Diabetes Mellitus.

TABLE 19-5 **Common Acute Complications of Diabetes Mellitus**

Hypoglycemia in Persons With Diabetes Mellitus	Diabetic Ketoacidosis	Hyperosmolar Hyperglycemic Syndrome
Synonyms		
Insulin shock, insulin reaction	Diabetic coma syndrome	Hyperosmolar hyperglycemia nonketotic syndrome
Persons at Risk		
Individuals taking insulin Individuals with rapidly fluctuating blood glucose levels Individuals with type 2 diabetes taking sulfonylurea agents	Individuals with type 1 diabetes Individuals with nondiagnosed diabetes	Older adults or very young individuals with type 2 diabetes, nondiabetic persons with predisposing factors, such as pancreatitis; individuals with undiagnosed diabetes
Predisposing Factors		
Excessive insulin or sulfonylurea agent intake, lack of sufficient food intake, excessive physical exercise, abrupt decline in insulin needs (e.g., renal failure, immediately postpartum), simultaneous use of insulin-potentiating agents or beta-blocking agents that mask symptoms	Stressful situation such as infection, accident, trauma, emotional stress; omission of insulin; medications that antagonize insulin	Infection, medications that antagonize insulin, comorbid condition
Typical Onset		
Rapid	Slow	Slowest
Presenting Symptoms		
Adrenergic reaction: pallor, sweating, tachycardia, palpitations, hunger, restlessness, anxiety, tremors Neurogenic reaction: fatigue, irritability, headache, loss of concentration, visual disturbances, dizziness, hunger, confusion, transient sensory or motor defects, convulsions, coma, death	Malaise, dry mouth, headache, polyuria, polydipsia, weight loss, nausea, vomiting, pruritus, abdominal pain, lethargy, shortness of breath, Kussmaul respirations, fruity or acetone odour to breath	Polyuria, polydipsia, hypovolemia, dehydration (parched lips, poor skin turgor), hypotension, tachycardia, hypoperfusion, weight loss, weakness, nausea, vomiting, abdominal pain, hypothermia, stupor, coma, seizures
Laboratory Analysis		
Serum glucose <1.7 mmol/L in newborn (first 2–3 days) and <3.0–3.4 mmol/L in adults	Glucose levels >14 mmol/L, reduction in bicarbonate concentration, increased anion gap, increased plasma levels of β-hydroxybutyrate, acetoacetate, and acetone	Glucose levels >33.6 mmol/L, lack of ketosis, serum osmolarity >320 mmol/L, elevated blood urea nitrogen and creatinine levels

catabolism. With insulin deficiency, lipolysis is enhanced and there is an increase in the amount of nonesterified fatty acids delivered to the liver. The consequence is increased glyconeogenesis contributing to hyperglycemia and production of ketone bodies (acetoacetate, hydroxybutyrate, and acetone) by the mitochondria of the liver at a rate that exceeds peripheral use. Accumulation of ketone bodies causes a drop in pH, resulting in metabolic acidosis. Symptoms of DKA include Kussmaul respirations (hyperventilation in an attempt to compensate for the acidosis), postural dizziness, central nervous system depression, ketonuria, anorexia, nausea, abdominal pain, thirst, and polyuria. DKA is managed with a combination of fluids, insulin, and electrolyte replacement.

HHS is an uncommon but significant complication of type 2 diabetes with a high overall mortality. It occurs more often in older adults who have other comorbidities, including infections or cardiovascular or renal disease. HHS differs from DKA in the degree of insulin deficiency (which is more profound in DKA) and the degree of fluid deficiency (which is more marked in HHS). The clinical features of HHS include a very high serum glucose concentration and osmolarity and a near-normal serum bicarbonate level and pH. Glucose levels are considerably higher in HHS than in DKA because of volume depletion. Because the amount of insulin required to inhibit fat breakdown is less than that needed for effective glucose transport, insulin levels are sufficient to prevent excessive lipolysis and ketosis (see Figure 19-13). Clinical manifestations include severe dehydration; loss of electrolytes, including potassium; and neurological changes, such as stupor. Management includes fluid, insulin, and electrolyte replacement.

Chronic Complications of Diabetes Mellitus

A number of serious complications are associated with any type of poorly controlled diabetes mellitus. Most complications are associated with insulin resistance or deficit, chronic hyperglycemia (also known as *glucose toxicity*), accumulation of advanced glycation end products, and activation of metabolic pathways that cause tissue damage and the chronic complications of diabetes mellitus. These complications include microvascular disease (damage to capillaries; **retinopathy**, **nephropathy**, and **neuropathy**) and macrovascular disease (damage to larger vessels; coronary artery, peripheral vascular, and cerebrovascular disease) (Table 19-6). Strict control of blood glucose level reduces some complications, particularly nonfatal myocardial infarction, but increases 5-year mortality. Strict control is not recommended for high-risk individuals with type 2 diabetes, but the individual risk–benefit profile should be considered.[73,74]

TABLE 19-6 Chronic Complications of Diabetes Mellitus

Complications	Pathological Mechanisms	Associated Symptoms
Microvascular		
Retinopathy		
Nonproliferative	Microaneurysms, capillary dilation, soft and hard exudates, dot and flame hemorrhages, arteriovenous shunts	May have no visual changes
Proliferative	Formation of new blood vessels, vitreal hemorrhage, scarring, retinal detachment	Loss of visual acuity
Maculopathy	Macular edema	Loss of central vision
Hyperglycemic lens edema	Shunting of glucose to polyol pathway: hyperosmolar fluid in lens	Blurring of vision
Cataract formation	Chronic hyperglycemia	Decreasing visual acuity
Nephropathy	Glomerular basement membrane thickening, mesangial expansion, glomerulosclerosis, focal tubular atrophy; hyperperfusion and hyperfiltration	Microalbuminuria and hypertension slowly progressing to end-stage kidney failure
Neuropathy	Oxidative stress, poor perfusion and ischemia, loss of nerve growth factor	Nerve dysfunction and degeneration
Peripheral neuropathy	Oxidative stress, poor perfusion and ischemia, loss of nerve growth factor	Distal symmetrical sensorimotor polyneuropathy with glove and stocking loss of sensation (pain, vibration, temperature, proprioception); loss of motor nerve function with clawed toes and small muscle wasting in hands and flexor muscles; Charcot joints (loss of sensation results in joint and ligament degeneration, particularly of foot) Acute painful neuropathy with burning pain in legs and feet
Autonomic neuropathy	Oxidative stress, poor perfusion and ischemia, loss of nerve growth factor	Heart rate variability and postural hypotension Gastroparesis (delayed gastric emptying) and diarrhea Loss of bladder tone, urinary retention, and risk for bladder infection Erectile dysfunction and impotence in men
Skin and foot lesions	Loss of sensation, poor perfusion, suppressed immunity, and increased risk for infection	High risk for pressure ulcers and delayed wound healing; abscess formation; development of necrosis and gangrene, particularly of toes and foot; infection and osteomyelitis
Macrovascular		
Cardiovascular	Endothelial dysfunction, dyslipidemia, accelerated atherosclerosis, coagulopathies	Hypertension, coronary artery disease, cardiomyopathy, and heart failure
Cerebrovascular	Endothelial dysfunction, dyslipidemia, accelerated atherosclerosis, coagulopathies	Increased risk for ischemic and thrombotic stroke
Peripheral vascular	Endothelial dysfunction, dyslipidemia, accelerated atherosclerosis, coagulopathies	Claudication, nonhealing ulcers, gangrene
Infection	Impaired immunity, decreased perfusion, recurrent trauma, delayed wound healing, urinary retention	Wound infections, urinary tract infections, increased risk for sepsis

Microvascular Disease

Diabetic microvascular complications (disease in capillaries) are a leading cause of blindness, end-stage kidney failure, and various neuropathies. Occlusion of capillaries is characteristic of diabetic microvascular disease. The frequency and severity of lesions appear to be proportional to the duration of the disease (more or less than 10 years) and the status of glycemic control. Hypoxia and ischemia accompany microvascular disease, especially in the eye, kidney, and nerves. Many individuals with type 2 diabetes will present with microvascular complications because of the long duration of asymptomatic hyperglycemia that generally precedes diagnosis. This evidence underscores the need to screen for diabetes.

Diabetic retinopathy. Diabetic retinopathy is a leading cause of blindness worldwide and is the most common cause of newly diagnosed blindness in people of working age.[75] Compared with that in type 1 diabetes, retinopathy seems to develop more rapidly in individuals with type 2 diabetes because of the likelihood of longstanding hyperglycemia before diagnosis. Most individuals with diabetes will eventually develop retinopathy, and they are also more likely to develop cataracts and glaucoma (see Chapter 14).

Diabetic retinopathy results from relative hypoxemia, damage to retinal blood vessels, red blood cell aggregation, and hypertension (Figure 19-14). The three stages of retinopathy that lead to loss of vision are *nonproliferative* (stage I), characterized by an increase in retinal capillary permeability, vein dilation, microaneurysm formation, and superficial (flame-shaped) and deep (blot) hemorrhages; *preproliferative* (stage II), a progression of retinal ischemia with areas of poor perfusion that culminate in infarcts; and *proliferative* (stage III), the result of neovascularization (angiogenesis) and fibrous tissue formation within the retina or optic disc. Traction of the new vessels on the vitreous humour may cause retinal detachment or hemorrhage into the vitreous humour with severe blurring or loss of vision. Macular edema is the leading cause of blurred vision among persons with diabetes. Blurring of vision also can be a consequence of hyperglycemia and sorbitol accumulation

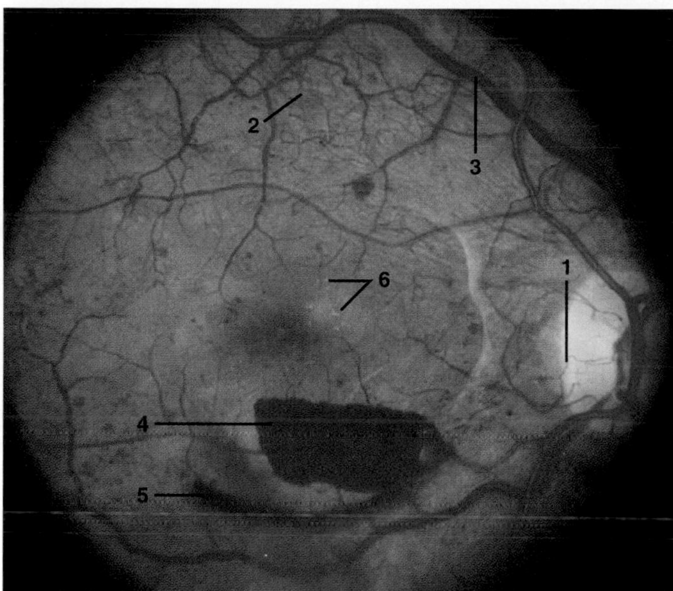

FIGURE 19-14 Diabetic Retinopathy. Neovascularization is present at the optic nerve (**1**) and along vascular pathways (**2**). Retinal veins are engorged (**3**) and a preretinal boat-shaped hemorrhage (**4**) is present below the fovea. A more diffuse mild vitreous hemorrhage (**5**) is present below the preretinal hemorrhage. A few small, hard exudates are visible in the fovea (**6**). (From Palay, D.A., & Krachmer, J.H. [2006]. *Primary care ophthalmology* [2nd ed.]. St. Louis: Mosby.)

in the lens. Dehydration of the lens, aqueous humour, and vitreous humour also reduces visual acuity.

Diabetic nephropathy. Diabetes is the most common cause of chronic kidney disease and end-stage kidney disease. Approximately 50% of individuals with diabetes mellitus develop diabetic kidney disease.[76]

Hyperglycemia, advanced glycation end products (AGEs), activation of metabolic pathways, and inflammation all contribute to kidney tissue injury; yet the exact process responsible for destruction of kidneys in diabetes is unknown. Renal glomerular changes occur early in diabetes mellitus, occasionally preceding the overt manifestation of the disease. The glomeruli are injured by hyperglycemia with high renal blood flow (hyperfiltration), by increases in proximal tubular reabsorption, and by intraglomerular hypertension exacerbated by systemic hypertension. There is progressive glomerulosclerosis and decreased glomerular blood flow and glomerular filtration. Alterations in glomerular membrane permeability occur with loss of negative charge and albuminuria. Ultimately, there can be tubular and interstitial fibrosis contributing to loss of function.[77]

Microalbuminuria is the first manifestation of diabetic kidney dysfunction. Before proteinuria, no clinical signs or symptoms of progressive glomerulosclerosis are likely to be evident. Later, hypoproteinemia, reduction in plasma oncotic pressure, fluid overload, anasarca (generalized body edema), and hypertension may occur. As renal function continues to deteriorate, individuals with type 1 diabetes may experience hypoglycemia (because of loss of renal insulin metabolism), which necessitates a decrease in insulin therapy. As the glomerular filtration rate drops below 10 mL/min, uremic signs, such as nausea, lethargy, acidosis, anemia, and uncontrolled hypertension, occur (see Chapter 30 for a discussion of renal failure). Proteinuria is strongly correlated with morbidity and mortality from cardiovascular disease.[78] Early diagnosis and control of hypertension and hyperglycemia decreases the severity of nephropathy and delays the onset of end-stage kidney disease.[79]

Diabetic neuropathies. Diabetic neuropathy is the most common cause of neuropathy in the Western world and is the most common complication of diabetes. The underlying pathological mechanism includes both metabolic and vascular factors related to chronic hyperglycemia with ischemia and demyelination contributing to neural changes and delayed conduction. Both somatic and peripheral nerve cells show diffuse or focal damage, resulting in polyneuropathy. Sensory neuropathies include distal symmetrical polyneuropathy, focal neuropathy (wristdrop, footdrop), and diabetic amyotrophy (muscle atrophy; weakness; and pain in the muscles of the hip, thigh, and buttocks). Loss of pain, temperature, and vibration sensation is more common than motor involvement and often involves the extremities first in the hands and feet. Motor neuropathies can affect muscle groups, particularly of the feet, contributing to deformity and unstable balance. Peripheral neuropathy can cause Charcot arthropathy, a progressive deterioration of weight-bearing joints, typically in the foot and ankle. Distal neuropathies combined with vascular complications, infection, or injury can lead to amputation[80] (Figures 19-15 and 19-16).

Autonomic neuropathies include delayed gastric emptying, diabetic diarrhea, altered bladder function (e.g., decreased sensation of bladder fullness, urge or overflow incontinence), impotence, orthostatic hypotension, and heart rate variability with both tachycardia and bradycardia.[81] Neuropathy may occur during periods of "good" glucose control and may be the initial clinical manifestation of type 2 diabetes. Chronic hyperglycemia also can cause cognitive dysfunction with alterations in learning and memory.[82]

Macrovascular Disease

Macrovascular disease (lesions in large- and medium-sized arteries) increases morbidity and mortality and increases risk for hypertension, accelerated atherosclerosis (Figure 19-17), cardiovascular disease, stroke, and peripheral vascular disease, particularly among individuals with type 2 diabetes. (Atherosclerosis is discussed in Chapter 24.) Children with poorly controlled diabetes have higher risk for macrovascular complications within one to two decades.[83] The process tends to be more severe and accelerated in the presence of other risk factors, including obesity, dyslipidemia, and smoking.[84]

Cardiovascular disease. Cardiovascular disease is the ultimate cause of death in up to 68% of people with diabetes, with higher risk for women.[85] Hypertension often coexists with diabetes mellitus, is more prevalent than in the nondiabetic population, and can have many causes. In type 1 diabetes, hypertension is associated with the development of microalbuminuria. In type 2 diabetes, hypertension is associated with metabolic syndrome. Hypertension increases the risk for coronary artery disease and stroke. Coronary artery disease is the most common cause of morbidity and mortality in individuals with diabetes mellitus. Mechanisms of disease include vessel injury related to insulin resistance and hyperglycemia oxidative stress, accelerated atherosclerosis associated with high levels of triglycerides, high levels of small low-density lipoproteins (LDLs), and low levels of high-density lipoproteins (HDLs); platelet activation and prothrombosis; and endothelial cell dysfunction.[86] In general, the prevalence of coronary artery disease increases with the duration but not the severity of diabetes and the onset can be silent.

The incidence of *heart failure* is higher in individuals with diabetes, even without myocardial infarction. This may be related to cardiomyopathy and the presence of increased amounts of collagen in the ventricular wall and ventricular hypertrophy. There is reduced mechanical adherence of the heart during filling with diastolic and, eventually, systolic failure.[87] (Heart disease is described in Chapter 24.) Guidelines have been developed to reduce the risk and improve treatment of cardiovascular and coronary artery disease in individuals with diabetes.[49,88,89]

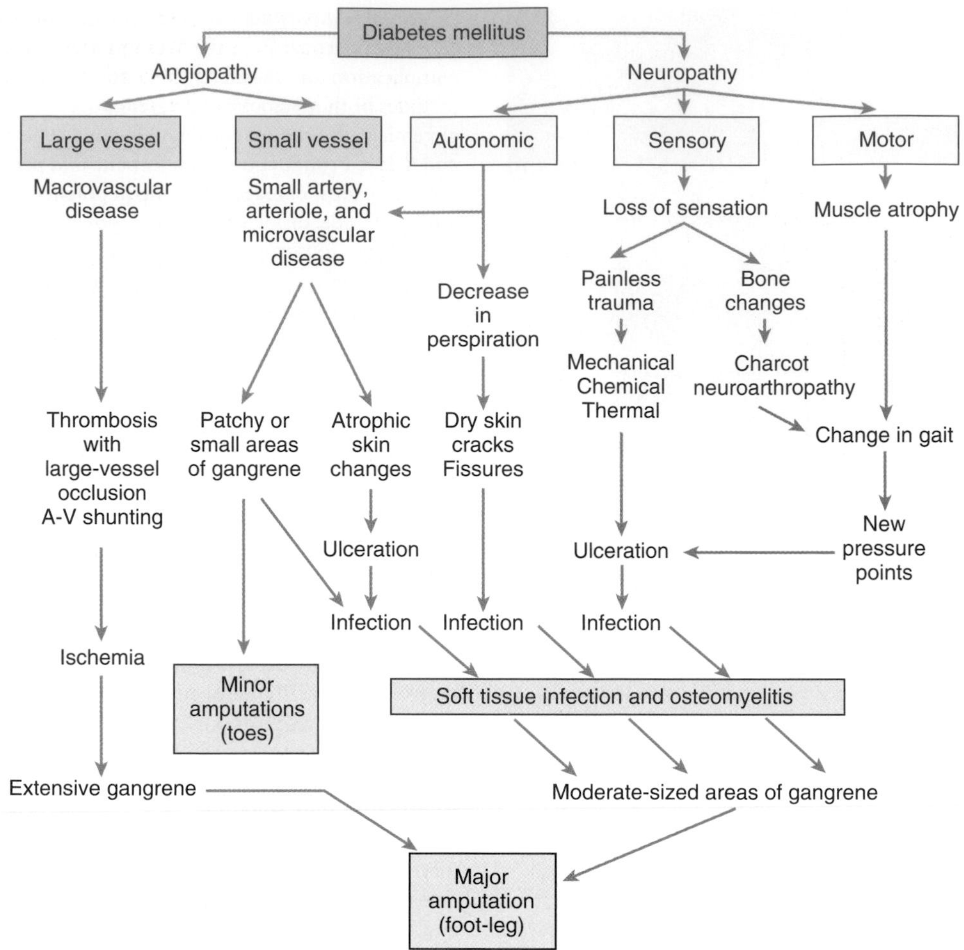

FIGURE 19-15 How Foot Lesions of Diabetes Lead to Amputation. (From Levin, M.E., O'Neal, L., & Bowker, J. [Eds.]. [1993]. *The diabetic foot* [5th ed.]. St. Louis: Mosby.)

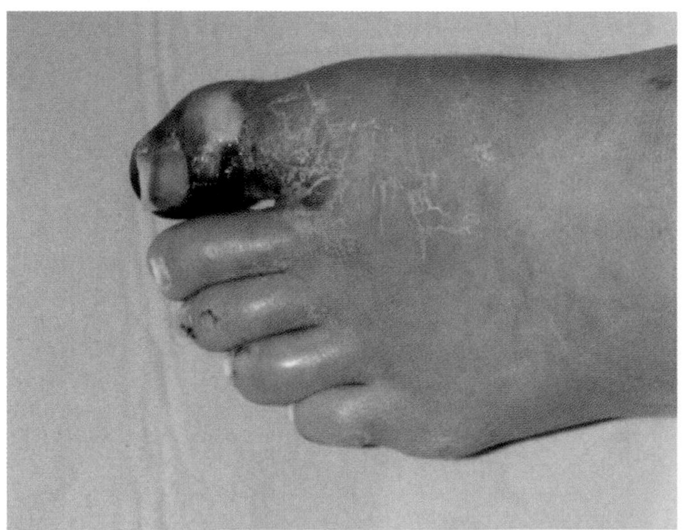

FIGURE 19-16 A Diabetic Foot. (Reprinted from *The Lancet,* 361(9368), Jeffcoate, W.J., & Harding, K.G., "Diabetic foot ulcers," Pages 1545–1551, Copyright 2003, with permission from Elsevier.)

Stroke. Stroke is twice as common in those with diabetes (particularly type 2 diabetes) as in the nondiabetic population.[90] The survival rate for individuals with diabetes after a massive stroke is typically shorter than that for nondiabetic individuals. Hypertension, hyperglycemia, dyslipidemia, and thrombosis are definite risk factors.

Peripheral vascular disease. Diabetes mellitus increases the incidence of peripheral vascular disease (PVD), with claudication (pain from reduced blood flow during exercise), ulcers, gangrene, and amputation.[84] Age, duration of diabetes, genetics, and additional risk factors (smoking, dyslipidemia, hypertension) influence the development and management of PVD. In those with diabetes, PVD is more diffuse and often involves arteries below the knee. Occlusions of the small arteries and arterioles cause most of the gangrenous changes of the lower extremities and occur in patchy areas of the feet and toes. The lesions begin as ulcers and progress to osteomyelitis or gangrene requiring amputation. Peripheral neuropathies and increased risk for infection advance the disease[80] (see Figure 19-15). Significant morbidity and mortality are associated with major amputation.

Infection

The individual with diabetes is at an increased risk for infection throughout the body for several reasons[91]:

- *The senses.* Impaired vision caused by retinal changes and impaired touch caused by neuropathy lead to loss of protection with injury

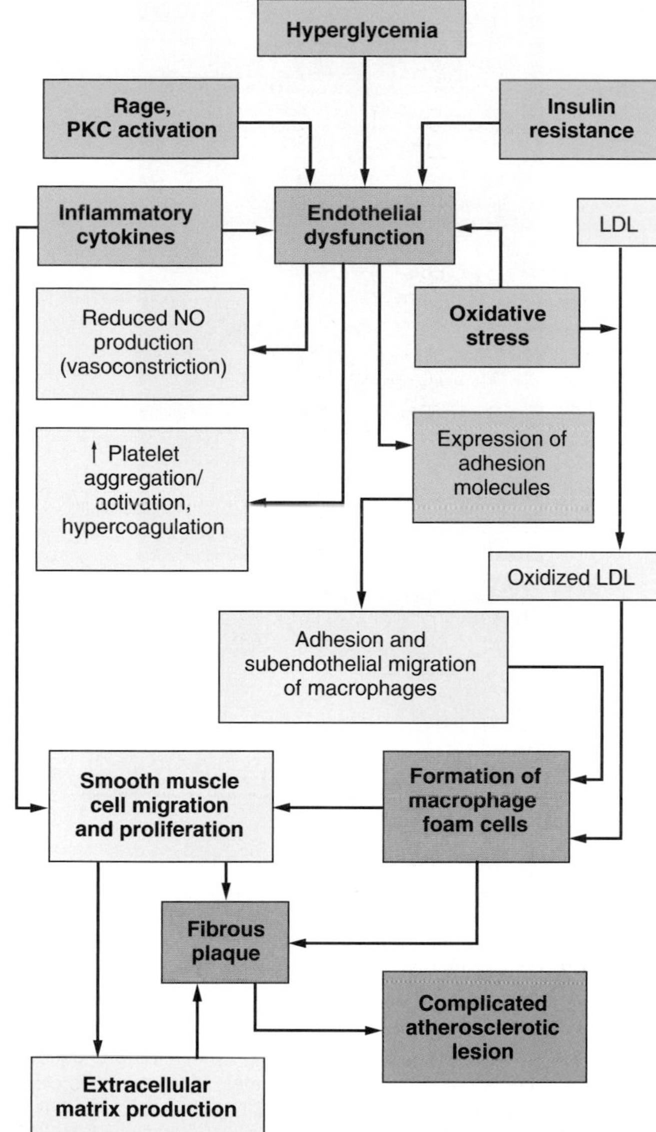

FIGURE 19-17 Diabetes Mellitus and Atherosclerosis. Diabetes with its associated hyperglycemia, relative hypoinsulinemia, oxidative stress, and proinflammatory state contributes to atherogenesis by causing arterial endothelial dysfunction (impaired vasodilation and adhesion of inflammatory cells), dyslipidemia, and smooth muscle proliferation. *LDL,* low-density lipoprotein; *NO,* nitric oxide; *PKC,* protein kinase C; *RAGE,* receptor advanced glycation end product. (Data from Plutzky, K., Zafrir, B., & Brown, J.D. [2015]. *Vascular biology of atherosclerosis in patients with diabetes, diabetes in cardiovascular disease: A companion to Braunwald's heart disease* [pp. 10, 111–126]. Philadelphia: Saunders; Zeadin, M.G., Petlura, C.I., & Werstuck, G.H. [2013]. *Can J Diabetes, 37*[5], 345–350.)

and repeated trauma, open wounds, and soft tissue or osseous infection, particularly in the legs and feet.

- *Hypoxia.* Once skin integrity is compromised, susceptibility to infection increases as a result of hypoxia. In addition, the glycosylated hemoglobin in the red blood cells impedes the release of oxygen to tissues.
- *Pathogens.* Some pathogens proliferate rapidly because of increased glucose in body fluids, which provides an excellent source of energy.
- *Blood supply.* Decreased blood supply results from vascular changes and reduces the supply of white blood cells to the affected area.
- *Suppressed immune response.* Chronic hyperglycemia impairs both innate and adaptive immune responses, including abnormal chemotaxis and vasoactive responses, and defective phagocytosis. Clinical signs of infection may be absent.

QUICK CHECK 19-4

1. What are the major differences between type 1 and type 2 diabetes mellitus in relation to insulin?
2. How does obesity contribute to the development of type 2 diabetes?
3. What are three metabolic alterations related to hyperglycemia that contribute to diabetic complications?
4. What is the single most important factor to address in the management of diabetes mellitus?

ALTERATIONS OF ADRENAL FUNCTION

Disorders of the Adrenal Cortex

Disorders of the adrenal cortex are related to hyperfunction or hypofunction. Hyperfunction that causes increased secretion of cortisol (hypercortisolism) leads to Cushing's disease or Cushing's syndrome. Hyperfunction that causes increased secretion of adrenal androgens or estrogens leads to virilization or feminization. Hyperfunction that causes increased levels of aldosterone leads to hyperaldosteronism, which may be primary or secondary. These syndromes often have overlapping features. Hypofunction of the adrenal cortex leads to Addison's disease.

Hypercortical Function (Cushing's Syndrome, Cushing's Disease)

Cushing's syndrome refers to the clinical manifestations resulting from chronic exposure to excess cortisol regardless of cause. Cushing's disease refers to excess endogenous secretion of ACTH. It is more common in women but men may have more severe symptoms.[92] *ACTH-dependent hypercortisolism* results from overproduction of pituitary ACTH by a pituitary adenoma (which can occur at any age) or by an ectopic-secreting nonpituitary tumour, such as a small cell carcinoma of the lung (more common in older adults). *ACTH-independent hypercortisolism* is caused by cortisol secretion from a rare benign or malignant tumour of one or both adrenal glands (more common in children). A Cushing's-like syndrome may develop as a side effect of long-term pharmacological administration of glucocorticoids.[93]

PATHOPHYSIOLOGY Whatever the cause, two observations consistently apply to individuals with hypercortisolism: (1) the normal diurnal or circadian secretion patterns of ACTH and cortisol are lost, and (2) there is no increase in ACTH and cortisol secretion in response to a stressor.[94] With ACTH-dependent hypercortisolism, the excess ACTH stimulates excess production of cortisol and there is loss of feedback control of ACTH secretion. In individuals with ACTH-dependent hypercortisolism, secretion of both cortisol and adrenal androgens is increased, and cortisol-releasing hormone is inhibited. ACTH-independent secreting tumours of the adrenal cortex, however, generally secrete only cortisol. When the secretion of cortisol by the tumour exceeds normal cortisol levels, symptoms of hypercortisolism develop.

CLINICAL MANIFESTATIONS Weight gain is the most common feature and results from the accumulation of adipose tissue in the trunk, facial, and cervical areas. These characteristic patterns of fat deposition have been respectively described as "truncal obesity," "moon face," and "buffalo hump" (Figures 19-18 and 19-19).

Glucose intolerance occurs because of cortisol-induced insulin resistance and increased gluconeogenesis and glycogen storage by the

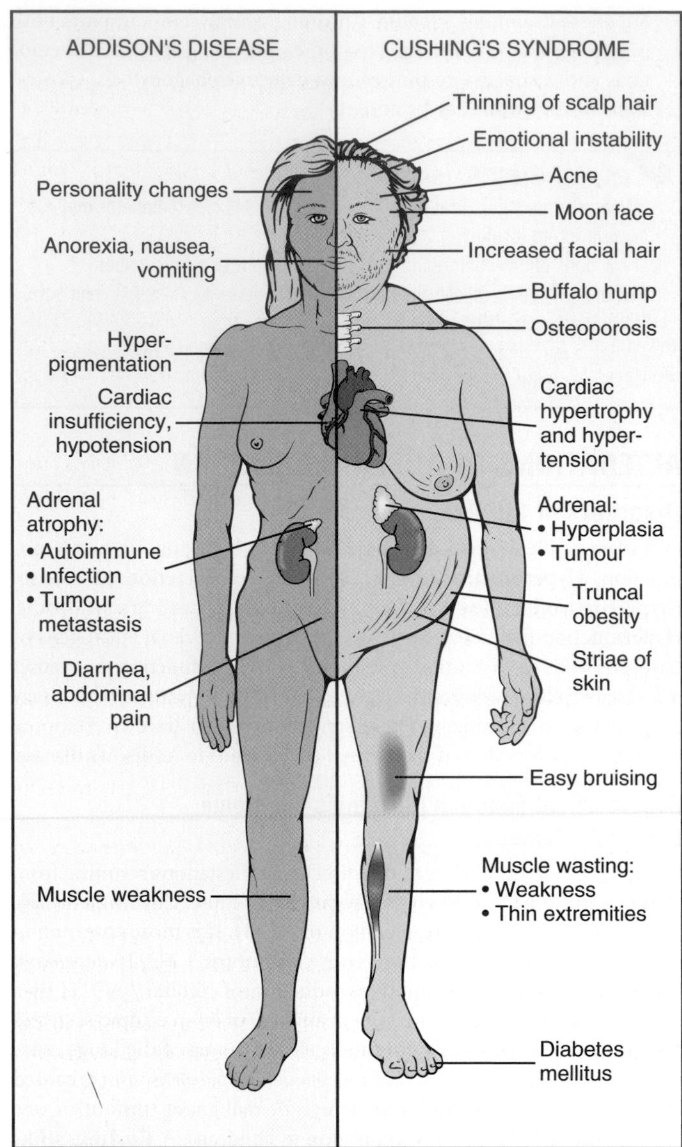

FIGURE 19-18 Symptoms of Addison's Disease and Cushing's Syndrome. (From Goodman, C.C., & Kelly Snyder, T.E. [2013]. *Differential diagnosis for physical therapists* [5th ed.]. Philadelphia: Saunders.)

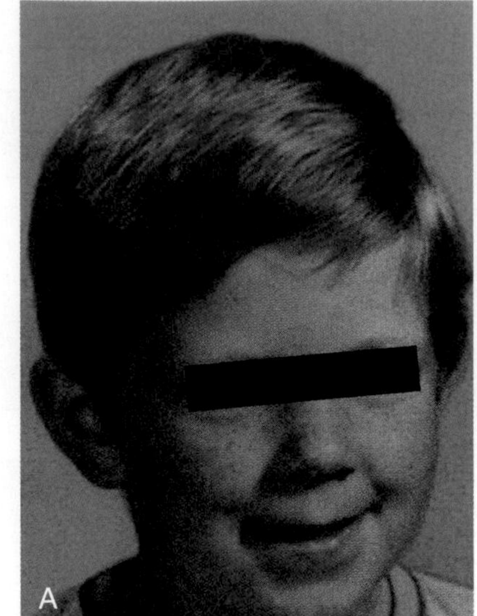

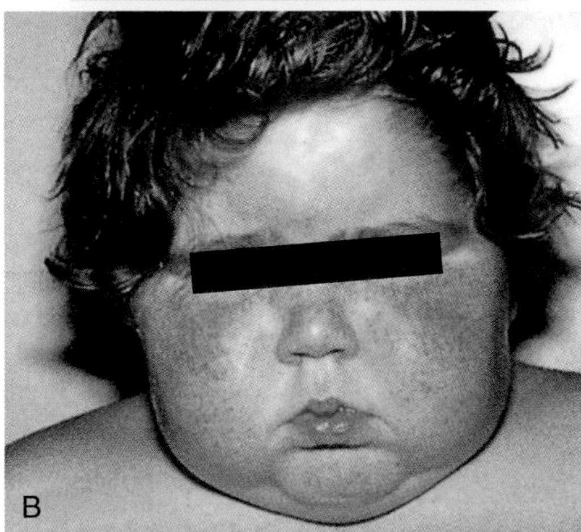

FIGURE 19-19 Cushing's Syndrome. A, Patient before onset of Cushing's syndrome. **B,** Patient 4 months later. Moon facies is clearly demonstrated. (From Zitelli, B.J., McIntire, S.C., & Nowalk, A.J. [2012]. *Zitelli and Davis' atlas of pediatric physical diagnosis* [6th ed.]. London: Saunders.)

liver. Overt diabetes mellitus develops in approximately 20% of individuals with hypercortisolism. Polyuria is a manifestation of hyperglycemia and resultant glycosuria.

Protein wasting is caused by the catabolic effects of cortisol on peripheral tissues. Muscle wasting leads to muscle weakness. In bone, loss of the protein matrix leads to osteoporosis, with pathological fractures, vertebral compression fractures, bone and back pain, kyphosis, and reduced height. Cortisol interferes with the action of GH in long bones; thus children who present with short stature may be experiencing growth delays related to Cushing's syndrome rather than GH deficiency. Bone disease may contribute to hypercalciuria and resulting renal stones.

In the skin, loss of collagen leads to thin, weakened integumentary tissues through which capillaries are more visible and are easily stretched by adipose deposits. Together, these changes account for the characteristic purple striae seen in the trunk area. Loss of collagenous support around small vessels makes them susceptible to rupture, leading to easy bruising, even with minor trauma. Thin, atrophied skin is also easily damaged, leading to skin breaks and ulcerations. Bronze or brownish hyperpigmentation of the skin, mucous membranes, and hair occurs when there are very high levels of ACTH.

With elevated cortisol levels, vascular sensitivity to catecholamines increases significantly, leading to vasoconstriction and hypertension. Mineralocorticoid effects promote hypokalemia and sodium and water retention with transient weight gain. Suppression of the immune system and increased susceptibility to infections also occur. Approximately 50% of individuals with Cushing's syndrome experience irritability and depression, disturbed sleep, difficulty concentrating, memory loss, and, rarely, schizophrenialike psychosis.[95] Females with ACTH-dependent hypercortisolism may experience symptoms of increased adrenal androgen levels (virilism), with increased hair growth (especially facial hair), acne, and oligomenorrhea. Rarely, unless an adrenal carcinoma is involved, do androgen levels become high enough to cause changes of the voice, recession of the hairline, and hypertrophy of the clitoris.

EVALUATION AND TREATMENT Routine laboratory examinations may reveal hyperglycemia, glycosuria, hypokalemia, and metabolic alkalosis. A variety of laboratory tests are used to confirm the diagnosis of hypercortisolism and to determine the underlying disorder. These include urinary free cortisol level higher than 138 nmol/day, abnormal dexamethasone suppressibility of either urinary or serum cortisol, and simultaneous measurement of ACTH and cortisol levels. Late-evening salivary cortisol levels are used as a screening test and to document alterations in the diurnal variation of cortisol level.[96] Tumours are diagnosed using imaging procedures.

Treatment is specific for the cause of hypercorticoadrenalism and includes surgery, medication, and radiation. Differentiation between pituitary ectopic and adrenal causes is essential for effective treatment. Without treatment, approximately 50% of individuals with Cushing's syndrome die within 5 years of onset as a result of overwhelming infection, suicide, complications from generalized arteriosclerosis, and hypertensive disease.

Congenital Adrenal Hyperplasia

Congenital adrenal hyperplasia results from an inherited deficiency of an enzyme that is critical in cortisol biosynthesis. Because cortisol is not produced efficiently, the concentration of ACTH increases and causes adrenal hyperplasia, which results in the overproduction of mineralocorticoids or androgens, or both. The most common form is a 21-hydroxylase deficiency, which involves both mineralocorticoid and cortisol synthesis. Affected female children are virilized and may have genital ambiguity. Infants of both genders exhibit salt wasting. Prenatal diagnosis is available and treatment guidelines have been developed. Disease management requires lifelong treatment with glucocorticoids and mineralocorticoids.[97,98]

Hyperaldosteronism

Hyperaldosteronism is characterized by excessive adrenal secretion of aldosterone. Both primary and secondary forms of hyperaldosteronism can occur.

Primary hyperaldosteronism (Conn's syndrome, primary aldosteronism) is caused by excessive secretion of aldosterone from an abnormality of the adrenal cortex, usually a single benign aldosterone-producing adrenal adenoma. Bilateral adrenal nodular hyperplasia and adrenal carcinomas account for the remainder of cases. The incidence is estimated to be about 10% of all hypertensive individuals; however, approximately 33% of people with resistant hypertension will have evidence of primary hyperaldosteronism.[99]

Secondary hyperaldosteronism results from an extra-adrenal stimulus of aldosterone secretion, most often by angiotensin II through a renin-dependent mechanism. Examples include decreased circulating blood volume (e.g., in dehydration, shock, or hypoalbuminemia) and decreased delivery of blood to the kidneys (e.g., renal artery stenosis, heart failure, or hepatic cirrhosis). Here, the activation of the renin-angiotensin system and subsequent aldosterone secretion may be seen as compensatory, although in some instances (e.g., heart failure) the increased circulating volume further worsens the condition. Other causes of secondary hyperaldosteronism are Bartter syndrome, a renal tubular defect causing hypokalemia, and renin-secreting tumours of the kidney.

PATHOPHYSIOLOGY In *primary hyperaldosteronism*, pathophysiological alterations are caused by excessive aldosterone secretion and the fluid and electrolyte imbalances that ensue. Hyperaldosteronism promotes (1) increased renal sodium and water reabsorption with corresponding hypervolemia (see Chapter 5) and hypertension and (2) renal excretion of hydrogen and potassium (see Chapter 5). The extracellular fluid volume overload, hypertension, and suppression of renin secretion are characteristic of primary disorders. Edema may not occur with primary aldosteronism because hypervolemia-induced atrial natriuretic factor release results in loss of sodium and water.[100] Hypokalemic alkalosis, changes in myocardial conduction, and skeletal muscle weakness may be seen, particularly with severe potassium depletion.

In *secondary hyperaldosteronism*, the effect of increased extracellular volume on renin secretion may vary. If renin secretion is being stimulated by variables other than pressure-initiated cellular changes at the juxtaglomerular apparatus (see Chapter 29), increased circulating blood volume may not decrease renin secretion through feedback mechanisms. This process occurs, for instance, in states of increased estrogen levels.

CLINICAL MANIFESTATIONS Hypertension, hypokalemia, and neuromuscular manifestations are the hallmarks of primary hyperaldosteronism. Hypertension is resistant to treatment and can lead to the development of left ventricular dilation and hypertrophy, vascular disease, and kidney disease.[101]

EVALUATION AND TREATMENT Various clinical and laboratory evaluations are useful in assessing hyperaldosteronism and include the following:

- Measurement of blood pressure: hypertension is usually present
- Measurement of serum and urinary electrolyte levels: serum sodium level is normal or elevated and serum potassium level is depressed, but urinary potassium level is elevated; metabolic alkalosis may be present
- Evaluation of the plasma aldosterone-to-renin ratio: an increased ratio may indicate hyperaldosteronism
- Aldosterone suppression testing: it is performed using either salt loading or fludrocortisone acetate (Florinef) if the aldosterone-to-renin ratio has increased
- Imaging techniques: they are used to localize an aldosterone-secreting adenoma

Treatment includes management of hypertension and hypokalemia, as well as correction of any underlying causal abnormalities. If an aldosterone-secreting adenoma is present, it must be surgically removed. Medical management with aldosterone receptor antagonists, such as spironolactone (Aldactone) or eplerenone (Inspra; a medication without the adverse effects of spironolactone) is a viable option in selected cases.

Hypersecretion of Adrenal Androgens and Estrogens

Hypersecretion of adrenal androgens and estrogens may be caused by adrenal tumours, either adenomas or carcinomas; Cushing's syndrome; or defects in steroid synthesis. The clinical syndrome that is manifested depends on the hormone secreted, the gender of the individual, and the age at which the hypersecretion is initiated. Hypersecretion of estrogens causes **feminization**, the development of female secondary sex characteristics. Hypersecretion of androgens causes **virilization**, the development of male secondary sex characteristics (Figure 19-20).

The effects of an estrogen-secreting tumour are most evident in males and result in gynecomastia (98% of cases), testicular atrophy, and decreased libido. In female children, such tumours may lead to early development of secondary sex characteristics. The changes caused by an androgen-secreting tumour are more easily observed in females and include excessive face and body hair growth (hirsutism), clitoral enlargement, deepening of the voice, amenorrhea, acne, and breast atrophy. In children, virilizing tumours promote precocious sexual development and bone aging. Treatment of androgen-secreting tumours usually involves surgical excision.

Adrenocortical Hypofunction

Hypocortisolism (low levels of cortisol secretion) develops either because of inadequate stimulation of the adrenal glands by ACTH or because of a primary inability of the adrenals to produce and secrete the adrenocortical hormones. Sometimes there is partial dysfunction of

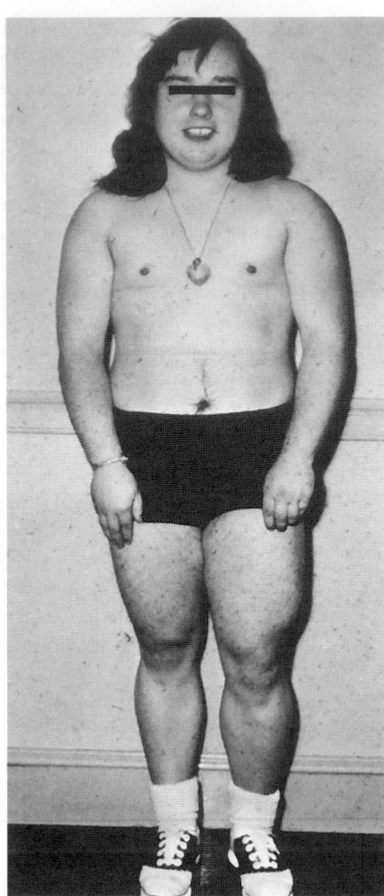

FIGURE 19-20 Virilization. Virilization of a young girl by an androgen-secreting tumour of the adrenal cortex. Masculine features include lack of breast development, increased muscle bulk, and hirsutism (excessive hair). (From Thibodeau, G.A., & Patton, K.T. [2010]. *The human body in health & disease* [4th ed.]. St. Louis: Mosby.)

the adrenal cortex, so only synthesis of cortisol and aldosterone or the adrenal androgens is affected. Hypofunction of the adrenal cortex may affect glucocorticoid or mineralocorticoid secretion, or both.

Addison's disease. Primary adrenal insufficiency is termed Addison's disease. It is relatively rare, occurring most often in adults aged 30 to 60 years, although it may appear at any time. Addison's disease is caused by autoimmune mechanisms that destroy adrenal cortical cells and is more common in women. Chronic infections, such as tuberculosis, account for the majority of cases of primary adrenal insufficiency in underdeveloped countries.

PATHOPHYSIOLOGY Addison's disease is characterized by inadequate corticosteroid and mineralocorticoid synthesis and elevated levels of serum ACTH (loss of negative feedback). Before clinical manifestations of hypocortisolism are evident, more than 90% of total adrenocortical tissue must be destroyed.

Idiopathic Addison's disease (organ-specific autoimmune adrenalitis) causes adrenal atrophy and hypofunction and is an organ-specific autoimmune disease. It may occur in childhood (type 1) or adulthood (type 2). 21-Hydroxylase autoantibodies and autoreactive T cells specific to adrenal cortical cells are present in 50 to 70% of individuals with idiopathic Addison's disease, and this percentage increases in younger persons and in those with other autoimmune diseases. This deficiency allows the proliferation of immunocytes directed against specific antigens within the adrenocortical cells.[102]

The adrenal glands in idiopathic Addison's disease are smaller than normal and may be misshapen. Idiopathic Addison's disease is often associated with other autoimmune diseases, especially Hashimoto's thyroiditis, pernicious anemia, and idiopathic hypoparathyroidism. In these cases, Addison's disease may be inherited as an autosomal recessive trait. (Mechanisms of inheritance are described in Chapter 2.)

CLINICAL MANIFESTATIONS The symptoms of Addison's disease are primarily a result of hypocortisolism and hypoaldosteronism and are often nonspecific. With mild to moderate hypocortisolism, symptoms begin with weakness and easy fatigability. Skin changes, including hyperpigmentation and vitiligo, may occur. As the condition progresses, anorexia, nausea, vomiting, and diarrhea may develop. Of greatest concern is the development of hypotension that can progress to complete vascular collapse and shock. This is known as *adrenal crisis*, or addisonian crisis, and develops with undiagnosed disease or acute withdrawal of glucocorticoid therapy.

EVALUATION AND TREATMENT Serum and urine levels of cortisol are depressed with primary hypocortisolism, and ACTH levels are increased. Because of dehydration, blood urea nitrogen levels may increase. Serum glucose level is low. Eosinophil and lymphocyte counts often are elevated. Hyperkalemia is seen in Addison's disease and may cause mild alkalosis (see Chapter 5). The ACTH stimulation test may be used to evaluate serum cortisol levels.

The treatment of Addison's disease involves lifetime glucocorticoid and possibly mineralocorticoid replacement therapy, together with dietary modifications and correction of any underlying disorders.[103] With acute stressors (e.g., infection, surgery, or trauma), additional cortisol must be administered to approximate the amount of cortisol that might be expected if normal adrenal function were present (approximately 100 to 300 mg/day). The individual's diet should include at least 150 mmol of sodium per day, and sodium intake should be increased if the individual experiences excessive sweating or diarrhea.

Secondary hypocortisolism. Secondary hypocortisolism commonly results from prolonged administration of exogenous glucocorticoids; they suppress ACTH secretion and cause adrenal atrophy, resulting in inadequate corticosteroidogenesis once the exogenous glucocorticoids are withdrawn. Decreased ACTH secretion also can result from pituitary infarction, pituitary tumours that compress ACTH-secreting cells, or hypophysectomy. In all instances of low ACTH levels, adrenal atrophy occurs and endogenous adrenal steroidogenesis is depressed. Clinical manifestations of secondary hypocortisolism are similar to those of Addison's disease, although hyperpigmentation usually does not occur. The renin-angiotensin system usually is normal, so aldosterone and potassium levels also tend to be normal.

Tumours of the Adrenal Medulla

Hyperfunction of the adrenal medulla is caused by pheochromocytomas (chromaffin cell tumours) or sympathetic paragangliomas of the adrenal medulla. They are rare, and about 10% are malignant and metastasize to the lungs, liver, bones, or para-aortic lymph nodes. The tumours are usually sporadic, although up to 40% of them can be inherited.[104]

PATHOPHYSIOLOGY Pheochromocytomas and sympathetic paragangliomas cause excessive production of norepinephrine, although large tumours secrete epinephrine and norepinephrine because of autonomous secretion of the tumour. Approximately 5% of people with these tumours have no symptoms, apparently because the tumour is nonfunctioning. Such tumours can, however, release catecholamines, especially in response to a stressor, such as surgery.

CLINICAL MANIFESTATIONS The clinical manifestations of a pheochromocytoma and sympathetic paragangliomas are related to the chronic effects of catecholamine secretion and include persistent hypertension, headache, pallor, diaphoresis, tachycardia, and palpitations. Hypertension results from increased peripheral vascular resistance and may be sustained or paroxysmal. An acute episode of hypertension related to hypersecretion of catecholamines may follow specific events, such as exercise, excessive ingestion of tyrosine-containing foods (aged cheese, red wine, beer, yogourt), ingestion of caffeine-containing foods, external pressure on the tumour, and induction of anaesthesia. Hypertension unresponsive to medication therapy is often the first indication of a pheochromocytoma. Headaches appear because of sudden changes in catecholamine levels in the blood, affecting cerebral blood flow. Hypermetabolism and sweating are related to chronic activation of sympathetic receptors in adipocytes, hepatocytes, and other tissues. Glucose intolerance may occur because of catecholamine-induced inhibition of insulin release by the pancreas. These tumours tend to be extremely vascular and can rupture, causing massive and potentially fatal hemorrhage.

EVALUATION AND TREATMENT Symptoms of pheochromocytoma can be insidious or intermittent and difficult to diagnose. A diagnosis is made when increased catecholamine production is found in the blood or urine. The site of the tumour is then determined using abdominal imaging techniques. Because of the possibility of metastasis, whole-body scanning may be done.

Management of catecholamine excess is essential to prevent hypertensive emergencies and requires the use of α- and β-adrenergic blockers. The usual treatment of pheochromocytoma is laparoscopic surgical excision of the tumour, although open resection is still completed for large tumours or when metastasis is suspected. Medical therapy is continued to stabilize blood pressure before, during, or after surgery.[105] Malignant pheochromocytoma is rarely curable and is usually managed by a combination of surgical debulking of the tumour combined with chemotherapy.[106]

QUICK CHECK 19-5

1. What are the symptoms of hyperaldosteronism?
2. What major diseases are classified as hypocortisolism?
3. What are pheochromocytomas?

DID YOU UNDERSTAND?

Mechanisms of Hormonal Alterations

1. Abnormalities in endocrine function may be caused by elevated or depressed hormone levels that result from (a) faulty feedback systems, (b) dysfunction of the gland, (c) altered metabolism of hormones, (d) dysfunction of carrier proteins, or (e) production of hormones from nonendocrine tissues.
2. Target cells may fail to respond to hormonal stimulation because of (a) cell surface receptor–associated disorders, (b) intracellular disorders, or (c) circulating hormone inhibitors.

Alterations of the Hypothalamic-Pituitary System

1. Dysfunction in the action of hypothalamic hormones is most commonly related to interruption of the connection between the hypothalamus and pituitary—the pituitary stalk.
2. Disorders of the posterior pituitary include syndrome of inappropriate antidiuretic hormone (SIADH) and diabetes insipidus (DI). SIADH is characterized by abnormally high ADH secretion; DI is characterized by abnormally low ADH secretion.
3. In SIADH, high ADH levels interfere with renal free water clearance, leading to hyponatremia and hypo-osmolality, and are associated with brain injury, surgical procedures with certain forms of cancer related to ectopic secretion of ADH by tumour cells, and medications.
4. DI may be neurogenic (caused by insufficient amounts of ADH) or nephrogenic (caused by an inadequate response to ADH). Its principal clinical features are polyuria and polydipsia.
5. Hypopituitarism can be primary (dysfunction of the pituitary) or secondary (dysfunction of the hypothalamus). Primary hypopituitarism can result from a pituitary tumour, trauma, infections, stroke, or surgical removal.
6. Hypopituitarism can affect any or all of the pituitary hormones, and symptoms may range from mild to life-threatening.
7. Hyperpituitarism is caused by pituitary adenomas, which are usually benign, slow-growing tumours that arise from cells of the anterior pituitary.
8. Expansion of a pituitary adenoma causes both neurological and secretory effects. Pressure from the expanding tumour causes hyposecretion of cells, dysfunction of the optic chiasma (leading to visual disturbances), and dysfunction of the hypothalamus and some cranial nerves.
9. Growth hormone (GH) deficiency causes increased body fat, decreased muscle mass, and psychological problems in adults, and hypopituitary dwarfism in children.
10. Hypersecretion of GH in adults causes acromegaly, in which GH secretion becomes high and unpredictable. Pituitary adenoma is the most common cause of acromegaly. Excessive GH secretion in children with open epiphyseal plates causes giantism.
11. Prolonged, abnormally high levels of GH lead to proliferation of body and connective tissue and slowly developing renal, thyroid, and reproductive dysfunction.
12. Prolactinomas result in galactorrhea, hirsutism, amenorrhea, hypogonadism, and osteopenia.

Alterations of Thyroid Function

1. Thyrotoxicosis is a general condition in which elevated thyroid hormone (TH) levels cause greater than normal physiological responses. The condition can be caused by a variety of specific diseases, each of which has its own pathophysiology and course of treatment.
2. In general, hyperthyroidism has a range of endocrine, reproductive, gastro-intestinal, integumentary, and ocular manifestations. These manifestations are caused by increased circulating levels of TH and by stimulation of the sympathetic division of the autonomic nervous system.
3. Graves' disease, the most common form of hyperthyroidism, is caused by an autoimmune mechanism that overrides normal mechanisms for control of TH secretion and is characterized by thyrotoxicosis, ophthalmopathy, and circulating thyroid-stimulating immunoglobulins.
4. Toxic nodular goitre and toxic multinodular goitre occur when TH-regulating mechanisms and abnormal hypertrophy of the thyroid gland cause hyperthyroidism. Toxic multinodular goitre is caused by independently functioning follicular cell adenomas.

5. Thyrotoxic crisis is a severe form of hyperthyroidism that is often associated with physiological or psychological stress. Without treatment, death occurs quickly.
6. Primary hypothyroidism is caused by deficient production of TH by the thyroid gland. Secondary hypothyroidism is caused by hypothalamic or pituitary dysfunction. Symptoms depend on the degree of TH deficiency. Common manifestations include decreased energy metabolism, decreased heat production, and myxedema.
7. Primary hypothyroidism is characterized by an increased level of TSH, which stimulates goitre formation.
8. Autoimmune thyroiditis (Hashimoto's disease) is associated with humoral (antibodies) and cellular autoimmune destruction of the thyroid gland and gradual loss of thyroid function. Autoimmune thyroiditis occurs in those individuals with genetic susceptibility to an autoimmune mechanism that causes thyroid damage and eventual hypothyroidism.
9. Subacute thyroiditis is a self-limiting nonbacterial inflammation of the thyroid gland that damages follicular cells, causing leakage of triiodothyronine (T_3) and thyroxine (T_4). Hyperthyroidism then is followed by transient hypothyroidism, which is corrected by cellular repair and a return to normal levels in the thyroid.
10. Congenital hypothyroidism is the absence of thyroid tissue during fetal development or defects in hormone synthesis.
11. Myxedema is a sign of hypothyroidism caused by alterations in connective tissue with water-binding proteins that lead to edema and thickened mucous membranes.
12. Myxedema coma is a severe form of hypothyroidism that may be life-threatening without emergency medical treatment.
13. Thyroid carcinoma is a relatively rare cancer associated with exposure to ionizing radiation, especially in childhood.

Alterations of Parathyroid Function

1. Hyperparathyroidism, which may be primary or secondary, is characterized by greater than normal secretion of parathyroid hormone (PTH).
2. Primary hyperparathyroidism is caused by an interruption of the normal mechanisms that regulate calcium and PTH levels. Manifestations include chronic hypercalcemia, increased bone resorption, and hypercalciuria.
3. Secondary hyperparathyroidism is a compensatory response to hypocalcemia and often occurs with chronic renal failure and vitamin D deficiency.
4. Tertiary hyperparathyroidism is persistent secretion of PTH after treatment of secondary hyperparathyroidism.
5. Hypoparathyroidism, defined by abnormally low PTH levels, is caused by thyroid surgery, autoimmunity, or genetic mechanisms.
6. The lack of circulating PTH in hypoparathyroidism causes hypocalcemia, hyperphosphatemia, decreased bone resorption, and hypocalciuria.

Dysfunction of the Endocrine Pancreas: Diabetes Mellitus

1. Diabetes mellitus is a group of metabollic disorders characterized by glucose intolerance, chronic hyperglycemia, and disturbances of carbohydrate, protein, and fat metabolism.
2. A diagnosis of diabetes mellitus is based on elevated plasma glucose concentrations and measurement of glycosylated hemoglobin. Classic signs and symptoms are often present as well.
3. The two most common types of diabetes mellitus are type 1 and type 2.
4. Type 1 diabetes mellitus is characterized by loss of beta cells, presence of islet cell antibody, lack of insulin, excess of glucagon, and altered metabolism of fat, protein, and carbohydrates.
5. Type 1 diabetes mellitus is caused by a gradual process of autoimmune destruction of beta cells in genetically susceptible individuals.
6. In type 1 diabetes, hyperglycemia causes polyuria and polydipsia resulting from osmotic diuresis.
7. Diabetic ketoacidosis (DKA) is caused by increased levels of circulating ketones without the inhibiting effects of insulin. Increased levels of circulating fatty acids and weight loss are both manifestations of type 1 uncontrolled diabetes mellitus.
8. Type 2 diabetes is caused by genetic susceptibility that is triggered by environmental factors. The most compelling environmental risk factor is obesity.
9. In the obese, many factors, including metabolic syndrome, altered adipokines, increased fatty acids, inflammation, and hyperinsulinemia, contribute to the development of insulin resistance and hyperglycemia.
10. Some insulin production continues in type 2 diabetes, but the weight and number of beta cells decrease. There are decreased levels of insulin, amylin, ghrelin, and incretins, and glucagon concentration is increased. All contribute to chronic hyperglycemia.
11. A rare monogenetic form of diabetes is called maturity-onset diabetes of youth (MODY).
12. Gestational diabetes mellitus is glucose intolerance during pregnancy.
13. Acute complications of diabetes mellitus include hypoglycemia, DKA, and hyperosmolar hyperglycemic syndrome (HHS).
14. Hypoglycemia in diabetes is a complication related to insulin treatment.
15. DKA develops when there is an absolute or relative deficiency of insulin and an increase in the insulin counter-regulatory hormones of catecholamines—cortisol, glucagon, and GH. DKA presents with hyperglycemia, acidosis, and ketonuria.
16. HHS is pathophysiologically similar to DKA, although levels of free fatty acids are lower in hyperosmolar nonacidotic diabetes, and a lack of ketosis indicates some level of insulin action. Severe dehydration and electrolyte imbalance are present.
17. Chronic complications of diabetes mellitus include microvascular disease (e.g., neuropathy, retinopathy, nephropathy), macrovascular disease (e.g., coronary artery disease, stroke, peripheral vascular disease), and infection.
18. Microvascular disease associated with diabetes mellitus is characterized by thickening of the capillary basement membrane, disruption of microcirculation, and decreased tissue perfusion.
19. Macrovascular disease associated with diabetes mellitus is most often related to the proliferation of atherosclerotic plaques in the arterial wall and coagulation defects.
20. The incidence of coronary heart disease, peripheral vascular disease, and stroke is greater in those with diabetes than in nondiabetic individuals.
21. Individuals with diabetes are at risk for a variety of infections. Infection may be related to sensory impairment and resulting injury, hypoxia, increased proliferation of pathogens in elevated concentrations of glucose, decreased blood supply associated with vascular damage, and impaired immune protection.

Alterations of Adrenal Function

1. Disorders of the adrenal cortex are related to hyperfunction or hypofunction. No known disorders are associated with hypofunction of the adrenal medulla, but medullary hyperfunction causes clinically defined syndromes.
2. Hypercorticol function, or hypercortisolism, causes Cushing's syndrome, which does not involve the pituitary gland, and Cushing's

disease, which is hypercortisolism with pituitary involvement. Congenital adrenal hyperplasia is a genetic disorder with deficient steroidogenesis and excess androgen synthesis.

3. Hypercortisolism is usually caused by Cushing's disease (pituitary-dependent) and very rarely can be caused by ectopic production of ACTH. Complications include obesity, diabetes, protein wasting, immune suppression, and mental status changes.
4. Excessive aldosterone secretion causes hyperaldosteronism, which may be primary or secondary. Primary hyperaldosteronism is caused by an abnormality of the adrenal cortex. Secondary hyperaldosteronism involves an extra-adrenal stimulus, often angiotensin.
5. Hyperaldosteronism promotes increased renal sodium and water reabsorption with corresponding hypervolemia, increased extracellular fluid volume (which is variable), hypokalemia related to renal reabsorption of sodium, and excrtion of potassium.
6. Hypersecretion of adrenal androgens and estrogens can be the result of adrenal tumours, either adenomas or carcinomas. Hypersecretion of estrogens causes feminization, the development of female secondary sexual characteristics. Hypersecretion of androgens causes virilization, the development of male secondary sexual characteristics.
7. Hypofunction of the adrenal cortex can affect glucocorticoid or mineralocorticoid secretion, or both. Hypofunction can be caused by a deficiency of ACTH or by a primary deficiency in the gland itself.
8. Hypocortisolism, or low levels of cortisol, is caused by inadequate adrenal stimulation by ACTH or by primary cortisol hyposecretion. Primary adrenal insufficiency is termed *Addison's disease.*
9. Addison's disease is characterized by elevated ACTH levels with inadequate corticosteroid synthesis and output.
10. Manifestations of Addison's disease are related to hypocortisolism and hypoaldosteronism. Symptoms include weakness, fatigability, hypoglycemia and related metabolic problems, lowered response to stressors, hyperpigmentation, vitiligo, and manifestations of hypovolemia and hyperkalemia.
11. Hyperfunction of the adrenal medulla is usually caused by a pheochromocytoma, a catecholamine-producing tumour. Symptoms of catecholamine excess are related to their sympathetic nervous system effects and include hypertension, palpitations, tachycardia, glucose intolerance, excessive sweating, and constipation.

KEY TERMS

Acromegaly, 469
Addison's disease (primary adrenal insufficiency), 490
Amylin, 477
Autoimmune thyroiditis (Hashimoto's disease, chronic lymphocyte thyroiditis), 473
Beta-cell dysfunction, 481
Central (secondary) thyroid disorders, 471
Congenital adrenal hyperplasia, 489
Cushing's disease, 487
Cushing's-like syndrome, 487
Cushing's syndrome, 487
Dawn phenomenon, 482
Diabetes insipidus (DI), 467
Diabetes mellitus, 476
Diabetic ketoacidosis (DKA), 478
Diabetic neuropathy, 485
Diabetic retinopathy, 484
Feminization, 489
Gestational diabetes mellitus (GDM), 482
Ghrelin, 481
Giantism, 469
Glucagon, 477
Glycosylated hemoglobin (A_{1C}), 476
Graves' disease, 471
Hyperaldosteronism, 489
Hypercortisolism, 487
Hyperosmolar hyperglycemic syndrome (HHS), 482
Hyperparathyroidism, 474
Hyperthyroidism, 471
Hypocortisolism, 489
Hypoglycemia, 482
Hypoparathyroidism, 475
Hypopituitarism, 468
Hypothyroidism, 473
Idiopathic Addison's disease (organ-specific autoimmune adrenalitis), 490
Incretin, 481
Insulin resistance, 479
Macular edema, 484
Maturity-onset diabetes of youth (MODY), 482
Metabolic syndrome, 479
Myxedema, 474
Myxedema coma, 474
Nephropathy, 483
Neuropathy, 483
Painless (silent) thyroiditis, 473
Panhypopituitarism, 468
Pheochromocytoma (chromaffin cell tumour), 490
Pituitary adenoma, 469
Postpartum thyroiditis, 473
Pretibial myxedema (Graves' dermopathy), 472
Primary hyperaldosteronism (Conn's syndrome, primary aldosteronism), 489
Primary hyperparathyroidism, 474
Primary thyroid disorder, 471
Prolactinoma, 470
Retinopathy, 483
Secondary hyperaldosteronism, 489
Secondary hyperparathyroidism, 475
Secondary hypocortisolism, 490
Somogyi effect, 482
Subacute thyroiditis (de Quervain's thyroiditis), 473
Subclinical hypothyroidism, 474
Subclinical thyroid disease, 471
Syndrome of inappropriate antidiuretic hormone (SIADH), 466
Tertiary hyperparathyroidism, 475
Thyroid carcinoma, 474
Thyrotoxic crisis (thyroid storm), 473
Thyrotoxicosis, 471
Toxic adenoma, 473
Toxic multinodular goitre, 472
Type 1 diabetes mellitus, 476
Type 2 diabetes mellitus, 479
Virilization, 489

REFERENCES

1. Sanchez, M., Picard, N., Sauvé, K., et al. (2013). Coordinate regulation of estrogen receptor β degradation by Mdm2 and CREB-binding protein in response to growth signals. *Oncogene, 32*(1), 117–126. doi:10.1038/onc.2012.19.
2. Janneck, M., Burkhardt, T., Rotermund, R., et al. (2014). Hyponatremia after trans-sphenoidal surgery. *Minerva Endocrinologica, 39*(1), 27–31.
3. Ramos-Levi, A. M., Duran Rodriguez-Hervada, A., Mendez-Bailon, M., et al. (2014). Drug-induced hyponatremia: An updated review. *Minerva Endocrinologica, 39*(1), 1–12.
4. Kortenoeven, M. L., & Fenton, R. A. (2014). Renal aquaporins and water balance disorders. *Biochimica et Biophysica Acta, 1840*(5), 1533–1549. doi:10.1016/j.bbagen.2013.12.002.
5. Peri, A., & Giuliani, C. (2014). Management of euvolemic hyponatremia attributed to SIADH in the hospital setting. *Minerva Endocrinologica, 39*(1), 33–41.
6. Bockenhauer, D., & Bichet, D. G. (2015). Pathophysiology, diagnosis and management of nephrogenic diabetes insipidus. *Nature Reviews. Nephrology, 11*(10), 576–588. doi:10.1038/nrneph.2015.89.
7. Wallia, A., Bizhanova, A., Huang, W., et al. (2013). Acute diabetes insipidus mediated by vasopressinase after placental abruption. *Journal of Clinical Endocrinology and Metabolism, 98*(3), 881–886. doi:10.1210/jc.2012-3548.
8. Oiso, Y., Robertson, G. L., Nørgaard, J. P., et al. (2013). Clinical review: Treatment of neurohypophyseal diabetes insipidus. *Journal of Clinical Endocrinology and Metabolism, 98*(10), 3958–3967. doi:10.1210/jc.2013-2326.
9. Kilicli, F., Dokmetas, H. S., & Acibucu, F. (2013). Sheehan's syndrome. *Gynecological Endocrinology, 29*(4), 292–295. doi:10.3109/09513590.2012.752454.
10. Tanriverdi, F., & Kelestimur, F. (2015). Pituitary dysfunction following traumatic brain injury: Clinical perspectives. *Neuropsychiatric Disease and Treatment, 11*, 1835–1843. doi:10.2147/NDT.S65814.
11. Andrikoula, M., Sertedaki, A., Andrikoula, S., et al. (2013). PROP-1 gene mutations in a 63-year-old woman presenting with osteoporosis and hyperlipidaemia. *Hormones, 12*(1), 128–134.

12. Audi, L., Fernández-Cancio, M., Camats, N., et al. (2013). Growth hormone deficiency: An update. *Minerva Endocrinologica, 38*(1), 1–16.
13. Kargi, A. Y., & Merriam, G. R. (2013). Diagnosis and treatment of growth hormone deficiency in adults. *Nature Reviews. Endocrinology, 9*(6), 335–345. doi:10.1038/nrendo.2013.77.
14. Erfurth, E. M., Siesjö, P., & Björk-Eriksson, T. (2013). Pituitary disease mortality: Is it fiction? *Pituitary, 16*(3), 402–412. doi:10.1007/s11102-013-0469-1.
15. Gadelha, M. R., Trivellin, G., Hernández Ramirez, L. C., et al. (2013). Genetics of pituitary adenomas. *Frontiers of Hormone Research, 41*, 111–140. doi:10.1159/000345673.
16. Samarasinghe, S., Emanuele, M. A., & Mazhari, A. (2014). Neurology of the pituitary. *Handbook of Clinical Neurology, 120*, 685–701. doi:10.1016/B978-0-7020-4087-0.00047-4.
17. Andersen, M. (2014). Management of endocrine disease: GH excess: Diagnosis and medical therapy. *European Journal of Endocrinology, 170*(1), R31–R41. doi:10.1530/EJE-13-0532.
18. Olarescu, N. C., Ueland, T., Godang, K., et al. (2014). Inflammatory adipokines contribute to insulin resistance in active acromegaly and respond differently to different treatment modalities. *European Journal of Endocrinology, 170*(1), 39–48. doi:10.1530/EJE-13-0523.
19. Arcopinto, M., Bobbio, E., Bossone, E., et al. (2013). The GH/IGF-1 axis in chronic heart failure. *Endocrine, Metabolic & Immune Disorders Drug Targets, 13*(1), 76–91. doi:10.2174/1871530311313010010.
20. Capatina, C., & Wass, J. A. (2015). 60 years of neuroendocrinology: Acromegaly. *Journal of Endocrinology, 226*(2), T141–T160. doi:10.1530/JOE-15-0109.
21. Glezer, A., & Bronstein, M. D. (2015). Prolactinomas. *Endocrinology and Metabolism Clinics of North America, 44*(1), 71–78. doi:10.1016/j.ecl.2014.11.003.
22. Vale, F. L., Deukmedjian, A. R., Hann, S., et al. (2013). Medically treated prolactin-secreting pituitary adenomas: When should we operate? *British Journal of Neurosurgery, 27*(1), 56–62. doi:10.3109/02688697.2012.714817.
23. Raverot, G., Jouanneau, E., & Trouilias, J. (2014). Management of endocrine disease: Clinicopathological classification and molecular markers of pituitary tumours for personalized therapeutic strategies. *European Journal of Endocrinology, 170*(4), R121–R132. doi:10.1530/EJE-13-1031.
24. Menconi, F., Marcocci, C., & Marinò, M. (2014). Diagnosis and classification of Graves' disease. *Autoimmunity Reviews, 13*(4–5), 398–402. doi:10.1016/j.autrev.2014.01.013.
25. Thyroid Foundation of Canada. (2016). *Health guides on thyroid disease: Hyperthyroidism (thyrotoxicosis)*. Retrieved from http://www.thyroid.ca/thyrotoxicosis.php.
26. Barrio-Barrio, J., Sabater, A. L., Bonet-Farriol, E., et al. (2015). Graves' ophthalmopathy: VISA versus EUGOGO classification, assessment, and management. *Journal of Ophthalmology, 2015*, 249125. doi:10.1155/2015/249125.
27. Dhali, T. K., & Chahar, M. (2015). Thyroid dermopathy—A diagnostic clue of hidden hyperthyroidism. *Dermatoendocrinol, 6*(1), e981078. doi:10.4161/19381980.2014.981078.
28. Sturniolo, G., Gagliano, E., Tonante, A., et al. (2013). Toxic multinodular goitre: Personal case histories and literature review. *Il Giornale Di Chirurgia, 34*(9–10), 257–259.
29. Klubo-Gwiezdzinska, J., & Wartofsky, L. (2012). Thyroid emergencies. *Medical Clinics of North America, 96*(2), 385–403. doi:10.1016/j.mcna.2012.01.015.
30. Pyzik, A., Grywalska, E., Matyjaszek-Matuszek, B., et al. (2015). Immune disorders in Hashimoto's thyroiditis: What do we know so far? *Journal of Immunology Research, 2015*, 979167. doi:10.1155/2015/979167.
31. Agrawal, P., Philip, R., Saran, S., et al. (2015). Congenital hypothyroidism. *Indian Journal of Endocrinology and Metabolism, 19*(2), 221–227. doi:10.4103/2230-8210.131748.
32. Puig-Domingo, M., & Vila, L. (2013). The implications of iodine and its supplementation during pregnancy in fetal brain development. *Current Clinical Pharmacology, 8*(2), 97–109. doi:10.2174/1574884711308020002.
33. Büyükgebiz, A. (2013). Newborn screening for congenital hypothyroidism. *Journal of Clinical Ressearch in Pediatric Endocrinology, 5*(Suppl. 1), 8–12. doi:10.4274/jcrpe.845.
34. Persani, L. (2012). Clinical review: Central hypothyroidism: Pathogenic, diagnostic, and therapeutic challenges. *Journal of Clinical Endocrinology and Metabolism, 97*(9), 3068–3078. doi:10.1210/jc.2012-1616.
35. Khandelwal, D., & Tandon, N. (2012). Overt and subclinical hypothyroidism: Who to treat and how. *Drugs, 72*(1), 17–33. doi:10.2165/11598070-000000000-00000.
36. Suh, S., & Kim, D. K. (2015). Subclinical hypothyroidism and cardiovascular disease. *Endocrinology and Metabolism, 30*(3), 246–251. doi:10.3803/EnM.2015.30.3.246.
37. Hirsch, D., Levy, S., Nadjer, V., et al. (2013). Pregnancy outcomes in women with severe hypothyroidism. *European Journal of Endocrinology, 169*(3), 313–320. doi:10.1530/EJE-13-0228.
38. Canadian Cancer Society. (2012). *Increased cancer rates studied*. Retrieved from http://www.cancer.ca/en/about-us/news/national/2012/increase-in-thyroid-cancer-rates-studied/?region=bc.
39. Brito, J. P., Glonfriddo, M. R., Al Nofal, A., et al. (2014). The accuracy of thyroid nodule ultrasound to predict thyroid cancer: Systematic review and meta-analysis. *Journal of Clinical Endocrinology and Metabolism, 99*(4), 1253–1263. doi:10.1210/jc.2013-2928.
40. Perri, F., Pezzullo, L., Chiofalo, M. G., et al. (2015). Targeted therapy: A new hope for thyroid carcinomas. *Critical Reviews in Oncology/Hematology, 94*(1), 55–63. doi:10.1016/j.critrevonc.2014.10.012.
41. Baloch, Z. W., & LiVolsi, V. A. (2013). Pathology of the parathyroid glands in hyperparathyroidism. *Seminars in Diagnostic Pathology, 30*(3), 165–177. doi:10.1053/j.semdp.2013.06.003.
42. Pasquali, D., Di Matteo, F. M., Renzullo, A., et al. (2012). Multiple endocrine neoplasia, the old and the new: A mini review. *Il Giornale Di Chirurgia, 33*(11–12), 370–373.
43. Jamal, S. A., & Miller, P. D. (2013). Secondary and tertiary hyperparathyroidism. *Journal of Clinical Densitometry, 16*(1), 64–68. doi:10.1016/j.jocd.2012.11.012.
44. Riccardi, D., & Brown, E. M. (2010). Physiology and pathophysiology of the calcium-sensing receptor in the kidney. *American Journal of Physiology – Renal Physiology, 298*(3), F485–F499. doi:10.1152/ajprenal.00608.2009.
45. Cunningham, J., Locatelli, F., & Rodriguez, M. (2011). Secondary hyperparathyroidism: Pathogenesis, disease progression, and therapeutic options. *Clinical Journal of the American Society of Nephrology : CJASN, 6*(4), 913–921. doi:10.2215/CJN.06040710.
46. Pyram, R., Mahajan, G., & Gliwa, A. (2011). Primary hyperparathyroidism: Skeletal and non-skeletal effects, diagnosis and management. *Maturitas, 70*(3), 246–255. doi:10.1016/j.maturitas.2011.07.021.
47. Betterle, C., Garelli, S., & Presotto, F. (2014). Diagnosis and classification of autoimmune parathyroid disease. *Autoimmunity Reviews, 13*(4–5), 417–422. doi:10.1016/j.autrev.2014.01.044.
48. Michels, T. C., & Kelly, K. M. (2013). Parathyroid disorders. *American Family Physician, 88*(4), 249–257.
49. Canadian Diabetes Association Clinical Practice Guidelines Expert Committee. (2013). Canadian Diabetes Association: Clinical practice guidelines for the prevention and management of diabetes in Canada. *Canadian Journal of Diabetes, 37*(Suppl. 1), S1–S212. Retrieved from http://guidelines.diabetes.ca/app_themes/cdacpg/resources/cpg_2013_full_en.pdf.
50. Canadian Diabetes Association. (2016). *Diabetes statistics in Canada*. Retrieved from http://www.diabetes.ca/how-you-can-help/advocate/why-federal-leadership-is-essential/diabetes-statistics-in-canada.
51. Public Health Agency of Canada. (2011). *Diabetes in Canada: Facts and figures from a public health perspective*. Retrieved from http://www.phac-aspc.gc.ca/cd-mc/publications/diabetes-diabete/facts-figures-faits-chiffres-2011/index-eng.php.
52. Atkinson, M. A., Eisenbarth, G. S., & Michels, A. W. (2014). Type 1 diabetes. *Lancet, 383*(9911), 69–82. doi:10.1016/S0140-6736(13)60591-7.
53. Chillarón, J. J., Flores Le-Roux, J. A., Benaiges, D., et al. (2014). Type 1 diabetes, metabolic syndrome and cardiovascular risk. *Metabolism: Clinical and Experimental, 63*(2), 181–187. doi:10.1016/j.metabol.2013.10.002.
54. Malik, F. S., & Taplin, C. E. (2014). Insulin therapy in children and adolescents with type 1 diabetes. *Paediatric Drugs, 16*(2), 141–150.
55. Cogger, K., & Nostro, M. C. (2015). Recent advances in cell replacement therapies for the treatment of type 1 diabetes. *Endocrinology, 156*(1), 8–15. doi:10.1210/en.2014-1691.
56. Ontario Ministry of Health. (1999). *Diabetes: Strategies for prevention*. Retrieved from http://health.gov.on.ca/en/common/ministry/publications/reports/diabetes/diabetes.aspx#identify.
57. Kahn, S. E., Cooper, M. E., & Del Prato, S. (2014). Pathophysiology and treatment of type 2 diabetes: Perspectives on the past, present, and future. *Lancet, 383*(9922), 1068–1083. doi:10.1016/S0140-6736(13)62154-6.
58. Pal, A., & McCarthy, M. I. (2013). The genetics of type 2 diabetes and its clinical relevance. *Clinical Genetics, 83*(4), 297–306. doi:10.1111/cge.12055.
59. Bruce, K. D. (2014). Maternal and in utero determinants of type 2 diabetes risk in the young. *Current Diabetes Reports, 14*(1), 446. doi:10.1007/s11892-013-0446-0.
60. Statistics Canada. (2015). *Metabolic syndrome in adults, 2012–2013*. Retrieved from http://www.statcan.gc.ca/pub/82-625-x/2014001/article/14123-eng.htm.
61. Naci, H., & Ioannidis, J. P. (2013). Comparative effectiveness of exercise and drug interventions on mortality outcomes: Metaepidemiological study. *British Medical Journal, 347*, f5577. doi:10.1136/bmj.f5577.
62. Blüher, M., & Mantzoros, C. S. (2015). From leptin to other adipokines in health and disease: Facts and expectations at the beginning of the 21st century. *Metabolism: Clinical and Experimental, 64*(1), 131–145. doi:10.1016/j.metabol.2014.10.016.
63. Winer, D. A., Winer, S., Chng, M. H., et al. (2014). B lymphocytes in obesity-related adipose tissue inflammation and insulin resistance. *Cellular and Molecular Life Sciences, 71*(6), 1033–1043. doi:10.1007/s00018-013-1486-y.
64. Vetere, A., Choudhary, A., Burns, S. M., et al. (2014). Targeting the pancreatic β-cell to treat diabetes. *Nature Reviews Drug Discovery, 13*(4), 278–289. doi:10.1038/nrd4231.
65. Gingell, J. J., Burns, E. R., & Hay, D. L. (2014). Activity of pramlintide, rat and human amylin but not Aβ1-42 at human amylin receptors. *Endocrinology, 155*(1), 21–26. doi:10.1210/en.2013-1658.
66. Gahete, M. D., Rincón-Fernández, D., Villa-Osaba, A., et al. (2014). Ghrelin gene products, receptors, and GOAT enzyme: Biological and pathophysiological insight. *Journal of Endocrinology, 220*(1), R1–R24. doi:10.1530/JOE-13-0391.
67. Lee, Y. S., & Jun, H. S. (2014). Anti-diabetic actions of glucagon-like peptide-1 on pancreatic beta-cells. *Metabolism: Clinical and Experimental, 63*(1), 9–19. doi:10.1016/j.metabol.2013.09.010.
68. White, J. R., Jr. (2015). Sodium glucose cotransporter 2 inhibitors. *Medical Clinics of North*

America, 99(1), 131–143. doi:10.1016/j.mcna.2014.08.020.
69. Tenzer-Iglesias, P. (2014). Type 2 diabetes mellitus in women. *Journal of Family Practice, 63*(2, Suppl.), S21–S26.
70. McDonald, T. J., & Ellard, S. (2013). Maturity onset diabetes of the young: Identification and diagnosis. *Annals of Clinical Biochemistry, 50*(Pt. 5), 403–415.
71. Moyer, V. A., & U.S. Preventive Services Task Force. (2014). Screening for gestational diabetes mellitus: U.S. Preventive Services Task Force recommendation statement. *Annals of Internal Medicine, 160*(6), 414–420. doi:10.7326/M13-2905.
72. Dabelea, D., Rewers, A., Stafford, J. M., et al. (2014). Trends in the prevalence of ketoacidosis at diabetes diagnosis: The SEARCH for diabetes in youth study. *Pediatrics, 133*(4), e938–e945.
73. ACCORD Study Group, Gerstein, H. C., Miler, M. E., et al. (2011). Long-term effects of intensive glucose lowering on cardiovascular outcomes. *New England Journal of Medicine, 364*(9), 818–828. doi:10.1056/NEJMoa1006524.
74. Giorgino, F., Leonardini, A., & Laviola, L. (2013). Cardiovascular disease and glycemic control in type 2 diabetes: Now that the dust is settling from large clinical trials. *Annals of the New York Academy of Sciences, 1281*, 36–50. doi:10.1111/nyas.12044.
75. Tarr, J. M., Kaul, K., Chopra, M., et al. (2013). Pathophysiology of diabetic retinopathy. *ISRN Ophthalmology, 2013*, 343560. doi:10.1155/2013/343560.
76. Tuttle, K. R., Bakris, G. L., Bilous, R. W., et al. (2014). Diabetic kidney disease: A report from an ADA consensus conference. *American Journal of Kidney Diseases, 64*(4), 510–533. doi:10.1053/j.ajkd.2014.08.001.
77. Blantz, R. C., & Singh, P. (2014). Glomerular and tubular function in the diabetic kidney. *Advances in Chronic Kidney Disease, 21*(3), 297–303. doi:10.1053/j.ackd.2014.03.006.
78. Parving, H. H., Persson, F., & Rossing, P. (2015). Microalbuminuria: A parameter that has changed diabetes care. *Diabetes Research and Clinical Practice, 107*(1), 1–8. doi:10.1016/j.diabres.2014.10.014.
79. Marshall, S. M. (2014). Natural history and clinical characteristics of CKD in type 1 and type 2 diabetes mellitus. *Advances in Chronic Kidney Disease, 21*(3), 267–272. doi:10.1053/j.ackd.2014.03.007.
80. DiPreta, J. A. (2014). Outpatient assessment and management of the diabetic foot. *Medical Clinics of North America, 98*(2), 353–373. doi:10.1016/j.mcna.2013.10.010.
81. Vinik, A. I., & Erbas, T. (2013). Diabetic autonomic neuropathy. *Handbook of Clinical Neurology, 117*, 279–294. doi:10.1016/B978-0-444-53491-0.00022-5.
82. Mayeda, E. R., Whitmer, R. A., & Yaffe, K. (2015). Diabetes and cognition. *Clinics in Geriatric Medicine, 31*(1), 101–115, ix. doi:10.1016/j.cger.2014.08.021.
83. Prendergast, C., & Gidding, S. S. (2014). Cardiovascular risk in children and adolescent with type 2 diabetes mellitus. *Current Diabetes Reports, 14*(2), 454. doi:10.1007/s11892-013-0454-0.
84. Gibbons, G. W., & Shaw, P. M. (2012). Diabetic vascular disease: Characteristics of vascular disease unique to the diabetic patient. *Seminars in Vascular Surgery, 25*(2), 89–92. doi:10.1053/j.semvascsurg.2012.04.005.
85. Norhammar, A., & Schenck-Gustafsson, K. (2013). Type 2 diabetes and cardiovascular disease in women. *Diabetologia, 56*(1), 1–9. doi:10.1007/s00125-012-2694-y.
86. Paneni, F., Beckman, J. A., Creager, M. A., et al. (2013). Diabetes and vascular disease: Pathophysiology, clinical consequences, and medical therapy, Part I. *European Heart Journal, 34*(31), 2436–2443. doi:10.1093/eurheartj/eht149.
87. Pappachan, J. M., Varughese, G. I., Sriraman, R., et al. (2013). Diabetic cardiomyopathy: Pathophysiology, diagnostic evaluation and management. *World Journal of Diabetes, 4*(5), 177–189.
88. Nathan, D. M. (2015). Diabetes: Advances in diagnosis and treatment. *JAMA: The Journal of the American Medical Association, 314*(10), 1052–1062. doi:10.1001/jama.2015.9536.
89. Task Force on Diabetes, Pre-diabetes, and Cardiovascular Diseases of the European Society of Cardiology (ESC), European Association for the Study of Diabetes (EASD), Rydén, L., et al. (2014). ESC guidelines on diabetes, pre-diabetes, and cardiovascular diseases developed in collaboration with the EASD—summary. *Diabetes and Vascular Disease Research, 11*(3), 133–173. doi:10.1177/1479164114525548.
90. Sander, D., & Kearney, M. T. (2009). Reducing the risk of stroke in type 2 diabetes: Pathophysiology and therapeutic perspectives. *Journal of Neurology, 256*(10), 1603–1619. doi:10.1007/s00415-009-5143-1.
91. Gupta, S., Koirala, J., Khardori, R., et al. (2007). Infections in diabetes mellitus and hyperglycemia. *Infectious Disease Clinics of North America, 21*(3), 617–638. doi:10.1016/j.idc.2007.07.003.
92. Zilio, M., Barbot, M., Ceccato, F., et al. (2014). Diagnosis and complications of Cushing's disease: Gender-related differences. *Clinical Endocrinology, 80*(3), 403–410. doi:10.1111/cen.12299.
93. Castinetti, F., Morange, I., Conte-Devolx, B., et al. (2012). Cushing's disease. *Orphanet Journal of Rare Diseases, 7*, 41. doi:10.1186/1750-1172-7-41.
94. Bansal, V., El Asmar, N., Selman, W. R., et al. (2015). Pitfalls in the diagnosis and management of Cushing's syndrome. *Neurosurgical Focus, 38*(2), E4. doi:10.3171/2014.11.FOCUS14704.
95. Starkman, M. N. (2013). Neuropsychiatric findings in Cushing syndrome and exogenous glucocorticoid administration. *Endocrinology and Metabolism Clinics of North America, 42*(3), 477–488. doi:10.1016/j.ecl.2013.05.010.
96. Elias, P., Martinez, E. Z., Barone, B. F., et al. (2014). Late-night salivary cortisol has a better performance than urinary free cortisol in the diagnosis of Cushing's syndrome. *Journal of Clinical Endocrinology and Metabolism, 99*(6), 2014–2051. doi:10.1210/jc.2013-4262.
97. Han, T. S., Walker, B. R., Arit, W., et al. (2014). Treatment and health outcomes in adults with congenital adrenal hyperplasia. *Nature Reviews. Endocrinology, 10*(2), 115–124. doi:10.1038/nrendo.2013.239.
98. Speiser, P. W., Azziz, R., Baskin, L. S., et al. (2010). Congenital adrenal hyperplasia due to steroid 21-hydroxylase deficiency: An Endocrine Society clinical practice guideline. *Journal of Clinical Endocrinology and Metabolism, 95*(9), 4133–4160. doi:10.1210/jc.2009-2631.
99. Chao, C. T., Wu, V. C., Kuo, C. C., et al. (2013). Diagnosis and management of primary aldosteronism: An updated review. *Annals of Medicine, 45*(4), 375–383. doi:10.3109/07853890.2013.785234.
100. Magill, S. B. (2014). Pathophysiology, diagnosis, and treatment of mineralocorticoid disorders. *Comprehensive Physiology, 4*(3), 1083–1119. doi:10.1002/cphy.c130042.
101. Harvey, A. M. (2014). Hyperaldosteronism: Diagnosis, lateralization, and treatment. *Surgical Clinics of North America, 94*(3), 643–656. doi:10.1016/j.suc.2014.02.007.
102. Brandão Neto, R. A., & de Carvalho, J. F. (2014). Diagnosis and classification of Addison's disease (autoimmune adrenalitis). *Autoimmunity Reviews, 13*(4–5), 408–411. doi:10.1016/j.autrev.2014.01.025.
103. Husebye, E. S., Allolio, B., Arit, W., et al. (2014). Consensus statement on the diagnosis, treatment and follow-up of patients with primary adrenal insufficiency. *Journal of Internal Medicine, 275*(2), 104–115. doi:10.1111/joim.12162.
104. Rana, H. Q., Rainville, I. R., & Vaidya, A. (2014). Genetic testing in the clinical care of patients with pheochromocytoma and paraganglioma. *Current Opinion in Endocrinology, Diabetes, and Obesity, 21*(3), 166–176. doi:10.1097/MED.0000000000000059.
105. Tsirlin, A., Oo, Y., Sharma, R., et al. (2014). Pheochromocytoma: A review. *Maturitas, 77*(3), 229–238. doi:10.1016/j.maturitas.2013.12.009.
106. Lenders, J. W., Duh, Q. Y., Eisenhofer, G., et al. (2014). Pheochromocytoma and paraganglioma: An Endocrine Society clinical practice guideline. *Journal of Clinical Endocrinology and Metabolism, 99*(6), 1915–1942. doi:10.1210/jc.2014-1498.

20

Structure and Function of the Hematological System

Neal S. Rote, Kathryn L. McCance, and Kelly Power-Kean

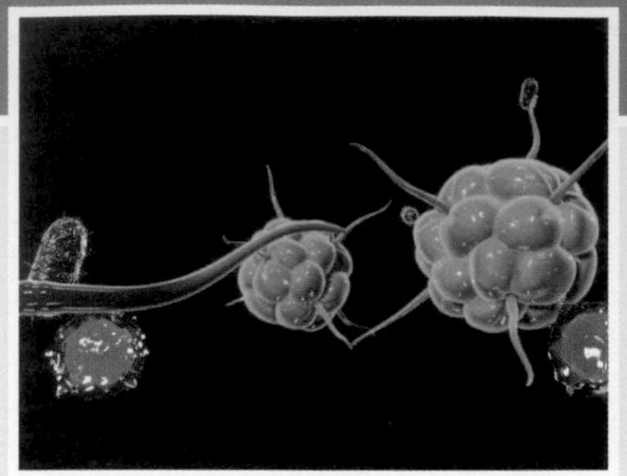

EVOLVE WEBSITE

http://evolve.elsevier.com/Canada/Huether/pathophysiology
Student Review Questions
Key Points
Case Studies
Animations
Quick Check Answers

CHAPTER OUTLINE

Components of the Hematological System, 496
Composition of Blood, 496
Lymphoid Organs, 500
The Mononuclear Phagocyte System, 503
Development of Blood Cells, 503
Hematopoiesis, 503
Development of Erythrocytes, 506
Development of Leukocytes, 509
Development of Platelets, 509
Mechanisms of Hemostasis, 510
Function of Platelets and Blood Vessels, 510
Function of Clotting Factors, 512
Retraction and Lysis of Blood Clots, 513
PEDIATRIC CONSIDERATIONS: **Hematological Value Changes, 516**
GERIATRIC CONSIDERATIONS: **Hematological Value Changes, 517**

All the body's tissues and organs require oxygen and nutrients to survive. These essential needs are provided by the blood that flows through kilometres of vessels throughout the human body. The red blood cells provide the oxygen, and the fluid portion of the blood carries the nutrients. The blood also cleans discarded waste from the tissues and transports cells (white blood cells) and other ingredients that are necessary for protecting the entire body from injury and infection.

COMPONENTS OF THE HEMATOLOGICAL SYSTEM

Composition of Blood

Blood consists of various cells that circulate suspended in a solution of protein and inorganic materials (plasma), which is approximately 92% water and 8% dissolved substances (solutes). The blood volume amounts to about 5.5 L in adults. The continuous movement of blood guarantees that critical components are available to all parts of the body to carry out their chief functions: (1) delivery of substances needed for cellular metabolism in the tissues, (2) removal of the wastes of cellular metabolism, (3) defence against invading microorganisms and injury, and (4) maintenance of acid-base balance.

Plasma and Plasma Proteins

In adults, plasma accounts for 50 to 55% of blood volume (Figure 20-1). **Plasma** is a complex aqueous liquid containing a variety of organic and inorganic elements (Table 20-1). The concentration of these elements varies depending on diet, metabolic demand, hormones, and vitamins. Plasma differs from serum in that **serum** is plasma that has been allowed to clot in the laboratory to remove fibrinogen and other clotting factors that may interfere with some diagnostic tests.

The plasma contains a large number of proteins (**plasma proteins**). These vary in structure and function and can be classified into two major groups: albumin and globulins. Most plasma proteins are produced by the liver. The major exception is antibodies, which are produced by plasma cells in the lymph nodes and other lymphoid tissues (see Chapter 7).

Albumin (about 60% of total plasma protein) serves as a carrier molecule for both normal components of blood and medications. Its most essential role is regulation of the passage of water and solutes through the capillaries. Albumin molecules are large and do not diffuse freely through the vascular endothelium, and thus they maintain the critical colloidal osmotic pressure (or oncotic pressure) that regulates the passage of fluids and electrolytes into the surrounding tissues (see Chapters 1 and 5). Water and solute particles tend to diffuse out of the arterial portions of the capillaries because blood pressure is greater in arterial than in venous blood vessels. Water and solutes move from tissues into the venous portions of the capillaries where the pressures are reversed, oncotic pressure being greater than intravascular pressure or hydrostatic pressure. In the case of decreased production (e.g., cirrhosis, other diffuse liver diseases, protein malnutrition) or excessive loss of albumin (e.g., certain kidney diseases), the reduced oncotic pressure leads to excessive movement of fluid and solutes into the tissue and decreased blood volume.

The remaining plasma proteins, or **globulins**, are often classified by their properties in an electric field (serum electrophoresis). Under the normal conditions used to perform serum electrophoresis, albumin is the most rapidly moving protein. The globulins are classified by their movement relative to albumin: alpha globulins (those moving most closely to albumin), beta globulins, and gamma globulins (those with the least movement). The alpha and beta globulins may be subdivided

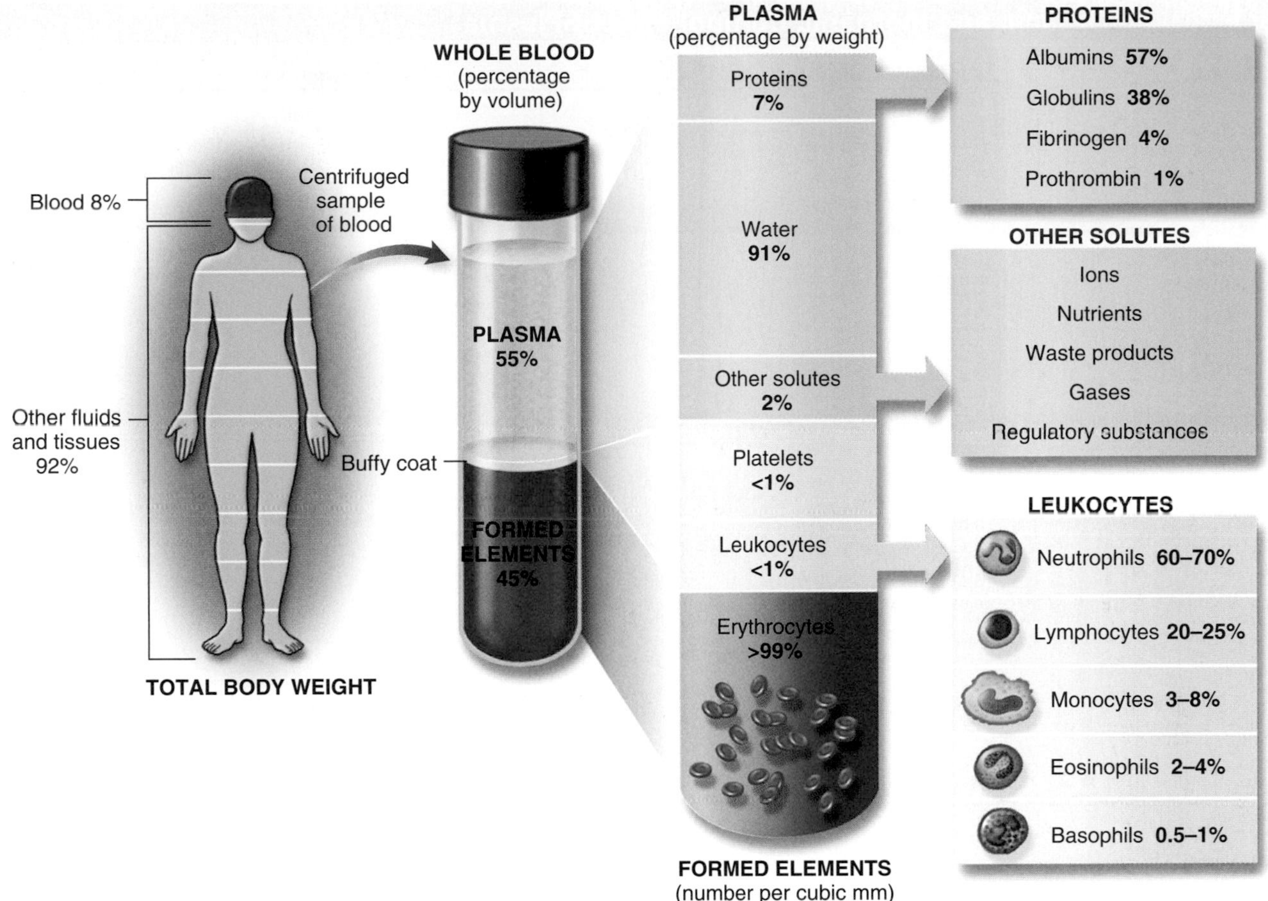

FIGURE 20-1 Composition of Whole Blood. Approximate values for the components of blood in a normal adult. (From Patton, K.T., & Thibodeau, G.A. [2016]. *Structure & function of the body* [15th ed.]. St. Louis: Mosby.)

into subregions (alpha-1, alpha-2, beta-1, or beta-2 globulins). Fibrinogen is a major plasma protein (about 4% of total plasma protein) that would move between the beta and gamma regions but is removed during the formation of serum. The gamma-globulin region consists primarily of antibodies (see Chapter 7).

Plasma proteins can also be classified by function: clotting, defence, transport, or regulation. The **clotting factors** promote coagulation and stop bleeding from damaged blood vessels. Fibrinogen is the most plentiful of the clotting factors and is the precursor of the fibrin clot (see Figure 20-18). Proteins involved in defence, or protection, against infection include antibodies and complement proteins (see Chapters 6 and 7). Transport proteins specifically bind and carry a variety of inorganic and organic molecules, including iron (transferrin), copper (ceruloplasmin), lipids and steroid hormones **(lipoproteins)** (see the discussion on membrane transport in Chapter 1), and vitamins (e.g., retinol-binding protein). Regulatory proteins include a variety of enzymatic inhibitors (e.g., α_1-antitrypsin) that protect the tissues from damage, precursor molecules (e.g., kininogen) that are converted into active biological molecules when needed, and protein hormones (e.g., cytokines) that communicate between cells.

Plasma also contains other solutes including nutrients, waste products, gases, regulatory substances and electrolytes. Several inorganic ions regulate cell function, osmotic pressure, and blood pH. These ions include electrolytes, sodium, potassium, calcium, chloride, and phosphate. (Electrolytes are described in Chapters 1 and 5.)

Cellular Components of the Blood

The cellular components of the blood are broadly classified as red blood cells (i.e., erythrocytes), white blood cells (i.e., leukocytes), and platelets. The components of the blood are listed in Table 20-2. Pathways of blood differentiation or maturation are shown in Figure 20-2.

Erythrocytes. **Erythrocytes** (red blood cells) are the most abundant cells of the blood, occupying about 48% of the blood volume in men and about 42% in women. Erythrocytes are primarily responsible for tissue oxygenation. Hemoglobin (Hb) carries the gases, and electrolytes regulate gas diffusion through the cell's plasma membrane. The mature erythrocyte lacks a nucleus and cytoplasmic organelles (e.g., mitochondria), so it cannot synthesize protein or carry out oxidative reactions. Because it cannot undergo mitotic division, the erythrocyte has a limited lifespan (approximately 80 to 120 days).

The erythrocyte's size and shape are ideally suited to its function as a gas carrier. It is a small disc with two unique properties: (1) a *biconcave* shape and (2) the capacity to be *reversibly deformed*. The flattened, biconcave shape provides a surface area/volume ratio that is optimal for gas diffusion into and out of the cell and for deformity. During its lifespan, the erythrocyte, which is 6 to 8 μm in diameter, repeatedly circulates through splenic sinusoids (Figure 20-3) and capillaries that are only 2 μm in diameter. Reversible deformity enables the erythrocyte to assume a more compact torpedolike shape, squeeze through the microcirculation, and return to normal.

TABLE 20-1 Organic and Inorganic Components of Plasma

Constituent	Amount/Concentration	Major Functions
Water (H_2O)	91% of plasma weight	A medium for carrying all other constituents
Electrolytes	Total >1% of plasma	Maintenance of H_2O in extracellular compartment; they act as buffers and function in membrane excitability
Sodium (Na^+)	136–145 mmol/L	
Potassium (K^+)	3.5–5.0 mmol/L	
Calcium (Ca^{++})	2.25–2.75 mmol/L	
Magnesium (Mg^{++})	0.74–1.07 mmol/L	
Chloride (Cl^-)	98–106 mmol/L	
Bicarbonate (HCO_3^-)	21–28 mmol/L	
Phosphate (PO_4^{3+})	0.97–1.45 mmol/L	
Proteins	64–83 g/L	Provision of colloid osmotic pressure of plasma; they act as buffers (see text for other functions)
Albumins	35–50 g/L	
Globulins	23–34 g/L	
Fibrinogen	5.8–11.8 mcmol/L	
Transferrin	Adult male: 2–5.0 g/L Adult female: 1.9–4.4 g/L	
Ferritin	Male: 12–300 mcg/L Female: 10–150 mcg/L	
Gases		
Carbon dioxide (CO_2) content	35–45 mm Hg	By-product of oxygenation; most CO_2 content is from HCO_3^- and acts as a buffer
Oxygen (O_2)	Pa_{O_2} 80–100 mm Hg (arterial); Pv_{O_2} 40–50 mm Hg (venous)	Oxygenation
Nitrogen gas (N_2)	0.64 mmol/L	By-product of protein catabolism
Nutrients		Provide nutrition and substances for tissue repair
Glucose and other carbohydrates	5.6 mmol/L	
Total amino acids	2.2 mmol/L	
Total lipids	7.5 mmol/L	
Cholesterol	<5.0 mmol/L	
Individual vitamins	0.000 07–1.79 mmol/L	
Individual trace elements	0.0007–0.2 mmol/L	
Iron	11–32 mcmol/L	
Waste Products		
Urea (BUN)	3.6–7.1 mmol/L	End product of protein catabolism
Creatinine (from creatine)	44–106 mcmol/L	End product of energy metabolism
Uric acid (from nucleic acids)	160–501 mcmol/L	End product of protein metabolism
Indirect bilirubin (from heme)	3.4–12.0 mcmol/L	End product of red blood cell destruction
Individual hormones	0.000 01–0.5 g/L	Functions specific to target tissue

PaO_2, partial pressure of oxygen in arterial blood; *PvO_2*, mixed venous oxygen tension.
Data from Pagana, KD., Pagana, T.J., Pike-MacDonald, S.A., et al. (2013). *Mosby's Canadian manual of diagnostic and laboratory tests.* Toronto: Elsevier; Vander, A.J., Luciano, D., & Sherman, J. (2001). *Human physiology: The mechanisms of body function* (8th ed.). New York: McGraw-Hill.

Leukocytes. Leukocytes (white blood cells) defend the body against organisms that cause infection and also remove debris, including dead or injured host cells of all kinds (Figure 20-4). The leukocytes act primarily in the tissues but are transported in the circulation. The average adult has approximately 5 to 10 × 10^9/L of blood.

Leukocytes are classified according to structure as either granulocytes or agranulocytes and according to function as either phagocytes or immunocytes. The granulocytes, which include neutrophils, basophils, and eosinophils, are all phagocytes. (Phagocytosis is described in Chapter 6.) Of the agranulocytes, the monocytes and macrophages are phagocytes, whereas the lymphocytes are immunocytes (cells that create immunity; see Chapter 7).

Granulocytes. The granulocytes have many membrane-bound granules in their cytoplasm. These granules contain enzymes capable of killing microorganisms and catabolizing debris ingested during phagocytosis. The granules also contain powerful biochemical mediators with inflammatory and immune functions. These mediators, along with the digestive enzymes, are released from granulocytes in response to specific stimuli and affect other cells in the circulation. Granulocytes are capable of amoeboid movement, by which they migrate through vessel walls (diapedesis) and then to sites where their action is needed.

The neutrophil (polymorphonuclear neutrophil [PMN]) is the most numerous and best understood of the granulocytes (Figure 20-5). Neutrophils constitute 60 to 70% of the total leukocyte count in adults.

TABLE 20-2 **Cellular Components of the Blood**

Cell	Structural Characteristics	Normal Amounts of Circulating Blood	Function	Lifespan
Erythrocyte (red blood cell [RBC])	Non-nucleated cytoplasmic disc containing hemoglobin	$4.2–6.1 \times 10^{12}$/L	Gas transport to and from tissue cells and lungs	80–120 days
Reticulocyte index	1.0	Immature erythrocyte		
Absolute reticulocyte count	0.5–2.0% of total number of RBCs			
Leukocyte (white blood cell)	Nucleated cell	$5–10 \times 10^9$/L	Body defence mechanisms	See below
Lymphocyte	Mononuclear immunocyte	20–40% of leukocyte count (leukocyte differential)	Humoral and cell-mediated immunity (see Chapter 7)	Days or years, depending on type
Natural killer cell	Large granular lymphocyte	5–10% circulatory pool (some in spleen)	Defence against some tumours and viruses (see Chapters 6 and 7)	Unknown
Monocyte and macrophage	Large mononuclear phagocyte	2–8% of leukocyte differential	Phagocytosis; mononuclear phagocyte system	Months or years
Eosinophil	Segmented polymorphonuclear granulocyte	1–4% of leukocyte differential	Control of inflammation, phagocytosis, defence against parasites, allergic reactions	Unknown
Neutrophil	Segmented polymorphonuclear granulocyte	55–70% of leukocyte differential	Phagocytosis, particularly during early phase of inflammation	4 days
Basophil	Segmented polymorphonuclear granulocyte	0.5–1.0% of leukocyte differential	Mast cell–like functions, associated with allergic reactions and mechanical irritation	Unknown
Platelet	Irregularly shaped cytoplasmic fragment (not a cell)	$150–400 \times 10^9$/L	Hemostasis after vascular injury; normal coagulation and clot formation/retraction	8–11 days

Neutrophils are the chief phagocytes of early inflammation. Soon after bacterial invasion or tissue injury, neutrophils migrate out of the capillaries and into the damaged tissue, where they ingest and destroy contaminating microorganisms and debris. Neutrophils are sensitive to the environment in damaged tissue (e.g., low pH, enzymes released from damaged cells) and die in 1 or 2 days. The breakdown of dead neutrophils releases digestive enzymes from their cytoplasmic granules. These enzymes dissolve cellular debris and prepare the site for healing.

Eosinophils, which have large, coarse granules, constitute only 2 to 4% of the normal leukocyte count in adults. Using a spectrum of pattern-recognition receptors, eosinophils are capable of amoeboid movement and phagocytosis. Unlike neutrophils, eosinophils ingest antigen-antibody complexes and are induced by immunoglobulin E (IgE)–mediated hypersensitivity reactions to attack parasites (see Chapters 7 and 8). Eosinophil secondary granules contain toxic chemicals (e.g., major basic protein, eosinophil cationic protein, eosinophil peroxidase, eosinophil-derived neurotoxin) that are highly destructive to parasites and viruses.[1] Eosinophil granules also contain a variety of enzymes (e.g., histaminase) that help to control inflammatory processes. Eosinophils also release leukotrienes, prostaglandins, platelet-activating factor (PAF), and a variety of cytokines (e.g., interleukin-1 [IL-1], IL-6, tumour necrosis factor-alpha [TNF-α], granulocyte-macrophage colony–stimulating factor [GM-CSF]) and chemokines (e.g., IL-8) that augment the inflammatory response. During type I hypersensitivity, allergic reactions and asthma are characterized by high eosinophil counts, which may be involved in a dual role of regulation of inflammation and contribute to the destructive inflammatory processes observed in the lungs of persons with asthma.

Basophils, which make up less than 1% of leukocytes, are structurally similar to the mast cells (see Figure 20-5). Basophils contain cytoplasmic granules with histamine, chemotactic factors, proteolytic enzymes (e.g., elastase, lysophospholipase), and an anticoagulant (heparin). Stimulation of basophils also induces synthesis of vasoactive lipid molecules (e.g., leukotrienes) and cytokines, including IL-6, which affects differentiation of Th1 cells and Th2 cells. Basophils also are a particularly rich source of the cytokine IL-4, which preferentially guides B-lymphocyte (B-cell) differentiation toward plasma cells that secrete IgE (see Chapter 7).

Agranulocytes. The agranulocytes—monocytes, macrophages, and lymphocytes—contain relatively fewer granules than granulocytes. Monocytes and macrophages make up the mononuclear phagocyte system (MPS) (see "The Mononuclear Phagocyte System" later in this chapter, and Chapter 6). Both monocytes and macrophages participate in the immune and inflammatory response, being powerful phagocytes. They also ingest dead or defective host cells, particularly blood cells.

Monocytes are immature macrophages (see Figure 20-5). Monocytes are formed and released by the bone marrow into the bloodstream. As they mature, monocytes migrate into a variety of tissues (e.g., liver, spleen, lymph nodes, peritoneum, gastro-intestinal tract) and fully mature into tissue **macrophages**. Other monocytes may mature into macrophages and migrate out of the vessels in response to infection or inflammation.

Lymphocytes constitute approximately 20 to 25% of the total leukocyte count and are the primary cells of the immune response (see Figure 20-5 and Chapter 7). Most lymphocytes transiently circulate in the blood and eventually reside in lymphoid tissues as mature T lymphocytes (T cells), B lymphocytes (B cells), or plasma cells. (Lymphocyte function and dysfunction are described in detail in Unit 2.)

Natural killer (NK) cells, which resemble lymphocytes, kill some types of tumour cells (in vitro) and some virus-infected cells without prior exposure (see Chapters 6 and 7). They develop in the bone marrow and circulate in the blood.

Platelets. **Platelets (thrombocytes)** are not true cells but platelike or disc-shaped anuclear cytoplasmic fragments that are essential for blood coagulation and control of bleeding. When platelets are stimulated

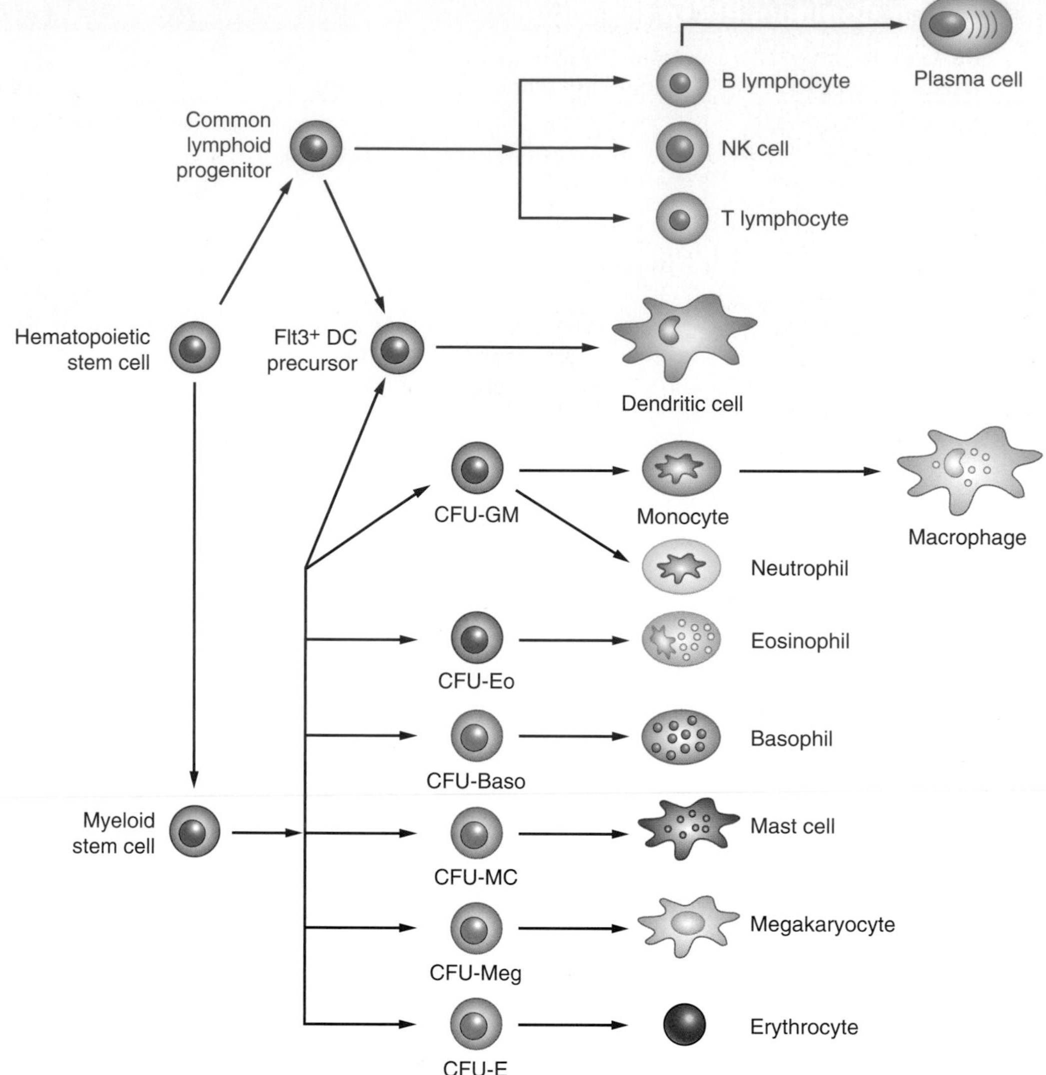

FIGURE 20-2 Differentiation of Hematopoietic Cells. *Arrows* indicate proliferation and expansion of prehematopoietic stem cell populations. *CFU*, colony-forming unit; *CFU-GM*, colony-forming unit–granulocyte-macrophage; *Flt3⁺ DC*, receptor-type tyrosine-protein kinase (Flt3+) dendritic cells (DC); NK, natural killer. (Mast cells are discussed in Chapter 6.)

by blood vessel injury, they have the ability to change shape to conform to the need of the injured site. They are formed by fragmentation of very large (40 to 100 μm in diameter) cells known as **megakaryocytes** and contain cytoplasmic granules capable of releasing potent mediators when stimulated by injury to a blood vessel (Figure 20-6).

The normal platelet concentration is approximately 150 to 400 × 10^9/L of circulating blood, although the normal ranges may vary slightly from laboratory to laboratory. An additional one-third of the body's available platelets are in a reserve pool in the spleen. A platelet circulates for approximately 8 to 11 days, ages, and is removed by macrophages, mostly in the spleen.

QUICK CHECK 20-1

1. What are the unique properties of the erythrocyte's shape?
2. Why are plasma proteins important to blood volume?
3. Which leukocytes are granulocytes?
4. Compare and contrast granulocytes, agranulocytes, phagocytes, and immunocytes.

Lymphoid Organs

The lymphoid system is closely integrated with the circulatory system. The lymphoid organs, some of which are merely aggregations of lymphoid tissue, are classified as primary or secondary. The **primary lymphoid organs** are the thymus and the bone marrow. The **secondary lymphoid organs** consist of the spleen, lymph nodes, tonsils, and Peyer patches of the small intestine. All of the lymphoid organs link the hematological and immune systems in that they are sites of residence, proliferation, differentiation, or function of lymphocytes and mononuclear phagocytes (monocytes and macrophages). (The liver, which also has hematological functions, is primarily a digestive organ and is described in Chapter 35.)

Spleen

The **spleen** is the largest of the lymphoid organs. It serves as a site of fetal hematopoiesis, filters and cleanses the blood by mononuclear phagocytes, initiates an immune response to bloodborne microorganisms, and serves as a reservoir for blood.

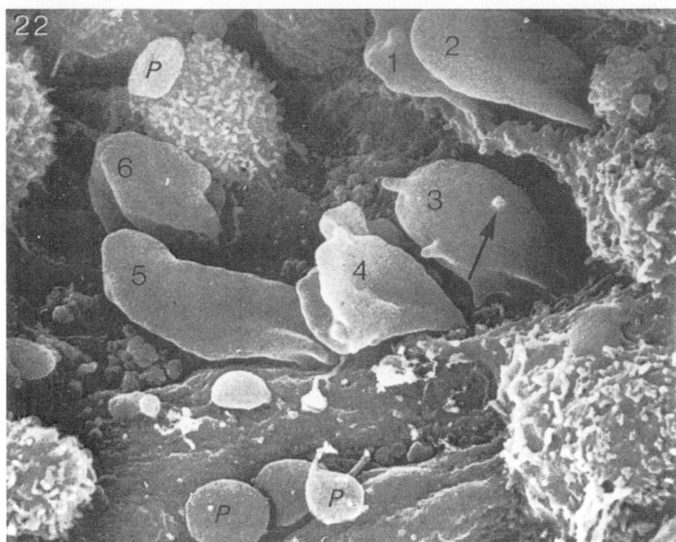

FIGURE 20-3 Red Blood Cells in the Spleen. Scanning electron micrograph of spleen, demonstrating erythrocytes (numbered *1* through *6*) squeezing through the fenestrated wall in transit from the splenic cord to the sinus. The view shows the endothelial lining of the sinus wall, to which platelets (*P*) adhere, along with "hairy" white blood cells, probably macrophages. The *arrow* shows a protrusion on a red blood cell (×5 000). (From Weiss, L. [1974]. *Blood, 43*, 665; reprinted with permission.)

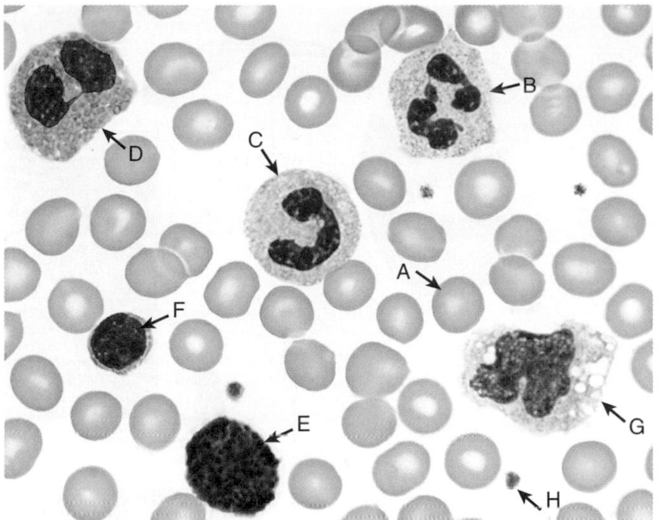

FIGURE 20-5 Leukocytes. Normal cells in peripheral blood: **A,** Erythrocyte (red blood cell); **B,** Neutrophil (segmented); **C,** Neutrophil (banded); **D,** Eosinophil; **E,** Basophil; **F,** Lymphocyte; **G,** Monocyte; **H,** Platelet. (From Keohane, E., Smith, L., & Walenga, J. [2016]. *Rodak's hemotology* [5th ed.]. St. Louis: Saunders.)

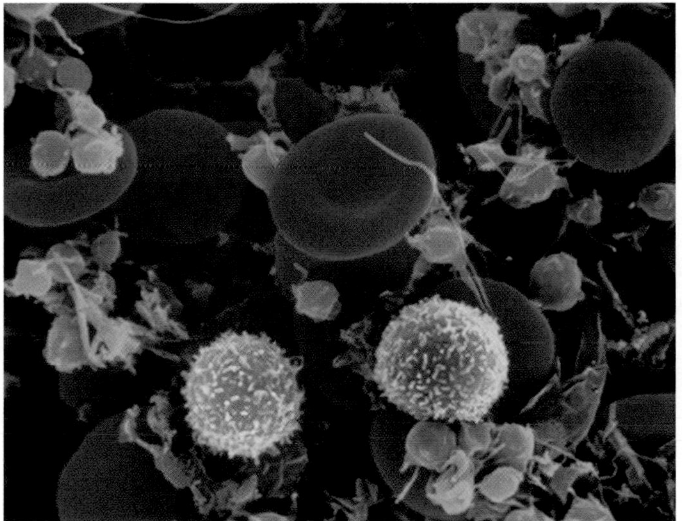

FIGURE 20-4 Blood Cells. Leukocytes are spherical and have irregular surfaces with numerous extending pili. Leukocytes are the cotton candy–like cells (*yellow*). Erythrocytes are flattened spheres with a depressed centre (*red*). (Dennis Kunkel Microscopy/Science Source.)

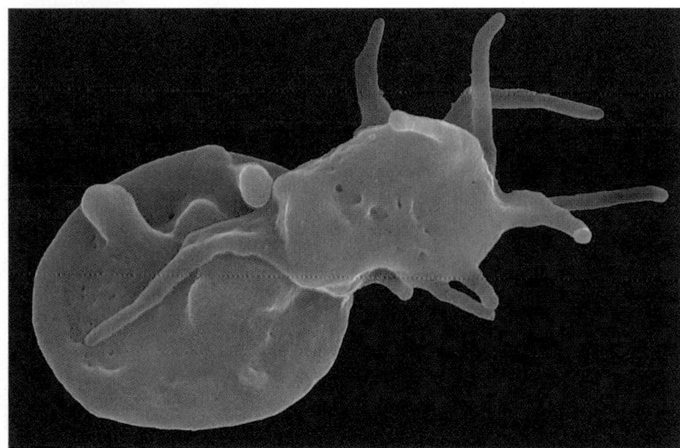

FIGURE 20-6 Coloured Micrograph of Platelets. The platelet on the left is moderately activated, with a generally round shape and the beginning of formation of pseudopodia (footlike extensions from the membrane). The platelet on the right is fully activated, with extensive pseudopodia. (Dennis Kunkel Microscopy/Science Source.)

The spleen is a concave, encapsulated organ that weighs about 150 g and is about the size of a fist. Strands of connective tissue (trabeculae) extend throughout the spleen from the splenic capsule, dividing it into compartments that contain masses of lymphoid tissue called *splenic pulp*. The spleen is interlaced with many blood vessels, some of which can distend to store blood.

Arterial blood that enters the spleen first encounters the white splenic pulp, which consists of masses of lymphoid tissue containing macrophages and lymphocytes, primarily T cells in proximity to the arterioles (Figure 20 7). Cellular clumps (lymphoid follicles) are formed in the white pulp around the splenic arterioles. The lymphoid follicles consist primarily of B cells and are the chief sites of immune function within the spleen. Here bloodborne antigens encounter lymphocytes, initiating the immune response and the conversion of lymphoid follicles into germinal centres (see Chapter 7).

Some of the blood continues through the microcirculation and enters highly distensible storage areas, called *venous sinuses*, in the red pulp of the spleen. The venous sinuses (and the red pulp) can store more than 300 mL of blood. Sudden reductions in blood pressure cause the sympathetic nervous system to stimulate constriction of the sinuses and expel as much as 200 mL of blood into the venous circulation, helping to restore blood volume or pressure in the circulation and increasing the hematocrit by as much as 4%.

The endothelial lining of the venous sinuses is discontinuous (having gaps between endothelial cells) and therefore extremely permeable so that blood cells are allowed to exit the circulation.[2] The red pulp contains a system of loosely interconnected resident macrophages that provide

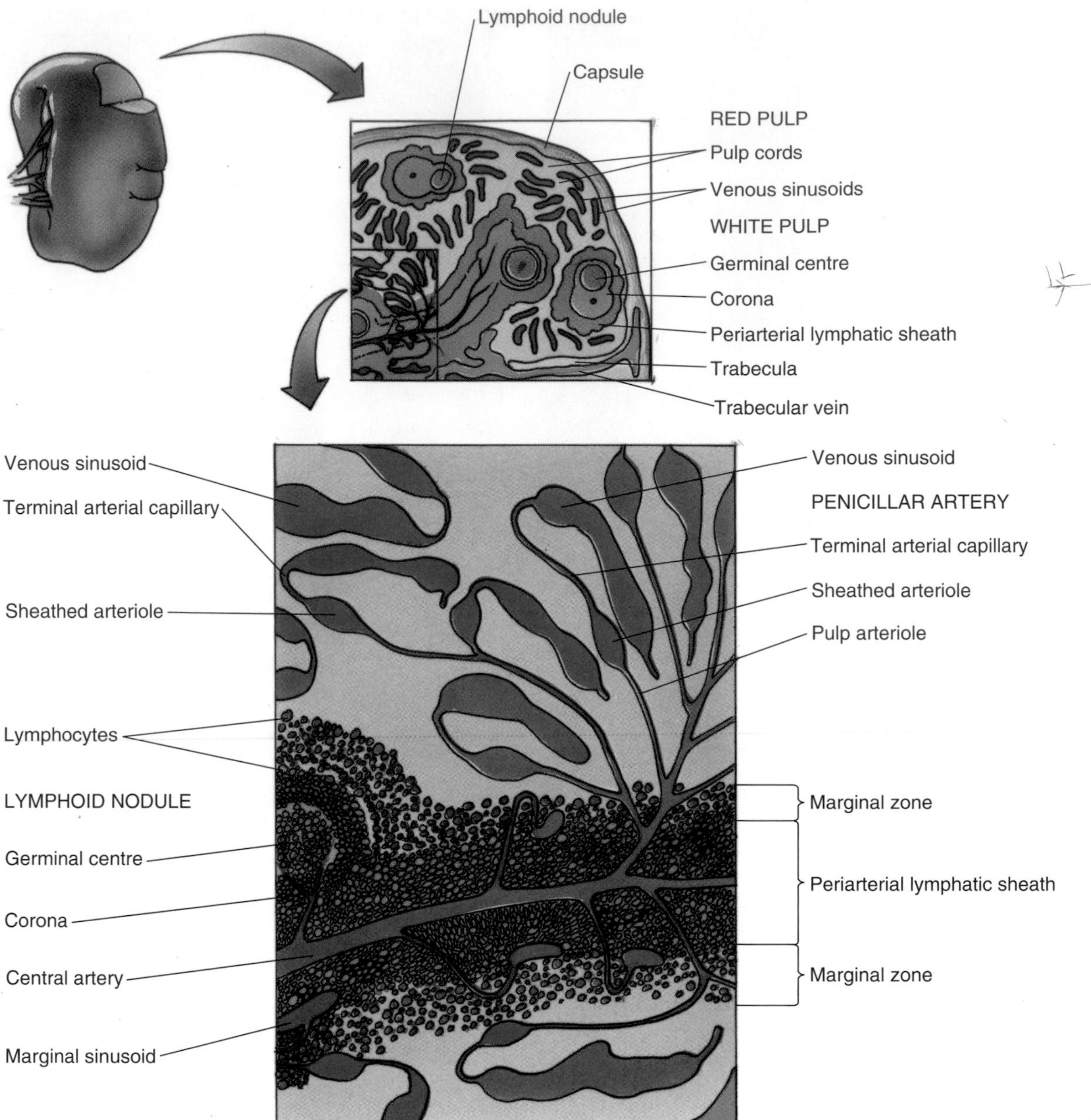

FIGURE 20-7 Diagram of the Spleen. (From Gartner, L.P., & Hiatt, J.L. [2007]. *Color textbook of histology* [3rd ed.]. Philadelphia: Elsevier.)

the principal site of splenic filtration. Because of the slow circulation in the sinuses, the macrophages easily phagocytose old, damaged, or dead blood cells of all kinds (but chiefly erythrocytes), microorganisms, macromolecules, and particles of debris. Hb from phagocytosed erythrocytes is catabolized, and heme (iron) is stored in the cytoplasm of the macrophages or released back into the blood. Blood that filters through the red pulp then moves through the venous sinuses and into the portal circulation.

The spleen is not absolutely necessary for life or for adequate hematological function. However, splenic absence from any cause (atrophy, traumatic injury, or removal because of disease) has several secondary effects on the body. For example, leukocytosis (high levels of circulating leukocytes) often occurs after splenectomy, suggesting that the spleen exerts some control over the rate of proliferation of leukocyte stem cells in the bone marrow or their release into the bloodstream. Circulating levels of iron also may decrease, reflecting the spleen's role in the iron cycle. The immune response to encapsulated bacteria (e.g., *Streptococcus pneumoniae* [pneumococcus], *Neisseria meningitidis* [meningococcus], *Haemophilus influenzae*), which is primarily an immunoglobulin M (IgM) response, may be severely diminished, resulting in increased susceptibility to disseminated infections. Loss of the spleen results in an increase in morphologically defective blood cells in the circulation, confirming the spleen's role in removing old or damaged cells.

Lymph Nodes

Structurally, **lymph nodes** are part of the lymphatic system. Lymphatic vessels collect interstitial fluid from the tissues and transport it, as lymph, through vessels of increasing size to the thoracic duct, which drains into the superior vena cava, returning the lymph to the circulation. Lymph nodes are distributed throughout the body and provide filtration of the lymph during its journey through the lymphatics. Each lymph

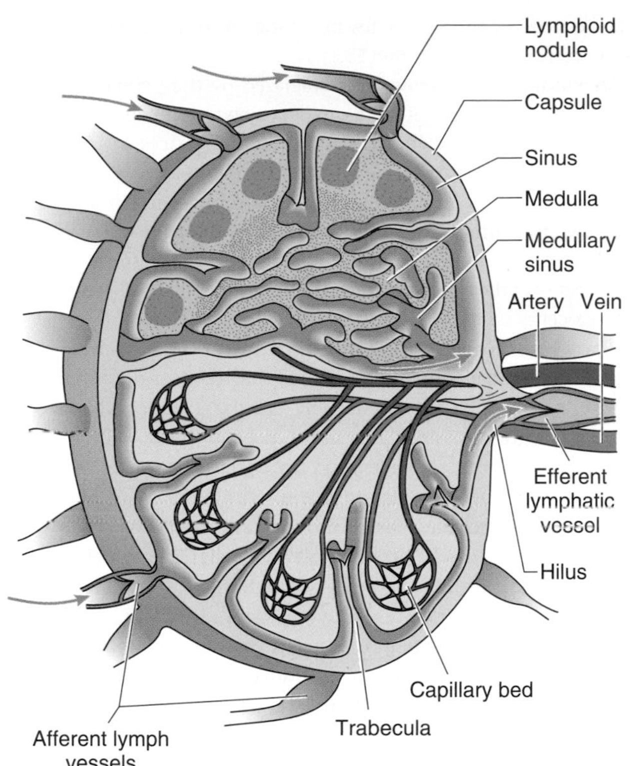

FIGURE 20-8 **Cross-Section of Lymph Node.** Several afferent valved lymphatics bring lymph to node. A single efferent lymphatic leaves the node at the hilus. Note that the artery and vein also enter and leave at the hilus. *Arrows* show direction of lymph flow. (Adapted from Gartner, L.P., & Hiatt, J.L. [2007]. *Color textbook of histology* [3rd ed.]. Philadelphia: Saunders.)

node is enclosed in a fibrous capsule, branches of which (trabeculae) extend inward to partition the node into several compartments (Figure 20-8). Reticular fibres of connective tissue divide the compartments into a meshwork throughout the lymph node. The node consists of outer (cortex) and inner (paracortex) cortical areas and an inner medulla. Lymph enters through multiple small afferent lymphatic vessels into the subcapsular sinus, just beneath the capsule, and drains into the cortical sinuses to the medullary sinuses, from which the lymph is collected and leaves the node by way of the efferent lymphatic vessel. Blood flows into the lymph nodes through the lymphatic artery, which ends in groups of postcapillary venules distributed throughout the outer cortex. The blood is drained through the lymphatic vein.

Functionally, lymph nodes are part of the hematological and immune systems and are the primary site for the first encounter between antigen and lymphocytes. Lymphocytes enter the lymph node from the blood through the postcapillary venules by means of diapedesis across the endothelial lining. B cells tend to migrate preferentially to the cortex and medulla of the nodes, whereas T cells predominantly migrate to the paracortex. Macrophages reside in the lymph node; help filter the lymph of debris, foreign substances, and microorganisms; and provide antigen-processing functions. The dendritic cells encounter and process antigens and microorganisms in other tissues, enter the lymph node through the afferent lymph vessels, and migrate throughout the nodes (see Chapter 6). The reticular network provides adhesive surfaces for trapping large numbers of phagocytes and lymphocytes and facilitates their organization into follicles or primary nodules. The presence of antigen, either removed from the lymph by macrophages or presented on the surface of dendritic cells, results in the production of secondary nodules containing germinal centres. In the germinal centres lymphocytes, particularly B cells, respond to antigenic stimulation by undergoing proliferation and further differentiation into memory cells and plasma cells (see Chapter 7). Plasma cells migrate to the medullary cords. The B-cell proliferation in response to a great deal of antigen (e.g., during infection) may result in lymph node enlargement and tenderness (reactive lymph node).

TABLE 20-3 Mononuclear Phagocyte System

Name of Cell	Location
Monocytes/macrophages	Bone marrow and peripheral blood
Kupffer cells (inflammatory macrophages)	Liver
Alveolar macrophages	Lung
Histiocytes	Connective tissue
Macrophages	Bone marrow
Fixed and free macrophages	Spleen and lymph nodes
Pleural and peritoneal macrophages	Serous cavities
Microglial cells	Nervous system
Mesangial cells	Kidney
Osteoclasts	Bone
Langerhans cells	Skin
Dendritic cells	Lymphoid tissue

The Mononuclear Phagocyte System

The **mononuclear phagocyte system (MPS)** (formerly called the *reticuloendothelial system*) consists of monocytes that differentiate without dividing and reside in the tissues for months or perhaps years.[3] Table 20-3 lists the various names given to macrophages localized in specific tissues.

Cells of the MPS play an important role in defence by ingesting and destroying (by phagocytosis) unwanted materials, such as foreign protein particles, circulating immune complexes, microorganisms, debris from dead or injured cells, defective or injured erythrocytes, and dead neutrophils. Recently, the osteoclast was classified as a true member of the MPS. *Osteoclasts* are multinucleated cells that originate from the monocyte cell lineage (see Figure 20-2) and are specialized for the function of lacunar bone resorption; however, they are also known to have phagocytic abilities.

QUICK CHECK 20-2

1. Why is the spleen considered a hematological organ? Why can humans live without it?
2. Why are lymph nodes considered part of the hematological system?
3. What is the mononuclear phagocyte system?

DEVELOPMENT OF BLOOD CELLS

Hematopoiesis

The typical human requires about 100 billion new blood cells per day. Blood cell production, termed **hematopoiesis**, is constantly ongoing, occurring in the liver and spleen of the fetus and only in bone marrow (*medullary hematopoiesis*) after birth. This process involves the biochemical stimulation of populations of relatively undifferentiated cells to undergo mitotic division (i.e., proliferation) and maturation (i.e., differentiation) into mature hematological cells. Although proliferation and differentiation are usually sequential, certain blood cells proliferate and differentiate simultaneously. Erythrocytes and neutrophils generally differentiate fully before entering the blood, but monocytes and lymphocytes continue to mature in the blood and in secondary lymphatic organs.

Hematopoiesis continues throughout life, increasing in response to a need to replenish destroyed circulating cells (e.g., during hemorrhage, hemolytic anemia [peripheral destruction of erythrocytes], consumptive thrombocytopenia) or in response to infection.[4] In general, long-term stimuli, such as chronic diseases, cause a greater increase in hematopoiesis than acute conditions, such as hemorrhage.

Various abnormalities in medullary hematopoiesis have been identified and are discussed in Chapter 21. **Extramedullary hematopoiesis**—blood cell production in tissues other than bone marrow—of apparently normal blood cells has been reported in the spleen, liver, and, less frequently, lymph nodes, adrenal glands, cartilage, adipose tissue, intrathoracic areas, and kidneys. Extramedullary hematopoiesis, however, is usually a sign of disease, occurring in pernicious anemia, sickle cell anemia, thalassemia, hemolytic disease of the newborn (erythroblastosis fetalis), hereditary spherocytosis, and certain leukemias.

Bone Marrow

Bone marrow is confined to the cavities of bone and is the primary residence of hematopoietic stem cells. It consists of blood vessels, nerves, mononuclear phagocytes, stromal cells, and blood cells in various stages of differentiation. Adults have two kinds of bone marrow: red, or active (hematopoietic), marrow (also called **myeloid tissue**); and yellow, or inactive, marrow. The large quantities of fat in inactive marrow make it yellow. Not all bones contain active marrow. In adults, active marrow is found primarily in the flat bones of the pelvis (36%), vertebrae (29%), cranium and mandible (13%), sternum and ribs (10%), upper limb girdle (8%), and in the extreme proximal portions of the femur (4%). Inactive marrow predominates in cavities of other bones. (Bones are discussed further in Chapter 38.)

Hematopoietic marrow is vascularized by the primary arteries of the bones, which terminate in a capillary network forming large venous sinuses. Hematopoietic marrow and fat fill the spaces surrounding the network of venous sinuses. Newly produced blood cells traverse narrow openings between endothelial cells in the venous sinus walls and thus enter the circulation. Normally, cells do not enter the circulation until they have differentiated (e.g., developed appropriate surface receptors to interact with the endothelium and enter the circulation), but premature release occurs in certain diseases.

The hematological compartment of the bone marrow consists of cellular microenvironments or **niches** that control differentiation of hematopoietic progenitor cells. The cellular composition of niches includes osteoblasts, osteoclasts, sinusoidal endothelial cells, fibroblasts, megakaryocytes, macrophages, and nerve cells. *Osteoblasts* are derived from fibroblasts and are responsible for construction of bone. *Osteoclasts* are multinucleate cells of monocytic origin that remodel bone by resorption. Both cells produce cytokines that affect proliferation of hematopoietic cells.[5] At least two populations of stem cells are found in bone marrow niches. **Mesenchymal stem cells (MSCs)** are **stromal cells** that can differentiate into a variety of cells, including osteoblasts, adipocytes, and chondrocytes (produce cartilage). **Hematopoietic stem cells (HSCs)** are progenitors of all hematological cells. Each type of blood cell originates from a parent stem cell. Both populations of stem cells undergo self-renewal in the bone marrow, so that additional MSCs and HSCs are produced to replace those undergoing differentiation.[6]

Two distinct types of niches have been identified—the osteoblastic (also called *endosteal*) niche and the vascular niche[7] (Figure 20-9). The **osteoblastic niche** is centralized around osteoblasts, which line the

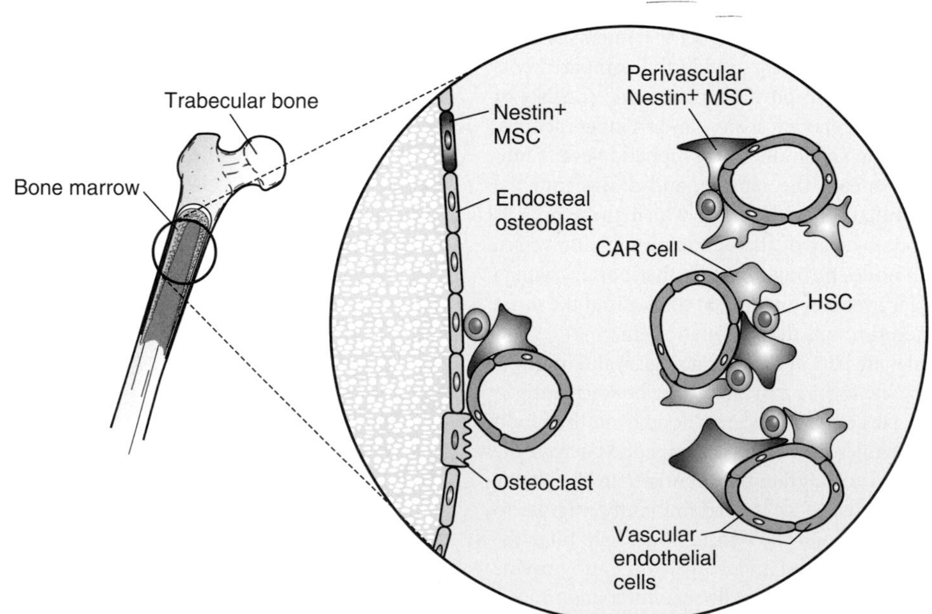

FIGURE 20-9 Bone Marrow Stem Cell Niches. Stem cell niches are microenvironments where stem cells undergo hematopoiesis into all forms of blood cells. Stem cell niches retain and maintain adult resting hematopoietic stem cells (*HSCs*) and are activated after cell injury to promote cell renewal or differentiation to form new tissues. The fate of individual HSCs is determined by interactions (intercellular adherence, cytokines, chemokines) with specialized cells within the niches. Within osteoblastic niches the HSC interacts primarily with the osteoblasts and specialized mesenchymal stem cells (*MSCs*) that include nestin-expressing (*Nestin*$^{+}$) MSCs and CXCL12-abundant reticular (*CAR*) cells. Within the vascular niches, the HSC interacts with vascular endothelial cells, Nestin^{+} MSC, and a more abundant population of CAR cells.

surface of bone, whereas the vascular niche is organized around sinusoidal endothelial cells. In both niches, HSCs are affected by direct cell-to-cell signalling and soluble mediators produced by cells within each niche. Each niche also contains two specialized cells derived from MSCs: CXCL12-abundant reticular (CAR) cells and nestin-expressing cells.[8]

CAR cells resemble reticular cells with long cellular processes and closely interact with HSCs to provide important intercellular signalling through HSC regulatory molecules, including chemokine ligand 12 (CXCL12), stem cell factor (SCF, also called *steel factor*), vascular cell adhesion molecule 1 (VCAM-1), and angiopoietin 1 (ANG1). CXCL12 is a chemokine that reacts with a chemokine receptor on HSCs. SCF is expressed as a cell-surface transmembrane protein or a soluble protein and reacts with the HSC KIT receptor (also called *stem cell growth factor receptor, proto-oncogene c-Kit*, or *CD117*). VCAM-1 mediates intercellular adhesion through its receptor, integrin $\alpha_4\beta_1$. ANG1 is secreted and reacts with a tyrosine kinase receptor. Nestin-expressing cells express large amounts of the intermediate filament protein, nestin, and particularly SCF and VCAM-1. Although both MSC-derived cells are present in the osteoblastic niche and vascular niche, the CAR cell is the predominant cell in the vascular niche.

Each bone marrow niche affects HSCs differently. In the osteoblastic niche, HSCs are in direct contact with osteoblasts, CAR cells, and nestin-expressing cells. The effect is retention of HSCs in the bone marrow in a quiescent (dormant) state. HSCs that traffic to the vascular niche directly contact endothelial cells, as well as nestin-expressing cells and larger numbers of perivascular CAR cells. The cumulative signalling events induce HSC proliferation and hematopoietic differentiation.

Cellular Differentiation

All humans originate from a single cell (the fertilized egg) that has the capacity to proliferate and eventually differentiate into the huge diversity of cells of the human body. After fertilization, the egg divides over a 5-day period to form a hollow ball (blastocyst) that implants on the uterus. Until about 3 days after fertilization, each cell (blastomere) is undifferentiated and retains the capacity to differentiate into any cell type. In the 5-day blastocyst, the outer layer of cells has undergone differentiation and commitment to become the placenta. Cells of the inner cell mass, however, continue to have unlimited differentiation potential (currently referred to as being *pluripotent*) and can grow into different kinds of tissue—blood, nerves, heart, bone, and so forth. After implantation, cells of the inner cell mass begin differentiation into other cell types. Differentiation is a multistep process and results in intermediate groups of stem cells with more limited, but still impressive, abilities to differentiate into many different types of cells.

Within the bone marrow niches, each type of blood cell originates from HSCs that proliferate and differentiate under control of a variety of cytokines and growth factors[9] (see Figure 20-2). As with all stem cells, the HSCs are self-renewing (they have the ability to proliferate without further differentiation) so that a relatively constant population of stem cells is available. Some HSCs will continue differentiation into hematopoietic progenitor cells. Progenitor cells retain proliferative capacity but are committed to possible further differentiation into particular types of hematological cells: lymphoid (lymphocytes, NK cells), granulocyte/monocyte (granulocytes, monocytes, macrophages), and megakaryocyte/erythroid (platelets, erythrocytes) progenitor cells.

Several cytokines participate in hematopoiesis, particularly colony-stimulating factors (CSFs or hematopoietic growth factors), which stimulate the proliferation of progenitor cells and their progeny and initiate the maturation events necessary to produce fully mature cells. Multiple cell types in hematopoietic organs, including endothelial cells, fibroblasts, and lymphocytes, produce the necessary CSFs.

Hematopoiesis in the bone marrow occurs in two separate pools—the stem cell pool and the bone marrow pool—with eventual release of mature cells into the peripheral circulation (Figure 20-10). The stem cell pool contains pluripotent stem cells and partially committed progenitor cells. The bone marrow pool contains cells that are proliferating and maturing in preparation for release into the circulation

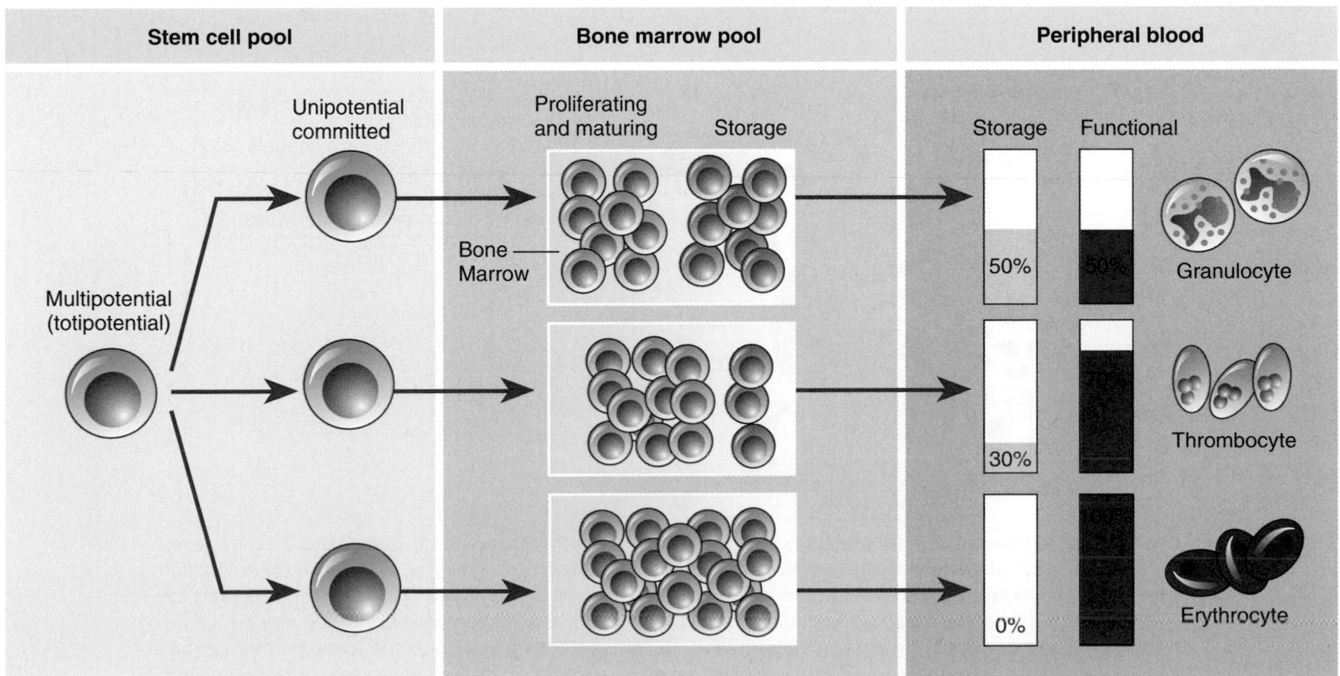

FIGURE 20-10 Hematopoiesis. Hematopoiesis from the stem cell pool; activity is mainly in the bone marrow and in the peripheral blood.

and mature cells that are stored for later release into the peripheral blood. The peripheral blood also contains two pools of cells: those circulating and those stored around the walls of the blood vessels (often called the **marginating storage pool**). The marginating storage pool primarily consists of neutrophils that adhere to the endothelium in vessels where the blood flow is relatively slow. These cells can rapidly move into tissues and mucous membranes when needed.

Under certain conditions, the levels of circulating hematological cells need to be rapidly replenished. Medullary hematopoiesis can be accelerated by any or all of three mechanisms: (1) conversion of yellow bone marrow, which does not produce blood cells, to red marrow, which does, by the actions of **erythropoietin** (a hormone that stimulates erythrocyte production); (2) faster differentiation of daughter cells; and, presumably, (3) faster proliferation of stem cells.

QUICK CHECK 20-3

1. Why is the stem cell system important to hematopoiesis?
2. What role do stromal cells play in hematopoiesis?
3. Why are some stem cells called pluripotent?

Development of Erythrocytes

For almost 100 years it was thought that erythrocytes developed in the spleen. It was not until the 1950s that the bone marrow was identified as the site of **erythropoiesis**, or development of red blood cells.

Erythropoiesis

In the confines of the bone marrow, erythroid progenitor cells proliferate and differentiate into large, nucleated **proerythroblasts**, which are committed into producing cells of the erythroid series. The proerythroblast differentiates through several intermediate forms of **erythroblast** (sometimes called **normoblast**), while progressively eliminating most intracellular structures (including the nucleus), synthesizing Hb, and becoming more compact, eventually assuming the shape and characteristics of an erythrocyte.

The last immature form is the **reticulocyte**, which contains a meshlike (reticular) network of ribosomal RNA that is visible microscopically after staining with certain dyes. Reticulocytes remain in the marrow approximately 1 day and are released into the venous sinuses. They continue to mature in the bloodstream and may travel to the spleen for several days of additional maturation. The normal reticulocyte count is 1% of the total red blood cell count. Approximately 1% of the body's circulating erythrocyte mass normally is generated every 24 hours. Therefore, the reticulocyte count is a useful clinical index of erythropoietic activity and indicates whether new red blood cells are being produced.

Most steps of erythropoiesis are primarily under the control of a feedback loop involving the glycoprotein erythropoietin. In healthy humans, the total volume of circulating erythrocytes remains surprisingly constant. In conditions of tissue hypoxia, erythropoietin is secreted primarily by the peritubular cells of the kidney (Figure 20-11). Rising levels of erythropoietin cause a compensatory increase in erythrocyte production if the oxygen content of blood decreases because of anemia, high altitude, or pulmonary disease. The normal steady-state rate of production (2.5 million erythrocytes per second) can increase (to 17 million per second) under anemic or low-oxygen states. Thus, the body responds to reduced oxygenation of blood in two ways: (1) by increasing the intake of oxygen through increased respiration and (2) by increasing the oxygen-carrying capacity of the blood through increased erythropoiesis.

Recombinant human erythropoietin (r-HuEPO) is used in individuals with anemia secondary to decreased erythropoietin from chronic renal failure. An immediate effect of erythropoietin administration is an increase in the blood reticulocyte count, followed by increasing levels of erythrocytes. The most significant side effect is increased blood pressure.

Hemoglobin Synthesis

Hemoglobin (Hb), the oxygen-carrying protein of the erythrocyte, constitutes approximately 90% of the cell's dry weight. Hb-packed blood cells take up oxygen in the lungs and exchange it for carbon dioxide in the tissues. Hb increases the oxygen-carrying capacity of blood by 100-fold. Each Hb molecule is composed of two pairs of polypeptide chains (the **globins**) and four colourful complexes of iron plus

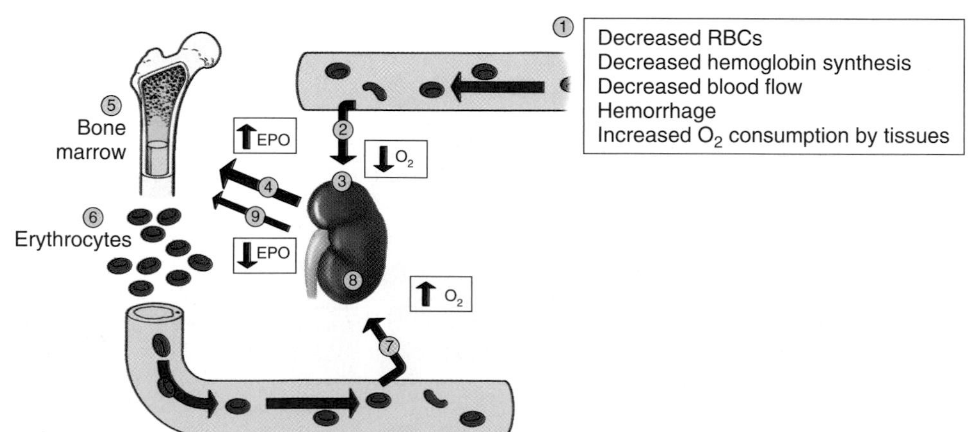

FIGURE 20-11 Role of Erythropoietin in Regulation of Erythropoiesis. (1) Decreased arterial oxygen levels result in (2) decreased tissue oxygen (hypoxia) that (3) stimulates the kidney to increase (4) production of erythropoietin. Erythropoietin is carried to the bone marrow (5) and binds to erythropoietin receptors on proerythroblasts, resulting in increased red blood cell production and maturation and expansion of the erythron (6). The increased release of red blood cells into the circulation frequently corrects the hypoxia in the tissues (7). (8) Perception of normal oxygen levels by the kidney causes (9) diminished production of erythropoietin (negative feedback) and return to normal levels of erythrocyte production. *EPO*, erythropoietin; *O_2*, oxygen (in the blood and tissue); *RBCs*, red blood cells.

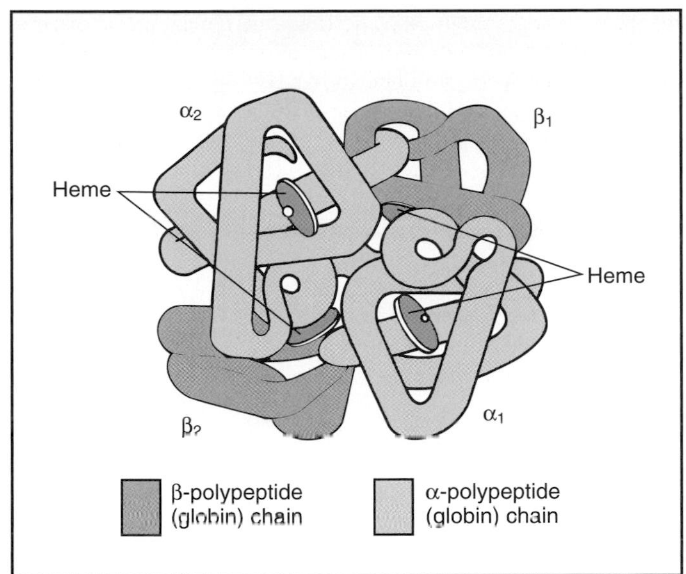

FIGURE 20-12 Molecular Structure of Hemoglobin. The molecule is a spherical tetramer weighing approximately 64 500 daltons. It contains a pair of α-polypeptide chains and a pair of β-polypeptide chains and several heme groups.

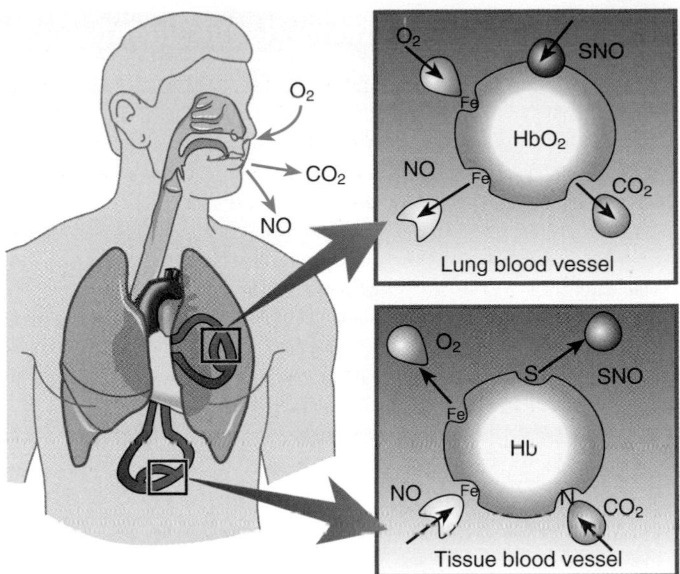

FIGURE 20-13 Hemoglobin Binding to Nitric Oxide. In the lungs, hemoglobin (*Hb*) binds to nitric oxide (*NO*) as *S*-nitrosothiol (*SNO*). In tissue, this SNO is released, and free, circulating NO is bound to a different site for exhalation. *CO_2*, carbon dioxide; *Fe*, iron; *N*, nitrogen; *O_2*, oxygen; *S*, sulphur.

protoporphyrin (the hemes), which is responsible for the blood's ruby-red colour (Figure 20-12).

Several variants of Hb exist, but they differ only slightly in primary structure based on the use of different polypeptide chains: alpha, beta, gamma, delta, epsilon, or zeta (α, β, γ, δ, ε, or ζ).[10] Hemoglobin A (Hb A), the most common type in adults, is composed of two α- and two β-polypeptide chains ($\alpha_2\beta_2$). A normal variant, fetal hemoglobin (Hb F), is a complex of two α- and two γ-polypeptide chains ($\alpha_2\gamma_2$) that binds oxygen with a much greater affinity than adult Hb.

Heme is a large, flat, iron-protoporphyrin disc that is synthesized in the mitochondria and can carry one molecule of oxygen.[11] Thus, an individual Hb molecule with its four hemes can carry four oxygen molecules. If all four oxygen-binding sites are occupied by oxygen, the molecule is said to be saturated. Through a series of biochemical reactions, **protoporphyrin**, a complex four-ringed molecule, is produced and bound with ferrous iron (Fe^{2+}). It is crucial that the iron be correctly charged; reduced Fe^{2+} can bind oxygen, whereas ferric iron (Fe^{3+}) cannot. Binding of oxygen to Fe^{2+} temporarily oxidizes Fe^{2+} to Fe^{3+} (**oxyhemoglobin**), but after the release of oxygen the body reduces the iron to Fe^{2+} and reactivates the Hb (**deoxyhemoglobin** [reduced Hb]). Without reactivation, the Fe^{3+}-containing Hb (**methemoglobin**) cannot bind oxygen. An excess of Fe^{3+} occurs with certain medications and chemicals, such as nitrates and sulphonamides.

Several other molecules can competitively bind to deoxyhemoglobin. Carbon monoxide directly competes with oxygen for binding to ferrous ion with an affinity that is about 200-fold greater than that of oxygen. Thus, even a small amount of carbon monoxide can dramatically decrease the ability of Hb to bind and transport oxygen. Hb also binds carbon dioxide, but at a binding site separate from where oxygen binds. In the lungs, carbon dioxide is released, allowing Hb to bind oxygen.

Erythrocytes may play a role in the maintenance of vascular relaxation. **Nitric oxide (NO)** produced by blood vessels is a major mediator of relaxation and dilation of the vessel walls. In the lungs, Hb can concurrently bind oxygen to the ferrous ion and NO to cysteine residues in the globins (Figure 20-13). As Hb transfers its oxygen to tissue, it may also shed small amounts of NO, contributing to dilation of the blood vessels and helping the transfer of oxygen into tissues.

Nutritional Requirements for Erythropoiesis

Normal development of erythrocytes and synthesis of Hb depend on an optimal biochemical state and adequate supplies of the necessary building blocks, including protein, vitamins, and minerals (Table 20-4). If these components are lacking for a prolonged time, erythrocyte production slows and anemia (insufficient numbers of functional erythrocytes) may result (see Chapter 21).

Erythropoiesis cannot proceed in the absence of vitamins, especially vitamin B_{12}, folate (folic acid), vitamin B_6, riboflavin, pantothenic acid, niacin, ascorbic acid, and vitamin E. Dietary vitamin B_{12} is a large molecule that requires a protein secreted by parietal cells into the stomach (intrinsic factor) for transport across the ileum. Vitamin B_{12} is stored in the liver and used as needed in erythropoiesis. Decreased B_{12} absorption may lead to pernicious anemia. Folate is necessary for DNA and RNA synthesis. Folate absorption occurs principally in the upper small intestine and is stored in the liver. Folate deficiency is more common than vitamin B_{12} deficiency and occurs more rapidly. Folate supplements are prescribed for pregnant women because pregnancy increases the demand for folate. Supplements can protect against neural tube defects and may prevent anemia.

Normal Destruction of Senescent Erythrocytes

Mature erythrocytes have cytoplasmic enzymes capable of glycolysis (anaerobic glucose metabolism) and production of small quantities of adenosine triphosphate (ATP). ATP provides the energy needed to maintain cell function and keep its plasma membrane pliable[12] (see Figure 1-1). Metabolic processes diminish as the erythrocyte ages, so less ATP is available to maintain plasma membrane function. The aged or senescent red blood cell becomes increasingly fragile and loses its reversible deformability, becoming susceptible to rupture while passing through narrowed regions of the microcirculation.

Additionally, the plasma membrane of senescent red blood cells undergoes phospholipid rearrangement with enrichment of surface phosphatidylserine that is recognized by receptors on macrophages (primarily in the spleen), which selectively remove and sequester the

TABLE 20-4 Nutritional Requirements for Erythropoiesis

Nutrient	Role in Erythropoiesis	Consequence of Deficiency (see Chapter 21)
Protein (amino acids)	Structural component of plasma membrane	Decreased strength, elasticity, and flexibility of membrane; hemolytic anemia
Synthesis of hemoglobin	Decreased erythropoiesis and lifespan of erythrocytes	
Intrinsic factor	Gastro-intestinal absorption of vitamin B_{12}	Pernicious anemia
Cobalamin (vitamin B_{12})	Synthesis of DNA, maturation of erythrocytes, facilitator of folate metabolism	Macrocytic (megaloblastic) anemia
Folate (folic acid)	Synthesis of DNA and RNA, maturation of erythrocytes	Macrocytic (megaloblastic) anemia
Vitamin B_6 (pyridoxine)	Heme synthesis, possibly increases folate metabolism	Hypochromic-microcytic anemia
Vitamin B_2 (riboflavin)	Oxidative reactions	Normochromic-normocytic anemia
Vitamin C (ascorbic acid)	Iron metabolism, acts as reducing agent to maintain iron in its ferrous (Fe^{++}) form	Normochromic-normocytic anemia
Pantothenic acid	Heme synthesis	Unknown in humans[a]
Niacin	None, but needed for respiration in mature erythrocytes	Unknown in humans
Vitamin E	Synthesis of heme; possible protection against oxidative damage in mature erythrocytes	Hemolytic anemia with increased cell membrane fragility; shortens lifespan of erythrocytes in individual with cystic fibrosis
Iron	Hemoglobin synthesis	Iron deficiency anemia
Copper	Structural component of plasma membrane	Hypochromic-microcytic anemia

[a]Although pantothenic acid is important for optimal synthesis of heme, experimentally induced deficiency failed to produce anemia or other hematopoietic disturbances.
Data from Harmening, D.M. (Ed.). (1997). *Clinical hematology and fundamentals of hemostasis* (3rd ed.). Philadelphia: FA Davis; Lee, G.R., Bithell, T.C., Foerster, J., et al. (1993). *Wintrobe's clinical hematology* (9th ed.). Philadelphia: Lee & Febiger.

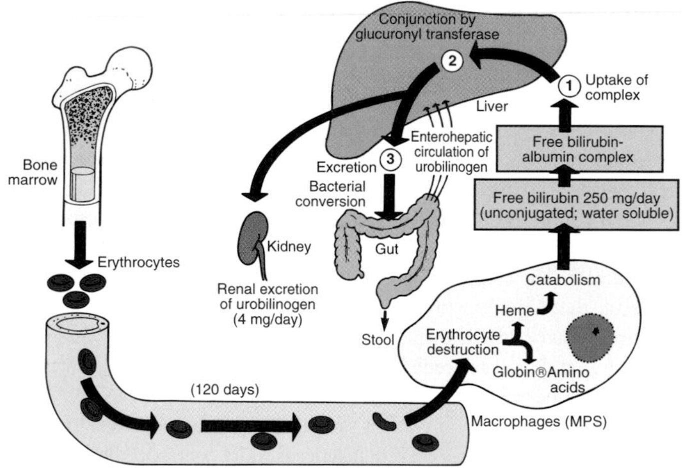

FIGURE 20-14 Metabolism of Bilirubin Released by Heme Breakdown. *MPS*, mononuclear phagocyte system.

red blood cells. If the spleen is dysfunctional or absent, macrophages in the liver (Kupffer cells) assume control. During digestion of Hb in the macrophage, porphyrin reduces to bilirubin, which is transported to the liver, conjugated, and finally excreted in the bile as glucuronide (Figure 20-14). Bacteria in the intestinal lumen transform conjugated bilirubin into urobilinogen. Although a small portion is reabsorbed, most urobilinogen is excreted in feces. Conditions causing accelerated erythrocyte destruction increase the load of bilirubin for hepatic clearance, leading to increased serum levels of unconjugated bilirubin and increased urinary excretion of urobilinogen. Gallstones (cholelithiasis) can result from a chronically elevated rate of bilirubin excretion.

Iron cycle. Approximately 67% of total body iron is bound to heme in erythrocytes (Hb) and muscle cells (**myoglobin**), and approximately 30% is stored in mononuclear phagocytes (i.e., macrophages) and hepatic parenchymal cells as either ferritin or hemosiderin.[13] The remaining 3% (less than 1 mg) is lost daily in urine, sweat, bile, sloughing of epithelial cells from the skin and intestinal mucosa, and minor bleeding. Approximately 25 mg of iron is required daily for erythropoiesis; only 1 to 2 mg of iron is dietary and the remainder is obtained from continual recycling of iron from erythrocytes.

The methemoglobin released from the breakdown of senescent or damaged erythrocytes is dissociated by the enzyme heme oxygenase, and the iron is released into the bloodstream where it is free to bind again to transferrin or be stored in the macrophage's cytoplasm as ferritin or hemosiderin (Figure 20-15). A minute amount of iron is stored in muscle cells by the heme-containing protein myoglobin. Unavailable stores of iron are present in cytochromes, catalases, and peroxidase enzymes.

The protein ferritin is the major intracellular iron storage protein. **Apoferritin**, which is ferritin without attached iron, can store thousands of atoms of iron. Several apoferritin complexes combine to form the micelle ferritin. Large aggregates of micelles (if a large amount of iron is present) produce large iron storage complexes, known as **hemosiderin**. Under a light microscope, hemosiderin is visible as an iron-based pigment in cell inclusions. The iron within deposits of hemosiderin is poorly available to supply iron when needed. The most common cause of hemosiderin deposition is simple bruising. Hemosiderin in small amounts within iron-rich tissues (i.e., spleen, liver, bone marrow) is considered normal. Large aggregates or its presence in tissue, such as the lungs or subcutaneous tissue, suggest a pathological condition.

Iron from either dietary sources, release of iron stores, or erythrocyte catabolism is transported in the blood bound to **apotransferrin**, thus becoming **transferrin**. Apotransferrin is a glycoprotein synthesized primarily by hepatocytes in the liver but also produced in small quantities by tissue macrophages, submaxillary and mammary glands, and ovaries or testes (see Figure 20-15). Transferrin is transported to the bone marrow, where it binds to transferrin receptors on erythroblasts. Transferrin receptors are on the plasma membrane of all nucleated cells, but at particularly high levels on erythroid precursors and rapidly proliferating cells (e.g., lymphocytes), and are thought to be the only

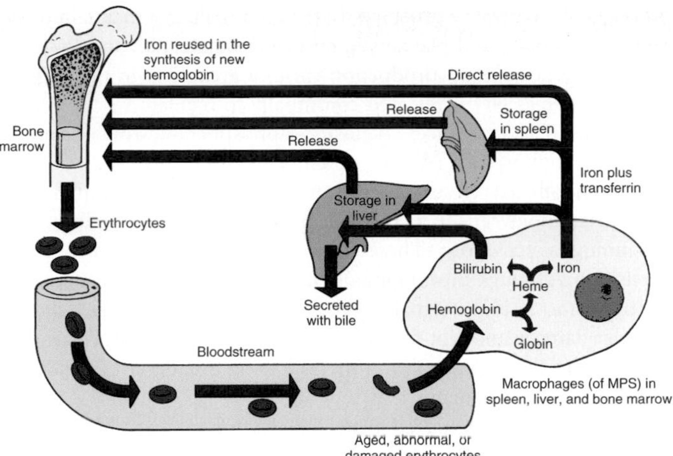

FIGURE 20-15 Iron Cycle. Iron released from gastro-intestinal epithelial cells circulates in the bloodstream associated with its plasma carrier, transferrin. It is delivered to erythroblasts in bone marrow, where most of it is incorporated into hemoglobin. Mature erythrocytes circulate for approximately 120 days, after which they become senescent and are removed by the mononuclear phagocyte system (*MPS*). Macrophages of MPS (mostly in the spleen) break down ingested erythrocytes and return iron to the bloodstream directly or after storing it as ferritin or hemosiderin.

route of cellular entry for transferrin-attached iron. Transferrin is recycled (transferrin cycle) by intracellular dissociation of the iron and secretion of the resultant apotransferrin to the bloodstream.

The iron is transported to the erythroblast's mitochondria (the site of Hb production), where the enzyme heme synthetase inserts ferrous iron into protoporphyrin to form heme. Heme then is bound to globin to form Hb. Iron not used in erythropoiesis is stored temporarily as ferritin or hemosiderin and later excreted.

The body's iron homeostasis is primarily controlled by the hormone **hepcidin**. Hepcidin is a 25–amino acid peptide synthesized in the liver and released into the plasma, where it is bound with high affinity to α_2-macroglobulin and with relatively lower affinity to albumin.[14] Hepatocellular hepcidin production is regulated physiologically by the levels of iron in the body, rate of erythropoiesis, and percentage of oxygen saturation. Hepatocytes (liver cells) sense levels of circulating iron by means of receptors for transferrin. Excess iron is stored in hepatocytes and macrophages, and hepatocytes sense these levels by means of receptors for bone morphogenetic protein (BMP), most likely BMP-6, which is a growth factor produced to a large extent by bone marrow sinusoid endothelial cells. Hepcidin production also can be induced by inflammation via IL-6.

Hepcidin regulates iron levels through its binding capacity to ferroportin, which is a transmembrane iron exporter found in the plasma membrane of cells that transport or store iron, including macrophages, hepatocytes, and enterocytes (intestinal cells).[15] The body's total iron balance is maintained through controlled absorption rather than excretion. Dietary iron (primarily as Fe^{2+}) is transported directly across the membranes of enterocytes in the duodenum and proximal jejunum. (Transport mechanisms are described in Chapter 1.) Hepcidin induces internalization and degradation of ferroportin, thus leading to increased intracellular iron stores, decreased dietary iron absorption, and decreased levels of circulating iron. Decreased production of hepcidin leads to release of stored iron and increased dietary absorption. Thus, if the body's iron stores are low or the demand for erythropoiesis increases, dietary iron is transported rapidly through the epithelial cell and into the plasma. If body stores are high and erythropoiesis is not increased, iron transport is stopped, although iron can cross the epithelial cells' plasma membrane passively and is stored as ferritin.

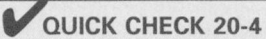

> **✔ QUICK CHECK 20-4**
> 1. Why is the reticulocyte count important?
> 2. Why is iron important to erythropoiesis?
> 3. What happens to aging erythrocytes?

Development of Leukocytes

Leukocytes consist of lymphocytes, granulocytes, and monocytes. Most leukocytes arise from HSCs in the bone marrow that differentiate into common lymphoid progenitors and common myeloid progenitors (their pathways of differentiation are shown in Figure 20-2). Lymphoid progenitor cells develop into lymphocytes, which are released into the bloodstream to undergo further maturation in the primary and secondary lymphoid organs (see Chapter 7). Common myeloid progenitors further differentiate into progenitors for erythrocytes, megakaryocytes, and mast cells, and into granulocyte/monocyte progenitors. The granulocyte/monocyte progenitors further differentiate into monocyte progenitors and granulocyte progenitors, which develop into monocytes/macrophages and granulocytes (neutrophils, basophils, eosinophils), respectively. Development from HSC to common granulocyte/monocyte progenitor primarily is under the control of SCF, IL-3, and GM-CSF, whereas further differentiation into granulocytic and monocytic progenitors is controlled by granulocyte colony-stimulating factor (G-CSF) and macrophage colony stimulating factor (M-CSF), respectively. The ultimate granulocytic phenotype is determined in the bone marrow by relative local concentrations of early and late-acting cytokines, including GM-CSF, G-CSF, IL-3, IL-5, SCF, and others. Granulocytes are released into the blood within 14 days of development. The bone marrow selectively retains immature granulocytes as a reserve pool that can be rapidly mobilized in response to the body's needs.

Monocytic progenitors differentiate into monocytes within 24 hours and are released into the circulation. Monocytes mature into various forms of macrophages, a process that is usually complete within 1 or 2 days after release.

Most leukocytes exist in the body from days to years, depending on type. Maintenance of optimal levels of granulocytes and monocytes in the blood depends on the availability of pluripotent stem cells in the marrow, induction of these into committed stem cells, timely release of new cells from the marrow, and mobilization of the granulocyte reserve pool. Leukocyte production increases in response to infection, to the presence of steroids, and to reduction or depletion of reserves in the marrow. It also is associated with strenuous exercise, convulsive seizures, heat, intense radiation, paroxysmal tachycardias (outbursts of rapid heart rate), pain, nausea and vomiting, and anxiety.

Development of Platelets

Platelets (thrombocytes) are derived from stem cells and progenitor cells that differentiate into megakaryocytes. During thrombopoiesis, the megakaryocyte progenitor is programmed to undergo an endomitotic cell cycle (**endomitosis**) during which DNA replication occurs, but anaphase and cytokinesis are blocked[16] (see Figures 20-2 and 20-6, and Chapter 1). Thus, the megakaryocyte nucleus enlarges and becomes extremely polyploidy (up to 100-fold or more of the normal amount of DNA) without cellular division. Concurrently, the numbers of cytoplasmic organelles (e.g., internal membranes, granules) increase, and the cell develops cellular surface elongations and branches that progressively fragment into platelets. A single large megakaryocyte (up to 100 μm) may produce thousands of smaller platelets (2 to

3 μm). Like erythrocytes, platelets released from the bone marrow lack nuclei.

About two-thirds of platelets enter the circulation, and the remainder resides in the splenic pool. Platelets circulate in the bloodstream for about 10 days before beginning to lose their ability to carry out biochemical reactions. Senescent platelets are sequestered and destroyed in the spleen by mononuclear cell phagocytosis. Thrombopoietin (TPO), a hormone growth factor, is the main regulator of the circulating platelet numbers. TPO is primarily produced by the liver and induces platelet production in the bone marrow.[17] Platelets express receptors for TPO and, when circulating platelet levels are normal, TPO is adsorbed onto the platelet surface and prevented from accessing the bone marrow and initiating further platelet production.[18] When platelet levels are low, however, the amount of TPO exceeds the number of available platelet TPO receptors, and free TPO can enter the bone marrow. During inflammation IL-6 induces increased production of TPO, which increases production of newly formed platelets, which are more thrombogenic.

MECHANISMS OF HEMOSTASIS

Hemostasis means arrest of bleeding. As a result of hemostasis, damaged blood vessels may maintain a relatively steady state of blood volume, pressure, and flow. Three equally important components of hemostasis are platelets, clotting factors, and the vasculature (endothelial cells and subendothelial matrix). The following list is the general sequence of events in hemostasis:

1. Vascular injury leads to a transient arteriolar vasoconstriction to limit blood flow to the affected site;
2. Damage to the endothelial cell lining of the vessel exposes prothrombogenic subendothelial connective tissue matrix leading to platelet adherence and activation and formation of a *hemostatic plug*, also referred to as a *platelet plug*, to prevent further bleeding (primary hemostasis);
3. Tissue factor, produced by the endothelium, collaborates with secreted platelet factors and activated platelets to activate the clotting (coagulation) system to form fibrin clots and further prevent bleeding (secondary hemostasis);
4. The fibrin/platelet clot contracts to form a more permanent plug; and
5. Regulatory pathways are activated (fibrinolysis) to limit the size of the plug and begin the healing process.

The relative importance of the hemostatic mechanisms clearly varies with vessel size. Damage to large vessels cannot easily be controlled by hemostasis but requires vascular contraction and dramatically decreased blood flow into the damaged vessels (Table 20-5).

Function of Platelets and Blood Vessels

Platelets normally circulate freely, suspended in plasma, in an unactivated state. Endothelial cells lining the vessels produce NO and the prostaglandin derivative prostacyclin (PGI_2), which help maintain blood flow and pressure and platelets in an inactive state. NO and PGI_2 are highly synergistic; PGI_2 production varies a great deal in response to stimuli, whereas NO is released continually to regulate vascular tone. Endothelium also produces adenosine diphosphatase, which degrades adenosine diphosphate (ADP; a potent activator of platelets).

The endothelial cell surface contains antithrombotic molecules, such as glycosaminoglycans (e.g., heparan sulphate), thrombomodulin, and plasminogen activators. These limit platelet activation and fibrin deposition. Although thrombomodulin and plasminogen activators help control hemostasis in normal vessels, their effects are magnified during vascular damage and clot formation; therefore, further information is provided on these molecules in the following text describing control of hemostatic mechanisms.

When a vessel is damaged, platelet activation may be initiated. The role of platelet activation is to (1) contribute to regulation of blood flow into a damaged site through induction of vasoconstriction (vasospasm); (2) initiate platelet-to-platelet interactions resulting in formation of a platelet plug to stop further bleeding; (3) activate the coagulation (or clotting) cascade to stabilize the platelet plug; and (4) initiate repair processes, including clot retraction and clot dissolution. The normal platelet count ranges from 150 to 400×10^9/L, and a count below 150 000/mm^3 is defined as thrombocytopenia. However, the thrombocytopenia is usually asymptomatic unless the count drops below 100×10^9/L, at which time the number of platelets may be inadequate and abnormal bleeding may occur in response to trauma. Spontaneous major bleeding episodes do not generally occur unless the platelet count falls below 20×10^9/L. However, these values are not absolute and their clinical significance will vary among individuals.

Platelet activation proceeds through a process of (1) increased adhesion to the damaged vascular wall; (2) platelet degranulation, which stimulates changes in platelet shape; (3) aggregation as platelet–vascular wall and platelet-platelet adherence increases; and (4) activation of the clotting system and development of an immobilizing meshwork of platelets and fibrin (Figure 20-16; and see *Health Promotion:* Sticky Platelets).

The platelet activation process can begin in several ways. If the vessel lining remains intact in an area of inflammation, the endothelial cells may become activated by cytokines and express new proteins on their surface. Several of these, particularly P-selectin, bind specifically yet weakly with receptors on the surface of inactive platelets (e.g., glycoprotein Ib [GPIb]) (Figure 20-17). As inflammation progresses, the platelets adhere more avidly through additional receptors that bind through a fibrinogen bridge with the endothelial cell surface. The principal fibrinogen receptor on platelets is the integrin $\alpha IIb\beta 3$ (also known as *glycoprotein PIIb/IIIa* [GPIIb/IIIa]).

During vessel damage, the endothelial layer is frequently compromised, resulting in exposure of the underlying matrix that contains collagen, fibronectin, and other components. The matrix also contains von

TABLE 20-5 Types of Bleeding: Sources, Vessel Size, and Sealing Requirements

Types and Sources of Bleeding	Involved Vessel	Size	Sealing Requirements
Pinpoint petechial hemorrhage (blood leakage from small vessels)	Capillary	Smallest	Generally direct-sealing
	Venule	↓	Mostly fused platelets
	Arteriole	↓	Mostly fused platelets
Ecchymosis (large, soft tissue bleeding)	Vein	↓	Vascular contraction, fused platelets, perivascular and intravascular hemostatic factor activation (see Figure 20-16)
Rapidly expanding "blowout" hemorrhage	Artery	Largest	Greater vascular contraction, more fused platelets, greater perivascular and intravascular hemostatic factor activation

Modified from Harmening, D.M. (Ed.). (1997). *Clinical hematology and fundamentals of hemostasis* (3rd ed.). Philadelphia: FA Davis.

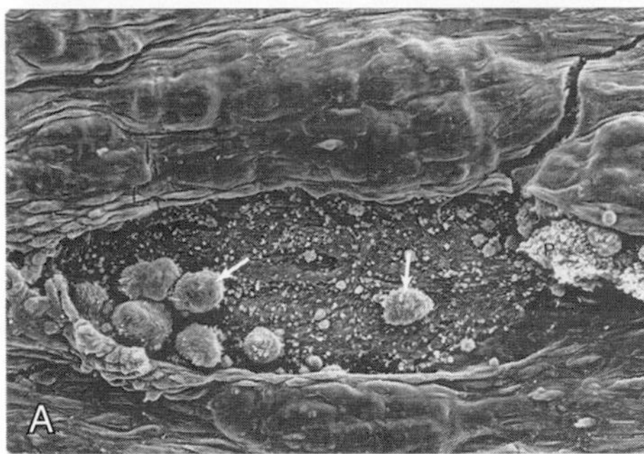

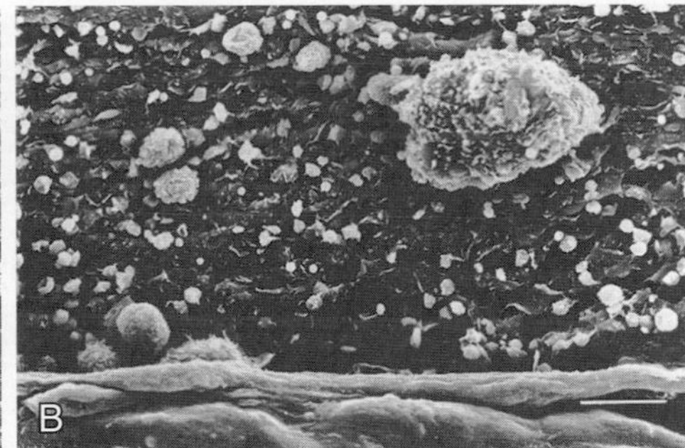

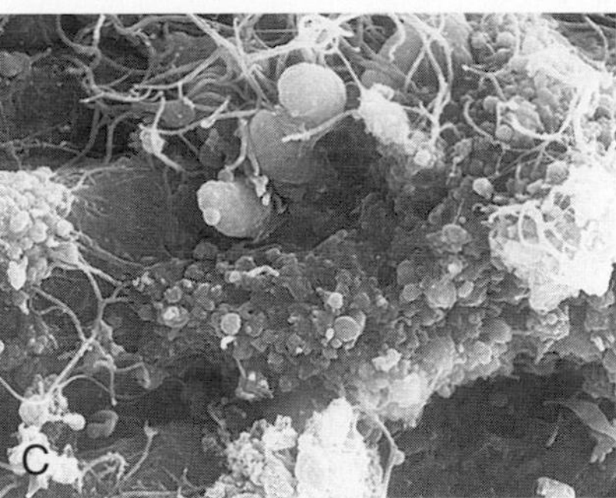

FIGURE 20-16 Platelet Activation. A, After endothelial denudation, platelets and leukocytes adhere to the subendothelium in a monolayer fashion. **B,** Higher-power view showing leukocytes and platelets adherent to the subendothelium. **C,** High magnification of a thrombus showing a mixture of red blood cells and platelets incorporated into the fibrin meshwork. (**A** and **B,** from Libby, P., Bonow R., Mann D.L., et al. [Eds.]. [2007]. *Braunwald's heart disease: A textbook of cardiovascular medicine* [8th ed.]. Philadelphia: Saunders; as reproduced from Faggiotto, A., & Ross, R. [1984]. *Arteriosclerosis, 4*[4], 341–356; **C,** from Damjanov, I., & Linder, J. [Eds.]. [1996]. *Anderson's pathology* [10th ed.]. St. Louis: Mosby.)

HEALTH PROMOTION

Sticky Platelets

Investigators report that a genetic trait induces some people to make sticky platelets. People with platelets that tend to stick together have an increased risk of forming deep arterial and venous thromboses, which can lead to myocardial infarction and cerebrovascular attacks. In pregnant women, sticky blood can result in the blockage of small blood vessels in the placenta, increasing the risk for miscarriage and late-term death of the fetus. In addition, people with this condition may also experience complications following cardiac procedures such as angioplasty.

It has been determined that testing for platelet stickiness could determine which people require anticlotting medications, and also the duration of their treatment, to prevent these complications. Treatment for persons who have not experienced significant blood clotting problems may include the administration of a daily baby Aspirin. Those persons with a history of venous thrombosis may require prescription anticoagulant medications such as warfarin (Coumadin). This treatment requires regular blood testing to ensure the blood remains at the required consistency to prevent the development of clots or excessive thinning of the blood and the risk of bleeding.

Data from Movva, S., Diamond, H.S., Carsons, S., et al. (2016). *Antiphospholipid syndrome*. Retrieved from http://emedicine.medscape.com/article/333221-overview#a5.

Willebrand factor (vWF), and the exposed collagen can bind additional vWF from the circulation (see Figure 20-17). Platelets adhere strongly to collagen through the action of several glycoprotein hormones that act as receptors (i.e., glycoprotein VI [GPVI] and integrin $\alpha_2\beta_1$) and to vWF through the receptor complex of platelet receptor GPIb and clotting factors IX and V. Progressively the platelets undergo further aggregation through platelet-to-platelet adhesion involving further fibrinogen bridging between receptors (particularly GPIIb/IIIa) on adjacent platelets.

As a result of interactions with the endothelium or the subendothelial matrix, as well as exposure to inflammatory mediators produced by the endothelium and other cells, the platelets are activated. Activation causes reorganization of the platelet cytoskeleton, leading to dynamic changes in platelet shape from smooth spheres to those with spiny projections and degranulation (also called the platelet-release reaction) and resulting in the release of various potent biochemicals.

Platelets contain three types of granules—lysosomes, dense bodies, and alpha granules. The contents of the dense bodies and alpha granules are particularly important in hemostasis. Dense bodies are generally proinflammatory (e.g., ADP, calcium, and serotonin). ADP recruits and activates other platelets through specific receptors. ADP also induces the platelet plasma membrane to undergo several important changes, including becoming ruffled and sticky; undergoing cellular spreading to make tight contacts between neighbouring platelets, causing the platelet plug to seal the injured endothelium; and undergoing externalization of the phospholipid phosphatidylserine, which provides a matrix for activation of clotting factors. Serotonin is a vasoactive amine with histaminelike properties to increase vasodilation and vascular permeability (see Chapter 6). Calcium is necessary for many of the intracellular signalling mechanisms that control platelet activation.

Alpha granules contain a mixture of clotting factors (fibrinogen, factor V), growth and angiogenic factors (e.g., platelet-derived growth factor [PDGF], vascular endothelial growth factor [VEGF], basic fibroblast growth factor [bFGF]), and angiogenesis inhibitors (e.g., platelet factor 4, thrombospondin, inhibitors of metalloproteinases). Platelet factor 4 also is a heparin-binding protein. Depending on the particular stimulus, platelets may selectively release promoters or inhibitors of angiogenesis. Many of these mediators also either promote or inhibit platelet activity and the eventual process of clot formation (see Figure 20-17). PDGF stimulates smooth muscle cells and promotes tissue repair. Heparin-binding proteins enhance clot formation at the site of injury.

Platelets also begin producing the prostaglandin derivative thromboxane A_2 (TXA_2), which counters the effects of PGI_2, produced by endothelial cells (see Figure 20-17). TXA_2 causes vasoconstriction and promotes the degranulation of platelets, whereas PGI_2 promotes vasodilation and inhibits platelet degranulation. In platelets, an isoform of cyclo-oxygenase-1 (COX-1) converts arachidonic acid to TXA_2. Aspirin, particularly at low doses, specifically and irreversibly inhibits COX-1, decreasing production of TXA_2 and decreasing platelet activation. Daily intake of low doses of Aspirin leads to more than 95% inhibition of TXA_2 in just a few days.

If blood vessel injury is minor, hemostasis is achieved temporarily by formation of the platelet plug, which usually forms within 3 to 5 minutes of injury. Platelet plugs seal the many minute ruptures that occur daily in the microcirculation, particularly in capillaries. With too few platelets, numerous small hemorrhagic areas called *purpuras* develop under the skin and throughout the tissues (see Chapter 21).

I. Subendothelial exposure

- Occurs after endothelial sloughing
- Platelets begin to fill endothelial gaps
- Promoted by thromboxane A_2 (TXA_2)
- Inhibited by prostacyclin (PGI_2)
- Platelet function depends on many factors, especially calcium

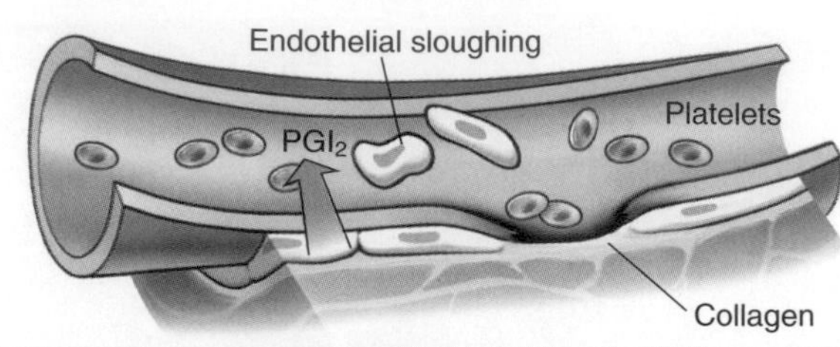

II. Adhesion

- Adhesion is initiated by loss of endothelial cells (or rupture or erosion of atherosclerotic plaque), which exposes adhesive glycoproteins such as collagen and von Willebrand factor (vWF) in the subendothelium. vWF and, perhaps, other adhesive glycoproteins in the plasma deposit on the damaged area. Platelets adhere to the subendothelium through receptors that bind to the adhesive glycoproteins (GPIb, GPIa/IIa, GPIIb/IIIa).

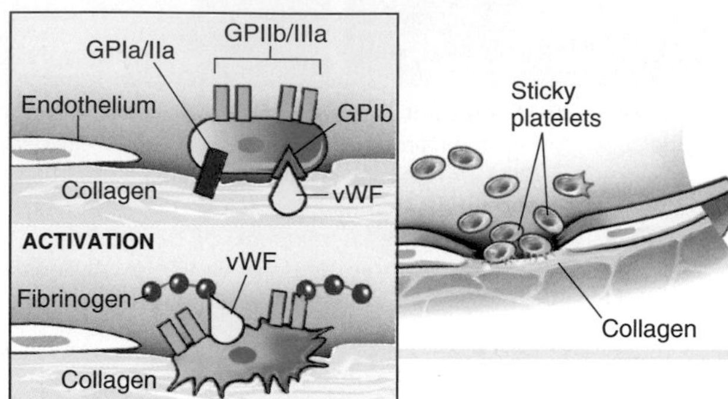

III. Activation

- After platelets adhere they undergo an activation process that leads to a conformational change in GPIIb/IIIa receptors, resulting in their ability to bind adhesive proteins, including fibrinogen and vWF
- Changes in platelet shape
- Formation of pseudopods
- Activation of arachidonic pathway

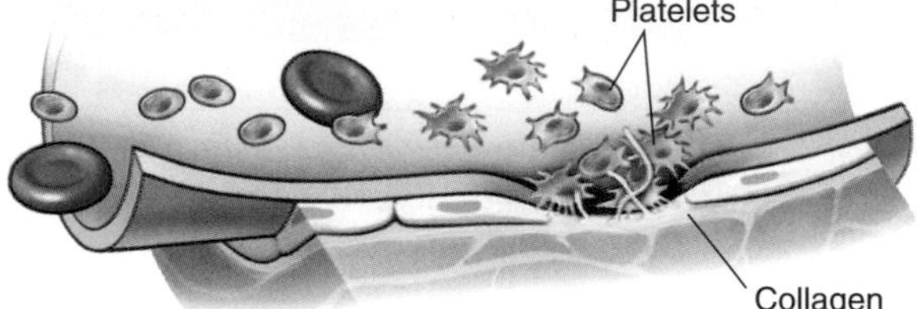

IV. Aggregation

- Induced by release of TXA_2
- Adhesive glycoproteins bind simultaneously to GPIIb/IIIa on two different platelets
- Stabilization of the platelet plug (blood clot) occurs by activation of coagulation factors, thrombin, and fibrin
- Heparin neutralizing factor enhances clot formation

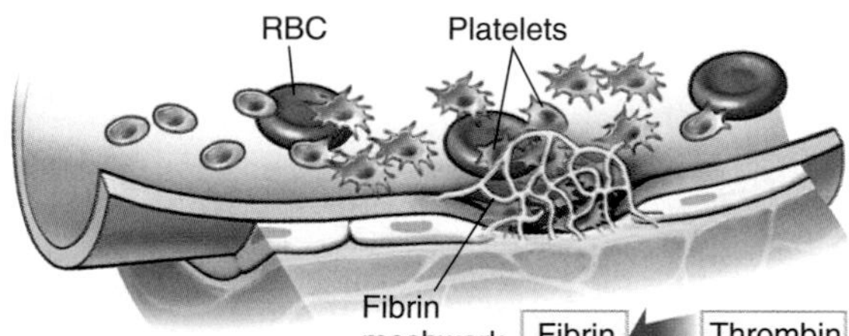

V. Platelet plug formation

- RBCs and platelets enmeshed in fibrin

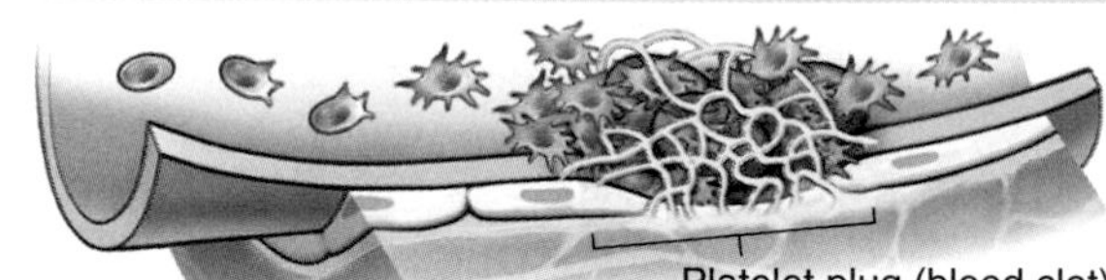

VI. Clot retraction and clot dissolution

- Clot retraction, using large number of platelets, joins the edges of the injured vessel
- Clot dissolution is regulated by thrombin and plasminogen activators

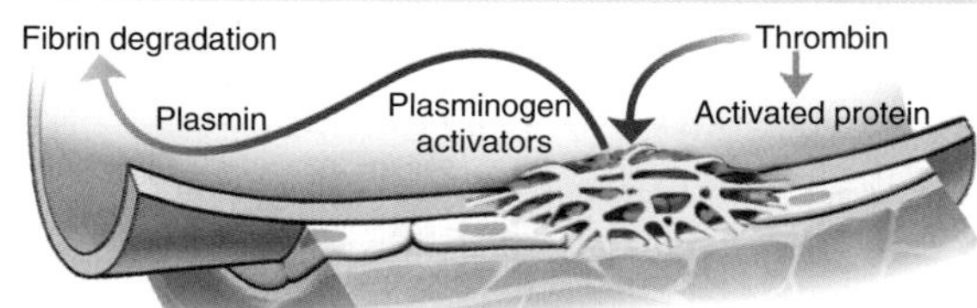

FIGURE 20-17 Blood Vessel Damage, Blood Clot, and Clot Dissolution. *RBC*, red blood cell.

Function of Clotting Factors

A **blood clot** is a meshwork of protein strands that stabilizes the platelet plug and traps other cells, such as erythrocytes, phagocytes, and microorganisms (Figure 20-18). The strands are made of fibrin, which is produced by the **clotting (coagulation) system**. The clotting system was described in Chapter 6 and consists of a family of proteins that circulate in the blood in inactive forms. Initiation of the system results in sequential activation (cascade) of multiple members of the system until a fibrin clot is created.

The clotting system is usually presented as two pathways of initiation (intrinsic and extrinsic pathways) that join in a common pathway. The intrinsic pathway is activated when Hageman factor (factor XII) in plasma contacts negatively charged subendothelial substances exposed by vascular injury. The extrinsic pathway is activated when **tissue thromboplastin**, a substance released by damaged endothelial cells, reacts with clotting factors, particularly factor VII. Both pathways lead to the common pathway and activation of factor X, which proceeds to clot formation.

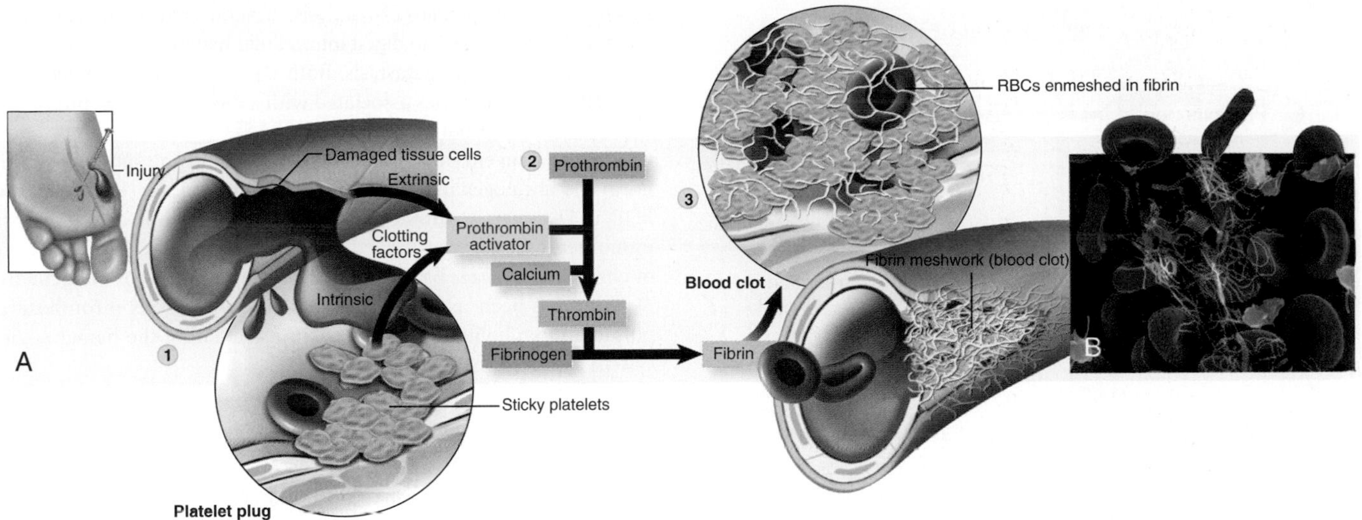

FIGURE 20-18 Blood Clotting Mechanism. **A,** The complex clotting mechanism can be summarized into three basic steps: **(1)** release of clotting factors from both injured tissue cells and sticky platelets at the injury site (which form temporary platelet plug); **(2)** series of chemical reactions that eventually result in the formation of thrombin; and **(3)** formation of fibrin and trapping of blood cells to form a clot. **B,** An electron micrograph showing entrapped red blood cells (*RBCs*) in a fibrin clot. (**A,** from Patton, K.T., & Thibodeau, G.A. [2012]. *Structure & function of the body* [14th ed.]. St. Louis: Mosby; **B,** Dennis Kunkel Microscopy/ Science Source.)

The extrinsic pathway is clearly predominant; individuals with deficiencies in intrinsic pathway components (i.e., factor XI, factor XII), surprisingly, do not have prolonged bleeding because these factors do not seem to be important for clotting. As with the complement cascade, the clotting system is complex with a large number of alternative activators and inhibitors, and the relative importance of particular factors may differ between in vivo hemostasis and in vitro testing of clotting or may depend on the particular mechanism by which the pathway is activated. There also is interaction between components of the intrinsic and extrinsic pathways so that an activated member of one pathway may activate a member of the other pathway (e.g., factor VIIa of the extrinsic pathway can directly activate factor IX of the intrinsic pathway).

Activated platelets are important participants in clotting. The phosphatidylserine-rich surface produced during platelet activation provides a matrix on which several important complexes of clotting factors are formed. These include the intrinsic pathway's *tenase complex* (factor X and activated factors VIII and IX) that activates factor X and the *prothrombinase complex* (prothrombin and activated factors X and V) that activates prothrombin into thrombin. Thrombin then converts fibrinogen into fibrin, which polymerizes into a fibrin clot. Thrombin has broad activity in the inflammatory response. In addition to producing fibrin, thrombin is an activator of other coagulation proteins (e.g., factors V, VIII, XI, XIII), platelets (e.g., aggregation, degranulation), endothelial cells (e.g., upregulation of adhesion molecules for leukocytes, increased NO, PGI_2, PDGF), and monocytes (e.g., cytokine secretion, increased receptors for endothelial cells).

Under normal conditions, spontaneous activation of hemostasis is prevented by factors residing on the endothelial cell surface. These include thrombin inhibitors (e.g., antithrombin III), tissue factor inhibitors (e.g., tissue factor pathway inhibitor), and mechanisms for degrading activated clotting factors (e.g., protein C). **Antithrombin III (AT-III)** is a circulating inhibitor of plasma serine proteases. AT-III is produced by the liver and binds to heparin sulphate found naturally on the surface of endothelial cells, or with heparin administered clinically to prevent thrombosis. Heparin induces a change in AT-III that greatly enhances its capacity to inhibit thrombin and other activated clotting factors. **Tissue factor pathway inhibitor (TFPI)** is produced by endothelial cells and platelets; complexes to, and reversibly inhibits, factor Xa in the prothrombinase complex; and also inhibits other activated clotting factors.

Thrombomodulin is a thrombin-binding protein on the surface of endothelial cells. **Protein C** in the circulation binds to thrombomodulin in a thrombin-dependent manner and is converted to activated protein C.[19] Activated protein C, in association with a cofactor (**protein S**), degrades factors Va and VIIIa. Deficiencies of AT-III, protein C, or protein S are important causes of hypercoagulation (increased clotting). Expression of thrombomodulin and the endothelial cell protein C receptor is downregulated by cytokines and other products of inflammation (e.g., IL-1α, TNF-α, endotoxin), thereby enhancing clot formation.

Retraction and Lysis of Blood Clots

After a clot is formed, it retracts, or "solidifies." Fibrin strands shorten, becoming denser and stronger, which approximates the edges of the injured vessel wall and seals the site of injury. Retraction is facilitated by the large numbers of platelets trapped within the fibrin meshwork. The platelets contract and "pull" the fibrin threads closer together while releasing a factor that stabilizes the fibrin. Contraction expels serum from the fibrin meshwork (see Figure 20-18). This process usually begins within a few minutes after a clot has formed, and most of the serum is expelled within 20 to 60 minutes.

Lysis (breakdown) of blood clots is carried out by the **fibrinolytic system** (Figure 20-19). Another plasma protein, plasminogen, is converted to **plasmin** by several products of coagulation and inflammation, especially by the enzymatic action of **tissue plasminogen activator (t-PA)**. Endothelial cells express t-PA, which is activated maximally after binding to fibrin. Another activator of plasminogen is **urokinaselike plasminogen activator (u-PA)**. The u-PA binds to a specific cellular urokinaselike plasminogen activator receptor (u-PAR), causing activation of plasminogen. This urokinase is the major activator of fibrinolysis in the *extravascular* or tissue compartment, whereas t-PA is largely

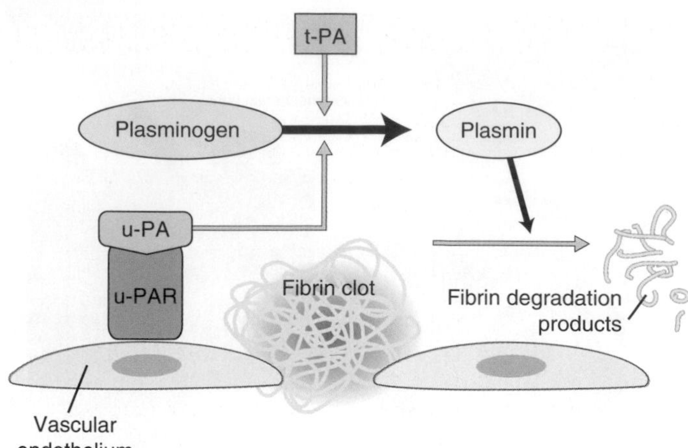

FIGURE 20-19 The Fibrinolytic System. Fibrinolysis is initiated by the binding of plasminogen to fibrin. Although tissue plasminogen activator (*t-PA*) initiates intravascular fibrinolysis, urokinaselike plasminogen activator (*u-PA*) is the major activator of fibrinolysis in tissue (extravascular). Plasmin digests the fibrin into smaller soluble pieces (fibrin degradation products). *u-PAR*, urokinaselike plasminogen activator receptor.

involved in *intravascular* fibrinolysis. Several cancers appear to use membrane-bound u-PA to digest intercellular matrix and greatly facilitate tumour invasion and metastasis. Both t-PA and u-PA have been used clinically to treat diseases associated with a blood clot (e.g., pulmonary embolism, myocardial infarction, stroke).[20]

Plasmin is an enzyme that dissolves clots (**fibrinolysis**) by degrading fibrin and fibrinogen into **fibrin degradation products (FDPs)**. A major FDP is D-dimer. **D-dimer** is two D domains from adjacent fibrin monomers that are cross-linked by factor XIIIa and released as a result of enzymatic cleavage by plasmin. Measurement of levels of circulating D-dimer has been used for diagnosis of deep venous thrombosis or pulmonary embolism.[21] Blood tests for evaluating the hematological system are listed in Table 20-6.

QUICK CHECK 20-5

1. What specific cells are involved in development of leukocytes?
2. Why are platelets necessary to stop bleeding?
3. Briefly describe the steps of platelet adhesion and aggregation.
4. How does plasminogen initiate fibrinolysis?

TABLE 20-6 Common Blood Tests for Hematological Disorders

Cell Type and Test	Property Evaluated by Test	Possible Hematological Cause of Abnormal Findings
Erythrocyte		
Red cell count	Number of erythrocytes in 1 mm^3 of peripheral blood	Altered erythropoiesis, anemias, hemorrhage, Hodgkin's disease, leukemia
Mean corpuscular volume (MCV)	Size of erythrocytes	Anemias, thalassemias
Mean corpuscular hemoglobin (MCH)	Amount of hemoglobin (Hb) in each erythrocyte (by weight)	Anemias, hemoglobinopathy
Mean corpuscular hemoglobin concentration (MCHC)	Concentration of Hb in each erythrocyte (percentage of erythrocyte occupied by Hb)	Anemias, hereditary spherocytosis
Hb determination	Amount of Hb (by weight)/L of blood	Anemias
Hematocrit determination	Percentage of a given volume of blood that is occupied by erythrocytes	Hemorrhage, polycythemia, erythrocytosis, anemias, leukemia
Reticulocyte count	Expressed as percentage of reticulocytes in total red blood cell count	Hyperactive or hypoactive bone marrow function
Erythrocyte osmotic fragility test	Cellular shape (biconcavity), structure of plasma membrane	Anemias, hemolytic disease caused by ABO or Rh incompatibility, Hodgkin's disease, polycythemia vera, thalassemia major
Hb electrophoresis	Relative percentage of different types of Hb in erythrocytes	Sickle cell disease, sickle cell trait, hemoglobin C (Hb C) disease, Hb C trait, thalassemias
Sickle cell test	Presence of hemoglobin S (Hb S) in erythrocytes	Sickle cell trait, sickle cell anemia
Glucose-6-phosphate dehydrogenase (G6PD) deficiency test	Deficiency of G6PD in erythrocytes	Hemolytic anemia
Hemoglobin Metabolism		
Serum ferritin determination	Depletion of body iron (potential deficiency of heme synthesis)	Iron deficiency anemias
Total iron-binding capacity (TIBC)	Amount of iron in serum plus amount of transferrin available in serum	Hemorrhage, iron deficiency anemia, hemochromatosis, hemosiderosis, iron overload, anemias, thalassemia
Transferrin saturation	Percentage of transferrin that is saturated with iron	Acute hemorrhage, hemochromatosis, hemosiderosis, sideroblastic anemia, iron deficiency anemia, iron overload, thalassemia
Porphyrin analysis (protoporphyrin analysis)	Concentration of protoporphyrin in erythrocytes, an indicator of iron-deficient erythropoiesis	Megaloblastic anemia, congenital erythropoietic porphyria

TABLE 20-6 Common Blood Tests for Hematological Disorders—cont'd

Cell Type and Test	Property Evaluated by Test	Possible Hematological Cause of Abnormal Findings
Direct antiglobulin test (DAT)	Antibody binding to erythrocytes	Hemolytic disease of newborn, autoimmune hemolytic anemia, medication-induced hemolytic anemia, transfusion reaction
Antibody screen test (indirect Coombs test)	Detection of antibodies to erythrocyte antigens (other than ABO antigens)	Same as for DAT
Leukocytes: Differential White Cell Count (Absolute Number of Leukocytes × 10^9/L of Blood)		
Neutrophil count	Neutrophils × 10^9/L	Myeloproliferative disorders, hematopoietic disorders, hemolysis, infection
Lymphocyte count	Lymphocytes × 10^9/L	Infectious lymphocytosis, infectious mononucleosis, hematopoietic disorders, anemias, leukemia, lymphosarcoma, Hodgkin's disease
Plasma cell count	Plasma cells × 10^9/L	Infectious mononucleosis, lymphocytosis, plasma cell leukemia
Monocyte count	Monocytes × 10^9/L	Hodgkin's disease, infectious mononucleosis, monocytic leukemia, non-Hodgkin's lymphoma, polycythemia vera
Eosinophil count	Eosinophils × 10^9/L	Hematopoietic disorders, parasitic infections, allergic reactions
Basophil count	Basophils × 10^9/L	Chronic myelogenous leukemia, hemolytic anemias, Hodgkin's disease, polycythemia vera
Platelets and Clotting Factors		
Platelet count	Number of circulating platelets per mm^3 of blood	Anemias, multiple myeloma, myelofibrosis, polycythemia vera, leukemia, disseminated intravascular coagulation (DIC), hemolytic disease of the newborn, transfusion reaction, lymphoproliferative disorders
Bleeding time	Duration of bleeding following a standardized superficial puncture wound of skin, integrity of platelet plug, measured in minutes following puncture	Leukemia, anemias, DIC, fibrinolytic activity, purpuras, hemorrhagic disease of the newborn, infectious mononucleosis, multiple myeloma, clotting factor deficiencies, thrombasthenia, thrombocytopenia, von Willebrand's disease
Clot retraction test	Platelet number and function, fibrinogen quantity and use, measured in hours required for expression of serum from a clot incubated in a test tube	Acute leukemia, aplastic anemia, factor XIII deficiency, increased fibrinolytic activity, Hodgkin's disease, hyperfibrinogenemia or hypofibrinogenemia, idiopathic thrombocytopenic purpura, multiple myeloma, polycythemia vera, secondary thrombocytopenia, thrombasthenia
Platelet adhesion studies	Ability of platelets to adhere to foreign surfaces	Anemia, macroglobulinemia, Bernard-Soulier syndrome, multiple myeloma, myeloid metaplasia, plasma cell dyscrasias, thrombasthenia, thrombocytopathy, von Willebrand's disease
Platelet aggregation tests	Ability of platelets to adhere to one another	Afibrinogenemia, Bernard-Soulier syndrome, thrombasthenia, hemorrhagic thrombocythemia, myeloid metaplasia, plasma cell dyscrasias, platelet-release defects, polycythemia vera, preleukemia, sideroblastic anemia, von Willebrand's disease, Waldenström macroglobulinemia, hypercoagulability
Whole blood clotting time (Lee-White coagulation time)	Overall ability of blood to clot, as measured in minutes in a test tube	Afibrinogenemia, clotting factor deficiencies, excessive fibrinolysis, hemorrhagic disease of the newborn, hypofibrinogenemia, hypoprothrombinemia, leukemia
Circulating anticoagulants (immunoglobulin G antibodies that inhibit coagulation)	Presence of antibodies that neutralize clotting factors and inhibit coagulation, as indicated by prolonged clotting time, prothrombin time, or partial thromboplastin time	Afibrinogenemia, presence of fibrin-fibrinogen degradation products, macroglobulinemia, multiple myeloma, DIC, plasma cell dyscrasias
Partial thromboplastin time (PTT)	Effectiveness of clotting factors (except factors VII and VIII), effectiveness of intrinsic pathway of coagulation cascade, as measured in a test tube (in seconds)	Presence of circulating anticoagulants, DIC, clotting factor deficiencies, excessive fibrinolysis, hemorrhagic disease of the newborn, hypofibrinogenemia and afibrinogenemia, prothrombin deficiency, von Willebrand's disease, acute hemorrhage

Continued

TABLE 20-6 Common Blood Tests for Hematological Disorders—cont'd

Cell Type and Test	Property Evaluated by Test	Possible Hematological Cause of Abnormal Findings
Prothrombin time	Effectiveness of activity of prothrombin, fibrinogen, and factors V, VII, and X; effectiveness of vitamin K–dependent coagulation factors of extrinsic and common pathways of coagulation cascade as measured in a test tube (in seconds)	Hypofibrinogenemia, dysfibrinogenemia, and afibrinogenemia; presence of circulating anticoagulants; DIC; deficiency of factors V, VII, or X; presence of fibrin degradation products, increased fibrinolytic activity, hemolytic jaundice, hemorrhagic disease of the newborn; acute leukemia, polycythemia vera, prothrombin deficiency, multiple myeloma
Thrombin time	Quantity and activity of fibrinogen as measured in a test tube (in seconds)	Hypofibrinogenemia, dysfibrinogenemia, and afibrinogenemia; presence of circulating anticoagulants; hemorrhagic disease of the newborn, polycythemia vera; increase in fibrinogen-fibrin degradation products; increased fibrinolytic activity
Fibrinogen assay	Amount of fibrinogen available for fibrin formation	Acute leukemia, congenital hypofibrinogenemia or afibrinogenemia, DIC, increased fibrinolytic activity, severe hemorrhage
Fibrin-fibrinogen degradation products (fibrin-fibrinogen split products)	Fibrinogenic activity as measured by levels of fibrin-fibrinogen degradation products (in mcmol/L of blood)	Transfusion reactions, DIC, internal hemorrhage in the newborn, deep venous thrombosis, pulmonary embolism

Data from Bick, R.L., Bennett, J.M., & Byrnes, R.K. (Eds.). (1993). *Hematology: Clinical and laboratory practice.* St. Louis: Mosby; Byrne, C.J., Saxton, D.F., Pelikan, P.K., et al. (1986). *Laboratory tests: Implications for nursing care.* Menlo Park, CA: Addison-Wesley; Pagana, K.D., Pagana, T.J., Pike-MacDonald, S.A., et al. (2013). *Mosby's Canadian manual of diagnostic and laboratory tests.* Toronto: Elsevier.

PEDIATRIC CONSIDERATIONS

Hematological Value Changes

Blood cell counts tend to rise above adult levels at birth and then decline gradually throughout childhood. Table 20-7 lists normal ranges during infancy and childhood. The immediate rise in values is the result of accelerated hematopoiesis during fetal life and the increased numbers of cells that result from the trauma of birth and cutting of the umbilical cord.

Average blood volume in the full-term neonate is 85 mL/kg of body weight. The premature infant has a slightly larger blood volume of 90 mL/kg of body weight. In both full-term and premature infants, blood volume decreases during the first few months. Thereafter the average blood volume is 75 to 77 mL/kg, which is similar to that of older children and adults.

The hypoxic intrauterine environment stimulates erythropoietin production in the fetus and accelerates fetal erythropoiesis, producing polycythemia (excessive proliferation of erythrocyte precursors) in the newborn. After birth, the oxygen from the lungs saturates arterial blood, and more oxygen is delivered to the tissues. In response to the change from a placental to a pulmonary oxygen supply during the first few days of life, levels of erythropoietin and the rate of blood cell formation decrease. The active rate of fetal erythropoiesis is reflected by the large numbers of immature erythrocytes (reticulocytes) in the peripheral blood of full-term neonates. After birth, the number of reticulocytes decreases by 50% every 12 hours, so it is rare to find an elevated reticulocyte count after the first week of life. During this period of rapid growth, the rate of erythrocyte destruction is greater than that in later childhood and adulthood. In full-term infants, the normal erythrocyte lifespan is 60 to 80 days; in premature infants, it may be as short as 20 to 30 days; and in children and adolescents, it is the same as that in adults—120 days.

The postnatal fall in hemoglobin and hematocrit values is more marked in premature infants than it is in full-term infants. In preschool and school-aged children, hemoglobin, hematocrit, and red blood cell counts gradually rise. Metabolic processes within the erythrocytes of neonates differ significantly from those found in erythrocytes of normal adults. The relatively young population of erythrocytes in newborns consumes greater quantities of glucose than do erythrocytes in adults.

The lymphocytes of children tend to have more cytoplasm and less compact nuclear chromatin than do the lymphocytes of adults. A possible explanation is that children tend to have more frequent viral infections, which are associated with atypical lymphocytes. Minor infections, in which the child fails to exhibit clinical manifestations of illness, and the administration of immunizations also may account for the lymphocyte changes.

At birth the lymphocyte count is high, and it continues to rise during the first year of life. Then it steadily declines until the lower value seen in adults is reached. It is unknown whether these developmental variations are physiological or a response to frequent viral infection and immunizations in children.

The neutrophil count, like the lymphocyte count, is high at birth and rises during the first days of life. After 2 weeks, the neutrophil count falls to within or below the normal adult range. Although the exact age can vary by approximately 7 years of age, the neutrophil count is the same as that of an adult.

The eosinophil count is higher in the first year of life and higher in children than in teenagers or adults. Monocyte counts also are high in the first year of life but then decrease to adult levels. Platelet counts in full-term neonates are comparable to those in adults and remain so throughout infancy and childhood.

TABLE 20-7 Mean Hematological Differential Counts From Birth to Adulthood

Hematological Differential	Newborn (Cord Blood)	2 Weeks of Age	3 Months of Age	6 Months to 6 Years of Age	7–12 Years of Age	Adult
Hemoglobin (g/L)	168	165	120	120	130	130
Hematocrit (%)	55	50	36	37	38	40
Reticulocytes (%)	5	1	1	1	1	1
Leukocytes WBC ($\times 10^9$/L)	9–30	5–20	5.0–19.5	6.0–17.5	4.5–13.5	5–10
Neutrophils (%)	61	40	30	45	55	55
Lymphocytes (%)	31	48	63	48	38	35
Eosinophils (%)	2	3	2	2	2	2
Monocytes (%)	6	9	5	5	5	5
Platelets ($\times 10^9$/L)	140–450	140–450	140–450	140–450	140–450	140–450

WBC, white blood cell

GERIATRIC CONSIDERATIONS

Hematological Value Changes

Blood composition changes little with age, although some components may be altered by iron deficiency. Total serum iron level, total iron-binding capacity, and intestinal iron absorption are all decreased somewhat in older adults. The erythrocyte lifespan is normal, although the erythrocytes are replenished more slowly after bleeding. Hemoglobin levels may be low, and the plasma membranes of erythrocytes become increasingly fragile, with portions being lost, presumably because of physical trauma inflicted during circulation.

Lymphocyte function appears to decrease with age (see Chapters 7 and 8), causing changes in cellular immunity and some decline in T-cell function. The humoral immune system is less able to respond to antigenic challenge.

No changes in platelet numbers or structure have been observed in older adults, yet platelet adhesiveness probably increases. Although fibrinogen levels and levels of factors V, VII, and IX tend to be increased, no major hypercoagulability has been confirmed.

DID YOU UNDERSTAND?

Components of the Hematological System

1. Blood consists of a variety of components—about 92% water and 8% solutes. In adults, the total blood volume is approximately 5.5 L.
2. Plasma, a complex aqueous liquid, contains two major groups of plasma proteins: albumins and globulins.
3. The cellular components of the blood are red blood cells (erythrocytes), white blood cells (leukocytes), and platelets.
4. Erythrocytes are the most abundant cells of the blood, occupying about 48% of the blood volume in men and about 42% in women. Erythrocytes are primarily responsible for tissue oxygenation.
5. Leukocytes are fewer in number than erythrocytes and constitute approximately 5 to 10 $\times 10^9$/L of blood. Leukocytes defend the body against infection and remove dead or injured host cells.
6. Leukocytes are classified as either granulocytes (neutrophils, eosinophils, basophils) or agranulocytes (monocytes/macrophages, lymphocytes).
7. Platelets are anuclear disc-shaped cytoplasmic fragments. Platelets are essential for blood coagulation and control of bleeding.
8. The lymphoid organs are sites of residence, proliferation, differentiation, or function of lymphocytes and mononuclear phagocytes.
9. The spleen is the largest lymphoid organ and functions as the site of fetal hematopoiesis, filters and cleanses the blood, and acts as a reservoir for lymphocytes and other blood cells.
10. The lymph nodes are the site of development or activity of large numbers of lymphocytes, monocytes, and macrophages.
11. The mononuclear phagocyte system (MPS) is composed of monocytes in bone marrow and peripheral blood and macrophages in tissue.
12. The MPS is an important line of defence against bacteria and other microorganisms in the bloodstream and cleanses the blood by removing old, injured, or dead blood cells; antigen-antibody complexes; and macromolecules.

Development of Blood Cells

1. Hematopoiesis, or blood cell production, occurs in the liver and spleen of the fetus and in the bone marrow after birth.
2. Hematopoiesis involves two stages: proliferation and differentiation (i.e., maturation). Each type of blood cell has parent cells called *stem cells.*
3. Hematopoiesis continues throughout life to replace blood cells that grow old and die, are killed by disease, or are lost through bleeding.
4. Bone marrow consists of red (hematopoietic) marrow (blood vessels, mononuclear phagocytes, stem cells, blood cells in various stages of differentiation, stromal cells) and yellow marrow (fatty tissue).
5. The bone marrow contains multiple populations of stem cells; mesenchymal stem cells develop into fibroblasts, osteoclasts, and adipocytes; and hematopoietic stem cells (HSCs) develop into blood cells.
6. Regulation of hematopoiesis occurs in bone marrow niches in which HSCs differentiate and are controlled by multiple cytokines and chemokines and through direct contact with osteoblasts (osteoblastic niche) or vascular endothelial cells (vascular niche), as well as several other specialized cells, including CXCL12-abundant reticular cells and nestin-expressing cells.
7. Specific hematopoietic growth factors (e.g., colony-stimulating factors) are necessary for the adequate production of myeloid, erythroid, lymphoid, and megakaryocytic lineages.
8. Hemoglobin, the oxygen-carrying protein of the erythrocyte, enables the blood to transport 100 times more oxygen than could be transported dissolved in plasma alone.

9. Regulation of erythropoiesis is mediated by erythropoietin, which is secreted by the kidneys in response to tissue hypoxia and causes a compensatory increase in erythrocyte production if the oxygen content of the blood decreases because of anemia, high altitude, or pulmonary disease.
10. Erythropoiesis depends on the presence of vitamins (especially vitamin B_{12}, folate, vitamin B_6, riboflavin, pantothenic acid, niacin, ascorbic acid, and vitamin E).
11. The iron cycle reutilizes iron released from old or damaged erythrocytes. Iron binds to transferrin in the blood, is transported to macrophages of the mononuclear phagocyte system, and is stored in the cytoplasm as ferritin.
12. Iron homeostasis is controlled by hepcidin, a small hormone produced by hepatocytes, which regulates ferroportin, the principal transporter of iron from stores in hepatocytes and macrophages and from intestinal cells that absorb dietary iron.
13. Maintenance of optimal levels of granulocytes and monocytes in the blood depends on the availability of pluripotent stem cells in the marrow, induction of these into committed stem cells, and timely release of new cells from the marrow.
14. Granulocytes and monocytes in the blood develop from common myeloid progenitor cells in the bone marrow under the direction of several growth factors, including stem cell factor, interleukin-3, and granulocyte-macrophage colony–stimulating factor.
15. Specific humoral colony-stimulating factors are necessary for the adequate growth of myeloid, erythroid, lymphoid, and megakaryocytic lineages.
16. Platelets develop from megakaryocytes by a process called *endomitosis*, which is controlled by thrombopoietin. During endomitosis the megakaryocytes undergo mitosis but not cell division and the cytoplasm and plasma membrane fragment into platelets.

Mechanisms of Hemostasis

1. Hemostasis, or arrest of bleeding, involves (a) vasoconstriction (vasospasm), (b) formation of a platelet plug, (c) activation of the clotting cascade, (d) formation of a blood clot, and (e) clot retraction and clot dissolution.
2. The normal vascular endothelium prevents spontaneous clotting by producing factors such as nitric oxide and prostacyclin that relax the vessels and prevent platelet activation.
3. Lysis of blood clots is the function of the fibrinolytic system. Plasmin, a proteolytic enzyme, splits fibrin and fibrinogen into fibrin degradation products that dissolve the clot.

Pediatric Considerations: Hematological Value Changes

1. Blood cell counts tend to rise above adult levels at birth and then decline gradually throughout childhood.
2. The lymphocytes of children tend to have more cytoplasm and less compact nuclear chromatin than do the lymphocytes of adults.

Geriatric Considerations: Hematological Value Changes

1. Blood composition changes little with age. Erythrocyte replenishment may be delayed after bleeding, presumably because of iron deficiency.
2. Lymphocyte function appears to decrease with age. Particularly affected is a decrease in cellular immunity.
3. Platelet adhesiveness probably increases with age.

KEY TERMS

Agranulocyte, 498
Albumin, 496
Antithrombin III (AT-III), 513
Apoferritin, 508
Apotransferrin, 508
Basophil, 499
Blood clot, 512
Bone marrow, 504
Clotting (coagulation) system, 512
Clotting factor, 497
Collagen, 510
Colony-stimulating factor (CSF, hematopoietic growth factor), 505
Cyclo-oxygenase-1 (COX-1), 511
D-dimer, 514
Deoxyhemoglobin, 507
Endomitosis, 509
Eosinophil, 499
Erythroblast (normoblast), 506
Erythrocyte, 497
Erythropoiesis, 506
Erythropoietin, 506
Extramedullary hematopoiesis, 504
Fibrin degradation product (FDP), 514
Fibrinolysis, 514
Fibrinolytic system, 513
Globin, 506
Globulin, 496
Granulocyte, 498
Hematopoiesis, 503
Hematopoietic stem cell (HSC), 504
Heme, 507
Hemoglobin (Hb), 506
Hemosiderin, 508
Hemostasis, 510
Hepcidin, 509
Immunocyte, 498
Integrin $\alpha_{IIb}\beta_3$ (GPIIb/IIIa), 510
Leukocyte, 498
Lipoprotein, 497
Lymph node, 502
Lymphocyte, 499
Macrophage, 499
Marginating storage pool, 506
Megakaryocytes, 500
Mesenchymal stem cells (MSCs), 504
Methemoglobin, 507
Monocyte, 499
Mononuclear phagocyte system (MPS), 503
Myeloid tissue, 504
Myoglobin, 508
Natural killer (NK) cells, 499
Neutrophil (polymorphonuclear neutrophil [PMN]), 498
Niche, 504
Nitric oxide (NO), 507
Osteoblastic niche, 504
Oxyhemoglobin, 507
Phagocyte, 498
Plasma, 496
Plasma protein, 496
Plasmin, 513
Platelet (thrombocyte), 499
Platelet-release reaction, 511
Primary lymphoid organs, 500
Proerythroblast, 506
Prostacyclin (PGI_2), 510
Protein C, 513
Protein S, 513
Protoporphyrin, 507
Reticulocyte, 506
Secondary lymphoid organs, 500
Serum, 496
Spleen, 500
Stromal cell, 504
Thrombomodulin, 513
Thrombopoietin (TPO), 510
Thromboxane A_2 (TXA_2), 511
Tissue factor pathway inhibitor (TFPI), 513
Tissue plasminogen activator (t-PA), 513
Tissue thromboplastin, 512
Transferrin, 508
Urokinaselike plasminogen activator (u-PA), 513
Vascular niche, 505
von Willebrand factor (vWF), 510

REFERENCES

1. Kita, H. (2013). Eosinophils: multifunctional and distinctive properties. *International Archives of Allergy and Immunology, 161*(Suppl. 2), 3–9. doi:10.1159/000350662.
2. Amon, T. I., & Cyster, J. G. (2014). Blood, sphintosine-1-phosphate and lymphocyte migration dynamics in the spleen. *Current Topics in Microbiology and Immunology, 378*(2014), 107–128. doi:10.1007/978-3-319-05879-5_5.
3. Jenkins, S. J., & Hume, D. A. (2014). Homeostasis in the mononuclear phagocyte system. *Trends in Immunology, 35*(8), 358–367. doi:10.1016/j.it.2014.06.006.
4. Glatman Zaretsky, A., Engiles, J. B., & Hunter, C. A. (2014). Infection-induced changes in hematopoiesis. *Journal of Immunology, 192*(1), 27–33. doi:10.4049/jimmunol.1302061.
5. Blin-Wakkach, C., Rouleau, M., & Wakkach, A. (2014). Roles of osteoclasts in the control of medullary hematopoietic niches. *Archives of Biochemistry and Biophysics, 561*, 29–37. doi:10.1016/j.abb.2014.06.032.
6. National Institutes of Health. (2016). *Stem cell information*. Retrieved from https://stemcells.nih.gov/.
7. He, N., Zhang, L., Cui, J., et al. (2014). Bone marrow vascular niche: Home for hematopoietic stem cells. *Bone Marrow Research, 2014*, 128436. doi:10.1155/2014/128436.
8. Morrison, S. J., & Scadden, D. T. (2014). The bone marrow niche for haematopoietic stem cells. *Nature, 505*(7483), 327–334. doi:10.1038/nature12984.
9. Endele, M., Etzrodt, M., & Schroeder, T. (2014). Instruction of hematopoietic lineage choice by cytokine signaling. *Experimental Cell Research, 329*(2), 207–213. doi:10.1016/j.yexcr.2014.07.011.
10. Thom, C. S., Dickson, C. F., Gell, D. A., et al. (2013). Hemoglobin variants: Biochemical properties and clinical correlates. *Cold Spring Harbor Perspectives in Medicine, 3*(3), a011858. doi:10.1101/cshperspect.a011858.
11. Chiabrando, D., Vinchi, F., Fiorito, V., et al. (2014). Heme in pathophysiology: A matter of scavenging, metabolism and trafficking across cell membranes. *Frontiers in Pharmacology, 5*, 61. doi:10.3389/fphar.2014.00061.
12. Simmonds, M. J., Meiselman, H. J., & Baskurt, O. K. (2013). Blood rheology and aging. *Journal of Geriatric Cardiology, 10*(3), 291–301. doi:10.3969/j.issn.1671-5411.2013.03.010.
13. Winter, W. E., Bazydio, L. A., & Harris, N. S. (2014). The molecular biology of human iron metabolism. *Laboratory Medicine, 45*(2), 92–102.
14. Loréal, O., Cavey, T., Bardou-Jacquet, E., et al. (2014). Iron, hepcidin, and the metal connection. *Frontiers in Pharmacology, 5*, 128. doi:10.3389/fphar.2014.00128.
15. Ganz, T. (2013). Systemic iron homeostasis. *Physiological Reviews, 93*(4), 1721–1741. doi:10.1152/physrev.00008.2013.
16. Machlus, K. R., Thon, J. N., & Italiano, J. E., Jr. (2014). Interpreting the development dance of the megakaryocyte: A review of the cellular and molecular processes mediating platelet formation. *British Journal of Haematology, 165*(2), 227–236. doi:10.1111/bjh.12758.
17. Hitchcock, I. S., & Kaushansky, K. (2014). Thrombopoietin from beginning to end. *British Journal of Haematology, 165*(2), 259–268. doi:10.1111/bjh.12772.
18. Kuter, D. J. (2014). Milestones in understanding platelet production: A historical overview. *British Journal of Haematology, 165*(2), 248–258. doi:10.1111/bjh.12781.
19. Spronk, H. M., Borissoff, J. I., & ten Cate, H. (2013). New insights into modulation of thrombin formation. *Current Atherosclerosis Reports, 15*(11), 363. doi:10.1007/s11883-013-0363-3.
20. Robertson, I., Kessel, D. O., & Berridge, D. C. (2013). Fibrinolytic agents for peripheral arterial occlusion. *Cochrane Database of Systematic Reviews*, (12), CD001099, doi:10.1002/14651858.CD001099.pub3.
21. Wells, P., & Anderson, D. (2013). The diagnosis and treatment of venous thromboembolism. *Hematology / the Education Program of the American Society of Hematology. American Society of Hematology. Education Program, 2013*(1), 457–463. doi:10.1182/asheducation-2013.1.457.

21

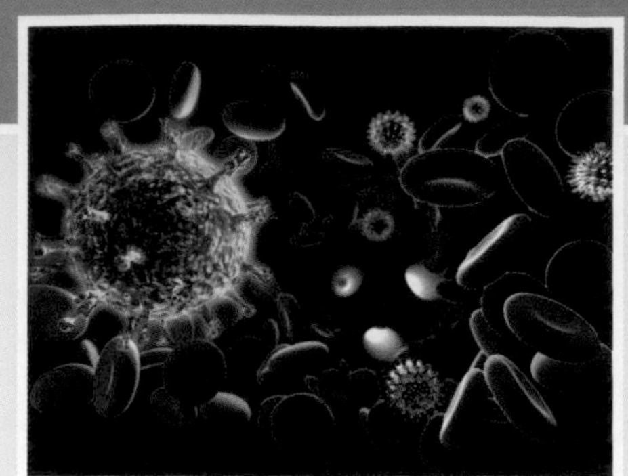

Alterations of Hematological Function

Anna Schwartz, Kathryn L. McCance, Neal S. Rote, and Kelly Power-Kean

EVOLVE WEBSITE

http://evolve.elsevier.com/Canada/Huether/pathophysiology
Student Review Questions
Key Points
Case Studies
Animations
Quick Check Answers

CHAPTER OUTLINE

Alterations of Erythrocyte Function, 520
- Classification of Anemias, 520
- Macrocytic-Normochromic Anemias, 522
- Microcytic-Hypochromic Anemias, 524
- Normocytic-Normochromic Anemias, 526

Myeloproliferative Red Blood Cell Disorders, 526
- Polycythemia Vera, 526
- Iron Overload, 529

Alterations of Leukocyte Function, 529
- Quantitative Alterations of Leukocytes, 529

Alterations of Lymphoid Function, 538
- Lymphadenopathy, 538
- Malignant Lymphomas, 538

Alterations of Splenic Function, 545

Hemorrhagic Disorders and Alterations of Platelets and Coagulation, 546
- Disorders of Platelets, 546
- Alterations of Platelet Function, 549
- Disorders of Coagulation, 550

Alterations of erythrocyte function involve either insufficient or excessive numbers of erythrocytes in the circulation or normal numbers of cells with abnormal components. Anemias are conditions in which there are too few erythrocytes or an insufficient volume of erythrocytes in the blood. Polycythemias are conditions in which erythrocyte numbers or volume is excessive. All of these conditions have many causes and are pathophysiological manifestations of a variety of disease states.

Many disorders involving leukocytes range from increased numbers of leukocytes (i.e., leukocytosis) in response to infections to proliferative disorders (such as leukemia). Many hematological disorders are malignancies, and many nonhematological malignancies metastasize to bone marrow, affecting leukocyte production. Thus a large portion of this chapter is devoted to malignant disease.

The primary role of clotting (hemostasis) is to stop bleeding through an interaction of endothelium lining the vessels, platelets, and clotting factors. A large number of disease states may be associated with a clinically significant increase or decrease in clotting resulting from alterations in any of the three main components of the clotting process.

ALTERATIONS OF ERYTHROCYTE FUNCTION

Classification of Anemias

Anemia is a reduction in the total number of erythrocytes in the circulating blood or a decrease in the quality or quantity of hemoglobin. Anemias commonly result from (1) impaired erythrocyte production, (2) blood loss (acute or chronic), (3) increased erythrocyte destruction, or (4) a combination of these three factors. Anemias are classified by their causes (e.g., anemia of chronic disease) or by the changes that affect the size, shape, or substance of the erythrocyte. The most common classification of anemias is based on the changes that affect the cell's size and hemoglobin content (Table 21-1). Terms used to identify anemias reflect these characteristics. Terms that end with *-cytic* refer to cell size, and those that end with *-chromic* refer to hemoglobin content. Additional terms describing erythrocytes found in some anemias are **anisocytosis** (assuming various sizes) and **poikilocytosis** (assuming various shapes).

CLINICAL MANIFESTATIONS The main alteration of anemia is a reduced oxygen-carrying capacity of the blood resulting in tissue hypoxia. Symptoms of anemia vary, depending on the body's ability to compensate for the reduced oxygen-carrying capacity. Anemia that is mild and starts gradually is usually easier to compensate and may cause problems for the individual only during physical exertion. As red blood cell reduction continues, symptoms become more pronounced and alterations in specific organs and compensation effects are more apparent. Compensation generally involves the cardiovascular, respiratory, and hematological systems (Figure 21-1).

A reduction in the number of red blood cells in the blood causes a reduction in the consistency and volume of blood. Initial compensation for cellular loss is movement of interstitial fluid into the blood, causing an increase in plasma volume. This movement maintains an adequate blood volume, but the viscosity (thickness) of the blood decreases. The "thinner" blood flows faster and more turbulently than normal blood, causing a hyperdynamic circulatory state. This hyperdynamic state creates cardiovascular changes—increased stroke volume and heart rate.

TABLE 21-1 Morphological Classification of Anemias

Structure of Erythrocytes	Name and Mechanism of Anemia	Primary Cause
Macrocytic-normochromic anemia: large, abnormally shaped erythrocytes, normal hemoglobin concentrations	Pernicious anemia: lack of vitamin B_{12}; abnormal DNA and RNA synthesis in erythroblast; premature cell death	Congenital or acquired deficiency of intrinsic factor; genetic disorder of DNA synthesis
	Folate deficiency anemia: lack of folate; premature cell death	Dietary folate deficiency
Microcytic-hypochromic anemia: small, abnormally shaped erythrocytes and reduced hemoglobin concentration	Iron deficiency anemia: lack of iron for hemoglobin; insufficient hemoglobin	Chronic blood loss, dietary iron deficiency, disruption of iron metabolism or iron cycle
	Sideroblastic anemia: dysfunctional iron uptake by erythroblasts and defective porphyrin and heme synthesis	Congenital dysfunction of iron metabolism in erythroblasts, acquired dysfunction of iron metabolism as result of medications or toxins
	Thalassemia: impaired synthesis of α- or β-chain of hemoglobin A; phagocytosis of abnormal erythroblasts in marrow	Congenital genetic defect of globin synthesis
Normocytic-normochromic anemia: normal size, normal hemoglobin concentration	Aplastic anemia: insufficient erythropoiesis	Depressed stem cell proliferation
	Posthemorrhagic anemia: blood loss	Increased erythropoiesis; iron depletion
	Hemolytic anemia: premature destruction (lysis) of mature erythrocytes in circulation	Increased fragility of erythrocytes
	Sickle cell anemia: abnormal hemoglobin synthesis, abnormal cell shape with susceptibility to damage, lysis, and phagocytosis	Congenital dysfunction of hemoglobin synthesis
	Anemia of chronic disease; abnormally increased demand for new erythrocytes	Chronic infection or inflammation; malignancy

DNA, Deoxyribonucleic acid; *RNA*, ribonucleic acid.

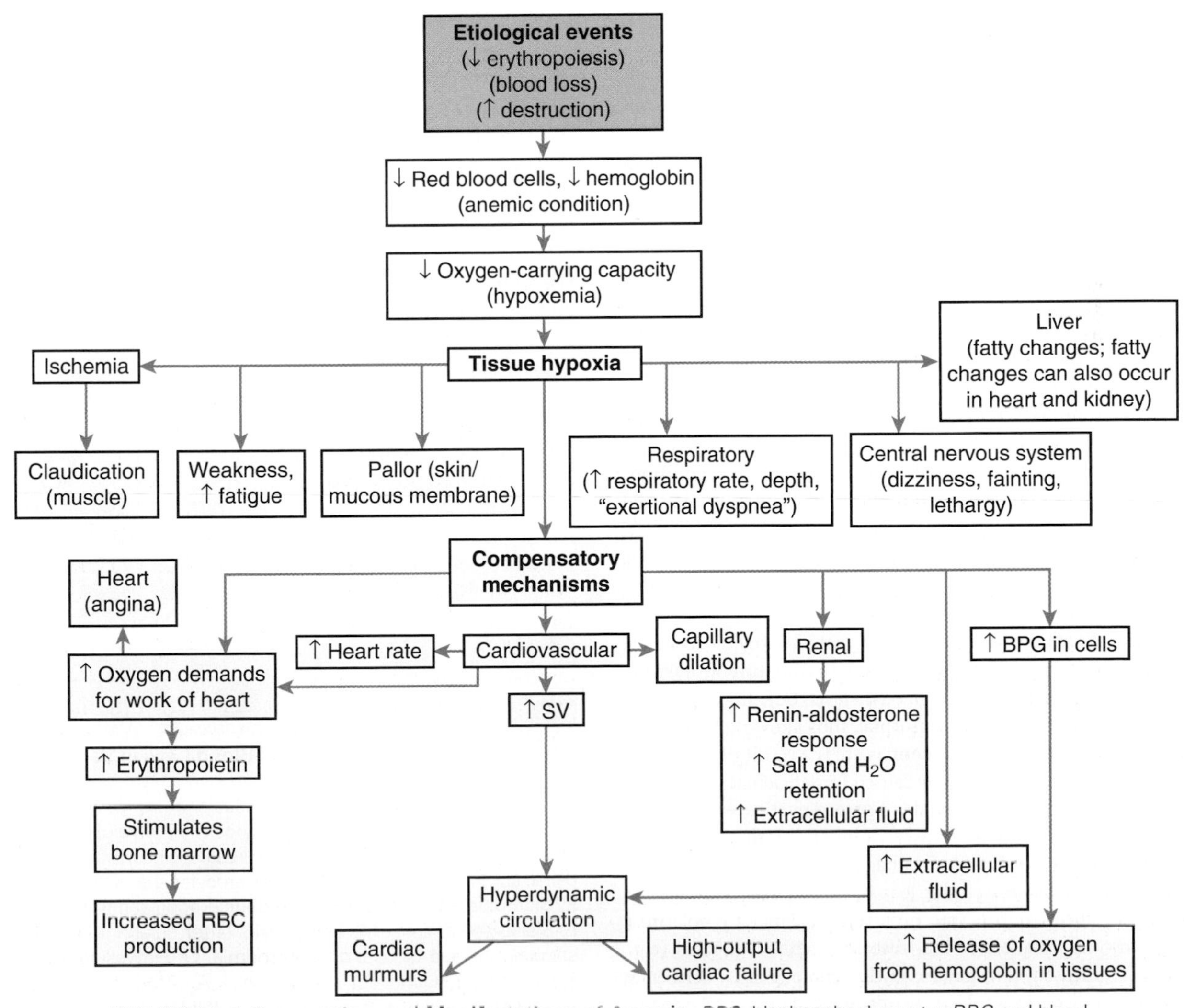

FIGURE 21-1 Progression and Manifestations of Anemia. *BPG*, bisphosphoglycerate; *RBC*, red blood cell; *SV*, stroke volume.

These changes may lead to cardiac dilation and heart valve insufficiency if the underlying anemic condition is not corrected.

Hypoxemia, reduced oxygen level in the blood, further contributes to cardiovascular dysfunction by causing dilation of arterioles, capillaries, and venules, thus increasing flow through them. Increased peripheral blood flow and venous return further contributes to an increase in heart rate and stroke volume in a continuing effort to meet normal oxygen demand and prevent cardiopulmonary congestion. These compensatory mechanisms may lead to heart failure.

Tissue hypoxia creates additional demands and effects on the pulmonary and hematological systems. The rate and depth of breathing increase in an effort to increase oxygen availability accompanied by an increase in the release of oxygen from hemoglobin. All of these compensatory mechanisms may cause individuals to experience shortness of breath (dyspnea), a rapid and pounding heartbeat, dizziness, and fatigue. In mild chronic cases, these symptoms may be present only when there is an increased demand for oxygen (e.g., during physical exertion), but in severe cases, symptoms may be experienced even at rest.

Manifestations of anemia may be seen in other parts of the body. The skin, mucous membranes, lips, nail beds, and conjunctivae become either pale because of reduced hemoglobin concentration or yellowish (jaundiced) because of accumulation of end products of red blood cell destruction (hemolysis) if that is the cause of the anemia. Tissue hypoxia of the skin results in impaired healing and loss of elasticity, as well as thinning and early greying of the hair. Nervous system manifestations may occur where the cause of anemia is a deficiency of vitamin B_{12}. Myelin degeneration occurs, causing a loss of nerve fibres in the spinal cord, resulting in paresthesias (numbness), gait disturbances, extreme weakness, spasticity, and reflex abnormalities. Decreased oxygen supply to the gastro-intestinal (GI) tract often produces abdominal pain, nausea, vomiting, and anorexia. Low-grade fever (less than 38.3°C [100.9°F]) occurs in some anemic individuals and may result from the release of leukocyte pyrogens from ischemic tissues.

When the anemia is severe or acute in onset (e.g., hemorrhage), the initial compensatory mechanism is peripheral blood vessel constriction, diverting blood flow to essential vital organs. Decreased blood flow detected by the kidneys activates the renin-angiotensin response, causing salt and water retention in an attempt to increase blood volume. These situations are considered to be emergencies and require immediate intervention to correct the underlying problem that caused the acute blood loss; therefore, long-term compensatory mechanisms do not develop.

Therapeutic interventions for slowly developing anemic conditions require treatment of the underlying condition and palliation of associated symptoms.[1] Therapies include transfusion, dietary correction, and administration of supplemental vitamins or iron.

Macrocytic-Normochromic Anemias

The macrocytic (megaloblastic) anemias are characterized by unusually large stem cells (megaloblasts) in the marrow that mature into erythrocytes that are unusually large in size (macrocytic), thickness, and volume.[2] The hemoglobin content is normal, thus allowing them to be classified as normochromic. These anemias are the result of ineffective erythrocyte DNA synthesis, commonly caused by deficiencies of vitamin B_{12} (cobalamin) or folate (folic acid). These defective erythrocytes die prematurely, which decreases their numbers in the circulation, causing anemia. Premature death of damaged erythrocytes, eryptosis, is a common mechanism of cellular loss in individuals with anemia secondary to deficiencies of iron, infections (e.g., malaria, mycoplasma), chronic diseases (e.g., diabetes, renal disease), genetic diseases (e.g., beta-thalassemia, glucose-6-phosphate dehydrogenase [G6PD] deficiency, sickle cell trait), and myelodysplastic syndrome.[3]

Defective DNA synthesis in megaloblastic anemias causes red blood cell growth and development to proceed at unequal rates. DNA synthesis and cell division are blocked or delayed. However, RNA replication and protein (hemoglobin) synthesis proceed normally. Asynchronous development leads to an overproduction of hemoglobin during prolonged cellular division, creating a larger than normal erythrocyte with a disproportionately small nucleus. With each cell division, the disproportion between RNA and DNA becomes more apparent.

Pernicious Anemia

Pernicious anemia (PA), the most common type of macrocytic anemia, is caused by vitamin B_{12} deficiency, which is often associated with the end stage of type A chronic atrophic (autoimmune) gastritis (Figure 21-2, *C*).[4] *Pernicious* means highly injurious or destructive and reflects the fact that this condition was once fatal. It most commonly affects individuals older than age 30 who are of Northern European descent;

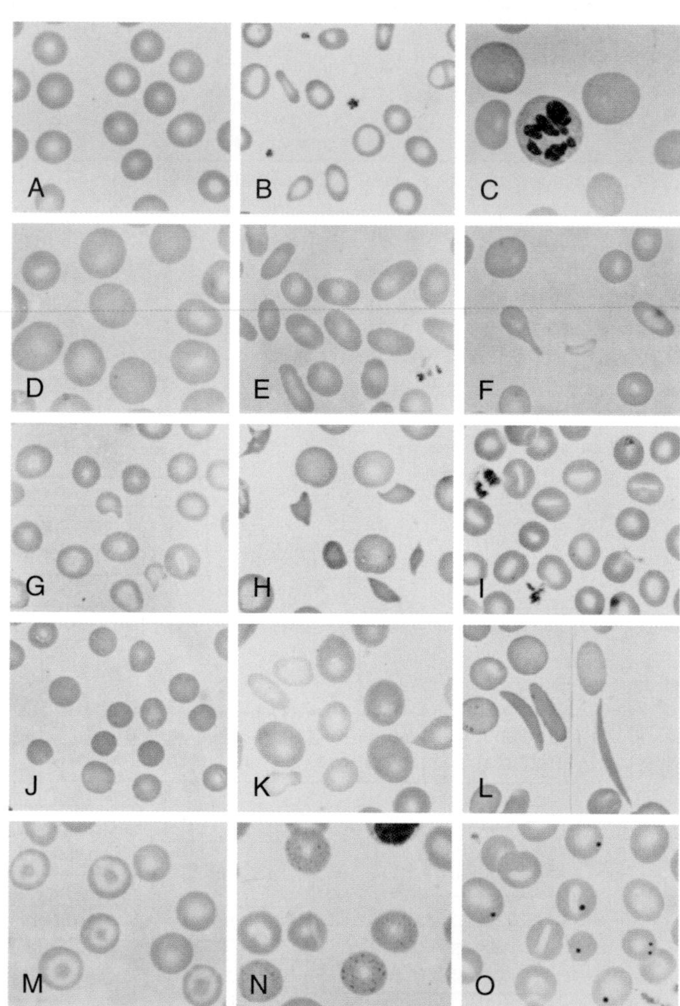

FIGURE 21-2 Appearance of Red Blood Cells in Various Disorders. **A,** Normal blood smear. **B,** Microcytic-hypochromic anemia (iron deficiency). **C,** Macrocytic anemia (pernicious anemia). **D,** Macrocytic anemia in pregnancy. **E,** Hereditary elliptocytosis. **F,** Myelofibrosis (teardrop). **G,** Hemolytic anemia associated with prosthetic heart valve. **H,** Microangiopathic anemia. **I,** Stomatocytes. **J,** Spherocytes (hereditary spherocytosis). **K,** Sideroblastic anemia; note the double population of red blood cells. **L,** Sickle cell anemia. **M,** Target cells (after splenectomy). **N,** Basophil stippling in case of unexplained anemia. **O,** Howell-Jolly bodies (after splenectomy). (John P. Greer, Daniel A. Arber, *Wintrobe's Clinical Hematology,* Wolters Kluwer Health, 2013.)

however, it has now been recognized in all populations and ethnic groups.

PATHOPHYSIOLOGY The underlying alteration in PA is the absence of **intrinsic factor (IF)**, a transporter required for gastric absorption of dietary vitamin B_{12}, a vitamin essential for nuclear maturation and DNA synthesis in red blood cells. Deficiency of IF may be congenital or, more often, an autoimmune process directed against gastric parietal cells. Congenital IF deficiency is a genetic disorder with an autosomal recessive inheritance pattern.[5] The autoimmune form of the disease also has a genetic component. Family clusters have been identified; 20 to 30% of individuals related to persons with PA also have PA. These relatives, particularly first-degree female relatives, also demonstrate a higher frequency of the presence of gastric autoantibodies. PA also is frequently a component of autoimmune polyendocrinopathy, which is a cluster of autoimmune diseases of endocrine organs (e.g., chronic autoimmune thyroiditis [Hashimoto's thyroiditis], type 1 diabetes mellitus, Addison's disease, primary hypoparathyroidism, Graves' disease, and myasthenia gravis) that frequently present as comorbidities. Autoimmune thyroiditis and type 1 diabetes mellitus, in particular, are associated with PA.

Most cases of PA result from an autoimmune gastritis (type A chronic gastritis) in which gastric atrophy results from destruction of parietal and zymogenic (relating to an enzyme) cells. Individuals with PA commonly have autoantibodies against the gastric H^+–K^+ ATPase, which is the major protein constituent of parietal cell membranes. Gastric mucosal atrophy, in which gastric parietal cells are destroyed, results in a deficiency of all secretions of the stomach—hydrochloric acid, pepsin, and IF. A direct correlation exists between the severity of the gastric lesion and the degree of malabsorption of vitamin B_{12}.[6,7] Additionally, autoantibodies against IF prevent the formation of the B_{12}–IF complex. Thus, PA is secondary to autoimmune destruction of parietal cells, diminishing the production of IF and the presence of autoantibodies that neutralize the capacity of remaining IF to transport vitamin B_{12}.

Initiation of the autoimmune process may be secondary to a past infection with *Helicobacter pylori*.[8] Although active infection with *H. pylori* is rare in individuals with PA, more than half of these individuals possess circulating antibodies against this microorganism, suggesting a history of infection. The current opinion is that in genetically prone individuals, antigens expressed by *H. pylori* mimic the parietal cell H^+–K^+ ATPase, resulting in production of an antibody that binds and damages the parietal cell (see Chapter 8 for a discussion of antigenic mimicry and autoimmune disease).

Environmental factors that may contribute to chronic gastritis include excessive alcohol or hot tea ingestion and smoking. Complete or partial removal of the stomach (gastrectomy) causes IF deficiency. Medications known as proton pump inhibitors (PPIs) are used to decrease gastric acidity and may decrease vitamin B_{12} absorption, but it is not thought that they actually cause PA. Although PA is a benign disorder, people with type A chronic gastritis also are at risk of developing gastric adenocarcinoma and gastric carcinoid type I. The incidence rate of carcinoma in these individuals is 2 to 3%.

CLINICAL MANIFESTATIONS PA develops slowly (over 20 to 30 years), so by the time an individual seeks treatment, it is usually severe. Early symptoms are often ignored because they are nonspecific and vague and include infections, mood swings, and GI, cardiac, or kidney ailments. When the hemoglobin level has decreased to 70 to 80 g/L, the individual experiences classic symptoms of PA: weakness, fatigue, paresthesias of feet and fingers, difficulty walking, loss of appetite, abdominal pain, weight loss, and a sore tongue that is smooth and beefy red. The skin may become "lemon yellow" (sallow), caused by a combination of pallor and jaundice. Hepatomegaly, indicating right-sided heart failure, may be present in the older adult along with splenomegaly, which is nonpalpable.

Neurological manifestations result from nerve demyelination that may produce neuronal death. The posterior and lateral columns of the spinal cord also may be affected, causing a loss of position and vibration sense, ataxia, and spasticity. These complications pose a serious threat because they are not reversible, even with appropriate treatment. The cerebrum also may be involved with manifestations of affective disorders, most commonly of the depressive types. Low levels of vitamin B_{12} have been associated with neurocognitive disorders. An increased prevalence of serum vitamin B_{12} deficiency has been reported among individuals with Alzheimer's disease.

EVALUATION AND TREATMENT Evaluation is based on blood tests, bone marrow aspiration, serological studies, gastric biopsy, and clinical manifestations. The Schilling test (no longer offered in most laboratories) indirectly evaluated vitamin B_{12} absorption by administering radioactive B_{12} and measuring excretion in the urine. Low urinary excretion was significant for PA. The Schilling test has been replaced with serological studies that measure methylmalonic acid and homocysteine levels, which are elevated early in PA, and this test is more sensitive. The presence of circulating antibodies against parietal cells and IF also is useful in diagnosis.[9] Autoimmune gastritis is a chronic progressive inflammatory disorder resulting in replacement of the parietal cell mass by atropic and metaplastic mucosa.[7] The interactions are very complex because of autoantibodies against IF that impair the absorption of vitamin B_{12} (cobalamin). The resulting cobalamin deficiency manifests with neurological and systemic symptoms of PA. The complexity increases with the underappreciated overlap with *H. pylori* infection. The risk for gastric cancer has not been adequately studied.[7] Gastric biopsy reveals total achlorhydria (absence of hydrochloric acid), which is diagnostic for PA because it occurs only in the presence of this gastric lesion.

Oral replacement of vitamin B_{12} (cobalamin) is the treatment of choice. Dosing for PA or food-bound cobalamin malabsorption is 1 000 mcg/day for the remainder of the individual's life. Monthly vitamin B_{12} injections are used by individuals whose deficiency is not corrected by the oral administration of the vitamin. The effectiveness of cobalamin replacement therapy is determined by a rising reticulocyte count. Blood counts return to normal within 5 to 6 weeks. PA cannot be cured, so maintenance therapy is lifelong.

Untreated PA is fatal, usually because of heart failure. With replacement therapy of vitamin B_{12}, mortality has decreased significantly. Death from PA is now rare, and relapses are often the result of nonadherence to therapy.

Folate Deficiency Anemias

Folate (folic acid) is an essential vitamin required for RNA and DNA synthesis within the maturing erythrocyte. Folates are coenzymes required for the synthesis of thymine and purines (adenine and guanine) and the conversion of homocysteine to methionine. Deficient production of thymine, in particular, affects cells undergoing rapid division (e.g., bone marrow cells undergoing erythropoiesis). Humans are totally dependent on dietary intake to meet the daily requirement of 50 to 200 mg/day. Increased amounts are required for lactating and pregnant females. Folate is absorbed from the upper small intestine and does not require any other element (i.e., IF) to facilitate absorption. After absorption, folate circulates through the liver, where it is stored. Folate deficiency occurs more often than B_{12} deficiency, particularly in alcoholics and individuals with chronic malnourishment. It is estimated that at least 10% of North Americans are folate deficient, but the incidence has been decreasing in Canada since the fortification of foods with folate and the increased use of folate supplements.

Clinical manifestations are similar to the malnourished appearance of individuals with PA. Specific manifestations include cheilosis (scales and fissures of the mouth), stomatitis (inflammation of the mouth), and painful ulcerations of the buccal mucosa and tongue characteristic of *burning mouth syndrome.* Burning mouth syndrome may be secondary to a large number of disorders (e.g., extremely dry mouth, infection, autoimmune disease, nutritional deficiencies, and other conditions). Dysphagia, flatulence, and watery diarrhea also may be present, as well as histological changes in the GI tract suggestive of sprue (chronic absorption disorder). Undiagnosed inflammatory bowel disease (e.g., Crohn's disease, ulcerative colitis) may be the underlying cause of folate malabsorption in some individuals, and folate deficiency may suppress proliferation of the intestinal mucosa, leading to an increase of GI damage. Neurological manifestations, if present, may be caused by thiamine deficiency, which often accompanies folate deficiency.

Evaluation of folate deficiency is based on blood tests, measurement of serum folate levels, and clinical manifestations. Treatment requires administration of oral folate preparations until adequate blood levels are obtained and manifestations are reduced or eliminated. Long-term therapy is not necessary if the appropriate dietary adjustments are made to maintain adequate intake. After administration of folate, the manifestations of anemia disappear within 1 to 2 weeks.

Microcytic-Hypochromic Anemias

The **microcytic-hypochromic anemias** are characterized by abnormally small erythrocytes that contain abnormally reduced amounts of hemoglobin (Figure 21-2, *B*). Hypochromia occurs even in cells of normal size. Microcytic-hypochromic anemias can result from (1) disorders of iron metabolism, (2) disorders of porphyrin and heme synthesis, or (3) disorders of globin synthesis. Specific conditions include iron deficiency anemia, sideroblastic anemia, and thalassemia.

Iron Deficiency Anemia

Iron deficiency anemia (IDA) is the most common type of anemia worldwide, occurring in both developing and developed countries.[2,10] Certain populations are at high risk of developing hypoferremia and IDA and include individuals living in poverty, women of childbearing age, and children. Iron deficiency in children is associated with numerous adverse health-related manifestations, especially cognitive impairment, which may be irreversible (see *Health Promotion:* Prevention of Iron Deficiency Anemia in Infants and Children in Chapter 22). Children in developing countries often are affected by chronic parasite infestations that result in blood and iron loss greater than dietary intake.[11] Treatment of helminth infections results in improvement in appetite, growth, and in the anemia. IDA also occurs in individuals with lead poisoning, and treatment is associated with a decrease in lead levels. An increased prevalence of iron deficiency has been observed in overweight children.

Females in Canada have a higher incidence than males for both hypoferremia and IDA, with the peak incidence occurring in the reproductive years and decreasing at menopause. Males have a higher incidence during childhood.

PATHOPHYSIOLOGY IDA can arise from one of two different etiologies or a combination of both inadequate dietary intake of iron or chronic blood loss. In both instances there is no intrinsic dysfunction in iron metabolism; however, both etiologies deplete iron stores and reduce hemoglobin synthesis. A second category is a metabolic or functional iron deficiency in which various metabolic disorders lead to either insufficient iron delivery to bone marrow or impaired iron use (or absorption) within the marrow. Paradoxically, iron stores may be sufficient but delivery is inadequate to maintain heme synthesis, thus producing a functional or relative iron deficiency.

In developed countries, pregnancy and a continuous loss of blood are the most common causes of IDA. A blood loss of 2 to 4 mL/day (1 to 2 mg of iron) is enough to cause IDA. Menorrhagia (excessive menstrual bleeding) causes primary IDA in females. Males may experience bleeding as a result of ulcers, hiatal hernia, esophageal varices, cirrhosis, hemorrhoids, ulcerative colitis, or cancer. Other causes of blood loss for both genders include the following: (1) use of medications that cause GI bleeding (such as Aspirin or nonsteroidal anti-inflammatory drugs [NSAIDs]); (2) surgical procedures that decrease stomach acidity, intestinal transit time, and absorption (e.g., gastric bypass); (3) insufficient dietary intake of iron; and (4) eating disorders such as pica—the craving and eating of non-nutritional substances, such as dirt, chalk, and paper. *H. pylori* infections also have been found to cause IDA of unknown origin, although *H. pylori* impairs iron uptake.

Iron in the form of hemoglobin is in constant demand by the body. An important attribute of iron is that it can be recycled; therefore, the body maintains a balance between iron that is in use as hemoglobin and iron that is stored and available for future hemoglobin synthesis (see Figure 21-2, *B*). Blood loss disrupts this balance by creating a need for more iron, thus depleting the iron stores more rapidly to replace the iron lost from bleeding. Iron contributes to immune function by regulating immune effector mechanisms (such as cytokine activities). The precise benefits or detriments of iron deficiency and immunity are controversial.

IDA develops slowly through three overlapping stages. In stage I, the body's iron stores for red blood cell production and hemoglobin synthesis are depleted. Red blood cell production proceeds normally with the hemoglobin content of red blood cells also remaining normal. In stage II, insufficient amounts of iron are transported to the marrow, and iron-deficient red blood cell production begins. Stage III begins when the hemoglobin-deficient red blood cells enter the circulation to replace normal, aged erythrocytes that have been destroyed. The manifestations of IDA appear in stage III when there is an insufficient iron supply and diminished hemoglobin synthesis.

CLINICAL MANIFESTATIONS The onset of symptoms is gradual, and individuals usually do not seek medical attention until hemoglobin levels drop to 70 or 80 g/L. Early symptoms are nonspecific and include fatigue, weakness, shortness of breath, and pale earlobes, palms, and conjunctivae (Figure 21-3).

As the condition progresses and becomes more severe, structural and functional changes occur in epithelial tissue. The fingernails become

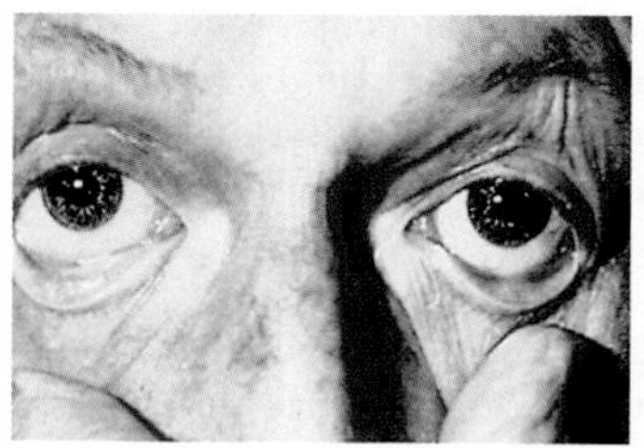

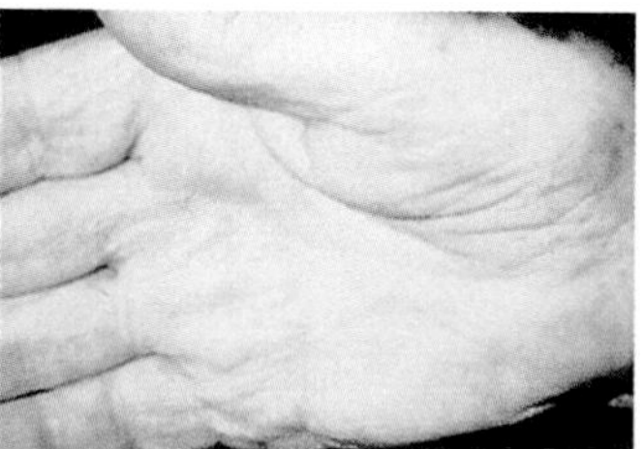

FIGURE 21-3 Pallor and Iron Deficiency. Pallor of the skin, mucous membranes, and palmar creases in an individual with a hemoglobin level of 90 g/L. Palmar creases become as pale as the surrounding skin when the hemoglobin level approaches 70 g/L. (From Hoffbrand, A.V., Pettit, J.E., & Vyas, P. [2009]. *Color atlas of clinical hematology* [4th ed.]. London: Mosby.)

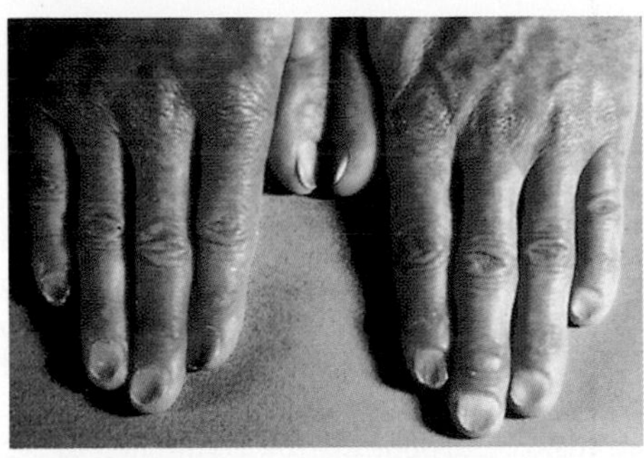

FIGURE 21-4 Koilonychia. The nails are concave, ridged, and brittle. (Courtesy Dr. S.M. Knowles. From Hoffbrand, A.V., Pettit, J.E., & Vyas, P. [2009]. *Color atlas of clinical hematology* [4th ed.]. London: Mosby.)

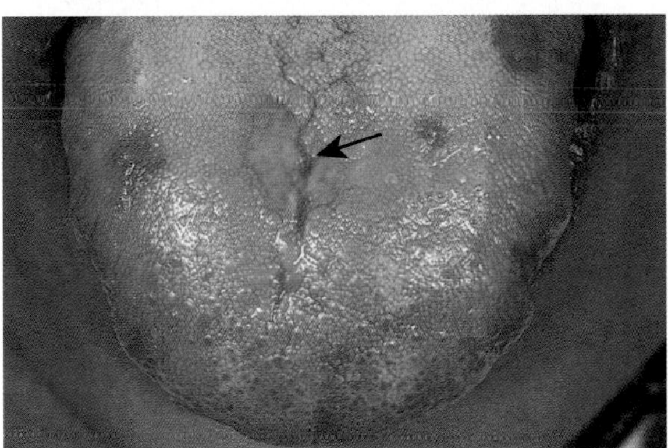

FIGURE 21-5 Glossitis. Tongue of individual with iron deficiency anemia has bald, fissured appearance (*arrow*) caused by loss of papillae and flattening. (From Hoffbrand, A.V., Pettit, J.E., & Vyas, P. [2009]. *Color atlas of clinical hematology* [4th ed.]. London: Mosby.)

brittle and "spoon shaped" or concave (koilonychia) (Figure 21-4). Tongue papillae atrophy can cause soreness along with redness and burning (Figure 21-5). These changes can be reversed within 1 to 2 weeks of iron replacement therapy. The corners of the mouth become dry and sore (angular stomatitis), and an individual may experience difficulty with swallowing because of a "web" that develops from mucus and inflammatory cells at the opening of the esophagus. These lesions have the potential to become cancerous.

Nonheme iron is a component of many enzymes in the body, and lack of iron may alter other physiological processes and contribute to the clinical manifestations. Individuals with IDA exhibit gastritis, neuromuscular changes, irritability, headache, numbness, tingling, and vasomotor disturbances. Gait disturbances are rare. In older adults, mental confusion, memory loss, and disorientation may be wrongly perceived as "normal" events associated with aging.

EVALUATION AND TREATMENT Evaluation is based on clinical manifestations and laboratory tests. Iron stores are measured directly, by bone marrow biopsy, or indirectly, by tests that measure serum ferritin level, transferrin saturation, or total iron-binding capacity. A sensitive indicator of heme synthesis is the amount of free erythrocyte protoporphyrin (FEP) within erythrocytes. A test that determines the concentration of soluble fragment transferrin receptor differentiates primary IDA from IDA that is associated with chronic disease.

The first step in treatment of IDA is to find and eliminate, or rule out, sources of blood loss. If this is not done, replacement therapy is ineffective. Iron replacement therapy is required and very effective. Initial doses are 150 to 200 mg/day and are continued until the serum ferritin level reaches 50 mcg/L, indicating that adequate replacement has occurred. A rapid decrease in fatigue, lethargy, and other associated symptoms is generally seen within the first month of therapy. Replacement therapy usually continues for 6 to 12 months after the bleeding has stopped but may continue for as long as 24 months. Menstruating females may need daily oral iron replacement therapy (325 mg/day) until menopause.

Sideroblastic Anemia

Sideroblastic anemia (SA) comprises a heterogeneous group of inherited and acquired disorders characterized by anemia of varying severity and the presence of ringed sideroblasts in the bone marrow (Figure 21-2, *K*). Ringed sideroblasts are erythroblasts that contain iron-laden mitochondria arranged in a circle around one-third or more of the nucleus. More simply, these are red blood cells that contain iron granules that have not been synthesized into hemoglobin but instead are arranged in a circle around the nucleus. Individuals with SA also have increased tissue levels of iron.

PATHOPHYSIOLOGY SAs have various causes, but all share the commonality of altered heme synthesis in the erythroid cells in bone marrow. Acquired sideroblastic anemias (ASAs), which are the most common, occur as a primary disorder with no known cause (idiopathic) or are associated with other myeloproliferative or myeloplastic disorders such as myeloma, polycythemia vera, and leukemias. Another form, referred to as reversible sideroblastic anemias (reversible SAs), is secondary to various conditions such as alcoholism, medication reactions, copper deficiency, and hypothermia. Reversible SA associated with alcoholism results from nutritional deficiencies of folate. Some medications also cause reversible SA and include antituberculous agents (isoniazid [isonicotinylhydrazide or INH], pyrazinamide [Tebrazid], cycloserine [Seromycin], and chloramphenicol [Pentamycetin]) that interfere with B_{12} metabolism or directly injure the mitochondria. Copper deficiency also causes reversible SA by interfering with conversion of ferric iron to ferrous iron. This occurrence is extremely rare and is associated with gastrectomy and prolonged parenteral nutrition without copper supplements. Hypothermia causes decreased heme synthesis and incorporation into hemoglobin.

Hereditary (congenital) sideroblastic anemias are rare and occur almost exclusively in males, supporting a recessive X-linked transmission; however, autosomal transmission affecting females has been reported. Other genetic, chromosomal, or enzyme dysfunctions also have been associated with hereditary SA, for example, mutations in *TRNT1* (transfer RNA nucleotidyl transferase 1) that lead to metabolic defects in both mitochondria and cytosol.[12] In all instances, SA anemia is present in infancy or childhood but may remain undetected until mid-life when other conditions, such as diabetes or cardiac failure from iron overload, cause its manifestation.

The leading known cause of primary ASA, myelodysplastic syndrome (MDS), is a group of disorders of hematopoietic stem cells with all three stem cell lines (erythrocytic, granulocytic, and megakaryocytic) demonstrating abnormal growth or cell characteristics.[13] Pure SA, or cellular features limited to the erythrocytic line, requires blood transfusions that may, over time, produce iron overload. With adequate chelation therapy, individuals are able to survive and thrive for many years. MDS, characterized by abnormalities of multiple cell lineages, may include alterations of neutrophils and platelets. Bleeding from thrombocytopenia and platelet dysfunction is prevalent. Of those who survive, 40% develop acute (myeloblastic) leukemia.

CLINICAL MANIFESTATIONS The anemias of SA are generally moderate to severe, with hemoglobin levels varying from 40 to 100 g/L. In addition to the cardiovascular and respiratory manifestations common to all anemias, individuals with SA may show signs of iron overload (hemochromatosis) and mild to moderate enlargement of the liver (hepatomegaly) and spleen (splenomegaly). However, liver function remains normal or only mildly affected. Occasionally, the skin may become abnormally coloured (bronze-tinted). Neurological and skin alterations associated with other anemias are absent. Hemosiderosis of cardiac tissue may result in heart rhythm disturbances, which is a significant but uncommon complication and generally occurs late in the course of the disease. Growth and development impairment may occur in infants and young children who are severely affected.

EVALUATION AND TREATMENT Initially, SA may be mistaken for deficiency of stem cells in the marrow (hypoplastic anemia) or IDA. The diagnosis of SA is established by bone marrow biopsy, which documents the presence of sideroblasts and confirms the diagnosis. The severity of the anemia is quite variable.

Initial treatment of SA is directed toward identification of a causative agent (i.e., medications or toxins).[14] Treatment is supportive, with transfusions being the primary intervention. Following removal of the agent, oral pyridoxine (100 mg/day) may be administered on a trial basis. Acquired SA related to alcohol abuse and pyridoxine antagonists often demonstrates a complete response to pyridoxine. SA caused by other etiologies does not demonstrate the same improvement.

Individuals with hereditary SA are initially treated with pyridoxine therapy (50 to 200 mg/day), which is effective in approximately one-third of individuals. An optimal response is reticulocytosis with blood hemoglobin levels and low FEP levels also returning to normal within 1 to 2 months. Structural abnormalities of cells (microcytosis), however, do not disappear. Hemoglobin levels also may increase in response to therapy but stabilize at less than normal levels. A therapeutic response to pyridoxine may be maintained with lifelong administration of a reduced dosage. Nonresponse to pyridoxine requires blood transfusions for symptom relief and to promote growth and development.

Evidence of iron overload requires iron depletion therapy to prevent or minimize organ damage. Phlebotomy, or removal of blood from the circulation, is used in individuals with mild to moderate anemia without other complications (e.g., heart disease). After iron removal, maintenance phlebotomies are continued. Severely anemic individuals who may require transfusions become extremely iron overloaded, which mandates use of deferoxamine, an iron-chelating agent, to reduce excess iron levels.

Individuals with acquired SA are less likely to respond to pyridoxine, but SA rarely incapacitates them. When SA is secondary to an identifiable cause, treatment or removal of the cause is essential. In the absence of blood cell abnormalities and iron overload, progression takes place over years. Transfusion and chelation therapy is the same as for hereditary SA when indicated.

Recent advances in treatment for SAs include prolonged administration of erythropoietin and stem cell transplant. Treatment with recombinant human erythropoietin improves anemia in 30% of those with myelodysplastic syndrome.[15] Individuals with the subset of MDS identified as refractory anemia have the overall best response rate. Congenital SA has been treated successfully with stem cell transplants; however, this treatment is in the early stages of use and long-term efficacy has not yet been established. Death from SA is rare and often secondary to complications, such as infection, bone marrow failure, liver failure, or cardiac failure or arrhythmias, or both.

Thalassemia

Thalassemias are inherited blood disorders characterized by abnormal hemoglobin production. The two main types of thalassemia are α-thalassemia and β-thalassemia. See Chapter 22 for detailed information regarding this disorder.

Normocytic-Normochromic Anemias

Normocytic-normochromic anemias (NNAs) are characterized by erythrocytes that are relatively normal in size and hemoglobin content but insufficient in number.[16] These types of anemia do not share any common etiology, pathological mechanism, or morphological characteristics. They are less common than the macrocytic-normochromic and the microcytic-hypochromic anemias. The four distinct anemias are (1) aplastic (damage to bone marrow erythropoiesis); (2) posthemorrhagic (acute blood loss); (3) hemolytic, which includes acquired (immune destruction of erythrocytes), heredity (e.g., sickle cell, see Figure 21-2, *L*), and hemolysis (destruction by eryptosis); and (4) anemia of chronic inflammation (multiple causes, e.g., chronic kidney disease). The diversity of the NNAs is summarized in Table 21-2. (Sickle cell anemia is discussed in Chapter 22.)

✔ QUICK CHECK 21-1

1. How do cell size and content determine classification of anemia?
2. Why is iron important to hemoglobin synthesis, and why is iron deficiency related to anemia?
3. Discuss the pathophysiology of iron deficiency anemia.
4. How is anemia diagnosed?

MYELOPROLIFERATIVE RED BLOOD CELL DISORDERS

Hematological dysfunction results from an overproduction of cells, as well as a deficiency. One or more hematopoietic lines may be overproduced in the marrow in response to exogenous (e.g., exposure to radiation, medications) or endogenous (e.g., physiological compensatory response, immune disorder) signals. Excessive red blood cell production is classified as polycythemia (Table 21-3). The two types of polycythemia are relative polycythemia and absolute polycythemia.

Relative polycythemia results from hemoconcentration of the blood associated with dehydration that may be caused by decreased water intake, diarrhea, excessive vomiting, or increased use of diuretics. Its development is usually of minor consequence and resolves with fluid administration or treatment of underlying conditions.

Absolute polycythemia consists of two forms: primary and secondary. *Secondary polycythemia*, the most common of the two, is a physiological response resulting from erythropoietin secretion caused by hypoxia. This hypoxia is noted in individuals living at higher altitudes (greater than 3 000 m), smokers with increased blood levels of carbon monoxide, and individuals with chronic obstructive pulmonary disease or heart failure, or both. Abnormal types of hemoglobin (e.g., San Diego, Chesapeake), which have a greater affinity for oxygen, also cause secondary polycythemia, as does inappropriate secretion of erythropoietin by certain tumours (e.g., renal cell carcinoma, hepatoma, and cerebellar hemangioblastomas).

Polycythemia Vera

Polycythemia vera (PV) (also known as primary polycythemia) is a stem cell disorder with hyperplastic and neoplastic bone marrow alterations. PV is characterized by an abnormal uncontrolled proliferation of red blood cells (frequently with increased levels of white blood cells [leukocytosis] and platelets [thrombocytosis]). The increase in red blood cells (polycythemia) is responsible for most of the clinical symptoms, including an increase in blood volume and viscosity. PV is one of several

TABLE 21-2 Normocytic-Normochromic Anemias

Anemia	Pathophysiology	Clinical Manifestations	Evaluation and Treatment
Aplastic	Rare; may result from infiltrative disorders of bone marrow, autoimmune diseases, renal failure, splenic dysfunction, vitamin B_{12} or folate deficiency, parvovirus infection, or exposure to radiation, medications, and toxins; also may be congenital Common stem cell population may be altered so it cannot proliferate or differentiate, or stem cell environment is altered to inhibit erythropoiesis Outcome ranges from death to minimal manifestations	Classic cardiovascular and respiratory manifestations with thrombocytopenia, hemorrhage into tissues, leukopenia, and infection	Bone marrow biopsy determines whether anemia is caused by pure RBC aplasia or hypoplasia Treatment of underlying disorder or prevent further exposure to causative agent Blood transfusions, marrow transplant, and pharmacological stimulation of bone marrow function
Posthemorrhagic	Cause is sudden blood loss with normal iron stores	Often obscured by cardiovascular manifestations of acute hemorrhage Severe shock, lactic acidosis, and death can occur if blood loss exceeds 40–50% of plasma volume	Restoration of blood volume by intravenous administration of saline, dextran, albumin, or plasma Transfusion of whole blood also required occasionally
Hemolytic	Acquired: caused by infection, systemic disease, medications or toxins, liver disease, kidney disease, abnormal immune responses Hereditary: caused by abnormalities of RBC membrane or cytoplasmic contents; present at birth Hemolysis: in blood vessels or lymphoid tissues that filter blood (e.g., spleen, liver) Erythrocytes: rigid, slowing their passage and making them vulnerable to phagocytosis Types: warm antibody disease (mediated by IgG antibody specific for erythrocyte antigens), cold antibody disease (mediated by IgM), and medication-induced	Splenomegaly, jaundice, aplastic hemolytic, or megaloblastic crises can develop with viral infection With severe disease, bones become deformed and pathological fractures occur Cardiovascular and respiratory manifestations correspond with severity of anemia	Blood and bone marrow studies Erythroid hyperplasia is found in marrow and blood smears Treatment of acquired disease involves removing cause or treating underlying disorder Other forms of treatment are transfusions, splenectomy, and steroids or folate
Anemia of chronic inflammation	Associated with chronic infections (e.g., AIDS), chronic inflammatory diseases (e.g., rheumatoid arthritis, SLE), and malignancies Causes are decreased erythrocyte lifespan, failure of mechanisms of compensatory erythropoiesis, or disturbance of iron cycle	Manifestations fewer and milder than most other anemias General disability caused by chronic disease limits physical activity so hemoglobin levels adequate; if they drop, signs of iron deficiency anemia develop	Blood tests show iron deficiency in marrow despite normal or increased iron stores elsewhere No treatment is needed unless anemia becomes symptomatic Erythropoietin may be used

AIDS, acquired immunodeficiency syndrome; *IgG*, immunoglobulin G; *IgM*, immunoglobulin M; *RBC*, red blood cell; *SLE*, systemic lupus erythematosus.

disorders collectively known as *myeloproliferative neoplasms* (MPNs). These disorders include certain leukemias, essential thrombocytosis, and chronic bone marrow fibrosis. The disorders all result from abnormal regulation of the hematopoietic stem cells. Specifically, the common pathogenic feature is the presence of a mutation in the Janus kinase 2 gene (*JAK2* gene) resulting in an overproduction of blood cells. Normally, the *JAK2* gene makes a protein that helps the body produce blood cells (see "Pathophysiology"). Because of numerous characteristics (e.g., overproduction of different blood cells, marrow hypercellularity, or fibrosis) shared by these disorders and a lack of specific molecular markers, the diagnosis can be quite challenging. The common features include (1) increased proliferative drive in the bone marrow, (2) hematopoiesis of neoplastic stem cells to secondary hematopoietic organs, (3) marrow fibrosis and peripheral deficiencies in blood cells (cytopenias), and (4) variable transformation to acute leukemia.

PV is quite rare, with an estimated incidence of 2.3 per 100 000 individuals; peak incidence is between the ages of 60 and 80 years, with a median incidence of 55 to 60. However, PV has been observed in individuals younger than the age of 40. Males are twice as likely as females to develop PV. It is more common in Whites of Eastern European Jewish ancestry. PV is rarely seen in children or in multiple members of a single family; however, an autosomal dominant form exists that causes increased secretion of erythropoietin.

PATHOPHYSIOLOGY Erythrocytosis is the essential component of PV. Proliferation of erythroid progenitors occurs in the bone marrow independent of the hormone erythropoietin, but the cells express a normal erythropoietin receptor. More than 95% of individuals with PV have an acquired mutation in the tyrosine kinase, Janus kinase 2 (JAK2).[17] Normal JAK2 increases the activity of the erythropoietin receptor and is self-regulatory so that JAK2 activity diminishes over time. The mutation associated with PV negates the self-regulatory activity of JAK2 so that the erythropoietin receptor is constantly active, regardless of the level of erythropoietin. Overall, the mutated tyrosine kinases

TABLE 21-3 Disorders Classified as Polycythemia

Type of Polycythemia	Mechanism of Increased Erythropoiesis	Cause of Associated Disorder
Primary polycythemia (polycythemia vera)	Excessive proliferation of erythroid precursors in marrow; *JAK2* mutation, increased sensitivity of stem cell to erythropoietin	Possible mutation in erythropoietin receptor
Secondary polycythemia	Physiological increase in erythropoietin secretion by kidneys in response to underlying systemic disorder	Tissue hypoxia caused by cardiopulmonary disorders (chronic obstructive pulmonary disease, heart failure), decreased barometric pressure, cardiovascular malformations causing mixing of arterial and venous blood, methemoglobinemia, carboxyhemoglobinemia, smoking, obesity
	"Nonphysiological"[a] increase in erythropoietin secretion	Renal disorders, cerebellar hemangioblastomas, hepatoma (liver tumour), ovarian carcinoma, uterine leiomyoma, pheochromocytoma, adrenocortical hypersecretion
Familial polycythemia	Genetically induced increase in erythroid precursors of marrow	Genetic defect
	Abnormal Hb with increased oxygen affinity	
	Decreased 2,3-DPG	
	Increased sensitivity of stem cells to erythropoietin	
	Increased erythropoietin secretion	

[a]*Nonphysiological* means that there is no obvious physiological explanation for hypersecretion of erythropoietin.
2,3-DPG, 2,3-Diphosphoglycerate; *Hb*, hemoglobin; *JAK2*, Janus kinase 2 gene.

bypass normal controls, causing growth factor–independent proliferation and survival of marrow progenitors or precursor cells. The cause of the mutation is unknown.

CLINICAL MANIFESTATIONS PV is uncommon and occurs insidiously. Clinical manifestations of PV are a result of the increased red blood cell mass and hematocrit. Usually there is an increase in blood volume. Together all of these factors cause abnormal blood flow that increases blood viscosity, creating a hypercoagulable state that results in clogging and occlusion of blood vessels. Tissue injury (ischemia) and death (infarction) are the outcome of blood vessel blockage. These outcomes are directly correlated with hematocrit levels. Increases in numbers of thrombocytes, as well as production of dysfunctional platelets, also contribute to this hypercoagulable condition.

Circulatory alterations caused by the thick, sticky blood give rise to other manifestations, such as plethora (ruddy, red colour of the face, hands, feet, ears, and mucous membranes) and engorgement of retinal and cerebral veins. Other symptoms may include headache, drowsiness, delirium, mania, psychotic depression, chorea, and visual disturbances. Individuals frequently have an enlarged spleen with abdominal pain and discomfort. Death from cerebral thrombosis is approximately five times greater in individuals with PV.[18,19]

Cardiovascular function, despite the vascular alterations, remains relatively normal. Cardiac workload and output remain constant; however, increased blood volume does increase blood pressure. Blood flow may be affected, precipitating angina, although cardiovascular infarctions are uncommon. Other cardiovascular manifestations include Raynaud phenomenon and thromboangiitis obliterans.

A unique feature of PV, and helpful in diagnosis, is the development of intense, painful itching that appears to be intensified by heat or exposure to water (aquagenic pruritus) so that individuals avoid exposure to water, particularly warm water when bathing or showering. The intensity of itching is related to the concentration of mast cells in the skin and is generally not responsive to antihistamines or topical lotions.

EVALUATION AND TREATMENT PV is frequently suspected because of clinical features, such as a thrombotic event, splenomegaly, or aquagenic pruritus. Blood and laboratory findings, characterized by an absolute increase in red blood cells and in total blood volume, confirm the diagnosis. Hematocrit levels increasing by one-third of normal levels, and a corresponding increase in hemoglobin and red blood cells, are used for diagnostic purposes. Erythrocytes appear normal, but anisocytosis may be present. There also may be moderate increases in white blood cells and platelets. A bone marrow examination may be done but is not very valuable unless performed in association with cytogenetic and molecular studies for relevant mutations in *JAK2*.[20] The presence of a *JAK2* mutation confirms the diagnosis.[21] Treatment of PV consists of reducing red blood cell proliferation and blood volume, controlling symptoms, and preventing clogging and clotting of the blood vessels. In low-risk individuals (e.g., those younger than age 60 or with no history of thrombosis and without risk factors for cardiovascular disease), the recommended therapy is phlebotomy (300 to 500 mL at a time to reduce erythrocytosis and blood volume) and low-dose Aspirin. Frequent phlebotomies also reduce iron levels, a condition that impedes erythropoiesis.

Hydroxyurea (Droxia), a nonalkylating myelosuppressive, is the medication of choice for myelosuppression because of a reduced incidence to cause leukemia and thrombosis. Radioactive phosphorus (^{32}P) also is used as an effective and easily tolerated intervention to suppress erythropoiesis. Its effects may last up to 18 months. Side effects of ^{32}P include suppression of hematopoiesis resulting in anemia, leukopenia, and thrombocytopenia. Acute leukemia is also a side effect, although most often it occurs only after 7 or more years of treatment, making its use in older adults more common. Interferon-alpha has been used when other forms of treatment have failed.

Survival for 10 to 15 years is common. However, without proper treatment, 50% of individuals with PV die within 18 months of the onset of initial symptoms because of thrombosis or hemorrhage. A significant potential outcome of PV is the conversion to acute myeloid (or myelogenous) leukemia (AML), occurring spontaneously in 10% of individuals and generally being resistant to conventional therapy. Conversion to AML is most likely related to treatment methods associated with cytotoxic myelosuppressive agents. Although PV is a chronic disorder, appropriate therapy results in remissions and prevention of significant pathological outcomes.

Iron Overload

Iron overload can be primary, as in hereditary hemochromatosis, or secondary. The secondary causes of iron overload include anemias with inefficient erythropoiesis (e.g., SA, aplastic anemia), dietary iron overload, or conditions that require repeated blood transfusions or iron dextran injections. Iron absorption is regulated by erythropoietin, tissue oxygenation, and iron stores (see Chapter 20).

Hereditary Hemochromatosis

Hemochromatosis is caused by excessive iron absorption. Hereditary hemochromatosis (HH) is a common inherited, autosomal recessive disorder of iron metabolism[22] and is characterized by increased GI iron absorption with subsequent tissue iron deposition. Excess iron is deposited first in the liver and pancreas, followed by the heart, joints, and endocrine glands. Excess iron causes tissue damage that can lead to diseases such as cirrhosis, diabetes, heart failure, arthropathies, and impotence. HH affects more males than females.

HH is caused by two genetic base pair alterations, C282Y and H63D. These are mutations in the *HFE* gene on chromosome 6. Homozygosity of C282Y is the most common genotype and accounts for 82 to 90% of HH cases. The remaining cases appear to be caused by environmental factors or other genotypes. *HFE* mutations are common in Canada, affecting an estimated 1 in 300 Canadians, primarily of Northern European descent.[23] A US study found that C282Y homozygosity is much lower among Latin Americans (0.27 in 1 000), Asian Americans (less than 0.001 per 1 000), Pacific Islanders (0.12 per 1 000), and Black persons (0.14 per 1 000).[24]

PATHOPHYSIOLOGY In HH, regulation of intestinal absorption of dietary iron is abnormal, causing iron accumulation. The *HFE* gene governs intestinal absorption of dietary iron by regulating the liver-derived protein hepcidin. Hepcidin lowers plasma iron level, and a deficiency in hepcidin, caused by genetic mutations, causes iron overload. The gene mutations in HH reduce hepcidin synthesis, thus reducing the level of circulating plasma hepcidin. The decreased hepcidin-ferroportin (iron transporter) interaction eventually leads to more iron outward flow (efflux) from cells in the small intestinal mucosa, causing a rise in iron concentration and a systemic overload. The iron overload leads to excess iron tissue deposits that can eventually result in liver fibrosis, cirrhosis, hepatocellular carcinoma, diabetes, hypothyroidism, arthritis, cardiomyopathies, and skin hyperpigmentation.

With HH there appears to be a long latent period with individual variation in biochemical expression modified by environmental factors, such as blood loss from menstruation or donation, alcohol intake, and diet. Cirrhosis is a late-stage development of HH that can shorten life expectancy. Cirrhosis also is a risk factor for hepatocellular carcinoma that occurs between 40 and 60 years of age. Cirrhosis prevention is a major goal of HH screening and treatment.

CLINICAL MANIFESTATIONS Clinical manifestations of HH include symptoms such as fatigue, malaise, abdominal pain, arthralgias, and impotence; and clinical findings of hepatomegaly, abnormal liver enzymes, bronzed skin, diabetes, and cardiomegaly. Many individuals are diagnosed as a result of serum iron studies as part of a health screening panel. Most affected individuals (greater than 75%) are asymptomatic and have a low frequency (less than 25%) of cirrhosis, diabetes, or skin pigmentation.

EVALUATION AND TREATMENT Laboratory findings in individuals with HH show elevations in serum iron levels, transferrin saturation, and ferritin levels. Documentation of iron overload relies on quantitative phlebotomy with calculation of the amount of iron removed or liver biopsy with determination of quantitative hepatic iron. With the advent of genetic testing, for individuals who are C282Y homozygous or compound heterozygous, less than 40 years old, and have normal liver functions, no further workup is necessary.

Treatment of HH is simple and consists of phlebotomy of 550 mL of whole blood, which is equivalent to 200 to 250 mg of iron. Frequency of phlebotomy depends on ferritin levels and should continue until the ferritin level is between 20 and 50 mcg/L. Initially, phlebotomy may be needed weekly but once therapeutic ferritin levels are reached, phlebotomy may only be needed every 2 to 3 months. Blood banks now accept blood donations from persons with documented HH. Iron-chelating agents are sometimes used in addition to phlebotomy, but this is not the mainstay of treatment. Individuals with HH should be instructed to refrain from taking iron and vitamin C supplements and consuming raw shellfish; in addition, alcohol should be used in moderation. Family screening is recommended and necessary for all first-degree relatives of a person with HH.

ALTERATIONS OF LEUKOCYTE FUNCTION

Leukocyte function is affected if too many or too few white blood cells are present in the blood or if the cells that are present are structurally or functionally defective. Phagocytic cells (granulocytes, monocytes, macrophages) may lose their ability to act as effective phagocytes, and the lymphocytes may lose their ability to respond to antigens. (Disruptions of inflammatory and immune processes caused by leukocyte disorders are described in Chapter 6.) Other leukocyte alterations include infectious mononucleosis (IM) and cancers of the blood—leukemia and multiple myeloma (MM).

Quantitative Alterations of Leukocytes

Quantitative alterations are increases or decreases in numbers and functions of leukocytes in the blood. Leukocytosis is present when the count is higher than normal; leukopenia is present when the count is lower than normal. Leukocytosis and leukopenia may affect a specific type of white blood cell and may result from a variety of physiological conditions and alterations.

Leukocytosis occurs as a normal protective response to physiological stressors, such as invading microorganisms, strenuous exercise, emotional changes, temperature changes, anaesthesia, surgery, pregnancy, and some medications, hormones, and toxins. It also is caused by pathological conditions, such as malignancies and hematological disorders. Unlike leukocytosis, leukopenia is never normal and is defined as an absolute blood cell count less than 4×10^9/L. Leukopenia is associated with a decrease in neutrophils, which increases risk for infection. When the neutrophil count falls below 1×10^9/L, the risk for infection increases drastically. With counts below 0.5×10^9/L, the possibility for life-threatening infections is high. Leukopenia may be caused by radiation, anaphylactic shock, autoimmune disease (e.g., systemic lupus erythematosus), immune deficiencies (see Chapter 8), and certain chemotherapeutic agents.

Granulocyte and Monocyte Alterations

Increased numbers of circulating granulocytes (neutrophils, eosinophils, basophils) and monocytes are chiefly a physiological response to infection. Increased numbers also occur as a result of myeloproliferative disorders that increase stem cell proliferation in the bone marrow.[25]

Decreased numbers occur when infectious processes deplete the supply of circulating granulocytes and monocytes, drawing them out of the circulation and into infected tissues faster than they can be replaced. Decreases also can be caused by disorders that suppress marrow function, such as severe congenital neutropenia, or immune-related neutropenia.[26]

Granulocytosis—an increase in granulocytes (neutrophils, eosinophils, or basophils)—begins when stored blood cells are released. **Neutrophilia** is another term that may be used to describe *granulocytosis* because neutrophils are the most numerous of the granulocytes (Table 21-4). Neutrophilia is seen in the early stages of infection or inflammation and is established when the absolute count exceeds 7.5×10^9/L. Release and depletion of stored neutrophils stimulates granulopoiesis to replenish neutrophil reserves. Specific conditions associated with neutrophilia and other white blood cells are identified in Table 21-4.

When the demand for circulating mature neutrophils exceeds the supply, immature neutrophils (and other leukocytes) are released from the bone marrow. Premature release of the immature cells is responsible for the phenomenon known as a **shift to the left**, or **leukemoid reaction**. This refers to the microscopic detection of disproportionate numbers

TABLE 21-4 Other Conditions Associated With Neutrophils, Eosinophils, Basophils, Monocytes, and Lymphocytes

Condition	Cause	Example
Neutrophil		
Neutrophilia (granulocytosis)	Inflammation or tissue necrosis	Surgery, burns, MI, pneumonitis, rheumatic fever, rheumatoid arthritis
	Infection	Bacterial: Gram-positive (staphylococci, streptococci, pneumococci), Gram-negative (*Escherichia coli, Pseudomonas* species)
	Physiological	Exercise, extreme heat or cold, third-trimester pregnancy, emotional distress
	Hematological	Acute hemorrhage, hemolysis, myeloproliferative disorder, chronic granulocytic leukemia
	Medications or chemicals	Epinephrine, steroids, heparin, histamine, endotoxin
	Metabolic	Diabetes (acidosis), eclampsia, gout, thyroid storm
	Neoplasm	Liver, GI tract, bone marrow
Neutropenia	Decreased marrow production	Radiation, chemotherapy, leukemia, aplastic anemia, abnormal granulopoiesis
	Increased destruction	Splenomegaly, hemodialysis, autoimmune disease
	Prolonged infection	Gram-negative (typhoid), viral (influenza, hepatitis B, measles, mumps, rubella), severe infections, protozoal infections (malaria)
Eosinophil		
Eosinophilia	Allergy	Asthma, hay fever, medication sensitivity
	Infection	Parasites (trichinosis, hookworm), chronic (fungal, leprosy, TB)
	Malignancy	CML, lung, stomach, ovary, Hodgkin's lymphoma
	Dermatosis	Pemphigus, exfoliative dermatitis (medication-induced)
	Medications	Digitalis, heparin, streptomycin, tryptophan (eosinophilia-myalgia syndrome), penicillins, propranolol
Eosinopenia	Stress response	Trauma, shock, burns, surgery, mental distress
	Medications	Steroids (Cushing's syndrome)
Basophil		
Basophilia	Inflammation	Infection (measles, chickenpox), hypersensitivity reaction (immediate)
	Hematological	Myeloproliferative disorders (CML, polycythemia vera, Hodgkin's lymphoma, hemolytic anemia)
	Endocrine	Myxedema, antithyroid therapy
Basopenia	Physiological	Pregnancy, ovulation, stress
	Endocrine	Graves' disease
Monocyte		
Monocytosis	Infection	Bacterial (subacute bacterial endocarditis, TB), recovery phase of infection
	Hematological	Myeloproliferative disorders, Hodgkin's lymphoma, agranulocytosis
	Physiological	Normal newborn
Monocytopenia	Rare	
Lymphocyte		
Lymphocytosis	Physiological	4 months to 4 years
	Acute infection	Infectious mononucleosis, CMV infection, pertussis, hepatitis, mycoplasma pneumonia, typhoid
	Chronic infection	Congenital syphilis, tertiary syphilis
	Endocrine	Thyrotoxicosis, adrenal insufficiency
	Malignancy	ALL, CLL, lymphosarcoma cell leukemia
Lymphocytopenia	Immunodeficiency syndrome	AIDS, agammaglobulinemia
	Lymphocyte destruction	Steroids (Cushing's syndrome), radiation, chemotherapy
		Hodgkin's lymphoma
		Heart failure, renal failure, TB, SLE, aplastic anemia

AIDS, acquired immunodeficiency syndrome; *ALL*, acute lymphocytic leukemia; *CLL*, chronic lymphocytic leukemia; *CML*, chronic myeloid (or myelogenous) leukemia; *CMV*, cytomegalovirus; *GI*, gastro-intestinal; *MI*, myocardial infarction; *SLE*, systemic lupus erythematosus; *TB*, tuberculosis.

of immature leukocytes in peripheral blood smears. To understand this phenomenon, visualize cellular differentiation, maturation, and release (see Figure 20-2) as progressing from left to right instead of vertically. The early release of immature white blood cells prevents the completion of the sequence and shifts the distribution of leukocytes in the blood toward those on the left side of the diagram. This phenomenon is also seen in the blood smear of individuals with leukemia, hence the term *leukemoid reaction*. As infection or inflammation diminishes, and granulopoiesis replenishes circulating granulocytes, a **shift to the right**, or return to normal, occurs.

Neutropenia is a condition associated with a reduction in circulating neutrophils and exists clinically when the neutrophil count is less than 2×10^9/L. Reduction in neutrophils occurs in severe prolonged infections when production of granulocytes cannot keep up with demand.[25,26]

Other causes of neutropenia, in the absence of infection, may be (1) decreased neutrophil production or ineffective granulopoiesis, (2) reduced neutrophil survival, and (3) abnormal neutrophil distribution and sequestration. Neutropenia also is classified as primary or secondary, and primary disorders are further identified as congenital or acquired. Primary acquired neutropenia is associated with multiple conditions, for example, hypoplastic anemia or aplastic anemia, leukemia (AML/chronic lymphocytic leukemia [CLL]), lymphomas (Hodgkin's, non-Hodgkin's), and MDS. The megaloblastic anemias (vitamin B_{12} and folate deficiency) as well as starvation and anorexia nervosa cause neutropenia because of an inadequate supply of vitamins and nutrients for protein production.

Congenital defects in neutrophil production include cyclic neutropenia, neutropenia with congenital immunodeficiencies, and multiple syndromes, such as Kostmann, Shwachman-Diamond, Diamond-Blackfan, and Barth syndromes. Reduced neutrophil survival and abnormal distribution and sequestration are usually secondary to other disorders. Neutropenia occurs in a variety of immunological disorders, particularly systemic lupus erythematosus, rheumatoid arthritis, Felty's and Sjögren's syndromes, splenomegaly, and medication-related causes.

Severe neutropenia, **granulocytopenia** (less than 0.5×10^9/L), or **agranulocytosis** (complete absence of granulocytes in blood) is usually secondary to arrested hematopoiesis in the bone marrow or massive cell destruction in the circulation. Chemotherapeutic agents used to treat hematological and other malignancies cause bone marrow suppression. Several other medications cause agranulocytosis, which occurs rarely but carries a high mortality of 10 to 50%. Clinical manifestations of agranulocytosis include severe infection (particularly of the respiratory system) leading to septicemia, general malaise, fever, tachycardia, and ulcers in the mouth and colon. If this condition remains untreated, sepsis caused by agranulocytosis results in death within 3 to 6 days. Other conditions associated with neutropenia are detailed in Table 21-4.

Eosinophilia is an absolute increase (greater than 4.5×10^9/L) in the total number of circulating eosinophils. Allergic disorders (type 1) associated with asthma, hay fever, parasitic infections, and medication reactions often cause eosinophilia. Hypersensitivity reactions trigger the release of eosinophil chemotactic factor of anaphylaxis (ECF-A), and histamine from mast cells attracts eosinophils to the area. Mast cells release interleukin-5 (IL-5), which stimulates the bone marrow to produce more eosinophils into the blood. Areas with abundant mast cells, such as the respiratory and GI tracts, are commonly affected. Eosinophilia also may occur in dermatological disorders, eosinophilia-myalgia syndrome, and parasitic invasion. Other conditions associated with eosinophilia are detailed in Table 21-4.

Eosinopenia, a decrease in the number of circulating eosinophils, generally is caused by migration of eosinophils into inflammatory sites. It may be seen in Cushing's syndrome and as a result of stress caused by surgery, shock, trauma, burns, or mental distress. Other conditions associated with eosinopenia are detailed in Table 21-4.

Basophilia, an increase in the number of circulating basophils, is rare and generally is a response to inflammation and immediate hypersensitivity reactions. Basophils contain histamine that is released during an allergic reaction. Increased numbers of basophils are seen in myeloproliferative disorders, such as chronic myeloid leukemia and myeloid metaplasia. Other conditions associated with basophilia are detailed in Table 21-4.

Basopenia (also known as *basophilic leukopenia*) is a decrease in circulating numbers of basophils. It is seen in hyperthyroidism, acute infection, ovulation and pregnancy, and long-term therapy with steroids. Other conditions associated with basopenia are detailed in Table 21-4.

Monocytosis is an increase in the number of circulating monocytes (generally greater than 8.0×10^9/L). It is often transient and not related to a dysfunction of monocyte production. If present, it is usually associated with neutropenia during bacterial infections, particularly in the late stages or recovery stage, when monocytes are needed to phagocytize surviving microorganisms and debris. Increased monocytes also may indicate marrow recovery from agranulocytosis. Monocytosis is often seen in chronic infections such as tuberculosis (TB), brucellosis, listeriosis, and subacute bacterial endocarditis (SBE). Monocytosis has been found to correlate with the extent of myocardial damage following myocardial infarctions. Other conditions associated with monocytosis are detailed in Table 21-4. **Monocytopenia**, a decrease in the number of circulating monocytes, is rare but has been identified with hairy cell leukemia and prednisone therapy.

Lymphocyte Alterations

Quantitative alterations of lymphocytes occur when lymphocytes are activated by antigenic stimuli, usually microorganisms (see Chapter 7). **Lymphocytosis** is an increase in the number **(absolute lymphocytosis)** or proportion of lymphocytes in the blood. It is rare in acute bacterial infections and is seen most commonly in acute viral infections, particularly those caused by the Epstein-Barr virus (EBV)—a causative agent in IM. Other specific disorders associated with lymphocytosis are detailed in Table 21-4.

Lymphocytopenia is a decrease in the number of circulating lymphocytes in the blood. It may be attributed to (1) abnormalities of lymphocyte production associated with neoplasias and immune deficiencies and (2) destruction by medications, viruses, or radiation. It is also known to occur without any detectable cause. Conditions associated with lymphocytopenia are detailed in Table 21-4. The lymphocytopenia associated with heart failure and other acute illnesses may be caused by elevated cortisol levels. Lymphocytopenia is a major problem in acquired immune deficiency syndrome (AIDS). AIDS-related lymphocytopenia is caused by human immunodeficiency virus (HIV), which destroys T-helper lymphocytes. (For a detailed discussion of AIDS, see Chapter 8.)

Infectious Mononucleosis

Infectious mononucleosis (IM) is a benign, acute, self-limiting, lymphoproliferative clinical syndrome characterized by acute infection of B lymphocytes (B cells). The most common cause is EBV.[27] EBV is a ubiquitous lymphotropic, herpesvirus and accounts for approximately 85% of IM cases. Other viruses that cause symptoms resembling IM include cytomegalovirus (CMV), adenovirus, HIV, hepatitis A, influenza A and B, and rubella, as well as the bacteria *Toxoplasma gondii*, *Corynebacterium diphtheriae*, and *Coxiella burnetii*. The classic symptoms are pharyngitis, lymphadenopathy, and fever. In individuals with immunodeficiency, the proliferation of infected B cells may be uncontrolled and can lead to the development of B-cell lymphomas.[28]

Individuals who are co-infected with malaria or HIV are at increased risk of developing EBV-associated lymphomas, including Burkitt lymphoma. EBV also is etiologically linked to subgroups of Hodgkin's lymphoma (HL). Approximately 50 to 85% of children are infected with EBV by age 4, and more than 90% of adults have indications of subclinical EBV infections. These early infections are usually asymptomatic and provide immunity to EBV; thus early EBV infections rarely develop into IM. IM may arise when the initial infection occurs during adolescence or later, but still only results in IM in 35 to 50% of these individuals. Symptomatic IM usually affects young adults between ages 15 and 35 years, with the peak incidences occurring between 15 and 24 years; males have a later peak (18 to 24 years) than females. The overall incidence rate for this age group is 6 to 8 cases per 1 000 persons per year. Children from low socioeconomic environments are particularly susceptible to infections with EBV. IM is uncommon in individuals older than age 40; however, if it does occur, it is commonly caused by CMV.

Transmission of EBV is usually through saliva from close personal contact (e.g., kissing, hence the term *kissing disease*). The virus also may be secreted in other mucosal secretions of the genital, rectal, and respiratory tracts, as well as blood. Transmission through sneezing or coughing has not been documented. The infection begins with widespread invasion of the B cells, which have receptors for EBV. The virus initially infects the oropharynx, nasopharynx, and salivary epithelial cells with later spread into lymphoid tissues and B cells.

In the immunocompetent individual, unaffected B cells produce antibodies (immunoglobulins IgG, IgA, IgM) against the virus. At the same time, there is a massive proliferation of T-cytotoxic cells (CD8) that are directed against EBV-infected cells (see Chapter 7). The immune response against EBV-infected cells is largely responsible for the cellular proliferation in the lymphoid tissue (lymph nodes, spleen, tonsils, and, occasionally, liver). Sore throat and fever are caused by inflammation at the site of initial viral entry (the mouth and throat).

CLINICAL MANIFESTATIONS The incubation period for IM is approximately 30 to 50 days. Early flulike symptoms, such as headache, malaise, joint pain, and fatigue, may appear during the first 3 to 5 days, although some individuals are without symptoms. At the time of diagnosis, the individual commonly presents with the classic group of symptoms: fever, sore throat (pharyngitis), cervical lymph node enlargement, and fatigue. The pharyngitis is usually diffuse with a whitish or greyish green, thick exudate. It can be painful, causing the individual to seek treatment. Characteristics with progression may include a generalized lymphadenopathy, enlarged spleen, and appearance in the blood of atypical activated T lymphocytes (mononucleosis cells). IM is usually self-limiting, and recovery occurs in a few weeks. Fatigue, however, may last for 1 to 2 months after resolution of the infection.

Severe clinical complications are rare. With progression of IM, general lymph node enlargement may develop with enlargement of the spleen and liver. Splenomegaly is clinically evident 50% of the time and is demonstrated radiologically 100% of the time. Difficulty in detecting splenomegaly with physical examination contributes to the underestimation of actual enlargement. Splenic rupture is rare (only 0.1 to 0.5% of all cases) and can occur spontaneously as a result of mild trauma, arising primarily in men younger than 25 years of age and between days 4 and 21 after the onset of symptoms. It is the most common cause of death related to IM. Other causes of fatalities are hepatic failure, extensive bacterial infection, or viral myocarditis. Other organ systems are rarely involved, but such involvement may be present with characteristic manifestations, such as fulminant hepatitis with jaundice and anemia, encephalitis, meningitis, Guillain-Barré syndrome, and Bell's palsy. Eye manifestations may include eyelid and periorbital edema, dry eyes, keratitis, uveitis, and conjunctivitis. Reye's syndrome has been known to develop in children with EBV infection. Pulmonary and respiratory failure has been documented, but it is more likely to occur in immunocompromised individuals. Approximately 3 to 10% of adults older than 40 years of age have never been infected with EBV and are susceptible to IM later in life. In these individuals, the classic symptoms are not generally present, making diagnosis more difficult.

EVALUATION AND TREATMENT The blood of affected individuals contains an increased number of white blood cells with many atypical forms. The diagnosis of IM depends on the following specific findings: (1) an increase in the number of lymphocytes, commonly based on Hoagland criteria of at least 50% lymphocytes and at least 10% atypical lymphocytes in the blood; (2) a positive heterophile antibody reaction (monospot test); and (3) a rising titer of specific antibodies for EBV antigens. **Heterophilic antibodies** are a heterogeneous group of IgM antibodies that are agglutinins against nonhuman red blood cells (e.g., horse, sheep) and are detected by qualitative (monospot test) or quantitative (heterophile antibody test) methods. Use of the monospot test is limited because other infections (e.g., CMV, adenovirus) and toxoplasmosis also produce heterophilic antibodies. Thus 5 to 15% of monospot tests yield false-positive results. Heterophilic antibodies in the blood increase as the condition progresses, although some individuals and children younger than 4 years of age do not produce them. Diagnosis of EBV infection specifically may be increased with newer viral-specific tests that identify EBV-specific antibodies.

Treatment is supportive and consists of rest and alleviation of symptoms with analgesics and antipyretics. Aspirin is avoided with children because of its association with Reye's syndrome. *Streptococcal pharyngitis*, which occurs in 20 to 30% of cases, is treated with penicillin or erythromycin (Erythrocin), not ampicillin (Principen)—ampicillin is known to cause a rash. Bed rest with avoidance of strenuous activity and contact sports is indicated. Steroids are used when severe complications, such as impending airway obstruction, or other organ involvement (central nervous system [CNS] manifestations, thrombocytopenic purpura, myocarditis, pericarditis) is evident. Acyclovir (Zovirax) has been used in immunocompromised individuals but is not considered standard therapy. In the rare event of splenic rupture, the treatment has been removal of the spleen and continues to be the choice in hemodynamically unstable individuals. Current research, however, is suggesting that it may be better to repair the spleen to avoid overwhelming postsplenectomy infection.

QUICK CHECK 21-2

1. What condition is manifested chiefly by an increase in the numbers of circulating granulocytes and monocytes?
2. What is the cause of infectious mononucleosis (IM)?
3. What are the classic symptoms of IM?

Leukemias

Leukemia is a clonal malignant disorder of the bone marrow and usually, but not always, of the blood. The common pathological feature of all forms of leukemia is an uncontrolled proliferation of malignant leukocytes, causing an overcrowding of bone marrow and decreased production and function of normal hematopoietic cells. Chromosomal abnormalities and translocations are common in the majority of leukemias. When genes become mutated, they create genomic aberrations that block cell maturation and activate pro-growth signalling pathways that prevent apoptotic cell death.

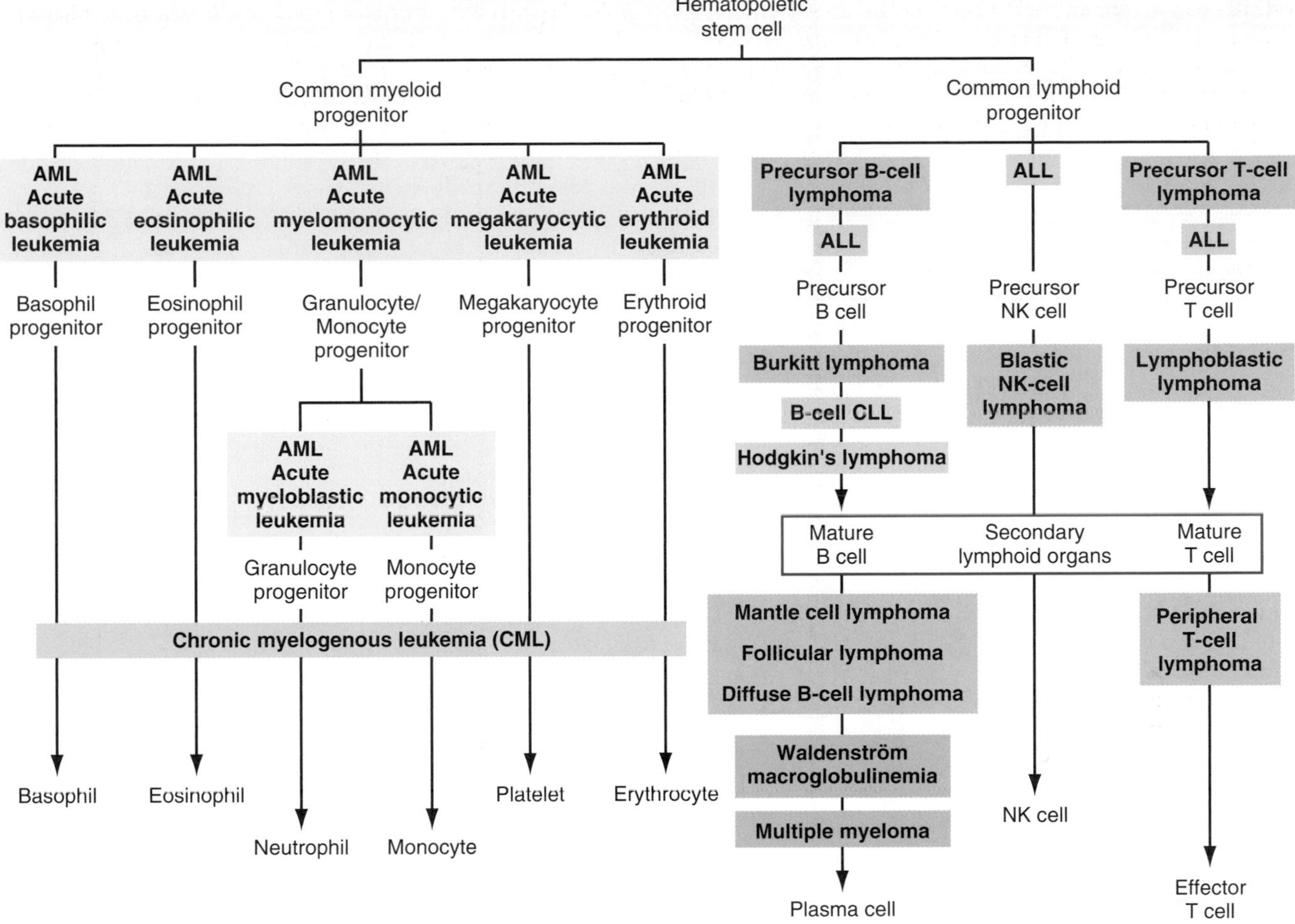

FIGURE 21-6 Origins of Leukemias and Lymphomas. Differentiation pathways of blood-forming cells and reported sites from which specific leukemias and lymphomas originate. Tumours of similar types are given the same background colouring. *ALL*, acute lymphocytic leukemia; *AML*, acute myeloid (or myelogenous) leukemia; *CLL*, chronic lymphocytic leukemia; *NK*, natural killer.

The classification of leukemia is based on (1) the predominant cell of origin (either myeloid or lymphoid) and (2) the rate of progression, which usually reflects the degree at which cell differentiation was arrested when the cell became malignant (acute or chronic) (Figure 21-6). **Acute leukemia** is characterized by undifferentiated or immature cells, usually a **blast cell**. The onset of disease is abrupt and rapid. Without treatment, disease progression results in a short survival time. In **chronic leukemia**, the predominant cell is more differentiated but does not function normally, with a relatively slow progression. There are four major types of leukemia: (1) acute lymphocytic leukemia (ALL), (2) acute myeloid (or myelogenous) leukemia (AML), (3) chronic lymphocytic leukemia (CLL), and (4) chronic myeloid (or myelogenous) leukemia (CML).[29-31] Further classification of acute leukemias is based on characteristics that may provide significant therapeutic prognostic information, such as structure, number of cells, genetics, identification of surface markers, and histochemical staining (see Figure 21-6).

Leukemia occurs with varying frequencies at different ages and is more common in adults than in children. In 2017, it was estimated that 6 200 Canadians would be diagnosed with leukemia, with males having a slightly higher incidence than females (Table 21-5). Leukemia accounts for about 34% of all childhood cancers; ALL accounts for almost 78% of all new cases of leukemia in children. CLL and AML are the most common types in adults. CML is found mostly in adults.

Over the past 2 decades, the rates of induced remission and survival in most forms of leukemia have increased. Current survival rates range from 24% for AML to 81% for CLL, and as high as 91% for children and adolescents younger than 15 years of age with ALL.[32]

PATHOPHYSIOLOGY Although the exact cause of leukemia is unknown, several risk factors and related genetic aberrations are associated with the onset of malignancy. The leukemias are clonal disorders driven by genetically abnormal stem-like cancer cells (SLCCs).[33] Abnormal immature white blood cells, called *blasts*, fill the bone marrow and spill into the blood. The leukemia blasts literally "crowd out" the marrow and cause cellular proliferation of the other cell lines to cease. Normal granulocytic-monocytic, lymphocytic, erythrocytic, and megakaryocytic progenitor cells cease to function, resulting in **pancytopenia** (a reduction in all cellular components of the blood). Almost 90% of ALLs have chromosomal changes that correlate with immunophenotyping and sometimes confer prognostic significance. Several genetic translocations (mitotic errors) are observed in leukemic cells. One of these translocations, the **Philadelphia chromosome**, is observed in 95% of those with CML and 30% of adults with ALL (Figure 21-7). The Philadelphia chromosome results from a reciprocal translocation between the long arms of chromosomes 9 and 22. A unique protein (BCR-ABL protein) is encoded from two genes (*BCR* from chromosome 22 and *ABL* from

TABLE 21-5 Estimated New Cases and Deaths From Leukemia in Canada

Types of Leukemia	TOTAL NEW CASES (Proportion of New Cases)	NEW CASES BY GENDER Male	NEW CASES BY GENDER Female	DEATHS BY GENDER Male	DEATHS BY GENDER Female
All types[a]	6 200 (100%)[a]	3 600[a]	2 600[a]	1 650[a]	1 250[a]
Acute lymphocytic leukemia (ALL)[b]	480 (7%)	255	220	72	66
Chronic lymphocytic leukemia (CLL)[b]	2 465 (35%)	1 495	965	396	212
Acute myeloid (or myelogenous) leukemia (AML)[b]	1 315 (20%)	740	575	589	458
Chronic myeloid (or myelogenous) leukemia (CML)[b]	675 (10%)	410	265	72	47

[a]Data for 2017.
[b]Data for 2013.
Data from Canadian Cancer Society. (2017). *Cancer information*. Retrieved from http://www.cancer.ca/en/?region=on; Canadian Cancer Society. (2017). Leukemia. Retrieved from http://www.cancer.ca/en/cancer-information/cancer-type/leukemia/leukemia/?region=on.

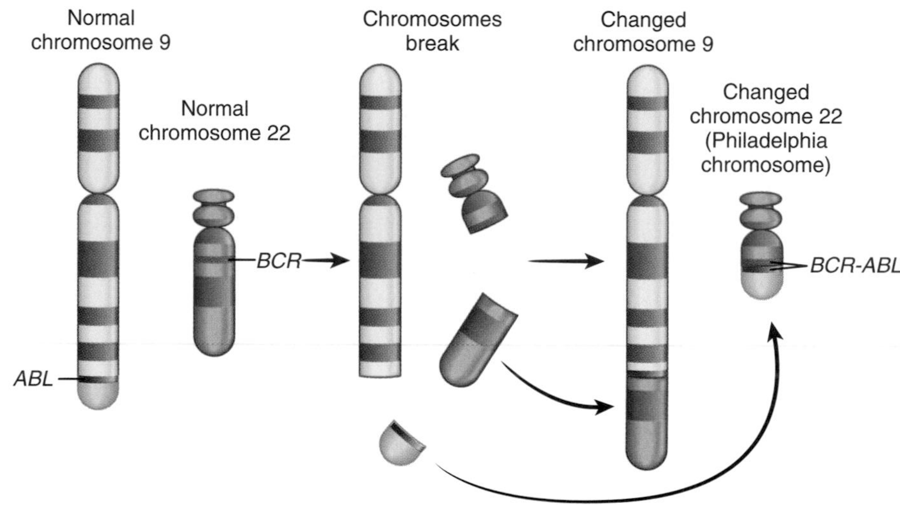

FIGURE 21-7 Philadelphia Chromosome. A piece of chromosome 9 and a piece of chromosome 22 break off and trade places. The *BCR-ABL* gene is formed on chromosome 22 where the piece of chromosome 9 attaches. The changed chromosome 22 is called *Philadelphia chromosome.* (Adapted from National Cancer Institute. [2014]. *Childhood acute lymphoblastic leukemia treatment.* Bethesda, MD: National Institutes of Health.)

chromosome 9) artificially linked at the junction of translocation. The BCR-ABL protein affects a variety of cell cycle control genes, leading to an increased rate of cellular division, inhibition of DNA repair, and other dysregulations of cell growth. Over time the original tumour becomes genetically unstable and diverse.

Risk factors for the onset of leukemia include environmental factors as well as other diseases. Increased risk for ALL has been linked to exposure to X-rays before birth, being exposed to ionizing radiation (postnatally), past treatment with chemotherapy, and certain genetic conditions including Down syndrome, neurofibromatosis type 1(NF1), Shwachman syndrome, Bloom's syndrome, and ataxia telangiectasia. There is growing concern about the effect of low-dose radiation on subsequent risk for leukemia.[34] There is a statistically significant tendency for leukemia to reappear in families. A unique characteristic of ALL, unlike other forms, is that ALL develops at different rates in different geographic locations, although the reason for this is unclear. Individuals in developed countries and in higher socioeconomic categories have an increased incidence of ALL. Acute leukemia also may develop secondary to certain acquired disorders, including CML, CLL, PV, myelofibrosis, HL, MM, ovarian cancer, and SA.

Potential risk factors for AML include smoking, previous chemotherapy, and exposure to ionizing radiation. AML is the most frequently reported secondary cancer after high doses of chemotherapy for HL, non-Hodgkin's lymphoma (NHL), MM, ovarian cancer, and breast cancer.

Acute leukemias. Acute leukemias consist of two types: acute lymphocytic leukemia (ALL) and acute myeloid (or myelogenous) leukemia (AML).[34] ALL is an aggressive, fast-growing leukemia with too many lymphoblasts or immature white blood cells found in blood and bone marrow. It also is called *acute lymphoblastic leukemia*. AML is an aggressive fast-growing leukemia with too many myeloblasts or immature white blood cells that are not lymphoblasts found in the bone marrow and blood. It also is called *acute myeloblastic leukemia* and *acute nonlymphocytic leukemia* (ANLL). Acute leukemias are seen in both genders and in all ages, with the incidence increasing dramatically in individuals older than 50 years. North American and Scandinavian countries have the highest mortality; Eastern European countries, Asia (except Japan), and Central America have the lowest mortality. Japan's higher mortality is the result of the atomic bombs dropped in World War II. Blacks have consistently shown a lower mortality than Whites. In 2013, 480 Canadians were diagnosed with ALL and 1 315 were diagnosed with AML. In the same year, 138 Canadians died from ALL and 1 047 died from AML.[35] As mentioned earlier, risk factors for ALL include being exposed to X-rays before birth,

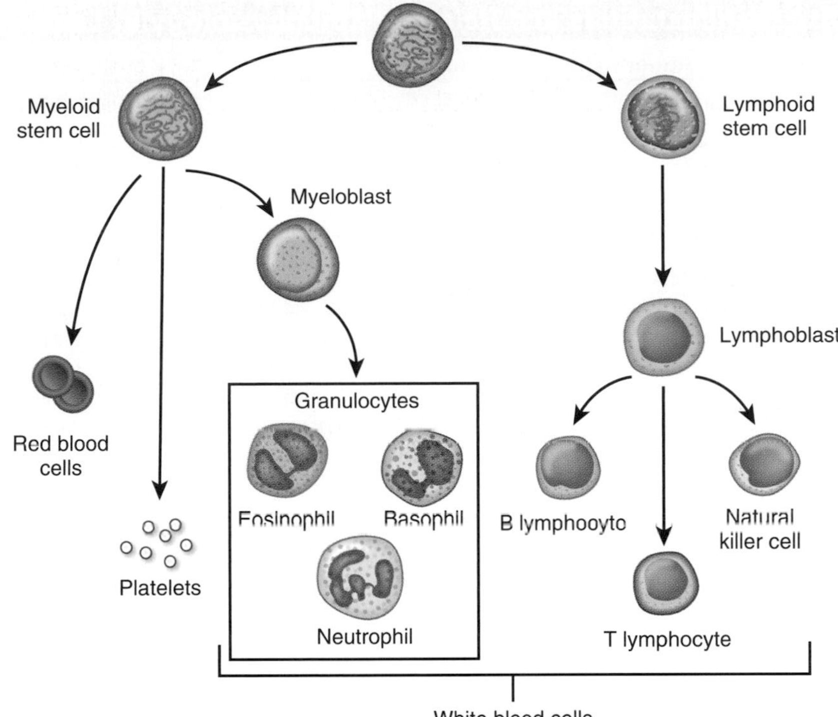

FIGURE 21-8 Leukemia Arises From Stemlike Cells. A blood stem cell undergoes multiple steps to finally become a red blood cell, platelet, or white blood cell. (Modified from National Cancer Institute. [2014]. *Adult acute lymphoblastic leukemia treatment (PDQ ®)*. Bethesda, MD: Author. Retrieved from http://www.cancer.gov/cancertopics/pdq/treatment/adultALL/HealthProfessional.)

exposure to ionizing radiation (postnatal), and past treatment with chemotherapy.

PATHOPHYSIOLOGY ALL presumably progresses from malignant transformation of B- or C-cell progenitor cells (like a stem cell) (Figure 21-8). Most cases of ALL occur in children and often in the first decade. Although adults account for about 20% of all cases, their mortality rate is significantly higher. The significant difference between the incidence of ALL in adults and children may be because of differences in the biology of the disease. Approximately 75% of ALL cases in children originate from transformed precursor B cells, whereas adult ALL is a mixture of cancers of precursor B-cell or precursor T-cell origin. Precursor B-cell ALL can be further divided into different phenotypes depending on their progression through the B-cell maturation process. The T-cell lineage ALL is distinguished by T-cell–associated markers.

B-cell ALL is strongly associated with aneuploidy of various types, with more than 50 chromosomes. T-cell ALL generally has fewer cytogenetic abnormalities, and the majority have genetic deletions. Several other translocations are commonly observed in ALL, including the Philadelphia chromosome and translocations involving the *ETV6* (formerly *TEL*) and *MLL* genes.

AML is the most common adult leukemia; the mean age of diagnosis is 67 years of age. AML results from an abnormal proliferation of myeloid precursor cells, a decreased rate of apoptosis, and an arrest in cellular differentiation. Therefore, the bone marrow and peripheral blood are characterized by leukocytosis and a predominance of blast cells. As these immature blast cells increase, they replace normal myelocytic cells, megakaryocytes, and erythrocytes. This displacement can lead to complications of bleeding, anemia, and infection. Several hereditary conditions are known to increase the risk for AML (e.g., Down syndrome, Fanconi anemia, Bloom's syndrome, and others). More than 150 structural chromosomal abnormalities and several duplications or deletions within genes have been identified in AML. Although ALL and AML are clinically very similar, they are genetically and immunologically distinct.[36]

CLINICAL MANIFESTATIONS Within days to a few weeks of the first symptoms is an abrupt stormy onset, which is more prevalent in ALL. The clinical manifestations of all varieties of acute leukemia are generally similar. Mechanisms associated with common manifestations are summarized in Table 21-6. Signs and symptoms related to bone marrow depression include fatigue caused by anemia, bleeding resulting from thrombocytopenia, and fever caused by infection. Bleeding may occur in the skin, gums, mucous membranes, and GI tract. Visible signs include petechiae and ecchymosis, as well as discoloration of the skin, gingival bleeding, hematuria, and mid-cycle or heavy menstrual bleeding.

Infection sites include the mouth, throat, respiratory tract, lower colon, urinary tract, and skin and may be caused by Gram-negative bacilli (*Escherichia coli*), *Pseudomonas aeruginosa*, and *K. pneumoniae*. Fever is an early sign often accompanied by chills.

Anorexia is accompanied by weight loss, diminished sensitivity to sour and sweet tastes, wasting of muscle, and difficulty swallowing. Liver, spleen, and lymph node enlargement occur more commonly in ALL than in AML. Liver and spleen enlargement commonly occur together. The leukemic individual often experiences abdominal pain and tenderness. Pain in the bones and joints is thought to result from leukemia infiltration with secondary stretching of the periosteum.

Neurological manifestations are common and may be caused by either leukemic infiltration or cerebral bleeding. Headache, vomiting, papilledema, facial palsy, blurred vision, auditory disturbances, and meningeal irritation can occur if leukemic cells infiltrate the cerebral or spinal meninges.

EVALUATION AND TREATMENT Because leukemia often is confused with other conditions, early detection may be difficult. Persistent

TABLE 21-6 Clinical Manifestations and Related Pathophysiology in Leukemia

Clinical Manifestations	Laboratory Abnormalities	Cause	Comments
Anemia	Relative *proportion* of erythroblasts to total count (decreased in anemia) is key	Decreased stem cell input or ineffective erythropoiesis, or both	In acute leukemia, anemia is usually present from beginning, often first symptom noticed, and severe; mild form without symptoms is common in CML and CLL; hemorrhage common in acute forms, occasional in CML, but rare in CLL
Bleeding (purpura, petechiae, ecchymosis, hemorrhage)	Decreased and possibly abnormal platelets	Reduction in megakaryocytes leading to thrombocytopenia	Bleeding more common in acute than in chronic leukemia
Infection	Increased multisegmented neutrophils	Opportunistic organisms; decreased protection resulting from granulocytopenia or immune deficiency secondary to chemotherapy, corticosteroids, and disease process	Major sites of infection: oral cavity, throat, lower colon, urinary tract, lungs, and skin; prevention of infection focuses on restoring host defences, decreasing invasive procedures, and reducing colonization of organisms
Weight loss	Decreased 24-hr urinary creatinine excretion; hypoalbuminemia	Condition can be attributed to pain, depression, chemotherapy, radiation therapy, loss of appetite, and alterations in taste	Severe weight loss may be related to excess production of TNF-α
Bone pain	Often no radiographic evidence of bone problems	Result of bone infiltration by leukemic cells or intramedullary infection	If combination medication regimens are ineffective, radiation therapy is used
Liver, spleen, and lymph node enlargement	Biopsy abnormal for liver and spleen	Leukemic cell infiltration	Lymph nodes also undergo leukemia proliferation in CLL
Elevated uric acid level	Normal excretion of uric acid is 300–500 mg/day; leukemic individual can excrete 50 times more	Increased catabolism of protein and nucleic acid; urate precipitation increased from dehydration caused by anorexia or fever and medication therapy	Hyperuricemia is present in both acute leukemia and CML; treatment focuses on increasing urine pH or decreasing acid production with medication allopurinol

CLL, chronic lymphocytic leukemia; *CML*, chronic myeloid (or myelogenous) leukemia; *TNF-α*, tumour necrosis factor-alpha.

symptoms need intensive medical investigation. The diagnosis is made through blood tests and examination of bone marrow.

Chemotherapy, used in various combinations, is the treatment of choice for leukemia. Supportive measures include blood transfusions, antibiotics, antifungals, and antivirals. Allopurinol (Zyloprim) is used to prevent uric acid production and elevation that occurs because of cellular death caused by treatment. Stem cell transplantation is now considered standard therapy for selected individuals with leukemia.

Advances in the treatment of AML have substantially improved the complete remission (CR) rates.[37] Attainment of CR requires fairly aggressive treatment. With appropriate induction therapy, approximately 60 to 70% of adults with AML will attain CR status. More than 25% of adults with AML (about 45% of those who attain CR) are expected to survive 3 or more years and may be cured.[37] Since the 1970s, 5-year survival rates for those with ALL have increased from 38 to 66% for adults and from 53 to 91% for children. Factors influencing increased survival rate include the use of combined and multimodality treatment methods; improved supportive services, such as blood banking and nutritional support; and antimicrobial treatment. The presence of the Philadelphia chromosome (observed in about 5% of children with ALL, in 30% of adults with ALL, and occasionally in AML) is a poor prognostic indicator.

Myelosuppression is both a consequence of leukemia and a treatment for the disease. Hematological support with blood products and granulocyte colony-stimulating factor (G-CSF) or granulocyte-macrophage colony–stimulating factor (GM-CSF) has effectively shortened the time of neutropenia and improved survival by reducing the risk for infection.

Chronic leukemias. The two main types of chronic leukemia are (1) **chronic myeloid (or myelogenous) leukemia (CML)** and (2) **chronic lymphocytic leukemia (CLL)**. CML is also called *chronic granulocytic leukemia*. Several forms of CML can occur, depending on the lineage of the malignant cells (e.g., chronic neutrophilic leukemia [CNL], chronic eosinophilic leukemia [CEL]). CML is a slowly progressing disease with too many blood cells (not lymphocytes) made in the bone marrow. CLL is a slow-growing cancer in which too many immature lymphocytes (white blood cells) are found mostly in the blood and bone marrow. Cancer cells also may be found in lymphoid tissues. In later stages of the disease, cancer cells are sometimes found in the lymph nodes and the disease is called **small lymphocytic lymphoma (SLL**; also known as **CLL/SLL)**. SLL cancer cells are found mostly in the lymph nodes; CLL/SLL also is classified as a NHL. In adults, CLL is the most common leukemia in the Western world.[36] Individuals with chronic leukemia have a longer life expectancy, usually extending several years from the time of diagnosis.

The chronic leukemias account for the majority of cases in adults (see Table 21-5). The incidences of CLL and CML increase significantly in individuals more than 40 years of age, with prevalence in the sixth through eighth decades. CML is one of a group of diseases called **myeloproliferative disorders**—acquired abnormalities in signalling pathways that lead to growth factor–independent proliferation—which also include PV, primary thrombocytosis, and idiopathic myelofibrosis (invasion of bone marrow by fibrous tissue).

PATHOPHYSIOLOGY CML is characterized from other myeloproliferative disorders by the presence of a *chimeric* (genetically distinct cells)

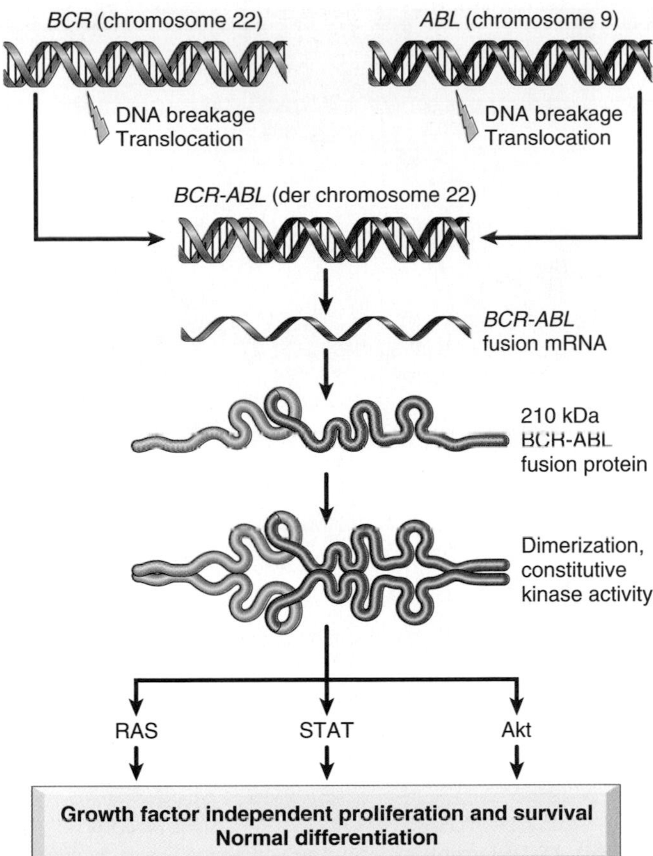

FIGURE 21-9 Pathogenesis of Chronic Myeloid Leukemia. The breakage and joining of *BCR* and *ABL* creates the chimeric fusion gene *BCR-ABL*. *BCR-ABL* genetically encodes an active BCR-ABL intracellular tyrosine kinase (an enzyme that controls intracellular "on–off" switches). The ABL kinase in turn induces signalling through the same pro-growth and pro-survival pathways that are activated by normal hematological growth factors. Altogether the activation of many downstream pathways drives growth factor–independent proliferation and survival of bone marrow progenitors. *Akt*, protein kinase B; *RAS*, renin-angiotensin system; *STAT*, signal transducer and activator of transcription. (From Kumar, V., Abbas, A.K., & Aster, J.C. [Eds.]. [2015]. *Robbins and Cotran pathologic basis of disease* [9th ed.]. Philadelphia: Saunders.)

BCR-ABL fusion gene derived from parts of the *BCR* gene on chromosome 22 and parts of the *ABL* gene on chromosome 9 (Figure 21-9).[36] In the majority of cases (i.e., over 90%), *BCR-ABL* is created by a reciprocal translocation of chromosomes 9 and 22 (the Philadelphia chromosome; see Figure 21-7). In the rest of the cases, the *BCR-ABL* fusion gene is made from complex genetic rearrangements and the cell of origin is a hematopoietic stem cell.[36] The *BCR-ABL* gene causes abnormal cell signalling resulting in pro-growth and pro-survival pathways of the leukemic cells. Much is still unknown about these cell-signalling abnormalities and why the *BCR-ABL* fusion gene preferentially drives proliferation of granulocytic and megakaryocytic blood cells. The only known cause of CML is exposure to ionizing radiation.

CLL involves transformation and progressive accumulation of monoclonal B cells; rarely (less than 5%) are CLL malignancies of T-cell origin. CLL is derived from a transformation of a partially mature B cell that has not yet encountered antigen. Investigations from the past two decades have classified CLL and predicted the outcome based on the immunoglobulin heavy chain variable region (*IGHV*) gene mutational status. Recent studies are addressing five epigenetic biomarkers to classify CLL, which could result in the use of more targeted therapies for specific subgroups.[38] Additionally, investigators report novel recurrent mutations in CLL, including *SF3B1* and *TP53* mutations, that are independent of *IGHV* mutational status, demanding the need for urgent standardization of detection methods.[39] The notch 1 (*NOTCH1*) gene also has been found recurrently mutated in a subset of individuals, not independent of *IGHV*, and these individuals had a shorter survival.[40] Chromosomal translocations (breakpoints) are rare in CLL. The cause of CLL is unknown.

CLINICAL MANIFESTATIONS Chronic leukemia advances slowly and insidiously. Approximately 70% of individuals with CLL are asymptomatic at the time of diagnosis. When symptoms do appear, the most common finding is lymphadenopathy. The most significant effect of CLL is suppression of humoral immunity and increased infection with encapsulated bacteria. Frequently, the level of neutrophils is depressed, which adds to the risk for infection. Invasion of most organ cells is uncommon but infiltration does occur in lymph nodes, liver, spleen, and salivary glands. CNS involvement is rare. Approximately 10% of individuals develop a more aggressive malignancy, usually a diffuse large B-cell lymphoma. In these individuals, extreme fatigue, weight loss, night sweats, low-grade fever, elevated levels of the enzyme lactic dehydrogenase, hypercalcemia, anemia, and thrombocytopenia are common.

Individuals with CML may progress through three phases of the disease: a chronic phase lasting 2 to 5 years, during which symptoms may not be apparent; an accelerated phase of 6 to 18 months, during which the primary symptoms develop; and a terminal blast phase ("blast crisis") with a survival of only 3 to 6 months. The accelerated phase is characterized by excessive proliferation and accumulation of malignant cells. Splenomegaly is prominent and becomes painful, but lymphadenopathy generally is not present. Liver enlargement also occurs, but liver function is rarely altered. Hyperuricemia is common and produces gouty arthritis. Infections, fever, and weight loss also are seen often. The terminal blast phase is characterized by rapid and progressive leukocytosis with an increase in basophils. In the later stages of the terminal phase, which then resembles AML, blast cells or promyelocytes predominate, and the individual experiences a "blast crisis."

The acute effects of CML resemble those of acute leukemia but with more prominent and painful splenomegaly. Liver function rarely is altered despite enlargement, and lymphadenopathy generally is found only in the acute phase of the disease. Hyperuricemia invariably is present and produces gouty arthritis. Infections, fever, and weight loss are common findings in individuals with CML.

EVALUATION AND TREATMENT Diagnosis of chronic leukemia depends on laboratory analyses of peripheral blood and bone marrow. Diagnosis of CLL is based on detection of a monoclonal B-cell lymphocytosis in the blood. The cells must have the characteristic immunophenotype (CD5+, and CD23-positive B cells) at levels in excess of 5 000 cells/mm^3 over a sustained period of time (usually 4 weeks). Confusion with other diseases may be avoided by determination of cell-surface markers. CLL lymphocytes co-express the B-cell antigens CD19 and CD20 along with the T-cell antigen CD5.[41] This co-expression only occurs in one other disease entity, mantle cell lymphoma.[41] Bone marrow may contain more than 30% lymphocytes and be normocellular or hypercellular. As assays have become more sensitive for detecting monoclonal B-CLL–like cells in peripheral blood, researchers have detected a monoclonal B-cell lymphocytosis (MBL) in 3% of adults older than 40 years and in 6% of adults older than 60 years.[42] Such early detection and diagnosis may falsely suggest improved survival for the group and may unnecessarily worry or result in therapy for some individuals who would have remained undiagnosed in their lifetime, a circumstance known in the literature as overdiagnosis or pseudodisease.[41,43]

Treatment of CLL ranges from periodic observation with treatment of infection, hemorrhage, or immunological complications to a variety of options including steroids, alkylating agents, purine analogue medications, combination chemotherapy, monoclonal antibodies, and transplant options.[41] For individuals with progressing CLL, treatment with conventional doses of chemotherapy is not curative; selected individuals treated with allogeneic stem cell transplantation have achieved prolonged disease-free survival.[41] Antileukemic therapy is frequently unnecessary in uncomplicated early disease.[41] From older clinical trials (1970s through the 1990s), the median survival for all individuals ranged from 8 to 12 years.[41] However, a large variation in survival exists, ranging from several months to a normal life expectancy. Treatment must be individualized on the basis of clinical behaviour of the disease.[41] Ongoing clinical trials are testing the concept of T lymphocytes (T cells) directed at specific antigen targets with engineered chimeric antigen receptors.[41] Complications of pancytopenia, including hemorrhage and infection, are a major cause of death for these individuals.

The development and introduction of the tyrosine kinase inhibitor imatinib mesylate (Gleevec) as a treatment modality have changed current management of CML. Imatinib mesylate is highly specific for CML and suppression of BCR-ABL kinase activity and produces a complete cytogenetic response in more than 80% of newly diagnosed persons. Although the *BCR-ABL* inhibitors markedly decrease the number of *BCR-ABL*–positive cells in the marrow and other places, they do not extinguish the CML stem cell, which persists at low levels.[36]

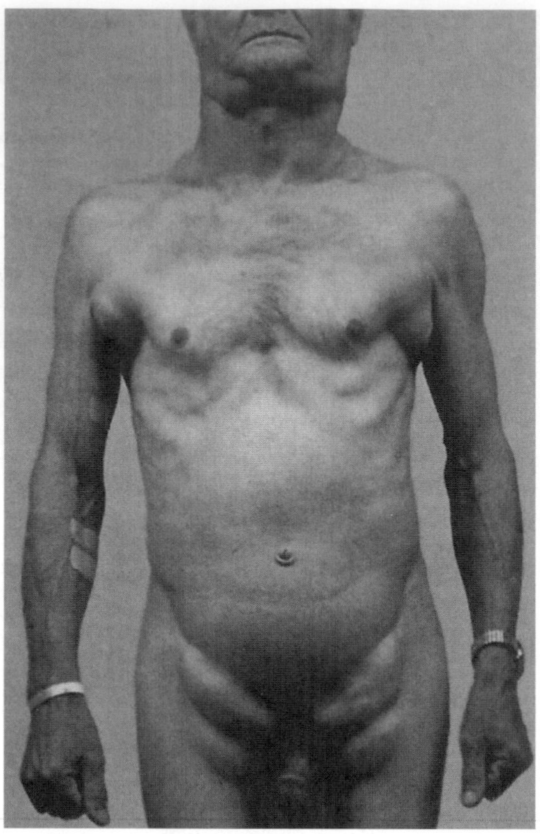

FIGURE 21-10 Lymphadenopathy. Individual with lymphocyte leukemia with extreme but symmetrical lymphadenopathy. (Courtesy Dr. A.R. Kagan, Los Angeles. From Ackerman, L.V., del Regato, J.A., Spjut, H.J., et al. [1985]. *Cancer: Diagnosis, treatment, and prognosis* [6th ed.]. St. Louis: Mosby.)

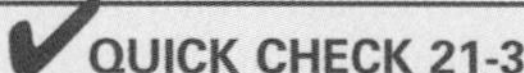

QUICK CHECK 21-3

1. How are leukemias classified?
2. What is the pathogenesis of acute lymphocytic leukemia?
3. What is the significance of the Philadelphia chromosome, and how is it related to leukemia?

ALTERATIONS OF LYMPHOID FUNCTION

Lymphadenopathy

Lymphadenopathy is characterized by enlarged lymph nodes (Figure 21-10). Lymph node enlargement occurs because of an increase in the size and number of its germinal centres caused by proliferation of lymphocytes and monocytes (immature phagocytes) or invasion by malignant cells. Normally, lymph nodes are not palpable or are barely palpable. Enlarged lymph nodes are characterized by being palpable and often also may be tender or painful to touch, although not in all situations.

Localized lymphadenopathy usually indicates drainage of an area associated with an inflammatory process or infection (reactive lymph node). *Generalized lymphadenopathy* occurs less often and is generally seen in the presence of malignant or nonmalignant disease, particularly in adults. Palpable nodes, however, do not always indicate serious disease and may indicate a minor trauma or infection. The location and size of the enlarged nodes are important factors in diagnosing the cause of the lymphadenopathy, as are the individual's age, gender, and geographic location. Generalized lymphadenopathy occurs with NHL, chronic lymphocytic leukemia, histiocytosis, and disorders that produce lymphocytosis. In general, lymphadenopathy results from four types of conditions: (1) neoplastic disease, (2) immunological or inflammatory conditions, (3) endocrine disorders, or (4) lipid storage diseases. Diseases of unknown cause, including autoimmune diseases and reactions to medications, also may lead to generalized lymphadenopathy.

Malignant Lymphomas

Lymphomas consist of a diverse group of neoplasms that develop from the proliferation of malignant lymphocytes in the lymphoid system (immune system). There are three major categories of lymphoid malignancies, based on morphology and cell lineage: (1) B-cell neoplasms; (2) T-cell and natural killer (NK)–cell neoplasms; and (3) the two general categories of HL and NHL. NHL can be further divided into cancers that have an indolent (slow-growing) course and those with an aggressive (fast-growing) course. These different subtypes progress and respond to treatment differently. Both HL and NHL occur in children and adults, and the overall treatment and prognosis depend on the stage and type of lymphoma.

Lymphoma is the most common blood cancer in Canada. Incidence rates of lymphoma differ with respect to age, gender, geographic location, and socioeconomic class. The incidence rate per 100 000 population reported in 2016 for NHL was 21, and that for HL was 3.[44] Since the early 1970s, the incidence of NHL has nearly doubled. The exact reason for this increase remains a mystery; however, a modest portion of the increase had been attributed to lymphomas developing in association with immune deficiencies, including AIDS and organ transplants. Conversely, the incidence of HL has declined over the same time period, especially among older adults.

In general, lymphomas are the result of genetic mutations or viral infection. Malignant transformation produces a cell with uncontrolled and excessive growth that accumulates in the lymph nodes and other sites, producing tumour masses.

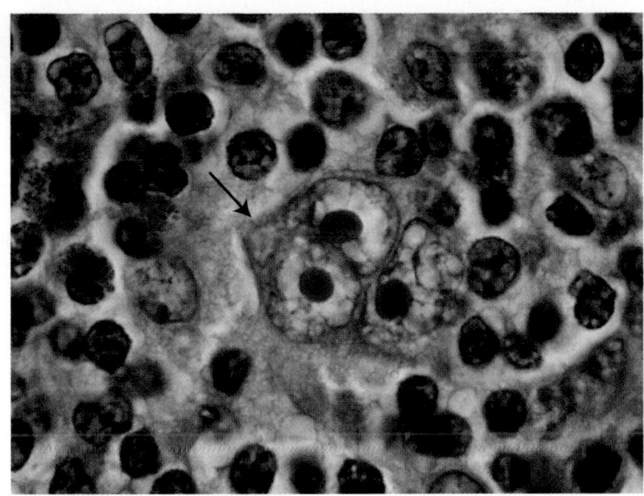

FIGURE 21-11 Lymph Nodes. Diagnostic Reed-Sternberg cell (*arrow*). A large multinucleated or multilobed cell with inclusion body–like nucleoli surrounded by a halo of clear nucleoplasm. (From Damjanov, I., & Linder, J. [Eds.]. [1996]. *Anderson's pathology* [10th ed.]. St. Louis: Mosby.)

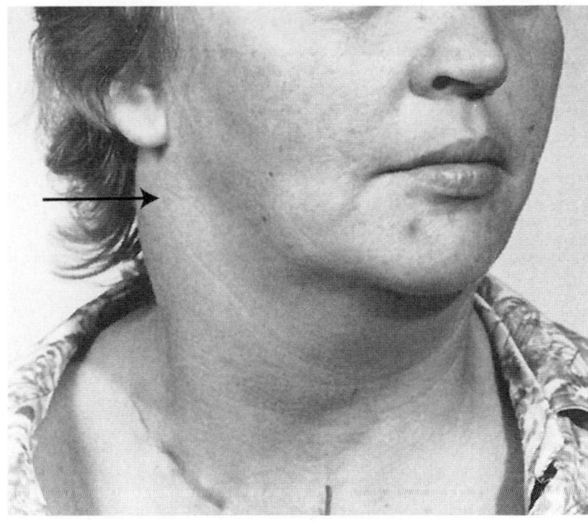

FIGURE 21-12 Hodgkin's Lymphoma and Enlarged Cervical Lymph Node. Typical enlarged cervical lymph node in the neck (*arrow*) of a 35-year-old woman with Hodgkin's lymphoma. (From Ackerman, L.V., del Regato, J.A., Spjut, H.J., et al. [1985]. *Cancer: Diagnosis, treatment, and prognosis* [6th ed.]. St. Louis: Mosby.)

Hodgkin's Lymphoma

Hodgkin's lymphoma (HL) is a malignant lymphoma that progresses from one group of lymph nodes to another, including the development of systemic symptoms, and the presence of B cells called **Reed-Sternberg (RS) cells**.[45,46] (see "Pathophysiology"). In about 70% of cases, RS cells are infected with EBV. The 2015 incidence of HL was approximately 3.0 per 100 000 males and 2.5 per 100 000 females; it peaks at two different times—during the second and third decades of life and later during the sixth and seventh decades.[47] The incidence is greater in Whites than in Blacks, with Denmark, the Netherlands, and the United States having the highest incidence and Japan and Australia having the lowest.

PATHOPHYSIOLOGY It is widely accepted that the RS cell represents the malignant transformed lymphocyte (Figure 21-11). RS cells are often large and binucleate with occasional mononuclear variants. RS cells are necessary for the diagnosis of HL; however, they are not specific to HL. In rare instances, cells resembling RS cells can be found in benign illnesses, as well as in other forms of cancer, including NHL and solid tissue cancers and in IM.

The triggering mechanism for the malignant transformation of cells remains unknown. Classic HL appears to be derived from a B cell in the germinal centre that has not undergone successful immunoglobulin gene rearrangement (see Chapter 7) and would normally be induced to undergo apoptosis. Survival of this cell may be linked to infection with EBV. Laboratory and epidemiological studies have linked HL with EBV infections, and EBV DNA, RNA, and proteins are frequently observed in HL cells.[48] The EBV epigenome poses a variety of viral-encoded and host-cell factors that control epigenetic regulation by expanding tissue growth, evading immune detection, and driving host-cell carcinogenesis. RS cells secrete and release cytokines (e.g., IL-10, transforming growth factor-beta [TGF-β]) that result in the accumulation of inflammatory cells, which produces local and systemic effects. HL is subcategorized into two main types: classic Hodgkin's and nodular lymphocyte–predominant Hodgkin's. Classic HL is subclassified into four types based on the morphology of RS cells and the characteristics of the inflammatory cell infiltrate in the tumour. Lymphocyte-predominant disease presents with earlier-stage disease, longer survival, and fewer treatment failures than classic HL.[49] However, despite a more favourable prognosis, lymphocyte-predominant HL has a tendency to histologically transform into diffuse large B-cell lymphoma by 10 years in approximately 10% of people.[50]

CLINICAL MANIFESTATIONS Many clinical features of HL can be explained by the complex action of cytokines and other growth factors that are secreted and released by the malignant cells. These substances induce infiltration and proliferation of inflammatory cells, resulting in an enlarged, painless lymph node in the neck (often the first sign of HL) (Figure 21-12). The discovery of an asymptomatic mediastinal mass on routine chest X-ray is not uncommon. The cervical, axillary, inguinal, and retroperitoneal lymph nodes are commonly affected in HL (Figure 21-13). Local symptoms caused by pressure and obstruction of the lymph nodes are the result of the lymphadenopathy.

About one-third of individuals will have some common systemic symptoms, such as intermittent fever, without other symptoms of infection, drenching night sweats, itchy skin (pruritus), and fatigue. These constitutional symptoms accompanied by weight loss are associated with a poor prognosis.

Although HL rarely arises in the lung, mediastinal and hilar node adenopathy can cause secondary involvement of the trachea, bronchi, pleura, or lungs. Retroperitoneal nodes can involve vertebral bodies and nerves and also can cause displacement of ureters. Spinal cord involvement is more common in the dorsal and lumbar regions than in the cervical region. Skin lesions, although uncommon, include psoriasis and eczematoid lesions, causing itching and scratching.

As a result of direct invasion from mediastinal lymph nodes, pericardial involvement can cause pericardial friction rub, pericardial effusion, and engorgement of neck veins. The GI tract and urinary tract are rarely involved. Anemia is often found in individuals with HL accompanied by a low serum iron level and reduced iron-binding capacity. Other laboratory findings include elevated sedimentation rate, leukocytosis, and eosinophilia. Leukopenia occurs in advanced stages of HL.

Splenic involvement in HL depends on histological type. In mixed cellularity and lymphocytic deletion types of HL, the spleen is involved in 60% of cases. With lymphocyte and nodular sclerosis types, 34% of cases involve the spleen.

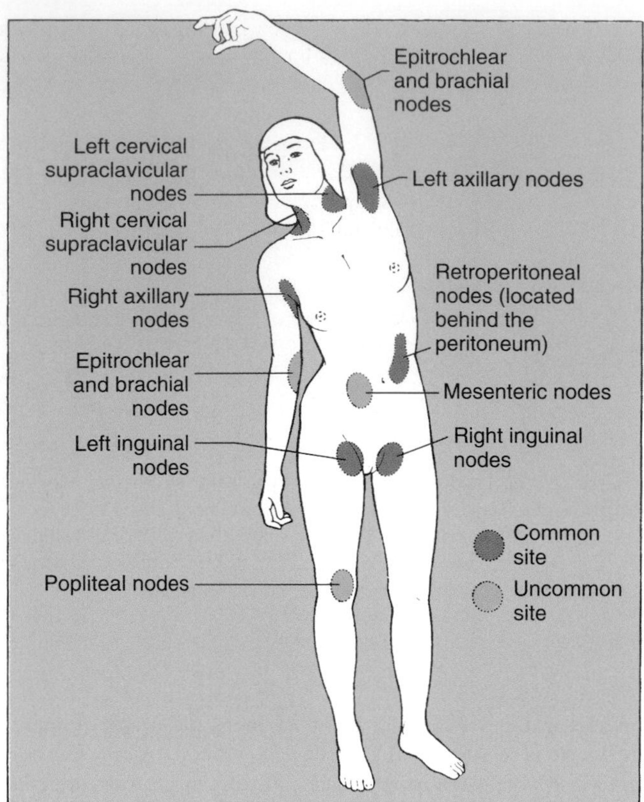

FIGURE 21-13 Common and Uncommon Involved Lymph Node Sites for Hodgkin's Lymphoma.

TABLE 21-7 Definitions of Stages of Hodgkin's Lymphoma

Stage	Criteria
I	Involvement of a single lymph node region (I) or localized involvement of a single extralymphatic organ or site (I_E)[a]
II	Involvement of two or more lymph node regions on same side of diaphragm (II) or localized involvement of a single associated extralymphatic organ or site and its regional lymph node(s), with or without involvement of other lymph node regions on same side of diaphragm (II_E)
III	Involvement of lymph node regions on both sides of diaphragm (III), which may also be accompanied by localized involvement of an associated extralymphatic organ or site (III_E), by involvement of the spleen (III_S), or by both (III_{E+S})
IV	Disseminated (multifocal) involvement of one or more extralymphatic organs, with or without associated lymph node involvement, or isolated extralymphatic organ involvement with distant (nonregional) nodal involvement
A: No systemic symptoms present	
B: Unexplained fevers >38°C [100.4°F], drenching night sweats, or weight loss >10% of body weight	

[a]The number of lymph node regions involved may be indicated by a subscript (e.g., II_3).

From National Comprehensive Cancer Network. (2014). Hodgkin lymphoma. In *NCCN practice guidelines, Version 2. 2014: Hodgkin lymphoma* (originally adapted from Carbono, P.P., Kaplan, H.S., Musshoff, K., et al. [1971]. *Cancer Res, 31*[11], 1860–1861).

EVALUATION AND TREATMENT Because of the variability in symptoms, early definitive detection may be challenging. Asymptomatic lymphadenopathy can progress undetected for several years. Diagnosis is made from physical examination and history, complete blood count (CBC), blood chemistry studies including sedimentation rate, lymph node biopsy, pathology review for RS cells, and immunophenotyping for disease markers.[51] Clinical staging for individuals with HL includes personal history; physical examination; laboratory studies, including sedimentation rate; and thoracic and abdominal/pelvic computed tomography (CT) scans[51] (Table 21-7). Positron emission tomography (PET) scans, usually combined with CT scans, have replaced gallium scans and lymphangiography for clinical staging.[52] Staging laparotomy is no longer recommended; it should be considered only when the results will allow substantial reduction in treatment. It should not be done in individuals who require chemotherapy. If the laparotomy is required for treatment decisions, the risks of potential morbidity should be considered.[52] Prognostic indicators include clinical stage, histological type, tumour cell concentration and tumour burden, constitutional symptoms, and age of the individual.

The effectiveness of treatment is related to the age, gender, and general health of the individual; signs and symptoms; stage of the disease; blood test results; type of HL; and classification of the disease as recurrent or progressive. Adult HL can usually be cured with early diagnosis and treatment.[51] Three types of treatment are used: chemotherapy, radiation therapy, and surgery. Treatment for pregnant women includes watchful waiting and steroid therapy. Newer treatments undergoing testing include chemotherapy and radiation therapy with stem cell transplant and monoclonal antibody therapy.[51] Treatment with chemotherapy or radiation therapy, or both, may increase the risk for secondary cancers, cardiovascular disease, and other health problems for many months or years after treatment.

Non-Hodgkin's Lymphoma

Non-Hodgkin's lymphoma (NHL) is not a single disease, but a heterogeneous group of proliferative lymphoid tissue neoplasms with differing clinical patterns of behaviour and responses to treatment. The generic classification of NHL that was used in the past has been reclassified into (1) B-cell neoplasms, a group that consists of a variety of lymphomas including myelomas that originate from B cells at various stages of differentiation; and (2) T-cell neoplasms and NK-cell neoplasms, a group that includes lymphomas that originate from either T or NK cells. These cancers are differentiated from HL by a lack of RS cells and other cellular changes not characteristic of HL.

In 2017, it was estimated that 8 300 Canadians would be diagnosed with NHL, and 2 700 Canadians would die from the disease.[35] The median age of diagnosis is 67 years and the highest incidences of NHL are in North America, Europe, Oceania, and several African countries.[53] The occurrence of NHL is higher in men than in women. For unknown reasons, incidence increased in many high-income countries between the 1950s and 1990s and no further increase has been observed during the last decade.[53] Part of the increased incidence has been attributed to diagnostic improvements as well as AIDS-related cancers following the HIV epidemic.[53] Conversely, the mortality has risen at a slower rate. It is thought that newer treatment modalities are improving survival rates.

PATHOPHYSIOLOGY NHL is best described as a progressive clonal expansion of B cells, T cells, or NK cells. B cells account for 85 to 90% of NHLs, with most of the remainder being T cells and rarely NK cells. Oncogenes may be activated by chromosomal translocations, or the tumour-suppressor loci may be inactivated by deletion or mutation of chromosomes. Certain subtypes may have altered genomes by oncogenic viruses. The various subtypes of NHL may be identified by specific diagnostic markers related to various cytogenetic lesions. The most common type of chromosomal alteration in NHL is translocation, which disrupts the genes encoded at the breakpoints. Unlike HL, NHL spreads in a less predictable way and spreads widely early.[36] Diffuse large B-cell lymphoma (DLBCL) is the most common form of NHL.

Risk factors for adult NHL include being older, male, or White and having one of the following: being afflicted by certain inherited immune disorders, an autoimmune disease, or HIV/AIDS; exposure to a variety of mutagenic chemicals or certain pesticides; infection with certain cancer-related viruses (e.g., EBV, HIV, human T-cell lymphotropic virus type 1 [HTLV-1]); consumption of a diet high in meats and fat; and use of immunosuppression medications after an organ transplant. Gastric infection with *H. pylori* increases the risk for gastric lymphomas. NHL is a disease of middle age, usually found in persons more than 50 years old.

CLINICAL MANIFESTATIONS Clinical manifestations of NHL usually begin as localized or generalized lymphadenopathy, similar to HL. Differences in clinical features are noted in Table 21-8. The cervical, axillary, inguinal, and femoral lymph node chains are the most commonly affected sites. Generally, the swelling is painless and the nodes have enlarged and transformed over a period of months or years. Other sites of involvement are the nasopharynx, GI tract, bone, thyroid, testes, and soft tissue. Some individuals have retroperitoneal and abdominal masses with symptoms of abdominal fullness, back pain, ascites (fluid in the peritoneal cavity), skin rash or itchy skin, fatigue, fever of unknown origin, drenching night sweats, and leg swelling.

Lymphomas are classified as low, intermediate, or high grade. A low-grade lymphoma, which also may be termed *indolent*, has a slow progression. Individuals with low-grade lymphoma commonly present with a painless, peripheral adenopathy. Spontaneous regression of these nodes may occur, mimicking the presence of an infection. Night sweats with an elevated temperature (more than 38°C [100.4°F]) and weight loss, as well as extranodular involvement, are not commonly present in the early stages but are common in advanced or end-stage disease. Cytopenia, or reduction in the number of blood cells, reflective of bone marrow involvement is often observed. Hepatomegaly is common; however, splenomegaly is present in approximately 40% of individuals. Fatigue and weakness are more prevalent with advanced stages.

TABLE 21-8 Clinical Differences Between Non-Hodgkin's Lymphoma and Hodgkin's Lymphoma

Characteristics	Non-Hodgkin's Lymphoma	Hodgkin's Lymphoma
Nodal involvement	Multiple peripheral nodes	Localized to single axial group of nodes (i.e., cervical, mediastinal, para-aortic)
	Mesenteric nodes and Waldeyer's tonsillar ring commonly involved	Mesenteric nodes and Waldeyer's tonsillar ring rarely involved
Spread	Noncontiguous	Orderly spread by contiguity
B symptoms[a]	Uncommon	Common
Extranodal involvement	Common	Rare
Extent of disease	Rarely localized	Often localized

[a]Fever, weight loss, night sweats.

Intermediate- and high-grade lymphomas, which are more aggressive, have a more varied clinical presentation. A high-grade lymphoma also may be termed *aggressive*.

EVALUATION AND TREATMENT The primary means for diagnosis of NHL is physical examination and history, blood tests, urine tests, flow cytometry, and bone marrow aspirate and biopsy. A common finding in NHL is noncontiguous lymph node involvement, which is not common in HL.

Treatment for NHL is quite diverse and depends on type (B cell or T cell), tumour stage, histological status (low, intermediate, or high grade), symptoms, age, and presence of comorbidities.[54] Depending on the type (B cell or T cell) of the tumour, stage of disease, and aggressiveness of the tumour, treatment is usually initiated at the time of diagnosis. However, because treatment is not curative for some low-grade indolent lymphomas that are widely disseminated, observation without treatment may be the most appropriate choice. These indolent tumours are often not symptomatic for the individual and this approach improves quality of life. In some cases, the disease may be so slow growing that treatment is not needed for an extended period of time.

Standard treatment for NHL includes radiation therapy, chemotherapy, target therapy (monoclonal antibody therapy, proteasome inhibitor therapy), plasmapheresis (if the blood becomes thick), biological therapy (e.g., interferon), and watchful waiting. Several factors affect prognosis, including the stage of the cancer, the type of NHL, the blood levels of lactate dehydrogenase, the amount of β_2-microglobulin in the blood (for Waldenström macroglobulinemia), the age and general health of the patient, and the properties of the lymphoma (i.e., whether it was recently diagnosed or is a recurrence). Indolent NHL types can have a median survival as long as 20 years but are not curable in advanced stages.[55] Those with the aggressive type of NHL have a more limited survival, but a significant number of individuals can achieve a cure with an intensive combination of chemotherapy. With modern treatments for NHL, the overall survival at 5 years for nonaggressive NHL is greater than 60%, and for aggressive types greater than 50%. High-grade NHL is seen with increasing frequency in persons with AIDS and has an extremely poor prognosis. New research suggests that a novel therapeutic approach may hold promise for individuals with chemotherapy-refractory advanced large B-cell lymphoma and indolent B-cell malignancies using engineered T cells that express an anti-CD19 chimeric antigen receptor.[56]

Burkitt lymphoma. **Burkitt lymphoma** is a B-cell tumour with unique clinical and epidemiological features. Although more common in Africa, Burkitt lymphoma is not confined to the African continent and is documented in Canada, the United States, Latin America, and other Western countries. Classification of Burkitt lymphoma includes (1) African (endemic) Burkitt lymphoma, (2) sporadic (nonendemic) Burkitt lymphoma, and (3) a subset of aggressive lymphomas in individuals infected with HIV. Burkitt lymphomas, in these classifications, are histologically identical but differ in some genetic, virological, and clinical characteristics.[36] Burkitt lymphoma is a fast-growing tumour that often appears as a large tumour mass in the jaw and sometimes the abdomen (Figure 21-14). It is now understood that Burkitt lymphoma is heterogeneous, and pathological confirmation is sometimes challenging.

PATHOPHYSIOLOGY Basically, all endemic Burkitt lymphomas are latently infected with EBV, which also is present in about 25% of HIV-associated tumours and 15 to 20% of sporadic cases.[36] It is suspected that suppression of the immune system by other illnesses (e.g., HIV infection, chronic malaria) increases the individual's susceptibility to EBV. B cells are particularly sensitive because of specific surface receptors

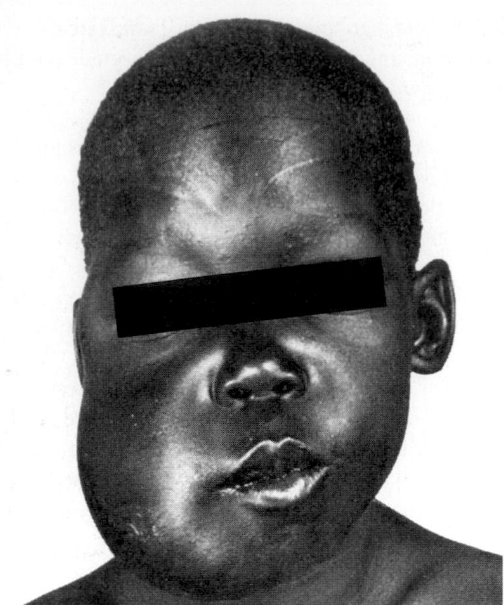

FIGURE 21-14 Burkitt Lymphoma. Burkitt lymphoma involving the jaw in a young African boy. (Courtesy I. Magrath, MD, Bethesda, MD. From Zitelli, B.J., McIntire, S.C., & Nowalk, A.J. [2012]. *Zitelli and Davis' atlas of pediatric physical diagnosis* [6th ed.]. Philadelphia: Saunders.)

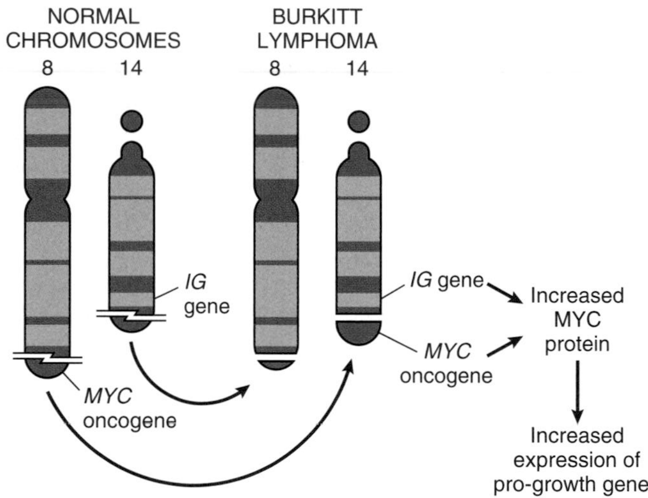

FIGURE 21-15 Burkitt Lymphoma Cells. The 8,14 chromosomal translocation and associated oncogenes in Burkitt lymphoma. *IG,* immunoglobulin; *MYC,* myelocytomatosis viral oncogene homologue.

for EBV. As a result, the B cell undergoes chromosomal translocations that result in overexpression of the *c-MYC* proto-oncogene and loss of control of cell growth (Figure 21-15). The most common translocation (75% of individuals) is between chromosomes 8 (containing the *c-MYC* gene) and 14 (containing the immunoglobulin heavy chain genes). When the t(8;14) translocation occurs, the *MYC* gene becomes regulated by the B-cell immunoglobulin gene (*IG*) on chromosome 14, and overproduction of MYC protein forces proliferation and blocks cellular differentiation. MYC is a transcriptional regulator that increases genes responsible for aerobic glycolysis (Warburg effect). When glucose and glutamine are available, the Warburg metabolism enables cells to synthesize nutrients that are needed for growth and cell division. Therefore, investigators believe that Burkitt lymphoma is the fastest-growing tumour.[36] Other translocations have been reported between chromosome 8 and chromosomes 2 or 22, which contain genes for immunoglobulin light chains.

CLINICAL MANIFESTATIONS The endemic (mainly occurring in Africa) and sporadic Burkitt lymphomas (the most common type in North America and European countries and without obvious infectious cofactors) are found mostly in children or young adults. Most tumours manifest at extranodal locations. Endemic Burkitt lymphoma usually presents as a mass of the mandible and an unusual tendency for involvement of the abdominal viscera, including the kidneys, ovaries, and adrenal glands. Sporadic Burkitt lymphoma usually appears as a mass involving the ileocecum and peritoneum. More advanced disease may involve other organs—eyes, ovaries, kidneys, glandular tissue (breast, thyroid, tonsil)—and presents with type B symptoms (night sweats, fever, weight loss).

EVALUATION AND TREATMENT The distribution of tumours and biopsies of enlarged lymph nodes or the bone marrow containing malignant B cells are usually indicative of Burkitt lymphoma. It is one of the most aggressive and quickly growing malignancies. Burkitt lymphoma, however, responds successfully to intensive chemotherapy in most children and adults. The outcome is more cautious in older adults.

Lymphoblastic lymphoma. Lymphoblastic lymphoma (LL) is a relatively rare variant of NHL overall (2 to 4%) but accounts for almost one-third of cases of NHL in children and adolescents, with a male predominance. The vast majority of LL (90%) is of T-cell origin; the remainder arises from B cells. LL is similar to acute lymphoblastic leukemia and may be considered a variant of that disease.

PATHOPHYSIOLOGY The disease arises from a clone of relatively immature T cells that becomes malignant in the thymus. As with most lymphoid tumours, LL is frequently associated with translocations, primarily of the chromosomes that encode for the T-cell receptor (chromosomes 7 and 14). These aberrations result in increased expression of a variety of transcription factors and loss of growth control.

CLINICAL MANIFESTATIONS The first sign of LL is usually a painless lymphadenopathy in the neck. Peripheral lymph nodes in the chest become involved in about 70% of individuals. Involved nodes are located mostly above the diaphragm. LL is a very aggressive tumour that presents as stage IV in most people. T-cell LL is associated with a unique mediastinal mass (up to 75%) because of the apparent origin of the tumour in the thymus. The mass results in dyspnea and chest pain and may cause compression of bronchi or the superior vena cava. The tumour may infiltrate the bone marrow in about half of those affected, and suppression of bone marrow hematopoiesis leads to increased susceptibility to infections. Other organs, including the liver, kidney, spleen, and brain, also may be affected. Many individuals express type B symptoms: fever, night sweats, and significant weight loss.

EVALUATION AND TREATMENT The most common therapeutic approach is combined chemotherapy (intensive therapy). Bulky tumour masses are sometimes treated with radiation therapy. In early stages of the disease, the response rate is high with increased survival; the 5-year survival in children is 80 to 90% and 45 to 55% in adults. Although LL is easily treated, there is a high relapse rate: 40 to 60% of adults.

Multiple myeloma. Multiple myeloma (MM) is a plasma cell (a white blood cell neoplasm called *myeloma cells*) cancer characterized by the slow proliferation of malignant cells, with tumour cell masses in the bone marrow usually resulting in destruction of the bone (Figure 21-16).[57] Myeloma cells reside in the bone marrow and are usually not found in the peripheral blood. As the number of myeloma cells increases, fewer red blood cells, white blood cells, and platelets are produced. Myeloma may spread to other tissues, especially in very advanced stages

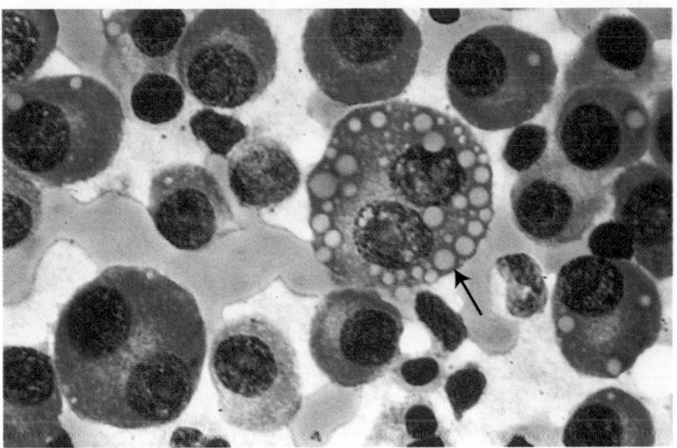

FIGURE 21-16 Multiple Myeloma, Bone Marrow Aspirate. Normal marrow cells are largely replaced by plasma cells, including atypical forms with multiple nuclei (*arrow*), and cytoplasmic droplets containing immunoglobulin. (From Kumar, V., Abbas, A.K., & Aster, J.C. [Eds.]. [2015]. *Robbins and Cotran pathologic basis of disease* [9th ed.]. Philadelphia: Saunders.)

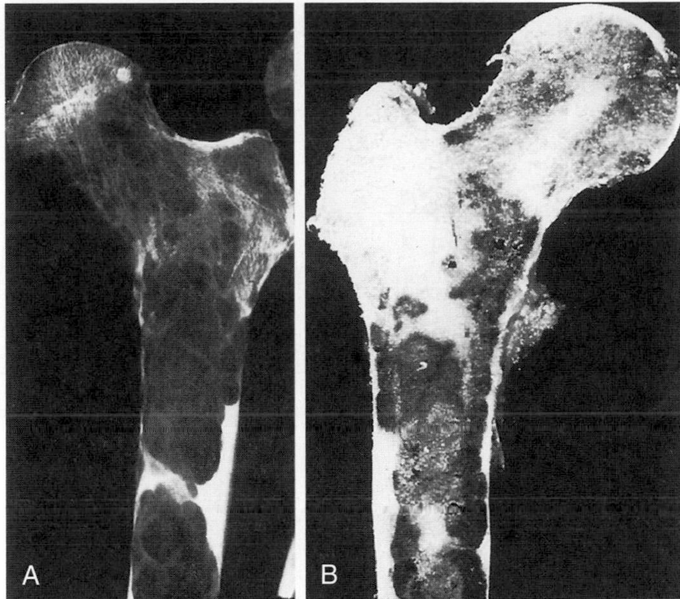

FIGURE 21-17 Multiple (Plasma Cell) Myeloma. A, Roentgenogram of femur showing extensive bone destruction caused by tumour. Note the absence of reactive bone formation. **B,** Gross specimen from the same individual; myelomatous sections appear as dark granular sections. (From Kissane, J.M. [Ed.]. [1990]. *Anderson's pathology* [9th ed.]. St. Louis: Mosby.)

of the disease. The reported incidence of MM has doubled in the past two decades, possibly as a result of more sensitive testing used for diagnosis. The annual incidence rate in Western industrialized countries is 4 per 100 000, and it was estimated that 2 900 new cases would be diagnosed in Canada in 2017.[35,58] MM occurs in all races, but in the United States the incidence in Blacks is about twice that of Whites. It rarely occurs before the age of 40 years—the peak age of incidence is between 65 and 70 years. It is slightly more common in men than in women. Other risk factors include exposure to radiation or certain chemicals and a history of monoclonal gammopathy of undetermined significance (MGUS; see "Clinical Manifestations") or plasmacytoma.

PATHOPHYSIOLOGY MM is a plasma cell neoplasia that causes lytic bone lesions (bony disease; radiologically appears as punched-out defects), hypercalcemia, renal failure, anemia, and immune abnormalities.[36,59] Multiple mutations in different pathways alter the intrinsic biology of the plasma cell, generating the features of myeloma.[60] MM tumours are highly heterogeneous.[61] Defining driver mutations and heterogeneity is essential for treatment decisions. Many myelomas are aneuploidy and, in most individuals with myeloma, chromosomal translocations are the most common. The primary translocation involves the immunoglobulin heavy chain on chromosome 14 and fibroblast growth factor receptor on chromosome 4.[62] Other reported chromosomal abnormalities include deletion of chromosome 13 and deletion of chromosome 17.[62] Development of further secondary genetic alterations causes progression to an aggressive MM. Investigators are studying various epigenetic alterations and interactions with extracellular matrix proteins. For example, myeloma cells interact and secrete peptides that adhere to stromal cells, inducing cytokines that possibly promote inflammation. Myeloma cells are prone to the accumulation of misfolded protein, such as unpaired immunoglobulin chains. Misfolded proteins activate apoptosis.

Malignant plasma cells arise from one clone of B cells that produce abnormally large amounts of one class of immunoglobulin (usually IgG, occasionally IgA, and rarely IgM, IgD, or IgE). The malignant transformation may begin early in B-cell development, possibly before encountering antigens in the secondary lymphoid organs. The myeloma cells return either to the bone marrow or to other soft tissue sites. Their return is aided by cell adhesion molecules that help them target favourable sites that promote continued expansion and maturation. Cytokines, particularly IL-6, have been identified as essential factors that promote the growth and survival of MM cells. (Lymphocytes and cytokines are described in Chapter 6.)

Myeloma cells in the bone marrow produce several cytokines themselves (e.g., IL-6, IL-1, IL-11, tumour necrosis factor-alpha [TNF-α]). IL-6 in particular acts as an osteoclast-activating factor and stimulates osteoclasts to reabsorb bone. This process results in bone lesions and hypercalcemia (high calcium levels in the blood) attributable to the release of calcium from the breakdown of bone.

The antibody produced by the transformed plasma cell is frequently defective, containing truncations, deletions, and other abnormalities, and is often referred to as a *paraprotein* (abnormal protein in the blood). Because of the large number of malignant plasma cells, the abnormal antibody, called the **M protein**, becomes the most prominent protein in the blood (as Figure 21-18 shows). Suppression of normal plasma cells by the myeloma results in diminished or absent normal antibodies. The excessive amount of M protein also may contribute to many of the clinical manifestations of the disease. Frequently, the myeloma produces free immunoglobulin light chain **(Bence Jones protein)** that is present in the blood and urine and contributes to damage of renal tubular cells.

CLINICAL MANIFESTATIONS The common presentation of MM is characterized by elevated levels of calcium in the blood (hypercalcemia), renal failure, anemia, and bone lesions. The hypercalcemia and bone lesions result from infiltration of the bone by malignant plasma cells and stimulation of osteoclasts to reabsorb bone. This process results in the release of calcium (hypercalcemia) and the development of "lytic lesions" (round, "punched-out" regions of bone) (Figure 21-17). Destruction of bone tissue causes pain, the most common presenting symptom, and pathological fractures. The bones most commonly involved, in decreasing order of frequency, are the vertebrae, ribs, skull, pelvis, femur, clavicle, and scapula. Spinal cord compression, because

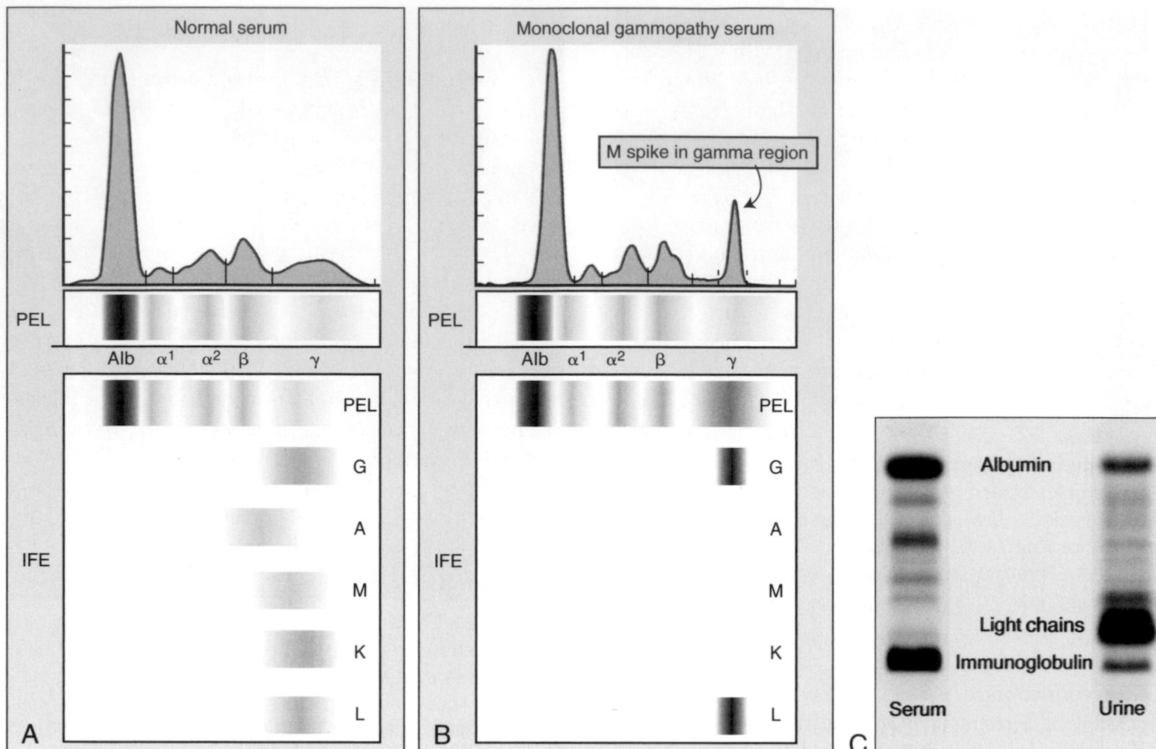

FIGURE 21-18 M Protein. Serum protein electrophoresis (*PEL*) is used to screen for M proteins in multiple myeloma. **A,** In normal serum the proteins separate into several regions between albumin (*Alb*) and a broad band in the gamma (γ) region, where most antibodies (gamma globulins) are found. Immunofixation (*IFE*) can identify the location of IgG (*G*), IgA (*A*), IgM (*M*), and kappa (κ) and lambda (*L*) light chains. **B,** Serum from an individual with multiple myeloma contains a sharp M protein (*M spike*). The M protein is monoclonal and contains only one heavy chain and one light chain. In this instance, the IFE identifies the M protein as an IgG containing a lambda light chain. **C,** Serum and urine protein electrophoretic patterns in an individual with multiple myeloma. Serum demonstrates an M protein (*Immunoglobulin*) in the gamma region, and the urine has a large amount of the smaller-sized light chains with only a small amount of the intact immunoglobulin. *Ig,* immunoglobulin. (**A** and **B,** from Abeloff, M., Armitage, J., Niederhuber, J., et al. [2008]. *Abeloff's clinical oncology* [4th ed.]. Philadelphia: Churchill Livingstone. **C,** from McPherson, R., & Pincus, M. [2012]. *Henry's clinical diagnosis and management by laboratory methods* [22nd ed.]. Edinburgh: Saunders.)

of the weakened vertebrae, occurs in about 10% of individuals. A condition called **amyloidosis** may occur, in which antibody proteins increase and stick together in peripheral nerves and organs, such as the kidney and heart. Signs and symptoms of amyloidosis include fatigue, purple spots on the skin, enlarged tongue, diarrhea, edema, and numbness or tingling in the legs and feet.

Proteinuria is observed in 90% of individuals. Renal failure may be either acute or chronic and is usually secondary to the hypercalcemia. Bence Jones protein may lead to damage of the proximal tubules. Anemia is usually normocytic and normochromic and results from inhibited erythropoiesis caused by tumour cell infiltration of the bone marrow.

The high concentration of paraprotein in the blood may lead to hyperviscosity syndrome. The increased viscosity interferes with blood circulation to various sites (brain, kidneys, extremities). Hyperviscosity syndrome is observed in up to 20% of persons. Additional neurological symptoms (e.g., confusion, headaches, blurred vision) may occur secondary to hypercalcemia or hyperviscosity.

Suppression of the humoral (antibody-mediated) immune response results in repeated infections, primarily pneumonias and pyelonephritis. The most commonly involved microorganisms are encapsulated bacteria that are particularly sensitive to the effects of antibody; pneumonia caused by *Streptococcus pneumoniae*, *Staphylococcus aureus*, or *K. pneumoniae*; or pyelonephritis caused by *E. coli* or other Gram-negative organisms. Cell-mediated (T-cell) function is relatively normal. Overwhelming infection is the leading cause of death from MM.

MM is a progressive disorder and is often preceded by a condition known as **monoclonal gammopathy of undetermined significance (MGUS)**. MGUS is diagnosed by the presence of an M protein in the blood or urine without additional evidence of MM.[63] MGUS is present in approximately 1% of the general population and in 3% of individuals older than 70 years. Although MGUS is considered nonpathological and requires no treatment, about 2% of individuals with MGUS progress to malignant plasma cell disorders. Progression of MM following MGUS advances to asymptomatic MM and finally symptomatic MM. Asymptomatic MM also may be referred to as **smouldering myeloma** and indolent myeloma.[63] Smouldering myeloma is usually characterized by the presence of an M protein and clonal bone marrow plasma cells, but with no indication of end-organ damage.

EVALUATION AND TREATMENT Diagnosis of MM is made by symptoms and radiographic and laboratory studies; a definitive diagnosis requires a bone marrow biopsy. The International Myeloma Working Group's new criteria[63] for the diagnosis of MM include biomarkers (monoclonal components in serum and urine; quantification of immunoglobulins IgG, IgA, and IgM; and characterization of the heavy and light chains by immunofixation) and the presence of hypercalcemia, renal failure, anemia, and bone lesions (CRAB). Other criteria include evaluation of bone marrow plasma cell infiltration by bone marrow biopsy and radiological evaluation of lytic bone lesions. Biomarkers based on quantitation of plasma cells (serum-free light chains) may help stratify risk for people with asymptomatic MM and identification, staging, prognosis, and monitoring of those with smouldering MM who are at an "ultra-high" risk of developing aggressive MM.

New techniques use microRNAs extracted from serum to measure immunoglobulins (IgG, IgM, IgA). Typically, one class of immunoglobulin (the M protein produced by the myeloma cell) is greatly increased, whereas the others are suppressed. Serum electrophoretic analysis shows increased levels of M protein (see Figure 21-18). Because the M protein is monoclonal, each molecule has the same electric charge and migrates at about the same site on electrophoresis, resulting in a highly concentrated protein (M spike) (see Figure 21-18). Bence Jones protein may be observed in the urine or serum by immunoelectrophoresis or in the serum using available enzyme-linked immunosorbent assays (ELISAs). Usually an intact antibody paraprotein coexists with Bence Jones protein. However, variants of MM include individuals in which free light chain only is produced and a rare variant that produces only free heavy chain; about 1% of cases are nonsecretory so that neither M protein nor Bence Jones protein is produced. Measurement of another protein, free **β2-microglobulin**, is used as an indicator of prognosis or effectiveness of therapy.

Although combinations of chemotherapy, radiation therapy, plasmapheresis (exchange), and stem cell transplant have been used for treatment, the prognosis for persons with MM remains poor. However, with the new high-sensitivity biomarkers that are associated with inevitable development of clinical symptoms, early diagnosis and treatment may be possible before individuals develop more advanced disease and organ damage. Conventional combinations of chemotherapeutic agents have included melphalan (Alkeran) and prednisone (Deltasone); prednisone with vincristine (Oncovin); carmustine (BiCNU) and cyclophosphamide (Procytox); vincristine, doxorubicin (Adriamycin), and dexamethasone (Decadron); and thalidomide (Thalomid) and dexamethasone. Thalidomide disrupts the stromal marrow–MM cell interaction by modulating cell-surface adhesion molecules and inhibiting angiogenesis. In addition, it increases apoptosis and G_1 growth arrest (i.e., the cell cycle gap 1; see Chapter 1) of MM cells. Hematopoietic stem cell transplantation has prolonged life but has not yet proven to be curative.[36] Controversy exists concerning whether tandem stem cell transplant offers the best outcome. Bisphosphonate therapy is the primary treatment for bone lesions. Individuals with multiple bone lesions, if untreated, rarely survive more than 6 to 12 months. Individuals with inactive (indolent) myeloma, however, can survive for many years. With chemotherapy and aggressive management of complications, the prognosis can improve significantly, with a median survival of 24 to 30 months and a 10-year survival rate of 3%. Promising new therapies include the use of proteasome inhibitors because proteasome degrades misfolded and unwanted proteins. The rates of new myeloma cases are increasing 0.7% each year and the death rates have decreased an average of 1.3% each year from 2002 to 2011. The 5-year survival for all stages of MM is 45.1%.

QUICK CHECK 21-4

1. Contrast the principal features of Hodgkin's lymphoma with those of non-Hodgkin's lymphoma.
2. What is Burkitt lymphoma?
3. Define what is meant by the following statement: Multiple myeloma (MM) is heterogeneous.
4. What are the main pathological features of MM?

ALTERATIONS OF SPLENIC FUNCTION

The complexities of splenic function are not totally understood, and its mysteries are still being studied. The normal functions of the spleen that may impact disease states include (1) phagocytosis of blood cells and particulate matter (e.g., bacteria), (2) antibody production, (3) hematopoiesis, and (4) sequestration of formed blood elements. The spleen is part of the mononuclear phagocyte system and is involved in all systemic inflammations, hematopoietic disorders, and many metabolic disorders.

In the past, **splenomegaly** (enlargement of the spleen) has been associated with various disease states. It is now recognized that splenomegaly is not necessarily pathological; an enlarged spleen may be present in certain individuals without any evidence of disease. Splenomegaly may be, however, one of the first physical signs of underlying conditions, and its presence should not be ignored. In conditions where splenomegaly is present, the normal functions of the spleen may become overactive, producing a syndrome known as **hypersplenism**. Hypersplenism is characterized by anemia, leukopenia, and thrombocytopenia alone or in combination. Some individuals may seek treatment for problems even though they have not met all the aforementioned clinical criteria; therefore, the relevance and significance of hypersplenism are still uncertain.

PATHOPHYSIOLOGY Specific conditions causing splenomegaly and resulting hypersplenism are many and are related to other categories of disease (Box 21-1). Different pathological processes that produce splenomegaly are described briefly next.

Acute inflammatory or infectious processes cause splenomegaly because of an increased demand for defensive activities. Acutely enlarged spleens secondary to infection may become so filled with erythrocytes that their natural rubbery resilience is lost and they become fragile and vulnerable to blunt trauma. Splenic rupture is a complication associated with IM; rupture occurs mostly in males between days 4 and 21 of acute illness.

Congestive splenomegaly is accompanied by ascites, portal hypertension, and esophageal varices and is most commonly seen in those

BOX 21-1 Diseases Related to Classification of Splenomegaly

Inflammation or Infection

Acute: viral (hepatitis, infectious mononucleosis, cytomegalovirus), bacterial (salmonella, Gram-negative), parasitic (typhoid)

Subacute or chronic: bacterial (subacute bacterial endocarditis, tuberculosis), parasitic (malaria), fungal (histoplasmosis), Felty's syndrome, systemic lupus erythematosus, rheumatoid arthritis, thrombocytopenia

Congestive

Cirrhosis, heart failure, portal vein obstruction (portal hypertension), splenic vein obstruction

Infiltrative

Gaucher's disease, amyloidosis, diabetic lipemia

Tumours or Cysts

Malignant: polycythemia rubra vera, chronic or acute leukemias, Hodgkin's lymphoma, metastatic solid tumours

Nonmalignant: Hamartoma

Cysts: true cysts (lymphangiomas, hemangiomas, epithelial, endothelial); false cysts (hemorrhagic, serous, inflammatory)

with hepatic cirrhosis. Splenic hyperplasia develops in disorders that increase splenic workload and is associated most commonly with various types of anemia (e.g., hemolytic) and chronic myeloproliferative disorders (i.e., PV).

Infiltrative splenomegaly is caused by engorgement by the macrophages with indigestible materials associated with various "storage diseases." Tumours and cysts cause actual growth of the spleen. Metastatic tumours in the spleen are rare and may result from primary tumours of the skin, lung, breast, and cervix.

CLINICAL MANIFESTATIONS Overactivity of the spleen results in hematological alterations that affect all blood components. Sequestering of red blood cells, granulocytes, and platelets results in a reduction of all circulating blood cells. The spleen may sequester up to 50% of the red blood cell population, thereby upsetting the normal physiological concentration of red blood cells in the circulation. The rate of splenic pooling is directly related to spleen size and the degree of increased blood flow through it. Sequestering exposes the red blood cells to splenic conditions that accelerate destruction, further contributing to the decreased red blood cell concentration. Anemia is the result of these combined activities. Anemia may be further potentiated by an increase in blood volume, which produces a dilutional effect on the already reduced concentration of red blood cells. The dilutional effect, as well as the removal and destruction of red blood cells, depends primarily on the degree of splenomegaly.

White blood cells and platelets also are affected by sequestering, although not to the same degree as the red blood cell. Again, the size of the spleen is the determining factor in the number of cells sequestered.

EVALUATION AND TREATMENT Treatment for hypersplenism is splenectomy; however, it may not always be indicated. A splenectomy is considered necessary to alleviate the destructive effects on red blood cells. Clinical indicators should determine the need for splenectomy, not necessarily specific conditions. Splenectomy for splenic rupture is no longer considered mandatory because of the possibility of overwhelming sepsis after removal. Repair and preservation are now considered before the decision to remove the spleen. Splenectomy also may be performed as treatment for hairy cell leukemia, Felty's syndrome, agnogenic myeloid metaplasia, thalassemia major, Gaucher's disease, hemodialysis, splenomegaly, splenic venous thrombosis, and thrombotic thrombocytopenic purpura (TTP).

Individuals are able to lead normal lives after splenectomy, but blood cell abnormalities often exist after removal of the spleen (i.e., red blood cells become thinner, broader, and wrinkled; white blood cell counts initially increase and then plateau; platelet counts rise after surgery and then stabilize). A major postoperative complication following splenectomy is overwhelming postsplenectomy infection. Unless treated in time, overwhelming postsplenectomy infection may rapidly progress to septic shock and possibly disseminated intravascular coagulation.

✔QUICK CHECK 21-5

1. Identify the major causes of splenomegaly.
2. How does splenomegaly differ from hypersplenism?

HEMORRHAGIC DISORDERS AND ALTERATIONS OF PLATELETS AND COAGULATION

The arrest of bleeding, or **hemostasis**, is dependent on adequate numbers of platelets, normal levels of coagulation factors, and absence of defects in vessels walls. The spectrum of abnormal bleeding varies widely from massive bleeds, such as rupture of large vessels like the aorta, to small bleeds in skin or mucosal membranes. Diminished or excessive levels of coagulation factors can lead to defective hemostasis or spontaneous and unnecessary clotting. (Hemostasis is discussed in Chapter 20.) Diminished hemostasis results in either internal or external hemorrhage. A classification of hemorrhagic disorders is presented in Table 21-9.

Purpuric disorders occur when there is a deficiency of normal platelets necessary to plug damaged vessels or prevent leakage from the tiny tears that occur daily in capillaries. More serious internal bleeding occurs from events that simply overwhelm hemostatic mechanisms, such as rupture of large blood vessels, trauma, and diseases associated with massive hemorrhage including abdominal aneurysm. Between these smaller bleeds and massive bleeds are deficiencies of coagulation factors found with the hemophilias (see Chapter 21). Disorders that result in spontaneous clotting can develop from genetic disorders of the clotting system components or from acquired diseases that activate clotting. These disorders are known collectively as **thromboembolic disease**. Additionally, any disorder of the blood that predisposes to clotting of blood or **thrombosis** is called *hypercoagulability* (thrombophilia).

Disorders of Platelets

Quantitative or qualitative abnormalities of platelets can interrupt normal blood coagulation and prevent hemostasis.[64] The quantitative abnormalities are thrombocytopenia, a decrease in the number of circulating platelets, and thrombocythemia, an increase in the number of platelets. Qualitative disorders affect the structure or function of individual platelets and can coexist with the quantitative disorders. Qualitative disorders usually prevent platelet adherence and aggregation, preventing formation of a platelet plug.

TABLE 21-9 Classification of Hemorrhagic Disorders

Type of Defect	Example	Manifestation
Defects of primary hemostasis	Platelet defects or von Willebrand's disease	Usually present with small bleeds in skin or mucosal membrane; bleeds are usually **petechiae** (<3-mm minute hemorrhages) or **purpuras** (>3-mm red-purple discolorations); common in capillaries; also includes **epistaxis** (nose bleeds), gastro-intestinal bleeds, or excessive menstruation
Defects of secondary hemostasis	Coagulation factor defects	Bleeds into soft tissue, muscle, or joints; intracranial bleeds may occur
Generalized defects of small vessels	Palpable purpura and ecchymoses	Extravasated blood creates a palpable mass (or **palpable purpura**), **ecchymoses** (simply called a *bruise*), or a larger palpable lesion (or **hematoma**); systemic disorders disrupt small blood vessels, called *vasculitis*

Thrombocytopenia

Thrombocytopenia is defined as a platelet count less than 150×10^9/L of blood, although most individuals do not consider the decrease significant unless it falls below 100×10^9/L of blood.[65] The risk for hemorrhage associated with minor trauma does not appreciably increase until the count falls below 50×10^9/L. Spontaneous bleeding without trauma can occur with counts ranging from 10 to 15×10^9/L, resulting in skin manifestations (i.e., petechiae, ecchymoses, and larger purpuric spots) or frank bleeding from mucous membranes. Severe spontaneous bleeding may result if the count is less than 10×10^9/L and can be fatal if it occurs in the GI tract, respiratory tract, or CNS.

Before the diagnosis of thrombocytopenia is made, pseudothrombocytopenia must be ruled out. This phenomenon occurs in approximately 1 in 1 000 to 1 in 10 000 laboratory samples and results from an error in platelet counting when a blood sample is analyzed by an automated cell counter. Platelets in the blood sample may become nonspecifically agglutinated by immunoglobulins in the presence of ethylenediaminetetraacetic acid (EDTA), a preservative in banked blood. The agglutinated platelets are not counted, thus giving an apparent, but false, thrombocytopenia. Thrombocytopenia also may be falsely diagnosed because of a dilutional effect observed after massive transfusion of platelet-poor packed cells to treat a hemorrhage. This occurs when more than 10 units of blood have been transfused within a 24-hour period. The hemorrhage that necessitated the transfusion also accelerates the loss of platelets, contributing to the pseudothrombocytopenic state. Splenic sequestering of platelets in hypersplenism (congestive) also induces an apparent thrombocytopenia, as does hypothermia (less than 25°C [77°F]), which is reversed when temperatures return to normal, suggesting an increased platelet sequestration in response to chilling.

PATHOPHYSIOLOGY Thrombocytopenia results from decreased platelet production, increased consumption, or both. The condition may also be either congenital or acquired and may be either primary or secondary to other acquired or congenital conditions.[66,67] Thrombocytopenia secondary to congenital conditions occurs in a large number of different diseases, although each is relatively rare.[68] These include thrombocytopenia–absent radius (TAR) syndrome, Wiskott-Aldrich syndrome (see Chapter 8), various forms of *MYH9* gene mutation (e.g., May-Hegglin anomaly), X-linked thrombocytopenia, and many other examples.

Acquired thrombocytopenia is more common and may occur as a result of decreased platelet production secondary to viral infections (e.g., EBV, rubella, CMV, HIV), medications (e.g., thiazides, estrogens, quinine-containing medications, chemotherapeutic agents, ethanol), nutritional deficiencies (vitamin B_{12} or folic acid in particular), chronic renal failure, bone marrow hypoplasia (e.g., aplastic anemia), radiation therapy, or bone marrow infiltration by cancer. Most common forms of thrombocytopenia are the result of increased platelet consumption. Examples include heparin-induced thrombocytopenia, idiopathic (immune) thrombocytopenia purpura, TTP, and DIC.

Heparin-induced thrombocytopenia. Heparin is the most common cause of medication-induced thrombocytopenia.[69] Approximately 4% of individuals treated with unfractionated heparin develop heparin-induced thrombocytopenia (HIT). The incidence is lower (about 0.1%) with the use of low-molecular-weight heparin. HIT is an immune-mediated, adverse drug reaction caused by IgG antibodies against the heparin–platelet factor 4 complex leading to platelet activation through platelet Fc γIIa receptors.[70] The release of additional platelet factor 4 from activated platelets and activation of thrombin lead to increased platelet consumption and a decrease in platelet counts beginning 5 to 10 days after administration of heparin.

CLINICAL MANIFESTATIONS The hallmark of HIT is thrombocytopenia. A decrease of approximately 50% in the platelet count is observed in more than 95% of individuals. However, 30% or more of those with thrombocytopenia are also at risk for venous or arterial thrombosis because a *prothrombotic state* is caused by antibody binding to platelets, inducing activation, aggregation, and consumption (thus the term *thrombocytopenia* in the syndrome name) of platelets. Venous thrombosis is more common and results in deep venous thrombosis (also called *deep vein thrombosis*) and pulmonary emboli. Arterial thrombosis affects the lower extremities, causing limb ischemia. Arterial thrombosis may lead to cerebrovascular accidents and myocardial infarctions. Other major arteries also may be affected (e.g., renal, mesenteric, upper limb). Although platelet counts are low, bleeding is uncommon.

EVALUATION AND TREATMENT Diagnosis is primarily based on clinical observations. The individual presents with dropping platelet counts after 5 days or longer of heparin treatment. On average, platelet counts may reach 60×10^9/L. Because most individuals are postsurgery and the onset of symptoms, including thrombosis, may be delayed until after release from the hospital, other possible causes of thrombocytopenia (e.g., infection, other medication reactions) must be considered. Tests are available to measure antiheparin-platelet factor 4 antibodies. The sensitivity of this test is extremely high (greater than 90%), but the specificity is less because of false-positive reactions (e.g., those receiving dialysis). Treatment is the withdrawal of heparin and use of alternative anticoagulants.

Immune thrombocytopenia purpura. The most common cause of thrombocytopenia, secondary to increased platelet destruction, is immune thrombocytopenic purpura (ITP). ITP, formerly known as *idiopathic thrombocytopenic purpura*, however, is widely recognized now as an immune process, hence the change from idiopathic to immune.[71] Although results and estimates are conflicting, the incidence of ITP is estimated to range from 9.5 to 20 per 100 000 in the general population and tends to increase with age. In individuals younger than 60 years, females have a higher incidence than males.[72] ITP may be acute or chronic. The acute form is frequently observed in children and typically lasts 1 to 2 months with a CR. In some instances it may last for up to 6 months, and some children (7 to 28%) may progress to the chronic condition (see Chapter 22). Acute ITP is usually secondary to infections (particularly viral) or other conditions that lead to large amounts of antigen in the blood, such as medication allergies or systemic lupus erythematosus. Under these conditions, the antigen usually forms immune complexes with circulating antibody, and it is thought that the immune complexes bind to Fc receptors on platelets, leading to their destruction in the spleen. The acute form of ITP usually resolves as the source of antigen is resolved (infection) or removed (medications). Recently, *H. pylori* has been implicated in various autoimmune disorders, including PA and ITP.[73-75] Similar to other autoimmune diseases, the epidemiology and gene–environment interactions and potential triggers for ITP need much study.

Chronic ITP is caused by autoantibody-mediated destruction against platelet-specific antigens. This form is more commonly observed in adults, being most prevalent in women between 20 and 40 years old, although it can be found in all ages. The chronic form tends to get progressively worse. It can occur from a variety of predisposing conditions or exposures (secondary) or have no known risk factors (primary). The autoantibodies are generally of the IgG class and are against one or more of several platelet glycoproteins (e.g., GPIIb/IIIa, GPIIb/IX, GPIa/IIa). The antibodies bind directly to the platelet antigens, after which the antibody-coated platelets are recognized and removed from the circulation by macrophages in the spleen. Autoreactive T cells also play a large role in the crosstalk between antigen-presenting cells and autoantibody-producing B cells and may play a role in ITP.[76]

CLINICAL MANIFESTATIONS Initial manifestations range from minor bleeding problems (development of petechiae and purpura) over the course of several days to major hemorrhage from mucosal sites (epistaxis, hematuria, menorrhagia, bleeding gums). Rarely will an individual present with intracranial bleeding or other sites of internal bleeding.

During pregnancy, a woman with ITP may have a newborn that is also thrombocytopenic. If the fetal platelets express the same antigen as the mother, the maternal antibody will coat the platelets, potentially resulting in thrombocytopenia in utero. A variant of neonatal thrombocytopenia (*neonatal alloimmune thrombocytopenia*) occurs when the mother does not have ITP but makes IgG antibodies against an antigen inherited from the father found on fetal platelets but not on maternal platelets.[77]

EVALUATION AND TREATMENT Diagnosis of ITP is based on a history of bleeding and associated symptoms (weight loss, fever, headache). Physical examination includes notations on the type, location, and severity of bleeding. In addition, evidence of infections (bacterial, HIV and other viral), medication history, family history, and evidence of thrombosis are assessed. Other diagnostic tests include CBC and peripheral blood smear. Unlike some other forms of thrombocytopenia, there is usually no evidence of splenectomy. Testing for antiplatelet antibodies is usually not helpful. Although most cases of ITP are associated with elevated levels of IgG on platelets, other forms of thrombocytopenia also have a high incidence of platelet-associated antibodies; thus, the specificity is low (50 to 65%).[78] In addition, some cases of ITP will not present with elevated platelet-associated antibodies; the sensitivity is 75 to 94%; therefore, a negative test does not rule out ITP.

The acute form of ITP usually resolves without major clinical consequences, but the chronic form (like many autoimmune diseases) is variable with multiple remissions and exacerbations. Treatment is palliative, not curative, and focuses on prevention of platelet destruction. Initial therapy for ITP is glucocorticoids (e.g., prednisone), which suppress the immune response and prevent sequestering and further destruction of platelets. If steroid therapy is ineffective, other reagents have been used. Treatment with intravenous immune globulin (IVIg) is used to prevent major bleeding. The response rate is 80%, but the effects are transient, lasting only days to a few weeks. Anti-Rh_o(D) (RhoGAM) has been used with limited success to treat individuals who are Rh-positive. The newer medications romiplostin (Nplate) and eltrombopag (Promacta) are now available and show promise in successfully treating ITP.

If platelet counts do not increase appropriately, splenectomy is considered to remove the site of platelet destruction. However, splenectomy is not without risks, and approximately 10 to 20% of individuals who undergo a splenectomy suffer a relapse and require further treatment. In that situation, it is believed that the liver has become the site for platelet destruction. If splenectomy is unsuccessful and life-threatening thrombocytopenia persists, more aggressive immunosuppressive medications (e.g., azathioprine [Nu-azathioprine], cyclophosphamide) are usually recommended. Because of potential complications, these medications are reserved for individuals who are severely thrombocytopenic and refractive to other therapies.

Thrombotic thrombocytopenic purpura. **Thrombotic thrombocytopenic purpura (TTP)** is a multisystem disorder characterized by thrombotic microangiopathy (TMA) (small or microvessel disease) in which platelets aggregate and cause occlusion of arterioles and capillaries within the microcirculation.[79,80] Aggregation may lead to increased platelet consumption and organ ischemia. TTP is relatively uncommon, occurring in about 5 per million individuals per year. The incidence is increasing and does appear to be an actual increase and not just the result of improved recognition. One suspected etiological factor for TMA, TTP, and hemolytic uremic syndrome (HUS) is medication-induced, and a recent report found definite evidence from three medications: quinine sulphate (Novo-Quinine), cyclosporine (Sandimmune), and tacrolimus (Advagraf, Prograf).[81]

There are two types of TTP: familial and acquired idiopathic. The familial type is the more rare type and is usually chronic, relapsing, and typically seen in children. Acquired TTP is more common and more acute and severe. It occurs mostly in females in their 30s and is rarely observed in infants and older adults.

The microthrombi formation is found throughout the entire vascular system, causing damage to multiple organs. The most susceptible organs for damage include the kidney, brain, and heart. Also affected are the pancreas, spleen, and adrenal glands. The thrombi are composed of platelets with minimal fibrin and red blood cells, differentiating them from thrombi secondary to intravascular coagulation (see p. 550).

CLINICAL MANIFESTATIONS **Chronic relapsing TTP** is a rare familial form of TTP observed in children and usually recognized and successfully treated. The acquired **acute idiopathic TTP** is much more common and more severe.[82] TTP is clinically related to and must be distinguished from other thrombotic microangiopathic conditions, including HUS, malignant hypertension, pre-eclampsia, and pregnancy-induced HELLP (*h*emolysis, *el*evated *l*iver enzymes, *l*ow *p*latelet count) syndrome. Early diagnosis and treatment is essential because TTP may prove fatal within 90 days.

Acute idiopathic TTP is characterized by a "pentad" of symptoms, including extreme thrombocytopenia (less than 20×10^9/L), intravascular hemolytic anemia, ischemic signs and symptoms most often involving the CNS (about 65% present with memory disturbances, behavioural irregularities, headaches, or coma), kidney failure (present in about 65%), and fever (present in about 33%).

EVALUATION AND TREATMENT A routine blood smear usually shows fragmented red blood cells (*schizocytes*) produced by shear forces when red blood cells are in contact with the fibrin mesh in clots that form in the vessels. As a result of tissue injury, serum levels of lactate dehydrogenase (LDH) may be very high, and low-density lipoprotein (LDL) levels may be elevated. Tests for antibody on red blood cells are negative, excluding immune hemolytic anemia.

Plasma exchange with fresh frozen plasma is the treatment of choice, achieving a 70 to 85% response rate. Additionally, steroids (glucocorticoids) are administered. In the absence of major organ damage, this approach may lead to complete recovery with no long-term complications. The anti-CD20 monoclonal antibody rituximab (Rituxan) has shown some success in people who are refractory to plasma exchange.[20] Relapses do occur at a rate of 13 to 36%, and recurrences have been reported, sometimes delayed until 9 years after treatment. Individuals who do not respond to conventional treatment may be candidates for splenectomy; however, postoperative hemorrhage remains a dangerous complication. Immunosuppression therapy has been successful in some individuals.

Thrombocythemia

Thrombocythemia (also called **thrombocytosis**) is characterized by a platelet count greater than 400×10^9/L of blood.[83] Thrombocythemia may be primary or secondary (reactive) and is usually asymptomatic until the count exceeds $1\,000 \times 10^9$/L. Then intravascular clot formation (thrombosis), hemorrhage, or other abnormalities can occur.

PATHOPHYSIOLOGY **Essential (primary) thrombocythemia** (ET) is a myeloproliferative neoplasm characterized by an increase in platelet production (or thrombocytosis) and often an increase in red blood cell production (or erythrocytosis).[84] Other disease features include leukocytosis, splenomegaly, thrombosis, bleeding, microcirculatory symptoms, itching (or pruritus), and risk for leukemic or bone marrow fibrotic transformation.[84] Myeloproliferative neoplasms (MPNs) are one of five categories of myeloid malignancies. ET is characterized by stem cell–derived clonal bone marrow proliferation (myeloproliferation) with a unique "gain-of-function" mutation that induces overactivity in cell signalling from JAK2. JAK2, a tyrosine kinase, is an essential player downstream of cytokine receptors, such as the thrombopoietin (affects platelet proliferation) and erythropoietin (affects erythrocyte proliferation) receptors, and a gain-of-function mutation contributes to the development of MPN. More simply, both erythropoietin and thrombopoietin convey their signals and consequent proliferation through JAK2. The alteration is a valine-to-phenylalanine (V617F) mutation that causes constant activation of the *JAK2* gene, leading to an increased responsiveness or production of platelets and other cells in the bone marrow. Along with increased platelets, there may be a concomitant increase in the number of red blood cells, indicating a myeloproliferative disorder; however, the increase in red blood cells is not to the extent seen in PV (see p. 526). Red blood cells in ET tend to aggregate and adhere to the endothelium and contribute to the blockage of flow in the microvasculature and altered interactions between platelets and the vascular endothelium.[85] The *JAK2* (V617F) mutation is present in 50 to 60% of persons with ET. Other mutually exclusive mutations found include calreticulin (CALR) or myeloproliferative leukemia virus oncogene (MPL) mutation. In Canada, the annual incidence rate for ET has been estimated to range from 0.1 to 1.5 per 100 000. The prevalence of ET has been estimated to be 24 per 100 000 people.[44] The overall incidence rate of ET is 0.8 per 100 000 in the United Kingdom, 2.53 per 100 000 in the United States, and 0.59 per 100 000 in Denmark. It is more common in middle-aged individuals, with the majority of cases occurring between ages 50 and 60 years. There is no known gender preference. There also is a rare hereditary type of ET called *familial essential thrombocythemia* (FET) that is inherited in an autosomal dominant pattern.

Secondary thrombocythemia may occur after splenectomy because platelets that normally would be stored in the spleen remain in circulating blood. The increase in platelets may be gradual, with thrombocythemia not occurring for up to 3 weeks after splenectomy. Reactive thrombocythemia may occur during some inflammatory conditions, such as rheumatoid arthritis and cancers. In these conditions, excessive production of some cytokines (e.g., IL-6, IL-11) may induce increased production of thrombopoietin in the liver, resulting in increased megakaryocyte proliferation. Reactive thrombocythemia also may occur during a variety of physiological conditions, such as after exercise.

CLINICAL MANIFESTATIONS Clinical manifestations vary among individuals. Those with ET are at risk for large-vessel arterial or venous thrombosis, although the most common complication is **microvasculature thrombosis** leading to ischemia in the fingers, toes, or cerebrovascular regions.[85] The primary presenting symptoms of microvasculature thrombosis are erythromyalgia, headache, and paresthesias. **Erythromyalgia** is characterized by unilateral or bilateral warm, congested, red hands and feet with painful burning sensations, particularly in the forefoot sole and one or more toes. The lower extremities are affected more often and only one side may be involved. The pain is initiated by standing, exercise, or warmth and relieved by elevation and cooling. In extreme situations, acrocyanosis and gangrene may result.

Arterial thrombosis is more common than venous thrombosis and may involve the coronary and renal arteries. Deep venous thrombosis of the lower extremities and pulmonary embolism are the major sites for venous involvement. Other common venous sites include intra-abdominal venous thrombosis (portal and hepatic). People older than 60 years of age or those with prior history of thrombotic events have as much as a 25% chance of developing a cerebral, cardiac, or peripheral arterial thrombus and, less often, developing a pulmonary embolism or deep venous thrombosis.[86,87] Conversion to acute leukemia is found in less than 10%.[88] Symptoms related to microvascular thrombosis in the CNS include headache, dizziness with paresthesias, transient ischemic attacks, strokes, visual disturbances, and seizures. Major thrombotic events, not directly related to the platelet count, occur in about 20 to 30% of individuals with ET. Prior history of thrombotic events, advanced age, and duration of thrombocytosis are predictors of future thrombotic complications. Individuals older than age 60 are at greatest risk.

Although thrombosis is the more common symptom, hemorrhage can also occur. Sites for bleeding include the GI tract, skin, mucous membranes, urinary tract, gums, teeth sockets after extraction, joints, eyes, and brain. GI bleeding may be mistaken for a duodenal ulcer. Hemorrhage is not severe and generally occurs in the presence of very high platelet counts; transfusions are required only occasionally. Bleeding and clotting may occur simultaneously, and individuals will not necessarily be "bleeders" or "clotters."

EVALUATION AND TREATMENT Initial diagnosis is not difficult; as many as two-thirds of cases are diagnosed from a routine CBC. Secondary thrombocytosis also may occur as a moderate rise in the platelet count that resolves with treatment or resolution of the underlying condition. The World Health Organization requires that the following four criteria be met for a diagnosis of ET: (1) sustained platelet count of at least 450×10^9/L; (2) bone marrow biopsy showing proliferation of enlarged mature megakaryocytes and no increase of granulocyte or erythrocyte precursors; (3) failure to meet the criteria of PV, myelofibrosis, CML, or other myelodysplastic syndrome; and (4) presence of JAK2 617F or another clonal marker or evidence of reactive thrombocytosis.[89] Since ET can be mistaken for CML, careful differentiation is necessary because treatment varies significantly.

Treatment of ET is directed toward preventing thrombosis or hemorrhage.[90] Reducing the platelet count remains a significant treatment issue. Hydroxyurea (Hydrea), a nonalkylating myelosuppressive agent, has been the medication of choice to suppress platelet production; however, long-term use may cause progression to other myeloplastic disorders, particularly AML or myelofibrosis.[90] Another medication used to treat ET is interferon (IFN). IFN has a response rate of 80% but may not be effective for everyone because of side effects. Anagrelide (Agrylin) is now the medication of choice. Anagrelide interferes with platelet maturation rather than production, thus not interfering with red and white blood cell growth and development. Low-dose Aspirin may be effective to alleviate erthromyalgia and transient neurological manifestations. ET is not necessarily considered life-threatening, but in those older than age 60 and who have had previous incidences of thrombosis, complications are more common and associated with a higher risk of mortality.

Alterations of Platelet Function

Qualitative alterations in platelet function are characterized by an increased bleeding time in the presence of a normal platelet count. Associated clinical manifestations include spontaneous petechiae and purpura, and bleeding from the GI tract, genitourinary tract, pulmonary mucosa, and gums. Congenital alterations in platelet function (thrombocytopathies) are quite rare.[91]

Acquired disorders of platelet function are more common than congenital disorders and may be categorized into three principal causes: (1) medications, (2) systemic inflammatory conditions, and (3) hematological alterations.

Multiple medications are known to interfere with platelet function in several ways: inhibition of platelet membrane receptors, inhibition of prostaglandin pathways, and inhibition of phosphodiesterase activity. Aspirin is the most commonly used medication that affects platelets. It irreversibly inhibits cyclo-oxygenase function for several days after administration. NSAIDs also affect cyclo-oxygenase, although in a reversible fashion.

Systemic disorders that affect platelet function are chronic renal disease, liver disease, cardiopulmonary bypass surgery, and severe deficiencies of iron or folate and antiplatelet antibodies associated with autoimmune disorders. Hematological disorders associated with platelet dysfunction include chronic myeloproliferative disorders, MM, leukemias, and myelodysplastic syndromes and dysproteinemias.

Disorders of Coagulation

Disorders of coagulation are usually caused by defects or deficiencies in one or more of the clotting factors. (The normal function of clotting factors is described in Chapter 20.) Qualitative or quantitative abnormalities interfere with or prevent the enzymatic reactions that transform clotting factors, circulating as plasma proteins, into a stable fibrin clot (see Figure 20-17). Some clotting factor defects are inherited and involve a deficiency in a single factor, such as the hemophilias and von Willebrand's disease. Other coagulation defects are acquired and tend to result from deficient synthesis of clotting factors by the liver. Causes include liver disease and dietary deficiency of vitamin K.

Other coagulation disorders are attributed to pathological conditions that trigger coagulation inappropriately, engaging the clotting factors and causing detrimental clotting within blood vessels. For example, any cardiovascular abnormality that alters normal blood flow by acceleration, deceleration, or obstruction can create conditions in which coagulation proceeds within the vessels. An example of cardiovascular-related coagulation pathology is thromboembolic disease, in which blood clots obstruct blood vessels. Coagulation is also stimulated by the presence of tissue factor (TF) that is released by damaged or dead tissues. Vasculitis, or inflammation of the blood vessels, along with vessel damage activates platelets, which in turn activates the coagulation cascade. In extensive or prolonged vasculitis, blood clot formation can suppress mechanisms that normally control clot formation and dissolution, leading to clogging of the vessels. In each of these acquired conditions, normal hemostatic function proves detrimental to the body by consuming coagulation factors excessively or by overwhelming normal control of clot formation and breakdown (fibrinolysis) (see Figure 20-19).

Impaired Hemostasis

Impaired hemostasis, or the inability to promote coagulation and the development of a stable fibrin clot, is commonly associated with liver dysfunction, which may be caused by either specific liver disorders or lack of vitamin K.

Vitamin K deficiency. Vitamin K, a fat-soluble vitamin, is required for the synthesis and regulation of prothrombin; the procoagulant factors (VII, IX, X); and the anticoagulant factors within the liver (proteins C and S).[92] Unknown is the contribution of vitamin K to the overall supply by the intestinal flora. The primary source of vitamin K is found in green leafy vegetables. The most common cause of vitamin deficiency is parenteral nutrition in combination with antibiotics that destroy normal gut flora. Rarely is the deficiency caused by a lack of dietary intake; however, bulimia can suppress vitamin K–dependent activity. Parenteral administration of vitamin K is the treatment of choice and usually results in correction of the deficiency within 8 to 12 hours. Fresh frozen plasma also may be administered but is usually reserved for individuals with life-threatening hemorrhages or those who require emergency surgery.

Liver disease. Individuals who have liver disease (e.g., acute or chronic hepatocellular diseases, cirrhosis, vitamin K deficiency, or liver surgery) present with a broad range of hemostatic derangements that may be characterized by defects in the clotting or fibrinolytic systems and by platelet function. The hepatic parenchyma cells produce most of the factors involved in hemostasis; therefore, damage to the liver frequently results in diminished production of factors involved in clotting. Factor VII level is the first to decline after liver damage because of its rapid turnover. Factor IX levels are less affected and do not decline until the liver destruction is well advanced. The liver also is a major site for production of plasminogen and α_2-antiplasmin of the fibrinolytic system, as well as thrombopoietin and the metalloprotease ADAMTS13. Diminished thrombopoietin may lead to thrombocytopenia from decreased platelet production. Decreased production of ADAMTS13 results in increased levels of large precursor molecules of von Willebrand factor, which leads to the formation of large aggregates of platelets.

With severe liver disease, such as cirrhosis, most clotting factors are significantly depressed. Levels of clotting system regulators, such as antithrombin, protein C, protein S, and fibrinogen, also are diminished. The fibrolytic system is commonly active because of plasmin inhibitor and unaffected other activators. Thrombocytopenia occurs in affected individuals because of diminished thrombopoietin and ADAMTS13, as well as increased sequestration (pooling) of platelets in the spleen, which is frequently enlarged in cirrhosis and is associated with portal hypertension. Thus, these individuals may appear to have a condition similar to DIC (see "Consumptive Thrombohemorrhagic Disorders").

Treatment of hemostasis alterations in liver disease must be comprehensive to cover all aspects of dysfunctions. Fresh frozen plasma administration is the treatment of choice; however, not all individuals tolerate the volume needed to adequately replace all deficient factors. Alternative modalities include the addition of exchange transfusions and platelet concentration to plasma administration.

Consumptive Thrombohemorrhagic Disorders

Consumptive thrombohemorrhagic disorders are a heterogeneous group of conditions that demonstrate the entire spectrum of hemorrhagic and thrombotic pathological findings. Symptoms range from the subtle to the devastating and generally are considered to be intermediary disease processes that complicate a vast number of primary disease states. These disorders are also characterized by confusion and controversy related to their diagnosis, treatment, and management. No one definition can cover all possible varieties of these disorders; however, in the clinical setting, DIC is most commonly used to describe a pathological condition that is associated with hemorrhage and thrombosis.

Disseminated intravascular coagulation. Disseminated intravascular coagulation (DIC) is an acquired clinical syndrome characterized by widespread activation of coagulation resulting in formation of fibrin clots in medium and small vessels or microvasculature throughout the body.[93] Widespread clotting may lead to blockage of blood flow to organs, resulting in multiple organ failure. The magnitude of clotting may result in consumption of platelets and clotting factors, leading to a tendency to bleed despite widespread clots.

The clinical course of DIC is largely determined by the stimulus intensity, host response, and comorbidities, and ranges from an acute, severe, life-threatening process that is characterized by massive hemorrhage and thrombosis to a chronic, low-grade condition. The chronic condition is characterized by subacute hemorrhage and diffuse microcirculatory thrombosis. DIC may be localized to one specific organ or generalized, involving multiple organs.

The diagnosis of DIC has been confusing and difficult because of the complexity and wide variations in clinical manifestations. Minimally acceptable diagnostic criteria have been established and include a systemic thrombohemorrhagic disorder with laboratory evidence of (1) clotting activation, (2) fibrinolytic activation, (3) coagulation inhibitor consumption, and (4) biochemical evidence of end-organ damage or failure.

DIC is secondary to a wide variety of well-defined clinical conditions, specifically those capable of activating the clotting cascade. Sepsis is the most common condition associated with DIC. Gram-negative microorganisms, as well as some Gram-positive microorganisms, fungi, protozoa (malaria), and viruses (influenza, herpes), are capable of precipitating DIC by causing damage to the vascular endothelium. Gram-negative endotoxins are the primary cause of endothelial damage; DIC may occur in up to 50% of individuals with Gram-negative sepsis. DIC occurs in approximately 10 to 20% of individuals with metastatic cancer or acute leukemia. The adenocarcinomas most frequently associated with DIC include the lung, pancreas, colon, and stomach.[36] Direct tissue damage (e.g., massive trauma, extensive surgery, severe burns) also results in release of TF, an initiator of DIC, by the endothelium. Severe trauma, especially to the brain, can induce DIC. DIC occurs in about two-thirds of individuals with a systemic inflammatory response to trauma. Some complications of pregnancy also are associated with DIC; incidences range from 50% for women with placental abruptions to less than 10% for severe pre-eclampsia. Other causes of DIC have been identified, most notably blood transfusion. Transfused blood dilutes the clotting factors, as well as circulating naturally occurring antithrombins. In hemolytic transfusion reactions, the endothelium is damaged by complement-mediated reactions.

PATHOPHYSIOLOGY The coagulation system is designed to function at local areas of vascular damage, resulting in cessation of bleeding and activation of repair to the vessels. The function of clotting is to prevent excessive blood loss, and the function of fibrinolysis is to ensure easy circulation within the vasculature (see Chapter 20). DIC results from abnormally widespread and ongoing activation of clotting—coagulopathy—in small and mid-size vessels that alters the microcirculation, leading to ischemic necrosis in various organs, particularly the kidney and lung. Concomitantly, DIC can be caused by the imbalance between the coagulant system and the fibrinolytic system (which generates plasmin) to maintain normal circulation. DIC can cause widespread deposition of fibrin in the microcirculation that leads to ischemia, microvascular thrombotic obstruction, and organ failure (Figure 21-19).

Seemingly paradoxical, DIC involves both widespread clotting and bleeding because of simultaneous procoagulant activation, fibrinolytic activation, and consumption of platelets and coagulation factors, which results directly in serious bleeding (see Figure 21-19).

DIC is not a disease but is secondary to a variety of conditions (Box 21-2) because of activation of the clotting cascade. The common pathway for DIC appears to be excessive and widespread exposure to TF. This may occur by several mechanisms: (1) damage to the vascular endothelium results in exposure to TF; (2) when stimulated by inflammatory cytokines, endothelial cells and monocytes express surface TF; (3) endotoxin triggers the release of many cytokines that can both promote and cause progression of DIC; (4) sepsis is associated with many cytokines, interleukins, and platelet-activating factor that promote DIC as well as activate endothelial cells that stimulate thrombi development; and (5) TF may be released directly into the bloodstream from circulating white blood cells.

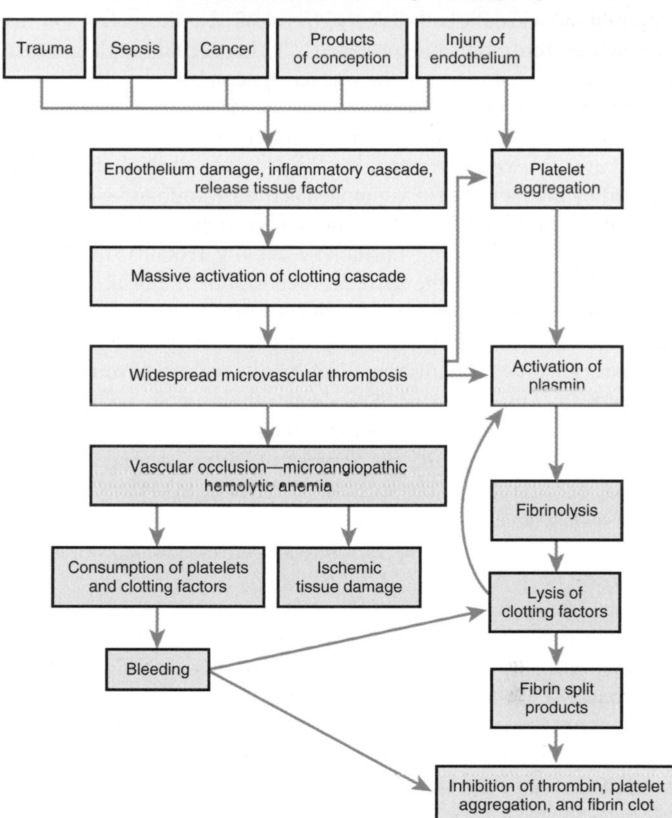

FIGURE 21-19 Pathophysiology of Disseminated Intravascular Coagulation. See text.

BOX 21-2 Conditions Associated With DIC

Malignancy: acute myelocytic leukemia, metastatic solid tumours (pancreas, prostate)

Infections: bacterial (Gram-negative endotoxin, Gram-positive mucopolysaccharides), viral (hepatitis, CMV, dengue, HIV), fungal, parasitic, rickettsial

Pregnancy complications: eclampsia/pre-eclampsia, placental abruption, amniotic fluid embolism, dead fetus syndrome

Severe trauma: head injury, burns, crush injuries, tissue necrosis, severe hypo- or hyperthermia

Liver disease: obstructive jaundice, acute liver failure, fatty liver of pregnancy

Intravascular hemolysis: transfusion reactions, medication-induced hemolysis, viper snake bites, graft versus host disease

Medical devices: aortic balloon, prosthetic devices

Hypoxia and low blood flow states: arterial hypotension secondary to shock, cardiopulmonary arrest

Vascular disorders: Giant hemangiomas (Kasabach-Merritt syndrome), aortic aneurysms

CMV, cytomegalovirus; *DIC*, disseminated intravascular coagulation; *HIV*, human immunodeficiency virus.

TF binds clotting factor VII, which leads to conversion of prothrombin to thrombin and formation of fibrin clots (see Figure 20-19). This pathway appears to be the primary route by which DIC is initiated.

Not only is the clotting system extensively activated in DIC, but also the activities of the predominant natural anticoagulants (TF pathway inhibitor, antithrombin III, protein C) are greatly diminished. During DIC, the activation of clotting is prolonged and is a result of certain conditions (e.g., bacteremia or endotoxemia); thrombin generation is increased and is insufficiently balanced by impaired anticoagulant systems, such as antithrombin and protein C.[94] The overall result is fibrin generation and deposition in the vascular system. In early DIC, plasmin (naturally occurring clot busting or fibrinolytic agent) produced from endothelial cells causes fibrinolysis to maintain circulation. Bleeding can occur with excess fibrinolytic activity. However, fibrinolysis becomes blunted by high levels of plasminogen activator inhibitor-1 (PAI-1), a fibrinolytic inhibitor.[94] Over time the activity of plasmin is diminished by PAI-1. Although some fibrinolytic activity remains, the level is inadequate to control the systemic deposition of fibrin. The slow breakdown of fibrin by plasmin produces **fibrin split products (FSPs)** (also known as **fibrin degradation products [FDPs]**). These products are powerful anticoagulants that are normally removed from blood by fibronectin and macrophages. FSPs, along with thrombin, induce further cytokine release from monocytes, contributing to endothelial damage and TF release. During DIC, the presence of FSPs is prolonged possibly because of diminished production of fibronectin. *Fibronectin* is a glycoprotein with adhesive properties that mediates removal of particulate matter, such as fibrin clumps. Low levels of fibronectin suggest a poor prognosis.

Although thrombosis is generalized and widespread, individuals with DIC are paradoxically at risk for hemorrhage. Hemorrhage is secondary to the abnormally high consumption of clotting factors and platelets, as well as the anticoagulant properties of FSPs, which interfere with fibrin mesh formation or polymerization. Both thrombin and FSPs have a high affinity for platelets and cause platelet activation and aggregation—an event that occurs early in the development of DIC—which facilitates microcirculatory coagulation and obstruction in the initial phase. However, platelet consumption exceeds production, resulting in a thrombocytopenia that increases bleeding.

Activation of clotting also leads to activation of other inflammatory pathways, including the kallikrein–kinin and complement systems (see Chapter 6). Factor XIIa, generated in DIC, converts prekallikrein to kallikrein, which then activates the vasoactive peptides bradykinin and kallidin. Activation of these systems contributes to increased vascular permeability, hypotension, and shock. Activated complement components also induce platelet destruction, which initially contributes to the thrombosis and later to the thrombocytopenia.

The deposition of fibrin clots in the circulation interferes with blood flow, causing widespread organ hypoperfusion. This condition may lead to ischemia, infarction, and necrosis, further potentiating and complicating the existing DIC process by causing further release of TF and eventually organ failure. Manifestations of multisystem organ dysfunction and failure ultimately result.

In addition to initiation of clotting by TF, DIC may be precipitated by direct proteolytic activation of factor X. The proteolytic activation of factor X has been described as "thrombin mimicry" and is the result of proteases directly converting fibrinogen to fibrin. These proteases may come from snake venom, some tumour cells, or the pancreas and liver, where they are respectively released during episodes of pancreatitis and various stages of liver disease. Direct proteolytic activity appears to be independent of any type of damage to the endothelium or tissue.

Whatever initiates the process of DIC, the cycle of thrombosis and hemorrhage persists until the underlying cause of the DIC is removed or appropriate therapeutic interventions are used.

CLINICAL MANIFESTATIONS Clinical signs and symptoms of DIC present a wide spectrum of possibilities, depending on the underlying disease process that initiates DIC and whether the DIC is acute or chronic in nature (Box 21-3). Most symptoms are the result of either bleeding or thrombosis. Acute DIC presents with rapid development of hemorrhaging (oozing) from venipuncture sites, arterial lines, or surgical wounds or development of ecchymotic lesions (purpura, petechiae) and hematomas. Other sites of bleeding include the eyes (sclera, conjunctiva), the nose, and the gums. Most individuals with DIC demonstrate bleeding at three or more unrelated sites, and any combination may be observed. Shock of variable intensity, out of proportion to the amount of blood loss, also may be observed. Hemorrhaging into closed compartments of the body also can occur and may precede the development of shock.

BOX 21-3 Clinical Manifestations Associated With DIC

Integumentary System
Widespread hemorrhage and vascular lesions
Oozing from puncture sites, incisions, mucous membranes
Acrocyanosis (irregular-shaped cyanotic patches)
Gangrene

Central Nervous System
Subarachnoid hemorrhage
Altered state of consciousness (slight confusion to convulsions and coma)

Gastro-Intestinal System
Occult bleeding to massive gastro-intestinal bleeding
Abdominal distension
Malaise
Weakness

Pulmonary System
Pulmonary infarctions
ARDS
Cyanosis
Tachypnea
Hypoxemia

Renal System
Hematuria
Oliguria
Renal failure

ARDS, acute respiratory distress syndrome; *DIC*, disseminated intravascular coagulation.

Manifestations of thrombosis are not always as evident, even though it is often the first pathological alteration to occur. The initial observations may be bleeding and sometimes very extensive hemorrhage. Several organ systems are susceptible to microvascular thrombosis associated with dysfunction: cardiovascular, pulmonary, central nervous, renal, and hepatic systems. Acute and accurate clinical interpretations are critical to preventing progression of DIC that may lead to multisystem organ dysfunction and failure. (Multiple organ dysfunction syndrome is discussed further in Chapter 24.) Indicators of multisystem dysfunction include changes in level of consciousness or behaviour, confusion, seizure activity, oliguria, hematuria, hypoxia, hypotension, hemoptysis, chest pain, and tachycardia. Symmetrical cyanosis of fingers and toes (blue finger/toe syndrome), nose, and breast may be observed and indicates macrovascular thrombosis. This may lead to infarction and gangrene that may require amputation. Jaundice also is observed and most likely results from red blood cell destruction rather than liver dysfunction.

Individuals with chronic or low-grade DIC do not present with the overt manifestations of hemorrhaging and thrombosis but instead have subacute bleeding and diffuse thrombosis; these individuals are described as having *compensated DIC*, or *nonovert DIC*. The major characteristic of this state is an increased turnover and decreased survival time of the components of hemostasis: platelets and clotting factors. Occasionally, diffuse or localized thrombosis develops, but this outcome is infrequent.

EVALUATION AND TREATMENT No single laboratory test can be used to effectively diagnose DIC. Diagnosis is based primarily on clinical symptoms and confirmed by a combination of laboratory tests. The person must present with a clinical condition that is known to be associated with DIC. The most commonly used combination of laboratory tests usually confirms thrombocytopenia or a rapidly decreasing platelet count on repeated testing, prolongation of clotting times, the presence of FSPs, and decreased levels of coagulation inhibitors. Platelet counts below 100×10^9/L or a progressive decrease in platelet counts is very sensitive for DIC, although not highly specific. These changes usually indicate consumption of platelets.

The standard coagulation tests (e.g., prothrombin time [PT], activated partial thromboplastin time [aPTT]) also have a high degree of sensitivity, but they are not highly specific for DIC. As a result of consumption of circulating clotting factors, these tests are usually abnormal, ranging from shortened to prolonged times. However, conditions other than DIC may prolong clotting times.

Detection of FSPs is more specific for DIC. Detection of D-dimers is a widely used test for DIC. A **D-dimer** is a molecule produced by plasmin degradation of cross-linked fibrin in clots. D-dimers in the blood can be quantified using ELISA tests that include commercially available and highly specific monoclonal antibody against the D-dimer. Agglutination tests for other FSPs are available. Levels of FSPs are elevated in the plasma in 95 to 100% of cases; however, they are less specific and only document the presence of plasmin and its action on fibrin. ELISAs for markers of thrombin activity are sometimes used.

Levels of coagulation inhibitors (e.g., antithrombin III [AT-III], protein C) can be measured by assays that rely on function or by ELISAs that quantify the amount of the specific inhibitor. AT-III levels can provide key information for diagnosing and monitoring therapy of DIC. Initial levels of functional AT-III are low in DIC because thrombin is irreversibly complexed with activated clotting factors and AT-III.

Treatment of DIC is directed toward (1) eliminating the underlying pathological condition, (2) controlling ongoing thrombosis, and (3) maintaining organ function. Elimination of the underlying pathological condition is the initial intervention in the treatment phase to remove the trigger for activation of clotting. Once the stimulus is gone, production of coagulation factors in the liver leads to restoration of normal plasma levels within 24 to 48 hours.

Control of thrombosis is more difficult to attain. Heparin has been used for this purpose; however, its use is controversial because its mechanism of action is binding to and activating AT-III, which is deficient in many types of DIC. Currently, heparin is only indicated in certain types of situations related to DIC. For instance, heparin seems to be effective in DIC caused by a retained dead fetus or associated with acute promyelocytic leukemia. Organ function is compromised by microthrombi, and there is a risk of losing an extremity because of vascular occlusion; thus heparin is also indicated in these conditions. However heparin's usefulness for DIC that is precipitated by septic shock has not been established and so is contraindicated in that instance; heparin is also contraindicated when there is evidence of postoperative bleeding, peptic ulcer, or CNS bleeding.

Replacement of deficient coagulation factors, platelets, and other coagulation elements is gaining recognition as an effective treatment modality. This treatment modality is not without controversy, however, because a major concern with replacement therapy is the possible risk of adding components that will increase the rate of thrombosis. Clinical judgement is the key factor in determining whether replacement is to be used as a treatment modality.

Several clinical trials are evaluating replacement of anticoagulants (i.e., AT-III, protein C). Replacement of AT-III appears to be effective in DIC caused by sepsis. Low levels of AT-III correlate with sepsis-initiated DIC, which makes a case for its use. AT-III inactivates thrombin, factor Xa, factor IXa, and other activated components of the clotting system. Heparin augments AT-III, but the effectiveness of the combination of heparin with AT-III replacement has not been established. Antifibrinolytic medications also are used in treatment but are limited to instances of life-threatening bleeding that have not been controlled by blood component replacement therapy.

Maintenance of organ function is achieved by fluid replacement to sustain adequate circulating blood volume and maintain optimal tissue and organ perfusion. Fluids may be required to restore blood pressure, cardiac output, and urine output to normal parameters.

Thromboembolic Disorders

Certain conditions within the blood vessels predispose an individual to develop clots spontaneously. A stationary clot attached to the vessel wall is called a **thrombus** (Figure 21-20). A thrombus is composed of fibrin and blood cells and can develop in either the arterial or the venous system. **Arterial thrombi** form under conditions of high blood flow and are composed mostly of platelet aggregates held together by fibrin strands. **Venous thrombi** form under conditions of low flow and are composed mostly of red blood cells with larger amounts of fibrin and few platelets.

A thrombus eventually reduces or obstructs blood flow to tissues or organs, such as the heart, brain, or lungs, depriving them of essential nutrients critical to survival. A thrombus also has the potential of detaching from the vessel wall and circulating within the bloodstream (referred to as an **embolus**). The embolus may become lodged in smaller blood vessels, blocking blood flow into the local tissue or organ and leading to ischemia. Whether episodes of thromboembolism are life-threatening depends on the site of vessel occlusion.

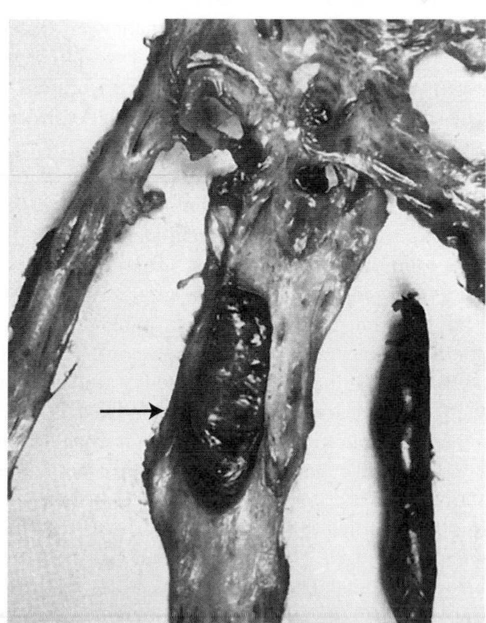

FIGURE 21-20 Thrombus. Thrombus arising in valve pocket at upper end of superficial femoral vein (*arrow*). Postmortem clot on the right is shown for comparison. (From McLachlin, J., & Paterson, J.C. [1951]. *Surg Gynecol Obstet, 93*[1], 1–8.)

Therapy consists of removal or dissolution of the clot and supportive measures. Anticoagulant therapy is effective in treating or preventing venous thrombosis; it is not as useful in treating or preventing arterial thrombosis. Parenteral heparin is the major anticoagulant used to treat thromboembolism. Oral warfarin (Coumadin) medications also are widely used, including a newer direct factor Xa inhibitor (rivaroxaban [Xarelto]). More aggressive therapy may be indicated for such conditions as pulmonary embolism, coronary thrombosis, or thrombophlebitis. Streptokinase (Kabikinase), tissue plasminogen activator (Alteplase) (t-PA), and urokinase (Kinlytic) activate the fibrinolytic system and are administered to accelerate the lysis of known thrombi. These medications are known as fibrinolytic or thrombolytic therapy and are prescribed with a high degree of caution because they can cause hemorrhagic complications.

The risk of developing spontaneous thrombi is related to several factors, referred to as the **Virchow triad**: (1) injury to the blood vessel endothelium, (2) abnormalities of blood flow, and (3) hypercoagulability of the blood. The role of estrogens as a cause of thrombi has received much attention.

Endothelial injury to blood vessels can result from atherosclerosis (plaque deposits on arterial walls) (see Chapter 24). Atherosclerosis initiates platelet adhesion and aggregation, promoting the development of atherosclerotic plaques that enlarge, causing further damage and occlusion. Other causes of vessel endothelial injury may be related to hemodynamic alterations associated with hypertension and turbulent blood flow. Injury also is caused by radiation injury, exogenous chemical agents (e.g., toxins from cigarette smoke), endogenous agents (e.g., cholesterol), bacterial toxins or endotoxins, or immunological mechanisms.

Sites of turbulent blood flow in the arteries and stasis of blood flow in the veins are at risk for thrombus formation. In areas of turbulence, platelets and endothelial cells may be activated, leading to thrombosis. In sites of stasis, platelets may remain in contact with the endothelium for prolonged lengths of time, and clotting factors that would normally be diluted with fresh flowing blood are not diluted and may become activated. The most common clinical conditions that predispose to venous stasis and subsequent thromboembolic phenomena are major surgery (e.g., orthopedic surgery), acute myocardial infarction, heart failure, limb paralysis, spinal injury, malignancy, advanced age, the postpartum period, and bed rest longer than 1 week. Turbulence and stasis occur with ulcerated atherosclerotic plaques (myocardial infarction), hyperviscosity (polycythemia), and conditions with deformed red blood cells (sickle cell anemia).

Hypercoagulability, or **thrombophilia**, is the condition in which an individual is at risk for thrombosis, but by itself it is a rare cause of thrombosis. Hypercoagulability is differentiated according to whether it results from primary (hereditary) or secondary (acquired) causes.

Hereditary thrombophilias. Thrombophilias can result from both inherited conditions and, more commonly, acquired conditions.[95] Several inherited conditions increase the risk of developing thrombosis, and most are autosomal dominant. Thus individuals who are homozygous for the mutation are at greatest risk for thrombosis. These inherited conditions include mutations in platelet receptors, coagulation proteins, fibrinolytic proteins, and other factors. The particular mutations that have been most strongly linked as risk factors for venous thrombosis or for arterial thrombosis leading to coronary artery disease or stroke include those that affect fibrinogen, prothrombin (G20210A variant), factor V (factor V Leiden) of the coagulation system, PAI-1 of the fibrinolytic system, the platelet receptor GPIIIa, and methylenetetrahydrofolate reductase (MTHFR), as well as mutations that result in excessive levels of homocysteine (hyperhomocysteinemia). Other inherited thrombophilias are risk factors mostly for venous thrombosis and include deficiencies in protein C, protein S, and AT-III.[95,96] Factor V Leiden results from a single nucleotide mutation that confers partial resistance to inactivation by activated protein C, resulting in prolonged high levels of activated factor V (factor Va) and overproduction of thrombin. Although this mutation increases the risk for thrombosis, most individuals with factor V Leiden do not have clinically relevant thrombotic events. It is the most common hereditary thrombophilia and is primarily observed in individuals of European ancestry. It is observed in about 5% of the White population and in about 30% of individuals presenting with deep venous thrombosis or pulmonary embolism.

Other hereditary thrombophilias are less common. Prothrombin mutation, which leads to high levels of circulating prothrombin, is observed in about 2 to 5% of individuals of European ancestry. It is, however, found in 5 to 10% of individuals presenting with thrombosis.

MTHFR mutation leads to alterations in the metabolism of the amino acid homocysteine into methionine and abnormally elevated levels of that amino acid in the blood (hyperhomocysteinemia). Acquired hyperhomocysteinemia may result from deficiencies in vitamins B_6 or B_{12}, endocrine diseases (e.g., diabetes mellitus, hypothyroidism), PA, inflammatory bowel disease, renal failure, and therapy with some medications. Individuals with homocysteine levels greater than the 95th percentile are 2.5 times more likely to experience an episode of deep venous thrombosis.

More than 100 different known mutations lead to defects of proteins C, protein S, and AT-III and increase the risk for venous thrombosis. Mutations may lead to either quantitative (low levels of protein) or qualitative (production of defective protein) changes.

Tests to diagnose inherited thrombophilias include PT; PTT; and levels of protein C, protein S, and AT-III. More elaborate tests to detect precise mutations in factor V, prothrombin, or MTHFR may be indicated.

Acquired hypercoagulability. Deficiencies in proteins S and C and AT-III may be acquired and contribute to a hypercoagulable state.[97] Conditions associated with an acquired protein deficiency include DIC, liver disease, infection, deep venous thrombosis, acute respiratory distress syndrome, L-asparaginase therapy, HUS, and TTP. The postoperative state also predisposes an individual to protein C or S deficiency; however, its role in contributing to deep venous thrombosis remains unclear.

Acquired hypercoagulable states include antiphospholipid syndrome (APS).[98] APS is an autoimmune syndrome characterized by autoantibodies against plasma membrane phospholipids and phospholipid-binding proteins. As with most autoimmune diseases, the predominantly affected individual is female and of reproductive age. Those with APS are at risk for both arterial and venous thrombosis and a variety of obstetrical complications, including pregnancy loss and pre-eclampsia/eclampsia. In severe cases the individual may die from recurrent major thrombus formation.[99] The pathophysiology is related to autoantibodies directly reacting with platelets or endothelial cells (increasing the risk for thrombosis) or the placental surface (resulting in damage to the placenta). The predominant diagnostic tests measure prolongation of laboratory blood coagulation tests related to an antibody inhibitor (lupus anticoagulant) and specific ELISAs for antibodies against phospholipids (e.g., anticardiolipin antibody) or proteins that bind to phospholipids (e.g., β_2-glycoprotein I). Highly effective therapy (i.e., unfractionated or low-molecular-weight heparin with low-dose Aspirin) is available to prevent the obstetrical complications.[100]

QUICK CHECK 21-6

1. Compare and contrast thrombocytopenia with thrombocytosis.
2. Why does vitamin K deficiency predispose an individual to a coagulation disorder?
3. Identify three pathological causes of DIC, and describe the manifestations associated with DIC.
4. Compare and contrast a thrombus with an embolus.

DID YOU UNDERSTAND?

Alterations of Erythrocyte Function

1. *Anemia* is defined as a reduction in the number or volume of circulating red blood cells or a decrease in the quality or quantity of hemoglobin.
2. The most common classification of anemias is based on changes in the cell size—represented by the cell suffix *-cytic*—and changes in the cell's hemoglobin content—represented by the suffix *-chromic*.
3. Clinical manifestations of anemia can be found in all organs and tissues throughout the body. Decreased oxygen delivery to tissues causes fatigue, dyspnea, syncope, angina, compensatory tachycardia, and organ dysfunction.
4. Macrocytic (megaloblastic) anemias are characterized by unusually large stem cells in the marrow that mature into very large erythrocytes. Macrocytic anemias are caused most commonly by deficiencies of vitamin B_{12} or folate. Pernicious anemia, the most common type of macrocytic anemia, can be fatal unless vitamin B_{12} replacement is given (lifelong replacement is required).
5. Microcytic-hypochromic anemias are characterized by abnormally small red blood cells with insufficient hemoglobin content. The most common cause is iron deficiency.
6. Iron deficiency anemia (IDA) is the most common type of anemia worldwide and usually develops slowly, with a gradual, insidious onset of symptoms, including fatigue, weakness, dyspnea, alteration of various epithelial tissues, and vague neuromuscular complaints.
7. IDA is usually a result of a chronic blood loss or decreased iron intake. Once the source of blood loss is identified and corrected, iron replacement therapy can be initiated.
8. Sideroblastic anemias (SAs) are a heterogeneous group of inherited and acquired disorders. SAs have various causes, but all share altered heme synthesis.
9. Normocytic-normochromic anemias are characterized by insufficient numbers of normal erythrocytes. Included in this category are aplastic, posthemorrhagic, hemolytic, and anemia of chronic inflammation.

Myeloproliferative Red Blood Cell Disorders

1. Polycythemia vera (PV) is a stem cell disorder with hyperplastic and neoplastic bone marrow alterations. It is characterized by excessive proliferation of erythrocyte precursors (frequently with increased white blood cells and platelets) in the bone marrow. Polycythemia is responsible for most of the clinical symptoms, including increased blood volume and viscosity. Frequent phlebotomies reduce iron levels, and hydroxyurea is the medication of choice for myelosuppression. Use of radioactive phosphorus has been helpful in decreasing the excessive red blood cell pool.
2. PV may spontaneously convert to acute myeloid (or myelogenous) leukemia.

Alterations of Leukocyte Function

1. Quantitative alterations of leukocytes (too many or too few) can be caused by bone marrow dysfunction or premature destruction of cells in the circulation. Many quantitative changes in leukocytes occur in response to invasion by microorganisms.
2. Leukocytosis is a condition in which the leukocyte count is higher than normal; it is usually a response to physiological stressors and invasion of microorganisms.
3. Leukopenia is present when the leukocyte count is lower than normal; it is caused by pathological conditions, such as malignancies and hematological disorders.
4. Granulocytosis (particularly as a result of an increase in neutrophils, eosinophils, or basophils) occurs in response to infection and inflammation.
5. Granulocytopenia, a significant decrease in the number of neutrophils, can be a life-threatening condition if sepsis occurs; it is often caused by chemotherapeutic agents, severe infection, and radiation.
6. Eosinophilia results most commonly from allergic disorders, parasitic invasion, and ingestion or inhalation of toxic foreign particles.
7. Basophilia is rare and generally is a response to inflammation and immediate hypersensitivity reactions. Basopenia is a decrease in circulating numbers of basophils.
8. Monocytosis is an increase in the number of circulating monocytes and is often transient. It occurs during the late or recuperative phase of infection. Monocytopenia is a decrease in the number of circulating monocytes.
9. Lymphocytopenia is a decrease in the number of circulating lymphocytes in the blood. It is associated with neoplasias, immune deficiencies, and destruction by medications, viruses, or radiation.
10. Infectious mononucleosis (IM) is an acute infection of B cells most commonly (85% of IM cases) associated with the Epstein-Barr virus (EBV). The classic symptoms are pharyngitis, lymphadenopathy, and fever. The proliferation of infected B cells may be uncontrolled and lead to B-cell lymphomas.
11. Transmission of EBV is usually through saliva from close personal contact. IM is self-limiting, and treatment consists of rest and symptomatic treatment.
12. The common pathological feature of all forms of leukemia is an uncontrolled proliferation of malignant leukocytes, causing an overcrowding of bone marrow and decreased production and function of normal hematopoietic cells.
13. The classification of leukemias is based on the cell type involved—myeloid or lymphoid—and the rate of progression—acute or chronic. There are four major types of leukemia: (a) acute lymphocytic leukemia (ALL), (b) acute myeloid (or myelogenous) leukemia (AML), (c) chronic lymphocytic leukemia (CLL), and (d) chronic myeloid (or myelogenous) leukemia (CML).
14. Although the exact cause of leukemia is unknown, several risk factors and related genetic aberrations are associated with the onset of malignancy. The leukemias are clonal disorders driven by genetically abnormal stem-like cancer cells.
15. Abnormal immature white blood cells, called *blasts*, fill the bone marrow and spill into the blood. The blasts overcrowd the marrow and cause cellular proliferation of the other cell lines to cease.
16. The major clinical manifestations of leukemia include fatigue caused by anemia, bleeding caused by thrombocytopenia, fever secondary to infection, anorexia, and weight loss.
17. Treatment varies depending on the type of leukemia and includes observation, steroids, chemotherapy, monoclonal antibodies, and transplant options.
18. Chronic leukemias progress slowly and insidiously, different from acute leukemias (which can have an abrupt stormy onset).

Alterations of Lymphoid Function

1. Lymphadenopathy is characterized by enlarged lymph nodes.
2. Lymphomas consist of a diverse group of neoplasms that develop from the proliferation of malignant lymphocytes in the lymphoid system. There are three major categories of lymphomas: (a) B-cell neoplasms, (b) T-cell and natural killer (NK)–cell neoplasms, and (c) the two general categories of Hodgkin's lymphoma (HL) and non-Hodgkin's lymphoma (NHL).

3. In general, lymphomas are the result of genetic mutations or viral infection. Malignant transformation produces a cell with uncontrolled and excessive growth that accumulates in the lymph nodes and other sites, producing tumour masses.
4. HL is characterized by the presence of B cells called the Reed-Sternberg cells.
5. The pathogenesis of HL may be linked to infection with EBV.
6. An enlarged, painless mass or swelling, most commonly in the neck, is an initial sign of HL; however, asymptomatic lymphadenopathy can progress undetected for years.
7. Treatment of HL includes chemotherapy, radiation therapy, and surgery. Treatment with chemotherapy or radiation therapy, or both, may increase the risk for secondary cancers, cardiovascular disease, and other health problems for many months or years after treatment.
8. NHL is not a single disease, but a heterogeneous group of proliferative lymphoid tissue neoplasms. Clonal expansion of B cells accounts for the majority of NHLs. Oncogenes may be activated by chromosomal translocation (most common alteration) or by deletion of tumour-suppressor genes. Certain subtypes may have altered genomes by oncogenic viruses.
9. Generally, with NHL, the swelling of lymph nodes is painless and the nodes enlarge and transform over a period of months or years.
10. Standard treatment for NHL includes radiation therapy, chemotherapy, target therapy (monoclonal antibody therapy, proteasome inhibitor therapy), plasmapheresis, biological therapy, and watchful waiting.
11. Burkitt lymphoma is a B-cell tumour and involves the jaw and facial bones and sometimes the abdomen. Although more common in Africa, it is documented in Canada, the United States, Latin America, and other Western countries. Burkitt lymphoma is heterogeneous and may involve infection with EBV and suppression of the immune system by other illnesses.
12. Treatment for Burkitt lymphoma is intensive chemotherapy.
13. Multiple myeloma (MM) is a neoplasm of plasma cells in the bone marrow and usually not found in the peripheral blood. It is characterized by multiple malignant tumour masses of plasma cells scattered throughout the skeletal system (lytic bone lesions) and sometimes found in soft tissue.
14. MM tumours are highly heterogeneous and involve mutations in different signalling pathways. Chromosomal translocations are common. The exact cause of MM is unknown, but risk factors include radiation, certain chemicals, and a history of monoclonal gammopathy of undetermined significance (MGUS).
15. The common presentation of MM is characterized by elevated levels of calcium in the blood, renal failure, anemia, and bone (lytic) lesions.
16. Treatment includes chemotherapy, radiation therapy, plasmapheresis, and stem cell transplant.

Alterations of Splenic Function

1. Splenomegaly (enlargement of the spleen) may be considered normal in certain individuals, but its presence is associated with various diseases.
2. Splenomegaly results from (a) acute inflammatory or infectious processes, (b) congestive disorders, (c) infiltrative processes, and (d) tumours or cysts.
3. Hypersplenism (overactivity of the spleen) results from splenomegaly. Hypersplenism results in sequestering of the blood cells, causing increased destruction of red blood cells, leukopenia, and thrombocytopenia.

Hemorrhagic Disorders and Alterations of Platelets and Coagulation

1. The arrest of bleeding is called *hemostasis.*
2. Thrombocytopenia is characterized by a platelet count below 150 $\times 10^9$/L of blood; the most significant count is less than 100 $\times 10^9$/L, and a count less than 50 $\times 10^9$/L increases the potential for hemorrhage associated with minor trauma.
3. Thrombocytopenia exists in primary or secondary forms and is associated with autoimmune diseases, viral infections, medications, nutritional deficiencies, chronic renal failure, cancer, radiation therapy, bone marrow hypoplasia, and disseminated intravascular coagulation (DIC).
4. Immune thrombocytopenic purpura (ITP) is the most common cause of thrombocytopenia, secondary to increased platelet destruction.
5. Thrombocythemia is characterized by a platelet count greater than 400 $\times 10^9$/L of blood and is symptomatic when the count exceeds 1 000 $\times 10^9$/L, at which time the risk for intravascular clot formation (thrombosis), hemorrhage, or other abnormalities can occur.
6. Essential (primary) thrombocythemia is a myeloproliferative neoplasm characterized by an increase in platelet production and often an increase in red blood cell production.
7. Qualitative alterations in normal platelet function prevent platelet plug formation and may result in prolonged bleeding times. Acquired disorders of platelet function are more common than congenital disorders.
8. Disorders of coagulation are usually caused by defects or deficiencies in one or more of the clotting factors. Coagulation is stimulated by the presence of tissue factor that is released by damaged or dead tissues.
9. Coagulation is impaired when there is a deficiency of vitamin K because of insufficient production of prothrombin and synthesis of clotting factors VII, IX, and X, often associated with liver diseases.
10. DIC is an acquired clinical syndrome characterized by widespread activation of coagulation, resulting in formation of fibrin clots in medium and small vessels or microvasculature throughout the body. Widespread clotting may lead to blockage of blood flow to organs, resulting in multiple organ failure. The magnitude of clotting may result in consumption of platelets and clotting factors, leading to a tendency to bleed despite widespread clots.
11. DIC is secondary to a wide variety of clinical conditions; sepsis is the most common condition associated with DIC.
12. For a diagnosis of DIC, the person must present with a clinical condition that is known to be associated with DIC. The most commonly used combination of laboratory tests usually confirms thrombocytopenia or a rapidly decreasing platelet count on repeated testing, prolongation of clotting times, the presence of fibrin split products, and decreased levels of coagulation inhibitors.
13. Treatment of DIC is directed toward (a) eliminating the underlying pathological condition, (b) controlling ongoing thrombosis, and (c) maintaining organ function.
14. Thromboembolic disorders result from a fixed (thrombus) or moving (embolus) clot that blocks flow within a vessel, denying nutrients to tissues distal to the occlusion; death can result when clots obstruct blood flow to the heart, brain, or lungs.
15. The term *Virchow triad* refers to three factors that can cause thrombus formation: (a) injury to the blood vessel endothelium, (b) abnormalities of blood flow, and (c) hypercoagulability of the blood.
16. Hypercoagulability, or thrombophilia, is a condition in which an individual is at risk for thrombosis.

KEY TERMS

Absolute lymphocytosis, 531
Absolute polycythemia, 526
Acquired sideroblastic anemia (ASA), 525
Acute idiopathic TTP, 548
Acute leukemia, 533
Acute lymphocytic leukemia (ALL), 534
Acute myeloid (or myelogenous) leukemia (AML), 534
Agranulocytosis, 531
Amyloidosis, 544
Anemia, 520
Anisocytosis, 520
Arterial thrombus (pl. *thrombi*), 553
Basopenia, 531
Basophilia, 531
B-cell neoplasm, 540
Bence Jones protein, 543
β_2-Microglobulin, 545
Blast cell, 533
Burkitt lymphoma, 541
Chronic leukemia, 533
Chronic lymphocytic leukemia (CLL), 536
Chronic myeloid (or myelogenous) leukemia (CML), 536
Chronic relapsing TTP, 548
Congestive splenomegaly, 545
Consumptive thrombohemorrhagic disorder, 550
D-dimer, 553
Disseminated intravascular coagulation (DIC), 550
Ecchymoses, 546
Embolus, 553
Eosinopenia, 531
Eosinophilia, 531
Epistaxis, 546
Eryptosis, 522
Erythromyalgia, 549
Essential (primary) thrombocythemia (ET), 549
Fibrin degranulation product (FDP), 552
Fibrin split product (FSP), 552
Folate (folic acid), 523
Granulocytopenia, 531
Granulocytosis, 530
Hematoma, 546
Hemochromatosis, 529
Hemolysis, 522
Hemostasis, 546
Heparin-induced thrombocytopenia (HIT), 547
Hereditary (congenital) sideroblastic anemia, 525
Hereditary hemochromatosis (HH), 529
Heterophilic antibody, 532
Hodgkin's lymphoma (HL), 539
Hypercoagulability (thrombophilia), 554
Hypersplenism, 545
Hypoplastic anemia, 526
Hypoxemia, 522
Immune thrombocytopenic purpura (ITP), 547
Impaired hemostasis, 550
Infectious mononucleosis (IM), 531
Infiltrative splenomegaly, 546
Intrinsic factor (IF), 523
Iron deficiency anemia (IDA), 524
Janus kinase 2 gene (*JAK2* gene), 527
Koilonychia, 525
Leukemia, 532
Leukocytosis, 529
Leukopenia, 529
Lymphadenopathy, 538
Lymphoblastic lymphoma (LL), 542
Lymphocytopenia, 531
Lymphocytosis, 531
M protein, 543
Macrocytic (megaloblastic) anemia, 522
Microcytic-hypochromic anemia, 524
Microvasculature thrombosis, 549
Monoclonal gammopathy of undetermined significance (MGUS), 544
Monocytopenia, 531
Monocytosis, 531
Multiple myeloma (MM), 542
Myelodysplastic syndrome (MDS), 525
Myeloproliferative disorder, 536
Neutropenia, 531
Neutrophilia, 530
NK-cell neoplasm, 540
Non-Hodgkin's lymphoma (NHL), 540
Normocytic-normochromic anemia (NNA), 526
Palpable purpura, 546
Pancytopenia, 533
Pernicious anemia (PA), 522
Petechia, 546
Philadelphia chromosome, 533
Phlebotomy, 526
Poikilocytosis, 520
Polycythemia, 526
Polycythemia vera (PV; also *primary polycythemia*), 526
Purpura, 546
Reed-Sternberg (RS) cell, 539
Relative polycythemia, 526
Reversible sideroblastic anemia (reversible SA), 525
Ringed sideroblast, 525
Secondary thrombocythemia, 549
Shift to the left (leukemoid reaction), 530
Shift to the right, 531
Sideroblastic anemia (SA), 525
Small lymphocytic lymphoma (SLL; also *CLL/SLL*), 536
Smouldering myeloma, 544
Splenomegaly, 545
T-cell neoplasm, 540
Thrombocythemia (thrombocytosis), 548
Thrombocytopenia, 547
Thromboembolic disease, 546
Thrombosis, 546
Thrombotic thrombocytopenic purpura (TTP), 548
Thrombus, 553
Vasculitis, 550
Venus thrombus (pl. *thrombi*), 553
Virchow triad, 554

REFERENCES

1. Sun, C. C., Vaja, V., Babitt, J. L., et al. (2012). Targeting the hepdicin-ferroportion axis to develop new treatment strategies for anemia of chronic disease and anemia of inflammation. *American Journal of Hematology, 87*, 392–400. doi:10.1002/ajh.23110.
2. Muñoz, M., García-Erce, J. A., & Remacha, A. F. (2011). Disorders of iron metabolism. Part II: Iron deficiency and iron overload. *Journal of Clinical Pathology, 64*(4), 287–296. doi:10.1136/jcp.2010.086991.
3. Lang, E., Qadri, S. M., & Lang, F. (2012). Killing me softly—Suicidal erythrocyte death. *International Journal of Biochemistry & Cell Biology, 44*(8), 1236–1243. doi:10.1016/j.biocel.2012.04.019.
4. den Elzen, W. P., van der Weele, G. M., Gussekloo, J., et al. (2010). Subnormal vitamin B_{12} concentrations and anaemia in older people: A systematic review. *BMC Geriatrics, 10*, 42. doi:10.1186/1471-2318-10-42.
5. Banka, S., Ryan, K., Thomson, W., et al. (2011). Pernicious anemia—Genetic insights. *Autoimmunity Reviews, 10*(8), 455–459. doi:10.1016/j.autrev.2011.01.009.
6. Annibale, B., Lahner, E., & Fave, G. D. (2011). Diagnosis and management of pernicious anemia. *Current Gastroenterology Reports, 13*(6), 518–524. doi:10.1007/s11894-011-0225-5.
7. Neumann, W. L., Coss, E., Rugge, M., et al. (2013). Autoimmune atropic gastritis-pathogenesis, pathology and management. *Nature Reviews. Gastroenterology & Hepatology, 10*, 529–541. doi:10.1038/nrgastro.2013.101.
8. Toh, B. H., Chan, J., Kyaw, T., et al. (2012). Cutting edge issues in autoimmune gastritis. *Clinical Reviews in Allergy & Immunology, 42*(3), 269–278. doi:10.1007/s12016-010-8218-y.
9. Vojdani, A. (2008). Antibodies as predictors of complex autoimmune diseases. *International Journal of Immunopathology and Pharmacology, 21*(2), 267–278.
10. Guidi, G. C., & Lechi Santonastaso, C. (2010). Advancements in anemias related to chronic conditions. *Clinical Chemistry and Laboratory Medicine, 48*(9), 1217–1226. doi:10.1515/CCLM.2010.264.
11. West, A. R., & Oates, P. S. (2008). Mechanisms of heme iron absorption: Current questions and controversies. *World Journal of Gastroenterology, 14*(26), 4101–4110.
12. Chakraborty, P. K., Schmitz-Abe, K., Kennedy, E. K., et al. (2014). Mutations in TRNT1 cause congenital sideroblastic anemia with immunodeficiency, fevers, and developmental delay (SIFD). *Blood, 124*(18), 2867–2871. doi:10.1182/blood-2014-08-591370.
13. Garcia-Manero, G. (2012). Myelodysplastic syndromes: 2012 update on diagnosis, risk-stratification, and management. *American Journal of Hematology, 87*(7), 693–701. doi:10.1002/ajh.23264.
14. Malcovati, L., & Nimer, S. D. (2008). Myelodysplastic syndromes: Diagnosis and staging. *Cancer Contr, 15*(Suppl.), 4–13.
15. Moyo, V., Lefebvre, P., Duh, M. S., et al. (2008). Erythropoiesis-stimulating agents in the treatment of anemia in myelodysplastic syndromes: A meta-analysis. *Annals of Hematology, 87*(7), 527–536. doi:10.1007/s00277-008-0450-7.
16. Scheinberg, P., & Chen, J. (2013). Aplastic anemia: What have we learned from animal models and from the clinic. *Seminars in Hematology, 50*(2), 156–164. doi:10.1053/j.seminhematol.2013.03.028.
17. Finazzi, G., & Barbui, T. (2008). Evidence and expertise in the management of polycythemia vera and essential thrombocythemia. *Leukemia, 22*(8), 1494–1502. doi:10.1038/leu.2008.177.
18. Tefferi, A. (2013). Polycythemia vera and essential thrombocythemia: 2013 update on diagnosis, risk

stratification and management. *American Journal of Hematology, 88*(6), 507–516. doi:10.1002/ajh.23417.
19. Tefferi, A., & Barbui, T. (2013). Personalized management of essential thrombocythemia—Application of recent evidence to clinical practice. *Leukemia, 27*(8), 1617–1620. doi:10.1038/leu.2013.99.
20. Scully, M., McDonald, V., Cavenagh, J., et al. (2011). A phase 2 study of the safety and efficacy of rituximab with plasma exchange in acute acquired thrombotic thrombocytopenic purpura. *Blood, 118*(7), 1746–1753. doi:10.1182/blood-2011-03-341131.
21. National Heart, Lung, and Blood Institute. (2008). *What are thrombocytopenia and thrombocytosis?* Bethesda, MD: National Institutes of Health, U.S. Department of Health and Human Services. Retrieved from www.nhlbi.nih.gov/health/dci/Diseases/thrm/thrm_all.html.
22. Crownover, B. K., & Covery, C. H. (2013). Hereditary hemochromatosis. *American Family Physician, 87*(3), 183–190.
23. Canadian Hemochromatosis Society. (n.d.). *How common is it?* Retrieved from https://www.toomuchiron.ca/hemochromatosis/how-common-is-it/.
24. Adams, P. C., Reboussin, D. M., Barton, J. C., et al. (2005). Hemochromatosis and iron-overload screening in a racially diverse population. *New England Journal of Medicine, 352*(17), 1769–1778.
25. Greenberg, P. L., Attar, E., Bennett, J. M., et al. (2011). Myelodysplastic syndromes. *Journal of the National Comprehensive Cancer Network, 9*(1), 30–56.
26. Weinzierl, E. P., & Arber, D. A. (2013). The differential diagnosis and bone marrow evaluation of new-onset pancytopenia. *American Journal of Clinical Pathology, 139*(1), 9–29. doi:10.1309/AJCP50AEEYGREWUZ.
27. Thorley-Lawson, D. A., Hawkins, J. B., Tracy, S. I., et al. (2013). The pathogenesis of Epstein-Barr virus persistent infection. *Current Opinion in Virology, 3*(3), 227–232. doi:10.1016/j.coviro.2013.04.005.
28. Thorley-Lawson, D. A., & Gross, A. (2004). Persistence of the Epstein-Barr virus and the origins of associated lymphomas. *New England Journal of Medicine, 350*(13), 1328–1337. doi:10.1056/NEJMra032015.
29. Konopleva, M. Y., & Jordan, C. T. (2011). Leukemia stem cells and microenvironment: Biology and therapeutic targeting. *Journal of Clinical Oncology, 29*(5), 591–599. doi:10.1200/JCO.2010.31.0904.
30. Pollyea, D. A., Gutman, J. A., Gore, L., et al. (2014). Targeting acute myeloid leukemia stem cells: A review and principles for the development of clinical trials. *Haematologica, 99*(8), 1277–1284. doi:10.3324/haematol.2013.085209.
31. Visco, C., Barcellini, W., Maura, F., et al. (2014). Autoimmune cytopenias in chronic lymphocutic leukemia. *American Journal of Hematology, 89*(11), 1055–1062. doi:10.1002/ajh.23785.
32. National Cancer Institute. (2011). *SEER cancer statistics review 1975–2008*. Bethesda, MD: National Institutes of Health, U.S. Department of Health and Human Services.
33. Radivoyevitch, T., Li, H., & Sachs, R. K. (2014). Etiology and treatment of hematological neoplasms: Stochastic mathematical models. *Advances in Experimental Medicine and Biology, 844*, 317–346. doi:10.1007/978-1-4939-2095-2_16.
34. Wakeford, R. (2013). The risk of childhood leukaemia following exposure to ionizing radiation—A review. *Journal of Radiological Protection, 33*(1), 1–25. doi:10.1088/0952-4746/33/1/1.
35. Canadian Cancer Society. (2017). *Cancer information*. Retrieved from http://www.cancer.ca/en/?region=on.
36. Kumar, V., Abbas, A. K., & Aster, J. C. (Eds.), (2015). *Robbins and Cotran pathologic basis of disease* (9th ed.). Philadelphia: Saunders.
37. National Cancer Institute. (2016). *Adult acute myeloid leukemia treatment (PDQ®)*. Bethesda, MD: Author. Retrieved from http://www.cancer.gov/cancertopics/pdq/treatment/adultAML/healthprofessional.
38. Queirós, A. C., Villamor, N., Clot, G., et al. (2015). A B-cell epigenetic signature defines three biologic subgroups of chronic lymphocytic leukemia with clinical impact. *Leukemia, 29*(3), 598–605. doi:10.1038/leu.2014.252.
39. Baliakas, P., Hadzidimitriou, A., Sutton, L. A., et al. (2015). Recurrent mutations refine prognosis in chronic lymphocytic leukemia. *Leukemia, 29*(2), 329–336. doi:10.1038/leu.2014.196.
40. Villamor, N., Conde, L., Martínez-Trillos, A., et al. (2013). NOTCH1 mutations identify a genetic subgroup of chronic lymphocytic leukemia patients with high risk of transformation and poor outcome. *Leukemia, 27*(5), 1100–1106. doi:10.1038/leu.2012.357.
41. National Cancer Institute. (2014). *Chronic lymphocytic leukemia treatment (PDQ®)*. Bethesda, MD: Author. Retrieved from http://cancer.gov/cancertopics/pdq/treatment/CLL/Patient. Date last modified July 28, 2016.
42. Rawstron, A. C., Bennett, F. L., O'Connor, S. J., et al. (2008). Monoclonal B-cell lymphocytosis and chronic lymphocytic leukemia. *New England Journal of Medicine, 359*(6), 575–583. doi:10.1056/NEJMoa075290.
43. Fazi, C., Scarfò, L., Pecciarini, L., et al. (2011). General population low-count CLL-like MBL persists over time without clinical progression, although carrying the same cytogenetic abnormalities of CLL. *Blood, 118*(25), 6618–6625. doi:10.1182/blood-2011-05-357251.
44. Leukemia and Lymphoma Society of Canada. (2017). *Blood cancer in Canada: Facts and stats, 2016*. Retrieved from http://www.llscanada.org/sites/default/files/National/CANADA/Pdf/InfoBooklets/Blood_Cancer_in_Canada_Facts_%26_Stats_2016.pdf.
45. Kreso, A., & Dick, J. E. (2014). Evolution of the cancer stem cell model. *Cell Stem Cell, 14*(3), 275–291. doi:10.1016/j.stem.2014.02.006.
46. Scott, D. W., & Gascoyne, R. D. (2014). The tumor microenvironment in B cell lymphomas. *Nature Reviews. Cancer, 14*(8), 517–534. doi:10.1038/nrc3774.
47. Canadian Cancer Society's Advisory Committee on Cancer Statistics. (2015). *Canadian cancer statistics 2015*. Toronto, ON: Canadian Cancer Society.
48. Mohamed, G., Vrzalikova, K., Cader, F. Z., et al. (2014). Epstein-Barr virus, the germinal centre and the development of Hodgkin's lymphoma. *Journal of General Virology, 95*(Pt. 9), 1861–1869. doi:10.1099/vir.0.066712-0.
49. Nogová, L., Reineke, T., Brillant, C., et al. (2008). Lymphocyte-predominant and classic Hodgkin's lymphoma: A comprehensive analysis from the German Hodgkin Study Group. *Journal of Clinical Oncology, 26*(3), 434–439. doi:10.1200/JCO.2007.11.8869.
50. Al-Mansour, M., Connors, J. M., Gascoyne, R. D., et al. (2010). Transformation to aggressive lymphoma in nodular lymphocyte-predominant Hodgkin's lymphoma. *Journal of Clinical Oncology, 28*(5), 793–799. doi:10.1200/JCO.2009.24.9516.
51. National Cancer Institute. (2016). *Adult Hodgkin lymphoma treatment (PDQ®)*. Bethesda, MD: Author. Retrieved from http://cancer.gov/cancertopics/pdq/treatment/adulthodgkins/HealthProfessional.
52. National Cancer Institute. (2015). *Adult Hodgkin lymphoma treatment (PDQ®)*. Bethesda, MD: Author. Retrieved from http:// cancer.gov/cancertopics/pdq/treatment/adulthodgkins/Patient.
53. Boffetta, P. (2011). Epidemiology of adult non-Hodgkin lymphoma. *Annals of Oncology, 22*(4), 1v27–1v31. doi:10.1093/annonc/mdr167.
54. National Cancer Institute. (2016). *Adult non-Hodgkin lymphoma treatment (PDQ®)*. Bethesda, MD: Author. Retrieved from http://cancer.gov/cancertopics/pdq/treatment/adult-non-hodgkins/Patient.
55. National Cancer Institute. (2016). *Adult non-Hodgkin lymphoma treatment (PDQ®)*. Bethesda, MD: Author. Retrieved from http://www.cancer.gov/cancertopics/pdq/treatment/adult-non-hodgkins/HealthProfessional.
56. Kochendorfer, J. N., Dudley, M. E., Kassim, S. H., et al. (2015). Chemotherapy-refractory diffuse large B-cell lymphoma and indolent B-cell malignancies can be effectively treated with autologous T cells expressing an anti-CD19 chimeric antigen receptor. *Journal of Clinical Oncology, 33*(6), 540–549. doi:10.1200/JCO.2014.56.2025.
57. Howlader, N., Noone, A. M., Krapcho, M., et al. (Eds.), (2013). *SEER cancer statistics review, 1975–2011*. Bethesda, MD: National Cancer Institute. Retrieved from http://seer.cancer.gov/csr/1975_2011/.
58. Myeloma Canada. (2017). *About multiple myeloma: Incidence and prevalence in Canada*. Retrieved from https://www.myelomacanada.ca/en/about-multiple-myeloma/what-is-myeloma/incidence-and-prevalence-in-canada.
59. Rajkumar, S. V., Dimopoulos, M. A., Palumbo, A., et al. (2014). International Myeloma Working Group updated criteria for the diagnosis of multiple myeloma. *Lancet Oncology, 15*(12), e528–e548. doi:10.1016/S1470-2045(14)70442-5.
60. Morgan, G. J., Walker, B. A., & Davies, F. E. (2012). The genetic architecture of multiple myeloma. *Nature Reviews. Cancer, 12*(5), 335–348. doi:10.1038/nrc3257.
61. Lohr, J. G., Stojanov, P., Carter, S. L., et al. (2014). Widespread genetic heterogeneity in multiple myeloma: Implications for targeted therapy. *Cancer Cell, 25*(1), 91–101. doi:10.1016/j.ccr.2013.12.015.
62. Hattori, Y., Du, W., Yamada, T., et al. (2013). A myeloma cell line established from a patient refractory to thalidomide therapy revealed high-risk cytogenetic abnormalities and produced vascular endothelial growth factor. *Blood Cancer J, 3*, e115. doi:10.1038/bcj.2013.13.
63. Rajkumar, S. V., Merlini, G., & San Migeul, J. F. (2012). Haematological cancer: Redefining myeloma. *Nature Reviews. Clinical Oncology, 9*(9), 494–496. doi:10.1038/nrclinonc.2012.128.
64. Ioannou, A., Kannan, L., & Tsokos, G. C. (2013). Platelets, complement and tissue inflammation. *Autoimmunity, 46*(1), 105. doi:10.3109/08916934.2012.722144.
65. National Heart, Lung, and Blood Institute. (2012).*What is thrombocytopenia*? Bethesda, MD: National Institutes of Health, U.S. Department of Health and Human Services. Retrieved from http://www.nhlbi.nih.gov/health/dci/Diseases/thcp/thcp_all.html.
66. Backmair, E. M., Ostertag, L. M., Zhang, X., et al. (2014). Dietary manipulation of platelet function. *Pharmacology & Therapeutics, 144*(2), 97–113. doi:10.1016/j.pharmthera.2014.05.008.
67. Paniccia, R., Priora, R., Liotta, A. A., et al. (2014). Assessment of platelet function: Laboratory and point-of-care methods. *World Journal of Translational Medicine, 3*(2), 69–83. doi:10.5528/wjtm.v3.i2.69.
68. Nurden, A. T., & Nurden, P. (2014). Congenital platelet disorders and understanding of platelet function. *British Journal of Haematology, 165*(2), 165–178. doi:10.1111/bjh.12662.
69. Bartholomew, J. R. (2014). Heparin-induced thrombocytopenia. In A. Lichtin & J. Bartholomew (Eds.), *The coagulation consult: A case-based guide*. New York: Springer.
70. Selleng, K., Selleng, S., & Greinacher, A. (2008). Heparin-induced thrombocytopenia in intensive care patients. *Seminars in Thrombosis and Hemostasis, 34*(5), 425–438. doi:10.1055/s-0028-1092872.
71. Lakshmanan, S., & Cuker, A. (2012). Contemporary management of primary immune thrombocytopenia (ITP) in adults. *Journal of Thrombosis and Haemostasis, 10*(10), 1988–1998. doi:10.1111/j.1538-7836.2012.04876.x.
72. Rodeghiero, F., & Ruggeri, M. (2015). Treatment of immune thrombocytopenia in adults: The role of thrombopoietin-receptor agonists. *Seminars in Hematology, 52*(1), 16–24. doi:10.1053/j.seminhematol.2014.10.006.

73. Kuwana, M. (2014). *Helicobacter pylori*-associated immune thrombocytopenia: Clinical features and pathogenic mechanisms. *World Journal of Gastroenterology, 20*(3), 714–723. doi:10.3748/wjg.v20.i3.714.
74. Stasi, R., & Provan, D. (2008). *Helicobacter pylori* and chronic ITP. *Hematology. American Society of Hematology. Education Program, 2008*, 206–211. doi:10.1182/asheducation-2008.1.206.
75. Veneri, D., De Matteis, G., Solero, P., et al. (2005). Analysis of B- and T-cell clonality and HLA class II alleles in patients with idiopathic thrombocytopenic purpura: Correlation with *Helicobacter pylori* infection and response to eradication treatment. *Platelets, 16*(5), 307–311. doi:10.1080/09537100400028685.
76. Xie, J., Cui, D., Liu, Y., et al. (2015). Changes in follicular helper T cells in idiopathic thrombocytopenic purpura patients. *International Journal of Biological Sciences, 11*(2), 220–229. doi:10.7150/ijbs.10178.
77. Kuhne, T., & Imback, P. (2013). Management of children and adolescents with primary immune thrombocytopenia: Controversies and solutions. *Vox Sanguinis, 104*(1), 55–66. doi:10.1111/j.1423-0410.2012.01636.x.
78. Bennett, C. M., de Jong, J. L., & Neufeld, E. J. (2006). Targeted ITP strategies: Do they elucidate the biology of ITP and related disorders? *Pediatric Blood & Cancer, 47*(Suppl. 5), 706–709. doi:10.1002/pbc.20974.
79. Kashiwagi, H., & Tomiyama, Y. (2013). Pathophysiology and management of primary immune thrombocytopenia. *International Journal of Hematology, 98*(1), 24–33. doi:10.1007/s12185-013-1370-4.
80. Lo, E., & Deane, S. (2014). Diagnosis and classification of immune-mediated thrombocytopenia. *Autoimmunity Reviews, 13*(3–5), 577–583. doi:10.1016/j.autrev.2014.01.026.
81. Al-Nouri, Z. L., Reese, J. A., Terrell, D. R., et al. (2015). Drug-induced thrombotic microangiopathy: A systematic review of published reports. *Blood, 125*(4), 616–618. doi:10.1182/blood-2014-11-611335.
82. Zöller, B., Li, X., Sundquist, J., et al. (2012). Autoimmune disease and venous thromboembolism: A review of the literature. *American Journal of Cardiovascular Disease, 2*(3), 171–183.
83. Rodeghiero, F., & Ruggeri, M. (2014). ITP and international guidelines: What do we know, what do we need? *La Presse Medicale, 43*(4), e61–e67. doi:10.1016/j.lpm.2014.02.004.
84. Tefferi, A., & Barbui, T. (2015). Polycythemia vera and essential thrombocytemia: 2015 update on diagnosis, risk-stratification and management. *American Journal of Hematology, 90*(2), 162–173. doi:10.1002/ajh.23895.
85. Landolfi, R., & Fi Gennaro, L. (2012). Thrombosis in myeloproliferative and myelodysplastic syndromes. *Hematology (Amsterdam, Netherlands), 17*(Suppl. 1), S174–S176. doi:10.1179/102453312X13336169156898.
86. Harrison, C., Kiladjian, J. J., Al-Ali, H. K., et al. (2012). JAK inhibition with ruxolitinib versus best available therapy for myelofibrosis. *New England Journal of Medicine, 366*(9), 787–798. doi:10.1056/NEJMoa1110556.
87. Passamonti, F., Thiele, J., Girodon, F., et al. (2012). A prognostic model to predict survival in 867 World Health Organization-defined essential thrombocythemia at diagnosis: A study by the international Working Group on Myelofibrosis Research and Treatment. *Blood, 120*(6), 1197–1201. doi:10.1182/blood-2012-01-403279.
88. Wolanskyj, A. P., Schwager, S. M., McClure, R. F., et al. (2006). Essential thrombocythemia beyond the first decade: Life expectancy, long-term complication rates, and prognostic factors. *Mayo Clinic Proceedings. Mayo Clinic, 81*(2), 159–166.
89. Tefferi, A., Thiele, J., & Vardiman, J. W. (2009). The 2008 World Health Organization classification system for myeloproliferative neoplasms: Order out of chaos. *Cancer, 115*(17), 3842–3847. doi:10.1002/cncr.24440.
90. Barbui, T., Finzzai, M. C., & Finzzai, G. (2012). Front-line therapy in polycythemia vera and essential thrombocythemia. *Blood Reviews, 26*(5), 205–211. doi:10.1016/j.blre.2012.06.002.
91. Salles, I. I., Feys, H. B., Iserbyt, B. F., et al. (2008). Inherited traits affecting platelet function. *Blood Reviews, 22*(3), 155–172. doi:10.1016/j.blre.2007.11.002.
92. Lisman, T., Caldwell, S. H., Burroughs, A. K., et al. (2010). Hemostasis and thrombosis in patients with liver disease: The ups and downs. *Journal of Hepatology, 53*(2), 362–371. doi:10.1016/j.jhep.2010.01.042.
93. Wada, H., Matsumoto, T., & Yamashita, Y. (2014). Diagnosis and treatment of disseminated intravascular coagulation (DIC) according to four DIC guidelines. *Journal of Intensive Care, 2*(1), 15. doi:10.1186/2052-0492-2-15.
94. Venugopal, A. (2014). Disseminated intravascular coagulation. *Indian Journal of Anaesthesia, 58*(5), 603–608. doi:10.4103/0019-5049.144666.
95. Nakashima, M. O., & Rogers, H. J. (2014). Hypercoagulable states: An algorithmic approach to laboratory testing and update on monitoring of direct oral anticoagulants. *Blood Research, 49*(2), 85–94. doi:10.5045/br.2014.49.2.85.
96. Bruce, A., & Massicotte, M. P. (2012). Thrombophilia screening: Whom to test. *Blood, 120*(7), 1353–1355. doi:10.1182/blood-2012-06-430678.
97. Baglin, T. (2012). Inherited and acquired risk factors for venous thromboembolism. *Seminars in Respiratory and Critical Care Medicine, 33*(2), 127–137. doi:10.1055/s-0032-1311791.
98. Giannakopoulos, B., & Krilis, S. A. (2013). The pathogenesis of the antiphospholipid syndrome. *New England Journal of Medicine, 368*(11), 1033–1044. doi:10.1056/NEJMra1112830.
99. Aksu, K., Donmez, A., & Keser, G. (2012). Inflammation-induced thrombosis: Mechanisms, disease associations and management. *Current Pharmaceutical Design, 18*(11), 1478–1493.
100. Heilmann, L., Schorch, M., Hahn, T., et al. (2008). Pregnancy outcome in women with antiphospholipid antibodies: Report on a retrospective study. *Seminars in Thrombosis and Hemostasis, 34*(8), 794–802. doi:10.1055/s-0029-1145261.

22

Alterations of Hematological Function in Children

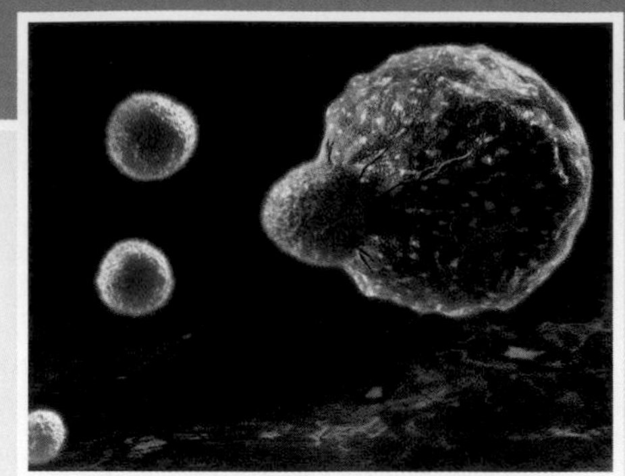

Joan Shea, Nancy E. Kline, Anna E. Roche, Kathryn L. McCance, and Kelly Power-Kean

EVOLVE WEBSITE

http://evolve.elsevier.com/Huether/
Student Review Questions
Key Points
Case Studies
Animations
Quick Check Answers

CHAPTER OUTLINE

Disorders of Erythrocytes, 560
Acquired Disorders, 560
Inherited Disorders, 564
Disorders of Coagulation and Platelets, 569
Inherited Hemorrhagic Disease, 569
Antibody-Mediated Hemorrhagic Disease, 569
Neoplastic Disorders, 570
Leukemia, 570
Lymphomas, 571

Among the diseases that affect erythrocytes in children are acquired disorders, such as iron deficiency anemia and hemolytic disease of the newborn, and inherited disorders, such as glucose-6-phosphate dehydrogenase deficiency, sickle cell disease, and the thalassemias.

Childhood disorders that involve the coagulation process and platelets include inherited hemorrhagic diseases, such as the hemophilias, and antibody-mediated hemorrhagic diseases, including immune thrombocytopenic purpura. Finally, leukocyte disorders, such as leukemia and the lymphomas (both Hodgkin's lymphoma [HL] and non-Hodgkin's lymphoma [NHL]), are discussed in this chapter.

DISORDERS OF ERYTHROCYTES

Anemia is the most common blood disorder in children. Like the anemias of adulthood, the anemias of childhood are caused by ineffective erythropoiesis or premature destruction of erythrocytes. The most common cause of insufficient erythropoiesis is iron deficiency, which may result from insufficient dietary intake or chronic loss of iron caused by bleeding. The hemolytic anemias of childhood may be divided into (1) disorders that result from premature destruction caused by intrinsic abnormalities of the erythrocytes and (2) disorders that result from damaging extraerythrocytic factors. The hemolytic anemias are either inherited or acquired.

The most dramatic form of acquired congenital hemolytic anemia is hemolytic disease of the newborn (HDN), also termed *erythroblastosis fetalis.* HDN is an alloimmunity (isoimmunity) disease in which maternal blood and fetal blood are incompatible, causing the mother's immune system to produce antibodies against fetal erythrocytes. Fetal erythrocytes attacked by (i.e., bound to) maternal antibodies are recognized as foreign or defective by the fetal mononuclear phagocyte system and are removed from the circulation by phagocytosis, usually in the fetal spleen. (For a complete examination of HDN, see the discussion in "Hemolytic Disease of the Newborn.") Other acquired hemolytic anemias—some of which begin in utero—include those caused by infections or the presence of toxic chemicals.

The inherited forms of hemolytic anemia result from intrinsic defects of the child's erythrocytes, any of which can lead to erythrocyte removal by the mononuclear phagocyte system. Structural defects include abnormal cellular size or shape and abnormalities of plasma membrane structure (spherocytosis). Intracellular defects include enzyme deficiencies, the most common of which is glucose-6-phosphate dehydrogenase (G6PD) deficiency, and defects of hemoglobin synthesis, which manifest as sickle cell disease or thalassemia, depending on which component of hemoglobin is defective. These and other causes of childhood anemia are listed in Table 22-1.

Acquired Disorders

Iron Deficiency Anemia

Iron is *critical* to the developing child, especially for normal brain development. Without it the damage from the periods of iron deficiency anemia (IDA) in children is irreversible. The prevalence of IDA in Canadian children among the general population is low (3.5 to 10.5%); however, there are certain Indigenous populations in Canada in whom the prevalence is very high (14 to 50%). IDA is the most common nutritional disorder worldwide, with the highest incidence occurring between 6 months and 2 years of age. IDA is common in Canada with prevalence higher in toddlers, adolescent girls, and women of childbearing age.[1] IDA causes clinical manifestations mostly related to inadequate hemoglobin synthesis.[2]

IDA can result from (1) dietary lack of iron, (2) problems with iron absorption, (3) blood loss, and (4) increased requirement for iron. Inadequate intake of iron is the most common cause of IDA during

TABLE 22-1 Anemias of Childhood

Cause	Anemic Condition
Deficient Erythropoiesis or Hemoglobin Synthesis	
Decreased stem cell population in marrow (congenital or acquired pure red cell aplasia)	Normocytic-normochromic anemia
Decreased erythropoiesis despite normal stem cell population in marrow (infection, inflammation, cancer, chronic renal disease, congenital dyserythropoiesis)	Normocytic-normochromic anemia
Deficiency of a factor or nutrient needed for erythropoiesis	
Cobalamin (vitamin B_{12}), folate	Megaloblastic anemia
Iron	Microcytic-hypochromic anemia
Increased or Premature Hemolysis	
Alloimmune disease (maternal–fetal Rh, ABO, or minor blood group incompatibility)	Autoimmune hemolytic anemia
Autoimmune disease (idiopathic autoimmune hemolytic anemia, symptomatic systemic lupus erythematosus, lymphoma, medication-induced autoimmune processes)	Autoimmune hemolytic anemia
Inherited defects of plasma membrane structure (spherocytosis, elliptocytosis, stomatocytosis) or cellular size or both (pyknocytosis)	Hemolytic anemia
Infection (bacterial sepsis, congenital syphilis, malaria, cytomegalovirus infection, rubella, toxoplasmosis, disseminated herpes)	Hemolytic anemia
Intrinsic and inherited enzymatic defects (deficiencies) of glucose-6-phosphate dehydrogenase, pyruvate kinase, 5′-nucleotidase, glucose phosphate isomerase	Hemolytic anemia
Inherited defects of hemoglobin synthesis	Sickle cell anemia Thalassemia
Disseminated intravascular coagulation (see Chapter 21)	Hemolytic anemia
Galactosemia	Hemolytic anemia
Prolonged or recurrent respiratory or metabolic acidosis	Hemolytic anemia
Blood vessel disorders (cavernous hemangiomas, large vessel thrombus, renal artery stenosis, severe coarctation of aorta)	Hemolytic anemia

the first few years of life. Blood loss is the most common cause during childhood and adolescence, and for adults in the Western world. Chronic IDA from occult (hidden) blood loss may be caused by a gastro-intestinal lesion, parasitic infestation, or hemorrhagic disease. A reasonable hypothesis for infants and young children who develop IDA is that it occurs because of chronic intestinal blood loss induced by exposure to a heat-labile protein in cow's milk. Such exposure causes an inflammatory gastro-intestinal reaction that damages the mucosa and results in diffuse microhemorrhage. Growing evidence indicates that cellular components of both innate and adaptive immunity play significant roles during the pathogenesis of cow's milk allergy.[3] Dietary lack of iron is not common in developed countries, where iron is in the readily absorbed form from heme found in meat. IDA was recently found in Israel, mainly in children 1.5 to 3 years old, and was associated with low red meat intake.[4] In developing countries, food may be less available and the iron found in plants is in the poorly absorbable inorganic form.[1] Infants are at increased risk for IDA because of very small amounts of iron in milk. Bioavailability of iron from breast milk is higher than that from cow's milk. Impaired absorption is found in chronic diarrhea, fat malabsorption, and sprue (see *Health Promotion:* Prevention of Iron Deficiency Anemia in Infants and Children).

Children in developing countries are often affected by chronic parasite infestations that result in blood and iron loss greater than dietary intake. Treatment of helminth (parasitic worm) infections results in improvement in both appetite and growth, as well as reduction of anemia. The association between IDA and lead poisoning is controversial. Newer areas of investigation include iron deficiency in overweight children and the association of *Helicobacter pylori* infection with IDA.[5]

PATHOPHYSIOLOGY No matter the cause, a deficiency of iron produces a hypochromic-microcytic anemia.[2] Progressive depletion of blood and low serum levels of ferritin and transferrin saturation eventually lead

HEALTH PROMOTION

Prevention of Iron Deficiency Anemia in Infants and Children

Studies have indicated that iron deficiency in infants and children is a public health concern within several Canadian populations. Certain Indigenous populations in Canada are affected by very high percentages of IDA, as are children of low socioeconomic status, children of Chinese background, low-birthweight infants, and children who consume whole cow's milk prior to 12 months of age. Risk factors associated with severe iron deficiency include high consumption of evaporated milk and cow's milk after 6 months of age, prolonged exclusive breastfeeding, and *Helicobacter pylori* infection. Chronic severe IDA in the first years of life increases the risk for irreversible cognition problems as well as affective and motor development issues.

IDA is a preventable disease that can be addressed through primary prevention efforts, including the promotion of breastfeeding or, alternatively, using fortified formula and infant cereal. It is recommended that healthy exclusively breastfed infants be supplemented with 1 mg/kg/day of oral iron beginning at 4 months of age until iron-containing foods are introduced. Whole milk should not be introduced before 12 months of age. In addition, the early introduction of red meat and higher iron content vegetables is recommended. Preterm infants who are fed human milk should receive an iron supplement of 2 mg/kg/day by 1 month of age until weaned to iron-fortified formula or beginning iron-containing foods.

Data from Canadian Pediatric Surveillance Program. (2011). *Iron deficiency anemia in children.* Retrieved from http://www.cpsp.cps.ca/uploads/publications/RA-iron-deficiency-anemia.pdf.

to a lowering of hemoglobin and hematocrit levels. In the early stages, an adaptive increase in red blood cell activity in the bone marrow may prevent the development of anemia. When the iron stores are depleted, with accompanying important laboratory indicators, anemia develops.

CLINICAL MANIFESTATIONS The symptoms of mild anemia—listlessness and fatigue—usually are not present or are undetectable in infants and young children, who are unable to describe these symptoms. Therefore, parents generally do not note any change in the child's behaviour or appearance until moderate anemia has developed. General irritability, decreased activity tolerance, weakness, and lack of interest in play are nonspecific indications of anemia. When hemoglobin levels fall below 50 mmol/L, pallor, anorexia, tachycardia, and systolic murmurs may occur.

Other symptoms and signs of chronic IDA include splenomegaly, widened skull sutures, decreased physical growth, developmental delays, pica (a behaviour in which nonfood substances, such as clay, are eaten), and altered neurological and intellectual functions, especially those involving attention span, alertness, and learning ability.

EVALUATION AND TREATMENT The diagnosis of IDA is confirmed by laboratory tests. These tests include measurement of hemoglobin, hematocrit, serum iron, and ferritin levels and determination of the total iron binding capacity. Most essential is obtaining a thorough history of present illness and dietary history in addition to performing a complete physical examination. Evaluation and treatment of iron deficiency anemia in children is similar to that used for adults with IDA (see Chapter 21). Oral administration of a simple ferrous salt is usually satisfactory and additional vitamin C helps promote absorption.[6] Iron in a liquid form should be administered through a straw because it can stain teeth. Dietary modification is required to prevent recurrences of IDA. Intake of iron-rich foods is increased, and the intake of cow's milk may be restricted.

Hemolytic Disease of the Newborn

The most common cause of hemolytic anemia in newborns is alloimmune disease. **Hemolytic disease of the newborn (HDN) (erythroblastosis fetalis)** can occur only if antigens on fetal erythrocytes differ from antigens on maternal erythrocytes. Maternal–fetal incompatibility exists if mother and fetus differ in ABO blood type or if the fetus is Rh-positive and the mother is Rh-negative. Some minor blood antigens also may be involved (see Chapter 7).

ABO incompatibility occurs in about 20 to 25% of all pregnancies, but only 1 in 10 cases of ABO incompatibility results in HDN. Rh incompatibility occurs in less than 10% of pregnancies and rarely causes HDN in the first incompatible fetus. Even after five or more pregnancies, only 5% of women have babies with hemolytic disease. Usually erythrocytes from the first incompatible fetus cause the mother's immune system to produce antibodies that affect the fetuses of subsequent incompatible pregnancies. Only one in three cases of HDN is caused by Rh incompatibility; most cases are caused by ABO incompatibility.

PATHOPHYSIOLOGY HDN will result (1) if the mother's blood contains preformed antibodies against fetal erythrocytes or produces them on exposure to fetal erythrocytes, (2) if sufficient amounts of antibody (usually immunoglobulin G [IgG]) cross the placenta and enter fetal blood, and (3) if IgG binds with sufficient numbers of fetal erythrocytes to cause widespread antibody-mediated hemolysis or splenic removal. (Antibody-mediated cellular destruction is described in Chapter 8.)

Maternal antibodies may be formed against type B erythrocytes if the mother is type A or against type A erythrocytes if the mother is type B. Usually, however, the mother is type O and the fetus is A or B. ABO incompatibility can cause HDN even if fetal erythrocytes do not escape into the maternal circulation during pregnancy. HDN occurs because the blood of most adults already contains anti-A or anti-B antibodies, which are produced on exposure to certain foods or infection by Gram-negative bacteria. (Anti-O antibodies do not exist because type O erythrocytes are not antigenic.) Therefore, IgG against type A or B erythrocytes is usually preformed in maternal blood and can enter the fetal circulation throughout the first incompatible pregnancy.

Anti-Rh antibodies, on the other hand, are formed only in response to the presence of incompatible (Rh-positive) erythrocytes from the fetus in the blood of an Rh-negative mother. Sources of exposure include fetal blood that is mixed with the mother's blood at the time of delivery, transfused blood, and, rarely, previous sensitization of the mother by her own mother's incompatible blood (Figure 22-1).

The first Rh-incompatible pregnancy generally presents no difficulties because few fetal erythrocytes cross the placental barrier during gestation. When the placenta detaches at birth, however, a large number of fetal erythrocytes usually enter the mother's bloodstream. If the mother is Rh-negative and the fetus is Rh-positive, the mother produces anti-Rh antibodies. Anti-Rh antibodies persist in the bloodstream for a long time, and if the next offspring is Rh-positive, the mother's anti-Rh antibodies can enter the bloodstream of the fetus and destroy the erythrocytes. Antibodies against Rh antigen D are of the IgG class and easily cross the placenta.

IgG-coated fetal erythrocytes usually are destroyed in the spleen. As hemolysis proceeds, the fetus becomes anemic. Erythropoiesis accelerates, particularly in the liver and spleen, and immature nucleated cells (erythroblasts) are released into the bloodstream (hence the name *erythroblastosis fetalis*). The degree of anemia depends on the length of time the antibody has been in the fetal circulation, the concentration of the antibody, and the ability of the fetus to compensate for increased hemolysis. Unconjugated (indirect) bilirubin, which is formed during breakdown of hemoglobin, is transported across the placental barrier into the maternal circulation and is excreted by the mother. Hyperbilirubinemia occurs in the neonate after birth because excretion of lipid-soluble unconjugated bilirubin through the placenta is no longer possible.

The pathophysiological effects of HDN are more severe in Rh incompatibility than in ABO incompatibility. ABO incompatibility may resolve after birth without life-threatening complications. Maternal–fetal incompatibility in which a mother with type O blood has a child with type A or B blood usually is so mild that it does not require treatment.

Rh incompatibility is more likely than ABO incompatibility to cause severe or even life-threatening anemia, death in utero, or damage to the central nervous system. Severe anemia alone can cause death as a result of cardiovascular complications. Extensive hemolysis also results in increased levels of unconjugated bilirubin in the neonate's circulation. If bilirubin levels exceed the liver's ability to conjugate and excrete bilirubin, some of it is deposited in the brain, causing cellular damage and, eventually, death if the neonate does not receive exchange transfusions.

Fetuses that do not survive anemia in utero usually are stillborn, with gross edema in the entire body, a condition called **hydrops fetalis**. Death can occur as early as 17 weeks' gestation and results in spontaneous abortion.

CLINICAL MANIFESTATIONS Neonates with mild HDN may appear healthy or slightly pale, with slight enlargement of the liver or spleen. Pronounced pallor, splenomegaly, and hepatomegaly indicate severe

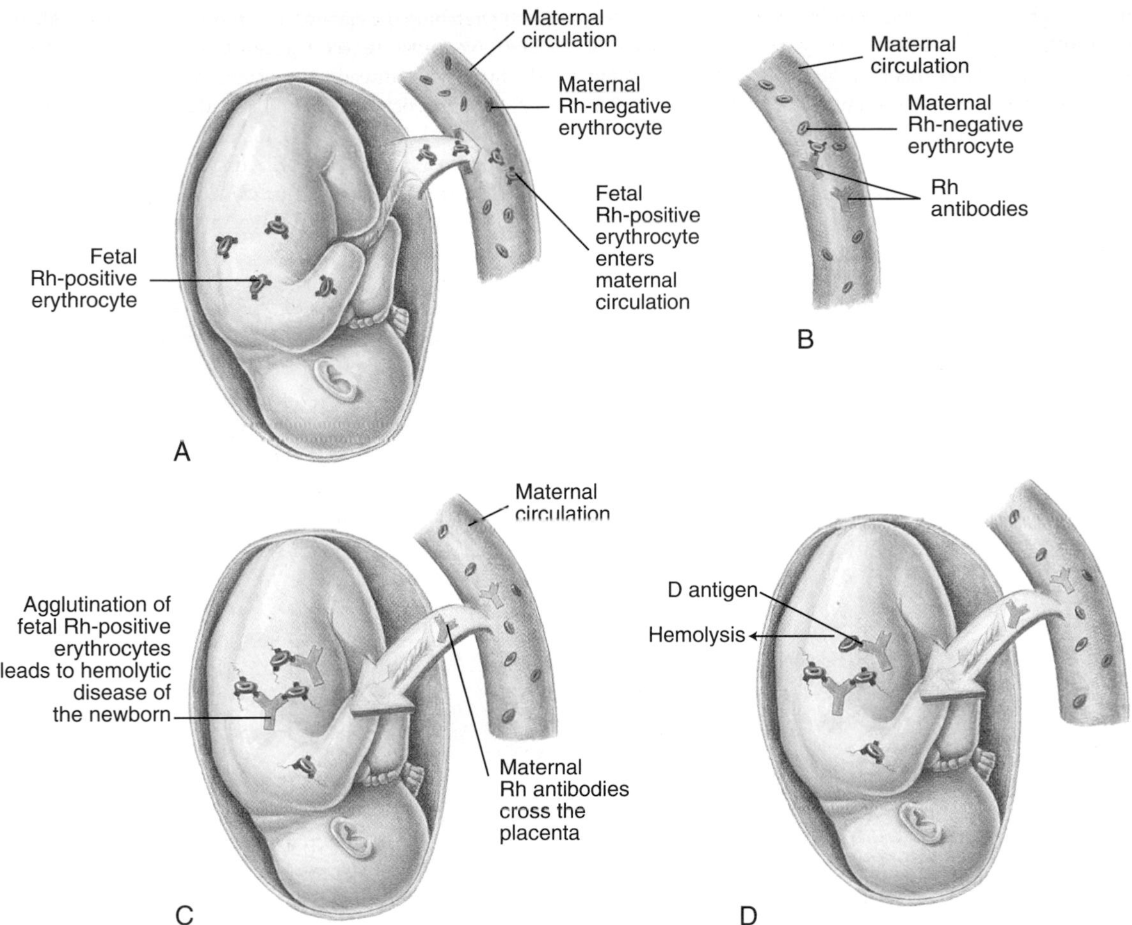

FIGURE 22-1 Hemolytic Disease of the Newborn. A, Before or during delivery, Rh-positive erythrocytes from the fetus enter the blood of an Rh-negative woman through a tear in the placenta. **B,** The mother is sensitized to the Rh antigen and produces Rh antibodies. Because this sensitization usually happens after delivery, there is no effect on the fetus in the first pregnancy. **C,** During a subsequent pregnancy with an Rh-positive fetus, Rh-positive erythrocytes cross the placenta, enter the maternal circulation, and **(D)** stimulate the mother to produce antibodies against the Rh antigen. (Modified from Seeley, R.R., Stephens, T.D., Tate, P., et al. [1995]. *Anatomy and physiology* [3rd ed.]. St. Louis: Mosby.)

anemia, which predisposes the neonate to cardiovascular failure and shock. Life-threatening Rh incompatibility is rare today, largely because of the routine use of Rh immunoglobulin.

Because the maternal antibodies remain in the neonate's circulatory system after birth, erythrocyte destruction can continue. This destruction causes **hyperbilirubinemia** and **icterus neonatorum (neonatal jaundice)** shortly after birth. Without replacement transfusions, in which the child receives Rh-negative erythrocytes, the bilirubin is deposited in the brain, a condition termed **kernicterus**. Kernicterus produces cerebral damage and usually causes death **(icterus gravis neonatorum)**. Infants who do not die may have intellectual disabilities, cerebral palsy, or high-frequency deafness.

EVALUATION AND TREATMENT Routine evaluation of fetuses at risk for HDN (i.e., fetuses resulting from Rh- or ABO-incompatible matings) includes the Coombs test. The indirect Coombs test measures antibodies in the mother's circulation and indicates whether the fetus is at risk for HDN. The direct Coombs test measures antibodies already bound to the surfaces of fetal erythrocytes and is used primarily to confirm the diagnosis of antibody-mediated HDN. With a prior history of fetal hemolytic disease, diagnostic tests are done to determine risk with the current pregnancy. These tests include maternal antibody titres, fetal blood sampling, amniotic fluid spectrophotometry, and ultrasound fetal assessment.

The key to treatment of HDN resulting from Rh incompatibility lies in prevention (immunoprophylaxis).[7,8] One of the success stories of immunology has been the result obtained with Rh immune globulin (RhoGAM), a preparation of antibodies against Rh antigen D (anti-D Ig). If an Rh-negative woman is given Rh immune globulin within 72 hours of exposure to Rh-positive erythrocytes, she will not produce antibodies against the D antigen, and the next Rh-positive baby she conceives will be protected. Updated recommendations also state that if anti-D Ig is not given within 72 hours, every effort should still be made to administer the anti-D Ig within 10 days. The newer updates on the use of anti-D Ig as prophylaxis to prevent sensitization to the D antigen *during* pregnancy or at *delivery* for the prevention of HDN can be found at the Canadian Blood Services website at https://professionaleducation.blood.ca/en/transfusion/clinical-guide/hemolytic-disease-fetus-and-newborn-and-perinatal-immune-thrombocytopenia. The British Society for Haematology (BSH) Guideline (previously known as *BCSH Guidelines*) also provides guidance on the use of anti-D Ig for Rh D prophylaxis.[8]

Inherited Disorders

Sickle Cell Disease

Sickle cell disease is a group of disorders characterized by the production of abnormal **hemoglobin S (Hb S)** within the erythrocytes. Hb S is formed by a genetic mutation in which one amino acid (valine) replaces another (glutamic acid) (Figure 22-2). Hb S, the so-called sickle hemoglobin, reacts to deoxygenation and dehydration by solidifying and stretching the erythrocyte into an elongated sickle shape, producing hemolytic anemia (see Figure 22-2).

Sickle cell disease is an inherited, autosomal recessive disorder expressed as sickle cell anemia, sickle cell–thalassemia disease, or sickle cell–hemoglobin C disease, depending on mode of inheritance (Table 22-2). (See Chapter 2 for a discussion of genetic inheritance of disease.) **Sickle cell anemia**, a homozygous form, is the most severe. **Sickle**

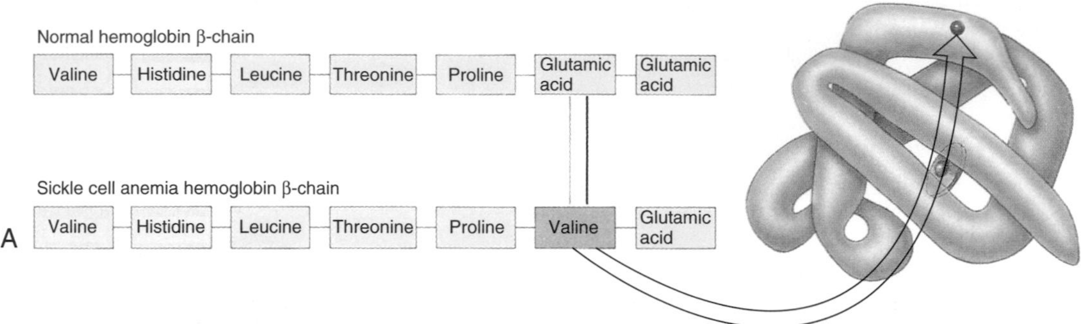

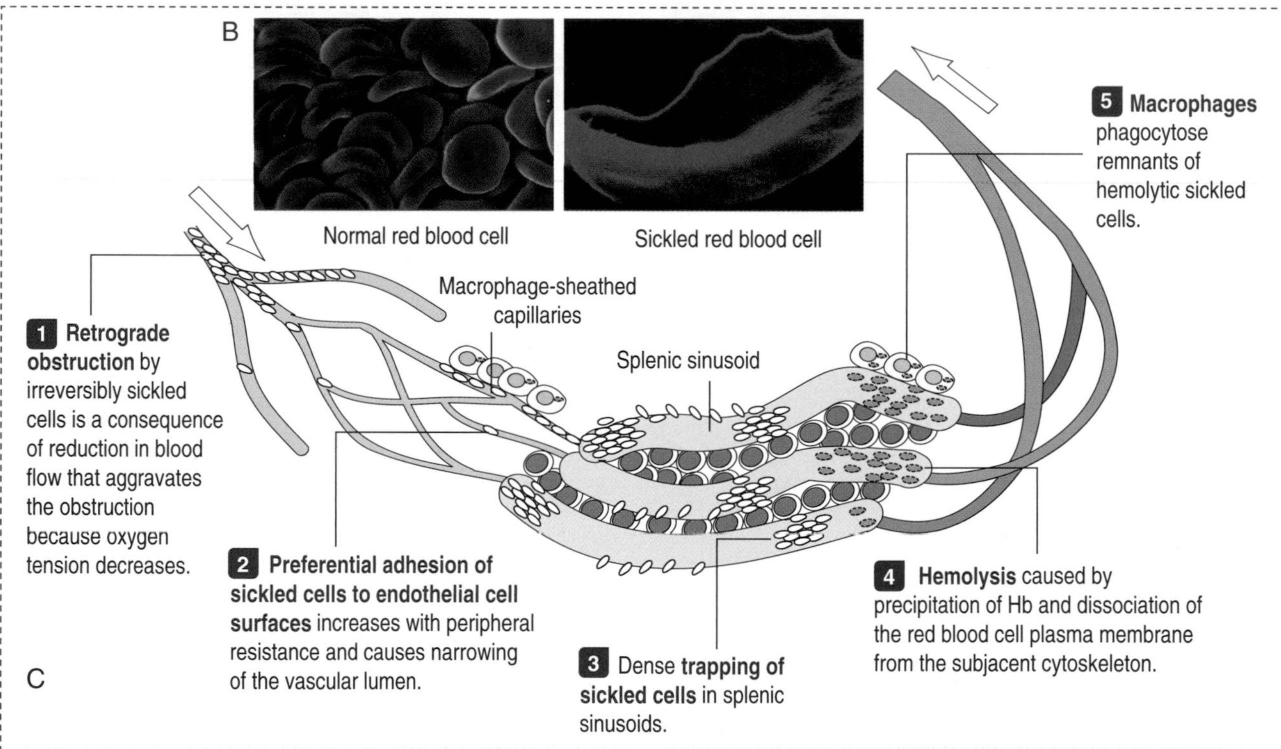

FIGURE 22-2 Sickle Cell Hemoglobin. A, Sickle cell hemoglobin is produced by a recessive allele of the gene encoding the β-chain of the protein hemoglobin. It represents a single amino acid change—from glutamic acid to valine at the sixth position of the chain. In this model of a hemoglobin molecule, the position of the mutation can be seen near the end of the upper arm. **B,** Colour-enhanced electron micrograph shows normal erythrocytes and sickled blood cell. **C,** Brief summary of sickle cell. (**A,** from Raven, P.H., & Johnson, G.B. [1992]. *Biology* [3rd ed.]. St. Louis: Mosby; **B,** Dennis Kunkel Microscopy/Science Source; **C,** from Kierszenbaum, A., & Tres, L. [2012]. *Histology and cell biology: An introduction to pathology* [3rd ed.]. St. Louis: Mosby.)

TABLE 22-2 Inheritance of Sickle Cell Disease

Hemoglobin Inherited From First Parent	Hemoglobin Inherited From Second Parent	Form of Sickle Cell Disease in Child
Hemoglobin (Hb) S (an abnormal hemoglobin)	Hb S	Sickle cell anemia: homozygous inheritance in which child's hemoglobin is mostly Hb S, with remainder Hb F (fetal hemoglobin)
Hb S	Defective or insufficient α- or β-chains of Hb A (α- or β-thalassemia)	Sickle cell–thalassemia disease (heterozygous inheritance of Hb S and α- or β-thalassemia)
Hb S	Hb C or D (both abnormal hemoglobins)	Sickle cell–hemoglobin C (or D) disease (heterozygous inheritance of hemoglobin S and either C or D)
Hb S	Normal hemoglobins (mostly Hb A)	Sickle cell trait, carrier state (heterozygous inheritance of Hb S and normal hemoglobin)

cell–thalassemia disease and sickle cell–hemoglobin C disease are heterozygous forms in which the child simultaneously inherits another type of abnormal hemoglobin from one parent. Sickle cell trait, in which the child inherits Hb S from one parent and normal hemoglobin (Hb A) from the other, is a heterozygous carrier state that rarely has clinical manifestations. All forms of sickle cell disease are lifelong conditions.

Sickle cell disease is a genetically linked disease that tends to occur in persons with ancestors from parts of Africa, the Mediterranean, the Caribbean, and India. In Canada, it is estimated that 3 000 to 7 000 people have been diagnosed with the disease.[9] The number of Canadian patients with sickle cell disease will continue to increase, related to high rates of immigration from countries with high prevalence. Improved outcomes for those affected by sickle cell disease are expected with advances in medical care. Sickle cell–hemoglobin C disease is less common (1 in 800 births), and sickle cell–thalassemia disease occurs in 1 in 1 700 births.

Sickle cell trait occurs in 7 to 13% of Blacks, whereas its incidence among East Africans may be as high as 45%. The sickle cell trait may provide protection against lethal forms of malaria, a genetic advantage to carriers who reside in endemic regions for malaria (Mediterranean and African zones), but it provides no advantage to carriers living in North America.

PATHOPHYSIOLOGY Hb S is soluble and usually causes no problem when properly oxygenated. When oxygen tension decreases, the single amino acid substitution in the β-globin chain of Hb S polymerizes, forming abnormal fluid polymers. As these polymers realign, they cause the red blood cell to deform into the sickle shape. Sickling depends on the degree of oxygenation, pH, and dehydration of the individual. A decrease in oxygenation (hypoxemia) and pH, as well as dehydration, increases sickling. Deoxygenation is probably the most important variable in determining the occurrence of sickling.[10] Sickle-trait cells sickle at oxygen tensions of about 15 mm Hg, whereas those from an individual with sickle cell disease begin to sickle at about 40 mm Hg. Sickled erythrocytes tend to plug the blood vessels, increasing the viscosity of the blood, which slows circulation and causes vascular occlusion, pain, and organ infarction. Viscosity increases the time of exposure to less oxygenation, promoting further sickling. Sickled cells undergo hemolysis in the spleen or become sequestered there, causing blood pooling and infarction of splenic vessels. The anemia that follows triggers erythropoiesis in the marrow and, in extreme cases, in the liver (Figure 22-3).

Sickling usually is not permanent; most sickled erythrocytes regain a normal shape after reoxygenation and rehydration. Irreversible sickling is caused by irreversible plasma membrane damage caused by sickling. In persons with sickle cell anemia, in which the erythrocytes contain a high percentage of Hb S (75 to 95%), up to 30% of the erythrocytes can become irreversibly sickled. Occasionally, irreversible sickling occurs in sickle cell disease but not in the carrier state (sickle cell trait). Sickling also can be triggered by increased plasma osmolality, decreased plasma volume, and low environmental temperature.

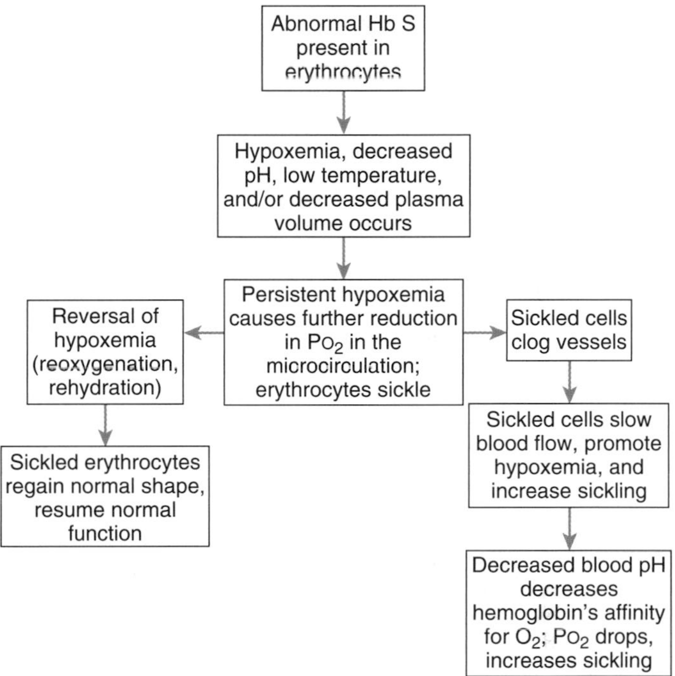

FIGURE 22-3 Sickling of Erythrocytes. *Hb S*, hemoglobin S; *O_2*, oxygen; *Po_2*, partial pressure of oxygen.

CLINICAL MANIFESTATIONS There is much variation in the clinical manifestations of sickle cell disease. Some individuals have mild symptoms, and others suffer from repeated vaso-occlusive crises.[2] When sickling occurs, the general manifestations of hemolytic anemia—pallor, fatigue, jaundice, and irritability—sometimes are accompanied by acute manifestations called *crises*. Extensive sickling can precipitate the following four types of crises:

1. Vaso-occlusive crisis (thrombotic crisis). This crisis begins with sickling in the microcirculation. As blood flow is obstructed by sickled cells, vasospasm occurs and a "logjam" effect blocks all blood flow through the vessel. Unless the process is reversed, thrombosis and infarction of local tissue follow. Vaso-occlusive crisis is extremely painful and may last for days or even weeks, with an average duration of 4 to 6 days. The frequency of this type of crisis is variable and

unpredictable. Vaso-occlusion in vessels to the brain can result in stroke. Chronic vaso-occlusion in vessels to the kidneys results in end-stage renal disease.

2. **Sequestration crisis.** Large amounts of blood become acutely pooled in the liver and spleen. This type of crisis is seen only in the young child. Because the spleen can hold as much as one-fifth of the body's blood supply at one time, up to 50% mortality has been reported, with death being caused by cardiovascular collapse.
3. **Aplastic crisis.** Profound anemia is caused by diminished erythropoiesis despite an increased need for new erythrocytes. In sickle cell anemia, erythrocyte survival is only 10 to 20 days. Normally a compensatory increase in erythropoiesis (five to eight times normal) replaces the cells lost through premature hemolysis. If this compensatory response is compromised, aplastic crisis develops in a very short time.
4. **Hyperhemolytic crisis.** Although unusual, this crisis may occur in association with certain medications or infections.

The clinical manifestations of sickle cell disease usually do not appear until the infant is at least 6 months old, at which time the postnatal decrease in concentrations of Hb F causes concentrations of Hb S to rise (Figure 22-4). Infection is the most common cause of death related to sickle cell disease. Sepsis and meningitis develop in as many as 10% of children with sickle cell anemia during the first 5 years of life. Survival time is unpredictable and has improved over the past decades.

Sickle cell–hemoglobin C disease is usually milder than sickle cell anemia. The main clinical problems are related to vaso-occlusive crises and are thought to result from higher hematocrit values and viscosity. In older children, sickle cell retinopathy, renal necrosis, and aseptic necrosis of the femoral heads occur along with obstructive crises.

Sickle cell–thalassemia disease has the mildest clinical manifestations of all the sickle cell diseases. The normal hemoglobins, particularly Hb F, inhibit sickling. In addition, the erythrocytes tend to be small (microcytic) and to contain relatively little hemoglobin (hypochromic), making them less likely to occlude the microcirculation, even when in a sickled state.

EVALUATION AND TREATMENT The sickle cell trait does not affect life expectancy or interfere with daily activities. However, on rare occasions, severe hypoxia caused by shock, vigorous exercising at high altitudes, flying at high altitudes in unpressurized aircraft, or undergoing anaesthesia is associated with vaso-occlusive episodes in persons with sickle cell trait. These cells form an ivy shape instead of a sickle shape.

The parents' hematological history and clinical manifestations may suggest that a child has sickle cell disease, but hematological tests are necessary for diagnosis. If the sickle solubility test confirms the presence of Hb S in peripheral blood, hemoglobin electrophoresis provides information about the amount of Hb S in erythrocytes. Prenatal diagnosis can be made after chorionic villus sampling as early as 8 to 10 weeks' gestation or by amniotic fluid analysis at 15 weeks' gestation (Figure 22-5). Newborn screening for sickle cell disease should be performed according to provincial recommendations.

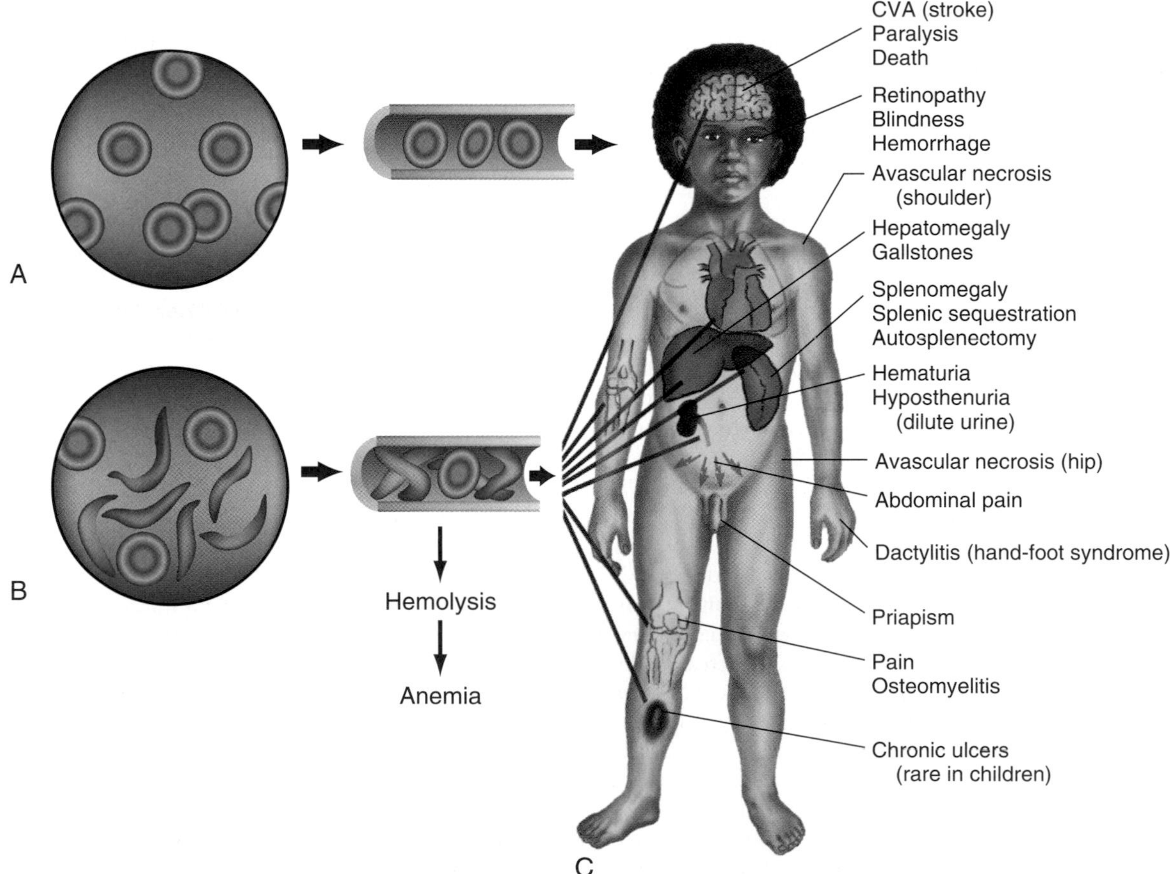

FIGURE 22-4 Differences Between Effects of (A) Normal and (B) Sickled Red Blood Cells on Blood Circulation, and Selected Consequences in a Child. C, Tissue Effects of Sickle Cell Anemia. *CVA,* cerebrovascular accident. (A and B, adapted from Hockenberry, M.J., & Wilson, D. [Eds.]. [2015]. *Wong's nursing care of infants and children* [10th ed.]. St. Louis: Mosby.)

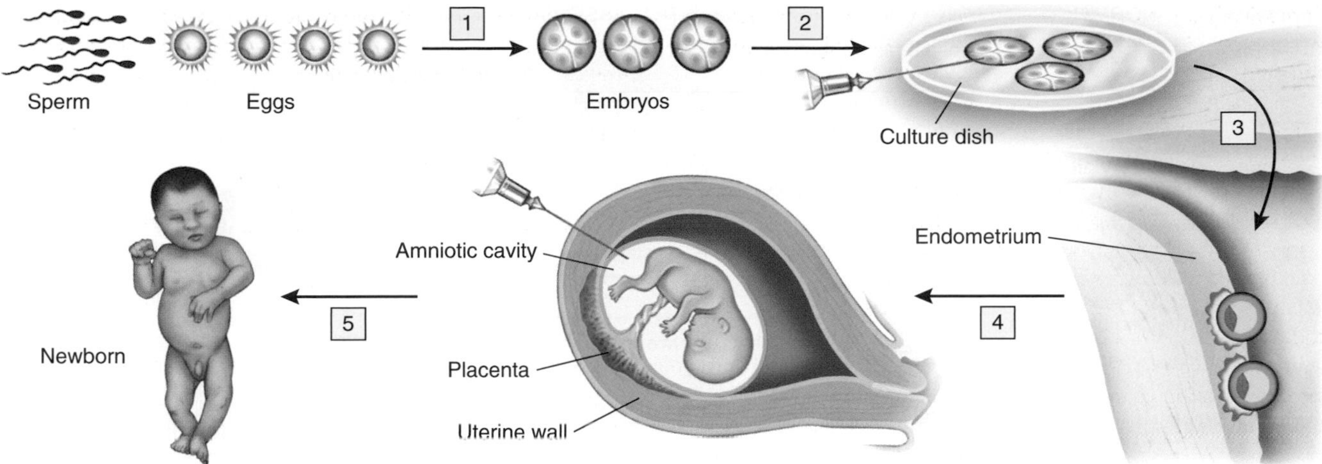

FIGURE 22-5 Prepregnancy Sickle Cell Test. This technique has potential for detection of other inherited diseases. **1,** Fertilization produces several embryos. **2,** The embryos are tested for the presence of the gene. **3,** The embryos without the gene are implanted. **4,** Amniocentesis confirms whether the fetus (or fetuses) has the sickle cell gene. **5,** Woman has a normal child.

The main treatment for sickle cell disease is hydroxyurea; it inhibits DNA synthesis, causes an increase in Hb F concentration, and results in an anti-inflammatory effect (decreases leukocyte production). These outcomes are thought to decrease crises. Treatment of sickle cell disease consists of supportive care aimed at preventing consequences of anemia and avoiding crises, including adequate hydration and pain management. Debate about transfusion therapy exists because of iron overload that can cause liver damage and fibrosis, delayed physical and sexual development, and heart disease; in addition, transfusion therapy requires chelation therapy to remove excess iron.[11] Genetic counselling and psychological support are important for the child and family.

Thalassemias

The α- and β-thalassemias are inherited autosomal recessive disorders that cause an impaired rate of synthesis of one of the two chains—α or β—of adult hemoglobin (Hb A). The disorder was named **thalassemia**, which is derived from the Greek word for *sea*, because it was discovered initially in persons with origins near the Mediterranean Sea. β-Thalassemia, in which synthesis of the β-globin chain is slowed or defective, is prevalent among Greeks, Italians, and some Arabs and Sephardic Jews. α-Thalassemia, in which the α-globin chain is affected, is most common among Chinese, Vietnamese, Cambodians, and Laotians. Both α- and β-thalassemias are common among Blacks.

Both α- and β-thalassemias are referred to as major or minor, depending on how many of the genes that control α- or β-chain synthesis are defective and whether the defects are inherited homozygously (thalassemia major) or heterozygously (thalassemia minor). Pathophysiological effects range from mild microcytosis to death in utero, depending on the number of defective genes and mode of inheritance. The anemic manifestation of thalassemia is microcytic-hypochromic hemolytic anemia.

PATHOPHYSIOLOGY The β-thalassemias are caused by mutations that decrease the synthesis of β-globin chains, leading to anemia, tissue hypoxia, and red blood cell hemolysis. β-Chain production is depressed—moderately in the heterozygous form, **β-thalassemia minor**, and severely in the homozygous form, **β-thalassemia major** (also called **Cooley's anemia**). This depressed production results in erythrocytes with a reduced amount of hemoglobin and an accumulation of free α-chains (Figure 22-6). The free α-chains are unstable and easily precipitate in the cell. Most erythroblasts that contain precipitates are destroyed by mononuclear phagocytes in the marrow, resulting in ineffective erythropoiesis and anemia. Some of the precipitate-carrying cells do mature and enter the bloodstream, but they are destroyed prematurely in the spleen, resulting in mild hemolytic anemia.

There are four forms of α-thalassemia: (1) **α-thalassemia trait** (the carrier state), in which a single α-chain–forming gene is defective; (2) **α-thalassemia minor**, in which two genes are defective; (3) **hemoglobin H disease**, in which three genes are defective; and (4) **α-thalassemia major**, a fatal condition in which all four α-forming genes are defective. Death is inevitable because α-chains are absent and oxygen cannot be released to the tissues.

CLINICAL MANIFESTATIONS β-Thalassemia occurs more commonly than does α-thalassemia. Occasionally, synthesis of γ- or δ-polypeptide chains is defective, resulting in γ- or δ-thalassemia. (Hemoglobin chains are described in Chapter 20.)

β-Thalassemia minor causes mild to moderate microcytic-hypochromic anemia, mild splenomegaly, bronze colouring of the skin, and hyperplasia of the bone marrow. The degree of reticulocytosis depends on the severity of the anemia and results in skeletal changes. Hemolysis of immature (and therefore fragile) erythrocytes may cause a slight elevation in serum iron and indirect bilirubin levels. Persons with β-thalassemia minor are usually asymptomatic.

Persons with β-thalassemia major may become quite ill. Anemia is severe and results in a significant cardiovascular burden with high-output heart failure. In the past, death resulted from heart failure. Today, blood transfusions can increase lifespan by one to two decades, and death usually is caused by hemochromatosis (from transfusions). Liver enlargement occurs as a result of progressive hemosiderosis, whereas enlargement of the spleen is caused by extramedullary hemopoiesis and increased destruction of red blood cells. Growth and maturation are developmentally delayed, and a characteristic chipmunk deformity develops on the face, caused by expansion of bones to accommodate hyperplastic marrow.

Persons who inherit the mildest form of α-thalassemia (the α-thalassemia trait) usually are symptom-free or have mild microcytosis. α-Thalassemia minor has clinical manifestations that are virtually identical to those of β-thalassemia minor: mild microcytic-hypochromic

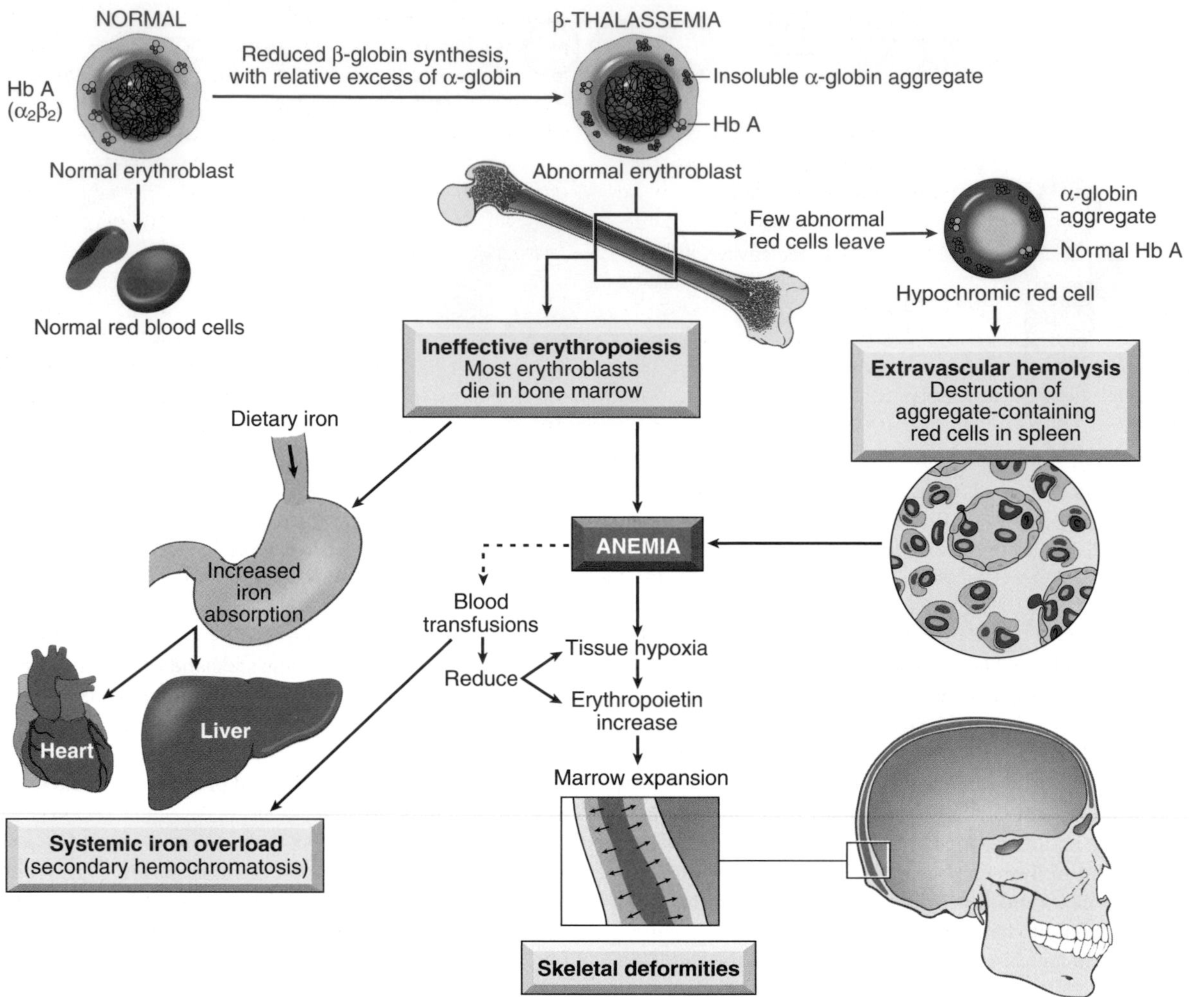

FIGURE 22-6 Pathogenesis of β-Thalassemia Major. The aggregates of unpaired α-globin chains are a hallmark of the disease. Blood transfusions can diminish the anemia, but they add to the systemic iron overload. *Hb A*, hemoglobin A. (From Kumar, V., Abbas, A.K., & Aster, J.C. [Eds.]. [2015]. *Robbins and Cotran pathologic basis of disease* [9th ed.]. Philadelphia: Saunders.)

reticulocytosis, bone marrow hyperplasia, increased serum iron concentrations, and moderate splenomegaly.

Signs and symptoms of α-thalassemia major are similar to those of β-thalassemia major, but milder. Moderate microcytic-hypochromic anemia, enlargement of the liver and spleen, and bone marrow hyperplasia are evident.

α-Thalassemia major causes hydrops fetalis, the most severe form of α-thalassemia, caused by deletion of all four α-globin genes. The infant suffers from severe tissue anoxia and may develop fulminant intrauterine heart failure. Signs of fetal distress became evident by the third trimester of pregnancy. In the past, severe tissue anoxia led to death in utero; now many such infants are saved by intrauterine transfusions.

Both α- and β-thalassemia major are life-threatening. Children with thalassemia major generally are weak, fail to thrive, show poor development, and experience cardiovascular compromise with high-output failure secondary to anemia. Untreated, they will die by 5 to 6 years of age.

EVALUATION AND TREATMENT Evaluation of thalassemia is based on familial disease history, clinical manifestations, and blood tests. Peripheral blood smears that show microcytosis and hemoglobin electrophoresis that demonstrates diminished amounts of α- or β-chains are used to make the diagnosis. Analysis of fetal DNA from withdrawn amniotic fluid is used as a screening test to detect hydrops fetalis (α-thalassemia major). Newborn screening for thalassemia should be done according to provincial recommendations.

Persons who are silent carriers or have thalassemia minor generally have few if any symptoms and require no specific treatment. However, therapies to support and prolong life are necessary for thalassemia major and include chronic blood transfusion therapy and management of resultant iron overload (see Figure 22-6). Allogeneic hematopoietic stem cell transplantation (HSCT) is the only cure. For both symptom-free carriers and those with the disease, prenatal diagnosis and genetic counselling may be the most important therapeutic measures that can be offered.

✔ QUICK CHECK 22-1

1. Why is Rh incompatibility rare today?
2. Why do clinical manifestations of sickle cell disease not appear until the infant is at least 6 months old?
3. Why do children with thalassemia major develop cardiovascular complications?

DISORDERS OF COAGULATION AND PLATELETS

Inherited Hemorrhagic Disease

Hemophilias

Hemophilia A is defined as factor VIII deficiency and is the most common hereditary disease associated with life-threatening bleeding. It is caused by a mutation in factor VIII, an essential cofactor for factor IX in the coagulation cascade. Factor IX deficiency is most often called hemophilia B (*Christmas disease*, after the first person identified and not the holiday) but is *clinically* indistinguishable from factor VIII deficiency because factors VIII and IX function together to activate factor X. Both hemophilia A and hemophilia B are inherited as X-linked recessive traits, thus affecting mainly males and homozygous females.[2] Excessive bleeding rarely occurs in heterozygous females. New mutations, not family history, are the cause of about 30% of cases. The incidence of hemophilia A is approximately 1 in 5000 male births, whereas hemophilia B is five times less common, with an incidence of approximately 1 in 30000 male births. The incidence worldwide of hemophilia is not well known, but it is estimated to be at more than 400 000 people.[12] Races are affected equally for both disorders.

Only hemophilias A and B will be discussed in this chapter. Of note is a third, less common hemophilia, called *hemophilia C*, which results from a deficiency of factor XI. Table 22-3 lists the coagulation factors and deficiencies associated with clinical bleeding.

PATHOPHYSIOLOGY Hemophilia may be inherited or caused by a spontaneous mutation of the factor gene. The genetic instructions for both factor VIII and factor IX lie on the long arm of the X chromosome. Deficiencies of factor VIII and factor IX are clinically manifested almost exclusively in males. Because a male's DNA contains only one X chromosome, hemophilia affects mostly males. Women have two X chromosomes, and if one X chromosome has a defective gene, the other X chromosome has the information needed to create clotting factors. A female can have hemophilia because of X-inactivation or lyonization (see Chapter 2). It is possible for one X chromosome to not express itself. If the X chromosome with the hemophilia gene is the active chromosome, the woman will have lower levels of clotting factors. Fifty percent of carriers have low clotting factor levels. There is a known family history of hemophilia A and B in about two-thirds of cases; the remaining third are new genetic mutations, either in the individual with hemophilia or in his unaffected carrier mother.

Numerous gene mutations and deletions have been identified at the molecular level in factor VIII and IX deficiency. The molecular defect that leads to hemophilia is identical among members of a given family; however, the deletion mutation has been unique in each family studied.[13]

TABLE 22-3 The Coagulation Factors and Associated Disorders

Clotting Factors	Synonym	Disorder
I	Fibrinogen	Congenital deficiency (afibrinogenemia) and dysfunction (dysfibrinogenemia)
II	Prothrombin	Congenital deficiency or dysfunction
V	Labile factor or proaccelerin	Congenital deficiency (parahemophilia)
VII	Stable factor or proconvertin	Congenital deficiency
VIII	Antihemophilic factor	Congenital deficiency is hemophilia A (classic hemophilia)
IX	Christmas factor	Congenital deficiency is hemophilia B
X	Stuart-Prower factor	Congenital deficiency
XI	Plasma thromboplastin antecedent	Congenital deficiency, sometimes referred to as *hemophilia C*
XII	Hageman factor	Congenital deficiency is *not* associated with clinical symptoms
XIII	Fibrin-stabilizing factor	Congenital deficiency

CLINICAL MANIFESTATIONS The clinical manifestations and severity of hemophilia depend largely on the level of factor VIII and IX activity. The severity designation of an individual's hemophilia will determine the characteristics of the resulting disorder and will direct treatment strategies.[14] Joint bleeding is the most characteristic type of bleeding in hemophilia. Bleeding into muscles, usually from trauma, also occurs with both hemophilia A and hemophilia B. Oral bleeding is common in the setting of dental surgery. Spontaneous painless hematuria, which is relatively common in hemophilia, generally does not result in significant blood loss but requires evaluation. Hematuria accompanied by pain requires prompt evaluation and treatment.

Intracranial bleeds, bleeding of internal organs, and bleeding into the tissues of the neck, chest, or abdomen are all life-threatening. Delayed or suboptimal treatment of these bleeds may lead to permanent brain injury, loss of organ function, or death.

EVALUATION AND TREATMENT Because hemophilia is most often an inherited disease, a positive family history may expedite a diagnosis of hemophilia. When a suspected carrier mother is pregnant, genetic testing in utero through amniocentesis or chorionic villus sampling (CVS) may reveal a hemophilia diagnosis before childbirth. In the absence of a positive family history, when a bleeding disorder is suspected, personal bleed history, laboratory testing, family history, and physical assessment contribute to a thorough evaluation and accurate diagnosis. In general, those with hemophilia A or B will have a prolonged partial thromboplastin time (PTT), and the prothrombin time (PT) will be normal. Measurement of factor VIII (hemophilia A) and factor IX (hemophilia B) levels is necessary for diagnosis.

The majority of children with hemophilia A (factor VIII deficiency) can be treated with recombinant factor VIII, and the majority of children with hemophilia B (factor IX deficiency) can be treated with recombinant factor IX. Recombinant factor is reconstituted in a small volume of diluent, administered by slow intravenous push, and raises the factor level almost immediately.

Antibody-Mediated Hemorrhagic Disease

The antibody-mediated hemorrhagic diseases are a group of disorders caused by the immune response. Antibody-mediated destruction of platelets or antibody-mediated inflammatory reactions to allergens damage blood vessels and cause seepage into tissues. The thrombocytopenic purpuras may be intrinsic or idiopathic, or they may be transient phenomena transmitted from mother to fetus. The inflammatory, or "allergic," purpuras, although rare, occur in response to allergens in the blood. All of these disorders first appear during infancy or childhood.

Immune Thrombocytopenic Purpura

Acute immune thrombocytopenic purpura (ITP; *autoimmune [primary] thrombocytopenic purpura*) is the most common disorder of platelet consumption. Autoantibodies bind to the plasma membranes of platelets, causing platelet sequestration and destruction by mononuclear phagocytes in the spleen and other lymphoid tissues at a rate that exceeds the ability of the bone marrow to produce them. The destruction of platelets is triggered by medications, infections, lymphomas, or an unknown cause.

PATHOPHYSIOLOGY The autoantibodies that produce the destruction are often of the IgG class and are usually against the platelet membrane glycoproteins (IIb-IIIa or Ib-IX). In approximately 70% of cases of ITP, there is an antecedent viral disease (e.g., cytomegalovirus [CMV], Epstein-Barr virus [EBV], parvovirus, or respiratory tract infection) that precedes the eruption of petechiae or purpura by 1 to 3 weeks.

CLINICAL MANIFESTATIONS Bruising and a generalized petechial rash often occur with acute onset. Petechiae can develop into ecchymoses. Asymmetrical bruising is typical and is found most often on the legs and trunk. Hemorrhagic bullae of the gums, lips, and other mucous membranes may be prominent, and epistaxis (nose bleeding) may be severe and difficult to control. Otherwise, the child appears well. The principal changes are found in the spleen, bone marrow, and blood.[2] The acute phase lasts 1 to 2 weeks, but thrombocytopenia often persists. Although the incidence is less than 1%, intracranial hemorrhage is the most serious complication of ITP. In some cases, the onset is more gradual, and clinical manifestations consist of moderate bruising and a few petechiae.

EVALUATION AND TREATMENT Laboratory examination reveals an isolated low platelet count, and the few platelets observed on a smear are large, reflecting increased bone marrow production. The Ivy test (a bleeding time test) is prolonged. Bone marrow aspiration is not recommended for children with typical features of ITP. The primary treatment for children with ITP is observation regardless of platelet count. When bleeding is present, primary treatment is with an infusion of intravenous immune globulin (IVIg) or a short course of corticosteroids.

Even without treatment, the prognosis for children with ITP is excellent: 75% recover completely within 3 months. After the initial acute phase, spontaneous clinical manifestations subside. By 6 months after onset, 80% of affected children have regained normal platelet counts.[15] ITP that persists longer than 12 months in children is considered chronic, and immunosuppressive therapies are utilized.[16,17]

QUICK CHECK 22-2

1. List the major disorders of coagulation and platelets found in children.
2. How do gene deletions differ from gene mutations?
3. Why are persons with hemophilia at risk of developing degenerative joint changes?
4. What is the major abnormality in immune thrombocytopenic purpura?

NEOPLASTIC DISORDERS

Leukemia

Leukemia is cancer of the blood-forming tissues, such as the bone marrow, that most often produces abnormal white blood cells called **leukemic cells**. Once in the blood, leukemic cells can spread to other organs, such as the lymph nodes, spleen, and brain. Leukemia is the most common malignancy in children and teens.

Among children and teens, about 75% of leukemias are acute lymphoblastic leukemia (ALL); the remaining cases are acute myeloid (or myelogenous) leukemia (AML). ALL is most common in early childhood, peaking between 2 and 4 years of age.[18] AML is slightly more common during the first 2 years of life and during the teenage years, and it occurs about equally among boys and girls of all races. ALL is more common in boys than girls and among Latin American and White children.[18]

The cause of most childhood cancer is unknown. About 5% of all childhood cancers are caused by inherited mutations. Genetic mutations can occur during fetal development. Other genetic conditions associated with leukemia include Down syndrome, neurofibromatosis, Shwachman-Diamond syndrome, Bloom's syndrome, and ataxia-telangiectasia. Many studies have shown that exposure to ionizing radiation (prenatal exposure to X-rays and postnatal exposure to high doses) can lead to the development of childhood leukemia and possibly other cancers.[19] There is recent concern for performing computed tomography (CT) scans in children because increased use combined with wide variability in radiation doses has resulted in many children receiving a high dose of radiation.[20] Studies of other possible environmental risk factors, including parental exposure to cancer-causing chemicals, prenatal exposure to pesticides, childhood exposure to common infectious agents, and living near a nuclear power plant, have so far produced inconsistent results. Higher risks of cancer have not been seen in children of individuals treated for sporadic cancer (cancer not caused by an inherited mutation).[21,22]

PATHOPHYSIOLOGY ALL is composed of immature B (pre-B) or T (pre-T) cells called **lymphoblasts**. The bone marrow is dense with lymphoblasts, considered hypercellular, that replace the normal marrow and disrupt normal function. Many of the chromosomal abnormalities documented in ALL cause dysregulation of the expression and function of transcription factors required for normal B-cell and T-cell development.[2] The mutations can include both gain of function and loss of function that are required for normal development.

AML is caused by acquired oncogenic mutations that impair differentiation, resulting in the accumulation of immature myeloid blasts in the marrow and other organs. Epigenetic alterations are frequent in AML and have a central role. The bone marrow crowding by blasts produces marrow failure and complications, including anemia, thrombocytopenia, and neutropenia. AML is very heterogeneous because myeloid cell differentiation is very complex. To be called *acute*, the bone marrow usually must include greater than 20% leukemic blasts.

CLINICAL MANIFESTATIONS The onset of leukemia may be abrupt or insidious, but the most common symptoms reflect the consequences of bone marrow failure: decreased levels of both red blood cells and platelets and changes in white blood cells. Pallor, fatigue, petechiae, purpura, bleeding, and fever generally are present. Approximately 45% of children have a hemoglobin level below 70 mmol/L. If acute blood loss occurs, characteristic symptoms of tachycardia, air hunger, restlessness, and thirst may be present. Epistaxis often occurs in children with severe thrombocytopenia.

Fever is usually present as a result of (1) infection associated with the decrease in functional neutrophils and (2) hypermetabolism associated with the ongoing rapid growth and destruction of leukemic cells. White blood cell counts greater than 200×10^9/L can cause leukostasis, an intravascular clumping of cells that results in infarction and hemorrhage, usually in the brain and lung.

Renal failure as a result of hyperuremia (high uric acid levels) can be associated with ALL, particularly at diagnosis or during active treatment. Extramedullary invasion with leukemic cells can occur in nearly all body tissue. The central nervous system (CNS) is a common site of infiltration of extramedullary leukemias, although less than 10% of children with ALL have CNS involvement at diagnosis. The most common symptoms of CNS involvement relate to increased intracranial pressure, causing early morning headaches, nausea, vomiting, irritability, and lethargy.

Gonadal involvement can occur, and leukemic infiltration into bones and joints is common. Reports of bone or joint pain actually lead to the diagnosis of leukemia in some children. In most children, bone pain is characterized as migratory, vague, and without areas of swelling or inflammation. However, if joint pain is the primary symptom and some swelling is associated with the pain, misdiagnoses of rheumatoid arthritis and rheumatic fever have occurred.

Other organs reported to be sites of leukemic invasion include the kidneys, heart, lungs, thymus, eyes, skin, and gastro-intestinal tract. Children with leukemia can show symptoms only 1 week before diagnosis.

EVALUATION AND TREATMENT The diagnosis of leukemia is made from blood tests and examination of peripheral blood smears. A bone marrow aspiration is usually performed to further characterize the leukemia. The **blast cell** is the hallmark of acute leukemia (Figure 22-7). Healthy children have less than 5% blast cells in the bone marrow and none in the peripheral blood. In ALL, the bone marrow often is replaced by 80 to 100% blast cells, with a reduction in normal developing red blood cells and granulocytes. Occasionally, the marrow appears hypocellular, making the diagnosis difficult to differentiate from aplastic anemia. When this difficulty occurs, bone marrow biopsy or biopsy of extramedullary sites is necessary to confirm the diagnosis.

Remarkable success has occurred with treatment of ALL in children. Chemotherapy is the treatment of choice for acute leukemia. Radiation has special considerations for use. In ALL, identification of various risk groups has led to the development of different intensities of medication protocols. Thus treatment is tailored specifically for a particular risk group.

Chronic myeloid (or myelogenous) leukemia (CML) accounts for less than 5% of childhood leukemias. In the past, it was treated with high-dose chemotherapy followed by allogeneic stem cell transplant, resulting in significant treatment-related mortality. However, targeted medications, known as tyrosine kinase inhibitors (TKIs), have revolutionized the treatment of CML. Several TKIs are now approved for use in children; treatment requires continued adherence to an oral regimen and the health impact of long-term TKI therapy is not yet known.[23]

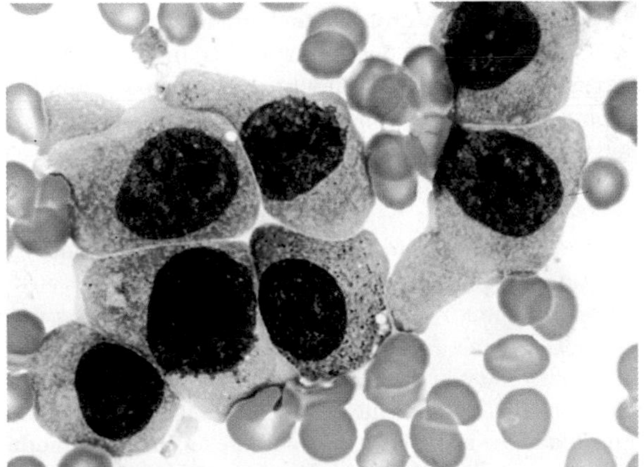

FIGURE 22-7 Monoblasts From Acute Monoblastic Leukemia. Monoblasts in a marrow smear from an individual with acute monoblastic leukemia. The monoblasts are larger than myeloblasts and usually have abundant cytoplasm, often with delicate scattered azurophilic granules (an element that stains well with blue aniline dyes). (From Damjanov, I., & Linder, J. [Eds.]. [1996]. *Anderson's pathology* [10th ed.]. St. Louis: Mosby.)

Lymphomas

Lymphoma (HL and NHL) develops from the proliferation of malignant lymphocytes (immune cells) in the lymphoid system (see Chapters 12 and 21). The four most common types of leukemia are (1) ALL, (2) AML, (3) chronic lymphocytic leukemia (CLL), and (4) CML (see Chapter 21). Most childhood leukemias are ALL. Chronic leukemias are rare in children.[24]

Lymphomas are malignant proliferations that arise from discrete tissue masses.[2] Lymphoid neoplasms involve some recognizable stage of lymphocyte B- or T-cell differentiation. With time and better understanding, it is clear that some lymphomas occasionally have leukemic presentations, and evolution to "leukemia" is not unusual during the progression of incurable "lymphomas." The terms, therefore, merely reflect the usual tissue distribution.[2] Much controversy has surrounded the classifications of lymphoma, and a consensus has been reached with the current World Health Organization classification scheme found at https://www.lymphoma.ca/lymphoma/lymphoma-101/types-lymphoma/classifying-nhl. NHL and HL constitute approximately 11% of all cases of childhood cancer. Approximately 100 children younger than 14 years of age are diagnosed with lymphoma in Canada each year.[25] NHL (including Burkitt lymphoma) occurs more often than HL (for newborns to children age 14 years, 5 to 6% versus 4%; and for ages 15 to 19 years, 8% versus 15% of all pediatric malignancies). Either group of diseases is rare before the age of 5 years, and the relative incidence increases throughout childhood. Boys are more likely to be diagnosed with a malignant lymphoma than are girls. At particular risk are children with inherited or acquired immune deficiency syndrome, who have increased rates of lymphoreticular cancers that range between 100 and 10 000 times the rate of normal children.

Non-Hodgkin's Lymphoma

Non-Hodgkin's lymphomas (NHLs) are neoplasms of immune cells. NHLs are a large and diverse group of tumours; some tumours have a slow-growing (indolent) course, whereas others have a fast-growing (aggressive) course. Almost without exception, childhood NHL becomes evident as a diffuse disease and can be further subdivided into four major types: (1) B-cell NHL (Burkitt and Burkitt-like lymphoma, and Burkitt leukemia); (2) diffuse large B-cell lymphoma; (3) lymphoblastic lymphoma; and (4) anaplastic large cell lymphoma.[26] The common types of NHL in children are different than those in adults. The most common types of NHL in children are Burkitt lymphoma (40%), lymphoblastic lymphoma (25 to 30%), and large cell lymphoma (10%).

PATHOPHYSIOLOGY Burkitt lymphoma will be discussed as an example of pathogenesis of NHL in children. All forms of Burkitt lymphoma are associated with translocations of the *MYC* gene on chromosome 8 that lead to increased MYC protein levels.[2] MYC is a transcriptional regulator that increases the expression of genes required for aerobic glycolysis, called the *Warburg effect* (see Chapter 10). Most Burkitt lymphomas are latently infected with EBV.[2] EBV is also present in about 25% of HIV-associated tumours and 15 to 20% of sporadic cases.[2] There is increased evidence of NHL in children with congenital immunodeficiency syndromes, such as Wiskott-Aldrich syndrome, ataxia-telangiectasia, and Bloom's syndrome.

CLINICAL MANIFESTATIONS NHL has been found to arise from any lymphoid tissue. Signs and symptoms therefore are specific for the site

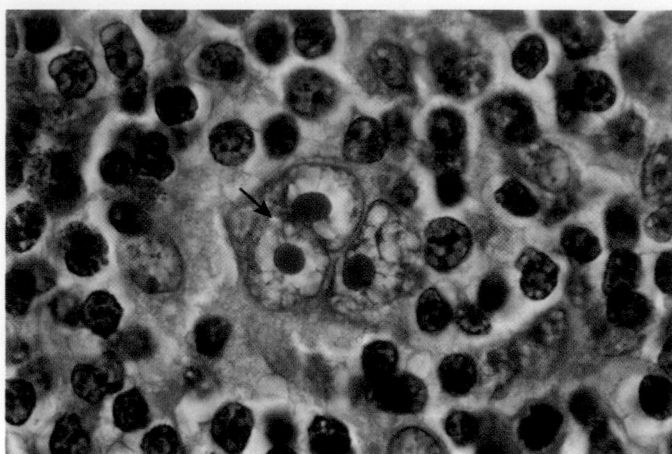

FIGURE 22-8 Diagnostic Reed-Sternberg Cell. A large multinucleated or multilobated cell with inclusion body–like nucleoli (*arrow*) surrounded by a halo of clear nucleoplasm. (From Damjanov, I., & Linder, J. [2000]. *Pathology: A color atlas.* St. Louis: Mosby.)

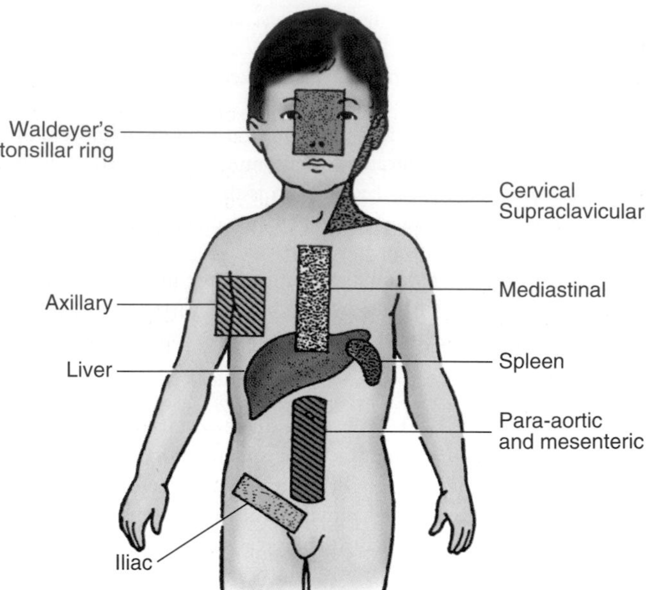

FIGURE 22-9 Main Areas of Lymphadenopathy and Organ Involvement in Hodgkin's Lymphoma. (From Hockenberry, M.J., & Wilson, D. [Eds.]. [2015]. *Wong's nursing care of infants and children* [10th ed.]. St. Louis: Mosby.)

involved. Associated signs of NHL include swelling of the lymph nodes in the neck, underarm, stomach, or groin; trouble swallowing; painless lump or swelling in a testicle; weight loss for unknown reason; night sweats; and possibly trouble breathing. Involvement of facial bones, particularly the jaw, is common in African Burkitt lymphoma.

EVALUATION AND TREATMENT Diagnosis is made by physical examination and health history, followed by biopsy of disease sites—usually the involved lymph nodes, tonsils, bone marrow, spleen, liver, bowel, or skin. Burkitt lymphoma is very aggressive and responds well to treatment. With intensive chemotherapy, most children and young adults can be cured.

Hodgkin's Lymphoma

Hodgkin's lymphoma (HL) is a group of lymphoid neoplasms that, unlike NHL, arises in a single chain of lymph nodes and spreads first in a contiguous way to lymphoid tissue. NHL frequently arises at extranodal sites and spreads in a noncontiguous or unpredictable way. HL is characterized by the presence of Reed-Sternberg cells, which are large cells derived from the germinal centre of B cells (Figure 22-8). The World Health Organization has identified five types of HL: (1) nodular sclerosis, (2) mixed cellularity, (3) lymphocyte rich, (4) lymphocyte depletion, and (5) lymphocyte predominance. The first four types are considered the *classic* types of HL with similar expression of Reed-Sternberg cells. In the lymphocyte predominance type, the Reed-Sternberg cell is distinctive but different than the others. HL is a common type of cancer in young adults and adolescents but rare in childhood. The average age at diagnosis is 32 years of age.

PATHOPHYSIOLOGY The Reed-Sternberg cells fail to express most of the B-cell normal genes, including the Ig genes. The causes of the genetic rearrangements or reprogramming are not fully known but are thought to be the result of widespread epigenetic changes. Activation of the transcription factor NF-κB, which controls transcription of DNA, is a very common event in classic HL.[2] NF-κB may be activated by EBV infection. EBV-infected B cells, resembling Reed-Sternberg cells, are found in lymph nodes in individuals with infectious mononucleosis, suggesting that the EBV proteins may have a role in changes of the B cells into Reed-Sternberg cells.[2] NF-κB is involved in many biological processes, including inflammation, immunity, cell growth, differentiation, and apoptosis. The cytoplasm is abundant with Reed-Sternberg cells and tissue is reactive with many inflammatory type cells and immune cells. These reactive cells crosstalk with Reed-Sternberg cells and support the growth and survival of the tumour cells.

CLINICAL MANIFESTATIONS Painless lymphadenopathy in the lower cervical chain, with or without fever, is the most common symptom in children. Other lymph nodes and organs also may be involved (Figure 22 9). Mediastinal involvement can cause pressure on the trachea or bronchi, leading to airway obstruction. Extranodal primary sites in HL are rare. Initial symptoms consist of anorexia, malaise, and lassitude. Intermittent fever is present in 30% of children, and weight loss also may accompany these symptoms. HL has a well-defined staging system that considers the extent and location of disease and the presence of fever, weight loss, or night sweats at diagnosis.

EVALUATION AND TREATMENT Treatment for HL includes chemotherapy and radiation therapy. Long-term survivors treated with radiotherapy had a much higher incidence of secondary cancers, including lung cancer, melanoma, and breast cancer. Individuals previously treated with chemotherapy alkylating agents also had a high incidence of secondary tumours. These results have changed the treatment protocols to minimize the use of radiotherapy and use less toxic chemotherapy. A promising target therapy is anti-CD30.

> **✔ QUICK CHECK 22-3**
> 1. List the childhood leukemias in order of rate of incidence.
> 2. Why do children with leukemia experience bone or joint pain?
> 3. What are the common types of non-Hodgkin's lymphoma in children?

DID YOU UNDERSTAND?

Disorders of Erythrocytes

1. Anemia is the most common blood disorder in children. Like the anemias of adulthood, the anemias of childhood are caused by ineffective erythropoiesis or premature destruction of erythrocytes.
2. Iron deficiency anemia (IDA) is the most common nutritional disorder worldwide. IDA has the highest incidence occurring between 6 months and 2 years of age. Iron is critical for the developing child. Without it the damage from the periods of IDA is irreversible.
3. No matter the cause of IDA, it produces a hypochromic-microcytic anemia, eventually lowering hemoglobin and hematocrit.
4. Hemolytic disease of the newborn (HDN) results from incompatibility between the maternal and the fetal blood, which may involve differences in Rh factors or blood type (ABO). Maternal antibodies (anti-Rh antibodies) form in response to the presence of fetal incompatible (Rh-positive) erythrocytes in the blood of an Rh-negative mother. The maternal antibodies then enter the fetal circulation and cause hemolysis of fetal erythrocytes. However, ABO incompatibility can cause HDN even if fetal erythrocytes do not escape into the maternal circulation during pregnancy.
5. The key to treatment of HDN resulting from Rh incompatibilities lies in prevention or immunoprophylaxis.
6. Sickle cell disease is a group of disorders characterized by the production of abnormal hemoglobin S (Hb S) within the erythrocytes.
7. Sickle cell disease is an inherited, autosomal recessive disorder expressed as sickle cell anemia, sickle cell–thalassemia disease, or sickle cell–hemoglobin C disease, depending on mode of inheritance. Sickle cell anemia, a homozygous form, is the most severe.
8. Sickle cell–thalassemia disease and sickle cell–hemoglobin C disease are heterozygous forms in which the child simultaneously inherits another type of abnormal hemoglobin from one parent. Sickle cell trait, in which the child inherits Hb S from one parent and normal hemoglobin (Hb A) from the other, is a heterozygous carrier state that rarely has clinical manifestations. All forms of sickle cell disease are lifelong conditions.
9. Sickle cell disease causes a change in the shape of red blood cells, resulting in deoxygenation or dehydration. It is most common among Blacks and those of Mediterranean descent.
10. The α- and β-thalassemias are inherited autosomal recessive disorders that cause an impaired rate of synthesis of one of the two chains—α or β—of adult hemoglobin (Hb A).

Disorders of Coagulation and Platelets

1. Hemophilia A is defined as factor VIII deficiency and is the most common hereditary disease associated with life-threatening bleeding. It is caused by a mutation in factor VIII, an essential cofactor for factor IX in the coagulation cascade. Factor IX deficiency is most often called *hemophilia B.*
2. Hemophilia may be inherited or caused by a spontaneous mutation of the factor gene.
3. The antibody-mediated hemorrhagic diseases are a group of disorders caused by the immune response. Antibody-mediated destruction of platelets or antibody-mediated inflammatory reactions to allergens damage blood vessels and cause seepage into tissues.
4. Immune thrombocytopenic purpura, the most common of the childhood thrombocytopenic purpuras, is a disorder of platelet consumption in which antiplatelet antibodies bind to the plasma membranes of platelets. This binding results in platelet sequestration and destruction by mononuclear phagocytes at a rate that exceeds the ability of the bone marrow to produce them.

Neoplastic Disorders

1. Leukemia is cancer of the blood-forming tissues, such as the bone marrow, that most often produces abnormal white blood cells called *leukemic cells.*
2. Among children and teens, about 75% of leukemias are acute lymphoblastic leukemia (ALL); the remaining cases are acute myeloid (or myelogenous) leukemia (AML). Chronic leukemias are rare in children.
3. The cause of childhood leukemia is unknown. About 5% of all childhood cancers are caused by inherited mutations. Genetic mutations can occur during fetal development.
4. Studies have shown that exposure to ionizing radiation can lead to the development of childhood leukemia and possibly other cancers.
5. ALL causes dysregulation of the expression and function of transcription factors required for normal B-cell and T-cell development.
6. Epigenetic alterations are frequent in AML and have a central role.
7. The onset of leukemia may be abrupt or insidious, but the most common symptoms reflect the consequences of bone marrow failure. These changes can include decreased levels of red blood cells and platelets and changes in white blood cells.
8. Lymphomas are malignant proliferations that arise from discrete tissue masses. Lymphoid neoplasms involve some recognizable stage of lymphocyte B- or T-cell differentiation.
9. With time and better understanding, it is now clear that some lymphomas occasionally have leukemic presentations.
10. The lymphomas of childhood are Hodgkin's lymphoma (HL) and non-Hodgkin's lymphoma (NHL).
11. NHL are neoplasms of immune cells. The most common types of NHL in children are Burkitt lymphoma (40%), lymphoblastic lymphoma (25 to 30%), and large cell lymphoma (10%).
12. Most Burkitt lymphomas are latently infected with the Epstein-Barr virus (EBV). There is increased evidence of NHL in children with congenital immunodeficiency syndromes.
13. Unlike NHL, HL arises in a single chain of lymph nodes and spreads first in a contiguous way to lymphoid tissue.
14. HL is characterized by the presence of Reed-Sternberg cells, which are large cells derived from the germinal centre of B cells.

KEY TERMS

α-Thalassemia major, 567
α-Thalassemia minor, 567
α-Thalassemia trait, 567
Aplastic crisis, 566
β-Thalassemia major (Cooley's anemia), 567
β-Thalassemia minor, 567
Blast cell, 571
Glucose-6-phosphate dehydrogenase (G6PD) deficiency, 560
Hemoglobin H disease, 567
Hemoglobin S (Hb S), 564
Hemolytic anemia, 560
Hemolytic disease of the newborn (HDN) (erythroblastosis fetalis), 562
Hemophilia A, 569
Hemophilia B, 569
Hodgkin's lymphoma (HL), 572
Hydrops fetalis, 562
Hyperbilirubinemia, 563
Hyperhemolytic crisis, 566
Icterus gravis neonatorum, 563
Icterus neonatorum (neonatal jaundice), 563
Immune thrombocytopenic purpura (ITP), 569

Kernicterus, 563
Leukemia, 570
Leukemic cell, 570
Lymphoblast, 570
Lymphoma, 571
Non-Hodgkin's lymphoma (NHL), 571
Sequestration crisis, 566
Sickle cell anemia, 564
Sickle cell disease, 564
Sickle cell–hemoglobin C disease, 565
Sickle cell–thalassemia disease, 564
Sickle cell trait, 565
Thalassemia, 567
Vaso-occlusive crisis (thrombotic crisis), 565

REFERENCES

1. Christofides, A., Schauer, C., & Zlotkin, S. H. (2005). Iron deficiency anemia among children: Addressing a global public health problem within a Canadian context. *Paediatrics & Child Health, 10*(10), 597–601.
2. Kumar, V., Abbas, A. K., & Aster, J. C. (Eds.), (2015). *Robbins and Cotran pathologic basis of disease* (9th ed.). Philadelphia: Saunders.
3. Jo, J., Garssen, J., Knippels, L., et al. (2014). Role of cellular immunity in cow's milk allergy: Pathogenesis, tolerance induction, and beyond. *Mediators of Inflammation, 2014*, 249784. doi:10.1155/2014/249784.
4. Moshe, G., Amitai, Y., Korchia, G., et al. (2013). Anemia and iron deficiency in children: Association with red meat and poultry consumption. *Journal of Pediatric Gastroenrology and Nutrition, 57*(6), 722–727. doi:10.1097/MPG.0b013e3182a80c42.
5. Gheibi, S. H., Farrokh-Eslamlou, H. R., Noroozi, M., et al. (2015). Refractory iron deficiency anemia and *Helicobacter pylori* infection in pediatrics: A review. *Iranian Journal of Pediatric Hematology and Oncology, 5*(1), 50–64.
6. Shah, M., Griffin, I. J., Lifschitz, C. H., et al. (2003). Effect of orange and apple juice on iron absorption in children. *Archives of Pediatrics and Adolescent Medicine, 157*(12), 1232–1236. doi:10.1001/archpedi.157.12.1232.
7. Crowther, C. A., Middleton, P., & McBain, R. D. (2013). Anti-D administration in pregnancy for preventing Rhesus alloimmunization. *Cochrane Database of Systematic Reviews*, (2), CD000020, doi:10.1002/14651858.CD000020.pub2.
8. Qureshi, H., Massey, E., Kirwan, D., et al. (2014). BCSH guideline for the use of anti-D immunoglobulin for the prevention of haemolytic disease of the fetus and newborn. *Transfusion Medicine (Oxford, England), 24*(1), 8–20.
9. Canadian Haemoglobinopathy Association. (2014). *Consensus statement on the care of patients with sickle cell disease in Canada.* Retrieved from https://emergencymedicinecases.com/wp-content/uploads/filebase/pdf/Canadian%20Sickle%20Cell%20Guidelines%202014.pdf.
10. Kyung, P. (2004). Sickle cell disease and other hemoglobinopathies. *International Anesthesiology Clinics, 42*(3), 77–93.
11. Yawn, B. P., Buchanan, G. R., Afenyi-Annan, A. N., et al. (2014). Management of sickle cell disease summary of the 2014 evidence-based report by Expert Panel Members. *JAMA: The Journal of the American Medical Association, 312*(10), 1033–1048. doi:10.1001/jama.2014.10517.
12. National Hemophilia Foundation. (2015). *National hemophilia foundation's information resource center.* New York: Author.
13. Mariani, G., & Bernardi, F. (2009). Factor II deficiency. *Seminars in Thrombosis and Hemostasis, 35*(4), 400–406. doi:10.1055/s-0029-1225762.
14. Blanchette, V. S., Breakey, V. R., & Revel-Vilk, S. (Eds.), (2013). *SickKids handbook of pediatric thrombosis and hemostasis* (pp. 59–78). Basel, Switzerland: Karger.
15. Gupta, V., Tilak, V., & Bhatia, B. D. (2008). Immune thrombocytopenic purpura. *Indian Journal of Pediatrics, 75*(7), 723–728. doi:10.1007/s12098-008-0137-z.
16. Neunert, C., Lim, W., Crowther, M., et al. (2011). The American Society of Hematology 2011 evidence-based practice guideline for immune thrombocytopenia. *Blood, 117*, 4190–4207. doi:10.1182/blood-2010-08-302984.
17. Provan, D., Stasi, R., Newland, A. C., et al. (2010). International consensus report on the investigation and management of primary immune thrombocytopenia. *Blood, 115*(2), 168–186. doi:10.1182/blood-2009-06-225565.
18. American Cancer Society. (2015). *What are the key statistics for childhood leukemia?* Atlanta, GA: Author.
19. National Cancer Institute. (2015). *Childhood acute lymphoblastic leukemia treatment PDQ®—Health professional version.* Bethesda, MD: Author. Retrieved from https://www.cancer.gov/types/leukemia/hp/child-all-treatment-pdq#link/_67_toc.
20. Miglioretti, D. L., Johnson, E., Williams, A., et al. (2013). The use of computed tomography in pediatrics and the associated radiation exposure and estimated cancer risk. *JAMA Pediatrics, 167*(8), 700–707. doi:10.1001/jamapediatrics.2013.311.
21. Hudson, M. M. (2010). Reproductive outcomes for survivors of childhood cancer. *Obstetrics and Gynecology, 116*(5), 1171–1183. doi:10.1097/AOG.0b013e3181f87c4b.
22. National Cancer Institute. (2014). *Cancer in children and adolescents.* Bethesda, MD: Author.
23. National Cancer Institute. (2015). *PDQ® childhood acute myeloid leukemia/other myeloid malignancies treatment.* Bethesda, MD: Author. Retrieved from http://cancer.gov/cancertopics/pdq/treatment/childAML/HealthProfessional.
24. American Cancer Society. (2015). *What you need to know about leukemia.* Bethesda, MD: National Cancer Institute.
25. Statistics Canada. (2015). *Health at a glance: Childhood cancer incidence and mortality in Canada.* Ottawa: Author. Retrieved from http://www.statcan.gc.ca/pub/82-624-x/2015001/article/14213-eng.pdf.
26. National Cancer Institute. *PDQ® childhood non-Hodgkin lymphoma treatment.* Bethesda, MD: Author. Retrieved from http://cancer.gov/cancertopics/pdq/treatment/child-non-hodgkins/Patient.

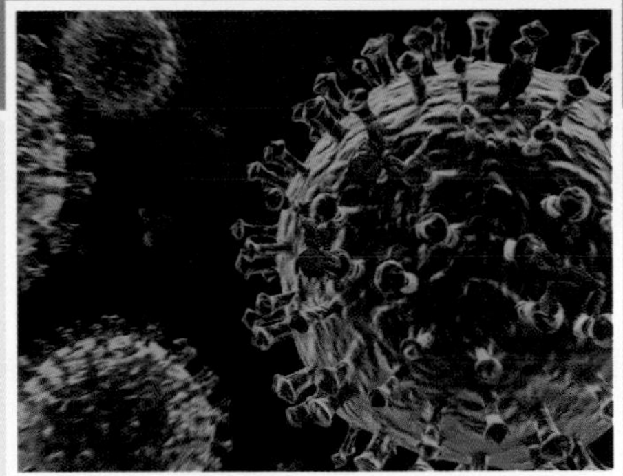

23

Structure and Function of the Cardiovascular and Lymphatic Systems

Susanna G. Cunningham, Valentina L. Brashers, Kathryn L. McCance, and Mohamed El-Hussein

EVOLVE WEBSITE

http://evolve.elsevier.com/Canada/Huether/pathophysiology
Student Review Questions
Key Points
Case Studies
Animations
Quick Check Answers

CHAPTER OUTLINE

The Circulatory System, 575
The Heart, 575
Structures That Direct Circulation Through the Heart, 576
Structures That Support Cardiac Metabolism: The Coronary Vessels, 578
Structures That Control Heart Action, 580
Factors Affecting Cardiac Output, 587
The Systemic Circulation, 589
Structure of Blood Vessels, 589
Factors Affecting Blood Flow, 593
Regulation of Blood Pressure, 595
Regulation of the Coronary Circulation, 598
The Lymphatic System, 599

The functions of the circulatory system include delivery of oxygen, nutrients, hormones, immune system components, and other substances to body tissues and removal of the waste products of metabolism. Delivery and removal are achieved by an extensive array of tubes—the blood and lymphatic vessels—connected to a pump, the heart. The heart continuously pumps blood through the blood vessels in collaboration with other systems, particularly the nervous and endocrine systems, which regulate the heart and blood vessels. Immune system components, nutrients, and oxygen are supplied by the immune, digestive, and respiratory systems; gaseous wastes of metabolism are expired through the lungs; and other wastes are removed by the kidneys and digestive tract.

The vascular endothelium also is a key component of the circulatory system and is sometimes considered a separate endocrine organ. This endothelium is a multifunctional tissue whose health is essential to normal vascular, immune, and hemostatic system function. Endothelial dysfunction is a critical factor in the development of vascular and other diseases.[1]

THE CIRCULATORY SYSTEM

The heart is composed of two conjoined pumps moving blood through two separate circulatory systems in sequence: one pump supplies blood to the lungs, whereas the second pump delivers blood to the rest of the body. Structures on the right side, or **right heart**, pump blood through the lungs. This system is termed the **pulmonary circulation** and is described in Chapter 26. The left side, or **left heart**, sends blood throughout the **systemic circulation**, which supplies all of the body except the lungs (Figure 23-1). These two systems are serially connected; thus the output of one becomes the input of the other.

Arteries carry blood from the heart to all parts of the body, where they branch into arterioles and even smaller vessels, ultimately becoming a fine meshwork of capillaries. Capillaries allow the closest contact and exchange between the blood and the interstitial space, or interstitium—the environment in which cells live. Venules and then veins next carry blood from the capillaries back to the heart. Some of the plasma or liquid part of the blood passes through the walls of the capillaries into the interstitial space. This fluid, lymph, is returned to the cardiovascular system by vessels of the lymphatic system. The lymphatic system is a critical component of the immune system as described in Chapters 6 and 7.

THE HEART

Adult hearts weigh between 200 and 350 grams and are about fist-sized. The heart lies obliquely (diagonally) in the **mediastinum**, the area above the diaphragm and between the lungs. Heart structures can be categorized by three functions:

1. *Structural support of heart tissues and circulation of pulmonary and systemic blood through the heart.* This category includes the heart wall and fibrous skeleton enclosing and supporting the heart and dividing it into four chambers: the valves directing flow through the chambers and the great vessels conducting blood to and from the heart.

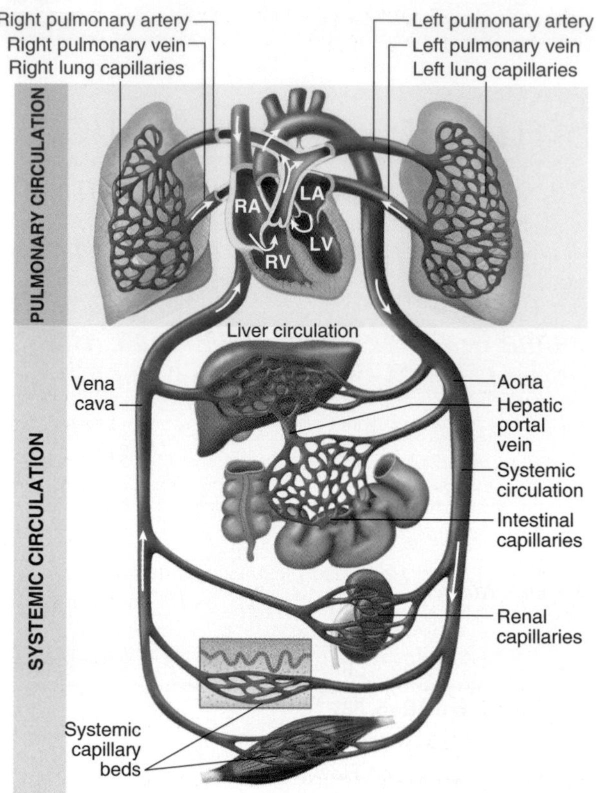

FIGURE 23-1 Diagram of the Pulmonary and Systemic Circulatory Systems. The right heart pumps unoxygenated blood (*blue*) through the pulmonary circulation, where oxygen enters the blood and carbon dioxide is exhaled, and the left heart pumps oxygenated (*red*) blood to and from all the other organ systems in the body. *LA*, left atrium; *LV*, left ventricle; *RA*, right atrium; *RV*, right ventricle. (From Patton, K.T., Thibodeau, G.A., & Douglas, M.M. [2012]. *Essentials of anatomy & physiology*. St. Louis: Elsevier.)

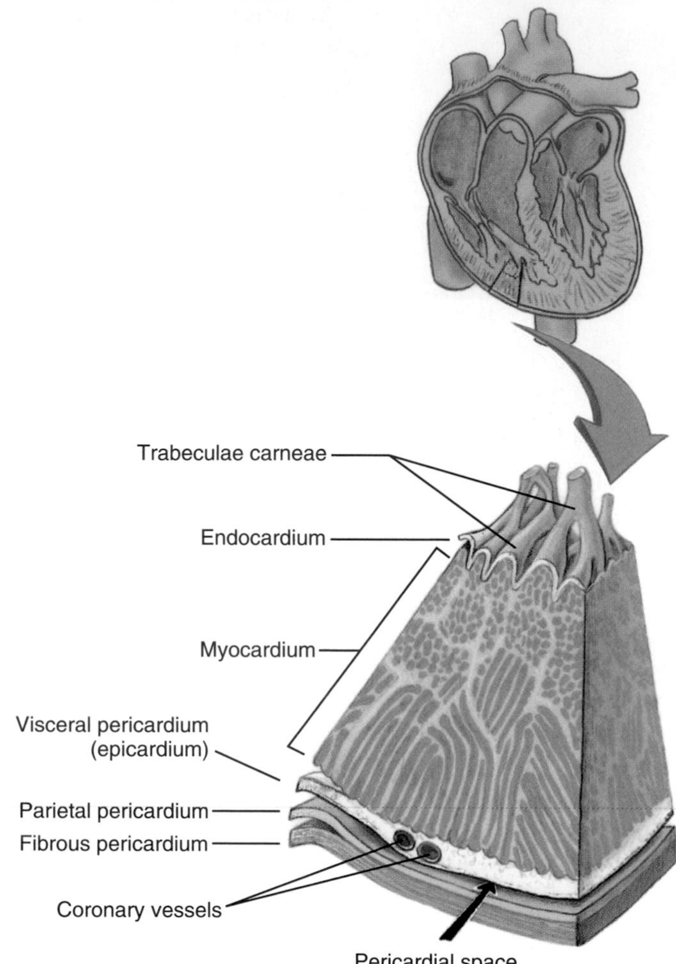

FIGURE 23-2 Wall of the Heart. This section of the heart wall shows the fibrous pericardium, the parietal and visceral layers of the serous pericardium (with the pericardial space between them), the myocardium, and the endocardium. Note the fatty connective tissue between the visceral layer of the serous pericardium (epicardium) and the myocardium. Note also that the endocardium covers tubular projections of myocardial muscle tissue called *trabeculae*. (Revised from Applegate, E. [2011]. *The anatomy and physiology learning system* [4th ed.]. St. Louis: Saunders.)

2. *Maintenance of heart cells.* This category includes all the vessels of the coronary circulation—the arteries and veins that serve the metabolic needs of all the heart cells—and the heart's lymphatic vessels.
3. *Stimulation and control of heart action.* Among these structures are the nerves and specialized muscle cells that direct the rhythmic contraction and relaxation of the heart muscles, propelling blood throughout the pulmonary and systemic circulatory systems.

Structures That Direct Circulation Through the Heart

The Heart Wall

The three layers of the heart wall—the epicardium, myocardium, and endocardium—are enclosed in a double-walled membranous sac, the **pericardium** (Figure 23-2). The **pericardial sac** has three main functions: (1) it prevents displacement of the heart during gravitational acceleration or deceleration, (2) it serves as a physical barrier to protect the heart against infection and inflammation coming from the lungs and pleural space, and (3) it contains pain receptors and mechanoreceptors that can cause reflex changes in blood pressure and **heart rate**. The two layers of the pericardium, the parietal and the visceral pericardia (see Figure 23-2), are separated by a fluid-containing space called the **pericardial cavity** (also referred to as *pericardial space*). The **pericardial fluid** (about 20 mL) is secreted by cells of the mesothelial layer of the pericardium and lubricates the membranes that line the pericardial cavity, enabling them to slide smoothly over one another with minimal friction as the heart beats. The amount and character of the pericardial fluid are altered if the pericardium is inflamed (see Chapter 24).

The smoothness of the outer layer of the heart, the epicardium, also minimizes the friction between the heart wall and the pericardial sac. The thickest layer of the heart wall, the **myocardium**, is composed of cardiac muscle and is anchored to the heart's fibrous skeleton. The heart muscle cells, **cardiomyocytes**, provide the contractile force needed for blood to flow through the heart and into the pulmonary and systemic circulations. About 0.5 to 1% of the cardiomyocytes are replaced annually; thus over a lifetime about half of these muscle cells are replaced.[2] There is great interest in finding therapies that will increase the rate of cardiomyocyte replacement for persons who have suffered a myocardial infarction or have heart failure from another cause.

The internal lining of the myocardium, the **endocardium**, is composed of connective tissue and squamous cells (see Figure 23-2). This lining is continuous with the endothelium that lines all the arteries, veins, and capillaries of the body, creating a continuous, closed circulatory system.

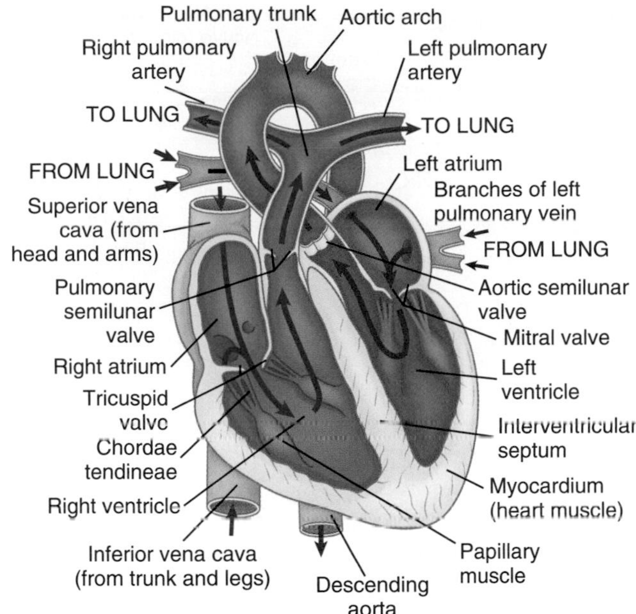

FIGURE 23-3 Structures That Direct Blood Flow Through the Heart. The blue and red arrows indicate the pathways of unoxygenated and oxygenated blood flow through chambers, valves, and major vessels.

Chambers of the Heart

The heart has four chambers: the **left atrium**, the **right atrium**, the **right ventricle**, and the **left ventricle**. These chambers form two pumps in series: the right heart is a low-pressure system pumping blood through the lungs, and the left heart is a high-pressure system pumping blood to the rest of the body (Figure 23-3). The atria are smaller than the ventricles and have thinner walls. The ventricles have a thicker myocardial layer and constitute much of the bulk of the heart. The ventricles are formed by a continuum of muscle fibres originating from the fibrous skeleton at the base of the heart.

The wall thickness of each cardiac chamber depends on the amount of pressure or resistance it must overcome to eject blood. The two atria have the thinnest walls because they are low-pressure chambers that serve as storage units and channels for blood that is emptied into the ventricles. Normally, there is little resistance to flow from the atria to the ventricles. The ventricles, on the other hand, must propel the blood all the way through the pulmonary or systemic vessels. The mean pulmonary artery pressure, the force the right ventricle must overcome, is only 15 mm Hg, whereas the mean arterial pressure the left ventricle must pump against is about 92 mm Hg. Because the pressure is markedly higher in the systemic circulation, the wall of the left ventricle is about three times thicker than that of the right ventricle.

The right ventricle is shaped like a crescent or triangle, enabling a bellowslike action that efficiently ejects large volumes of blood through the pulmonary semilunar valve into the low-pressure pulmonary system. The larger left ventricle is bullet shaped, which allows it to generate enough pressure to eject blood through a relatively larger aortic semilunar valve into the high-pressure systemic circulation.

The septal membrane separates the right and left sides of the heart and prevents blood from crossing between the two circulatory systems. The atria are separated by the interatrial septum, and the ventricles are separated by the interventricular septum. Because the fetus does not depend on the lungs for oxygenation, there is an opening before birth between the right and left atria called the *foramen ovale* that facilitates circulation. This opening closes functionally at the time of birth as the higher pressure in the left atrium pushes a flap, the septum primum, over the hole. In 75 to 80% of infants, these septa are permanently fused within the first year of life[3,4] (see Chapter 25).

Fibrous Skeleton of the Heart

Four rings of dense fibrous connective tissue provide a firm anchorage for the attachments of the atrial and ventricular musculature, as well as the valvular tissue (Figure 23-4). The fibrous rings are adjacent and form a central, fibrous supporting structure collectively termed the *annuli fibrosi cordis*.

Valves of the Heart

Four heart valves and the pressure gradients they maintain ensure that blood only flows one way through the heart. When the ventricles are relaxed, the two **atrioventricular valves (AV valves)** open and blood flows from the relatively higher pressure in the atria to the lower pressure in the ventricles. As the ventricles contract, ventricular pressure increases and causes these valves to close and prevent backflow into the atria. The **semilunar valves** of the heart open when intraventricular pressure exceeds aortic and pulmonary pressures, and blood flows out of the ventricles and into the pulmonary and systemic circulations. After ventricular contraction and ejection, intraventricular pressure falls and the **pulmonic semilunar valve** and **aortic semilunar valve** close when the pressure in the vessels is greater than the pressure in the ventricles, thus preventing backflow into the right and left ventricles, respectively. The actions of the heart valves are shown in Figures 23-3 and 23-4.

The AV (tricuspid and mitral) valve openings are composed of tissue flaps called *leaflets* or *cusps*, which are attached at the upper margin to a ring in the heart's fibrous skeleton and by the **chordae tendineae** at the lower end to the papillary muscles (see Figure 23-3). The **papillary muscles**, extensions of the myocardium, help hold the cusps together and downward at the onset of ventricular contraction, thus preventing their backward expulsion or **prolapse** into the atria.

The AV valve in the right heart is called the **tricuspid valve** because it has three cusps. The left AV valve is a bicuspid (two-cusp) valve called the **mitral valve (left atrioventricular valve, bicuspid valve)**. The tricuspid and mitral valves function as a unit because the atria, fibrous rings, valvular tissue, chordae tendineae, papillary muscles, and ventricular walls are connected. Collectively, these six structures are known as the **mitral and tricuspid complex**. Damage to any one of the six components of this complex can alter function significantly and contribute to heart failure.

Blood leaves the right ventricle through the pulmonic semilunar valve, and it leaves the left ventricle through the aortic semilunar valve (see Figures 23-3 and 23-4). Both the pulmonic and aortic semilunar valves have three cup-shaped cusps that arise from the fibrous skeleton.

The Great Vessels

Blood moves in and out of the heart through several large veins and arteries (see Figure 23-3). The right heart receives venous blood from the systemic circulation through the **superior vena cava** and **inferior vena cava**, which join and then enter the right atrium. Blood leaving the right ventricle enters the pulmonary circulation through the **pulmonary artery**, which divides into right and left branches to transport unoxygenated blood from the right heart to the lungs. The pulmonary arteries branch further into the pulmonary capillary beds, where oxygen and carbon dioxide exchange occurs.

Four **pulmonary veins**, two from the right lung and two from the left lung, carry oxygenated blood from the lungs to the left side of the heart. The oxygenated blood moves through the left atrium and ventricle, out into the **aorta** that subsequently branches into the systemic arteries that supply the body.

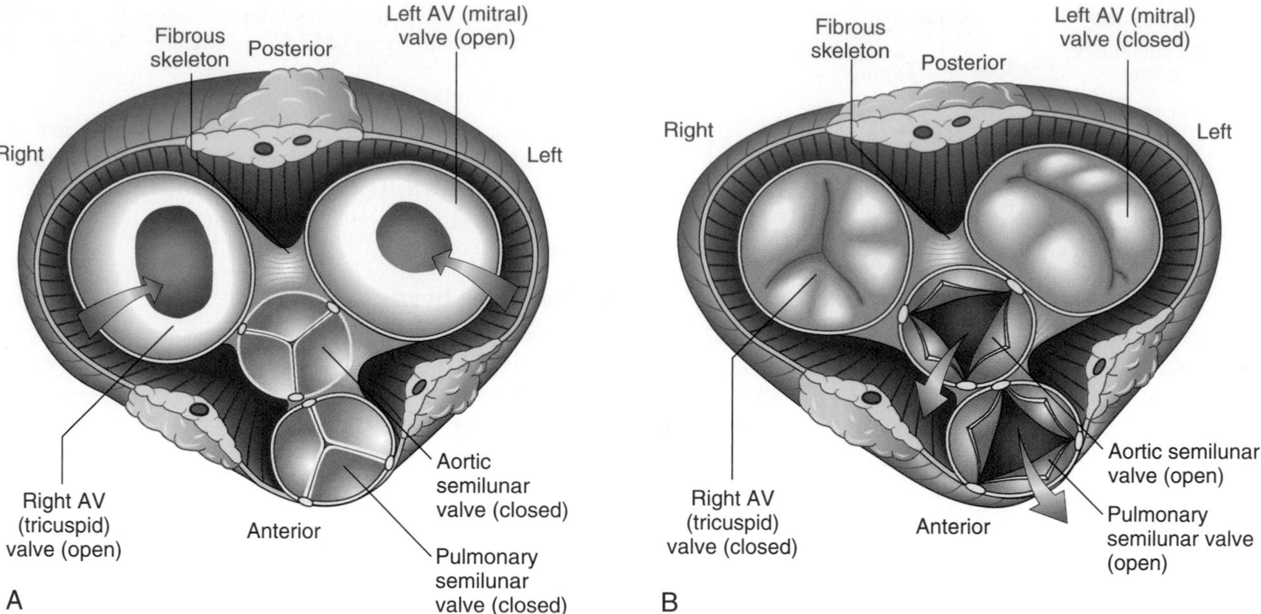

FIGURE 23-4 Transverse Section of the Heart Showing the Atrioventricular (Mitral and Tricuspid) and Semilunar (Aortic and Pulmonary) Valves. Superior view with the atria and vessels removed. *Arrows* indicate direction of blood flow. **A,** When the heart is filling with blood, the AV valves are open and the semilunar valves are closed. **B,** When blood is leaving the heart, the semilunar valves are open and the AV valves are closed. *AV,* atrioventricular. (From Naish, J. [2015]. *Medical sciences* [2nd ed.]. London: Saunders.)

Blood Flow During the Cardiac Cycle

The pumping action of the heart consists of contraction and relaxation of the heart muscle, or myocardium. Each ventricular contraction and the relaxation that follows it constitute one cardiac cycle. (Blood flow through the heart during a single cardiac cycle is illustrated in Figure 23-5.) During the period of relaxation, termed diastole, blood fills the ventricles. The ventricular contraction that follows, termed systole, propels the blood out of the ventricles and into the pulmonary and systemic circulations. Contraction of the left ventricle occurs slightly earlier than contraction of the right ventricle.

The five phases of the cardiac cycle are said to begin with the opening of the mitral and tricuspid valves and atrial contraction (Figures 23-6 and 23-7). Closing of the mitral and tricuspid valves as passive ventricular filling begins marks the end of one cardiac cycle.

Normal Intracardiac Pressures

Normal intracardiac pressures are shown in Table 23-1.

QUICK CHECK 23-1

1. Why are the two separate circulatory systems said to be "serially connected"?
2. What are the functions of the pericardial sac?
3. Why is the thickness of the myocardium different in the right and left ventricles?
4. Trace the flow of blood through the heart during one cardiac cycle.

Structures That Support Cardiac Metabolism: The Coronary Vessels

The myocardium and other heart structures are supplied with oxygen and nutrients by the coronary circulation, which is part of the systemic circulation. The coronary arteries originate at the upper edge of the aortic semilunar valve cusps (Figure 23-8, *B*) and receive blood through openings in the aorta called the coronary ostia. The cardiac veins empty into the right atrium through another ostium, the opening of a large vein called the coronary sinus (Figure 23-8, *C*). (Regulation of the coronary circulation, which is similar to regulation of flow through systemic and pulmonary vessels, is described in "Regulation of the Coronary Circulation," p. 598.)

TABLE 23-1 Normal Intracardiac Pressures

	Mean (mm Hg)	Range (mm Hg)
Right atrium	4	0–8
Right ventricle		
Systolic	24	15–28
End-diastolic	4	0–8
Left atrium	7	4–12
Left ventricle		
Systolic	130	90–140
End-diastolic	7	4–12

Coronary Arteries

The major coronary arteries, the right coronary artery (RCA) and the left coronary artery (LCA) (Figure 23-8, *A*), traverse the epicardium, myocardium, and endocardium and branch to become arterioles and then capillaries. Their main branches are outlined in Box 23-1. The coronary arteries are smaller in women than in men because women's hearts weigh proportionately less than men's hearts.

Collateral Arteries

Collateral arteries are anastomoses or connections between branches of the same coronary artery or connections of branches of the RCA with branches of the left. The epicardium contains more collateral vessels

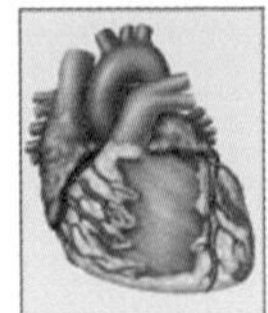

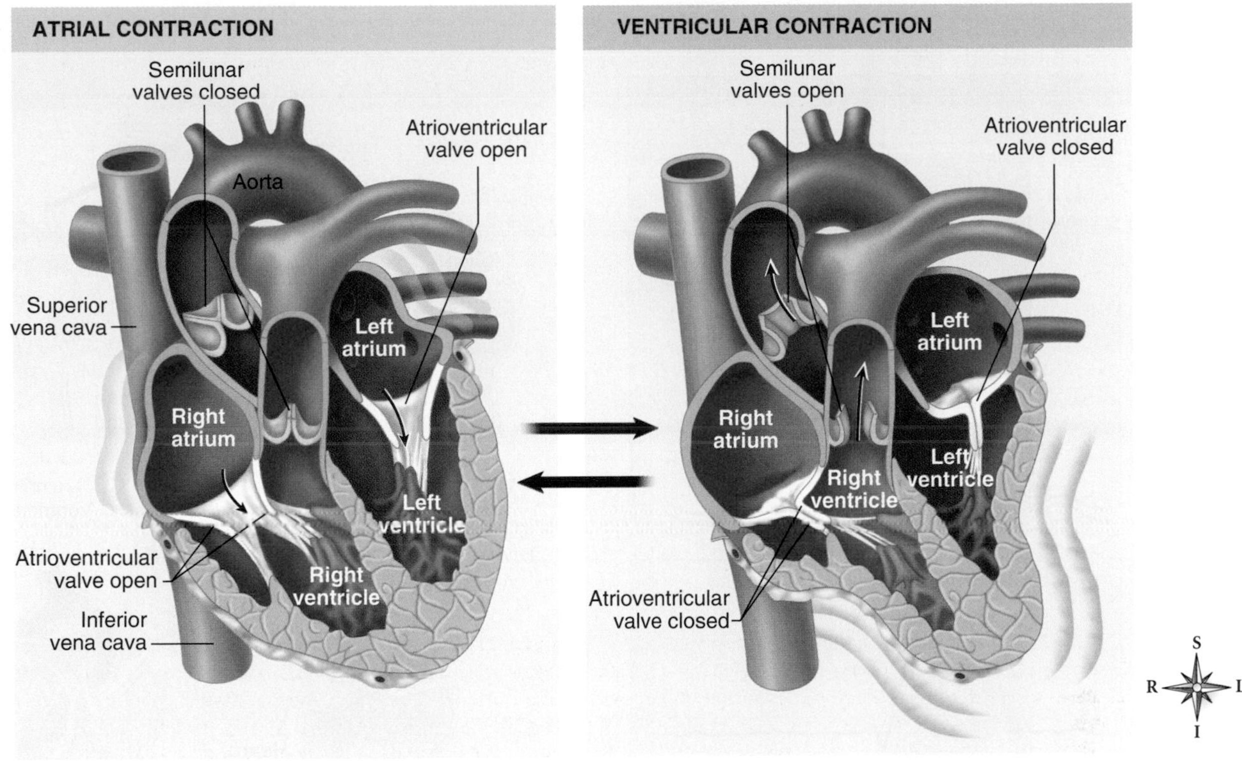

FIGURE 23-5 Blood Flow Through the Heart During a Single Cardiac Cycle. A, During diastole, blood flows into atria, atrioventricular valves are pushed open, and blood begins to fill ventricles. Atrial systole squeezes blood remaining in the atria into the ventricles. **B,** During ventricular systole, the ventricles contract, pushing blood out through semilunar valves into the pulmonary artery (right ventricle) and the aorta (left ventricle). (From Patton, K.T., & Thibodeau, G.A. [2016]. *Structure & function of the body* [15th ed.]. St. Louis: Elsevier.)

BOX 23-1 Main Branches of the Coronary Arteries

Left coronary artery. Arises from single ostium behind left cusp of aortic semilunar valve; ranges from a few millimetres to a few centimetres long; passes between left arterial appendage and pulmonary artery and generally divides into two branches: the left anterior descending artery and the circumflex artery; other branches are distributed diagonally across the free wall of the left ventricle.

Left anterior descending artery (or anterior interventricular artery). Delivers blood to portions of left and right ventricles and much of interventricular septum; travels down the anterior surface of the interventricular septum toward apex of the heart.

Circumflex artery. Travels in a groove (*coronary sulcus*) that separates left atrium from left ventricle and extends to left border of heart; supplies blood to left atrium and lateral wall of left ventricle; often branches to posterior surfaces of left atrium and left ventricle.

Right coronary artery. Originates from an ostium behind the right aortic cusp, travels from behind the pulmonary artery, and extends around the right heart to the heart's posterior surface, where it branches to atrium and ventricle; three major branches are conus (supplies blood to upper right ventricle), right marginal branch (supplies right ventricle to the apex), and posterior descending branch (lies in posterior interventricular sulcus and supplies smaller branches to both ventricles).

than the endocardium. New collateral vessels are formed through two processes: **arteriogenesis** (new artery growth branching from pre-existing arteries) and **angiogenesis** (growth of new capillaries within a tissue).[5] This collateral growth is stimulated by **shear stress** that results from increased blood flow speed within and just beyond areas of stenosis, as well as the production of growth factors and cytokines, including monocyte chemoattractant protein-1 (MCP-1) and vascular endothelial growth factor (VEGF).[6] The collateral circulation assists in supplying blood and oxygen to myocardium that has become ischemic following gradual narrowing, or **stenosis**, of one or more major coronary arteries (coronary artery disease). Unfortunately, diabetes, which predisposes to coronary artery disease, also impedes collateral formation because of increased production of antiangiogenic factors, such as endostatin and angiostatin. Current research is focused on identifying whether some factors that stimulate collateral growth might be useful treatments for myocardial ischemia; so far, none have been demonstrated to be effective.[6]

Coronary Capillaries

The heart requires an extensive capillary network to function. Blood travels from the arteries to the arterioles and then into the capillaries, where oxygen and other nutrients enter the myocardium while waste products enter the blood. At rest, the heart extracts 50 to 80% of the oxygen delivered to it, and coronary blood flow is directly correlated with myocardial oxygen consumption.[7] Any alteration of the cardiac muscles dramatically affects blood flow in the capillaries.

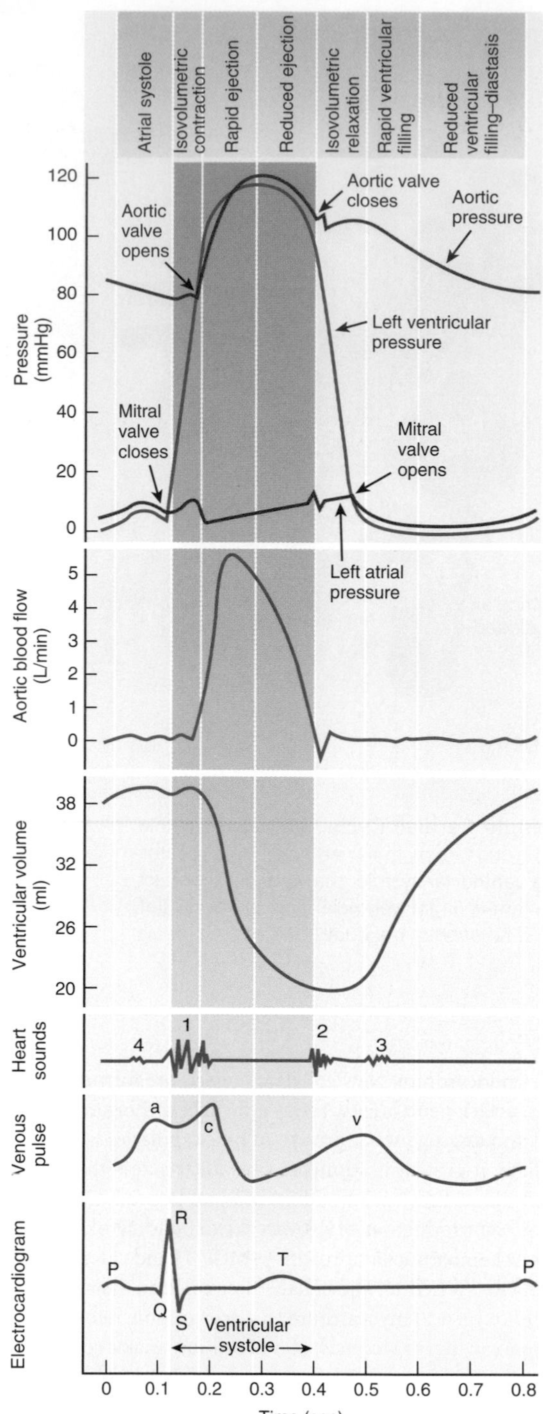

FIGURE 23-6 Composite Chart of Heart Function. This chart is a composite of several diagrams of heart function (cardiac pumping cycle, blood pressure, blood flow, volume, heart sounds, venous pulse, and electrocardiogram [ECG]), all on the same time scale.

Coronary Veins and Lymphatic Vessels

After passing through the capillary network, blood from the coronary arteries drains into the cardiac veins located alongside the arteries. Most of the venous drainage of the heart occurs through veins in the visceral pericardium. The veins then feed into the great cardiac vein (see Figure 23-8, *C*) and coronary sinus on the posterior surface of the heart, between the atria and ventricles, in the coronary sulcus.

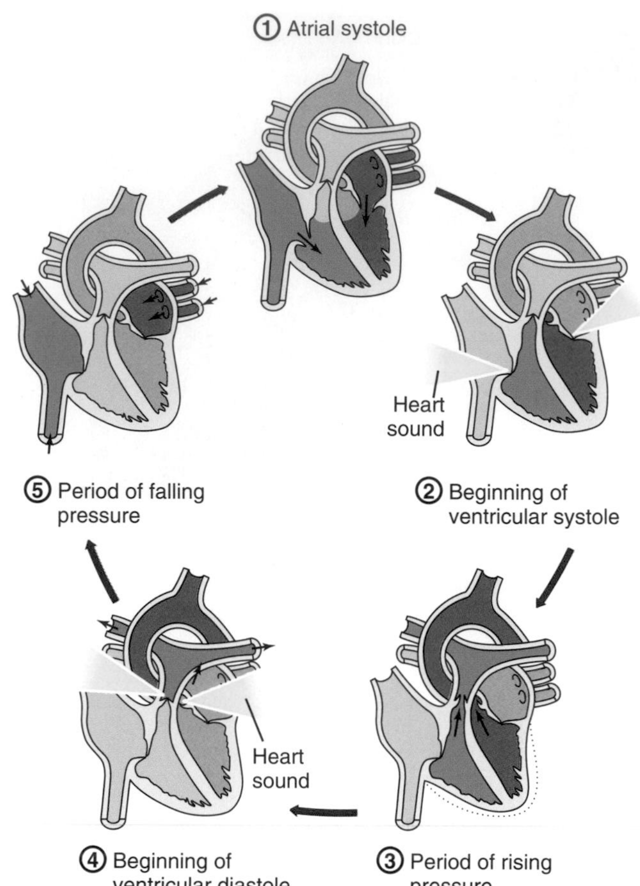

FIGURE 23-7 The Five Phases of the Cardiac Cycle. 1, Atrial systole: Atria contract, pushing blood through the open tricuspid and mitral valves into the ventricles. Semilunar valves are closed. **2,** Beginning of ventricular systole. Ventricles contract, increasing pressure within the ventricles. The tricuspid and mitral valves close, causing the first heart sound. **3,** Period of rising pressure: semilunar valves open when pressure in the ventricle exceeds that in the arteries. Blood spurts into the aorta and pulmonary arteries. **4,** Beginning of ventricular diastole: pressure in the relaxing ventricles drops below that in the arteries. Semilunar valves snap shut, causing the second heart sound. **5,** Period of falling pressure: blood flows from veins into the relaxed atria. Tricuspid and mitral valves open when pressure in the ventricles falls below that in the atria. (Adapted from Solomon, E. [2016]. *Introduction to human anatomy and physiology* [4th ed.]. St. Louis: Saunders.)

The myocardium has an extensive system of lymphatic capillaries and collecting vessels within the layers of the myocardium and the valves. With cardiac contraction, the lymphatic vessels drain fluid to lymph nodes in the anterior mediastinum that empty into the superior vena cava. The lymphatics are important for protecting the myocardium against infection and injury.

Structures That Control Heart Action

Life depends on continuous repetition of the cardiac cycle (systole and diastole), which requires the transmission of electrical impulses, termed cardiac action potentials, through the myocardium.[7] (Action potentials are described in Chapters 1 and 5.) The muscle fibres of the myocardium are electrically coupled so that action potentials pass from cell to cell rapidly and efficiently.

The myocardium contains its own pacemakers and conduction system—specialized cells that enable it to generate and transmit action potentials without input from the nervous system (Figure 23-9). The

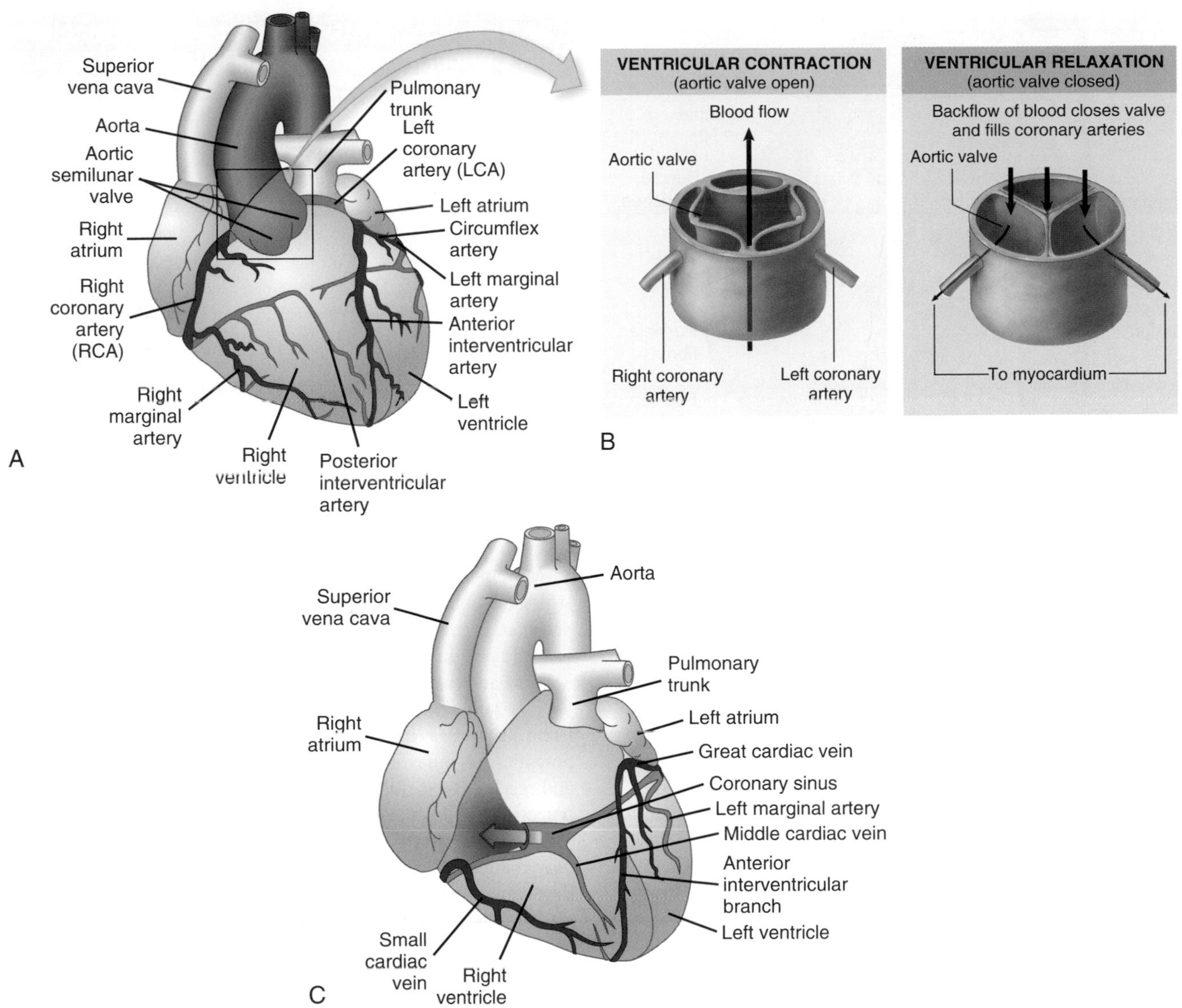

FIGURE 23-8 Coronary Circulation. **A**, Arteries. **B**, Coronary artery openings from the aorta. **C**, Veins. Both **A** and **C** are anterior views of the heart. Vessels near the anterior surface are more darkly coloured than vessels of the posterior surface seen through the heart. **B**, Placement of the coronary artery opening behind the leaflets of the aortic valve allows the coronary arteries to fill during ventricular relaxation. (**A** and **C**, from Patton, K.T., & Thibodeau, G.A. [2010]. *Anatomy & physiology* [7th ed.]. St. Louis: Mosby. **B**, Patton, K.T., & Thibodeau, G.A. [2014]. *The human body in health & disease* [6th ed.]. St. Louis: Mosby.)

pacemaker cells are concentrated at two sites, or nodes, in the myocardium. The cardiac cycle is stimulated by these nodes of specialized cells. Although the heart is innervated by the autonomic nervous system (both sympathetic and parasympathetic fibres), neural impulses are not needed to maintain the cardiac cycle. Thus the heart will beat in the absence of any innervation, one of the many factors that allow heart transplantation to be successful.

Heart action is also influenced by substances delivered to the myocardium in coronary blood. Nutrients and oxygen are needed for cellular survival and normal function. Hormones and biochemical substances, including medications, can affect the strength and duration of myocardial contraction and the degree and duration of myocardial relaxation. Normal or appropriate function depends on the supply of these substances, which is why coronary artery disease can seriously disrupt heart function.

The Conduction System

Normally, electrical impulses arise in the **sinoatrial node (SA node, sinus node)**, the usual pacemaker of the heart. The SA node is located at the junction of the right atrium and superior vena cava, just superior to the tricuspid valve. The SA node is heavily innervated by both sympathetic and parasympathetic nerve fibres.[8] In the resting adult, the SA node generates about 60 to 100 action potentials per minute, depending on age and physical condition. Each action potential travels rapidly from cell to cell and through the atrial myocardium, carrying the action potential onward to the **atrioventricular node (AV node)**, as well as causing both atria to contract, beginning systole.[8]

The AV node, located in the right atrial wall superior to the tricuspid valve and anterior to the ostium of the coronary sinus, conducts the action potentials onward to the ventricles. It is innervated by nerves from the autonomic parasympathetic ganglia that serve as receptors

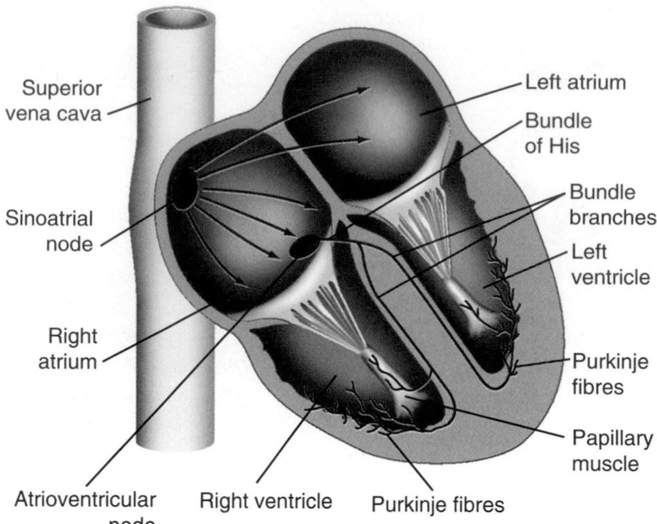

FIGURE 23-9 The Cardiac Conduction System. Specialized cardiac muscle cells in the heart wall rapidly conduct an electrical impulse throughout the myocardium. The signal is initiated by the sinoatrial node (pacemaker) and spreads through the atrial myocardium to the atrioventricular node. The atrioventricular node then initiates a signal that is conducted through the ventricular myocardium by way of the atrioventricular bundle (of His) and Purkinje fibres. (From Koeppen, B.M. [Ed.]. [2010]. *Berne & Levy physiology* [6th ed.]. St. Louis: Mosby.)

for the vagus nerve and cause slowing of impulse conduction through the AV node.

Conducting fibres from the AV node converge to form the **bundle of His (atrioventricular bundle [AV bundle])**, within the posterior border of the interventricular septum. The bundle of His then gives rise to the right and left bundle branches. The **right bundle branch (RBB)** is thin and travels without much branching to the right ventricular apex. Because of its thinness and relative lack of branches, the RBB is susceptible to interruption of impulse conduction by damage to the endocardium. The **left bundle branch (LBB)** in some hearts divides into two branches, or fascicles. The left anterior bundle branch (LABB) passes the left anterior papillary muscle and the base of the left ventricle and crosses the aortic outflow tract. Damage to the aortic valve or the left ventricle can interrupt this branch. The left posterior bundle branch (LPBB) travels posteriorly, crossing the left ventricular inflow tract to the base of the left posterior papillary muscle. This branch spreads diffusely through the posterior inferior left ventricular wall. Blood flow through this portion of the left ventricle is relatively nonturbulent, so the LBB is somewhat protected from injury caused by wear and tear.

The **Purkinje fibres** are the terminal branches of the RBB and LBB. They extend from the ventricular apexes to the fibrous rings and penetrate the heart wall to the outer myocardium. The first areas of the ventricles to be excited are portions of the interventricular septum. The septum is activated from both the RBB and the LBB. The extensive network of Purkinje fibres promotes the rapid spread of the impulse to the ventricular apexes. The basal and posterior portions of the ventricles are the last to be activated.

QUICK CHECK 23-2

1. Draw a diagram of the conduction system of the heart.
2. Why are the left and right coronary vessels considered the major coronary vessels?

TABLE 23-2 Intracellular and Extracellular Ion Concentrations in the Myocardium

	Intracellular Concentration (mmol/L)	Extracellular Concentration (mmol/L)
Sodium (Na^+)	5	135–145
Potassium (K^+)	150	3.5–5.0
Chloride (Cl^-)	5	98–106
Calcium (Ca^{++})	10^{-7}	Total Ca: 2.25–2.75 Ionized: 1.05–1.30

Propagation of cardiac action potentials. Electrical activation of the muscle cells, termed **depolarization**, is caused by the movement of ions, including sodium, potassium, calcium, and chloride, across cardiac cell membranes. Deactivation, called **repolarization**, occurs the same way. (Movement of ions across cell membranes is described in Chapter 1; electrical activation of muscle cells is described in Chapter 38.)

Movement of ions into and out of the cell creates an electrical (voltage) difference across the cell membrane, called the *membrane potential.* The resting membrane potential of myocardial cells is between −80 and −90 mV, whereas that of the SA node is between −50 and −60 mV and that of the AV node is between −60 and −70 mV.[8] During depolarization, the inside of the cell becomes less negatively charged. In cardiac cells, as in other excitable cells, when the resting membrane potential (in millivolts) becomes more negative with depolarization and reaches the threshold potential for cardiac cells, a cardiac action potential is fired. Table 23-2 summarizes the intracellular and extracellular ionic concentrations of cardiac muscle. Medications that alter the movement of these ions (e.g., calcium) have profound effects on the action potential and can alter heart rate. The various phases of the cardiac action potential are related to changes in the permeability of the cell membrane to sodium, potassium, chloride, and calcium. Threshold is the point at which the cell membrane's selective permeability to these ions is temporarily disrupted, leading to an "all or nothing" depolarization. If the resting membrane potential becomes more negative because of a decrease in extracellular potassium concentration (hypokalemia), it is termed *hyperpolarization.*

A **refractory period**, during which no new cardiac action potential can be initiated by a stimulus, follows depolarization. This effective or absolute refractory period corresponds to the time needed for the reopening of channels that permit sodium and calcium influx into the cells. A relative refractory period occurs near the end of repolarization, following the effective refractory period. During this time, the membrane can be depolarized again but only by a greater-than-normal stimulus. Abnormal refractory periods as a result of disease can cause abnormal heart rhythms or dysrhythmias, including ventricular fibrillation and cardiac arrest (see Chapter 24).

The electrocardiogram. An electrocardiogram originates from myocardial cell electrical activity as recorded by skin electrodes and is the summation of all the cardiac action potentials (Figure 23-10). The **P wave** represents atrial depolarization. The **PR interval** is a measure of time from the onset of atrial activation to the onset of ventricular activation (normally 0.12 to 0.20 second). The PR interval represents the time necessary for electrical activity to travel from the sinus node through the atrium, AV node, and His–Purkinje system to activate ventricular myocardial cells. The **QRS complex** represents the sum of all ventricular muscle cell depolarization. The configuration and amplitude of the QRS complex may vary considerably among individuals.

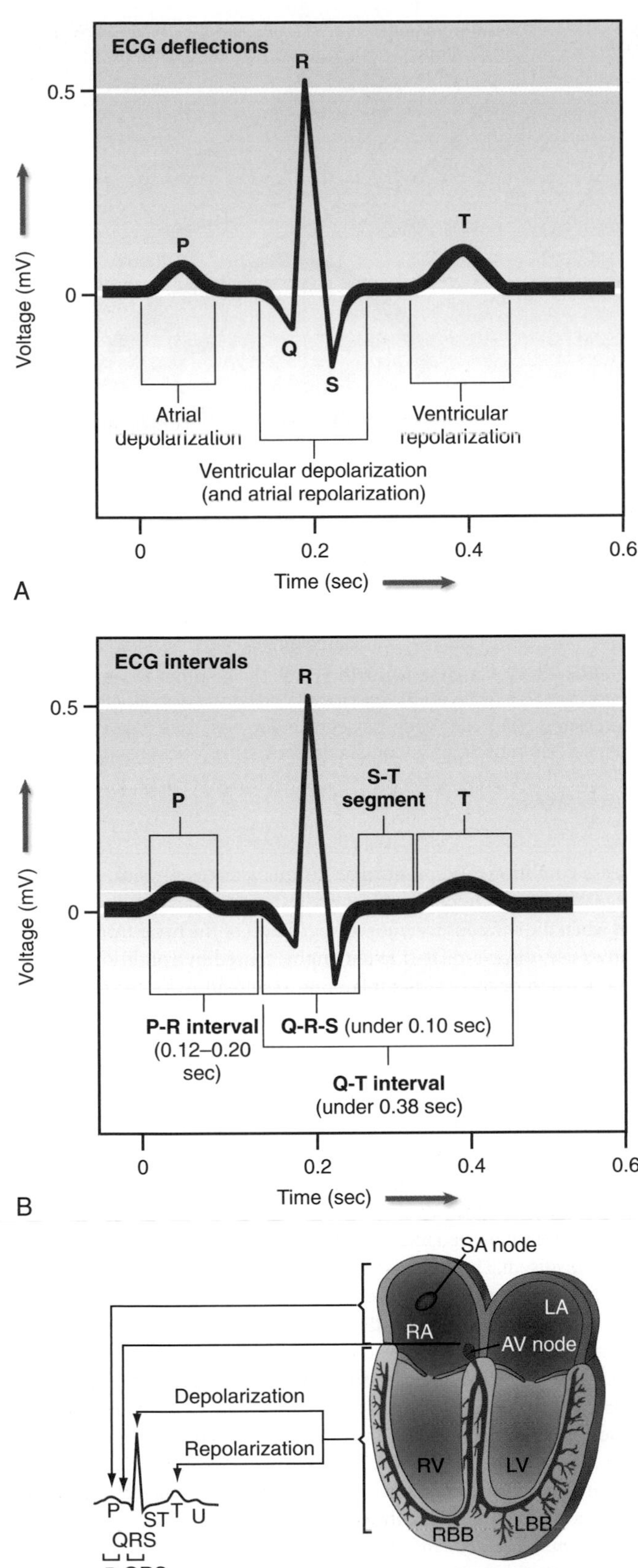

FIGURE 23-10 Electrocardiogram, and Cardiac Electrical Activity. **A,** Normal ECG. Depolarization and repolarization. **B,** ECG intervals among P, QRS, and T waves. **C,** Schematic representation of ECG and its relationship to cardiac electrical activity. *AV,* atrioventricular; *ECG,* electrocardiogram; *LA,* left atrium; *LBB,* left bundle branch; *LV,* left ventricle; *RA,* right atrium; *RBB,* right bundle branch; *RV,* right ventricle.

The duration is normally between 0.06 and 0.10 second. During the ST interval, the entire ventricular myocardium is depolarized. The QT interval is sometimes called the "electrical systole" of the ventricles. It lasts about 0.4 second but varies inversely with the heart rate. The T wave represents ventricular repolarization.

Automaticity. Automaticity, or the property of generating spontaneous depolarization to threshold, enables the SA and AV nodes to generate cardiac action potentials without any external stimulus. Cells capable of spontaneous depolarization are called automatic cells. The automatic cells of the cardiac conduction system can stimulate the heart to beat even when it is transplanted and thus has no innervation. Spontaneous depolarization is possible in automatic cells because the membrane potential of these special cells does not actually "rest" during return to the resting membrane potential. Instead, it slowly depolarizes toward threshold during the diastolic phase of the cardiac cycle. Because threshold is approached during diastole, return to the resting membrane potential in automatic cells is called diastolic depolarization. The electrical impulse normally begins in the SA node because its cells depolarize more rapidly than other automatic cells.

Rhythmicity. Rhythmicity is the regular generation of an action potential by the heart's conduction system. The SA node sets the pace because normally it has the fastest rate. The SA node depolarizes spontaneously 60 to 100 times per minute. If the SA node is damaged, the AV node can become the heart's pacemaker at a rate of about 40 to 60 spontaneous depolarizations per minute. Eventually, however, conduction cells in the atria usually take over from the AV node. Purkinje fibres are capable of spontaneous depolarization but at an even slower rate than the AV node.

> **QUICK CHECK 23-3**
> 1. What are the pathways of conduction through the heart?
> 2. What does each of the electrocardiogram waves (P, Q, R, S, T) represent?
> 3. Define *automaticity* and *rhythmicity*.

Cardiac Innervation

Although the heart's nodes and conduction system are able to generate action potentials independently, the autonomic nervous system influences both the rate of impulse generation (firing), depolarization, and repolarization of the myocardium, and the strength of atrial and ventricular contraction. Autonomic neural transmission produces changes in the heart and circulatory system faster than metabolic or humoral agents. Speed is important, for example, in stimulating the heart to increase its pumping action during times of stress and fear—the so-called fight-or-flight response—or with increased physical activity. Although increased delivery of oxygen, glucose, hormones, and other bloodborne factors sustains increased cardiac activity, the rapid initiation of increased activity depends on the sympathetic and parasympathetic fibres of the autonomic nervous system.

Sympathetic and parasympathetic nerves. Sympathetic and parasympathetic nerve fibres innervate all parts of the atria and ventricles and the SA and AV nodes. In general, sympathetic stimulation increases electrical conductivity and the strength of myocardial contraction, and vagal parasympathetic nerve activity does the opposite, slowing the conduction of action potentials through the heart and reducing the strength of contraction. Thus the sympathetic and parasympathetic nerves affect the speed of the cardiac cycle (heart rate, or beats per minute), and the sympathetic nerves also influence the diameter of the coronary vessels (Figure 23-11). Sympathetic nervous activity enhances myocardial performance. Stimulation of the SA node by the sympathetic

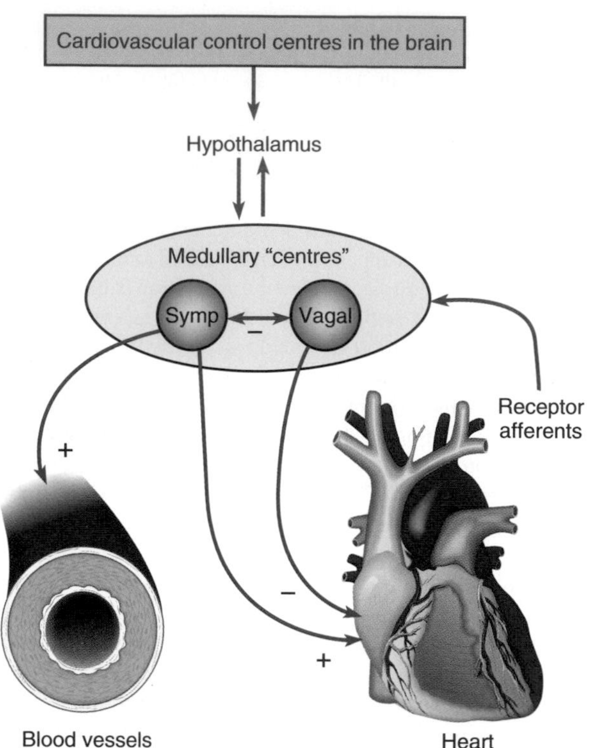

FIGURE 23-11 Autonomic Innervation of Cardiovascular System. Inhibition (–); activation (+).

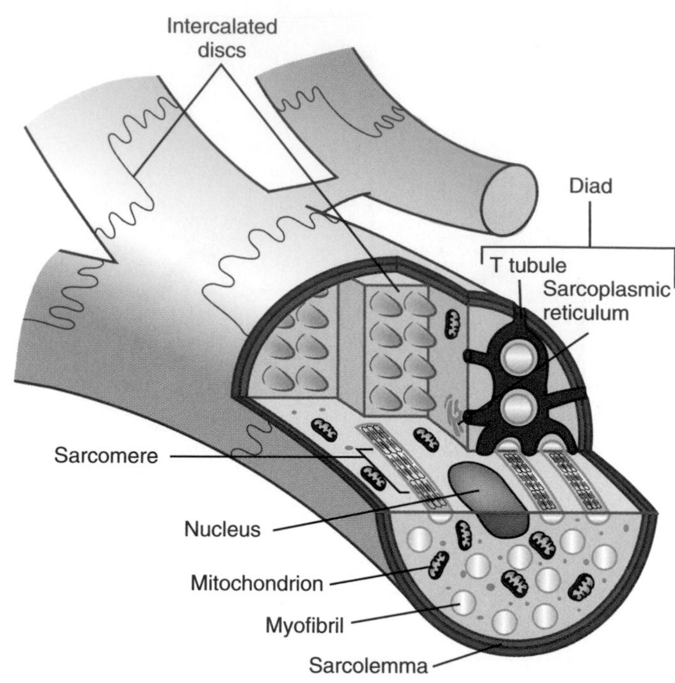

FIGURE 23-12 Cardiac Muscle Fibre. Unlike other types of muscle fibres, cardiac muscle fibres are typically branched with junctions, called *intercalated discs*, between adjacent myocytes. Like skeletal muscle cells, cardiac muscle cells contain sarcoplasmic reticula and T tubules, although these structures are not as highly organized as in skeletal muscle fibres.

nervous system rapidly increases heart rate. Furthermore, neurally released norepinephrine or circulating catecholamines interact with β-adrenergic receptors on the cardiac cell membranes. The overall effect is an increased influx of calcium (Ca^{++}), which increases the contractile strength of the heart and increases the speed of electrical impulses through the heart muscle and the nodes.[8] Finally, increased sympathetic discharge dilates the coronary vessels by causing the release of vasodilating metabolites resulting from increased myocardial contraction.[7]

The parasympathetic nervous system affects the heart through the vagus nerve, which releases acetylcholine. Acetylcholine causes decreased heart rate and slows conduction through the AV node.

Myocardial Cells

Cardiomyocytes are composed of long, narrow fibres that contain bundles of longitudinally arranged myofibrils; a nucleus (cardiac muscle); mitochondria; an internal membrane system (the sarcoplasmic reticulum); cytoplasm (sarcoplasm); and a plasma membrane (the sarcolemma), which encloses the cell. Cardiac and skeletal muscle cells also have an "external" membrane system made up of transverse tubules (T tubules) formed by inward pouching of the sarcolemma. The sarcoplasmic reticulum forms a network of channels that surrounds the muscle fibre.

Because the myofibrils in both cardiac and skeletal fibres consist of alternating light and dark bands of protein, the fibres appear striped, or striated. The dark and light bands of the myofibrils create repeating longitudinal units, called *sarcomeres*, which are between 1.6 and 2.2 μm long (Figures 23-12 and 23-13). The length of these sarcomeres determines the limits of myocardial stretch at the end of diastole and subsequently the force of contraction during systole. Alterations in sarcomere size are seen in both physiological and pathological myocardial hypertrophy.

Hypertrophy, or enlargement, of the heart may occur through growth in either the length or the width of the sarcomeres in both normal and disease conditions. When normal stimuli, such as physical activity or pregnancy, cause hypertrophy, myocardial contractility is increased; and when the stimulus is removed, regression of the hypertrophy occurs. Conversely, disease-related hypertrophy caused by conditions such as hypertension or myocardial infarction results in reduced contractility and often heart failure. It has long been thought that this pathological hypertrophy was not reversible, but new research has shown that reversal may be possible.

When patients with hypertrophic heart failure awaiting a heart transplant were treated by the placement of a left ventricular assist device, regression of the ventricular hypertrophy was observed, occasionally to the point that heart transplant was not required. Research on the mechanisms involved in regression has shown that gene activation, several signalling pathways, angiogenesis, and autophagy are all involved. The hope is that identification of these mechanisms will lead to new and more effective pharmaceutical treatments for heart failure that currently is associated with a poor long-term prognosis.[9-11]

Differences between cardiac and skeletal muscle reflect heart function. Cardiac cells are arranged in branching networks throughout the myocardium, whereas skeletal muscle cells tend to be arranged in parallel units throughout the length of the muscle. Cardiac fibres have only one nucleus, whereas skeletal muscle cells have many nuclei. Other differences enable cardiac fibres to do the following:

- *Transmit action potentials quickly from cell to cell.* Electrical impulses are transmitted rapidly from cardiac fibre to cardiac fibre because the network of fibres connects at **intercalated discs**, which are thickened portions of the sarcolemma. The intercalated discs contain three junctions: desmosomes or macula adherens; fascia adherens, which mechanically attach one cell to another; and gap junctions, also known as *tight junctions*, which allow the electrical impulse to spread from cell to cell through a low-resistance pathway (see Chapter 1).

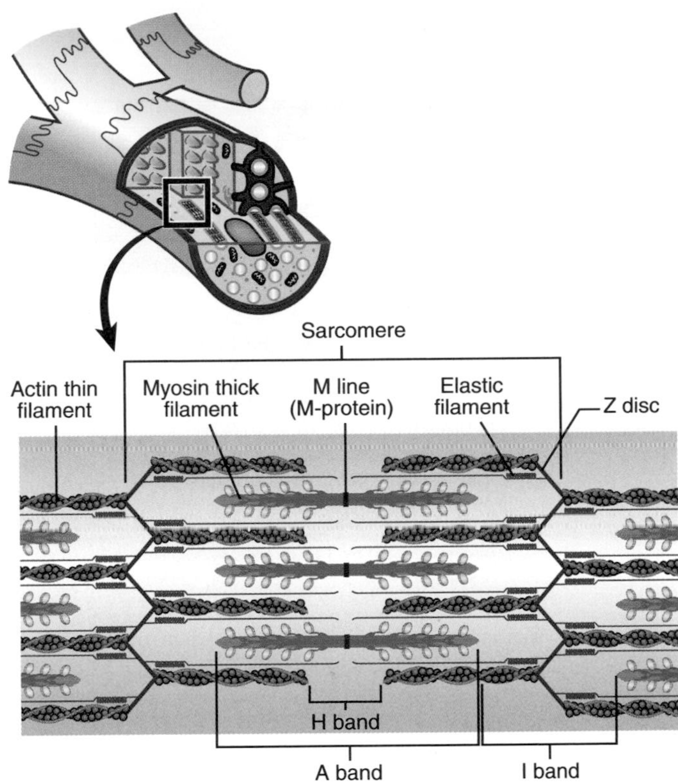

FIGURE 23-13 Structure of a Sarcomere. The sarcomere is the basic contractile unit of a muscle cell. The Z disc is the anchor for the contractile elements actin and myosin. Actin attaches directly to the Z disc, whereas myosin is attached to it by elastic titin filaments. The myosin filaments are connected to each other by M-protein at the M line. The A, H, and I bands refer to parts of the sarcomere as they were originally seen by light microscopy.

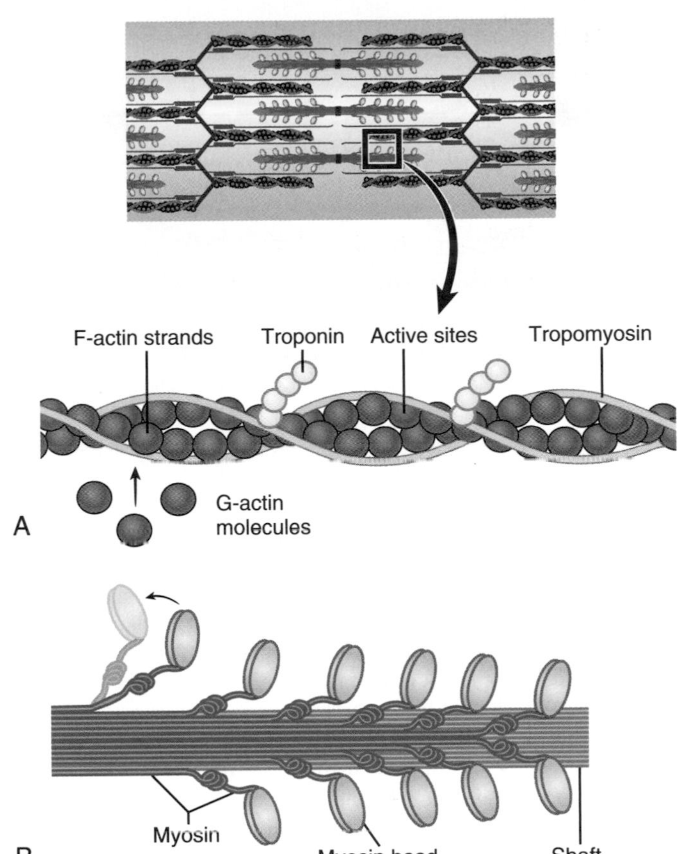

FIGURE 23-14 Structure of Myofilaments. A, Thin myofilament. **B,** Thick myofilament.

Changes in the function of these junctional elements may cause an increased risk for arrhythmias.[8]

- *Maintain high levels of energy synthesis.* Unlike skeletal muscle, the heart cannot rest and is in constant need of energy, which is supplied by molecules such as adenosine triphosphate (ATP). Therefore, the cytoplasm surrounding the bundles of myofibrils in each cardiomyocyte contains a large number of mitochondria (25 to 33% of cell volume). Cardiac muscle cells have more mitochondria than do skeletal muscle cells to provide the necessary respiratory enzymes for aerobic metabolism and supply quantities of ATP sufficient for the constant action of the myocardium.[12]
- *Gain access to more ions, particularly sodium and potassium, in the extracellular environment.* Cardiac fibres contain more T tubules than do skeletal muscle fibres (see Figure 23-12). This increased closeness to the T tubules gives each myofibril in the myocardium faster access to molecules needed for the transmission of action potentials, a process that involves transport of sodium and potassium through the walls of the T tubules. Because the T tubule system is continuous with the extracellular space and the interstitial fluid, it facilitates the rapid transmission of the electrical impulses from the surface of the sarcolemma to the myofibrils inside the fibre. This rapid transmission activates all the myofibrils of one fibre simultaneously. The sarcoplasmic reticulum is located around the myofibrils. As an action potential is transmitted through the T tubules, it induces the sarcoplasmic reticulum to release its stored calcium, thus activating the contractile proteins actin and myosin.

Actin, myosin, and the troponin–tropomyosin complex. Within each myocardial sarcomere are myosin molecules that resemble golf clubs with two large, ovoid heads at one end of the shaft (Figure 23-14, *B*). The two heads contain an actin binding site and a site of adenosinetriphosphatase (ATPase) activity. Thick filaments of myosin overlapping with thinner actin molecules form the central dark band of the sarcomere called the anisotropic band, or A band (see Figures 23-13 and 23-14). A thick filament has about 200 myosin molecules bundled together with their outward-facing heads named *cross-bridges* because they can form force-generating bridges by binding with exposed actin molecules, resulting in contraction (Figure 23-14, *A*). Actin molecules are part of the thin filaments (see Figures 23-13 and 23-14). The light bands, called isotropic bands (or I bands), of the sarcomere contain only actin molecules and no myosin (see Figure 23-13). Thin filaments of actin extend from each side of the Z line, a dense fibrous structure at the centre of each I band. The area from one dark Z line to the next Z line defines one sarcomere. The centre of the sarcomere is the H zone, a less dense region with a central thin, dark M line.[12]

A single tropomyosin molecule (a relaxing protein) lies alongside seven actin molecules. Troponin, another relaxing protein, associates with the tropomyosin molecule, forming the troponin–tropomyosin complex (see Figures 23-14, *A*, and 23-15). The troponin complex itself has three components. Troponin T aids in the binding of the troponin complex to actin and tropomyosin; troponin I inhibits the ATPase of actomyosin; and troponin C contains binding sites for the calcium ions involved in contraction. Troponin T and I molecules are released into

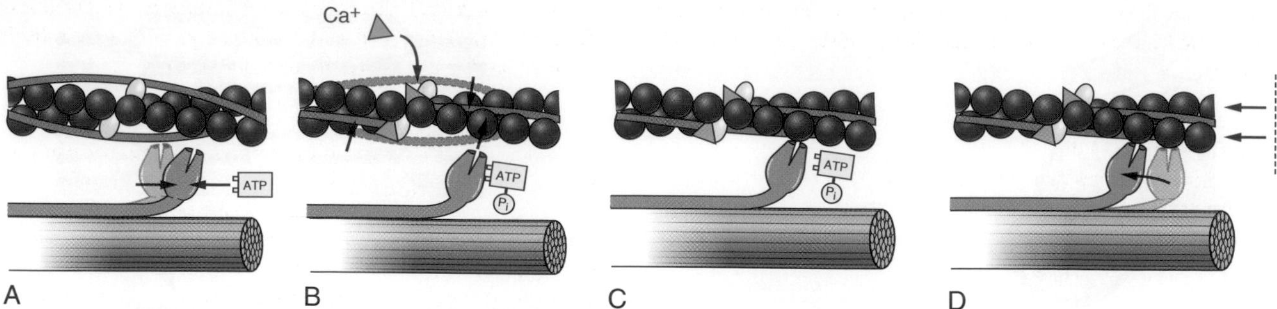

FIGURE 23-15 Cross-Bridge Theory of Muscle Contraction. A, Each myosin cross-bridge in the thick filament moves into a resting position after an adenosine triphosphate (*ATP*) molecule binds and transfers its energy. **B,** Calcium ions (*Ca*⁺) released from the sarcoplasmic reticulum bind to troponin in the thin filament, allowing tropomyosin to shift from its position blocking the active sites of actin molecules. **C,** Each myosin cross-bridge then binds to an active site on a thin filament, displacing the remnants of ATP hydrolysis—adenosine diphosphate and inorganic phosphate (*Pi*). **D,** The release of stored energy from step A provides the force needed for each cross-bridge to move back to its original position, pulling actin along with it. Each cross-bridge will remain bound to actin until another ATP molecule binds to it and pulls it back into its resting position **(A)**. (Adapted from Thibodeau, G.A., & Patton, K.T. [1999]. *Anatomy & physiology* [4th ed.]. St. Louis: Mosby.)

the bloodstream during myocardial injury and are measured to evaluate if a myocardial infarction or other damage has occurred. When troponin and tropomyosin cover the myosin binding sites on actin, the cross-bridges release calcium and the myocardium relaxes. The sarcomere also contains a giant elastic protein, titin, which attaches myosin to the Z line, acts as a spring, and influences myocardial stiffness.[12] Titin structure impacts myocardial diastolic filling and has been found to play a role in heart failure.[13]

Myocardial metabolism. Cardiomyocytes depend on the constant production of ATP, which is synthesized within the mitochondria mainly from glucose, fatty acids, and lactate. If the myocardium is underperfused because of coronary artery disease, anaerobic metabolism must be used for energy (see Chapter 1). Energy produced by metabolic processes fuels muscle contraction and relaxation, electrical excitation, membrane transport, and synthesis of large molecules. Normally, the amount of ATP produced supplies sufficient energy to pump blood throughout the system.

Cardiac work is expressed as myocardial oxygen consumption ($M\dot{V}O_2$), which is closely correlated with total cardiac energy requirements. $M\dot{V}O_2$ is determined by three major factors: (1) amount of wall stress during systole, estimated by measuring the systolic blood pressure; (2) duration of systolic wall tension, measured indirectly by the heart rate; and (3) contractile state of the myocardium, which is not measured clinically.

The coronary arteries deliver oxygen to the myocardium. Approximately 70 to 75% of this oxygen is used immediately by cardiac muscle, leaving little oxygen in reserve. Since the oxygen content of the blood and the amount of oxygen extracted from the blood cannot be increased under normal circumstances, any increased energy needs can be met only by increasing coronary blood flow. $M\dot{V}O_2$ increases with exercise and decreases with hypotension and hypothermia. As myocardial metabolism and consumption of oxygen increase, the local concentration of local vasoactive metabolic factors increases. Some of these factors—such as adenosine, nitric oxide, and prostaglandins—dilate coronary arterioles, thus increasing coronary blood flow.[14]

Myocardial Contraction and Relaxation

Myocardial contractility is a change in developed tension at a given resting fibre length, which basically is the ability of the heart muscle to shorten. At the molecular level, thin filaments of actin slide over thick filaments of myosin, called the cross-bridge theory of muscle contraction. Anatomically, contraction occurs when the sarcomere shortens, so adjacent Z lines move closer together (see Figure 23-13). The degree of shortening depends on the amount of overlap between the thick and thin filaments.

Calcium and excitation–contraction coupling. Excitation–contraction coupling is the process by which an action potential arriving at the muscle fibre plasma membrane triggers the cycle, leading to cross-bridge formation and contraction. Cycle activation depends on calcium availability, and the amount of force developed is regulated by how much the concentration of calcium ions increases within the cardiomyocytes. Calcium enters the myocardial cell from the interstitial fluid after electrical excitation that increases membrane calcium permeability. Two types of calcium channels (L-type, T-type) are found in cardiac tissues.[12] The L-type, or long-lasting, channels predominate and are the channels blocked by calcium channel–blocking medications (verapamil [Isoptin], nifedipine [Adalat], diltiazem [Cardizem]).[12] The T-type, or transient, channels are much less abundant in the heart. T-type channels are not blocked by currently available calcium channel–blocking medications; therefore T-type channel blockers are being investigated.[15] Calcium entering the cell triggers the release of additional calcium from the two storage sites within the sarcomere—the sarcoplasmic reticulum and tubule system. Calcium ions then diffuse toward the myofibrils, where they bind with troponin.

The calcium–troponin complex interaction facilitates the contraction process. In the resting state, troponin I is bound to actin and the tropomyosin molecule covers the sites where the myosin heads bind to actin, thereby preventing interaction between actin and myosin. Calcium binds to troponin C, which ultimately results in tropomyosin moving troponin I, thus uncovering the binding sites on the myosin heads. Myosin and actin can now form cross-bridges, and ATP can be dephosphorylated to adenosine diphosphate (ADP). Under these circumstances, sliding of the thick and thin filaments can occur, and the muscle contracts.[12]

Myocardial relaxation. Relaxation is as vital to optimal cardiac function as contraction; and calcium, troponin, and tropomyosin also facilitate relaxation. After contraction, free calcium ions are actively pumped out of the cell back into the interstitial fluid or taken back into storage by the sarcoplasmic reticulum and tubule system. As the concentration of calcium within the sarcomere decreases, troponin releases its bound calcium. The tropomyosin complex moves and blocks the active sites on the actin molecule, preventing cross-bridge formation with the myosin heads. If the ability of the myocardium to relax is impaired, it can lead to increased diastolic filling pressures and eventually heart failure.[16]

QUICK CHECK 23-4

1. What features distinguish myocardial cells from skeletal cells?
2. Describe the interactions of actin, myosin, and the troponin–tropomyosin complex in controlling heart function.
3. Define *excitation–contraction coupling.*

Factors Affecting Cardiac Output

Cardiac performance can be evaluated by measuring the cardiac output. **Cardiac output** is calculated by multiplying heart rate in beats per minute (beats/min) by **stroke volume** in litres per beat. Normal adult cardiac output is about 5 L/min at rest given a heart rate of about 70 beats/min and a normal stroke volume of about 70 mL.[7]

With each heartbeat, the ventricles eject much of their blood volume, and the amount ejected per beat is called the **ejection fraction**. The ejection fraction is estimated by echocardiography, computed tomography (CT) scan, nuclear medicine scan, or cardiac catheterization and is calculated by dividing stroke volume by end-diastolic volume. The end-diastolic volume of the normal ventricle is about 70 to 80 mL/m^2, and the normal ejection fraction of the resting heart measured with gated myocardial perfusion imaging is 66% ± 8% for women and 58% ± 8% for men.[17]

The ejection fraction is increased by factors that increase contractility, such as increased sympathetic nervous system activity. A decrease in ejection fraction may indicate ventricular failure. The effects of aging on cardiovascular function are summarized in Table 23-3.

TABLE 23-3 Cardiovascular Function in Older Adults

Determinant	Resting Cardiac Performance	Exercise Cardiac Performance[a]
Cardiac output	Unchanged	Decreases because of a decrease in maximum heart rate
Heart rate	Slight decrease	Increases less than in younger people
Stroke volume	Slight increase	No change
Ejection fraction	Unchanged	Decreased
Afterload	Increased	Increased
End-diastolic volume	Unchanged	Increased
End-systolic volume	Unchanged	Increased
Contraction	Decreased velocity	Decreased
Myocardial wall stiffness	Increased	Increased
Maximum oxygen consumption	Not applicable	Decreased
Plasma catecholamines	—	Increased

[a]Changes in healthy men and women up to age 80 years as compared with those who are 20 years of age.

Data from Lakatta, E.G., Najjar, S.S., Schulman, S.P., et al. (2011). Aging and cardiovascular disease in the elderly. In V. Fuster, R.A. Walsh, R.A. Harrington, et al. (Eds.), *Hurst's the heart* (13th ed., pp. 2196–2225). Philadelphia: McGraw-Hill.

The factors that determine cardiac output are (1) preload, (2) afterload, (3) myocardial contractility, and (4) heart rate. Preload, afterload, and contractility all affect stroke volume.

Preload

Preload is the volume and pressure inside the ventricle at the end of diastole (**ventricular end-diastolic volume [VEDV]** and **ventricular end-diastolic pressure [VEDP]**). Preload is determined by two primary factors: (1) the amount of venous blood returning to the ventricle during diastole and (2) the amount of blood left in the ventricle after systole (end-systolic volume). Venous return is dependent on blood volume and flow through the venous system and the AV valves. End-systolic volume is dependent on the strength of ventricular contraction and the resistance to ventricular emptying. Clinically, preload is estimated by measuring the central venous pressure (CVP) for the right side of the heart and the pulmonary artery wedge pressure for the left side. Normal values for these two estimates are 1 to 5 mm Hg and 4 to 12 mm Hg, respectively.[18]

Laplace's law states that wall tension generated in the wall of the ventricle (or any chamber or vessel) to produce a given intraventricular pressure depends directly on ventricular size or internal radius and inversely on ventricular wall thickness. VEDV, which determines the size of the ventricle and the stretch of the cardiac muscle fibres, therefore affects the tension (or force) for contraction. **Starling's law of the heart** indicates that the volume of blood in the heart at the end of diastole determines the length of its muscle fibres and is directly related to the force of contraction during the next systole. Muscle fibres have an optimal resting length from which to generate the maximum amount of contractile strength. Within a physiological range of muscle stretching, increased preload increases stroke volume (and therefore cardiac output and stroke work) (Figure 23-16, curve *B*). Excessive ventricular filling and preload (increased VEDV) stretches the heart muscle beyond optimal length and stroke volume begins to fall. Factors that increase contractility cause the heart to operate on a higher length-tension curve (see Figure 23-16, curve *A*). Factors that decrease contractility (see Figure 23-16, curve *C*) cause the heart to operate at a lower length-tension curve. Figure 23-17 illustrates the relationship between VEDV and stroke volume, cardiac output, and stroke work.

Increases in preload (VEDV) may not only cause a decline in stroke volume but also result in increases in VEDP. These changes can lead to heart failure (see Chapter 24). Increased VEDP causes pressures to increase or "back up" into the pulmonary or systemic venous circulation,

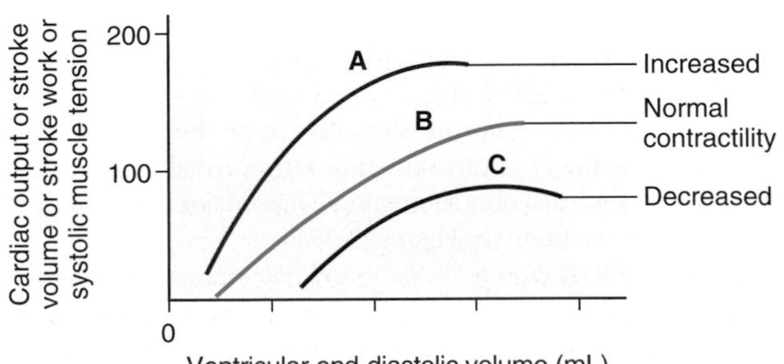

FIGURE 23-16 Starling's Law of the Heart. The relationship between length and tension in the heart. End-diastolic volume determines end-diastolic length of ventricular muscle fibres and is proportional to tension generated during systole, as well as to cardiac output, stroke volume, and stroke work. A change in myocardial contractility causes the heart to perform on a different length-tension curve. *A,* Increased contractility; *B,* normal contractility; *C,* heart failure or decreased contractility. (See text for further explanation.)

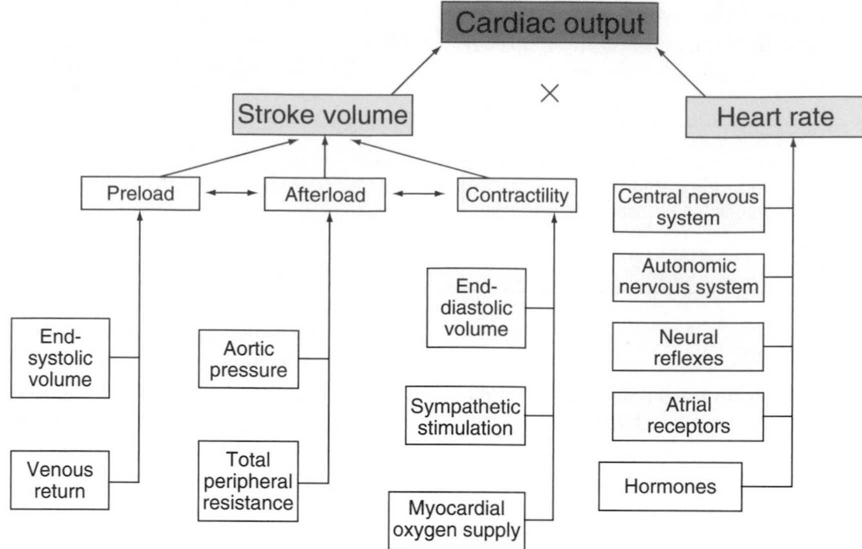

FIGURE 23-17 Factors Affecting Cardiac Performance. Cardiac output, the amount of blood (in litres) ejected by the heart per minute, depends on heart rate (beats per minute) and stroke volume (millilitres of blood ejected during ventricular systole).

thus increasing the movement of plasma out through vessel walls, causing fluid to accumulate in lung tissues (pulmonary edema; see Chapter 27) or in peripheral tissues (peripheral edema).

Afterload

Left ventricular **afterload** is the resistance to ejection of blood from the left ventricle. It is the load the muscle must move during contraction (see Figure 23-17). Aortic systolic pressure is an index of afterload. Pressure in the ventricle must exceed aortic pressure before blood can be pumped out during systole. Low aortic pressures (decreased afterload) enable the heart to contract more rapidly and efficiently, whereas high aortic pressures (increased afterload) slow contraction and cause higher workloads against which the heart must function to eject blood. Increased aortic pressure is usually the result of increased **systemic vascular resistance (SVR)**, sometimes referred to as **total peripheral resistance (TPR)**. In individuals with hypertension, increased TPR means that afterload is chronically elevated, resulting in increased ventricular workload and hypertrophy of the myocardium. In some individuals, changes in afterload are the result of aortic valvular disease. SVR is calculated by dividing mean arterial pressure by cardiac output; the normal range is 700 dyne/sec/cm^{-5}.[7,18]

Myocardial Contractility

Stroke volume, or the volume of blood ejected per beat during systole, also depends on the *force* of contraction, myocardial contractility, or the degree of myocardial fibre shortening. Three major factors determine the force of contraction (see Figure 23-17):

1. *Changes in the stretching of the ventricular myocardium caused by changes in VEDV (preload).* As discussed previously, increased venous return to the heart distends the ventricle, thus increasing preload, which increases the stroke volume and, subsequently, cardiac output, up to a certain point. However, an excessive increase in preload leads to decreased stroke volume.
2. *Alterations in the inotropic stimuli of the ventricles.* Hormones, neurotransmitters, or medications that affect contractility are called **inotropic agents**. The most important endogenous positive inotropic agents are **epinephrine** and norepinephrine released from the sympathetic nervous system. Other positive inotropes include thyroid hormone and dopamine. The most important negative inotropic agent is acetylcholine released from the vagus nerve. Many medications have positive or negative inotropic properties that can have profound effects on cardiac function. In sepsis, a variety of cytokines, including tumour necrosis factor-alpha (TNF-α) and interleukin-1β, have been shown to impair myocardial contractility.[19]
3. *Adequacy of myocardial oxygen supply.* Oxygen and carbon dioxide levels (tensions) in the coronary blood also influence contractility. With severe hypoxemia (arterial oxygen saturation of less than 50%), contractility is decreased. With less severe hypoxemia (arterial oxygen saturation of more than 50%), contractility is stimulated. Moderate degrees of hypoxemia may increase contractility by enhancing the myocardial response to circulating catecholamines.[20]

Preload, afterload, and contractility all interact with one another to determine stroke volume and cardiac output. Changes in any one of these factors can result in deleterious effects on the others, resulting in heart failure (see Chapter 24).

Heart Rate

As described previously, SA node activity is the primary determinant of the heart rate. The average heart rate in healthy adults is about 70 beats/min. This rate diminishes by 10 to 20 beats/min during sleep and can accelerate to more than 100 beats/min during muscular activity or emotional excitement. In well-conditioned athletes, resting heart rate is normally about 50 to 60 beats/min. In highly trained or elite athletes, the resting heart rate can be below 50 beats/min; these athletes also have a greater stroke volume and lower peripheral resistance in active muscles than they had before training. The control of heart rate includes activity of the central nervous system, autonomic nervous system, neural reflexes, atrial receptors, and hormones (see Figure 23-17).

Cardiovascular control centres in the brain. The **cardiovascular vasomotor control centre** is in the medulla and pons areas of the brainstem, with additional areas in the hypothalamus, cerebral cortex, and thalamus.[21] The hypothalamic centres regulate cardiovascular responses to changes in temperature, the cerebral cortex centres adjust cardiac reaction to a variety of emotional states, and the brainstem control centre regulates heart rate and blood pressure (see Figure 23-11).

The nerve fibres from the cardiovascular control centre synapse with autonomic neurons that influence the rate of firing of the SA node. As previously discussed, increased heart rate occurs with sympathetic (adrenergic) stimulation. When the parasympathetic nerves to the heart are stimulated (primarily via the vagus nerve), heart rate slows and the sympathetic nerves to the heart, arterioles, and veins are inhibited.[8] At rest, the heart rate in healthy individuals is primarily under the control of parasympathetic stimulation. Administration of medications that block parasympathetic function (anticholinergic) or physical interruption of the vagus nerve causes significant tachycardia (abnormally fast heart rate) because this inhibitory parasympathetic influence is lost.

Neural reflexes. Output from the baroreceptor reflexes influences short-term regulation of the vascular smooth muscle of resistance arteries, myocardial contractility, and heart rate, all components of blood pressure control. The baroreceptors or pressoreceptors are located in the aortic arch and carotid arteries. If blood pressure decreases, the baroreceptor reflex accelerates heart rate, increases myocardial contractility, and increases vascular smooth muscle contraction in the arterioles, thus raising blood pressure. This reflex is critical to maintaining adequate tissue perfusion. When blood pressure increases, the baroreceptors increase their rate of discharge, sending neural impulses over a branch of the glossopharyngeal nerve (ninth cranial nerve) and through the vagus nerve to the cardiovascular control centres in the medulla. These reflexes increase parasympathetic activity and decrease sympathetic activity, causing the resistance arteries to dilate, decreasing myocardial contractility and heart rate. The role of baroreceptors in influencing blood pressure is discussed in more detail in "Baroreceptors" later in this chapter.

Atrial receptors. Mechanoreceptors that influence heart rate exist in both atria.[21] They are located where the veins, venae cavae, and pulmonary veins enter their respective atria. Bainbridge reflex is the name for the changes in the heart rate that may occur after intravenous infusions of blood or other fluid. The change in heart rate is thought to be caused by a reflex mediated by these atrial volume receptors that are innervated by the vagus nerve (volume receptors are thought to respond to increased plasma volume). Although this reflex can be elicited in humans, its relevance is uncertain at this time.[22]

Stimulation of these atrial receptors also increases urine volume, presumably because of a neurally mediated reduction in antidiuretic hormone. In addition, peptides of the atrial natriuretic family are released from atrial tissue in response to the increases in blood volume. These peptides have diuretic and natriuretic (salt excretion) properties, resulting in decreased blood volume and pressure. The atrial natriuretic peptides also have been shown to relax vascular smooth muscle and oppose myocardial hypertrophy, leading to measurement of blood levels to evaluate clinical status and raising interest in their use as therapeutic agents.[23]

Hormones and biochemicals. Hormones and other biochemically active substances affect the arteries, arterioles, venules, capillaries, and contractility of the myocardium. Norepinephrine, mainly released as a neurotransmitter from the adrenal medulla, dilates vessels of the liver and skeletal muscle and also causes an increase in myocardial contractility. Some adrenocortical hormones, such as hydrocortisone, potentiate the effects of the catecholamines—norepinephrine and epinephrine.

Thyroid hormones enhance sympathetic activity and increase cardiac output. Growth hormone, working together with insulinlike growth factor 1 (IGF-1), also has been shown to increase myocardial contractility.[24] Decreases in levels of growth hormone or thyroid hormone may result in bradycardia (heart rate below 60 beats/min), reduced cardiac output, and low blood pressure. (Other hormones are discussed in "Regulation of Blood Pressure," later in this chapter.)

✔ QUICK CHECK 23-5

1. Explain four ways that aging impacts the cardiovascular system.
2. Why is Starling's law of the heart important to the understanding of heart failure?
3. Discuss the baroreceptor reflex and explain its influence on blood pressure and heart rate.

THE SYSTEMIC CIRCULATION

The arteries and veins of the systemic circulation are illustrated in Figure 23-18. Oxygenated blood leaves the left side of the heart through the aorta and flows into the systemic arteries. These arteries branch into small arterioles, which branch into the smallest vessels, the capillaries, where nutrient and waste product exchange between the blood and tissues occurs. Blood from the capillaries then enters tiny venules that join to form the larger veins, which return venous blood to the right heart. Peripheral vascular system is the term used to describe the part of the systemic circulation that supplies the skin and the extremities, particularly the legs and feet.

Structure of Blood Vessels

Blood vessel walls are composed of three layers: (1) the tunica intima (innermost, or intimal, layer); (2) the tunica media (middle, or medial, layer); and (3) the tunica externa or adventitia (outermost, or external, layer), which also contains nerves and lymphatic vessels. These layers are illustrated in Figure 23-19. Blood vessel walls vary in thickness depending on the thickness or absence of one or more of these three layers. Cells of the larger vessel walls are nourished by the vasa vasorum, small vessels located in the tunica externa.

Arterial Vessels

An *artery* is a thick-walled pulsating blood vessel transporting blood away from the heart. In the systemic circulation, arteries carry oxygenated blood. Arterial walls are composed of elastic connective tissue, fibrous connective tissue, and smooth muscle. Elastic arteries, such as the aorta, the branches of the aorta, and the trunk of the pulmonary artery, have a thick tunica media with more elastic fibres than smooth muscle fibres. Elasticity allows the vessel to absorb energy and stretch as blood is ejected from the heart during systole. During diastole, elasticity promotes recoil of the arteries, maintaining blood pressure within the vessels.

Muscular arteries, medium- and small-sized arteries, are farther from the heart than the elastic arteries. They contain more muscle fibres and fewer elastic fibres than the elastic arteries and they function to distribute blood to arterioles throughout the body. Because their smooth muscle can contract or relax, they play a role in blood flow control and in directing flow to body parts with the highest need at any point in time. Contraction narrows the vessel lumen (the internal cavity of the vessel), which diminishes flow through the vessel (vasoconstriction). When the smooth muscle layer relaxes, more blood flows through the vessel lumen (vasodilation).

An artery becomes an arteriole where the diameter of its lumen narrows to less than 0.5 mm. Arterioles are mainly composed of smooth muscle and regulate the flow of blood into the capillaries by constricting or dilating to either slow or increase the flow of blood into the capillaries (Figure 23-20). The thick smooth muscle layer of the arterioles is a major determinant of the resistance blood encounters as it flows through the systemic circulation.

The capillary network is composed of connective channels called metarterioles, and "true" capillaries (see Figure 23-20). Metarterioles have discontinuous smooth muscle cells in their tunica media, whereas capillaries have no smooth muscle cells. There is a ring of smooth muscle called the precapillary sphincter at the point where capillaries branch from metarterioles. As the sphincters contract and relax, they regulate blood flow through the capillary beds. The precapillary sphincters help to maintain arterial pressure and regulate selective flow to vascular beds.

Capillaries are composed solely of a layer of endothelial cells surrounded by a basement membrane. Their thin walls and unique structure make possible the rapid exchange of water; small (low molecular weight) soluble molecules; some larger molecules, such as albumin; and cells of the innate and adaptive components of the immune system between the blood and the interstitial fluid. In some capillaries, the endothelial cells contain oval windows or pores termed fenestrations covered by a thin diaphragm.

Substances pass between the capillary lumen and the interstitial fluid (1) through junctions between endothelial cells, (2) through fenestrations in endothelial cells, (3) in vesicles moved by active transport across the endothelial cell membrane, or (4) by diffusion through the endothelial cell membrane. A single capillary may be only 0.5 to 1 mm in length and 0.01 mm in diameter, but the capillaries are so numerous their total surface area may be more than 600 m^2 (about 100 football fields).

Endothelium

The vascular endothelium is important to several body functions and is sometimes considered a separate endocrine organ. All tissues depend on a blood supply, and the blood supply depends on endothelial cells, which form the lining (or endothelium) of the blood vessel

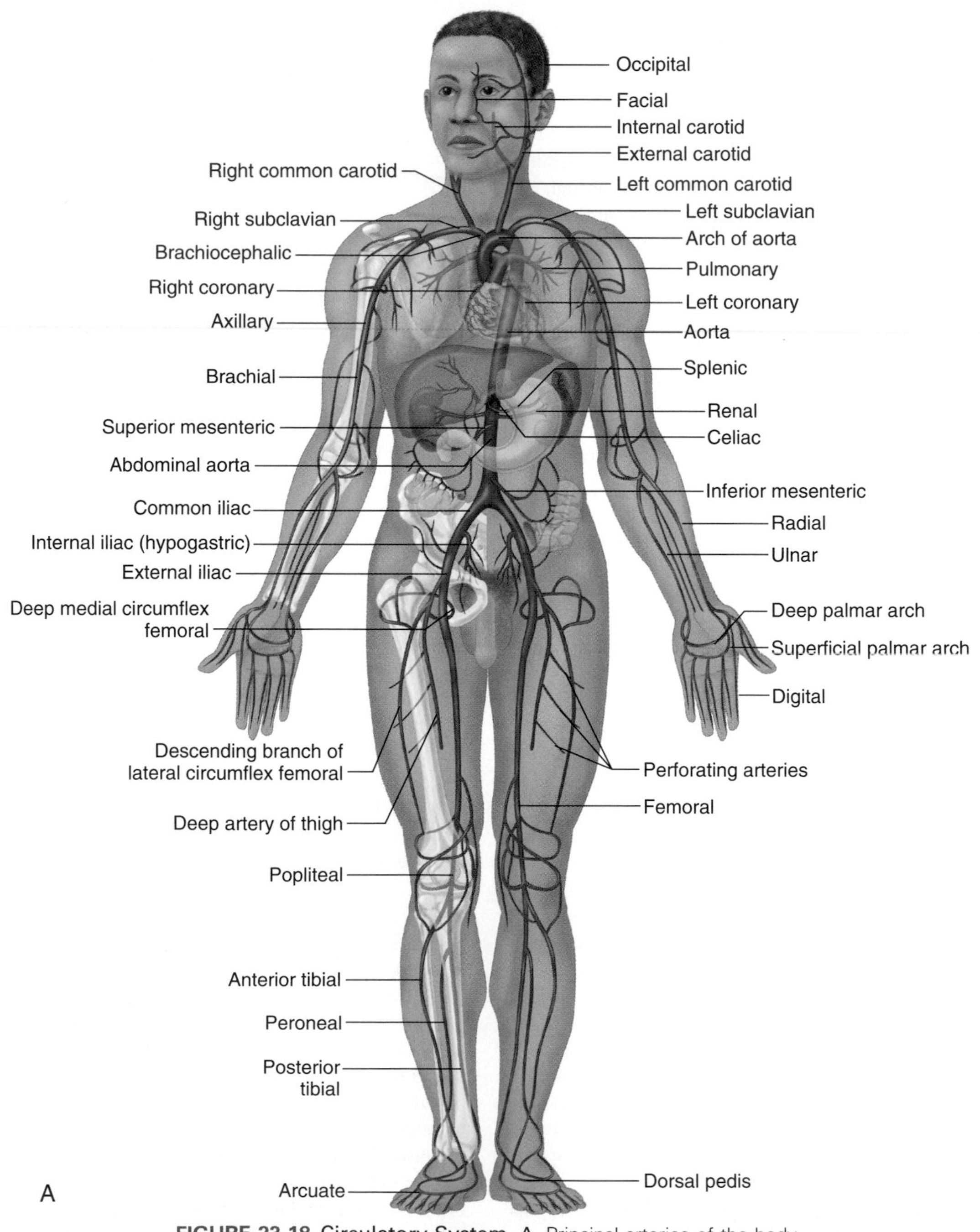

FIGURE 23-18 Circulatory System. **A,** Principal arteries of the body.

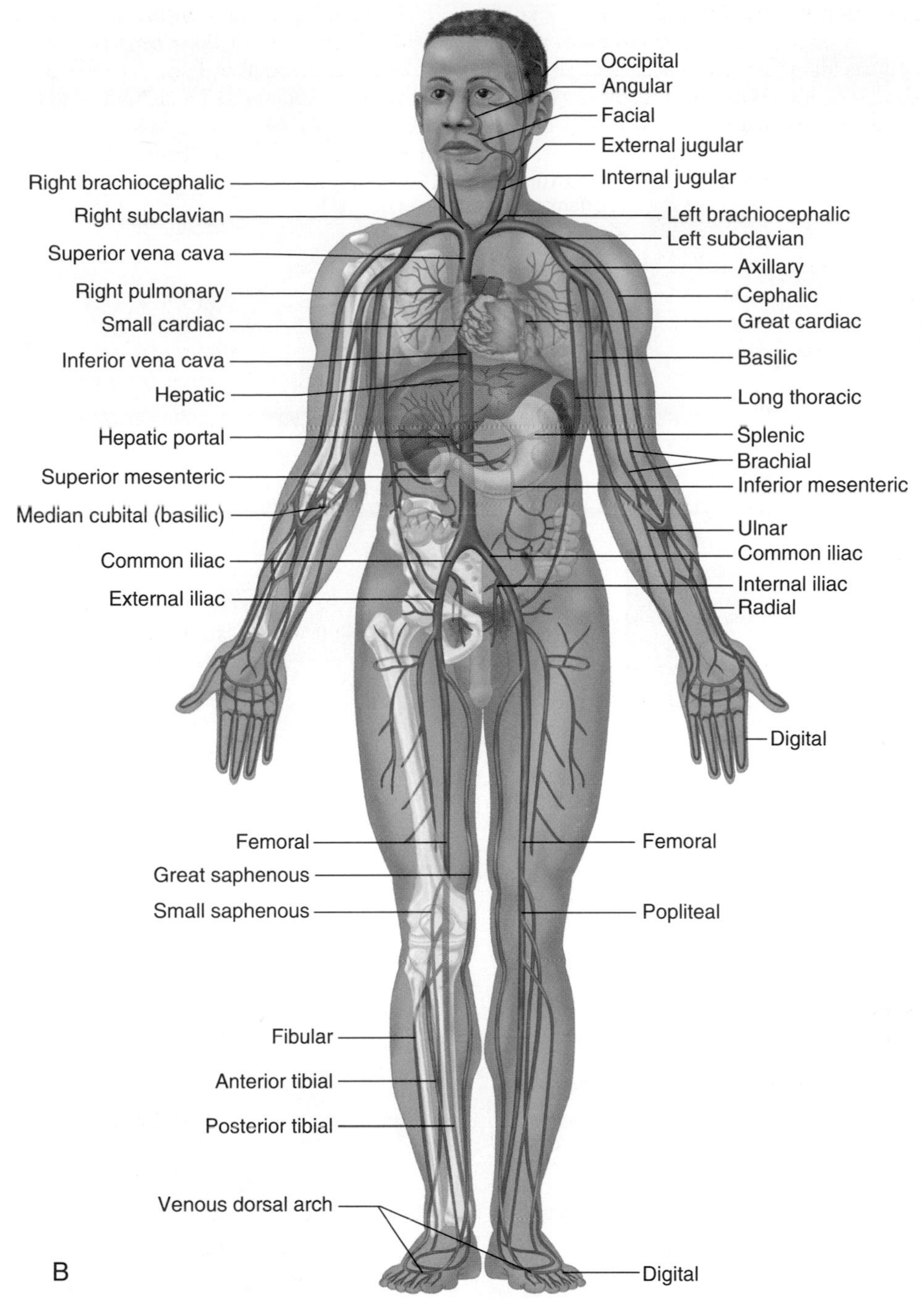

FIGURE 23-18, cont'd B, Principal veins of the body. (From Patton, K.T., Thibodeau, G.A., & Douglas, M.M. [2012]. *Essentials of anatomy & physiology*. St. Louis: Elsevier.)

(Figure 23-21). In addition to substance transport, the vascular endothelium has important roles in coagulation, antithrombogenesis, and fibrinolysis; immune system function; tissue and vessel growth and wound healing; and vasomotion, the contraction and relaxation of vessels.[25] Table 23-4 summarizes some of the more important endothelial functions. Endothelial injury and dysfunction are central processes in many of the most common and serious cardiovascular disorders, including hypertension and atherosclerosis (see Chapter 24).

Veins

Compared with arteries, **veins** are thin walled with more fibrous connective tissue and have a larger diameter (see Figure 23-19). Veins also are more numerous than arteries. The smallest venules downstream from the capillaries have an endothelial lining and are surrounded by connective tissue. The largest venules have some smooth muscle fibres in their thin tunica media. The venous tunica externa has less elastic tissue than that in arteries, so veins do not recoil as much or as rapidly after distension. Like arteries, veins receive nourishment from tiny vasa vasorum.

Veins contain valves to facilitate the one-way flow of blood toward the heart (Figure 23-22). These valves are folds of the tunica intima and resemble the semilunar valves of the heart. When a person stands up, contraction of the skeletal muscles of the legs compresses the deep veins of the legs and assists the flow of blood toward the heart. This

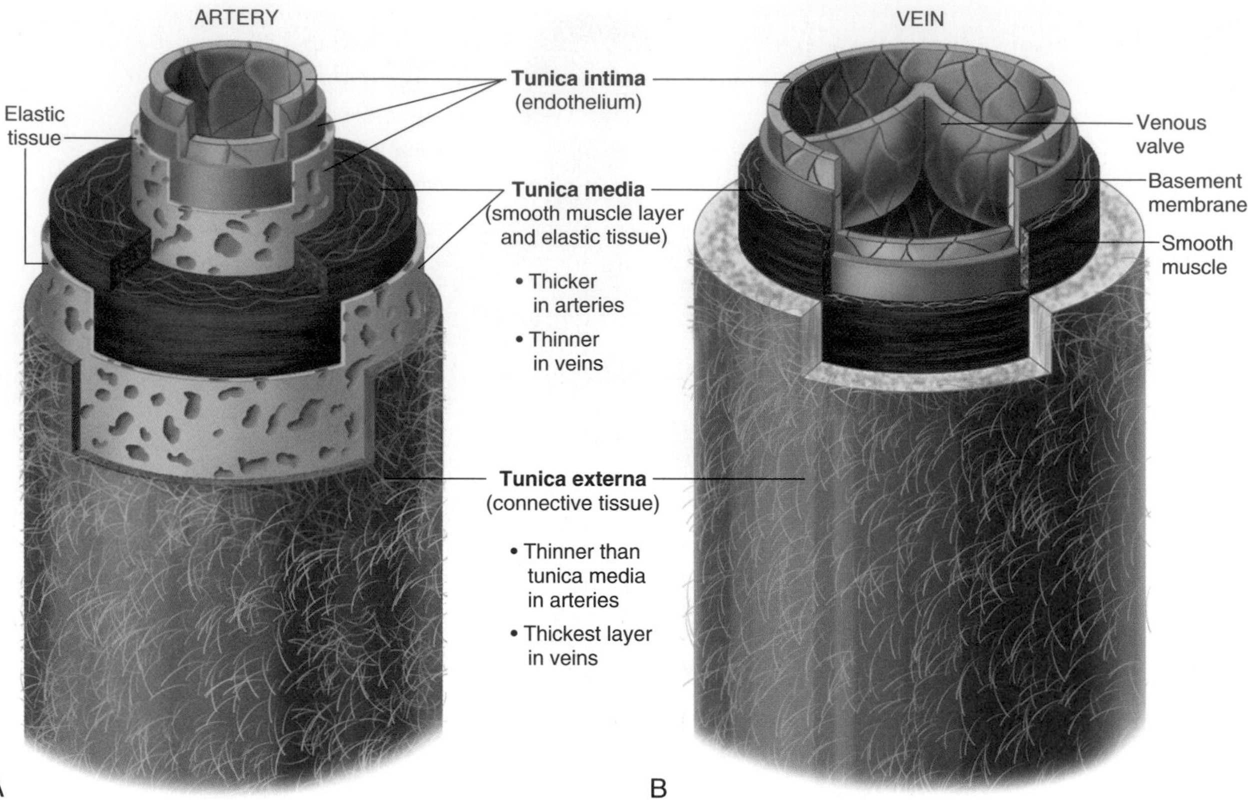

FIGURE 23-19 Structure of the Blood Vessels. The tunica externa of the veins is colour-coded blue and the arteries red. (From Patton, K.T., & Thibodeau, G.A. [2016]. *Structure & function of the body* [15th ed.]. St. Louis: Elsevier.)

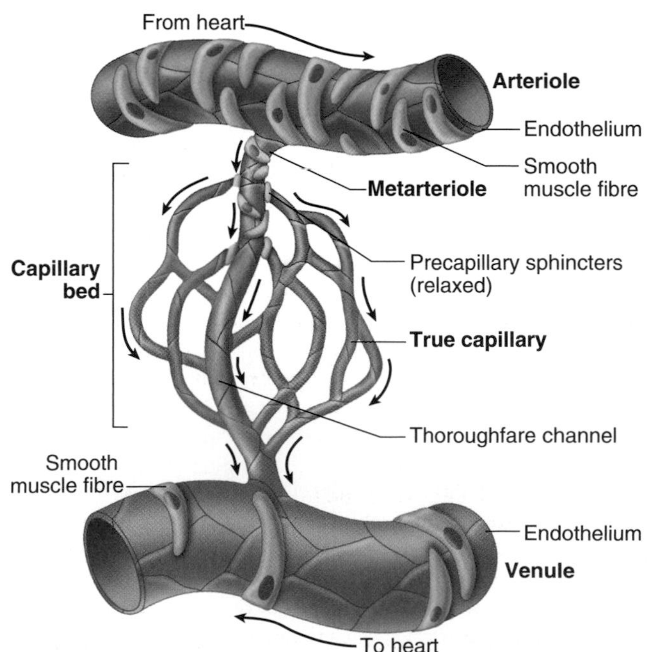

FIGURE 23-20 Microcirculation. Control of local blood flow through a capillary network is regulated by altering the tone of precapillary sphincters surrounding arterioles and metarterioles. In the diagram, the sphincters are relaxed, permitting blood flow to enter the capillary bed. (From Patton, K.T., Thibodeau, G.A., & Douglas, M.M. [2012]. *Essentials of anatomy & physiology*. St. Louis: Elsevier.)

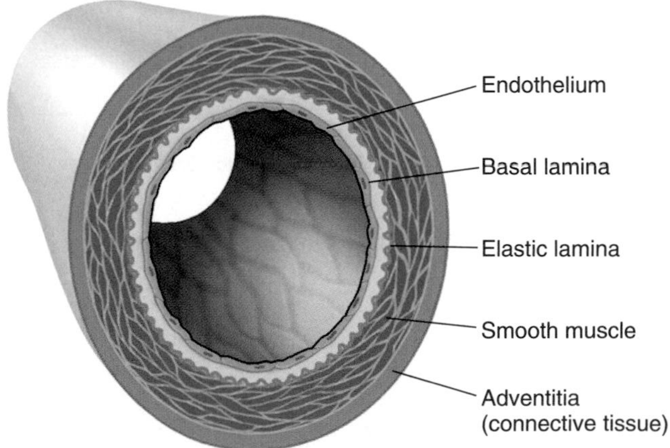

FIGURE 23-21 Vascular Endothelium. The endothelial cells arrange themselves as a single-layer lining that has numerous critical functions (see Table 23-4).

TABLE 23-4 **Functions of the Endothelium**

Function	Actions Involved
Filtration and permeability	Facilitates transport of large molecules via vesicular transport movement through intercellular junctions
	Facilitates transport of small molecules via movement of vesicles, through opening of tight junctions, and across cytoplasm
Vasomotion	Stimulates vascular relaxation through production of nitric oxide, prostacyclin, and other vasodilators
	Stimulates vascular constriction through production of endothelin-1 and of angiotensin II by the action of endothelial angiotensin-converting enzyme on angiotensin I
Hemostatic balance	Maintains a balance between procoagulant and anticoagulant factors, as well as profibrinolytic and antifibrinolytic factors; endothelial surface is normally antithrombotic
	Counteracts coagulation through anticoagulant factors, including prostacyclin, nitric oxide, antithrombin, thrombomodulin, tissue factor pathway inhibitor, and heparins
	Activates coagulation through procoagulant factors, including tissue factor (factor VII), factor VIII, factor V, and plasminogen activator inhibitor-1 (PAI-1)
	Controls coagulation through profibrinolytic factors: tissue- and urokinase-type plasminogen activating factor and plasminogen activator inhibitor-1 (PAI-1)
	Breaks down blood clots through antifibrinolytic factor: tissue plasminogen activator
Inflammation/immunity	Expresses chemotactic agents and adhesion molecules that support white blood cells (including monocytes, neutrophils, and lymphocytes) moving into tissues
	Expresses receptors for oxidized lipoproteins, allowing them to enter vascular intima
Angiogenesis/vessel growth	Releases growth factors such as endothelin-1 and heparins for vascular smooth muscle cells
Lipid metabolism	Expresses receptors for lipoprotein lipase and low-density lipoproteins

From Griendling, K.K., Harrison, D.G., & Alexander, R.W. (2011). Biology of the vessel wall. In V. Fuster, R.A. Walsh, R.A. Harrington, et al. (Eds.), *Hurst's the heart* (13th ed., pp. 153–171). Philadelphia: McGraw-Hill; Rajendran, P., Rengarajan, T., Thangavel, J., et al. (2013). *Int J Biol Sci, 9*(10), 1057–1069.

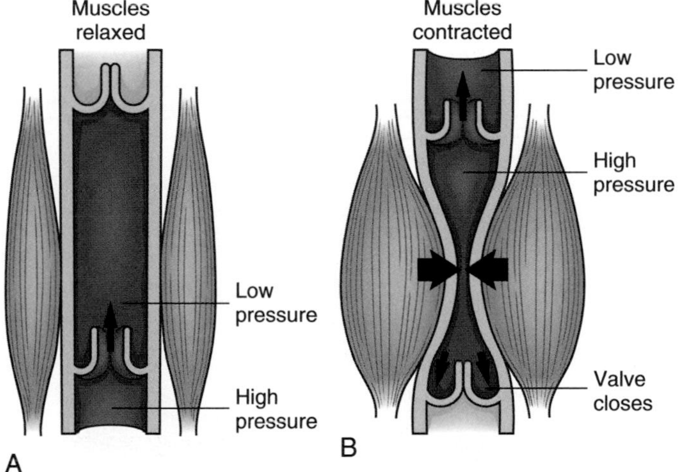

FIGURE 23-22 Venous Valves and the Muscle Pump. In veins, one-way valves aid circulation by preventing backflow of venous blood when pressure in a local area is low. **A,** Blood is moved toward the heart as valves in the veins are forced open by pressure from volume of blood downstream and the neighbouring muscles are relaxed. **B,** When pressure below the valve drops, blood begins to flow backward but fills the "pockets" formed by the valve flaps, pushing the flaps together and thus blocking further backward flow. Contraction in the adjacent muscles and the valves of the systemic veins assist in the return of unoxygenated blood to the right heart.

important mechanism of venous return is called the muscle pump (Figure 23-22, *B*).

Factors Affecting Blood Flow

Blood flow, the amount of fluid moved per unit of time, is usually expressed as litres or millilitres per minute (L/min or mL/min). Factors that influence blood flow include pressure, resistance, velocity, turbulent versus laminar flow, and compliance, with the most important of these being pressure and resistance.

Pressure and Resistance

Pressure in a liquid system is the force exerted on the liquid per unit area and is expressed clinically as millimetres of mercury (mm Hg), or torr (1 torr = 1 mm Hg). Blood flow to an organ depends partly on the pressure difference between the arterial and venous vessels supplying that organ. Fluid moves from the arterial "side" of the capillaries where the pressure is higher to the venous side where the pressure is lower.

Resistance is the opposition to blood flow. Most opposition to blood flow results from the diameter and length of the vessels. Changes in blood flow through an organ result from changes in the vascular resistance within the organ because of increases or decreases in vessel diameter and the opening or closing of vascular channels. Resistance in a vessel is inversely related to blood flow—that is, increased resistance leads to decreased blood flow. Poiseuille's law indicates that resistance is directly related to tube length and blood viscosity and inversely related to the radius of the tube to the fourth power (r^4). Because blood flow is inversely related to resistance, the greater the resistance the lower the blood flow will be. Resistance to flow cannot be measured directly, but it can be calculated if the pressure difference and flow volumes are known. Resistance to blood flow in a single vessel is determined by the radius and length of the blood vessel and by the blood viscosity.

Clinically, the most important factor determining resistance *in a single vessel* is the radius or diameter of the vessel's lumen. Small changes in the lumen's radius or diameter lead to large changes in vascular resistance. Clinically, vasoconstriction will contribute to an increase in resistance whereas vasodilation will cause a decrease in resistance that may be reflected by a fall in blood pressure. Because vessel length is relatively constant, whereas lumen size is quite variable, length is not as important as lumen size in determining flow through a single vessel. Because viscosity is relatively constant, blood vessel radius is usually the key factor in determining TPR. An exception to this rule is when red blood cell volume, measured as hematocrit, is elevated, which is relatively rare. Conditions with elevated hematocrits include a lack of body water, cyanotic congenital heart disease (see Chapter 25), or polycythemia (see Chapter 21), and can lead to increased cardiac work as a result of increased vascular resistance.

Resistance to flow through a *system of vessels*, or **total resistance**, depends not only on characteristics of individual vessels but also on whether the vessels are arranged in series or in parallel and on the total cross-sectional area of the system. Vessels arranged in parallel provide less resistance than vessels arranged in series. Blood flowing through the distributing arteries, beginning with branches off the aorta and ending at arterioles in the capillary bed, encounters more resistance than blood flowing through the capillary bed itself, where flow is distributed among many short, tiny branches arranged in parallel (Figure 23-23). The total cross-sectional area of the arteriolar system is greater than that of the arterial system, yet the greater number of arterioles arranged in series leads to great resistance to flow in the arteriolar system. In contrast, the capillary system has a larger number of vessels arranged in parallel than the arteriolar system, and the total cross-sectional area is much greater; thus there is lower resistance overall through the capillary system. The resulting slow velocity of flow in each capillary is optimal for capillary–tissue exchange.

Velocity

Blood velocity or speed is the *distance* blood travels in a unit of time, usually centimetres per second. It is directly related to blood flow (*amount* of blood moved per unit of time) and inversely related to the cross-sectional area of the vessel in which the blood is flowing (see Figure 23-23). As blood moves from the aorta to the capillaries, the total cross-sectional area of the vessels increases and the velocity decreases.

Laminar Versus Turbulent Flow

Flow through a tubular system can be either laminar or turbulent. Blood flow through the vessels, except where vessels split or branch, is usually laminar. In **laminar flow**, concentric layers of molecules move "straight ahead," with each layer flowing at a slightly different velocity (Figure 23-24). The cohesive attraction between the fluid and the vessel wall prevents the molecules of blood that are in contact with the wall from moving at all. The next thin layer of blood is able to slide slowly past the stationary layer and so on until, at the centre, the blood velocity is greatest. Large vessels have room for a large centre layer; therefore, they have less resistance to flow and greater flow and velocity than smaller vessels.

Where flow is obstructed, the vessel turns, or blood flows over rough surfaces, the flow becomes **turbulent** with whorls or eddy currents that produce noise, causing a murmur to be heard on auscultation. Resistance increases with turbulence, which frequently occurs in areas with atherosclerotic plaque (see Chapter 24).

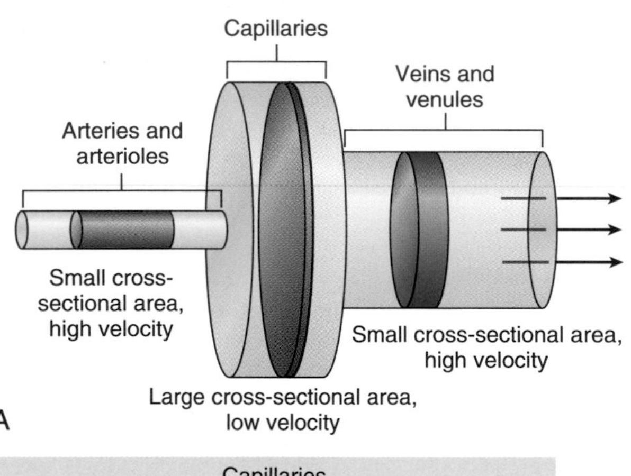

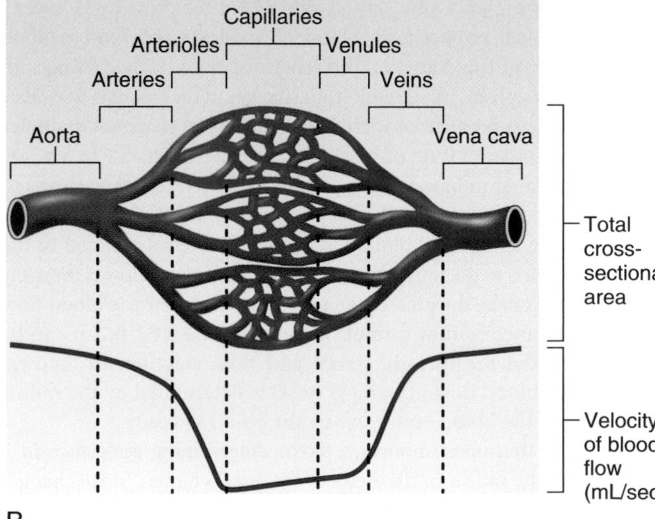

FIGURE 23-23 Relationship Between Cross-Sectional Area and Velocity of Blood Flow. Blood flows with great speed in the large arteries. However, branching of arterial vessels increases the total cross-sectional area of the arterioles and capillaries, reducing the flow rate. When capillaries merge into venules and venules merge into veins, the total cross-sectional area decreases, causing the flow rate to increase. (From Patton, K.T., & Thibodeau, G.A. [2016]. *Anatomy & physiology* [9th ed.]. St. Louis: Elsevier.)

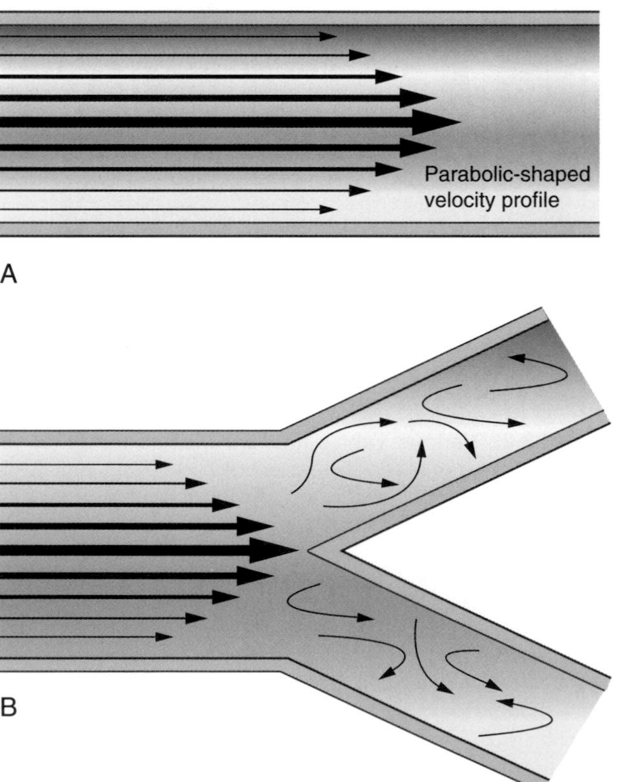

FIGURE 23-24 Laminar and Turbulent Blood Flow. A, Laminar flow. Fluid flows in long, smooth-walled tubes as if it were composed of a large number of concentric layers. **B,** Turbulent flow. Turbulent flow is caused by numerous small currents flowing cross-wise or oblique to the long axis of the vessel, resulting in flowing whorls and eddy currents.

Vascular Compliance

Vascular compliance is the increase in volume a vessel can accommodate for a given increase in pressure. Compliance depends on factors related to the nature of a vessel wall, such as the ratio of elastic fibres to muscle fibres in the wall. Elastic arteries are more compliant than muscular arteries. The veins are more compliant than either type of artery, and they can serve as storage areas for the circulatory system.

Compliance determines a vessel's response to pressure changes. For example, a large volume of blood can be accommodated by the venous system with only a small increase in pressure. In the less compliant arterial system, where smaller volumes and higher pressures are normal, even small changes in blood volume can cause significant changes in arterial pressure.

Stiffness is the opposite of compliance. Several conditions and disorders can cause stiffness, with the most common being aging and atherosclerosis (see Chapter 24).

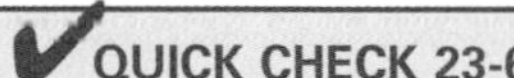
QUICK CHECK 23-6

1. What is the function of the arterioles?
2. Identify the functions of the endothelium.
3. Why does the total cross-sectional area in the capillary system lower the resistance to flow?

Regulation of Blood Pressure

Arterial Pressure

Arterial blood pressure is determined by the cardiac output multiplied by the peripheral resistance (Figure 23-25). The systolic blood pressure is the highest arterial blood pressure following ventricular contraction or systole. The diastolic blood pressure is the lowest arterial blood pressure that occurs during ventricular filling or diastole. The mean arterial pressure (MAP), which is the average pressure in the arteries throughout the cardiac cycle, depends on the elastic properties of the arterial walls and the mean volume of blood in the arterial system. MAP can be approximated from the measured values of the systolic (P_s) and diastolic (P_d) pressures as follows:

$$MAP = P_d + \frac{1}{3}(P_s - P_d)$$

The normal range for MAP is 70 to 110 mm Hg.[26] The difference between the systolic pressure and diastolic pressure ($P_s - P_d$) is called the pulse pressure and typically is between 40 and 50 mm Hg.[7] Pulse pressure is directly related to arterial wall stiffness and stroke volume.

During a wide range of physiological conditions, including changes in body position, muscular activity, and circulating blood volume, arterial pressure is regulated within a fairly narrow range to maintain tissue perfusion, or blood supply to the capillary beds. The major factors and relationships that regulate arterial blood pressure are summarized in Figure 23-25.

Effects of Cardiac Output

The cardiac output (minute volume) of the heart can be changed by alterations in heart rate, stroke volume (volume of blood ejected during each ventricular contraction), or both. An increase in cardiac output without a decrease in peripheral resistance will cause MAP and flow rate to increase. The higher arterial pressure increases blood flow through the arterioles. On the other hand, a decrease in the cardiac output causes a drop in the mean arterial blood pressure and arteriolar flow if peripheral resistance stays constant.

Effects of Total Peripheral Resistance

Total resistance in the systemic circulation, known as either *SVR* or *TPR*, is primarily a function of arteriolar diameter. If cardiac output

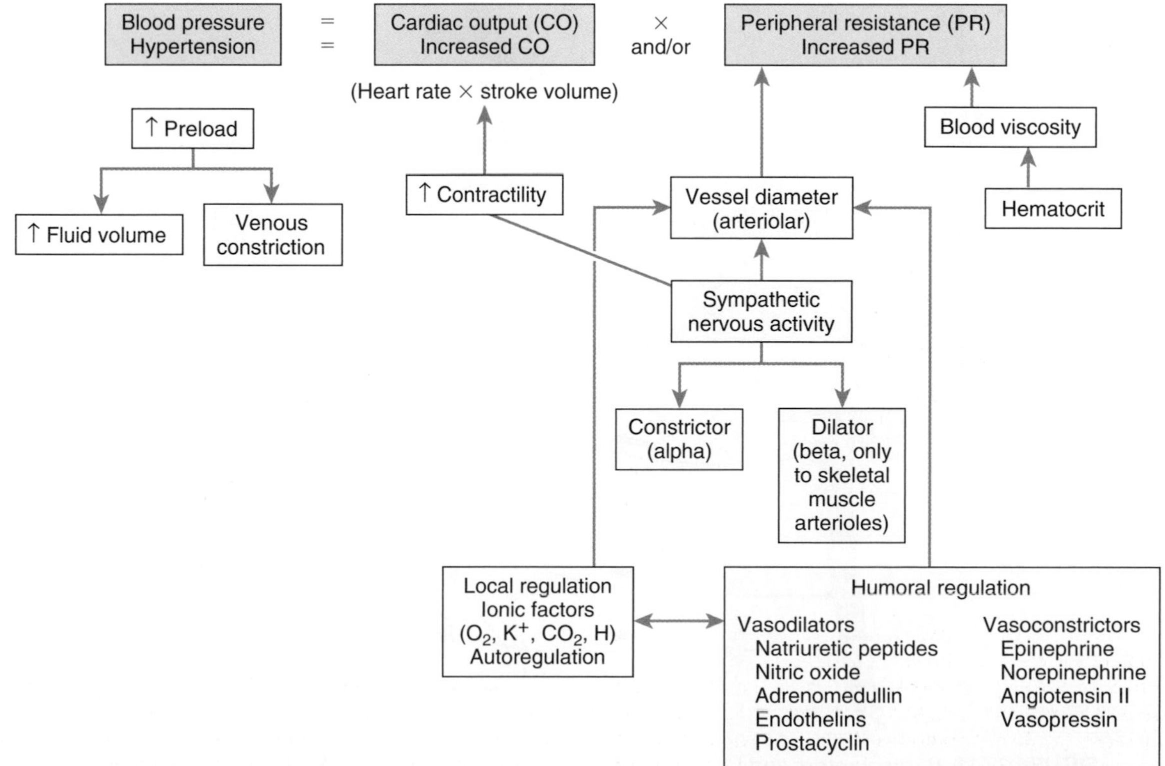

FIGURE 23-25 Factors and Relationships Regulating Blood Pressure. CO_2, carbon dioxide; *H*, hydrogen; *K+*, potassium; O_2, oxygen.

remains constant, arteriolar constriction raises MAP by reducing the flow of blood into the capillaries, whereas arteriolar dilation has the opposite effect. Reflex control of total cardiac output and peripheral resistance includes (1) sympathetic stimulation of heart, arterioles, and veins; and (2) parasympathetic stimulation of the heart (Figure 23-26). The cardiovascular centre in the medulla receives input from arterial baroreceptors and chemoreceptors throughout the vascular system and then modifies vagal and sympathetic output to control heart rate and contractility, plus vascular diameter. Vasoconstriction is regulated by an area of the brainstem that maintains a constant (tonic) output of norepinephrine from sympathetic fibres in the peripheral arterioles. This tonic activity is essential for maintenance of blood pressure.

Baroreceptors. As discussed previously, baroreceptors are stretch receptors located predominantly in the aorta and in the carotid sinus (Figure 23-26, *A*). They respond to changes in smooth muscle fibre length by altering their rate of discharge and supplying sensory information to the cardiovascular centre in the brainstem. When activated (stretched), the baroreceptors decrease cardiac output (by lowering heart rate and stroke volume) and peripheral resistance, and thus lower blood pressure. (Postural changes and the baroreceptor reflex are discussed in Chapter 24.)

Arterial chemoreceptors. Specialized areas within the aortic arch and carotid arteries are sensitive to concentrations of oxygen, carbon dioxide, and hydrogen ions (pH) in the blood (Figure 23-26, *B*). Although these chemoreceptors are most important for respiratory control, they also transmit impulses to the medullary cardiovascular centres that regulate blood pressure. A decrease in arterial oxygen concentration or an increase in carbon dioxide concentration contributes to an increase in heart rate, stroke volume, and blood pressure, whereas an increase in carbon dioxide concentration causes decreases in these variables. The major chemoreceptive reflex is caused by alterations in arterial oxygen concentration. The effects of altered pH or carbon dioxide levels are minor.[21]

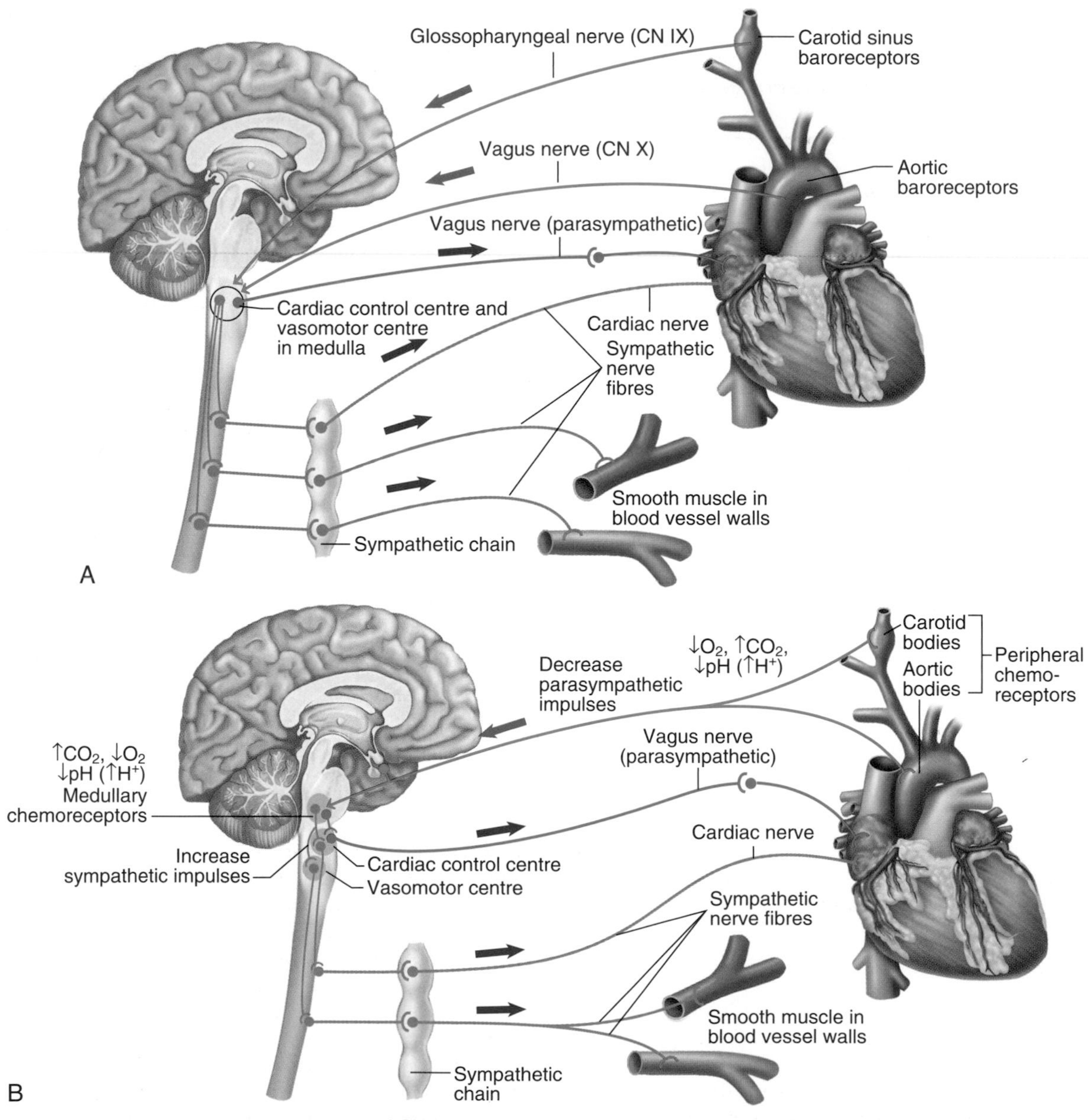

FIGURE 23-26 Baroreceptors and Chemoreceptor Reflex Control of Blood Pressure. A, Baroreceptor reflexes. **B,** Vasomotor chemoreflexes. *CN,* cranial nerve; CO_2, carbon dioxide; H^+, hydrogen; O_2, oxygen. (Modified from Patton, K.T., & Thibodeau, G.A. [2016]. *Anatomy & physiology* [9th ed.]. St. Louis: Elsevier.)

Effect of Hormones

Hormones influence blood pressure regulation through their effects on vascular smooth muscle and blood volume. By constricting or dilating the arterioles in organs, hormones can (1) increase or decrease the flow in response to the body's needs, (2) redistribute blood volume during hemorrhage or shock, and (3) regulate heat loss. The key vasoconstrictor hormones include angiotensin II, vasopressin (or antidiuretic hormone), epinephrine, and norepinephrine. The main vasodilator hormones are the atrial natriuretic hormones. By causing fluid retention or loss, aldosterone, vasopressin, and the natriuretic hormones can influence stroke volume and thus blood pressure.

A variety of other factors, including adipokines and insulin, may be related to the hypertension that occurs with chronic conditions, such as adiposity and diabetes mellitus; but these factors have not been clearly demonstrated to play a role in blood pressure regulation in healthy individuals.[27] Some research has suggested that the risk for cardiovascular disease and hypertension that often co-occurs with diabetes mellitus is more closely related to insulin resistance than to insulin levels.[28] Adrenomedullin (ADM) is a vasodilating peptide present in cardiovascular, pulmonary, renal, and other tissues. Because increases in ADM levels are associated with heart failure and myocardial infarction, ADM levels may be useful for risk categorization in people with these conditions.[29]

Vasoconstrictor hormones. The vasoconstrictor hormones include epinephrine; norepinephrine; angiotensin II, which is part of the renin-angiotensin-aldosterone system; and vasopressin (also known as *antidiuretic hormone*). Epinephrine, the catecholamine hormone released from the adrenal medulla, causes vasoconstriction in most vascular beds except the coronary, liver, and skeletal muscle circulations. Norepinephrine mainly acts as a neurotransmitter; however, some norepinephrine also is released from the adrenal medulla. When released into the circulation, it is a more potent vasoconstrictor than epinephrine. Although angiotensin II and vasopressin are vasoconstrictors, they are not thought to have a major role in blood pressure control in normal circumstances.

Vasopressin and aldosterone also affect blood pressure by increasing blood volume through their influence on fluid reabsorption in the kidney and by stimulating thirst. Vasopressin causes the reabsorption of water from tubular fluid in the distal tubule and collecting duct of the nephron. Aldosterone, the end product of the renin-angiotensin-aldosterone system, stimulates the reabsorption of sodium, chloride, and water from the same locations in the kidney (Figure 23-27; also see Chapters 5 and 18).

Vasodilator hormones. The natriuretic peptides (NPs) or hormones (see Figure 23-27), including atrial natriuretic peptide (ANP), B-type natriuretic peptide (BNP), C-type natriuretic peptide (CNP), and urodilatin, function as both vasodilators and regulators of sodium and water excretion (natriuresis and diuresis). Increased pressure or diastolic volume in the heart stimulates the release of these peptide hormones. Increased levels of BNP predict increased risk for a poor outcome in heart failure (see *Health Promotion:* B-type Natriuretic Peptide and Heart Failure), pulmonary embolism, valvular heart disease, and chronic coronary artery disease.[30]

Effects of Other Mediators

A variety of other mediators have been demonstrated to cause arteriolar vasodilation or vasoconstriction. Some of the vasodilating mediators include nitric oxide, ADM, the endothelins, and prostacyclin. These mediators are being investigated to determine whether they or their inhibitors might be useful medications for the treatment of cardiovascular diseases or whether their levels might be useful in determining the prognosis of persons with known disease.

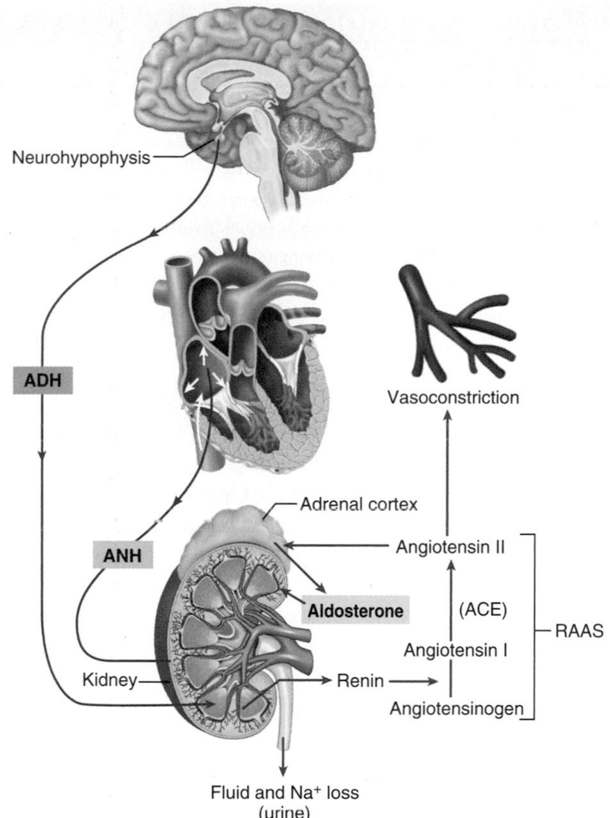

FIGURE 23-27 Three Mechanisms That Influence Total Plasma Volume. The antidiuretic hormone (*ADH*) mechanism and renin-angiotensin-aldosterone system (*RAAS*) tend to increase water, sodium, and chloride retention and thus increase total plasma volume. The atrial natriuretic hormone (*ANH*) mechanism antagonizes these mechanisms by promoting water, sodium, and chloride loss, thus promoting a decrease in total plasma volume. *ACE*, angiotensin-converting enzyme. (Modified from Patton, K.T., & Thibodeau, G.A. [2016]. *Anatomy & physiology* [9th ed.]. St. Louis: Elsevier.)

Nitric oxide (NO), an intercellular and intracellular signalling molecule produced in endothelial cells, has a variety of roles in vascular function, including acting as a vasodilator and inhibitor of smooth muscle proliferation. Nitric oxide also has been referred to as *endothelium-derived relaxing factor* (EDRF). One way that diabetes may contribute to hypertension is through inhibition of nitric oxide production by impeding a family of enzymes—the nitric oxide synthases.[31] Understanding the role of nitric oxide in producing vasodilation explains why sublingual nitroglycerine has been a useful treatment for coronary artery spasm.[32]

ADM, a peptide with powerful vasodilatory activity, is present in numerous tissues. It is a member of the calcitonin gene–related peptide family. Although it has been found to have numerous cardiovascular effects, including a role in fetal cardiovascular system development and vasodilation, its exact role in adult human cardiovascular function and disease is unclear. Some research indicates that elevated ADM levels may be useful disease indicators.[33]

The endothelins are a family of three peptides (ET-1, ET-2, and ET-3) and four receptors produced in cells in the vascular smooth muscle, the endothelium, the kidneys, and other organs. Understanding the physiological and pathological roles of these peptides has been complicated by the fact that endothelin binding to the type-A receptor causes vasodilation and natriuresis, whereas binding to type-B receptor causes the opposite response—vasoconstriction plus sodium and water

HEALTH PROMOTION

B-type Natriuretic Peptide and Heart Failure

Heart failure occurs due to chronic and progressive loss of functioning cardiac myocytes and a disruption of the ability of the myocardium to contract normally, which triggers a variety of compensatory mechanisms. Compensatory mechanisms such as an increase in adrenergic nervous system activity and excessive activation of the renin-angiotensin-aldosterone system will initially restore cardiovascular contractility. However, over time, continual activation of these systems can lead to detrimental dysfunction in myocardial pumping ability, left ventricular remodelling, and subsequent cardiac decompensation.

B-type natriuretic peptide (BNP) is a hormone that was initially identified in the brain but is now recognized as being released primarily from the heart, particularly the ventricles. The normal reference range for BNP is less than 100 ng/L. Values increase with age and weight, and are higher in women than men. The production of BNP increases in response to ventricular volume expansion and pressure overload. It also increases to counteract the possible deleterious effects of the compensatory mechanisms. BNP has diuretic, natriuretic, and vasodilator actions. It also inhibits the renin-angiotensin-aldosterone system, the secretion of endothelin, and systemic and renal sympathetic activity. BNP may protect against collagen formation and accumulation, and the pathological cardiac remodelling that contributes to the worsening of heart failure. As such, elevated BNP serum levels is a marker of ventricular distress and useful in diagnosing and monitoring the severity of heart failure. BNP levels higher than 400 correlate with heart failure. The severity of heart failure is directly correlated with the level of BNP. That is, the higher the BNP level, the greater the severity of heart failure.

In 2015, Lourenço, Ribeiro, Pintalhão, and colleagues established that BNP is the gold standard for heart failure prognostic prediction. They also concluded that a decrease in BNP levels independently predicts better survival and lower mortality. For example, patients in whom BNP decreased by greater than 30% had a hazard ratio of death of 0.57 (0.37 to 0.89). Also in 2015, Egom suggested that a linear relationship exists between plasma BNP levels and cardiovascular mortality. It should be noted that elevated BNP does not differentiate between ventricular systolic or ventricular diastolic dysfunction.

Studies reveal that BNP is a marker that is highly sensitive and specific. The greater value of BNP is in repeated measurement to monitor the progression of disease and in evaluating the response to medical therapy. As a marker, BNP is particularly useful in the emergency department setting for patients who present with acute dyspnea. BNP measurement is also a valuable tool in differentiating cardiac from noncardiac causes of respiratory distress. Several studies have shown that concentrations of BNP are substantially higher in patients with acute heart failure when compared with those with dyspnea due to other causes.

Data from Egom, E.E. (2015). *J Cardiovasc Transl Res, 8*(3), 149–157. doi:10.1007/s12265-015-9619-3; Kessenich, C.R. (2011). *Nurse Pract, 36*(1), 13–14. doi:10.1097/01.npr.0000391180.55502.18; Lourenço, P., Ribeiro, A., Pintalhão, M., et al. (2015). *Am J Cardiol, 116*(5), 744–748. doi:10.1016/j.amjcard.2015.05.046.

retention.[34] Inhibitors to ET-1 have been approved for the treatment of pulmonary hypertension.[35]

Prostacyclin is a vasodilator that is produced by the actions of cyclo-oxygenases (COX-1 and COX-2) on arachidonic acid. It also has the additional properties of opposing clot formation (antithrombotic), decreasing platelet activity, and inhibiting the release of growth factors from macrophages and the endothelial cells.[32] Nonsteroidal anti-inflammatory drugs (NSAIDs) that inhibit these cyclo-oxygenases have been associated with cardiovascular disease risk in healthy people and in those with a known cardiovascular disease.[36,37]

Venous Pressure

The main determinants of venous blood pressure are (1) the volume of fluid within the veins and (2) the compliance (distensibility) of the vessel walls. The venous system typically accommodates about 66% of the total blood volume at any time, with venous pressure averaging less than 10 mm Hg. The systemic arteries accommodate about 11% of the total blood volume, with an average arterial pressure (blood pressure) of about 100 mm Hg; the remainder of the blood volume is within the heart, capillaries, and pulmonary circulation.[26]

The sympathetic nervous system controls venous compliance. The walls of the veins are highly innervated by sympathetic fibres that control venous smooth muscle. Rather than constriction that would occur in the arteries, smooth muscle contraction in the veins results in stiffening of the vessel walls. This stiffening reduces venous distensibility and increases venous blood pressure, thus forcing more blood through the veins and into the right heart.

Two other mechanisms that increase venous pressure and venous return to the heart are (1) the skeletal muscle pump and (2) the respiratory pump. During skeletal muscle contraction, the veins within the muscles are partially compressed, causing decreased venous capacity and increased return to the heart (see Figure 23-26). The respiratory pump acts during inspiration, when the veins of the abdomen are partially compressed by the downward movement of the diaphragm. Increased abdominal pressure moves blood toward the heart.

Regulation of the Coronary Circulation

Coronary blood flow is directly proportional to the perfusion pressure and inversely proportional to the vascular resistance of the coronary bed. **Coronary perfusion pressure** is the difference between pressure in the aorta and pressure in the coronary vessels. Thus, aortic pressure is the driving pressure for the arteries and arterioles that perfuse the myocardium. Vasodilation and vasoconstriction maintain coronary blood flow despite stresses imposed by the constant contraction and relaxation of the heart muscle and despite shifts (within a physiological range) of coronary perfusion pressure.

Several unique anatomical factors influence coronary blood flow. Because of their anatomical location, the aortic valve cusps can obstruct coronary blood flow by occluding the openings of the coronary arteries during systole. Also during systole, the coronary arteries are compressed by ventricular contraction. The resulting **systolic compressive effect** is particularly evident in the subendocardial layers of the left ventricular wall and can greatly increase resistance to coronary blood flow with the result that most left ventricular coronary blood flow occurs during diastole. During the period of systolic compression, when flow is slowed or stopped, **myoglobin**, a protein in heart muscle that binds oxygen, provides the supply of oxygen to the myocardium. Myoglobin's oxygen levels are replenished during diastole.

Autoregulation

Autoregulation (automatic self-regulation) enables organs to regulate blood flow by altering the resistance (diameter) in their arterioles. Autoregulation in the coronary circulation maintains the blood flow at a nearly constant rate at perfusion pressures (MAP) between 60 and

140 mm Hg when other influencing factors are held constant.[21] Thus autoregulation helps to ensure constant coronary blood flow despite shifts in the perfusion pressure within the stated range.

Given that blood flow is directly related to pressure and inversely related to resistance, for flow to stay constant as pressure decreases resistance also has to decrease; therefore, the mechanisms underlying autoregulation must be related to control of smooth muscle contraction in the arteriolar walls. Although the exact mechanisms underlying autoregulation are unknown, research has indicated that factors influencing calcium release with the myocardium are involved and perhaps also the accumulation of vasodilatory products of metabolism, such as adenosine.[21,38]

Autonomic Regulation

Although the coronary vessels, themselves, contain sympathetic (α- and β-adrenergic) and parasympathetic neural receptors, coronary blood flow during regular activity is regulated locally by the factors that cause autoregulation. During exercise, however, the vasodilating effects of β_2-receptors on the smaller coronary resistance arteries are responsible for about 25% of any increase in blood flow. At the same time, α-adrenergic receptors in larger arteries cause vasoconstriction to direct the blood flow to the inner layers of the myocardium.[21]

> **QUICK CHECK 23-7**
> 1. Identify the factors and relationships regulating blood pressure.
> 2. Why is capillary flow increased with increased mean arterial pressure?
> 3. Why is angiotensin significant in blood flow?
> 4. Define *natriuretic peptides* and *adrenomedullin.*

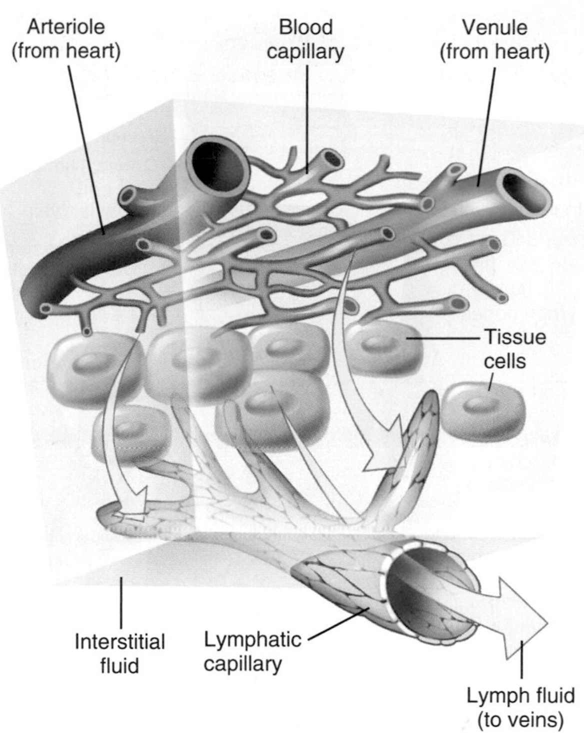

FIGURE 23-28 Role of the Lymphatic System in Fluid Balance. Fluid from plasma flowing through the capillaries moves into interstitial spaces. Although most of this interstitial fluid is either absorbed by tissue cells or reabsorbed by blood capillaries, some of the fluid tends to accumulate in the interstitial spaces. This lymph then diffuses into the lymphatic vessels that carry it to the lymph nodes and then into the systemic venous blood. Green is used to diagram the lymphatic vessels, although the lymphatic vessels, particularly the smaller ones, are almost transparent. (Modified from Thibodeau, G.A., & Patton, K.T. [2008]. *Structure & function of the body* [13th ed.]. St. Louis: Elsevier.)

THE LYMPHATIC SYSTEM

The lymphatic system is a one-way network of lymphatic vessels and the lymph nodes (Figures 23-28 and 23-29) that is important for immune function, fluid balance, and transport of lipids, hormones, and cytokines. Every day about 3 litres of fluid filters out of venous capillaries in body tissues and is not reabsorbed. This fluid becomes the lymph that is carried by the lymphatic vessels to the chest, where it enters the venous circulation. The lymphatic vessels run in the same sheaths with the arteries and veins. (Lymph nodes and lymphoid tissues are described in Chapters 6 and 8.) In this pumpless system, a series of valves ensures one-way flow of the excess interstitial fluid (now called *lymph*) toward the heart. The lymphatic capillaries are closed at the distal ends, as shown in Figure 23-30.

Lymph consists primarily of water and small amounts of dissolved proteins, mostly albumin, that are too large to be reabsorbed into the less permeable blood capillaries. Lymph also carries two types of immune system cells: lymphocytes and antigen-presenting cells. The antigen-presenting cells are carried to the next lymph node in the system while lymphocytes traffic between lymph nodes. Once within the lymphatic system, lymph travels through **lymphatic venules** and **lymphatic veins** that drain into one of two large ducts in the thorax: the right lymphatic duct and the thoracic duct. The **right lymphatic duct** drains lymph from the right arm and the right side of the head and thorax, whereas the larger **thoracic duct** receives lymph from the rest of the body (see Figure 23-29). The right lymphatic duct and the thoracic duct drain lymph into the right and left subclavian veins, respectively.

Lymphatic veins are thin walled like the veins of the cardiovascular system. In larger lymphatic veins, endothelial flaps form valves similar to those in blood-carrying veins (see Figure 23-30). The valves allow lymph to flow in only one direction as lymphatic vessels are compressed intermittently by skeletal muscle contraction, pulsatile expansion of the artery in the same sheath, and contraction of the smooth muscles in the walls of the lymphatic vessels.

As lymph is transported toward the heart, it is filtered through thousands of bean-shaped **lymph nodes** clustered along the lymphatic vessels (see Figure 23-29). Lymph enters the nodes through **afferent lymphatic vessels**, filters through the sinuses in the node, and leaves by way of **efferent lymphatic vessels**. Lymph flows slowly through a node, allowing phagocytosis of foreign substances within the node and delivery of lymphocytes. (Phagocytosis is described in Chapter 7.)

> **QUICK CHECK 23-8**
> 1. Why is the lymphatic system considered a circulatory system?
> 2. What happens to lymph in lymph nodes?

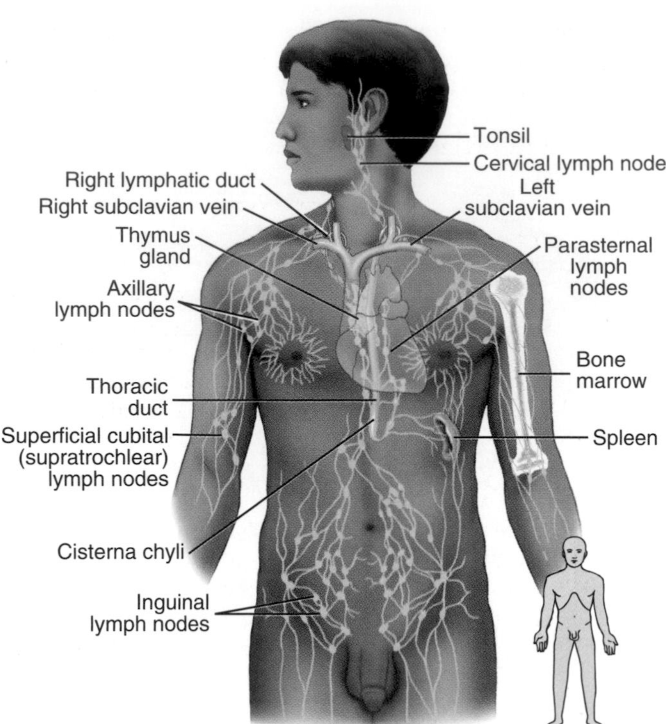

FIGURE 23-29 Principle Organs of the Lymphatic System. (From VanMeter, K.C., & Hubert, R.J. [2010]. *Microbiology for the healthcare professional.* St. Louis: Mosby.)

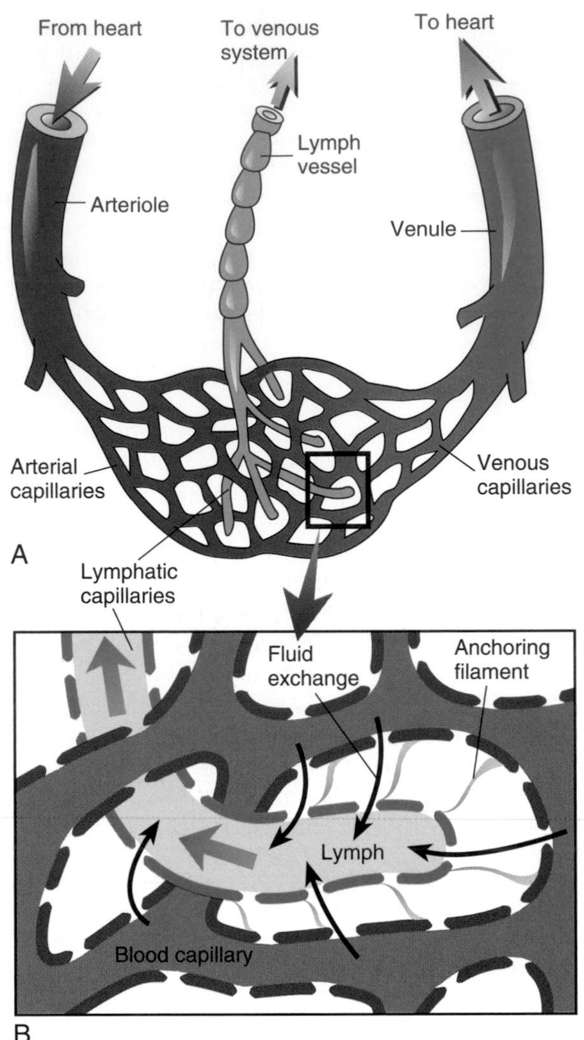

FIGURE 23-30 Lymphatic Capillaries. **A,** Schematic representation of lymphatic capillaries. **B,** Anatomical components of microcirculation.

DID YOU UNDERSTAND?

Overview

1. The circulatory system is part of the body's transport and communication systems. It delivers oxygen, nutrients, metabolites, hormones, neurochemicals, proteins, and blood cells including lymphocytes and leukocytes throughout the body and carries metabolic wastes to the kidneys, lungs, and liver for excretion.

The Circulatory System

1. The circulatory system consists of the heart and the blood and lymphatic vessels and is made up of two separate, but conjoined serially connected pump systems: the pulmonary circulation and the systemic circulation. The lymphatic system is a one-way network consisting of lymphatic vessels and lymph nodes.
2. The low-pressure pulmonary circulation is driven by the right side of the heart; its function is to deliver blood to the lungs for oxygenation.
3. The higher pressure systemic circulation is driven by the left side of the heart and functions to provide oxygenated blood, nutrients, and other key substances to body tissues and transport waste products to the lungs, kidneys, and liver for excretion.
4. The lymphatic vessels collect fluids from the interstitium and return the fluids to the circulatory system; lymphatic vessels also deliver antigens, microorganisms, and cells to the lymph nodes.

The Heart

1. The heart consists of four chambers (two atria and two ventricles), four valves (two atrioventricular valves [AV valves] and two semilunar valves), a muscular wall, a fibrous skeleton, a conduction system, nerve fibres, systemic vessels (the coronary circulation), and openings where the great vessels enter the atria and ventricles.
2. The heart wall, which encloses the heart and divides it into chambers, is made up of three layers: the epicardium (outer layer), the myocardium (muscular layer), and the endocardium (inner lining). The heart lies within the pericardium, a double-walled membranous sac.

3. The myocardial layer of the two atria, which receive blood entering the heart, is thinner than the myocardial layer of the ventricles, which have to be stronger to squeeze blood out of the heart.
4. The right and left sides of the heart are separated by portions of the heart wall called the *interatrial septum* and the *interventricular septum*.
5. Deoxygenated (venous) blood from the systemic circulation enters the right atrium through the superior and inferior venae cavae. From the right atrium, the blood passes through the right AV (tricuspid) valve into the right ventricle. In the ventricle, the blood flows from the inflow tract to the outflow tract and then through the pulmonary semilunar valve (pulmonary valve) into the pulmonary artery, which delivers it to the lungs for oxygenation.
6. Oxygenated blood from the lungs enters the left atrium through the four pulmonary veins (two from the left lung and two from the right lung). From the left atrium, the blood passes through the left AV valve (mitral valve) into the left ventricle. In the ventricle, the blood flows from the inflow tract to the outflow tract and then through the aortic semilunar valve (aortic valve) into the aorta, which delivers it to systemic arteries of the entire body.
7. There are four heart valves. The AV valves ensure one-way flow of blood from the atria to the ventricles. The semilunar valves ensure one-way blood flow from the right ventricle to the pulmonary artery and from the left ventricle to the aorta.
8. Oxygenated blood enters the coronary arteries through openings from the aorta, and deoxygenated blood from the coronary veins enters the right atrium through the coronary sinus.
9. The pumping action of the heart consists of two phases: diastole, during which the myocardium relaxes and the ventricles fill with blood; and systole, during which the myocardium contracts, forcing blood out of the ventricles. A cardiac cycle includes one systolic contraction and the diastolic relaxation that follows it. Each cardiac cycle represents one heartbeat.
10. The conduction system of the heart generates and transmits electrical impulses (cardiac action potentials) that stimulate systolic contractions. The autonomic nerves (sympathetic and parasympathetic fibres) can adjust heart rate and force of contraction, but they do not originate the heartbeat.
11. Each cardiac action potential travels from the SA node to the AV node to the bundle of His (atrioventricular bundle [AV bundle]), through the bundle branches, and finally to the Purkinje fibres and ventricular myocardium, where the impulse stops. It is prevented from reversing its path by the refractory period of cells that have just been polarized. The refractory period ensures that diastole (relaxation) will occur, thereby completing the cardiac cycle.
12. The normal electrocardiogram is the sum of all cardiac action potentials. The P wave represents atrial depolarization; the QRS complex is the sum of all ventricular cell depolarizations. The ST interval occurs when the entire ventricular myocardium is depolarized.
13. Cells of the cardiac conduction system possess the properties of automaticity and rhythmicity. Automatic cells return to threshold and depolarize rhythmically without an outside stimulus. The cells of the SA node depolarize faster than other automatic cells, making it the natural pacemaker of the heart. If the SA node is disabled, the next fastest pacemaker, the atrioventricular node (AV node), takes over.
14. Cardiac action potentials are generated by the sinoatrial node (SA node) at a rate of 60 to 100 impulses per minute. The impulses can travel through the conduction system of the heart, stimulating myocardial contraction as they go.
15. Adrenergic receptor number, type, and function govern autonomic (sympathetic) regulation of heart rate, contractile strength, and the dilation or constriction of coronary arteries. The presence of specific receptors on the myocardium and coronary vessels determines the effects of the neurotransmitters norepinephrine and epinephrine.
16. Unique features that distinguish myocardial cells from skeletal cells enable myocardial cells to transmit action potentials faster (through intercalated discs), synthesize more adenosine triphosphate (because of a large number of mitochondria), and have readier access to ions in the interstitium (because of an abundance of transverse tubules). These combined differences enable the myocardium to work constantly, which is not required by skeletal muscle.
17. Cross-bridges between actin and myosin enable contraction. Calcium ions interacting with the troponin complex help initiate the contraction process. Subsequently, myocardial relaxation begins as troponin releases calcium ions.
18. Cardiac performance is affected by preload, afterload, myocardial contractility, and heart rate.
19. Preload, or pressure generated in the ventricles at the end of diastole, depends on the amount of blood in the ventricle. Afterload is the resistance to ejection of the blood from the ventricle. Afterload depends on pressure in the aorta.
20. Myocardial stretch determines the force of myocardial contraction; thus the greater the stretch, the stronger the contraction up to a certain point. This relationship is known as Starling's law of the heart.
21. Contractility is the potential for myocardial fibre shortening during systole. It is determined by the amount of stretch during diastole (i.e., preload) and by sympathetic stimulation of the ventricles.
22. Heart rate is determined by the SA node and by components of the autonomic nervous system, including cardiovascular control centres in the brain, receptors in the aorta and carotid arteries, and hormones, including catecholamines (epinephrine, norepinephrine).

The Systemic Circulation

1. Blood flows from the left ventricle into the aorta and from the aorta into arteries that eventually branch into arterioles and capillaries, the smallest of the arterial vessels. Oxygen, nutrients, and other substances needed for cellular metabolism pass from the capillaries into the interstitium, where they are taken up by the cells. Capillaries also absorb metabolic waste products from the interstitium.
2. Venules, the smallest veins, receive capillary blood. From the venules, the venous blood flows into larger and larger veins until it reaches the venae cavae, through which it enters the right atrium.
3. Blood vessel walls have three layers: (1) the tunica intima (inner layer), (2) the tunica media (middle layer), and (3) the tunica externa (the outer layer).
4. Layers of the blood vessel wall differ in thickness and composition from vessel to vessel, depending on the vessel's size and location within the circulatory system. In general, the tunica media of arteries close to the heart has more elastic fibres because these arteries must be able to distend during systole and recoil during diastole. Distributing arteries farther from the heart contain more smooth muscle fibres because they constrict and dilate to control blood pressure and volume within specific capillary beds.
5. Blood flow into the capillary beds is controlled by the contraction and relaxation of smooth muscle bands (precapillary sphincters) at junctions between metarterioles and capillaries.
6. Endothelial cells line the blood vessels. The endothelium is a life-support tissue; it functions as a filter (altering permeability),

changes in vasomotion (constriction and dilation), and is involved in clotting and inflammation.

7. Blood flow through the veins is assisted by the contraction of skeletal muscles (the muscle pump), and backward flow is prevented by one-way valves, which are particularly important in the deep veins of the legs.
8. Blood flow is affected by blood pressure, resistance to flow within the vessels, blood consistency (which affects velocity), anatomical features that may cause turbulent or laminar flow, and compliance (distensibility) of the vessels.
9. Poiseuille's law describes the relationship of blood flow, pressure, and resistance as the difference between pressure at the inflow end of the vessel and pressure at the outflow end divided by resistance within the vessel.
10. The greater a vessel's length and the blood's viscosity and the narrower the radius of the vessel's lumen, the greater the resistance within the vessel.
11. Total peripheral resistance, or the resistance to flow within the entire systemic circulatory system, depends on the combined lengths and radii of all the vessels within the system and on whether the vessels are arranged in series (greater resistance) or in parallel (lesser resistance).
12. Blood flow is also influenced by neural stimulation (vasoconstriction or vasodilation) and by autonomic features that cause turbulence within the vascular lumen (e.g., protrusions from the vessel wall, twists and turns, vessel branching).
13. Arterial blood pressure is influenced and regulated by factors that affect cardiac output (heart rate, stroke volume), total resistance within the system, and blood volume.
14. Antidiuretic hormone, the renin-angiotensin-aldosterone system, and natriuretic peptides can all alter blood volume and thus blood pressure.
15. Venous blood pressure is influenced by blood volume within the venous system and compliance of the venous walls.
16. Blood flow through the coronary circulation is governed by the same principles as flow through other vascular beds plus two adaptations dictated by cardiac dynamics. First, blood flows into the coronary arteries during diastole rather than systole, because during systole the cusps of the aortic semilunar valve block the openings of the coronary arteries. Second, systolic contraction inhibits coronary artery flow by compressing the coronary arteries.
17. Myoglobin in heart muscle stores oxygen for use during the systolic phase of the cardiac cycle.
18. Autoregulation enables the coronary vessels to maintain optimal perfusion pressure despite systolic compression.

The Lymphatic System

1. The vessels of the lymphatic system run in the same sheaths as the arteries and veins.
2. Lymph (interstitial fluid) is absorbed by lymphatic venules in the capillary beds and travels through ever larger lymphatic veins until it empties through the right lymphatic duct or thoracic duct into the right or left subclavian veins, respectively.
3. As lymph travels toward the thoracic ducts, it passes through thousands of lymph nodes clustered around the lymphatic veins. The lymph nodes are sites of immune function and are ideally placed to sample antigens and cells carried by the lymph from the periphery of the body into the central circulation.

KEY TERMS

Actin, 585
Adrenomedullin (ADM), 597
Afferent lymphatic vessel, 599
Afterload, 588
Angiogenesis, 579
Anisotropic band (A band), 585
Aorta, 577
Aortic semilunar valve, 577
Arteriogenesis, 579
Arteriole, 589
Artery, 589
Atrioventricular node (AV node), 581
Atrioventricular valve (AV valve), 577
Automatic cell, 583
Automaticity, 583
Autoregulation, 598
Bainbridge reflex, 589
Baroreceptor reflex, 589
Blood flow, 593
Blood velocity, 594
Bundle of His (atrioventricular bundle [AV bundle]), 582
Capillary, 589
Cardiac action potential, 580
Cardiac cycle, 578
Cardiac output, 587
Cardiac vein, 578
Cardiomyocyte, 576
Cardiovascular vasomotor control centre, 588
Chordae tendineae, 577
Collateral artery, 578
Conduction system, 580
Coronary artery, 578
Coronary ostium (*pl.*, ostia), 578
Coronary perfusion pressure, 598
Coronary sinus, 578
Cross-bridge theory of muscle contraction, 586
Depolarization, 582
Diastole, 578
Diastolic blood pressure, 595
Diastolic depolarization, 583
Efferent lymphatic vessel, 599
Ejection fraction, 587
Elastic artery, 589
Endocardium, 576
Endothelial cell, 590
Endothelium, 590
Epinephrine, 588
Excitation–contraction coupling, 586
Fenestration, 590
Great cardiac vein, 580
Heart rate, 576
Inferior vena cava, 577
Inotropic agent, 588
Intercalated disc, 584
Isotropic band (I band), 585
Laminar flow, 594
Laplace's law, 587
Left atrium, 577
Left bundle branch (LBB), 582
Left coronary artery (LCA), 578
Left heart, 575
Left ventricle, 577
Lumen, 589
Lymph, 599
Lymph node, 599
Lymphatic vein, 599
Lymphatic venule, 599
Mean arterial pressure (MAP), 595
Mediastinum, 575
Metarteriole, 589
Mitral and tricuspid complex, 577
Mitral valve (left atrioventricular valve, bicuspid valve), 577
M line, 585
Muscle pump, 593
Muscular artery, 589
Myocardial contractility, 586
Myocardial oxygen consumption ($M\dot{V}O_2$), 586
Myocardium, 576
Myoglobin, 598
Myosin, 585
Natriuretic peptide (NP), 597
Nitric oxide (NO), 597
Papillary muscle, 577
Perfusion, 595
Pericardial cavity, 576
Pericardial fluid, 576
Pericardial sac, 576
Pericardium, 576
Peripheral vascular system, 589
Poiseuille's law, 593
PR interval, 582
Precapillary sphincter, 590
Preload, 587
Pressure, 593
Prolapse, 577
Pulmonary artery, 577
Pulmonary circulation, 575
Pulmonary vein, 577
Pulmonic semilunar valve, 577
Pulse pressure, 595
Purkinje fibre, 582
P wave, 582
QRS complex, 582
QT interval, 583
Radius (diameter), 593
Refractory period, 582

Repolarization, 582
Resistance, 593
Rhythmicity, 583
Right atrium, 577
Right bundle branch (RBB), 582
Right coronary artery (RCA), 578
Right heart, 575
Right lymphatic duct, 599
Right ventricle, 577
Semilunar valve, 577
Shear stress, 579
Sinoatrial node (SA node, sinus node), 581
Starling's law of the heart, 587
Stenosis, 579
ST interval, 583
Stroke volume, 587
Superior vena cava, 577
Systemic circulation, 575
Systemic vascular resistance (SVR), 588
Systole, 578
Systolic blood pressure, 595
Systolic compressive effect, 598
Thoracic duct, 599
Titin, 586
Total peripheral resistance (TPR), 588
Total resistance, 594
Tricuspid valve, 577
Tropomyosin, 585
Troponin C, 585
Troponin I, 585
Troponin T, 585
Troponin–tropomyosin complex, 585
Tunica externa (adventitia), 589
Tunica intima, 589
Tunica media, 589
Turbulent (flow), 594
T wave, 583
Vasa vasorum, 589
Vascular compliance, 595
Vasoconstriction, 589
Vasodilation, 589
Vein, 591
Ventricular end-diastolic pressure (VEDP), 587
Ventricular end-diastolic volume (VEDV), 587
Venule, 589
Z line, 585

REFERENCES

1. Rajendran, P., Rengarajan, T., Thangavel, J., et al. (2013). The vascular endothelium and human diseases. *International Journal of Biological Sciences, 9*(10), 1057–1069. doi:10.7150/ijbs.7502.
2. Lin, Z., & Pu, W. T. (2014). Strategies for cardiac regeneration and repair. *Science Translational Medicine, 6*(239), 239rv1. doi:10.1126/scitranslmed.3006681.
3. Kutty, S., Sengupta, P. P., & Khandheria, B. K. (2012). Patent foramen ovale: The known and the to be known. *Journal of the American College of Cardiology, 59*(19), 1665–1671. doi:10.1016/j.jacc.2011.09.085.
4. Tobis, J., & Shenoda, M. (2012). Percutaneous treatment of patent foramen ovale and atrial septal defects. *Journal of the American College of Cardiology, 60*(19), 1722–1732. doi:10.1016/j.jacc.2012.01.086.
5. Faber, J. E., Chilian, W. M., Deindl, E., et al. (2014). A brief etymology of the collateral circulation. *Arteriosclerosis, Thrombosis, and Vascular Biology, 34*(9), 1854–1859. doi:10.1161/ATVBAHA.114.303929.
6. Fung, E., & Helisch, A. (2012). Macrophages in collateral arteriogenesis. *Frontiers in Physiology, 3*, 353. doi:10.3389/fphys.2012.00353.
7. Klabunde, R. E. (2012). *Cardiovascular physiology concepts* (2nd ed.). Baltimore: Lippincott, Williams & Wilkins.
8. Rubart, M., & Zipes, D. P. (2015). Genesis of cardiac arrhythmias. In D. L. Mann, D. P. Zipes, P. Libby, et al. (Eds.), *Braunwald's heart disease: A textbook of cardiovascular medicine* (10th ed., p. 33). Philadelphia: Saunders.
9. Hariharan, N., Ikeda, Y., Hong, C., et al. (2013). Autophagy plays an essential role in mediating regression of hypertrophy during unloading of the heart. *PLoS ONE, 8*(1), e51632. doi:10.1371/journal.pone.0051632.
10. Hou, J., & Kang, Y. J. (2012). Regression of pathological cardiac hypertrophy: Signaling pathways and therapeutic targets. *Pharmacology & Therapeutics, 135*(3), 337–354. doi:10.1016/j.pharmthera.2012.06.006.
11. Narula, N., Agozzino, M., Gazzoli, F., et al. (2014). *Heart Failure Clinics, 10*(1, Suppl.), S63–S74. doi:10.1016/j.hfc.2013.09.001.
12. Opie, L. H., & Bers, D. M. (2015). Mechanisms of cardiac contraction and relaxation. In D. L. Mann, D. P. Zipes, P. Libby, et al. (Eds.), *Braunwald's heart disease: A textbook of cardiovascular medicine* (10th ed., pp. 429–453). Philadelphia: Saunders.
13. Linke, W. A., & Hamdani, N. (2014). Gigantic business: Titin properties and function through thick and thin. *Circulation Research, 114*, 1052–1068. doi:10.1161/CIRCRESAHA.114.301286.
14. Deussen, A., Ohanyan, V., Jannasch, A., et al. (2012). Mechanisms of metabolic coronary flow regulation. *Journal of Molecular and Cellular Cardiology, 52*(4), 794–801. doi:10.1016/j.yjmcc.2011.10.001.
15. Hansen, P. B. (2015). Functional importance of T-type voltage-gated calcium channels in the cardiovascular and renal system: News from the world of knockout mice. *American Journal of Physiology – Regulatory Integrative and Comparative Physiology, 308*(4), R227–R237. doi:10.1152/ajpregu.00276.2014.
16. Sakata, Y., Ohtani, T., Takeda, Y., et al. (2013). Left ventricular stiffening as therapeutic target for heart failure with preserved ejection fraction. *Circulation Journal, 77*(4), 886–892. doi:10.1253/circj.CJ-13-0214.
17. Ababneh, A. A., Sciacca, R. R., Kim, B., et al. (2000). Normal limits for left ventricular ejection fraction and volumes estimated with gated myocardial perfusion imaging in patients with normal exercise test results: Influence of tracer, gender, and acquisition camera. *Journal of Nuclear Cardiology, 7*(6), 661–668. doi:10.1067/mnc.2000.109861.
18. Davidson, C. J., Bonow, R. O., et al. (2015). Cardiac catheterization. In D. L. Mann, D. P. Zipes, & P. Libby (Eds.), *Braunwald's heart disease: A textbook of cardiovascular medicine* (10th ed., pp. 364–391). Philadelphia: Saunders.
19. Sato, R., & Nasu, M. (2015). A review of sepsis-induced cardiomyopathy. *Journal of Intensive Care, 3*, 48. doi:10.1186/s40560-015-0112-5.
20. Goegel, B., Handrick, V., Lauten, A., et al. (2013). Impact of acute normobaric hypoxia on regional and global myocardial function: A speckle tracking echocardiography study. *International Journal of Cardiovascular Imaging, 29*(3), 561–567. doi:10.1007/s10554-012-0117-2.
21. Hoit, B. D., & Walsh, R. A. (2011). Normal physiology of the cardiovascular system. In V. Fuster, R. A. Walsh, R. A. Harrington, et al. (Eds.), *Hurst's the heart* (13th ed.). Philadelphia: McGraw-Hill.
22. Crystal, G. J., & Salem, M. R. (2012). The Bainbridge and the "reverse" Bainbridge reflexes: History, physiology, and clinical relevance. *Anesthesia and Analgesia, 114*(3), 520–532. doi:10.1213/ANE.0b013e3182312e21.
23. Volpe, M., Rubattu, S., & Burnett, J., Jr. (2014). Natriuretic peptides in cardiovascular diseases: Current use and perspectives. *European Heart Journal, 35*(7), 419–425. doi:10.1093/eurheartj/eht466.
24. Perkel, D., Naghi, J., Agarwal, M., et al. (2012). The potential effects of IGF-1 and GH on patients with chronic heart failure. *Journal of Cardiovascular Pharmacology and Therapeutics, 17*(1), 72–78. doi:10.1177/1074248411402078.
25. Girard, J.-P., Moussion, C., & Förster, R. (2012). HEVs, lymphatics and homeostatic immune cell trafficking in lymph nodes. *Nature Reviews. Immunology, 12*(11), 762–773. doi:10.1038/nri3298.
26. Patton, K. T., & Thibodeau, G. A. (2016). *Anatomy & physiology online package* (9th ed.). St. Louis: Elsevier.
27. Kim, D. H., Kim, C., Ding, E. L., et al. (2013). Adiponectin levels and the risk of hypertension: A systematic review and meta-analysis. *Hypertension, 62*(1), 27–32. doi:10.1161/HYPERTENSIONAHA.113.01453.
28. Younk, L. M., Lamos, E. M., & Davis, S. N. (2014). The cardiovascular effects of insulin. *Expert Opinion on Drug Safety, 13*(7), 955–966. doi:10.1517/14740338.2014.919256.
29. Yuyun, M. F., Narayan, H. K., & Ng, L. L. (2015). Prognostic significance of adrenomedullin in patients with heart failure and with myocardial infarction. *American Journal of Cardiology, 115*(7), 986–991. doi:10.1016/j.amjcard.2015.01.027.
30. Bergler-Klein, J., Gyöngyösi, M., & Maurer, G. (2014). The role of biomarkers in valvular heart disease: Focus on natriuretic peptides. *Canadian Journal of Cardiology, 30*(9), 1027–1034. doi:10.1016/j.cjca.2014.07.014.
31. Lei, J., Vodovotz, Y., Tzeng, E., et al. (2013). Nitric oxide, a protective molecule in the cardiovascular system. *Nitric Oxide: Biology and Chemistry, 35*, 175–185. doi:10.1016/j.niox.2013.09.004.
32. Griendling, K. K., Harrison, D. G., & Alexander, R. W. (2011). Biology of the vessel wall. In V. Fuster, R. A. Walsh, R. A. Harrington, et al. (Eds.), *Hurst's the heart* (13th ed., pp. 153–171). Philadelphia: McGraw-Hill.
33. Nishikimi, T., Kuwahara, K., Nakagawa, Y., et al. (2013). Adrenomedullin in cardiovascular disease: A useful biomarker, its pathological roles and therapeutic application. *Current Protein and Peptide Science, 14*(4), 256–267. doi:10.2174/13892037113149990045.
34. Kohan, D. E., Rossi, N. F., Inscho, E. W., et al. (2011). Regulation of blood pressure and salt homeostasis by endothelin. *Physiological Reviews, 91*(1), 1–77. doi:10.1152/physrev.00060.2009.
35. Nasser, S. A., & El-Mas, M. M. (2014). Endothelin ETA receptor antagonism in cardiovascular disease. *European Journal of Pharmacology, 737*, 210–213. doi:10.1016/j.ejphar.2014.05.046.
36. Schjerning Olsen, A. M., Fosbøl, E. L., & Gislason, G. H. (2014). The impact of NSAID treatment on cardiovascular risk—Insight from Danish observational data. *Basic and Clinical Pharmacology and Toxicology, 115*(2), 179–184. doi:10.1111/bcpt.12244.
37. Singh, B. K., Haque, S. E., & Pillai, K. K. (2014). Assessment of nonsteroidal anti-inflammatory drug-induced cardiotoxicity. *Expert Opinion on Drug Metabolism and Toxicology, 10*(2), 143–156. doi:10.1517/17425255.2014.856881.
38. Izzard, A. S., & Haegerty, A. M. (2014). Myogenic properties of brain and cardiac vessels and their relation to disease. *Current Vascular Pharmacology, 12*(6), 829–835. doi:10.2174/15701611113116660150.

24

Alterations of Cardiovascular Function

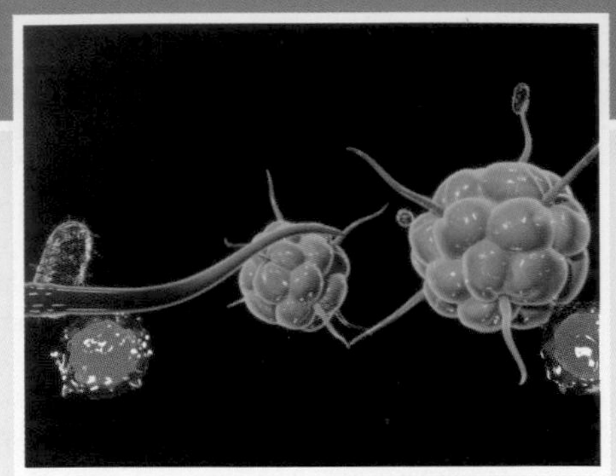

Valentina L. Brashers and Mohamed El-Hussein

EVOLVE WEBSITE

http://evolve.elsevier.com/Canada/Huether/pathophysiology

Student Review Questions
Key Points
Case Studies
Animations
Quick Check Answers

CHAPTER OUTLINE

Diseases of the Veins, 604
- Varicose Veins and Chronic Venous Insufficiency, 604
- Thrombus Formation in Veins, 605
- Superior Vena Cava Syndrome, 605

Diseases of the Arteries, 606
- Hypertension, 606
- Orthostatic (Postural) Hypotension, 611
- Aneurysm, 611
- Thrombus Formation, 612
- Embolism, 613
- Peripheral Vascular Disease, 613
- Atherosclerosis, 614
- Peripheral Artery Disease, 617
- Coronary Artery Disease, Myocardial Ischemia, and Acute Coronary Syndromes, 617

Disorders of the Heart Wall, 629
- Disorders of the Pericardium, 629
- Disorders of the Myocardium: The Cardiomyopathies, 630
- Disorders of the Endocardium, 632
- Cardiac Complications in AIDS, 638

Manifestations of Heart Disease, 638
- Heart Failure, 638
- Dysrhythmias, 643

Shock, 643
- Impairment of Cellular Metabolism, 643
- Clinical Manifestations of Shock, 648
- Treatment for Shock, 648
- Types of Shock, 648
- Multiple Organ Dysfunction Syndrome, 653

Our understanding of the pathophysiology of cardiovascular diseases is evolving rapidly. Neurohumoral, genetic, inflammatory, and metabolic factors are now the focus. This new information is leading to improvements in prevention and treatment.

DISEASES OF THE VEINS

Varicose Veins and Chronic Venous Insufficiency

A varicose vein is a vein in which blood has pooled, producing distended, tortuous, and palpable vessels (Figure 24-1). Veins are thin-walled, highly distensible vessels with valves to prevent backflow and pooling of blood (see Figure 23-26). Varicose veins typically involve the saphenous veins of the leg and are caused by (1) trauma to the saphenous veins that damages one or more valves or (2) gradual venous distension caused by the action of gravity on blood in the legs.

If a valve is damaged, a section of the vein is subjected to the pressure of a larger volume of blood under the influence of gravity. Altered connective tissue proteins and proteolytic enzyme activity also play a role in remodelling of the vessel wall.[1] The vein swells as it becomes engorged and surrounding tissue becomes edematous because increased hydrostatic pressure pushes plasma through the stretched vessel wall. Venous distension can develop over time in individuals who habitually stand for long periods, wear constricting garments, or cross the legs at the knees, which diminishes the action of the muscle pump (see Figure 23-27). Risk factors also include age, female gender, a family history of varicose veins, obesity, pregnancy, deep venous thrombosis (DVT), and previous leg injury. Eventually the pressure in the vein damages venous valves, rendering them incompetent and unable to maintain normal venous pressure.

Varicose veins and valvular incompetence can progress to chronic venous insufficiency, especially in obese individuals. Chronic venous insufficiency (CVI) is inadequate venous return over a long period. Venous hypertension, circulatory stasis, and tissue hypoxia cause an inflammatory reaction in vessels and tissue leading to fibrosclerotic remodelling of the skin and then to ulceration. Symptoms include edema of the lower extremities and hyperpigmentation of the skin of the feet and ankles. Edema in these areas may extend to the knees. Circulation to the extremities can become so sluggish that the metabolic demands of the cells to obtain oxygen and nutrients and to remove wastes are barely met. Any trauma or pressure can therefore lower the oxygen supply and cause cell death and necrosis (venous stasis ulcers) (Figure 24-2). Infection can occur because poor circulation impairs the delivery of the cells and biochemicals necessary for the immune and inflammatory responses. This same sluggish circulation makes infection following reparative surgery a significant risk.

Treatment of varicose veins and CVI begins conservatively, and excellent wound healing results have followed noninvasive treatments

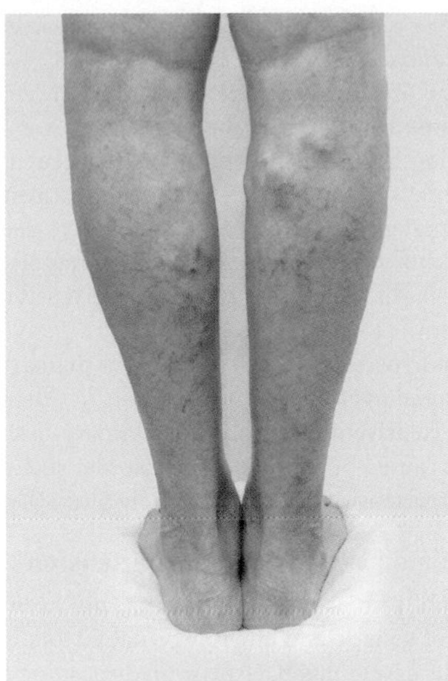

FIGURE 24-1 Varicose Veins of the Leg. (Solarisys/Shutterstock .com.)

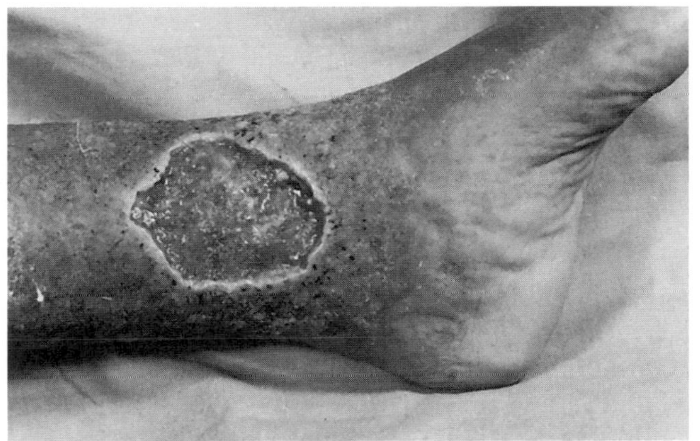

FIGURE 24-2 Venous Stasis Ulcer. (From Rosai, J. [1989]. *Ackerman's surgical pathology* [7th ed., vol. 2]. St. Louis: Mosby.)

such as elevating the legs, wearing compression stockings, and performing physical exercise.[2] Invasive management includes endovenous ablation, sclerotherapy or surgical ligation, conservative vein resection, and vein stripping.[3]

Thrombus Formation in Veins

A **thrombus** is a blood clot that remains attached to a vessel wall (see Figure 21-20). A detached thrombus is a **thromboembolus**. Venous thrombi are more common than arterial thrombi because flow and pressure are lower in the veins than in the arteries. **Deep venous thrombosis (DVT)** occurs primarily in the lower extremity. Three factors (Virchow triad) promote venous thrombosis: (1) venous stasis (e.g., immobility, age, heart failure), (2) venous endothelial damage (e.g., trauma, intravenous medications), and (3) hypercoagulable states (e.g., inherited disorders, malignancy, pregnancy, use of oral contraceptives or hormone replacement therapy). Orthopedic trauma or surgery, spinal cord injury, and obstetric/gynecological conditions can be associated with up to a 100% likelihood of DVT. Numerous genetic abnormalities are associated with an increased risk for venous thrombosis primarily related to states of hypercoagulability. These inherited abnormalities include factor V Leiden mutation, prothrombin mutations, and deficiencies of protein C, protein S, and antithrombin; these abnormalities are commonly found in individuals who develop thrombi in the absence of the usual risk factors.[4]

Accumulation of clotting factors and platelets leads to thrombus formation in the vein, often near a venous valve. Inflammation around the thrombus promotes further platelet aggregation, and the thrombus propagates or grows proximally. This inflammation may cause pain and redness, but because the vein is deep in the leg, it is usually not accompanied by clinical symptoms or signs. If the thrombus creates significant obstruction to venous blood flow, increased pressure in the vein behind the clot may lead to edema of the extremity. Most thrombi will eventually dissolve without treatment; however, untreated DVT is associated with a high risk for embolization of a part of the clot to the lung (pulmonary embolism) (see Chapter 27). Persistent venous obstruction may lead to CVI and post-thrombotic syndrome with associated pain, edema, and ulceration of the affected limb.[5]

Because DVT is usually asymptomatic and difficult to detect clinically, prevention is important in at-risk individuals and includes early ambulation, pneumatic devices, and prophylactic anticoagulation. If thrombosis does occur, diagnosis is confirmed by a combination of serum D-dimer measurement and Doppler ultrasonography. Management most often consists of anticoagulation therapy using heparin (low-molecular-weight heparin) and warfarin (Coumadin).[6] New oral anticoagulant therapies, such as factor Xa inhibitors and direct thrombin inhibitors, have been shown to have a more favourable benefit-to-risk ratio and are rapidly becoming the treatments of choice.[7] Thrombolytic therapy or placement of an inferior vena cava filter may be indicated in selected individuals.[4,6]

Superior Vena Cava Syndrome

Superior vena cava syndrome (SVCS) is a progressive occlusion of the superior vena cava (SVC) that leads to venous distension in the upper extremities and head. Causes include bronchogenic cancer (75% of cases) followed by lymphomas and metastasis of other cancers.[8] Other less common causes include tuberculosis, mediastinal fibrosis, and cystic fibrosis. Invasive therapies (pacemaker wires, central venous catheters, and pulmonary artery catheters) with associated thrombosis now account for nearly 40% of cases.[9] The SVC is a relatively low-pressure vessel that lies in the closed thoracic compartment; therefore, tissue expansion can easily compress the SVC. The right mainstem bronchus abuts the SVC so that cancers occurring in this bronchus may exert pressure on the SVC. Additionally, the SVC is surrounded by lymph nodes and lymph chains that commonly become involved in thoracic cancers and compress the SVC during tumour growth. Because onset of SVCS is most often slow, collateral venous drainage to the azygos vein usually has time to develop.

Clinical manifestations of SVCS are edema and venous distension in the upper extremities and face, including the ocular beds. Affected persons complain of a feeling of fullness in the head or tightness of shirt collars, necklaces, and rings. Cerebral edema may cause headache, visual disturbance, and impaired consciousness. The skin of the face and arms may become purple and taut, and capillary refill time is prolonged. Respiratory distress may be present because of edema of bronchial structures or compression of the bronchus by a carcinoma. In infants, SVCS can lead to hydrocephalus.

Diagnosis is made by chest X-ray, Doppler studies, computed tomography (CT), magnetic resonance imaging (MRI), and ultrasound. Because of its slow onset and the development of collateral venous drainage, SVCS is generally not a vascular emergency, but it is an oncological emergency. Treatment for malignant disorders can include radiation therapy, surgery, chemotherapy, and the administration of diuretics, steroids, and anticoagulants, as necessary. Treatment for nonmalignant causes may include bypass surgery using various grafts, thrombolysis (both locally and systemically), balloon angioplasty, and placement of intravascular stents.[8]

> **QUICK CHECK 24-1**
> 1. What is chronic venous insufficiency, and how does it present clinically?
> 2. What are the major risk factors for deep venous thrombosis?
> 3. Name three causes of superior vena cava syndrome.

DISEASES OF THE ARTERIES

Hypertension

Hypertension is consistent elevation of systemic arterial blood pressure.[10] Approximately 7.5 million Canadians have hypertension. Hypertension is considered to be the main factor contributing to mortality, disability-adjusted life years (DALYs), and years of life lost (YLL) in Canada. About 90% of Canadians are expected to develop hypertension if they live an average lifespan.[11]

The chance of developing primary hypertension increases with age. Although hypertension is usually considered an adult health problem, it is important to remember that hypertension does occur in children and is being diagnosed with increasing frequency (see Chapter 25). The prevalence of hypertension is higher in those of African descent and in those with diabetes. *Hypertension* is defined by Hypertension Canada as a mean systolic blood pressure greater than or equal to 140 mm Hg or diastolic blood pressure greater than or equal to 90 mm Hg when a nonautomated office blood pressure measurement is used (Table 24-1). Alternately, hypertension is also defined as a mean systolic blood pressure greater than or equal to 135 mm Hg or diastolic blood pressure greater than or equal to 85 mm Hg when an automated office blood pressure measurement is used.[12] Figure 24-3 presents a hypertension diagnostic algorithm for adults.

According to Hypertension Canada, all Canadian adults should have their blood pressure checked each time they visit a clinic, regardless of the reason. It is recommended that health care providers use automated measurement of blood pressure rather than manual measurement. It is also recommended that these measurements be done multiple times and be unattended. Patients are also encouraged to record and report out-of-office blood pressure measurements to confirm the initial diagnosis of hypertension. Optimum management of the hypertensive patient requires thorough assessment and evaluation. Patients should be reminded that modification of health behaviour is effective in preventing hypertension, treating hypertension, and reducing cardiovascular risk. However, a combination of both health behaviour changes and medications is often necessary to achieve target blood pressures. Patients should be taught how to measure blood pressure at home to be involved in self-monitoring and self-management, and to promote adherence to medications and a healthy diet.[13]

Normal blood pressure is associated with the lowest cardiovascular risk, whereas those who fall into the prehypertension category are at risk of developing hypertension and many associated cardiovascular complications unless lifestyle modification and treatment are instituted. All stages of hypertension are associated with increased risk for target organ disease events, such as myocardial infarction (MI), kidney disease, and stroke; thus both stage I and stage II hypertension need effective long-term therapy.

Most cases of hypertension are diagnosed as **primary hypertension** (also called *essential hypertension* or *idiopathic hypertension*). From 92 to 95% of hypertensive individuals have primary disease. **Secondary hypertension** is caused by an underlying disorder such as renal disease. This form of hypertension accounts for only 5 to 8% of cases.

Factors Associated With Primary Hypertension

A specific cause of primary hypertension has not been identified, and a combination of genetic and environmental factors is thought to be responsible for its development. Genetic predisposition to hypertension

TABLE 24-1 Classification of Blood Pressure for Adults Age 18 Years and Older

Category	Systolic (mm Hg)		Diastolic (mm Hg)
Normal	<120	AND	<80
Prehypertension	120–139	OR	80–89
Stage 1 hypertension	140–159	OR	90–99
Stage 2 hypertension	≥160	OR	≥100

Data from James, P.A., Oparil, S., Carter, B., et al. (2014). *JAMA, 311*(5), 507–520.

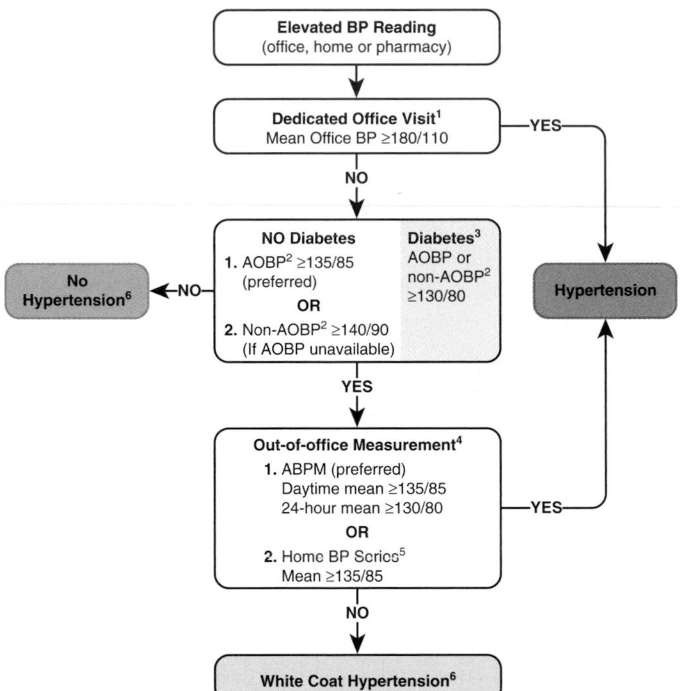

FIGURE 24-3 Hypertension Diagnostic Algorithm. [1]If AOBP is used, use the mean calculated and displayed by the device. If non-AOBP (see note 2) is used, take at least three readings, discard the first, and calculate the mean of the remaining measurements. A history and physical exam should be performed and diagnostic tests ordered. [2]AOBP is performed with the patient unattended in a private area. Non-AOBP is performed using an electronic upper arm device with the provider in the room. [3]Diagnostic thresholds for AOBP, ABPM, and home BP in patients with diabetes have yet to be established (and might be lower than 13/80 mm Hg). [4]Serial office measurements over 3–5 visits can be used if ABPM or home measurement is not available. [5]For a home BP series, two readings are taken each morning and evening for 7 days (28 total). Discard the first day readings and average the last 6 days. [6]Annual BP measurement is recommended to detect progression to hypertension. *ABPM*, ambulatory blood pressure measurement; *AOBP*, automated office blood pressure; BP, blood pressure. (Reprinted from *Can J Card,* 33(5), Leung, A., Daskalopoulou, S.S., Dasgupta, K., et al, "Hypertension Canada's 2017 Guidelines for Diagnosis, Risk Assessment, Prevention, and Treatment of Hypertension in Adults," Pages 557–576, Copyright 2017, with permission from Elsevier.)

is thought to be polygenic and associated with epigenetic changes influenced by diet and lifestyle.[14] Inherited defects are associated with renal sodium excretion, insulin and insulin sensitivity, activity of the sympathetic nervous system (SNS) and the renin-angiotensin-aldosterone system (RAAS), and cell membrane sodium or calcium transport.[15] Factors associated with primary hypertension relate to age, gender, race, and dietary factors (see *Risk Factors:* Primary Hypertension). Many of these factors are also risk factors for other cardiovascular disorders. In fact, obesity, hypertension, dyslipidemia, and glucose intolerance often are found together in a condition called *metabolic syndrome* (see Chapter 19).

RISK FACTORS

Primary Hypertension

- Family history
- Advancing age
- Cigarette smoking
- Obesity
- Heavy alcohol consumption
- Gender (men greater than women before age 55; women greater than men after 55)
- Being of African descent
- Being of Indigenous descent
- Immigration-related change in socioeconomic status
- High dietary sodium intake
- Low dietary intake of potassium, calcium, magnesium
- Glucose intolerance

The Indigenous population in Canada and primary hypertension. In Canada, the rate of developing and dying of heart disease and stroke among Indigenous people is twice that in the rest of the population. Moreover, Indigenous people are three to four times more likely to experience type 2 diabetes mellitus than non-Indigenous people, and they are 10.5 times more likely to die from coronary heart disease. About 40% of the Indigenous population in Canada lives on reserves, thus they do not have prompt access to health care facilities and their standard of living is often lower than that of the average Canadian.[16] A lower standard of living is linked to unhealthy behaviours such as smoking, eating mostly processed, high-salt, and cholesterol diets.[17] Indigenous people typically have heart attacks earlier in life than non-Indigenous people. The Indigenous population has a higher prevalence of physical inactivity, smoking, overweight, obesity, high blood pressure, and diabetes—all of which are risk factors for cardiovascular disease and hypertension. Indigenous people are more likely to have high blood pressure than the non-Indigenous population. As well, smoking rates among Indigenous people are, on average, twice as high as those of non-Indigenous people (39% versus 20.5%).[18]

New immigrants and primary hypertension. New immigrants to Canada often have fewer chronic conditions upon arrival compared with the native-born population. This trend is referred to as the *healthy immigrant effect* and reflects that fact that when immigrants first arrive in their new homeland, they tend to be healthier than the native-born population. However, new immigrants to Canada tend to experience a rapid deterioration in their general health status after living in Canada for several years due to lifestyle changes that impact their physical activity and dietary habits.[19] Dietary acculturation, which is the process by which immigrants adopt the dietary practices of the host country, has been associated with obesity, diabetes, and hypertension.[20] Dietary acculturation for immigrant groups has largely been attributed to the "Westernization" of immigrant diets, as characterized by an increased consumption of unhealthy north American foods (e.g., fast food, junk food).[20] In addition, immigrants may also be eating the foods of their festivals ("festival foods") more regularly. Festival foods are calorically rich foods that are typically consumed only a few times a year, during festivals or special occasions in the home country, and usually in limited amounts. After immigration, immigrants tend to prepare these festival foods more frequently and eat them in larger quantities. As such, in the process of acculturation, festival foods become "traditional foods" that are eaten on a more regular basis.[20] Immigration-related cultural changes have been found to be independently associated with high blood pressure.[19]

PATHOPHYSIOLOGY Hypertension results from a sustained increase in peripheral resistance (arteriolar vasoconstriction), an increase in circulating blood volume, or both.

Primary Hypertension

Primary hypertension is the result of an extremely complicated interaction of genetics and the environment mediated by a host of neurohumoral effects. Multiple pathophysiological mechanisms mediate these effects, including the SNS, the RAAS, and natriuretic peptides. Inflammation, endothelial dysfunction, obesity-related hormones, and insulin resistance also contribute to both increased peripheral resistance and increased blood volume. Increased vascular volume is related to a decrease in renal excretion of salt, often referred to as a shift in the **pressure–natriuresis relationship** (Figure 24-4). This shift means that for a given blood pressure, individuals with hypertension tend to secrete less salt in their urine.

The SNS has been implicated in both the development and the maintenance of elevated blood pressure and plays a role in hypertensive end-organ damage.[21] Increased SNS activity causes increased heart rate and systemic vasoconstriction, thus raising the blood pressure. Additional mechanisms of SNS-induced hypertension include structural changes in blood vessels (vascular remodelling), renal sodium retention (shift in the pressure–natriuresis curve), insulin resistance, increased renin and angiotensin levels, and procoagulant effects.[22]

The renin-angiotensin-aldosterone system and cardiovascular disease. In hypertensive individuals, overactivity of the RAAS contributes

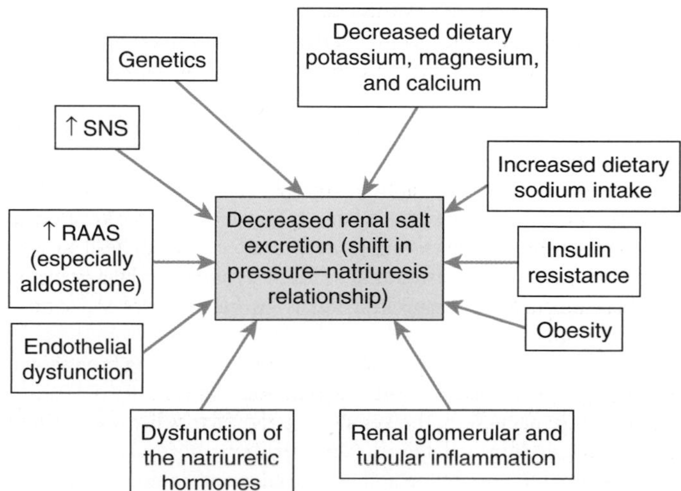

FIGURE 24-4 Factors That Cause a Shift in the Pressure–Natriuresis Relationship. Numerous factors have been implicated in the pathogenesis of sodium retention in individuals with hypertension. These factors cause less renal excretion of salt than would normally occur with increased blood pressure. This is called a shift in the pressure–natriuresis relationship and is thought to be a central process in the pathogenesis of primary hypertension. *RAAS*, renin-angiotensin-aldosterone system; *SNS*, sympathetic nervous system.

to salt and water retention and increased vascular resistance (see Figure 23-27). There are two primary renin-angiotensin-aldosterone systems. The best known includes the release of renin, the synthesis of angiotensin II (Ang II) through angiotensin-converting enzyme (ACE), stimulation of the angiotensin II type 1 receptor (AT1R), and secretion of aldosterone. The RAAS has multiple effects on the cardiovascular system. Ang II and aldosterone contribute to hypertensive hypertrophy and fibrosis of heart muscle, decreased contractility, and an increased susceptibility to arrhythmias and heart failure (HF). Further, Ang II causes systemic vasoconstriction and renal salt and water retention, and stimulates tissue growth and inflammation.[23-34] High levels of Ang II contribute to endothelial dysfunction (decreased release of endothelial vasodilators and anticoagulants), insulin resistance, remodelling of blood vessels, atherogenesis, and platelet aggregation and play an important role in the complications associated with metabolic syndrome (MetS).[29] In the kidney, these hormones cause a shift in the pressure–natriuresis curve, inflammation, and glomerular remodelling and are a major contributor to renal failure in individuals with hypertension and diabetes.

Further, Ang II mediates **arteriolar remodelling**, which is structural change in the vessel wall that results in permanent increases in peripheral resistance and contributes to atherogenesis[28] (see Figure 23-33). Ang II is associated with end-organ effects of hypertension, including atherosclerosis, renal disease, cardiac hypertrophy, and HF.[23,34] Finally, aldosterone not only contributes to sodium retention by the kidney but also has other deleterious effects on the cardiovascular system and contributes to insulin resistance.[35]

In contrast, the second RAAS serves a counter-regulatory system. Activation of a second ACE pathway (ACE2) leads to the synthesis of angiotensin 1-7 (Ang [1-7]) from Ang II. Ang (1-7) stimulates Mas receptors in the brain, blood vessels, heart, kidney, gut, pancreas, and inflammatory cells and has vasodilatory, antiproliferative, antifibrotic, and antithrombotic effects. These protective effects lead to lower blood pressure, less vascular inflammation and clotting, and decreased tissue remodelling and damage to target organ tissues. This pathway appears to be especially important in protecting renal tissue and improving insulin sensitivity in those with diabetes and hypertension. Research is under way to develop pharmacological interventions, such as synthetic Mas agonists, Ang (1-7) formulations, and ACE2 activators that will stimulate these protective RAAS pathways. More recently, additional RAAS pathways have been identified that play a role in proto-oncogene stimulation, hypothalamic function, and central nervous system function.[23-34]

Medications, such as ACE inhibitors and angiotensin receptor blockers (ARBs), oppose the activity of the RAAS and are effective in reducing blood pressure and protecting against target organ damage.[32] Also, the use of ACE2 to create Ang (1-7), which has cardiovascular, cerebrovascular, and metabolic protective effects,[31] may lead to new and more effective medications.[26] *Health Promotion:* Hypertension provides information on how individuals can help prevent and control hypertension.

Populations with high dietary sodium intake have long been shown to have an increased incidence of hypertension.[36] Low dietary potassium, calcium, and magnesium intakes also are risk factors because without their intake, sodium is retained. The natriuretic hormones modulate renal sodium (Na^+) excretion and require adequate potassium, calcium, and magnesium to function properly. The natriuretic hormones include atrial natriuretic peptide (ANP), B-type natriuretic peptide (BNP), C-type natriuretic peptide (CNP), and urodilatin. Dysfunction of these hormones, along with alterations in the RAAS and the SNS, causes an increase in vascular tone and a shift in the pressure–natriuresis relationship. When there is inadequate natriuretic function, serum levels of the natriuretic peptides increase. In hypertension, increased ANP and BNP levels are linked to an increased risk for ventricular hypertrophy, atherosclerosis, and HF.[37] Salt retention leads to water retention and increased blood volume, which contributes to an increase in blood pressure. Subtle renal injury results, with renal vasoconstriction and tissue ischemia. Tissue ischemia causes inflammation of the kidney and contributes to dysfunction of the glomeruli and tubules, which promotes additional sodium retention. Salt restriction combined with adequate intake of dietary potassium, magnesium, and calcium has been linked to improved natriuretic peptide function.[38]

Inflammation plays a role in the pathogenesis of hypertension. One proposed mechanism for initiating hypertension-related inflammation is *peripheral vascular resistance–mediated ischemic cellular injury* and the release of **damage-associated molecular patterns (DAMPs)** that activate Toll-like receptors on immune cells[39] (see Chapter 6). Activation of innate and adaptive immunity results in damage to endothelial cells.[40] Endothelial injury and tissue ischemia result in the release of vasoactive inflammatory cytokines. Although many of these cytokines (e.g., histamine, prostaglandins) have vasodilatory actions in acute inflammatory injury, chronic inflammation leads to decreased production of vasodilators (such as nitric oxide), vascular remodelling, and smooth muscle contraction. Inflammation also contributes to insulin resistance, decreased natriuresis, and autonomic dysfunction (increased SNS activity).[41-43]

Obesity is recognized as an important risk factor for hypertension in both adults and children and contributes to many of the neurohumoral, metabolic, renal, and cardiovascular processes that cause hypertension (see *Health Promotion:* Obesity and Hypertension).[44] Obesity causes changes in the adipokines (i.e., leptin and adiponectin) and also is associated with increased activity of the SNS and the RAAS.[45] Obesity is linked to inflammation, endothelial dysfunction, and insulin resistance and an increased risk for cardiovascular complications from hypertension.[44]

Finally, insulin resistance is common in hypertension, even in individuals without clinical diabetes. Insulin resistance is associated with decreased endothelial release of nitric oxide and other vasodilators.[46]

HEALTH PROMOTION

Hypertension

According to Hypertension Prevention and Control and Hypertension Canada, adjusting modifiable risk factors such as excess body fat, low dietary potassium (low fruit and vegetable intake), physical inactivity, and high alcohol intake can help prevent and control hypertension for most individuals.

Hypertension is related to eating an unhealthy diet, specifically one that is high in sodium. It is estimated that high sodium intake causes 32% of all cases of hypertension in Canada. Current national guidelines recommend consuming less than 2 300 mg of sodium per day. Reducing sodium intake at a population level has been shown repeatedly to be cost saving, effective, and efficient in preventing early cardiovascular disease.

Canada has the highest rate of hypertension awareness, treatment, and control worldwide. However, Hypertension Prevention and Control and Hypertension Canada recommend public policies for the prevention and control of hypertension. For example, they recommend screening for high blood pressure and providing education about healthy behaviours. These strategies have proven to be cost-effective in recognizing adults at increased risk for cardiovascular disease due to high blood pressure, and for initiating early treatment to prevent future complications.

Data from Hypertension Prevention and Control, & Hypertension Canada. (2016). *Fact sheet: Hypertension in Canada.* Retrieved from http://www.hypertensiontalk.com/wp-content/uploads/2016/05/HTN-Fact-Sheet-2016_FINAL.pdf.

It also affects renal function and causes renal salt and water retention. Insulin resistance is associated with overactivity of the SNS and the RAAS. It is interesting to note that in many individuals with diabetes treated with medications that increase insulin sensitivity, blood pressure often declines, even in the absence of antihypertensive medications. The interactions between obesity, hypertension, insulin resistance, and lipid disorders in MetS result in a high risk for cardiovascular disease.[46]

It is likely that primary hypertension is an interaction between many of these factors leading to sustained increases in blood volume and peripheral resistance. The pathophysiology of primary hypertension is summarized in Figure 24-5.

HEALTH PROMOTION

Obesity and Hypertension

According to a 2016 report of The Standing Senate Committee on Social Affairs, Science and Technology, each year 48 000 to 66 000 Canadians die from conditions linked to excess weight. Moreover, it is estimated that two-thirds of adults and one-third of children are obese or overweight, costing Canada between $4.6 billion and $7.1 billion per year in health care and lost productivity.

The same report notes the role of the social determinants of health within the context of increasing obesity rates, establishing that socioeconomic status (which relates to household income, education level, and occupation) is linked to obesity. The report concludes that men of higher socioeconomic status and women of lower socioeconomic status have the highest obesity rates.

Food insecurity, due to an individual's or a household's inability to buy an adequate supply of food on an ongoing basis, is directly related to income. In Canada, 1 in 8 households is food insecure due to lack of income, which deprives people of the opportunity to purchase healthy foods and limits their options to food they can afford. The food available to low-income Canadians is often highly processed and ready to eat, but is also the least healthy.

Data from Hypertension Canada. (2016). *Key messages.* Markham, ON: Author. Retrieved from http://www.hypertension.ca/images/CHEP_2016/2016_KeyMessages_EN.pdf; The Standing Senate Committee on Social Affairs, Science and Technology. (2016). *Obesity in Canada: A whole-of-society approach for a healthier Canada.* Ottawa: Author. Retrieved from https://sencanada.ca/content/sen/committee/421/SOCI/Reports/2016-02-25_Revised_report_Obesity_in_Canada_e.pdf.

Secondary Hypertension

Secondary hypertension is caused by an underlying disease process or medication that raises peripheral vascular resistance or cardiac output. Examples include renal vascular or parenchymal disease, adrenocortical tumours, adrenomedullary tumours (pheochromocytoma), and medications (oral contraceptives, corticosteroids, antihistamines). If the cause is identified and removed before permanent structural changes occur, blood pressure returns to normal.

Complicated Hypertension

As hypertension becomes more severe and chronic, tissue damage can occur in the blood vessels and tissues leading to target organ damage in the heart, kidney, brain, and eyes. Cardiovascular complications of sustained hypertension include left ventricular hypertrophy, angina pectoris, HF, coronary artery disease (CAD), MI, and sudden death. Myocardial hypertrophy in response to hypertension is mediated by several neurohormonal substances, including catecholamines from the SNS and Ang II. Hypertrophy is characterized by changes in the myocyte proteins, apoptosis of myocytes, and deposition of collagen in heart muscle, which causes it to become thickened, scarred, and less able to relax during diastole, leading to HF with preserved ejection fraction.[47] In addition, the increased size of the heart muscle increases demand for oxygen delivery over time, the contractility of the heart is impaired, and the individual is at increased risk for MI and HF with reduced ejection fraction. Vascular complications include the formation, dissection, and rupture of aneurysms (outpouchings in vessel walls) and atherosclerosis leading to vessel occlusion.

Renal complications of complicated hypertension include parenchymal damage, nephrosclerosis, renal arteriosclerosis, and renal insufficiency or failure. Microalbuminuria (small amounts of protein in the urine) occurs in 10 to 25% of individuals with primary hypertension and is now recognized as an early sign of impending renal dysfunction and significantly increased risk for cardiovascular events, especially in those who also have diabetes.[48] Complications specific to the retina include retinal vascular sclerosis, exudation, and hemorrhage. Cerebrovascular complications include transient ischemia, stroke, cerebral thrombosis, aneurysm, hemorrhage, and dementia.[49] The pathological effects of complicated hypertension are summarized in Table 24-2.

Hypertensive crisis (or **malignant hypertension**) is rapidly progressive hypertension in which diastolic pressure is usually greater than 140 mm Hg. It can occur in those with primary hypertension, but the

TABLE 24-2 Pathological Effects of Sustained, Complicated Primary Hypertension

Site of Injury	Mechanism of Injury	Potential Pathological Effect
Heart		
Myocardium	Increased workload combined with diminished blood flow through coronary arteries	Left ventricular hypertrophy, myocardial ischemia, heart failure
Coronary arteries	Accelerated atherosclerosis (coronary artery disease)	Myocardial ischemia, myocardial infarction, sudden death
Kidneys	Reduced blood flow, increased arteriolar pressure, RAAS and SNS stimulation, and inflammation	Glomerulosclerosis and decreased glomerular filtration, end-stage renal disease
Brain	Reduced blood flow and oxygen supply; weakened vessel walls, accelerated atherosclerosis	Transient ischemic attacks, cerebral thrombosis, aneurysm, hemorrhage, acute brain infarction
Eyes (retinas)	Retinal vascular sclerosis, increased retinal artery pressures	Hypertensive retinopathy, retinal exudates and hemorrhages
Aorta	Weakened vessel wall	Dissecting aneurysm
Arteries of lower extremities	Reduced blood flow and high pressures in arterioles, accelerated atherosclerosis	Intermittent claudication, gangrene

RAAS, renin-angiotensin-aldosterone system; *SNS*, sympathetic nervous system.

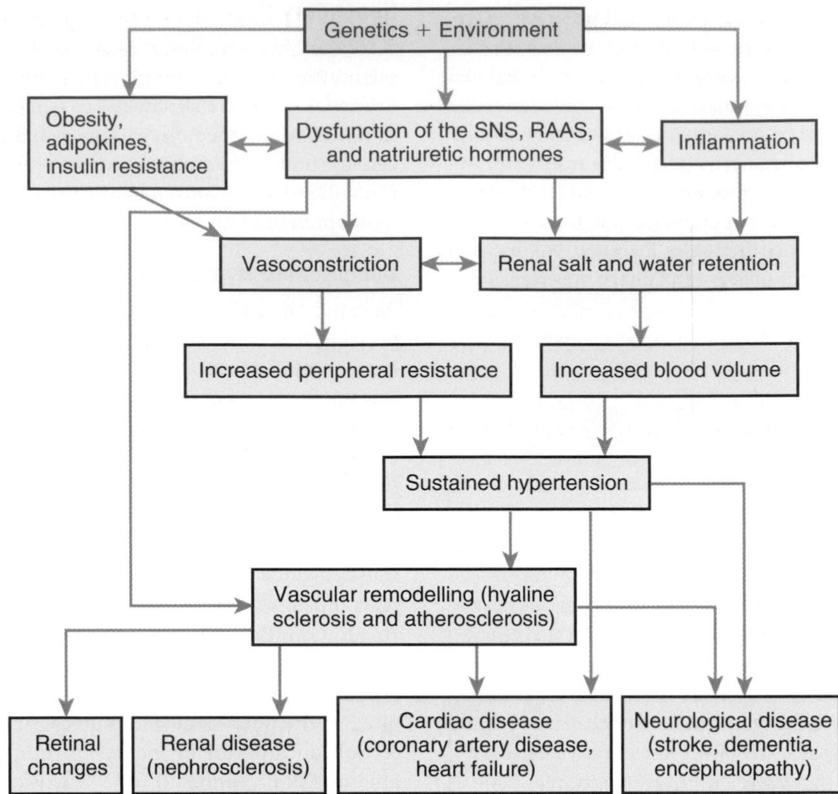

FIGURE 24-5 Pathophysiology of Hypertension. Numerous genetic vulnerabilities have been linked to hypertension and these, in combination with environmental risks, cause neurohumoral dysfunction (sympathetic nervous system [*SNS*], renin-angiotensin-aldosterone system [*RAAS*], and natriuretic hormones) and promote inflammation and insulin resistance. Insulin resistance and neurohumoral dysfunction contribute to sustained systemic vasoconstriction and increased peripheral resistance. Inflammation contributes to renal dysfunction, which, in combination with the neurohumoral alterations, results in renal salt and water retention and increased blood volume. Increased peripheral resistance and increased blood volume are two primary causes of sustained hypertension.

reason why some people develop this complication and others do not is unknown. Other causes include complications of pregnancy, cocaine or amphetamine use, reaction to certain medications, adrenal tumours, and alcohol withdrawal. High arterial pressure renders the cerebral arterioles incapable of regulating blood flow to the cerebral capillary beds. High hydrostatic pressures in the capillaries cause vascular fluid to exude into the interstitial space. If blood pressure is not reduced, cerebral edema and cerebral dysfunction (encephalopathy) increase until death occurs. Organ damage resulting from malignant hypertension is life-threatening. Besides encephalopathy, hypertensive crisis can cause papilledema, cardiac failure, uremia, retinopathy, and cerebrovascular accident and is considered a medical emergency.[50]

CLINICAL MANIFESTATIONS The early stages of hypertension have no clinical manifestations other than elevated blood pressure; for this reason, hypertension is called a silent disease. Some hypertensive individuals never have signs, symptoms, or complications, whereas others become very ill, and hypertension can be a cause of death. Still other individuals have anatomical and physiological damage caused by past hypertensive disease, despite current blood pressure measurements being within normal ranges. If elevated blood pressure is not detected and treated, it becomes established and may begin to accelerate its effects on tissues when the individual is 30 to 50 years of age. This sets the stage for the complications of hypertension that begin to appear during the fourth, fifth, and sixth decades of life.

Most clinical manifestations of hypertensive disease are caused by complications that damage organs and tissues outside the vascular system. Besides elevated blood pressure, the signs and symptoms therefore tend to be specific for the organs or tissues affected. Evidence of heart disease, renal insufficiency, central nervous system dysfunction, impaired vision, impaired mobility, vascular occlusion, or edema can all be caused by sustained hypertension.

EVALUATION AND TREATMENT A single elevated blood pressure reading does not mean that a person has hypertension. Diagnosis requires the measurement of blood pressure on at least two separate occasions, averaging two readings at least 2 minutes apart, with the following conditions: the person is seated, the arm is supported at heart level, the person must be at rest for at least 5 minutes, and the person should not have smoked or ingested any caffeine in the previous 30 minutes.[12] Diagnostic tests for further evaluation of hypertension include 24-hour blood pressure monitoring in selected individuals, complete blood count, urinalysis, biochemical blood profile (measures levels of plasma glucose, sodium, potassium, calcium, magnesium, creatinine, cholesterol, and triglycerides), and an electrocardiogram (ECG). Individuals who have elevated blood pressure are assumed to have primary hypertension unless their history, physical examination, or initial diagnostic screening indicates secondary hypertension. Once the diagnosis is made, a careful evaluation for other cardiovascular risk factors and for end-organ damage should be done.

Treatment of primary hypertension depends on its severity. Hypertension Canada recommends beginning with lifestyle modification in preventing and treating hypertension.[12] Important lifestyle modifications include following an exercise program, making dietary modifications, stopping smoking, and losing weight. Reducing salt intake is an important dietary modification and has been shown to significantly reduce blood pressure in both hypertensive and normotensive individuals.[36,51] Pharmacological treatment of hypertension reduces the risk for end-organ damage and prevents major diseases, such as MI and stroke. Hypertension Canada recommends that treatment begin with thiazide diuretics alone or in combination with Ang II blockers (ACE inhibitors or ARBs) or calcium channel blockers.[52] Beta-blockers were found to have a higher rate of stroke than Ang II blockers and are no longer recommended as first-line medications. Individuals with HF, chronic kidney disease, or a history of MI or stroke should begin antihypertensive treatment with an ACE inhibitor or ARB. Some individuals require two or more medications for blood pressure control.

Hypertension Canada also recommends that antihypertensive therapy be prescribed for average diastolic blood pressure measurements of greater than or equal to 100 mm Hg or average systolic blood pressure measurements of greater than or equal to 160 mm Hg in patients without macrovascular target organ damage or other cardiovascular risk factors. It also strongly recommends that antihypertensive therapy be considered for average diastolic blood pressure readings greater than or equal to 90 mm Hg or for average systolic blood pressure readings greater than or equal to 140 mm Hg in the presence of macrovascular target organ damage or other independent cardiovascular risk factors.[52]

In individuals with refractive hypertension, catheter-based renal denervation can result in significant reductions in blood pressure,[53] but many questions remain pertaining to long-term safety, mechanisms of action, and selection of appropriate candidates for the procedure.[54] Careful follow-up to support continued adherence, determine the response, and monitor for potential adverse effects of these medications is important.

Orthostatic (Postural) Hypotension

The term **orthostatic (postural) hypotension (OH)** refers to a decrease in systolic blood pressure of at least 20 mm Hg or a decrease in diastolic blood pressure of at least 10 mm Hg within 3 minutes of moving to a standing position.[55] *Idiopathic*, or primary, OH implies no known initial cause. This kind of OH is often called *neurogenic* and is usually the result of primary neurological disorders or secondary to conditions that affect autonomic function.[56] It affects men more often than women and usually occurs between the ages of 40 and 70 years. Up to 18% of older adults may be affected by primary OH, and it is a significant risk factor for falls and associated injury, with increased mortality.[57] Recently, OH has been implicated in contributing to depression and dementia.[58]

Normally when an individual stands, the gravitational changes on the circulation are compensated by such mechanisms as baroreceptor-mediated reflex arteriolar and venous constriction and increased heart rate. Other compensatory mechanisms include mechanical factors, such as the closure of valves in the venous system, contraction of the leg muscles, and a decrease in intrathoracic pressure.[58] The normally increased sympathetic activity during upright posture is mediated through a stretch receptor (baroreceptor) reflex that responds to shifts in volume caused by postural changes. This reflex promptly increases heart rate and constricts the systemic arterioles. Thus, arterial blood pressure is maintained. These mechanisms are dysfunctional or inadequate in individuals with OH; consequently, upon standing, blood pools and normal arterial pressure cannot be maintained.

OH may be acute or chronic. Acute OH is caused when the normal regulatory mechanisms are sluggish as a result of (1) altered body chemistry, (2) medication action (e.g., antihypertensives, antidepressants), (3) prolonged immobility caused by illness, (4) starvation, (5) physical exhaustion, (6) any condition that produces volume depletion (e.g., dehydration, diuresis, potassium or sodium depletion), or (7) any condition that results in venous pooling (e.g., pregnancy, extensive varicosities of the lower extremities). Older adults are particularly susceptible to this type of OH.

Chronic orthostatic hypotension may be (1) secondary to a specific disease or (2) idiopathic or primary. The diseases that cause secondary OH are endocrine disorders (e.g., adrenal insufficiency, diabetes), metabolic disorders (e.g., porphyria), or diseases of the central or peripheral nervous systems (e.g., Parkinson's disease, multiple system atrophy, intracranial tumours, cerebral infarcts, Wernicke encephalopathy, peripheral neuropathies). Cardiovascular autonomic neuropathy is a common cause of OH in persons with diabetes and is a serious and often overlooked complication. In addition to cardiovascular symptoms, associated impotence and bowel and bladder dysfunction are common.

OH is often accompanied by dizziness, blurring or loss of vision, and syncope or fainting caused by insufficient vasomotor compensation and reduction of blood flow through the brain. Although no curative treatment is available for idiopathic OH, often it can be managed adequately with a combination of nondrug and medication therapies—increasing fluid and salt intake, wearing thigh-high stockings, and taking mineralocorticoids and vasoconstrictors.[56,58]

QUICK CHECK 24-2

1. What are the major risk factors for hypertension?
2. Summarize the pathophysiology of primary hypertension.
3. What is malignant hypertension?
4. What are the causes of orthostatic hypotension?

Aneurysm

An **aneurysm** is a localized dilation or outpouching of a vessel wall or cardiac chamber (Figure 24-6). Laplace's law (discussed in detail in Chapter 23) can provide an understanding of the hemodynamics of an aneurysm. **True aneurysms** involve all three layers of the arterial wall and are best described as a weakening of the vessel wall (Figure 24-7, *A*). Most are fusiform and circumferential, whereas *saccular aneurysms* are basically spherical in shape. A **false aneurysm** is an extravascular hematoma that communicates with the intravascular space. A common cause of this type of lesion is a leak between a vascular graft and a natural artery.

Aneurysms most commonly occur in the thoracic or abdominal aorta. The aorta is particularly susceptible to aneurysm formation because of constant stress on the vessel wall and the absence of penetrating vasa vasorum in the media layer. Genetic and environmental risk factors (such as smoking and diet) are implicated in the pathogenesis of aortic aneurysms.[59] Atherosclerosis is the most common cause of arterial aneurysms because plaque formation erodes the vessel wall and contributes to inflammation and release of proteinases that can further weaken the vessel. Hypertension also contributes to aneurysm formation by increasing wall stress. Collagen vascular disorders (e.g., Marfan's syndrome), syphilis, and other infections that affect arterial walls also can cause aneurysms.

Cardiac aneurysms most commonly form after MI when intraventricular tension stretches the noncontracting infarcted muscle. The stretching produces infarct expansion, a weak and thin layer of necrotic muscle, and fibrous tissue that bulges with each systole.

Clinical manifestations depend on where the aneurysm is located. Aortic aneurysms often are asymptomatic until they rupture, and then cause severe pain and hypotension. Thoracic aortic aneurysms can cause dysphagia (difficulty swallowing) and dyspnea (breathlessness). An aneurysm that impairs flow to an extremity causes symptoms of ischemia. Cerebral aneurysms, which often occur in the circle of Willis, are associated with signs and symptoms of increased intracranial pressure.

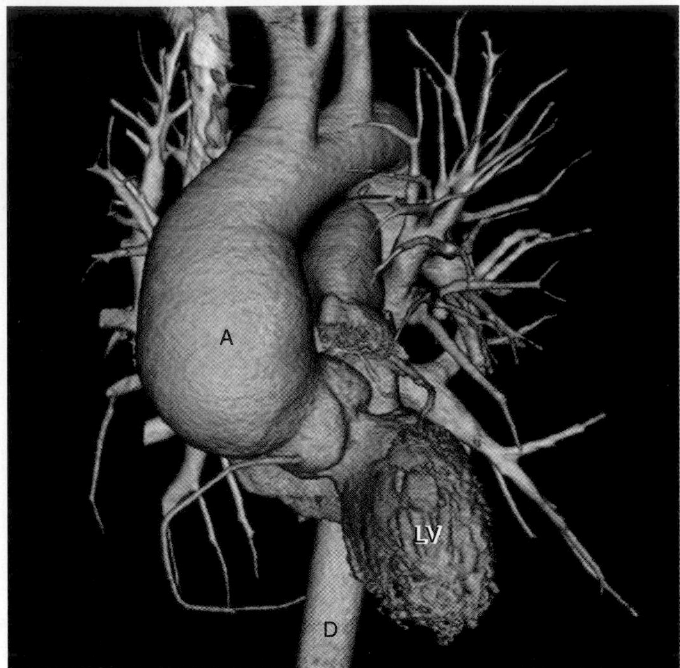

FIGURE 24-6 Aneurysm. A three-dimensional CT scan shows the aneurysm (*A*) involving the ascending thoracic aorta. *D*, descending aorta; *LV*, left ventricle.

Signs and symptoms of stroke occur when cerebral aneurysms leak. (Cerebral aneurysms are described in Chapter 16.) Aneurysms in the heart present with dysrhythmias, HF, and embolism of clots to the brain or other vital organs.

Aortic aneurysms can be complicated by acute aortic syndromes, which include aortic dissection, hemorrhage into the vessel wall, or vessel rupture. Dissection of the layers of the arterial wall occurs when there is a tear in the intima and blood enters the wall of the artery (Figure 24-7, *B*). Dissections can involve any part of the aorta (ascending, arch, or descending) and can disrupt flow through arterial branches, thus creating a surgical emergency.

The diagnosis of an aneurysm is usually confirmed by ultrasonography, CT, MRI, or angiography. Medical treatment is indicated for slow-growing aortic aneurysms, particularly in early stages, and includes cessation of smoking, reduction of blood pressure and blood volume, and implementation of β-adrenergic blockade. For those aneurysms that are dilating rapidly or have become large, surgical treatment is indicated and usually includes replacement with a prosthetic graft. Endovascular surgical techniques are commonly used for aneurysm repair and management of acute aortic rupture.[60]

Thrombus Formation

As in venous thrombosis, arterial thrombi tend to develop when intravascular conditions promote activation of coagulation, or when there is stasis of blood flow. These conditions include those in which there is intimal irritation or roughening (such as in surgical procedures), inflammation, traumatic injury, infection, low blood pressures, or obstructions that cause blood stasis and pooling within the vessels. (Mechanisms of coagulation are described in Chapter 20.) Inflammation of the endothelium leads to activation of the clotting cascade, causing platelets to adhere readily. An anatomical change in an artery (such as an aneurysm) can contribute to thrombus formation, particularly if

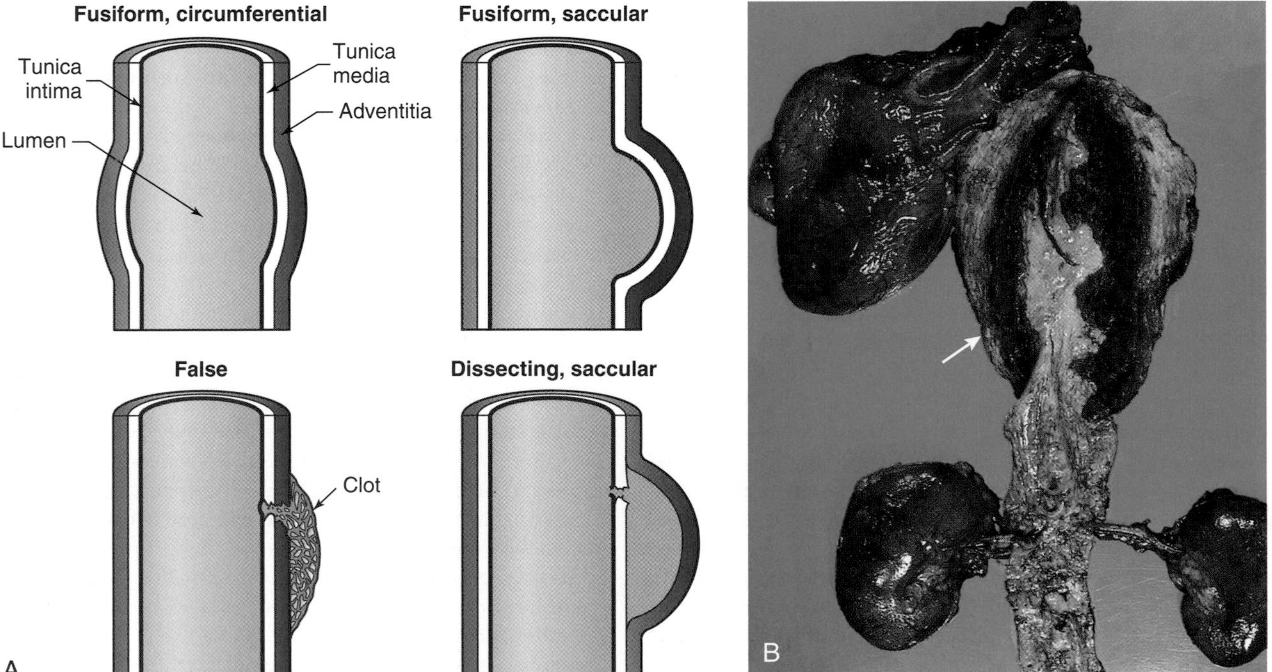

FIGURE 24-7 Longitudinal Sections Showing Types of Aneurysms. A, The fusiform circumferential and fusiform saccular aneurysms are true aneurysms, caused by weakening of the vessel wall. False and saccular aneurysms involve a break in the vessel wall, usually caused by trauma. **B,** Dissecting aneurysm of thoracic aorta (*arrow*). (**B,** from Damjanov, I., & Linder, J. [Eds.]. [1996]. *Anderson's pathology* [10th ed.]. St. Louis: Mosby.)

the change results in a pooling of arterial blood. Thrombi also form on heart valves altered by calcification or bacterial vegetation. Valvular thrombi are most commonly associated with inflammation of the endocardium (endocarditis) and rheumatic heart disease. Widespread arterial thrombus formation can occur in shock, particularly shock resulting from septicemia. In septic shock, systemic inflammation activates the intrinsic and extrinsic pathways of coagulation, resulting in microvascular thrombosis throughout the systemic arterial circulation.

Arterial thrombi pose two potential threats to the circulation. First, the thrombus may grow large enough to occlude the artery, causing ischemia in tissue supplied by the artery. Second, the thrombus may dislodge, becoming a thromboembolus that travels through the vascular system until it occludes flow into a distal systemic vascular bed.

Diagnosis of arterial thrombi is usually accomplished through the use of Doppler ultrasonography and angiography. Pharmacological treatment involves the administration of heparin, warfarin derivatives, thrombin inhibitors, or thrombolytics. A balloon-tipped catheter also can be used to remove or compress an arterial thrombus. Various combinations of medication and catheter therapies are sometimes used concurrently.

Embolism

Embolism is the obstruction of a vessel by an **embolus**—a bolus of matter circulating in the bloodstream. The embolus may consist of a dislodged thrombus; an air bubble; an aggregate of amniotic fluid; an aggregate of fat, bacteria, or cancer cells; or a foreign substance. An embolus travels in the bloodstream until it reaches a vessel through which it cannot pass. No matter how tiny it is, an embolus will eventually lodge in a systemic or pulmonary vessel determined by its source. Pulmonary emboli originate on the venous side (mostly from the deep veins of the legs) of the systemic circulation or in the right heart; arterial emboli most commonly originate in the left heart and are associated with thrombi after MI, valvular disease, left ventricular failure, endocarditis, and dysrhythmias.

Embolism causes ischemia or infarction in tissues distal to the obstruction, producing organ dysfunction and pain. Infarction and subsequent necrosis of a central organ are life-threatening. For example, occlusion of a coronary artery will cause an MI, whereas occlusion of a cerebral artery causes a stroke (see Chapter 16). The types of emboli are summarized in Table 24-3.

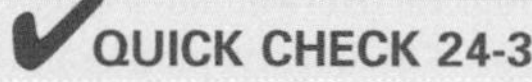
QUICK CHECK 24-3

1. How does Laplace's law function in aneurysms?
2. What is a thrombus?
3. Why are emboli dangerous?

TABLE 24-3 Types of Emboli

Type	Characteristics
Arteries	
Arterial thromboembolism	Dislodged thrombus; source is usually from heart; most common sites of obstruction are lower extremities (femoral and popliteal arteries), coronary arteries, and cerebral vasculature
Veins	
Venous thromboembolism	Dislodged thrombus; source is usually from lower extremities; obstructs branches of pulmonary artery
Air embolism	Bolus of air displaces blood in vasculature; source usually room air entering circulation through intravenous (IV) lines; trauma to chest also may allow air from lungs to enter vascular space
Amniotic fluid embolism	Bolus of amniotic fluid; extensive intra-abdominal pressure attending labour and delivery can force amniotic fluid into bloodstream of mother; introduces antigens, cells, and protein aggregates that trigger inflammation, coagulation, and immune responses
Bacterial embolism	Aggregates of bacteria in bloodstream; source is subacute bacterial endocarditis or abscess
Fat embolism	Globules of fat floating in bloodstream associated with trauma to long bones; lungs in particular are affected
Foreign matter	Small particles or fibres introduced during trauma or through an IV or intra-arterial line; coagulation cascade is initiated and thromboemboli form around particles

Peripheral Vascular Disease

Thromboangiitis Obliterans (Buerger's Disease)

Thromboangiitis obliterans (Buerger's disease) is an inflammatory disease of the peripheral arteries. It is strongly associated with smoking. Buerger's disease is an autoimmune condition characterized by the formation of thrombi filled with inflammatory and immune cells.[61] Inflammatory cytokines and toxic oxygen free radicals contribute to accompanying vasospasm.[62] Over time, these thrombi become organized and fibrotic and result in permanent occlusion and obliteration of portions of small- and medium-sized arteries in the feet and sometimes in the hands. Although collateral vessels develop in Buerger's disease, they are inadequate to supply the extremities with blood. These collateral vessels have a characteristic corkscrew shape, thought to be a result of dilated vasa vasorum in the affected artery.

The chief symptom of Buerger's disease is pain and tenderness of the affected part, usually affecting more than one extremity. Clinical manifestations are caused by sluggish blood flow and include rubor (redness of the skin), which is caused by dilated capillaries under the skin, and cyanosis, which is caused by tissue ischemia. Chronic ischemia causes the skin to thin and become shiny and the nails to become thickened and malformed. In advanced disease, profound ischemia of the extremities resulting from vessel obliteration can cause gangrene necessitating amputation. Buerger's disease has also been associated with cerebrovascular disease (stroke), mesenteric disease, and rheumatic symptoms (joint pain).

Diagnosis of Buerger's disease is made by identification of the following common features—age less than 45 years, smoking history, evidence of peripheral ischemia—and by exclusion of other causes of arterial insufficiency. The most important part of treatment is cessation of cigarette smoking. If the person continues to smoke, the likelihood of recurrence of the disease and gangrene requiring amputation is high. Other measures are aimed at improving circulation to the foot or hand. Vasodilators are prescribed to alleviate vasospasm, and the individual receives instruction in exercises that use gravity to improve blood flow.

Raynaud Phenomenon

Raynaud phenomenon is characterized by attacks of vasospasm in the small arteries and arterioles of the fingers and, less commonly, the toes. Primary Raynaud phenomenon is a common primary vasospastic disorder of unknown origin. Secondary Raynaud phenomenon is associated with systemic diseases, particularly collagen vascular disease (scleroderma), vasculitis, malignancy, pulmonary hypertension, chemotherapy, cocaine use, hypothyroidism, thoracic outlet syndrome, trauma, serum sickness, or long-term exposure to environmental conditions such as cold temperatures or vibrating machinery in the workplace. Blood vessels in affected individuals demonstrate endothelial dysfunction with an imbalance in endothelium-derived vasodilators (e.g., nitric oxide) and vasoconstrictors (e.g., endothelin-1).[63] Platelet activation also may play a role, and autoantibodies have been identified in some individuals. Secondary Raynaud phenomenon tends to affect young women and is characterized by vasospastic attacks triggered by brief exposure to cold, vibration, or emotional stress. Genetic predisposition may play a role in its development.

The clinical manifestations of the vasospastic attacks of either disorder are changes in skin colour and sensation caused by ischemia. Vasospasm occurs with varying frequency and severity and causes pallor, numbness, and the sensation of coldness in the digits. Attacks tend to be bilateral, and manifestations usually begin at the tips of the digits and progress to the proximal phalanges. Sluggish blood flow resulting from ischemia may cause the skin to appear cyanotic. Rubor, throbbing pain, and paresthesias follow as blood flow returns. Skin colour returns to normal after the attack, but frequent, prolonged attacks interfere with cellular metabolism, causing the skin of the fingertips to thicken and the nails to become brittle. In severe, chronic Raynaud phenomenon, ischemia can eventually cause ulceration and gangrene.

Once evident, the clinical manifestations confirm the diagnosis of Raynaud phenomenon; however, nailfold capillaroscopy is a more sensitive method of diagnosis and can improve management and follow-up of individuals with associated collagen vascular disorders.[64] Treatment for Raynaud phenomenon consists of removing the stimulus or treating the primary disease process. Treatment of Raynaud phenomenon begins with avoidance of stimuli that trigger attacks (e.g., cold temperatures, emotional stress) and cessation of cigarette smoking to eliminate the vasoconstricting effects of nicotine. If attacks of vasospasm become frequent or prolonged, vasodilators, such as calcium channel blockers, nitric oxide agonists, alpha-blockers, prostaglandin analogues, or endothelin antagonists, are administered.[63] Sympathectomy may be indicated in severe cases, but may not be effective. If ischemia leads to ulceration and gangrene, amputation may be necessary.

QUICK CHECK 24-4

1. What is Buerger's disease, and why does it occur?
2. Compare the physical manifestations of Buerger's disease and Raynaud phenomenon.

Atherosclerosis

Arteriosclerosis is a condition characterized by thickening and hardening of the vessel wall. **Atherosclerosis** is a form of arteriosclerosis that is caused by the accumulation of lipid-laden macrophages within the arterial wall, which leads to the formation of a lesion called a **plaque**. Atherosclerosis is not a single disease entity but rather a pathological process that can affect vascular systems throughout the body, resulting in ischemic syndromes that can vary widely in their severity and clinical manifestations. It is the leading cause of CAD and cerebrovascular disease. (Atherosclerosis of the coronary arteries is described in "Coronary Artery Disease, Myocardial Ischemia, and Acute Coronary Syndromes," later in this chapter, and atherosclerosis of the cerebral arteries is described in Chapter 16.)

PATHOPHYSIOLOGY Atherosclerosis begins with injury to the endothelial cells that line artery walls. Pathologically, the lesions progress from endothelial injury and dysfunction to fatty streak to fibrotic plaque to complicated lesion (Figure 24-8). Possible causes of **endothelial injury** include the common risk factors for atherosclerosis, such as smoking, hypertension, diabetes, increased levels of low-density lipoprotein (LDL), decreased levels of high-density lipoprotein (HDL), and autoimmunity. Other "nontraditional" risk factors include increased serum markers for inflammation and thrombosis (such as **high-sensitivity C-reactive protein [hs-CRP]**, troponin I, adipokines, infection, and air pollution). These risk factors are discussed in more detail in "Coronary Artery Disease, Myocardial Ischemia, and Acute Coronary Syndromes," later in this chapter.

Injured endothelial cells become inflamed. Inflammation plays a fundamental role in mediating the steps in the initiation and progression of atherogenesis.[65] Inflamed endothelial cells cannot make normal amounts of antithrombic and vasodilating cytokines. Evidence is accumulating that microRNAs (short pieces of RNA that regulate post-transcriptional gene expression) are activated by many of the risk factors for atherosclerosis and impact endothelial cell responses to injury.[66]

The next step in atherogenesis occurs when inflamed endothelial cells express adhesion molecules that bind macrophages and other inflammatory and immune cells (Figure 24-9). Macrophages are activated by binding to DAMPs released from injured cells, and release numerous inflammatory cytokines (e.g., tumour necrosis factor-alpha [TNF-α], interferons, interleukins, and C-reactive protein [CRP]) and enzymes that further injure the vessel wall.[65,67] Toxic oxygen free radicals generated by the inflammatory process cause oxidation (i.e., addition of oxygen) of LDL that has accumulated in the vessel intima. Dyslipidemia, diabetes, smoking, and hypertension contribute to LDL oxidation and its accumulation in the vessel wall.[68] Oxidized LDL causes additional adhesion molecule expression with the recruitment of monocytes that differentiate into macrophages. These macrophages penetrate into the intima, where they engulf oxidized LDL. These lipid-laden macrophages are now called **foam cells**, and when they accumulate in significant amounts, they form a lesion called a **fatty streak** (see Figures 24-8 and 24-9). These lesions can be found in the walls of arteries of most people, even young children. Once formed, fatty streaks produce more toxic oxygen free radicals, recruit T lymphocytes (T cells) leading to autoimmunity, and secrete additional inflammatory mediators resulting in progressive damage to the vessel wall.[65]

Macrophages also release growth factors that stimulate smooth muscle cell proliferation.[67] Smooth muscle cells in the region of endothelial injury proliferate, produce collagen, and migrate over the fatty streak, forming a **fibrous plaque** (see Figure 24-10). The fibrous plaque may calcify, protrude into the vessel lumen, and obstruct blood flow to distal tissues (especially during exercise), which may cause symptoms (e.g., angina or intermittent claudication).

Many plaques, however, are "unstable," meaning they are prone to rupture even before they affect blood flow significantly and are clinically silent until they rupture. Plaque rupture occurs because of innate and adaptive immune responses to tissue injury, including activation of proteinases (matrix metalloproteinases and cathepsins) and apoptosis of cells within the plaque, and can be accelerated by bleeding within the lesion (plaque hemorrhage).[65] Plaques that have ruptured are called **complicated plaques**. Once rupture occurs, exposure of underlying tissue results in platelet adhesion, initiation of the clotting cascade, and rapid thrombus formation. The thrombus may suddenly occlude the affected vessel, resulting in ischemia and infarction. Aspirin or other antithrombotic agents are used to prevent this complication of atherosclerotic disease.

CLINICAL MANIFESTATIONS Atherosclerosis presents with symptoms and signs that result from inadequate perfusion of tissues because of

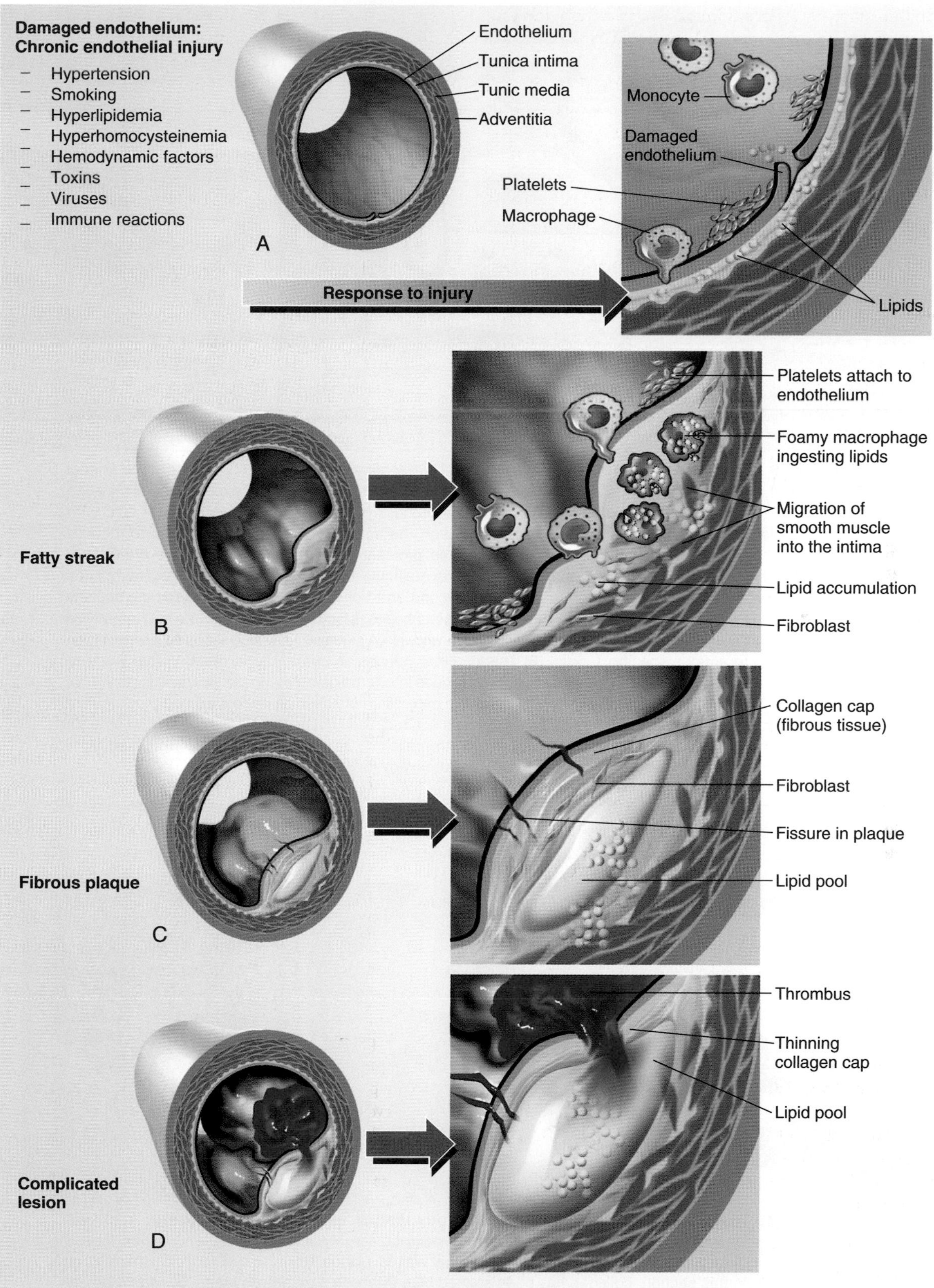

FIGURE 24-8 Progression of Atherosclerosis. A, Damaged endothelium. **B,** Diagram of fatty streak and lipid core formation (see Figure 24-9 for a diagram of oxidized low-density lipoprotein [LDL]). **C,** Diagram of fibrous plaque. Raised plaques are visible: some are yellow; others are white. **D,** Diagram of complicated lesion; thrombus is red; collagen is blue. Plaque is complicated by red thrombus deposition.

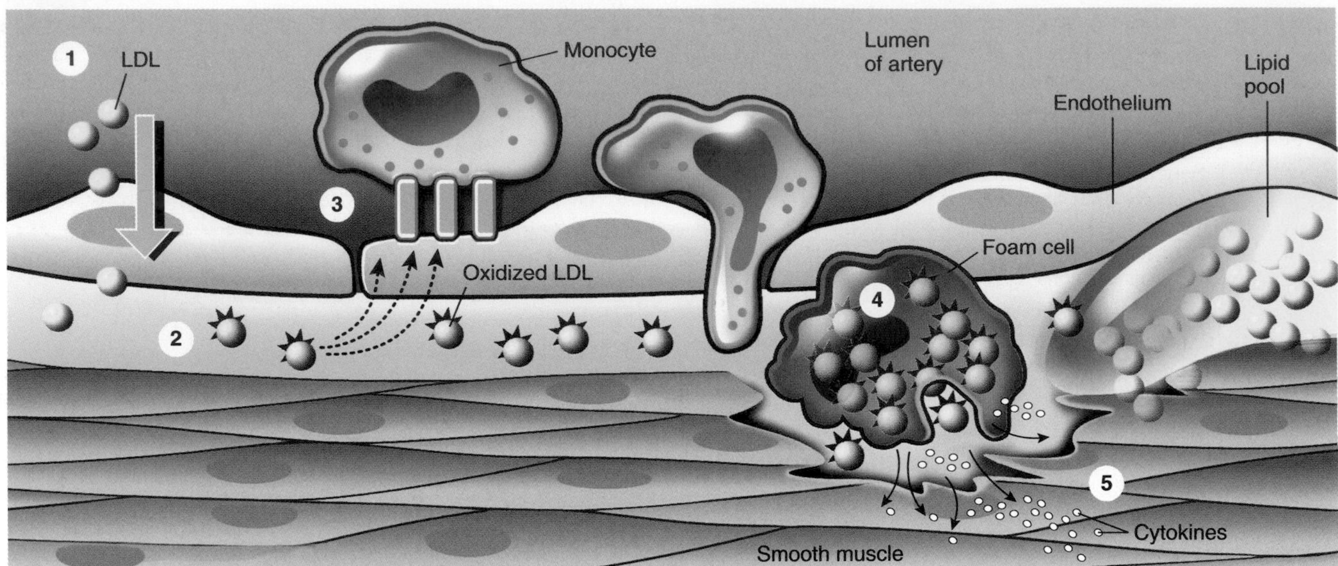

FIGURE 24-9 Low-Density Lipoprotein Oxidation. (1) Low-density lipoprotein (*LDL*) enters the arterial tunica intima through an intact endothelium. In hypercholesterolemia, the influx of LDL exceeds the eliminating capacity and an extracellular pool of LDL is formed. This process is enhanced by association of LDL with the extracellular matrix. **(2)** Intimal LDL is oxidized through the action of oxygen free radicals formed by enzymatic or nonenzymatic reactions. **(3)** This generates proinflammatory lipids that induce endothelial expression of the adhesion molecule; vascular cell adhesion molecule-1 activates complement and stimulates chemokine secretion. All of these factors cause adhesion and entry of mononuclear leukocytes, particularly monocytes and T cells. **(4)** Monocytes differentiate into macrophages. Macrophages upregulate and internalize oxidized LDL and transform into foam cells. Macrophage update of oxidized LDL also leads to presentation of its fragments to antigen-specific T cells. **(5)** This process induces an autoimmune reaction that leads to production of proinflammatory cytokines. Such cytokines include interferon-gamma, tumour necrosis factor-alpha, and interleukin-1, which act on endothelial cells to stimulate expression of adhesion molecules and procoagulant activity; on macrophages to activate proteases, endocytosis, nitric oxide (NO), and cytokines; and on smooth muscle cells to induce NO production and inhibit growth, collagen, and actin expression. (Modified from Crawford, M.H., DiMarco, J.P., & Paulus, W.J. [2010]. *Cardiology* [3rd ed.]. London: Mosby.)

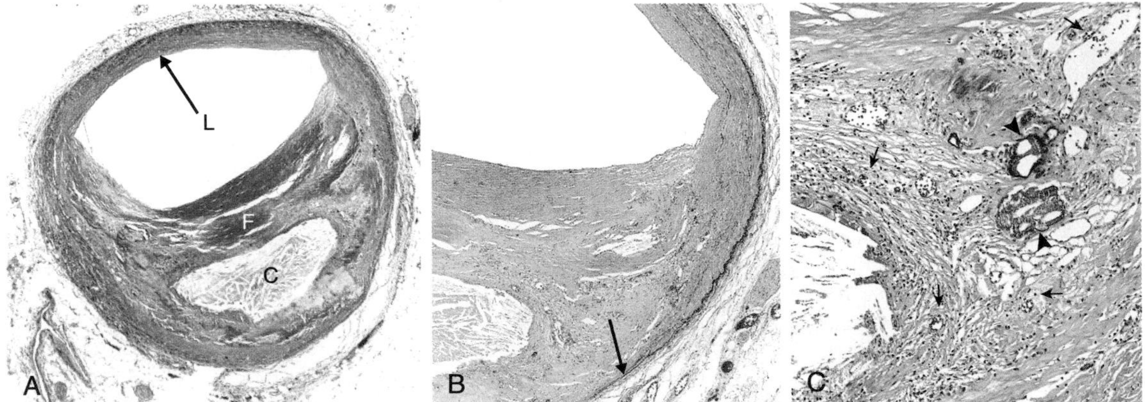

FIGURE 24-10 Histological Features of Atheromatous Plaque in the Coronary Artery. A, Overall architecture demonstrating fibrous cap (*F*) and a central necrotic (largely lipid) core (*C*). The lumen (*L*) has been moderately narrowed. Note that a segment of the wall is plaque free (*arrow*), so that there is an eccentric lesion. In this section, collagen has been stained blue (Masson's trichrome stain). **B,** Higher power photograph of a section of the plaque shown in **A,** stained for elastin (*black*), demonstrating that the internal and external elastic membranes are destroyed and the media of the artery is thinned under the most advanced plaque (*arrow*). **C,** Higher magnification photomicrograph at the junction of the fibrous cap and core, showing scattered inflammatory cells, calcification (*arrowhead*), and neovascularization (*small arrows*). (From Kumar, V., Abbas, A., & Aster J. [2007]. *Robbins Basic Pathology* [9th ed.]. St. Louis: Saunders.)

obstruction of the vessels that supply them. Partial vessel obstruction may lead to transient ischemic events, often associated with exercise or stress. As the lesion becomes complicated, increasing obstruction with superimposed thrombosis may result in tissue infarction. Obstruction of peripheral arteries can cause significant pain and disability. CAD caused by atherosclerosis is the major cause of myocardial ischemia. Atherosclerotic obstruction of the vessels supplying the brain is the major cause of stroke. Similarly, any part of the body may become ischemic when its blood supply is compromised by atherosclerotic lesions. Often, more than one vessel will become involved with this disease process such that an individual may present with symptoms from several ischemic tissues at the same time, and disease in one area may indicate that the individual is at risk for ischemic complications elsewhere.

EVALUATION AND TREATMENT In evaluating individuals for the presence of atherosclerosis, obtaining a complete health history (including risk factors and symptoms of ischemia) is essential. Physical examination may reveal arterial bruits and evidence of decreased blood flow to tissues. Laboratory data that include measurement of levels of lipids, blood glucose, and hs-CRP are also indicated. Judicious use of X-ray films, electrocardiography, ultrasonography, nuclear scanning, CT, MRI, and angiography may be necessary to identify affected vessels, particularly coronary vessels.[69] New modalities aimed at identifying vulnerable plaques before the rupture are being evaluated.[70]

Current management of atherosclerosis is focused on detection and treatment of preclinical lesions with medications aimed at stabilizing and reversing plaques before they rupture. Once a lesion obstructs blood flow, the primary goal in the management of atherosclerosis is to restore adequate blood flow to the affected tissues. If an individual has presented with acute ischemia (e.g., MI, stroke), interventions are specific to the diseased area (discussed further under those topics). In situations in which the disease process does not require immediate intervention, management focuses on reduction of risk factors and prevention of plaque progression. Management strategies include implementation of an exercise program, cessation of smoking, and control of hypertension and diabetes where appropriate while reducing LDL cholesterol level by diet or medications, or both. Management of atherosclerotic risk factors is discussed further starting on p. 621.

Peripheral Artery Disease

Peripheral artery disease (PAD) refers to atherosclerotic disease of arteries that perfuse the limbs, especially the lower extremities. PAD affects an estimated 800 000 Canadians over 40 years of age.[71] The risk factors for PAD are the same as those previously described for atherosclerosis, but it is especially prevalent in older adults with diabetes and has a very strong link with smoking.[72]

Lower extremity ischemia resulting from arterial obstruction in PAD can be gradual or acute. In most individuals, gradually increasing obstruction to arterial blood flow to the legs caused by atherosclerosis in the iliofemoral vessels can result in pain with ambulation called intermittent claudication. If a thrombus forms over the atherosclerotic lesion, complete obstruction of blood flow can occur acutely, causing severe pain, loss of pulses, and skin colour changes in the affected extremity.

Although individuals with PAD have an increased mortality, more than two-thirds of adults with PAD are asymptomatic even in severe cases.[10] Therefore, evaluation for PAD requires a careful history and physical examination that focuses on finding evidence of atherosclerotic disease (e.g., bruits), determining a difference in blood pressure measured at the ankle versus the arm (ankle-brachial index), and measuring blood flow using noninvasive Doppler.[73] Treatment includes risk factor reduction (smoking cessation and treatment of diabetes, hypertension, and dyslipidemia) and antiplatelet therapy. Symptomatic PAD should be managed with vasodilators in combination with antiplatelet or antithrombotic medications (Aspirin, ticlopidine [Ticlid], or clopidogrel [Plavix]), and cholesterol-lowering medications.[74] Aerobic exercise is a crucial part of therapy.[10] If acute or refractory symptoms occur, emergent percutaneous or surgical revascularization may be indicated. Newer treatment modalities that are being explored include autologous stem cell therapies and angiogenesis.[75]

Coronary Artery Disease, Myocardial Ischemia, and Acute Coronary Syndromes

Coronary artery disease (CAD), myocardial ischemia, and MI form a pathophysiological continuum that impairs the pumping ability of the heart by depriving the heart muscle of bloodborne oxygen and nutrients. The earliest lesions of the continuum are those of CAD, which is usually caused by atherosclerosis (see Figure 24-10). CAD can diminish the myocardial blood supply until deprivation impairs myocardial metabolism enough to cause ischemia, a local state in which the cells are temporarily deprived of blood supply. The cells remain alive but cannot function normally. Persistent ischemia or the complete occlusion of a coronary artery causes the acute coronary syndromes including infarction, or irreversible myocardial damage. Infarction constitutes the potentially fatal event known as a *heart attack*.

Development of Coronary Artery Disease

More than 1.4 million Canadians have heart disease. It is also one of the leading causes of death in Canada, claiming more than 33 600 lives per year.[76] Fortunately, the incidence and mortality statistics for CAD have been decreasing over the past 15 years because of more aggressive recognition, prevention, and treatment. Risk factors for CAD are the same as those for atherosclerosis and can be categorized as conventional (major) versus nontraditional (novel), and as modifiable versus non-modifiable. The plethora of new information obtained about the conventional risk factors has markedly improved prevention and management of CAD. In addition, nontraditional risk factors have been identified that have provided insight into the pathogenesis of CAD and may lead to more effective interventions in the future.

Conventional or major risk factors for CAD that are nonmodifiable include (1) advanced age, (2) male gender or women after menopause, and (3) family history. Aging and menopause are associated with increased exposure to risk factors and poor endothelial healing. Family history may contribute to CAD through genetics and shared environmental exposures. Many gene polymorphisms have been associated with CAD and its risk factors. Modifiable major risks include (1) dyslipidemia, (2) hypertension, (3) cigarette smoking, (4) diabetes mellitus (insulin resistance), (5) obesity, (6) sedentary lifestyle, and (7) atherogenic diet. Fortunately, modification of these factors can dramatically reduce the risk for CAD.[77]

Dyslipidemia. The link between CAD and abnormal levels of lipoproteins is well documented. The term lipoprotein refers to lipids, phospholipids, cholesterol, and triglycerides bound to carrier proteins. Lipids (cholesterol in particular) are required by most cells for the manufacture and repair of plasma membranes. Cholesterol is also a necessary component for the manufacture of such essential substances as bile acids and steroid hormones. Although cholesterol can easily be obtained from dietary fat intake, most body cells also can manufacture cholesterol.

The cycle of lipid metabolism is complex. Dietary fat is packaged into particles known as *chylomicrons* in the small intestine. Chylomicrons are required for absorption of fat and function by transporting exogenous lipid from the intestine to the liver and peripheral cells. Chylomicrons

TABLE 24-4 Criteria for Dyslipidemia

	Optimal	Near-Optimal	Desirable	Low	Borderline	High	Very High
Total cholesterol			<5 mmol/L	4.15–5.19 mmol/L	5.2–6.19 mmol/L	≥6.2–7.2 mmol/L	>7.21 mmol/L
LDL	<2.59 mmol/L	2.59–3.34 mmol/L			3.37–4.11 mmol/L	4.14–4.90 mmol/L	≥4.92 mmol/L
Triglycerides			<0.45–1.81 mmol/L		150–199	200–499	≥5.6 mmol/L
HDL				<1.036 mmol/L		≥1.55 mmol/L	

HDL, high-density lipoprotein; *LDL*, low-density lipoprotein.
Data from Expert Panel on Detection, Evaluation, and Treatment of High Blood Cholesterol in Adults. (2001). *JAMA, 285*(19), 2486–2497.

are the least dense of the lipoproteins and primarily contain triglyceride. Some of the triglyceride may be removed and either stored by adipose tissue or used by muscle as an energy source. The chylomicron remnants, composed mainly of cholesterol, are taken up by the liver. A series of chemical reactions in the liver results in the production of several lipoproteins that vary in density and function. These include very-low-density lipoproteins (VLDLs), primarily triglyceride and protein; LDLs, mostly cholesterol and protein; and HDLs, mainly phospholipids and protein.

Dyslipidemia (or **dyslipoproteinemia**) refers to abnormal concentrations of serum lipoproteins. It has been defined by the Third Report of the National Cholesterol Education Program in the United States[78] (Table 24-4), although more recent Canadian guidelines place less emphasis on specific serum lipoprotein levels.[79] These abnormalities are the result of a combination of genetic and dietary factors. Primary or familial dyslipoproteinemias result from genetic defects that cause abnormalities in lipid-metabolizing enzymes and abnormal cellular lipid receptors. Secondary causes of dyslipidemia include the existence of several common systemic disorders, such as diabetes, hypothyroidism, pancreatitis, and renal nephrosis, as well as the use of certain medications, such as some diuretics, glucocorticoids, interferons, and antiretrovirals.

LDL is responsible for the delivery of cholesterol to the tissues, and an increased serum concentration of LDL is a strong indicator of coronary risk. Serum levels of LDL are normally controlled by hepatic receptors that bind LDL and limit liver synthesis of this lipoprotein. High dietary intake of cholesterol and saturated fats, in combination with a genetic predisposition to accumulations of LDL in the serum (e.g., dysfunction of the hepatic LDL receptor), results in high levels of LDL in the bloodstream. LDL migration into the vessel wall, oxidation, and phagocytosis by macrophages are key steps in the pathogenesis of atherosclerosis (see Figure 24-9). LDL also plays a role in endothelial injury, inflammation, and immune responses that have been identified as being important in atherogenesis.[68] The term *LDL* actually describes several types of LDL molecules. Measurement of LDL subfractions allows for a better prediction of coronary risk. For example, LDL cholesterol measurements enable the detection of the small, dense LDL particles that are the most atherogenic, and apolipoprotein B (structural protein found in both LDL and VLDL) levels are a very strong predictor of future coronary events. Recent guidelines from the Canadian Cardiovascular Society focus on treating dyslipidemia in the context of other risk factors.[79] (See *Health Promotion*: Recommendations for Managing Cholesterol.)

Low levels of HDL cholesterol also are a strong indicator of coronary risk. HDL is responsible for "reverse cholesterol transport," which returns excess cholesterol from the tissues to the liver for processing or elimination in the bile. HDL also participates in endothelial repair and decreases thrombosis. It can be fractionated into several particle densities (HDL-2 and HDL-3) that have different effects on vascular function. Exercise, weight loss, fish oil consumption, and moderate alcohol use result in modest increases in HDL level. Despite the wealth of evidence that HDL plays an important role in preventing atherosclerotic coronary disease, studies have suggested that raising overall levels of HDL is not adequate to prevent cardiovascular disease. Niacin and fibrates are medications that can cause modest increases in HDL levels that are not correlated with an improvement in cardiovascular risk in individuals without documented coronary disease (primary prevention). Medications that are aimed specifically at increasing HDL levels include recombinant apolipoprotein A-I (ApoA-I) mimetics, thiazolidinediones (used to treat diabetes), and cholesteryl ester transfer protein inhibitors, but they have not been shown to be effective in preventing heart disease. Recent studies suggest that it is not the serum levels of HDL that are key to determining CAD risk, but rather HDL functionality, which is harder to measure.[80,81]

Other lipoproteins associated with increased cardiovascular risk include elevated levels of serum VLDLs (triglycerides) and increased **lipoprotein(a) (Lp[a])** levels. Triglycerides are associated with an increased risk for CAD, especially in combination with other risk factors such as diabetes. Lp(a) is a genetically determined molecular complex between LDL and a serum glycoprotein called *apolipoprotein A* and has been shown to be an important risk factor for atherosclerosis, especially in women.

Hypertension. Hypertension is responsible for a twofold to threefold increased risk for atherosclerotic cardiovascular disease. It contributes to endothelial injury, a key step in atherogenesis. It also can cause myocardial hypertrophy, which increases myocardial demand for coronary flow. Overactivity of the SNS and RAAS commonly found in hypertension also contributes to the genesis of CAD.

Cigarette smoking. Both direct and passive (environmental) smoking increase the risk for CAD. Smoking has a direct effect on endothelial cells and the generation of oxygen free radicals that contribute to atherogenesis.[82] Nicotine stimulates the release of catecholamines (epinephrine and norepinephrine), which increase heart rate and peripheral vascular constriction. As a result, blood pressure increases, as do cardiac workload and oxygen demand. Cigarette smoking is associated with an increase in LDL levels and a decrease in HDL levels. The risk for CAD increases with heavy smoking and decreases when smoking is stopped.

Diabetes mellitus (insulin resistance). Insulin resistance and diabetes mellitus are extremely important risk factors for CAD. Insulin resistance and diabetes have multiple effects on the cardiovascular system, including damage to the endothelium, thickening of the vessel wall, increased inflammation, increased thrombosis, glycation of vascular proteins, and decreased production of endothelial-derived vasodilators, such as nitric oxide.[83] Diabetes also is associated with dyslipidemia (see Chapter 19). Good diabetic control is linked to reduced risk for CAD.

Obesity or a sedentary lifestyle. In Canada, 14.9% of adults have a combination of obesity, dyslipidemia, hypertension, and insulin resistance, called **metabolic syndrome (MetS)**, which is associated with an even higher risk for CAD events. The importance of MetS for public health is demonstrated by its significant association with chronic disease relative to the general population. The 10-year incidence estimate for diabetes and mean percent risk for a fatal cardiovascular disease event were higher in those with MetS compared to those without (18.0% versus 7.1% for diabetes, and 4.1% versus 0.8% for cardiovascular

HEALTH PROMOTION

Recommendations for Managing Cholesterol

The Heart and Stroke Foundation of Canada recommends that cholesterol be tested in the following individuals:

- Men over 40 years of age
- Women who are over 50 years of age, postmenopausal, or both
- Individuals with heart disease, diabetes, or high blood pressure
- Individuals with a waist circumference greater than 94 cm (37 in.) for men and 80 cm (31.5 in.) for women
- Individuals who smoke or have smoked within the last year
- Men with erectile dysfunction
- Individuals with family history of heart disease or stroke

It also recommends that individuals prevent or manage cholesterol levels by doing the following:

1. **Eat a healthy balanced diet.**
   - Choose a variety of whole and minimally processed foods at every meal. This means foods that are not packaged or that have few ingredients.
   - Fill half your plate with vegetables and fruit at every meal. Choose vegetables and fruit for snacks. Select fresh, frozen, or canned vegetables and fruit. You want them to be plain, without sauce, sugar, or salt added.
   - Choose whole grains. Look for whole-grain breads, barley, oats (including oatmeal), quinoa, brown rice, bulgur, farro, etc.
   - Mix up the centre of your plate. Choose more vegetarian options such as beans, lentils, tofu, and nuts. Include vegetarian options as often as possible in your weekly meal plan. Make sure your meat is lean and poultry is without the skin, and include fish a couple of times per week. Limit your portion sizes.
   - Choose lower fat dairy products or alternatives with no added sugar. Select 1% or skim milk, plain yogurt, and lower fat cheeses.
   - Plan healthy snacks with at least two different types of food. For example, try hummus and baby carrots, apple wedges and lower fat cheese, or plain yogurt with berries.
   - Drink water or lower fat plain milk to satisfy thirst. Avoid sugary drinks, including soft drinks, sports drinks, sweetened milk or alternatives, fruit drinks, 100% fruit juice, and ready-to-drink sweetened coffees and teas.
2. **Cook and eat more meals at home.** Cooking at home allows you to select whole and minimally processed foods.
   - Develop and share skills in food preparation and cooking with your family.
   - Buy a healthy cookbook or use the healthy recipes at http://www.heartandstroke.ca/recipes. Select the top 10 recipes your family loves and get everyone involved in the meal preparation.
   - Reduce the amount of sugar, salt, and solid fats used in your favourite recipes.
3. **Make eating out a special occasion.** Eating out usually results in you consuming large amounts of food and more fat, salt, and sugar.
   - Try to limit the number of times you eat in a restaurant per month.
   - When you do eat out, choose restaurants that serve freshly made dishes using whole and minimally processed foods and provide nutrition information.
   - Share meals or ask for half the meal to be packed up to eat the next day.
4. **Achieve and maintain a healthy weight.** Being overweight or obese increases your LDL or bad cholesterol level, lowers your HDL or good cholesterol level, and raises your triglyceride levels. Reducing your weight is a positive way to reduce your blood cholesterol levels. Help is available at heartandstroke.ca/hwplan.
5. **Physical activity.** Being physically active will help improve your cholesterol levels and general heart health. Aim for 150 minutes a week. That is less than 25 minutes per day! Choose activities you like. Cycling, swimming, gardening, and walking are great ways to keep active.
6. **Be smoke-free.** Smoking is a risk factor for heart disease. It reduces the level of your HDL "good" cholesterol. Once you quit, within a few weeks your HDL levels will start to rise.

From Heart & Stroke Foundation of Canada. (2017). *How to Manage Your Cholesterol.* Ottawa: Author. Retrieved from http://www.heartandstroke.ca/-/media/pdffiles/canada/heart/how-to-manage-your-cholesterolen.ashx?la=en&hash=48EBF71E615142114D3F49A19CDA8A36BD079F6E. © 2017, Heart and Stroke Foundation of Canada. Reproduced with the permission of the Heart and Stroke Foundation of Canada. www.heartandstroke.ca.

disease). MetS is prevalent in Canadian adults, and a high proportion of individuals with MetS have diagnosed or undiagnosed chronic conditions. Projection estimates for the incidence of chronic disease associated with MetS demonstrate higher rates in individuals with this condition. Thus, MetS may be a relevant risk factor in the development of chronic disease.[84]

Abdominal obesity has the strongest link with increased CAD risk and is related to inflammation, insulin resistance, decreased HDL level, increased blood pressure, and fewer changes in hormones called adipokines (leptin and adiponectin).[85] A sedentary lifestyle not only increases the risk for obesity but also has an independent effect on increasing CAD risk. Physical activity and weight loss offer substantial reductions in risk factors for CAD.[86] There is emerging evidence that bariatric surgery procedures, such as gastric bypass, can provide sustained improvement in risk factors for cardiovascular disease, such as hypertension, dyslipidemia, and diabetes.[87]

Atherogenic diet. Diet plays a complex role in atherogenic risk. Diets high in salt, fats, trans fats, and carbohydrates have all been implicated. There are many recommendations regarding diet modification to reduce coronary risk; one of the most effective is called the *Mediterranean Diet.*

Nontraditional risk factors. Nontraditional, or novel, risk factors for CAD include increased serum markers for inflammation and thrombosis (troponin I, adipokines, infection, and air pollution). The amount of risk conferred by these relatively newly identified factors is still being explored.

Markers of inflammation and thrombosis. Of the numerous markers of inflammation that have been linked to an increase in CAD risk (hs-CRP, fibrinogen, protein C, plasminogen activator inhibitor), the relationship between serum levels of hs-CRP and CAD has been explored in the greatest depth. Hs-CRP is a protein mostly synthesized in the liver and is used as an indirect measure of atherosclerotic plaque–related inflammation. An elevated serum level of hs-CRP is strongly correlated with an increased risk for coronary events,[88] but it is a nonspecific measure of inflammation and may indicate the presence of other inflammatory conditions. The primary use of hs-CRP is as an aid to decision making about pharmacological interventions for individuals with other risk factors for coronary disease.[89] Other markers of inflammation associated with CAD include the erythrocyte sedimentation rate and concentrations of von Willebrand factor, interleukin-6 (IL-6), IL-18, tumour necrosis factor, fibrinogen, and cluster of differentiation (CD) 40 ligand. Interestingly, the long-term use of some anti-inflammatories, such as ibuprofen (Advil), has been linked to increased (rather than decreased) risk for CAD because of their potentiation of clotting in certain tissues.[90]

Troponin I. Troponin I (TnI) is a serum protein whose measurement is used as a sensitive and specific diagnostic test to help identify myocardial injury during acute coronary syndromes. Highly sensitive TnI assays are used in individuals without a history of CAD to assess risk for future CHD events, mortality, and HF.

Adipokines. Adipokines are a group of hormones released from adipose cells. Obesity causes increased levels of leptin, which is implicated in hypertension and diabetes, and decreased levels of adiponectin, which is a hormone that functions to protect the vascular endothelium and is anti-inflammatory.[91,92] Other adipokines also have been linked to inflammation in endothelial cells.[93] Weight loss, exercise, and healthy diet improve adipokine levels.

Infection. Infections with various microorganisms, including *Chlamydia pneumoniae*, *Helicobacter pylori*, and cytomegalovirus, have been linked to an increased risk for CAD, although cause and effect have not been proven. Periodontal disease also has been linked to an increased risk for CAD. One hypothesis is that systemic infection results in increased inflammation of vessels and, therefore, contributes to vascular disease. Unfortunately, the use of antibiotics for the prevention and treatment of CAD has not yielded consistently positive results.

Air pollution. Exposure to air pollution, especially roadway exposures, is strongly correlated with coronary risk. It is postulated that toxins in pollution contribute to macrophage activation, oxidation of LDL, thrombosis, and inflammation of vessel walls.[94]

Myocardial Ischemia

PATHOPHYSIOLOGY The coronary arteries normally supply blood flow sufficient to meet the demands of the myocardium as it labours under varying workloads. Oxygen is extracted from these vessels with maximal efficiency. If demand increases, healthy coronary arteries can dilate to increase the flow of oxygenated blood to the myocardium. Narrowing of a major coronary artery by more than 50% impairs blood flow enough to hamper cellular metabolism when myocardial demand increases.

Myocardial ischemia develops if the flow or oxygen content of coronary blood is insufficient to meet the metabolic demands of myocardial cells (Figure 24-11). Imbalances between coronary blood supply and myocardial demand can result from a number of conditions. The most common cause of decreased coronary blood flow and resultant myocardial ischemia is the formation of atherosclerotic plaques in the coronary circulation. As the plaque increases in size, it may partially occlude the vessel lumina, thus limiting coronary flow and causing ischemia, especially during exercise. As discussed earlier in this chapter, some plaques are "unstable," meaning they are prone to ulceration or rupture. When this ulceration or rupture occurs, underlying tissues of the vessel wall are exposed, resulting in platelet adhesion and thrombus formation (see Figures 24-7 and 24-15). Thrombus formation can suddenly stop blood supply to the heart muscle, resulting in acute myocardial ischemia, and if the vessel obstruction cannot be reversed rapidly, ischemia will progress to infarction. Myocardial ischemia also can result from other causes of decreased blood and oxygen delivery to the myocardium, such as coronary spasm, hypotension, dysrhythmias, and decreased oxygen-carrying capacity of the blood (e.g., anemia, hypoxemia). Common causes of increased myocardial demand for blood include tachycardia, exercise, hypertension (hypertrophy), and valvular disease.

Myocardial cells become ischemic within 10 seconds of coronary occlusion, thus hampering pump function and depriving the myocardium of a glucose source necessary for aerobic metabolism. Anaerobic processes take over, and lactic acid accumulates. After several minutes, the heart cells lose the ability to contract and cardiac output decreases. Cardiac cells remain viable for approximately 20 minutes under ischemic conditions. If blood flow is restored, aerobic metabolism resumes, contractility is restored, and cellular repair begins. If perfusion is not restored, then MI occurs (see Figure 24-11).

CLINICAL MANIFESTATIONS Individuals with reversible myocardial ischemia present clinically in several ways. Chronic coronary obstruction results in recurrent predictable chest pain called *stable angina.* Abnormal vasospasm of coronary vessels results in unpredictable chest pain called *Prinzmetal angina.* Myocardial ischemia that does not cause detectable symptoms is called *silent ischemia.*

1. **Stable angina pectoris.** Angina is chest pain caused by myocardial ischemia. Stable angina is caused by gradual luminal narrowing and hardening of the arterial walls, with associated inflammation, endothelial cell dysfunction, and a decrease in endogenous vasodilators. These changes are more prevalent in individuals with obesity, diabetes, and dyslipidemia.[95] Affected vessels cannot dilate in response to increased myocardial demand associated with physical exertion or emotional stress. With rest, blood flow is restored and necrosis of myocardial cells does not occur. Angina pectoris is typically experienced as transient substernal chest discomfort, ranging from a sensation of heaviness or pressure to moderately severe pain. Individuals often describe the sensation by clenching a fist over the left sternal border. The discomfort may be mistaken for indigestion. The pain is caused by the buildup of lactic acid or abnormal stretching of the ischemic myocardium that irritates myocardial nerve fibres. These afferent sympathetic fibres enter the spinal cord from levels C3 to T4, accounting for a variety of locations and radiation patterns

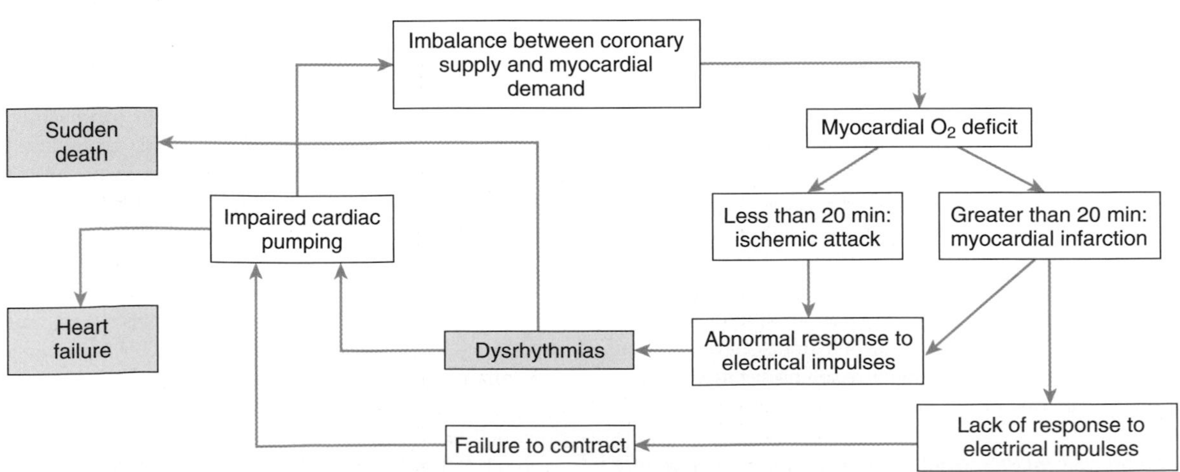

FIGURE 24-11 Cycle of Ischemic Events. O_2, oxygen.

of anginal pain. Discomfort may radiate to the neck, lower jaw, left arm, and left shoulder, or occasionally to the back or down the right arm. Pallor, diaphoresis, and dyspnea may be associated with the pain. The pain is usually relieved by rest and nitrates. However, myocardial ischemia in women may not present with typical anginal pain. Common symptoms in women include atypical chest pain, palpitations, sense of unease, and severe fatigue. In addition, it is estimated that half of women with stable angina do not have obstructive CAD, but rather have "microvascular angina" that results from vasoconstriction of small coronary arterioles deep in the myocardium[96] (see *Health Promotion:* Women and Microvascular Angina).

2. **Prinzmetal angina**. Prinzmetal angina (also called *variant angina*) is chest pain attributable to transient ischemia of the myocardium that occurs unpredictably and often at rest. Pain is caused by vasospasm of one or more major coronary arteries with or without associated atherosclerosis. The pain often occurs at night during rapid eye movement sleep and may have a cyclic pattern of occurrence. The angina may result from decreased vagal activity, hyperactivity of the SNS, or decreased nitric oxide activity. Other causes include altered calcium channel function in arterial smooth muscle or impaired production or release of inflammatory mediators, such as serotonin, histamine, endothelin, or thromboxane.[97] Serum markers of inflammation, such as CRP and IL-6, are elevated in individuals with this form of angina. Prinzmetal angina is usually a benign condition, but it can occasionally cause serious dysrhythmias, especially if treatment is withdrawn; therefore calcium channel blockers or long-acting nitrates, or both, should be continued even if clinical remission is achieved.[98]
3. **Silent ischemia** and **mental stress–induced ischemia**. Myocardial ischemia may not cause detectable symptoms such as angina. Ischemia can be totally asymptomatic (and referred to as *silent ischemia*), or individuals may complain of fatigue, dyspnea, or a feeling of unease. Some individuals only have silent ischemia, and episodes of silent ischemia are common in individuals who also experience angina. One proposed mechanism for the absence of angina in silent myocardial ischemia is the presence of a global or regional abnormality in left ventricular sympathetic afferent innervation. The most common cause of autonomic dysfunction leading to silent ischemia is diabetes mellitus. Other causes include surgical denervation during coronary artery bypass grafting (CABG) or cardiac transplantation, or following ischemic local nerve injury by MI. Also of interest is silent ischemia occurring in some individuals during mental stress (Figures 24-12 and 24-13). Chronic stress has been linked to an increase in the number of inflammatory cytokines and a hypercoagulable state that may contribute to acute ischemic events.[99,100] Silent ischemia can be detected by stress radionucleotide imaging. Detection and management of silent ischemia caused by coronary disease is important because it is an indicator of increased risk for serious cardiovascular events.[101]

EVALUATION AND TREATMENT Many individuals with reversible myocardial ischemia will have a normal physical examination between events. Physical examination of those experiencing myocardial ischemia

HEALTH PROMOTION

Women and Microvascular Angina

Heart disease and stroke are the leading cause of death among Canadian women, with more women dying from heart disease than from all cancers combined. Heart disease and stroke kill seven times as many women as does breast cancer.

Overall, 42% of women suffering a heart attack do not experience chest pain. Women with myocardial ischemia often have either no symptoms or atypical symptoms, such as palpitations, anxiety, weakness, and fatigue. Additionally, many women with angina are found to have cardiac ischemia yet no evidence of obstructive CAD on cardiac catheterization, a condition sometimes called *cardiac syndrome x*. Evidence is accumulating that nearly half of women with myocardial ischemia suffer from coronary microvascular disease, a condition often called **microvascular angina (MVA)**. Small intramyocardial arterioles constrict in MVA, causing ischemic pain that is less predictable than with typical epicardial CAD. The pathophysiology is complex and still being elucidated, but there is strong evidence that endothelial dysfunction, decreased endogenous vasodilators, inflammation, changes in adipokines, and platelet activation are contributing factors. Managing MVA can be challenging; for example, women with this condition have less coronary microvascular dilation in response to nitrates than do those without MVA. Aggressive interventions to reduce modifiable risk factors for CAD are an important component of management, especially smoking cessation, exercise, and diabetes management. The combination of non-nitrate vasodilators, such as calcium channel blockers with HMG-CoA reductase inhibitors (statins), also has been shown to be effective in many women, and new medications, such as ranolazine (Ranexa) and ivabradine (Lancora), have shown promise in the treatment of MVA.

Data from: Arthur, H.M., Campbell, P., Harvey, P.J., et al. (2012). *Can J Cardiol, 28*(2, Suppl.), S42–S49; Ashley, K.E., & Geraci, S.A. (2013). *South Med J, 106*(7), 427–433; Heart Research Institute (CAN). (n.d.). *Women and heart disease*. Retrieved from http://www.hricanada.org/about-heart-disease/women-and-heart-disease; Luo, C., Long, M., Hu, X., et al. (2014). *Circulation, 7*(1), 43–48; Recio-Mayoral, A., Rimoldi, O.E., Camici, P.G., et al. (2013). *JACC Cardiovasc Imaging, 6*(6), 660–667; Russo, G., Di Franco, A., Lamendola, P., et al. (2013). *Cardiovasc Drugs Ther, 27*(3), 229–234; Taqueti, V.R., & Ridker, P.M. (2013). *JACC Cardiovasc Imaging, 6*(6), 668–671; Zhang, X., Li, Q., Zhao, J., et al. (2014). *Coron Artery Dis, 25*(1), 40–44; Zuchi, C., Tritto, I., Ambrosio, G., et al. (2013). *Int J Cardiol, 163*(2), 132–140.

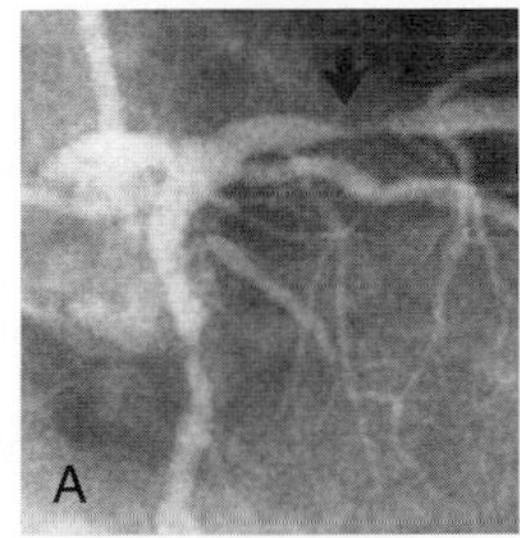

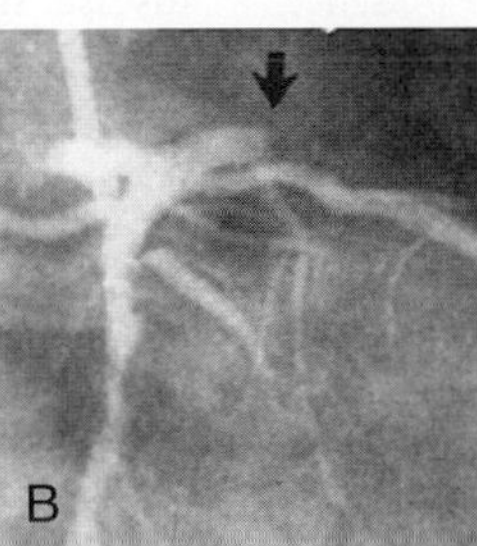

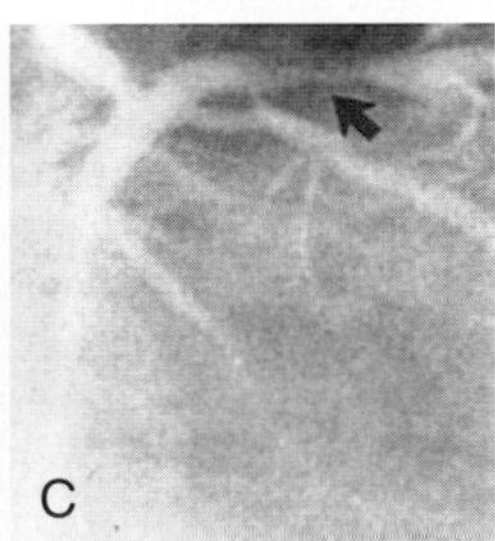

FIGURE 24-12 Mental Stress and Angiogram of Coronary Arteries. A, Baseline. **B,** Transient total occlusion of left anterior descending branch of the left coronary artery after mental stress. **C,** After nitrates and nifedipine, artery reopened to same diameter as baseline. (Modified from Stern, S. [Ed.]. [1998]. *Silent myocardial ischemia.* St. Louis: Mosby.)

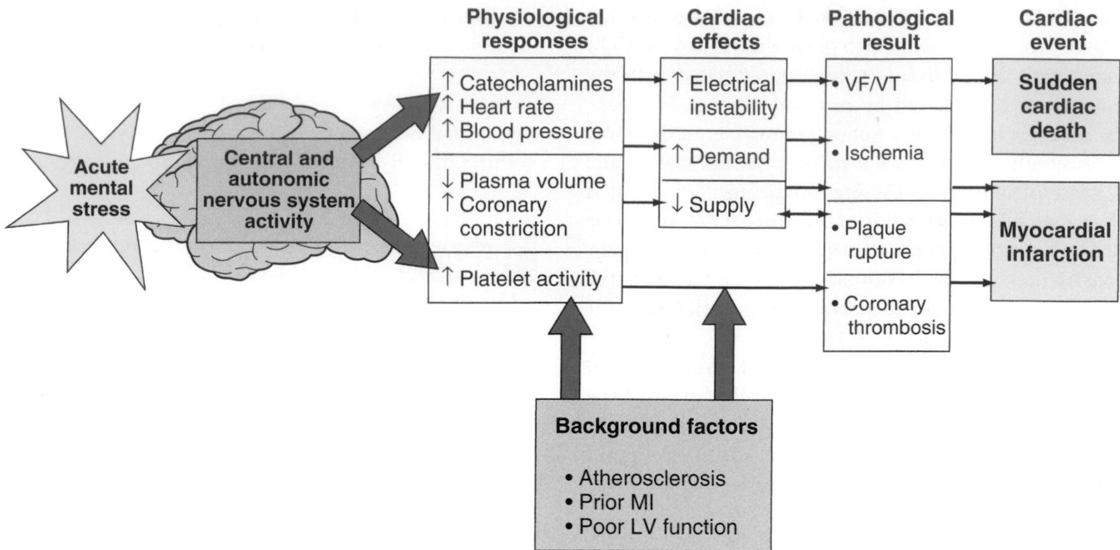

FIGURE 24-13 Pathophysiological Model of the Effects of Acute Stress as a Trigger of Cardiac Clinical Events. Acting via the central and autonomic nervous systems, stress can produce a cascade of physiological responses that may lead to myocardial ischemia, especially in persons with coronary artery disease, potentially fatal dysrhythmia, plaque rupture, or coronary thrombosis. *LV*, left ventricular; *MI*, myocardial infarction; *VF*, ventricular fibrillation; *VT*, ventricular tachycardia. (From Krantz, D.S., Kop, W.J., Santiago, H.T., et al. [1996]. Mental stress as a trigger of myocardial ischemia and infarction. In P.C. Deedwania, & G.H. Tofler, [Eds.], *Triggers and timing of cardiac events* [2nd ed.]. London: Saunders.)

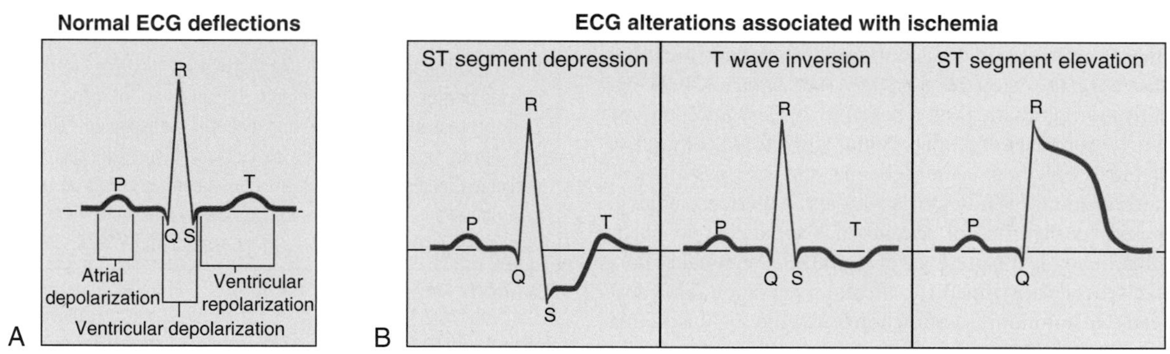

FIGURE 24-14 Electrocardiogram and Ischemia. A, Normal electrocardiogram (*ECG*). **B,** Electrocardiographic alterations associated with ischemia.

may disclose rapid pulse rate or extra heart sounds (gallops or murmurs), and pulmonary congestion indicating impaired left ventricular function. The presence of xanthelasmas (small fat deposits) around the eyelids or arcus senilis of the eyes (a yellow lipid ring around the cornea) suggests severe dyslipidemia and possible atherosclerosis. The presence of peripheral or carotid artery bruits suggests probable atherosclerotic disease and increases the likelihood that CAD is present.

Electrocardiography is a critical tool for the diagnosis of myocardial ischemia. Ischemic cells distort the electrical impulses that are measured across the myocardium during an ECG. Because many individuals have normal ECGs when there is no pain, diagnosis requires that an ECG be performed during an attack of angina or during exercise stress testing. The ST segment and the T wave segments of the ECG respectively correlate with ventricular contraction and relaxation (see Figure 23-10). Transient ST segment depression and T wave inversion are characteristic signs of ischemia that involves only the inner wall of the myocardium (subendocardial ischemia). ST elevation is indicative of ischemia involving the full myocardial wall (transmural ischemia) (Figure 24-14). The ECG tracings correlate with different parts of the myocardium and, therefore, can give some indication of which coronary artery is involved.

Stress radionucleotide imaging is indicated to detect ischemic changes in asymptomatic individuals with multiple risk factors for coronary disease, such as diabetes and dyslipidemia, and for older individuals who plan to start vigorous exercise. Currently, the diagnostic modality of choice for the diagnosis of myocardial ischemia is single-photon emission computed tomography (SPECT), which is effective at identifying ischemia and estimating coronary risk.[102] Stress echocardiography is another technique used to diagnose CAD. Unfortunately, these tests cannot detect the presence of vulnerable plaques that are the cause of the majority of acute coronary syndromes; therefore, new diagnostic techniques are being evaluated.[70] Noninvasive tests for evaluating coronary atherosclerotic lesions include measurement of coronary artery calcium concentration by CT, noninvasive coronary angiography using electron beam CT, protein-weighted MRI, and intravascular ultrasound; however, the sensitivity and specificity of these tests vary widely.[102] Coronary angiography helps determine the anatomical extent of CAD, but the procedure is expensive and carries some risk. It is used primarily to determine whether possible percutaneous coronary intervention (PCI) or CABG surgery is warranted for individuals whose noninvasive studies suggest severe disease.

The primary aims of therapy for myocardial ischemia and stable angina are to increase coronary blood flow and to reduce myocardial oxygen consumption. Recommendations for appropriate diet, exercise, and risk reduction strategies have been widely distributed, and the use of lipid-lowering statins has been shown to be effective for both primary and secondary prevention of CAD.[79,103] Coronary blood flow is improved by reversing vasoconstriction, reducing plaque growth and rupture, and preventing clotting. Myocardial oxygen demand is reduced by manipulation of blood pressure, heart rate, contractility, and left ventricular volume. Several classes of medications are useful for increasing coronary flow and decreasing myocardial demand, especially nitrates, beta-blockers, and calcium channel blockers.[102,104] Ranolazine represents a relatively new class of antianginal medications known as sodium ion channel inhibitors and has been found to improve exercise tolerance, lessen anginal symptoms, and reduce the need for nitrates in many individuals with chronic stable angina.[105]

Percutaneous coronary intervention (PCI) is a procedure whereby stenotic (narrowed) coronary vessels are dilated with a catheter. Indications for PCI in stable angina include persistent symptoms despite optimal medical therapy or severe disease that indicates a high risk for infarction.[102] Restenosis of the artery is the major complication of the procedure; however, placement of a coronary stent can reduce this risk. Pharmacological treatment with antithrombotics, such as Aspirin, clopidogrel, or glycoprotein IIb/IIIa receptor antagonists, after stenting also can improve outcomes.

Severe CAD can be surgically treated by a CABG, usually using the saphenous vein from the lower leg. In selected individuals, a modified CABG procedure called minimally invasive direct coronary artery bypass (MIDCAB) can be used with much less surgical morbidity and more rapid recovery.

> **QUICK CHECK 24-5**
> 1. Define *atherosclerosis,* and briefly describe how it develops.
> 2. Why do hypertension and dyslipidemia increase the likelihood of developing coronary artery disease?
> 3. Describe the relationships among myocardial ischemia, angina, and silent ischemia.

Acute Coronary Syndromes

The process of atherosclerotic plaque progression can be gradual. However, when there is sudden coronary obstruction caused by thrombus formation over a ruptured or ulcerated atherosclerotic plaque, acute coronary syndromes result (Figure 24-15). **Unstable angina** is the result of reversible myocardial ischemia and is a harbinger of impending infarction. **Myocardial infarction (MI)** results when there is prolonged ischemia causing irreversible damage to the heart muscle. MI can be further subdivided into **non-ST elevation myocardial infarction (non-STEMI)** and **ST elevation myocardial infarction (STEMI)**. Sudden cardiac death can occur as a result of any of the acute coronary syndromes.

An atherosclerotic plaque that is prone to rupture is called "unstable" and has a core that is especially rich in deposited oxidized LDL and a thin fibrous cap (Figure 24-16). These unstable plaques may not extend into the lumen of the vessel and may be clinically silent until they rupture. Plaque disruption (ulceration or rupture) occurs because of the effects of shear forces, inflammation with release of multiple inflammatory mediators, secretion of macrophage-derived degradative

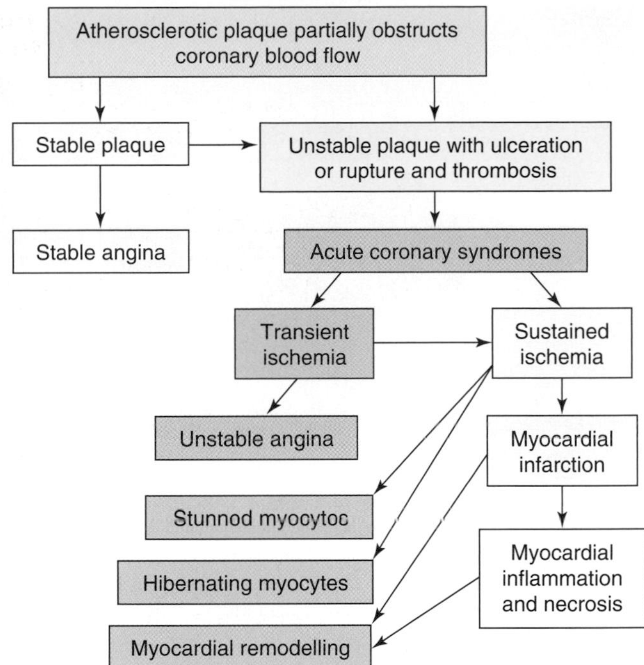

FIGURE 24-15 Pathophysiology of Acute Coronary Syndromes. The atherosclerotic process can lead to stable plaque formation and stable angina or can result in unstable plaques that are prone to rupture and thrombus. Thrombus formation on a ruptured plaque that disperses in less than 20 minutes leads to transient ischemia and unstable angina. If the vessel obstruction is sustained, myocardial infarction with inflammation and necrosis of the myocardium results. In addition, myocardial infarction is associated with other structural and functional changes, including myocyte stunning and hibernation and myocardial remodelling (see Figure 24-34).

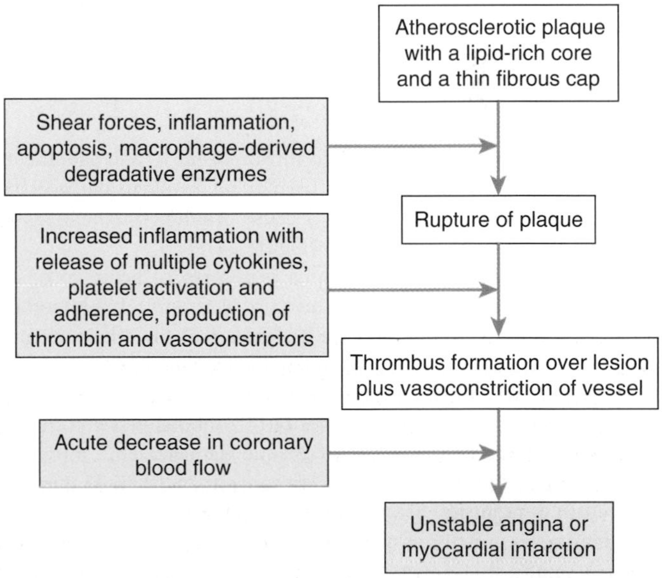

Atherosclerotic plaque with a lipid-rich core and a thin fibrous cap
Shear forces, inflammation, apoptosis, macrophage-derived degradative enzymes
Rupture of plaque
Increased inflammation with release of multiple cytokines, platelet activation and adherence, production of thrombin and vasoconstrictors
Thrombus formation over lesion plus vasoconstriction of vessel
Acute decrease in coronary blood flow
Unstable angina or myocardial infarction

FIGURE 24-16 Pathogenesis of Unstable Plaques and Thrombus Formation.

enzymes, and apoptosis of cells at the edges of the lesions. Exposure of the plaque substrate activates the clotting cascade. In addition, platelet activation results in the release of coagulants and exposure of platelet glycoprotein IIb/IIIa surface receptors, resulting in further platelet aggregation and adherence. The resulting thrombus can form very quickly (Figure 24-17, *A*). Vessel obstruction is further exacerbated by

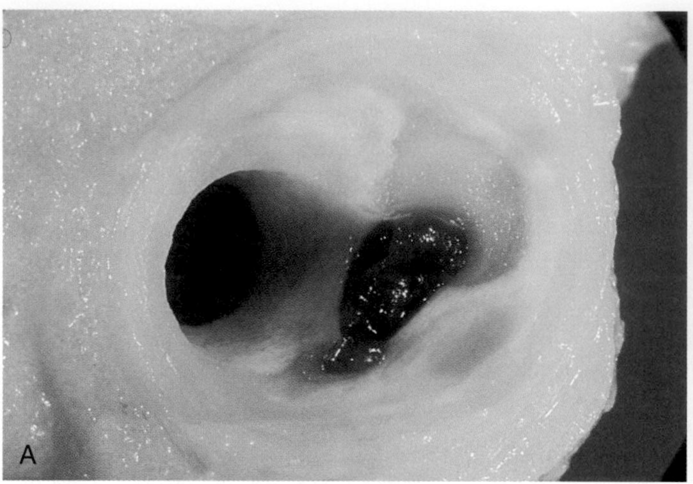

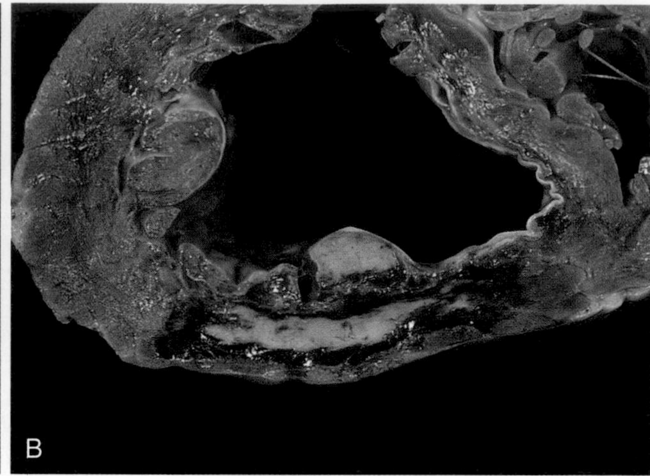

FIGURE 24-17 Plaque Disruption and Myocardial Infarction. A, Plaque disruption. The cap of the lipid-rich plaque has become torn with the formation of a thrombus, mostly inside the plaque. **B,** Myocardial infarction. This infarct is 6 days old. The centre is yellow and necrotic with a hemorrhagic red rim. The responsible arterial occlusion is probably in the right coronary artery. The infarct is on the posterior wall. (From Damjanov, I., & Linder, J. [Eds.]. [1996]. *Anderson's pathology* [10th ed.]. St. Louis: Mosby.)

BOX 24-1 Three Principal Presentations of Unstable Angina

1. Rest angina: Angina occurring at rest and prolonged, usually >20 minutes
2. New-onset angina: New-onset angina of at least CCS Class III severity
3. Increasing angina: Previously diagnosed angina that has become distinctly more frequent, longer in duration, or lower in threshold (i.e., increased by ≥1 CCS class to at least CCS Class III severity)

CCS, Canadian Cardiovascular Society.
From Anderson, J., Adams, C.D., Antman, E.M., et al. (2007). *J Am Coll Cardiol, 50,* e1–e157; originally adapted from Braunwald, E. (1989). *Circulation, 80,* 410–414.

the release of vasoconstrictors, such as thromboxane A_2 and endothelin. The thrombus may shatter before permanent myocyte damage has occurred (unstable angina) or it may cause prolonged ischemia with infarction of the heart muscle (MI) (Figure 24-17, *B*).

Unstable angina. Unstable angina is a form of acute coronary syndrome that results from reversible myocardial ischemia. It is important to recognize this syndrome because it signals that the atherosclerotic plaque has become complicated, and infarction may soon follow. Unstable angina occurs when a fairly small fissuring or superficial erosion of the plaque leads to transient episodes of thrombotic vessel occlusion and vasoconstriction at the site of plaque damage. This thrombus is labile and occludes the vessel for no more than 10 to 20 minutes, with return of perfusion before significant myocardial necrosis occurs. Unstable angina presents as new-onset angina, angina that is occurring at rest, or angina that is increasing in severity or frequency (Box 24-1). Individuals may experience increased dyspnea, diaphoresis, and anxiety as the angina worsens. Physical examination may reveal evidence of ischemic myocardial dysfunction such as pulmonary congestion. The ECG most commonly shows ST segment depression and T wave inversion during pain that resolve as the pain is relieved. Unstable angina has traditionally been diagnosed by ECG changes without serum cardiac isoenzyme evidence of myocyte necrosis. However, the advent of highly sensitive measurements of myocardial damage (high-sensitive cardiac troponin T [hs-cTnT]) that can identify tiny amounts of enzymes released from damaged myocytes has blurred the distinction between unstable angina and MI.[106] Therefore, the current guidelines for the management of unstable angina and non-STEMI are identical.[107] Management of unstable angina requires immediate hospitalization with administration of oxygen, Aspirin (if not contraindicated), nitrates, and morphine if pain is still present. Additional antithrombotic therapy with clopidogrel or glycoprotein IIb/IIIa platelet receptor antagonists may be indicated. Beta-blockers and ACE inhibitors also may be used. Anticoagulants (such as low-molecular-weight heparin) or direct thrombin inhibitors (e.g., fondaparinux [Arixtra]) also can be given. Rapid intervention with PCI also may be indicated.[107]

Myocardial infarction. When coronary blood flow is interrupted for an extended period of time, myocyte necrosis occurs. This results in MI. Plaque progression, disruption, and subsequent clot formation are the same for MI as they are for unstable angina (see Figures 24-14, 24-15, and 24-16). In this case, however, the thrombus is less labile and occludes the vessel for a prolonged period, such that myocardial ischemia progresses to myocyte necrosis and death. Pathologically, there are two major types of MI: subendocardial infarction and transmural infarction. Clinically, however, MI is categorized as non-STEMI or STEMI.

If the thrombus disintegrates before complete distal tissue necrosis has occurred, the infarction will involve only the myocardium directly beneath the endocardium (subendocardial MI) (Figure 24-18). This infarction will usually present with ST segment depression and T wave inversion without Q waves; therefore it is termed *non-STEMI.* It is especially important to recognize this form of acute coronary syndrome because recurrent clot formation on the disrupted atherosclerotic plaque is likely. If the thrombus lodges permanently in the vessel, the infarction will extend through the myocardium all the way from endocardium to epicardium, resulting in severe cardiac dysfunction (**transmural myocardial infarction**) (see Figure 24-18). Transmural MI will usually result in marked elevations in the ST segments on ECG, and these individuals are categorized as having STEMI. Clinically, it is important to identify those individuals with STEMI because they are at highest risk for serious complications and should receive definitive intervention without delay.

PATHOPHYSIOLOGY After 8 to 10 seconds of decreased blood flow, the affected myocardium becomes cyanotic and cooler. Myocardial

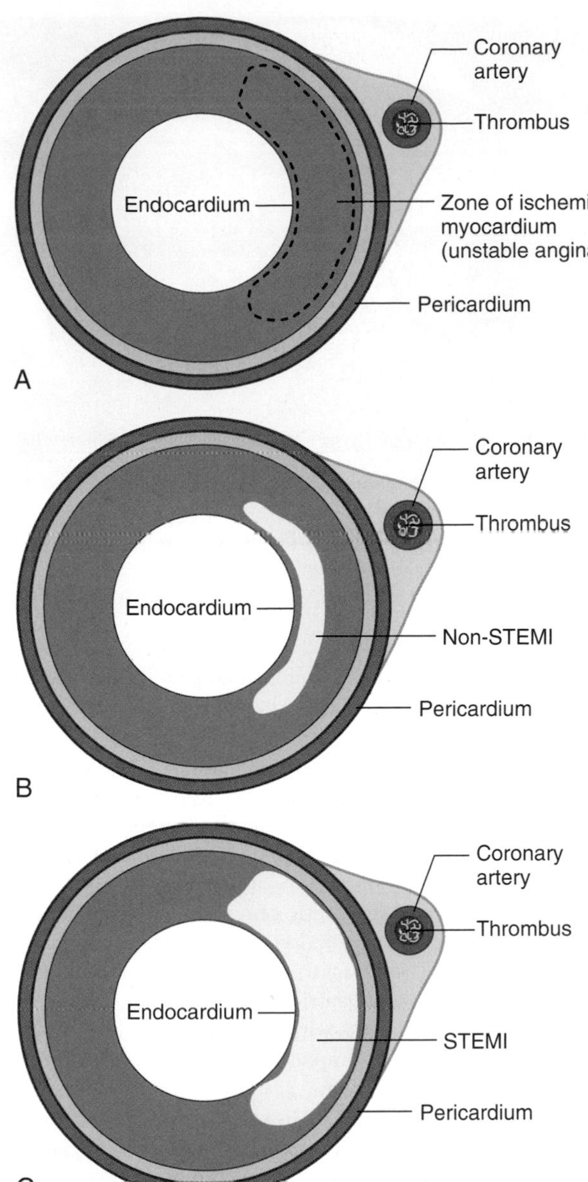

FIGURE 24-18 Unstable Angina, non-STEMI, and STEMI. **A,** Unstable angina. Coronary thrombosis leads to myocardial ischemia. **B,** Non-STEMI. Persistent coronary occlusion leads to infarction of the myocardium closest to the endocardium. **C,** STEMI. Continued coronary occlusion leads to transmural infarction extending from endocardium to pericardium. *Non-STEMI,* non-ST elevation myocardial infarction; *STEMI,* ST elevation myocardial infarction.

oxygen reserves are used quickly (within about 8 seconds) after complete cessation of coronary flow. Glycogen stores decrease as anaerobic metabolism begins. Unfortunately, glycolysis can supply only 65 to 70% of the total myocardial energy requirement and produces much less adenosine triphosphate (ATP) than aerobic processes. Hydrogen ions and lactic acid accumulate. Because myocardial tissues have poor buffering capabilities and myocardial cells are sensitive to low cellular pH, accumulation of these products further compromises the myocardium. Acidosis may make the myocardium more vulnerable to the damaging effects of lysosomal enzymes and may suppress impulse conduction and contractile function, thereby leading to HF.

Oxygen deprivation also is accompanied by electrolyte disturbances, specifically the loss of potassium, calcium, and magnesium from cells. Myocardial cells deprived of necessary oxygen and nutrients lose contractility, thereby diminishing the pumping ability of the heart. Ischemia causes the myocardial cells to release catecholamines, predisposing the individual to serious imbalances of sympathetic and parasympathetic function, irregular heartbeats (dysrhythmia), and HF. Catecholamines mediate the release of glycogen, glucose, and stored fat from body cells. Therefore, plasma concentrations of free fatty acids and glycerol rise within 1 hour after the onset of acute MI. Excessive levels of free fatty acids can have a harmful detergent effect on cell membranes. Norepinephrine elevates blood glucose levels through stimulation of liver and skeletal muscle cells and suppresses pancreatic beta-cell activity, which reduces insulin secretion and elevates blood glucose concentration further. Infiltration of inflammatory cells contributes to tissue injury.[108] Ang II is released during myocardial ischemia and contributes to the pathogenesis of MI in several ways. First, it results in the systemic effects of peripheral vasoconstriction and fluid retention, which increase myocardial workload. Second, it is a growth factor for vascular smooth muscle cells, myocytes, and cardiac fibroblasts, resulting in structural changes in the myocardium called *remodelling*. Finally, Ang II promotes catecholamine release and causes coronary artery spasm.

Ischemic injury can be exacerbated by reperfusion injury once blood flow is restored. This process involves the release of toxic oxygen free radicals, calcium flux, and pH changes that cause a sustained opening of mitochondrial permeability transition pores (mPTPs) and contribute to resultant cellular death. Many innovative therapies are being explored to reduce reperfusion injury.[108]

Cardiac cells can withstand ischemic conditions for about 20 minutes before irreversible hypoxic injury causes cellular death (apoptosis) and tissue necrosis. This results in the release of intracellular enzymes such as creatine phosphokinase-myocardial bound (CPK-MB) and myocyte proteins such as the troponins through the damaged cell membranes into the interstitial spaces. The lymphatics absorb the enzymes and transport them into the bloodstream, where they can be detected by serological tests.

MI results in both structural and functional changes of cardiac tissues (Figure 24-19). Gross tissue changes at the area of infarction may not become apparent for several hours, despite almost immediate onset (within 30 to 60 seconds) of electrocardiographic changes. Cardiac tissue surrounding the area of infarction also undergoes changes. **Myocardial stunning** is a temporary loss of contractile function that persists for hours to days after perfusion has been restored. This pathophysiological state can occur both with MI and in individuals who suffer ischemia during cardiovascular procedures or during central nervous system trauma. Stunning is caused by the alterations in electrolyte pumps and calcium homeostasis and by the release of toxic oxygen free radicals; it can contribute to HF, shock, and dysrhythmias. Recurrent episodes of transient myocardial ischemia (angina) before MI can result in myocyte adaptation to oxygen deprivation with reduced stunning and preservation of myocardium.[109] This process, termed *ischemic preconditioning*, is being studied to determine whether it has potential prophylactic or therapeutic uses.[110] **Hibernating myocardium** describes tissue that is persistently ischemic and undergoes metabolic adaptation to prolong myocyte survival until perfusion can be restored. PCI or surgery aimed at reperfusion of hibernating myocardium can restore significant cardiac function.[111] **Myocardial remodelling** is a process mediated by Ang II, aldosterone, catecholamines, adenosine, and inflammatory cytokines that causes myocyte hypertrophy and loss of contractile function in the areas of the heart distant from the site of infarction. Remodelling can be limited through rapid restoration of coronary flow and the use of renin-angiotensin-aldosterone blockers and beta-blockers after MI.[112]

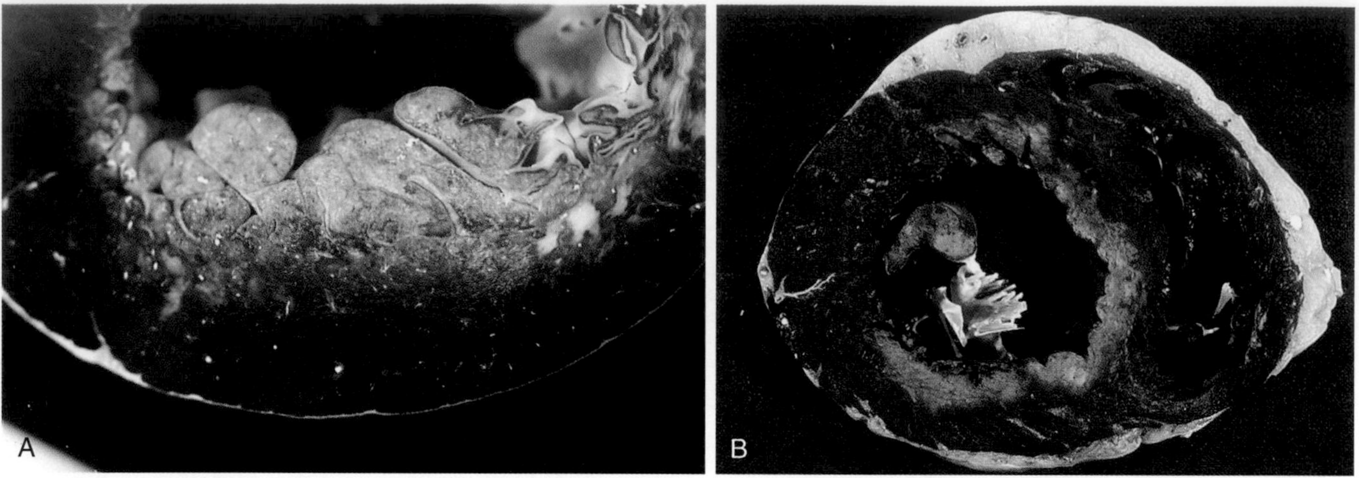

FIGURE 24-19 Myocardial Infarction. A, Local infarct confined to one region. **B,** Massive large infarct caused by occlusion of three coronary arteries. (From Damjanov, I., & Linder, J. [Eds.]. [1996]. *Anderson's pathology* [10th ed.]. St. Louis: Mosby.)

The severity of functional impairment depends on the size of the lesion and the site of infarction. Functional changes can include (1) decreased cardiac contractility with abnormal wall motion, (2) altered left ventricular compliance, (3) decreased stroke volume, (4) decreased ejection fraction, (5) increased left ventricular end-diastolic pressure (LVEDP), and (6) sinoatrial node malfunction. Life-threatening dysrhythmias and HF often follow MI.

With infarction, ventricular function is abnormal and the ejection fraction falls, resulting in increases in ventricular end-diastolic volume (VEDV). If the coronary obstruction involves the perfusion to the left ventricle, pulmonary venous congestion ensues; if the right ventricle is ischemic, increases in systemic venous pressures occur.

MI causes a severe inflammatory response that ends with wound repair (see Chapter 6). Damaged cells undergo degradation, fibroblasts proliferate, and scar tissue is synthesized. Many cell types, hormones, and nutrient substrates must be available for optimal healing to proceed. Within 24 hours, leukocytes infiltrate the necrotic area, and proteolytic enzymes from scavenger neutrophils degrade necrotic tissue. The collagen matrix that is deposited is initially weak, mushy, and vulnerable to re-injury. Unfortunately, it is at this time in the recovery period (10 to 14 days after infarction) that individuals feel more like increasing activities and may stress the newly formed scar tissue. After 6 weeks, the necrotic area is completely replaced by scar tissue, which is strong but cannot contract and relax like healthy myocardial tissue.

CLINICAL MANIFESTATIONS The first symptom of acute MI is usually sudden, severe chest pain. The pain is similar to that of angina pectoris but more severe and prolonged. It may be described as heavy and crushing, such as a "truck sitting on my chest." Radiation to the neck, jaw, back, shoulder, or left arm is common. Some individuals, especially those who are older adults or have diabetes, experience no pain, thereby having a "silent" infarction. Infarction often simulates a sensation of unrelenting indigestion. Nausea and vomiting may occur because of reflex stimulation of vomiting centres by pain fibres. Vasovagal reflexes from the area of the infarcted myocardium also may affect the gastro-intestinal tract.

Various cardiovascular changes are found on physical examination:

- The SNS is reflexively activated to compensate, resulting in a temporary increase in heart rate and blood pressure.
- Abnormal extra heart sounds reflect left ventricular dysfunction.
- Pulmonary findings of congestion including dullness to percussion and inspiratory crackles at the lung bases can occur if the individual develops HF.
- Peripheral vasoconstriction may cause the skin to become cool and clammy.

The number and severity of postinfarction complications depend on the location and extent of necrosis, the individual's physiological condition before the infarction, and the availability of swift therapeutic intervention. Sudden cardiac death can occur in individuals with myocardial ischemia even if infarction is absent or minimal, and is a multifactorial problem. Risk factors for sudden death are related to three factors: ischemia, left ventricular dysfunction, and electrical instability. These factors interact with each other (Figure 24-20). Table 24-5 lists the most common complications.

EVALUATION AND TREATMENT The diagnosis of acute MI is made on the basis of history, physical examination, ECG results, and serial cardiac troponin elevations (Box 24-2). The cardiac troponins (troponin I and troponin T) are the most specific indicators of MI. A transient rise in these plasma enzyme levels can confirm the occurrence of MI and indicate its severity. Blood is drawn for troponin level determination as soon as possible after the onset of symptoms, and serial serum levels are assessed for several days. If serological tests show abnormally high levels of troponin, acute MI has occurred. Elevation of troponin level may not occur immediately after infarction and laboratory confirmation that an infarction has occurred may be delayed up to 12 hours.

MI can occur in various regions of the heart wall and may be described as anterior, inferior, posterior, lateral, subendocardial, or transmural, depending on the anatomical location and extent of tissue damage from infarction. Twelve-lead ECGs help localize the affected area through identification of changes in ST segments and T waves (Figure 24-21). The infarcted myocardium is surrounded by a zone of hypoxic injury, which may progress to necrosis or return to normal, and adjacent to this zone of hypoxic injury is a zone of reversible ischemia (see Figure 24-21). A characteristic Q wave often develops on ECG some hours later in STEMI.

Cardiac troponin I (cTnI) is the most specific indicator of MI, and measurement of its level should be performed on admission to the emergency department. cTnI level elevation is detectable 2 to 4 hours after onset of symptoms. Additional measurements within 6 to 9 hours

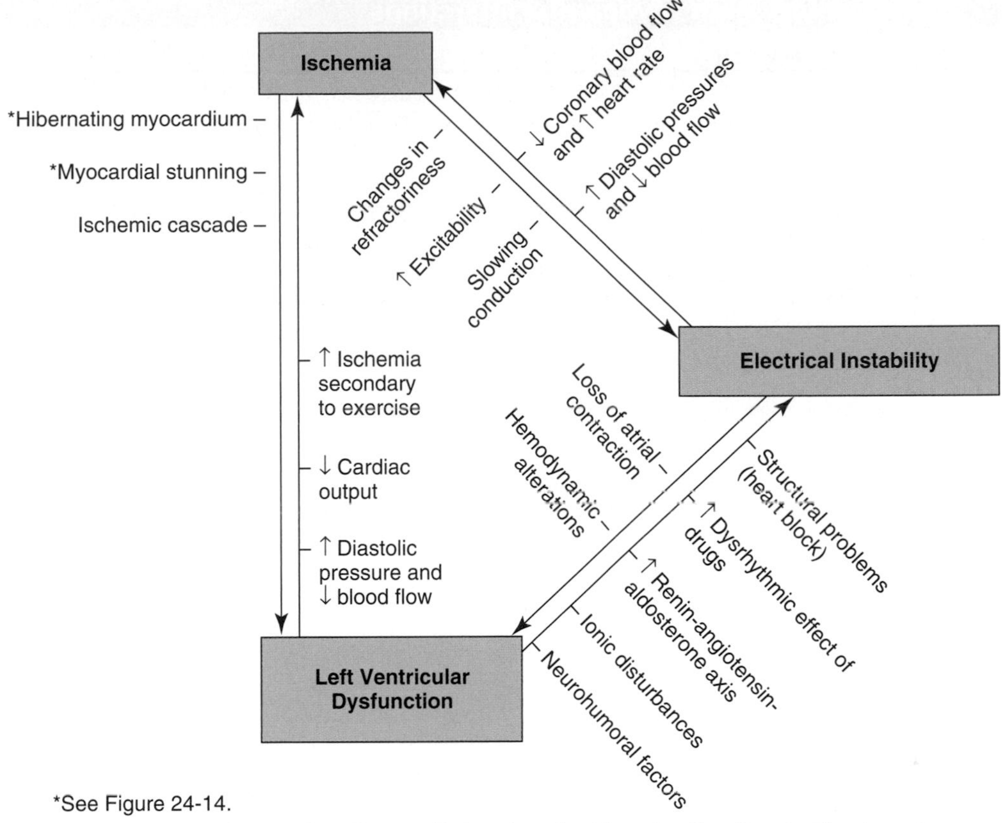

FIGURE 24-20 Three Interacting Factors Related to Sudden Cardiac Death. The three factors are ischemia, left ventricular dysfunction, and electrical instability.

BOX 24-2 Universal Definition of Myocardial Infarction

The term *myocardial infarction* should be used when there is evidence of myocardial necrosis in a clinical setting with myocardial ischemia. Under these conditions any one of the following criteria meets the diagnosis for myocardial infarction:

- Detection of rise and/or fall of cardiac biomarkers (preferably troponin) with at least one value above the 99th percentile of the upper reference limit (URL) together with evidence of myocardial ischemia with at least one of the following:
  - Symptoms of ischemia
  - Electrocardiogram (ECG) changes indicative of new ischemia (new ST–T changes or new left bundle branch block [LBBB])
  - Development of pathological Q waves in the ECG
  - Imaging evidence of new loss of viable myocardium or new regional wall motion abnormality
- Sudden, unexpected cardiac death, involving cardiac arrest, often with symptoms suggestive of myocardial ischemia, and accompanied by presumably new ST elevation, or new LBBB, and/or evidence of fresh thrombus by coronary angiography and/or at autopsy; but death occurring before blood samples could be obtained, or at a time before the appearance of cardiac biomarkers in the blood.
- For percutaneous coronary interventions (PCIs) in persons with normal baseline troponin values, elevations of cardiac biomarkers greater than the 99th percentile URL are indicative of periprocedural myocardial necrosis. By convention, increases of biomarkers greater than 3 × 99th percentile URL have been designated as defining PCI-related myocardial infarction. A subtype related to a documented stent thrombosis is recognized.
- For coronary artery bypass grafting (CABG) in persons with normal baseline troponin values, elevations of cardiac biomarkers greater than the 99th percentile URL are indicative of periprocedural myocardial necrosis. By convention, increases of biomarkers greater than 5 × 99th percentile URL plus either new pathological Q waves or new LBBB, or angiographically documented new graft or native coronary artery occlusion, or imaging evidence of new loss of viable myocardium have been designated as defining CABG-related myocardial infarction.
- Pathological findings of an acute myocardial infarction.

Data from Linden, B. (2013). *BJCN, 8*(1), 8–9. doi:10.12968/bjca.2013.8.1.8; Thygesen, K., Alpert, J.S., Jaffe, A.S., et al. (2012). *Circulation, 126*(16), 2020–2035; Thygesen, K., Alpert, J.S., Jaffe, A.S., et al. (2015). The universal definition of myocardial infarction. In M. Tubaro, P. Vranckx, S. Price, et al. (Eds.), *The ESC textbook of intensive and acute cardiovascular care* (2nd ed., pp. 356–364). Oxford: Oxford University Press; Thygesen, K., Alpert, J.S., White, H.D., et al. (2007). *J Am Coll Cardiol,* 50, 2173–2195.

and again at 12 to 24 hours are recommended if clinical suspicion is high and previous samples were negative. Troponin levels also can be used to estimate infarct size and, therefore, the likelihood of complications. Additional laboratory data may reveal leukocytosis and elevated CRP, both of which indicate inflammation. The individual's blood glucose level is usually elevated, and the glucose tolerance level may remain abnormal for several weeks.

Acute MI requires admission to the hospital, often directly into a coronary care unit. Most guidelines continue to recommend the use of oxygen in acute MI; however, a recent review did not demonstrate

TABLE 24-5 Complications With Myocardial Infarctions

Type	Characteristics
Dysrhythmias	Disturbances of cardiac rhythm that affect 90% of persons with cardiac infarction
	Causes are ischemia, hypoxia, autonomic nervous system imbalances, lactic acidosis, electrolyte abnormalities, alterations of impulse conduction pathways or conduction abnormalities, medication toxicity, or hemodynamic abnormalities
Left ventricular failure (heart failure)	Characterized by pulmonary congestion, reduced myocardial contractility, and abnormal heart wall motion
	Cardiogenic shock can develop
Inflammation of pericardium (pericarditis)	Pericardial friction rubs
	Often noted 2 to 3 days later and associated with anterior chest pain that worsens with respiratory effort
Dressler postinfarction syndrome	Essentially a delayed form of pericarditis that occurs 1 week to several months after acute myocardial infarction (MI) syndrome
	Thought to be immunological response to necrotic myocardium marked by pain, fever, friction rub, pleural effusion, and arthralgias
Organic brain syndrome	Occurs if blood flow to brain is impaired secondary to MI
Transient ischemic attacks or cerebrovascular accident	Occur if thromboemboli detach from clots that form in cardiac chambers or on cardiac valves
Rupture of heart structures	Cause is necrosis of tissue in or around papillary muscles
	Papillary muscles of chordae tendineae cordis affected
	Predisposing factors include thinning of wall, poor collateral flow, shearing effect of muscular contraction against stiffened necrotic area, marked necrosis at terminal end of blood supply, and aging of myocardium with laceration of myocardial microstructure
Rupture of wall of infarcted ventricle	Can be caused by aneurysm formation when pressure becomes too great
Left ventricular aneurysm	Late (month to years) complication of MI that can contribute to heart failure and thromboemboli
Infarctions around septal structures	Occur in those structures that separate heart chambers and lead to septal rupture
	Associated with audible, harsh cardiac murmurs; increased left ventricular end-diastolic pressure; and decreased systemic blood pressure
Systemic thromboembolism	May disseminate from debris and clots that collect inside dilated aneurysmal sacs or from infarcted endocardium
Pulmonary thromboembolism	Usually from deep venous thrombi of legs
	Reduced incidence associated with early mobilization and prophylactic anticoagulation therapy
Sudden death	Dysrhythmias frequently causative, particularly ventricular fibrillation
	Risk for death increased by age more than 65 years, previous angina pectoris, hypotension or cardiogenic shock, acute systolic hypertension at time of admission, diabetes mellitus, dysrhythmias, and previous MI

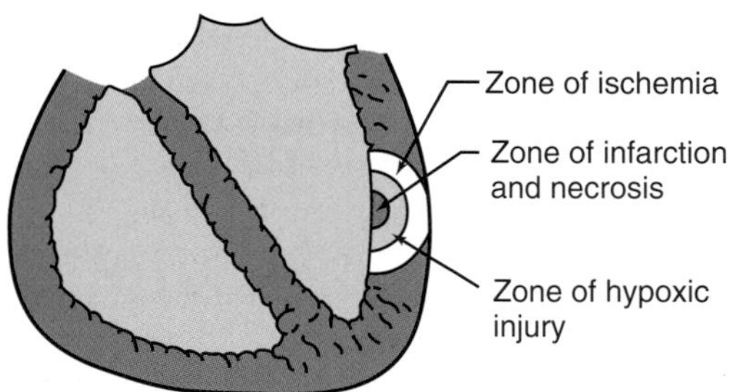

FIGURE 24-21 Electrocardiographic Alterations Associated With the Three Zones of Myocardial Infarction.

a clear benefit of oxygen therapy.[113] The individual should be given an Aspirin immediately (ticlopidine if allergic to Aspirin). Pain relief is of utmost importance and involves the use of sublingual nitroglycerine and morphine sulphate. Continuous monitoring of cardiac rhythms and enzymatic changes is essential, because the first 24 hours after onset of symptoms is the time of highest risk for sudden death. Non-STEMI is treated in the same way as unstable angina, including antithrombotics, anticoagulation or PCI, or both.[107] STEMI is best managed with emergent PCI and antithrombotics.[114] Thrombolytics may be used if PCI is not readily available. Hyperglycemia is treated with insulin. Once the person is stabilized, further management includes ACE inhibitors, beta-blockers, and statins.[114] Individuals who are in shock require aggressive fluid resuscitation, ionotropic medications, and possible emergent invasive procedures.

Bed rest, followed by gradual return to activities of daily living, reduces the myocardial oxygen demands of the compromised heart. Individuals not receiving thrombolytic or heparin infusion must receive DVT prophylaxis as long as their activity is significantly limited. Stool softeners are given to eliminate the need for straining, which can precipitate bradycardia and can be followed by increased venous return to the heart, causing possible cardiac overload. Education regarding appropriate diet and caffeine intake, smoking cessation, exercise, and other aspects of risk factor reduction is crucial for secondary prevention of recurrent myocardial ischemia.

QUICK CHECK 24-6

1. Describe the coronary artery disease–myocardial ischemia continuum.
2. Describe the pathophysiology of myocardial infarction.
3. What complications are associated with the period after infarction?

DISORDERS OF THE HEART WALL

Disorders of the Pericardium

Pericardial disease is a localized manifestation of another disorder, such as infection (bacterial, viral, fungal, rickettsial, or parasitic); trauma or surgery; neoplasm; or a metabolic, immunological, or vascular disorder (uremia, rheumatoid arthritis, systemic lupus erythematosus, periarteritis nodosa). The pericardial response to injury from these diverse causes may consist of acute pericarditis, pericardial effusion, or constrictive pericarditis.

Acute Pericarditis

Acute pericarditis is acute inflammation of the pericardium. The etiology of acute pericarditis is most often idiopathic or caused by viral infection by coxsackie, influenza, hepatitis, measles, mumps, or varicella viruses. It also is the most common cardiovascular complication of human immunodeficiency virus (HIV) infection. Other causes include MI, trauma, neoplasm, surgery, uremia, bacterial infection (especially tuberculosis), connective tissue disease (especially systemic lupus erythematosus and rheumatoid arthritis), or radiation therapy.[115] The pericardial membranes become inflamed and roughened, and a pericardial effusion may develop that can be serous, purulent, or fibrinous (Figure 24-22). Possible sequelae of pericarditis include recurrent pericarditis, pericardial constriction, and cardiac tamponade.

Symptoms may follow several days of fever and usually begin with the sudden onset of severe retrosternal chest pain that worsens with respiratory movements and when assuming a recumbent position. The pain may radiate to the back as a result of irritation of the phrenic nerve (innervates the trapezius muscles) as it traverses the pericardium. Individuals with acute pericarditis also report dysphagia, restlessness, irritability, anxiety, weakness, and malaise.

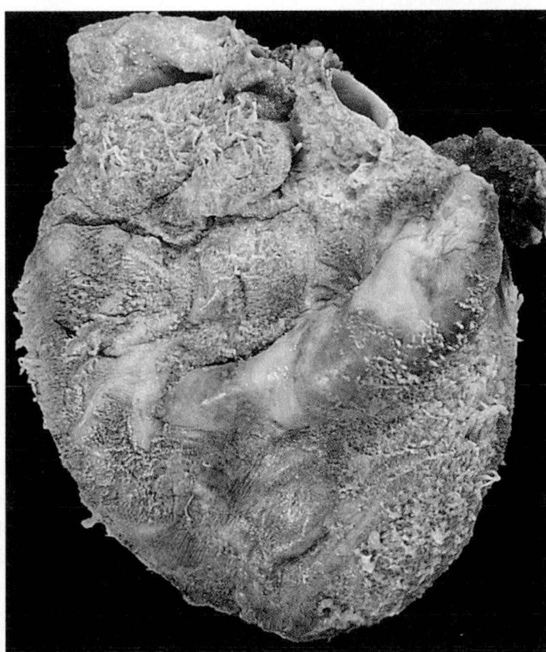

FIGURE 24-22 Acute Pericarditis. Note shaggy coat of fibres covering the surface of heart. (From Damjanov, I., & Linder, J. [2000]. *Pathology: A color atlas.* St. Louis: Mosby.)

Physical examination often discloses low-grade fever (less than 38°C [100.4°F]) and sinus tachycardia. A friction rub—a scratchy, grating sound—may be heard at the cardiac apex and left sternal border and is highly suggestive of pericarditis. The rub is caused by the roughened pericardial membranes rubbing against each other. Friction rubs are not always present and may be intermittently heard and transient. Hypotension or the presence of a pulsus paradoxus (a decrease in systolic blood pressure of greater than 10 mm Hg with inspiration) is suggestive of cardiac tamponade, which can be life-threatening. Electrocardiographic changes may reflect inflammatory processes through PR segment depression and diffuse ST segment elevation without Q waves, and they may remain abnormal for days or even weeks.[115] Ultrasound, CT scanning, and MRI may be used as diagnostic modalities. Acute pericarditis requires at least two of the following four criteria for diagnosis: (1) chest pain characteristics of pericarditis, (2) pericardial rub, (3) characteristic electrocardiographic changes, and (4) new or worsening pericardial effusion.[115]

Treatment for uncomplicated acute pericarditis consists of relieving symptoms and includes administration of anti-inflammatory agents, such as salicylates and nonsteroidal anti-inflammatory drugs (NSAIDs), and colchicine. Approximately one-third of cases will be complicated by the development of idiopathic recurrent pericarditis.[116] Exploration of the underlying cause is important. If pericardial effusion develops, aspiration of the excessive fluid may be necessary.

Pericardial Effusion

Pericardial effusion is the accumulation of fluid in the pericardial cavity and can occur in all forms of pericarditis. Most are idiopathic (20%), but other causes (such as neoplasm and infection) must be considered.[115] Analysis of the fluid obtained through pericardiocentesis allows for identification of the likely source of the fluid.[117] The fluid may be a transudate, such as the serous effusion that develops with left ventricular failure, overhydration, or hypoproteinemia. More often, however, the fluid is an exudate, which reflects pericardial inflammation like that seen with acute pericarditis, heart surgery, some chemotherapeutic agents, infections, and autoimmune disorders such as systemic lupus erythematosus. (Types of exudate are described in Chapter 6.) Exudative effusions also are found in up to 12% of individuals with STEMI.[118] If the fluid is serosanguineous, the underlying cause is likely to be tuberculosis, neoplasm, uremia, or radiation. Idiopathic serosanguineous (cause unknown) effusion is possible, however. Effusions of frank blood are generally related to aneurysms, trauma, or coagulation defects (Figure 24-23). If chyle leaks from the thoracic duct, it may enter the pericardium and lead to cholesterol pericarditis.

Pericardial effusion, even in large amounts, is not necessarily clinically significant, except that it indicates an underlying disorder. If an effusion develops gradually, the pericardium can stretch to accommodate large quantities of fluid without compressing the heart. If the fluid accumulates rapidly, however, even a small amount (50 to 100 mL) may create sufficient pressure to cause cardiac compression, a serious condition known as tamponade. The danger is that pressure exerted by the pericardial fluid eventually will equal diastolic pressure within the heart chambers, which will interfere with right atrial filling during diastole. The decrease in right atrial filling causes increased venous pressure, systemic venous congestion, and signs and symptoms of right ventricular failure (distension of the jugular veins, edema, hepatomegaly). Decreased atrial filling leads to decreased ventricular filling, decreased stroke volume, and reduced cardiac output. Life-threatening circulatory collapse may occur.

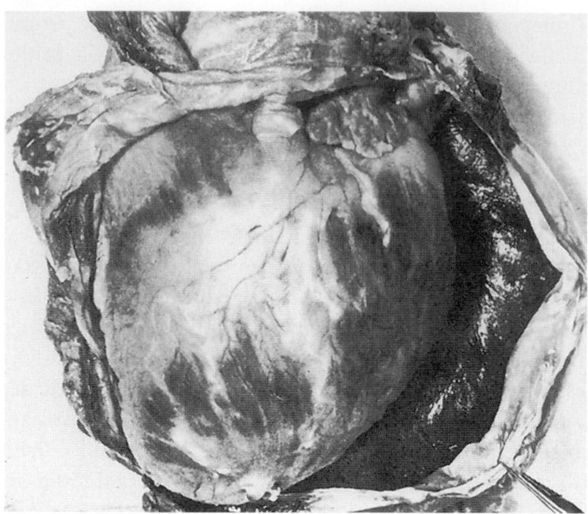

FIGURE 24-23 Exudate of Blood in the Pericardial Sac From Rupture of Aneurysm. (From Damjanov, I., & Linder, J. [2000]. *Pathology: A color atlas.* St. Louis: Mosby.)

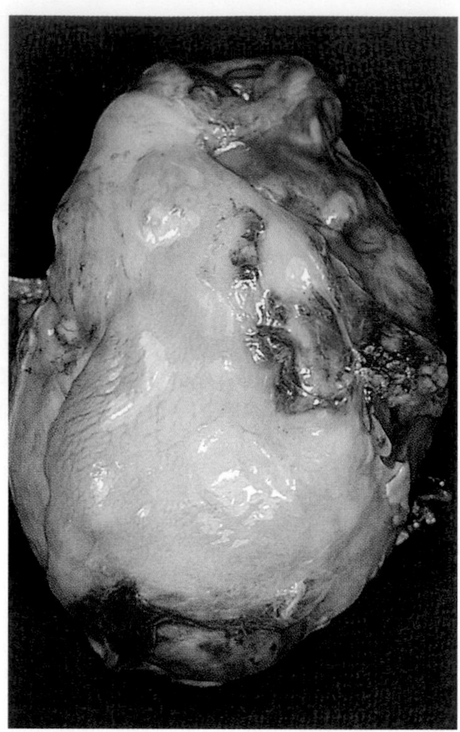

FIGURE 24-24 Constrictive Pericarditis. The fibrotic pericardium encases the heart in a rigid shell. (From Damjanov, I., & Linder, J. [2000]. *Pathology: A color atlas.* St. Louis: Mosby.)

An important clinical finding is pulsus paradoxus, in which arterial blood pressure during expiration exceeds arterial pressure during inspiration by more than 10 mm Hg. Pulsus paradoxus in the setting of a pericardial effusion indicates tamponade and reflects impairment of diastolic filling of the left ventricle plus reduction of blood volume within all four cardiac chambers. The presence of a large pericardial effusion or tamponade magnifies the normally insignificant effect of inspiration on intracardiac flow and volume.

Other clinical manifestations of pericardial effusion are distant or muffled heart sounds, poorly palpable apical pulse, dyspnea on exertion, and dull chest pain. A chest X-ray film may disclose a "water-bottle configuration" of the cardiac silhouette. An echocardiogram can detect an effusion as small as 20 mL and is a reliable and accurate diagnostic test, although CT scans also may be done.[115]

Treatment of pericardial effusion or tamponade generally consists of pericardiocentesis (aspiration of excessive pericardial fluid) and treatment of the underlying condition. Persistent pain may be treated with analgesics, anti-inflammatory medications, or steroids. Surgery may be required if the underlying cause of tamponade is trauma or aneurysm. A pericardial "window" may be surgically created to prevent tamponade.[119]

Constrictive Pericarditis

Constrictive pericarditis, or restrictive pericarditis (chronic pericarditis), was synonymous with tuberculosis years ago, and tuberculosis continues to be an important cause of pericarditis in immunocompromised individuals. Currently, this form of pericardial disease is more commonly idiopathic or associated with viral infection, radiation exposure, collagen vascular disorders, sarcoidosis, neoplasm, uremia, or cardiac surgery.[115] In constrictive pericarditis, fibrous scarring with occasional calcification of the pericardium causes the visceral and parietal pericardial layers to adhere, obliterating the pericardial cavity. The fibrotic lesions encase the heart in a rigid shell (Figure 24-24). Like tamponade, constrictive pericarditis compresses the heart and eventually reduces cardiac output. Unlike tamponade, however, constrictive pericarditis always develops gradually.

Symptoms tend to be exercise intolerance, dyspnea on exertion, fatigue, and anorexia. Clinical assessment shows edema, distension of the jugular vein, hepatic congestion, and systemic hypotension. Restricted ventricular filling may cause a pericardial knock (early diastolic sound). ECG findings include nonspecific ST and T wave abnormalities and atrial fibrillation (AF). Chest X-ray films often disclose prominent pulmonary vessels and calcification of the pericardium. CT, MRI, and transesophageal echocardiography are used to detect pericardial thickening and constriction and to distinguish constrictive pericarditis from restrictive cardiomyopathy. Pericardial biopsy may be needed to determine the etiology.

Initial treatment for constrictive pericarditis consists of restriction of dietary sodium intake and administration of diuretics to improve cardiac output. Management also may include use of anti-inflammatory medications and treatment of any underlying disorder. If these modalities are unsuccessful, surgical excision of the restrictive pericardium is indicated (pericardial decortication).[115]

Disorders of the Myocardium: The Cardiomyopathies

The cardiomyopathies are a diverse group of diseases that primarily affect the myocardium itself. They may, however, be secondary to infectious disease, toxin exposure, systemic connective tissue disease, infiltrative and proliferative disorders, or nutritional deficiencies. Many cases are idiopathic; others are caused by ischemia, hypertension, inherited disorders, infections, toxins, or systemic inflammatory disorders. Some are preceded by myocarditis; however, most individuals with acute myocarditis recover without sequelae.[115] The cardiomyopathies are categorized as dilated (formerly, congestive), hypertrophic, or restrictive, depending on their physiological effects on the heart (Figure 24-25).

Dilated cardiomyopathy is usually the result of ischemic heart disease, valvular disease, diabetes, renal failure, alcohol or medication toxicity, peripartum complications, or infection.[115] There is a strong genetic basis for dilated cardiomyopathy, and it can be associated with inherited disorders, such as muscular dystrophy. It is characterized by impaired systolic function leading to increases in intracardiac volume, ventricular dilation, and HF with reduced ejection fraction (Figure 24-26).

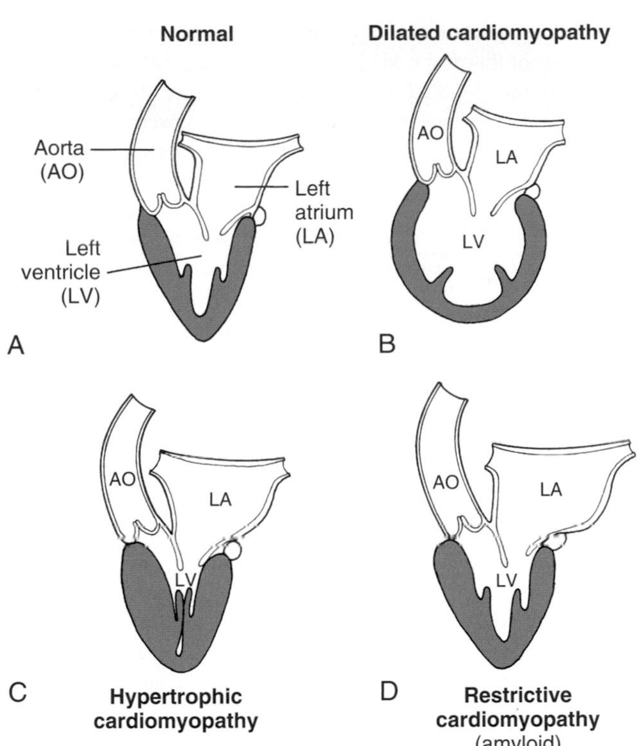

FIGURE 24-25 Diagram Showing Major Distinguishing Pathophysiological Features of the Three Types of Cardiomyopathy. **A,** The normal heart. **B,** In the dilated type of cardiomyopathy, the heart has a globular shape and the largest circumference of the left ventricle is not at its base but midway between apex and base. **C,** In the hypertrophic type, the wall of the left ventricle is greatly thickened; the left ventricular cavity is small, but the left atrium may be dilated because of poor diastolic relaxation of the ventricle. **D,** In the restrictive (constrictive) type, the left ventricular cavity is normal size, but, again, the left atrium is dilated because of the reduced diastolic compliance of the ventricle. (From Kissane, J.M. [Ed.]. [1990]. *Anderson's pathology* [9th ed.]. St Louis: Mosby.)

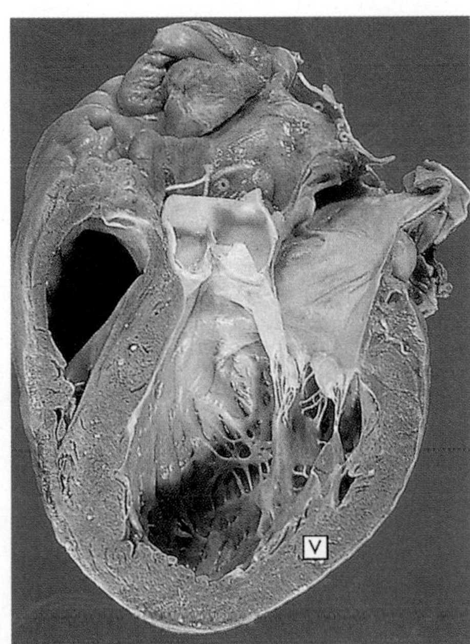

FIGURE 24-26 Dilated Cardiomyopathy. The dilated left ventricle has a thin wall (*V*). (From Stevens, A., Lowe, J.S., & Scott, I. [2009]. *Core pathology* [3rd ed.]. London: Mosby.)

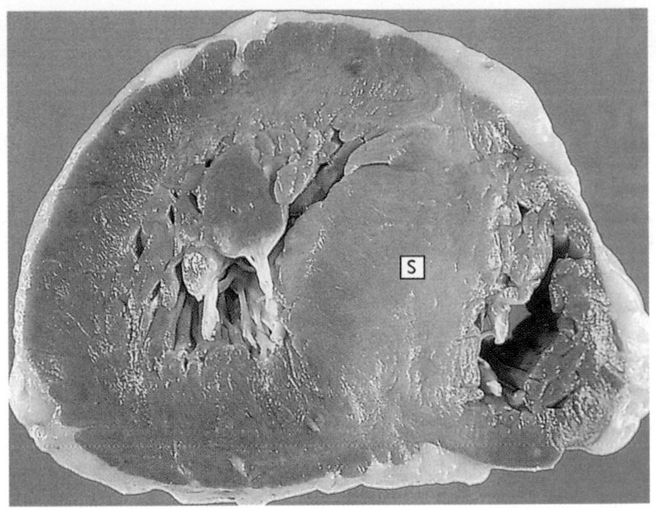

FIGURE 24-27 Hypertrophic Cardiomyopathy. There is marked left ventricular hypertrophy, which often affects the septum (*S*). (From Stevens, A., Lowe, J.S., & Scott, I. [2009]. *Core pathology* [3rd ed.]. London: Mosby.)

Individuals complain of dyspnea, fatigue, and pedal edema. Findings on examination include a displaced apical pulse, S_3 gallop, peripheral edema, jugular venous distension, and pulmonary congestion. Diagnosis is confirmed by chest X-ray and echocardiogram, and management is focused on reducing blood volume, increasing contractility, and reversing the underlying disorder if possible.[115] Heart transplant is required in severe cases.

Hypertrophic cardiomyopathy refers to two major categories of thickening of the myocardium: (1) hypertrophic obstructive cardiomyopathy (asymmetric septal hypertrophic cardiomyopathy or subaortic stenosis) and (2) hypertensive or valvular hypertrophic cardiomyopathy. **Hypertrophic obstructive cardiomyopathy** is the most commonly inherited cardiac disorder. It is characterized by thickening of the septal wall (Figure 24-27), which may cause outflow obstruction to the left ventricle outflow tract.[115] Obstruction of left ventricular outflow can occur when the heart rate is increased and the intravascular volume is decreased. This type of hypertrophic cardiomyopathy is a significant risk factor for serious ventricular dysrhythmias and sudden death.[115,120] There are other conditions that cause hypertrophic changes in the ventricles; **hypertensive hypertrophic cardiomyopathy** and **valvular hypertrophic cardiomyopathy** are the most common.[121] These conditions occur because of increased resistance to ventricular ejection, which is commonly seen in individuals with hypertension or valvular stenosis (usually aortic). In this case, hypertrophy of the myocytes is an attempt to compensate for increased myocardial workload. Long-term dysfunction of the myocytes develops over time, with diastolic dysfunction appearing first and leading eventually to systolic dysfunction of the ventricle. Individuals with hypertrophic cardiomyopathy may be asymptomatic or may complain of angina, syncope, dyspnea on exertion, and palpitations. Examination may reveal extra heart sounds and murmurs. Echocardiography and cardiac catheterization can confirm the diagnosis.

Restrictive cardiomyopathy is characterized by restrictive filling and increased diastolic pressure of either or both ventricles with normal or near-normal systolic function and wall thickness. It may occur idiopathically or as a cardiac manifestation of systemic diseases, such as amyloidosis, scleroderma, sarcoidosis, lymphoma, and hemochromatosis, or a number of inherited storage diseases.[115] The myocardium becomes rigid and noncompliant, impeding ventricular filling and raising filling pressures during diastole. The most common clinical manifestation of restrictive cardiomyopathy is right ventricular failure with systemic venous congestion. Cardiomegaly and dysrhythmias are common. A thorough evaluation for the underlying cause should be initiated (and may include myocardial biopsy). Treatment is aimed at the underlying cause. Death occurs as a result of HF or dysrhythmias.

QUICK CHECK 24-7

1. Why does pericarditis develop?
2. What are the cardiomyopathies? List the major disorders.
3. Briefly describe the pathophysiological effects of the cardiomyopathies.

Disorders of the Endocardium

Valvular Dysfunction

Disorders of the endocardium (the innermost lining of the heart wall) damage the heart valves, which are composed of endocardial tissue. Endocardial damage can be either congenital or acquired. The acquired forms result from inflammatory, ischemic, traumatic, degenerative, or infectious alterations of valvular structure and function. One of the most common causes of acquired valvular dysfunction is degeneration or inflammation of the endocardium secondary to rheumatic heart disease (Table 24-6). Structural alterations of the heart valves are caused by remodelling changes in the valvular extracellular matrix and lead to stenosis, incompetence, or both.

In **valvular stenosis**, the valve orifice is constricted and narrowed, so blood cannot flow forward and the workload of the cardiac chamber proximal to the diseased valve increases (Figure 24-28). Pressure (intraventricular or atrial) rises in the chamber to overcome resistance to flow through the valve, necessitating greater exertion by the myocardium and producing myocardial hypertrophy.

Although all four heart valves may be affected, in adults those of the left heart (mitral and aortic valves) are far more commonly affected than those of the right heart (tricuspid and pulmonic valves). In **valvular regurgitation** (also called **valvular insufficiency** or **valvular incompetence**), the valve leaflets, or cusps, fail to shut completely, permitting blood flow to continue even when the valve is presumably closed (see Figure 24-28). During systole or diastole, some blood leaks back into the chamber proximal to the diseased valve, which increases the volume of blood the heart must pump and increases the workload of both the atrium and the ventricle. Increased volume leads to chamber dilation, and increased workload leads to hypertrophy, both of which are compensatory mechanisms intended to increase the pumping capability of the heart but that lead to cardiac dysfunction over time. Eventually, myocardial contractility diminishes, ejection fraction drops, and diastolic pressure increases, and the ventricles fail from being overworked. Depending on the severity of the valvular dysfunction and the capacity of the heart to compensate, valvular alterations cause a range of symptoms and some degree of incapacitation (see Table 24-6).

In general, valvular disease is diagnosed by transthoracic echocardiography (TTE), which can be used to assess the severity of valvular

TABLE 24-6 Clinical Manifestations of Valvular Stenosis and Regurgitation

Manifestation	Aortic Stenosis	Mitral Stenosis	Aortic Regurgitation	Mitral Regurgitation	Tricuspid Regurgitation
Most common cause	Congenital bicuspid valve, degenerative (calcific) changes with aging, rheumatic heart disease	Rheumatic heart disease	Infective endocarditis; aortic root disease (connective tissue diseases, Marfan's syndrome); dilation of aortic root from hypertension and aging	Myxomatous degeneration (mitral valve prolapse)	Congenital
Cardiovascular outcome (untreated)	Left ventricular hypertrophy followed by left ventricular failure; decreased coronary blood flow with myocardial ischemia	Left atrial hypertrophy and dilation with fibrillation, followed by right ventricular failure	Left ventricular hypertrophy and dilation, followed by left ventricular failure	Left atrial hypertrophy and dilation, followed by left ventricular failure	Right ventricular failure
Pulmonary effects	Pulmonary edema: dyspnea on exertion	Pulmonary edema: dyspnea on exertion, orthopnea, paroxysmal nocturnal dyspnea, predisposition to respiratory tract infections, hemoptysis, pulmonary hypertension	Pulmonary edema with dyspnea on exertion	Pulmonary edema with dyspnea on exertion	Dyspnea
Central nervous system effects	Syncope, especially on exertion	Neural deficits only associated with emboli (e.g., hemiparesis)	Syncope	None	None
Pain	Angina pectoris	Atypical chest pain	Angina pectoris	Atypical chest pain	Palpitations
Heart sounds	Systolic murmur heard best at right parasternal second intercostal space and radiating to neck	Low, rumbling diastolic murmur heard best at apex and radiating to axilla; accentuated first heart sound, opening snap	Diastolic murmur heard best at right parasternal second intercostal space and radiating to neck	Murmur throughout systole heard best at apex and radiating to axilla	Murmur throughout systole heard best at left lower sternal border

With data from Mann, D.L., Zipes, D.P., Libby, P., et al. (Eds.). (2014). *Braunwald's heart disease: A textbook of cardiovascular medicine* (10th ed.). Philadelphia: Saunders.

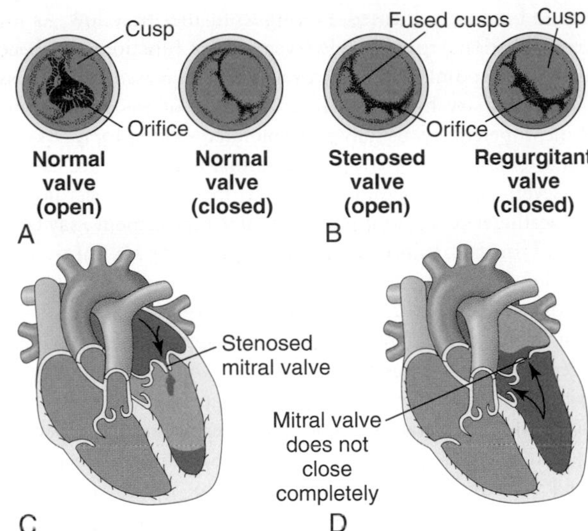

FIGURE 24-28 **Valvular Stenosis and Regurgitation.** **A,** Normal position of the valve leaflets, or cusps, when the valve is open and closed. **B,** Open position of a stenosed valve (*left*) and open position of a closed regurgitant valve (*right*). **C,** Hemodynamic effect of mitral stenosis. The stenosed valve is unable to open sufficiently during left atrial systole, inhibiting left ventricular filling. **D,** Hemodynamic effect of mitral regurgitation. The mitral valve does not close completely during left ventricular systole, permitting blood to re-enter the left atrium.

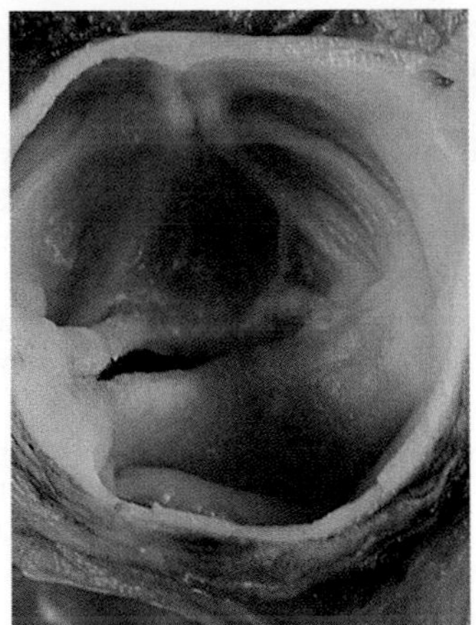

FIGURE 24-29 **Aortic Stenosis.** Mild stenosis in valve leaflets of a young adult. (From Damjanov, I., & Linder, J. [2000]. *Pathophysiology: A color atlas.* St. Louis: Mosby.)

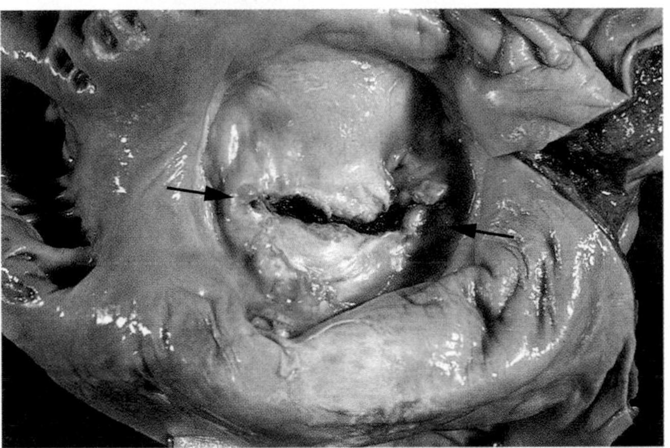

FIGURE 24-30 **Mitral Stenosis With Classic "Fish Mouth" Orifice.** (From Kumar, V., Abbas, A.K., & Aster, J.C. [Eds.]. [2015]. *Robins and Cotran pathologic basis of disease* [9th ed.]. Philadelphia: Saunders.)

obstruction or regurgitation before the onset of symptoms. CT or MRI may be indicated in certain settings. Valvular lesions are staged and appropriate management is determined by using four general categories: (1) at risk, (2) progressive, (3) asymptomatic severe, and (4) symptomatic severe.[122] Management almost always includes careful medical management, valvular repair, or valve replacement followed by long-term anticoagulation therapy and prophylaxis for endocarditis as needed. The purpose of valvular intervention is to improve symptoms and prolong survival, as well as to minimize complications, such as asymptomatic irreversible ventricular dysfunction, pulmonary hypertension, stroke, and AF.[122]

Stenosis

Aortic stenosis. **Aortic stenosis** is the most common valvular abnormality, affecting nearly 2% of adults older than 65 years of age.[123] It has three common causes: (1) congenital bicuspid valve, (2) degeneration with aging, and (3) inflammatory damage caused by rheumatic heart disease. Aortic stenosis also is associated with many risk factors for CAD, including hypertension, smoking, and dyslipidemia. Aortic valve degeneration with aging is associated with chronic inflammation, lipoprotein deposition in the tissue, and leaflet calcification. The orifice of the aortic valve narrows, causing resistance to blood flow from the left ventricle into the aorta (Figure 24-29). Outflow obstruction increases pressure within the left ventricle as it tries to eject blood through the narrowed opening. Left ventricular hypertrophy develops to compensate for the increased workload. Eventually, hypertrophy increases myocardial oxygen demand, which the coronary arteries may not be able to supply, leading to attacks of angina. In addition, aortic stenosis is frequently accompanied by atherosclerotic coronary disease, further contributing to inadequate coronary perfusion. Untreated aortic stenosis can lead to hypertrophic cardiomyopathy, dysrhythmias, MI, and HF.[123]

Aortic stenosis usually develops gradually. Classic symptoms include angina, syncope, and dyspnea. Clinical manifestations include decreased stroke volume and narrowed pulse pressure (the difference between systolic and diastolic pressures). Heart rate is often slow, and pulses are delayed. Resistance to flow leads to a crescendo-decrescendo systolic heart murmur heard best at the right parasternal second intercostal space, and may radiate to the neck. Echocardiography can be used to assess the severity of valvular obstruction before the onset of symptoms. Medical management includes vasodilator therapy. Surgical valve replacement with either a mechanical or a bioprosthetic valve is indicated for both symptomatic and asymptomatic individuals with severe stenosis.[122] Percutaneous placement of a prosthetic valve avoids major heart surgery in selected individuals.[122,124] Once individuals become symptomatic from aortic stenosis, the prognosis is poor.

Mitral stenosis. **Mitral stenosis** impairs the flow of blood from the left atrium to the left ventricle. Mitral stenosis is the most common form of rheumatic heart disease. Autoimmunity in response to group A β-hemolytic streptococcal M protein antigens leads to inflammation and scarring of the valvular leaflets. Scarring causes the leaflets to become fibrous and fused, and the chordae tendineae cordis become shortened (Figure 24-30).

Impedance to blood flow results in incomplete emptying of the left atrium and elevated atrial pressure as the chamber tries to force blood through the stenotic valve. Continued increases in left atrial volume and pressure cause atrial dilation and hypertrophy. The risk of developing AF and dysrhythmia-induced thrombi is high. As mitral stenosis progresses, symptoms of decreased cardiac output occur, especially during exertion. Continued elevation of left atrial pressure and volume causes pressure to rise in the pulmonary circulation. If untreated, chronic mitral stenosis develops into pulmonary hypertension, pulmonary edema, and right ventricular failure.

Blood flow through the stenotic valve results in a rumbling decrescendo diastolic murmur heard best over the cardiac apex and radiating to the left axilla. If the mitral valve is forced open during diastole, it may make a sharp noise called an opening snap. The first heart sound (S_1) is often accentuated and somewhat delayed because of increased left atrial pressure. Other signs and symptoms are generally those of pulmonary congestion and right ventricular failure. Atrial enlargement and valvular obstruction are demonstrated by chest X-ray films, electrocardiography, and echocardiography. Management includes use of anticoagulation therapy and control of heart rate. Mitral stenosis can often be repaired with percutaneous balloon commissurotomy, but may require valve replacement in advanced cases.[122]

Regurgitation

Aortic regurgitation. **Aortic regurgitation** results from an inability of the aortic valve leaflets to close properly during diastole because of abnormalities of the leaflets, the aortic root and annulus, or both. It can be primary, caused by congenital bicuspid valve or degeneration in older adults; or secondary, resulting from chronic hypertension, rheumatic heart disease, bacterial endocarditis, syphilis, connective tissue disorders (e.g., Marfan's syndrome and ankylosing spondylitis), appetite-suppressing medications, trauma, or atherosclerosis.[123] During systole, blood is ejected from the left ventricle into the aorta. During diastole, some of the ejected blood flows back into the left ventricle through the leaking valve. Volume overload occurs in the ventricle because it receives blood both from the left atrium and from the aorta during diastole. The hemodynamic abnormalities depend on the amount of regurgitation. As the end-diastolic volume of the left ventricle increases, myocardial fibres stretch to accommodate the extra fluid. Compensatory dilation permits the left ventricle to increase its stroke volume and maintain cardiac output. Ventricular hypertrophy also occurs as an adaptation to the increased volume and because of increased afterload created by the high stroke volume and resultant systolic hypertension. Over time, ventricular dilation and hypertrophy eventually cannot compensate for aortic incompetence, and HF develops.

Clinical manifestations include widened pulse pressure resulting from increased stroke volume and diastolic backflow. Turbulence across the aortic valve during diastole produces a decrescendo murmur in the second, third, or fourth intercostal spaces parasternally and may radiate to the neck. Large stroke volume and rapid runoff of blood from the aorta cause prominent carotid pulsations and bounding peripheral pulses (Corrigan's pulse). Other symptoms are usually associated with HF that occurs when the ventricle can no longer pump adequately. Dysrhythmias are a common complication of aortic regurgitation. The severity of regurgitation can be estimated by echocardiography, and valve replacement surgery may be delayed for many years through careful use of vasodilators and inotropic agents.[122]

Mitral regurgitation. **Mitral regurgitation** can be primary because of mitral valve prolapse, rheumatic heart disease, infective endocarditis, MI, connective tissue diseases (Marfan's syndrome), and dilated cardiomyopathy. It can also be secondary because of ischemic or nonischemic myocardial disease, which damages the chordae tendineae or the mitral annulus.[122] Mitral regurgitation permits backflow of blood from the left ventricle into the left atrium during ventricular systole, producing a holosystolic (throughout systole) murmur heard best at the apex, which radiates into the back and axilla. Because of increased volume from the left atrium, the left ventricle becomes dilated and hypertrophied to maintain adequate cardiac output. The volume of backflow re-entering the left atrium gradually increases, causing atrial dilation and associated AF. As the left atrium enlarges, the valve structures stretch and become deformed, leading to further backflow. As mitral valve regurgitation progresses, left ventricular function may become impaired to the point of failure. Eventually, increased atrial pressure leads to pulmonary hypertension and failure of the right ventricle. Mitral incompetence is usually well tolerated—often for years—until ventricular failure occurs. Most clinical manifestations are caused by HF. The severity of regurgitation can be estimated by echocardiography, and transcatheter or surgical repair or valve replacement may become necessary.[125] In acute mitral regurgitation caused by MI, surgical repair must be done emergently.

Tricuspid regurgitation. **Tricuspid regurgitation** is more common than tricuspid stenosis. Primary tricuspid regurgitation is caused by congenital defects, rheumatic heart disease, endocarditis, or trauma.[123] However, 80% of the cases of tricuspid regurgitation are functional because of annular dilatation and leaflet tethering abnormalities related to dilation of the right ventricle secondary to pulmonary hypertension.[122] Tricuspid valve incompetence leads to volume overload in the right atrium and ventricle, increased systemic venous blood pressure, and right ventricular failure. Pulmonic valve dysfunction can have the same consequences as tricuspid valve dysfunction.

Mitral Valve Prolapse Syndrome

In **mitral valve prolapse syndrome (MVPS)**, one or both of the cusps of the mitral valve billow upward (prolapse) into the left atrium during systole (Figure 24-31). The most common cause of MVPS is myxomatous degeneration of the leaflets in which the cusps are redundant, thickened, and scalloped because of changes in tissue proteoglycans, increased levels of proteinases, and infiltration by myofibroblasts. Mitral regurgitation occurs if the ballooning valve permits blood to leak into the atrium.

Because mitral valve prolapse can be associated with other inherited connective tissue disorders (Marfan's syndrome, Ehlers-Danlos syndrome, osteogenesis imperfecta), it has been suggested that it results from a genetic or environmental disruption of valvular development during the fifth or sixth week of gestation. There also may be a relationship between symptomatic mitral valve prolapse and hyperthyroidism.

Many cases of mitral valve prolapse are completely asymptomatic. Cardiac auscultation on routine physical examination may disclose a regurgitant murmur or midsystolic click in an otherwise healthy individual, or echocardiography may demonstrate the condition in the absence of auscultatory findings. Symptomatic mitral valve prolapse can cause palpitations related to dysrhythmias, tachycardia, lightheadedness, syncope, fatigue (especially in the morning), lethargy, weakness, dyspnea, chest tightness, hyperventilation, anxiety, depression, panic attacks, and atypical chest pain. Many symptoms are vague and puzzling and are unrelated to the degree of prolapse. Most individuals with mitral valve prolapse have an excellent prognosis, do not develop symptoms, and do not require any restriction in activity or medical management. Occasionally, beta-blockers are needed to alleviate syncope, severe chest pain, or palpitations.

Acute Rheumatic Fever and Rheumatic Heart Disease

Rheumatic fever is a systemic, inflammatory disease caused by a delayed exaggerated immune response to infection by group A β-hemolytic streptococcus in genetically predisposed individuals. In its acute form, rheumatic fever is a febrile illness characterized by inflammation of the joints, skin, nervous system, and heart.[126] If untreated, rheumatic fever can cause scarring and deformity of cardiac structures, resulting in **rheumatic heart disease**. While acute rheumatic fever (ARF) is now considered to be a disease of the past in Canada, its incidence in First Nations communities is 21.3 per 100 000, which is 75 times greater than the overall Canadian estimated incidence.[127]

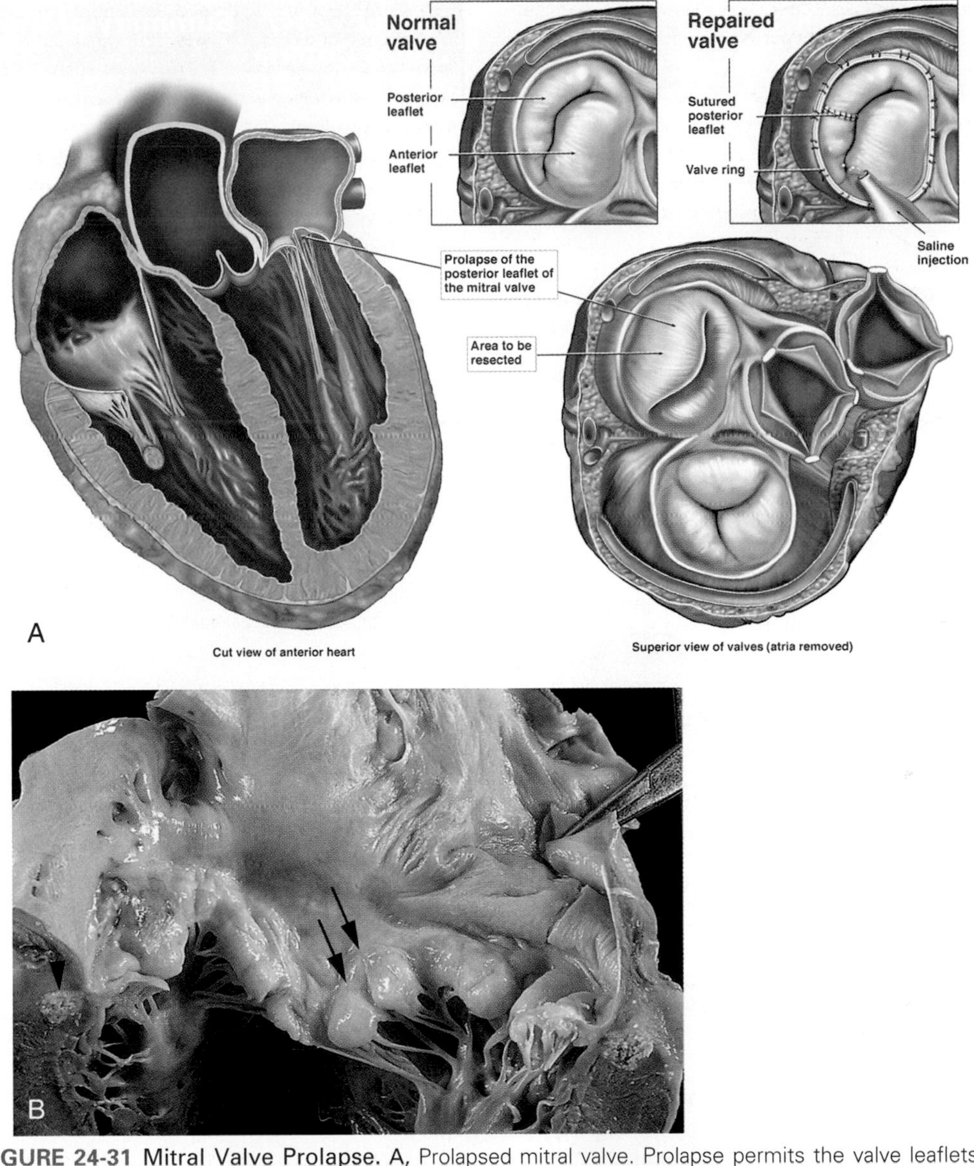

FIGURE 24-31 Mitral Valve Prolapse. A, Prolapsed mitral valve. Prolapse permits the valve leaflets to billow back (*arrow*) into the atrium during left ventricular systole. The billowing causes the leaflets to part slightly, permitting regurgitation into the atrium. **B,** Looking down into the mitral valve, the ballooning (*arrows*) of the leaflets is seen. (From Kumar, V., Abbas, A.K., & Aster, J.C. [Eds.]. [2015]. *Robins and Cotran pathologic basis of disease* [9th ed.]. Philadelphia: Saunders. **A,** Nucleus Medical Media Inc./Alamy Stock Photo.)

PATHOPHYSIOLOGY ARF can develop only as a sequel to pharyngeal infection by group A β-hemolytic streptococcus. Streptococcal skin infections do not progress to ARF because the strains of the microorganism that affect the skin do not have the same antigenic molecules in their cell membranes as those that cause pharyngitis and, therefore, do not elicit the same kind of immune response. However, both skin and pharyngeal infections can cause acute glomerulonephritis.

ARF is the result of an abnormal humoral and cell-mediated immune response to group A streptococcal cell membrane antigens called M proteins (Figure 24-32).[128,129] This immune response cross-reacts with molecularly similar self-antigens in heart, muscle, brain, and joints, causing an autoimmune response that results in diffuse, proliferative, and exudative inflammatory lesions in these tissues. The inflammation may subside before treatment, leaving behind damage to the heart valves. Repeated attacks of ARF cause chronic proliferative changes in the previously mentioned organs with resultant tissue scarring, granuloma formation, and thrombosis.

Approximately 10% of individuals with rheumatic fever develop rheumatic heart disease. In developed countries, the peak incidence of the development of rheumatic heart disease occurs in adults between the ages of 25 and 34. Although rheumatic fever can cause carditis in all three layers of the heart wall, the primary lesion usually involves the endocardium. Endocardial inflammation causes swelling of the valve leaflets, with secondary erosion along the lines of leaflet contact. Small, beadlike clumps of vegetation containing platelets and fibrin are deposited on eroded valvular tissue and on the chordae tendineae cordis. These lesions can become progressively adherent. Scarring and shortening of the involved structures occur over time. The valves lose their elasticity, and the leaflets may adhere to each other.

If inflammation penetrates the myocardium, called *myocarditis*, localized fibrin deposits develop that are surrounded by areas of necrosis. These fibrinoid necrotic deposits are called *Aschoff bodies*. Pericardial inflammation is usually characterized by serofibrinous effusion within the pericardial cavity. Cardiomegaly and left ventricular failure may

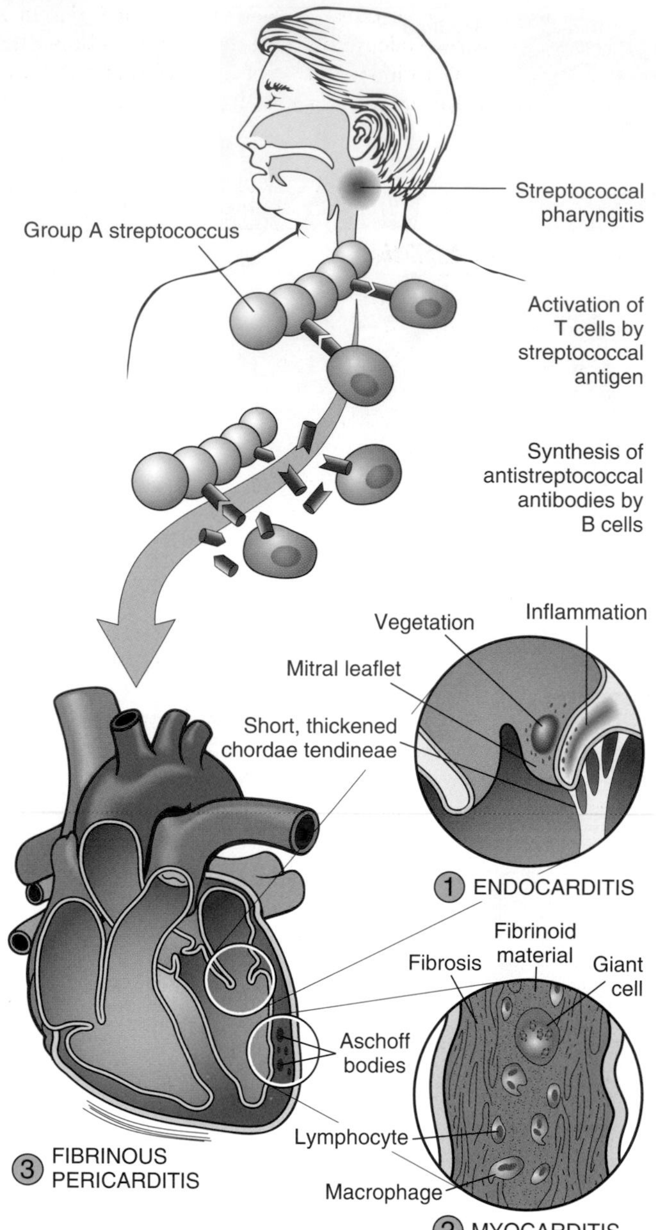

FIGURE 24-32 Pathogenesis and Structural Alterations of Acute Rheumatic Heart Disease. Beginning usually with a sore throat, rheumatic fever can develop only as a sequel to pharyngeal infection by group A β-hemolytic streptococcus. Suspected as a hypersensitivity reaction, it is proposed that antibodies directed against the M proteins of certain strains of streptococci cross-react with tissue glycoproteins in the heart, joints, and other tissues. The exact nature of cross-reacting antigens has been difficult to define, but it appears that the streptococcal infection causes an autoimmune response against self-antigens. Inflammatory lesions are found in various sites; the most distinctive within the heart are called *Aschoff bodies*. The chronic sequelae result from progressive fibrosis because of healing of the inflammatory lesions and the changes induced by valvular deformities. (From Damjanov, I. [2012]. *Pathology for the health professions* [4th ed.]. Philadelphia: Saunders.)

occur during episodes of untreated acute or recurrent rheumatic fever. Conduction defects and AF often are associated with rheumatic heart disease.

CLINICAL MANIFESTATIONS The common symptoms of ARF are fever, lymphadenopathy, arthralgia, nausea, vomiting, epistaxis (nosebleed), abdominal pain, and tachycardia. The major clinical manifestations of ARF usually occur singly or in combination 1 to 5 weeks after streptococcal infection of the pharynx. They are carditis, acute migratory polyarthritis, chorea, erythema marginatum, and subcutaneous nodules.

ARF is a clinical diagnosis and has no single confirmatory test. The most common approach to diagnosis is to use the Jones criteria (Table 24-7). The Jones criteria were first proposed in 1944 and modified in 2015. The main modifications were the inclusion of echocardiography for the diagnosis of carditis, risk stratification based on two sets of criteria, and the establishment of specific recommendations for diagnosis of recurrent ARF.[130] The diagnosis of the initial episode of ARF requires documentation of a recent streptococcal infection and at least two major or one major and two minor criteria (see Table 24-7).

TABLE 24-7 Summary of the 2015 Jones Criteria

Evidence of Preceding GAS Infection (at Least One of the Following)

1. Increased or rising anti-streptolysin O titer or other streptococcal antibodies (anti-DNase B). A rise in titre is better evidence than a single titre result
2. A positive throat culture for group A β-hemolytic streptococci
3. A positive rapid group A streptococcal carbohydrate antigen test in a child whose clinical presentation suggests a high pretest probability of streptococcal pharyngitis

Risk Stratification	
Low-Risk Population	Moderate/High Risk Population
ARF incidence ≤2 per 100 000 school-aged children or all-age RHD prevalence of ≤2 per 1 000 population year	Children not clearly from a low-risk population
Major Criteria	
Clinical and/or subclinical carditis	Clinical and/or subclinical carditis
Polyarthritis	Monoarthritis, polyarthritis, and/or polyarthralgia
Chorea	Chorea
Erythema marginatum	Erythema marginatum
Subcutaneous nodules	Subcutaneous nodules
Minor Criteria	
Prolonged PR interval	Prolonged PR interval
Polyarthralgia	Monoarthralgia
≥38.5°C	≥38°C
Peak ESR ≥60 mm in 1 hour and/or CRP ≥3.0 mg/dL	Peak ESR ≥30 mm in 1 hour and/or CRP ≥3.0 mg/dL

ARF, acute rheumatic fever; *CRP*, C-reactive protein; *ESR*, erythrocyte sedimentation rate; *GAS*, group A streptococcal; *RHD*, rheumatic heart disease.
From Zühlke, L., Beaton, A., Engel, M.A., et al. (2017). *Curr Treat Options Cardiovasc Med*, 19(2), 15.

EVALUATION AND TREATMENT Supportive evidence for group A β-hemolytic streptococci includes positive throat cultures and measurement of serum antibodies against the hemolytic factor streptolysin O. Cultures may be negative when the rheumatic attack begins, however. Several other antibody tests are sensitive prognosticators of streptococcal infection, including antideoxyribonuclease B (anti-DNase B), antihyaluronidase, and antistreptozyme (ASTZ). Elevated measurements of white blood cell count, erythrocyte sedimentation rate, and C-reactive protein indicate inflammation. All three are usually increased at the time cardiac or joint symptoms begin to appear. Echocardiographic screening for rheumatic heart disease in children with a history of rheumatic fever is controversial because not all detectable abnormalities are clinically relevant.[131]

Therapy for ARF is aimed at eradicating the streptococcal infection and involves a 10-day regimen of oral penicillin or erythromycin administration. NSAIDs are used as anti-inflammatory agents for both rheumatic carditis and arthritis. Serious carditis may require corticosteroids and diuretics. Because recurrent rheumatic fever occurs in more than half of affected children, continuous prophylactic antibiotic therapy may be necessary for as long as 5 years. Several potential group A β-hemolytic streptococcus vaccines are being developed. Rheumatic heart disease may require surgical repair of damaged valves.

QUICK CHECK 24-8

1. Compare the effect of aortic stenosis with mitral stenosis on the left ventricle and atrium.
2. Describe aortic regurgitation, mitral regurgitation, and tricuspid regurgitation.
3. What are the common symptoms of mitral valve prolapse?
4. What is the cause of rheumatic heart disease?

Infective Endocarditis

Infective endocarditis is a general term used to describe infection and inflammation of the endocardium—especially the cardiac valves. Bacteria are the most common cause of infective endocarditis, especially streptococci, staphylococci, and enterococci, which account for more than 80% of cases.[132] Other causes include viruses, fungi, rickettsia, and parasites. Infective endocarditis was once a lethal disease, but morbidity and mortality diminished significantly with the advent of antibiotics and improved diagnostic techniques (see *Risk Factors:* Infective Endocarditis).

RISK FACTORS

Infective Endocarditis

- Acquired valvular heart disease
- Implantation of prosthetic heart valves
- Congenital lesions associated with highly turbulent flow (e.g., ventricular septal defect)
- Previous attack of infective endocarditis
- Intravenous medication use
- Long-term indwelling intravenous catheterization (e.g., for pressure monitoring, feeding, hemodialysis)
- Implantable cardiac pacemakers
- Heart transplant with defective valve

PATHOPHYSIOLOGY The pathogenesis of infective endocarditis requires at least three critical elements (Figure 24-33):

1. *Endocardial damage.* Trauma, congenital heart disease, valvular heart disease, and the presence of prosthetic valves are the most common risk factors for endocardial damage that lead to infective endocarditis. Turbulent blood flow caused by these abnormalities usually affects the atrial surface of atrioventricular valves or the ventricular surface of semilunar valves. Endocardial damage exposes the endothelial

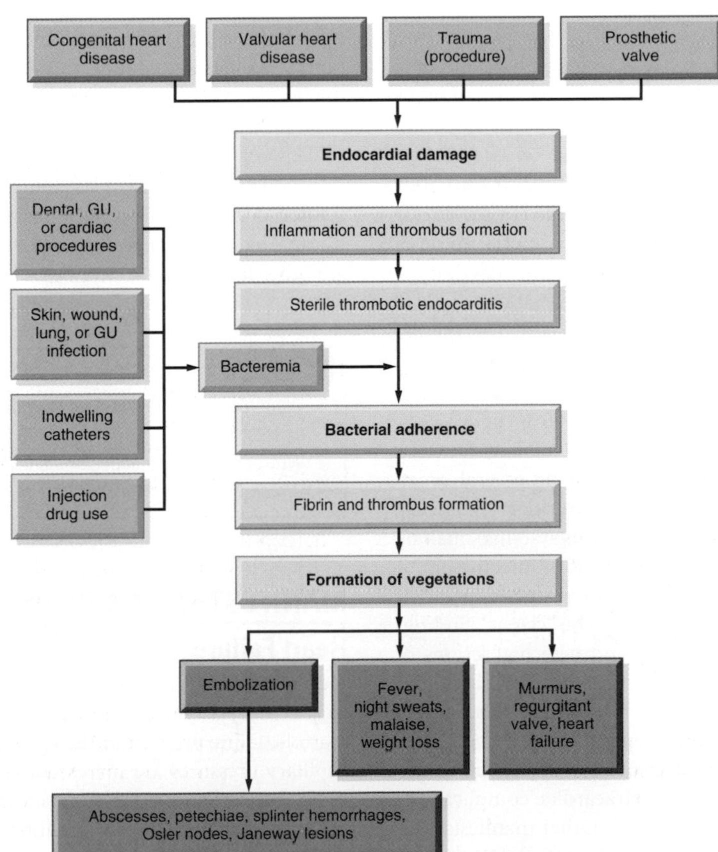

FIGURE 24-33 Pathogenesis of Infective Endocarditis. *GU,* genitourinary.

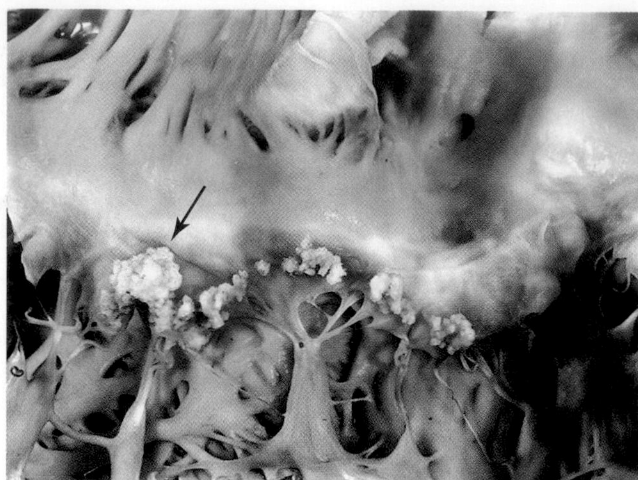

FIGURE 24-34 Bacterial Endocarditis of Mitral Valve. The valve is covered with large, irregular vegetations (*arrow*). (From Damjanov, I., & Linder, J. [2000]. *Pathology: A color atlas*. St. Louis: Mosby.)

basement membrane, which contains a type of collagen that attracts platelets, triggers the inflammatory process, and stimulates sterile thrombus formation on the membranes (**nonbacterial thrombotic endocarditis**).

2. *Adherence of bloodborne microorganisms to the damaged endocardial surface.* Bacteria may enter the bloodstream during injection drug use, trauma, dental procedures that involve manipulation of the gingiva, cardiac surgery, genitourinary procedures and indwelling catheters in the presence of infection, or gastro-intestinal instrumentation, or they may spread from uncomplicated upper respiratory tract or skin infections. Bacteria adhere to the damaged endocardium using adhesins.[132]
3. *Formation of infective endocardial vegetations* (Figure 24-34). Bacteria infiltrate the sterile thrombi and accelerate fibrin formation by activating the clotting cascade. These vegetative lesions can form anywhere on the endocardium but usually occur on heart valves and surrounding structures. Although endocardial tissue is constantly bathed in antibody-containing blood and is surrounded by scavenging monocytes and polymorphonuclear leukocytes, bacterial colonies are inaccessible to host defences because they are embedded in the protective fibrin clots. Embolization from these vegetations can lead to abscesses and characteristic skin changes, such as petechiae, splinter hemorrhages, Osler nodes, and Janeway lesions.

CLINICAL MANIFESTATIONS Fever occurs in 80% of cases.[132] Infective endocarditis causes varying degrees of valvular dysfunction and may be associated with manifestations involving several organ systems (respiratory [lungs], sensory [eyes], genitourinary [kidneys], musculo-skeletal [bones, joints], and central nervous systems), making diagnosis exceedingly difficult. Signs and symptoms of infective endocarditis are caused by infection and inflammation, systemic spread of microemboli, and immune complex deposition. The "classic" findings are fever; new or changed cardiac murmur; and petechial lesions of the skin, conjunctiva, and oral mucosa. Characteristic physical findings include Osler nodes (painful erythematous nodules on the pads of the fingers and toes) and Janeway lesions (nonpainful hemorrhagic lesions on the palms and soles). Central nervous system complications are the most frequent and the most severe extracardiac complications and include stroke, abscess, and meningitis.[132,133] Other manifestations include weight loss, back pain, night sweats, and HF. Splenic, renal, pulmonary, peripheral arterial, coronary, and ocular emboli may lead to a wide variety of signs and symptoms.

EVALUATION AND TREATMENT The criteria for the diagnosis of infective endocarditis are called the *Duke criteria* and include repetitive blood cultures positive for bacteria and evidence for endocardial involvement (murmurs or documented regurgitation) along with recognized risk factors, fever, and vascular complications.[132] Serum measures, such as C-reactive protein, also are elevated. Echocardiography should be performed immediately. Antimicrobial therapy is generally given for several weeks, beginning with intravenous and ending with oral administration. In some cases, two different antibiotics are given simultaneously to eliminate the offending microorganism and prevent the development of medication resistance.[122,132] Other medications may be necessary to treat left ventricular failure secondary to valvular dysfunction. Surgery that involves excision of infected tissue with or without valve replacement improves outcomes in many persons with infective endocarditis, especially those with severe HF or persistent bacteremia despite antibiotic therapy.

Antibiotic prophylaxis to prevent infective endocarditis is indicated for those with prosthetic valves, a history of infective endocarditis, unrepaired cyanotic congenital heart disease, and heart transplant with valvular defect in the setting of gingival procedures or in the presence of documented acute gastro-intestinal or genitourinary infection.[122]

Cardiac Complications in AIDS

Individuals with HIV infection and acquired immune deficiency syndrome (AIDS) are at risk for cardiac complications including dilated cardiomyopathy, myocarditis, pericardial effusion, endocarditis, pulmonary hypertension, and nonantiretroviral medication–related cardiotoxicity. In addition, cardiac involvement may be induced by various bacterial, viral, protozoal, mycobacterial, and fungal pathogens that complicate AIDS. Malignancies, such as lymphoma and Kaposi sarcoma, are seen often in individuals with AIDS and can affect the heart. HIV has been found to cause immune activation that increases the risk for coronary atherosclerosis.[134,135] Furthermore, treatment with antiretroviral therapy can cause dyslipidemia and atherosclerotic disease.

Left ventricular failure is the most common complication of HIV infection and is related to left ventricular dilation and dysfunction and sudden death.[136] Pericardial effusion, ventricular dysrhythmias, electrocardiographic changes, and right ventricular dilation and hypertrophy are other less common findings.

QUICK CHECK 24-9

1. What three critical elements are required for the pathogenesis of infective endocarditis?
2. Why does infective endocarditis involve several organ systems?
3. What effect does AIDS have on the heart?

MANIFESTATIONS OF HEART DISEASE

Heart Failure

Heart failure (HF) is when the heart is unable to generate an adequate cardiac output, causing inadequate perfusion of tissues or increased diastolic filling pressure of the left ventricle, or both, so that pulmonary capillary pressures are increased. It affects nearly 10% of individuals older than age 65 and is the most common reason for admission to the hospital in that age group. Ischemic heart disease and hypertension are the most important predisposing risk factors.[10] Other risk factors include age, obesity, diabetes, renal failure, valvular heart disease, cardiomyopathies, myocarditis, congenital heart disease, and excessive alcohol use. Numerous genetic polymorphisms have been linked to an increased risk for HF, including genes for cardiomyopathies, myocyte contractility, and neurohumoral receptors. Most causes of HF result from dysfunction of the left ventricle (HF with reduced ejection fraction and HF with preserved ejection fraction). The right ventricle also may be dysfunctional, especially in pulmonary disease (right ventricular failure). Finally, some conditions cause inadequate perfusion despite normal or elevated cardiac output (high-output failure). (See *Health Promotion:* Canadian Heart Failure Statistics.)

HEALTH PROMOTION

Canadian Heart Failure Statistics

In Canada, the annual direct costs of heart failure (HF) are estimated to be more than $2.8 billion, due to hospitalizations and the associated costs. According to data from the Canadian Institute for Health Information (CIHI), 60 000 patients were hospitalized between 2013 and 2014 as a consequence of HF. Unfortunately, the number of visits due to HF has been increasing over the last couple of years, reaching a 13% increase in the last 6 years. Currently, 600 000 Canadians are living with HF, and these numbers are expected to increase as the Canadian population gets older, placing an increased burden on the Canadian health care system.

Living conditions play an important role in the longevity of Canadians and their cardiovascular health. Studies have shown that low-income Canadians tend to experience more heart attacks than Canadians with better incomes. Job insecurity plays a significant role in contributing to undue stress, increasing the physiological and psychological load, eventually overwhelming the body, and leading to sleep deprivation, high blood pressure, and heart disease. Job insecurity also has a negative impact on personal relationships, parenting effectiveness, and children's behaviour.

The following health care interventions can help patients prevent and manage HF:

- Promoting healthy lifestyle behaviours that preserve and maintain the current capacity and potentially improve cardiovascular fitness and future health status
- Promoting activities that strengthen mind–body interactions
- Empowering patients and families to understand HF symptoms and collaborating with them to manage those symptoms using health-promoting behaviours
- Promoting opportunities for social networking and interaction to overcome patients' barriers to socialization to enhance quality of life
- Promoting an atmosphere that focuses on wellness rather than illness, eventually creating hope for people living with HF
- Encouraging and rewarding health-promoting behaviours and lifestyle changes that emphasize health

Although health-promoting behaviours may not change the course of the disease, they can influence the patient's response to the illness condition, thereby mitigating its effect on quality of life.

Data from Clark, A.P., Stuifbergen, A., Gottlieb, N.H., et al. (2006). *Holist Nurs Pract, 20*(2), 73–79; Heart and Stroke Foundation. (2016). *Canada is failing our heart failure patients* [Press release]. Retrieved from http://www.heartandstroke.ab.ca/site/apps/nlnet/content2.aspx?c=lqIRL1PJJtI&b=3651445&ct=14817815&printmode=1; Mikkonen, J., & Raphael, D. (2010). *Social determinants of health: The Canadian facts.* Toronto: York University School of Health Policy and Management. Retrieved from http://www.thecanadianfacts.org/the_canadian_facts.pdf.

Left Ventricular Failure

Left ventricular failure is further categorized as HF with reduced ejection fraction or HF with preserved ejection fraction. It is possible for these two types of HF to occur simultaneously in one individual.

Heart failure with reduced ejection fraction (HFrEF), or **systolic heart failure**, is defined as an ejection fraction of less than 40% and an inability of the heart to generate an adequate cardiac output to perfuse vital tissues. Cardiac output depends on the heart rate and stroke volume. Stroke volume is influenced by three major determinants: contractility, preload, and afterload (see Chapter 23).

Contractility is reduced by diseases that disrupt myocyte activity. MI is the most common primary cause of decreased contractility. Other primary causes include myocarditis and cardiomyopathies. Secondary causes of decreased contractility, such as recurrent myocardial ischemia and increased myocardial workload, contribute to inflammatory, immune, and neurohumoral changes (activation of the SNS and RAAS) that mediate a process called ventricular remodelling.[34] **Ventricular remodelling** results in disruption of the normal myocardial extracellular structure with resultant dilation of the myocardium and causes progressive myocyte contractile dysfunction over time (Figure 24-35). When contractility is decreased, stroke volume falls and left ventricular end-diastolic volume (LVEDV) increases. This decreased contractility causes dilation of the heart and an increase in preload.

Preload, or LVEDV, increases with decreased contractility or an excess of plasma volume (intravenous fluid administration, renal failure, mitral valvular disease). Increases in LVEDV can actually improve cardiac output up to a certain point, but as preload continues to rise, it causes a stretching of the myocardium that eventually can lead to dysfunction of the sarcomeres and decreased contractility. This relationship is described by Starling's law of the heart (see Figure 23-16). Decreased contractility leads to further increases in preload (Figure 24-36).

Increased afterload is most commonly a result of increased peripheral vascular resistance, such as that seen with hypertension. Nearly 75% of cases of HF have antecedent hypertension.[10] Although much less common, it also can be the result of aortic valvular disease. With increased afterload, there is resistance to ventricular emptying and more workload for the ventricle; and the ventricle responds with hypertrophy, which is a form of myocardial remodelling. This process differs from the physiological myocyte response to increased workload (exercise) in which the workload is intermittent rather than sustained, resulting in an increase in muscle mass but no distortion of the cardiac architecture. Sustained afterload leads to pathological hypertrophy mediated by Ang II and catecholamines and results in an increase in oxygen demand by the thickened myocardium.[137] A state of relative ischemia develops that further contributes to changes in the myocytes themselves and ventricular remodelling (Figure 24-37). In addition, hypertrophic remodelling results in alteration of the cardiac extracellular matrix and deposition of collagen between the myocytes, which can disrupt the integrity of the muscle, decrease contractility, and increase the likelihood that the ventricle will dilate and fail.[138] These changes in ventricular structure and function are referred to as *hypertensive hypertrophic cardiomyopathy*.

As cardiac output falls, renal perfusion diminishes with activation of the RAAS, which acts to increase peripheral vascular resistance and plasma volume, thus further increasing afterload and preload. In addition, baroreceptors in the central circulation detect the decrease in perfusion and stimulate the SNS to cause yet more vasoconstriction and the hypothalamus to produce antidiuretic hormone (ADH). This vicious cycle of decreasing contractility, increasing preload, and increasing afterload causes progressive worsening of left ventricular failure.

In addition to these hemodynamic interactions, HFrEF is characterized by a complex constellation of neurohumoral, inflammatory, and metabolic processes. Ang II and aldosterone have direct toxicity to the

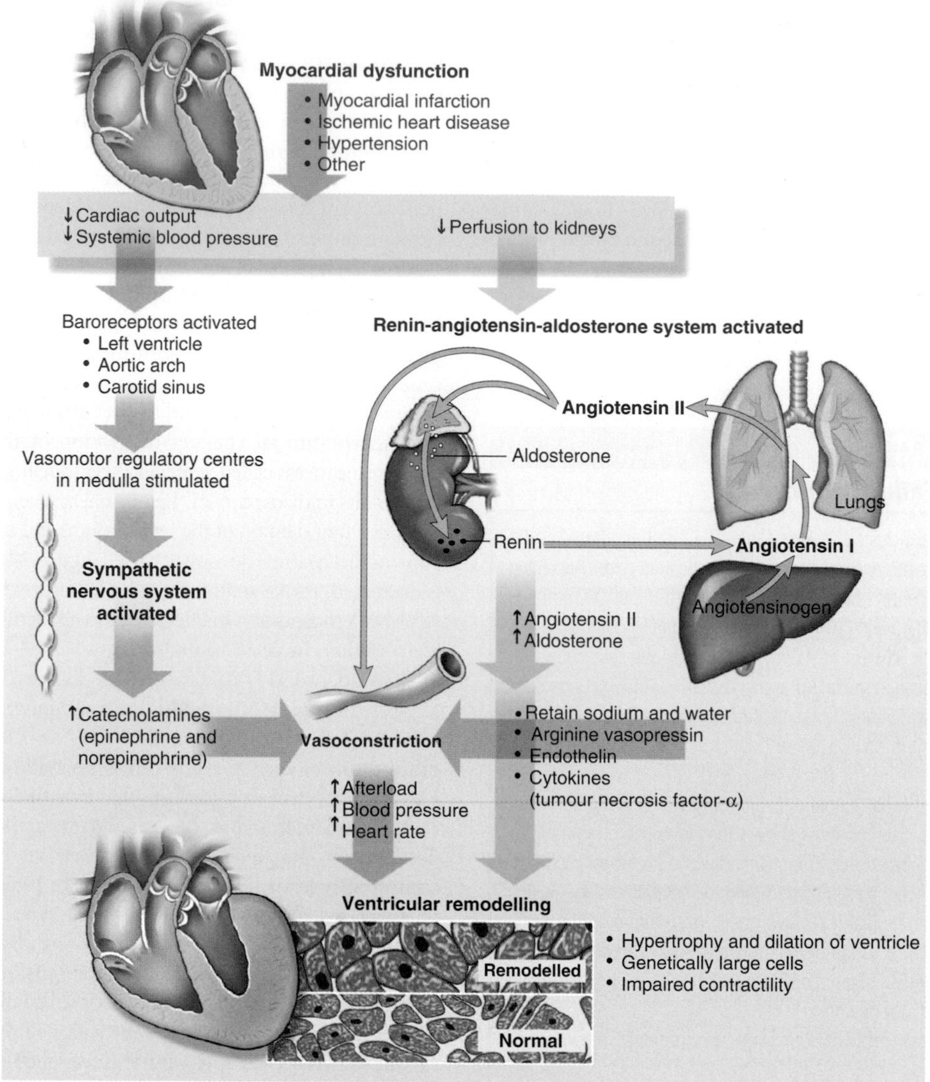

FIGURE 24-35 Pathophysiology of Ventricular Remodelling. Myocardial dysfunction activates the renin-angiotensin-aldosterone and sympathetic nervous systems, releasing neurohormones (angiotensin II, aldosterone, catecholamines, and cytokines). These neurohormones contribute to ventricular remodelling. (Carelock, J., & Clark, A.P., "Heart Failure: Pathophysiologic Mechanisms: The same neurohormonal actions that initially preserve cardiac output subsequently cause functional deterioration. New drug breakthroughs may provide a solution," *Am J Nurs,* 101[12]: 26–33, http://journals.lww.com/ajnonline/Citation/2001/12000/Heart_Failure__Pathophysiologic_Mechanisms__The.17.aspx?trendmd-shared=0.)

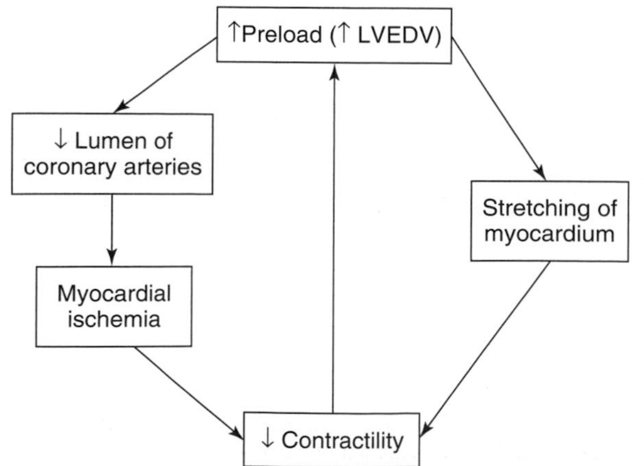

FIGURE 24-36 Effect of Elevated Preload on Myocardial Oxygen Supply and Demand. *LVEDV,* left ventricular end-diastolic volume.

myocardium, contributing to remodelling, myocyte death, and fibrosis. Catecholamines released by the SNS also are toxic to the myocardium and contribute to remodelling.[34] Natriuretic peptides are released in an effort to improve renal salt and water excretion but are inadequate to compensate for these neurohumoral perturbations.[139] Insulin resistance and diabetes not only contribute to HF but also are a complication of HF with changes in myocyte metabolism. Inflammatory cytokines, such as TNF-α, are released in HF, contributing to myocardial damage as well as systemic weight loss (cardiac cachexia). Finally, changes in the metabolic processes within the myocardium also are affected with a decreased ability of the heart to produce energy and an increase in release of toxic metabolites.[140] These neurohumoral, inflammatory, and metabolic aspects of left HFrEF have led to the routine use of combinations of medications that inhibit angiotensin, aldosterone, and catecholamines and increase salt excretion in an effort to prevent long-term damage to the myocardium, as well as the exploration of new treatment

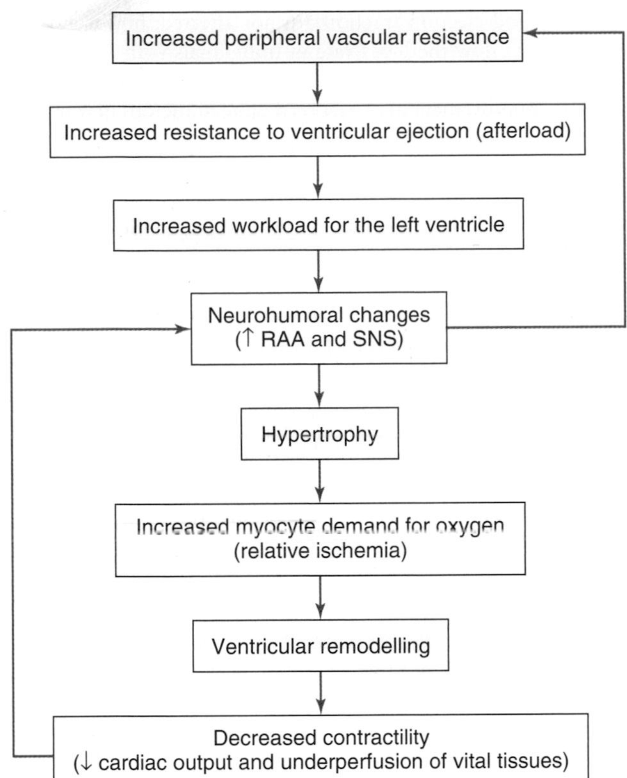

FIGURE 24-37 Role of Increased Afterload in the Pathogenesis of Heart Failure. *RAAS*, renin-angiotensin-aldosterone system; *SNS*, sympathetic nervous system.

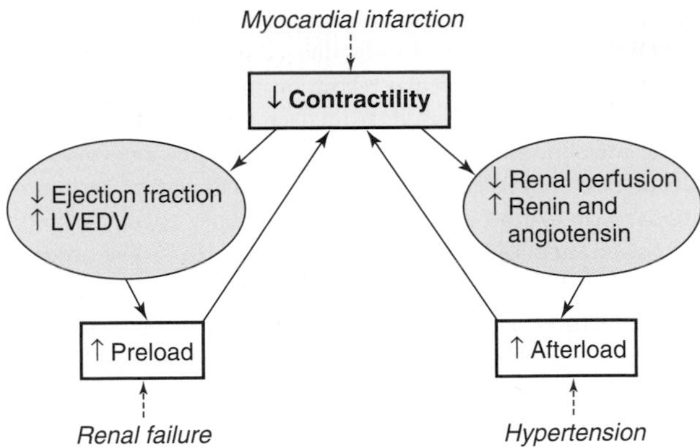

FIGURE 24-38 Vicious Cycle of Heart Failure With Reduced Ejection Fraction. Although the initial insult may be one of primary decreased contractility (e.g., myocardial infarction), increased preload (e.g., renal failure), or increased afterload (e.g., hypertension), all three factors play a role in the progression of left ventricular failure. *LVEDV*, left ventricular end-diastolic volume.

modalities focused on reducing inflammation and improving myocardial metabolic function.[140,141]

The interaction of these hemodynamic, neurohumoral, inflammatory, and metabolic processes results in a steady decline in myocardial function. Pathologically, the heart muscle exhibits gradual changes in myocyte structure and function, with apoptosis of cells, deposition of fibrin, and remodelling of the myocardium such that contractility and cardiac output decline. A vicious cycle of decreasing contractility, increasing preload, and increasing afterload develops, causing the progressive worsening of symptoms associated with left ventricular failure (Figure 24-38).

The clinical manifestations of left ventricular failure are the result of pulmonary vascular congestion and inadequate perfusion of the systemic circulation. Individuals experience dyspnea, orthopnea, cough of frothy sputum, fatigue, decreased urine output, and edema. Physical examination often reveals pulmonary edema (cyanosis, inspiratory crackles, pleural effusions), hypotension or hypertension, an S_3 gallop, and evidence of underlying CAD or hypertension. The diagnosis can be further confirmed with echocardiography showing decreased cardiac output and cardiomegaly. The level of serum BNP can also help make the diagnosis of HF and give some insight into its severity.[142]

Management of HFrEF is aimed at interrupting the worsening cycle of decreasing contractility, increasing preload, and increasing afterload. The acute onset of left ventricular failure is most often the result of acute myocardial ischemia and must be managed in conjunction with management of the underlying coronary disease. Oxygen, nitrate, and morphine administration improves myocardial oxygenation and helps relieve coronary spasm while lowering preload through systemic venodilation. Inotropic medications, such as dopamine, dobutamine (Dobutrex), and milrinone, increase contractility and can help raise the blood pressure in hypotensive individuals but must be monitored carefully.[143] Diuretics reduce preload. ACE inhibitors, ARBs, and aldosterone blockers reduce both preload and afterload by decreasing aldosterone levels and reducing peripheral vascular resistance. Finally, individuals with severe HFrEF failure may benefit from acute coronary bypass or PCI. These people often are supported with the intra-aortic balloon pump (IABP) or left ventricular assist devices (LVADs) until surgery can be performed.

Management of chronic left ventricular failure is based on current clinical guidelines and clinical severity.[144] The overall goals are to reduce preload and afterload. Salt restriction and diuretics (loop diuretics) are effective in reducing preload. ACE inhibitors (or Ang II receptor blockers) reduce preload and afterload and have been shown to significantly reduce mortality in individuals with chronic left ventricular failure. Aldosterone blockers, such as spironolactone, also are associated with improved outcomes.[145] Beta-blockers improve symptoms and increase survival but must be used carefully to avoid hypotension. The inotropic medication digoxin (Toloxin) may be considered in selected individuals, especially those with refractory HF or AF.[144] Although many individuals with left ventricular failure die suddenly from dysrhythmias, prophylactic administration of antidysrhythmics has not been shown to improve survival. In individuals with sustained ventricular tachycardia, implantable cardioverter-defibrillators should be considered. Cardiac resynchronization therapy is proving to be an important modality in selected individuals.[146] For those individuals with CAD, coronary bypass surgery or PCI may improve perfusion to ischemic myocardium (hibernating myocardium) and improve cardiac output. Surgical interventions may be performed (including improving ventricular geometry, implanting assist devices) or heart transplantation may need to be considered. Experimental therapies, including natriuretic peptide analogues, gene transfer, and stem cell therapies, are being explored.[147] Gene therapy offers some exciting new hope for severe HF.

Heart failure with preserved ejection fraction (HFpEF), or **diastolic heart failure**, can occur singly or along with HFrEF. Isolated HFpEF is defined as pulmonary congestion despite a normal stroke volume and cardiac output. Accurate estimation of the prevalence of HFpEF in Canada is challenging due to lack of standardization in diagnostic criteria and inherent difficulties in its diagnosis. However, a recent study estimated that the overall prevalence of HFpEF in the general population ranges between 1.1 and 5.5%.[148]

HFpEF is preceded by a condition called *preclinical diastolic dysfunction* (PDD) in which affected individuals do not have symptoms, but have early changes in ventricular relaxation and a high untreated risk of developing HF.[149] HFpHF results from decreased compliance of the left ventricle and abnormal diastolic relaxation such that a normal LVEDV results in an increased LVEDP. This pressure is reflected back into the pulmonary circulation and results in pulmonary edema, pulmonary hypertension, and right ventricular hypertrophy.[150] The amount of left ventricle stiffness and right venrticle hypertrophy are the strongest pathophysiological predictors of complications from HFpEF.[151] The major causes of diastolic dysfunction include hypertension-induced myocardial hypertrophy and myocardial ischemia–induced ventricular remodelling. Hypertrophy and ischemia cause a decreased ability of the myocytes to actively pump calcium from the cytosol, resulting in impaired relaxation. Other causes include aortic valvular disease, mitral valve disease, pericardial diseases, and cardiomyopathies. Diabetes also increases the risk for diastolic dysfunction. Like HFrEF, HFpEF is characterized by sustained activation of the RAAS and the SNS.

Individuals with diastolic dysfunction present with dyspnea on exertion and fatigue. Evidence of pulmonary edema (inspiratory crackles on auscultation, pleural effusions) is usually not present in resting individuals without tachycardia. Late in diastole, atrial contraction with rapid ejection of blood into the noncompliant ventricle may give rise to an S_4 gallop. Electrocardiography often reveals evidence of left ventricular hypertrophy, and chest X-ray may show pulmonary congestion without cardiomegaly (Table 24-8). There also may be evidence of underlying coronary disease, hypertension, or valvular disease. Diagnosis is based on three factors: signs and symptoms of HF, normal left ventricular ejection fraction, and evidence of diastolic dysfunction. The diagnosis is confirmed by clinical Doppler echocardiography, which demonstrates poor ventricular filling with normal ejection fractions.[152]

Management is aimed at improving ventricular relaxation and prolonging diastolic filling times to reduce diastolic pressure. No therapy has been shown to improve survival, and calcium channel blockers, beta-blockers, ACE inhibitors, and ARBs have been used with only varying success.[153] Treatment with the 3-hydroxy-3-methyl-glutaryl-coenzyme A (HMG-CoA) reductase inhibitors (statins) has consistently resulted in improvements in left ventricle diastolic function.[153,154] Inotropic medications are not indicated in isolated HFpEF because contractility and ejection fraction are not affected; however, digoxin may be used to slow the heart rate in individuals with AF. Outcomes for individuals with HFpEF are as poor as those with HFrEF, and there has been no improvement in prognosis despite numerous new treatment trials.[155]

TABLE 24-8 Comparison of HFrEF and HFpEF

Characteristic	HFrEF	HFpEF
Gender	Males greater than females	Females greater than males
Left ventricular ejection fraction	Decreased	Normal
Left ventricular chamber size	Increased	Decreased
Left ventricular hypertrophy on electrocardiogram	Possible	Probable
Chest radiography	Pulmonary congestion with cardiomegaly	Pulmonary congestion without cardiomegaly
Gallop	S_3	S_4

HFpEF, heart failure with preserved ejection fraction; *HFrEF*, heart failure with reduced ejection fraction.
Adapted from Jessup, M., & Brozena, S. (2003). *N Engl J Med, 348*(20), 2007–2018.

Right Ventricular Failure

Right ventricular failure is defined as the inability of the right ventricle to provide adequate blood flow into the pulmonary circulation at a normal central venous pressure. It can result from left ventricular failure when an increase in left ventricular filling pressure is reflected back into the pulmonary circulation. As pressure in the pulmonary circulation rises, the resistance to right ventricular emptying increases (Figure 24-39). The right ventricle is poorly prepared to compensate for this increased afterload and will dilate and fail. As a result, pressure will rise in the systemic venous circulation, leading to peripheral edema and hepatosplenomegaly. Treatment relies on management of the left ventricular dysfunction as just outlined. When right ventricular failure occurs in the absence of left ventricular failure, it is typically attributable to diffuse hypoxic pulmonary disease such as chronic obstructive pulmonary disease (COPD), cystic fibrosis, and acute respiratory distress syndrome (ARDS). These disorders result in an increase in right ventricular afterload. The mechanisms for this type of right ventricular failure (cor pulmonale) are discussed in Chapter 27. Finally, MI, cardiomyopathies, and pulmonic valvular disease interfere with right ventricular contractility and can lead to right ventricular failure.

High-Output Failure

High-output failure is the inability of the heart to adequately supply the body with bloodborne nutrients, despite adequate blood volume

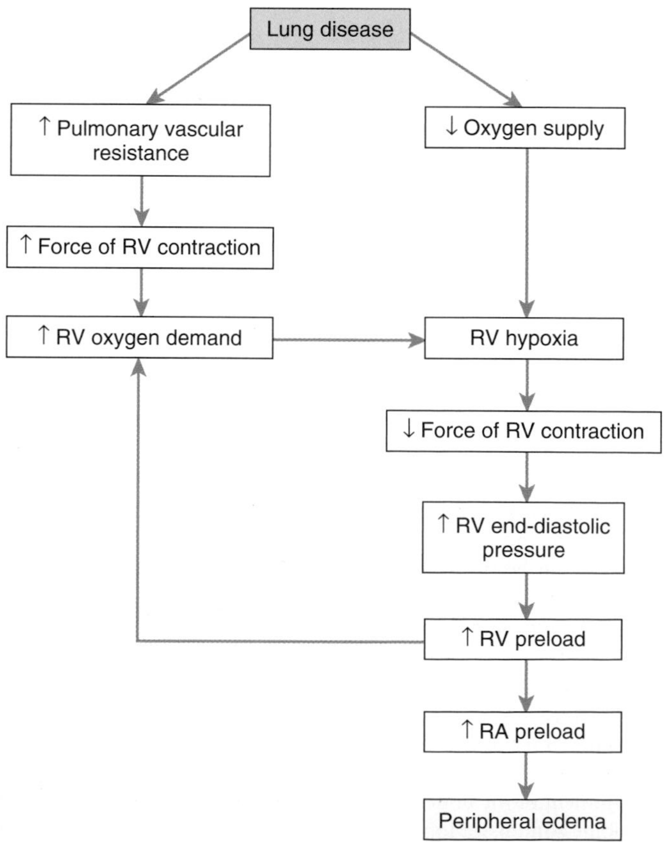

FIGURE 24-39 Right Ventricular Failure. *RA*, right atrial; *RV*, right ventricular.

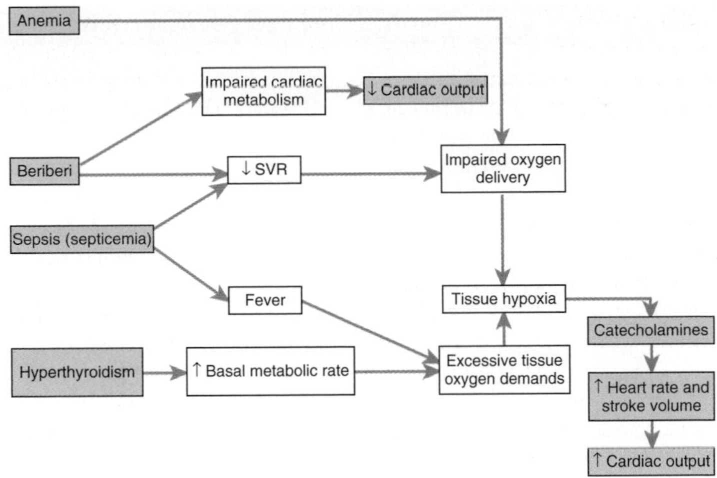

FIGURE 24-40 High-Output Failure. *SVR*, systemic vascular resistance.

and normal or elevated myocardial contractility. In high-output failure, the heart increases its output but the body's metabolic needs are still not met. Common causes of high-output failure are anemia, septicemia, hyperthyroidism, and beriberi (Figure 24-40).

Anemia decreases the oxygen-carrying capacity of the blood. Metabolic acidosis occurs as the body's cells switch to anaerobic metabolism (see Chapter 5). In response to metabolic acidosis, heart rate and stroke volume increase in an attempt to improve tissue perfusion. If anemia is severe, however, even maximum cardiac output does not supply the cells with enough oxygen for metabolism.

In septicemia, disturbed metabolism, bacterial toxins, and the inflammatory process cause systemic vasodilation and fever. Faced with a lowered systemic vascular resistance (SVR) and an elevated metabolic rate, cardiac output increases to maintain blood pressure and prevent metabolic acidosis. In overwhelming septicemia, however, the heart may not be able to raise its output enough to compensate for vasodilation. Body tissues show signs of inadequate blood supply despite a high cardiac output.

Hyperthyroidism accelerates cellular metabolism through the actions of elevated levels of thyroxine from the thyroid gland. This may occur chronically (thyrotoxicosis) or acutely (thyroid storm). Because the body's increased demand for oxygen threatens to cause metabolic acidosis, cardiac output increases. If blood levels of thyroxine are high and the metabolic response to thyroxine is vigorous, even an abnormally elevated cardiac output may be inadequate.

In North America, beriberi (thiamine deficiency) usually is caused by malnutrition secondary to chronic alcoholism. Beriberi actually causes a mixed type of HF. Thiamine deficiency impairs cellular metabolism in all tissues, including the myocardium. In the heart, impaired cardiac metabolism leads to insufficient contractile strength. In blood vessels, thiamine deficiency leads to peripheral vasodilation, which decreases SVR. HF ensues as decreased SVR triggers increased cardiac output, which the impaired myocardium is unable to deliver. The strain of demands for increased output in the face of impaired metabolism may deplete cardiac reserves until low-output failure begins.

Dysrhythmias

A **dysrhythmia**, or **arrhythmia**, is a disturbance of heart rhythm. Normal heart rhythms are generated by the sinoatrial node and travel through the heart's conduction system, causing the atrial and ventricular myocardium to contract and relax at a regular rate that is appropriate to maintain circulation at various levels of physical activity (see Chapter 23). Dysrhythmias range in severity from occasional "missed" or rapid beats to serious disturbances that impair the pumping ability of the heart, contributing to HF and death. Dysrhythmias can be caused either by an abnormal rate of impulse generation (Table 24-9) from the sinoatrial node or other pacemaker or by the abnormal conduction of impulses (Table 24-10) through the heart's conduction system, including the myocardial cells themselves.

QUICK CHECK 24-10
1. What is ventricular remodelling?
2. Why are changes in left ventricular end-diastolic volume important for left ventricular failure?
3. What is the vicious cycle of heart failure with preserved ejection fraction?

SHOCK

In **shock** the cardiovascular system fails to perfuse the tissues adequately, resulting in widespread impairment of cellular metabolism. Because tissue perfusion can be disrupted by any factor that alters heart function, blood volume, or blood pressure, shock has many causes and various clinical manifestations. Ultimately, however, shock progresses to organ failure and death, unless compensatory mechanisms reverse the process or clinical intervention succeeds. Untreated severe shock overwhelms the body's compensatory mechanisms through positive feedback loops that initiate and maintain a downward physiological spiral.

The term *multiple organ dysfunction syndrome* (MODS) describes the failure of two or more organ systems after severe illness and injury and is a frequent complication of severe shock. The disease process is initiated and perpetuated by uncontrolled inflammatory and stress responses. It is progressive and is associated with significant mortality.

Impairment of Cellular Metabolism

The final common pathway in shock of any type is impairment of cellular metabolism. Figure 24-41 illustrates the pathophysiology of shock at the cellular level.

Impairment of Oxygen Use

In all types of shock, the cell either is not receiving an adequate amount of oxygen or is unable to use oxygen. Without oxygen, the cell shifts from aerobic to anaerobic metabolism. Anaerobic metabolism is a less

TABLE 24-9 Disorders of Impulse Formation

Type	Electrocardiogram	Effect	Pathophysiology	Treatment
Sinus bradycardia	P rate 60 or less PR interval normal QRS for each P	Increased preload Decreased mean arterial pressure	Hyperkalemia: slows depolarization Vagal hyperactivity: unknown Digoxin toxicity common Late hypoxia: lack of adenosine triphosphate (ATP)	If hypotensive, treat cause Sympathomimetics, anticholinergics Pacemaker placement
Simple sinus tachycardia	P rate 100–150 PR interval normal QRS for each P	Decreased filling times Decreased mean arterial pressure Increased myocardial demand	Catecholamines: rise in resting potential and calcium influx Fever: unknown Early heart failure: compensatory response to decreased stroke volume Lung disease: hypoxic cell metabolism Hypercalcemia	Oxygen, bed rest Calcium blockers
Premature atrial contractions (PACs) or beats[a]	Early P waves that may have morphological changes PR interval normal QRS for each P	Occasional decreased filling time and mean arterial pressure	Electrolyte disturbances (especially hypercalcemia): alter action potentials Hypoxia and elevated preload: cell membrane disturbances	Treat underlying cause Digoxin
Sinus dysrhythmias	Rate varies P–P regularly irregular, short with inspiration, long with exhalation PR interval normal QRS for each P	Variable filling times Variable mean arterial pressure Variable oxygen demand	Unknown Common in young children and young adults	None
Atrial tachycardia (includes premature atrial tachycardia if onset is abrupt)	P rate 151–250 P morphology may differ from sinus P PR interval normal P/QRS ratio variable	Decreased filling time Decreased mean arterial pressure Increased myocardial demand	Same as PACs: leads to increased atrial automaticity, atrial re-entry Digoxin toxicity: common Aging	Control ventricular rate Digoxin, calcium channel blockers, vagus stimulation Pacemaker to override atrial conduction Cardioversion
Atrial flutter[a]	P rate 251–300, morphology may vary from sinus P PR interval usually not observable P/QRS ratio variable	Decreased filling time Decreased mean arterial pressure	Same as atrial tachycardia	Same as atrial tachycardia
Atrial fibrillation[a]	P rate >300 and usually not observable No PR interval QRS rate variable and rhythm irregular	Same as atrial flutter	Same as atrial tachycardia	Same as atrial tachycardia
Idiojunctional rhythm	P absent or independent QRS normal, rate 41–59, regular	Decreased cardiac output from loss of atrial contribution to ventricular preload	Atrial and sinus bradycardia, standstill, or block	Same as sinus bradycardia
Junctional bradycardia	P absent or independent QRS normal, rate 40 or less	Same as idiojunctional rhythm	Same as idiojunctional rhythm Vagal hyperactivity	Same as sinus bradycardia
Premature junctional contractions (PJCs) or beats	Early beats without P waves QRS morphology normal	Decreased cardiac output from loss of atrial contribution to ventricular preload for that beat	Hyperkalemia (5.4–6 mmol/L) Hypercalcemia, hypoxia, and elevated preload (see PACs)	Same as PAC
Accelerated junctional rhythm	P absent or independent QRS morphology normal, rate 60–99	Decreased cardiac output from loss of atrial contribution to ventricular preload	Same as PJCs	Same as PAC

TABLE 24-9 Disorders of Impulse Formation—cont'd

Type	Electrocardiogram	Effect	Pathophysiology	Treatment
Junctional tachycardia	P absent or independent QRS morphology normal, rate 100 or more	Decreased cardiac output from loss of atrial contribution to ventricular preload Increased myocardial demand because of tachycardia	Same as PJCs	Same as PAC
Idioventricular rhythm[b]	P absent or independent QRS >0.11 and rate 20–39	Same as idiojunctional rhythm	Sinus, atrial, and junctional bradycardia, standstill, or block	Same as sinus bradycardia
Ventricular bradycardia[b]	P absent or independent QRS >0.11 and rate 60 or less	Same as idiojunctional rhythm	Same as idiojunctional rhythm	Same as sinus bradycardia
Agonal rhythm/ electromechanical dissociation[b]	P absent or independent QRS >0.11 and rate 20 or less	Absent or barely present cardiac output and pulse Not compatible with life	Depolarization and contraction not coupled: electrical activity present with little or no mechanical activity Usually caused by profound hypoxia	Vigorous pharmacological treatment aimed at restoring rate and force Usually ineffective May attempt to use pacemaker
Ventricular standstill or asystole[b]	P absent or independent QRS absent	No cardiac output Not compatible with life	Profound ischemia, hyperkalemia, acidosis	Same as agonal rhythm, plus electrical defibrillation
Premature ventricular contractions (PVCs) or depolarizations[a]	Early beats with P waves QRS occasionally opposite in deflection from usual QRS	Same as premature junctional contractions	Same as PJCs, aging and induction of anaesthesia Impulse originates in cell outside normal conduction system and spreads through intercalated disks	Pharmacological interventions to change thresholds, refractory periods; reduce myocardial demand, increase supply
Accelerated ventricular rhythm	P absent or independent QRS >0.11 and rate of 41–99	Same as accelerated junctional rhythm	Same as PVCs	Removal of cause Same as PVCs
Ventricular tachycardia[b]	P absent or independent QRS >0.11 and rate 100 or more	Same as junctional tachycardia	Same as PVCs	Same as PVCs, plus electrical cardioversion
Ventricular fibrillation[b]	P absent QRS >300 and usually not observable	Same as ventricular standstill	Same as PVCs Rapid infusion of potassium	Same as PVCs, plus electrical cardioversion

[a]Most common in adults.
[b]Life-threatening in adults.

TABLE 24-10 Disorders of Impulse Conduction

Type	Electrocardiogram	Effect	Pathophysiology	Treatment
Sinus block	Occasionally absent P, with loss of QRS for that beat	Occasional decrease in cardiac output Increase in preload for following beat	Local hypoxia, scarring of intra-atrial conduction pathways, electrolyte imbalances Increased atrial preload	Conservative Usually do not progress in severity Pharmacological treatment includes vagolytics, sympathomimetics, pacing
First-degree block[a]	PRI >0.2 sec	None	Same as sinus block Hyperkalemia (>7 mmol/L) Hypokalemia (<3.5 mmol/L) Formation of myocardial abscess in endocarditis	Conservative Discovery and correction of cause
Second-degree block, Mobitz I, or Wenckebach[a]	Progressive prolongation of PRI until one QRS is dropped Pattern of prolongation resumes	Same as sinus block	Hypokalemia (<3.5 mmol/L) Faulty cell metabolism in AV node Severity increases as heart rate increases Supports theory that AV node is fatiguing Digoxin toxicity, beta blockade CAD, MI, hypoxia, increased preload, valvular surgery and disease, diabetes	Same as sinus block

Continued

TABLE 24-10 Disorders of Impulse Conduction—cont'd

Type	Electrocardiogram	Effect	Pathophysiology	Treatment
Second-degree block or Mobitz II	Same as sinus block	Same as sinus block	Hypokalemia (<3.5 mmol/L) Faulty cell metabolism below AV node Antidysrhythmics, tricyclic antidepressants CAD, MI, hypoxia, increased preload, valvular surgery and disease, diabetes	More aggressively than Mobitz I, because can progress to type III Pacemaker after pharmacological treatment
Third-degree block[b]	P waves present and independent of QRS No observed relationship between P and QRS Always AV dissociation	Same as idiojunctional rhythm	Hypokalemia (<3.5 mmol/L) Faulty cell metabolism low in bundle of His MI, especially inferior wall, as nodal artery interrupted; results in ischemia of AV node	Pacemaker after pharmacological treatment Temporary pacing if caused by inferior MI, because ischemia usually resolves
Atrioventricular dissociation	P waves present and independent of QRS, but not always because of block (e.g., ventricular tachycardia) AV dissociation not always third-degree block	Decreased cardiac output from loss of atrial contribution to ventricular preload Variable effect on myocardial demand, depending on ventricular rate	May result from third-degree block or accelerated junctional or ventricular rhythm or be caused by sinus, atrial, and junctional bradycardias	Treat according to cause Pacemaker or reducing rate of AV or ventricular discharge, or increasing rate of sinus or AV node discharge
Ventricular block	QRS >0.11 sec R-S-R″ in V_1, V_2, V_5, V_6	None	Faulty cell metabolism in right and left bundle branches RBBB more common than LBBB because of dual blood supply to left bundle branch HF, MR, especially anterior MI, because of infarct of fascicles Left anterior hemiblock more common than left posterior hemiblock because posterior fascicles have dual blood supply	Isolated RBBB or LBBB or hemiblock not treated If acute and/or associated with acute anterior MI, treated with permanent pacer and vigorous pharmacological therapy
Aberrant conduction	QRS >0.11 sec	None, unless ventricular rate abnormalities present	Conduction of impulse through intercalated disks because conduction system transiently blocked as a result of hypoxia, electrolyte imbalances, digoxin toxicity, excessively rapid rate of discharge	Correct underlying cause
Pre-excitation syndromes (Wolff-Parkinson-White and Lown-Ganong-Levine)	P present with QRS for each PPRI <0.12 sec and QRS <0.11 sec because of delta wave in PRI	None	Congenital presence of accessory pathways (bundle of Kent and fibre of Mahaim) that conduct very rapidly and bypass AV node, causing early ventricular depolarization in relation to atrial depolarization Prone to tachycardias and atrial fibrillation that can result in very rapid ventricular rates (reason unknown)	Aimed at aligning refractory periods of accessory pathway and AV node to prevent re-entry May slow rate with medication therapy May surgically cut pathways

[a]Most common in adults.
[b]Life-threatening in adults.
AV, atrioventricular; *CAD*, coronary artery disease; *HF*, heart failure; *LBBB*, left bundle branch block; *MI*, myocardial infarction; *MR*, mitral regurgitation; *PRI*, PR interval; *RBBB*, right bundle branch block.

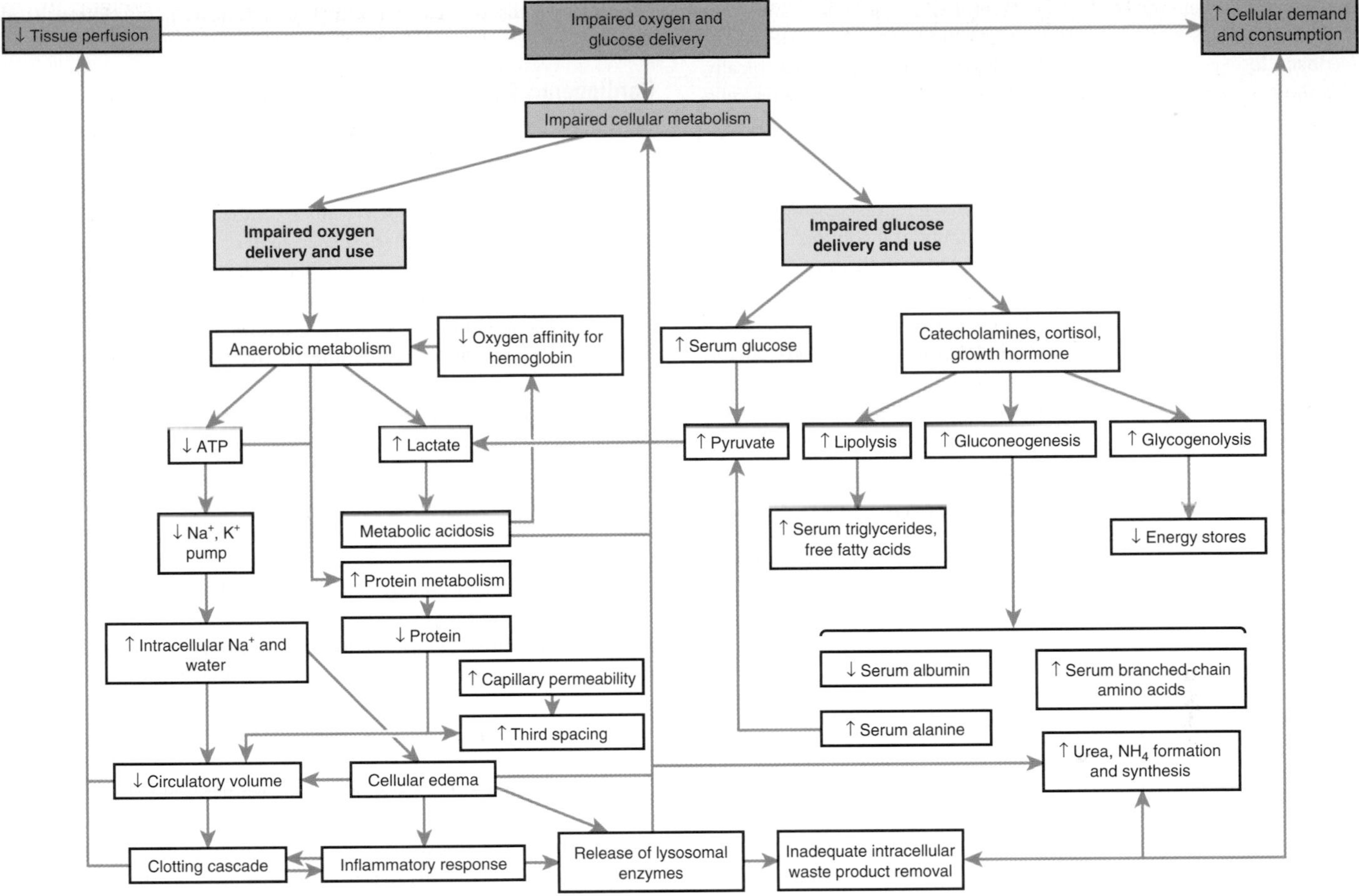

FIGURE 24-41 Impaired Cellular Metabolism in Shock. *ATP,* adenosine triphosphate.

efficient method of extracting energy from carbon bonds, and the cell begins to use its stores of ATP faster than stores can be replaced. Without ATP, the cell cannot maintain an electrochemical gradient across its selectively permeable membrane. Specifically, the cell cannot operate the sodium–potassium pump. Sodium and chloride accumulate inside the cell, and potassium exits the cell. Cells of the nervous system and myocardium are profoundly and immediately affected. The resting potentials of these cells are reduced, and action potentials decrease in amplitude. Various clinical manifestations of impaired central nervous system and myocardial function result.

As sodium moves into the cell, water follows. Throughout the body, the water drawn from the interstitium into the cells is "replaced" by water that is, in turn, drawn out of the vascular space. This decreases circulatory volume. Within the cells, water causes cellular edema that disrupts cellular membranes, releasing lysosomal enzymes that injure the cells internally and then leak into the interstitium. Compensatory mechanisms, including inflammation and activation of the clotting cascade, further impair oxygen use and contribute to the complications of shock, such as acute tubular necrosis (ATN), ARDS, and disseminated intravascular coagulation (DIC).

In addition to decreasing ATP stores, anaerobic metabolism affects the pH of the cell, and metabolic acidosis develops. A compensatory mechanism enables cardiac and skeletal muscles to use lactic acid as a fuel source, but only for a limited time. The decreasing pH of the cell that is functioning anaerobically has serious consequences. Enzymes necessary for cellular function dissociate under acid conditions. Enzyme dissociation stops cell function, repair, and division. As lactic acid is released systemically, blood pH drops, reducing the oxygen-carrying capacity of the blood (see Chapter 4). Therefore, less oxygen is delivered to the cells. Further acidosis triggers the release of more lysosomal enzymes because the low pH disrupts lysosomal membrane integrity.

Impairment of Glucose Use

Impaired glucose use can be caused by either impaired glucose delivery or impaired glucose uptake by the cells (see Figure 24-41). The reasons for inadequate glucose delivery are the same as those enumerated for inadequate oxygen delivery. In addition, in septic and anaphylactic shock, glucose metabolism may be increased or disrupted because of fever or bacteria, and glucose uptake can be prevented by the presence of vasoactive toxins, endotoxins, histamine, and kinins.

Some compensatory mechanisms activated by shock contribute to decreased glucose uptake by the cells. High serum levels of cortisol, thyroid hormone, and catecholamines account for hyperglycemia and insulin resistance, tachycardia, increased SVR, and increased cardiac contractility. Cells shift to glycogenolysis, gluconeogenesis, and lipolysis to generate fuel for survival (see Chapter 1). Except in the liver, kidneys, and muscles, the body's cells have extremely limited stores of glycogen. In fact, total body stores can fuel the metabolism for only about 10 hours. The depletion of fat and glycogen stores is not itself a cause of organ failure, but the energy costs of glycogenolysis and lipolysis are considerable and contribute to cell failure.

The depletion of protein also is a cause of organ failure. When gluconeogenesis causes proteins to be used for fuel, these proteins are no longer available to maintain cellular structure, function, repair, and replication. The breakdown of protein occurs in starvation states, hyperdynamic metabolic states, and septic shock. During anaerobic metabolism, protein metabolism liberates alanine, which is converted to pyruvate. In sepsis, pyruvic acid is changed into lactic acid, and a positive feedback loop is formed. As proteins are broken down anaerobically, ammonia and urea are produced. Ammonia is toxic to living cells. Uremia develops, and uric acid further disrupts cellular metabolism. Serum albumin and other plasma proteins are consumed for fuel first. Serum protein consumption decreases capillary osmotic pressure and contributes to the development of interstitial edema, creating another positive feedback loop that decreases circulatory volume. In septic shock, plasma protein breakdown includes metabolism of immunoglobulins, thereby impairing immune system function when it is most needed.

Muscle wasting caused by protein breakdown weakens skeletal and cardiac muscle. Skeletal muscle wasting impairs the muscles that facilitate breathing. Muscle wasting therefore alters the actions of both the heart and the lungs. The delivery of oxygen and glucose to the cells is directly reduced, as is the removal of waste products, forming another positive feedback loop.

A final outcome of impaired cellular metabolism is the buildup of metabolic end products in the cell and interstitial spaces. Waste products are toxic to the cells and further disrupt cellular function and membrane integrity. Once a sufficiently large number of cells from vital organs have damage to cellular membranes, leakage of lysosomal enzymes, and depletion of ATP, shock can be irreversible.

Clinical Manifestations of Shock

The clinical manifestations of shock are variable depending on the type of shock, and observable and measurable signs and symptoms are often conflicting in nature. Subjective complaints in shock are usually nonspecific. The individual may report feeling sick, weak, cold, hot, nauseated, dizzy, confused, afraid, thirsty, and short of breath. Hypotension, characterized by a mean arterial pressure below 60 mm Hg, is common to almost all shock states; however, it is a late sign of decreased tissue perfusion. Cardiac output and urinary output are usually variable early in shock states but generally become decreased as the shock syndrome progresses. Respiratory rate is usually increased, and respiratory alkalosis may be an important early indicator of impending shock. Other variable indicators of shock include alterations of heart rate, core body temperature, skin temperature, SVR, and skin colour. Altered sensorium may be another indicator of poor tissue perfusion. Decreased mixed venous oxygen saturation indicates poor tissue oxygenation and an alteration in cellular oxygen extraction and can be used to monitor response to therapy.

Treatment for Shock

The first treatment for shock is to discover and correct or remove the underlying cause. Simultaneously, management should begin directed at improvement in microcirculatory tissue perfusion. General supportive treatment includes administration of intravenous fluids to expand intravascular volume, use of vasopressors and supplemental oxygen, and control of glucose levels. Further treatment depends on the cause and severity of the shock syndrome, which is discussed with each type of shock. Once positive feedback loops are established, intervention in shock is difficult. Prevention and very early treatment offer the best prognosis.

Types of Shock

Shock is classified by cause as cardiogenic (caused by HF), hypovolemic (caused by insufficient intravascular fluid volume), neurogenic (caused by neural alterations of vascular smooth muscle tone), anaphylactic (caused by immunological processes), or septic (caused by infection). As described previously, each of these share similar effects on tissues and cells but can vary in their clinical manifestations and severity.

Cardiogenic Shock

Cardiogenic shock is defined as decreased cardiac output and evidence of tissue hypoxia in the presence of adequate intravascular volume. Most cases of cardiogenic shock follow MI, but shock also can follow left ventricular failure, dysrhythmias, acute valvular dysfunction, ventricular or septal rupture, myocardial or pericardial infections, massive pulmonary embolism, cardiac tamponade, and medication toxicity. Microcirculation changes within the myocardium contribute to decreased contractility and worsening cardiac output.[156] Compensatory neurohumoral responses contribute to the overall pathophysiology (Figure 24-42).

The clinical manifestations of cardiogenic shock are caused by widespread impairment of cellular metabolism. They include impaired mentation, dyspnea and tachypnea, systemic venous and pulmonary edema, dusky skin colour, marked hypotension, oliguria, and ileus. Management of cardiogenic shock includes careful fluid and vasopressor administration followed by early angiography, IABP counterpulsation, ventricular assist devices, extracorporeal membrane oxygenation, and early revascularization (PCI or bypass surgery).[157] Cardiogenic shock is often unresponsive to treatment, with a mortality of more than 70% reported. New therapies being explored include anti-inflammatory medications and nitric oxide synthase inhibitors.

Hypovolemic Shock

Hypovolemic shock is caused by loss of whole blood (hemorrhage), plasma (burns), or interstitial fluid (diaphoresis, diabetes mellitus, diabetes insipidus, emesis, diarrhea, or diuresis) in large amounts. Hypovolemic shock begins to develop when intravascular volume has decreased by about 15%.

Hypovolemia is offset initially by compensatory mechanisms (Figure 24-43). Heart rate and SVR increase, boosting both cardiac output and tissue perfusion pressures. Interstitial fluid moves into the vascular compartment. The liver and spleen add to blood volume by disgorging stored red blood cells and plasma. In the kidneys, renin stimulates aldosterone release and the retention of sodium (and hence water), whereas ADH from the posterior pituitary gland increases water retention. However, if the initial fluid or blood loss is great or if loss continues, compensation fails, resulting in decreased tissue perfusion. As in cardiogenic shock, oxygen and nutrient delivery to the cells is impaired and cellular metabolism fails. Anaerobic metabolism and lactate production result in lactic acidosis and serum and cellular electrolyte abnormalities.

The clinical manifestations of hypovolemic shock include high SVR, poor skin turgor, thirst, oliguria, low systemic and pulmonary preloads, rapid heart rate, thready pulse, and mental status deterioration. The differences between the signs and symptoms of hypovolemic shock and those of cardiogenic shock are mainly caused by differences in fluid volume and cardiac muscle health. Management begins with rapid fluid replacement with crystalloids and blood products.[158] For hemorrhagic hypovolemic shock, the administration of pharmacological doses of ADH can improve blood pressure. Hypothermia and coagulopathies frequently complicate treatment.[158] If adequate tissue perfusion cannot be restored promptly, systemic inflammation and multiple organ dysfunction are likely.

Neurogenic Shock

Neurogenic shock (sometimes called vasogenic shock) is the result of widespread and massive vasodilation that results from parasympathetic overstimulation and sympathetic understimulation (Figure 24-44) (see

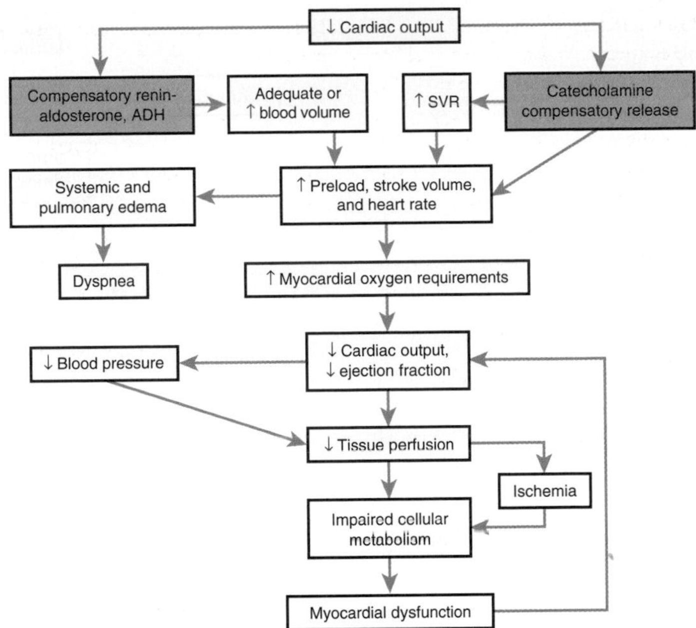

FIGURE 24-42 Cardiogenic Shock. Shock becomes life-threatening when compensatory mechanisms (in *orange boxes*) cause increased myocardial oxygen requirements. Renal and hypothalamic adaptive responses (i.e., renin-angiotensin-aldosterone and antidiuretic hormone [*ADH*]) maintain or increase blood volume. The adrenal gland releases catecholamines (e.g., mostly epinephrine, some norepinephrine), causing vasoconstriction and increases in contractility and heart rate. These adaptive mechanisms, however, increase myocardial demands for oxygen and nutrients. These demands further strain the heart, which can no longer pump an adequate volume, resulting in shock and impaired metabolism. *SVR*, systemic vascular resistance.

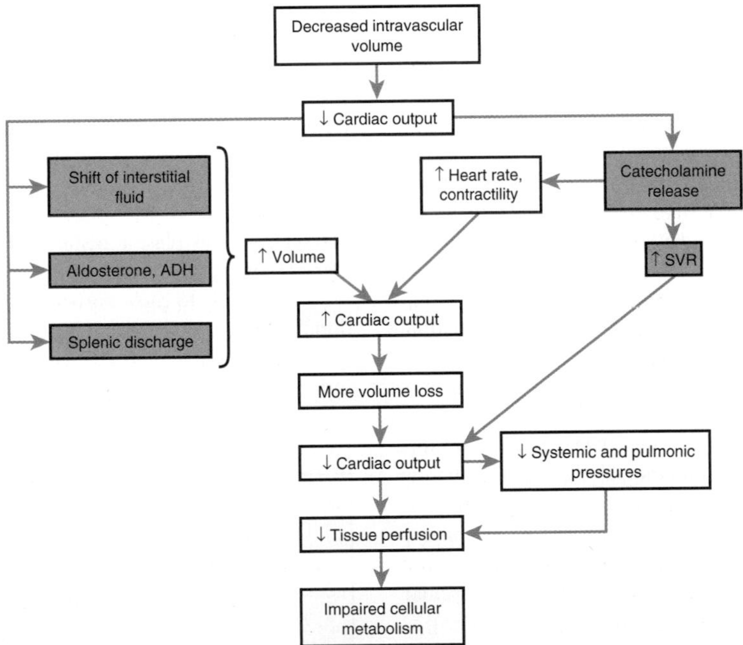

FIGURE 24-43 Hypovolemic Shock. This type of shock becomes life-threatening when compensatory mechanisms (in *orange boxes*) are overwhelmed by continued loss of intravascular volume. *ADH*, antidiuretic hormone; *SVR*, systemic vascular resistance.

Chapter 23). This type of shock can be caused by any factor that stimulates parasympathetic or inhibits sympathetic stimulation of vascular smooth muscle. Trauma to the spinal cord or medulla and conditions that interrupt the supply of oxygen or glucose to the medulla can cause neurogenic shock by interrupting sympathetic activity. Depressive medications, anaesthetic agents, and severe emotional stress and pain are other causes. The loss of vascular tone results in "relative hypovolemia," in which blood volume has not changed but SVR decreases drastically so that the amount of space containing the blood has increased.[159] The pressure in the vessels falls below that which is needed to drive nutrients across capillary membranes to the cells. In addition, neurological insult may cause bradycardia, which decreases cardiac

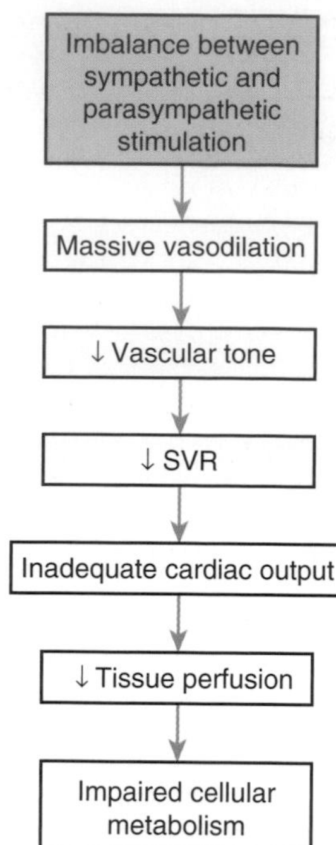

FIGURE 24-44 Neurogenic Shock. *SVR,* systemic vascular resistance.

output and further contributes to hypotension and underperfusion of tissues. As with other types of shock, neurogenic shock leads to impaired cellular metabolism. Management includes the careful use of fluids and vasopressors until blood pressure stabilizes.

Anaphylactic Shock

Anaphylactic shock results from a widespread hypersensitivity reaction known as **anaphylaxis**. The lifetime prevalence of anaphylaxis is 0.5 to 2%.[160] The basic physiological alteration is the same as that of neurogenic shock: vasodilation and relative hypovolemia, leading to decreased tissue perfusion and impaired cellular metabolism (Figure 24-45). Anaphylactic shock is characterized by other effects that rapidly involve the entire body.

Anaphylactic shock begins with exposure of a sensitized individual to an allergen. Common allergens known to cause these reactions are insect venoms, shellfish, peanuts, latex, and medications such as penicillin. In genetically predisposed individuals, these allergens initiate a vigorous humoral immune response (type I hypersensitivity reaction) that results in the production of large quantities of immunoglobulin E (IgE) antibody (see Chapter 8). Allergen bound to IgE causes degranulation of mast cells. Mast cells release a large number of vasoactive and inflammatory cytokines. The released substances mediate an extensive immune and inflammatory response, including vasodilation and increased vascular permeability, resulting in peripheral pooling and tissue edema. Extravascular effects include constriction of extravascular smooth muscle, often causing laryngospasm and bronchospasm (see Chapter 27) and cramping abdominal pain with diarrhea.

The onset of anaphylactic shock is usually sudden, and progression to death can occur within minutes unless emergency treatment is given. The primary clinical manifestations of anaphylaxis include anxiety, dizziness, difficulty breathing, stridor, wheezing, pruritus with hives (urticaria), swollen lips and tongue, and abdominal cramping. A precipitous fall in blood pressure occurs, followed by impaired mentation. Other signs include decreased SVR, with high or normal cardiac output, and oliguria. The diagnosis can be confirmed by a number of serum

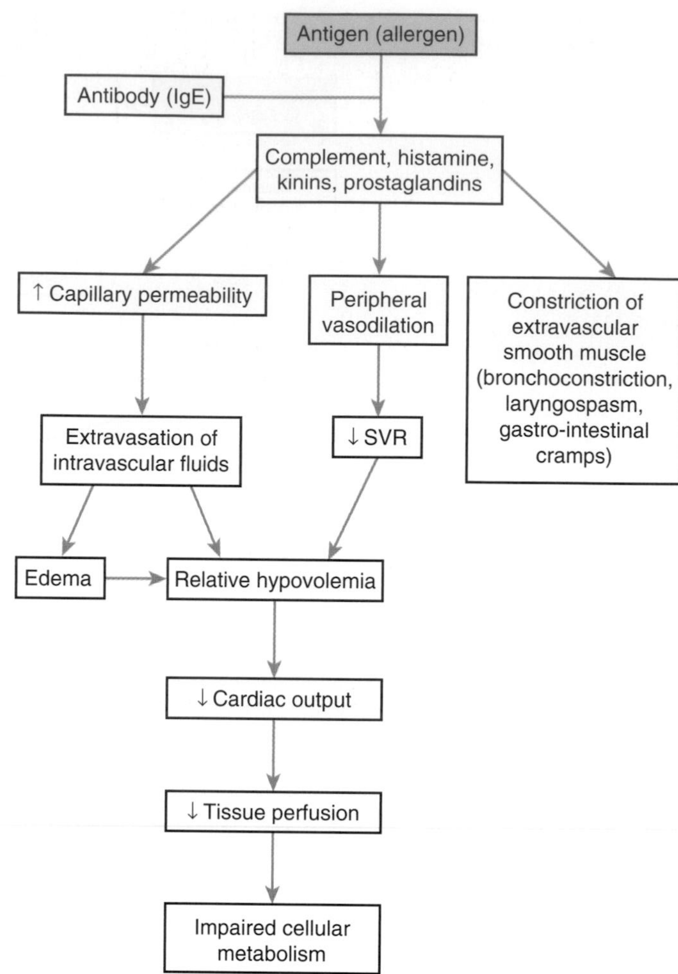

FIGURE 24-45 Anaphylactic Shock. *IgE,* immunoglobulin E; *SVR,* systemic vascular resistance.

markers, such as plasma histamine and tryptase.[161] Treatment begins with removal of the antigen (if possible). Epinephrine is administered intramuscularly to cause vasoconstriction and reverse airway constriction.[162] Fluids are given intravenously to reverse the relative hypovolemia, and antihistamines and corticosteroids are administered to stop the inflammatory reaction. Vasopressors and inhaled β-adrenergic agonist bronchodilators may also be necessary.

✔ QUICK CHECK 24-11

1. Describe the mechanisms operative in shock.
2. Why does myocardial infarction often cause cardiogenic shock?
3. How is hypovolemic shock manifested?
4. Why is anaphylactic shock considered a medical emergency?

Septic Shock

Septic shock begins with an infection that progresses to bacteremia, then **systemic inflammatory response syndrome (SIRS)** with sepsis, then severe sepsis, then septic shock, and finally MODS. Causes and definitions of each component of septic shock are presented in Table 24-11.[163]

In 2011, 1 in 18 deaths in Canada involved sepsis, a serious medical condition caused by an overwhelming immune response to an infection. Deaths involving sepsis increased significantly between 2000 and 2007

TABLE 24-11 Causes and Definitions of Septic Shock

Cause	Definition
Infection	Microbial phenomenon characterized by inflammatory response to presence of microorganisms or invasion of normally sterile host tissue by those microorganisms
Bacteremia	Presence of viable bacteria in blood
Systemic inflammatory response syndrome (SIRS)	Systemic inflammatory response to a variety of severe clinical insults manifested by two or more of the following signs: Temperature >38°C (100.4°F) or <36°C (96.8°F) Heart rate >90 beats/min Respiratory rate >20 breaths/min or arterial blood carbon dioxide level <32 mm Hg White blood cell count >12 000 cells/mm³, <4 000 cells/mm³, or containing <10% immature forms (bands)
Sepsis	Systemic response to infection characterized by two or more of SIRS criteria
Severe sepsis	Sepsis associated with organ dysfunction
Septic shock	Severe sepsis complicated by persistent hypotension refractory to early fluid therapy
Multiple organ dysfunction syndrome	Presence of altered organ function in an acutely ill individual such that homeostasis cannot be maintained without intervention

Data adapted from American College of Chest Physicians/Society of Critical Care Medicine Consensus Conference. (1992). *Crit Care Med, 20*(6), 864–874; Levy, M.M., Fink, M.P., Marshall, J.C., et al. (2003). *Crit Care Med, 31*(4), 1250–1256.

and then remained stable between 2007 and 2011. Between 2000 and 2007, deaths involving sepsis were higher among males than females, although between 2007 and 2011 the difference between the sexes narrowed. From 2009 to 2011, sepsis contributed to 53.4% of all deaths from infectious diseases and 5.5% of all deaths in Canada.[164]

Although death rates from septic shock have been declining, septic shock remains a highly lethal condition.[165] Septic shock can be caused by community-acquired or health care–associated infections, especially pneumonia and intra-abdominal and urinary tract infections. Indwelling arterial and central venous catheters also are an important source of infection (see *Health Promotion:* Sepsis Prevention: Central Line–Associated Bloodstream Infection).[156] Most often, sepsis is caused by bacteria, with *Staphylococcus aureus* and *Streptococcus pneumoniae* as the most common Gram-positive causes; and *Escherichia coli, Klebsiella* species, and *Pseudomonas aeruginosa* as the most common Gram-negative causes.[166] Septic shock also can be caused by fungi and viruses, and in almost one-third of cases, the infectious organism is never identified. The source and virulence of the infectious microorganism, as well as the underlying health of the affected individual, significantly affect prognosis. Risk factors for septic shock include the individual's genetic composition, underlying chronic diseases, immune deficiency states, and timeliness of therapeutic interventions for infection.

Most septic shock begins when bacteria enter the bloodstream to produce bacteremia. These bacteria and their associated toxins initiate an innate immune response. Gram-negative microorganisms release endotoxins, and Gram-positive microorganisms release exotoxins, lipoteichoic acids, and peptidoglycans. These pathogen-associated molecular patterns (PAMPs), as well as molecules released from injured cells (damage-associated molecular patters), trigger the septic syndrome by interacting with pattern-associated receptors on macrophages, such as Toll-like receptor 2 (TLR-2) for Gram-positive PAMPs and Toll-like receptor 4 (TLR-4) for Gram-negative PAMPs (Figure 24-46).[166,167] These microbial molecules also activate complement, coagulation, kinins, and inflammatory cells.

The release of inflammatory mediators triggers intense cellular responses and the subsequent release of secondary mediators, including cytokines, complement fragments, prostaglandins, platelet-activating factor, oxygen free radicals, nitric oxide, and proteolytic enzymes (see *Risk Factors:* Proinflammatory Mediators Contributing to Septic Shock). Chemotaxis, activation of granulocytes, and reactivation of the phagocytic cells and inflammatory cascades result. This systemic inflammation, especially through the action of nitric oxide, leads to widespread vasodilation with compensatory tachycardia and increased cardiac output in the early stages of septic shock (hyperdynamic phase).[167] Later in the course of disease, inflammatory mediators, such as complement and interleukins, depress myocardial contractility such that cardiac output falls and tissue perfusion decreases. Tissue perfusion and cellular oxygen extraction also are affected by activation of the clotting cascade through the action of platelet-activating factor and depletion of the endogenous anticoagulant protein C.[166,167] Furthermore, unresponsiveness to or depletion of vasoactive factors such as vasopressin contributes to hypotension and tissue hypoperfusion. The inflammatory response can become overwhelming, leading to the SIRS.[168] SIRS can progress to widespread tissue hypoxia, necrosis, and apoptosis, leading to septic shock and MODS. It has been determined that there is a parallel release of anti-inflammatory mediators and impairment of phagocytic and adaptive immune cell function that accompanies SIRS, causing a depression in the immune response to infection that contributes to the overall shock syndrome.[166,168]

Clinical manifestations of septic shock are the result of inflammation, decreased perfusion of vital tissues, and an alteration in oxygen extraction

HEALTH PROMOTION

Sepsis Prevention: Central Line–Associated Bloodstream Infection

Central line–associated bloodstream infection (CLABSI) is an important cause of sepsis and septic shock and occurs in more than 40 000 people each year. Central lines are most commonly placed in the central venous circulation for administering medications, performing hemodialysis, and monitoring hemodynamics. Catheters can be placed in several ways, including surgical and percutaneous access methods, depending on the purpose of the catheter. Risk factors for CLABSI include extremes of age, underlying systemic and immunocompromising conditions, and catheter-related factors, such as number of catheters, site of catheter insertion, and length of time the catheter has been in place. The Centers for Disease Control and Prevention (CDC) has determined that nearly one in four individuals who contracts CLABSI dies from associated complications, and it has been active in educating health care providers in CLABSI prevention. Prevention consists of appropriate patient selection and guideline-driven placement and management techniques.

Data from Centers for Disease Control and Prevention. (2014). Bloodstream infection event (central line–associated bloodstream infection and non-central line–associated bloodstream infection). Retrieved from http://www.cdc.gov/nhsn/pdfs/pscmanual/4psc_clabscurrent.pdf; Huber, K., Zenilman, J., Blanding, R., et al. (2014). *Am J Infect Control, 42*(6, Suppl.), S166; The Joint Commission. (2012). *Preventing central line–associated bloodstream infections: a global challenge, a global perspective.* Oak Brook, IL: Joint Commission Resources. Retrieved from http://www.PreventingCLABSIs.pdf.

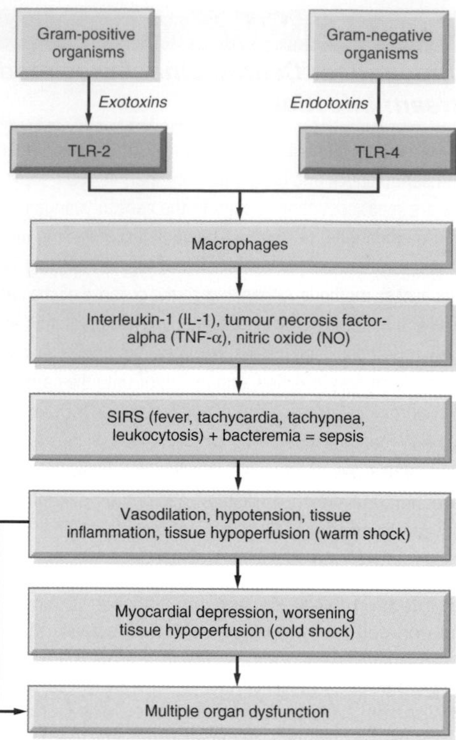

FIGURE 24-46 Septic Shock. *SIRS*, systemic inflammatory response syndrome; *TLR*, Toll-like receptor.

by all cells. In early shock, tachycardia causes cardiac output to remain normal or become elevated, although myocardial contractility is reduced. Temperature instability is present, ranging from hyperthermia to hypothermia. Effects on other organ systems may result in deranged renal function, jaundice, clotting abnormalities with DIC, deterioration of mental status, and ARDS. Gastro-intestinal mucosa changes cause the translocation of bacteria from the gut into the bloodstream. Increased permeability of the gut also can lead to increased inflammation and immune reactions attributable to toxins carried by the intestinal lymphatics.

The diagnosis of septic shock rests on the recognition of the systemic manifestations of overwhelming inflammation (SIRS) in individuals with suspected or documented infection. Determining the cause and severity of septic shock can be aided by measurement of levels of serum lactate, troponin[169] C-reactive protein, and procalcitonin.[170] The management of septic shock has improved outcomes[171] by following the Surviving Sepsis Guidelines (see *Health Promotion:* The Surviving Sepsis Guidelines). These guidelines include rapid goal-directed resuscitation with fluids and vasopressors, antibiotic administration, and respiratory support.[171] Control of hyperglycemia with insulin, treatment of complications associated with MODS, careful nutritional support, and prevention of stress ulcers and DVT are also essential. Despite improvements in septic shock–related mortality in recent years, mortality remains high and new treatments are being explored.[172]

✔ QUICK CHECK 24-12

1. What are some of the important causes of septic shock?
2. What is the systemic inflammatory response syndrome?
3. Why is correction of the underlying problem the most important treatment for all kinds of shock?

RISK FACTORS

Proinflammatory Mediators Contributing to Septic Shock

More than 100 inflammatory mediators have been implicated in the pathogenesis of septic shock. The following are some of the most important contributors:

Tumour Necrosis Factor-Alpha (TNF-α)

Produced from macrophages, natural killer cells, and mast cells in response to endotoxin and interleukins

Net effect: generates same symptoms of septic shock as those seen with interleukins; thus is redundant

Interleukin-1β (IL-1β)

Released by macrophages and lymphocytes in septic shock in response to bacterial toxins

Net effect: produces fever, vasodilation and hypotension, edema, myocardial depression, and elevated white blood count

Interleukin-6 (IL-6)

Released by macrophages and lymphocytes during infection

Net effect: fever, elevated white blood count

Nitric Oxide (NO)

Released by activated macrophages and neutrophils

Net effect: damages tissues and causes systemic vasodilation and hypotension

Platelet-Activating Factor (PAF)

Released from mononuclear phagocytes, platelets, and some endothelial cells in response to endotoxin

Net effect: contributes to widespread clotting, generates same symptoms of shock as those seen with interleukins and TNF-α, and may initiate multiple organ failure

Complement

Activated by bacterial products and antigen/antibody complexes

Net effect: damages tissues and amplifies the inflammatory process by cellular chemotaxis and promotion of phagocytosis

HEALTH PROMOTION

The Surviving Sepsis Guidelines

Mortality rates for severe sepsis and septic shock have declined because of more rapid recognition of systemic infection and more effective management. Current Surviving Sepsis Guidelines for the management of sepsis were developed on the basis of an in-depth analysis of the pathophysiology, clinical manifestations, and management outcomes reported over a decade of sepsis care. The guidelines provide a prioritized list of interventions that seek to quickly restore tissue perfusion, control infection, and support adequate oxygenation and ventilation. Intravenous infusion of fluids along with vasopressors, such as norepinephrine and vasopressin, is implemented quickly. Blood cultures, imaging modalities to determine the source of infection, and administration of appropriate antimicrobials are essential components of care. Respiratory support often includes mechanical ventilation, proper patient positioning, and careful monitoring of outcomes. Sedation is implemented as needed, and general supportive care includes glucose management with insulin, stress ulcer prevention, and nutrition. These Surviving Sepsis Guidelines have improved morbidity and mortality outcomes for individuals with septic shock.

Data from Dellinger, R.P., Levy, M.M., Rhodes, A., et al. (2013). *Crit Care Med, 41*(2), 580–637.

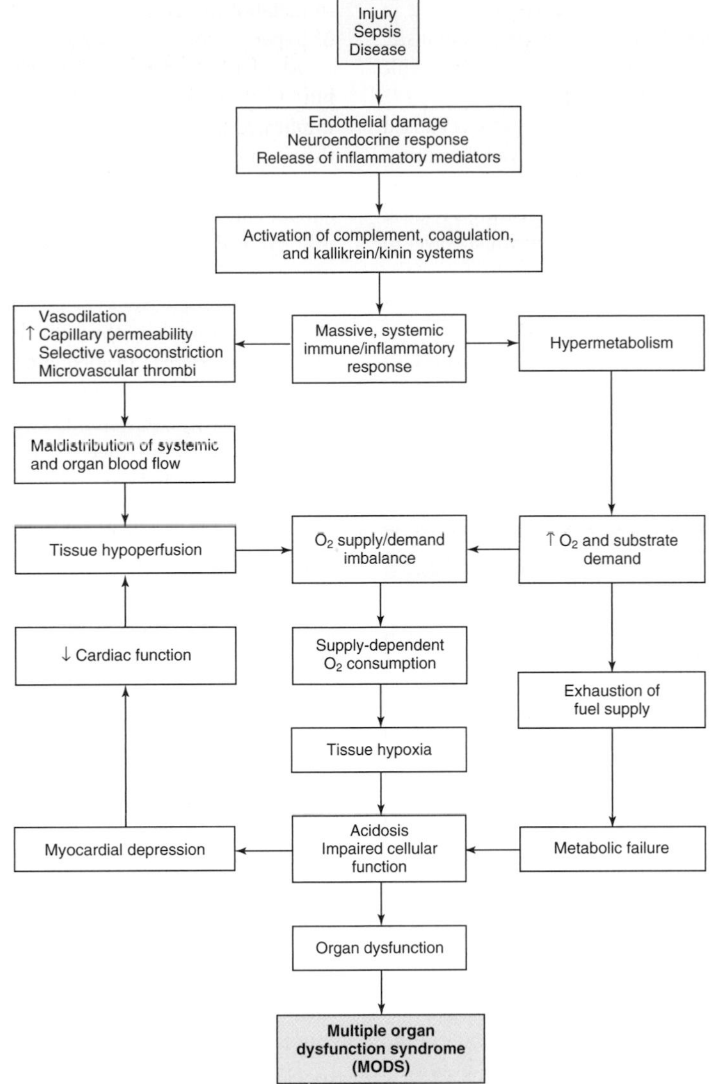

FIGURE 24-47 Pathogenesis of Multiple Organ Dysfunction Syndrome. *O_2,* oxygen.

Multiple Organ Dysfunction Syndrome

Multiple organ dysfunction syndrome (MODS) is the progressive dysfunction of two or more organ systems resulting from an uncontrolled inflammatory response to a severe illness or injury. The organ dysfunction can progress to organ failure and death (Figure 24-47). Although sepsis and septic shock are the most common causes, any severe injury or disease process that activates a massive systemic inflammatory response in the host can initiate MODS. These triggers include severe trauma, burns, acute pancreatitis, obstetrical complications, major surgery, circulatory shock, some medications, and gangrenous or necrotic tissue.

MODS is a common cause of mortality in Critical Care Units. Mortality for individuals ranges from 36 to 100% if there is failure of five or more organs, with liver and kidney failure being the most common.[173] People at greatest risk of developing MODS are older adults and persons with significant tissue injury or pre-existing disease (Box 24-3).

PATHOPHYSIOLOGY As a result of the initiating insult (sepsis, injury, or disease), the neuroendocrine system is activated with the release of the stress hormones cortisol, epinephrine, and norepinephrine into the bloodstream (see Chapter 8). Vascular endothelial damage occurs as a direct result of injury or from damage by bacterial toxins and inflammatory mediators, such as nitric oxide, tumour necrosis factor, and IL-1, which are released into the circulation. The vascular endothelium becomes permeable, allowing fluid and protein to leak into the interstitial spaces, contributing to hypotension and hypoperfusion. Leakage of fluid into the lungs causes ARDS. When the endothelium is damaged, platelets and tissue thromboplastin are activated, resulting in systemic microvascular coagulation that may lead to DIC (see Chapter 21).[174]

Because of the release of inflammatory mediators, four major plasma enzyme cascades are activated: complement, coagulation, fibrinolytic, and kallikrein/kinin. The overall effect of the activation of these cascades is a hyperinflammatory and hypercoagulant state that maintains the interstitial edema formation, cardiovascular instability, endothelial damage, and clotting abnormalities characteristic of MODS.[175] A massive systemic immune and inflammatory response then develops involving neutrophils, macrophages, and mast cells (Table 24-12). The inflammatory process initiated is the same as that described in septic shock and SIRS and sets the stage for MODS.

The numerous inflammatory and clotting processes operating in MODS cause maldistribution of blood flow and hypermetabolism. Oxygen delivery to the tissues decreases despite the supranormal systemic blood flow for several reasons:

- Shunting of blood past selected regional capillary beds is caused when inflammatory mediators override the normal vascular tone.
- Interstitial edema, resulting from microvascular changes in permeability, contributes to decreased oxygen delivery by creating a relative hypovolemia and by increasing the distance oxygen must travel to reach the cells.
- Capillary obstruction occurs because of formation of microvascular thrombi and the aggregation of white blood cells.

Hypermetabolism in MODS with accompanying alterations in carbohydrate, fat, and lipid metabolism is initially a compensatory measure to meet the body's increased demands for energy. The alterations in metabolism affect all aspects of substrate utilization. The net result of hypermetabolism is depletion of oxygen and fuel supplies.

Myocardial depression also accompanies MODS. The cause is unclear but inflammatory cytokines, bacterial products, and ischemia have been implicated. Decreased cardiac output contributes to poor perfusion of tissues and exacerbation of MODS.

Maldistribution of blood flow, coagulation, myocardial depression, ARDS, and the hypermetabolic state combine to create an imbalance in oxygen supply and demand. This imbalance is critical in the pathogenesis of MODS because it results in a pathological condition known as **supply-dependent oxygen consumption**. Ordinarily, the amount of oxygen consumed by the cells depends only on the demands of the cells, because there is an adequate reserve of oxygen that can be delivered if needed. The reserve, however, has been exhausted in MODS, and the amount of oxygen consumed becomes dependent on the amount the circulation is able to deliver; this amount is inadequate in MODS. Therefore, tissue hypoxia with cellular acidosis and impaired cellular function ensue and result in multiple organ failure.

BOX 24-3 Other Common Triggers of MODS

Severe trauma	Heat stroke
Major surgery	Liver failure
Burns	Mesenteric ischemia
Circulatory shock	Propofol infusion syndrome
Acute pancreatitis	Persistent inflammatory foci
Acute renal failure	Necrotic tissue
Acute respiratory distress syndrome	Disseminated intravascular coagulation
Blood transfusion	

MODS, multiple organ dysfunction syndrome.

Data from Abboud, B., Daher, R., & Boujaoude, J. (2008). *World J Gastroenterol, 14*(35), 5361–5370; Adukauskienė, D., Dockiene, I., Naginiene, R., et al. (2008). *Medicina (Kaunas), 44*(7): 536–540; Beger, H.G., & Rau, B.M. (2007). *World J Gastroenterol, 13*(38), 5043–5051; Bouchama, A., & Knochel, J.P. (2002). *N Engl J Med, 346*, 1978–1988; Broessner, G., Beer, R., Franz, G., et al. (2005). *Crit Care, 9*(5), R498–R501; Carnovale, A., Rabitti, P.G., Manes, G., et al. (2005). *J Pancreas (Online), 6*(5), 438–444; Ciesla, D.J., Moore, E.E., Johnson, J.L., et al. (2005). *Arch Surg, 140*(5), 432–440; Gando, S. (2010). *Crit Care Med, 38*(2), S35–S42; Kam, P.C.A., & Cardone, D. (2007). *Anesthesia, 62*(1), 690–701; Oeckler, R.A., & Hubmayr, R.D. (2007). *Eur Respir J, 30*(6), 1216–1226; Shaheem, M.A., & Akhtar, A.J. (2007). *J Nat Med Assoc, 99*(12), 1402–1406; Varghese, G.M., John, G., Thomas, K., et al. (2005). *Emerg Med J, 22*, 185–187; Vincent, J.L., Nelson, D.R., & Williams, M.D. (2011). *Crit Care Med, 39*(5), 1050–1055; Zaccheo, M.M., & Bucher, D.H. (2008). *Crit Care Nurse, 28*(3), 18–26.

CLINICAL MANIFESTATIONS There may be a lag time between the inciting event and the onset of symptoms that may last for as long as 24 hours. The individual develops a low-grade fever, tachycardia, dyspnea, altered mental status, and hyperdynamic and hypermetabolic states. ARDS is often an early manifestation of MODS (see Chapter 27) and is characterized by tachypnea, pulmonary edema with crackles and diminished breath sounds, use of accessory muscles, and hypoxemia.

As the syndrome continues, hypermetabolic and hyperdynamic states intensify and signs of liver and kidney failure appear. Liver failure presents with jaundice, abdominal distension, liver tenderness, muscle wasting, and hepatic encephalopathy. All facets of metabolism, substance detoxification, and immune response are impaired; albumin and clotting factor synthesis decreases; protein wastes accumulate; and liver tissue macrophages (Kupffer cells) no longer function effectively. Progressive oliguria, azotemia, and edema mark the development of renal failure. Anuria, hyperkalemia, and metabolic acidosis may occur if renal shutdown is severe.

The gastro-intestinal system also shows evidence of dysfunction. The gastro-intestinal system is sensitive to ischemic and inflammatory injury. Clinical manifestations of bowel involvement are hemorrhage, ileus, malabsorption, diarrhea or constipation, vomiting, anorexia, and abdominal pain. Stress ulceration of the stomach lining is a common complication of shock and MODS and, although usually painless, can result in massive blood loss and death. Compounding the damage caused by injury to the bowel is the phenomenon of bacterial translocation. When mediators and severe ischemia injure the mucosal epithelium, bacteria and toxins pass from the gut into the portal circulation. The

TABLE 24-12 Cells of Inflammation and Multiple Organ Dysfunction

Cell	Activators	Contribution to Multiple Organ Dysfunction
Neutrophils	Complement, kinins, endotoxin, clotting factors	Release of phagocytic products: toxic oxygen free radicals, superoxide ion, hydrogen peroxide, hydroxyl radicals, proteases, platelet-activating factor (PAF), arachidonic acid metabolites (prostaglandins, thromboxane, leukotrienes) Endothelial damage, vasodilation, vasopermeability, microvascular coagulation, selective vasoconstriction, hypotension, shock
Macrophages	Complement, endotoxin, chemotactic factors	Release of same phagocytic products as neutrophils Release of monokines: tumour necrosis factor (TNF), interleukin-1 (IL-1) TNF produces fever, anorexia, hyperglycemia, weight loss
Mast cells	Direct injury, endotoxin, complement	Release of histamine, PAF, arachidonic acid metabolites Vasodilation, vasopermeability, hypotension, shock

overwhelmed liver is unable to clear these products and they move into the systemic circulation. Thus, whether infection or some other injury was the precipitating cause of MODS, sepsis occurs once the gut barrier is damaged.

Hematological failure and myocardial failure are usually later manifestations. The signs and symptoms of cardiac failure in the hypermetabolic, hyperdynamic phase of MODS are similar to those of septic shock: tachycardia, bounding pulse, increased cardiac output, decreased SVR, and hypotension. In the terminal stages, hypodynamic circulation with bradycardia, profound hypotension, and ventricular dysrhythmias may develop. Encephalopathy, characterized by mental status changes ranging from confusion to deep coma, may occur at any time. Ischemia and inflammation are responsible for the central nervous system manifestations, which include apprehension, confusion, disorientation, restlessness, agitation, headache, decreased cognitive ability and memory, and decreased level of consciousness. When ischemia is severe, seizures and coma can occur. Death may occur as early as 14 days or after a period of several weeks.

EVALUATION AND TREATMENT Early detection of organ failure is extremely important so that supportive measures can be initiated immediately. Frequent assessment of the clinical status of individuals at known risk is essential. The Acute Physiology and Chronic Health Evaluation (APACHE) II and III systems are used to assess for severity and progression of MODS. Once organ failure develops, monitoring of laboratory values and hemodynamic parameters also can be used to assess the degree of impairment.

There is no specific treatment for MODS, and therapeutic management consists of prevention and support. Prevention consists of controlling the initial insult, treating infections quickly, and supporting healing. Management goals include controlling infection, restoring oxygenation and perfusion, and supporting organ function. Sources of infection are removed and antimicrobials are administered. Ventilatory support is initiated to maintain adequate oxygen saturation, and fluids are administered to maintain vascular volume. Nutritional support must be provided to meet metabolic demand. Dialysis also may be required.

QUICK CHECK 24-13

1. Why can multiple organ dysfunction syndrome be initiated by either a septic or a nonseptic insult?
2. Why are inflammation and clotting triggered when the vascular endothelium is injured?
3. Describe the mechanisms that result in decreased oxygen delivery to the tissues in MODS.

DID YOU UNDERSTAND?

Diseases of the Veins

1. Varicosities are areas of veins in which blood has pooled, usually in the saphenous veins. Varicosities may be caused by damaged valves as a result of trauma to the valve or by chronic venous distension involving gravity and venous constriction.
2. Chronic venous insufficiency (CVI) is inadequate venous return over a long period that causes pathological ischemic changes in the vasculature, skin, and supporting tissues.
3. Venous stasis ulcers follow the development of CVI and probably develop as a result of the borderline metabolic state of the cells in the affected extremities.
4. Deep venous thrombosis (DVT) results from stasis of blood flow, endothelial damage, or hypercoagulability. The most serious complication of DVT is pulmonary embolism.
5. Superior vena cava syndrome is a progressive occlusion of the superior vena cava that leads to venous distension in the upper extremities and head. Because this syndrome is usually caused by bronchogenic cancer, it is generally considered an oncological emergency rather than a vascular emergency.

Diseases of the Arteries

1. Hypertension is the elevation of systemic arterial blood pressure resulting from increases in cardiac output (blood volume), total peripheral resistance, or both.
2. Hypertension can be primary (without a known cause) or secondary (caused by an underlying disease).
3. The risk factors for hypertension include family history; gender (men greater than women before age 55; women greater than men after 55); advancing age; being of African descent; being of Indigenous descent; recent immigration; obesity; high dietary sodium intake; dietary intake of potassium, calcium, and magnesium; glucose intolerance; cigarette smoking; and heavy alcohol consumption.
4. The exact cause of primary hypertension is unknown, although several hypotheses are proposed, including overactivity of the sympathetic nervous system (SNS); overactivity of the renin-angiotensin-aldosterone system (RAAS); sodium and water retention by the kidneys; hormonal inhibition of sodium–potassium transport across cell walls; and complex interactions involving insulin resistance, inflammation, and endothelial function.
5. Clinical manifestations of hypertension result from damage of organs and tissues outside the vascular system. These include retinal changes, heart disease, renal disease, and central nervous system disorders, such as stroke and dementia.
6. Hypertension is managed with both pharmacological and non-pharmacological methods that lower the blood volume and the total peripheral resistance.
7. Orthostatic hypotension (OH) is a drop in blood pressure that occurs on standing. The compensatory vasoconstriction response to standing is replaced by a marked vasodilation and blood pooling in the muscle vasculature.
8. The clinical manifestations of OH include fainting and may involve cardiovascular symptoms, as well as impotence and bowel and bladder dysfunction.
9. An aneurysm is a localized dilation of a vessel wall; the aorta is particularly susceptible.
10. A thrombus is a clot that remains attached to a vascular wall. An embolus is a mobile aggregate of a variety of substances that occludes the vasculature. Sources of emboli include clots, air, amniotic fluid, bacteria, fat, and foreign matter. These emboli cause ischemia and necrosis when a vessel is totally blocked.
11. The most common source of arterial emboli is the heart as a result of mitral and aortic valvular disease and atrial fibrillation, followed by myxomas. Tissues affected include the lower extremities, the brain, and the heart.
12. Emboli to the central organs cause tissue death in lungs, kidneys, and mesentery.
13. Peripheral vascular diseases include Buerger's disease and Raynaud phenomenon, involving arterioles of the extremities.

14. Atherosclerosis is a form of arteriosclerosis and is the leading contributor to coronary artery disease (CAD) and cerebrovascular disease.
15. Atherosclerosis is an inflammatory disease that begins with endothelial injury.
16. Important steps in atherogenesis include vasoconstriction, adherence of macrophages, release of inflammatory mediators, oxidation of low-density lipoprotein, formation of foam cells and fatty streaks, and development of fibrous plaque.
17. Once a plaque has formed, it can rupture, resulting in clot formation and instability and vasoconstriction, which lead to obstruction of the lumen and inadequate oxygen delivery to tissues.
18. Ischemic heart disease is most commonly the result of CAD and the ensuing decrease in myocardial blood supply.
19. Peripheral artery disease is the result of atherosclerotic plaque formation in the arteries that supply the extremities, and it causes pain and ischemic changes in the nerves, muscles, and skin of the affected limb.
20. CAD is the result of an atherosclerotic plaque that gradually narrows the coronary arteries or that ruptures and causes sudden thrombus formation.
21. Many risk factors contribute to the onset and escalation of CAD, including traditional risk factors such as dyslipidemia, cigarette smoking, hypertension, diabetes mellitus (insulin resistance), obesity, and sedentary lifestyle, and nontraditional risk factors such as elevated C-reactive protein levels, hyperhomocysteinemia, and changes in adipokines.
22. Atherosclerotic plaque progression can be gradual and cause stable angina pectoris, which is predictable chest pain caused by myocardial ischemia in response to increased demand (e.g., exercise) without infarction.
23. Prinzmetal angina results from coronary artery vasospasm.
24. Myocardial ischemia may be asymptomatic, which is called *silent ischemia*, and is a risk factor for the development of the acute coronary syndromes.
25. Sudden coronary obstruction because of thrombus formation causes the acute coronary syndromes. These syndromes include unstable angina, non-ST elevation myocardial infarction (non-STEMI), and ST elevation myocardial infarction (STEMI).
26. Unstable angina results in reversible myocardial ischemia.
27. Myocardial infarction (MI) is caused by prolonged, unrelieved ischemia that interrupts blood supply to the myocardium. After about 20 minutes of myocardial ischemia, irreversible hypoxic injury causes cellular death and tissue necrosis.
28. Dysrhythmias and cardiac failure are the most common complications of acute MI.
29. MI is clinically classified as non-STEMI or STEMI based on electrocardiographic findings that suggest the extent of myocardial damage (subendocardial versus transmural).
30. An increase in plasma enzyme levels is used to diagnose the occurrence of MI as well as indicate its severity. Elevations of the isoenzymes creatine kinase-myocardial bound (CK-MB), troponins, and lactate dehydrogenase 1 (LDH-1) are most predictive of an MI.
31. Treatment of an MI includes revascularization (thrombolytics or PCI) and administration of antithrombotics, angiotensin-converting enzyme (ACE) inhibitors, and beta-blockers. Pain relief and fluid management also are key components of care.

Disorders of the Heart Wall

1. Inflammation of the pericardium, or *pericarditis*, may result from several sources (e.g., infection, trauma or surgery, neoplasm). Pericarditis presents with symptoms that are physically troublesome, but in and of themselves they are not life-threatening.
2. Fluid may collect within the pericardial sac (pericardial effusion). Cardiac function may be severely impaired if the accumulation of fluid occurs rapidly and involves a large volume.
3. Cardiomyopathies are a diverse group of primary myocardial disorders that are usually the result of remodelling, neurohumoral responses, and hypertension. The cardiomyopathies are categorized as dilated (formerly, congestive), hypertrophic (asymmetric), or restrictive (rigid and noncompliant). The size of the cardiac muscle walls and chambers may increase or decrease depending on the type of cardiomyopathy, thereby altering contractile activity.
4. The hemodynamic integrity of the cardiovascular system depends to a great extent on properly functioning cardiac valves. Congenital or acquired disorders that result in stenosis, regurgitation, or both can structurally alter the valves.
5. Characteristic heart sounds, cardiac murmurs, and systemic complaints assist in identification of an abnormal valve. If severely compromised function exists, a prosthetic heart valve may be surgically implanted to replace the faulty one.
6. Mitral valve prolapse syndrome (MVPS) describes the condition in which the mitral valve leaflets do not position themselves properly during systole. MVPS may be a completely asymptomatic condition or can result in unpredictable symptoms.
7. Rheumatic fever is an inflammatory disease that results from a delayed immune response to a streptococcal infection in genetically predisposed individuals. The disorder usually resolves without sequelae if treated early.
8. Severe or untreated cases of rheumatic fever may progress to rheumatic heart disease, a potentially disabling cardiovascular disorder.
9. Infective endocarditis is a general term for infection and inflammation of the endocardium, especially the cardiac valves. In the mildest cases, valvular function may be slightly impaired by vegetations that collect on the valve leaflets. If left unchecked, severe valve abnormalities, chronic bacteremia, and systemic emboli may occur as vegetations detach from the valve surface and travel through the bloodstream. Antibiotic therapy can limit the extension of this disease.
10. Human immunodeficiency virus (HIV) infection and acquired immune deficiency syndrome (AIDS) are associated with cardiac abnormalities, including myocarditis, endocarditis, pericarditis, and cardiomyopathy.

Manifestations of Heart Disease

1. Heart failure (HF) can be divided into HF with reduced ejection fraction (systolic) and HF with preserved ejection fraction (diastolic).
2. The most common causes of left ventricular failure are MI and hypertension.
3. HF with reduced ejection fraction (systolic) is caused by increased preload, decreased contractility, or increased afterload. These processes result in an increased left ventricular end-diastolic volume and an increased left ventricular end-diastolic pressure (LVEDP) that cause increased pulmonary venous pressures and pulmonary edema.
4. In addition to the hemodynamic changes of left ventricular failure, there is a neuroendocrine response that tends to exacerbate and perpetuate the condition.
5. The neuroendocrine mediators of HF include the SNS and the RAAS; thus diuretics, beta-blockers, and ACE inhibitors are important components of pharmacological therapy.

6. HF with preserved ejection fraction (diastolic HF) is a clinical syndrome characterized by the symptoms and signs of HF, a preserved ejection fraction, and abnormal diastolic function.
7. Diastolic dysfunction means that the LVEDP is increased, even if volume and cardiac output are normal.
8. Right ventricular failure can result from left ventricular failure or pulmonary disease.
9. A dysrhythmia (arrhythmia) is a disturbance of heart rhythm. Dysrhythmias range in severity from occasional missed beats or rapid beats to disturbances that impair myocardial contractility and are life-threatening.
10. Dysrhythmias can occur because of an abnormal rate of impulse generation or an abnormal conduction of impulses.

Shock

1. Shock is a widespread impairment of cellular metabolism involving positive feedback loops that places the individual on a downward physiological spiral leading to multiple organ dysfunction syndrome (MODS).
2. Types of shock are cardiogenic, hypovolemic, neurogenic, anaphylactic, and septic. MODS can develop from all types of shock.
3. The final common pathway in all types of shock is impaired cellular metabolism—cells switch from aerobic to anaerobic metabolism. Energy stores drop, and cellular mechanisms relative to membrane permeability, action potentials, and lysozyme release fail.
4. Anaerobic metabolism results in activation of the inflammatory response, decreased circulatory volume, and decreasing pH.
5. Impaired cellular metabolism results in cellular inability to use glucose because of impaired glucose delivery or impaired glucose intake, resulting in a shift to glycogenolysis, gluconeogenesis, and lipolysis for fuel generation.
6. Glycogenolysis is effective for only about 10 hours. Gluconeogenesis results in the use of proteins necessary for structure, function, repair, and replication that leads to more impaired cellular metabolism.
7. Gluconeogenesis contributes to lactic acid, uric acid, and ammonia buildup, interstitial edema, and impairment of the immune system, as well as general muscle weakness, leading to decreased respiratory function and cardiac output.
8. Cardiogenic shock is decreased cardiac output, tissue hypoxia, and the presence of adequate intravascular volume.
9. Hypovolemic shock is caused by loss of blood or fluid in large amounts. The use of compensatory mechanisms may be vigorous, but tissue perfusion ultimately decreases and results in impaired cellular metabolism.
10. Neurogenic shock results from massive vasodilation, causing a relative hypovolemia even though cardiac output may be high, and leads to impaired cellular metabolism.
11. Anaphylactic shock is caused by physiological recognition of a foreign substance. The inflammatory response is triggered, and a massive vasodilation with fluid shift into the interstitium follows. The relative hypovolemia leads to impaired cellular metabolism.
12. Septic shock begins with impaired cellular metabolism caused by uncontrolled septicemia. The infecting agent triggers the inflammatory and immune responses. This inflammatory response is accompanied by widespread changes in tissue and cellular function.
13. MODS is the progressive failure of two or more organ systems after a severe illness or injury. It can be triggered by chronic inflammation, necrotic tissue, severe trauma, burns, adult respiratory distress syndrome, acute pancreatitis, and other severe injuries.
14. MODS involves the stress response; changes in the vascular endothelium resulting in microvascular coagulation; release of complement, coagulation, and kinin proteins; and numerous inflammatory processes. Consequences of all these mediators are a maldistribution of blood flow, hypermetabolism, hypoxic injury, and myocardial depression.
15. Clinical manifestations of MODS include inflammation, tissue hypoxia, and hypermetabolism. All organs can be affected including the kidney, lung, liver, gastro-intestinal tract, and central nervous system.

KEY TERMS

Acute coronary syndrome, 617
Acute pericarditis, 629
Anaphylactic shock, 650
Anaphylaxis, 650
Aneurysm, 611
Aortic regurgitation, 634
Aortic stenosis, 633
Arteriolar remodelling, 608
Arteriosclerosis, 614
Atherosclerosis, 614
Cardiogenic shock, 648
Cardiomyopathy, 630
Chronic orthostatic hypotension, 611
Chronic venous insufficiency (CVI), 604
Chylomicron, 617
Complicated plaque, 614
Constrictive pericarditis (restrictive pericarditis [chronic pericarditis]), 630
Coronary artery disease (CAD), 617
Damage-associated molecular pattern (DAMP), 608
Deep venous thrombosis (DVT), 605
Diastolic heart failure, 641
Dilated cardiomyopathy, 630
Dyslipidemia (dyslipoproteinemia), 618
Dysrhythmia (arrhythmia), 643
Electrocardiogram (ECG), 610
Embolism, 613
Embolus, 613
Endothelial injury, 614
False aneurysm, 611
Fatty streak, 614
Fibrous plaque, 614
Foam cell, 614
Heart failure (HF), 638
Heart failure with preserved ejection fraction (HFpEF), 641
Heart failure with reduced ejection fraction (HFrEF), 639
Hibernating myocardium, 625
High-output failure, 642
High-sensitivity C-reactive protein (hs-CRP), 614
Hypertension, 606
Hypertensive crisis (malignant hypertension), 609
Hypertensive hypertrophic cardiomyopathy, 631
Hypertrophic cardiomyopathy, 631
Hypertrophic obstructive cardiomyopathy, 631
Hypovolemic shock, 648
Infarction, 617
Infective endocarditis, 637
Intermittent claudication, 617
Ischemia, 617
Left ventricular failure, 639
Lipoprotein, 617
Lipoprotein(a) (Lp[a]), 618
Mental stress–induced ischemia, 621
Metabolic syndrome (MetS), 618
Microvascular angina (MVA), 621
Mitral regurgitation, 634
Mitral stenosis, 633
Mitral valve prolapse syndrome (MVPS), 634
Multiple organ dysfunction syndrome (MODS), 653
Myocardial infarction (MI), 623
Myocardial remodelling, 625
Myocardial stunning, 625

Neurogenic shock (vasogenic shock), 648
Nonbacterial thrombotic endocarditis, 638
Non-ST elevation myocardial infarction (non-STEMI), 623
Orthostatic (postural) hypotension (OH), 611
Percutaneous coronary intervention (PCI), 623
Pericardial effusion, 629
Peripheral artery disease (PAD), 617
Plaque, 614
Pressure–natriuresis relationship, 607
Primary hypertension, 606
Prinzmetal angina, 621
Raynaud phenomenon, 613
Restrictive cardiomyopathy, 631
Rheumatic fever, 634
Rheumatic heart disease, 634
Right ventricular failure, 642
Secondary hypertension, 606
Septic shock, 650
Shock, 643
Silent ischemia, 621
Stable angina pectoris, 620
ST elevation myocardial infarction (STEMI), 623
Superior vena cava syndrome (SVCS), 605
Supply-dependent oxygen consumption, 654
Systemic inflammatory response syndrome (SIRS), 650
Systolic heart failure, 639
Tamponade, 629
Thromboangiitis obliterans (Buerger's disease), 613
Thromboembolus, 605
Thrombus, 605
Transmural myocardial infarction, 624
Tricuspid regurgitation, 634
True aneurysm, 611
Unstable angina, 623
Valvular hypertrophic cardiomyopathy, 631
Valvular regurgitation (valvular insufficiency or valvular incompetence), 632
Valvular stenosis, 632
Varicose vein, 604
Venous stasis ulcer, 604
Ventricular remodelling, 639

REFERENCES

1. Pfisterer, L., König, G., Hecker, M., et al. (2014). Pathogenesis of varicose veins—Lessons from biomechanics. *VASA. Zeitschrift für Gefässkrankheiten, 43*(2), 88–99. doi:10.1024/0301-1526/a000335.
2. Poynter, E., Andrews, M., & Ackerman, W. (2013). Clinical inquiry what is the best initial treatment for venous stasis ulcers? *Journal of Family Practice, 62*(8), 433–434.
3. Gohel, M. (2013). Which treatments are cost-effective in the management of varicose veins? *Phlebology/Venous Forum of the Royal Society of Medicine, 28*(Suppl. 1), 153–157. doi:10.1177/0268355513477003.
4. Bates, S. M., Jaeschke, R., Stevens, S. M., et al. (2012). Diagnosis of DVT: Antithrombotic therapy and prevention of thrombosis (9th ed.): American College of Chest Physicians Evidence-Based Clinical Practice Guidelines. *Chest, 1431*(2, Suppl.), e35IS–e418S. doi:10.1378/chest.11-2299.
5. Baldwin, M. J., Moore, H. M., Rudarakanchana, N., et al. (2013). Post-thrombotic syndrome: A clinical review. *Journal of Thrombosis and Haemostasis, 11*(5), 795–805. doi:10.1111/jth.12180.
6. Pollak, A. W., & McBane, R. D. (2014). Succinct review of the new VTE prevention and management guidelines. *Mayo Clinic Proceedings, 89*(3), 394–408. doi:10.1016/j.mayocp.2013.11.015.
7. Prandoni, P. (2014). Venous thromboembolism in 2013: The advent of the novel oral anticoagulants. *Nature Reviews. Cardiology, 11*(2), 70–72. doi:10.1038/nrcardio.2013.210.
8. Shaheen, K., & Alraies, M. (2012). Superior vena cava syndrome. *Cleveland Clinic Journal of Medicine, 79*(6), 410–412. doi:10.3949/ccjm.79a.11106.
9. Quinn, K. L., & Smith, C. A. (2013). Nonmalignant superior vena cava syndrome. *Journal of General Internal Medicine, 28*(7), 970–971. doi:10.1007/s11606-013-2362-z.
10. Go, A. S., Mozaffarian, D., Roger, V. L., et al. (2014). Heart disease and stroke statistics—2014 update: A report from the American Heart Association. *Circulation, 129*(3), e28–e292. doi:10.1161/01.cir.0000441139.02102.80.
11. Hypertension Prevention and Control, & Hypertension Canada. (2016). *Fact sheet: Hypertension in Canada.* Retrieved from http://www.hypertensiontalk.com/wp-content/uploads/2016/05/HTN-Fact-Sheet-2016_FINAL.pdf.
12. Hypertension Canada. (2015). *Diagnosis and assessment.* Retrieved from http://guidelines.hypertension.ca/diagnosis-assessment/.
13. Hypertension Canada. (2016). *Key messages.* Markham, ON: Author. Retrieved from http://www.hypertension.ca/images/. CHEP_2016/2016_KeyMessages_EN.pdf.
14. Friso, S., Carvajal, C. L., Fardella, C. E., et al. (2015). Epigenetics and arterial hypertension: The challenge of emerging evidence. *Translational Research: The Journal of Laboratory and Clinical Medicine, 165*(1), 154–165. doi:10.1016/j.trsl.2014.06.007.
15. Lind, J. M., & Chiu, C. L. (2013). Genetic discoveries in hypertension: Steps on the road to therapeutic translation. *Heart (British Cardiac Society), 99*(22), 1645–1651. doi:10.1136/heartjnl-2012-302883.
16. Statistics Canada. (2015). *Aboriginal fact sheet for Canada.* http://www.statcan.gc.ca/pub/89-656-x/89-656-x2015001-eng.htm.
17. Pampel, F. C., Krueger, P. M., & Denney, J. T. (2010). Socioeconomic disparities in health behaviors. *Annual Review of Sociology, 36,* 349–370.
18. Heart Research Institute. (2017). *First Nations people and heart disease.* Retrieved from http://www.hricanada.org/about-heart-disease/first-nations-people-and-heart-disease.
19. Sanou, D., O'Reilly, E., Ngnie-Teta, I., et al. (2014). Acculturation and nutritional health of immigrants in Canada: A scoping review. *Journal of Immigrant and Minority Health, 16*(1), 24–34. doi:10.1007/s10903-013-9823-7.
20. Azar, K. M. J., Chen, E., Holland, A. T., et al. (2013). Festival foods in the immigrant diet. *Journal of Immigrant and Minority Health, 15*(5), 953–960. doi:10.1007/s10903-012-9705-4.
21. DiBona, G. F. (2013). Sympathetic nervous system and hypertension. *Hypertension, 61*(3), 556–560. doi:10.1097/MNH.0b013e32834db45d.
22. Grassi, G., Bertoli, S., & Seravalle, G. (2012). Sympathetic nervous system: Role in hypertension and in chronic kidney disease. *Current Opinion in Nephrology and Hypertension, 21*(1), 46–51. doi:10.1097/MNH.0b013e32834db45d.
23. Clarke, C., Flores-Muñoz, M., McKinney, C. A., et al. (2013). Regulation of cardiovascular remodeling by the counter-regulatory axis of the renin-angiotensin system. *Future Cardiology, 9*(1), 23–38. doi:10.2217/fca.12.75.
24. Dominici, F. P., Burghi, V., Munoz, M. C., et al. (2014). Modulation of the action of insulin by angiotension-(1-7). *Clinical Science (London, England: 1979), 126*(9), 613–630. doi:10.1042/CS20130333.
25. Farag, E., Maheshwari, K., Morgan, J., et al. (2015). An update of the role of rennin angiotensin in cardiovascular homeostasis. *Anesthesia and Analgesia, 120*(2), 275–292. doi:10.1213/ANE.0000000000000528.
26. Fraga-Silva, R. A., Ferreira, A. J., & Dos Santos, R. A. (2013). Opportunities for targeting the angiotensin-converting enzyme 2/angiotensin-(1-7)/mas receptor pathway in hypertension. *Current Hypertension Reports, 15*(1), 31–38. doi:10.1007/s11906-012-0324-1.
27. Henriksen, E. J., & Prasannarong, M. (2013). The role of the renin-angiotensin system in the development of insulin resistance in skeletal muscle. *Molecular and Cellular Endocrinology, 378*(1–2), 15–22. doi:10.1016/j.mce.2012.04.011.
28. McKinney, C. A., Fattah, C., Loughrey, C. M., et al. (2014). Angiotensin-(1-7) and angiotensin-(1-9): Function in cardiac and vascular remodeling. *Clinical Science (London, England: 1979), 126*(12), 815–827. doi:10.1042/CS20130436.
29. Ohishi, M., Yamamoto, K., & Rakugi, H. (2013). Angiotensin (1-7) and other angiotensin peptides. *Current Pharmaceutical Design, 19*(17), 3060–3064. doi:10.2174/1381612811319170013.
30. Regenhardt, R. W., Bennion, D. M., & Sumners, C. (2014). Cerebroprotective action of angiotensin peptides in stroke. *Clinical Science (London, England: 1979), 126*(3), 195–205. doi:10.1042/CS20130324.
31. Santos, R. A., Ferreira, A. J., Verano-Braga, T., et al. (2013). Angiotensin-converting enzyme 2, angiotensin-(1-7) and mas: New players of the renin-angiotensin system. *Journal of Endocrinology, 216*(2), R1–R17. doi:10.1530/JOE-12-0341.
32. Sevá Pessôa, B., van der Lubbe, N., Verdonk, K., et al. (2013). Key developments in renin-angiotensin-aldosterone system inhibition. *Nature Reviews. Nephrology, 9*(1), 26–36. doi:10.1038/nrneph.2012.249.
33. Wang, Y., Tikellis, C., Thomas, M. C., et al. (2013). Angiotenin coverting enzyme 2 and atherosclerosis. *Atherosclerosis, 226*(1), 3–8. doi:10.1016/j.atherosclerosis.2012.08.018.
34. Zucker, I. H., Xiao, L., & Haack, K. K. (2014). The central renin-angiotensin system and sympathetic nerve activity in chronic heart failure. *Clinical Science (London, England: 1979), 126*(10), 695–706. doi:10.1042/CS20130294.
35. Bender, S. B., McGraw, A. P., Jaffe, I. Z., et al. (2013). Mineralocorticoid receptor-mediated vascular insulin resistance: An early contributor to diabetes-related vascular disease? *Diabetes, 62*(2), 313–319. doi:10.2337/db12-0905.
36. Bibbins-Domingo, K. (2014). The Institute of Medicine report sodium intake in populations: Assessment of evidence: Summary of primary findings and implications for clinicians. *Journal of the American Medical Association Internal Medicine, 174*(1), 136–137. doi:10.1001/jamainternmed.2013.11818.
37. Rubattu, S., Calvieri, C., Pagliaro, B., et al. (2013). Atrial natriuretic peptide and regulation of vascular function in hypertension and heart failure: Implications for novel therapeutic strategies. *Journal of Hypertension, 31*(6), 1061–1072. doi:10.1097/HJH.0b013e32835ed5eb.
38. Koliaki, C., & Katsilambros, N. (2013). Dietary sodium, potassium, and alcohol: Key players in the pathophysiology, prevention, and treatment of human hypertension. *Nutrition Reviews, 71*(6), 402–411. doi:10.1111/nure.12036.
39. McCarthy, C. G., Goulopoulou, S., Wenceslau, C. F., et al. (2014). Toll-like receptors and damage-associated molecular patterns: Novel links between inflammation and hypertension. *American Journal of Physiology, Heart and Circulatory*

Physiology, 306(2), H184–H196. doi:10.1152/ajpheart.00328.2013.
40. Schiffrin, E. L. (2014). Immune mechanisms in hypertension and vascular injury. *Clinical Science (London, England: 1979), 126*(4), 267–274. doi:10.1042/CS20130407.
41. Aroor, A. R., McKarns, S., Demarco, V. G., et al. (2013). Maladaptive immune and inflammatory pathways lead to cardiovascular insulin resistance. *Metabolism: Clinical and Experimental, 62*(11), 1543–1552. doi:10.1016/j.metabol.2013.07.001.
42. Johns, E. J., & Abdulla, M. H. (2013). Renal nerves in blood pressure regulation. *Current Opinion in Nephrology and Hypertension, 22*(5), 504–510. doi:10.1097/MNH.0b013e3283641a89.
43. Santisteban, M. M., Zubcevic, J., Baekey, D. M., et al. (2013). Dysfunctional brain-bone marrow communication: A paradigm shift in the pathophysiology of hypertension. *Current Hypertension Reports, 15*(4), 377–389. doi:10.1007/s11906-013-0361-4.
44. Landsberg, L., Aronne, L. J., Beilin, L. J., et al. (2013). Obesity-related hypertension: Pathogenesis, cardiovascular risk, and treatment—A position paper of the Obesity Society and the American Society of Hypertension. *Obesity, 21*(1), 8–24. doi:10.1002/oby.20181.
45. Van de Voorde, J., Pauwels, B., Boydens, C., et al. (2013). Adipocytokines in relation to cardiovascular disease. *Metabolism: Clinical and Experimental, 62*(11), 1513–1521. doi:10.1016/j.metabol.2013.06.004.
46. Kovacic, J. C., Castellano, J. M., Farkouh, M. E., et al. (2014). The relationships between cardiovascular disease and diabetes: Focus on pathogenesis. *Endocrinology and Metabolism Clinics of North America, 43*(1), 41–57. doi:10.1016/j.ecl.2013.09.007.
47. Ishizu, T., Seo, Y., Kameda, Y., et al. (2014). Left ventricular strain and transmural distribution of structural remodeling in hypertensive heart disease. *Hypertension, 63*(3), 500–506. doi:10.1161/HYPERTENSIONAHA.113.02149.
48. Lioudaki, E., Florentin, M., Ganotakis, E. S., et al. (2013). Microalbuminuria: A neglected cardiovascular risk factor in non-diabetic individuals? *Current Pharmaceutical Design, 19*(27), 4964–4980. doi:10.2174/13816128113199270019.
49. Köhler, S., Baars, M. A., Spauwen, P., et al. (2014). Temporal evolution of cognitive changes in incident hypertension: Prospective cohort study across the adult age span. *Hypertension, 63*(2), 245–251. doi:10.1161/HYPERTENSIONAHA.113.02096.
50. Johnson, W., Nguyen, M. L., & Patel, R. (2012). Hypertension crisis in the emergency department. *Cardiology Clinics, 30*(4), 533–543. doi:10.1016/j.ccl.2012.07.011.
51. He, F. J., Li, J., & Macgregor, G. A. (2013). Effect of longer term modest salt reduction on blood pressure: Cochrane systematic review and meta-analysis of randomised trials. *British Medical Journal, 346*, f1325. doi:10.1136/bmj.f1325.
52. Hypertension Canada. (2015). *Prevention and treatment.* Retrieved from http://guidelines.hypertension.ca/prevention-treatment/.
53. Krum, H., Schlaich, M. P., Sobotka, P. A., et al. (2014). Percutaneous renal denervation in patients with treatment-resistant hypertension: Final 3-year report of the Symplicity HTN-1 study. *Lancet, 383*(9917), 622–629. doi:10.1016/S0140-6736(13)62192-3.
54. Bhatt, D. L., Kandzari, D. E., O'Neill, W. W., et al. (2014). A controlled trial of renal denervation for resistant hypertension. *New England Journal of Medicine, 370*(15), 1393–1401. doi:10.1056/NEJMoa1402670.
55. Freeman, R., Wieling, W., Axelrod, F. B., et al. (2011). Consensus statement on the definition of orthostatic hypotension, neurally mediated syncope and the postural tachycardia syndrome. *Clinical Autonomic Research, 21*(2), 69–72. doi:10.1007/s10286-011-0119-5.
56. Metzler, M., Duerr, S., Granata, R., et al. (2013). Neurogenic orthostatic hypotension: Pathophysiology, evaluation, and management. *Journal of Neurology, 260*(9), 2212–2219. doi:10.1007/s00415-012-6736-7.
57. Xin, W., Lin, Z., & Mi, S. (2014). Orthostatic hypotension and mortality risk: A meta-analysis of cohort studies. *Heart (British Cardiac Society), 100*(5), 406–413. doi:10.1136/heartjnl-2013-304121.
58. Perlmuter, L. C., Sarda, G., Casavant, V., et al. (2013). A review of the etiology, associated comorbidities, and treatment of orthostatic hypotension. *American Journal of Therapeutics, 20*(3), 279–291. doi:10.1097/MJT.0b013e31828bfb7f.
59. Björck, M., & Wanhainen, A. (2013). Pathophysiology of AAA: Heredity vs environment. *Progress in Cardiovascular Diseases, 56*(1), 2–6. doi:10.1016/j.pcad.2013.05.003.
60. Singh, M. J., Hager, E., Mapara, K., et al. (2014). Ruptured abdominal aortic aneurysms: Is open surgery an outdated operation? *Journal of Cardiovascular Surgery, 55*(2), 137–149.
61. Ketha, S. S., & Cooper, L. T. (2013). The role of autoimmunity in thromboangiitis obliterans (Buerger's disease). *Annals of the New York Academy of Sciences, 1285*, 15–25. doi:10.1111/nyas.12048.
62. Alamdari, D. H., Ravarit, H., Tavallaie, S., et al. (2014). Oxidative and antioxidative pathways might contribute to thromboangiitis obliterans pathophysiology. *Vascular, 22*(1), 46–50. doi:10.1177/1708538112473979.
63. Prete, M., Fatone, M. C., Favoino, E., et al. (2014). Raynaud's phenomenon: From molecular pathogenesis to therapy. *Autoimmunity Reviews, 13*(6), 655–667. doi:10.1016/j.autrev.2013.12.001.
64. Cutolo, M., & Smith, V. (2013). State of the art on nailfold capillaroscopy: A reliable diagnostic tool and putative biomarker in rheumatology? *Rheumatology (Oxford, England), 52*(11), 1933–1940. doi:10.1093/rheumatology/ket153.
65. Witztum, J. L., & Lichtman, A. H. (2014). The influence of innate and adaptive immune responses on atherosclerosis. *Annual Review of Pathology, 9*, 73–102. doi:10.1146/annurev-pathol-020712-163936.
66. Madrigal-Matute, J., Rotllan, N., Aranda, J. F., et al. (2013). MicroRNAs and atherosclerosis. *Current Atherosclerosis Reports, 15*(5), 322. doi:10.1007/s11883-013-0322-z.
67. Jaipersad, A. S., Lip, G. Y., Silverman, S., et al. (2014). The role of monocytes in angiogenesis and atherosclerosis. *Journal of the American College of Cardiology, 63*(1), 1–11. doi:10.1016/j.jacc.2013.09.019.
68. Arai, H. (2014). Oxidative modification of lipoproteins. *Sub-Cellular Biochemistry, 77*, 103–114. doi:10.1007/978-94-007-7920-4_9.
69. Pattanayak, P., & Bluemke, D. A. (2014). New era of evidence-based medicine with noninvasive imaging. *Nature Reviews. Cardiology, 11*, 74–76. doi:10.1038/nrcardio.2013.215.
70. Bourantas, C. V., Garcia-Garcia, H. M., Diletti, R., et al. (2013). Early detection and invasive passivation of future culprit lesions: A future potential or an unrealistic pursuit of chimeras? *American Heart Journal, 165*(6), 869–881.e4. doi:10.1016/j.ahj.2013.02.015.
71. Lovell, M., Harris, K., Forbes, T., et al. (2009). Peripheral arterial disease: Lack of awareness in Canada. *Canadian Journal of Cardiology, 25*(1), 39–45.
72. Lu, L., Mackay, D. F., & Pell, J. P. (2014). Meta-analysis of the association between cigarette smoking and peripheral arterial disease. *Heart (British Cardiac Society), 100*(5), 414–423. doi:10.1136/heartjnl-2013-304082.
73. Wennberg, P. W. (2013). Approach to the patient with peripheral arterial disease. *Circulation, 128*(20), 2241–2250. doi:10.1161/CIRCULATIONAHA.113.000502.
74. Tattersall, M. C., Johnson, H. M., & Mason, P. J. (2013). Contemporary and optimal medical management of peripheral arterial disease. *Surgical Clinics of North America, 93*(4), 761–778, vii. doi:10.1016/j.suc.2013.04.009.
75. Szabó, G. V., Kövesd, Z., Cserepes, J., et al. (2013). Peripheral blood-derived autologous stem cell therapy for the treatment of patients with late-stage peripheral artery disease—Results of the short- and long-term follow-up. *Cytotherapy, 15*(10), 1245–1252. doi:10.1016/j.jcyt.2013.05.017.
76. Government of Canada. (2015). *Heart disease—Heart health.* Retrieved from http://healthycanadians.gc.ca/diseases-conditions-maladies-affections/disease-maladie/heart-disease-eng.php.
77. Jhamnani, S., Patel, D., Heimlich, L., et al. (2015). Meta-analysis of the effects of lifestyle modifications on coronary and carotid atherosclerotic burden. *American Journal of Cardiology, 115*(2), 268–375. doi:10.1016/j.amjcard.2014.10.035.
78. Expert Panel on Detection, Evaluation, and Treatment of High Blood Cholesterol in Adults. (2001). Executive summary of the third report of the National Cholesterol Education Program (NCEP) Expert Panel on Detection, Evaluation, and Treatment of High Blood Cholesterol in Adults (Adult Treatment Panel III). *Journal of the American Medical Association, 285*(19), 2486–2497. doi:10.1001/jama.285.19.2486.
79. Anderson, T. J., Grégoire, J., Pearson, G. J., et al. (2016). 2016 Canadian Cardiovascular Society guidelines for the management of dyslipidemia for the prevention of cardiovascular disease in the adult. *Canadian Journal of Cardiology, 32*(11), 1263–1282. doi:10.1016/j.cjca.2016.07.510.
80. Feig, J. E., Hewing, B., Smith, J. D., et al. (2014). High-density lipoprotein and atherosclerosis regression: Evidence from preclinical and clinical studies. *Circulation Research, 114*(1), 205–213. doi:10.1161/CIRCRESAHA.114.300760.
81. Rosenson, R. S., Brewer, H. B., Jr., Ansell, B., et al. (2013). Translation of high-density lipoprotein function into clinical practice: Current prospects and future challenges. *Circulation, 128*(11), 1256–1267. doi:10.1161/CIRCULATIONAHA.113.000962.
82. Messner, B., & Bernhard, D. (2014). Smoking and cardiovascular disease: Mechanisms of endothelial dysfunction and early atherogenesis. *Arteriosclerosis, Thrombosis, and Vascular Biology, 34*(3), 509–515. doi:10.1161/ATVBAHA.113.300156.
83. Bornfeldt, K. E. (2014). 2013 Russell Ross Memorial Lecture in vascular biology: Cellular and molecular mechanisms of diabetes mellitus-accelerated atherosclerosis. *Arteriosclerosis, Thrombosis, and Vascular Biology, 34*(4), 705–714. doi:10.1161/ATVBAHA.113.301928.
84. Rao, D. P., Dai, S., Lagacé, C., et al. (2014). Metabolic syndrome and chronic disease. *Chronic Diseases and Injuries in Canada, 34*(1). Retrieved from http://www.phac-aspc.gc.ca/publicat/hpcdp-pspmc/34-1/ar-06-eng.php.
85. Bastien, M., Poirier, P., Lemieux, I., et al. (2014). Overview of epidemiology and contribution of obesity to cardiovascular disease. *Progress in Cardiovascular Diseases, 56*(4), 369–381. doi:10.1016/j.pcad.2013.10.016.
86. Ades, P. A., & Savage, P. D. (2014). Potential benefits of weight loss in coronary heart disease. *Progress in Cardiovascular Diseases, 56*(4), 448–456. doi:10.1016/j.pcad.2013.09.009.
87. Tschoner, A., Sturm, W., Gelsinger, C., et al. (2013). Long-term effects of weight loss after bariatric surgery on functional and structural markers of atherosclerosis. *Obesity, 21*(10), 1960–1965. doi:10.1002/oby.20357.
88. Goff, D. C., Jr., Lloyd-Jones, D. M., Bennett, G., et al. (2014). 2013 ACC/AHA guideline on the assessment of cardiovascular risk: A report of the American College of Cardiology/American Heart Association Task Force on Practice Guidelines. *Journal of the American College of Cardiology, 63*(25, Pt. B), 3026. doi:10.1016/j.jacc.2013.11.005.
89. The Emerging Risk Factors Collaboration. (2012). C-reactive protein, fibrinogen, and cardiovascular disease prediction. *New England Journal of Medicine, 367*(14), 1310–1320. doi:10.1056/NEJMoa1107477.
90. Coxib and traditional NSAID Trialists' (CNT) Collaboration. (2013). Vascular and upper gastrointestinal effects of non-steroidal anti-inflammatory drugs: Meta-analyses of

individual participant data from randomised trials. *Lancet*, *382*(9894), 769. doi:10.1016/S0140-6736(13)60900-9.

91. Van de Voorde, J., Pauwels, B., Boydens, C., et al. (2013). Adipocytokines in relation to cardiovascular disease. *Metabolism: Clinical and Experimental*, *62*(11), 1513–1521. doi:10.1016/j.metabol.2013.06.004.
92. Yanai, H., & Hirowatari, Y. (2013). Serum adiponectin levels are significantly associated with favorable metabolic parameters and elevation of atherosclerotic markers. *International Journal of Cardiology*, *167*(6), 3065–3066. doi:10.1016/j.ijcard.2012.11.079.
93. Ntaios, G., Gatselis, N. K., Makaritsis, K., et al. (2013). Adipokines as mediators of endothelial function and atherosclerosis. *Atherosclerosis*, *227*(2), 216–221. doi:10.1016/j.atherosclerosis.2012.12.029.
94. Adar, S. D., Sheppard, L., Vedal, S., et al. (2013). Fine particulate air pollution and the progression of carotid intima-medial thickness: A prospective cohort study from the multi-ethnic study of atherosclerosis and air pollution. *PLoS Medicine*, *10*(4), e1001430. doi:10.1371/journal.pmed.1001430.
95. Thomsen, M., & Nordestgaard, B. G. (2014). Myocardial infarction and ischemic heart disease in overweight and obesity with and without metabolic syndrome. *Journal of the American Medical Association Internal Medicine*, *174*(1), 15–22. doi:10.1001/jamainternmed.2013.
96. Zuchi, C., Tritto, I., & Ambrosio, G. (2013). Angina pectoris in women: Focus on microvascular disease. *International Journal of Cardiology*, *163*(2), 132–140. doi:10.1016/j.ijcard.2012.07.001.
97. Moukarbel, G. V., & Weinrauch, L. A. (2012). Disruption of coronary vasomotor function: The coronary spasm syndrome. *Cardiovascular Therapeutics*, *30*(2), e66–e73. doi:10.1111/j.1755-5922.2010.00235.x.
98. Seo, S. M., Kim, P. J., Shin, D. I., et al. (2013). Persistent coronary artery spasm documented by follow-up coronary angiography in patients with symptomatic remission of variant angina. *Heart and Vessels*, *28*(3), 301–307. doi:10.1007/s00380-012-0249-2.
99. Chen, H., Zhang, L., Zhang, M., et al. (2013). Relationship of depression, stress and endothelial function in stable angina patients. *Physiology and Behavior*, *118*, 152–158. doi:10.1016/j.physbeh.2013.05.024.
100. Paine, N. J., Bosch, J. A., & Van Zanten, J. J. (2012). Inflammation and vascular responses to acute mental stress: Implications for the triggering of myocardial infarction. *Current Pharmaceutical Design*, *18*(11), 1494–1501. doi:10.2174/138161212799504713.
101. Conti, C. R., Bavry, A. A., & Petersen, J. W. (2012). Silent ischemia: Clinical relevance. *Journal of the American College of Cardiology*, *59*(5), 435–441. doi:10.1016/j.jacc.2011.07.050.
102. Fihn, S. D., Gardin, J. M., Abrams, J., et al. (2012). ACCF/AHA/ACP/AATS/PCNA/SCAI/STS guideline for the diagnosis and management of patients with stable ischemic heart disease: A report of the American College of Cardiology Foundation/American Heart Association Task Force on Practice Guidelines, and the American College of Physicians, American Association for Thoracic Surgery, Preventive Cardiovascular Nurses Association, Society for Cardiovascular Angiography and Interventions, and Society of Thoracic Surgeons. *Circulation*, *126*, e354–e471. doi:10.1161/CIR.0b013e318277d6a0.
103. Taylor, F., Huffman, M. D., Macedo, A. F., et al. (2013). Statins for the primary prevention of cardiovascular disease. *Cochrane Database of Systematic Reviews*, (1), CD004816. doi:10.1002/14651858.
104. Wilson, J. F. (2014). In the clinic. Stable ischemic heart disease. *Annals of Internal Medicine*, *160*(1), ITC1-1-16, quiz ITC1-16. doi:10.7326/0003-4819-160-1-201401070-01001.
105. Banon, D., Filion, K. B., Budiovsky, T., et al. (2014). The usefulness of ranolazine for the treatment of refractory chronic stable angina pectoris as determined from a systematic review of randomized controlled trials. *American Journal of Cardiology*, *113*(6), 1075–1082. doi:10.7326/0003-4819-160-1-201401070-01001.
106. Braunwald, E., & Morrow, D. A. (2013). Unstable angina: Is it time for a requiem? *Circulation*, *127*(24), 2452–2457. doi:10.1161/CIRCULATIONAHA.113.001258.
107. 2012 Writing Committee Members, Jneid, H., Anderson, J. L., et al. (2012). 2012 ACCF/AHA focused update of the guideline for the management of patients with unstable angina/non-ST-elevation myocardial infarction (updating the 2007 guideline and replacing the 2011 focused update): A report of the American College of Cardiology Foundation/American Heart Association Task Force on Practice Guidelines. *Circulation*, *126*(7), 875–910. doi:10.1161/CIR.0b013e318256f1e0.
108. Lin, L., & Knowlton, A. A. (2014). Innate immunity and cardiomyocytes in ischemic heart disease. *Life Sciences*, *100*(1), 1–8. doi:10.1016/j.lfs.2014.01.062.
109. Reiter, R., Henry, T. D., & Traverse, J. H. (2013). Preinfarction angina reduces infarct size in ST-elevation myocardial infarction treated with percutaneous coronary intervention. *Circulation. Cardiovascular Interventions*, *6*(1), 52–58. doi:10.1161/CIRCINTERVENTIONS.112.973164.
110. Schevchuck, A., & Laskey, W. K. (2013). Ischemic conditioning as an adjunct to percutaneous coronary intervention. *Circulation. Cardiovascular Interventions*, *6*(4), 484–492. doi:10.1161/CIRCINTERVENTIONS.113.000146.
111. Shah, B. N., Khattar, R. S., & Senior, R. (2013). The hibernating myocardium: Current concepts, diagnostic dilemmas, and clinical challenges in the post-STICH era. *European Heart Journal*, *34*(18), 1323–1336. doi:10.1093/eurheartj/eht018.
112. Ozaki, Y., Imanishi, T., Tanimoto, T., et al. (2014). Effect of direct renin inhibitor on left ventricular remodeling in patients with primary acute myocardial infarction. *International Heart Journal*, *55*(1), 17–21. doi:10.1536/ihj.13-212.
113. Cabello, J. B., Buris, A., Emparanza, J. I., et al. (2013). Oxygen therapy for acute myocardial infarction. *Cochrane Database of Systematic Reviews*, (8), CD007160. doi:10.1002/14651858.CD007160.pub2.
114. O'Gara, P. T., Kushner, F. G., Ascheim, D. D., et al. (2013). 2013 ACCF/AHA guideline for the management of ST-elevation myocardial infarction: A report of the American College of Cardiology Foundation/American Heart Association Task Force on Practice Guidelines. *Circulation*, *127*, e362–e425. doi:10.1161/CIR.0b013e3182742cf6.
115. Shammas, N. W., Padaria, R. F., & Coyne, E. P. (2013). Pericarditis, myocarditis, and other cardiomyopathies. *Primary Care*, *40*(1), 213–236. doi:10.1016/j.pop.2012.11.009.
116. Cantarini, L., Imazio, M., Brizi, M. G., et al. (2013). Role of autoimmunity and autoinflammation in the pathogenesis of idiopathic recurrent pericarditis. *Clinical Reviews in Allergy and Immunology*, *44*(1), 6–13. doi:10.1007/s12016-010-8219-x.
117. Kopcinovic, L. M., & Culej, J. (2014). Pleural, peritoneal and pericardial effusions—A biochemical approach. *Biochemical Medicine*, *24*(1), 123–237. doi:10.11613/BM.2014.014.
118. Figueras, J., Barrabés, J. A., Lidón, R. M., et al. (2014). Predictors of moderate-to-severe pericardial effusion, cardiac tamponade, and electromechanical dissociation in patients with ST-elevation myocardial infarction. *American Journal of Cardiology*, *113*(8), 1291–1296. doi:10.1016/j.amjcard.2013.11.071.
119. Imazio, M., & Adler, Y. (2013). Management of pericardial effusion. *European Heart Journal*, *34*(16), 1186–1197. doi:10.1093/eurheartj/ehs372.
120. Smith, K. M., & Squiers, J. (2013). Hypertrophic cardiomyopathy: An overview. *Critical Care Nursing Clinics of North America*, *25*(2), 263–272. doi:10.1016/j.ccell.2013.02.011.
121. Yilmaz, A., & Sechtem, U. (2014). Diagnostic approach and differential diagnosis in patients with hypertrophied left ventricles. *Heart (British Cardiac Society)*, *100*(8), 662–671. doi:10.1136/heartjnl-2011-301528.
122. Nishimura, R. A., Otto, C. M., Bonow, R. O., et al. (2014). 2014 AHA/ACC guideline for the management of patients with valvular heart disease: Executive summary: A report of the American College of Cardiology/American Heart Association Task Force on Practice Guidelines. *Journal of the American College of Cardiology*, *63*(22), 2438–2488. doi:10.1016/j.jacc.2014.02.537.
123. Brinkley, D. M., & Gelfand, E. V. (2013). Valvular heart disease: Classic teaching and emerging paradigms. *American Journal of Medicine*, *126*(12), 1035–1042. doi:10.1016/j.amjmed.2013.05.022.
124. Holmes, D. R., Jr., Brennan, J. M., Rumsfield, J. S., et al. (2015). Clinical outcomes at 1 year following transcatheter aortic valve replacement. *Journal of the American Medical Association*, *313*(10), 1019–1028. doi:10.1001/jama.2015.1474.
125. O'Gara, P. T., Calhoon, J. H., Moon, M. R., et al. (2014). Transcatheter therapies for mitral regurgitation: A professional society overview from the American College of Cardiology, the American Association for Thoracic Surgery, Society for Cardiovascular Angiography and Interventions Foundation, and the Society of Thoracic Surgeons. *Journal of the American College of Cardiology*, *63*(8), 840–852. doi:10.1016/j.jacc.2013.11.014.
126. Burke, R. J., & Chang, C. (2014). Diagnostic criteria of acute rheumatic fever. *Autoimmunity Reviews*, *13*(4–5), 503–507. doi:10.1016/j.autrev.2014.01.036.
127. Gordon, J., Kirlew, M., Schreiber, Y., et al. (2015). Acute rheumatic fever in First Nations communities in northwestern Ontario: Social determinants of health "bite the heart". *Canadian Family Physician*, *61*(10), 881–886.
128. Nitsche-Schmitz, D. P., & Chhatwal, G. S. (2013). Host-pathogen interactions in streptococcal immune sequelae. *Current Topics in Microbiology and Immunology*, *368*, 155–171. doi:10.1007/82_2012_296.
129. Nussinovitch, U., & Shoenfeld, Y. (2013). The clinical and diagnostic significance of anti-myosin autoantibodies in cardiac disease. *Clinical Reviews in Allergy and Immunology*, *44*(1), 98–108. doi:10.1007/s12016-010-8229-8.
130. Zühlke, L., Beaton, A., Engel, M. A., et al. (2017). Group A streptococcus, acute rheumatic fever and rheumatic heart disease: Epidemiology and clinical considerations. *Current Treatment Options in Cardiovascular Medicine*, *19*(2), 15.
131. Roberts, K., Colquhoun, S., Steer, A., et al. (2013). Screening for rheumatic heart disease: Current approaches and controversies. *Nature Reviews. Cardiology*, *10*(1), 49–58. doi:10.1038/nrcardio.2012.157.
132. Hoen, B., & Duval, X. (2013). Clinical practice. Infective endocarditis. *New England Journal of Medicine*, *368*(15), 1425–1433. doi:10.1056/NEJMcp1206782.
133. Ferro, J. M., & Fonseca, A. C. (2014). Infective endocarditis. *Handbook of Clinical Neurology*, *119*, 75–91. doi:10.1016/B978-0-7020-4086-3.00007-2.
134. Fitch, K. V., Srinivasa, S., Abbara, S., et al. (2013). Noncalcified coronary atherosclerotic plaque and immune activation in HIV-infected women. *Journal of Infectious Diseases*, *208*(11), 1737–1746. doi:10.1093/infdis/jit508.
135. Gupta, M., Miller, C. J., Baker, J. V., et al. (2013). Biomarkers and electrocardiographic evidence of myocardial ischemia in patients with human immunodeficiency virus infection. *American Journal of Cardiology*, *111*(5), 760–764. doi:10.1016/j.amjcard.2012.11.032.
136. Moyers, B. S., Secemsky, E. A., Vittinghoff, E., et al. (2014). Effect of left ventricular dysfunction and viral load on risk of sudden cardiac death in patients with human immunodeficiency virus. *American Journal of Cardiology*, *113*(7), 1260–1265. doi:10.1016/j.amjcard.2013.12.036.
137. Oka, T., Akazawa, H., Naito, A. T., et al. (2014). Angiogenesis and cardiac hypertrophy:

Maintenance of cardiac function and causative roles in heart failure. *Circulation Research, 114*(3), 565–571. doi:10.1161/CIRCRESAHA.114.300507.
138. Li, A. H., Liu, P. P., Villarreal, F. J., et al. (2014). Dynamic changes in myocardial matrix and relevance to disease: Translational perspectives. *Circulation Research, 114*(5), 916–927. doi:10.1161/CIRCRESAHA.114.302819.
139. D'Alessandro, R., Masarone, D., Buono, A., et al. (2013). Natriuretic peptides: Molecular biology, pathophysiology and clinical implications for the cardiologist. *Future Cardiology, 9*(4), 519–534. doi:10.2217/fca.13.32.
140. Turer, A. T. (2013). Using metabolomics to assess myocardial metabolism and energetics in heart failure. *Journal of Molecular and Cellular Cardiology, 55*, 12–18. doi:10.1016/j.yjmcc.2012.08.025.
141. Dominic, E. A., Ramezani, A., Anker, S. D., et al. (2014). Mitochondrial cytopathies and cardiovascular disease. *Heart (British Cardiac Society), 100*(8), 611–618. doi:10.1136/heartjnl-2013-304657.
142. Reddy, P., & Samson, R. (2013). Clinical utility of natriuretic peptides in left ventricular failure. *Southern Medical Journal, 106*(2), 182–187. doi:10.1097/SMJ.0b013e3182804b66.
143. Charisopoulou, D., Leaver, N., & Banner, N. R. (2014). Milrinone in advanced heart failure: Dose and therapeutic monitor outside intensive care unit. *Angiology, 65*(4), 343–349. doi:10.1177/0003319713485808.
144. Writing Committee Members, Yancy, C. W., Jessup, M., et al. (2013). 2013 ACCF/AHA guideline for the management of heart failure: A report of the American College of Cardiology Foundation/American Heart Association Task Force on practice guidelines. *Circulation, 128*(16), e240–e327. doi:10.1161/CIR.0b013e31829e8776.
145. Vizzardi, E., Nodari, S., Caretta, G., et al. (2014). Effects of spironolactone on long-term mortality and morbidity in patients with heart failure and mild or no symptoms. *American Journal of the Medical Sciences, 347*(4), 271–276. doi:10.1097/MAJ.0b013e31829dd6b1.
146. Kosmala, W., & Marwick, T. H. (2014). Meta-analysis of effects of optimization of cardiac resynchronization therapy on left ventricular function, exercise capacity, and quality of life in patients with heart failure. *American Journal of Cardiology, 113*(6), 988–994. doi:10.1016/j.amjcard.2013.12.006.
147. Braunwald, E. (2015). The war against heart failure: The Lancet lecture. *Lancet, 385*(9970), 812–824. doi:10.1016/S0140-6736(14)61889-4.
148. Lam, C. S., Donal, E., Kraigher-Krainer, E., et al. (2011). Epidemiology and clinical course of heart failure with preserved ejection fraction. *European Journal of Heart Failure, 13*(1), 18–28.
149. Wan, S. H., Vogel, M. W., & Chen, H. H. (2014). Pre-clinical diastolic dysfunction. *Journal of the American College of Cardiology, 63*(5), 407–416. doi:10.1016/j.jacc.2013.10.063.
150. Guazzi, M. (2014). Pulmonary hypertension in heart failure preserved ejection fraction: Prevalence, pathophysiology, and clinical perspectives. *Circulation. Heart Failure, 7*(2), 367–377. doi:10.1161/CIRCHEARTFAILURE.113.000823.
151. Burke, M. A., Katz, D. H., Beussink, L., et al. (2014). Prognostic importance of pathophysiologic markers in patients with heart failure and preserved ejection fraction. *Circulation. Heart Failure, 7*(2), 288–299. doi:10.1161/CIRCHEARTFAILURE.113.000854.
152. Penicka, M., Vanderheyden, M., & Bartunek, J. (2014). Diagnosis of heart failure with preserved ejection fraction: Role of clinical Doppler echocardiography. *Heart (British Cardiac Society), 100*(1), 68–76. doi:10.1136/heartjnl-2011-301321.
153. Liu, G., Zheng, X. X., Xu, Y. L., et al. (2014). Meta-analysis of the effect of statins on mortality in patients with preserved ejection fraction. *American Journal of Cardiology, 113*(7), 1198–1204. doi:10.1016/j.amjcard.2013.12.023.
154. Athyros, V. G., Katsiki, N., & Karagiannis, A. (2014). Treating heart failure with preserved ejection fraction: Statins could make the difference. *Angiology, 65*(4), 328–329. doi:10.1177/0003319713507629.
155. Quiroz, R., Doros, G., Shaw, P., et al. (2014). Comparison of characteristics and outcomes of patients with heart failure preserved ejection fraction versus reduced left ventricular ejection fraction in an urban cohort. *American Journal of Cardiology, 113*(4), 691–696. doi:10.1016/j.amjcard.2013.11.014.
156. Ashruf, J. F., Bruining, H. A., & Ince, C. (2013). New insights into the pathophysiology of cardiogenic shock: The role of the microcirculation. *Current Opinion in Critical Care, 19*(5), 381–386. doi:10.1097/MCC.0b013e328364d7c8.
157. Tharmaratnam, D., Nolan, J., & Jain, A. (2013). Management of cardiogenic shock complicating acute coronary syndromes. *Heart (British Cardiac Society), 99*(21), 1614–1623. doi:10.1136/heartjnl-2012-302028.
158. Gann, D. S., & Drucker, W. R. (2013). Hemorrhagic shock. *Journal of Trauma and Acute Care Surgery, 75*(5), 888–895. doi:10.1097/TA.0b013e3182a686ed.
159. Summers, R. L., Baker, S. D., Sterling, S. A., et al. (2013). Characterization of the spectrum of hemodynamic profiles in trauma patients with acute neurogenic shock. *Journal of Critical Care, 28*(4), 531.e1–531.e5. doi:10.1016/j.jcrc.2013.02.002.
160. Samant, S. A., Campbell, R. L., & Li, J. T. (2013). Anaphylaxis: Diagnostic criteria and epidemiology. *Allergy and Asthma Proceedings, 34*(2), 115–119. doi:10.2500/aap.2013.34.3630.
161. Sicherer, S. H., & Leung, D. Y. (2014). Advances in allergic skin disease, anaphylaxis, and hypersensitivity reactions to foods, drugs, and insects in 2013. *Journal of Allergy and Clinical Immunology, 133*(2), 324–334. doi:10.1016/j.jaci.2013.11.013.
162. Lieberman, P. L. (2014). Recognition and first-line treatment of anaphylaxis. *American Journal of Medicine, 127*(1, Suppl.), S6–S11. doi:10.1016/j.amjmed.2013.09.008.
163. Levy, M. M., Fink, M. P., Marshall, J. C., et al. (2003). 2001 SCCM/ESICM/ACCP/ATS/SIS International Sepsis Definitions Conference. *Critical Care Medicine, 31*(4), 1250–1256. doi:10.1097/01.CCM.0000050454.01978.3B.
164. Statistics Canada. (2016). *Health at a glance: Deaths involving sepsis in Canada.* Ottawa: Author. Retrieved from http://www.statcan.gc.ca/pub/82-624-x/2016001/article/14308-eng.htm.
165. Stevenson, E. K., Rubenstein, A. R., Radin, G. T., et al. (2014). Two decades of mortality trends among patients with severe sepsis: A comparative meta-analysis. *Critical Care Medicine, 42*(3), 625–631. doi:10.1097/CCM.0000000000000026.
166. Angus, D. C., & van der Poll, T. (2013). Severe sepsis and septic shock. *New England Journal of Medicine, 369*(9), 840–851. doi:10.1056/NEJMra1208623.
167. King, E. G., Bauza, G. J., Mella, J. R., et al. (2014). Pathophysiologic mechanisms in septic shock. *Laboratory Investigation, 94*(1), 4–12. doi:10.1038/labinvest.2013.110.
168. Bosmann, M., & Ward, P. A. (2013). The inflammatory response in sepsis. *Trends in Immunology, 34*(3), 129–136. doi:10.1016/j.it.2012.09.004.
169. Landesberg, G., Jaffe, A. S., Gilon, D., et al. (2014). Troponin elevation in severe sepsis and septic shock: The role of left ventricular diastolic dysfunction and right ventricular dilatation. *Critical Care Medicine, 42*(4), 790–800. doi:10.1097/CCM.0000000000000107.
170. Corona, A., & De Iaco, M. (2014). Procalcitonin or C-reactive protein: That is the question? *Critical Care Medicine, 42*(4), e310–e311. doi:10.1097/CCM.0000000000000116.
171. Dellinger, R. P., Levy, M. M., Rhodes, A., et al. (2013). Surviving Sepsis Campaign: International guidelines for management of severe sepsis and septic shock: 2012. *Critical Care Medicine, 41*(2), 580–637. doi:10.1097/CCM.0b013e31827e83af.
172. Huet, O., & Chin-Dusting, J. P. (2014). Septic shock: Desperately seeking treatment. *Clinical Science (London, England: 1979), 126*(1), 31–39. doi:10.1042/CS20120668.
173. Sauaia, A., Moore, E. E., Johnson, J. L., et al. (2014). Temporal trends of postinjury multiple-organ failure: Still resource intensive, morbid, and lethal. *Journal of Trauma and Acute Care Surgery, 76*(3), 582–592, discussion 592–593. doi:10.1097/TA.0000000000000147.
174. Levi, M., Schultz, M., & van der Poll, T. (2013). Sepsis and thrombosis. *Seminars in Thrombosis and Hemostasis, 39*(5), 559–566. doi:10.1055/s-0033-1343894.
175. Bosmann, M., & Ward, P. A. (2013). The inflammatory response in sepsis. *Trends in Immunology, 34*(3), 129–136. doi:10.1016/j.it.2012.09.004.

25

Alterations of Cardiovascular Function in Children

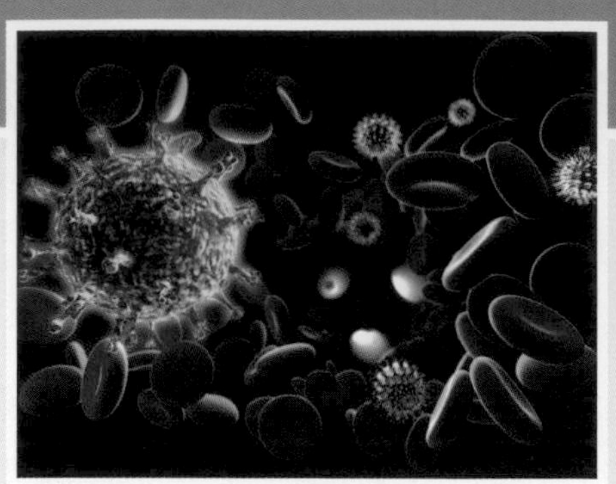

Nancy Pike, Nancy L. McDaniel, and Mohamed El-Hussein

EVOLVE WEBSITE

http://evolve.elsevier.com/Canada/Huether/pathophysiology
Student Review Questions
Key Points
Case Studies
Animations
Quick Check Answers

CHAPTER OUTLINE

Congenital Heart Disease, 662
- Obstructive Defects, 664
- Defects With Increased Pulmonary Blood Flow, 667
- Defects With Decreased Pulmonary Blood Flow, 668
- Mixing Defects, 670
- Heart Failure, 672

Acquired Cardiovascular Disorders, 673
- Kawasaki Disease, 673
- Systemic Hypertension, 674

Cardiovascular disorders in children are classified as congenital or acquired. Congenital heart disease is the most common. The diagnosis and management of congenital heart disease continue to improve with the use of fetal echocardiography and early interventional catheterization or surgical repair. Acquired heart disease in children continues to present challenges to the practitioner. Although guidelines for diagnosing acquired diseases are available, work is still needed in developing standards of treatment and long-term follow-up protocols.

CONGENITAL HEART DISEASE

The incidence of **congenital heart disease (CHD)** varies from 4 to 8 per 1 000 live births and is the major cause of death in the first year of life other than prematurity. Several environmental and genetic risk factors are associated with the incidence of different types of CHD. Among the environmental risk factors are (1) maternal conditions, such as intrauterine viral infections (especially rubella), diabetes mellitus, phenylketonuria, alcoholism, hypercalcemia, medications (e.g., thalidomide, phenytoin [Dilantin]), and complications of advanced maternal age; (2) antepartal bleeding; and (3) prematurity (Table 25-1).[1,2]

Genetic risk factors also have been implicated in the incidence of CHD, although the mechanism of causation is often unknown (Table 25-2). The incidence of CHD is three to four times higher in siblings of affected children, and chromosomal defects account for about 6% of all cases of CHD. Down syndrome, trisomies 13 and 18, Turner's syndrome, and cri du chat syndrome (chromosome 5p deletion syndrome) have been associated with a relatively high incidence of heart defects. Only a small percentage of cases of CHD are clearly linked solely to genetic or environmental factors. There also are multiple hereditary and nonhereditary syndromes that are associated with cardiovascular abnormalities in children.[2] However, the cause of most defects is multifactorial.[1,2]

According to the Canadian Congenital Heart Alliance (CCHA), CHD is the leading birth defect around the world. In Canada, 1 in 80 to 100 Canadian children are born with CHD. Sixty years ago only about 20% of children survived to adulthood; that number has since increased to about 90%, resulting in a growing population of young adults who require lifelong cardiac care.[3]

There are approximately 257 000 Canadians living with CHD; two-thirds are adults and at least half face the prospect of complications, multiple surgeries, and/or premature or sudden death. The limited availability of resources for the care of adult CHD patients means that CHD patients experience excessive wait times for clinical visits and surgical intervention compared with other cardiac patients. The result for CHD patients can be increased anxiety, added risk, and sometimes death.[3]

A congenital heart defect can be categorized according to (1) whether the defect causes cyanosis, (2) whether the defect causes increased or decreased blood flow into the pulmonary circulation, and (3) whether the defect causes obstruction of blood flow from the ventricles (Figure 25-1). The normal movement of blood through the right side of the heart and into the pulmonary system is separate from the blood flow through the left side of the heart into the systemic circulation (Figure 25-2, *A*). Abnormal movement from one side of the heart to the other is termed a **shunt**. Shunting of blood flow from the left heart into the right heart is called a **left-to-right shunt** and occurs in conditions such as atrial septal defect (ASD) and ventricular septal defect (Figure 25-2, *B*). This left-to-right shunt increases blood flow into the pulmonary circulation. Because blood continues to flow through the lungs before passing into the systemic circulation, there is no decrease in tissue oxygenation or cyanosis. Thus defects that cause left-to-right shunt are termed **acyanotic heart defects**. Other types of acyanotic heart defects obstruct blood flow from the ventricles but do not cause shunting. **Cyanotic heart defects** frequently cause shunting of blood from the right side of the heart directly into the left side of the heart (**right-to-left shunt**). This type of shunt decreases blood flow through the pulmonary system, causing less than normal oxygen delivery to the tissues and resultant cyanosis (see Chapter 27). Tetralogy of Fallot (TOF) occurs in 5 to 10% of all CHD and is the most common cyanotic heart defect.[2] In this condition, narrowing of the pulmonary outflow tract increases right heart pressures, thus forcing blood through a defect in the ventricular septum into the left heart (Figure 25-2, *C*). **Cyanosis**, a bluish discoloration of the skin indicating that tissues are not receiving normal amounts of oxygen, also can be caused by other types of heart defects that result in the mixing of venous and arterial blood that enter the systemic circulation.

Most congenital heart defects are named to describe the underlying defect (e.g., valvular abnormalities; abnormal openings in the septa, including persistence of the foramen ovale; continued patency of the ductus arteriosus; and malformation or abnormal placement of the great vessels). Descriptions of the most common defects follow.

TABLE 25-1 Maternal Conditions and Environmental Exposures and the Associated Congenital Heart Defects

Cause	Type of Congenital Heart Defect
Infection	
Intrauterine	Patent ductus arteriosus (PDA), pulmonary stenosis (PS), coarctation of the aorta (COA)
Systemic viral	PDA, PS, COA
Rubella	PDA, PS, COA
Coxsackie B5	Endocardial fibroelastosis
Radiation	Specific cardiovascular effect not known
Metabolic Disorders	
Diabetes	Ventricular septal defect (VSD), cardiomegaly, transposition of the great vessels
Phenylketonuria	COA, PDA
Hypercalcemia	Supravalvular aortic stenosis, PS; aortic hyperplasia
Medications	
Thalidomide (Thalomid)	No specific lesion
Dextroamphetamine (Dexedrine)	One case of reported transposition
Alcohol	Tetralogy of Fallot (TOF), atrial septal defect (ASD), VSD
Peripheral Conditions	
Increased maternal age	VSD, TOF (relationship unclear)
Antepartal bleeding	Various defects (relationship unclear)
Prematurity	PDA, VSD
High altitude	PDA, ASD (increased incidence)

TABLE 25-2 Congenital Heart Disease in Selected Fetal Chromosomal Aberrations

Conditions	Incidence of CHD (%)	Common Defects (in Decreasing Order of Frequency)
Chromosome 5p deletion syndrome (cri du chat syndrome)	25	VSD, PDA, ASD
Trisomy 13 syndrome	90	VSD, PDA, dextrocardia
Trisomy 18 syndrome	99	VSD, PDA, PS
Trisomy 21 (Down syndrome)	50	AVSD, VSD
Turner's syndrome (XO)	35	COA, AS, ASD
Klinefelter's variant (XXXXY)	15	PDA, ASD

AS, aortic stenosis; *ASD*, atrial septal defect; *AVSD*, atrioventricular septal defect; *CHD*, congenital heart disease; *COA*, coarctation of the aorta; *PDA*, patent ductus arteriosus; *PS*, pulmonary stenosis; *VSD*, ventricular septal defect.

From Park, M.K. (2014). *Pediatric cardiology for practitioners* (6th ed.). St. Louis: Mosby.

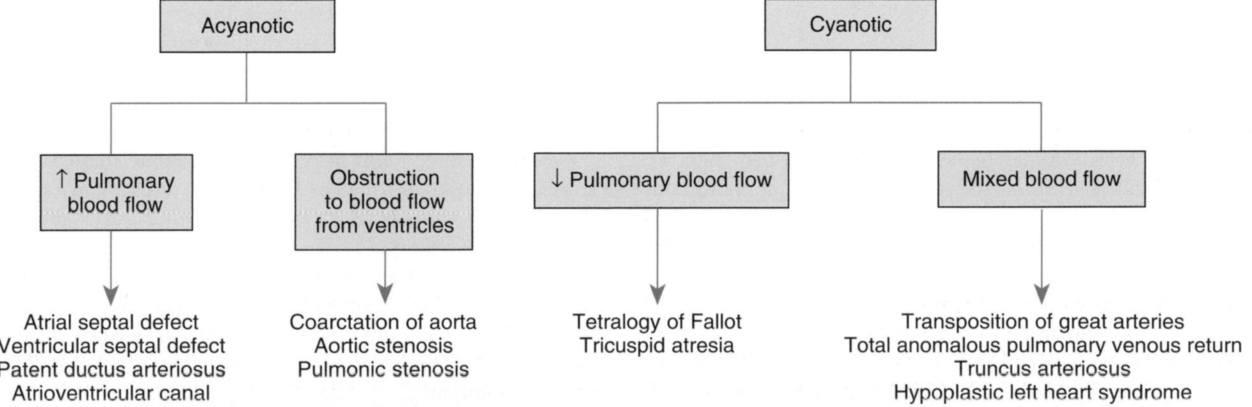

FIGURE 25-1 Comparison of Acyanotic–Cyanotic and Hemodynamic Classification Systems of Congenital Heart Disease. (From Hockenberry, M.J., & Wilson, D. [2015]. *Wong's nursing care of infants and children* [10th ed.]. St. Louis: Mosby.)

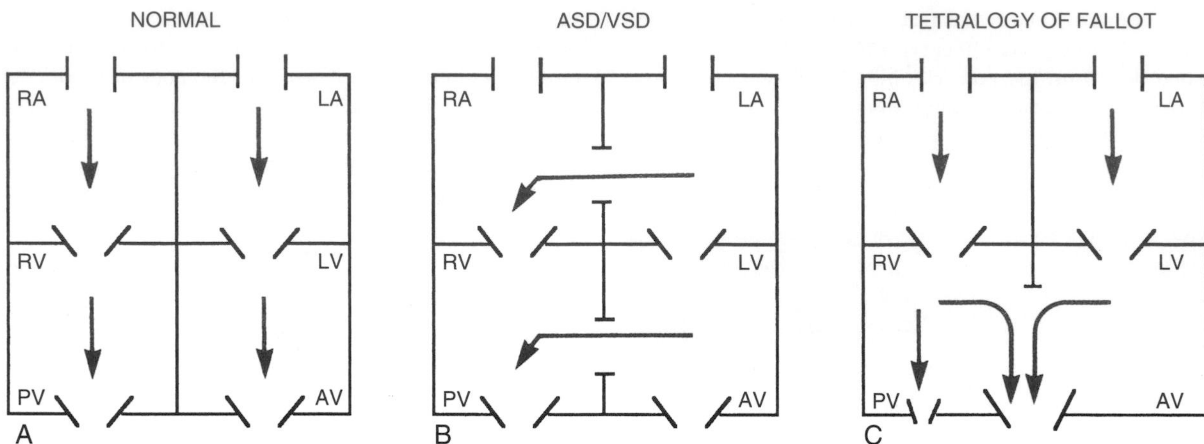

FIGURE 25-2 Shunting of Blood in Congenital Heart Disease. A, Normal. **B,** Acyanotic defect. **C,** Cyanotic defect. *ASD*, atrial septal defect; *AV*, aortic valve; *LA*, left atrium; *LV*, left ventricle; *PV*, pulmonic valve; *RA*, right atrium; *RV*, right ventricle; *VSD*, ventricular septal defect. (From Hockenberry, M.J., & Wilson, D. [2015]. *Wong's nursing care of infants and children* [10th ed.]. St. Louis: Mosby.)

Obstructive Defects

Coarctation of the Aorta

PATHOPHYSIOLOGY **Coarctation of the aorta (COA)** is an abnormal localized narrowing of the aorta just proximal to the insertion of the ductus arteriosus. Before birth, the ductus arteriosus bypasses this obstruction and allows for blood to flow from the pulmonary artery into the distal aorta. However, once the ductus functionally closes within 15 hours after birth, blood flow to the lower extremities is then restricted by the coarctation. Clinically, there is increased blood pressure proximal to the defect (head and upper extremities, right greater than left) and decreased blood pressure distal to the obstruction (torso and lower extremities) (Figure 25-3).

CLINICAL MANIFESTATIONS The location and severity of the COA determine whether an infant will become symptomatic after the ductus arteriosus closes. If the COA is severe, infants will present with low cardiac output, poor tissue perfusion, acidosis, and hypotension. Physical examination of the infant will reveal weak or absent femoral pulses. Some infants with COA will remain asymptomatic after the closure of the ductus arteriosus. As they age, children with undiagnosed COA will present with unexplained upper extremity hypertension. Children may complain of leg pain or cramping with exercise. Although rare, they also may experience dizziness, headaches, fainting, or epistaxis from hypertension.[1,2]

EVALUATION AND TREATMENT Physical examination and measurement of upper and lower extremity blood pressures will often suggest the diagnosis. Echocardiography, magnetic resonance imaging (MRI), and cardiac catheterization may be needed to confirm the diagnosis. Initial treatment in the symptomatic newborn consists of continuous intravenous infusion of prostaglandin E_1 to maintain the patency of the ductus arteriosus. Once the symptomatic newborn is stabilized, surgical correction is indicated.[4]

Surgical correction consists of either resection of the narrowed portion of the aorta with an end-to-end anastomosis or enlargement of the constricted section using a graft taken from a portion of the left subclavian artery. Because this defect is outside the heart and pericardium, cardiopulmonary bypass usually is not required and a thoracotomy incision is used. However, coarctation repair may be part of a more complex operation, which might require a sternotomy incision and cardiopulmonary bypass. Postoperative hypertension is treated with intravenous medication, often a short-acting beta-blocker, followed by oral medications, such as an angiotensin-converting enzyme inhibitor. Residual hypertension after repair of COA seems to be related to age and time of repair.

Studies have shown percutaneous balloon angioplasty with or without the use of a stent to be an effective, less invasive option for treating native COA or for reducing residual postoperative coarctation in most children.[1,2,5] Balloon angioplasty of COA as an initial intervention can also be considered. However, in infants younger than 6 months of age, most will experience recoarctation in only a short period of time after primary angioplasty. Other complications include aneurysm formation and blood vessel injury from arterial access. Data exist that support balloon angioplasty as an effective therapy in selected infants older than 6 months of age with a decreased risk for aneurysm formation as compared with younger infants.[5]

Aortic Stenosis

PATHOPHYSIOLOGY **Aortic stenosis (AS)** is a narrowing or stricture of the left ventricular outlet, causing resistance of blood flow from the left ventricle into the aorta (Figure 25-4). The physiological consequence of severe AS is hypertrophy of the left ventricular wall, which eventually leads to increased end-diastolic pressure, resulting in pulmonary venous and pulmonary arterial hypertension. If severe, there may be decreased cardiac output and pulmonary vascular congestion. Left ventricular hypertrophy impedes coronary artery perfusion and may result in subendocardial ischemia and associated papillary muscle dysfunction that cause mitral insufficiency.

There are three types of AS. **Valvular aortic stenosis** occurs as a consequence of malformed or fused cusps, resulting in a unicuspid or bicuspid valve. Valvular AS is a serious defect because (1) the obstruction tends to be progressive; (2) there may be sudden episodes of myocardial ischemia or low cardiac output that, on rare occasions, can result in sudden death in late childhood or adolescence; and (3) surgical repair will not result in a normal valve. This is one of the rare forms of CHD in which strenuous physical activity may be curtailed because of the cardiac condition.[1,2]

Subvalvular aortic stenosis is a stricture caused by a fibrous ring below a normal valve. It can also be caused by a narrowed left ventricular outflow tract in combination with a small aortic valve annulus.

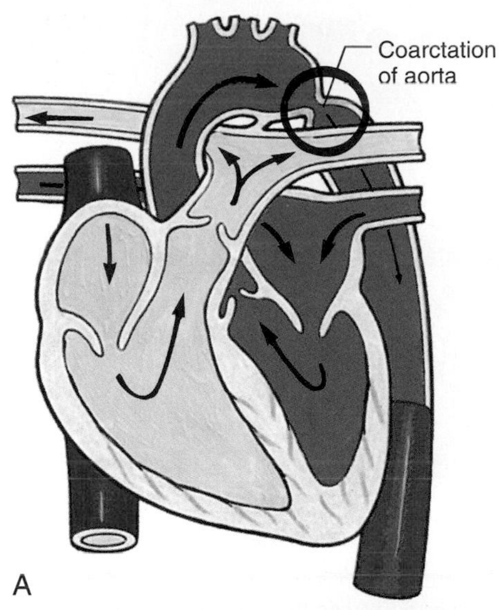

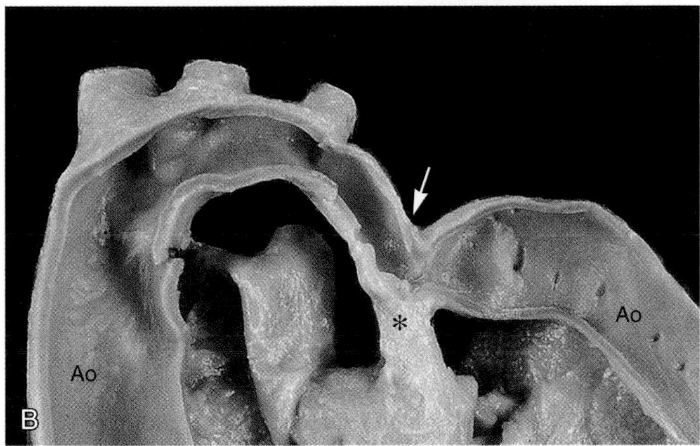

FIGURE 25-3 Postductal and Preductal Coarctation of the Aorta. **A,** Postductal coarctation occurs distal to ("after") the insertion of the closed ductus arteriosus into the aortic arch. Preductal coarctation occurs proximal to ("before") the insertion of the patent ductus arteriosus. The coarctation consists of a flap of tissue that protrudes from the tunica media of the aortic wall. **B,** Coarctation of the aorta with typical indentation of the aortic wall (*arrow*) opposite the ductal arterial ligament (*asterisk*). *Ao,* aorta. (**A,** from Hockenberry, M.J., & Wilson, D. [2013]. *Wong's essentials of pediatric nursing* [9th ed.]. St. Louis: Mosby; **B,** from Damjanov, I., & Linder, J. [Eds.]. [1996]. *Anderson's pathology* [10th ed.]. St. Louis: Mosby.)

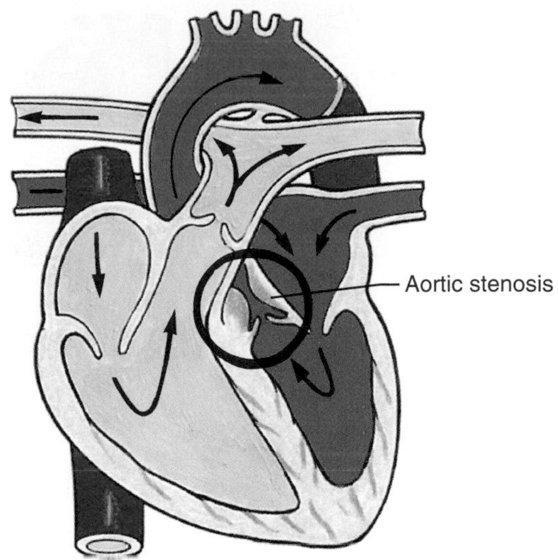

FIGURE 25-4 Aortic Stenosis. Narrowing of the aortic valve causing resistance to blood flow in the left ventricle, decreased cardiac output, left ventricular hypertrophy, and pulmonary congestion. (From Hockenberry, M.J., & Wilson, D. [Eds.]. [2013]. *Wong's essentials of pediatric nursing* [9th ed.]. St. Louis: Mosby.)

Supravalvular aortic stenosis, a narrowing of the aorta just above the valve, occurs infrequently. It can occur as a single defect (familial supravalvular stenosis syndrome) or as a part of Williams syndrome, which also is characterized by unusual elfinlike facial appearance and mental disability.[6]

CLINICAL MANIFESTATIONS Infants with significant AS demonstrate signs of decreased cardiac output with faint pulses, hypotension, tachycardia, and poor feeding. A loud, harsh systolic ejection murmur is expected. Older children also may have complaints of exercise intolerance and, rarely, chest pain. Children are at risk for bacterial endocarditis, although prophylaxis with antibiotics is no longer routinely recommended (see *Health Promotion:* Endocarditis Risk). AS, when severe, also can be complicated by coronary insufficiency, ventricular dysfunction, and, rarely, sudden death.

EVALUATION AND TREATMENT Valvular AS diagnosis is confirmed by echocardiography. Mild to moderate valvular AS does not usually require intervention or restriction of activity. Treatment of severe valvular AS varies, with nonsurgical palliation the initial treatment of choice by many interventional cardiologists. Dilation of the stenotic valve with balloon angioplasty, which is performed in the cardiac catheterization laboratory, still carries a high morbidity and mortality in the critically ill neonate; however, in older infants and children it compares favourably with surgical valvotomy.[5] Balloon angioplasty is, however, associated with the risk for aortic regurgitation (insufficiency). Children undergoing this procedure almost always require surgical intervention at some time to relieve recurrent narrowing or worsening regurgitation.[5]

Surgical treatment for valvular AS depends on the severity of the stenosis, previous interventions, and age of the child. Aortic valve commissurotomy or valvotomy may be used as an early intervention. Aortic valve replacement may be required if the valve is severely dysplastic. The Ross procedure, which involves moving the native pulmonary valve (autograft) into the aortic position and replacing the pulmonary valve with an allograft (cadaver), and coronary artery reimplantation have become an option. The advantage of the Ross procedure over mechanical valve replacement, especially in a young child, is that there is no requirement for long-term anticoagulation therapy; however, the valve may fail with time. Mechanical valve replacement is usually deferred as long as possible to minimize the number of valve replacements related to growth. AS requires lifelong evaluation and treatment. Multiple surgical or catheterization interventions are expected. Mortality for sick infants and young children is higher than that for older children.

Subvalvular aortic stenosis. Surgical correction for subvalvular AS involves incising the constricting fibromuscular ring. If the obstruction results from a narrow left ventricular outflow tract and a small aortic valve annulus, a patch may be required to enlarge the entire left ventricular outflow tract and annulus and replace the aortic valve, an approach known as the Konno procedure. An aortic homograft with a valve also may be used (extended aortic root replacement).

Supravalvular aortic stenosis. Surgery is usually required for management of moderate-to-severe supravalvular AS. Balloon angioplasty and stent insertion have been successful but carry a higher risk for

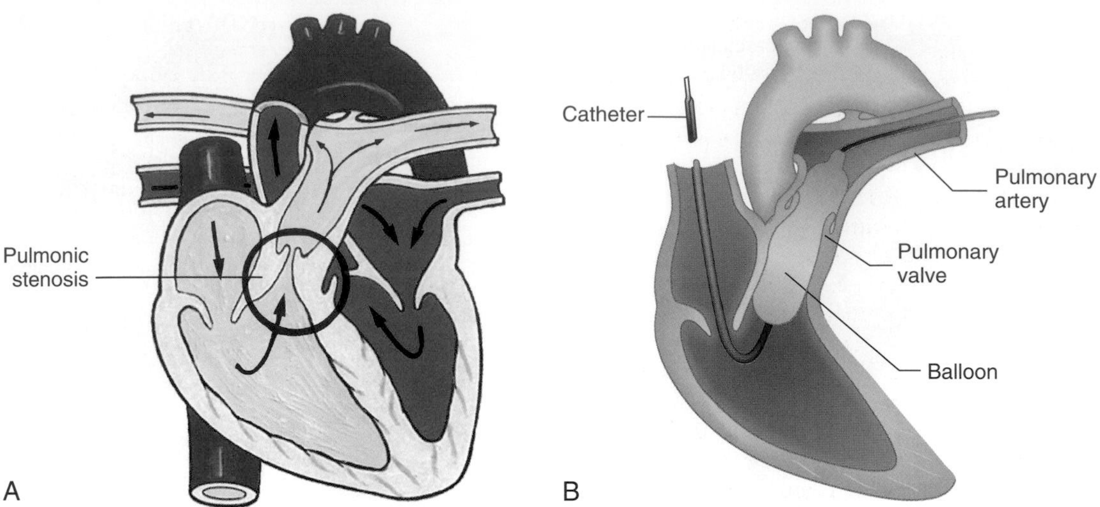

FIGURE 25-5 Pulmonary Stenosis. A, The pulmonary valve narrows at the entrance of the pulmonary artery. **B,** Balloon angioplasty is used to dilate the valve. A catheter is inserted across the stenotic pulmonic valve into the pulmonary artery, and a balloon at the end of the catheter is inflated while it is positioned across the narrowed valve opening. (**A,** from Hockenberry, M.J., & Wilson, D. [Eds.]. [2013]. *Wong's essentials of pediatric nursing* [9th ed.]. St. Louis: Mosby.)

HEALTH PROMOTION

Endocarditis Risk

Children with CHD are at risk of developing endocarditis. Although the risk is low, a transient bacteremia has been noted to follow dental and surgical procedures and instrumentation involving mucosal surfaces.

According to the Canadian Dental Association (CDA), only those patients at greatest risk of developing infective endocarditis must receive short-term prophylactic antibiotics before common, routine dental and surgical procedures, because the risks of taking prophylactic antibiotics outweigh the benefits for most patients. The CDA supports the growing body of evidence that promotes dental hygiene and care rather than prophylactic antibiotics and emphasizes the importance of achieving and maintaining excellent oral health and practising daily oral hygiene. Administering antibiotics can potentially lead to antibiotics-resistant bacteria and other mild to severe adverse effects.

In Canada, dental plans are available to only 26% of low-income workers. Among the 74% of these lower-income workers without plans, only 39% are seen by a dentist on a yearly basis. By contrast, dental care is part of the national health plan in several Europeans nations. Provincial health insurance plans should provide access to dental care to families living on low incomes.

The CDA recommends that people with the following should take prophylactic antibiotics before routine dental and surgical procedures:

- Prosthetic cardiac valve
- History of infective endocarditis
- Serious congenital heart conditions
- Repaired congenital heart defect with prosthetic material or device
- Repaired congenital heart defect with residual defect at the site or adjacent to the site of a prosthetic patch or a prosthetic device
- A cardiac transplant that develops a problem in a heart valve

The CDA suggests that prophylactic antibiotics are no longer needed for patients with the following conditions:

- Mitral valve prolapse
- Rheumatic heart disease
- Bicuspid valve disease
- Calcified aortic stenosis
- Congenital heart conditions such as ventricular septal defect, atrial septal defect, and hypertrophic cardiomyopathy

A bloodborne pathogen can inhabit areas of the heart following dental procedures or oral surgery. Good dental hygiene with daily brushing and flossing is critically important along with regular dental check-ups.

Data from American Heart Association. (2017). *What is infective endocarditis?* Retrieved from http://www.heart.org/idc/groups/heart-public/@wcm/@hcm/documents/downloadable/ucm_300297.pdf; Canadian Dental Association. (2014). *CDA position on prevention of infective endocarditis*. Retrieved from https://www.cda-adc.ca/_files/position_statements/infectiousEndocarditis.pdf; Mikkonen, J., & Raphael, D. (2010). *Social determinants of health: The Canadian facts*. Toronto: York University School of Health Policy and Management, p. 39. Retrieved from http://www.thecanadianfacts.org/the_canadian_facts.pdf.

rupture.[1,2,5] An extended graft with coronary reimplantation may be needed if narrowing is severe.

Pulmonary Stenosis

PATHOPHYSIOLOGY **Pulmonary stenosis (PS)** is a narrowing or stricture of the pulmonary valve that causes resistance to blood flow from the right ventricle to the pulmonary artery (Figure 25-5). Generally, moderate to severe stenosis causes right ventricular hypertrophy. **Pulmonary atresia** is an extreme form of PS with total fusion of the valve leaflets (blood cannot flow to the lungs); the right ventricle may be hypoplastic. In some cases of right ventricular outflow obstruction, the narrowing is below the valve (infundibular or subvalve PS).

CLINICAL MANIFESTATIONS Most infants are asymptomatic if the PS is mild to moderate. Newborns with severe PS or pulmonary atresia will be cyanotic (from a right-to-left shunt through an ASD) and may have signs of decreased cardiac output. A harsh systolic murmur is expected with PS. Pulmonary atresia produces a continuous murmur.

EVALUATION AND TREATMENT Echocardiography confirms the diagnosis and determines the severity of the PS. The treatment of choice for infants with moderate-to-severe PS is balloon angioplasty (Figure 25-5, *B*). A catheter with a special balloon device is used to dilate the area of narrowing. Multiple studies have proven the effectiveness and safety of balloon angioplasty in reducing the pressure gradient across the pulmonic valve.[5] In rare cases, surgical valvotomy may be required. Pulmonary blood flood is supported with prostaglandin E_1 infusion to maintain the patency of the ductus arteriosus in cases of pulmonary atresia with right ventricle–dependent coronary circulation in the neonatal period until surgery is performed to supply pulmonary blood flow.[5]

Both balloon dilation and surgical valvotomy leave the pulmonary valve incompetent (insufficient); however, most children are usually able to tolerate pulmonary valve incompetence and are asymptomatic. Long-term problems with restenosis are rare for uncomplicated PS.[1,2,5] However, clinically significant valve incompetence that results in right ventricle dilation and dysfunction may occur, requiring surgical intervention.[1,2,5]

Defects With Increased Pulmonary Blood Flow

Patent Ductus Arteriosus

PATHOPHYSIOLOGY **Patent ductus arteriosus (PDA)** is failure of the fetal ductus arteriosus (artery connecting the aorta and pulmonary artery) to functionally close within the first 15 hours after birth. However, several weeks after birth (Figure 25-6) may be needed for attainment of true anatomical closure, in which the ductus loses the ability to reopen. The continued patency of this vessel allows blood to flow from the higher-pressure aorta to the lower-pressure pulmonary artery, causing a left-to-right shunt.

CLINICAL MANIFESTATIONS Infants may be asymptomatic or show signs of pulmonary overcirculation, such as dyspnea, fatigue, and poor feeding. There is a characteristic machinerylike murmur in both systole and diastole. Aortic flow (run-off) into the lower pressure pulmonary circulation produces low diastolic blood pressure, widened pulse pressure, and bounding pulses. Children are at risk for bacterial endocarditis and may develop pulmonary hypertension in later life from chronic excessive pulmonary blood flow.

EVALUATION AND TREATMENT Diagnosis is confirmed with echocardiography. Administration of indomethacin (Indocin; a prostaglandin inhibitor) has proved successful in closing a PDA in premature infants and some newborns. Surgical division of the PDA through a left thoracotomy also may be done; in some cases the procedure can be performed with thoracoscopy. Closure with an occlusion device during cardiac catheterization is performed in select children older than 6 months of age. Both surgical and nonsurgical procedures are considered low risk.[2,5]

Atrial Septal Defect

PATHOPHYSIOLOGY An **atrial septal defect (ASD)** is an opening in the septal wall between the two atria. This opening allows blood to shunt from the left atrium to the right atrium. There are three types of ASDs. An **ostium primum atrial septal defect** is an opening low in the atrial septum and may be associated with abnormalities of the mitral valve. An **ostium secundum atrial septal defect** is an opening in the middle of the atrial septum and is the most common type. A **sinus venosus atrial septal defect** is an opening usually high in the atrial wall near the junction of the superior vena cava and may be associated with partial anomalous pulmonary venous connection.[7] Left-to-right shunting of blood can occur with a large ASD.

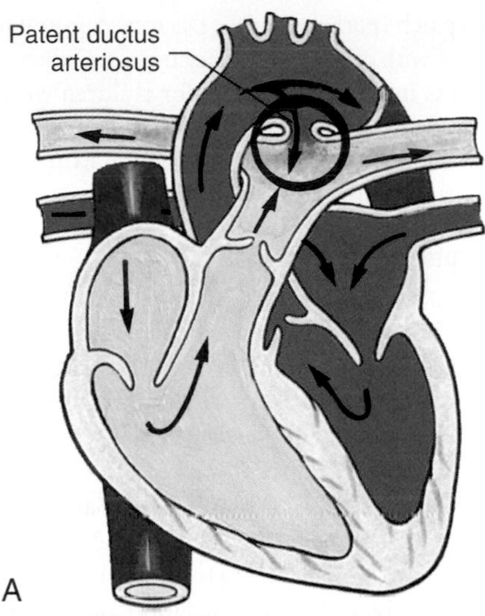

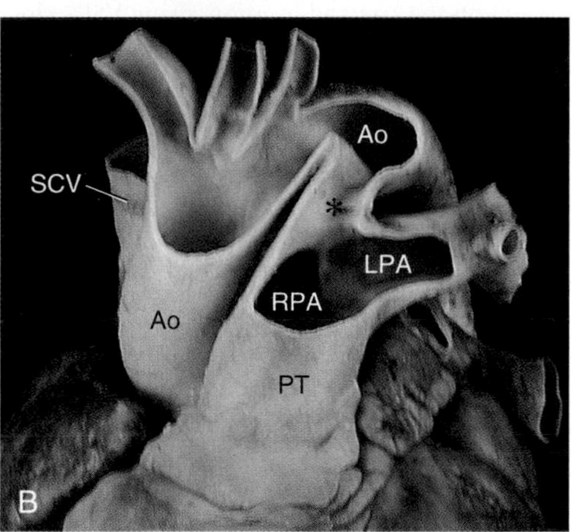

FIGURE 25-6 Patent Ductus Arteriosus. A, Patent ductus arteriosus (PDA) with left-to-right shunt. **B,** PDA in an adult with pulmonary hypertension. *Ao,* aorta; *LPA,* left pulmonary artery; *PT,* pulmonary trunk; *RPA,* right pulmonary artery; *SCV,* subclavian vein. (**A,** from Hockenberry, M.J., & Wilson, D. [2013]. *Wong's essentials of pediatric nursing* [9th ed.]. St. Louis: Mosby; **B,** from Damjanov, I., & Linder, J. [Eds.]. [1996]. *Anderson's pathology* [10th ed.]. St. Louis: Mosby.)

Another opening in the atrial septal wall that is part of normal fetal communication, which usually closes after birth, is the **foramen ovale.** When the lungs become functional at birth, the pulmonary pressure decreases and the left atrial pressure exceeds that of the right. The pressure change forces the septum to functionally close the foramen ovale. If it does not close, it is called a **patent foramen ovale (PFO).** About one out of four adults has a PFO without CHD; however, in children with CHD, the foramen ovale often remains open.

CLINICAL MANIFESTATIONS Children with an ASD are usually asymptomatic. Infants with a large ASD may, in rare cases, develop pulmonary overcirculation and slow growth. Some older children and adults will experience shortness of breath with activity as the right ventricle becomes less compliant with age. Pulmonary hypertension and stroke are associated rare complications. A systolic ejection murmur and a widely split second heart sound are the expected findings on physical examination.

EVALUATION AND TREATMENT Diagnosis is confirmed by echocardiography. The ASD may be closed surgically with primary repair (sutured closed) or with a patch (pericardium or Dacron). Surgical repair involves open-heart surgery with cardiopulmonary bypass. Catheterization device closure offers a less invasive alternative for children with an ASD that meets anatomical and size criteria.[8] All options have low morbidity and mortality. Atrial dysrhythmias persist in about 5 to 10% of individuals in both groups after closure.[8]

Ventricular Septal Defect

PATHOPHYSIOLOGY A **ventricular septal defect (VSD)** is an opening of the septal wall between the ventricles. VSDs are the most common type of congenital heart defect and account for 15 to 20% of all such defects.[2] VSDs are classified by location. **Perimembranous ventricular septal defects** are located high in the ventricular septal wall underneath the atrioventricular valves, and VSDs located under the aortic valve are subarterial. **Muscular ventricular septal defects** are located low in the septal wall. VSDs also can be located in the inlet or outlet portion of the ventricle. VSDs are similar to ASDs in that blood will shunt from left to right. Left-to-right shunting of blood can occur with a large VSD. Depending on the size and location, many VSDs close spontaneously, most often within the first 2 years of life.

CLINICAL MANIFESTATIONS Depending on the size, location, and degree of shunting and pulmonary vascular resistance (PVR), children may have no symptoms or have clinical effects from excessive pulmonary blood flow. In the infant, excessive pulmonary blood flow from left-to-right shunting causes dyspnea and tachypnea symptoms, commonly referred to as *heart failure* (HF), even though the heart muscle functions well with a VSD. A holosystolic (pansystolic) murmur is expected.

If the degree of shunting is significant and not corrected, the child is at risk of developing pulmonary hypertension. Irreversible pulmonary hypertension can result in **Eisenmenger's syndrome**, a condition in which shunting of blood is reversed because of high pulmonary pressure and resistance (right-to-left shunt with cyanosis).

EVALUATION AND TREATMENT Diagnosis is confirmed by echocardiography. Cardiac catheterization may be needed to calculate the degree of shunting and to directly measure the pressures in the heart. Smaller VSDs require minimal treatment and may close completely or become small enough that surgical closure is not required. If the infant has severe HF or failure to thrive that is unmanageable with medical therapy, early surgical repair is performed. Surgical repair involves open-heart surgery with cardiopulmonary bypass. The opening is either sutured closed (primary) or covered with a patch (pericardium or Dacron). Nonsurgical device closure is available but only under restricted conditions.[5,9] Endocarditis prophylaxis is only recommended for 6 months after surgical or device closure and indefinitely with a residual VSD after patch closure.[9]

Atrioventricular Canal Defect

PATHOPHYSIOLOGY **Atrioventricular canal (AVC) defect**, also known as **atrioventricular septal defect (AVSD)** or by the traditional term **endocardial cushion defect (ECD)**, is the result of incomplete fusion of endocardial cushions (Figure 25-7). AVC defect consists of an ostium primum ASD and inlet VSD with associated abnormalities of the atrioventricular valve tissue. These valve abnormalities range from a cleft in the mitral valve to a common mitral and tricuspid valve. The directions and pathways of flow are determined by pulmonary and systemic resistance, left and right ventricular pressures, and the compliance of each chamber. Flow is generally from left to right. AVC defect is a common cardiac defect in children with Down syndrome. However, children with this defect can have a normal karyotype.

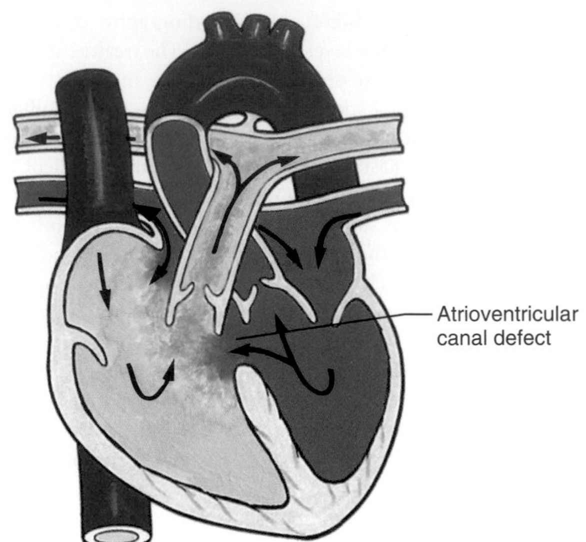

FIGURE 25-7 Atrioventricular Canal Defect. (From Hockenberry, M.J., & Wilson, D. [2013]. *Wong's essentials of pediatric nursing* [9th ed.]. St. Louis: Mosby.)

CLINICAL MANIFESTATIONS Infants with this defect often display moderate to severe HF attributable to left-to-right shunting and pulmonary overcirculation. Infants with pulmonary hypertension and high pulmonary resistance have less shunting and therefore minimal signs of HF. There may be mild cyanosis that increases with crying. Those with a large left-to-right shunt will have a murmur, and those with minimal shunt may not have a murmur. Children with AVC defect are at risk of developing irreversible pulmonary hypertension if left surgically untreated.

EVALUATION AND TREATMENT AVC defect is one of the most frequent diagnoses made with fetal echocardiography. Cardiac catheterization usually is not needed. Initial treatment goals include aggressive medical management of HF and nutritional supplementation. Infants are followed closely for signs or symptoms of failure to thrive. Pulmonary artery banding is occasionally performed in small infants with severe symptoms. However, complete surgical repair is most common and typically performed between 3 and 6 months of age to prevent irreversible pulmonary hypertension. This procedure consists of patch closure of the septal defects and reconstruction of the atrioventricular (AV) valve tissue (either repair of the mitral valve cleft or fashioning of two AV valves). If the mitral valve defect is severe, valve replacement may be needed. A potential problem following repair is mitral regurgitation, which may later require valve replacement.

Defects With Decreased Pulmonary Blood Flow

Tetralogy of Fallot

PATHOPHYSIOLOGY The classic form of **tetralogy of Fallot (TOF)** includes four defects: (1) VSD, (2) PS, (3) overriding aorta, and (4) right ventricular hypertrophy (Figure 25-8). The pathophysiology varies widely, depending not only on the degree of PS but also on the pulmonary and systemic vascular resistance to flow. If total resistance to pulmonary flow is greater than systemic resistance, the shunt is from right to left. If systemic resistance is more than pulmonary resistance, the shunt is from left to right. PS decreases blood flow to the lungs and, consequently, the amount of oxygenated blood that returns to the left heart. Physiological compensation to chronic, severe hypoxia includes production of more red blood cells (polycythemia), development of collateral bronchial vessels, and enlargement of the nail beds (clubbing).

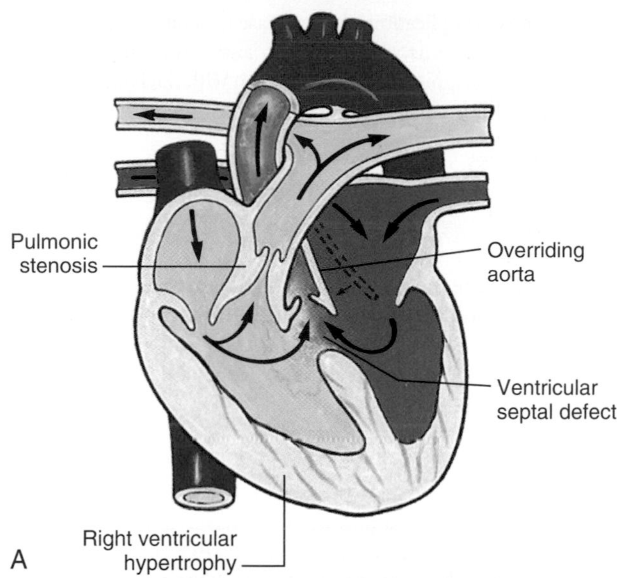

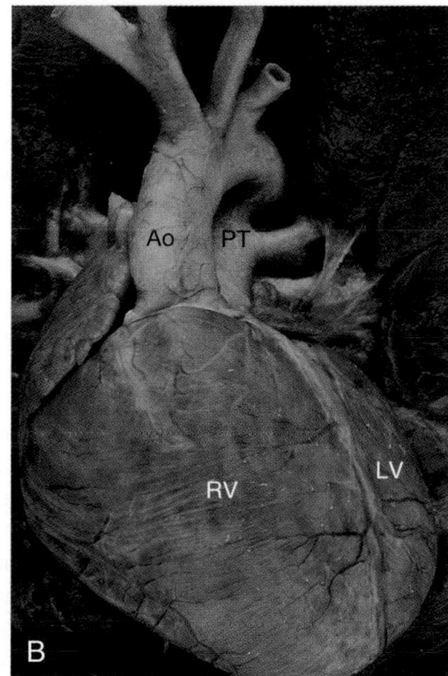

FIGURE 25-8 Tetralogy of Fallot. A, Tetralogy of Fallot hemodynamics. **B,** Right ventricular hypertrophy and overriding aorta (*Ao*). *LV,* left ventricle; *PT,* pulmonary trunk; *RV,* right ventricle. (**A,** from Hockenberry, M.J., & Wilson, D. [2013]. *Wong's essentials of pediatric nursing* [9th ed.]. St. Louis: Mosby; **B,** from Damjanov, I., & Linder, J. [Eds.]. [1996]. *Anderson's pathology* [10th ed.]. St. Louis: Mosby.)

CLINICAL MANIFESTATIONS Some infants may be acutely cyanotic at birth. In others, progression of hypoxia and cyanosis may be more gradual over the first year of life as the PS worsens. Acute episodes of cyanosis and hypoxia can occur, called *hypercyanotic spells, blue spells,* or *"tet" spells.* These spells (increased right-to-left shunt) may occur during crying or after feeding. Oxygen has little effect in improving hypoxemia, but placing the infant in a knee–chest position (Figure 25-9) and administering morphine sulphate subcutaneously or intravenously is most commonly used to treat "tet" spells. If prolonged or frequent, these spells are an indication for emergent evaluation and surgical treatment.

Chronic cyanosis may cause clubbing of the fingers and poor growth in children. Squatting or the knee–chest position can help with cyanosis

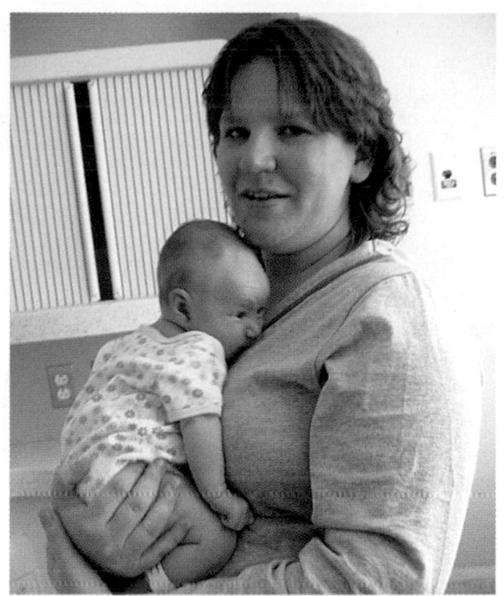

FIGURE 25-9 Infant Held in a Knee–Chest Position. (From Hockenberry, M.J., & Wilson, D. [2013]. *Wong's essentials of pediatric nursing* [9th ed.]. St. Louis: Mosby.)

in these children because it increases peripheral resistance in the systemic circulation, which causes an increase in pressures in the left heart and consequent reduction in right-to-left shunting and improvement in pulmonary perfusion. Children with unrepaired TOF are at risk for emboli, stroke, brain abscess, seizures, and loss of consciousness or sudden death following a "tet" spell.

EVALUATION AND TREATMENT Diagnosis is confirmed with echocardiography. Elective surgical repair is usually performed in the first year of life. Indications for earlier repair include increasing cyanosis or the development of hypercyanotic spells. Complete repair involves closure of the VSD, resection of the infundibular stenosis, and application of a pericardial patch to enlarge the right ventricular outflow tract that can extend across the pulmonary valve annulus (transannular patch).

In very small infants who cannot undergo primary repair, a palliative procedure to increase pulmonary blood flow and increase oxygen saturation may be performed. This systemic artery to pulmonary artery anastomosis is the Blalock-Taussig or the modified Blalock-Taussig shunt, which provides blood flow to the pulmonary arteries.

Tricuspid Atresia

PATHOPHYSIOLOGY **Tricuspid atresia** is failure of the tricuspid valve to develop; consequently, there is no communication from right atrium to right ventricle (Figure 25-10). Blood flows through an ASD or a PFO to the left atrium and through a VSD to the right ventricle. This condition is often associated with PS or transposition of the great arteries. There is complete mixing of unoxygenated and oxygenated blood in the left side of the heart, resulting in systemic desaturation and mild cyanosis. The physiological process that causes lesion development is variable, depending on the great vessel anatomy and amount of PS.

CLINICAL MANIFESTATIONS A murmur is noted, and cyanosis is usually seen in the newborn period. Tachycardia, dyspnea, fatigue, and poor feeding may be noted with excessive pulmonary blood flow. Older children may have signs of chronic hypoxemia with clubbing. Children are at risk for bacterial endocarditis, brain abscess, and stroke.

EVALUATION AND TREATMENT After diagnosis is confirmed by echocardiography, the neonate with decreased pulmonary blood flow

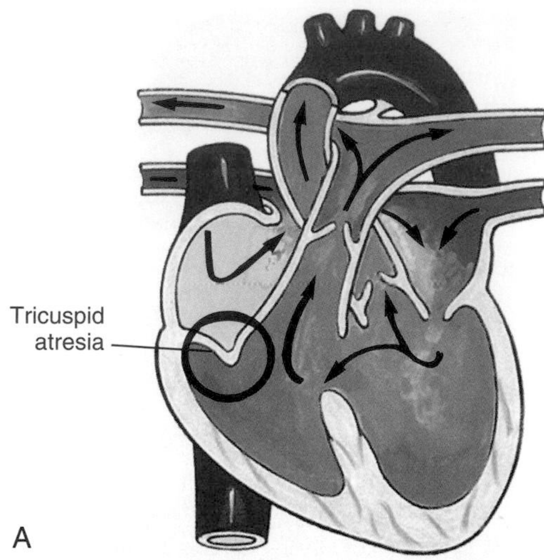

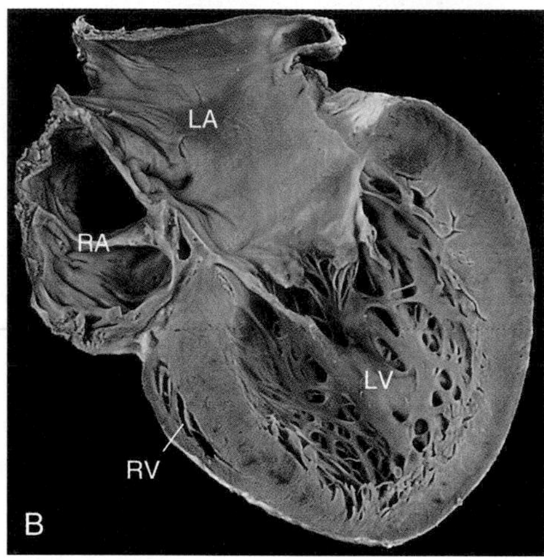

FIGURE 25-10 Tricuspid Atresia. **A,** Tricuspid atresia hemodynamics. **B,** Small right ventricle *(RV)* slit of ventricular septal defect; left ventricle *(LV)* is enlarged. *LA,* left atrium; *RA,* right atrium. (**A,** from Hockenberry, M.J., & Wilson, D. [2013]. *Wong's essentials of pediatric nursing* [9th ed.]. St. Louis: Mosby; **B,** from Damjanov, I., & Linder, J. [Eds.]. [1996]. *Anderson's pathology* [10th ed.]. St. Louis: Mosby.)

is treated with a continuous infusion of prostaglandin E_1 to maintain the patency of the ductus arteriosus until surgical intervention. If the ASD is restrictive, an atrial septostomy is performed during cardiac catheterization or under echocardiographic guidance.[10] Treatment is accomplished in staged procedures. Once the infant is stabilized, a Blalock-Taussig shunt (systemic to pulmonary artery anastomosis) is placed to increase blood flow to the lungs.

Further surgery is undertaken between 4 and 8 months of age, depending on the child's growth and degree of cyanosis. The second-stage procedure is the bidirectional Glenn shunt, in which the superior vena cava is anastomosed to the pulmonary artery. At that time, the pulmonary artery may be ligated and the Blalock-Taussig shunt is removed. The final separation of the pulmonary circulation from the systemic circulation is the modified Fontan procedure. In this stage, the inferior vena cava blood flow is routed to the pulmonary artery using an intra- or extracardiac tube graft or baffle. The procedure is typically performed between 2 and 4 years of age. Surgical outcomes are best in the child with normal ventricular function and low PVR. For children with borderline PVR, a fenestration (opening) can be created in the baffle or graft to relieve high systemic pulmonary venous pressures if needed.

Postoperative complications that increase hospital stay include pleural and pericardial effusions, elevated PVR, and ventricular dysfunction. Exercise tolerance is limited in many children with the Fontan procedure, but general health is considered good.

Mixing Defects

Transposition of the Great Arteries or Transposition of the Great Vessels

PATHOPHYSIOLOGY In **transposition of the great arteries (TGA)** or **transposition of the great vessels (TGV)**, the pulmonary artery leaves the left ventricle and the aorta exits the right ventricle (Figure 25-11). Associated defects, such as ASD, VSD, or PDA, permit mixing of saturated and desaturated blood, which maintains adequate tissue oxygenation for a limited time.

CLINICAL MANIFESTATIONS Clinical manifestations depend on the type and size of the associated defects. Children with limited communication between cardiac chambers are severely cyanotic, acidotic, and ill at birth. Those with large septal defects or a PDA may be less severely cyanotic but may have symptoms of pulmonary overcirculation. Classically, no murmur is heard unless there is an associated VSD.

EVALUATION AND TREATMENT Diagnosis is suspected by physical examination and confirmed with echocardiography. Administration of intravenous prostaglandin E_1 to maintain the patency of the ductus arteriosus may be initiated to temporarily increase oxygen delivery. Enlargement of the PFO by balloon atrial septostomy may be performed during cardiac catheterization or under echocardiographic guidance to increase mixing and maintain cardiac output.[5,10]

The most preferred type of surgical repair for TGA performed in the first weeks of life is the arterial switch procedure. It involves transecting the great arteries and anastomosing the main pulmonary artery to the native proximal aorta (just above the aortic valve) and anastomosing the ascending aorta to the native proximal pulmonary artery. The coronary arteries are moved with a "button" of tissue from the proximal aorta to the proximal pulmonary artery, creating a new aorta. Reimplantation of the coronary arteries is critical to the infant's survival, and the arteries must be reattached without torsion or kinking to provide the heart with its supply of oxygen. The advantage of the arterial switch procedure is the re-establishment of normal circulation with the left ventricle acting as the systemic pump. Potential complications of the arterial switch include narrowing at the great artery anastomoses, neoaortic valve regurgitation, or coronary artery insufficiency.[2] Long-term results for the arterial switch operation are usually good.

Total Anomalous Pulmonary Venous Connection

PATHOPHYSIOLOGY **Total anomalous pulmonary venous connection (TAPVC)** is a rare defect characterized by failure of the pulmonary veins to join the left atrium during cardiac development. TAPVC is also called *total anomalous pulmonary venous return* (TAPVR) or *total anomalous pulmonary venous drainage* (TAPVD) (Figure 25-12). The pulmonary venous return is connected to the right side of the circulation rather than to the left atrium. The type of TAPVC is classified according to the pulmonary venous point of attachment:

- *Supracardiac:* Attachment above the diaphragm, usually to the superior vena cava (most common form)
- *Cardiac:* Direct attachment to the heart, usually to the right atrium or coronary sinus
- *Infracardiac:* Attachment below the diaphragm, such as to the inferior vena cava (most severe and least common form)

The right atrium receives all the blood that normally would flow into the left atrium. As a result, the right side of the heart is enlarged

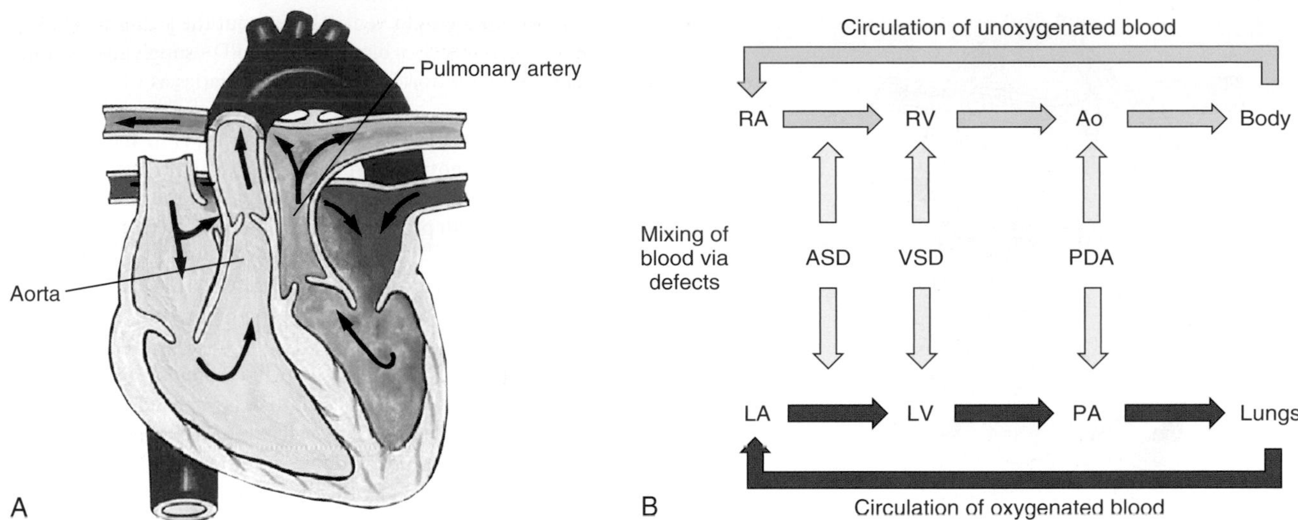

FIGURE 25-11 **Hemodynamics in Transposition of the Great Vessels. A,** Complete transposition of the great vessels with an intact interventricular septum. The aorta arises from the right ventricle and the pulmonary artery from the left ventricle. **B,** Oxygen saturation in the two, parallel circuits. *Ao,* aorta; *ASD,* atrial septal defect; *LA,* left atrium; *LV,* left ventricle; *PA,* pulmonary artery; *PDA,* patent ductus arteriosus; *RA,* right atrium; *RV,* right ventricle; *VSD,* ventricular septal defect. (**A,** from Hockenberry, M.J., & Wilson, D. [2013]. *Wong's essentials of pediatric nursing* [9th ed.]. St. Louis: Mosby.)

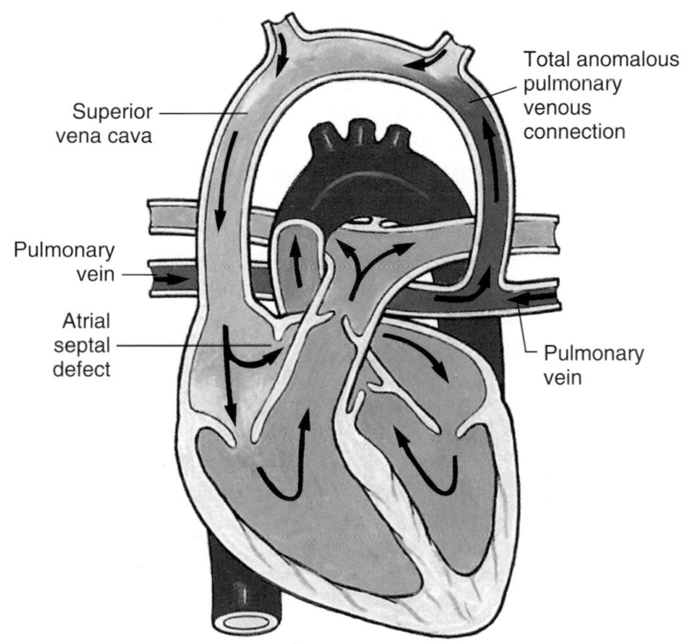

FIGURE 25-12 Total Anomalous Pulmonary Venous Connection.

and the left side, especially the left atrium, is smaller than normal. An associated ASD or PFO allows systemic venous blood to shunt from the right atrium to the left side of the heart. As a result, the oxygen saturation of the blood in both sides of the heart (and, ultimately, in the systemic arterial circulation) is the same. If the pulmonary blood flow is increased, pulmonary venous return is also large, and the amount of saturated blood is relatively high. However, if there is obstruction to pulmonary venous drainage, the infant has severe cyanosis and low cardiac output. Infracardiac TAPVC often is associated with obstruction of pulmonary venous drainage and is a surgical emergency with higher mortality than the unobstructed types.

CLINICAL MANIFESTATIONS Most infants develop cyanosis early in life. The degree of cyanosis is inversely related to the amount of pulmonary blood flow. Children with unobstructed TAPVC may be asymptomatic until PVR decreases during infancy, increasing pulmonary blood flow, with resulting signs of pulmonary overcirculation. Cyanosis becomes worse with pulmonary vein obstruction; once obstruction occurs, the infant's condition usually deteriorates rapidly. Without intervention, cardiac failure will progress to death. Murmur is not a common feature of TAPVC.

EVALUATION AND TREATMENT Diagnosis is suspected with echocardiography but may require confirmative angiography. Corrective repair is usually required in early infancy. The surgical approach varies with the anatomical defect. In general, however, the common pulmonary vein (venous confluence) is sutured to the left atrium, the ASD is closed, and the anomalous pulmonary venous connection or vertical vein may be ligated.

Truncus Arteriosus

PATHOPHYSIOLOGY Truncus arteriosus (TA) is failure of normal septation and division of the embryonic outflow tract into a pulmonary artery and an aorta, resulting in a single vessel that exits the heart. There is always an associated VSD with mixing of the systemic and arterial circulations (Figure 25-13), causing some degree of cyanosis. Blood ejected from the heart flows preferentially to the lower-pressure pulmonary arteries, causing increased pulmonary blood flow. The three types are as follows:

- *Type I:* A single pulmonary trunk arises near the base of the truncus and divides into the left and right pulmonary arteries.
- *Type II:* The left and right pulmonary arteries arise separately from the posterior aspect of the truncus.
- *Type III:* The pulmonary arteries arise independently and from the lateral aspect of the truncus.

CLINICAL MANIFESTATIONS Most infants are symptomatic with moderate HF and variable cyanosis, poor growth, and activity intolerance. Children are at risk for brain abscess and bacterial endocarditis.

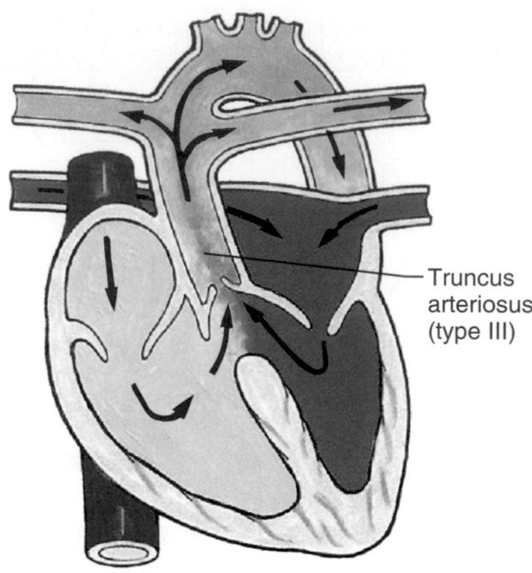

FIGURE 25-13 Truncus Arteriosus. The truncus arteriosus (TA) fails to divide into the pulmonary artery and aorta, and the interventricular septum fails to close at the top. Blood from both ventricles mixes in the TA and then enters the pulmonary and systemic circuits. (From Hockenberry, M.J., & Wilson, D. [2013]. *Wong's essentials of pediatric nursing* [9th ed.]. St. Louis: Mosby.)

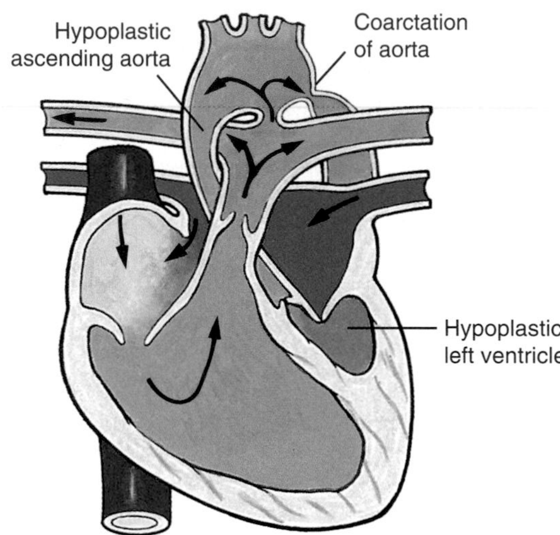

FIGURE 25-14 Hypoplastic Left Heart Syndrome. (From Hockenberry, M.J., & Wilson, D. [Eds.]. [2009]. *Wong's essentials of pediatric nursing* [8th ed.]. St. Louis: Mosby.)

EVALUATION AND TREATMENT Diagnosis is made by echocardiography. Corrective repair is a modification of the Rastelli procedure and is performed in the first few weeks or months of life. It involves closing the VSD so that the TA receives the outflow from the left ventricle, and excising the pulmonary arteries from the aorta and attaching them to the right ventricle by means of a homograft (cadaver) conduit. These children require additional procedures to replace the conduit since its size becomes inadequate in relation to growth or narrows because of calcification over time.

Hypoplastic Left Heart Syndrome

PATHOPHYSIOLOGY **Hypoplastic left heart syndrome (HLHS)** is underdevelopment of the left side of the heart. Features include small left atrium, small or absent mitral valve, small or absent left ventricle, and small or absent aortic valve. Coarctation also is expected (Figure 25-14). Most blood from the left atrium flows across the PFO to the right atrium, to the right ventricle, and out the pulmonary artery. The descending aorta receives blood from the PDA supplying systemic blood flow and filling the aorta and coronary arteries as well.

CLINICAL MANIFESTATIONS HLHS presents in the early newborn period as mild cyanosis, tachypnea, and low cardiac output if not already detected by fetal echocardiography. Support of the systemic circulation is accomplished with prostaglandin E_1 infusion. If HLHS is not suspected and the PDA closes, there is progressive deterioration with cyanosis and decreased cardiac output, leading to cardiovascular collapse. If untreated, HLHS is usually fatal in the first months of life.

EVALUATION AND TREATMENT Echocardiography shows all of the features of HLHS. Cardiac catheterization is rarely required. A multistage repair approach is used. The first stage is the *Norwood procedure*, which is anastomosis of the main pulmonary artery to the aorta to create a new aorta, construction of either a modified Blalock-Taussig (systemic to pulmonary artery) or Sano (right ventricle to pulmonary artery) shunt to provide pulmonary blood flow, creation of a large ASD, and repair of the coarctation. The second stage is a bidirectional Glenn shunt performed at 3 to 6 months of age by connecting the superior vena cava to the pulmonary artery, which minimizes cyanosis and reduces the volume load on the right ventricle. The final stage is a modified Fontan procedure that relieves cyanosis by connecting the inferior vena cava blood to the pulmonary artery using an intra- or extracardiac tube graft or baffle. Few centres perform heart transplantation in the newborn period rather than the staged procedure (Norwood, Glenn, Fontan) because of the scarcity of newborn donor hearts. Disadvantages of neonatal transplantation include shortage of newborn organ donors, risk of rejection, long-term problems with chronic immunosuppression, and infection. For infants who are not candidates for staged procedures or transplantation, the family is then offered palliative care.

Infants successfully treated for HLHS have improved survival rates related to advances in surgical and medical technology. Long-term (10 to 15 years) health problems after the Fontan procedure related to reduced right ventricular function and high central venous pressures have been reported to impact quality of life.[11,12]

QUICK CHECK 25-1

1. What are the three principal classifications of congenital heart disease?
2. Describe the different characteristics that determine whether the defects are cyanotic or acyanotic.
3. What is the most common type of congenital heart defect?

Heart Failure

Heart failure (HF) is a common complication of many congenital heart defects. HF occurs when the heart is unable to maintain sufficient cardiac output to meet the metabolic demands of the body. The most common congenital causes of HF in infancy and childhood are listed in Table 25-3. Classic HF in children also can be acquired, usually resulting from cardiomyopathies, dysrhythmias, or electrolyte disturbances. Pulmonary overcirculation from a large left-to-right shunt is often called *heart failure* but is not usually associated with decreased ventricular function and failure to meet metabolic demands. However, the clinical manifestations are similar, such as failure to thrive, tachypnea, tachycardia, and exercise intolerance.[2]

In general, the pathophysiological mechanisms of HF in infants and children are similar to those in adults. It is most often a result of decreased left ventricular systolic function and the associated left atrial and pulmonary venous hypertension and pulmonary venous

TABLE 25-3 Causes of Heart Failure Resulting From Congenital Heart Disease

Age of Onset	Cause
At birth	HLHS
	Volume overload lesions
	Severe tricuspid or pulmonary insufficiency
	Large systemic AV fistula
First week	TGA
	PDA in small premature infants
	HLHS (with more favourable anatomy)
	TAPVR, particularly those with pulmonary venous obstruction
	Others
	Systemic AV fistula
	Critical AS or PS
1–4 weeks	COA with associated anomalies
	Critical AS
	Large left-to-right shunt lesions (VSD, PDA) in premature infants
	All other lesions previously listed
4–6 weeks	Some left-to-right shunt lesions, such as AVSD
6 weeks to 4 months	Large VSD
	Large PDA
	Others, such as anomalous left coronary artery from PA

AS, aortic stenosis; *AV*, atrioventricular; *AVSD*, atrioventricular septal defect; *COA*, coarctation of the aorta; *HLHS*, hypoplastic left heart syndrome; *PA*, pulmonary artery; *PDA*, patent ductus arteriosus; *PS*, pulmonary stenosis; *TAPVR*, total anomalous pulmonary venous return; *TGA*, transposition of the great arteries; *VSD*, ventricular septal defect.

Modified from Park, M.K. (2014). *Pediatric cardiology for practitioners* (6th ed.). St. Louis: Mosby.

BOX 25-1 Clinical Manifestations of Heart Failure

Impaired Myocardial Function
Tachycardia
Sweating (inappropriate)
Decreased urinary output
Fatigue
Weakness
Restlessness
Anorexia
Pale, cool extremities
Weak peripheral pulses
Decreased blood pressure
Gallop rhythm
Cardiomegaly

Pulmonary Congestion
Tachypnea
Dyspnea
Retractions (infants)
Flaring nares
Exercise intolerance
Orthopnea
Cough, hoarseness
Cyanosis
Wheezing
Grunting

Systemic Venous Congestion
Weight gain
Hepatomegaly
Peripheral edema, especially periorbital
Ascites
Neck vein distension

From Hockenberry, M.J., & Wilson, D. (Eds.). (2013). *Wong's essentials of pediatric nursing* (9th ed.). St. Louis: Mosby.

congestion. The same compensatory mechanisms are activated in the face of inadequate cardiac output. Right ventricular failure is rare in childhood.

Left ventricular failure in infants is manifested as poor feeding and sucking, often leading to failure to thrive. In left ventricular failure, dyspnea, tachypnea, and diaphoresis may be accompanied by retractions, grunting, and nasal flaring. Wheezing, coughing, and rales are rare in childhood HF.[1,2,13] Common skin changes, such as pallor or mottling, are often present (Box 25-1). Signs of systemic venous congestion, such as hepatomegaly, weight gain, ascites, and peripheral edema, can be present but could be suggestive of other medical conditions such as renal or nutritional deficiencies.

A thorough physical examination with emphasis on cardiac and pulmonary findings will often reveal the degree of HF. Plotting a child's growth (height, weight, head circumference) is an important method of assessing a child's health. Infants with HF or pulmonary overcirculation usually have low weight with normal length and head circumference measurements. The failure to thrive is usually the result of increased metabolic expenditure relative to caloric intake. An electrocardiogram (ECG) also should be performed to determine the presence of dysrhythmia or hypertrophy. A chest X-ray is useful in assessing the presence of cardiomegaly and signs of increased pulmonary circulation or pulmonary edema with echocardiography to assess impaired function and possible etiology. B-type natriuretic peptide (BNP) has emerged as another diagnostic test of HF in children to confirm or exclude a cardiac cause for the symptoms.[2,14]

Treatment is aimed at decreasing cardiac workload and increasing the efficiency of heart function. Severe CHD is typically managed with surgical repair if applicable. Medical management initially consists of diuretics, such as furosemide (Lasix). Depending on the degree of HF, other diuretics can be used in combination with furosemide to counteract potassium losses. Agents that reduce afterload, such as captopril (Capoten) or enalapril (Vasotec) and beta-blockers, are employed to further manage severe HF.[1,2,13] Children with end-stage HF on maximal medical therapy can be supported on a ventricular assist device (VAD) while awaiting cardiac transplantation in severe cases that meet eligibility.[13]

ACQUIRED CARDIOVASCULAR DISORDERS

Acquired heart diseases refer to disease processes or abnormalities that occur after birth. They result from various causes, such as infection, genetic disorders, autoimmune processes in response to infection, environmental factors, or autoimmune diseases. Examples of acquired heart diseases include Kawasaki disease (KD), myocarditis, rheumatic heart disease, cardiomyopathy, and systemic hypertension. This chapter discusses KD and systemic hypertension. Myocarditis, rheumatic heart disease, and cardiomyopathy are discussed in Chapter 24.

Kawasaki Disease

Kawasaki disease (KD), formerly known as *mucocutaneous lymph node syndrome*, is an acute, usually self-limiting systemic vasculitis that may result in cardiac sequelae without treatment. Although KD occurs throughout the world, the greatest number of cases are seen in Japan.[1,2] KD's high prevalence in Japan reflects the genetic component of KD, with the case rate being highest among Asians and lower among White and Black children.

KD is primarily a condition of young children. Eighty percent of cases are seen in children younger than 5 years of age, with the incidence peaking in the toddler age group. Males are affected slightly more than females. The peak incidence is in the winter and spring.[1,2]

The etiology of KD remains unknown. Current etiological theories centre on an immunological response to an infectious, toxic, or antigenic substance.[2,14]

PATHOPHYSIOLOGY KD progresses pathologically and clinically in the following stages. In the early or acute phase, small capillaries, arterioles, and venules become inflamed, as does the heart itself. In the subacute state, inflammation spreads to larger vessels and aneurysms of the coronary arteries may develop. In the convalescent stage, medium-sized arteries begin the granulation process and may cause coronary artery thickening with increased risk for thrombosis. After the convalescent stage, inflammation wanes with potential scarring, calcification, and stenosis of the affected vessels.

CLINICAL MANIFESTATIONS The clinical course of KD progresses in three stages: acute, subacute, and convalescent. In the acute phase, the child with classic or typical KD has fever, conjunctivitis, oral changes ("strawberry" tongue), rash, erythema of the palms and soles, and lymphadenopathy, and is often irritable. During this phase, myocarditis may develop. The subacute phase begins when the fever ends and continues until the clinical signs have resolved. It is at this time that the child is most at risk for coronary artery aneurysm development. Desquamation of the palms and soles occurs at this time, as well as marked thrombocytosis. The convalescent phase is marked by the elevation of the erythrocyte sedimentation rate and C-reactive protein level, as well as by an increased platelet count. Arthritis or arthralgia of the joints may be present. This phase continues until all laboratory values return to normal—usually about 6 to 8 weeks after onset.[1,2] Atypical or "incomplete" KD can be seen in infants and children who lack the diagnostic criteria (have fewer than four signs) or "classic" physical findings. Recognition can be difficult and often results in delay of treatment with possible cardiovascular sequelae.[2,14]

EVALUATION AND TREATMENT The diagnostic criteria for KD are based on clinical features, which state that the child must exhibit fever for more than 5 days along with four of five criteria (Box 25-2). Children diagnosed with KD usually have leukocytosis, increased erythrocyte sedimentation rates, thrombocytosis, and elevated liver enzymes. An echocardiogram is obtained at the time of diagnosis as a baseline measurement to assess for coronary aneurysms or inflammation. Serial echocardiograms are obtained after treatment to assess for development of coronary aneurysms or regression of those present early in the course of the disease. Treatment includes oral administration of Aspirin and intravenous infusion of gamma globulin (most often only one dose). Aspirin is continued until the manifestations of inflammation are resolved but may be used indefinitely in children with residual coronary artery abnormalities.

Treatment with Aspirin and intravenous immunoglobulin during the acute phase has decreased the morbidity of KD and has reduced the incidence of coronary abnormalities from approximately 20% to less than 10% at 6 to 8 weeks after initiation of therapy. Most children recover completely from KD, including regression of aneurysms. The most common cardiovascular sequela is coronary thrombosis.[14]

BOX 25-2 Diagnostic Criteria for Kawasaki Disease

The child must exhibit five of the following six criteria, including fever:

1. Fever for 5 or more days (often diagnosed with shorter duration of fever if other symptoms are present)
2. Bilateral conjunctival infection without exudation
3. Changes in the oral mucous membranes, such as erythema, dryness, and fissuring of the lips; oropharyngeal reddening; or "strawberry tongue"
4. Changes in the extremities, such as peripheral edema, peripheral erythema, and desquamation of palms and soles, particularly periungual peeling
5. Polymorphous rash, often accentuated in the perineal area
6. Cervical lymphadenopathy (one lymph node >1.5 cm)

Modified from Hockenberry, M.J., & Wilson, D. (Eds.). (2013). *Wong's essentials of pediatric nursing* (9th ed.). St. Louis: Mosby.

Systemic Hypertension

Systemic hypertension in children is defined as systolic and diastolic blood pressure levels greater than the 95th percentile for age and gender on at least three occasions (Tables 25-4 and 25-5). The Fourth Task Force on Blood Pressure Control in Children uses height as an additional criterion to the blood pressure guidelines.[1,15]

Hypertension is classified into two categories: primary (or essential) hypertension, in which a specific cause cannot be identified; and secondary hypertension, in which a cause *can* be identified (Box 25-3). Hypertension in children differs from adult hypertension in etiology

TABLE 25-4 Normative Blood Pressure Levels (Systolic/Diastolic [Mean]) by DINAMAP Monitor in Children 5 Years Old and Younger

Age	Mean BP Levels (mm Hg)	90th Percentile	95th Percentile
1–3 days	64/41 (50)	75/49 (50)	78/52 (62)
1 month to 2 years	95/58 (72)	106/68 (83)	110/71 (86)
2–5 years	101/57 (74)	112/66 (82)	115/68 (85)

BP, blood pressure.
Data from Park, M.K. (2014). *Pediatric cardiology for practitioners* (6th ed.). St Louis: Mosby; modified from Park, M.K., & Menard, S.M. (1989). *Am J Dis Children, 143*, 860.

TABLE 25-5 Auscultatory Blood Pressure Values for Boys and Girls Aged 6 to 17 Years (Systolic/Diastolic K5)

Age and Gender	Mean BP Levels (mm Hg)	90th Percentile	95th Percentile
6–7 years			
Boys	95–96 / 53–55	105–107 / 64–66	108–110 / 67–70
Girls	94–94 / 52–54	103–104 / 63–65	106–107 / 66–68
8–9 years			
Boys	97–99 / 56–57	108–109 / 68–68	111–113 / 71–71
Girls	96–98 / 56–56	106–108 / 67–67	109–111 / 70–70
10–11 years			
Boys	100–102 / 57–57	111–113 / 68–68	114–116 / 71–71
Girls	100–102 / 57–57	110–112 / 68–68	113–115 / 71–71
12–13 years			
Boys	105–108 / 56–56	116–118 / 68–68	119–122 / 71–71
Girls	104–105 / 57–57	113–115 / 68–68	116–118 / 71–71
14–15 years			
Boys	110–113 / 57–57	121–124 / 68–69	122–127 / 71–72
Girls	106–107 / 58–58	116–117 / 68–69	119–119 / 72–72
16–17 years			
Boys	114–114 / 59–62	125–125 / 71–73	128–128 / 74–77
Girls	107–108 / 59–59	117–118 / 69–70	120–121 / 73–73

BP, blood pressure; *K5*, Korotkoff phase 5.
From Park, M.K. (2014). *Pediatric cardiology for practitioners* (6th ed.). St. Louis: Mosby.

BOX 25-3 Conditions Associated With Secondary Hypertension in Children

Renal

Renal parenchymal disease
- Glomerulonephritis, acute and chronic
- Pyelonephritis, acute and chronic
- Congenital anomalies (polycystic or dysplastic kidneys)
- Obstructive uropathies (hydronephrosis)
- Hemolytic-uremic syndrome
- Collagen disease (periarteritis, lupus)
- Renal damage from nephrotoxic medications, trauma, or radiation

Renovascular disease
- Renal artery disorders (e.g., stenosis, polyarteritis, thrombosis)
- Renal vein thrombosis

Cardiovascular

Coarctation of the aorta

Conditions with large stroke volume (patent ductus arteriosus, aortic insufficiency, systemic arteriovenous fistula, complete heart block) (these conditions cause only systolic hypertension)

Endocrine

Hyperthyroidism (systolic hypertension)

Excessive catecholamine levels
- Pheochromocytoma
- Neuroblastoma

Adrenal dysfunction
- Congenital adrenal hyperplasia
  - 11-β-Hydroxylase deficiency
  - 17-Hydroxylase deficiency
- Cushing's syndrome
- Hyperaldosteronism
  - Primary
    - Conn's syndrome
    - Idiopathic nodular hyperplasia
    - Dexamethasone-suppressible hyperaldosteronism
  - Secondary
    - Renovascular hypertension
    - Renin-producing tumour (juxtaglomerular cell tumour)

Hyperparathyroidism (and hypercalcemia)

Neurogenic

Increased intracranial pressure (any cause, especially tumours, infections, trauma)

Poliomyelitis

Guillain-Barré syndrome

Dysautonomia (Riley-Day syndrome)

Medications and Chemicals

Sympathomimetic medications (nose drops, cough medications, cold preparations, theophylline [Uniphyl])

Amphetamines

Corticosteroids

Nonsteroidal anti-inflammatory drugs

Oral contraceptives

Heavy-metal poisoning (mercury, lead)

Cocaine, acute or chronic use

Cyclosporine

Thyroxine

Tacrolimus

Miscellaneous

Hypervolemia and hypernatremia

Stevens-Johnson syndrome

Bronchopulmonary dysplasia (newborns)

From Park, M.K. (2014). *Pediatric cardiology for practitioners* (6th ed.). St. Louis: Mosby.

and presentation. Young children, when diagnosed with hypertension, are often found to have secondary hypertension caused by some underlying disease, such as renal disease or COA (see Box 25-3). An increased prevalence of primary hypertension in older children has been noted. Researchers are now focusing on primary hypertension in older children in relation to morbidity and the presence of early atherosclerotic disease. Certain factors influence blood pressure in children. Children who are overweight are often hypertensive (see *Health Promotion:* Childhood Obesity in Canada). Smoking also is associated with an increased risk for hypertension.[16-18]

PATHOPHYSIOLOGY In infants and children, a cause of hypertension is almost always found. In general, the younger the child with significant hypertension, the more likely a correctable cause can be determined. Therefore, a thorough evaluation needs to be performed.[2,16]

The pathophysiology of primary hypertension in children is not clearly understood but may result from a complex interaction of a strong predisposing genetic component with disturbances in sympathetic vascular smooth muscle tone, humoral agents (angiotensin, catecholamines), renal sodium excretion, and cardiac output. New studies have shown that an increased level of leptin, a hormone produced by adipose tissue, is associated with hypertension in obese children.[18] Ultimately, these factors impair the ability of the peripheral vascular bed to relax.

CLINICAL MANIFESTATIONS Most children with systemic hypertension are asymptomatic. It is necessary that a thorough history and physical examination be obtained. The examination should include an accurate blood pressure measurement obtained in the right arm with the arm supported at the level of the heart; three separate measurements using an appropriate-size cuff also are needed for an accurate blood pressure reading.[16-18]

EVALUATION AND TREATMENT In children, the history and physical examination should be directed at determining the etiology of hypertension, such as COA or renal disease (Table 25-6). A complete blood count, serum chemistry levels (including blood urea nitrogen and creatinine), uric acid level, urinalysis, urine culture, lipid profile, and renal ultrasound are part of the routine evaluation for renal disease (Table 25-7). Blood pressure differential between upper and lower extremities and echocardiography can be used to identify COA. If COA is found, surgical correction or balloon angioplasty with or without a stent is initiated, depending on the child's age and the severity of the coarctation. If hypertension is determined to be essential, or primary, in nature, nonpharmacological therapy is used initially. Moderate weight loss and exercise can decrease systolic and diastolic pressures in many children. Appropriate diet, regular physical activity, and avoidance of smoking have been shown to be effective in reducing blood pressure.[1]

HEALTH PROMOTION

Childhood Obesity in Canada

In 2016, the Standing Senate Committee on Social Affairs, Science and Technology reported that approximately 13% of children between the ages of 5 and 17 were obese, while another 20% were overweight. These numbers reflect a three-fold increase in the proportion of obese children since 1980. The Heart and Stroke Foundation of Canada's *2017 Report on the Health of Canadians* concluded that obesity in Canadian children can be linked to the marketing strategies used by food and beverages companies for unhealthy, low-cost choices. These easily accessible and heavily marketed food and beverages are often energy-dense and nutrient-poor, such as processed foods and sugary drinks. The report added that sugary drinks are the single largest provider of sugar in diets, as one can of pop contributes to about the recommended daily maximum. It is estimated that 90% of food and beverages marketed on TV are high in salt, fat, or sugar. Children tend to be directly impacted by these ads because the average child watches about 2 hours of TV a day and sees four to five food and beverage ads per hour. Canadian children and youth spend almost 8 hours a day in front of screens.

Before 5 years of age, most children cannot distinguish ads from unbiased programming. Children younger than 8 years of age do not understand the intent of marketing messages and believe what they see. By age 10 to 12, children understand that ads are designed to sell products, but they are not always able to be critical of these ads.

Another factor contributing to childhood obesity is the weight of the mother when she enters pregnancy. Studies have shown that regardless of the mother's prepregnancy weight, the risk of childhood obesity increases by 30 to 40% when a woman enters pregnancy overweight or obese, or when she gains excessive weight during pregnancy. Overweight and obese mothers are three times more likely to exceed the recommended weight gain guidelines during pregnancy than are healthy weight women, leading to the delivery of larger babies. Larger infants are more likely than healthy weight babies to become overweight children, who grow into overweight and obese adolescents. The cycle continues when these overweight young women become pregnant.

Notably, Quebec has the lowest obesity rate among children ages 6 to 11 and the highest rate of vegetable and fruit consumption in Canada. In Quebec, a law enacted in 1980 banned commercial advertising of all goods and services to children under 13, which has resulted in a 13% reduction (compared with Ontario) in the likelihood to purchase fast food.

The Heart and Stroke Foundation of Canada suggests that parents apply the following recommendations to protect their children from childhood obesity:

- Limit children's screen time.
- Provide a balanced diet including a variety of natural, whole, and minimally processed foods.
- Encourage children to eat more vegetables and fruit and choose whole grains.
- Avoid buying processed and prepackaged foods and sugary drinks.
- Prepare meals at home as much as possible.
- Involve children and youth in planning and preparing meals.
- Promote, encourage, and support policies that create healthier environments for children, including restrictions around food and beverage marketing.

Heart and Stroke Foundation of Canada. (2017). *2017 report on the health of Canadians: The kids are not alright.* Ottawa: Author. Retrieved from https://www.heartandstroke.ca/-/media/pdf-files/canada/2017-heart-month/heartandstroke-reportonhealth2017.ashx; The Standing Senate Committee on Social Affairs, Science and Technology. (2016). *Obesity in Canada: A whole-of-society approach for a healthier Canada.* Ottawa: Author, pp. 1–2, 18. Retrieved from https://sencanada.ca/content/sen/committee/421/SOCI/Reports/2016-02-25_Revised_report_Obesity_in_Canada_e.pdf.

TABLE 25-6 Most Common Causes of Chronic Sustained Hypertension

Age Group	Causes
Newborn	Renal artery thrombosis, renal artery stenosis, congenital renal malformation, COA, bronchopulmonary dysplasia
<6 years	Renal parenchymal disease, COA, renal artery stenosis
6–10 years	Renal artery stenosis, renal parenchymal disease, primary hypertension
>10 years	Primary hypertension, renal parenchymal disease

COA, coarctation of the aorta.
From Park, M.K. (2014). *Pediatric cardiology for practitioners* (6th ed.). St. Louis: Mosby.

TABLE 25-7 Routine and Special Laboratory Tests for Hypertension

Laboratory Tests	Significance of Abnormal Results
Urinalysis, urine culture, blood urea nitrogen, and creatinine levels	Renal parenchymal disease
Serum electrolyte levels (hypokalemia)	Hyperaldosteronism, primary or secondary Adrenogenital syndrome Renin-producing tumours
ECG, chest X-ray studies	Cardiac cause of hypertension, also baseline function
Intravenous pyelography (or ultrasonography, radionuclide studies, computed tomography of kidneys)	Renal parenchymal diseases Renovascular hypertension Tumours (neuroblastoma, Wilms tumour)
Plasma renin activity, peripheral	High-renin hypertension Renovascular hypertension Renin-producing tumours Some caused by Cushing's syndrome Some caused by essential hypertension Low-renin hypertension Adrenogenital syndrome Primary hyperaldosteronism
24-hr urine collection for 17-ketosteroids and 17-hydroxycorticosteroids	Cushing's syndrome Adrenogenital syndrome
24-hr urine collection for catecholamine levels and vanillylmandelic acid	Pheochromocytoma Neuroblastoma
Aldosterone	Hyperaldosteronism, primary or secondary Renovascular hypertension Renin-producing tumours
Renal vein plasma renin activity	Unilateral renal parenchymal disease Renovascular hypertension
Abdominal aortogram	Renovascular hypertension Abdominal COA Unilateral renal parenchymal diseases Pheochromocytoma
Intra-arterial digit subtraction angiography	Renovascular hypertension

COA, coarctation of the aorta; *ECG*, electrocardiogram.
From Park, M.K. (2014). *Pediatric cardiology for practitioners* (6th ed.). St. Louis: Mosby.

Ambulatory blood pressure monitoring (ABPM) has the potential to become an important tool in the evaluation and management of childhood hypertension.[19]

Medication therapy is controversial in children with primary hypertension; however, when nonpharmacological therapy fails, the approach is similar to the treatment of hypertension in adults with the use of angiotensin-converting enzyme inhibitors or angiotensin receptor blocker medications.[2,17] The current emphasis on preventive cardiology, especially for children, is significant because many investigators believe signs of atherosclerosis are present during childhood.[1,16-18]

QUICK CHECK 25-2

1. Why are the infant's height, weight, and head circumference important in the assessment of heart failure?
2. Why is it critical to recognize and treat children during the acute phase of Kawasaki disease?
3. Discuss the causes of obesity in children and the cardiovascular effects.

DID YOU UNDERSTAND?

Congenital Heart Disease

1. Most instances of congenital heart disease (CHD) have begun to develop by the eighth week of gestation, and some are associated with environmental and genetic risk factors.
2. Environmental risk factors associated with the incidence of CHD typically are (a) maternal conditions, including intrauterine viral infections, diabetes mellitus, medications, and complications of advanced maternal age; (b) antepartal bleeding; and (c) prematurity.
3. Genetic risk factors associated with CHD include, but are not limited to, Down syndrome, trisomies 13 and 18, cri du chat syndrome, and Turner's syndrome.
4. Classification of a congenital heart defect is based on (a) whether the defect causes cyanosis, (b) whether the defect causes increased or decreased blood flow into the pulmonary circulation, and (c) whether the defect causes obstruction of blood flow from the ventricles.
5. Cyanosis, a bluish discoloration of the skin, indicates that the tissues are not receiving normal amounts of oxygenated blood. Cyanosis can be caused by defects that (a) restrict blood flow into the pulmonary circulation; (b) overload the pulmonary circulation, causing pulmonary overcirculation, pulmonary edema, and respiratory difficulty; or (c) cause large amounts of unoxygenated blood to shunt from the pulmonary to the systemic circulation.
6. Congenital heart defects that maintain or create direct communication between the pulmonary and systemic circulatory systems cause blood to shunt from one system to another, mixing oxygenated and unoxygenated blood and increasing blood volume and, occasionally, pressure on the receiving side of the shunt.
7. The direction of shunting through an abnormal communication depends on differences in pressure and resistance between the two systems. Flow is always from an area of high pressure to an area of low pressure.
8. Acyanotic heart defects that increase pulmonary blood flow consist of abnormal openings (atrial septal defect, ventricular septal defect, patent ductus arteriosus, or atrioventricular canal defect) that permit blood to shunt from left (systemic circulation) to right (pulmonary circulation). Cyanosis does not occur because the left-to-right shunt does not interfere with the flow of oxygenated blood through the systemic circulation.
9. Obstruction of ventricular outflow is commonly caused by aortic stenosis (left ventricle) or pulmonary stenosis (right ventricle).
10. In less severe obstruction, ventricular outflow remains normal because of compensatory ventricular hypertrophy stimulated by increased afterload and, in postductal coarctation of the aorta (COA), development of collateral circulation around the coarctation.
11. If the abnormal communication between the left and right circuits is large, volume and pressure overload in the pulmonary circulation can lead to left ventricular failure.
12. Cyanotic congenital defects in which saturated and desaturated blood mix within the heart or great arteries include tetralogy of Fallot (TOF), transposition of the great arteries, total anomalous pulmonary venous connection, truncus arteriosus, and hypoplastic left heart syndrome.
13. In cyanotic heart defects that decrease pulmonary blood flow (TOF), myocardial hypertrophy cannot compensate for restricted right ventricular outflow. Flow to the lungs decreases, and cyanosis is caused by an insufficient volume of oxygenated blood and right-to-left shunt.
14. Heart failure (HF) is usually the result of congenital heart defects that increase blood volume in the pulmonary circulation. A clinical manifestation of HF unique to children is failure to thrive.
15. Initial treatment for CHD, depending on the defect, is aimed at controlling the level of HF symptoms or cyanosis. Interventional procedures in the cardiac catheterization laboratory and surgical palliation or repair are performed to establish a source of pulmonary blood flow or restore normal circulation.

Acquired Cardiovascular Disorders

1. Two examples of acquired heart disease in children are Kawasaki disease (KD) and systemic hypertension.
2. KD is an acute systemic vasculitis that also may result in the development of coronary artery aneurysms and thrombosis if untreated.
3. Systemic hypertension in children differs from hypertension in adults in etiology and presentation. When significant hypertension is found in a young child, the examiner should evaluate for the presence of secondary hypertension, most commonly renal disease or COA.

KEY TERMS

Acyanotic heart defect, 663
Aortic stenosis (AS), 664
Atrial septal defect (ASD), 667
Atrioventricular canal (AVC) defect (atrioventricular septal defect [AVSD], endocardial cushion defect [ECD]), 668
Coarctation of the aorta (COA), 664
Congenital heart disease (CHD), 662
Cyanosis, 663
Cyanotic heart defect, 663
Eisenmenger's syndrome, 668
Foramen ovale, 667
Heart failure (HF), 672
Hypoplastic left heart syndrome (HLHS), 672
Kawasaki disease (KD), 673
Left-to-right shunt, 662
Muscular ventricular septal defect, 668

Ostium primum atrial septal defect, 667
Ostium secundum atrial septal defect, 667
Patent ductus arteriosus (PDA), 667
Patent foramen ovale (PFO), 667
Perimembranous ventricular septal defect, 668
Pulmonary atresia, 666
Pulmonary stenosis (PS), 666
Right-to-left shunt, 663
Shunt, 662
Sinus venosus atrial septal defect, 667
Subvalvular aortic stenosis, 664
Supravalvular aortic stenosis, 665
Systemic hypertension, 674
Tetralogy of Fallot (TOF), 668
Total anomalous pulmonary venous connection (TAPVC), 670
Transposition of the great arteries (TGA; transposition of the great vessels [TGV]), 670
Tricuspid atresia, 669
Truncus arteriosus (TA), 671
Valvular aortic stenosis, 664
Ventricular septal defect (VSD), 668

REFERENCES

1. Allen, H. D. (Ed.), (2012). *Moss and Adams' heart disease in infants, children, and adolescents including the fetus and young adults* (8th ed.). Philadelphia: Lippincott Williams & Wilkins.
2. Park, M. K. (2014). *Pediatric cardiology for practitioners* (6th ed.). St Louis: Mosby. Retrieved from http://mdconsult/book.
3. Canadian Congenital Heart Alliance. (2016). *CHD facts and issues.* Retrieved from http://www.cchaforlife.org/facts-issues.
4. Vergales, J. E., Gangemi, J. J., Rhueban, K. S., et al. (2013). Coarctation of the aorta—The current state of surgical and transcatheter therapies. *Current Cardiology Reviews, 9*(3), 211–219. doi:10.2174/1573403X113099990032.
5. Feltes, T. F., Bacha, E., Beekman, R. H., 3rd., et al. (2011). Indications for cardiac catheterization and intervention in pediatric heart disease: A scientific statement from the American Heart Association. *Circulation, 123*(22), 2607–2625. doi:10.1161/CIR.0b013e31821b1f10.
6. Ng, R., Järvinen, A., & Bellugi, U. (2014). Characterizing associations and dissociations between anxiety, social and cognitive phenotypes of Williams syndrome. *Research in Developmental Disabilities, 35*(10), 2403–2415. doi:10.1016/j.ridd.2014.06.010.
7. Hockenberry, M. J., & Wilson, D. (Eds.), (2011). *Wong's nursing care of infants and children* (9th ed.). St. Louis: Mosby.
8. Geva, T., Martins, J. D., & Wald, R. M. (2014). Atrial septal defects. *Lancet, 383*(9932), 1921–1932. doi:10.1016/S0140-6736(13)62145-5.
9. Penny, D. J., & Vick, G. W. (2011). Ventricular septal defect. *Lancet, 377*(9771), 1103–1112. doi:10.1016/S0140-6736(10)61339-6.
10. Schranz, D., & Michel-Behnke, I. (2013). Advances in interventional and hybrid therapy in neonatal congenital heart disease. *Seminars in Fetal and Neonatal Medicine, 18*(5), 311–321. doi:10.1016/j.siny.2013.05.005.
11. Pike, N. A., Evangelista, L. S., Doering, L. V., et al. (2011). Clinical profile of the adolescent/adult Fontan survivor. *Congenital Heart Disease, 6*(1), 9–17. doi:10.1111/j.1747-0803.2010.00475.x.
12. Pike, N. A., Evangelista, L. S., Doering, L. V., et al. (2012). Quality of life, health status and depression in adolescents and adults after the Fontan procedure compared to healthy counterparts. *Journal of Cardiovascular Nursing, 27*(6), 539–546. doi:10.1097/JCN.0b013e31822ce5f6.
13. Rossano, J. W., & Shaddy, R. E. (2014). Heart failure in children: Etiology and treatment. *Journal of Pediatrics, 165*(2), 228–233. doi:10.1016/j.jpeds.2014.04.055.
14. Eleftheriou, D., Levin, M., Shingadia, D., et al. (2014). Management of Kawasaki disease. *Archives of Disease in Childhood, 99*(1), 74–83. doi:10.1136/archdischild-2012-302841.
15. National High Blood Pressure Education Program Working Group on High Blood Pressure in Children and Adolescents. (2004). The fourth report on the diagnosis, evaluation and treatment of high blood pressure in children and adolescents. *Pediatrics, 114*(Suppl. 2, 4th rep.), 555–576.
16. Gauer, R., Belprez, M., & Rerucha, C. (2014). Pediatric hypertension: Often missed and mismanaged. *Journal of Family Practice, 63*(3), 129–136.
17. Riley, M., & Bluhm, B. (2012). High blood pressure in children and adolescents. *American Family Physician, 85*(7), 693–700.
18. Flynn, J. T. (2012). The changing face of pediatric hypertension in the era of the childhood obesity epidemic. *Pediatric Nephrology (Berlin, Germany), 28*(7), 1059–1066. doi:10.1007/s00467-012-2344-0.
19. Flynn, J. T., Daniels, S. R., Hayman, L. L., et al. (2014). Update: ambulatory blood pressure monitoring in children and adolescents: A scientific statement from the American Heart Association. *Hypertension, 63*(5), 1116–1135. doi:10.1161/HYP.0000000000000007.

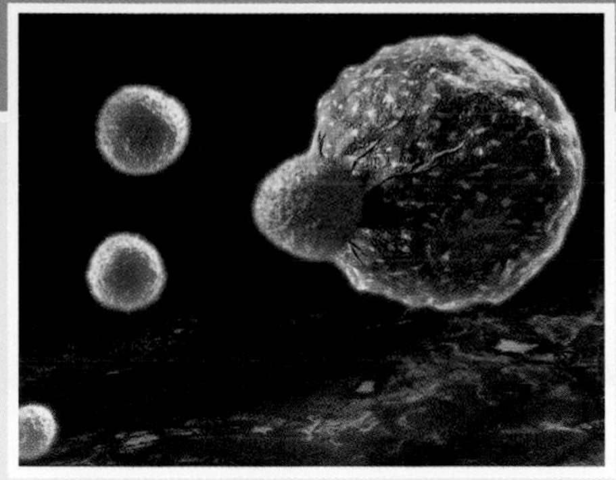

26

Structure and Function of the Pulmonary System

Valentina L. Brashers and Mohamed El-Hussein

EVOLVE WEBSITE

http://evolve.elsevier.com/Canada/Huether/pathophysiology

Student Review Questions
Key Points
Case Studies
Animations
Quick Check Answers

CHAPTER OUTLINE

Structures of the Pulmonary System, 679
- Conducting Airways, 679
- Gas-Exchange Airways, 680
- Pulmonary and Bronchial Circulation, 681
- Control of the Pulmonary Circulation, 683
- Chest Wall and Pleura, 683

Function of the Pulmonary System, 684
- Ventilation, 684
- Neurochemical Control of Ventilation, 684
- Mechanics of Breathing, 686
- Gas Transport, 688

***GERIATRIC CONSIDERATIONS:* Aging and the Pulmonary System, 692**

The primary function of the pulmonary system is the exchange of gases between the environmental air and the blood. The three steps in this process are (1) ventilation, the movement of air into and out of the lungs; (2) diffusion, the movement of gases between air spaces in the lungs and the bloodstream; and (3) perfusion, the movement of blood into and out of the capillary beds of the lungs to body organs and tissues. The first two steps are carried out by the pulmonary system and the third by the cardiovascular system (see Chapter 23). Normally the pulmonary system functions efficiently under a variety of conditions and with little energy expenditure.

STRUCTURES OF THE PULMONARY SYSTEM

The pulmonary system includes two lungs, the upper and lower airways, the blood vessels that serve these structures (Figure 26-1), the diaphragm, and the chest wall or thoracic cage. The lungs are divided into lobes: three in the right lung (upper, middle, lower) and two in the left lung (upper, lower). Each lobe is further divided into segments and lobules. The **mediastinum** is the space between the lungs and contains the heart, great vessels, and esophagus. A set of conducting airways, or bronchi, delivers air to each section of the lung. The lung tissue that surrounds the airways supports them, preventing distortion or collapse of the airways as gas moves in and out during ventilation. The diaphragm is a dome-shaped muscle that separates the thoracic and abdominal cavities and is involved in ventilation.

The lungs are protected from exogenous contaminants by a series of mechanical barriers (Table 26-1). These defence mechanisms are so effective that, in the healthy individual, contamination of the lung tissue itself, particularly by infectious agents, is rare.

Conducting Airways

The conducting airways allow air into and out of the gas-exchange structures of the lung. The **nasopharynx**, **oropharynx**, and related structures are often called the *upper airway* (Figure 26-2). These structures are lined with a ciliated mucosa that warms and humidifies inspired air and removes foreign particles from it. The mouth and oropharynx are used for ventilation when the nose is obstructed or when increased flow is required (e.g., during exercise). Filtering and humidifying are not as efficient with mouth breathing.

The **larynx** connects the upper and lower airways and consists of the endolarynx and its surrounding triangular-shaped bony and cartilaginous structures. The endolarynx encompasses two pairs of folds: the false vocal cords (supraglottis) and the true vocal cords. The slit-shaped space between the true cords forms the glottis (see Figure 26-2). The vestibule is the space above the false vocal cords. The laryngeal box is formed of three large cartilages (epiglottis, thyroid, cricoid) and three smaller cartilages (arytenoid, corniculate, cuneiform) connected by ligaments. The supporting cartilages prevent collapse of the larynx during inspiration and swallowing. The internal laryngeal muscles control vocal cord length and tension, and the external laryngeal muscles move the larynx as a whole. Both sets of muscles are important to swallowing, ventilation, and vocalization.[1] The internal muscles contract during swallowing to prevent aspiration into the trachea. These muscles also contribute to voice pitch.

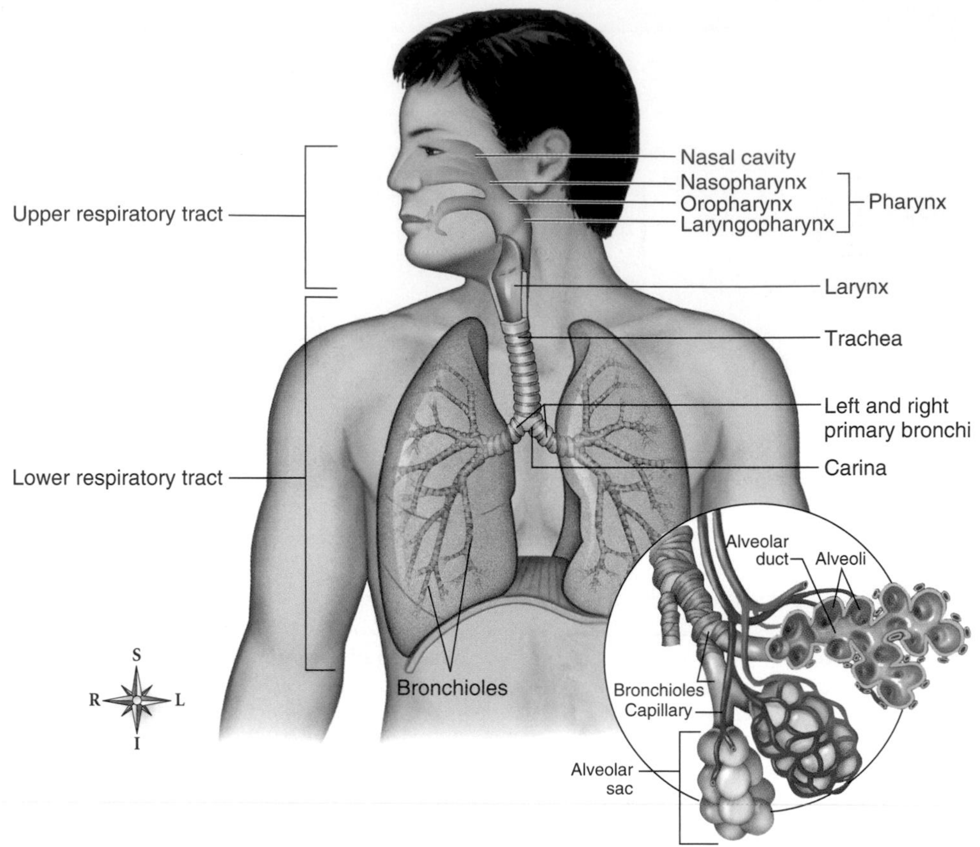

FIGURE 26-1 Structure of the Pulmonary System. The upper and lower respiratory tracts (airways) are illustrated. The enlargement in the circle depicts the acinus, where oxygen and carbon dioxide are exchanged. (From Patton, K.T., & Thibodeau, G.A. [2016]. *Structure & function of the body* [15th ed.]. St. Louis: Mosby.)

TABLE 26-1 Pulmonary Defence Mechanisms

Structure or Substance	Mechanism of Defence
Upper respiratory tract mucosa	Maintains constant temperature and humidification of gas entering lungs; traps and removes foreign particles, some bacteria, and noxious gases from inspired air
Nasal hairs and turbinates	Trap and remove foreign particles, some bacteria, and noxious gases from inspired air
Mucous blanket	Protects trachea and bronchi from injury; traps most foreign particles and bacteria that reach lower airways
Cilia	Propel mucous blanket and entrapped particles toward oropharynx, where they can be swallowed or expectorated
Irritant receptors in nares (nostrils)	Trigger sneeze reflex when stimulated by chemical or mechanical irritants, resulting in the rapid removal of irritants from nasal passages
Irritant receptors in trachea and large airways	Trigger cough reflex when stimulated by chemical or mechanical irritants, resulting in the removal of irritants from lower airways
Alveolar macrophages	Ingest and remove bacteria and other foreign material from alveoli by phagocytosis (see Chapters 6 and 7)

The trachea, which is supported by U-shaped cartilage, connects the larynx to the bronchi, the conducting airways of the lungs. The trachea branches into two main airways, or bronchi (*sing.*, bronchus), at the carina (see Figure 26-1). The right and left main bronchi enter the lungs at the hila (*sing.*, hilum), or "roots" of the lungs, along with the pulmonary blood and lymphatic vessels. From the hila the main bronchi branch further, as shown in Figure 26-3.

The bronchial walls have three layers: an epithelial lining, a smooth muscle layer, and a connective tissue layer. The epithelial lining of the bronchi contains single-celled exocrine glands—the mucous-secreting goblet cells—and ciliated cells. The goblet cells produce a mucous blanket that protects the airway epithelium, and the ciliated epithelial cells rhythmically beat this mucous blanket toward the trachea and pharynx where it can be swallowed or expectorated by coughing. The layers of epithelium that line the bronchi become thinner with each successive branching (see Figure 26-3).

Gas-Exchange Airways

The conducting airways terminate in the respiratory bronchioles, alveolar ducts, and alveoli (*sing.*, alveolus). These thin-walled structures together are sometimes called the acinus (see Figures 26-1 and 26-3), and all of them participate in gas exchange.[2]

The alveoli are the primary gas-exchange units of the lung, where oxygen (O_2) enters the blood and carbon dioxide (CO_2) is removed

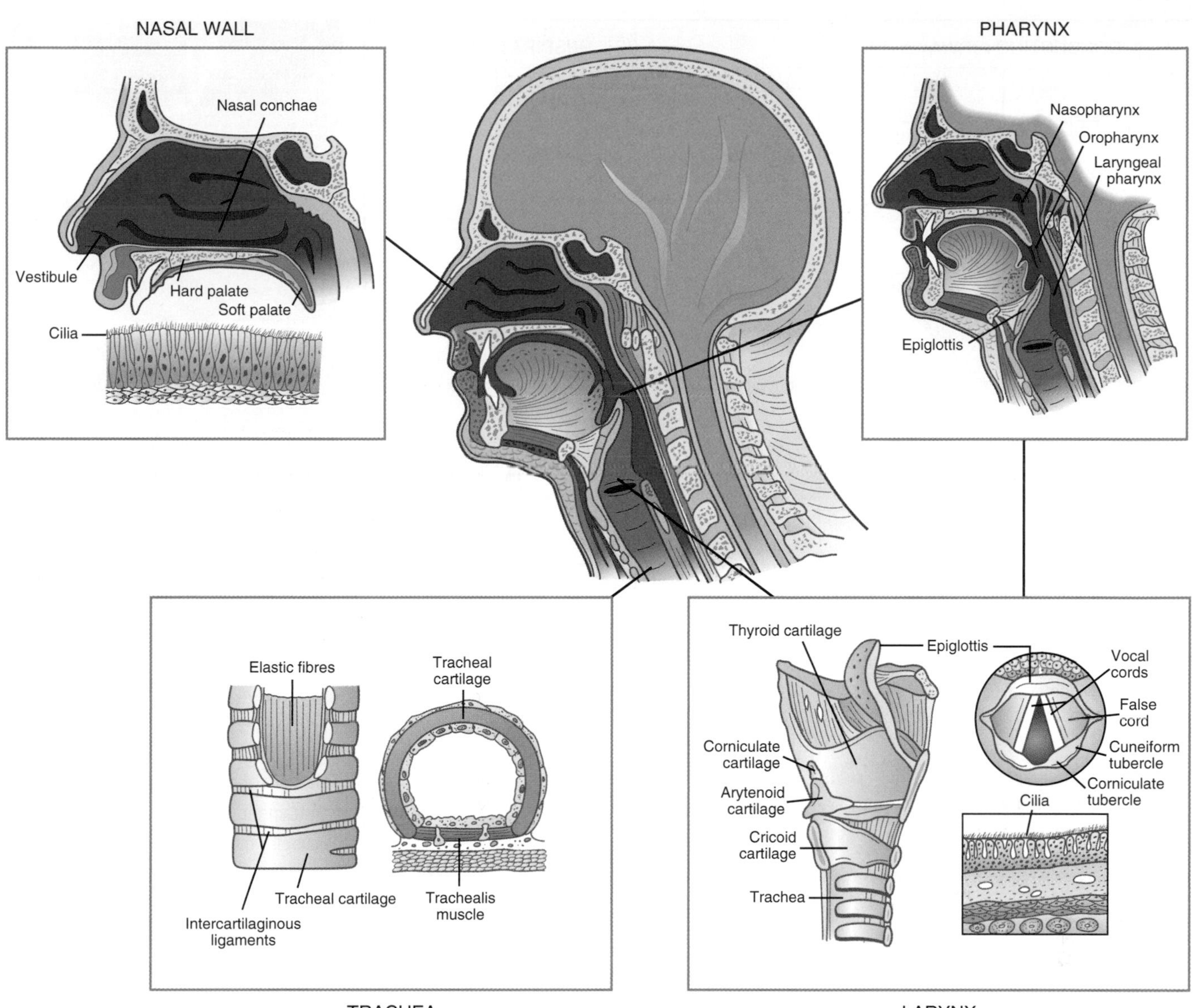

FIGURE 26-2 Structures of the Upper Airway. (Redrawn from Thompson, J.M., McFarland, G.K., Hirsch, J.E., et al. [2002]. *Mosby's clinical nursing* [5th ed.]. St. Louis: Mosby.)

(Figure 26-4). Tiny passages called *pores of Kohn* permit some air to pass through the septa from alveolus to alveolus, promoting collateral ventilation and even distribution of air among the alveoli. The lungs contain approximately 25 million alveoli at birth and 300 million by adulthood.

Lung epithelial cells provide a protective interface with the environment and are essential for adequate gas exchange, preventing entry of foreign agents, regulating ion and water transport, and maintaining mechanical stability of the alveoli.[3] Two major types of epithelial cells appear in the alveolus. Type I alveolar cells provide structure, and type II alveolar cells secrete **surfactant**, a lipoprotein that coats the inner surface of the alveolus and lowers alveolar surface tension at end-expiration, thereby preventing lung collapse.[1,2,4,5]

Like the bronchi, alveoli contain cellular components of immunity and inflammation, particularly the mononuclear phagocytes (called *alveolar macrophages*). These cells ingest foreign material that reaches the alveolus and prepare it for removal through the lymphatics. (Phagocytosis and the mononuclear phagocyte system are described in Chapters 6 and 7.)

QUICK CHECK 26-1

1. List the major components of the pulmonary system.
2. Which components of the pulmonary system contribute to the body's defence?
3. What are conducting airways?
4. Describe an alveolus.

Pulmonary and Bronchial Circulation

The pulmonary circulation facilitates gas exchange, delivers nutrients to lung tissues, acts as a reservoir for the left ventricle, and serves as a filtering system that removes clots, air, and other debris from the circulation.

Although the entire cardiac output from the right ventricle goes into the lungs, the pulmonary circulation has a lower pressure and resistance than the systemic circulation. Pulmonary arteries are exposed to about one-fifth of the pressure of the systemic circulation. Usually about one-third of the pulmonary vessels are filled with blood (perfused) at any given time. More vessels become perfused when right

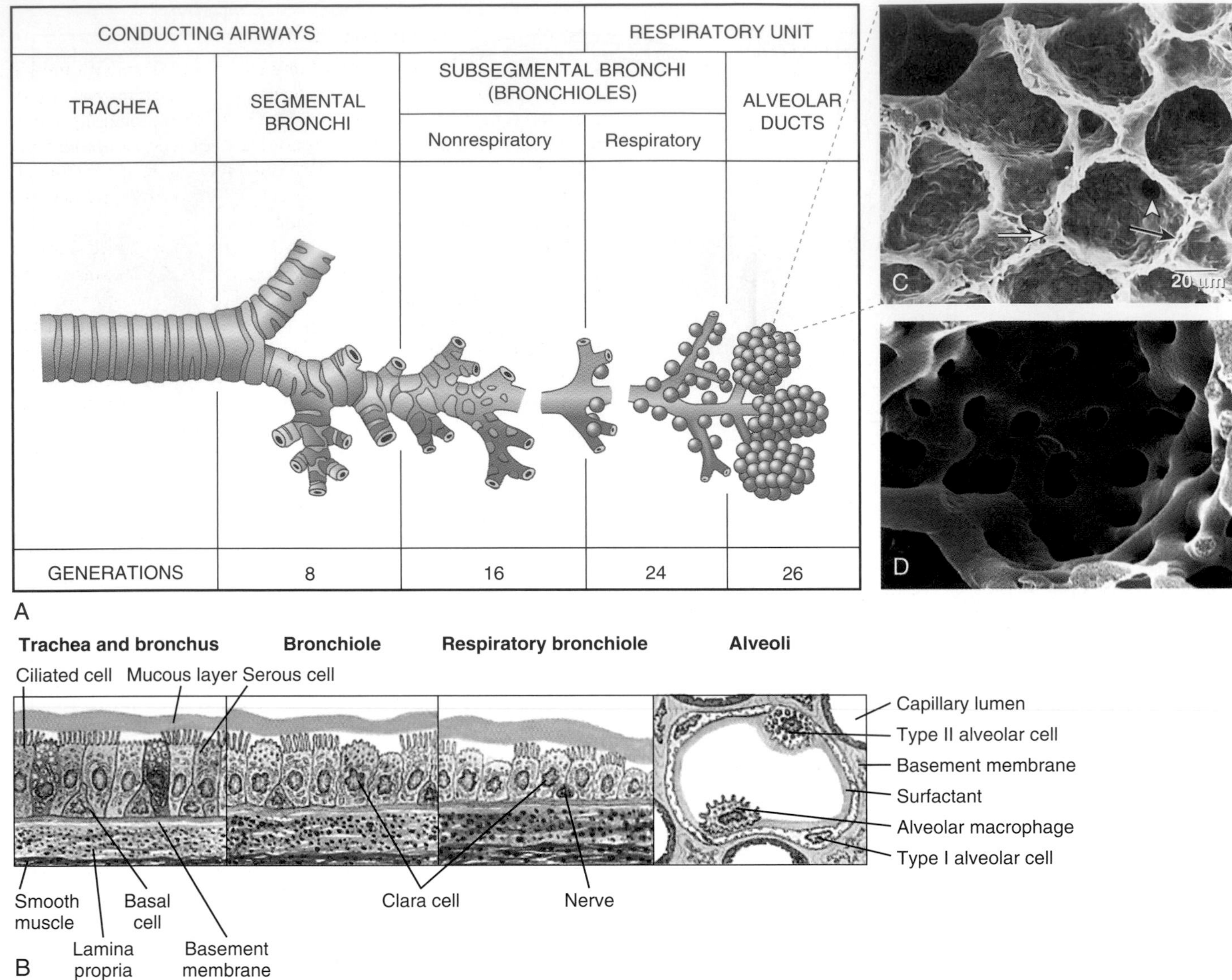

FIGURE 26-3 Structures of the Lower Airway. **A,** Structures of lower respiratory airway. **B,** Changes in bronchial wall with progressive branching. **C,** Electron micrograph of alveoli: *long white arrow* identifies type II pneumocyte (secretes surfactant); *white arrowhead* identifies pores of Kohn; *red arrow* identifies alveolar capillary. **D,** Plastic cast of pulmonary capillaries at high magnification. (**A,** Redrawn from Thompson, J.M., McFarland, G.K., Hirsch, J.E., et al. [2002]. *Mosby's clinical nursing* [5th ed.]. St. Louis: Mosby; **B,** from Wilson, S.F., & Thompson, J.M. [1990]. *Respiratory disorders.* St. Louis: Mosby; **C,** from Mason, R.J., Broaddus, M.D., Martin, T.R., et al. [2010]. *Murray and Nadel's textbook of respiratory medicine* [5th ed.]. Philadelphia: Saunders; **D,** courtesy A. Churg, MD, and J. Wright, MD, Vancouver, Canada. From Leslie, K.O., & Wick, M.R. [2011]. *Practical pulmonary pathology: a diagnostic approach* [2nd ed.]. Philadelphia: Saunders.)

ventricular cardiac output increases. Therefore, increased delivery of blood to the lungs does not normally increase mean pulmonary artery pressure.

The pulmonary artery divides and enters the lung at the hila, branching with each main bronchus and with all bronchi at every division. Thus, every bronchus and bronchiole has an accompanying artery or arteriole. The arterioles divide at the terminal bronchioles to form a network of pulmonary capillaries around the acinus. Capillary walls consist of an endothelial layer and a thin basement membrane, which often fuses with the basement membrane of the alveolar septum. Consequently, there is very little separation between blood in the capillary and gas in the alveolus.

The shared alveolar and capillary walls compose the **alveolocapillary membrane** (respiratory membrane) (Figure 26-5). Gas exchange occurs across this membrane. With normal perfusion, approximately 100 mL of blood in the pulmonary capillary bed is spread very thinly over 70 to 100 m^2 of alveolar surface area. Any disorder that thickens the membrane impairs gas exchange.

Each pulmonary vein drains several pulmonary capillaries. Unlike the pulmonary arteries, pulmonary veins are dispersed randomly throughout the lung and then leave the lung at the hila and enter the left atrium. They have no valves.

The bronchial circulation is part of the systemic circulation, and it both moistens inspired air and supplies nutrients to the conducting airways, large pulmonary vessels, and membranes (pleurae) that surround the lungs. Not all of its capillaries drain into its own venous system. Some empty into the pulmonary vein and contribute to the normal venous mixture of oxygenated and deoxygenated blood or right-to-left

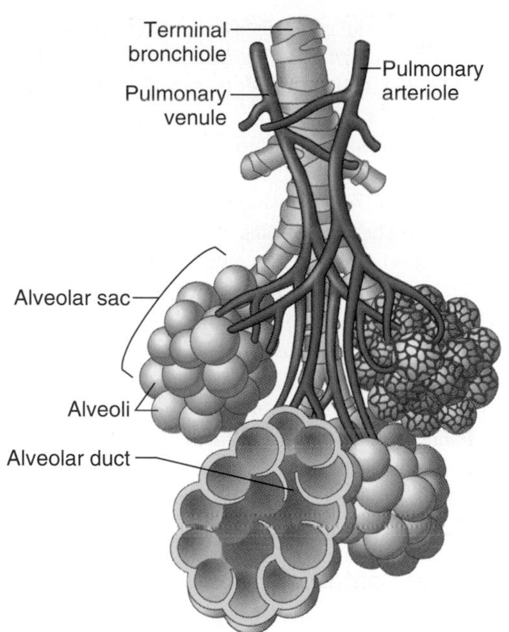

FIGURE 26-4 Alveoli. Bronchioles subdivide to form tiny tubes called *alveolar ducts*, which end in clusters of alveoli called *alveolar sacs*. (From Patton, K.T., & Thibodeau, G.A. [2014]. *The human body in health & disease* [6th ed.]. St. Louis: Mosby.)

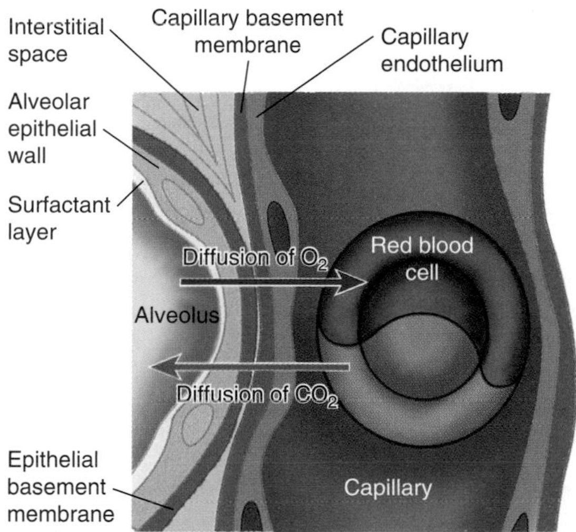

FIGURE 26-5 Cross-Section Through an Alveolus Showing Histology of the Alveolar-Capillary Membrane (Respiratory Membrane). The dense network of capillaries forms an almost continuous sheet of blood in the alveolar walls, providing a very efficient arrangement for gas exchange. CO_2, carbon dioxide; O_2, oxygen. (Adapted from Montague, S.E., Watson, R., & Herbert, R. [2005]. *Physiology for nursing practice* [3rd ed.]. London: Elsevier.)

shunt (right-to-left shunts are described in Chapter 27). The bronchial circulation does not participate in gas exchange.[6]

Lung vasculature also includes deep and superficial pulmonary lymphatic capillaries. Fluid and alveolar macrophages migrate from the alveoli to the terminal bronchioles, where they enter the lymphatic system. Both deep and superficial lymphatic vessels leave the lung at the hilum through a series of mediastinal lymph nodes. The lymphatic system plays an important role in both providing immune defence and keeping the lung free of fluid. (The lymphatic system is described in Chapter 23.)

Control of the Pulmonary Circulation

The calibre of pulmonary artery lumina decreases as smooth muscle in the arterial walls contracts. Contraction increases pulmonary artery pressure. Calibre increases as these muscles relax, decreasing blood pressure. Contraction (vasoconstriction) and relaxation (vasodilation) primarily occur in response to local humoral conditions, even though the pulmonary circulation is innervated by the autonomic nervous system (ANS), as is the systemic circulation.

The most important cause of pulmonary artery constriction is a low alveolar partial pressure of oxygen (Po_2). Vasoconstriction is caused by alveolar and pulmonary venous hypoxia, often termed **hypoxic pulmonary vasoconstriction**, and results from an increase in intracellular calcium levels in vascular smooth muscle cells in response to low O_2 concentration and the presence of charged O_2 molecules called *oxygen radicals*.[7] It can affect only one portion of the lung (i.e., one lobe that is obstructed, decreasing its partial pressure of oxygen in alveolar gas [P_AO_2]) or the entire lung. If only one segment of the lung is involved, the arterioles to that segment constrict, shunting blood to other, well-ventilated portions of the lung. This reflex improves the lung's efficiency by better matching ventilation and perfusion. If all segments of the lung are affected, however, vasoconstriction occurs throughout the pulmonary vasculature and pulmonary hypertension (elevated pulmonary artery pressure) can result. The pulmonary vasoconstriction caused by low alveolar Po_2 is reversible if the alveolar Po_2 is corrected. Chronic alveolar hypoxia can result in structural changes in pulmonary arterioles causing permanent pulmonary artery hypertension, which eventually leads to right ventricular failure (cor pulmonale).[7]

Acidemia also causes pulmonary artery constriction. If the acidemia is corrected, the vasoconstriction is reversed. (Respiratory acidosis and metabolic acidosis are described in Chapter 5.) An elevated partial pressure of carbon dioxide in arterial blood ($PaCO_2$) value without a drop in pH does not cause pulmonary artery constriction. Other biochemical factors that affect the calibre of vessels in pulmonary circulation are histamine, prostaglandins, serotonin, nitric oxide, and bradykinin (see the *Geriatric Considerations:* Aging and the Pulmonary System box).

Chest Wall and Pleura

The chest wall (skin, ribs, intercostal muscles) protects the lungs from injury. The intercostal muscles of the chest wall, along with the diaphragm, accessory muscles, and abdominal muscles, perform the muscular work of breathing. The **thoracic cavity** is contained by the chest wall and encases the lungs (Figure 26-6). A serous membrane called the **pleura** (*pl.*, **pleurae**) adheres firmly to the lungs and then folds over itself and attaches firmly to the chest wall. The membrane covering the lungs is the *visceral pleura*; that lining the thoracic cavity is the *parietal pleura*. The area between the two pleurae is called the **pleural space**, or **pleural cavity**. Normally, only a thin layer of fluid secreted by the pleura (pleural fluid) fills the pleural space, lubricating the pleural surfaces and allowing the two layers to slide over each other without separating. Pressure in the pleural space is usually negative or subatmospheric (−4 to −10 mm Hg).

QUICK CHECK 26-2

1. What are the functions of the pulmonary circulation and of the bronchial circulation?
2. What is the most important factor causing pulmonary artery constriction? What other factors are involved?
3. What are the visceral and parietal pleurae?
4. What are the characteristics of the pleural space?

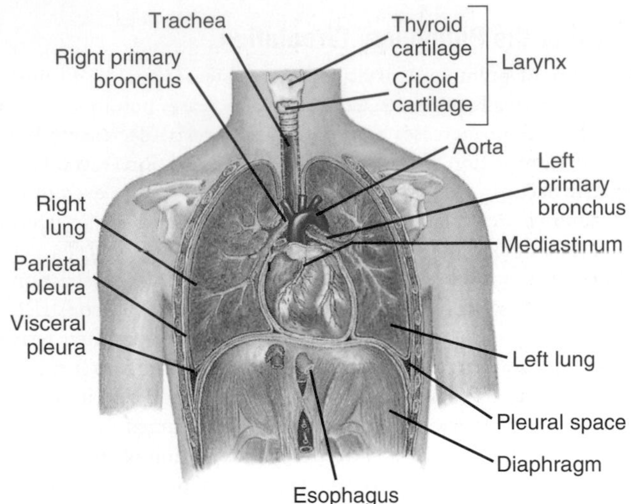

FIGURE 26-6 Thoracic (Chest) Cavity and Related Structures. The thoracic (chest) cavity is divided into three subdivisions (left and right pleural divisions and mediastinum) by a partition formed by a serous membrane called the *pleura.* (From Thibodeau, G.A., & Patton, K.T. [1996]. *Anatomy & physiology* [3rd ed.]. St. Louis: Mosby.)

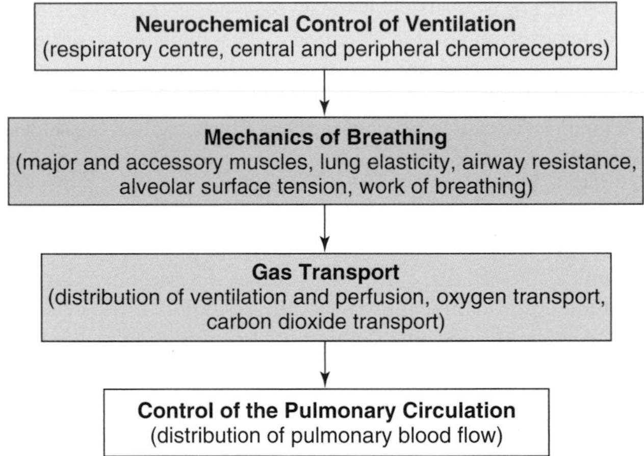

FIGURE 26-7 Functional Components of the Respiratory System. The central nervous system responds to neurochemical stimulation of ventilation and sends signals to the chest wall musculature. The response of the respiratory system to these impulses is influenced by several factors that impact the mechanisms of breathing and, therefore, affect the adequacy of ventilation. Gas transport between the alveoli and pulmonary capillary blood depends on a variety of physical and chemical activities. Finally, the control of the pulmonary circulation plays a role in the appropriate distribution of blood flow.

FUNCTION OF THE PULMONARY SYSTEM

The pulmonary system (1) ventilates the alveoli, (2) diffuses gases into and out of the blood, and (3) perfuses the lungs so that the organs and tissues of the body receive blood that is rich in O_2 and deficient in CO_2. Each component of the pulmonary system contributes to one or more of these functions (Figure 26-7).

Ventilation

Ventilation is the mechanical movement of gas or air into and out of the lungs. It is often misnamed *respiration,* which is actually the exchange of O_2 and CO_2 during cellular metabolism. "Respiratory rate" is actually the ventilatory rate, or the number of times gas is inspired and expired per minute. The amount of effective ventilation is calculated by multiplying the ventilatory rate (breaths per minute) by the volume or amount of air per breath (litres per breath or tidal volume). This is called the **minute volume** (or **minute ventilation**) and is expressed in litres per minute.

CO_2, the gaseous form of carbonic acid (H_2CO_3), is produced by cellular metabolism. The lung eliminates about 10 000 mmol of carbonic acid per day in the form of CO_2, which is produced at the rate of approximately 200 mL/min. CO_2 is eliminated to maintain a normal arterial CO_2 pressure ($PaCO_2$) of 40 mm Hg and normal acid-base balance (see Chapter 5 for a discussion of acid-base regulation). Adequate ventilation is necessary to maintain normal $PaCO_2$ levels. Diseases that limit ventilation result in CO_2 retention. The adequacy of **alveolar ventilation** *cannot* be accurately determined by observation of ventilatory rate, pattern, or effort. If a health care provider needs to determine the adequacy of ventilation, an arterial blood gas analysis must be performed to measure $PaCO_2$.

Neurochemical Control of Ventilation

Breathing is usually involuntary, because homeostatic changes in ventilatory rate and volume are adjusted automatically by the nervous system to maintain normal gas exchange. Voluntary breathing is necessary for talking, singing, laughing, and deliberately holding one's breath. The mechanisms that control respiration are complex (Figure 26-8).

The **respiratory centre** in the brainstem controls respiration by transmitting impulses to the respiratory muscles, causing them to contract and relax. The respiratory centre is composed of several groups of neurons: the dorsal respiratory group (DRG), the ventral respiratory group (VRG), the pneumotaxic centre, and the apneustic centre.[1,2,4]

The basic automatic rhythm of respiration is set by the DRG, which receives afferent input from **peripheral chemoreceptors** in the carotid and aortic bodies; from mechanical, neural, and chemical stimuli; and from receptors in the lungs.[8] The VRG contains both inspiratory and expiratory neurons and is almost inactive during normal, quiet respiration, becoming active when increased ventilatory effort is required. The pneumotaxic centre and apneustic centre, situated in the pons, do not generate primary rhythm but, rather, act as modifiers of the rhythm established by the medullary centres. The pattern of breathing can be influenced by emotion, pain, and disease.

Lung Receptors

Three types of lung receptors send impulses from the lungs to the DRG:

1. **Irritant receptors** (C fibres) are found in the epithelium of all conducting airways. They are sensitive to noxious aerosols (vapours), gases, and particulate matter (e.g., inhaled dusts), which cause them to initiate the cough reflex.[9] When stimulated, irritant receptors also cause bronchoconstriction and increased ventilatory rate.
2. **Stretch receptors** are located in the smooth muscles of airways and are sensitive to increases in the size or volume of the lungs. They decrease ventilatory rate and volume when stimulated, an occurrence sometimes referred to as the *Hering-Breuer reflex.* This reflex is active in newborns and assists with ventilation. In adults, this reflex is active only at high tidal volumes (such as with exercise) and may protect against excess lung inflation. Bronchopulmonary C fibres and a subset of stretch-sensitive, acid-sensitive myelinated sensory nerves mediate the cough reflex.[10]
3. **J-receptors** (juxtapulmonary capillary receptors) are located near the capillaries in the alveolar septa. They are sensitive to increased pulmonary capillary pressure, which stimulates them to initiate rapid, shallow breathing; hypotension; and bradycardia.[5]

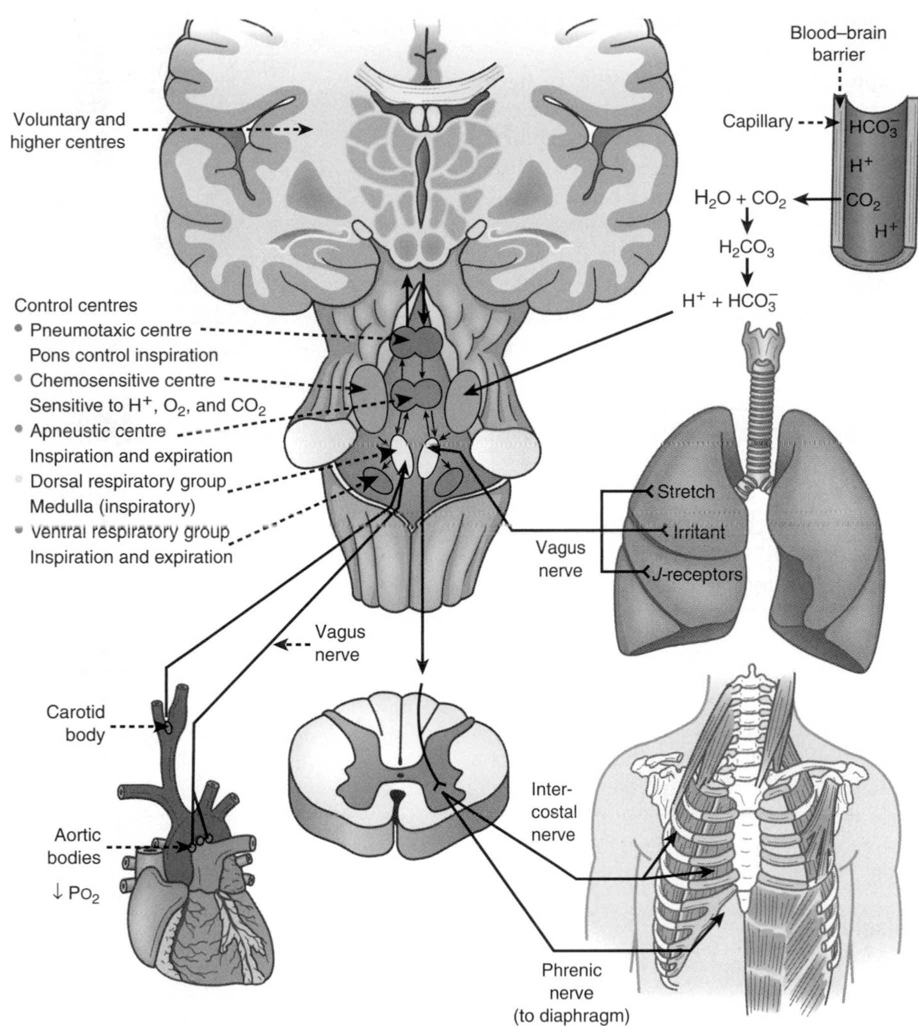

FIGURE 26-8 Neurochemical Respiratory Control System. *CO_2*, carbon dioxide; *H+*, hydrogen; *H_2CO_3*, carbonic acid; *H_2O*, water; *HCO_3^-*, bicarbonate; *O_2*, oxygen; *PO_2*, partial pressure of oxygen.

The lung is innervated by the ANS. Fibres of the sympathetic division in the lung branch from the upper thoracic and cervical ganglia of the spinal cord. Fibres of the parasympathetic division of the ANS travel in the vagus nerve to the lung. (Structures and function of the ANS are discussed in detail in Chapter 13.) The parasympathetic and sympathetic divisions control airway calibre (interior diameter of the airway lumen) by stimulating bronchial smooth muscle to contract or relax. The parasympathetic receptors cause smooth muscle to contract, whereas sympathetic receptors cause it to relax. Bronchial smooth muscle tone depends on equilibrium—that is, equal stimulation of contraction and relaxation. The parasympathetic division of the ANS is the main controller of airway calibre under normal conditions. Constriction occurs if the irritant receptors in the airway epithelium are stimulated by irritants in inspired air, by inflammatory mediators (e.g., histamine, serotonin, prostaglandins, leukotrienes), by many medications, and by humoral substances.

Chemoreceptors

Chemoreceptors monitor the pH, $PaCO_2$, and PaO_2 (partial pressure of oxygen in arterial blood) of arterial blood. **Central chemoreceptors** monitor arterial blood indirectly by sensing changes in the pH of cerebrospinal fluid (CSF) (see Figure 26-8).[11] They are located near the respiratory centre and are sensitive to hydrogen ion concentration in the CSF. (Chapter 5 describes the relationship between ions and the pH, or acid-base status, of body fluids.) The pH of the CSF reflects arterial pH because CO_2 in arterial blood can diffuse across the blood–brain barrier (the capillary wall separating blood from cells of the central nervous system) into the CSF until the partial pressure of carbon dioxide (PCO_2) is equal on both sides. CO_2 that has entered the CSF combines with water (H_2O) to form carbonic acid, which subsequently dissociates into hydrogen ions that are capable of stimulating the central chemoreceptors. In this way, $PaCO_2$ regulates ventilation through its impact on the pH (hydrogen ion content) of the CSF.[1,2,4,11]

If alveolar ventilation is inadequate, $PaCO_2$ increases. CO_2 diffuses across the blood–brain barrier until PCO_2 values in the blood and the CSF reach equilibrium. As the central chemoreceptors sense the resulting decrease in pH (increase in hydrogen ion concentration), they stimulate the respiratory centre to increase the depth and rate of ventilation. Increased ventilation causes the PCO_2 of arterial blood to decrease below that of the CSF, and CO_2 diffuses out of the CSF, returning its pH to normal.

The central chemoreceptors are sensitive to very small changes in the pH of CSF (equivalent to a 1 to 2 mm Hg change in PCO_2) and can maintain a normal $PaCO_2$ under many different conditions, including strenuous exercise.[11] If inadequate ventilation, or hypoventilation, is long term (e.g., in chronic obstructive pulmonary disease), these receptors become insensitive to small changes in $PaCO_2$ ("reset") and regulate ventilation poorly.[12]

The peripheral chemoreceptors are somewhat sensitive to changes in $PaCO_2$ and pH but are sensitive primarily to O_2 levels in arterial blood (PaO_2). As PaO_2 and pH decrease, peripheral chemoreceptors, particularly in the carotid bodies, send signals to the respiratory centre to increase ventilation. However, the PaO_2 must drop well below normal (to approximately 60 mm Hg) before the peripheral chemoreceptors have much influence on ventilation. If $PaCO_2$ is elevated as well, ventilation increases much more than it would in response to either abnormality alone. The peripheral chemoreceptors become the major stimulus to ventilation when the central chemoreceptors are reset by chronic hypoventilation.[13]

QUICK CHECK 26-3

1. What are the functions of the pulmonary system?
2. How do ventilation and respiration differ?
3. Describe three functions of the respiratory centre in the brainstem.
4. What are the three types of lung receptors?
5. How do the functions of central and peripheral chemoreceptors differ?

Mechanics of Breathing

The mechanical aspects of inspiration and expiration are known collectively as the *mechanics of breathing* and involve (1) major and accessory muscles of inspiration and expiration, (2) elastic properties of the lungs and chest wall, and (3) resistance to airflow through the conducting airways. Alterations in any of these properties increase the work of breathing or the metabolic energy needed to achieve adequate ventilation and oxygenation of the blood.

Major and Accessory Muscles

The major muscles of inspiration are the diaphragm and the external intercostal muscles (muscles between the ribs) (Figure 26-9). The diaphragm is a dome-shaped muscle that separates the abdominal and thoracic cavities. When it contracts and flattens downward, it increases the volume of the thoracic cavity, creating a negative pressure that draws gas into the lungs through the upper airways and trachea. Contraction of the external intercostal muscles elevates the anterior portion of the ribs and increases the volume of the thoracic cavity by increasing its front-to-back (anterior–posterior [AP]) diameter. Although the external intercostals may contract during quiet breathing, inspiration at rest is usually assisted by the diaphragm only.

The accessory muscles of inspiration are the sternocleidomastoid and scalene muscles. Like the external intercostals, these muscles enlarge the thorax by increasing its AP diameter. The accessory muscles assist inspiration when the minute volume (volume of air inspired and expired per minute) is high, as during strenuous exercise, or when the work of breathing is increased because of disease. The accessory muscles do not increase the volume of the thorax as efficiently as the diaphragm does.

There are no major muscles of expiration because normal, relaxed expiration is passive and requires no muscular effort. The accessory muscles of expiration, the abdominal and internal intercostal muscles, assist expiration when minute volume is high, during coughing, or when airway obstruction is present. When the abdominal muscles contract, intra-abdominal pressure increases, pushing up the diaphragm and decreasing the volume of the thorax. The internal intercostal muscles pull down the anterior ribs, decreasing the AP diameter of the thorax.

Alveolar Surface Tension

Surface tension occurs at any gas–liquid interface and refers to the tendency for liquid molecules that are exposed to air to adhere to one another. This phenomenon can be seen in the way liquids "bead" when splashed on a waterproof surface.

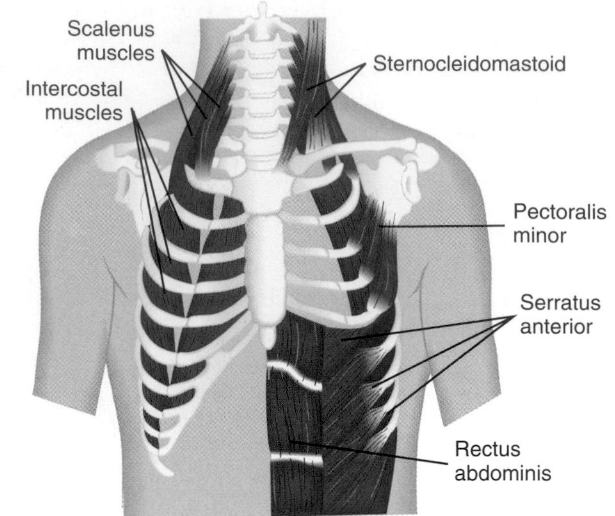

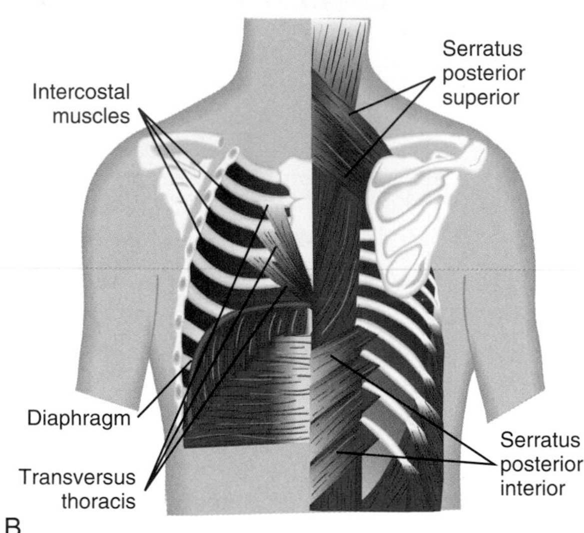

FIGURE 26-9 Muscles of Ventilation. A, Anterior view. **B,** Posterior view. (Modified from Thompson, J.M., McFarland, G.K., Hirsch, J.E., et al. [2002]. *Mosby's clinical nursing* [5th ed.]. St. Louis: Mosby.)

Within a sphere, such as an alveolus, surface tension tends to make expansion difficult. According to Laplace's law, the pressure (P) required to inflate a sphere is equal to two times the surface tension ($2T$) divided by the radius (r) of the sphere, or $P = 2T/r$. As the radius of the sphere (or alveolus) decreases, more and more pressure is required to inflate it. If the alveoli were lined only with a waterlike fluid, taking breaths would be extremely difficult.

Alveolar ventilation, or distension, is made possible by surfactant, which lowers surface tension by coating the air–liquid interface in the alveoli. Surfactant, a lipoprotein (90% lipids and 10% protein) produced by type II alveolar cells, includes two groups of *surfactant* proteins. One group consists of small hydrophobic molecules that have a detergentlike effect that separates the liquid molecules, thereby decreasing alveolar surface tension.[2,14] The second group of surfactant proteins consists of large hydrophilic molecules called **collectins** that are capable of inhibiting foreign pathogens (see Chapter 6).[15]

As the radius of an alveolus shrinks, the surface tension of the surfactant-lined sphere decreases, and as the radius expands, the surface tension increases. Thus, normal alveoli are much easier to inflate at low lung volumes (i.e., after expiration) than at high volumes (i.e., after inspiration). The decrease in surface tension caused by surfactant also is responsible for keeping the alveoli free of fluid. If surfactant is not produced in adequate quantities, alveolar surface tension increases, causing alveolar collapse, decreased lung expansion, increased work of breathing, and severe gas-exchange abnormalities.

Elastic Properties of the Lung and Chest Wall

The lung and chest wall have elastic properties that permit expansion during inspiration and return to resting volume during expiration. The elasticity of the lung is caused both by elastin fibres in the alveolar walls and surrounding the small airways and pulmonary capillaries, and by surface tension at the alveolar air–liquid interface.[13] The elasticity of the chest wall is the result of the configuration of its bones and musculature.

Elastic recoil is the tendency of the lungs and chest wall to return to the resting state after inspiration. Normal elastic recoil permits passive expiration, eliminating the need for major muscles of expiration. Passive elastic recoil may be insufficient during laboured breathing (high minute volume), when the accessory muscles of expiration may be needed. The accessory muscles are used also if disease compromises elastic recoil (e.g., in emphysema) or blocks the conducting airways.

Normal elastic recoil depends on an equilibrium between opposing forces of recoil in the lungs and chest wall. Under normal conditions, the chest wall tends to recoil by expanding outward. The tendency of the chest wall to recoil by expanding is balanced by the tendency of the lungs to recoil or inward collapse around the hila. The opposing forces of the chest wall and lungs create the small negative intrapleural pressure.

Balance between the outward recoil of the chest wall and inward recoil of the lungs occurs at the resting level, the end of expiration, where the functional residual capacity (FRC) is reached. However, muscular effort is needed to overcome lung resistance to expansion. During inspiration, the diaphragm and intercostal muscles contract, air flows into the lungs, and the chest wall expands. During expiration, the muscles relax and the elastic recoil of the lungs causes the thorax to decrease in volume until, once again, balance between the chest wall and lung recoil forces is reached (Figure 26-10).

Compliance is the measure of lung and chest wall distensibility and is defined as volume change per unit of pressure change. It represents the relative ease with which these structures can be stretched and is, therefore, the opposite of elasticity. Compliance is determined by the alveolar surface tension and the elastic recoil of the lung and chest wall.

Increased compliance indicates that the lungs or chest wall is abnormally easy to inflate and has lost some elastic recoil. A decrease

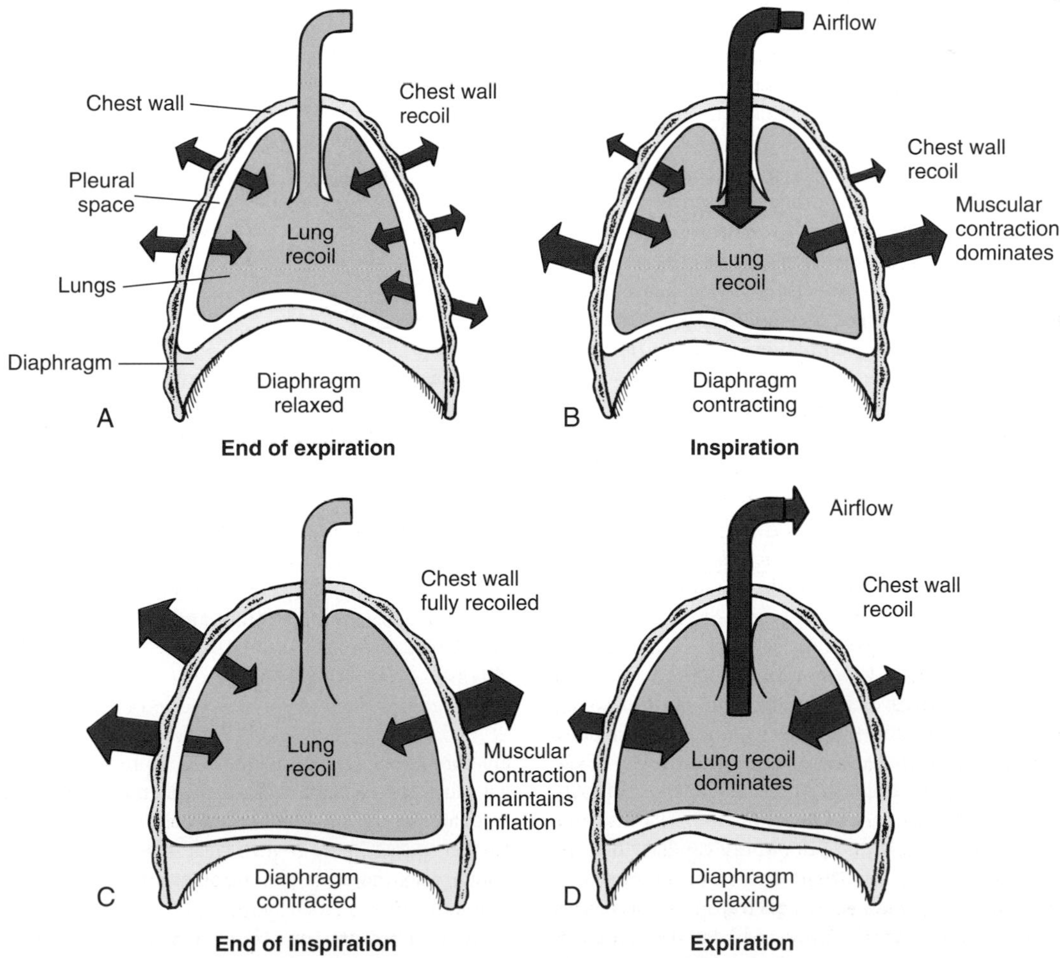

FIGURE 26-10 Interaction of Forces During Inspiration and Expiration. **A,** Outward recoil of the chest wall equals inward recoil of the lungs at the end of expiration. **B,** During inspiration, contraction of respiratory muscles, assisted by chest wall recoil, overcomes the tendency of lungs to recoil. **C,** At the end of inspiration, respiratory muscle contraction maintains lung expansion. **D,** During expiration, respiratory muscles relax, allowing elastic recoil of the lungs to deflate the lungs.

in compliance indicates that the lungs or chest wall is abnormally stiff or difficult to inflate. Compliance increases with normal aging and with disorders such as emphysema; it decreases in individuals with acute respiratory distress syndrome, pneumonia, pulmonary edema, and pulmonary fibrosis. (These disorders are described in Chapter 27.)

Airway Resistance

Airway resistance, which is similar to resistance to blood flow (described in Chapter 23), is determined by the length, radius, and cross-sectional area of the airways and by the density, viscosity, and velocity of the gas (Poiseuille's law). Resistance (R) is computed by dividing change in pressure (P) by rate of flow (F), or $R = P/F$ (Ohm's law). Airway resistance is normally very low. One-half to two-thirds of total airway resistance occurs in the nose. The next highest resistance is in the oropharynx and larynx. There is very little resistance in the conducting airways of the lungs because of their large cross-sectional area. Airway resistance is affected by the diameter of the airways. Bronchodilation, which decreases resistance to airflow, is caused by β_2-adrenergic receptor stimulation. Bronchoconstriction, which increases airway resistance, can be caused by stimulation of parasympathetic receptors in the bronchial smooth muscle and by numerous irritants and inflammatory mediators.[2] Airway resistance can also be increased by edema of the bronchial mucosa and by airway obstructions such as mucus, tumours, or foreign bodies. Pulmonary function tests (PFTs) measure lung volumes and flow rates and can be used to diagnose lung disease.

Work of Breathing

The work of breathing is determined by the muscular effort (and therefore O_2 and energy) required for ventilation. Normally very low, the work of breathing may increase considerably in diseases that disrupt the equilibrium between forces exerted by the lung and chest wall. More muscular effort is required when lung compliance decreases (e.g., in pulmonary edema), chest wall compliance decreases (e.g., in spinal deformity or obesity), or airways are obstructed by bronchospasm or mucous plugging (e.g., in asthma or bronchitis). An increase in the work of breathing can result in a marked increase in O_2 consumption and an inability to maintain adequate ventilation (Figure 26-11).

QUICK CHECK 26-4

1. Describe the work of the diaphragm in ventilation.
2. What is surfactant? What is its function?
3. How is elastic recoil related to compliance?
4. What causes changes in airway resistance?

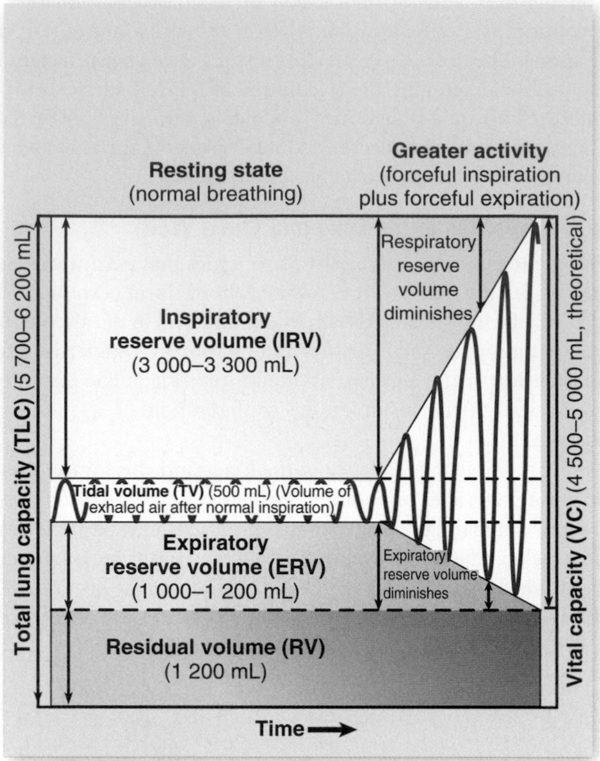

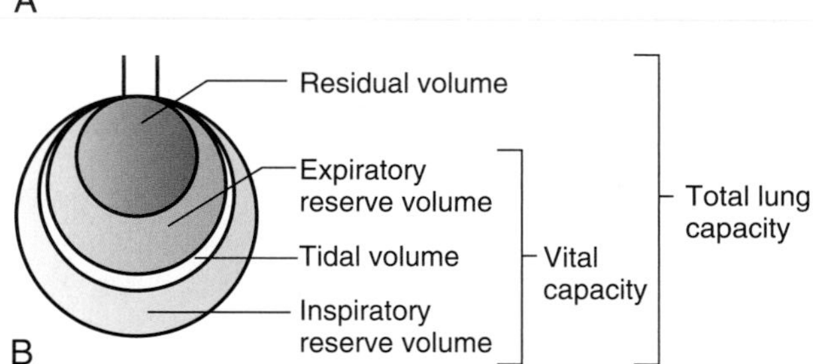

FIGURE 26-11 Pulmonary Ventilation and Lung Volumes. The chart in **A** shows a tracing like that produced with a spirometer. The diagram in **B** shows the pulmonary volumes as relative proportions of an inflated balloon. During normal, quiet breathing, about 500 mL of air is moved into and out of the respiratory tract (*TV*). During forceful breathing (like that during and after heavy exercise), an extra 3300 mL can be inspired (*IRV*), and an extra 1 000 mL or so can be expired (*ERV*). The largest volume of air that can be moved in and out during ventilation is called the vital capacity (*VC*). Air that remains in the respiratory tract after a forceful expiration is called the residual volume (*RV*). (From Patton, K.T., & Thibodeau, G.A. [2010]. *The human body in health & disease* [4th ed.]. St. Louis: Mosby.)

Gas Transport

Gas transport is the delivery of O_2 to the cells of the body and the removal of CO_2. It has four steps: (1) ventilation of the lungs, (2) diffusion of O_2 from the alveoli into the capillary blood, (3) perfusion of systemic capillaries with oxygenated blood, and (4) diffusion of O_2 from systemic capillaries into the cells. Steps in the transport of CO_2 occur in reverse order: (1) diffusion of CO_2 from the cells into the systemic capillaries, (2) perfusion of the pulmonary capillary bed by venous blood, (3) diffusion of CO_2 into the alveoli, and (4) removal of CO_2 from the lung by ventilation. If any step in gas transport is impaired by a respiratory or cardiovascular disorder, gas exchange at the cellular level is compromised.

Measurement of Gas Pressure

A gas is composed of millions of molecules moving randomly and colliding with each other and with the wall of the space in which they are contained. These collisions exert pressure. If the same number of gas molecules is contained in a small and a large container, the pressure is greater in the small container because more collisions occur in the smaller space (Figure 26-12). Heat increases the speed of the molecules, which also increases the number of collisions and, therefore, the pressure.

Barometric pressure (P_B) (atmospheric pressure) is the pressure exerted by gas molecules in air at specific altitudes. At sea level, P_B is 760 mm Hg and is the sum of the pressures exerted by each gas in the air at sea level. The portion of the total pressure exerted by any individual gas is its partial pressure (see Figure 26-12). At sea level, the air consists of O_2 (20.9%), nitrogen (78.1%), and a few other trace gases. The

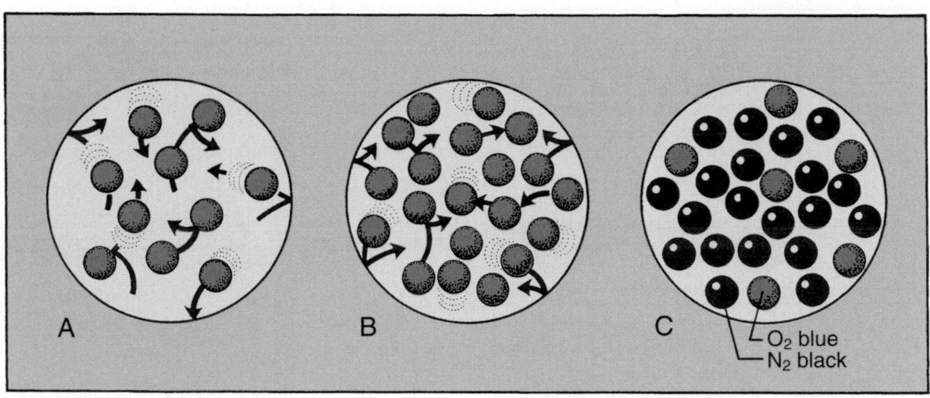

FIGURE 26-12 Relationship Between Number of Gas Molecules and Pressure Exerted by the Gas in an Enclosed Space. A, Theoretically, 10 molecules of the same gas exert a total pressure of 10 within the space. **B,** If the number of molecules is increased to 20, total pressure is 20. **C,** If there are different gases in the space, each gas exerts a partial pressure: here the partial pressure of nitrogen (*N_2*) is 20, that of oxygen (*O_2*) is 6, and the total pressure is 26.

TABLE 26-2 Common Pulmonary Abbreviations

Symbol	Definition
FEV_1	Forced expiratory volume in 1 second
FiO_2	Fraction of inspired oxygen
FRC	Functional residual capacity
FVC	Forced vital capacity
P	Pressure (usually partial pressure) of a gas
PaO_2	Partial pressure of oxygen in arterial blood
P_AO_2	Partial pressure of oxygen in alveolar gas
$P(A–a)O_2$	Difference between alveolar and arterial partial pressure of oxygen (A–a gradient)
$PaCO_2$	Partial pressure of carbon dioxide in arterial blood
P_B	Barometric or atmospheric pressure
$PvCO_2$	Venous partial pressure of carbon dioxide
PvO_2	Partial pressure of oxygen in mixed venous or pulmonary artery blood
Q	Perfusion or blood flow
SaO_2	Saturation of hemoglobin (in arterial blood) with oxygen
SvO_2	Saturation of hemoglobin (in mixed venous blood) with oxygen
V	Volume or amount of gas
V_A	Alveolar ventilation
V_D	Dead-space ventilation
V_E	Minute capacity
V_T	Tidal volume or average breath
$\dot{V}/\dot{Q}$	Ratio of ventilation to perfusion (the overhead dot means measurement over time, usually 1 minute)

partial pressure of O_2 is equal to the percentage of O_2 in the air (20.9%) times the total P_B (760 mm Hg at sea level), or 159 mm Hg ($760 \times 0.209 = 158.84$ mm Hg). (Symbols used in the measurement of gas pressures and pulmonary ventilation are defined in Table 26-2.)

The amount of water vapour contained in a gas mixture is determined by the temperature of the gas and is unrelated to P_B. Gas that enters the lungs becomes saturated with water vapour (humidified) as it passes through the upper airway. At body temperature (37°C [98.6°F]), water vapour exerts a pressure of 47 mm Hg regardless of total P_B. The partial pressure of water vapour must be subtracted from the P_B before the partial pressures of other gases in the mixture can be determined. In saturated air at sea level, the partial pressure of O_2 is therefore $(760 - 47) \times 0.209 = 149$ mm Hg. All pressure and volume measurements made in pulmonary function laboratories specify the temperature and humidity of a gas at the time of measurement.

Many pressure measurements are stated as variations from P_B, rather than percentages of it. On such scales, P_B is considered zero, and pressure varies up or down from zero. Physiological pressure measurements that involve fluids, rather than gases, are measured as variations from P_B. For example, a systolic blood pressure of 120 mm Hg indicates that the systolic pressure is 120 mm Hg higher than P_B.

Distribution of Ventilation and Perfusion

Effective gas exchange depends on an approximately even distribution of gas (ventilation) and blood (perfusion) in all portions of the lungs.[1] The lungs are suspended from the hila in the thoracic cavity. When an individual is in an upright position (sitting or standing), gravity pulls the lungs down toward the diaphragm and compresses their lower portions or bases. The alveoli in the upper portions, or apices, of the lungs contain a greater residual volume of gas and are larger and less numerous than those in the lower portions. Because surface tension increases as the alveoli become larger, the larger alveoli in the upper portions of the lung are more difficult to inflate (less compliant) than the smaller alveoli in the lower portions of the lung. Therefore, during ventilation most of the tidal volume is distributed to the bases of the lungs, where compliance is greater.

The heart pumps against gravity to perfuse the pulmonary circulation. As blood is pumped into the lung apices of a sitting or standing individual, some blood pressure is dissipated in overcoming gravity. As a result, blood pressure at the apices is lower than that at the bases. Because greater pressure causes greater perfusion, the bases of the lungs are better perfused than the apices (Figure 26-13). Thus, ventilation and perfusion are greatest in the same lung portions—the lower lobes—and depend on body position. If a standing individual assumes a supine or side-lying position, the areas of the lungs that are then most dependent become the best ventilated and perfused.

Distribution of perfusion in the pulmonary circulation also is affected by alveolar pressure (gas pressure in the alveoli). The pulmonary capillary bed differs from the systemic capillary bed in that it is surrounded by gas-containing alveoli. If the gas pressure in the alveoli exceeds the blood pressure in the capillary, the capillary collapses and flow ceases.

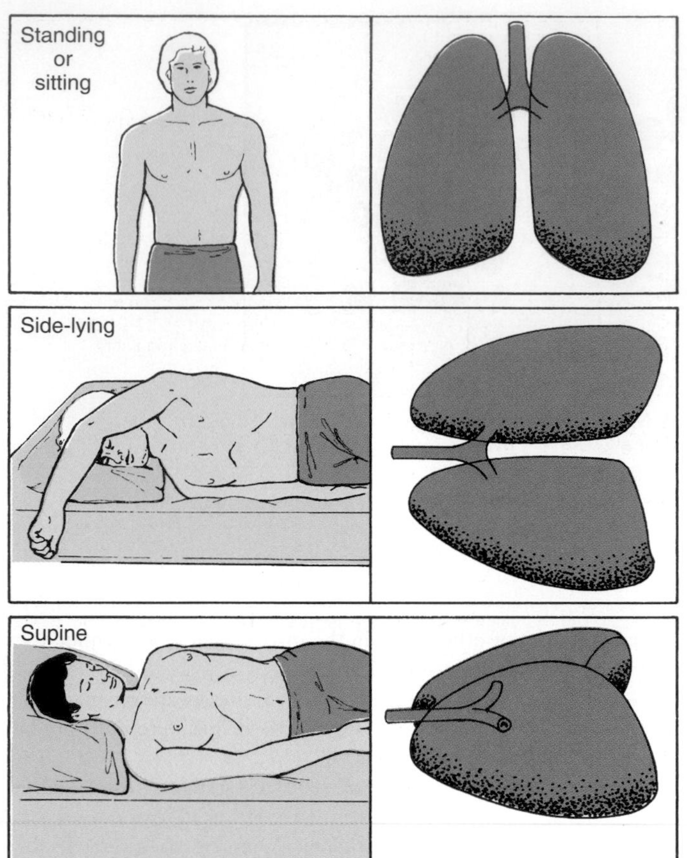

FIGURE 26-13 Pulmonary Blood Flow and Gravity. The greatest volume of pulmonary blood flow normally will occur in the gravity-dependent areas of the lung. Body position has a significant effect on the distribution of pulmonary blood flow. Shaded areas represent gravity-dependent pulmonary blood flow.

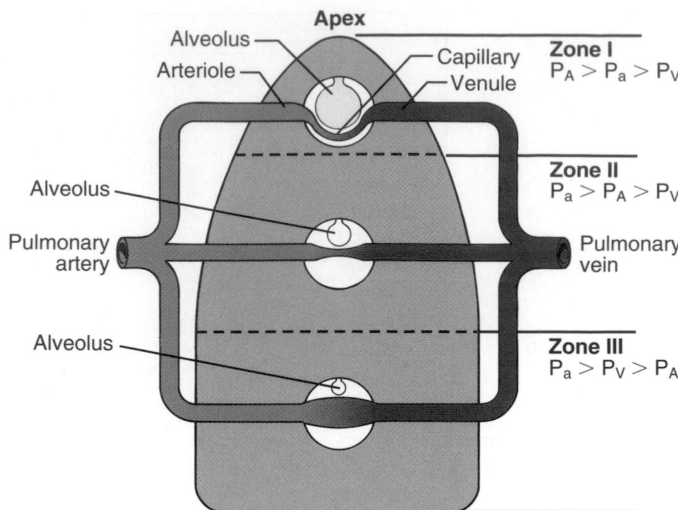

FIGURE 26-14 Gravity and Alveolar Pressure. Effects of gravity and alveolar pressure on pulmonary blood flow in the three lung zones. In zone I, alveolar pressure (P_A) is greater than arterial pressure (P_a) and venous pressure (P_V), and no blood flow occurs. In zone II, arterial pressure exceeds alveolar pressure, but alveolar pressure exceeds venous pressure. Blood flow occurs in this zone, but alveolar pressure compresses the venules (venous ends of the capillaries). In zone III, both arterial and venous pressures are greater than alveolar pressure and blood flow fluctuates depending on the difference between arterial pressure and venous pressure.

This outcome is most likely to occur in portions of the lung where blood pressure is lowest and alveolar gas pressure is greatest—that is, at the apex of the lung.

The lungs are divided into three zones on the basis of relationships among all the factors affecting pulmonary blood flow. Alveolar pressure and the forces of gravity, arterial blood pressure, and venous blood pressure affect the distribution of perfusion, as shown in Figure 26-14.

In zone I, alveolar pressure exceeds pulmonary arterial and venous pressures. The capillary bed collapses, and normal blood flow ceases. Normally zone I is a very small part of the lung at the apex. In zone II, alveolar pressure is greater than venous pressure but not arterial pressure. Blood flows through zone II, but it is impeded to a certain extent by alveolar pressure. Zone II is normally above the level of the left atrium. In zone III, both arterial and venous pressures are greater than alveolar pressure and blood flow is not affected by alveolar pressure. Zone III is in the base of the lung. Blood flow through the pulmonary capillary bed increases in regular increments from the apex to the base.

Although both blood flow and ventilation are greater at the base of the lungs than at the apices, they are not perfectly matched in any zone. Perfusion exceeds ventilation in the bases, and ventilation exceeds perfusion in the apices of the lung. The relationship between ventilation and perfusion is expressed as a ratio called the **ventilation–perfusion ratio** ($\dot{V}/\dot{Q}$).[1] The normal $\dot{V}/\dot{Q}$ is 0.8. This is the amount by which perfusion exceeds ventilation under normal conditions.

Oxygen Transport

Approximately 1 000 mL (1 L) of O_2 is transported to the cells of the body each minute. O_2 is transported in the blood in two forms: a small amount dissolves in plasma, and the remainder binds to hemoglobin molecules. Without hemoglobin, O_2 would not reach the cells in amounts sufficient to maintain normal metabolic function. (Hemoglobin is discussed in detail in Chapter 20, and cellular metabolism is explored in Chapter 1.)

Diffusion across the alveolocapillary membrane. The alveolocapillary membrane is ideal for O_2 diffusion because it has a large total surface area (70 to 100 m^2) and is very thin (0.5 μm). In addition, the partial pressure of oxygen molecules in alveolar gas (P_AO_2) is much greater than that in capillary blood, a condition that promotes rapid diffusion down the concentration gradient from the alveolus into the capillary. The partial pressure of oxygen (oxygen tension) in mixed venous or pulmonary artery blood (PvO_2) is approximately 40 mm Hg as it enters the capillary, and alveolar oxygen tension (P_AO_2) is approximately 100 mm Hg at sea level. Therefore, a pressure gradient of 60 mm Hg facilitates the diffusion of O_2 from the alveolus into the capillary (Figure 26-15).

Blood remains in the pulmonary capillary for about 0.75 second, but only 0.25 second is required for O_2 concentration to equilibrate (equalize) across the alveolocapillary membrane. Therefore, O_2 has ample time to diffuse into the blood, even during increased cardiac output, which speeds blood flow and shortens the time the blood remains in the capillary.

Determinants of arterial oxygenation. As O_2 diffuses across the alveolocapillary membrane, it dissolves in the plasma, where it exerts pressure (PaO_2). As the PaO_2 increases, O_2 moves from the plasma into the red blood cells (erythrocytes) and binds with hemoglobin molecules. O_2 continues to bind with hemoglobin until the hemoglobin-binding sites are filled or *saturated.* O_2 then continues to diffuse across the alveolocapillary membrane until the PaO_2 (O_2 dissolved in plasma) and

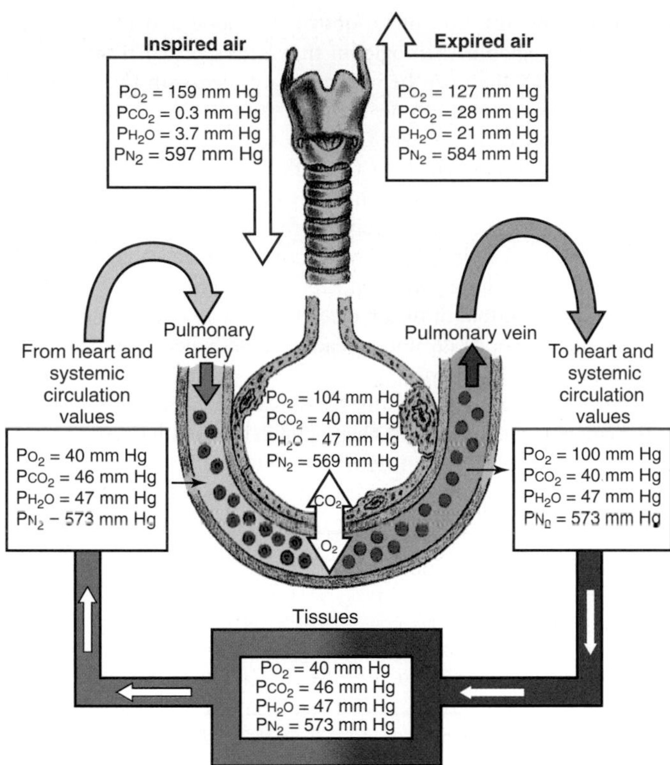

FIGURE 26-15 Partial Pressure of Respiratory Gases in Normal Respiration. The numbers shown are average values near sea level. The values of Po_2, Pco_2, and P_{N_2} fluctuate from breath to breath. *CO_2*, Carbon dioxide; *O_2*, oxygen; *Pco_2*, partial pressure of carbon dioxide; *P_{H_2O}*, partial pressure of water; *P_{N_2}*, partial pressure of nitrogen; *Po_2*, partial pressure of oxygen. (Modified from Thompson, J.M., McFarland, G.K., Hirsch, J.E., et al. [2002]. *Mosby's clinical nursing* [5th ed.]. St. Louis: Mosby.)

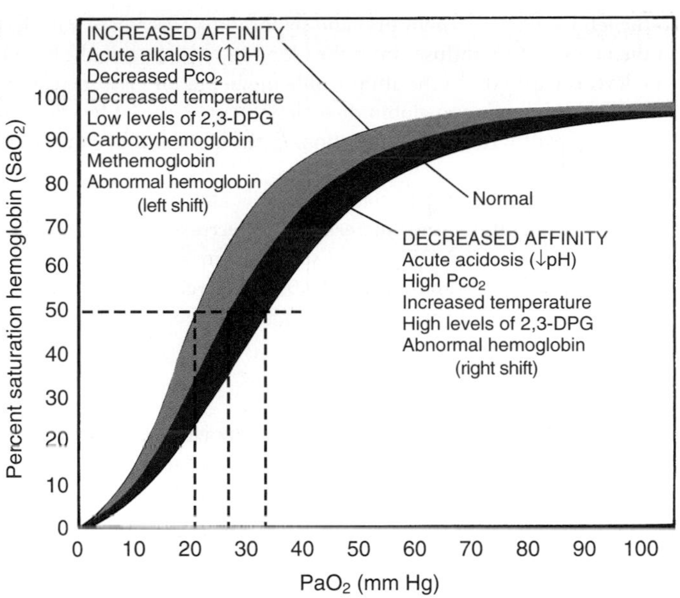

FIGURE 26-16 Oxyhemoglobin Dissociation Curve. The horizontal or flat segment of the curve at the top of the graph is the arterial or association portion, or that part of the curve where oxygen (O_2) is bound to hemoglobin and occurs in the lungs. This portion of the curve is flat because partial pressure changes of O_2 between 60 and 100 mm Hg do not significantly alter the percentage saturation of hemoglobin with O_2 and allow adequate hemoglobin saturation at a variety of altitudes. If the relationship between SaO_2 and PaO_2 was linear (in a downward sloping straight line) instead of flat between 60 and 100 mm Hg, there would be inadequate saturation of hemoglobin with O_2. The steep part of the oxyhemoglobin dissociation curve represents the rapid dissociation of O_2 from hemoglobin that occurs in the tissues. During this phase there is rapid diffusion of O_2 from the blood into tissue cells. The P_{50} is the PaO_2 at which hemoglobin is 50% saturated, normally 26.6 mm Hg. A lower than normal P_{50} represents increased affinity of hemoglobin for O_2; a high P_{50} is seen with decreased affinity. Note that variation from the normal is associated with decreased (low P_{50}) or increased (high P_{50}) availability of O_2 to tissues (*dashed lines*). The shaded area shows the entire oxyhemoglobin dissociation curve under the same circumstances. *2,3-DPG*, 2,3-Diphosphoglycerate; *PaO_2*, partial pressure of oxygen in arterial blood; *Pco_2*, partial pressure of carbon dioxide; *SaO_2*, saturation of hemoglobin (in arterial blood) with oxygen. (From Lane, E.E., & Walker, J.F. [1987]. *Clinical arterial blood gas analysis*. St. Louis: Mosby.)

P_AO_2 (O_2 in the alveolus) equilibrate, eliminating the pressure gradient across the alveolocapillary membrane. At this point, diffusion ceases (see Figure 26-15).

The majority (97%) of the O_2 that enters the blood is bound to hemoglobin. The remaining 3% stays in the plasma and creates PaO_2. The PaO_2 can be measured in the blood by obtaining an arterial blood gas measurement. **Oxygen saturation (SaO_2)** is the percentage of the available hemoglobin that is bound to O_2 and can be measured using a device called an *oximeter*.

Because hemoglobin transports all but a small fraction of the O_2 carried in arterial blood, changes in hemoglobin concentration affect the O_2 content of the blood. Decreases in hemoglobin concentration below the normal value of 150 g/L of blood reduce O_2 content, and increases in hemoglobin concentration may increase O_2 content, minimizing the impact of impaired gas exchange. In fact, increased hemoglobin concentration is a major compensatory mechanism in pulmonary diseases that impair gas exchange. For this reason, measurement of hemoglobin concentration is important in assessing individuals with pulmonary disease. If cardiovascular function is normal, the body's initial response to low O_2 content is to accelerate cardiac output. In individuals who also have cardiovascular disease, this compensatory mechanism is ineffective, making increased hemoglobin concentration an even more important compensatory mechanism. (Hemoglobin structure and function are described in Chapter 20.)

Oxyhemoglobin association and dissociation. When hemoglobin molecules bind with O_2, **oxyhemoglobin (HbO_2)** forms. Binding occurs in the lungs and is called *oxyhemoglobin association* or *hemoglobin saturation with oxygen* (SaO_2). The reverse process, where O_2 is released from hemoglobin, occurs in the body tissues at the cellular level and is called *hemoglobin desaturation*. When hemoglobin saturation and desaturation are plotted on a graph, the result is a distinctive S-shaped curve known as the **oxyhemoglobin dissociation curve** (Figure 26-16).

Several factors can change the relationship between PaO_2 and SaO_2, causing the oxyhemoglobin dissociation curve to shift to the right or left (see Figure 26-16). A shift to the right depicts hemoglobin's decreased affinity for O_2 or an increase in the ease with which oxyhemoglobin dissociates and O_2 moves into the cells. A shift to the left depicts hemoglobin's increased affinity for O_2, which promotes association in the lungs and inhibits dissociation in the tissues.

The oxyhemoglobin dissociation curve is shifted to the right by acidosis (low pH) and hypercapnia (increased $PaCO_2$). In the tissues, the increased levels of CO_2 and hydrogen ions produced by metabolic activity decrease the affinity of hemoglobin for O_2. The curve is shifted to the left by alkalosis (high pH) and hypocapnia (decreased $PaCO_2$). In the lungs, as CO_2 diffuses from the blood into the alveoli, the blood CO_2 level is reduced and the affinity of hemoglobin for O_2 is increased. The shift in the oxyhemoglobin dissociation curve caused by changes in CO_2 and hydrogen ion concentrations in the blood is called the **Bohr effect**.

The oxyhemoglobin dissociation curve is also shifted by changes in body temperature and increased or decreased levels of 2,3-diphosphoglycerate (2,3-DPG), a substance normally present in erythrocytes. Hyperthermia and increased 2,3-DPG levels shift the curve to the right. Hypothermia and decreased 2,3-DPG levels shift the curve to the left.

Carbon Dioxide Transport

CO_2 is carried in the blood in three ways: (1) dissolved in plasma (PCO_2), (2) as bicarbonate (HCO_3^-), and (3) as carbamino compounds. As CO_2 diffuses out of the cells into the blood, it dissolves in the plasma. Approximately 10% of the total CO_2 in venous blood and 5% of the CO_2 in arterial blood are transported dissolved in the plasma (venous partial pressure of carbon dioxide [$PvCO_2$] and $PaCO_2$, respectively). As CO_2 moves into the blood, it diffuses into the red blood cells. Within the red blood cells, CO_2, with the help of the enzyme carbonic anhydrase, combines with water to form carbonic acid and then quickly dissociates into hydrogen and bicarbonate. As carbonic acid dissociates, the hydrogen binds to hemoglobin, where it is buffered, and the bicarbonate moves out of the red blood cell into the plasma. Approximately 60% of the CO_2 in venous blood and 90% of the CO_2 in arterial blood are carried in the form of bicarbonate. The remainder combines with blood proteins, hemoglobin in particular, to form carbamino compounds. Approximately 30% of the CO_2 in venous blood and 5% of the CO_2 in arterial blood are carried as carbamino compounds.

CO_2 is 20 times more soluble than O_2 and diffuses quickly from the tissue cells into the blood. The amount of CO_2 able to enter the blood is enhanced by diffusion of O_2 out of the blood and into the cells. Reduced hemoglobin (hemoglobin that is dissociated from O_2) can carry more CO_2 than can hemoglobin saturated with O_2. Therefore, the drop in oxygen saturation (SO_2) at the tissue level increases the ability of hemoglobin to carry CO_2 back to the lung.

The diffusion gradient for CO_2 in the lung is only approximately 6 mm Hg (venous PCO_2 = 46 mm Hg; alveolar PCO_2 = 40 mm Hg) (see Figure 26-15). Yet CO_2 is so soluble in the alveolocapillary membrane that the CO_2 in the blood quickly diffuses into the alveoli, where it is removed from the lung with each expiration. Diffusion of CO_2 in the lung is so efficient that diffusion defects that cause hypoxemia (low O_2 content of the blood) do not as readily cause hypercapnia (excessive CO_2 in the blood).

The diffusion of CO_2 out of the blood is also enhanced by O_2 binding with hemoglobin in the lung. As hemoglobin binds with O_2, the amount of CO_2 carried by the blood decreases. Thus, in the tissue capillaries, O_2 dissociation from hemoglobin facilitates the pickup of CO_2, and the binding of O_2 to hemoglobin in the lungs facilitates the release of CO_2 from the blood. This effect of O_2 on CO_2 transport is called the **Haldane effect**.

QUICK CHECK 26-5

1. What are the eight steps of gas transport?
2. What is barometric pressure? How is it related to physiological pressure measurements?
3. Describe the relationship between ventilation and pulmonary blood flow.
4. What is the alveolocapillary membrane? How does it function in ventilation and perfusion?
5. Describe the process of oxyhemoglobin association and dissociation.

GERIATRIC CONSIDERATIONS

Aging and the Pulmonary System

Elasticity/Chest Wall

- Chest wall compliance decreases because ribs become ossified and joints are stiffer, which results in increased work of breathing.
- Kyphoscoliosis may curve the vertebral column, decreasing lung volumes.
- Intercostal muscle strength decreases.
- Elastic recoil diminishes, possibly the result of loss of elastic fibres.

Result: Lung compliance increases and vital capacity (VC) declines, residual volume (RV) increases, total lung capacity (TLC) is unchanged, ventilatory reserves decline, and ventilation–perfusion ratios fall.

Gas Exchange

- Pulmonary capillary network decreases.
- Alveoli dilate, and peripheral airways lose supporting tissues.
- Surface area for gas exchange decreases.
- pH and PCO_2 do not change much, but PO_2 declines.
- Sensitivity of respiratory centres to hypoxia or hypercapnia decreases.
- Ability to initiate an immune response against infection decreases.

NOTE: Maximum PaO_2 at sea level can be estimated by multiplying the person's age by 0.3 and subtracting the product from 100.

Exercise

- Decreased PaO_2 and diminished ventilatory reserve lead to decreased exercise tolerance.
- Early airway closure inhibits expiratory flow.
- Changes depend on activity and fitness levels earlier in life.
- An active, physically fit individual has fewer changes in function at any age than does a sedentary individual.
- Respiratory muscle strength and endurance decrease but can be enhanced by exercise.

Lung Immunity

- Alterations in alveolar complement and surfactant and an increase in proinflammatory cytokines increase the risk for pulmonary disease and infection.

GERIATRIC CONSIDERATIONS—cont'd

Aging and the Pulmonary System

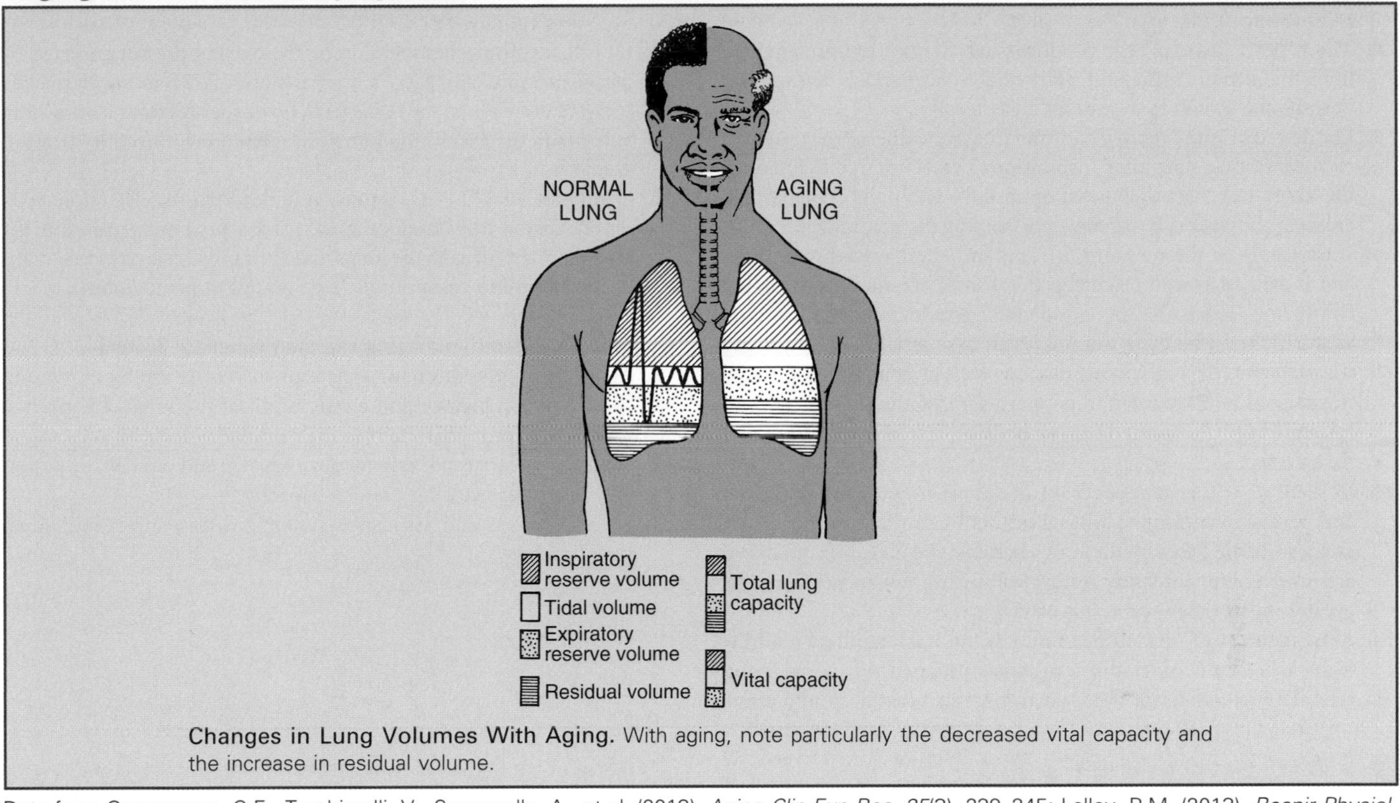

Changes in Lung Volumes With Aging. With aging, note particularly the decreased vital capacity and the increase in residual volume.

Data from Carpagnano, G.E., Turchiarelli, V., Spanevello, A., et al. (2013). *Aging Clin Exp Res, 25*(3), 239–245; Lalley, P.M. (2013). *Respir Physiol Neurobiol, 187*(3), 199–210; Lowery, E.M., Brubaker, A.L., Kuhlmann, E., et al. (2013). *Clin Interv Aging, 8*, 1489–1496; Miller, M.R. (2010). *Semin Respir Crit Care Med, 31*(5), 521–527; Moliva, J.I., Rajaram, M.V., Sasindran, S.J., et al. (2014). *Age (Dordr), 36*(3), 9633; Ramly, E., Kaafarani, H.M., & Velmahos, G.C. (2015). *Surg Clin North Am, 95*(1), 53–69; Weiss, C.O., Hoenig, H.H., Varadhan, R., et al. (2010). *J Gerontol A Biol Sci Med Sci, 65*(3), 287–294.

DID YOU UNDERSTAND?

Structures of the Pulmonary System

1. The pulmonary system consists of two lungs, the upper and lower airways, chest wall, and pulmonary and bronchial circulation.
2. Air is inspired and expired through the conducting airways: nasopharynx, oropharynx, trachea, bronchi, and bronchioles.
3. Gas exchange occurs in structures beyond the respiratory bronchioles: in the alveolar ducts and the alveoli. Together these structures compose the acinus.
4. The primary gas-exchange units of the lungs are the alveoli. The membrane that surrounds each alveolus and contains the pulmonary capillaries is called the *alveolocapillary membrane.*
5. The gas-exchange airways are perfused by the pulmonary circulation, a separate division of the circulatory system. The bronchi and other lung structures are perfused by a branch of the systemic circulation called the *bronchial circulation.*
6. The pulmonary circulation is innervated by the autonomic nervous system (ANS), but vasodilation and vasoconstriction are controlled mainly by local and humoral factors, particularly arterial oxygenation and acid-base status.
7. The chest wall, which contains and protects the contents of the thoracic cavity, consists of the skin, ribs, and intercostal muscles (which lie between the ribs).
8. The chest wall is lined by a serous membrane called the *parietal pleura*; the lungs are encased in a separate membrane called the *visceral pleura*. The *pleural space* is the area where these two pleurae contact and slide over one another.

Function of the Pulmonary System

1. The pulmonary system enables oxygen (O_2) to diffuse into the blood and carbon dioxide (CO_2) to diffuse out of the blood.
2. Ventilation is the process by which air flows into and out of the gas-exchange airways.
3. Most of the time, ventilation is involuntary. It is controlled by the sympathetic and parasympathetic divisions of the ANS, which adjust airway calibre (by causing bronchial smooth muscle to contract or relax) and control the rate and depth of ventilation.
4. Neuroreceptors in the lungs (lung receptors) monitor the mechanical aspects of ventilation. Irritant receptors sense the need to expel unwanted substances, stretch receptors sense lung volume (lung expansion), and J-receptors sense pulmonary capillary pressure.
5. Chemoreceptors in the circulatory system and brainstem sense the effectiveness of ventilation by monitoring the pH status of cerebrospinal fluid and the O_2 content (partial pressure of oxygen) of arterial blood.
6. Successful ventilation involves the mechanics of breathing: the interaction of forces and counterforces involving the muscles of inspiration and expiration, alveolar surface tension, elastic properties of the lungs and chest wall, and resistance to airflow.

7. The major muscles of inspiration are the diaphragm and the external intercostal muscles. When the diaphragm contracts, it moves downward in the thoracic cavity, creating a vacuum that causes air to flow into the lungs.
8. The type II alveolar cells produce surfactant, a lipoprotein that lines the alveoli. Surfactant reduces alveolar surface tension and permits the alveoli to expand as air enters.
9. Elastic recoil is the tendency of the lungs and chest wall to return to their resting state after inspiration. The elastic recoil forces of the lungs and chest wall are in opposition and pull on each other, creating the normally negative pressure of the pleural space.
10. Compliance is the measure of lung and chest wall distensibility and is defined as volume change per unit of pressure change. Lung compliance is ensured by an adequate production of surfactant, whereas chest wall expansion depends on elasticity.
11. Gas transport depends on ventilation of the alveoli, diffusion across the alveolocapillary membrane, perfusion of the pulmonary and systemic capillaries, and diffusion between systemic capillaries and tissue cells.
12. Efficient gas exchange depends on an even distribution of ventilation and perfusion within the lungs. Both ventilation and perfusion are greatest in the bases of the lungs because the alveoli in the bases are more compliant (their resting volume is low) and perfusion is greater in the bases as a result of gravity.
13. Almost all the O_2 that diffuses into pulmonary capillary blood is transported by hemoglobin, a protein contained within red blood cells. The remainder of the O_2 is transported dissolved in plasma.
14. O_2 enters the body by diffusing down the concentration gradient, from high concentrations in the alveoli to lower concentrations in the capillaries. Diffusion ceases when alveolar and capillary O_2 pressures equilibrate.
15. O_2 is loaded onto hemoglobin by the driving pressure exerted by partial pressure of oxygen in arterial blood (PaO_2) in the plasma. As pressure decreases at the tissue level, O_2 dissociates from hemoglobin and enters tissue cells by diffusion, again down the concentration gradient.
16. Compared with O_2, CO_2 is more soluble in plasma. Therefore, CO_2 diffuses readily from tissue cells into plasma and from plasma into the alveoli. CO_2 returns to the lungs dissolved in plasma, as bicarbonate, or in carbamino compounds (e.g., bound to hemoglobin).

Geriatric Considerations: Aging and the Pulmonary System

1. Aging affects the mechanical aspects of ventilation by decreasing chest wall compliance and elastic recoil of the lungs. Changes in these elastic properties reduce the ventilatory reserve.
2. With aging, the surface area for gas exchange and capillary perfusion may decrease, reducing exercise capacity.
3. Level of fitness and associated systemic disease affect individual lung function.

KEY TERMS

Acinus, 680
Alveolar duct, 680
Alveolar ventilation, 684
Alveolocapillary membrane, 682
Alveolus (*pl.*, alveoli), 680
Bohr effect, 692
Bronchus (*pl.*, bronchi), 680
Carina, 680
Central chemoreceptor, 685
Collectin, 686
Compliance, 687
Elastic recoil, 687
Goblet cell, 680
Haldane effect, 692
Hilum (*pl.*, hila), 680
Hypoxic pulmonary vasoconstriction, 683
Irritant receptor, 684
J-receptor, 684
Larynx, 679
Mediastinum, 679
Minute volume (minute ventilation), 684
Nasopharynx, 679
Oropharynx, 679
Oxygen saturation (SaO_2), 691
Oxyhemoglobin (HbO_2), 691
Oxyhemoglobin dissociation curve, 691
Partial pressure (of a gas), 689
Peripheral chemoreceptor, 684
Pleura (*pl.*, pleurae), 683
Pleural space (pleural cavity), 683
Respiratory bronchiole, 680
Respiratory centre, 684
Stretch receptor, 684
Surface tension, 686
Surfactant, 681
Thoracic cavity, 683
Trachea, 680
Ventilation, 684
Ventilation–perfusion ratio ($\dot{V}/\dot{Q}$), 690

REFERENCES

1. Lumb, A. (2011). *Nunn's applied respiratory physiology* (7th ed.). St. Louis: Mosby.
2. Barrett, K. E., Barman, S. M., Boitano, S., et al. (2015). *Ganong's review of medical physiology* (25th ed.). New York: McGraw-Hill.
3. Guillot, L., Nathan, N., Tabary, O., et al. (2013). Alveolar epithelial cells: Master regulators of lung homeostasis. *International Journal of Biochemistry & Cell Biology, 45*(11), 2568–2573. doi:10.1016/j.biocel.2013.08.009.
4. Clouter, M., & Thrall, R. (2010). The respiratory system. In B. M. Koeppen & B. A. Stanton (Eds.), *Berne and Levy physiology* (6th ed.). St. Louis: Mosby.
5. West, J. B., & Luks, A. M. (2015). *West's respiratory physiology: The essentials* (10th ed.). Philadelphia: Lippincott, Wolters Kluwer.
6. Osiro, S., Wear, C., Hudson, R., et al. (2012). A friend to the airways: Review of the emerging clinical importance of the bronchial arterial circulation. *Surgical and Radiologic Anatomy, 34*(9), 791–798. doi:10.1007/s00276-012-0974-3.
7. Ariyaratnam, P., Loubani, M., & Morice, A. H. (2013). Hypoxic pulmonary vasoconstriction in humans. *BioMed Research International, 2013*, 623684. doi:10.1155/2013/623684.
8. Urfy, M. Z., & Suarez, J. I. (2014). Breathing and the nervous system. *Handbook of Clinical Neurology, 119*, 241–250. doi:10.1016/B978-0-7020-4086-3.00017-5.
9. Nattie, E. (2011). Julius H. Comroe, Jr., distinguished lecture: Central chemoreception: Then … and now. *Journal of Applied Physiology, 110*(1), 1–8. doi:10.1152/japplphysiol.01061.2010.
10. Canning, B. J., Chang, A. B., Bolser, D. C., et al. (2014). Anatomy and neurophysiology of cough: CHEST Guideline and Expert Panel report. *Chest, 146*(6), 1633–1648. doi:10.1378/chest.14-1481.
11. Guyenet, P. G., Abbott, S. B., & Stornetta, R. L. (2013). The respiratory chemoreception conundrum: Light at the end of the tunnel? *Brain Research, 1511*, 126–137. doi:10.1016/j.brainres.2012.10.028.
12. Jacono, F. J. (2013). Control of ventilation in COPD and lung injury. *Respiratory Physiology and Neurobiology, 189*(2), 371–376. doi:10.1016/j.resp.2013.07.010.
13. Kacmarek, R., Stoller, J., & Heuer, A. (2013). *Egan's fundamentals of respiratory care* (10th ed.). St. Louis: Mosby.
14. Brown, L. K. (2010). Hypoventilation syndromes. *Clinics in Chest Medicine, 31*(2), 249–270. doi:10.1016/j.ccm.2010.03.002.
15. Jakel, A., Qaseem, A. S., Kishore, U., et al. (2013). Ligands and receptors of lung surfactant proteins SP-A and SP-D. *Frontiers in Bioscience (Landmark Edition), 18*, 1129–1140. doi:10.2741/4168.

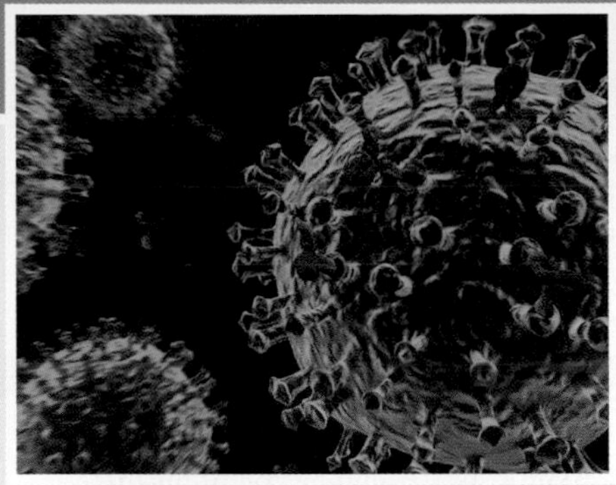

27

Alterations of Pulmonary Function

Valentina L. Brashers, Sue E. Huether, and Mohamed El-Hussein

EVOLVE WEBSITE

http://evolve.elsevier.com/Canada/Huether/pathophysiology
Student Review Questions
Key Points
Case Studies
Animations
Quick Check Answers

CHAPTER OUTLINE

Clinical Manifestations of Pulmonary Alterations, 695
Signs and Symptoms of Pulmonary Disease, 695
Conditions Caused by Pulmonary Disease or Injury, 697
Disorders of the Chest Wall and Pleura, 699
Chest Wall Restriction, 699
Pleural Abnormalities, 699
Pulmonary Disorders, 701
Restrictive Lung Diseases, 701
Obstructive Lung Diseases, 705
Respiratory Tract Infections, 711
Pulmonary Vascular Disease, 715
Malignancies of the Respiratory Tract, 717

Pulmonary disease is often classified as acute or chronic, obstructive or restrictive, or infectious or noninfectious. Symptoms of lung disease are common and associated not only with primary lung disorders but also with diseases of other organ systems, particularly the heart.

CLINICAL MANIFESTATIONS OF PULMONARY ALTERATIONS

Signs and Symptoms of Pulmonary Disease

Pulmonary disease is associated with many signs and symptoms, the most common of which are dyspnea and cough. Others include abnormal sputum, hemoptysis, altered breathing patterns, hypoventilation and hyperventilation, cyanosis, clubbing, and chest pain.

Dyspnea

Dyspnea is a subjective experience of breathing discomfort that comprises qualitatively distinct sensations that vary in intensity. Dyspnea is an individual experience and derives from interactions among multiple physiological, psychological, social, and environmental factors, and it may induce secondary physiological and behavioural responses.[1] It is often described as breathlessness, air hunger, shortness of breath, laboured breathing, and preoccupation with breathing. Dyspnea may be the result of pulmonary disease or many other conditions, such as pain, heart disease, trauma, and psychogenic disorders.[2]

The severity of the experience of dyspnea may not directly correlate with the severity of underlying disease. Either diffuse or focal disturbances of ventilation, gas exchange, or ventilation–perfusion relationships can cause dyspnea, as can the increased work of breathing or any disease that damages lung tissue (lung parenchyma). Neurophysiological mechanisms of dyspnea involve an impaired sense of effort in which the perceived work of breathing is greater than the actual motor response that is generated. Stimulation of many receptors can contribute to the sensation of dyspnea, including afferent receptors in the cortex and medulla and mechanoreceptors in the chest wall, upper airway receptors, and central and peripheral chemoreceptors.[3]

The more severe signs of dyspnea include flaring of the nostrils and use of accessory muscles of respiration. Retraction (pulling back) of the supercostal or intercostal muscles is predominant in children. Dyspnea can be quantified by the use of both ordinal rating scales and visual analogue scales and is frequently associated with significant anxiety.

Dyspnea may occur transiently or can become chronic. Dyspnea first presents during exercise and is called *dyspnea on exertion*. **Orthopnea** is dyspnea that occurs during heart failure when an individual lies flat, which causes the abdominal contents to exert pressure on the diaphragm, and decreases the efficiency of the respiratory muscles. **Paroxysmal nocturnal dyspnea (PND)** occurs when individuals with pulmonary or cardiac disease awake at night gasping for air and have to sit or stand to relieve the dyspnea. Dyspnea may be unrecognized in mechanically ventilated individuals and is often accompanied by pain and anxiety. A focused assessment and change in ventilator settings may be required.[4]

Cough

Cough is a protective reflex that helps clear the airways by an explosive expiration. Inhaled particles, accumulated mucus, inflammation, or the presence of a foreign body initiates the cough reflex by stimulating the irritant receptors in the airway. There are few such receptors in the most distal bronchi and the alveoli; thus it is possible for significant amounts of secretions to accumulate in the distal respiratory tree without cough being initiated. The cough reflex consists of inspiration, closure of the glottis and vocal cords, contraction of the expiratory muscles, and reopening of the glottis, causing a sudden, forceful expiration that removes the offending matter. The effectiveness of the cough depends on the depth of the inspiration and the degree to which the airways narrow, increasing the velocity of expiratory gas flow. Those with an inability to cough effectively are at greater risk for pneumonia.

Acute cough is cough that resolves within 2 to 3 weeks of the onset of illness or resolves with treatment of the underlying condition. It is most commonly the result of upper respiratory tract infections, allergic rhinitis, acute bronchitis, pneumonia, heart failure, pulmonary embolus, or aspiration. *Chronic cough* is defined as cough that is persistent and in individuals who do not smoke. Chronic cough is commonly caused or triggered by postnasal drainage syndrome, asthma, eosinophilic bronchitis, laryngeal hypersensitivity, and gastroesophageal reflux disease or there may be no identifiable underlying cause.[5] In persons who smoke, chronic bronchitis is the most common cause of chronic cough, although lung cancer must always be considered. Individuals taking angiotensin-converting enzyme inhibitors for cardiovascular disease may develop chronic cough that resolves with discontinuation of the medication.

Abnormal Sputum

Changes in the amount, colour, and consistency of sputum provide information about progression of disease and effectiveness of therapy. The gross and microscopic appearances of sputum enable the clinician to identify cellular debris or microorganisms, which aids in diagnosis and choice of therapy.

Hemoptysis

Hemoptysis is the coughing up of blood or bloody secretions. Hemoptysis is sometimes confused with hematemesis, which is the vomiting of blood. Blood produced with coughing is usually bright red, has an alkaline pH, and is mixed with frothy sputum. Blood that is vomited is dark, has an acidic pH, and is mixed with food particles.

Hemoptysis usually indicates infection or inflammation that damages the bronchi (bronchitis, bronchiectasis) or the lung parenchyma (pneumonia, tuberculosis, lung abscess). Other causes include cancer, pulmonary infarction, or pulmonary venous stenosis. The amount and duration of bleeding provide important clues about its source. Bronchoscopy, combined with chest computed tomography (CT), is used to confirm the site of bleeding.

Abnormal Breathing Patterns

Normal breathing (eupnea) is rhythmic and effortless. The resting ventilatory rate is 8 to 16 breaths per minute, and tidal volume ranges from 400 to 800 mL. A short expiratory pause occurs with each breath, and the individual takes an occasional deeper breath, or sighs. Sigh breaths, which help to maintain normal lung function, are usually 1.5 to 2 times the normal tidal volume and occur approximately 10 to 12 times per hour.

The rate, depth, regularity, and effort of breathing undergo characteristic alterations in response to physiological and pathophysiological conditions. Patterns of breathing automatically adjust to minimize the work of respiratory muscles. Strenuous exercise or metabolic acidosis induces **Kussmaul respiration (hyperpnea)**, which is characterized by a slightly increased ventilatory rate, very large tidal volumes, and no expiratory pause.

Laboured breathing occurs whenever there is an increased work of breathing, especially if the airways are obstructed. In large airway obstruction, a slow ventilatory rate, large tidal volume, increased effort, prolonged inspiration and expiration, and stridor or audible wheezing (depending on the site of obstruction) are typical. In small airway obstruction, such as that seen in asthma and chronic obstructive pulmonary disease (COPD), a rapid ventilatory rate, small tidal volume, increased effort, prolonged expiration, and wheezing are often present. *Restricted breathing* is commonly caused by disorders, such as pulmonary fibrosis, that stiffen the lungs or chest wall and decrease compliance, resulting in small tidal volumes and rapid ventilatory rate (tachypnea).

Shock and severe cerebral hypoxia (insufficient oxygen [O_2] in the brain) contribute to gasping respirations that consist of irregular, quick inspirations with an expiratory pause. Anxiety can cause sighing respirations, which consist of irregular breathing characterized by frequent, deep sighing inspirations. **Cheyne-Stokes respiration** is characterized by alternating periods of deep and shallow breathing. Apnea lasting from 15 to 60 seconds is followed by ventilations that increase in volume until a peak is reached; then ventilation (tidal volume) decreases again to apnea. Cheyne-Stokes respiration results from any condition that reduces blood flow to the brainstem, which in turn slows impulses sending information to the respiratory centres of the brainstem. Neurological impairment above the brainstem is also a contributing factor (see Figure 15-1).

Hypoventilation and Hyperventilation

Hypoventilation is inadequate alveolar ventilation in relation to metabolic demands. Hypoventilation occurs when minute volume (tidal volume × respiratory rate) is reduced. It is caused by alterations in pulmonary mechanics or in the neurological control of breathing.[6] When alveolar ventilation is normal, carbon dioxide (CO_2) is removed from the lungs at the same rate as it is produced by cellular metabolism and arterial and alveolar partial pressure of carbon dioxide (P_{CO_2}) values remain at normal levels (40 mm Hg). With hypoventilation, CO_2 removal does not keep up with CO_2 production and partial pressure of carbon dioxide in arterial blood ($PaCO_2$) increases, causing hypercapnia ($PaCO_2$ greater than 44 mm Hg) (see Table 26-2 for a definition of gas partial pressures and other pulmonary abbreviations). This increase in $PaCO_2$ results in respiratory acidosis that can affect the function of many tissues throughout the body. Hypoventilation is often overlooked until it is severe because breathing pattern and ventilatory rate may appear to be normal and changes in tidal volume can be difficult to detect clinically. Blood gas analysis (i.e., measurement of the $PaCO_2$ of arterial blood) reveals the hypoventilation. Pronounced hypoventilation can cause secondary hypoxemia, somnolence, or disorientation.

Hyperventilation is alveolar ventilation exceeding metabolic demands. The lungs remove CO_2 faster than it is produced by cellular metabolism, resulting in decreased $PaCO_2$, or **hypocapnia** ($PaCO_2$ less than 36 mm Hg). Hypocapnia results in a respiratory alkalosis that also can interfere with tissue function. Like hypoventilation, hyperventilation can be determined by arterial blood gas analysis. Hyperventilation commonly occurs with severe anxiety, acute head injury, pain, and in response to conditions that cause hypoxemia.

Cyanosis

Cyanosis is a bluish discoloration of the skin and mucous membranes caused by increasing amounts of desaturated or reduced hemoglobin (which is bluish) in the blood. It generally develops when 5 g of hemoglobin is desaturated, regardless of hemoglobin concentration.

Peripheral cyanosis (slow blood circulation in fingers and toes) is most often caused by poor circulation resulting from intense peripheral vasoconstriction, like that observed in persons who have Raynaud disease, are in cold environments, or are severely stressed. Peripheral cyanosis is best seen in the nail beds. *Central cyanosis* is caused by decreased arterial oxygenation (low PaO_2) from pulmonary diseases or pulmonary or cardiac right-to-left shunts. Central cyanosis is best detected in buccal mucous membranes and lips.

Lack of cyanosis does not necessarily indicate that oxygenation is normal. In adults, cyanosis is not evident until severe hypoxemia is present and, therefore, is an insensitive indication of respiratory failure. For example, severe anemia (inadequate hemoglobin concentration)

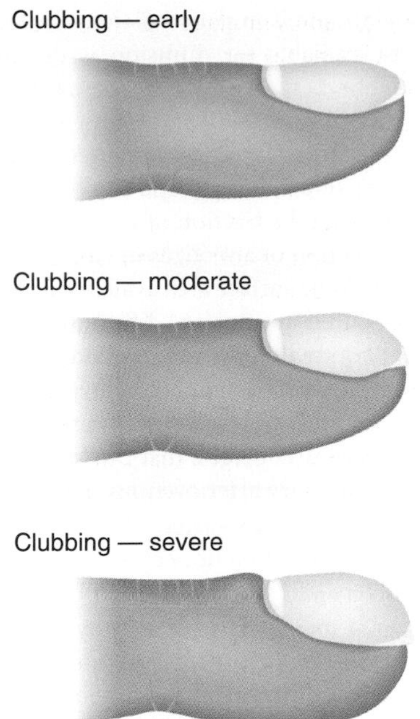

FIGURE 27-1 Clubbing of Fingers Caused by Chronic Hypoxemia. (Modified from Seidel, H.M., Stewart, R.W., Ball, J.W., et al. [2011]. *Mosby's guide to physical examination* [7th ed.]. St. Louis: Mosby.)

and carbon monoxide poisoning (in which hemoglobin binds to carbon monoxide instead of to O_2) can cause inadequate oxygenation of tissues without causing cyanosis. Individuals with polycythemia (an abnormal increase in numbers of red blood cells), however, may have cyanosis when oxygenation is adequate. Therefore, cyanosis must be interpreted in relation to the underlying pathophysiological condition. If cyanosis is suggested, the PaO_2 should be measured.

Clubbing

Clubbing is the selective bulbous enlargement of the end (distal segment) of a digit (finger or toe) (Figure 27-1); its severity can be graded from 1 to 5 based on the extent of nail bed hypertrophy and the amount of changes in the nails themselves. It is usually painless. Clubbing is commonly associated with diseases that disrupt the normal pulmonary circulation and cause chronic hypoxemia, such as bronchiectasis, cystic fibrosis, pulmonary fibrosis, lung abscess, and congenital heart disease, and is rarely reversible. It is proposed that whole megakaryocytes enter the systemic circulation and become impacted in the fingertip circulation. Megakaryocytes and megakaryocyte fragments are activated to release platelet-derived growth factor (PDGF). PDGF promotes growth, vascular permeability, and monocyte and neutrophil chemotaxis and leads to an increased number of vascular smooth muscle cells and fibroblasts, all of which are seen in the pathology of clubbing.[7] It can sometimes be seen in individuals with lung cancer even without hypoxemia because of the effects of inflammatory cytokines and growth factors (hypertrophic osteoarthropathy).[8]

Pain

Pain caused by pulmonary disorders originates in the pleurae, airways, or chest wall.[9] Infection and inflammation of the parietal pleura cause sharp or stabbing pain (pleurodynia) when the pleura stretches during inspiration. The pain is usually localized to a portion of the chest wall, where a unique breath sound called a *pleural friction rub* may be heard over the painful area. Laughing or coughing makes pleural pain worse. Pleural pain is common with pulmonary infarction (tissue death) caused by pulmonary embolism (PE) and emanates from the area around the infarction.

Infection and inflammation of the trachea or bronchi (tracheitis or tracheobronchitis, respectively) can cause central chest pain that is pronounced after coughing. It can be difficult to differentiate from cardiac pain. High blood pressure in the pulmonary circulation (pulmonary hypertension) can cause pain during exercise that is often mistaken for cardiac pain (angina pectoris).

Pain in the chest wall is muscle pain or rib pain. Excessive coughing (which makes the muscles sore) and rib fractures or thoracic surgery produce such pain. Inflammation of the costochondral junction (costochondritis) also can cause chest wall pain. Chest wall pain can often be reproduced by pressing on the sternum or ribs.

Conditions Caused by Pulmonary Disease or Injury

Hypercapnia

Hypercapnia, or increased CO_2 concentration in the arterial blood (increased $PaCO_2$), is caused by hypoventilation of the alveoli. As discussed in Chapter 26, CO_2 is easily diffused from the blood into the alveolar space; thus minute volume (respiratory rate × tidal volume) determines not only alveolar ventilation but also $PaCO_2$. Hypoventilation is often overlooked because the breathing pattern and ventilatory rate may appear to be normal; therefore, it is important to obtain blood gas analysis to determine the severity of hypercapnia and resultant respiratory acidosis (acid-base balance is described in Chapter 5).

There are many causes of hypercapnia. Most are a result of a decreased drive to breathe or an inadequate ability to respond to ventilatory stimulation. Some of these causes include (1) depression of the respiratory centre by medications; (2) diseases of the medulla, including infections of the central nervous system or trauma; (3) abnormalities of the spinal conducting pathways, as in spinal cord disruption or poliomyelitis; (4) diseases of the neuromuscular junction or of the respiratory muscles themselves, as in myasthenia gravis or muscular dystrophy; (5) thoracic cage abnormalities, as in chest injury or congenital deformity; (6) large airway obstruction, as in tumours or sleep apnea; and (7) increased work of breathing or physiological dead space, as in emphysema.

Hypercapnia and the associated respiratory acidosis result in electrolyte abnormalities that may cause dysrhythmias. Individuals also may present with somnolence and even coma because of changes in intracranial pressure associated with high levels of arterial CO_2, which causes cerebral vasodilation. Alveolar hypoventilation with increased alveolar CO_2 concentration limits the amount of O_2 available for diffusion into the blood, thereby leading to secondary hypoxemia.

Hypoxemia

Hypoxemia, or reduced oxygenation of arterial blood (reduced PaO_2), is caused by respiratory alterations, whereas hypoxia (or ischemia) is reduced oxygenation of cells in tissues. Although hypoxemia can lead to tissue hypoxia, tissue hypoxia can result from other abnormalities unrelated to alterations of pulmonary function, such as low cardiac output or cyanide poisoning.

Hypoxemia results from problems with one or more of the major mechanisms of oxygenation:

1. O_2 delivery to the alveoli
   a. O_2 content of the inspired air (fraction of inspired oxygen [FiO_2])
   b. Ventilation of alveoli
2. Diffusion of O_2 from the alveoli into the blood
   a. Balance between alveolar ventilation and perfusion ($\dot{V}/\dot{Q}$ match)
   b. Diffusion of O_2 across the alveolar capillary barrier
3. Perfusion of pulmonary capillaries

The amount of O_2 in the alveoli is called the P_AO_2 and is dependent on two factors. The first factor is the presence of adequate O_2 content of the inspired air. The amount of O_2 in inspired air is expressed as the percentage or fraction of air that is composed of O_2, called the FiO_2. The FiO_2 of air at sea level is approximately 21%, or 0.21. Anything that decreases the FiO_2 (such as high altitude) decreases the P_AO_2. A second factor is the amount of alveolar minute volume (tidal volume × respiratory rate). Hypoventilation results in an increase in partial pressure of carbon dioxide in alveolar gas and a decrease in P_AO_2 such that there is less O_2 available in the alveoli for diffusion into the blood. This type of hypoxemia can be completely corrected if alveolar ventilation is improved by increases in the rate and depth of breathing. Hypoventilation causes hypoxemia in unconscious persons; in persons with neurological, muscular, or bone diseases that restrict chest expansion; and in individuals who have COPD.

Diffusion of O_2 from the alveoli into the blood is also dependent on two factors. The first is the balance between the amount of air that enters alveoli ($\dot{V}$) and the amount of blood perfusing the capillaries around the alveoli ($\dot{Q}$). An abnormal ventilation–perfusion ratio ($\dot{V}/\dot{Q}$) is the most common cause of hypoxemia (Figure 27-2). The normal $\dot{V}/\dot{Q}$ is 0.8 because perfusion is somewhat greater than ventilation in the lung bases and because some blood is normally shunted to the bronchial circulation. *$\dot{V}/\dot{Q}$ mismatch* refers to an abnormal distribution of ventilation and perfusion. Hypoxemia can be caused by inadequate ventilation of well-perfused areas of the lung (low $\dot{V}/\dot{Q}$). Mismatching of this type, called **shunting**, occurs in atelectasis, in asthma as a result of bronchoconstriction, and in pulmonary edema and pneumonia when alveoli are filled with fluid. When blood passes through portions of the pulmonary capillary bed that receive no ventilation, the pulmonary capillaries in that area constrict and a right-to-left shunt occurs, resulting in decreased systemic PaO_2 and hypoxemia. Hypoxemia also can be caused by poor perfusion of well-ventilated portions of the lung (high $\dot{V}/\dot{Q}$), resulting in wasted ventilation. The most common cause of high $\dot{V}/\dot{Q}$ is a pulmonary embolus that impairs blood flow to a segment of the lung. An area where alveoli are ventilated but not perfused is termed **alveolar dead space**.

The second factor affecting diffusion of O_2 from the alveoli into the blood is the alveolocapillary membrane. Diffusion of O_2 through the alveolocapillary membrane is impaired if the membrane is thickened or the surface area available for diffusion is decreased. Thickened alveolocapillary membranes, as occur with edema (tissue swelling) and fibrosis (formation of fibrous lesions), increase the time required for O_2 to diffuse from the alveoli into the capillaries. If diffusion is slowed enough, the PO_2 levels of alveolar gas and capillary blood do not have time to equilibrate during the fraction of a second that blood remains in the capillary. Destruction of alveoli, as in emphysema, decreases the alveolocapillary membrane surface area available for diffusion. Hypercapnia is seldom produced by impaired diffusion because CO_2 diffuses so easily from capillary to alveolus that the individual with impaired diffusion would die from hypoxemia before hypercapnia could occur.

Hypoxemia can result from blood flow bypassing the lungs. It can occur because of intracardiac defects that cause right-to-left shunting or because of intrapulmonary arteriovenous malformations.

Hypoxemia is most often associated with a compensatory hyperventilation and the resultant respiratory alkalosis (i.e., decreased $PaCO_2$ and increased pH). However, in individuals with associated ventilatory difficulties, hypoxemia may be complicated by hypercapnia and respiratory acidosis. Hypoxemia results in widespread tissue dysfunction and, when severe, can lead to organ infarction. In addition, hypoxic pulmonary vasoconstriction can contribute to increased pressures in the pulmonary artery (pulmonary artery hypertension [PAH]) and lead to right ventricular failure or cor pulmonale. Clinical manifestations of acute hypoxemia may include cyanosis, confusion, tachycardia, edema, and decreased renal output.

QUICK CHECK 27-1

1. List the primary signs and symptoms of pulmonary disease.
2. What abnormal breathing patterns are seen with pulmonary disease?
3. What mechanisms produce hypercapnia?
4. What mechanisms produce hypoxemia?

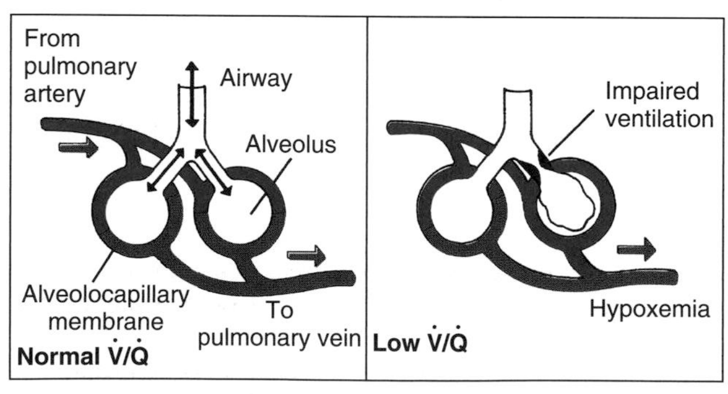

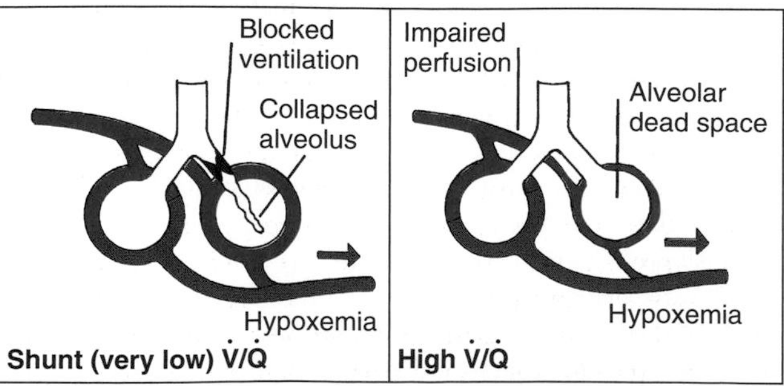

FIGURE 27-2 Ventilation–Perfusion Abnormalities. *$\dot{V}/\dot{Q}$*, ventilation–perfusion ratio.

Acute Respiratory Failure

Respiratory failure is defined as inadequate gas exchange such that PaO_2 is less than or equal to 60 mm Hg or $PaCO_2$ is greater than or equal to 50 mm Hg, with pH less than or equal to 7.25.[10] Respiratory failure can result from direct injury to the lungs, airways, or chest wall or indirectly because of disease or injury involving another body system, such as the brain, spinal cord, or heart. It can occur in individuals who have an otherwise normal respiratory system or in those with underlying chronic pulmonary disease. Most pulmonary diseases can cause episodes of acute respiratory failure. If the respiratory failure is primarily hypercapnic, it is the result of inadequate alveolar ventilation and the individual must receive ventilatory support, such as with a bag-valve mask, noninvasive positive pressure ventilation, or intubation and placement on mechanical ventilation. If the respiratory failure is primarily hypoxemic, it is the result of inadequate exchange of O_2 between the alveoli and the capillaries and the individual must receive supplemental O_2 therapy. Many people will have combined hypercapnic and hypoxemic respiratory failure and will require both kinds of support.

Respiratory failure is an important potential complication of any major surgical procedure, especially those that involve the central nervous system, thorax, or upper abdomen. The most common postoperative pulmonary problems are atelectasis, pneumonia, pulmonary edema, and pulmonary emboli. People who smoke are at risk, particularly if they have pre-existing lung disease. Limited cardiac reserve, neurological disease, chronic renal failure, chronic hepatic disease, and infection also increase the tendency to develop postoperative respiratory failure.

Prevention of postoperative respiratory failure includes frequent turning and position changes, deep-breathing exercises, and early ambulation to prevent atelectasis and accumulation of secretions. Humidification of inspired air can help loosen secretions. Incentive spirometry gives individuals immediate feedback about tidal volumes, which encourages them to breathe deeply. Supplemental O_2 is given for hypoxemia, and antibiotics are given as appropriate to treat infection. If respiratory failure develops, the individual may require mechanical ventilation or extracorporeal membrane oxygenation.

DISORDERS OF THE CHEST WALL AND PLEURA

There are many conditions that can affect the chest wall or pleura, or both, and influence the function of the respiratory system. Chest wall disorders primarily affect tidal volume and, therefore, result in hypercapnia. Pleural diseases impact both ventilation and oxygenation.

Chest Wall Restriction

If the chest wall is deformed, traumatized, immobilized, or heavy from the accumulation of fat, the work of breathing increases and ventilation may be compromised because of a decrease in tidal volume. The degree of ventilatory impairment depends on the severity of the chest wall abnormality. Grossly obese individuals are often dyspneic on exertion or when recumbent. Individuals with severe kyphoscoliosis (lateral bending and rotation of the spinal column, with distortion of the thoracic cage) often present with dyspnea on exertion that can progress to respiratory failure. Obesity and kyphoscoliosis are risk factors for respiratory failure or infections in individuals admitted to the hospital for other problems, particularly those who require surgery. Other musculo-skeletal abnormalities that can impair ventilation are ankylosing spondylitis (see Chapter 39) and pectus excavatum (a deformity characterized by depression of the sternum).

Impairment of respiratory muscle function caused by neuromuscular diseases such as poliomyelitis, muscular dystrophy, myasthenia gravis, and Guillain-Barré syndrome (see Chapter 16) also can restrict the chest wall and impair pulmonary function. Muscle weakness can result in hypoventilation, inability to remove secretions, and hypoxemia.

Pain from chest wall injury, surgery, or disease can cause significant hypoventilation, especially in those with underlying lung disease. Trauma to the thorax can not only restrict chest expansion because of pain but also cause structural and mechanical changes that impair the ability of the chest to expand normally. **Flail chest** results from the fracture of several consecutive ribs in more than one place or fracture of the sternum and several consecutive ribs. These multiple fractures result in instability of a portion of the chest wall, causing paradoxical movement of the chest with breathing. During inspiration, the unstable portion of the chest wall moves inward and during expiration it moves outward, impairing movement of gas in and out of the lungs (Figure 27-3).

Chest wall restriction results in a decrease in tidal volume. An increase in respiratory rate can compensate for small decreases in tidal volume, but many individuals will progress to hypercapnic respiratory failure. Diagnosis of chest wall restriction is made by pulmonary function testing (reduction in forced vital capacity [FVC]), arterial blood gas measurement (hypercapnia), and radiographs. Treatment is aimed at any reversible underlying cause but is otherwise supportive. In severe cases, mechanical ventilation may be indicated.

Pleural Abnormalities

Pneumothorax

Pneumothorax is the presence of air or gas in the pleural space caused by a rupture in the visceral pleura (which surrounds the lungs) or the parietal pleura and chest wall. As air separates the visceral and parietal pleurae, it destroys the negative pressure of the pleural space and disrupts the equilibrium between elastic recoil forces of the lung and chest wall. The lung then tends to recoil by collapsing toward the hilum (Figure 27-4).

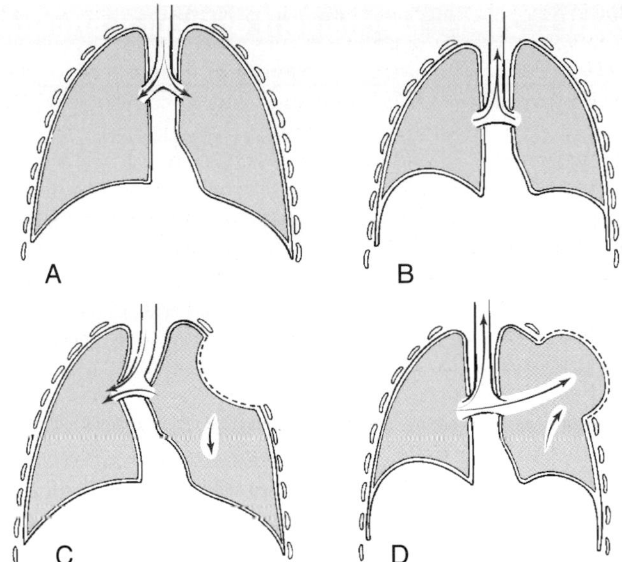

FIGURE 27-3 Flail Chest. Normal respiration: **A,** inspiration; **B,** expiration. Paradoxical motion: **C,** inspiration, area of lung underlying unstable chest wall flattens on inspiration; **D,** expiration, unstable area inflates. Note movement of mediastinum toward opposite lung during inspiration.

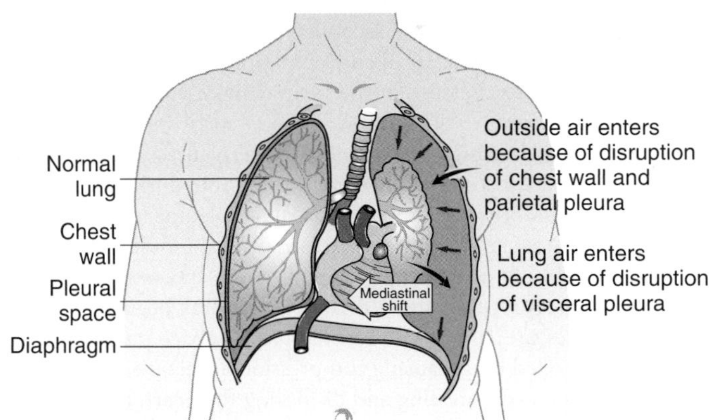

FIGURE 27-4 Pneumothorax. Air in the pleural space causes the lung to collapse around the hilus and may push mediastinal contents (heart and great vessels) toward the other lung.

Primary (spontaneous) pneumothorax occurs unexpectedly in healthy individuals (usually men) between 20 and 40 years of age and is caused by the spontaneous rupture of blebs (blisterlike formations) on the visceral pleura. Bleb rupture can occur during sleep, rest, or exercise. The ruptured blebs are usually located in the apexes of the lungs. The cause of bleb formation is not known, although more than 80% of these individuals have been found to have emphysemalike changes in their lungs even if they have no history of smoking or no known genetic disorder. Approximately 10% of affected individuals have a significant family history of primary pneumothorax that has been linked to mutations in the folliculin gene.[11] *Secondary pneumothorax* can be caused by chest trauma (such as a rib fracture or stab and bullet wounds that tear the pleura; rupture of a bleb or bulla [larger vesicle], as occurs in emphysema; or mechanical ventilation, particularly if it includes positive

TABLE 27-1 Mechanism of Pleural Effusion[a]

Type of Fluid/Effusion	Source of Accumulation	Primary or Associated Disorder
Transudate (hydrothorax)	Watery fluid that diffuses out of capillaries beneath pleura (i.e., capillaries in lung or chest wall)	Cardiovascular disease that causes high pulmonary capillary pressures; liver or kidney disease that disrupts plasma protein production, causing hypoproteinemia (decreased oncotic pressure in blood vessels)
Exudate	Fluid rich in cells and proteins (leukocytes, plasma proteins of all kinds; see Chapter 5) that migrates out of capillaries	Infection, inflammation, or malignancy of pleura that stimulates mast cells to release biochemical mediators that increase capillary permeability
Pus (empyema)	Microorganisms and debris of infection (leukocytes, cellular debris) accumulate in pleural space	Pulmonary infections, such as pneumonia; lung abscesses; infected wounds
Blood (hemothorax)	Hemorrhage into pleural space	Traumatic injury, surgery, rupture, or malignancy that damages blood vessels
Chyle (chylothorax)	Chyle (milky fluid containing lymph and fat droplets) that moves from lymphatic vessels into pleural space instead of passing from gastro-intestinal tract to thoracic duct	Traumatic injury, infection, or disorder that disrupts lymphatic transport

[a]The principles of diffusion are described in Chapter 1; mechanisms that increase capillary permeability and cause exudation of cells, proteins, and fluid are discussed in Chapter 5.

end-expiratory pressure [PEEP]). *Iatrogenic pneumothorax* is most commonly caused by transthoracic needle aspiration.

Primary pneumothorax and secondary pneumothorax can present as either open or tension. In **open pneumothorax (communicating pneumothorax)**, air pressure in the pleural space equals barometric pressure because air that is drawn into the pleural space during inspiration (through the damaged chest wall and parietal pleura or through the lungs and damaged visceral pleura) is forced back out during expiration. In **tension pneumothorax**, however, the site of pleural rupture acts as a one-way valve, permitting air to enter on inspiration but preventing its escape by closing during expiration. As more and more air enters the pleural space, air pressure in the pneumothorax begins to exceed barometric pressure. Air pressure in the pleural space pushes against the already recoiled lung, causing compression atelectasis, and against the mediastinum, compressing and displacing the heart, great vessels, and trachea (*mediastinal shift*). The pathophysiological effects of tension pneumothorax are life-threatening (see Figure 27-4).

Clinical manifestations of spontaneous or secondary pneumothorax begin with sudden pleural pain, tachypnea, and dyspnea. Depending on the size of the pneumothorax, physical examination may reveal absent or decreased breath sounds and hyper-resonance to percussion on the affected side. Tension pneumothorax may be complicated by severe hypoxemia, tracheal deviation away from the affected lung, and hypotension (low blood pressure). Deterioration occurs rapidly and immediate treatment is required. Diagnosis of pneumothorax is made with chest radiographs, ultrasound, and CT. Pneumothorax is treated by aspiration, usually with insertion of a chest tube that is attached to a water-seal drainage system with suction or a small-bore catheter with a one-way valve.[12] After the pneumothorax is evacuated and the pleural rupture is healed, the chest tube is removed. For individuals with persistent air leaks, other interventions may be needed including thoracoscopic surgical techniques or pleurodesis (instillation of a caustic substance, such as talc, into the pleural space).

Pleural Effusion

Pleural effusion is the presence of fluid in the pleural space. The source of the fluid is usually from blood vessels or lymphatic vessels lying beneath the pleural space, but occasionally an abscess or other lesion may drain into the pleural space. Pleural effusions that enter the pleural space from intact blood vessels can be **transudative** (watery) or **exudative** (high concentrations of white blood cells and plasma proteins). Other types of pleural effusion are characterized by the presence of pus (empyema), blood (hemothorax), or chyle (chylothorax). Mechanisms of pleural effusion are summarized in Table 27-1.

Small collections of fluid may not affect lung function and remain undetected. Most will be removed by the lymphatic system once the underlying condition is resolved. In larger effusions, dyspnea, compression atelectasis with impaired ventilation, and pleural pain are common. Mediastinal shift and cardiovascular manifestations occur in a large, rapidly developing effusion. Physical examination shows decreased breath sounds and dullness to percussion on the affected side. A pleural friction rub can be heard over areas of inflamed pleura.

Diagnosis is confirmed by chest X-ray and thoracentesis (needle aspiration), which can determine the type of effusion and provide symptomatic relief. If the effusion is large, drainage usually requires the placement of a chest tube and surgical interventions may be needed to prevent recurrence of the effusion.

Empyema

Empyema (infected pleural effusion) is the presence of pus in the pleural space and develops when the pulmonary lymphatics become blocked, leading to an outpouring of contaminated lymphatic fluid into the pleural space. Empyema occurs most commonly in older adults and children and usually develops as a complication of pneumonia, surgery, trauma, or bronchial obstruction from a tumour. Commonly documented infectious organisms include *Staphylococcus aureus*, *Escherichia coli*, anaerobic bacteria, and *Klebsiella pneumoniae*.

Individuals with empyema present clinically with cyanosis, fever, tachycardia (rapid heart rate), cough, and pleural pain. Breath sounds are decreased directly over the empyema. Diagnosis is made by chest radiographs, thoracentesis, and sputum culture. The treatment for empyema includes the administration of appropriate antimicrobials and drainage of the pleural space with a chest tube. In severe cases, ultrasound-guided pleural drainage, instillation of fibrinolytic agents, or introduction of deoxyribonuclease (DNase) into the pleural space is needed for adequate drainage. Surgical debridement may be required.[13]

QUICK CHECK 27-2

1. How does chest wall restriction affect ventilation?
2. How does pneumothorax differ from pleural effusion?
3. What causes empyema?

PULMONARY DISORDERS

Restrictive Lung Diseases

Restrictive lung diseases are characterized by decreased compliance of the lung tissue. This decrease in lung compliance means that it takes more effort to expand the lungs during inspiration, which increases the work of breathing. Individuals with lung restriction have dyspnea, an increased respiratory rate, and a decreased tidal volume. Pulmonary function testing reveals a decrease in FVC. Restrictive lung diseases can cause $\dot{V}/\dot{Q}$ mismatch and affect the alveolocapillary membrane, which reduces the diffusion of O_2 from the alveoli into the blood and results in hypoxemia. Some of the most common restrictive lung diseases in adults are aspiration, atelectasis, bronchiectasis, bronchiolitis, pulmonary fibrosis, inhalation disorders (e.g., pneumoconiosis and allergic alveolitis), pulmonary edema, and acute lung injury (ALI)/acute respiratory distress syndrome (ARDS).

Aspiration

Aspiration is the passage of fluid and solid particles into the lung. It tends to occur in individuals whose normal swallowing mechanism and cough reflex are impaired by central or peripheral nervous system abnormalities. Predisposing factors include an altered level of consciousness caused by substance abuse, sedation, or anaesthesia; seizure disorders; stroke; neuromuscular disorders that cause dysphagia; and feeding through a nasogastric tube. The right lung, particularly the right lower lobe, is more susceptible to aspiration than the left lung because the branching angle of the right mainstem bronchus is straighter than the branching angle of the left mainstem bronchus.

Aspiration of large food particles or gastric fluid with pH of less than 2.5 has serious consequences. Solid food particles can obstruct a bronchus, resulting in bronchial inflammation and collapse of airways distal to the obstruction. If the aspirated solid is not identified and removed by bronchoscopy, a chronic, local inflammation develops that may lead to recurrent infection and bronchiectasis (permanent dilation of the bronchus).

Aspiration of oral or pharyngeal secretions can lead to aspiration pneumonia. Intubation of the trachea also can cause aspiration and bacterial pneumonia. Aspiration of acidic gastric fluid may cause severe pneumonitis. Bronchial damage includes inflammation, loss of ciliary function, and bronchospasm. In the alveoli, acidic fluid damages the alveolocapillary membrane. This damage to the alveolocapillary membrane allows plasma and blood cells to move from capillaries into the alveoli, resulting in hemorrhagic pneumonitis. The lung becomes stiff and noncompliant as surfactant production is disrupted, leading to further edema and collapse. Hypoventilation may develop as this process progresses and systematic complications, such as hypotension, may occur.

Clinical manifestations of aspiration include the sudden onset of choking and intractable cough with or without vomiting, fever, dyspnea, and wheezing. Some individuals have no symptoms acutely; instead, they have recurrent lung infections, chronic cough, or persistent wheezing over months and even years.

Preventive measures for individuals at risk are more effective than treatment of known aspiration. The most important preventive measures include use of a semirecumbent position, surveillance of enteral feeding, use of promotility agents, and avoidance of excessive sedation. Nasogastric tubes, which are often used to remove stomach contents, are used to prevent aspiration but also can cause aspiration if fluid and particulate matter are regurgitated as the tube is being placed.

Treatment of aspiration pneumonitis includes use of supplemental O_2 and mechanical ventilation with PEEP and administration of corticosteroids. Fluids are restricted to decrease blood volume and minimize pulmonary edema. Bacterial pneumonia may develop as a complication of aspiration pneumonitis and must be treated with broad-spectrum antimicrobials.

Atelectasis

Atelectasis is the collapse of lung tissue. There are three types of atelectasis:

1. Compression atelectasis is caused by external pressure exerted by tumour, fluid, or air in the pleural space or by abdominal distension pressing on a portion of lung, causing alveoli to collapse.
2. Absorption atelectasis results from removal of air from obstructed or hypoventilated alveoli or from inhalation of concentrated O_2 or anaesthetic agents.
3. Surfactant impairment results from decreased production or inactivation of surfactant, which is necessary to reduce surface tension in the alveoli and thus prevent lung collapse during expiration. Surfactant impairment can occur because of premature birth, ARDS, anaesthesia induction, or mechanical ventilation.

Atelectasis tends to occur after surgery, especially in those who have been administered general anaesthetics.[14] Postoperative individuals are often in pain, breathe shallowly, are reluctant to change position, and produce viscous secretions that tend to pool in dependent portions of the lung, especially following thoracic or upper abdominal surgery. Atelectasis increases shunt, decreases compliance, and may lead to perioperative hypoxemia.

Clinical manifestations of atelectasis are similar to those of pulmonary infection including dyspnea, cough, fever, and leukocytosis. Prevention and treatment of postoperative atelectasis usually include deep-breathing exercises (often with the aid of an incentive spirometer), frequent position changes, and early ambulation. Deep breathing promotes ciliary clearance of secretions, stabilizes the alveoli by redistributing surfactant, and promotes collateral ventilation through the pores of Kohn, promoting expansion of collapsed alveoli (Figure 27-5). Postoperative noninvasive positive-pressure ventilation (NIPPV) has been shown to improve oxygenation and ventilation for high-risk individuals (i.e., individuals who are obese or in respiratory distress).

Bronchiectasis

Bronchiectasis is persistent abnormal dilation of the bronchi. There may be a genetic predisposition or a defect in host defence.[15] It usually occurs in conjunction with other respiratory conditions that are associated with chronic bronchial inflammation, such as obstruction of an airway with mucous plugs, atelectasis, aspiration of a foreign body, infection, cystic fibrosis (see Chapter 28), tuberculosis, congenital weakness of the bronchial wall, or immunocompromised health status. Chronic inflammation of the bronchi leads to destruction of elastic and muscular components of their walls, obstruction of the bronchial lumen, traction from adjacent fibrosis, and permanent dilation. Bronchiectasis also is associated with a number of systemic disorders, such as rheumatological disease, inflammatory bowel disease, and immunodeficiency syndromes (e.g., acquired immune deficiency syndrome [AIDS]). There may be no known cause.

The primary symptom of bronchiectasis is a chronic productive cough that may date back to a childhood illness or infection. The disease is commonly associated with recurrent lower respiratory tract infections and expectoration of voluminous amounts of foul-smelling purulent

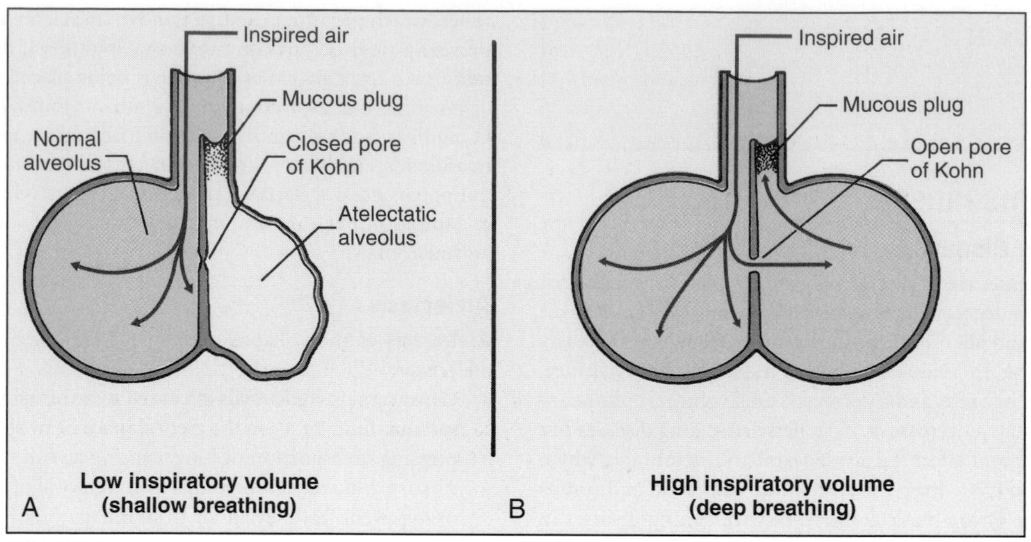

FIGURE 27-5 Pores of Kohn. **A,** Absorption atelectasis caused by lack of collateral ventilation through pores of Kohn. **B,** Restoration of collateral ventilation during deep breathing.

sputum (measured in cupfuls). Hemoptysis and clubbing of the fingers (from chronic hypoxemia) are common. Pulmonary function studies show decreases in FVC and expiratory flow rates. Hypoxemia eventually leads to cor pulmonale. Diagnosis is usually confirmed by the use of high-resolution CT. Bronchiectasis is treated with sputum culture, antibiotics, anti-inflammatory medications, bronchodilators, chest physiotherapy, and supplemental O_2.

Bronchiolitis

Bronchiolitis is a diffuse, inflammatory obstruction of the small airways or bronchioles occurring most commonly in children. In adults it usually occurs with chronic bronchitis but can occur in otherwise healthy individuals in association with an upper or lower respiratory tract viral infection or with inhalation of toxic gases, or be of unknown etiology.[16] Bronchiolitis also is a serious complication of stem cell and lung transplantation and can progress to **bronchiolitis obliterans**, a fibrotic process that occludes airways and causes permanent scarring of the lungs. **Bronchiolitis obliterans organizing pneumonia (BOOP)** is a complication of bronchiolitis obliterans in which the alveoli and bronchioles become filled with plugs of connective tissue.

Clinical manifestations include a rapid ventilatory rate; marked use of accessory muscles; low-grade fever; dry, nonproductive cough; and hyperinflated chest. A decrease in the $\dot{V}/\dot{Q}$ results in hypoxemia. Diagnosis is made by spirometry and bronchoscopy with biopsy. Bronchiolitis is treated with appropriate antibiotics, corticosteroids, immunosuppressive agents, and chest physiotherapy (humidified air administration, coughing and deep-breathing exercises, postural drainage).

Pulmonary Fibrosis

Pulmonary fibrosis is an excessive amount of fibrous or connective tissue in the lung. Pulmonary fibrosis can be caused by formation of scar tissue after active pulmonary disease (e.g., ARDS, tuberculosis), in association with a variety of autoimmune disorders (e.g., rheumatoid arthritis, progressive systemic sclerosis, sarcoidosis), or by inhalation of harmful substances (e.g., coal dust, asbestos). Chronic inflammation leads to fibrosis and causes a marked loss of lung compliance. The lung becomes stiff and difficult to ventilate, and the diffusing capacity of the alveolocapillary membrane may decrease, causing hypoxemia. Diffuse pulmonary fibrosis has a poor prognosis.

Pulmonary fibrosis is known as idiopathic pulmonary fibrosis when there is no specific cause. **Idiopathic pulmonary fibrosis (IPF)** is the most common idiopathic interstitial lung disorder. It is more common in men than in women and most cases occur after age 60. Although IPF is characterized by chronic inflammation, recent studies suggest that it results from multiple injuries at different lung sites with aberrant healing responses to alveolar epithelial cell injury, which probably occurs in response to a combination of environmental insults and genetic predispositions.[17] Fibroproliferation of the interstitial lung tissue around the alveoli causes decreased O_2 diffusion across the alveolocapillary membrane and hypoxemia. As the disease progresses, decreased lung compliance leads to increased work of breathing, decreased tidal volume, and resultant hypoventilation with hypercapnia.

The primary symptom of IPF is increasing dyspnea on exertion. Physical examination reveals diffuse inspiratory crackles. The diagnosis is confirmed by pulmonary function testing (decreased FVC), high-resolution CT, and lung biopsy. Treatment includes O_2, corticosteroids, and cytotoxic medications, although success rates are low and toxicities are high. Newer therapies include antifibrotic medications (*N*-acetylcysteine [Mucomyst], pirfenidone [Esbriet]), nintedanib (Ofev; an angiogenesis inhibitor), interferon alfa-2 (Intron A), and anticoagulation therapy.[18] Selected individuals may benefit from lung transplantation.

Inhalation Disorders

Exposure to toxic gases. Inhalation of gaseous irritants can cause significant respiratory dysfunction. Commonly encountered toxic gases include smoke, ammonia, hydrogen chloride, sulphur dioxide, chlorine, phosgene, and nitrogen dioxide. Inhalation injuries in burns can include toxic gases from household or industrial combustants, heat, and smoke particles. Inhaled toxic particles cause damage to the airway epithelium and promote mucus secretion, inflammation, mucosal edema, ciliary damage, pulmonary edema, and surfactant inactivation. The cellular effects of toxic gases and polluted air are described in Chapter 4. Acute toxic inhalation is frequently complicated by ARDS and pneumonia. Initial symptoms include burning of the eyes, nose, and throat; coughing; chest tightness; and dyspnea. Hypoxemia is common. Treatment includes administration of supplemental O_2, mechanical ventilation with PEEP, and support of the cardiovascular system. Corticosteroids are sometimes used, although their effectiveness has not been well documented. Most individuals respond quickly to therapy. Some, however, may improve initially and then deteriorate as a result of bronchiectasis or bronchiolitis.

Prolonged exposure to high concentrations of supplemental O_2 can result in a relatively rare condition known as oxygen toxicity. The basic underlying mechanism of injury is a severe inflammatory response mediated by O_2 free radicals. Damage to alveolocapillary membranes results in disruption of surfactant production, production of interstitial and alveolar edema, and a reduction in lung compliance. In infants this can lead to a condition known as bronchopulmonary dysplasia in which there is severe scarring of the lung. Treatment involves ventilatory support and a reduction of inspired O_2 concentration to less than 60% as soon as tolerated.

Pneumoconiosis. Pneumoconiosis represents any change in the lung caused by inhalation of inorganic dust particles, usually occurring in the workplace. As in all cases of environmentally acquired lung disease, the individual's history of exposure is important in determining the diagnosis. Pneumoconiosis often occurs after years of exposure to the offending dust, with progressive fibrosis of lung tissue.

The dusts of silica, asbestos, and coal are the most common causes of pneumoconiosis. Others include talc, fibreglass, clays, mica, slate, cement, cadmium, beryllium, tungsten, cobalt, aluminum, and iron. Deposition of these materials in the lungs causes the release of proinflammatory cytokines. This leads to chronic inflammation with scarring of the alveolocapillary membrane, resulting in pulmonary fibrosis and progressive pulmonary deterioration. Clinical manifestations with advancement of disease include cough, chronic sputum production, dyspnea, decreased lung volumes, and hypoxemia. In most cases, diagnosis is confirmed by performing chest X-ray or CT and obtaining a complete occupational history. Treatment is usually palliative and focuses on preventing further exposure and improving working conditions, along with pulmonary rehabilitation and management of associated hypoxemia and bronchospasm.

Hypersensitivity pneumonitis. Hypersensitivity pneumonitis (extrinsic allergic alveolitis) is an allergic, inflammatory disease of the lungs caused by inhalation of organic particles or fumes. Many allergens can cause this disorder, including grains, silage, bird droppings or feathers, wood dust (particularly redwood and maple), cork dust, animal pelts, coffee beans, fish meal, mushroom compost, and moulds that grow on sugarcane, barley, and straw. The lung inflammation is a hypersensitivity response that occurs after repeated, prolonged exposure to the allergen causing pneumonitis. Lymphocytes and inflammatory cells infiltrate the interstitial lung tissue, releasing a variety of autoimmune and inflammatory cytokines.[19]

Hypersensitivity pneumonitis can be acute, subacute, or chronic. The acute form causes fever, cough, and chills a few hours after exposure. With continued exposure, the disease becomes chronic and pulmonary fibrosis develops. Diagnosis is made by obtaining a history of allergen exposure and by performing serum antibody testing, chest X-ray, bronchoalveolar lavage, CT, and, in some cases, lung biopsy. Treatment consists of removal of the offending agent and administration of corticosteroids.[20]

Pulmonary Edema

Pulmonary edema is excess water in the lung. The normal lung is kept dry by lymphatic drainage and a balance among capillary hydrostatic pressure, capillary oncotic pressure, and capillary permeability. In addition, surfactant lining the alveoli repels water, keeping fluid from entering the alveoli. Predisposing factors for pulmonary edema include heart disease, ARDS, and inhalation of toxic gases. The pathogenesis of pulmonary edema is shown in Figure 27-6.

The most common cause of pulmonary edema is left-sided heart disease. When the left ventricle fails, filling pressures on the left side of the heart increase and cause a concomitant increase in pulmonary capillary hydrostatic pressure. When the hydrostatic pressure exceeds the oncotic pressure (which holds fluid in the capillary), fluid moves from the capillary into the interstitial space (the space within the alveolar septum between the alveolus and capillary). When the flow of fluid out of the capillaries exceeds the lymphatic system's ability to remove it, pulmonary edema develops.

Another cause of pulmonary edema is capillary injury that increases capillary permeability, as in cases of adult respiratory distress syndrome or inhalation of toxic gases, such as ammonia. Capillary injury and

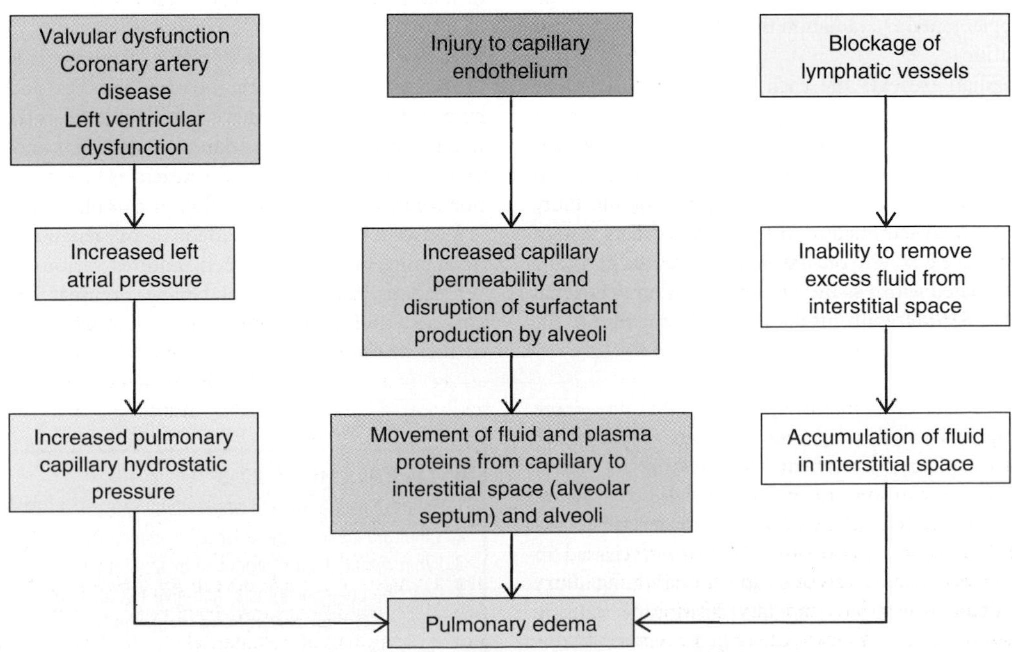

FIGURE 27-6 Pathogenesis of Pulmonary Edema.

inflammation causes water and plasma proteins to leak out of the capillary and move into the interstitial space, increasing the interstitial oncotic pressure (which is usually very low). As the interstitial oncotic pressure begins to exceed the capillary oncotic pressure, water moves out of the capillary and into the lung. (Mechanisms of edema are discussed in Chapter 5, Figures 5-1 and 5-2.) Pulmonary edema also can result from obstruction of the lymphatic system by tumours and fibrotic tissue and by increased systemic venous pressure.

Clinical manifestations of pulmonary edema include dyspnea, hypoxemia, and increased work of breathing. Physical examination may disclose inspiratory crackles (rales) and dullness to percussion over the lung bases. In severe edema, pink frothy sputum is expectorated, hypoxemia worsens, and hypoventilation with hypercapnia may develop.

The treatment of pulmonary edema depends on its cause. If the edema is caused by increased hydrostatic pressure resulting from heart failure, therapy is directed toward improving cardiac output with diuretics, vasodilators, and medications that improve the contraction of the heart muscle. If edema is the result of increased capillary permeability resulting from injury, the treatment is focused on removing the offending agent and implementing supportive therapy to maintain adequate ventilation and circulation. Individuals with either type of pulmonary edema require supplemental O_2. Mechanical ventilation may be needed if edema significantly impairs ventilation and oxygenation.

Acute Lung Injury/Acute Respiratory Distress Syndrome

Acute lung injury (ALI)/acute respiratory distress syndrome (ARDS) represents a spectrum of acute lung inflammation and diffuse alveolocapillary injury. Both ALI and ARDS are defined as (1) the acute onset of bilateral infiltrates on chest radiograph, (2) a low ratio of PaO_2 to the fraction of inhaled O_2 under positive airway pressure, and (3) is not derived from hydrostatic pulmonary edema. Biomarkers that can be used to diagnose ARDS are under investigation.[21] Advances in therapy have decreased overall mortality in people younger than 60 years to approximately 40%, although mortality in older adults and those with severe infections remains much higher. The most common predisposing factors are genetic factors, sepsis, and multiple trauma. There are many other causes, including pneumonia, burns, aspiration, cardiopulmonary bypass surgery, pancreatitis, blood transfusions, drug overdose, inhalation of smoke or noxious gases, fat emboli, high concentrations of supplemental O_2, radiation therapy, and disseminated intravascular coagulation.

Over 10 000 Canadian patients die each year from ARDS. The mortality rate from ALI/ARDS is close to 50%. Often patients are so sick that they need to be on mechanical ventilation, which itself may result in ventilator-induced lung injury (VILI). Studies have reported that lung stretch due to cyclical stretching can increase the mortality rate by nearly 10%. In Canada, annually, thousands of patients sustain a severe injury to the lung (e.g., severe pneumonia) that results in ARDS. The estimated cost associated with a single patient admission to hospital with ARDS approaches $15 000, putting the national expenditure for this condition at over $2 billion annually.[22]

PATHOPHYSIOLOGY All disorders causing ALI/ARDS cause acute injury to the alveolocapillary membrane, producing massive pulmonary inflammation, increased capillary permeability, severe pulmonary edema, shunting, $\dot{V}/\dot{Q}$ mismatch, and hypoxemia. ARDS can occur directly (from aspiration of highly acidic gastric contents, inhalation of toxic gases) or indirectly (from circulating inflammatory mediators released in response to systemic disorders, such as sepsis and trauma). Lung injury and inflammation damage the alveolocapillary membrane, causing pulmonary edema, often referred to as *noncardiogenic pulmonary edema*. ARDS progresses through three overlapping phases characterized by histological changes in the lung: exudative (inflammatory), proliferative, and fibrotic[23,24] (Figure 27-7). The three phases are described as follows:

1. *Exudative phase (within 72 hours):* Neutrophils and other cells (platelets, macrophages, lung epithelial, and endothelial cells) that release a cascade of inflammatory cytokines are activated, causing damage to the alveolocapillary membrane and greatly increasing capillary membrane permeability. Fluids, proteins, and blood cells leak from the capillary bed into the pulmonary interstitium and flood the alveoli (hemorrhagic exudate). Surfactant is inactivated. The resulting pulmonary edema and hemorrhage severely reduce lung compliance and impair alveolar ventilation. The inflammatory mediators also cause pulmonary vasoconstriction, contributing to ventilation–perfusion mismatch. The inflammatory mediators causing the alveolocapillary damage of ARDS often cause inflammation, endothelial damage, and capillary permeability throughout the body, resulting in systemic inflammatory response syndrome (SIRS). SIRS then leads to multiple organ dysfunction syndrome (MODS) and may cause death (see Chapter 24 and Figure 24-46).
2. *Proliferative phase (within 4 to 21 days):* Resolution of the pulmonary edema and proliferation of type II pneumocytes, fibroblasts, and myofibroblasts take place. The intra-alveolar hemorrhagic exudate becomes a cellular granulation tissue appearing as hyaline membranes and there is progressive hypoxemia.
3. *Fibrotic phase (within 14 to 21 days):* Remodelling and fibrosis of lung tissue take place. The fibrosis progressively obliterates the alveoli, respiratory bronchioles, and interstitium, leading to a decrease in functional residual capacity (FRC) and continuing $\dot{V}/\dot{Q}$ mismatch with severe right-to-left shunt. The result of this overwhelming inflammatory response by the lungs is acute respiratory failure.

CLINICAL MANIFESTATIONS The clinical manifestations of ARDS are progressive, as follows:

1. Dyspnea and hypoxemia with poor response to O_2 supplementation
2. Hyperventilation and respiratory alkalosis
3. Decreased tissue perfusion, metabolic acidosis, and organ dysfunction
4. Increased work of breathing, decreased tidal volume, and hypoventilation
5. Hypercapnia, respiratory acidosis, and worsening hypoxemia
6. Respiratory failure, decreased cardiac output, hypotension, and death

EVALUATION AND TREATMENT Diagnosis is based on a history of the lung injury, physical examination, blood gas analysis, and radiological examination. Measurement of serum biomarkers (i.e., surfactant proteins, mucin-associated antigens and interleukins) may aid in the diagnosis and prognosis of ARDS.[25] Treatment is based on early detection, supportive therapy, and prevention of complications. Supportive therapy is focused on maintaining adequate oxygenation and ventilation while preventing infection. It often requires various modes of mechanical ventilation. Pharmacological therapy continues to be explored. Low-dose corticosteroids may improve survival in selected individuals but needs further investigation.[26]

QUICK CHECK 27-3

1. Contrast *aspiration* and *atelectasis.*
2. What are some of the causes of pulmonary fibrosis?
3. What symptoms are produced by inhalation of toxic gases?
4. Describe pneumoconiosis, and give two examples.
5. Briefly describe the role of neutrophils in acute respiratory distress syndrome.

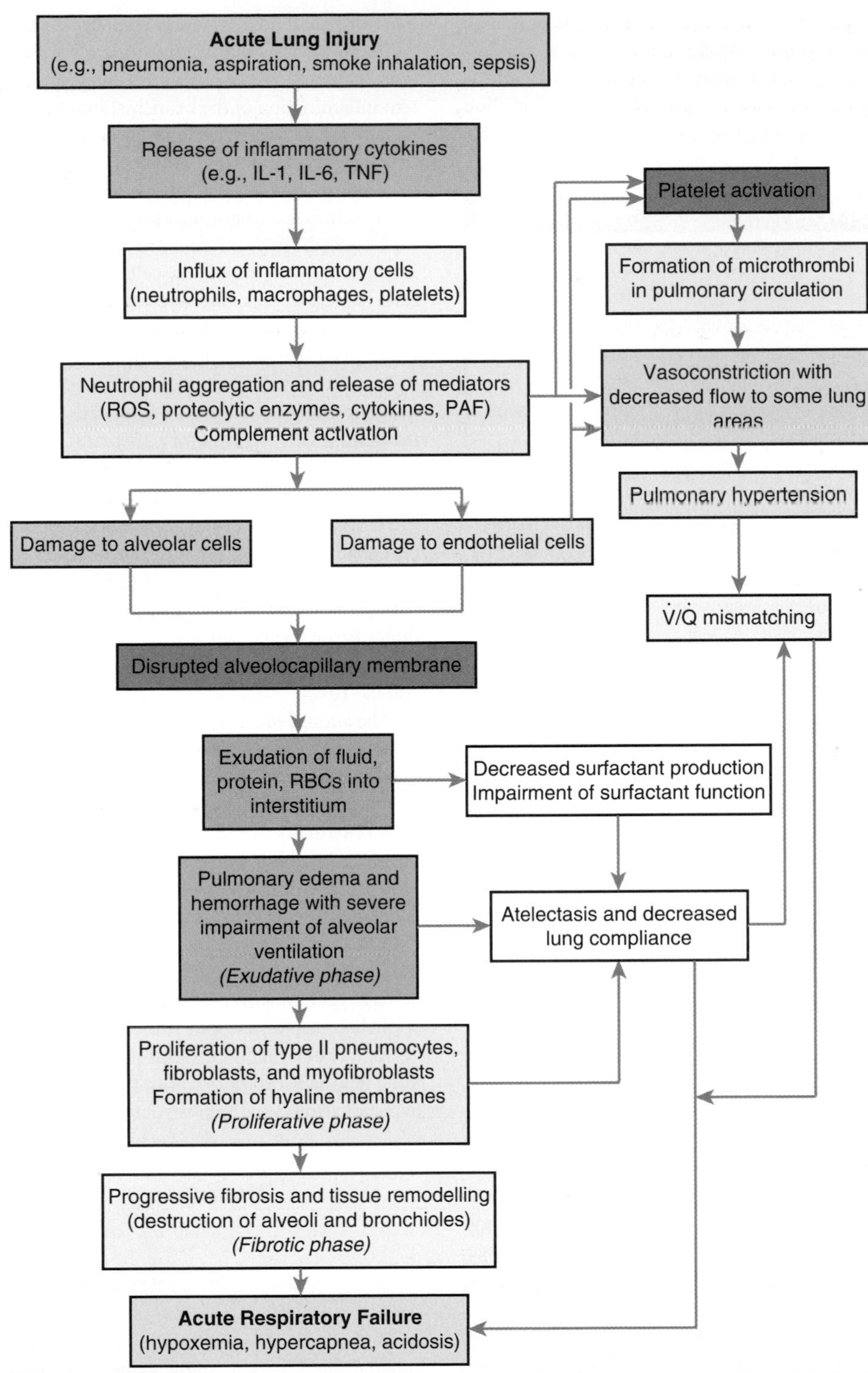

FIGURE 27-7 Pathogenesis of Acute Respiratory Distress Syndrome. *IL*, interleukin; *PAF*, platelet-activating factor; *RBCs*, red blood cells; *ROS*, reactive oxygen species; *TNF*, tumour necrosis factor; $\dot{V}/\dot{Q}$, ventilation–perfusion ratio.

Obstructive Lung Diseases

Obstructive lung disease is characterized by airway obstruction that is worse with expiration. More force (i.e., use of accessory muscles of expiration) is required to expire a given volume of air and emptying of the lungs is slowed. The unifying symptom of obstructive lung diseases is dyspnea, and the unifying sign is wheezing. Individuals have an increased work of breathing, ventilation–perfusion mismatching, and a decreased forced expiratory volume in 1 second (FEV_1). The most common obstructive diseases are asthma, chronic bronchitis, and emphysema. Because many individuals have chronic bronchitis with emphysema, these diseases together are often called *chronic obstructive pulmonary disease* (COPD).

Asthma

Asthma is a chronic inflammatory disorder of the bronchial mucosa that causes bronchial hyper-responsiveness, constriction of the airways, and variable airflow obstruction that is reversible. Asthma occurs at all ages and is the third-most common chronic disease in Canada (see *Health Promotion:* Asthma).[27] In the United States, asthma affects approximately 6.8 million children (see Chapter 28) and 18.7 million adults. The prevalence of asthma is increasing.[28]

HEALTH PROMOTION

Asthma

Asthma affects 2.4 million Canadians over the age of 12 (8.5% of the population) and another 490 000 children between the ages of 4 and 11 (15.6% of children in this age bracket).

It is estimated that between 150 000 and 250 000 Canadians who have asthma suffer from *severe asthma*, a more severe form of asthma and a greater threat to the health of these Canadians.

In Canada, many asthma patients do not have control over their asthma; 53% of Canadians with asthma have what doctors call "poorly controlled" asthma. This designation means that the asthma treatment is ineffective. Those who have poorly controlled asthma have poorer health outcomes and quality of life as compared with individuals with well-controlled asthma.

Indigenous people in Canada are highly impacted by asthma. Asthma is 40% more prevalent among First Nations, Inuit, and Métis communities than in the general Canadian population.

It is estimated that 250 Canadians die each year from asthma. Around the world, approximately 250 000 people die prematurely each year because of asthma. Asthma is the leading cause of hospital admission in Canada. In 2011, Canadian emergency departments dealt with 64 526 asthma-related events.

Asthma is a billion-dollar problem in Canada. According to the Conference Board of Canada, the cost of hospitalization for asthma in 2010 was $250 728 024. The physicians who cared for these patients cost $196 321 334. The cost of asthma medication in 2010 was $535 681 566. Indirect costs associated with asthma, including decreased productivity, are estimated at $646 million.

From Asthma Society of Canada. (2014). *Severe asthma: The Canadian patient journey.* Toronto: Author. Retrieved from https://asthma.ca/living-with-severe-asthma.

Asthma is a familial disorder, and more than 100 genes have been identified that may play a role in the susceptibility, pathogenesis, and treatment response of asthma. Specific gene expressions may impart associated *phenotypes* with specific inflammatory markers (i.e., cells, cytokines, or exhaled nitric oxide) or *endotypes* including clinical characteristics, biomarkers, lung physiology, genetics, histopathology, epidemiology, and treatment response.[29] Other risk factors include age at onset of disease, levels of allergen exposure, urban residence, exposure to indoor and outdoor air pollution, tobacco smoke, recurrent respiratory tract viral infections, gastroesophageal reflux disease, and obesity (which promotes a proinflammatory state).[30-32] Exposure to inhaled irritants can cause inflammation and damage to airways independent of allergen sensitivity. This exposure leads to irritant (or nonallergic) asthma, as well as increases the hyper-responsiveness of the airways to allergens in those with a history of atopy (allergy).[33] Inhaled irritants affect both the epigenetics of asthma and asthma presentation, including age of onset, symptoms, and gender differences.[34]

Exposure to high levels of certain allergens during childhood increases the risk for asthma. Furthermore, decreased exposure to certain infectious organisms appears to create an immunological imbalance that favours the development of allergy and asthma. This complex relationship has been called the *hygiene hypothesis*.[35] Recently, the relationship between the microbiome and asthma risk is shedding light on these complex interactions.[36]

PATHOPHYSIOLOGY Airway epithelial exposure to antigen initiates both an innate and an adaptive immune response in sensitized individuals[37] (see Chapter 8). Many cells and cellular elements contribute to the persistent inflammation of the bronchial mucosa and hyper-responsiveness of the airways, including dendritic cells (antigen-presenting macrophages), T-helper 2 lymphocytes (Th2 cells), B lymphocytes (B cells), mast cells, neutrophils, eosinophils, and basophils. There is both an immediate (early asthmatic response) and a late (delayed) response.

During the *early asthmatic response*, antigen exposure to the bronchial mucosa activates dendritic cells, which present antigen to T-helper cells. T-helper cells differentiate into Th2 cells, releasing inflammatory cytokines and interleukins that activate B cells (plasma cells) and eosinophils. Plasma cells produce antigen-specific immunoglobulin E (IgE), which binds to the surface of mast cells. Subsequent cross-linking of IgE molecules with the antigen causes mast cell degranulation with the release of inflammatory mediators, including histamine, bradykinins, leukotrienes and prostaglandins, platelet-activating factor, and interleukins[38] (see Figures 8-11 and 8-12 for additional details). These inflammatory mediators cause vasodilation, increased capillary permeability, mucosal edema, bronchial smooth muscle contraction (bronchospasm), and mucus secretion from mucosal goblet cells with narrowing of the airways and obstruction to airflow. Eosinophils cause direct tissue injury and release of toxic neuropeptides that contribute to increased bronchial hyper-responsiveness[39] (Figures 27-8, 27-9, and 27-10).

The *late asthmatic response* begins 4 to 8 hours after the early response. Chemotactic recruitment of eosinophils, neutrophils, and lymphocytes during the acute response causes a latent release of inflammatory mediators, again inciting bronchospasm, edema, and mucus secretion with obstruction to airflow. Synthesis of leukotrienes contributes to prolonged smooth muscle contraction. Eosinophils cause direct tissue injury with fibroblast proliferation and airway scarring. Damage to ciliated epithelial cells contributes to impaired mucociliary function, with the accumulation of mucus and cellular debris forming plugs in the airways. Untreated inflammation can lead to long-term airway damage that is irreversible and is known as *airway remodelling* (subepithelial fibrosis, smooth muscle hypertrophy).[40]

Airway obstruction increases resistance to airflow and decreases flow rates, especially expiratory flow. Impaired expiration causes air trapping, hyperinflation distal to obstructions, and increased work of breathing.

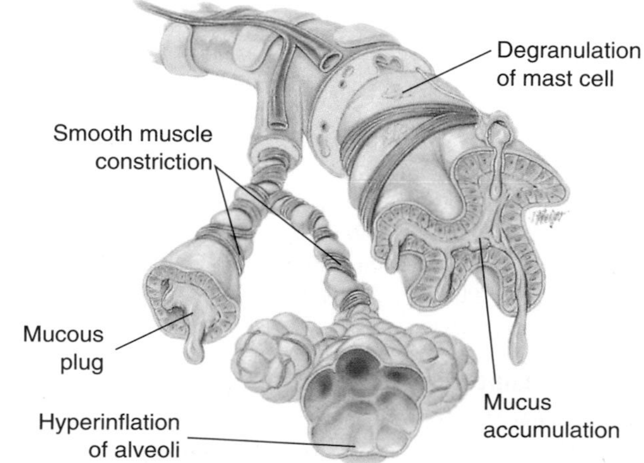

FIGURE 27-8 Bronchial Asthma. Thick mucus, mucosal edema, and smooth muscle spasm cause obstruction of small airways; breathing becomes laboured and expiration is difficult. (Modified from Des Jardins, T., & Burton, G.G. [1995]. *Clinical manifestations and assessment of respiratory disease* [3rd ed.]. St. Louis: Mosby.)

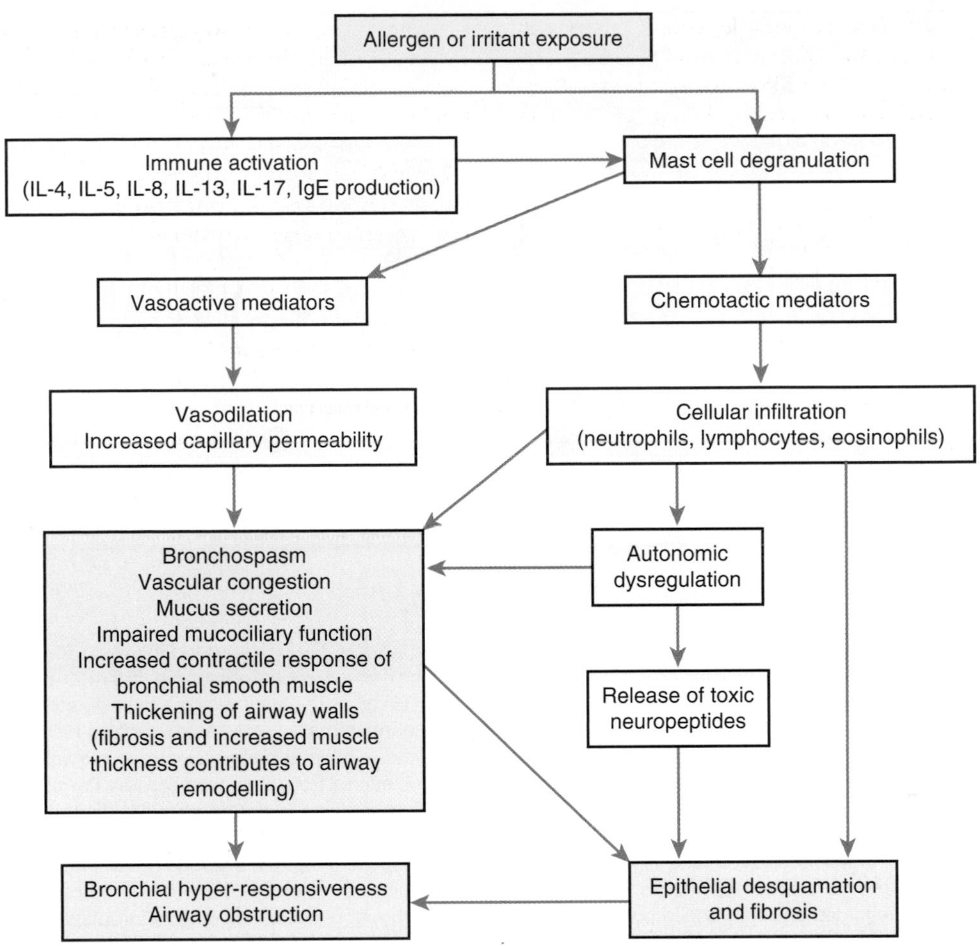

FIGURE 27-9 Pathophysiology of Asthma. Allergen or irritant exposure results in a cascade of inflammatory events leading to acute and chronic airway dysfunction. *IgE,* immunoglobulin E; *IL,* interleukin.

Changes in resistance to airflow are not uniform throughout the lungs and the distribution of inspired air is uneven, with more air flowing to the less resistant portions. Continued air trapping increases intrapleural and alveolar gas pressures and causes decreased perfusion of the alveoli. Increased alveolar gas pressure, decreased ventilation, and decreased perfusion lead to variable and uneven ventilation–perfusion relationships within different lung segments. Hyperventilation is triggered by lung receptors responding to increased lung volume and obstruction. The result is early hypoxemia without CO_2 retention. Hypoxemia further increases hyperventilation through stimulation of the respiratory centre, causing $PaCO_2$ to decrease and pH to increase (respiratory alkalosis). With progressive obstruction of expiratory airflow, air trapping becomes more severe and the lungs and thorax become hyperexpanded, positioning the respiratory muscles at a mechanical disadvantage. This leads to a decrease in tidal volume with increasing CO_2 retention and respiratory acidosis. Respiratory acidosis signals respiratory failure, especially when left ventricular filling, and thus cardiac output, becomes compromised because of severe hyperinflation.

CLINICAL MANIFESTATIONS Individuals are asymptomatic between attacks, and pulmonary function tests are normal. At the beginning of an attack, the individual experiences chest constriction, expiratory wheezing, dyspnea, nonproductive coughing, prolonged expiration, tachycardia, and tachypnea. Severe attacks involve the accessory muscles of respiration, and wheezing is heard during both inspiration and expiration. A **pulsus paradoxus** (decrease in systolic blood pressure during inspiration of more than 10 mm Hg) may be noted. Peak flow measurements should be obtained. Because the severity of blood gas alterations is difficult to evaluate by clinical signs alone, arterial blood gas tensions should be measured if O_2 saturation falls below 90%. Usual findings are hypoxemia with an associated respiratory alkalosis. In the *late asthma response*, symptoms can be even more severe than the initial attack.

If bronchospasm is not reversed by usual treatment measures, the individual is considered to have acute severe bronchospasm or **status asthmaticus**.[41] If status asthmaticus continues, hypoxemia worsens, expiratory flows and volumes decrease further, and effective ventilation decreases. Acidosis develops as the $PaCO_2$ level begins to rise. Asthma becomes life-threatening at this point if treatment does not reverse this process quickly. A silent chest (no audible air movement) and a $PaCO_2$ of greater than 70 mm Hg are ominous signs of impending death.

EVALUATION AND TREATMENT The diagnosis of asthma is supported by a history of allergies and recurrent episodes of wheezing, dyspnea, and cough or exercise intolerance. Further evaluation includes spirometry, which may document reversible decreases in FEV_1 during an induced attack.

The evaluation of an acute asthma attack requires the rapid assessment of arterial blood gases and expiratory flow rates (using a peak flow meter) and a search for underlying triggers, such as infection. Hypoxemia and respiratory alkalosis are expected early in the course of an acute attack. The development of hypercapnia with respiratory acidosis signals the need for mechanical ventilation. Management of the acute asthma attack requires immediate administration of O_2 and inhaled beta-agonist

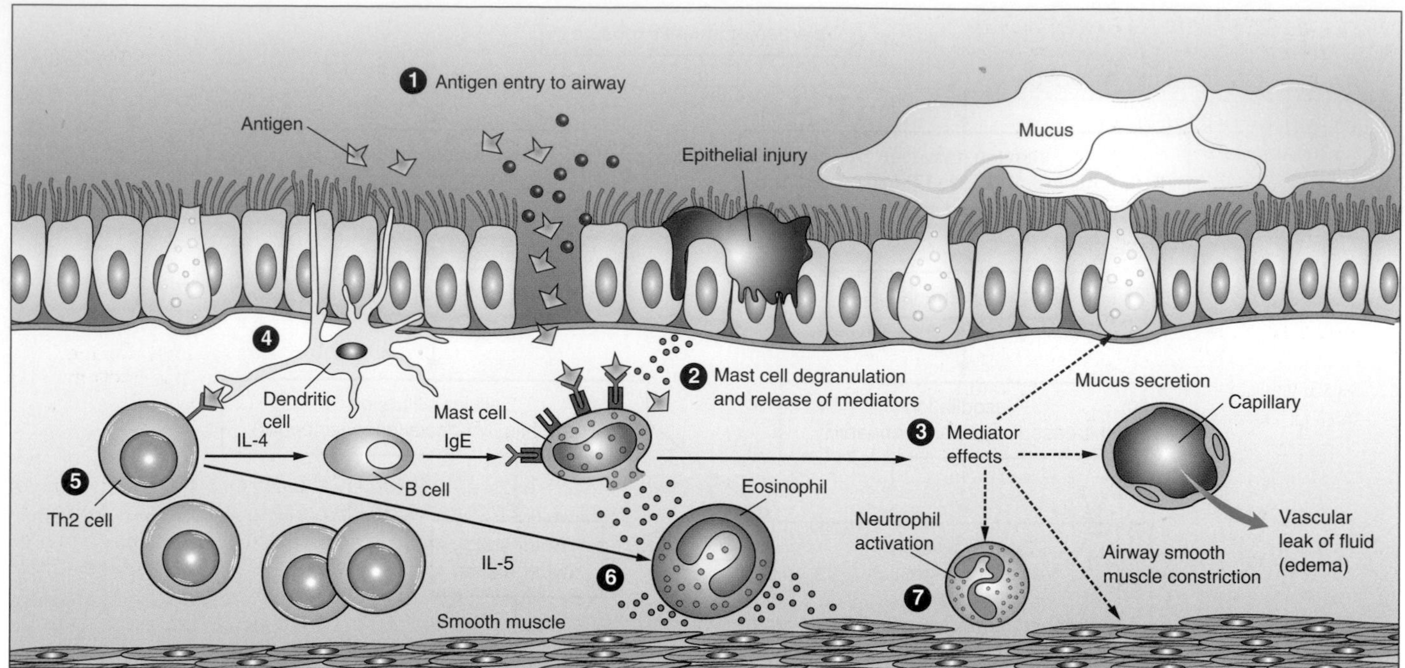

FIGURE 27-10 Acute Asthmatic Responses. Inhaled antigen **(1)** binds to mast cells covered with preformed immunoglobulin E (*IgE*). Mast cells degranulate **(2)** and release inflammatory mediators such as histamine, bradykinins, leukotrienes, prostaglandins, platelet-activating factor, and interleukins. Secreted mediators **(3)** induce active bronchospasm (airway smooth muscle constriction), edema from increased capillary permeability, and airway mucus secretion from goblet cells. At the same time, antigen is detected by **(4)** dendritic cells that process and present it to Th2 cells **(5)**, which produce interleukin-4 (*IL-4*) and many other interleukins (see text). IL-4 promotes switching of B cells to favour IgE production. Th2 cells also produce interleukin-5 (*IL-5*) **(6)**, which activates eosinophils. Eosinophil products, such as major basic protein and eosinophilic cationic protein, damage the respiratory epithelium. Many inflammatory cells, including neutrophils **(7)**, also contribute to the inflammatory process and airway obstruction.

bronchodilators. In addition, oral corticosteroids should be administered early in the course of management.[42] Careful monitoring of gas exchange and airway obstruction in response to therapy provides information necessary to determine whether hospitalization is necessary. Antibiotics are not indicated for acute asthma unless there is a documented bacterial infection.

Management of asthma begins with avoidance of allergens and irritants. Individuals with asthma tend to underestimate the severity of their asthma and extensive education is important, including use of a peak flow meter and adherence to an action plan. In the mildest form of asthma (intermittent), short-acting beta-agonist inhalers are prescribed. For all categories of persistent asthma, anti-inflammatory medications are essential, and inhaled corticosteroids are the mainstay of therapy. In individuals who are not adequately controlled with inhaled corticosteroids, leukotriene antagonists can be considered. In more severe asthma, long-acting beta agonists can be used to control persistent bronchospasm; however, these agonists can actually worsen asthma in some individuals with certain genetic polymorphisms.[43] Immunotherapy has been shown to be an important tool in reducing asthma exacerbations and can now be given sublingually.[44] Monoclonal antibodies to IgE (omalizumab [Xolair]) have been found to be helpful as adjunctive therapy to inhaled steroids.[45] Biomarkers and epigenetic markers are being evaluated to personalize treatment and reduce mortality.[46,47]

Asthma Canada (formerly Asthma Society of Canada) has issued stepwise guidelines for the diagnosis and management of chronic asthma based on clinical severity (see https://www.asthma.ca/get-help/community/publications/). The Canadian Paediatric Society and the Canadian Thoracic Society have issued age-specific guidelines for diagnosis and management of asthma in preschoolers (see http://www.cps.ca/en/documents/position/asthma-in-preschoolers).

Chronic Obstructive Pulmonary Disease

Chronic obstructive pulmonary disease (COPD) is defined as a common preventable and treatable disease characterized by persistent airflow limitation that is usually progressive and associated with an enhanced chronic inflammatory response in the airways and the lung to noxious particles or gases. Exacerbations and comorbidities contribute to the overall severity of disease.[48] COPD is the most common chronic lung disease in the world, and the fourth-leading cause of death globally. However, COPD prevalence in women is higher throughout the lifespan. Risk factors for COPD include tobacco smoke (cigarette, pipe, cigar, and environmental tobacco smoke), occupational dusts and chemicals (vapours, irritants, and fumes), indoor air pollution from biomass fuel used for cooking and heating (in poorly vented dwellings), outdoor air pollution (see *Health Promotion*: Tips to Keep Lungs Healthy), and any factor that affects lung growth during gestation and childhood (low birth weight, respiratory tract infections).[49] Genetic and epigenetic susceptibilities have been identified including polymorphisms of genes that code for tumour necrosis factor, surfactant, proteases, and antiproteases and acquired failure of DNA repair.[50] The clinical phenotypes of COPD discussed here are chronic bronchitis and emphysema. An inherited mutation in the α_1-antitrypsin gene results in the development of COPD at an early age, even in individuals who do not smoke.

According to Statistics Canada, 4% of Canadians aged 35 to 79 self-reported being diagnosed with COPD, whereas direct measurements

HEALTH PROMOTION

Tips to Keep Lungs Healthy

1. **Get help to quit smoking.** Smoke from cigarettes, cigars, and pipes contains over 4 000 harmful chemicals, 50 of which are known to cause cancer. As such, smoking can cause lung cancer and chronic obstructive pulmonary disease (COPD).
2. **Stay away from second hand smoke.** Second hand smoke is a mix of chemicals produced by burning tobacco. Two-thirds of the smoke from a cigarette is not inhaled by the smoker. Instead, it enters the air around the smoker and is sometimes inhaled by people sharing the same space, increasing their risk of developing a disease and even dying.
3. **Wash your hands well with soap and water.** Around 80% of common infectious respiratory diseases like colds and flu are spread through touch. Avoid excessive use of antibacterial soaps and cleaners to prevent antibiotic resistance. Also, use an alcohol-based hand sanitizer in cases where you do not have access to soap and water.
4. **Take part in minimizing air pollution.** Avoid idling your car engine and open-air burning. Avoid using pesticides and other chemicals on your lawn and garden. Walk or use public transit. Do not forget to ventilate your house to make sure that you are getting a lot of fresh, clean air. Always open your windows when cleaning, painting, installing new carpet, or doing other household projects.
5. **Wear protective gear if you work around dust and asbestos.** By protecting your lungs from potential health hazards at work, you can decrease the risk of developing lung diseases such as lung cancer, asthma, and COPD.

© All rights reserved. *How do I keep my lungs healthy?* Public Health Agency of Canada, 2008. Adapted and reproduced with permission from the Minister of Health, 2017. Retrieved from http://www.phac-aspc.gc.ca/cd-mc/crd-mrc/healthy_lungs-poumons_en_sante-eng.php.

of lung function from the Canadian Health Measures Survey (CHMS) indicate that 13% of Canadians had a lung function score indicative of COPD; that is, a FEV_1/FVC ratio of less than 0.70. The disparity between self-reported and measured COPD in the CHMS suggests that COPD is underdiagnosed in Canada. Further, Canadians aged 60 to 79 (19%) were more likely to have measured COPD than those aged 40 to 59 (11%). Despite the gravity of COPD, 60 to 85% of patients (most with mild to moderately severe COPD) are thought to remain undiagnosed.[51]

Chronic Bronchitis

Chronic bronchitis is defined as hypersecretion of mucus and chronic productive cough for at least 3 months of the year (usually the winter months) for at least 2 consecutive years.

PATHOPHYSIOLOGY Inspired irritants result in airway inflammation with infiltration of neutrophils, macrophages, and lymphocytes into the bronchial wall. Continual bronchial inflammation causes bronchial edema, an increase in the size and number of mucous glands and goblet cells in the airway epithelium, smooth muscle hypertrophy with fibrosis, and narrowing of airways. Thick, tenacious mucus is produced and cannot be cleared because of impaired ciliary function (Figure 27-11). The lung's defence mechanisms are, therefore, compromised, increasing susceptibility to pulmonary infection and injury and ineffective repair. Frequent infectious exacerbations from bacterial colonization of damaged airways are complicated by bronchospasm with dyspnea and productive cough.[52,53] The pathogenesis of chronic bronchitis is shown in Figure 27-12.

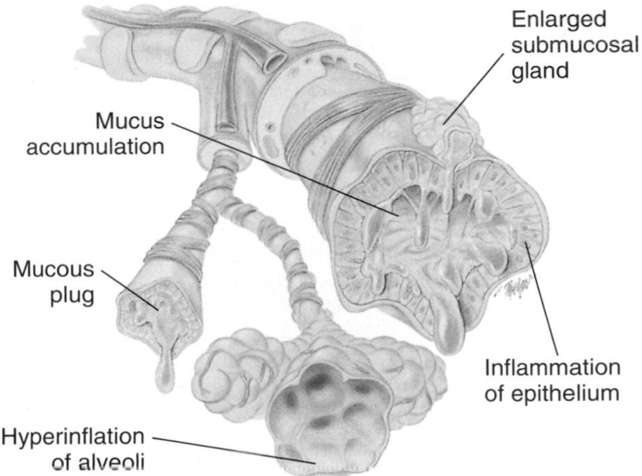

FIGURE 27-11 Chronic Bronchitis. Inflammation and thickening of mucous membrane with accumulation of mucus and pus leading to obstruction characterized by productive cough. (Modified from Des Jardins, T., & Burton, G.G. [1995]. *Clinical manifestations and assessment of respiratory disease* [3rd ed.]. St. Louis: Mosby.)

TABLE 27-2 Clinical Manifestations of Chronic Obstructive Lung Disease

Clinical Manifestations	Chronic Bronchitis	Emphysema
Productive cough	Classic sign	With infection
Dyspnea	Late in course	Common
Wheezing	Intermittent	Common
History of smoking	Common	Common
Barrel chest	Occasionally	Classic
Prolonged expiration	Always present	Always present
Cyanosis	Common	Uncommon
Chronic hypoventilation	Common	Late in course
Polycythemia	Common	Late in course
Cor pulmonale	Common	Late in course

This process initially affects only the larger bronchi, but eventually all airways are involved. The thick mucus and hypertrophied bronchial smooth muscle constrict the airways and lead to obstruction, particularly during expiration when the airways are narrowed (Figure 27-13). Obstruction eventually leads to ventilation–perfusion mismatch with hypoxemia. The airways collapse early in expiration, trapping gas in the distal portions of the lung (hyperinflation).[54] Air trapping expands the thorax and positions the respiratory muscles at a mechanical disadvantage. This air trapping leads to decreased tidal volume, hypoventilation, and hypercapnia.

CLINICAL MANIFESTATIONS Table 27-2 lists the common clinical manifestations of chronic bronchitis and emphysema.

EVALUATION AND TREATMENT Diagnosis is based on history of symptoms, physical examination, chest imaging, pulmonary function tests (i.e., a FEV_1/FVC ratio less than 0.7), and blood gas analyses. These tests reflect the progressive nature of the disease. Prevention of chronic bronchitis is essential because pathological changes are not reversible. By the time an individual seeks medical care for symptoms, considerable airway damage is present. If the individual stops smoking, disease progression can be halted.[55] Influenza and pneumococcal vaccinations should be up to date.

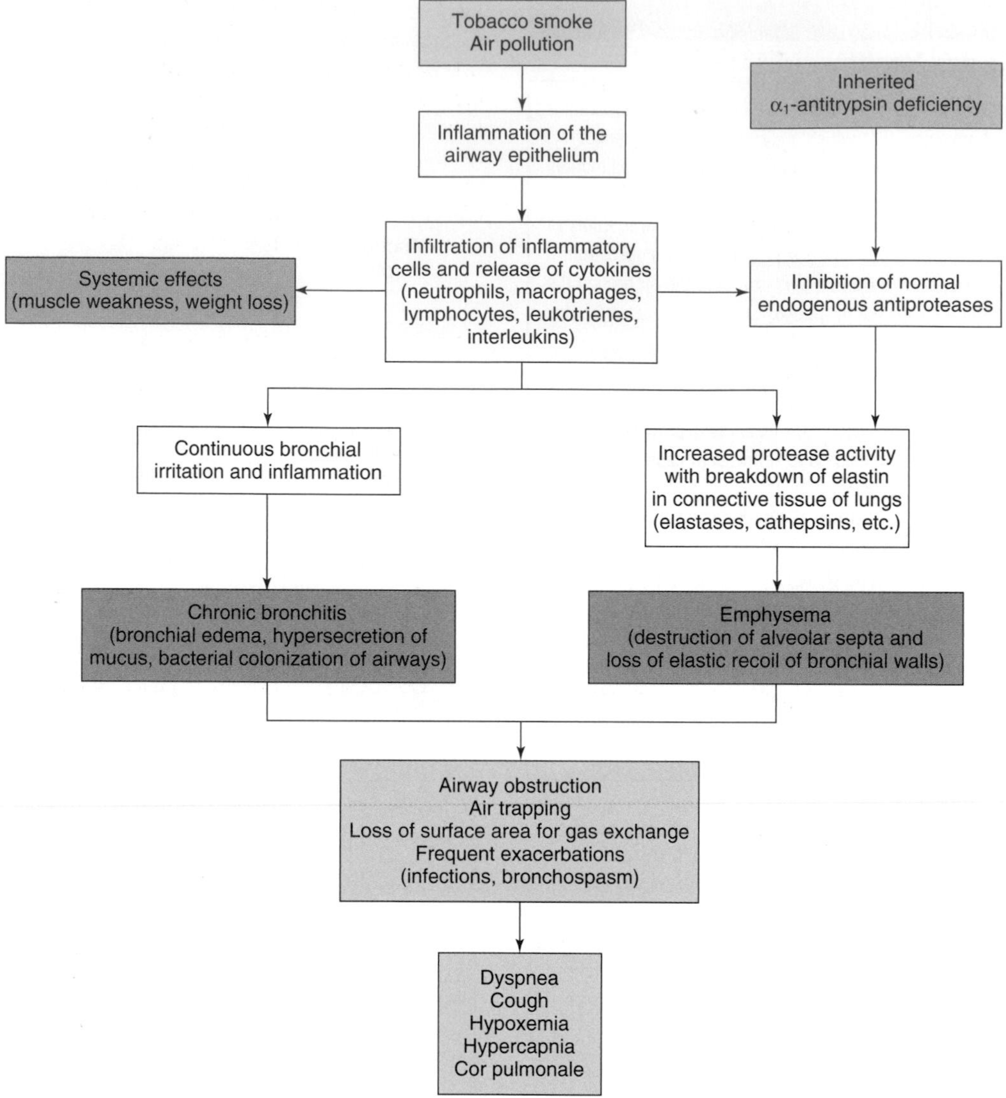

FIGURE 27-12 Pathogenesis of Chronic Bronchitis and Emphysema (Chronic Obstructive Pulmonary Disease).

Bronchodilators, mucolytics, antioxidants, and anti-inflammatory medications are prescribed as needed to control cough and reduce dyspnea. Chest physiotherapy may be helpful and includes deep breathing and postural drainage. During acute exacerbations (infection and bronchospasm), individuals require treatment with antibiotics and steroids and may need mechanical ventilation.[56] Chronic use of oral steroids may be needed late in the course of the disease but should be considered a last resort. Individuals with severe hypoxemia will require home O_2 therapy. O_2 is administered with care to individuals with severe hypoxemia and CO_2 retention. Chronic elevation of $PaCO_2$ diminishes the sensitivity of central chemoreceptors, and they no longer act as the primary stimulus for breathing. Teaching includes nutritional counselling, respiratory hygiene, recognition of the early signs of infection, and techniques that relieve dyspnea, such as pursed-lip breathing. In addition, many comorbidities accompany COPD and require monitoring and therapy, including cardiovascular disorders, metabolic diseases, bone disease, stroke, lung cancer, cachexia, skeletal muscle weakness, anemia, depression, and cognitive decline. Chronic low-grade systemic inflammation may be associated with these conditions.[57]

Emphysema

Emphysema is abnormal permanent enlargement of gas-exchange airways (acini) accompanied by destruction of alveolar walls without obvious fibrosis. Obstruction results from changes in lung tissues rather than mucus production and inflammation, as in chronic bronchitis. The major mechanism of airflow limitation is loss of elastic recoil.

Primary emphysema, which accounts for 1 to 3% of all cases of emphysema, is commonly linked to an inherited deficiency of the enzyme α_1-antitrypsin. Normally α_1-antitrypsin inhibits the action of many proteolytic enzymes (i.e., elastases released by neutrophils); therefore, α_1-antitrypsin deficiency (an autosomal recessive trait) increases the likelihood of developing emphysema because proteolysis in lung tissues is not inhibited.[58] α_1-Antitrypsin deficiency is suggested in individuals who develop emphysema before 40 years of age and in individuals who do not smoke but still develop the disease. The major cause of secondary emphysema is the inhalation of tobacco smoke, although air pollution, occupational exposures, and childhood respiratory tract infections are known to be contributing factors.

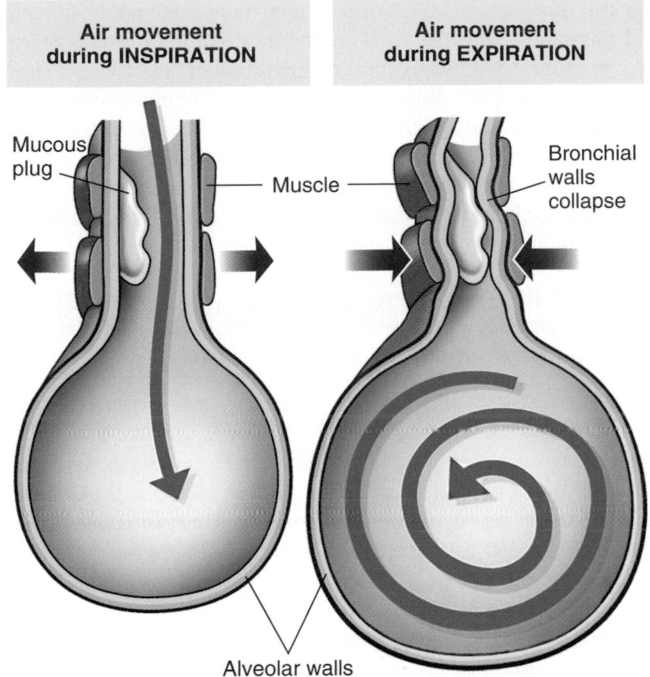

FIGURE 27-13 Mechanisms of Air Trapping in Chronic Obstructive Pulmonary Disease. Mucous plugs and narrowed airways cause air trapping and hyperinflation of alveoli on expiration. During inspiration, the airways are pulled open, allowing gas to flow past the obstruction. During expiration, decreased elastic recoil of the bronchial walls results in collapse of the airways and prevents normal expiratory airflow.

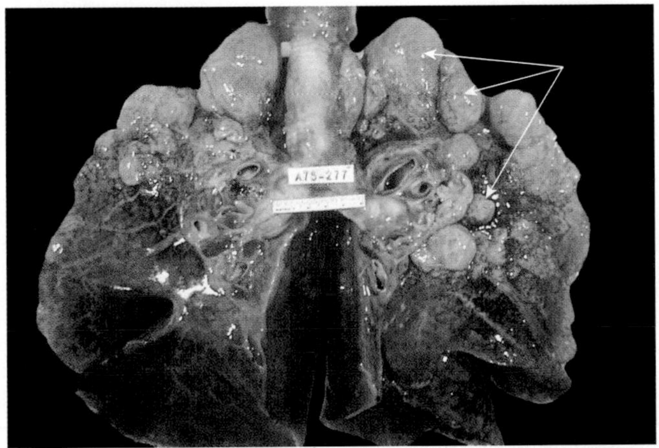

FIGURE 27-14 Bullous Emphysema With Large Apical and Subpleural Bullae (*arrows*). (From Kumar, V., Abbas, A.K., Fausto, N., et al. [Eds.]. [2007]. *Robbins basic pathology* [8th ed.]. Philadelphia: Saunders.)

PATHOPHYSIOLOGY Emphysema is characterized by destruction of alveoli through the breakdown of elastin within the septa by an imbalance between proteases and antiproteases, oxidative stress, and apoptosis of lung structural cells (see Figure 27-12).[59] Alveolar destruction also produces large air spaces within the lung parenchyma (bullae) and air spaces adjacent to pleurae (blebs) (Figure 27-14). Bullae and blebs are not effective in gas exchange and result in significant ventilation–perfusion mismatching and hypoxemia. Expiration becomes difficult because loss of elastic recoil reduces the volume of air that can be expired passively and air is trapped in the lungs (see Figure 27-13). Air trapping causes hyperexpansion of the chest, placing the muscles of respiration at a mechanical disadvantage. It results in increased workload of breathing, so that late in the course of disease, many individuals will develop hypoventilation and hypercapnia. Persistent inflammation in the airways can result in hyper-reactivity of the bronchi with bronchoconstriction, which may be partially reversible with bronchodilators. Destruction of alveolar walls and pulmonary capillaries also causes PAH and cor pulmonale. Chronic inflammation also can have significant systemic effects including weight loss, muscle weakness, and increased susceptibility to comorbidities, such as infection.

CLINICAL MANIFESTATIONS The clinical manifestations of emphysema are listed in Table 27-2.

EVALUATION AND TREATMENT Emphysema is usually diagnosed and staged by pulmonary function measures. In COPD, pulmonary function tests indicate obstruction to gas flow during expiration with a marked decrease in FEV_1. Chronic management of emphysema begins with smoking cessation. Pharmacological management is based on clinical severity (mild, moderate, severe, or very severe). Inhaled anticholinergic agents and beta agonists should be prescribed. Inhaled corticosteroids are indicated for severe COPD, although long-term therapy with oral steroids should be avoided if possible. Pulmonary rehabilitation, improved nutrition, and breathing techniques can improve symptoms. Progressive pulmonary dysfunction with hypoxemia and hypercapnia may require long-term O_2 therapy and ventilation, if indicated.[60] A class of medications called *phosphodiesterase E4* (PDE4) inhibitors is proving to be effective in selected individuals with severe COPD.[56] α_1-Antitrypsin augmentation may be indicated for primary emphysema.[61] Selected individuals with severe emphysema can benefit from lung volume reduction surgery.[62]

QUICK CHECK 27-4
1. What mechanisms cause airway obstruction in asthma?
2. Define *chronic bronchitis.*
3. How does emphysema affect oxygenation and ventilation?

Respiratory Tract Infections

Respiratory tract infections are a common cause of short-term disability in Canada and the United States. Most of these infections—the common cold, pharyngitis (sore throat), and laryngitis—involve only the upper airways. Although the lungs have direct contact with the atmosphere, they usually remain sterile. Infections of the lower respiratory tract occur most often in the very young and very old or those with impaired immunity.

Acute Bronchitis

Acute bronchitis is acute infection or inflammation of the airways or bronchi and is usually self-limiting. The vast majority of cases of acute bronchitis are caused by viruses. Many of the clinical manifestations are similar to those of pneumonia (i.e., fever, cough, chills, malaise), but physical examination does not reveal signs of pulmonary consolidation and chest radiographs do not show infiltrates. Individuals with viral bronchitis usually have a nonproductive cough that often occurs in paroxysms and is aggravated by cold, dry, or dusty air. In some cases, purulent sputum is produced. Chest pain often develops from the effort of coughing. Treatment consists of rest, Aspirin, humidity, and a cough suppressant, such as codeine. Bacterial bronchitis is treated with rest, antipyretics, humidity, and antibiotics.

Pneumonia

Pneumonia is infection of the lower respiratory tract caused by bacteria, viruses, fungi, protozoa, or parasites. It is the eighth leading cause of death in Canada and the United States.[63,64] The incidence and mortality of pneumonia are highest in older adults. Risk factors for pneumonia include advanced age, compromised immunity, underlying lung disease, alcoholism, altered consciousness, impaired swallowing, smoking, endotracheal (ET) intubation, malnutrition, immobilization, underlying cardiac or liver disease, and residence in a long-term care facility. The causative microorganism influences the clinical presentation of the individual, the treatment plan, and the prognosis.

Pneumonia can be categorized as community-acquired pneumonia (CAP), health care–associated pneumonia (HCAP), hospital-acquired pneumonia (HAP), or ventilator-associated pneumonia (VAP). CAP is a significant cause of morbidity, mortality, and health care costs. As many as 36% of patients with CAP require Critical Care Unit (CCU) admission, and these patients have mortality ranging from 21 to 58%. Moreover, patients with CAP in the CCU have longer durations of stay compared with those that are not in the CCU, which is associated with higher hospital costs.[65] CAP is the eighth leading cause of death in Canada and the United States and the leading cause of infection-related hospitalization.[66]

HCAP is defined as occurring in individuals with recent hospitalization, residence in a long-term care facility or extended care facility, home infusion therapy, chronic dialysis, or home wound care, although more recent studies suggest nonambulatory status, tube feedings, and the use of gastric acid suppressive agents also should be considered as criteria for HCAP.[67] It is estimated that nearly one-third of all hospital admissions for pneumonia are now considered HCAP.

HAP is the second most common health care–associated infection (urinary tract infection [UTI] is the most common) but has the greatest mortality (overall 20 to 50% mortality). VAP is a health care–associated infection that occurs in 9 to 27% of individuals who require intubation and mechanical ventilation.[68-70]

The microorganisms that most commonly cause CAP are different from those that cause HCAP, HAP, and VAP (Box 27-1). The most common CAP is caused by *Streptococcus pneumoniae* (also known as *pneumococcus*), which results in hospitalization in more than half of affected individuals and an overall hospital mortality of about 10%.[71] *Mycoplasma pneumoniae* is a common cause of atypical pneumonia in young people, especially those living in group housing such as dormitories and army barracks. Community-acquired methicillin-resistant *Staphylococcus aureus* (MRSA) is becoming more common.[72,73] Influenza and respiratory syncytial virus are the most common causes of viral CAP in adults.[74] VAP is a frequent complication in the CCU (see *Health Promotion:* Ventilator-Associated Pneumonia). Immunocompromised individuals (e.g., those with human immunodeficiency virus [HIV] or those undergoing organ transplantation) are especially susceptible to *Pneumocystis jirovecii* (formerly called *Pneumocystis carinii*), mycobacterial infections, and fungal infections of the respiratory tract. These infections can be difficult to treat and have a high mortality.

BOX 27-1 Etiological Microorganisms for Pneumonia in Adults

CAP	HCAP/HAP/VAP	Immunocompromised Individuals
Streptococcus pneumoniae	*Pseudomonas aeruginosa*	*Pneumocystis jirovecii*
Moraxella catarrhalis	*Staphylococcus aureus*	*Mycobacterium tuberculosis*
Haemophilus influenzae	*Klebsiella pneumoniae*	Atypical mycobacteria
Oral anaerobic bacteria	*Escherichia coli*	Fungi
Influenza virus		Respiratory viruses
Respiratory syncytial virus		Protozoa
Staphylococcus aureus		Parasites
Chlamydia pneumoniae		
Legionella pneumophila		
Mycoplasma pneumoniae		

CAP, community-acquired pneumonia; *HAP*, hospital-acquired pneumonia; *HCAP*, health care–associated pneumonia; *VAP*, ventilator-associated pneumonia.

HEALTH PROMOTION

Ventilator-Associated Pneumonia

Ventilator-associated pneumonia (VAP) is a common complication of mechanical ventilation and is the most serious infection in the Critical Care Unit. VAP is associated with higher mortality, morbidity, and costs. Although there are many risk factors, including age greater than 65 years, presence of comorbidities, use of sedation, supine posture, poor oral hygiene, and immunocompromised status, the principal determinant of VAP development is the presence of the ET tube. Common etiological microorganisms include *Staphylococcus aureus* and *Pseudomonas aeruginosa*; multidrug-resistant strains are common. Bacterial colonization of the oropharynx occurs soon after placement of the ET tube with subsequent aspiration and pooling of bacteria near the ET tube cuff. Many bacteria are capable of forming a protective coating, called a *biofilm*, on the surface of the ET tube that contributes to bacterial replication and makes microorganisms less vulnerable to antibiotics. Injury to the tracheal mucosa and decreased mucociliary clearance contribute to lower airway infection. Analgesic and sedation agents alter cellular function and reduce the immune response. Implementation of certain treatment protocols has shown improved outcomes regarding VAP prevention and mortality reduction, especially the use of a "bundle" of techniques including raising the head of the bed, improving oral hygiene, providing continuous suction of subglottic secretions by antimicrobial-impregnated ET tubes, using checklists, and encouraging effective team communication. Recent studies have suggested that surveillance cultures could improve the prescribing of appropriate antibiotics and that the addition of aerosolized antibiotics may improve treatment outcomes.

According to the Canadian Patient Safety Institute, VAP is the leading cause of death among hospital-acquired infections in Canada. Hospital mortality of ventilated patients who developed VAP in Canadian hospitals is 46%, compared with 32% for ventilated patients who do not develop VAP.

In Canada, it is estimated that VAP is associated with an increase of 7.6 days of ventilation, an increase of 8.7 days in the CCU, and an increase in total stay of 11.5 days. It also plays a role in 6 to 30% of additional deaths in critically ill patients.

Data from Canadian Patient Safety Institute. (2016). *Ventilator-associated pneumonia (VAP)*. Retrieved from http://www.patientsafetyinstitute.ca/en/Topic/Pages/Ventilator-Associated-Pneumonia-(VAP).aspx; Kallet, R.H. (2015). *Respir Care, 60*(10), 1495–1508; Klompas, M., Speck, K., Howell, M.D., et al. (2014). *JAMA Intern Med, 174*(5), 751–761; Kollef, M.H., Hamilton, C.W., & Montgomery, A.B. (2013). *Curr Opin Infect Dis, 26*(6), 538–544; Luna, C.M., Bledel, I., & Raimondi, A. (2014). *Curr Opin Infect Dis, 27*(2), 184–193; Mietto, C., Pinciroli, R., Patel, N., et al. (2013). *Resp Care, 58*(6), 990–1007; Rouze, A., & Nseir, S. (2013). *Curr Opin Crit Care, 19*(5), 440–447; Smith, M.A., Hibino, M., Falcione, B.A., et al. (2014). *Ann Pharmacother, 48*(1), 77–85.

PATHOPHYSIOLOGY Aspiration of oropharyngeal secretions is the most common route of lower respiratory tract infection; thus, the nasopharynx and oropharynx constitute the first line of defence for most infectious agents. Another route of infection is through the inhalation of microorganisms that have been released into the air when an infected individual coughs, sneezes, or talks, or from aerosolized water such as that from contaminated respiratory therapy equipment. This route of infection is most important in viral and mycobacterial pneumonias and in *Legionella* outbreaks. ET tubes become colonized with bacteria that form biofilms (i.e., protected colonies of bacteria that are resistant to host defences and treatment with antibiotics) and can seed the lung with microorganisms, especially during ET suctioning. Pneumonia also can occur when bacteria are spread to the lung in the blood from bacteremia that can result from infection elsewhere in the body or from intravenous drug abuse.

In healthy individuals, pathogens that reach the lungs are expelled or controlled by mechanisms of self-defence (see Chapters 6, 7, and 8). If a microorganism evades the upper airway defence mechanisms, such as the cough reflex and mucociliary clearance, the next line of defence is the airway epithelial cell. Airway epithelial cells can recognize some pathogens directly (e.g., *P. aeruginosa* and *S. aureus*). The most important guardian cell of the lower respiratory tract is the alveolar macrophage; it recognizes pathogens through its pattern-recognition receptors (e.g., Toll-like receptors). Macrophages present infectious antigens to the adaptive immune system, activating T cells and B cells with the induction of both cellular and humoral immunity. Release of tumour necrosis factor-alpha (TNF-α) and interleukin-1 (IL-1) from macrophages and chemokines and chemotactic signals from mast cells and fibroblasts contributes to widespread inflammation in the lung and recruitment of neutrophils from the capillaries of the lungs into the alveoli. The resulting inflammatory mediators and immune complexes can damage bronchial mucous membranes and alveolocapillary membranes, causing the acini and terminal bronchioles to fill with infectious debris and exudate. Some microorganisms release toxins from their cell walls that can cause further lung damage and consolidation of lung tissue. The accumulation of exudate in the acinus leads to dyspnea and to $\dot{V}/\dot{Q}$ mismatching and hypoxemia.

Pneumococcus (*S. pneumoniae*) is the most common and lethal cause of outpatient and inpatient pneumonias.[75] Pneumococci can infect the lungs through inhalation of aerosolized bacteria or, more commonly, by aspiration of colonized oropharyngeal secretions. These bacteria have several virulence factors; most important, they have capsules that make phagocytosis by alveolar macrophages more difficult, and they have the ability to release a variety of toxins (including pneumolysin, which damages airway and alveolar cells).[76] An intense inflammatory response is initiated with release of TNF-α and IL-1.[77] Neutrophils and inflammatory exudates cause alveolar edema, which leads to the other changes shown in Figure 27-15.

Viral pneumonia is a seasonal and usually mild and self-limiting CAP. It can set the stage for a secondary bacterial infection by damaging ciliated epithelial cells, which normally prevent pathogens from reaching the lower airways. Immunocompromised individuals are at risk for very serious viral infections, such as pneumonia caused by cytomegalovirus. Viral pneumonia also can be a complication of another viral illness, such as chickenpox or measles (spread from the blood). New or atypical forms of viral infection, such as swine influenza A (H1N1) virus, avian influenza A (H5N1) virus, and the coronavirus that causes severe acute respiratory syndrome (SARS), are affecting previously healthy populations and pose a considerable threat for pandemics.[78]

Viruses destroy the ciliated epithelial cells and invade the goblet cells and bronchial mucous glands. Sloughing of destroyed bronchial epithelium occurs throughout the respiratory tract, preventing mucociliary clearance. Bronchial walls become edematous and infiltrated with leukocytes. In severe cases, the alveoli are involved with decreased compliance and increased work of breathing.

CLINICAL MANIFESTATIONS Most cases of pneumonia are preceded by a viral upper respiratory tract infection. Individuals then develop fever, chills, productive or dry cough, malaise, pleural pain, and sometimes

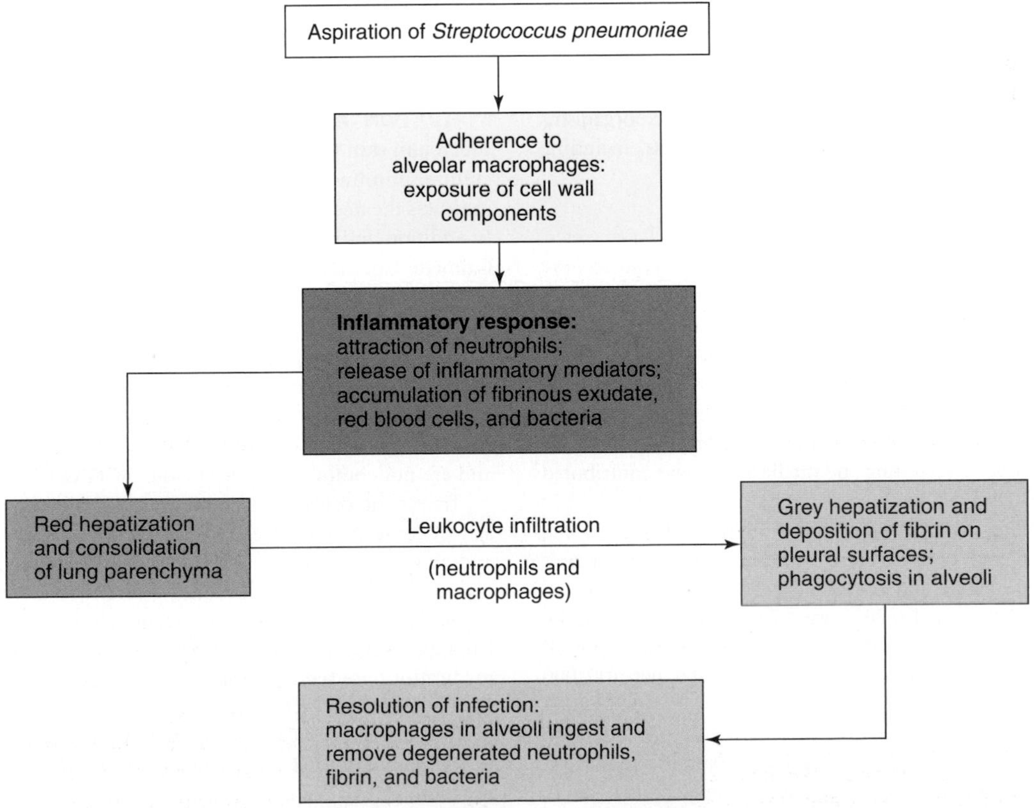

FIGURE 27-15 Pathophysiological Course of Pneumococcal Pneumonia.

dyspnea and hemoptysis. Physical examination may show signs of pulmonary consolidation, such as dullness to percussion, inspiratory crackles, increased tactile fremitus, egophony, and whispered pectoriloquy. Individuals also may demonstrate symptoms and signs of underlying systemic disease or sepsis.

EVALUATION AND TREATMENT Diagnosis is made on the basis of history and physical examination (tachypnea, tachycardia, crackles, bronchial breath sounds, findings of pleural effusion), white blood cell count, oxygenation and pH, chest X-rays, stains and cultures of respiratory tract secretions, and blood cultures before starting antibiotics. The white blood cell count is usually elevated, although it may be low if the individual is debilitated or immunocompromised. Serum procalcitonin level can be used to help differentiate bacterial from viral infection and guide therapy. Chest radiographs show infiltrates that may involve a single lobe of the lung or may be more diffuse. Once the diagnosis of pneumonia has been made, the pathogen is identified by means of sputum characteristics (Gram stain, colour, odour) and cultures or, if sputum is absent, blood cultures. Because many pathogens exist in the normal oropharyngeal flora, the specimen may be contaminated with pathogens from oral secretions. If sputum studies fail to identify the pathogen, the individual is immunocompromised, or the individual's condition worsens, further diagnostic studies may include thoracentesis, bronchoscopy, or lung biopsy. Urine antigen testing offers rapid pathogen identification for *Legionella pneumophila*, *S. pneumoniae*, and *Histoplasma capsulatum* but requires culture for microbial specificity.[79]

Prevention of pneumonia includes avoidance of aspiration, respiratory isolation of immunocompromised individuals, and vaccination. The first step in the management of pneumonia is establishing adequate ventilation and oxygenation. Adequate hydration and good pulmonary hygiene (e.g., deep breathing, coughing, chest physiotherapy) also are important. Antibiotics are given within 4 hours to treat bacterial pneumonia; however, resistant strains of microorganisms are becoming more prevalent and require secondary antibiotics.[79] When a specific microorganism is not identified, empirical antibiotics are chosen on the basis of the likely causative microorganism.[67] Viral pneumonia is usually treated with supportive therapy alone; however, antivirals may be needed in severe cases. Infections with opportunistic microorganisms may be polymicrobial and require multiple medications, including antifungals.

Tuberculosis

Tuberculosis (TB) is an infection caused by *Mycobacterium tuberculosis*, an acid-fast bacillus that usually affects the lungs but may invade other body systems. TB is a leading cause of death from a curable infectious disease in the world. TB cases increased greatly during the mid-1990s as a result of AIDS, but incidence of both diseases has decreased since 2000.[80] Emigration of infected individuals from high-prevalence countries, transmission in crowded institutional settings, homelessness, substance abuse, and lack of access to screening and medical care have contributed to the spread of TB.

For most Canadians, the risk of developing TB is very low. However, there are about 1 600 new cases of TB reported in Canada every year.[81] In Canada, 1 640 new active and retreatment TB cases were reported in 2013, and the incidence rate for 2013 was 4.7 per 100 000 population. These figures are comparable to both the number of TB cases reported in 2012 (1 699) and the incidence rate for 2012 (4.9 per 100 000 population).[82]

PATHOPHYSIOLOGY TB is highly contagious and is transmitted from person to person in airborne droplets. In immunocompetent individuals, the microorganism is usually contained by the inflammatory and immune response systems. This results in latent TB infection (LTBI) and is associated with no clinical evidence of disease.

Once the bacilli are inspired, they lodge in the lung periphery, usually in the upper lobe, and cause localized nonspecific pneumonitis (lung inflammation). Some bacilli migrate through the lymphatics and become lodged in the lymph nodes, where they encounter lymphocytes and initiate the immune response. Inflammation in the lung causes activation of alveolar macrophages and neutrophils. These phagocytes engulf the bacilli and begin the process by which the body's defence mechanisms isolate the bacilli, preventing them from spreading. However, the bacterium is successful as a pathogen because it can survive and multiply within macrophages and resist lysosomal killing, forming a granulomatous lesion (see Chapter 6) called a *tubercle*. Infected tissues within the tubercle die, forming cheeselike material called *caseation necrosis*. Collagenous scar tissue then grows around the tubercle, completing the isolation of the bacilli. The immune response is complete after about 10 days, preventing further multiplication of the bacilli.

Once the bacilli are isolated in tubercles and immunity develops, TB may remain dormant for life. If the immune system is impaired, reactivation with progressive disease occurs and may spread through the blood and lymphatics to other organs. Infection with HIV is the single greatest risk factor for reactivation of TB infection. Cancer, immunosuppressive medications (e.g., corticosteroids), poor nutritional status, and renal failure can also reactivate disease.

CLINICAL MANIFESTATIONS LTBI is asymptomatic. Symptoms of active disease often develop so gradually that they are not noticed until the disease is advanced. Common clinical manifestations include fatigue, weight loss, lethargy, anorexia (loss of appetite), and a low-grade fever that usually occurs in the afternoon. A cough that produces purulent sputum develops slowly and becomes more frequent over several weeks or months. Night sweats and general anxiety are often present. Dyspnea, chest pain, and hemoptysis may occur as the disease progresses. Extrapulmonary TB disease is common in HIV-infected individuals and may cause neurological deficits, meningitis symptoms, bone pain, and urinary symptoms.

EVALUATION AND TREATMENT TB is diagnosed by a positive tuberculin skin test (TST; purified protein derivative [PPD]), sputum culture, immunoassays, and chest radiographs.[83] A positive skin test indicates the need for yearly chest radiographs to detect active disease. In addition, individuals who have received the TB vaccine with bacille Calmette-Guérin (BCG) will have a positive TST even if they have never had TB. When active pulmonary disease is present, the tubercle bacillus can be cultured from the sputum and may be seen with an acid-fast stain. However, sputum culture can take up to 6 weeks to become positive. Two immunoassays (enzyme-linked immunospot and quantitative blood interferon-gamma assay) are available. These new tests are more sensitive and specific than TST for the diagnosis of latent TB and are not confounded by previous BCG vaccination.[84]

Treatment consists of combination antibiotic therapy to control active disease or prevent reactivation of LTBI. Adverse effects are common and new medications are being explored.[85] Two worrisome treatment categories of TB have become more prevalent in recent years. "Multidrug-resistant TB" and "extensively resistant TB" now account for approximately 2 to 5% of cases worldwide. Multiple second-line medications are required for treatment success.[86] The BCG vaccine is used in countries where TB is endemic.

In Canada, the BCG vaccine is not recommended for routine use in the population. However, BCG may be recommended for certain populations in Canada; for example, infants in high-incidence communities and travellers who are returning for an extended stay to a high-incidence country where BCG is routinely given. For infants born in Canada who will be moving to and staying for an extended period in a country with high TB incidence and where BCG vaccination is still standard practice, vaccination is recommended soon after arrival in the high-incidence country.[87] New vaccines are in clinical trials.[88] Treatment of TB HIV co-infection requires monitoring of medication interactions and toxicities.[89]

Abscess Formation and Cavitation

An **abscess** is a circumscribed area of suppuration and destruction of lung parenchyma. Abscess formation follows consolidation of lung tissue, in which inflammation causes alveoli to fill with fluid, pus, and microorganisms. Aspiration abscess can occur from aspiration of anaerobes, such as those found in individuals who have pneumonia or who are infected with *Klebsiella* or *Staphylococcus*. Aspiration abscess is usually associated with alcohol misuse, seizure disorders, general anaesthesia, and swallowing disorders. Necrosis (death and decay) of consolidated tissue may progress proximally until it communicates with a bronchus. **Cavitation** is the process of the abscess emptying into a bronchus and cavity formation. Abscess communication with a bronchus causes production of copious amounts of often foul-smelling sputum, and occasionally hemoptysis. Other clinical manifestations include fever, cough, chills, and pleural pain. The diagnosis is made by chest radiography. Treatment includes appropriate antibiotics and chest physiotherapy (chest percussion and postural drainage). Bronchoscopy may be performed to drain the abscess.

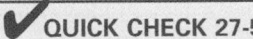

QUICK CHECK 27-5

1. Compare pneumococcal and viral pneumonia as to severity of disease.
2. Describe the pathophysiological features of tuberculosis.
3. How does lung abscess present clinically?

Pulmonary Vascular Disease

Blood flow through the lungs can be disrupted by disorders that occlude the vessels, increase pulmonary vascular resistance, or destroy the vascular bed. Effects of altered pulmonary blood flow may range from insignificant dysfunction to severe and life-threatening changes in ventilation–perfusion ratios. Major disorders include PE, pulmonary hypertension, and cor pulmonale.

Pulmonary Embolism

Pulmonary embolism (PE) is occlusion of a portion of the pulmonary vascular bed by an embolus. PE most commonly results from embolization of a clot from deep venous thrombosis involving the lower leg (see Chapter 24). Other less common emboli include tissue fragments, lipids (fats), a foreign body, an air bubble, or amniotic fluid. Risk factors for PE include conditions and disorders that promote blood clotting as a result of venous stasis (immobilization, heart failure), hypercoagulability (inherited coagulation disorders, malignancy, hormone replacement therapy, oral contraceptives), and injuries to the endothelial cells that line the vessels (trauma, infection, caustic intravenous infusions). Genetic risks include factor V Leiden, antithrombin II, protein S, protein C, and prothrombin gene mutations. No matter its source, a blood clot becomes an embolus when all or part of it detaches from the site of formation and begins to travel in the bloodstream.

PATHOPHYSIOLOGY The effect of the embolus depends on the extent of pulmonary blood flow obstruction, the size of the affected vessels, the nature of the embolus, and the secondary effects. Pulmonary emboli can result in any of the following:

- *Embolus with infarction:* an embolus that causes infarction (death) of a portion of lung tissue
- *Embolus without infarction:* an embolus that does not cause permanent lung injury (perfusion of the affected lung segment is maintained by the bronchial circulation)
- *Massive occlusion:* an embolus that occludes a major portion of the pulmonary circulation (i.e., main pulmonary artery embolus)
- *Multiple pulmonary emboli:* multiple emboli may be chronic or recurrent

Significant obstruction of the pulmonary vasculature leads to increased pulmonary artery vasoconstriction, pulmonary hypertension, and right ventricular dilation and afterload.[90] The pathogenesis of massive PE caused by a thrombus is summarized in Figure 27-16.

If the embolus does not cause infarction, the clot is dissolved by the fibrinolytic system and pulmonary function returns to normal. If pulmonary infarction occurs, shrinking and scarring develop in the affected area of the lung.

CLINICAL MANIFESTATIONS In most cases, the clinical manifestations of PE are nonspecific; therefore, evaluation of risk factors and predisposing factors is an important aspect of diagnosis. Although most emboli originate from clots in the lower extremities, deep venous thrombosis

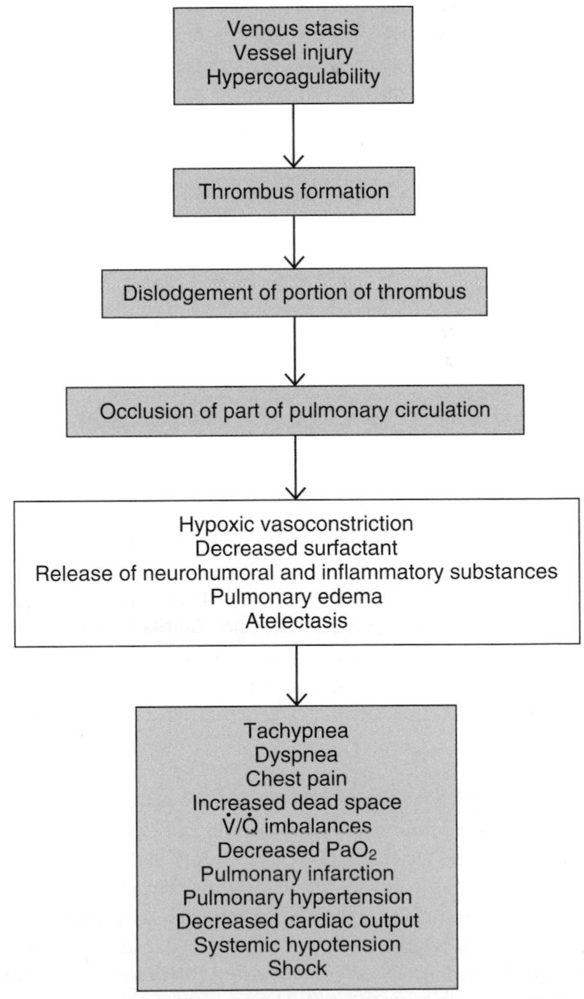

FIGURE 27-16 Pathogenesis of Massive Pulmonary Embolism Caused by a Thrombus (Pulmonary Thromboembolism). PaO_2, partial pressure of oxygen in arterial blood; $\dot{V}/\dot{Q}$, ventilation–perfusion ratio.

is often asymptomatic, and clinical examination has low sensitivity for the presence of clot, especially in the thigh and pelvis.

An individual with PE usually presents with the sudden onset of pleuritic chest pain, dyspnea, tachypnea, tachycardia, and unexplained anxiety. Occasionally syncope (fainting) or hemoptysis occurs. With large emboli, a pleural friction rub, pleural effusion, fever, and leukocytosis may be noted. Recurrent small emboli may not be detected until progressive incapacitation, precordial pain, anxiety, dyspnea, and right ventricular enlargement are exhibited. Massive occlusion causes severe pulmonary hypertension and shock.

EVALUATION AND TREATMENT Routine chest radiographs and pulmonary function tests are not definitive for PE in the first 24 hours. Arterial blood gas analyses usually demonstrate hypoxemia and hyperventilation (respiratory alkalosis). The diagnosis is made by measuring elevated levels of D-dimer in the blood (a product of thrombus degradation) in combination with CT scanning or magnetic resonance imaging (MRI). Measurement of the levels of brain natriuretic peptide and troponin is useful in PE associated with right ventricular dysfunction.[91]

Prevention of PE includes elimination of predisposing factors for individuals at risk. Venous stasis in hospitalized persons is minimized by leg elevation, bed exercises, position changes, early postoperative ambulation, and pneumatic calf compression. Clot formation is also prevented by prophylactic low-dose anticoagulant therapy.

Anticoagulant therapy is the primary treatment for PE. Initial anticoagulant therapy usually includes low-molecular-weight heparins (e.g., enoxaparin [Lovenox]) and factor Xa inhibitors. If a massive life-threatening embolism occurs, a fibrinolytic agent, such as streptokinase (Kabikinase), is sometimes used, and some individuals will require catheter-directed therapies or surgical thrombectomy. A filter in the inferior vena cava can prevent emboli from reaching the lungs. After stabilization, anticoagulation is continued for several months.[92]

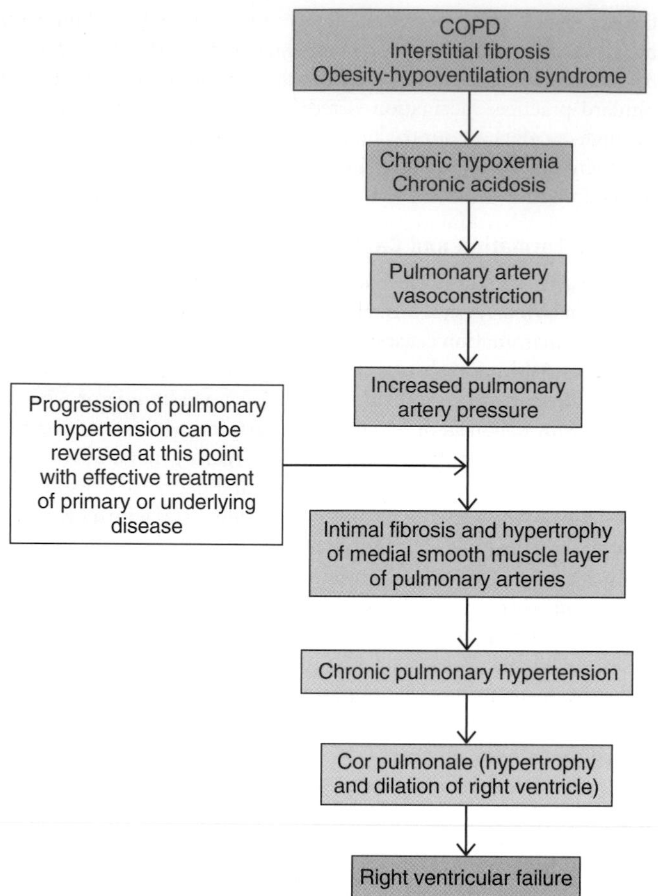

FIGURE 27-17 Pathogenesis of Pulmonary Hypertension and Cor Pulmonale. *COPD,* chronic obstructive pulmonary disease.

Pulmonary Artery Hypertension

Pulmonary artery hypertension (PAH) is defined as a mean pulmonary artery pressure greater than 25 mm Hg at rest. PAH is classified into several groups[93]:

- No known cause or associated with inheritance, medications or toxins, connective tissue disease, or infection
- Pulmonary hypertension attributable to left ventricular disease (see Chapter 24)
- Pulmonary hypertension caused by chronic lung disease or hypoxia, or both
- Chronic thromboembolic pulmonary hypertension
- Pulmonary hypertension caused by other multifactorial mechanisms including blood, metabolic, and systemic disorders.

COPD is the most common lung disease associated with PAH, but any condition that causes chronic hypoxemia can result in pulmonary hypertension.

PATHOPHYSIOLOGY Idiopathic pulmonary arterial hypertension (IPAH) (also called *pulmonary hypertension caused by unclear multifactorial mechanisms*) is characterized by endothelial dysfunction with overproduction of vasoconstrictors, such as thromboxane and endothelin, and decreased production of vasodilators, such as prostacyclin and nitric oxide. Vascular growth factors are released, causing fibrosis and thickening of vessel walls (called *remodelling*) with luminal narrowing and abnormal vasoconstriction.[94] These changes cause resistance to pulmonary artery blood flow, thus increasing the pressure in the pulmonary arteries and right ventricle. Gas exchange is reduced with restriction in lung volumes. As resistance and pressure increase, the workload of the right ventricle increases and subsequent right ventricular hypertrophy, followed by failure, may occur (cor pulmonale). The pathogenesis of PAH and cor pulmonale resulting from disease of the respiratory system or hypoxia is shown in Figure 27-17.

Pulmonary hypertension associated with lung respiratory disease or hypoxia, or both, is a serious complication of many acute and chronic pulmonary disorders, such as COPD and hypoventilation associated with obesity. These conditions are complicated by hypoxic pulmonary vasoconstriction, which further increases pulmonary artery pressure.

CLINICAL MANIFESTATIONS Pulmonary hypertension may not be detected until it is quite severe. The symptoms are often masked by other forms of pulmonary or cardiovascular disease. The first indication of PAH may be an abnormality seen on a chest radiograph (enlarged right heart border) or an electrocardiogram that shows right ventricular hypertrophy. Manifestations of fatigue, chest discomfort, tachypnea, and dyspnea (particularly with exercise) are common. Examination may reveal peripheral edema, jugular venous distension, a precordial heave, and accentuation of the pulmonary component of the second heart sound.

EVALUATION AND TREATMENT Definitive diagnosis of PAH can be made only with right heart catheterization. Common diagnostic modalities used to determine the cause include chest X-ray, echocardiography, and CT. The diagnosis of IPAH is made when all other causes of pulmonary hypertension have been ruled out.

General therapies for PAH include administration of O_2, diuretics, and anticoagulants and avoidance of contributing factors, such as air travel, decongestant medications, nonsteroidal anti-inflammatory drugs, pregnancy, and tobacco use. Medications used in the treatment of PAH include prostacyclin and its analogues, endothelin antagonists, phosphodiesterase-5 inhibitors, and a soluble guanylate cyclase activator. None of these medications are curative, but there is improved morbidity and mortality.[95] Percutaneous catheter-based therapies are under development.[96] Individuals who do not achieve adequate clinical remission may require lung transplantation.

The most effective treatment for pulmonary hypertension associated with lung respiratory disease or hypoxia, or both, is treatment of the primary disorder. Supplemental O_2 may be indicated to reverse hypoxic vasoconstriction.

Cor Pulmonale

Cor pulmonale is defined as right ventricular enlargement (hypertrophy, dilation, or both) caused by PAH (see Figure 27-17).[97]

PATHOPHYSIOLOGY Cor pulmonale develops as PAH exerts chronic pressure overload in the right ventricle. Pressure overload increases the work of the right ventricle and causes hypertrophy of the normally thin-walled heart muscle. This pressure overload eventually progresses to dilation and failure of the ventricle.

CLINICAL MANIFESTATIONS The clinical manifestations of cor pulmonale may be obscured by underlying respiratory or cardiac disease and appear only during exercise testing. The heart may appear normal at rest, but with exercise, cardiac output falls. The electrocardiogram may show right ventricular hypertrophy. The pulmonary component of the second heart sound, which represents closure of the pulmonic valve, may be accentuated, and a pulmonic valve murmur also may be present. Tricuspid valve murmur may accompany the development of right ventricular failure. Increased pressures in the systemic venous circulation cause jugular venous distension, hepatosplenomegaly, and peripheral edema.

EVALUATION AND TREATMENT Diagnosis is based on physical examination, imaging, and electrocardiography or echocardiography, or both. The goal of treatment for cor pulmonale is to decrease the workload of the right ventricle by lowering pulmonary artery pressure. Treatment is the same as that for pulmonary hypertension, and its success depends on reversal of the underlying lung disease.

QUICK CHECK 27-6

1. What factors influence the impact of an embolus?
2. List three causes of pulmonary hypertension.
3. What is cor pulmonale?

Malignancies of the Respiratory Tract

Laryngeal Cancer

According to the Canadian Cancer Society, in 2017 an estimated 1 150 Canadians were diagnosed with laryngeal cancer and 440 would die from it. In 2017, an estimated greater number of men (970) than women (180) were diagnosed with laryngeal cancer. Moreover, an estimated greater number of men (350) than women (95) would die from it.[98] In Canada, the incidence rates of laryngeal cancer decreased significantly from 1992 to 2013 for both males (3.2% per year) and females (3.4% per year).[99]

The primary risk factor for laryngeal cancer is tobacco smoking; risk is further heightened with the combination of smoking and alcohol consumption. The human papillomavirus (HPV 6 and 11) also has been linked to both benign and malignant disease of the larynx.[100] The highest incidence is in men between 50 and 75 years of age.

PATHOPHYSIOLOGY Carcinoma of the true vocal cords (glottis) is more common than that of the supraglottic structures (epiglottis, aryepiglottic folds, arytenoids, false cords). Tumours of the subglottic area are rare. Squamous cell carcinoma is the most common cell type, although small cell carcinomas also occur (Figure 27-18). Metastasis develops by spread to the draining lymph nodes, and distant metastasis is rare.

CLINICAL MANIFESTATIONS The presenting symptoms of laryngeal cancer include hoarseness, dyspnea, and cough. Progressive hoarseness can result in voice loss. Dyspnea is rare with supraglottic tumours but can be severe in subglottic tumours. Cough may follow swallowing. Laryngeal pain is likely with supraglottic lesions.

EVALUATION AND TREATMENT Evaluation of the larynx includes external inspection and palpation of the larynx and the lymph nodes of the neck. Indirect laryngoscopy provides a stereoscopic view of the structure and movement of the larynx. A biopsy also can be obtained

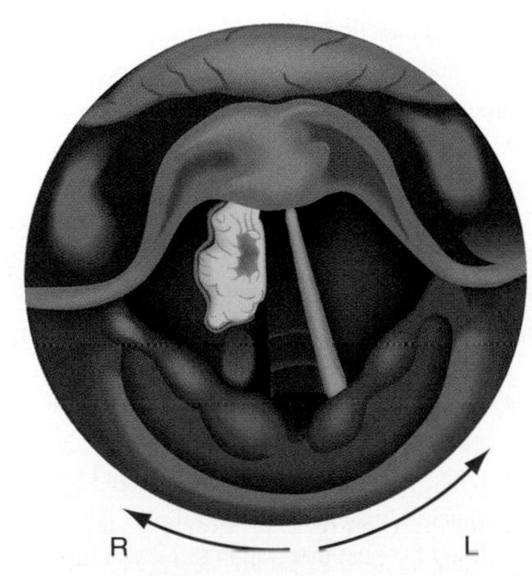

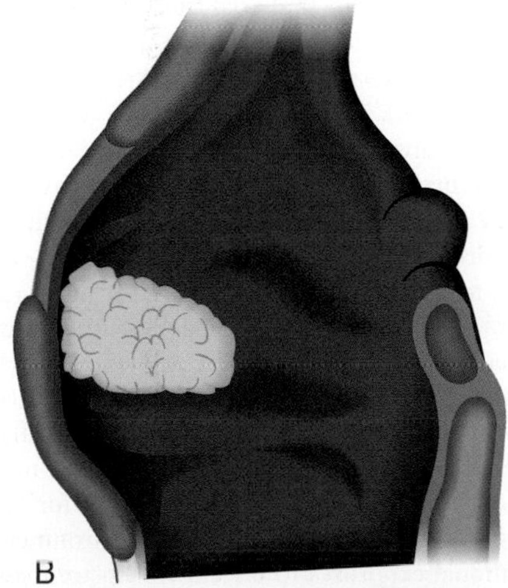

FIGURE 27-18 Laryngeal Cancer. A, Mirror view of carcinoma of the right false cord partially hiding the true cord. **B,** Lateral view. (Redrawn from Ackerman, L.V., del Regato, J.A., Spjut, H.J., et al. [1985]. *Ackerman and del Regato's cancer* [2nd ed.]. St. Louis: Mosby.)

TABLE 27-3 Characteristics of Lung Cancers

Tumour Type	Growth Rate	Metastasis	Means of Diagnosis	Clinical Manifestations and Treatment
Non–Small Cell Carcinoma				
Squamous cell carcinoma	Slow	Late; mostly to hilar lymph nodes	Biopsy, sputum analysis, bronchoscopy, electron microscopy, immunohistochemistry	Cough, hemoptysis, sputum production, airway obstruction, hypercalcemia; treated surgically, chemotherapy and radiation as adjunctive therapy
Adenocarcinoma	Moderate	Early; to lymph nodes, pleura, bone, adrenal glands, and brain	Radiography, fibre-optic bronchoscopy, electron microscopy	Pleural effusion; treated surgically, chemotherapy as adjunctive therapy
Large cell carcinoma	Rapid	Early and widespread	Sputum analysis, bronchoscopy, electron microscopy (by exclusion of other cell types)	Chest wall pain, pleural effusion, cough, sputum production, hemoptysis, airway obstruction resulting in pneumonia; treated surgically
Neuroendocrine Tumours of the Lung				
Small cell carcinoma	Very rapid	Very early; to mediastinum, lymph nodes, brain, bone marrow	Radiography, sputum analysis, bronchoscopy, electron microscopy, immunohistochemistry	Cough, chest pain, dyspnea, hemoptysis, localized wheezing, airway obstruction, signs and symptoms of excessive hormone secretion; treated by chemotherapy and ionizing radiation to thorax and central nervous system
Other Pulmonary Tumours				
Malignant pleural mesothelioma (MPM)	Rapid	Early; to lymph nodes, lungs, heart, bone	Radiography, thoracentesis	Chest pain, chronic cough, signs of pleural effusion

during this procedure. Direct laryngoscopy provides more thorough visualization of the tumour. Imaging procedures facilitate the identification of tumour boundaries and the degree of extension to surrounding tissue.

Combined chemotherapy and radiation or surgical resection can result in cure in selected cases; however, sequelae such as swallowing and speech difficulties may result.[101] Total laryngectomy is required when lesions are extensive and involve the cartilage. Swallowing and speech therapy after treatment can significantly improve recovery.

Lung Cancer

The term lung cancer refers to tumours that arise from the epithelium of the respiratory tract (bronchogenic carcinomas). Other pulmonary tumours, such as mesotheliomas (associated with asbestos exposure), occur less commonly (Table 27-3).

Lung cancer is the leading cause of cancer death in Canada; it causes more cancer deaths among Canadians than breast, colorectal, and prostate cancer combined. Despite its prevalence, the lung cancer death rate (especially for men) has dropped substantially over the past 25 years in Canada, which has led to a decline in the overall cancer death rate. In 2010, lung cancer was responsible for 27% of the premature deaths caused by cancer in Canada.[102]

The most common cause of lung cancer is tobacco smoking (see Figure 11-5) (see *Health Promotion:* Facts on Tobacco Use). Smokers with obstructive lung disease (low FEV_1 measurements) are at a much greater risk of developing lung cancer. Other risk factors for lung cancer include radon gas exposure, secondhand smoke (environmental tobacco smoke), occupational exposures to certain workplace toxins, radiation, and air pollution (see Chapter 11 and Figures 11-1, 18, and 19). Genetic risks include polymorphisms of the genes responsible for growth factor receptors, angiogenesis, apoptosis, DNA repair, and detoxification of inhaled smoke.[103] Lung cancers are classified by cell type

HEALTH PROMOTION

Facts on Tobacco Use

According to the Registered Nurses' Association of Ontario (RNAO), smoking cigarettes is mentally and physically addictive. It is estimated that 45 000 Canadians over the age of 35 die every year as a result of smoking. Smoking cigarettes increases the risk for heart disease, cancer, lung disease, pregnancy complications, stomach problems, and gum problems.

Passive or secondhand smoke can cause cancer due to the presence of many chemicals in secondhand smoke, and at least 50 of them are known to be associated with cancer. Passive smoking leads to 1 100 and 7 800 deaths per year in Canada, with at least one-third of them in Ontario. Children are also impacted by secondhand smoke and become more prone to breathing problems and lung infections.

For smokers who want to quit smoking, the RNAO recommends the following tips:

- Using a calendar, pick a "quit date" to stop smoking. This date should make sense to you in your busy life. Stick to this date!
- Prepare yourself for situations that you know will be difficult without smoking.
- Take it one day at a time. When you first stop, try to change the places where you do your daily routine.
- Keep busy, try to increase your level of activity. Congratulate yourself often: think positive.
- Ask at least one friend and some family members to help support you through the process.
- Count or save the money you would have spent on cigarettes and treat yourself to something special.
- Don't try "just one" cigarette, it will take you back to the start.

From Registered Nurses Association of Ontario (2009). *Deciding to Quit Smoking Health Education Fact Sheet.* Toronto, ON: Registered Nurses Association of Ontario. Retrieved from http://rnao.ca/sites/rnao-ca/files/Deciding_to_Quit_Smoking.pdf.

and molecular profiling. The most common types of lung cancer are presented here.

Types of lung cancer. Primary lung cancers arise from cells that line the bronchi within the lungs and are therefore called *bronchogenic carcinomas*. Although there are many types of lung cancer, they can be divided into two major categories: non–small cell lung carcinoma (NSCLC) and neuroendocrine tumours of the lung. The category of non–small cell lung carcinoma accounts for 75 to 85% of all lung cancers and can be subdivided into three types of lung cancer: squamous cell carcinoma, adenocarcinoma, and large cell undifferentiated carcinoma. They are further described by genotyping (i.e., epidermal growth factor receptor *[EGFR]* gene or anaplastic lymphoma kinase *[ALK]* gene mutations and rearrangements), which is important for targeted personalized therapy.[104] Neuroendocrine tumours of the lung arise from the bronchial mucosa and include small cell carcinoma, large cell neuroendocrine carcinoma, and typical carcinoid and atypical carcinoid tumours. Small cell carcinoma is the most common of these neuroendocrine tumours, accounting for 15 to 20% of all lung cancers. Characteristics of these tumours, including clinical manifestations, are listed in Table 27-3. Many cancers that arise in other organs of the body metastasize to the lungs; however, these are not considered lung cancers and are categorized by their primary site of origin.

Non–small cell lung cancer. Squamous cell carcinoma accounts for about 30% of bronchogenic carcinomas and is associated with smoking and COPD. These tumours are typically located near the hila and project into bronchi (Figure 27-19, *A*). Because of this central location, symptoms of nonproductive cough or hemoptysis are common. Pneumonia and atelectasis are often associated with squamous cell carcinoma (see Figure 27-19, *A*). Chest pain is a late symptom associated with large tumours. These tumours are often fairly well localized and tend not to metastasize until late in the course of the disease.

Adenocarcinoma (tumour arising from glands) of the lung constitutes 35 to 40% of all bronchogenic carcinomas (Figure 27-19, *B*). Pulmonary adenocarcinoma develops in a stepwise fashion through atypical adenomatous hyperplasia, adenocarcinoma in situ, and minimally invasive adenocarcinoma to invasive carcinoma.[105] These tumours, which are usually smaller than 4 cm, more commonly arise in the peripheral regions of the pulmonary parenchyma. They may be asymptomatic and discovered by routine chest roentgenogram in the early stages, or the individual may present with pleuritic chest pain and shortness of breath from pleural involvement by the tumour.

Included in the category of adenocarcinoma is bronchioloalveolar cell carcinoma. These tumours arise from terminal bronchioles and alveoli and are now being referred to as *adenocarcinoma in situ* or *minimally invasive adenocarcinoma*.[106] They are slow-growing tumours with an unpredictable pattern of metastasis through the pulmonary arterial system and mediastinal lymph nodes.

Large cell carcinoma (undifferentiated). Large cell carcinomas constitute approximately 10% of bronchogenic carcinomas. These transformed epithelial cells have lost all evidence of differentiation and are considered an undifferentiated non–small cell carcinoma. Recent studies have confirmed that these tumours arise from squamous, glandular, or neuroendocrine precursor cells, and molecular analyses have made it possible to target some of these aggressive cancers for immunological therapy.[107] These tumours commonly arise centrally and can grow to distort the trachea and cause widening of the carina.

Neuroendocrine tumours. Small cell (oat cell) carcinomas are the most common type of neuroendocrine lung tumours and have the

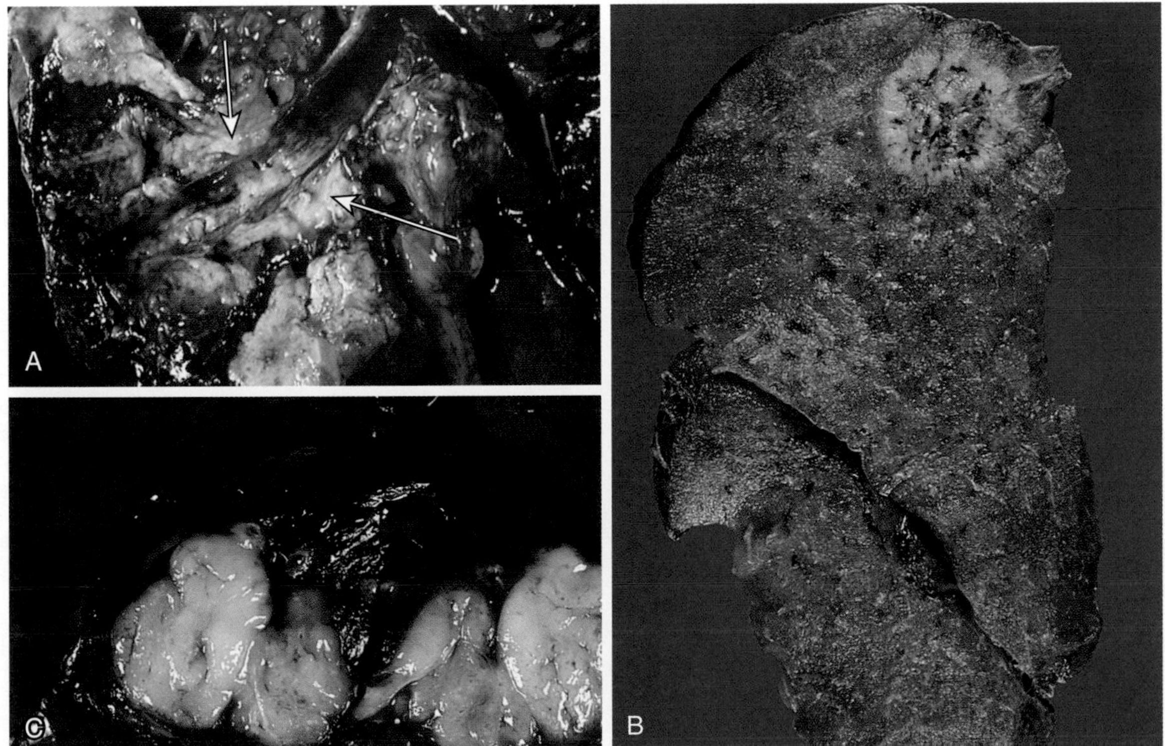

FIGURE 27-19 Lung Cancer. A, Squamous cell carcinoma. This hilar tumour originates from the main bronchus. **B,** Peripheral adenocarcinoma. The tumour shows prominent black pigmentation, suggestive of having evolved in an anthracotic scar. **C,** Small cell carcinoma. The tumour forms confluent nodules. On cross section, the nodules have an encephaloid appearance. (From Damjanov, I., & Linder, J. [Eds.]. [1996]. *Anderson's pathology* [10th ed.]. St. Louis: Mosby.)

highest correlation with tobacco smoking. Small cell carcinoma arises from neuroendocrine cells that contain neurosecretory granules. Most of these tumours are central in origin (hilar and mediastinal) (Figure 27-19, *C*). Cell sizes range from 6 to 8 μm, have a rapid rate of growth, and tend to metastasize early and widely.[108] Small cell carcinomas tend to present at tumour-nodes-metastasis (TNM) stage IV and have the worst prognosis. They are often associated with ectopic hormone production. Ectopic hormone production is important to the clinician because resulting signs and symptoms called *paraneoplastic syndromes* may be the first manifestation of the underlying cancer. Examples include hyponatremia (antidiuretic hormone), Cushing's syndrome (adrenocorticotropic hormone), hypocalcemia (calcitonin), gynecomastia (gonadotropins), carcinoid syndrome (serotonin), and Lambert-Eaton myasthenic syndrome (paneoplastic cerebellar degeneration).

PATHOPHYSIOLOGY Tobacco smoke contains more than 30 carcinogens and is responsible for causing 80 to 90% of lung cancers. These carcinogens, along with inherited genetic predisposition to cancers, result in tumour development. Once lung cancer is initiated by these carcinogen-induced mutations, further tumour development is promoted by growth factors that alter cell growth and differentiation, such as epidermal growth factor, and by production of inflammatory mediators, such as toxic O_2 free radicals. The bronchial mucosa suffers multiple carcinogenic "hits" because of repetitive exposure to tobacco smoke and, eventually, epithelial cell changes begin to be visible on biopsy. These changes progress from metaplasia to carcinoma in situ and finally to invasive carcinoma. Further tumour progression includes invasion of surrounding tissues and finally metastasis to distant sites including the brain, bone marrow, and liver (see Chapter 10 for details of cancer biology).

CLINICAL MANIFESTATIONS Table 27-3 summarizes the characteristic clinical manifestations of neuroendocrine tumours of the lung. Symptoms are often attributed to side effects of smoking; and when they are severe enough to motivate the individual to seek medical advice, the disease is usually advanced.

EVALUATION AND TREATMENT Screening for lung cancer remains controversial, but use of low-dose spiral CT scanning decreases the risk of dying from lung cancer by 20% in heavy smokers.[109] Diagnostic tests for the evaluation of lung cancer include sputum cytological studies, chest imaging, virtual bronchoscopy, radial probe endobronchial ultrasound, electromagnetic navigational bronchoscopy, and biopsy. Biopsy determines the cell type, and the evaluation of lymph nodes and other organ systems is used to determine the stage of the cancer.[110] The histological cell type, the genotype, and the stage of the disease are major factors that influence choice of therapy. The current accepted system for the staging of non–small cell cancer is the TNM classification (*T* indicates the extent of the primary tumour, *N* indicates nodal involvement, and *M* indicates the extent of distant metastasis) (see Chapter 10). In contrast, small cell lung cancers are only staged as either limited (confined to the area of origin in the lung) or extensive.

The only proven way of reducing the risk for lung cancer is the cessation of smoking and avoidance of environmental toxins.[111] For all types of early-stage lung carcinoma, the preferred treatment is surgical resection. Once metastasis has occurred, total surgical resection is more difficult and survival rates dramatically decrease. For individuals with non–small cell carcinoma with metastasis at diagnosis, adjunctive radiation and chemotherapy and treatment based on molecular markers may improve outcomes.[112] Treatment modalities, including dose-intensified radiation, radiofrequency ablation, microwave ablation, cryotherapy, and brachytherapy, may be available as primary or palliative treatment for those for whom surgical removal is not an option. Research is in progress to advance personalized genetic and immunological approaches to treatment[113,114] (see *Health Promotion:* Lung Cancer).

HEALTH PROMOTION

Lung Cancer

Lung cancer is estimated to be the most commonly diagnosed form of cancer in Canada (an estimated 25 500 new cases in 2013) as well as the leading cause of cancer death in Canada (an estimated 20 200 deaths in 2013). Almost all (97%) of the estimated new cases of lung cancer in 2013 were adults aged 50 years and older. In the same year, the age-standardized incidence rate of lung cancer in men was estimated at 60 cases per 100 000, compared with 46.8 cases per 100 000 in women.

While the incidence rate of lung cancer is currently higher in men than women, the rate for men became stable about 30 years ago (approximately 20 years after a reduction in smoking prevalence among men) and has been showing a significant ($p < .01$) annual decrease since the late 1990s. By contrast, the incidence rate for women has been increasing steadily ($p < .01$) and has not yet reached a similar plateau following a general decline in tobacco consumption in the mid-1980s. Lung cancer has a poor prognosis, and the 5-year relative survival ratio is among the lowest for all types of cancer in Canada (17% in 2013).

Cigarette smoking is the main risk factor for developing lung cancer and is associated with over 85% of the cases of this disease in Canada. The 2012 Canadian Tobacco Use Monitoring Survey (CTUMS) reported that 44% of adults (4.6 million Canadians) were current or ever smokers (16% are current smokers). Other factors that increase risk for lung cancer include secondhand exposure to tobacco smoke, exposure to radon and other toxic substances (e.g., asbestos, arsenic, diesel exhaust, silica, and chromium), having a first-degree relative with lung cancer, and undergoing radiation therapy to the chest.

The Canadian Task Force on Preventive Health Care (CTFPHC) recommendations for lung-cancer screening are as follows:

- Low-dose computed tomography (LDCT) screening is recommended for adults aged 55 to 74 years with at least a 30 pack-year* smoking history who currently smoke or quit less than 15 years ago. Screening should take place every year for up to three consecutive years. Screening should ONLY be carried out in health care settings with expertise in early diagnosis and treatment of lung cancer.
- No screening with LDCT is recommended for all other adults, regardless of age, smoking history, or other risk factors.
- No screening with chest X-ray, with or without sputum cytology, is recommended.

*"Pack-year" is defined as the (average number of cigarette packs smoked daily) × (number of years smoking).

Data from Canadian Cancer Society. (2014). *Risk factors for lung cancer 2014.* Retrieved from http://www.cancer.ca/en/cancer-information/cancer-type/lung/risks/?region=on; Canadian Task Force on Preventive Health Care. (2014). *CTFPHC Guidelines: Lung cancer.* Retrieved from http://canadiantaskforce.ca/ctfphc-guidelines/2015-lung-cancer/; Canadian Task Force on Preventive Health Care. (2014). *CTFPHC guidelines: Lung cancer—protocol.* Retrieved from http://canadiantaskforce.ca/ctfphc-guidelines/2015-lung-cancer/protocol/; Health Canada. (2012). *Canadian Tobacco Use Monitoring Survey (CTUMS) 2012.* Retrieved from http://www.hc-sc.gc.ca/hc-ps/tobac-tabac/research-recherche/stat/ctums-esutc_2012-eng.php.

QUICK CHECK 27-7

1. Describe squamous cell carcinoma of the vocal cords.
2. Differentiate the two types of non–small cell lung cancer.
3. What are paraneoplastic syndromes?

DID YOU UNDERSTAND?

Clinical Manifestations of Pulmonary Alterations

1. Dyspnea is the feeling of breathlessness and increased respiratory effort.
2. Coughing is a protective reflex that expels secretions and irritants from the lower airways.
3. Changes in the sputum volume, consistency, or colour may indicate underlying pulmonary disease.
4. Hemoptysis is expectoration of bloody mucus.
5. Abnormal breathing patterns are adjustments made by the body to minimize the work of respiratory muscles. They include Kussmaul, obstructed, restricted, gasping, and Cheyne-Stokes respirations as well as sighing.
6. Hypoventilation is decreased alveolar ventilation caused by airway obstruction, chest wall restriction, or altered neurological control of breathing and results in increased partial pressure of carbon dioxide in arterial blood ($PaCO_2$), or hypercapnia.
7. Hyperventilation is increased alveolar ventilation produced by anxiety, head injury, or severe hypoxemia and causes decreased $PaCO_2$ (hypocapnia).
8. Cyanosis is a bluish discoloration of the skin caused by desaturation of hemoglobin, polycythemia, or peripheral vasoconstriction.
9. Clubbing of the fingertips is associated with diseases that interfere with oxygenation of the tissues.
10. Chest pain can result from inflamed pleurae, trachea, bronchi, ribs, or respiratory muscles.
11. Hypoxemia is a reduced PaO_2 caused by (a) decreased O_2 content of inspired gas, (b) hypoventilation, (c) O_2 diffusion abnormality, (d) ventilation–perfusion mismatch, or (e) shunting.

Disorders of the Chest Wall and Pleura

1. Chest wall compliance is diminished by obesity and kyphoscoliosis (which compress the lungs), and by neuromuscular diseases that impair chest wall muscle function.
2. Flail chest results from rib or sternal fractures that disrupt the mechanics of breathing.
3. Pneumothorax is the accumulation of air in the pleural space. It can be caused by spontaneous rupture of weakened areas of the pleura or can be secondary to pleural damage caused by disease, trauma, or mechanical ventilation.
4. Tension pneumothorax is a life-threatening condition caused by trapping of air in the pleural space, producing displacement of the great vessels and heart.
5. Pleural effusion is the accumulation of fluid in the pleural space resulting from disorders that promote transudation or exudation from capillaries underlying the pleura or from blockage or injury to lymphatic vessels that drain into the pleural space.
6. Empyema is the presence of pus in the pleural space (infected pleural effusion); it usually occurs because of lymphatic drainage from sites of bacterial pneumonia.

Pulmonary Disorders

1. Pulmonary disorders can be restrictive (limiting lung volumes) or obstructive (limiting airflow) or both.
2. Aspiration of food particles or pharyngeal or gastric secretions can cause obstruction, inflammation, or pneumonitis.
3. Atelectasis is the collapse of alveoli resulting from compression of lung tissue or absorption of gas from obstructed alveoli.
4. Bronchiectasis is abnormal dilation of the bronchi secondary to another pulmonary disorder, usually infection or inflammation.
5. Bronchiolitis is the inflammatory obstruction of small airways. It occurs most commonly in children.
6. Pulmonary fibrosis is excessive connective tissue in the lung that diminishes lung compliance; it may be idiopathic or caused by disease and is associated with chronic inflammation.
7. Inhalation of toxic gases or prolonged exposure to high concentrations of oxygen (O_2) can damage the bronchial mucosa or alveolocapillary membrane and cause inflammation or acute respiratory failure.
8. Pneumoconiosis, which is caused by inhalation of dust particles in the workplace, can cause pulmonary fibrosis, increase susceptibility to lower airway infection, and initiate tumour formation.
9. Hypersensitivity pneumonitis (extrinsic allergic alveolitis) is an allergic or hypersensitivity reaction to many allergens causing lung inflammation.
10. Pulmonary edema is excess water in the lung caused by increased capillary hydrostatic pressure, decreased capillary oncotic pressure, or increased capillary permeability. Causes include left ventricular failure that increases capillary hydrostatic pressure in the pulmonary circulation, inflammation of alveoli, or lymphatic obstruction.
11. Acute lung injury (ALI)/acute respiratory distress syndrome (ARDS) results from an acute, diffuse injury to the alveolocapillary membrane and decreased surfactant production, which increases membrane permeability and causes edema, atelectasis, and hypoxemia.
12. Obstructive lung disease is characterized by airway obstruction that causes difficult expiration. Obstructive disease can be acute or chronic and includes asthma, chronic bronchitis, and emphysema.
13. Asthma is an inflammatory disease of the airways resulting from a type I hypersensitivity immune response involving the activity of antigen, immunoglobulin E, mast cells, eosinophils, and other inflammatory cells and mediators.
14. In asthma, airway obstruction is caused by episodic attacks of bronchospasm, bronchial inflammation, mucosal edema, and increased mucus production.
15. Chronic obstructive pulmonary disease (COPD) is the coexistence of chronic bronchitis and emphysema and is an important cause of hypoxemic and hypercapnic respiratory failure.
16. Chronic bronchitis causes airway obstruction resulting from inflammation, bronchial smooth muscle hypertrophy, and production of thick, tenacious mucus.
17. In emphysema, destruction of the alveolar septa and loss of passive elastic recoil lead to alveolar enlargement, airway collapse, obstruction of gas flow, and air trapping during expiration.
18. Acute bronchitis is usually a self-limiting viral infection.
19. Pneumococcal pneumonia (*Streptococcus pneumoniae*) is the most common acute lung infection, resulting in an inflammatory response with four phases: (a) consolidation, (b) red hepatization, (c) grey hepatization, and (d) resolution.
20. Viral pneumonia can be severe, but is more often an acute, self-limiting lung infection usually caused by the influenza virus. Atypical forms and new forms can cause severe acute respiratory syndrome (SARS).
21. Tuberculosis (TB) is a lung infection caused by *Mycobacterium tuberculosis* (tubercle bacillus). In TB, the inflammatory response proceeds to isolate colonies of bacilli by enclosing them in tubercles and surrounding the tubercles with scar tissue. TB bacilli escape immune defences by surviving within macrophages.
22. Pulmonary vascular diseases are caused by embolism or hypertension in the pulmonary circulation.

23. Pulmonary embolism is most often the result of embolism of part of a clot from deep venous thrombosis and causes vascular obstruction, $\dot{V}/\dot{Q}$ mismatch, hypoxemia, and pulmonary hypertension; it may or may not cause infarction.
24. Pulmonary artery hypertension (pulmonary artery pressure greater than 25 mm Hg at rest) can be idiopathic or associated with left ventricular failure, lung disease, or recurrent pulmonary emboli that increase resistance to blood flow in the pulmonary artery or its branches.
25. Cor pulmonale is right ventricular enlargement or failure caused by pulmonary hypertension.
26. In Canada, the incidence rates of laryngeal cancer decreased significantly from 1992 to 2013 for both males (3.2% per year) and females (3.4% per year). Squamous cell carcinoma of the true vocal cords is most common and presents with a clinical symptom of progressive hoarseness.
27. Lung cancer, the most common cause of cancer death in Canada, is commonly caused by tobacco smoking.
28. Lung cancer (bronchogenic carcinomas) cell types include non–small cell carcinoma (squamous cell carcinoma, adenocarcinoma, and large cell undifferentiated carcinoma) and, less commonly, neuroendocrine tumours (small cell carcinoma, large cell neuroendocrine carcinoma, and typical carcinoid and atypical carcinoid tumours). Each type arises in a characteristic site or type of tissue, causes distinctive clinical manifestations, and differs in likelihood of metastasis and prognosis.

KEY TERMS

Abscess, 715
Absorption atelectasis, 701
Acute bronchitis, 711
Acute lung injury (ALI), 704
Acute respiratory distress syndrome (ARDS), 704
Adenocarcinoma, 719
Air trapping, 711
Alveolar dead space, 698
Aspiration, 701
Asthma, 705
Atelectasis, 701
Bronchiectasis, 701
Bronchiolitis, 702
Bronchiolitis obliterans, 702
Bronchiolitis obliterans organizing pneumonia (BOOP), 702
Cavitation, 715
Cheyne-Stokes respiration, 696
Chronic bronchitis, 709
Chronic obstructive pulmonary disease (COPD), 708
Clubbing, 697
Compression atelectasis, 701
Consolidation, 713
Cor pulmonale, 717
Cough, 695
Cyanosis, 696
Dyspnea, 695
Emphysema, 710
Empyema (infected pleural effusion), 700
Extrinsic allergic alveolitis (hypersensitivity pneumonitis), 703
Exudative effusion, 700
Flail chest, 699
Hemoptysis, 696
Hypercapnia, 697
Hypersensitivity pneumonitis (extrinsic allergic alveolitis), 703
Hyperventilation, 696
Hypocapnia, 696
Hypoventilation, 696
Hypoxemia, 697
Hypoxia, 697
Idiopathic pulmonary fibrosis (IPF), 702
Ischemia, 697
Kussmaul respiration (hyperpnea), 696
Large cell carcinoma, 719
Laryngeal cancer, 717
Latent TB infection (LTBI), 714
Lung cancer, 718
Open pneumothorax (communicating pneumothorax), 700
Orthopnea, 695
Oxygen toxicity, 703
Paroxysmal nocturnal dyspnea (PND), 695
Pleural effusion, 700
Pneumoconiosis, 703
Pneumonia, 711
Pneumothorax, 699
Pulmonary artery hypertension (PAH), 716
Pulmonary edema, 703
Pulmonary embolism (PE), 715
Pulmonary fibrosis, 702
Pulsus paradoxus, 707
Respiratory failure, 698
Shunting, 698
Small cell (oat cell) carcinoma, 719
Squamous cell carcinoma, 719
Status asthmaticus, 707
Surfactant impairment, 701
Tension pneumothorax, 700
TNM classification, 720
Transudative effusion, 700
Tuberculosis (TB), 714

REFERENCES

1. Hayen, A., Herigstad, M., & Pattinson, K. T. (2013). Understanding dyspnea as a complex individual experience. *Maturitas, 76*(1), 45–50. doi:10.1016/j.maturitas.2013.06.005.
2. Peters, S. P. (2013). When the chief complaint is (or should be) dyspnea in adults. *Journal of Allergy and Clinical Immunology: In Practice, 1*(2), 129–136. doi:10.1016/j.jaip.2013.01.004.
3. Parshall, M. B., Schwartzstein, R. M., Adams, L., et al. (2012). An official American Thoracic Society statement: Update on the mechanisms, assessment, and management of dyspnea. *American Journal of Respiratory and Critical Care Medicine, 185*(4), 435–452. doi:10.1164/rccm.201111-2042ST.
4. Schmidt, M., Banzett, R. B., Raux, M., et al. (2014). Unrecognized suffering in the ICU: Addressing dyspnea in mechanically ventilated patients. *Intensive Care Medicine, 40*(1), 1–10. doi:10.1007/s00134-013-3117-3.
5. Gibson, P. G., Simpson, J. K., Ryan, N. M., et al. (2014). Mechanisms of cough. *Current Opinion in Allergy and Clinical Immunology, 14*(1), 55–61. doi:10.1097/ACI.0000000000000027.
6. Guyton, A. C., & Hall, J. E. (Eds.), (2015). *Textbook of medical physiology* (13th ed.). Philadelphia: Saunders.
7. Spicknall, K. E., Zirwas, M. J., & English, J. C., 3rd. (2005). Clubbing: An update on diagnosis, differential diagnosis, pathophysiology, and clinical relevance. *Journal of the American Academy of Dermatology, 52*(6), 1020–1028. doi:10.1016/j.jaad.2005.01.006.
8. Nguyen, S., & Hojjati, M. (2011). Review of current therapies for secondary hypertrophic pulmonary osteoarthropathy. *Clinical Rheumatology, 30*(1), 7–13. doi:10.1007/s10067-010-1563-7.
9. Brims, F. J., Davies, H. E., & Lee, Y. C. (2010). Respiratory chest pain: Diagnosis and treatment. *Medical Clinics of North America, 94*(2), 217–232. doi:10.1016/j.mcna.2010.01.003.
10. Oana, S., & Mukherji, J. (2014). Acute and chronic respiratory failure. *Handbook of Clinical Neurology, 119*, 273–288. doi:10.1016/B978-0-7020-4086-3.00019-9.
11. Sundaram, S., Tasker, A. D., & Morrell, N. W. (2009). Familial spontaneous pneumothorax and lung cysts due to a Folliculin exon 10 mutation. *European Respiratory Journal, 33*(6), 1510–1512. doi:10.1183/09031936.00062608.
12. Repanshek, Z. D., Ufberg, J. W., Vilke, G. M., et al. (2013). Alternative treatments of pneumothorax. *Journal of Emergency Medicine, 44*(2), 457–466. doi:10.1016/j.jemermed.2012.02.049.
13. Psallidas, I., Corcoran, J. P., & Rahman, N. M. (2014). Management of parapneumonic effusions and empyema. *Seminars in Respiratory and Critical Care Medicine, 35*(6), 715–722. doi:10.1055/s-0034-1395503.
14. O'Brien, J. (2013). Absorption atelectasis: Incidence and clinical implications. *AANA Journal, 81*(3), 205–208.
15. McDonnell, M. J., Ward, J. C., Lordan, J. L., et al. (2013). Non-cystic fibrosis bronchiectasis. *QJM: Monthly Journal of the Association of Physicians, 106*(8), 709–715. doi:10.1093/qjmed/hct109.
16. Papiris, S. A., Malagari, K., Manali, E. D., et al. (2013). Bronchiolitis: Adopting a unifying definition and a comprehensive etiological classification. *Expert Review of Respiratory Medicine, 7*(3), 289–306. doi:10.1586/ers.13.21.
17. Wolters, P. J., Collard, H. R., & Jones, K. D. (2014). Pathogenesis of idiopathic pulmonary fibrosis. *Annual Review of Pathology, 9*, 157–179. doi:10.1146/annurev-pathol-012513-104706.
18. Ahluwalia, N., Shea, B. S., & Tager, A. M. (2014). New therapeutic targets in idiopathic pulmonary fibrosis. Aiming to rein in runaway wound-healing responses. *American Journal of Respiratory and Critical Care Medicine, 190*(8), 867–878. doi:10.1164/rccm.201403-0509PP.

19. Grunes, D., & Beasley, M. B. (2013). Hypersensitivity pneumonitis: A review and update of histologic findings. *Journal of Clinical Pathology, 66*(10), 888–895. doi:10.1136/jclinpath-2012-201337.
20. Ohshimo, S., Bonella, F., Guzman, J., et al. (2012). Hypersensitivity pneumonitis. *Immunology and Allergy Clinics of North America, 32*(4), 537–556. doi:10.1016/j.iac.2012.08.008.
21. Fujishima, S. (2014). Pathophysiology and biomarkers of acute respiratory distress syndrome. *Journal of Intensive Care, 2*(1), 32. doi:10.1186/2052-0492-2-32.
22. Ontario Lung Association. (2015). *Research and education grants and awards 2010–2011.* Retrieved from http://www.on.lung.ca/page.aspx?pid=716.
23. Bakowitz, M., Bruns, M., & McCunn, M. (2012). Acute lung injury and the acute respiratory distress syndrome in the injured patient. *Scandinavian Journal of Trauma, Resuscitation and Emergency Medicine, 20*, 54. doi:10.1186/1757-7241-20-54.
24. Matthay, M. A., Ware, L. B., & Zimmerman, G. A. (2012). The acute respiratory distress syndrome. *Journal of Clinical Investigation, 122*(8), 2731–2740. doi:10.1172/JCI60331.
25. Fujishima, S. (2014). Pathophysiology and biomarkers of acute respiratory distress syndrome. *Journal of Intensive Care, 2*(1), 32. doi:10.1186/2052-0492-2-32.
26. Ruan, S. Y., Lin, H. H., Huang, C. T., et al. (2014). Exploring the heterogeneity of effects of corticosteroids on acute respiratory distress syndrome: A systematic review and meta-analysis. *Critical Care, 18*(2), R63. doi:10.1186/cc13819.
27. Asthma Society of Canada. (2014). *Severe asthma: The Canadian patient journey.* Toronto: Author. Retrieved from https://asthma.ca/living-with-sever e-asthma.
28. Centers for Disease Control and Prevention. (2014). *FastStats: Asthma.* Retrieved from http://www.cdc.gov/nchs/fastats/asthma.htm.
29. Corren, J. (2013). Asthma phenotypes and endotypes: An evolving paradigm for classification. *Discovery Medicine, 15*(83), 243–249.
30. Guarnieri, M., & Balmes, J. R. (2014). Outdoor air pollution and asthma. *Lancet, 383*(9928), 1581–1592. doi:10.1016/S0140-6736(14)60617-6.
31. Mackenzie, K. J., Anderton, S. M., & Schwarze, J. (2014). Viral respiratory tract infections and asthma in early life: Cause and effect? *Clinical and Experimental Allergy, 44*(1), 9–19. doi:10.1111/cea.12246.
32. Sutherland, E. R. (2014). Linking obesity and asthma. *Annals of the New York Academy of Sciences, 1311*, 31–41.
33. Yoo, Y., & Perzanowski, M. S. (2014). Allergic sensitization and the environment: Latest update. *Current Allergy and Asthma Reports, 14*(10), 465. doi:10.1007/s11882-014-0465-1.
34. Kabesch, M. (2014). Epigenetics in asthma and allergy. *Current Opinion in Allergy and Clinical Immunology, 14*(1), 62–68. doi:10.1097/ACI.0000000000000025.
35. Kramer, A., Bekeschus, S., Bröker, B. M., et al. (2013). Maintaining health by balancing microbial exposure and prevention of infection: The hygiene hypothesis versus the hypothesis of early immune challenge. *Journal of Hospital Infection, 83*(Suppl. 1), S29–S34. doi:10.1016/S0195-6701(13)60007-9.
36. Beigelman, A., Weinstock, G. M., & Bacharier, L. B. (2014). The relationships between environmental bacterial exposure, airway bacterial colonization, and asthma. *Current Opinion in Allergy and Clinical Immunology, 14*(2), 137–142. doi:10.1097/ACI.0000000000000036.
37. Holgate, S. T. (2012). Innate and adaptive immune responses in asthma. *Nature Medicine, 18*(5), 673–683. doi:10.1038/nm.2731.
38. Deckers, J., Branco Madeira, F., & Hammad, H. (2013). Innate immune cells in asthma. *Trends in Immunology, 34*(11), 540–547. doi:10.1016/j.it.2013.08.004.
39. Busse, W. W. (2010). The relationship of airway hyperresponsiveness and airway inflammation: Airway hyperresponsiveness in asthma: Its measurement and clinical significance. *Chest, 138*(Suppl. 2), 4S–10S. doi:10.1378/chest.10-0100.
40. Bai, T. R. (2010). Evidence for airway remodeling in chronic asthma. *Current Opinion in Allergy and Clinical Immunology, 10*(1), 82–86. doi:10.1097/ACI.0b013e32833363b2.
41. Shah, R., & Saltoun, C. A. (2012). Chapter 14: Acute severe asthma (status asthmaticus). *Allergy and Asthma Proceedings, 33*(Suppl. 1), S47–S50. doi:10.2500/aap.2012.33.3547.
42. Murata, A., & Ling, P. M. (2012). Asthma diagnosis and management. *Emergency Medicine Clinics of North America, 30*(2), 203–222, vii. doi:10.1016/j.emc.2011.10.004.
43. Fajt, M. L., & Wenzel, S. E. (2015). Asthma phenotypes and the use of biologic medications in asthma and allergic disease: The next steps toward personalized care. *Journal of Allergy and Clinical Immunology, 135*(2), 299–310. doi:10.1016/j.jaci.2014.12.1871.
44. Penagos, M., Passalacqua, G., Compalati, E., et al. (2008). Meta-analysis of the efficacy of sublingual immunotherapy in the treatment of allergic asthma in pediatric patients, 3 to 18 years of age. *Chest, 133*(3), 599–609. doi:10.1378/chest.06-1425.
45. Normansell, R., Walker, S., Milan, S. J., et al. (2014). Omalizumab for asthma in adults and children. *Cochrane Database of Systematic Reviews,* (1), CD003559, doi:10.1002/14651858.CD003559.pub4.
46. Apter, A. J. (2014). Advances in adult asthma diagnosis and treatment in 2013. *Journal of Allergy and Clinical Immunology, 133*(1), 49–56. doi:10.1016/j.jaci.2013.11.005.
47. Lovinsky-Desir, S., & Miller, R. L. (2012). Epigenetics, asthma, and allergic diseases: A review of the latest advancements. *Current Allergy and Asthma Reports, 12*(3), 211–220. doi:10.1007/s11882-012-0257-4.
48. Vestbo, J., Hurd, S. S., Agusti, A. G., et al. (2013). Global strategy for the diagnosis, management and prevention of chronic obstructive pulmonary disease, GOLD executive summary. *American Journal of Respiratory and Critical Care Medicine, 187*, 347–365. doi:10.1164/rccm.201204-0596PP.
49. Diaz-Guzman, E., & Mannino, D. M. (2014). Epidemiology and prevalence of chronic obstructive pulmonary disease. *Clinics in Chest Medicine, 35*(1), 7–16. doi:10.1016/j.ccm.2013.10.002.
50. Tzortzaki, E. G., Papi, A., Neofytou, E., et al. (2013). Immune and genetic mechanisms in COPD: Possible targets for therapeutic interventions. *Current Drug Targets, 14*(2), 141–148. doi:10.2174/1389450111314020002.
51. Statistics Canada. (2013). *Chronic obstructive pulmonary disease in Canadians, 2009 to 2011 (Health Fact Sheets, 82-625-X).* Retrieved from http://www.statcan.gc.ca/pub/82-625-x/2012001/article/11709-eng.htm.
52. Kim, V., & Criner, G. J. (2013). Chronic bronchitis and chronic obstructive pulmonary disease. *American Journal of Respiratory and Critical Care Medicine, 187*(3), 228–237. doi:10.1164/rccm.201210-1843CI.
53. Vijayan, V. K. (2013). Chronic obstructive pulmonary disease. *Indian Journal of Medical Research, 137*(2), 251–269.
54. Gagnon, P., Guenette, J. A., Langer, D., et al. (2014). Pathogenesis of hyperinflation in chronic obstructive pulmonary disease. *International Journal of Chronic Obstructive Pulmonary Disease, 9*, 187–201. doi:10.2147/COPD.S38934.
55. Csikesz, N. G., & Gartman, E. J. (2014). New developments in the assessment of COPD: Early diagnosis is key. *International Journal of Chronic Obstructive Pulmonary Disease, 9*, 277–286. doi:10.2147/COPD.S46198.
56. Kim, V., & Criner, G. J. (2013). Chronic bronchitis and chronic obstructive pulmonary disease. *American Journal of Respiratory and Critical Care Medicine, 187*(3), 228–237. doi:10.1164/rccm.201210-1843CI.
57. Martinez, C. H., & Han, M. K. (2012). Contribution of the environment and comorbidities to chronic obstructive pulmonary disease phenotypes. *Medical Clinics of North America, 96*(4), 713–727. doi:10.1016/j.mcna.2012.02.007.
58. Stockley, R. A. (2014). Alpha1-antitrypsin review. *Clinics in Chest Medicine, 35*(1), 39–50. doi:10.1016/j.ccm.2013.10.001.
59. Tuder, R. M., & Petrache, I. (2012). Pathogenesis of chronic obstructive pulmonary disease. *Journal of Clinical Investigation, 122*(8), 2749–2755. doi:10.1172/JCI60324.
60. Kent, B. D., Mitchell, P. D., & McNicholas, W. T. (2011). Hypoxemia in patients with COPD: Cause, effects, and disease progression. *International Journal of Chronic Obstructive Pulmonary Disease, 6*, 199–208. doi:10.2147/COPD.S10611.
61. Stockley, R. A., & Turner, A. M. (2014). α-1-Antitrypsin deficiency: Clinical variability, assessment, and treatment. *Trends in Molecular Medicine, 20*(2), 105–115. doi:10.1016/j.molmed.2013.11.006.
62. Murphy, P. B., Zoumot, Z., & Polkey, M. I. (2014). Noninvasive ventilation and lung volume reduction. *Clinics in Chest Medicine, 35*(1), 251–269. doi:10.1016/j.ccm.2013.10.011.
63. Statistics Canada. (2015). *The 10 leading causes of death, 2011.* Retrieved from http://www.statcan.gc.ca/pub/82-625-x/2014001/article/11896-eng.htm.
64. Heron, M. (2016). Deaths: Leading causes for 2014. *National Vital Statistics Reports, 65*(5), 1–95. Retrieved from https://www.cdc.gov/nchs/data/nvsr/nvsr65/nvsr65_05.pdf.
65. Antimicrobial Stewardship Program (ASP) in Intensive Care Units (ICU) ARTIC Project. (2012). *Community-acquired pneumonia educational module, p. 3.* Retrieved from http://www.antimicrobialstewardship.com/sites/default/files/article_files/community-acquired_pneumonia_educational_module.pdf.
66. Asadi, L., Sligl, W. I., Eurich, D. T., et al. (2012). Macrolide-based regimens and mortality in hospitalized patients with community-acquired pneumonia: A systematic review and meta-analysis. *Clinical Infectious Diseases, 55*, 371–380.
67. Wunderink, R. G., & Waterer, G. W. (2014). Clinical practice. Community-acquired pneumonia. *New England Journal of Medicine, 370*(6), 543–551. doi:10.1056/NEJMcp1214869.
68. Ashraf, M., & Ostrosky-Zeichner, L. (2012). Ventilator-associated pneumonia: A review. *Hospital Practice (1995), 40*(1), 93–105. doi:10.3810/hp.2012.02.950.
69. Charles, M. P., Kali, A., Easow, J. M., et al. (2014). Ventilator-associated pneumonia. *Australasian Medical Journal, 7*(8), 334–344. doi:10.4066/AMJ.2014.2105.
70. Lobdell, K. W., Stamou, S., & Sanchez, J. A. (2012). Hospital-acquired infections. *Surgical Clinics of North America, 92*(1), 65–77. doi:10.1016/j.suc.2011.11.003.
71. Remington, L. T., & Sligl, W., I. (2014). Community-acquired pneumonia. *Current Opinion in Pulmonary Medicine, 20*(3), 215–224. doi:10.1097/MCP.0000000000000052.
72. Hidron, A. I., Low, C. E., Honig, E. G., et al. (2009). Emergence of community-acquired methicillin-resistant *Staphylococcus aureus* strain USA3 00 as a cause of necrotising community-onset pneumonia. *Lancet Infectious Diseases, 9*(6), 384–392. doi:10.1016/S1473-3099(09)70133-1.
73. Klevens, R. M., Morrison, M. A., Nadle, J., et al. (2007). Invasive methicillin-resistant *Staphylococcus aureus* infections in the United States. *JAMA: The Journal of the American Medical Association, 298*, 1763–1771. doi:10.1001/jama.298.15.1763.
74. Lieberman, D., Shimoni, A., Shemer-Avni, Y., et al. (2010). Respiratory viruses in adults with community-acquired pneumonia. *Chest, 138*(4), 811–816. doi:10.1378/chest.09-2717.
75. Vernatter, J., & Pirofski, L. A. (2013). Current concepts in host-microbe interaction leading to pneumococcal pneumonia. *Current Opinion in Infectious Diseases, 26*(3), 277–283. doi:10.1097/QCO.0b013e3283608419.

76. Mitchell, T. J., & Dalziel, C. E. (2014). The biology of pneumolysin. *Sub-Cellular Biochemistry, 80*, 145–160. doi:10.1007/978-94-017-8881-6_8.
77. Ramsey, C. D., & Kumar, A. (2013). Influenza and endemic viral pneumonia. *Critical Care Clinics, 29*(4), 1069–1086. doi:10.1016/j.ccc.2013.06.003.
78. Couturier, M. R., Graf, E. H., & Griffin, A. T. (2014). Urine antigen tests for the diagnosis of respiratory infections: Legionellosis, histoplasmosis, pneumococcal pneumonia. *Clinics in Laboratory Medicine, 34*(2), 219–236. doi:10.1016/j.cll.2014.02.002.
79. Yayan, J. (2014). The comparative development of elevated resistance to macrolides in community-acquired pneumonia caused by *Streptococcus pneumoniae. Drug Design, Development and Therapy, 8*, 1733–1743. doi:10.2147/DDDT.S71349.
80. Murray, C. J., Ortblad, K. F., Guinovart, C., et al. (2014). Global, regional, and national incidence and mortality for HIV, tuberculosis, and malaria during 1990–2013: A systematic analysis for the Global Burden of Disease Study 2013. *Lancet, 384*(9947), 1005–1070. doi:10.1016/S0140-6736(14)60844-8.
81. Health Canada. (2013). *Tuberculosis*. Retrieved from http://www.hc-sc.gc.ca/hc-ps/dc-ma/tuberculos-eng.php.
82. Public Health Agency of Canada. (2015). *Tuberculosis in Canada, 2013*. Ottawa: Author. Retrieved from http://www.phac-aspc.gc.ca/tbpc-latb/pubs/tbcan13pre/assets/pdf/tbcan13pre-eng.pdf.
83. Pai, M., Minion, J., Steingart, K., et al. (2010). New and improved tuberculosis diagnostics: Evidence, policy, practice, and impact. *Current Opinion in Pulmonary Medicine, 16*(3), 271–284. doi:10.1097/MCP.0b013e328338094f.
84. Moon, H. W., & Hur, M. (2013). Interferon-gamma release assays for the diagnosis of latent tuberculosis infection: An updated review. *Annals of Clinical and Laboratory Science, 43*(2), 221–229.
85. Zumla, A. I., Gillespie, S. H., Hoelscher, M., et al. (2014). New antituberculosis drugs, regimens, and adjunct therapies: Needs, advances, and future prospects. *Lancet Infectious Diseases, 14*(4), 327–340. doi:10.1016/S1473-3099(13)70328-1.
86. Günther, G. (2014). Multidrug-resistant and extensively drug-resistant tuberculosis: A review of current concepts and future challenges. *Clinical Medicine (London), 14*(3), 279–285. doi:10.7861/clinmedicine.14-3-279.
87. Public Health Agency of Canada, The Lung Association, & Canadian Thoracic Society. (2014). *Canadian tuberculosis standards* (7th ed.). Ottawa: Public Health Agency of Canada. Retrieved from http://strauss.ca/OEMAC/wp-content/uploads/2013/11/Canadian_TB_Standards_7th-edition_English.pdf.
88. Weiner, J., 3rd, & Kaufmann, S. H. (2014). Recent advances towards tuberculosis control: Vaccines and biomarkers. *Journal of Internal Medicine, 275*(5), 467–480. doi:10.1111/joim.12212.
89. Regazzi, M., Carvalho, A. C., Villani, P., et al. (2014). Treatment optimization in patients co-infected with HIV and Mycobacterium tuberculosis infections: Focus on drug–drug interactions with rifamycins. *Clinical Pharmacokinetics, 53*(6), 489–507. doi:10.1007/s40262-014-0144-3.
90. Konstantinides, S. V., Torbicki, A., Agnelli, G., et al. (2014). 2014 ESC guidelines on the diagnosis and management of acute pulmonary embolism. *European Heart Journal, 35*(43), 3033–3069, 3069a–3069k. doi:10.1093/eurheartj/ehu283.
91. Moorjani, N., & Price, S. (2013). Massive pulmonary embolism. *Cardiology Clinics, 31*(4), 503–518, vii. doi:10.1016/j.ccl.2013.07.005.
92. Wells, P. S., Forgle, M. A., & Rodger, M. A. (2014). Treatment of venous thromboembolism. *JAMA: The Journal of the American Medical Association, 311*(7), 717–728. doi:10.1001/jama.2014.65.
93. National Heart Lung and Blood Institute. (2011). *Types of pulmonary hypertension*. Retrieved from http://www.nhlbi.nih.gov/health/health-topics/topics/pah/types.
94. Roden, A. C. (2014). Pulmonary pathology: LC22-1 PULMONARY HYPERTENSION. *Pathology, 46*(Suppl. 2), S37. doi:10.1097/01.PAT.0000454213.97350.b1.
95. Zamanian, R. T., Kudelko, K. T., Sung, Y. K., et al. (2014). Current clinical management of pulmonary arterial hypertension. *Circulation Research, 115*(1), 131–147. doi:10.1161/CIRCRESAHA.115.303827.
96. Rosanio, S., Pelliccia, F., Gaudio, C., et al. (2014). Pulmonary arterial hypertension in adults: Novel drugs and catheter ablation techniques show promise? Systematic review on pharmacotherapy and interventional strategies. *BioMedical Research International, 2014*, 743868. doi:10.1155/2014/743868.
97. Rich, S. (2012). Right ventricular adaptation and maladaptation in chronic pulmonary arterial hypertension. *Cardiology Clinics, 30*(2), 257–269. doi:10.1016/j.ccl.2012.03.004.
98. Canadian Cancer Society. (2017). *Laryngeal cancer*. Retrieved from http://www.cancer.ca/en/cancer-information/cancer-type/laryngeal/statistics/?region=on.
99. Canadian Cancer Society's Advisory Committee on Cancer Statistics. (2017). *Canadian cancer statistics 2017*. Toronto: Canadian Cancer Society. Retrieved from http://www.cancer.ca/~/media/cancer.ca/CW/cancer%20information/cancer%20101/Canadian%20cancer%20statistics/Canadian-Cancer-Statistics-2017-EN.pdf?la=en.
100. Grce, M., & Mravak-Stipetić, M. (2014). Human papillomavirus-associated diseases. *Clinics in Dermatology, 32*(2), 253–258. doi:10.1016/j.clindermatol.2013.10.006.
101. Agra, I. M., Ferlito, A., Takes, R. P., et al. (2012). Diagnosis and treatment of recurrent laryngeal cancer following initial nonsurgical therapy. *Head and Neck, 34*(5), 727–735. doi:10.1002/hed.21739.
102. Statistics Canada, & Canadian Cancer Society. (2015). *Canadian cancer statistics, 2015* (p. 6). Ottawa: Author. Retrieved from https://www.cancer.ca/~/media/cancer.ca/CW/cancer%20information/cancer%20101/Canadian%20cancer%20statistics/Canadian-Cancer-Statistics-2015-EN.pdf.
103. Sakashita, S., Sakashita, M., & Sound Tsao, M. (2014). Genes and pathology of non-small cell lung carcinoma. *Seminars in Oncology, 41*(1), 28–39. doi:10.1053/j.seminoncol.2013.12.008.
104. Hensing, T., Chawia, A., Batra, R., et al. (2014). A personalized treatment for lung cancer: Molecular pathways, targeted therapies, and genomic characterization. *Advances in Experimental Medicine and Biology, 799*, 85–117. doi:10.1007/978-1-4614-8778-4_5.
105. Noguchi, M. (2010). Stepwise progression of pulmonary adenocarcinoma—Clinical and molecular implications. *Cancer Metastasis Reviews, 29*(1), 15–21. doi:10.1007/s10555-010-9210-y.
106. Kerr, K. M. (2013). Clinical relevance of the new IASLC/ERS/ATS adenocarcinoma classification. *Journal of Clinical Pathology, 66*(10), 832–838. doi:10.1136/jclinpath-2013-201519.
107. Rossi, G., Mengoli, M. C., Cavazza, A., et al. (2014). Large cell carcinoma of the lung: Clinically oriented classification integrating immunohistochemistry and molecular biology. *Virchows Archiv, 464*(1), 61–68. doi:10.1007/s00428-013-1501-6.
108. Detterbeck, F. C. (2014). Clinical presentation and evaluation of neuroendocrine tumors of the lung. *Thoracic Surgery Clinics, 24*(3), 267–276. doi:10.1016/j.thorsurg.2014.04.002.
109. Nanavaty, P., Alvarez, M. S., & Alberts, W. M. (2014). Lung cancer screening: Advantages, controversies, and applications. *Cancer Control: Journal of the Moffitt Cancer Center, 21*(1), 9–14.
110. Rivera, M. P., Mehta, A. C., & Wahidi, M. M. (2013). Establishing the diagnosis of lung cancer: Diagnosis and management of lung cancer 3rd ed.: American College of Chest Physicians evidence-based clinical practice guidelines. *Chest, 143*(5, Suppl.), e142S–e165S. doi:10.1378/chest.12-2353.
111. Groot, P., & Munden, R. F. (2012). Lung cancer epidemiology, risk factors, and prevention. *Radiologic Clinics of North America, 50*(5), 863–876. doi:10.1016/j.rcl.2012.06.006.
112. Carnio, S., Novello, S., Mele, T., et al. (2014). Extending survival of stage IV non-small cell lung cancer. *Seminars in Oncology, 41*(1), 69–92. doi:10.1053/j.seminoncol.2013.12.013.
113. Declerck, S., & Vansteenkiste, J. (2014). Immunotherapy for lung cancer: Ongoing clinical trials. *Future Oncology (London, England), 10*(1), 91–105. doi:10.2217/fon.13.166.
114. Freitas, D. P., Teixeira, C. A., Santos-Silva, F., et al. (2014). Therapy-induced enrichment of putative lung cancer stem-like cells. *International Journal of Cancer. Journal International du Cancer, 134*(6), 1270–1278. doi:10.1002/ijc.28478.

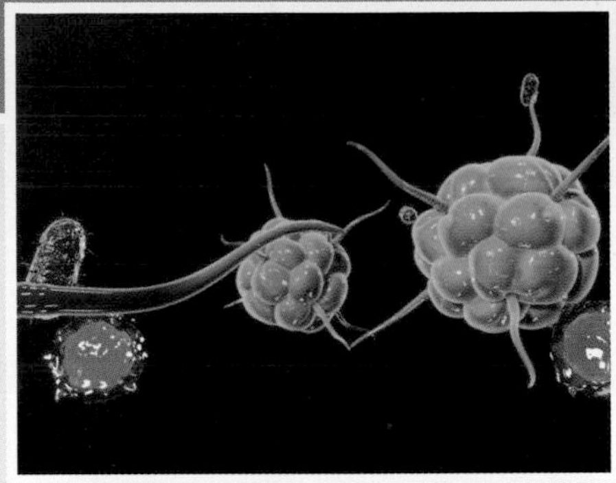

28

Alterations of Pulmonary Function in Children

Valentina L. Brashers, Sue E. Huether, and Mohamed El-Hussein

EVOLVE WEBSITE

http://evolve.elsevier.com/Canada/Huether/pathophysiology
Student Review Questions
Key Points
Case Studies
Animations
Quick Check Answers

CHAPTER OUTLINE

Disorders of the Upper Airways, 725
- Infections of the Upper Airways, 725
- Aspiration of Foreign Bodies, 727
- Obstructive Sleep Apnea Syndrome, 727

Disorders of the Lower Airways, 728
- Respiratory Distress Syndrome of the Newborn, 728
- Bronchopulmonary Dysplasia, 730
- Respiratory Tract Infections, 730
- Aspiration Pneumonitis, 733
- Bronchiolitis Obliterans, 733
- Asthma, 733
- Acute Lung Injury/Acute Respiratory Distress Syndrome, 735
- Cystic Fibrosis, 735

Sudden Unexpected Infant Death, 737

Alterations of respiratory function in children are influenced by physiological maturation, which is determined by age, genetics, and environmental conditions. Infants, especially premature infants, may present special problems because of incomplete development of the airways, circulation, chest wall, and immune system. A variety of upper and lower airway infections can cause respiratory compromise or play a role in the pathogenesis of more chronic pulmonary disease. Pulmonary dysfunction can be categorized into disorders of either the upper or the lower airways.

DISORDERS OF THE UPPER AIRWAYS

Disorders of the upper airways can cause significant obstruction to airflow. Common causes of **upper airway obstruction** in children are infections, foreign body aspiration, obstructive sleep apnea, and trauma.

Infections of the Upper Airways

Table 28-1 compares some of the more common upper airway infections.

Croup

Croup illnesses can be divided into two categories: (1) acute laryngotracheobronchitis (croup) and (2) spasmodic croup.[1] Diphtheria can also be considered a croup illness but is now rare because of vaccinations. Croup illnesses are all characterized by infection and obstruction of the upper airways.

Croup is an acute laryngotracheitis and almost always occurs in children between 6 months and 5 years of age, with a peak incidence at 2 years of age. In 85% of cases, croup is caused by a virus, most commonly parainfluenza. Other causes include respiratory syncytial virus (RSV), rhinovirus, adenovirus, rubella virus, or atypical bacteria. The incidence of croup is higher in males and is most common during the winter months. Approximately 15% of affected children have a strong family history of croup.[2] *Spasmodic croup* usually occurs in older children. The etiology is unknown but can be triggered by cold, allergy, or viral infection.[2,3] Spasmodic croup develops acutely, usually without fever, and tends to recur.

PATHOPHYSIOLOGY The pathophysiology of viral croup is caused primarily by subglottic inflammation and edema from the infection. The mucous membranes of the larynx are tightly adherent to the underlying cartilage, whereas those of the subglottic space are looser and thus allow accumulation of mucosal and submucosal edema (Figure 28-1). Furthermore, the cricoid cartilage is structurally the narrowest point of the airway, making edema in this area critical. Spasmodic croup also causes obstruction but with less inflammation and edema. As illustrated in Figure 28-2, increased resistance to airflow leads to increased work of breathing, which generates more negative intrathoracic pressure that, in turn, may exacerbate dynamic collapse of the upper airway.

CLINICAL MANIFESTATIONS Typically, the child experiences rhinorrhea, sore throat, and low-grade fever for a few days, and then develops a harsh (seal-like) barking cough, inspiratory stridor, and hoarse voice. The quality of voice, cough, and stridor may suggest the location of the obstruction (Figure 28-3). Most cases resolve spontaneously within 24 to 48 hours and do not warrant hospital admission. A child with severe croup usually displays deep retractions (Figure 28-4), stridor, agitation, tachycardia, and sometimes pallor or cyanosis.

TABLE 28-1 Comparison of Upper Airway Infections

Condition	Age	Onset	Etiology	Pathophysiology	Symptoms
Acute laryngotracheobronchitis	6 months to 3 years	Usually gradual	Viral	Inflammation from larynx to bronchi	Harsh cough; stridor; low-grade fever; may have nasal discharge, conjunctivitis
Acute tracheitis	1 to 12 years	Abrupt or following viral illness	*Staphylococcus aureus*	Inflammation of upper trachea	High fever; toxic appearance; harsh cough; purulent secretions
Acute epiglottitis	2 to 6 years	Abrupt	*Haemophilus influenzae*, group A streptococci	Inflammation of supraglottic structures	Severe sore throat; dysphagia; high fever; toxic appearance; muffled voice; may drool; dyspnea; sits erect and quietly

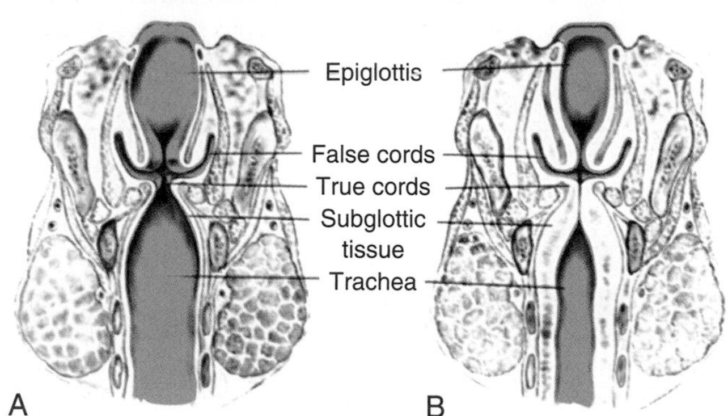

FIGURE 28-1 The Larynx and Subglottic Trachea. A, Normal trachea. **B,** Narrowing and obstruction from edema caused by croup. (From Hockenberry, M.J., & Wilson, D. [Eds.]. [2015]. *Wong's nursing care of infants and children* [10th ed.]. St. Louis: Mosby.)

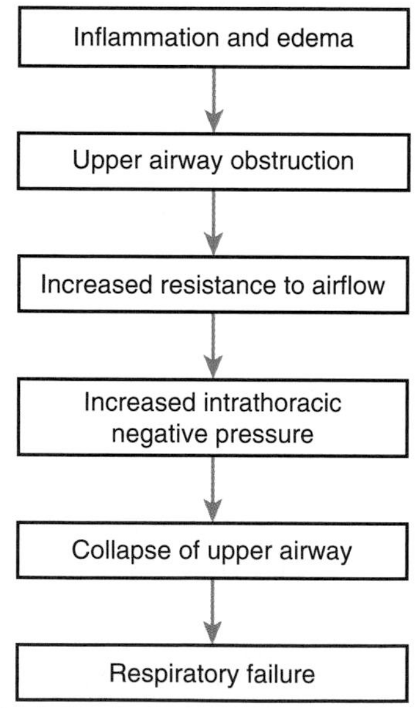

FIGURE 28-2 Upper Airway Obstruction With Croup.

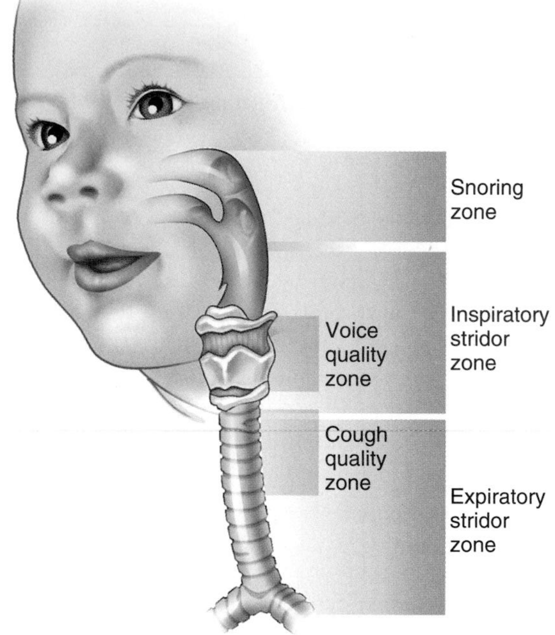

FIGURE 28-3 Listening Can Help Locate the Site of Airway Obstruction. A loud, gasping snore suggests enlarged tonsils or adenoids. In inspiratory stridor, the airway is compromised at the level of the supraglottic larynx, vocal cords, subglottic region, or upper trachea. Expiratory stridor results from a narrowing or collapse in the trachea or bronchi. Airway noise during both inspiration and expiration often represents a fixed obstruction of the vocal cords or subglottic space. Hoarseness or a weak cry is a by-product of obstruction at the vocal cords. If a cough is croupy, suspect constriction below the vocal cords. (Redrawn from Eavey, R.D. [1986]. *Contemp Ped, 3*[6]: 79; original illustration by Paul Singh-Roy.)

Spasmodic croup is characterized by similar hoarseness, barking cough, and stridor. It is of sudden onset and usually occurs at night and without prodromal symptoms. It usually resolves quickly.

EVALUATION AND TREATMENT The degree of symptoms determines the level of treatment. The most common tool for estimating croup severity is the Westley croup score.[4] Most children with croup require no treatment; however, some cases require outpatient treatment. These children usually have only mild stridor or retractions and appear alert, playful, and able to eat. There has been much debate about the most effective outpatient treatments for croup. Humidified air does not improve symptoms in mild to moderate croup.[5]

Glucocorticoids—either injected, oral (dexamethasone [Dexasone]), or nebulized (budesonide [Pulmicort])—have been shown to improve symptoms.[6] The presence of stridor at rest, moderate or severe retractions of the chest, or agitation suggests more severe disease and does require inpatient observation and treatment. For acute respiratory distress, nebulized epinephrine (Adrenalin) stimulates α- and β-adrenergic receptors and decreases mucosal edema and airway secretions.[7]

Oxygen should be administered. Heliox (helium–oxygen mixture) also can be used in severe cases although it is not yet considered a mainstay of routine treatment. Heliox works by improving gas flow and thus decreasing the flow resistance of the narrowed airway.[8] In rare cases, croup and spasmodic croup may require placement of an endotracheal tube.

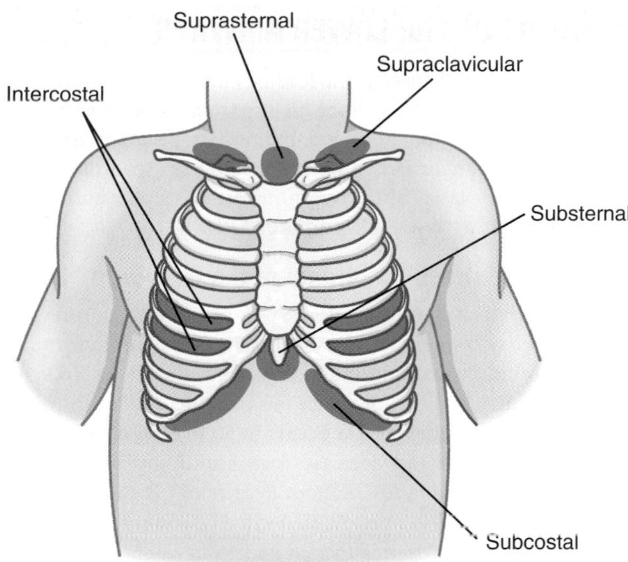

FIGURE 28-4 Areas of Chest Muscle Retraction.

Bacterial tracheitis. Bacterial tracheitis (pseudomembranous croup) is the most common potentially life-threatening upper airway infection in children. It is most often caused by *Staphylococcus aureus* (including methicillin-resistant *Staphylococcus aureus* [MRSA] strains), *Haemophilus influenzae*, or group A beta-hemolytic *Streptococcus* (GABHS). Treatment of viral croup with corticosteroids has increased the risk for bacterial tracheitis. The presence of airway edema and copious purulent secretions leads to airway obstruction that can be worsened by the formation of a tracheal pseudomembrane and mucosal sloughing. Bacterial tracheitis is treated with immediate administration of antibiotics and endotracheal intubation to prevent total upper airway obstruction.[9]

Acute Epiglottitis

Historically, acute epiglottitis was caused by *Haemophilus influenzae* type b (Hib). Since the advent of *H. influenzae* vaccine, the overall incidence of acute epiglottitis has been reduced; however, up to 25% of epiglottitis cases are still caused by Hib, which is now more common in adults.[10] Current cases in children usually are related to vaccine failure or are caused by other pathogens.

PATHOPHYSIOLOGY The epiglottis arises from the posterior tongue base and covers the laryngeal inlet during swallowing. Bacterial invasion of the mucosa with associated inflammation leads to the rapid development of edema, causing severe, life-threatening obstruction of the upper airway.[10]

CLINICAL MANIFESTATIONS In the classic form of the disease, a child between 2 and 7 years of age suddenly develops high fever, irritability, sore throat, inspiratory stridor, and severe respiratory distress. The child appears anxious and has a voice that sounds muffled ("hot potato" voice). Drooling, absence of cough, preference to sit, and dysphagia (inability to swallow) are common.[11] In addition to appearing ill, the child will generally adopt a position of leaning forward (tripoding) to try to improve breathing. Death can occur in a few hours. Pneumonia, cervical lymph node inflammation, otitis, and, rarely, meningitis or septic arthritis may occur concomitantly because of bacterial sepsis.

EVALUATION AND TREATMENT Acute epiglottitis is a life-threatening emergency. Efforts should be made to keep the child calm and undisturbed. Examination of the throat should not be attempted because it may trigger laryngospasm and cause respiratory collapse. With severe airway obstruction, the airway may be secured with intubation, and antibiotics are administered promptly. Racemic epinephrine and corticosteroids may be given until definitive management of the airway can be achieved.[12] Resolution with treatment is usually rapid. Postexposure prophylaxis with rifampin (Rifadin) is recommended for all household unvaccinated contacts after a child is diagnosed.

Tonsillar Infections

Tonsillar infections (tonsillitis) are occasionally severe enough to cause upper airway obstruction. As with other infections of the upper airway, the incidence of tonsillitis secondary to GABHS and MRSA has risen in the past 15 years. Upper airway obstruction because of tonsillitis is a well-known complication of infectious mononucleosis, especially in a young child. Tonsillitis may be complicated by formation of a tonsillar abscess, which can further contribute to airway obstruction. Peritonsillar abscess is usually unilateral and is most often a complication of acute tonsillitis.[13] The abscess must be drained and the child given antibiotics.[14] The development of significant obstruction in tonsillar infections may require the use of corticosteroids, especially in the case of mononucleosis. The management of severe bacterial tonsillitis requires the use of antibiotics. Some children with recurrent tonsillitis benefit from adenotonsillectomy.[15]

Aspiration of Foreign Bodies

Aspiration of foreign bodies (FBs) into the airways usually occurs in children 1 to 4 years of age. More than 100 000 cases and 100 deaths occur each year.[16] Most objects are expelled by the cough reflex, but some objects may lodge in the larynx, trachea, or bronchi. Large objects (e.g., hard candy, a bite of hotdog, nuts, popcorn, grapes, beans, toy pieces, fragments of popped balloons, or coins) may occlude the airway and become life-threatening. Items of particular concern would be batteries and magnets. The aspiration event commonly is not witnessed or is not recognized when it happens because the coughing, choking, or gagging symptoms may resolve quickly. FBs lodged in the larynx or upper trachea cause cough, stridor, hoarseness or inability to speak, respiratory distress, and agitation or panic; the presentation is often dramatic and frightening. If the child is acutely hypoxic and unable to move air, immediate action such as sweeping the oral airway or performing abdominal thrusts (formerly called the *Heimlich manoeuvre*) may be required to prevent tragedy. Otherwise, bronchoscopic removal should be performed urgently. If an aspirated FB is small enough, it will be transferred to a bronchus before becoming lodged. If the FB is lodged in the airway for a notable period of time, local irritation, granulation, obstruction, and infection will ensue. Thus children may present with cough or wheezing, atelectasis, pneumonia, lung abscess, or blood-streaked sputum. These children are treated by prompt bronchoscopic removal of the object and administration of antibiotics as necessary.[17]

Obstructive Sleep Apnea Syndrome

Obstructive sleep apnea syndrome (OSAS) is defined by partial or intermittent complete upper airway obstruction during sleep with disruption of normal ventilation and sleep patterns. Childhood OSAS is common, with an estimated prevalence of 2 to 3% of children 12 to 14 years of age and up to 13% of children between 3 and 6 years of age.[18,19] Prevalence is estimated to be two to four times higher in vulnerable populations (Blacks, Latin Americans, and preterm infants).[18] In children, unlike adults, OSAS occurs equally among girls and boys. Possible influences early in life may include passive smoke inhalation, socioeconomic status, and snoring together with genetic modifiers that promote airway inflammation.

PATHOPHYSIOLOGY Reduced airway diameter and increased upper airway collapsibility are the common causes of OSAS. Obstruction of the upper airway during sleep results in cyclic episodes of increasing respiratory effort and changes in intrathoracic pressures with oxygen desaturation, hypercapnia, and arousal. The child goes back to sleep and the cycle repeats. Adenotonsillar hypertrophy, obesity, and craniofacial anomalies are associated with decreased airway diameter. Infants are at risk because they have both anatomical and physiological predispositions toward airway obstruction and gas exchange abnormalities.[20]

Reduced motor tone of the upper airways may be seen in neurological disorders, such as cerebral palsy and Down syndrome. Upper airway inflammation and altered neurological reflexes involving respiratory control of upper airway muscles are significant factors in reducing airway diameter. Allergy and asthma may contribute to inflammation, and children who have a history of a clinically significant episode of RSV bronchiolitis in infancy may exhibit altered neuroimmunomodulatory pathways toward inflammation in the upper airway.[21] In obese children, current research links OSAS with airway inflammation and elevated levels of C-reactive protein, which also contribute to increased risk for cardiovascular and metabolic disease.[22,23] OSAS also may cause pulmonary disease, insulin resistance, and growth failure.[24]

CLINICAL MANIFESTATIONS Common manifestations of OSAS include snoring and laboured breathing, sweating, and restlessness during sleep, which may be continuous or intermittent. There may be episodes of increased respiratory effort but no audible airflow, often terminated by snorting, gasping, repositioning, or arousal. Daytime sleepiness/napping is occasionally reported, as well as nocturnal enuresis. There is no correlation between sleep position and OSAS in children, except for those children who are notably obese. Obese children may adopt the prone position to attempt improved ventilation. Cognitive and neurobehavioural impairment, excessive daytime sleepiness, impaired school performance, and poor quality of life are consequences of OSAS.[25]

EVALUATION AND TREATMENT All parents should be asked if their child exhibits snoring, followed by a careful history and physical examination. A variety of screening tools are available. Imaging of the upper airway may be used to rule out adenoidal hypertrophy or upper airway narrowing.[26] The most definitive evaluation is the polysomnographic sleep study, which documents obstructed breathing and physiological impairment. If obstructive sleep apnea is documented or strongly suspected clinically, children are most often referred for tonsillectomy and adenoidectomy (*T & A*) on the basis of described symptoms and physical findings, such as enlarged tonsils, adenoidal facies, and mouth breathing. For severely affected children who do not respond to T & A or who have different problems, such as obesity, continuous positive airway pressure (CPAP), anti-inflammatories, dental treatments, high-flow nasal cannula, and weight loss can be considered. Treatment is important to minimize associated morbidities.[27,28]

✔ QUICK CHECK 28-1

1. Compare and contrast pathology, clinical presentations, and severity of croup and epiglottitis.
2. What symptoms indicate aspiration of a foreign body?
3. What signs and symptoms suggest obstructive sleep apnea syndrome?

DISORDERS OF THE LOWER AIRWAYS

Lower airway disease is one of the leading causes of morbidity in the first year of life and continues to be an important component of other illnesses progressing into childhood. Pulmonary disorders commonly observed include neonatal respiratory distress syndrome, bronchopulmonary dysplasia (BPD), infections, asthma, cystic fibrosis (CF), and acute respiratory distress syndrome (ARDS).

Respiratory Distress Syndrome of the Newborn

Respiratory distress syndrome (RDS) of the newborn (previously known as *hyaline membrane disease* [HMD]) is a significant cause of neonatal morbidity and mortality. It occurs almost exclusively in premature infants, and the incidence has increased in North America over the past two decades.[29] RDS occurs in 50 to 60% of infants born at 29 weeks' gestation and decreases significantly by 36 weeks. Risk factors are summarized in *Risk Factors:* Respiratory Distress Syndrome of the Newborn. Death rates have declined significantly since the introduction of antenatal steroid therapy and postnatal surfactant therapy.

RISK FACTORS

Respiratory Distress Syndrome of the Newborn

- Premature birth or low birth weight
- Male gender
- Caesarean delivery without labour
- Diabetic mother
- Perinatal asphyxia

PATHOPHYSIOLOGY RDS is caused by surfactant deficiency, which decreases the alveolar surface area available for gas exchange. Surfactant is a lipoprotein with a detergentlike effect that separates the liquid molecules inside the alveoli, thereby decreasing alveolar surface tension. Without surfactant, alveoli collapse at the end of each exhalation. Surfactant normally is not secreted by the alveolar cells until approximately 30 weeks' gestation. In addition to surfactant deficiency, premature infants are born with underdeveloped and small alveoli that are difficult to inflate and have thick walls and inadequate capillary blood supply such that gas exchange is significantly impaired. Furthermore, the infant's chest wall is weak and highly compliant and, thus, the rib cage tends to collapse inward with respiratory effort. The net effect is atelectasis (collapsed alveoli), resulting in significant hypoxemia. Atelectasis is difficult for the neonate to overcome because it requires a significant negative inspiratory pressure to open the alveoli with each breath. This increased work of breathing may result in hypercapnia. Hypoxia and hypercapnia cause pulmonary vasoconstriction and increase intrapulmonary resistance and shunting. This pulmonary vasoconstriction results in hypoperfusion of the lung and a decrease in effective pulmonary blood flow. Increased pulmonary vascular resistance may even cause a partial return to fetal circulation, with right-to-left shunting of blood through the ductus arteriosus and foramen ovale. Inadequate perfusion of tissues and hypoxemia contribute to metabolic acidosis.

Inadequate alveolar ventilation can be further complicated by increased pulmonary capillary permeability. Many premature infants with RDS will require mechanical ventilation, which damages the alveolar epithelium. Together these conditions result in the leakage of plasma proteins into the alveoli. Fibrin deposits in the air spaces create the appearance of "hyaline membranes," for which the disorder was originally named. The plasma proteins leaked into the air space have the additional adverse effect of inactivating any surfactant that may be present. The pathogenesis of RDS is summarized in Figure 28-5.

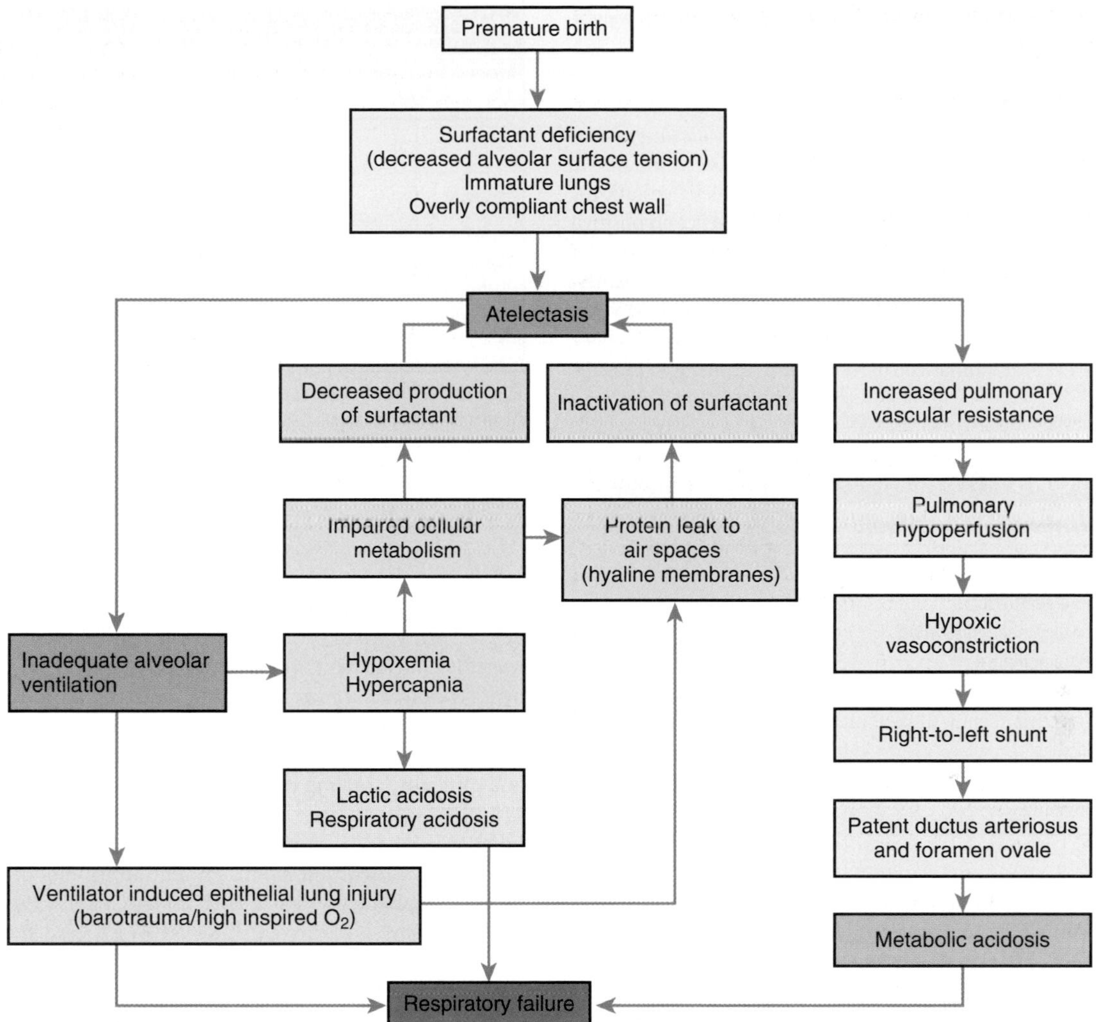

FIGURE 28-5 Pathogenesis of Respiratory Distress Syndrome of the Newborn.

CLINICAL MANIFESTATIONS Signs of RDS appear within minutes of birth and include tachypnea (respiratory rate greater than 60 breaths/min), expiratory grunting, intercostal and subcostal retractions, nasal flaring, and cyanosis. Severity tends to increase over the first 2 days of life. Apnea and irregular respirations occur as the infant tires. Severity of hypoxemia and difficulty in providing supplemental oxygenation have resulted in the Vermont Oxford Neonatal Network definition of RDS: a partial pressure of oxygen in arterial blood (PaO_2) less than 50 mm Hg in room air, central cyanosis in room air, or a need for supplemental oxygen to maintain PaO_2 greater than 50 mm Hg, as well as classic chest film appearance.[30] The typical chest radiograph shows diffuse, fine granular densities within the first 6 hours of life. This "ground glass" appearance is associated with alveolar flooding. Ventilatory support is often required. In most cases the clinical manifestations reach a peak within 3 days, after which there is gradual improvement.

EVALUATION AND TREATMENT Diagnosis is made on the basis of premature birth or other risk factors, chest radiographs, pulse oximetry measurements, and, if needed, analysis of amniotic fluid or tracheal aspirates to estimate lung maturity (lecithin/sphingomyelin ratio [L/S ratio]). Some neonates require immediate resuscitation because of asphyxia or severe respiratory distress. The ultimate treatment for RDS would be prevention of premature birth. For women at risk for preterm birth, antenatal treatment with glucocorticoids induces a significant and rapid acceleration of lung maturation and stimulation of surfactant production in the fetus and significantly reduces the incidence of RDS and death.[31,32]

Current recommendations for infants weighing less than 1 000 g include prophylaxis beginning within 15 to 30 minutes of birth by administration of exogenous surfactant (either synthetic or natural) through nebulizer or nasal CPAP ventilation. Repeat doses are given every 12 hours for the first few days. There is usually a dramatic improvement in oxygenation as well as a decreased incidence of RDS death, pneumothorax, and pulmonary interstitial emphysema. For infants weighing more than 1 000 g, surfactant replacement is based on clinical need. Surfactant therapy should be considered complementary to antenatal glucocorticoids. The two therapies together appear to have an additive effect on improving lung function.[33]

Supportive care includes oxygen administration and often such measures as mechanical ventilation. Mechanical ventilation can result in a proinflammatory state that may contribute to the development of chronic lung disease (CLD), such as BPD. Strategies that are lung protective include greater reliance on nasal CPAP, permissive hypercapnia, lower oxygen saturation targets, modulation of tidal volume (V_T) settings, and use of high-frequency oscillation. Further studies are needed to evaluate the effectiveness of inhaled nitric oxide (iNO) in preterm infants.[34] Most infants survive RDS and, in many cases, recovery may be complete within 10 to 14 days. However, the incidence of subsequent CLD (i.e., BPD) is significant among very low–birth weight infants.[35]

Bronchopulmonary Dysplasia

Bronchopulmonary dysplasia (BPD), also known as *chronic lung disease of prematurity*, is the major cause of pulmonary disease in infants. It is associated with premature birth (usually before 28 weeks' gestation), prolonged (at least 28 days) perinatal supplemental oxygen, and positive pressure ventilation. In 2013 in Canada, 7.5% of the babies born to mothers aged 35 to 49 years were considered low–birth weight babies, compared with 5.9% of the babies born to mothers aged 20 to 34 years and 6.6% of the babies born to mothers younger than 20 years of age.[36] Risk factors for BPD[37] are summarized in *Risk Factors:* Bronchopulmonary Dysplasia.

RISK FACTORS

Bronchopulmonary Dysplasia

- Premature birth (especially ≤28 weeks)
- Positive-pressure ventilation
- Supplemental oxygen administration
- Antenatal chorioamnionitis
- Postnatal sepsis or pneumonia
- Patent ductus arteriosus
- Nutritional deficiencies
- Early adrenal insufficiency
- Genetic susceptibility

The widespread use of antenatal glucocorticoids and postnatal surfactant has lessened the incidence and severity of RDS, and BPD is occurring primarily in the smallest premature infants (23 to 28 weeks' gestation) who have received mechanical ventilation. The presence of antenatal chorioamnionitis with fetal involvement, postnatal sepsis, a patent ductus arteriosus, and genetic susceptibility confer additional risks of developing BPD.[37] Surprisingly, some of these tiny infants who develop BPD have shown few or no clinical signs of RDS at birth or have initially received only low levels of supplemental oxygen or ventilatory support, sometimes for other reasons, such as apnea.

PATHOPHYSIOLOGY Lung immaturity and inflammation contribute to the development of BPD. Before the widespread use of surfactant therapy, BPD was a disease characterized by airway injury, inflammation, and parenchymal fibrosis (*classic BPD*). With the initiation of surfactant therapy, what is called the *new BPD* is most common and is a form of arrested lung development. There is poor formation of the alveolar structure with fewer and larger alveoli and decreased surface area for gas exchange. Persistent inflammation contributes to pulmonary capillary fibrosis, ventilation–perfusion mismatch, pulmonary hypertension, and decreased exercise capacity.[38,39] The predominant mediators of new BPD are profibrotic and angiogenic cytokines rather than proinflammatory cytokines, which contribute to pulmonary hypertension.[40] Table 28-2 and Figure 28-6 illustrate the pathophysiology of BPD.

CLINICAL MANIFESTATIONS The clinical definition of BPD includes need for supplemental oxygen at 36 weeks' postmenstrual age or gestational age (the time elapsed between the first day of the last normal menstrual period and the day of birth), and for at least 28 days after birth. It also details a graded severity dependent on required respiratory support at term (mild, moderate, and severe, based on oxygen requirements and ventilatory needs). Clinically, the infant exhibits hypoxemia

TABLE 28-2 Comparison of Classic and New Bronchopulmonary Dysplasia

Classic BPD	New BPD
Metaplasia of respiratory epithelium	Less severe squamous metaplasia
Smooth muscle hypertrophy	Less smooth muscle hypertrophy
Significant fibrosis	Less fibrosis
Large vascular modifications	Abnormal pulmonary vascular structure Small number and increased diameter of alveoli Increase in elastic tissue

BPD, bronchopulmonary dysplasia.
Adapted from Monte, L.F., Silva Filho, L.V., Miyoshi, M.H., et al. (2005). *J Pediatr (Rio J), 81*(2), 99–110, Table 3. Retrieved from http://www.scielo.br/scielo.php?pid=s0021-75572005000300004&script=sci_arttext&tlng=en.

and hypercapnia caused by ventilation–perfusion mismatch and diffusion defects. The work of breathing increases and the ability to feed may be impaired. Intermittent bronchospasm, mucus plugging, and pulmonary hypertension characterize the clinical course. Of the most severely affected infants, dusky spells may occur with agitation, feeding, or gastroesophageal reflux. Infants with mild BPD may demonstrate only mild tachypnea and difficulty handling respiratory tract infections.

EVALUATION AND TREATMENT Infants with severe BPD require prolonged assisted ventilation. Prevention of lung damage with noninvasive respiratory support, such as early nasal CPAP or nasal intermittent positive-pressure ventilation (IPPV), is used in clinical situations when permitted. When compared with mechanical ventilation, use of CPAP has resulted in fewer days of oxygen and ventilator requirement by reducing the amount of lung injury.[41] Diuretics are used to control pulmonary edema. Bronchodilators reduce airway resistance. Inhaled corticosteroids improve the rate of extubation and reduce the time that mechanical ventilation is required.[42] Prophylactic caffeine citrate administration, vitamin A supplementation, and careful fluid and nutritional support are routinely used and have resulted in improved outcomes.[43] Children with BPD will need to be monitored into adulthood for the development of CLD.

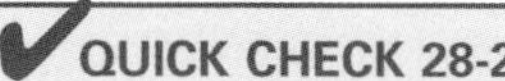
QUICK CHECK 28-2
1. Why are premature infants susceptible to respiratory distress syndrome?
2. Describe the pathological findings of "new bronchopulmonary dysplasia."

Respiratory Tract Infections

Respiratory tract infections are common in children and are a frequent cause for emergency department visits and hospitalizations. Clinical presentation, age of the child, and season of the year can often provide clues to the etiological agent, even when the agent cannot be proved.

Bronchiolitis

Bronchiolitis is a common, viral respiratory tract infection of the small airways that occurs almost exclusively in infants and young toddlers and is a major reason for hospitalization. It has a seasonal, yearly incidence, from approximately November to April, and is the leading cause of hospitalization for infants during the winter season. The most

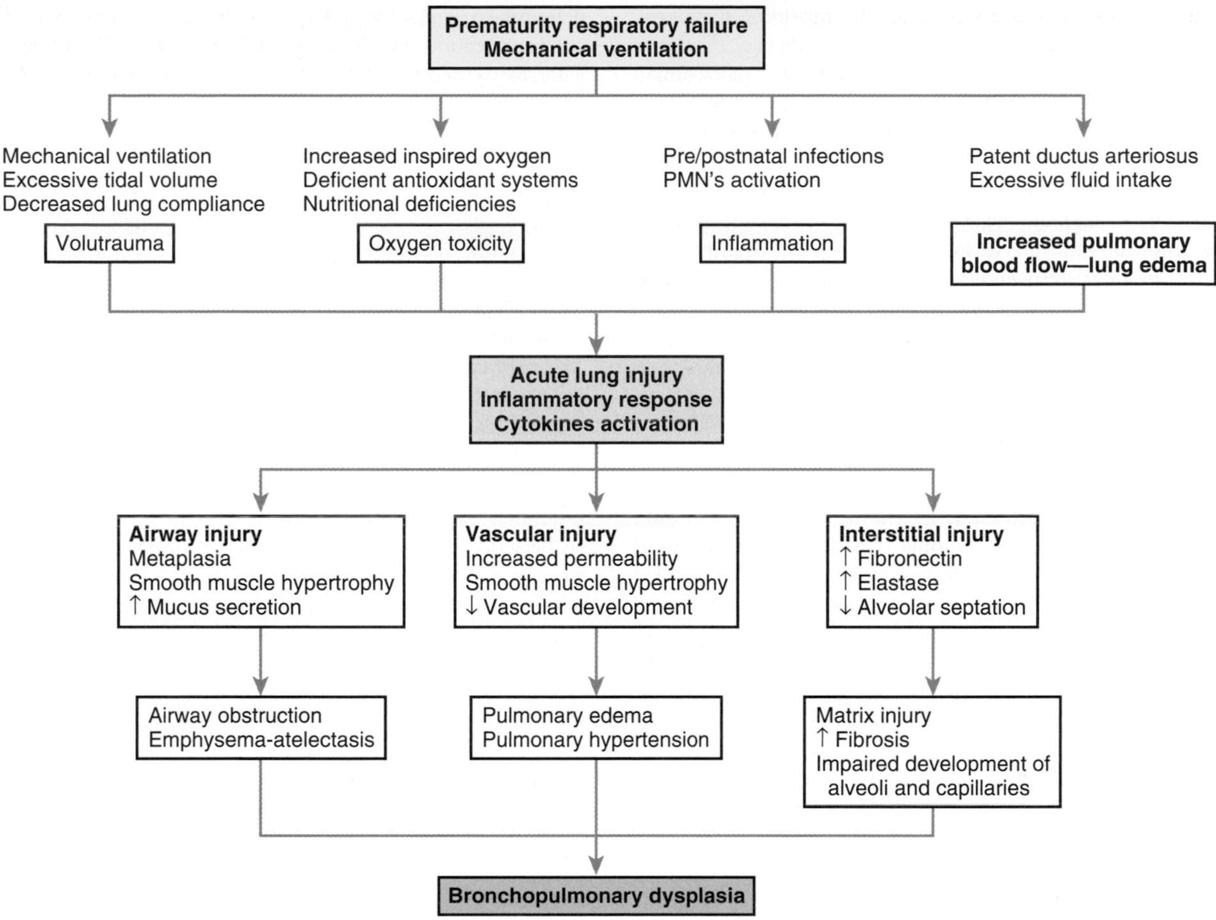

FIGURE 28-6 Pathophysiology of Bronchopulmonary Dysplasia. *PMN,* polymorphonuclear leukocyte.

common associated pathogen is RSV, but bronchiolitis also may be associated with human metapneumovirus and human bocavirus. Healthy infants usually make a full recovery from RSV bronchiolitis, but infants who were premature (birth weight less than 2 500 g) or who have underlying BPD or heart disease may have a much higher risk for a more severe or even deadly course. Bronchiolitis has been linked to an increased risk for asthma later in childhood.[44] Associations with rhinovirus and low vitamin D levels also are being investigated because they appear to correlate with the increased likelihood that children develop asthma after they have experienced bronchiolitis.[45]

PATHOPHYSIOLOGY Viral infection causes necrosis of the bronchial epithelium and destruction of ciliated epithelial cells. There is infiltration with lymphocytes around the bronchioles and a cell-mediated hypersensitivity to viral antigens with release of lymphokines causing inflammation, as well as activation of eosinophils, neutrophils, and monocytes. The submucosa becomes edematous and cellular debris and fibrin form plugs within the bronchioles. Edema of the bronchiolar wall, accumulation of mucus and cellular debris, and bronchospasm narrow many peripheral airways. Other airways become partially or completely occluded. Atelectasis occurs in some areas of the lung and hyperinflation in others.

The mechanics of breathing are disrupted by bronchiolitis. Airway narrowing causes obstruction of airflow that is worse on expiration. This airway narrowing leads to air trapping, hyperinflation, and increased functional residual capacity (FRC). Airway resistance and hyperinflation result in increased work of breathing and the development of hypercapnia in severe cases.

CLINICAL MANIFESTATIONS Symptoms usually begin with significant rhinorrhea followed by a tight cough over the next several days, along with systemic signs of decreased appetite, lethargy, and fever. Infants typically have tachypnea, variable degrees of respiratory distress, and abnormal auscultatory findings of the chest. Wheezing is most common, but rales or rhonchi also may be present. Chest radiographs often reveal hyperexpanded lungs, patchy or peribronchial infiltrates, and, sometimes, atelectasis of the right upper lobe. Very young infants may present with severe apnea before lower respiratory tract symptoms appear, and these apneas frequently require mechanical ventilation. Many children also may present with conjunctivitis or otitis media.

EVALUATION AND TREATMENT According to the Canadian Paediatric Society, bronchiolitis is a clinical diagnosis. Typically, diagnosis is made by review of history, signs, and symptoms (e.g., rhinitis, cough, wheezing, chest retractions, tachypnea). Laboratory, radiological examination (chest X-ray), blood tests, and viral or bacterial cultures are not routinely performed.

The decision to admit a child with bronchiolitis to the hospital depends on the risk for progression to severe disease, respiratory status, ability to maintain adequate hydration, the family's ability to cope at home, and the age of the child. The use of antibiotics is not recommended, unless there is suspicion of an underlying bacterial infection.[46] Most cases are mild and require no specific treatment and may be monitored as outpatients. Continuous oxygen saturation monitoring may be indicated for high-risk children in the acute phase of illness, and intermittent monitoring or spot checks are appropriate for lower-risk children and patients who are improving clinically. When treatment is indicated, it is primarily supportive in nature, including hydration, minimal handling, gentle nasal suctioning, and oxygen therapy. Preventive treatment with RSV-specific monoclonal antibody (palivizumab [Synagis]), provided as a monthly injection for 5 months through the RSV season, is recommended for high-risk infants younger than 2 years who meet specific criteria (e.g., hemodynamically significant heart disease and chronic lung disease of prematurity). Other preventive measures include use of hand hygiene and alcohol-based decontamination, prevention of exposure to tobacco smoke, and promotion of infant breastfeeding. If intravenous fluids are used for hydration, an isotonic solution (0.9% sodium chloride/5% dextrose) is recommended, together with routine monitoring of serum sodium. Current evidence from the Canadian Paediatric Society does not support the use of salbutamol (Ventolin), corticosteroids, or epinephrine. The use of chest physiotherapy is also not recommended.[46]

Pneumonia

Pneumonia is infection and inflammation in the terminal airways and alveoli. Community-acquired pneumonia (CAP) is a major cause of morbidity and mortality in children, particularly in developing countries. The most common agents are viruses, followed by bacteria and atypical microorganisms (e.g., mycoplasma) (Table 28-3), and clinical symptoms often do not differentiate viral from bacterial or atypical pneumonia. Risk factors for developing CAP are age younger than 2 years, overcrowded living conditions, winter season, recent antibiotic treatment, day-care attendance, and passive smoke exposure. Nutritional status, age, and underlying disease process influence morbidity and mortality rates related to CAP.

PATHOPHYSIOLOGY **Viral pneumonia** is two to three times more likely to occur in children than in adults, and incidence generally follows a seasonal pattern. Bacterial co-infections are common. RSV is the most common viral pneumonia in young children. A number of other viruses are important, including parainfluenza, influenza, human rhinovirus, human metapneumovirus, adenoviruses, and *Mycoplasma pneumoniae*.[47] Acquisition of these viruses is by direct contact, droplet transmission, or aerosol exposure. There is initial destruction of the ciliated epithelium of the distal airway with sloughing of cellular material. A mononuclear-predominant inflammatory response occurs, in the interstitium initially, and later may involve the alveoli as well. Early in the course of the disease, it is often difficult to determine whether the pneumonia is viral or bacterial. Viral pneumonia often presents with cough and no fever. Differences in the clinical presentation can help to determine origin, such as degree of elevation of temperature, absolute neutrophil counts, and percentage of bands. Ultimately, diagnosis requires laboratory confirmation using immunofluorescence tests. Development of safe drugs to treat and prevent viral pneumonia continues to be a focus of much research.[48]

Bacterial pneumonia beyond the neonatal period is most commonly the result of infection with streptococci and staphylococci microorganisms. Pneumococcal (*Streptococcus pneumoniae*) pneumonia is the most common cause of community-acquired bacterial pneumonia and presents acutely and with variable severity.[49] Childhood immunization with polyvariant pneumococcal conjugate vaccine appears to decrease the incidence of pneumococcal pneumonia in children younger than 2 years of age.[50] Staphylococcal pneumonia and group A streptococcal pneumonia can be particularly fulminant (sudden, severe) and necrotizing (causing cell death) with a high incidence of accompanying empyema, pneumatocele (a lung lesion filled with air), and sepsis. *H. influenzae* pneumonia has become rare because of widespread immunization.

Bacterial pneumonia usually begins with aspiration of nasopharyngeal bacteria. A preceding viral infection sometimes sets the stage for bacterial infection by causing epithelial damage, reduced mucociliary clearance in the trachea and major bronchi, and a reduced immune response. Once in the alveolar region, bacteria encounter local host defences, such as antibodies, complement, and cytokines, which prepare bacteria for ingestion by alveolar macrophages. Alveolar macrophages recognize bacteria with their surface receptors and phagocytose them. If these mechanisms fail, macrophages release numerous inflammatory cytokines and neutrophils will be recruited into the lung.[51] An intense, cytokine-mediated inflammation will ensue. Vascular engorgement, edema, and a fibrinopurulent exudate occur. Alveolar filling precludes gas exchange and, if extensive, can lead to respiratory failure. If sepsis occurs at the same time, shock and end-organ hypoperfusion will cause metabolic acidosis.

The clinical presentation of bacterial pneumonia, particularly pneumococcal, may include a preceding viral illness followed by fever with chills and rigors, shortness of breath, and an increasingly productive cough. Occasionally, there is blood streaking of the sputum. Respiratory rate and oxygen saturation also are important clinical indicators. Auscultation usually shows such abnormalities as crackles or decreased breath sounds. Other, less specific findings may include malaise, emesis, abdominal pain, and chest pain. Chest films will usually present with a lobar pattern in older children and adolescents but may appear patchier with a bronchopneumonic pattern in younger children.

TABLE 28-3 Common Types of Pneumonia in Children

Type	Causal Agent	Age	Onset	Signs/Symptoms
Viral pneumonia	Respiratory syncytial virus (RSV), influenza, adenovirus, others	Infants for RSV, all ages for others	Acute or gradual, winter and early spring	Mild to high fever, cough, rhinorrhea, malaise, rales, rhonchi, wheezing, or apnea; variable radiographic pattern
Pneumococcal pneumonia	Pneumococci (*Streptococcus pneumoniae*)	Usually 1 to 4 years	Acute, follows an upper respiratory tract infection, winter and early spring	High fever, productive cough, pleuritic pain, increased respiration rate, decreased breath sounds in area of consolidation; lobar infiltrate or "round pneumonia" on radiograph
Staphylococcal pneumonia	*Staphylococcus aureus* (including methicillin-resistant strains)	1 weeks to 2 years	Acute, winter	High fever, cough, respiratory distress; empyema or pneumatoceles common
Streptococcal pneumonia	Group A beta-hemolytic streptococci	All ages	Acute, any season	High fever, chills, respiratory distress, sepsis, or shock
Mycoplasmal and chlamydial pneumonia	*Mycoplasma pneumoniae*, *Chlamydophila pneumonia*	School-age and adolescents	Gradual	Low-grade fever, cough

Atypical pneumonia (*Mycoplasma pneumoniae, Chlamydophila pneumoniae*) is the most common cause of CAP for school-age children and young adults. *Chlamydophila* pneumonia is clinically indistinguishable from and is typically grouped with *Mycoplasma* as "atypical pneumonia." Transmission is from person to person with a 2- to 3-week incubation period.

Mycoplasmic microorganisms lack cell walls but have a limiting membrane and a specialized receptor for attaching to ciliated respiratory epithelial cells. Local sloughing of cells occurs. Peribronchial lymphocytic infiltration develops, along with neutrophil recruitment to the airway lumen. The pattern resembles bronchitis or bronchopneumonia. Onset is usually gradual, resembling a typical upper respiratory tract infection but with low-grade fever, cough, and chest pain.[52] *Mycoplasma* can cause a wide spectrum of disease and is more extensive as a cause of complications than previously noted. It also is occurring more frequently in infants and younger children. Most cases are not clinically severe and full recovery should be expected. Complications, when they do occur, can include bronchopneumonia, parapneumonic effusions, and necrotizing pneumonitis.

EVALUATION AND TREATMENT Guidelines have been developed to improve and aid assessment and management of pediatric pneumonia.[53,54] Diagnosis of pneumonia is based on clinical and laboratory findings. The etiological agent can sometimes be inferred from the age of the child and clinical scenario.[55] Chest X-ray in bacterial pneumonia often will initially produce a patchy infiltration and later reveal a segmental or lobar disease. A viral infection is more likely to be associated with an interstitial pattern. Biomarkers (i.e., procalcitonin) facilitate more rapid diagnosis and guide antibiotic therapy. The high-sensitivity C-reactive protein (hs-CRP) is less specific, and its level is elevated in both viral and bacterial infections.[56] Several microbiological tests are available, such as polymerase chain reaction (PCR) and nucleic acid amplification tests (NAATs).

Some pneumonias may be treated on an outpatient basis; however, many children require oxygen supplementation and, occasionally, assisted ventilation. This requirement is particularly true with infants who have a viral interstitial pneumonia, such as RSV. In addition, adequate hydration, proper nutrition, and supportive pulmonary therapy are required to reduce the duration and severity of illness. Many infants are markedly tachypneic and unable to coordinate their breathing with swallowing; they may require enteral feeding. Aspiration is always a risk with infants in respiratory distress.

Appropriate antibiotic administration for bacterial pneumonias is dependent on age and severity assessment. Local patterns of resistance must be considered when choosing appropriate antibiotics. Pneumococcal and mycoplasmal pneumonias present some unique treatment obstacles and may need a multifaceted approach to care including vaccine antigens and immune adjuvant therapies in addition to antibiotics.[57] Children should be vaccinated against influenza and pneumococcus.

QUICK CHECK 28-3

1. Describe the typical presentation of respiratory syncytial virus bronchiolitis.
2. What clinical features distinguish bacterial pneumonia from atypical pneumonia?

Aspiration Pneumonitis

Aspiration pneumonitis is caused by a foreign substance, such as food, meconium, secretions (saliva or gastric), or environmental compounds, entering the lung and resulting in inflammation of the lung tissue. The aspiration of meconium from amniotic fluid can occur at birth.[58] Neurologically compromised children or children with CLD may have chronic pulmonary aspiration (CPA), which can cause progressive lung disease, bronchiectasis, and respiratory failure. CPA is the leading cause of death in children who are neurologically compromised because of failure of protective reflexes and difficulty swallowing.[59] Children undergoing sedation or anaesthesia also may aspirate oral secretions contaminated with anaerobic bacteria or acidic stomach contents. The severity of lung injury after an aspiration incident is determined by the volume and pH of the material aspirated and the presence of pathogenic bacteria. Very low pH or extremely high pH will cause a significant inflammatory response. With hydrocarbon ingestions, lung injury is determined by the volatility and viscosity of the aspirated substance. A low-viscosity substance, such as gasoline or lighter fluid, is the most toxic, and high-viscosity hydrocarbons, such as petroleum jelly or mineral oil, are much less likely to cause a pneumonitis. Treatment for aspiration pneumonitis depends on the material aspirated but can include broad-spectrum antibiotics with failure to improve after 48 hours. Children with CPA and a large amount of upper respiratory tract secretions may benefit from salivary gland injection with botulinum toxin A (BTX-A) to suppress secretion.[60]

Bronchiolitis Obliterans

Bronchiolitis obliterans (BO) is fibrotic obstruction of the respiratory bronchioles and alveolar ducts secondary to intense inflammation. It is relatively rare in children. There are two types: proliferative and constrictive (obstructive), with the latter being the more common form. BO most often occurs as a sequela of a severe viral pulmonary infection (e.g., influenza, adenovirus, pertussis [whooping cough], or measles). Other cases may be secondary to parainfluenza, RSV, human immunodeficiency virus (HIV), *M. pneumoniae* infection, or lung transplant. It also may occur after lung, heart–lung, or bone marrow transplantation, or be associated with collagen vascular disease, toxic fume inhalation, chronic hypersensitivity pneumonitis, Crohn's disease, and Stevens-Johnson syndrome.[61,62] Although the child may initially improve after the acute insult, the progression of disease is then reflected by increasing tachypnea, dyspnea, cough, sputum production, crackles, wheezing, increased chest anteroposterior diameter (APD), and hypoxemia.

There is no specific treatment for bronchiolitis obliterans and, because it is so rare, there have been no randomized clinical trials. Therapeutic options include inhaled corticosteroids, bronchodilators, antibiotics, and oxygen supplementation. Mechanical ventilation may contribute to the progression of the disease. Some children deteriorate rapidly and die within weeks, whereas others follow a more chronic course. Antiviral agents may assist in blunting the initial viral response but otherwise have limited effect on the illness. Anti-inflammatory agents are showing promise in reducing airway inflammation and improving pulmonary function. For those children having undergone lung transplantation, increased immunosuppressive regimens are sometimes helpful.[63,64]

Asthma

Asthma is a chronic inflammatory disease characterized by bronchial hyper-reactivity and reversible airflow obstruction, usually in response to an allergen (see Chapter 27). It is the most prevalent chronic disease in childhood, affecting 490 000 Canadian children between the ages of 4 and 11.[65,66] Populations most affected include those living in an urban setting, and those of low socioeconomic status.[66]

Childhood asthma results from a complex interaction between *genetic* susceptibility and *environmental* factors. Many genotypes are associated with susceptibility and phenotypes of asthma, including early-onset mild allergic asthma, asthma with severe exacerbations, later-onset asthma associated with obesity, severe nonatopic asthma, and corticosteroid-dependent asthma. Important risk factors include early exposure to allergens (e.g., air pollution, dust mites, cockroach antigen, cat exposure, and tobacco smoke), respiratory tract infections, preterm birth, and childhood obesity.[67-70] The *hygiene hypothesis* proposes that infants and children exposed to a highly hygienic environment and who receive vaccinations to prevent certain infections lack adequate exposure to common pathogens and therefore do not achieve balanced immune responses as they mature[71] (see Chapter 27).

About 70 to 80% of acute wheezing episodes in children with asthma are associated with viral respiratory tract infection (i.e., RSV, human rhinoviruses, and parainfluenza viruses). In infants and toddlers less than 2 years old, the most common of these is RSV. In older children and adults, the major viral trigger is rhinovirus (the "common cold" virus). Bacterial respiratory tract infections also can trigger asthma.[72] Vitamin D insufficiency may be a risk factor for airway inflammation and wheezing in children because vitamin D suppresses T-helper 2 (Th2)-mediated allergic disease.[73]

PATHOPHYSIOLOGY The pathophysiology of asthma in children is similar to that for adults and is described in Chapter 27. Asthma is initiated by a type I hypersensitivity reaction primarily mediated by Th2 lymphocytes whose cytokines activate mast cells, eosinophilia, leukocytosis, and enhanced B-lymphocyte immunoglobulin E (IgE) production (see Chapter 8; see also Figures 27-8, 27-9, 27-10). As in adults, inflammation, bronchospasm, and mucus production in the airways lead to ventilation–perfusion mismatch with hypoxemia and expiratory airway obstruction with air trapping and increased work of breathing. In young children, airway obstruction can be more severe because of the smaller diameter of their airways.

CLINICAL MANIFESTATIONS Clinical manifestations of an acute asthma attack include coughing, expiratory wheezing, and shortness of breath. Breath sounds may become faint when air movement is poor. The child may speak in clipped sentences or not at all because of dyspnea. Sometimes hyperinflation (barrel chest) is visible. Respiratory rate and heart rate are elevated. Nasal flaring and use of accessory muscles with retractions in the substernal, subcostal, intercostal, suprasternal, or sternocleidomastoid areas are evident. Infants may appear to be "head bobbing" because of sternocleidomastoid muscle use. Pulsus paradoxus (decrease in systolic blood pressure of more than 10 mm Hg during inspiration) may be present. The child may appear anxious or diaphoretic, important signs of respiratory compromise.

Findings in chronic asthma may include hyperinflation of the thorax or pectus excavatum. Clubbing should not be seen with asthma and, if present, should trigger evaluation for other conditions such as CF. Exercise intolerance may indicate underlying asthma (see *Health Promotion:* Exercise-Induced Bronchoconstriction).

EVALUATION AND TREATMENT Asthma is often underdiagnosed and undertreated, especially in preschool-age children because asthma symptoms overlap with other respiratory illnesses, such as bronchitis or upper respiratory tract infections. Diagnosis of asthma is based on episodes of wheezing as well as a variety of risk factors including parental history of asthma, atopic dermatitis, sensitization to aeroallergens or foods, blood eosinophilia, or wheezing not associated with upper respiratory tract illnesses. Confirmation of the diagnosis of asthma relies on pulmonary function testing using spirometry, which can be accomplished only after the child is 5 to 6 years of age. For younger children, an empirical trial of asthma medications is commonly initiated.

The Canadian Thoracic Society and the Canadian Paediatric Society have made several recommendations for diagnosing asthma in children 1 to 5 years of age. Diagnosis should be based on observation of signs or symptoms of airflow obstruction and reversibility of airflow obstruction (i.e., improvement in signs or symptoms with asthma therapy). Moreover, there should be no clinical suspicion of an alternative diagnosis (e.g., bronchiolitis, which often presents as wheezing in a child less than 1 year of age).[74] For children with recurrent (two or more) episodes of asthmalike symptoms *and wheezing* on presentation, direct observation of improvement with an inhaled bronchodilator should be made by a physician to confirm the diagnosis. An alternative diagnostic method for children with recurrent (two or more) episodes of asthmalike symptoms, *no wheezing* on presentation, *frequent symptoms*, or any *moderate or severe exacerbation* is a 3-month therapeutic trial with a medium daily dose of inhaled corticosteroid (with short-acting β_2-agonists, as needed). Clear and consistent improvement in the frequency and severity of symptoms, exacerbations, or both confirms the diagnosis. To adequately interpret a therapeutic trial, physicians should ensure adherence to asthma therapy, use of proper inhalation technique, and timely parental report of symptoms.[74]

HEALTH PROMOTION

Exercise-Induced Bronchoconstriction

According to Statistics Canada, 8.1% of Canadians aged 12 and older were diagnosed with asthma by a health care provider in 2014. Females were more likely than males to report that they had asthma. In the same year, the rate was 9.2% for females compared with 7.0% for males. The Asthma Society of Canada estimates that approximately 3 million Canadians live with asthma: 66.6% experience asthma symptoms during exercise and 45% choose not to engage in regular exercise. Roughly 60% of people with asthma view their asthma as a barrier to participating in physical activity.

Exercise-induced bronchoconstriction (EIB) occurs in 90% of children diagnosed with asthma. A proposed mechanism for EIB is epithelial injury and inflammation, which results from drying of the mucosa and changes in the osmolarity in the airway epithelium leading to degranulation of mast cells. Another contributing factor is the inhalation of particles and toxins at high flow rates; this is of particular importance in urban areas and in swimmers in chlorinated pools. These changes result in increased type I hypersensitivity and airway hyper-responsiveness (AHR) in those with asthma and are associated with an increase in leukotriene release. Eosinophil activation also plays a role in airway hyper-reactivity and tissue damage. Finally, it has been found that obese children who have high levels of the inflammatory adipokine leptin are more likely to develop EIB than nonobese children. Symptoms are a poor indicator of the severity of bronchoconstriction, especially in obese children, and spirometry with exercise challenge testing is needed to make the diagnosis. Warm-up exercises and cooling down slowly after exercise, along with the use of facemasks in cold weather, can be helpful. A recent study reported that yoga training can markedly improve EIB in children aged 6 to 17. Although bronchodilators remain the most commonly used medications for EIB, studies suggest that inhaled corticosteroids or leukotriene inhibitors are more effective and safer in children with EIB and asthma.

Data from Asthma Society of Canada. (n.d.). *Breathe easy: A guide for being active and health with asthma.* Toronto: Author. Retrieved from http://www.asthma.ca/pdfs/ExerciseGuideEN.pdf; Baek, H.-S., Choi, J.-H., Oh, J.-W., et al. (2013). *Ann Allergy Asthma Immunol, 111*(2), 112–117; Lazarinis, N., Jørgensen, L., Ekström, T., et al. (2014). *Thorax, 69*(2), 130–136; Molphy, J., Dickinson, J., Hu, J., et al. (2014). *J Asthma, 51*(1), 44–50; Pasnick, S.D., Carlos, 3rd., W.G., Arunachalam, A., et al. (2014). *Ann Am Thorac Soc, 11*(10), 1651–1652; Randolph, C. (2013). *Curr Allergy Asthma Rep, 13*(6), 662–671; Statistics Canada. (2015). *Asthma 2014 (Health Fact Sheets: 82-625-X).* Retrieved from http://www.statcan.gc.ca/pub/82-625-x/2015001/article/14179-eng.htm; Tahan, F., Eke Gungor, H., & Bicici, E. (2014). *Altern Ther Health Med, 20*(2), 18–23.

The goal of asthma therapy is to achieve long-term control by reduction in impairment and risk.[74,75] Child and family education and appropriate allergen avoidance techniques should begin immediately. Care providers need to periodically assess asthma control in children. Key features for assessment include nighttime awakenings, interference with normal activities, use of short-acting β_2 agonists, pulmonary function testing, and exacerbations requiring steroids. Peak flow meters are often used to help guide treatment. Before therapy is augmented, care providers need to assess medication administration techniques, environmental controls, and comorbidities. For reduction in therapy, the asthma needs to be under good control for a minimum of 3 months.[75]

The pharmacological treatment of asthma in children is essentially the same as that for adults and is initiated in a stepwise sequence based on asthma severity and response to treatment (see Chapter 27). Management of asthma medications in children is often difficult because fluctuation in severity of symptoms is common.

QUICK CHECK 28-4

1. What are the key features of the early and late asthmatic responses?
2. Explain the full progression of blood gas abnormalities in a severe asthma attack.
3. What is air trapping and how is it manifested in children?

Acute Lung Injury/Acute Respiratory Distress Syndrome

Acute respiratory distress syndrome (ARDS) can occur in children and is a dramatic, life-threatening condition resulting from a direct acute lung injury (ALI) such as pneumonia, aspiration, near drowning, or smoke inhalation; or from a systemic insult, such as sepsis or multiple trauma, either of which activates an inflammatory response that causes alveolocapillary injury. ARDS accounts for approximately 10% of total patient days and one-third of all deaths in pediatric Critical Care Units. Mortality in pediatric ARDS remains high, at approximately 40%.[76]

PATHOPHYSIOLOGY The pathophysiology of ARDS in children is the same as that described for adults in Chapter 27 (see Figure 27-7).

CLINICAL MANIFESTATIONS ARDS develops acutely after ALI, usually within 24 hours, although occasionally it is delayed by up to a few days. ARDS is characterized by progressive respiratory distress, severe hypoxemia, decreased pulmonary compliance, and diffuse densities on chest radiograph. Initially, hyperventilation occurs, but carbon dioxide retention may ultimately occur as well because of inadequate functional air space and respiratory muscle fatigue. The severity of the overall picture is modified by comorbid factors, such as the presence of sepsis or multiorgan failure, and by the presence or absence of complications, such as health care–associated pneumonia. Some children who recover have residual pulmonary abnormalities.

EVALUATION AND TREATMENT Treatment for ARDS remains supportive in nature, and the goals are to maintain adequate tissue oxygenation, minimize ALI, and avoid iatrogenic pulmonary complications. Most individuals with ARDS require mechanical ventilation and often relatively high levels of positive end-expiratory pressure (PEEP) to promote alveolar ventilation and stabilization, and redistribution of alveolar edema fluid into the interstitium. Lung-protective ventilation strategies may include low tidal volume and permissive hypercapnia, permissive hypoxemia to prevent oxygen toxicity, prone positioning, high-frequency oscillatory ventilation, and airway pressure release ventilation. Use of corticosteroids in children with ARDS is controversial and remains at the discretion of the clinician. Extracorporeal membrane oxygenation (ECMO) can provide cardiac or respiratory support, or both, but does not heal the underlying condition.[77]

Cystic Fibrosis

Cystic fibrosis (CF) is an autosomal recessive inherited disease that results from defective epithelial chloride ion transport. The CF gene is located on chromosome 7. There are more than 1 800 known mutations of this gene divided into six classes with varying severity of disease expression. Classes 1 through 3 are associated with more severe disease and 4 through 6 with milder pulmonary disease and pancreatic sufficiency. Mortality correlates respectively with the aforementioned classes.[78] CF primarily affects Whites (approximately 1 in 3 000). There are approximately 1 000 new cases of CF diagnosed each year, and the median age at diagnosis is 6 months. The projected mean age of survival is the early 40s.[79]

PATHOPHYSIOLOGY CF is a multiorgan disease that affects the lungs, digestive tract (see Chapter 37), and reproductive organs. The cystic fibrosis transmembrane conductance regulator (*CFTR*) gene mutation results in the abnormal expression of cystic fibrosis transmembrane conductance regulator (CFTR) protein, which is an activated chloride channel present on the surface of many types of epithelial cells, including those lining airways, bile ducts, pancreas, sweat ducts, and vas deferens. The most important effects are on the lungs, and respiratory failure is almost always the cause of death. The typical features of CF lung disease are mucus plugging, chronic inflammation, and chronic infection of the small airways. The mucus plugging results from both increased production and altered physicochemical properties of the mucus. Mucus-secreting airway cells (goblet cells and submucosal glands) are increased in number and size. CF mucus is dehydrated and viscous because of defective chloride secretion and excess sodium absorption. The periciliary fluid layer is depleted in volume, impairing the mobility of the cilia and thereby allowing mucus to adhere to the airway epithelium, along with bacteria and injurious by-products from neutrophils. Neutrophils are present in great excess in the airways and release damaging oxidants and proteases (i.e., elastase) that cause direct damage to lung structural proteins, induce airway cells to produce interleukin-8 (IL-8) (which attracts more neutrophils and stimulates mucus secretion), and destroy immunoglobulin G (IgG) and complement components important for opsonization and phagocytosis of pathogens[80] (Figure 28-7).

The CF airway microenvironment favours bacterial colonization. *S. aureus* and *H. influenzae* are common in younger children, and *Pseudomonas aeruginosa* ultimately colonizes airways in at least 75% of children with CF.[81] Their biofilm resists β-lactam antibiotics, and rapid mutation of the biofilm makes these children antibiotic resistant.[82] Persistence of these microorganisms incites chronic local inflammation and airway damage with microabscess formation, bronchiectasis, patchy consolidation and pneumonia, peribronchial fibrosis, and cyst formation (Figure 28-8).[83] Peripheral bullae may develop and pneumothorax may occur. Hemoptysis, sometimes life-threatening, may occur because of the erosion of enlarged bronchial arteries. Over time, pulmonary vascular remodelling occurs because of localized hypoxia and arteriolar vasoconstriction. Pulmonary hypertension and cor pulmonale may develop in the late stages of disease.

CLINICAL MANIFESTATIONS The most common presenting symptoms of CF are respiratory or gastro-intestinal (see Chapter 37). Respiratory symptoms include persistent cough or wheeze, excessive sputum production, and recurrent or severe pneumonia. Physical signs that develop over time include barrel chest and digital clubbing. More subtle presentations include chronic sinusitis and nasal polyps. (See *Health Promotion:* Cystic Fibrosis).

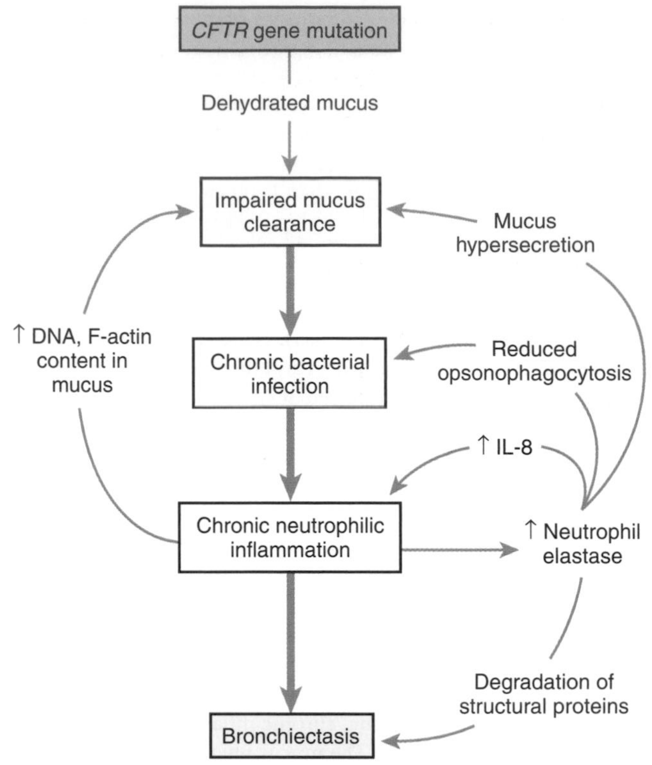

FIGURE 28-7 Pathogenesis of Cystic Fibrosis Lung Disease. *CFTR*, cystic fibrosis transmembrane conductance regulator, *IL-8*, interleukin-8.

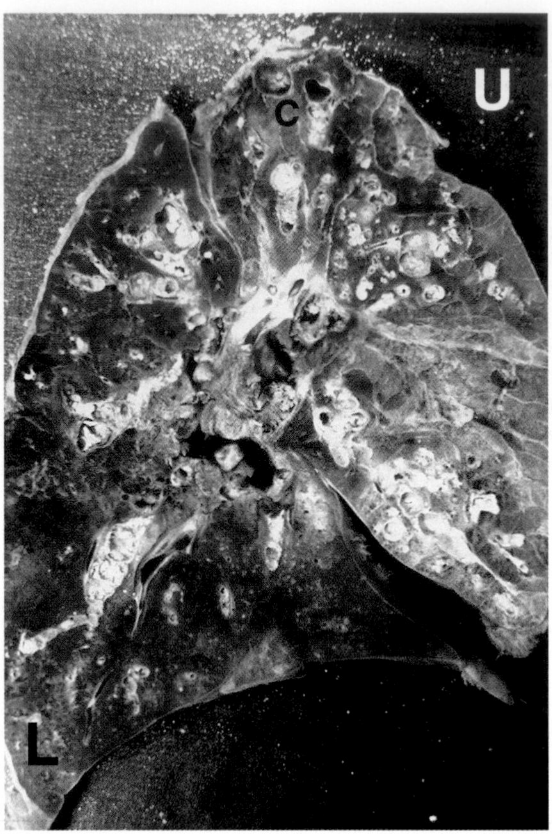

FIGURE 28-8 Pathology of the Lung in End-Stage Cystic Fibrosis. Key features are widespread mucus impaction of airways and bronchiectasis, especially from the upper lobe (*U*), with hemorrhagic pneumonia in the lower lobe (*L*). Small cysts (*C*) are present at the apex of the lung. (From Kleinerman, J., & Vauthy, P. [1976]. *Pathology of the lung in cystic fibrosis*. Atlanta: Cystic Fibrosis Foundation.)

HEALTH PROMOTION

Cystic Fibrosis

Approximately 1 in 25 Canadians is a cystic fibrosis (CF) carrier, with one abnormal version of the gene responsible for this life-altering disease. Many people are unaware that they are carriers. Over 1 900 different mutations in the cystic fibrosis transmembrane conductance regulator (*CFTR*) gene have been identified. However, 87.5% of individuals with CF in Canada carry at least one copy of the most common CF-causing mutation, deltaF508. When two individuals who are carriers have a child, there is a 25% chance that the child will be born with CF. There is also a 50% chance that the child will be a carrier, and a 25% chance that the child will neither be a carrier nor have CF. It is estimated that 1 in every 3 600 children born in Canada has CF; 58.9% of people with CF are diagnosed in the first year of life, and 88.7% by 10 years of age.

According to Cystic Fibrosis Canada, in 2014 the median age of Canadians with CF was 21.9 years of age, and their median age of survival was 51.8 years of age. In 2014, 120 new cases of CF were diagnosed, 52 of them were through newborn screening and 18 were over 18 years of age. Almost 60% of all people with CF in Canada are adults. Cumulatively, CF patients underwent 867 courses of home intravenous therapy, spent almost 25 000 days in hospital, and attended over 15 500 clinic visits in 2014. The forced expiratory volume in 1 second (FEV_1) percent predicted for persons with CF is improving: half of all 30-year-olds with CF had an FEV_1 greater than 62.3% in 2014 compared with 47.4% 20 years ago. It is estimated that 86.2% of Canadians with CF must take pancreatic enzymes to digest food and absorb nutrients. Moreover, 28.7% of female adults with CF and 18.9% of male adults with CF are classified as underweight. However, 42.3% of female children and 41.9% of male children with CF are above the national goal of 50th body mass index percentile. In 2014, 33 CF patients underwent lung transplants. In terms of bacterial species and respiratory infections, in 2014, 47.4% of all CF patients had *Staphylococcus aureus* bacteria and 37.4% had *Pseudomonas aeruginosa* bacteria in their lungs. In addition, 24% of all CF patients had CF-related diabetes, and 40% of these individuals were 35 years of age and older. Of the 54 patients who died in 2014, half were under 32.4 years of age.

On January 26, 2016, Health Canada approved the medication ivacaftor/lumacaftor (ORKAMBI™) for use in Canada. This approval has given Canadians with CF who are age 12 and older and have two copies of the deltaF508 mutation a chance to gain access to this breakthrough treatment.

In addition to medication therapy, the Canadian Paediatric Society recommends that children with CF should be encouraged to participate in any physical activity and should have individualized exercise programs that include strength training. Moreover, children are required to engage in home exercises that elevate their heart rate by 70 to 80% of maximum heart rate to increase aerobic exercise tolerance. If coughing happens during exercise, children should be encouraged not to stop activity. Scuba diving is not recommended for children with CF as well as contact or collision sports, especially in those with an enlarged spleen or diseased liver. Children with CF should drink flavoured sodium chloride–containing fluids above thirst levels to prevent hyponatremia dehydration. Those with diabetes mellitus require additional carbohydrates during prolonged exercise.

Data from Cystic Fibrosis Canada. (2014). *The Canadian Cystic Fibrosis Registry 2015 Annual Report*. Toronto: Author; Philpott, J., Houghton, K., & Luke, A. (2010). *Paediatr Child Health, 15*(4), 213–218.

EVALUATION AND TREATMENT The standard method of diagnosis (screening) are the immunoreactive trypsinogen (IRT) blood test and the sweat test, which reveal sweat chloride concentration in excess of 60 mmol/L. Alternative or supplemental methods include genotyping for *CFTR* mutations. Every province and territory in Canada, except Quebec, has committed to newborn screening for CF. In 2015, Cystic Fibrosis Canada continued to engage the Quebec government regarding the importance of newborn screening. Canadian researchers used data from the Canadian Cystic Fibrosis Registry to evaluate the impact of newborn screening on long-term health outcomes. They demonstrated that those identified with CF at birth have fewer lung infections, reduced hospitalizations, and better nutritional status.[84] Another health economics study revealed that it is also more cost-effective, from the perspective of the public health system, than not implementing newborn screening.

Treatment is primarily focused on pulmonary health and nutrition (see Chapter 37). Common pulmonary therapies include techniques to promote mucus clearance, such as chest physiotherapy and related mechanical devices; use of bronchodilators; and administration of aerosolized dornase alfa (Pulmozyme) and hypertonic saline, which liquefy mucus.[85,86] Oral, inhaled, or intravenous antibiotics are used to treat exacerbations of pulmonary infection. Different classes of antibiotics are used to treat different pathogens and to overcome antibiotic resistance.[87,88] Recombinant human growth hormone has been shown to improve lung function, height, and weight in children with severe CF.[89] Individuals with end-stage lung disease may consider lung transplantation.[90] Newer approaches to gene therapy are being explored, including mutation-specific targets.[91]

SUDDEN UNEXPECTED INFANT DEATH

Sudden unexpected infant death (SUID) remains a disease of unknown cause and is the most common cause of unexplained infant death in Western countries. It is defined as "sudden death of an infant under 1 year of age which remains unexplained after a thorough case investigation, including performance of a complete autopsy, examination of the death scene, and review of the clinical history."[92]

The incidence of SUID is low during the first month of life, with the peak incidence at 2 to 4 months of age. It is unusual after 6 months of age. SUID almost always occurs during nighttime sleep, when infants are least likely to be observed. A seasonal variation has been noted, with higher frequencies during the winter months. This has been related to a higher rate of respiratory tract infections during those months, and such infections are often reported to have preceded the death. The sleeping room also may be overheated or the infant overwrapped.

In 1993, the Government of Canada, along with other international organizations, recommended that infants be placed on their backs to sleep, and in 1999 it reinforced this message by launching the Back to Sleep campaign. The rate of SUID has been declining since the late 1980s. In Canada, between 1999 and 2004, the rate of SUID decreased by 50%. This decline may be attributable, in part, to changes in parental behaviour such as placing infants on their backs to sleep and decreasing maternal smoking during pregnancy.[93]

According to an American Academy of Pediatrics policy statement, infants should be placed on a separate surface specifically made for infants in the same room with parents until the age of 1. While there is no evidence supporting moving an infant to his or her own room before 1 year of age, keeping the infant in the parents' bedroom during the first 6 months of age is highly recommended because the rates of SUID and other sleep-related deaths, especially those occurring in bed-sharing situations, are highest in the first 6 months. Placing the infant's especially designed bed close to the parents' bed so that the parents can view and reach the infant can facilitate feeding, comforting, and monitoring. Room-sharing reduces SUID risk and removes the possibility of suffocation, strangulation, and entrapment that can occur when the infant is sleeping in the adult bed.[94,94a]

Clinical risk groups are summarized in *Risk Factors*: Sudden Unexpected Infant Death. About 75% of all SUID victims have no known predisposing clinical risk factor.[95]

RISK FACTORS

Sudden Unexpected Infant Death

- Prone and side-lying sleeping positions
- Sleeping on soft bedding
- Overheated sleeping environment
- Lower socioeconomic status
- Mothers younger than 20
- Low birth weight or growth-restricted infants
- Male infants
- Preterm birth
- Multiple gestations
- Sibling who died of SUID
- Smoking during pregnancy
- Exposure to tobacco smoke
- Lack of prenatal care
- Parent's illicit drug use or binge drinking
- Larger family size

Data from Bergman, N.J. (2015). *Pediatr Res, 77*(1–1), 10–19; Blackwell, C., Moscovis, S., Hall, S., et al. (2015). *Front Immunol, 6*, 44; Hakeem, G.F., Oddy, L., Holcroft, C.A., et al. (2015). *World J Pediatr, 11*(1), 41–47; Van Nguyen, J.M., & Abenhaim, H.A. (2013). *Am J Perinatol, 30*(9), 703–714.

The etiology of SUID remains unknown but probably involves a combination of predisposing factors, including a vulnerable infant and environmental stressors. There has been longstanding interest in hypotheses involving impaired autonomic regulation and failure of cardiovascular, ventilatory, and arousal responses to hypoxemia or hypercapnia. There also is a potential relationship between SUID, auditory function, and central chemosensitivity to carbon dioxide.[96,97]

Alternative theories involve airway obstruction events, such as control of tongue movements related to inspiratory activity, increased vagal tone, sudden intrapulmonary shunting because of abnormalities of surfactant or pulmonary vessels, exaggerated inflammation, or exaggerated inflammation in response to bacterial pathogens from the nasopharynx or viral respiratory tract infections.[98] Genetic factors may predispose certain individuals to SUID. The most important risk factor genes include those involved in the regulation of the immune system, cardiac abnormalities, and brainstem function.[99-102]

Currently, the best strategies for reducing SUID seem to be avoidance of all the controllable risk factors. Parents of infants with clinical risk should be taught cardiopulmonary resuscitation (CPR) as a precaution. Home monitoring has not been demonstrated to decrease the incidence of SUID, and more research is needed.[103] Some at-risk infants may warrant cardiorespiratory monitoring after careful consideration of the individual situation.

QUICK CHECK 28-5

1. How are the alveoli and capillaries affected by the inflammation of acute respiratory distress syndrome?
2. What aspects of lung disease in cystic fibrosis are the focus of current therapies?
3. What are the risk factors for sudden unexpected infant death?

DID YOU UNDERSTAND?

Disorders of the Upper Airways

1. Croup is an acute laryngotracheobronchitis, usually caused by parainfluenza virus. This infection causes swelling of the upper trachea. The typical sign is a seal-like barking cough, which appears after a few days of rhinorrhea, sore throat, and low-grade fever.
2. Spasmodic croup is characterized by a similar barking cough but occurs in older children, is of sudden onset at night and without fever, and has unknown etiology.
3. Acute epiglottitis is a potentially life-threatening airway infection whose incidence in children has decreased dramatically since the advent of *Haemophilus influenzae* vaccine. Now other pathogens, such as group A beta-hemolytic *Streptococcus* (GABHS), *Candida* species, *Staphylococcus aureus*, methicillin-resistant *Staphylococcus aureus*, or viral pathogens, are usually the causative agents.
4. Tonsillar infections are usually caused by GABHS and can be complicated by tonsillar abscesses.
5. Aspiration of foreign bodies (FBs) that lodge in the airways may cause cough, hoarseness, stridor or wheezing, and dyspnea. The severity depends on the location of the FB within the airway and the degree of obstruction. Blockage of the larynx or trachea can be fatal, whereas bronchial obstruction may not be diagnosed immediately.
6. Obstructive sleep apnea syndrome (OSAS) is defined by partial or intermittent upper airway obstruction during sleep with disruption of normal ventilation and normal sleep patterns.

Disorders of the Lower Airways

1. Respiratory distress syndrome (RDS) of the newborn usually occurs in premature infants who are born before surfactant production and alveolocapillary development are complete. Atelectasis and hypoventilation cause shunting, hypoxemia, and hypercapnia. Prenatal steroids and postnatal surfactant are beneficial preventive therapies.
2. Bronchopulmonary dysplasia (BPD) is the result of tissue injury and repair and disrupted alveolar development in the lungs of infants who required ventilatory support during a time when their lungs were underdeveloped because of their prematurity. Surfactant therapy has improved outcomes. Infants with BPD may require oxygen and additional therapies for many months.
3. Bronchiolitis is a viral lower respiratory tract infection that presents with runny nose, wheezing, cough, and tachypnea in infants and is usually caused by infection with respiratory syncytial virus (RSV). Infants with risk factors of prematurity or underlying lung or heart disease are at high risk and may receive RSV-specific monoclonal antibody to prevent RSV disease.
4. Viral pneumonia and bacterial pneumonia cause varying degrees of illness in children. Viral pneumonia is the most common type of pneumonia and frequently precedes bacterial pneumonia. Community-acquired bacterial pneumonia is one of the leading causes of hospitalization and is prevented with polyvariant pneumococcal conjugate vaccine.
5. Aspiration pneumonitis is caused by inhalation of a foreign substance, such as food, milk, secretions, or environmental compounds, into the lung, and results in inflammation.
6. Bronchiolitis obliterans is a rare postinflammatory condition in which the bronchioles and some small bronchi are partially or completely obliterated by fibrous tissue, causing pulmonary impairment and disability.
7. Asthma is a chronic inflammatory disease characterized by bronchial hyper-reactivity and reversible airflow obstruction, and is usually a type I hypersensitivity response to an antigen. Its origins are multifactorial, including genetic, allergic, and viral-triggered mechanisms.
8. Acute respiratory distress syndrome results from acute lung injury and can occur when there is an insult to the lung that activates an inflammatory response causing alveolar capillary injury, usually within 24 hours. There is progressive respiratory distress with severe hypoxemia and respiratory failure.
9. Cystic fibrosis (CF) is an autosomal recessive genetic disease that affects the epithelial lining of many organ systems, especially the respiratory and gastro-intestinal systems. Airway secretions are particularly thick and tenacious, and the airways develop chronic bacterial infection with pathogens such as *Pseudomonas aeruginosa* and *Staphylococcus aureus*. Chronic infection, plugged airways, and severe inflammation cause long-term lung damage and ultimately death. However, the prognosis is improving, and most children with CF now survive to adulthood.

Sudden Unexpected Infant Death

1. Sudden unexpected infant death (SUID) is the leading cause of postnatal death for infants outside of the hospital setting and is associated with low birth weight, prone sleeping position, and other environmental factors. There has been a significant reduction in SUID since widespread adoption of recommendations for supine positioning of infants during sleep.

KEY TERMS

Acute epiglottitis, 727
Acute respiratory distress syndrome (ARDS), 735
Aspiration pneumonitis, 733
Asthma, 733
Atypical pneumonia (*Mycoplasma pneumoniae, Chlamydophila pneumoniae*), 733
Bacterial pneumonia, 732
Bacterial tracheitis, 727
Bronchiolitis, 730
Bronchiolitis obliterans (BO), 733
Bronchopulmonary dysplasia (BPD), 730
Croup, 725
Cystic fibrosis (CF), 735
Cystic fibrosis transmembrane conductance regulator (CFTR) protein, 735
Obstructive sleep apnea syndrome (OSAS), 727
Peritonsillar abscess, 727
Pneumonia, 732
Respiratory distress syndrome (RDS) of the newborn, 728
Sudden unexpected infant death (SUID), 737
Tonsillar abscess, 727
Tonsillar infections, 727
Upper airway obstruction, 725
Viral pneumonia, 732

REFERENCES

1. Choi, J., & Lee, G. L. (2012). Common pediatric respiratory emergencies. *Emergency Medicine Clinics of North America, 30*(2), 529–563, x. doi:10.1016/j.emc.2011.10.009.
2. Zoorob, R., Sidani, M., & Murray, J. (2011). Croup: An overview. *American Family Physician, 83*(9), 1067–1073.
3. Sammer, M., & Pruthi, S. (2010). Membranous croup (exudative tracheitis or membranous laryngotracheobronchitis). *Pediatric Radiology, 40,* 781. doi:10.1007/s00247-009-1397-0.
4. Li, S. F. (2003). The Westley croup score. *Academic Emergency Medicine, 10*(3), 289. author reply 289.
5. Pitluk, J. D., Uman, H., & Safranek, S. (2011). Clinical inquiries. What's best for croup? *Journal of Family Practice, 60*(11), 680–681.
6. Dobrovoljac, M., & Geelhoed, G. C. (2012). How fast does oral dexamethasone work in mild to moderately severe croup? A randomized double-blinded clinical trial. *Emergency Medicine Australasia : EMA, 24*(1), 79–85. doi:10.1111/j.1742-6723.2011.01475.x.
7. Bjornson, C., Russell, K., Vandermeer, B., et al. (2011). Nebulized epinephrine for croup in children. *Cochrane Database of Systematic Reviews,* (2), CD006619, doi:10.1002/14651858.
8. Moraa, I., Sturman, N., McGuire, T., et al. (2013). Heliox for croup in children. *Cochrane Database of Systematic Reviews,* (12), CD006822, doi:10.1002/14651858.
9. Kuo, C. Y., & Parikh, S. R. (2014). Bacterial tracheitis. *Pediatrics in Review, 35*(11), 497–499. doi:10.1542/pir.35-11-497.
10. Cirilli, A. R. (2013). Emergency evaluation and management of the sore throat. *Emergency Medicine Clinics of North America, 31*(2), 501–515. doi:10.1016/j.emc.2013.01.002.
11. Tibballs, J., & Watson, T. (2011). Symptoms and signs differentiating croup and epiglottitis. *Journal of Paediatrics and Child Health, 47*(3), 77–82. doi:10.1111/j.1440-1754.2010.01892.x.
12. Shah, R. K., & Stocks, C. (2010). Epiglottitis in the United States: National trends, variances, prognosis, and management. *Laryngoscope, 120*(6), 1256–1262. doi:10.1002/lary.20921.
13. Kordeluk, S., Novack, L., Puterman, M., et al. (2011). Relation between peritonsillar infection and acute tonsillitis: Myth or reality? *Otolaryngology–Head and Neck Surgery, 145*(6), 940–945. doi:10.1177/0194599811415802.
14. Powell, J., & Wilson, J. A. (2012). An evidence-based review of peritonsillar abscess. *Clinical Otolaryngology, 37*(2), 136–145. doi:10.1111/j.1749-4486.2012.02452.x.
15. Yenigun, A. (2015). The efficacy of tonsillectomy in chronic tonsillitis patients as demonstrated by the neutrophil-to-lymphocyte ratio. *Journal of Laryngology and Otology, 129*(4), 386–391. doi:10.1017/S0022215115000559.
16. Kim, I. A., Shapiro, N., & Bhattacharyya, N. (2015). The national cost burden of bronchial foreign body aspiration in children. *Laryngoscope, 125*(5), 1221–1224. doi:10.1002/lary.25002.
17. Shlizerman, L., Mazzawi, S., Rakover, Y., et al. (2010). Foreign body aspiration in children: The effects of delayed diagnosis. *American Journal of Otolaryngology, 31*(5), 320–324. doi:10.1016/j.amjoto.2009.03.007.
18. Katz, E. S., & D'Ambrosio, C. M. (2010). Pediatric obstructive sleep apnea syndrome. *Clinics in Chest Medicine, 31,* 221–234. doi:10.1016/j.ccm.2010.02.002.
19. Snow, A., Dayyat, E., Montgomery-Downs, H. E., et al. (2009). Pediatric obstructive sleep apnea: A potential late consequence of respiratory syncytial virus bronchiolitis. *Pediatric Pulmonology, 44,* 1186–1191. doi:10.1002/ppul.21109.
20. Katz, E. S., Mitchell, R. B., & D'Ambrosio, C. M. (2012). Obstructive sleep apnea in infants. *American Journal of Respiratory and Critical Care Medicine, 185*(8), 805–816. doi:10.1164/rccm.201108-1455CI.
21. Tan, H. L., Gozal, D., & Kheirandish-Gozal, L. (2013). Obstructive sleep apnea in children: A critical update. *Nature and Science of Sleep, 5,* 109–123. doi:10.2147/NSS.S51907.
22. Gozal, D., Kheirandish-Gozal, L., Bhattacharjee, R., et al. (2012). C-reactive protein and obstructive sleep apnea syndrome in children. *Frontiers in Bioscience (Elite Edition), 4,* 2410–2422. doi:10.2741/553.
23. Kim, J., Hakim, F., Kheirandish-Gozal, L., et al. (2011). Inflammatory pathways in children with insufficient or disordered sleep. *Respiratory Physiology and Neurobiology, 178*(3), 465–474. doi:10.1016/j.resp.2011.04.024.
24. Alexander, N. S., & Schroeder, J. W., Jr. (2013). Pediatric obstructive sleep apnea syndrome. *Pediatric Clinics of North America, 60*(4), 827–840. doi:10.1016/j.pcl.2013.04.009.
25. Lal, C., Strange, C., & Bachman, D. (2012). Neurocognitive impairment in obstructive sleep apnea. *Chest, 141*(6), 1601–1610. doi:10.1378/chest.11-2214.
26. Donnelly, L. F. (2010). Magnetic resonance sleep studies in the evaluation of children with obstructive sleep apnea. *Seminars in Ultrasound, CT, and MR, 31*(2), 107–115. doi:10.1053/j.sult.2009.12.001.
27. Marcus, C. L., Brooks, L. J., Draper, K. A., et al. (2012). Diagnosis and management of childhood obstructive sleep apnea syndrome. *Pediatrics, 130*(3), e714–e755. doi:10.1542/peds.2012-1672.
28. Tapia, I. E., & Marcus, C. L. (2013). Newer treatment modalities for pediatric obstructive sleep apnea. *Paediatric Respiratory Reviews, 14*(3), 199–203. doi:10.1016/j.prrv.2012.05.006.
29. Shapiro-Mendoza, C. K., & Lackritz, E. M. (2012). Epidemiology of late and moderate preterm birth. *Seminars in Fetal and Neonatal Medicine, 17*(3), 120–125. doi:10.1016/j.siny.2012.01.007.
30. Sweet, D., Bevilacqua, G., Carnielli, V., et al. (2007). European consensus guidelines on the management of neonatal respiratory distress syndrome. *Journal of Perinatal Medicine, 35,* 175–186. doi:10.1515/JPM.2007.048.
31. Kamath-Rayne, B. D., DeFranco, E. A., & Marcotte, M. P. (2012). Antenatal steroids for treatment of fetal lung immaturity after 34 weeks of gestation: An evaluation of neonatal outcomes. *Obstetrics and Gynecology, 119*(5), 909–916. doi:10.1097/AOG.0b013e31824ea4b2.
32. McKinlay, C. J., Crowther, C. A., Middleton, P., et al. (2012). Repeat antenatal glucocorticoids for women at risk of preterm birth: A Cochrane Systematic Review. *American Journal of Obstetrics and Gynecology, 206*(3), 187–941. doi:10.1016/j.ajog.2011.07.042.
33. Smolarova, S., Kocvarova, L., Matasova, K., et al. (2015). Impact of updated European Consensus Guidelines on the management of neonatal respiratory distress syndrome on clinical outcome of preterm infants. *Advances in Experimental Medicine and Biology, 835,* 61–66. doi:10.1007/5584_2014_39.
34. Dani, C., & Pratesi, S. (2013). Nitric oxide for the treatment of preterm infants with respiratory distress syndrome. *Expert Opinion on Pharmacotherapy, 14*(1), 97–103. doi:10.1517/14656566.2013.746662.
35. Bhandari, A., & McGrath-Morrow, S. (2013). Long-term pulmonary outcomes of patients with bronchopulmonary dysplasia. *Seminars in Perinatology, 37*(2), 132–137. doi:10.1053/j.semperi.2013.01.010.
36. Statistics Canada. (2016). *Health fact sheets: Low birth weight newborns in Canada, 2000 to 2013.* Retrieved from http://www.statcan.gc.ca/pub/82-625-x/2016001/article/14674-eng.htm.
37. Trembath, A., & Laughon, M. M. (2012). Predictors of bronchopulmonary dysplasia. *Clinics in Perinatology, 39*(3), 585–601. doi:10.1016/j.clp.2012.06.014.
38. Berkelhamer, S. K., Mestan, K. K., & Steinhorn, R. H. (2013). Pulmonary hypertension in bronchopulmonary dysplasia. *Seminars in Perinatology, 37*(2), 124–131. doi:10.1053/j.semperi.2013.01.009.
39. Simpson, S. J., Hall, G. L., & Wilson, A. C. (2015). Lung function following very preterm birth in the era of "new" bronchopulmonary dysplasia. *Respirology (Carlton, Vic.), 20*(4), 535–540. doi:10.1111/resp.12503.
40. Viscardi, R. M. (2012). Perinatal inflammation and lung injury. *Seminars in Fetal and Neonatal Medicine, 17*(1), 30–35. doi:10.1016/j.siny.2011.08.002.
41. Pfister, R. H., & Soll, R. F. (2012). Initial respiratory support of preterm infants: The role of CPAP, the INSURE method, and noninvasive ventilation. *Clinics in Perinatology, 39*(3), 459–481. doi:10.1016/j.clp.2012.06.015.
42. Picone, S., Bedetta, M., & Paolillo, P. (2012). Caffeine citrate: When and for how long. A literature review. *Journal of Maternal-Fetal and Neonatal Medicine, 25*(Suppl. 3), 11–14. doi:10.3109/14767058.2012.712305.
43. Lodha, A., Seshia, M., McMillan, D. D., et al. (2015). Association of early caffeine administration and neonatal outcomes in very preterm neonates. *Journal of the American Medical Association Pediatrics, 169*(1), 33–38. doi:10.1001/jamapediatrics.2014.2223.
44. Teshome, G., Gattu, R., & Brown, R. (2013). Acute bronchiolitis. *Pediatric Clinics of North America, 60*(5), 1019–1034. doi:10.1016/j.pcl.2013.06.005.
45. Beigelman, A., & Bacharier, L. B. (2013). The role of early life viral bronchiolitis in the inception of asthma. *Current Opinion in Allergy and Clinical Immunology, 13*(2), 211–216. doi:10.1097/ACI.0b013e32835eb6ef.
46. Friedman, J. N., Rieder, M. J., Walton, J. M., et al. (2014). Bronchiolitis: Recommendations for diagnosis, monitoring and management of children one to 24 months of age. *Paediatrics & Child Health, 19*(9), 485–491.
47. Jain, S., Williams, D. J., Arnold, S. R., et al. (2015). Community-acquired pneumonia requiring hospitalization among U.S. children. *New England Journal of Medicine, 372*(9), 835–845. doi:10.1056/NEJMoa1405870.
48. Pavia, A. T. (2013). What is the role of respiratory viruses in community-acquired pneumonia? What is the best therapy for influenza and other viral causes of community-acquired pneumonia? *Infectious Disease Clinics of North America, 27*(1), 157–175. doi:10.1016/j.idc.2012.11.007.
49. Yamada, M., Buller, R., Bledsoe, S., et al. (2012). Rising rates of macrolide-resistant *Mycoplasma pneumoniae* in the central United States. *Pediatric Infectious Disease Journal, 31*(4), 409–410. doi:10.1097/INF.0b013e318247f3e0.
50. Durando, P., Alicino, C., De Florentiis, D., et al. (2012). Improving the protection against *Streptococcus pneumoniae* with the new generation 13-valent pneumococcal conjugate vaccine. *Journal of Preventive Medicine and Hygiene, 53*(2), 68–77.
51. van der Sluijs, K. F., van der Poll, T., Lutter, R., et al. (2010). Bench-to-bedside review: Bacterial pneumonia with influenza—pathogenesis and clinical implications. *Critical Care, 14*(2), 219. doi:10.1186/cc8893.
52. Wang, K., Gill, P., Perera, R., et al. (2012). Clinical symptoms and signs for the diagnosis of *Mycoplasma pneumoniae* in children and adolescents with community-acquired pneumonia. *Cochrane Database of Systematic Reviews,* (10), CD009175, doi:10.1002/14651858.CD009175.pub2.
53. Bradley, J. S., Byington, C. L., Shah, S. S., et al. (2011). The management of community-acquired pneumonia in infants and children older than 3 months of age: Clinical practice guidelines by the Pediatric Infectious Diseases Society and the Infectious Diseases Society of America. *Clinical*

Infectious Diseases, *53*, e25–e76. doi:10.1093/cid/cir531.
54. Schauner, S., Erickson, C., Fadara, K., et al. (2013). Community-acquired pneumonia in children: A look at the IDSA guidelines. *Journal of Family Practice*, *62*(1), 9–15.
55. Patria, F., Longhi, B., Tagliabue, C., et al. (2013). Clinical profile of recurrent community-acquired pneumonia in children. *BMC Pulmonary Medicine*, *13*, 60. doi:10.1186/1471-2466-13-60.
56. Krüger, S., & Welte, T. (2012). Biomarkers in community-acquired pneumonia. *Expert Review of Respiratory Medicine*, *6*(2), 203–214. doi:10.1586/ers.12.6.
57. Mulholland, S., Gavranich, J. B., Billies, M. B., et al. (2012). Antibiotics for community-acquired lower respiratory tract infections secondary to *Mycoplasma pneumoniae* in children. *Cochrane Database of Systematic Reviews*, (9), CD004875, doi:10.1002/14651858.CD004875.pub4.
58. Swarnam, K., Soraisham, A. S., & Sivanandan, S. (2012). Advances in the management of meconium aspiration syndrome. *International Journal of Pediatrics*, *2012*, 359571. doi:10.1155/2012/359571.
59. Boesch, R. P., Daines, C., Willging, J. P., et al. (2006). Advances in the diagnosis and management of chronic pulmonary aspiration in children. *European Respiratory Journal*, *28*, 847–861. do i:10.1183/09031936.06.00138305.
60. Pena, A. H., Cahill, A. M., Gonzalez, L., et al. (2009). Botulinum toxin A injection of salivary glands in children with drooling and chronic aspiration. *Journal of Vascular and Interventional Radiology*, *20*(3), 368–373. doi:10.1016/j.jvir.2008.11.011.
61. Fischer, G. B., Sarria, E. E., Mattiello, R., et al. (2010). Post infectious bronchiolitis obliterans in children. *Paediatric Respiratory Reviews*, *11*(4), 233–239. doi:10.1016/j.prrv.2010.07.005.
62. Moonnumakal, S. P., & Fan, L. L. (2008). Bronchiolitis obliterans in children. *Current Opinion in Pediatrics*, *20*(3), 272–278. doi:10.1097/MOP.0b013e3282ff62e9.
63. Champs, N. S., Lasmar, L. M., Camargos, P. A., et al. (2011). Post-infectious bronchiolitis obliterans in children. *Jornal de Pediatria*, *87*(3), 187–198. doi:10.2223/JPED.2083.
64. Sacher, V. Y., Fertel, D., Srivastava, K., et al. (2014). Effects of prophylactic use of sirolimus on bronchiolitis obliterans syndrome development in lung transplant recipients. *Annals of Thoracic Surgery*, *97*(1), 268–274. doi:10.1016/j.athoracsur.2013.07.072.
65. Asthma Society of Canada. (2014). *Severe asthma: The Canadian patient journey*. Toronto: Author. Retrieved from https://asthma.ca/wp-content/uploads/2017/06/SAstudy.pdf.
66. Akinbami, L. J., Moorman, J. E., Bailey, C., et al. (2012). *Trends in asthma prevalence, health care use, and mortality in the United States, 2001–2010 (NCHS Data Brief Number 94)*. Hyattsville, MD: Author. Retrieved from http://www.cdc.gov/nchs/data/databriefs/db94.htm.
67. Been, J. V., Lugtenberg, M. J., Smets, E., et al. (2014). Preterm birth and childhood wheezing disorders: A systematic review and meta-analysis. *PLoS Medicine*, *11*(1), e1001596. doi:10.1371/journal.pmed.1001596.
68. Blumenthal, M. N. (2012). Genetic, epigenetic, and environmental factors in asthma and allergy. *Annals of Allergy, Asthma and Immunology*, *108*(2), 69–73. doi:10.1016/j.anai.2011.12.003.
69. Hakimeh, D., & Tripodi, S. (2013). Recent advances on diagnosis and management of childhood asthma and food allergies. *Italian Journal of Pediatrics*, *39*, 80. doi:10.1186/1824-7288-39-80.
70. Papoutsakis, C., Priftis, K. N., Drakouli, M., et al. (2013). Childhood overweight/obesity and asthma: Is there a link? A systematic review of recent epidemiologic evidence. *Journal of the Academy of Nutrition and Dietetics*, *113*(1), 77–105. doi:10.1016/j.jand.2012.08.025.
71. Prokopakis, E., Vardouniotis, A., Kawauchi, H., et al. (2013). The pathophysiology of the hygiene hypothesis. *International Journal of Pediatric Otorhinolaryngology*, *77*(7), 1065–1071. doi:10.1016/j.ijporl.2013.04.036.
72. Fuchs, O., & von Mutius, E. (2013). Prenatal and childhood infections: Implications for the development and treatment of childhood asthma. *Lancet. Respiratory Medicine*, *1*(9), 743–754. doi:10.1016/S2213-2600(13)70145-0.
73. Keating, P., Munim, A., & Hartmann, J. X. (2014). Effect of vitamin D on T-helper type 9 polarized human memory cells in chronic persistent asthma. *Annals of Allergy, Asthma and Immunology*, *112*(2), 154–162. doi:10.1016/j.anai.2013.11.015.
74. Ducharme, F. M., Dell, S. D., Radhakrishnan, D., et al. (2015). Diagnosis and management of asthma in preschoolers: A Canadian Thoracic Society and Canadian Paediatric Society Position Paper. *Canadian Respiratory Journal*, *22*(3), 135–143. doi:10.1155/2015/101572.
75. Agency for Healthcare Quality and Research. (2015). *National Guideline Clearing House and the Institute for Clinical Systems Improvement (ICSI): Diagnosis and management of asthma*. Retrieved from http://www.guideline.gov/content.aspx?id=38255#Section420.
76. Willson, D. F., Chess, P. R., & Notter, R. H. (2008). Surfactant for pediatric acute lung injury. *Pediatric Clinics of North America*, *55*(3), 545–575, ix. doi:10.1016/j.pcl.2008.02.016.
77. Cheifetz, I. M. (2013). Advances in monitoring and management of pediatric acute lung injury. *Pediatric Clinics of North America*, *60*(3), 621–639. doi:10.1016/j.pcl.2013.02.015.
78. CFTR.INFO. (2014). *Classification of CFTR mutations*. Retrieved from www.cftr.info/about-cf/role-of-ctfr-in-cf/cftr-mutations/the-six-classes-o f-cftr-defects/.
79. MacKenzie, T., Gifford, A. H., Sabadosa, K. A., et al. (2014). Longevity of patients with cystic fibrosis in 2000 to 2010 and beyond: Survival analysis of the Cystic Fibrosis Foundation Patient Registry. *Annals of Internal Medicine*, *161*(4), 233–241. doi:10.7326/M13-0636.
80. Gifford, A. M., & Chalmers, J. D. (2014). The role of neutrophils in cystic fibrosis. *Current Opinion in Hematology*, *21*(1), 16–22. doi:10.1097/MOH.0000000000000009.
81. Lobo, J., Rojas-Balcazar, J. M., & Noone, P. G. (2012). Recent advances in cystic fibrosis. *Clinics in Chest Medicine*, *33*(2), 307–328. doi:10.1016/j.ccm.2012.02.006.
82. López-Causapé, C., Rojo-Molinero, E., Macià, M. D., et al. (2015). The problems of antibiotic resistance in cystic fibrosis and solutions. *Expert Review of Respiratory Medicine*, *9*(1), 73–88. doi:10.1586/17476348.2015.995640.
83. O'Sullivan, B. P., & Freedman, S. D. (2009). Cystic fibrosis. *Lancet*, *373*(9678), 1891–1904. doi:10.1016/S0140-6736(09)60327-5.
84. Mak, D. Y. F., Sykes, J., Stephenson, A. L., et al. (2016). The benefits of newborn screening for cystic fibrosis: The Canadian experience. *Journal of Cystic Fibrosis*, *15*(3), 302–308. doi:10.1016/j.jcf.2016.04.001.
85. Dentice, R., & Elkins, M. (2013). Timing of dornase alfa inhalation for cystic fibrosis. *Cochrane Database of Systematic Reviews*, (6), CD007923, doi:10.1002/14651858.
86. Elkins, M., & Dentice, R. (2012). Timing of hypertonic saline inhalation for cystic fibrosis. *Cochrane Database of Systematic Reviews*, (2), CD008816, doi:10.1002/14651858.CD008816.pub2.
87. Chmiel, J. F., Aksamit, T. R., Chotirmall, S. H., et al. (2014). Antibiotic management of lung infections in cystic fibrosis. I. The microbiome, methicillin-resistant *Staphylococcus aureus*, Gram-negative bacteria, and multiple infections. *Annals of the American Thoracic Society*, *11*(7), 1120–1129. doi:10.1513/AnnalsATS.201402-050AS.
88. Chmiel, J. F., Aksamit, T. R., Chotirmall, S. H., et al. (2014). Antibiotic management of lung infections in cystic fibrosis. II. Nontuberculous mycobacteria, anaerobic bacteria, and fungi. *Annals of the American Thoracic Society*, *11*(8), 1298–1306. doi:10.1513/AnnalsATS.201405-203AS.
89. Thaker, V., Haagensen, A. L., Carter, B., et al. (2013). Recombinant growth hormone therapy for cystic fibrosis in children and young adults. *Cochrane Database of Systematic Reviews*, (6), CD008901, doi:10.1002/14651858.CD008901.pub2.
90. Lynch, J. P., 3rd., Sayah, D. M., Belperio, J. A., et al. (2015). Lung transplantation for cystic fibrosis: Results, indications, complications, and controversies. *Seminars in Respiratory and Critical Care Medicine*, *36*(2), 299–320. doi:10.1055/s-0035-1547347.
91. Amaral, M. D. (2015). Novel personalized therapies for cystic fibrosis: Treating the basic defect in all patients. *Journal of Internal Medicine*, *277*(2), 155–166. doi:10.1111/joim.12314.
92. Centers for Disease Control and Prevention. (2015). *Sudden unexpected infant death and sudden infant death syndrome*. Retrieved from http://www.cdc.gov/sids/index.htm.
93. Public Health Agency of Canada. (2011). *Joint statement on safe sleep: Preventing sudden infant deaths in Canada*. Ottawa: Author. Retrieved from http://www.phac-aspc.gc.ca/hp-ps/dca-dea/stages-etapes/childhood-enfance_0-2/sids/pdf/jsss-ecss2011-eng.pdf.
94. Task Force on Sudden Infant Death Syndrome. (2016). SIDS and other sleep-related infant deaths: Updated 2016 recommendations for a safe infant sleeping environment. *Pediatrics*, *138*(5), e20162938. doi:10.1542/peds.2016-2938.
94a. Government of Canada. (2012). *Is Your Child Safe? Sleep Time*. Retrieved from https://www.canada.ca/en/health-canada/services/consumer-product-safety/reports-publications/consumer-education/your-child-safe/sleep-time.html#a31.
95. Bergman, N. J. (2015). Proposal for mechanisms of protection of supine sleep against sudden infant death syndrome: An integrated mechanism review. *Pediatric Research*, *77*(1–1), 10–19. doi:10.1038/pr.2014.140.
96. Garcia, A. J., 3rd., Koschnitzky, J. E., & Ramirez, J. M. (2013). The physiological determinants of sudden infant death syndrome. *Respiratory Physiology and Neurobiology*, *189*(2), 288–300. doi:10.1016/j.resp.2013.05.032.
97. Rubens, D., & Sarnat, H. B. (2013). Sudden infant death syndrome: An update and new perspectives of etiology. *Handbook of Clinical Neurology*, *112*, 867–874. doi:10.1016/B978-0-444-52910-7.00008-8.
98. Alfelali, M., & Khandaker, G. (2014). Infectious causes of sudden infant death syndrome. *Paediatric Respiratory Reviews*, *15*(4), 307–311. doi:10.1016/j.prrv.2014.09.004.
99. Kinney, H. C., Cryan, J. B., Haynes, R. L., et al. (2015). Dentate gyrus abnormalities in sudden unexplained death in infants: Morphological marker of underlying brain vulnerability. *Acta Neuropathologica*, *129*(1), 65–80. doi:10.1007/s00401-014-1357-0.
100. Klaver, E. C., Versluijs, G. M., & Wilders, R. (2011). Cardiac ion channel mutations in the sudden infant death syndrome. *International Journal of Cardiology*, *152*(2), 162–170. doi:10.1016/j.ijcard.2010.12.051.
101. Salomonis, N. (2014). Systems-level perspective of sudden infant death syndrome. *Pediatric Research*, *76*(3), 220–229. doi:10.1038/pr.2014.90.
102. Sweeting, J., & Semsarian, C. (2014). Cardiac abnormalities and sudden infant death syndrome. *Paediatric Respiratory Reviews*, *15*(4), 301–306. doi:10.1016/j.prrv.2014.09.006.
103. Strehle, E. M., Gray, W. K., Gopisetti, S., et al. (2012). Can home monitoring reduce mortality in infants at increased risk of sudden infant death syndrome? A systematic review. *Acta Paediatrica*, *101*(1), 8–13. doi:10.1111/j.1651-2227.2011.02464.x.

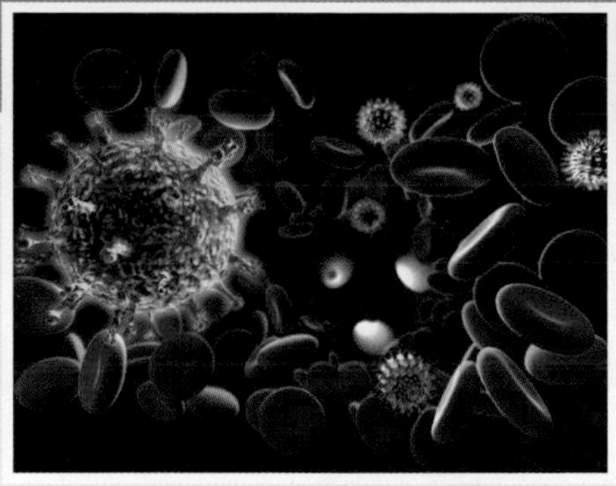

29

Structure and Function of the Renal and Urological Systems

Sue E. Huether and Mohamed El-Hussein

EVOLVE WEBSITE

http://evolve.elsevier.com/Canada/Huether/pathophysiology
Student Review Questions
Key Points
Case Studies
Animations
Quick Check Answers

CHAPTER OUTLINE

Structures of the Renal System, 741
- Structures of the Kidney, 741
- Urinary Structures, 745

Renal Blood Flow, 746
- Autoregulation of Intrarenal Blood Flow, 746
- Neural Regulation of Renal Blood Flow, 747
- Hormones and Other Factors Regulating Renal Blood Flow, 747

Kidney Function, 747
- Nephron Function, 747
- Hormones and Nephron Function, 752
- Renal Hormones, 752

Tests of Renal Function, 753
- Renal Clearance, 753
- Plasma Creatinine Concentration, 754
- Blood Urea Nitrogen, 754

PEDIATRIC CONSIDERATIONS: **Pediatrics and Renal Function, 756**

GERIATRIC CONSIDERATIONS: **Aging and Renal Function, 756**

The primary function of the kidney is to maintain a stable internal environment for optimal cell and tissue metabolism. The kidneys accomplish these life-sustaining tasks by balancing solute and water transport, excreting metabolic waste products, conserving nutrients, and regulating acids and bases. The kidney also has an endocrine function and secretes the hormones renin, erythropoietin (EPO), and 1,25-dihydroxy-vitamin D_3 for regulation of blood pressure, erythrocyte production, and calcium metabolism, respectively. The kidney also can release glucose into the circulation by the processes of glycogenolysis and gluconeogenesis. The formation of urine is achieved through the processes of glomerular filtration, tubular reabsorption, and secretion within the kidney. The bladder stores the urine received from the kidney by way of the ureters. Urine is then released from the bladder through the urethra.

STRUCTURES OF THE RENAL SYSTEM

Structures of the Kidney

The **kidneys** are paired organs located in the posterior region of the abdominal cavity behind the peritoneum. They lie on either side of the vertebral column, with their upper and lower poles extending from the twelfth thoracic vertebra to the third lumbar vertebra (Figure 29-1). The right kidney is slightly lower and is displaced downward by the overlying liver. Each kidney is approximately 11 cm long, 5 to 6 cm wide, and 3 to 4 cm thick. A tightly adhering capsule (the **renal capsule**) surrounds each kidney, which is embedded in a mass of perirenal fat. The capsule and fatty layer are covered with a double layer of **renal fascia** composed of fibrous tissue. The cushion of adipose tissue (paranephric fat) and the position of the kidney between the abdominal organs and muscles of the back protect it from trauma. The **hilum** is a medial indentation in the kidney and is the location of the entry and exit for the renal blood vessels, nerves, lymphatic vessels, and ureter.

The structures of the kidney are summarized in Figure 29-2. The outer layer of the kidney is called the **cortex** and contains all of the glomeruli, most of the proximal tubules, and some segments of the distal convoluted tubule. The **medulla** forms the inner part of the kidney and consists of regions call **pyramids. Renal columns** are an extension of the cortex and extend between the pyramids to the renal pelvis. The pyramids extend into the renal pelvis and contain the loops of Henle and collecting ducts. The minor and major **calyces** are chambers receiving urine from the collecting ducts and form the entry into the renal pelvis, which is an extension of the upper ureter. The structural unit of the kidney is the lobe. Each **lobe** is composed of a pyramid and the overlying cortex. There are about 14 to 18 lobes in each kidney.

Nephron

The **nephron** is the functional unit of the kidney. Each kidney contains approximately 1.2 million nephrons. The nephron is a tubular structure with subunits that include the renal corpuscle, proximal convoluted tubule, loop of Henle, distal convoluted tubule, and collecting duct, all of which contribute to the formation of final urine (Figure 29-3). The different structures of the epithelial cells lining various segments of the tubule facilitate the special functions of secretion and reabsorption (Figure 29-4).

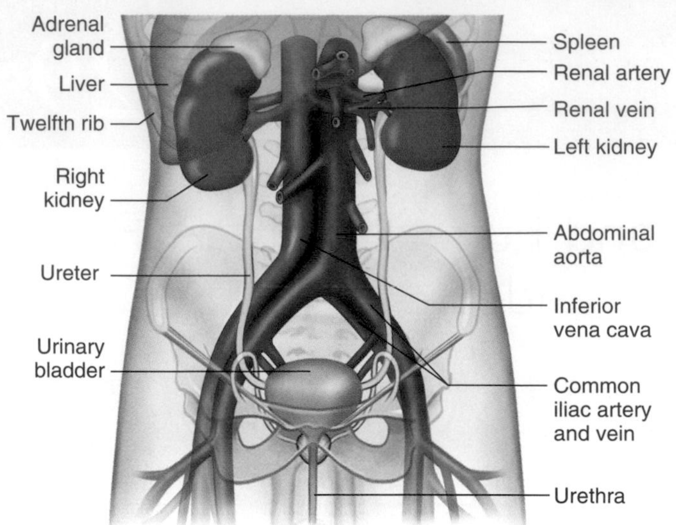

FIGURE 29-1 **Organs of the Urinary System.** (From Patton, K.T., & Thibodeau, G.A. [2014]. *The human body in health & disease* [6th ed.]. St. Louis: Mosby.)

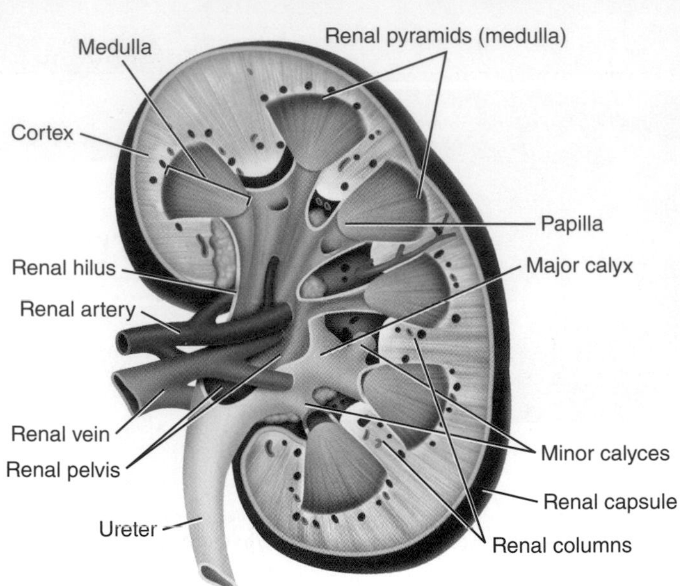

FIGURE 29-2 **Internal Structure of the Kidney.** (From Solomon, E. [2016]. *Introduction to human anatomy and physiology* [4th ed.]. St. Louis: Saunders.)

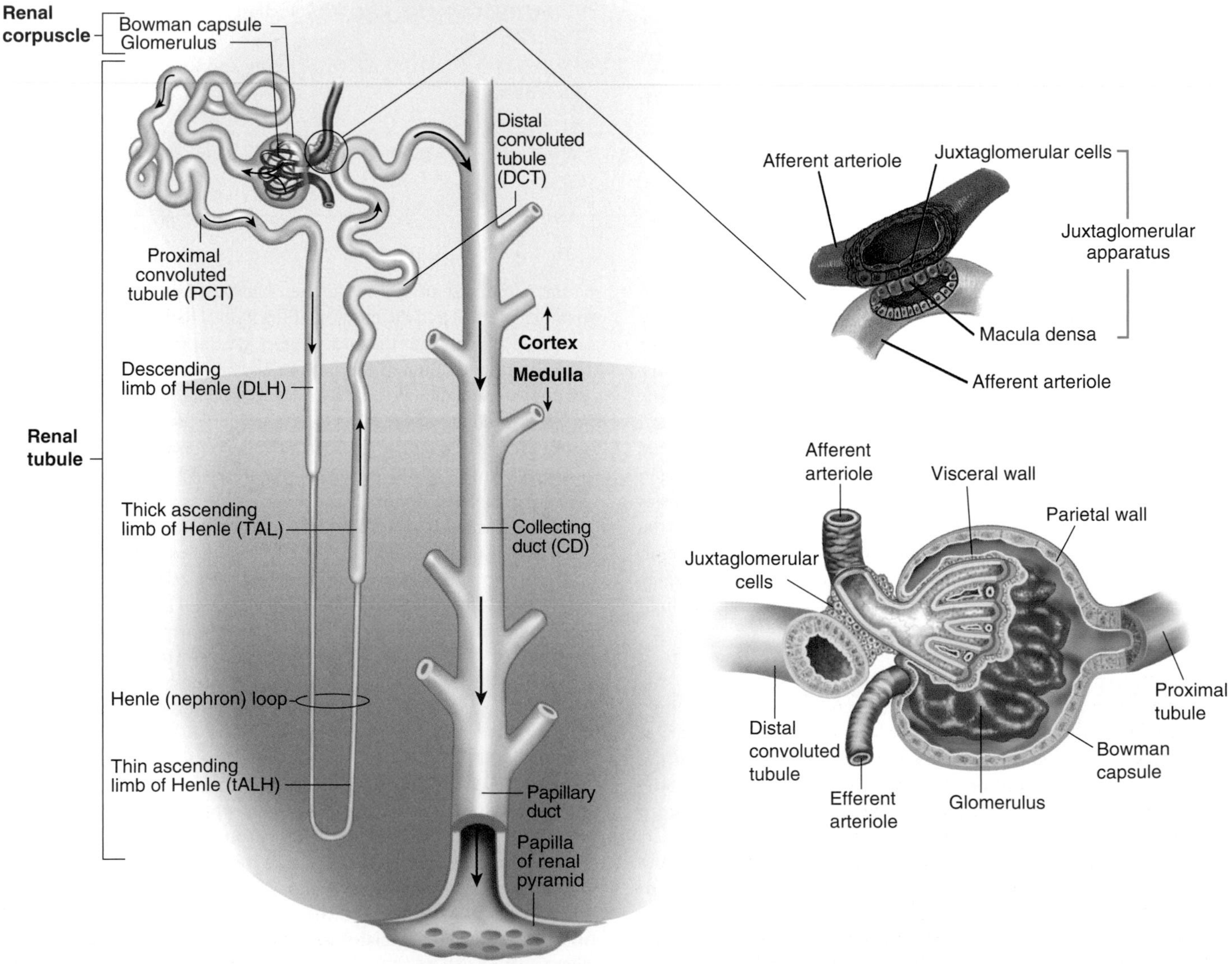

FIGURE 29-3 **Components of the Nephron.** (From Damjanov, I. [2012]. *Pathology for the health professions* [4th ed.]. St. Louis: Mosby; Patton, K.T., Thibodeau, G.A., & Douglas, M.M. [2012]. *Essentials of anatomy & physiology*. St. Louis: Mosby.)

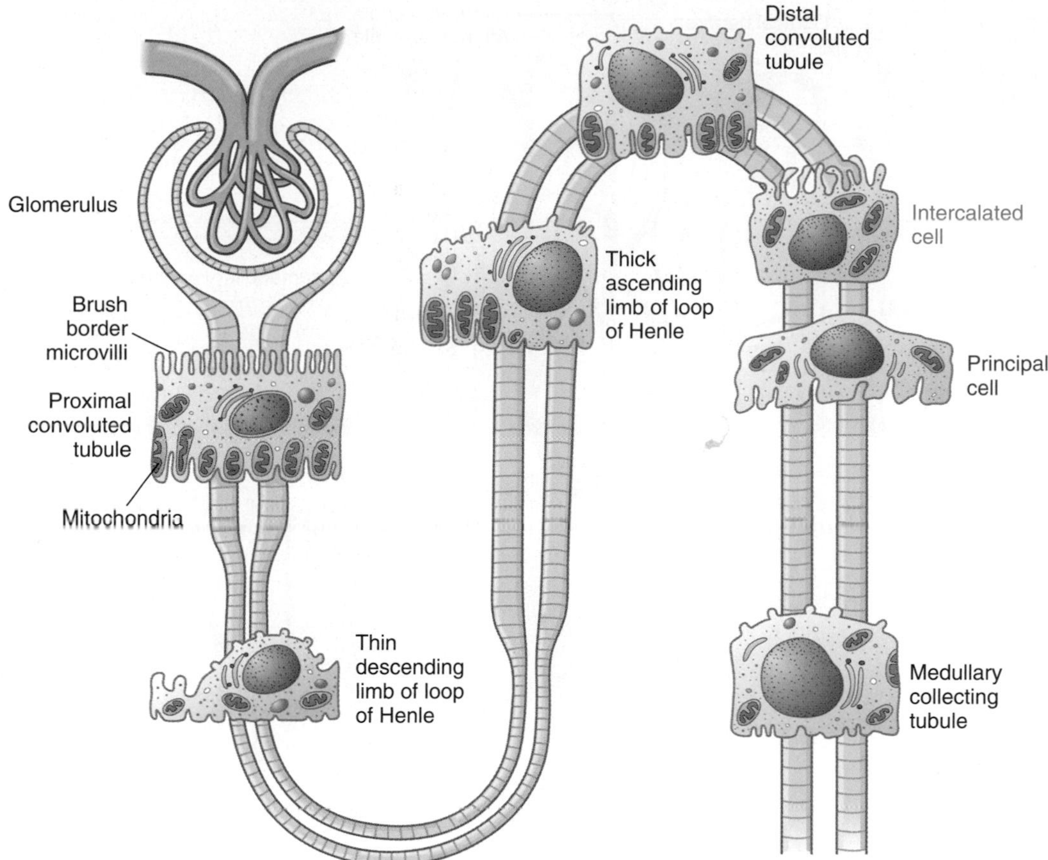

FIGURE 29-4 Epithelial Cells of the Various Segments of Nephron Tubules. The brush border and high number of mitochondria in cells of the proximal tubule promote reabsorption of 50% of the glomerular filtrate. Intercalated cells secrete H^+ (through K^+ exchange) or reabsorb HCO_3^-. Principal cells are influenced by aldosterone and reabsorb Na^+ and water and secrete K^+. *H^+*, hydrogen; *HCO_3^-*, bicarbonate; *K^+*, potassium; *Na^+*, sodium.

The kidney has three kinds of nephrons: (1) superficial **cortical nephrons** (85% of all nephrons), which extend partially into the medulla; (2) **midcortical nephrons** with short or long loops; and (3) **juxtamedullary nephrons** (about 12% of nephrons), which lie close to and extend deep into the medulla (about 40 mm) and are important for the concentration of urine (Figure 29-5). The **glomerulus** is a tuft of capillaries that loop into the **Bowman capsule (Bowman space)**, like fingers pushed into bread dough. **Mesangial cells** (shaped like smooth muscle cells) secrete the **mesangial matrix** (a type of connective tissue) and lie between and support the capillaries (Figure 29-6). Mesangial cells also have phagocytic abilities similar to monocytes, release inflammatory cytokines, and can contract to regulate glomerular capillary blood flow.[1] Together, the glomerulus, the Bowman capsule, and mesangial cells are called the **renal corpuscle**.

The **glomerular filtration membrane** filters blood components through its three layers: (1) an inner capillary endothelium, (2) a middle basement membrane, and (3) an outer layer of capillary epithelium. The capillary endothelium is composed of cells in continuous contact with the basement membrane and contains pores. The middle basement membrane is a selectively permeable network of glycoproteins and mucopolysaccharides. The epithelium has specialized cells called **podocytes** from which pedicles (foot projections) radiate and adhere to the basement membrane. The pedicles interlock with the pedicles of adjacent podocytes, forming an elaborate network of intercellular clefts (**filtration slits**, or slit membranes). The endothelium, basement membrane, and podocytes are covered with protein molecules bearing anionic (negative) charges that retard the filtration of anionic proteins and prevent proteinuria. The glomerular filtration membrane separates the blood of the glomerular capillaries from the fluid in the Bowman space and allows all components of the blood to be filtered, with the exception of blood cells and plasma proteins with a molecular weight greater than 70 000. The glomerular filtrate passes through the three layers of the glomerular membrane and forms the primary urine.

The glomerulus is supplied by the afferent arteriole and drained by the efferent arteriole. A group of specialized cells known as **juxtaglomerular cells** (renin-releasing cells) are located around the afferent arteriole where it enters the glomerulus (see Figure 29-3). Between the afferent and efferent arterioles is the **macula densa** (sodium-sensing cells) of the distal convoluted tubule (see Figure 29-6). Together the juxtaglomerular cells and macula densa cells form the **juxtaglomerular apparatus** (see Figure 29-3). Control of renal blood flow (RBF), glomerular filtration, and renin secretion occurs at this site.[2]

The **proximal convoluted tubule** continues from the Bowman space and has an initial convoluted segment (pars convoluta) and then a straight segment (pars recta) that descends toward the medulla (see Figure 29-3). The wall of the proximal tubule consists of one layer of cuboidal epithelial cells with a surface layer of microvilli (a brush border) that increases reabsorptive surface area. This is the only surface inside the nephron where the cells are covered with a brush border of microvilli (see Figure 29-4). The proximal convoluted tubule joins the **loop of Henle**, which extends into the medulla. The cells of the thick segment

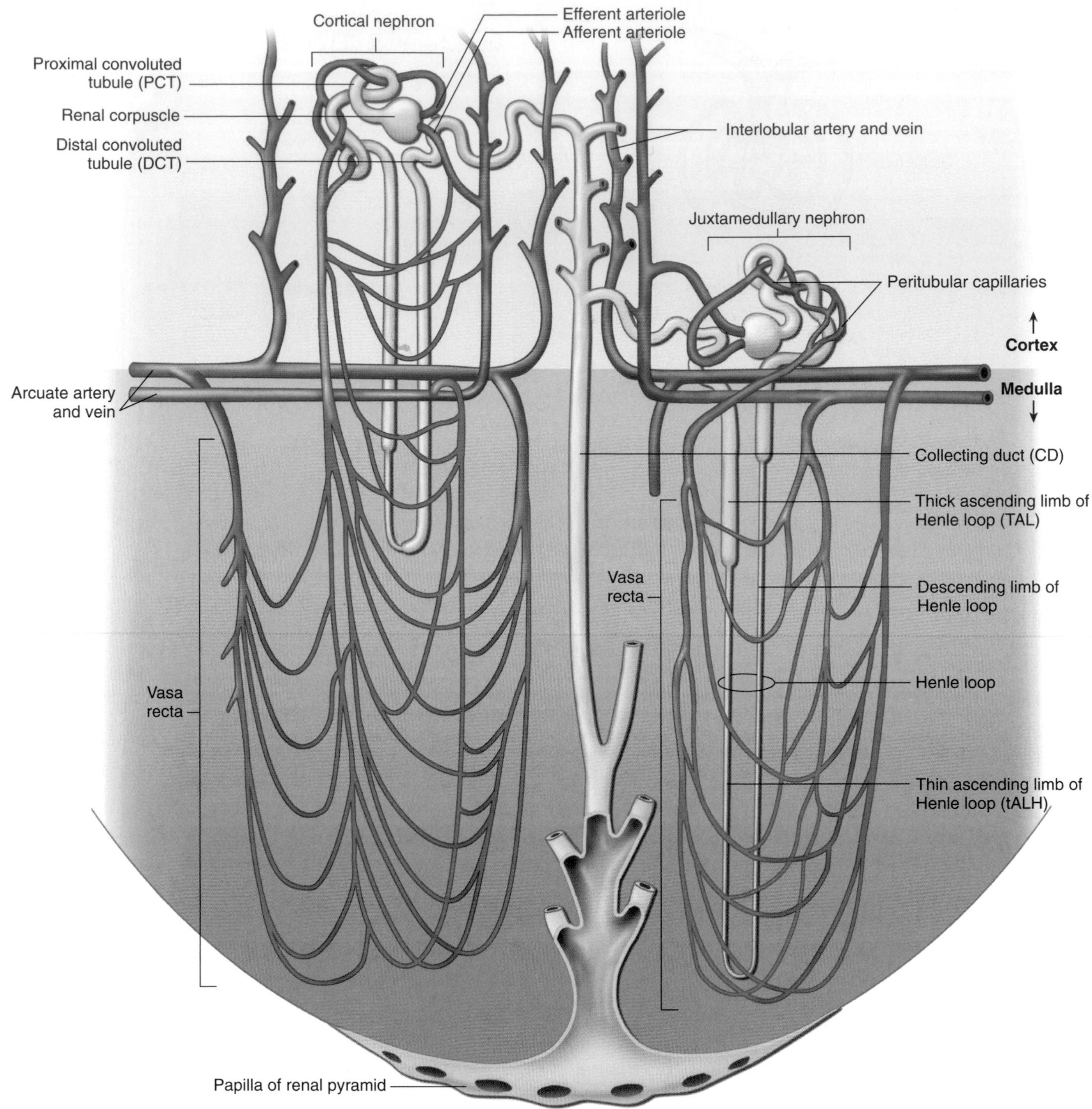

FIGURE 29-5 Nephron Unit With Its Blood Vessels. Blood flows through nephron vessels as follows: interlobular artery, afferent arteriole, glomerulus, efferent arteriole, peritubular capillaries (around the tubules), venules, interlobular vein. (From Patton, K.T., Thibodeau, G.A., & Douglas, M.M. [2012]. *Essentials of anatomy & physiology*. St. Louis: Mosby.)

are cuboidal and actively transport several solutes, but not water. The thin ascending segment of the loop of Henle narrows and is composed of thin squamous cells with no active transport function.

The **distal convoluted tubule** has straight and convoluted segments. It extends from the macula densa to the **collecting duct**, a large tubule that descends down the cortex and through the renal pyramids of the inner and outer medullae, draining urine into the minor calyx. In the distal convoluted tubule, **principal cells** reabsorb sodium and secrete potassium, and **intercalated cells** secrete hydrogen and reabsorb potassium and bicarbonate.

Blood Vessels of the Kidney

The blood vessels of the kidney closely parallel nephron structure. The major vessels are as follows:

1. **Renal arteries** arise as the fifth branches of the abdominal aorta, divide into anterior and posterior branches at the renal hilum, and

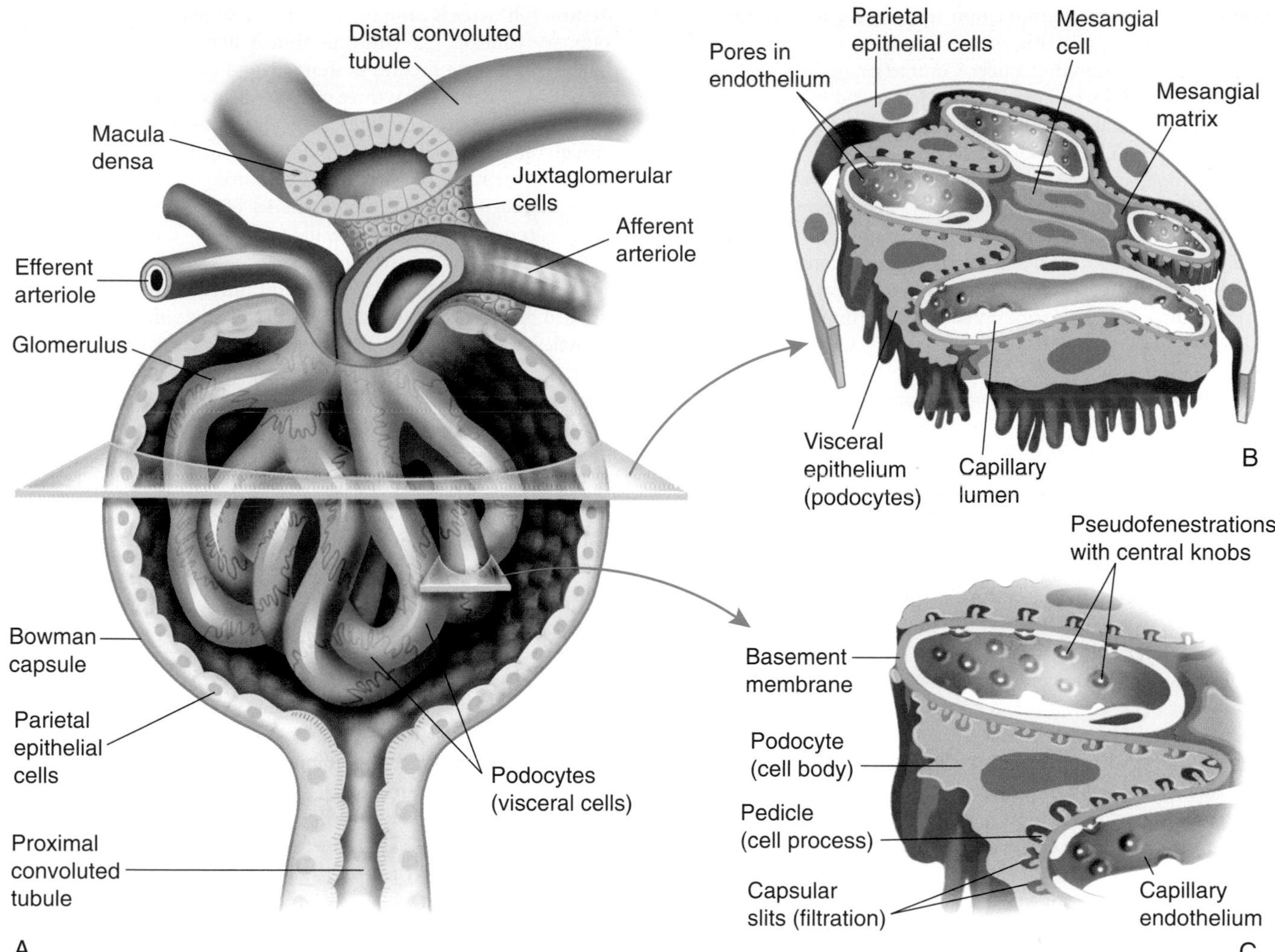

FIGURE 29-6 Anatomy of the Glomerulus and Juxtaglomerular Apparatus. **A,** Longitudinal cross section of glomerulus and juxtaglomerular apparatus. **B,** Horizontal cross section of glomerulus. **C,** Enlargement of glomerular capillary filtration membrane.

then subdivide into lobar arteries supplying blood to the lower, middle, and upper thirds of the kidney.

2. **Interlobar artery** subdivisions travel down renal columns and between pyramids and form afferent glomerular arteries.
3. **Arcuate arteries** consist of branches of interlobar arteries at the cortical-medullary junction; they arch over the base of the pyramids and run parallel to the surface.
4. **Glomerular capillaries** consist of four to eight vessels and are arranged in a fistlike structure; they arise from the **afferent arteriole** and empty into the **efferent arteriole**, which carries blood to the peritubular capillaries. They are the major resistance vessels for regulating intrarenal blood flow (see "Autoregulation of Intrarenal Blood Flow," p. 746).
5. **Peritubular capillaries** surround convoluted portions of the proximal and distal convoluted tubules and the loop of Henle; they are adapted for cortical and juxtamedullary nephrons.
6. **Vasa recta** is a network of capillaries that forms loops and closely follow the loops of Henle; it is the only blood supply to the medulla (important for formation of concentrated urine).
7. **Renal veins** follow the arterial path in reverse direction and have the same names as the corresponding arteries; they eventually empty into the inferior vena cava. The lymphatic vessels also tend to follow the distribution of the blood vessels.

QUICK CHECK 29-1

1. What is the major structural difference between the cortex and medulla of the kidney?
2. What is the function of the nephron?
3. Why are proteins not filtered at the glomerulus?

Urinary Structures

Ureters

The urine formed by the nephrons flows from the distal convoluted tubules and collecting ducts through the papillary ducts to the **renal papillae** (projections of the ducts) into the calyces, where it is collected in the renal pelvis (see Figures 29-2 and 29-5), and then funnelled into the **ureters**. Each adult ureter is approximately 30 cm long and is composed of long, intertwining smooth muscle bundles. The lower ends pass obliquely through the posterior aspect of the bladder wall. The close approximation of smooth muscle cells permits the direct transmission of electrical stimulation from one cell to another. The resulting downward peristaltic contraction from intrinsic pacemaker activity propels urine into the bladder. Contraction of the bladder during **micturition** (urination) compresses the lower end of the ureter, preventing reflux. Peristalsis is maintained even when the ureter is denervated, so ureters can be transplanted.

Sensory innervation for the upper part of the ureter arises from sympathetic inputs from the tenth thoracic nerve roots, with referred pain to the umbilicus. The innervation of lower segments arises from the parasympathetic sacral nerves, with referred pain to the vulva or penis. The ureters have a rich blood supply. The primary arteries come from the kidney, with contributions from the lumbar and superior vesical arteries.

Bladder and Urethra

The **bladder** is a bag composed of smooth muscle fibres that forms the **detrusor muscle** and its smooth lining of uroepithelium (also called *transitional epithelium*). As the bladder fills with urine, it distends and the layers of uroepithelium within the lining slide past each other and become thinner as bladder volume increases. The uroepithelium forms the interface between the urinary space and the underlying vasculature and connective, nervous, and muscle tissue. Uroepithelium also lines the urinary tract from the renal pelvis to the urethra. The uroepithelium maintains an important barrier function to prevent movement of water and solutes between the urine and the blood. It communicates information about urine pressure and composition to surrounding nerve and muscle cells.[3] The **trigone** is a smooth triangular area between the openings of the two ureters and the urethra (Figure 29-7). The position of the bladder varies with age and sex. The bladder has a profuse blood supply, accounting for the bleeding that readily occurs with trauma, surgery, or inflammation.

The **urethra** extends from the inferior side of the bladder to the outside of the body. A ring of smooth muscle forms the **internal urethral sphincter** at the junction of the urethra and bladder. The **external urethral sphincter** is composed of striated skeletal muscle and is under voluntary control. The entire urethra is lined with mucus-secreting glands. The female urethra is short (3 to 4 cm). The male urethra is long (18 to 20 cm) and has three main segments: prostatic, membranous, and penile. The prostatic urethra is closest to the bladder. It passes through the prostate gland and contains the openings of the ejaculatory ducts. The membranous urethra passes through the floor of the pelvis. The penile segment forms the remainder of the tube. It is surrounded by the corpous spongiosum erectile tissue and contains the openings of the bulbourethral mucous glands.

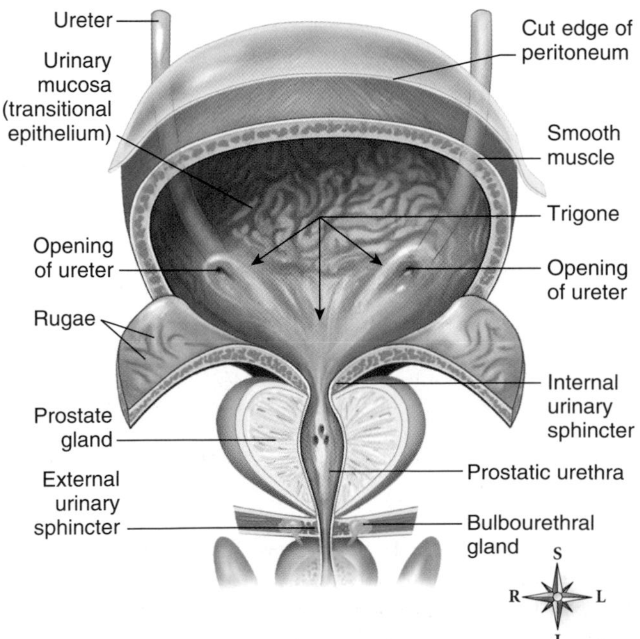

FIGURE 29-7 Structure of the Urinary Bladder. Frontal view of a dissected urinary bladder (male) in a fully distended position. (From Patton, K.T., & Thibodeau, G.A. [2014]. *The human body in health & disease* [6th ed.]. St. Louis: Mosby.)

The innervation of the bladder and internal urethral sphincter is supplied by parasympathetic fibres of the autonomic nervous system. The reflex arc required for micturition is stimulated by mechanoreceptors that respond to stretching of tissue, sensing bladder fullness and sending impulses to the sacral level of the cord. When the bladder accumulates 250 to 300 mL of urine, the bladder contracts and the internal urethral sphincter relaxes through activation of the spinal reflex arc (known as the *micturition reflex*). At this time, a person feels the urge to void. The reflex can be inhibited or facilitated by impulses coming from the brain, resulting in voluntary control of micturition by the relaxation or contraction of the external sphincter.

RENAL BLOOD FLOW

The kidneys are highly vascular organs and usually receive 1 000 to 1 200 mL of blood per minute, or about 20 to 25% of the cardiac output. With a normal hematocrit of 45%, about 600 to 700 mL of blood flowing through the kidney per minute is plasma. From the renal plasma flow (RPF), 20% (approximately 120 to 140 mL/min) is filtered at the glomerulus and passes into the Bowman capsule. The filtration of the plasma per unit of time is known as the **glomerular filtration rate (GFR)**, which is directly related to the perfusion pressure of the glomerular capillaries.

The remaining 80% (about 480 mL/min) of plasma flows through the efferent arterioles to the peritubular capillaries. The ratio of glomerular filtrate to RPF per minute (125/600 = 0.20) is called the *filtration fraction*. Normally all but 1 to 2 mL/min of the glomerular filtrate is reabsorbed from nephron tubules and returned to the circulation by the peritubular capillaries.

The GFR is directly related to RBF, which is regulated by intrinsic autoregulatory mechanisms, by neural regulation, and by hormonal regulation. In general, blood flow to any organ is determined by the arteriovenous pressure differences across the vascular bed. If mean arterial pressure decreases or vascular resistance increases, RBF declines and urinary output decreases. Normal urinary output is about 30 mL/hour minimum in adults or 0.5 to 1.0 mL/kg/hr.

Autoregulation of Intrarenal Blood Flow

In the kidney, a local mechanism tends to keep the rate of glomerular perfusion and, therefore, the GFR fairly constant over a range of arterial pressures between 80 and 180 mm Hg (Figure 29-8). Changes in afferent arteriolar resistance occur in the same direction. Therefore, RBF and GFR are relatively constant, a relationship maintained by an intrinsic autoregulatory myogenic mechanism of contraction when blood vessels are stretched. The purpose of **autoregulation of intrarenal blood flow** is to keep RBF and GFR constant when there are increases or decreases in systemic blood pressure. Solute and water excretion, and thus blood volume, are regulated despite arterial pressure changes.[4]

A second mechanism of autoregulation is **tubuloglomerular feedback**. Because the GFR in an individual nephron increases or decreases, the macula densa cells in the distal convoluted tubule sense the increasing or decreasing amounts of filtered sodium. When GFR and sodium

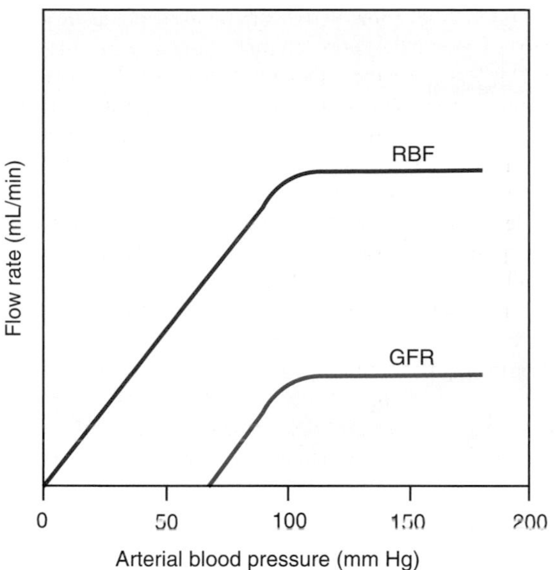

FIGURE 29-8 Renal Autoregulation. Renal blood flow (*RBF*) and glomerular filtration rate (*GFR*) are stabilized in the face of changes in perfusion pressure. (From Koeppen, B.M., & Stanton, B.A. [2010]. *Berne and Levy physiology* [6th ed., updated]. St. Louis: Mosby.)

concentration increase, the macula densa cells stimulate afferent arteriolar vasoconstriction and decrease GFR. The opposite occurs with decreases in GFR and sodium concentration at the macula densa. This mechanism prevents large fluctuations in body water and salt.[5]

Neural Regulation of Renal Blood Flow

The blood vessels of the kidney are innervated by sympathetic nerve fibres located primarily on afferent arterioles. When systemic arterial pressure decreases, increased renal sympathetic nerve activity is mediated reflexively through the carotid sinus and the baroreceptors of the aortic arch. The sympathetic nerves release catecholamines. This release stimulates afferent renal arteriolar vasoconstriction and decreases RBF and GFR, increases renal tubular sodium and water reabsorption, and increases blood pressure. Decreased afferent renal sympathetic nerve activity produces the opposite effects. The integrated response regulates water and sodium balance. **Renalase** is a hormone released by the kidney and heart that promotes the metabolism of catecholamines, and in this way participates in blood pressure regulation.[6] The sympathetic nervous system also participates in hormonal (i.e., angiotensin II) regulation of RBF. There is no significant parasympathetic innervation. The innervation of the kidney arises primarily from the celiac ganglion and greater splanchnic nerve.

Hormones and Other Factors Regulating Renal Blood Flow

Hormones and other mediators can alter the resistance of the renal vasculature by stimulating vasodilation or vasoconstriction. A major hormonal regulator of RBF is the **renin-angiotensin-aldosterone system (RAAS)**, which can increase systemic arterial pressure and change RBF. Renin is an enzyme formed and stored in the cells of the arterioles of the juxtaglomerular apparatus (see Figure 29-3). Renin release is triggered by decreased blood pressure in the afferent arterioles, decreased sodium chloride concentration in the distal convoluted tubule, sympathetic nerve stimulation of β-adrenergic receptors on the juxtaglomerular cells, and the release of prostaglandins.[7] Numerous physiological effects of the RAAS stabilize systemic blood pressure and preserve the extracellular fluid volume during hypotension or hypovolemia. Actions include sodium reabsorption, systemic vasoconstriction, sympathetic nerve stimulation, and thirst stimulation with increased fluid intake. The effects of aldosterone combine with those of antidiuretic hormone (ADH) in regulating blood volume are summarized in Figure 29-9 (see also Figures 5-4 and 18-18).

Natriuretic peptides are synthesized and released from the heart and are natural antagonists to the RAAS. Natriuretic peptides cause vasodilation and increase sodium and water excretion and decrease blood pressure. They assist in protecting the heart from volume overload. **Urodilatin** is renal natriuretic peptide produced by cells in the distal convoluted tubule and collecting duct. It increases RBF, causing diuresis.

> **QUICK CHECK 29-2**
> 1. Where is pain from the ureters referred?
> 2. How do the bladder and urethra function in urine regulation?
> 3. What is autoregulation in the kidney? What other regulatory mechanisms are at work in renal function?

KIDNEY FUNCTION

Nephron Function

The nephron can perform many functions simultaneously (Figure 29-10), as follows:

1. Filters plasma at glomerulus.
2. Reabsorbs and secretes different substances along tubular structures.
3. Forms a filtrate of protein-free fluid (ultrafiltration).
4. Regulates the filtrate to maintain body fluid volume, electrolyte composition, and pH within narrow limits.

Glomerular filtration is the movement of fluid and solutes across the glomerular capillary membrane into the Bowman space. **Tubular reabsorption** is the movement of fluids and solutes from the tubular lumen to the peritubular capillary plasma. **Tubular secretion** is the transfer of substances from the plasma of the peritubular capillary to the tubular lumen. The transport mechanisms are both active and passive (processes defined in Chapter 1). **Excretion** is the elimination of a substance in the final urine (Figure 29-11).

Glomerular Filtration

The fluid filtered by the glomerular capillary filtration membrane and released into the proximal convoluted tubule is protein-free but contains electrolytes (such as sodium, chloride, and potassium) and organic molecules (such as creatinine, urea, and glucose) in the same concentrations as found in plasma. Like other capillary membranes, the glomerulus is freely permeable to water and relatively impermeable to large colloids, such as plasma proteins. The molecule's size and electrical charge and the small size of the filtration slits in the glomerular epithelium affect the permeability of substances crossing the glomerulus and entering the proximal convoluted tubule.

Capillary pressures also affect glomerular filtration. The hydrostatic pressure within the capillary is the major force for moving water and solutes across the filtration membrane and into the Bowman capsule. Two forces oppose the filtration effects of the glomerular capillary hydrostatic pressure (P_{GC}): (1) the Bowman capsule hydrostatic pressure (P_{BC}) and (2) the effective glomerular capillary oncotic pressure (π_{GC}). Because the fluid in the Bowman space normally contains only minute amounts of protein, it does not usually have an oncotic influence on the plasma of the glomerular capillary (Figure 29-12).

The combined effect of forces favouring and forces opposing filtration determines the filtration pressure. The **net filtration pressure (NFP)**

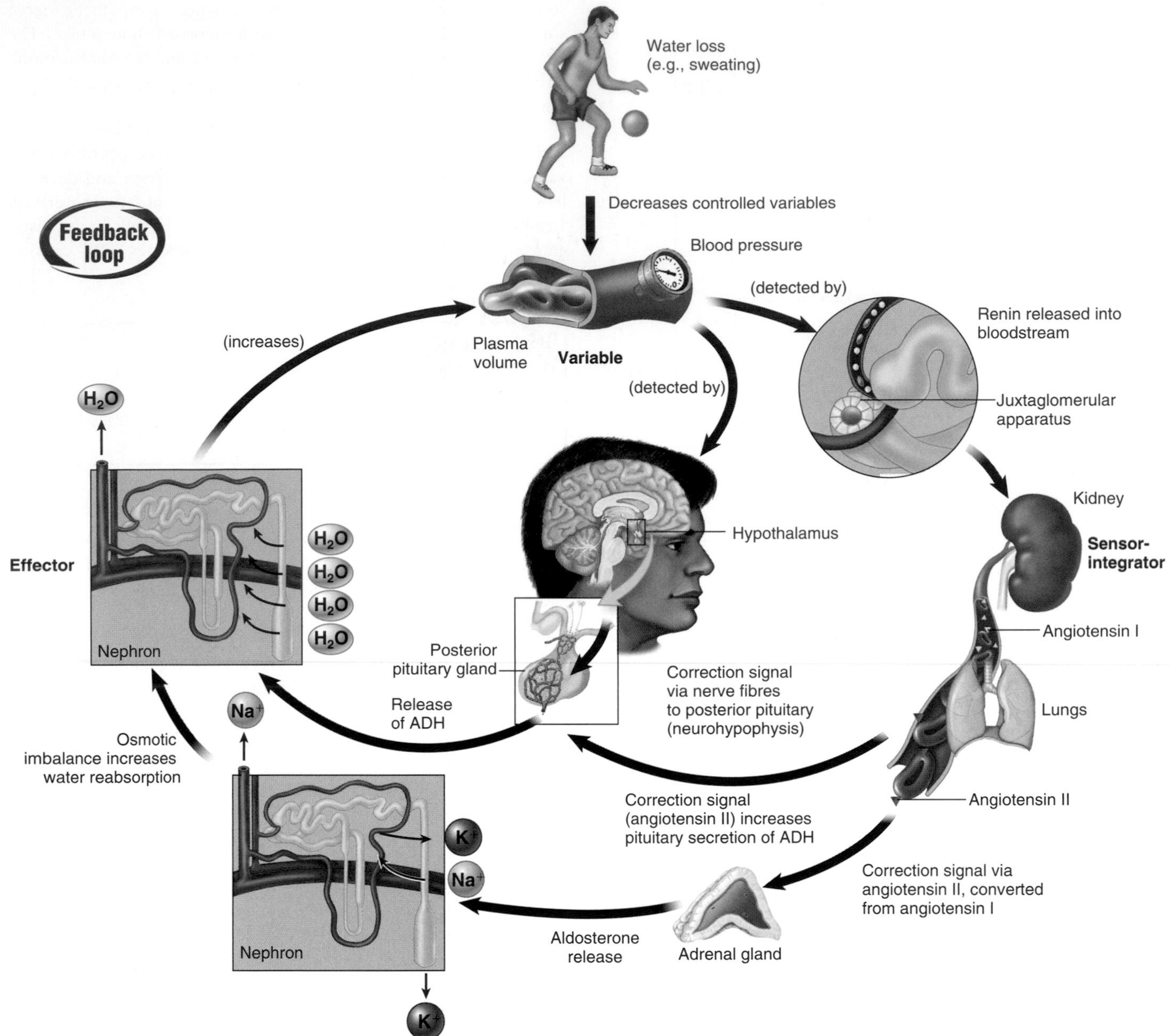

FIGURE 29-9 Cooperative Roles of Antidiuretic Hormone and Aldosterone in Regulating Urine and Plasma Volume. The drop in blood pressure that accompanies loss of fluid from the internal environment triggers the hypothalamus to rapidly release antidiuretic hormone (*ADH*) from the posterior pituitary gland. ADH increases water reabsorption by the kidney by increasing water permeability of the distal convoluted tubules and collecting ducts. The drop in blood pressure also is detected by each nephron's juxtaglomerular apparatus, which responds by secreting renin. Renin triggers the formation of angiotensin II, which stimulates release of aldosterone from the adrenal cortex. Aldosterone then slowly boosts water (H_2O) reabsorption by the kidneys by increasing reabsorption of sodium (Na^+). Because angiotensin II also stimulates secretion of ADH, it serves as an additional link between the ADH and aldosterone mechanisms. K^+, potassium. (From Patton, K.T., & Thibodeau, G.A. [2016]. *Anatomy & physiology* [9th ed.]. St. Louis: Mosby.)

is the sum of forces favouring and opposing filtration. The estimated values contributing to the forces of net filtration are presented in Table 29-1.

As the protein free fluid is filtered into the Bowman capsule, the plasma oncotic pressure increases and the hydrostatic pressure decreases. The increase in glomerular capillary oncotic pressure is great enough to reduce the NFP to zero at the efferent end of the capillary and to stop the filtration process effectively. The low hydrostatic pressure and the increased oncotic pressure in the efferent arteriole then are transferred to the peritubular capillaries and facilitate reabsorption of fluid from the proximal convoluted tubules.

Filtration rate. The total volume of fluid filtered by the glomeruli averages 180 L/day, or approximately 120 mL/min, a phenomenal amount considering the size of the kidneys. Because only 1 to 2 L of urine is excreted per day, 99% of the filtrate is reabsorbed into the peritubular capillaries and returned to the blood. The factors determining the GFR

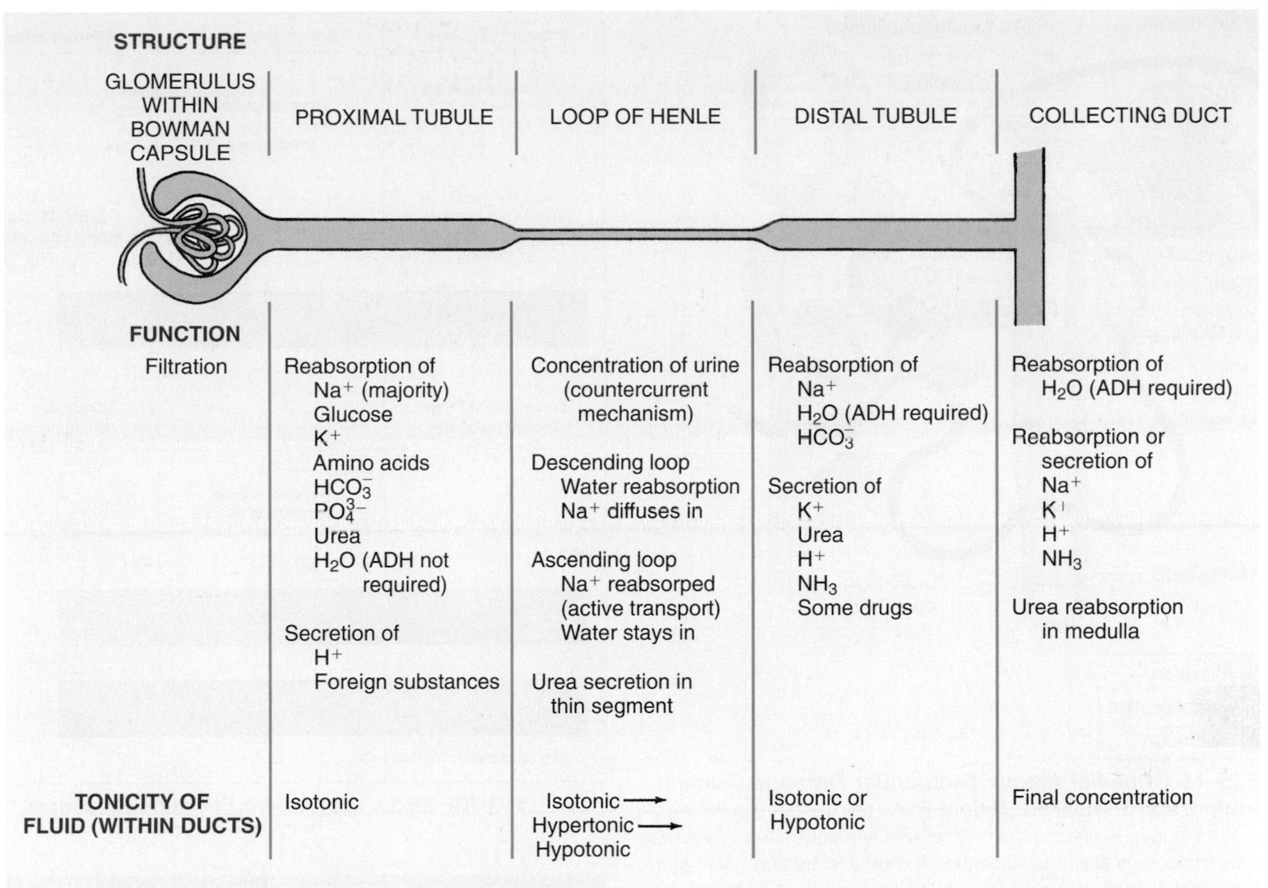

FIGURE 29-10 Major Functions of Nephron Segments. *ADH*, antidiuretic hormone; *H^+*, hydrogen; *H_2O*, water; *HCO_3^-*, bicarbonate; *K^+*, potassium; *Na^+*, sodium; *NH_3*, ammonia; *PO_4^{3-}*, phosphate. (Modified from Hockenberry, M.J., & Wilson, D. [Eds.]. [2007]. *Wong's nursing care of infants and children* [8th ed.]. St. Louis: Mosby.)

TABLE 29-1 Glomerular Filtration Pressures

Forces	Pressures	PRESSURES (mm Hg) Beginning of Capillary	End of Capillary
Promoting Filtration			
Glomerular capillary hydrostatic pressure	P_{GC}	47	45
Bowman capsule oncotic pressure	π_{BC}	Negligible effect	Negligible effect
Opposing Filtration			
Bowman capsule hydrostatic pressure	P_{BC}	10	10
Glomerular capillary oncotic pressure	π_{GC}	25	35
Net filtration pressure		12	0

are directly related to the pressures that favour or oppose filtration (see Figure 29-12 and Table 29-1).

Obstruction to the outflow of urine (caused by strictures, stones, or tumours along the urinary tract) can cause a retrograde increase in hydrostatic pressure at the Bowman space and a decrease in GFR. Low levels of plasma protein in the blood can result in a decrease in glomerular capillary oncotic pressure, which increases GFR. Excessive loss of *protein-free fluid* from vomiting, diarrhea, use of diuretics, or excessive sweating can increase glomerular capillary oncotic pressure and decrease the GFR. Renal disease also can cause changes in pressure relationships by altering capillary permeability and the surface area available for filtration (see Chapter 30).

Proximal convoluted tubule. By the end of the proximal tubule, approximately 60 to 70% of filtered sodium and water and about 50% of urea have been actively reabsorbed, along with 90% or more of potassium, glucose, bicarbonate, calcium, phosphate, amino acids, and uric acid. Chloride, water, and urea are reabsorbed passively but linked to the active transport of sodium (a co-transport mechanism). For some molecules, active transport in the renal tubules is limited as the carrier molecules become saturated, a phenomenon known as **transport maximum (T_m)**. For example, when the carrier molecules for glucose reabsorption in the proximal convoluted tubule become saturated (i.e., with the development of hyperglycemia), the excess will be excreted in the urine.

Active reabsorption of sodium is the primary function of the proximal convoluted tubule. Water, most other electrolytes, and organic substances are co-transported with sodium. The osmotic force generated by active sodium transport promotes the passive diffusion of water out of the tubular lumen and into the peritubular capillaries. Passive transport of water is further enhanced by the elevated oncotic pressure of the blood in the peritubular capillaries, which is created by the previous

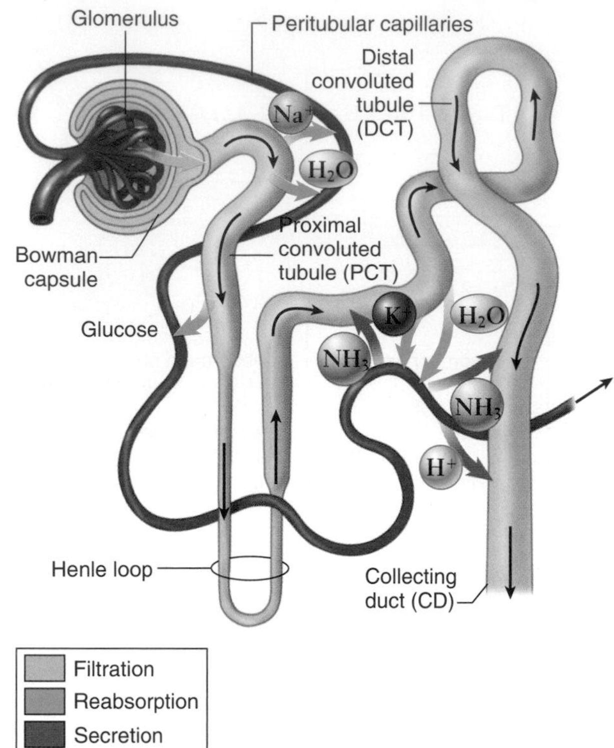

FIGURE 29-11 Urine Formation: Glomerular Filtration, Tubular Reabsorption, and Tubular Secretion. These are the three processes by which the kidneys excrete urine. Water (*H_2O*), electrolytes, glucose, and organic molecules are filtered at the glomerulus. Sodium (*Na^+*) and glucose are reabsorbed into peritubular capillaries by active transport from the proximal convoluted tubules, and H_2O reabsorption follows by osmosis. Na^+ is reabsorbed by active transport from distal convoluted tubules; more Na^+ is conserved when aldosterone is secreted. Osmotic reabsorption of H_2O from the distal convoluted tubules occurs when antidiuretic hormone is present. Secretion of ammonia (*NH_3*), hydrogen (*H^+*), and potassium (*K^+*) occurs from peritubular capillaries into distal convoluted tubules by active transport. (From Patton, K.T., & Thibodeau, G.A. [2014]. *The human body in health & disease* [6th ed.]. St. Louis: Mosby.)

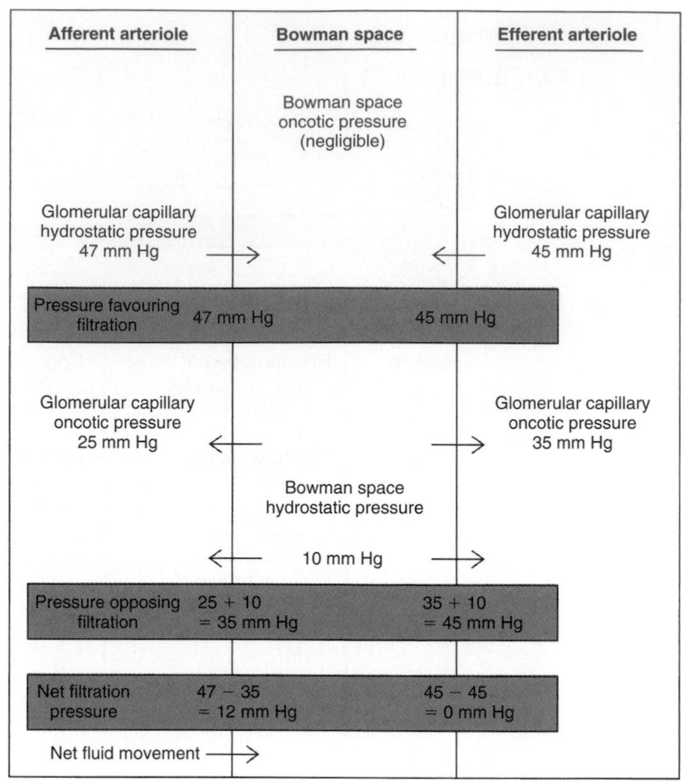

FIGURE 29-12 Glomerular Filtration Pressures.

filtration of water at the glomerulus. The reabsorption of water leaves an increased concentration of urea within the tubular lumen, creating a gradient for its passive diffusion to the peritubular plasma. As the positively charged sodium ions leave the tubular lumen, negatively charged chloride ions passively follow to maintain electroneutrality. Because the inner membrane of the proximal tubular cell has a limited permeability to chloride, chloride reabsorption lags behind sodium.

Hydrogen ions are actively exchanged for sodium ions in the tubular lumen. The hydrogen ions (H^+) then combine with bicarbonate.

Bicarbonate is completely filtered at the glomerulus, and approximately 90% is reabsorbed in the proximal tubule. In the tubular lumen, hydrogen and bicarbonate ions form carbonic acid (H_2CO_3), which rapidly breaks down, or dissociates, to carbon dioxide (CO_2) and water (H_2O). These then diffuse into the tubular cell, where carbonic anhydrase again catalyzes the CO_2 and H_2O to form bicarbonate (HCO_3^-) and H^+. The H^+ is secreted again, and bicarbonate combines with sodium and is transported to the peritubular capillary blood as $NaHCO_3$ (a sodium bicarbonate buffer). Bicarbonate is thus conserved, and the hydrogen is reabsorbed as water. Therefore, these ions normally do not contribute to the urinary excretion of acid or the addition of acid to the blood.

In addition to the proximal tubular secretion of hydrogen ions, secretory transport mechanisms exist for creatinine, other organic bases, and endogenous and exogenous organic acids including *para*-aminohippurate (PAH) and penicillin (Box 29-1). These secretory mechanisms eliminate medications and other exogenous chemical products from the body, often after first conjugating them with sulphate and glucuronic acid in the liver. Many medications and their metabolites are eliminated from the body in this way. When the renal tubules are damaged, metabolic by-products and medications may accumulate, causing toxic levels in the body.

BOX 29-1 Substances Transported by Renal Tubules

Reabsorption	Secretion
Albumin	Choline
Ascorbate	Creatinine
Fructose	Histamine
Galactose	Methylguanidine
Glutamate	*para*-Aminohippurate
Glucose	Penicillin and many other medications
Phosphate	Steroid glucuronides
Sulphate	Thiamine
Xylose	

Normally, 99% of the glomerular filtrate is reabsorbed. When the GFR spontaneously decreases or increases, the renal tubules, primarily the proximal tubules, automatically adjust their rate of reabsorption of sodium and water to balance the change in GFR. This prevents wide fluctuations in the excretion of sodium and water into the urine and is known as **glomerulotubular balance**.

Loop of Henle and distal convoluted tubule. Urine can be hypotonic, isotonic, or hypertonic. **Urine concentration** or **urine dilution** occurs principally in the loop of Henle, distal convoluted tubules, and collecting

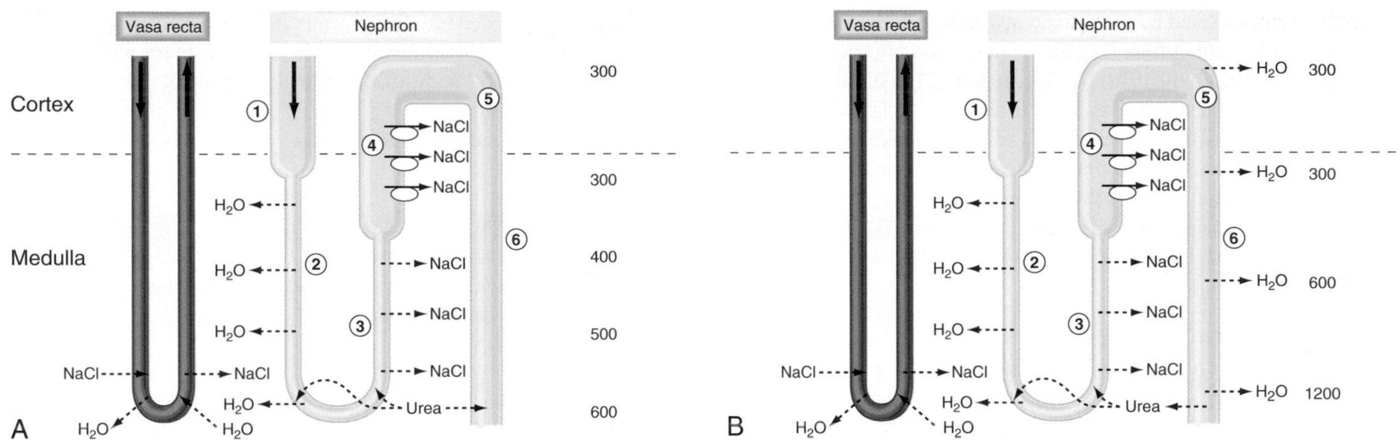

FIGURE 29-13 Countercurrent Mechanism for Concentrating and Diluting Urine. **A,** Urine dilution; **B,** urine concentration. **1,** Filtrate isotonic to plasma. **2,** Descending thin limb permeable to water (*H_2O*). **3,** Ascending thin limb impermeable to H_2O; permeable to ions. **4,** Ascending thick limb actively transports sodium chloride (*NaCl*); impermeable to H_2O and urea. **5,** Distal convoluted tubule actively resorbs NaCl; resorbs H_2O in presence of antidiuretic hormone. **6,** Medullary collecting duct actively resorbs NaCl, and slightly permeable to H_2O and urea. (NOTE: Numbers on illustration represent milliosmoles [mOsm]). See text for details. (From Koeppen, B.M., & Stanton, B.A. [2010]. *Berne and Levy physiology* [6th ed., updated]. St. Louis: Mosby.)

ducts. The structural features of the medullary hairpin loops allow the kidney to concentrate urine and conserve water for the body. The transition of the filtrate into the final urine reflects the concentrating ability of the loops. Final adjustments in urine composition are made by the distal convoluted tubule and collecting duct according to body needs.

Production of concentrated urine involves a countercurrent exchange system, in which fluid flows in opposite directions through the parallel tubes of the loop of Henle. A concentration gradient causes fluid to be exchanged across the parallel pathways. The longer the loop, the greater the concentration gradient; the concentration gradient increases from the cortex to the tip of the medulla. The loops of Henle multiply the concentration gradient, and the vasa recta blood vessels act as a countercurrent exchanger for maintaining the gradient. The process is initiated in the thick ascending limb of the loop of Henle with the active transport of chloride and sodium out of the tubular lumen and into the medullary interstitium (Figure 29-13). Because the lumen of the ascending limb is impermeable to water, water cannot follow the sodium–chloride transport. This impermeability to water causes the ascending tubular fluid to become hypo-osmotic and the medullary interstitium to become hyperosmotic. The descending limb of the loop, which receives fluid from the proximal tubule, is highly permeable to water but it is the only place in the nephron that does not actively transport either sodium or chloride. Sodium and chloride may, however, diffuse into the descending tubule from the interstitium. The hyperosmotic medullary interstitium causes water to move out of the descending limb, and the remaining fluid in the descending tubule becomes increasingly concentrated while it flows toward the tip of the medulla. While the tubular fluid rounds the loop and enters the ascending limb, sodium and chloride are removed and water is retained. The fluid then becomes more and more dilute as it encounters the distal convoluted tubule.

The slow rate of blood flow and the hairpin structure of the vasa recta blood vessels allow blood to flow through the medullary tissue without disturbing the osmotic gradient. When blood flows into the descending limb of the vasa recta, it encounters the increasing osmotic concentration gradient of the medullary interstitium. Water moves out and sodium and chloride diffuse into the descending vasa recta. The plasma becomes increasingly concentrated as it flows toward the tip of the medulla.

As blood flows away from the tip of the medulla and toward the cortex, the surrounding interstitial fluid becomes comparatively more dilute. Water then moves back into the vasa recta, and sodium and chloride diffuse out and the plasma again becomes more dilute. The net result is a preservation of the medullary osmotic gradient. If blood were to flow rapidly through the vasa recta, as occurs in some renal diseases, the medullary concentration gradient would be washed away and the ability to concentrate urine and conserve water would be lost. The efficiency of water conservation is related to the length of the loops of Henle: the longer the loops, the greater the ability to concentrate the urine.

Urea is the major constituent of urine along with water. The glomerulus freely filters urea, and tubular reabsorption depends on urine flow rate, with less reabsorption at higher flow rates. Approximately 50% of urea is excreted in the urine, and 50% is recycled within the kidney. This recycling contributes to the osmotic gradient within the medulla and is necessary for the concentration and dilution of urine (see Figure 29-13). Because urea is an end product of protein metabolism, individuals with protein deprivation cannot maximally concentrate their urine.[8]

Another function of the loop of Henle is the production of uromodulin (also known as Tamm-Horsfall protein [THP]), the most abundant protein in human urine. This protein binds to uropathogens to prevent urinary tract infection, protects the uroepithelium from injury, protects against kidney stone formation, and is associated with progression of kidney disease.[9]

The convoluted portion of the distal convoluted tubule is poorly permeable to water but readily reabsorbs ions and contributes to the dilution of the tubular fluid. The later, straight segment of the distal convoluted tubule and the collecting duct are permeable to water as controlled by ADH released from the posterior pituitary gland. Sodium is readily reabsorbed by the later segment of the distal convoluted tubule and collecting duct under the regulation of the hormone aldosterone (see Chapter 18). Potassium is actively secreted in these segments and is also controlled by aldosterone and other factors related to the concentration of potassium in body fluids (see Chapter 5).

Hydrogen is secreted by the distal convoluted tubule and combines with nonbicarbonate buffers (i.e., ammonium and phosphate) for the elimination of acids in the urine (see Figure 5-11). The distal convoluted tubule thus contributes to the regulation of acid–base balance by excreting hydrogen ions into the urine and by adding new bicarbonate to the plasma. The mechanism is similar to the conservation of bicarbonate by the proximal tubule, except that the hydrogen ion is excreted in the urine and influences acid–base balance (see Figure 5-11). The specific mechanisms of acid–base balance and acid excretion are described in Chapter 5.

Urine Composition

Urine is normally clear yellow or amber in colour. Cloudiness may indicate the presence of bacteria, cells, or high solute concentration. The pH ranges from 4.6 to 8.0, but it is normally acidic, providing protection against bacteria. Specific gravity ranges from 1.001 to 1.035. Normal urine does not contain glucose or blood cells and only occasionally contains traces of protein, usually in association with rigorous exercise.

Hormones and Nephron Function

Antidiuretic Hormone

The distal convoluted tubule in the cortex receives the hypo-osmotic urine from the ascending limb of the loop of Henle. The concentration of the final urine is controlled by **antidiuretic hormone (ADH)**, which is secreted from the posterior pituitary or neurohypophysis. ADH increases water permeability and reabsorption in the last segment of the distal convoluted tubule and along the entire length of the collecting ducts, which pass through the inner and outer zones of the medulla. The water diffuses into the ascending limb of the vasa recta and returns to the systemic circulation. The excreted urine can have a high osmotic concentration, up to 1 400 mOsm. The volume is normally reduced to about 1% of the amount filtered at the glomerulus. (The mechanism for the regulation of ADH and plasma osmolality is described in Chapters 5 and 18.)

Aldosterone

Aldosterone is synthesized and secreted by the adrenal cortex under the regulation of the RAAS (see Chapter 18). Aldosterone stimulates the epithelial cells of the distal convoluted tubule and collecting duct to reabsorb sodium (promoting water reabsorption) and increases the excretion of potassium and hydrogen ion.

Natriuretic Peptides

Natriuretic peptides are a group of peptide hormones, including **atrial natriuretic peptide (ANP)**, secreted from myocardial cells in the atria, and B-type natriuretic peptide (BNP), secreted from myocardial cells in the cardiac ventricles.[10] When the heart dilates during volume expansion or heart failure, ANP and BNP inhibit sodium and water absorption by kidney tubules, inhibit secretion of renin and aldosterone, vasodilate the afferent arterioles, and constrict the efferent arterioles. The result is increased urine formation leading to a decrease in blood volume and blood pressure. C-type natriuretic peptide is secreted from the vascular endothelium and causes vasodilation in the nephron. Urodilatin is secreted by the distal convoluted tubules and collecting ducts and causes vasodilation and natriuretic and diuretic effects.

Diuretics as a Factor in Urine Flow

A **diuretic** is any agent enhancing the flow of urine. Clinically, diuretics interfere with renal sodium reabsorption and reduce extracellular fluid volume. Diuretics are commonly used to treat hypertension and edema caused by heart failure, cirrhosis, and nephrotic syndrome.

Diuretics are divided into five general categories: (1) osmotic diuretics, (2) carbonic anhydrase inhibitors (inhibitors of urinary acidification), (3) inhibitors of loop sodium or chloride transport, (4) aldosterone antagonists (potassium-sparing diuretics), and (5) aquaretics. (The physiological mechanism related to each category is summarized in Table 29-2.)

Renal Hormones

Certain hormones are either activated or synthesized by the kidney. These hormones have significant systemic effects and include urodilatin, the active form of vitamin D, and EPO.

Vitamin D

Vitamin D is a hormone that can be obtained in the diet or synthesized by the action of ultraviolet radiation (sun exposure) on cholesterol in the skin. These forms of vitamin D_3 (cholecalciferol) are inactive and require two hydroxylations to establish a metabolically active form. The first step occurs in the liver and the second in the kidneys.

Vitamin D is necessary for the absorption of calcium and phosphate by the small intestine (see *Health Promotion:* Vitamin D Supplementation). The renal hydroxylation step is stimulated by parathyroid hormone (see Chapter 18). A decreased plasma calcium level (less than 2.25 mmol/L) stimulates the secretion of parathyroid hormone. Parathyroid hormone then stimulates a sequence of events to help restore plasma calcium concentration toward normal levels (2.25 to 2.75 mmol/L):

1. Calcium mobilization from bone
2. Synthesis of 1,25-dihydroxy-vitamin D_3
3. Absorption of calcium from the intestine
4. Increased renal calcium reabsorption
5. Decreased renal phosphate reabsorption

Serum phosphate concentration fluctuations also influence the renal hydroxylation of vitamin D. Decreased levels stimulate active 1,25-dihydroxy-vitamin D_3 formation, and increased levels inhibit formation. The formation of 1,25-dihydroxy-vitamin D_3 results in compensatory changes in phosphate absorption from bone and intestine. Individuals with renal disease have a deficiency of 1,25-dihydroxy-vitamin D_3 and manifest symptoms of disturbed calcium and phosphate balance (see Chapters 5, 18, and 30).

HEALTH PROMOTION

Vitamin D Supplementation

Most Canadians (68%) have blood concentrations of vitamin D over 50 nmol/L—a level that is sufficient for healthy bones in most people. However, about 32% of Canadians fall below this cut-off. Children aged 3 to 5 have the highest rates above the cut-off (89%), while 20- to 39-year-olds have the lowest (59%).

A minority of Canadians (34%) take a supplement containing vitamin D, but a larger percentage of those taking supplements are above the cut-off (85%), compared with nonsupplement users (59%). About 40% of Canadians fall below the cut-off in winter, compared with 25% in the summer.

On average, females have a higher concentration of vitamin D in their blood than males.

Adding vitamin D to cow's milk and margarine is mandatory in Canada as a preventive measure against rickets, osteomalacia, and osteoporosis. It is also added to some foods, such as goat's milk, fortified plant-based beverages (such as fortified soy beverages), and calcium-fortified orange juice.

Data from Statistics Canada. (2015). *Health at a glance: Vitamin D blood levels of Canadians.* Retrieved from http://www.statcan.gc.ca/pub/82-624-x/2013001/article/11727-eng.htm.

TABLE 29-2 **Action of Diuretics**

Diuretic	Site of Action	Action	Common Side Effects
Osmotic Diuretics			
Mannitol (Osmitrol) Glycerol Urea (Ureaphil)	Proximal tubule	Freely filtered but not reabsorbed; osmotically attract water and diminish sodium reabsorption	Hypokalemia, dehydration
Carbonic Anhydrase Inhibitors			
Acetazolamide (Diamox)	Proximal tubule	Inhibits carbonic anhydrase; blocks hydrogen ion secretion and reabsorption of sodium and bicarbonate	Hypokalemia, systemic acidosis, alkaline urine
Inhibitors of Sodium or Chloride Reabsorption			
Thiazides Hydrochlorothiazide (HCTZ, Urozide)	Distal convoluted tubules	Inhibit sodium and chloride reabsorption; mildly suppress carbonic anhydrase; reduce calcium excretion	Hypokalemia, metabolic alkalosis
Furosemide (Lasix) Ethacrynic acid (Edecrin)	Thick ascending limb of loop of Henle	Inhibit active transport of chloride, sodium, and potassium	Hypokalemia, uric acid retention
Torsemide (Demadex) Bumetanide (Burinex)	Cortical vasodilation	Increase rate of urine formation	Hypokalemia, uric acid retention
Potassium-Sparing Diuretics			
Spironolactone (Aldactone)	Distal convoluted tubule/ collecting duct	Inhibits aldosterone, blocks sodium reabsorption, and results in potassium retention	Hyperkalemia, nausea, confusion, gynecomastia
Triamterene (APO Triazide) and amiloride (Midamor)	Distal convoluted tubule/ collecting duct	Inhibit sodium reabsorption and inhibit potassium excretion	Nausea, vomiting, headache, granulocytopenia, skin rash
Aquaretics			
Vasopressin (V_2) blockers (e.g., conivaptan [Vaprisol])	Distal convoluted tubule/ collecting ducts	Block action of antidiuretic hormone	Dehydration

Erythropoietin

Erythropoietin (EPO) stimulates the bone marrow to produce red blood cells in response to tissue hypoxia and may have tissue-protective effects.[11] Erythrocyte production is discussed in Chapter 20. The stimulus for EPO release is decreased oxygen delivery in the kidneys. Oxygen-sensing EPO-producing cells are peritubular fibroblasts located in the juxtamedullary cortex.[12] The anemia of chronic kidney disease, in which kidney cells have become nonfunctional, can be related to the lack of this hormone (see Chapter 30).

Kidney function changes throughout the lifespan, and major changes are summarized in the following boxes: *Health Promotion:* Kidney Failure in Canada, *Pediatric Considerations:* Pediatrics and Renal Function, and *Geriatric Considerations:* Aging and Renal Function.

✔ QUICK CHECK 29-3

1. Outline the process of glomerular filtration.
2. What types of absorption/reabsorption take place in the proximal tubule, the loops of Henle, and the distal convoluted tubule?
3. What is the countercurrent exchange system? What substances are involved?
4. What hormones are activated or synthesized by the kidney?

TESTS OF RENAL FUNCTION

Renal Clearance

A number of specific renal functions can be measured by renal clearance. Renal clearance techniques determine how much of a substance can be cleared from the blood by the kidneys per given unit of time. The application of this principle permits an indirect measure of GFR, tubular secretion, tubular reabsorption, and RBF.

Clearance and Renal Blood Flow

A clearance formula also can be used to estimate RPF and RBF using a molecule called *para*-aminohippuric acid (PAH). Some PAH is filtered at the glomerulus, and most of the remainder is secreted into the tubules in one circulation through the kidney. If all the PAH were removed from the plasma during a single pass through the kidney, total RPF could be determined. Because the supporting and nonsecreting structures of the kidney receive 10 to 15% of the effective renal blood flow (ERBF), clearance of PAH measures only what is known as the effective renal plasma flow (ERPF), which is 85 to 90% of the true RPF.

Clearance and Glomerular Filtration Rate

The GFR provides the best estimate of functioning renal tissue and is important for assessing or monitoring kidney damage and medication dosing. Damage to the glomerular membrane or loss of nephrons leads to a corresponding decrease in GFR. The measurement of GFR requires the use of a substance that has a stable plasma concentration; is freely filtered at the glomerulus; is not secreted, reabsorbed, or metabolized by the tubules; and is easy to measure. Inulin (a fructose polysaccharide) is one substance that meets the criteria for measurement of GFR.

The accurate determination of inulin clearance requires constant infusion to maintain a stable plasma level. This is time-consuming and inconvenient. Therefore, the clearance of creatinine, a natural substance produced by muscle and released into the blood at a relatively constant rate, is commonly used as an estimate clinically. It is freely filtered at the glomerulus, but a small amount is secreted by the renal tubules.

HEALTH PROMOTION

Kidney Failure in Canada

An estimated 1 in 10 Canadians has kidney disease, and millions more are at risk of developing the disease. Each day, an average of 15 people (nearly 5500 per year) are told that their kidneys have failed. The two leading causes of kidney failure in new patients are diabetes (38%) and renal vascular disease (including high blood pressure) (14%). In 2012, kidney disease was the 10th leading cause of death in Canada.

The number of Canadians being treated for kidney failure has tripled over the past 20 years. A full 47% of new kidney failure patients starting renal replacement therapy are under age 65. Among the 36 251 people being treated for kidney failure in Canada in 2015, 58.5% (21 214) were on dialysis and 41.5% (15 037) had a functioning transplant.

Hemodialysis is the treatment used in the majority of dialysis cases, and it costs roughly $56 000–$107 000 per patient per year. The one-time cost for a kidney transplant in Canada, including donor costs, is approximately $100 000, plus $20 000 in care costs for year two and decreasing annually each year thereafter. Over a 5-year period, a transplant is approximately $250 000 less expensive per patient than dialysis and improves the patient's quality of life.

Nearly 76% of the over 4585 Canadians on the waiting list for an organ transplant are waiting for a kidney. In 2015, nearly one-third of the people who died while waiting for organs were waiting for a kidney (73 people). There were 1513 kidney transplants performed in 2015. Nearly 46.5% of kidney transplants are made possible by living donors. Donor rates have stagnated since 2006 (14 to 17 donors per million population). Kidney patients waited a median time of 4 years in 2017 for a deceased-donor kidney transplant. Median wait times for 2013–2015 were longest in Saskatchewan (5.4 years) and Manitoba (5.3 years), and shortest in Nova Scotia (2.5 years).

Diabetes is the leading cause of kidney disease. Screening for kidney disease in people with diabetes involves an assessment of urinary albumin excretion and a measurement of the overall level of kidney function through an estimation of the glomerular filtration rate (GFR). Patients with type 1 diabetes often do not have kidney disease at the time of onset of diabetes, so screening can be postponed until the duration of diabetes exceeds 5 years (5 years after the initial diagnosis). For patients with type 2 diabetes, the delay between onset and diagnosis can be several years. As such, significant renal disease can be present at the time of diagnosis, so screening should be initiated immediately at the time of diagnosis in type 2 diabetes. In adults, screening for chronic kidney disease (CKD) in diabetes should be conducted using a random urine albumin-to-creatinine ratio (ACR) and a serum creatinine converted into a GFR. A diagnosis of CKD should be made in patients with a random urine ACR greater than or equal to 2 mg/mmol and/or an estimated glomerular filtration rate (eGFR) of less than 60 mL/min in at least two of three samples over a 3-month period. Adults with diabetes and CKD with either hypertension or albuminuria should receive an angiotensin-converting enzyme (ACE) inhibitor or an angiotensin receptor blocker (ARB) to delay progression of CKD. People with diabetes who are on an ACE inhibitor or an ARB should have their serum creatinine and potassium levels checked at baseline and within 1 to 2 weeks of initiation or titration of therapy and during times of acute illness.

Data from The Kidney Foundation of Canada. (2017). *Facing the facts.* Montreal: Author. Data for the report taken from multiple sources. Retrieved from https://kidney.ca/file/kidney.ca_nat/news-press-releases/Facing-the-Facts-2017_final.pdf; Canadian Diabetes Association Clinical Practice Guidelines Expert Committee. (2013). Canadian Diabetes Association 2013 Clinical Practice Guidelines for the Prevention and Management of Diabetes in Canada. *Can J Diabetes,* 37(suppl 1): S1–S212.

Therefore, creatinine clearance overestimates the GFR, but within tolerable limits. Creatinine clearance provides a good clinical measure of GFR because only one blood sample is required in addition to an accurately collected 24-hour volume of urine. **Cystatin C** is a stable protein in serum filtered at the glomerulus and metabolized in the tubules. Serum levels of cystatin C also are a marker for estimating GFR, particularly for mild to moderate impaired renal function.[13] A combined creatinine and cystatin C estimate of GFR was developed in 2012 and considers age, race, and sex.[14]

Formulas are used to estimate GFR.[15] The Cockcroft–Gault formula is commonly used and considers age, body weight, and plasma creatinine (P_{cr}) values. The National Kidney Foundation in the United States recommends using the Modification of Diet in Renal Disease (MDRD) equation.[16] The Chronic Kidney Disease Epidemiology Collaboration (2009 CKD-EPI) equation has been developed as a more precise estimate of GFR than the MDRD and considers age, sex, and ethnicity.[17] In 2012, cystatin C and combined creatinine and cystatin C equations were developed. Calculators for estimates of GFR using these formulas are readily available on the Internet (e.g., see http://touchcalc.com/ip_epi_gfr/ip_ckd_epi). Normal GFR values are 90 to 120 mL/min.

Plasma Creatinine Concentration

A chronic decline in the GFR over weeks or months is reflected in the **plasma creatinine (P_{cr}) concentration** (normal value = 44 to 97 mcmol/L for females; 53 to 106 mcmol/L for males). The P_{cr} concentration has a stable value when the GFR is stable, because creatinine has a constant rate of production as a product of muscle metabolism. The amount filtered is approximately equal to the amount excreted. When the GFR declines, the P_{cr} increases proportionately. Thus the GFR and P_{cr} are inversely related. If the GFR were to decrease by 50%, the filtration and excretion of creatinine would be reduced by 50% and creatinine would accumulate in plasma to twice the normal value. Therefore, elevated P_{cr} values represent decreasing GFR. In the new steady state, however, the total amount of creatinine excreted in the urine would remain the same because of the proportionate decrease in GFR and increase in P_{cr}.

The application of this principle is simple and useful for monitoring progressive changes in renal function. The test is most valuable for monitoring the progress of chronic rather than acute renal disease because it takes 7 to 10 days for the plasma creatinine level to stabilize when GFR declines. Serial measures can be obtained over a long time and plotted as a curve of glomerular function. The P_{cr} also becomes elevated during trauma or the breakdown of muscle tissue. In such instances, the value is then not useful for estimating GFR.

Blood Urea Nitrogen

The concentration of urea nitrogen in the blood reflects glomerular filtration and urine-concentrating capacity. Because urea is filtered at the glomerulus, blood urea nitrogen (BUN) levels increase as glomerular filtration drops. Because urea is reabsorbed by the blood through the permeable tubules, the BUN value rises in states of dehydration and with acute and chronic kidney disease when passage of fluid through the tubules slows. BUN values also change as a result of altered protein intake and protein catabolism. The normal range for BUN level in the adult is 3.6 to 7.1 mmol/L of blood.

Urinalysis

Urinalysis is a noninvasive and relatively inexpensive diagnostic pro cedure. The best results are obtained from a fresh, cleanly voided specimen because decay permits changes in the composition of urine. Urinalysis includes evaluation of colour, turbidity, protein, pH, specific gravity, sediment, and supernatant. Urine tests are listed in Table 29-3, and bladder function tests are listed in Table 29-4.

TABLE 29-3 Normal Renal Function Tests

Test	Normal Value	Interpretation
Urine		
Colour	Amber-yellow	Medications and foods may change urine colour
Turbidity	Clear	Purulent matter will make urine cloudy
pH	4.6–8.0	Bacteria create an alkaline urine
Specific gravity (density of water = 1.000)		Gravity represents concentrating ability or density of urine in relation to density of water (i.e., higher when contains glucose or protein; lower with dilute urine)
Adults	1.010–1.025	
Infants	1.010–1.018	
Blood	Negative	Blood indicates bleeding along urinary tract
Microscopic Urine		
Bacteria	None	Bacteria indicates infection
Red blood cells	Negative	Red blood cells indicate bleeding along urinary tract
White blood cells	Negative	White blood cells indicate urinary tract infection
Crystals	Negative	Crystals may indicate stones
Fat	Negative	Fat can be associated with nephrosis
Casts	Occasional	A few casts are normal; many may represent renal disease
Urinary Chemistry		
Bilirubin	Negative	An increase may cause dark orange colour
Urobilinogen	0.5–4 mg/24 hours	An increase may indicate red blood cell hemolysis
Ketones	Negative	Ketones represent an increase in fat metabolism
Glucose	Negative	Glucose usually signifies hyperglycemia
Sodium	40–220 mmol/day	Sodium can increase or decrease with renal disease
Potassium	25–120 mmol/day	Potassium can increase or decrease with renal disease, potassium intake, aldosteronism, or diuretic use
Protein	Negative-trace	Protein indicates dysfunction of glomerulus
Normal Serum Values		
BUN	3.6–7.1 mmol/L	Blood urea nitrogen (BUN) is elevated with diseased kidneys
Creatinine	Elevated with decreased GFR	
Male	53–106 mcmol/L	
Female	44–97 mcmol/L	
Cystatin C	0.0444–0.11667 mmol/L	This test provides early detection of decreased glomerular filtration rate (GFR)
Potassium		Potassium is elevated in kidney failure

TABLE 29-4 Bladder Function Tests

Procedure	Description
Urodynamic Tests	
Cystometry (cystometrogram)	Measures bladder pressure using a pressure-measuring catheter; fluid volume and pressures are measured as bladder is filled with fluid; simultaneous pressures may be measured in rectum; sensations of bladder fullness are also recorded; coughing or straining can lead to involuntary bladder contractions Bladder capacity: male, 350–750 mL; female, 350–550 mL Intrabladder pressure with empty bladder: 40 cm H_2O Detrusor pressure: <10 cm H_2O Residual urine: <30 mL
Uroflowmetry	Measures time it takes to empty a full bladder of urine; flow rates may be faster with urge incontinence or slower with prostatic obstruction
Postvoid residual urine	Measures residual urine in bladder after voiding; urine can be removed with catheter and measured, or ultrasound imaging can be used to measure urine; postvoid residual of more than 200 mL is abnormal and requires further evaluation
Measurement of leak point pressure	Measures pressure at which bladder fluid will leak from bladder without warning
Pressure flow study	Measures pressure required to empty bladder; pressure flow study identifies bladder outlet obstruction such as that occurring with prostate enlargement
Electromyography	Measures nerve impulses and muscle activity in urethral sphincter by placing sensors on skin near urethra and rectum or by placing sensors on catheter placed in urethra or rectum
Video urodynamics	Takes pictures and videos during filling and emptying of bladder; imaging equipment uses X-rays or ultrasound waves; this test shows size and shape of urinary tract
Direct Visualization Diagnostic Procedures	
Cystoscopy	Cystoscope (a type of endoscope) is inserted through urethra and is used to visualize inside of bladder
Ureteroscopy	Ureteroscope is inserted through urethra and bladder and directly into ureter and upper urinary tract to visualize upper urinary tract

H_2O, water.

✔ QUICK CHECK 29-4

1. Why is creatinine clearance a good estimate of glomerular filtration rate (GFR)?
2. What is the relationship between plasma creatinine concentration and GFR?

PEDIATRIC CONSIDERATIONS

Pediatrics and Renal Function

Glomerular filtration rate (GFR) in infants does not reach adult levels until 1 to 2 years of age, and newborns have a decreased ability to efficiently remove excess water and solutes. Their shorter loops of Henle also decrease concentrating ability and produce a more dilute urine than that produced by adults. Risks for metabolic acidosis are increased during the first few months of life while the mechanisms for excreting acid and retaining bicarbonate are maturing. These normal developmental processes result in a narrow safety margin for fluid and electrolyte balance when there is any disturbance such as diarrhea, infection, fever, fasting for diagnostic tests, improper feeding, fluid replacement, or medication administration. Newborns diurese 2 to 3 days after birth, which is reflected by a decrease in total body water and body weight. An increased risk of toxicity accompanies medication administration. Low–birth weight infants have a delay in achieving full renal function and may not have full GFR until 8 years of age. They also are at a greater risk for low nephron numbers and chronic kidney disease as adults.

Data from Filler, G., Yasin, A., & Medeiros, M. (2014). *Pediatr Nephrol, 29*(2), 183–192; Hoseini, R., Otukesh, H., Rahimzadeh, et al. (2012). *Iran J Kidney Dis, 6*(3), 166–172; Lankadeva, Y.R., Singh, R.R., Tare, M., et al. (2014). *Am J Physiol Renal Physiol, 306*(8), F791–F800; Sulemanji, M., & Vakili, K. (2013). *Semin Pediatr Surg, 22*(4), 195–198.

GERIATRIC CONSIDERATIONS

Aging and Renal Function

- Structural changes commonly occur in the kidney with aging, including loss of renal mass, arterial sclerosis, an increased number of sclerotic glomeruli, loss of tubules, and interstitial fibrosis. These changes contribute to a slow decline in glomerular filtration rate (GFR) and a reduction in creatinine clearance in most individuals, but it generally is not significant enough to lead to severe loss of renal function. As the number of nephrons decreases and degenerative changes occur, nephrons are less able to concentrate urine and less able to tolerate dehydration, excessive water loads, or electrolyte imbalances, particularly with physiological stress. Up to 45% of people older than 70 years of age have chronic kidney disease.
- The presence of comordid conditions, such as hypertension and diabetes mellitus, accelerates the decline of renal function. Obesity does not accelerate a decline in GFR.
- Response to acid–base changes and reabsorption of glucose may be delayed.
- Medications eliminated by the kidney can accumulate in the plasma, causing toxic reactions; GFR and medication dosage should be carefully evaluated.
- Decreased thirst sensation and diminished water intake may alter water balance.
- Impairment in renal blood flow, hormonal regulatory systems, and metabolism of medications may alter sodium and water balance.
- Older donor kidneys show decreased regenerative capacity.

Data from Baldea, A.J. (2009). *Surg Clin North Am, 95*(1), 71–83; Bolignano, D., Mattace-Raso, F., Sijbrands, E.J., et al. (2014). *Ageing Res Rev, 14*, 65–80; Karam, Z., & Tuazon, J. (2013). *Clin Geriatr Med, 29*(3), 555–564; Presta, P., Lucisano, G., Fuiano, L., et al. (2012). *Int Urol Nephrol, 44*(2), 625–632; Sands, J.M. (2012). *J Gerontol A Biol Sci Med Sci, 67*(12), 1352–1357; Schmitt, R., & Melk, A. (2012). *Am J Transplant, 12*(11), 2892–2900; Tonelli, M., & Riella, M.C. (2014). *Nat Rev Nephrol, 10*(3), 127–128.

DID YOU UNDERSTAND?

Structures of the Renal System

1. The kidneys are paired structures lying bilaterally between the twelfth thoracic and third lumbar vertebrae and behind the peritoneum of the abdominal cavity.
2. The kidney is composed of an outer cortex and an inner medulla.
3. The calyces receive urine from the distal convoluted tubules and join to form the renal pelvis, which is continuous with the upper end of the ureter.
4. The nephron is the urine-forming unit of the kidney and is composed of the glomerulus, proximal convoluted tubule, hairpin loops of Henle, distal convoluted tubule, and collecting duct.
5. The glomerulus contains loops of capillaries supported by mesangial cells. The capillary walls serve as a filtration membrane for the formation of the primary urine.
6. The proximal tubule is lined with microvilli to increase surface area and enhance reabsorption of water, solutes, and electrolytes.
7. The hairpin loops of Henle transport solutes and water, contributing to the hypertonic state of the medulla, and are important for the concentration and dilution of urine.
8. The distal convoluted tubule adjusts acid–base balance by excreting acid into the urine and forming new bicarbonate ions. It reabsorbs water with the influence of antidiuretic hormone and reabsorbs sodium and excretes potassium with the influence of aldosterone.
9. The ureters extend from the renal pelvis to the posterior wall of the bladder. Urine flows through the ureters and into the bladder by means of peristaltic contraction of the ureteral muscles.
10. The bladder is a bag composed of the detrusor and trigone muscles and innervated by parasympathetic fibres. When accumulation of urine reaches 250 to 300 mL, mechanoreceptors, which respond to stretching of tissue, stimulate the micturition reflex.

Renal Blood Flow

1. Renal blood flows at about 1 000 to 1 200 mL/min, or 20 to 25% of the cardiac output.
2. Blood flow through the glomerular capillaries is maintained at a constant rate in spite of a wide range of arterial pressures by autoregulation of the glomerular capillaries.
3. The glomerular filtration rate (GFR) is the filtration of plasma per unit of time and is directly related to the perfusion pressure of renal blood flow (RBF).
4. Renin is an enzyme secreted from the juxtaglomerular apparatus in response to decreased blood pressure and causes the generation of angiotensin II, a potent vasoconstrictor. The renin-angiotensin-aldosterone system is thus a regulator of RBF.

Kidney Function

1. The major function of the nephron is urine formation, which involves the processes of glomerular filtration, tubular reabsorption, tubular secretion, and excretion.
2. Glomerular filtration is favoured by capillary hydrostatic pressure and opposed by oncotic pressure in the capillary and hydrostatic pressure in the Bowman capsule. The balance of favouring and opposing filtration forces is known as net filtration pressure.
3. The GFR is approximately 120 mL/min, and 99% of the filtrate is reabsorbed.
4. The proximal convoluted tubule reabsorbs about 60 to 70% of the filtered sodium and water and 90% or more of other electrolytes.
5. Because most molecules are reabsorbed by active transport, the carrier mechanism can become saturated at a point known as the transport maximum (T_m). Molecules not reabsorbed are excreted with the urine.
6. The concentration or specific gravity of the final urine is a function of the level of antidiuretic hormone (ADH). This hormone stimulates the distal convoluted tubules and collecting ducts to reabsorb water. The countercurrent exchange system of the long loops of Henle and their accompanying capillaries establishes a concentration gradient within the renal medulla to facilitate the reabsorption of water from the collecting duct.
7. The kidney secretes or activates a number of hormones having systemic effects, including vitamin D, erythropoietin, and the natriuretic hormone urodilatin.

Tests of Renal Function

1. Creatinine, a substance produced by muscle, is measured in both plasma and urine to calculate a commonly used clinical measurement of GFR.
2. Plasma creatinine concentration, cystatin C level, and blood urea nitrogen (BUN) level are estimates of glomerular function. BUN value also is an indicator of hydration status.
3. Formulas for estimating GFR can be helpful clinical indicators of renal function.
4. Urinalysis involves evaluation of colour, turbidity, protein, pH, specific gravity, sediment, and supernatant. Presence of bacteria, red blood cells, white blood cells, casts, or crystals in the urine sediment may indicate a renal or bladder disorder.

Pediatric Considerations: Pediatrics and Renal Function

1. Compared with adults, infants and children have more dilute urine because of higher blood flow and shorter loops of Henle.
2. Children are more affected than adults by fluid imbalances resulting from diarrhea, infection, or improper feeding because of their limited ability to quickly regulate changes in pH or osmotic pressure.

Geriatric Considerations: Aging and Renal Function

1. Older adults have a decreased ability to concentrate urine and are less able to tolerate dehydration or water loads because they have fewer nephrons.
2. Responses to acid–base changes and reabsorption of glucose are delayed in older adults.
3. In older adults, medications eliminated by the kidney can accumulate in the plasma, causing toxic reactions.

KEY TERMS

Afferent arteriole, 745
Aldosterone, 752
Antidiuretic hormone (ADH), 752
Arcuate artery, 745
Atrial natriuretic peptide (ANP), 752
Autoregulation of intrarenal blood flow, 746
Bladder, 746
Bowman capsule, 743
Bowman space, 743
Calyx (*pl.*, calyces), 744
Collecting duct, 744
Cortex, 741
Cortical nephron, 743
Countercurrent exchange system, 751
Cystatin C, 754
Detrusor muscle, 746
Distal convoluted tubule, 744
Diuretic, 752
Effective renal blood flow (ERBF), 753
Effective renal plasma flow (ERPF), 753
Efferent arteriole, 745
Erythropoietin (EPO), 753
Excretion, 747
External urethral sphincter, 746
Filtration slit, 743
Glomerular capillary, 745
Glomerular filtration, 747
Glomerular filtration membrane, 743
Glomerular filtration rate (GFR), 746
Glomerulotubular balance, 750
Glomerulus, 743
Hilum, 741
Intercalated cell, 744
Interlobar artery, 745
Internal urethral sphincter, 746
Juxtaglomerular apparatus, 743
Juxtaglomerular cell, 743
Juxtamedullary nephron, 743
Kidney, 741
Lobe, 741
Loop of Henle, 743
Macula densa, 743
Medulla, 741
Mesangial cell, 743
Mesangial matrix, 743
Micturition, 746
Midcortical nephron, 743
Natriuretic peptides, 752
Nephron, 741
Net filtration pressure (NFP), 747
Peritubular capillary, 745
Plasma creatinine (P_{cr}) concentration, 754
Podocyte, 743
Principal cell, 744
Proximal convoluted tubule, 743
Pyramid, 741
Renal artery, 744
Renal capsule, 741
Renal columns, 741
Renal corpuscle, 743
Renal fascia, 741
Renal papilla (*pl.*, papillae), 745
Renal vein, 745
Renalase, 747
Renin-angiotensin-aldosterone system (RAAS), 747
Tamm-Horsfall protein (THP), 751
Transport maximum (T_m), 749
Trigone, 746
Tubular reabsorption, 747
Tubular secretion, 747
Tubuloglomerular feedback, 746
Urea, 751
Ureter, 745
Urethra, 746
Urinalysis, 754
Urine concentration, 750
Urine dilution, 750
Urodilatin, 747
Uromodulin, 751
Vasa recta, 745
Vitamin D, 752

REFERENCES

1. Abboud, H. E. (2012). Mesangial cell biology. *Experimental Cell Research, 318*(9), 979–985. doi:10.1016/j.yexcr.2012.02.025.
2. Friis, U. G., Madsen, K., Stubbe, J., et al. (2013). Regulation of renin secretion by renal juxtaglomerular cells. *Pflugers Archiv: European Journal of Physiology, 465*(1), 25–37. doi:10.1007/s00424-012-1126-7.
3. Birder, L. A., Kanai, A. J., Cruz, F., et al. (2010). Is the urothelium intelligent? *Neurourology and Urodynamics, 29*(4), 598–602. doi:10.1002/nau.20914.
4. Guan, Z., Fellner, R. C., Van Beusecum, J., et al. (2014). P2 receptors in renal autoregulation. *Current Vascular Pharmacology, 12*(6), 818–828. doi:10.2174/15701611113116660152.
5. Singh, P., & Thomson, S. C. (2010). Renal homeostasis and tubuloglomerular feedback. *Current Opinion in Nephrology and Hypertension, 19*(1), 59–64. doi:10.1097/MNH.0b013e3283331ffd.
6. Desir, G. V., Wang, L., & Peixoto, A. J. (2012). Human renalase: A review of its biology, function, and implications for hypertension. *Journal of the American Society of Hypertension: JASH, 6*(6), 417–426. doi:10.1016/j.jash.2012.09.002.
7. Castrop, H., Höcherl, K., Kurz, A., et al. (2010). Physiology of kidney renin. *Physiological Reviews, 90*(2), 607–673. doi:10.1152/physrev.00011.2009.
8. Benabe, J. E., & Martinez-Maldonado, M. (1998). The impact of malnutrition on kidney function. *Mineral and Electrolyte Metabolism, 24*(1), 20–26.
9. Iorember, F. M., & Vehaskari, V. M. (2014). Uromodulin: Old friend with new roles in health and disease. *Pediatric Nephrology (Berlin, Germany), 29*(7), 1151–1158. doi:10.1007/s00467-013-2563-z.
10. Januzzi, J. L., Jr. (2013). Natriuretic peptides as biomarkers in heart failure. *Journal of Investigative Medicine, 61*(6), 950–955. doi:10.2310/JIM.0b013e3182946b69.
11. Bartnicki, P., Kowalczyk, M., & Rysz, J. (2013). The influence of the pleiotropic action of erythropoietin and its derivatives on nephroprotection. *Medical Science Monitor, 19*, 599–605. doi:10.12659/MSM.889023.
12. Bunn, H. F. (2013). Erythropoietin. *Cold Spring Harbor Perspectives in Medicine, 3*(3), aD11619. doi:10.1101/cshperspect.a011619.
13. Shlipak, M. G., Mattes, M. D., & Peralta, C. A. (2013). Update on cystatin C: Incorporation into clinical practice. *American Journal of Kidney Diseases, 62*(3), 595–603. doi:10.1053/j.ajkd.2013.03.027.
14. Kidney Disease Improving Global Outcomes Work Group. (2013). KDIGO 2012 clinical practice guideline for the evaluation and management of chronic kidney disease. *Kidney International, 3*(1), 1–150. doi:10.1038/kisup.2012.73. Retrieved from http://www.kdigo.org/clinical_practice_guidelines/pdf/CKD/KDIGO_2012_CKD_GL.pdf.
15. Levey, A. S., Inker, L. A., & Coresh, J. (2014). GFR estimation: From physiology to public health. *American Journal of Kidney Diseases, 63*(5), 820–834. doi:10.1053/j.ajkd.2013.12.006.
16. Botev, R., Mallié, J. P., Couchoud, C., et al. (2009). Estimating glomerular filtration rate: Cockcroft-Gault and modification of diet in renal disease formulas compared to renal insulin clearance. *Clinical Journal of the American Society of Nephrology : CJASN, 4*(5), 899–906. doi:10.2215/CJN.05371008.
17. Levey, A. S., Stevens, L. A., Schmid, C. H., et al. (2009). A new equation to estimate glomerular filtration rate. *Annals of Internal Medicine, 150*(9), 604–612.

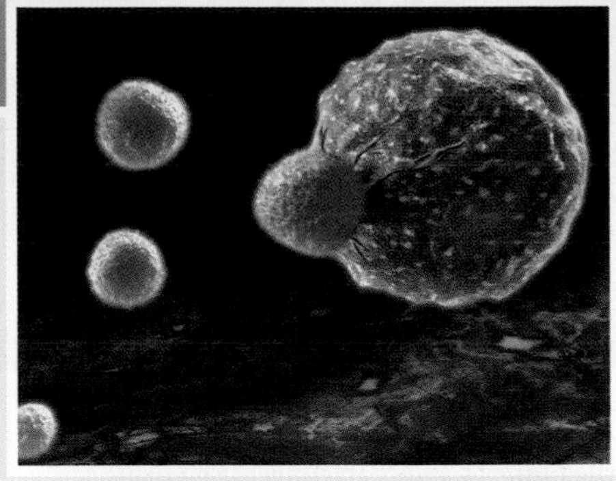

30

Alterations of Renal and Urinary Tract Function

Sue E. Huether and Mohamed El-Hussein

EVOLVE WEBSITE

http://evolve.elsevier.com/Canada/Huether/pathophysiology

Student Review Questions
Key Points
Case Studies
Animations
Quick Check Answers

CHAPTER OUTLINE

Urinary Tract Obstruction, 759
- Upper Urinary Tract Obstruction, 759
- Lower Urinary Tract Obstruction, 761
- Tumours, 763

Urinary Tract Infection, 765
- Causes of Urinary Tract Infection, 765
- Types of Urinary Tract Infection, 765

Glomerular Disorders, 767
- Glomerulonephritis, 767
- Nephrotic and Nephritic Syndromes, 771

Acute Kidney Injury, 772
- Classification of Kidney Dysfunction, 772
- Classification of Acute Kidney Injury, 772

Chronic Kidney Disease, 775
- Creatinine and Urea Clearance, 777
- Fluid and Electrolyte Balance, 777
- Calcium, Phosphate, and Bone, 778
- Protein, Carbohydrate, and Fat Metabolism, 778
- Cardiovascular System, 778
- Pulmonary System, 779
- Hematological System, 779
- Immune System, 779
- Neurological System, 779
- Gastro-intestinal System, 779
- Endocrine and Reproductive Systems, 779
- Integumentary System, 779

Renal and urinary function can be affected by a variety of disorders. The most common type of urinary dysfunction is infection of the bladder. Stones, tumours, or inflammation also can obstruct the urinary tract. Renal function can be impaired by disorders of the kidney itself or by systemic diseases and may ultimately result in acute kidney injury (AKI) or chronic kidney disease (CKD). Because the kidney filters the blood, it is directly linked to every other organ system. Kidney failure, whether acute or chronic, is therefore a life-threatening condition.

URINARY TRACT OBSTRUCTION

Urinary tract obstruction is an interference with the flow of urine at any site along the urinary tract (Figure 30-1). An obstruction may be anatomical or functional. The obstruction impedes flow proximal to the blockage, dilates structures distal to the obstruction, increases the risk for infection, and compromises renal function. Anatomical changes in the urinary system caused by obstruction are referred to as **obstructive uropathy**. The severity of an obstructive uropathy is determined by (1) the location of the obstructive lesion, (2) the involvement of ureters and kidneys, (3) the severity (completeness) of the blockage, (4) the duration of the blockage, and (5) the nature of the obstructive lesion.[1,2] Obstructions may be relieved or partially alleviated by correction of the obstruction, although permanent impairments occur if a complete or partial obstruction persists over a period of weeks to months or longer.

Upper Urinary Tract Obstruction

Common causes of upper urinary tract obstruction include stricture or congenital compression of a calyx at the ureteropelvic–ureterovesical junction (e.g., stones [calculi], or vesicoureteral reflux) (see Chapter 31); compression from an aberrant vessel, tumour, or abdominal inflammation and scarring (retroperitoneal fibrosis); or ureteral blockage from stones or a malignancy of the renal pelvis or ureter.

Obstruction of the upper urinary tract causes dilation of the ureter, renal pelvis, calyces, and renal parenchyma proximal to the site of urinary blockage resulting from a "backing up" of urine. The increased pressure is transmitted to the glomerulus, which decreases filtration. Dilation of the ureter is referred to as **hydroureter** (accumulation of urine in the ureter), and dilation of the renal pelvis and calyces proximal to a blockage is referred to as **hydronephrosis** or **ureterohydronephrosis** (dilation of both the ureter and the pelvicaliceal system) (Figure 30-2). Dilation of the upper urinary tract is an early response to obstruction and includes smooth muscle hypertrophy and accumulation of urine above the level of blockage (urinary stasis). Unless the obstruction is relieved, the dilation leads to enlargement and **tubulointerstitial fibrosis** with deposition of excessive amounts of collagen and other proteins. These changes occur in the distal nephrons and affect renal function within approximately 7 days. By 14 days, obstruction has adversely affected both distal and proximal tubular aspects of the nephron units. Within 28 days, the glomeruli of the kidney have been damaged and

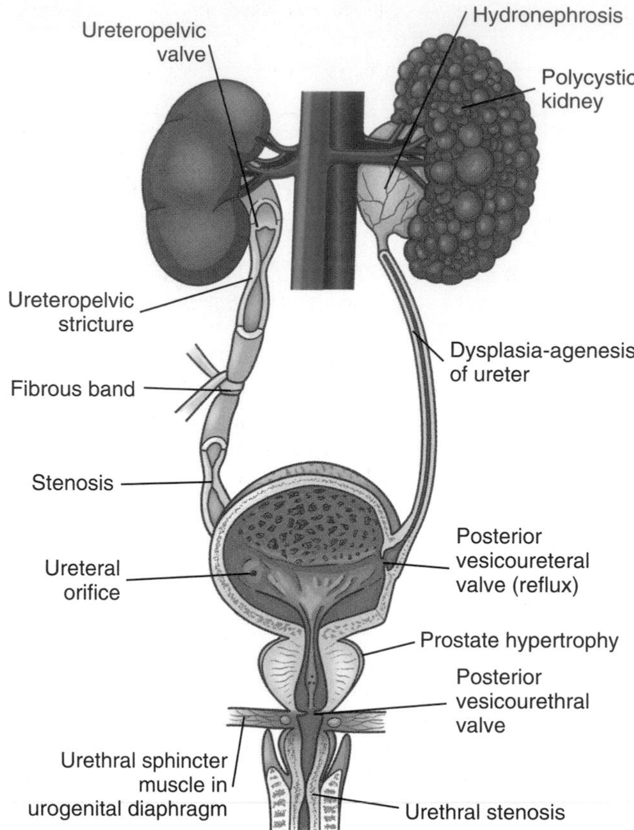

FIGURE 30-1 Major Sites of Urinary Tract Obstruction.

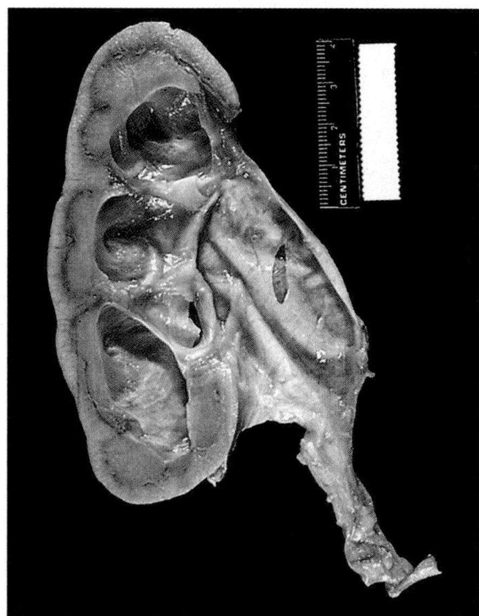

FIGURE 30-2 Hydronephrosis of the Kidney. There is marked dilation of the renal pelvis and calyces with thinning of the overlying cortex and medulla due to compression atrophy. (From Kumar, V., Abbas, A.K., & Aster, J.C. [Eds.]. [2015]. *Robbins and Cotran pathologic basis of disease* [9th ed.]. Philadelphia: Saunders.)

the renal cortex and medulla are reduced in size (thinned). Tubular damage initially decreases the kidney's ability to concentrate urine, causing an increase in urine volume despite a decrease in glomerular filtration rate (GFR). The affected kidney is unable to conserve sodium, bicarbonate, and water or to excrete hydrogen or potassium, leading to metabolic acidosis and dehydration. The magnitude of this damage, and the kidney's ability to recover normal regulatory function, is affected by the severity and duration of the obstruction. With complete obstruction and compression of the renal vasculature, damage to the renal tubules occurs in a matter of hours, and irreversible damage occurs within 4 weeks. Nevertheless, even in the face of a complete obstruction, the human kidney may recover at least partial function provided that the blockage is removed within 56 to 69 days.[3] This recovery requires a period of approximately 4 months. Partial obstruction (in the absence of renal infection) leads to subtler but ultimately permanent impairments, including loss of the kidney's ability to concentrate urine, reabsorb bicarbonate, excrete ammonia, or regulate metabolic acid–base balance.

The body is able to partially counteract the negative consequences of unilateral obstruction by a process called **compensatory hypertrophy** and **hyperfunction**.[4] Compensatory response is the result of two growth processes: obligatory growth occurs under the influence of somatomedins, and compensatory growth occurs under the influence of still unidentified hormone(s). These processes cause the unobstructed kidney to increase the size of individual glomeruli and tubules but not the total number of functioning nephrons. The ability of the body to engage in compensatory hypertrophy and hyperfunction diminishes with age, and the process is reversible when relief of obstruction results in recovery of function by the obstructed kidney.

Relief of bilateral, partial urinary tract obstruction or complete obstruction of one kidney is usually followed by a brief period of diuresis (commonly called **postobstructive diuresis**).[5] Postobstructive diuresis is a physiological response and is typically mild, representing a restoration of fluid and electrolyte imbalance caused by the obstructive uropathy. Occasionally, relief of obstruction will cause rapid excretion of large volumes of water, sodium, or other electrolytes, resulting in a urine output of 10 L/day or more. Rapid postobstructive diuresis causes dehydration and fluid and electrolyte imbalances that must be promptly corrected. Risk factors for severe postobstructive diuresis include chronic, bilateral obstruction; impairment of one or both kidneys' ability to concentrate urine or reabsorb sodium (acquired nephrogenic diabetes insipidus); hypertension; edema and weight gain; heart failure; and uremic encephalopathy.

Kidney Stones

Calculi, or **urinary stones**, are masses of crystals, protein, or other substances that are a common cause of urinary tract obstruction in adults. Calculi can be located in the kidneys, ureters, and urinary bladder.[6] Most renal stones are unilateral. The risk for urinary calculi formation is influenced by a number of factors, including age, sex, ethnicity, geographical location, seasonal factors, fluid intake, diet, and occupation. Most persons develop their first stone before age 50 years. Geographical location influences the risk for stone formation because of indirect factors, including average temperature, humidity, and rainfall, and their influence on fluid intake and dietary patterns. Persons who regularly consume an adequate volume of water and those who are physically active are at reduced risk when compared with persons who are inactive or consume lower volumes of water.

Urinary calculi can be classified according to the primary minerals (salts) that make up the stones. The most common stone types include calcium oxalate or phosphate (70 to 80%), struvite (magnesium-ammonium-phosphate) (15%), and uric acid (7%). Cystine stones are rare (<1%).[7]

PATHOPHYSIOLOGY Calculus formation is complex and related to (1) supersaturation of one or more salts in the urine, (2) precipitation of the salts from a liquid to a solid state, (3) growth through crystallization or agglomeration (sometimes called *aggregation*), and (4) the presence or absence of stone inhibitors (e.g., uromodulin [Tamm-Horsfall protein]).[8] *Supersaturation* is the presence of a higher concentration of a salt within a fluid (in this case, the urine) than the volume is able to dissolve to maintain equilibrium.

Human urine contains many ions capable of *precipitating* from solution and forming a variety of salts. The salts form crystals that are retained and grow into stones. *Crystallization* is the process by which crystals grow from a small *nidus* or nucleus to larger stones in the presence of supersaturated urine. Although supersaturation is essential for free stone formation, the urine need not remain continuously supersaturated for a calculus to grow once its nidus has precipitated from solution. Intermittent periods of supersaturation after the ingestion of a meal or during times of dehydration from limited oral intake or secondary to continued use of diuretics are sufficient for stone growth in many individuals. In addition, the renal tubules and papillae have many surfaces that may attract a crystalline nidus (Randall plaque) and add biological material (matrix) forming a stone.[9] *Matrix* is an organic material (i.e., mucoprotein) in which the components of a kidney stone are embedded.

The temperature and pH of the urine also influence the risk for precipitation and calculus formation, and pH is most important. An alkaline urinary pH (pH >7.0) significantly increases the risk for calcium phosphate stone formation, whereas acidic urine (pH <5.0) increases the risk for uric acid stone formation. Cystine and xanthine also precipitate more readily in acidic urine.

Stone or *crystal growth-inhibiting substances*, such as potassium citrate, Tamm-Horsfall protein, pyrophosphate, and magnesium, are capable of crystal growth inhibition, thereby reducing the risk for calcium phosphate or calcium oxalate precipitation in the urine and preventing subsequent stone formation.

The size of a stone determines the likelihood that it will pass through the urinary tract and be excreted through micturition.[10] Stones smaller than 5 mm have about a 50% chance of spontaneous (painful) passage, whereas stones that are 1 cm have almost no chance of spontaneous passage.

Retention of crystal particles occurs primarily at the papillary collecting ducts. Although most crystals are flushed from the tract through antegrade urine flow, urinary stasis (i.e., from benign prostatic hyperplasia, neurogenic bladder), anatomical abnormalities (strictures), or inflamed epithelium within the urinary tract may prevent prompt flushing of crystals from the system, thus increasing the risk for calculus formation.

Calcium stones account for 70 to 80% of all stones requiring treatment. Calcium oxalate accounts for about 80% of these stones and calcium phosphate about 15%. Most individuals have idiopathic calcium urolithiasis (ICU), a condition whose exact etiology has not yet been defined. Stones can form freely in supersaturated urine or detach from interstitial sites within the tubules (Randall plaque formation) near the tip of the renal papillae. Hypercalciuria, hyperoxaluria, hyperuricosuria, hypocitraturia, mild renal tubular acidosis, or crystal growth inhibitor deficiencies and alkaline urine are associated with calcium stones. Hypercalciuria is attributable to intestinal hyperabsorption of dietary calcium and decreased renal calcium reabsorption. Hyperparathyroidism and bone demineralization associated with prolonged immobilization are also known to cause hypercalciuria. Although oxalate in the diet influences the risk of developing calcium stones, primary hyperoxaluria is a rare, inherited disorder.

Struvite stones primarily contain magnesium-ammonium-phosphate as well as varying levels of matrix. Matrix forms in an alkaline urine and during infection with a urease-producing bacterial pathogen, such as a *Proteus*, *Klebsiella*, or *Pseudomonas*. Struvite calculi may grow quite large and branch into a staghorn configuration (**staghorn calculus**) that approximates the pelvicaliceal collecting system.

Uric acid stones occur in persons who excrete excessive uric acid in the urine, such as those with gouty arthritis. Uric acid is primarily a product of biosynthesis of endogenous purines and is secondarily affected by consumption of purines (e.g., meat and beer) in the diet. A consistently acidic urine (pH <5.0) greatly increases this risk. Cystine and xanthine are amino acids that precipitate more readily in acidic urine. Cystinuria and xanthinuria are both genetic disorders of amino acid metabolism, and excess of these amino acids in urine can cause **cystinuric (xanthine) stone** formation in the presence of a low urine pH of 5.5 or less.

CLINICAL MANIFESTATIONS **Renal colic**, described as moderate to severe pain often originating in the flank and radiating to the groin, usually indicates obstruction of the renal pelvis or proximal ureter.[11] Colic that radiates to the lateral flank or lower abdomen typically indicates obstruction in the midureter, and bothersome lower urinary tract symptoms (urgency, frequent voiding, urge incontinence) indicate obstruction of the lower ureter or ureterovesical junction. The pain can be severe and incapacitating and may be accompanied by nausea and vomiting. Gross or microscopic hematuria may be present.

EVALUATION AND TREATMENT The evaluation and diagnosis of urinary calculi is based on presenting symptoms and history combined with a focused physical assessment. Imaging studies determine the location of the calculi, the severity of obstruction, and associated obstructive uropathy. The history queries dietary habits, the age of the first stone episode, stone analysis, and presence of complicating factors including hyperparathyroidism or recent gastro-intestinal or genito-urinary surgery. Urinalysis (including pH) is obtained, and a 24-hour urine is completed to identify calcium oxalate, calcium citrate, and other significant constituents. In addition, every effort is made to retrieve and analyze calculi that are passed spontaneously or retrieved through aggressive intervention. To diagnose and manage underlying metabolic disorders, additional tests are completed for those with suspected hyperparathyroidism (elevated serum calcium levels) or cystine or uric acid (high purine diet) stones.

The goals of treatment are to manage acute pain, promote stone passage, reduce the size of stones already formed, and prevent new stone formation. The components of treatment include (1) managing pain, (2) reducing the concentration of stone-forming substances by increasing urine flow rate with high fluid intake, (3) adjusting the pH of the urine (e.g., make it more alkaline with potassium citrate administration), (4) decreasing the amount of stone-forming substances in the urine by decreasing dietary intake or endogenous production or by altering urine pH, and (5) removing stones using percutaneous nephrolithotomy, ureteroscopy, or ultrasonic or laser lithotripsy to fragment stones for excretion in the urine. Prevention of recurrent stones includes increasing fluid intake to generate 2.5 L of urine per day, avoiding intake of colas and other soft drinks acidified with phosphoric acid, avoiding dietary oxalate (e.g., chocolate, beets, nuts, rhubarb, spinach, strawberries, tea, wheat bran), eating less animal protein, limiting sodium intake, and, for calcium stone prevention, maintaining a dietary calcium intake of 1 000 to 1 200 mg/day. Potassium citrate may be used to raise urinary pH.[12,13]

Lower Urinary Tract Obstruction

Obstructive disorders of the lower urinary tract are primarily related to storage of urine in the bladder or emptying of urine through the bladder outlet. The causes of obstruction include both neurogenic and anatomical alterations or, in some instances, a combination of both.

TABLE 30-1 Types of Incontinence

Type	Description
Urge incontinence (most common in older adults)	Involuntary loss of urine associated with abrupt and strong desire to void (urgency); often associated with involuntary contractions of detrusor; when associated with neurological disorder, this is called detrusor hyper-reflexia; when no neurological disorder exists, this is called detrusor instability; may be associated with decreased bladder wall compliance
Stress incontinence (most common in women <60 years and men who have had prostate surgery)	Involuntary loss of urine during coughing, sneezing, laughing, or other physical activity associated with increased abdominal pressure
Overflow incontinence	Involuntary loss of urine with overdistension of bladder; associated with neurological lesions below S1, polyneuropathies, and urethral obstruction (e.g., enlarged prostate)
Mixed incontinence (most common in older women)	Combination of both stress and urge incontinence
Functional incontinence	Involuntary loss of urine attributable to dementia or immobility

Data from Agency for Health Care Policy and Research, National Guideline Clearing House. (2014). *Assessment and diagnosis: Guidelines on urinary incontinence.* Retrieved from https://www.ahrq.gov/; Khandelwal, C., & Kistler, C. (2013). *Am Fam Physician, 87*(8), 543–550.

TABLE 30-2 Neurogenic Bladder

Site of Lesion	Cause (Symptoms)	Diseases
Lesions above C2 involve pontine micturition centre (UMN disorder)	Detrusor hyper-reflexia (urgency and urine leakage)	Stroke, traumatic brain injury, multiple sclerosis (MS), hydrocephalus, cerebral palsy, Alzheimer's disease, brain tumours
Lesions between C2 and S1 (UMN disorder)	Detrusor hyper-reflexia with vesicosphincter dyssynergia (functional bladder outlet obstruction)	Spinal cord injury C2–T12, MS, transverse myelitis, Guillain-Barré syndrome, disc problems
Lesions below S1 (cauda equina syndrome) (LMN disorder)	Acontractile detrusor, with or without urethral sphincter incompetence (stress urinary incontinence)	Myelodysplasia, peripheral polyneuropathies, MS, tabes dorsalis, spinal injury T12–S1, cauda equina syndrome, herpes simplex/zoster

LMN, lower motor neuron; *UMN*, upper motor neuron.

Incontinence is a common symptom, and types of incontinence are reviewed in Table 30-1.

In Canada, the continence care community generally agrees that incontinence affects about 10% of the population. That translates into approximately 3.5 million Canadians who experience some form of incontinence.[14] Individual research estimates for the prevalence of incontinence in Canada range from 2 to 50% of the population, depending on the study, the research method, and the questions posed. For example, asking the question "Are you incontinent?" will collect a dramatically lower rate of positive responses than the question "Do you suffer from occasional leakage of urine?" There tends to be a greater prevalence of incontinence among women than men. It is assumed that this difference is related to childbearing and other consequences of being female.[14]

Neurogenic Bladder

Neurogenic bladder is a general term for bladder dysfunction caused by neurological disorders (Table 30-2). The types of dysfunction are related to the sites in the nervous system controlling sensory and motor bladder function. Lesions developing in upper motor neurons of the brain and spinal cord result in **dyssynergia** (loss of coordinated neuromuscular contraction) and overactive or hyper-reflexive bladder function. Lesions in the sacral area of the spinal cord or peripheral nerves result in underactive, hypotonic, or atonic (flaccid) bladder function, often with loss of bladder sensation.

Neurological disorders that develop above the pontine micturition centre result in **detrusor hyper-reflexia (overactivity)**, also known as an uninhibited or reflex bladder. This is an upper motor neuron disorder in which the bladder empties automatically when it becomes full and the external sphincter functions normally. Because the pontine micturition centre remains intact, there is coordination between detrusor muscle contraction and relaxation of the urethral sphincter. Stroke, traumatic brain injury, dementia, and brain tumours are examples of disorders that result in detrusor hyper-reflexia. Symptoms include urine leakage and incontinence.

Neurological lesions that occur below the pontine micturition centre but above the sacral micturition centre (between C2 and S1) are also upper motor neuron lesions and result in **detrusor hyper-reflexia with vesicosphincter dyssynergia**. There is loss of pontine coordination of detrusor muscle contraction and external sphincter relaxation, so both the bladder and the sphincter are contracting at the same time, causing a functional obstruction of the bladder outlet.[15] Spinal cord injury, multiple sclerosis, Guillain-Barré syndrome, and vertebral disc problems are causes of this disorder. There is diminished bladder relaxation during storage with small urine volumes and high intravesicular (inside the bladder) pressures. The result is an overactive bladder syndrome with symptoms of frequency, urgency, urge incontinence, and increased risk for urinary tract infection (UTI).

Lesions involving the sacral micturition centre (below S1; may also be termed *cauda equina syndrome*) or peripheral nerve lesions result in **detrusor areflexia** (acontractile detrusor), a lower motor neuron disorder. The result is an acontractile detrusor or atonic bladder with retention of urine and distension. If the sensory innervation of the bladder is intact, the full bladder will be sensed but the detrusor may not contract. This is an *underactive bladder syndrome* and may have symptoms of stress and overflow incontinence. Myelodysplasia, multiple sclerosis, tabes dorsalis, and peripheral polyneuropathies are associated with this disorder.

Overactive Bladder Syndrome

Overactive bladder (OAB) syndrome is a syndrome of detrusor overactivity characterized by urgency with involuntary detrusor contractions during the bladder filling phase that may be spontaneous or provoked.[16] There is coordination between the contracting bladder and the external sphincter, but the detrusor is too weak to empty the bladder, resulting in urinary retention with overflow or stress incontinence. *Overactive bladder* is defined by the International Continence Society as a symptom syndrome of urgency, with or without urge incontinence and usually associated with frequency and nocturia.[17] OAB syndrome affects millions of adults and children. Adults are often reluctant to discuss this syndrome with their health care provider.

Anatomical Obstructions to Urine Flow

Anatomical causes of resistance to urine flow include urethral stricture, prostatic enlargement in men, pelvic organ prolapse in women, and tumour compression. Symptoms of obstruction are more common in men and include (1) frequent daytime voiding (urination more than every 2 hours while awake); (2) nocturia (awakening more than once each night to urinate for adults younger than 65 years of age or more than twice for older adults); (3) poor force of stream; (4) intermittency of urinary stream; (5) bothersome urinary urgency, often combined with hesitancy; and (6) feelings of incomplete bladder emptying despite micturition.

A **urethral stricture** is a narrowing of its lumen and occurs when infection, injury, or surgical manipulation produces a scar that reduces the calibre of the urethra. The vast majority of urethral strictures occur in men; they are rare in women. The severity of obstruction is influenced by its location within the urethra, its length, and the minimum calibre of urethral lumen within the stricture. Specifically, proximal urethral strictures cause more severe obstruction than do strictures of the distal urethra, longer strictures tend to be more obstructive, and the magnitude of blockage is inversely proportional to the urethral calibre.[18,19]

Prostate enlargement is caused by acute inflammation, benign prostatic hyperplasia, or prostate cancer (see Chapter 33). Each of these disorders can cause encroachment on the urethra with obstruction to urine flow and the symptoms summarized previously.

Severe **pelvic organ prolapse** (see Chapter 33) in a woman causes bladder outlet obstruction when a cystocele (the downward protrusion or herniation of the bladder into the vagina) descends below the level of the urethral outlet. A cystocele reaching or protruding beyond the vaginal introitus creates the greatest risk for obstruction, particularly if the bladder neck has been surgically repaired without simultaneous repair of the cystocele. In men the bladder may rarely herniate into the scrotum, causing a similar type of obstruction.

Partial obstruction of the bladder outlet or urethra initially causes an increase in the force of detrusor contraction. If the blockage persists, afferent nerves within the bladder wall are adversely affected, leading to urinary urgency and, in some cases, overactive detrusor contractions (a myogenic cause of OAB). When obstruction persists, there is an increased deposition of collagen within the smooth muscle bundles of the detrusor muscle (trabeculation), possibly in an attempt to increase the force of its contraction strength. Ultimately, the bladder wall loses its ability to stretch and accommodate urine, a condition called **low bladder wall compliance**, and the detrusor loses its ability to contract efficiently. Low bladder wall compliance chronically elevates intravesicular pressure, greatly increasing the likelihood of hydroureter, hydronephrosis, and impaired renal function.

EVALUATION AND TREATMENT Although the history and physical examination are critical to the evaluation of lower urinary tract disorders, it must be remembered that no symptom or cluster of symptoms has been identified that accurately differentiates the various causes of these disorders. For example, symptoms such as urgency, urge incontinence, frequent urination, and nocturia may develop because of OAB or either increased or decreased bladder outlet resistance. Reduced resistance is associated with the symptom of stress incontinence (incontinence with coughing or sneezing) and symptoms of increased resistance are similar to bladder outlet obstruction, including poor force of urinary stream, hesitancy, and feelings of incomplete bladder emptying.

Various diagnostic tests assist with evaluation. The *postvoid urine* is measured by catheterization within 5 to 15 minutes of urination or through a bladder ultrasound machine that measures bladder height and width to provide an approximation of urine within the vesicle. This measurement may be combined with *uroflowmetry*, a graphic representation of the force of the urinary stream expressed as millilitres voided per second. A *cystometric test* uses a catheter and manometer to evaluate bladder urine volume and pressure in relation to involuntary bladder contraction (the leak point pressure) and the urge to void. Each of these measurements assesses the lower urinary tract's efficiency in evacuating urine through micturition, but neither differentiates poor detrusor contraction strength from obstruction as a cause of urinary retention. Instead, *multichannel urodynamic testing* is used to identify obstruction, quantify its severity, and measure detrusor contraction strength (Figure 30-3). *Video urodynamic* recordings can also demonstrate OAB and detrusor sphincter dyssynergia. An evaluation of renal function, including functional imaging studies and measurement of serum creatinine level, is completed particularly when obstruction is severe and associated with elevated residuals or UTI.

Because the bladder neck consists of circular smooth muscle with adrenergic innervation, OAB and detrusor sphincter dyssynergia may be managed by α-adrenergic blocking (antimuscarinic) medications. In intractable cases, botulinum toxin type A (Botox) injections or surgery is recommended.[20] Detrusor sphincter dyssynergia may be managed by intermittent catheterization in combination with higher-dose antimuscarinic medications to prevent overactive detrusor contractions and associated dyssynergia while ensuring regular, complete bladder evacuation by catheterization. Alternatively, men with dyssynergia may be managed by condom catheter containment, supplemented by an α-adrenergic-blocking medication or transurethral sphincterotomy (surgical incision of the striated sphincter) to relieve obstruction. Low bladder wall compliance may be managed by antimuscarinic medications and intermittent catheterization; however, more severe cases may require augmentation enterocystoplasty (enlargement of the low compliant bladder wall using a detubularized piece of small bowel), urinary diversion, or long-term in-dwelling catheterization. Untreated OAB impairs health and quality of life, causes depression, leads to social isolation, and causes significant economic burden. In the older adult, OAB may cause risk for falls and UTI.[21]

Prostate enlargement is managed by treating the underlying cause of the prostate enlargement with medication or surgery. Urinary retention may require transient placement of a suprapubic catheter. Urethral stricture is treated with urethral dilation accomplished by using a steel instrument shaped like a catheter (urethral sound) or a series of incrementally increasing catheterlike tubes (filiforms and followers). Long, dense strictures typically require surgical repair to prevent recurrence.

Tumours

Renal Tumours

There are a number of different types of kidney tumours. **Renal adenomas** (benign tumours) are uncommon but are increasing in number. The tumours are encapsulated and are usually located near the cortex of the kidney. Because the tumours can become malignant, they are usually surgically removed. **Renal cell carcinoma (RCC)** is the most common renal neoplasm. **Renal transitional cell carcinoma (RTCC)** is rare and primarily arises in the renal parenchyma and renal pelvis.

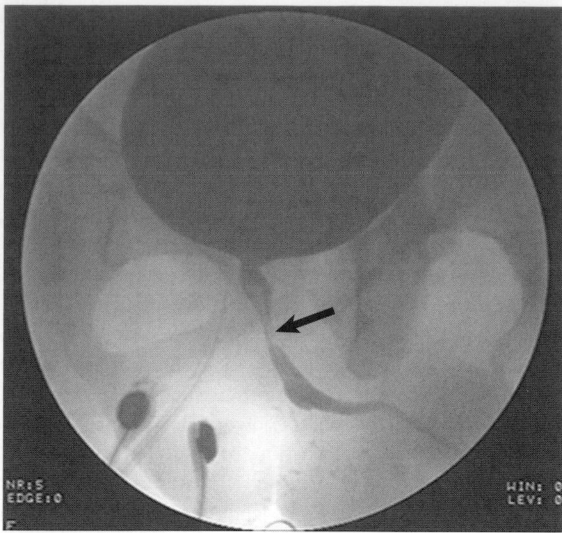

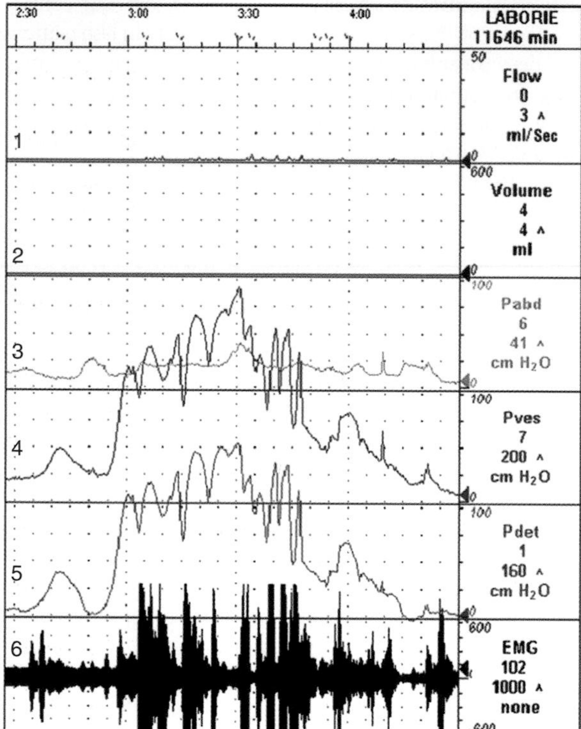

FIGURE 30-3 Neurogenic Detrusor Overactivity With Detrusor Sphincter Dyssynergia. The *arrow* indicates narrowing of the striated sphincter consistent with electromyographic activity (*line 6*) noted on the urodynamic tracing. Note the characteristic poor flow pattern (*line 1*) with elevated voiding pressures (*lines 4 and 5*) indicating obstruction. *Line 1*, urine flow rate; *line 2*, urine volume; *line 3*, abdominal pressure (*Pabd*); *line 4*, intravesicular (inside bladder) pressure (*Pves*); *line 5*, detrusor muscle pressure (*Pdet*); *line 6*, bladder electromyelogram (*EMG*).

Risk factors include cigarette smoking, obesity, and uncontrolled hypertension. With surgical resection 5-year survival is about 90% for stage I (encapsulated) cancer.[22]

The Canadian Cancer Society estimated that in 2017, 6 600 Canadians (4 200 men and 2 400 women) were diagnosed with kidney cancer. It also estimated that close to 1 900 Canadians (1 200 men and 670 women) died from this disease in 2017. RCC usually occurs in men (two times more often than in women) between 50 and 60 years of age.[23]

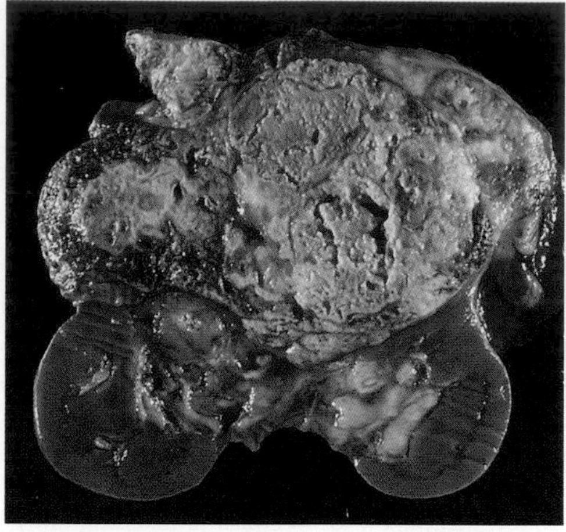

FIGURE 30-4 Renal Cell Carcinoma. Renal cell carcinomas usually are spheroidal masses composed of yellow tissue mottled with hemorrhage, necrosis, and fibrosis. (From Damjanov, I., & Linder, J. [Eds.]. [1996]. *Anderson's pathology* [10th ed.]. St. Louis: Mosby.)

PATHOGENESIS RCCs are adenocarcinomas that usually arise from the tubular epithelium, commonly in the renal cortex. The etiology is unknown. They are classified according to cell type and extent of metastasis. *Clear cell tumours*, the most common, present a better prognosis than granular cell or spindle tumours. Confinement within the renal capsule, together with treatment, is associated with a better survival rate. The tumours usually occur unilaterally (Figure 30-4). About 25% of individuals with RCC present with metastasis.[24]

CLINICAL MANIFESTATIONS The classic clinical manifestations of renal tumours are hematuria, dull and aching flank pain, palpable flank mass, and weight loss, but all of these symptoms occur in fewer than 10% of cases. Further, they represent an advanced stage of disease, whereas earlier stages are often silent (painless hematuria). The most common sites of distant metastasis are the lung, lymph nodes, liver, bone, thyroid gland, and central nervous system.

EVALUATION AND TREATMENT Diagnosis is based on the clinical symptoms, plain X-ray films of the abdomen, intravenous pyelography, renal angiography, computed tomography (CT) or positron emission tomography using ^{124}I-girentuximab, and a radiolabelled monoclonal antibody that binds to clear cell cancer cells. The tumour-nodes-metastasis (TNM) classification is used to stage RCC.[25] Staging systems using molecular tumour markers are rapidly improving.[26] Treatment for localized disease is surgical removal of the affected kidney (radical nephrectomy) or partial nephrectomy for smaller tumours, with combined use of chemotherapeutic agents. Radiofrequency ablation also may be used for early stage tumours when surgery is not an option. Metastatic disease is treated with immunotherapy (i.e., bevacizumab [angiogenesis inhibitor such as sunitinib (Sutent) or sorafenib (Nexavar)], T-cell activators, interferon-alpha, and interleukin-2) and target therapies including vascular endothelial growth factor (VEGF) or the mammalian target of rapamycin (mTOR) pathways, or both. Cell-based vaccines are showing promise.[27,28] Survival is related to tumour grade, tumour cell type, and extent of metastasis.

Bladder Tumours

The development of bladder cancer is most common in men older than 60 years. *Transitional cell (urothelial) carcinoma* is the most common bladder malignancy, and tumours are usually superficial. More advanced tumours are muscle invasive. Less common forms are squamous cell and adenocarcinoma (cells that produce mucus). The Canadian Cancer Society estimated that in 2017, 8 900 Canadians (6 700 men and 2 200 women) were diagnosed with bladder cancer. It also estimated that 2 400 Canadians (1 700 men and 680 women) died from this disease in 2017.[29]

PATHOGENESIS The risk for primary bladder cancer is greater among people who smoke or are exposed to metabolites of aniline dyes, high levels of arsenic in drinking water, heavy consumption of phenacetin, or have uroepithelial schistosomiasis infection. Bladder cancer results from a genetic alteration in normal bladder epithelium.[30] Metastasis is usually to lymph nodes, liver, bones, or lungs. The TNM classification is used for staging bladder carcinoma.[31] Secondary bladder cancer develops by invasion of cancer from bordering organs, such as cervical carcinoma in women or prostatic carcinoma in men.

CLINICAL MANIFESTATIONS Gross painless hematuria is the archetypal clinical manifestation of bladder cancer. Episodes of hematuria tend to recur, and they are often accompanied by bothersome lower urinary tract symptoms including daytime voiding frequency, nocturia, urgency, and urge urinary incontinence, particularly for carcinoma in situ. Flank pain may occur if tumour growth obstructs one or both ureterovesical junctions.

EVALUATION AND TREATMENT Cystoscopy with tissue biopsy confirms the diagnosis of bladder cancer. Urine cytological study (pathological analysis of sloughed cells within the urine) is used for screening high-risk individuals. Use of biological markers for bladder cancer diagnosis and treatment prognosis are under investigation.[32] Transurethral resection or laser ablation, combined with intravesical chemotherapy or biological therapy, is effective for superficial tumours. Radical cystectomy with urinary diversion and adjuvant chemotherapy is required for locally invasive tumours.[33]

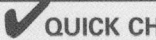

QUICK CHECK 30-1

1. List two typical complications of urinary tract obstruction, and briefly describe them.
2. How do kidney stones form?
3. Which population group is at greatest risk for bladder tumours?

URINARY TRACT INFECTION

Causes of Urinary Tract Infection

A **urinary tract infection (UTI)** is an inflammation of the urinary epithelium usually caused by bacteria from gut flora. A UTI can occur anywhere along the urinary tract, including the urethra, prostate, bladder, ureter, or kidney. At risk are premature newborns; prepubertal children; sexually active and pregnant women; women treated with antibiotics that disrupt vaginal flora; spermicide users; estrogen-deficient post-menopausal women; individuals with in-dwelling catheters; and persons with diabetes mellitus, neurogenic bladder, or urinary tract obstruction. Cystitis is more common in women because of the shorter urethra and the closeness of the urethra to the anus (increasing the possibility of bacterial contamination). Up to 50% of women may have a lower UTI at some time in their life.[34] Canadian women make about 500 000 visits to doctors per year due to UTIs.[35] Generally, UTIs are mild and without complications, and they occur in individuals with a normal urinary tract; these infections are termed *uncomplicated UTIs*. A *complicated UTI* develops when there is an abnormality in the urinary system or a health problem that compromises host defences, such as human immunodeficiency virus (HIV), kidney transplant, diabetes mellitus, or spinal cord injury. UTI may occur alone or in association with pyelonephritis, prostatitis, or kidney stones.[36] Up to 40% of cases of septic shock are caused by urosepsis.[37] Factors associated with UTI are summarized in Figure 30-5.

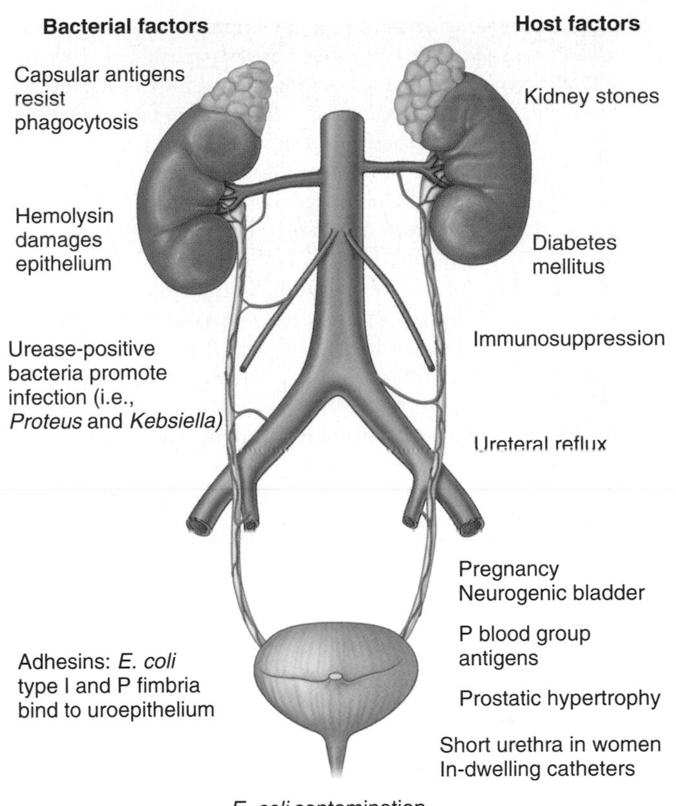

FIGURE 30-5 Mechanisms of Urinary Tract Infection.

Several factors normally combine to protect against UTIs. Most bacteria are washed out of the urethra during micturition. The low pH and high osmolality of urea, the presence of Tamm-Horsfall protein or uromodulin (secreted by renal tubular cells in the distal loop of Henle), and secretions from the uroepithelium provide a bactericidal effect. The ureterovesical junction closes during bladder contraction, preventing reflux of urine to the ureters and kidneys. Both the longer urethra and the presence of prostatic secretions decrease the risk for infection in men. A UTI occurs when a pathogen circumvents or overwhelms the host's defence mechanisms and rapidly reproduces.

Types of Urinary Tract Infection

Acute Cystitis

Acute cystitis is an inflammation of the bladder and is the most common site of UTI. The morphological appearance of the bladder through cystoscopy describes different types of cystitis. With mild inflammation, the mucosa is hyperemic (red). More advanced cases may show diffuse hemorrhage (termed *hemorrhagic cystitis*), pus formation, or suppurative exudates (termed *suppurative cystitis*) on the epithelial surface of the bladder. Prolonged infection may lead to sloughing of the bladder mucosa with ulcer formation (termed *ulcerative cystitis*). The most severe infections may cause necrosis of the bladder wall (termed *gangrenous cystitis*).

PATHOPHYSIOLOGY The most common infecting microorganisms are uropathic strains of *Escherichia coli* and the second most common is *Staphylococcus saprophyticus*. Less common microorganisms include *Klebsiella*, *Proteus*, *Pseudomonas*, fungi, viruses, parasites, or tubercular bacilli. Schistosomiasis is the most common cause of parasitic invasion of the urinary tract on a global basis; it infects more than 200 million people and has a strong association with bladder cancer.[38]

Bacterial contamination of the normally sterile urine usually occurs by retrograde movement of Gram-negative bacilli into the urethra and bladder and then to the ureter and kidney. Uropathic strains of *E. coli* have type-1 fimbriae that bind to latex catheters and receptors on the uroepithelium. They resist flushing during normal micturition. These strains also have P fimbriae (pyelonephritis-associated fimbriae) that bind to the uroepithelium of individuals with P blood group antigen and readily ascend the urinary tract (see Figure 30-5). Some women may be genetically susceptible to certain strains of *E. coli* attachment.[39] Hematogenous infections are uncommon and often preceded by septicemia. Infection initiates an inflammatory response and the symptoms of cystitis. The inflammatory edema in the bladder wall stimulates discharge of stretch receptors, initiating symptoms of bladder fullness with small volumes of urine and producing the urgency and frequency of urination associated with cystitis.

CLINICAL MANIFESTATIONS Many individuals with bacteriuria are asymptomatic, and older adults have the highest risk. Clinical manifestations of cystitis are related to the inflammatory response and usually include frequency, urgency, dysuria (painful urination), and suprapubic and low back pain. Hematuria, cloudy urine, and flank pain are more serious symptoms. Approximately 10% of individuals with bacteriuria have no symptoms, and 30% of individuals with symptoms are abacteriuric. Older adults with cystitis may be asymptomatic or demonstrate confusion or vague abdominal discomfort. Older adults who have recurrent UTIs and other concurrent illness have a higher risk for mortality.[40]

EVALUATION AND TREATMENT Infections in symptomatic individuals are diagnosed by urine culture of specific microorganisms with counts of 10 000/mL or more from freshly voided urine. Urine dipstick testing that is positive for leukocyte esterase or nitrite reductase can be used for the diagnosis of uncomplicated UTI. Risk factors, such as urinary tract obstruction, should be identified and treated. Evidence of bacteria from urine culture and antibiotic sensitivity warrants treatment with a microorganism-specific antibiotic. Acute uncomplicated cystitis in nonpregnant women can be diagnosed without an office visit or urine culture. If a urine culture and sensitivity are ordered, the urine specimen must be obtained before the initiation of any antibiotic therapy; 3 to 7 days of treatment is most common.[41] Complicated UTI requires 7 to 14 days of treatment. From 20 to 25% of women have relapsing infection within 7 to 10 days, requiring prolonged antibiotic treatment. Follow-up urine cultures should be obtained 1 week after initiation of treatment and at monthly intervals for 3 months. Clinical symptoms are frequently relieved, but bacteriuria may still be present. Repeat cultures should be obtained every 3 to 4 months until 1 year after treatment for evaluation and treatment of recurrent infection[42] (see *Health Promotion:* Urinary Tract Infection and Antibiotic Resistance).

Painful Bladder Syndrome/Interstitial Cystitis

Painful bladder syndrome/interstitial cystitis (PBS/IC) is a condition that includes **nonbacterial infectious cystitis** (viral, mycobacterial, chlamydial, fungal), **noninfectious cystitis** (radiation injury, chemical, autoimmune, hypersensitivity), and interstitial cystitis. It occurs most commonly in women ages 20 to 30 years who have symptoms of cystitis, such as frequency, urgency, dysuria, and nocturia, but with negative urine cultures and no other known etiology. Nonbacterial infectious cystitis is most common among those who are immunocompromised. Noninfectious cystitis is associated with radiation or chemotherapy treatment for pelvic and urogenital cancers.

The cause of PBS/IC is unknown. An autoimmune reaction may be responsible for the inflammatory response, which includes mast cell

HEALTH PROMOTION

Urinary Tract Infection and Antibiotic Resistance

Uncomplicated urinary tract infection (UTI) is one of the most common bacterial infections. Of major concern is the worldwide emergence of bacterial strains resistant to specific antibiotics in both hospital- and community-acquired UTIs, causing increased cost, hospitalization, morbidity, and mortality. The resistance is caused in part by overuse of antibiotics. Risks for resistance are highest in regions with the highest rates of prescription and in those who have received trimethoprim-sulfamethoxazole (TMP-SMX [Bactrim]) treatment within the last 3 months, have a diagnosis of diabetes mellitus, have been recently hospitalized, and have community-specific antibiotic resistance rates of greater than 20%. The leading cause of UTI is *Escherichia coli*, followed by *Klebsiella pneumoniae* and *Proteus mirabilis*, and antibiotics are the mainstay of treatment. These bacteria and other Gram-negative species produce β-lactamases and carbapenemases, causing resistance to penicillins, cephalosporins, and carbapenems (used for complicated UTI). TMP-SMX and fluoroquinolone (such as ciprofloxacin [Cipro] and levofloxacin [Levaquin]) have a high rate of resistance. Multidrug-resistant extended-spectrum β-lactamase (ESBL)–producing *E. coli* are occurring with no known risk factors. First-time uncomplicated UTI can be treated empirically with a 3-day regimen. Complicated infection requires individualized assessment of risk factors for medication resistance and medication tolerability and includes history, physical examination, urine culture and sensitivity, and possible radiological evaluation. Asymptomatic bacteriuria only requires treatment in exceptional cases. Awareness of medication resistance and knowledgeable prescribing are essential to prevent inappropriate use of antibiotics. New medications are being discovered that overcome bacterial resistance, and old medications in new combinations are being tested.

The North American Urinary Tract Infection Collaborative Alliance (NAUTICA) study indicates that antibiotic resistance rates for UTIs are higher in the United States than in Canada for four out of the five antibiotics tested. The study analyzed 813 isolates obtained from 586 patients in the United States and 227 patients in Canada. Overall, most of the bacteria found in the isolates were *E. coli* (54.4%), followed by *K. pneumoniae* (11.8%), Enterococcus species (7%), *P. mirabilis* (5.1%), *Pseudomonas aeruginosa* (2.9%), *Staphylococcus aureus* (2.3%), and *Enterobacter cloacae* (2.2%) (other bacteria accounted for the remaining 14.3% of the isolates). The antibiotic resistance rates were as follows: TMP-SMX, 20.8% among the US isolates and 16.7% among the Canadian isolates; nitrofurantoin (MacroBid), 13.7% among the US isolates and 11% among the Canadian isolates; levofloxacin, 8.9% among the US isolates and 5.3% among the Canadian isolates; and ciprofloxacin, 9.9% among the US isolates and 5.7% among the Canadian isolates. Only ampicillin had a higher antibiotic resistance rate among the Canadian isolates compared with the US isolates (44.9% versus 40.8%).

Data from Bush, K., Courvalin, P., Dantas, G., et al. (2011). *Nat Rev Microbiol, 9*(12), 894–896; Grigoryan, L., Trautner, B.W., & Gupta, K. (2014). *JAMA, 312*(16), 1677–1684; Gupta, K., & Bhadelia, N. (2014). *Infect Dis Clin North Am, 28*(1), 49–59; Ling, L.L., Schneider, T., Peoples, A.J., et al. (2015). *Nature, 517*(7535), 455–459; National Guideline Clearinghouse. (2008). *Guideline synthesis: Diagnosis and management of lower urinary tract infection.* Rockville, MD: Author and Agency for Healthcare Research and Quality. Retrieved from https://www.guideline.gov; Splete, H. (2003). UTI patients show antibiotic resistance: Lower resistance in Canada. *Internal Medicine News, 1*(39); Trautner, B.W., & Grigoryan, L. (2014). *Infect Dis Clin North Am, 28*(1), 15–31.

TABLE 30-3 Common Causes of Pyelonephritis

Predisposing Factor	Pathological Mechanisms
Kidney stones	Obstruction and stasis of urine contributing to bacteriuria and hydronephrosis; irritation of epithelial lining with entrapment of bacteria
Vesicoureteral reflux	Chronic reflux of urine up the ureter and into kidney during micturition, contributing to bacterial infection
Pregnancy	Dilation and relaxation of ureter with hydroureter and hydronephrosis; partly caused by obstruction from enlarged uterus and partly from ureteral relaxation caused by higher progesterone levels
Neurogenic bladder	Neurological impairment interfering with normal bladder contraction with residual urine and ascending infection
Instrumentation	Introduction of organisms into urethra and bladder by catheters and endoscopes introduced into urinary tract for diagnostic purposes
Female sexual trauma	Movement of organisms from urethra into bladder with infection and retrograde spread to kidney

activation, altered uroepithelial permeability, and increased sensory nerve sensitivity. Inflammation and fibrosis of the bladder wall are accompanied by the presence of hemorrhagic ulcers (Hunner ulcers), and bladder volume may decrease as a result of fibrosis. Alteration of the bladder uroepithelial proteoglycan layer makes it more susceptible to penetration by bacteria. Characteristic symptoms of PBS/IC include bladder fullness, urinary frequency (including nocturia), small urine volume, and chronic pelvic pain with symptoms lasting longer than 9 months. Diagnosis of PBS/IC requires the exclusion of other diagnoses, and extensive evaluations are completed. No single treatment is effective. Oral and intravesical therapies, sacral nerve stimulation, and botulinum toxin type A are used for symptom relief. Surgery is used in refractory cases.[43,44]

Acute Pyelonephritis

Pyelonephritis is an infection of one or both upper urinary tracts (ureter, renal pelvis, and interstitium). Common causes are summarized in Table 30-3. Urinary obstruction and reflux of urine from the bladder (vesicoureteral reflux) are the most common underlying risk factors. One or both kidneys may be involved. Most cases occur in women.

PATHOPHYSIOLOGY Microorganisms usually associated with acute pyelonephritis include *E. coli*, *Proteus*, or *Pseudomonas*. The latter two microorganisms are more commonly associated with infections after urethral instrumentation or urinary tract surgery. These microorganisms also split urea into ammonia, making alkaline urine that increases the risk for stone formation. The infection is probably spread by ascending uropathic microorganisms along the ureters, but dissemination also may occur by way of the bloodstream. The inflammatory process is usually focal and irregular, primarily affecting the pelvis, calyces, and medulla. The infection causes medullary infiltration of white blood cells with renal inflammation, renal edema, and purulent urine. In severe infections, localized abscesses may form in the medulla and extend to the cortex. Primarily affected are the tubules; the glomeruli usually are spared. Necrosis of renal papillae can develop. After the acute phase, healing occurs with fibrosis and atrophy of affected tubules. The number of bacteria decreases until the urine again becomes sterile. Acute pyelonephritis rarely causes kidney failure.[45]

CLINICAL MANIFESTATIONS The onset of symptoms is usually acute, with fever, chills, and flank or groin pain. Symptoms characteristic of a UTI, including frequency, dysuria, and costovertebral tenderness, may precede systemic signs and symptoms. Older adults may have nonspecific symptoms, such as low-grade fever and malaise.

EVALUATION AND TREATMENT Differentiating symptoms of cystitis from those of pyelonephritis by clinical assessment alone is difficult. The specific diagnosis is established by urine culture, urinalysis, and clinical signs and symptoms. White blood cell casts indicate pyelonephritis, but they are not always present in the urine. Complicated pyelonephritis requires blood cultures and urinary tract imaging.[46] Uncomplicated acute pyelonephritis responds well to 2 to 3 weeks of microorganism-specific antibiotic therapy. Follow-up urine cultures are obtained at 1 and 4 weeks after treatment if symptoms recur. Antibiotic-resistant microorganisms or re-infection may occur in cases of urinary tract obstruction or reflux. Intravenous pyelography and voiding cystourethrography identify surgically correctable lesions.

Chronic Pyelonephritis

Chronic pyelonephritis is a persistent or recurrent infection of the kidney leading to scarring of one or both kidneys. The specific cause of chronic pyelonephritis is difficult to determine. Recurrent infections from acute pyelonephritis may be associated with chronic pyelonephritis. Generally, chronic pyelonephritis is more likely to occur in individuals who have renal infections associated with some type of obstructive pathological condition, such as renal stones and vesicoureteral reflux.

PATHOPHYSIOLOGY Chronic urinary tract obstruction prevents elimination of bacteria and starts a process of progressive inflammation, alterations of the renal pelvis and calyces, destruction of the tubules, atrophy or dilation and diffuse scarring, and, finally, impaired urine-concentrating ability, leading to CKD. The lesions of chronic pyelonephritis are sometimes termed *chronic interstitial nephritis* because the inflammation and fibrosis are located in the interstitial spaces between the tubules.

CLINICAL MANIFESTATIONS The early symptoms of chronic pyelonephritis are often minimal and may include hypertension, frequency, dysuria, and flank pain. Progression can lead to kidney failure, particularly in the presence of obstructive uropathy or diabetes mellitus.

EVALUATION AND TREATMENT Urinalysis, intravenous pyelography, and ultrasound are used diagnostically. Treatment is related to the underlying cause. Obstruction must be relieved. Antibiotics may be given, with prolonged antibiotic therapy for recurrent infection.

✔ QUICK CHECK 30-2

1. Why is cystitis more common in women?
2. What is interstitial cystitis?
3. How does pyelonephritis differ from cystitis?

GLOMERULAR DISORDERS

Glomerulonephritis

Acute glomerulonephritis is an inflammation of the glomerulus caused by *primary glomerular injury*, including immunological responses, ischemia, free radicals, medications, toxins, vascular disorders, and infection. *Secondary glomerular injury* is a consequence of systemic diseases, including diabetes mellitus, hypertension, bacterial toxins, systemic lupus erythematosus, heart failure, and HIV-related kidney disease.

PATHOPHYSIOLOGY Immune mechanisms are a major cause of injury for primary and secondary causes of glomerulonephritis (Figure 30-6). The injury damages the glomerular capillary filtration membrane, including the endothelium, basement membrane, and epithelium (podocytes). The most common types of immune injury are (1) deposition of circulating antigen–antibody immune complexes into the glomerulus (type III hypersensitivity) and (2) reaction of antibodies in situ against planted antigens within the glomerulus (type II hypersensitivity, cytotoxic) (see Chapter 8). Nonimmune glomerular injury is related to ischemia, metabolic disorders (e.g., diabetes mellitus), toxin exposure, medications, vascular disorders (e.g., vasculitis), and infection with direct injury to glomerular cells. Different causes of injury may result in more than one type of glomerular lesion; thus lesions are not necessarily disease specific (Table 30-4).

Immune injury is caused by activation of biochemical mediators of inflammation (i.e., complement and cytokines from leukocytes) and begins after the antigen–antibody complexes have deposited or formed in the glomerular capillary wall or mesangium. Complement is deposited with the antibodies, and activation can cause cell lysis or serve as a chemotactic stimulus for attraction of neutrophils, monocytes, and T cells. These phagocytes, along with activated platelets, further the inflammatory reaction by releasing mediators that injure the glomerular filtration membrane, including epithelial cells, glomerular basement membrane, and endothelial cells (podocytes and filtration slits).[47] The injury increases glomerular membrane permeability and reduces glomerular membrane surface area. The GFR decreases, resulting in increased serum creatinine levels. There also may be swelling and proliferation of mesangial cells and expansion of the extracellular matrix

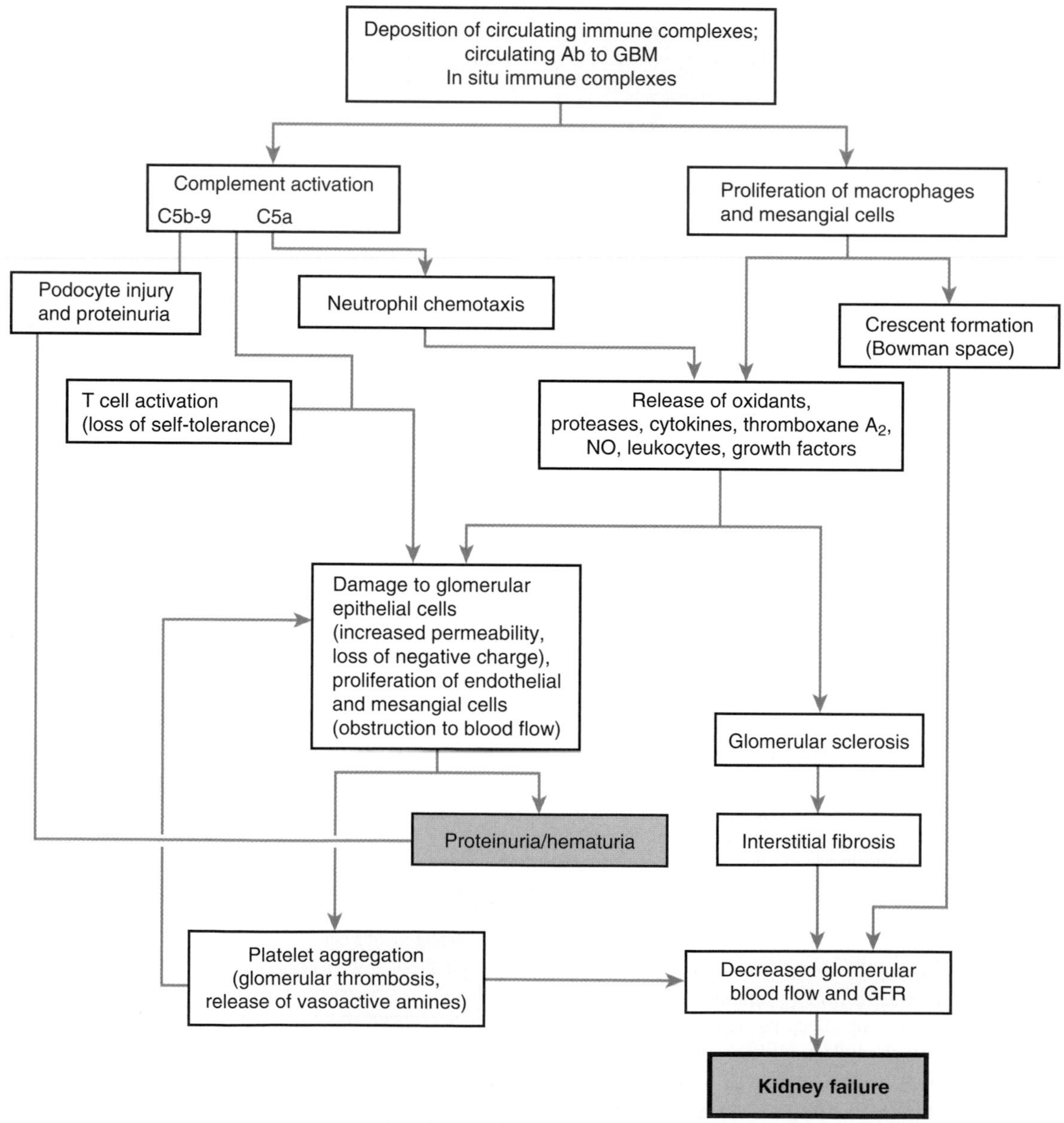

FIGURE 30-6 Mechanisms of Glomerular Injury. *Ab*, antibody; *C5a*, small fragment produced from complement component C5; *C5b-9*, a complement complex; *GBM*, glomerular basement membrane; *GFR*, glomerular filtration rate; *NO*, nitric oxide.

in the Bowman space, contributing to crescent formation (deposition of substances in the Bowman space, forming the shape of a crescent moon). The result is decreased glomerular blood flow, decreased driving hydrostatic pressure, decreased GFR, and hypoxic injury.[48]

Loss of negative electrical charge across the glomerular filtration membrane and increase in filtration pore size enhance movement of proteins into the urine. Proteins are normally repelled because they also have a negative charge. Red blood cells also escape if pore size is large enough. Proteinuria or hematuria, or both, develops. The severity of glomerular damage and decline in glomerular function is related to the size, number, and location (focal or diffuse) of cells injured, duration of exposure, and type of antigen–antibody complexes.

CLINICAL MANIFESTATIONS The onset of glomerulonephritis may be sudden or insidious, and significant loss of nephron function can occur before symptoms develop. Acute glomerulonephritis may be silent, mild, moderate, or severe in symptom presentation. Severe or progressive glomerular disease causes oliguria (urine output of 30 mL/hour or less), hypertension, and kidney failure. Focal lesions tend to produce less severe clinical symptoms. Salt and water are reabsorbed, contributing to fluid volume expansion, edema, and hypertension.

TABLE 30-4 Types of Glomerular Lesions

Lesion	Characteristics
Glomerular Lesions	
Diffuse	Relatively uniform involvement of most or all glomeruli; most common form of glomerulonephritis
Focal	Changes in only some glomeruli, whereas others are normal
Segmental-local	Changes in one part of glomerulus with other parts unaffected
Lesion Characteristics	
Mesangial	Deposits of immunoglobulins in mesangial matrix, mesangial cell proliferation
Membranous	Thickening of glomerular capillary wall with immune deposits
Proliferative	Increase in number of glomerular cells
Sclerotic	Glomerular scarring from previous glomerular injury
Crescentic	Accumulation of proliferating cells within Bowman space, making crescent appearance
Interstitial fibrosis	Scarring between glomerulus and tubules

Two major symptoms distinctive of more severe glomerulonephritis (i.e., associated with rapidly progressive glomerulonephritis) are (1) hematuria with red blood cell casts and (2) proteinuria exceeding 3 to 5 g/day with albumin (macroalbuminuria) as the major protein. Different types of acute glomerulonephritis may be associated with different patterns of urinary sediment and nephrotic or nephritic syndrome.

EVALUATION AND TREATMENT The diagnosis of glomerular disease is confirmed by the progressive development of clinical manifestations and laboratory findings of abnormal urinalysis with proteinuria, red blood cells, white blood cells, and casts. Microscopic evaluation from renal biopsy provides a specific determination of renal injury and type of pathological condition. Patterns of antigen–antibody complex deposition within the glomerular capillary filtration membrane have been established using light, electron, and immunofluorescent microscopy for different disease processes. The findings with light microscopy provide information about the distribution and extent of immune response injury (Table 30-5). Electron microscopy differentiates morphological changes within the glomerular capillary wall. Staining with fluorescein identifies different antibodies (i.e., immunoglobulin G [IgG] or immunoglobulin A [IgA]) and their configurations when viewed under ultraviolet (black) light with a microscope.

Reduced GFR during glomerulonephritis is evidenced by elevated plasma urea, cystatin C, and creatinine concentrations, or by reduced creatinine clearance (see Chapter 29). Edema, caused by excessive sodium and water retention, may require the use of diuretics or dialysis.

Management principles for treating glomerulonephritis are related to treating the primary disease, preventing or minimizing immune responses, and correcting accompanying problems, such as edema, hypertension, hypoalbuminemia, and dyslipidemia. Specific treatment regimens are necessary for particular types of glomerulonephritis. Antibiotic therapy is essential for the management of underlying infections that may be contributing to ongoing antigen–antibody responses. Corticosteroids decrease antibody synthesis and suppress inflammatory responses. Cytotoxic agents (e.g., cyclophosphamide) may be used to suppress the immune response in corticosteroid-resistant cases. Anticoagulants may be useful for controlling fibrin crescent formation in rapidly progressive glomerulonephritis.

Types of Glomerulonephritis

The classification of glomerulonephritis can be described according to cause, pathological lesions, disease progression (acute, rapidly progressive, chronic), or clinical presentation (nephrotic syndrome, nephritic

TABLE 30-5 Immunological Pathogenesis of Glomerulonephritis

Glomerular Injury	Mechanism
Soluble immune-complex glomerulonephritis (90%)	Formation of antibodies stimulated by presence of endogenous or exogenous antigens; results in circulating soluble antigen–antibody complexes deposited in glomerular capillaries or formation of complexes within the glomerular membrane; glomerular injury occurs with complement activation and release of immunological substances that lyse cells and increase membrane permeability; severity of glomerular injury related to number of complexes formed; type III hypersensitivity reaction
Anti–glomerular basement membrane glomerulonephritis (5%)	Antibodies are formed and act directly against glomerular basement membrane; immune response causes accumulation of inflammatory cells in Bowman space (in shape of a crescent moon) surrounding and compressing glomerular capillaries; generally associated with rapidly progressive kidney failure, such as Goodpasture's syndrome; type II hypersensitivity reaction
Alternative complement pathway	Relatively rare, mechanism associated with low levels of complement and membranoproliferative glomerulonephritis; type III hypersensitivity reaction
Cell-mediated immunity	Delayed hypersensitivity response that damages glomerulus; actual cellular mechanism not clearly understood; type IV hypersensitivity reaction

syndrome, AKI, or CKD). In nearly all types of glomerulonephritis, the epithelial or podocyte layer of the glomerular capillary membrane is disturbed with loss of negative charges and changes in membrane permeability; the mesangial matrix may be expanded or the basement membrane thickened. Features of the patterns of glomerular injury are summarized in Table 30-6. Many types of glomerular injury occur most often in children or young adults, including acute postinfectious glomerulonephritis and minimal change nephropathy (lipoid nephrosis). Details of these diseases are presented in Chapter 31.

Complications of diabetic nephropathy and systemic lupus erythematosus can affect the entire nephron and glomerular injury is significant. Different patterns of injury develop over the course of these diseases. **Diabetic nephropathy** develops from metabolic and vascular complications (see Chapter 19). Changes in the glomerulus are characterized by progressive thickening and fibrosis of the glomerular basement membrane, and nodular expansion of the mesangial matrix with albuminuria, podocyte loss, tubular epithelial cell atrophy, and progression to CKD (Figure 30-7). Diabetic nephropathy is the most common cause of CKD and end-stage kidney disease (ESKD; also called *end-stage renal failure*). Glomerular structure and function can return to normal after pancreatic transplantation and years of normoglycemia.[49] **Lupus nephritis** is caused by the formation of autoantibodies against double-stranded DNA with glomerular deposition of the immune complexes and alteration in B-cell and T-cell subsets. There is complement activation and a cascade of inflammatory events resulting in damage to the glomerular membrane with mesangial expansion.[50]

Chronic Glomerulonephritis

Chronic glomerulonephritis encompasses several glomerular diseases with a progressive course leading to CKD. There may be no history of kidney disease before the diagnosis. Hypercholesterolemia and proteinuria have been associated with progressive glomerular and tubular injury. The proposed mechanism is related to those observed in glomerulosclerosis and interstitial injury, such as hyperfiltration and inflammatory processes.[51] The primary cause may be difficult to establish because advanced pathological changes may obscure specific disease characteristics (see Figure 30-7). Diabetes mellitus and lupus erythematosus are examples of secondary causes of chronic glomerular injury.[52] Renal insufficiency

TABLE 30-6 Features of the Common Types of Glomerulonephritis

Type and Cause	Pathophysiology
Associated With Nephritic Syndrome	
Acute postinfectious/infection-related glomerulonephritis (group A β-hemolytic streptococcus or staphylococcus)	Diffuse deposits of immune complexes (IgG and complement) in glomerular capillary wall; infiltration of leukocytes; endocapillary proliferation and mesangial proliferation
• Occurs with untreated primary infection in throat or skin	Decreased capillary blood flow and GFR
Crescentic or rapidly progressive glomerulonephritis	Accumulation of immune deposits and inflammatory cells and debris that proliferate into Bowman space and form crescent-shaped lesions
• In situ formation of anti–glomerular basement membrane antibodies or immune complex deposition	Decreased capillary blood flow and GFR
• Nonspecific response to glomerular injury; can occur in any severe glomerular disease	Can result in kidney failure within 3 months Formation of Ab against both pulmonary capillary and GBM
• Can be associated with Goodpasture's syndrome	
Mesangial proliferative glomerulonephritis	Deposits of immune complexes in mesangium with mesangial proliferation
• IgA nephropathy	Decreased glomerular blood flow and GFR Abnormal glycosylated IgA-1 and complement bind to mesangial cells causing proliferation
Associated With Nephrotic Syndrome	
Minimal change disease (lipoid nephrosis)	Uniform diffuse thinning of epithelial (podocyte) foot processes; loss of negative charge in basement membrane and increased permeability
• Glomerular basement membrane appears normal	
• Usually idiopathic	Severe proteinuria and nephrotic syndrome
• No immune deposits	
Focal segmented glomerulosclerosis	Similar to minimal change disease
• Usually idiopathic	
Membranous nephropathy (autoimmune response to unknown renal antigen)	Thickening of glomerular capillary wall caused by antibody and complement deposition and release of inflammatory cytokines with focal segmental sclerosis and increased permeability, proteinuria, and nephrotic syndrome
• Usually idiopathic	
• Can be associated with systemic diseases (i.e., hepatitis B virus, systemic lupus erythematous, solid malignant tumours)	
Membranoproliferative glomerulonephritis	Mesangial cell proliferation; thickening of basement membrane; subendothelial deposits of immune complex occlude glomerular capillary blood flow
• Usually idiopathic; associated with low complement levels	Decreased GFR
IgA nephropathy (Berger's disease) Usually idiopathic; elevated IgA plasma levels	Mesangial deposits of IgA and proliferation of inflammatory cells into Bowman space, with sclerosis and fibrosis of glomerulus and crescent formation Decreased GFR and hematuria; usually focal, some diffuse lesions
Chronic glomerulonephritis	Glomerular fibrosis and scarring, interstitial and tubular fibrosis and vascular sclerosis; original glomerular lesions may not be definable; progression to end-stage kidney disease with uremia
• Can be a consequence of any type of glomerulonephritis; more common with crescentic or rapidly progressive glomerulonephritis	

Ab, antibody; *GBM*, glomerular basement membrane; *GFR*, glomerular filtration rate; *IgA*, immunoglobulin A; *IgG*, immunoglobulin G.

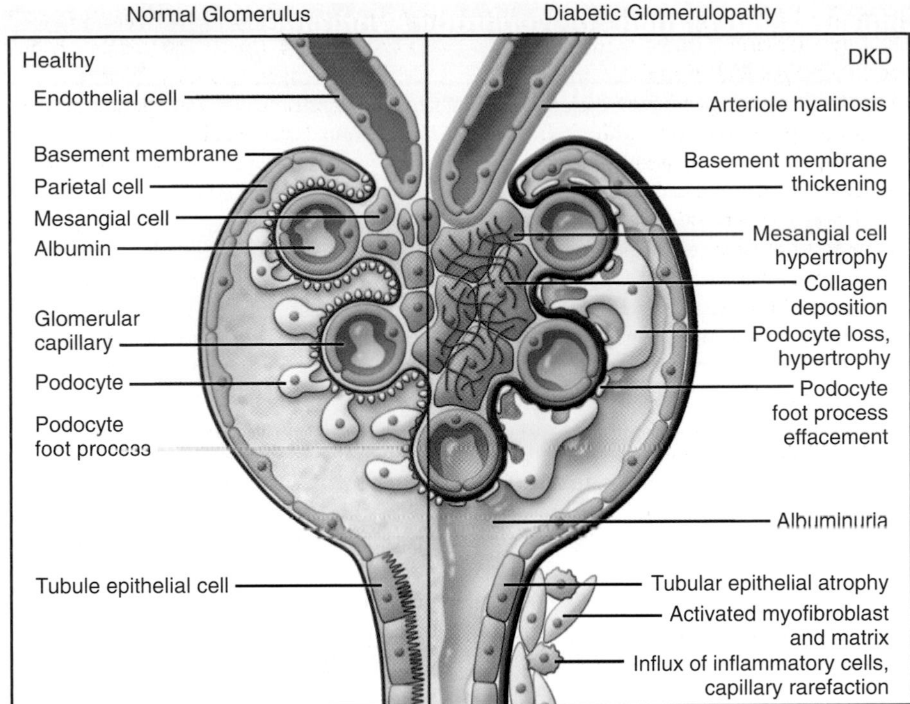

FIGURE 30-7 Diabetic Glomerulopathy. *DKD,* diabetic kidney disease. (From Reidy, K., Kang, H.M., Hostetter, T., et al. [2014]. *J Clin Invest, 124*[6], 2333–2340. JOURNAL OF CLINICAL INVESTIGATION. ONLINE by AMERICAN SOCIETY FOR CLINICAL INVESTIGATION. Reproduced with permission of AMERICAN SOCIETY FOR CLINICAL INVESTIGATION in the format Republish in a book via Copyright Clearance Center.)

usually begins to develop after 10 to 20 years, followed by nephrotic syndrome and an accelerated progression to ESKD. Symptom patterns vary depending on the underlying cause. The specific pathological condition is identified by renal biopsy and is best performed in early stages of CKD to identify specific treatment options.[53] Use of steroids and immunosuppressive agents can prolong remissions and preserve renal function. Dialysis or kidney transplantation ultimately may be needed.

Nephrotic and Nephritic Syndromes

Nephrotic syndrome is the excretion of 3.5 grams or more of protein in the urine per day and is characteristic of glomerular injury. It occurs when filtration of proteins exceeds tubular reabsorption. *Primary causes of nephrotic syndrome* include minimal change nephropathy (lipoid nephrosis) (see Chapter 31), membranous glomerulonephritis, and focal segmental glomerulosclerosis.[54] *Secondary forms of nephrotic syndrome* occur in systemic diseases, including diabetes mellitus (see Chapter 19), amyloidosis, systemic lupus erythematosus, and Henoch-Schönlein purpura (see Chapter 31). Nephrotic syndrome also is associated with certain medications (e.g., nonsteroidal anti-inflammatory drugs [NSAIDs]), infections, malignancies, and vascular disorders. When present as a secondary complication with renal diseases, nephrotic syndrome often signifies a more serious prognosis.[54] Nephrotic syndrome is more common in children than adults (see Chapter 31).

Nephritic syndrome is characterized by hematuria and red blood cell casts in the urine. Proteinuria is usually less severe than in nephrotic syndrome. It occurs primarily with infection-related glomerulonephritis and rapidly progressive crescentic glomerulonephritis.

PATHOPHYSIOLOGY In nephrotic syndrome, disturbances in the glomerular basement membrane and podocyte injury lead to increased permeability to protein and loss of electrical negative charge. Loss of plasma proteins, particularly albumin and some immunoglobulins, occurs across the injured glomerular filtration membrane. Loss of plasma proteins decreases plasma oncotic pressure, resulting in edema. The predominant cause of nephrotic syndrome is minimal change nephropathy, which is common in children (see Chapter 31). Hypoalbuminemia results from urinary loss of albumin combined with a diminished synthesis of replacement albumin by the liver. Albumin is lost in the greatest quantity because of its high plasma concentration and low molecular weight. Decreased dietary intake of protein from anorexia or malnutrition or accompanying liver disease may also contribute to lower levels of plasma albumin. Loss of albumin stimulates lipoprotein synthesis by the liver and dyslipidemia and can promote progression of glomerular disease. Loss of immunoglobulins may increase susceptibility to infections. Sodium retention is common.[55]

In nephritic syndrome, hematuria (usually microscopic) is present and red blood cell casts are present in the urine in addition to proteinuria, which is not severe. It is caused by increased permeability of the glomerular filtration membrane with pore sizes large enough to allow the passage of red blood cells and protein. Nephritic syndrome is associated with postinfectious glomerulonephritis, rapidly progressive (crescentic) glomerulonephritis, IgA nephropathy, lupus nephritis, and diabetic nephropathy. The pathophysiology is related to immune injury of the glomerulus as previously described. Hypertension and uremia occur in advanced stages of disease.

CLINICAL MANIFESTATIONS Many clinical manifestations of nephrotic and nephritic syndrome are related to loss of serum proteins and associated sodium retention (Table 30-7). They include edema, hypoproteinemia, proteinuria, dyslipidemia, lipiduria, vitamin D deficiency, and hypothyroidism.[56] Vitamin D deficiency is related to loss of serum transport proteins and decreased vitamin D activation by the kidney. Hypothyroidism can result from urinary loss of thyroid-binding protein and thyroxine. Alterations in coagulation factors can cause hypercoagulability and may lead to thromboembolic events.[57]

TABLE 30-7 Clinical Manifestations of Nephrotic Syndrome

Manifestation	Contributing Factors	Result
Significant proteinuria	Increased glomerular permeability, decreased proximal tubule reabsorption	Edema, increased susceptibility to infection from loss of immunoglobulins
Hypoalbuminemia	Increased urinary losses of protein	Edema
Edema	Hypoalbuminemia (decreased plasma oncotic pressure, sodium and water retention, increased aldosterone and antidiuretic hormone [ADH] secretion), unresponsiveness to atrial natriuretic peptides	Soft, pitting, generalized edema
Dyslipidemia	Decreased serum albumin level; increased hepatic synthesis of very low–density lipoproteins; increased levels of cholesterol, phospholipids, triglycerides	Increased atherogenesis
Lipiduria	Sloughing of tubular cells containing fat (oval fat bodies); free fat from dyslipidemia	Fat droplets that may float in urine

EVALUATION AND TREATMENT Nephrotic syndrome is diagnosed when the protein level in a 24-hour urine collection is greater than 3.5 g. Serum albumin level decreases (to less than 30 g/L), and concentrations of serum cholesterol, phospholipids, and triglycerides increase. Fat bodies may be present in the urine.

Nephrotic syndrome is commonly treated by consuming a moderate protein restriction (i.e., 0.8 g/kg body weight/day), low-fat, salt-restricted diet, as well as by prescribing diuretics. Diuretics are used to control hypertension and eliminate fluid. Care must be taken to observe for hypovolemia and hypokalemia or potassium toxicity in the presence of renal insufficiency. Spironolactone may be combined with loop diuretics to suppress aldosterone activity to conserve potassium. Heparinoids are used for prophylactic anticoagulation. Glucocorticoids are used to control immune-mediated disease or may be combined with immunosuppressive medications. Angiotensin-converting enzyme (ACE) inhibitors or angiotensin receptor blockers (ARBs) lower urine protein excretion.[58]

The evaluation and treatment of nephritic syndrome are similar to those described for nephrotic syndrome. The course of glomerulonephritis is usually more severe with nephritic syndrome. High-dose corticosteroids and cyclophosphamide represent the standard therapy for rapidly progressive crescentic glomerulonephritis. The addition of plasma exchange (plasmapheresis) also may be helpful.[59]

✔QUICK CHECK 30-3
1. What is glomerulonephritis? List two types.
2. What immune mechanisms are operative in glomerulonephritis?
3. Why is edema present in individuals with nephrotic syndrome?

ACUTE KIDNEY INJURY

Classification of Kidney Dysfunction

Kidney injury may be acute and rapidly progressive (within hours), and the process may be reversible. **Acute kidney injury (AKI)** commonly occurs as a result of ischemic damage to renal tubular epithelial cells (RTECs). The term **acute tubular necrosis (ATN)**, which signifies a sudden deterioration in kidney function resulting from ischemic or toxin-related insult to the RTECs, was the common term in use. Recently, clinicians and researchers have debated the precision in using *ATN* because of the limited number of necrotic cells found on kidney biopsy. The term *acute tubular injury* has commonly been used instead of *acute tubular necrosis*, as it offers a broader and more inclusive definition that extends beyond the pathology of necrosis.[60] In this chapter we will continue to use *ATN* until a consensus on new terminology is reached.

Kidney failure also can be chronic, progressing to ESKD over a period of months or years. The terms *renal insufficiency, kidney failure, uremia*, and *azotemia* are associated with decreasing renal function but are not specific in relation to the cause of kidney disease. They are often used synonymously, although with some distinctions. Generally, **renal insufficiency** refers to a decline in renal function to about 25% of normal or a GFR of 25 to 30 mL/min. Levels of serum creatinine and urea are mildly elevated. The term *acute kidney injury* is preferred to the term *acute renal failure* because it captures the diverse nature of this syndrome, ranging from minimal or subtle changes in renal function to complete kidney failure requiring renal replacement therapy. **Kidney failure** refers to significant loss of renal function. When less than 10% of renal function remains, the term used is **end-stage kidney disease (ESKD)**. Specific criteria for acute renal dysfunction are discussed in the next section. **Uremia (uremic syndrome)** is a syndrome of kidney failure and includes elevated blood urea and creatinine levels accompanied by fatigue, anorexia, nausea, vomiting, pruritus, and neurological changes. Uremia represents numerous consequences related to kidney failure, including retention of toxic wastes, deficiency states, electrolyte disorders, and immune activation promoting a proinflammatory state. **Azotemia** is characterized by increased blood urea nitrogen (BUN) levels (normal is 3.6-7.1 mmol/L) and frequently increased serum creatinine levels (normal is male 53–106 mcmol/L, female 44–97 mcmol/L). Renal insufficiency or kidney failure causes azotemia. Both azotemia and uremia indicate an accumulation of nitrogenous waste products in the blood, a common characteristic that explains the overlap in definitions of terms.

Classification of Acute Kidney Injury

AKI is a sudden decline in kidney function with a decrease in glomerular filtration and urine output with accumulation of nitrogenous waste products in the blood as demonstrated by an elevation in plasma creatinine and BUN levels. Classification criteria have been developed to guide the diagnosis of acute kidney dysfunction or failure and are described by the acronym RIFLE (*R* = risk, *I* = injury, *F* = failure, *L* = loss, and *E* = end-stage kidney disease [ESKD]), representing three levels of renal dysfunction of increasing severity (Table 30-8). A similar set of criteria has been published by the Acute Kidney Injury Network (AKIN) and Kidney Disease, Improving Global Outcomes (KDIGO).[61]

PATHOPHYSIOLOGY AKI results from ischemic injury related to extracellular volume depletion and decreased renal blood flow, toxic injury from chemicals, or sepsis-induced injury. The injury initiates an inflammatory response, vascular responses, and cell death. Alterations in renal function may be minimal or severe.[62] AKI can be categorized as prerenal (renal hypoperfusion), intrarenal (disorders involving renal parenchymal or interstitial tissue), or postrenal (urinary tract obstructive disorders) (Table 30-9 and Figure 30-8).

Prerenal acute kidney injury is the most common reason for AKI and is caused by inadequate kidney perfusion. Poor perfusion can result from hypotension, hypovolemia associated with hemorrhage or fluid loss (e.g., burns), sepsis, inadequate cardiac output (e.g., myocardial infarct [heart attack]), or renal vasoconstriction (e.g., caused by NSAIDs or radiocontrast agents) or renal artery stenosis. The GFR declines because of the decrease in filtration pressure. Failure to restore blood volume or blood pressure and oxygen delivery can cause ischemic cell injury and ATN or acute interstitial necrosis, a more severe form of AKI. Reperfusion injury with cell death also can occur[63] (see Figure 4-11). AKI can occur during CKD if a sudden stress is imposed on already marginally functioning kidneys.

Intrarenal (intrinsic) acute kidney injury can result from ischemic ATN related to prerenal AKI, nephrotoxic ATN (e.g., exposure to radiocontrast media), acute glomerulonephritis, vascular disease

TABLE 30-8 RIFLE Criteria for Acute Kidney Dysfunction or Failure

Category	GFR Criteria	Urine Output (UO) Criteria
Risk	Increased creatinine × 1.5 or GFR decrease >25%	UO <0.5 mL/kg/hr × 6 hr
Injury	Increased creatinine × 2 or GFR decrease >50%	UO <0.5 mL/kg/hr × 12 hr
Failure	Increased creatinine × 3 or GFR decrease >75%	UO <0.3 mL/kg/hr × 24 hr or anuria × 12 hr
Loss	Persistent ARF = complete loss of kidney function >4 weeks	
ESKD	End-stage kidney disease (>3 months)	

ARF, acute renal failure; *GFR*, glomerular filtration rate.
Adapted from Bellomo, R., Kellum, J.A., Mehta, R., et al. (2002). *Curr Opin Crit Care, 8*(6), 505–508; Bellomo, R., Ronco, C., Kellum, J.A., et al. (2004). *Crit Care, 8*(4). R204–R212.

TABLE 30-9 Categories of Acute Kidney Injury

Area of Dysfunction	Possible Causes
Prerenal	*Hypovolemia*
	Hemorrhagic blood loss (trauma, gastro-intestinal bleeding, complications of childbirth)
	Loss of plasma volume (burns, peritonitis)
	Water and electrolyte losses (severe vomiting or diarrhea, intestinal obstruction, uncontrolled diabetes mellitus, inappropriate use of diuretics)
	Hypotension or hypoperfusion
	Septic shock
	Cardiac failure or shock
	Massive pulmonary embolism
	Stenosis or clamping of renal artery
Intrarenal	*Acute tubular necrosis (postischemic or nephrotoxic)*
	Glomerulopathies
	Acute interstitial necrosis (tumours or toxins)
	Vascular damage
	Malignant hypertension, vasculitis
	Coagulation defects
	Renal artery/vein occlusion
	Bilateral acute pyelonephritis
Postrenal	*Obstructive uropathies (usually bilateral)*
	Ureteral destruction (edema, tumours, stones, clots)
	Bladder neck obstruction (enlarged prostate)
	Neurogenic bladder

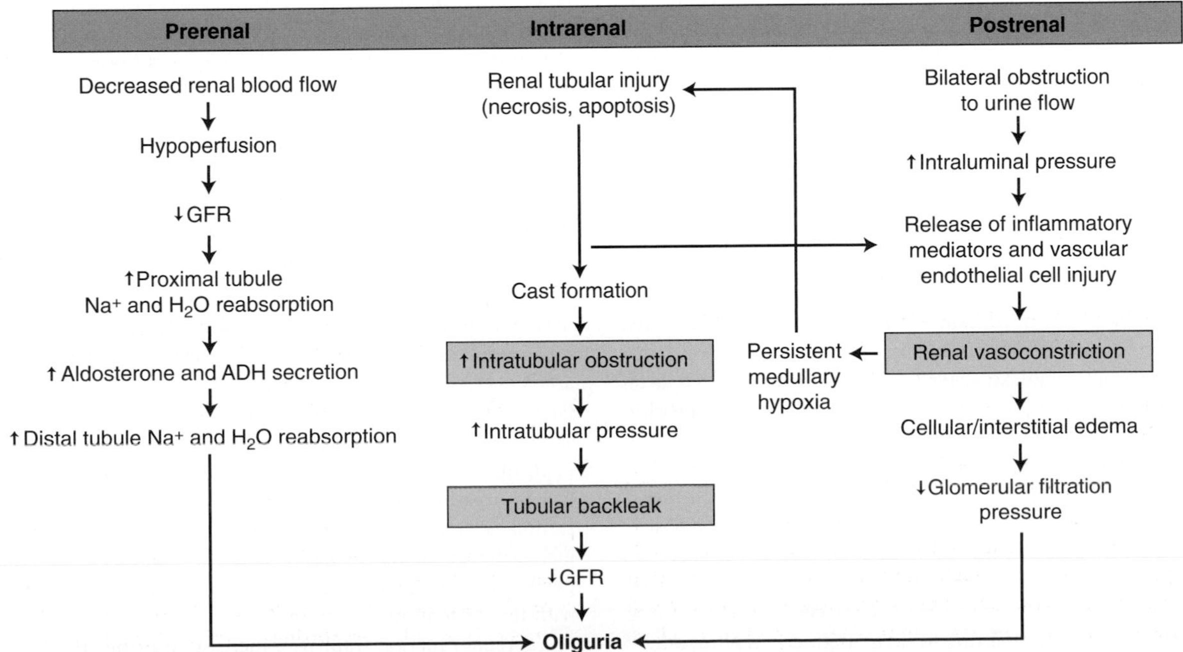

FIGURE 30-8 Acute Kidney Injury and Mechanisms of Oliguria. *ADH*, antidiuretic hormone; *GFR*, glomerular filtration rate; *H_2O*, water; *Na^+*, sodium.

(malignant hypertension, disseminated intravascular coagulation, and renal vasculitis), allograft rejection, or interstitial disease (medication allergy, infection, tumour growth). When ATN results from ischemia, it is often associated with necrosis of the tubular epithelium and the basement membrane. Moreover, because of normal discrepancies in regional blood flow and differences in energy and oxygen consumption in different areas of the nephron, tubular necrosis tends to be patchy. In the hospital setting, ATN is the most common cause of AKI, attributable to half of all cases.[60]

ATN caused by ischemia occurs most often after surgery (40 to 50% of cases) but also is associated with sepsis, obstetric complications, and severe hemorrhagic trauma or severe burns. Septic shock creates a hostile environment for the kidney because of changes in renal perfusion from systemic vasodilatation and intrarenal vasoconstriction. The decrease in renal perfusion is associated with a decrease in oxygen delivery and impairment of cellular waste removal. Moreover, sepsis can result in direct tubular damage from endotoxins and inflammatory cytokines. Hence sepsis-related tubular injury can occur in the absence of hypoperfusion and may be related to inflammation and changes in microcirculation and mitochondrial function.[60]

Abrupt cessation of blood supply to the kidney is rare but can result in kidney infarction. The culprits are usually atrial fibrillation, cardiac thrombus following myocardial infarction, paradoxical emboli from a patent foramen ovale, or thromboemboli from complex atherosclerotic plaques in the aorta.[60]

Hypotension associated with hypovolemia or shock produces ischemia and the inflammatory response, generating toxic oxygen free radicals that cause cellular swelling, injury, and necrosis. Under normal conditions, the kidney receives 20 to 25% of the total cardiac output. In response to shock and failure of peripheral circulation, the body will react by triggering the increased activity of the sympathetic nervous system and renin-angiotensin-aldosterone system. This reaction in turn causes severe vasoconstriction, particularly within the renal vasculature.[64]

Nephrotoxic ATN can be produced by radiocontrast media and numerous antibiotics, particularly the aminoglycosides (neomycin [Neosporin], gentamicin [Garamycin], tobramycin [Nebcin]) because these medications accumulate in the renal cortex. Medications that interfere with the autoregulation of renal blood flow can also contribute to ATN. For instance, over-the-counter medications (i.e., NSAIDs) can decrease blood flow through the afferent arteriole and can impair medullary blood flow in patients who are prostaglandin-dependent. Other classes of medications that can potentially lead to ATN are ACE inhibitors and ARBs.[60]

Other substances, such as excessive myoglobin (oxygen-transporting substance from muscles released with crush injuries), can also contribute to ATN. Free circulating hemoglobin occurs in the setting of intravascular hemolysis. In small quantities, circulating hemoglobin will be completely bound by plasma haptoglobin to form a hemoglobin–haptoglobin compound that is then cleared by monocytes and macrophages. However, when significant quantities of hemoglobin are present in the plasma, the haptoglobin supply is quickly depleted. Filtered hemoglobin is taken up by proximal tubule cells, or it contributes to cast formation within the lumen. Numerous causes of hemolysis can lead to hemoglobinuria. Common etiologies include transfusion reactions, autoimmune hemolytic anemia, mechanical shearing from prosthetic valves, and glucose-6 phosphate dehydrogenase deficiency. The term **rhabdomyolysis** specifically refers to the clinical syndrome associated with muscle necrosis and the release of intracellular contents into the extracellular space. The clinical spectrum can range from a relatively benign course to severe systemic illness with AKI due to heme pigment nephropathy.[60]

Other substances that can lead to ATN are carbon tetrachloride, heavy metals (mercury, arsenic), or methoxyflurane anaesthetic, and bacterial toxins may promote kidney failure. Dehydration, advanced age, concurrent renal insufficiency, and diabetes mellitus tend to enhance nephrotoxicity. Necrosis caused by nephrotoxins is usually uniform and limited to the proximal tubules.

Postrenal acute kidney injury is rare and usually occurs with urinary tract obstruction that affects the kidneys bilaterally (e.g., bladder outlet obstruction, prostatic hypertrophy, bilateral ureteral obstruction), tumours, or neurogenic bladder. A pattern of several hours of anuria with flank pain followed by polyuria is a characteristic finding. The obstruction causes an increase in intraluminal pressure upstream from the site of obstruction with a gradual decrease in GFR. This type of kidney failure can occur after diagnostic catheterization of the ureters, a procedure that may cause edema of the tubular lumen.

Oliguria (urine output of less than 400 mL/24 hours) can occur in AKI, and three mechanisms have been proposed to account for the decrease in urine output.[65] All three mechanisms probably contribute to oliguria in varying combinations and degrees throughout the course of the disease (see Figure 30-8). These mechanisms are as follows:

1. *Alterations in renal blood flow.* Efferent arteriolar vasoconstriction may be produced by intrarenal release of angiotensin II or there may be redistribution of blood flow from the cortex to the medulla. Autoregulation of blood flow may be impaired, resulting in decreased GFR. Changes in glomerular permeability and decreased GFR also may result from ischemia.
2. *Tubular obstruction.* Necrosis of the tubules causes sloughing of cells, cast formation, or ischemic edema that results in tubular obstruction, which in turn causes a retrograde increase in pressure and reduces the GFR. Kidney failure can occur within 24 hours.
3. *Tubular backleak.* Glomerular filtration remains normal, but tubular reabsorption of filtrate is accelerated as a result of permeability caused by ischemia and increased tubular pressure from obstruction.

CLINICAL MANIFESTATIONS The clinical progression of AKI with recovery of renal function occurs in three overlapping phases: initiation phase, maintenance phase, and recovery phase. The *initiation phase* is the phase of reduced perfusion or toxicity in which kidney injury is evolving. Prevention of injury is possible during this phase. The *maintenance* or *oliguric phase* is the period of established kidney injury and dysfunction after the initiating event has been resolved, and may last from weeks to months. Urine output is lowest during this phase and serum creatinine and BUN levels both increase. The *recovery* or *polyuric phase* is the interval when glomerular function returns but the regenerating tubules cannot concentrate the filtrate. Diuresis is common during this phase, with a decline in serum creatinine and urea concentrations and an increase in creatinine clearance.

Oliguria begins within 1 day after a hypotensive event and lasts 1 to 3 weeks, but it may regress in several hours or extend for several weeks, depending on the duration of ischemia or the severity of injury or obstruction. **Anuria** (urine output of less than 50 mL/day) is uncommon in ATN, involves both kidneys, and suggests bilateral renal artery occlusion, obstructive uropathy, or acute cortical necrosis. Kidney failure can present with **nonoliguric renal failure** and represents less severe injury, particularly with intrinsic kidney injury associated with nephrotoxins. The urine output may vary in volume, but the BUN and plasma creatinine concentrations increase (plasma creatinine concentration is inversely proportional to the GFR). Other manifestations include hyperkalemia, hyperphosphatemia, and metabolic acidosis from decreased urine excretion. Edema and heart failure can be associated with fluid retention.

As renal function improves, increase in urine volume (diuresis) is progressive. The tubules are still damaged early in the recovery phase but are recovering function. Polyuria can result in excessive loss of

TABLE 30-10 Differentiation of Acute Oliguric Kidney Failure

	Urine Volume	Urine Specific Gravity	Urine Osmolality	Urine Sodium Concentration	BUN/Plasma Creatinine Ratio	FE_{Na}
Prerenal failure	<400 mL	1.016–1.020	>500 mOsm	<10 mmol/L	>15:1	<1% (also seen in acute glomerulonephritis)
Intrarenal failure (i.e., acute tubular necrosis)	<400 mL	1.010–1.012	<400 mOsm	>30 mmol/L	<15:1	>1% (also seen in acute urinary tract obstruction and renal parenchymal disease)

NOTE: $FE_{Na} = \frac{\text{Urine Na/plasma Na}}{\text{Urine creatinine/plasma creatinine}} = 100.$

BUN, blood urea nitrogen.

sodium, potassium, and water. Fluid and electrolyte balance must be carefully monitored and excessive urinary losses replaced.

Serial measurements of plasma creatinine concentration provide an index of renal function during the *recovery phase*. Return to normal status may take from 3 to 12 months, and some individuals do not have full recovery of a normal GFR or tubular function.

EVALUATION AND TREATMENT The diagnosis of AKI is related to the cause of the disease. A history of surgery, trauma, or cardiovascular disorders is common, and exposure to nephrotoxins, obstructive uropathies (e.g., an enlarged prostate), or infection must be considered. The diagnostic challenge is to differentiate prerenal AKI from intrarenal AKI, and some evidence is available from urinalysis and measurement of plasma creatinine and BUN levels (Table 30-10). However, more than 50% of glomerular filtration must be lost before there is elevation of serum creatinine level. *Cystatin C*, a serum protein freely filtered at the glomerulus, can serve as a measure of GFR. Biomarkers are being developed to assess the extent of kidney injury before elevation of serum creatinine level.[66] Prevention of AKI is the most important therapeutic approach and involves avoidance of hypotension, hypovolemia, and nephrotoxicity.

The primary goal of therapy is to maintain the individual's life until renal function has recovered. Management principles directly related to physiological alterations generally include (1) correcting fluid and electrolyte disturbances, particularly hyperkalemia; (2) managing blood pressure; (3) preventing and treating infections; (4) maintaining nutrition; and (5) remembering that certain medications or their metabolites are not excreted and can be toxic. Renal replacement therapy (hemodialysis or peritoneal dialysis) may be indicated for uncontrollable hyperkalemia, acidosis, or severe fluid overload.[67,68]

CHRONIC KIDNEY DISEASE

Chronic kidney disease (CKD) is the progressive loss of renal function associated with systemic diseases, such as diabetes mellitus (most significant risk factor), hypertension, or systemic lupus erythematosus, or with intrinsic kidney diseases, such as AKI, chronic glomerulonephritis, chronic pyelonephritis, obstructive uropathies, or vascular disorders. AKI can progress to CKD. The Canadian Medical Association and the US National Kidney Foundation define *kidney damage* as a GFR less than 60 mL/min/1.73 m^2 for 3 months or more, irrespective of cause. *Chronic kidney disease* is the preferred terminology to describe gradual loss of kidney function and declining GFR. Although the terms *renal insufficiency* and *chronic renal failure* are still often used to describe declining renal function, they do not have the specificity of the stages based on GFR recommended by the US National Kidney Foundation and the Kidney Foundation of Canada (Table 30-11). CKD decreases

TABLE 30-11 Stages of Chronic Kidney Disease

Stage	Description	Signs/Symptoms
I	Normal kidney function Normal or high GFR (>90 mL/min)	*Usually none* Hypertension common
II	Mild kidney damage, mild reduction in GFR (60–89 mL/min)	*Subtle* Hypertension Increasing creatinine and urea levels
III	Moderate kidney damage GFR 30–59 mL/min	*Mild* As above
IV	Severe kidney damage GFR 15–29 mL/min	*Moderate* As above Erythropoietin deficiency anemia Hyperphosphatemia Increased triglycerides Metabolic acidosis Hyperkalemia Salt or water retention
V	End-stage kidney disease Established kidney failure GFR <15 mL/min	*Severe* As above

GFR, glomerular filtration rate.

GFR and tubular functions with changes manifested throughout all organ systems (Table 30-12 and Figure 30-9).[69]

PATHOPHYSIOLOGY The kidneys have a remarkable ability to adapt to a loss of nephron mass. Symptomatic changes result from increased levels of creatinine, urea, and potassium. Alterations in salt and water balance usually do not become apparent until renal function declines to less than 25% of normal when adaptive renal reserves have been exhausted.

Different theories have been proposed to account for the adaptation to loss of renal function. The *intact nephron hypothesis* proposes that loss of nephron mass with progressive kidney damage causes the surviving nephrons to sustain normal kidney function. These nephrons are capable of a compensatory hypertrophy and expansion or hyperfunction in their rates of filtration, reabsorption, and secretion and can maintain a constant rate of excretion in the presence of overall declining GFR.[70] The intact nephron hypothesis explains adaptive changes in solute and water regulation that occur with advancing kidney failure. Although

TABLE 30-12 Systemic Effects of Chronic Kidney Disease

System	Manifestations	Mechanisms	Treatment
Skeletal	Spontaneous fractures and bone pain Deformities of long bones	Osteitis fibrosa: bone inflammation with fibrous degeneration related to hyperparathyroidism Osteomalacia: bone resorption associated with vitamin D and calcium deficiency	Control of hyperphosphatemia to reduce hyperparathyroidism; administration of calcium and aluminum hydroxide antacids, which bind phosphate in the gut, together with a phosphate-restricted diet; vitamin D replacement; avoidance of magnesium antacids because of impaired magnesium excretion
Cardiopulmonary	Pulmonary edema, Kussmaul respirations	Fluid overload associated with pulmonary edema and metabolic acidosis leading to Kussmaul respirations	ACE inhibitors; combination of propranolol (Apo-Propranolol), hydralazine (Apo-Hydralazine), and minoxidil (Loniten) for those with high levels of renin; bilateral nephrectomy with dialysis or transplantation
Cardiovascular	Left ventricular hypertrophy, cardiomyopathy, and ischemic heart disease; hypertension, dysrhythmias, accelerated atherosclerosis; pericarditis with fever, chest pain, and pericardial friction rub	Extracellular volume expansion and hypersecretion of renin associated with hypertension; anemia increases cardiac workload; dyslipidemia promotes atherosclerosis; toxins precipitate into pericardium	Volume reduction with diuretics that are not potassium sparing (to avoid hyperkalemia); dialysis
Neurological	Encephalopathy (fatigue, reduced attention span, difficulty with problem solving); peripheral neuropathy (pain and burning in legs and feet, loss of vibration sense and deep tendon reflexes); loss of motor coordination, twitching, fasciculations, stupor, and coma with advanced uremia	Progressive accumulation of uremic toxins associated with end-stage kidney disease (ESKD) Stroke or intracerebral hemorrhage associated with chronic dialysis	Dialysis or successful kidney transplantation
Hematological	Anemia, usually normochromic–normocytic; platelet disorders with prolonged bleeding times	Reduced erythropoietin secretion and reduced red cell production; uremic toxins shorten red blood cell survival and alter platelet function	Dialysis; recombinant human erythropoietin and iron supplementation; conjugated estrogens; DDAVP (1-desamino-8-D-arginine vasopressin); transfusion
Gastro-intestinal	Anorexia, nausea, vomiting; mouth ulcers, stomatitis, urine odour of breath (uremic fetor), hiccups, peptic ulcers, gastro-intestinal bleeding, and pancreatitis associated with ESKD	Retention of metabolic acids and other metabolic waste products	Protein-restricted diet for relief of nausea and vomiting
Integumentary	Abnormal pigmentation and pruritus	Retention of urochromes, contributing to sallow yellow colour; high plasma calcium levels and neuropathy associated with pruritus	Dialysis with control of serum calcium levels
Immunological	Increased risk for infection that can cause death; increased risk for carcinoma	Suppression of cell-mediated immunity; reduction in number and function of lymphocytes, diminished phagocytosis	Routine dialysis
Reproductive	Sexual dysfunction: menorrhagia, amenorrhea, infertility, and decreased libido in women; decreased testosterone levels, infertility, and decreased libido in men	Dysfunction of ovaries and testes; presence of neuropathies	No specific treatment

With data from Almeras, C., & Argilés, A. (2009). *Semin Dial, 22*(4), 329–333; Keane, W.F. (2000). *Kidney Int Suppl, 75*, S27–S31; Thomas, R., Kanso, A., & Sedor, J.R. (2008). *Prim Care, 35*(2), 329–344.

the urine of an individual with CKD may contain abnormal amounts of protein and red and white blood cells or casts, the major end products of excretion are similar to those of normally functioning kidneys until the advanced stages of kidney failure, when there is a significant reduction of functioning nephrons.[71]

With severe or repeated injury, epithelial cells have an impaired proliferative response resulting in interstitial capillary loss and fibroblast proliferation. The progressive process of glomerulosclerosis and tubulointerstitial fibrosis contributes to CKD and ESRD.[72] The *particular location of kidney damage* also influences loss of kidney function. For example, tubular interstitial diseases damage primarily the tubular or medullary parts of the nephron, producing problems such as renal tubular acidosis, salt wasting, and difficulty diluting or concentrating the urine. When the damage is primarily vascular or glomerular, proteinuria, hematuria, and nephrotic syndrome are more prominent.

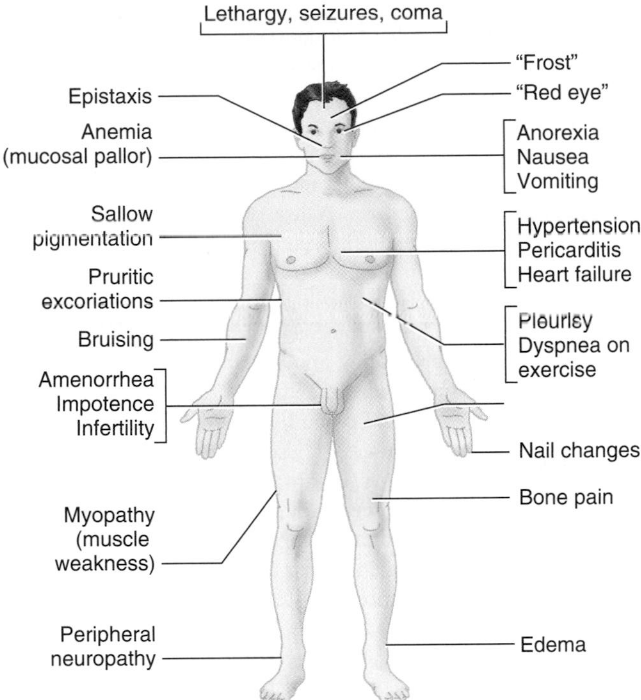

FIGURE 30-9 Common Signs and Symptoms of Kidney Failure. (From Goldman, L., & Schafer, A.I. [2012]. *Goldman's Cecil medicine* [24th ed.]. Philadelphia: Saunders; redrawn from Forbes, C.D., & Jackson, W.F. [2003]. *Color atlas and text of clinical medicine* [3rd ed.]. London: Mosby.)

A summary of factors involved in the progression of CKD is outlined in Table 30-13 and Figure 30-10.

Two factors that have consistently been recognized to advance renal disease are proteinuria and angiotensin II activity. Glomerular hyperfiltration and increased glomerular capillary permeability and loss of negative charge lead to proteinuria. *Proteinuria* contributes to tubulointerstitial injury by accumulating in the interstitial space of the nephron tubules and activating complement proteins and other mediators and cells, such as macrophages, that promote inflammation and progressive fibrosis.[73] Angiotensin II (from activation of the renin-angiotensin-aldosterone system) promotes glomerular hypertension and hyperfiltration caused by efferent arteriolar vasoconstriction and also promotes systemic hypertension. The chronically high intraglomerular pressure increases glomerular capillary permeability, contributing to proteinuria. Angiotensin II also may promote the activity of inflammatory cells and growth factors that participate in tubulointerstitial fibrosis and scarring.[74]

CLINICAL MANIFESTATIONS The clinical manifestations of CKD include uremia and azotemia with many systemic effects.[75] The many systemic manifestations associated with CKD are discussed in the following sections and summarized in Table 30-12 and Figure 30-9.

Creatinine and Urea Clearance

Creatinine is constantly released from muscle and excreted primarily by glomerular filtration. In CKD, as GFR declines, the plasma creatinine level increases by a reciprocal amount to maintain a constant rate of excretion. As GFR continues to decline, plasma creatinine concentration increases. The clearance of urea follows a similar pattern, but urea is both filtered and reabsorbed and its level varies with the state of hydration; therefore, urea concentration is not a good index of GFR. However, as the GFR decreases, plasma urea concentration also increases.

Fluid and Electrolyte Balance

Fluid and electrolyte and acid–base balance is significantly disturbed with CKD. When the GFR decreases to 25%, there is an adaptive loss

TABLE 30-13 Factors Representing Progression of Chronic Kidney Disease

Factor	Characteristics
Proteinuria	Glomerular hyperfiltration of protein contributes to tubular interstitial injury by accumulating in interstitial space and promoting inflammation and progressive fibrosis.
Creatinine and urea clearance	In chronic kidney disease (CKD), the glomerular filtration rate (GFR) falls and the plasma creatinine concentration increases by a reciprocal amount; because there is no regulatory adjustment for creatinine, plasma levels continue to rise and serve as an index of changing glomerular function. As GFR declines, urea clearance increases. (**NOTE:** Urea is both filtered and reabsorbed and varies with state of hydration.)
Sodium and water balance	In CKD, sodium load delivered to nephrons exceeds normal, so excretion must increase; thus less is reabsorbed. Obligatory loss occurs, leading to sodium deficits and volume depletion. As GFR is reduced, ability to concentrate and dilute urine diminishes.
Phosphate and calcium balance	Changes in acid–base balance affect phosphate and calcium balance. Major disorders associated with CKD are reduced renal phosphate excretion, decreased renal synthesis of 1,25-dihydroxy-vitamin D_3, and hypocalcemia. Hypocalcemia leads to secondary hyperparathyroidism, GFR falls, and progressive hyperphosphatemia, hypocalcemia, and dissolution of bone result.
Hematocrit	Because of anemia that accompanies CKD, lethargy, dizziness, and low hematocrit are common.
Potassium balance	In CKD, tubular secretion of potassium increases until oliguria develops. Use of potassium-sparing diuretics also may precipitate elevated serum potassium levels. As disease progresses, total body potassium levels can rise to life-threatening levels and dialysis is required.
Acid–base balance	In early renal insufficiency, acid excretion and bicarbonate reabsorption are increased to maintain normal pH. Metabolic acidosis begins when GFR reaches 30–40%. Metabolic acidosis and hyperkalemia may be severe enough to require dialysis when end-stage kidney disease develops.
Dyslipidemia	Chronic dyslipidemia may induce glomerular and tubulointerstitial injury, contributing to progression of CKD.

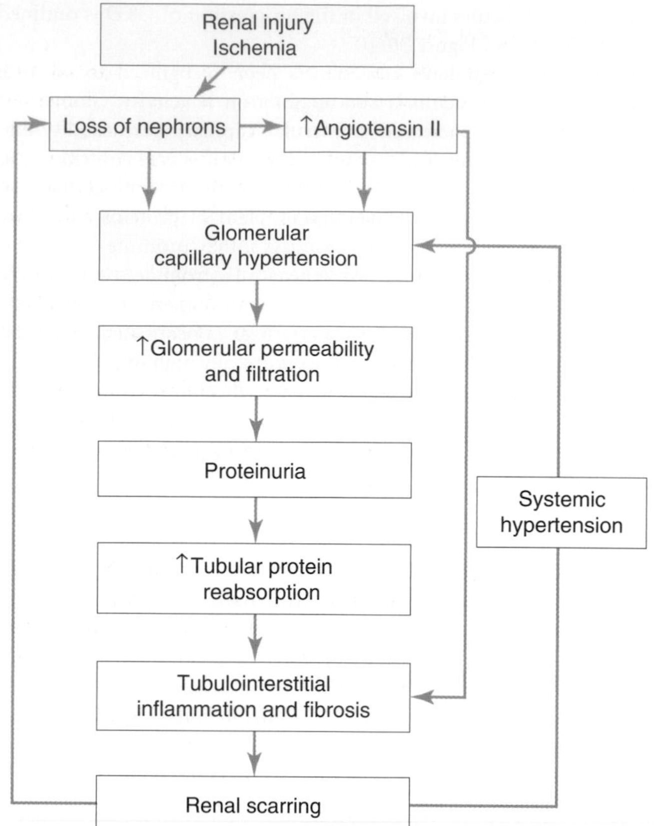

FIGURE 30-10 Mechanisms Related to the Progression of Chronic Kidney Disease.

of 20 to 40 mmol of sodium per day with osmotic loss of water. Dietary intake must be maintained to prevent sodium deficits and volume depletion. As GFR continues to decline, there also is loss of tubular function to dilute and concentrate the urine and urine-specific gravity becomes fixed at about 1.010. Ultimately the kidney loses its ability to regulate sodium and water balance. Both sodium and water are retained, contributing to edema, proteinuria, and hypertension.

In early kidney failure, tubular secretion of potassium is maintained, and larger amounts of potassium are lost through the bowel. With the onset of oliguria, total body potassium concentration can increase to life-threatening levels and must be controlled by dialysis.

Metabolic acidosis develops when the GFR decreases to less than 20 to 25% of normal. The causes of acidosis are primarily related to decreased hydrogen ion elimination and decreased bicarbonate reabsorption. With ESRD, metabolic acidosis may be severe enough to require alkali therapy and dialysis.[76]

Calcium, Phosphate, and Bone

Bone and skeletal changes develop with alterations in calcium and phosphate metabolism. These changes begin when the GFR decreases to 25% or less. Hypocalcemia is accelerated by impaired renal synthesis of 1,25-dihydroxy-vitamin D_3 (calcitriol) with decreased intestinal absorption of calcium. Renal phosphate excretion also decreases and the increased serum phosphate binds calcium, further contributing to hypocalcemia. Acidosis also contributes to a negative calcium balance. Decreased serum calcium level stimulates parathyroid hormone secretion with mobilization of calcium from bone. The combined effect of hyperparathyroidism related to elevated phosphate levels and vitamin D deficiency can result in renal osteodystrophies (i.e., osteoporosis, osteomalacia, and osteitis fibrosa) with increased risk for fractures.[77]

A recent Canadian study established that adequate vitamin D is an essential factor in the prevention of osteoporosis. To improve clinical outcomes such as fracture risk, an optimal serum level of 25-hydroxyvitamin D is probably above 75 nmol/L. In Canada, some vitamin D is obtained with safe exposure to the sun during the summer months, but exposure to sunlight and dietary intake are insufficient to maintain average serum 25-hydroxyvitamin D concentration above 75 nmol/L throughout the year.[78] For most Canadians, supplementation is needed to achieve this level. A daily intake of 25 mcg of vitamin D_3 (1 000 units)—a safe, commonly available dose—will raise the average serum level of 25-hydroxyvitamin D by 15 to 25 nmol/L. The recommended vitamin D intake is 10 to 25 mcg (400 to 1 000 units) daily for low-risk adults under 50 years of age and 20 to 50 mcg (800 to 2 000 units) for high-risk adults and older adults, with the potential for consideration of higher doses. A dose of up to 50 mcg (2 000 units) is safe and does not require monitoring, but if a higher dose is needed, closer monitoring is recommend.

The benefits of calcium supplementation are closely linked to adequate vitamin D intake.[79] Calcium is a mineral available in the food we consume and is instrumental for building and maintaining strong bones and teeth. Dietitians of Canada recommends that Canadian adults 19 to 50 years of age intake 1 000 mg of calcium per day (through two servings of milk or other calcium sources). It also recommends that adults age 51 and older intake 1 200 mg of calcium per day (through three servings of milk or other calcium sources).[79] Supplementation with vitamin D and calcium increases bone density in postmenopausal women and in men over age 50 years of age. Further, a daily dose of 20 mcg (800 IU) of vitamin D_3 in combination with calcium (1 000 mg) reduces the risk for hip and nonvertebral fractures in older adults living in institutions. There is evidence that supplementation with 20 mcg (800 units) of vitamin D_3 daily reduces the risk for falls.[78]

Osteoporosis Canada recommends that adults obtain their calcium through nutrition whenever possible, adding that excess calcium from diet is not harmful. If a person finds it difficult to obtain the recommended amounts of calcium through diet alone, a low-dose calcium supplement is recommended. The supplement label should state the amount of *elemental* calcium in each tablet (e.g., 400 mg of elemental calcium in a 1 000 mg tablet of calcium carbonate). It is the amount of elemental calcium that determines the true daily intake from a supplement.[80]

Protein, Carbohydrate, and Fat Metabolism

Protein, carbohydrate, and fat metabolism are altered in CKD. Proteinuria, metabolic acidosis, inflammation, and a catabolic state contribute to a negative nitrogen balance. Levels of serum proteins diminish, including albumin, complement, and transferrin, and there is loss of muscle mass. Insulin resistance and glucose intolerance are common and may be related to proinflammatory cytokines, and alterations in adipokines (high leptin and low adiponectin levels) that interfere with insulin action.[81]

Dyslipidemia is common among individuals with CKD. There is a high ratio of low-density lipoprotein (LDL) to high-density lipoprotein (HDL), a high level of triglycerides, and an accumulation of LDL particles with accelerated atherosclerosis and vascular calcification. Uremia causes a deficiency in lipoprotein lipase and a decreased level of hepatic triglyceride lipase. Decreased lipolytic activity results in a reduction in HDL level. The concentration of apolipoprotein B is also elevated, thereby accelerating atherogenesis.[82]

Cardiovascular System

Cardiovascular disease is a major cause of morbidity and mortality in CKD. Proinflammatory cytokines, oxidative stress, metabolic derangements, and uremic toxins are significant contributors. Hypertension is the result of excess sodium and fluid volume and arteriosclerosis. Endothelial cell dysfunction and calcium deposits lead to a loss of vessel elasticity and vascular calcification. Elevated renin concentration also stimulates the secretion of aldosterone, increasing sodium reabsorption. Dyslipidemia promotes atheromatous plaque formation. The resulting vascular disease increases the risk for ischemic heart disease, left ventricular hypertrophy, heart failure, stroke, and peripheral vascular disease in individuals with uremia. Declining erythropoietin production causes anemia, thereby increasing demands for cardiac output and adding to the cardiac workload. Pericarditis can develop from inflammation caused by the presence of uremic toxins. Accumulation of fluid in the pericardial space can compromise ventricular filling and cardiac output.[83] Fluid overload and hypertension can promote heart failure (cardiorenal syndrome).

Pulmonary System

Pulmonary complications are associated with fluid overload, heart failure, and dyspnea. Pulmonary edema develops and metabolic acidosis can cause Kussmaul respirations. Pulmonary hypertension can develop because of left ventricular dysfunction or uremic-associated vascular changes.[84]

Hematological System

Hematological alterations include normochromic–normocytic anemia, impaired platelet function, and hypercoagulability. Inadequate production of erythropoietin decreases red blood cell production, and uremia decreases red blood cell lifespan. Lethargy, dizziness, and low hematocrit values are common findings. Defective platelet aggregation, decreased platelet numbers, and altered vascular endothelium promote an increased bleeding tendency, increased risk for bruising, epistaxis, gastro-intestinal bleeding, or cerebrovascular hemorrhage. Alterations in thrombin and other clotting factors contribute to hypercoagulability; thus control of coagulation is essential during dialysis.[85]

Immune System

Immune system dysregulation develops with the uremia of CKD. Chemotaxis, phagocytosis, antibody production, and cell-mediated immune responses are suppressed. Malnutrition, metabolic acidosis, and hyperglycemia may amplify immunosuppression. Release of inflammatory cytokines results in systemic inflammation. Failure of antioxidant systems also promotes inflammation. There are deficient responses to vaccination, increased risk for infection, and virus-associated cancers (e.g., human papillomavirus, hepatitis B and C viruses, Epstein-Barr virus).[75]

Neurological System

Neurological symptoms are common and progressive with CKD. Symptoms may include headache, pain, drowsiness, sleep disorders, impaired concentration, memory loss, and impaired judgement (known as *uremic encephalopathy*). In advanced stages of kidney failure, symptoms may progress to seizures and coma. Neuromuscular irritation can cause hiccups, muscle cramps, and muscle twitching. Peripheral neuropathies associated with uremic toxins also can develop with impaired sensations, particularly in the lower limbs. Symptoms improve with hemodialysis.[86]

Gastro-intestinal System

Gastro-intestinal complications are common in individuals with CKD. Uremic gastroenteritis can cause bleeding ulcers and significant blood loss. Nonspecific symptoms include anorexia, nausea, vomiting, constipation, or diarrhea. Uremic fetor is a form of bad breath caused by the breakdown of urea by salivary enzymes. Malnutrition is common.[87]

Endocrine and Reproductive Systems

Endocrine and reproductive alterations develop with progression of CKD. Both males and females have a decrease in levels of circulating sex steroids. Males often experience a reduction in testosterone levels and may have erectile dysfunction. Oligospermia and germinal cell dysplasia can result in infertility. Females have reduced estrogen levels, amenorrhea, and difficulty maintaining a pregnancy to term.[88] A decrease in libido and fertility can occur in both genders.[89]

Insulin resistance is common in uremia, and as CKD progresses the ability of the kidney to degrade insulin is reduced and the half-life of insulin is prolonged. Individuals with diabetes mellitus and CKD need to carefully manage their insulin dosages.[90]

CKD also causes alterations in thyroid hormone metabolism, particularly hypothyroidism, known as *nonthyroidal illness syndrome*. Uremia delays the response of thyroid-stimulating hormone receptors and triiodothyronine (T_3) levels are often low.[91]

Integumentary System

Skin changes are associated with other complications that develop with CKD. Anemia can cause pallor and bleeding into the skin and results in hematomas and ecchymosis. Retained urochromes manifest as a sallow skin colour. Hyperparathyroidism and uremic skin residues (known as *uremic frost*) are associated with inflammation, irritation, and pruritus with scratching, excoriation, and increased risk for infection. Half-and-half nails (half white and half red or brown) are common. Local bullous lesions and nephrogenic systemic fibrosis are less common.[92]

EVALUATION AND TREATMENT Early screening and evaluation of CKD is based on the risk factors, history, presenting signs and symptoms, and diagnostic testing. Elevated serum creatinine and serum urea nitrogen concentrations are consistent with CKD. Markers of kidney damage include measurement of urine protein level, particularly albumin, and examination of urine sediment. Ultrasound, CT scan, or plain X-ray films will show small kidney size. Renal biopsy confirms the diagnosis.

Management involves dietary restriction of protein, sodium, potassium, and phosphate; supplementation with vitamin D or vitamin D–receptor activators; maintenance of sodium and fluid balance; promotion of adequate caloric intake; management of dyslipidemias; and use of erythropoietin as needed. ACE inhibitors or ARBs are often used to control systemic hypertension, reduce proteinuria, provide renoprotection, and prevent progressive renal damage.[93,94]

ESKD related to diabetic nephropathy can be significantly reduced with glycemic control.[90] ESKD is treated with conservative care, continuous renal replacement therapy, supportive therapy, and kidney transplantation.[95,96] Portable and wearable dialysis devices are in clinical trials.[97]

QUICK CHECK 30-4

1. What mechanisms cause prerenal acute kidney injury (AKI)?
2. How does intrarenal AKI differ from postrenal AKI?
3. Briefly describe the causes of anemia, cardiovascular disease, and bone and neurological changes associated with CKD.

DID YOU UNDERSTAND?

Urinary Tract Obstruction

1. Obstruction can occur anywhere in the urinary tract, and it may be anatomical or functional, including renal stones, an enlarged prostate gland, urethral strictures, or neurogenic bladder. The most serious complications are hydronephrosis, hydroureter, ureterohydronephrosis, and infection caused by the accumulation of urine behind the obstruction.
2. Hypertrophy of the opposite kidney compensates for loss of function of the kidney with obstructive disease.
3. Relief of obstruction is usually followed by postobstructive diuresis and may cause fluid and electrolyte imbalance.
4. Persistent obstruction of the bladder outlet leads to residual urine volumes, low bladder wall compliance, and risk for vesicoureteral reflux and infection.
5. Kidney stones are caused by supersaturation of the urine with precipitation of stone-forming substances, changes in urine pH, or urinary tract infection (UTI).
6. The most common kidney stone is formed from calcium oxalate and most often causes obstruction by lodging in the ureter.
7. Obstructions of the bladder are a consequence of neurogenic or anatomical alteration of the bladder, or both.
8. A neurogenic bladder is caused by a neural lesion that interrupts innervation of the bladder.
9. Upper motor neuron lesions result in overactive or hyper-reflexive bladder function.
10. Lower motor neuron lesions result in underactive, hypotonic, or atonic bladder function.
11. Underactive bladder (UAB) syndrome is a condition in which the duration or strength of contraction is inadequate to empty the bladder, resulting in distension and overflow incontinence.
12. Overactive bladder (OAB) syndrome is an uncontrollable or premature contraction of the bladder that results in urgency with or without incontinence, frequency, and nocturia.
13. Detrusor sphincter dyssynergia is failure of the urethrovesical junction smooth muscle to release urine during bladder contraction and causes a functional obstruction.
14. Other causes of lower urinary tract obstruction include urethral stricture, prostate enlargement, and pelvic organ prolapse in women.
15. Partial obstruction of the bladder can result in OAB contractions with urgency. There is deposition of collagen in the bladder wall over time, resulting in decreased bladder wall compliance and ineffective detrusor muscle contraction.
16. Renal cell carcinoma is the most common renal neoplasm and usually presents with hematuria. The larger neoplasms tend to metastasize to the lung, liver, and bone.
17. Bladder tumours are commonly composed of transitional cells with a papillary appearance and a high rate of recurrence.

Urinary Tract Infection

1. UTIs are commonly caused by the retrograde movement of bacteria into the urethra and bladder. UTIs are uncomplicated when the urinary system is normal or complicated when there is an abnormality.
2. Cystitis is an inflammation of the bladder commonly caused by bacteria and may be acute or chronic.
3. Painful bladder syndrome/interstitial cystitis includes nonbacterial infectious cystitis (viral, mycobacterial, chlamydial, fungal), noninfectious cystitis (e.g., radiation injury), and interstitial cystitis, which is related to autoimmune injury.
4. Pyelonephritis is an infection of one or both upper urinary tracts (ureter, renal pelvis, and interstitium) often related to obstructive uropathies and may cause abscess formation and scarring with an alteration in renal function.

Glomerular Disorders

1. Glomerular disorders are a group of related diseases of the glomerulus that can be caused by immune responses, toxins or medications, vascular disorders, and other systemic diseases.
2. Acute glomerulonephritis commonly results from inflammatory damage to the glomerular filtration membrane as a consequence of immune reactions (e.g., after a streptococcal infection).
3. Immune mechanisms in glomerulonephritis include the deposition of circulating antigen–antibody complexes often with complement components or the in situ formation of antibodies, or both, specific for the glomerular basement membrane.
4. Diabetic nephropathy is the most common cause of glomerular injury progressing to chronic kidney disease (CKD) as well as end-stage kidney disease (ESKD).
5. Chronic glomerulonephritis is related to a variety of diseases that cause deterioration of the glomerulus and a progressive loss of renal function.
6. Nephrotic syndrome is the excretion of 3.5 grams or more of protein (primarily albumin) in the urine per day because of glomerular injury with increased capillary permeability and loss of membrane negative charge. Its principal signs are hypoproteinuria, dyslipidemia, and edema. The liver cannot produce enough protein to adequately compensate for urinary loss.
7. Nephritic syndrome is characterized by hematuria and red blood cell casts with less severe proteinuria.

Acute Kidney Injury

1. Acute kidney injury (AKI) is a sudden decline in kidney function with a decrease in glomerular filtration rate (GFR) and urine output and with an elevation in plasma creatinine and blood urea nitrogen levels.
2. Prerenal AKI is caused by inadequate kidney perfusion with a decreased GFR, ischemia, and tubular necrosis.
3. Intrarenal AKI is associated with several systemic diseases but is commonly related to acute tubular necrosis.
4. Postrenal AKI is associated with diseases that obstruct the flow of urine from the kidneys.
5. Oliguria is urine output of less than 400 mL/24 hours.

Chronic Kidney Disease

1. CKD is the progressive loss of renal function. Plasma creatinine levels gradually become elevated as GFR declines; sodium is lost in the urine; potassium is retained; acidosis develops; calcium and phosphate metabolism are altered; and erythropoietin production is diminished. All organs systems are affected by CKD.

KEY TERMS

Acute cystitis, 765
Acute glomerulonephritis, 767
Acute kidney injury (AKI), 772
Acute tubular necrosis (ATN), 772
Anuria, 774
Azotemia, 772
Calcium stone, 761
Calculus (*pl.*, calculi) (urinary stone), 760
Chronic glomerulonephritis, 770
Chronic kidney disease (CKD), 775
Chronic pyelonephritis, 767
Compensatory hypertrophy, 760
Cystinuric (xanthine) stone, 761
Detrusor areflexia, 762
Detrusor hyper-reflexia (overactivity), 762
Detrusor hyper-reflexia with vesicosphincter dyssynergia, 762
Diabetic nephropathy, 770
Dyssynergia, 762
End-stage kidney disease (ESKD), 772
Hydronephrosis, 759
Hydroureter, 759
Hyperfunction, 760
Intrarenal (intrinsic) acute kidney injury, 773
Kidney failure, 772
Low bladder wall compliance, 763
Lupus nephritis, 770
Nephritic syndrome, 771
Nephrotic syndrome, 771
Neurogenic bladder, 762
Nonbacterial infectious cystitis, 766
Noninfectious cystitis, 766
Nonoliguric renal failure, 774
Obstructive uropathy, 759
Oliguria, 774
Overactive bladder (OAB) syndrome, 762
Painful bladder syndrome/interstitial cystitis (PBS/IC), 766
Partial obstruction of the bladder outlet or urethra, 763
Pelvic organ prolapse, 763
Postobstructive diuresis, 760
Postrenal acute kidney injury, 774
Prerenal acute kidney injury, 773
Prostate enlargement, 763
Pyelonephritis, 767
Renal adenoma, 763
Renal cell carcinoma (RCC), 763
Renal colic, 761
Renal insufficiency, 772
Renal transitional cell carcinoma (RTCC), 763
Rhabdomyolysis, 774
Staghorn calculus, 761
Struvite stone, 761
Tubulointerstitial fibrosis, 759
Uremia (uremic syndrome), 772
Ureterohydronephrosis, 759
Urethral stricture, 763
Uric acid stone, 761
Urinary tract infection (UTI), 765

REFERENCES

1. Siddiqui, M. M., & McDougal, W. S. (2011). Urologic assessment of decreasing renal function. *Medical Clinics of North America, 95*(1), 161–168. doi:10.1016/j.mcna.2010.08.031.
2. Tseng, T. Y., & Stoller, M. L. (2009). Obstructive uropathy. *Clinics in Geriatric Medicine, 25*(3), 437–443. doi:10.1016/j.cger.2009.06.003.
3. Klatt, E. C. (2015). *Robbins and Cotran atlas of pathology* (3rd ed.). Philadelphia: Saunders.
4. Maarten, T. W., & Brenner, B. M. (2012). Adaptation to nephron loss and mechanisms of progression chronic kidney disease. In B. M. Brenner (Ed.), *Brenner and Rector's the kidney* (9th ed.). Philadelphia: Saunders.
5. Frokiaer, J., & Zeidel, M. L. (2008). Urinary tract obstruction. In B. M. Brenner (Ed.), *Brenner and Rector's the kidney* (8th ed.). Philadelphia: Saunders.
6. Lotan, Y., Buendia Jimènez, I., Lenoir-Wijnkoop, I., et al. (2012). Primary prevention of nephrolithiasis is cost-effective for a national healthcare system. *BJU International, 110*(11 Pt. C), E1060–E1067. doi: 10.1111/j.1464-410X.2012.11212.x.
7. Sakhaee, K., Maalouf, N. M., & Sinnott, B. (2012). Clinical review. Kidney stones 2012: Pathogenesis, diagnosis, and management. *Journal of Clinical Endocrinology and Metabolism, 97*(6), 1847–1860. doi:10.1210/jc.2011-3492.
8. Argade, S., Chen, T., Shaw, T., et al. (2015). An evaluation of Tamm-Horsfall protein glycans in kidney stone formers using novel techniques. *Urolithiasis, 43*(4), 303–312. doi:10.1007/s00240-015-0775-3.
9. Daudon, M., Bazin, D., & Letavernier, E. (2015). Randall's plaque as the origin of calcium oxalate kidney stones. *Urolithiasis, 43*(Suppl. 1), 5–11. doi:10.1007/s00240-014-0703-y.
10. Matlaga, B. R., & Lingeman, J. E. (2012). Surgical management of upper urinary tract calculi. In W. S. McDougall, A. J. Wein, L. R. Kavoussi, et al. (Eds.), *Campbell-Walsh urology* (10th ed.). Philadelphia: Saunders.
11. Dalziel, P. J., & Noble, V. E. (2013). Bedside ultrasound and the assessment of renal colic: A review. *Emergency Medicine Journal, 30*(1), 3–8. doi:10.1136/emermed-2012-201375.
12. Pearle, M. S., Goldfarb, D. S., Assimos, D. G., et al. (2014). Medical management of kidney stones: AUA guideline. *Journal of Urology, 192*(2), 316–324. doi:10.1016/j.juro.2014.05.006.
13. Qaseem, A., Dallas, P., Forciea, M. A., et al. (2014). Dietary and pharmacologic management to prevent recurrent nephrolithiasis in adults: A clinical practice guideline from the American College of Physicians. *Annals of Internal Medicine, 161*, 659–667. doi:10.7326/M13-2908.
14. The Canadian Continence Foundation. (2014). *Incontinence: The Canadian perspective.* Peterborough, ON: Author. Retrieved from http://www.canadiancontinence.ca/pdfs/en-incontinence-a-canadian-perspective-2014.pdf.
15. Unger, C. A., Tunitsky-Bitton, E., Muffly, T., et al. (2014). Neuroanatomy, neurophysiology, and dysfunction of the female lower urinary tract: A review. *Female Pelvic Medicine & Reconstructive Surgery, 20*(2), 65–75. doi:10.1097/SPV.0000000000000058.
16. Banakhar, M. A., Al-Shaiji, T. F., & Hassouna, M. M. (2012). Pathophysiology of overactive bladder. *International Urogynecology Journal, 23*(8), 975–982. doi:10.1007/s00192-012-1682-6.
17. Abrams, P., Cardozo, L., Fall, M., et al. (2002). The standardisation of terminology of lower urinary tract function: Report from the Standardisation Sub-committee of the International Continence Society. *American Journal of Obstetrics and Gynecology, 187*(1), 116–126.
18. Hampson, L. A., McAninch, J. W., & Breyer, B. N. (2014). Male urethral strictures and their management. *Nature Reviews. Urology, 11*(1), 43–50. doi:10.1038/nrurol.2013.275.
19. Osman, N. I., Mangera, A., & Chapple, C. R. (2013). A systematic review of surgical techniques used in the treatment of female urethral stricture. *European Urology, 64*(6), 965–973. doi:10.1016/j.eururo.2013.07.038.
20. Chibelean, C., & Nechifor-Boila, I. A. (2015). Botulinum neurotoxin A for overactive bladder treatment: Advantages and pitfalls. *Canadian Journal of Urology, 22*(2), 7681–7689.
21. Coyne, K. S., Wein, A., Nicholson, S., et al. (2013). Comorbidities and personal burden of urgency urinary incontinence: A systematic review. *International Journal of Clinical Practice, 67*(10), 1015–1033. doi:10.1111/ijcp.12164.
22. American Cancer Society (2015). *Cancer facts & figures—2015*. Atlanta: Author.
23. Canadian Cancer Society. (2017). *Kidney cancer statistics*. Retrieved from http://www.cancer.ca/en/cancer-information/cancer-type/kidney/kidney-cancer/?region=on.
24. Bhatt, J. R., & Finelli, A. (2014). Landmarks in the diagnosis and treatment of renal cell carcinoma. *Nature Reviews. Urology, 11*(9), 517–525. doi:10.1038/nrurol.2014.194.
25. National Cancer Institute. (2015). *Renal cell cancer treatment (PDQ®)*. Retrieved from http://www.cancer.gov/types/kidney/patient/kidney-treatment-pdq#section/all.
26. Ridge, C. A., Pua, B. B., & Madoff, D. C. (2014). Epidemiology and staging of renal cell carcinoma. *Seminars in Interventional Radiology, 31*(1), 3–8. doi: 10.1055/s-0033-1363837.
27. Bedke, J., Gouttefangeas, C., Singh-Jasuja, H., et al. (2014). Targeted therapy in renal cell carcinoma: Moving from molecular agents to specific immunotherapy. *World Journal of Urology, 32*(1), 31–38. doi:10.1007/s00345-013-1033-3.
28. Su, D., Stamatakis, L., Singer, E. A., et al. (2014). Renal cell carcinoma: Molecular biology and targeted therapy. *Current Opinion in Oncology, 26*(3), 321–327. doi:10.1097/CCO.0000000000000069.
29. Canadian Cancer Society. (2017). *Bladder cancer statistics*. Retrieved from http://www.cancer.ca/en/cancer-information/cancer-type/bladder/statistics/?region=on.
30. Sapre, N., Anderson, P. D., Costello, A. J., et al. (2014). Gene-based urinary biomarkers for bladder cancer: An unfulfilled promise? *Urologic Oncology, 32*(1), 48.e9–48.e17. doi:10.1016/j.urolonc.2013.07.002.
31. National Cancer Institute. (2015). *Bladder cancer treatment (PDQ®)*. Retrieved from http://www.cancer.gov/types/bladder/patient/bladder-treatment-pdq#section/all.
32. Sonpavde, G., Jones, B. S., Bellmunt, J., et al. (2015). Future directions and targeted therapies in bladder cancer. *Hematolgy/Oncology Clinics of North America, 29*(2), 361–376. doi:10.1016/j.hoc.2014.10.008.
33. Lee, R. K., Abol-Enein, H., Artibani, W., et al. (2014). Urinary diversion after radical cystectomy for bladder cancer: Options, patient selection, and

outcomes. *BJU International, 113*(1), 11–23. doi:10.1111/bju.12121.
34. Dielubanza, E. J., & Schaeffer, A. J. (2011). Urinary tract infections in women. *Medical Clinics of North America, 95*(1), 27–41. doi:10.1016/j.mcna.2010.08.023.
35. The Kidney Foundation of Canada. (2007). *Urinary tract infections.* Retrieved from http://www.kidney.ca/document.doc?id=316.
36. Dielubanza, E. J., Mazur, D. J., & Schaeffer, A. J. (2014). Management of non-catheter-associated complicated urinary tract infection. *Infectious Disease Clinics of North America, 28*(1), 121–123. doi:10.1016/j.idc.2013.10.005.
37. Nicolle, L. E. (2013). Urinary tract infection. *Critical Care Clinics, 29*(3), 699–715. doi:10.1016/j.ccc.2013.03.014.
38. Rinaldi, G., Young, N. D., Honeycutt, J. D., et al. (2015). New research tools for urogenital schistosomiasis. *Journal of Infectious Diseases, 211*(6), 861–869. doi:10.1093/infdis/jiu527.
39. Stapleton, A. E. (2014). Urinary tract infection pathogenesis: Host factors. *Infectious Disease Clinics of North America, 28*(1), 149–159. doi:10.1016/j.idc.2013.10.006.
40. Rowe, T. A., & Juthani-Mehta, M. (2014). Diagnosis and management of urinary tract infection in older adults. *Infectious Disease Clinics of North America, 28*(1), 75–89. doi:10.1016/j.idc.2013.10.004.
41. Grigoryan, L., Trautner, B. W., & Gupta, K. (2014). Diagnosis and management of urinary tract infections in the outpatient setting: A review. *JAMA: The Journal of the American Medical Association, 312*(16), 1677–1684.
42. National Guideline Clearinghouse (2008). *Guideline synthesis: Diagnosis and management of lower urinary tract infection.* Rockville, MD: National Guideline Clearinghouse, Agency for Healthcare Research and Quality. Retrieved from http://www.guideline.gov.
43. Dyer, A. J., & Twiss, C. O. (2014). Painful bladder syndrome: An update and review of current management strategies. *Current Urology Reports, 15*(2), 384. doi:10.1007/s11934-013-0384-z.
44. Hanno, P. M., Erickson, D., Moldwin, R., et al. (2015). Diagnosis and treatment of interstitial cystitis/bladder pain syndrome: AUA guideline amendment. *Journal of Urology, 193*(5), 1545–1553. doi:10.1016/j.juro.2015.01.086.
45. Hooton, T. (2015). Bacterial urinary tract infections. In R. J. Johnson, J. Feehally, & J. Floege (Eds.), *Comprehensive clinical nephrology* (5th ed., pp. 632–643). Philadelphia: Saunders.
46. Takhar, S. S., & Moran, G. F. (2014). Diagnosis and management of urinary tract infection in the emergency department and outpatient settings. *Infectious Disease Clinics of North America, 28*(1), 33–48. doi:10.1016/j.idc.2013.10.003.
47. Kościelska-Kasprzak, K., Bartoszek, D., Myszka, M., et al. (2014). The complement cascade and renal disease. *Archivum Immunologiae et Therapiae Experimentalis, 62*(1), 47–57. doi:10.1007/s00005-013-0254-x.
48. Hénique, C., Papista, C., Guyonnet, L., et al. (2014). Update on crescentic glomerulonephritism. *Seminars in Immunopathology, 36*(4), 479–490. doi:10.1007/s00281-014-0435-7.
49. Fioretto, P., Barzon, I., & Mauer, M. (2014). Is diabetic nephropathy reversible? *Diabetes Research and Clinical Practice, 104*(3), 323–328. doi:10.1016/j.diabres.2014.01.017.
50. Yap, D. Y., & Lai, K. N. (2015). Pathogenesis of renal disease in systemic lupus erythematosus—The role of autoantibodies and lymphocytes subset abnormalities. *International Journal of Molecular Sciences, 16*(4), 7917–7931. doi:10.3390/ijms16047917.
51. Reidy, K., Kang, H. M., Horstetter, T., et al. (2014). Molecular mechanisms of diabetic kidney disease. *Journal of Clinical Investigation, 124*(6), 2333–2340. doi:10.1172/JCI72271.
52. Sun, Y. M., Su, Y., Li, J., et al. (2013). Recent advances in understanding the biochemical and molecular mechanism of diabetic nephropathy. *Biochemical and Biophysical Research Communications, 433*(4), 359–361. doi:10.1016/j.bbrc.2013.02.120.
53. Haider, D. G., Friedl, A., Peric, S., et al. (2012). Kidney biopsy in patients with glomerulonephritis: Is the earlier the better? *BMC Nephrology, 13,* 34. doi:10.1186/1471-2369-13-34.
54. Kodner, C. (2009). Nephrotic syndrome in adults: Diagnosis and management. *American Family Physician, 80*(10), 1129–1134.
55. Siddall, E. C., & Radhakrishnan, J. (2012). The pathophysiology of edema formation in the nephrotic syndrome. *Kidney International, 82*(6), 635–642. doi:10.1038/ki.2012.180.
56. Yee, J. (2014). Treatment of nephrotic syndrome: Retrospection. *Advances in Chronic Kidney Disease, 21*(2), 115–118. doi:10.1053/j.ackd.2014.01.012.
57. Gigante, A., Barbano, B., Sardo, L., et al. (2014). Hypercoagulability and nephrotic syndrome. *Current Vascular Pharmacology, 12*(3), 512–517. doi:10.2174/15701611120314051817 2048.
58. Ponticelli, C., & Glassock, R. J. (2014). Glomerular diseases: Membranous nephropathy—A modern view. *Clinical Journal of the American Society of Nephrology : CJASN, 9*(3), 609–616. doi:10.2215/CJN.04160413.
59. Moroni, G., & Ponticelli, C. (2014). Rapidly progressive crescentic glomerulonephritis: Early treatment is a must. *Autoimmunity Reviews, 13*(7), 723–729. doi:10.1016/j.autrev.2014.02.007.
60. Turner, J. M., & Coca, S. G. (2014). Acute tubular injury and acute tubular necrosis. In S. Gilbert (Ed.), *National Kidney Foundation primer on kidney diseases* (6th ed., pp. 304–311). Amsterdam: Elsevier.
61. Thomas, M. E., Blaine, C., Dawnay, A., et al. (2014). The definition of acute kidney injury and its use in practice. *Kidney International, 87*(1), 62–73. doi:10.1038/ki.2014.328.
62. Tögel, F., & Westenfelder, C. (2014). Recent advances in the understanding of acute kidney injury. *F1000prime Reports, 6,* 83. doi:10.12703/P6-83.
63. Chatauret, N., Badet, L., Barrou, B., et al. (2014). Ischemia-reperfusion: From cell biology to acute kidney injury. *Progres En Urologie: Journal de l'Association Francaise D'urologie et de la Societe Francaise D'urologie, 24*(Suppl. 1), S4–S12. doi:10.1016/S1166-7087(14)70057-0.
64. Gomez, H., Ince, C., De Backer, D., et al. (2014). A unified theory of sepsis-induced acute kidney injury: Inflammation, microcirculatory dysfunction, bioenergetics, and the tubular cell adaptation to injury. *Shock (Augusta, Ga.), 41*(1), 3–11. doi:10.1097/SHK.0000000000000052.
65. Glodowski, S. D., & Wagener, G. (2014). New insights into the mechanisms of acute kidney injury in the intensive care unit. *Journal of Clinical Anesthesia, 27*(2), 175–180. doi:10.1016/j.jclinane.2014.09.011.
66. Obermüller, N., Geiger, H., Weipert, C., et al. (2014). Current developments in early diagnosis of acute kidney injury. *International Urology and Nephrology, 46*(1), 1–7. doi:10.1007/s11255-013-0448-5.
67. Chionh, C. Y., Soni, S. S., Finkelstein, F. O., et al. (2013). Use of peritoneal dialysis in AKI: A systematic review. *Clinical Journal of the American Society of Nephrology : CJASN, 8*(10), 1649–1660. doi:10.2215/CJN.01540213.
68. Macedo, E., & Mehta, R. L. (2013). Timing of dialysis initiation in acute kidney injury and acute-on-chronic renal failure. *Seminars in Dialysis, 26*(6), 675–681. doi:10.1111/sdi.12128.
69. Thomas, R., Kanso, A., & Sedor, J. R. (2008). Chronic kidney disease and its complications. *Primary Care, 35*(2), 329–344, vii. doi:10.1016/j.pop.2008.01.008.
70. Cleper, R. (2012). Mechanisms of compensatory renal growth. *Pediatric Endocrinology Reviews, 10*(1), 152–163.
71. Fong, D., Denton, K. M., Moritz, K. M., et al. (2014). Compensatory responses to nephron deficiency: Adaptive or maladaptive? *Nephrology (Carlton, Vic.), 19*(3), 119–128. doi:10.1111/nep.12198.
72. Grgic, I., Campanholie, G., Bijol, V., et al. (2012). Targeted proximal tubule injury triggers interstitial fibrosis and glomerulosclerosis. *Kidney International, 82*(2), 172–183. doi:10.1038/ki.2012.20.
73. Gorriz, J. L., & Martinez-Castelao, A. (2012). Proteinuria: Detection and role in native renal disease progression. *Transplantation Reviews (Orlando, Fla.), 26*(1), 3–13. doi:10.1016/j.trre.2011.10.002.
74. Navar, L. G. (2014). Intrarenal renin-angiotensin system in regulation of glomerular function. *Current Opinion in Nephrology and Hypertension, 23*(1), 38–45. doi:10.1097/01.mnh.0000436544.86508.f1.
75. Betjes, M. G. (2013). Immune cell dysfunction and inflammation in end-stage renal disease. *Nature Reviews. Nephrology, 9*(5), 255–265. doi:10.1038/nrneph.2013.44.
76. Dobre, M., Rahman, M., & Hostetter, T. H. (2015). Current status of bicarbonate in CKD. *Journal of the American Society of Nephrology, 26*(3), 515–523. doi:10.1681/ASN.2014020205.
77. Kazama, J. J., Matsuo, K., Iwasaki, Y., et al. (2015). Chronic kidney disease and bone metabolism. *Journal of Bone and Mineral Metabolism, 33*(3), 245–252. doi:10.1007/s00774-014-0639-x.
78. Hanley, D. A., Cranney, A., Jones, G., et al. (2010). Vitamin D in adult health and disease: A review and guideline statement from Osteoporosis Canada (summary). *CMAJ : Canadian Medical Association Journal, 182*(12), 1315–1319. doi:10.1503/cmaj.091062.
79. Dietitians of Canada. (2016). *Calcium.* Retrieved from http://www.dietitians.ca/Your-Health/Nutrition-A-Z/Calcium.aspx.
80. Osteoporosis Canada. (2016). *How do I know if I need a calcium supplement?* Retrieved from http://www.osteoporosis.ca/osteoporosis-and-you/nutrition/supplements/.
81. Liao, M. T., Sung, C. C., Hung, K. C., et al. (2012). Insulin resistance in patients with chronic kidney disease. *Journal of Biomedicine & Biotechnology, 2012,* 691369. doi:10.1155/2012/691369.
82. Keane, W. F., Tomassini, J. E., & Neff, D. R. (2013). Lipid abnormalities in patients with chronic kidney disease: Implications for the pathophysiology of atherosclerosis. *Journal of Atherosclerosis and Thrombosis, 20*(2), 123–133. doi:10.5551/jat.12849.
83. Stenvinkel, P., & Herzog, C. A. (2015). Cardiovascular disease in chronic kidney disease. In R. J. Johnson, J. Feehally, & J. Floege (Eds.), *Comprehensive clinical nephrology* (5th ed., pp. 949–966). Philadelphia: Saunders.
84. Kawar, B., Ellam, T., Jackson, C., et al. (2013). Pulmonary hypertension in renal disease: Epidemiology, potential mechanisms and implications. *American Journal of Nephrology, 37*(3), 281–290. doi:10.1159/000348804.
85. Leung, N. (2013). Hematologic manifestations of kidney disease. *Seminars in Hematology, 50*(3), 207–215. doi:10.1053/j.seminhematol.2013.06.002.
86. Baumgaertel, M. W., Kraemer, M., & Berlit, P. (2014). Neurologic complications of acute and chronic renal disease. *Handbook of Clinical Neurology, 119,* 383–393. doi:10.1016/B978-0-7020-4086-3.00024-2.
87. Thomas, R., Panackal, C., John, M., et al. (2013). Gastrointestinal complications in patients with chronic kidney disease—A 5-year retrospective study from a tertiary referral center. *Renal Failure, 35*(1), 49–55. doi:10.3109/0886022X.2012.731998.
88. Vellanki, K. (2013). Pregnancy in chronic kidney disease. *Advances in Chronic Kidney Disease, 20*(3), 223–228. doi:10.1053/j.ackd.2013.02.001.
89. Holley, J. L., & Schmidt, R. J. (2013). Changes in fertility and hormone replacement therapy in kidney disease. *Advances in Chronic Kidney Disease, 20*(3), 240–245. doi:10.1053/j.ackd.2013.01.003.
90. Williams, M. E., & Garg, R. (2014). Glycemic management in ESRD and earlier stages of CKD. *American Journal of Kidney Diseases, 63*(2, Suppl. 2), S22–S38. doi:10.1053/j.ajkd.2013.10.049.
91. Mohamedali, M., Reddy Maddika, S., Vyas, A., et al. (2014). Thyroid disorders and chronic kidney disease. *International Journal of Nephrology, 2014,* 520281. doi:10.1155/2014/520281.

92. Galperin, T. A., Cronin, A. J., & Leslie, K. S. (2014). Cutaneous manifestations of ESRD. *Clinical Journal of the American Society of Nephrology : CJASN, 9*(1), 201–218. doi:10.2215/CJN.05900513.
93. Levey, A. S., & Coresh, J. (2012). Chronic kidney disease. *Lancet, 379*(9811), 165–180. doi:10.1016/S0140-6736(11)60178-5.
94. Ruggenenti, P., Cravedi, P., & Remuzzi, G. (2012). Mechanisms and treatment of CKD. *Journal of the American Society of Nephrology, 23*(12), 1917–1928. doi:10.1681/ASN.2012040390.
95. Kane, P. M., Vinen, K., & Murtagh, F. E. (2013). Palliative care for advanced renal disease: A summary of the evidence and future direction. *Palliative Medicine, 27*(9), 817–821. doi:10.1177/0269216313491796.
96. Legendre, C., Canaud, G., & Martinez, F. (2014). Factors influencing long-term outcome after kidney transplantation. *Transplant International, 27*(1), 19–27. doi:10.1111/tri.12217.
97. Davenport, A. (2015). Portable and wearable dialysis devices for the treatment of patients with end-stage kidney failure: Wishful thinking or just over the horizon? *Pediatric Nephrology (Berlin, Germany), 30*(12), 2053–2060. doi:10.1007/s00467-014-2968-3.

31

Alterations of Renal and Urinary Tract Function in Children

Patricia Ring, Sue E. Huether, and Mohamed El-Hussein

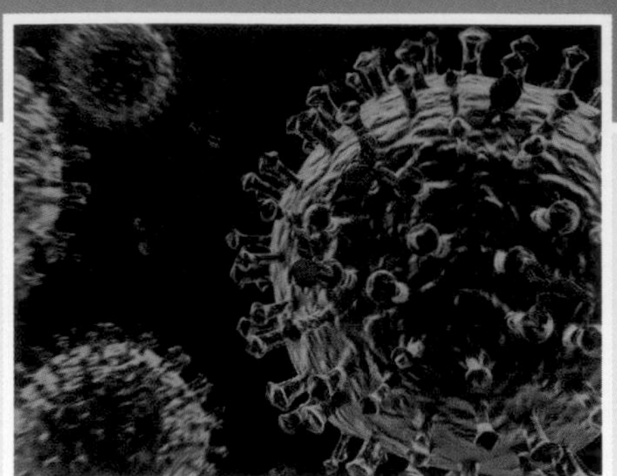

EVOLVE WEBSITE

http://evolve.elsevier.com/Canada/Huether/pathophysiology
Student Review Questions
Key Points
Case Studies
Animations
Quick Check Answers

CHAPTER OUTLINE

Structural Abnormalities, 784
Hypospadias, 784
Epispadias and Exstrophy of the Bladder, 785
Bladder Outlet Obstruction, 785
Ureteropelvic Junction Obstruction, 785
Hypoplastic or Dysplastic Kidneys, 786
Polycystic Kidney Disease, 786
Renal Agenesis, 786
Glomerular Disorders, 786
Glomerulonephritis, 786
Immunoglobulin A Nephropathy, 787
Nephrotic Syndrome, 787
Hemolytic Uremic Syndrome, 787
Nephroblastoma, 788
Bladder Disorders, 788
Urinary Tract Infections, 788
Vesicoureteral Reflux, 789
Urinary Incontinence, 790
Types of Incontinence, 790

The incidence and type of renal and urinary tract disorders experienced by children vary with age and maturation. Newborn disorders may involve congenital malformations. During childhood, the kidney and genitourinary structures continue to develop, so renal dysfunction may be associated with mechanisms and manifestations that differ from those found in adults.

STRUCTURAL ABNORMALITIES

Congenital abnormalities of the kidney and urinary tract occur in about 1 to 2% of newborns.[1] These abnormalities range from minor, non-pathological, or easily correctable anomalies to those that are incompatible with life. For example, the kidneys may fail to ascend from the pelvis to the abdomen, causing ectopic kidneys—which usually function normally. The kidneys may fuse as they ascend, causing a single, U-shaped **horseshoe kidney**. Approximately one-third of individuals with horseshoe kidneys are asymptomatic, with the most common problems being hydronephrosis, infection, stone formation, and, rarely, renal malignancies.[2] Collectively, structural anomalies of the renal system account for approximately 45% of cases of kidney failure in children in developed countries.[3] Many are linked to gene defects.[4] Certain structural anomalies are associated with urinary tract malformations,[4,5] including the following:

- Low-set, malformed ears
- Sensorineural deafness
- Chromosomal disorders, including trisomy 13 (Patau's syndrome) and trisomy 18 (Edwards' syndrome)
- Absent abdominal muscles (prune-belly syndrome)
- Anomalies of the spinal cord and lower and upper extremities
- Imperforate anus and Hirschsprung's disease
- Optic nerve coloboma (hole)
- Nephroblastoma (Wilms tumour)
- Cystic disease of the liver

Hypospadias

Hypospadias is a congenital condition in which the urethral meatus is located on the ventral side or undersurface of the penis. The meatus can be located anywhere on the glans, on the penile shaft, at the base of the penis, at the penoscrotal junction, or on the perineum (Figure 31-1). Hypospadias is the most common anomaly of the penis; it occurs in about 1 in 300 infant boys.[6] The cause of this condition is multifactorial and includes genetic, endocrine, and environmental factors. Advanced maternal age and low birth weight also have been implicated.[7,8] **Chordee (penile torsion)** may accompany cases of hypospadias. In chordee, skin tethering and shortening of subcutaneous tissue cause the penis to bend or "bow ventrally" (Figure 31-2). Penile torsion is rotation of the penile shaft to either the right or the left. Partial absence of the foreskin and cryptorchidism (undescended testes; see Chapter 32) are associated with the anomaly.

The goals for corrective surgery on the child with hypospadias are (1) a straight penis when erect to facilitate intercourse as an adult, (2) a uniform urethra of adequate calibre to prevent spraying during urination, (3) a cosmetic appearance satisfactory to the individual, and (4) repair completed in as few procedures as possible. Surgery is most

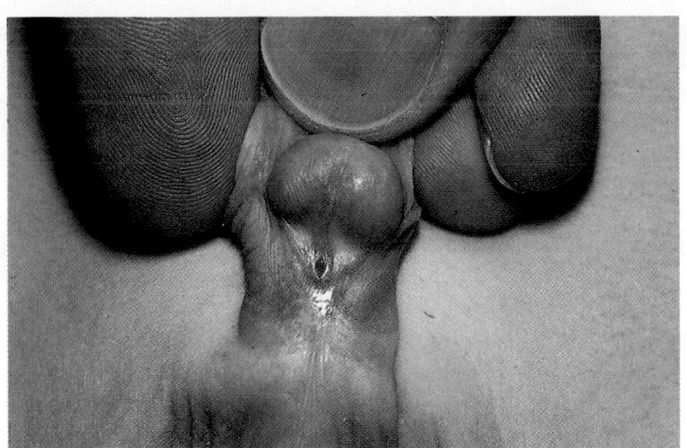

FIGURE 31-1 Hypospadias. (Courtesy H. Gil Rushton, MD, Children's National Medical Center, Washington, DC; from Hockenberry, M.J., & Wilson, D. [2015]. *Wong's nursing care of infants and children.* [10th ed.]. St. Louis: Mosby.)

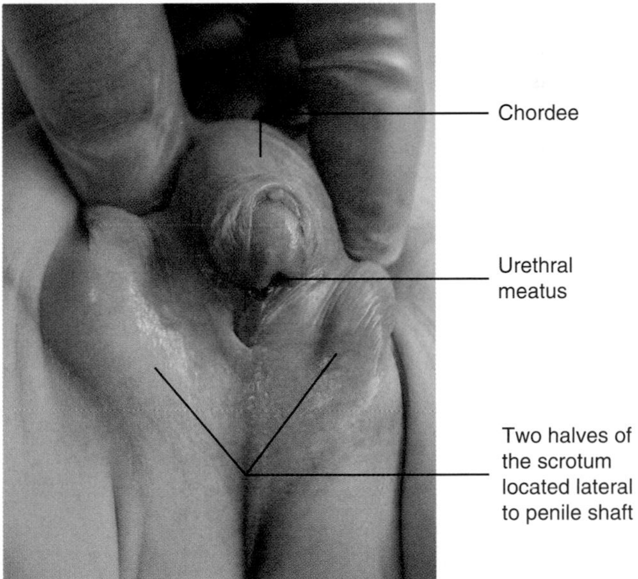

FIGURE 31-2 Hypospadias With Significant Chordee. (From Kliegman, R.M., Stanton, B.F., Gemell, J.W., et al. [Eds.]. [2011]. *Nelson textbook of pediatrics* [19th ed.]. Philadelphia: Saunders.)

effective, psychologically as well as physically, when performed between 6 and 12 months of age.[9]

Epispadias and Exstrophy of the Bladder

Epispadias and exstrophy of the bladder are the same congenital defect expressed to differing degrees. In male epispadias, the urethral opening is on the dorsal surface of the penis. In females, a cleft along the ventral urethra usually extends to the bladder neck. The incidence of epispadias is about 9.25 per 100 000 in-hospital live births.[10] Epispadias is seen predominantly in males.

In boys, the urethral opening may be small and situated behind the glans (anterior epispadias), or a fissure may extend the entire length of the penis and into the bladder neck (posterior epispadias). Continence is determined in part by the location of the defect, with urinary incontinence rates of up to 75% in children with distal epispadias.[11] Treatment is surgical reconstruction.

Exstrophy of the bladder is a rare, extensive congenital anomaly of herniation of the bladder through the abdominal wall. The bony part

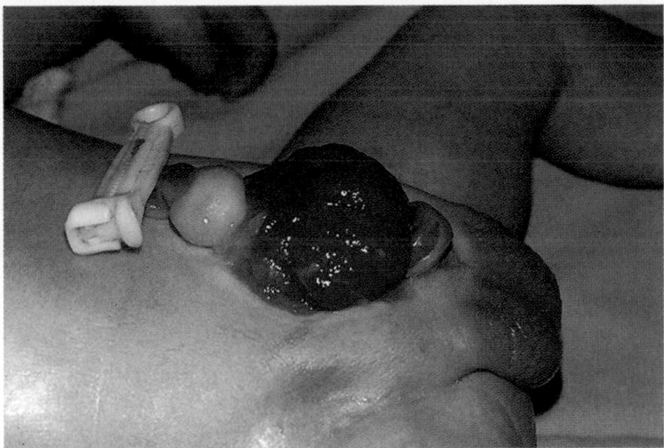

FIGURE 31-3 Exstrophy of Bladder. (Courtesy H. Gil Rushton, MD, Children's National Medical Center, Washington, DC; from Hockenberry, M.J., & Wilson, D. [2015]. *Wong's nursing care of infants and children.* [10th ed.]. St. Louis: Mosby.)

of the pelvis remains open (Figure 31-3), and the posterior portion of the bladder mucosa is exposed through the abdominal opening and appears bright red. Studies vary widely concerning male versus female prevalence.[12]

Exstrophy of the bladder is caused by intrauterine failure of the abdominal wall and the mesoderm of the anterior bladder to fuse. The rectus muscles below the umbilicus are separated, and the pubic rami (bony projections of the pubic bone) are not joined. This causes a waddling gait when the child first learns to walk, but most children quickly learn to compensate. The clitoris in girls is divided into two parts with the urethra between each half. The penis in boys is epispadiac. Urine seeps onto the abdominal wall from the ureters, causing a constant odour of urine and excoriation of the surrounding skin. Because the exposed bladder mucosa becomes hyperemic and edematous, it bleeds easily and is painful.

The unrepaired exstrophic bladder is prone to cancerous changes as soon as 1 year after birth. Ideally, the bladder and pubic defect should be closed before the infant is 72 hours old. Surgical reconstruction is usually performed within the first year either as a complete primary repair or as staged procedures. Staged procedures may include bladder augmentation, bladder neck reconstruction, and epispadias repair.[13] Objectives of management include preservation of renal function, attainment of urinary control, prevention of infection, and improvement of sexual function. Diagnosis is often made by prenatal ultrasound.

Cloacal exstrophy is the most rare and severe form of bladder exstrophy. The intestine and spine may be involved, and reconstruction with restored urine and fecal control is difficult.

Bladder Outlet Obstruction

Congenital causes of bladder outlet obstruction are rare and include urethral valves and polyps. A urethral valve is a thin membrane of tissue that occludes the urethral lumen and obstructs urinary outflow in males. Most valves occur in the posterior urethra, although a few arise from the embryologically distinct anterior urethra. Urethral polyps are rare.[14] The timing and presentation of these conditions depend on the degree of obstruction they cause. Severe obstruction may impair renal embryogenesis and lead to kidney failure.[15] Urethral valves or polyps are resected as soon as they are diagnosed.

Ureteropelvic Junction Obstruction

Ureteropelvic junction (UPJ) obstruction is a blockage of the tapered point where the renal pelvis transitions into the ureter. UPJ obstruction is the most common cause of hydronephrosis in neonates. An intrinsic malformation of smooth muscle or urothelial development produces obstruction in the majority of cases. Extrinsic compression abnormalities are less common.[16] Secondary ureteropelvic junction (UPJ) obstruction is caused by kinking or secondary scarring in the presence of high-grade vesicoureteral reflux. There is an increased risk for VUR in children with UPJ obstruction in the obstructed or contralateral kidney, or both; whether this increased risk represents a sequela of the embryonic defect leading to the UPJ defect is not known. Diagnosis of a UPJ obstruction can be made by ultrasound. Obstruction of the distal ureter (ureterovesical junction obstruction) causes dilation of the entire ureter, renal pelvis, and calyceal system. An ureterocele is a cystic dilation of the intravesical ureter. Open or endoscopic surgery to relieve an obstruction occurs if there is decline of renal drainage or function.[17]

Hypoplastic or Dysplastic Kidneys

During embryological development, the ureteric duct grows into the metanephric tissue, triggering the formation of the kidneys. If this growth does not occur, the kidney is absent—a condition called renal aplasia. A hypoplastic kidney is small with a decreased number of nephrons. These conditions may be unilateral or bilateral; the occurrence may be incidental or familial. Bilateral hypoplastic kidneys are a common cause of chronic kidney disease in children.[18] Segmental hypoplasia—the Ask-Upmark kidney—may be congenital or secondary to VUR. Systemic hypertension is a common presentation.[19]

Renal dysplasia usually results from abnormal differentiation of the renal tissues; for example, primitive glomeruli and tubules, cysts, and nonrenal tissue (such as cartilage) are found in the dysplastic kidney. Dysplasia may be secondary to antenatal obstruction of the urinary tract from ureteroceles, posterior urethral valves, or prune-belly syndrome (congenital absence of abdominal muscles).

Polycystic Kidney Disease

Polycystic kidney disease (PKD) is an autosomal dominant disease (*PDK1* or *PDK2* gene) occurring in 1 of 1 000 live births, or an autosomal recessive inherited disorder (*PKHD1* gene) with an incidence of 1 in 20 000 to 1 in 40 000.[20] Affected kidneys have multiple cysts that interfere with renal function. Autosomal dominant polycystic kidney disease (ADPKD) usually presents in late childhood or adulthood with the development of cysts. Defects in the formation of epithelial cells and their cilia result in cyst formation in all parts of the nephron. Cysts in other organs, including the liver, pancreas, and ovaries, may occur. Hypertension, aortic and intracranial aneurysms, and heart valve defects may develop. Autosomal recessive polycystic kidney disease (ARPKD) is often first suspected on a prenatal ultrasound. Epithelial hyperplasia and fluid secretion result in collecting duct cysts. Hepatic disease and hypertension typically accompany PKD. Clinical trials for various potential treatment modalities are ongoing.[21]

Renal Agenesis

Renal agenesis (the absence of one or both kidneys) may be unilateral or bilateral, and may occur randomly or be hereditary. It may be an isolated entity or be associated with anomalies in other organs.

Unilateral renal agenesis occurs in approximately 1 in 1 000 live births. Males are more often affected, and it is usually the left kidney that is absent. The single remaining kidney is often completely normal so that the child can expect a normal, healthy life. By the time the child is several years old, the volume of this kidney may approach twice the normal size to compensate for the absence of a second kidney. In some instances, however, the single kidney is abnormally formed and associated with abnormalities of its collecting system. Because the child has a decreased number of nephrons, there is a risk for "hyperfiltration injury," increasing the chance of developing proteinuria, hypertension, and chronic kidney disease.[22] Extrarenal congenital abnormalities of the urogenital, skeletal, cardiac, and other systems may coexist.

Bilateral renal agenesis is a rare disorder incompatible with extrauterine life. Approximately 75% of affected children are males. Oligohydramnios (low amount of amniotic fluid) resulting from inadequate fetal urine production leads to underdeveloped lungs and Potter syndrome (wide-set eyes, parrot-beak nose, low-set ears, and receding chin). Approximately 40% of affected infants are stillborn. Infants with this condition rarely live more than 24 hours because of pulmonary insufficiency.[23] Renal agenesis can be detected prenatally by ultrasound.

✔ QUICK CHECK 31-1

1. Describe hypospadias.
2. Why does bladder exstrophy occur?
3. Contrast dysplastic kidney and hypoplastic kidney.

GLOMERULAR DISORDERS

Common glomerular disorders in children are glomerulonephritis, nephrotic syndrome, immunoglobulin A (IgA) nephropathy, and hemolytic uremic syndrome (HUS). Most glomerular diseases are acquired and immunologically mediated (see Chapter 30, Figure 30-6, and Table 30-5). The disease can be acute or chronic. The likelihood of developing kidney failure depends on the specific condition.

Glomerulonephritis

Glomerulonephritis includes a number of renal disorders in which proliferation and inflammation of the glomeruli are secondary to an immune mechanism (the pathophysiology is described in Chapter 30) and is the causative factor for 9 to 35% of end-stage kidney disease in children worldwide.[24]

Acute Poststreptococcal Glomerulonephritis

Acute poststreptococcal glomerulonephritis (APGN) is one of the most common immune complex–mediated renal diseases in children. It most commonly occurs after a throat or skin infection with a nephritogenic strain of group A beta-hemolytic streptococci, although other bacteria and viruses also may be responsible.[25] Occurrences have been observed after bacterial endocarditis, which may be associated with streptococcal or staphylococcal microorganisms, or after viral diseases, such as varicella-zoster virus and hepatitis B and C. Glomerulonephritis develops with the deposition of antigen–antibody complexes in the glomerulus. The antigen–antibody complex activates complement and the release of inflammatory mediators that damage endothelial and epithelial cells lying on the glomerular basement membrane. Damage to the glomerular basement membrane leads to hematuria and proteinuria.

Symptoms usually begin 1 to 2 weeks after an upper respiratory tract infection (more common during cold weather) and up to 6 weeks after skin infections such as impetigo (more common during warm weather).

The onset of symptoms is abrupt, varying with disease severity. The child typically has gross or microscopic hematuria, proteinuria, edema, and renal insufficiency. Oliguria may be present. Hypertension occurs because of increased vascular volume. Acute hypertension may cause headache, vomiting, somnolence, and other central nervous system manifestations. Cardiovascular symptoms are related to circulatory overload and are compounded by hypertension. These include dyspnea, tachypnea, and an enlarged, tender liver. The most severely affected children develop acute kidney injury with oliguria. As many as half of affected children are asymptomatic.

The disease usually runs its course in 1 month, but urine abnormalities may be found for up to 1 year or longer after the onset. Prolonged proteinuria and abnormal glomerular filtration rate (GFR) indicate an unfavourable prognosis. More than 95% of affected children recover completely. Less than 1% of children develop end-stage kidney disease.[26] Treatment is supportive and symptom specific.

Immunoglobulin A Nephropathy

Immunoglobulin A (IgA) nephropathy is the most common form of glomerulonephritis worldwide and occurs more often in males. It is characterized by deposition primarily of immunoglobulin A and complement proteins in the mesangium of the glomerulus. Children with the disease have recurrent gross hematuria concurrent with a respiratory tract infection. Most continue to have microscopic hematuria between the attacks of gross hematuria and have a mild proteinuria as well. Treatment is supportive. Some children recover completely, whereas 20% or more will eventually require dialysis and transplantation.[27] IgA nephropathy may recur following transplantation.[28]

Henoch-Schönlein purpura nephritis is a particular form of IgA nephropathy that involves a systemic vasculitis. Symptoms vary widely. In addition to palpable purpura, children may experience abdominal pain, arthralgia, hematuria, and/or proteinuria. Complete recovery may occur, but some children progress to end-stage kidney disease.[29]

Nephrotic Syndrome

Nephrotic syndrome is characterized by severe proteinuria, hypoalbuminemia, dyslipidemia, and edema. The syndrome is more common in children than in adults. When no identifiable cause is found, the condition is **primary (idiopathic) nephrotic syndrome**. If it results from a systemic disease or other causes (e.g., medications, toxins), it is called **secondary nephrotic syndrome**. Primary nephrotic syndrome is found predominantly in the preschool-age child, with a peak incidence of onset between 2 and 3 years of age. It is rare after 8 years of age. Boys are affected more often than girls. No prevalent ethnic or geographical distributions are evident. The incidence is approximately 3 per 100 000 children per year.

Since childhood nephrotic syndrome meets the Canadian Institutes of Health Research definition of a "rare" disease (it affects 1 person out of 2 000 or fewer), almost no single centre or region in Canada has a sufficient number of patients to produce generalizable knowledge regarding effective treatments.[30]

PATHOPHYSIOLOGY The most common causes of primary nephrotic syndrome in children are minimal change nephropathy and focal segmental glomerulosclerosis. **Minimal change nephropathy (MCN) (lipoid nephrosis)** is characterized by fusion of the glomerular podocyte foot processes, which are seen by electron microscopy. The glomeruli appear normal by light microscopy. A systemic immune mechanism is a likely cause of the disease, but the true etiology is unknown. An unidentified circulating permeability factor released by T lymphocytes has been proposed.[31] Loss of the electrical negative charge and increased permeability within the glomerular capillary wall lead to albuminuria. Hypoalbuminemia (causing decreased plasma oncotic pressure) and sodium retention contribute to edema.[32] Dyslipidemia leads to hyperlipiduria and primarily results from increased hepatic lipid synthesis and decreased plasma lipid catabolism.

In idiopathic **focal segmental glomerulosclerosis (FSGS)**, there is segmental loss of glomerular capillaries with proliferation of the mesangial matrix and adhesion of the capillaries to the Bowman capsule.

CLINICAL MANIFESTATIONS The onset of nephrotic syndrome can be insidious, with periorbital edema as the usual first sign. The edema is most noticeable in the morning and subsides during the day as fluid shifts to the abdomen, genitalia, and lower extremities. Parents may notice diminished, frothy, or foamy urine output; or when edema becomes pronounced with ascites, respiratory difficulty from pleural effusion or labial or scrotal swelling may occur. Edema of the intestinal mucosa may cause diarrhea, anorexia, and poor absorption. Edema often masks the malnutrition caused by malabsorption and protein loss. Pallor, with shiny skin and prominent veins, also is common. Blood pressure is usually normal. The child has an increased susceptibility to infection, especially pneumonia, peritonitis, cellulitis, and septicemia. Irritability, fatigue, and lethargy are common. **Congenital nephrotic syndrome (Finnish type)** is caused by an autosomal recessive mutation of the *NPHS1* gene that encodes an immunoglobulinlike protein—nephrin—at the podocyte slit membrane.[33] Congenital nephrotic syndrome (Finnish type) presents with heavy proteinuria, hypoproteinemia, and edema in the first 3 months of life. These babies do not respond to steroid treatment and require albumin infusion and diuretics.[34]

EVALUATION AND TREATMENT The diagnosis of nephrotic syndrome is evident from the findings of proteinuria, dyslipidemia, and edema. Diagnostic testing, including kidney biopsy, may be required to determine whether the cause is an intrinsic kidney disease or a consequence of systemic disease. Basic management of nephrotic syndrome includes administering glucocorticosteroids (prednisone [Deltasone]); adhering to a low-sodium, well-balanced diet; performing good skin care; and, if edema becomes problematic, prescribing diuretics (furosemide [Lasix], metolazone [Zaroxolyn]). Immunosuppressive agents (i.e., cyclophosphamide [Procytox]) may be used with children who have frequent relapses or who are resistant to steroid therapy. Long-term outcomes depend on the underlying cause of the nephrotic syndrome. Children with minimal change disease tend to do very well, whereas those with other conditions may develop end-stage kidney disease.

Hemolytic Uremic Syndrome

Hemolytic uremic syndrome (HUS) is an acute disorder characterized by hemolytic anemia, thrombocytopenia, and acute kidney injury. HUS is the most common cause of acute kidney injury in children. The disease occurs most often in infants and children younger than 4 years of age but has been known to occur in adolescents and adults.

PATHOPHYSIOLOGY HUS has been associated with bacterial and viral agents, as well as endotoxins, especially that from *Escherichia coli* 0157:H7 and, more recently, *E. coli* 0104:H4 (Shiga toxins).[35] In HUS, the endothelial lining of the glomerular arterioles becomes swollen and occluded with platelets and fibrin clots. Narrowed vessels damage passing erythrocytes. These damaged red blood cells are removed by the spleen, causing acute hemolytic anemia. Fibrinolysis, the process of dissolution of a clot, acts on precipitated fibrin, causing the fibrin split products to appear in serum and urine. Platelet thrombi develop within damaged vessels, and platelet removal produces thrombocytopenia. Varying degrees of vascular occlusion cause altered renal perfusion and renal insufficiency or failure.[36]

CLINICAL MANIFESTATIONS A prodromal gastro-intestinal illness (fever, vomiting, diarrhea) or, less frequently, an upper respiratory tract infection often precedes the onset of HUS by 1 to 2 weeks. After a symptom-free 1- to 5-day period, the sudden onset of pallor, bruising or purpura, irritability, and oliguria heralds the commencement of the disease. Slight fever, anorexia, vomiting, diarrhea (with the stool characteristically watery and blood stained), abdominal pain, mild jaundice, and circulatory overload are accompanying symptoms. Seizures and lethargy indicate central nervous system involvement. Kidney failure is apparent within the first days of onset. The kidney failure causes metabolic acidosis, azotemia, hyperkalemia, and often hypertension.

EVALUATION AND TREATMENT Clinical evaluation includes history of pre-existing illness, presenting symptoms, and urine and blood analysis. Management is supportive. When kidney failure occurs, dialysis is indicated. Blood transfusions with packed red cells are needed to maintain reasonable hemoglobin levels. Seventy percent of children recover completely. Potential long-term sequelae include renal (hypertension, proteinuria, chronic kidney disease, and end-stage kidney disease) and nonrenal abnormalities (diabetes mellitus, neurological manifestations). In cases unresponsive to treatment, splenectomy may be indicated.[37]

NEPHROBLASTOMA

Nephroblastoma (Wilms tumour) is a rare embryonal tumour of the kidney arising from undifferentiated mesoderm. The peak incidence occurs between 2 and 3 years of age. Nephroblastoma is slightly more common in black children than in white children. Maternal preconception toxin exposure (e.g., pesticides) may be associated with increased risk in offspring.[38]

PATHOGENESIS Nephroblastoma has both sporadic and inherited origins. The sporadic form occurs in children with no known genetic predisposition. Inherited cases, which are relatively rare, are transmitted in an autosomal dominant fashion. Syndromic and nonsyndromic causes of nephroblastoma have been linked to mutation of several tumour-suppressor genes (i.e., *WT1* and *WT2* mutations).[39]

Eighteen percent of children who have nephroblastoma also have other congenital anomalies. The anomalies associated with nephroblastoma include aniridia (lack of an iris in the eye), hemihyperplasia (an asymmetry of the body), and genitourinary malformations (i.e., horseshoe kidneys, hypospadias, ureteral duplication, polycystic kidneys).[40] Children with both congenital anomalies and nephroblastoma are more likely to have the inherited bilateral form of the disease.

CLINICAL MANIFESTATIONS Most children with nephroblastoma present with an enlarging asymptomatic abdominal mass before the age of 5 years. Many tumours are actually discovered by the child's parent, who feels or notices an abdominal swelling, usually while dressing or bathing the child. The child appears healthy and thriving. Other presenting complaints include vague abdominal pain, hematuria, anemia, and fever. Hypertension may be present, often as a result of excessive renin secretion by the tumour.[41]

Nephroblastoma may occur in any part of the kidney and varies greatly in size at the time of diagnosis. The tumour generally appears as a solitary mass surrounded by a smooth, fibrous external capsule and also may contain cystic or hemorrhagic areas. A pseudocapsule generally separates the tumour from the renal parenchyma.

EVALUATION AND TREATMENT On physical examination, the tumour feels firm, nontender, and smooth, and is generally confined to one side of the abdomen. If the tumour is palpable past the midline of the abdomen, it may be large or may be arising from a horseshoe or ectopic kidney. Once an abdominal mass is detected, diagnostic imaging demonstrates a solid intrarenal mass.

Diagnosis is based on surgical biopsy. Imaging studies are used to evaluate the presence or absence of metastasis.[42] The most common sites of metastasis are regional lymph nodes and the lungs, and less common sites are the liver, brain, and bone.

TABLE 31-1 Staging of Nephroblastoma Tumour[a]

Stage	Tumour Characteristics
I	Tumour limited to kidney; can be completely resected
II	Tumour ascending beyond kidney but is totally resected
III	Residual nonhematogenous tumour confined to abdomen
IV	Hematogenous metastases to organs such as lungs, liver, bone, or brain
V	Bilateral disease either at diagnosis or later, then staged for each kidney

[a]Staging system of the National Wilms Tumor Study Group.

Several staging systems for nephroblastoma have been developed and serve as guides to treatment. The most widely accepted system was developed by the National Wilms Tumor Study Group (Table 31-1). Primary treatment is usually surgical exploration and resection or chemotherapy and then surgical resection. Radiation therapy may be used for children with higher stages of disease and metastases. Survival is greater than 90% for localized disease and up to 80% for higher stages, although heart failure, kidney failure, and hypertension occur more frequently in long-term survivors than in the general population.[43]

✔ QUICK CHECK 31-2
1. What is the cause of proteinuria?
2. What is Wilms tumour and what cellular components are involved?

BLADDER DISORDERS

Urinary Tract Infections

Urinary tract infections (UTIs) are rare in newborns, and children with congenital renal abnormalities and noncircumcised males are at increased risk.[44] UTIs in children are most common in 7- to 11-year-old girls as a result of perineal bacteria, especially *E. coli*, ascending the urethra. Susceptibility, bacterial virulence, and, perhaps, genetics affect the severity of the disease.[45] An abnormal urinary tract (presence of reflux, obstruction, stasis, or stones) is particularly susceptible to infection. Sexually active female adolescents are at increased risk to have a UTI.

Cystitis, or infection of the bladder, results in mucosal inflammation and congestion. This causes detrusor muscle hyperactivity and thus a decrease in bladder capacity, resulting in urgency and frequency. It may also cause distortion of the ureterovesical junction, leading to transient reflux of infected urine up the ureters, causing acute or chronic pyelonephritis.

Differentiating whether an infection is in the bladder or in the kidneys is difficult based on symptoms alone. Infants may be asymptomatic or develop fever, lethargy, abdominal pain, vomiting, diarrhea, or asymptomatic jaundice. Children may present with fever of undetermined origin, frequency, urgency, dysuria, enuresis or incontinence in a previously dry child, flank or back pain, and sometimes hematuria. Acute pyelonephritis usually causes chills, high fever, and flank or abdominal pain, along with enlarged kidney(s) caused by inflammatory edema. Chronic pyelonephritis may be asymptomatic.

Diagnosis of UTIs is by urine culture. Dipstick analyses for nitrite, leukocyte esterase, and blood may be used as a screening tool. Any positive or strong suspicion of a UTI, including unexplained jaundice in infants,[46] requires urine culture. Diagnostic imaging may be necessary to rule out obstructions, renal scarring, or functional abnormalities. With treatment, UTI symptoms are usually relieved in 1 to 2 days, and the urine becomes sterile. A 2- to 4-day course of oral antibiotics is effective for uncomplicated UTI.[47] Longer treatment may be required if the child has a history of recurrent UTIs or has congenital abnormalities of the urinary tract. If there is no improvement in 2 days, the child should be re-evaluated (see *Health Promotion:* Childhood Urinary Tract Infections).

HEALTH PROMOTION

Childhood Urinary Tract Infections

Childhood urinary tract infections (UTIs) are often seen in primary care settings and can cause significant longer-term morbidity if not treated. Children younger than 2 years often have few, nonspecific signs of infection, including fever, irritability, poor feeding, failure to thrive, and diarrhea. Obtaining a proper urine sample and culture is vital because true infections require further examination. Antibiotic prophylaxis may be considered because of the link between vesicoureteral reflux (VUR), recurrent UTIs, and renal scarring and hypertension; however, this issue is controversial because of the risk for antibiotic resistance. Current recommendations are to *consider* prophylaxis for children younger than 1 year of age with VUR and a history of febrile UTIs, and other children as indicated.

Although recent studies have shown a decreased rate of UTIs in circumcised boys, the benefits and risks of circumcision are controversial. The circumcision of newborn males in Canada has become a less frequent practice over the past few decades. This change has been significantly influenced by past recommendations by the Canadian Paediatric Society and the American Academy of Pediatrics, who have both affirmed that the procedure is not medically indicated. Recent evidence suggesting the potential benefit of circumcision in preventing UTIs (and some sexually transmitted infections, including HIV) has prompted the Canadian Paediatric Society to review the current medical literature in this regard. While there may be a benefit for some boys in high-risk populations and circumstances where the procedure could be considered for disease reduction or treatment, the Canadian Paediatric Society does not recommend the routine circumcision of every newborn male.

The Canadian Paediatric Society recommends that UTI be ruled out in preverbal children with unexplained fever and in older children with symptoms suggestive of UTI (dysuria, urinary frequency, hematuria, abdominal pain, back pain, or new daytime incontinence). A midstream urine sample should be collected for urinalysis and culture in toilet-trained children; others should have urine collected by catheter or by suprapubic aspirate. UTI is unlikely if the urinalysis is completely normal. A bagged urine sample may be used for urinalysis but should not be used for urine culture. Antibiotic treatment for 7 to 10 days is recommended for febrile UTI. Oral antibiotics may be offered as initial treatment when the child is not seriously ill and is likely to receive and tolerate every dose. Children younger than 2 years of age should be investigated after their first febrile UTI with a renal and bladder ultrasound to identify any significant renal abnormalities. A voiding cystourethrogram is not required for children with a first UTI unless the renal and bladder ultrasound reveals findings suggestive of VUR, selected renal anomalies, or obstructive uropathy.

Abnormalities in bowel and bladder function must be addressed because they can impact the development of UTIs and affect the resolution of VUR. Surgical management of VUR is considered on the basis of failure of medical management to prevent recurrent infections, VUR grade, and degree of renal scarring.

Data from American Academy of Pediatrics. (2012). *Pediatrics, 130*(3), 585–586; Arshad, M., & Seed, P.C. (2015). *Clin Perinatol, 42*(1), 17–28, vii; Canadian Paediatric Society. (2015). *Position statement: Newborn male circumcision.* Retrieved from http://www.cps.ca/documents/position/circumcision; Paintsil, E. (2013). *Curr Opin Pediatr, 25*(1), 88–94; Robinson, J.L., Finlay, J.C., Lang, M.E., et al. (2014). *Paediatr Child Health, 19*(6), 1; Saperston, K.N., Shapiro, D.J., Hersh, A.L., et al. (2014). *J Urol, 191*(5, Suppl.), 1608–1613.

Vesicoureteral Reflux

Vesicoureteral reflux (VUR) is the retrograde flow of urine from the bladder into the kidney or ureters, or both. This allows infected urine from the bladder to reach the kidneys. VUR occurs more often in girls by a ratio of 10 : 1 and is uncommon in Blacks. The actual incidence is unknown because VUR is often undiagnosed. An estimated 30 to 40% of children younger than 5 years who develop a UTI have VUR. Siblings of those affected have about a 27 to 51% chance of having reflux, and children with parents who had childhood reflux have almost a 70% chance of reflux.[48] Although reflux is considered abnormal at any age, the shortness of the submucosal tunnel of the ureter during infancy and childhood renders the antireflux mechanism relatively inefficient and delicate. Thus reflux is seen commonly in association with infections during early childhood but rarely in older children and adults.

PATHOPHYSIOLOGY The normal distal ureter enters the bladder through the detrusor muscle and passes through a submucosal tunnel before opening into the bladder lumen via the ureteral orifice. As the bladder fills with urine, the ureter is compressed within the bladder wall, preventing reflux. Primary VUR results from a congenital abnormally short submucosal tunnel and ureter that permits reflux by the rising pressure of the filling bladder (Figure 31-4). Urine sweeps up into the ureter and then flows back into the empty bladder. The reflux perpetuates infection by preventing complete emptying of the bladder and providing a reservoir for infection. With bladder filling, the maximal intravesical pressure can be transmitted up the ureter to the renal pelvis and calyces. The combination of reflux and infection is an important cause of pyelonephritis. Renal parenchymal injury, scarring, hypertension, and chronic renal insufficiency can occur many years later, making early diagnosis and treatment important. Secondary reflux develops in association with acquired conditions (e.g., neurogenic bladder dysfunction, ureteral obstruction, voiding disorders, or surgery on the ureterovesical junction). Reflux may be unilateral or bilateral, and is graded using the International Reflux Grading System[49] (Figure 31-5):

- *Grade I:* reflux into a nondilated distal ureter
- *Grade II:* reflux into the upper collecting system without dilation
- *Grade III:* reflux into a dilated ureter or blunting of calyceal fornices
- *Grade IV:* reflux into a grossly dilated ureter and calyces

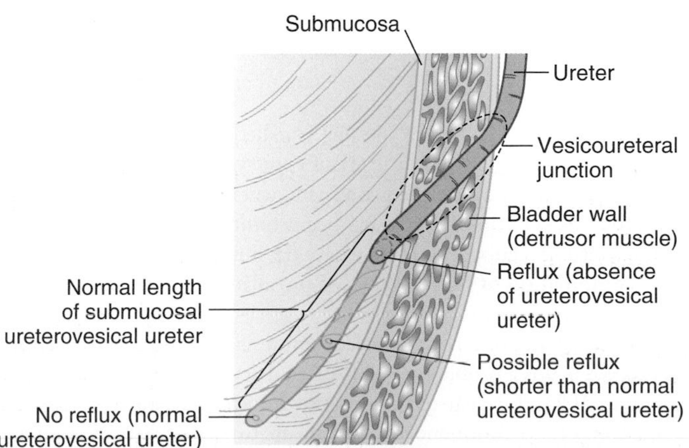

FIGURE 31-4 Normal and Abnormal Configurations of the Ureterovesical Ureter. A refluxing ureterovesical ureter has the same anatomical features as a nonrefluxing ureter, except for the shorter length of the intravesical ureter, which allows reflux of urine during filling of the bladder.

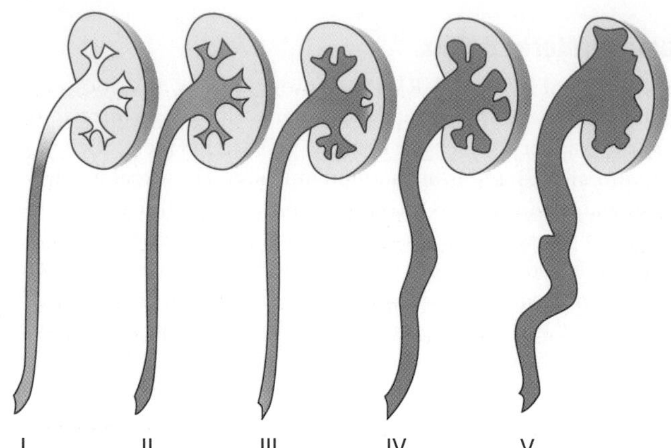

FIGURE 31-5 Grades of Vesicoureteral Reflux. (From Johnson, J.R., Feehally, J., & Floege, J. [2015]. *Comprehensive clinical nephrology* [5th ed.]. Philadelphia: Saunders.)

- *Grade V:* massive reflux with urethral dilation and tortuosity and effacement of the calyceal details

CLINICAL MANIFESTATIONS Children with reflux may be asymptomatic or have recurrent UTIs, unexplained fevers, poor growth and development, irritability, and feeding problems. The family history may reveal VUR or UTIs.

EVALUATION AND TREATMENT In addition to the history of recurrent UTI and other symptoms, a voiding cystourethrogram is the primary diagnostic procedure. Most children with VUR respond to nonoperative management aimed at prevention and treatment of infection. Spontaneous remission of grades I, II, and III reflux may occur in 50 to 80% of children younger than 5 years. Approximately 20% of grades IV and V will resolve.[50] Recurrent infection may require endoscopic, open, laparoscopic, and robotic procedures to stop the refluxing ureter.[51]

URINARY INCONTINENCE

Urinary incontinence refers to the involuntary passage of urine by a child who is beyond the age when voluntary bladder control should have been acquired. Bladder control is accomplished by most children before the age of 5 years, although it is largely influenced by cultural beliefs and parental toilet-training practices.

Types of Incontinence

Wetness that occurs during the day is called **daytime incontinence**. Nighttime wetting is called **enuresis**. **Primary incontinence** (enuresis) means the child has never been continent, whereas **secondary incontinence** (enuresis) means the child has been continent for at least 6 months before wetting recurs. A child may have daytime incontinence, enuresis, or a combination of both. (Types of incontinence and clinical manifestations are defined in Table 31-2.)

The incidence of incontinence (or enuresis) is difficult to determine because it is not a problem parents often discuss. Enuresis occurs in as many as 10% of 7-year-old males and resolves at a rate of 15% per year. Daytime incontinence occurs in up to 9% of early school-age children.[52]

PATHOGENESIS A combination of factors is likely responsible for incontinence or enuresis. Organic causes account for a minority of cases and include UTIs; neurological disturbances; congenital defects of the meatus, urethra, or bladder neck; and allergies. Disorders that increase the normal output of urine, such as diabetes mellitus and diabetes insipidus, or disorders that impair the concentrating ability of the kidney, such as chronic kidney disease or sickle cell disease, should be considered during evaluation. Other conditions that may be associated with incontinence include perinatal anoxia, central nervous system trauma, seizures, attention-deficit/hyperactivity disorder,[53] developmental delay, imperforate anus, bladder trauma or surgery, obesity,[54] and occult spinal dysraphism. Altered sleep arousal or obstructive sleep apnea[55] may be associated with enuresis. Stressful psychological situations, such as a new sibling, may cause incontinence or enuresis to develop. Constipation is frequently present in children with urinary incontinence.[56] Incontinence or enuresis in which no structural or neurological abnormality is identified is common in children.

Genetic factors contribute to some types of incontinence. At least four gene loci associated with enuresis have been identified. Enuresis occurs with high frequency among parents, siblings, and other near relatives of symptomatic children. There is a high concordance rate in monozygotic twins with enuresis.[57]

TABLE 31-2 Classification of Incontinence

Type	Definition
Daytime voiding frequency	Decreased: 3 or fewer voids per day Increased: 8 or more voids per day
Dysfunctional voiding	Habitual contraction of urethral sphincter during voiding; observed by uroflow measurements
Enuresis	Incontinence of urine while sleeping
Incontinence, continuous	Continuous leakage, not in discrete portions
Incontinence, stress	Leakage with raised intra-abdominal pressure
Urgency	Sudden, unexpected, immediate need to void
Overactive bladder	Child with urgency; increased voiding frequency, incontinence, or both may or may not be present
Underactive bladder	Decreased voiding frequency with use of raised intra-abdominal pressure to void
Urge incontinence	Incontinence in children with urgency

From Nevéus, T., von Gontard, A., Hoebeke, P., et al. (2006). *J Urol, 176*(1), 314–324.

EVALUATION AND TREATMENT Diagnostic evaluation of childhood incontinence includes a thorough history, voiding dairy, physical examination, and urinalysis. Urodynamic flow studies or imaging may be required on the basis of history and physical findings. Therapeutic management of incontinence or enuresis begins with education. If the child and family understand the probably etiology of the child's condition, they are better able to choose and participate in therapies that are most likely to succeed. Treatment of daytime incontinence includes behavioural therapy, including timed voiding; fluid management; treatment of constipation, UTIs, and other coexisting conditions if present; and medication (anticholinergic or alpha-blocker medications). Enuresis treatment also may include enuresis alarms or other medications (e.g., desmopressin acetate).[58]

QUICK CHECK 31-3

1. How does the cause of urinary tract infections (UTIs) in newborns differ from that in older children?
2. How does vesicoureteral reflux occur?
3. What organic causes are operative in enuresis?

DID YOU UNDERSTAND?

Structural Abnormalities

1. Congenital renal disorders affect about 10 to 15% of the population. These disorders range in severity from minor conditions that need no treatment to those incompatible with life.
2. Hypospadias is a congenital condition in which the urethral meatus is located anywhere on the ventral surface of the glans, the penile shaft, the midline of the scrotum, or the perineum.
3. Exstrophy of the bladder is a congenital malformation in which the pubic bones are separated, the lower portion of the abdominal wall and anterior wall of the bladder are missing, and the posterior wall of the bladder is everted through the opening.
4. Urethral valves and polyps are congenital formations of tissue that block the urethra.
5. Ureteropelvic junction obstruction is blockage where the renal pelvis joins the ureter and is often caused by smooth muscle or urothelial malformation or by scarring that leads to hydronephrosis.
6. A dysplastic kidney is the result of abnormal differentiation of renal tissues. A hypoplastic kidney is small with a decreased number of nephrons.
7. Polycystic kidney disease is a cystic genetic disorder resulting in multiple, bilateral renal cysts.
8. Renal agenesis is the failure of a kidney to grow or develop. The condition may be unilateral or bilateral and may occur as an isolated entity or in association with other disorders.

Glomerular Disorders

1. Glomerulonephritis is an inflammation of the glomeruli characterized by hematuria, edema, and hypertension. The cause is unknown but is often immune mediated. Glomerulonephritis may follow infections, especially those of the upper respiratory tract caused by strains of group A beta-hemolytic streptococcus. Increases in glomerular capillary permeability lead to hematuria and proteinuria.
2. Immunoglobulin A (IgA) nephropathy occurs with deposition of IgA in the glomerulus, causing glomerular injury with gross hematuria.
3. *Nephrotic syndrome* is a term used to describe a symptom complex characterized by proteinuria, hypoproteinemia, dyslipidemia, and edema. Metabolic, biochemical, or physiochemical disturbances in the glomerular basement membrane may lead to increased permeability to protein.
4. Hemolytic uremic syndrome is an acute disorder characterized by hemolytic anemia, acute kidney injury, and thrombocytopenia.

Nephroblastoma

1. Nephroblastoma (Wilms tumour) is an embryonal tumour of the kidney that usually presents before the age of 5 years. Survival is high following treatment by surgery, a combination of medications, and, sometimes, radiation therapy.

Bladder Disorders

1. Urinary tract infections (UTIs) can result from general sepsis in the newborn but are caused by bacteria ascending the urethra in older children. The bladder alone is infected in cystitis. The infection ascends to one or both kidneys in pyelonephritis. Urinary tract anomalies may require surgical correction to prevent frequent recurrent infections.
2. Vesicoureteral reflux is the retrograde flow of bladder urine into the kidney or ureter, or both, increasing the risk for pyelonephritis. It can be unilateral or bilateral; primary or secondary.

Urinary Incontinence

1. Urinary incontinence is the involuntary passage of urine. It may occur during the day (incontinence) or at night (enuresis), or both. Maturational delay, UTIs, constipation, and many other factors may contribute.

KEY TERMS

Acute poststreptococcal glomerulonephritis (APGN), 786
Acute pyelonephritis, 788
Ask-Upmark kidney, 786
Chordee (penile torsion), 784
Chronic pyelonephritis, 788
Congenital nephrotic syndrome (Finnish type), 787
Cystitis, 788
Daytime incontinence, 790
Enuresis, 790
Epispadias, 785
Exstrophy of the bladder, 785
Focal segmental glomerulosclerosis (FSGS), 787
Glomerulonephritis, 786
Hemolytic uremic syndrome (HUS), 787
Henoch-Schönlein purpura nephritis, 787
Horseshoe kidney, 784
Hypoplastic kidney, 786
Hypospadias, 784
Immunoglobulin A (IgA) nephropathy, 787
Minimal change nephropathy (MCN) (lipoid nephrosis), 787
Nephroblastoma (Wilms tumour), 788
Oligohydramnios, 786
Polycystic kidney disease (PKD), 786
Potter syndrome, 786
Primary incontinence, 790
Primary (idiopathic) nephrotic syndrome, 787
Renal agenesis, 786
Renal aplasia, 786
Renal dysplasia, 786
Secondary incontinence, 790
Secondary nephrotic syndrome, 787
Secondary ureteropelvic junction (UPJ) obstruction, 786
Ureterocele, 786
Ureteropelvic junction (UPJ) obstruction, 785
Ureterovesical junction obstruction, 786
Urethral polyp, 785
Urethral valve, 785
Urinary incontinence, 790
Urinary tract infection (UTI), 788
Vesicoureteral reflux (VUR), 789

REFERENCES

1. Caiulo, V. A., Caiulo, S., Gargasole, C., et al. (2012). Ultrasound mass screening for congenital anomalies of the kidney and urinary tract. *Pediatric Nephrology (Berlin, Germany)*, *27*(6), 949–953. doi:10.1007/s00467-011-2098-0.
2. Natsis, K., Piagkou, M., Skotsimara, A., et al. (2013). Horseshoe kidney: A review of anatomy and pathology. *Surgical and Radiologic Anatomy*, *36*(6), 517–526. doi:10.1007/s00276-013-1229-7.
3. Harambat, J., van Stralen, K. J., Kim, J. J., et al. (2012). Epidemiology of chronic kidney disease in children. *Pediatric Nephrology (Berlin, Germany)*, *27*(3), 363–373. doi:10.1007/s00467-011-1939-1.
4. Vivante, A., Kohl, S., Hwang, D. Y., et al. (2014). Single-gene causes of congenital anomalies of the kidney and urinary tract (CAKUT) in humans. *Pediatric Nephrology (Berlin, Germany)*, *29*(4), 695–704. doi:10.1007/s00467-013-2684-4.
5. Yosypiv, I. V. (2012). Congenital anomalies of the kidney and urinary tract: A genetic disorder?

International Journal of Nephrology, *2012*, 909083. doi:10.1155/2012/909083.

6. Montag, S., & Palmer, L. S. (2011). Abnormalities of penile curvature: Chordee and penile torsion. *Scientific World Journal*, *11*, 1470–1478. doi:10.1100/tsw.2011.136.
7. Carmichael, S. L., Shaw, G. M., & Lammer, E. J. (2012). Environmental and genetic contributors to hypospadias: A review of the epidemiologic evidence. *Birth Defects Research. Part A, Clinical and Molecular Teratology*, *94*(7), 499–510. doi:10.1002/bdra.23021.
8. Gill, S. K., Broussard, C., Devine, O., et al. (2012). National Birth Defects Prevention Study: Association between maternal age and birth defects of unknown etiology: United States, 1997–2007. *Birth Defects Research. Part A, Clinical and Molecular Teratology*, *94*(12), 1010–1018. doi:10.1002/bdra.23049.
9. Springer, A., & Baskin, L. S. (2014). Timing of hypospadias repair in patients with disorders of sex development. *Endocrine Development*, *27*, 197–202. doi:10.1159/000363662.
10. Lloyd, J. C., Wiener, J. S., Gargolio, P. C., et al. (2013). Contemporary epidemiological trends in complex congenital genitourinary anomalies. *Journal of Urology*, *190*(4, Suppl.), 1590–1595. doi:10.1016/j.juro.2013.04.034.
11. Frimberger, D. (2011). Diagnosis and management of epispadias. *Seminars in Pediatric Surgery*, *20*(2), 85–90. doi:10.1053/j.sempedsurg.2011.01.003.
12. Siffel, C., Correa, A., Amar, E., et al. (2011). Bladder exstrophy: An epidemiologic study from the International Clearinghouse for Birth Defects Surveillance and Research, and an overview of the literature. *American Journal of Medical Genetics. Part C, Seminars in Medical Genetics*, *157C*(4), 321–332. doi:10.1002/ajmg.c.30316.
13. Inouye, B. M., Massanyi, E. Z., Di Carlo, H., et al. (2013). Modern management of bladder exstrophy repair. *Current Urology Reports*, *14*(4), 359–365. doi:10.1007/s11934-013-0332-y.
14. Akbarzadeh, A., Khorramirouz, R., Kajbafzadeh, A. M., et al. (2014). Congenital urethral polyps in children: Report of 18 patients and review of literature. *Journal of Pediatric Surgery*, *49*(5), 835–839. doi:10.1016/j.jpedsurg.2014.02.080.
15. Lopez Pereira, P., Martinez Urrutia, M. J., Espinosa, L., et al. (2013). Long-term consequences of posterior urethral valves. *Journal of Pediatric Urology*, *9*(5), 590–596. doi:10.1016/j.jpurol.2013.06.007.
16. Alberti, C. (2012). Congenital ureteropelvic junction obstruction: Physiopathology, decoupling of tout court pelvic dilatation-obstruction semantic connection, biomarkers to predict renal damage evolution. *European Review for Medical and Pharmacological Sciences*, *16*(2), 213–219.
17. Pohl, H. G. (2011). Recent advances in the management of ureteroceles in infants and children: Why less may be more. *Current Opinion in Urology*, *21*(4), 3227. doi:10.1097/MOU.0b013e328346d455.
18. Cain, J. E., Di Giovanni, V., Smeeton, J., et al. (2010). Genetics of renal hypoplasia: Insights into the mechanisms controlling nephron endowment. *Pediatric Research*, *68*(2), 91–98. doi:10.1203/00006450-201011001-00175.
19. Prasad, S., Kaler, A. K., & Shariff, S. (2013). Ask-Upmark kidney: A report of 2 cases. *IJHSR*, *3*(1), 61–64. Retrieved from http://www.ijhsr.org.
20. Sweeney, W. E., Jr., & Avner, E. D. (2014). Pathophysiology of childhood polycystic kidney diseases: New insights into disease-specific therapy. *Pediatric Research*, *75*(1–2), 148–157. doi:10.1038/pr.2013.191.
21. Ong, A. C., Devuyst, O., Knebelmann, B., et al. (2015). ERA-EDTA Working Group for Inherited Kidney Diseases: Autosomal dominant polycystic kidney disease: The changing face of clinical management. *Lancet*, *385*(9981), 1993–2002. doi:10.1016/S0140-6736(15)60907-2.
22. Westland, R., Schreuder, M. F., van Goudoever, J. B., et al. (2014). Clinical implications of the solitary functioning kidney. *Clinical Journal of the American Society of Nephrology : CJASN*, *9*(5), 978–986. doi:10.2215/CJN.08900813.
23. Shastry, S. M., Kolte, S. S., & Sanagapati, P. R. (2012). Potter's sequence. *Journal of Clinical Neonatology*, *1*(3), 157–159. doi:10.4103/2249-4847.101705.
24. Rizvi, S. A., Sultan, S., Zafar, M. N., et al. (2013). Pediatric kidney transplantation in the developing world: Challenges and solutions. *American Journal of Transplantation*, *13*(9), 2441–2449. doi:10.1111/ajt.12356.
25. Stratta, P., Musetti, C., Barreca, A., et al. (2014). New trends of an old disease: The acute post infectious glomerulonephritis at the beginning of the new millennium. *Journal of Nephrology*, *27*(3), 229–239. doi:10.1007/s40620-013-0018-z.
26. Nast, C. C. (2012). Infection-related glomerulonephritis: Changing demographics and outcomes. *Advances in Chronic Kidney Disease*, *19*(2), 68–75. doi:10.1053/j.ackd.2012.02.014.
27. Wyatt, R. J., & Julian, B. A. (2013). IgA nephropathy. *New England Journal of Medicine*, *368*(25), 2402–2414. doi:10.1056/NEJMra1206793.
28. Floege, J., & Gröne, H. J. (2013). Recurrent IgA nephropathy in the renal allograft: Not a benign condition. *Nephrology, Dialysis, Transplantation*, *28*(5), 1070–1073. doi:10.1093/ndt/gft077.
29. Davin, J. C., & Coppo, R. (2014). Henoch-Schönlein purpura nephritis in children. *Nature Reviews. Nephrology*, *10*(10), 563–573. doi:10.1038/nrneph.2014.126.
30. Samuel, S., Scott, S., Morgan, C., et al. (2014). The Canadian Childhood Nephrotic Syndrome (CHILDNEPH) Project: Overview of design and methods. *Canadian Journal of Kidney Health and Disease*, *1*(1), 1–8. doi:10.1186/2054-3581-1-17.
31. Sinha, A., & Bagga, A. (2012). Nephrotic syndrome. *Indian Journal of Pediatrics*, *79*(8), 1045–1055. doi:10.1007/s12098-012-0776-y.
32. Cadnapaphornchai, M. A., Tkachenko, O., Shchekochikhin, D., et al. (2014). The nephrotic syndrome: Pathogenesis and treatment of edema formation and secondary complications. *Pediatric Nephrology (Berlin, Germany)*, *29*(7), 1159–1167. doi:10.1007/s00467-013-2567-8.
33. Avni, E. F., Vandenhoute, K., Devriendt, A., et al. (2011). Update on congenital nephrotic syndromes and the contribution of US. *Pediatric Radiology*, *41*(1), 76–81. doi:10.1007/s00247-010-1793-5.
34. Rheault, M. N. (2014). Nephrotic and nephritic syndrome in the newborn. *Clinics in Perinatology*, *41*(3), 605–618. doi:10.1016/j.clp.2014.05.009.
35. Petruzziello-Pellegrini, T. N., & Marsden, P. A. (2012). Shiga toxin-associated hemolytic uremic syndrome: Advances in pathogenesis and therapeutics. *Current Opinion in Nephrology and Hypertension*, *21*(4), 433–440. doi:10.1097/MNH.0b013e328354a62e.
36. Trachtman, H. (2013). HUS and TTP in children. *Pediatric Clinics of North America*, *60*(6), 1513–1526. doi:10.1016/j.pcl.2013.08.007.
37. Rosales, A., Hofer, J., Zimmerhackl, L. B., et al. (2012). Need for long-term follow-up in enterohemorrhagic *Escherichia coli*-associated hemolytic uremic syndrome due to late-emerging sequelae. *Clinical Infectious Diseases*, *54*(10), 1413–1421. doi:10.1093/cid/cis196.
38. Chu, A., Heck, J. E., Ribeiro, K. B., et al. (2010). Wilms' tumour: A systematic review of risk factors and meta-analysis. *Paediatric and Perinatal Epidemiology*, *24*(5), 449–469. doi:10.1111/j.1365-3016.2010.01133.x.
39. National Cancer Institute. (2015). *Wilms tumor and other childhood kidney tumors treatment–for health professionals (PDQ®)*. Retrieved from http://www.cancer.gov/types/kidney/hp/wilms-treatment-pdq#section/_1.
40. Dumoucel, S., Gauthier-Villars, M., Stoppa-Lyonnet, D., et al. (2014). Malformations, genetic abnormalities, and Wilms tumor. *Pediatric Blood & Cancer*, *61*(1), 140–144. doi:10.1002/pbc.24709.
41. Davidoff, A. M. (2012). Wilms tumor. *Advances in Pediatrics*, *59*(1), 247–267. doi:10.1016/j.yapd.2012.04.001.
42. Kembhavi, S. A., Qureshi, S., Vora, T., et al. (2013). Understanding the principles in management of Wilms' tumour: Can imaging assist in patient selection? *Clinical Radiology*, *68*(7), 646–653. doi:10.1016/j.crad.2012.11.012.
43. Termuhlen, A. M., Tersak, J. M., Liu, Q., et al. (2011). Twenty-five year follow-up of childhood Wilms tumor: A report from the Childhood Cancer Survivor Study. *Pediatric Blood & Cancer*, *57*(7), 1210–1216. doi:10.1002/pbc.23090.
44. Becknell, B., Schober, M., Korbel, L., et al. (2015). The diagnosis, evaluation and treatment of acute and recurrent pediatric urinary tract infections. *Expert Review of Anti-infective Therapy*, *13*(1), 81–90. doi:10.1586/14787210.2015.986097.
45. Ragnarsdóttir, B., & Svanborg, C. (2012). Susceptibility to acute pyelonephritis or asymptomatic bacteriuria: Host-pathogen interaction in urinary tract infections. *Pediatric Nephrology (Berlin, Germany)*, *7*(11), 2017–2029. doi:10.1007/s00467-011-2089-1.
46. Mutlu, M., Cayir, Y., & Aslan, Y. (2014). Urinary tract infections in neonates with jaundice in their first two weeks of life. *World Journal of Pediatrics*, *10*(2), 164–167. doi:10.1007/s12519-013-0433-1.
47. Fitzgerald, A., Mori, R., Lakhanpaul, M., et al. (2012). Antibiotics for treating lower urinary tract infection in children. *Cochrane Database of Systematic Reviews*, (8), CD006857, doi:10.1002/14651858.CD006857.pub2.
48. Hunziker, M., & Puri, P. (2012). Familial vesicoureteral reflux and reflux related morbidity in relatives of index patients with high grade vesicoureteral reflux. *Journal of Urology*, *188*(4, Suppl.), 1463–1466. doi:10.1016/j.juro.2012.02.024.
49. Lebowitz, R. L., Olbing, H., Parkkulainen, K. V., et al. (1985). International system of radiographic grading of vesicoureteric reflux. International Reflux Study in Children. *Pediatric Radiology*, *15*(2), 105–109.
50. Tullus, K. (2015). Vesicoureteric reflux in children. *Lancet*, *385*(9965), 371–379. doi:10.1016/S0140-6736(14)60383-4.
51. Altobelli, E., Gerocarni Nappo, S., Guidotti, M., et al. (2014). Vesicoureteral reflux in pediatric age: Where are we today? *Urologia*, *81*(2), 76–87.
52. Buckley, B. S., Lapitan, M. C., & Epidemiology Committee of the Fourth International Consultation on Incontinence. (2010). Prevalence of urinary incontinence in men, women, and children—current evidence: Findings of the Fourth International Consultation on Incontinence. *Urology*, *76*(2), 265–270. doi:10.1016/j.urology.2009.11.078.
53. Mellon, M. W., Natchev, B. E., Katusic, S. K., et al. (2013). Incidence of enuresis and encopresis among children with attention-deficit/hyperactivity disorder in a population-based birth cohort. *Academic Pediatrics*, *13*(4), 322–327. doi:10.1016/j.acap.2013.02.008.
54. Weintraub, Y., Singer, S., Alexander, D., et al. (2013). Enuresis—An unattended comorbidity of childhood obesity. *International Journal of Obesity (2005)*, *37*(1), 75–78. doi:10.1038/ijo.2012.108.
55. Su, M. S., Li, A. M., So, H. K., et al. (2011). Nocturnal enuresis in children: Prevalence, correlates, and relationship with obstructive sleep apnea. *Journal of Pediatrics*, *159*(2), 238–242. doi:10.1016/j.jpeds.2011.01.036.
56. Burgers, R. E., Mugie, S. M., Chase, J., et al. (2013). Management of functional constipation in children with lower urinary tract symptoms: Report from the Standardization Committee of the International Children's Continence Society. *Journal of Urology*, *190*(1), 29–36. doi:10.1016/j.juro.2013.01.001.
57. von Gontard, A., Heron, J., & Joinson, C. (2011). Family history of nocturnal enuresis and urinary incontinence: Results from a large epidemiological study. *Journal of Urology*, *185*(6), 2303–2306. doi:10.1016/j.juro.2011.02.040.
58. Maternik, M., Krzeminska, K., & Zurowska, A. (2014). The management of childhood urinary incontinence. *Pediatric Nephrology (Berlin, Germany)*, *30*(1), 41–50. doi:10.1007/s00467-014-2791-x.

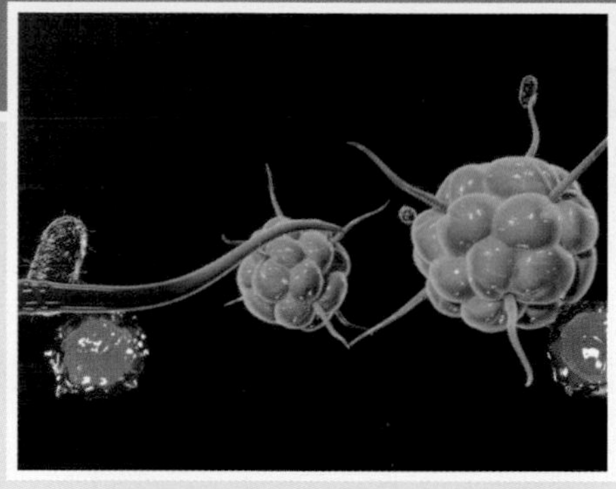

32

Structure and Function of the Reproductive Systems

Afsoon Moktar, George W. Rodway, Sue E. Huether, and Kelly Power-Kean

EVOLVE WEBSITE

http://evolve.elsevier.com/Canada/Huether/pathophysiology
Student Review Questions
Key Points
Case Studies
Animations
Quick Check Answers

CHAPTER OUTLINE

Development of the Reproductive Systems, 793
Sexual Differentiation in Utero, 793
Puberty and Reproductive Maturation, 795
The Female Reproductive System, 796
External Genitalia, 796
Internal Genitalia, 798
Female Sex Hormones, 801
Menstrual Cycle, 802
Structure and Function of the Breast, 805
Female Breast, 805
Male Breast, 807
The Male Reproductive System, 807
External Genitalia, 807
Internal Genitalia, 809
Spermatogenesis, 810
Male Sex and Reproductive Hormones, 810
Aging and Reproductive Function, 811
Aging and the Female Reproductive System, 811
Aging and the Male Reproductive System, 812

The male and female reproductive systems have several anatomical and physiological features in common. Most obvious is their major function—reproduction—through which a 23-chromosome female gamete, the ovum, and a 23-chromosome male gamete, the **spermatozoon (sperm cell)**, unite to form a 46-chromosome zygote that is capable of developing into a new individual. The male reproductive system produces sperm that can be transferred to the female reproductive tract. The female reproductive system produces the **ovum** (*pl.*, **ova**), and if the ovum is fertilized it is then called the *embryo* and *developing fetus*. These functions are determined not only by anatomical structures but also by complex hormonal and neurological factors.[1,2]

DEVELOPMENT OF THE REPRODUCTIVE SYSTEMS

The structure and function of both male and female reproductive systems depend on steroid hormones called **sex hormones** and their precursors. Cholesterol is the precursor for steroid hormones, including the sex hormones. Other hormones support reproduction. The actions of both sex and reproductive hormones are summarized in Table 32-1. Sex hormones, like all hormones, act on target tissues by binding with cellular receptors (see Chapter 18). Hormonal effects on the reproductive systems begin during embryonic development and continue in varying degrees throughout life.

Sexual Differentiation in Utero

Initially, in embryonic development, the reproductive structures of male and female embryos are homologous (the same) or undifferentiated. They consist of one pair of primary sex organs, or **gonads**, and two pairs of ducts—the mesonephric ducts (wolffian ducts) and the paramesonephric ducts (müllerian ducts) (Figure 32-1). The müllerian ducts are the precursor of the internal female sex organs (oviducts, uterus, cervix, and upper vagina). Müllerian ducts are initially formed regardless of genotypic sex and require no *SRY* signalling for development. *SRY* signalling is required in males to cause regression of the müllerian ducts, which in turn prevents the development of the female reproductive tract. The wolffian ducts are the precursor of male internal sex organs (secrete testosterone and promote development of the male sex organs).

The first sign of development of reproductive organs (male or female) occurs during the fifth week of gestation. Between 6 to 8 weeks of gestation, the male embryo will differentiate under the influence of testes-determining factor (TDF), a protein expressed by a gene in the sex-determining region on the Y chromosome (*SRY*). When the *SRY* gene is expressed, male gonadal development prevails. TDF stimulates the male gonads to develop into the two testes, and between 8 to 9 weeks' gestation testosterone secretion begins. Müllerian inhibitory hormone (MIF), secreted by Sertoli cells in the testes, promotes

TABLE 32-1 Summary of Female and Male Sex and Reproductive Hormones

Hormone (Source)	Action in Females	Action in Males
Dehydroepiandrosterone (DHEA) (adrenal gland, ovary, other tissues)	Converted to androstenedione and then to estrogens, testosterone, or both	Converted to androstenedione and then to estrogens, testosterone, or both
Estrogens (estrone, estradiol, estriol) function through estrogen receptors alpha and beta (ovary and placenta, small amounts in other tissues)	Stimulates development of female sexual characteristics: maturation of breast, uterus, and vagina; promotes proliferative development of endometrium during menstrual cycle; during pregnancy promotes mammary gland development, fetal adrenal gland function, and uteroplacental blood flow (see Box 32-1)	Growth at puberty, growth plate fusion in bone, prevention of apoptosis of germ cells
Testosterone (adrenal glands from DHEA, ovaries)	Contributes to libido, learning, sleep, protein anabolism, growth of muscle and bone; growth of pubic and axillary hair; activation of sebaceous glands, accounting for some cases of acne during puberty	Stimulates spermatogenesis, stimulates development of primary and secondary sexual characteristics, promotes growth of muscle and bone (anabolic effect); growth of pubic and axillary hair; activates sebaceous glands, accounting for some cases of acne during puberty; maintains libido
Gonadotropin-releasing hormone (GnRH) (hypothalamus-neuroendocrine cells)	Stimulates secretion of gonadotropins (FSH and LH) from anterior pituitary	Stimulates secretion of gonadotropins (FSH and LH) from anterior pituitary
Follicle-stimulating hormone (FSH) (anterior pituitary, gonadotroph cells)	Gonadotropin; promotes development of ovarian follicle; stimulates estrogen secretion	Gonadotropin; promotes development of testes and stimulates spermatogenesis by Sertoli cells
Luteinizing hormone (LH) (anterior pituitary, gonadotroph cells)	Gonadotropin; triggers ovulation; promotes development of corpus luteum	Gonadotropin; stimulates testosterone production by Leydig cells of testis
Inhibin (ovary and testes)	Inhibits FSH production in anterior pituitary (perhaps by limiting GnRH)	Inhibits FSH production in anterior pituitary
Human chorionic gonadotropin (hCG) (placenta)	Supports corpus luteum, which secretes estrogen and progesterone during first 7 weeks of pregnancy	
Activin (ovary)	Stimulates secretion of FSH and pituitary response to GnRH and FSH binding in dominant granulosa cells	
Progesterone (ovary and placenta)	Promotes secretory changes in endometrium during luteal phase of menstrual cycle; quiets uterine myometrium (muscle) activity and prevents lactogenesis during pregnancy	
Relaxin (corpus luteum, myometrium and placenta)	Inhibits uterine contractions during pregnancy and softens pelvic joints and cervix to facilitate childbirth	

degeneration of the müllerian ducts. Without MIF, the müllerian ducts would develop and the wolffian ducts would degenerate with loss of male sex organ development. By 9 months' gestation, the male gonads (testes) have descended into the scrotum. The testes produce sperm after puberty.

Female gonadal development occurs in the absence of *SRY* expression and with the expression of other genes.[3] The presence of estrogen and the absence of testosterone and MIF cause a loss in the wolffian system, and at 6 to 8 weeks' gestation the two female gonads develop into ovaries, which will produce ova. In females, the mesonephric ducts deteriorate and the upper ends of paramesonephric ducts become the fallopian tubules, whereas the lower ends join to become the uterus, cervix, and upper two-thirds of the vagina (see Figure 32-1). The fallopian tubes will carry ova from the ovaries to the uterus during a woman's reproductive years. Lack of testosterone and the presence of estrogen promote the development of external genitalia (lower end of vagina, labia, and clitoris).

Like the internal reproductive structures, the external structures develop from homologous embryonic tissues. During the first 7 to 8 weeks' gestation, both male and female embryos develop an elevated structure called the *genital tubercle* (Figure 32-2). **Testosterone** is necessary for the genital tubercle to differentiate into external male genitalia; otherwise, female genitalia develop, which may occur even in the absence of ovaries, possibly because of the presence of placental estrogens.

Anterior pituitary development begins between the fourth and fifth weeks of fetal life, and the vascular connection between the hypothalamus and the pituitary is established by the twelfth week. **Gonadotropin-releasing hormone (GnRH)** is produced in the hypothalamus by 10 weeks' gestation and controls the production of two gonadotropins, **luteinizing hormone (LH)** and **follicle-stimulating hormone (FSH)**, by the anterior pituitary gland. In the female fetus, high levels of FSH and LH are excreted. FSH and LH stimulate the production of estrogen and progesterone by the ovary. The production of FSH and LH increases until about 28 weeks' gestation, when the production of estrogen and progesterone by the ovaries and placenta is high enough to result in the decline of gonadotropin production.[4] Production of primitive female gametes (ova) occurs solely during fetal life. From puberty to menopause, one female gamete matures per menstrual cycle. Production of the male gametes (sperm) begins at puberty; after that, millions are produced daily, usually for life.

By the end of pregnancy, a sensitive negative feedback system, which includes the **gonadostat** (also known as the **gonadotropin-releasing hormone pulse generator**), is operative in the human fetus. The gonadostat responds to high levels of placental estrogens by releasing low levels of GnRH. Soon after birth, steroid hormone levels drop

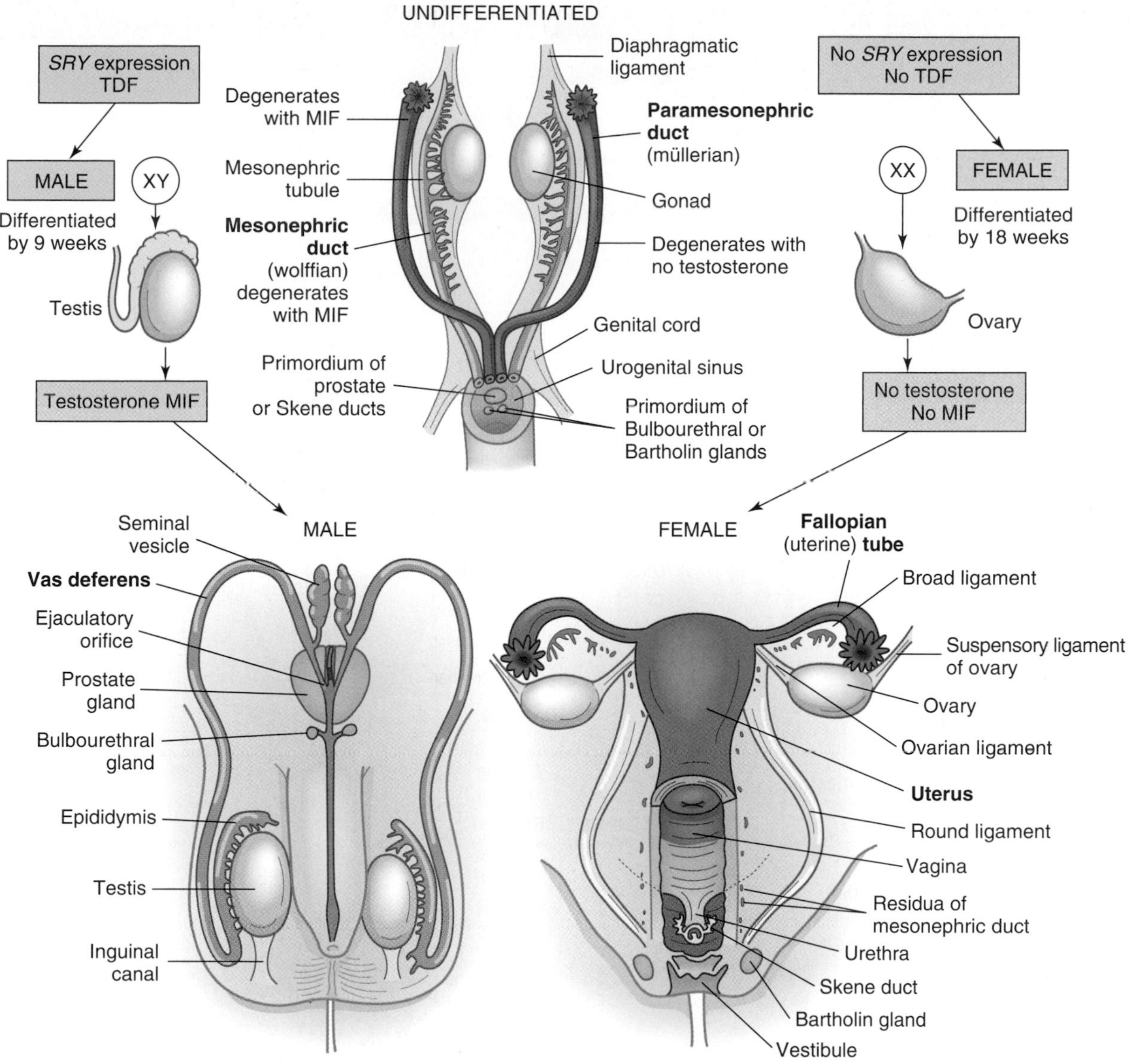

FIGURE 32-1 Internal Genitalia Development. Embryonic and fetal development of the internal genitalia. *MIF*, Müllerian inhibitory factor; *SRY*, sex-determining region on the Y chromosome (it produces TDF); *TDF*, testes-determining factor; see text for additional details.

because of the loss of maternal placental hormones. Hypothalamic pulsatile GnRH is secreted and gonadotropins LH and FSH are released; their levels peak at 3 to 6 months for boys and at 12 to 18 months for girls and then fall steadily. The gonadotropins will be suppressed until the onset of puberty.

Puberty and Reproductive Maturation

Puberty is the onset of sexual maturation and differs from adolescence. Adolescence is the stage of human development between childhood and adulthood and includes social, psychological, and biological changes. In girls, puberty begins at about age 8 to 9 years with **thelarche** (breast development). In boys, puberty begins later—at about age 11 years and occurs earlier with increased weight and body mass index.[5] Genetics, environment, ethnicity, general health, and nutrition can influence the timing of puberty. There is an association between obesity and earlier puberty in girls perhaps from higher estrogen levels related to leptin, gonadotropin, and estrogen secretion.[6] Girls who have low body fat and reduced body weight and perform intense exercise may experience delayed maturation.[7]

Reproductive maturation involves the hypothalamic-pituitary-gonadal axis, the central nervous system, and the endocrine system (Figure 32-3). There is a sequential series of hormonal events that promote sexual maturation as puberty approaches. About 1 year before puberty in girls, nocturnal pulses of gonadotropin secretion (i.e., LH and FSH) and an increased response in the pituitary to GnRH occur. This gonadotropin secretion and increased pituitary response, in turn, stimulates gonadal maturation (**gonadarche**) with estradiol secretion in girls and testosterone secretion in boys. Estradiol causes development of the breasts (thelarche), maturation of the reproductive organs (vagina, uterus, ovaries), and deposition of fat in the female's hips. Estrogen and increased production of growth factors cause rapid skeletal growth in both boys and girls. Testosterone causes growth of the testes, scrotum, and penis. A positive feedback loop is created with gonadotropins stimulating the gonads to produce more sex hormones. The most important hormonal effects occur in the gonads. In males, the testes begin to produce mature sperm that are capable of fertilizing an ovum. Male puberty is complete with the first ejaculation that contains mature sperm. In females, the ovaries begin to release mature ova. Female puberty is complete at the time of

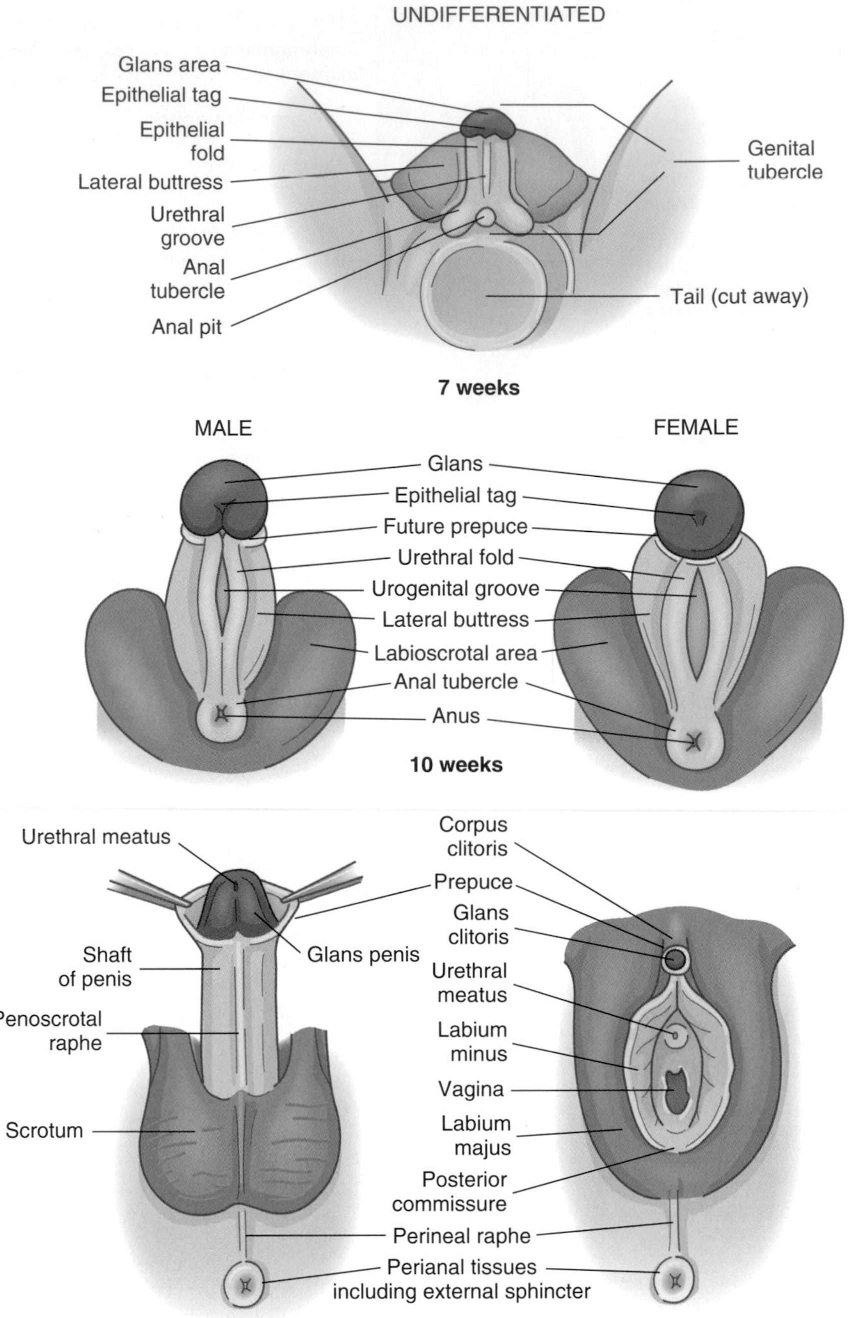

FIGURE 32-2 External Genitalia Development. Embryonic and fetal development of the external genitalia.

the first ovulatory menstrual period; however, puberty can take up to 1 to 2 years to complete after menarche. **Adrenarche** is the increased production of adrenal **androgens** (dehydroepiandrosterone [DHEA] and androstenedione, which are converted to testosterone and estrogen) before puberty, which occurs in both sexes and is manifested by growth of axillary and pubic hair and activation of sweat and sebaceous glands. Puberty is complete when an individual is capable of reproduction.

> **QUICK CHECK 32-1**
> 1. When do sex hormones first exhibit an effect on sexual development?
> 2. Why are sex hormones necessary for reproduction?

THE FEMALE REPRODUCTIVE SYSTEM

The function of the female reproductive system is to produce mature ova; if fertilization occurs, the female reproductive system provides protection and nourishment of the fetus until it is expelled at birth. The most important internal reproductive organs in females are the ovaries, fallopian tubes, uterus, and vagina. The external genitalia protect body openings and play an important role in sexual functioning.

External Genitalia

Figure 32-4 shows the external female genitalia, known collectively as the **vulva**, or pudendum. The major structures are as follows:

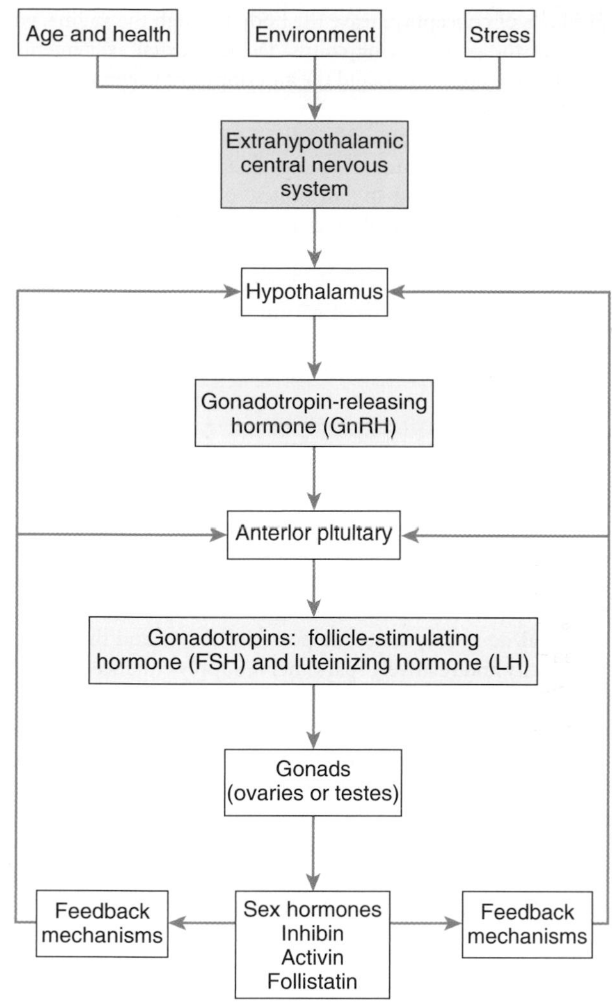

FIGURE 32-3 Hormonal Stimulation of the Gonads. The hypothalamic-pituitary-gonadal axis.

Mons pubis: Fatty layer of tissue over pubic symphysis (joint formed by union of the pubic bones). During puberty it becomes covered with pubic hair, and sebaceous and sweat glands become more active. Estrogen causes fat to be deposited under the skin, gives the mons pubis a moundlike shape, and protects the pubic symphysis during sexual intercourse.

Labia majora (sing., labium majus): Two folds of skin arising at the mons pubis and extending back to the fourchette, forming a cleft. During puberty the amount of fatty tissue increases, pubic hair grows on lateral surfaces, and sebaceous glands on hairless medial surfaces secrete lubricants. This structure is highly sensitive to temperature, touch, pressure, and pain; it is homologous to the male scrotum; and it protects the inner structures of the vulva.

Labia minora (sing., labium minus): Two smaller, thinner, asymmetrical folds of skin within the labia majora that form the clitoral hood (prepuce) and frenulum, then split to enclose the vestibule, and converge near the anus to form the fourchette. The labia minora are hairless, pink, and moist; they are well supplied by nerves, blood vessels, and sebaceous glands that secrete bactericidal fluid with a distinctive odour that lubricates and waterproofs vulvar skin. The labia swell with blood during sexual arousal.

Clitoris: Richly innervated erectile organ between the labia minora. It is a small, cylindrical structure having a visible glans and a shaft that lies beneath the skin; the clitoris is homologous to the penis. It secretes smegma, which has a unique odour that may be sexually arousing to the male. Like the penis, the clitoris is a major site of sexual stimulation and orgasm. With sexual arousal, erectile tissue fills with blood, causing the clitoris to enlarge slightly.

Vestibule: An area protected by the labia minora that contains the external opening of the vagina, called the *introitus* or vaginal orifice. A thin, perforated membrane, the *hymen*, may cover the introitus. The vestibule also contains the opening of the urethra, or *urinary meatus* (orifice). These structures are lubricated by

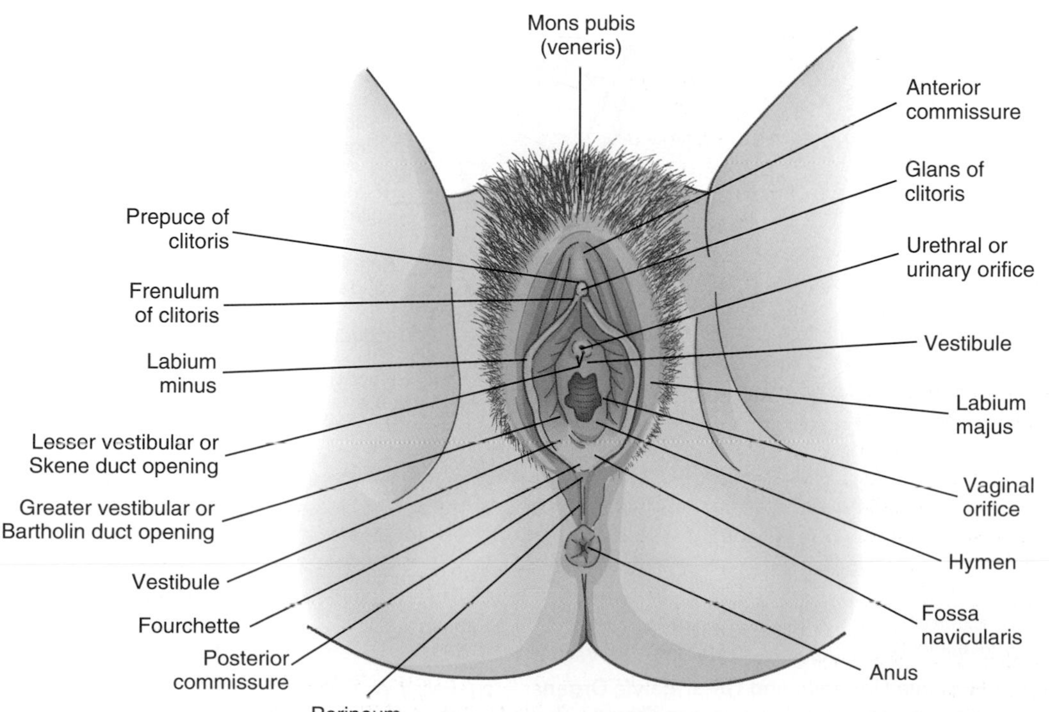

FIGURE 32-4 External Female Genitalia.

two pairs of glands: Skene glands and Bartholin glands. The ducts of the *Skene glands* (also called the *lesser vestibular* or *paraurethral glands*) open on both sides of the urinary meatus. The ducts of the *Bartholin glands* (*greater vestibular* or *vulvovaginal glands*) open on either side of the introitus. In response to sexual stimulation, Bartholin glands secrete mucus that lubricates the inner labial surfaces, as well as enhances the viability and motility of sperm. Skene glands help lubricate the urinary meatus and the vestibule. Secretions from both sets of glands facilitate coitus. In response to sexual excitement, the highly vascular tissue just beneath the vestibule also fills with blood and becomes engorged.

Perineum: An area with less hair, skin, and subcutaneous tissue lying between the vaginal orifice and anus. Unlike the rest of the vulva, this area has little subcutaneous fat so the skin is close to the underlying muscles. The perineum covers the muscular *perineal body*, a fibrous structure that consists of elastic fibres and connective tissue and serves as the common attachment for the bulbocavernosus, external anal sphincter, and levator ani muscles. The perineum varies in length from 2 to 5 cm or more and has elastic properties. The length of the perineum and the elasticity of the perineal body influence tissue resistance and injury during childbirth.

Internal Genitalia

Vagina

The **vagina** is an elastic, fibromuscular canal that is 9 to 10 cm long in a reproductive-age female. It extends up and back from the introitus to the lower portion of the uterus. As Figure 32-5 shows, the vagina lies between the urethra (and part of the bladder) and the rectum. Mucosal secretions from the upper genital organs, menstrual fluids, and products of conception leave the body through the vagina, which also receives the penis during coitus. During sexual excitement, the vagina lengthens and widens and the anterior third becomes congested with blood.

The vaginal wall is composed of four layers:

1. Mucous membrane lining of squamous epithelial cells that thickens and thins in response to hormones, particularly estrogen. The squamous epithelial membrane is continuous with the membrane that covers the lower part of the uterus. In women of reproductive age, the mucosal layer is arranged in transverse wrinkles, or folds, called **rugae** (*sing.*, **ruga**) that permit stretching during coitus and childbirth
2. Fibrous connective tissue containing numerous blood and lymphatic vessels
3. Smooth muscle
4. Connective tissue and a rich network of blood vessels

The upper part of the vagina surrounds the cervix, the lower end of the uterus (see Figure 32-5). The recessed space around the cervix is called the **fornix** of the vagina. The posterior fornix is "deeper" than the anterior fornix because of the angle at which the cervix meets the vaginal canal. In most women, this angle is about 90 degrees. A pouch called the **cul-de-sac** separates the posterior fornix and the rectum.

Its elasticity and relatively sparse nerve supply enhance the vagina's function as the birth canal. During sexual arousal, the vaginal wall becomes engorged with blood, like the labia minora and clitoris. Engorgement pushes some fluid to the surface of the mucosa, enhancing lubrication. The vaginal wall does not contain mucus-secreting glands; rather, secretions drain into the vagina from the endocervical glands or from the Bartholin and Skene glands of the vestibule.

Two factors help to maintain the self-cleansing action of the vagina and to defend it from infection, particularly during the reproductive

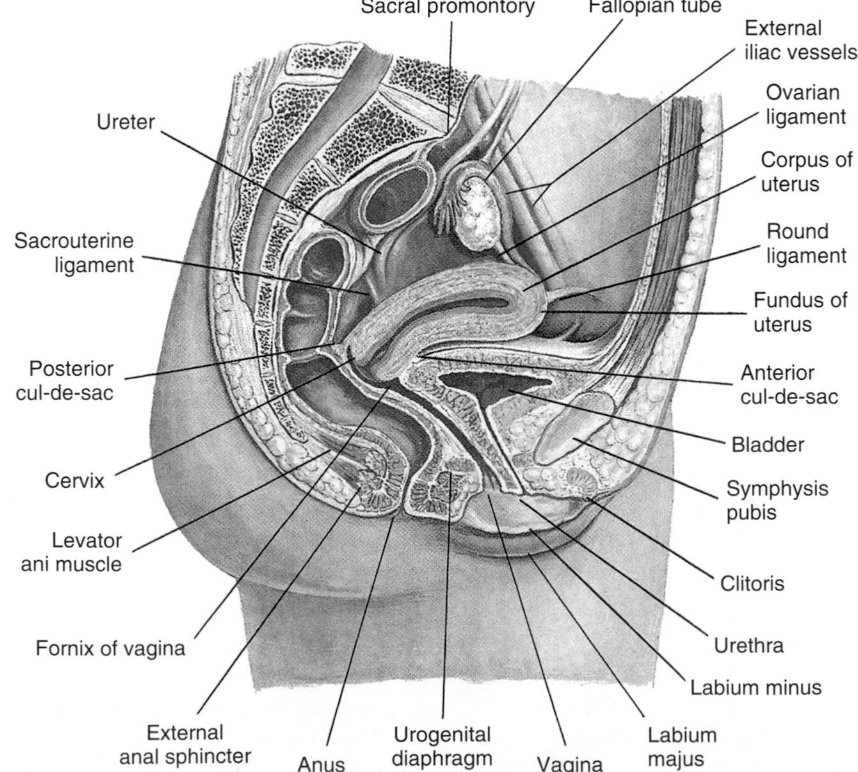

FIGURE 32-5 Internal Female Genitalia and Other Pelvic Organs. (From Ball, J.W., Dains, J.E., Flynn, J.A., et al. [2015]. *Seidel's guide to physical examination* [8th ed.]. St. Louis: Mosby.)

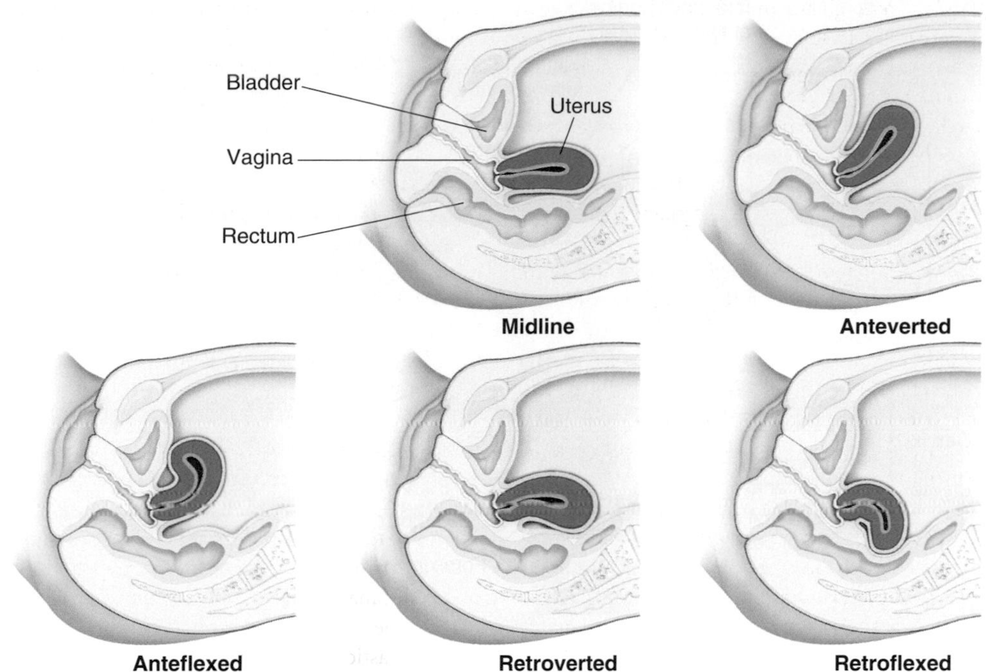

FIGURE 32-6 Variations in Uterine Positions.

years. They are (1) an acid–base balance that discourages the proliferation of most pathogenic bacteria and (2) the thickness of the vaginal epithelium. Before puberty, vaginal pH is about 7.0 (neutral) and the vaginal epithelium is thin. At puberty, the pH becomes more acidic (4.0 to 5.0) and the squamous epithelial lining thickens. These changes are maintained until menopause (cessation of menstruation), when the pH rises again to more alkaline levels and the epithelium thins. Therefore, protection from infection is greatest during the years when a woman is most likely to be sexually active. Both defence factors are greatest when estrogen levels are high and the vagina contains a normal population of *Lactobacillus acidophilus*, a harmless resident bacterium that helps to maintain pH at acidic levels. Any condition that causes vaginal pH to rise—such as douching or use of vaginal sprays or deodorants, the presence of low estrogen levels, or destruction of *L. acidophilus* by antibiotics—lowers vaginal defences against infection.

Uterus

The **uterus** is a hollow, pear-shaped organ whose lower end opens into the vagina. It anchors and protects a fertilized ovum, provides an optimal environment while the ovum develops, and pushes the fetus out at birth. In addition, the uterus plays an important role in sexual response and conception. During sexual excitement, the opening of the lower uterus (the cervix) dilates slightly. At the same time, the uterus increases in size and moves upward and backward, creating a tenting effect in the midvagina that results in the cervix "sitting" in a pool of semen. During orgasm, rhythmic contractions facilitate movement of sperm through the cervical os while also enhancing physical pleasure.

At puberty, the uterus attains its adult size and proportions and descends from the abdomen to the lower pelvis, between the bladder and the rectum (see Figure 32-5). The uterus of a mature, nonpregnant female is approximately 7 to 9 cm long and 6.5 cm wide, with muscular walls 3.5 cm thick, and enlarges about 1 cm in all dimensions after pregnancy.[8] It is loosely held in position by ligaments, peritoneal tissue folds, and the pressure of adjacent organs, especially the urinary bladder, sigmoid colon, and rectum. In most women, the uterus is tipped forward (anteverted) so that it rests on the urinary bladder; however, it may be tipped backward (retroverted). Various degrees of flexion are normal (Figure 32-6).

The uterus has two major parts: the body, or **corpus**, and the cervix (Figure 32-7). The top of the corpus, above the insertion of the fallopian tubes, is called the **fundus**. The diameter of the uterine cavity is widest at the fundus and narrowest at the **isthmus**, just above the **cervix** (see Figure 32-5). The cervix, or "neck of the uterus," extends from the isthmus to the vagina. The passageway between the upper opening (the internal os) and the lower opening (the external os) of the cervix is called the **endocervical canal** (see Figure 32-7). The entire uterus, like the upper vagina, is innervated exclusively by motor and sensory fibres of the autonomic nervous system.

The uterine wall is composed of three layers (see Figure 32-7). The **perimetrium (parietal peritoneum)** is the outer serous membrane that covers the uterus. The **myometrium** is the thick, muscular middle layer. It is thickest at the fundus, apparently to facilitate birth. The **endometrium**, or uterine lining, is composed of a functional layer (superficial compact layer and spongy middle layer) and a basal layer. The functional layer of the endometrium responds to the sex hormones estrogen and progesterone. Between puberty and menopause, this layer proliferates and is shed monthly. The basal layer, which is attached to the myometrium, regenerates the functional layer after shedding (menstruation).

The endocervical canal does not have an endometrial layer but is lined with columnar epithelial cells. It is continuous with the lining of the outer cervix and vagina, which are lined with squamous epithelial cells. The point where the two types of cells meet is called the *transformation zone*, or **squamocolumnar junction**. The transformation zone is vulnerable to the human papillomavirus, which can lead to cervical dysplasia or carcinoma in situ (see Figure 33-16). Cells of the transformation zone are removed for examination during a Papanicolaou (Pap test) smear.[8]

The cervix acts as a mechanical barrier to infectious microorganisms from the vagina. The external cervical os is a very small opening that contains thick, sticky mucus (the mucous "plug") during the luteal phase of the menstrual cycle and throughout pregnancy. During ovulation, the mucus changes under the influence of estrogen and forms

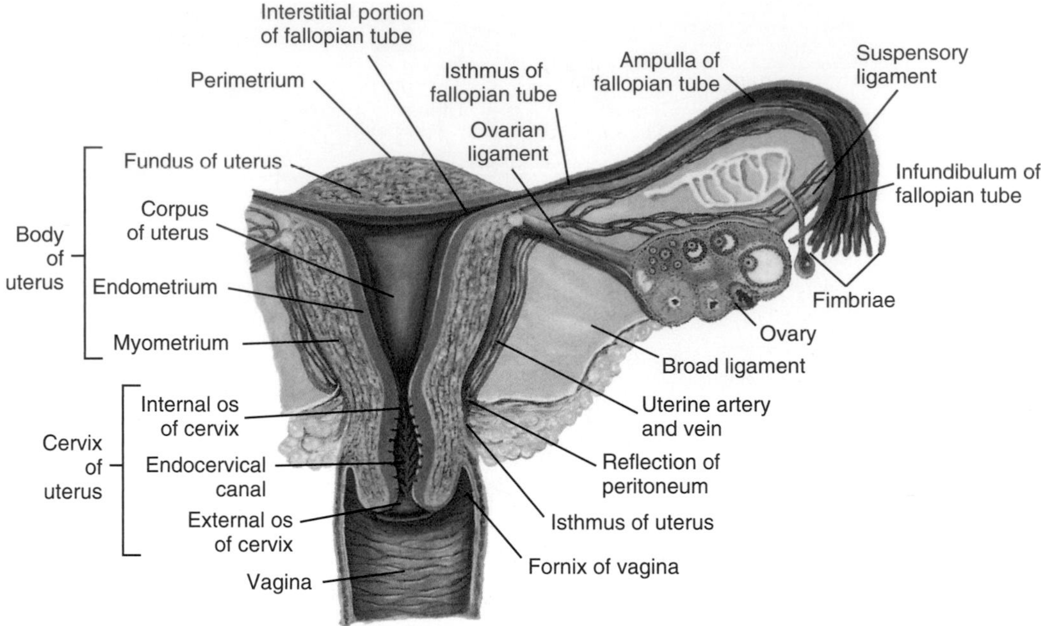

FIGURE 32-7 Cross Section of Uterus, Fallopian Tube, and Ovary. (From Ball, J.W., Dains, J.E., Flynn, J.A., et al. [2015]. *Seidel's guide to physical examination* [8th ed.]. St. Louis: Mosby.)

watery strands, or **spinnbarkeit mucus**, to facilitate the transport of sperm into the uterus. In addition, the downward flow of cervical secretions moves microorganisms away from the cervix and uterus. In women of reproductive age, the pH of these secretions is inhospitable to many bacteria. Further, mucosal secretions contain enzymes and antibodies (mostly immunoglobulin A [IgA]) of the secretory immune system. Uterine pathophysiological disorders include infection, displacement of the uterus within the pelvis, benign growths (fibroids) of the uterine wall, hyperplasia of the endometrium, endometriosis, and cancer (see Chapter 33).

QUICK CHECK 32-2

1. Where are the Bartholin glands located? What is their function?
2. Name three functions of the uterus.
3. What is the name of the cells in which cervical cancer is most likely to grow?

Fallopian Tubes

The two **fallopian tubes** (oviducts, **uterine tubes**) enter the uterus bilaterally just beneath the fundus (see Figure 32-7). They direct the ova from the spaces around the ovaries to the uterus. From the uterus, the fallopian tubes curve up and over the two ovaries. Each tube is 8 to 12 cm long and about 1 cm in diameter, except at its ovarian end, which resembles the bell of a trumpet and is fringed or fimbriated (**infundibulum**). The **fimbriae** (fringes) move, creating a current that draws the ovum into the infundibulum. Once the ovum enters the fallopian tube, cilia (hairlike structures) and peristalsis (muscle contractions) keep it moving toward the uterus.

The ampulla, or distal third, of the fallopian tube is the usual site of fertilization (see Figure 32-7). Sperm released into the vagina travel upward through the endocervical canal and uterine cavity and enter the fallopian tubes. If an ovum is present in either tube, fertilization can occur. Whether or not the ovum encounters sperm, it continues to travel through the fallopian tube to the uterus. If fertilized, the ovum (then called a *blastocyst*) implants itself in the endometrial layer of the uterine wall. If not fertilized, the ovum fragments and leaves the uterus with menstrual fluids. Disorders that affect the fallopian tubes (e.g., congenital malformations, infection, and inflammation) block the path of both sperm and the ovum and may cause infertility or ectopic (tubal) pregnancy.

Ovaries

The **ovaries**, the female gonads, are the primary female reproductive organs (Figure 32-8). Their two main functions are secretion of female sex hormones and development and release of female gametes, or ova.

The almond-shaped ovaries are located on both sides of the uterus and are suspended and supported by the mesovarium portions of the broad ligament, ovarian ligaments, and suspensory ligaments (see Figure 32-7). The ovaries are smaller than their male homologues, the testes. In women of reproductive age, each ovary is about 3 to 5 cm long, 2.5 cm wide, and 2 cm thick and weighs 4 to 8 g. Size and weight vary slightly during each phase of the menstrual cycle.

At birth, the cortex of each ovary contains approximately 1 to 2 million ova within primordial (immature) **ovarian follicles**. By puberty, the number ranges between 300 000 and 500 000, and some of the follicles and the ova within them begin to mature. Between puberty and menopause, the ovarian cortex always contains follicles and ova in various stages of development (primary and secondary follicles). Once every menstrual cycle (about every 28 days), one of the follicles reaches maturation and discharges its ovum through the ovary's outer covering, the germinal epithelium. During the reproductive years, 400 to 500 ovarian follicles mature completely and release an ovum (ovulation). The remaining follicles either fail to develop at all or degenerate without maturing completely and are known as atretic follicles[8] (see Figure 32-8).

After release of the mature ovum (ovulation), the follicle develops into another structure, the **corpus luteum** (see Figure 32-8). If fertilization occurs, the corpus luteum enlarges and begins to secrete hormones that maintain and support pregnancy. If fertilization does not occur, the corpus luteum secretes these hormones for approximately 14 days

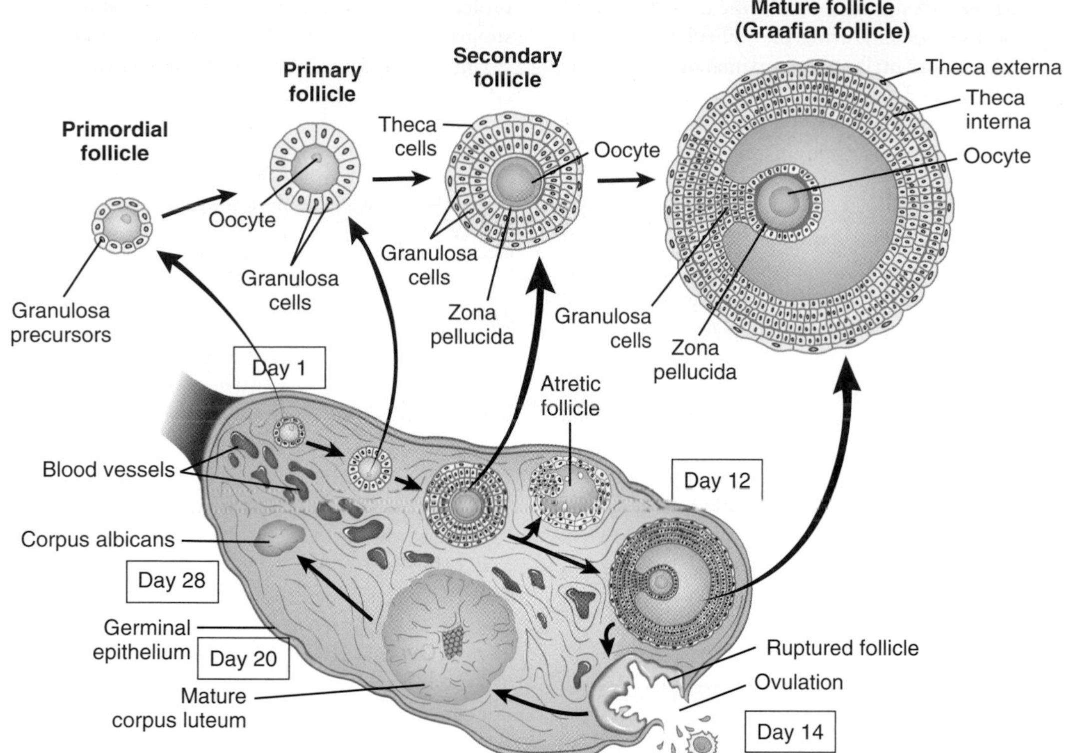

FIGURE 32-8 Cross Section of Ovary and Development of an Ovarian Follicle. Schematic representation (not to scale) of the structure of the ovary, showing the various stages in the development of the follicle and its successor structure, the corpus luteum. (Adapted from Berne, R.M., & Levy, M.N. [Eds.]. [2003]. *Physiology* [5th ed.]. St. Louis: Mosby.)

and then degenerates, which triggers the maturation of another follicle. The **ovarian cycle**—the process of follicular maturation, ovulation, corpus luteum development, and corpus luteum degeneration—is continuous from puberty to menopause, except during pregnancy or hormonal contraceptive use. At menopause, this process ceases and the ovaries atrophy to the point that they cannot be felt during a pelvic examination.

Sex hormones are secreted by cells present within the ovarian cortex, including two types of cells in the ovarian follicle—**theca cells** (produce androgens that migrate to granulosa cells) and **granulosa cells** (convert androgens to estradiol)—and cells of the corpus luteum (secrete primarily progesterone, estrogen, and inhibin) (see Figure 32-8). These cells all contain receptors for the gonadotropins (LH, FSH) or for the sex hormones, which are discussed in the next section.

Female Sex Hormones

The sex hormones are all steroid hormones and are synthesized from cholesterol (see Chapter 18). Both male and female sex hormones are present in all adults (see Table 32-1). However, the female body contains low levels of testosterone and other androgens, and the male body contains low levels of estrogen. Individual effects of sex hormones depend on the amount and concentration in the blood.

Estrogens and Androgens

Estrogen is a generic term for any of three similar hormones derived from cholesterol: estradiol, estrone, and estriol. **Estradiol (E_2)** is the most potent and plentiful of the three and is principally produced (95%) by the ovaries (ovarian follicle and corpus luteum). Limited amounts are secreted by the cortices of the adrenal glands and the placenta during pregnancy. Androgens are converted to estrone in ovarian and adipose tissue; estriol is the peripheral metabolite of estrone and estradiol.

Estrogen has numerous biological effects, many of which involve interactions with other hormones. It is needed for maturation of reproductive organs, development of secondary sex characteristics, growth, and maintenance of pregnancy, as well as the many nonreproductive effects of estrogen, including closure of long bones after the pubertal growth spurt (in both males and females), maintenance of bone and skin, and systemic organ function (see Table 32-1 and Box 32-1). After menopause, the ovaries dramatically reduce production of estradiol and secretion of estrone is markedly diminished (see "Aging and the Female Reproductive System," p. 811). At this time, the majority of estradiol is derived from intracellular synthesis in peripheral tissues. Estradiol acts locally to meet physiological needs according to cell type and is then inactivated without systemic effects.[9]

Although androgens are primarily male sex hormones produced in the testes, small amounts are produced in the adrenal cortex in both men and women, and in the ovaries in women. Some androgens (DHEA and its metabolite androstenedione) are precursors of estrogens (estrone, estradiol) (see Table 32-1). At puberty, androgens contribute to the skeletal growth spurt and cause growth of pubic and axillary hair. Androgens also activate sebaceous glands, accounting for some cases of acne during puberty, and play a role in libido.

Progesterone

LH from the anterior pituitary stimulates the corpus luteum to secrete **progesterone**, the second major female sex hormone. With estrogen, progesterone controls the ovarian menstrual cycle. LH surge occurs when there is a peak level of estrogen, about 24 to 36 hours before ovulation. LH promotes luteinization of the granulosa in the dominant follicle, resulting in progesterone production and the development of blood vessels and connective tissue. During the follicular phase, the ovary and adrenal glands each contribute approximately 50% of the progesterone production. Conversely, large amounts are cyclically secreted from the ovary while the corpus luteum is active for about 9 to 13 days after ovulation. The complementary and opposing effects of progesterone and estrogen are listed in Table 32-2. Progesterone secreted by the corpus luteum stimulates the thickened endometrium to become more complex in preparation for implantation of a blastocyte. If conception and implantation do occur, the corpus luteum persists and secretes progesterone (and estrogen) until the placenta is well established at approximately 8 to 10 weeks' gestation and undertakes progesterone production.

Progesterone is sometimes called the *hormone of pregnancy.* Progesterone's effects in pregnancy include (1) maintaining the thickened endometrium; (2) relaxing smooth muscle in the myometrium, which prevents premature contractions and helps the uterus to expand; (3) thickening (hypertrophy) the myometrium, which prepares it for the muscular work of labour; (4) promoting growth of lobules and alveoli in the breast in preparation for lactation, but preventing lactation until the fetus is born and then promoting lactation in collaboration with prolactin after birth[10]; (5) preventing additional maturation of ova by suppressing FSH and LH, thereby stopping the menstrual cycle; and (6) providing immune modulation, allowing tolerance against fetal antigens (the mother's immune system does not attack the fetus).[11]

BOX 32-1 Summary of Nonreproductive Effects of Estrogen

Estrogens (including estrone, estradiol, estriol) function through estrogen receptors alpha and beta, have different roles in different cells and tissues, and have paracrine or intracrine function. Estrogen has the following nonreproductive effects:

- Maintains bone density
- Acts in liver to decrease cholesterol level, increase high-density lipoprotein (HDL) level, and decrease low-density lipoprotein (LDL) level (antiatherosclerotic); promotes fat deposition
- Maintains nervous system (neurotrophic and neuroprotective); facilitates memory and cognition
- Increases collagen content, dermal thickness, elasticity, water content, and healing ability of skin
- Protects against chronic kidney disease in individuals without diabetes
- Prevents vascular injury and early atheroma formation through endothelial mechanisms
- Inhibits platelet adhesiveness
- Can promote inflammation and have variable effects on immunity

Estrogen associated with pregnancy or use in contraceptive pills promotes clotting and increased risk of thromboembolism.

✔ QUICK CHECK 32-3

1. What hormones does the ovary produce?
2. Why is the ovary the most essential female reproductive organ?

Menstrual Cycle

In addition to pregnancy, the obvious manifestation of female reproductive functioning is menstrual bleeding (the menses), which starts with **menarche** (first menstruation) and ends with **menopause** (cessation of menstrual flow for 1 year). The median age of first menarche varies on the basis of ethnicity and country. Studies indicate a median age of 12.7 years in Canada; 12.3 years in the United States; in Europe, a range from 12.3 years in Greece to 13.3 years in Finland; 13.0 years in Australia; and 13.0 years in Russia.[12] Menarche appears to be related to body weight, especially percentage of body fat (ratio of fat-to-lean tissue), which may trigger a change in the metabolic rate and lead to hormonal changes associated with early menarche (age 11 years or younger).[13] There is an increased sensitivity to leptin (a regulatory hormone of appetite and energy metabolism) during puberty and, in theory, the adolescent consumes more calories to meet the caloric needs of the pubertal growth spurt.[14]

Cycles are anovulatory at first and may vary in length from 10 to 60 days or more. As adolescence proceeds, regular patterns of menstruation and ovulation are established at intervals ranging from 21 to 45 days.[15] Menstruation continues to recur in a recognizable and characteristic pattern during adulthood, with the length of the menstrual cycle varying considerably among women. The commonly accepted cycle average is 28 (25 to 30) days, with rhythmic intervals of 21 to 35 days considered normal (Figure 32-9). Approximately 2 to 8 years before menopause, cycles begin to lengthen again. Menstrual cyclicity and regular ovulation are dependent on (1) the activity of GnRH; (2) the initial pituitary secretion of the gonadotropin FSH; and (3) the estrogen (estradiol) positive feedback mechanism for preovulatory FSH and LH surge, oocyte maturation, corpus luteum formation, and progesterone production.[16]

Phases of the Menstrual Cycle

The menstrual cycle (see Figure 32-9) consists of three phases: the ischemic/menstrual phase (menstruation), the follicular/proliferative phase (postmenstrual), and the luteal/secretory phase (premenstrual).

TABLE 32-2 Complementary and Opposing Effects of Estrogen and Progesterone

Structure	Effect of Estrogen	Effect of Progesterone
Vaginal mucosa	Proliferation of squamous epithelium; increase in glycogen content of cells; layering (cornification) of cells	Thinning of squamous epithelium; decornification
Cervical mucosa	Production of abundant fluid secretions that favour survival and enhance motility of sperm	Production of thick, sticky secretions that tend to plug cervical os
Fallopian tube	Increase of motility and ciliary action	Decrease of motility and ciliary action
Uterine muscle	Increase of blood flow; increase of contractile proteins; increase of uterine muscle and myometrial excitability to action potential; increase of sensitization to oxytocin	Relaxation of myometrium; decrease of sensitization to oxytocin
Endometrium	Stimulation of growth; increase in number of progesterone receptors	Activation of glands and blood vessels; decrease in number of estrogen receptors
Breasts	Growth of ducts; promotion of prolactin effects	Growth of lobules and alveoli; inhibition of prolactin effects

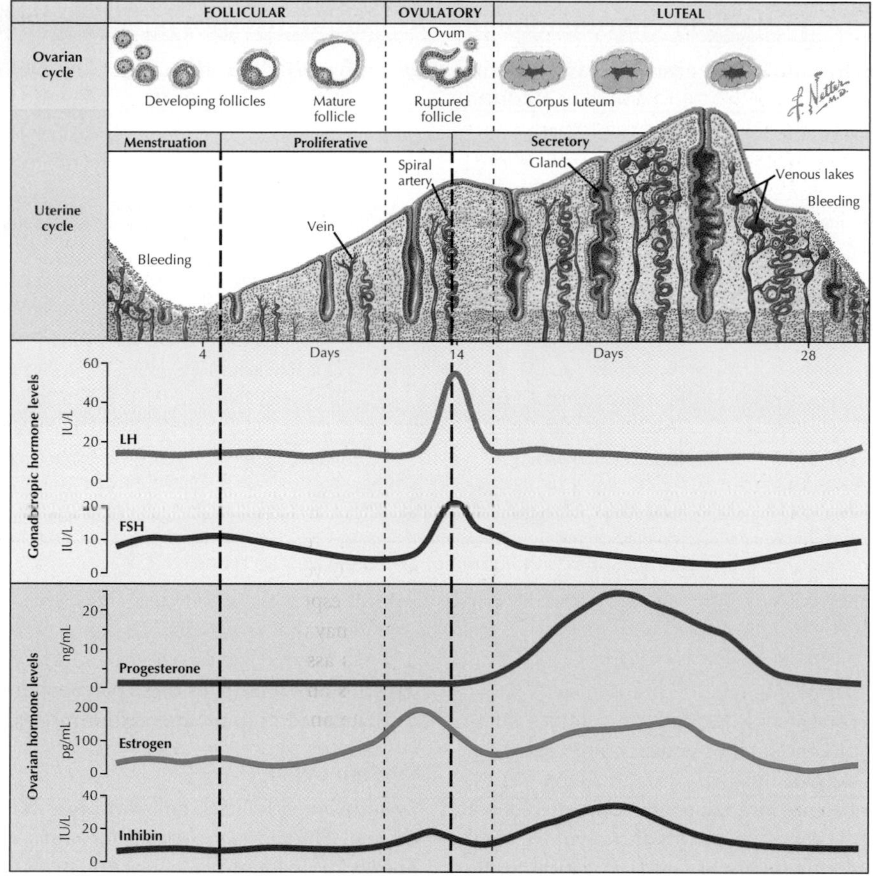

FIGURE 32-9 Female Reproductive Cycle. Correlation of events in follicular development, ovulation, hormonal interrelationships, and the menstrual cycle. Note: levels of estrogen (from ovarian follicle) and luteinizing hormone (*LH*) (from pituitary) are highest at the time of ovulation; progesterone from corpus luteum is highest during postovulation. *FSH*, follicle-stimulating hormone. (From Mulroney, S.E., & Myers, A.K. (2009). *Netter's Essential Physiology*. Philadelphia: Saunders. Copyright © 2009 Elsevier Inc. All rights reserved. www.netterimages.com.)

During **menstruation (menses)**, the functional layer of the endometrium disintegrates and is discharged through the vagina. Menstruation is followed by the **follicular/proliferative phase**. This phase is named for two simultaneous processes: maturation of an ovarian follicle and proliferation of the endometrium (see Figure 32-9). During this phase, GnRH contributes to the increase of FSH level, which stimulates a number of follicles. The pulsatile secretion of FSH from the anterior pituitary gland rescues a dominant ovarian follicle from apoptosis by days 5 to 7 of the cycle. Together, estrogen and FSH increase the number of FSH receptors in the granulosa cells of the primary follicle, making them more sensitive to FSH. FSH and estrogen combine to induce production of LH receptors on the granulosa cells, thus promoting LH stimulation to combine with FSH stimulation and cause a more rapid secretion of follicular estrogen. As estrogen level increases FSH level drops. This drop in FSH concentration decreases the growth of less developed follicles (see Figure 32-8). Estrogen causes cells of the endometrium to proliferate and stimulates production of LH. A surge in the levels of both FSH and LH is required for final follicular growth and ovulation.

Ovulation is the release of an ovum from a mature follicle and marks the beginning of the **luteal/secretory phase** of the menstrual cycle. The ovarian follicle begins its transformation into a corpus luteum (see Figure 32-8), hence the name *luteal phase*. Pulsatile secretion of LH from the anterior pituitary stimulates the corpus luteum to secrete progesterone, which in turn initiates the secretory phase of endometrial development. Glands and blood vessels in the endometrium branch and curl throughout the functional layer, and the glands begin to secrete a thin, glycogen-containing fluid, hence the name *secretory phase*. If conception occurs, the nutrient-laden endometrium is ready for implantation. Human chorionic gonadotropin (hCG) is secreted 3 days after fertilization and maintains the corpus luteum once implantation occurs at about day 6 or 7. hCG can be detected in maternal blood and urine 8 to 10 days after ovulation. The production of estrogen and progesterone will continue until the placenta can adequately maintain hormonal production. If conception and implantation do not occur, the corpus luteum degenerates and ceases its production of progesterone and estrogen. Without progesterone or estrogen to maintain it, the endometrium enters the ischemic ("blood-starved") phase and disintegrates, hence the name **ischemic/menstrual phase**. Then menstruation occurs, marking the beginning of another cycle.

Ovulatory cycles appear to have a minimum length of 24 to 26.5 days: the ovarian follicle requires 10 to 12.5 days to develop, and the luteal phase appears fixed at 14 days (±3 days). Menstrual blood flow usually lasts 3 to 7 days but may last as long as 8 days or stop after 2 days and still be considered within normal limits. Bleeding is consistently scant to heavy and varies from 30 to 80 mL, with most blood loss occurring during the first 3 days of menses. Menstrual discharge consists of blood, mucus, and desquamated endometrial tissue and does not clot under normal circumstances. It is usually dark and produces a characteristic musty odour on oxidation. Environmental factors, such as severe emotional stress, illness, malnutrition, obesity, and seasonal variation, may affect the length of the menstrual cycle.[17-19]

TABLE 32-3 Hormonal Feedback Mechanism in the Menstrual Cycle

Phase of Cycle and Ovarian Hormone Levels	Feedback to Hypothalamus and Anterior Pituitary	Resultant GnRH, FSH, and LH Levels	Ovarian and Menstrual Events
Early follicular phase: estrogen levels low; minute amount of progesterone secreted	Negative and inhibitory	All low	Ovarian follicle develops; endometrium proliferates
Late follicular (preovulatory) phase: estrogen levels high; progesterone level increases with small surge before ovulation	Positive and stimulatory	All surge; LH dominates	Process of ovulation begins; endometrial proliferation complete
Ovulatory phase: estrogen levels dip; progesterone levels begin to rise	Negative and inhibitory	All fall sharply	Corpus luteum begins to develop; endometrium enters secretory phase
Early luteal phase: estrogen and progesterone levels high; progesterone dominates	Negative and inhibitory	All continue to decline, but gradually	Corpus luteum fully developed; endometrium ready for implantation
Late luteal phase: estrogen and progesterone levels fall sharply	Negative and inhibitory; feedback lessens slightly	All rise slightly	Corpus luteum regresses; endometrium disintegrates; menstruation begins
Menstrual phase: estrogens levels low; minute amount of progesterone secreted	Negative and inhibitory	All low	More ovarian follicles begin to develop; functional layer of endometrium is shed

FSH, follicle-stimulating hormone; *GnRH*, gonadotropin-releasing hormone; *LH*, luteinizing hormone.

Hormonal Controls

Hormonal control of the menstrual cycle depends on complex interactions among the hypothalamus, the anterior pituitary, and the ovaries (or hypothalamic-pituitary-ovarian [H-P-O] axis)[20] (Table 32-3). Hormonal control is dependent on negative and positive ovarian feedback mechanisms. GnRH controls the gonadotropin production of FSH and LH, and the constant and pulsatile release of GnRH is critical to the timing of the menstrual cycle. GnRH is secreted by the hypothalamus and travels to the anterior pituitary, where it stimulates the secretion of FSH and LH. FSH and LH are released from the anterior pituitary in pulses that correspond to the secretion of GnRH.

During the early follicular phase, estrogen levels rise steadily and, through negative feedback, suppress FSH production and positively increase the production of LH. During the late follicular phase, the preovulatory rise in progesterone level facilitates a positive feedback loop whereby estrogen levels begin to increase, stimulating a surge of FSH and LH secretion from the anterior pituitary. The midcycle surge of LH and FSH induces ovulation.[21] Rising estrogen and progesterone levels during the luteal phase may inhibit the anterior pituitary and thus reduce LH and FSH secretion. Just before menstruation, FSH and LH levels begin to increase slightly, probably because of declining estrogen and progesterone levels (see Figure 32-9).

A variety of growth factors and autocrine/paracrine peptides influence hormonal control and follicular response. During the early follicular stage, FSH stimulates FSH receptors, LH receptors and release of insulinlike growth factor 1 as well as the production of inhibin and activin in the ovary. **Activin** from granulosa cells stimulates the secretion of FSH, increases the pituitary response to GnRH, and increases FSH binding in the granulosa cells in the dominant follicle. FSH stimulates **inhibin** secretion from granulosa cells and it, in turn, suppresses FSH synthesis. Inhibin B is primarily secreted in the follicular phase of the cycle but sharply spikes when ovulation occurs. Inhibin A is secreted in the luteal phase and further suppresses FSH. Inhibin also restrains prolactin and growth hormone release, interferes with GnRH receptors, and promotes breakdown of intracellular gonadotropins. In summary, the balance between activin and inhibin regulates FSH secretion and **follistatin** inhibits activin and boosts inhibin activity. Inhibin and activin also regulate LH stimulation of androgen synthesis in theca cells.[22] Research continues to advance understanding of the function and structural complexity of these polypeptides and their interaction with GnRH, gonadotropins, and sex hormones.

Ovarian Cycle

By stimulating follicles, gonadotropins initiate their growth and maturation. The most important hormonal event is a rise in FSH level. The decline in luteal-phase estrogen, progesterone, and inhibin secretion allows FSH level to rise; concurrently there is a slight increase in LH levels (see Figure 32-9). FSH stimulates granulosa cell growth and initiates estrogen production in these cells. At this time, a group of ovarian follicles is recruited and begins to mature; the exact number depends on the remaining pool of inactive follicles. As the follicles mature, granulosa cells multiply, increasing estradiol secretion. Within a few days of the cycle, one follicle becomes dominant and the others atrophy. The mechanism for follicular recruitment or dominance is unknown. The dominant follicle begins to secrete progressively larger amounts of estrogen (estradiol), which exerts an increase in GnRH receptor concentration and an increase in pituitary sensitivity to GnRH, creating a positive feedback effect that causes a FSH and LH surge. Ovulation occurs 1 to 2 hours before the final progesterone surge, or about 12 to 36 hours after the onset of the FSH and LH surge. Progesterone, proteolytic enzymes, and prostaglandins trigger mechanisms controlling follicular rupture and release of the ovum.[23] The FSH and LH surge also transforms the granulosa cells of the ovulatory follicle into the corpus luteum. The corpus luteum secretes both estrogen and progesterone in amounts that depend, in part, on adequate development of the follicle before ovulation. Progesterone acts both centrally and locally within the ovary to suppress new follicular growth during the early to midluteal phases. If pregnancy does not occur, the corpus luteum persists for 11 to 14 days and then regresses and eventually disappears. An increase in pulse frequency of GnRH from a low level reactivates hormonal control of the menstrual cycle.

Uterine Phases

Uterine phases of the menstrual cycle—the follicular/proliferative phase, the luteal/secretory phase, and menstruation—involve the cyclic changes that occur in the endometrium controlled by estrogen and progesterone. Hormonal effects are influenced by the presence of receptors and numerous growth factors, peptides, and enzymes that act as intermediaries between the sex steroids and the endometrium.[23] During the midfollicular/proliferative phase, increasing levels of estrogen contribute to endometrial repair and proliferation, thus increasing endometrial thickness (luteal phase). Once ovulation occurs and serum progesterone levels increase, the endometrial tissue develops secretory characteristics (secretory phase). If implantation of a fertilized ovum does not take place, endometrial tissue begins to break down approximately 11 days after ovulation (ischemic phase of menstruation; see Figure 32-9). Shedding of tissue (menstrual bleeding) begins about 14 days after ovulation.

Cervical mucus also undergoes cyclic changes. During the proliferative phase, the cervical mucus is thin and watery. Peak estrogen levels occur just before ovulation and maximally stimulate the cervical glands to produce mucus. Cervical mucus becomes abundant and more elastic (spinnbarkeit). Increasing estrogen levels apparently contribute to the development of tiny channels in cervical mucus, providing access for sperm into the interior of the uterus. Changes in the consistency of cervical mucus can be used to identify fertile intervals.[24]

Vaginal Response

The vaginal endothelium also responds to the cyclic hormonal changes of the menstrual cycle. Under the influence of estrogen, cells of the vaginal epithelium grow maximally during the follicular/proliferative phase. After ovulation, layers of keratinized cells overgrow the basal epithelium, a process known as **cornification**. Near the end of the luteal phase, leukocytes invade vaginal epithelium, removing the outer layers in a process termed **decornification**.

Body Temperature

Basal body temperature (BBT) undergoes characteristic biphasic changes during menstrual cycles in which ovulation occurs. During the follicular phase, the BBT fluctuates around 37°C (98°F). During the luteal phase, the average temperature increases by 2° to 0.5°C (0.4° to 1.0°F). At the end of the luteal phase, 1 to 3 days before the onset of menstruation, BBT declines to follicular-phase levels. The shift in temperature is related to ovulation, corpus luteum formation, and increased serum progesterone levels. Progesterone probably acts on the thermoregulatory centre of the hypothalamus to increase body temperature. Changes in BBT are used to document ovulatory cycles but when used alone are not the best method to predict the exact timing of ovulation.[25]

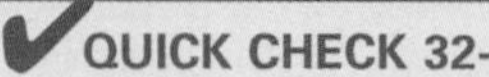

QUICK CHECK 32-4

1. Why does menstruation occur?
2. What event is associated with the luteal/secretory phase of the menstrual cycle?

STRUCTURE AND FUNCTION OF THE BREAST

The **breasts** are modified sebaceous glands that lie on the ventral surface of the thorax, within the superficial fascia of the chest wall. They extend vertically from the second rib to the sixth or seventh intercostal space and laterally from the side of the sternum to the midaxillary line. Breast tissue also may extend into the axilla; this tissue is known as the *tail of Spence.*

Female Breast

The female breast is composed of 15 to 20 pyramid-shaped lobes that are separated and supported by Cooper ligaments (Figure 32-10). Each lobe contains 20 to 40 lobules (alveoli), which subdivide further into many functional units called **acini** (*sing.*, **acinus**). Each acinus is lined with a layer of epithelial cells capable of secreting milk and a layer of subepithelial cells capable of contracting to squeeze milk from the acinus. Biochemical signalling and density within the extracellular matrix is essential for differentiation and function of the acini glandular epithelium. The acini empty into a network of lobular collecting ducts, which empty into interlobular collecting and ejecting ducts. Collagen fibre alignment is required for ductal elongation and organized branching.[26] The ducts reach the skin through openings (pores) in the nipple. The lobes and lobules are surrounded and separated by muscle strands and fatty connective tissue. The amount of fatty connective tissue varies among individuals, depending on weight and genetic and endocrine factors, and contributes to the diversity of breast size and shape and the function of the mammary epithelium. Fat increases in the breast after menopause.[27]

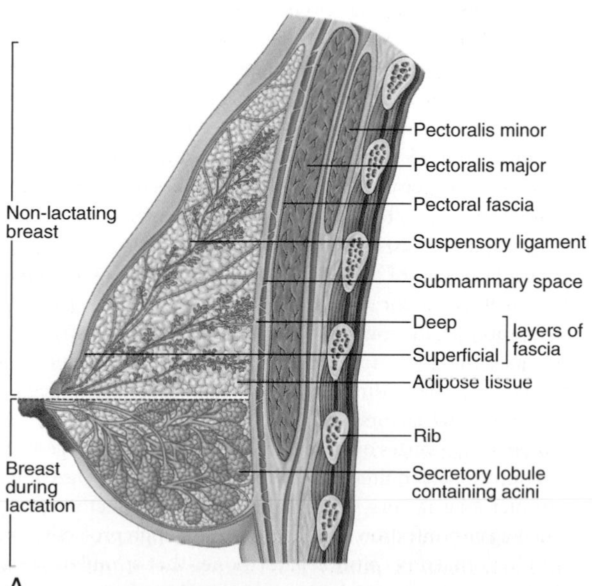

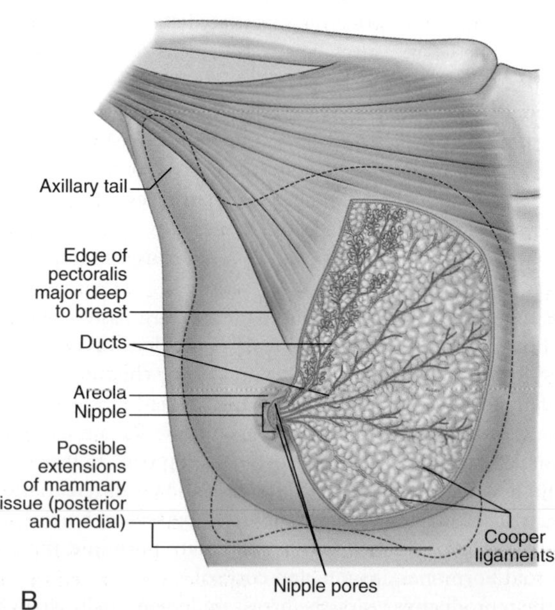

FIGURE 32-10 Schematic Diagram of the Breast. (From Standring, S. [2009]. *Gray's anatomy* [40th ed.]. London: Churchill Livingstone.)

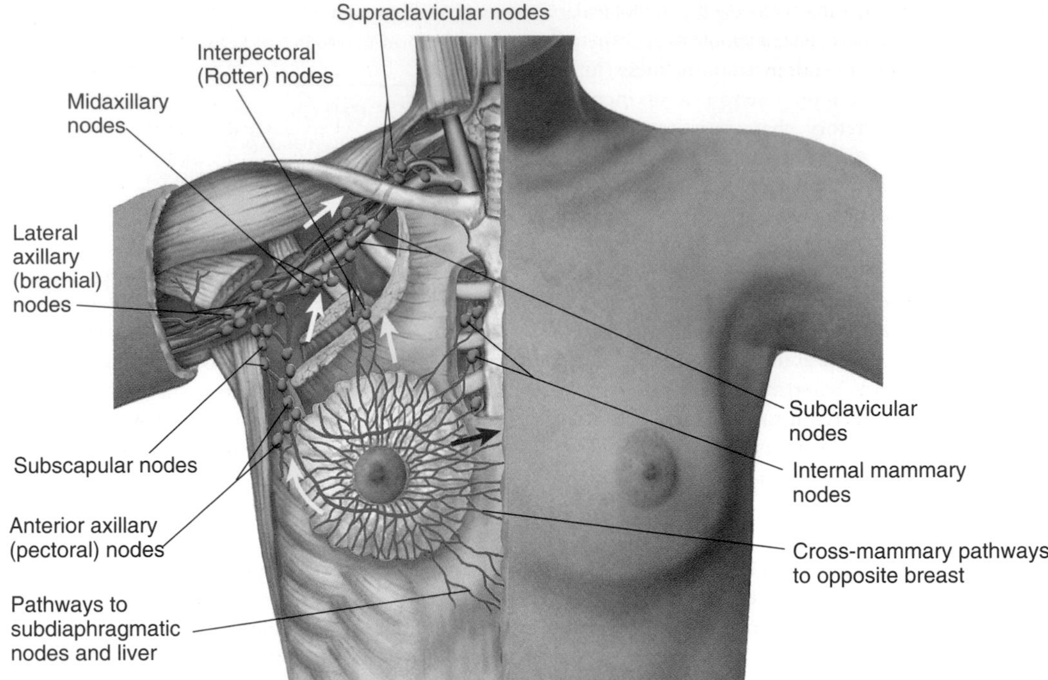

FIGURE 32-11 Lymphatic Drainage of the Female Breast. (From Ball, J.W., Dains, J.E., Flynn, J.A., et al. [2015]. *Seidel's guide to physical examination* [8th ed.]. St. Louis: Mosby.)

An extensive capillary network surrounds the acini and is supplied by the internal and lateral thoracic arteries and the intercostal arteries. Venous return follows arterial supply, with relatively rapid emptying into the superior vena cava. The breasts receive sensory innervation from branches of the second through sixth intercostal nerves and the cervical plexus. As a result, breast pain may be referred to the chest, back, scapula, medial arm, and neck. Lymphatic drainage of the breast occurs largely through axillary nodes, but there may be predominance of superficial mammary routes with resultant asymmetry between a person's breasts[27] (Figure 32-11).

The **nipple** is a pigmented cylindrical structure usually located at the fourth or fifth intercostal space. On its surface lie multiple openings, one from each lobe. It measures 0.5 to 1.3 cm in diameter and is approximately 10 to 12 mm in height when erect. The **areola** is the pigmented circular area around the nipple. It may be 15 to 60 mm in diameter. A number of sebaceous glands, the **glands of Montgomery**, are located within the areola and aid in lubrication of the nipple during lactation. The nipple and areola contain smooth muscles, which receive motor innervation from the sympathetic nervous system. Sexual stimulation, breastfeeding, and exposure to cold cause the nipple to become erect.

The fetal and early postnatal development of breast tissue does not depend on hormones, although fetal breast tissue does become progressively responsive to hormonal stimulation. During childhood, breast growth is latent and growth of the nipple and areola keeps pace with body surface growth. At the onset of puberty in the female, estrogen secretion stimulates mammary growth. Breast development, or thelarche, is usually the first sign of puberty in the female. Full differentiation and development of breast tissue are mediated by several hormones, including estrogen, progesterone, prolactin, growth hormone, thyroid and parathyroid hormones, insulin, and cortisol.

During the reproductive years, the breast undergoes cyclic changes in response to changes in the levels of estrogen and progesterone associated with the menstrual cycle. Estrogen promotes development of the lobular ducts; progesterone stimulates development of cells lining the acini. Lactation (milk production) occurs after childbirth in response to increased levels of prolactin. Prolactin secretion, in turn, increases by continued breastfeeding. **Oxytocin**, another hormone released after delivery, controls milk ejection (let down) from acini cells. During the follicular/proliferative phase of the menstrual cycle, high estradiol levels increase the vascularity of breast tissue and stimulate proliferation of ductal and acinar tissue. This effect is sustained into the luteal/secretory phase of the cycle. During this phase, progesterone levels increase and contribute to the breast changes induced by estradiol. Specific effects of progesterone include dilation of the ducts and conversion of the acinar cells into secretory cells. Most women experience some degree of premenstrual breast fullness, tenderness, and increased breast nodularity. Breast volume may increase as much as 10 to 30 mL. Because the length of the menstrual cycle does not allow for complete regression of new cell growth, breast growth continues at a slow rate until approximately 35 years of age. Because of the cyclic changes that occur in breast tissue, breast examination should be conducted at the conclusion of or a few days after the menstrual cycle, when hormonal effects are minimal and breasts are at their smallest.

The function of the female breast is primarily to provide a source of nourishment for the newborn. Physiologically, breast milk is the most appropriate nourishment for newborns. Colostrum, produced in low quantities in the first few days postpartum, is rich in immunological components, including secretory IgA, lactoferrin, leukocytes, and developmental factors, such as epidermal growth factor. The nutrient composition changes over time to meet the changing digestive capabilities and nutritional requirements of the infant. Secretory IgA and nonspecific antimicrobial factors, such as lysosomes and lactoferrin, protect the infant against infection.[28] During lactation, high prolactin levels interfere with hypothalamic-pituitary hormones that stimulate ovulation. This mechanism suppresses the menstrual cycle and can prevent ovulation.[29] In some parts of the world, breastfeeding is the major means of contraception (lactational amenorrhea method).[30,31] However, it is not absolute that ovulation will not occur, and this method will not ensure that pregnancy will not occur. Breasts are also a source of pleasurable sexual sensation and in Western cultures have become a sexual symbol.

Male Breast

Until puberty, development of the male breast is similar to that of the female breast. In the absence of sufficiently high levels of estrogen and progesterone, and with antagonistic effects of androgens, the male breast does not develop any further. The normal male breast consists mostly of fat with a small, underdeveloped nipple and a few ductlike structures in the subareolar area. The male breast may appear enlarged in obese men because of accumulation of fatty tissue. During puberty, some males experience benign gynecomastia (benign proliferation of male breast glandular tissue), a condition in which the breasts enlarge temporarily as a result of hormonal fluctuations, and should be differentiated from any underlying systemic disorders.[32]

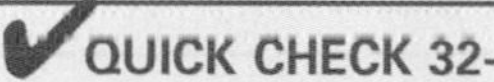

QUICK CHECK 32-5

1. How does breast development differ between adult men and women?

THE MALE REPRODUCTIVE SYSTEM

The external genitalia in men perform the major functions of reproduction. Sperm are produced in the male gonads and the testes, and delivered by the penis. The internal male genitalia consist of conducting tubes and fluid-producing glands, all of which aid in the transport of sperm from the testes to the urethral opening of the penis. The male reproductive and urinary structures are shown in Figure 32-12.

External Genitalia

Testes

The testes are the essential organs of male reproduction. Like the ovaries, the testes have two functions: (1) production of gametes (i.e., sperm) and (2) production of sex hormones (i.e., androgens and testosterone).

During embryonic and fetal life, the testes develop within the abdomen (see Figure 32-1). About 3 months before birth, the testes start to descend toward the developing scrotum. About 1 month before birth, they enter twin passageways called **inguinal canals**. The inguinal canals are vaginal processes created by outpouchings of the peritoneum (lining of the abdominal cavity). The descent of a testis is shown in Figure 32-13. When descent is complete, the abdominal end of each vaginal process closes and the inguinal canal disappears. Failure of the testes to descend through the inguinal canal is known as *cryptorchidism*. The scrotal end of each vaginal process becomes the outer covering of the testis, the **tunica vaginalis**.

Figure 32-14 shows a sagittal section of a mature testis. The adult **testis** is oval and varies considerably in length (3 to 6 cm), width (2 to 3.5 cm), depth (3 to 4 cm), and weight (10 to 40 g). The testis is almost entirely surrounded by the tunica vaginalis, which separates the testis from the scrotal wall, and the **tunica albuginea**. Inward extensions of the tunica albuginea separate the testis into about 250 compartments, or lobules, each of which contains several tortuously coiled ducts called **seminiferous tubules**. Sperm are produced in these tubules. Tissue surrounding these ducts contains **Leydig cells**, which occur in clusters and produce androgens, chiefly testosterone.

The two ends of each seminiferous tubule join and leave the lobule through the **tubulus rectus**, which leads to the central portion of the testis, the **rete testis**. The sperm then move through the **efferent tubules**, or vasa efferentia, to the epididymis, where they mature.

The testes are innervated by adrenergic fibres whose sole function apparently is to regulate blood flow to the Leydig cells. Arterial blood

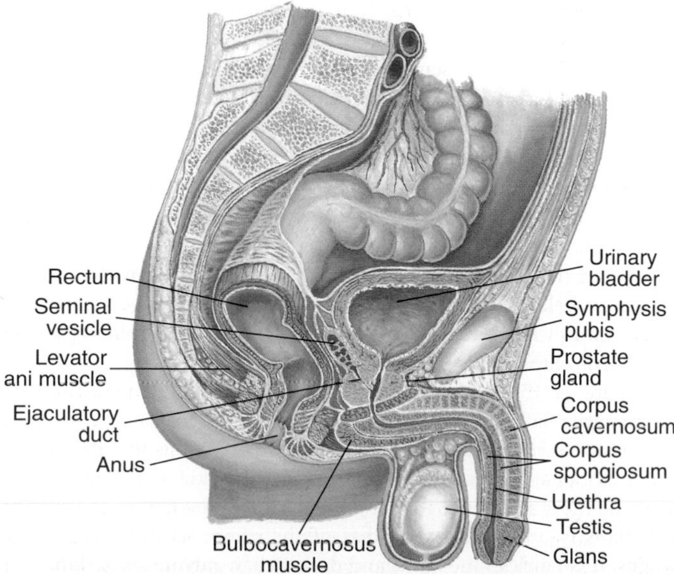

FIGURE 32-12 Structure of the Male Reproductive Organs. (From Ball, J.W., Dains, J.E., Flynn, J.A., et al. [2015]. *Seidel's guide to physical examination* [8th ed.]. St. Louis: Mosby.)

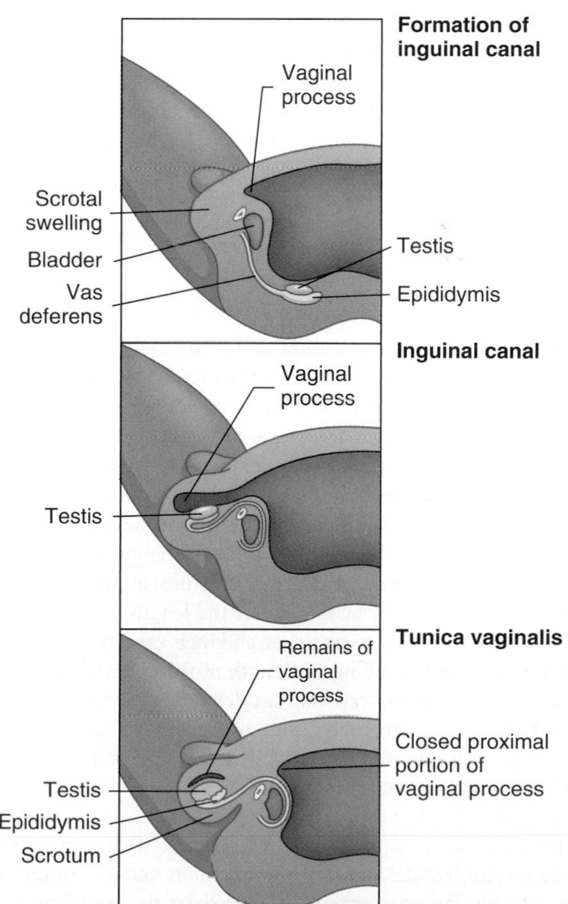

FIGURE 32-13 Descent of a Testis. The testes descend from the abdominal cavity to the scrotum during the last 3 months of fetal development.

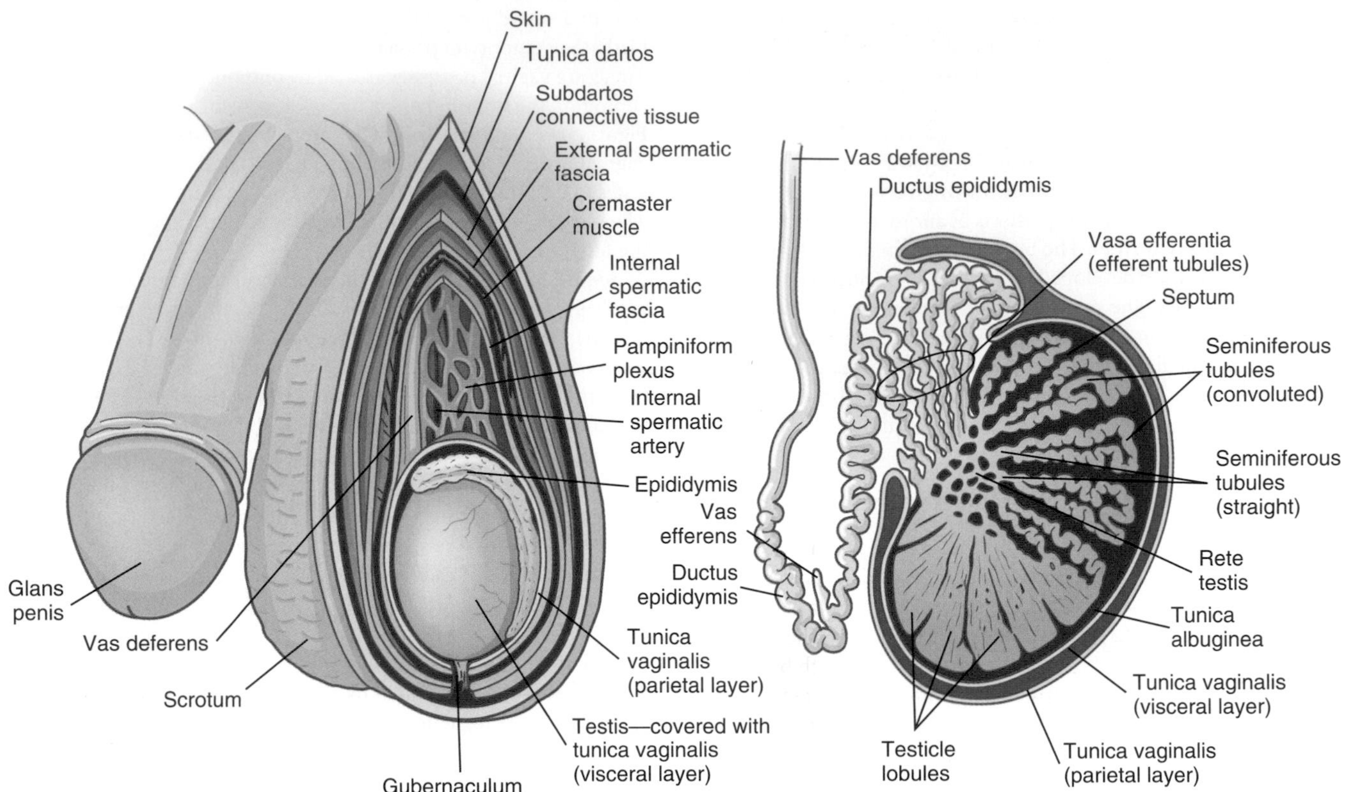

FIGURE 32-14 The Testes. External and sagittal views showing interior anatomy.

from the internal spermatic and differential arteries flows over the surface of the testes before entering the parenchyma (functional tissues). Surface flow cools the blood to temperatures that promote spermatogenesis, approximately 1° to 7°C (33.8° to 44.6°F) below body core temperature.[33] Additionally, the testes are suspended outside the pelvic cavity to facilitate cooling.

Epididymis

The **epididymis** (*pl.*, **epididymides**) is a comma-shaped structure that curves over the posterior portion of each testis (see Figure 32-14). It consists of a single, densely packed and markedly coiled duct measuring 5 to 7 cm in length (but about 6 m in length when uncoiled). The epididymis has structural and physiological functions. Its structural function is to conduct sperm from the efferent tubules to the vas deferens, whereas physiological functions include sperm maturation, mobility, and fertility. When sperm enter the head of the epididymis, they are not fully mature or motile, nor can they fertilize an ovum. During the 12 days (or more) sperm take to travel the length of the epididymis, they receive nutrients and testosterone and their capacity for fertilization is enhanced.[34] After travelling the length of the epididymis, sperm are stored in the epididymal tail and vas deferens. The **vas deferens** is a duct with muscular layers capable of powerful peristalsis that transports sperm toward the urethra. The vas deferens enters the pelvic cavity through the spermatic cord (see Figure 32-14).

Scrotum

The testes, epididymides, and spermatic cord are enclosed and protected by the **scrotum**, a skin-covered, fibromuscular sac homologous to the female labia majora (see Figure 32-2). The skin of the scrotum is thin and has rugae (wrinkles or folds), which enable it to enlarge or relax away from the body. At puberty the scrotal skin darkens, develops active sebaceous glands, and becomes sparsely covered with hair. Just under the skin lies a layer of connective tissue (fascia) and smooth muscle, the **tunica dartos** (see Figure 32-14). The tunica dartos also forms a septum that separates the two testes. Exposure to cold temperatures causes the tunica dartos to contract, pulling the testes close to the warm body. In warm temperatures, the tunica dartos relaxes, suspending the testes away from body heat. These mechanisms promote optimal temperatures (about 1° to 2°C lower than body temperature) for spermatogenesis. In addition, scrotal sensitivity to touch, pressure, temperature, and pain protects the testes from potential harm. During sexual excitement, the scrotal skin and tunica thicken, the scrotum tightens and lifts, and the spermatic cords shorten, partially elevating the testes toward the body. As excitement plateaus, the engorged testes increase 50% in size, rotate anteriorly, and flatten against the body, signalling impending ejaculation.

Penis

The **penis** has two main functions: delivery of sperm to the female vagina and elimination of urine. (Urine formation and excretion are discussed in Chapter 29.) Embryonically, the penis is homologous to the female clitoris (see Figure 32-2).

Figure 32-15 shows a sagittal section of the adult penis and its anatomical relation to other urogenital structures. Externally, the penis consists of a shaft with a tip (the **glans**) that contains the opening of the urethra (see Figures 32-14 and 32-15). The skin of the glans folds over the tip of the penis, forming the **prepuce (foreskin)**. The skin of the penis is continuous with that of the groin, scrotum, and inner thighs. It is hairless, movable, and darker than surrounding skin.

Internally, the penis consists of the urethra and three compartments or sinusoids: two **corpora cavernosa** and the **corpus spongiosum** (see Figure 32-15) separated by Buck fascia. Like the testes, these compartments are

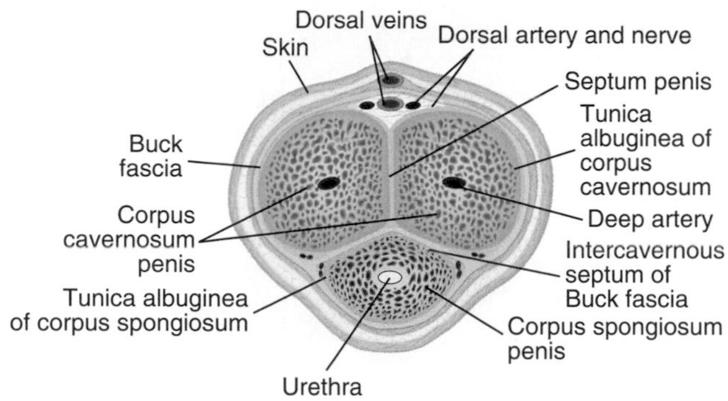

FIGURE 32-15 Cross Section of the Penis. (From Thompson, J.M., McFarland, G.K., Hirsch, J.E., et al. [Eds.]. [2002]. *Mosby's clinical nursing* [5th ed.]. St. Louis: Mosby.)

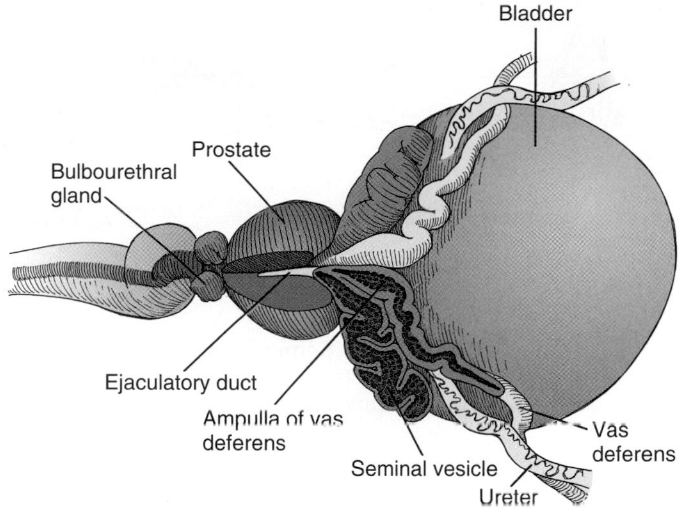

FIGURE 32-16 Prostate Gland, Seminal Vesicles, and Vas Deferens. (From Huguet, J. [2012]. *Hinman's atlas of urosurgical anatomy* [2nd ed., pp. 249–286]. Philadelphia: Saunders.)

enclosed by the fibrous tunica albuginea. The **urethra** passes through the corpus spongiosum and ends at a sagittal slit in the glans.

Penetration of the female vagina is made possible by the **erectile reflex**, a process in which erectile tissues within the corpora cavernosa and corpus spongiosum become engorged with blood. The erectile tissues consist of vascular spaces, or chambers, supplied with blood by arterioles (small arteries). Usually, the arterioles are constricted, so that not much blood flows through the erectile tissues. Sexual stimulation, however, causes the arterioles to dilate and fill with blood, expanding the erectile tissues and causing an erection. Erection apparently is maintained by compression or constriction of veins that drain the corpora cavernosa and corpus spongiosum. When sexual stimulation ceases or orgasm and ejaculation occur, these veins open, blood flows out of the arterioles, and the penis becomes flaccid (soft and pendulous). Erection is under the control of the autonomic nervous system but can be stimulated or inhibited by central nervous system input.

Erections begin in utero and continue throughout life, but ejaculation does not occur until sperm production begins at puberty. Growth of the penis and scrotal contents continues well past puberty, however, and may not be complete until the late teens or early twenties. Penis size, when flaccid, varies considerably; with an erection, difference in penis size diminishes. Sexual excitement causes the corpora cavernosa to increase in length and width and become rigid; the penis becomes erect. Stimulation of the glans, which is endowed with copious sensitive nerve endings, provides maximum erotic sensation. With sexual arousal, skin colour deepens, the glans doubles in size, and the urethral meatus dilates. Ejaculation occurs with frequent, strong contractions of the vas deferens, epididymis, seminal vesicles, prostate, urethra, and penis. Erection and ejaculation can occur independently of each other.[35,36]

Internal Genitalia

Figure 32-12 shows the anatomy of the internal genitalia and their relation to other pelvic organs. The internal genitalia consist of ducts and glands, as follows:

Ducts: consist of two vasa deferentia, ejaculatory duct, and urethra; conduct sperm and glandular secretions from the testes to the urethral opening of the penis

Glands: consist of prostate gland, two seminal vesicles, and two bulbourethral glands (Cowper glands); secrete fluids that serve as a vehicle for sperm transport and create nutritious alkaline medium that promotes sperm motility and survival

Together the sperm and the glandular fluids compose **semen**.

Sperm leave the epididymides and travel rapidly through the internal ducts (**emission**). Emission occurs just seconds before ejaculation, at the moment when sexual arousal peaks. It always leads to ejaculation.

Emission occurs as smooth muscle in the walls of the epididymides and vasa deferentia begins to contract rhythmically, pushing sperm and epididymal secretions through the vasa deferentia. Each vas deferens is a firm, elastic, fibromuscular tube that begins at the tail of the epididymis, enters the pelvic cavity within the spermatic cord, loops up and over the bladder, and ends in the prostate gland (Figure 32-16). Sperm are conducted by peristaltic contractions of smooth muscle in the walls of the vas deferens.

As sperm leave the ampulla (wide portion) of the vas deferens, the seminal vesicles secrete a nutritive, glucose-rich fluid into the ejaculate (semen). The **seminal vesicles** are glands about 4 to 6 cm long that lie behind the urinary bladder and in front of the rectum. The ducts of the seminal vesicles join the ampulla of the vas deferens to become the **ejaculatory duct**, which contracts rhythmically during emission and ejaculation. As seen in Figures 32-13 and 32-16, the ejaculatory duct joins the urethra, where both pass through the prostate gland. During emission and ejaculation, a sphincter (muscle surrounding a duct) closes, preventing urine from entering the prostatic urethra.

The **prostate gland** is about the size of a walnut, surrounds the urethra, and is composed of glandular alveoli and ducts embedded in fibromuscular tissue. Nerves required for penile erection travel along the posterolateral surface of the prostate. While semen moves through the prostatic portion of the urethra, the prostate gland contracts rhythmically and secretes prostatic fluid (a thin, milky substance with an alkaline pH that helps sperm to survive in the acidic environment of the female reproductive tract) into the mixture. In addition, substances in seminal and prostatic fluids help to mobilize sperm after ejaculation.

Bulbourethral glands (Cowper glands) are the last pair of glands to add fluid to the ejaculate; their ducts secrete mucus into the urethra near the base of the penis. Ejaculation occurs as semen reaches the base of the penis, where muscles rhythmically contract and expel semen. Normally a man ejaculates between 2 and 6 mL of semen, containing 75 million to 400 million sperm. About 98% of the ejaculate consists of glandular fluids; 60% to 70% of the volume originates from the seminal vesicles and 20% from the prostate. Therefore, the ejaculate of a man who has undergone a vasectomy (a surgical procedure for permanent male birth control) is reduced by only about 2%.

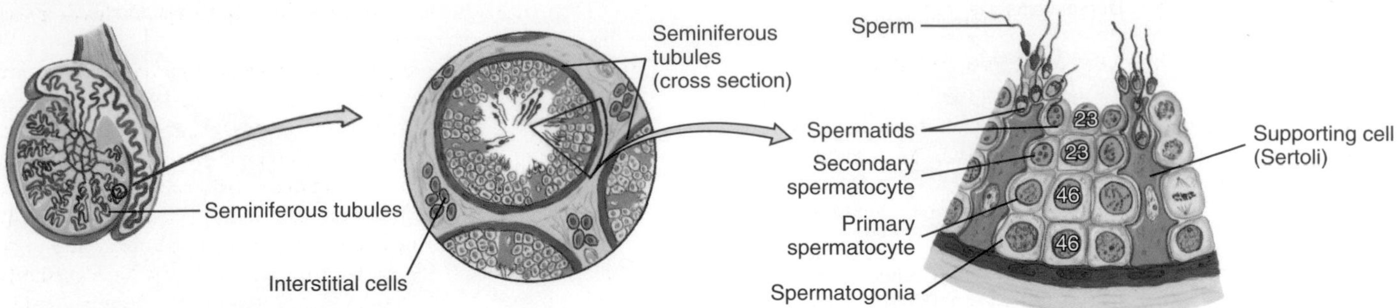

FIGURE 32-17 Seminiferous Tubule and Spermatogenesis. Cross section of a seminiferous tubule showing the different cell types. Interstitial cells that produce testosterone are between the seminiferous tubules. Spermatids in the lumen become sperm by a process called *spermiogenesis*. The numbers in white represent the number of chromosomes. (From Applegate, E. [2011]. *The anatomy and physiology learning system* [4th ed.]. St. Louis: Saunders.)

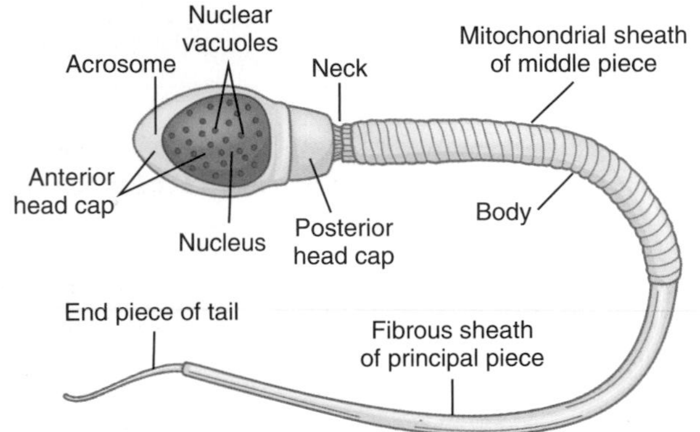

FIGURE 32-18 Mature Sperm Cell (Spermatozoon). Anatomy of mature sperm cell.

Spermatogenesis

Spermatogenesis begins at puberty and continues for life. In this respect, spermatogenesis differs markedly from oogenesis (production of primordial ova), which occurs during fetal life only. Spermatogenesis takes place within the seminiferous tubules of the testes (see Figures 32-14 and 32-17). The basement membrane of each seminiferous tubule is lined with diploid (46-chromosome) germ cells called spermatogonia (*sing.*, spermatogonium). These cells undergo continuous mitotic division (division into two identical cells, see Chapter 1.) Some spermatogonia move away from the basement membrane and mature, becoming primary spermatocytes (Figure 32-17). These spermatogonia undergo meiosis, cell division that results in two haploid (23-chromosome) cells called secondary spermatocytes. (Meiosis is described and illustrated in Chapter 2.) The secondary spermatocytes also undergo meiosis, resulting in four spermatids. The spermatids differentiate into spermatozoa, or sperm, each of which contains 23 chromosomes (Figure 32-18).

The development of spermatids into sperm depends on the presence of Sertoli cells (nondividing support cells) within the seminiferous tubules. Spermatids attach themselves to the Sertoli cells (see Figure 32-17), where they receive nutrients and hormonal signals necessary to develop into sperm.[37]

The process of spermatogenesis, from mitotic division of a spermatogonium to maturation of the spermatids, takes about 70 to 80 days. Mature sperm migrate from the seminiferous tubules to the epididymides, where their capacity for fertilization continues to develop. Although they are completely mature by the time they are ejaculated, the sperm do not become motile (capable of movement) until they are activated by biochemicals in semen and in the female reproductive tract (known as *sperm capacitation*).[38]

Male Sex and Reproductive Hormones

The male sex hormones are androgens. Testosterone, the primary male sex hormone, and other androgens are produced mainly by Leydig cells of the testes, but they are also produced by the adrenal glands (see Table 32-1 and discussion about adrenarche under "Puberty and Reproductive Maturation," p. 795). In men, sex hormone production is relatively constant and does not occur in a cyclic pattern, as it does in women.

The physiological actions of androgen are related to the growth and development of male tissues and organs.[39] Androgens are responsible for the fetal differentiation and development of the male urogenital system and have some effects on the fetal brain. After birth, the Leydig cells become quiescent until activated by the gonadotropins during puberty. Then androgens cause the sex organs to grow and secondary sex characteristics to develop.

Testosterone affects nervous and skeletal tissues, bone marrow, skin and hair, and sex organs. It has an anabolic effect on skeletal muscle tissue, thereby contributing to the difference in body weight and composition between men and women. Testosterone also stimulates growth of the musculature and cartilage of the larynx, causing a permanent deepening of the voice. Testosterone directly stimulates the bone marrow and indirectly stimulates renal erythropoietin production to achieve increased hemoglobin and hematocrit levels. Because sebaceous gland activity is stimulated by testosterone, acne may develop. Hair becomes coarser in texture, and facial, axillary, and pubic hair grows in male patterns. Later in life, testosterone causes baldness in genetically susceptible individuals. Testosterone is required for spermatogenesis and for secretion of fluid by the prostate gland, seminal vesicles, and Cowper glands. Testosterone is also associated with libido (sex drive). Other, less-understood effects of testosterone include alterations in fatty acid and cholesterol metabolism.

The regulation of androgen production and spermatogenesis is achieved by a complex feedback system involving the extrahypothalamic central nervous system, the hypothalamus, the anterior pituitary, the testes, and the androgen-sensitive end organs. These relationships are essentially the same in women (see Figure 32-3).

QUICK CHECK 32-6

1. Why do sperm take 12 days to travel the length of the epididymis?2. What is the purpose of prostatic secretion?
3. Which cells produce testosterone?

AGING AND REPRODUCTIVE FUNCTION

Aging and the Female Reproductive System

Menopause is a normal developmental and transitional event that is universally experienced by the average age of about 51 years with a range of 40 to 60 years. Genetics are associated with timing of menopause and menopause can occur 2 years sooner on average for smokers. Findings from studies of body mass index, physical activity, and ethnicity are inconsistent in relation to timing of menopause.[40] Changes are caused primarily by declining ovarian function and a resulting decrease in ovarian hormone secretion. The primary changes of menopause are as follows:[41]

Perimenopause: This is the transitional period between reproductive and nonreproductive years and can last 1 to 8 years. About 5 to 10 years before menopause, approximately 90% of women note mild to extreme variability in frequency and quality of menstrual flow. Symptoms usually begin with a shortening of the menstrual cycle, which correlates with a shorter follicular phase, followed by unpredictable or irregular ovulation and a lengthening of the menstrual cycle. The perimenopause varies between women and from cycle to cycle in the same woman.

Menopause: Menopause is defined by the point that marks 12 consecutive months of amenorrhea. This means that it is determined retrospectively after a woman has not had a menstrual period for 1 year. It is characterized by loss of ovarian function, low estrogen and progesterone levels, and high FSH and LH levels (Figure 32-19).[42] Early menopause is the 5 years after menopause onset. Late menopause follows and continues until death.[43]

Ovarian changes: Around 37 to 38 years of age, women experience accelerated follicular loss, which ends when the supply of follicles is depleted at menopause. This accelerated loss is correlated with increased FSH stimulation, declining inhibin production, and slightly elevated estradiol levels (see Figure 32-19). The ovarian response to high FSH level recruits increasing numbers of follicles; these follicles only partially develop, with a net effect of irregular ovulation, lower progesterone levels, and depleted follicle reserve.

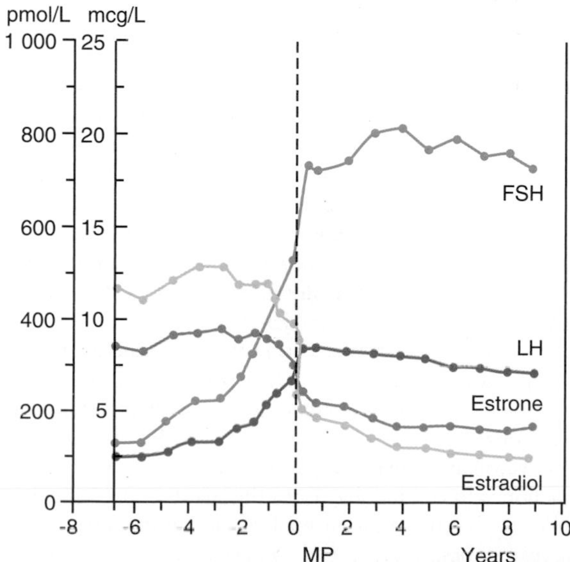

FIGURE 32-19 Perimenopausal Hormone Transition. Mean circulating hormone levels. *FSH,* follicle-stimulating hormone; *LH,* luteinizing hormone; *MP,* menopause.

The ovaries begin to decrease in size around age 30; this decrease accelerates after age 60.

Uterine changes: The increase in anovulatory cycles allows for proliferative growth of the endometrium. With this longer exposure to unopposed estrogen and greater thickness of the endometrium, 50% of perimenopausal women will experience dysfunctional uterine bleeding that is heavy and unpredictable. In the past, this has put women at high risk for hysterectomy. Newer treatment includes progesterone administration or endometrial ablation by laser or electrocautery. New methods of decreasing the function of the endometrial tissue are being developed.

Breast tissue changes: Breast tissue becomes involuted, fat deposits and connective tissue increase, and breasts are reduced in size and firmness.

Urogenital tract changes: The ovaries shrink; the uterus atrophies; and the vagina shortens, narrows, and loses some elasticity. Lubrication of the vagina diminishes and vaginal pH increases, creating higher incidence of vaginitis. The cervix atrophies; the cervical os shrinks; vaginal epithelium atrophies; labia major and minora become less prominent; some pubic hair is lost; urethral tone declines along with muscle tone throughout the pelvic area; urinary frequency or urgency, urinary tract infections, and incontinence may occur. Regular sexual activity and orgasm may diminish some of these changes. Sexually active women have less vaginal atrophy.

Skeletal changes: Bone mass is lost, leading to increased brittleness and porosity and possibly osteoporosis particularly in the lumbar spine and femoral neck (see Chapter 39).

Cardiac changes: The risk for coronary heart disease increases significantly with an increase in total and LDL-cholesterol and a decrease in HDL-cholesterol (see Chapter 24).

Systemic changes: **Vasomotor flushes** are characterized by a rise in skin temperature, dilation of peripheral blood vessels, increased blood flow in the hands, increased skin conductance, and transient increase in heart rate followed by a temperature drop and profuse perspiration over the area of flush distribution. This usually occurs in the face and neck and may radiate into the chest and other parts of the body. Dizziness, nausea, headaches, and palpitations may accompany the flush.[44] These flushes can vary in frequency, intensity, and duration and are experienced for 1 to 15 years (mean 1 to 5 years) by up to 85% of perimenopausal to postmenopausal women. Flushes are believed to be caused by rapid decreases in estrogen levels; estrogen replacement therapy can ameliorate these symptoms. Rapid changes in estrogen levels also can increase emotional stress with unpredictable mood swings, depression and anxiety, weight gain, migraine headaches, and insomnia. Lower estrogen levels will decrease skin thickness and diminish skin elasticity, thereby causing increased skin dryness and wrinkling.

Menopause increases the risk for ovarian, breast, and uterine cancers. The risk is greater in women who began menstruating before age 12 or experience menopause after age 55. Women who menstruate longer than normal during a lifetime are exposed to more estrogen and have more ovulations. A longer exposure to estrogen increases a woman's risk for uterine and breast cancers, and having more ovulations than normal increases a woman's risk for ovarian cancer.[45,46]

Hormone therapy can be considered to relieve severe menopausal symptoms. However, risk and benefits of such therapy must be carefully evaluated. There is increased risk for serious disorders for some women including breast cancer, heart disease, and stroke. Risks vary depending on age, timing of menopause, health history, dosage, and route of delivery (oral versus patch). Nonhormonal therapy also may be an option for symptom relief. An individualized management plan considering risks and benefits of available alternatives can improve quality of life.[47,48]

Aging and the Male Reproductive System

Men maintain reproductive capacity longer than women. No known discrete event, comparable to menopause, characterizes aging of the male reproductive system. Changes do occur, however, in testicular structure and function and sexual behaviour.[49] Emotional and physical changes associated with androgen deficiency in the aging male are known as **andropause**, but it occurs in only a small percentage of men.[50] Contributing factors include decreased levels of testosterone, change in responsiveness of target tissues, decreased levels of sex hormone binding globulin, and changes in the hypothalamus and pituitary gland. Obesity also contributes to decreased testosterone production in aging men.[51,52]

Male sexual behaviour encompasses both sexual drive and erectile and ejaculatory capacity. Libido, or sexual drive, is a complex phenomenon that requires a baseline hormonal milieu and is significantly influenced by health status and environmental, social, and psychological factors. However, in men older than 40 years of age, organic factors are involved in more than half of cases of male sexual dysfunction. Chronic disease and also vascular, endocrine, and neurological disorders are common causes of organically based dysfunction of sexual capability. Primary changes[53] are summarized as follows:

Sexual drive (libido): influenced by changes in health status and testosterone levels

Erectile/ejaculatory capacity: longer stimulation needed to achieve full erection, slower and less forceful ejaculation, less pelvic muscle involvement; decreased vasocongestive response; longer refractory time, up to 24 hours

Testicular changes: decreased weight, atrophy, softening of testes; seminiferous tubules thicken in basement membrane area, have germ cell arrest, decrease in spermatogenic activity, and collapse; then sclerosis and fibrosis cause complete obstruction; semen volume, sperm concentration, total sperm count, sperm motility, and number of motile sperm decrease; morphological appearance of sperm changes; decreased fertility[54]

Hormonal changes: hormone synthesis decreases and target tissues decline in responsiveness; testosterone levels decline as number of Leydig cells decreases; gonadotropin levels increase

Associated change: functional deterioration of accessory sex organs occurs; loss of muscle mass, strength, and endurance and decrease in libido develop

QUICK CHECK 32-7

1. What happens to estradiol levels in perimenopausal women?
2. What are the physical changes associated with menopausal decreases in estrogen level?
3. How does andropause affect muscle mass?

DID YOU UNDERSTAND?

Development of the Reproductive Systems

1. Differentiation of female and male genitalia begins around 6 to 8 weeks of embryonic development, when the gonads of genetically male embryos begin to secrete male sex hormones, primarily testosterone, under the influence of *SRY* gene expression and testes-determining factor. Female gonadal development occurs in the absence of *SRY* gene expression. Until that time, the primitive reproductive organs of males and females are homologous (the same).
2. The structure and function of both male and female reproductive systems depend on interactions among the central nervous system (hypothalamus), the endocrine system (anterior pituitary), the gonads (ovaries, testes), and the hypothalamic-pituitary-gonadal axis. A set of complex neurological and hormonal interactions accelerate at puberty and lead to sexual maturation and reproductive capability.
3. Production of primitive female gametes (ova) occurs solely during fetal life. From puberty to menopause, one female gamete matures per menstrual cycle. Production of the male gametes (sperm) begins at puberty; after that, millions are produced daily, usually for life.
4. Puberty is the onset of sexual maturation. Adolescence is a stage of human development between childhood and adulthood and includes social, psychological, and biological changes.
5. At puberty, extrahypothalamic factors cause the hypothalamus to secrete gonadotropin-releasing hormone, which stimulates the anterior pituitary to secrete the gonadotropins follicle-stimulating hormone (FSH) and luteinizing hormone (LH) that stimulate the gonads (ovaries and testes) to secrete female (estrogen and progesterone) or male sex hormones (testosterone). Puberty is complete in females with the first ovulatory menstrual period and is complete in males with the first ejaculation that contains mature sperm.

The Female Reproductive System

1. The function of the female reproductive system is to produce mature ova; if fertilization occurs, the female reproductive system provides protection and nourishment of the fetus until it is expelled at birth.
2. The external female genitalia are the mons pubis, labia majora, labia minora, clitoris, vestibule (urinary and vaginal openings), and perineum. They protect body openings and may play a role in sexual functioning.
3. The internal female genitalia are the vagina, uterus, fallopian tubes, and ovaries. Although all these organs are needed for reproduction, the ovaries are the most essential because they produce the female gametes and female sex hormones.
4. The vagina is a fibromuscular canal that receives the penis during sexual intercourse and is the exit route for menstrual fluids and products of conception. The vagina leads from the introitus (its external opening) to the cervical portion of the uterus.
5. The uterus is the hollow, muscular organ in which a fertilized ovum develops until birth. The uterine walls have three layers: the endometrium (lining), myometrium (muscular layer), and perimetrium (outer covering, which is continuous with the pelvic peritoneum). The endometrium proliferates (thickens) and is shed in response to cyclic changes in levels of female sex hormones. The cervix is the narrow, lower portion of the uterus that opens into the vagina.
6. The two fallopian tubes extend from the uterus to the ovaries. Their function is to conduct ova from the spaces around the ovaries to the uterus. Fertilization normally occurs in the distal third of the fallopian tubes.
7. From puberty to menopause, the ovaries are the site of (a) ovum maturation and release and (b) production of female sex hormones (estrogen, progesterone) and androgens. The female sex hormones

are involved in sexual differentiation and development, the menstrual cycle, pregnancy, and lactation. Although they are primarily male sex hormones, androgens in women are precursors of female sex hormones and contribute to the prepubertal growth spurt, pubic and axillary hair growth, and activation of sebaceous glands.

8. Estrogen (primarily estradiol) is produced by cells in the developing ovarian follicle (structure that encloses the ovum). Progesterone is produced by cells of the corpus luteum, the structure that develops from the ruptured ovarian follicle after ovulation (ovum release). Androgens are produced within the ovarian follicle, adrenal glands, and adipose tissue.
9. The average menstrual cycle lasts 25 to 30 days and consists of three phases, which are named for ovarian and endometrial changes: the ischemic/menstrual phase (menstruation), the follicular/proliferative phase (postmenstrual), and the luteal/secretory phase (premenstrual).
10. Ovarian events of the menstrual cycle are controlled by gonadotropins and follicular secretion of inhibin. High FSH levels stimulate follicle and ovum maturation (follicular phase); then a surge of LH causes ovulation, which is followed by development of the corpus luteum (luteal phase).
11. Uterine (endometrial) phases of the menstrual cycle are caused by ovarian hormones. During the follicular phase of the ovarian cycle, estrogen produced by the follicle causes the endometrium to proliferate (proliferative phase). During the luteal phase, estrogen maintains the thickened endometrium, and progesterone causes it to develop blood vessels and secretory glands (secretory phase). During the ischemic/menstrual phase, the corpus luteum degenerates, production of both hormones drops sharply, and the "starved" endometrium degenerates and is shed, causing menstruation.
12. Cyclic changes in hormone levels also cause thinning and thickening of the vaginal epithelium, thinning and thickening of cervical secretions, and changes in basal body temperature.

Structure and Function of the Breast

1. Until puberty, the female and male breasts are similar, consisting of a small, underdeveloped nipple, some fatty and fibrous tissue, and a few ductlike structures under the areola. At puberty, however, a variety of hormones (estrogen, progesterone, prolactin, growth hormone, insulin, cortisol) cause the female breast to develop into a system of glands and ducts that is capable of producing and ejecting milk.
2. The basic functional unit of the female breast is the lobe, a system of ducts that branches from the nipple to milk-producing units called *lobules*. Each breast contains 15 to 20 lobes, which are separated and supported by Cooper ligaments. The lobules contain *acini cells*, which are convoluted spaces lined with epithelial cells. Contraction of the subepithelial cells of each acinus moves milk into the system of ducts that leads to the nipple.
3. Milk production occurs in response to prolactin, a hormone that is secreted in larger amounts after childbirth. Milk ejection is under the control of oxytocin, another hormone of pregnancy and lactation.
4. During the reproductive years, breast tissue undergoes cyclic changes in response to hormonal changes of the menstrual cycle. At menopause, the tissue involutes, fat deposits and connective tissue increase, and the breasts reduce in size and firmness.
5. The male breast does not develop because of the absence of sufficiently high levels of estrogen and progesterone, and antagonistic effects of androgens.

The Male Reproductive System

1. The function of the male reproductive system is to produce male gametes (sperm) and deliver them to the female reproductive tract.
2. The external male genitalia are the testes, epididymides, scrotum, and penis.
3. The testes (male gonads) are paired glands suspended within the scrotum. The testes have two functions: spermatogenesis (sperm production) and production of male sex hormones (androgens, chiefly testosterone).
4. The epididymis is a long, coiled tube arranged in a comma-shaped compartment that curves over the top and rear of the testis. The epididymis receives sperm from the testis and stores them while they develop further. Sperm travel the length of the epididymis and then are ejaculated into the vas deferens, which transports sperm to the urethra.
5. The scrotum is a skin-covered, fibromuscular sac that encloses the testes and epididymides, which are suspended within the scrotum by the spermatic cord. The scrotum keeps these organs at optimal temperatures for sperm survival (about 1° to 2°C lower than body temperature) by contracting in cold environments and relaxing in warm environments.
6. The penis is a cylindrical organ consisting of three longitudinal compartments (two corpora cavernosa and one corpus spongiosum) and the urethra. The urethra runs through the corpus spongiosum. The corpora cavernosa and corpus spongiosum consist of erectile tissue. Externally the penis consists of a shaft and a tip, which is called the *glans*.
7. The penis has two functions: delivery of sperm and elimination of urine.
8. Sexual intercourse is made possible by the erectile reflex, in which tactile or psychogenic stimulation of the parasympathetic nerves causes arterioles in the corpora cavernosa and corpus spongiosum to dilate and fill with blood, causing the penis to enlarge and become firm.
9. The internal genitalia are the vas deferens, ejaculatory duct, prostatic and membranous sections of the urethra, seminal vesicles, prostate gland, and bulbourethral glands.
10. Emission, which occurs at the peak of sexual arousal, is the movement of semen from the epididymides to the penis. Ejaculation, which is a continuation of emission, is the pulsatile ejection of semen from the penis.
11. Spermatogenesis is a continuous process because spermatogonia, the primitive male gametes, undergo continuous mitosis within the seminiferous tubules of the testes. Some spermatogonia develop into primary spermatocytes, which divide meiotically into secondary spermatocytes and then spermatids. The spermatids develop into sperm with the help of nutrients and hormonal signals from Sertoli cells.
12. Production of the male sex hormones (androgens) is controlled by interactions among the hypothalamus, anterior pituitary, and gonads. The male hormones are produced steadily rather than cyclically, however.

Aging and Reproductive Function

1. Perimenopause is the transitional period between reproductive and nonreproductive years in women.
2. Menopause, the point that marks 12 consecutive months of amenorrhea, includes atrophic changes in the ovaries, vagina, and breast; loss of bone mass; and increased risk for cardiovascular disease.
3. Andropause is androgen deficiency in the aging male and occurs in only a small percentage of men. There is a decrease in testosterone production with testicular atrophy, decreased fertility, and some loss of muscle mass and strength.

KEY TERMS

Acinus (*pl.*, acini) of breast, 805
Activin, 804
Adrenarche, 796
Androgen, 796
Andropause, 812
Areola, 806
Breast, 805
Bulbourethral gland (Cowper gland), 809
Cervix, 799
Cornification, 805
Corpus (body of uterus), 799
Corpus cavernosum (*pl.*, corpora cavernosa), 808
Corpus luteum, 800
Corpus spongiosum, 808
Cul-de-sac, 798
Decornification, 805
Efferent tubule, 807
Ejaculatory duct, 809
Emission, 809
Endocervical canal, 799
Endometrium, 799
Epididymis (*pl.*, epididymides), 808
Erectile reflex, 809
Estradiol (E_2), 801
Estrogen, 801
Fallopian tube (uterine tube), 800
Fimbriae, 800
Follicle-stimulating hormone (FSH), 794
Follicular/proliferative phase, 803
Follistatin, 804
Fornix, 798
Fundus, 799
Glands of Montgomery, 806
Glans, 808
Gonad, 793
Gonadarche, 795
Gonadostat (gonadotropin-releasing hormone pulse generator), 794
Gonadotropin-releasing hormone (GnRH), 794
Granulosa cell, 801
Infundibulum, 800
Inguinal canal, 807
Inhibin, 804
Ischemic/menstrual phase, 803
Isthmus, 799
Leydig cell, 807
Libido, 810
Luteal/secretory phase, 803
Luteinizing hormone (LH), 794
Menarche, 802
Menopause, 802
Menstruation (menses), 803
Myometrium, 799
Nipple, 806
Ovarian cycle, 801
Ovarian follicle, 800
Ovary, 800
Ovulation, 803
Ovum (*pl.*, ova), 793
Oxytocin, 806
Penis, 808
Perimetrium (parietal peritoneum), 799
Prepuce (foreskin), 808
Primary spermatocyte, 810
Progesterone, 801
Prostate gland, 809
Puberty, 795
Rete testis, 807
Ruga (*pl.*, rugae), 798
Scrotum, 808
Secondary spermatocyte, 810
Semen, 809
Seminal vesicle, 809
Seminiferous tubule, 807
Sertoli cell (nondividing support cell), 810
Sex hormone, 793
Spermatid, 810
Spermatogenesis, 810
Spermatogonium (*pl.*, spermatogonia), 810
Spermatozoon (sperm cell), 793
Spinnbarkeit mucus, 800
Squamocolumnar junction, 799
Testis, 807
Testosterone, 794
Theca cell, 801
Thelarche, 795
Tubulus rectus, 807
Tunica albuginea, 807
Tunica dartos, 808
Tunica vaginalis, 807
Urethra, 809
Uterus, 799
Vagina, 798
Vas deferens, 808
Vasomotor flush, 811
Vulva, 796

REFERENCES

1. Alves, M. G., Rato, L., Carvalho, R. A., et al. (2013). Hormonal control of Sertoli cell metabolism regulates spermatogenesis. *Cellular and Molecular Life Sciences, 70*(5), 777–793. doi:10.1007/s00018-012-1079-1.
2. Berga, S., & Naftolin, F. (2012). Neuroendocrine control of ovulation. *Gynecological Endocrinology, 28*(Suppl. 1), 9–13. doi:10.3109/09513590.2012.651929.
3. Larney, C., Bailey, T. L., & Koopman, P. (2014). Switching on sex: Transcriptional regulation of the testis-determining gene *SRY*. *Development (Cambridge, England), 141*(11), 2195–2205. doi:10.1242/dev.107052.
4. Martin, R. J., Fanaroff, A. A., & Walsh, M. C. (2014). *Fanaroff and Martin's neonatal-perinatal medicine* (10th ed.). Philadelphia: Saunders.
5. Tomova, A., Robeva, R., & Kumanov, P. (2015). Influence of the body weight on the onset and progression of puberty in boys. *Journal of Pediatric Endocrinology & Metabolism : JPEM, 28*(7–8), 859–865. doi:10.1515/jpem-2014-0363.
6. Biro, F. M., Greenspan, L. C., & Galvez, M. P. (2012). Puberty in girls of the 21st century. *Journal of Pediatric and Adolescent Gynecology, 25*(5), 289–294. doi:10.1016/j.jpag.2012.05.009.
7. Burt Solorzano, C. M., & McCartney, C. R. (2010). Obesity and the pubertal transition in girls and boys. *Reproduction (Cambridge, England), 140*(3), 399–410. doi:10.1530/REP-10-0119.
8. Lentz, G. M., Lobo, R., Gershenson, D., et al. (2012). *Comprehensive gynecology* (6th ed.). St. Louis: Mosby.
9. Labrie, F. (2015). All sex steroids are made intracellularly in peripheral tissues by the mechanisms of intracrinology after menopause. *Journal of Steroid Biochemistry and Molecular Biology, 145C*, 133–138. doi:10.1016/j.jsbmb.2014.06.001.
10. Macias, H., & Hinck, L. (2012). Mammary gland development. *Wiley Interdisciplinary Reviews. Developmental Biology, 1*(4), 533–557. doi:10.1002/wdev.35.
11. Schumacher, A., Costa, S. D., & Zenclussen, A. C. (2014). Endocrine factors modulating immune responses in pregnancy. *Frontiers in Immunology, 5*, 196. doi:10.3389/fimmu.2014.00196.
12. The Sex Information and Education Council of Canada. (2013). *Early menarche: Trends, risks and possible causes.* Retrieved from http://studylib.net/doc/8125998/early-menarche--trends--risks-and-possible-causes.
13. Karapanou, O., & Papadimitriou, A. (2010). Determinants of menarche. *Reproductive Biology and Endocrinology, 8*, 115. doi:10.1186/1477-7827-8-115.
14. Rogol, A. D. (2010). Sex steroids, growth hormone, leptin and the pubertal growth spurt. *Endocrine Development, 17*, 77–85. doi:10.1159/000262530.
15. Rosenfield, R. L. (2013). Clinical review: Adolescent anovulation: Maturational mechanisms and implications. *Journal of Clinical Endocrinology and Metabolism, 98*(9), 3572–3583. doi:10.1210/jc.2013-1770.
16. Adams Hillard, P. J., & Deitch, H. R. (2005). Menstrual disorders in the college age female. *Pediatric Clinics of North America, 52*(1), 179–197, ix–x. doi:10.1016/j.pcl.2004.10.004.
17. Pandey, S., & Bhattacharya, S. (2010). Impact of obesity on gynecology. *Womens Health (London), 6*(1), 107–117. doi:10.2217/whe.09.77.
18. Scheid, J. L., & De Souza, M. J. (2010). Menstrual irregularities and energy deficiency in physically active women: The role of ghrelin, PYY and adipocytokines. *Medicine and Sport Science, 55*, 82–102. doi:10.1159/000321974.
19. Yamanoto, K., Okazaki, A., Sakamoto, Y., et al. (2009). The relationship between premenstrual symptoms, menstrual pain, irregular menstrual cycles, and psychosocial stress among Japanese college students. *Journal of Physiological Anthropology, 28*(3), 129–136.
20. Richards, J. S., & Pangas, S. A. (2010). The ovary: Basic biology and clinical implications. *Journal of Clinical Investigation, 120*(4), 963–972. doi:10.1172/JCI41350.
21. Messinis, I. E. (2006). Ovarian feedback, mechanism of action and possible clinical implications. *Human Reproduction Update, 12*(5), 557–571. doi:10.1093/humupd/dml020.
22. Makanji, Y., Harrison, C. A., & Robertson, D. M. (2011). Feedback regulation by inhibins A and B of the pituitary secretion of follicle-stimulating hormone. *Vitamins and Hormones, 85*, 299–321. doi:10.1016/B978-0-12-385961-7.00014-7.
23. Henriet, P., Gaide Chevronnay, H. P., & Marbaix, E. (2012). The endocrine and paracrine control of menstruation. *Molecular and Cellular Endocrinology, 358*(2), 197–207. doi:10.1016/j.mce.2011.07.042.
24. Curlin, M., & Bursac, D. (2013). Cervical mucus: From biochemical structure to clinical implications. *Frontiers in Bioscience (Scholar Edition), 5*, 507–515.
25. Pallone, S. R., & Bergus, G. R. (2009). Fertility awareness-based methods: Another option for family planning. *Journal of the American Board of Family Medicine : JABFM, 22*(2), 147–157. doi:10.3122/jabfm.2009.02.080038.
26. Barnes, C., Speroni, L., Quinn, K. P., et al. (2014). From single cells to tissues: Interactions between the matrix and human breast cells in real time. *PLoS ONE, 9*(4), e93325. doi:10.1371/journal.pone.0093325.
27. Jesinger, R. A. (2014). Breast anatomy for the interventionalist. *Techniques in Vascular and Interventional Radiology, 17*(1), 3–9. doi:10.1053/j.tvir.2013.12.002.
28. Ballard, O., & Morrow, A. L. (2013). Human milk composition: Nutrients and bioactive factors.

Pediatric Clinics of North America, 60(1), 49–74. doi:10.1016/j.pcl.2012.10.002.

29. Bachelot, A., & Binart, N. (2007). Reproductive role of prolactin. *Reproduction (Cambridge, England), 133*(2), 361–369. doi:10.1530/REP-06-0299.
30. Buitrón-García-Figueroa, R., Malanco-Hernández, L. M., Lara-Ricalde, R., et al. (2014). [Contraception and breast feeding. Spacing of pregnancies. Present concepts] [Article in Spanish]. *Ginecologia Y Obstetricia de Mexico, 82*(6), 389–393.
31. Romero-Gutiérrez, G., Vaca-Ortiz, N., Ponce-Ponce de Léon, A. L., et al. (2007). Actual use of the lactational amenorrhoea method. *European Journal of Contraception and Reproductive Health Care, 12*(4), 340–344. doi:10.1080/13625180701536656.
32. Limony, Y., Friger, M., & Hochberg, Z. (2013). Pubertal gynecomastia coincides with peak height velocity. *Journal of Clinical Research in Pediatric Endocrinology, 5*(3), 142–144. doi:10.4274/Jcrpe.958.
33. Reyes, J. G., Farias, J. G., Henriquez-Olavarrieta, S., et al. (2012). The hypoxic testicle: Physiology and pathophysiology. *Oxidative Medicine and Cellular Longevity, 2012*, 929285. doi:10.1155/2012/929285.
34. Dacheux, J. L., & Dacheux, F. (2013). New insights into epididymal function in relation to sperm maturation. *Reproduction (Cambridge, England), 147*(2), R27–R42. doi:10.1530/REP-13-0420.
35. Giuliano, F. (2010). Neurophysiology of erection and ejaculation. *Journal of Sexual Medicine, 8*(Suppl. 4), 310–315. doi:10.1111/j.1743-6109.2011.02450.x.
36. Hsieh, C. H., Liu, S. P., Hsu, G. L., et al. (2012). Advances in understanding of mammalian penile evolution, human penile anatomy and human erection physiology: Clinical implications for physicians and surgeons. *Medical Science Monitor, 18*(7), RA118–RA125.
37. Hogarth, C. A., & Griswold, M. D. (2010). The key role of vitamin A in spermatogenesis. *Journal of Clinical Investigation, 120*(4), 956–962. doi:10.1172/JCI41303.
38. Aitken, R. J., & Nixon, B. (2013). Sperm capacitation: A distant landscape glimpsed but unexplored. *Molecular Human Reproduction, 19*(12), 785–793. doi:10.1093/molehr/gat067.
39. Hiort, O. (2013). The differential role of androgens in early human sex development. *BMC Medicine, 11*, 152. doi:10.1186/1741-7015-11-152.
40. Forman, M. R., Mangini, L. D., Thelus-Jean, R., et al. (2013). Life-course origins of the ages at menarche and menopause. *Adolescent Health, Medicine and Therapeutics, 4*, 1–21. doi:10.2147/AHMT.S15946.
41. Hale, G. E., Robertson, D. M., & Burger, H. G. (2014). The perimenopausal woman: Endocrinology and management. *Journal of Steroid Biochemistry and Molecular Biology, 142*, 121–131. doi:10.1016/j.jsbmb.2013.08.015.
42. Su, H. I., & Freeman, E. W. (2009). Hormone changes associated with the menopausal transition. *Minerva Ginecologica, 61*(6), 483–489.
43. Gold, E. B. (2011). The timing of the age at which natural menopause occurs. *Obstetrics and Gynecology Clinics of North America, 38*(3), 425–440. doi:10.1016/j.ogc.2011.05.002.
44. Freedman, R. R. (2014). Menopausal hot flashes: Mechanisms, endocrinology, treatment. *Journal of Steroid Biochemistry and Molecular Biology, 142*, 115–120. doi:10.1016/j.jsbmb.2013.08.010.
45. Collaborative Group on Hormonal Factors in Breast Cancer. (2012). Menarche, menopause, and breast cancer risk: Individual participant meta-analysis, including 118,964 women with breast cancer from 117 epidemiological studies. *Lancet Oncology, 13*(11), 1141–1151. doi:10.1016/S1470-2045(12)70425-4.
46. Cramer, D. W. (2012). The epidemiology of endometrial and ovarian cancer. *Hematology/Oncology Clinics of North America, 26*(1), 1–12. doi:10.1016/j.hoc.2011.10.009.
47. Grant, M. D., Marbella, A., Wang, A. T., et al. (2015). *Comparative effectiveness review: Number 147. Menopausal symptoms: Comparative effectiveness of therapies.* Rockville, MD: Agency for Healthcare Research and Quality. Retrieved from http://effectivehealthcare.ahrq.gov/search-for-guides-reviews-and-reports/?pageaction=displayproduct&productID=2051.
48. Neves-E-Castro, M., Birkhauser, M., Samsioe, G., et al. (2015). EMAS position statement: The ten-point guide to the integral management of menopausal health. *Maturitas, 81*(1), 88–92. doi:10.1016/j.maturitas.2015.02.003.
49. Paul, C., & Robaire, B. (2013). Ageing of the male germ line. *Nature Reviews. Urology, 10*(4), 227–234. doi:10.1038/nrurol.2013.18.
50. Pines, A. (2011). Male menopause: Is it a real clinical syndrome? *Climacteric, 14*(1), 15–17. doi:10.3109/13697137.2010.507442.
51. Basaria, S. (2013). Reproductive aging in men. *Endocrinology and Metabolism Clinics of North America, 42*(2), 255–270. doi:10.1016/j.ecl.2013.02.012.
52. Corona, G., Rastrelli, G., Maseroli, E., et al. (2013). Sexual function of the ageing male. *Best Practice and Research. Clinical Endocrinology and Metabolism, 27*(4), 581–601. doi:10.1016/j.beem.2013.05.007.
53. Zirkin, B. R., & Tenover, J. L. (2012). Aging and declining testosterone: Past, present, and hopes for the future. *Journal of Andrology, 33*(6), 1111–1118. doi:10.2164/jandrol.112.017160.
54. Crosnoe, L. E., & Kim, E. D. (2013). Impact of age on male fertility. *Current Opinion in Obstetrics and Gynecology, 25*(3), 181–185. doi:10.1097/GCO.0b013e32836024cb.

33

Alterations of the Female Reproductive System

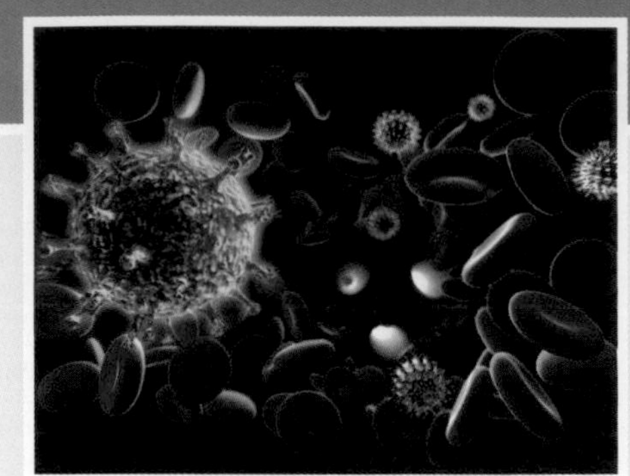

Kathryn L. McCance, Afsoon Moktar, and Kelly Power-Kean

EVOLVE WEBSITE

http://evolve.elsevier.com/Canada/Huether/pathophysiology
Student Review Questions
Key Points
Case Studies
Animations
Quick Check Answers

CHAPTER OUTLINE

Abnormalities of the Female Reproductive Tract, 816
Alterations of Sexual Maturation, 817
- Delayed or Absent Puberty, 818
- Precocious Puberty, 818

Disorders of the Female Reproductive System, 819
- Hormonal and Menstrual Alterations, 819
- Infection and Inflammation, 823
- Pelvic Organ Prolapse, 827
- Benign Growths and Proliferative Conditions, 829
- Cancer, 833
- Sexual Dysfunction, 842
- Impaired Fertility, 843

Disorders of the Female Breast, 843
- Galactorrhea, 843
- Benign Breast Disease and Conditions, 844
- Breast Cancer, 845

Alterations of the reproductive system span a wide range of concerns—from delayed sexual development and suboptimal sexual performance to structural and functional abnormalities. Many common reproductive disorders carry potentially serious physiological or psychological consequences. For example, sexual or reproductive dysfunction, such as impotence or infertility, can dramatically affect self-concept, relationships, and overall quality of life. Conversely, organic and psychosocial problems, such as alcoholism, depression, situational stressors, chronic illness, and medications, can affect ovulation and menstruation, sexual performance, and fertility and may be risk factors for the development of some types of reproductive tract cancers. Diagnosis and treatment of reproductive system disorders, however, are often complicated by the stigma and symbolism associated with the reproductive organs and emotion-laden beliefs and behaviours related to reproductive health.[1] Treatment or diagnosis for any problem may be delayed because of embarrassment, guilt, fear, or denial.

ABNORMALITIES OF THE FEMALE REPRODUCTIVE TRACT

Normal development of the female reproductive tract requires absence of testosterone during embryonic and fetal life (see Chapter 32). The resulting fusion of the two paramesonephric (müllerian) ducts produces the normal cervix and the uterus with an internal cavity. The distal portions of the paramesonephric ducts remain independent and form the two fallopian/uterine tubes. Alterations in the normal process include errors in cellular sensitivity to testosterone (androgen insensitivity) or failures of cell line migration resulting in changes in the structure of the reproductive organs.

Androgen insensitivity occurs in its most extreme form in about 1 in 20 000 people[2] and is discussed briefly in this chapter because of the often-resulting female phenotype despite a male genotype. **Androgen insensitivity syndrome (AIS)** is a disorder of hormone resistance characterized by a female phenotype in an individual with an XY karyotype or male genotype, and with testes producing age-appropriate normal concentrations of androgens.[3] To date, more than 1 000 mutations have been reported in the androgen receptor, with most of these being associated with AIS.[4] Children with complete androgen insensitivity may have testes palpable within the labia majora, but are often not diagnosed until puberty.[5] Breast development may be normal but pubic and axillary hair is often sparse and menarche does not occur because of the absence of a cervix, uterus, and ovaries.[5] A short vagina that ends blindly also may be present. Milder forms of androgen insensitivity (also a common cause of male infertility)[2] are much more common and have less dramatic phenotypic manifestations with many having normal male genitalia.

Other abnormalities of the uterus, cervix, and fallopian/uterine tubes have multifactorial origins, often the result of an interaction between genetic predisposition and environmental factors. Such interactions result in müllerian duct abnormalities.[6] Some medications, chemicals, and toxins have been implicated as a direct cause of uterine abnormalities.

About 5% of the general female population has some sort of uterine abnormality, but the rate is much higher in populations of women who have experienced infertility or miscarriage.[7] Most uterine abnormalities stem from abnormal cell migration in the müllerian ducts during key moments in fetal development (Figure 33-1). Uterine abnormalities are rarely diagnosed until the woman has trouble becoming pregnant

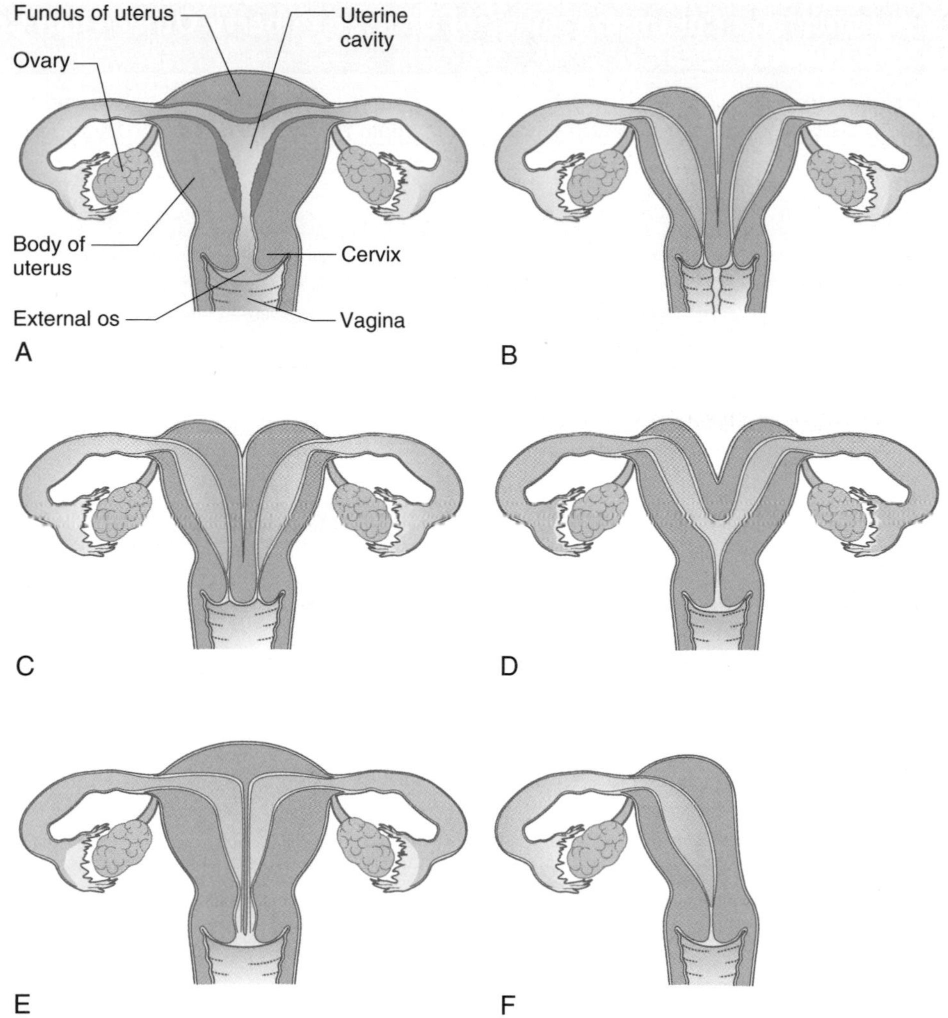

FIGURE 33-1 Uterine Malformations. Congenital uterine abnormalities. **A,** The normal configuration of the uterus and the ovaries. **B,** Double uterus with a double vagina and, **C,** a single vagina. **D,** Bicornuate uterus. **E,** A uterus with a midline septum. **F,** Unicornuate uterus. (From de Bruyn, R. [2010]. *Pediatric ultrasound* [2nd ed.]. London: Churchill Livingstone.)

or carrying a baby to term because the uterus is capable of menstruation but may have difficulty supporting a growing fetus.[6] Uterine malformations are usually diagnosed by ultrasound during pregnancy or with magnetic resonance imaging (MRI). Their prognosis depends on the severity of the malformation and the location and size of the placenta and fetus. Some abnormalities can be surgically corrected to improve the outcome of subsequent pregnancies.[6] Abnormalities of the lower genital tract also can result in women having two vaginas or a vaginal septum (a thin membrane dividing the vaginal vault). For most women, these structural abnormalities do not create functional problems but can be surgically corrected if needed.

ALTERATIONS OF SEXUAL MATURATION

The process of sexual maturation, or **puberty**, is marked by the development of secondary sex characteristics, rapid growth, and, ultimately, the ability to reproduce. A variety of congenital and endocrine disorders can disrupt the timing of puberty. These disorders may cause puberty to occur too late (*delayed puberty*) or too early (*precocious puberty*). Both types involve an inappropriate onset of sex hormone production by the gonads.

The age of puberty is multifactorial, involving genetic and environmental components. The study of epigenetics and the regulation of puberty is only beginning.[8,9] A Canadian-based study revealed that variations related to menarch were statistically significant related to the province of residence, household income, and family type. The provinces of New Brunswick, Prince Edward Island, and Quebec had the highest proportions of early menarche, while Ontario had the highest proportions of late menarch. As there are limited Canadian studies related to this topic, it is speculated that these variations are associated with ethnic background diversity, lifestyle variations, and disparity in socioeconomic classes.[10] Research has also shown that obesity decreases the age at onset of puberty by about 6 months. Although many factors are associated with obesity, much research is being done on leptin-responsive pathways in the regulation of eating behaviours and the onset of puberty, follicle-stimulating hormone (FSH), and luteinizing hormone (LH).[11,12] A recent genetic study found that pubertal onset in girls is strongly influenced by genetic variation affecting FSH.[13] FSH stimulates ovarian follicle maturation and estradiol synthesis, which is responsible for breast development.[13] The normal range for the onset of puberty is now 8 to 13 years of age. Although there are conflicting and inconsistent reports, the age of pubertal onset appears to be decreasing for girls.[14]

TABLE 33-1 Frequency and Common Causes of Delayed Puberty Other Than Constitutional Delay of Growth and Puberty

Delayed Puberty	Hypergonadotropic Hypogonadism	Permanent Hypogonadotropic Hypogonadism	Functional Hypogonadotropic Hypogonadism
Frequency (%)			
Boys	5–10	10	20
Girls	25	20	20
Common causes	Turner's syndrome, gonadal dysgenesis, chemotherapy, or radiation therapy	Tumours or infiltrative diseases of the central nervous system, GnRH deficiency (isolated hypogonadotropic hypogonadism, Kallmann's syndrome), combined pituitary-hormone deficiency, chemotherapy, or radiation therapy	Systemic illness (inflammatory bowel disease, celiac disease, anorexia nervosa, or bulimia), hypothyroidism, excessive exercise

GnRH, gonadotropin-releasing hormone.
From Palmert, M.R., & Dunkel, L. (2012). *N Engl J Med,* 366(5), 443–453.

This earlier onset appears primarily in breast development, not age of menarche.

Delayed or Absent Puberty

About 3% of children living in North America experience delayed development of secondary sex characteristics.[15] One of the first signs of puberty in girls is **thelarche**, or breast development; it should begin by 13 years of age. Normally, boys tend to mature later than girls, around 14 to 14.5 years of age. In boys, the first sign of maturity is enlargement of the testes and thinning of the scrotal skin. In **delayed puberty**, these secondary sex characteristics develop later.

In about 95% of cases, delayed puberty is a normal physiological event. Hormonal levels are normal, the hypothalamic-pituitary-gonadal (HPG) axis is intact, and maturation is slowly occurring. Treatment is seldom needed unless the delayed puberty is causing psychosocial problems.[16]

The other 5% of cases are caused by the disruption of the HPG axis or by the outcomes of a systemic disease. Treatment depends on the cause (Table 33-1 and Box 33-1), and referral to a pediatric endocrinologist is recommended.[17]

Precocious Puberty

Precocious puberty is a rare event, affecting about 1 in 10 000 girls and fewer than 1 in 50 000 boys. Precocious puberty has been defined as sexual maturation occurring before age 6 in black girls or age 7 in white girls and before age 9 in boys. Precocious puberty for boys of all ethnic or racial groups is defined as sexual maturation occurring before age 9. Precocious puberty may be caused by many conditions (Box 33-2), including obesity, an increase in protein consumption, and endocrine disruptors in common household products, pesticides, plasticizers, and pharmaceuticals,[18,19] as well as lethal central nervous system (CNS) tumours. All cases of precocious puberty require thorough evaluation.

All forms of precocious puberty are treated by identifying and removing the underlying cause or administering appropriate hormones (see Boxes 33-2 and 33-3). In many cases, precocious puberty can be reversed. However, **complete precocious puberty**, the onset and progression of all pubertal features (i.e., thelarche, pubarche, and menarche), is a challenge to treat and causes long bones to stop growing before the child has reached normal height.

QUICK CHECK 33-1

1. Why does puberty occur too late or too early in some individuals?
2. Define the normal age range for the onset of puberty.

BOX 33-1 Causes of Delayed Puberty

Hypergonadotropic Hypogonadism (Increased Follicle-Stimulating Hormone [FSH] and Luteinizing Hormone [LH])

1. Gonadal dysgenesis, most commonly Turner's syndrome (45,X/46,XX; structural X or Y abnormalities; or mosaicism)
2. Klinefelter's syndrome (47,XXY)
3. Bilateral gonadal failure
   a. Traumatic or infectious
   b. Postsurgical, postirradiation, or postchemotherapy
   c. Autoimmune
   d. Idiopathic empty-scrotum or vanishing-testes syndrome (congenital anorchia) or resistant-ovary syndrome

Hypogonadotropic Hypogonadism (Decreased LH, Depressed FSH)

1. Reversible
   a. Physiological delay
   b. Weight loss or anorexia
   c. Strenuous exercise
   d. Severe obesity
   e. Illegal drug use, especially marihuana
   f. Primary hypothyroidism
   g. Congenital adrenal hyperplasia
   h. Cushing's syndrome
   i. Prolactinomas
2. Irreversible
   a. Gonadotropin-releasing hormone deficiency (Kallmann's syndrome) or idiopathic hypogonadotropic hypogonadism
   b. Hypopituitarism
   c. Congenital central nervous system defects
   d. Other pituitary adenomas
   e. Craniopharyngioma
   f. Malignant pituitary tumours

Eugonadism

These conditions are associated with amenorrhea but may have otherwise normal pubertal development:

1. Congenital anomalies
   a. Müllerian agenesis
   b. Vaginal septum or imperforate hymen
2. Androgen insensitivity syndrome
3. Inappropriate positive feedback

BOX 33-2 Primary Forms of Precocious Puberty

Complete Precocious Puberty

Premature development of appropriate characteristics for the child's gender
Hypothalamic-pituitary-ovarian axis functioning normally but prematurely
In about 10% of cases, lethal central nervous system tumour may be the cause

Partial Precocious Puberty

Partial development of appropriate secondary sex characteristics
Premature thelarche (breast budding) seen in girls between 6 months and 2 years of age
Does not progress to complete puberty (ovulation and menstruation)
Premature adrenarche (growth of axillary and pubic hair) tends to occur between 5 and 8 years of age
Can progress to complete precocious puberty; may be caused by estrogen-secreting neoplasms or may be a variant of normal pubertal development

Mixed Precocious Puberty

Causes the child to develop some secondary sex characteristics of the opposite gender
Common causes: adrenal hyperplasia or androgen-secreting tumours

Data from Burns, C.E., Dunn, A.M., Brady, M.A., et al. (Eds.). (2009). *Pediatric primary care* (4th ed.). St. Louis: Saunders; Osborn, L.M., DeWitt, T.G., First, L.R., et al. (Eds.). (2005). *Pediatrics.* Philadelphia: Mosby.

BOX 33-3 Causes of Mixed Precocious Puberty

Female (Virilization)	Male (Feminization)
Congenital adrenal hyperplasia	Estrogen-producing tumours
Androgen-secreting tumours	Adrenal
Adrenal	Teratoma
Ovarian	Hepatoma
Teratoma	Testicular
Exogenous androgens	Exogenous estrogens
	Increased peripheral conversion of androgens to estrogens

From Jospe, N. (2005). Disorders of pubertal development. In L.M. Osborn, T.G. DeWitt, L.R. First, et al. (Eds.), *Pediatrics.* Philadelphia: Mosby.

DISORDERS OF THE FEMALE REPRODUCTIVE SYSTEM

Hormonal and Menstrual Alterations

Dysmenorrhea

Primary dysmenorrhea is painful menstruation associated with the release of prostaglandins in ovulatory cycles, but not with pelvic disease. Approximately 50% of all women experience dysmenorrhea, and 10% are incapacitated for 1 to 3 days because of pain severity. Primary dysmenorrhea begins with the onset of ovulatory cycles, and prevalence is highest during adolescence.[20] The incidence steadily rises, peaks in women in the late teens and early twenties, and decreases slowly thereafter. **Secondary dysmenorrhea** is related to pelvic pathological conditions, manifests later in the reproductive years, and may occur any time in the menstrual cycle.

PATHOPHYSIOLOGY Primary dysmenorrhea results mostly from excessive prostaglandin $F_2\alpha$ ($PGF_2\alpha$), a potent myometrial stimulant and vasoconstrictor, found in secretory endometrium. Elevated levels of prostaglandins, especially $PGF_2\alpha$ and $PGE_2\alpha$, increase myometrial contractions, constrict endometrial blood vessels, and enhance nerve hypersensitivity, resulting in pain.[21] These changes can lead to ischemia and endometrial shedding. Increased synthesis of prostaglandins may result from increased cyclo-oxygenase (COX) enzyme activity. Inflammatory mediators produced in leukocytes (leukotrienes) also contribute to increased levels of pain.[21] The first 48 hours of menstruation correlate with higher prostaglandin levels. Women who are anovulatory because they use oral contraceptives rarely have primary dysmenorrhea. Secondary dysmenorrhea results from disorders such as endometriosis (most common cause), endometritis (infection), pelvic inflammatory disease, adhesions, obstructive uterine or vaginal anomalies, inflammation, uterine fibroids, polyps, tumours, cysts, or intrauterine devices (IUDs).[21]

CLINICAL MANIFESTATIONS The chief symptom of dysmenorrhea is pelvic pain associated with the onset of menses. The severity is directly related to length and amount of menstrual flow. The pain often radiates into the groin and may be accompanied by backache, anorexia, vomiting, diarrhea, syncope, and headache. The latter symptoms are caused by the entry of prostaglandins and their metabolites into the systemic circulation. The discomfort commonly begins shortly before the onset of menstruation and rarely persists 1 to 3 days during menstrual flow.[21]

EVALUATION AND TREATMENT Primary dysmenorrhea can be differentiated from secondary dysmenorrhea by obtaining a thorough medical history and performing a pelvic examination. Nonsteroidal anti-inflammatory drugs (NSAIDs, e.g., ibuprofen) are the treatment of choice because they reduce COX enzyme activity and thus prostaglandin production. NSAIDs are effective in the majority of women with primary dysmenorrhea and are most effective if started at the first sign of bleeding or cramping. In women who desire contraception, dysmenorrhea may be relieved with hormonal contraceptives. Hormonal contraception stops ovulation and creates an atrophic endometrium, thereby decreasing prostaglandin synthesis and myometrial contractility. Regular exercise and stress reduction are thought to prevent or reduce symptoms. Other palliative approaches with some evidence of effectiveness in pain relief include local application of heat; acupuncture; high-frequency transcutaneous electrical nerve stimulation (TENS); supplements, such as thiamine and vitamin E; and Chinese herbal treatment.[22]

Amenorrhea

Amenorrhea means lack of menstruation; and the most common causes (aside from pregnancy) include hypothalamic dysfunction, polycystic ovarian syndrome, hyperprolactinemia, and ovarian failure. **Primary amenorrhea** is the failure of menarche and the absence of menstruation by age 13 years without the development of secondary sex characteristics or by age 15 years, regardless of the presence of secondary sex characteristics[23]. **Secondary amenorrhea** is the absence of menstruation for a time equivalent to three or more cycles in women who have previously menstruated.

PATHOPHYSIOLOGY One approach to understanding the pathophysiology is to compartmentalize. *Compartment I disorders* are anatomical defects, including absence of the vagina and uterus. *Compartment II disorders* involve the ovary, primarily genetic disorders (such as Turner's syndrome) and AIS. The target organs (e.g., ovaries) in AIS are completely resistant to the action of androgens, resulting in a lack of estrogen. *Compartment III disorders* are of the anterior pituitary gland, including tumours, and result in failure of signalling to the ovaries through FSH

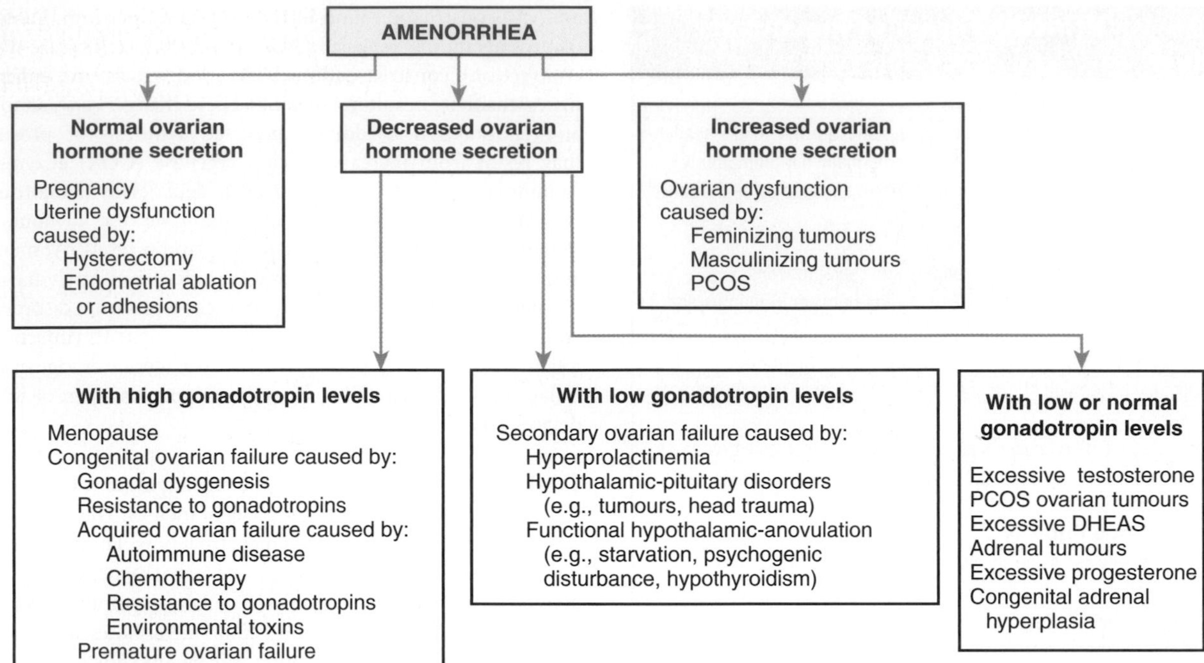

FIGURE 33-2 Causes of Secondary Amenorrhea. Of note, hypothyroidism is a relatively common condition and should be ruled out as the cause of hyperprolactinemia before more extensive evaluation (i.e., computed tomography or magnetic resonance imaging) occurs. *DHEAS*, dehydroepiandrosterone sulphate; *PCOS*, polycystic ovary syndrome.

and LH secretion. *Compartment IV disorders* include CNS disorders and primarily involve hypothalamic defects that prevent secretion of gonadotropin-releasing hormone (GnRH); thus, there is no signalling to the pituitary to release FSH and LH.

CLINICAL MANIFESTATIONS The major clinical manifestation of primary amenorrhea is the absence of the first menstrual period. The cause of the amenorrhea determines whether secondary sex characteristics and height are affected.

EVALUATION AND TREATMENT Diagnosis of primary amenorrhea is based on the results of a history and physical examination and determination of the presence or absence of secondary sexual characteristics. Laboratory studies may be required to document abnormal levels of gonadotropins or ovarian hormones or the presence of genetic conditions. Diagnostic imaging, including ultrasonography and MRI, is used to document structural abnormalities.

Treatment involves correction of any underlying disorders and implementation of hormone replacement therapy (HRT) to induce the development of secondary sex characteristics. Although surgical alteration of the genitalia may be undertaken to correct abnormalities, it should be postponed until the individual can make a truly informed decision.

Secondary Amenorrhea

Many disorders and physiological conditions are associated with secondary amenorrhea. Secondary amenorrhea is common (normal) during early adolescence, pregnancy, lactation, and the perimenopausal period, primarily because of anovulation. The most common causes (after pregnancy) are thyroid disorders (e.g., hypothyroidism); hyperprolactinemia; hypothalamic-pituitary-ovarian (HPO) interruption secondary to excessive exercise, stress, or weight loss; and polycystic ovary syndrome (PCOS).

PATHOPHYSIOLOGY The pathophysiology is dependent on the causes of secondary amenorrhea. These causes are summarized in Figure 33-2.

CLINICAL MANIFESTATIONS The major manifestation of secondary amenorrhea is the absence of menses after previous menstrual periods. Depending on the underlying cause of the amenorrhea, infertility, vasomotor flushes, vaginal atrophy, acne, osteopenia, and **hirsutism** (abnormal hairiness) may be present.

EVALUATION AND TREATMENT Pregnancy is the most common cause of secondary amenorrhea and must be ruled out before any further evaluation. A thorough history and physical examination is important because the menstrual cycle may stop or become irregular in response to stress, extreme exercise, large dietary changes, eating disorders, or sleep abnormalities. Hypothyroidism also is a common cause and should be ruled out as well. Diagnosis of secondary amenorrhea involves identifying underlying hormonal or anatomical alterations. Evaluation of thyroid-stimulating hormone (TSH) or prolactin levels may be indicated. Depending on the cause of the amenorrhea, treatment may involve HRT or a corrective procedure, such as surgical removal of a pituitary tumour. The choice of treatment may be influenced by the woman's child-bearing plans.

Abnormal Uterine Bleeding

Menstrual irregularity or abnormal bleeding patterns (Table 33-2) account for approximately 33% of all gynecological visits. The most common cause of cycle irregularity is failure to ovulate related to age, stress, or endocrinopathy. Common causes of abnormal bleeding based on age group and frequency are presented in Table 33-3.

Dysfunctional uterine bleeding (DUB) is heavy or irregular bleeding in the absence of organic disease (i.e., uterine fibroids, polyps, infection, or systemic disease). DUB is a diagnosis of exclusion made only after other causes have been ruled out. DUB accounts for 70% of all

TABLE 33-2 Abnormal Menstrual Bleeding Patterns

Term	Definition
Polymenorrhea	Cycles shorter than 3 weeks; may indicate disturbance in endocrine control of ovulation
Oligomenorrhea	Cycles longer than 6–7 weeks; may indicate disturbance in endocrine control of ovulation
Metrorrhagia	Intermenstrual bleeding or bleeding of light character occurring irregularly between cycles; may be a sign of an underlying physiological tissue/organ disorder
Hypermenorrhea	Excessive flow; may be a sign of an underlying physiological tissue/organ disorder
Menorrhea	Increased amount and duration of flow
Menorrhagia	Increased amount and duration of flow
Menometrorrhagia	Prolonged flow associated with irregular and intermittent spotting between bleeding episodes

hysterectomies, and almost all endometrial ablation procedures.[24] Perimenopausal women are by far the most affected by DUB.

PATHOPHYSIOLOGY The majority of DUB is associated with lack of ovulation.[25] Although DUB may occur at any time during the reproductive years and many conditions are associated with irregular ovulation, more than 50% of cases occur in perimenopausal women ages 40 to 50 years when they are more likely to ovulate irregularly. Women who fail to ovulate experience irregularities in their menstrual bleeding because of a lack of progesterone and, in some cases, an excess of estrogen. This results in excessive and irregular endometrial thickness and subsequent excessive and irregular bleeding. PCOS, obesity, and thyroid disease also are common contributors. Abnormal bleeding can result from defects of the corpus luteum resulting in progesterone deficiencies or from abnormalities of the uterus or cervix, such as endometrial polyps, uterine fibroids, or uterine or cervical cancers.

Abnormal menstrual bleeding in ovulatory cycles is less common, and mechanisms underlying the bleeding are unclear but can include defects of the corpus luteum and abnormalities of the uterus or cervix, such as polyps, fibroids, or cancer. Excessive fibrinolytic activity, use of anticoagulants, diseases of coagulation, infection, and changes in prostaglandin production may be implicated.

CLINICAL MANIFESTATIONS DUB is characterized by unpredictable and variable bleeding in terms of amount and duration. Especially during perimenopause, dysfunctional bleeding also may involve flooding and the passing of large clots, leading to excessive blood loss. Excessive bleeding can lead to iron deficiency anemia and associated symptoms, including fatigue or shortness of breath.

EVALUATION AND TREATMENT DUB is diagnosed after other organic conditions that could cause abnormal bleeding are eliminated. If no cause is found it is usually assumed that the bleeding is caused by lack of regular ovulation. NSAIDs are often first-line treatments for excessive menstrual bleeding because they reduce prostaglandin synthesis within the endometrial tissues, leading to vasoconstriction and decreased bleeding. For the best effect they should be taken in the few days preceding the beginning of the menstrual period and be continued through the days of heaviest bleeding. NSAIDs are not as effective in controlling menstrual blood loss as hormonal therapies but they are readily available without a prescription.

TABLE 33-3 Common Causes of Abnormal (Vaginal/Genital) Bleeding in Descending Order of Frequency

Age Group	Cause
Prepubescence	Sexual assault
	Trauma
	Foreign bodies
	Precocious puberty
Adolescence	Anovulation (immature hypothalamic-pituitary-ovarian axis)
	Trauma and sexual abuse
Reproductive years	Pregnancy
	Pelvic inflammatory disease
	Coagulation disorder
	Hormonal contraceptives
	Endometriosis
	Anovulation
	Intrauterine device
	Ovarian cysts
	Uterine polyps or tumours
	Polycystic ovary syndrome
	Bleeding disorders (e.g., von Willebrand's disease)
	Trauma/rape
Perimenopause	Anovulation
	Malignancy
	Pregnancy
	Endometriosis
	Benign neoplasms (myomas, adenomyosis)
Postmenopause	Malignancy
Other: non–age-specific	Chronic conditions
	Adrenal conditions
	Thyroid disorders
	Liver disease
	Diabetes mellitus
	Obesity
	Hypertension

Goals of therapy are to control bleeding, prevent hyperplasia, prevent or treat anemia, and treat concurrent endocrine problems if present. Common treatments include administration of oral contraceptive pills that contain estrogen and progesterone, prescription of long-term therapy with medroxyprogesterone (Provera) (although the Health Canada black box warning about potential bone loss has greatly curtailed the use of this therapy), and placement of a levonorgestrel intrauterine device (LNG-IUD). The LNG-IUD has a dual indication from Health Canada for both birth control and suppression of abnormal menstrual bleeding. The device releases a steady amount of progesterone directly into the uterus to stabilize and suppress the uterine lining. In addition, the progesterone works to suppress the HPG axis and prevent ovulation.

Women who do not wish to have future pregnancies also can opt for treatments that permanently suppress their uterine lining. These treatments include ablation, where the lining is burned to prevent future proliferation of the endometrial cells, and complete removal of the uterus in hysterectomy. If a woman is menopausal and has not had a menstrual period for greater than 1 year, all vaginal bleeding should be investigated to rule out uterine and other cancers.

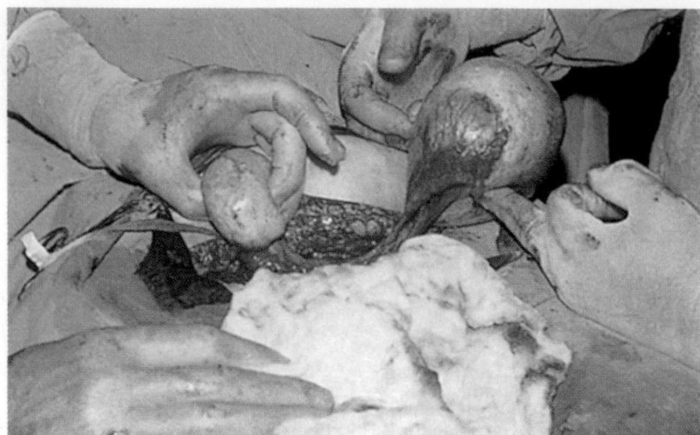

FIGURE 33-3 Polycystic Ovary. Surgical view of polycystic ovaries. (From Symonds, E.M., & Macpherson, M.B.A. [1997]. *Diagnosis in color: Obstetrics and gynecology.* London: Mosby-Wolfe.)

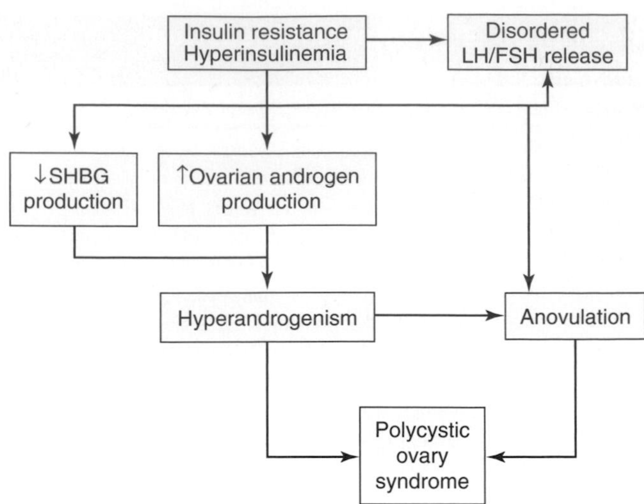

FIGURE 33-4 Insulin Resistance and Hyperinsulinemia in Polycystic Ovary Syndrome. See text for explanation. *FSH,* follicle-stimulating hormone; *LH,* luteinizing hormone; *SHBG,* sex hormone–binding globulin.

Polycystic Ovary Syndrome

Polycystic ovary syndrome (PCOS) remains one of the most common endocrine disturbances affecting women (Figure 33-3). International criteria for the diagnosis of PCOS require at least two of the following conditions: few or anovulatory menstrual cycles, elevated levels of androgens, and polycystic ovaries. Thus polycystic ovaries do not have to be present to diagnose PCOS and their presence alone does not establish the diagnosis. Furthermore, PCOS should not be confused with benign ovarian cysts, which are common during the reproductive years and have a different etiology (see "Benign Ovarian Cysts," p. 829). PCOS is a leading cause of infertility in the United States. PCOS has a large incidence of inheritability. Signs and symptoms of PCOS can vary over time, with metabolic syndrome becoming more prominent with age.[26]

PATHOPHYSIOLOGY The direct cause of PCOS is related to a genetic predisposition and an obesity-prone lifestyle related to insulin resistance and an excess of insulin and androgens. A hyperandrogenic state is a cardinal feature in the pathogenesis of PCOS. However, glucose intolerance or insulin resistance and hyperinsulinemia often occur concurrently and markedly aggravate the hyperandrogenic state, thus contributing to the severity of signs and symptoms of PCOS.[26] PCOS predisposes to obesity, and pre-existing obesity predisposes to more severe PCOS.

Insulin resistance and resultant compensatory hyperinsulinemia overstimulates androgen secretion by the ovarian stroma and reduces hepatic secretion of serum sex hormone–binding globulin (SHBG). The net effect is an increase in free testosterone levels. Excessive androgens affect follicular growth, and insulin affects follicular decline by suppressing apoptosis and enabling the survival of follicles that would normally disintegrate (Figure 33-4). Further, there seems to be a genetic ovarian defect in PCOS that makes the ovary either more susceptible to or more sensitive to insulin's stimulation of androgen production in the ovary.

Inappropriate gonadotropin secretion triggers the beginning of a vicious cycle that perpetuates anovulation. Typically, levels of FSH are low or below normal and the LH level is elevated. Persistent LH level elevation causes an increase in the concentration of androgens (dehydroepiandrosterone sulphate [DHEAS] from the adrenal glands, and testosterone, androstenedione, and dehydroepiandrosterone [DHEA] from the ovary). Androgens are converted to estrogen in peripheral tissues, and increased testosterone levels cause a significant reduction (approximately 50%) in SHBG level, which, in turn, causes increased levels of free estradiol. Elevated estrogen levels trigger a positive feedback response in LH and a negative feedback response in FSH. Because FSH levels are not totally depressed, new follicular growth is continuously stimulated, but not to full maturation and ovulation (see Figure 33-4).[26,27]

CLINICAL MANIFESTATIONS Clinical manifestations of PCOS usually appear within 2 years of puberty, but may appear after a period of normal menstrual function and pregnancy. Symptoms are related to anovulation and hyperandrogenism and include DUB or amenorrhea, hirsutism, acne, and infertility (Box 33-4). Hypertension and dyslipidemia also are frequently found in association with PCOS. PCOS is often found in association with other endocrine disorders.[27]

EVALUATION AND TREATMENT Diagnosis of PCOS is based on evidence of androgen excess (hirsutism, male pattern hair distribution, acne), chronic anovulation (as evidenced by irregular menstrual patterns, amenorrhea, and infertility), insulin resistance (obesity may be an indication, as well as abnormal glucose tolerance testing), and inappropriate gonadotropin secretion (low serum FSH concentration, and elevated levels of LH and DHEA). Treatment of PCOS often includes use of combined oral contraceptives to control irregular menstrual cycles and to oppose estrogens and androgens. Insulin sensitizers, such as metformin (Glucophage), may be used to decrease insulin resistance, prevent diabetes and heart disease, and restore fertility. Insulin sensitizers combined with clomiphene citrate (Clomid) may be effective for ovulation induction for women who are trying to become pregnant. Reductions in weight can dramatically improve insulin sensitivity and return of ovulatory cycles.

Premenstrual Disorders Syndrome

Premenstrual syndrome (PMS) and premenstrual dysphoric disorder (PMDD) are the cyclic recurrence (in the luteal phase of the menstrual cycle) of distressing physical, psychological, or behavioural changes that impair interpersonal relationships or interfere with usual activities. The luteal phase of ovulatory cycles is linked with complex hormonal changes of the menstrual cycle. PMDD is often considered a severe, sometimes disabling extension of PMS. The prevalence of PMS and PMDD is difficult to determine, possibly because of the wide-ranging nature of accepted symptoms. Symptoms for PMS and PMDD begin after ovulation during the luteal phase and persist up to 4 days into

BOX 33-4 Clinical Manifestations of Polycystic Ovary Syndrome

Presenting Signs and Symptoms (% of Women Affected)
Obesity (41%)
Menstrual disturbance (70% [e.g., dysfunctional uterine bleeding])
Oligomenorrhea (47%)
Amenorrhea (19%)
Regular menstruation (48%)
Hyperandrogenism (69–74%)
Infertility (73% of anovulatory infertility)
Asymptomatic (20% of those with polycystic ovary syndrome)

Hormonal Disturbances
Increased insulin (independent of obesity)
Decreased SHBG
Increased androgens (testosterone, androstenedione)
Increased DHEA (occurs in 50% of women)
Increased LH (genetic variant LH-β subunit)
Increased prolactin
Increased leptin, especially in obesity (independent of insulin)
Suggested decreased IGF-1 receptors on theca cells
Possible decreased estrogen receptors (intraovarian and along hypothalamic-pituitary axis)

Possible Late Sequelae
Dyslipidemia: increased low-density lipoproteins, decreased high-density lipoproteins, increased triglycerides
Diabetes mellitus (30% of women with or without obesity will develop type 2 diabetes mellitus by age 30)
Cardiovascular disease; hypertension
Endometrial hyperplasia and carcinoma (anovulatory women are hyperestrogenic)

Other
Women with PCOS are at increased risk for gestational diabetes mellitus, pregnancy-induced hypertension, preterm birth, and perinatal mortality

DHEA, dehydroepiandrosterone; *IGF-1*, insulinlike growth factor 1; *LH*, luteinizing hormone; *PCOS*, polycystic ovary syndrome; *SHBG*, sex hormone–binding globulin.
Adapted from Azziz, R., Carmina, E., Dewailly, D., et al. (2009). *Fertil Steril, 91*(2), 456–488; Boomsma, C.M., Fauser, B.C., & Macklon, N.S. (2008). *Semin Reprod Med, 26*(1), 72–84; Diamanti-Kandarakis, E. (2008). *Expert Rev Mol Med, 10*(2), e3; Spritzer, P.M., & Motta, A.B. (2015). *Int J Clin Pract, 69*(11), 1236–1246.

the menstrual cycle.[28] It has been estimated that 91% of women experience some form of distress around their menstrual period; 30% experience enough distress to interrupt their daily routine; but a much smaller number, as low as 3.1%, meet the criteria for PMDD.

PATHOPHYSIOLOGY There are many theories to explain PMS/PMDD, and their mechanisms, including an increased vulnerability to *fluctuations* in ovarian-derived hormones, and hypothalamic-pituitary-adrenal (HPA) axis changes.[29] Poorly understood are the neuroendocrine mechanisms of the hormonal environment of the menopausal transition that might trigger depression.[29] Erratic ovarian hormone fluctuation may be a mediator of risk for both vasomotor symptoms (hot flashes) and perimenopausal depression. Under investigation are the effects of changes in estradiol concentrations and the altered anti-inflammatory and neuroprotective consequences and modulation of limbic processing and memory.[29] Neurotransmitters, such as serotonin, gamma-aminobutyric acid (GABA), and norepinephrine, have demonstrated interactions with estrogen and progesterone and have established mood and behaviour effects, including negative mood, irritability, aggression, and impulse control. Additionally, neurotransmitters may have mediating or moderating roles on symptom manifestation. Sex steroids also interact with the renin-angiotensin-aldosterone system (RAAS), which could explain some PMS/PMDD signs and symptoms (e.g., water retention, bloating, weight gain). Levels of inflammatory mediators may be elevated with menstrual symptom severity and PMS.[30]

A predisposition to PMS occurs in families, perhaps because of genetics or shared environment. A woman's menstrual experience is often similar to her mother's or her sister's experience. Evidence supports a relationship between severity and frequency of PMS/PMDD and reports of low well-being, major affective disorder, and personal characteristics, such as increased stress, poor nutrition, lack of exercise, low self-esteem, perfectionism, history of sexual abuse, and family conflict. In turn, when PMS/PMDD is distressing, the quality of interpersonal relationships and self-image are negatively affected.

CLINICAL MANIFESTATIONS The pattern of symptom frequency and severity is more important than specific complaints. Nearly 300 physical, emotional, and behavioural symptoms have been attributed to PMS/PMDD. Emotional symptoms, particularly depression, anger, irritability, and fatigue, have been reported as the most prominent and the most distressing, whereas physical symptoms seem to be the least prevalent and problematic. The presence of underlying physical or psychological disease may be aggravated premenstrually and must be diagnosed and treated independently of PMS/PMDD.

EVALUATION AND TREATMENT Diagnosis of PMS/PMDD is based on health history and symptoms. Current treatment is symptomatic because the cause is complex and cannot be reduced to a single biological explanation and occurrence and severity are mediated by lifestyle, social, and psychological factors. For many women, nonpharmacological therapies, with or without medication, can be as effective in controlling symptoms as medication alone.[31] Approaches may include stress reduction, exercise, family or individual counselling, biofeedback, diet (see *Health Promotion:* Nutrition and Premenstrual Syndrome), imagery, acupuncture, and rest. Two major forms of treatment include the use of hormonal cycle regulation and use of selective serotonin reuptake inhibitor (SSRI) antidepressants.[32] If a woman does not desire immediate fertility, the oral contraceptive pill containing estrogen and progesterone has shown benefits in decreasing PMS/PMDD. In severe cases, menses can be abolished using GnRH agonists.

✔ QUICK CHECK 33-2
1. Why does amenorrhea occur?
2. Why do anovulatory menstrual cycles lead to dysfunctional uterine bleeding?
3. Discuss insulin resistance, hyperinsulinemia, anovulation, and androgen production in polycystic ovary syndrome.
4. What are the current theories of pathophysiology for premenstrual syndrome/premenstrual dysphoric disorder?

Infection and Inflammation

Infections of the genital tract may result from exogenous or endogenous microorganisms. Exogenous pathogens are most often sexually transmitted. Endogenous causes of infection include microorganisms that are normally resident in the vagina, bowel, or vulva. Infection occurs if these microorganisms migrate to a new location or overproliferate when the immune system and other defence mechanisms are impaired.

HEALTH PROMOTION

Nutrition and Premenstrual Syndrome

Women who are affected by premenstrual syndrome (PMS) often look for ways to decrease or prevent their symptoms. Dietary interventions that can help are multiple: eating six small meals each day; increasing intake of complex carbohydrates, fibre, and water; and decreasing caffeine, alcohol, refined sugar, and animal fat consumption. A low-fat vegetarian diet has been associated with decreased symptoms, possibly because of an increase in serum sex hormone–binding globulin concentration that lowers serum estrogen levels. It also may be helpful to limit sodium intake, and some limited evidence suggests that moderate doses (50 mg/day) of vitamin B_6 may reduce emotional symptoms of depression, irritability, and fatigue. This finding needs to be confirmed.

High food intake of thiamine and riboflavin was observed to lower risk for PMS. Thiamine, riboflavin, niacin, vitamin B_6, folate, and vitamin B_{12} are required to synthesize neurotransmitters. Limited data suggest that dietary minerals may be useful in preventing PMS. Prospective analyses suggest that higher plasma vitamin D levels may be inversely related to the development of specific menstrual symptoms. Vitamin D deficiency is associated with increased renin-angiotensin-aldosterone system activity, a system that regulates fluid balance and blood pressure. Vitamin D may lower the risk for unipolar depression. More research needs to confirm all of these findings.

Some researchers have suggested links between serotonin, endorphins, and high sugar intake and PMS risk. One interesting craving is chocolate. Some researchers suggest that a craving for chocolate is an unconscious desire for a compound called *phenylethylamine* in chocolate that stimulates the release of the neurotransmitter dopamine, which regulates mood.

Data from Bernard, N.D., Scialli, A.R., Hurlock, D., et al. (2000). *Obstet Gynecol, 95*(2), 245; Bertone-Johnson, E., Hankinson, S.E., Forger, N.G., et al. (2014). *BMC Womens Health, 14,* 56; Chocano-Bedoya, P.O., Manson, J.E., Hankinson, S.E., et al. (2011). *Am J Clin Nutr, 93*(5), 1080–1086; Chocano-Bedoya, P.O., Manson, J.E., Hankinson, S.E., et al. (2013). *Am J Epidemiol, 177*(10): 1118–1127; Eyles, D.W., Burne, T.H., & McGrath, J.J. (2012). *Front Neuroendocrinol, 34,* 47–64; Mahan, L.K., & Escott-Stump, S. (2000). *Krause's food, nutrition, and diet therapy* (10th ed.). Philadelphia: Saunders; Murakami, K., Sasaki, S., Takahashi, Y., et al. (2008). *Nutrition, 24*(6), 554–561.

Skin disorders that can affect the vulva include reactive dermatitis, contact dermatitis, psoriasis, and impetigo. (For a discussion of skin disorders, see Chapter 41.) Most infectious disorders, however, that affect the vulva and vagina are sexually transmitted. These currently recognized sexually transmitted infections (STIs) are described in Table 34-1, on p. 892.

Pelvic Inflammatory Disease

Pelvic inflammatory disease (PID) is an acute inflammatory process caused by infection (Figure 33-5). PID may involve any organ, or combination of organs, of the upper genital tract—the uterus, fallopian tubes, or ovaries—and, in its most severe form, the entire peritoneal cavity. Many infectious disorders that affect the vulva and vagina are sexually transmitted, such as chlamydia and gonorrhea that migrate from the vagina to the uterus, fallopian tubes, and ovaries.[33] However, microorganisms that comprise the vaginal flora (e.g., anaerobes, *Gardnerella vaginalis, Haemophilus influenzae,* enteric Gram-negative rods, and *Streptococcus agalactiae*) also are implicated with PID. Additionally, cytomegalovirus (CMV), *Mycoplasma hominis, Ureaplasma urealyticum,* and *Mycoplasma genitalium* may be associated with PID. The risk factors for PID include infection by a *previous* STI that was not treated (delaying treatment increases complications from PID); having multiple sex partners or a sex partner who has had multiple sex partners or a previous PID; being sexually active at age 25 or younger; using douches; and using an IUD for birth control.[33] Other causes of infection include spontaneous or induced abortions, normal or abnormal deliveries (called *puerperal infections*), or other surgical procedures; these infections are often polymicrobial.[34]

PATHOPHYSIOLOGY The development of upper genital tract infections is mediated by a number of defence mechanisms, including virulence of the microorganism, size of the inoculum, and immune defence status of the individual. PID develops when pathological microbes ascend from an infected cervix to infect the uterus and adnexae (uterine appendages). The initial infection usually involves the endocervical mucosa, but it can start in the Bartholin gland and other glands. From these sites the infection can move upward to involve the fallopian tubes and tubo-ovarian region (Figure 33-6). STIs from gonorrhea and chlamydia are the main infectious causes of PID; however, other infections not sexually transmitted (e.g., induced abortion, dilation and curettage of the uterus, and other surgical procedures) also can cause PID.[34] Many

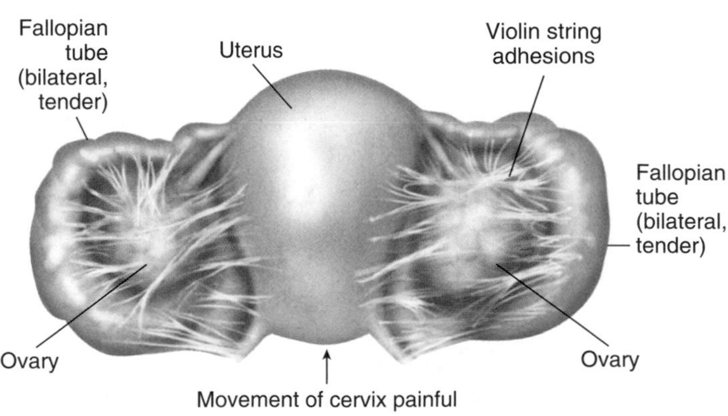

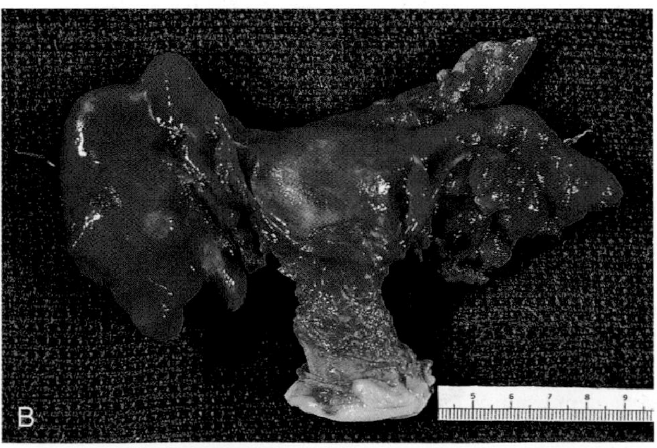

FIGURE 33-5 Pelvic Inflammatory Disease. A, Drawing depicting involvement of both ovaries and fallopian tubes. **B,** Total abdominal hysterectomy and bilateral salpingo-oophorectomy specimen showing unilateral pyosalpinx. (**A,** from Ball, J.W., Dains, J.E., Flynn, J.A., et al. [2015]. *Seidel's guide to physical examination* [8th ed.]. St. Louis: Mosby; **B,** from Morse, S.A., Holmes, K.K., & Ballard, R.C. [2010]. *Atlas of sexually transmitted diseases and AIDS* [4th ed.]. Edinburgh: Mosby.)

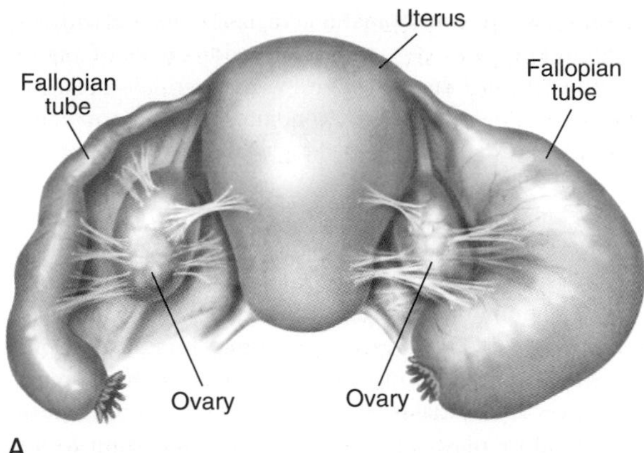

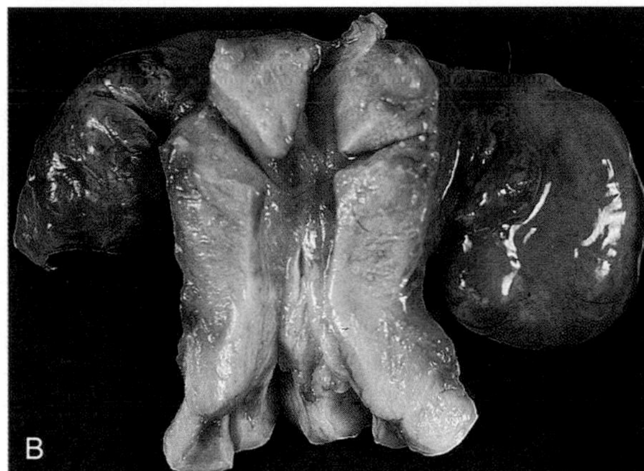

FIGURE 33-6 Salpingitis. A, Advanced pyosalpinx. Note the swollen fallopian tubes. **B,** Bilateral, retort-shaped, swollen, sealed tubes and adhesions of ovaries are typical of salpingitis. (**A,** from Ball, J.W., Dains, J.E., Flynn, J.A., et al. [2015]. *Seidel's guide to physical examination* [8th ed.]. St. Louis: Mosby; **B,** from Damjanov, I., & Linder, J. [Eds.]. [1996]. *Anderson's pathology* [10th ed.]. St. Louis: Mosby.)

anaerobic bacteria have been implicated in increasing the risk for PID because they alter the pH of the vaginal environment and may decrease the integrity of the mucus blocking the cervical canal. Bacterial vaginosis (BV) is present in up to 66% of women with PID, and other anaerobes, such as *Bacteroides*, and *G. vaginalis*, *H. influenzae*, and genital tract mycoplasmas (*M. hominis*, *M. genitalis*, and *U. urealyticum*) are frequently isolated from women with PID. *Escherichia coli* may contribute to pelvic infections in older women. Therefore, although gonorrhea and chlamydia are the main pathogens in PID, the infection is actually polymicrobial in origin and is treated with a broad spectrum of antibiotics to ensure that all the causative agents are eliminated.[33]

Salpingitis

Salpingitis is inflammation of the fallopian tubes (see Figure 33-6). The inflammatory process develops after the infection has been established and induces changes in the columnar epithelia that line the upper reproductive tract. The inflammation causes localized edema and sometimes necrosis of the area. Gonorrhea gonococci attach to the fallopian tubes and excrete a substance toxic to the tubal mucosa, causing further inflammation and damage. Chlamydia enters the tubal cells and replicates, bursting the cell membrane as it reproduces, causing permanent scarring. Gonorrhea and chlamydia can spread to the abdominal cavity through the openings of the fallopian/uterine tubes. Other mechanisms that may contribute to PID include lymphatic drainage with parametrial spread of the infection. The acute complications of PID include peritonitis and bacteremia, which can increase the risk for endocarditis, meningitis, and infectious arthritis. The chronic consequences of PID include infertility and tubal obstruction, ectopic pregnancy, pelvic pain of varying degrees, and intestinal obstruction from adhesions between the bowel and pelvic organs.[34]

BOX 33-5 Diagnostic Criteria for Pelvic Inflammatory Disease

Minimum Criteria (One or More Needed for Diagnosis)
Cervical motion tenderness, *or*
Uterine tenderness, *or*
Adnexal tenderness

Additional Criteria That Increase Specificity of Diagnosis
Body temperature >38.3°C (>101°F)
Mucopurulent cervical or vaginal discharge
Numerous white blood cells on saline wet prep
Elevated C-reactive protein
Elevated erythrocyte sedimentation rate
Documented infection with *Chlamydia trachomatis* or *Neisseria gonorrhoeae*

Definitive Criteria (Not Needed for Treatment)
Transvaginal ultrasound, magnetic resonance imaging, *or*
Doppler studies showing thickened and fluid-filled tubes
Laparoscopic visualization of PID-related abnormalities

PID, pelvic inflammatory disease.
Data from Centers for Disease Control and Prevention. (2010). *MMWR Morb Mortal Wkly Rep, 59*(RR-12); Yudin, M.H., & Ross, J.D.C. (2012). Pelvic inflammatory disease. In J.M. Zenilman, & M. Shahmansesh (Eds.), *Sexually transmitted diseases* (pp. 67–76). Sudbury, MA: Jones & Bartlett Learning.

CLINICAL MANIFESTATIONS The clinical manifestations of PID vary from sudden, severe abdominal pain with fever to no symptoms at all. An asymptomatic cervicitis may be present for some time before PID develops. The first sign of the ascending infection may be the onset of low bilateral abdominal pain, often characterized as dull and steady with a gradual onset. Symptoms are more likely to develop during or immediately after menstruation. The pain of PID may worsen with walking, jumping, or intercourse. Other manifestations of PID include dysuria (difficult or painful urination) and irregular bleeding.

EVALUATION AND TREATMENT PID often has limited or vague clinical symptoms, leading to undertreatment and long-term health effects.[35] Because PID is a substantial health risk to a woman, the Centers for Disease Control and Prevention (CDC) encourages clinicians to consider PID as a likely diagnosis when a sexually active woman has abdominal or pelvic tenderness and *one* of the following: cervical motion tenderness, uterine tenderness, or adnexal tenderness.[33] Box 33-5 lists the diagnostic criteria for PID. No laboratory results or studies are needed to begin treatment; however, additional information can improve the specificity of diagnosis. Abdominal pain in women can have many causes, and it is important to rule out other diagnoses, which can be done while treating for PID.[33]

The complications of PID can be significant; therefore, rapid treatment is recommended even before the causative pathogen can be identified. Because treatment is empirical, it needs to be effective against a broad range of pathogens, especially chlamydia, gonorrhea, and anaerobic bacteria.[33] Treatment is usually done on an outpatient basis unless the woman has symptoms of advanced infection, cannot take oral medications, is pregnant, or exhibits other pathologies that cannot be excluded. The CDC-recommended outpatient regimen is shown in Box 33-6.

BOX 33-6 PHAC Outpatient Recommended Regimen for Pelvic Inflammatory Disease

1. **Ceftriaxone** (Rocephin) 250 mg intramuscularly (IM) in a single dose
   OR
   Cefoxitin (Mefoxin Pws) 2 g IM in a single dose
   PLUS
   Probenecid (Benuryl) 1 g orally administered concurrently in a single dose
   OR
   Other parenteral third-generation cephalosporin (e.g., ceftizoxime [Cefizox] or cefotaxime [Cefotaxime Sodium])
   PLUS
   Doxycycline (Teva-Doxycycline) 100 mg orally twice a day for 14 days
   With or without
   Metronidazole (Flagyl) 500 mg orally twice a day for 14 days
   Or
2. **Ofloxaxin** 400 mg orally twice a day for 14 days
   OR
   Levofloxacin 500 mg orally once a day for 14 days
   With or without
   Metronidazole 500 mg orally twice a day for 14 days

PHAC, Public Health Agency of Canada.
© All rights reserved. From Public Health Agency of Canada. (2013). *Canadian Guidelines on Sexually Transmitted Infections* (Section 4-4: Management and treatment of specific syndrome – Pelvic Inflammatory Disease [PID], Table 5). Ottawa: Author. Retrieved from https://www.canada.ca/en/public-health/services/infectious-diseases/sexual-health-sexually-transmitted-infections/canadian-guidelines/sexually-transmitted-infections/canadian-guidelines-sexually-transmitted-infections-22.html. Public Health Agency of Canada, Modified: 2017. Adapted and reproduced with permission from the Minister of Health, 2017.

Although alternative treatment regimens are available, the growing antibiotic resistance of gonorrhea limits antibiotic choices. The CDC is closely monitoring gonorrhea's antibiotic sensitivity and updates treatment guidelines periodically to reflect new information.[33] To prevent recurrence, sexual partners of women with PID should also receive treatment, even if they are asymptomatic. Women receiving treatment should be re-evaluated by their care provider in 3 days to ensure antibiotic treatment is effective.[33] Because women with a history of PID are at increased risk for ectopic pregnancy, they should seek care as soon as they know they are pregnant because ectopic pregnancy is a major cause of maternal mortality.[36]

The diagnosis of PID is based on history, abdominal tenderness, the presence of uterine and cervical movement tenderness on bimanual pelvic examination, mucopurulent discharge at the cervical os, white blood cells on Gram stain or wet mount of cervical discharge, leukocytosis, and increased erythrocyte sedimentation rate. To support the diagnosis, tests for chlamydia and gonorrhea are done; sonography, laparoscopy, and culdocentesis are indicated when a woman has recurrent symptoms or symptoms unresponsive to outpatient treatment regimens, a temperature greater than 38°C (100.4°F), or an adnexal mass. Other conditions that cause pelvic pain must be excluded, including ectopic pregnancy, threatened abortion, ovarian torsion, ovarian cyst, or appendicitis. Recommendations for physical rest and avoidance of intercourse are often given as precautionary and comfort measures during initial recovery (i.e., 1 to 2 weeks).

Vaginitis

Vaginitis is irritation or inflammation of the vagina, typically caused by infection. Vaginitis is characterized by an increase in white blood cells on saline wet prep examination. Vaginal irritation without white blood cells is known as vaginosis. The major causes of vaginitis are overgrowth of normal flora, STIs, and vaginal irritation related to low estrogen levels during menopause (a condition known as *atropic vaginitis*). The incidence of sexually transmitted vaginitis remains highest in women 15 to 24 years of age.

The development of vaginitis is related to alterations in the vaginal environment and includes changes with complications in local defence mechanisms, such as skin integrity, immune reaction, and particularly vaginal pH. The pH of the vagina (normally 4.0 to 4.5) depends on cervical secretions and the presence of normal flora that help maintain an acidic environment. Changes in the vaginal pH may predispose a woman to infection. Variables that affect the vaginal pH and thus the bactericidal nature of secretions and the predisposition to infection include douching; using soaps, spermicides, feminine hygiene sprays, and deodorant menstrual pads or tampons; and having conditions associated with increased glycogen content of vaginal secretions, such as pregnancy and diabetes.

Antibiotics often destroy normal vaginal flora, facilitating overgrowth of *Candida albicans* and causing a yeast infection. Increased vaginal alkalinity also may enhance susceptibility to trichomoniasis and BV.

Diagnosis is based on history, physical examination, and microscopic examination of the discharge using a wet mount technique. Infection is suggested with a marked change in colour or if the discharge becomes copious, malodorous, or irritating.

Treatment involves developing and maintaining an acidic environment, relieving symptoms (usually pruritus and irritation), and administering antimicrobial or antifungal medications to eradicate the infectious organism. If the infection can be sexually transmitted, the woman's partner will also need to be treated. Research suggests that probiotics, especially *Lactobacillus crispatus*, can encourage proliferation of normal vaginal flora and decrease the incidence of vaginitis in women at risk for this disease.[37,38] A probiotic bacterial strain, *Lactobacillus plantarum* P17630, can attach to vaginal epithelium and reduce the adhesion of *C. albicans*, and may help reduce *Candida* recurrence.[39]

Cervicitis

Cervicitis is a nonspecific term used to describe inflammation of the cervix. The CDC defines *cervicitis* as having two major diagnostic signs: a purulent or mucopurulent discharge from the cervical os or endocervical bleeding induced by gently introducing a cotton swab into the cervix.[40] Either sign or both may be present. Cervicitis can have infectious or noninfectious causes. Chemicals and substances introduced into the vagina can cause cervicitis as well as disruptions in the normal vaginal flora. However, there are conflicting definitions of *cervicitis* used clinically and in research. Age and risk factors are important in assessing a woman with cervicitis. Younger women are at risk for STIs and should be tested for chlamydia, gonorrhea, and trichomoniasis. Older women with cervicitis may have STIs but are at risk for irritation from abnormal vaginal flora related to low vaginal estrogen levels.

Mucopurulent cervicitis (MPC) is usually caused by one or more sexually transmitted pathogens, such as *Trichomonas*, *Neisseria*, *Chlamydia*, *Mycoplasma*, or *Ureaplasma*. Infection causes the cervix to become red and edematous. A mucopurulent (mucus- and pus-containing) exudate drains from the external cervical os, and the individual may report vague pelvic pain, bleeding, or dysuria. Bleeding can occur during sexual intercourse or with pelvic examinations, or both, and Papanicolaou (Pap) Pap smears. Because mucopurulent cervicitis is a symptom of PID, women at risk for STIs, especially those less than 26 years old, should receive treatment for PID while awaiting results of microbial testing.[41] If the woman is not at risk for STIs, a thorough evaluation often reveals another cause for the inflammation. Partners should be notified and examined if chlamydia, gonorrhea, or trichomoniasis was identified or suspected in the affected woman; these partners should then be treated for the STIs. To avoid re-infection, women and their sex partners should abstain from sexual intercourse until therapy is completed (i.e., 7 days after a single-dose regimen or after completion of a 7-day regimen).[41] The infectious microorganisms are cultured or identified by immunoassay. Definitive diagnosis is followed by oral antibiotic therapy.

Vulvodyniavestibulitis

Vulvodyniavestibulitis (VV) (also referred to as *vulvitis, vestibulitis*, or *vulvovestibulitisdynia*) is chronic vulvar pain lasting 3 months or longer without visible dermatosis; inflammation of the vulva or vaginal vestibule, or both; infection; neoplasia; or identifiable neurological disorder.[42,43] The classification of vulvodynia is based on the location of the pain, whether it is localized or generalized, and whether the pain is provoked, unprovoked, or mixed.[42] *Localized* is characterized by pain from a cause that usually does not cause pain (allodynia) to the vulvar vestibule (entrance of vagina) area. *Generalized* is a diffuse pain pattern involving all of the pudendal nerve distribution and beyond. *Provoked* means any touch or stimulation that elicits pain, *unprovoked* is pain that occurs in the absence of touch or stimulation, and *mixed* is pain that varies with or without touch or stimulation. Individuals describe the pain as burning, stinging, irritation, or rawness. In many cases, it may represent several disorders without an identifiable cause. Vulvodynia is fairly common with lifetime estimates of prevalence ranging from 10 to 28% among reproductive-aged women; in addition, it can affect girls.[44] It occurs across ethnicities, and the incidence seems to decrease with increasing age.

The cause of vulvodynia is unknown. Theories suggest that it is multifactorial in origin and may include embryonic factors, chronic inflammation, genetic immune factors, nerve pathways, increased sensitivity to environmental factors (infection, trauma, irritants), hormonal changes, human papillomavirus (HPV), and oxalates.[42] Although the inflammation of VV may be caused by contact dermatitis (i.e., exposure to soaps, detergents, lotions, sprays, shaving, menstrual pads/tampons, perfumed toilet paper, tight-fitting clothes), the condition may be more complex and represent abnormalities in three interdependent systems: vestibular mucosa, pelvic floor musculature, and CNS pain regulatory pathways. The condition also may represent an autoimmune reaction. The suggested pathophysiology of vulvodynia is a chronic disorder of the nerves that supply the vulva. Some evidence has documented nerve fibre proliferation or neural hyperplasia in the affected tissue.[42] An important trigger is chronic inflammation caused by contact irritants, recurrent infections, hormonal changes, and chronic skin conditions. Overall, with normal sensations there is a heightened sensitivity. Vulvodynia often occurs in the context of other pain conditions and includes irritable bowel syndrome, interstitial cystitis, recurrent yeast infections, and fibromyalgia.[43] Because the mechanisms of vulvodynia are poorly understood, it is often a difficult condition to evaluate and treat.

After ruling out and treating conditions that can contribute to or cause vulvar inflammation (e.g., *Candida*, STIs, seborrhea, psoriasis), there are few treatment options. Cotton swab testing is used to identify painful areas. Studies on treatments are limited but suggest that women may benefit from topical lidocaine (Xylocaine), topical or systemic antidepressants, behavioural treatment, botulinum toxin type A (Botox) injections into the affected nerve, or vestibulectomy. Bathing in lukewarm water in a mild baking soda solution can be soothing, and ice packs may help.[42] Hot water may incite vulvar symptoms. Suggested approaches include use of hydrocortisone cream, application of a water barrier (such as thick skin cream or solid vegetable shortening) during a period of healing, behavioural treatment (35 to 83% of women benefit), or vestibulectomy (61 to 94% success rate), which is a procedure that is understandably unacceptable to many women. Women also are advised to avoid irritants, wear loose cotton clothing, and use appropriate antimicrobial or antifungal treatments for any recurrent vaginitis.

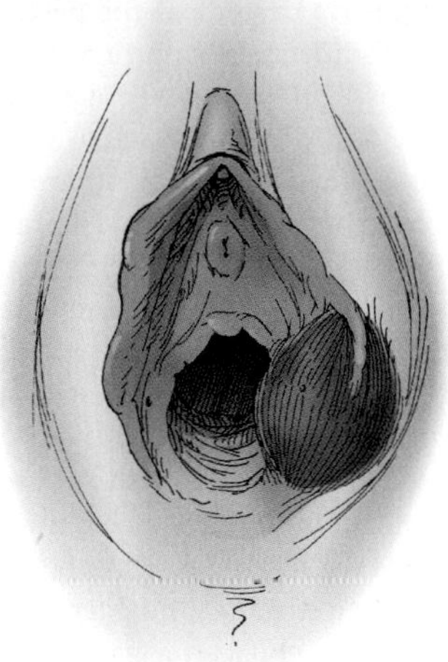

FIGURE 33-7 Inflammation of Bartholin Gland. (Modified from Fuller, J.K. [2013]. *Surgical technology* [6th ed.]. Philadelphia: Saunders; Gershenson, D.M., DeCherney, A.H., Curry, S.L., et al. [2001]. *Operative gynecology* [2nd ed.]. Philadelphia: Saunders.)

Bartholinitis

Bartholinitis, or Bartholin cyst, is an acute inflammation of one or both of the ducts that lead from the introitus (vaginal opening) to the Bartholin/greater vestibular glands (Figure 33-7). Most lesions of the Bartholin gland are cysts or abscesses. The usual causes are microorganisms that infect the lower female reproductive tract, such as streptococci, staphylococci, and sexually transmitted pathogens. Acute bartholinitis may be preceded by an infection, such as cervicitis, vaginitis, or urethritis.

Infection or trauma causes inflammatory changes that narrow the distal portion of the duct, leading to obstruction and stasis of glandular secretions. The obstruction, or cyst, varies from 1 to 8 cm in diameter and is located in the posterolateral portion of the vulva. The affected area is usually red and painful, and pus may be visible at the opening of the duct. This exudate should be cultured. The individual may have fever and malaise. Diagnosis is based on the clinical manifestations and the identification of infectious microorganisms.

Chronic bartholinitis is characterized by the presence of a small cyst that is slightly tender but otherwise is asymptomatic. Most Bartholin cysts require no treatment. Symptoms only occur if an exacerbation of infection causes an abscess to form in the gland itself.

Diagnosis is based on the clinical manifestations and the identification of infectious microorganisms. Treatment is controversial but involves broad-spectrum antibiotics. Some clinicians attempt to drain the cyst using hot soaks, needle aspiration, insertion of a catheter, or marsupialization (cutting a slit and suturing the edges) of the infected gland. No single treatment has proved superior for both relief and prevention of recurrence. Pain is relieved with analgesics and warm sitz baths. If an abscess forms, it may be surgically drained.

Pelvic Organ Prolapse

The bladder, urethra, and rectum are supported by the endopelvic fascia and perineal muscles. This muscular and fascial tissue loses tone and strength with aging and may fail to maintain the pelvic organs in the proper position. Progressive descent of the pelvic support structures may cause pelvic floor disorders, such as urinary and fecal incontinence, and pelvic organ prolapse. **Pelvic organ prolapse (POP)** is the descent of one or more of the following: the vaginal wall, the uterus, or the apex of the vagina (after a hysterectomy). Although more than 50% of women have some version of POP on physical examination, most women have no symptoms. When prolapse becomes severe, the function of the surrounding organs can be altered. POP is thought be caused by direct trauma (such as childbirth); pelvic floor surgery; or damage to pelvic innervation, particularly the pudendal nerve. Risk factors in nulliparous women, however, include occupational activities that require heavy lifting or chronic medical conditions, such as chronic lung disease or refractory constipation (chronically increased intra-abdominal pressure). The most frequently cited risk factors are aging, obesity, and hysterectomy. Other risk factors include a strong familial tendency (from family and twin studies) and possibly a multifactorial genetic component.[45] Prolapse of the bladder, urethra, rectum, or uterus may occur many years after an initial injury to the supporting structure.

Uterine prolapse is descent of the cervix or entire uterus into the vaginal canal, and in severe cases the uterus falls completely through the vagina and protrudes from the introitus, creating ulceration and obvious discomfort. Figure 33-8 illustrates the different degrees (grades) of uterine prolapse, showing descent of the cervix or the entire uterus into the vaginal canal. Grade 1 prolapse is not treated unless it causes discomfort. Grades 2 and 3 prolapse usually cause feelings of fullness, heaviness, and collapse through the vagina. Symptoms of other pelvic floor disorders also may be present.

A common first-line treatment is a **pessary**, which is a removable mechanical device that holds the uterus in position. The pelvic fascia may be strengthened through Kegel exercises (repetitive isometric tightening and relaxing of the pubococcygeal muscles) or by estrogen therapy in menopausal women. Maintaining a healthy body mass index (BMI), preventing constipation, and treating chronic cough may help prevent prolapse. Surgical repair, with or without hysterectomy, is the treatment of last resort.

Figure 33-9 shows POP associated with cystocele and rectocele. **Cystocele** is descent of a portion of the posterior bladder wall and trigone into the vaginal canal and is usually caused by childbirth. In severe cases, the bladder and anterior vaginal wall bulge outside the introitus. Symptoms are usually insignificant in mild to moderate cases. Increased bulging and descent of the anterior vaginal wall and urethra can be aggravated by vigorous activity, prolonged standing, sneezing, coughing, or straining and can be relieved by rest or by assumption of a recumbent or prone position. If the prolapse is large, women may state symptoms of vaginal pressure. Medical management can include vaginal pessary, Kegel exercises, and estrogen therapy for postmenopausal women (see *Health Promotion:* Nonsurgical Management of Vaginal Prolapse). Surgical treatment is used for severe injury unresponsive to medical treatment.

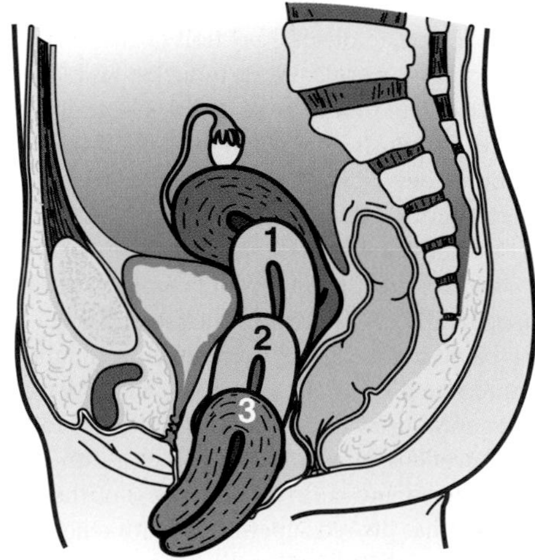

FIGURE 33-8 Degrees of Uterine Prolapse. Grade 1 is minimal and rarely requires correction. Grade 2 prolapse has moderate symptoms, and grade 3 prolapse is severe. The uterus is so low that the cervix protrudes from the vagina. (From Phillips, N. [2013]. *Berry & Kohn's operating room technique* [12th ed.]. Philadelphia: Mosby.)

HEALTH PROMOTION

Nonsurgical Management of Vaginal Prolapse

Women with very mild symptoms of vaginal prolapse (mild pelvic discomfort and urinary symptoms) do not require treatment but may benefit from the recommendations made for women with moderate symptoms (increased pelvic discomfort, bowel and urinary symptoms, and sexual dysfunction), including weight loss if necessary, refraining from heavy lifting, and smoking cessation.

Other strategies may be employed to improve symptoms, including performing regular Kegel exercises and the use of a pessary. Kegel exercises are a series of contractions that strengthen the pelvic floor. The woman is instructed to squeeze, at the same time, the two sets of pelvic floor muscles that are used to prevent the passage of gas and urine. It is recommended to complete 30 to 40 contractions spread over the duration of the day, holding the contraction for 3 seconds, gradually increasing to 10 seconds. Rest periods are recommended in between contractions. A second option is the utilization of a pessary (a removable device that is inserted into the vagina to assist in uterine support, similar to a diaphragm). These two less invasive treatments may diminish symptoms enough to delay the woman from seeking more aggressive surgical treatment.

Data from Harvard University. (2005). *What to do about pelvic organ prolapse.* Retrieved from http://www.health.harvard.edu/family-health-guide/what-to-do-about-pelvic-organ-prolapse.

A **rectocele** is the bulging of the rectum and posterior vaginal wall into the vaginal canal. Childbirth may increase damage, ultimately leading to a rectocele, but symptoms may not appear until after menopause. Genetic and familial predisposition and bowel habits contribute to rectocele development. Lifelong chronic constipation and straining may produce or aggravate a rectocele. A large rectocele may cause vaginal pressure, rectal fullness, and incomplete bowel evacuation. Defecation may be difficult and can be facilitated by applying manual pressure to the posterior vaginal wall. Medical treatment focuses on the management and prevention of constipation and, if needed, the use of a pessary. Rectocele alone (without associated enterocele, uterine prolapse, and cystocele) seldom requires surgery.

An **enterocele** is a herniation of the rectouterine pouch into the rectovaginal septum (between the rectum and the posterior vaginal wall). It can be congenital or acquired. Although congenital enterocele rarely causes symptoms or progresses in size, those acquired can result from muscular weakness caused by previous surgery, especially those through the vagina, or from pelvic relaxation disorders, such as uterine prolapse, cystocele, and rectocele. Most large enteroceles are often found in grossly obese adults and older adults. Treatment is surgical. Box 33-7 summarizes the symptoms and treatment of POP.

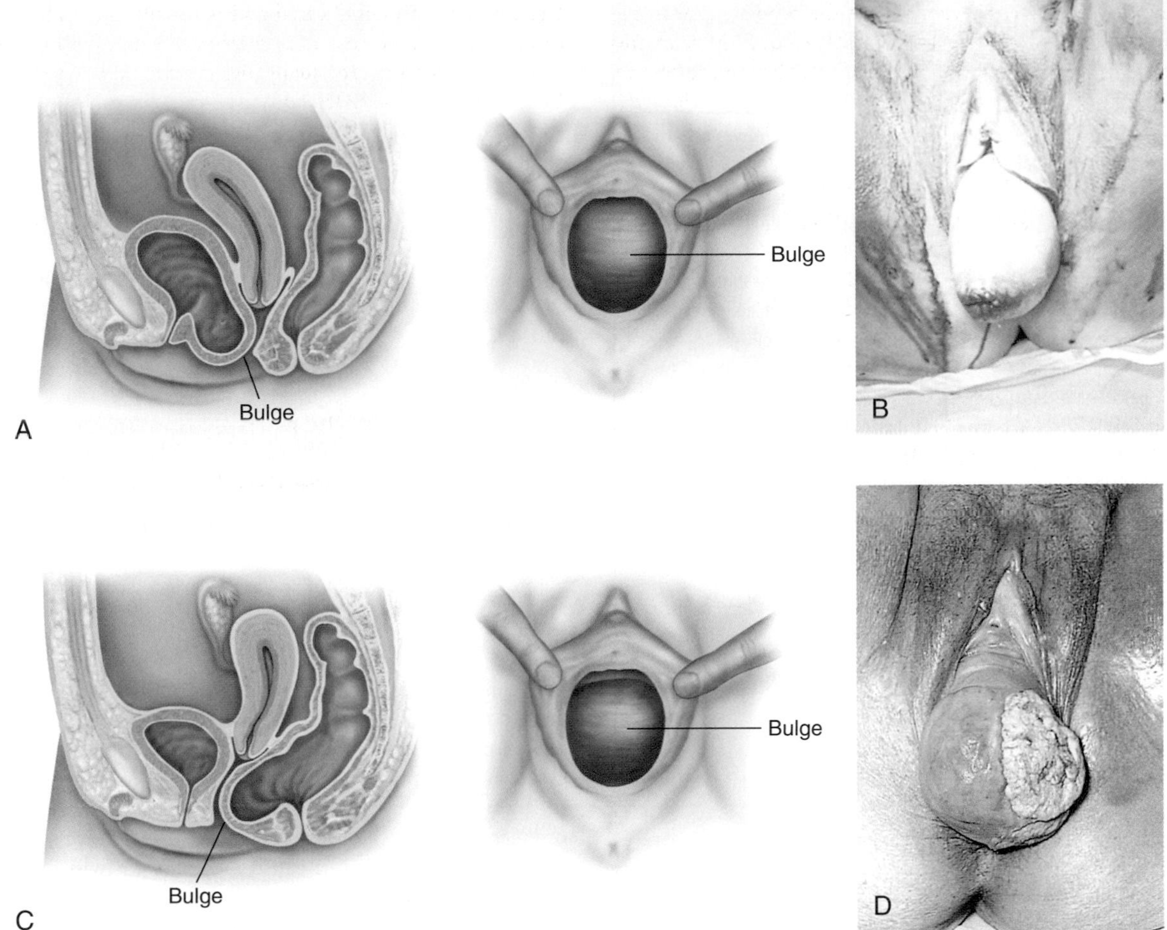

FIGURE 33-9 Cystocele and Rectocele. A, Grade 2: anterior vaginal wall prolapse (i.e., cystocele). B, Grade 4: prolapse. C, Grade 2: posterior wall prolapse (i.e., rectocele). D, Grade 4: associated with ulceration of vaginal wall. Grades 1 and 3 not shown. (A and C, from Seidel, H.M., Ball, J.W., & Dains, J.E. [1999]. *Mosby's guide to physical examination* [4th ed.]. St. Louis: Mosby; B and D, from Symonds, E.M., & Macpherson, M.B.A. [1994]. *Color atlas of obstetrics and gynecology.* London: Mosby-Wolfe.)

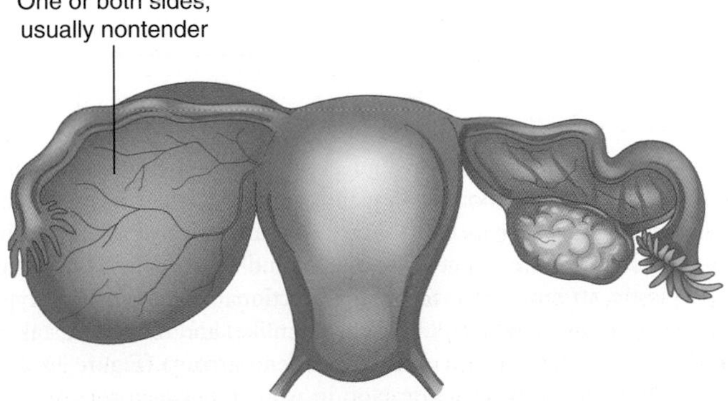

FIGURE 33-10 Depiction of Ovarian Cyst.

Benign Growths and Proliferative Conditions

Benign Ovarian Cysts

Benign cysts of the ovary may occur at any time during the lifespan, but are most common during the reproductive years and, in particular, at the extremes of those years (Figure 33-10). An increase in benign ovarian cysts occurs when hormonal imbalances are more common, around puberty and menopause.[46] Benign ovarian cysts are quite common, comprising one-third of gynecological hospital admissions. Two common causes of benign ovarian enlargement in ovulating women are follicular cysts and corpus luteum cysts. These cysts are called **functional cysts** because they are caused by variations of normal physiological events. Follicular and corpus luteum cysts are unilateral. They are typically 5 to 6 cm in diameter but can grow as large as 8 to 10 cm. Most women are asymptomatic.

Benign cysts of the ovary are produced when a follicle or a number of follicles are stimulated but no dominant follicle develops and completes the maturation process. Every month about 120 follicles are stimulated, and generally, only 1 succeeds in ovulation of a mature ovum. Normally, in the early follicular phase of the menstrual cycle, follicles of the ovary respond to hormonal signals from the brain. The pituitary gland produces FSH to mature follicles in the ovary. If the dominant follicle develops properly before ovulation, the corpus luteum becomes vascularized and secretes progesterone. Progesterone arrests development of other follicles in both ovaries in that cycle. LH, proteolytic enzymes, and prostaglandins trigger follicular rupture and release of the ovum.

Follicular cysts (also called *ovarian cysts* or *functional cysts*) are filled with fluid and can be caused by a transient condition in which the dominant follicle fails to rupture or one or more of the nondominant follicles fails to regress. This disturbance is not well understood. It may be that the hypothalamus does not receive or send a message strong

BOX 33-7 Pelvic Organ Prolapse: Symptoms and Treatments

Symptoms	Treatment
Urinary	Depending on age of woman and cause and severity of condition:
Sensation of incomplete emptying of bladder	Isometric exercises to strengthen pubococcygeal muscles (Kegel exercises)
Urinary incontinence	Estrogen to improve tone and vascularity of fascial support (postmenopausal)
Urinary frequency/urgency	Pessary (a removable device) to hold pelvic organs in place
Bladder "splinting" to accomplish voiding	**Surgical**
Bowel	Reconstructive: autologous grafts; synthetic mesh/sling
Constipation or feeling of rectal fullness or blockage	Obliterative (most extreme)
Difficult defecation	Weight loss
Stool or flatus incontinence	Avoidance of constipation
Urgency	Treatment of cough/lung conditions
Manual "splinting" of posterior vaginal wall to accomplish defecation	
Pain and Bulging	
Vaginal, bladder, rectum	
Pelvic pressure, bulging, pain	
Lower back pain	
Sexual	
Dyspareunia	
Decreased sensation, lubrication, arousal	

enough to increase FSH levels to the degree necessary to develop or mature a dominant follicle. The hypothalamus monitors blood levels of estradiol and progesterone; when FSH level is low, estradiol concentration does not increase enough to stimulate LH surge. Research indicates that when progesterone is not being produced, the hypothalamus releases GnRH to increase the FSH level. FSH continues to stimulate follicles to mature, and the granulosa cells grow and, presumably, estradiol level increases. This abnormal cycle continues to stimulate follicular size and causes follicular cysts to develop. Although individuals may experience no symptoms, some have pelvic pain, a sensation of feeling bloated, tender breasts, and heavy or irregular menses. After several subsequent cycles in which hormone levels once again follow a regular cycle and progesterone levels are restored, cysts usually will be absorbed or will regress. Follicular cysts can be random or recurrent events.

A **corpus luteum cyst** may normally form by the granulosa cells left behind after ovulation. This cyst is highly vascularized but usually limited in size, and with the normal menstrual cycle it spontaneously regresses. With an imbalance in hormones, low LH and progesterone levels may cause an abnormal or hemorrhagic cyst. In some cases, large cysts can rupture and cause hemorrhage.

Corpus luteum cysts are less common than follicular cysts, but luteal cysts typically cause more symptoms, particularly if they rupture. Manifestations include dull pelvic pain and amenorrhea or delayed menstruation, followed by irregular or heavier-than-normal bleeding. Rupture occasionally occurs and can cause massive bleeding with excruciating pain; immediate surgery may be required. Corpus luteum cysts usually regress spontaneously in nonpregnant women. Oral contraceptives may be used to prevent cysts from forming in the future.

Dermoid cysts are ovarian teratomas that contain elements of all three germ layers; they are common ovarian neoplasms. These growths may contain mature tissue including skin, hair, sebaceous and sweat glands, muscle fibres, cartilage, and bone. Dermoid cysts are usually asymptomatic and are found incidentally on pelvic examination. Dermoid cysts have malignant potential and should be removed.

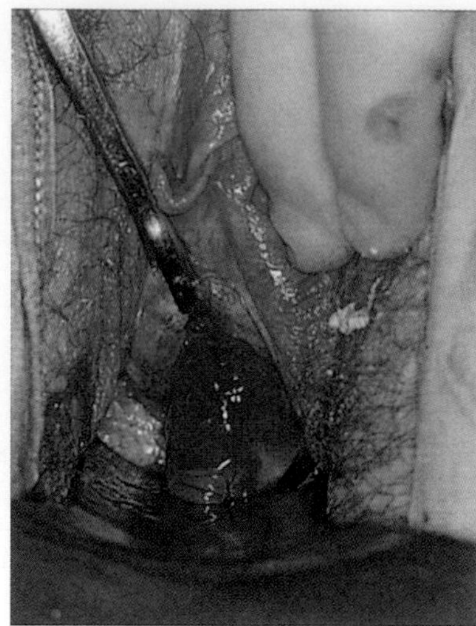

FIGURE 33-11 Endometrial Polyp. Polyp is protruding through the cervical os. (From Symonds, E.M., & Macpherson, M.B.A. [1994]. *Color atlas of obstetrics and gynecology*. London: Mosby.)

Torsion of the ovary is a rare complication of ovarian cysts or tumours or enlargement of the ovary; it can occur in girls or women. If a cyst is sufficiently large, it can cause the ovary to twist on its ligaments, decreasing blood supply to the ovary and causing extreme pain. **Ovarian torsion** is rare but is a gynecological emergency when present. It usually presents with acute, severe unilateral abdominal or pelvic pain and is treated surgically.

QUICK CHECK 33-3

1. Why is prompt treatment of pelvic inflammatory disease critical to reproductive health?
2. Why do benign ovarian cysts develop in women who ovulate?
3. What is the difference between a follicular cyst and a corpus luteum cyst?

Endometrial Polyps

An **endometrial polyp** is a benign mass of endometrial tissue and contains a variable amount of glands, stroma, and blood vessels. Endometrial polyps are usually solitary and can occur anywhere within the uterus. Polyps are structurally diverse and are usually classified as hyperplastic, atrophic (or inactive), or functional. Hyperplastic polyps are often pedunculated (stalk or mushroomlike) and may be mistaken for endometrial hyperplasia or, if large, adenosarcoma (Figure 33-11). Although polyps most often develop in women between ages 40 and 50 years, they can occur at all ages. Hyperestrogenic states, obesity, use of tamoxifen (Nolvadex; a medication that blocks the actions of estrogen), and hypertension are risk factors for developing polyps.

Most polyps are asymptomatic; however, they are a common cause of intermenstrual bleeding or even excessive menstrual bleeding. Diagnosis is made by hysteroscopy or ultrasonography. The lesions can be removed with small, curved forceps but there is a high rate of spontaneous resolution. Coexistence of a separate endometrial atypical hyperplasia (AH) or adenocarcinoma is possible but malignancy is extremely rare.

Leiomyomas

Leiomyomas, commonly called myomas or uterine fibroids, are benign tumours that develop from smooth muscle cells in the myometrium. Leiomyomas are the most common benign tumours of the uterus, affecting 70 to 80% of all women, and most remain small and asymptomatic. Prevalence increases in women ages 30 to 50 years but decreases with menopause. The incidence of leiomyomas in black and Asian women is two to five times higher than that in white women.

The cause of uterine leiomyomas is unknown, although the size of the tumour appears to be related to hormonal fluctuations, including estrogen and progesterone, growth factors, and reduced apoptosis. Because leiomyomas are estrogen and progesterone sensitive, uterine leiomyomas are not seen before menarche, are common during the reproductive years, and generally shrink after menopause if present. Tumours in pregnant women enlarge rapidly but often decrease in size after the end of the pregnancy. Risk factors include heredity, nulliparity, obesity, PCOS, diabetes, being of African descent, and hypertension.

PATHOPHYSIOLOGY Most leiomyomas occur in multiples in the fundus of the uterus, although they often occur singly and throughout the uterus. Leiomyomas are classified as subserous, submucous, or intramural, according to location within the various layers of the uterine wall (Figure 33-12). Most leiomyomas have normal karyotypes, but some have simple chromosomal abnormalities. Recently, mutations in the Mediator Subcomplex 12 (*MED12*) gene have been identified in about 70% of uterine leiomyomas.[47] Uterine leiomyomas are usually firm and surrounded by a connective tissue layer. Degeneration and necrosis may occur when the leiomyoma outgrows its blood supply, which is more common in larger tumours and is frequently accompanied by pain.

CLINICAL MANIFESTATIONS The major clinical manifestations of leiomyomas are abnormal vaginal bleeding, pain, and symptoms related to pressure on nearby structures. Fibroids also may contribute to infertility and subfertility, as well as obstruction during birth if large enough. The leiomyoma can make the uterine cavity larger, thereby increasing the endometrial surface area. This enlargement may account for the increased menstrual bleeding associated with leiomyomas. Although pain is not an early symptom, it occurs with the devascularization of larger leiomyomas and is associated with blood vessel compression that limits blood supply to adjacent structures. Because the fibroid is relatively slow growing, enabling adjacent structures to adapt to pressure, symptoms of abdominal pressure develop slowly. Pressure on the bladder may contribute to urinary frequency, urgency, and dysuria. Pressure on the ureter may cause it to become distended "upstream" from the pressure point; rectosigmoid pressure may lead to constipation. Larger fibroids may cause a sensation of abdominal or genital heaviness.

EVALUATION AND TREATMENT Uterine leiomyomas are suspected when bimanual examination discloses irregular, nontender nodularity of the uterus. Pelvic sonography or MRI confirms the diagnosis. Treatment depends on symptoms, tumour size, age, reproductive status, and overall health of the individual. Most leiomyomas are asymptomatic and can be managed by observation only. Medical treatment is aimed at shrinking the myoma or reducing the symptoms. Use of hormonal contraceptives may shrink or enhance growth and should be closely monitored. Mifepristone (Mifegymiso; called *RU-486* in other countries), a progesterone receptor agonist, may be useful as a conservative treatment, while GnRH agonists may provide temporary management. Myomectomy or removal of the fibroid from the muscle of the uterus may be less invasive than a full hysterectomy and remains the standard of cure for women wishing to preserve their fertility. Other treatments, such as uterine artery embolization (UAE), laser ablation, and levonorgestrel intrauterine system (LNG-IUS), all hold promise. A Cochrane review found UAE appears to have an overall satisfaction rate similar to hysterectomy and myomectomy.[48] UAE is associated with a higher rate of minor complications and a much higher risk of requiring future surgical intervention within 2 to 5 years of the initial procedure.[48] Benefits and risks of all treatments should be carefully considered, as well as a woman's desire for future pregnancy.

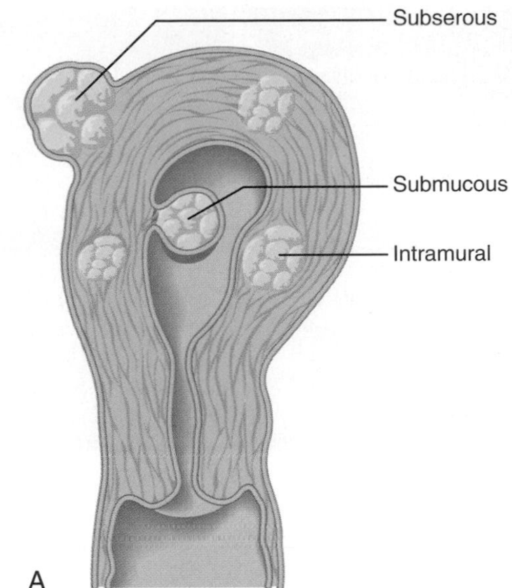

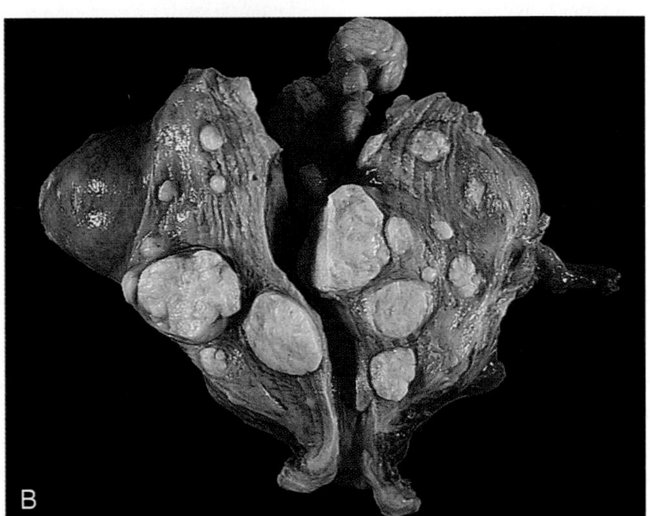

FIGURE 33-12 Leiomyomas. A, Uterine section showing whorl-like appearance and locations of leiomyomas, which are also called *uterine fibroids*. **B,** Multiple leiomyomas in sagittal section. Typical, well-circumscribed, solid, light grey nodules distort uterus. (**B,** from Damjanov, I., & Linder, J. [2000]. *Pathology: A color atlas*. St. Louis: Mosby.)

Adenomyosis

Adenomyosis is the presence of islands of endometrial glands surrounded by benign endometrial stroma within the uterine myometrium. It commonly develops during the late reproductive years, with the highest incidence among women in their 40s and in women taking tamoxifen. Parity also increases the risk for adenomyosis. Adenomyosis may be asymptomatic or may be associated with abnormal menstrual bleeding, anemia, dysmenorrhea, uterine enlargement, and uterine tenderness during menstruation. Secondary dysmenorrhea becomes increasingly

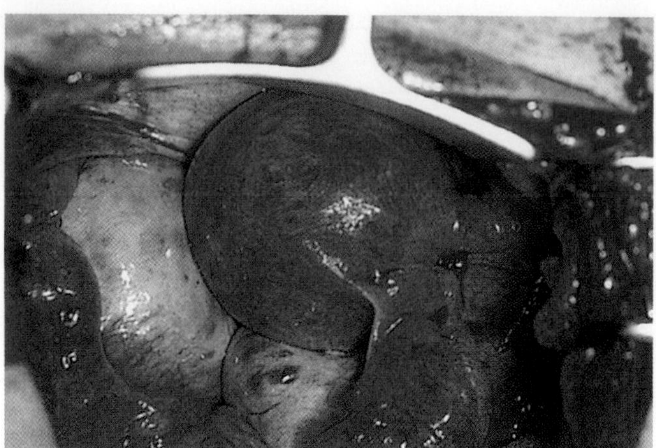

FIGURE 33-13 Endometriosis. The uterus is distended, and retrograde spill of menstrual loss has led to the development of endometriosis (*dark purple patches*). (From Symonds, E.M., & Macpherson, M.B.A. [1994]. *Color atlas of obstetrics and gynecology.* London: Mosby-Wolfe.)

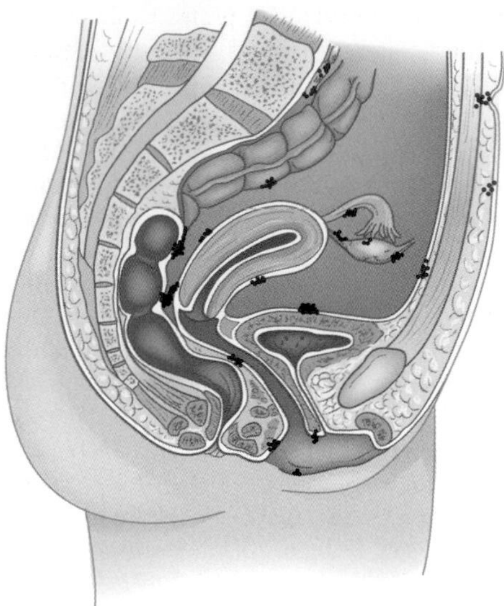

FIGURE 33-14 Pelvic Sites of Endometrial Implantation in Endometriosis. Endometrial cells may enter the pelvic cavity during retrograde menstruation.

severe as disease progresses. On examination, the uterus is enlarged, globular, and most tender just before or after menstruation. Diagnosis is confirmed with ultrasonography or MRI. Treatment is symptomatic, and similar to that for dysmenorrhea (i.e., NSAIDs, hormonal contraceptives, or LNG-IUS). Other options include surgical resection or, in severe cases, hysterectomy. UAE and LNG-IUDs have shown good initial results but need further testing.

Endometriosis

Endometriosis is the presence of functioning endometrial tissue or implants outside the uterus. Like normal endometrial tissue, the ectopic (out-of-place) endometrium responds to the hormonal fluctuations of the menstrual cycle. The incidence of endometriosis is difficult to determine, especially in asymptomatic adolescent and fertile women. About 50% of women evaluated for pelvic pain, infertility, or pelvic mass are diagnosed with endometriosis. Additionally, the frequency and severity of symptoms do not correlate with the extent or site of lesions. Many theories exist on the cause of endometriosis, including the implantation of endometrial cells during *retrograde menstruation*, in which menstrual fluids move through the fallopian tubes and into the pelvic cavity. It is now known, however, that retrograde menstruation occurs in almost all women, but not all women develop endometriosis. The main theories include coelomic metaplasia (peritoneal mesothelium, the müllerian ducts, and the germinal epithelium of the ovary are all derived from coelomic wall epithelium), retrograde menstruation, embryonic cell rest (primitive "at rest" embryonic cells become activated), iatrogenic mechanical transplantation, and lymphatic and vascular dissemination.[49] A genetic predisposition to endometriosis has been documented. Some genetic polymorphisms have been identified.

PATHOPHYSIOLOGY Endometriosis is a multifactorial estrogen-dependent condition that may affect 5 to 10% of women of child-bearing age in developed countries (Figure 33-13).[49] Emerging evidence suggests that endometriosis can have heterogeneous characteristics; therefore, the pathogenesis is modulated by many factors, including genetic, epigenetic, environmental, and cellular factors.[49] The endometrium is highly dynamic tissue with regenerative tissue undergoing cyclic processes of growth, differentiation, shedding, and regeneration as part of the menstrual cycle. These processes depend on steroid hormones, growth factors, and leukocytes that affect the balance between proliferation and apoptosis. Although endometriosis is considered benign, approximately 1.0% of affected women have an increased risk for malignant transformation involving multiple pathways of development.[49] The defining feature of endometriosis is the presence and proliferation of endometrial-like tissue (implants), including stromal and glandular tissue, in locations outside of the uterine cavity, primarily in the ovaries, fallopian tubes, bladder, rectosigmoid colon, and uterine myometrium (adenomyosis), often causing infertility and pain (Figure 33-14).[49]

The pathophysiology of endometriosis remains poorly understood, but several characteristics are being investigated, including the following:

- High levels of estrogen production are observed in endometriosis, and a key enzyme in estrogen production is aromatase, which has been correlated with the severity of endometriosis.
- There is evidence of switching of cell fates during development, where epithelial and mesenchymal markers highlight a contribution of the mesenchymal–epithelial transition (MET) and of the epithelial–mesenchymal transition (EMT) in endometriosis (see Chapter 10).
- The roles of inflammation and of peritoneal leukocytes and their mediators may facilitate the progression of endometriotic lesions.
- Some components of the innate immune system are involved in endometriosis (dendritic cells, macrophages, Toll-like receptors), and components of the adaptive immune system (T- and B-cell functions) can promote apoptosis, tissue damage, and multiorgan involvement.
- The development of lesions is dependent on new blood vessel development (angiogenesis).
- Genetic and epigenetic roles are present in endometriotic lesions and some ovarian cancers (clear cell carcinoma, endometrioid adenocarcinoma).
- Stem cells play a role in the development of endometriotic lesions. Changes in stem cell populations of endometriotic lesions are associated with genetic and epigenetic alterations.

Cyclic changes depend on the blood supply of the lesions (implants) and the presence of glandular and stromal cells. Given that the blood supply is sufficient, the ectopic endometrium proliferates, breaks down, and bleeds with the normal menstrual cycle. The bleeding is one cause of inflammation, triggering a cascade of cellular inflammatory mediators, including cytokines, chemokines, growth factors, and protective factors such as secretory leukocyte protease inhibitor and superoxide dismutase.[50] The inflammation may lead to fibrosis, scarring, adhesions, and pain.

CLINICAL MANIFESTATIONS The clinical manifestations of endometriosis vary in frequency and severity and can mimic other pelvic disease (i.e., PID, ovarian cysts, irritable bowel syndrome). Symptoms include infertility, pelvic pain, dyschezia (pain on defecation), dyspareunia, (pain on intercourse), and, less commonly, constipation and abnormal vaginal bleeding. If implants are located within the pelvis, an asymptomatic pelvic mass having irregular, movable nodules and a fixed, retroverted uterus are found on examination. Most symptoms can be explained by the proliferation, breakdown, and bleeding of the ectopic endometrial tissue with subsequent formation of adhesions. In most instances, however, the degree of endometriosis is not related to the frequency or severity of symptoms. Dysmenorrhea, for example, does not appear to be related to the degree of endometriosis. With involvement of the rectovaginal septum or the uterosacral ligaments, dyspareunia develops. Dyschezia, a hallmark symptom of endometriosis, occurs with bleeding of ectopic endometrium in the rectosigmoid musculature and subsequent fibrosis.

Up to 25 to 40% of women with infertility have endometriosis. The relationship between endometriosis and infertility is strong; however, the *degree* of disease is not as closely associated. More simply, women with untreated minimal to mild disease may have high pregnancy rates or may experience infertility. The exact reason for infertility in women with endometriosis is unknown.

EVALUATION AND TREATMENT A presumptive diagnosis is based on the previously described symptoms, but pelvic laparoscopy is required for a definitive diagnosis. A uniform classification system that includes both extent and severity has been developed including stage I, minimal; stage II, mild; and stage III, moderate. The classification, however, still does not correlate well with a woman's symptoms. Treatment is based on preventing progression of the disease, alleviating pain, and restoring fertility. Medical therapies include suppression of ovulation with various medications, such as noncyclic estrogen-progestin–combined oral contraceptive pills (COCs), depot medroxyprogesterone acetate (DMPA), danazol (Cyclomen), GnRH agonists, or mifepristone, and promotion of atrophy of the endometrium with progestins or an LNG-IUD. Conservative surgical treatment includes laparoscopic removal of endometrial implants with conventional or laser techniques and presacral neurectomy for severe dysmenorrhea. All treatments have risks or side effects and recurrent symptoms will develop in the majority of women within a few years, even with surgical treatments. Women should be fully informed of all options and understand the risk-to-benefit ratio of treatments, especially nonreversible treatments.

Cancer

Malignant tumours of the female reproductive system are common. Because the pelvis and abdomen are poorly innervated and designed to accommodate a growing fetus, cancers of the female reproductive tract can often grow large before causing pain. Reproductive cancers are likely to be diagnosed early if there are symptoms; for example, vaginal bleeding prompts women to seek treatment. Cervical cancer has minimal symptoms until late in the process, but is easy to detect early with Pap smears. Globally, cervical cancer is ranked third in incidence. However, in Canada this cancer is ranked eleventh in incidence. This significant difference is attributed to the advent of improved screening techniques, increased uptake of testing, and the universality of the Canadian health care system.[51] Investigators are researching new biomarkers for the screening, diagnosis, and surveillance for ovarian cancer. Obtaining an early diagnosis for ovarian cancer is very challenging.

Cervical Cancer

Cervical cancer is the fourth most common cancer in women worldwide, and has the fourth highest death rate among cancers in women.[52,53] The Canadian Cancer Society estimated that 1 550 Canadian women were diagnosed with invasive cervical cancer in 2017. It also estimated that 400 Canadian women died of this disease in 2017.[51] In Canada, female populations identified less likely to participate in regular cervical cancer screening include recent immigrants, Indigenous people, those of lower socioeconomic status, and those living in rural areas. The rates of invasive cervical cancer in Canada have steadily decreased since the 1960s, and death rates have declined significantly in Canada (and other developed countries)—a decline mainly attributable to the prevalence and frequency of screening with Pap tests.[51,54,55] (See *Health Promotion:* Screening With the Papanicolaou Test and With the Human Papillomavirus DNA Test.) Deaths related to cervical cancer in Canada have declined by 83% between 1952 and 2006, with older adult women experiencing the greatest decline.[51]

It is now widely known that HPV infection is a necessary condition in the development of almost all precancerous and cancerous cervical lesions. There are multiple subtypes of HPV, and the "high-risk" (oncogenic) types of HPV (predominantly 16 and 18) have been most closely associated with high-grade dysplasia and cancer (also see Chapters 10 and 11). The precancerous lesion or dysplasia, also called *cervical intraepithelial neoplasia* (CIN) and *cervical carcinoma in situ* (CIS), is a more advanced form of the cell changes and can progress to become invasive cancer. This process can be very slow. About 30 to 70% of those untreated for in situ carcinoma will develop invasive carcinoma over 10 to 12 years; but in about 10% of women, progression from in situ to invasive cancer can occur in less than 1 year.[56] Other risk factors for cervical cancer include multiple sexual partners, a male partner with multiple previous or current sexual partners, young age at first sexual intercourse, high parity, persistent infection with HPV-16 or HPV-18, immunosuppression, use of oral contraceptives, certain human leukocyte antigen (HLA) subtypes, and use of nicotine.[34,56]

PATHOGENESIS As discussed earlier, HPV-16 and HPV-18 are the most important risk factors for cervical disease progression and cancer. HPV-16 accounts for about 60% of cervical cancer cases and HPV-18 for about another 10%; other types contribute less than 5% of cases. The cervix is lined by two types of epithelial cells: squamous cells at the outer aspect and columnar glandular cells along the inner canal (Figure 33-15). The site of the cellular transformation zone, called the *squamous-columnar junction,* is illustrated in Figure 33-16. HPVs infect immature basal cells of the squamous epithelium in the areas of epithelial breaks or injury, or immature metaplastic squamous cells present at the squamous-columnar junction. Establishing HPV infection in the mature squamous cells that cover the ectocervix, vagina, or vulva requires damage to the surface epithelium. The cervix, with its large areas of immature epithelium, is very vulnerable to HPV infection.[34] The ability of HPV to act as a carcinogen depends on the viral proteins E6 and E7 because they interfere with the activity of tumour-suppressor proteins that regulate cell growth and survival.[34] Replication of HPV occurs in the maturing squamous cells, and studies have shown that HPV activates the cell cycle by interfering with two tumour-suppressor genes, *Rb* and *p53*.[34] Although HPV is a causative factor for cervical cancer, it is not the *only* factor. Other important cocarcinogens must play a role because in spite of the high percentage of young women infected with one or more HPV types during their reproductive years, only a few develop cancer. The other factors that appear to be associated include immune

HEALTH PROMOTION

Screening With the Papanicolaou Test and With the Human Papillomavirus DNA Test

Evidence shows that regular screening of appropriate women for cervical cancer with the Papanicolaou (Pap) test reduces mortality from cervical cancer. The benefits of screening women younger than 21 years are small because of the low prevalence of lesions that will progress to invasive cancer. Screening is not beneficial in women older than 65 years if they have had a history of recent negative tests.[*,†,‡] Regular Pap screening decreases cervical cancer incidence and mortality by at least 80%.[§]

When considering the harmful effects of Pap screening, evidence shows that regular screening leads to additional diagnostic procedures (e.g., colposcopy) and treatment for low-grade squamous intraepithelial lesions (LSILs), with long-term consequences for fertility and pregnancy. These harms are greatest for younger women, who have a higher prevalence of LSILs—lesions that often regress without treatment. Harms are also increased in younger women because they have a higher rate of false-positive results.

Additional cervical screening may be undertaken with the human papillomavirus (HPV) DNA test (also called *HPV RNA* and *HPV test*). Evidence shows that screening with the HPV DNA test detects high-grade cervical dysplasia, a precursor lesion for cervical cancer. Additional clinical trials show that HPV testing is superior to other cervical cancer screening strategies. The HPV test is available in Canada but is not used in all provinces and is not used as a part of regular cervical cancer screening.[**] This test is used only for women 30 years of age and older as a follow-up to abnormal Pap test results.[§]

Routine HPV testing may have harmful consequences. Evidence shows that HPV testing identifies numerous infections that will not lead to cervical dysplasia or cervical cancer. This point is especially true for women younger than 30 years, in whom rates of HPV infection may be higher. A positive test may expose these women to additional unnecessary examinations and testing.

Regarding the combined use of the Pap test and the HPV DNA test, evidence shows that screening every 5 years with the Pap test and the HPV DNA test (cotesting) in women 30 years and older is more sensitive in detecting cervical abnormalities, compared with the Pap test alone. Screening with the Pap test and HPV DNA test reduces the incidence of cervical cancer.[‡]

There are also potential harmful consequences of combined testing, with evidence revealing that co-testing is associated with more false-positive results than the Pap test alone. Abnormal test results can lead to more frequent testing and invasive diagnostic procedures.[‡]

Regarding women who present for screening without a cervix, evidence shows that screening is not helpful in these women if the hysterectomy was performed for a benign condition.

*Sasieni, P., Castanon, A., & Cuzick, J. (2009). *BMJ, 339,* b2968; †Sawaya, G.F., McConnell, K.J., Kulasingam, S.L., et al. (2003). *N Engl J Med, 349*(16), 1501–1509; ‡Moyer, V.A. (2012). *Ann Intern Med, 156*(12), 880–891, W312; §National Cancer Institute. (2015). *PDQ® cervical cancer screening.* Retrieved from https://www.cancer.gov/types/cervical/hp/cervical-screening-pdq#link/_115_toc; **Canadian Cancer Society. (2016). *HPV testing.* Retrieved from http://www.cancer.ca/en/prevention-and-screening/be-aware/viruses-and-bacteria/human-papillomavirus-hpv/hpv-testing/?region=on.

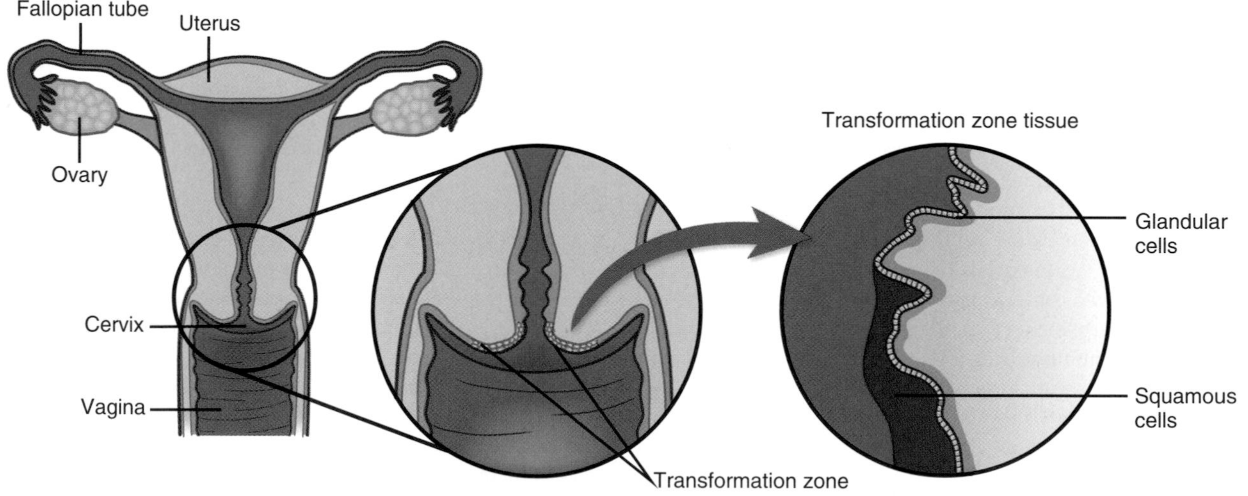

FIGURE 33-15 Cervix Is Lined by Two Types of Epithelial Cells: Squamous Cells and Columnar Glandular Cells.

responses, hormonal responses, and other environmental factors that determine regression or persistence of the HPV infection.[34] Cervical cancer is a slowly progressive disease and moves from normal cervical epithelial cells to dysplasia to carcinoma in situ and, eventually, to invasive cancer (see Figure 33-16, *B*). Table 33-4 summarizes the staging of cervical cancer. Testing for high-risk HPV is often positive for many years (10 years or more) before dysplasia progresses to high-grade squamous intraepithelial lesions (HSILs) that can develop into invasive cervical cancer (CIN III, Table 33-5).

CLINICAL MANIFESTATIONS Because cervical neoplasms are predominantly asymptomatic, about 90% of cervical cancers can be detected early through the use of Pap and HPV testing. If symptoms exist, they may include a change in vaginal discharge or bleeding. Bleeding varies and may occur after intercourse or between menstrual periods. At times, women will complain of abnormal menses or postmenopausal bleeding. A less common symptom may be a serosanguineous or yellowish vaginal discharge. A new or foul odour also may be present. Advanced disease may cause urinary or rectal symptoms and pelvic or back pain.

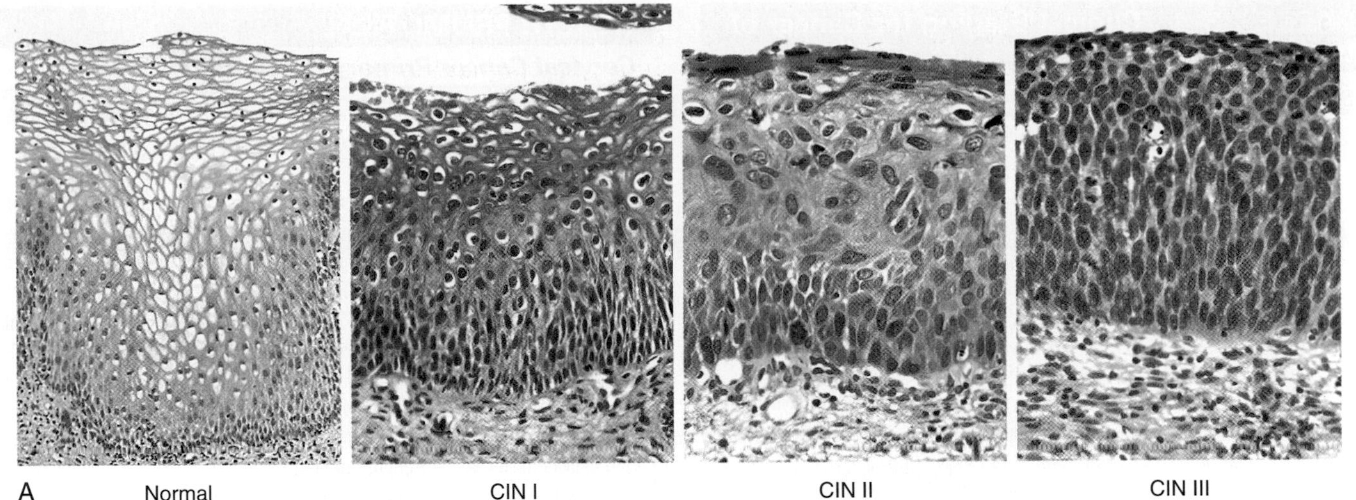

Cervical Disease Progression[1-6]

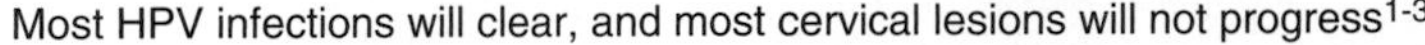
Most HPV infections will clear, and most cervical lesions will not progress[1-3]

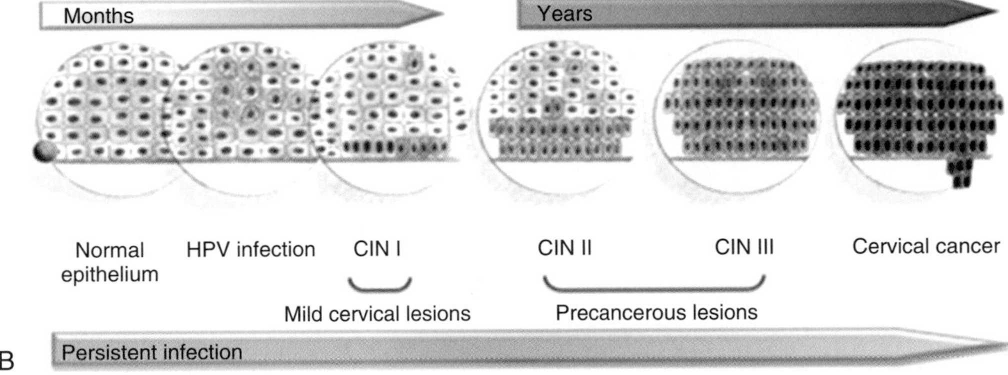

• CIN 2/3 lesions are more likely to progress to cervical cancer than CIN 1 lesions[1]

1. Oster A. *Int J of Gynecol Path*, 1993, 12:186-92. 2. Moscicki A et al, *Vaccine*, 2006, 2453:42-51. 3. Einstein M. *Cancer Immunol Immunother*, 2008, 57:443-51. 4. Winer R. et al. *J Int Dis*, 2005, 191:731-38. 5. Holowaty P. et al. *J Natl Cancer Inst*, 1999, 91:252-58. 6. Solomon D. et al. *JAMA*, 2002, 287:2114-19.

FIGURE 33-16 Cervical Intraepithelial Neoplasia. **A,** Normal multiparous cervix including the transformation zone where precancerous and cancerous changes occur. CIN stage I, note the white appearance of part of the anterior lip of the cervix associated with neoplastic changes; CIN stage II, lesions also are reflected in distant capillaries; CIN stage III, lesions are predominantly around the external os. **B,** Normal epithelium, HPV infection progressing to CIN stage I, and then with more time persistent HPV infections progressing to precancerous lesions CIN II and CIN III and eventually cervical cancer. Most cervical lesions do not progress to cervical cancer. *CIN,* cervical intraepithelial neoplasia; *HPV,* human papillomavirus. (**A,** from Kumar, V., Abbas, A.K., & Aster, J.C. [Eds.]. [2015]. *Robbins and Cotran pathologic basis of disease* [9th ed.]. Philadelphia: Saunders; **B,** from Symonds, E.M., & Macpherson, M.B.A. [1994]. *Color atlas of obstetrics and gynecology.* London: Mosby.)

EVALUATION AND TREATMENT When dysplasia is detected, colposcopy is usually indicated to identify lesions and obtain needed biopsies. If invasive carcinoma is found, lymphangiography, computed tomography (CT) scan, MRI, ultrasonography, or radioimmunodetection methods are used to further assess tissue involvement.

Treatment depends on the degree of neoplastic change, the size and location of the lesion, and the extent of metastatic spread. Treatment for invasive carcinoma depends on the stage of the tumour and includes surgery, radiation therapy, chemotherapy, and targeted treatment. Prognosis is excellent with early detection and treatment. The prevention of HPV infection appears to be key for substantially reducing the risk for cervical cancer, and the Health Canada–approved vaccines for two of the high-risk types of HPV show excellent promise (see *Health Promotion:* Cervical Cancer Primary Prevention).

Vaginal Cancer

Cancer of the vagina is the rarest (about 0.6 per 100 000 women yearly) of the female genital cancers. It can occur at any age but is found predominantly in women 50 years of age and older. More than 90% of women with vaginal cancer have squamous cell carcinoma. Most squamous cell carcinomas of the vagina are associated with high-risk HPVs. Risk factors include being age 60 or older; diethylstilbestrol (DES) exposure in utero; HPV-16 (cause); human immunodeficiency virus (HIV); genital warts (associated most often with nononcogenic types HPV-6 and HPV-11, which can infect female and male genital organs and the anal area); and previous carcinoma of the cervix or vulva. The relationship between vaginal cancer and developing precancerous cell changes (called *vaginal intraepithelial neoplasia* [VAIN]) is controversial because these changes are associated with oncogenic HPV.[57,58]

TABLE 33-4 Clinical Staging for Cancer of the Cervix

Stage	Characteristics
0	Cancer in situ, intraepithelial carcinoma; earliest stage of cancer; cancer confined to its original site
I	Carcinoma confined to cervix (extension to corpus disregarded)
IA	Earliest form of stage I; there is very small amount of cancer, which is visible only under a microscope
IA1	Area of invasion is <3 mm deep and <7 mm wide
IA2	Area of invasion is between 3 and 5 mm deep, and <7 mm wide
IB	Includes cancers that can be seen without a microscope; also includes cancers seen only with a microscope that have spread deeper than 5 mm into connective tissue of the cervix or are wider than 7 mm
IB1	IB cancer that is no larger than 4 cm
IB2	IB cancer that is >4 cm
II	Cancer has spread beyond the cervix to the upper part of the vagina; cancer does not involve the lower third of the vagina
IIA	Cancer has spread beyond the cervix to the upper part of the vagina; cancer does not involve the lower third of the vagina
IIB	Cancer has spread to the tissue next to the cervix, called the *parametrial tissue*
III	Cancer has spread to the lower part of the vagina or the pelvic wall; cancer may be blocking the ureters (tubes that carry urine from the kidneys to the bladder)
IIIA	Cancer has spread to the lower third of the vagina but not to the pelvic wall
IIIB	Cancer extends to the pelvic wall, blocks urine flow to the bladder, or both
IV	Most advanced stage of cervical cancer; cancer has spread to other parts of the body
IVA	Cancer has spread to the bladder or rectum, which are organs close to the cervix
IVB	Cancer has spread to distant organs beyond the pelvic area, such as the lungs

TABLE 33-5 Classification System for Squamous Cervical Precursor Lesions

Dysplasia/ Carcinoma in Situ	Cervical Intraepithelial Neoplasia	Squamous Intraepithelial Lesion, Current Classification
Mild dysplasia	CIN I	Low-grade SIL (LSIL)
Moderate dysplasia	CIN II	High-grade SIL (HSIL)
Severe dysplasia	CIN III	High-grade SIL (HSIL)
Carcinoma in situ	CIN III	High-grade SIL (HSIL)

CIN, cervical intraepithelial neoplasia; *SIL*, squamous intraepithelial lesion.
From Kumar, V., Abbas, A.K., & Aster, J.C. (Eds.). (2015). *Robbins and Cotran pathologic basis of disease* (9th ed.). Philadelphia: Saunders.

A large proportion (30 to 50%) of women with vaginal carcinomas have had a prior hysterectomy for benign, premalignant, or malignant disease.[59]

Vaginal cancer can be asymptomatic. Therefore, regular pelvic examinations, particularly for women with a history of intrauterine DES exposure, are extremely important. Clinical manifestations that occur include abnormal vaginal bleeding or discharge not related to menstrual periods, pain during intercourse, pain in the pelvic area, pain when urinating, and constipation.

Very careful biopsy techniques confirm the tumour type and determine its size, location, and extent. Treatment depends on these findings and on the age of the individual. Treatments include surgery, chemotherapy, and radiation therapy.

HEALTH PROMOTION

Cervical Cancer Primary Prevention

Individuals not sexually active rarely develop genital HPV infections. HPV vaccination before sexual activity can reduce the risk for infection by HPV types targeted by the vaccine.

Health Canada has approved three vaccines to prevent HPV infection: Gardasil, Gardasil 9, and Cervarix. These vaccines provide strong protection against the HPV-targeted infections, but they are not effective for treating established infections or disease caused by HPV. All three vaccines prevent infections with HPV-16 and HPV-18, the two high-risk HPVs that cause about 70% of cervical cancers. Gardasil also prevents infection with HPV-6 and HPV-11, which causes about 90% of genital warts. Gardasil 9 prevents infection with the same four high-risk HPV types plus five additional high-risk types (31, 33, 45, 52, and 58). All three vaccines are given as a series of three injections into muscle tissue over a 6-month period.

Importantly, consistent and correct condom use is associated with reduced HPV transmission, and less frequent use is not. The virus can infect areas not covered by the condom.

From National Cancer Institute. (2016). *Human papillomavirus (HPV) vaccines*. Retrieved from https://www.cancer.gov/about-cancer/causes-prevention/risk/infectious-agents/hpv-vaccine-fact-sheet; Public Health Agency of Canada. (2011). *Human papillomavirus (HPV) prevention and HPV vaccines: Questions and answers*. Retrieved from https://www.canada.ca/en/public-health/services/infectious-diseases/sexual-health-sexually-transmitted-infections/hpv-prevention-vaccines-questions-answers.html.

Vulvar Cancer

Cancer of the vulva most often affects the labia majora and less often the labia minora, clitoris, or vaginal glands.[60] In Canada, 955 women were diagnosed with unspecified female genital organ cancers in 2013, which includes vulvar cancer.[61] Risk factors for vulvar cancer include HPV-16 (cause), HIV, HPV-18 (probable cause), increasing age, previous cancer (untreated high-grade vulvar intraepithelial neoplasia [VIN]), cervical cancer survivor, previous CIN, women with certain autoimmune conditions (increased risk for HPV-associated tumours), organ transplant recipients (perhaps because of immunosuppression to clear HPV), and tobacco use (may relate to inability to clear HPV infection).[62] The development of vulvar cancer is preceded by condyloma or squamous dysplasia.[63] Other possible risk factors include having many sexual partners, having first sexual intercourse at a young age, and having a history of abnormal Pap tests.[63] Risk factors for STIs are risk factors for vulvar cancer. Early detection is critical. Treatment includes surgery, radiation, chemotherapy, and biological therapy.

Endometrial Cancer

Carcinoma of the endometrium is the most common type of uterine cancer and the most prevalent gynecological malignancy (Figure 33-17). The Canadian Cancer Society estimated that 7 300 Canadian women were diagnosed with uterine cancer (which includes endometrial cancer) in 2017. It also estimated that 1 150 Canadian women died of this disease in 2017.[51] In Canada, the 5-year net survival for uterine cancer

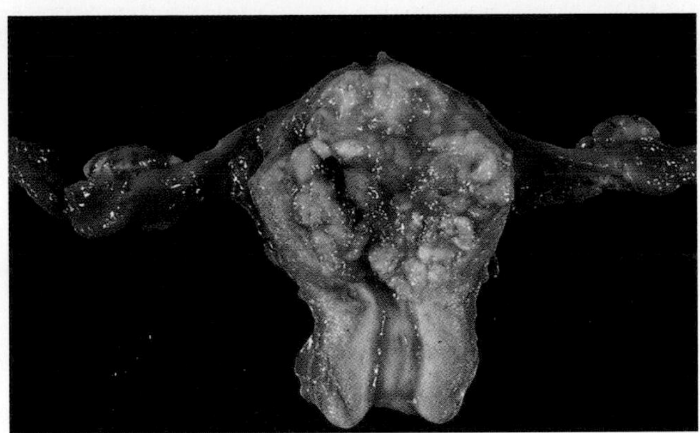

FIGURE 33-17 Endometrial Cancer. Tumour fills the endometrial cavity. Obvious myometrial invasion is shown. (From Damjanov, I., & Linder, J. [Eds.]. [1996]. *Anderson's pathology* [10th ed.]. St. Louis: Mosby.)

is 84%.[64] It is the sixth most common cancer worldwide, and the incidence is highest in high-income countries in North America and in Northern and Western Europe.[65]

The primary risk factor for endometrial cancer is unopposed estrogen exposure (without progesterone). Exposure to unopposed estrogen includes estrogen-only HRT, tamoxifen, early menarche, late menopause, never having children, and a failure to ovulate (i.e., PCOS and anovulatory cycles typical of the late reproductive years). Less is known about the association between endometrial cancer and other types of hormone therapy. Chronic hyperinsulinemia, hyperglycemia, body fatness and adult weight gain, chronic inflammation, and lack of physical activity represent an increased risk for endometrial cancer[66] (Figure 33-18).

Epidemiological studies suggest an association between type 2 diabetes mellitus and endometrial cancer, as well as other cancers, and that type 2 diabetes mellitus increases mortality.[67-69] Diabetes mellitus and cancer share several mechanisms, including insulin and insulinlike growth factor (IGF) signalling, dysregulation of ovarian steroid hormones, and chronic inflammation.[69] Some studies have shown an elevated risk for endometrial cancer with PCOS and insulin resistance.[70] Additionally, another cause may be epigenetic silencing of the tumour-suppressor gene *PTEN*.[71]

Investigators recently found the use of long-cycle estrogen and progestin HRT was related to a tendency toward an elevated risk of developing endometrial cancer for exposure less than 5 years or more.[72] For exposure of more than 10 years, the risk for endometrial cancer was elevated among users of long-cycle HRT and sequential HRT. Norethisterone acetate and medroxyprogesterone acetate (MPA) (HRT) did not differ in their endometrial cancer risk.[73,74] The use of continuous HRT or estradiol plus a LNG-IUD system (Mirena) showed a decreased risk for endometrial cancer.[72] Other risk factors not directly related to estrogen include gallbladder disease and hypertension, although being overweight may be a mediating factor for these risks. A family history of colon, endometrial, or ovarian cancer could signal hereditary nonpolyposis colorectal cancer (HNPCC; also known as *Lynch syndrome*); women with this family history may wish to explore genetic testing and more aggressive screening.[75]

Ninety-five percent of endometrial cancers occur in postmenopausal women, with the peak incidence occurring in the late 50s to early 60s. Although incidence rates are slightly higher in White women than in Black women, death rates in Black women are nearly twice as high as those for other ethnic or racial groups. Factors related to reductions in risk for endometrial cancer include delayed menarche; history of pregnancy or breastfeeding, or both; use of combined hormonal contraception; use of progestin-containing IUDs; and engagement in

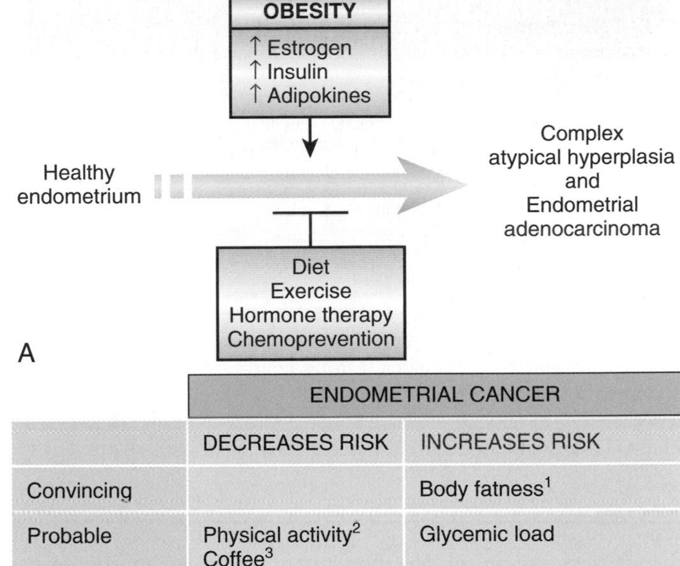

ENDOMETRIAL CANCER		
	DECREASES RISK	INCREASES RISK
Convincing		Body fatness[1]
Probable	Physical activity[2] Coffee[3]	Glycemic load

1 The panel interpreted BMI (including BMI at age 18–25 years), measures of abdominal girth, and adult weight gain as interrelated aspects of body fatness as well as fat distribution
2 Physical activity of all types; occupational, household, transport, and recreational
3 The effect is found in both caffeinated and decaffeinated coffee and cannot be attributed to caffeine

B

FIGURE 33-18 Food, Nutrition, Physical Activity, and Endometrial Cancer. A, Overview of the contribution of obesity to endometrial cancer progression and preventive strategies. The T-shaped bar indicates factors that decrease the risk for endometrial cancer. See text for full discussion. **B,** Convincing and probable data for decreases and increases of endometrial cancer. *BMI*, body mass index. (**A,** Reprinted from *Am J Obstet Gynecol*, 205(6), Schmandt, R.E., et al, "Understanding obesity and endometrial cancer risk: opportunities for prevention," Pages 518–525, Copyright 2011, with permission from Elsevier. **B,** from World Cancer Research Fund/American Institute for Cancer Research. [2013]. *Continuous update project report: Food, nutrition, physical activity, and the prevention of endometrial cancer.* Retrieved from http://www.dietandcancerreport.org.)

physical activity. So far, the lone dietary factor that may lower risk for endometrial cancer is drinking coffee regularly.[66] A large European study[76] first investigated the link between coffee and endometrial cancer risk. Then researchers looked at dietary factors in two US studies—the Nurses' Health Studies I and II.[77] For those in the European study, the average high coffee intake was about 3 cups per day, and in the United States it was 4.5 cups of coffee per day.

PATHOGENESIS Endometrial hyperplasia is associated with prolonged estrogenic stimulation of the endometrium. Endometrial hyperplasia and carcinoma share acquired genetic alterations in genes linked to carcinogenesis.[34] Frequent alterations in endometrial cancer include (1) altered estrogen receptor (ER) and progesterone receptor (PR) expression; (2) genetic mutation causing loss of function (inactivation) of the tumour-suppressor gene *PTEN*, which may enhance (3) the PI3K/AKT signalling pathway to become overactive, increasing the ability of the ER to "turn on" the expression of target genes; and (4) mutations to several genes, including fibroblast growth factor receptor (FGFR) and tumour protein 53 (TP53).[78] All of these events are predicted to affect PR actions in cancer pathogenesis. Progesterone inhibits estrogen-driven

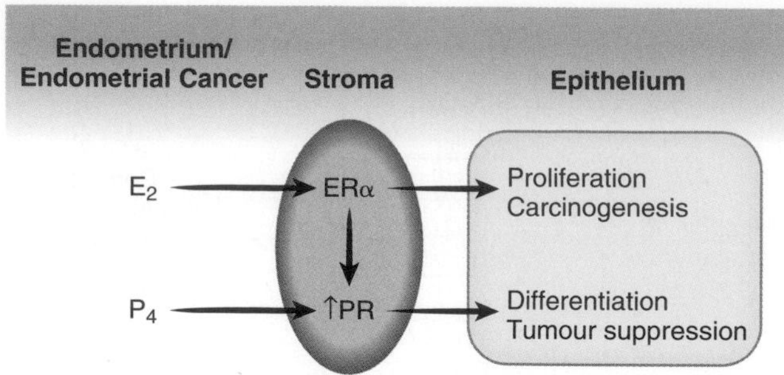

FIGURE 33-19 Actions of Estradiol and Progesterone in the Development of Endometrial Cancer. Estradiol (*E_2*) action through stromal estrogen receptor alpha (*ERα*) is critical for the development of endometrial cancer. Progesterone (*P_4*) acts through stromal progesterone receptor (*PR*) to oppose this carcinogenic effect of E_2. (From Kim, J.J., Kurita, T., & Bulun, S.E. [2013]. *Endocr Rev, 34*[1], 130–162.)

growth in the uterus.[78] The antagonistic effects of progesterone on the estrogen-induced proliferation and growth occur mostly during the luteal phase and are dependent on the presence of functional PR expression.[78] Investigators are studying the importance of stromal PR and its role in progesterone inhibition of epithelial proliferation (Figure 33-19). The interactions between the epithelial and stromal cells of the endometrium may determine the eventual role in the actions of progesterone.[78] PR has two isoforms: PR-A and PR-B. These isoforms are both expressed in the epithelial and stromal cells of the endometrium, and their expression fluctuates during the menstrual cycle as well as during pregnancy. The delicate balance of the PR isoforms can tip the scales to foster endometrial hyperplasia and atypia and enhance expression of uterine growth factors.[78] Overall, depending on isoform expression, progesterone can be either an anti- or a pro-proliferative force on the endometrium. Misregulation of isoform expression can lead to abnormal function and precancerous changes.[78]

Two broad categories of endometrial carcinoma include type I and type II. About 80% of cases are type I. Type I and type II endometrial carcinoma are summarized in Table 33-6.

TABLE 33-6 Type I and Type II Endometrial Carcinoma

Characteristics	Type I	Type II
Age	55–65 years	65–75 years
Clinical setting	Unopposed estrogen Obesity Hypertension Diabetes	Atrophy Thin physique
Morphology	Endometrioid	Serous Clear cell Mixed müllerian tumour
Precursor	Hyperplasia	Serous endometrial intraepithelial carcinoma
Mutated genes/ genetic abnormalities	*PTEN* *ARID1A* (regulator of chromatin) *PIK3CA* (PI3K) *KRAS* *FGF2* (growth factor) MSI *CTNNB1* (beta-catenin gene involved in Wnt signalling) *TP53*	*TP53* Aneuploidy *PIK3CA* (PI3K) *FBXW7* (regulator of MYC, cyclin E) *CHD4* (regulator of chromatin) *PPP2R1A* (PP2A)
Behaviour	Indolent Spreads via lymphatics	Aggressive Intraperitoneal and lymphatic spread

MSI, microsatellite instability, *MYC*, myelocytomatosis viral oncogene homologue; *PI3K*, phosphatidylinositol-3-kinase; *PP2A*, protein phosphatase 2A.
From Kumar, V., Abbas, A.K., & Aster, J.C. (Eds.). (2015). *Robbins and Cotran pathologic basis of disease* (9th ed.). Philadelphia: Saunders.

CLINICAL MANIFESTATIONS, EVALUATION, AND TREATMENT Abnormal vaginal bleeding is the most common clinical manifestation of endometrial cancer. Postmenopausal women, obese women, and women with unopposed estrogenic conditions (i.e., anovulatory cycles) should be evaluated in the event of unscheduled or persistent, irregular vaginal bleeding. Pain and weight loss are symptoms of more advanced disease. Transvaginal ultrasound (TVUS) may be used to measure endometrial thickness. If the endometrium is abnormally thick (defined as greater than 5 mm), then further testing, such as an endometrial biopsy, is done. Treatment is based on the extent of the disease and may include curettage for carcinoma in situ, total abdominal hysterectomy, chemotherapy, radiation, and (although controversial) progestins. The data supporting the use of metformin in the prevention and treatment of cancers are increasing, including those for endometrial cancer.[79,80]

Ovarian Cancer

Among gynecological malignancies, ovarian cancer is the leading cause of mortality in developed countries, with 239 000 new cases and 152 000 estimated deaths worldwide[53] (Figure 33-20). Globally, ovarian cancer is the seventh most common cancer and the eighth cause of death from cancer in women.[53] Incidence rates are highest in more developed regions and lowest in sub-Saharan Africa.[53] The Canadian Cancer Society estimated that 2 800 Canadian women were diagnosed with ovarian cancer in 2017. It also estimated that 1 800 Canadian women died of this disease in 2017.[51] An understanding of incidence patterns both within and between populations is essential to revealing potential causes of and risk factors for ovarian cancer (Figure 33-21). Worldwide, ovarian cancer is responsible for more deaths than all other gynecological malignancies combined.[53] Risk factors for ovarian cancer are summarized in Table 33-7.

Despite study limitations, several factors related to ovulation have been consistently associated with increased or decreased risk of developing ovarian cancer. Risk is reduced by factors that suppress ovulation (pregnancy, breastfeeding, and combined hormonal contraceptive use). Ovarian cancer has been a very difficult disease to diagnose early and treat. The high mortality reflects a lack of early symptoms and a lack of effective screening tests.

PATHOGENESIS The biology of ovarian cancer is changing, and it is clear that ovarian cancer is diverse in character, or *heterogeneous*. Many genetic and epigenetic changes are evident in ovarian tumours. Previously, the majority of ovarian cancers were thought to arise from just epithelial cells that cover the ovarian surface or line subserosal cysts. Newer evidence suggests that tumours arise from three ovarian components: (1) from the fimbriae of fallopian tubes and from deposits of endometriosis; (2) from germ cells, which are pluripotent and migrate to the ovary from the yolk sac; and (3) from stromal cells, including the sex cords, which precede endocrine changes of the postnatal ovary.[34,81] Some ovarian tumours remain too difficult to classify. The normal ovary contains

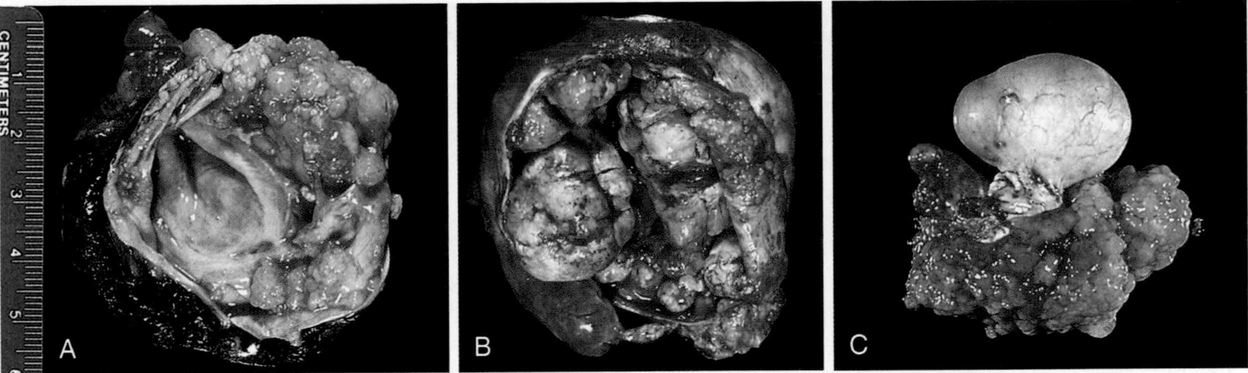

FIGURE 33-20 Ovarian Tumours. A serous borderline tumour displays a cyst cavity lined by papillary tumour growths **(A)**. The cyst is opened **(B)** to reveal a large bulky tumour mass called *cystadenocarcinoma* **(C)**, a tumour on the ovarian surface. Bilaterality of tumours is common, occurring in 20% of benign tumours, 30% of serous borderline tumours, and approximately 66% of serous carcinomas. A significant proportion of both borderline malignant and malignant tumours involve the surface of the ovary **(C)**. (From Kumar, V., Abbas, A.K., & Aster, J.C. [Eds.]. [2015]. *Robbins and Cotran pathologic basis of disease* [9th ed.]. Philadelphia: Saunders.)

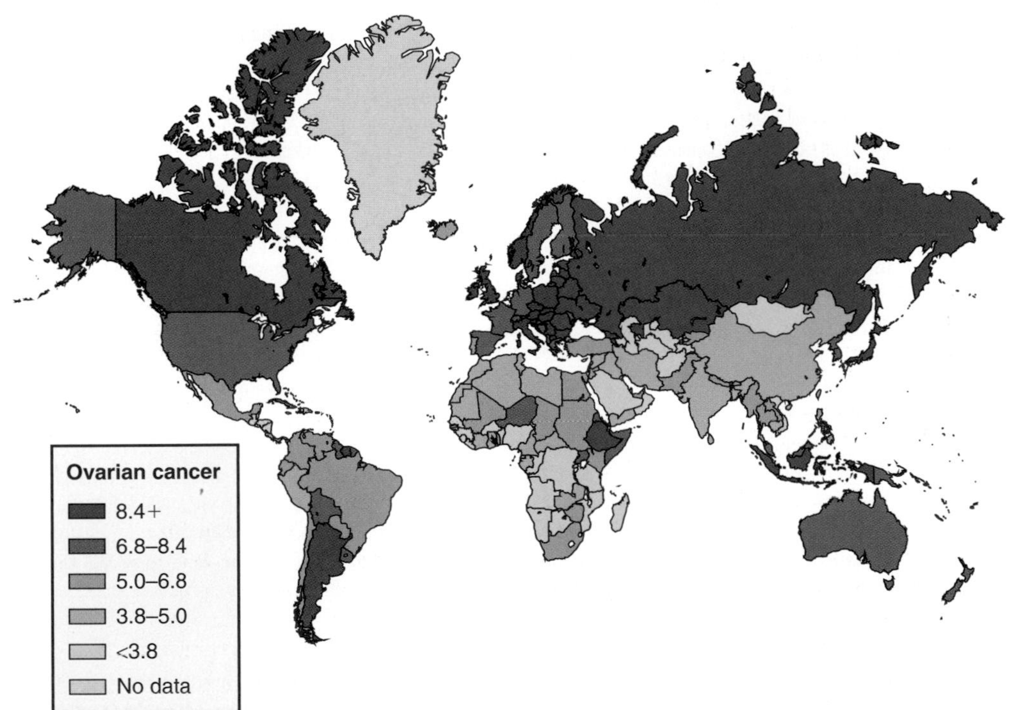

FIGURE 33-21 Map of Ovarian Cancer Worldwide. Rates are per 100 000 women and are age-standardized to the 1960 world standard population. Data were not included for white areas on the map. (Reproduced with permission from Ferlay J, Soerjomataram I, Ervik M, Dikshit R, Eser S, Mathers C, Rebelo M, Parkin DM, Forman D, Bray, F. GLOBOCAN 2012 v1.0, Cancer Incidence and Mortality Worldwide: IARC CancerBase No. 11 [Internet]. Lyon, France: International Agency for Research on Cancer; 2013. Available from: http://globocan.iarc.fr, accessed on 28 September 2017.)

three major cell types: (1) germ cells that are derived from the endoderm and migrate to the gonadal ridge, where they proliferate and differentiate into oocytes; (2) the endocrine and interstitial hormone producing cells that produce estrogen and progesterone; and (3) epithelial cells derived from the müllerian duct that cover the ovary and line inclusion cysts just beneath the ovarian surface. During normal ovulation, oocytes released from mature follicles enter the fallopian tube where fertilization usually occurs. The fimbriae of the fallopian tube cover the ruptured follicle and promote uptake of oocytes.[82] Both benign and malignant tumours come from each of the three ovarian cell types[83] (Figure 33-22). Epithelial ovarian cancers constitute about 90% of malignant ovarian tumours and generally develop after age 40. Sex cord–stromal tumours arise from connective tissue, often secrete hormones, can occur in women of all ages, and comprise about 7% of ovarian tumours.[82] Tumours that arise from germ cells occur in the second and third decades and account for about 3 to 5% of ovarian tumours.[82] Borderline tumours of low malignant potential can contain structural and molecular evidence of transformed epithelial cells that do not invade the underlying stromal tissue. Approximately 10% of borderline tumours can recur after surgical resection and prove lethal.[82]

There are three major histological types of epithelial tumours: serous, mucinous, and endometrioid. These types all have a benign, borderline,

TABLE 33-7 Risk Factors for Ovarian Cancer

Risk Factor	Description
Advancing age	Incidence of ovarian cancer increases with advancing age. Most cases occur in postmenopausal women.
Genetic factors	About 5–15% of all ovarian cancers are inherited. Of these, the majority are related to mutations in *BRCA1/BRCA2* genes, and others include mismatch repair genes (e.g., Lynch syndrome), *TP53* in the germ line (e.g., Li-Fraumeni syndrome), and Peutz-Jeghers syndrome. Fallopian tube cancer and peritoneal carcinomas also are part of the *BRCA*-associated disease spectrum.
Family history	A family history of ovarian cancer in a first-degree relative (e.g., mother, daughter, or sister) is the most important risk factor. The highest risk appears in women who have two or more first-degree relatives with ovarian cancer. Risk may be higher if the affected relative was diagnosed at a younger age, had previous breast cancer diagnosed before the age of 40, and had previous breast cancer and a history of ovarian cancer. A cohort study showed ovarian cancer risk is higher in women whose sibling has or had liver, stomach, breast, prostate, connective tissue cancer, or melanoma; or whose parent has or had breast or liver cancer.
Overweight and obesity (BMI)	Meta-analysis found higher risk for ovarian cancer in premenopausal women with a body mass index (BMI) >30 and no effect in postmenopausal women. Another meta-analysis found a link between high BMI and ovarian cancer risk in women who had never used menopausal hormone therapy (MHT).
Height	Greater adult attained height (reflects factors that promote childhood growth) is classified by World Cancer Research Fund (WCRF) and the American Institute for Cancer Research (AICR) as a probable cause of ovarian cancer. A pooled analysis of Nordic data and meta-analyses showed ovarian cancer risk is 7–10% higher per 5-cm increment in height.
Reproductive/hormonal factors	Ovarian cancer risk is associated with factors affecting lifetime ovulations (and breaks between) or sex hormone levels (estrogens, progesterone, and androgens), or both. Structural changes to the ovary can occur with ovulation that may stimulate cancer development. These changes may be affected and enhanced by hormonal factors. Having more children, breastfeeding, or using oral contraceptives deceases the number of ovulations and therefore reduces the risk for ovarian cancer.
Menopausal hormone therapy	Current use of postmenopausal hormone replacement therapy (HRT, also known as *menopausal hormone therapy* [MHT]) is classified by the International Agency for Research on Cancer (IARC) as a cause of ovarian cancer (see Table 11-1). A meta-analysis found women using MHT for just a few years were more likely to develop ovarian cancer than women who had never used MHT. For every 1 000 women who take MHT for 5 years from about age 50, there will be 1 extra case of ovarian cancer. An estimated 1% of cases of ovarian cancer in the United Kingdom are linked to MHT use. In long-term (5+ years) users of estrogen-only MHT, compared with never-users, ovarian cancer risk is 53% higher. From a cohort study, ovarian cancer risk is 17% higher in long-term (5+ years) estrogen–progesterone MHT users when compared with never-users.
Endometriosis	Recent studies have shown that women with endometriosis have an increase in ovarian cancer risk.
Diabetes	Meta-analyses have shown ovarian cancer risk is 20–55% higher in women with diabetes compared with those without diabetes.
Previous cancer	Ovarian cancer risk is 24% higher in breast cancer survivors compared with the general population (possibly reflects *BRCA* mutations and Lynch syndrome or shared hormonal factors). It is higher in those diagnosed with breast cancer at a younger age versus those diagnosed older; the higher risk is limited to estrogen receptor (ER)–negative or ER-unknown breast cancer.
Smoking	An analysis showed an increased risk for mucinous ovarian tumours in current smokers. The risk decreased to normal after cessation of smoking. Recent results from the European Prospective Investigation into Cancer and Nutrition (EPIC) study showed smoking increases the risk for mucinous ovarian tumours.
Asbestos (occupational exposure)	Asbestos is classified by IARC as a cause of ovarian cancer (see Table 11-1).
Talc-based powder	Talc-based powder used peritoneally is classified by IARC as a probable cause of ovarian cancer (see Table 11-1). The risk for ovarian cancer with talc-based powders has been based on meta-analyses and pooled analyses of case-control studies. Not all body powders contain talc.
Ionizing radiation	Use of X-radiation and gamma radiation is classified by IARC as a probable cause of ovarian cancer (see Table 11-1). A small number of individuals with ovarian cancer may be associated with radiotherapy for previous cancer.
Factors that reduce risk for ovarian cancer	Taking contraceptives is classified by IARC as protective against ovarian cancer. Breastfeeding is classified by WCRF/AICR as possibly protective against ovarian cancer. Ovarian cancer risk is lower in women with the following factors supported by meta-analyses and pooled analyses: higher parity, hysterectomy, tubal ligation, and use of statins; there is controversial evidence linking systemic lupus erythematosus.

From Cancer Research UK. (n.d.). *Ovarian cancer risk factors.* Retrieved from http://www.cancerresearchuk.org/health-professional/cancer-statistics/statistics-by-cancer-type/ovarian-cancer/risk-factors; Cogliano, V.J., Baan, R., Straif, K., et al. (2011). *J Natl Cancer Inst, 103,* 1827–1839; Ferlay, J., Shin, H.R., Bray, F., et al. (2010). *GLOBOCAN 2008 v1.2, Cancer incidence and mortality worldwide: IARC CancerBase no. 10.* Lyon, France: International Agency for Research on Cancer; International Agency for Research on Cancer. (2017). *List of classifications by cancer sites with sufficient or limited evidence in humans, Volumes 1 to 119.* Retrieved from http://monographs.iarc.fr/ENG/Classification/latest_classif.php; National Cancer Institute. (2015). *Ovarian epithelial, fallopian tube, and primary peritoneal cancer treatment (PDQ®)—Health professional version.* Retrieved from http://cancer.gov/cancertopics/pdq/treatment/ovarianepithelial/HealthProfessional; Parkin, D.M., Boyd, L., & Walker, L.C. (2011). *Cancer, 105*(Suppl. 2), S77–S81; World Cancer Research Fund/American Institute for Cancer Research. (2007). *Food, nutrition, physical activity, and the prevention of cancer: A global perspective.* Washington, DC: American Institute for Cancer Research.

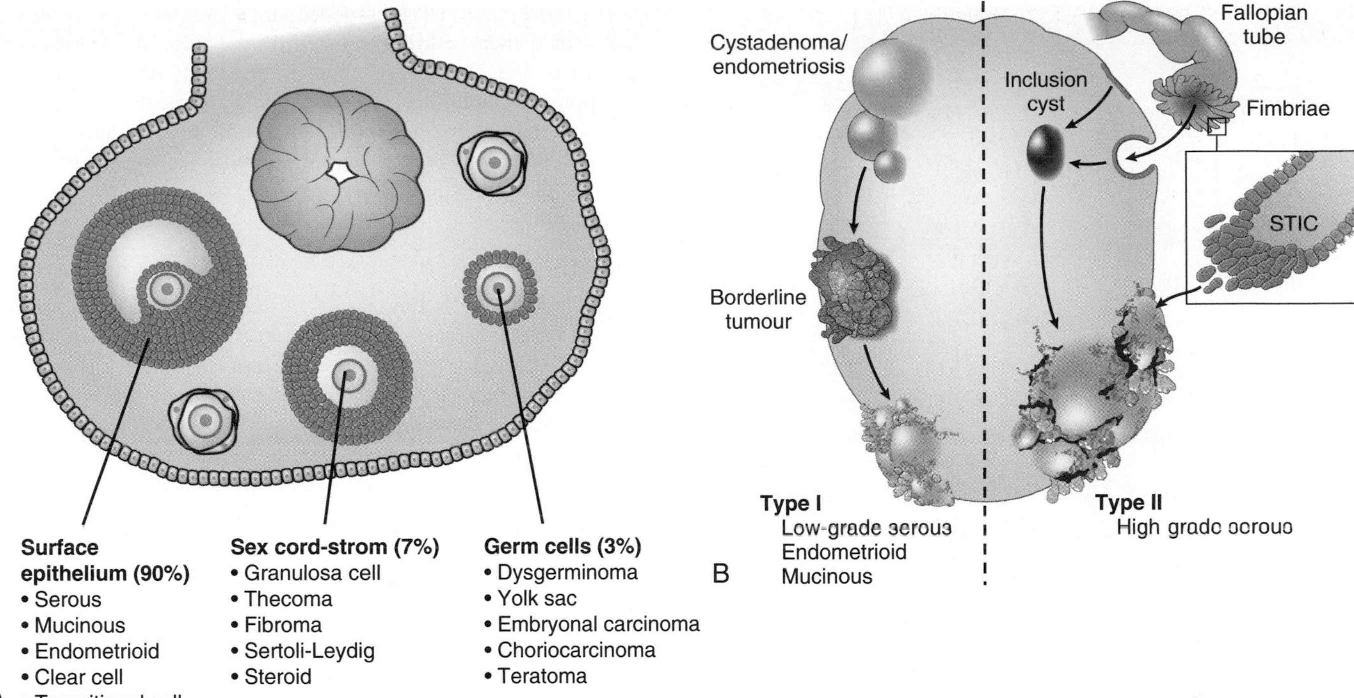

FIGURE 33-22 Heterogeneous Ovarian Tumours. **A,** Diverse ovarian tumours originate from different cell subtypes. **B,** Type I and type II ovarian tumours. Type I tumours progress from benign tumours through borderline tumours that give rise to low-grade carcinoma, and type II tumours arise from inclusion cysts/fallopian tube epithelium through intraepithelial precursors that often are unidentifiable. These tumours demonstrate high-grade features and are commonly of serous histology. *STIC,* serous tubal intraepithelial carcinoma. (**B,** from Kumar, V., Abbas, A.K., & Aster, J.C. [Eds.]. [2015]. *Robbins and Cotran pathologic basis of disease* [9th ed.]. Philadelphia: Saunders.)

and malignant category.[34] The most common histological subtype is high-grade serous cancers, and they may originate from a precursor lesion that arises from the fimbriae of the fallopian tubes. In women who underwent prophylactic salpingo-oophorectomies, studies showed that fallopian tubal lesions were present in almost 100% of women with early serous cancers associated with familial *BRCA* (breast cancer gene) mutations. Investigators recently proposed that the fallopian tube *is* the primary site of most serous carcinomas.[83] Although historically investigators proposed that the vast majority of serous carcinomas arose from cortical inclusion cysts, a newer hypothesis is that the cysts arise from implantation of detached fallopian tube epithelium at sites where ovulation has disrupted the surface of the ovary.[34] These findings have led to changes in management of women at high risk for ovarian cancer (*BRCA* mutation carriers and women with a strong family history of breast or ovarian cancer); they are now recommended to have salpingo-oophorectomy and not just a simple oophorectomy.[34]

Additionally, histologically similar cancers diagnosed as primary peritoneal carcinomas share molecular findings (i.e., inactivation of *p53* and BRCA1 and BRCA2 proteins). Therefore, tumours arising from fallopian tube and other locations from the peritoneal cavity, together with most ovarian epithelial cancers, are classified as "extrauterine adenocarcinomas of Müllerian epithelial origin" and are included, staged, and treated similarly to ovarian cancer.[84]

The defining characteristics of malignant tumours are stromal invasion and increased epithelial atypia. Ovarian tumours are now classified as type I (low-grade) and type II (high-grade) (see Figure 33-22, *B*). Low-grade tumours arising in serous borderline tumours have several oncogene mutations, whereas high-grade tumours have a high frequency of *TP53* mutations. Gene amplifications are noted in many tumours, as well as deletions of tumour-suppressor genes. The majority of *BRCA* mutations are high-grade serous carcinomas with *TP53* mutations. *BRCA*-associated cancer risks are determined by the mutation location and variation of the *BRCA1/BRCA2* gene function.[81] Endometrioid ovarian carcinomas may arise in the setting of endometriosis and are sometimes associated with borderline tumour.[34]

CLINICAL MANIFESTATIONS Generally, individuals with ovarian cancer have no early symptoms. Because there are no effective screening techniques to detect it, the disease is usually advanced by the time treatment is sought. Some women may experience vague symptoms that include abdominal distension, loss of appetite, early satiety, and pelvic pain. These symptoms are important as *nonspecific* symptoms and can lead to delays in treatment. Symptoms of advanced disease include pain, abdominal swelling and distension, dyspepsia, vomiting, and alterations in bowel habits. Abnormal vaginal bleeding may occur if the postmenopausal endometrium is stimulated by a hormone-secreting tumour. The tumour also may cause ulcerations through the vaginal wall that result in bleeding. There also can be a feeling of pressure in the pelvis and leg pain. Given the location of the ovaries, assessing abnormalities on routine gynecological examination poses difficulty, especially in obese women. Ovarian cancer is generally considered a silent disease.

Tumour obstruction of vascular channels can cause venous and, occasionally, arterial thrombosis. Alterations in coagulation also occur, contributing to clot formation. Metastasis often causes pleural effusion (Figure 33-23).

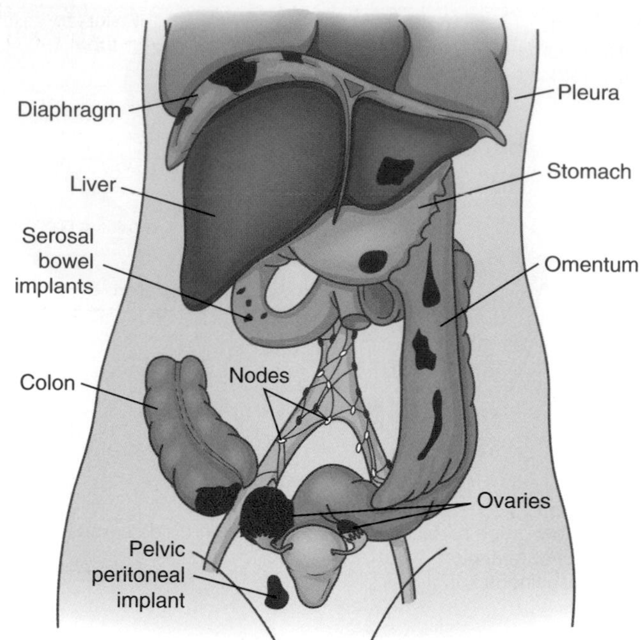

FIGURE 33-23 Metastasis of Ovarian Cancer. Pattern of spread for epithelial cancer of the ovary.

TABLE 33-8 FIGO[a] Staging of Carcinoma of the Ovary

Stage	Characteristics
I	Growth limited to ovaries
II	Growth involves one or both ovaries and involvement of other organs (i.e., uterus, bladder, colon)
III	Cancer involves one or both ovaries, and one or both of following are present: (1) cancer has spread beyond pelvis to lining of abdomen, (2) cancer has spread to lymph nodes
IV	Growth involves one or both ovaries with distant metastases to lungs, liver, or other organs outside peritoneal cavity
Recurrent	Cancer recurs after completion of treatment

[a]The International Federation of Gynecology and Obstetrics.

EVALUATION AND TREATMENT There is no sensitive and specific test for ovarian cancer for screening low-risk women, and routine screening of women without risk factors has not been shown to be beneficial and may cause harm because more women have unnecessary surgical procedures.[85] Solid evidence indicates that screening with a CA-125 blood test and TVUS does not result in a decrease in ovarian cancer mortality, after a research follow-up of 12.4 years.[84] Importantly, ovarian cancer deaths were higher in the screened group than in the usual care group (3.1 deaths versus 2.6 deaths per 10 000 women). These effects are attributed to false-positive test results, higher rates of oophorectomy, and surgical complications. Pelvic examination may detect advanced disease.[84] Several biomarkers with potential application to screening are under investigation. A malignant tumour is confirmed by biopsy and extent of disease evaluated with imaging techniques. The International Federation of Gynecology and Obstetrics (FIGO) staging system is described in Table 33-8.

The initial approach to treatment is surgery, which is performed to determine the stage of disease and to remove as much of the tumour as possible. Survival increases with the expertise of the surgeon. Understanding the biology of cancers and decreasing tumour implantation (seeding) have mandated highly skilled surgical and biopsy techniques.[86,87] Treatment is then customized based on the stage of the cancer, the woman's desires, the cell type, and the sensitivity of the cancer cells. Radiation and chemotherapy are common treatments. New therapies under investigation include monoclonal antibodies, epidermal growth factor receptor, gene therapy, and small-molecular-weight inhibitors. Research into prevention and treatment of ovarian cancer is ongoing and expanding.

Sexual Dysfunction

Sexual dysfunction is the lack of satisfaction with sexual function resulting from pain or a deficiency in sexual desire, arousal, or orgasm/climax.[88,89] Sexual function and dysfunction result from a complex set of personal and biological factors that interact with culture. Both organic and psychosocial disorders can be implicated in sexual dysfunction. Additionally, studies have shown that up to 45% of adult women have some form of sexual dysfunction, and adequate research is still needed.[90] Chronic medical conditions can greatly affect both sexual desire and sexual function (Table 33-9).

Disorders of desire (hypoactive sexual desire, decreased libido) are the most common sexual dysfunction in women.[90] The prevalence of hypoactive sexual desire increases with age and may be a biological manifestation of depression, dissatisfaction with partner relationships, a history of sexual or physical abuse, alcohol or other substance abuse, prolactin-secreting pituitary tumours, or testosterone deficiency.[91] Medications, such as β-adrenergic blockers used for heart disease, may inhibit sexual desire. Treatment may include counselling, psychotherapy, and antidepressants.

Anorgasmia (orgasmic dysfunction) is the inability of a woman to reach or achieve orgasm and ranges from difficulty in arousal to lack of orgasm. Any chronic illness may affect arousal. Specific disorders that may block orgasm are diabetes, alcoholism, neurological disturbances, hormonal deficiencies, and pelvic disorders, such as infections, trauma, and surgical scarring. Other inhibitors include medications, such as narcotics, tranquilizers, antidepressants (especially SSRIs), and anti-hypertensive medications.

Dyspareunia (painful intercourse) is common. Women may experience pain at any time from the beginning of arousal to after intercourse. The pain may have a burning, sharp, searing, or cramping quality and may be described as external, vaginal, deep abdominal, or pelvic. A variety of psychosocial and organic causes have been identified. Inadequate lubrication may make penetration or intercourse difficult or painful. Medications with a drying effect (such as antihistamines, certain tranquilizers, and marihuana) and disorders (such as diabetes, vaginal infections, and estrogen deficiency) can decrease lubrication. Other causes include skin problems around the introitus or affecting the vulva; irritation or infection of the clitoris; disorders of the vaginal opening and disorders of the urethra or anus; disorders of the vagina, such as infections, thinning of the walls caused by aging or decreased estrogen level, or irritation caused by spermicides or douches; and pelvic disorders, such as infection, tumours, and cervical or uterine abnormalities.

Vaginismus is an involuntary muscle spasm in response to attempted penetration. Common psychological causes include prior sexual trauma and fear of sex. Organic causes are similar to those that cause dyspareunia, including vulvovestibulitis. Even after the underlying organic problem is detected and successfully treated, vaginismus may persist.

Sexual dysfunction may develop as a coping mechanism. Women with a history of sexual trauma—rape, incest, or molestation—often have problems with desire, arousal, or orgasm or experience pain with sexual activity. In extreme cases, total sexual aversion may develop. At other times, sexual dysfunction may be a symptom of marital or

TABLE 33-9 Possible Effects of Chronic Disease on Sexual Functioning in Women

Disease	Sexual Function
Cerebral palsy	Intact genital sensations, decreased lubrication; difficulty with sexual activity/positioning because of muscle spasticity, rigidity, or weakness; pain with positioning caused by contracture of knees and hips or because of increased spasms with arousal
Cerebrovascular accident	Difficulties in sexual positioning and sensitivity because of impaired motor strength, coordination, or paralysis; decreased libido with stroke on dominant side of brain
Diabetes	Diminished intensity of orgasm and gradual decline in ability to achieve orgasm; decreased lubrication or recurrent vaginal infections with resultant dyspareunia
Chronic kidney disease	Decreased arousal; increasingly rare and less intense orgasms; decreased lubrication
Rheumatoid arthritis	Painful sexual activity/positions because of swollen, painful joints, muscular atrophy, and joint contracture; decreased libido because of pain, fatigue, or medication; genital sensations remain intact
Systemic lupus erythematosus	Similar to rheumatoid arthritis; decreased lubrication and vaginal lesions result in painful penetration
Myocardial infarction	Most literature male-oriented; problems related to medications
Multiple sclerosis	Diminished genital sensitivity; decreased lubrication; declining orgasmic ability; difficulty with sexual activity because of muscle weakness, pain, or incontinence
Spinal cord injury	Reflex sexual response with injury above sacral area; disrupted response with lesion at or below sacrum; loss of sensation, decreased lubrication; spasticity, incontinence, or pain with arousal; continued orgasmic sensations or sensations diffused in general or to specific body parts, such as breast or lips

relationship problems. Because sexual dysfunction has many causes, assessment and treatment should be holistic and culturally sensitive.

Impaired Fertility

Infertility affects approximately 16% (or 1 in 6) of all couples in Canada and is defined as the inability to conceive over 1 year of unprotected intercourse.[92] Fertility can be impaired by factors in the man or woman, or in both partners. Female infertility results from dysfunction of the normal reproductive process: menses and ovulation, fallopian tube function (transport of the egg to the uterus and as a site of fertilization), and implantation of the fertilized egg into a receptive endometrium. Ovarian dysfunction includes defective ovulation because of hormonal effects (e.g., PCOS, depressed hypothalamic activity, secondary physical or emotional stress), diminished ovarian reserve (lack of immature eggs secondary to congenital, medical, or unexplained factors), or premature ovarian insufficiency (failure of ovarian function before the age of 40). Fallopian tube dysfunction may result from acute pelvic infections with chlamydia or gonorrhea. Adhesions from pelvic infection, abdominal surgery, or endometriosis may cause blockage of one or both fallopian tubes, preventing access of the sperm to the ovum. The fertilized ovum must implant on a receptive endometrium.[93] Receptivity may be greatly diminished by fibroids or inadequate molecular or cellular preparation of the implantation site.

A number of diagnostic procedures are required in the routine investigation of the infertile couple.[94] Initial workup includes analysis of semen, determination of ovulation, and hysterosalpingography of the fallopian tubes. Treatment of infertility is aimed toward correction of problems identified during diagnostic workup. Male infertility may be corrected surgically (varicoceles) or by artificial insemination with the husband's or donor's sperm. Anovulation can be treated with hormonal medications that induce ovulation (e.g., clomiphene citrate, FSH, GnRH). Women with fallopian tube defects, who have failed other approaches or have no identifiable cause of their infertility, are frequently treated by assisted reproductive technology (ART).[95] The basic ART procedure is in vitro fertilization (IVF), which involves collecting eggs directly from the ovary, performing fertilization and early embryonic development in the laboratory, and then transferring the eggs into the uterus. Many variations of this procedure are available. Depending on the potential cause of infertility, appropriate modifications allow for the use of donor sperm, egg, or uterus (in the case of surrogacy). An essential treatment for infertility is prevention of STI, which can result in scarring and adhesion formation in the reproductive tract of either the man or the woman.

QUICK CHECK 33-4

1. Why is cervical cancer considered a sexually transmitted infection?
2. What are the risk factors and pathogenesis for endometrial cancer?
3. What factors reduce the risk for ovarian cancer?
4. Discuss the new hypothesis for pathogenesis of ovarian cancer.

DISORDERS OF THE FEMALE BREAST

Galactorrhea

Galactorrhea (inappropriate lactation) is the persistent and sometimes excessive secretion of a milky fluid from the breasts of a woman who is not pregnant or nursing an infant. Galactorrhea, which also can occur in men, may involve one or both breasts, and is not associated with breast cancer.

The incidence of galactorrhea is difficult to estimate because of differences among definitions of the condition, examination techniques, and populations of women who have been studied. Prevalence has been documented as 0.1 to 32% of all women.

PATHOPHYSIOLOGY Galactorrhea is a manifestation of pathophysiological processes elsewhere in the body, rather than a primary breast disorder. These processes are chiefly hormone imbalances caused by hypothalamic-pituitary disturbances, pituitary tumours, or neurological damage. Exogenous causes include medications, estrogen, and manipulation of the nipples.

The most common cause of galactorrhea is nonpuerperal hyperprolactinemia, or excessive amounts of prolactin in the blood not related to pregnancy or childbirth. Nonpuerperal hyperprolactinemia can be caused by any factor that (1) stimulates or overstimulates the prolactin-secreting units of the pituitary gland; (2) interferes with production of prolactin-inhibiting factor (PIF), a neurotransmitter (probably dopamine) that inhibits prolactin secretion; or (3) interferes with pituitary receptors for PIF.

Certain medications can cause nonpuerperal hyperprolactinemia. They include the phenothiazines, reserpine (Serpasil), and methyldopa (Aldomet); exogenous estrogens, particularly in oral contraceptives; morphine; and the tricyclic antidepressants.

Hypothyroidism causes increased secretion of hypothalamic TSH, which stimulates prolactin release from the pituitary. Hypothyroidism also is associated with reduced metabolic clearance of prolactin, which prolongs its effects.

Many types of pituitary tumours cause hyperprolactinemia, particularly prolactinoma. Prolactinomas cause hyperprolactinemia by secreting prolactin, decreasing production of PIF, or applying pressure to the pituitary stalk, thus preventing delivery of PIF to the anterior pituitary. Growth hormone–secreting pituitary tumours may cause galactorrhea through the intrinsic lactogenic effect that growth hormone appears to have on mammary tissue. Prolactin-secreting lung and kidney tumours also cause hyperprolactinemia.

Chronic stress may cause hyperprolactinemia by inhibiting PIF release. Head trauma, cervical spinal injuries, encephalitis, meningitis, herpes zoster, or thoracotomy scars may stimulate the suckling reflex. The suckling reflex increases prolactin secretion.

CLINICAL MANIFESTATIONS Inappropriate lactation is manifested by the appearance of a milky breast secretion from one or both breasts of nonpregnant, nonlactating women. Most women with galactorrhea experience menstrual abnormality. If a pituitary process is involved, the woman usually experiences hirsutism and infertility; if a hypothalamic lesion is present, she may report CNS symptoms, such as intractable headache, visual field disturbances, sleep disturbances, and abnormal temperature, thirst, or appetite.

EVALUATION AND TREATMENT Galactorrhea in nulliparous women (women who have never been pregnant) or in parous women who have not breastfed for 12 months must be thoroughly evaluated. Evaluation includes a variety of diagnostic tests. Serum prolactin levels are measured, and at least two positive results are needed to diagnose hyperprolactinemia. Prolactin levels higher than 25 to 30 mcg/L (measured by radioimmunoassay) are considered elevated. Those in the range of 75 to 100 mcg/L are possibly caused by a pituitary tumour until proven otherwise. Serum thyroxine (T_4) and TSH levels are measured to rule out hypothyroidism, and LH and FSH levels are obtained if the individual is amenorrheic. MRI may assist in locating adenomas.

Treatment for galactorrhea consists of identification and treatment of the cause. Medical therapy is typical and surgical or radiation therapy is rarely required.

Benign Breast Disease and Conditions

Benign breast disease (BBD) is a spectrum of noncancerous changes in the breast. Numerous benign alterations in ducts and lobules occur in the breast, including lumps, cysts, sensitive nipples, and itching. The most common symptoms reported by women are pain, palpable mass, or nipple discharge; the majority of these prove to have a benign cause. Major determinants of the risk for breast cancer after a diagnosis of BBD include histological or biological features, or both; previous biopsy; and degree of family history.[96] Benign epithelial lesions can be broadly classified as (1) nonproliferative breast lesions, (2) proliferative breast disease without atypia, and (3) atypical (atypia) hyperplasia. The majority of nonproliferative benign lesions are not precursors of cancer and generally not associated with an increased risk for breast cancer.[96,97] Some benign breast lesions (e.g., AH) confer an increase in risk for development of breast cancer, and these women are recommended for counselling about screening recommendations and risk reduction.[96]

Nonproliferative Breast Lesions

Nonproliferative epithelial breast lesions are usually not associated with an increased risk for breast cancer. The nonproliferative lesions include (1) simple breast cysts, (2) papillary apocrine change, and (3) mild hyperplasia of the usual type. Terms such as fibrocystic changes (FCCs; or physiological nodularity and cysts), fibrocystic disease, chronic cystic mastitis, and mammary dysplasia refer to nonproliferative lesions but are not definitive because they are a heterogeneous group of diagnoses.[96] Simple cysts (fluid-filled sacs) are the most common nonproliferative breast lesion and are a specific type of lump that commonly occurs in women in their 30s, 40s, and early 50s. Cysts feel "squishy" when they occur close to the surface of the breast but when deeply embedded, they can feel hard. An estimated 50 to 80% of women normally experience some of these changes. The prevalence of fibrocystic lesions is probably related to hormonal changes, which in turn are affected by genetic background, age, parity, history of lactation, and use of caffeine and exogenous hormones. Cystic changes can be induced in experimental animals by altering ratios of estrogens and progesterone. It is assumed, therefore, that breast cysts are the result of ovarian alterations, but the exact mechanism is unknown. Cysts also can be associated with unilateral nipple discharge. Cysts often rupture with release of secretory material into the adjacent tissue. The resulting chronic inflammation and scarring fibrosis contribute to the palpable firmness of the breast. Fibrous tissue increases progressively until menopause and regresses thereafter.

Papillary apocrine change is an increase in ductal epithelial cells that has apocrine changes or an eosinophilic cytoplasm. Mild hyperplasia of the usual type is an increase in the number of epithelial cells within a duct that is more than two cells, but not more than four cells, in depth.[96]

Proliferative Breast Lesions Without Atypia

Proliferative breast lesions without atypia are characterized by proliferation of ductal epithelium or stroma, or both, without cellular signs of abnormality (atypia or deviation from normal). The following structurally diverse lesions are included and discussed next: (1) usual ductal hyperplasia, (2) intraductal papillomas, (3) sclerosing adenosis, (4) radial scar, and (5) simple fibroadenoma.[96]

1. Usual ductal hyperplasia (UDH) is additional or proliferating epithelial cells that fill and distend the ducts and lobules and are usually found as an incidental finding from mammography. The cells can vary in size and shape, but they retain features of benign cells.[96] No additional treatment is needed and chemoprevention is not recommended.[96]
2. Intraductal papillomas can occur as solitary or multiple lesions. *Solitary papillomas* are a monotonous (sameness) array of papillary cells that grow from the wall of the cyst into the lumen of the duct. Growth occurs within a dilated duct often near or beside the nipple, causing benign nipple discharge. These papillomas *can* harbour areas of atypia requiring surgical excision. Diffuse papillomatosis (multiple papillomas) may present as breast masses, nodules on ultrasound, or the cause of nipple discharge. Diffuse papillomatosis is defined as a minimum of five papillomas within a localized segment of breast tissue.[96] Although the breast cancer risk is small, these lesions require surgical excision.
3. Sclerosing adenosis is a lobular lesion with increased fibrous tissue and scattered glandular cells.[96] It is a common but poorly understood benign breast lesion.[98] A recent study found increased Ki-67 expression (a proliferation marker) carried an approximate twofold increased chance of subsequent breast cancer.[99] It is usually found as a suspicious lesion on mammography.
4. Radial scar (RS) refers to an irregular, radial proliferation of ductlike small tubules entrapped in a dense central fibrosis. The term *scar*

refers to the structural appearance only because these lesions are not associated with prior injury, biopsy, or surgery. *Radial scar* also has been called *radial sclerosing lesions* and *sclerosing papillary proliferation*. RSs are usually discovered when a breast lesion or radiological abnormality is biopsied or removed. Controversy exists about the need for surgical excision.[96]

5. Simple fibroadenomas are benign solid tumours that contain glandular and fibrous lesions.[96] In about 20% of cases, multiple fibroadenomas can occur in the same breast or bilaterally.[96] The etiology for fibroadenomas is unknown but appears to be hormonal because they can persist during the reproductive years and can increase in size during pregnancy or with estrogen therapy. They usually regress after menopause.[96] They are more common among women between 15 and 35 years of age. Fibroadenomas are now considered proliferative lesions and the histological features influence the risk for breast cancer. There is no increased risk for breast cancer in the majority of women with a simple fibroadenoma. It is not necessary to excise all biopsy-proven fibroadenomas.[96] Disadvantages of excisional surgery include scarring at the incision site, dimpling of the breast from the removal of the tumour, damage to the breast's duct system, and mammographic changes (e.g., architectural distortion, skin thickening, increased focal density).[96] If a biopsy-proven fibroadenoma is asymptomatic, it can then be left in place, although some women wish to have the mass excised so that they will not worry further.[96]

Proliferative Breast Lesions With Atypia

Atypical hyperplasia (AH) is an increase in the number of cells (or proliferation) with the cells having some variation in structure—*atypia*. AH is a high-risk benign lesion found in about 10% of biopsies with benign findings.[97,100] These proliferative breast lesions with some atypia include atypical ductal hyperplasia and atypical lobular hyperplasia.[97] Atypical ductal hyperplasia (ADH) refers to abnormal proliferating cells in breast ducts. Atypical lobular hyperplasia (ALH) refers to proliferation of cells in the lumen of lobular units.

Much of the next discussion will refer to just "atypical hyperplasia (AH)." Studies indicate that women with AH have an increased risk (about fourfold) of breast cancer compared with women who have nonproliferative lesions.[101-103] Ongoing studies will further determine risk estimates with such factors, for example, as breast density[97,101] (Figure 33-24). About 60% of the subsequent breast cancers in women with AH occur in the ipsilateral breast (same side) as the biopsy.[101,104,105] From long-term studies mentioned earlier, AH has been shown to confer a relative risk of 4 for future breast cancer, and recently the *absolute risk* has been better defined with a cumulative incidence of breast cancer of about 30% at 25 years of follow-up.[102,106] This high cumulative risk is not widely appreciated and, therefore, women with AH are not included in many high-risk guidelines, for example, screening with MRI and use of chemopreventive agents.[100] Because some studies have shown a lack of concordance (agreement) among pathologists in differentiating AH from carcinoma in situ,[107] it is important that pathologists follow standardized, published criteria; and a diagnosis of either conditions may be a factor for women to seek a second opinion. It appears that menopausal status at the time of benign breast biopsy influences the magnitude of subsequent breast cancer risk. For women who were premenopausal at the time of their breast biopsy, the risk for breast cancer was greater in those with ALH than among women with ADH.[105] Overall, the younger a woman is when she receives a diagnosis of AH, the higher the risk that breast cancer will develop.[102-104] Among women who were postmenopausal at the time of benign breast biopsy, the risk was similar with ALH and women with ADH.[105] Overall, ADH and ALH are viewed best as "markers" of a generalized bilateral increase in breast cancer risk.[96,105]

EVALUATION AND TREATMENT Breast problems are diagnosed from a multimodal approach that combines physical examination, mammography, ultrasonography, thermography, possibly MRI, and biopsy. The dense breast tissue often seen in young women can make mammographic interpretation extremely difficult (see *Health Promotion:* Breast Cancer Screening Mammography).

Treatment consists largely of relieving symptoms. Decreased consumption of caffeinated beverages (e.g., cola, root beer) and chocolate, which can cause overstimulation for some women, may reduce pain and nodularity. Given time, the cysts may disappear without treatment.

Although still controversial, isoflavone exposure was associated with a decreased risk for proliferative benign fibrocystic changes, nonproliferative changes, and breast cancer.[108] Genistein, a soy isoflavone, has been reported to downregulate an enzyme important in cancer progression (i.e., telomerase) and contributes to inhibition in both breast benign and cancer cells.[109] Toxicologists, in perhaps the first in vitro study quantifying the proliferative effects of isoflavone metabolites, have concluded that soy supplement intake will not induce proliferation of normal breast tissue and may even inhibit proliferation.[110] The North American Menopause Society found that soy foods generally appear to be breast protective and recommended moderate lifelong soy consumption.[111] Although quite controversial, another preventive factor may be iodine.[112]

Breast Cancer

In 2012, 1.7 million women were diagnosed with breast cancer, and there were 6.3 million women alive who had been diagnosed with breast cancer in the previous 5 years (Figure 33-25).[53] Mortality has increased by 14%. Breast cancer is the most common cause of cancer death among women (522 000 deaths in 2012) and the most frequently diagnosed cancer among women in 140 of 184 countries worldwide.[53] It now represents one in four of all cancers in women.

Breast cancer is the most common cancer in Canadian women, excluding nonmelanoma skin cancers. It is the leading cause of death in women 40 to 44 years of age and the second leading cause of cancer death in women of all ages after lung cancer. The Canadian Cancer Society estimated that 26 300 Canadian women were diagnosed with breast cancer in 2017. It also estimated that 5 000 women died of this disease in 2017.[51] Breast cancer is more common in high-income, developed countries such as Canada, the United States, and some European countries. The risk of developing breast cancer increases with age, and it occurs most often in women between the ages of 50 and 69.[113] Because DCIS is almost exclusively detected by mammography, the large increase in incidence of DCIS over the past 20 years can be attributed to screening.

Although breast cancer is a multifactorial disease involving a complex web of interacting factors, risk is related to timing, duration, and pattern of exposures. Risk factors and possible causes of breast cancer can be classified broadly as reproductive, hormonal, environmental, and familial (Table 33-10). However, two factors emerging as important are involution of the mammary gland and breast density, which are not as easily classified (see the following discussion).

Reproductive Factors: Pregnancy

A clearer understanding of mammary gland structure (morphology) and function from fetal development to puberty, pregnancy, and aging will help elucidate fundamental changes to breast development and disease. A key element in that process is "branching morphogenesis," in which the mammary gland fulfills its function by producing and

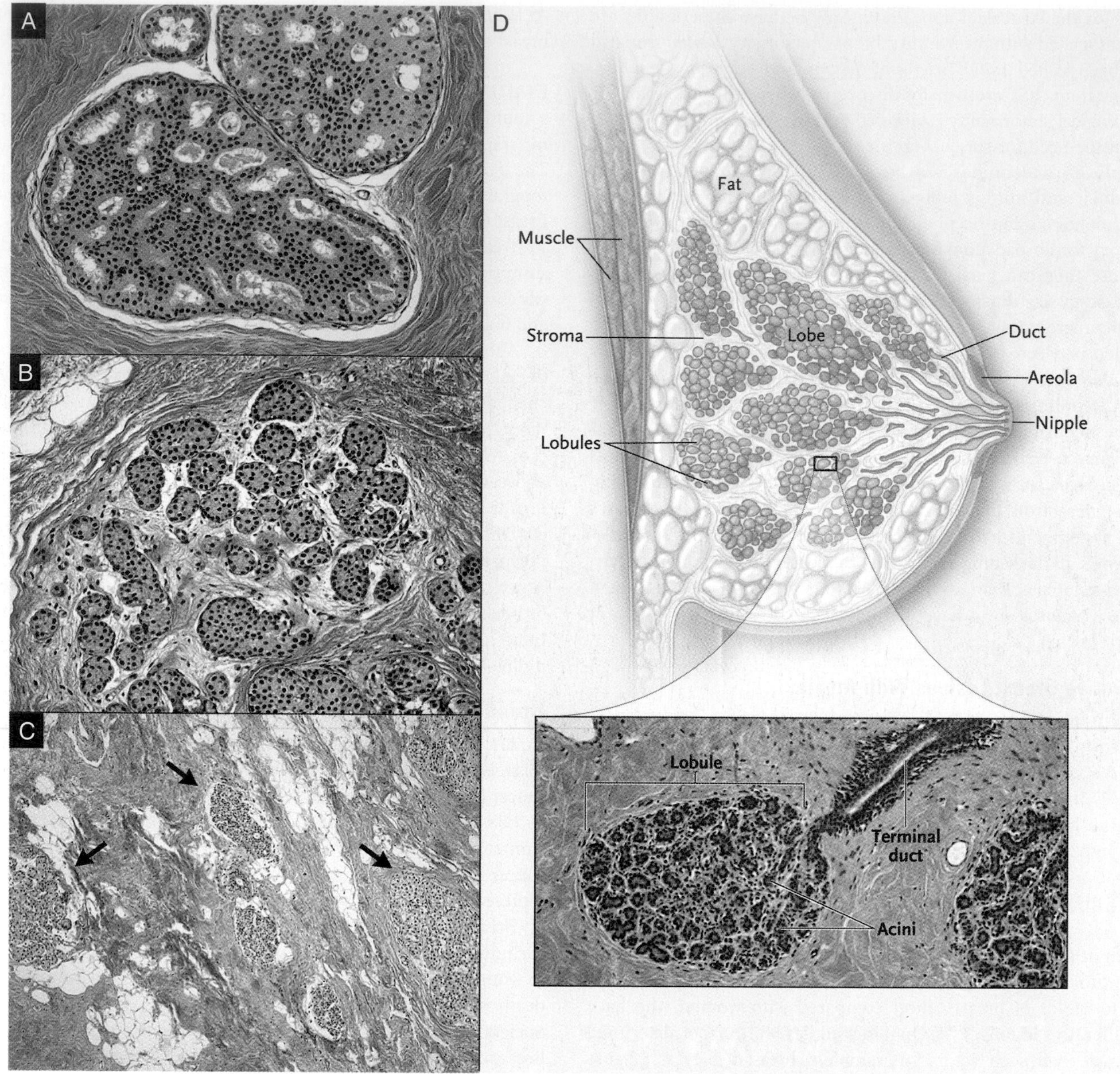

FIGURE 33-24 Anatomical and Histological Features of Atypical Hyperplasia. Panel **A** shows atypical ductal hyperplasia with proliferation of monotonous cells in architecturally complex patterns, including secondary lumens and micropapillary formations. Panel **B** shows atypical lobular hyperplasia (ALH), with expanded acini filled with monotonous polygonal cells and a loss of acinar lumen. Panel **C** shows multifocal atypical hyperplasia (in this case ALH). ALH is present in more than one terminal duct lobular unit (TDLU), and units are clearly separated from one another by interlobular mammary stroma (*arrows*). Panel **D** is an illustration of the microanatomy of the breast, including a photomicrograph of a TDLU. (From *N Engl J Med,* Hartmann, L.C., Degnim, A.C., Santen, R.J., Dupont, W.D., & Ghosh, K., "Atypical hyperplasia of the breast—risk assessment and management options," 372[1]: 1271–1272. Copyright © 2015 Massachusetts Medical Society. Reprinted with permission from Massachusetts Medical Society.)

delivering copious amounts of milk by forming a rootlike network of branched ducts from a rudimentary epithelial bud.[114] Branching morphogenesis begins in fetal development, pauses after birth, starts again in response to estrogens at puberty, and is modified by cyclic ovarian hormonal action. This systemic hormonal action elicits local paracrine interactions between the developing epithelial ducts and their adjacent mesenchyme (embryonic) or postnatal stroma.[114] The local cellular crosstalk then directs the tissue remodelling, ultimately producing a mature ductal tree.[114]

A woman's age when her first child is born affects her risk of developing breast cancer—the younger she is, the lower the risk. Overall, lifetime risk for breast cancer is reduced in parous women compared with nulliparous women, but pregnancy must occur at a young age.[115] The influence of pregnancy on the risk for breast cancer also depends on family history, lactation postpartum, and overall parity.[116] Findings from a large prospective study found a *dual effect* from pregnancy—a transient postpartum increase in breast cancer risk followed by a long-term reduction in risk (compared with nulliparous women).[117]

HEALTH PROMOTION

Breast Cancer Screening Mammography

The idea behind screening healthy individuals for disease is the hope that we can diagnose disease early, when more treatment options are available and when we can positively impact the life of the individual. Screening programs that cover the entire population of a country are a large undertaking and usually require extensive resources. Therefore, we need to make certain that the test has a high level of accuracy with reasonable costs and disadvantages, the disease is not too rare, and the treatment is effective for individuals who are diagnosed because of the screening.

Women have been encouraged to undergo breast cancer screening for many decades. Early screening programs encouraged women to perform self-breast examinations and also to have their clinician perform a breast examination in the office—subsequent data have shown that these screening techniques lead to false-positive examinations and are not associated with a reduction in mortality.

Breast cancer screening with mammography continues to be recommended by many groups, although the benefits are less than we had hoped, and we are learning more about the harms. Mammography is an X-ray examination that takes views of each breast (see figure). The recommended age of first mammogram and the frequency of screening vary among guidelines and countries. The Canadian Task Force on Preventive Health periodically reviews the evidence and issues guidelines to help aid discussions with women about screening.

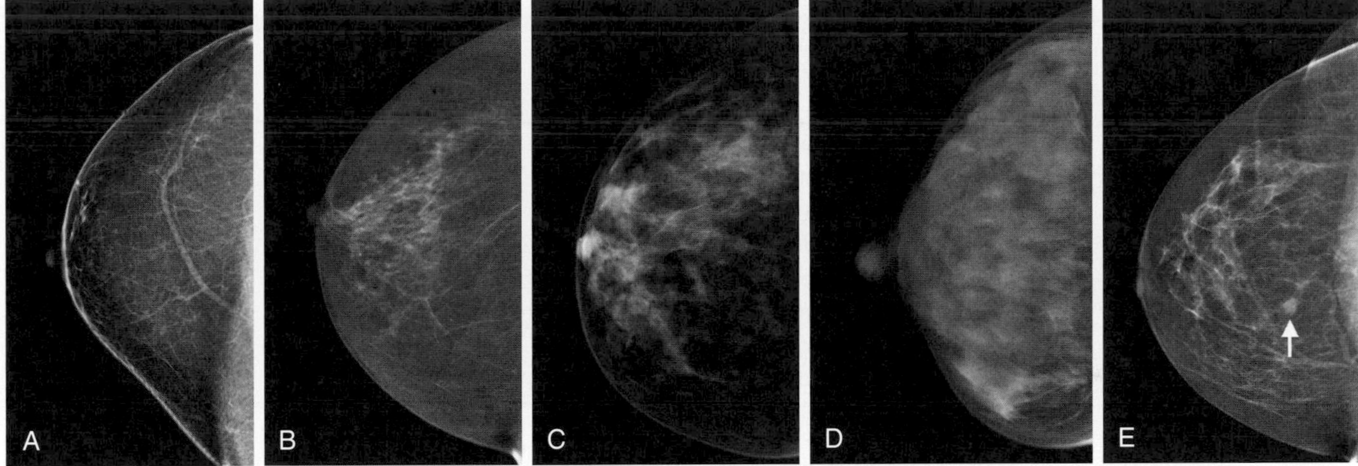

Mammograms. A–D, Mammograms depicting varying breast densities from a craniocaudal view: **A,** almost entirely fat; **B,** scattered fibroglandular densities; **C,** heterogeneously dense; and **D,** extremely dense. **E,** Mammogram showing invasive cancer. (Images provided by Christoph I. Lee, MD, MSHS. Reprinted from Fuller, M.S., et al. [2015]. Breast cancer screening: An evidence-based update. *Med Clin North Am,* 99[3]: 451–468, with permission from Elsevier.)

The benefits, risks, and accuracy of mammography screening depend on numerous factors, including women's age, breast density, and time interval between screening examinations. Possible risks of screening are important to consider because screening at a population level involves testing healthy individuals; we are to "first, do no harm."

No medical test is perfect. The US National Cancer Institute reports that about 10% of screening mammograms are interpreted as "abnormal," requiring additional testing. The great majority of women with these "abnormal" examinations do not have breast cancer; this is called a false-positive result. The false-positive results lead to additional diagnostic testing, which can result in anxiety and morbidity to women. It is estimated that at least 50% of women who are screened annually for a decade will have experienced at least one false-positive examination.

Another harm of screening mammography is overdiagnosis—a *diagnosis* that would never have harmed the woman during her lifetime; such diagnoses can be either of a pre-invasive lesion, such as ductal carcinoma in situ (DCIS), or of invasive breast cancer. With more women undergoing screening with mammography, we have seen a sharp increase in the number of women *diagnosed* with DCIS and early stage breast cancer. By definition, DCIS is not an invasive carcinoma and not an immediate life-threatening cancer—it is confined to the duct; but DCIS is almost always treated as if it is an invasive early stage breast cancer. Women with DCIS are at increased risk for a subsequent, invasive breast cancer diagnosis; however, the majority of women with DCIS are never subsequently diagnosed with invasive cancer, and treatment of DCIS does not alter mortality. Women with DCIS have the same death rates as women without DCIS. Some discussion has centred on changing the name of DCIS lesions to better differentiate preinvasive DCIS from invasive cancer because the term *carcinoma* is similar to the term *cancer.* However, it is not likely that the name will be changed because of its current common usage.

Unfortunately, we are not able to identify which women with a new diagnosis of DCIS or invasive breast cancer have the type of lesion that is so low risk that it will never harm them during their lifetime. Thus, most women undergo treatment with either lumpectomy and radiation therapy or mastectomy. This is overtreatment if the DCIS or invasive cancer was overdiagnosed. Estimates of the prevalence of overdiagnosis vary in the literature from less than 10 to 50%; more research is clearly needed.

Women with abnormalities noted on screening mammography are often offered the option of a breast biopsy versus watchful waiting with follow-up mammograms in 6 to 12 months. Some women think that a breast biopsy will provide an immediate and definitive diagnosis; however, this is not always the case. Pathologists have been noted to disagree on the diagnoses of atypia and DCIS.

Balancing the benefits and harms of breast cancer screening is not an easy task for women or their clinicians. Every woman should be encouraged to make an informed decision.

Joann G. Elmore, MD, MPH

From Elmore, J.G., Longton, G.M., Carney, P.A., et al. (2015). *JAMA, 313*(11), 1122–1132; Fuller, M.S., Lee, C.I., & Elmore, J.G. (2015). *Med Clin North Am, 99*(3), 451–468; Katz, D.L., Wild, D., Elmore, J., et al. (2013). *Jekel's epidemiology, biostatistics, preventive medicine, and public health* (4th ed.). Philadelphia: Saunders; National Guideline C: *Breast cancer screening.* Retrieved from https://www.guideline.gov; National Care Institute. (2016). *Breast cancer screening: (PDQ®)–Health professional version.* Retrieved from https://www.cancer.gov/types/breast/hp/breast-screening-pdq; Pace, L.E., & Keating, N.L. (2015). *JAMA, 311*(13), 1327–1335; US Preventive Services Task Force. (2009). *Ann Intern Med, 151*(10), 716–726.

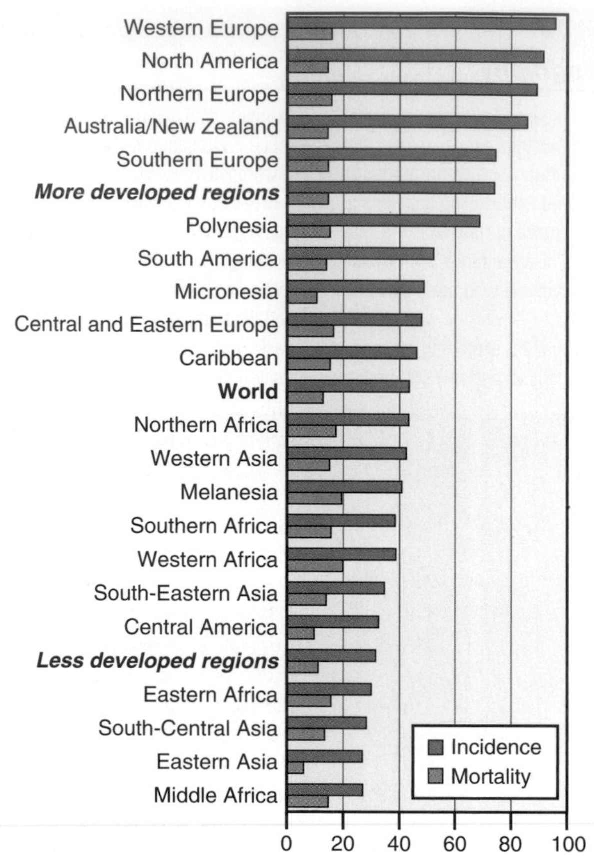

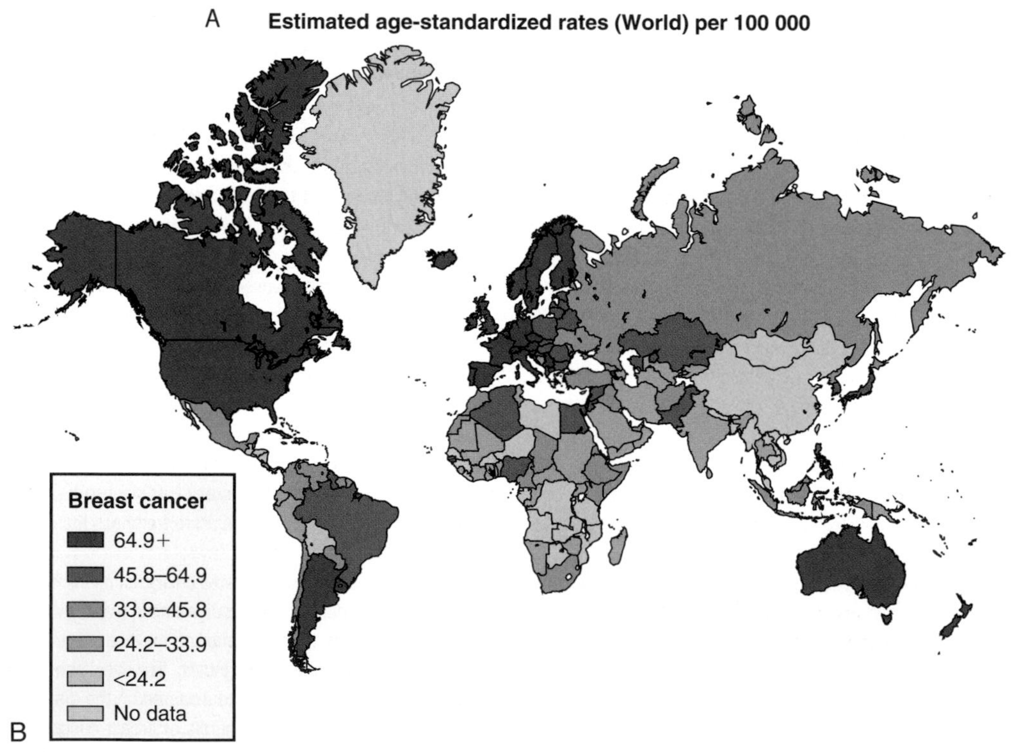

FIGURE 33-25 Breast Cancer Estimated Incidence and Mortality Worldwide in 2012. A, Estimated age-standardized rates (world) per 100 000 population. **B,** Incidence and mortality estimated age-standardized rates (world) per 100 000. These numbers represent a sharp rise in breast cancer incidence since the 2008 estimates by more than 20%. It is the most common cancer in women both in more and in less developed regions, with slightly more cases in less developed (883 000 cases) than in more developed (794 000) regions. Incidence rates vary nearly fourfold across the world regions. (Reproduced with permission from Ferlay J, Soerjomataram I, Ervik M, Dikshit R, Eser S, Mathers C, Rebelo M, Parkin DM, Forman D, Bray, F. *GLOBOCAN 2012 v1.0, Cancer Incidence and Mortality Worldwide: IARC CancerBase No. 11* [Internet]. Lyon, France: International Agency for Research on Cancer; 2013. Available from: http://globocan.iarc.fr, accessed on 28 September 2017.)

TABLE 33-10 Established Risk Factors for Breast Cancer

Relative Risk	Risk Factor
>4.0	Female
	Age
	Family history of breast cancer
	Personal history of breast cancer
	Inherited genetic mutations (*BRCA1/BRCA2* and others)
	High breast density
	Atypical hyperplasia
2.1–4.0	Family history (one first-degree relative)
	High-dose radiation to chest/breast
	Prior benign breast disease
1.1–2.0	No full-term pregnancies
	Late age at first full-term pregnancy (>30 years)
	Early menarche (<12 years)
	Late menopause (>55 years)
	Never breastfed children
	High alcohol consumption
	Smoking
	Recent oral contraceptive use
	Recent or current use of combined hormone replacement therapy
	Physical inactivity
	Obesity or adult weight gain (postmenopausal)

Data from American Cancer Society. (2010). *Cancer facts & figures 2010.* Atlanta: Author.

Pregnancy-associated breast cancer (PABC) is defined as breast cancer that occurs during pregnancy, and risk may persist for at least 5 years postpartum and longer.[118,119] Delayed child-bearing, observed in Canada, the United States, and all developing countries, is expected to show a rise in diagnosed breast cancers.[116] A recent hypothesis for risk at any age is that gland *involution* after pregnancy and lactation uses some of the same tissue remodelling pathways activated during wound healing (i.e., proinflammatory pathways).[120] The proinflammatory environment, although physiologically normal, promotes tumour progression. The presence of macrophages in the involuting mammary gland may be contributing to carcinogenesis, and the normal involuting gland may be in an immunosuppressed state with T-cell suppression.[120,121] Involution is discussed in the following section.

Although many mechanisms have been proposed for the *protective* effect of pregnancy, newer data on the genomic profile of parous women have shown pregnancy induces a long-lasting "genomic signature" that reveals chromatin remodelling derived from the early first pregnancy. The chromatin modifications are accompanied by higher expression of genes related to cell adhesion and differentiation, and genes only activated during the first 5 years after pregnancy may contribute to increased risk, but the long-lasting genetic signature may explain pregnancy's preventive effect.[122]

Lobular Involution and Age and Postlactational Involution

Part of the uniqueness of the mammary gland is its profound physiological changes throughout the phases of a woman's life. These phases include puberty, pregnancy, lactation, postlactational involution, and aging. The human breast is organized into 15 to 20 major lobes, each with terminal lobules containing milk-forming acini (see Figure 32-10, p. 805). **Terminal duct lobular units (TDLUs)**, structures of the breast that are responsible for lactation, are the predominant source of breast cancers.[123] With aging, breast lobules regress or involute with a decrease in the number and size of acini per lobule and with replacement of the intralobular stroma with the denser collagen of connective tissue.[124] With time, the glandular elements and collagen are replaced with fatty tissue. This process is called **lobular involution**, and over many years the parenchymal elements progressively atrophy and disappear. The first study of its kind found lobular involution was associated with reduced risk for breast cancer.[124] Breast cancer risk decreased with increasing *extent* of involution in both high- and low-risk subgroups defined by family history of breast cancer, epithelial atypia, reproductive history, and age.[124] Based on pathological and epidemiological factors, these investigators propose that *delayed* involution (persistent glandular epithelium) is a major risk factor for breast cancer.[124] Tissue involution involves massive epithelial cell death, recruitment and activation of fibroblasts, stromal remodelling, and immune cell infiltration, including macrophages with similarities to microenvironments present during wound healing and tumour progression.[125]

Investigators suggest that the effect of lobular involution on breast cancer risk is a reduction in tissue from the involuting process, or the issue may be aging. Widely appreciated is that as women age, their risk for breast cancer increases. But, the *rate* of increase of breast cancer *slows* at about 50 years of age. This decline has been attributed to a reduction in ovarian hormone production; however, involution may contribute to this slowing rate. Importantly, investigators found an inverse association between lobular involution and parity.[124] Other investigators have reported that the more children a woman has, the more likely she is to have persistent lobular tissue,[126,127] which Milanese and colleagues[124] found was associated with increased risk for breast cancer. However, multiparity also has been found to reduce the risk for breast cancer. This apparent contradiction may be explained by studies documenting that full-term pregnancies after 35 years of age are correlated with an increased risk for breast cancer.[128] In the Milanese study, the age of the mother at each child's birth was unknown.

Henson and colleagues[129] proposed that late pregnancy with its concomitant increase in the proliferation of the ductal-alveolar epithelium is likely to interrupt the process of involution, which typically begins between 30 and 40 years of age. Failure to undergo TDLU involution among women with BBD has been associated with progression to breast cancer, independent of other breast cancer risk factors.[123] The activated stromal environment (with the influx of immune cells similar to that which occurs during wound healing) in the process of involution is the "ideal niche" for carcinogenesis.

Major signalling pathways involved in mammary gland involution also are involved in breast cancer.[130] Certain proteases activated during involution modify the extracellular matrix (ECM) and are implicated in loss of cell anchoring, providing a microenvironment for tumour growth.[130] Further, the normal involuting gland may be in an immunosuppressed state with the transient presence of immune-regulating cells that promote T-cell suppression.[121] Overall, for breast cancer, the long-term protective effects of pregnancy from hormones released (with consequent genetic and epigenetic changes) during pregnancy affect remodelling of the stromal microenvironment by causing apoptosis and involution. However, a transient increase in breast cancer risk following pregnancy may be caused by the *process* of mammary gland involution, which returns the tissue to its prepregnant state and is co-opted by the process of wound healing, resulting in a proinflammatory environment that, although physiologically normal, can promote carcinogenesis.[120] In postlactational involution, the mammary gland regresses and remodels to its prepregnant state whereby fibroblasts secrete proteases that degrade the ECM proteins. Consequently, the increased release of bioactive matrix fragments can promote tumour growth, motility, and invasion.[131] The ECM is very different between nulliparous, lactating, and involuting glands, as shown in Figure 33-26.

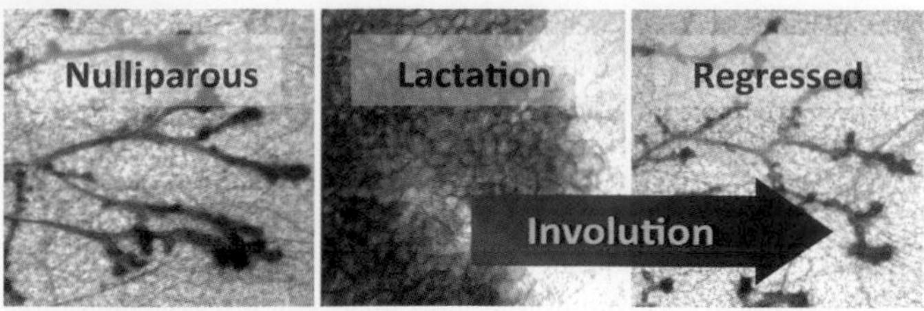

FIGURE 33-26 Extracellular Matrix Is Different in Nulliparous, Lactating, and Involuting Glands. Several extracellular matrix (ECM) differences between nulliparous, lactational, and involuting mammary glands are related to collagen-fibre organization, cell motility and attachment, and cytokine regulation in a rodent model. Many protumourigenic ECM proteins are mediators of breast cancer progression specific to the involutional window, and systemic ibuprofen experimental treatment during involution decreases its tumour promotional changes. (Reprinted with permission from O'Brien, J.H., et al. [2012]. Rat Mammary Extracellular Matrix Composition and Response to Ibuprofen Treatment During Postpartum Involution by Differential GeLC–MS/MS Analysis. *J Proteome Res,* 11: 4894–4905. Copyright 2012 American Chemical Society.)

Oophorectomy, which is associated with a decrease in risk for breast cancer, leads to atrophy of breast parenchyma in young women, as is noted in older women.[129] Thus the risk reduction of oophorectomy may be caused by an accelerated involution.[129]

Investigators have shown that a benign biopsy demonstrating histological changes consistent with incomplete or nonexistent involution or a mammogram classified as high density is independently associated with breast cancer risk, and that these factors combined are associated with an even greater risk.[132] The assessment of these "phenotypes" shows promise for improving risk prediction, particularly because they reflect the cumulative interaction of numerous genetic and environmental breast cancer risk factors over time.

Hormonal Factors

The link between breast cancer and hormones is based on six factors that affect risk: (1) the protective effect of an early (i.e., in the 20s) first pregnancy; (2) the protective effect of removal of the ovaries and pituitary gland; (3) the increased risk associated with early menarche, late menopause, and nulliparity; (4) the relationship between types of fat, free estrogen levels, and oxidative changes in estrogen metabolism; (5) the hormone-dependent development and differentiation of mammary gland structures; and (6) the efficacy of antihormone therapies for treatment and prevention of breast cancer. Throughout its existence, the mammary gland epithelium proceeds through critical "exposure periods" of rapid growth or cycles of proliferation, including neonatal growth, pubertal development, pregnancy lactation, and involution (after pregnancy and postmenopause).[120] Importantly, lack of TDLU involution has been associated with increased breast cancer risk, but the role of sex hormone levels and TDLU assessments has only begun to be studied. Investigators suggest that hormone levels may act, in part, to delay age-appropriate TDLU involution, resulting in a higher quantity of at-risk epithelium.[123] These investigators found significant associations between higher TDLU counts, representing less involution, with higher levels of prolactin and lower levels of progesterone among premenopausal women, and higher levels of estradiol among postmenopausal women.[123] Higher testosterone levels were suggestively associated with higher TDLU counts among postmenopausal women.

The understanding of the role of systemic hormones as powerful regulators of mammary gland development is shifting. Evidence is pointing to the wide-ranging effects of systemic hormones, possibly not because of their *direct* hormone action but rather because of their *induced* actions from multiple secondary paracrine effectors—thus the term *hierarchical.* Unravelling is a complex model of hormone, paracrine, and adhesion molecule signalling pathways affecting both epithelial and stromal cell fate in both breast development and carcinogenesis (Figure 33-27). Key is *tissue remodelling* that applies not only to pubertal growth but also immediately after pregnancy and during involution (see the previous section).

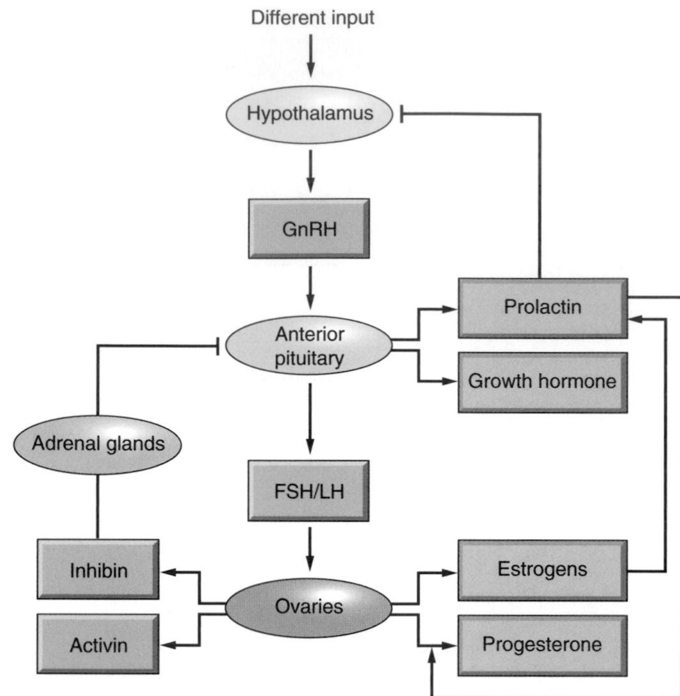

FIGURE 33-27 Female Endocrine System. The different mammary growth (mammotropic) hormone sites are shown in ovals, hormones are noted in blue boxes, and mammotropic hormones are noted in red boxes. *FSH,* follicle-stimulating hormone; *GnRH,* gonadotropin-releasing hormone; *LH,* luteinizing hormone.

The female reproductive hormones (estrogens, progesterone, and prolactin) have a major role and effect on mammary gland development and breast cancer. A vast majority of breast cancers are *initially* hormone dependent (estrogen positive [ER+], progesterone positive [PR+], or both), with estrogens playing a crucial role in their development.[133] Estrogens control processes critical for cellular functions by regulating activities and expression of key signalling molecules. These processes include regulation of receptor activity and receptor interaction with other intracellular proteins and DNA.[133] Estrogens thus play prominent roles in cellular proliferation, differentiation, and apoptosis.[133] Estrogens affect microtubules that are essential for establishing cell shape and cell polarity, processes necessary for epithelial gland organization.[133]

It is possible to consider four major hormonal hypotheses for breast cancer: (1) ovarian androgen excess (e.g., testosterone); (2) estrogen and progesterone levels (ovarian and hormone replacement); (3) elevated estrogen levels alone (ovarian and hormone replacement); and (4) local biosynthesis of estrogens in breast tissue. These hypotheses, however, may not be mutually exclusive. HRT, or the newer term menopausal hormone therapy (MHT), is discussed in the following section; the present discussion is concerned with endogenous levels of hormones.

The first hypothesis that breast cancer risk is increased among women who have an ovarian androgen excess also includes chronic anovulation and reduction of luteal phase (menstrual cycle) progesterone production. Therefore, it is also called the "ovarian hyperandrogenism/luteal inadequacy hypothesis." This hypothesis was based on the observation that women with breast cancer also exhibit hyperplasia of the

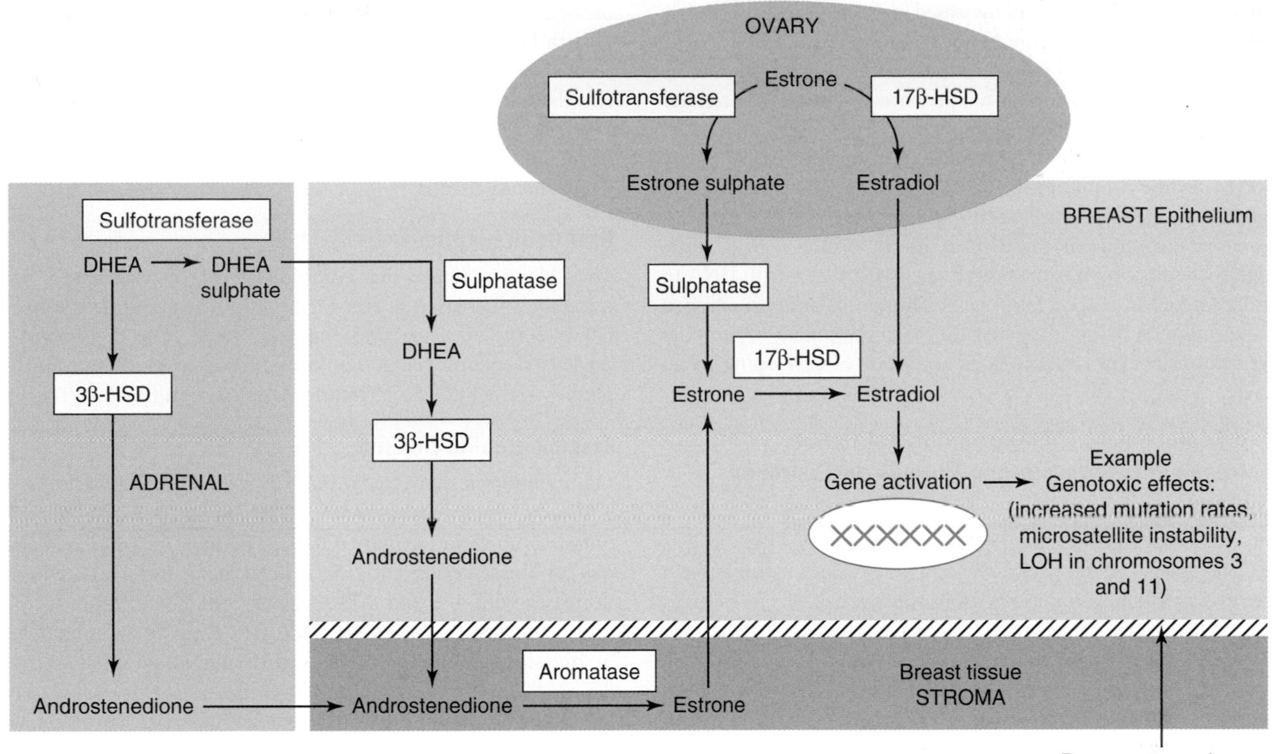

FIGURE 33-28 Local Biosynthesis of Estrogens. Four main enzyme complexes (*yellow*) are involved in estrogen formation in breast tissue: aromatase, sulphatase, 17β-estradiol hydroxysteroid dehydrogenase (*17β-HSD*), and 3β-hydroxysteroid dehydrogenase (*3β-HSD*). Data suggest that most abundant is sulphatase in both premenopausal and postmenopausal women with breast cancer. Numerous agents can block the aromatase action. Exploration of progesterone and various progestins to inhibit sulphatase and 17β-HSD or stimulate sulfotransferase (i.e., breast cancer cells cannot inactivate estrogens because they lack sulfotransferase) may provide new possibilities for treatment. *LOH*, loss of heterozygosity (see Chapter 10). (Adapted from Russo, J., & Russo, I. [2004]. *Molecular basis of breast cancer: Prevention and treatment.* Berlin: Springer-Verlag.)

endometrium—a common symptom of ovarian androgen excess chronic anovulation and progesterone deficiency.[134] From the combination of prospective studies, case-control studies, and laboratory data, the association between circulating testosterone levels in postmenopausal women and subsequent risk for breast cancer is now well established. Unclear is whether the association with testosterone levels is direct or indirect (i.e., enzyme conversion by aromatase of testosterone to estradiol) (Figure 33-28).

The androgen receptor has been implicated in prostate cancer and now in the development and progression of breast cancer.[135] Investigators used breast cancer cell lines and found that treatment of the breast cancer cells with 5α-dihydrotestosterone (DHT) promotes cell proliferation and decreases apoptosis.[135] The reduction of testosterone levels in women with oophorectomy or hysterectomy also may be a protective factor.[136]

The second hypothesis is that breast cancer risk is increased among women with blood elevations of both estrogens and androgens—the "estrogen-plus-progesterone hypothesis." Evidence has revealed increased proliferation rates of breast epithelium during the luteal phase of the menstrual cycle when the ovaries produce both estradiol and progesterone. Substantial evidence supports a positive association of circulating estrogens, androgens, and prolactin with postmenopausal breast cancer risk.[137] New data identify mammary stem cells (MaSCs) as critical targets for ovarian hormones, especially during the normal reproductive cycle when progesterone levels surge and during pregnancy when the proliferation of MaSCs is increased. Higher levels of progesterone among premenopausal women have been associated with lower TDLU counts.[123] Among postmenopausal women, higher levels of estradiol and testosterone have been associated with higher TDLU counts.[123] Select hormones may influence breast cancer risk through delaying TDLU involution.

The third hypothesis is often called the "estrogen-alone hypothesis." Substantial prospective data have accrued on the relationship between levels of circulating estrogens and breast cancer risk in postmenopausal women.[138,139] Overall, the positive association between levels of circulating estrogens in postmenopausal women and subsequent risk for breast cancer is now well established.

The fourth hypothesis suggests that *local* (in situ; paracrine) formation of estrogens in breast tumours may be more significant than circulating estrogens in *plasma* for the growth and survival of estrogen-dependent breast cancer in postmenopausal women.[133] Investigators measured breast sex steroids in both benign and cancerous tissue.[140] Estrogen and androgen concentrations varied greatly in both tissue and blood levels in benign and cancerous tissue.[140] The estradiol-to-estrone ratio was lowest in premenopausal benign tissue and much higher in premenopausal cancerous tissue and postmenopausal benign and cancerous tissue. Estradiol and estrone levels were substantially higher in tissue than in plasma in both premenopausal and postmenopausal women.[140] Hormone levels in breast adipose tissue revealed high levels of androstenedione and testosterone and significant estrone and estradiol levels in breast adipocytes from postmenopausal breast cancer patients consistent with an obesity-inflammation-aromatase axis (obesity with inflammation, COX elevation, and increased aromatase, which converts androgens to estrogen) occurring locally in breast tissue.[140]

Overall, two main mechanisms of carcinogenicity of estrogens involve (1) a receptor-mediated hormonal activity shown to stimulate cellular proliferation, resulting in increased opportunities for accumulation of genetic damage; and (2) oxidative catabolism of estrogens mediated by various cytochrome complexes (cytochrome P-450 [CYP] system) that eventually activate and generate reactive oxygen species (ROS) that can cause oxidative stress and genomic damage directly. Oxidative metabolites of estrogens can develop ultimate carcinogens that react with DNA to cause mutations leading to carcinogenesis. Thus, imbalances in estrogen metabolites in breast tissue correlate with the development of tumours and suggest possible biomarkers related to the risk of developing breast cancer.

Hormone Replacement Therapy and Breast Cancer Risk: Estrogen Plus Progesterone Therapy and Estrogen Only Therapy

The International Agency for Research on Cancer (IARC) lists estrogen-progestogen menopausal therapy and estrogen-progestogen contraceptives as carcinogenic agents with sufficient evidence in humans for breast cancer[141] (see Table 11-1). Evidence from the US Agency for Healthcare Research and Quality (AHRQ) published a systematic review from 283 trials comparing effectiveness of treatments for menopausal symptoms.[142] In this report they state, "Over the long term, estrogen combined with progestogen has both beneficial effects (fewer osteoporotic fractures) and harmful effects (increased risk for breast cancer, gallbladder disease, venous thromboembolic events, and stroke). Estrogens given alone do not appear to increase breast cancer risk, although endometrial cancer risk is increased."[142] Evidence on the route of administration of MHT, oral versus transdermal (gel or patch), and the risk for breast cancer has limited research.

Insulin and Insulinlike Growth Factors

IGFs regulate cellular functions involving cell proliferation, migration, differentiation, and apoptosis. Insulinlike growth factor 1 (IGF-1) is a protein hormone with a structure similar to that of insulin. IGF-1 is a potent mitogen and after binding to the IGF-1R (receptor) triggers a signalling cascade leading to proliferation and antiapoptosis.[143]

Diabetes is associated with complex physiology of insulin resistance, increased insulin level, estrogen and growth hormone levels, inflammation, and signalling pathways leading to an increased risk for breast cancer.[144] Insulin therapy and sulphonylureas were found to be mildly associated with increased breast cancer risk.[144] A UK study showed that women treated with insulin glargine were not associated with breast cancer risk in the first 5 years; however, longer use may increase the risk.[145] Metformin appears to have a protective role. Much more investigation is needed to understand the role of insulin, IGFs, and diabetes mellitus and the risk for breast cancer and recurrence of breast cancers.

Melatonin as a regulator of circadian rhythm is the main focus of shift work and light at night and breast cancer risk. However, tumour growth (in vivo) can be accelerated by light at night in part from continuous activation of IGF-1R signalling.[146] A recent case-control study of 1 679 women indicated that exposure to light at night during sleep is significantly associated with breast cancer risk.[146] Although inconclusive, shift work and its disruptive effects on circadian rhythms and sleep deprivation at night have been suggested as risk factors for breast cancer.[147,148]

Prolactin and Growth Hormone

Growth hormone induces the production of IGFs in the liver; IGF signalling is important for breast development and is implicated in breast carcinogenesis. Two studies, however, have reported a link between growth hormone level and breast cancer risk.[149,150] In the largest prospective analysis comparing circulating prolactin levels and breast cancer risk, those with the highest levels had the highest risk.[151] From a European Prospective Investigation into Cancer and Nutrition (EPIC) cohort, higher circulating prolactin level was associated with increased risk for in situ breast cancer.[152]

Oral Contraceptives

The IARC confirmed that combined estrogen-progestogen oral contraceptives increase the risk for breast, cervix, and liver cancers.[141,153] However, the efficacy of oral contraceptives in protecting against ovarian cancer and endometrial cancer is well established. Hormones are discussed further in the following "Pathogenesis" section (p. 855).

Mammographic Density

Mammographic density (MD; also called *mammographic breast density*) is the radiological appearance of the breast, reflecting variations in breast composition (Figure 33-29). MD appears white or dense on a risk for breast, cervix, and liver cancers factor for breast cancer.[132] MD decreases with age and is associated with BMI, family history, and postmenopausal hormone use.[154,155] IGF-1R may play an important role in breast cancer in individuals with mammographic breast tissue density.[156] Investigators are studying whether MD is related to reduced lobular involution of breast tissue in dense breasts (reduced involution increases cancer risk). Having a combination of dense breasts and no lobular involution was found to be associated with higher breast cancer risk than having nondense or fatty breasts and complete involution.[132] Women with dense breasts whose percentage of MD is more than 60 to 75% of the breast have a fourfold to sixfold increased risk for breast cancer compared with those with little or no density.[155,157] Dense area percentage is a stronger breast cancer risk factor than absolute dense area.[158] Mammographic dense tissue has been thought to represent both epithelial and stromal components. One hypothesis is that the stromal-rich environment in MD may have an abundance of growth factors that could stimulate the epithelium in a noninvoluted breast, thereby increasing the risk for malignant transformation.[132] Finding

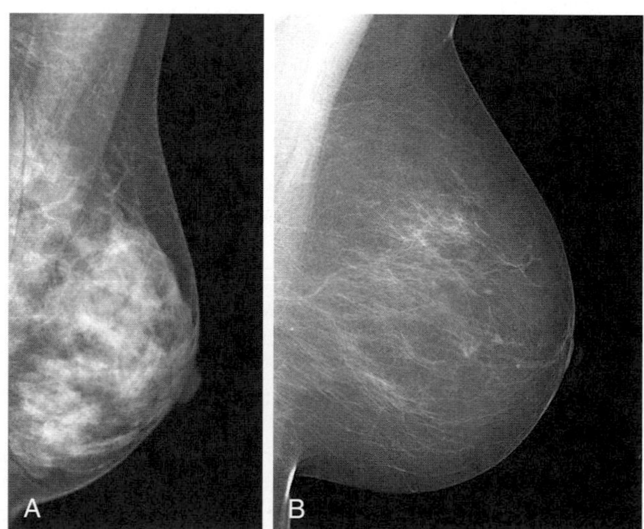

FIGURE 33-29 Breast Density Varies Among Women. The sensitivity of mammography for detecting malignancy is significantly reduced if the breast consists of a high proportion of fibroglandular (dense) breast tissue **(A)** compared with a breast that is fatty **(B)**. (From O'Malley, F.P., Pinder, S.E., & Mulligan, A.M. [Eds.]. [2011]. *Breast pathology* [2nd ed.]. Philadelphia: Saunders.)

tumours in women with MD is a challenge because they both appear white; as breast cancer surgeon Dr. Susan Love states, it is "… like trying to find a polar bear in a snow storm."

Environmental Factors

The environmental causes of breast cancer possibly affect the breast the most during critical phases or "windows" of development including early differential stages—that is, undifferentiated cells to alveolar buds and then lobules, puberty, pregnancy and lactation, involution, and menopause. During these early phases, mitotic activity and cell division are greater than later in life.

Radiation. Ionizing radiation is a known mutagen and established carcinogen for breast cancer. To date, only accidentally or medically induced radiation has been demonstrated to exert a carcinogenic effect on the breast. According to the US Institute of Medicine (IOM), the two most strongly associated environmental factors are exposure to ionizing radiation and combined postmenopausal HRT.[159] There are many sources of ionizing radiation, including X-rays, CT scans, fluoroscopy, and other medical radiological procedures (see Chapter 11). The IOM conclusion of a causal relationship between radiation exposure in the same range as CT and cancer is consistent from a large varied literature.[160] The IOM makes it clear that *avoidance* of medical imaging is an important and concrete step that women (girls) can take to reduce their risk for breast cancer.[161] Scientists and clinicians also have expressed concern about the increasing number of CT scans performed, including those performed on children.[161,162] Radiological exposure of the upper spine, heart, ribs, lungs, shoulders, and esophagus also exposes breast tissue to radiation. Breast tissue may be exposed from abdominal CT scans; X-rays and fluoroscopy of infants may constitute whole-body irradiation. The duration of increased risk from radiation is unknown, but increased risk appears to have lasted at least 35 years in women treated for mastitis, those treated with fluoroscopy, and those who survived the atomic bombs during World War II. Breast cancer rates in atomic bomb survivors in Japan were highest among women younger than 20 years of age at time of exposure; importantly, those who had early full-term pregnancies were at significantly lower risk than those who did not. Thus, interacting factors can modulate the risks from radiation.

An important topic currently is the effect of low-dose ionizing radiation. The debate is that low-energy X-rays may be more hazardous per unit dose than previously reported. Conventional X-ray mammography is one of the most valuable diagnostic tools for imaging of the breast. Currently, full-field digital mammography (FFDM) is frequently used. Continuous technical development has led to several new imaging techniques, including digital breast tomosynthesis (DBT), phase contrast X-ray imaging, and CT of the breast, as well as ultrasound and MRI. Despite technical innovations, except for ultrasound and MRI, these modalities require exposure of breast tissue to ionizing radiation, and the breast is considered a very radiosensitive organ.[163] Therefore, it is critical to compare delivered radiation doses to the breast and measure X-ray–induced DNA damage. A new technique for the detection and quantification of in vivo DNA damage has been developed. DNA double-strand breaks (DSBs) are the most relevant lesion induced by ionizing irradiation.[163] After the induction of DSBs, phosphorylation of the histone variant H2AX (named *γ-H2AX*) occurs. Phosphorylated γ-H2AX forms visible foci, which are a reliable and sensitive tool for the determination of DNA damage. Recently, investigators found that mammography induces a slight but significant increase of γ-H2AX foci in systemic blood lymphocytes. A clear induction of DNA lesions was found both by FFDM and by DBT.[163] These data will be important in the comparison of different breast imaging techniques. Investigators are studying mammographic radiation–induced DNA damage in mammary epithelial cells from women with low or high family risk for breast cancer, including comparisons of the number of views performed during screening.[164] Radiobiological effects have been found in both low-risk and high-risk women, but they are greater in high-risk women.[164-166] Investigators are looking for markers that are activated by DNA damage. One new marker may be CAV1 (caveolin 1 protein, see Chapter 1). Caveolin protein acts as a sensor and early mediator in response to DNA damage and may be important as a biomarker for radiosensitivity.[167] New biological understandings of low doses of radiation are presented in Chapter 11.

Women treated with chest radiation for a pediatric or young adult type of cancer have a substantially increased risk for breast cancer. Investigators from international studies have concluded that diagnostic chest irradiation or radiation therapy for benign or malignant diseases increases the risk for breast cancer for cumulative doses as low as 130 mGy. The breast cancer risk did not decrease when increasing the number of radiological treatment fractions for delivering the same total dose, but risk decreased greatly with increasing age of exposure to ionizing radiation.[168] International agencies are assessing the utility of screening MRI and mammography in these high-risk populations. The risk for secondary lung malignancy is an important concern for women treated with whole-breast radiation therapy after breast-conserving surgery for early-stage breast cancer.[169] Investigators studied secondary lung malignancy risk associated with several common methods of delivering whole-breast radiation therapy. Compared with supine whole-breast irradiation, prone breast irradiation is associated with a significantly lower predicted risk for secondary lung malignancy.[169]

The Canadian Task Force on Preventive Health Care has updated the recommendations for mammography because of overdiagnosis and overtreatment issues related to screening mammography (see *Health Promotion:* Breast Cancer Screening Mammography).

Diet. Prospective epidemiological studies on diet and breast cancer risk fail to show an association that is consistent, strong, and statistically significant except for alcohol intake, being overweight, and weight gain after menopause (see the following section). Diet has been postulated as important for breast cancer risk because of the international correlations of consumption of specific dietary factors (e.g., fats) and breast cancer incidence and mortality and because of migrant studies showing greater incidence of breast cancer among descendants who relocated to another country compared with those in the country of origin. International variations also can occur because of differences in reproductive history, physical activity, obesity, and other factors.

Dietary fat and breast cancer risk is the subject of much study, controversy, and debate.[170] Potential biological mechanisms between fat intake and breast cancer risk include the following: (1) fat may stimulate endogenous steroid hormone production (also affects weight gain, age of menarche), (2) fat interferes with immune or inflammatory function, and (3) fat influences gene expression. Although prospective studies and case-control studies on fat and breast cancer risk have been inconsistent, concern has been raised that any association with fat intake may be because of total energy intake. Moreover, there is limited evidence that modest reductions in fat intake (less than 20% of caloric intake) reduce breast cancer risk. Despite extensive investigation, there is no conclusive evidence overall that *adult* consumption of macronutrients including fat, carbohydrate, or fibre is strongly related to breast cancer incidence.

The association between individual foods and breast cancer is inconsistent, and new data on *dietary patterns* are emerging. The Mediterranean diet includes high intake of vegetables, legumes, fruits, nuts, and minimally processed cereals; moderately high intake of fish; and high intake of monounsaturated lipids coupled with low intake of saturated fat, low to moderate intake of dairy products, low intake of meat products, and moderate intake of alcohol. The Mediterranean diet may favourably influence the risk for breast cancer.[171] The Western pattern includes higher intake of red and processed meats, refined grains, sweets and desserts, and high-fat dairy products.

Most prospective studies have not supported a link between fibre intake and breast cancer. Carbohydrate quality, however, rather than absolute amount, may be important for breast cancer risk, especially for premenopausal women.

Evidence exists that alcohol consumption increases breast cancer risk. Beer, wine, and liquor all contributed to the positive association, and risks did not differ by menopausal status. In large prospective studies, high intake of folic acid appeared to decrease the enhanced risk for breast cancer caused by alcohol. The mechanisms by which alcohol intake increases the risk for breast cancer are unknown; however, physiological studies have reported that alcohol intake leads to an estrogen level increase in women taking HRT as well as IGF-1 level increases. Alcohol may increase breast cancer risk through increasing MD, especially in women at high risk.[172] It is not known whether reducing or discontinuing alcohol consumption in midlife decreases the risk for breast cancer.

The relationship between fruit and vegetable intake and reduction in breast cancer risk has been studied over three decades. To date, no protective effects have been firmly established.[173]

Soybeans are the main source of isoflavones. The isoflavone compounds, including daidzein and genistein, can bind ERs but are far less potent than estradiol. Soy may act like other antiestrogens (e.g., tamoxifen) by blocking the action of endogenous estrogens to reduce breast cancer risk. Thus, depending on the estradiol concentration, soy exhibits weak estrogenic or antiestrogenic activity. Many other mechanisms of action are proposed for isoflavones, including apoptosis and inhibition of angiogenesis. In 2011 the North American Menopause Society held a symposium to review the latest evidence-informed science on the role of soy and found that soy foods generally appear to be breast protective and recommended moderate lifelong soy consumption.[111] A recent large study of both American and Chinese women suggested that moderate intake of soy (equal to or greater than 10 mg of isoflavones per day) contributed to a significant reduction in breast cancer recurrence but was not significant in reduction of overall breast cancer mortality.[174] In addition, soy may optimize extrarenal 1,25-dihydroxycholecalciferol or vitamin D_3 (a prodifferentiating vitamin D metabolite), which could result in growth control and, conceivably, inhibition of tumour progression.

Iodine deficiency is hypothesized as contributing to the development of breast pathology and cancer.[112,175] Iodine plays a significant role in breast health.[175-178] Evidence reveals that iodine is an antioxidant and antiproliferative agent contributing to the integrity of normal mammary tissue.[179] Seaweed, which is iodine-rich, is an important dietary item in Asian communities and has been associated with the *low* evidence of BBD and breast cancer disease in Japanese women.[179] Molecular iodine (I_2) supplementation exerts an inhibitory effect on the development and size of benign and cancerous tissue.[180] Nutrition remains an important area of study.

Obesity. Excess body fatness is known to increase cancer risk from cellular pathways that involve hormonal regulation, cellular proliferation, and immunity.[181] Obesity, measured as BMI, has been associated with a *reduced* risk for *premenopausal* breast cancer. Recently reported (from the Nurses' Health Study I and II), however, was that weight gain or weight loss since age 18 did not significantly decrease the risk for premenopausal breast cancer.[182] Other data measuring adiposity using the waist–hip ratio (WHR) have not shown a reduced risk but rather no association (null) or an increased risk. Excess adiposity is positively associated with breast cancer recurrence and breast cancer–specific mortality among both premenopausal and postmenopausal women.[183]

In 2002, the IARC concluded that excess body weight (EBW) increased the risk of developing postmenopausal breast, colorectum, endometrium, kidney, and esophageal adenocarcinoma.[184] World Cancer Research Fund (now *World Cancer Research Fund International*) used a more standardized approach to evaluate studies and concluded that evidence is convincing and that a probable association exists between body fat and postmenopausal breast cancer.[185]

Despite strong links with endogenous estrogen levels, body fat has been consistently but *weakly* related to increased postmenopausal risk.[186] This observation (i.e., weakly) has been surprising because obese postmenopausal women have endogenous estrogen levels (estrone and estradiol) nearly double those of lean women.[186,187] This weak association is possibly related to two factors. First, the premenopausal reduction in breast cancer risk related to being overweight possibly persists, opposing the adverse effect of elevated levels of estrogens after menopause. Thus, *weight gain* should be more strongly related to postmenopausal breast cancer risk than attained weight. In two case-control studies and prospective studies, this was indeed true.[188-191]

Obesity is associated with poor survival among women with breast cancer, and the association of obesity with mortality from breast cancer appears to be stronger than its association with incidence.[186,190] The increase in breast cancer risk with increasing BMI among postmenopausal women is most likely the result of increases in levels of estrogens by aromatase activity in adipose tissue.[181] However, studies of hormones secreted by adipose tissue, *leptin* and *adiponectin*, may underlie the association between obesity and breast cancer risk. Increasing BMI and central fat deposition are associated with increased risk for breast cancer in prospective studies, and in vitro studies have shown leptin-stimulated breast carcinogenesis.[192,193] From molecular mechanism studies, leptin enhances breast cancer cell proliferation by inhibiting cell death (pro-apoptosis) signalling pathways and by increasing in vitro sensitivity to estrogens.[194] Leptin secreted by adipocytes and fibroblasts in the microenvironment act on breast cancer cells in a paracrine fashion.[195] Adiponectin has been shown to exert antiproliferative effects in vitro on human breast cancer cells.[194] Additionally, factors that may be related to recurrence of breast cancer in women with excess adiposity at the time of diagnosis include cytokines, IGF, and/or immune function.[181]

Environmental chemicals. Evidence linking chemicals to the cause of breast cancer is difficult to obtain. It is challenging because it is a life history of exposure that is important—not just a single chemical but complex mixtures of chemicals and their interaction with endogenous hormones. With industrial development, breast cancer rates increase. An estimated 23 000 chemical substances that were manufactured, imported, or used in Canada on a commercial scale since the mid-1980s have been identified, and approximately 600 new chemical substances are added each year.[196] In 2006, Canada established the Chemicals Management Plan (CMP), a national science-based program that aims to reduce the risks posed by chemicals to Canadians and their environment through various risk-management strategies.

Chemicals persist in the environment, accumulate in adipose tissue, interact with local adipose tissue physiology in an endocrine/paracrine manner, and remain in breast tissue for decades. ERs are some of the main targets of endocrine-disrupting chemicals (EDCs), including the plasticizer bisphenol A and the flame retardant tetrachlorobisphenol A.[197] Women who immigrate to North America from Asian countries experience an enormous percentage increase in risk for breast cancer within one generation. A generation later, the rate of their daughters' risk approaches that of women born in North America. This change in risk suggests that *in utero* exposures affect subsequent disease risk.

It is difficult to know whether these changes in risk emanate from nutritional content, pollutants, food additives, or other factors.

Xenoestrogens are synthetic chemicals that mimic the actions of estrogens and are found in many pesticides, fuels, plastics, detergents, and medications. Because many factors correlated with breast cancer (e.g., early menarche, delayed pregnancy and breastfeeding, late menopause) are associated with lifetime exposure to estrogens, investigators have reasoned that environmental chemicals affect estrogen metabolism and contribute to breast cancer. The most significant chemicals may be polychlorinated biphenyls (PCBs), such as dichlorodiphenyltrichloroethane (DDT), pesticides (dieldrin, aldrin, heptachlor, and others), bisphenol A (pervasive in polycarbonate plastics), tobacco smoke (active and passive), dioxins (vehicle exhaust, incineration, contaminated food supply), alkylphenols (detergents and cleaning products), metals, phthalates (makes plastics flexible, some cosmetics), parabens (antimicrobials), food additives (recombinant bovine somatotropin [rBST] and zeranol to enhance growth in cattle and sheep), MHT (i.e., HRT), and others.

Physical activity. Regular physical activity may reduce overall risk for breast cancer, especially in premenopausal or young postmenopausal women. Activity also may reduce the invasiveness of breast cancer.[198] A sedentary lifestyle may increase cancer risk through several mechanisms including increased insulin resistance, increased inflammation, and decreased immune function.[199] Epidemiological studies demonstrate that physical activity lowered the risk for breast cancer mortality in breast cancer survivors and improved their physiological and immune functions.[199]

Inherited Cancer Syndromes, Genes, Epigenetic Considerations

The causes of breast cancer have been difficult to define because each woman has a different genetic profile, which is called genetic heterogeneity.[200] Genetic heterogeneity is common not only among individuals but also at the level of the tumour itself, involving both genetic and epigenetic processes. These genetic factors interact with environmental factors. These facts are sobering and make an understanding of the genetic driving force behind tumour initiation, progression, and metastasis very complicated. However, recently, an experiment using a mouse model of breast tumour heterogeneity allowed investigators to probe the molecular basis of stable differences in cell (clonal) populations to contribute to various aspects of the cancer process, including the ability to form circulating tumour cells (CTCs) and ultimately metastases[201] (see the following "Pathogenesis" section).

A history of breast cancer in first-degree relatives (mother or sister) increases a woman's risk about two to three times. Risk increases even more if two first-degree relatives are involved, especially if the disease occurred before menopause and was bilateral. A small total proportion of breast cancers (5 to 10%, although the prevalence is significant) are the result of highly penetrant dominant genes (i.e., hereditary breast cancers). The most important of the dominant genes are the breast cancer susceptibility genes (*BRCA1* [breast cancer 1], *BRCA2* [breast cancer 2]). *BRCA1*, located on chromosome 17, is a tumour-suppressor gene; therefore, any mutation in the gene may inhibit or retard its suppressor function, leading to uncontrolled cell proliferation. *BRCA2* is located on chromosome 13. A family history of both breast cancer and ovarian cancer increases the risk that an individual with breast cancer carries a *BRCA1* mutation.[202] Carriers of the *BRCA1* gene also are at higher risk for ovarian cancer. The risks for breast or ovarian cancer, or both, however, are not equal in all mutation carriers and have been found to vary by several factors, including type of cancer, age at onset, and mutation position.[202] This observed variation in penetrance has led to the hypothesis that other genetic factors, environmental factors, or both modify cancer risk in mutation carriers. Men who develop breast cancer are more likely to have a *BRCA2* mutation than a *BRCA1* mutation (see Chapter 34). Options for those who have a positive test for *BRCA1* or *BRCA2* mutation include surveillance to find cancers early, prophylactic surgery (i.e., bilateral salpingo-oophorectomy), risk factor avoidance, promotion of breastfeeding, and chemoprevention. Several other genetic alterations can increase the risk for breast cancer.

PATHOGENESIS Most breast cancers are adenocarcinomas and first arise from the ductal/lobular epithelium as carcinoma in situ. Carcinoma in situ is a proliferation of epithelial cells that is confined to the ducts and lobules by the basement membrane. Tumours of the infiltrating (invasive) ductal type do not grow to a large size, but they metastasize early. This type accounts for 70% of breast cancers. Table 33-11 summarizes some types of breast cancer. Breast cancer is a heterogeneous—not a single—disease with diverse molecular, biological, phenotypic, and pathological changes.[203] Heterogeneity is an important concept because the biological attributes of a tumour as a whole are strongly influenced by its subpopulation of cells, as well as by the tumour's surrounding neighbourhood or microenvironment.[204] Recent research suggests that breast cancer is heterogeneous from its initial pre-invasive stages[205] and within the same tumour.

The many genetic and epigenetic changes drive the sequential expansion of progressively more and more malignant cell populations.[206] Breast tissue stem cells are thought to be the cell of origin for all breast cancers. Gene expression profiling studies have identified at least four major subtypes classified as luminal A, luminal B, HER2+, and basal-like.[207] Mounting evidence shows that there are "subtypes within subtypes," and emerging evidence suggests that the biology of specific subtypes reflects contributions from the microenvironment.[208] Many models of breast carcinogenesis have been suggested, and three interrelated themes related to breast cancer initiation also have emerged: (1) gene addiction, (2) phenotype plasticity, and (3) cancer stem cells.

Cancer gene addiction includes oncogene addiction, whereby these driver genes play key roles in breast cancer development and progression, and nononcogene addiction, whereby these genes may not initiate cancer but play roles in cancer development and progression.[209] Examples of key driver genes include *HER2* and *MYC*, and examples of tumour-suppressor genes are *TP53*, *BRCA1*, and *BRCA2*. Once a founding tumour clone is established, genomic instability may assist through the establishment of other subclones and contribute to both tumour progression and therapy resistance.[97] Phenotypic plasticity is exemplified by a distinctive phenotype called epithelial–mesenchymal transition (EMT) (see Chapter 10). EMT is involved in the generation of tissues and organs during embryogenesis, is essential for driving tissue plasticity during development, and is an unintentional process during cancer progression. The EMT-associated reprogramming is involved in many cancer cell characteristics, including suppression of cell death or apoptosis and senescence, is reactivated during wound healing, and is resistant to chemotherapy and radiation therapy.[210] Remodelling or reprogramming of the breast during postpregnancy involution is important because it involves inflammatory and "wound healing–like" tissue reactions known as *reactive stroma*. These tissue reactions increase the risk for tumour invasion and may facilitate the transition of carcinoma in situ to invasive carcinoma. Activation of an EMT program during cancer development often requires signalling between cancer cells and neighbouring stromal cells.[211] In advanced primary carcinomas, cancer cells recruit a variety of cell types into the surrounding stroma, including fibroblasts, myofibroblasts, granulocytes, macrophages, mesenchymal stem cells, and lymphocytes (Figure 33-30). Overall, increasing evidence suggests that interactions of cancer cells with adjacent tumour-associated stromal cells induce malignant cell phenotypes (Figure 33-31).

TABLE 33-11 Types of Breast Carcinomas and Major Distinguishing Features

Histological Type	Distinguishing Features
Carcinoma of Mammary Ducts	
Papillary	Well-delineated cystic masses in multiple areas; hemorrhage often present; majority appear in 40- to 60-year age group; often involves skin
Intraductal (comedo)	Often accompanied by evidence of inflammation; well-circumscribed tumours within duct; well-differentiated tumour cells; rarely ulcerates skin
Infiltrating Carcinoma	
Ductal (no specific type)	Fibrous, firm, glistening, grey-tan mass with chalky streaks, mixture of patterns; may cause discharge from nipple; represents about 70–80% of all breast cancers
Mucinous	Usually large (>3 cm in diameter), circumscribed, and encapsulated, glistening appearance, varies in colour; two types: pure and mixed; pure tumour is surrounded by mucin; infrequent; found in lateral half of breast; tends to occur in women after age 70 years
Medullary	Encapsulated and grows very large (7–8 cm in diameter); commonly surrounded by lymphocytic inflammatory infiltrate; occurs after age 50 years
Tubular	Well-differentiated with orderly tubules in centre (stroma) of mass; can be associated with noninfiltrating ductal carcinoma; occurs in women about 50 years of age; nodal metastasis infrequent; occurrence rare
Adenoid cystic	Very rare; well-circumscribed, painless mass arising from nipple and areola
Metaplastic	Involves cartilage or bone, mixed tumours or osteogenic sarcomas
Squamous cell	Frequent in Blacks; originates in ductal epithelium
Carcinoma of Mammary Lobules	
Lobular carcinoma in situ	Found in individuals with fibrocystic disease; localized to upper breast quadrants; 15–35% risk of becoming invasive; occurs frequently in mid-40s; infiltrating variety occurs in early 50s
Infiltrating lobular	Infiltrates from duct; firm mass with chalky streaks
Paget's disease	Eczema of nipple that extends to areola; cancer usually found underneath nipple; poorly circumscribed; large Paget cells arise from duct and directly invade nipple; history of scaly, red rash spreading from nipple; lesion palpable beneath nipple, often bilateral; occurs in middle age
Inflammatory carcinoma	Not a histological type; fairly diffuse within breast tissue, diffuse edema of overlying skin; extremely undifferentiated, very rare; most metastasize to axilla
Sarcoma of the Breast	
Cystosarcoma phyllodes	Usually large (>17 cm in diameter); mostly localized but can rupture through skin; rarely metastasizes to lymph nodes; history of painless nodule present for years before it forms a large mass; ulceration and bleeding of skin often present; occurs in wide age range (13–77 years)
Fibrosarcoma	Well-circumscribed, firm, and usually does not involve skin or nipple; well-differentiated to extremely undifferentiated; arises from connective tissue; extremely rare (e.g., liposarcoma, angiosarcoma)

Research is ongoing to define cancer stem cells in breast carcinogenesis, including cancer stem cell origin and renewability properties. Studies have begun to identify the role of MaSCs and to describe how they drive development of the gland and maintain homeostasis, maintain the many cycles of proliferation and apoptosis needed to expand and maintain the breast during pregnancy, and return it to a quiet (quiescent) state after involution.[212] EMT generates multiple epithelial cell subsets with different states of stemness relative to more differentiated cells.[213] The ECM and the basement membrane, in particular, are no longer just considered the "bricks and mortar" of a tissue but now a place where stem cells reside; and correct tissue architecture, together with the reservoir of growth factors, cytokines, and proteinases, is critical for mammary tissue to develop and function properly.[212] Many of the biological traits of high-grade malignancy—motility, invasiveness, and self-renewal—have been traced to subpopulations of stem cells within carcinomas.[214,215] Hormones may act as accelerators as well as initiators, delay involution, and influence the susceptibility of the breast epithelium to environmental carcinogens because hormones control the differentiation of the mammary gland epithelium and, thereby, regulate the rate of stem cell division.

Two new concepts being investigated as important to metastases are tumour dormancy and vascular mimicry. **Tumour dormancy** has been noted in the care of people with cancer, whereby microscopic and occult cancerous lesions enter a latent or dormant phase in various stages of tumour progression. In fact, these microscopic and occult cancerous lesions are often found in healthy people.[216] Ironically, in healthy people these are the slow-growing tumours (some called "pseudodisease") detected by present screening methods that would not advance to routine clinical presentation over the individual's lifetime.[216] Current debates surround the concern that individuals often undergo unnecessary treatment for a disease they were never destined to experience.[216] Evidence exists that organ-specific molecular signalling can determine whether a metastatic lesion will expand or remain dormant. Significant to different signalling profiles that may determine this outcome are stress-activated kinases, transcription factors (such as p53), and cell cycle inhibitors. Thus, cell stress–activated signalling may be increased, for example, with certain treatment modalities such as surgery. Evidence has been accumulating that removal of a malignant tumour from a host is curative for many but—in some circumstances—is insufficient to prevent the cancer from recurring and can lead to rapid cancer recurrence.[217,218]

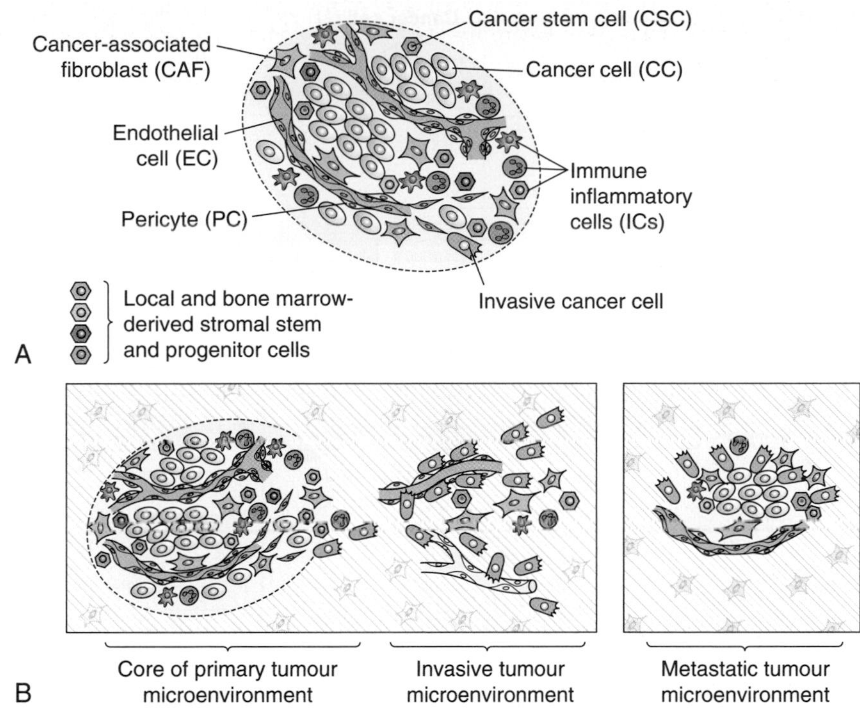

FIGURE 33-30 Cells of the Tumour Microenvironment. A, Distinct cell types constitute most solid tumours including breast tumours. Both the main cellular tissue, called *parenchyma,* and the surrounding tissue, or stroma, of tumours contain cell types that enable tumour growth and progression. For example, the immune-inflammatory cells present in tumours can include both tumour-promoting and tumour-killing subclasses of cells. **B,** The microenvironment of tumours. Multiple stromal cell types create a succession of tumour microenvironments that change as tumours invade normal tissue, eventually seeding and colonizing distant tissues. The organization, numbers, and phenotypic characteristics of the stromal cell types and the extracellular matrix (*hatched background*) evolve during progression and enable primary, invasive, and metastatic growth.(Not shown are the premalignant stages.) (Data from Hanahan, D., & Weinberg, R. [2011]. *Cell, 144,* 646–674.)

Immune cells in the ECM or stroma and the overall immune response have been recognized for their role in regulating tumour growth and are being investigated for their role in tumour dormancy.

Cancer metastases require that primary tumour cells evolve the ability to intravasate into the lymphatic system or vasculature, and extravasate into and colonize secondary sites.[201] Investigators developed a mouse model of breast tumour heterogeneity and isolated a distinct clone of specialized cells that efficiently enter the vasculature and express two proteins, Serpine2 and SLPI, which were necessary and sufficient to program these cells for vascular mimicry. Vascular mimicry is a blood supply pathway in tumours that is formed by tumour cells and is independent of endothelial cell–lined blood vessels—thus it *mimics* real blood vessels (Figure 33-32). This blood supply pathway facilitates perfusion of the primary tumours and correlates with poor clinical outcome. The increase in these blood supply pathways was associated with an increase in CTCs and a subsequent increase in lung metastases. Additionally, treatment with the anticoagulant warfarin (Coumadin) increased the number of CTCs and lung metastases, suggesting that the anticoagulant function of Serpine2 and SLPI both maintains blood flow through the extravascular network and promotes intravasation. These remarkable findings identify Serpine2- and SLPI-driven vascular mimicry as a critical mechanism or driver of metastatic progression in cancer.[201]

Ductal and Lobular Carcinoma in Situ

Ductal carcinoma in situ (DCIS) is a heterogeneous group of proliferations limited to breast ducts and lobules without invasion of the basement membrane. About 84% of all in situ disease is DCIS; the remainder is mostly lobular carcinoma in situ (LCIS). DCIS occurs predominantly in females but can occur in males. Since 1980, the widespread adoption of screening mammography has led to an epidemic of diagnoses of DCIS.[219] DCIS presents as microcalcifications (low grade) (Figure 33-33, *B*) or rod-shaped branching (high grade) on a mammogram (Figure 33-33, *A*).

Still controversial, DCIS does not appear to progress from sequential steps of low grade or risk types to higher grade or risk types during its route to cancer or cancer recurrence.[205,220] This property, therefore, suggests a stable population.[205] Because of these findings, some argue that the term is misleading and should be replaced by *ductal intraepithelial neoplasia*, similar to the term used in prostate cancer, and that breast cancer statistics should exclude these DCIS cases with invasive breast cancer statistics.[221] DCIS is a very common type of noninvasive cancer, with one in five breast cancers diagnosed as DCIS.[222] Because of the large numbers of cases diagnosed yearly in Canada, the debate is whether mammography is causing the overdiagnosis of potential pseudodisease; for example, the Canadian National Breast Screening Study-2 of women aged 50 to 59 years found a fourfold increase in DCIS cases in those screened by clinical breast examination (CBE) plus mammography compared with those screened by CBE alone, with no difference in breast cancer mortality.[219,222] The difficulty for this clinical dilemma is that the natural history of DCIS is poorly understood because nearly all cases are treated. More directed research is needed on DCIS with genetic expression profiling, best treatment to achieve disease regression, and studies of tumour characteristics and risk profiling. An important,

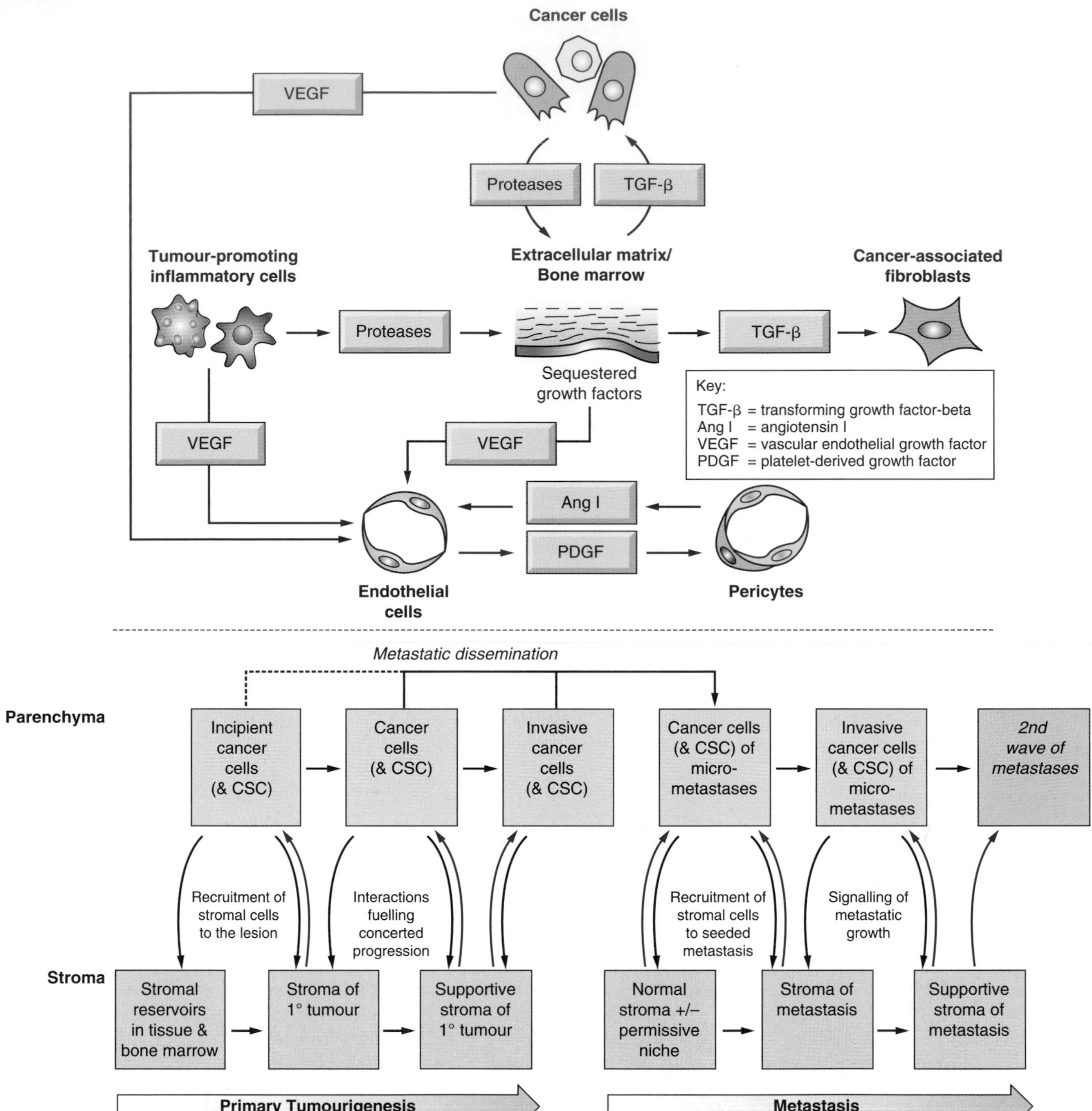

FIGURE 33-31 Signalling Interactions in the Tumour Microenvironment During Malignant Progression. *Upper panel:* Numerous cell types constitute the tumour microenvironment and are orchestrated and maintained by reciprocal interactions. *Lower panel:* The reciprocal interactions between the breast main tissue or parenchyma and the surrounding stroma are important for cancer progression and growth. Certain organ sites of "fertile soil" or "metastasis niches" facilitate metastatic seeding and colonization. Cancer stem cells are involved in some or all stages of tumour development and progression. *CSC,* cancer stem cell. (Adapted from Hanahan, D., & Weinberg, R. [2011]. *Cell, 144,* 646–674.)

newer mission of the DCIS Discovery Enterprise at MD Anderson Cancer Center in Houston, Texas, is to prevent invasive disease while also reducing unnecessary surgery or radiation.

Key to understanding the progression of breast cancer after treatment of DCIS are the characteristics of the lesion and the delivered treatment. According to the US National Cancer Institute, the best evidence indicates that most lesions of DCIS will not evolve to invasive cancer, and those that do can be managed successfully, even after that transition.[221] The detection and treatment of nonpalpable DCIS often represents overdiagnosis and overtreatment.[221] Surprisingly, the overall death rate for

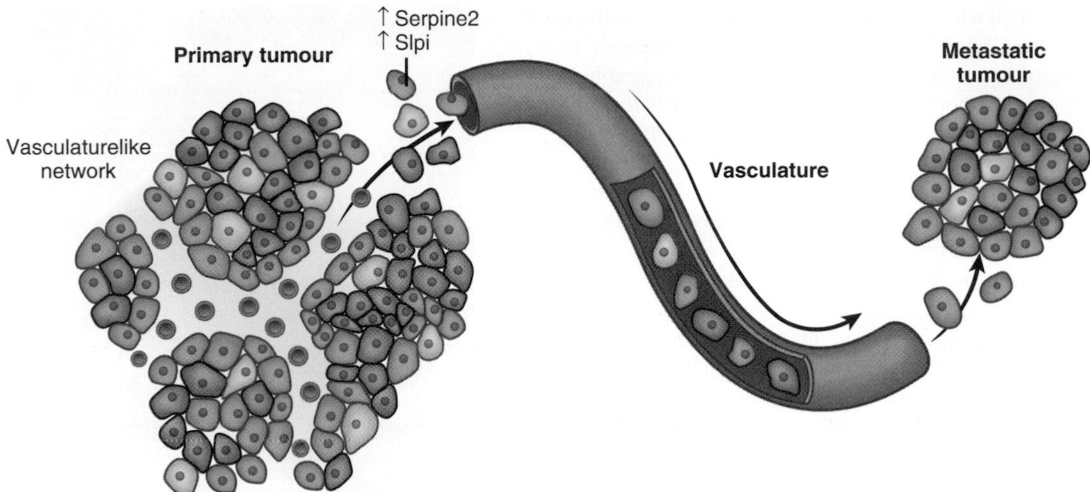

FIGURE 33-32 Vascular Mimicry Drives Metastasis. The steps to accomplish metastasis include *intravasation*, in which tumour cells escape from the primary tumour into the vasculature and move through the bloodstream; or *extravasation*, in which tumour cells escape from the vasculature to colonize in distant tissue. Metastasis is promoted by vascular mimicry, whereby tumour cells adopt characteristics similar to those of the endothelial cells that line blood vessels, and mimic vascularlike networks within tumours and between tumours and blood vessels. Wagenblast and colleagues found that two proteins, Serpine2 and SLPI, promoted metastasis by stimulating vascular mimicry. Tumour cells expressing these proteins (*green*) form the vascularlike network that allows other tumour cells (*purple, blue*) to move to secondary sites. (Adapted from Hendrix, M.J.C. [2015]. *Nature, 520*, 300–302; Wagenblast, E., Soto, M., Gutiérrez-Ángel, C.A., et al. [2015]. *Nature, 520*, 358–362.)

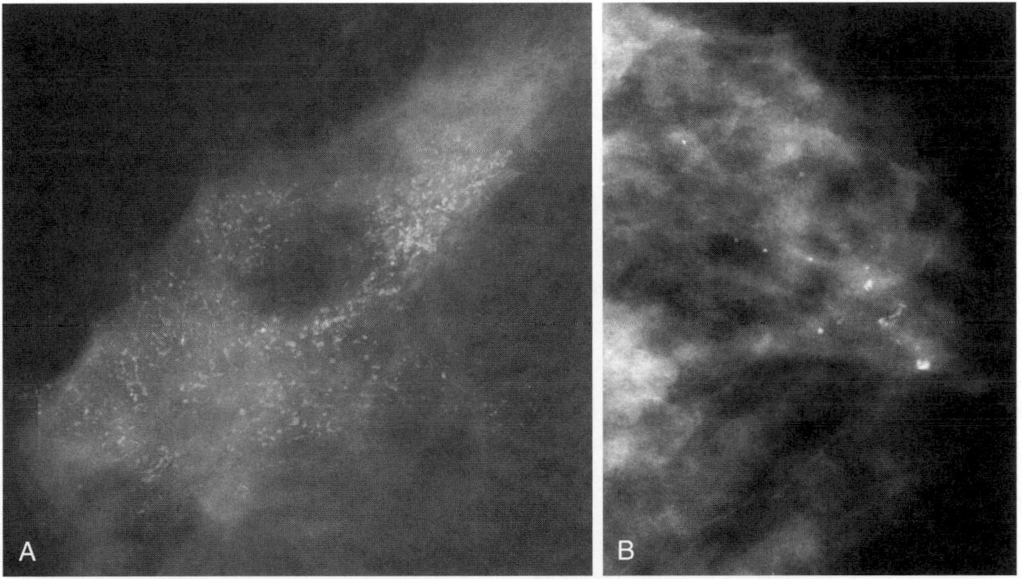

FIGURE 33-33 Ductal Carcinoma in Situ. A, Malignant microcalcifications. Extensive area of pleomorphic microcalcifications; granular, rod-shaped, and branching microcalcifications can be identified. The appearances are typical of high-grade ductal carcinoma in situ (DCIS). **B,** Craniocaudal mammography reveals fine and coarse granular calcifications. Histopathological analysis revealed low-grade DCIS. (**A,** from O'Malley, F.P., Pinder, S.E., & Mulligan, A.M. [Eds.]. [2011]. *Breast pathology* [2nd ed.]. Philadelphia: Saunders; **B,** from Donegan, W.L., & Spratt, J.S. [2002]. *Cancer of the breast* [5th ed.]. Philadelphia: Saunders.)

women with DCIS is lower than that for women in the population as a whole.[97,221] This favourable outcome may reflect the benign nature of the condition or the benefits of treatment, or it may be a marker for socioeconomic factors associated with longevity.[97,221] Attempts to define low-risk DCIS cases that can be managed with fewer therapies are critical.[221]

Lobular carcinoma in situ (LCIS) originates from the TDLU. Unlike DCIS, LCIS has a uniform appearance—the cells expand but do not distort involved spaces; thus the lobular structure is preserved. The cells grow in a noncohesive (discohesive) fashion usually because of a loss of the tumour-suppressive adhesion protein E-cadherin.[97] LCIS is found as an incidental lesion from a biopsy and not from mammography because it is not associated with calcifications or stromal reactions that produce mammographic densities. LCIS has an incidence of about 1 to 6% of all carcinomas and did not increase with mammographic screening.[97] With biopsies in both breasts, LCIS is bilateral in 20 to 40% of cases, compared with 10 to 20% of cases of DCIS.[97] The cells of AH, LCIS, and invasive lobular carcinoma are structurally identical.[97] Loss of cellular adhesion because of dysfunction of E-cadherin results in a rounded shape without attachment to adjacent cells, increasing the risk for invasion. E-cadherin functions as a tumour-suppressor protein and may be lost in neoplastic proliferations from various mechanisms, including mutation.

LCIS is a risk factor for invasive carcinoma and develops in 25 to 35% of women over a period of 20 to 30 years. Unlike DCIS, the risk is almost as high in the contralateral breast as in the ipsilateral breast. Treatments include close clinical follow-up and mammographic screening, tamoxifen, and bilateral prophylactic mastectomy.

CLINICAL MANIFESTATIONS The majority of carcinomas of the breast occur in the upper outer quadrant, where most of the glandular tissue of the breast is located. The lymphatic spread of cancer to the opposite breast, to lymph nodes in the base of the neck, and to the abdominal cavity is caused by obstruction of the normal lymphatic pathways or destruction of lymphatic vessels by surgery or radiotherapy (see Figure 32-11). The less common inner quadrant tumours may spread to mediastinal nodes or Rotter nodes, which are located between the pectoral muscles (see Figure 32-11). Internal mammary chain nodes also are common sites of metastasis. Metastases from the vertebral veins can involve the vertebrae, pelvic bones, ribs, and skull. The lungs, kidneys, liver, adrenal glands, ovaries, and pituitary gland are also sites of metastasis.

The first sign of breast cancer is usually a painless lump. Lumps caused by breast tumours do not have any classic characteristics. Other presenting signs include palpable nodes in the axilla, retraction of tissue (dimpling) (Figure 33-34), or bone pain caused by metastasis to the vertebrae. Table 33-12 summarizes the clinical manifestations of breast cancer. Manifestations vary according to the type of tumour and stage of disease.

EVALUATION AND TREATMENT CBE, mammography, ultrasound, thermography, MRI, biopsy, hormone receptor assays, and gene expression profiling are used in evaluating breast alterations and cancer.

Treatment is based on the extent or stage of the cancer. The extent of the tumour at the primary site, the presence and extent of lymph node metastases, and the presence of distant metastases are all evaluated to determine the stage of disease. Treatment includes surgery, radiation, chemotherapy, hormone therapy, and biological therapy.

QUICK CHECK 33-5

1. What types of fibrocystic breast changes increase the risk for breast cancer?
2. What is the role of hormones and growth factors in the pathophysiology of breast cancer?
3. Why are reproductive factors, such as early menarche and late menopause, important for the pathogenesis of breast cancer?
4. Why is complete breast involution important for reducing risk for breast cancer?
5. Discuss the role of the microenvironment or stromal tissue on breast cancer development.

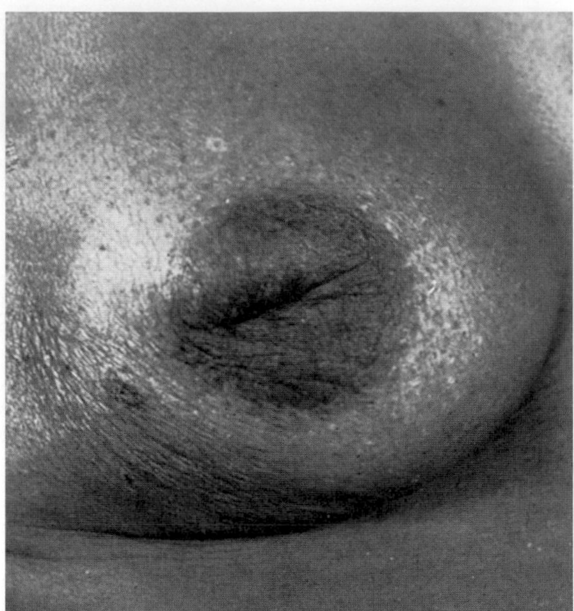

FIGURE 33-34 Retraction of Nipple Caused by Carcinoma. (From Ackerman, L.V., del Regato, J.A., Spjut, H.J., et al. [1985]. *Cancer: Diagnosis, treatment, and prognosis* [6th ed.]. St. Louis: Mosby.)

TABLE 33-12 Clinical Manifestations of Breast Cancer

Clinical Manifestation	Pathophysiology
Local pain	Local obstruction caused by tumour
Dimpling of skin	Can occur with invasion of dermal lymphatics because of retraction of Cooper ligament or involvement of pectoralis fascia
Nipple retraction	Shortening of mammary ducts
Skin retraction	Involvement of suspensory ligament
Edema	Local inflammation or lymphatic obstruction
Nipple/areolar eczema	Paget's disease
Pitting of skin (similar to surface of an orange [*peau d'orange*])	Obstruction of subcutaneous lymphatics, resulting in accumulation of fluid
Reddened skin, local tenderness, and warmth	Inflammation
Dilated blood vessels	Obstruction of venous return by a fast-growing tumour; obstruction dilates superficial veins
Nipple discharge in a nonlactating woman	Spontaneous and intermittent discharge caused by tumour obstruction
Ulceration	Tumour necrosis
Hemorrhage	Erosion of blood vessels
Edema of arm	Obstruction of lymphatic drainage in axilla
Chest pain	Metastasis to lung

DID YOU UNDERSTAND?

Abnormalities of the Female Reproductive Tract

1. Normal development of the female reproductive tract requires absence of testosterone during embryonic and fetal life.
2. Alterations in the normal process include errors in cellular sensitivity to testosterone (androgen insensitivity) or failures of cell line migration resulting in changes in the structure of the reproductive organs.
3. Androgen insensitivity syndrome is a disorder of hormone resistance characterized by a female phenotype in an individual with an XY karyotype or male genotype.
4. Other abnormalities of the uterus, cervix, and fallopian/uterine tubes have multifactorial origins and are often the result of an interaction between genetic predisposition and environmental factors.

Alterations of Sexual Maturation

1. Sexual maturation, or puberty, is marked by the development of secondary sex characteristics, rapid growth, and, ultimately, the ability to reproduce. The normal range for the onset of puberty is now 8 to 13 years of age but can vary geographically.
2. Delayed puberty is the onset of sexual maturation after these ages; precocious puberty is the onset before these ages. Treatment for delayed and precocious puberty depends on the cause.

Disorders of the Female Reproductive System

1. The female reproductive system can be altered by hormonal imbalances, infectious microorganisms, inflammation, structural abnormalities, and benign or malignant proliferative conditions.
2. Primary dysmenorrhea is painful menstruation not associated with pelvic disease. It results from excessive synthesis of prostaglandin $F_2\alpha$. Secondary dysmenorrhea results from endometriosis, pelvic adhesions, inflammatory disease, uterine fibroids, or adenomyosis.
3. Primary amenorrhea is the continued absence of menarche and menstrual function by 13 years of age without the development of secondary sex characteristics or by 15 years of age if these changes have occurred.
4. Secondary amenorrhea is the absence of menstruation for a time equivalent to three or more cycles in women who have previously menstruated. Secondary amenorrhea is associated with many disorders and physiological conditions.
5. Dysfunctional uterine bleeding is heavy or irregular bleeding in the absence of organic disease.
6. Polycystic ovary syndrome is a condition in which excessive androgen production is triggered by inappropriate secretion of gonadotropins. This hormonal imbalance prevents ovulation and causes enlargement and cyst formation in the ovaries, excessive endometrial proliferation, and often hirsutism. Insulin resistance and hyperinsulinemia play a key role in androgen excess.
7. Premenstrual syndrome is the cyclic recurrence of physical, psychological, or behavioural changes distressing enough to disrupt normal activities or interpersonal relationships. Emotional symptoms, particularly depression, anger, irritability, and fatigue, are reported as the most distressing symptoms; physical symptoms tend to be less problematic. Treatment is symptomatic and includes stress reduction, exercise, biofeedback, lifestyle changes, counselling, and medication.
8. Infection and inflammation of the female genitalia can result from microorganisms that are present in the environment and often sexually transmitted or from overproliferation of microorganisms that normally populate the genital tract.
9. Pelvic inflammatory disease (PID) is an acute inflammatory process caused by infection. Many infections are sexually transmitted and microorganisms that comprise the vaginal flora are implicated. PID is a substantial health risk to women, and untreated PID can lead to infertility.
10. Vaginitis is irritation or inflammation of the vagina, typically caused by infection. It is usually caused by sexually transmitted pathogens or *Candida albicans*, which causes candidiasis.
11. Cervicitis, which is infection of the cervix, can be acute (mucopurulent cervicitis) or chronic. Its most common cause is a sexually transmitted pathogen.
12. Vulvodyniavestibulitis (VV) is chronic vulvar pain lasting 3 months or longer without visible dermatosis. The cause of VV is unknown and theories include embryonic factors, chronic inflammation, genetic immune factors, nerve pathways, increased sensitivity to environmental factors, human papillomavirus (HPV), and hormonal changes.
13. Bartholinitis, also called *Bartholin cyst*, is an infection of the ducts that lead from the Bartholin glands to the surface of the vulva. Infection blocks the glands, preventing the outflow of glandular secretions.
14. The pelvic relaxation disorders—uterine displacement, uterine prolapse, cystocele, rectocele, and urethrocele—are caused by the relaxation of muscles and fascial supports, usually a result of advancing age or following childbirth or other trauma, and are more likely to occur in women with a familial or genetic predisposition.
15. Benign ovarian cysts develop from mature ovarian follicles that do not release their ova (follicular cysts) or from a corpus luteum that persists abnormally instead of degenerating (corpus luteum cyst). Cysts usually regress spontaneously.
16. Endometrial polyps consist of benign overgrowths of endometrial tissue and often cause abnormal bleeding in the premenopausal woman.
17. Leiomyomas, also called *myomas* or *uterine fibroids*, are benign tumours arising from the smooth muscle layer of the uterus, the myometrium.
18. Adenomyosis is the presence of endometrial glands and stroma within the uterine myometrium.
19. Endometriosis is the presence of functional endometrial tissue (i.e., tissue that responds to hormonal stimulation) at sites outside the uterus. Endometriosis causes an inflammatory reaction at the site of implantation and is a cause of infertility. Emerging is the relationship between endometriosis and ovarian cancer.
20. Cancers of the female genitalia involve the uterus (particularly the endometrium), the cervix, and the ovaries. Cancer of the vagina is rare.
21. Cervical cancer arises from the cervical epithelium and is triggered by HPV. The cellular transformational zone is called the *squamous-columnar junction*. The progressively serious neoplastic alterations are cervical intraepithelial neoplasia (CIN) (cervical dysplasia), cervical carcinoma in situ, and invasive cervical carcinoma. Cocarcinogens include immune responses, hormonal responses, and other environmental factors that determine regression or persistence of the HPV infection.
22. Primary cancer of the vagina is rare. Risk factors include being 60 or older, diethylstilbestrol exposure in utero, HPV-16, human immunodeficiency virus (HIV), genital warts, and previous carcinoma of the cervix or vulva. The relationship between cancer of the vagina and developing precancerous cell changes called *vaginal intra-epithelial neoplasia* is controversial.

23. Risk factors for vulvar cancer include HPV-16 (cause), HIV, HPV-18 (probable cause), increasing age, previous cancer (untreated high-grade vulvar intraepithelial neoplasia), cervical cancer survivor, previous CIN, certain autoimmune conditions, organ transplant recipient (perhaps because of immunosuppression to clear HPV), and tobacco use (may relate to inability to clear HPV infection).
24. Carcinoma of the endometrium is the most common type of uterine cancer and the most prevalent gynecological malignancy. Primary risk factors for endometrial cancer include exposure to unopposed estrogen (e.g., estrogen-only hormone replacement therapy [HRT], tamoxifen, early menarche, late menopause, nulliparity, failure to ovulate), chronic hyperinsulinemia, hyperglycemia, body fatness and adult weight gain, chronic inflammation, and lack of physical exercise.
25. Risk factors for ovarian cancer include advancing age, genetic factors, family history, overweight and obesity, height, reproductive or hormonal factors, HRT, endometriosis, diabetes, previous cancer, smoking, asbestos, talc-based powder, and ionizing radiation. Ovarian cancer causes more deaths than any other genital cancer in women.
26. The biology of ovarian cancer is changing, and ovarian cancer is heterogeneous.
27. Sexual dysfunction is the lack of satisfaction with sexual function resulting from pain or a deficiency in sexual desire, arousal, or orgasm/climax.
28. Sexual function and dysfunction result from a complex set of personal and biological factors that interact with culture. Both organic and psychosocial disorders can be implicated in sexual dysfunction.
29. Infertility, or the inability to conceive after 1 year of unprotected intercourse, affects approximately 16% of all couples. Fertility can be impaired by factors in the male, female, or both partners.
30. Female infertility results from dysfunction of the normal reproductive process: menses and ovulation, fallopian tube function (transport of the egg to the uterus and as a site of fertilization), ovarian dysfunction, and implantation of the fertilized egg into a receptive endometrium.

Disorders of the Female Breast

1. Most disorders of the breast are disorders of the mammary gland—that is, the female breast.
2. Galactorrhea, or *inappropriate lactation*, is the persistent secretion of a milky substance by the breasts of a woman who is not in the postpartum state or nursing an infant. Its most common cause is nonpuerperal hyperprolactinemia—a rise in serum prolactin levels.
3. Benign breast conditions are numerous and involve both ducts and lobules. Benign epithelial lesions can be broadly classified according to their future risk of developing breast cancer as (a) nonproliferative breast lesions, (b) proliferative breast disease, and (c) atypical (atypia) hyperplasia.
4. Nonproliferative breast lesions include simple breast cysts, papillary apocrine change, and mild hyperplasia of the usual type.
5. Proliferative breast lesions without atypia are diverse and include usual ductal hyperplasia, intraductal papillomas, sclerosing adenosis, radial scar, and simple fibroadenoma.
6. Proliferative breast lesions with atypia include atypical ductal hyperplasia and atypical lobular hyperplasia.
7. Ductal carcinoma in situ (DCIS) refers to a heterogeneous group of proliferations limited to breast ducts and lobules without invasion of the basement membrane. Lobular carcinoma in situ (LCIS) originates from the duct lobular unit.
8. Breast cancer is the most common form of cancer in women and second to lung cancer as the most common cause of cancer death. However, the inclusion of DCIS with invasive breast cancer statistics is controversial. Breast cancer is a heterogeneous disease with diverse molecular, phenotypic, and pathological changes.
9. The major risk factors for breast cancer are reproductive factors, such as nulliparity; hormonal factors and growth factors, such as excessive estradiol and insulinlike growth factor 1; familial factors, such as a family history of breast cancer; and environmental factors, such as ionizing radiation. Two factors emerging as important are delayed involution of the mammary gland and breast density. Physical activity and lack of postmenopausal weight gain may be risk-reducing factors.
10. A dominating movement in the field of cancer research is that epithelial function depends on the *entire* tissue including the stroma or microenvironment. Breast cancer is now known as a tissue-based disease with a possible abnormal, aberrant wound healing and inflammatory stromal (reactive stroma) component.
11. Models of breast carcinogenesis include three interrelated themes: gene addiction, phenotype plasticity, and cancer stem cells. The exact molecular events leading to breast cancer invasion are complex and not completely understood. These events involve genetic and epigenetic alterations and cancer cell and stromal interactions. New concepts for breast cancer metastases include tumour dormancy and vascular mimicry.
12. Most breast cancers arise from the ductal epithelium and then may metastasize to the lymphatics, opposite breast, abdominal cavity, lungs, bones, kidneys, liver, adrenal glands, ovaries, and pituitary glands.
13. The first clinical manifestation of breast cancer is usually a small, painless lump in the breast. Other manifestations include palpable lymph nodes in the axilla, dimpling of the skin, nipple and skin retraction, nipple discharge, ulcerations, reddened skin, and bone pain associated with bony metastases.

KEY TERMS

Adenomyosis, 831
Amenorrhea, 819
Androgen insensitivity syndrome (AIS), 816
Anorgasmia (orgasmic dysfunction), 842
Atypia, 844
Atypical ductal hyperplasia (ADH), 845
Atypical hyperplasia (AH), 845
Atypical lobular hyperplasia (ALH), 845
Bartholinitis (Bartholin cyst), 827
Benign breast disease (BBD), 844
Carcinoma in situ, 855
Cervicitis, 826
Complete precocious puberty, 818
Corpus luteum cyst, 830
Cyst, 844
Cystocele, 828
Delayed puberty, 818
Dermoid cyst, 830
Diffuse papillomatosis, 844
Disorder of desire (hypoactive sexual desire, decreased libido), 842
Ductal carcinoma in situ (DCIS), 857
Dysfunctional uterine bleeding (DUB), 820
Dyspareunia (painful intercourse), 842
E-cadherin, 859
Endometrial polyp, 830
Endometriosis, 832
Enterocele, 828

Epithelial–mesenchymal transition (EMT), 855
Fibrocystic change (FCC), 844
Follicular cyst, 829
Functional cyst, 829
Galactorrhea (inappropriate lactation), 843
Genetic heterogeneity, 855
Hirsutism, 820
Infertility, 843
Intraductal papilloma, 844
Leiomyoma (myoma, uterine fibroid), 831
Lobular carcinoma in situ (LCIS), 859
Lobular involution, 849
Mammographic density (MD), 852
Menopausal hormone therapy (MHT), 850
Mild hyperplasia of the usual type, 844
Mucopurulent cervicitis (MPC), 826
Nonpuerperal hyperprolactinemia, 843
Ovarian torsion, 830
Papillary apocrine change, 844
Pelvic inflammatory disease (PID), 824
Pelvic organ prolapse (POP), 828
Pessary, 828
Polycystic ovary syndrome (PCOS), 822
Precocious puberty, 818
Pregnancy-associated breast cancer (PABC), 849
Premenstrual dysphoric disorder (PMDD), 822
Premenstrual syndrome (PMS), 822
Primary amenorrhea, 819
Primary dysmenorrhea, 819
Prolactin-inhibiting factor (PIF), 843
Puberty, 817
Radial scar (RS), 844
Rectocele, 828
Salpingitis, 825
Sclerosing adenosis, 844
Secondary amenorrhea, 819
Secondary dysmenorrhea, 819
Sexual dysfunction, 842
Simple fibroadenoma, 845
Terminal duct lobular unit (TDLU), 849
Thelarche, 818
Tumour dormancy, 856
Usual ductal hyperplasia (UDH), 844
Uterine prolapse, 828
Vaginismus, 842
Vaginitis, 826
Vaginosis, 826
Vascular mimicry, 857
Vulvodyniavestibulitis (VV), 827
Xenoestrogen, 855

REFERENCES

1. Greil, A. L., Shreffler, K. M., Schmidt, L., et al. (2011). Variation in distress among women with infertility: Evidence from a population-based sample. *Human Reproduction*, *26*(8), 2101–2112. doi:10.1093/humrep/der148.
2. Geffner, M. E. (2011). Androgen insensitivity syndrome (AIS). In S. Yazdano, S. A. McGhee, & R. Stiehm (Eds.), *Chronic complex diseases of childhood: A practical guide for clinicians*. Boca Raton, FL: Universal Publishers.
3. Hughes, I. A., Davies, J. D., Bunch, T. I., et al. (2012). Androgen insensitivity syndrome. *Lancet*, *380*(9851), 1419–1428. doi:10.1016/S0140-6736(12)60071-3.
4. Eisermann, K., Wang, D., Jing, Y., et al. (2013). Androgen receptor gene mutation, rearrangement, polymorphism. *Translational Andrology and Urology*, *2*(3), 137–147. doi:10.3978/j.issn.2223-4683.2013.09.15.
5. Galani, A., Kitsiou-Tzeli, S., Sofokleous, C., et al. (2008). Androgen insensitivity syndrome: Clinical features and molecular defects. *Hormones (Athens, Greece)*, *7*(3), 217–299.
6. Reichman, D. E., & Laufer, M. R. (2010). Congenital uterine anomalies affecting reproduction. *Best Practice and Research. Clinical Obstetrics and Gynaecology*, *24*(2), 193–208. doi:10.1016/j.bpobgyn.2009.09.006.
7. Chan, Y. Y., Jayaprakasan, K., Zamora, J., et al. (2011). The prevalence of congenital uterine anomalies in unselected and high-risk populations: A systematic review. *Human Reproduction Update*, *17*(6), 761–771. doi:10.1093/humupd/dmr028.
8. Lomniczi, A., Loche, A., Castellano, J. M., et al. (2013). Epigenetic control of female puberty. *Nature Neuroscience*, *16*(3), 281–289. doi:10.1038/nn.3319.
9. Rzeczkowska, P. A., Hou, H., Wilson, M. D., et al. (2014). Epigenetics: A new player in the regulation of mammalian puberty. *Neuroendocrinology*, *99*(3–4), 139–155. doi:10.1159/000362559.
10. Al-Sahab, B., Ardern, C. I., Mazen, J. H., et al. (2010). Age at menarche in Canada: Results from the National Longitudinal Survey of Children & Youth. *BMC Public Health*, *10*, 736.
11. Farooqi, I. S., & O'Rahilly, S. (2014). 20 years of leptin: Human disorders of leptin action. *Journal of Endocrinology*, *223*(1), T63–T70. doi:10.1530/JOE-14-0480.
12. Addo, O. Y., Miller, B. S., Lee, P. A., et al. (2014). Age at hormonal onset of puberty based on luteinizing hormone, inhibin B, and body composition in preadolescent US girls. *Pediatric Research*, *76*(6), 564–570. doi:10.1038/pr.2014.131.
13. Hagen, C. P., Sørensen, K., Aksglaede, L., et al. (2014). Pubertal onset in girls is strongly influenced by genetic variation affecting FSH action. *Scientific Reports*, *4*, 6412. doi:10.1038/srep06412.
14. Neeley, E. K., & Crossen, S. S. (2014). Precocious puberty. *Current Opinion in Obstetrics and Gynecology*, *26*(5), 332–338. doi:10.1097/GCO.0000000000000099.
15. Jospe, N. (2005). Disorders of pubertal development. In L. M. Osborn, T. G. DeWitt, L. R. First, et al. (Eds.), *Pediatrics*. Philadelphia: Mosby.
16. Whittemore, B. J., Smaldone, A., & Steiner, R. D. (2012). Endocrine and metabolic disorders. In C. E. Burns, A. M. Dunn, M. A. Brady, et al. (Eds.), *Pediatric primary care*. St. Louis: Saunders.
17. Foster, D. L., Jackson, L. M., & Padmanabhan, V. (2006). Programming of GnRH feedback controls timing puberty and adult reproductive activity. *Molecular and Cellular Endocrinology*, *254–255*, 109–119. doi:10.1016/j.mce.2006.04.004.
18. Baker, M. E., & Hardiman, G. (2014). Transcriptional analysis of endocrine disruption using zebrafish and massively parallel sequencing. *Journal of Molecular Endocrinology*, *52*(3), R241–R256. doi:10.1530/JME-13-0219.
19. Toppari, J., & Juul, A. (2010). Trends in puberty timing in humans and environmental modifiers. *Molecular and Cellular Endocrinology*, *324*(1–2), 39–44. doi:10.1016/j.mce.2010.03.011.
20. Fedorowicz, Z., Nasser, M., Jagannath, V. A., et al. (2012). Beta2-adrenoceptor agonists for dysmenorrhoea. *Cochrane Database of Systematic Reviews*, (5), CD008585, doi:10.1002/14651858.CD008585.pub2.
21. Rapkin, A., & Nathan, L. (2012). Pelvic pain and dysmenorrhea. In J. Berek (Ed.), *Berek & Novak's gynecology*. Philadelphia: Lippincott Williams & Wilkins.
22. Khan, K. S., Champaneria, R., & Latthe, P. M. (2012). How effective are non-drug, non-surgical treatments for primary dysmenorrhoea? *BMJ (Clinical Research Ed.)*, *344*, e3011. doi:10.1136/bmj.e3011.
23. Baker, V. L., Schillings, W. J., & McClamrock, H. D. (2012). Amenorrhea. In J. Berek (Ed.), *Berek & Novak's gynecology*. Philadelphia: Lippincott Williams & Wilkins.
24. Pitkin, J. (2007). Dysfunctional uterine bleeding. *BMJ (Clinical Research Ed.)*, *334*(7603), 1110–1111. doi:10.1136/bmj.39203.399502.BE.
25. Munro, M. G. (2011). FIGO classification system (PALM-COEIN) for causes of abnormal uterine bleeding in nongravid women of reproductive age. *International Journal of Gynaecology and Obstetrics*, *113*(1), 3–13. doi:10.1016/j.ijgo.2010.11.011.
26. Azziz, R., Carmina, E., Dewally, D., et al. (2009). The Androgen Excess and PCOS Society criteria for the polycystic ovary syndrome: The complete task force reports. *Fertility and Sterility*, *91*(2), 456–488. doi:10.1016/j.fertnstert.2008.06.035.
27. Diamanti-Kandarakis, E. (2008). Polycystic ovarian syndrome: Pathophysiology, molecular aspects and clinical implications. *Expert Reviews in Molecular Medicine*, *10*(2), e3. doi:10.1017/S1462399408000598.
28. Hartlage, S., Freels, S., Gotman, N., et al. (2012). Criteria for premenstrual dysphoric disorder: Secondary analyses of relevant data sets. *Archives of General Psychiatry*, *69*(3), 300. doi:10.1001/archgenpsychiatry.2011.1368.
29. Gordon, J. L., Girdler, S. S., Meltzer-Brody, S. E., et al. (2015). Ovarian hormone fluctuation, neurosteroids, and HPA axis dysregulation in perimenopausal depression: A novel heuristic model. *American Journal of Psychiatry*, *172*(3), 227–236. doi:10.1176/appi.ajp.2014.14070918.
30. Berone-Johnson, E. R., Ronnenberg, A. G., Houghton, S. C., et al. (2014). Association of inflammation markers with menstrual symptom severity and premenstrual syndrome in young women. *Human Reproduction*, *29*(9), 1987–1994. doi:10.1093/humrep/deu170.
31. Jarvis, C. I., Lynch, A. M., & Morin, A. K. (2008). Management strategies for premenstrual syndrome/premenstrual dysphoric disorder. *Annals of Pharmacotherapy*, *42*(7), 967–978. doi:10.1345/aph.1K673.
32. Majorbanks, J., Brown, J., O'Brien, P. M., et al. (2013). Selective serotonin reuptake inhibitors for premenstrual syndrome. *Cochrane Database of Systematic Reviews*, (6), CD001396, doi:10.1002/14651858.CD001396.pub3.
33. Centers for Disease Control and Prevention (2015). *Sexually transmitted diseases (STDs)*. Atlanta: Author.
34. Kumar, V., Abbas, A. K., & Aster, J. C. (Eds.), (2015). *Robbins and Cotran pathologic basis of disease* (9th ed.). Philadelphia: Saunders.
35. Wiesenfeld, H. C., Hillier, S. L., Meyn, L. A., et al. (2012). Subclinical pelvic inflammatory disease and infertility. *Obstetrics and Gynecology*, *120*(1), 37–43. doi:10.1097/AOG.0b013e31825a6bc9.
36. Bender, N., Herrmann, B., Anderson, B., et al. (2011). Chlamydia infection, pelvic inflammatory disease, ectopic pregnancy and infertility: Cross-national study. *Sexually Transmitted Infections*, *87*(7), 601–608. doi:10.1136/sextrans-2011-050205.
37. Nyirjesy, P., Robinson, J., Mathew, L., et al. (2011). Alternative therapies in women with chronic

vaginitis. *Obstetrics and Gynecology, 117*(4), 856. doi:10.1097/AOG.0b013e31820b07d5.
38. Ray, A., George, A. T., & Swaminathan, N. (2011). Interventions for prevention and treatment of vulvovaginal candidiasis in women with HIV infection. *Cochrane Database of Systematic Reviews*, (8), CD008739, doi:10.1002/14651858.CD008739.pub2.
39. De Seta, F., Parazzinin, F., De Leo, R., et al. (2014). *Lactobacillus plantarum P17630* for preventing *Candida* vaginitis recurrence: A retrospective comparative study. *European Journal of Obstetrics, Gynecology, and Reproductive Biology, 182*, 136–139. doi:10.1016/j.ejogrb.2014.09.018.
40. Centers for Disease Control and Prevention (2014). *Diseases characterized by urethritis and cervicitis, STD sexually transmitted disease treatment guidelines*. Atlanta: Author.
41. Centers for Disease Control and Prevention (2014). *STD treatment guidelines*. Atlanta: Author.
42. Shah, M., & Hoffstetter, S. (2014). Vulvodynia. *Obstetrics and Gynecology Clinics of North America, 41*(3), 453–464. doi:10.1016/j.ogc.2014.05.005.
43. Wesselmann, U., Bonham, A., & Foster, D. (2014). Vulvodynia: Current state of the biological science. *Pain, 155*, 1696–1701. doi:10.1016/j.pain.2014.05.010.
44. Sadownik, L. A. (2014). Etiology, diagnosis, and clinical management of vulvodynia. *International Journal of Women's Health, 6*, 437–449. doi:10.2147/IJWH.S37660.
45. Cartwright, R., Kirby, A. C., Tikkinen, K. A., et al. (2014). Systematic review and meta-analysis of genetic association studies of urinary symptoms and prolapse in women. *American Journal of Obstetrics and Gynecology, 212*(2), 199, e1–e14. doi:10.1016/j.ajog.2014.08.005.
46. Hoffman, B. L., et al. (2008). Pelvic mass. In B. L. Hoffman, J. O. Schorge, & K. D. Bradshaw (Eds.), *Williams gynecology* (pp. 187–224). New York: McGraw-Hill.
47. Mäkinen, N., Mehine, M., Tolvanen, J., et al. (2011). MED12, the mediator complex subunit 12 gene, is mutated at high frequency in uterine leiomyomas. *Science, 334*(6053), 252–255. doi:10.1126/science.1208930.
48. Gupta, J. K., Sinha, A., Lumsden, M. A., et al. (2014). Uterine artery embolization for symptomatic uterine fibroids. *Cochrane Database of Systematic Reviews*, (12), CD005073, doi:10.1002/14651858.
49. Forte, A., Cipollaro, M., & Galderisi, U. (2014). Genetic, epigenetic and stem cell alterations in endometriosis: New insights and potential therapeutic perspectives. *Clinical Science, 126*(2), 123–138. doi:10.1042/CS20130099.
50. Giudice, L. C. (2010). Endometriosis. *New England Journal of Medicine, 362*(25), 2389–2398. doi:10.1056/NEJMcp1000274.
51. Canadian Cancer Society, & Government of Canada (2017). *Canadian cancer statistics 2017*. Toronto: Author. Retrieved from http://www.cancer.ca/~/media/cancer.ca/CW/publications/Canadian%20Cancer%20Statistics/Canadian-Cancer-Statistics-2017-EN.pdf.
52. Dickinson, J. A., Stankiewicz, A., Popadiuk, C., et al. (2012). Reduced cervical cancer incidence and mortality in Canada: National data from 1932 to 2006. *BMC Public Health, 12*, 992. doi:10.1186/1471-2458-12-992.
53. Ferlay, J., Soerjomataram, I., Ervik, M., et al. (2013). *GLOBOCAN 2012: Estimated cancer incidence, mortality and prevalence worldwide in 2012 v1.0: IARC CancerBase No. 11*. Lyon, France: International Agency for Research on Cancer. Retrieved from http://globocan.iarc.fr.
54. Centers for Disease Control and Prevention (2014). *Cervical cancer statistics*. Atlanta: Author.
55. National Cancer Institute. (2015). *PDQ® cervical cancer screening*. Retrieved from http://cancer.gov/cancertopics/pdq/screening/cervical/HealthProfessional.
56. National Cancer Institute. (2015). *PDQ® cervical cancer treatment*. Retrieved from http://cancer.gov/cancertopics/pdq/treatment/cervical/HealthProfessional.
57. Blomberg, M., Friis, S., Munk, C., et al. (2012). Genital warts and risk of cancer: A Danish study of nearly 50 000 patients with genital warts. *Journal of Infectious Diseases, 205*(10), 1544–1553. doi:10.1093/infdis/jis228.
58. Cancer Research UK (2013). *Risks and causes of vaginal cancer*. London: Author.
59. National Cancer Institute. (2015). *PDQ® vaginal cancer treatment*. Retrieved from http://cancer.gov/cancertopics/pdq/treatment/vaginal/HealthProfessional.
60. National Cancer Institute. (2015). *Vulvar cancer treatment (PDQ®)—Patient version*. Retrieved from http://cancer.gov/cancertopics/pdq/treatment/vulvar/Patient.
61. Canadian Cancer Society. (2017). *Vulvar cancer statistics*. Retrieved from http://www.cancer.ca/en/cancer-information/cancer-type/vulvar/statistics/?region=on.
62. Cancer Research UK (2015). *Vulval cancer risk factors*. London: Author.
63. National Cancer Institute. (2015). *Vulvar cancer treatment (PDQ®)—Health professional version*. Retrieved from http://cancer.gov/cancertopics/pdq/treatment/vulvar/HealthProfessional.
64. Canadian Cancer Society. (2017). *Survival statistics for uterine cancer*. Retrieved from http://www.cancer.ca/en/cancer-information/cancer-type/uterine/prognosis-and-survival/survival-statistics/?region=on.
65. Ferlay, J., Soerjomataram, I., Dikshit, R., et al. (2015). Cancer incidence and mortality worldwide: Sources, methods and major patterns in GLOBOCAN 2012. *International Journal of Cancer. Journal International du Cancer, 136*(5), E359–E386.
66. World Cancer Research Fund/American Institute for Cancer Research. (2013). *Continuous update project report. Food, nutrition, physical activity, and the prevention of endometrial cancer*. Retrieved from http://www.dietandcancerreport.org.
67. Campbell, P. T., Newton, C. C., Patel, A. V., et al. (2012). Diabetes and cause-specific mortality in a prospective cohort of one million U.S. adults. *Diabetes Care, 35*(9), 1835–1844. doi:10.2337/dc12-0002.
68. Chen, H.-F., Liu, M. D., Chen, P., et al. (2013). Risks of breast and endometrial cancer in women with diabetes: A population-based cohort study. *PLoS ONE, 8*(6), e67420. doi:10.1371/journal.pone.0067420.
69. Joung, K. H., Jeong, J. W., & Ku, B. J. (2015). The association between type 2 diabetes mellitus and women cancer: The epidemiological evidences and putative mechanisms. *BioMed Research International, 2015*, 920610. doi:10.1155/2015/920618.
70. Gottschau, M., Kjaer, S. K., Jensen, A., et al. (2015). Risk of cancer among women with polycystic ovary syndrome: A Danish cohort study. *Gynecologic Oncology, 136*(1), 99–103. doi:10.1016/j.ygyno.2014.11.012.
71. Yoneyama, K., Ishibashi, O., Kawase, R., et al. (2015). miR-200a, miR-200b and miR-429 are onco-miRs that target the PTEN gene in endometrioid endometrial carcinoma. *Anticancer Research, 35*(3), 1401–1410.
72. Jaakkola, S., Lyytinen, H. K., Dyba, T., et al. (2011). Endometrial cancer associated with various forms of postmenopausal hormone therapy: A case control study. *International Journal of Cancer. Journal International du Cancer, 128*(7), 1644–1651. doi:10.1002/ijc.25762.
73. SGO Clinical Practice Endometrial Cancer Working Group, Burke, W. M., Orr, J., et al. (2014). Endometrial cancer: A review and current management strategies: Part II. *Gynecologic Oncology, 134*(2), 393–402. doi:10.1016/j.ygyno.2014.06.003.
74. Allen, N. E., Tsilidis, K. K., Key, T. J., et al. (2010). Menopausal hormone therapy and risk of endometrial carcinoma among postmenopausal women in the European Prospective Investigation into cancer and nutrition. *American Journal of Epidemiology, 172*(12), 1394–1403. doi:10.1093/aje/kwq300.
75. Yurgelun, M. B., Mercado, R., Rosenblatt, M., et al. (2012). Impact of genetic testing on endometrial cancer risk-reducing practices in women at risk for Lynch syndrome. *Gynecologic Oncology, 127*(3), 544–551. doi:10.1016/j.ygyno.2012.08.031.
76. Riboli, E., Hunt, K. J., Silmani, N., et al. (2002). European Prospective Investigation into Cancer and Nutrition (EPIC): Study populations and data collection. *Public Health Nutrition, 5*(6B), 1113–1124. doi:10.1079/PHN2002394.
77. Merritt, M. A., Tzoulaki, I., Tworoger, S. S., et al. (2015). Investigation of dietary factors and endometrial cancer risk using a nutrient-wide association study approach in the EPIC and Nurses' Health Study (NHS) and NHSII. *Cancer Epidemiology, Biomarkers and Prevention, 24*(2), 466–471. doi:10.1158/1055-9965.EPI-14-0970.
78. Diep, C., Daniel, A. R., Mauro, L. J., et al. (2015). Progesterone action in breast, uterine, and ovarian cancers. *Journal of Molecular Endocrinology, 54*(2), R31–R53. doi:10.1530/JME-14-0252.
79. Banno, K., Iida, M., Yanokura, M., et al. (2015). Drug repositioning for gynecologic tumors: A new therapeutic strategy for cancer. *Scientific World Journal, 2015*, 341362. doi:10.1155/2015/341362.
80. Stine, J. E., & Bae-Jump, V. (2014). Metformin and gynecologic cancers. *Obstetrical and Gynecological Survey, 69*(8), 477–489. doi:10.1097/OGX.0000000000000092.
81. Desai, A., Xu, J., Aysola, K., et al. (2014). Epithelial ovarian cancer: An overview. *World Translational Medicine, 3*(1), 1–8. doi:10.5528/wjtm.v3.i1.1.
82. Romero, I., & Bast, R. C. (2012). Minireview: Human ovarian cancer biology, current management, and paths to personalizing therapy. *Endocrinology, 153*(4), 1593–1602. doi:10.1210/en.2011-2123.
83. Nik, N. N., Wang, R., Shih, I., et al. (2014). Origin and pathogenesis of pelvic (ovarian, tubal, and primary peritoneal) serous carcinoma. *Annual Review of Pathology, 9*, 27–45. doi:10.1146/annurev-pathol-020712-163949.
84. National Cancer Institute. (2015). *PDQ® ovarian, fallopian tube, and primary peritoneal cancer screening*. Retrieved from http://www.cancer.gov/types/ovarian/hp/ovarian-screening-pdq.
85. U.S. Preventive Services Task Force. (2012). Screening for ovarian cancer: U.S. Preventive Services Task Force reaffirmation recommendation statement. *Annals of Internal Medicine, 157*(12), 900–904. doi:10.7326/0003-4819-157-11-201212040-00539.
86. Giede, K. C., Kieser, K., Dodge, J., et al. (2005). Who should operate on patients with ovarian cancer? An evidence-based review. *Gynecologic Oncology, 99*(2), 447–461. doi:10.1016/j.ygyno.2005.07.008.
87. Mercado, C., Zingmond, D., Karlan, B. Y., et al. (2010). Quality of care in advanced ovarian cancer: The importance of provider specialty. *Gynecologic Oncology, 117*(1), 18–22. doi:10.1016/j.ygyno.2009.12.033.
88. American College of Obstetricians and Gynecologists (2011). *Female sexual dysfunction*. Washington, DC: Author.
89. Hatzichristou, D., Rosen, R. C., Derogatis, L. R., et al. (2010). Recommendations for the clinical evaluation of men and women with sexual dysfunction. *Journal of Sexual Medicine, 7*(1 Pt. 2), 337–348. doi:10.1111/j.1743-6109.2009.01619.x.
90. Lewis, R. W., Fugl-Meyer, K. S., Corona, G., et al. (2010). Definitions/epidemiology/risk factors for sexual dysfunction. *Journal of Sexual Medicine, 7*(4 Pt. 2), 1598–1607. doi:10.1111/j.1743-6109.2010.01778.x.
91. Kingsberg, S. A., & Woodard, T. (2015). Female sexual dysfunction: Focus on low desire. *Obstetrics and Gynecology, 125*(2), 477–486. doi:10.1097/AOG.0000000000000620.
92. Government of Canada. (2013). *Fertility*. Retrieved from http://healthycanadians.gc.ca/

healthy-living-vie-saine/pregnancy-grossesse/fertility-fertilite/fert-eng.php.
93. Timeva, T., Shterev, A., & Kyurkchiev, S. (2014). Recurrent implantation failure: The role of the endometrium. *Journal of Reproduction & Infertility, 15*(4), 173–183.
94. Marshburn, P. B. (2015). Counseling and diagnostic evaluation for the infertile couple. *Obstetrics and Gynecology Clinics of North America, 42*(1), 1–14. doi:10.1016/j.ogc.2014.10.001.
95. Farquhar, C., Rishworth, J. R., Brown, J., et al. (2014). Assisted reproductive technology: An overview of Cochrane reviews. *Cochrane Database of Systematic Reviews,* (12), CD010537, doi:10.1002/14651858.CD010537.pub3.
96. Sabel, M. S. (2015). *Overview of benign breast disease.* Retrieved from http://www.uptodate.com.
97. Lester, S. (2015). The breast. In V. Kumar, A. K. Abbas, & J. C. Aster (Eds.), *Robbins and Cotran pathologic basis of disease* (9th ed.). Philadelphia: Saunders.
98. Visscher, D. W., Nassar, A., Degnim, A. C., et al. (2014). Sclerosing adenosis and risk of breast cancer. *Breast Cancer Research and Treatment, 144*(1), 205–212. doi:10.1007/s10549-014-2862-5.
99. Nasser, A., Hoskin, T. L., Stallings-Mann, M. L., et al. (2015). Ki-67 expression in sclerosing adenosis and adjacent normal breast terminal ductal lobular units: A nested case-control study from the Mayo Benign Breast Disease Cohort. *Breast Cancer Research and Treatment, 151*(1), 89–97. doi:10.1007/s10549-015-3370-y.
100. Hartmann, L. C., Degnim, A. C., Santen, R. J., et al. (2015). Atypical hyperplasia of the breast—Risk assessment and management options. *New England Journal of Medicine, 372*(1), 78–89. doi:10.1056/NEJMsr1407164.
101. Dupont, W. D., & Page, D. L. (1985). Risk factors for breast cancer in women with proliferative breast disease. *New England Journal of Medicine, 312*(3), 146–151. doi:10.1056/NEJM198501173120303.
102. Hartmann, L. C., Sellers, T. A., Frost, M. H., et al. (2005). Benign breast disease and the risk of breast cancer. *New England Journal of Medicine, 353*(3), 229–237.
103. Hartmann, L. C., Radisky, D. C., Frost, M. H., et al. (2014). Understanding the premalignant potential of atypical hyperplasia through its natural history: A longitudinal cohort study. *Cancer Prevention Research, 7*(2), 211–217. doi:10.1158/1940-6207.CAPR-13-0222.
104. Page, D. L., Dupont, W. D., Rogers, L. W., et al. (1985). Atypical hyperplastic lesions of the female breast. A long-term follow-up study. *Cancer, 55*(11), 2698–2708.
105. Sanders, M., Schuyler, P. A., Simpson, J. F., et al. (2015). Continued observation of the natural history of low-grade ductal carcinoma in situ reaffirms proclivity for local recurrence even after more than 30 years of follow-up. *Modern Pathology, 28*(5), 662–669. doi:10.1038/modpathol.2014.141.
106. Page, D. L., Schuyler, P. A., Dupont, W. D., et al. (2003). Atypical lobular hyperplasia as a unilateral predictor of breast cancer risk: A retrospective cohort study. *Lancet, 361*(9352), 125–129. doi:10.1016/S0140-6736(03)12230-1. [Erratum: *Lancet, 361*(9373), 1994.].
107. Elmore, J. G., Longton, G. M., Carney, P. A., et al. (2015). Diagnostic concordance among pathologists interpreting breast biopsy specimens. *JAMA: The Journal of the American Medical Association, 313*(11), 1122–1132. doi:10.1001/jama.2015.1405.
108. Hollowell, J. G., Staehling, N. W., Hannon, W. H., et al. (1998). Iodine nutrition in the United States. Trends and public health implications: Iodine excretion data from National Health and Nutrition Examination Surveys I and II (1971–1974 and 1988–1994). *Journal of Clinical Endocrinology and Metabolism, 83*(10), 3401–3408. doi:10.1210/jcem.83.10.5168.
109. Li, Y., Andrews, L. G., & Tollefsbol, T. O. (2009). Genistein depletes telomerase activity through cross-talk between genetic and epigenetic mechanism. *International Journal of Cancer. Journal International du Cancer, 125*(2), 286–296. doi:10.1002/ijc.24398.
110. Islam, M. A., Bekele, R., Vanden Berg, J. H., et al. (2015). Deconjugation of soy isoflavone glucuronides needed for estrogenic activity. *Toxicology In Vitro, 29*(4), 706–715. doi:10.1016/j.tiv.2015.01.013.
111. North American Menopause Society. (2011). The role of soy isoflavones in menopausal health: Report of The North American Menopause Society/Wulf H. Utian Translational Science Symposium in Chicago, IL. *Menopause (New York, N.Y.), 18*(7), 732–753. doi:10.1097/gme.0b013e31821fc8e0.
112. Iodine monograph. (2010). *Alternative Medicine Review, 15*(3), 273–278.
113. Canadian Cancer Society. (2017). *Breast cancer in Canada, 2016.* Retrieved from http://www.cbcf.org/ontario/AboutBreastCancerMain/FactsStats/Pages/Breast-Cancer-Canada.aspx.
114. Sternlicht, M. D., Kouros-Mehr, H., Lu, P., et al. (2006). Hormonal and local control of mammary branching morphogenesis. *Differentiation; Research in Biological Diversity, 74*(7), 365–381. doi:10.1111/j.1432-0436.2006.00105.x.
115. Lyons, T. R., O'Brien, J., Borges, V. F., et al. (2011). Postpartum mammary gland involution drives progression of ductal carcinoma in situ through collagen and COX-2. *Nature Medicine, 17*(9), 1109–1115. doi:10.1038/nm.2416.
116. Lyons, T. R., Schedin, P. J., & Borges, V. F. (2009). Pregnancy and breast cancer: When they collide. *Journal of Mammary Gland Biology and Neoplasia, 14*(2), 87–98. doi:10.1007/s10911-009-9119-7.
117. Albrektsen, G., Heuch, I., & Kvale, G. (1995). The short-term and long-term effect of pregnancy on breast cancer risk: A prospective study of 802,457 parous Norwegian women. *British Journal of Cancer, 72*(2), 480–484.
118. Callihan, E. B., Gao, D., Jindal, S., et al. (2013). Postpartum diagnosis demonstrates a high risk for metastasis and merits an expanded definition of pregnancy-associated breast cancer. *Breast Cancer Research and Treatment, 138*(2), 549–559. doi:10.1007/s10549-013-2437-x.
119. Johansson, A. L., Andersson, T. M., Hsieh, C. C., et al. (2011). Increased mortality in women with breast cancer detected during pregnancy and different periods postpartum. *Cancer Epidemiology, Biomarkers and Prevention, 20*(9), 1865–1872. doi:10.1158/1055-9965.EPI-11-0515.
120. Schedin, P., O'Brien, J., Rudolph, M., et al. (2007). Microenvironment of the involuting mammary gland mediates mammary cancer progression. *Journal of Mammary Gland Biology and Neoplasia, 12*(1), 71–82. doi:10.1007/s10911-007-9039-3.
121. Martinson, H. A., Jindal, S., Durand-Rougely, C., et al. (2015). Wound healing-like immune program facilitates postpartum mammary gland involution and tumor progression. *International Journal of Cancer. Journal International du Cancer, 136*(8), 1803–1813. doi:10.1002/ijc.29181.
122. Barton, M., Santucci-Pereira, J., & Russo, J. (2014). Molecular pathways involved in pregnancy-induced prevention against breast cancer. *Frontiers in Endocrinology (Lausanne), 5,* 213. doi:10.3389/fendo.2014.00213.
123. Khodr, Z. G., Sherman, M. E., Pfeiffer, R. M., et al. (2014). Circulating sex hormones and terminal duct lobular unit involution of the normal breast cancer. *Cancer Epidemiology and Biomarkers Prevention, 23*(12), 2765–2773. doi:10.1158/1055-9965.EPI-14-0667.
124. Milanese, T. R., Hartmann, L. C., Sellers, T. A., et al. (2006). Age-related lobular involution and risk of breast cancer. *Journal of the National Cancer Institute, 98*(2), 1600–1607. doi:10.1093/jnci/djj439.
125. Jindal, S., Gao, D., Bell, P., et al. (2014). Postpartum breast involution reveals regression of secretory lobules mediated by tissue-remodeling. *Breast Cancer Research : BCR, 16*(2), R31. doi:10.1186/bcr3633.
126. Vorherr, H. (Ed.), (1974). *The breast: Morphology, physiology, and lactation.* New York: Academic Press.
127. Geschickter, C. D. (1945). *Diseases of the breast* (2nd ed.). Philadelphia: Lippincott.
128. Trichopoulos, D., Hsieh, C. C., MacMahon, B., et al. (1983). Age at any birth and breast cancer risk. *International Journal of Cancer. Journal International du Cancer, 31*(6), 701–704.
129. Henson, D. E., Tarone, R. E., & Nsouli, H. (2006). Lobular involution: The physiological prevention of breast cancer. *Journal of the National Cancer Institute, 98*(22), 1589–1590. doi:10.1093/jnci/djj454.
130. Zaragozá, R., Garcia-Trevijano, E. R., Lluch, A., et al. (2015). Involvement of different networks in mammary gland involution after the pregnancy/lactation cycle: Implications in breast cancer. *IUBMB Life, 67*(4), 227–238. doi:10.1002/iub.1365.
131. Schedin, P. (2006). Pregnancy-associated breast cancer and metastasis. *Nature Reviews. Cancer, 6*(4), 281–291. doi:10.1038/nrc1839.
132. Ghosh, K., Vachon, C. M., Pankratz, V. S., et al. (2010). Independent association of lobular involution and mammographic breast density with breast cancer risk. *Journal of the National Cancer Institute, 102*(22), 1716–1723. doi:10.1093/jnci/djq414.
133. Russo, J., & Russo, I. (2004). *Molecular basis of breast cancer: Prevention and treatment.* Berlin: Springer-Verlag.
134. Kaaks, R., Rinaldi, S., Key, T. J., et al. (2005). Postmenopausal serum androgens, oestrogens, and breast cancer risk: The European prospective investigation into cancer and nutrition. *Endocrine-Related Cancer, 12*(4), 1017–1082. doi:10.1677/erc.1.01038.
135. Mehta, J., Asthana, S., Mandal, C. C., et al. (2015). A molecular analysis provides novel insights into androgen receptor signaling in breast cancer. *PLoS ONE, 10*(3), e0120622. doi:10.1371/journal.pone.0120622.
136. Kotsopoulos, J., Shafrir, A. L., Rice, M., et al. (2015). The relationship between bilateral oophorectomy and plasma hormone levels in postmenopausal women. *Hormones & Cancer, 6*(1), 54–63. doi:10.1007/s12672-014-0209-7.
137. Tworoger, S. S., Zhang, X., Eliassen, A. H., et al. (2014). Inclusion of endogenous hormone levels in risk prediction models of postmenopausal breast cancer. *Journal of Clinical Oncology, 32*(28), 3111–3117. doi:10.1200/JCO.2014.56.1068.
138. Hankinson, S. E., & Eliassen, H. (2007). Endogenous estrogen, testosterone, and progesterone levels in relation to breast cancer risk. *Journal of Steroid Biochemistry and Molecular Biology, 106*(1–5), 24–30. doi:10.1016/j.jsbmb.2007.05.012.
139. Key, T., Appleby, P., Barnes, I., et al. (2002). Endogenous sex hormones and breast cancer in postmenopausal women; reanalysis of nine prospective studies. *Journal of the National Cancer Institute, 94*(8), 606–616.
140. Stanczyk, F. Z., Mathews, B. W., & Sherman, M. E. (2015). Relationships of sex steroid hormone levels in benign and cancerous breast tissue and blood: A critical appraisal of current science. *Steroids, 99*(Pt. A), 91–102. doi:10.1016/j.steroids.2014.12.011.
141. World Health Organization (2015). *A review of human carcinogens. B. Biological agents IARC monographs on the evaluation of carcinogenic risks to humans, IARC Monographs* (Vol 100(B)). Geneva, Switzerland: Author.
142. Grant, M. D., Marbella, A., Wang, A. T., et al. (2015). *Menopausal symptoms: Comparative effectiveness of therapies.* Rockville, MD: Agency for Healthcare Research and Quality.
143. Christopoulos, P. F., Msaouei, P., & Koutsilieris, M. (2015). The role of insulin-like growth factor-1 system in breast cancer. *Molecular Cancer, 14*(1), 43. doi:10.1186/s12943-015-0291-7.
144. Ahmadieh, H., & Azar, S. T. (2013). Type 2 diabetes oral diabetic medications, insulin therapy, and overall breast cancer risk. *ISRN Endocrinology, 2013,* 181240. doi:10.1155/2013/181240.
145. Suissa, S., Azoulay, L., Dell'Aniello, S., et al. (2011) Long-term effects of insulin glargine on the risk of

breast cancer. *Diabetologia, 54*(9), 2254–2262. doi:10.1007/s00125-011-2190-9.
146. Wu, J., Dauchy, R. T., Tirrell, P. C., et al. (2011). Light at night activates IGF-1R/PDK1 signaling and accelerates tumor growth in human breast cancer xenografts. *Cancer Research, 71*(7), 2622–2631. doi:10.1158/0008-5472.CAN-10-3837.
147. Akerstedt, T., Knutsson, A., Narusyte, J., et al. (2015). Night work and breast cancer in women: A Swedish cohort study. *BMJ (Clinical Research Ed.), 5*(4), e008127. doi:10.1136/bmjopen-2015-008127.
148. Wang, X. S., Armstrong, M. E., Cairns, B. J., et al. (2011). Shift work and chronic disease: The epidemiological evidence. *Occupational Medicine (Oxford, England), 61*(2), 78–89. doi:10.1093/occmed/kqr001.
149. Renehen, A. G., & Brennan, B. M. (2008). Acromegaly, growth hormone and cancer risk. *Best Practice and Research. Clinical Endocrinology and Metabolism, 22*(4), 639–657. doi:10.1016/j.beem.2008.08.011.
150. Schernhammer, E. S., Holly, J. J., Hunter, D. J., et al. (2006). Insulin-like growth factor-I, its binding protein (IGFBP-1 and IBFBP-3), and growth hormone and breast cancer risk in The Nurses' Health Study II. *Endocrine-Related Cancer, 13*, 583–592. doi:10.1677/erc.1.01149.
151. Tworoger, S. S., Eliassen, H., Sluss, P., et al. (2007). A prospective study of plasma prolactin concentrations and risk of premenopausal and postmenopausal breast cancer. *Journal of Clinical Oncology : Official Journal of the American Society of Clinical Oncology, 25*(12), 1482–1488. doi:10.1200/JCO.2006.07.6356.
152. Tikk, K., Sookthai, D., Fortner, R. T., et al. (2015). Circulating prolactin and in situ breast cancer risk in the European EPIC cohort: A case-control study. *Breast Cancer Research : BCR, 17*(1), 49. doi:10.1186/s13058-015-0563-6.
153. Grosse, Y., Baan, R., Straif, K., et al. (2009). A review of human carcinogens—Part A: Pharmaceuticals. *Lancet Oncology, 10*(1), 13–14.
154. Boyd, N. F., Rommens, J. M., Vogt, K., et al. (2005). Mammographic breast density as an intermediate phenotype for breast cancer. *Lancet Oncology, 6*(10), 798–808. doi:10.1016/S1470-2045(05)70390-9.
155. Vachon, C. M., van Gils, C. H., Sellers, T. A., et al. (2007). Mammographic density, breast cancer risk and risk prediction breast. *Cancer Research, 9*(6), 217. doi:10.1186/bcr1829.
156. Sun, W. Y., Yun, H. Y., Song, Y. J., et al. (2015). Insulin-like growth factor 1 receptor expression in breast cancer tissue and mammographic density. *Molecular and Clinical Oncology, 3*(3), 572–580. doi:10.3892/mco.2015.497.
157. Boyd, N. F., Guo, H., Martin, L. J., et al. (2007). Mammographic density and the risk and detection of breast cancer. *New England Journal of Medicine, 56*(3), 227–236. doi:10.1056/NEJMoa062790.
158. Pettersson, A., Graff, R. E., Ursin, G., et al. (2014). Mammographic density phenotypes and risk of breast cancer: A meta-analysis. *Journal of the National Cancer Institute, 106*(5), doi:10.1093/jnci/dju078. pii: dju078.
159. Institute of Medicine of the National Academies (2011). *Breast cancer and the environment: A life course approach.* Washington, DC: The National Academies Press.
160. Ginsburg, O. N., Martin, L. J., & Boyd, N. F. (2008). Mammographic density, lobular involution, and risk of breast cancer. *British Journal of Cancer, 4*(99), 1369–1374. doi:10.1038/sj.bjc.6604635.
161. Smith-Bindman, R. (2012). Environmental causes of breast cancer and radiation from medical imaging. *Archives of Internal Medicine, 172*(13), 1023–1027. doi:10.1001/archinternmed.2012.2329.
162. Brenner, D. J., & Hall, E. J. (2007). Computed tomography—An increasing source of radiation exposure. *New England Journal of Medicine, 357*(22), 2277–2284. doi:10.1056/NEJMra072149.
163. Schwab, S. A., Brand, M., Schlude, I. K., et al. (2013). X-ray induced formation of γ-H2AX foci after full-field digital mammography and digital breast tomosynthesis. *PLoS ONE, 8*(7), e70660. doi:10.1371/journal.pone.0070660.
164. Colin, C., Devic, C., Noël, A., et al. (2011). DNA double-strand breaks induced by mammographic screening procedures in human mammary epithelial cells. *International Journal of Radiation Biology, 87*(11), 1103–1112. doi:10.3109/09553002.2011.608410.
165. Colin, C., & Foray, N. (2012). DNA damage induced by mammography in high family risk patients: Only one single view in screening. *The Breast, 21*(3), 409–410. doi:10.1016/j.breast.2011.12.003.
166. Frankenberg-Schwager, M., & Gregus, A. (2012). Chromosomal instability carriers. *International Journal of Radiation Biology, 88*(11), 846–857. doi:10.3109/09553002.2012.711500.
167. Pucci, M., Bravata, V., Forte, G. I., et al. (2015). Caveolin-1, breast cancer and ionizing radiation. *Cancer Genomics & Proteomics, 12*(3), 143–152.
168. Colin, C., de Vathaire, F., Noël, A., et al. (2012). Updated relevance of mammographic screening modalities in women previously treated with chest irradiation for Hodgkin disease. *Radiology, 265*(3), 669–676. doi:10.1148/radiol.12120794.
169. Ng, J., Shuryak, I., Xu, Y., et al. (2012). Predicting the risk of secondary lung malignancies associated with whole-breast radiation therapy. *International Journal of Radiation Oncology, Biology, Physics, 83*(4), 1101–1106. doi:10.1016/j.ijrobp.2011.09.052.
170. Mourouti, N., Kontogianni, M. D., Papvagelis, C., et al. (2015). Diet and breast cancer. *International Journal of Food Sciences and Nutrition, 66*(1), 1–42. doi:10.3109/09637486.2014.950207.
171. Demetriou, C. A., Hadjisavvas, A., Loizidou, M. A., et al. (2012). The Mediterranean dietary pattern and breast cancer risk in Greek-Cypriot women: A case-control study. *BMC Cancer, 12*, 113. doi:10.1186/1471-2407-12-113.
172. Trinh, T., Christensen, S. E., Brand, J. S., et al. (2015). Background risk of breast cancer influences the association between alcohol consumption and mammographic density. *British Journal of Cancer, 113*(1), 159–165. doi:10.1038/bjc.2015.185.
173. Key, T. J. (2011). Minireview: Fruit and vegetables and cancer risk. *British Journal of Cancer, 104*(1), 6–11. doi:10.1038/sj.bjc.6606032.
174. Nechuta, S. J., Caan, B. J., Chen, W. Y., et al. (2012). Soy food intake after diagnosis of breast cancer and survival: An in-depth analysis of combined evidence from cohort studies of U.S. and Chinese women. *American Journal of Clinical Nutrition, 96*(1), 123–132. doi:10.3945/ajcn.112.035972.
175. Aceves, C., Anguiano, B., & Delgado, G. (2005). Is iodine a gatekeeper of the integrity of the mammary gland? *Journal of Mammary Gland Biology and Neoplasia, 10*(2), 189–196. doi:10.1007/s10911-005-5401-5.
176. Cann, S. A., van Netten, J. P., & van Netten, C. (2000). Hypothesis: Iodine, selenium and the development of breast cancer. *Cancer Causes and Control, 11*(2), 121–127.
177. Eskin, B. A., Grotkowski, C. E., Connolly, C. P., et al. (1995). Different tissue responses for iodine and iodide in rat thyroid and mammary glands. *Biological Trace Element Research, 49*(1), 9–19. doi:10.1007/BF02788999.
178. Ghent, W. R., Eskin, B. A., Low, D. A., et al. (1993). Iodine replacement in fibrocystic disease of the breast. *Canadian Journal of Surgery. Journal Canadien de Chirurgie, 36*(5), 453–460.
179. Funahashi, H., Imai, T., Mase, T., et al. (2001). Seaweed prevents breast cancer. *Japanese Journal of Cancer Research: Gann, 92*(5), 483–487.
180. Smyth, P. P. (2003). Role of iodine in antioxidant defense in thyroid and breast disease. *Biofactors (Oxford, England), 19*(3–4), 121–130.
181. Byers, T., & Sedjo, R. L. (2015). Body fatness as a cause of cancer: Epidemiologic clues to biologic mechanisms. *Endocrine-Related Cancer, 22*(3), R125–R134. doi:10.1530/ERC-14-0580.
182. Michels, K. B., Terry, K. L., Eliassen, A. H., et al. (2012). Adult weight change and incidence of premenopausal breast cancer. *International Journal of Cancer. Journal International du Cancer, 130*(4), 902–909. doi:10.1002/ijc.26069.
183. Protani, M., Coory, M., & Martin, J. H. (2010). Effect of obesity on survival of women with breast cancer: Systematic review and meta-analysis. *Breast Cancer Research and Treatment, 123*(3), 627–635. doi:10.1007/s10549-010-0990-0.
184. Vaino, H., & Bianchini, F. (Eds.), (2002). *IARC. International Agency for Research on Cancer. Weight control and physical activity.* Lyon, France: IARC Press.
185. World Cancer Research Fund (2007). *Food, nutrition, physical activity, and the prevention of cancer; a global perspective* (2nd ed.). Washington, DC: American Institute for Cancer Research.
186. Holmes, M. D., & Willett, W. C. (2004). Does diet affect breast cancer risk? *Breast Cancer Research : BCR, 6*(4), 170–178. doi:10.1186/bcr909.
187. Wenten, M., Gilliland, F. D., Baumgartner, K., et al. (2002). Associations of weight, weight change, and body mass with breast cancer risk in Hispanic and non-Hispanic white women. *Annals of Epidemiology, 12*(6), 435–444.
188. Trentham-Diaz, A., Newcomb, P. A., Egan, K. M., et al. (2000). Weight change and risk of postmenopausal breast cancer (United States). *Cancer Causes and Control, 11*(6), 533–542.
189. Le Marchand, L., Kolonei, L. N., Earle, M. E., et al. (1998). Body size at different periods of life and breast cancer risk. *American Journal of Epidemiology, 128*(1), 137–152.
190. Morimoto, L. M., White, E., Chen, Z., et al. (2002). Obesity, body size, and risk of postmenopausal breast cancer: The Women's Health Initiative (United States). *Cancer Causes and Control, 13*(8), 741–751.
191. Endogenous Hormones Breast Cancer Collaborative Group. (2003). Body mass index, serum sex hormones, and breast cancer risk in postmenopausal women. *Journal of the National Cancer Institute, 95*(6), 1218–1226.
192. Korner, A., Pazaitou-Panayiotou, K., Kelesidis, T., et al. (2007). Total and high molecular weight adiponectin in breast cancer: In vitro and in vivo studies. *Journal of Clinical Endocrinology and Metabolism, 92*(3), 1041–1048. doi:10.1210/jc.2006-1858.
193. Surmacz, E. (2007). Obesity hormone leptin: A new target in breast cancer? *Breast Cancer Research : BCR, 9*(1), 301. doi:10.1186/bcr1638.
194. Jarde, T., Perrier, S., Vasson, M. P., et al. (2011). Molecular mechanism of leptin and adiponectin in breast cancer. *European Journal of Cancer, 47*(1), 33–43. doi:10.1016/j.ejca.2010.09.005.
195. Andó, S., Barone, I., Giordano, C., et al. (2014). The multifaceted mechanism of leptin signaling within tumor microenvironment in driving breast cancer growth and progression. *Frontiers in Oncology, 4*, 340. doi:10.3389/fonc.2014.00340.
196. UN Department of Economic and Social Affairs. (n.d.). *Canada national reporting to CSD-18/19 thematic profile on chemicals.* Retrieved from https://sustainabledevelopment.un.org/dsd_aofw_ni/ni_pdfs/NationalReports/canada/Chemicals.pdf.
197. Barrett, J. R. (2014). EDCs and estrogen receptor activity: A pathway to safer chemical design. *Environmental Health Perspectives, 122*(12), A339. doi:10.1289/ehp.122-A339.
198. Sprague, B. L., Trentham-Dietz, A., Newcomb, P. A., et al. (2007). Lifetime recreational and occupational physical activity and risk of in situ and invasive breast cancer. *Cancer Epidemiology, Biomarkers and Prevention, 16*(2), 236–243. doi:10.1158/1055-9965.EPI-06-0713.
199. Kim, J., Choi, W. J., & Jeong, S. H. (2013). The effects of physical activity on breast cancer survivors after diagnosis. *Cancer Prevention, 18*(3), 193–200.
200. Stephens, P. J., Tarpey, P. S., Davies, H., et al. (2012). The landscape of cancer genes and mutational processes in breast cancer. *Nature, 486*(7403), 400–404. doi:10.1038/nature11017.
201. Wagenblast, E., Soto, M., Gutierrez-Angel, S., et al. (2015). A model of breast cancer heterogeneity reveals vascular mimicry as a driver of metastasis.

Nature, 520(7547), 358–362. doi:10.1038/nature14403.
202. National Cancer Institute. (2015). *PDQ® genetics of breast and gynecologic cancers*. Retrieved from http://www.cancer.gov/types/breast/hp/breast-ovarian-genetics-pdq.
203. Marusyk, A., Tabassum, D. P., Altrock, P. M., et al. (2014). Non-cell autonomous tumor-growth driving supports sub-clonal heterogeneity. *Nature, 514*(7520), 54–58. doi:10.1038/nature13556.
204. Hanahan, D., & Weinberg, R. (2011). Hallmarks of cancer: The next generation. *Cell, 144*(5), 646–674. doi:10.1016/j.cell.2011.02.013.
205. Damonte, P., Hodgson, J. G., Chen, J. Q., et al. (2008). Mammary carcinoma behavior is programmed in the precancer stem cell. *Breast Cancer Research : BCR, 10*(3), R50. doi:10.1186/bcr2104.
206. Janiszewska, M., & Polyak, K. (2015). Clonal evolution in cancer: A tale of twisted twines. *Cell Stem Cell, 16*(1), 11–12. doi:10.1016/j.stem.2014.12.011.
207. Sorlie, T., Perou, C. M., Tibshirani, R., et al. (2001). Gene expression patterns of breast carcinomas distinguish tumor subclasses with clinical implications. *Proceedings of the National Academy of Sciences of the United States of America, 98*(19), 10869–10874. doi:10.1073/pnas.191367098.
208. Boudreau, A., van't Veer, L. J., & Bissell, M. J. (2012). An "elite hacker:" Breast tumors exploit the normal microenvironment program to instruct their progression and biological diversity. *Cell Adhesion & Migration, 6*(3), 236–248. doi:10.4161/cam.20880.
209. Cardiff, R. D., Couto, S., & Bolon, B. (2011). Three interrelated themes in current breast cancer research: Gene addiction, phenotypic plasticity, and cancer stem cells. *Breast Cancer Research : BCR, 13*(5), 216. doi:10.1186/bcr2887.
210. Craene, D. B., & Berx, G. (2013). Regulatory networks defining EMT during cancer initiation and progression. *Nature Reviews. Cancer, 13*(2), 97–110. doi:10.1038/nrc3447.
211. Chaffer, C. L., & Weinberg, R. A. (2011). A perspective on cancer cell metastasis. *Science, 331*(6024), 1559–1564. doi:10.1126/science.1203543.
212. Inman, J. L., Robertson, C., Mott, J. D., et al. (2015). Mammary gland development: Cell fates specification, stem cells and the microenvironment. *Development (Cambridge, England), 142*(6), 1028–1042. doi:10.1242/dev.087643.
213. Mani, S. A., Guo, W., Liao, M. J., et al. (2008). The epithelial-mesenchymal transition generates cells with properties of stem cells. *Cell, 133*(4), 704–715. doi:10.1016/j.cell.2008.03.027.
214. Charafe-Jauffret, E., Ginestier, C., Iovino, F., et al. (2009). Breast cancer cell lines contain functional cancer stem cells with metastatic capacity and a distinct molecular signature. *Cancer Research, 69*(4), 1302–1313. doi:10.1158/0008-5472.CAN-08-2741.
215. Marcato, P., Dean, C. A., Pan, D., et al. (2011). Aldehyde dehydrogenase activity of breast cancer stem cells is primarily due to isoform ALDH1A3 and its expression is predictive of metastasis. *Stem Cell, 29*(1), 32–45. doi:10.1002/stem.563.
216. Almog, N. (2013). Genes and regulatory pathways involved in persistence of dormant micro-tumors. In H. Enderling, N. Almog, & L. Hlatky (Eds.), *System biology of tumor dormancy advances in experimental medicine and biology*. New York: Springer Science.
217. Enderling, H., Almog, N., & Hlatky, L. (2013). *System biology of tumor dormancy advances in experimental medicine and biology*. New York: Springer Science.
218. Kim, Y., & Boushaba, K. (2013). Regulation of tumor dormancy and role of microenvironment: A mathematical model. In H. Enderling, N. Almog, & L. Hlatky (Eds.), *System biology of tumor dormancy advances in experimental medicine and biology*. New York: Springer Science.
219. Kerlikowske, K. (2010). Epidemiology of ductal carcinoma in situ. *Journal of the National Cancer Institute. Monographs, 2010*(41), 139–141. doi:10.1093/jncimonographs/lgq027.
220. Bombonati, A., & Sgroi, D. C. (2011). The molecular pathology of breast cancer progression. *Journal of Pathology, 223*(2), 307–317. doi:10.1002/path.2808.
221. National Cancer Institute. (2015). *PDQ® breast cancer screening*. Retrieved from http://www.cancer.gov/types/breast/hp/breast-screening-pdq.
222. Miller, A. B., Baines, C. J., To, T., et al. (1992). Canadian National Breast Screening Study: 2. Breast cancer detection and death rates among women aged 50 to 59 years. *CMAJ : Canadian Medical Association Journal, 147*(10), 1477–1488.

34

Alterations of the Male Reproductive System

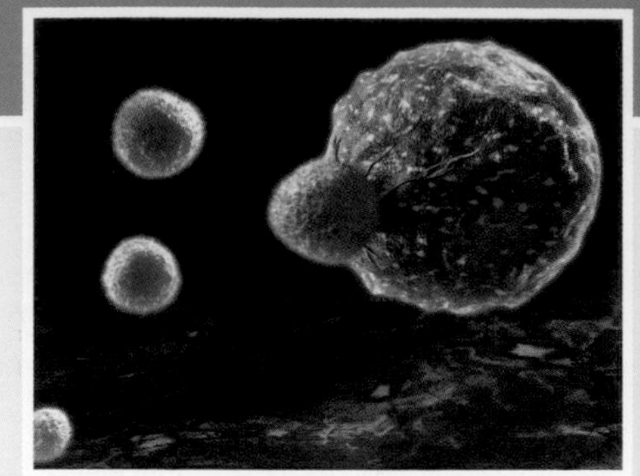

George W. Rodway, Kathryn L. McCance, and Kelly Power-Kean

EVOLVE WEBSITE

http://evolve.elsevier.com/Canada/Huether/pathophysiology
Student Review Questions
Key Points
Case Studies
Animations
Quick Check Answers

CHAPTER OUTLINE

Alterations of Sexual Maturation, 868
Delayed or Absent Puberty, 868
Precocious Puberty, 868
Disorders of the Male Reproductive System, 869
Disorders of the Urethra, 869
Disorders of the Penis, 869
Disorders of the Scrotum, Testis, and Epididymis, 872
Disorders of the Prostate Gland, 876
Sexual Dysfunction, 888
Disorders of the Male Breast, 890
Gynecomastia, 890
Carcinoma, 891
Sexually Transmitted Infections, 891

Alterations of the reproductive system span a wide range of concerns, from delayed sexual development and suboptimal sexual performance to structural and functional abnormalities. Many common male reproductive disorders carry potentially serious physiological or psychological consequences. For example, sexual or reproductive dysfunction, such as erectile dysfunction or infertility, can dramatically affect self-concept, relationships, and overall quality of life. Conversely, organic and psychosocial problems, such as alcoholism, depression, situational stressors, chronic illness, and medications, can affect sexual performance and may be risk factors for the development of some types of reproductive tract cancers. Aside from skin cancer, prostate cancer is the second leading cause of cancer deaths and is the most frequently diagnosed cancer in men. Incidence rates for prostate cancer changed substantially between the mid-1980s and mid-1990s and have since fluctuated widely from year to year, in large part reflecting changes in prostate cancer screening with the prostate-specific antigen (PSA) blood test.[1] Diagnosis and treatment of male reproductive system disorders are, like female reproductive system disorders, often complicated by the stigma and symbolism associated with the reproductive organs and emotion-laden beliefs and behaviours related to reproductive health. Treatment or diagnosis for any problem may be delayed because of embarrassment, guilt, fear, or denial.

ALTERATIONS OF SEXUAL MATURATION

The process of sexual maturation, or puberty, is marked by the development of secondary sex characteristics, rapid growth, and, ultimately, the ability to reproduce. A variety of congenital and endocrine disorders can disrupt the timing of puberty. Puberty that occurs too late (delayed puberty) or too early (precocious puberty) is caused by the inappropriate onset of sex hormone production. While the mean age of pubertal onset appears to be decreasing for girls, the age of pubertal onset has remained essentially unchanged for boys.

Delayed or Absent Puberty

About 3% of children living in North America experience delayed development of secondary sex characteristics.[2] Normally, boys tend to mature later than girls, around 14 to 14.5 years of age. In boys, the first sign of maturity is the enlargement of testes and thinning of the scrotal skin. In **delayed puberty**, these secondary sex characteristics develop later.

In about 95% of cases, delayed puberty is a normal physiological event. Hormonal levels are normal, the hypothalamic-pituitary-gonadal axis is intact, and maturation is slowly occurring. Treatment is seldom needed unless the delayed puberty is causing psychosocial problems.[3]

The other 5% of cases are caused by the disruption of the hypothalamic-pituitary-gonadal axis or by the outcomes of a systemic disease. Treatment depends on the cause (Box 34-1), and referral to a pediatric endocrinologist is necessary.[4]

Precocious Puberty

Precocious puberty is a rare event, affecting fewer than 1 in 50 000 boys. Precocious puberty for boys of all ethnic/racial groups is defined as sexual maturation occurring before age 9.[5] A recent study observed that the mean ages of beginning male genital and pubic hair growth and early testicular volumes are leaning toward younger ages than earlier studies have suggested, although this seems to be dependent on race/ethnicity.[6] Precocious puberty may be caused by many conditions (Box 34-2), including lethal central nervous system tumours. All cases of precocious puberty require thorough evaluation.

All forms of precocious puberty are treated by identifying and removing the underlying cause or administering appropriate hormones.

BOX 34-1 Causes of Delayed Puberty

Hypergonadotropic Hypogonadism (Low Testosterone, Increased Follicle-Stimulating Hormone [FSH] and Luteinizing Hormone [LH])

1. Gonadal dysgenesis, most commonly Turner syndrome (45,X/46,XX; structural X or Y abnormalities, or mosaicism)
2. Klinefelter's syndrome (47,XXY)
3. Bilateral gonadal failure
   a. Traumatic or infectious
   b. Postsurgical, postirradiation, or postchemotherapy
   c. Autoimmune
   d. Idiopathic empty-scrotum or vanishing-testes syndrome (congenital anorchia)

Hypogonadotropic Hypogonadism (Low Testosterone, Decreased LH, Depressed FSH)

1. Reversible
   a. Physiological delay
   b. Weight loss/anorexia
   c. Strenuous exercise
   d. Severe obesity
   e. Illegal drug use, especially marihuana
   f. Primary hypothyroidism
   g. Congenital adrenal hyperplasia
   h. Cushing's syndrome
   i. Prolactinomas
2. Irreversible
   a. Gonadotropin-releasing hormone (GnRH) deficiency (Kallmann's syndrome) or idiopathic hypogonadotropic hypogonadism (IHH)
   b. Hypopituitarism
   c. Congenital central nervous system defects
   d. Other pituitary adenomas
   e. Craniopharyngioma
   f. Malignant pituitary tumours

BOX 34-2 Primary Forms of Precocious Puberty

Complete Precocious Puberty

Appropriate characteristics for the child's gender develop prematurely.

Hypothalamic-pituitary-gonadal axis functions normally but prematurely.

In about 10% of cases, lethal central nervous system tumour may be the cause.

Partial Precocious Puberty

Appropriate secondary sex characteristics develop partially.

Premature adrenarche (growth of axillary and pubic hair) tends to occur between 5 and 8 years of age.

It can progress to complete precocious puberty; it may be caused by estrogen-secreting neoplasms or may be a variant of normal pubertal development.

Mixed Precocious Puberty

It causes the child to develop some secondary sex characteristics of the opposite gender.

Common causes are adrenal hyperplasia or androgen-secreting tumours.

Data from Burchett, M.L.R., Hanna, C.E., & Steiner, R.D. (2009). Endocrine and metabolic diseases. In C.E. Burns, A.M. Dunn, M.A. Brady, et al. (Eds.), *Pediatric primary care* (4th ed.). St. Louis: Saunders; Jospe, N. (2005). Disorders of pubertal development. In L.M. Osborn, T.G. DeWitt, L.R. First, et al. (Eds.), *Pediatrics*. Philadelphia: Mosby.

In many cases, precocious puberty can be reversed. However, **complete precocious puberty** (development consistent with the gender of the individual) is difficult to treat and can cause long bones to stop growing before the child has reached normal height.

✔ QUICK CHECK 34-1

1. Why does puberty occur too late or too early in some individuals?
2. Why do all forms of precocious puberty require evaluation?

DISORDERS OF THE MALE REPRODUCTIVE SYSTEM

Disorders of the Urethra

Urethritis and urethral strictures are common disorders of the male urethra. Urethral carcinoma, an extremely rare form of cancer, can occur in men older than 60 years.

Urethritis

Urethritis is an inflammatory process that is usually, but not always, caused by a sexually transmitted microorganism. Infectious urethritis caused by *Neisseria gonorrhoeae* is often called *gonococcal urethritis* (GU); urethritis caused by other microorganisms is called *nongonococcal urethritis* (NGU). Nonsexual origins of urethritis include inflammation or infection as a result of urological procedures, insertion of foreign bodies into the urethra, anatomical abnormalities, or trauma.

Noninfectious urethritis is rare and is associated with the ingestion of wood or ethyl alcohol or turpentine. It is also seen with reactive arthritis.[7]

Symptoms of urethritis include urethral tingling or itching or a burning sensation, and frequency and urgency with urination. The individual may note a purulent or clear mucouslike discharge from the urethra. Nucleic acid detection amplification tests allow early detection of *N. gonorrhoeae* and *Chlamydia trachomatis* in urine studies.[8] Treatment consists of appropriate antibiotic therapy for infectious urethritis and avoidance of future exposure or mechanical irritation.

Urethral Strictures

A **urethral stricture** is a narrowing of the urethra caused by scarring. The scars may be congenital but can be present at any age and have a wide range of etiological factors, including untreated urethral infection, trauma, and urological instrumentation. Infections also can occur from long-term use of indwelling catheters. Prostatitis and infection secondary to urinary stasis are common complications. Severe and prolonged obstruction can result in hydronephrosis and kidney failure.

The clinical manifestations of urethral stricture are caused by bladder outlet obstruction. Urethral stricture often manifests itself as lower urinary tract symptoms (LUTS) or urinary tract infections with significant impairment in the quality of life. The primary symptom is diminished force and calibre of the urinary system; other symptoms include urinary frequency and hesitancy, mild dysuria, double urinary stream or spraying, and dribbling after voiding. Urethral stricture is diagnosed on the basis of history, physical examination, flow rates, and cystoscopy. Treatment is usually surgical and may involve urethral dilation, urethrotomy, or a variety of open surgical techniques. The choice of surgical intervention depends on the age of the individual and the severity of the problem.

Disorders of the Penis

Phimosis and Paraphimosis

Phimosis and paraphimosis are both disorders in which the foreskin (prepuce) is "too tight" to move easily over the glans penis. **Phimosis**

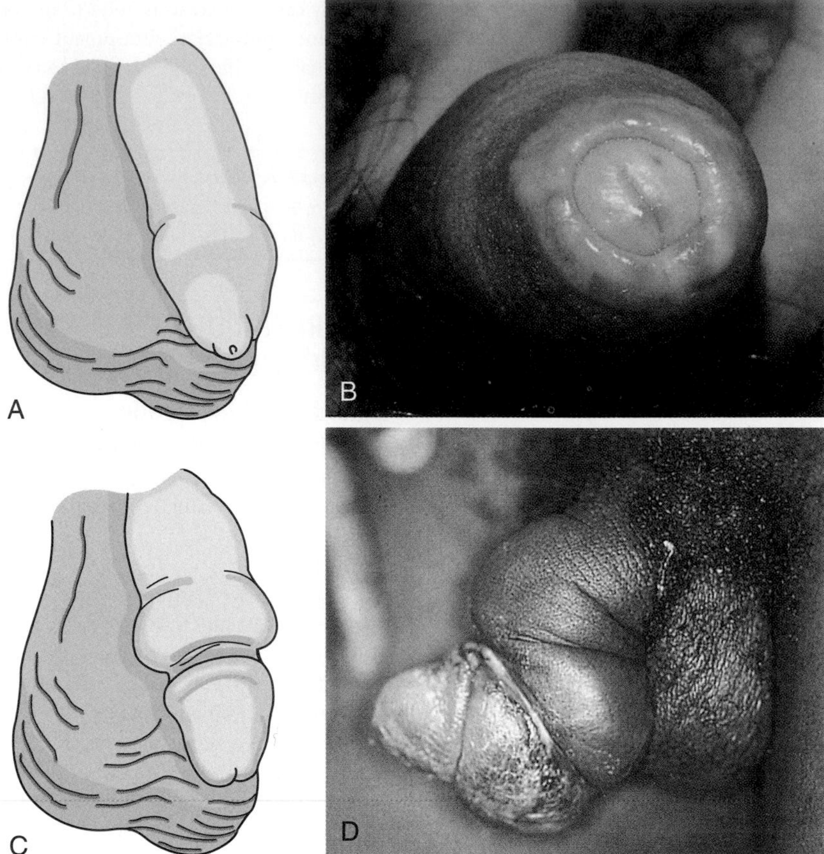

FIGURE 34-1 Phimosis and Paraphimosis. A, Phimosis: the foreskin has a narrow opening that is not large enough to permit retraction over the glans. **B,** Lesions on the prepuce secondary to infection cause swelling, and retraction of foreskin may be impossible. Circumcision is usually required. **C,** Paraphimosis: the foreskin is retracted over the glans but cannot be reduced to its normal position. Here it has formed a constricting band around the penis. **D,** Ulcer on the retracted prepuce with edema. (**A** and **C,** from Monahan, F.D., Sands, J., Neighbors, M., et al. [2007]. *Phipps' medical-surgical nursing: Health and illness perspectives* [8th ed.]. St. Louis: Mosby; **B,** from Taylor, P.K. [1995]. *Diagnostic picture tests in sexually transmitted diseases.* St. Louis: Mosby; **D,** from Morse, S.A., Holmes, K.K., & Ballard, R.C. [2011]. *Atlas of sexually transmitted diseases and AIDS* [4th ed.]. London: Saunders.)

is a condition in which the foreskin cannot be retracted back over the glans, whereas **paraphimosis** is the opposite: the foreskin is retracted and cannot be moved forward (reduced) to cover the glans (Figure 34-1). Both conditions can cause penile pathological conditions.

The inability to retract the foreskin is normal in infancy and is caused by congenital adhesions. During the first 3 years of life, congenital adhesions (between the foreskin and glans) separate naturally with penile erections and are not an indication for circumcision. Phimosis can occur at any age and is most commonly caused by poor hygiene and chronic infection.[9] It rarely occurs with normal foreskin.

Reasons for seeking treatment include edema, erythema, and tenderness of the prepuce and purulent discharge; inability to retract the foreskin is a less common complaint. Circumcision, if needed, is performed after infection has been eradicated. Complications of phimosis include inflammation of the glans (balanitis) or prepuce (posthitis) and paraphimosis. There is a higher incidence of penile carcinoma in uncircumcised males, but chronic infection and poor hygiene are usually the underlying factors in such cases. Approximately 40 to 63% of invasive penile carcinomas are attributable to human papillomavirus (HPV).[10,11]

Paraphimosis, in which the foreskin is retracted, can constrict the penis, causing edema of the glans. If the foreskin cannot be reduced manually, surgery must be performed to prevent necrosis of the glans caused by constricted blood vessels. Severe paraphimosis is a surgical emergency.

Peyronie Disease

Peyronie disease ("bent nail syndrome") is a fibrotic condition that causes lateral curvature of the penis during erection (Figure 34-2). Peyronie disease develops slowly and is characterized by tough, fibrous thickening of the fascia in the erectile tissue of the corpora cavernosa. A dense, fibrous plaque is usually palpable on the dorsum of the penile shaft. The problem usually affects middle-aged men and is associated with painful erection, painful intercourse (for both partners), and poor erection distal to the involved area.[12] In some cases, erectile dysfunction or unsatisfactory penetration occurs. When the penis is flaccid, there is no pain.

A local vasculitislike inflammatory reaction occurs, and decreased tissue oxygenation results in fibrosis and calcification. The exact cause is unknown. Peyronie disease is associated with Dupuytren's contracture (a flexion deformity of the fingers or toes caused by shortening or fibrosis of the palmar or plantar fascia), diabetes, tendency to develop keloids, and, in rare cases, use of beta-blocker medications.[9]

There is no definitive treatment for Peyronie disease; however, treatment can include pharmacological agents and surgery. Spontaneous

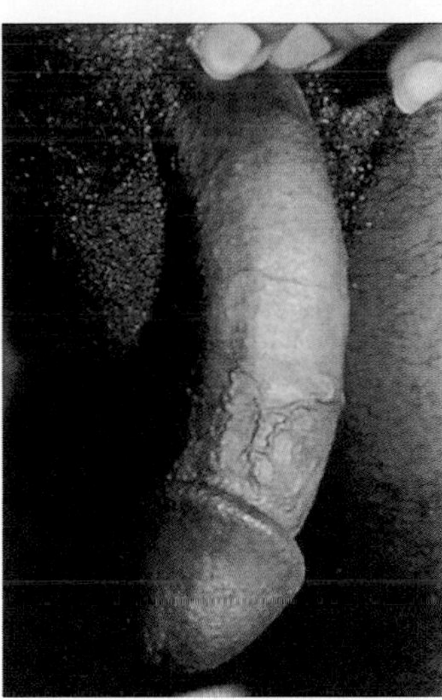

FIGURE 34-2 Peyronie Disease. This person complained of pain and deviation of his penis to one side on erection. (From Taylor, P.K. [1995]. *Diagnostic picture tests in sexually transmitted diseases.* London: Mosby.)

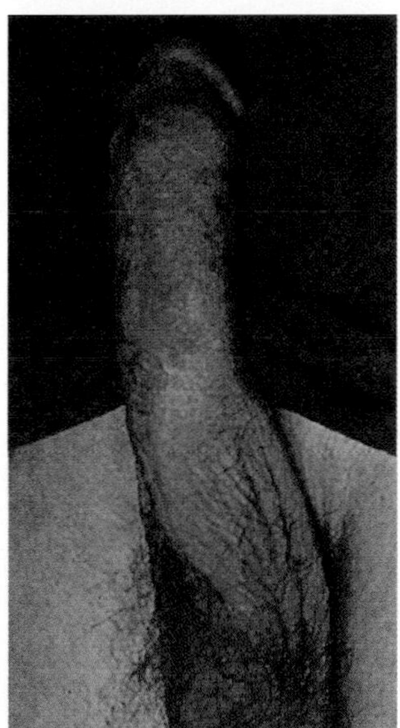

FIGURE 34-3 Priapism. (From Lloyd-Davies, R.W., Parkhouse, H., Crow, J., et al. [1994]. *Color atlas of urology* [2nd ed.]. London: Wolfe Medical.)

remissions occur in as many as 50% of individuals. However, men suffering with Peyronie disease and who have significant penile deformity precluding successful coitus should be appraised for surgical correction.[9]

Priapism

Priapism is an uncommon condition of prolonged penile erection. It is usually painful and is not associated with sexual arousal (Figure 34-3). Priapism is idiopathic in 60% of cases; the remaining 40% of cases can be associated with spinal cord trauma, sickle cell disease, leukemia, pelvic tumours, infections, or penile trauma.

Priapism must be considered a urological emergency. Treatment within hours is effective and prevents erectile dysfunction. Conservative approaches include iced saline enemas, ketamine administration, and spinal anaesthesia. Needle aspiration of blood from the corpus through the dorsal glans is often effective and is followed by catheterization and pressure dressings to maintain decompression. More aggressive surgical treatments include the creation of vascular shunts to maintain blood flow. Erectile dysfunction results in up to 50% of prolonged cases.

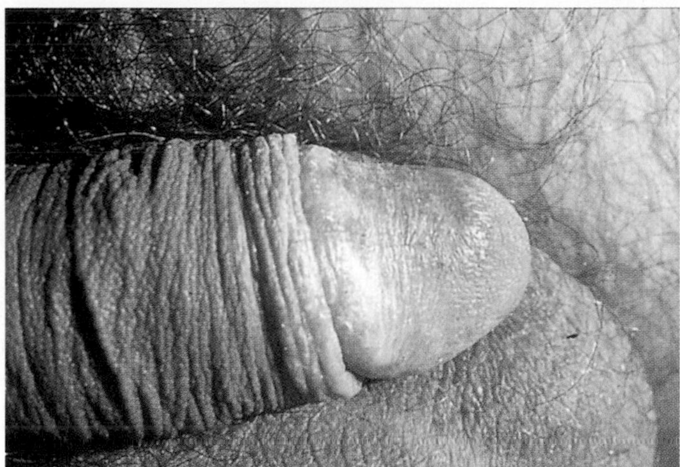

FIGURE 34-4 Balanitis. (From Taylor, P.K. [1995]. *Diagnostic picture tests in sexually transmitted diseases.* London: Mosby.)

Balanitis

Balanitis is an inflammation of the glans penis (Figure 34-4) and usually occurs in conjunction with posthitis, an inflammation of the prepuce. (Inflammation of the glans and the prepuce is called *balanoposthitis.*) It is associated with poor hygiene and phimosis. The accumulation under the foreskin of glandular secretions (smegma), sloughed epithelial cells, and *Mycobacterium smegmatis* can irritate the glans directly or lead to infection. Skin disorders (e.g., psoriasis, lichen planus, eczema) and candidiasis must be differentiated from inflammation resulting from poor hygienic practices. Balanitis is most commonly seen in men with poorly controlled diabetes mellitus and candidiasis. The infection is treated with antimicrobials. After the inflammation has subsided, circumcision can be considered to prevent recurrences.

Tumours of the Penis

Tumours of the penis are not common. The most frequent are the benign epithelial tumour condyloma acuminatum and penile carcinomas.

Condyloma acuminatum is a benign tumour caused by HPV, a sexually transmitted infection (STI). HPV type 6 and, less often, type 11 are the most frequent types and can cause a common wart and moist surface of the external genitalia. Giant condylomata (Buschke-Löwenstein tumour) affect older men and may be 5 to 10 cm in size.[13] Atypia may be evident in longstanding, giant condylomata, and assessment of other HPV subtypes may be indicated to distinguish from a noninvasive warty carcinoma.[13,14]

Penile Cancer

Carcinoma of the penis is rare in Canada. The Canadian Cancer Society estimated that 220 Canadian men were diagnosed with penile cancer in 2013. It also estimated that 41 Canadian men died of this disease in 2013.[15] It does account, however, for about 10% of cancers in African and South American men. It can affect men 40 to 70 years of age, with two-thirds of men diagnosed at 65 years of age and older. Although the exact cause is unknown, risk factors include HPV infection, smoking, low socioeconomic status, poor personal hygiene, and psoriasis (possibly autoimmune diseases linked to the lack of clearance of HPV). Circumcision at birth decreases the risk for penile cancer, and penile cancer is more common in men with phimosis and those with acquired immune deficiency syndrome (AIDS).[16]

Squamous cell carcinoma accounts for 95% of invasive penile cancers. Other premalignant lesions, or in situ forms of epidermal carcinoma, that occur on the penis include leukoplakia (white plaque), Paget's disease (red, inflamed areas), erythroplasia of Queyrat (raised red areas), and Buschke-Löwenstein patches (large venous areas). Recently, penile intraepithelial neoplasia (PeIN; atypical cells) has been redesignated into two subcategories: differentiated PeIN and undifferentiated PeIN, including warty basaloid and mixed warty-basaloid subtypes.[13] HPV-6 and HPV-11 associated with genital warts (condylomata acuminata) have low cancer risks.[17] At times, the penis might be the site of metastatic spread of solid tumours from the bladder, prostate, rectum, or kidney. Early squamous cell carcinoma and premalignant epidermal lesions are easily treated, but delays in seeking treatment are attributed to denial, embarrassment, failure to detect lesions under a phimotic foreskin, fear, guilt, and ignorance.

Squamous cell carcinoma usually begins as a small, flat, ulcerative or papillary lesion on the glans or foreskin that grows to involve the entire penile shaft. Extensive lesions are associated with metastases and a poor prognosis.[18,19] The regional femoral and iliac lymph nodes are common metastatic sites; the urethra and bladder are rarely involved. Weight loss, fatigue, and malaise accompany chronic suppurative lesions.

The specific diagnosis is made by biopsy after examination to document the location, size, and fixation of the lesion. After a positive biopsy, the extent of cancer spread is determined by imaging studies. Distant metastases are uncommon. Stages of carcinoma of the penis are presented in Box 34-3.

Penile carcinoma is managed primarily with surgery. Newer, innovative surgical techniques can preserve as much penile tissue as possible without compromising cancer control. A multimodal approach with chemotherapy is under study.[20,21] Palliative treatment with radiation or chemotherapy may be used when the disease is inoperable and bulky inguinal metastases have occurred. Options for individuals with carcinoma in situ include local excision, radiation, laser surgery, cryosurgery, chemosurgery, or chemotherapy with topical (5%) 5-fluorouracil (Efudex).[18]

✔QUICK CHECK 34-2

1. Why are priapism and severe paraphimosis considered urological emergencies?
2. What are the risk factors for cancer of the penis?

BOX 34-3 Staging for Penile Cancer

Stage 0: Tis or Ta, N0, M0

The cancer has not grown into tissue below the top layers of skin and has not spread to lymph nodes or distant sites.

Stage I: T1a, N0, M0

The cancer has grown into tissue just below the superficial layer of skin but has not grown into blood or lymph vessels. It is a grade 1 or 2. It has not spread to lymph nodes or distant sites.

Stage II: Any of the Following:

T1b, N0, M0

The cancer has grown into tissue just below the superficial layer of skin and is high grade or has grown into blood or lymph vessels. It has not spread to lymph nodes or distant sites.

Or

T2, N0, M0

The cancer has grown into one of the internal chambers of the penis (the corpus spongiosum or corpora cavernosa). The cancer has not spread to lymph nodes or distant sites.

Or

T3, N0, M0

The cancer has grown into the urethra. It has not spread to lymph nodes or distant sites.

Stage IIIA: T1 to T3, N1, M0

The cancer has grown into tissue below the superficial layer of skin (T1). It also may have grown into the corpus spongiosum, the corpora cavernosa, or the urethra (T2 or T3). The cancer has spread to a single groin lymph node (N1). It has not spread to distant sites.

Stage IIIB: T1 to T3, N2, M0

The cancer has grown into the tissues of the penis and may have grown into the corpus spongiosum, the corpora cavernosa, or the urethra (T1 to T3). It has spread to two or more groin lymph nodes. It has not spread to distant sites.

Stage IV: Any of the Following:

T4, any N, M0

The cancer has grown into the prostate or other nearby structures. It may or may not have spread to groin lymph nodes. It has not spread to distant sites.

Or

Any T, N3, M0

The cancer has spread to lymph nodes in the pelvis or spread in the groin lymph nodes and grown through the lymph nodes' outer covering and into surrounding tissue. The cancer has not spread to distant sites.

Or

Any T, any N, M1

The cancer has spread to distant sites.

T, Primary tumour size; *N*, regional lymph nodes; *M*, distant metastasis.

Disorders of the Scrotum, Testis, and Epididymis

Disorders of the Scrotum

Men may seek treatment for painful or painless scrotal masses. Masses may be serious (cancer or torsion) or benign (hydrocele or cyst), and may require immediate surgical intervention or allow for careful observation. Varicocele, hydrocele, and spermatocele are common intrascrotal disorders. A varicocele is an abnormal dilation of the testicular veins and the pampiniform plexus within the scrotum, and is classically described as a "bag of worms" (Figure 34-5). Varicoceles are one of the most commonly identified scrotal abnormalities and abnormal findings among infertile men. Advancements in diagnostic techniques indicate that the incidence of varicoceles is significantly greater than previously reported.[22] Most (90%) occur on the left side because of discrepancies in venous drainage and may be painful or tender. Varicocele occurs in 10 to 15% of males and is seen most often after puberty.[23] Because most develop in adolescence, physiological changes in testosterone level may contribute to increasing blood flow to the testicle, causing venous dilation.[24] Unilateral right-sided varicoceles are rare and result from compression or obstruction of the inferior vena cava by a tumour or thrombus. Varicoceles may be less likely to be diagnosed among obese men.[25]

The cause of varicocele is poorly understood. Blood pools in the veins rather than flowing into the venous system. Varicocele decreases blood flow through the testis, interfering with spermatogenesis and causing infertility. Varicoceles can alter testosterone and follicle-stimulating

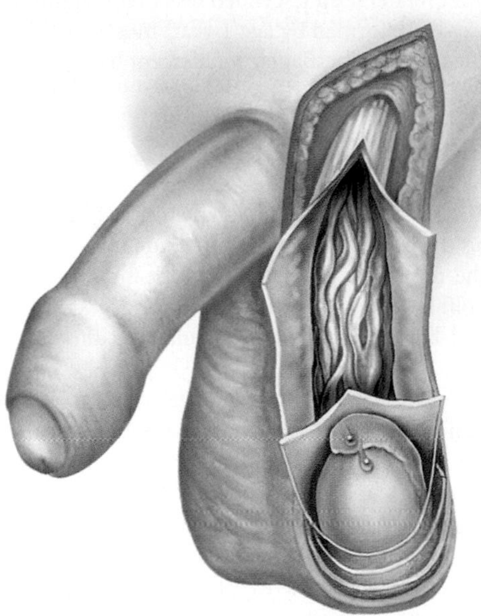

FIGURE 34-5 Depiction of a Varicocele. Dilation of veins within the spermatic cord. (From Ball, J.W., Dains, J.E., Flynn, J.A., et al. [2015]. *Seidel's guide to physical examination* [8th ed.]. St. Louis: Mosby.)

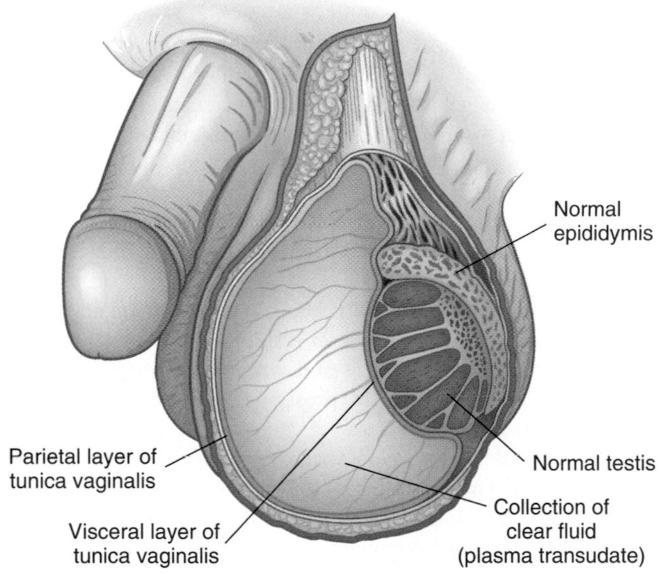

FIGURE 34-6 Depiction of a Hydrocele. Accumulation of clear fluid between the visceral (inner) and parietal (outer) layers of the tunica vaginalis.

hormone (FSH) levels, cause oxidative stress, decrease sperm count, and affect sperm quality.[26] Varicocele surgical repair is generally done when the male has a grade II or III varicocele and an abnormal semen analysis and the female has no known cause of infertility. If varicocele is mild and fertility is not an issue, a scrotal support is usually sufficient to relieve symptoms of scrotal heaviness or "dragging." Colour doppler ultrasonography is used to confirm diagnosis.[26]

A **hydrocele** is a collection of fluid between the layers of the tunica vaginalis (Figure 34-6). It is the most common cause of scrotal swelling. Hydroceles occur in 6% of male newborns and are congenital malformations that often resolve spontaneously in the first year of life.[27] In North America, common infectious causes include epididymitis and

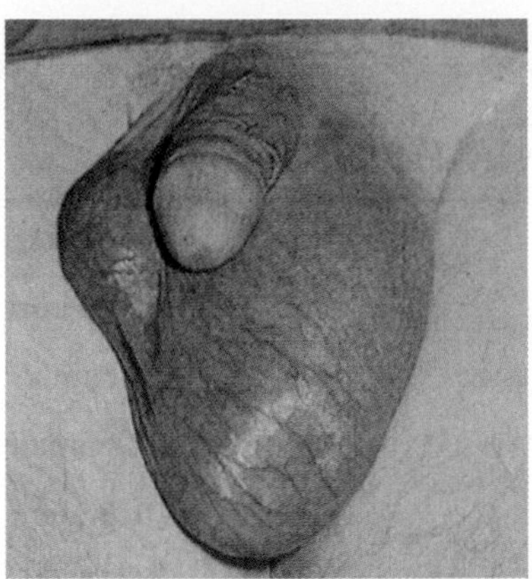

FIGURE 34-7 Spermatocele. Retention cyst of the head of the epididymis or of an aberrant tubule or tubules of the rete testis. The spermatocele lies outside the tunica vaginalis; therefore, on palpation it can be readily distinguished and separated from the testis. (From Lloyd-Davies, R.W., Parkhouse, H., Crow, J., et al. [1994]. *Color atlas of urology* [2nd ed.]. London: Wolfe Medical.)

viruses. Worldwide, however, filariasis is a major cause, especially with recent travel to tropical countries.[22] Other causes include trauma, torsion of the testicle or testicular appendage, and recent scrotal surgery. A man presenting with a hydrocele in his third or fourth decade needs careful evaluation for testicular cancer.[28]

Hydroceles vary in size, and most are asymptomatic. The most important feature on physical examination is a tense, smooth, scrotal mass that easily transilluminates. Transillumination, or holding a light behind the scrotum, can help distinguish a hydrocele from a hernia or a solid mass. Treatment includes watchful waiting in infants and for those older than 1 year; 75% of hydroceles resolve within 6 months.[27,28] Symptomatic or communicating hydroceles need definitive treatment. Treatment includes surgical resection, aspiration, and sclerotherapy (injection of a sclerosing agent into the scrotal sac [cystic dilation]) to excise the tunica vaginalis.[22]

Spermatoceles (epididymal cysts) are benign cystic collections of fluid of the epididymis located between the head of the epididymis and the testis. Spermatoceles are filled with a milky fluid containing sperm and are usually painless (Figure 34-7). Spermatoceles that cause significant pain or discomfort are excised. Both spermatoceles and epididymal cysts present clinically as discrete, firm, freely mobile masses distinct from the testis that may be transilluminated. Usually, however, spermatoceles are asymptomatic or produce mild discomfort that is relieved by scrotal support. Neither hydroceles nor spermatoceles are associated with infertility.

Cryptorchidism and Ectopy

Cryptorchidism is a group of abnormalities in which the testis fails to descend completely, whereas an **ectopic testis** has strayed from the normal pathway of descent. Ectopy may be caused by an abnormal connection at the distal end of the gubernaculum testis that leads the gonad to an abnormal position, usually at the superficial inguinal site. In cryptorchidism, the descent of one or both testes is arrested, with unilateral arrest occurring more often than bilateral arrest. The testes may remain in the abdomen, or testicular descent may be arrested in the inguinal canal or the puboscrotal junction. Cryptorchidism is a common congenital anomaly, with an incidence of approximately 3% in full-term infants. However, this rate increases significantly with low birth weight; for instance, the rate of cryptorchidism at 3 months has been found to be 7.7% for infants with birth weights less than 2 000 grams, 2.5% for birth weights of 2 000 to 2 500 grams, and 1.41% for birth weights of 2 500 grams or more.[29,30] The incidence of cryptorchidism in adults is 0.7 to 0.8%.[26] Cryptorchidism is commonly associated with vasal or epididymal abnormalities. These congenital anomalies affect about 33 to 66% of newborns with cryptorchidism. Other structural anomalies include posterior urethral valves (less than 5%), upper genital tract abnormalities (less than 5%), and hypospadias. The presence of both hypospadias and cryptorchidism raises the suspicion of mixed gonadal dysgenesis (intersex infant). It has been hypothesized that cryptorchidism may result from an absence or abnormality of the gubernaculum—a cordlike structure that extends from the lower pole of the testis to the scrotum; a congenital gonadal or dysgenetic defect that makes the testis insensitive to gonadotropins (a likely explanation for unilateral cryptorchidism); or lack of maternal gonadotropins (a likely explanation for bilateral cryptorchidism of prematurity).[26]

Mechanical possibilities include a short spermatic cord, fibrous bands or adhesions in the normal path of the testes, or a narrowed inguinal canal. Chromosomal studies do not support a genetic component. Physiological cryptorchidism, also called *retractile testis* or *migratory testis*, is an involuntary retraction of the testes out of the scrotum that occurs with excitement, physical activity, or exposure to cold and is caused by the small mass of prepubertal testis and the strength of the cremaster muscle. This phenomenon is common and self-limiting (descent occurs at puberty).

Physical examination discloses the absence of one or both testes in the scrotum and an atrophic scrotum on the affected side. If the undescended testis is in a vulnerable position, over the pubic bone for example, an individual may complain of severe pain secondary to trauma. The adult male with bilateral cryptorchidism may be infertile.

Testicular cancer also is a well-established complication of cryptorchidism. In men with a history of unilateral cryptorchidism, neoplasms also develop more commonly in the contralateral testis. This finding suggests that cryptorchidism affects the testes and is a process more significant than simply the position of the testis in childhood. The risk for testicular cancer is 35 to 50 times greater for men with cryptorchidism or a history of cryptorchidism than for the general male population. Because definite histological change occurs in the cryptorchid testis by 1 year of age, surgical correction is recommended around that age.[29,31] Treatment often begins with administration of gonadotropin-releasing hormone (GnRH) or human chorionic gonadotropin (hCG), hormones that may initiate descent and make surgery unnecessary. GnRH is available as a nasal spray in Europe and may enhance germ cell counts even when the testis does not descend.[31] If hormonal therapy is not successful (success rates range from 6 to 75%), the testis is located and moved surgically (orchiopexy) in young children or removed (orchiectomy) in adults and children more than 10 years of age.[26] The testis that is properly placed in the scrotum provides adequate hormonal function and gives the scrotum a normal appearance. A successful operation does not ensure fertility if the testis is congenitally defective. Approximately 20% of males with unilateral undescended testis remain infertile even though orchiopexy is performed by age 1 year; most individuals with treated or untreated bilateral testicular maldescent have poor fertility.

Torsion of the Testis and Testicular Appendages

In **torsion of the testis**, the testis rotates on its vascular pedicle, interrupting its blood supply (Figure 34-8). Torsion of the testis is one of several conditions that cause an acute scrotum, which is testicular pain and swelling. **Testicular appendages** include the appendix testis (a remnant of the müllerian duct) and the appendix epididymis (a remnant of the wolffian duct). Torsion of the appendages can also cause acute scrotum and be confused with testicular torsion, a urological emergency.

Torsion of the testis can occur at any age but is most common among neonates and adolescents, particularly at puberty.[27] Onset may be spontaneous or follow physical exertion or trauma. Torsion twists the arteries and veins in the spermatic cord, reducing or stopping circulation to the testis. Vascular engorgement and ischemia develop, causing scrotal swelling and pain not relieved by rest or scrotal support. Diagnostic testing includes urinalysis (to determine infection) and colour doppler ultrasonography.[26] Torsion of the testis is a surgical emergency. If it cannot be reduced manually (scrotal elevation), surgery must be performed within 6 hours after the onset of symptoms to preserve normal testicular function.

Orchitis

Orchitis is an acute inflammation of the testes (Figure 34-9) and is uncommon except as a complication of systemic infection or as an extension of an associated epididymitis[32]. Infectious organisms may reach the testes through the blood or the lymphatics or, most commonly, by ascent through the urethra, vas deferens, and epididymis. Most cases of orchitis are actually cases of epididymo-orchitis (inflammation of both the epididymis and testis). Occasionally in middle-aged men, a nonspecific, apparently noninfectious inflammatory process (called *granulomatous orchitis*) can occur, presumably a granulomatous response to spermatozoa.

Mumps is the most common infectious cause of orchitis and usually affects postpubertal males. The onset is sudden, occurring 3 to 4 days after the onset of parotitis. Signs and symptoms include high fever, reaching 40°C (104°F), marked prostration, bilateral or unilateral erythema, edema and tenderness of the scrotum, and leukocytosis. An acute hydrocele may develop. Urinary signs and symptoms, which accompany epididymitis, are absent. Atrophy with irreversible damage to spermatogenesis may result in 30% of affected testes. Bilateral orchitis does not affect hormonal function but may cause permanent sterility.

Treatment is supportive and includes bed rest, scrotal support, elevation of the scrotum, hot or cold compresses, and analgesic agents

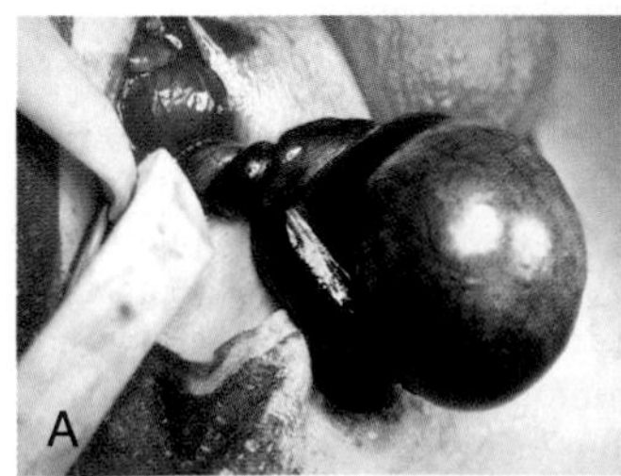

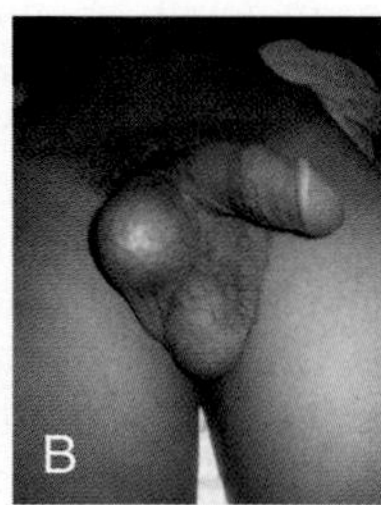

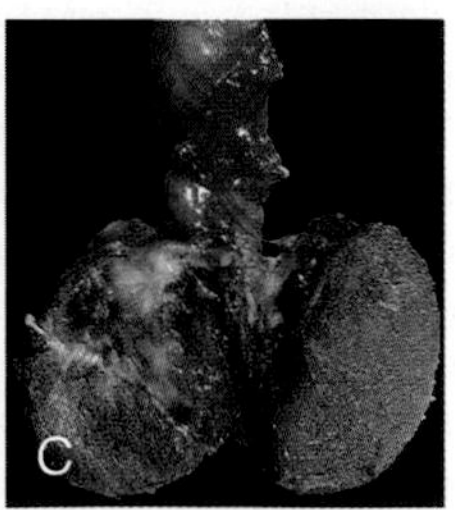

FIGURE 34-8 Torsion of the Testis. (**A** and **B**, from Kliegman, R.M., Stanton, B.F., Gemell, J.W., et al. [Eds.]. [2011]. *Nelson textbook of pediatrics* [19th ed.]. Philadelphia: Saunders; **C**, from Damjanov, I., & Linder, J. [Eds]. [1996]. *Anderson's pathology* [10th ed.]. St. Louis: Mosby.)

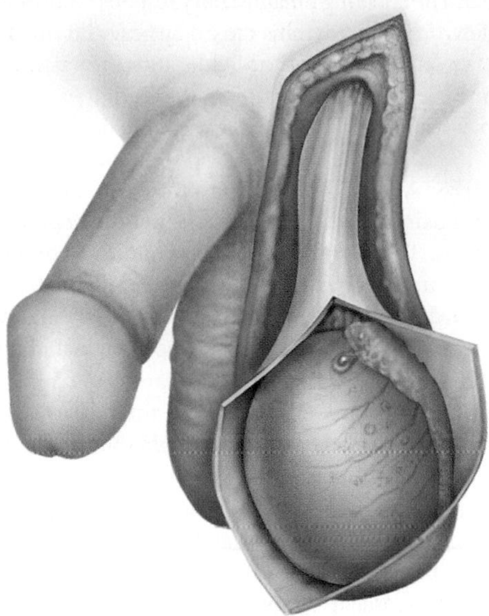

FIGURE 34-9 Depiction of Orchitis. (From Ball, J.W., Dains, J.E., Flynn, J.A., et al. [2015]. *Seidel's guide to physical examination* [8th ed.]. St. Louis: Mosby.)

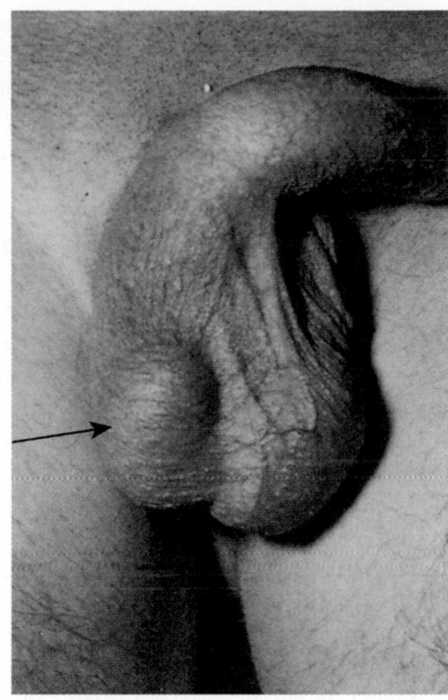

FIGURE 34-10 Testicular Tumour. (From Wolfe, J. [1984]. *400 self-assessment picture tests in clinical medicine.* London: Wolfe Medical.)

for relief of pain. If an acute hydrocele develops, it is aspirated. Testicular abscess usually requires orchiectomy (removal of the testis). Appropriate antimicrobial medications should be used for bacterial orchitis, and corticosteroids are indicated in proven cases of nonspecific granulomatous orchitis.

Cancer of the Testis

Testicular cancer is a highly treatable, usually curable cancer that most often develops in young and middle-aged men. For men with seminoma (all stages combined), the cure rate exceeds 90%. For men with low-stage seminoma or nonseminoma, the cure rate approaches 100%.[33] Overall, testicular cancers are uncommon, accounting for approximately 1% of all male cancers; yet they are the most common solid tumour of young adult men.[33] Cancer of the testis occurs most commonly in men between the ages of 15 and 35 years. The Canadian Cancer Society estimated that 1 100 Canadian men were diagnosed with testicular cancer in 2017. It also estimated that 41 Canadian men died of this disease in 2017.[34] Testicular cancer is more common in White men than in men of African or Asian ancestry, and occurs more often in men with a higher socioeconomic status.[33] Testicular tumours are slightly more common on the right side than on the left, a pattern that parallels the occurrence of cryptorchidism, and they are bilateral in 1 to 3% of cases (Figure 34-10).

PATHOPHYSIOLOGY Ninety percent of testicular cancers are germ cell tumours, arising from the male gametes. Germ cell tumours include seminomas (most common), embryonal carcinomas, teratomas, and choriosarcomas. Testicular tumours also can arise from specialized cells of the gonadal stroma (Leydig, Sertoli, granulosa, theca cells).

The cause of testicular neoplasms is unknown (see *Risk Factors:* Cancer of the Testis). A genetic predisposition is suggested by the fact that the incidence is higher among brothers, identical twins, and other close male relatives. Genetic predisposition is supported statistically, showing that the disease is relatively rare among Africans, Blacks, Asians, and native New Zealanders. Risk factors include history of cryptorchidism, abnormal testicular development, human immunodeficiency virus (HIV) and AIDS, Klinefelter's syndrome, and history of testicular cancer.[33]

RISK FACTORS

Cancer of the Testis

- HIV and AIDS
- History of cryptorchidism
- Abnormal testicular development
- Klinefelter's syndrome
- History of testicular cancer

CLINICAL MANIFESTATIONS Painless testicular enlargement commonly is the first sign of testicular cancer. Occurring gradually, it may be accompanied by a sensation of testicular heaviness or a dull ache in the lower abdomen. Occasionally acute pain occurs because of rapid growth, resulting in hemorrhage and necrosis. Ten percent of affected men have epididymitis, 10% have hydroceles, and 5% have breast enlargement (gynecomastia). The testicular mass is usually discovered by the individual or by his sexual partner. At the time of initial diagnosis, approximately 10% of individuals already have symptoms related to metastases. Lumbar pain also may be present and usually is caused by retroperitoneal node metastasis. Signs of metastasis to the lungs include cough, dyspnea, and bloody sputum (hemoptysis). Supraclavicular node involvement may cause difficulty swallowing (dysphagia) and neck swelling. With metastasis to the central nervous system, alterations in vision or mental status, papilledema, and seizures may be experienced.

EVALUATION AND TREATMENT An incorrect diagnosis at the initial examination occurs in as many as 25% of men with testicular cancer. Epididymitis and epididymo-orchitis are the most common misdiagnoses; others include hydrocele and spermatocele. Evaluation begins with careful physical examination, including palpation of the scrotal contents with the individual in the erect and supine positions. Signs of testicular cancer include abnormal consistency, induration, nodularity, or irregularity of the testis. The abdomen and lymph nodes are palpated to seek evidence of metastasis, and tumour type is identified after orchiectomy. The Canadian Cancer Society recommends that all males over the age of 15 should know how their testicles normally look and feel, and should talk to their primary health care provider if they notice any changes in their testicles.[35] Testicular biopsy is not recommended because it may cause dissemination of the tumour and increase the risk for local recurrence. Primary testicular cancer can be assessed rapidly and accurately by scrotal ultrasonography. Tumour markers are higher than normal in the presence of a tumour and may help detect a tumour that is too small to be palpated during physical examination or to be visualized on imaging. Radiological imaging and measurement of serum markers are used in clinical staging of the disease. Besides surgery, treatment involves radiation and chemotherapy singly or in combination. Factors influencing the prognosis include histological studies of the tumour stage of the disease and selection of appropriate treatment. Most individuals treated for cancer of the testis can expect a normal lifespan; some have persistent paresthesias, Raynaud phenomenon, or infertility. Approximately 10% of men treated for testicular cancer will experience a relapse; if the relapse is discovered early and treated, 99% can be cured. Orchiectomy does not affect sexual function.

Epididymitis

Epididymitis, or inflammation of the epididymis, generally occurs in sexually active young males (younger than 35 years) and is rare before puberty (Figure 34-11). In young men, the usual cause is a sexually transmitted microorganism, such as *N. gonorrhoeae* or *C. trachomatis*. Coliform bacteria are the common pathogens in other age groups.[36] Men who practise unprotected anal intercourse may acquire sexually transmitted epididymitis that results from infection with *Escherichia coli*, *Haemophilus influenzae*, tuberculosis, or *Cryptococcus* or *Brucella* species. In men older than 35 years, Enterobacteriaceae (intestinal bacteria) and *Pseudomonas aeruginosa* associated with urinary tract infections and prostatitis also may cause epididymitis. Epididymitis also may result from a chemical inflammation caused by the reflux of sterile urine into the ejaculatory ducts, which is then called chemical epididymitis.[36] It is associated with urethral strictures, congenital posterior valves, and excessive physical straining in which increased abdominal pressure is transmitted to the bladder. Chemical epididymitis is usually self-limiting and does not require evaluation or intervention unless it persists.

PATHOPHYSIOLOGY The pathogenic microorganism usually reaches the epididymis by ascending the vasa deferentia from an already infected urethra or bladder. The resulting inflammatory response causes symptoms of bacterial epididymitis. Epididymitis caused by heavy lifting or straining results from reflux of urine from the bladder into the vas deferens and epididymis. Urine is extremely irritating to the epididymis and initiates the inflammatory response called *chemical epididymitis*.

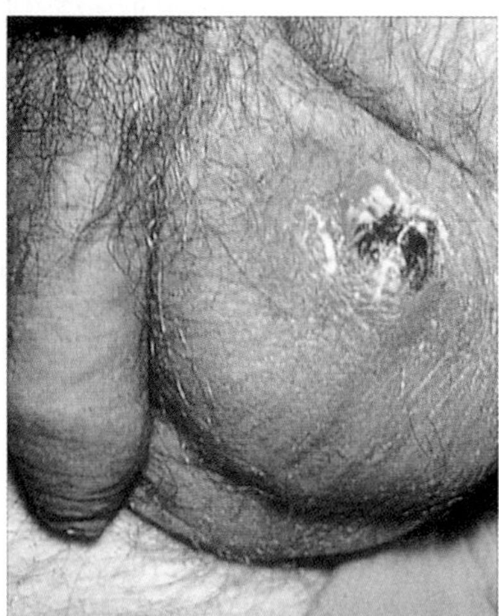

FIGURE 34-11 Epididymitis Secondary to Gonorrhea or Nongonococcal Urethritis. This infection spread to the testes, and rupture through the scrotal wall is threatened. (From Taylor, P.K. [1995]. *Diagnostic picture tests in sexually transmitted disease.* London: Mosby.)

CLINICAL MANIFESTATIONS The main symptom of epididymitis is scrotal or inguinal pain caused by inflammation of the epididymis and surrounding tissues. The pain is usually acute and severe. Flank pain may occur if, as the urethra passes over the spermatic cord, edematous swelling of the cord obstructs the urethra. The individual may have pyuria, bacteriuria, and a history of urinary symptoms, including urethral discharge. The scrotum on the involved side is red and edematous. The tail of the epididymis near the lower pole of the testis usually swells first; then swelling ascends to the head of the epididymis. The spermatic cord also may be swollen and tender.

Complications include abscess formation, infarction of the testis, recurrent infection, and infertility. Infarction is probably caused by thrombosis (obstruction by blood clots) of the prostatic vessels secondary to severe inflammation. Recurrent epididymitis may result from inadequate initial treatment or failure to identify or treat predisposing factors. Chronic epididymitis can cause scarring of the epididymal endothelium and infertility. Once scarring has occurred, treatment with antibiotics is ineffective because adequate antibiotic levels cannot be achieved within the epididymis.

EVALUATION AND TREATMENT A history of recent urinary tract infections or urethral discharge suggests the diagnosis of epididymitis. Common physical findings include a swollen, tender epididymis or testis located in the normal anatomical position with an intact same-side cremasteric reflex.[37] The relief of pain when the inflamed testis and epididymis are elevated (Prehn sign) is also diagnostic. Definitive diagnosis is based on culture or Gram stain of a urethral swab. Epididymal aspiration may be necessary to obtain a specimen, especially if the individual has been taking antibiotics and has sterile urine.

Treatment includes antibiotic therapy for the infection itself. Analgesics, ice, and scrotal elevation can provide symptomatic relief. If the individual does not steadily improve, he should be re-evaluated for possible complications, such as abscess formation, sepsis, or continued infection. Complete resolution of swelling and pain may take several weeks to months. The individual's sexual partner should be treated with antibiotics if the causative microorganism is a sexually transmitted pathogen.

QUICK CHECK 34-3

1. Why is a genetic predisposition suggested for testicular cancer?
2. Why is testicular torsion considered a urological emergency?
3. Why is epididymitis rare in prepubescent males?

Disorders of the Prostate Gland

Benign Prostatic Hyperplasia

Benign prostatic hyperplasia (BPH), also called benign prostatic hypertrophy, is the enlargement of the prostate gland (Figure 34-12). (Because the major prostatic changes are caused by hyperplasia, not hypertrophy, *benign prostatic hyperplasia* is the preferred term.) This condition becomes problematic when prostatic tissue compresses the urethra, where it passes through the prostate, resulting in frequency of LUTS. Similar to prostate cancer, BPH occurs more often in Westernized countries (e.g., Canada, the United States, and the United Kingdom). BPH appears to be more common in Black men than White men, and

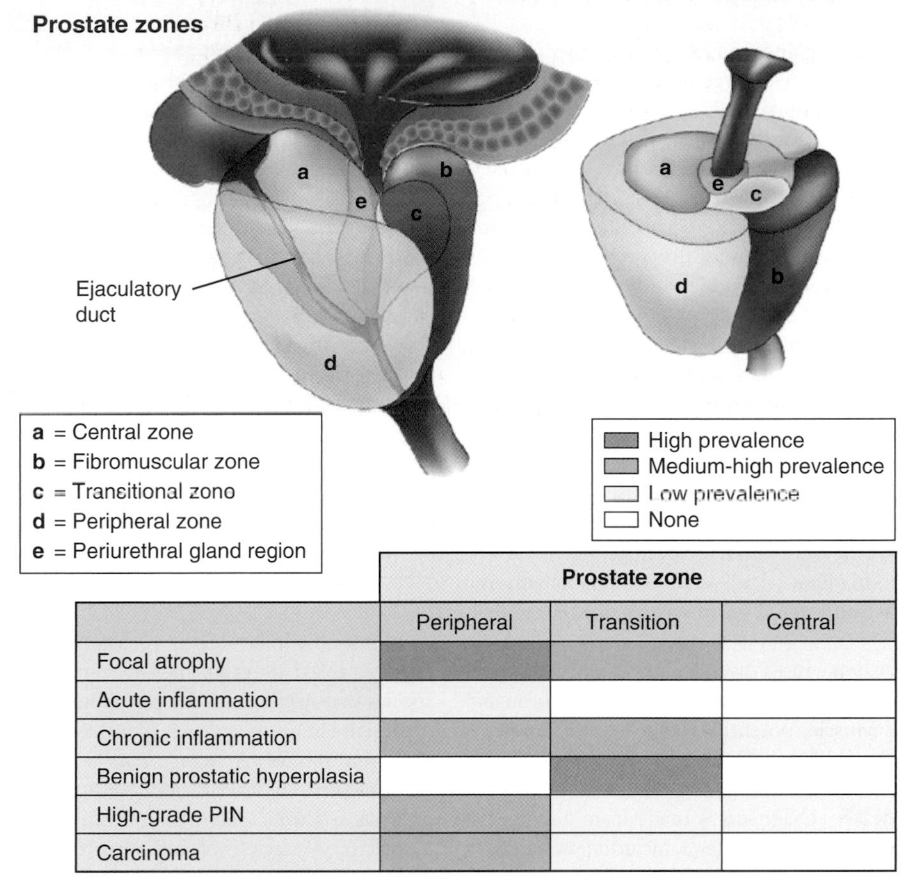

FIGURE 34-12 Prostate Zones, Benign Prostatic Hyperplasia (BPH), and Prostate Cancer Locations. Benign prostatic hyperplasia (BPH) occurs in the peripheral zone of the prostate gland that can enlarge (not shown). BPH nodules and atrophy are associated with inflammation in the transition zone. Most cancer lesions occur in the peripheral zone. Carcinoma can involve the central zone but rarely occurs in isolation, suggesting that prostatic intraepithelial neoplasia (PIN) lesions do not easily progress to carcinoma in this region. (Adapted from De Marzo, A.M., Platz, E.A., Sutcliffe, S., et al. [2007]. *Nat Rev Cancer, 7,* 256–269.)

family history may increase the risk. Being overweight or obese with central fat distribution (i.e., around the abdomen) increases the risk of developing BPH. The global prevalence is approximately 8% for men in their 40s, 50% for men in their 60s, and 80% for men in their 90s.[38] BPH is common and involves a complex pathophysiology with several endocrine and local factors and remodelled microenvironment. Its relationship to aging is well documented. At birth, the prostate is pea sized, and growth of the gland is gradual until puberty. At that time, there is a period of rapid development that continues until the third decade of life when the prostate reaches adult size (see Chapter 32). Around 40 to 45 years of age, benign hyperplasia begins and continues slowly until death. Although androgens, such as dihydrotestosterone (DHT), are necessary for normal prostatic development, their role in BPH remains unclear. Among all the androgen-metabolizing enzymes within the prostate, 5α-reductase is the most powerful. This reductase corresponds to an age-dependent DHT level. Therefore, although levels of 5α-reductase and DHT in the epithelium decrease with age, they remain constant in the stroma (microenvironment) of the prostate gland.

PATHOGENESIS Current causative theories of BPH focus on aging and levels and ratios of endocrine factors such as androgens and estrogens (androgen/estrogen ratio), the role of chronic inflammation, and the effects of autocrine/paracrine growth-stimulating and growth-inhibiting factors. These factors include insulinlike growth factors (IGFs), epidermal growth factors, fibroblast factors, and transforming growth factor-beta (TGF-β), and several others. Recent data show that human prostate stromal cells can actively contribute to the inflammatory process from the induction of inflammatory cytokines and chemokines[39] (see "Cancer of the Prostate," p. 879).

With aging, circulating androgens are associated with BPH and enlargement. Other effects related to estrogens include apoptosis, aromatase expression, and paracrine regulation that may be important for stimulating inflammation.[40] BPH is a multifactorial disease and not all men respond well to currently available treatments, suggesting factors are involved other than androgens. Testosterone, the primary circulating androgen in men, also can be metabolized through aromatase cytochrome P450 (CYP19) into the potent estrogen estradiol-17β. The prostate is an estrogen target tissue, and estrogens directly and indirectly affect growth and differentiation of the prostate. The precise role of endogenous and exogenous estrogens in directly affecting prostate growth and differentiation in the context of BPH is an understudied area. Estrogens and selective estrogen receptor modulators have been shown to promote or inhibit prostate proliferation, signifying potential roles in BPH.[41,42] Taken together, these interactions lead to an increase in prostate volume. The remodelled stroma promotes local inflammation with altered cytokine, reactive oxygen or nitrogen species, and chemoattractants.[43] The resultant increased oxygen demands of proliferating cells cause a local hypoxia that induces angiogenesis and changes to fibroblasts.

BPH begins in the periurethral glands, which are the inner glands or layers of the prostate. The prostate enlarges as nodules form and grow (nodular hyperplasia) and glandular cells enlarge (hypertrophy). The development of BPH occurs over a prolonged period of time, and changes within the urinary tract are slow and insidious.

CLINICAL MANIFESTATIONS As nodular hyperplasia and cellular hypertrophy progress, tissues that surround the prostatic urethra compress it, usually, but not always, causing bladder outflow obstruction. These symptoms are sometimes called the spectrum of LUTS. Symptoms include the urge to urinate often, some delay in starting urination, and decreased force of the urinary stream. As the obstruction progresses, often over several years, the bladder cannot empty all the urine, and the increasing volume leads to long-term urine retention. The volume of urine retained may be great enough to produce uncontrolled "overflow incontinence" with any increase in intra-abdominal pressure. At this stage, the force of the urinary stream is significantly reduced, and much more time is required to initiate and complete voiding.[44] Hematuria, bladder or kidney infection, bladder calculi, acute urinary retention hydroureter, hydronephrosis, and renal insufficiency are common complications.[44]

Progressive bladder distension causes diverticular outpouchings of the bladder wall. The ureters may be obstructed where they pass through the hypertrophied detrusor muscle, potentially causing hydroureter, hydronephrosis, and bladder or kidney infection.

EVALUATION AND TREATMENT Diagnosis is made from a medical history, physical examination, and laboratory tests, including urinalysis. Careful review of symptoms is necessary. Digital rectal examination (DRE) and measurement of PSA level are conducted to determine hyperplasia. PSA level alone, however, cannot confirm symptoms attributable to BPH because PSA level is elevated in both BPH and prostate cancer. Annual DREs are used to screen men older than 40 years for BPH, sooner in high-risk men.[45] If marked enlargement, moderate to severe symptoms, or complications are present, transrectal ultrasound (TRUS) is used to determine bladder and prostate volume and residual urine. Urinalysis, serum creatinine and blood urea nitrogen levels, uroflowmetry, postvoid residual (PVR) urine, pressure-flow study, cystometry, and cystourethroscopy are used to determine kidney and bladder function.[44] BPH has been treated successfully with medications. α_1-Adrenergic blockers (prazosin [Minipress] and tamsulosin [Flomax CR]) are used to relax the smooth muscle of the bladder and prostate. Antiandrogen agents, such as finasteride (Proscar), selectively block androgens at the prostate cellular level and cause the prostate gland to shrink.[46] By shrinking the prostate, these medications have been shown to improve BPH-related symptoms and reduce the risk for future urinary retention and BPH-related surgery. α_1-Adrenergic blockers do not affect PSA and have no effect on prostate cancer risk; however, antiandrogen agents lower PSA by 50% after 6 months of therapy.[47] Newer, minimally invasive treatments include interstitial laser treatment, transurethral radiofrequency procedures (such as transurethral needle ablation [TUNA]), and Cooled ThermoTherapy™.

Prostatitis

Prostatitis is an inflammation of the prostate. The incidence and prevalence of prostatitis is not known. Inflammation is usually limited to a few of the gland's excretory ducts.

Prostatitis syndromes have been classified by the US National Institutes of Health as (1) acute bacterial prostatitis (ABP), (2) chronic bacterial prostatitis (CBP), (3) chronic pelvic pain syndrome (CPPS), and (4) asymptomatic inflammatory prostatitis (Box 34-4). ABP and CBP are mostly caused by gram-negative Enterobacteriaceae and *Enterococci* species that originate in the gastro-intestinal flora. The most common organism is *E. coli*, which is identified in the majority of infections.[48] *Klebsiella* species, *P. aeruginosa*, and *Serratia* species are common gram-negative cultured microorganisms. Nonbacterial prostatitis (chronic prostatitis/chronic pelvic pain syndrome [CP/CPPS]) syndromes are caused by a cascade of inflammatory, immunological, neuroendocrine, and neuropathic mechanisms whereby the initiating cause is unknown.

BOX 34-4 NIH Classification of Prostatitis Syndrome

This system, developed for clinical research purposes, can be simplified for use in primary care practice (see text).

Category I, or acute bacterial prostatitis (ABP), is an acute infection of the prostate and is manifested by systemic signs of infection and positive urine culture.

Category II, or chronic bacterial prostatitis (CBP), is a chronic bacterial infection in which bacteria are received in significant numbers from a purulent prostatic fluid. These bacteria are thought to be the most common cause of recurrent urinary tract infection in men.

Category III, or chronic pelvic pain syndrome (CPPS), is diagnosed when no pathological bacteria can be localized to the prostate (culture of expressed prostatic fluid or postprostatic massage urine specimen) and is further divided into IIIa and IIIb. Category IIIa refers to inflammatory CPPS, where a significant number of white blood cells (WBCs) are localized to the prostate, whereas category IIIb is noninflammatory.

Category IV refers to asymptomatic inflammatory prostatitis in which bacteria or WBCs are localized to the prostate, but individuals are asymptomatic.

Bacterial prostatitis. Acute bacterial prostatitis (ABP, category I) is an ascending infection of the urinary tract that tends to occur in men between the ages of 30 and 50 years but is also associated with BPH in older men. Infection stimulates an inflammatory response in which the prostate becomes enlarged, tender, firm, or boggy. The onset of prostatitis may be acute and unrelated to previous illnesses, or it may follow catheterization or cystoscopy.

Clinical manifestations of ABP are those of urinary tract infection or pyelonephritis. Sudden onset of malaise, low back and perineal pain, high fever (up to 40°C [104°F]), and chills is common, as are dysuria, inability to empty the bladder, nocturia, and urinary retention. The individual also may have symptoms of lower urinary tract obstruction, such as slow, small, "narrowed" urinary stream, which may be a medical emergency. Acute inflammatory prostatic edema can compress the urethra, causing urinary obstruction. Systemic signs of infection include sudden onset of a high fever, fatigue, arthralgia, and myalgia. Prostatic pain may occur, especially when the individual is in an upright position, because the pelvic floor muscles tighten with standing and compression of the prostate gland occurs. Some individuals experience low back pain, painful ejaculation, and rectal or perineal pain. Palpation discloses an enlarged, extremely tender and swollen prostate that is firm, indurated, and warm to the touch.

Because ABP is usually associated with a bladder infection caused by the same microorganism, urine cultures disclose its identity. Prostatic massage may express enough secretions from the urethra for direct bacterial examination, but massage may be painful and increases the risk that the infection will ascend to adjacent structures or enter the bloodstream and cause septicemia.

To resolve the infection and control its spread, individuals may require antibiotics. In severe cases, the individual is hospitalized and treated with intravenous antibiotics, followed by oral antibiotics. Analgesics, antipyretics, bed rest, and adequate hydration are also therapeutic. Complications include urinary retention that resolves with antibiotic therapy; prostatic abscess that may rupture into the urethra, rectum, or perineum; epididymitis; bacteremia; and septic shock. Urinary retention requiring drainage is best managed with a suprapubic catheter; Foley catheterization is contraindicated during acute infection.

Chronic bacterial prostatitis (CBP, category II) is characterized by recurrent urinary tract symptoms and persistence of pathogenic bacteria (usually gram negative) in urine or prostatic fluid. This form of prostatitis is the most common recurrent urinary tract infection in men. Symptoms may be similar to those of an acute bladder infection: frequency, urgency, dysuria, perineal discomfort, low back pain, myalgia, arthralgia, and sexual dysfunction. The prostate may be only slightly enlarged or boggy, but it may be fibrotic because repeated infections can cause it to be firm and irregular in shape.

When the initial urine sample is bacteria-free, prostatic massage is used to express secretions. Subsequently, the first 10 mL of voided urine is collected and examined microscopically. Prostatic secretions showing more than 10 white blood cells (WBCs) per high-power field (hpf) and macrophages containing fat are indicative of bacterial infection; diagnosis is confirmed by culture. A pelvic X-ray or transurethral ultrasound (TRUS) may show prostatic calculi.

Treatment of CBP is difficult because it is often caused by prostatic calculi. Calculi are silent and are found in up to 50% of men with prostatitis, and infected calculi can serve as a source of bacterial persistence and relapsing urinary tract infection. Calculi harbour pathogens within the stone and, consequently, pathogens cannot be eradicated from the urinary tract. Permanent cure is achieved by surgical intervention.[49]

Chronic prostatitis/chronic pelvic pain syndrome. **Chronic prostatitis/chronic pelvic pain syndrome (CP/CPPS, category III)** is diagnosed when no pathogenic bacteria can be localized to the prostate, and is further subdivided into categories IIIa and IIIb (see Box 34-4). Category IIIa refers to inflammatory CPPS in which WBC count is elevated and localized to the prostate. Compared with category III, symptoms tend to be milder but are persistent and annoying. Presumably, noninfectious prostatitis or pain is caused by reflux of sterile urine into the ejaculatory ducts because of high-pressure voiding.[49] Reflux may be triggered by spasms of the external or internal sphincters. Category IIIb is noninflammatory. Category IV exists when individuals are asymptomatic but have an increase in bacteria and WBCs localized to the prostate. Microorganisms suspected of causing CP/CPPS include *E. coli*, *Enterobacter*, *P. aeruginosa*, and, a new suspect, *Helicobacter pylori*.[50]

Men with **nonbacterial prostatitis** may complain of pain or a dull ache that is continuous or spasmodic in the suprapubic, infrapubic, scrotal, penile, or inguinal area. Other symptoms are pain on ejaculation and urinary symptoms, such as frequency of urination. The prostate gland generally feels normal on palpation.

Nonbacterial prostatitis is a diagnosis of exclusion. Digital examination of the prostate, bacterial cultures of the urogenital tract, microscopic examination of expressed prostatic fluid, urethroscopy, and urodynamic studies are used to verify the diagnosis of nonbacterial prostatitis.

There is no generally accepted treatment for nonbacterial prostatitis. Hot sitz baths, bed rest, and pharmacological therapies, including anti-inflammatory medications, can relieve symptoms.

Cancer of the Prostate

Prostate cancer is the most commonly diagnosed, nonskin cancer in men in Canada, with an incidence rate of 99 per 100 000 persons.[51] The incidence varies greatly worldwide (Figure 34-13), but it is still considered to be the second most frequently diagnosed cancer in men and the sixth leading cause of death worldwide.[52] An estimated 1.1 million cases of prostate cancer were diagnosed worldwide in 2012, accounting for 15% of the cancers diagnosed in men. Almost 70% of diagnosed cases of prostate cancer (759 000) occurred in more developed regions.[53] Importantly, incidence rates vary by more than 25-fold worldwide, with the highest rates recorded mostly in developed countries in regions such as Oceania, Europe, and North America, largely because of wide

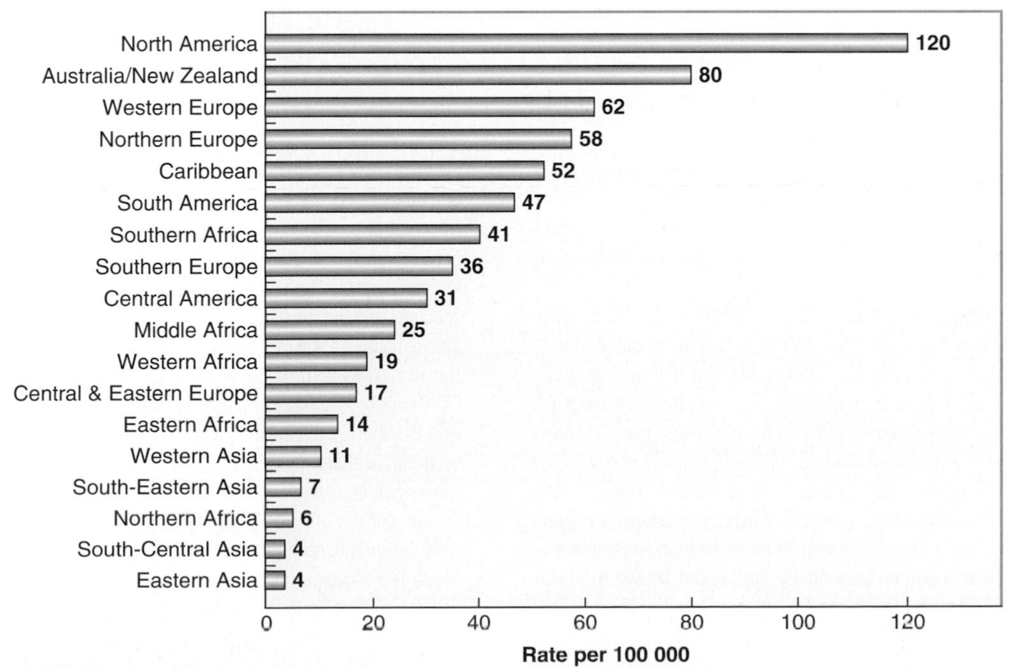

FIGURE 34-13 Selected World Population Age-Standardized (to the World Population) Incidence Rates of Prostate Cancer. (From Jemal, A., Center, M.M., DeSantis, C., et al. [2010]. *Cancer Epidemiol Biomarkers Prev, 19*[8], 1893–1907.)

use or overuse of PSA testing. Screening with PSA can amplify the incidence of prostate cancer by allowing detection of prostate lesions that, although meeting the pathological criteria for malignancy, may have low potential (e.g., latent, indolent, preclinical) for growth and metastasis. In countries with higher use of PSA testing, such as Canada, the United States, Australia, and the Nordic countries, trends in incidence rates follow similar patterns.[53]

Different from Western countries, incidence and death rates are rising in several Asian and Central and Eastern European countries, including Japan. Death rates have been decreasing in several countries, including Australia, Canada, the United Kingdom, the United States, Italy, and Norway, in part because of improved treatment. Males of African descent in the Caribbean region have the highest mortality from prostate cancer in the world.[53] Most cases of prostate cancer have a good prognosis even without treatment, but some cases are aggressive; the lifetime risk of dying of prostate cancer is 2.8%. Prostate cancer is rare before age 50 years, and very few men die from this cancer before 60 years of age. Indeed, more than 75% of all prostate cancer is diagnosed in men older than 65.[51] With aging, most of the androgen-metabolizing enzymes undergo significant alteration and older age, race (Black), and family history remain the well-established risk factors.

Dietary factors. Although evidence exists for a dietary role in prostate cancer, the epidemiological evidence is inconsistent.[54] The problem has been confounded by the lack of biomarkers for certain nutrients, difficulties in measuring and quantifying diet, and a limitation of clinical trials to study diet over time. Important are the effects of diet on signalling pathways, hormones, oxidative stress, and reactive oxygen species (ROS). Obesity seems to be negatively associated with more indolent prostate cancer and positively associated with more aggressive disease and a worse outcome.[55] The nutrients in the epidemiology of prostate cancer that have received the most attention include carotenoids, fat, vitamin E, vitamin D, calcium, and selenium (Box 34-5).

BOX 34-5 Summary of Diet for Prostate Cancer

- Lower rates of prostate cancer are found in countries whose residents consume a low-fat and high-vegetable diet. When men from a low-risk country move to North America and eat a Western diet, their rates of prostate cancer increase significantly. Inconclusive are the exact culprits that increase this risk, including fat and sugar intake.
- Obesity is linked to advanced and aggressive prostate cancer.
- High body mass index (BMI) is associated with more aggressive disease and a worse outcome.
- Calorie-dense or excessive carbohydrate intake and obesity, independent of dietary fat intake, may increase the risk of developing prostate cancer.
- Dietary fat may increase levels of androgens, increase oxidative stress, and increase reactive oxygen species (ROS).
- Monounsaturated fats may decrease the risk for prostate cancer.
- High levels of linoleic acid (found in corn oil) act as a proinflammatory eicosanoid, which is implicated in promotion of cell proliferation and angiogenesis as well as inhibition of apoptosis.
- The Western diet has increased omega-6 to omega-3 ratios and therefore is proinflammatory. Carcinogenic nitrosamines are formed after consumption of processed meat that contains nitrites and from heme iron present in large quantities of red meat.
- Even given the preceding knowledge, it is important to realize that studies showing an association between meat intake and prostate cancers have been largely inconclusive. Some studies reveal red meat is positively associated with increased prostate cancer risk with an association with more aggressive disease states. Despite some studies showing a 43% elevation in prostate cancer risk with high consumption of red meat, others show no association with prostate cancer risk.
- Although the role of red meat in prostate and breast cancer remains inconclusive, one explanation for the possible associations reported is the accumulation of carcinogens during the cooking process. Cooking meat at high temperatures produces heterocyclic amines and aromatic hydrocarbons that are carcinogenic.
- Vitamin E has long been considered a candidate for prostate cancer prevention based on in vitro and in vivo animal studies. Vitamin E belongs to the family of tocopherols and tocotrienols that exist as α, β, γ, and δ isoforms. Among these, δ-tocopherol is the major dietary isoform, whereas supplements contain α-tocopherol. Vitamin E is a fat-soluble vitamin obtained from vegetable oils, nuts, and egg yolk. It is a potent intracellular antioxidant known to inhibit peroxidation and DNA damage. The Alpha-Tocopherol, Beta-Carotene Cancer Prevention Study (ATBC) showed that supplementation with vitamin E could reduce the incidence of prostate cancer among men who smoked. In vitro studies demonstrate that α-tocopherol succinate induces cell cycle arrest in human prostate cancer cells (i.e., induces apoptosis) and inhibits the androgen receptor (AR). Mouse studies show vitamin E can inhibit the growth-promoting effects of a high-fat diet; however, vitamin E in combination with selenium does not reduce the incidence of prostate cancer in Lady mice models. A prospective large clinical trial, the Selenium and Vitamin E Cancer Prevention Trial (SELECT), showed no reduction in prostate cancer period prevalence but an increased risk for prostate cancer with vitamin E alone.
- Selenium is a trace mineral and exists in food as selenomethionine and selenocysteine. It is essential for the functioning of many antioxidant enzymes and proteins in the body. Humans receive selenium in their diet through plant (dependent on soil concentrations) and animal products. SELECT showed that neither selenium nor vitamin E, taken alone or together, helped to prevent prostate cancer.
- Vitamin D may play an important role in prostate cancer prevention.
- Soy anticancer properties include inhibition of cell proliferation and angiogenesis and reduction in prostate-specific antigen (PSA) and AR levels. Countries whose residents have a high intake of soy have much lower rates of prostate cancer.
- Tomatoes or tomato products ingested daily seem to reduce prostate cancer risk. In vitro studies show lycopene found in tomatoes inhibits DNA strand breaks. Unresolved is whether lycopene itself or a metabolic product is responsible for its biological effect. In clinical studies tomato paste, which is high in lycopene, reduced plasma PSA levels in those men with benign prostatic hyperplasia. Lycopene administration is associated with cell cycle arrest (apoptosis) and growth factor signalling. In 2007 the US Food and Drug Administration evaluated 13 available studies and found the relationship between lycopene and reduced risk for prostate cancer inadequate.
- Vegetables including broccoli, cabbage, cauliflower, Brussels sprouts, Chinese cabbage, and turnips (all crucifers) may be protective (several epidemiological studies) against prostate cancer. In particular, a diet high in broccoli reduced cancer risk. By contrast, four studies revealed no cancer-preventive effects. Cruciforms have anticancer properties mediated by the phytochemicals phenethyl isothiocyanate, sulforaphane, and indole-3-carbinol. Sulforaphane is a naturally occurring isothiocyanate that was first isolated in broccoli. It protects against carcinogen-induced cancer in many rodents. Mice given 240 mg of broccoli sprouts per day showed a significant reduction in growth of prostate cancer cells. Sulforaphane treatment lowered AR protein and gene expression.
- Green tea contains polyphenols, including epigallocatechin gallate (EGCG). Green tea consumption has been associated with a reduced incidence of several cancers, including prostate cancer. Green tea consumed within a balanced controlled diet in humans improved overall antioxidant potential. The potential anticancer effect of green tea from in vitro and experimental studies shows these compounds bind directly to carcinogens and induce phase

BOX 34-5 Summary of Diet for Prostate Cancer—cont'd

II enzymes that inhibit heterocyclic amines. EGCG administration decreased NF-κβ activity. Green tea was shown to inhibit insulinlike growth factor 1 (IGF-1) and increase IGF-binding protein 3 (IGFBP3), leading to inhibition of prostate cancer development and progression. Yet, in two small randomized studies in individuals with high-grade prostatic neoplasia, it showed no effects. However, treatment with a mixture of bioactive compounds that share molecular anticarcinogenic targets may enhance the effect on these targets at low concentrations of individual compounds.

- Epidemiological studies have consistently shown that regular consumption of fruits and vegetables is strongly associated with reduced risk of developing chronic diseases, such as cancer. It is now accepted that the actions of any specific phytonutrient alone do not explain the observed health benefits of diets rich in fruits and vegetables; also, clinical trials demonstrated that consumption of phytonutrients did not show consistent preventive effects. Synergistic inhibition of prostate cancer cell growth has been evident when using combinations of low concentrations of various carotenoids or carotonoids with retinoic acid and the active metabolite of vitamin D. Combinations of several carotenoids (e.g., lycopene, phytoene, and phytofluene) or carotenoids and polyphenols (e.g., carnosic acid and curcumin) and/or other compounds (e.g., vitamin E) synergistically inhibit the androgen receptor activity and activate the electrophile/antioxidant response element (EpRE/ARE) transcription system. The activation of EpRE/ARE is up to fourfold higher than the sum of activities of single ingredients.
- Examples of important potential processes that can be targeted in the regulation of tumourigenesis include cholesterol synthesis and metabolites, ROS and hypoxia, macrophage activation and conversion, indoleamine 2,3-dioxygenase regulation of dendritic cells, vascular endothelial growth factor regulation of angiogenesis, fibrosis inhibition, and endoglin and Janus kinase signalling.
- Curcumin has anticarcinogenic potential with well-characterized anti-inflammatory, antiangiogenic, and antioxidant properties. Recent studies report curcumin modulates the Wingless signalling pathway (Wnt) that supports its antiproliferative potential. Curcumin is characteristic of regulating multiple targets, a desirable feature in current medication design and medication development. Together with its potential in treating castration-resistant prostate cancer and its safety profile, this feature enables curcumin to serve as an ideal compound for the design and syntheses of agents with improved potential for enhancing clinical therapies used to treat prostate cancer.
- Overall, multiple signalling pathways are involved in prostate cancer development and progression, many of which are affected by dietary and lifestyle factors.

References

Alexander, D. D., Mink, P. J., Cushing, C. A., et al. (2010). A review and meta-analysis of prospective studies of red and processed meat intake and prostate cancer. *Nutrition Journal, 9,* 50. doi:10.1186/1475-2891-9-50.

Astorg, P. (2004). Dietary N-6 and N-3 polyunsaturated fatty acids and prostate cancer risk: A review of epidemiological and experimental evidence. *Cancer Causes and Control, 15*(4), 367–386. doi:10.1023/B:CACO.0000027498.94238.a3.

Beier, R., Bürgin, A., Kiermaier, A., et al. (2000). Induction of cyclin E-cdk2 kinase activity, E2F-dependent transcription and cell growth by Myc are genetically separable events. *The EMBO Journal, 19*(21), 5813–5823. doi:10.1093/emboj/19.21.5813.

Casey, S. C., Amedei, A., Aquilano, K., et al. (2015). Cancer prevention and therapy through the modulation of the tumor microenvironment. *Seminars in Cancer Biology, 35*(Suppl.), S199–S223. doi:10.1016/j.semcancer.2015.02.007.

Chen, Q. H. (2015). Curcumin-based anti-prostate cancer agents. *Anti-cancer Agents in Medicinal Chemistry, 15*(2), 138–156.

Dagnelie, P. C., Schuurman, A. G., Goldbohm, R. A., et al. (2004). Diet, anthropometric measures and prostate cancer risk: A review of prospective cohort and intervention studies. *BJU International, 93*(8), 1139–1150. doi:10.1111/j.1464-410X.2004.04795.x.

Demark-Wahnefried, W., & Moyad, M. A. (2007). Dietary intervention in the management of prostate cancer. *Current Opinion in Urology, 17*(3), 168–174. doi:10.1097/MOU.0b013e3280eb10fc.

Freedland, S. J., & Aronson, W. J. (2005). Obesity and prostate cancer. *Urology, 65*(3), 433–439. doi:10.1016/j.urology.2004.08.035.

Giovannucci, E., Liu, Y., Platz, E. A., et al. (2007). Risk factors for prostate cancer incidence and progression in the health professionals follow-up study. *International Journal of Cancer, 121*(7), 1571–1578. doi:10.1002/ijc.22788.

Greenwald, P. (2004). Clinical trials in cancer prevention: Current results and perspectives for the future. *The Journal of Nutrition, 134*(12, Suppl.), 3507S–3512S.

Hill, P., Wynder, E. L., Barbaczewski, L., et al. (1979). Diet and urinary steroids in black and white North American men and black South African men. *Cancer Research, 39*(12), 5101–5105.

Kim, D. J., Gallagher, R. P., Hislop, T. G., et al. (2000). Premorbid diet in relation to survival from prostate cancer (Canada). *Cancer Causes and Control, 11*(1), 65–77.

Kobayashi, N., Barnard, R. J., Henning, S. M., et al. (2006). Effect of altering dietary omega-6/omega-3 fatty acid ratios on prostate cancer membrane composition, cyclooxygenase-2, and prostaglandin E2. *Clinical Cancer Research, 12*(15), 4660–4670. doi:10.1158/1078-0432.CCR-06-0459.

Kolonel, L. N. (2001). Fat, meat, and prostate cancer. *Epidemiologic Reviews, 23*(1), 72–81.

Kristal, A. R., Arnold, K. B., Schenk, J. M., et al. (2008). Dietary patterns, supplement use, and the risk of symptomatic benign prostatic hyperplasia: Results from the prostate cancer prevention trial. *American Journal of Epidemiology, 167*(8), 925–934. doi:10.1093/aje/kwm389.

Linnewiel-Hermoni, K., Khanin, M., Danilenko, M., et al. (2015). The anti-cancer effects of carotenoids and other phytonutrients resides in their combined activity. *Archives of Biochemistry and Biophysics, 572,* 28–35. doi:10.1016/j.abb.2015.02.018.

Lloyd, J. C., Antonelli, J. A., Phillips, T. E., et al. (2010). Effect of isocaloric low fat diet on prostate cancer xenograft progression in a hormone deprivation model. *The Journal of Urology, 183*(4), 1619–1624. doi:10.1016/j.juro.2009.12.003.

Matsumara, K., Tanaka, T., Kawashima, H., et al. (2008). Involvement of the estrogen receptor beta in genistein-induced expression of p21 (waf1/cip1) in PC-3 prostate cancer cells. *Anticancer Research, 28*(2A), 709–714.

Ngo, T. H., Barnard, R. J., Cohen, P., et al. (2003). Effect of isocaloric low-fat diet on human LAPC-4 prostate cancer xenografts in severe combined immunodeficient mice and the insulin-like growth factor axis. *Clinical Cancer Research, 9*(7), 2734–2743.

Ngo, T. H., Barnard, R. J., Tymchuk, C. N., et al. (2002). Effect of diet and exercise on serum insulin, IGF-1, and IGFBP-1 levels and growth of LNCaP cells in vitro (United States). *Cancer Causes and Control, 13*(10), 929–935.

Ni, J., & Yeh, S. (2007). The roles of alpha-vitamin E and its analogues in prostate cancer. *Vitamins and Hormones, 76,* 493–518. doi:10.1016/S0083-6729(07)76019-3.

Punnen, S., Hardin, J., Cheng, I., et al. (2011). Impact of meat consumption, preparation, and mutagens on aggressive prostate cancer. *PLoS ONE, 6*(11), e27711. doi:10.1371/journal.pone.0027711.

Rodriguez, C., Freedland, S. J., Deka, A., et al. (2007). Body mass index, weight change, and risk of prostate cancer in the Cancer Prevention Study II Nutrition Cohort. *Cancer Epidemiology, Biomarkers and Prevention, 16*(1), 63–69. doi:10.1158/1055-9965.EPI-06-0754.

Salem, S., Salahi, M., Mohseni, M., et al. (2011). Major dietary factors and prostate cancer risk: A prospective multicenter case-control study. *Nutrition and Cancer, 63*(1), 21–27. doi:10.1080/01635581.2010.516875.

Sinha, R., Park, Y., Graubard, B. I., et al. (2009). Meat and meat-related compounds and risk of prostate cancer in a large prospective cohort study in the United States. *American Journal of Epidemiology, 170*(9), 1165–1177. doi:10.1093/aje/kwp280.

Teiten, M., Gaascht, F., Cronauer, M., et al. (2011). Anti-proliferative potential of curcumin in androgen dependent prostate cancer cells occurs through modulation of the Wingless signaling pathway. *International Journal of Oncology, 38*(3), 603–611. doi:10.3892/ijo.2011.905.

Wang, P., Wang, B., Chung, S., et al. (2014). Increased chemopreventive effect by combining arctigenin, green tea polyphenol and curcumin in prostate and breast cancer cells. *RSC Advance, 4*(66), 35242–35250. doi:10.1039/C4RA06616B.

Wright, J. L., Neuhouser, M. L., Lin, D. W., et al. (2011). AMACR polymorphisms, dietary intake of red meat and dairy and prostate cancer risk. *The Prostate, 71*(5), 498–506. doi:10.1002/pros.21267.

Zhou, D. Y., Ding, N., Du, Z. Y., et al. (2014). Curcumin analogues with high activity for inhibiting human prostate cancer cell growth and androgen receptor activation. *Molecular Medicine Reports, 10*(3), 1315–1322. doi:10.3892/mmr.2014.2380.

Hormones. Prostate cancer develops in an androgen-dependent epithelium and is usually androgen sensitive. Androgens are synthesized not only in the testis, accounting for 50 to 60% of the total testosterone in the prostate, but also in the prostate gland itself. In a process called **intraprostatic conversion**, the hormone dehydroepiandrosterone (DHEA) produced by the adrenal glands[56] is converted to testosterone and then into DHT in the prostate (Figure 34-14). Additionally, prostate cancer cells have been reported to make androgens from cholesterol (i.e., de novo).[57] However, these overall relative contributions from intratumoural sources remain to be determined. Population studies have not, however, provided clear and convincing patterns involving associations between circulating (e.g., not tissue concentrations) hormone concentrations and prostate cancer risk.[58] Thus, there is universal agreement that androgens are important for prostatic growth, development, and maintenance of tissue balance; however, their role in cancer is controversial. Evidence in support of the involvement of androgens in prostate cancer development is derived from clinical trials with 5α-reductase inhibitors. However, the involvement of 5α-reductase, which is critical in androgen activity in the prostate, is contradictory and inconsistent[58,59] (see Figure 34-14). A prevention study has provided some of the strongest hormonal data with the medication finasteride (Apo-Finasteride), which inhibits 5α-reductase. The 7-year intervention study reduced prostate cancer risk in healthy men by about 25%.[60] Important, however, was that more high-grade tumours were found in those men who developed prostate cancer while on the medication. In men younger than 50 years, circulating levels of androgens and estrogens appear to be higher in men of African descent than in North American men of European descent.

Despite the well-documented importance of androgens, their pathophysiological process in prostate diseases is incomplete.[61] Androgens also are metabolized to estrogens (Figure 34-14, *B*) through the action of the enzyme aromatase, and a growing body of evidence implicates estrogens in the etiology of prostate disease (see the following "Pathogenesis" section).

Vasectomy. Vasectomy has been identified as a possible risk factor for prostate cancer in both case-controlled studies and cohort studies.[62,63]

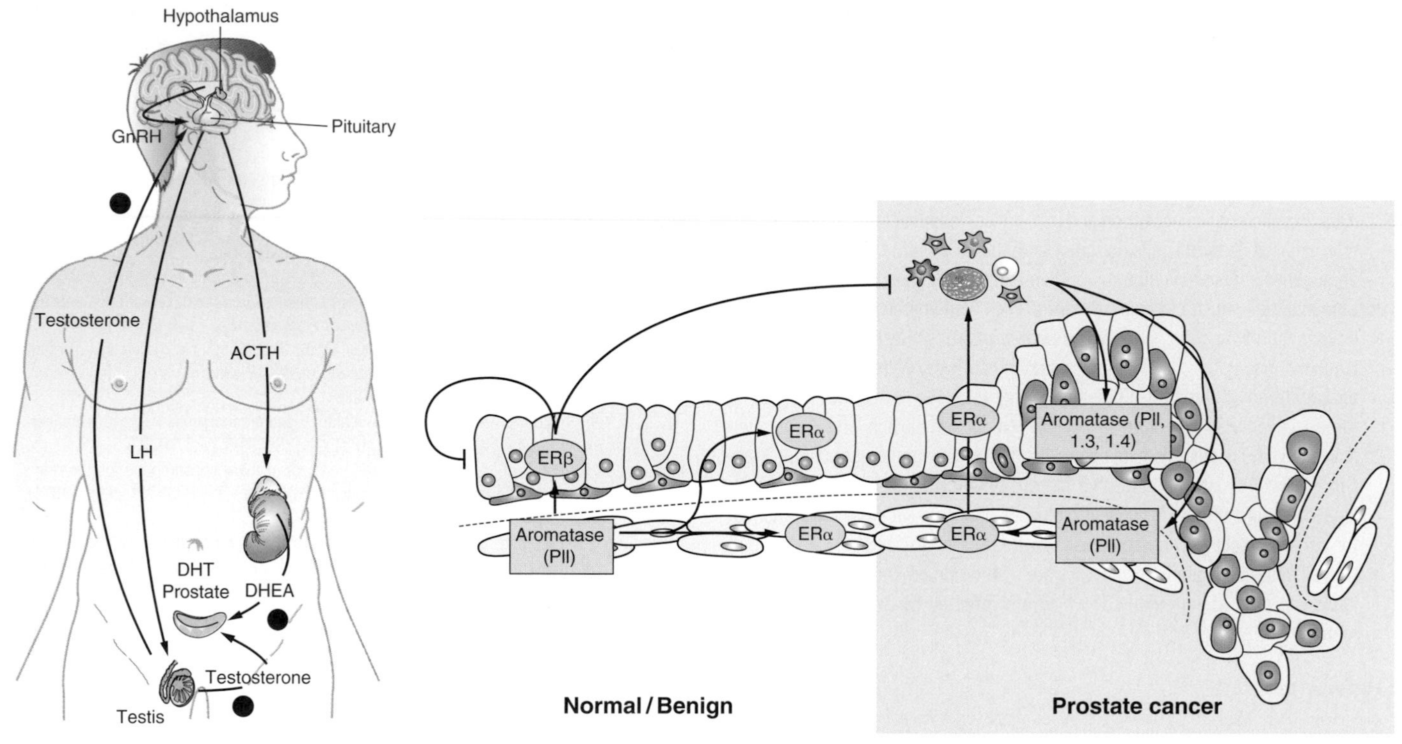

FIGURE 34-14 Sources of Androgens and Aromatase and Estrogen Signalling in the Prostate. **A,** Body sources of androgens in the prostate gland. Hypothalamic GnRH causes the release of LH from the anterior pituitary gland. LH stimulates the testes to produce testosterone, which then accumulates in the blood. Pituitary ACTH release stimulates the adrenal glands, which secrete the androgen precursor DHEA into the blood. DHEA is converted into testosterone and then into DHT in the prostate. **B,** Aromatase and estrogen signalling in the prostate. In normal and benign tissue, aromatase is expressed within the stroma and regulated by promoter PII. Estrogen then exerts its effects in an autocrine fashion through the stromal ERα receptor and also in a paracrine fashion through both ERα and ERβ receptors. With prostate cancer, aromatase is now expressed within the tumour cells and in stromal cells, and regulated by aromatase promoters 1.3, 1.4, and PII. Thus estrogen exerts its effects in an autocrine way through stromal and epithelial ERα and ERβ. Consequently, the increased levels of estrogen and abnormal ERα signalling promote inflammation, which increases aromatase expression and the development of a positive feedback cycle. Inflammation drives aromatase expression, thus increasing estrogen, which in turn promotes further inflammation. *ACTH,* Adrenocorticotropic hormone; *DHEA,* dehydroepiandrosterone; *DHT,* dihydrotestosterone; *ERα,* estrogen receptor alpha; *ERβ,* estrogen receptor beta; *GnRH,* gonadotropin-releasing hormone; *LH,* luteinizing hormone. (**A,** adapted from Labrie, F. [2011]. *Nat Rev Urol, 8,* 73–80; **B,** from Ellem, S.J., & Risbridger, G.P. [2010]. *J Steroid Biochem Mol Biol, 118*[4–5], 246–251.)

Three mechanisms by which vasectomy could increase risk are (1) elevation of circulating androgens; (2) activation of immunological mechanisms involving antisperm antibodies; and (3) reduction of seminal fluid levels of 5α-DHT, the active metabolite of testosterone in the prostate, in vasectomized men. These results suggest an elevation of circulating free testosterone level following vasectomy. However, with these combined mechanisms, it is unlikely that vasectomy plays a causal role.[64]

Chronic inflammation. A 5-year longitudinal study of the influence of chronic inflammation and prostate cancer was undertaken with 144 men, 33 of whom presented with chronic inflammation in their initial biopsy.[65] Biopsies revealed prostatic hyperplasia and proliferative inflammatory atrophy (PIA) in those with chronic inflammation. Upon repeat biopsy, 29 new cancers were diagnosed, representing a new cancer incidence of 20%.[65] In contrast, of the 33 men initially showing no inflammation, 2 (6%) were found to have adenocarcinoma. Certain metabolic comorbidities, including obesity, diabetes, sleep apnea, and erectile dysfunction, may be linked to both BPH and inflammation.[66] The causes of chronic inflammation are emerging (possible causes are shown in Figure 34-15). Thus, chronic inflammation may be an important risk factor for prostatic adenocarcinoma.[67] Chronic inflammation involves autocrine/paracrine growth-stimulating and growth-inhibiting factors. These factors include IGFs, epidermal growth factors, fibroblast factors, and TGF-β, as well as several others. Recent data show that human prostate stromal cells can actively contribute to the inflammatory process from the induction of inflammatory cytokines and chemokines.[39,68] Importantly, a continuous input from TGF-β and IGF in the tumour microenvironment or stroma will result in cancer progression. Understanding of these events can help prevention, diagnosis, and therapy of prostate cancer[68] (Figure 34-16).

Genetic and epigenetic factors. Other possible causes are those of genetic predisposition (familial and hereditary forms). Genetic studies suggest that strong familial predisposition may be responsible for 5 to 10% of prostate cancers.[1] Compared with men with no family history, those with one first-degree relative with prostate cancer have twice the risk, and those with two first-degree relatives have five times the risk.[69] Germline mutations in the breast cancer predisposition gene 2 (*BRCA2*) are the genetic events known to date that confer the highest risk for prostate cancer (8.6-fold in men 65 years of age and younger). Although the role of *BRCA2* and *BRCA1* in prostate tumourigenesis remains unrevealed, deleterious mutations in both genes have been associated with more aggressive disease and poor clinical outcomes.[70,71] Men with *BRCA2* (tumour suppressor) germline mutations have a 20-fold increase in risk for prostate cancer. Using previously estimated population carrier frequencies, investigators have recently found that deleterious *BRCA1* mutations confer a relative risk for prostate cancer of approximately 3.75-fold, translating to 8.6% cumulative risk by age 65.[72] A common type of somatic mutation that develops into chromosomal rearrangements

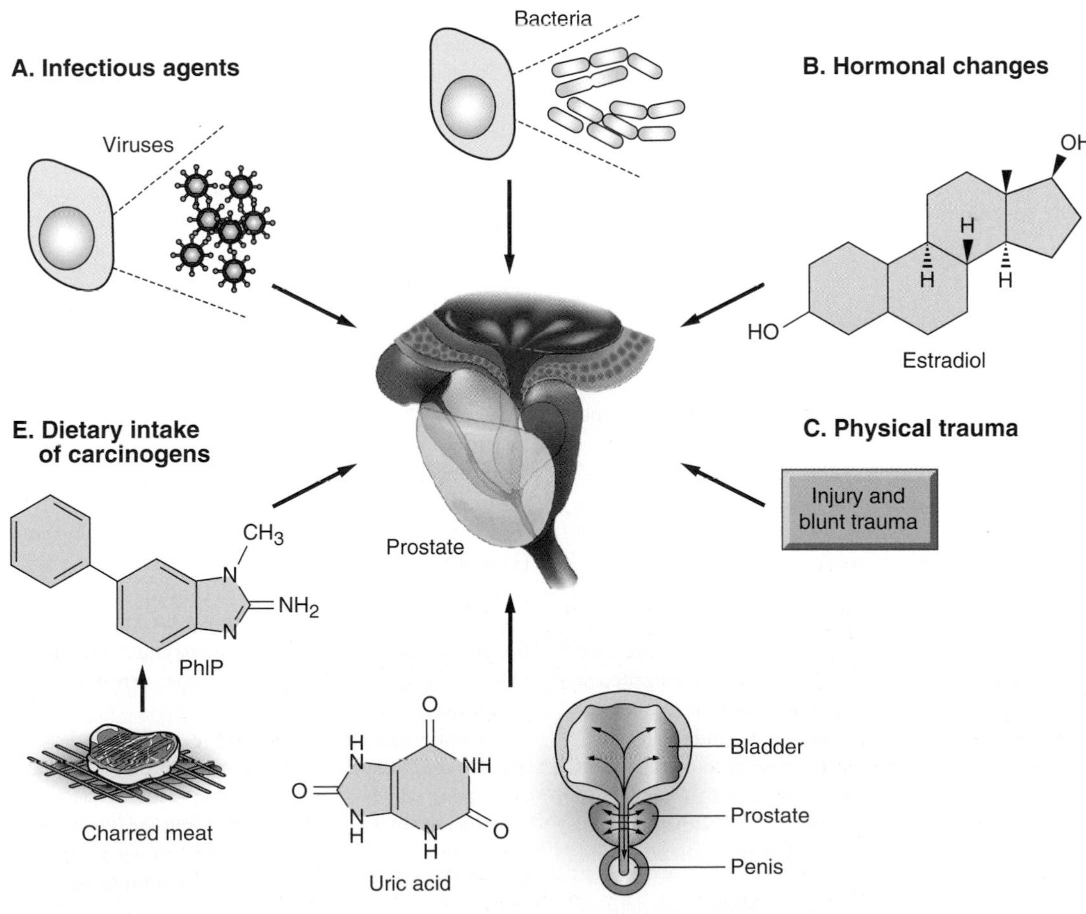

FIGURE 34-15 **Possible Causes of Prostate Inflammation.** **A,** Infection, including viruses, bacteria, fungi, and parasites. **B,** Hormones, for example, estrogen at key times during development. **C,** Physical trauma, any type of blunt physical injury. **D,** Urine reflex. **E,** Certain dietary factors (see text).

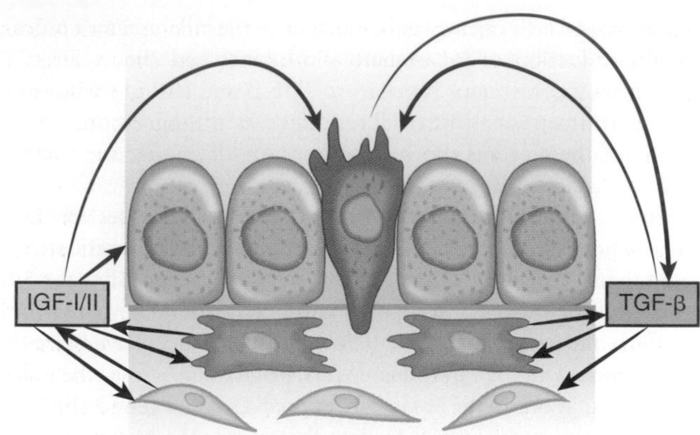

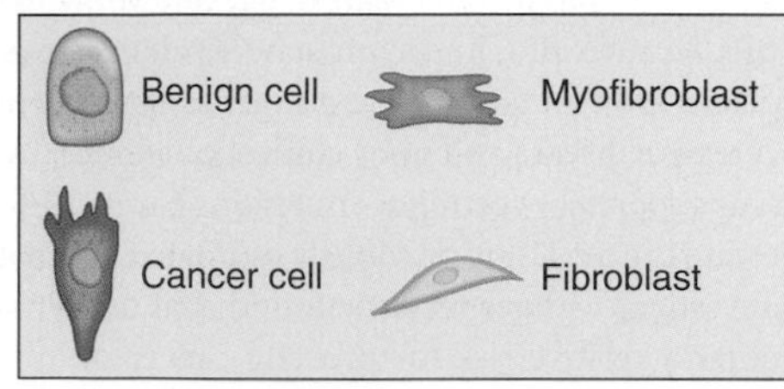

FIGURE 34-16 Working Model Stromal–Epithelial Interaction in Prostate Cancer Development and Progression. Normally, signalling events between transforming growth factor-beta (*TGF-β*) and insulinlike growth factor (*IGF*) are tightly regulated, keeping the epithelial cells under homeostatic balance. TGF-β binds to receptors on the cell surface known as receptor type I (TBR-I) and type II (TBR-II). A reduction in TBRs in the stromal cells will result in an increase in IGF production. The increase in IGF has a proliferative effect on the prostate epithelial cells (which have already undergone a cancer initiation process as a result of the hormones testosterone and estradiol). TGF-β and IGF in the stromal cells adjacent to prostate epithelial cells will perpetuate a vicious cycle to promote cancer progression. (Adapted from Lee, C., Jia, Z., Rahmatpanah, F., et al. [2014]. *Biomed Res Int, 2014*, 502093.)

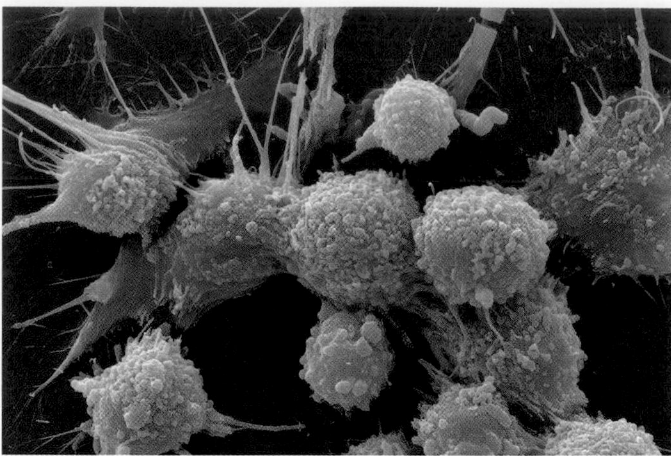

FIGURE 34-17 Photomicrograph of Prostate Cancer Cells. Pink ruffled cells are prostate cancer cells. (Dr. Gopal Murti/Science Source.)

BOX 34-6 Determining the Grade of Prostate Cancer With the Gleason Score

Grade 1. The cancer cells closely resemble normal cells. They are small, uniform in shape, evenly spaced, and well differentiated (i.e., they remain separate from one another).

Grade 2. The cancer cells are still well differentiated, but they are arranged more loosely and are irregular in shape and size. Some of the cancer cells have invaded the neighbouring prostate tissue.

Grade 3. This grade is the most common. The cells are less well differentiated (some have fused into clumps) and are more variable in shape.

Grade 4. The cells are poorly differentiated and highly irregular in shape. Invasion of the neighbouring prostate tissue has progressed further.

Grade 5. The cells are undifferentiated. They have merged into large masses that no longer resemble normal prostate cells. Invasion of the surrounding tissue is extensive.

is the *ETS* gene. The most common epigenetic alteration in prostate cancer is hypermethylation of the glutathione-*S*-transferase (*GSTP1*) gene located on chromosome 11. More than 30 independent, peer-reviewed studies have reported a consistently high sensitivity and specificity of *GSTP1* hypermethylation in prostatectomy or biopsy tissue.[73] There is no clear evidence of a causal link between BPH and prostate cancer, even though they may often occur together. Variations in several other genes related to inflammatory pathways might affect the probability of developing prostate cancer.

PATHOGENESIS More than 95% of prostatic neoplasms are adenocarcinomas,[74] and most occur in the periphery of the prostate (see Figures 34-12 and 34-17). Prostatic adenocarcinoma is a heterogeneous group of tumours with a diverse spectrum of molecular and pathological characteristics and, therefore, diverse clinical behaviours and challenges.[75] The biological aggressiveness of the neoplasm appears to be related to the degree of differentiation rather than the size of the tumour (Box 34-6). Several genetic alterations have been found for prostate carcinoma, including acquired genomic structural changes, somatic mutations, and epigenetic alterations.[76]

Hormonal factors. Just as the testicles are the male equivalent of the female ovaries, the prostate is the male equivalent of the female uterus; in both situations, they originate from the same embryonic cells. This correspondence may be important in understanding the role of the associated hormones testosterone, DHT, and estrogens in prostate cancer development. Testicular testosterone synthesis and serum testosterone levels fall as men age, but the levels of estradiol do not decline, remaining unchanged or increasing with age.[77,78] The relationship between hormones and the pathophysiology of prostate carcinogenesis is incomplete and controversial.[79] The main issues and controversies include (1) sources of androgen production outside of the testes, or extratesticular sources (e.g., from adrenal DHEA and from prostate tissue cholesterol [de novo] itself); (2) the role of prostatic androgen receptor (AR); (3) the role of estrogens, aromatase enzyme, and the estrogen receptors (ERα and ERβ); and (4) the role of the surrounding microenvironment or stroma.

Prostate cancer is considered a hormone-dependent disease; cell growth and survival of early-stage prostate cancer can respond to androgens, which is the background evidence for androgen-deprivation therapy (ADT). However, evidence thus far is lacking to associate *plasma* androgens with prostate cancer progression. Prostatic tissue has the ability to produce its own steroids, including androgens and estrogens.[80] Therefore, the local tissue levels of sex steroids have become a major focus of intraprostatic hormonal profiles. Prostate tissue contains many metabolizing enzymes for the local production of active androgens and estrogens. Carcinogenesis can alter these intraprostatic enzymes and alter the normal balance.

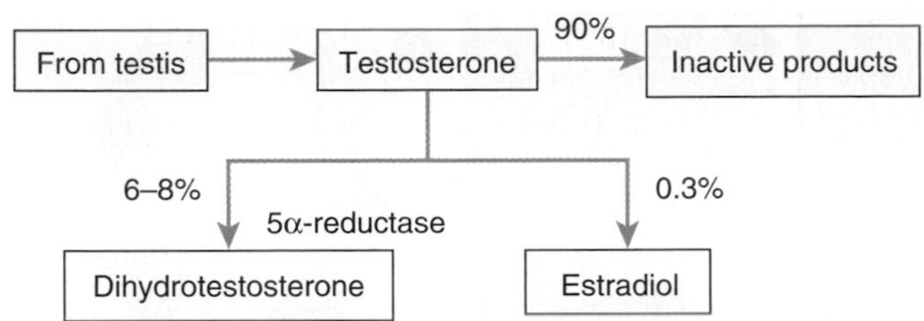

FIGURE 34-18 Testosterone and Conversion to Dihydrotestosterone.

The androgenic hormone responses in the normal prostate and prostate cancer are mediated by **androgen receptor (AR) signalling.**[81] Exactly how AR drives the growth of prostate cancer cells is not fully known. Several mechanisms have been suggested,[81] and specific pathways of signalling are important because they can provide novel therapeutic targets. A recent study using animal models found that loss of AR function prevented prostatic carcinogenesis, malignant transformation, and metastasis. Tissue-specific evaluation of androgen hormone action demonstrated that epithelial AR was not necessary for prostate cancer progression, whereas the stromal AR was essential for prostate cancer progression, malignant transformation, and metastasis.[82]

Testicular testosterone provides the main source of androgens in the prostate (see Figure 34-14) and is the major *circulating* androgen, whereas DHT predominates in prostate tissue and binds to the AR with greater affinity than does testosterone.[83] The adrenal cortex contributes the far less potent DHEA, which promotes synthesis of androgens in the prostate. In the target tissues and, to a lesser extent, in the testes themselves, testosterone is converted to DHT by the enzyme 5α-reductase (Figure 34-18). Thus, DHT is the most potent intraprostatic androgen.

Normally, a small amount of estrogen is produced daily—estrone and estradiol—by the aromatization of androstenedione and testosterone, respectively. This reaction is catalyzed by the enzyme aromatase. A small quantity of estradiol is released by the testes (see Figure 34-18); the rest of the estrogens in males are produced by adipose tissue, liver, skin, brain, and other nonendocrine tissue. Thus, testosterone is a precursor of two hormones—DHT and estradiol.

Recent studies show that aromatase is expressed in stromal tissue in the benign human prostate gland.[78] Thus, it appears that both normal prostate and benign prostate have the capacity to locally metabolize androgens to estrogens through aromatase. This finding leads to the following question: How does aromatase gene expression contribute to the etiology and progression of prostate cancer? Investigators have demonstrated altered aromatase expression in prostate cancer[78,84,85] (Figure 34-14, *B*).

Accumulating evidence shows that estrogens participate in the pathogenesis and development of BPH and prostate cancer by activating estrogen receptor alpha (ERα). In contrast, estrogen receptor beta (ERβ) is involved in the differentiation and maturation of prostatic epithelial cells, and thus possesses antitumour effects in prostate cancer.[86] The effect of estrogen is determined by the two receptors ERα and ERβ. ERα leads to abnormal proliferation, inflammation, and the development of premalignant lesions.[78] In contrast, ERβ leads to antiproliferative, anti-inflammatory, and potentially anticarcinogenic effects that act in concert or balance the actions of ERα and androgens.[78] Increased expression of ERα has been found to be associated with prostate cancer progression, metastasis, and the so-called castration-resistant (medical treatment that suppresses androgens) phenotype.[87] A specific oncogene is regulated by ERs, and those hormones that stimulate the ERα receptorlike (i.e., agonists) endogenous estrogens can stimulate oncogene expression.[88]

Most of the androgen-metabolizing enzymes undergo a significant age-dependent alteration. In epithelium, both the blood levels of 5α-reductase activity and the DHT level decrease with age, whereas in stroma (prostate), not only the 5α-reductase activity but also the stromal DHT level is rather constant over the lifetime. In contrast to the relatively unaltered DHT level over time, the estrogen concentration follows an age-dependent increase. Thus, the age-dependent decrease of the DHT accumulation in epithelium and the concomitant increase of the estrogen accumulation in stroma lead to a tremendous increase with age of the estrogen/androgen ratio in the human prostate. In animal studies, chronic exposure to testosterone plus estradiol is strongly carcinogenic, whereas testosterone alone is weakly carcinogenic.[59] In mice studies, elevated testosterone level in the absence of estrogen leads to the development of hypertrophy and hyperplasia but not malignancy.[78] High estrogen and low testosterone levels have been shown to lead to inflammation with aging and the emergence of precancerous lesions.[78] The mechanism is not clearly understood and may involve estrogen-generated oxidative stress and DNA toxicity, and it requires androgen-mediated and estrogen receptor–mediated processes, such as changes in sex steroid metabolism and receptor status. In addition, there are changes in the balance between autocrine/paracrine growth-stimulatory and growth-inhibitory factors, such as the IGFs.[59]

Investigators have summarized the following key findings on hormones and prostate cancer: (1) androgens are clearly involved in the progression of prostate cancer; (2) it is only with the addition of estrogen to testosterone in rats that cancer can be reliably induced; (3) in vivo and in vitro studies have identified multiple mechanisms involving hormonal involvement with genotoxicity, epigenetic toxicity, hyperprolactinemia, chronic inflammation, and estrogen receptor–mediated changes.[79]

Prostate epithelial neoplasia. A precursor lesion, **prostatic intraepithelial neoplasia (PIN)**, has been described. PIN may be more concentrated in prostates containing cancer and is noted in proximity to cancer.[89] However, the final fate of PIN is unknown, including the possibilities of latency, invasion, and even regression. The current working model of prostate carcinogenesis suggests that repeated cycles of injury and cell death occur to the prostate epithelium as a result of damage (i.e., from oxidative stress) from inflammatory responses.[90] The direct injury is hypothesized as a response to infections; autoimmune disease; circulating carcinogens or toxins, or both, from the diet; or urine that has refluxed into the prostate (see Figure 34-15). The resultant manifestation of this injury is focal atrophy or PIA. Biological responses cause an increase in proliferation and a massive increase in epithelial cells that possess a phenotype intermediate between basal cells and mature luminal cells[90] (Figure 34-19). In a small subset of cells, some may contain "stem cell" or tumour-initiating properties and telomere shortening (see Chapter 10). A subset of PIN cells may activate telomerase enzyme, causing the cells to become immortal.[91] Molecular genetic and epigenetic changes can increase genetic instability that might progress to high-grade PIN and early prostate cancer formation. This model of prostate carcinogenesis needs much more research.

Stromal environment. The prostate gland is composed of secretory luminal epithelium, basal epithelium, neuroendocrine cells, and various cell types comprising supportive tissue or stroma. **Stroma**, or tissue microenvironment, produces autocrine/paracrine factors as well as structural supporting molecules that help regulate normal cell behaviour and organ homeostasis.[92] Stromal components in the tumour microenvironment are important contributions to tumour progression and metastasis.[93] Reciprocal interactions between tumour cells and stromal components influence the metastatic, dormancy-related, and stem cell–like potential of tumour cells.[94] The stromal compartment of the tumour is complex and includes inflammatory/immune cells, vascular

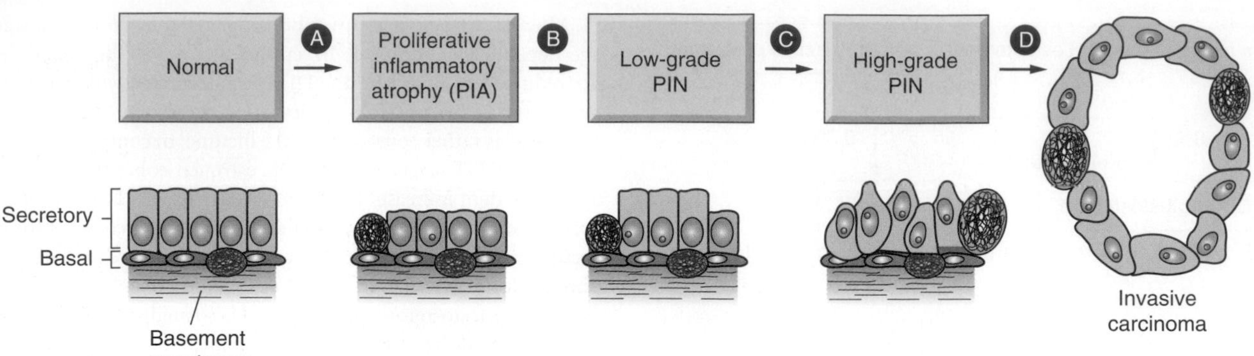

FIGURE 34-19 Cellular and Molecular Model of Early Prostate Neoplasia Progression. A, This stage includes infiltration of lymphocytes, macrophages, and neutrophils caused by repeated infections, dietary factors, urine reflux, injury, onset of autoimmunity (which triggers inflammation), and wound healing. **B,** Epigenetic alterations mediate telomere shortening. **C,** Genetic instability and accumulation of genetic alterations. **D,** Continued proliferation of genetically unstable cells leading to cancer progression. *PIN,* Prostatic intraepithelial neoplasia.

endothelial cells, pericytes, fibroblasts, adipocytes, and components of the extracellular matrix.[93,95] Tumour-infiltrating inflammatory cells release a host of growth factors, chemokines, cytokines, and proinvasive matrix-degrading enzymes to promote tumour growth and progression.[93] Angiogenesis occurs in response to factors secreted from tumour cells, resulting in continued growth and progression. Adipocytes in the tumour microenvironment produce adipokines, which are important for tumour growth.[93] **Fibroblasts** in the tumour microenvironment provide the structural framework of the stroma; they remain quiet or dormant, but proliferate during wound healing, inflammation, and cancer.[93] Tumour cells release paracrine factors that activate fibroblasts to become "cancer-associated fibroblasts" (CAFs). CAFs secrete factors that modulate tumour growth and modify the stroma to enhance metastasis and dampen responses to anticancer therapies.[93] These findings suggest that alteration in the prostate microenvironment with therapeutic agents and approaches—in particular, natural products such as berberine, resveratrol, onionin A, epigallocatechin gallate, genistein, curcumin, naringenin, desoxyrhapontigenin, piperine, and zerumbone—warrants further investigation to target the tumour microenvironment for the treatment and prevention of cancer.[95]

Epithelial–mesenchymal transition (EMT) was first described in embryonic development, and it is observed in a number of solid tumours[96] (see Chapter 10). Cells that undergo EMT become more migratory and invasive and gain access to vascular vessels.[97] Numerous studies have shown that these transition states (EMT and mesenchymal–epithelial transition [MET]) are a consequence of tumour–stromal interactions.[97,98] Investigators studying prostate cancer cells in vitro correlated EMT with increased growth, migration, and invasion.[99] These investigators demonstrated that the microenvironment is a critical site for the transition of human prostate cancer cells from epithelial to mesenchymal structure, resulting in increased metastatic potential for bone and adrenal gland.[99]

Prostate cancer is known to be diverse and composed of multiple genetically distinct cancer cell clones. Recent studies, however, indicate that most metastatic cancers arise from a single precursor cancer cell.[100]

From all of these observations, the following multifactorial general hypothesis of prostate carcinogenesis emerges: (1) androgens act as strong tumour promoters through AR-mediated mechanisms to enhance the carcinogenic activity of strong endogenous DNA toxic carcinogens, including reactive estrogen metabolites and estrogen, and prostate-generated ROS; (2) reciprocal interactions between tumour cells and the stromal microenvironment promote prostate cancer pathogenesis; and (3) possibly unknown environmental–lifestyle carcinogens may contribute to prostate cancer. All of these factors are modulated by diet and genetic determinants, such as hereditary susceptibility genes and polymorphic genes, which encode receptors and enzymes involved in the metabolism and action of steroid hormones.[59]

The most common sites of distant metastasis are the lymph nodes, bones, lungs, liver, and adrenals. The pelvis, lumbar spine, femur, thoracic spine, and ribs are the most common sites of bone metastasis. Local extension is usually posterior, although late in the disease the tumour may invade the rectum or encroach on the prostatic urethra and cause bladder outlet obstruction (Figure 34-20). The spread of cancer through blood vessels is illustrated in Figure 34-21.

CLINICAL MANIFESTATIONS Prostatic cancer often causes no symptoms until it is far advanced. The first manifestations of disease are those of bladder outlet obstruction: slow urinary stream, hesitancy, incomplete emptying, frequency, nocturia, and dysuria. Unlike the symptoms of obstruction caused by BPH, the symptoms of obstruction caused by prostatic cancer are progressive and do not remit. Local extension of prostatic cancer can obstruct the upper urinary tract ureters as well. Rectal obstruction also may occur, causing the individual to experience large bowel obstruction or difficulty in defecation. Symptoms of late disease include bone pain at sites of bone metastasis, edema of the lower extremities, enlargement of lymph nodes, liver enlargement, pathological bone fractures, and mental confusion associated with brain metastases. Prostatic cancer and its treatment can affect sexual functioning.

EVALUATION AND TREATMENT Screening for prostatic cancer includes digital rectal examination (DRE) and PSA blood tests. There is lack of evidence, however, whether screening with PSA or DRE reduces mortality from prostate cancer.[101] It is unclear whether detection of prostate cancer at an early stage leads to any change in the natural history or outcome.[101] Observational studies in some countries show a trend toward lower mortality, but the relationship between the intensity and trends of screening is not clear and the associations with screening are inconsistent.[101] The observed trends may be a result of screening or improved treatment. Two randomized trials show no effect on mortality through 7 years and are inconsistent beyond 7 to 10 years.[102] Strong evidence shows implementation of PSA or DRE detects some prostate cancers that would never have caused significant clinical problems.[101] These screening tests lead to some degree of overtreatment. The screening

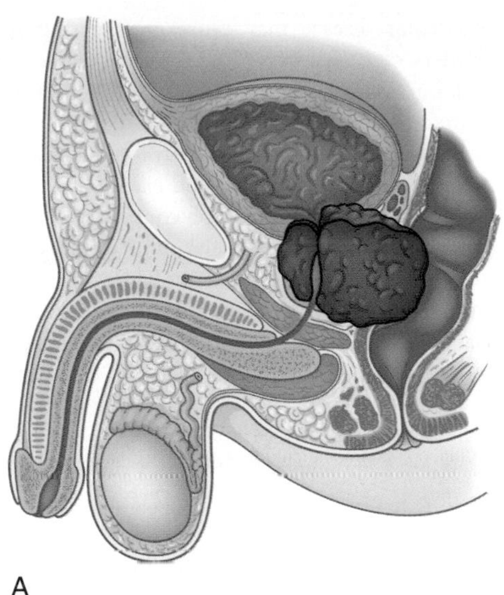

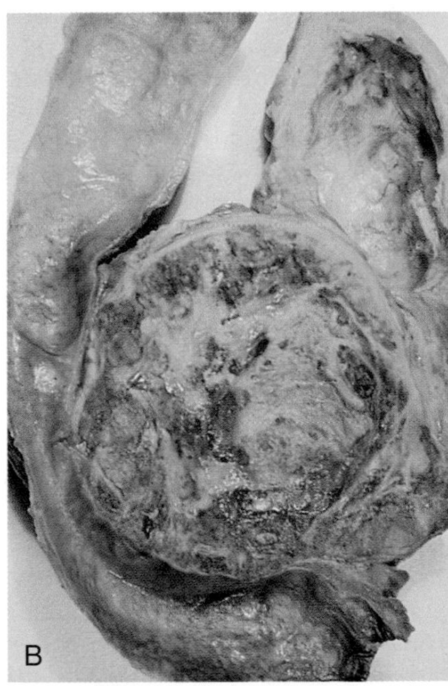

FIGURE 34-20 Carcinoma of Prostate. A, Schematic of carcinoma of the prostate. **B,** Carcinoma of the prostate extending into the rectum and urinary bladder. (**B** from Damjanov, I., & Linder, J. [Eds]. [2000]. *Pathology: A color atlas.* St. Louis: Mosby.)

tests can harm patients; for example, they may lead to radical prostatectomy and radiation therapy that result in irreversible side effects in many men.[101] The most common side effects are ED and urinary incontinence. The screening process can cause considerable anxiety, especially in men who have a prostate biopsy but no identified prostate cancer. Screening can lead to biopsies, which are associated with complications, including fever, pain, hematuria, hematospermia, positive urine cultures for bacteria, and, rarely, sepsis. About 20 to 70% of men who had no problems before radical prostatectomy or external-beam radiation therapy will have reduced sexual function or urinary problems, or both.

Prostate cancer usually grows very slowly and is predominantly a tumour of older men, with the median age at diagnosis of 72 years.[101] Until recently, many physicians and organizations encouraged yearly PSA screening for men beginning at age 50; however, with more

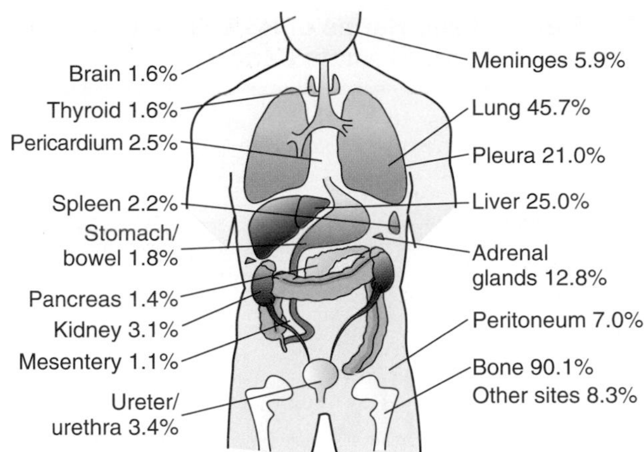

FIGURE 34-21 Distribution of Hematogenous Metastases in Prostate Cancer. Based on an autopsy study of 1 589 patients with metastatic prostate cancer. (Adapted from Budendorf, L., Schöpfer, A., Wagner, U., et al. [2000]. *Hum Pathol, 31*(5), 578–583.)

understanding about the benefits and detriments, a number of organizations have cautioned men against routine population screening (Figure 34-22). Some organizations continue to recommend PSA screening. Some tumours found through PSA screening do not cause symptoms, grow slowly, and are unlikely to threaten a man's life. The PSA screening test often suggests that prostate cancer may be present when there is no cancer. This is called a "false positive" result. False-positive results lead to unnecessary follow-up tests. Detecting these benign tumours is called overdiagnosis.

Across age ranges, Black men and men with a family history of prostate cancer have an increased risk of developing and dying of prostate cancer. Black men are approximately twice as likely to die of prostate cancer compared with men of other races in North America, and the reason for this disparity is unknown. Black men represent a very small minority of participants in randomized clinical trials of screening, and thus no firm conclusions can be made about the balance of benefits and harms of PSA-based screening in this population. As such, it is questionable practice to selectively recommend PSA-based screening for Black men in the absence of data that support a more favourable balance of risks and benefits.[103] Because of this "overtreatment" phenomenon, active surveillance with delayed intervention is gaining traction as a viable management approach in contemporary practice.

Treatment of prostatic cancer depends on the stage of the neoplasm, the anticipated effects of treatment, and the age, general health, and life expectancy of the individual. Options include no treatment; surgical treatments, such as total prostatectomy, transurethral resection of the prostate (TURP), or cryotherapy; nonsurgical treatments, such as radiation therapy, hormone therapy, or chemotherapy; watchful waiting; and any combination of these treatment modalities.[103] In addition, new approaches are using immunotherapy. Palliative treatment is aimed at relieving urinary, bladder outlet, or colon obstruction; spinal cord compression; and pain. Box 34-7 shows staging for prostate cancer. Prognosis and survival rates have improved steadily over the past 50 years. Over the past 25 years, the 5-year relative survival rate for all stages combined has increased from 68% to almost 100%. According to the most recent data, 10- and 15-year relative survival rates are 98% and 94%, respectively.[1]

Stress incontinence can occur after surgery and mild urge incontinence can occur after radiation therapy. Prostate cancer and its treatment can affect sexual functioning. Sensation of orgasm is not usually affected, but smaller amounts of ejaculate will be produced or men may experience a "dry" ejaculate because of retrograde ejaculation.

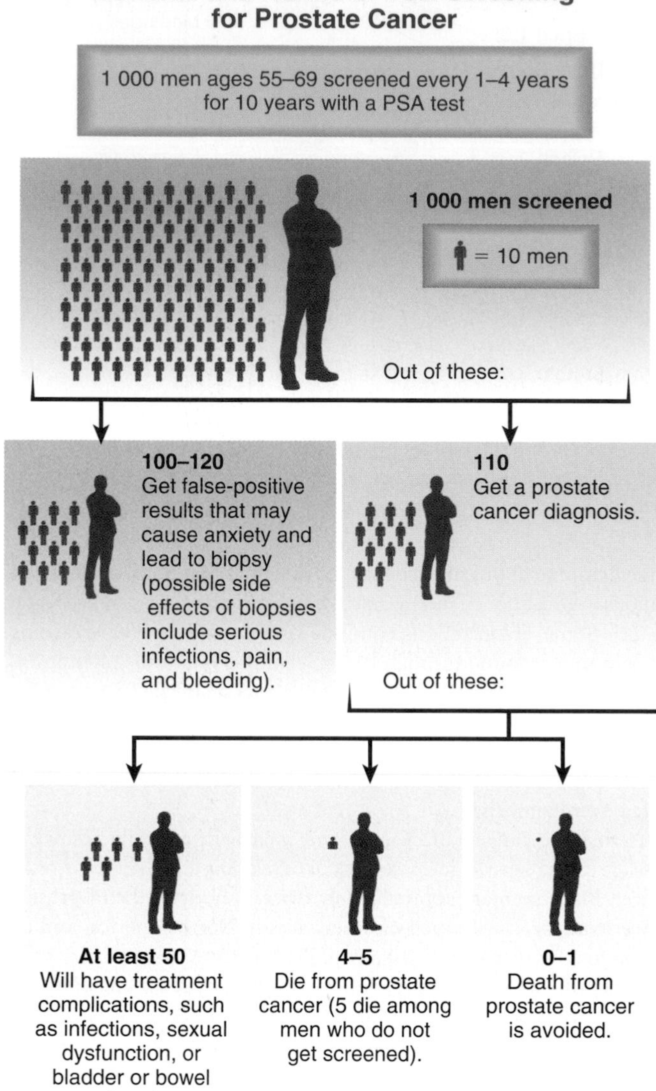
Benefits and Harms of PSA Screening for Prostate Cancer
1 000 men ages 55–69 screened every 1–4 years for 10 years with a PSA test
1 000 men screened
= 10 men
Out of these:
100–120
Get false-positive results that may cause anxiety and lead to biopsy (possible side effects of biopsies include serious infections, pain, and bleeding).
110
Get a prostate cancer diagnosis.
Out of these:
At least 50
Will have treatment complications, such as infections, sexual dysfunction, or bladder or bowel control problems.
4–5
Die from prostate cancer (5 die among men who do not get screened).
0–1
Death from prostate cancer is avoided.

FIGURE 34-22 Benefits and Harms of PSA Screening for Prostate Cancer. The US Preventive Services Task Force (PSTF) recommends against PSA-based screenings for prostate cancer (grade D recommendation). *PSA*, Prostate-specific antigen. (Adapted from USPSTF Recommendation Statement, Annals of Internal Medicine, 2012.)

Sexual Dysfunction

In males, the normal sexual response involves erection, emission, and ejaculation. **Sexual dysfunction** is the impairment of any or all of these processes and can be caused by various physiological, psychological, and emotional factors.

Until the late 1970s, most cases of male sexual dysfunction were considered psychogenic. Now there is evidence that 89 to 90% of cases involve organic factors and include (1) vascular, endocrine, and neurological disorders; (2) chronic disease, including kidney failure and diabetes mellitus; (3) penile diseases and penile trauma; and (4) iatrogenic factors, such as surgery and pharmacological therapies. Most of these disorders cause erectile dysfunction.[104]

PATHOPHYSIOLOGY Sexual dysfunction can have a specific physiological cause, can be associated with many chronic diseases and their treatment, or may be related to low energy levels, stress, or depression. For example, vascular disease may cause erectile dysfunction, and endocrine disorders or conditions that cause decreased testosterone levels or testicular atrophy can diminish sexual functioning or libido. In addition, neurological disorders and spinal cord injuries can interfere with sympathetic, parasympathetic, and central nervous system mechanisms required for erection, emission, and ejaculation.

Medication-induced sexual dysfunction consists of decreased desire, decreased erectile ability, or decreased ejaculatory ability. Alcohol and other central nervous system depressants, antihypertensives, antidepressants, antihistamines, and hormonal preparations are commonly used medications that affect sexual functioning. Other pharmacological agents may diminish the quality or quantity of sperm or cause priapism.

CLINICAL MANIFESTATIONS AND TREATMENT Evaluation of sexual dysfunction includes a thorough history and physical examination. Particular attention is given to medication history and examination of the genitalia, prostate, and nervous system. Basic laboratory tests are used to identify the presence of endocrinopathies or other underlying disorders that can cause dysfunction. Psychological evaluation is indicated for younger men with a sudden onset of sexual dysfunction or for men of any age who can achieve but not maintain an erection. If no physiological cause is found and the condition does not improve with psychotherapy, the man is referred for further investigation of organic causes.

Treatments for organic sexual dysfunction include both medical and surgical approaches. The advent of phosphodiesterase type 5 inhibitors (PDE5i) has revolutionized the erectile dysfunction treatment landscape and provided effective, minimally invasive therapies to restore male sexual function. The original PDE5i, sildenafil (Viagra), has created much enthusiasm over its ability to help a man maintain an erection. For a small percentage of men (1%), however, this improvement in sexual function is accompanied by heart attacks and death. Whether these effects are the result of sexual performance or sildenafil has been controversial. Research has shown that sildenafil increases blood concentrations of the enzyme cyclic guanosine monophosphate (cGMP)–dependent protein kinase G (PKG), which increases blood flow to the penis. PKG, however, plays a dual role: first, it increases platelet aggregation; and then, minutes later, it decreases clot size. The initial clot could cause some men with heart disease to experience cardiac arrest.

Currently available PDE5i medications in Canada include sildenafil, vardenafil (Levitra), tadalafil (Cialis), and avanafil (Stendra), each of which has unique side effect profiles. For instance, sildenafil is associated with (in addition to the previously mentioned cardiac issues) an increased rate of visual changes, vardenafil with QT prolongation, and tadalafil with lower back pain.[105] Nonsurgical approaches include correction of underlying disorders, particularly medication-induced dysfunction and endocrinopathy-related (e.g., reduced testosterone level associated with chronic kidney disease) dysfunction. Use of vasodilators and cessation of smoking can benefit individuals with vasculogenic ED. Surgical approaches include penile implants, penile revascularization, and correction of other anatomical defects contributing to sexual dysfunction.

Impairment of Sperm Production and Quality

Spermatogenesis requires adequate secretion of FSH and luteinizing hormone (LH) by the pituitary and sufficient secretion of testosterone by the testes. Inadequate secretion of gonadotropins may be caused by numerous alterations (e.g., hypothyroidism, hyperadrenocortisolism, hyperprolactinemia, or hypogonadotropic hypogonadism). In the absence of adequate gonadotropin levels, the Leydig cells are not stimulated to secrete testosterone, and sperm maturation is not promoted in the Sertoli cells. Spermatogenesis also depends on an appropriate response by the testes. Defects in testicular response to the gonadotropins result

BOX 34-7 Staging for Prostate Cancer

Stage I

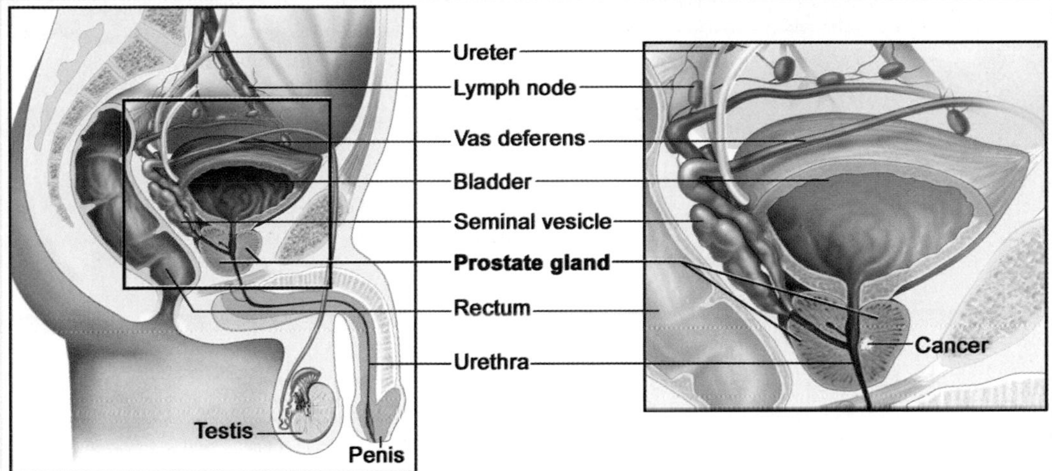

In stage I, cancer is found in the prostate only. In this stage, cancer:

- Is found by performing a needle biopsy (done for a high prostate-specific antigen [PSA] level) or by examining a small amount of tissue during surgery for other reasons (such as benign prostatic hyperplasia). The PSA level is lower than 10, and the Gleason score is 6 or lower; *or*
- Is found on half or less of one lobe of the prostate. The PSA level is lower than 10, and the Gleason scores is 6 or lower; *or*
- Cannot be felt during a digital rectal examination and cannot be seen in imaging tests. Cancer is found in half or less of one lobe of the prostate. The PSA level and the Gleason score are not known.

Stage II

In stage II, cancer is more advanced than in stage I, but has not spread outside the prostate. Stage II is divided into stages IIA and IIB.

Stage IIA

In stage IIA, cancer:

- Is found by performing a needle biopsy (done for a high PSA level) or by examining a small amount of tissue during surgery for other reasons (such as benign prostatic hyperplasia). The PSA level is lower than 20, and the Gleason score is 7; *or*
- Is found by performing a needle biopsy (done for a high PSA level) or by examining a small amount of tissue during surgery for other reasons (such as benign prostatic hyperplasia). The PSA level is at least 10 but lower than 20, and the Gleason score is 6 or lower; *or*
- Is found in half or less of one lobe of the prostate. The PSA level is at least 10 but lower than 20, and the Gleason score is 6 or lower; *or*
- Is found in half or less of one lobe of the prostate. The PSA level is lower than 20, and the Gleason score is 7; *or*
- Is found in more than half of one lobe of the prostate.

Stage IIB

In stage IIB, cancer:

- Is found on opposite sides of the prostate. The PSA can be any level, and the Gleason score can range from 2 to 10; *or*
- Cannot be felt during a digital rectal examination (DRE) and cannot be seen in imaging tests. The PSA level is 20 or higher, and the Gleason score can range from 2 to 10; *or*
- Cannot be felt during a DRE and cannot be seen in imaging tests. The PSA can be any level, and the Gleason score is 8 or higher.

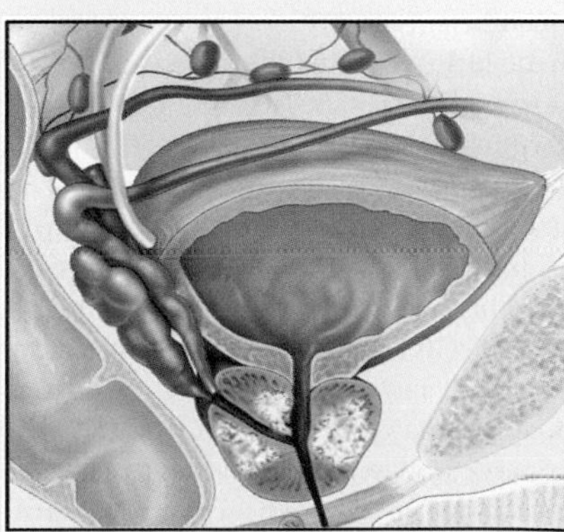

Continued

BOX 34-7 Staging for Prostate Cancer—cont'd

Stage III

In stage III, cancer has spread beyond the outer layer of the prostate and may have spread to the seminal vesicles. The PSA can be any level, and the Gleason score can range from 2 to 10.

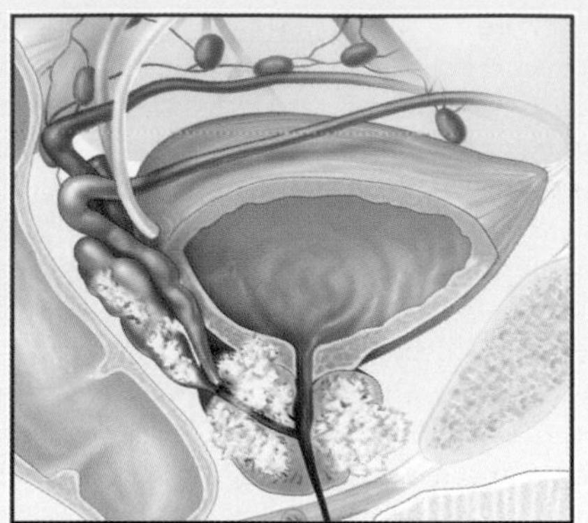

Stage IV

In stage IV, the PSA can be any level, and the Gleason score can range from 2 to 10. Also, in this stage, cancer:

- Has spread beyond the seminal vesicles to nearby tissue or organs, such as the rectum, bladder, or pelvic wall; *or*
- May have spread to the seminal vesicles or to nearby tissue or organs, such as the rectum, bladder, or pelvic wall. Cancer has spread to nearby lymph nodes; *or*
- Has spread to distant parts of the body, which may include lymph nodes or bones. Prostate cancer often spreads to the bones.

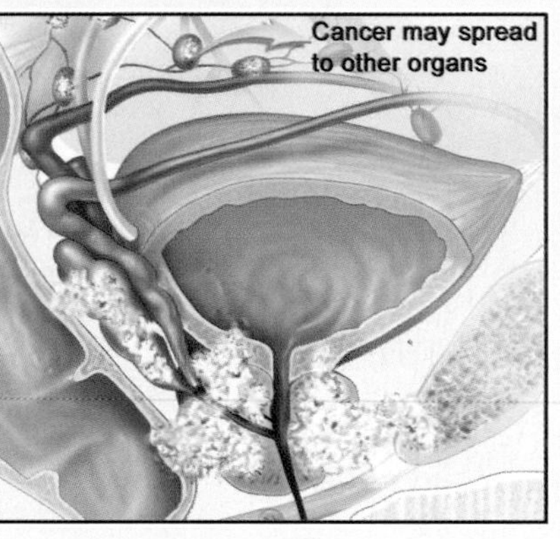
Cancer may spread to other organs

Data from National Cancer Institute. (2016). Prostate cancer treatment (PDQ®)—Patient version. Retrieved from https://www.cancer.gov/types/prostate/patient/prostate-treatment-pdq. Figures © 2010 Terese Winslow; U.S. Government has certain rights.

in decreased secretion of testosterone and inhibin B and occur as a result of normal feedback mechanisms and high levels of circulating gonadotropins. In the absence of adequate testosterone levels, spermatogenesis is impaired. Newer studies demonstrate the importance of inhibin B as a valuable marker of the competence of Sertoli cells and spermatogenesis.[26,106] Impaired spermatogenesis also can be caused by testicular trauma, infection, atrophy of the testes, systemic illness involving high fever, ingestion of various medications, exposure to environmental toxins, and cryptorchidism.

Fertility is adversely affected if spermatogenesis is normal but the sperm are chromosomally or morphologically abnormal or are produced in insufficient quantities. Chromosomal abnormalities are caused by genetic factors and by external variables, such as exposure to radiation or toxic substances. Because the Y chromosome plays a key role in testis determination and control of spermatogenesis, understanding how the genes interact can elucidate exact causes of infertility. The most common mutations are microdeletion of the Y chromosome (AZ [azoospermia] a, b, and c).[107] Research related to mapping the critical genes and gene pathways is the current focus of male infertility. Common mechanisms may be involved in infertility and testicular cancer. In utero environmental exposure to endocrine disruptors modulates the genetic makeup of the gonad and may result in both infertility and testicular cancer.[26]

Sperm motility also may affect fertility. Motility appears to be affected by the characteristics of the semen. Dysfunction of the prostate, excessive viscosity of the semen, presence of medications or toxins in the semen, and presence of antisperm antibodies are associated with impaired sperm motility. However, new data show that motile density may not be a good indicator of infertility.[108] Approximately 17% of infertile males have antisperm antibodies in their semen. These antibodies may be (1) cytotoxic antibodies, which attack sperm and reduce their number in the semen, or (2) sperm-immobilizing antibodies, which impair sperm motility and reduce their ability to traverse the endocervical canal.

Treatment for impaired spermatogenesis involves correcting any underlying disorders, avoiding radiation and possibly electromagnetic radiation (hypothesis from cellphones) and toxins, and using hormones to enhance spermatogenesis. In addition, semen can be modified to improve sperm motility; modifications are followed by artificial insemination.

QUICK CHECK 34-4

1. Why is the worldwide variation of prostate cancer incidence important?
2. What is the current understanding of hormones in the pathophysiology of prostate cancer?
3. Describe what is meant by prostate cancer cell and stromal interactions for carcinogenesis.
4. What causes impaired spermatogenesis?

DISORDERS OF THE MALE BREAST

Gynecomastia

Gynecomastia is the overdevelopment of breast tissue in a male. Gynecomastia accounts for approximately 85% of all masses that develop in the male breast and affects 32 to 40% of the male population. If only one breast is involved, it is typically the left. Incidence is greatest among adolescents and men older than 50 years.

Gynecomastia results from hormonal alterations, which may be idiopathic or caused by systemic disorders, medications, or neoplasms. Gynecomastia usually involves an imbalance of the estrogen/testosterone ratio. The normal estrogen/testosterone ratio can be altered in one of two ways. First, estrogen levels may be excessively high, although testosterone levels are normal. This is the case in medication-induced and tumour-induced hyperestrogenism. Second, testosterone levels may be extremely low, although estrogen levels are normal, as is the case in hypergonadism. Gynecomastia also can be caused by alterations in breast tissue responsiveness to hormonal stimulation. Breast tissue may have increased responsiveness to estrogen or decreased responsiveness to androgen. Alterations of responsiveness may cause many cases of idiopathic gynecomastia.

Besides puberty and aging, estrogen/testosterone imbalances are associated with hypogonadism, Klinefelter's syndrome, and testicular neoplasms. Hormone-induced gynecomastia is usually bilateral. Pubertal gynecomastia is a self-limiting phenomenon that usually disappears within 4 to 6 months. Senescent gynecomastia usually regresses spontaneously within 6 to 12 months.

Systemic disorders associated with gynecomastia include cirrhosis of the liver, infectious hepatitis, chronic kidney disease, chronic obstructive lung disease, hyperthyroidism, tuberculosis, and chronic malnutrition. It may be that these disorders ultimately alter the estrogen/testosterone ratio, initiating the gynecomastia.

Gynecomastia is often seen in males receiving estrogen therapy, either in preparation for a gender-change operation or in the treatment of prostatic carcinoma. Other medications that can cause gynecomastia include digitalis (Digoxin), cimetidine (Tagamet), spironolactone (Aldactone), reserpine (Serpasil), thiazide (Hydrochlorothiazide), isoniazid (Rifater), ergotamine (Bellergal Spacetabs), tricyclic antidepressants, amphetamines, vincristine (Oncovin), and busulfan (Busulfex). Gynecomastia is usually unilateral in these instances.

Malignancies of the testes, adrenals, or liver can cause gynecomastia if they alter the estrogen/testosterone ratio. Pituitary adenomas and lung cancer also are associated with gynecomastia.

PATHOPHYSIOLOGY The enlargement of the breast consists of hyperplastic stroma and ductal tissue. Hyperplasia results in a firm, palpable mass that is at least 2 cm in diameter and located beneath the areola.

EVALUATION AND TREATMENT The diagnosis of gynecomastia is based on physical examination. Identification and treatment of the cause are likely to be followed by resolution of the gynecomastia. The man should be taught to perform breast self-examination and is re-examined at 6- and 12-month intervals if the gynecomastia persists.

Carcinoma

Breast cancer in males accounts for 0.26% of all male cancers and 1.1% of all breast cancers.[1] The Canadian Cancer Society estimated that 230 men were diagnosed with breast cancer in 2017. It also estimated that 60 men died of this disease in 2017.[109] Global incidence rates were generally less than 1 per 100 000 man-years, in contrast to much higher rates in females.[110] The highest incidence rate for male breast cancer (MBC) was reported in Israel (1.24 per 100 000), and the lowest incidence rates for males (0.16 per 100 000) and females (18.0 per 100 000) were observed in Thailand.[110] MBC is seen most commonly after the age of 60 years, with the peak incidence between 60 and 69 years (men tend to be diagnosed at an older age than women). It has, however, been reported in males as young as 6 years old and in adolescents. Klinefelter's syndrome is the strongest risk factor for developing MBC. Other risk factors include germline mutation in *BRCA1* or *BRCA2*, but familial cases usually have *BRCA2* rather than *BRCA1* mutations.[111-113] Obesity increases the risk for MBC. Testicular disorders, including cryptorchidism, mumps, orchitis, and orchiectomy, are related to risk.[114] The relationship between these factors and the risk for disease is not clearly defined.

Recent data on the most frequent molecular subtypes of MBC appear to be different than those for female breast cancers. Luminal A and luminal B are most common; and basal-like, unclassifiable triple-negative, and *HER2*-driven MBCs are rare.[115,116] Male breast tumours often resemble carcinoma of the breast in women. The majority of MBCs express estrogen and progesterone receptors. The malignant male breast lesion is usually a unilateral solid mass located near the nipple. Because the nipple is commonly involved, crusting and nipple discharge are typical clinical manifestations. Other findings include skin retraction, ulceration of the skin over the tumour, and axillary node involvement. Patterns of metastasis are similar to those in females.

The diagnosis of cancer is confirmed by biopsy. Because of delays in seeking treatment, MBC tends to be advanced at the time of diagnosis and therefore is likely to have a poor prognosis. Treatment protocols are similar to those for female breast cancer, but endocrine therapy is used more often for males because a higher percentage of male tumours are hormone dependent. The mainstay of treatment is modified mastectomy with axillary node dissection to assess stage and prognosis. Because 90% of tumours are hormonal-receptor positive, tamoxifen (Nolvadex) is standard adjuvant therapy. Orchiectomy is performed to treat metastatic disease. For metastatic disease, hormonal therapy is the main treatment, but chemotherapy also can provide palliation.[111]

SEXUALLY TRANSMITTED INFECTIONS

Sexually transmitted infections (STIs) are a variety of clinical syndromes and infections caused by pathogens that can be acquired and transmitted through sexual activity.[117] Trends in reportable STIs in Canada have revealed steady increases since 1998. Similar increases in reportable STI rates have been observed in Australia, England, and the United States.[118] Young Canadians have the highest reported rates of STIs; however, increased rates have been reported among middle-aged and older adults[118] (Table 34-1). STIs can lead to severe reproductive health problems, for example, infertility and ectopic pregnancy.[119] Untreated or undertreated chlamydial infections are the primary cause of preventable infertility and ectopic pregnancy. In addition to ectopic pregnancy and infertility, other complications of STIs include pelvic inflammatory disease (PID), chronic pelvic pain, neonatal morbidity and mortality, genital cancer, and epidemiological synergy with HIV transmission (Table 34-2). Long-term sequelae of untreated or undertreated STIs may be disastrous and can affect a person's physical, emotional, and financial well-being. Treatment guidelines for STIs can be found on the Centers for Disease Control and Prevention website (http://www.cdc.gov/std/tg2015/2015-poster-press.pdf).

Anyone can become infected with an STI, but young people and gay and bisexual men are at greatest risk.[118] Young people between the ages of 20 and 24 years have the highest reported rates of chlamydia, and females between the ages of 15 and 24 years and males between the ages of 20 and 29 years account for the highest rates of gonorrhea. Both young men and women are negatively affected by STIs, but young women have the most serious long-term health consequences. Undiagnosed STIs may cause PID, which may lead to chronic abdominal pain, infertility, and ectopic pregnancy.[118] In Canada, it has been suggested that recent increases in the incidence of syphilis is largely related to transmission among men who have sex with men (MSM) who engage in high-risk sexual practices. The majority (65.6%) of all reported cases of infectious

TABLE 34-1 Currently Recognized Sexually Transmitted Infections

Causal Microorganism	Infection
Bacteria	
Campylobacter	Campylobacter enteritis
Calymmatobacterium granulomatis	Granuloma inguinale
Chlamydia trachomatis	Urogenital infections; lymphogranuloma venereum
Polymicrobial	
Gardnerella vaginalis interaction with anaerobes (*Bacteroides* and *Mobiluncus* spp.) and genital mycoplasmas	Bacterial vaginosis
Haemophilus ducreyi	Chancroid
Mycoplasma	Mycoplasmosis
Neisseria gonorrhoeae	Gonorrhea
Shigella	Shigellosis
Treponema pallidum	Syphilis
Viruses	
Cytomegalovirus	Cytomegalic inclusion disease
Hepatitis B virus (HBV)	Hepatitis
Hepatitis C virus (HCV)	Hepatitis
Herpes simplex virus (HSV)	Genital herpes
Human immunodeficiency virus (HIV)	Acquired immune deficiency syndrome (AIDS)
Human papillomavirus (HPV)	Condylomata acuminata, cervical dysplasia, and cervical cancer
Molluscum contagiosum virus	Molluscum contagiosum
Protozoa	
Entamoeba histolytica	Amebiasis; amebic dysentery
Giardia lamblia	Giardiasis
Trichomonas vaginalis	Trichomoniasis
Ectoparasites	
Phthirus pubis	Pediculosis pubis
Sarcoptes scabiei	Scabies
Fungus	
Candida albicans	Candidiasis

TABLE 34-2 Photographs of Sexually Transmitted Infections and Precursors to Sexually Transmitted Infections

Bacterial Sources

Gonococcal Infections

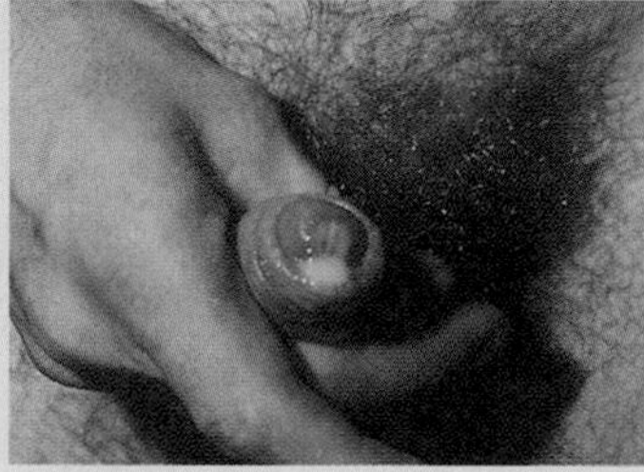

Symptomatic Gonococcal Urethritis.[a]

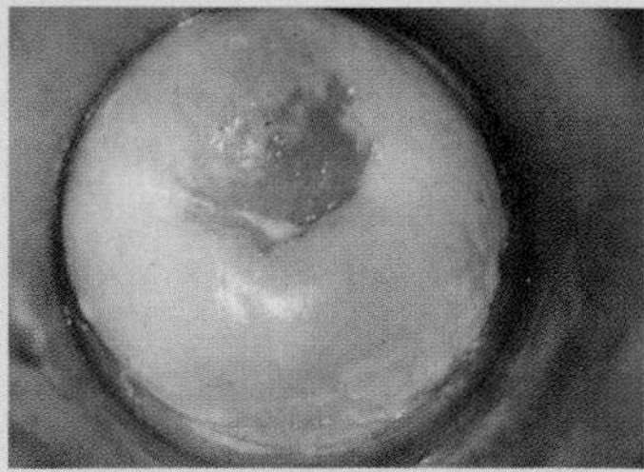

Endocervical Gonorrhea.[a]

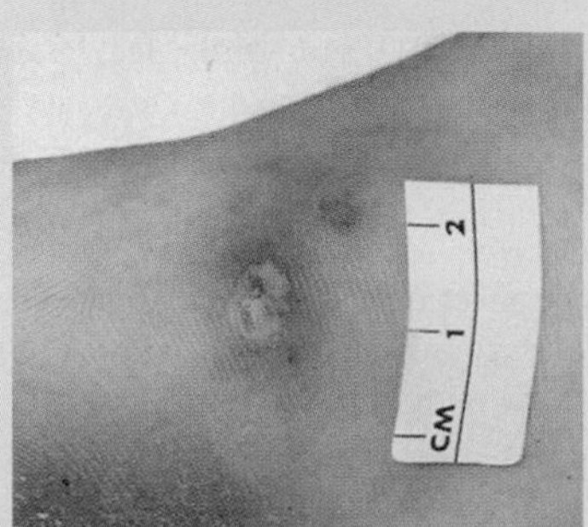

Skin Lesions of Disseminated Gonococcal Infection.[a]

Bacterial Vaginosis

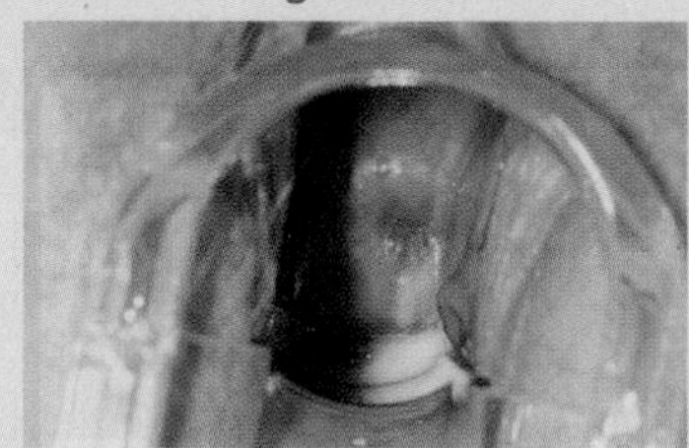

Vaginal Examination Showing Mild Bacterial Vaginosis.[a]

Syphilis

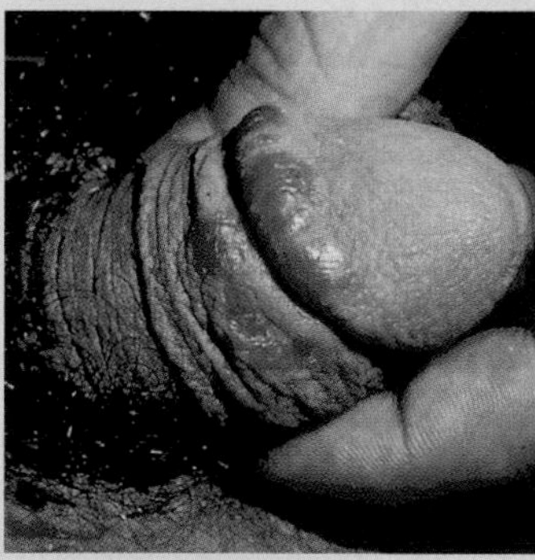

Erythematous Penile Plaques of Secondary Syphilis.[b]

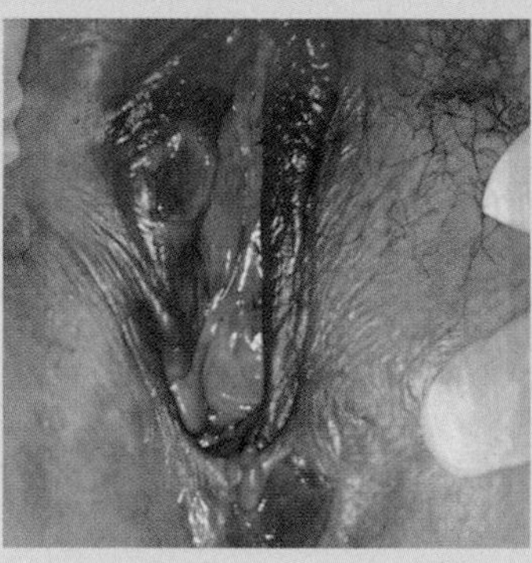

Multiple Primary Syphilitic Chancres of Labia and Perineum. Courtesy Barbara Romanowski, MD.[a]

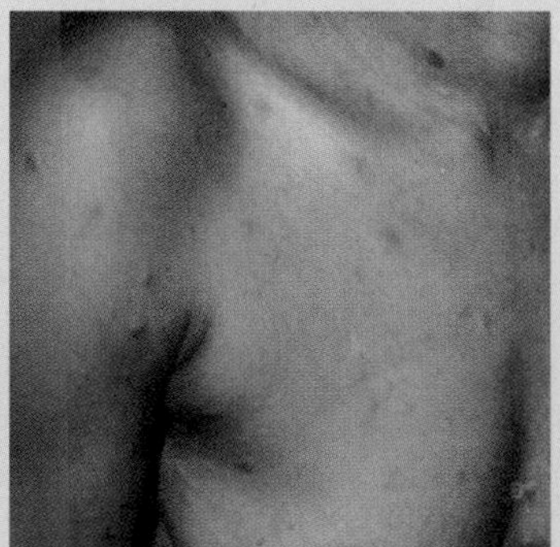

Papular Secondary Syphilis.[a]

TABLE 34-2 Photographs of Sexually Transmitted Infections and Precursors to Sexually Transmitted Infections—cont'd

Lymphogranuloma

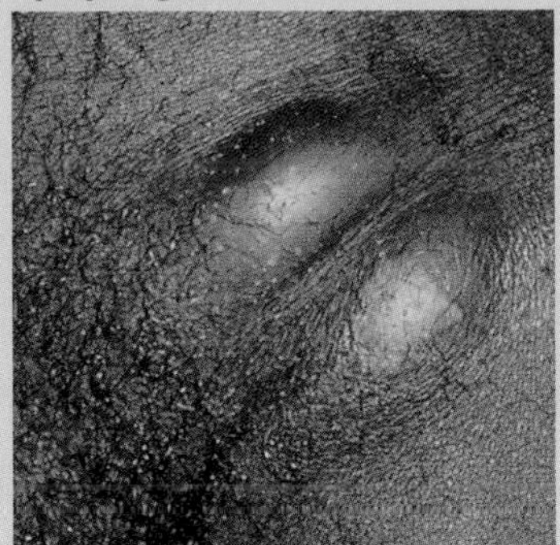

"Groove Sign" in Man With Lymphogranuloma Vonoroum (LV).[b]

Chlamydial Infections

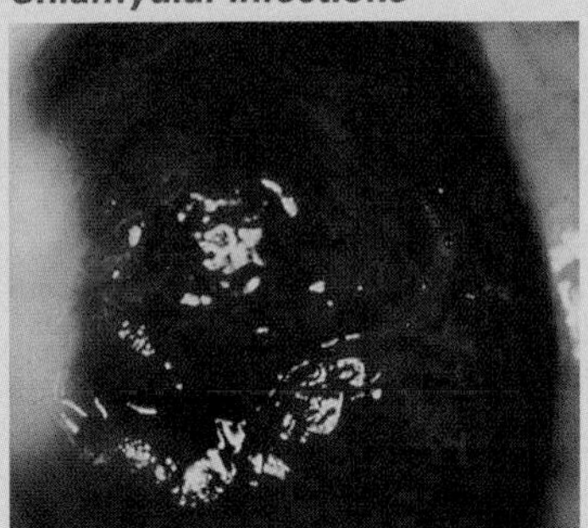

Beefy Red Mucosa in Chlamydial Infection.[a]

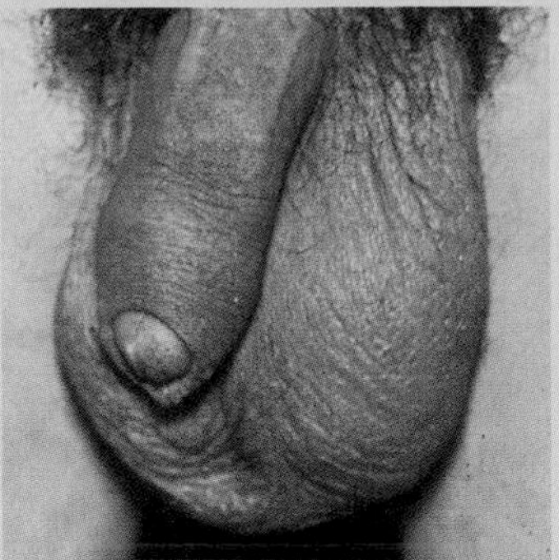

Chlamydial Epididymitis. Courtesy Richard E. Berger.[a]

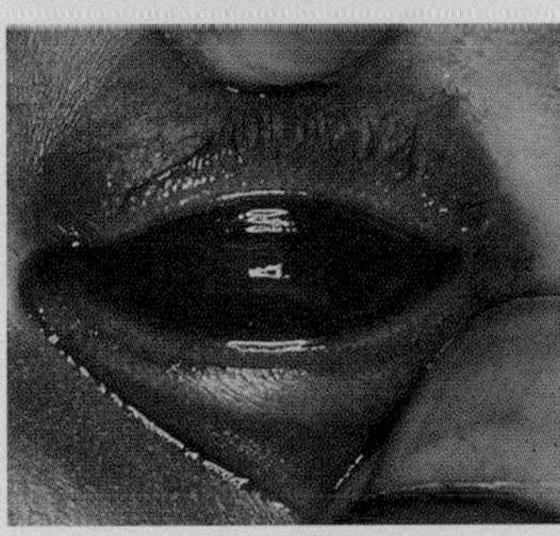

Chlamydial Ophthalmia: Erythematous Conjunctiva in Infant.[a]

Viral Sources

Genital Herpes

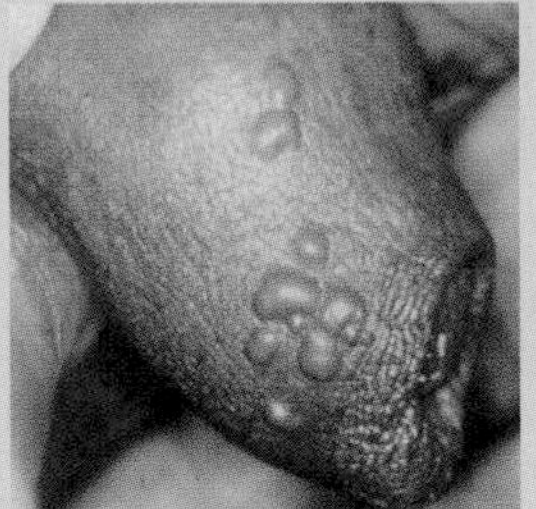

Early Lesions of Primary Genital Herpes.[a]

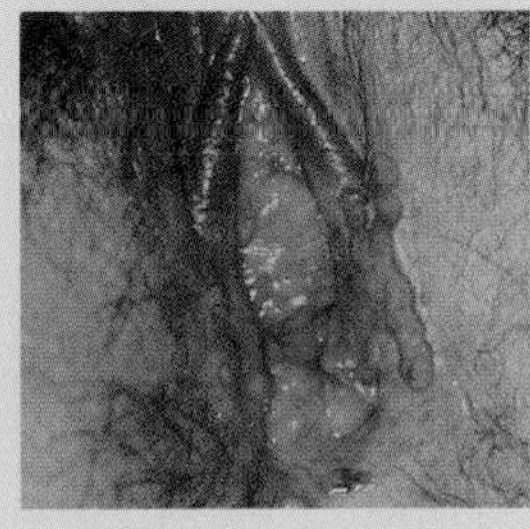

Primary Vulvar Herpes. Courtesy Barbara Romanowski, MD.[a]

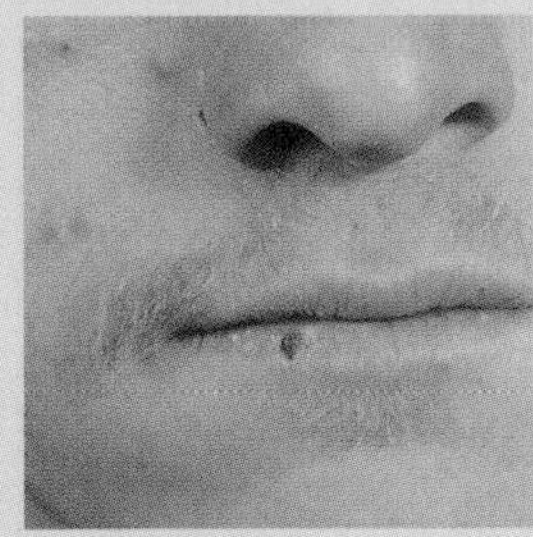

Generalized Herpes Simplex in Patient With Atopic Dermatitis. Courtesy David Mandeville and Peter Lane, MD.[a]

Human Papillomavirus

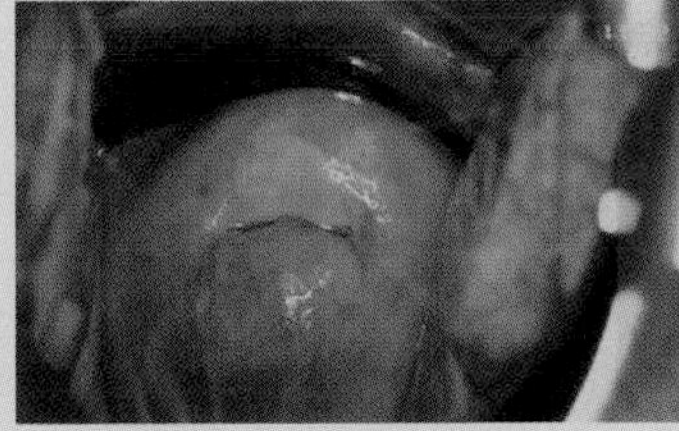

Human Papillomavirus (HPV) Infection of the Cervix.[b]

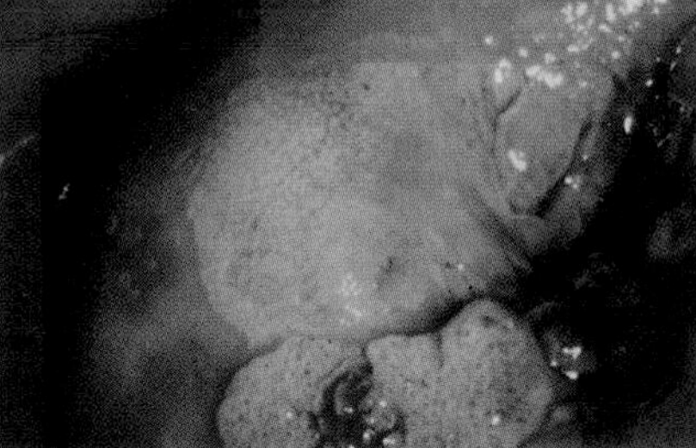

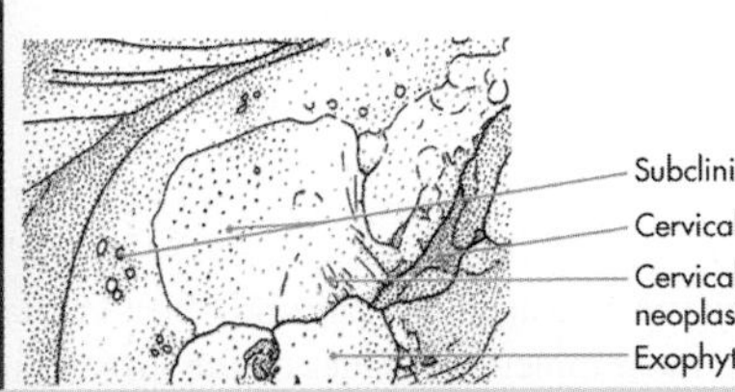

Exophytic (Outward-Growing) Condyloma, Subclinical Human Papillomavirus (HPV) Infection, and High-Grade Cervical Intraepithelial Neoplasia (CIN).[b]

Continued

TABLE 34-2 Photographs of Sexually Transmitted Infections and Precursors to Sexually Transmitted Infections—cont'd

Condylomata Acuminata

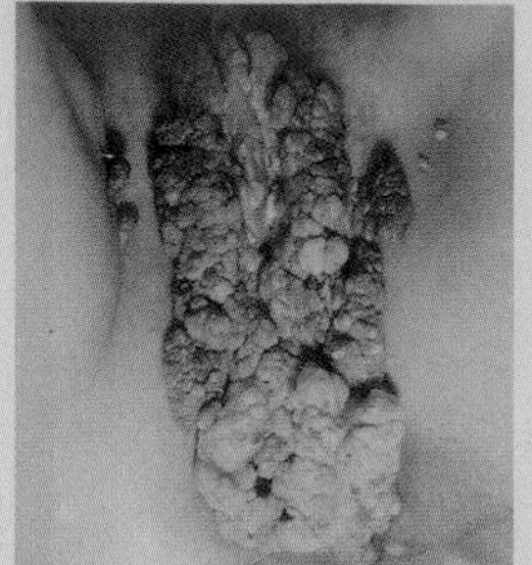

Condylomata Acuminata: Vulva and Perineum.[a]

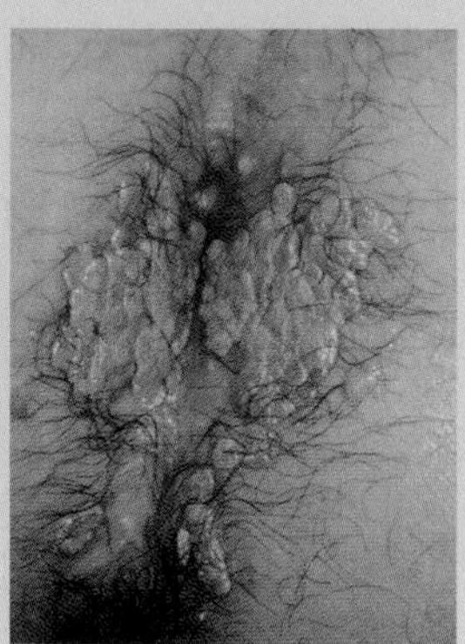

Condylomata Acuminata: Perianal.[a]

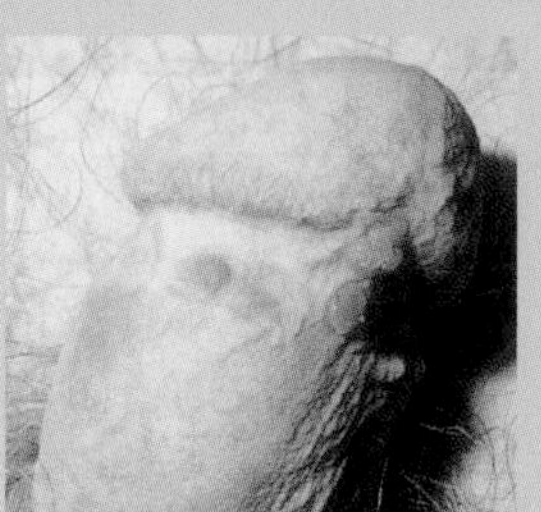

Condylomata Acuminata: Penile.[a]

Parasite Sources

Trichomonisasis

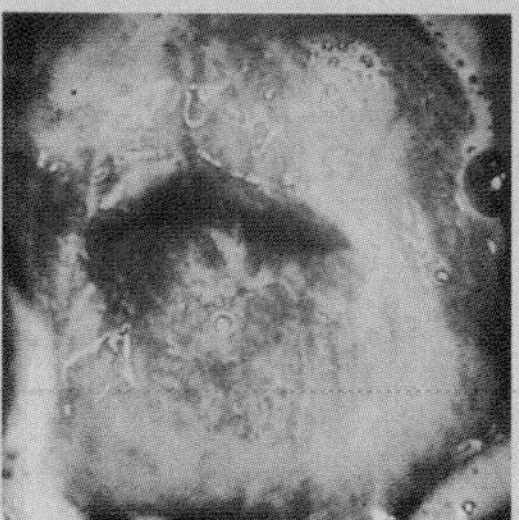

"Strawberry Cervix" Seen With Trichomoniasis.[a]

Scabies

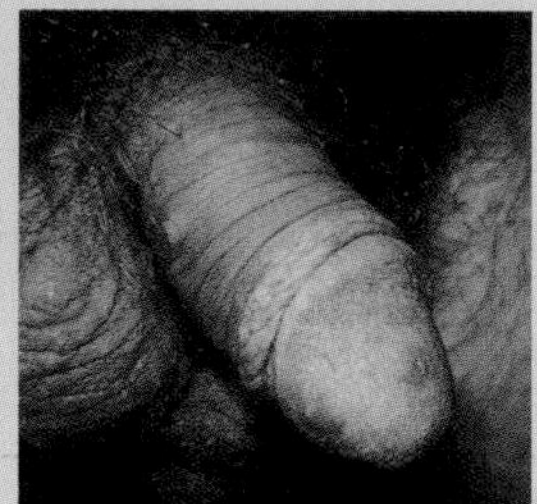

Nodular Lesions of Scabies on Male Genitalia.[b]

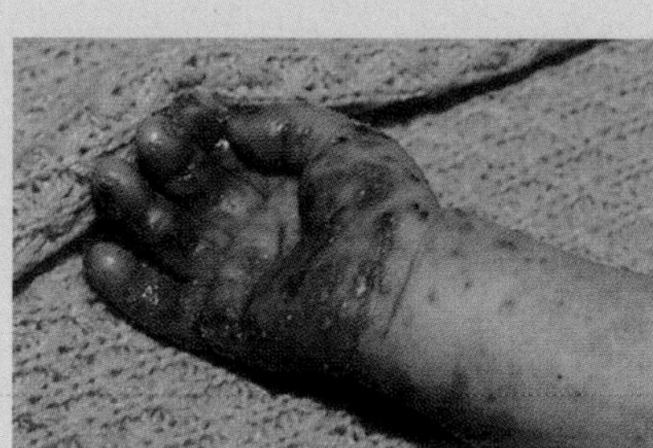

Scabies of Palm With Secondary Pyoderma in Infant.[a]

***Pediculosis Pubis* (Phthirus pubis *[Crablouse]*)**

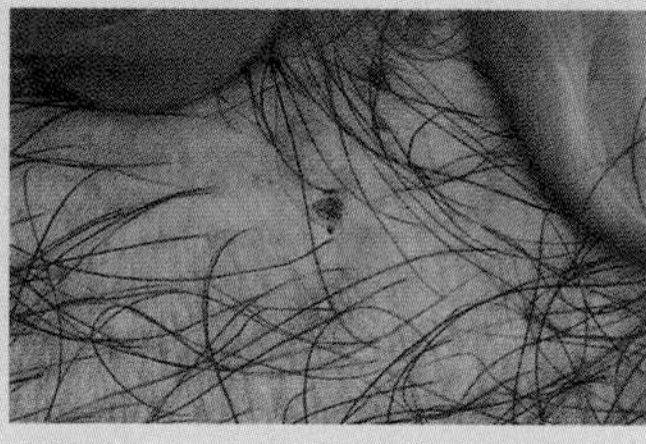

Phthirus pubis Feeding on Its Host.[a]

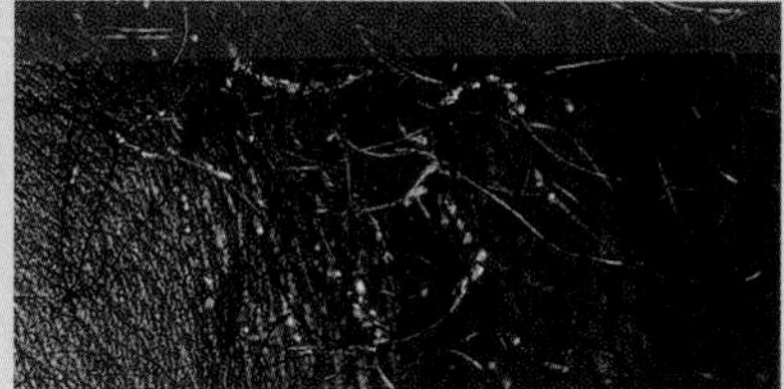

Pubic Hair With Multiple Nits.[a]

[a]From Morse, S.A., Holmes, K.K., & Ballard, R.C. (2010). *Atlas of sexually transmitted diseases and AIDS* (4th ed.). London: Elsevier.
[b]From Morse, S.A., Moreland, A.A., & Holmes, K.K. (1996). *Atlas of sexually transmitted diseases and AIDS* (2nd ed.). London: Elsevier.

syphilis were among men aged 30 years and older. Primary and secondary syphilis are the most infectious stages of the disease and, if not treated adequately, can lead to visual impairment and stroke.[118] Syphilis infection raises the risk of acquiring and transmitting HIV infection and is a common and concerning occurrence.[118]

Individual risk behaviours, such as higher numbers of lifetime sex partners and environmental, social, and cultural factors, contribute to health disparities of MSM, for example, difficulty accessing health care. Homophobia and stigma also can make it difficult for gay and bisexual men to find culturally sensitive and appropriate care and treatment.[118] STI screening is critical. It is recommended that women who are sexually active and younger than 25 years of age or have multiple sex partners be tested annually for chlamydia and gonorrhea. A woman should request syphilis, HIV, chlamydia, and hepatitis B testing early in her pregnancy. These tests also should be requested if a woman has a new partner or multiple sex partners.[118] Recommended tests include syphilis, chlamydia, gonorrhea, and HIV once a year for gay, bisexual, or other MSM. More frequent testing is recommended for men at high risk.

QUICK CHECK 34-5

1. What is the cause of male gynecomastia?
2. What are the risk factors for male breast cancer?
3. What factors increase the incidence of sexually transmitted infections (STIs)?
4. What are the serious long-term health consequences of STIs for young women?
5. What are the long-term health consequences of acquiring syphilis for men who have sex with men?

DID YOU UNDERSTAND?

Alterations of Sexual Maturation

1. Sexual maturation, or puberty, begins in boys between the ages of 9 and 14.5 years.
2. Delayed puberty is the onset of sexual maturation after 14.5 years; precocious puberty is sexual maturation occurring before age 9. Treatment for delayed, precocious, or absent puberty depends on the cause.

Disorders of the Male Reproductive System

1. Disorders of the urethra include urethritis (infection of the urethra) and urethral strictures (narrowing or obstruction of the urethral lumen caused by scarring).
2. Most cases of urethritis result from sexually transmitted pathogens. Urological instrumentation, foreign body insertion, trauma, or an anatomical abnormality can cause urethral inflammation with or without infection.
3. Urethritis causes urinary symptoms, including a burning sensation during urination (dysuria), frequency, urgency, urethral tingling or itching, and clear or purulent discharge.
4. The scarring that causes urethral stricture can be attributed to trauma or severe untreated urethritis.
5. Manifestations of urethral stricture include those of bladder outlet obstruction: urinary frequency and hesitancy, diminished force and calibre of the urinary stream, dribbling after voiding, and nocturia.
6. Phimosis and paraphimosis are penile disorders involving the foreskin (prepuce). In phimosis, the foreskin cannot be retracted over the glans. In paraphimosis, the foreskin is retracted and cannot be reduced (returned to its normal anatomical position over the glans). Phimosis is caused by poor hygiene and chronic infection and can lead to paraphimosis. Paraphimosis can constrict the penile blood vessels, preventing circulation to the glans.
7. Peyronie disease consists of fibrosis affecting the corpora cavernosa, which causes penile curvature during erection. Fibrosis prevents engorgement on the affected side, causing a lateral curvature that can prevent intercourse.
8. Priapism is a prolonged, painful erection that is not stimulated by sexual arousal. The corpora cavernosa (but not the corpus spongiosum) fill with blood that will not drain from the area, probably because of venous obstruction. Priapism is associated with spinal cord trauma, sickle cell disease, leukemia, and pelvic tumours. It can also be idiopathic.
9. Balanitis is an inflammation of the glans penis. It is associated with phimosis, inadequate cleansing under the foreskin, skin disorders, and pathogens (e.g., *Candida albicans*).
10. Carcinoma of the penis is rare in Canada. Penile carcinoma in situ tends to involve the glans; invasive carcinoma of the penis involves the shaft as well.
11. A varicocele is an abnormal dilation of the testicular veins within the spermatic cord caused either by congenital absence of valves in the internal spermatic vein or by acquired valvular incompetence.
12. A hydrocele is a collection of fluid between the testicular and scrotal layers of the tunica vaginalis. Hydroceles can be idiopathic or caused by trauma or infection of the testes.
13. A spermatocele is a cyst located between the testis and epididymis that is filled with fluid and sperm.
14. Cryptorchidism is a congenital condition in which one or both testes fail to descend into the scrotum. Uncorrected cryptorchidism is associated with infertility and significantly increased risk for testicular cancer.
15. Testicular torsion is the rotation of a testis, which twists blood vessels in the spermatic cord. This rotation interrupts the blood supply to the testis, resulting in edema and, if not corrected within 6 hours, necrosis and atrophy of testicular tissues.
16. Orchitis is an acute inflammation of the testes. Complications of orchitis include hydrocele and abscess formation.
17. Testicular cancer is the most common malignancy in males 15 to 35 years of age. Although its cause is unknown, high androgen levels, genetic predisposition, and history of cryptorchidism, trauma, or infection may contribute to tumourigenesis.
18. Epididymitis, an inflammation of the epididymis, is usually caused by a sexually transmitted pathogen that ascends through the vasa deferentia from an already infected urethra or bladder.
19. Benign prostatic hyperplasia (BPH), also called *benign prostatic hypertrophy*, is the enlargement of the prostate gland. This condition becomes symptomatic as the enlarging prostate compresses the urethra, causing symptoms of bladder outlet obstruction and urine retention.
20. Prostatitis is an inflammation of the prostate. Prostatitis syndromes have been classified by the US National Institutes of Health as (a) acute bacterial prostatitis (ABP), (b) chronic bacterial prostatitis (CBP), (c) chronic pelvic pain syndrome (CPPS), and (d) asymptomatic inflammatory prostatitis.
21. Prostate cancer is the most commonly diagnosed nonskin cancer in men in Canada. Its incidence varies greatly worldwide. Possible causes include genetic predisposition, environmental and dietary factors, inflammation, and alterations in levels of hormones (testosterone, dihydrotestosterone, and estradiol) and growth factors. Incidence is greatest in men in developed countries in regions such as Oceania, Europe, and North America, men older than 65 years, and Black men.
22. Most cancers of the prostate are adenocarcinomas that develop at the periphery of the gland.
23. Sexual dysfunction in males can be caused by any physical or psychological factor that impairs erection, emission, or ejaculation.
24. Spermatogenesis (sperm production by the testes) can be impaired by disruptions of the hypothalamic-pituitary-testicular axis that reduce testosterone secretion and by testicular trauma, infection, or atrophy from any cause. Sperm production is also impaired by neoplastic disease, cryptorchidism, or any factor that causes testicular temperature to rise (e.g., circulatory impairment, wearing tight clothing).

Disorders of the Male Breast

1. Gynecomastia is the overdevelopment (hyperplasia) of breast tissue in a male. It is first seen as a firm, palpable mass at least 2 cm in diameter and is located in the subareolar area.
2. Gynecomastia affects 32 to 40% of the male population. The incidence is greatest among adolescents and men older than 50 years of age.
3. Gynecomastia is caused by hormonal or breast tissue alterations that cause estrogen to dominate. These alterations can result from systemic disorders, medications, neoplasms, or idiopathic causes.
4. Breast cancer is relatively uncommon in males, but it has a poor prognosis because men tend to delay seeking treatment until the disease is advanced. The incidence is greatest in men in their 60s.
5. Most breast cancers in men are estrogen-receptor positive.

Sexually Transmitted Infections

1. Sexually transmitted infections (STIs) are contracted through intimate as well as sexual contact and include systemic infections, such as tuberculosis and hepatitis, which can spread to a sexual partner.
2. The etiology of an STI may be bacterial, viral, protozoan, parasitic, or fungal.

KEY TERMS

Acute bacterial prostatitis (ABP, category I), 878
Androgen receptor (AR) signalling, 885
Balanitis, 871
Benign prostatic hyperplasia (BPH, benign prostatic hypertrophy), 876
Bladder outflow obstruction, 878
Chemical epididymitis, 876
Chronic bacterial prostatitis (CBP, category II), 879
Chronic prostatitis/chronic pelvic pain syndrome (CP/CPPS, category III), 879
Complete precocious puberty, 869
Condyloma acuminatum, 871
Cryptorchidism, 873
Delayed puberty, 868
Ectopic testis, 873
Epididymitis, 876
Fibroblast, 886
Gynecomastia, 890
Hydrocele, 873
Intraprostatic conversion, 882
Nonbacterial prostatitis, 879
Orchitis, 874
Paraphimosis, 870
Penile intraepithelial neoplasm (PeIN), 872
Peyronie disease ("bent nail syndrome"), 870
Phimosis, 869
Precocious puberty, 868
Priapism, 871
Prostatic intraepithelial neoplasia (PIN), 885
Prostatitis, 878
Sexual dysfunction, 888
Sexual transmitted infections (STIs), 891
Spermatocele (epididymal cyst), 873
Stroma, 885
Testicular appendage, 874
Torsion of the testis, 874
Urethral stricture, 869
Urethritis, 869
Varicocele, 872

REFERENCES

1. American Cancer Society (2015). *Cancer facts & figures 2015*. Atlanta: Author.
2. Jospe, N. (2005). Disorders of pubertal development. In L. M. Osborn, T. G. DeWitt, L. R. First, et al. (Eds.), *Pediatrics*. Philadelphia: Mosby.
3. Whittemore, B. J., Smaldone, A., & Steiner, R. D. (2012). Endocrine and metabolic disorders. In C. E. Burns, A. M. Dunn, M. A. Brady, et al. (Eds.), *Pediatric primary care*. St. Louis: Saunders.
4. Foster, D. L., Jackson, L. M., & Padmanabhan, V. (2006). Programming of GnRH feedback controls timing puberty and adult reproductive activity. *Molecular and Cellular Endocrinology, 254–255*, 109–119. doi:10.1016/j.mce.2006.04.004.
5. Euling, S. Y., Herman-Giddens, M. E., Lee, P. A., et al. (2008). Examination of US puberty-timing data from 1940 to 1994 for secular trends: Panel findings. *Pediatrics, 12*(Suppl. 3), S172–S191. doi:10.1542/peds.2007-1813D.
6. Herman-Giddens, M. E., Steffes, J., Harris, D., et al. (2012). Secondary sexual characteristics in boys: Data from the Pediatric Research in Office Settings Network. *Pediatrics, 130*(5), e1058–e1068. doi:10.1542/peds.2011-3291.
7. Kwiatkowska, B., & Filipowicz-Sosnowska, A. (2009). Reactive arthritis. *Polskie Archiwum Medycyny Wewnetrznej, 119*(1–2), 60–65.
8. Brill, J. R. (2010). Diagnosis and treatment of urethritis in men. *American Family Physician, 81*(7), 873–878.
9. McAninch, J. W. (2012). Disorders of the penis and male urethra. In J. W. McAninch & T. F. Lue (Eds.), *Smith and Tanagho's general urology* (18th ed.). Norwalk, CT: McGraw-Hill Lange.
10. Anic, G. M., & Giuliano, A. R. (2011). Genital HPV infection and related lesions in men. *Preventive Medicine, 53*(Suppl. 1), S36–S41. doi:10.1016/j.ypmed.2011.08.002.
11. Centers for Disease Control and Prevention (2014). *How many cancers are linked with HPV each year?* Atlanta: Author.
12. Gur, S., Limin, M., & Hellstrom, W. J. (2011). Current status and new developments in Peyronie's disease: Medical, minimally invasive and surgical treatment options. *Expert Opinion on Pharmacotherapy, 12*(6), 931–944. doi:10.1517/14656566.2011.544252.
13. Downes, M. R. (2015). Review of in situ and invasive penile squamous cell carcinoma and associated non-neoplastic dermatological conditions. *Journal of Clinical Pathology, 68*(5), 333–340. doi:10.1136/jclinpath-2015-202911.
14. Chaux, A., & Cubilla, A. L. (2012). Advances in pathology of penile carcinoma. *Human Pathology, 43*(6), 771–789. doi:10.1016/j.humpath.2012.01.014.
15. Canadian Cancer Society. (2017). *Penile cancer statistics*. Retrieved from http://www.cancer.ca/en/cancer-information/cancer-type/penile/statistics/?region=bc.
16. American Cancer Society. (2015). *Penile cancer resource center*. Retrieved from http://www.cancer.org/cancer/penilecancer/index.
17. Trottler, H., & Burchell, A. N. (2009). Epidemiology of mucosal human papillomavirus infection and associated diseases. *Public Health Genomics, 12*(5–6), 291–307. doi:10.1159/000214920.
18. Blais, N., & Kassouf, E. (2014). Managing advanced penile cancer in 2014. *Current Opinion in Supportive and Palliative Care, 8*(3), 241–249. doi:10.1097/SPC.0000000000000075.
19. Letendre, J., Saad, F., & Lattouf, J. B. (2011). Penile cancer: What's new? *Current Opinion in Supportive and Palliative Care, 5*(3), 185–191. doi:10.1097/SPC.0b013e32834903d9.
20. Pagliaro, L. C., Williams, D. L., Daliani, D., et al. (2010). Neoadjuvant paclitaxel, ifosfamide, and cisplatin chemotherapy for metastatic penile cancer: A phase II study. *Journal of Clinical Oncology, 28*(24), 3851. doi:10.1200/JCO.2010.29.5477.
21. Zou, B., Han, Z., Wang, Z., et al. (2014). Neoadjuvant therapy combined with a BMP regimen for treating penile cancer patients with lymph node metastasis: A retrospective study in China. *Journal of Cancer Research and Clinical Oncology, 140*(10), 1733–1738. doi:10.1007/s00432-014-1720-5.
22. Wampler, S. M., & Llanes, M. (2010). Common scrotal and testicular problems. *Primary Care, 37*(3), 613–626. doi:10.1016/j.pop.2010.04.009.
23. Chen, S. S. (2012). Differences in the clinical characteristics between young and elderly men with varicocele. *International Journal of Andrology, 35*(5), 695–699. doi:10.1111/j.1365-2605.2012.01257.x.
24. Montgomery, J. S., & Bloom, D. A. (2011). The diagnosis and management of scrotal masses. *The Medical Clinics of North America, 95*(1), 235–244. doi:10.1016/j.mcna.2010.08.029.
25. Davis, J. E., & Silverman, M. (2011). Scrotal emergencies. *Emergency Medicine Clinics of North America, 29*(3), 469–484. doi:10.1016/j.emc.2011.04.011.
26. Walsh, T. J., & Smith, J. F. (2012). Male infertility. In J. W. McAninch & T. F. Lue (Eds.), *Smith and Tanagho's general urology* (18th ed.). Norwalk, CT: McGraw-Hill Lange.
27. Günther, P., & Rübben, I. (2012). The acute scrotum in childhood and adolescence. *Deutsches Ärzteblatt International, 109*(25), 449–457. doi:10.3238/arztebl.2012.0449.
28. Rioja, J., Sánchez-Margallo, F. M., Usón, J., et al. (2011). Adult hydrocele and spermatocele. *BJU International, 107*(11), 1852–1864. doi:10.1111/j.1464-410X.2011.10353.x.
29. John Radcliffe Hospital Cryptorchidism Study Group. (1992). Cryptorchidism: A prospective study of 7500 consecutive male births, 1984–8. *Archives of Disease in Childhood, 67*(7), 892–899.
30. Jensen, M. S., Wilcox, A. J., Olsen, J., et al. (2012). Cryptorchidism and hypospadias in a cohort of 934 538 Danish boys: The role of birth weight, gestational age, body dimensions, and fetal growth. *American Journal of Epidemiology, 175*(9), 917–925. doi:10.1093/aje/kwr421.
31. Walsh, T. J., Dall'Era, M. A., Croughan, M. S., et al. (2007). Prepubertal orchiopexy for crytorchidism may be associated with lower risk of testicular cancer. *The Journal of Urology, 178*(4 Pt. 1), 1440–1446. doi:10.1016/j.juro.2007.05.166.
32. Nguyen, H. T. (2012). Bacterial infections of the genitourinary tract. In J. W. McAninch & T. F. Lue (Eds.), *Smith and Tanagho's general urology* (18th ed.). Norwalk, CT: McGraw-Hill Lange.
33. National Cancer Institute. (2014). *Testicular cancer incidence and mortality*. Retrieved from http://seer.cancer.gov/statfacts/html/testis.html.
34. Canadian Cancer Society. (2017). *Testicular cancer statistics*. Retrieved from http://www.cancer.ca/en/cancer-information/cancer-type/testicular/statistics/?region=on.
35. Canadian Cancer Society. (2016). *Finding testicular cancer early*. Retrieved from http://www.cancer.ca/en/cancer-information/cancer-type/testicular/finding-cancer-early/?region=on.
36. Raynor, M. C., & Carson, C. C. (2011). Urinary infections in men. *The Medical Clinics of North America, 95*(1), 43–54. doi:10.1016/j.mcna.2010.08.015.
37. Trojian, T. H., Lishnak, T. S., & Helman, D. (2009). Epididymitis and orchitis: An overview. *American Family Physician, 79*(7), 583–587.
38. Patel, N. D., & Parsons, J. K. (2014). Epidemiology and etiology of benign prostatic hyperplasia and bladder outlet obstruction. *Indian Journal of Urology, 30*(2), 170–176. doi:10.4103/0970-1591.126900.
39. Timms, B. G., & Hofkamp, L. E. (2011). Prostate development and growth in benign prostatic hyperplasia. *Differentiation; Research in Biological Diversity, 82*(4–5), 173–183. doi:10.1016/j.diff.2011.08.002.
40. Ho, C. K., & Habib, F. K. (2011). Estrogen and androgen signaling in the pathogenesis of BPH. *Nature Reviews: Urology, 8*(1), 29–41. doi:10.1038/nrurol.2010.207.
41. Nicholson, T. M., & Ricke, W. A. (2011). Androgens and estrogens in benign prostatic hyperplasia: Past, present and future. *Differentiation; Research in Biological Diversity, 82*(4–5), 184–199. doi:10.1016/j.diff.2011.04.006.

42. Nicholson, T. M., Sehgal, P. D., Drew, S. A., et al. (2013). Sex steroid receptor expression and localization in benign prostatic hyperplasia varies with tissue compartment. *Differentiation; Research in Biological Diversity, 85*(4–5), 140–149. doi:10.1016/j.diff.2013.02.006.
43. Chughtai, B., Lee, R., Te, A., et al. (2011). Inflammation and benign prostatic hyperplasia: Clinical implications. *Current Urology Reports, 12*(4), 274–277. doi:10.1007/s11934-011-0191-3.
44. Bachmann, A., & de la Rosette, J. (2012). *Benign prostatic hyperplasia and lower urinary tract symptoms in men.* New York: Oxford University Press.
45. Pearson, R., & Williams, P. M. (2014). Common questions about the diagnosis and management of benign prostatic hyperplasia. *American Family Physician, 90*(11), 769–774.
46. Schauer, I., & Madersbacher, S. (2015). Medical treatment of lower urinary tract symptoms/benign prostatic hyperplasia: Anything new in 2015. *Current Opinion in Urology, 25*(1), 6–11. doi:10.1097/MOU.0000000000000120.
47. Kapoor, A. (2012). Benign prostatic hyperplasia (BPH) management in the primary care setting. *The Canadian Journal of Urology, 19*(5, Suppl. 1), 10–17.
48. Touma, N. J., & Nickel, J. C. (2011). Prostatitis and chronic pelvic pain in men. *The Medical Clinics of North America, 95*(1), 75–86. doi:10.1016/j.mcna.2010.08.019.
49. Wagenlehner, F. M., Weidner, W., Pilatz, A., et al. (2014). Urinary tract infections and bacterial prostatitis in men. *Current Opinion in Infectious Diseases, 27*(1), 97–101. doi:10.1097/QCO.0000000000000024.
50. Karatas, O. F., Turkay, C., Bayrak, O., et al. (2010). Helicobacter pylori seroprevalence in patients with chronic prostatitis: A pilot study. *Scandinavian Journal of Urology and Nephrology, 44*(2), 91–94. doi:10.3109/00365590903535981.
51. Canadian Cancer Society. (2016). *Prostate cancer statistics.* Retrieved from http://www.cancer.ca/en/cancer-information/cancer-type/prostate/statistics/?region=bc.
52. Torre, L. A., Bray, F., Siegel, R. L., et al. (2015). Global cancer statistics, 2012. *CA: A Cancer Journal for Clinicians, 65*(2), 87–108. doi:10.3322/caac.21262.
53. Ferlay, J., Soerjomataram, I., Dikshit, R., et al. (2015). Cancer incidence and mortality worldwide: Sources, methods and major patterns in GLOBOCAN 2012. *International Journal of Cancer, 136*(5), E359–E386. doi:10.1002/ijc.29210.
54. Labbé, D. P., Zadra, G., Ebot, E. M., et al. (2015). Role of diet in prostate cancer: The epigenetic link. *Oncogene, 34*(36), 4683–4691. doi:10.1038/onc.2014.422.
55. Allott, E. H., Masko, E. M., & Freedland, S. J. (2013). Obesity and prostate cancer: Weighing the evidence. *European Urology, 63*(5), 800–809. doi:10.1016/j.eururo.2012.11.013.
56. Labrie, F. (2011). Blockage of testicular and adrenal androgens in prostate cancer treatment. *Nature Reviews: Urology, 8*, 73–80.
57. Titus, M. A., Zeithaml, B., Kantor, B., et al. (2012). Dominant-negative androgen receptor inhibition of intracrine androgen-dependent growth of castration-recurrent prostate cancer. *PLoS ONE, 7*(1), e30192. doi:10.1371/journal.pone.0030192.
58. Bosland, M. C. (2006). Sex steroids and prostate carcinogenesis: Integrated, multifactorial working hypothesis. *Annals of the New York Academy of Sciences, 1089*, 168–176. doi:10.1196/annals.1386.040.
59. Bosland, M. C., & Mahmoud, A. M. (2011). Hormones and prostate carcinogenesis: Androgens and estrogens. *Journal of Carcinogenesis, 10*, 33. doi:10.4103/1477-3163.90678.
60. Thompson, I. M., Goodman, P. J., Tangen, C. M., et al. (2003). The influence of finasteride on the development of prostate cancer. *The New England Journal of Medicine, 349*(3), 215–224. doi:10.1056/NEJMoa030660.
61. Ellem, S. J., & Risbridger, G. P. (2009). The dual, opposing roles of estrogen in the prostate. *Annals of the New York Academy of Sciences, 1155*, 174–186. doi:10.1111/j.1749-6632.2009.04360.x.
62. Ganesh, B., Saoba, S. L., Sarade, M. N., et al. (2011). Risk factors for prostate cancer: A hospital-based case-control study from Mumbai, India. *Indian Journal of Urology, 27*(3), 345–350. doi:10.4103/0970-1591.85438.
63. van Leeuwen, P. J., van den Bergh, R. C., Wolters, T., et al. (2011). Critical assessment of prebiopsy parameters for predicting prostate cancer metastasis and mortality. *The Canadian Journal of Urology, 18*(6), 6018–6024.
64. Köhler, T. S., Fazili, A. A., & Brannigan, R. E. (2009). Putative health risks associated with vasectomy. *The Urologic Clinics of North America, 36*(3), 337–345. doi:10.1016/j.ucl.2009.05.004.
65. MacLennan, G. T., Eisenberg, R., Fleshman, R. L., et al. (2006). The influence of chronic inflammation in prostatic carcinogenesis: A 5-year follow-up study. *The Journal of Urology, 176*(3), 1012–1016. doi:10.1016/j.juro.2006.04.033.
66. Jiang, M., Strand, D. W., Franco, O. E., et al. (2011). PPARγ: A molecular link between systemic metabolic disease and benign prostate hyperplasia. *Differentiation; Research in Biological Diversity, 82*(4–5), 220–236. doi:10.1016/j.diff.2011.05.008.
67. Elkahwaji, J. E. (2012). The role of inflammatory mediators in the development of prostatic hyperplasia and prostate cancer. *Research and Reports in Urology, 5*, 1–10. doi:10.2147/RRU.S23386.
68. Lee, C., Jia, Z., Rahmatpanah, F., et al. (2014). Role of the adjacent stroma cells in prostate cancer development and progression: Synergy between TGF-β and IGF signaling. *BioMed Research International, 2014*, 502093. doi:10.1155/2014/502093.
69. Albright, F., Teerlink, C., Werner, T. L., et al. (2012). Significant evidence for a heritable contribution to cancer predisposition: A review of cancer familiality by site. *BMC Cancer, 12*, 138. doi:10.1186/1471-2407-12-138.
70. Akbari, M. R., Wallis, C. J., Toi, A., et al. (2014). The impact of a BRCA2 mutation on mortality from screen-detected prostate cancer. *British Journal of Cancer, 111*(6), 1238–1240. doi:10.1038/bjc.2014.428.
71. Castro, E., & Eeles, R. (2012). The role of BRCA1 and BRCA2 in prostate cancer. *Asian Journal of Andrology, 14*(3), 409–414. doi:10.1038/aja.2011.150.
72. Leongamornlert, D., Mahmud, N., Tymrakiewicz, M., et al. (2012). Germline BRCA1 mutations increase prostate cancer risk. *British Journal of Cancer, 106*(10), 1697–1701. doi:10.1038/bjc.2012.146.
73. Van Neste, L., Herman, J. G., Otto, G., et al. (2012). The epigenetic promise for prostate cancer diagnosis. *The Prostate, 72*(11), 1248–1261. doi:10.1002/pros.22459.
74. Lumen, N., Fonteyne, V., De Meerleer, G., et al. (2012). Screening and early diagnosis of prostate cancer: An update. *Acta Clinica Belgica, 67*(4), 270–275. doi:10.2143/ACB.67.4.2062671.
75. Mackinnon, A. C., Yan, B. C., Joseph, L. J., et al. (2009). Molecular biology underlying the clinical heterogeneity of prostate cancer: An update. *Archives of Pathology & Laboratory Medicine, 133*(7), 1033–1040. doi:10.1043/1543-2165-133.7.1033.
76. Kumar, V., Abbas, A. K., & Aster, J. C. (Eds.). (2015). *Robbins and Cotran pathologic basis of disease* (9th ed.). Philadelphia: Saunders.
77. Bonkoff, H., & Berges, R. (2009). The evolving role of oestrogens and their receptors in the development and progression of prostate cancer. *European Urology, 55*(3), 533–542. doi:10.1016/j.eururo.2008.10.035.
78. Ellem, S. J., & Risbridger, G. P. (2010). Aromatase and regulating the estrogen:androgen ratio in the prostate gland. *The Journal of Steroid Biochemistry and Molecular Biology, 118*(4–5), 246–251. doi:10.1016/j.jsbmb.2009.10.015.
79. Nellies, J. L., Hu, W.-Y., & Prins, G. S. (2011). Estrogen action and prostate cancer. *Expert Review of Endocrinology & Metabolism, 6*(3), 437–451. doi:10.1586/eem.11.20.
80. Labrie, A., Dupont, A., Simard, J., et al. (1993). Intracrinology: The basis for the rational design of endocrine therapy at all stages of prostate cancer. *European Urology, 24*(Suppl. 2), 94–105.
81. Vander Griend, D. J., D'Antonio, J., Gurel, B., et al. (2010). Cell autonomous intracellular androgen signaling drives the growth of human prostate cancer-initiating cells. *The Prostate, 70*(1), 90–99. doi:10.1002/pros.21043.
82. Ricke, E. A., Williams, K., Lee, Y. F., et al. (2012). Androgen hormone action in prostatic carcinogenesis: Stromal androgen receptors mediate prostate cancer progression, malignant transformation and metastasis. *Carcinogenesis, 33*(7), 1391–1398. doi:10.1093/carcin/bgs153.
83. Nakagawa, H., Akamatsu, S., Takata, R., et al. (2012). Prostate cancer genomics, biology, and risk assessment through genome-wide association studies. *Cancer Science, 103*(4), 607–613. doi:10.1111/j.1349-7006.2011.02193.x.
84. Santen, R. J., Brodie, H., Simpson, E. R., et al. (2009). History of aromatase: Saga of an important biological mediator and therapeutic target. *Endocrine Reviews, 30*(4), 343–375. doi:10.1210/er.2008-0016.
85. Risbridger, G. P., Davis, I. D., Birrell, S. N., et al. (2010). Breast and prostate cancer: More similar than different. *Nature Reviews: Cancer, 10*(3), 205–212. doi:10.1038/nrc2795.
86. Kawashima, H., & Nakatani, T. (2012). Involvement of estrogen receptors in prostatic diseases. *International Journal of Urology, 19*(6), 512–522. doi:10.1111/j.1442-2042.2012.02987.x.
87. Yu, Y., Yang, O., Fazil, L., et al. (2015). Progesterone receptor expression during prostate cancer progression suggests a role of this receptor in stromal cell differentiation. *The Prostate, 75*(10), 1043–1050. doi:10.1002/pros.22988.
88. Setlur, S. R., Mertz, K. D., Hoshida, Y., et al. (2008). Estrogen-dependent signaling in a molecularly distinct subclass of aggressive prostate cancer. *Journal of the National Cancer Institute, 100*(11), 815–825. doi:10.1093/jnci/djn150.
89. Epstein, J. I. (2009). The lower urinary tract and male genital system. In V. Kumar, A. K. Abbas, N. Fausto, et al. (Eds.), *Robbins and Cotran pathologic basis of disease* (8th ed., pp. 971–1004). Philadelphia: Saunders.
90. Taverna, G., Pedretti, E., Di Caro, G., et al. (2015). Inflammation and prostate cancer: Friends or foe? *Inflammation Research, 64*(5), 275–286. doi:10.1007/s00011-015-0812-2.
91. Marian, C. O., & Shay, J. W. (2009). Prostate tumor initiating cells: A new target for telomerase inhibition therapy? *Biochimica et Biophysica Acta, 1792*(4), 289–296. doi:10.1016/j.bbadis.2009.02.012.
92. Bianchi-Frias, D., Vakar-Lopez, F., Coleman, I. M., et al. (2010). The effects of aging on the molecular and cellular composition of the prostate microenvironment. *PLoS ONE, 5*(9), e12501. doi:10.1371/journal.pone.0012501.
93. Feitelson, M. A., Arzumanyan, A., Kulathinal, R. J., et al. (2015). Sustained proliferation in cancer: Mechanisms and novel therapeutic targets. *Seminars in Cancer Biology, 35*(Suppl.), S25–S54. doi:10.1016/j.semcancer.2015.02.006.
94. Polyak, K., Haviv, I., & Campbell, I. G. (2009). Co-evolution of tumor cells and their microenvironment. *Trends in Genetics, 25*(1), 30–38. doi:10.1016/j.tig.2008.10.012.
95. Casey, S. C., Amedei, A., Aquilano, K., et al. (2015). Cancer prevention and therapy through the modulation of the tumor microenvironment. *Seminars in Cancer Biology, 35*(Suppl.), S199–S223. doi:10.1016/j.semcancer.2015.02.007.
96. Thiery, J. P. (2002). Epithelial-mesenchymal transitions in tumor progression. *Nature Reviews: Cancer, 2*(6), 442–454. doi:10.1038/nrc822.
97. Josson, S., Sharp, S., Sung, S. Y., et al. (2010). Tumor-stromal interaction influence radiation sensitivity in epithelial versus mesenchymal-like

prostate cancer cell. *Journal of Oncology, 2010*, doi:10.1155/2010/232831.
98. Bhowmick, N. A., & Moses, H. L. (2005). Tumor–stroma interactions. *Current Opinion in Genetics & Development, 15*(1), 97–101. doi:10.1016/j.gde.2004.12.003.
99. Xu, J., Wang, R., Xie, Z. H., et al. (2006). Prostate cancer metastasis: Role of the host microenvironment in promoting epithelial to mesenchymal transition and increased bone adrenal gland metastasis. *The Prostate, 66*(15), 1664–1673.
100. Liu, W., Laitinen, S., Khan, S., et al. (2009). Copy number analysis indicates monoclonal origin of lethal metastatic prostate cancer. *Nature Medicine, 15*(5), 559–565. doi:10.1038/nm.1944.
101. National Cancer Institute. (2015). *PDQ® prostate cancer treatment*. Retrieved from http://www.cancer.gov/types/prostate/hp/prostate-treatment-pdq.
102. Ilic, D., Neuberger, M. M., Djulbegovic, M., et al. (2013). Screening for prostate cancer. *The Cochrane Database of Systematic Reviews*, (1), CD004720, doi:10.1002/14651858.CD004720.pub3.
103. Moyer, V. A. (2012). US Preventive Services Task Force: Screening for prostate cancer: US Preventive Services Task Force recommendation statement. *Annals of Internal Medicine, 157*(2), 120–134.
104. Matsui, H., Sopko, N. A., Hannan, J. L., et al. (2015). Mini review: Pathophysiology of erectile dysfunction. *Current Drug Targets, 16*(5), [Epub ahead of print].
105. Smith, W. B., McCaslin, I. R., Gokce, A., et al. (2013). PDE5 inhibitors: Considerations for preference and long-term adherence. *International Journal of Clinical Practice, 67*(8), 768–780. doi:10.1111/ijcp.12074.
106. Toulis, K. A., Iliadou, P. K., Venetis, C. A., et al. (2010). Inhibin B and anti-Mullerian hormone as markers of persistent spermatogenesis in men with non-obstructive azoospermia: A meta-analysis of diagnostic accuracy studies. *Human Reproduction Update, 16*(6), 713–724. doi:10.1093/humupd/dmq024.
107. Zhang, F., Li, L., Wang, L., et al. (2013). Clinical characteristics and treatment of azoospermia and severe oligospermia patients with Y-chromosome microdeletions. *Molecular Reproduction and Development, 80*(11), 908–915. doi:10.1002/mrd.22226.
108. Check, J. H. (2006). The infertile male: Diagnosis. *Clinical and Experimental Obstetrics & Gynecology, 33*(3), 133–139.
109. Canadian Cancer Society. (2017). *Breast cancer statistics*. Retrieved from http://www.cancer.ca/en/cancer-information/cancer-type/breast/statistics/?region=on.
110. Ly, D., Forman, D., Ferlay, J., et al. (2012). An international comparison of male and female breast cancer incidence rates. *International Journal of Cancer, 132*(8), 1918–1926. doi:10.1002/ijc.27841.
111. Gómez-Raposo, C., Zambrana Tévar, F., Sereno Moyano, M., et al. (2010). Male breast cancer. *Cancer Treatment Reviews, 36*(6), 451–457. doi:10.1016/j.ctrv.2010.02.002.
112. Johansen Taber, K. A., Morisy, L. R., Osbahr, A. J., 3rd, et al. (2010). Male breast cancer: Risk factors, diagnosis, and management. *Oncology Reports, 24*(5), 1115–1120.
113. Ottini, L., Palli, D., Rizzo, S., et al. (2010). Male breast cancer. *Critical Reviews in Oncology/Hematology, 73*(2), 141–155. doi:10.1016/j.critrevonc.2009.04.003.
114. Zygogianni, A. G., Kyrgias, G., Gennatas, C., et al. (2012). Male breast carcinoma: Epidemiology, risk factors and current therapeutic approaches. *Asian Pacific Journal of Cancer Prevention : APJCP, 13*(1), 15–19.
115. Kornegoor, R., Verschuur-Maes, A. H., Buerger, H., et al. (2012). Molecular subtyping of male breast cancer by immunochemistry. *Modern Pathology, 25*(3), 398–404. doi:10.1038/modpathol.2011.174.
116. Sanchez-Munoz, A., Roman-Jobacho, A., Perez-Villa, L., et al. (2012). Male breast cancer: Immunohistochemical subtypes and clinical outcome characterization. *Oncology, 83*(4), 228–233. doi:10.1159/000341537.
117. Centers for Disease Control and Prevention. (2015). Sexually transmitted diseases treatment guidelines. *Morbidity and Mortality Weekly Report, 64*(3), 1–140.
118. Public Health Agency of Canada. (2011). *Report on sexually transmitted infections in Canada: 2012*. Retrieved from http://www.phac-aspc.gc.ca/sti-its-surv-epi/rep-rap-2012/note-eng.php.
119. Centers for Disease Control and Prevention. (2014). *Fact sheet reported STDs in the United States 2013 national data for chlamydia, gonorrhea, and syphilis*. Atlanta, GA: Author.

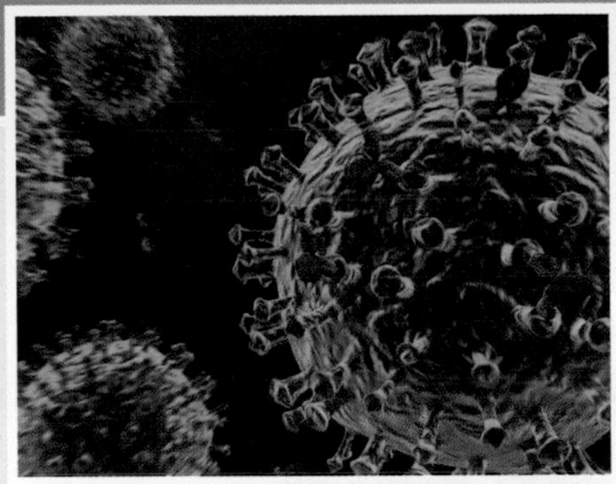

35

Structure and Function of the Digestive System

Sue E. Huether and Mohamed El-Hussein

EVOLVE WEBSITE

http://evolve.elsevier.com/Canada/Huether/pathophysiology
Student Review Questions
Key Points
Case Studies
Animations
Quick Check Answers

CHAPTER OUTLINE

The Gastro-Intestinal Tract, 899
Mouth and Esophagus, 899
Stomach, 902
Small Intestine, 905
Large Intestine, 909
Intestinal Microbiome, 910
Splanchnic Blood Flow, 910
Accessory Organs of Digestion, 910
Liver, 911
Gallbladder, 914
Exocrine Pancreas, 915
***GERIATRIC CONSIDERATIONS:* Aging and the Gastro-Intestinal System, 918**

The digestive system includes the gastro-intestinal (GI) tract and accessory organs of digestion: the salivary glands, liver, gallbladder, and exocrine pancreas (Figure 35-1). The digestive system breaks down ingested food, prepares it for uptake by the body's cells, absorbs fluid, and eliminates wastes. Food breakdown begins in the mouth with chewing and continues in the stomach, where food is churned and mixed with acid, mucus, enzymes, and other secretions. From the stomach, the fluid and partially digested food pass into the small intestine, where biochemical agents and enzymes secreted by the intestinal cells, liver, gallbladder, and exocrine pancreas break it down into absorbable components of proteins, carbohydrates, and fats. These nutrients pass through the walls of the small intestine into blood vessels and lymphatics that carry them to the liver for storage or further processing.

Ingested substances and secretions that are not absorbed in the small intestine pass into the large intestine, where fluid continues to be absorbed. Fluid wastes travel to the kidneys and are eliminated in the urine. Solid wastes pass into the rectum and are eliminated from the body through the anus. Except for chewing, swallowing, and defecation of solid wastes, the movements of the digestive system (peristalsis) are all controlled by hormones and the autonomic nervous system. The autonomic innervation, both sympathetic and parasympathetic, is controlled by centres in the brain and by local stimuli that are mediated at plexuses (networks of nerve fibres) within the GI walls. The GI tract and gut microbiome provide important immune and protective functions. Aging can alter the structure and function of the GI tract (see *Geriatric Considerations:* Aging and the Gastro-Intestinal System).

THE GASTRO-INTESTINAL TRACT

The **gastro-intestinal (GI) tract** (alimentary canal) consists of the mouth, esophagus, stomach, small intestine, large intestine, rectum, and anus (see Figure 35-1). It carries out the following digestive processes:

- Ingestion of food
- Propulsion of food and wastes from the mouth to the anus
- Secretion of mucus, water, and enzymes
- Mechanical digestion of food particles
- Chemical digestion of food particles
- Absorption of digested food
- Elimination of waste products by defecation
- Immune and microbial protection against infection

Histologically, the GI tract consists of four layers. From the inside out they are the mucosa, submucosa, muscularis, and serosa (or adventitia). These concentric layers vary in thickness, and each layer has sublayers (Figure 35-2). A network of intrinsic nerves that controls mobility, secretion, sensation, and blood flow is located solely within the GI tract and controlled by local and autonomic nervous system stimuli through the **enteric (intramural) plexus** located in different layers of the GI walls (see Figure 35-2).

Mouth and Esophagus

The **mouth** is a reservoir for the chewing and mixing of food with saliva. There are 32 permanent teeth in the adult mouth, and they are important for speech and mastication. As food particles become smaller and move around in the mouth, the taste buds and olfactory nerves are continuously stimulated, adding to the satisfaction of eating. The tongue's surface contains thousands of chemoreceptors, or taste buds, which can distinguish salty, sour, bitter, sweet, and savoury (umami) tastes. Tastes and food odours help to initiate salivation and the secretion of gastric juice in the stomach.

Salivation

The three pairs of **salivary glands**—the submandibular, sublingual, and parotid glands (Figure 35-3)—secrete about 1 L of saliva per day. **Saliva** consists mostly of water with mucus, sodium, bicarbonate, chloride,

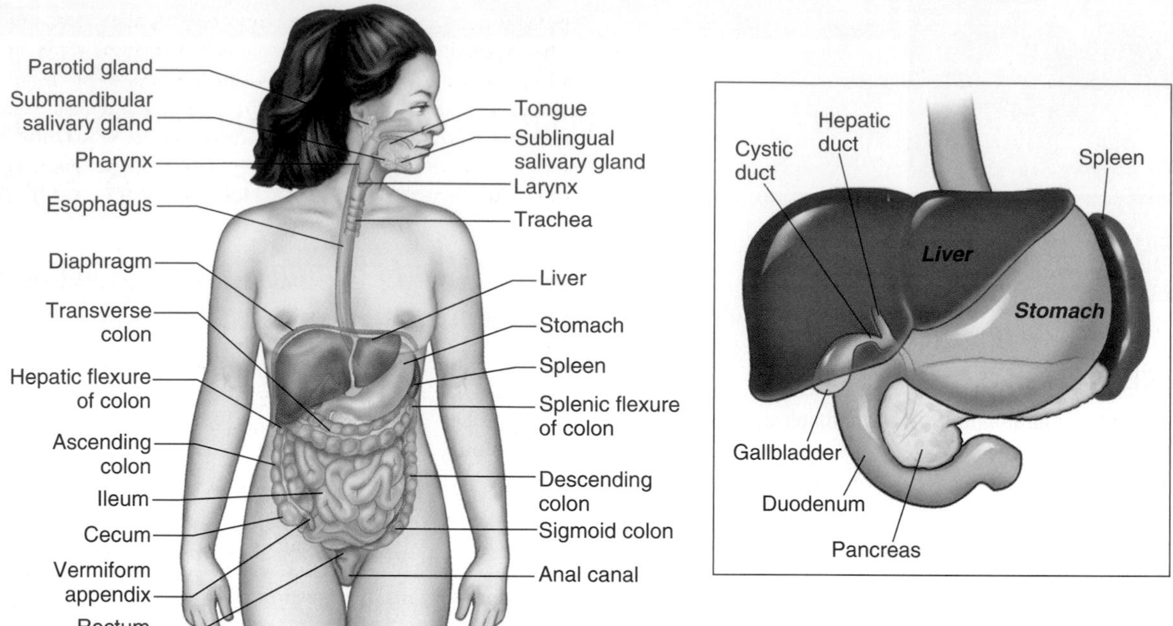

FIGURE 35-1 Structures of the Digestive System. (From Patton, K.T., & Thibodeau, G.A. [2014]. *The human body in health & disease* [6th ed.]. St. Louis: Mosby.)

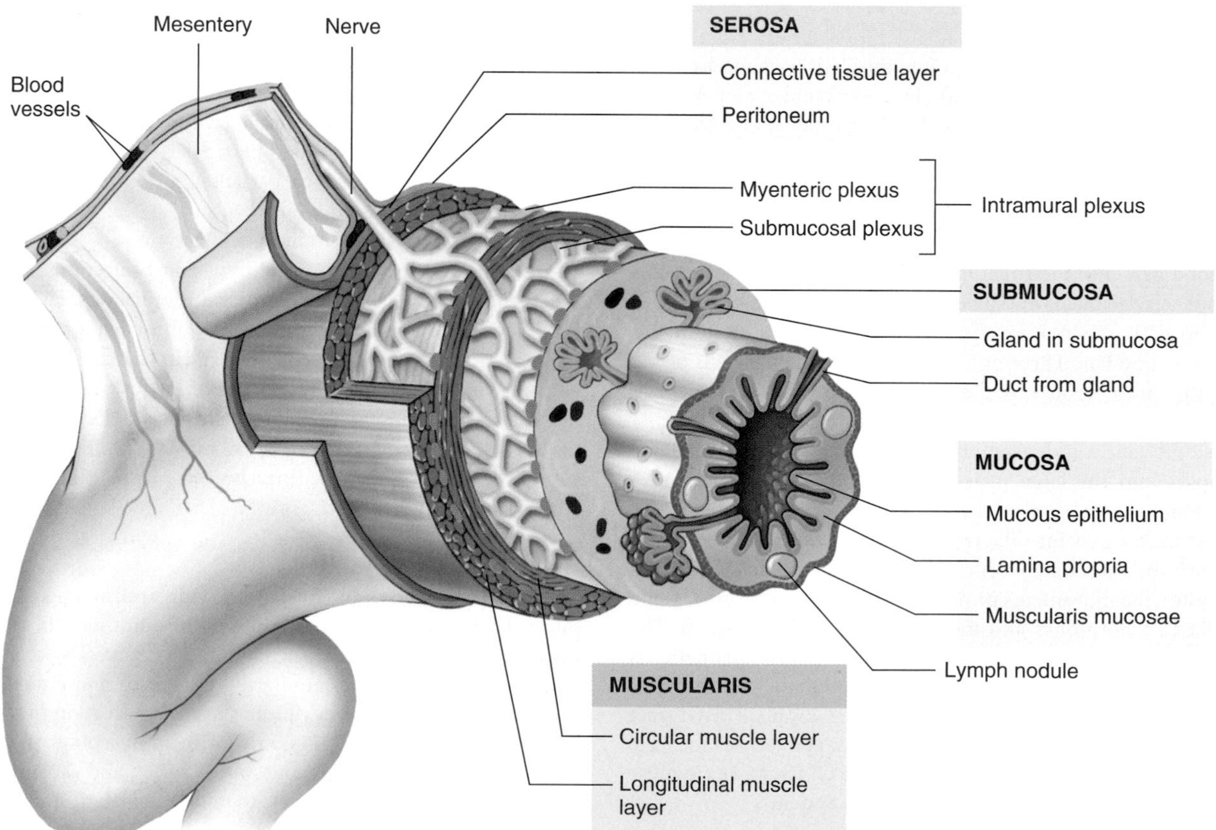

FIGURE 35-2 Wall of the Gastro-Intestinal Tract. The wall of the gastro-intestinal (GI) tract is made up of four layers with a network of nerves between the layers. This generalized diagram shows a segment of the GI tract. Note that the serosa is continuous with a fold of serous membrane called the *mesentery*. Note also that digestive glands may empty their products into the lumen of the GI tract by way of ducts. (From Patton, K.T., & Thibodeau, G.A. [2016]. *Anatomy & physiology* [9th ed.]. St. Louis: Mosby.)

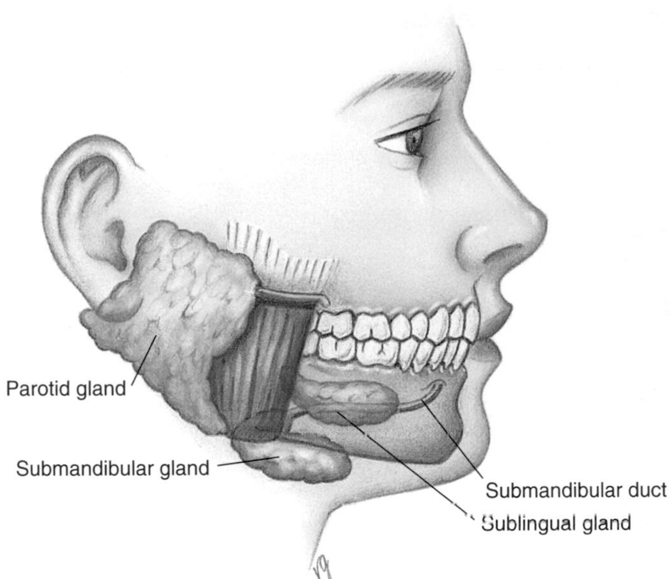

FIGURE 35-3 **Salivary Glands.** (From Gerdin, J. [2012]. *Health careers today* [5th ed.]. St. Louis: Mosby.)

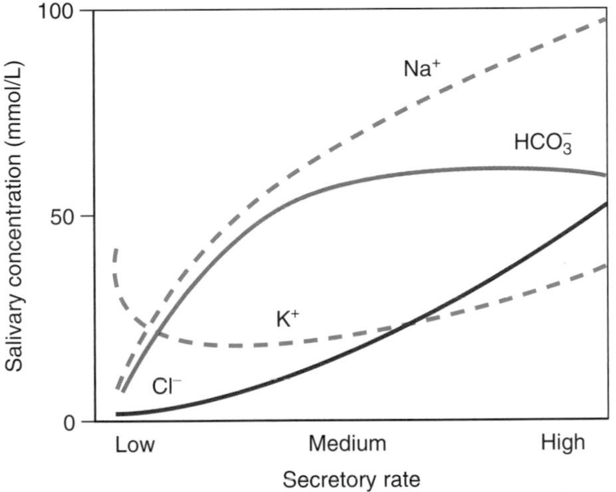

FIGURE 35-4 **Salivary Electrolyte Concentrations and Flow Rate.** Changes in concentrations of sodium (Na^+), potassium (K^+), chloride (Cl^-), and bicarbonate (HCO_3^-) increase flow rate of saliva. *Green line*, sodium; *orange line*, bicarbonate; *red line*, chloride; *blue line*, potassium. At low rates of salivary flow (i.e., between meals), sodium, chloride, and bicarbonate are reabsorbed in the collecting ducts of the salivary glands, and the saliva contains fewer of these electrolytes (i.e., is more hypotonic). At higher flow rates (i.e., stimulated by food), reabsorption decreases and saliva is hypertonic. By this mechanism, sodium, chloride, and bicarbonate are recycled until they are released to help with digestion and absorption.

potassium, and salivary α-amylase (ptyalin), an enzyme that initiates carbohydrate digestion in the mouth and stomach.

Both sympathetic and parasympathetic divisions of the autonomic nervous system control salivation. Cholinergic parasympathetic fibres stimulate the salivary glands, and atropine (an anticholinergic agent) inhibits salivation and makes the mouth dry. β-Adrenergic stimulation from sympathetic fibres also increases salivary secretion. The salivary gland secretion is not regulated by hormones.

The composition of saliva depends on the rate of secretion (Figure 35-4). Aldosterone can increase epithelial exchange of sodium for potassium, increasing sodium conservation and potassium excretion. The bicarbonate concentration of saliva sustains a pH of about 7.4, which neutralizes bacterial acids and prevents tooth decay. Saliva also contains mucin, immunoglobulin A (IgA), and other antimicrobial substances, which help prevent infection. Mucin provides lubrication. Exogenous fluoride (e.g., fluoride in drinking water) is also secreted in the saliva, providing additional protection against tooth decay.

Swallowing

The esophagus is a hollow, muscular tube approximately 25 cm long that conducts substances from the oropharynx to the stomach (see Figure 35-1). Swallowed food is moved to the stomach by peristalsis, the coordinated sequential contraction and relaxation of outer longitudinal and inner circular layers of muscles. The pharynx and upper third of the esophagus contain striated muscle (voluntary) that is directly innervated by skeletal motor neurons that control swallowing. The lower two-thirds contain smooth muscle (involuntary) that is innervated by preganglionic cholinergic fibres from the vagus nerve. The fibres are activated in a downward sequence and coordinated by the swallowing centre in the medulla. Peristalsis is stimulated when afferent fibres distributed along the length of the esophagus sense changes in wall tension caused by stretching as food passes. The greater the tension, the greater the intensity of esophageal contraction. Occasionally, intense contractions cause pain similar to "heartburn" or angina.

Each end of the esophagus is opened and closed by a sphincter. The upper esophageal sphincter keeps air from entering the esophagus during respiration. The lower esophageal sphincter (cardiac sphincter) prevents regurgitation from the stomach and caustic injury to the esophagus.

Swallowing is coordinated primarily by the swallowing centre in the medulla. During the oropharyngeal (voluntary) phase of swallowing, the following steps occur:

1. Food is segmented into a bolus by the tongue and forced posteriorly toward the pharynx.
2. The superior constrictor muscle of the pharynx contracts so the food cannot move into the nasopharynx.
3. Respiration is inhibited, and the epiglottis slides down to prevent the food from entering the larynx and trachea.

This entire sequence takes place in less than 1 second.

The esophageal phase of swallowing proceeds as follows:

1. The bolus of food enters the esophagus.
2. Waves of relaxation travel the esophagus, preparing for the movement of the bolus.
3. Peristalsis, the sequential waves of muscular contractions that travel down the esophagus, transports the food to the lower esophageal sphincter, which is relaxed at that point.
4. The bolus enters the stomach, and the sphincter muscles return to their resting tone.

This phase takes 5 to 10 seconds, with the bolus moving 2 to 6 cm/sec.

Peristalsis that immediately follows the oropharyngeal phase of swallowing is called primary peristalsis. If a bolus of food becomes stuck in the esophageal lumen, secondary peristalsis—a wave of contraction and relaxation independent of voluntary swallowing—occurs. This secondary peristalsis occurs in response to stretch receptors (stimulated by increased wall tension) that activate impulses from the swallowing centre of the brain.

The lower esophageal sphincter is normally constricted and serves as a barrier between the stomach and esophagus. The muscle tone of the lower sphincter changes with neural and hormonal stimulation and relaxes with swallowing. Cholinergic vagal input and the digestive hormone gastrin increase sphincter tone. Nonadrenergic, noncholinergic

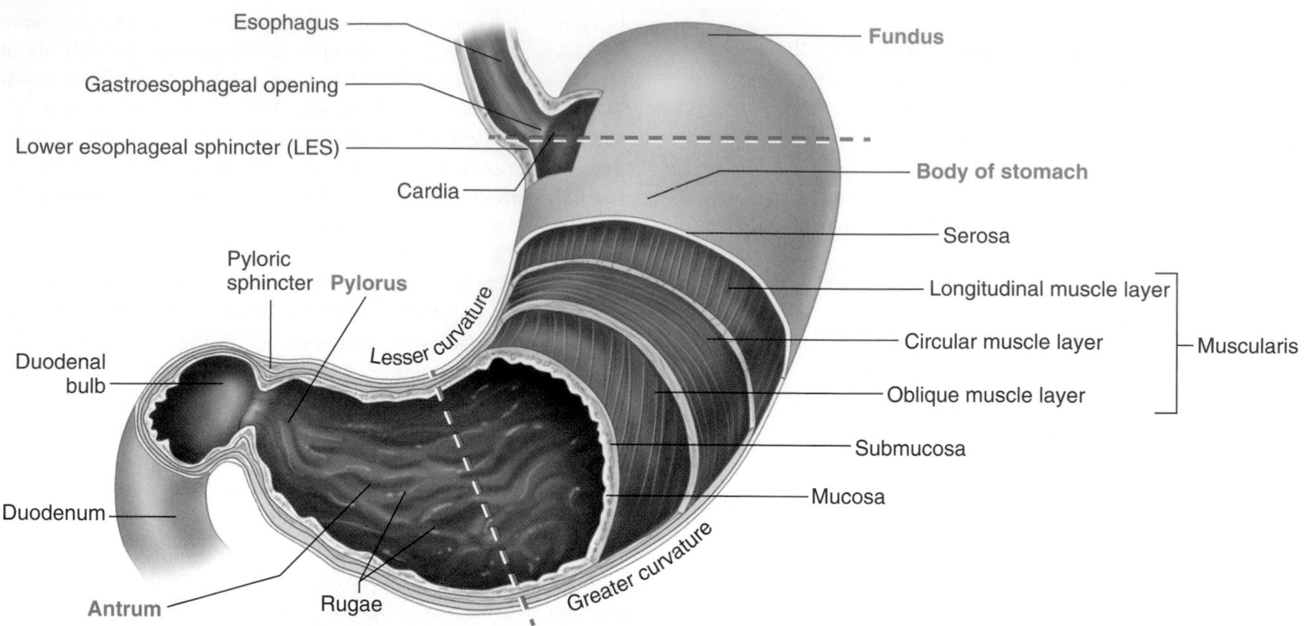

FIGURE 35-5 Stomach. A portion of the anterior wall has been excised to reveal the muscle layers of the stomach wall. Note that the mucosa lining the stomach forms folds called *rugae*. The dashed lines distinguish the fundus, body, and antrum of the stomach. (Modified from Patton, K.T., & Thibodeau, G.A. [2014]. *The human body in health & disease* [6th ed.]. St. Louis: Mosby.)

vagal impulses relax the lower esophageal sphincter, as do the hormones progesterone, secretin, and glucagon.[1]

QUICK CHECK 35-1

1. What are the functions of saliva?
2. What are the phases of swallowing and how are they controlled?

Stomach

The **stomach** is a hollow, muscular organ just below the diaphragm that stores food during eating, secretes digestive juices, mixes food with these juices, and propels partially digested food, called **chyme**, into the duodenum of the small intestine. The anatomy of the stomach is presented in Figure 35-5. The stomach's major anatomical boundaries are the lower esophageal sphincter, where food passes through the **cardiac orifice** at the gastroduodenal junction into the stomach, and the **pyloric sphincter**, which relaxes as food is propelled through the **pylorus (gastroduodenal junction)** into the duodenum. Functional areas are the **fundus** (upper portion), **body of the stomach** (middle portion), and **antrum** (lower portion).

The stomach has three layers of smooth muscle: an outer, longitudinal layer; a middle, circular layer; and an inner, oblique layer (the most prominent) (see Figure 35-5). These layers become progressively thicker in the body and antrum where food is mixed and pushed into the duodenum. The glandular epithelium is discussed under "Gastric Secretion" (see p. 904).

The stomach's blood supply comes from a branch of the celiac artery (Figure 35-6) and is so abundant that nearly all arterial vessels must be occluded before ischemic changes occur in the stomach wall. A series of small veins drain blood from the stomach toward the hepatic portal vein.

Sympathetic and parasympathetic divisions of the autonomic nervous system innervate the stomach. Some of the autonomic fibres are extrinsic—that is, they originate outside of the stomach and are controlled by nerve centres in the brain. The vagus nerve provides parasympathetic innervation, and branches of the celiac plexus innervate the stomach sympathetically. The **myenteric plexus (Auerbach plexus)** and the **submucosal plexus (Meissner plexus)** are intrinsic and part of the enteric (intramural) nervous system. They originate within the stomach and respond to local stimuli.

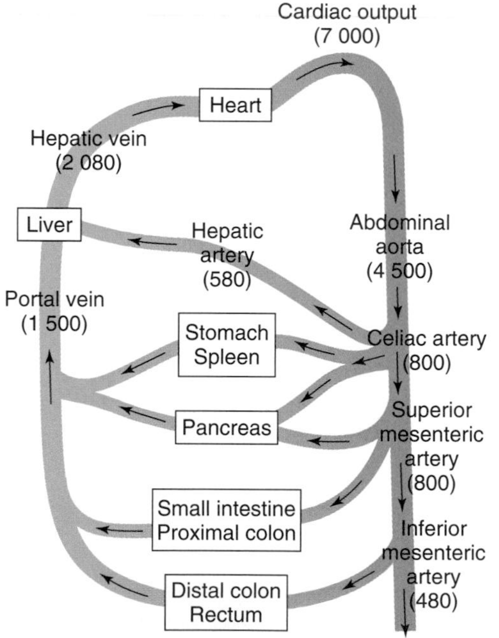

FIGURE 35-6 Major Blood Vessels and Organs Supplied With Blood in the Splanchnic Circulation. Numbers in parentheses reflect approximate blood flow values (mL/min) for each major vessel in an 80-kg normal, resting, adult human subject. Arrows indicate the direction of blood flow. (Modified from Johnson, L.R. [2001]. *Gastrointestinal pathophysiology*. St. Louis: Mosby.)

Gastric Motility

In its resting state, the stomach is small and contains about 50 mL of fluid. There is no wall tension, and the muscle layers in the fundus contract very little. Swallowing causes the fundus to relax (receptive relaxation) to receive a bolus of food from the esophagus (see "Swallowing," p. 901). Relaxation is coordinated by efferent, nonadrenergic, noncholinergic vagal fibres and is facilitated by **gastrin** and **cholecystokinin**—two polypeptide hormones secreted by the GI mucosa. (The actions of digestive hormones are summarized in Table 35-1.) Food is stored in vertical or oblique layers as it arrives in the fundus, whereas fluids flow relatively quickly down to the antrum.

Gastric (stomach) motility increases with the initiation of peristaltic waves, which sweep over the body of the stomach toward the antrum. The rate of peristaltic contractions is approximately three per minute and is influenced by neural and hormonal activity. Gastrin, **motilin** (an intestinal hormone), and the vagus nerve increase the rate of contraction by lowering the threshold potential of muscle fibres. (The neural and biochemical mechanisms of muscle contraction are described in Chapter 38.) Sympathetic activity and **secretin** (another intestinal hormone) are inhibitory and raise the threshold potential. The rate of peristalsis is mediated by pacemaker cells that initiate a wave of depolarization (basic electrical rhythm), which moves from the upper part of the stomach to the pylorus.

Gastric mixing and emptying of gastric contents (chyme) from the stomach take several hours. Mixing occurs as food is propelled toward the antrum. As food approaches the pylorus, the velocity of the peristaltic wave increases, forcing the contents back toward the body of the stomach. This **retropulsion** effectively mixes food with digestive juices, and the oscillating motion breaks down large food particles. With each peristaltic wave, a small portion of the gastric contents (chyme) passes through the pylorus and into the duodenum. The pyloric sphincter is about 1.5 cm long and is always open about 2.0 mm. It opens wider during antral contraction. Normally there is no regurgitation from the duodenum into the antrum.

The rate of **gastric emptying** (movement of gastric contents into the duodenum) depends on the volume, osmotic pressure, and chemical

TABLE 35-1 Selected Hormones[a] and Neurotransmitters of the Digestive System

Source	Hormone/ Neurotransmitter	Stimulus for Secretion	Action
Mucosa of stomach	Gastrin	Presence of partially digested proteins in stomach	Stimulates gastric glands to secrete hydrochloric acid, pepsinogen, and histamine; growth of gastric mucosa
	Histamine	Gastrin	Stimulates acid secretion
	Somatostatin	Acid in stomach	Inhibits acid, pepsinogen, and histamine secretion and release of gastrin
	Acetylcholine	**Vagus and local nerves in stomach**	**Stimulates release of pepsinogen and acid secretion**
	Gastrin-releasing peptide (bombesin)	Vagus and local nerves in stomach	Stimulates gastrin and release of pepsinogen and acid secretion
	Ghrelin	High during fasting	Stimulates growth hormone secretion and hypothalamus to increase appetite
Mucosa of small intestine	Motilin	Presence of acid and fat in duodenum	Increases gastro-intestinal (GI) motility
	Secretin	Presence of chyme (acid, partially digested proteins, fats) in duodenum	Stimulates pancreas to secrete alkaline pancreatic juice and liver to secrete bile; decreases GI motility; inhibits gastrin and gastric acid secretion
	Serotonin (5-hydroxytryptamine)	**Intestinal distension; vagal stimulation; presence of acids, amino acids, or hypertonic fluids; released from enterochromaffin cells throughout intestine**	**Stimulates intestinal secretion, motility and sensation (i.e., pain and nausea), vasodilation; activates gut immune responses**
	Cholecystokinin	Presence of chyme (acid, partially digested proteins, fats) in duodenum	Stimulates gallbladder to eject bile and pancreas to secrete alkaline fluid; decreases gastric motility; constricts pyloric sphincter; inhibits gastrin
	Enteroglucagon	Intraluminal fats and carbohydrates	Weakly inhibits gastric and pancreatic secretion and enhances insulin release, lipolysis, ketogenesis, and glycogenolysis
	Gastric inhibitory peptide (GIP)	Fat and glucose in small intestine	Inhibits gastric secretion and emptying; stimulates insulin release
	Peptide YY	Intraluminal fat and bile acids	Inhibits postprandial gastric acid and pancreatic secretion and delays gastric and small bowel emptying
	Pancreatic polypeptide	Protein, fat, and glucose in small intestine	Decreases pancreatic and enzyme secretion
	Vasoactive intestinal peptide	Intestinal mucosa and muscle	Relaxes intestinal smooth muscle

[a]The digestive hormones are not secreted into the gastro-intestinal (GI) lumen but instead into the bloodstream, where they travel to target tissues. There are more than 30 peptide hormone genes expressed in the GI tract and more than 100 hormonally active peptides.
Modified from Johnson, L.R. (2014). *Gastrointestinal physiology* (8th ed.). St. Louis: Mosby. Data from Feldman, M., Friedman, L.S., & Brandt, L.J. (2015). *Sleisenger and Fordtran's gastrointestinal and liver disease* (10th ed.). Philadelphia: Saunders.

composition of the gastric contents. Larger volumes of food increase gastric pressure, peristalsis, and rate of emptying. Solids, fats, and nonisotonic solutions (i.e., hypertonic or hypotonic gastric tube feedings) delay gastric emptying. (Osmotic pressure and tonicity are described in Chapters 1 and 5.) Products of fat digestion, which are formed in the duodenum by the action of bile from the liver and enzymes from the pancreas, stimulate the secretion of cholecystokinin. This hormone inhibits food intake, reduces gastric motility, and decreases gastric emptying so that fats are not emptied into the duodenum at a rate that exceeds the rate of bile and enzyme secretion. Osmoreceptors in the wall of the duodenum are sensitive to the osmotic pressure of duodenal contents. The arrival of hypertonic or hypotonic gastric contents activates the osmoreceptors, which delay gastric emptying to facilitate formation of an isosmotic duodenal environment. The rate at which acid enters the duodenum also influences gastric emptying. Secretions from the pancreas, liver, and duodenal mucosa neutralize gastric hydrochloric acid in the duodenum. The rate of emptying is adjusted to the duodenum's ability to neutralize the incoming acidity.[2]

Gastric Secretion

The secretion of gastric juice is influenced by numerous stimuli that together facilitate the process of digestion. The phases of gastric secretion are the *cephalic phase* (stimulated by the thought, smell, and taste of food), the *gastric phase* (stimulated by distension of the stomach), and the *intestinal phase* (stimulated by histamine and digested protein). All phases promote the secretion of acid by the stomach.

Gastric secretion is stimulated by the process of eating (gastric distension), by the actions of the hormone gastrin and paracrine pathways (e.g., histamine, ghrelin, somatostatin), and by the effects of the neurotransmitter acetylcholine (ACh) and other chemicals (e.g., ethanol, coffee, protein). The stomach secretes large volumes of gastric juices or gastric secretions, including mucus, acid, enzymes, hormones, intrinsic factor, and gastroferrin. **Intrinsic factor** is necessary for the intestinal absorption of vitamin B_{12}, and gastroferrin facilitates small intestinal absorption of iron. The hormones are secreted into the blood and travel to target tissues. The other gastric secretions are released directly into the stomach lumen.[3]

In the fundus and body of the stomach, the **gastric glands** of the mucosa are the primary secretory units (Figure 35-7). The composition of gastric juice depends on volume and flow rate (Figure 35-8). Potassium level remains relatively constant, but its concentration is greater in gastric juice than in plasma. The rate of secretion varies with the time of day. Generally, the rate and volume of secretion are lowest in the morning and highest in the afternoon and evening. Loss of gastric juices through vomiting, drainage, or suction may decrease body stores of sodium and potassium and result in fluid, electrolyte (e.g., hyponatremia, hypokalemia, dehydration), and acid–base imbalances (e.g., metabolic alkalosis) (see Chapters 5 and 36).[4]

Gastric secretion is inhibited by somatostatin, by unpleasant odours and tastes, and by rage, fear, or pain. A discharge of sympathetic impulses inhibits parasympathetic impulses. Increased secretions are associated with aggression or hostility and may contribute to some forms of gastric pathology.

Gastric acid. The major functions of gastric hydrochloric acid are to dissolve food fibres, act as a bactericide against swallowed microorganisms, and convert pepsinogen to pepsin. The production of acid by the **parietal cells** requires the transport of hydrogen and chloride from the parietal cells to the stomach lumen. Acid is formed in the parietal cells, primarily through the hydrolysis of water (Figure 35-9). At a high rate of gastric secretion, bicarbonate moves into the plasma, producing an "alkaline tide" in the venous blood, which also may result in a more alkaline urine.[4]

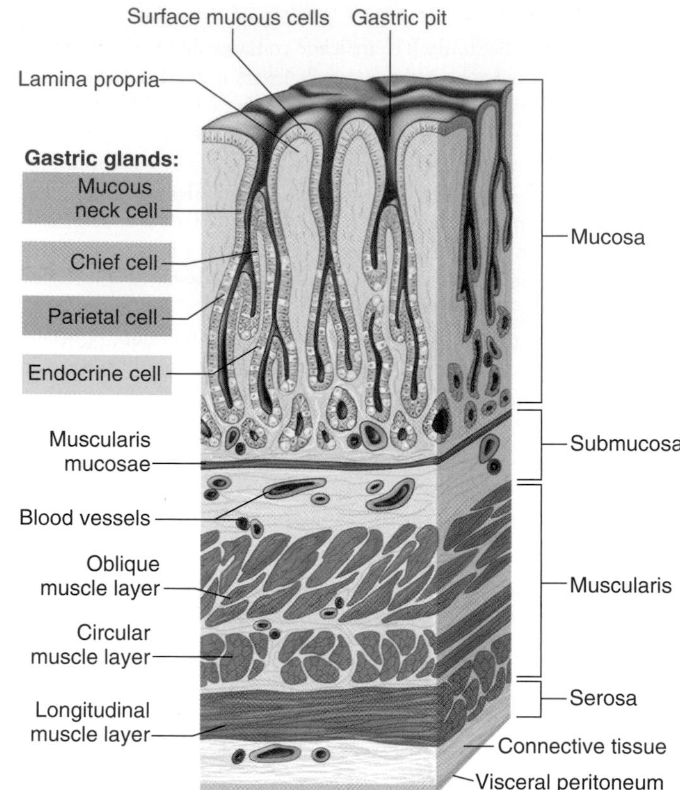

FIGURE 35-7 Gastric Pits and Gastric Glands. Gastric pits are depressions in the epithelial lining of the stomach. At the bottom of each pit are one or more tubular *gastric glands*. Chief cells produce pepsinogen, which is converted to pepsin (a proteolytic enzyme); parietal cells secrete hydrochloric acid and intrinsic factor; G cells produce gastrin; endocrine cells (enterochromaffinlike cells and D cells) secrete histamine and somatostatin. (From Patton, K.T., Thibodeau, G.A., & Douglas, M.M. [2012]. *Essentials of anatomy & physiology*. St. Louis: Mosby.)

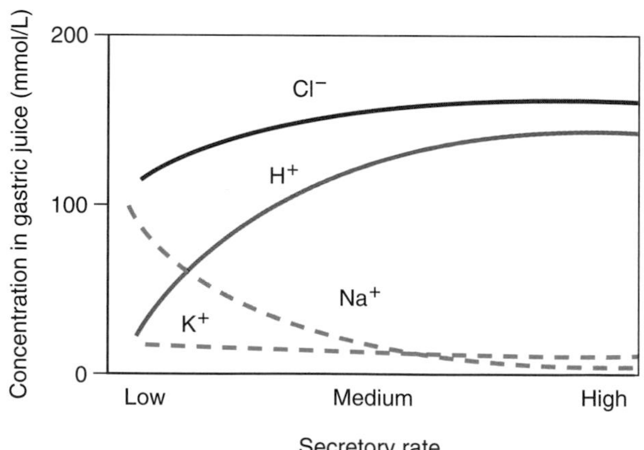

FIGURE 35-8 Gastric Electrolyte Concentrations and Flow Rate. Sodium (*Na*⁺) concentration is lower in the gastric juice than in the plasma, whereas hydrogen (*H*⁺), potassium (*K*⁺), and chloride (*Cl*⁻) concentrations are higher. *Red line*, chloride; *orange line*, hydrogen; *green line*, sodium; *blue line*, potassium.

Acid secretion is stimulated by the vagus nerve, which releases ACh and stimulates the secretion of gastrin; then gastrin stimulates the release of histamine from enterochromaffin cells (mast cells; see Chapter 6) in the gastric mucosa. Histamine stimulates acid secretion by activating histamine receptors (H2 receptors) on acid-secreting parietal cells.

Caffeine stimulates acid secretion, as does calcium. Acid secretion is inhibited by somatostatin, secretin, and other intestinal hormones.[3]

Pepsin. ACh, gastrin, and secretin stimulate the **chief cells** to release pepsinogen during eating. Pepsinogen is quickly converted to **pepsin** in the acidic gastric environment (optimum pH for pepsin activation = 2.0). Pepsin is a proteolytic enzyme—that is, it breaks down protein and forms polypeptides in the stomach. Once chyme has entered the duodenum, the alkaline environment of the duodenum inactivates pepsin.

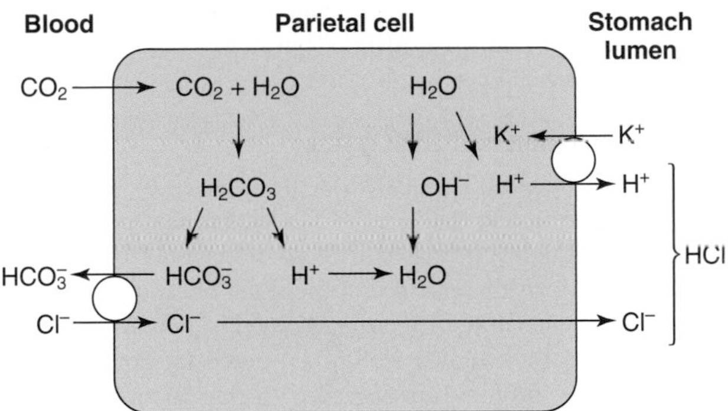

FIGURE 35-9 Hydrochloric Acid Secretion by Parietal Cell. *Cl^-*, Chloride; CO_2, carbon dioxide; *H^+*, hydrogen; *H_2CO_3*, carbonic acid; *H_2O*, water; *HCl*, hydrochloric acid; *HCO_3^-*, bicarbonate; *K^+*, potassium; *OH^-*, hydroxyl ion.

Mucus. The gastric mucosa is protected from the digestive actions of acid and pepsin by intercellular tight junctions, a coating of mucus called the **mucosal barrier**, and gastric mucosal blood flow. Prostaglandins protect the mucosal barrier by stimulating the secretion of mucus and bicarbonate and by inhibiting the secretion of acid. A break in the protective barrier may occur from ischemia or by exposure to *H. pylori*, Aspirin, nonsteroidal anti-inflammatory drugs (which inhibit prostaglandin synthesis), ethanol, or regurgitated bile. Breaks cause inflammation and ulceration.

Few substances are absorbed in the stomach. The stomach mucosa is impermeable to water, but the stomach can absorb alcohol and Aspirin.

QUICK CHECK 35-2

1. Why are there three layers of stomach muscle and how do they function?
2. What hormones stimulate gastric motility?
3. What are the phases of gastric secretion?

Small Intestine

The **small intestine** is coiled within the peritoneal cavity and is about 5 to 6 m long. Functionally, it is divided into three segments: the **duodenum, jejunum,** and **ileum** (Figure 35-10). The duodenum begins at the pylorus and ends where it joins the jejunum at a suspensory ligament called the *Treitz ligament.* The end of the jejunum and beginning of the ileum are not distinguished by an anatomical marker. These

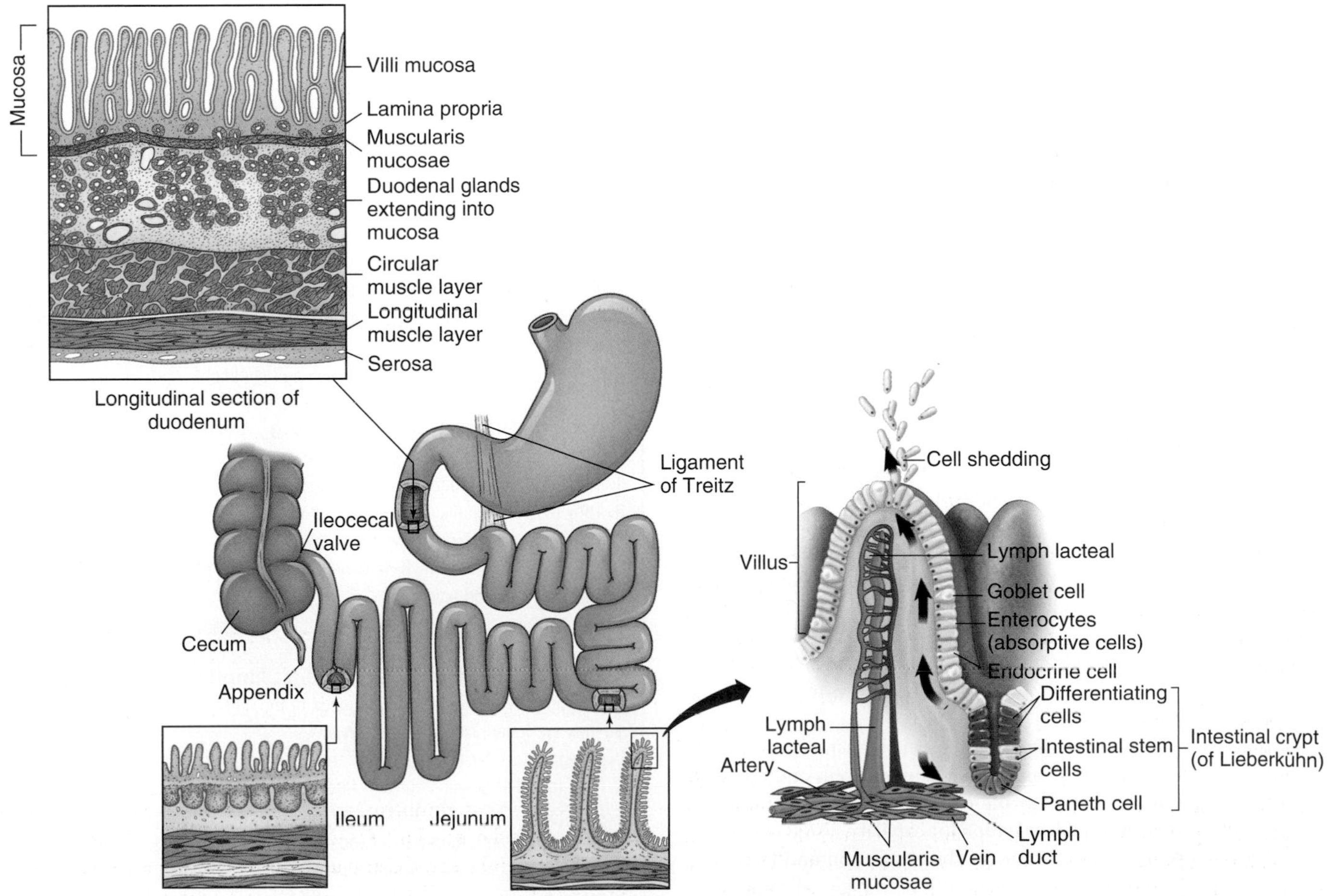

FIGURE 35-10 The Small Intestine.

structures are not grossly different, but the jejunum has a slightly larger lumen than the ileum. The ileocecal valve, or sphincter, controls the flow of digested material from the ileum into the large intestine and prevents reflux into the small intestine.

The duodenum lies behind the peritoneum, or retroperitoneally, and is attached to the posterior abdominal wall. The ileum and jejunum are suspended in loose folds from the posterior abdominal wall by a peritoneal membrane called the mesentery. The mesentery facilitates intestinal motility and supports blood vessels, nerves, and lymphatics.

The peritoneum is the serous membrane surrounding the organs of the abdomen and pelvic cavity. It is analogous to the pericardium around the heart and the pleura around the lungs. The visceral peritoneum lies on the surface of the organs, and the parietal peritoneum lines the wall of the body cavity. The space between these two layers is called the peritoneal cavity and normally contains just enough fluid to lubricate the two layers and prevent friction during organ movement.

The arterial supply to the duodenum arises primarily from the gastroduodenal artery, a branch of the celiac artery. The jejunum and ileum are supplied by branches of the superior mesenteric artery. The superior mesenteric vein drains blood from the entire small intestine and empties into the hepatic portal circulation. The regional lymph nodes and lymphatics drain into the thoracic duct.

Enteric nerves from both divisions of the autonomic nervous system innervate the small intestine. Secretion, motility, pain sensation, and intestinal reflexes (e.g., relaxation of the lower esophageal sphincter) are mediated parasympathetically by the vagus nerve. Sympathetic activity inhibits motility and produces vasoconstriction. Intrinsic reflexive activity is mediated by the myenteric plexus (Auerbach plexus) and the submucosal plexus (Meissner plexus) of the enteric nervous system.

The smooth muscles of the small intestine are arranged in two layers: a longitudinal outer layer and a thicker inner circular layer (see Figures 35-2 and 35-10). Circular folds of the small intestine slow the passage of food, thereby providing more time for digestion and absorption. The folds are most numerous and prominent in the jejunum and proximal ileum (see Figure 35-10).

Absorption occurs through villi (*sing.*, villus), which cover the circular folds and are the functional units of the intestine. A villus is composed of absorptive columnar cells (enterocytes) and mucus-secreting goblet cells of the mucosal epithelium. Each villus (see Figure 35-10) secretes some of the enzymes necessary for digestion and absorbs nutrients. Near the surface, columnar cells closely adhere to each other at sites called *tight junctions.* Water and electrolytes are absorbed through these intercellular spaces. The surface of each columnar epithelial cell on the villus contains tiny projections called microvilli (*sing.*, microvillus) (see Figure 35-10). Together the microvilli create a mucosal surface known as the brush border. The villi and microvilli greatly increase the surface area available for absorption. Coating the brush border is an "unstirred" layer of water that is important for the absorption of water-soluble substances, including emulsified micelles of fat. The lamina propria (a connective tissue layer of the mucous membrane) lies beneath the epithelial cells of the villi and contains lymphocytes and plasma cells, which produce immunoglobulins (see "The Gastro-Intestinal Tract and Immunity," p. 910).

Central arterioles ascend within each villus and branch into a capillary array that extends around the base of the columnar cells and cascades down to the venules that lead to the hepatic portal circulation (see Figure 35-10). A central lacteal, or lymphatic capillary, also is contained within each villus and is important for the absorption and transport of fat molecules. Contents of the lacteals flow to regional nodes and channels that eventually drain into the thoracic duct.[5]

Between the bases of the villi are the crypts of Lieberkühn, which extend to the submucosal layer. Undifferentiated cells arise from stem cells at the base of the crypt and move toward the tip of the villus, maturing to become columnar epithelial secretory cells (water, electrolytes, and enzymes) and goblet cells (mucus). After completing their migration to the tip of the villus, they function for a few days and then are shed into the intestinal lumen and digested. Discarded epithelial cells are an important source of endogenous protein. The entire epithelial population is replaced about every 4 to 7 days. Many factors can influence this process of cellular proliferation. Starvation, vitamin B_{12} deficiency, and cytotoxic medications or irradiation suppress cell division and shorten the villi. Decreased absorption across the epithelial membrane can cause diarrhea and malnutrition. Nutrient intake and intestinal resection stimulate cell production.

Intestinal Digestion and Absorption

The process of digestion is initiated in the stomach by the actions of gastric hydrochloric acid and pepsin. The chyme that passes into the duodenum is a liquid with small particles of undigested food. Digestion continues in the proximal portion of the small intestine by the action of pancreatic enzymes, intestinal enzymes, and bile salts. In the proximal small intestine, carbohydrates are broken down to monosaccharides and disaccharides; proteins are degraded further to amino acids and peptides; and fats are emulsified and reduced to fatty acids (Box 35-1)

BOX 35-1 Dietary Fat

Saturated Fatty Acids (e.g., Palmitic Acid [$C_{16}H_{32}O_2$])

Each carbon atom in the chain is linked by single bonds to adjacent carbon and hydrogen atoms.

1. They are solid at room temperature; they include animal fat and tropical oils (coconut and palm oils).
2. They increase low-density lipoprotein (LDL) cholesterol ("bad" cholesterol) blood levels.
3. They increase the risk of coronary artery disease.

Unsaturated Fatty Acids

1. They are soft or liquid at room temperature.
2. Omega-6 fatty acids are found in plants and vegetables (olive, canola, and peanut oils).
3. Omega-3 fatty acids are found in fish and shellfish.

Monounsaturated Fatty Acids (e.g., Oleic Acid [$C_{18}H_{34}O_2$])

They contain one double bond in the carbon chain.

1. They are found in both plants and animals.
2. They may be beneficial in reducing blood cholesterol level, glucose level, and systolic blood pressure.
3. They do not lower high-density lipoprotein (HDL) cholesterol ("good" cholesterol) blood levels.
4. Low HDL levels have been associated with coronary heart disease.

Polyunsaturated Fatty Acids (e.g., Linoleic Acid [$C_{18}H_{32}O_2$])

They contain two or more double bonds in the carbon chain.

1. They are found in plants and fish oils.
2. Omega-6 fatty acids lower total and LDL cholesterol blood levels.
3. High levels of polyunsaturated fatty acids may lower LDL levels.
4. Omega-3 fatty acids lower blood triglyceride levels and reduce platelet aggregation and, therefore, blood coagulation.
5. They are necessary for growth and development and may prevent coronary artery disease, hypertension, and inflammatory and immune disorders.

and monoglycerides (Figure 35-11). These nutrients, along with water, vitamins, and electrolytes, are absorbed across the intestinal mucosa by active transport, diffusion, or facilitated diffusion. Products of carbohydrate and protein breakdown move into villus capillaries and then to the liver through the hepatic portal vein. Digested fats move into the lacteals and eventually reach the liver through the systemic circulation. Intestinal motility exposes nutrients to a large mucosal surface area by mixing chyme and moving it through the lumen. Different segments of the GI tract absorb different nutrients. Digestion and absorption of all major nutrients and many medications occur in the small intestine. Sites of absorption are shown in Figure 35-12. Box 35-2 outlines the major nutrients involved in this process.

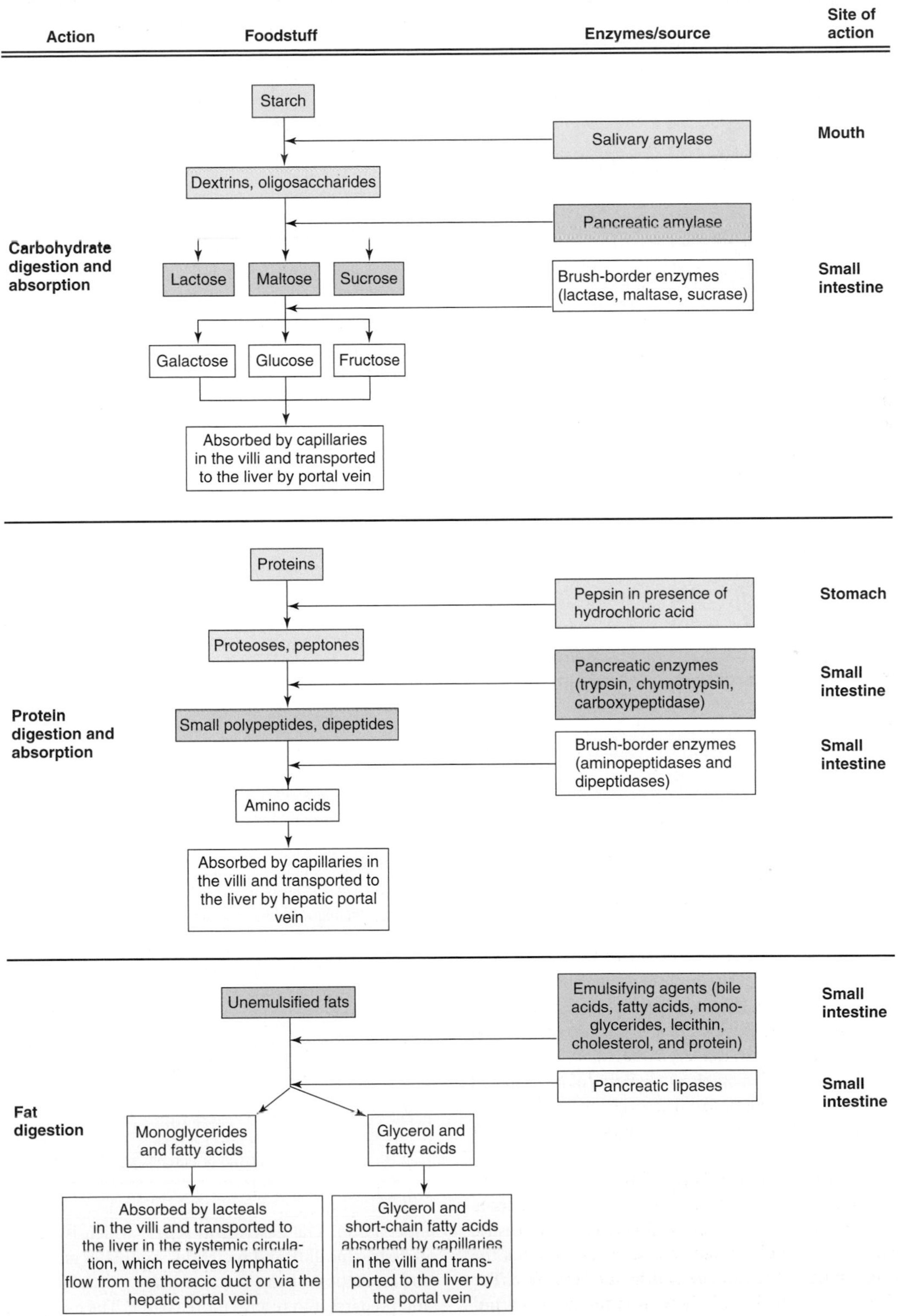

FIGURE 35-11 Digestion and Absorption of Foodstuffs.

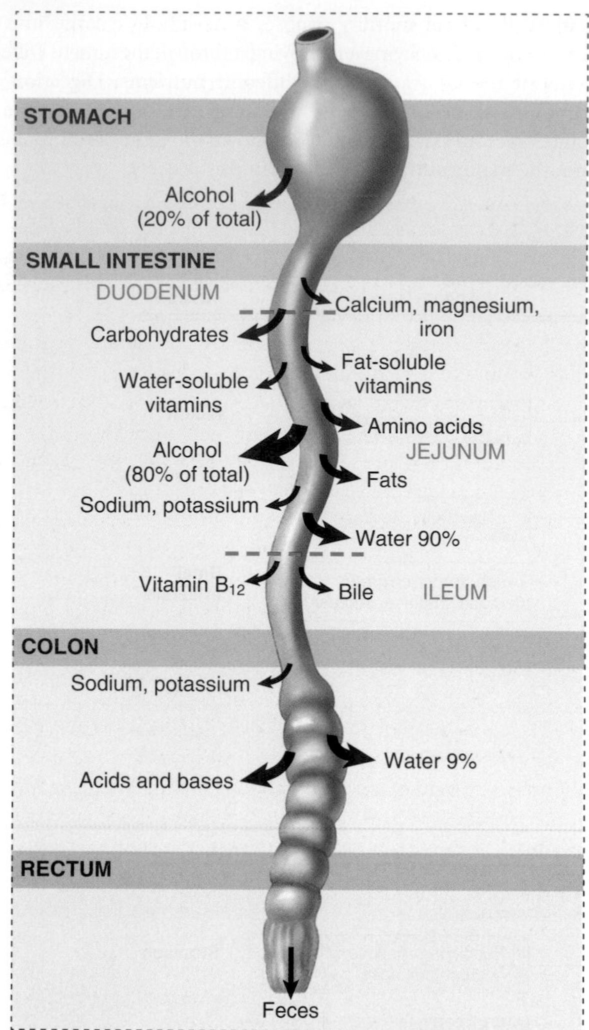

FIGURE 35-12 Sites of Absorption of Major Nutrients.

Intestinal Motility

The movements of the small intestine facilitate digestion and absorption. Chyme leaving the stomach and entering the duodenum stimulates intestinal movements that help blend secretions from the liver, gallbladder, pancreas, and intestinal glands. A churning motion brings the luminal contents into contact with the absorbing cells of the villi. Propulsive movements then advance the chyme toward the large intestine.

Intestinal motility is affected by the following two movements:

1. **Haustral segmentation.** Localized rhythmic contractions of circular smooth muscles divide and mix the chyme, enabling the chyme to have contact with digestive enzymes and the absorbent mucosal surface, and then propel it toward the large intestine.
2. **Peristalsis.** Waves of contraction along short segments of longitudinal smooth muscle allow time for digestion and absorption. The intestinal villi move with contractions of the muscularis mucosae, a thin layer of muscle separating the mucosa and submucosa, with absorption promoted by the swaying of the villi in the luminal contents.

Neural reflexes along the length of the small intestine facilitate motility, digestion, and absorption. The **ileogastric reflex** inhibits gastric motility when the ileum becomes distended. This reflex prevents the continued movement of chyme into an already distended intestine. The **intestinointestinal reflex** inhibits intestinal motility when one part of the intestine is overdistended. Both of these reflexes require extrinsic innervation. The **gastroileal reflex**, which is activated by an increase in gastric motility and secretion, stimulates an increase in ileal motility and relaxation of the ileocecal valve (sphincter). It empties the ileum and prepares it to receive more chyme. The gastroileal reflex is probably regulated by the hormones gastrin and cholecystokinin.

BOX 35-2 Major Nutrients Absorbed in the Small Intestine

Water and Electrolytes

- Approximately 85 to 90% of the water that enters the gastro-intestinal tract is absorbed in the small intestine.
- Sodium passes through tight junctions and is actively transported across cell membranes; it is exchanged for bicarbonate to maintain electroneutrality in the ileum; sodium absorption is enhanced by co-transport with glucose.
- Potassium moves passively across tight junctions with changes in the electrochemical gradient.

Carbohydrates

- Only monosaccharides are absorbed by intestinal mucosa; therefore complex carbohydrates must be hydrolyzed to simplest form.
- Salivary and pancreatic amylases break down starches to oligosaccharides (sucrose, maltose, lactose) in stomach and duodenum; brush-border enzymes hydrolyze them in intestine so they can pass through the unstirred water layer by diffusion.
- Fructose diffuses into the bloodstream; glucose and galactose diffuse or are actively transported.
- Cellulose remains undigested and stimulates large intestine motility.

Proteins

- From 90 to 95% of protein is absorbed; major hydrolysis is accomplished in the small intestine by the pancreatic enzymes trypsin, chymotrypsin, and carboxypeptidase.
- Brush-border enzymes break down proteins into smaller peptides that can cross cell membranes. In the cytosol, they are metabolized into amino acids, specifically neutral amino acids, basic amino acids, and proline and hydroxyproline.

Fats

Digestion and absorption occur in four phases:

1. *Emulsification and lipolysis:* agents cover small fat particles and prevent them from re-forming into fat droplets; then lipolysis divides them into diglycerides, monoglycerides, free fatty acids, and glycerol.
2. *Micelle formation:* products are made water soluble.
3. *Fat absorption:* fat products move from micelle to absorbing surface of intestinal epithelium and diffuse through resynthesis.
4. *Triglycerides and phospholipids:* they then become chylomicrons that eventually enter the systemic circulation.

Minerals

- *Calcium:* it is absorbed by passive diffusion and transported actively across cell membranes bound to a carrier protein; absorption primarily in ileum.
- *Magnesium:* 50% is absorbed by active transport or passive diffusion in jejunum and ileum.
- *Phosphate:* it is absorbed by passive diffusion and active transport in small intestine.
- *Iron:* it is absorbed by epithelial cells of duodenum and jejunum; vitamin C facilitates iron absorption.

Vitamins

- They are absorbed mainly by sodium-dependent active transport, with vitamin B_{12} bound to intrinsic factor and absorbed in terminal ileum.

During prolonged fasting or between meals, particularly overnight, slow waves sweep along the entire length of the intestinal tract from the stomach to the terminal ileum. This interdigestive myoelectric complex appears to propel residual gastric and intestinal contents into the colon.

The ileocecal valve (sphincter) marks the junction between the terminal ileum and the large intestine. This valve is intrinsically regulated and is normally closed. The arrival of peristaltic waves from the last few centimetres of the ileum causes the ileocecal valve to open, allowing a small amount of chyme to pass. Distension of the upper large intestine causes the sphincter to constrict, preventing further distension or retrograde flow of intestinal contents.

QUICK CHECK 35-3

1. What cells arise from the crypts of Lieberkühn?
2. How are fats absorbed from the small intestine?
3. Which reflexes inhibit intestinal motility? Which promote it?

Large Intestine

The **large intestine** is approximately 1.5 m long and consists of the cecum, appendix, colon (ascending, transverse, descending, and sigmoid), rectum, and anal canal (Figure 35-13). The **cecum** is a pouch that receives chyme from the ileum. Attached to it is the **vermiform appendix**, an appendage having little or no physiological function. From the cecum, chyme enters the **colon**, which loops upward, traverses the abdominal cavity, and descends to the anal canal. The four parts of the colon are the **ascending colon**, **transverse colon**, **descending colon**, and **sigmoid colon**. Two sphincters control the flow of intestinal contents through the cecum and colon: the ileocecal valve, which admits chyme from the ileum to the cecum, and the **rectosigmoid (O'Beirne) sphincter**, which controls the movement of wastes from the sigmoid colon into the rectum. A thick (2.5 to 3 cm) portion of smooth muscle surrounds the anal canal, forming the **internal anal sphincter**. Overlapping it distally is the striated skeletal muscle of the **external anal sphincter** (anus).

In the cecum and colon, the longitudinal muscle layer consists of three longitudinal bands called **teniae coli** (see Figure 35-13). They are shorter than the colon and give it a gathered appearance. The circular muscles of the colon separate the gathers into outpouchings called **haustra** (*sing.*, **haustrum**). The haustra become more or less prominent with the contractions and relaxations of the circular muscles. The mucosal surface of the colon has rugae (folds), particularly between the haustra, and Lieberkühn crypts but no villi. Columnar epithelial cells and mucus-secreting goblet cells form the mucosa throughout the large intestine. The columnar epithelium absorbs fluid and electrolytes, and the mucus-secreting cells lubricate the mucosa.

The enteric nervous system regulates motor and secretory activity independently of the extrinsic nervous system. Extrinsic parasympathetic innervation occurs through the vagus nerve and extends from the cecum up to the first part of the transverse colon. Vagal stimulation increases rhythmic contraction of the proximal colon. Extrinsic parasympathetic fibres reach the distal colon through the sacral parasympathetic splanchnic nerves. The internal anal sphincter is usually contracted, and its reflex response is to relax when the rectum is distended. The myenteric plexus provides the major innervation of the internal anal sphincter, but responds to sympathetic stimulation to maintain contraction and parasympathetic stimulation that facilitates relaxation when the rectum is full. Sympathetic innervation of this sphincter arises from the celiac and superior mesenteric ganglia and the sphincter nerve. The

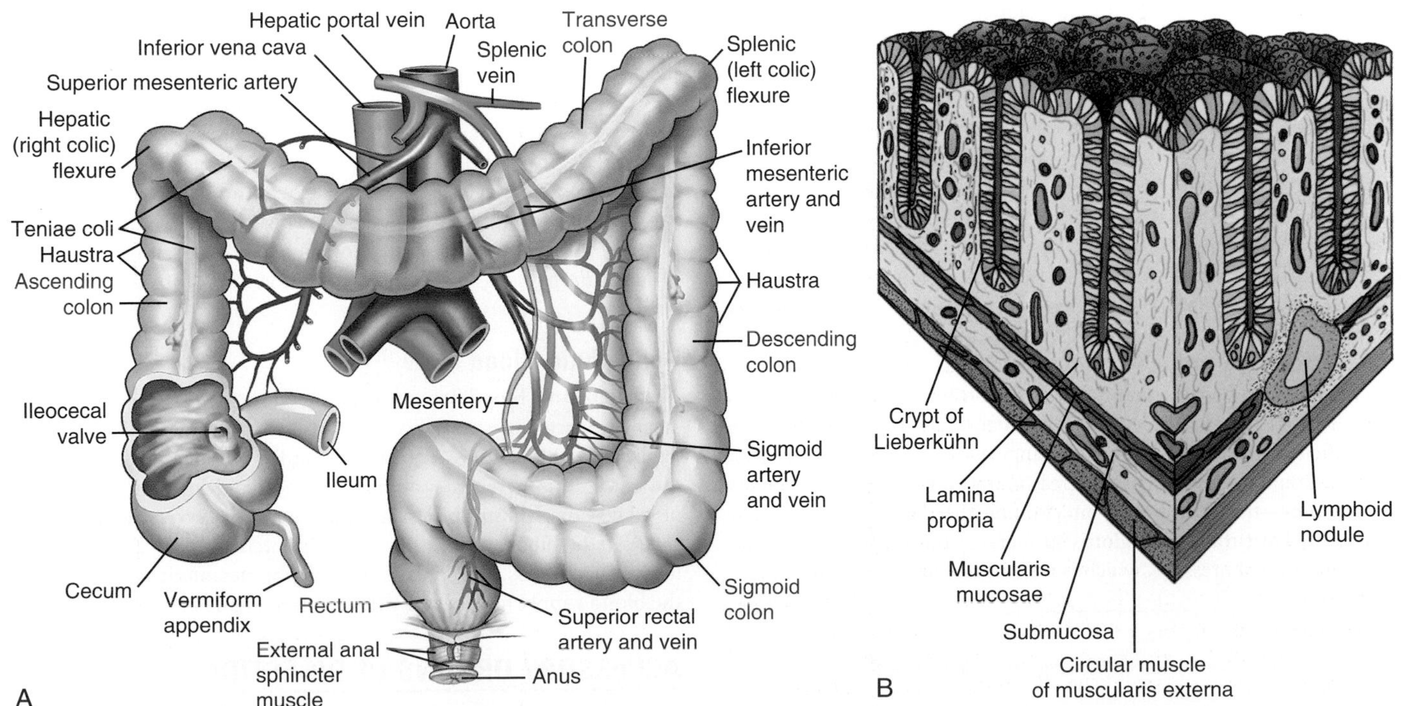

FIGURE 35-13 Large Intestine. **A,** Structure of the large intestine. **B,** Microscopic cross-section illustrating cellular structures of the large intestine. The wall of the large intestine is lined with columnar epithelium in contrast to the villi characteristics of the small intestine. The longitudinal layer of muscularis is reduced to become the teniae coli. (**A,** modified from Patton, K.T., & Thibodeau, G.A. [2014]. *The human body in health & disease* [6th ed.]. St. Louis: Mosby; **B,** from Gartner, L.P., & Hiatt, J.L. [2007]. *Color textbook of histology* [3rd ed.]. Philadelphia: Saunders.)

external anal sphincter is innervated by the pudendal nerve arising from sacral levels of the spinal cord. Sympathetic activity in the entire large intestine modulates intestinal reflexes, conveys somatic sensations of fullness and pain, participates in the defecation reflex, and constricts blood vessels. The blood supply of the large intestine and rectum is derived primarily from branches of the superior and inferior mesenteric arteries[6] (see Figure 35-6), and venous blood drains through the inferior mesenteric vein.

The primary type of colonic movement is segmental. The circular muscles contract and relax at different sites, shuttling the intestinal contents back and forth between the haustra, most commonly during fasting. The movements massage the intestinal contents, called the **fecal mass** at that point, and facilitate the absorption of water. Propulsive movement occurs with the proximal-to-distal contraction of several haustral units. Peristaltic movements also occur and promote the emptying of the colon. The **gastrocolic reflex** initiates propulsion in the entire colon, usually during or immediately after eating, when chyme enters from the ileum. The gastrocolic reflex causes the fecal mass to pass rapidly into the sigmoid colon and rectum, stimulating defecation. Gastrin may participate in stimulating this reflex. Epinephrine inhibits contractile activity.

Approximately 500 to 700 mL of chyme flows from the ileum to the cecum per day. Most of the water is absorbed in the colon by diffusion and active transport. Aldosterone increases membrane permeability to sodium, thereby increasing both the diffusion of sodium into the cell and the active transport of sodium to the interstitial fluid. (See Chapters 5 and 18 for a discussion of aldosterone secretion.) The colon does not absorb monosaccharides and amino acids, but some short-chain free fatty acids, which are produced by fermentation, are absorbed.

Absorption and epithelial transport occur in the cecum, ascending colon, transverse colon, and descending colon. By the time the fecal mass enters the sigmoid colon, the mass consists entirely of wastes and is called the *feces*, composed of food residue, unabsorbed GI secretions, shed epithelial cells, and bacteria.

The movement of feces into the sigmoid colon and **rectum** stimulates the **defecation reflex (rectosphincteric reflex)**. The rectal wall stretches, and the tonically constricted internal anal sphincter (smooth muscle with autonomic nervous system control) relaxes, creating the urge to defecate. The defecation reflex can be overridden voluntarily by contraction of the external anal sphincter and muscles of the pelvic floor. The rectal wall gradually relaxes, reducing tension, and the urge to defecate passes. Retrograde contraction of the rectum may displace the feces out of the rectal vault until a more convenient time for evacuation. Pain or fear of pain associated with defecation (e.g., rectal fissures or hemorrhoids) can inhibit the defecation reflex.

Squatting and sitting facilitate defecation because these positions straighten the angle between the rectum and anal canal and increase the efficiency of straining (increasing intra-abdominal pressure). Intra-abdominal pressure is increased by initiating the **Valsalva manoeuvre**—that is, inhaling and forcing the diaphragm and chest muscles against the closed glottis to increase both intrathoracic and intra-abdominal pressure, which is transmitted to the rectum.

QUICK CHECK 35-4

1. What is the major arterial blood supply to the large intestine?
2. What is the function of haustra?
3. What is the Valsalva manoeuvre?

The Gastro-Intestinal Tract and Immunity

The GI tract plays a major role in immune defences by killing many microorganisms.[7] The mucosa of the intestine covers a large surface area, and muscosal secretions produce antibodies, particularly IgA, and enzymes that provide defences against microorganisms. Small intestinal **Paneth cells**, located near the base of the crypts of Leiberkühn, produce defensins and other antimicrobial peptides and lysozymes important to mucosal immunity. Small intestinal **Peyer patches** (lymph nodules containing collections of lymphocytes, plasma cells, and macrophages) are most numerous in the ileum and produce antimicrobial peptides and IgA as a component of the gut-associated lymph tissue in the small intestine (see Figures 35-2 and 7-3). Peyer patches are important for antigen processing and immune defence (see Chapter 7).

Intestinal Microbiome

The type and number of bacterial flora vary greatly throughout the normal GI tract and among individuals. There are an increasing number of bacteria from the proximal to the distal GI tract, with the highest number in the colon. Genetics, diet, environmental pollution, personal hygiene, vaccination, and antibiotics and other medications affect the normal composition of bacterial flora. The intestinal bacteria do not have major digestive or absorptive functions but do play a role in metabolism of bile salts, estrogens, androgens, lipids, carbohydrates, various nitrogenous substances, and medications. They produce antimicrobial peptides, hormones, neurotransmitters, anti-inflammatory metabolites, and vitamins; destroy toxins; prevent pathogen colonization; and alert the immune system to protect against infection. They are important to overall health and when altered (dysbiosis) or translocated, they cause disease.[8]

The intestinal tract is sterile at birth but becomes colonized within a few hours. Within 3 to 4 weeks after birth, the normal flora are established. The number and diversity of bacteria decrease with aging, increasing the risk for infection. The normal flora do not have the virulence factors associated with pathogenic microorganisms, thus permitting immune tolerances.[9]

Bacteria in the stomach are relatively sparse because of the secretion of acid that kills ingested pathogens or inhibits bacterial growth (with the exception of *H. pylori*). Bile acid secretion, intestinal motility, and antibody production suppress bacterial growth in the duodenum. In the duodenum and jejunum, there is a low concentration of aerobes (10^{-1} to 10^{-4}/mL), primarily streptococci, lactobacilli, staphylococci, and other enteric bacteria. Anaerobes are found distal to the ileocecal valve but not proximal to the ileum. They constitute about 95% of the fecal flora in the colon and contribute one-third of the solid bulk of feces. *Bacteroides* and *Firmicutes* are the most common intestinal bacteria.

Splanchnic Blood Flow

The **splanchnic blood flow** provides blood to the esophagus, stomach, small and large intestines, liver, gallbladder, pancreas, and spleen (see Figure 35-6). Blood flow is regulated by cardiac output and blood volume, the autonomic nervous system, hormones, and local autoregulatory blood flow mechanisms. The splanchnic circulation serves as an important reservoir of blood volume to maintain circulation to the heart and lungs when needed. The superior and inferior mesenteric arteries provide the blood supply to the large intestine (see Figures 35-6 and 35-13).

ACCESSORY ORGANS OF DIGESTION

The liver, gallbladder, and exocrine pancreas all secrete substances necessary for the digestion of chyme. These secretions are delivered to the duodenum through the **sphincter of Oddi** at the **major duodenal papilla** (of Vater) (Figure 35-14). The liver produces bile, which contains salts necessary for fat digestion and absorption. Between meals, bile is stored in the gallbladder. The exocrine pancreas produces (1) enzymes needed for the complete digestion of carbohydrates, proteins, and fats and (2) an alkaline fluid that neutralizes chyme, creating a duodenal pH that supports enzymatic action.

The liver also receives nutrients absorbed by the small intestine and metabolizes or synthesizes them into forms that can be absorbed by the body's cells. It then releases the nutrients into the bloodstream or stores them for later use.

Liver

The **liver** weighs 1 200 to 1 600 g. It is located under the right diaphragm and is divided into right and left lobes. The larger right lobe is divided further into the caudate and quadrate lobes (Figure 35-15). The *falciform ligament* separates the right and left lobes and attaches the liver to the anterior abdominal wall. The *round ligament (ligamentum teres)* extends along the free edge of the falciform ligament, extending from the umbilicus to the inferior surface of the liver. The *coronary ligament* branches from the falciform ligament and extends over the superior surface of the right and left lobes, binding the liver to the inferior surface of the diaphragm. The liver is covered by the **Glisson capsule**, which contains blood vessels, lymphatics, and nerves. When the liver is diseased or swollen, distension of the capsule causes pain because it is innervated by sensory neurons.

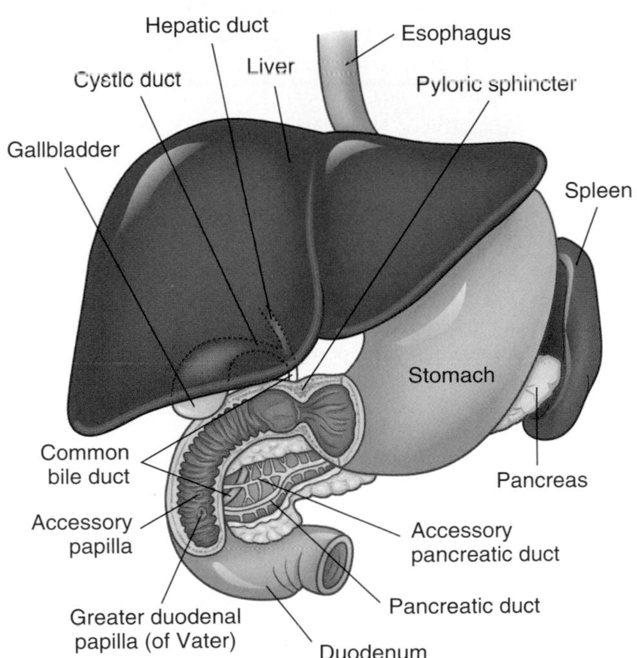

FIGURE 35-14 Location of the Liver, Gallbladder, and Exocrine Pancreas, Which Are the Accessory Organs of Digestion.

The metabolic functions of the liver require a large amount of blood. The liver receives blood from both arterial and venous sources. The **hepatic artery** branches from the celiac artery and provides oxygenated blood at the rate of 400 to 500 mL/min (about 25% of the cardiac output). The **hepatic portal vein** receives deoxygenated blood from the inferior and superior mesenteric veins, the splenic vein, and the gastric and esophageal veins, and delivers about 1 000 to 1 500 mL/min to the liver. The hepatic portal vein, which carries 70% of the blood supply to the liver, is rich in nutrients that have been absorbed from the intestinal tract (Figure 35-16).

Within the liver lobes are multiple, smaller anatomical units called **liver lobules** (Figure 35-17). They are formed of cords or plates of **hepatocytes**, which are the functional cells of the liver. These cells can regenerate; therefore damaged or resected liver tissue can regrow. Small capillaries, or **sinusoids**, are located between the plates of hepatocytes. They receive a mixture of venous and arterial blood from branches of the hepatic artery and portal vein. Blood from the sinusoids drains to a central vein in the middle of each liver lobule. Venous blood from all the lobules then flows into the **hepatic vein**, which empties into the inferior vena cava. Small channels **(bile canaliculi)** conduct bile, which is produced by the hepatocytes, outward to bile ducts and eventually drain into the **common bile duct** (see Figure 35-17). This duct empties bile into the ampulla of Vater, and then into the duodenum through an opening called the *major duodenal papilla* (which is surrounded by the sphincter of Oddi).

The sinusoids of the liver lobules are lined with highly permeable endothelium. This permeability enhances the transport of nutrients from the sinusoids into the hepatocytes, where they are metabolized. Immune functions of the liver are carried out by various cells. The sinusoids are lined with phagocytic **Kupffer cells (tissue macrophages)** and are part of the mononuclear phagocyte system. Kupffer cells are important for healing of liver injury, are bactericidal, and are important

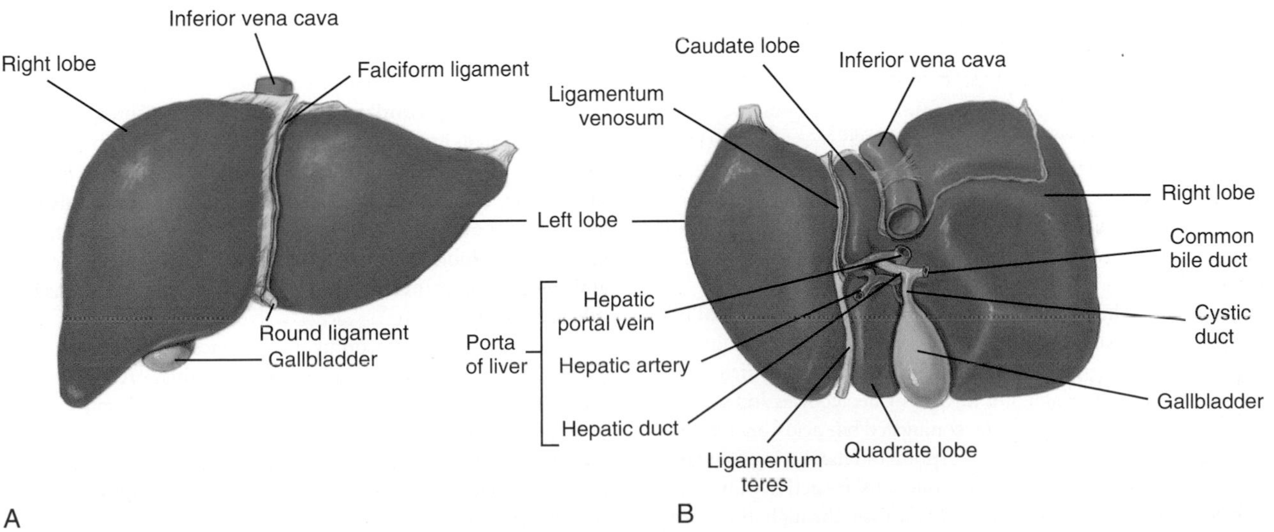

FIGURE 35-15 Gross Structure of the Liver. **A**, Anterior surface. **B**, Visceral surface. (From Applegate, E. [2011]. *The anatomy and physiology learning system* [4th ed.]. St. Louis: Saunders.)

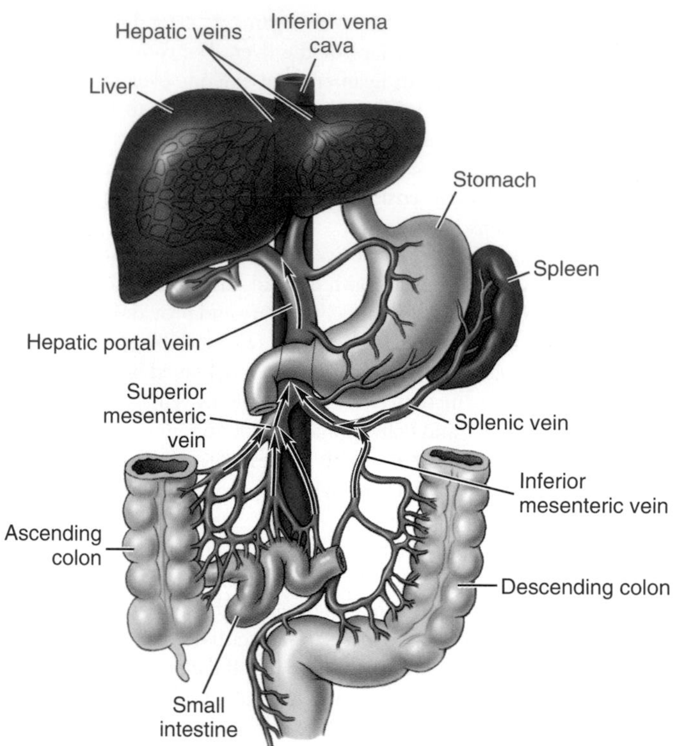

FIGURE 35-16 Hepatic Portal Circulation. In this unusual circulatory route, a vein is located between two capillary beds. The hepatic portal vein collects blood from capillaries in visceral structures located in the abdomen and empties into the liver. Hepatic veins return blood to the inferior vena cava. (From Herlihy, B. [2015]. *The human body in health and illness* [5th ed.]. St. Louis: Saunders.)

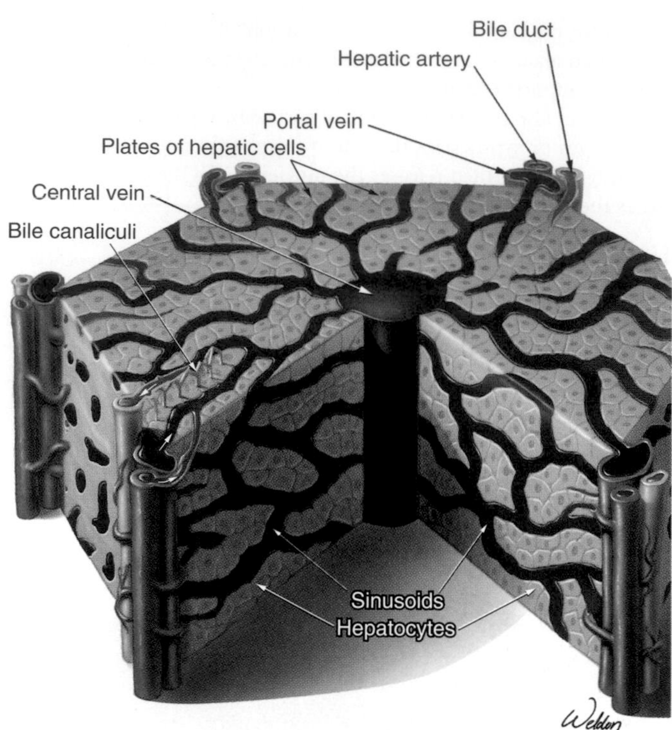

FIGURE 35-17 Schematic View of the Liver Lobule. The central vein is shown in the centre of the lobule, separated by cords of hepatocytes forming sinusoids from six portal areas at the periphery. The portal areas contain a portal vein, hepatic artery, and bile duct. Blood flow is toward the centre of the lobule, while bile flows toward the portal triads at the margins. Note the hepatic artery providing oxygenated blood to the hepatic sinusoids as well as the peribiliary plexus. (From Polin, R.A., Fox, W.W., & Abman, S.H. [2011]. *Fetal and neonatal physiology* [4th ed.]. St. Louis: Saunders.)

for bilirubin production and lipid metabolism.[10] **Stellate cells** contain retinoids (vitamin A), are contractile in liver injury, regulate sinusoidal blood flow, may proliferate into myofibroblasts, participate in liver fibrosis, produce erythropoietin, can act as antigen-presenting cells, remove foreign substances from the blood, and trap bacteria.[11] **Natural killer cells (pit cells)** also are found in the sinusoidal lumen; they produce interferon gamma and are important in tumour defence.[12] Between the endothelial lining of the sinusoid and the hepatocyte is the **Disse space**, which drains interstitial fluid into the hepatic lymph system.

QUICK CHECK 35-5
1. Where does blood in the hepatic portal vein originate?
2. What is the function of hepatocytes?
3. What is the function of Kupffer cells?

Secretion of Bile

The liver assists intestinal digestion by secreting 700 to 1 200 mL of bile per day. **Bile** is an alkaline, bitter-tasting, yellowish green fluid that contains bile salts (conjugated bile acids), cholesterol, bilirubin (a pigment), electrolytes, and water. It is formed by hepatocytes and secreted into the canaliculi. **Bile salts**, which are conjugated bile acids, are required for the intestinal emulsification and absorption of fats. Having facilitated fat emulsification and absorption, most bile salts are actively absorbed in the terminal ileum and returned to the liver through the portal circulation for resecretion. The pathway for recycling of bile salts is termed the **enterohepatic circulation** (Figure 35-18).

Bile has two fractional components: the acid-dependent fraction and the acid-independent fraction. Hepatocytes secrete the **bile acid–dependent fraction**, which consists of bile acids, cholesterol, lecithin (a phospholipid), and bilirubin (a bile pigment). The **bile acid–independent fraction**, which is secreted by the hepatocytes and epithelial cells of the bile canaliculi, is a bicarbonate-rich aqueous fluid that gives bile its alkaline pH.

Bile salts are conjugated in the liver from primary and secondary bile acids. The **primary bile acids** are cholic acid and chenodeoxycholic (chenic) acid. These acids are synthesized from cholesterol by the hepatocytes. The **secondary bile acids** are deoxycholic and lithocholic acid. These acids are formed in the small intestine by intestinal bacteria, after which they are absorbed and flow to the liver (see Figure 35-18). Both forms of bile acids are conjugated with amino acids (glycine or taurine) in the liver to form bile salts. Conjugation makes the bile acids more water soluble, thus restricting their diffusion from the duodenum and ileum. The primary and secondary bile acids together form the **bile acid pool**.

Some bile salts are deconjugated by intestinal bacteria to secondary bile acids. These acids diffuse passively into the portal blood from both the small and large intestines. An increase in the plasma concentration of bile acids accelerates the uptake and resecretion of bile acids and salts by the hepatocytes. The cycle of hepatic secretion, intestinal absorption, and hepatic resecretion of bile acids completes the enterohepatic circulation.

Bile secretion is called **choleresis**. A **choleretic agent** stimulates the liver to secrete bile. One strong stimulus is a high concentration of bile

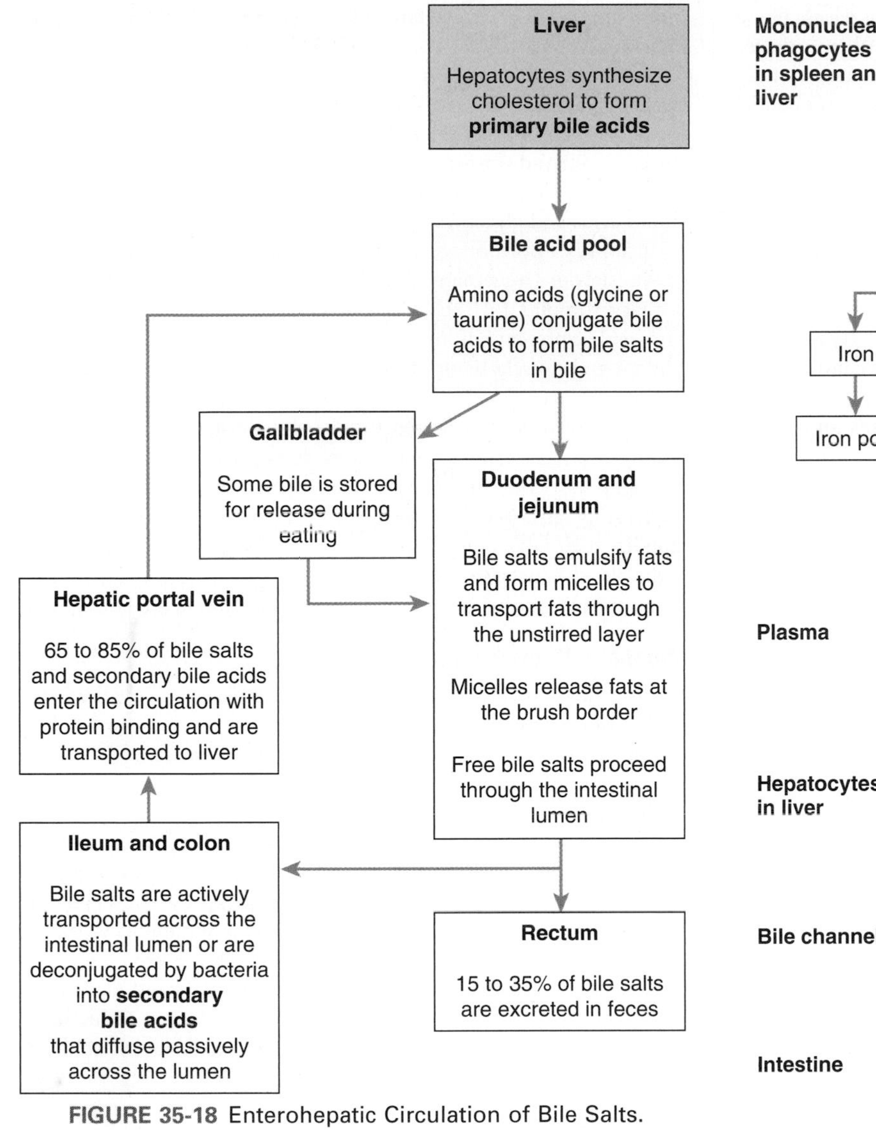

FIGURE 35-18 Enterohepatic Circulation of Bile Salts.

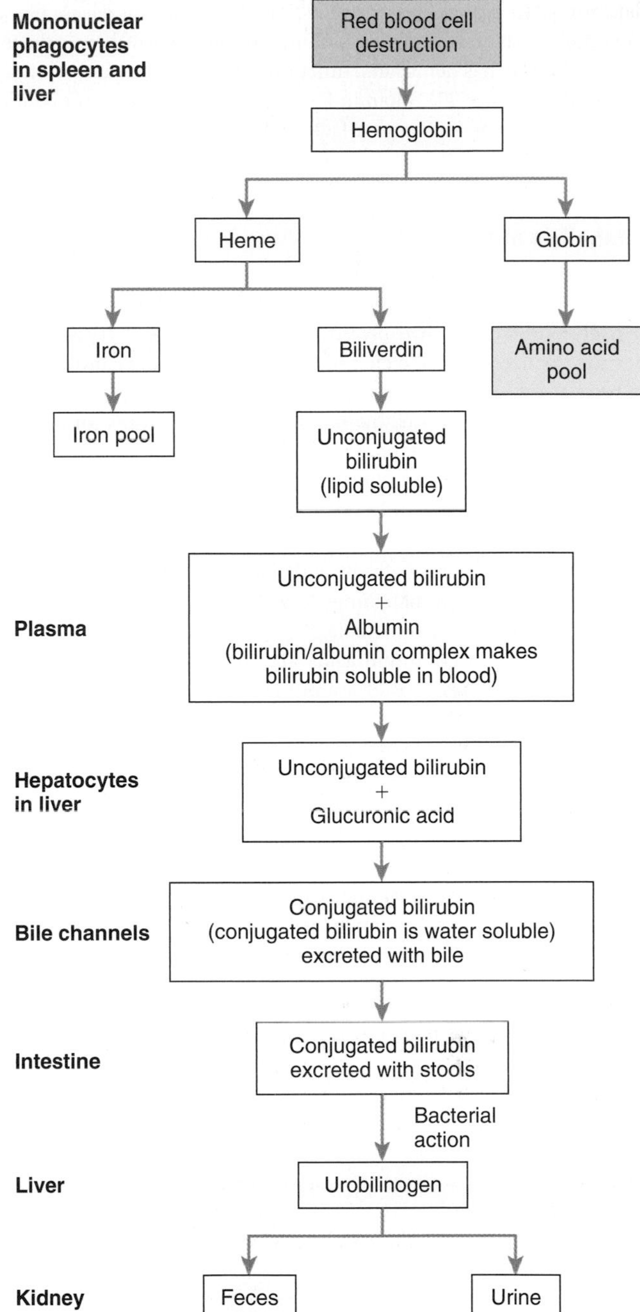

FIGURE 35-19 Bilirubin Metabolism. See text for explanation.

salts. Other choleretics include cholecystokinin, vagal stimulation, and secretin, which increases the rate of bile flow by promoting the secretion of bicarbonate from canaliculi and other intrahepatic bile ducts.

Metabolism of Bilirubin

Bilirubin is a byproduct of the destruction of aged red blood cells. It gives bile a greenish black colour and produces the yellow tinge of jaundice. Aged red blood cells are absorbed and destroyed by macrophages (Kupffer cells) of the mononuclear phagocyte system (also called the **reticuloendothelial system**), primarily in the spleen and liver. Within these cells, hemoglobin is separated into its component parts: heme and globin (Figure 35-19). The globin component is further degraded into its constituent amino acids, which are recycled to form new protein. The heme moiety is converted to biliverdin by the enzymatic (heme oxygenase) cleavage of iron. The iron attaches to transferrin in the plasma and can be stored in the liver or used by the bone marrow to make new red blood cells. The biliverdin is enzymatically converted to bilirubin in the Kupffer cell and then is released into the plasma, where it binds to albumin and is known as **unconjugated bilirubin**, or free bilirubin, which is lipid soluble. Bilirubin also may have a role as an antioxidant and provide cytoprotection.[12]

In the liver, unconjugated bilirubin moves from plasma in the sinusoids into the hepatocyte. Within hepatocytes, unconjugated bilirubin joins with glucuronic acid to form **conjugated bilirubin**, which is water soluble and is secreted in the bile. When conjugated bilirubin reaches the distal ileum and colon, it is deconjugated by bacteria and converted to **urobilinogen**. Urobilinogen is then reabsorbed in the intestines and excreted in the urine as urobilin. A small amount is eliminated in feces, as stercobilin, which contributes to the stool's brown pigmentation.

Vascular and Hematological Functions

Because of its extensive vascular network, the liver can store a large volume of blood. The amount stored at any one time depends on pressure relationships in the arteries and veins. The liver also can release blood to maintain systemic circulatory volume in the event of hemorrhage.

The liver also has hemostatic functions. It synthesizes most clotting factors (see Chapter 20). Vitamin K, a fat-soluble vitamin, is essential for the synthesis of the clotting factors. Because bile salts are needed for reabsorption of fats, vitamin K absorption depends on adequate bile production in the liver.

Metabolism of Nutrients

Fats. Ingested fat absorbed by lacteals in the intestinal villi enters the liver through the lymphatics, primarily as triglycerides. In the liver the triglycerides can be hydrolyzed to glycerol and free fatty acids and used to produce metabolic energy (adenosine triphosphate), or they can be released into the bloodstream bound to proteins (lipoproteins). The lipoproteins are carried by the blood to adipose cells for storage. The liver also synthesizes phospholipids and cholesterol, which are needed for the hepatic production of bile salts, steroid hormones, components of plasma membranes, and other special molecules.

Proteins. Protein synthesis requires the presence of all the essential amino acids (obtained only from food), as well as nonessential amino acids. Proteins perform many important functions in the body; these functions are summarized in Table 35-2.

Within hepatocytes, amino acids are converted to carbohydrates (keto acids) by the removal of ammonia (NH_3), a process known as **deamination**. The ammonia is converted to urea by the liver and passes into the blood to be excreted by the kidneys. Depending on the nutritional status of the body, the keto acids either are converted to fatty acids for fat synthesis and storage or are oxidized by the Krebs cycle (also called the *tricarboxylic acid cycle*; see Chapter 1) to provide energy for the liver cells.

The plasma proteins, including albumins and globulins (with the exception of gamma globulin, which is formed in lymph nodes and lymphoid tissue), are synthesized by the liver. They play an important role in preserving blood volume and pressure by maintaining plasma oncotic pressure. The liver also synthesizes several nonessential amino acids and serum enzymes, including aspartate aminotransferase (AST; previously *serum glutamic oxaloacetic transaminase [SGOT]*), alanine aminotransferase (ALT; previously *serum glutamic pyruvic transaminase [SGPT]*), lactate dehydrogenase (LDH), and alkaline phosphatase (ALP).

Carbohydrates. The liver contributes to the stability of blood glucose levels by releasing glucose during hypoglycemia (low blood glucose level) and absorbing glucose during hyperglycemia (high blood glucose level) and storing it as glycogen (glycogenesis) or converting it to fat. When all glycogen stores have been used, the liver can convert amino acids and glycerol to glucose (gluconeogenesis).

Insulin is a hormone synthesized in the pancreas by the beta cells of the islets of Langerhans and plays a vital role in glycogenesis. The primary stimulus for the secretion of insulin from the beta cells is glucose. The presence of insulin stimulates the diffusion of glucose into adipose and muscle tissue, and inhibits the production of glucagon. Declining glucose levels, on the other hand, stimulate the alpha cells of the pancreatic islets to secrete insulin antagonist, glucagon. Glucagon is a hyperglycemic hormone because it raises blood glucose levels. Glucagon works on the liver and fat tissue. Liver cells respond by accelerating glycogenolysis and gluconeogenesis, whereas fats cells mobilize their fatty stores (lipolysis) and release fatty acid and glycerol to the blood. Glucagon-stimulated glycogenolysis and gluconeogenesis are responsible for up to 75% of glucose production in the fasting state.

TABLE 35-2 Importance of Proteins in the Body

Function	Example
Contraction	Actin and myosin enable muscle contraction and cellular movement.
Energy	Proteins can be metabolized for energy.
Fluid balance	Albumin is a major source of plasma oncotic pressure.
Protection	Antibodies and complement protect against infection and foreign substances.
Regulation	Enzymes control chemical reactions; hormones regulate many physiological processes.
Structure	Collagen fibres provide structural support to many parts of body; keratin strengthens skin, hair, and nails.
Transport	Hemoglobin transports oxygen and carbon dioxide in blood; plasma proteins, particularly albumin, serve as transport molecules (i.e., for hormones, cations, bilirubin, and medications); proteins in cell membranes control movement of materials into and out of cells.
Coagulation	Hemostasis is regulated by clotting factors and proteins that balance coagulation and anticoagulation.

Metabolic Detoxification

The liver alters exogenous and endogenous chemicals (e.g., medications), foreign molecules, and hormones to make them less toxic or less biologically active. This process, called **metabolic detoxification** or **biotransformation**, diminishes intestinal or renal tubular reabsorption of potentially toxic substances and facilitates their intestinal and renal excretion. In this way alcohol, barbiturates, amphetamines, steroids, and hormones (including estrogens, aldosterone, antidiuretic hormone, and testosterone) are metabolized or detoxified, preventing excessive accumulation and side effects. Although metabolic detoxification is usually protective, the end products of metabolic detoxification sometimes become toxins (see *Health Promotion:* Acetaminophen and Acute Liver Failure) or active metabolites. Toxins of alcohol metabolism, for example, are acetaldehyde and hydrogen, which can damage the liver's ability to function (see Chapter 4 and Figure 4-19).

Storage of Minerals and Vitamins

The liver stores certain vitamins and minerals, including iron and copper, in times of excessive intake and releases them in times of need. The liver can store vitamins B_{12} and D for several months and vitamin A for several years. The liver also stores vitamins E and K. Iron is stored in the liver as ferritin, an iron–protein complex, and is released as needed for red blood cell production. Common tests of liver function are listed in Table 35-3.

Gallbladder

The **gallbladder** is a saclike organ on the inferior surface of the liver (Figure 35-20). Its primary function is to store and concentrate bile between meals. During the interdigestive period, bile flows from the liver through the right or left hepatic duct into the common hepatic duct and meets resistance at the closed sphincter of Oddi, which controls flow into the duodenum and prevents backflow of duodenal contents into the pancreatobiliary system. Bile then flows through the **cystic duct** into the gallbladder, where it is concentrated and stored. The mucosa of the gallbladder wall readily absorbs water and electrolytes, leaving a high concentration of bile salts, bile pigments, and cholesterol. The gallbladder holds about 90 mL of bile.

Within 30 minutes after eating, the gallbladder begins to contract, forcing stored bile through the cystic duct and into the common bile duct. The sphincter of Oddi relaxes, and bile flows into the duodenum

HEALTH PROMOTION

Acetaminophen and Acute Liver Failure

Acetaminophen (Tylenol) is an over-the-counter analgesic and antipyretic that is considered by most users to be a safe medication. Acetaminophen has been misused by patients to the extent that it is now the most common cause of acute live failure in Canada. While the maximum daily dose is 4 grams, some patients exceed this dose (unintentionally, in one in five cases) due to the established safe profile and good reputation of this medication. Another cause of misuse is extending the duration of acetaminophen's intended use: acetaminophen is intended to be used for 5 days for pain and 3 days for fever, but some patients use it for months or even years to treat persistent pain. In addition, prescription analgesics that combine acetaminophen with a strong analgesic (e.g., codeine) are more likely to be misused because patients tend to use them for longer periods.

In Canada, the number of patients admitted to hospital with acetaminophen overdose exceeds 4000 per year, and the number of unintentional cases is increasing. Overdose on acetaminophen products has been shown to be prevalent among adolescents and young adults, primarily among females.

In 2015, Health Canada made the following recommendations to the pharmaceutical industry to decrease the number of unintentional acetaminophen overdoses:

- Improve product labelling and packaging (Health Canada imposed new labelling rules in 2016)
- Reduce the amount of acetaminophen in over-the-counter products
- Reduce the maximum recommended daily dose
- Reconsider the practice of adding acetaminophen to narcotic products
- Provide accurate and easy-to-use dosing devises for children's acetaminophen liquid products

Acetaminophen toxicity from chronic use or overdose is the leading cause of acute liver failure in the developed world (see Figure 4-16). Concomitant alcohol use or abuse, medications, genetics, and nutritional status can influence the susceptibility and severity of hepatotoxicity. Hepatoxicity should be suspected when doses exceed 4 grams per day. Liver injury occurs in 17% of adults who have unintentionally overdosed on acetaminophen. The onset of toxicity is sudden and lasts for up to 24 hours. Symptoms include gastro-intestinal upset, nausea, vomiting, anorexia, diaphoresis, and pallor. Elevated levels of serum aminotransferase (AT) appear after 48 hours accompanied by hypoprothrombinemia, metabolic acidosis, and kidney failure. Early treatment (within 8 hours) with *N*-acetylcysteine (NAC) provides a 66% chance of recovery. The acetaminophen–aminotransferase multiplication product (APAP × AT) and the Psi parameter (acetaminophen level at 4 hours postingestion and the time-to-initiation of NAC) are predictors of acetaminophen toxicity in NAC-treated individuals. Liver transplant is lifesaving, and there is about 70% survival at 1 year after liver transplantation.

APAP, Acetaminophen. Data from Blieden, M., Paramore, C., Shah, D., et al. (2014). *Expert Rev Clin Pharmacol, 7*(3), 341–348; Bunchorntavakul, C., & Reddy, K.R. (2013). *Clin Liver Dis, 17*(4), 587–607, viii; Chomchai, S., & Chomchai, C. (2014). *Clin Toxicol (Phila), 52*(5), 506–511; Craig, D.G., Bates, C.M., Davidson, J.S., et al. (2011). *Br J Clin Pharmacol, 71*(2), 273–282; Government of Canada. (2016). *Revised guidance document: Acetaminophen labelling standard.* Retrieved from https://www.canada.ca/en/health-canada/services/drugs-health-products/drug-products/applications-submissions/guidance-documents/revised-guidance-document-acetaminophen-labelling-standard.html; Health Canada. (2015). *Summary safety review—acetaminophen—liver injury.* Retrieved from http://www.hc-sc.gc.ca/dhp-mps/medeff/reviews-examens/acetamino-eng.php; Hodgman, M.F., & Garrard, A.R. (2012). *Crit Care Clin, 28*(4), 499–516.

through the major duodenal papilla. During the cephalic and gastric phases of digestion, gallbladder contraction is mediated by cholinergic branches of the vagus nerve. Hormonal regulation of gallbladder contraction is derived primarily from the release of *cholecystokinin* secreted by the duodenal and jejunal mucosa in the presence of fat. Vasoactive intestinal peptide, pancreatic polypeptide, and sympathetic nerve stimulation relax the gallbladder.

Exocrine Pancreas

The **pancreas** is approximately 20 cm long, with its head tucked into the curve of the duodenum and its tail touching the spleen. The body of the pancreas lies deep in the abdomen, behind the stomach (see Figure 35-20). The pancreas is unique in that it has both endocrine and exocrine functions. The endocrine pancreas secretes hormones: insulin, glucagon, somatostatin, and pancreatic polypeptide (see Chapter 18).

The **exocrine pancreas** is composed of acinar cells that secrete enzymes and networks of ducts that secrete alkaline fluids. Both have important digestive functions. The acinar cells are organized into spherical lobules around small secretory ducts (see Figure 35-20). Secretions drain into a system of ducts that leads to the **pancreatic duct (Wirsung duct)**, which empties into the common bile duct at the **ampulla of Vater**, and then into the duodenum. In some individuals, an accessory duct (the duct of Santorini) branches off the pancreatic duct and drains directly into the duodenum at the minor duodenal papilla.

Arterial blood is supplied to the pancreas by branches of the celiac and superior mesenteric arteries. Venous blood leaves the head of the pancreas through tributaries to the portal vein, with the body and tail being drained through the splenic vein. All hormonal pancreatic secretions also pass through the hepatic portal vein into the liver.

Pancreatic innervation arises from parasympathetic neurons of the vagus nerve. These fibres activate postganglionic fibres, which stimulate enzymatic and hormonal secretion. Sympathetic postganglionic fibres from the celiac and superior mesenteric plexuses innervate the blood vessels, cause vasoconstriction, and inhibit pancreatic secretion.

The aqueous secretions of the exocrine pancreas are isotonic and contain potassium, sodium, bicarbonate, and chloride. The highly alkaline pancreatic juice neutralizes the acidic chyme that enters the duodenum from the stomach and provides the alkaline medium needed for the actions of digestive enzymes and intestinal absorption of fat.

In the pancreas, transport of water and electrolytes through the ductal epithelium involves both active and passive mechanisms. The ductal cells actively transport hydrogen into the blood and bicarbonate into the duct lumen. Potassium and chloride are secreted by diffusion according to changes in electrochemical potential gradients. As the secretion flows down the duct, water is osmotically transported into the juice until it becomes isosmotic. At low flow rates bicarbonate is exchanged passively for chloride, but at higher flow rates there is less time for this exchange and bicarbonate concentration increases. Because eating stimulates the flow of pancreatic juice, the juice is most alkaline when it needs to be: during digestion.

The pancreatic enzymes can hydrolyze proteins (proteases), carbohydrates (amylases), and fats (lipases) (see Figure 35-11). The proteolytic (protein-digesting) enzymes include trypsin, chymotrypsin, carboxypeptidase, and elastase. These enzymes are secreted in their inactive

TABLE 35-3 **Common Tests of Liver Function**

Test	Normal Value	Interpretation
Serum Enzymes		
Alkaline phosphatase (ALP)	35–120 units/L	It increases with biliary obstruction and cholestatic hepatitis.
Gamma-glutamyltranspeptidase (GGT)	Males: 8–38 units/L Females: 5–31 units/L	It increases with biliary obstruction and cholestatic hepatitis.
Aspartate aminotransferase (AST)	0–35 units/L	It increases with hepatocellular injury (and injury in other tissues, such as skeletal and cardiac muscle).
Alanine aminotransferase (ALT)	4–36 units/L	It increases with hepatocellular injury and necrosis.
Lactate dehydrogenase (LDH)	100–190 units/L	Isoenzyme LD_5 is elevated with hypoxic and primary liver injury.
5′-Nucleotidase	2–16 units/L	It increases with an increase in ALP and in cholestatic disorders.
Bilirubin Metabolism		
Serum bilirubin		
Unconjugated (indirect)	3.4–120 mcmol/L	It increases with hemolysis (lysis of red blood cells).
Conjugated (direct)	1.7–5.1 mcmol/L	It increases with hepatocellular injury or obstruction.
TOTAL	5.1–17 mcmol/L	It increases with biliary obstruction.
Urine bilirubin	0	It increases with biliary obstruction.
Urine urobilinogen	0–34 mcmol/L	It increases with hemolysis or shunting of portal blood flow.
Serum Proteins		
Albumin	35–50 g/L	It decreases with hepatocellular injury.
Globulin	23–34 g/L	It increases with hepatitis.
TOTAL	64–83 g/L	
Albumin/globulin (A/G) ratio	1.5:1 to 2.5:1	The ratio reverses with chronic hepatitis or other chronic liver disease.
Transferrin	Males: 2–5 g/L Females: 1.9–4.4 g/L	Liver damage occurs with decreased values; iron deficiency with increased values.
Alpha fetoprotein (AFP)	0–40 mcg/L	Elevated values occur in primary hepatocellular carcinoma.
Blood-Clotting Functions		
Prothrombin time (PT)	11–12.5 sec or 85–100% of control	It increases with chronic liver disease (cirrhosis) or vitamin K deficiency.
Activated partial thromboplastin time (aPTT)	30–40 sec	It increases with severe liver disease or heparin therapy.
Bromosulfophthalein (BSP) excretion	<6% retention in 45 min	Increased retention occurs with hepatocellular injury.

forms—that is, as trypsinogen, chymotrypsinogen, procarboxypeptidase, and proelastase, respectively—to protect the pancreas from the digestive effects of its own enzymes. For further protection, the pancreas produces **trypsin inhibitor**, which prevents the activation of proteolytic enzymes while they are in the pancreas. Once in the duodenum, the inactive forms (proenzymes) are activated by **enterokinase**, an enzyme secreted by the duodenal mucosa. Trypsinogen is the first proenzyme to be activated. Its conversion to trypsin stimulates the conversion of chymotrypsinogen to chymotrypsin and procarboxypeptidase to carboxypeptidase. Each of these enzymes cleaves specific peptide bonds to reduce polypeptides to smaller peptides.

Secretion of the aqueous and enzymatic components of pancreatic juice is controlled by hormonal and vagal stimuli. Secretin stimulates the acinar and duct cells to secrete the bicarbonate-rich fluid that neutralizes chyme and prepares it for enzymatic digestion. As chyme enters the duodenum, its acidity (pH of 4.5 or less) stimulates the **S cells** (secretin-producing cells) of the duodenum to release secretin, which is absorbed by the intestine and delivered to the pancreas in the bloodstream. In the pancreas, secretin causes ductal and acinar cells to release alkaline fluid. Secretin also inhibits the actions of gastrin, thereby decreasing gastric hydrochloric acid secretion and motility. The overall effect is to neutralize the contents of the duodenum.

Enzymatic secretion follows, stimulated by cholecystokinin, which activates ACh from the vagus nerve and release of ACh from pancreatic stellate cells. Cholecystokinin is released in the duodenum in response to the essential amino acids and fatty acids already present in chyme. Once in the small intestine, activated pancreatic enzymes inhibit the release of more cholecystokinin and ACh. This feedback mechanism inhibits the secretion of more pancreatic enzymes. Pancreatic polypeptide is released after eating and inhibits postprandial pancreatic exocrine secretion. (See Table 35-1 for a summary of hormonal stimulation of pancreatic secretions.) Selected tests of pancreatic function are listed in Table 35-4.

QUICK CHECK 35-6

1. Trace the route of bile salts and acids from formation to recycling.
2. What are the sources of the two types of bilirubin?
3. What is the function of the gallbladder?
4. How do pancreatic beta cells differ from acinar cells?

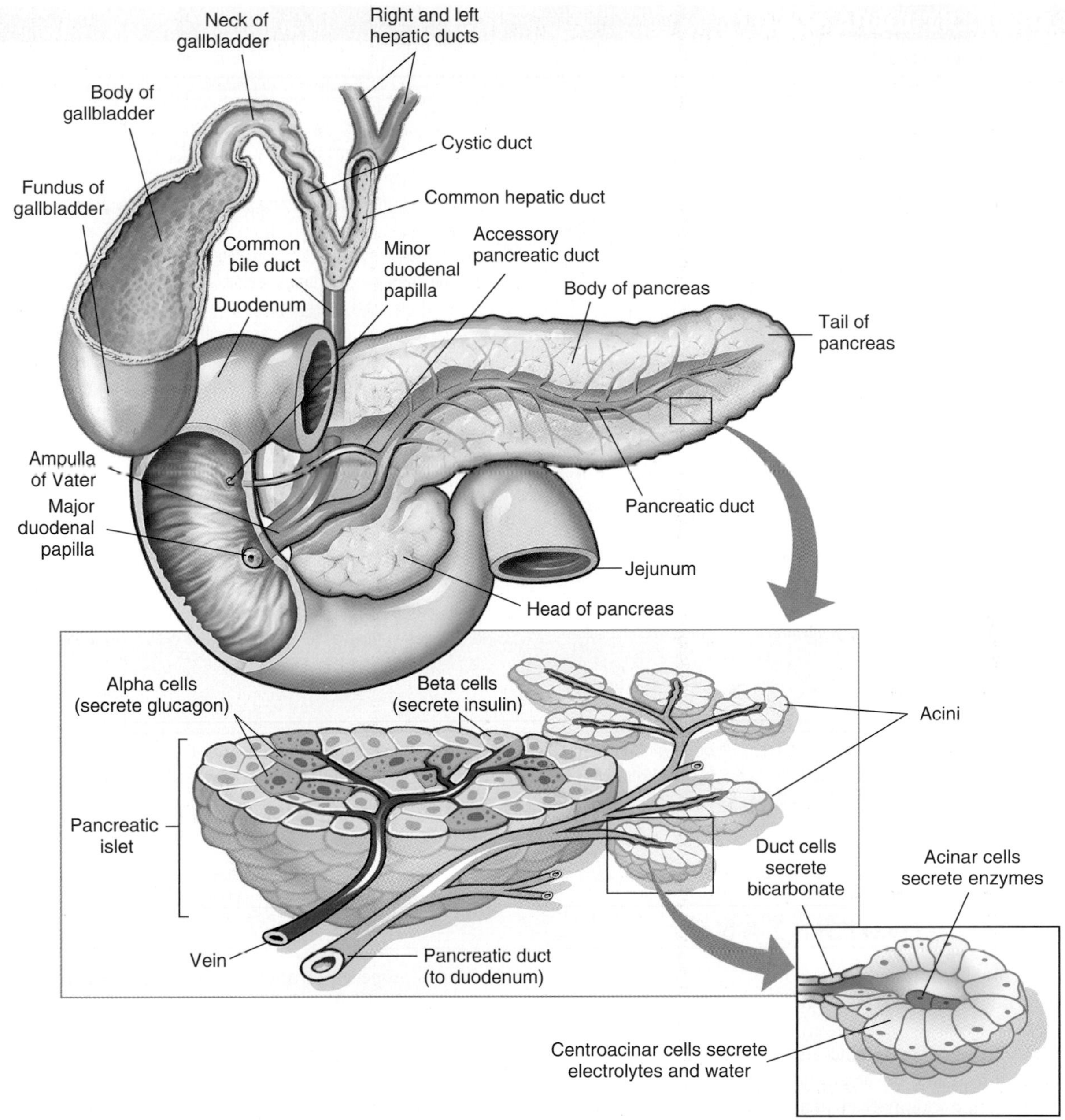

FIGURE 35-20 Associated Structures of the Gallbladder, Pancreas, and Pancreatic Acinar Cells and Duct. (Modified from Thibodeau, G.A., & Patton, K.T. [2007]. *Anatomy & physiology* [6th ed.]. St. Louis: Mosby.)

TABLE 35-4 Common Laboratory Tests of Exocrine Pancreatic Function

Test	Normal Value	Clinical Significance
Serum amylase	31–107 units/L	Elevated levels occur with pancreatic inflammation.
Serum lipase	0–160 units/L	Elevated levels occur with pancreatic inflammation (may be elevated with other conditions; differentiates pancreatitis from other condition by measuring amylase isoenzyme study).
Urine amylase	2–19 units/hr 24–408 units/24 hr	Elevated levels occur with pancreatic inflammation.
Secretin test	Volume 1.8 mL/kg/hr	Decreased volume occurs with pancreatic disease because a secretin stimulates pancreatic secretion.
	Bicarbonate concentration: >80 mmol/l	Decreased concentration or secretion can occur with pancreatic injury related to pancreatitis; lack of buffering of gastric acid can lead to intestinal ulcers and decrease activation of digestive enzymes and medications that require a higher pH.
	Bicarbonate output: >10 mmol/L/30 sec	See above.
Stool fat	2–5 g/24 hr	This test measures fatty acids; decreased pancreatic lipase increases stool fat.

GERIATRIC CONSIDERATIONS

Aging and the Gastro-Intestinal System

Age-related changes in gastro-intestinal (GI) function vary among individuals and within organ systems. Changes can include the following:

Oral Cavity and Esophagus

1. Tooth enamel and dentin deteriorate, so cavities are more likely.
2. Teeth are lost as a result of periodontal disease and brittle roots that break easily.
3. Taste buds decline in number.
4. Sense of smell diminishes.
5. Salivary secretion decreases.
6. Dysphagia is much more common.
7. Eating is less pleasurable, appetite is reduced, and food is not sufficiently chewed or lubricated; therefore swallowing is difficult.

Stomach

1. Gastric motility, blood flow, and volume and acid content of gastric juice may be reduced, particularly with gastric atrophy, and gastric emptying may be delayed.
2. Protective mucosal barrier decreases.

Intestines

1. There is a change in the composition of the intestinal microbiota and resultant increased susceptibility to disease.
2. Size of Peyer patches and degree of mucosal immunity decline, which increases the risk for infection and inflammation.
3. The brain–gut axis (bidirectional neuroendocrine communication) may be disrupted, and enteric neurons may degenerate with changes in GI motility, secretion, and absorption as well as the older adult's appetite and overall nutritional status.
4. Intestinal villi may become shorter and more convoluted, with diminished reparative capacity.
5. Intestinal absorption, motility, and blood flow may decrease, prolonging transit time and altering nutrient absorption.
6. Rectal muscle mass decreases and the anal sphincter weakens.
7. Constipation, fecal impaction, and fecal incontinence may develop and are related to immobility, low-fibre diet, and changes in enteric nervous system structure and functions.

Liver

1. There is decreased hepatic regeneration; size and weight of liver decrease.
2. The ability to detoxify medications decreases.
3. Blood flow decreases, influencing the efficiency of medication metabolism.

Pancreas and Gallbladder

1. Fibrosis, fatty acid deposits, and pancreatic atrophy occur.
2. Secretion of digestive enzymes, particularly proteolytic enzymes, decreases.
3. No changes in gallbladder and bile ducts occur, but there is an increased prevalence of gallstones and cholecystitis.

Data from Britton, E., & McLaughlin, J.T. (2013). *Proc Nutr Soc, 72*(1), 173–177; Lakshminarayanan, B., Stanton, C., O'Toole, P.W., et al. (2014). *J Nutr Health Aging, 18*(9), 773–786; Rayner, C.K., & Horowitz, M. (2013). *Curr Opin Clin Nutr Metab Care, 16*(1), 33–38; Saffrey, M.J. (2013). *Dev Biol, 382*(1), 344–355; Saffrey, M.J. (2014). *Age (Dordr), 36*(3), 9603.

DID YOU UNDERSTAND?

The Gastro-Intestinal Tract

1. The gastro-intestinal (GI) tract is a hollow tube that extends from the mouth to the anus.
2. The major functions of the GI tract are the mechanical and chemical breakdown of food and the absorption of digested nutrients.
3. The wall of the GI tract is made up of four layers: mucosa, muscularis, submucosa, and serosa.
4. The peritoneum is a double layer of membranous tissue. The visceral layer covers the abdominal organs, and the parietal layer extends along the abdominal wall. The peritoneal cavity is the space between the two layers.
5. Except for swallowing and defecation, which are controlled voluntarily, the functions of the GI tract are controlled by extrinsic and intrinsic autonomic nerves and intestinal hormones.
6. Digestion begins in the mouth, with chewing and salivation. The digestive component of saliva is α-amylase, which initiates carbohydrate digestion.
7. The esophagus is a hollow, muscular tube that transports food from the mouth to the stomach. The tunica muscularis in the upper part of the esophagus is striated muscle, and that in the lower part is smooth muscle.
8. Swallowing is controlled by the swallowing centre in the reticular formation of the brain. The two phases of swallowing are the oropharyngeal phase (voluntary swallowing) and the esophageal phase (involuntary swallowing).
9. Food is propelled through the esophagus by peristalsis: waves of sequential relaxations and contractions of the tunica muscularis.
10. The lower esophageal sphincter opens to admit swallowed food into the stomach and then closes to prevent regurgitation of food back into the esophagus.
11. The stomach is a hollow, baglike structure that secretes digestive juices, mixes and stores food, and propels partially digested food (chyme) through the pylorus into the duodenum.
12. The hormones gastrin and motilin stimulate gastric emptying; the hormones secretin and cholecystokinin delay gastric emptying.
13. The vagus nerve stimulates gastric (stomach) secretion and motility.
14. The three phases of acid secretion by the stomach are the cephalic phase (anticipation and swallowing), the gastric phase (food in the stomach), and the intestinal phase (chyme in the intestine).
15. Gastric glands in the fundus and body of the stomach secrete intrinsic factor, which is needed for vitamin B_{12} absorption, and hydrochloric acid, which dissolves food fibres, kills microorganisms, and activates the enzyme pepsin.
16. Acid secretion is stimulated by the vagus nerve, gastrin, and histamine and is inhibited by sympathetic stimulation and cholecystokinin.
17. Chief cells in the stomach secrete pepsinogen, which is converted to pepsin in the acidic environment created by hydrochloric acid.
18. Mucus is secreted throughout the stomach and protects the stomach wall from acid and digestive enzymes.

19. The small intestine is 5 to 6 m long and has three segments: the duodenum, jejunum, and ileum.
20. The ileocecal valve connects the small and large intestines and prevents reflux into the small intestine.
21. Villi are small fingerlike projections that extend from the small intestinal mucosa and increase its absorptive surface area.
22. The duodenum receives chyme from the stomach through the pyloric valve. The presence of chyme stimulates the liver and gallbladder to deliver bile and the pancreas to deliver digestive enzymes. Bile and enzymes flow through an opening guarded by the sphincter of Oddi.
23. Enzymes secreted by the small intestine (maltase, sucrase, lactase), pancreatic enzymes, and bile salts act in the small intestine to digest proteins, carbohydrates, and fats.
24. Digested substances are absorbed across the intestinal wall and then transported to the liver, where they are metabolized further.
25. Carbohydrates, amino acids, and fats are absorbed primarily by the duodenum and jejunum; bile salts and vitamin B_{12} are absorbed by the ileum. Vitamin B_{12} absorption requires the presence of intrinsic factor.
26. Minerals and water-soluble vitamins are absorbed by both active and passive transport throughout the small intestine.
27. Peristaltic movements created by longitudinal muscles propel the chyme along the intestinal tract, and contractions of the circular muscles (haustral segmentation) mix the chyme.
28. The ileogastric reflex inhibits gastric motility when the ileum is distended.
29. The intestinointestinal reflex inhibits intestinal motility when one intestinal segment is overdistended.
30. The gastroileal reflex increases intestinal motility when gastric motility increases.
31. The large intestine consists of the cecum, appendix, colon (ascending, transverse, descending, and sigmoid), rectum, and anal canal.
32. The teniae coli are three bands of longitudinal muscle that extend the length of the colon.
33. Haustra are pouches of colon formed with alternating contraction and relaxation of the circular muscles.
34. The mucosa of the large intestine contains mucus-secreting cells and mucosal folds, but no villi.
35. The large intestine massages the fecal mass and absorbs water and electrolytes.
36. Distension of the ileum with chyme causes the gastrocolic reflex, or the mass propulsion of feces to the rectum.
37. Defecation is stimulated when the rectum is distended with feces. The tonically contracted internal anal sphincter relaxes, and if the voluntarily regulated external sphincter relaxes, defecation occurs.
38. The immune system of the GI tract consists of Paneth cells, which produce defensins and other antimicrobial peptides and lysozymes; and the lymph nodes of Peyer patches, which contain lymphocytes, plasma cells, and macrophages.
39. There are an increasing number of bacteria from the proximal to the distal GI tract, with the highest number in the colon. Intestinal bacteria are important for metabolism of bile salts, metabolism of selected medications and hormones, and prevention of pathogen colonization.
40. The intestinal tract is sterile at birth and becomes totally colonized within 3 to 4 weeks.
41. The most numerous anaerobes in the colon are *Bacteroides* and *Firmicutes*.
42. The splanchnic blood flow provides blood to the esophagus, stomach, small and large intestines, gallbladder, pancreas, and spleen.

Accessory Organs of Digestion

1. The liver is the second largest organ in the body. It has digestive, metabolic, hematological, vascular, and immunological functions.
2. The liver is divided into the right and left lobes and smaller units called *liver lobules*. The liver is supported by the falciform, round, and coronary ligaments.
3. Liver lobules consist of plates of hepatocytes, which are the functional cells of the liver.
4. Bile is produced by the liver and is necessary for fat digestion and absorption. Bile's alkalinity helps to neutralize chyme, thereby creating a pH that enables the pancreatic enzymes to digest proteins, carbohydrates, and fats.
5. Bile salts emulsify and hydrolyze fats and incorporate them into water-soluble micelles, which are then transported through the unstirred water layer to the brush border of the intestinal mucosa. The fat content of the micelles readily diffuses through the epithelium into lacteals (lymphatic ducts) in the villi. From there, fats flow into lymphatics and into the systemic circulation, which delivers them to the liver.
6. The hepatocytes synthesize 700 to 1 200 mL of bile per day and secrete it into the bile canaliculi, which are small channels between the hepatocytes. The bile canaliculi drain bile into the common bile duct and then into the duodenum through an opening called the *major duodenal papilla* (which is surrounded by the sphincter of Oddi).
7. Sinusoids are capillaries located between the plates of hepatocytes. Blood from the portal vein and hepatic artery flows through the sinusoids to a central vein in each lobule and then to the hepatic vein and inferior vena cava.
8. Kupffer cells, which are part of the mononuclear phagocyte system, line the sinusoids and destroy microorganisms in sinusoidal blood; they are important in bilirubin production and lipid metabolism.
9. The primary bile acids are synthesized from cholesterol by the hepatocytes. The primary acids are then conjugated to form bile salts. The secondary bile acids are the product of bile salt deconjugation by bacteria in the intestinal lumen.
10. Most bile salts and acids are recycled. The absorption of bile salts and acids from the terminal ileum and their return to the liver are known as the *enterohepatic circulation of bile*.
11. Bilirubin is a pigment liberated by the lysis of aged red blood cells in the liver and spleen. Unconjugated bilirubin is fat soluble and can cross cell membranes. Unconjugated bilirubin is converted to water-soluble, conjugated bilirubin by hepatocytes and is secreted with bile.
12. The liver produces clotting factors and can store a large volume of blood.
13. The liver plays a major role in the metabolism of fats, proteins, and carbohydrates; and it stores minerals, vitamin B_{12}, and fat-soluble vitamins.
14. The liver metabolically transforms or detoxifies hormones, toxic substances, and medications to less active substances.
15. The gallbladder is a saclike organ located on the inferior surface of the liver. The gallbladder stores bile between meals and ejects it when chyme enters the duodenum.
16. Stimulated by cholecystokinin, the gallbladder contracts and forces bile through the cystic duct and into the common bile duct. The sphincter of Oddi relaxes, enabling bile to flow through the major duodenal papilla into the duodenum.

17. The pancreas is a gland located behind the stomach. The endocrine pancreas produces hormones (glucagon, insulin) that facilitate the formation and cellular uptake of glucose. The exocrine pancreas secretes an alkaline solution and the enzymes (trypsin, chymotrypsin, carboxypeptidase, α-amylase, lipase) that digest proteins, carbohydrates, and fats.

18. Secretin stimulates pancreatic secretion of alkaline fluid, and cholecystokinin and acetylcholine stimulate secretion of enzymes. Pancreatic secretions originate in acini and ducts of the pancreas and empty into the duodenum through the common bile duct or an accessory duct that opens directly into the duodenum.

KEY TERMS

Ampulla of Vater, 915
Antrum, 902
Ascending colon, 909
Bile, 912
Bile acid pool, 912
Bile acid–dependent fraction, 912
Bile acid–independent fraction, 912
Bile canaliculi, 911
Bile salt, 912
Bilirubin, 913
Body of the stomach, 902
Brush border, 906
Cardiac orifice, 902
Cecum, 909
Chief cell, 905
Cholecystokinin, 903
Choleresis, 912
Choleretic agent, 912
Chyme, 902
Colon, 909
Common bile duct, 911
Conjugated bilirubin, 913
Crypts of Lieberkühn, 906
Cystic duct, 914
Deamination, 914
Defecation reflex (rectosphincteric reflex), 910
Descending colon, 909
Disse space, 912
Duodenum, 905
Enteric (intramural) plexus, 899
Enterocytes, 906
Enterohepatic circulation, 912
Enterokinase, 916
Esophageal phase of swallowing, 901
Esophagus, 901
Exocrine pancreas, 915
External anal sphincter, 909
Fecal mass, 910
Fundus, 902
Gallbladder, 914
Gastric emptying, 903
Gastric gland, 904
Gastrin, 903
Gastrocolic reflex, 910
Gastroileal reflex, 908
Gastro-Intestinal (GI) tract, 000
Glisson capsule, 911
Haustral segmentation, 908
Haustrum (*pl.*, haustra), 909
Hepatic artery, 911
Hepatic portal vein, 911
Hepatic vein, 911
Hepatocyte, 911
Ileocecal valve (sphincter), 906
Ileogastric reflex, 908
Ileum, 905
Internal anal sphincter, 909
Intestinointestinal reflex, 908
Intrinsic factor, 904
Jejunum, 905
Kupffer cell (tissue macrophage), 911
Lacteal, 906
Lamina propria, 906
Large intestine, 909
Liver, 911
Liver lobule, 911
Lower esophageal sphincter (cardiac sphincter), 901
Major duodenal papilla, 910
Mesentery, 906
Metabolic detoxification (biotransformation), 914
Microvillus (*pl.*, microvilli), 906
Motilin, 903
Mouth, 899
Mucosal barrier, 905
Myenteric plexus (Auerbach plexus), 902
Natural killer cells (pit cells), 912
Oropharyngeal (voluntary) phase of swallowing, 901
Pancreas, 915
Pancreatic duct (Wirsung duct), 915
Paneth cell, 910
Parietal cell, 904
Pepsin, 905
Peristalsis, 908
Peritoneal cavity, 906
Peritoneum, 906
Peyer patch, 910
Primary bile acid, 912
Primary peristalsis, 901
Pyloric sphincter, 902
Pylorus (gastroduodenal junction), 902
Rectosigmoid (O'Beirne) sphincter, 909
Rectum, 910
Reticuloendothelial system, 913
Retropulsion, 903
S cell, 916
Saliva, 899
Salivary α-amylase (ptyalin), 901
Salivary gland, 899
Secondary bile acid, 912
Secondary peristalsis, 901
Secretin, 903
Sigmoid colon, 909
Sinusoid, 911
Small intestine, 905
Sphincter of Oddi, 910
Splanchnic blood flow, 910
Stellate cells, 912
Stomach, 902
Submucosal plexus (Meissner plexus), 902
Swallowing, 901
Teniae coli, 909
Transverse colon, 909
Trypsin inhibitor, 916
Unconjugated bilirubin, 913
Upper esophageal sphincter, 901
Urobilinogen, 913
Valsalva manoeuvre, 910
Vermiform appendix, 909
Villus (*pl.*, villi), 906

REFERENCES

1. Woodland, P., Sifrim, D., Krarup, A. L., et al. (2013). The neurophysiology of the esophagus. *Annals of the New York Academy of Sciences, 1300*, 53–70. doi:10.1111/nyas.12238.
2. Hellström, P. M., Gryback, P., & Jacobsson, H. (2006). The physiology of gastric emptying. *Best Practice and Research: Clinical Anaesthesiology, 20*(3), 397–407.
3. Chu, S., & Schuberft, M. L. (2012). Gastric secretion. *Current Opinion in Gastroenterology, 28*(6), 587–593. doi:10.1097/MOG.0b013e328358e5cc.
4. Niv, Y., & Fraser, G. M. (2002). The alkaline tide phenomenon. *Journal of Clinical Gastroenterology, 35*(1), 5–8.
5. Miller, M. J., McDole, J. R., & Newberry, R. D. (2010). Microanatomy of the intestinal lymphatic system. *Annals of the New York Academy of Sciences, 1207*(Suppl. 1), E21–E28. doi:10.1111/j.1749-6632.2010.05708.x.
6. Bobadilla, J. L. (2013). Mesenteric ischemia. *The Surgical Clinics of North America, 93*(4), 925–940, ix. doi:10.1016/j.suc.2013.04.002.
7. Mowat, A. M., & Agace, W. W. (2014). Regional specialization within the intestinal immune system. *Nature Reviews: Immunology, 14*(10), 667–685. doi:10.1038/nri3738.
8. Schippa, S., & Conte, M. P. (2014). Dysbiotic events in gut microbiota: Impact on human health. *Nutrients, 6*(12), 5786–5805. doi:10.3390/nu6125786.
9. Khanna, S., & Tosh, P. K. (2014). A clinician's primer on the role of the microbiome in human health and disease. *Mayo Clinic Proceedings, 89*(1), 107–114. doi:10.1016/j.mayocp.2013.10.011.
10. Dixon, L. J., Barnes, M., Tang, H., et al. (2013). Kupffer cells in the liver. *Comprehensive Physiology, 3*(2), 785–797. doi:10.1002/cphy.c120026.
11. Weiskirchen, R., & Tacke, F. (2014). Cellular and molecular functions of hepatic stellate cells in inflammatory responses and liver immunology. *Hepatobiliary Surgery & Nutrition, 3*(6), 344–363. doi:10.3978/j.issn.2304-3881.2014.11.03.
12. Tian, Z., Chen, Y., & Gao, B. (2013). Natural killer cells in liver disease. *Hepatology (Baltimore, Md.), 57*(4), 1654–1662. doi:10.1002/hep.26115.
13. Jansen, T., & Daiber, A. (2012). Direct antioxidant properties of bilirubin and biliverdin. Is there a role for biliverdin reductase? *Frontiers in Pharmacology, 3*, 30. doi:10.3389/fphar.2012.00030.

36

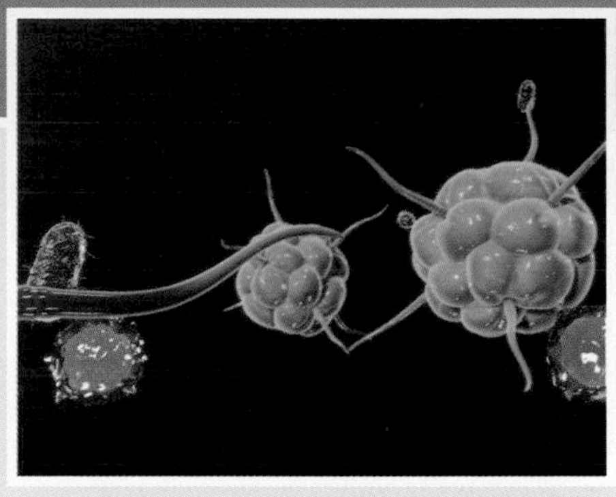

Alterations of Digestive Function

Sue E. Huether and Mohamed El-Hussein

EVOLVE WEBSITE

http://evolve.elsevier.com/Canada/Huether/pathophysiology
Student Review Questions
Key Points
Case Studies
Animations
Quick Check Answers

CHAPTER OUTLINE

Disorders of the Gastro-Intestinal Tract, 921
- Clinical Manifestations of Gastro-Intestinal Dysfunction, 921
- Disorders of Motility, 925
- Gastritis, 930
- Peptic Ulcer Disease, 931
- Malabsorption Syndromes, 935
- Inflammatory Bowel Disease, 935
- Diverticular Disease of the Colon, 938
- Appendicitis, 939
- Mesenteric Vascular Insufficiency, 939
- Disorders of Nutrition, 940

Disorders of the Accessory Organs of Digestion, 943
- Common Complications of Liver Disorders, 943
- Disorders of the Liver, 947
- Disorders of the Gallbladder, 951
- Disorders of the Pancreas, 952

Cancer of the Digestive System, 953
- Cancer of the Gastro-Intestinal Tract, 953
- Cancer of the Accessory Organs of Digestion, 957

The gastro-intestinal (GI) tract is a continuous, hollow organ that extends from the mouth to the anus. It includes the esophagus, stomach, small intestine, large intestine, and rectum. The accessory organs of digestion include the salivary glands, liver, gallbladder, and pancreas.

Disorders of the GI tract disrupt one or more of its functions. Structural and neural abnormalities can slow, obstruct, or accelerate the movement of intestinal contents at any level of the GI tract. Inflammatory and ulcerative conditions of the GI wall disrupt secretion, motility, and absorption. Inflammation or obstruction of the liver, pancreas, or gallbladder can alter metabolism and result in local and systemic symptoms. Many clinical manifestations of GI tract disorders are nonspecific and can be caused by a variety of impairments.

DISORDERS OF THE GASTRO-INTESTINAL TRACT

Clinical Manifestations of Gastro-Intestinal Dysfunction

Anorexia

Anorexia is lack of a desire to eat despite physiological stimuli that would normally produce hunger. This nonspecific symptom is often associated with nausea, abdominal pain, diarrhea, and psychological stress. Side effects of medications and disorders of other organ systems, including cancer, heart disease, and kidney disease, are often accompanied by anorexia.

Vomiting

Vomiting (emesis) is the forceful emptying of stomach and intestinal contents (chyme) through the mouth.[1] The vomiting centre lies in the medulla oblongata. Stimuli initiating the vomiting reflex include severe pain; distension of the stomach or duodenum; the presence of ipecac or copper salts in the duodenum; stimulation of the vestibular system through the eighth cranial nerve (motion sickness); side effects of many medications; torsion or trauma affecting the ovaries, testes, uterus, bladder, or kidney; motion; and activation of the chemoreceptor trigger zone (CTZ) (area postrema) in the medulla (e.g., morphine). Nausea and retching (dry heaves) are distinct events that usually precede vomiting. **Nausea** is a subjective experience associated with various conditions, including abnormal pain and labyrinthine stimulation (i.e., spinning movement). Specific neural pathways have not been identified, but hypersalivation and tachycardia are common associated symptoms. **Retching** is the muscular event of vomiting without the expulsion of vomitus.

Vomiting begins with deep inspiration. The glottis closes, the intrathoracic pressure falls, and the esophagus becomes distended. Simultaneously, the abdominal muscles contract, creating a pressure gradient from abdomen to thorax. The lower esophageal sphincter (LES) and body of the stomach relax, but the duodenum and antrum of the stomach spasm. The reverse peristalsis and pressure gradient force chyme from the stomach and duodenum up into the esophagus. Because the upper esophageal sphincter is closed, chyme does not enter the mouth. As the abdominal muscles relax, the contents of the esophagus drop back into the stomach. This process may be repeated several times before vomiting occurs. A diffuse sympathetic discharge causes the tachycardia, tachypnea, and diaphoresis that accompany retching and vomiting. The parasympathetic system mediates copious salivation, increased gastric motility, and relaxation of the upper and lower esophageal sphincters.

With vomiting, the duodenum and antrum of the stomach produce reverse peristalsis, while the body of the stomach and the esophagus relax. When the stomach is full of gastric contents, the diaphragm is forced high into the thoracic cavity by strong contractions of the abdominal muscles. The higher intrathoracic pressure forces the upper esophageal sphincter to open, and chyme is expelled from the mouth. Then the stomach relaxes and the upper part of the esophagus contracts, forcing the remaining chyme back into the stomach. The LES then closes. The cycle is repeated if there is a volume of chyme remaining in the stomach.

Spontaneous vomiting not preceded by nausea or retching is called projectile vomiting. It is caused by direct stimulation of the vomiting centre by neurological lesions (e.g., increased intracranial pressure, tumours, or aneurysms) involving the brainstem or can be a symptom of GI obstruction (pyloric stenosis). The metabolic consequences of vomiting are fluid, electrolyte, and acid–base disturbances, including hyponatremia, hypokalemia, hypochloremia, and metabolic alkalosis (see Chapter 5).

Constipation

Constipation is difficult or infrequent defecation. It is a common problem, particularly among older adults, and usually means a decrease in the number of bowel movements per week, hard stools, and difficult evacuation. The definition of *constipation* must be individually determined since normal bowel habits range from one to three evacuations per day to one per week. Constipation is not significant until it causes health risks or impairs quality of life.

PATHOPHYSIOLOGY Constipation can occur as a primary or secondary condition.[2] Primary constipation is generally classified into three categories. *Normal transit (functional) constipation* involves a normal rate of stool passage, but there is difficulty with stool evacuation. *Functional constipation* is associated with a sedentary lifestyle, low-residue diet (the habitual consumption of highly refined foods), or low fluid intake. *Slow-transit constipation* involves impaired colonic motor activity with infrequent bowel movements, straining to defecate, mild abdominal distension, and palpable stool in the sigmoid colon. *Pelvic floor dysfunction* or *outlet dysfunction* refers to an inability or difficulty expelling stool because of dysfunction of the pelvic floor muscles or anal sphincter. Examples include pelvic floor dyssynergia, rectal fissures, strictures, or hemorrhoids.

Secondary constipation can be caused by diet, medications, or neurogenic disorders (e.g., stroke, Parkinson's disease, spinal cord lesions, multiple sclerosis, Hirschsprung's disease) in which neural pathways or neurotransmitters are altered and colon transit time delayed. Opiates (particularly codeine), antacids containing calcium carbonate or aluminum hydroxide, anticholinergics, iron, and bismuth tend to inhibit bowel motility. Endocrine or metabolic disorders associated with constipation include hypothyroidism, diabetes mellitus, hypokalemia, and hypercalcemia. Pelvic hiatal hernia (herniation of the bowel through the floor of the pelvis), diverticuli, irritable bowel syndrome (constipation predominant), and pregnancy are associated with constipation. Aging may result in decreased mobility, changes in neuromuscular function, use of medications, and comorbid medical conditions causing constipation.[2] Constipation as a notable change in bowel habits can be an indication of colorectal cancer.

CLINICAL MANIFESTATIONS Indicators of constipation include two of the following for at least 3 months: (1) straining with defecation at least 25% of the time; (2) lumpy or hard stools at least 25% of the time; (3) sensation of incomplete emptying at least 25% of the time; (4) manual manoeuvres to facilitate stool evacuation for at least 25% of defecations; and (5) fewer than three bowel movements per week.[3] Changes in bowel evacuation patterns, such as less frequent defecation, smaller stool volume, hard stools, difficulty passing stools (straining), or a feeling of bowel fullness and discomfort, require investigation. Fecal impaction (hard, dry stool retained in the rectum) is associated with rectal bleeding, abdominal or cramping pain, nausea and vomiting, weight loss, and episodes of diarrhea. Straining to evacuate stool may cause engorgement of the hemorrhoidal veins and hemorrhoidal disease or thrombosis with rectal pain, bleeding, and itching. Passage of hard stools can cause painful anal fissures.

EVALUATION AND TREATMENT The history, current use of medications, physical examination, and stool diaries provide precise clues regarding the nature of constipation. The individual's description of frequency, stool consistency, associated pain, and presence of blood or whether evacuation was stimulated by enemas or cathartics (laxatives) is important. Palpation may disclose colonic distension, masses, and tenderness. Digital examination of the rectum and anorectal manometry are performed to assess sphincter tone and detect anal lesions. Colonic transit time and imaging techniques can assist in identifying the cause of constipation. Colonoscopy is used to visualize the lumen directly.

The treatment for constipation is to manage the underlying cause or disease for each individual. Management of constipation usually consists of bowel retraining, in which the individual establishes a satisfactory bowel evacuation routine without becoming preoccupied with bowel movements. The individual also may need to engage in moderate exercise, drink more fluids, and increase fibre intake. Fibre supplements, stool softeners, and laxative agents are useful for some individuals. Enemas can be used to establish bowel routine, but they should not be used habitually. Biofeedback may be beneficial in some instances for forming new bowel evacuation habits. When there is failure to respond to dietary or medical therapies, surgery (colectomy) is considered as a last resort.[4]

Diarrhea

Diarrhea is the presence of loose, watery stools. Acute diarrhea is more than three loose stools developing within 24 hours and lasting less than 14 days. Persistent diarrhea lasts longer than 14 to 30 days, and chronic diarrhea lasts longer than 4 weeks.[5,6] Diarrhea can have high rates of morbidity and mortality in children younger than 5 years of age, particularly in developing countries (see Chapter 37) and in older adults. Many factors determine stool volume, including water content of the colon, diet, the presence of nonabsorbed food, nonabsorbable material, and intestinal secretions. Stool volume in the normal adult averages less than 200 g per day. Stool volume in children depends on age and size. An infant may pass up to 100 g per day. The adult intestine processes approximately 9 L of luminal contents per day: 2 L are ingested and the remaining 7 L consist of intestinal secretions. Of this volume, 99% of the fluid is absorbed: 90% (7 to 8 L) in the small intestine and 9% (1 to 2 L) in the colon. Normally, approximately 150 mL of water is excreted daily in the stool.

PATHOPHYSIOLOGY Diarrhea in which the volume of feces is increased is called *large-volume diarrhea*. It generally is caused by excessive amounts of water or secretions or both in the intestines. *Small-volume diarrhea*, in which the volume of feces is not increased, usually results from excessive intestinal motility.

The three major mechanisms of diarrhea are osmotic, secretory, and motile:

1. Osmotic diarrhea. A nonabsorbable substance in the intestine draws excess water into the intestine and increases stool weight and volume, producing large-volume diarrhea. Causes include lactase and

pancreatic enzyme deficiency; excessive ingestion of synthetic, nonabsorbable sugars; full-strength tube-feeding formulas; or dumping syndrome associated with gastric resection.

2. **Secretory diarrhea**. Excessive mucosal secretion of fluid and electrolytes produces large-volume diarrhea. Infectious causes include viruses (e.g., rotavirus), bacterial enterotoxins (e.g., *Escherichia coli* and *Vibrio cholerae*), exotoxins from overgrowth of *Clostridium difficile* following antibiotic therapy (see *Health Promotion: Clostridium difficile* and Diarrhea), and small bowel bacterial overgrowth.[7] Small-volume diarrhea is usually caused by an inflammatory disorder of the intestine, such as ulcerative colitis (UC), Crohn's disease (CD), or microscopic colitis, but also can result from colon cancer or fecal impaction.
3. **Motility diarrhea** is caused by resection of the small intestine (short bowel syndrome), surgical bypass of an area of the intestine or fistula formation between loops of intestine, irritable bowel syndrome–diarrhea predominant, diabetic neuropathy, hyperthyroidism, and laxative abuse. Excessive motility decreases transit time and opportunity for fluid absorption, resulting in diarrhea.

CLINICAL MANIFESTATIONS Diarrhea can be acute or chronic, depending on its cause. Systemic effects of prolonged diarrhea are dehydration, electrolyte imbalance (hyponatremia, hypokalemia), and weight loss. Manifestations of acute bacterial or viral infection include fever, with or without vomiting or cramping pain. Most infectious diarrhea usually lasts less than 2 weeks. The exceptions are *C. difficile*, *Aeromonas*, or *Yersinia enterocolitica*.[8] Fever, cramping pain, and bloody stools accompany chronic diarrhea caused by inflammatory bowel disease (IBD) or dysentery. **Steatorrhea** (fat in the stools), bloating, and diarrhea are common signs of malabsorption syndromes. (Steatorrhea can also indicate alterations in liver and pancreatic functions.) Anal and perineal skin irritation can occur.

EVALUATION AND TREATMENT A thorough history is taken to document the onset, frequency, and duration of diarrhea, the volume of stools, and the presence of blood in the stools. Malabsorption syndromes usually manifest as steatorrhea. Exposure to contaminated food or water is indicated if the individual has travelled in foreign countries or areas where drinking water might be contaminated. Iatrogenic diarrhea is suggested if the individual has undergone abdominal radiation therapy, intestinal resection, or treatment with selected medications (e.g., antibiotics, diuretics, antihypertensives, laxatives, anticoagulants or chemotherapy). Physical examination helps identify underlying systemic disease. Stool studies, abdominal imaging, endoscopy, and

HEALTH PROMOTION

Clostridium difficile and Diarrhea

Clostridium difficile is a gram-positive, spore-forming, anaerobic bacillus that causes infectious diarrhea by producing toxins. *C. difficile* is the most frequent cause of health care–associated infectious diarrhea in Canada and other developed countries.

The reported incidence of health care–associated *C. difficile* infection in Canada has risen over the last decade. *C. difficile* infection manifestations range from uncomplicated diarrhea to life-threatening pseudomembranous colitis, bowel perforation, and sepsis. In Canadian hospitals, the mortality rate associated with *C. difficile* infection increased almost fourfold from 1997 to 2005 (1.5% of cases to 5.7% of cases, respectively, $p < .001$).

The main mode of transmission for *C. difficile* in health care settings is person-to-person spread through the fecal–oral route. Momentary contamination of the hands of health care personnel with *C. difficile* spores and environmental contamination play an important role in the transmission of *C. difficile* in health care settings. *C. difficile*, unlike other bacterial pathogens, persists longer in the environment and resists routine disinfection processes. For this reason, environmental contamination is a significant factor in cross-transmission between patients and health care providers.

Often a *C. difficile* infection is associated with previous antibiotic use. Judicious administration of antibiotics is believed to have a role in preventing and terminating the incidence of *C. difficile* infection.

Measures to Prevent *C. difficile* Infections in Health Care Facilities

- Facility design should include single rooms for the routine care of inpatients that includes private toilets inside the room, designated patient sinks, alcohol-based hand rub dispensers, and designated handwashing sinks for staff.
- Special disposal systems should be used to manage the disposal of fecal matter when bedpans or commodes are required to avoid environmental contamination with *C. difficile* spores.
- For patients with acute diarrhea due (suspected or confirmed) to *C. difficile* infection, contact precautions must be implemented immediately until the diarrhea is resolved or its cause is determined not to be infectious.
- Patients with uncontrolled diarrhea or fecal incontinence should be given preference for single private rooms where possible.
- Signage should be placed at the entrance to the infected patient's room, cubicle, and designated bed space to indicate the need to apply contact precautions.
- Frequent hand hygiene should be performed using effective techniques:
  - Following patient care or contact with patient's environment
  - After removing gloves at point of care and just prior to leaving the patient's room
  - Following contact with fecal matter, bedpans, and commodes.
- Handwashing with soap and water should be performed at the point of care and at an assigned staff handwashing sink. If an assigned staff handwashing sink is not available at the point of care, alcohol-based hand rub (with an alcohol concentration between 60 and 90%) must be used, and hand hygiene with soap and water must be performed as soon as a staff handwashing sink is available.
- Hand wipes (impregnated with plain soap, antimicrobials, or alcohol) may be used as an alternative to soap and water when an assigned staff handwashing sink is not readily available, or when the handwashing sink is not appropriate (e.g., contaminated, no running water, no soap), when hands are not visibly soiled. When hands are visibly soiled, alcohol-based hand rub should be used after the use of hand wipes, and hands should be washed with soap and water once a suitable staff handwashing sink is available.
- Unless medically indicated (e.g., for essential diagnostic and therapeutic tests or treatment) the transfer of patients suspected or confirmed to have *C. difficile* infection within and between facilities should be avoided.
- The number of visitors for a patient on contact precautions must be restricted to essential visitors (e.g., immediate family member or parent, guardian, or primary caretaker) only.

From Public Health Agency of Canada. (2013). *Clostridium difficile* infection: Infection prevention and control guidance for management in acute care settings. Retrieved from http://www.phac-aspc.gc.ca/nois-sinp/guide/c-dif-acs-esa/index-eng.php.

intestinal biopsies provide more specific data, particularly for persistent diarrhea.

Treatment for diarrhea includes restoration of fluid and electrolyte balance, administration of antimotility (e.g., loperamide [Imodium]) medication, water absorbent medication (e.g., attapulgite [Kaopectate] and polycarbophil [Equalactin]), or both, and treatment of causal factors. Nutritional deficiencies need to be corrected in cases of chronic diarrhea or malabsorption.[9]

Abdominal Pain

Abdominal pain is the presenting symptom of a number of GI diseases and can be acute or chronic.[10] The causal mechanisms of abdominal pain are *mechanical*, *inflammatory*, or *ischemic*. Generally, the abdominal organs are not sensitive to mechanical stimuli, such as cutting, tearing, or crushing. These organs are, however, sensitive to stretching and distension, which activate nerve endings in both hollow and solid structures. Pain accompanies rapid distension rather than gradual distension. Traction on the peritoneum caused by adhesions, distension of the common bile duct, or forceful peristalsis resulting from intestinal obstruction causes pain because of increased tension. Capsules that surround solid organs, such as the liver and gallbladder, contain pain fibres that are stimulated by stretching if these organs swell. Abdominal pain may be generalized to the abdomen or localized to a particular abdominal quadrant. The nature of the pain is often described as sharp, dull, or colicky.

Abdominal pain is usually associated with tissue injury and inflammation. Biochemical mediators of the inflammatory response, such as histamine, bradykinin, and serotonin, stimulate organic nerve endings and produce abdominal pain. The edema and vascular congestion that accompany chemical, bacterial, or viral inflammation also cause painful stretching. Hindrance of blood flow from the distension of bowel obstruction or mesenteric vessel thrombosis produces the pain of ischemia, and increased concentrations of tissue metabolites stimulate pain receptors.

Abdominal pain can be parietal (somatic), visceral, or referred. **Parietal pain**, from the parietal peritoneum, is more localized and intense than visceral pain, which arises from the organs themselves. Parietal pain lateralizes because, at any particular point, the parietal peritoneum is innervated from only one side of the nervous system.

Visceral pain arises from a stimulus (distension, inflammation, ischemia) acting on an abdominal organ. Inflammatory mediators associated with chronic low-grade inflammation can cause pain hypersensitivity.[11] The pain is usually poorly localized, diffuse, or vague with a radiating pattern, because nerve endings in abdominal organs are sparse and multisegmented. Pain arising from the stomach, for example, is experienced as a sensation of fullness, cramping, or gnawing in the midepigastric area. **Referred pain** is visceral pain felt at some distance from a diseased or affected organ. It is usually well localized and is felt in the skin dermatomes or deeper tissues that share a central afferent pathway with the affected organ. For example, acute cholecystitis may have pain referred to the right shoulder or scapula.

Gastro-Intestinal Bleeding

Upper gastro-intestinal bleeding is bleeding in the esophagus, stomach, or duodenum, and is characterized by frank, bright-red bleeding or dark, grainy digested blood ("coffee grounds") that has been affected by stomach acids (Table 36-1). Upper GI bleeding is commonly caused by bleeding varices (varicose veins) in the esophagus, peptic ulcers, arteriovenous malformations, or a Mallory-Weiss tear at the esophageal-gastric junction caused by severe retching.[12] **Lower gastro-intestinal bleeding**, or bleeding from the jejunum, ileum, colon, or rectum, can be caused by polyps, diverticulitis, inflammatory disease, cancer, or hemorrhoids.

TABLE 36-1 Presentations of Gastro-Intestinal Bleeding

Presentations	Definition
Acute Bleeding	
Hematemesis	Bloody vomitus; either fresh, bright-red blood or dark, grainy digested blood with "coffee grounds" appearance
Melena	Black, sticky, tarry, foul-smelling stools caused by digestion of blood in gastro-intestinal tract; should be distinguished from black stools caused by dietary iron supplements, blackberries, or bismuth (e.g., Pepto-Bismol)
Hematochezia	Fresh, bright-red blood passed from rectum
Occult Bleeding	Trace amounts of blood in normal-appearing stools or gastric secretions; detectable only with positive fecal occult blood test (guaiac test)

Occult bleeding is usually caused by slow, chronic blood loss that is not obvious and results in iron deficiency anemia as iron stores in the bone marrow are slowly depleted.[13] Acute, severe GI bleeding is life-threatening depending on the volume and rate of blood loss, associated disease and age of the affected individual, and effectiveness of treatment.

Physiological response to GI bleeding depends on the amount and rate of the loss (Figure 36-1). Changes in blood pressure and heart rate are the best indicators of massive blood loss in the GI tract. During the early stages of blood volume depletion, the peripheral arteries and arterioles constrict to shunt blood to vital organs, including the brain. Signs of large-volume blood loss are postural hypotension (a drop in blood pressure that occurs with a change from the recumbent position to a sitting or upright position), lightheadedness, and loss of vision. Tachycardia develops as a compensatory response to maintain cardiac output and tissue perfusion. If blood loss continues, hypovolemic shock develops (see Chapter 24). Diminished blood flow to the kidneys causes decreased urine output and may lead to oliguria (low urine output), tubular necrosis, and kidney failure. Ultimately, insufficient cerebral and coronary blood flow causes irreversible anoxia and death.

The presentations of GI bleeding are summarized in Table 36-1. The accumulation of blood in the GI tract is irritating and increases peristalsis, causing vomiting or diarrhea, or both. If bleeding is from the lower GI tract, the diarrhea is frankly bloody. Bleeding from the upper GI tract also can be rapid enough to produce **hematochezia** (bright-red stools), but generally some digestion of the blood components will have occurred, producing **melena**—black or tarry stools that are sticky and have a characteristic foul odour. The digestion of blood proteins originating from massive upper GI bleeding is reflected by an increase in blood urea nitrogen (BUN) levels (see Figure 36-1).

The hematocrit and hemoglobin values are not the best indicators of acute GI bleeding because plasma volume and red cell volume are lost proportionately. As the plasma volume is replaced, the hematocrit and hemoglobin values begin to reflect the extent of blood loss. The interpretation of these values is modified to account for exogenous replacement of fluids and the hydration status of the tissues.

QUICK CHECK 36-1

1. How does osmotic diarrhea differ from secretory diarrhea?
2. How is visceral pain "referred"?
3. What are the best clinical indicators of acute GI bleeding blood loss?

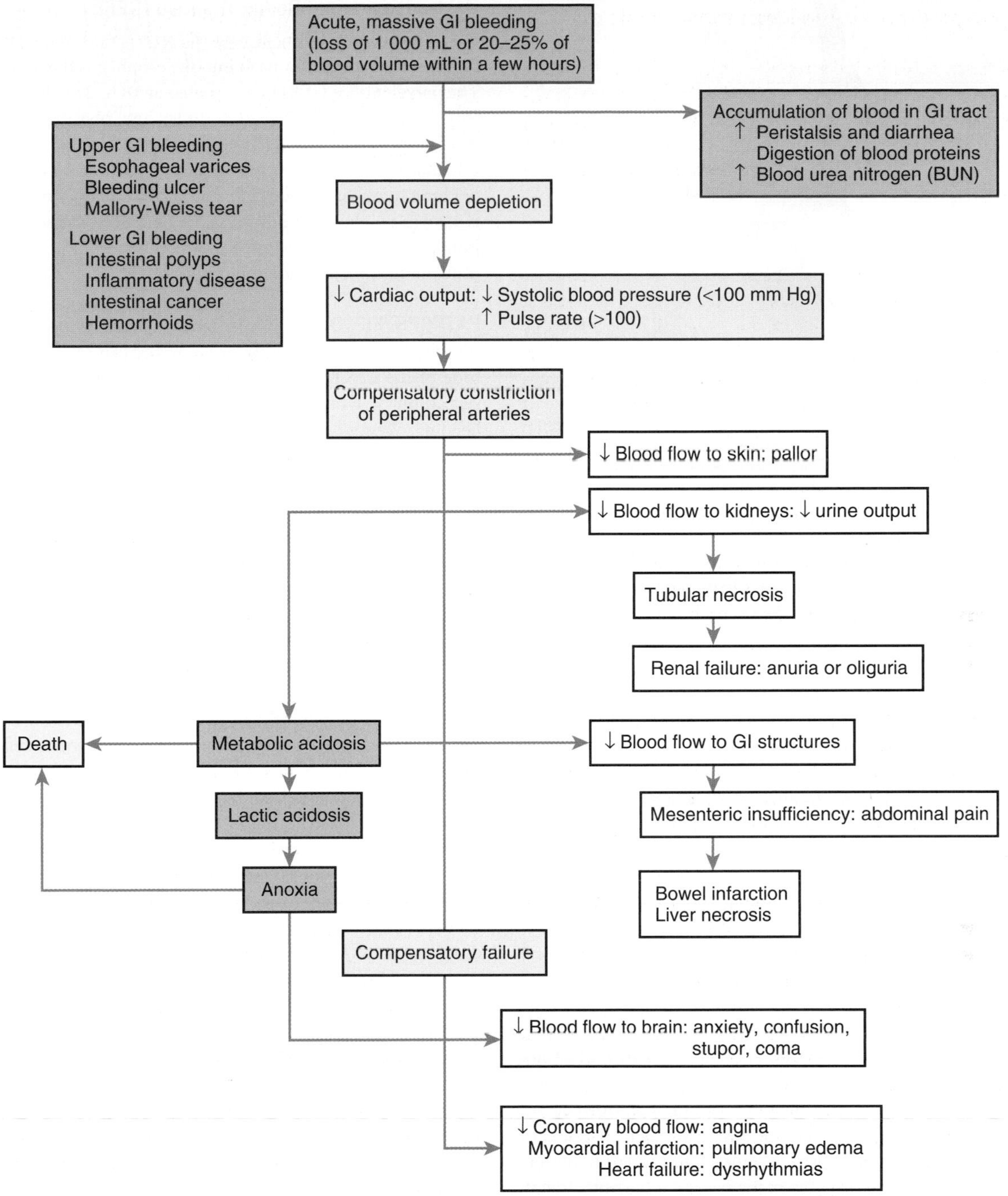

FIGURE 36-1 **Pathophysiology of Gastro-Intestinal Bleeding.** *GI,* Gastro-Intestinal.

Disorders of Motility

Dysphagia

PATHOPHYSIOLOGY **Dysphagia** is difficulty swallowing. It can result from *mechanical obstruction* of the esophagus or a functional disorder that impairs esophageal motility. Intrinsic obstructions originate in the wall of the esophageal lumen (esophageal dysphagia) and include tumours, strictures, and diverticular herniations (outpouchings). Extrinsic mechanical obstructions originate outside the esophageal lumen and narrow the esophagus by pressing inward on the esophageal wall. The most common cause of extrinsic mechanical obstruction is tumour.

Functional dysphagia is caused by neural or muscular disorders that interfere with voluntary swallowing or peristalsis. Disorders that affect the striated muscles of the hypopharyngeal area and upper esophagus interfere with the oropharyngeal (voluntary) phase of swallowing (oropharyngeal dysphagia). Typical causes are dermatomyositis (a muscle disease) and neurological impairments caused by cerebrovascular accidents, Parkinson's disease, multiple sclerosis, muscular dystrophy, or achalasia.[14]

Achalasia is a rare form of dysphagia related to loss of inhibitory neurons in the myenteric plexus with smooth muscle atrophy in the middle and lower portions of the esophagus. The myenteric neurons are attacked by a cell-mediated and antibody-mediated immune response against an unknown antigen. This leads to altered esophageal peristalsis and failure of the LES to relax, causing functional obstruction of the lower esophagus with varying severity.[15] Food accumulates above the

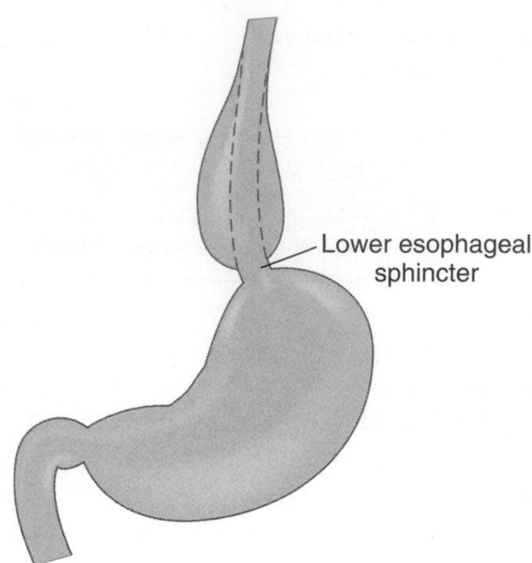

FIGURE 36-2 Achalasia. Increased lower esophageal sphincter muscle tone and loss of peristaltic function prevent food from entering the stomach, causing esophageal distension.

obstruction, distends the esophagus, and causes dysphagia (Figure 36-2). Cough and aspiration can occur. As hydrostatic pressure increases, food is slowly forced past the obstruction into the stomach. Chronic esophageal distension requires dilation or surgical myotomy of the LES.

CLINICAL MANIFESTATIONS Distension and spasm of the esophageal muscles during eating or drinking may cause a mild or severe stabbing pain at the level of obstruction. Discomfort occurring 2 to 4 seconds after swallowing is associated with upper esophageal obstruction. Discomfort occurring 10 to 15 seconds after swallowing is more common in obstructions of the lower esophagus. If obstruction results from a growing tumour, dysphagia begins with difficulty swallowing solids and advances to difficulty swallowing semisolids and liquids. If motor function is impaired, both solids and liquids are difficult to swallow. Regurgitation of undigested food, unpleasant taste sensation, vomiting, aspiration, and weight loss are common manifestations of all types of dysphagia. Aspiration of esophageal contents can lead to cough and pneumonia.

EVALUATION AND TREATMENT Knowledge of the person's history and clinical manifestations contributes significantly to a diagnosis of dysphagia. Further evaluation of swallowing should be performed by a speech language pathologist to determine what the person can eat/drink, and whether the swallowing reflex is intact, to prevent potential aspiration. Recommendations are then made based on the outcome of this assessment. (Note that this evaluation is *not* performed by the nurse).

Imaging is used to visualize the contours of the esophagus and identify structural defects. High-resolution manometry and intraluminal impedance monitoring document the duration and amplitude of abnormal pressure changes associated with obstruction or loss of neural regulation. Esophageal endoscopy is performed to examine the esophageal mucosa and obtain biopsy specimens.

The individual is taught to manage symptoms by eating small meals slowly, taking fluid with meals, and sleeping with the head elevated to prevent regurgitation and aspiration. Food and medications may need to be formulated so they can be swallowed. Anticholinergic medications (e.g., botulinum toxin type A [Botox]) may relieve symptoms of dysphagia. Mechanical dilation of the esophageal sphincter and surgical separation of the lower esophageal muscles with a longitudinal incision (myotomy) are the most effective treatments for achalasia.[16]

Gastroesophageal Reflux Disease (GERD)

Gastroesophageal reflux disease (GERD) is the reflux of acid and pepsin or bile salts from the stomach into the esophagus that causes esophagitis. The prevalence of GERD is estimated at 18 to 27% in North America.[17] Risk factors for GERD include older age, obesity, hiatal hernia, and medications or chemicals that relax the LES (anticholinergics, nitrates, calcium channel blockers, nicotine).[18] GERD may be a trigger for asthma or chronic cough. Gastroesophageal reflux that does not cause symptoms is known as *physiological reflux*. In *nonerosive reflux disease (NERD)*, individuals have symptoms of reflux disease but no visible esophageal mucosal injury (functional heartburn).[19]

PATHOPHYSIOLOGY Abnormalities in LES function, esophageal motility, and gastric motility or emptying can cause GERD. The resting tone of the LES tends to be lower than normal from either transient relaxation or weakness of the sphincter. Vomiting, coughing, lifting, bending, obesity, or pregnancy increases abdominal pressure, contributing to the development of reflux esophagitis. Hiatal hernia can weaken the LES. Delayed gastric emptying can contribute to reflux esophagitis by (1) lengthening the period during which reflux is possible and (2) increasing gastric acid content. Disorders that delay emptying include gastroparesis, gastric or duodenal ulcers, which can cause pyloric edema and strictures that narrow the pylorus.

The severity of the esophagitis depends on the composition of the gastric contents and the esophageal mucosa exposure time. An acid pocket is an area of postprandial unbuffered gastric acid immediately distal to the gastroesophageal junction. It is enlarged in hiatal hernia and can contribute to GERD. If the gastric content is highly acidic or contains bile salts and pancreatic or intestinal enzymes, reflux esophagitis can be severe. In individuals with weak esophageal peristalsis, refluxed chyme remains in the esophagus longer than usual. The prolonged presence of refluxed chime in the esophagus increases the amount of time the esophageal mucosa is exposed to acids, enzymes, and bile. The refluxate causes mucosal injury and inflammation with hyperemia, increased capillary permeability, edema, tissue fragility, and erosion. Fibrosis and thickening may develop. Precancerous lesions (Barrett esophagus) can be a long-term consequence. Precancerous lesions can progress to adenocarcinoma.[20]

CLINICAL MANIFESTATIONS The clinical manifestations of erosive reflux esophagitis are heartburn (pyrosis), acid regurgitation, dysphagia, chronic cough, asthma attacks (see Chapter 27), laryngitis, and upper abdominal pain within 1 hour of eating. The symptoms worsen if the individual lies down or if intra-abdominal pressure increases (e.g., as a result of coughing, vomiting, or straining at stool). Edema, strictures, esophageal spasm, or decreased esophageal motility may result in dysphagia with weight loss. Alcohol or acid-containing foods, such as citrus fruits, can cause discomfort during swallowing.

EVALUATION AND TREATMENT Diagnosis of GERD is based on history and clinical manifestations. Esophageal endoscopy shows hyperemia, edema, erosion, and strictures. Dysplastic changes (Barrett esophagus) can be identified by tissue biopsy. Impedance or pH monitoring measures the movement of stomach contents upward into the esophagus and the acidity of the refluxate. Because heartburn also may be experienced as chest pain, cardiac ischemia must be ruled out.

Proton pump inhibitors are the agents of choice for controlling symptoms and healing esophagitis. Other therapies include H2 receptor antagonists or prokinetics and antacids. Weight reduction, smoking cessation, elevation of the head of the bed 15 cm, and avoiding tight clothing also help to alleviate symptoms. Laparoscopic fundoplication is the most common surgical intervention when medical treatment fails.[21]

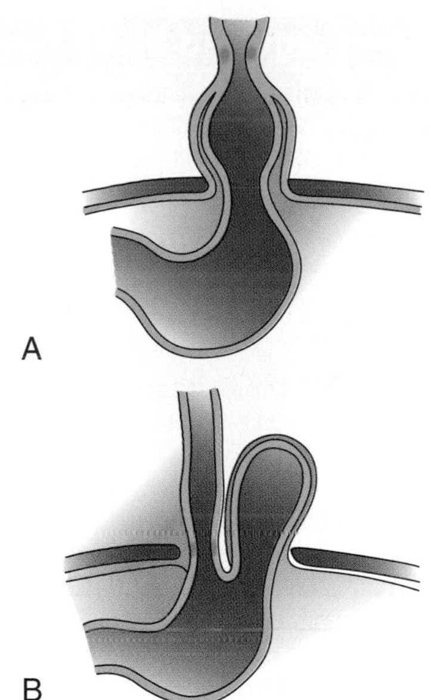

FIGURE 36-3 Types of Hiatal Hernia. A, Sliding hiatal hernia (type 1). B, Paraesophageal hiatal hernia (type 2). Not shown is mixed hiatal hernia (type 3).

Eosinophilic esophagitis is an idiopathic inflammatory disease of the esophagus characterized by infiltration of eosinophils associated with atopic disease, including asthma and food allergies. It occurs in adults and children. Dysphagia, food impaction, vomiting, and weight loss are common symptoms. Endoscopy with biopsy identifies the eosinophilc infiltration and differentiation from GERD. Treatment is symptomatic, including elimination diets and steroids.

Hiatal Hernia

PATHOPHYSIOLOGY Hiatal hernia is a type of diaphragmatic hernia with protrusion (herniation) of the upper part of the stomach through the diaphragm and into the thorax (Figure 36-3).[22] Sliding hiatal hernia (type 1) is the most common. With this type of hernia, the proximal portion of the stomach moves into the thoracic cavity through the esophageal hiatus, an opening in the diaphragm for the esophagus and vagus nerves. A congenitally short esophagus, fibrosis or excessive vagal nerve stimulation, or weakening of the diaphragmatic muscles at the gastroesophageal junction contributes to the hernia. GERD is associated with this type of herniation. Coughing, bending, tight clothing, ascites, obesity, and pregnancy accentuate the hernia.

Paraesophageal hiatal hernia (type 2) is the herniation of the greater curvature of the stomach through a secondary opening in the diaphragm alongside the esophagus. The position of a portion of the stomach above the diaphragm causes congestion of mucosal blood flow, leading to gastritis and ulcer formation. Strangulation of the hernia is a major complication. It can present with vomiting and epigastric and retrosternal epigastric pain and is a surgical emergency.[23]

Mixed hiatal hernia (type 3) is less common and is a combination of sliding and paraesophageal hiatal hernias. It tends to occur in conjunction with several other diseases, including reflux esophagitis, peptic ulcer, cholecystitis (gallbladder inflammation), cholelithiasis (gallstones), chronic pancreatitis, and diverticulosis.

CLINICAL MANIFESTATIONS Hiatal hernias are often asymptomatic. Generally, a wide variety of symptoms develop later in life and are associated with other GI disorders, including GERD. Symptoms include heartburn, regurgitation, dysphagia, and epigastric pain. Ischemia from hernia strangulation causes acute, severe chest or epigastric pain, nausea, vomiting, and GI bleeding.

EVALUATION AND TREATMENT Diagnostic procedures include radiology with barium swallow, endoscopy, and high-resolution manometry. A chest X-ray film often will show the protrusion of the stomach into the thorax, indicating paraesophageal hiatal hernia.

Treatment for sliding hiatal hernia is usually conservative. The individual can diminish reflux by eating small, frequent meals and avoiding the recumbent position after eating. Abdominal supports and tight clothing should be avoided, and weight control is recommended for obese individuals. Antacids alleviate reflux esophagitis. Individuals who are uncomfortable at night benefit from sleeping with the head of the bed elevated 15 cm. Surgery (fundoplication) is performed if medical management fails to control symptoms.

Gastroparesis is delayed gastric emptying in the absence of mechanical gastric outlet obstruction. It is most commonly associated with diabetes mellitus, surgical vagotomy, or fundoplication. It can be idiopathic. The pathophysiology is not well understood but involves abnormalities of the autonomic nervous system, smooth muscle cells, enteric neurons, and GI hormones. Diabetic gastroparesis represents a form of neuropathy involving the vagus nerve. Symptoms include nausea, vomiting, abdominal pain, and postprandial fullness or bloating. Treatment options include dietary management; prokinetic medications; and, in some cases, gastric electrical stimulation or surgical venting gastrostomy.[24]

Pyloric Obstruction

PATHOPHYSIOLOGY Pyloric obstruction (gastric outlet obstruction) is the narrowing or blocking of the opening between the stomach and the duodenum. This condition can be congenital (e.g., infantile hypertrophic pyloric stenosis; see Chapter 37) or acquired. Acquired obstruction is caused by peptic ulcer disease or carcinoma near the pylorus. Duodenal ulcers are more likely than gastric ulcers to obstruct the pylorus. Ulceration causes obstruction resulting from inflammation, edema, spasm, fibrosis, or scarring. Tumours cause obstruction by growing into the pylorus.

CLINICAL MANIFESTATIONS Early in the course of pyloric obstruction, the individual experiences vague epigastric fullness, which becomes more distressing after eating and at the end of the day. Nausea and epigastric pain may occur as the muscles of the stomach contract in attempts to force chyme past the obstruction. These symptoms disappear when the chyme finally moves into the duodenum. As obstruction progresses, anorexia develops, sometimes accompanied by weight loss. Severe obstruction causes gastric distension and atony (lack of muscle tone and gastric motility). Gastric distension stimulates gastric secretion, which increases the feeling of fullness. Rolling or jarring of the abdomen produces a sloshing sound called the *succussion splash.* At this stage, vomiting is a cardinal sign of obstruction. It is usually copious and occurs several hours after eating. The vomitus contains undigested food but no bile. Prolonged vomiting leads to dehydration, which is accompanied by a hypokalemic and hypochloremic metabolic alkalosis caused by loss of gastric potassium and acid, respectively. Because food does not enter the intestine, stools are infrequent and small. Prolonged pyloric obstruction causes severe malnutrition, dehydration, and extreme debilitation.

EVALUATION AND TREATMENT Diagnosis is based on clinical manifestations, a history of ulcer disease, and examination of residual gastric contents. Endoscopy is performed if gastric carcinoma is the suggested cause of pyloric obstruction.

TABLE 36-2 Common Causes of Intestinal Obstruction

Cause	Pathophysiology
Hernia	Protrusion of intestine through weakness in abdominal muscles or through inguinal ring
Intussusception	Telescoping of one part of intestine into another; this usually causes strangulation of blood supply; more common in infants 10–15 months of age than in adults (see Figure 36-4, *D*)
Torsion (volvulus)	Twisting of intestine on its mesenteric pedicle, with occlusion of blood supply; often associated with fibrous adhesions; occurs most often in middle-aged and older adult men
Diverticulosis	Inflamed saccular herniations (diverticuli) of mucosa and submucosa through tunica muscularis of colon; diverticuli are interspersed between thick, circular, fibrous bands; most common in obese individuals older than 60 years (see Figure 36-9)
Tumour	Tumour growth into intestinal lumen; adenocarcinoma of colon and rectum is most common tumoural obstruction; most common in individuals older than 60 years
Paralytic (adynamic) ileus	Loss of peristaltic motor activity in intestine; associated with abdominal surgery, peritonitis, hypokalemia, ischemic bowel, spinal trauma, or pneumonia
Fibrous adhesions	Peritoneal irritation from surgery, trauma, or Crohn's disease leads to formation of fibrin and adhesions that attach to intestine, omentum, or peritoneum and can cause obstruction; most common in small intestine
Fecal mass (impaction)	Hardened stool impacted in the rectum or distal sigmoid colon, with subsequent obstruction; associated with lack of mobility due to aging or spinal cord injury; fecal impaction is related to reduction of colonic mass movements and an inability to use abdominal muscles to assist in defecation

Obstructions resulting from ulceration often resolve with conservative management. A large-bore nasogastric tube is used to aspirate stomach contents and relieve distension. Then nasogastric suction is maintained for 2 to 3 days to decompress the stomach and restore normal motility. Gastric secretions that contribute to inflammation and edema can be suppressed with proton pump inhibitors or H2 receptor antagonists. Fluids and electrolytes (saline and potassium) are given intravenously to promote rehydration and correct hypokalemia and alkalosis (see Chapter 5). Severely malnourished individuals may require parenteral hyperalimentation (intravenous nutrition). Surgery or the placement of pyloric stents may be required to treat gastric carcinoma or persistent obstruction caused by fibrosis and scarring.[25]

Intestinal Obstruction and Paralytic Ileus

Intestinal obstruction can be caused by any condition that prevents the normal flow of chyme through the intestinal lumen (Table 36-2).[26] Obstructions can occur in either the small or the large intestine (Table 36-3). The small intestine is more commonly obstructed because of its narrower lumen. Classifications of intestinal obstruction are summarized in Table 36-4. Intestinal obstruction is classified by cause as simple or

TABLE 36-3 Large and Small Bowel Obstruction

Type of Obstruction	Cause
Small bowel obstruction	Adhesions: secondary to previous abdominal surgeries—75% Hernia: inguinal, ventral, or femoral—10% Tumours: may be associated with intussusception—10% Mesenteric ischemia—3–5% Crohn's disease—<1%
Large bowel obstruction	Colon/rectal cancer—90% Volvulus—4–5% Diverticular disease—3–5% Other causes (inflammatory bowel disease, adhesions, hernia)

Data from Mizell, J.S., & Turnage, R.H. (2016). Intestinal obstruction. In M. Feldman, L.S. Friedman, & L.J. Brandt (Eds.), *Sleisenger & Fordtran's gastrointestinal and liver disease: Pathophysiology, diagnosis, management* (10th ed., pp. 2154–2170). Philadelphia: Saunders.

functional. *Simple obstruction* is mechanical blockage of the lumen by a lesion and it is the most common type of intestinal obstruction. Paralytic ileus, or *functional obstruction*, is a failure of intestinal motility often occurring after intestinal or abdominal surgery, acute pancreatitis, or hypokalemia. Acute obstructions usually have mechanical causes, such as adhesions or hernias (Figure 36-4). Chronic or partial obstructions are more often associated with tumours or inflammatory disorders, particularly of the large intestine.

PATHOPHYSIOLOGY The major pathophysiological alterations are presented in Figure 36-5. Postoperative paralytic ileus results from inhibitory neural reflexes associated with inflammatory mediators and the influence of exogenous (i.e., meperidine [Demerol] or morphine) and endogenous opioids (endorphins) that affect the entire GI tract. Small bowel obstruction (SBO) is caused by postoperative adhesions, tumours, CD, and hernias. SBO leads to distension caused by impaired absorption and increased secretion with accumulation of fluid and gas inside the lumen proximal to the obstruction.[27] Distension decreases the intestine's ability to absorb water and electrolytes and increases the net secretion of these substances into the lumen. Copious vomiting or sequestration of fluids in the intestinal lumen prevents their reabsorption and produces severe fluid and electrolyte disturbances. Extracellular fluid volume and plasma volume decrease, causing dehydration, increased hematocrit level, hypotension, and tachycardia. Severe dehydration leads to hypovolemic shock. Metabolic alkalosis initially develops as a result of excessive loss of hydrogen ions that would normally be reabsorbed from the gastric juice and vomiting. With prolonged obstruction or obstruction lower in the intestine, metabolic acidosis is more likely to occur because bicarbonate from pancreatic secretions and bile cannot be reabsorbed. Hypokalemia from vomiting and decreased potassium absorption can be extreme, promoting acidosis and atony of the intestinal wall. Metabolic acidosis also may be accentuated by ketosis, the result of declining carbohydrate stores caused by starvation. Lack of circulation permits the buildup of significant amounts of lactic acid, which worsen the metabolic acidosis. If pressure from the distension is severe enough, it occludes the arterial circulation and causes ischemia, necrosis, perforation, and peritonitis. Fever and leukocytosis are often associated with overgrowth of bacteria, ischemia, and bowel necrosis. Bacterial proliferation and translocation across the mucosa to the systemic

TABLE 36-4 Classifications of Intestinal Obstruction

Criteria for Classification	Definition
Onset	
Acute	Sudden onset; often caused by torsion, intussusception, or herniation
Chronic	Protracted onset; more commonly from tumour growth or progressive formation of strictures
Extent of Obstruction	
Partial	Incomplete obstruction of intestinal lumen
Complete	Complete obstruction of intestinal lumen
Location of Obstructing Lesion	
Intrinsic	Obstruction develops within intestinal lumen; examples: gut wall edema or hemorrhage, foreign bodies (gallstones), tumours, or gut wall fibrosis
Extrinsic	Obstruction originates outside intestine; examples: tumours, torsion, fibrosis, hernia, intussusception
Effects on Intestinal Wall	
Simple	Luminal obstruction without impairment of blood supply
Strangulated	Luminal obstruction with occlusion of blood supply
Closed loop	Obstruction at each end of a segment of intestine
Casual Factors	
Mechanical	Blockage of intestinal lumen by intrinsic or extrinsic lesions; usually treated surgically
Functional (paralytic ileus)	Paralysis of intestinal musculature caused by trauma, peritonitis, electrolyte imbalances, or spasmolytic agents; usually treated by decompression with suction or surgery if death of tissue occurs

circulation cause peritonitis or sepsis. The release of inflammatory mediators into the circulation causes remote organ failure.

Large bowel obstruction is less common and often related to cancer. Diverticulitis, IBD, and other causes of obstruction are less common. Acute colonic pseudo-obstruction (Ogilvie syndrome) is a rare massive dilation of the large bowel that is related to excessive sympathetic motor input or decreased parasympathetic motor input with absence of mechanical obstruction. It occurs primarily in people who are critically ill and immobilized older adults.

CLINICAL MANIFESTATIONS Signs and symptoms of *small intestine obstruction* include colicky pains caused by intestinal distension followed by nausea and vomiting. Pain intensifies for seconds or minutes as a peristaltic wave of muscle contraction meets the obstruction. Pain may be continuous with severe distension and then diminish in intensity. If ischemia occurs, the pain loses its colicky character and becomes more constant and severe. Sweating and tachycardia occur as a sympathetic nervous system response to hypotension. Fever, severe leukocytosis, abdominal distension, and rebound tenderness develop as ischemia progresses to necrosis, perforation, and peritonitis.

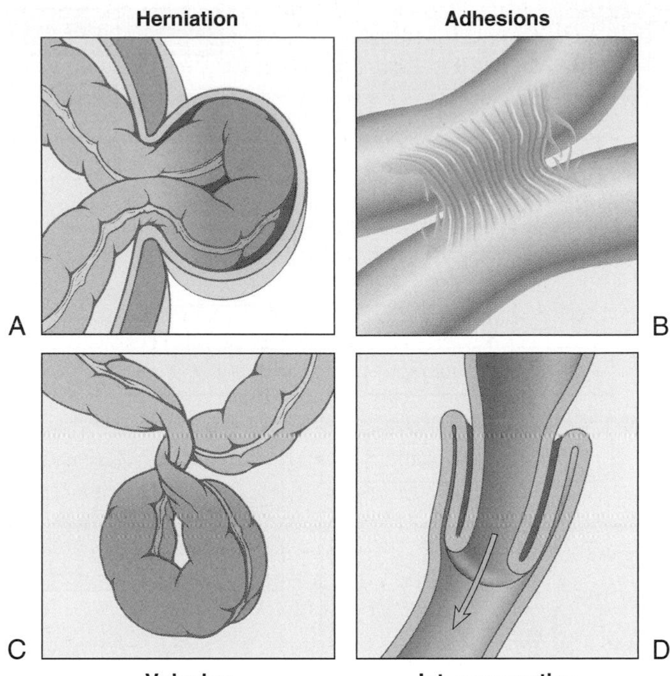

FIGURE 36-4 Intestinal Obstructions. **A,** Hernia. **B,** Constrictions from adhesions. **C,** Volvulus. **D,** Intussusception. (From Kumar, V., Abbas, A., & Aster, J. [2013]. *Robbins basic pathology* [9th ed.]. Philadelphia: Saunders.)

Obstruction at the pylorus causes early, profuse vomiting. Obstruction in the proximal small intestine causes mild distension and vomiting of bile-stained fluid. Lower obstruction in the small intestine causes more pronounced distension because a greater length of intestine is proximal to the obstruction. In this case, vomiting may not occur early but may occur later and contain fecal material. Partial obstruction can cause diarrhea or constipation, but complete obstruction usually causes constipation only. Complete obstruction increases the number of bowel sounds, which may be tinkly and accompanied by peristaltic rushes and crampy abdominal pain. Signs of hypovolemia and metabolic acidosis may be observed as early as 24 hours after the occurrence of complete obstruction. Distension may be severe enough to push against the diaphragm and decrease lung volume. It can also lead to atelectasis and pneumonia, particularly in debilitated individuals.

Large intestine obstruction usually presents with hypogastric pain and abdominal distension. Pain can vary from vague to excruciating, depending on the degree of ischemia and the development of peritonitis. Vomiting occurs late in the obstructive process. Small and large intestinal perforation presents the same with acute, persistent abdominal pain, nausea, vomiting, and fever.[28] *Acute colonic pseudo-obstruction* is characterized by abdominal distension, abdominal pain, and nausea and vomiting. Bowel sounds are usually present.

EVALUATION AND TREATMENT Evaluation is based on clinical manifestations and imaging studies. Successful management requires early identification of the site and type of obstruction. Replacement of fluid and electrolytes and decompression of the lumen with gastric or intestinal suction are essential forms of therapy. Laparoscopic procedures can release adhesions. Immediate surgical intervention is required for strangulation, complete obstruction, or perforation. Colonic stents may be placed for malignant obstruction. Neostigmine (Prostigmin), a parasympathomimetic, is used for colonic pseudo-obstruction and colonoscopic decompression may be required.[29]

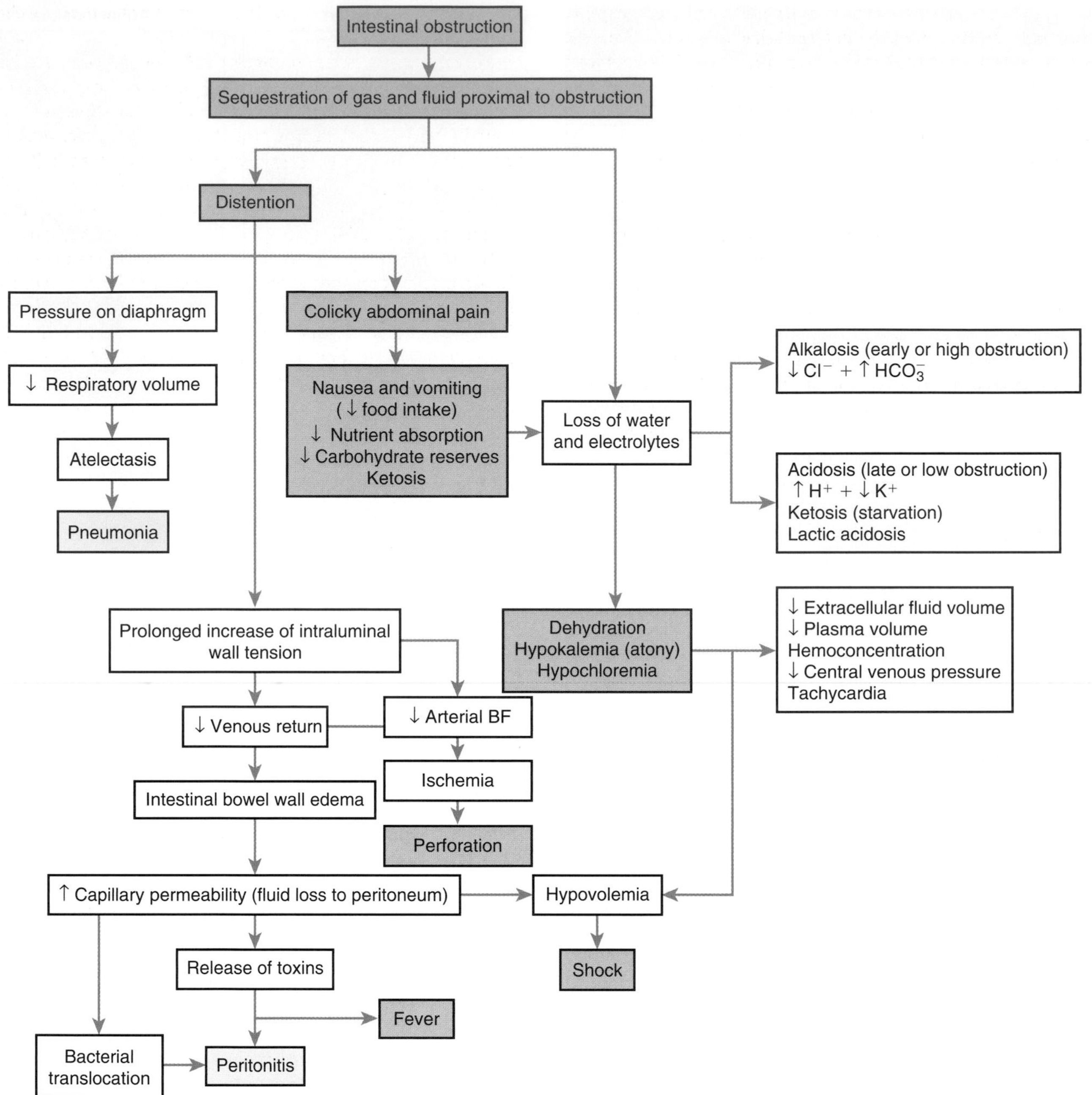

FIGURE 36-5 **Pathophysiology of Intestinal Obstruction.** *BF*, Blood flow, *Cl⁻*, Chloride; *H⁺*, hydrogen; HCO_3^-, bicarbonate; *K⁺*, potassium.

> **QUICK CHECK 36-2**
> 1. Why is heartburn associated with gastroesophageal reflux?
> 2. What causes postoperative paralytic ileus?
> 3. How does peritonitis develop with bowel obstruction?

Gastritis

Gastritis is an inflammatory disorder of the gastric mucosa. It can be acute or chronic and affect the superficial mucosa of the fundus or antrum, or both.

Acute gastritis is caused by injury of the protective mucosal barrier caused by medications, chemicals, or *Helicobacter pylori* infection. Nonsteroidal anti-inflammatory drugs (NSAIDs; e.g., ibuprofen [Advil], naproxen [Apo-Naproxren], indomethacin [Indocin], and Aspirin) inhibit the action of cyclooxygenase-1 (COX-1) and cause gastritis because they inhibit prostaglandin synthesis, which normally stimulates the secretion of mucus. Alcohol, histamine, digitalis, and metabolic disorders, such as uremia, are contributing factors. *H. pylori*–associated acute gastritis causes inflammation, increased gastric secretion in antral gastritis, decreased gastric section in fundal gastritis, pain, nausea, and vomiting. The clinical manifestations of acute gastritis can include vague abdominal discomfort, epigastric tenderness, and bleeding. Healing usually occurs spontaneously within a few days. Discontinuing injurious medications, using antacids, or decreasing acid secretion with H2 receptor antagonists facilitates healing.

Chronic gastritis tends to occur in older adults and causes chronic inflammation, mucosal atrophy, and epithelial metaplasia. Chronic gastritis is classified as type A, immune (fundal), or type B, nonimmune (antral), depending on the pathogenesis and location of the lesions. When both types of chronic gastritis occur, it is known as type AB, or pangastritis, and the antrum is more severely involved. Type C gastritis is associated with reflux of bile and pancreatic secretions into the stomach, causing chemical injury.

Chronic immune (fundal) gastritis is the rarest form of gastritis and is associated with loss of T lymphocyte (T cell) tolerance and development of autoantibodies to gastric H^+–K^+ ATPase. The gastric mucosa degenerates extensively in the body and fundus of the stomach, leading to gastric atrophy. Loss of parietal cells diminishes acid and intrinsic factor secretion. Pernicious anemia can develop from decreased vitamin B_{12} absorption (see Chapter 21). The feedback mechanism that normally inhibits gastrin secretion is impaired, causing elevated plasma levels of gastrin. Chronic fundal gastritis occurs in association with other autoimmune diseases (e.g., rheumatoid arthritis, autoimmune thyroid disease, or type 1 diabetes mellitus) and is a risk factor for gastric carcinoma, particularly in individuals who develop pernicious anemia.

Chronic nonimmune (antral gastritis) generally involves the antrum only and is more common than fundal gastritis. It is caused by *H. pylori* bacteria and it also is associated with use of alcohol, tobacco, and NSAIDs.[30] There are high levels of hydrochloric acid secretion with an increased risk for duodenal ulcers. *H. pylori* also can progress to autoimmune atrophic gastritis and involves the fundus, thus becoming pangastritis. There is greater risk for the development of gastric cancer in these cases.[31]

Signs and symptoms of chronic gastritis often include vague symptoms: anorexia, fullness, nausea, vomiting, and epigastric pain. Gastric bleeding may be the only clinical manifestation of gastritis. Gastroscopic examination and biopsy may show a longstanding inflammatory process and gastric atrophy in an individual with no history of abdominal distress. Failure to stimulate acid secretion confirms achlorhydria (diminished secretion of hydrochloric acid). The gastric secretions also can be evaluated for the presence of intrinsic factor. Symptoms can usually be managed by eating smaller meals in conjunction with a soft, bland diet and by avoiding alcohol and Aspirin. *H. pylori* infection is treated with antibiotics, and vitamin B_{12} is administered to correct pernicious anemia.

Peptic Ulcer Disease

A **peptic ulcer** is a break or ulceration in the protective mucosal lining of the lower esophagus, stomach, or duodenum. Ulcers develop when mucosal protective factors are overcome by erosive factors commonly caused by NSAIDs and *H. pylori* infection. Risk factors for peptic ulcer disease are summarized in *Risk Factors:* Peptic Ulcer. Psychological stress may be a risk factor for peptic ulcer disease, but the exact mechanism of causation is not known.[32]

In Canada, it is estimated that 8 to 10 million people are infected with *H. pylori*. In First Nations communities, approximately 75% of people are infected with *H. pylori*. *H. pylori* eradication therapy costs around $90 per person in Canada and is 80 to 90% effective. A second round of therapy in instances of resistance costs around $275.[33]

The *H. pylori* infection rate increases with age in Canada. The infection rate for 30-year-olds is 1 in 5 people, or 1 million people. The infection rate for people 80 years or older is 1 in 2 people, or 0.5 million people.[33]

H. pylori infection is one of the causes of functional dyspepsia. The Canadian population groups considered to be at a high risk for *H. pylori* infection number over 4.1 million; these groups have been identified based on origin of birth, area of residence, or both. Testing and eradication costs for these groups are estimated to be $350 million.[33]

H. pylori infection is considered to be a carcinogen by World Health Organization because it is associated with the development of stomach cancer. In communities with a high prevalence of *H. pylori* infection, treated individuals have a 1 in 10 chance of re-infection after one year.[33]

RISK FACTORS
Peptic Ulcer

- Infection of the gastric and duodenal mucosa with *Helicobacter pylori*
- Chronic use of nonsteroidal anti-inflammatory drugs
- Alcohol
- Smoking
- Advanced age
- Chronic diseases, such as emphysema, rheumatoid arthritis, cirrhosis, obesity, and diabetes
- Type O blood
- Psychological stress

Peptic ulcers can be single or multiple, acute or chronic, and superficial or deep. Superficial ulcerations are called *erosions* because they erode the mucosa but do not penetrate the muscularis mucosae (Figure 36-6). True ulcers extend through the muscularis mucosae and damage blood vessels, causing hemorrhage, or perforate the GI wall.

Zollinger-Ellison syndrome is a rare syndrome that also is associated with peptic ulcers caused by a gastrin-secreting neuroendocrine tumour or multiple tumours (gastrinoma) of the pancreas or duodenum. Increased secretion of gastrin causes excess secretion of gastric acid, resulting in gastric and duodenal ulcers, gastroesophageal reflux with abdominal pain, and diarrhea.[34]

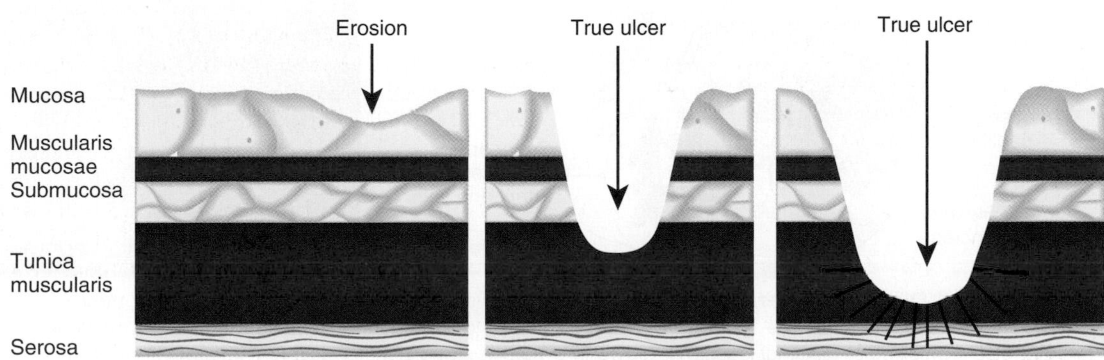

FIGURE 36-6 Lesions Caused by Peptic Ulcer Disease.

Duodenal Ulcers

Duodenal ulcers occur with greater frequency than other types of peptic ulcers and are commonly caused by *H. pylori* infection and NSAID use.[35] Idiopathic duodenal ulcers are rare and can be associated with altered mucosal defences, rapid gastric emptying, elevated serum gastrin levels, or acid production stimulated by smoking.[36]

PATHOPHYSIOLOGY Causative factors, singly or in combination, cause acid and pepsin concentrations in the duodenum to penetrate the mucosal barrier and cause ulceration (Figure 36-7). The host response to *H. pylori* infection is activation of T and B lymphocytes (T and B cells) with infiltration of neutrophils. Release of inflammatory cytokines damages the gastric epithelium. An *H. pylori* virulence factor (cytotoxin-associated gene A [CagA]) produces vacuolating cytotoxin A (VacA), causing apoptosis of gastric epithelial cells and promoting inflammation. *H. pylori* mucosal infection underlies gastric and duodenal ulcer and gastric cancer.[37]

CLINICAL MANIFESTATIONS The characteristic manifestation of a duodenal ulcer is chronic intermittent pain in the epigastric area. The pain begins 2 or 3 hours after eating, when the stomach is empty. It is not unusual for pain to occur in the middle of the night and disappear by morning. Pain is relieved rapidly by ingestion of food or antacids, creating a typical pain-food-relief pattern. Some individuals with duodenal ulcer may have no symptoms; the first manifestation may be hemorrhage or perforation, particularly with a history of NSAID or anticoagulant use.

Complications of duodenal ulcer include bleeding, perforation, and obstruction of the duodenum or outlet of the stomach. Bleeding is the most common cause of mortality, particularly among older adults. Perforation occurs with destruction of all layers of the duodenal wall and causes sudden, severe epigastric pain.[38] Obstruction may be the result of edema from inflammation or scarring from chronic injury. It is not clear why individuals infected with *H. pylori* duodenal ulcers are negatively associated with gastric cancer.[39]

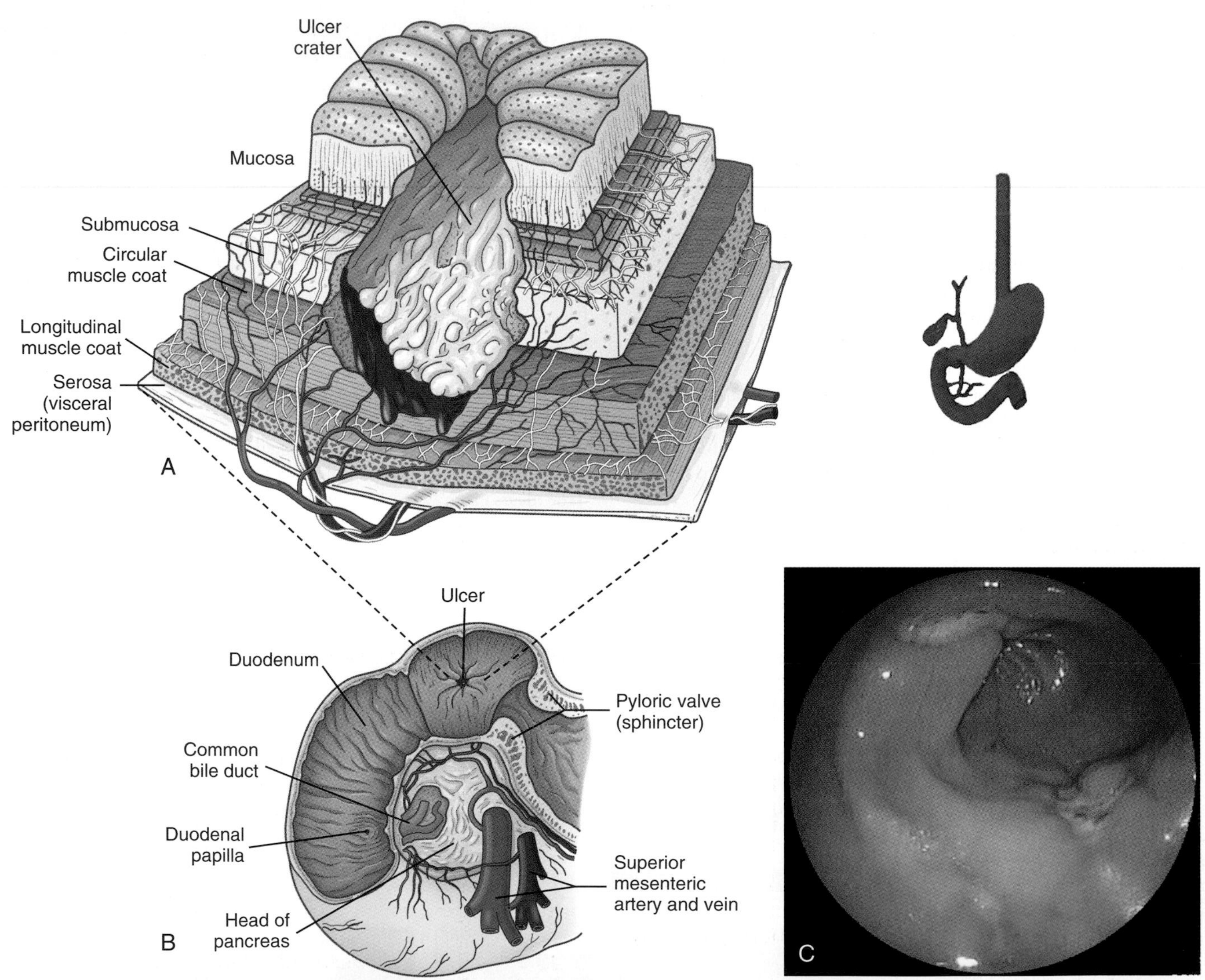

FIGURE 36-7 Duodenal Ulcer. A, A deep ulceration in the duodenal wall extending as a crater through the entire mucosa and into the muscle layers. **B,** Sequence of ulcerations from normal mucosa to duodenal ulcer. **C,** Bilateral (kissing) duodenal ulcers in a person using nonsteroidal anti-inflammatory drugs. (**C,** Med_Chaos.)

Duodenal ulcers often heal spontaneously but recur within months without treatment. Exacerbations tend to develop in the spring and fall. Relief of pain accompanies healing. Constant, unremitting pain may be caused by complications, such as intestinal obstruction or perforation. Bleeding from duodenal ulcers causes hematemesis or melena.[40]

EVALUATION AND TREATMENT Several diagnostic approaches are used to differentiate duodenal ulcers from gastric ulcers or gastric carcinoma. Endoscopic evaluation allows visualization of lesions and biopsy. Radioimmune assays of gastrin levels are evaluated to identify ulcers associated with gastric carcinomas. *H. pylori* is detected using the urea breath test, *H. pylori*–specific serum immunoglobulin G (IgG) and immunoglobulin A (IgA) antibodies, and measurement of *H. pylori* stool antigen levels. Findings from gastric biopsy detect *H. pylori* infection and confirm eradication after treatment.[41]

Management of duodenal ulcers is aimed at relieving the causes and effects of hyperacidity and preventing complications. Antacids neutralize gastric contents and relieve pain. Acid secretion can be suppressed with medications that block H2 receptors and inhibit the secretion of acid. Proton pump inhibitors inhibit acid production. *H. pylori* is treated with a combination of antibiotics and proton pump inhibitors, but antibiotic resistance is an increasing problem.[42] Surgical resection may be required for bleeding or perforating ulcers, obstruction, or peritonitis.

Gastric Ulcers

Gastric ulcers are ulcers of the stomach and occur about equally in males and females, usually between the ages of 55 and 65 years. They are about one-fourth as common as duodenal ulcers (Table 36-5).

PATHOPHYSIOLOGY Generally, gastric ulcers develop in the antral region, adjacent to the acid-secreting mucosa of the body. The primary defect is an abnormality that increases the mucosal barrier's permeability to hydrogen ions. Gastric secretion may be normal or less than normal, and there may be a decreased mass of parietal cells. Chronic gastritis is often associated with development of gastric ulcers and may precipitate ulcer formation by limiting the mucosa's ability to secrete a protective layer of mucus (Figure 36-8). Other factors include the following:

- Decreased mucosal synthesis of prostaglandins
- Duodenal reflux of bile and pancreatic enzymes damage the mucosal membrane
- Use of NSAIDs (decreases prostaglandin synthesis)
- *H. pylori* infection

A break in the mucosal barrier permits hydrogen ions to diffuse into the mucosa, where they disrupt permeability and cellular structure. A vicious cycle can be established as the damaged mucosa liberates histamine, which stimulates the increase of acid and pepsinogen production, blood flow, and capillary permeability. The disrupted mucosa becomes edematous and loses plasma proteins. Destruction of small vessels causes bleeding.

CLINICAL MANIFESTATIONS The clinical manifestations of gastric ulcers are similar to those of duodenal ulcers (see Table 36-5). The pattern of pain is common but the pain of gastric ulcers also occurs immediately after eating. Gastric ulcers also tend to be chronic rather than alternating between periods of remission and exacerbation and cause more anorexia, vomiting, and weight loss than duodenal ulcers. The evaluation and treatment of gastric ulcers are similar to the evaluation and treatment of duodenal ulcers.

TABLE 36-5 Characteristics of Gastric and Duodenal Ulcers

Characteristics	Gastric Ulcer	Duodenal Ulcer
Incidence		
Age at onset	50–70 years	20–50 years
Family history	Usually negative	Positive
Gender (prevalence)	Equal in women and men	Greater in men
Stress factors	Increased	Average
Ulcerogenic medications	Normal use	Increased use
Cancer risk	Increased	Not increased
Pathophysiology		
Abnormal mucus	May be present	May be present
Parietal cell mass	Normal or decreased	Increased
Acid production	Normal or decreased	Increased
Serum gastrin	Increased	Normal
Serum pepsinogen	Normal	Increased
Associated gastritis	More common	Usually not present
Helicobacter pylori	May be present (60–80%)	Often present (95–100%)
	Stimulates reduced acid secretion, gastric atrophy, and risk for gastric cancer	Stimulates acid hypersecretion
Clinical Manifestations		
Pain	Located in upper abdomen	Located in upper abdomen
	Intermittent	Intermittent
	Pain-antacid-relief pattern	Pain-antacid/food-relief pattern
	Food–pain pattern (when food in stomach)	Pain when stomach empty
		Nocturnal pain common
Clinical course	Chronic ulcer without pattern of remission and exacerbation	Pattern of remissions and exacerbation for years
	Heals more slowly	Heals more quickly

Stress-Related Mucosal Disease

A **stress-related mucosal disease (stress ulcer)** is an acute form of peptic ulcer that tends to accompany the physiological stress of severe illness or major trauma. Usually multiple sites of ulceration are distributed within the stomach or duodenum. Stress ulcers may be classified as ischemic ulcers or Cushing ulcers.

Ischemic ulcers develop within hours of an event such as hemorrhage, multisystem trauma, severe burns, heart failure, or sepsis. Shock, anoxia, inflammation, and sympathetic responses cause ischemia of the stomach and duodenal mucosa, disrupting the mucosal barrier. Stress ulcers that develop as a result of burn injury are often called **Curling ulcers**. **Cushing ulcer** is a stress ulcer associated with severe brain trauma or brain surgery. Decreased mucosal blood flow and hypersecretion of acid caused by overstimulation of the vagal nuclei damage the mucosal barrier, causing erosions and ulceration.

The primary clinical manifestation of stress-related mucosal disease is bleeding, which is uncommon, but occurs more readily with the presence of coagulopathy and more than 48 hours of mechanical ventilation. Prophylactic treatment regimens are used to prevent this disease.[43] Stress ulcers seldom become chronic.

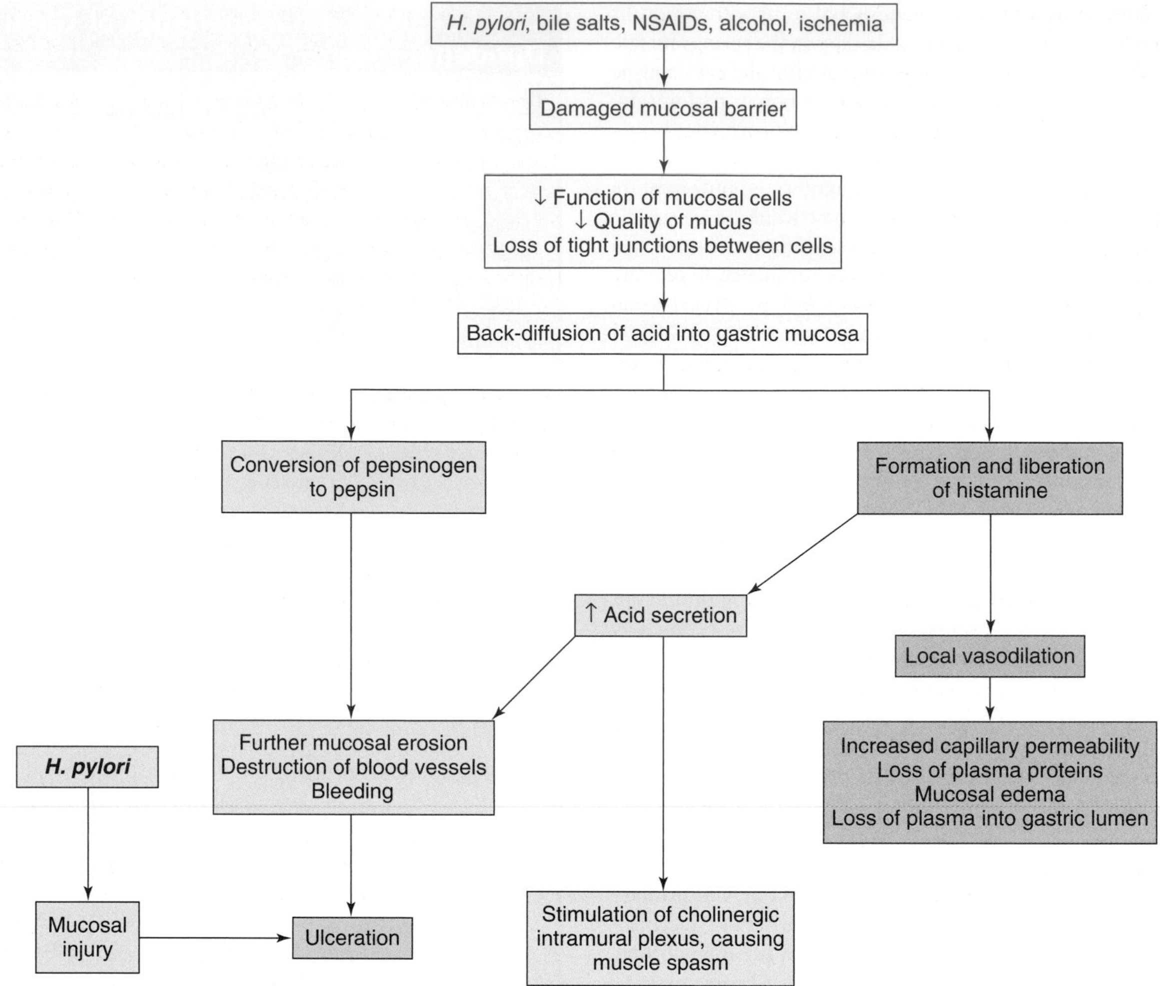

FIGURE 36-8 Pathophysiology of Gastric Ulcer Formation. *NSAIDs,* Nonsteroidal anti-inflammatory drugs.

Surgical Treatment of Ulcer

Advances in the medical treatment of peptic ulcer disease with acid suppression and eradication of *H. pylori* have reduced the number of cases requiring surgery. The most common indications for ulcer surgery are recurrent or uncontrolled bleeding and perforation of the stomach or duodenum. The primary objectives of surgical treatment are to reduce stimuli for acid secretion, decrease the number of acid-secreting cells in the stomach, and correct complications of ulcer disease.

Acute complications of gastrectomy or anastomosis are relatively uncommon except in debilitated persons. Chronic complications, however, are likely to develop if a large portion of the stomach has been removed. These complications and their pathophysiological mechanisms are described in the next section.

QUICK CHECK 36-3

1. What is the most common cause of chronic gastritis?
2. Compare the three types of peptic ulcers.
3. What causes a stress ulcer?

Postgastrectomy Syndromes

Postgastrectomy syndromes are a group of signs and symptoms that occur after gastric resection for the treatment of peptic ulcer, gastric carcinoma, or bariatric surgery for extreme obesity. They are caused by anatomical and functional changes in the stomach and upper small intestine[44] and include the following:

- **Dumping syndrome.** Rapid emptying of hypertonic chyme from the surgically residual stomach (the stomach component remaining after surgical resection following gastric or bariatric surgery) into the small intestine 10 to 20 minutes after eating; promoted by loss of gastric capacity, loss of emptying control when pylorus is removed, and loss of feedback control by duodenum when it is removed; responds to dietary management. Symptoms include cramping pain, nausea, vomiting, osmotic diarrhea, weakness, pallor, and hypotension.
- **Alkaline reflux gastritis.** Stomach inflammation caused by reflux of bile and alkaline pancreatic secretions containing proteolytic enzymes that disrupt the mucosal barrier in the remnant stomach. Symptoms include nausea, bilious vomiting, and sustained epigastric pain that worsens after eating and is not relieved by antacids; responds somewhat to avoidance of Aspirin and alcohol,[45] but surgical correction may be required.
- **Afferent loop obstruction.** Intermittent severe pain and epigastric fullness after eating as a result of volvulus, hernia, adhesion, or stenosis of the duodenal stump on the proximal side of the gastrojejunostomy; vomiting relieves symptoms; management includes low-fat diet, but decompression or surgery revision is required for complete obstruction.[46]

- Diarrhea. Either frequent, persistent elimination of loose stools or intermittent, precipitous, and unpredictable elimination of a large volume of stool; related to rapid gastric emptying and osmotic attraction of water into the gut, especially after large intake of high-carbohydrate liquids; small, dry meals and anticholinergic medications are effective control measures.
- Weight loss. Commonly caused by inadequate caloric intake because individual cannot tolerate carbohydrates or a normal-sized meal; stomach is also less able to mix, churn, and break down food. In the case of bariatric surgery for extreme obesity, weight loss is the intended outcome, but nutrient deficiencies, including vitamins and minerals, must be supplemented.[47]
- Anemia. Iron malabsorption may result from decreased acid secretion or lack of duodenum after Billroth II procedure (gastrojejunostomy); deficiencies of iron and vitamin B_{12} or folate may result.
- Bone and mineral disorders. Related to altered calcium absorption and metabolism, with increased risk for fractures and deformity and malabsorption of vitamins and nutrients, such as vitamin D.

Malabsorption Syndromes

Malabsorption syndromes interfere with nutrient absorption in the small intestine. Historically they have been classified as maldigestion or malabsorption. Maldigestion is failure of the chemical processes of digestion that take place in the intestinal lumen or at the brush border of the intestinal mucosa. Malabsorption is failure of the intestinal mucosa to absorb (transport) the digested nutrients. Often these two syndromes are interrelated, or occur together, making classification difficult. Generally, however, maldigestion is caused by deficiencies of the enzymes needed for digestion or inadequate secretion of bile salts and inadequate reabsorption of bile in the ileum. Malabsorption is the result of mucosal disruption caused by gastric or intestinal resection, vascular disorders, or intestinal disease.

Pancreatic Exocrine Insufficiency

The pancreatic enzymes (lipase, amylase, trypsin, chymotrypsin) are required for the digestion of proteins, carbohydrates, and fats. Pancreatic insufficiency is the deficient production of these enzymes, particularly lipase, by the pancreas. Causes include chronic pancreatitis, pancreatic carcinoma, pancreatic resection, and cystic fibrosis. Significant damage to or loss of pancreatic tissue must occur before enzyme levels decrease sufficiently to cause maldigestion. Although pancreatic insufficiency causes poor digestion of all nutrients, fat maldigestion is the chief problem. Absence of pancreatic bicarbonate in the duodenum and jejunum causes an acidic pH that worsens maldigestion by precipitating bile salts and preventing activation of the pancreatic enzymes that are present. A large amount of fat in the stool (steatorrhea) is the most common sign of pancreatic insufficiency. There is also a deficit of fat-soluble vitamins (A, D, E, and K) and weight loss.[48]

Lactase Deficiency (Lactose Intolerance)

Deficiency of disaccharidase at the brush border of the small intestine is caused by a genetic defect in which a single enzyme, usually lactase, is lacking. Lactase deficiency inhibits the breakdown of lactose (milk sugar) into monosaccharides and therefore prevents lactose digestion and absorption across the intestinal wall. Secondary (acquired) lactase deficiency can be caused by several diseases of the intestine, including gluten-sensitive enteropathy, enteritis, and bacterial overgrowth.

The undigested lactose remains in the intestine, where bacterial fermentation causes formation of gases. Undigested lactose also increases the osmotic gradient in the intestine, causing irritation and osmotic diarrhea. Clinical manifestations of lactose consumption with lactase deficiency are bloating, crampy pain, diarrhea, and flatulence. The disorder is diagnosed by a lactose-tolerance test. Avoiding milk products (more than 250 mL of milk) and adhering to a lactose-free diet relieve symptoms.[49]

According to a 2013 study, no data exist on the prevalence, correlates, and potential impact of perceived lactose intolerance among Canadians. To address this lack of data, the study's author undertook an online survey of 2 251 Canadians aged 19 years and older on whether they perceive themselves to be lactose intolerant. In all, 16% of respondents self-reported as lactose intolerant. Lactose intolerance was more common in women and in non-Whites and less common in those older than 50 years of age.[50]

Bile Salt Deficiency

Conjugated bile acids (bile salts) are necessary for the digestion and absorption of fats. Bile salts are conjugated in the bile that is secreted from the liver. When bile enters the duodenum, the bile salts aggregate with fatty acids and monoglycerides to form micelles. Micelle formation makes fat molecules more soluble and allows them to pass through the unstirred layer at the brush border of the small intestinal villi (see Chapter 35). A minimum concentration of bile salts, termed the *critical micelle concentration*, is required to allow formation of micelles. Therefore, conditions that decrease the production or secretion of bile result in decreased micelle formation and fat malabsorption. These conditions include advanced liver disease, which decreases the production of bile salts; obstruction of the common bile duct, which decreases flow of bile into the duodenum (cholestasis); intestinal stasis (lack of motility), which permits overgrowth of intestinal bacteria that deconjugate bile salts; and diseases of the ileum, which prevent the reabsorption and recycling of bile salts (enterohepatic circulation).[51]

Clinical manifestations of bile salt deficiency are related to poor intestinal absorption of fat and fat-soluble vitamins (A, D, E, and K). The absence of bile secretion can cause the feces to turn grey or pale. Increased fat in the stools (steatorrhea) leads to diarrhea and decreased levels of plasma proteins. The losses of fat-soluble vitamins and their effects include the following:

- Vitamin A deficiency results in night blindness.
- Vitamin D deficiency results in decreased calcium absorption with bone demineralization (osteoporosis), bone pain, and fractures.
- Vitamin K deficiency prolongs prothrombin time, leading to spontaneous development of purpura (bruising) and petechiae.
- Vitamin E deficiency has uncertain effects but may cause testicular atrophy and neurological defects in children.

The most effective treatment for fat-soluble vitamin deficiency is to increase consumption of medium-chain triglycerides in the diet, for example, by using coconut oil for cooking. Vitamins A, D, and K are given parenterally. Oral bile salts are an effective therapy.

Inflammatory Bowel Disease

UC and CD are chronic relapsing IBDs. The disease is more prevalent among White populations and Ashkenazi Jews.[52] In addition to the disease processes that impact the bowels, patients with IBD suffer from financial and nonfinancial costs due to their illness (see *Health Promotion:* The Impact of Inflammatory Bowel Disease in Canada). Risk factors and theories of causation include susceptibility genes, environmental factors, alterations in epithelial cell barrier functions, and an altered immune response to intestinal microflora[53,54] (Table 36-6). Environmental factors or infections are thought to alter the barrier function of the mucosal epithelium, leading to loss of immune tolerance to normal intestinal antigens. There is possible loss of discrimination of potentially harmful pathogens from commensal microorganisms in the intestinal mucosa. The loss of tolerance activates dendritic cells, triggering their transport to mesenteric lymph nodes, where they promote differentiation

TABLE 36-6 Features of Ulcerative Colitis and Crohn's Disease

Feature	Ulcerative Colitis	Crohn's Disease
Incidence		
Age at onset	Any age; 10–40 years most common	Any age; 10–30 years most common
Family history	Less common	More common
Gender	Prevalence equal in women and men	Prevalence about equal in women and men
Cancer risk	Increased	Increased
Nicotine use	Later and less severe disease; nicotine withdrawal may cause exacerbation	Increases disease risk and greater disease severity
Pathophysiology		
Location of lesions	Large intestine, continuous lesions Left side more common	Mouth to anus, "skip" lesions common Right side more common
Inflammation	Mucosal layer involved	Entire intestinal wall involved
Granulomata	Rare	Transmural granulomata common; cobblestone appearance
Ulceration	Friable mucosa, superficial ulcers, crypt abscesses common	Deep fissuring ulcers and fistulae common
Anal and perianal fistulae	Rare	Common; abscesses
Narrowed lumen and possible obstruction	Rare	Common; obstruction
Clinical Manifestations		
Abdominal pain	Mild to severe	Moderate to severe
Diarrhea	Common; 4 times/day	May or may not be present
Bloody stools	Common	Less common
Weight loss	Less common	Common
Abdominal mass	Rare	Common
Small intestine malabsorption	None	Common
Clinical course	Remissions and exacerbations	Remissions and exacerbations
Comorbidities	Extraintestinal manifestations	Extraintestinal manifestations

HEALTH PROMOTION

The Impact of Inflammatory Bowel Disease in Canada

The Crohn's and Colitis Foundation of Canada estimates that 18 employed Canadians with Crohn's disease (CD) die per year, at an average age of 49 years. The productivity loss associated with these deaths is $9.4 million.

In 2012, the economic costs of inflammatory bowel disease (IBD) in Canada were estimated at $2.8 billion (over $11 900 per person with IBD every year). Direct medical costs added up to over $1.2 billion and are dominated by medications ($521 million), followed by hospitalizations ($395 million), and physician visits ($132 million). Costs are higher for CD than for ulcerative colitis (UC) because CD leads to more frequent hospitalizations and greater use of newer, expensive medications. Indirect costs (to society and to the patient, including loss of productivity) are greater than direct medical costs: they were over $1.6 billion in 2012. Indirect costs are dominated by lower labour participation rates (long-term work losses of $979 million), followed by patient out-of-pocket expenses ($300 million) and then short-term work absences ($181 million). Indirect costs are similar for CD and UC.

In Canada, 43% of employed persons with IBD required time off due to IBD. Further, the short-term work losses were estimated at 7.2 days per employed person with IBD per year, strictly due to IBD. In 2012, IBD cost $181 million in short-term work losses in Canada for the 140 000 actively employed individuals with the disease.

People with IBD have a lower labour participation rate (3 to 13%) than the general population. The costs of reduced labour participation could range from $326 million (with 3% nonparticipation) to $1.4 billion (with 13% nonparticipation due to IBD). The best estimate is a minimum of $979 million (9% nonparticipation—21 000 individuals).

Limited data exist with which to estimate caregiver costs. At a minimum, parental caregiving for pediatric cases of IBD could cost $7 million a year. Potentially, caregiving for severely ill people with IBD costs $86 million per year.

IBD causes nonfinancial costs to individuals who bear the burden of disease and to their families. Those costs include reduced quality of life, loss of leisure time, and limited choices in relation to career, travel, and other personal options. CD and UC have a comparable effect in the reduction of quality of life. Individuals with IBD have a lower quality of life, compared with the general population, and even those in remission have a quality of life that is below the population average. Quality of life can be improved significantly with effective treatment, including both surgery and medication therapy. Treatment-improved quality of life often leads to restored productivity.

It is difficult to quantify the cost of loss of quality of life, but, based on Australian research, the cost of IBD in Canada for loss of quality of life may be more than $4 billion.

From Crohn's and Colitis Foundation of Canada. (2012) *The impact of inflammatory bowel disease in Canada: 2012 final report and recommendations*. Toronto: Author. Retrieved from http://crohnsandcolitis.ca/Crohns_and_Colitis/documents/reports/ccfc-ibd-impact-report-2012.pdf.

of naive T cells to T-helper 1 (Th1), Th2, and Th17 cells, or T-regulatory cells. Production of proinflammatory cytokines and chemokines, including tumour necrosis factor (TNF), interleukins, toxic oxygen free radicals, and interferon gamma (IFN-γ), damages the intestinal epithelium.[55] The risk for colon cancer increases significantly after 30 to 35 years of IBD, particularly in untreated disease.[56] Future research is directed at an integration of these factors to refine our understanding of disease cause and trajectory, particularly interactions between genetics, the microflora, mucosa, and immune responses.[57,58]

In Canada, it is estimated that 233 000 individuals are living with IBD. Among them, 129 000 have CD and 104 000 have UC. Over 10 200 new cases of IBD are diagnosed every year in Canada: 5 700 with CD and 4 500 with UC. Canada has among the highest reported prevalence (number of people with CD or UC) and incidence rates (number of new cases per year) of IBD in the world. The prevalence of IBD in Canada is estimated to be 0.7%, equating to more than 1 in every 150 Canadians. IBD can be diagnosed at any age, but has a typical age of onset in the 20s. Incidence of IBD has been rising, particularly since 2001, and significantly so in children under the age of 10 years. Approximately 5 900 Canadian children have IBD. Individuals with IBD have an increased risk of developing colorectal cancer. Further, individuals with CD face a significantly elevated risk for premature death (47% higher) than the general public.[59]

Compared with the general population, quality of life with IBD is low across all dimensions of health.

Ulcerative Colitis

Ulcerative colitis (UC) is a chronic inflammatory disease that causes ulceration of the colonic mucosa, most commonly in the rectum and sigmoid colon. The lesions appear in susceptible individuals between 20 and 40 years of age. UC is less common in people who smoke.[60]

PATHOPHYSIOLOGY The primary lesion of UC begins with inflammation at the base of the crypt of Lieberkühn in the large intestine. The disease begins in the rectum (proctitis) and may extend proximally to the entire colon (pancolitis). The mucosa is hyperemic and may appear dark red and velvety, and is involved in a continuous fashion. Small erosions form and coalesce into ulcers. Abscess formation, necrosis, and ragged ulceration of the mucosa ensue. Edema and thickening of the muscularis mucosae may narrow the lumen of the involved colon. Mucosal destruction and inflammation causes bleeding, cramping pain, and an urge to defecate. Frequent diarrhea, with passage of small amounts of blood and purulent mucus, is common. Loss of the absorptive mucosal surface and rapid colonic transit time cause large volumes of watery diarrhea.

CLINICAL MANIFESTATIONS The course of UC consists of intermittent periods of remission and exacerbation. Mild UC involves less mucosa, so that the frequency of bowel movements, bleeding, and pain is minimal. Severe forms may involve the entire colon and are characterized by abdominal pain, fever, elevated pulse rate, frequent diarrhea (10 to 20 stools/day), urgency, obviously bloody stools, and continuous, crampy pain. Dehydration, weight loss, anemia, and fever result from fluid loss, bleeding, and inflammation. Complications include anal fissures, hemorrhoids, and perirectal abscess. Severe hemorrhage is rare. Edema, strictures, or fibrosis can obstruct the colon. Perforation is an unusual but possible complication. Extraintestinal manifestations include cutaneous lesions (erythema nodosum), polyarthritis, episcleritis, uveitis, disorders of the liver, and alterations in coagulation.[61]

EVALUATION AND TREATMENT Diagnosis of UC is based on the medical history, clinical manifestations, and laboratory, serological, radiological, endoscopic, and biopsy findings. Infectious causes are ruled out by stool culture. The symptoms of UC may be similar to those of CD, making differential diagnosis challenging.[62] Treatment is individualized and depends on the severity of symptoms and the extent of mucosal involvement. A goal is to promote mucosal healing and avoid surgery. Mild to moderate disease is treated with 5-aminosalicylate therapy followed by steroids. Thioprine and immunomodulatory agents (cyclosporine [Sandimmune] and TNF-blocking agents [i.e., tacrolimus (Advagraf, Prograf)]) or vedolizumab (Entyvio) are used for serious disease.[63] New immunotherapies are emerging.[64] Severe, unremitting disease can require hospital admission for administration of intravenous fluids and steroids. Extreme malnutrition may require total parenteral nutrition (TPN). Surgical resection of the colon may be performed if other forms of therapy are unsuccessful or if there are acute serious complications (sepsis, hemorrhage, perforation, or obstruction). Surgical approaches for severe UC include total proctocolectomy, with end ileostomy or ileorectal anastomosis, or ileal pouch anal anastomosis (IPAA).[65] *Pouchitis* is a complication of restorative proctocolectomy with ileal pouch–anal anastomosis performed as surgical treatment for both UC and CD. Antibiotic treatment is usually successful.[66]

Crohn's Disease

Crohn's disease (CD) (granulomatous colitis, ileocolitis, or regional enteritis) is an idiopathic inflammatory disorder that affects any part of the GI tract from the mouth to the anus. In a small percentage of cases, CD is difficult to differentiate from UC (see Table 36-6). The distal small intestine and proximal large colon are most commonly involved.[53]

PATHOPHYSIOLOGY Inflammation begins in the intestinal submucosa and spreads with discontinuous transmural involvement ("skip lesions"). The ascending colon and the transverse colon are the most common sites of the disease, but both the large and small intestines may be involved, particularly the ileum. One side of the intestinal wall may be affected and not the other. The ulcerations of CD can produce fissures that extend inflammation into lymphoid tissue. The typical lesion is a granuloma (granulomas are described in Chapter 6) with a cobblestone appearance from projections of inflamed tissue surrounded by ulceration. Fistulae may form in the perianal area between loops of intestine or extend into the bladder, rectum, or vagina. Strictures may develop, promoting obstruction. Smoking increases the risk of developing severe disease, and may cause a poorer response to treatment.[67]

CLINICAL MANIFESTATIONS Individuals with CD may have no specific symptoms for several years. Symptoms vary according to the location of the disease but are similar to those for UC. Diarrhea is one of the most common symptoms and, occasionally, rectal bleeding if the colon is involved. Weight loss and abdominal pain accompany CD. If the ileum is involved, the individual may be anemic as a result of malabsorption of vitamin B_{12}. There also may be deficiencies in folic acid and vitamin D absorption. In addition, proteins may be lost, leading to hypoalbuminemia. Extraintestinal complications are similar to those occurring in UC.

EVALUATION AND TREATMENT The diagnosis and treatment of CD are similar to the diagnosis and treatment of UC; however, imaging of the small intestine is used in the diagnosis of CD, including either a small bowel series or a capsule endoscopy (camera pill). There are no specific biomarkers or definitive treatments. Smoking cessation is a component of therapy. Immunomodulators (i.e., anti-TNF) are effective for initial therapy or for resistance to other medications.[68] Surgery may be performed to manage complications such as fistula, abscess, or obstruction. Routine colonoscopy for cancer screening should be performed for longstanding colonic disease.

Microscopic Colitis

Microscopic colitis is a relatively common cause of diarrhea primarily in females and older adults. Although the mucosa appears normal, there are two histological forms: lymphocytic and collagenous. Lymphocytic colitis shows an increase in the number of intraepithelial lymphocytes. Collagenous colitis is characterized by a thickened subepithelial collagen layer, alteration of the vascular mucosal pattern, and mucosal nodularity. The cause is unknown. Risk factors include age (50 years or older), female gender, weight loss, absence of abdominal pain, and use of proton pump inhibitors or NSAIDs.[69]

The symptoms of frequent, chronic daily watery diarrhea are the same for both types and can be accompanied by abdominal pain and weight loss. Antidiarrheal agents and budesonide (an anti-inflammatory steroid) are the best documented treatments. The disease is negatively associated with colorectal cancer.[70]

Irritable Bowel Syndrome

Irritable bowel syndrome (IBS) currently is a symptom-based disease characterized by recurrent abdominal pain with altered bowel habits. There is increasing evidence of organic causes of disease. In North America the prevalence is about 12% and is probably underestimated.[71] It is more common in women (1.5 to 3 times greater than in men) with a higher prevalence during youth and middle age. Individuals with symptoms of IBS also are more likely to have anxiety, depression, and reduced quality of life.[72]

The pathophysiology of IBS is unknown and there are no specific biomarkers for the disease. There is increasing evidence to explain the varying symptom presentations, particularly in relation to altered gut microflora, gut immune responses, gut neuroendocrine cell function, the brain–gut axis, genetic susceptibility, and epigenetic factors.[73,74] The presentations are summarized as follows:

- *Visceral hypersensitivity or hyperalgesia*, particularly with distension of the rectum but also other areas of the gut, may originate in either the peripheral or the central nervous system. The mechanism may be related to dysregulation of the bidirectional "brain–gut axis" (alterations in gut or central nervous system processing of gut nociceptive information).[75] Factors include genetic-related changes in the function of serotonin-secreting cells of gut–brain pain modulation, alterations in gut microbiota metabolite production with activation of the gut immune system, increased visceral sensitivity and permeability, and altered motility.[76]
- *Abnormal GI permeability, motility, and secretion* are associated with IBS. Individuals with diarrhea-type IBS have more rapid colonic transit times and increased intestinal permeability. Those with bloating and constipation have delayed transit times and decreased intestinal permeability. The mechanism may be related to dysregulation of the brain–gut axis, alterations in the function of gut neuroendocrine cells or dorsal root ganglion neurons, or changes in the activity of mast cells.[77]
- *Postinflammatory (infectious or noninfectious) IBS* is diagnosed if two or more of the following occur: fever, vomiting, diarrhea, and a positive stool culture. Intestinal infection (bacterial enteritis) and low-grade inflammation have been associated with symptoms of IBS and appear to be related to alteration of gut microbiota, immune activation in gut tissues, and changes in intestinal permeability.[78,79]
- *Alteration in gut microbiota (dysbiosis)* influences the sensory, motor, and immune systems of the gut and interacts with higher brain centres and may contribute to symptoms of IBS.[80] Small intestine overgrowth of normal gut bacteria may be associated with IBS symptoms in some cases.[81] Nonabsorbable antibiotics and prebiotics and probiotics may be helpful in some individuals.
- *Food allergy or food intolerance* is associated with IBS in some cases. Food antigens may activate the mucosal immune system, alter intestinal flora, or mediate hypersensitivity reactions and IBS symptoms. Food elimination approaches are helpful in some cases.[82]
- *Psychosocial factors (epigenetic factors)*—including early life trauma or abuse or emotional stress interacting with neuroendocrine, neuroimmune, autonomic nervous system, and pain modulatory responses—contribute to the symptoms of IBS.[74,83]

CLINICAL MANIFESTATIONS IBS is characterized by lower abdominal pain or discomfort and bloating. Women report more abdominal pain and constipation, and men report more diarrhea.[84] IBS can be grouped as diarrhea-predominant, constipation-predominant, or alternating diarrhea and constipation. Symptoms including gas, bloating, and nausea are usually relieved with defecation and do not interfere with sleep.

EVALUATION AND TREATMENT The diagnosis of IBS is based on signs, symptoms, and personal history and includes the exclusion of structural or biochemical causes of disease. Diagnostic procedures to rule out other causes of symptoms may include endoscopic evaluations, computed tomography (CT) scans or abdominal ultrasound, blood tests, and tests for lactose intolerance, celiac disease (see Chapter 37), or other disorders. The person may be evaluated for food allergies, parasites, or bacterial growth. The Rome III criteria for diagnosing IBS guide evaluation (Box 36-1).

There is no cure for IBS and treatment is individualized. Treatment of symptoms may include laxatives and fibre, antidiarrheals, antispasmodics, prosecretory medications, low-dose antidepressants, visceral analgesics, and serotonin agonists or antagonists. Alternative therapies include prebiotics and probiotics to manipulate the microflora, hypnosis, acupuncture, yoga, cognitive-behavioural therapy, and dietary interventions. Research continues to advance the management and understanding of the pathophysiology of this complex syndrome.[85,86]

Diverticular Disease of the Colon

Diverticula are herniations or saclike outpouchings of the mucosa and submucosa through the muscle layers, usually in the wall of the sigmoid colon (Figure 36-9). They rarely occur in the small intestine.[87] Diverticulosis is asymptomatic diverticular disease. Diverticulitis represents inflammation. The cause of diverticular disease is unknown. It is associated with increased intracolonic pressure, abnormal neuromuscular function, and alterations in intestinal motility. Approximately 300 000 hospital admissions per year are related to diverticular disease.[88]

BOX 36-1 Rome III—Diagnostic Criteria for Irritable Bowel Syndrome

Recurrent abdominal pain or discomfort* at least 3 days/month in the last 3 months associated with two or more of the following:

- Improvement with defecation
- Onset associated with a change in frequency of stool
- Onset associated with a change in form (appearance) of stool[†]
- Onset of symptoms more than 6 months before diagnosis

*"Discomfort" means an uncomfortable sensation not described as pain.
[†]Diagnostic criterion.
From Rome Foundation. (n.d.). *Rome III diagnostic criteria for functional gastrointestinal disorders.* Retrieved from http://www.romecriteria.org/assets/pdf/19_RomeIII_apA_885-898.pdf.

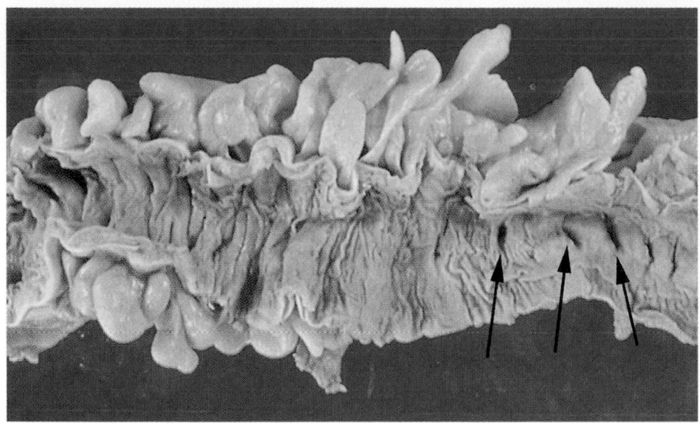

FIGURE 36-9 Diverticular Disease. In diverticular disease, the outpouches (*arrows*) of mucosa seen in the sigmoid colon appear as slitlike openings from the mucosal surface of the opened bowel. (From Stevens, A., Lowe, J., & Scott, I. [2009]. *Core pathology* [3rd ed.]. London: Mosby.)

Predisposing factors include older age, genetic predisposition, obesity, smoking, diet, lack of physical activity, and medication use, such as Aspirin and NSAIDs.[89] Lack of dietary fibre may or may not contribute to diverticular disease.[90]

PATHOPHYSIOLOGY Diverticula can occur anywhere in the GI tract, particularly at weak points in the colon wall, usually where arteries penetrate the tunica muscularis. The most common sites are the left sigmoid colon (prevalent in Western countries) and the right colon (prevalent in Asian countries). A common associated finding is thickening of the circular muscles and shortening of the longitudinal (teniae coli) muscles surrounding the diverticula. Increased collagen and elastin deposition, not muscle hypertrophy, is associated with muscle thickening, which contributes to increased intraluminal pressure and herniation. According to Laplace's law (see Chapter 23), wall pressure increases as the diameter of a cylindrical structure decreases. Therefore, pressure within the narrow lumen can increase enough to rupture the diverticula, causing inflammation and diverticulitis. Bacteria and local ischemia also may be contributing factors. Complicated diverticulitis includes abscess, fistula, obstruction, bleeding, or perforation.

CLINICAL MANIFESTATIONS Symptoms of uncomplicated diverticular disease may be vague or absent. Cramping pain of the lower abdomen can accompany constriction of the thickened colonic muscles. Diarrhea, constipation, distension, or flatulence may occur. If the diverticula become inflamed or abscesses form, the individual develops fever, leukocytosis (increased white blood cell count), and tenderness of the lower-left quadrant.

EVALUATION AND TREATMENT Diverticula are often discovered during diagnostic procedures performed for other problems. Ultrasound, sigmoidoscopy, or colonoscopy permits direct observation of the lesions. Abdominal CT is used for diagnosis of complicated cases.

An increase of dietary fibre intake often relieves symptoms, and probiotics and mesalazine (Pentasa) are being evaluated. Uncomplicated diverticulitis is usually treated with bowel rest and analgesia. Antibiotics are not required.[91] Laparoscopic resection and other minimally invasive approaches are implemented for more severe complications.[92]

Appendicitis

Appendicitis is an inflammation of the vermiform appendix, which is a projection from the apex of the cecum. It is the most common surgical emergency of the abdomen, usually occurs between 10 and 19 years of age (although it may develop at any age), and has an incidence in the United States of 7 to 10 per 10 000 persons.[93]

PATHOPHYSIOLOGY The exact mechanism of the cause of appendicitis is controversial. Obstruction of the lumen with stool, tumours, or foreign bodies with consequent bacterial infection is the most common theory. The obstructed lumen does not allow drainage of the appendix, and as mucosal secretion continues, intraluminal pressure increases. The increased pressure decreases mucosal blood flow, and the appendix becomes hypoxic. The mucosa ulcerates, promoting bacterial or other microbial invasion with further inflammation and edema. Inflammation may involve the distal or entire appendix. Gangrene develops from thrombosis of the luminal blood vessels, followed by perforation.[94]

CLINICAL MANIFESTATIONS Gastric or periumbilical pain is the typical symptom of an inflamed appendix. The pain may be vague at first and in the periumbilical area, increasing in intensity over 3 to 4 hours. It may subside and then migrate to the right lower quadrant, indicating extension of the inflammation to the surrounding tissues. Nausea, vomiting, and anorexia follow the onset of pain, and a low-grade fever is common. Diarrhea occurs in some individuals, particularly children; others have a sensation of constipation. Perforation, peritonitis, and abscess formation are the most serious complications of appendicitis.

EVALUATION AND TREATMENT In addition to clinical manifestations, there is pain with abdominal palpation and rebound tenderness, usually referred to the lower-right quadrant. The white blood cell count is greater than 10 000 cells/mm^3 with increased neutrophils and C-reactive protein. Abdominal ultrasound, CT scans, and magnetic resonance imaging (MRI) (particularly for pregnant women and children) assist with diagnostic accuracy and help rule out nonappendiceal disease.[95] Antibiotics and appendectomy are the treatment for simple or perforated appendicitis. There is controversy regarding antibiotics first, then surgery.[96] Laparoscopic surgery provides quick recovery for simple appendicitis. Recovery is more complicated in cases of perforation, abscess formation, peritonitis, or older age.

Mesenteric Vascular Insufficiency

Mesenteric vascular insufficiency is rare, with an incidence of about 2 to 3 cases per 100 000 persons.[97] Three branches of the abdominal aorta supply the stomach and intestines: the celiac artery and the superior and inferior mesenteric arteries (see Figure 35-6). The inferior mesenteric vein drains into the splenic vein, and the splenic vein and superior mesenteric vein join the portal vein. *Mesenteric venous thrombosis* is the least common of the causes of mesenteric vascular insufficiency. Malignancies, right ventricular failure, and deep vein thrombosis are risk factors. Mesenteric venous thrombosis presents with abdominal pain and is treated with anticoagulants.[98]

Acute mesenteric arterial insufficiency results in a significant reduction in mucosal blood flow to the large and small intestines and can be acute or chronic.[99] Pre-existing morbidities include dissecting aortic aneurysms, arterial thrombi, or emboli. Embolic obstruction is associated with atrial fibrillation, mitral valve disease, heart valve prostheses, and myocardial infarction. The superior mesenteric artery has a more direct line of flow from the aorta; therefore, emboli enter it more readily than the inferior branch, causing ischemia and necrosis of the small intestine. Ischemia and necrosis (intestinal infarction) alter membrane permeability. Initially, there is increased motility, nausea and vomiting, urgent bowel evacuation, and severe abdominal pain. Ischemia leads to decreased motility and distension. The damaged intestinal mucosa cannot produce enough mucus to protect itself from digestive enzymes. Mucosal alteration causes fluid to move from the blood vessels into the bowel wall and peritoneum. Fluid loss causes hypovolemia, and further decreases intestinal blood flow. As intestinal infarction progresses, shock, fever, bloody diarrhea, and leukocytosis develop. Bacteria invade the necrotic intestinal wall, causing gangrene and peritonitis.

Chronic mesenteric ischemia is rare but can develop with atherosclerotic stenosis or occlusion[100] or secondary to heart failure, acute myocardial infarction, hemorrhage, thrombus formation, or any condition that decreases arterial blood flow. Chronic occlusion is often accompanied by formation of collateral circulation. The collateral vessels may be able to nourish the resting intestine, but after eating, when the intestine requires more blood, the arterial supply may be insufficient. Ischemia develops, causing cramping abdominal pain (abdominal angina), a cardinal symptom. Some individuals suffer significant weight loss because they stop eating to control the pain. Progressive vascular obstruction eventually causes continuous abdominal pain and necrosis of the intestinal tissue.

Diagnosis of acute and chronic mesenteric ischemia is based on clinical manifestations, laboratory findings, and imaging studies. A bruit can often be heard over a partially occluded artery. Treatment includes aggressive rehydration and the use of antibiotics, anticoagulants, vasodilators, and inhibitors of reperfusion injury. Surgery, including endovascular techniques, is required to remove necrotic tissue, repair sclerosed vessels, and revascularize affected tissue. Acute occlusion is a surgical emergency and mortality is high (50 to 90%). Early diagnosis and aggressive treatment result in the best survival rates.[101]

Disorders of Nutrition

Obesity

Obesity is an increase in body fat mass and a metabolic disorder that has become an epidemic worldwide, with no sex differences. According to the obesity report published in 2011 by the Public Health Agency of Canada (PHAC) and the Canadian Institute for Health Information (CIHI), 1 in 4 Canadian adults are obese, and 8.6% of children and youth aged 6 to 17 are obese (see *Health Promotion:* Promotion of Physical Activity in Canadian Schools). The incidence is rapidly increasing among children and adolescents, and they tend to become obese adults.[102] Obesity is associated with higher all-cause mortality.[103]

Obesity is defined as a body mass index (BMI = kg/m^2) that exceeds 30 and generally develops when caloric intake exceeds caloric expenditure.[104] Obesity is a major risk factor for morbidity, death, and high health care costs.[105] Three leading causes of death associated with obesity are coronary artery disease, type 2 diabetes mellitus, and cancer (colorectal, breast in postmenopausal women, endometrial, prostate, renal, and esophageal). Obesity also is a risk factor for hypertension, stroke, dyslipidemia, gallstones, nonalcoholic steatohepatitis (NASH), gastroesophageal reflux, osteoarthritis, infectious disease, and sleep apnea.[106]

The causes and consequences of obesity are multiple and complex. Rapidly advancing research regarding risk factors, causal mechanisms, complications, and treatment is in progress. Obesity is known to occur in families and genotypes, and gene–environment interactions are important predisposing factors.[107] Environmental factors include culture, socioeconomic status, food intake habits, and level of physical activity. Metabolic abnormalities associated with obesity include Cushing's syndrome, Cushing's disease, polycystic ovarian syndrome, hypothyroidism, and hypothalamic injury.

PATHOPHYSIOLOGY The pathophysiology of obesity involves the interaction of peripheral and central pathways and numerous cytokines, hormones, and neurotransmitters. In the periphery, white adipocytes (fat cells) store triglycerides and increase in size and number. Adipocytes also secrete hormones and cytokines, known as *adipocytokines*.[108] These adipocytokines and other hormones (Box 36-2) participate in regulation of food intake, lipid storage, insulin sensitivity, vascular homeostasis, blood pressure regulation, angiogenesis, coagulation, bone metabolism,

HEALTH PROMOTION

Promotion of Physical Activity in Canadian Schools

Many Canadian children and youth have a risk of developing cardiovascular disease, obesity, and diabetes because they do not get enough physical activity. Moreover, several studies have concluded that children who do not get enough physical activity are more likely to struggle with cognitive and academic challenges. The Canadian Physical Activity Guidelines recommend that children between the ages of 5 and 17 years get at least 60 minutes of moderate-to-vigorous physical activity daily.

School occupies the major portion of a student's day. As such, schools can provide ample opportunities for students to improve both health and academic outcomes by promoting physical activity, healthy behaviours, and healthy eating as part of a Comprehensive School Health (CSH) approach. CSH is an internationally recognized approach that was created to improve students' educational outcomes without neglecting students' health. The CSH framework is designed in an integrated and holistic way, taking into consideration four categories: (1) teaching and learning; (2) social and physical environments; (3) healthy school policy; and (4) partnerships and services. Schools can apply several interventions to help children improve their levels of physical activity within these categories. Factors such as geography and socioeconomic status should also be considered to address the needs of individual school communities.

The Heart and Stroke Foundation of Canada also recommends that children and youth accumulate at least 60 minutes of daily physical activity through a variety of activities and programs (both structured and unstructured). It recommends that schools integrate knowledge into physical activities to develop positive attitudes toward physical activity; for example, it suggests incorporating physical activity into lesson plans for subjects other than physical education (e.g., math, science, languages etc.). As well, it recommends that schools encourage students to engage in physical activity and active play during recess and lunch breaks, and provide students with incentives such as free healthy drinks and fruits. By promoting active transportation (e.g., walking and cycling), schools can also increase students' level of physical activity.

Schools should be located in areas that are accessible to large numbers of students. Municipalities must take into consideration ways to help students use active transportation by developing active and safe routes to school and by providing amenities like bike racks and crossing guards. The benefits of these measures extend beyond children and youth to families and the community as a whole.

School facilities should be available during nonschool hours to provide additional programs (e.g., child care, cooking classes) for the whole community, giving parents the opportunity to engage in supporting the healthy development of their children.

Given that health, well-being, and learning are intimately connected, schools have the ability to make a dramatic difference in the lives of Canadian children and youth. However, to accomplish this goal, schools need funding and policies for the delivery of programs that foster physical activity.

Data from Heart and Stroke Foundation of Canada. (n.d.). *Fact sheet: Schools and heart healthy children and youth.* Retrieved from http://www.heartandstroke.ns.ca; Heart and Stroke Foundation of Canada. (2013). *Position statement: Schools and physical activity.* Retrieved from http://www.heartandstroke.ca/-/media/pdf-files/canada/2017-position-statements/schoolsand-physical-activity-ps-eng.ashx?la=en;

BOX 36-2 Examples of Adipocytokines and Other Hormones Related to Complications of Obesity

Cytokines From Adipose Cells

Adipocytokines

Leptin: Suppresses appetite at hypothalamus; promotes insulin sensitivity

Adiponectin: Insulin sensitizing for regulation of blood glucose level; promotes anti-inflammatory and antihypertensive vascular effects; reduces atherosclerosis and oncogenesis; increases metabolic rate

Resistin: Promotes insulin resistance and increases blood glucose levels

Visfatin: Mimics insulin and binds to insulin receptors

Proinflammatory Cytokines

Tumour necrosis factor-alpha: A proinflammatory hormone; suppresses appetite; induces insulin resistance

Interleukin-6, -8, and -10: Proinflammatory mediators; suppress appetite; induce insulin resistance

Monocyte chemotactic protein-1: Involved in macrophage recruitment

Plasminogen activator inhibitor-1: Promotes clot formation by inhibiting plasminogen and urokinase (also released by endothelial cells)

Retinol binding protein 4: Promotes insulin resistance

Other Hormones

Insulin: Secreted from pancreatic beta cells; suppresses appetite at hypothalamus; promotes glucose utilization in muscle and fat

Amylin: Secreted from pancreatic beta cells; suppresses appetite and postprandial glucagon secretion

Ghrelin: Secreted from stomach; stimulates appetite and controls gastric motility and acid secretion

Peptide YY: Secreted from intestine; reduces appetite and inhibits gastric motility

Incretin: Stimulates insulin release; inhibits glucagon release; slows gastric emptying to reduce postprandial hyperglycemia

Glucagonlike peptide 1: Gastric inhibitory peptide (glucose-dependent insulinotropic peptide)

inflammatory and immune responses, female reproduction, and regulation of energy metabolism. Visceral white fat accumulation causes dysfunction in the regulation and interaction of these cytokines and hormones and contributes to the complications and consequences of obesity.

Neuroendocrine regulation of appetite, eating behaviour, energy metabolism, and body fat mass are controlled by a dynamic circuit of signalling mediators from the periphery acting centrally on the hypothalamus and brainstem to regulate hunger and satiety.[109] Peripheral sources of mediators include insulin from the beta cells of the pancreas; ghrelin from the stomach; peptide YY from the intestines; glucagonlike peptide-1 from intestinal endocrine cells; and the adipokines leptin, adiponectin, and resistin. Obesity is associated with increased circulating plasma levels of leptin, insulin, resistin, and ghrelin. There are decreased levels of adiponectin and peptide YY (see Box 36-2).

Within the hypothalamus are the orexigenic neurons (increase food intake and decrease metabolism) and the anorexigenic neurons (decrease food intake and increase metabolism). They interact with peripheral mediators to control food intake and energy expenditure. The hypothalamus also communicates with higher brain centres related to reward, pleasure, and addictive behaviour. These centres can override hypothalamic control of food intake and satiety, increasing consumption of highly palatable foods and resulting in increased fat stores.[110,111] Interaction of altered levels of hormones and adipocytokines with hypothalamic neurons is an important determinant of excessive fat mass and the complications of obesity.

Leptin, a product of the obesity gene (*Ob* gene), acts on the hypothalamus to suppress appetite and functions to regulate body weight within a fairly narrow range. Leptin levels increase as the number of adipocytes increases; however, for unknown reasons, high leptin levels are ineffective at decreasing appetite and energy expenditure, a condition known as **leptin resistance**.[112] Leptin resistance fails to inhibit orexigenic hypothalamic satiety signalling and promotes overeating and excessive weight gain. Leptin resistance is also associated with insulin resistance (hyperinsulinemia or glucose intolerance) and the cardiovascular complications of obesity. Simultaneously there is an increase in **ghrelin**, which stimulates orexigenic neurons and increases appetite. Decreased levels of **adiponectin** and **peptide YY** decrease stimulation of anorexigenic neurons. Adiponectin also is insulin sensitizing, promotes glucose uptake, and has anti-inflammatory actions. A decrease in adiponectin is associated with insulin resistance, coronary artery disease, and hypertension, contributing to the complications of obesity.

Enlarged adipocytes increase lipolysis (with release of fatty acids) and secrete proinflammatory adipokines from T cells and activated macrophages. The result is a low-grade systemic inflammation. The inflammatory state and accelerated lipolysis contribute to the development of insulin resistance and metabolic syndrome (hypertriglyceridemia, reduced high-density lipoproteins, increased low-density lipoproteins, hypertension, and insulin resistance).[113,114] Figure 36-10 summarizes the pathophysiology and major consequences of obesity.

CLINICAL MANIFESTATIONS Obesity usually presents with two different forms of adipose tissue distribution, visceral and peripheral.[115] Visceral obesity (also known as *intra-abdominal, central,* or *masculine obesity*) occurs when the distribution of body fat is localized around the abdomen and upper body, resulting in an apple shape.[116] Visceral obesity has an increased risk for systemic inflammation, metabolic syndrome, obstructive sleep apnea syndrome, cardiovascular complications, nonalcoholic steatohepatitis cancer, osteoarthritis, and type 2 diabetes mellitus.[117,118] (Diabetes mellitus is discussed in Chapter 19.)

Peripheral obesity (also known as *gluteal-femoral, feminine,* or *subcutaneous obesity*) occurs when the distribution of body fat is extraperitoneal and distributed around the thighs and buttocks and through the muscle, resulting in a pear shape, and is more common in women. Peripheral and subcutaneous fat is less metabolically active, is less lipolytic, and releases fewer adipocytokines (particularly adiponectin) than visceral fat. Risk factors are still present for the complications of obesity but they are less severe than those for visceral obesity.

Normal weight obesity (NWO) describes individuals with normal body weight and BMI with percentage of body fat greater than 30%. These individuals are at risk for metabolic dysregulation, increases in inflammatory cytokines, insulin resistance, increased risk for cardiovascular disease, and higher mortality.[119] NWO is estimated to occur in 2 to 28% of women and 3% of men.[120]

Metabolically healthy obesity (MHO) describes about 10 to 30% of individuals who are obese but have no metabolic-obesity–associated complications and decreased risk for morbidity and mortality. MHO is more prevalent among women and declines with age with adverse long-term outcomes.[121] Research is in progress to better understand the genetics, body fat distribution patterns, metabolic pathways, lifestyle practices, and therapeutic options for these individuals.

EVALUATION AND TREATMENT There are several methods for measuring or estimating body fat mass, including CT and MRI techniques; bioimpedance analysis; underwater weighing; and anthropometric measurements, such as skinfold thickness, circumferences, and various

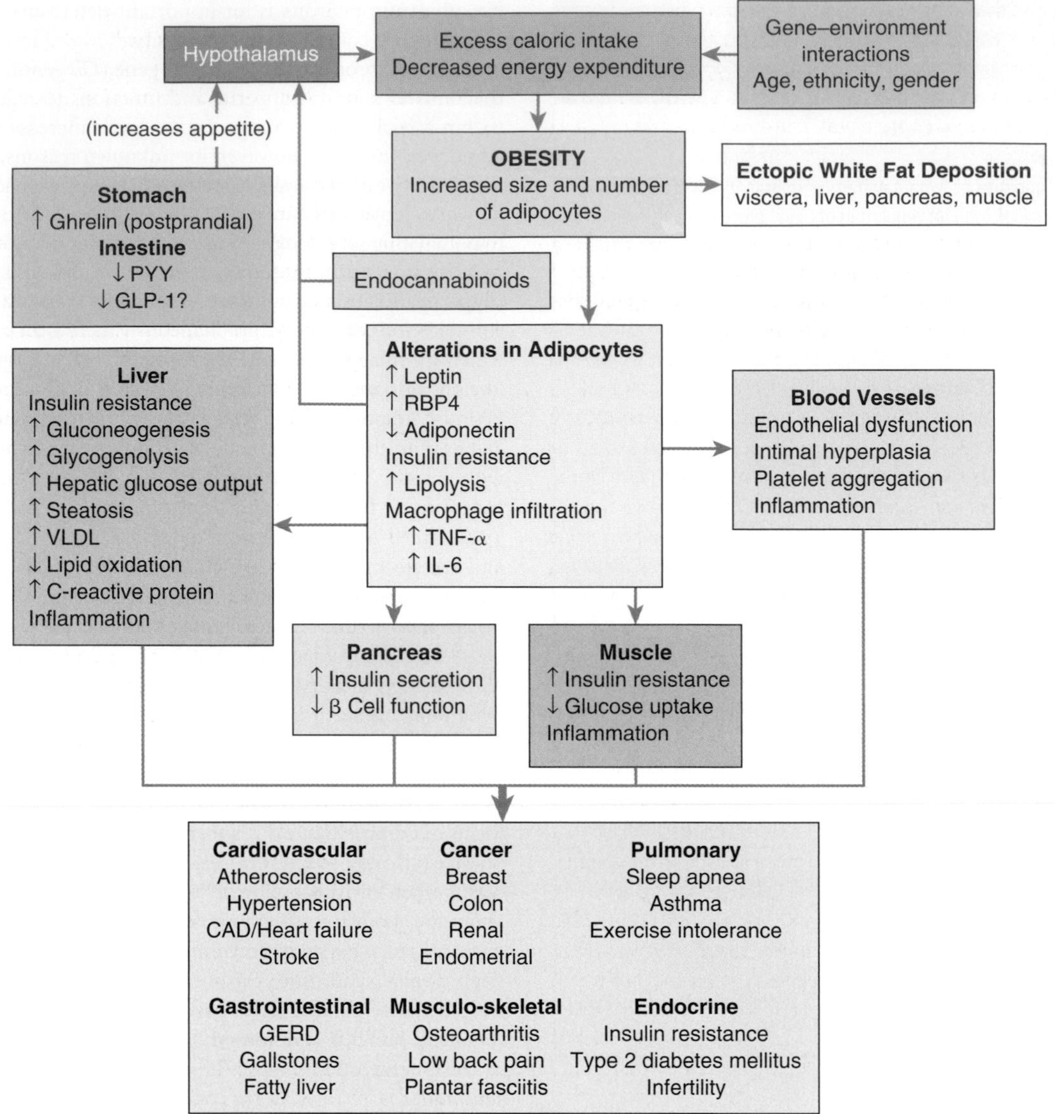

FIGURE 36-10 Pathophysiology and Common Complications of Obesity. See text for details. *CAD*, Coronary artery disease; *GERD*, gastroesophageal reflux disease; *GLP-1*, glucagonlike peptide-1; *IL-6*, interleukin-6; *PYY*, intestinal peptide YY; *RBP4*, retinol-binding protein 4; *TNF-α*, tumour necrosis factor-alpha; *VLDL*, very-low-density lipoprotein.

body diameters (i.e., waist-to-hip ratios and waist circumference; BMI tables).[122] The BMI and waist-to-hip ratios are most commonly used because they are the easiest to measure and are most cost effective. *Overweight* is defined as a BMI greater than 25 kg/m^2, and *obesity* is defined as a BMI greater than 30 kg/m^2. BMI charts are available for children ages 2 to 20 years; they can be used for comparison during adulthood because obese children generally become obese adults.[123] No specific diagnostic criteria for obesity have been established. The complications of obesity affect nearly every body system (see Figure 36-10).

Obesity is a chronic disease for which various approaches to treatment have been used; these include correction of metabolic abnormalities, individually tailored weight reduction diets and exercise programs, psychotherapy, behavioural modification, and antiobesity medications.[124,125] Weight loss (bariatric) surgery is the most effective treatment for decreasing obesity-related morbidity.[126,127] Unravelling the causes of obesity will lead to more specific prevention and pharmacotherapeutic strategies.

Malnutrition and Starvation

Malnutrition is lack of nourishment from inadequate amounts of calories, protein, vitamins, or minerals and is caused by improper diet, alterations in digestion or absorption, chronic disease, or a combination of these factors. **Starvation** is a reduction in energy intake leading to weight loss. Short-term starvation and long-term starvation have different effects. Therapeutic short-term starvation is part of many weight-reduction programs because it causes an initial rapid weight loss that reinforces the individual's motivation to diet. Therapeutic long-term starvation is used in medically controlled environments to facilitate rapid weight loss in morbidly obese individuals. Pathological long-term starvation can be caused by poverty (particularly in developing countries); chronic diseases of the cardiovascular, pulmonary, hepatic, renal, and digestive systems; malabsorption syndromes; and cancer.

Short-term starvation, or extended fasting, consists of several days of total dietary abstinence or deprivation. Once all available energy has been absorbed from the intestine, glycogen in the liver is converted to glucose through **glycogenolysis**, the metabolism of glycogen into glucose.

This process peaks within 4 to 8 hours, and gluconeogenesis begins. Gluconeogenesis is the formation of glucose from noncarbohydrate molecules: lactate, pyruvate, amino acids, and the glycerol portion of fats. Like glycogenolysis, gluconeogenesis takes place within the liver. Both of these processes deplete stored nutrients and thus cannot meet the body's energy needs indefinitely. Proteins continue to be catabolized to a minimal degree, providing carbon for the synthesis of glucose needed by brain and blood cells.

Long-term starvation begins after several days of dietary abstinence and eventually causes death. The major characteristics of long-term starvation are decreased energy expenditure, a decreased dependence on gluconeogenesis, and an increased use of ketone bodies (products of lipid and pyruvate metabolism) as a cellular energy source. Depressed insulin and glucagon levels promote lipolysis in adipose tissue. Lipolysis liberates fatty acids, which supply energy to cardiac and skeletal muscle cells, as well as ketone bodies, which sustain brain tissue. Fatty acid or ketone body oxidation meets most energy needs of the cells. (Some glucose is still needed as fuel for brain tissue.) Once the supply of adipose tissue is depleted, proteolysis begins. The breakdown of muscle protein is the last process to supply energy for life. Death results from severe alterations in electrolyte balance and loss of renal, pulmonary, and cardiac function.[128]

Adequate ingestion of appropriate nutrients is the obvious treatment for starvation. In medically induced starvation, the body is maintained in a ketotic state until the desired amount of adipose tissue has been lysed. Starvation imposed by chronic disease, long-term illness, or malabsorption is treated with enteral or parenteral nutrition. Care must be taken to prevent refeeding syndrome during the treatment of long-term starvation.[129] With refeeding, insulin release, hypophosphatemia, hypomagnesemia, and hypokalemia can cause life-threatening complications.

Cachexia (also known as *cytokine-induced malnutrition*) is physical wasting with loss of weight and muscle atrophy, fatigue, and weakness. Inflammatory cytokines induce skeletal muscle wasting and a blunted response to ghrelin. Adiponectin suppresses appetite. Cancer, acquired immune deficiency syndrome (AIDS), tuberculosis, and other major chronic progressive diseases contribute to cachexia (see Chapter 10).[130]

✔ QUICK CHECK 36-4

1. Why are Crohn's disease and ulcerative colitis called *inflammatory bowel diseases*?
2. How is leptin resistance associated with obesity?
3. When does proteolysis begin in long-term starvation?

DISORDERS OF THE ACCESSORY ORGANS OF DIGESTION

The accessory organs of digestion (liver, gallbladder, pancreas) secrete substances necessary for digestion and, in the case of the liver, carry out metabolic functions needed to maintain life. Disorders of these organs include inflammatory disease, obstruction of ducts, and tumours. (Cancer of the digestive system is described at the end of this chapter.)

Common Complications of Liver Disorders

Of all the accessory organ disorders, acute or chronic liver disease leads to the most significant systemic, life-threatening complications. These complications are common to all liver disorders and include portal hypertension, ascites, hepatic encephalopathy, jaundice, and hepatorenal syndrome.

Portal Hypertension

Portal hypertension is abnormally high blood pressure in the portal venous system caused by resistance to blood flow. Pressure in this system is normally 3 mm Hg; portal hypertension is an increase to at least 10 mm Hg.

PATHOPHYSIOLOGY Portal hypertension is caused by disorders that obstruct or impede blood flow through any component of the portal venous system or vena cava. *Intrahepatic causes* result from vascular remodelling with shunts, thrombosis, inflammation, or fibrosis of the sinusoids, as occurs in cirrhosis of the liver, biliary cirrhosis, viral hepatitis, or schistosomiasis (a parasitic infection). *Posthepatic causes* occur from hepatic vein thrombosis or cardiac disorders that impair the pumping ability of the right side of the heart. The impaired ability of the right side of the heart causes blood to collect and increases pressure in the veins of the portal system. The most common cause of portal hypertension is fibrosis and obstruction caused by cirrhosis of the liver. Long-term portal hypertension causes several pathophysiological problems that are difficult to treat and can be fatal. These problems include varices, splenomegaly, ascites, hepatic encephalopathy, and hepatopulmonary syndrome.[131]

Varices are distended, tortuous collateral veins. Prolonged elevation of pressure in the portal vein cause collateral veins to open between the portal vein and systemic veins and their transformation into varices, particularly in the lower esophagus and stomach, but also over the abdominal wall (known as the *caput medusae* [Medusa head]) and rectum (hemorrhoidal varices) (Figure 36-11). Rupture of varices can cause life-threatening hemorrhage.[132]

Splenomegaly is enlargement of the spleen caused by increased pressure in the splenic vein, which branches from the portal vein. Thrombocytopenia is the most common symptom of congestive splenomegaly. The enlarged spleen can be palpated. Hepatopulmonary syndrome (vasodilation, intrapulmonary shunting, and hypoxia) and portopulmonary hypertension (pulmonary vasoconstriction and vascular remodelling) are complications of liver disease and portal hypertension. The pathophysiology is complex and involves different effects of vasoactive substances. There may be no clinical manifestations, although dyspnea, cyanosis, and clubbing may occur.[133]

CLINICAL MANIFESTATIONS Vomiting of blood (hematemesis) from bleeding esophageal varices is the most common clinical manifestation of portal hypertension. Bleeding is usually from varices that have developed slowly over a period of years. Slow, chronic bleeding from varices causes anemia or melena. Rupture of esophageal varices causes hemorrhage and voluminous vomiting of dark-coloured blood. The ruptured varices are usually painless. Rupture is caused by a combination of erosion by gastric acid and elevated venous pressure. Mortality from ruptured esophageal varices ranges from 30 to 60%. Recurrent bleeding of esophageal varices indicates a poor prognosis. Hemorrhoidal varices present as hematochezia and copious rectal bleeding. Most individuals die within 1 year.

EVALUATION AND TREATMENT Portal hypertension is often diagnosed at the time of variceal bleeding and confirmed by upper GI endoscopy and evaluation of portal venous pressure. The individual usually has a history of jaundice, hepatitis, alcoholism, or cirrhosis. Pressure in the portal venous system can be reduced with nonselective beta-blocking medications to assist in preventing variceal bleeding.[134]

Emergency management of bleeding varices includes use of vasopressors and compression of the varices with an inflatable tube or balloon, sclerotherapy, variceal ligation, or portacaval shunt. Surgical construction of transjugular intrahepatic portosystemic shunts (TIPS procedure:

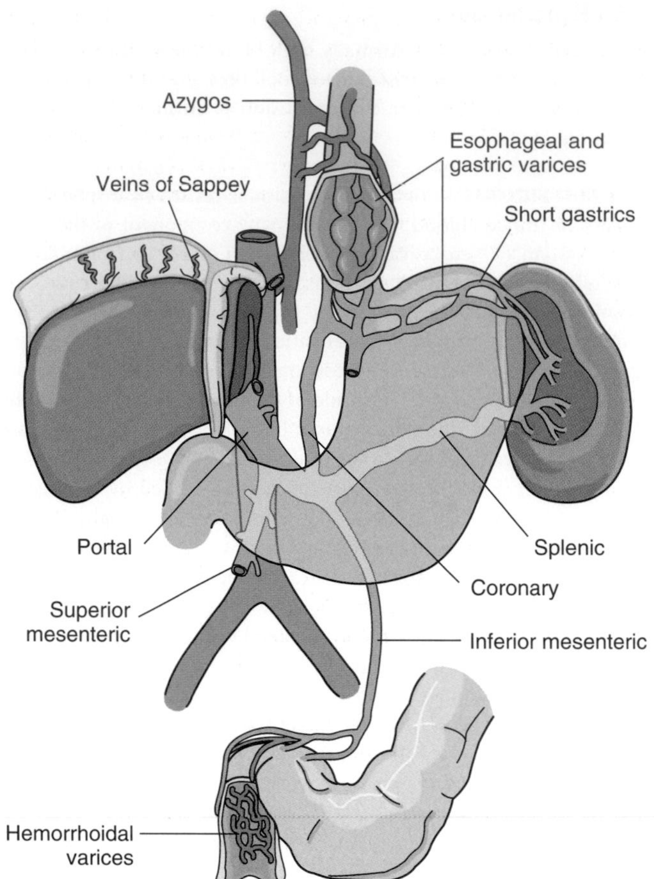

FIGURE 36-11 Varices Related to Portal Hypertension. Portal vein, its major tributaries, and the most important shunts (collateral veins) between the portal and caval systems. The shunted blood returns to the systemic venous system, bypassing the liver. (From Monahan, F.D., Sands, J.K., Neighbors, M., et al. [2007]. *Phipps' medical-surgical nursing: Concepts and clinical practice* [8th ed.]. St. Louis: Mosby.)

anastomosis of the portal vein to the inferior vena cava) may decompress the varices. This treatment can precipitate encephalopathy. Liver transplant is the most successful option for liver failure.[135]

Ascites

Ascites is the accumulation of fluid in the peritoneal cavity. Ascites traps body fluid in the peritoneal space, from which it cannot escape. The effect is to reduce the amount of fluid available for normal physiological functions. Cirrhosis is the most common cause of ascites, but other causes include heart failure, constrictive pericarditis, abdominal malignancies, nephrotic syndrome, and malnutrition.[136] Of individuals who develop ascites caused by cirrhosis, 25% die within 1 year. Continued heavy drinking of alcohol is associated with this mortality and is related to cirrhosis.

PATHOPHYSIOLOGY Several factors contribute to the development of ascites, including portal hypertension, decreased synthesis of albumin by the liver, splanchnic arterial vasodilation, and renal sodium and water retention. Portal hypertension and reduced serum albumin levels cause capillary hydrostatic pressure to exceed capillary osmotic pressure (see Chapter 5), pushing water into the peritoneal cavity. Portal hypertension also increases the production of hepatic lymph, which "weeps" into the peritoneal cavity. Splanchnic arterial vasodilation, associated with increased nitric oxide produced by the diseased liver, can decrease effective circulating blood volume, activating aldosterone and antidiuretic hormone, which promote renal sodium and water retention. The sodium and water retention expands plasma volume, thereby accelerating portal hypertension and ascites formation. Translocation of bacteria and release of endotoxin cause peritonitis with an inflammatory response that increases mesenteric capillary permeability and fluid movement into the peritoneal cavity, promoting ascites. Figure 36-12 summarizes the mechanisms by which cirrhosis of the liver cause ascites.

CLINICAL MANIFESTATIONS The accumulation of ascitic fluid causes abdominal distension, increased abdominal girth, and weight gain (Figure 36-13). Large volumes of fluid (10 to 20 L) displace the diaphragm and

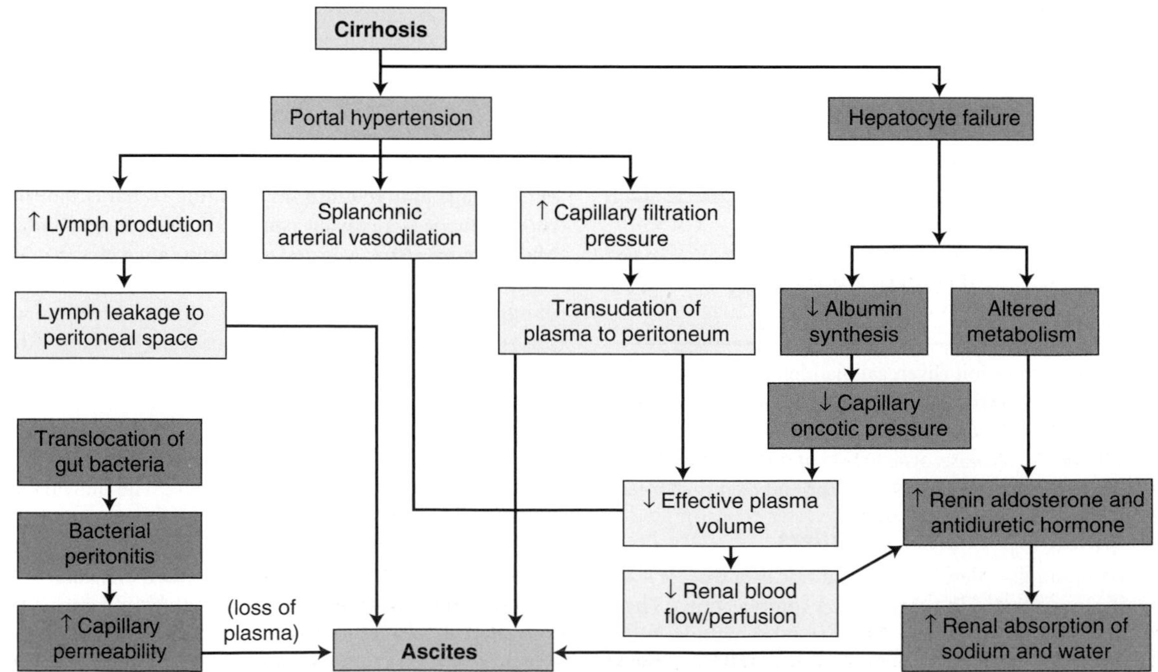

FIGURE 36-12 Mechanisms of Ascites Caused by Cirrhosis.

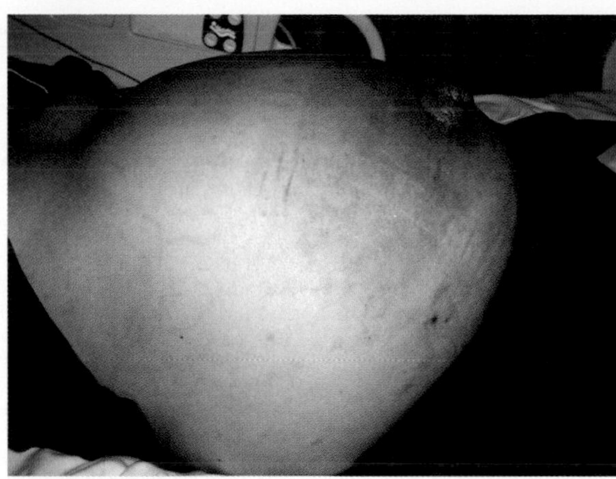

FIGURE 36-13 Massive Ascites in an Individual With Cirrhosis. Distended abdomen, dilated upper abdominal veins, and inverted umbilicus are classic manifestations. (From Goldman, L., & Schafer, A.I. [2012]. *Goldman's Cecil medicine* [24th ed.]. Philadelphia: Saunders.)

cause dyspnea by decreasing lung capacity. Respiratory rate increases, and the individual assumes a semi-Fowler position to relieve the dyspnea. Some peripheral edema is usually present. Approximately 10% of individuals with ascites develop bacterial peritonitis, which causes fever, chills, abdominal pain, decreased bowel sounds, and cloudy ascitic fluid.

EVALUATION AND TREATMENT Diagnosis is usually based on clinical manifestations and identification of liver disease. Dietary salt restriction and use of potassium-sparing diuretics can reduce ascites. Stronger diuretics, such as furosemide (Lasix) or ethacrynic acid (Edecrin), may be used, and vasopressin receptor 2 antagonists are effective for dilutional hyponatremia. Albumin may be given. Paracentesis is used to aspirate ascitic fluid for bacterial culture, biochemical analysis, and microscopic examination. The goal of treatment is to relieve discomfort. If the restoration of liver function is possible, the ascites diminishes spontaneously. Levels of serum electrolytes are monitored carefully because the individual is at risk for hyponatremia and hypokalemia.

Palliative measures include paracentesis to remove 1 or 2 L of ascitic fluid and relieve respiratory distress. However, the removal of too much fluid relieves pressure on blood vessels and carries the risk for hypotension, shock, or death. Despite repeated paracentesis, ascitic fluid reaccumulates because of the persistent portal hypertension and reduced plasma albumin levels associated with irreversible disease. Peritonitis is treated with antibiotics. Other procedures include peritoneovenous shunt (peritoneal fluid into veins) and TIPS (bypass of blood flow from the portal venous branch to the hepatic venous branch).[137] Individuals with ascites and portal hypertension have a poor prognosis, and liver transplant is the best treatment option.[137]

Hepatic Encephalopathy

Hepatic encephalopathy (portal-systemic encephalopathy) is a complex neurological syndrome characterized by impaired behavioural, cognitive, and motor function. The syndrome may develop rapidly during acute fulminant hepatitis or slowly during the course of cirrhosis and the development of portal hypertension or after portosystemic bypass or shunting.

PATHOPHYSIOLOGY Hepatic encephalopathy results from a combination of biochemical alterations that affect neurotransmission and brain function. Liver dysfunction and the development of collateral vessels that shunt blood around the liver to the systemic circulation permit toxins absorbed from the GI tract and normally removed by the liver to accumulate and circulate freely to the brain. The accumulated toxins alter cerebral energy metabolism, interfere with neurotransmission, and cause edema. The most hazardous substances are end products of intestinal protein digestion, particularly ammonia, which cannot be converted to urea by the diseased liver. Other substances include inflammatory cytokines, short-chain fatty acids, serotonin, tryptophan, and manganese. These substances cause astrocyte swelling and alter the blood–brain barrier, promoting cerebral edema. Infection, hemorrhage, electrolyte imbalance (including zinc deficiency), constipation, and use of sedatives and analgesics can precipitate hepatic encephalopathy in the presence of liver disease.[138]

CLINICAL MANIFESTATIONS Subtle changes in personality, memory loss, irritability, disinhibition, lethargy, and sleep disturbances are common initial manifestations of hepatic encephalopathy. Symptoms then can progress to confusion, disorientation to time and space, flapping tremor of the hands (asterixis), slow speech, bradykinesia, stupor, convulsions, and coma. Coma is usually a sign of liver failure and ultimately results in death. Variceal bleeding and ascites may develop concurrently. Symptoms may be episodic, recurrent, or persistent.[139] Hepatic encephalopathy is often associated with bleeding varices and ascites.

EVALUATION AND TREATMENT Diagnosis of hepatic encephalopathy is based on a history of liver disease, clinical manifestations, psychometric tests, and exclusion of other causes of brain dysfunction. Electroencephalography and blood chemistry tests provide supportive data. Tracking levels of serum ammonia assesses treatment effectiveness and liver function.

Correction of fluid and electrolyte imbalances and withdrawal of depressant medications metabolized by the liver are the first steps in the treatment of hepatic encephalopathy. Dietary protein is maintained to prevent malnutrition, but at levels that reduce blood ammonia levels.[140] Lactulose (Apo-Lactulose) prevents ammonia absorption in the colon. Neomycin (Neosporin) eliminates ammonia-producing intestinal bacteria but can be nephrotoxic. Glutamase inhibitors reduce gut ammonia. Rifaximin (Xifaxan) decreases intestinal production of ammonia and is used for lactulose nonresponders. Extracorporeal liver support systems remove toxins from the blood and are an option for managing overt hepatic encephalopathy.[141]

Jaundice

Jaundice, or icterus, is a yellow or greenish pigmentation of the skin caused by hyperbilirubinemia (plasma bilirubin concentrations greater than 42.5 to 51 mcmol/L. Hyperbilirubinemia and jaundice can result from (1) extrahepatic (posthepatic) obstruction to bile flow, (2) intrahepatic obstruction, or (3) prehepatic excessive production of unconjugated bilirubin (i.e., excessive hemolysis of red blood cells)[142] (Figure 36-14). Jaundice in newborns is caused by impaired bilirubin uptake and conjugation (see Chapter 37).

PATHOPHYSIOLOGY Obstructive jaundice can result from extrahepatic or intrahepatic obstruction.[143] *Extrahepatic obstructive jaundice* develops if the common bile duct is occluded (e.g., by a gallstone, tumour, or inflammation). Bilirubin conjugated by the hepatocytes cannot flow through the obstructed common bile duct into the duodenum. Therefore, it accumulates in the liver and enters the bloodstream, causing hyperbilirubinemia and jaundice. *Intrahepatic obstructive jaundice* involves disturbances in hepatocyte function and obstruction of bile canaliculi. The uptake, conjugation, or excretion of bilirubin can be affected, with elevated levels of both conjugated and unconjugated bilirubin.

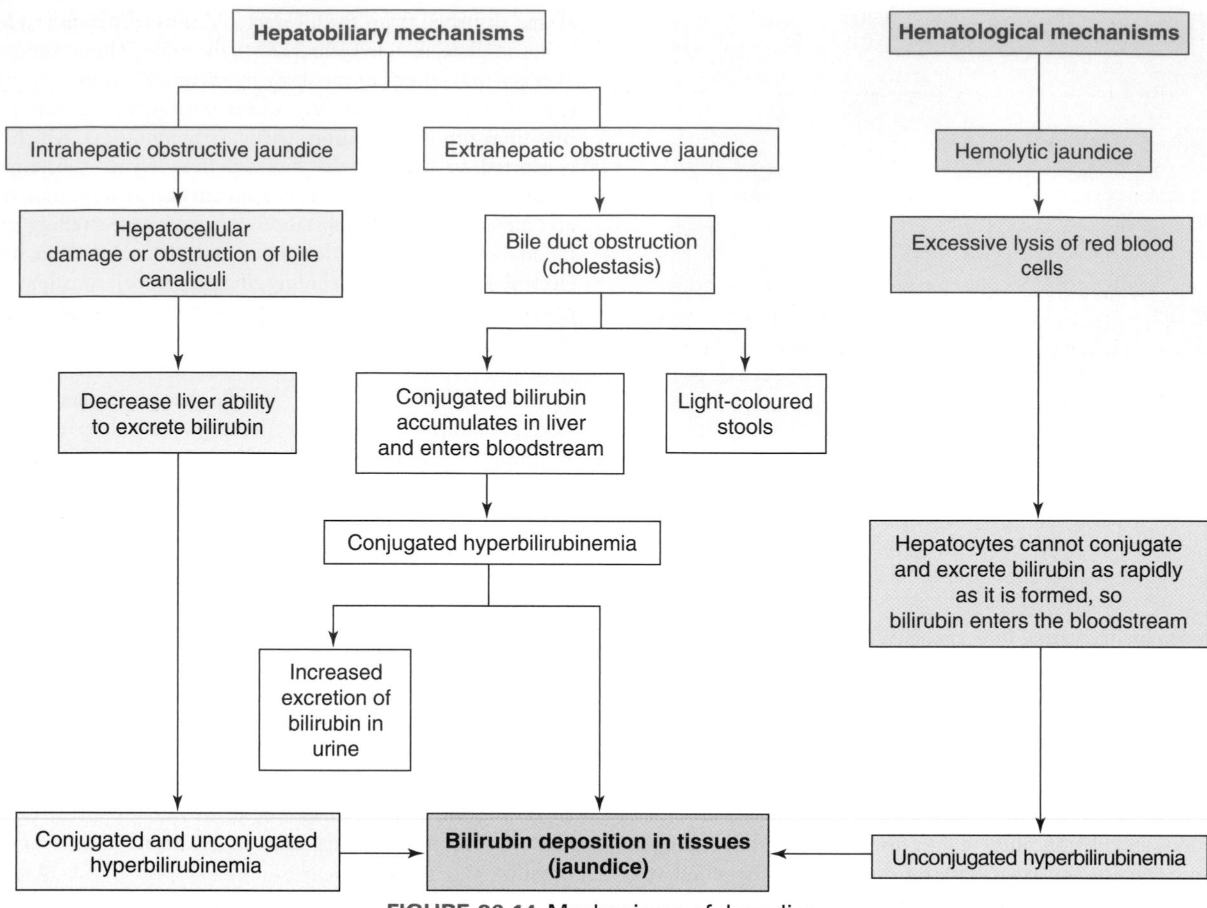

FIGURE 36-14 Mechanisms of Jaundice.

Obstruction of bile canaliculi diminishes flow of conjugated bilirubin into the common bile duct. In mild cases, some of the bile canaliculi open. Consequently, the amount of bilirubin in the intestinal tract may be only slightly decreased.

Excessive hemolysis (destruction) of red blood cells can cause hemolytic jaundice (*prehepatic* or *nonobstructive jaundice*). Increased unconjugated bilirubin is formed through metabolism of the heme component of destroyed red blood cells and exceeds the conjugation ability of the liver, causing blood levels of unconjugated bilirubin to rise. Decreased bilirubin uptake or conjugation also causes unconjugated hyperbilirubinemia, as occurs with reaction to some medications (e.g., rifampin [Rifadin]) and in genetic disorders such as Gilbert's syndrome. Because unconjugated bilirubin is not water soluble, it is not excreted in the urine. The causes of jaundice are summarized in Table 36-7.

CLINICAL MANIFESTATIONS Conjugated bilirubin is water soluble and appears in the urine. The urine may darken several days before the onset of jaundice. The complete obstruction of bile flow from the liver to the duodenum causes grey or light-coloured stools. With partial obstruction, the stools are normal in colour and bilirubin is present in the urine.

Fever, chills, and pain often accompany jaundice resulting from viral or bacterial inflammation of the liver (e.g., viral hepatitis). Yellow discoloration may first occur in the sclera of the eye and then progress to the skin as bilirubin attaches to elastic fibres. Pruritus (itching) often accompanies jaundice because bilirubin accumulates in the skin.

EVALUATION AND TREATMENT Laboratory evaluation of serum establishes whether elevated plasma bilirubin is conjugated, unconjugated, or both. The history and physical examination identify underlying disorders, such as cirrhosis, exposure to hepatitis virus, and gallbladder or pancreatic disease. The treatment for jaundice consists of correcting the cause.

Hepatorenal Syndrome

Hepatorenal syndrome is functional kidney failure that develops as a complication of advanced liver disease. The kidney failure is not caused by primary kidney disease or other extrinsic factors but rather by portal hypertension, cardiac impairment, and other circulatory alterations associated with advanced liver disease, such as cirrhosis or fulminant hepatitis with portal hypertension. Manifestations include oliguria, sodium and water retention (usually with ascites and peripheral edema), hypotension, and peripheral vasodilation.[144] The kidney usually has a normal structure.

PATHOPHYSIOLOGY *Type 1 hepatorenal syndrome* accompanies a sudden decrease in blood volume secondary to massive GI or variceal bleeding and hypotension caused by bleeding and peripheral vasodilation associated with failing liver function. Hypotension also can be caused by the excessive use of diuretics to treat ascites or decreased cardiac output. The decrease in blood volume and hypotension result in decreased renal perfusion, decreased glomerular filtration, and oliguria (see Chapter 30). *Type 2 hepatorenal syndrome* develops slowly and is related to ascites. Ineffective circulating blood volume causes decreased glomerular filtration and oliguria. Intrarenal vasoconstriction may result from the selective effects of vasoactive substances that accumulate in the blood because of liver failure or a compensatory response to portal hypertension and the pooling of blood in the splanchnic circulation.[145]

TABLE 36-7 Common Types of Jaundice

Type	Mechanism	Causes
Hemolytic (prehepatic) jaundice (predominantly unconjugated bilirubin)	Destruction of erythrocytes (increased bilirubin production)	Hemolytic anemias (e.g., sickle cell) Severe infection Toxic substances in circulation (e.g., snake venom) Transfusion of incompatible blood
Disorders of bilirubin metabolism (unconjugated bilirubin)	Decreased bilirubin uptake Decreased bilirubin conjugation	Medication induced (e.g., rifampin [Rifadin] and cyclosporine [Sandimmune]) Hereditary disorder (e.g., Gilbert's syndrome)
Obstructive (posthepatic) jaundice (predominantly conjugated bilirubin)	Obstruction of passage of conjugated bilirubin from liver to intestine	Obstruction of bile duct by gallstones or tumour (extrahepatic obstructive jaundice) Obstruction of bile flow through liver (intrahepatic obstructive jaundice) Medications
Hepatocellular (intrahepatic) jaundice (both conjugated and unconjugated bilirubin)	Failure of liver cells (hepatocytes) to conjugate bilirubin and of bilirubin to pass from liver to intestine	Genetic defect of hepatocytes (decreased enzymes), such as occurs in premature infants (see Chapter 37) Severe infections (e.g., hepatitis) Alcoholic liver disease or biliary cirrhosis

CLINICAL MANIFESTATIONS The onset of hepatorenal manifestations may be acute or gradual. Oliguria and complications of advanced liver disease, including jaundice, ascites, peripheral edema, hypotension, and GI bleeding, are usually present. Systolic blood pressure is usually below 100 mm Hg. Nonspecific symptoms of hepatorenal syndrome include anorexia, weakness, and fatigue.[144]

EVALUATION AND TREATMENT Despite oliguria, serum potassium levels do not become dangerously elevated until the terminal stages of the hepatorenal syndrome. Blood urea level increases, followed by an increase in creatinine concentration. Urine osmolality increases, but urine sodium concentrations are below normal. Urine specific gravity is greater than 1.015.

The prognosis is usually poor and is related to a failing liver requiring liver transplant. Bridge treatments include albumin administration and a vasopressin analogue (Pressyn).[144]

QUICK CHECK 36-5

1. How does portal hypertension cause varices and promote formation of ascites?
2. What are two factors that cause hepatic encephalopathy?
3. Why is the concentration of unconjugated bilirubin elevated in hemolytic jaundice?
4. Describe how failure of liver function causes kidney failure (hepatorenal syndrome).

Disorders of the Liver

Liver disease is the fourth leading cause of death in Canada. The most common cause of liver failure is a condition known as fatty liver disease, but hepatitis B and C are also major causes of chronic liver disease. The causes of liver disease are different in children as compared with adults. In children, the leading causes of acute liver failure include acetaminophen toxicity, metabolic disorders, and autoimmune disease. It is estimated that more than 2 million Canadians—regardless of age, sex, ethnic origin, or lifestyle—will be affected by a liver or biliary tract disease in their lifetime.[146]

Acute Liver Failure

Acute liver failure (fulminant liver failure) is a rare clinical syndrome resulting in severe impairment or necrosis of liver cells without pre-existing liver disease or cirrhosis (see *Health Promotion:* Acetaminophen and Acute Liver Failure in Chapter 35). Acute liver failure also can occur with concurrent liver disease (acute or chronic liver failure),[147] including complication of viral hepatitis, particularly hepatitis B virus (HBV) infection; compounded by infection with the delta virus; as well as metabolic liver disorders. Edematous hepatocytes and patchy areas of necrosis and inflammatory cell infiltrates disrupt the parenchyma. The death of hepatocytes may be caused by viral or toxic injury or immunological and inflammatory damage with necrosis or apoptosis.

Acute liver failure usually develops 6 to 8 weeks after the initial symptoms of viral hepatitis or a metabolic liver disorder, or within 5 days to 8 weeks of acetaminophen (Tylenol) overdose. Anorexia, vomiting, abdominal pain, and progressive jaundice are initial signs followed by ascites and GI bleeding. Hepatic encephalopathy is manifested as lethargy and altered motor functions. Coma is related to cerebral edema, ischemia, and brainstem herniation. Liver function tests show elevations in the levels of both direct and indirect serum bilirubin, serum transaminases, and blood ammonia. Prothrombin time is prolonged. Kidney failure and pulmonary distress can occur.[148] Treatment of acute liver failure requires rapid evaluation and critical care. The hepatic necrosis is irreversible, and 60 to 90% of affected children die. Liver transplantation may be lifesaving;[149] in Canada, over 400 liver transplant operations are performed every year.[146] Artificial liver support devices are being evaluated. Survivors usually do not develop cirrhosis or chronic liver disease.

Cirrhosis

Cirrhosis is an irreversible inflammatory and fibrotic liver disease. Many disorders can cause cirrhosis and are listed in Box 36-3. The process of cellular injury depends on the cause of cirrhosis, and the pathological mechanisms are not all clearly understood. Structural changes result from injury (e.g., viruses or toxicity from alcohol) and fibrosis, which is a consequence of infiltration of leukocytes, release of inflammatory mediators, and activation of hepatic stellate cells and myofibroblasts.[150] Chaotic fibrosis alters or obstructs biliary channels and blood flow, producing jaundice and portal hypertension. New vascular channels form shunts, and blood from the portal vein bypasses the liver, contributing to portal hypertension, metabolic alterations, and toxin accumulation. The process of regeneration is disrupted by hypoxia, necrosis, atrophy, and (ultimately) liver failure. The formation of fibrous bands and regenerating nodules distorts the architecture of the liver

BOX 36-3 Causes of Cirrhosis

Hepatitis virus: B and C (common)
Excessive alcohol intake (common)
Idiopathic (common)
Nonalcoholic fatty liver disease, also known as *nonalcoholic steatohepatitis*
Autoimmune disorders
- Autoimmune hepatitis
- Primary biliary cirrhosis
- Primary sclerosing cholangitis

Hereditary metabolic disorder
- α_1-Antitrypsin deficiency
- Hemochromatosis
- Wilson's disease
- Glycogen or lipid storage diseases

Prolonged exposure to chemicals or toxins (e.g., carbon tetrachloride, cleaning and industrial solvents, copper salts)
Hepatic venous outflow obstruction
- Budd-Chiari syndrome
- Right ventricular failure

parenchyma and gives the liver a cobbly appearance. The liver may be larger or smaller than normal and is usually firm or hard when palpated.

There is no data on the prevalence of cirrhosis in Canada. However, from 2000 to 2007, noncancer liver–related deaths increased from 2 673 to 3 227 per year, an increase of 20.7%. Over the same period, all deaths from chronic liver disease increased from 3 964 to 5 049 per year, an increase of 27.9%. This significant increase in mortality occurred over only 8 years.[151]

Cirrhosis develops slowly over a period of years. Its severity and rate of progression depend on the cause. If toxins, such as alcohol metabolites, are involved, the rate of cell death and the severity of inflammation depend on the amount of toxin present. Removal of the toxin slows the progression of liver damage and enhances the process of regeneration.[152]

Alcoholic liver disease. Alcoholic liver disease is related to the toxic effects of alcohol (see Chapter 4) and coexisting liver disease. The incidence of alcoholic cirrhosis is greatest in middle-aged men; however, women develop more severe liver injury than men.[153] Although alcoholic cirrhosis is the most prevalent of the various types of cirrhosis, the occurrence of cirrhosis among persons with alcoholism is relatively low (approximately 25%). The spectrum of alcoholic liver disease includes alcoholic fatty liver, alcoholic steatohepatitis, and alcoholic cirrhosis.

PATHOPHYSIOLOGY Alcoholic fatty liver (steatosis) is the mildest form of alcoholic liver disease. It can be caused by relatively small amounts of alcohol, may be asymptomatic, and is reversible with cessation of drinking.[154] Fat deposition (deposition of triglycerides) within the liver is caused primarily by increased lipogenesis, cholesterol synthesis, and decreased fatty acid oxidation by hepatocytes. Lipids mobilized from adipose tissue or dietary fat intake may contribute to fat accumulation.

Alcoholic steatohepatitis (alcoholic hepatitis) is a precursor of cirrhosis characterized by increased hepatic fat storage, inflammation, and degeneration and necrosis of hepatocytes with infiltration of neutrophils and lymphocytes. The injured hepatocytes contain Mallory bodies (hyaline endoplasmic reticulum), indicating the onset of fibrosis. The inflammation and necrosis caused by alcoholic steatohepatitis stimulate the irreversible fibrosis characteristic of the cirrhotic stage of disease.[155]

Alcoholic cirrhosis is caused by the toxic effects of alcohol metabolism on the liver, immunological alterations, inflammatory cytokines, oxidative stress from lipid peroxidation, and malnutrition. Alcohol is transformed to acetaldehyde, and excessive amounts significantly alter hepatocyte function and activate hepatic stellate cells, a primary cell involved in liver fibrosis. Mitochondrial function is impaired, decreasing oxidation of fatty acids. Enzyme and protein synthesis may be depressed or altered, and hormone and ammonia degradation is diminished. Acetaldehyde inhibits export of proteins from the liver, alters metabolism of vitamins and minerals, and induces malnutrition.[156,157] Kupffer cell (macrophage) activation attracts neutrophils, promoting inflammation; endotoxins accumulate from translocation of gut bacteria; and cell-mediated immunity is suppressed. Cellular damage initiates an inflammatory response that, along with necrosis, results in activation of hepatic stellate cells and excessive collagen formation. Fibrosis and scarring alter the structure of the liver and obstruct biliary and vascular channels.

CLINICAL MANIFESTATIONS Fatty infiltration causes no specific symptoms or abnormal liver function test results. The liver is usually enlarged, however, and the individual has a history of continuous alcohol intake during the previous weeks or months. Anorexia, nausea, jaundice, and edema develop with advanced fatty infiltration or the onset of alcoholic steatohepatitis (Figure 36-15).

The clinical manifestations of alcoholic steatohepatitis can be mild or severe. Nonspecific symptoms include fatigue, weight loss, and anorexia. Manifestations of acute illness include nausea, anorexia, fever, abdominal pain, and jaundice. Cirrhosis is a multiple-system disease and causes hepatomegaly, splenomegaly, ascites, portal hypertension, GI hemorrhage, hepatic encephalopathy, and esophageal varices. Anemia results from blood loss, malnutrition, and hypersplenism. Kidney failure is often a late complication of hepatorenal syndrome. Toxic effects of alcohol also can cause testicular atrophy, reduced libido, azoospermia, and decreased testosterone levels in men. The presence of numerous and severe manifestations increases the risk for death. Cirrhosis increases the risk for hepatocellular carcinoma.

EVALUATION AND TREATMENT The diagnosis of alcoholic steatohepatitis or cirrhosis is based on the individual's history and clinical manifestations. The results of liver function tests are abnormal, and serological studies show elevated levels of serum enzymes and bilirubin, decreased levels of serum albumin, and prolonged prothrombin time that is not easily corrected with vitamin K therapy. Liver biopsy can confirm the diagnosis of cirrhosis, but biopsy is not necessary if clinical manifestations of cirrhosis are evident.

There is no specific treatment for alcoholic steatohepatitis or cirrhosis. Rest, vitamin supplements, a nutritious diet, corticosteroids, antioxidants, medications that slow fibrosis, and management of complications (such as ascites, GI bleeding, and encephalopathy) slow disease progression. Cessation of alcohol consumption slows the progression of liver damage, improves clinical symptoms, and prolongs life. Although the liver damage is irreversible, measures that halt the inflammation and destruction of liver cells prolong life. Liver transplantation is the treatment of end-stage liver disease. Artificial liver support systems continue to be evaluated and hepatocyte transplantation is being explored.[158,159]

Nonalcoholic fatty liver disease and nonalcoholic steatohepatitis. Nonalcoholic fatty liver disease (NAFLD) is infiltration of hepatocytes with fat, primarily in the form of triglycerides, but it occurs in the absence of alcohol intake. It is associated with obesity (including obese children), high levels of cholesterol and triglycerides, metabolic syndrome, and type 2 diabetes mellitus. Some individuals with NAFLD will develop nonalcoholic steatohepatitis (NASH) with hepatocellular injury, inflammation, and fibrosis. NASH is difficult to distinguish from

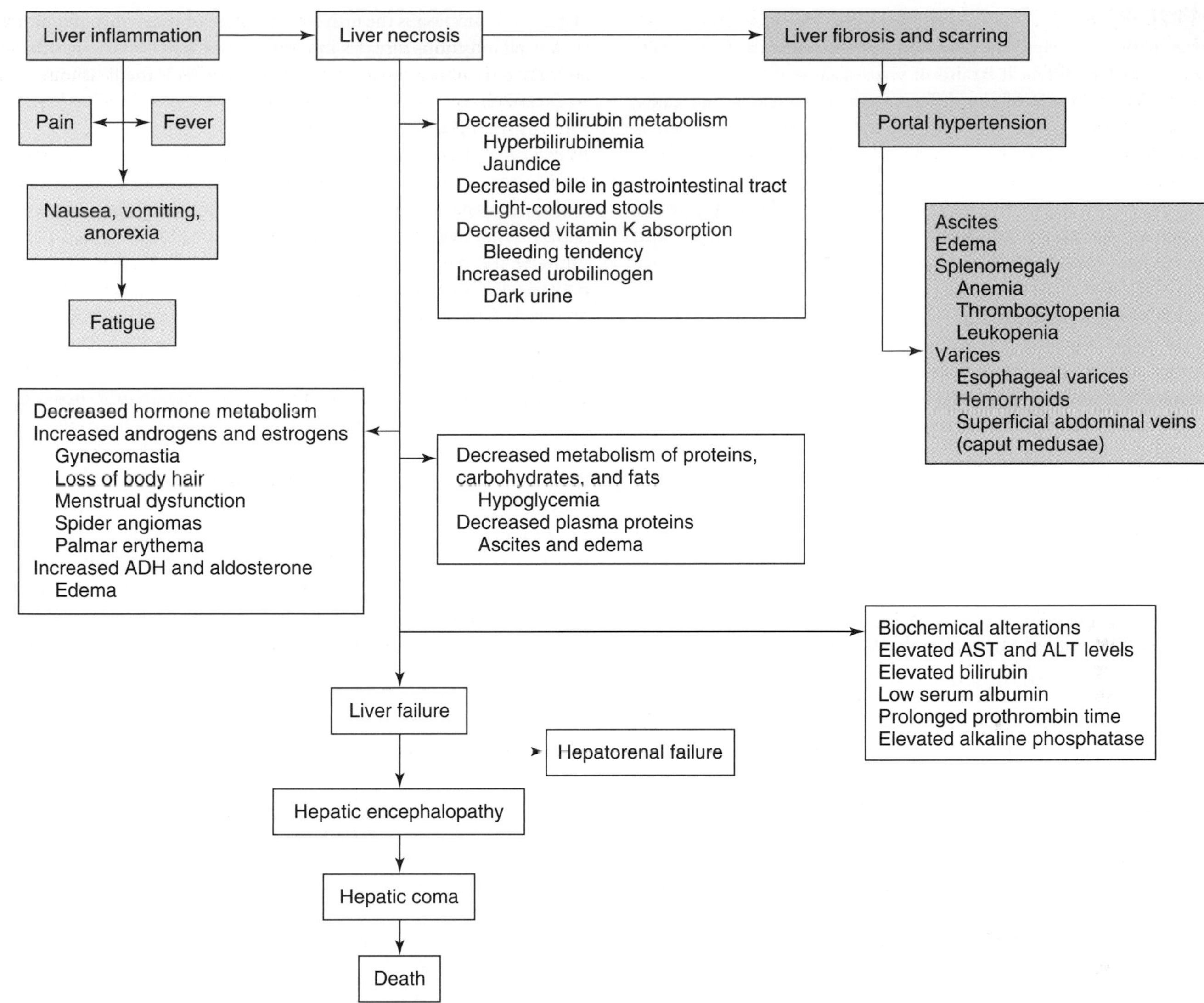

FIGURE 36-15 Clinical Manifestations of Cirrhosis. *ADH,* Antidiuretic hormone; *ALT,* alanine transaminase; *AST,* aspartate transaminase.

alcohol-induced liver fibrosis. NAFLD is usually asymptomatic and may remain undetected for years. The most severe forms of NASH progress to cirrhosis and end-stage liver disease. Treatment is individualized and includes the use of behavioural modification, dietary counselling, and regular exercise.[160,161]

Biliary cirrhosis. **Biliary cirrhosis** differs from alcoholic cirrhosis in that the damage and inflammation leading to cirrhosis begin in bile canaliculi and bile ducts, rather than in the hepatocytes. The two types of biliary cirrhosis are *primary* and *secondary.* Although both involve bile duct pathological changes, they differ with respect to cause, risk factors, and mechanisms of obstruction and inflammation.

Primary biliary cirrhosis is a chronic, autoimmune, cholestatic liver disease. It is caused by autoimmune T-cell and highly specific antimitochondrial antibody destruction of the small intrahepatic bile ducts and primarily affects middle-aged women. Primary biliary cirrhosis often accompanies other autoimmune diseases. Pathogenesis includes inflammation, destruction, fibrosis, and obstruction of the intrahepatic bile ducts. Primary biliary cirrhosis can be detected by biochemical evidence of cholestatic liver disease. Test findings include the presence of antinuclear antibodies, anticentromere antibodies, and the GP210 antinuclear antibody as well as elevated alkaline phosphatase levels for at least 6 months' duration. Ultrasound imaging of the liver, or liver biopsy, assists with diagnosis. Manifestations progress insidiously from pruritus, hyperbilirubinemia, jaundice, and light or clay-coloured stools to cirrhosis, portal hypertension, and encephalopathy. Life expectancy is 5 to 10 years after onset of symptoms if not treated. Treatment with ursodeoxycholic acid (Usrodiol) slows disease progression, and pruritus may be relieved by cholestyramine (Olestyr), which binds bile salts in the intestine. Liver transplant is highly effective.[162]

Secondary biliary cirrhosis is caused by prolonged partial or complete obstruction of the common bile duct or branches by gallstones, tumours, fibrotic strictures, or chronic pancreatitis; biliary atresia and cystic fibrosis are causative in children. Necrotic areas develop and lead to proliferation and inflammation of portal ducts, producing edema, fibrosis, and cirrhosis if not treated. Surgery or endoscopy relieves obstruction, prolongs survival, and diminishes or resolves symptoms.

QUICK CHECK 36-6

1. How does alcohol damage the liver?
2. What kind of liver changes are common to alcoholic cirrhosis and nonalcoholic fatty liver disease?
3. What are the major pathological differences between alcoholic and primary biliary cirrhosis?

Viral Hepatitis

Viral hepatitis is a relatively common systemic disease that affects primarily the liver. Different strains of viruses cause different types of hepatitis. Characteristics of the different types of viruses that cause hepatitis are presented in Table 36-8. Viral hepatitis in children is presented in Chapter 37.

Hepatitis B infection is a reportable disease. All public health jurisdictions record all positive hepatitis B blood tests (HBsAg-positive is the marker for active infection) and report data on acute and "indeterminate" cases to the Canadian Notifiable Disease Surveillance System (CNDSS).[151]

Canada draws a large proportion of its immigrants from areas of the world where hepatitis B is highly prevalent, including China, the Philippines, and other areas of South East Asia, as well as the Middle East and Africa. Based on the size and origin of the immigrant population in the 2006 census, the estimated number of people infected with hepatitis B in Canada ranges from 242 749 to 444 500, which corresponds to 0.81 to 1.44% of the Canadian population.[151]

As the province with the highest proportion of hepatitis B carriers in Canada (50%), Ontario is the only province that has attempted to determine the effect of hepatitis B on population morbidity and mortality. Hepatitis B infection is the fifth leading cause of morbidity and mortality among all infectious diseases in Ontario. And yet, Ontario has the most restrictive reimbursement criteria for hepatitis B medications.[151]

PATHOPHYSIOLOGY All five types of viral hepatitis (A, B, C, D, and E) can cause acute, icteric illness. The pathological lesions of hepatitis include hepatic cell necrosis, scarring (with chronic disease), and Kupffer cell hyperplasia, and infiltration by mononuclear phagocytes occurs with varying severity. Cellular injury is promoted by cell-mediated immune mechanisms (i.e., T-cytotoxic cells, T-regulatory cells, and natural killer cells). Regeneration of hepatic cells begins within 48 hours of injury. The inflammatory process can damage and obstruct bile canaliculi, leading to cholestasis and obstructive jaundice. In milder cases, the liver parenchyma is not damaged. Damage tends to be most severe in cases of hepatitis B and C. Acute fulminating hepatitis can cause acute liver failure and severe hepatic encephalopathy, which is manifested as confusion, stupor, coma, and coagulopathy. Hepatitis B and C are the most common causes as well as hepatitis E in pregnant women.[163]

Co-infection of hepatitis B virus (HBV), hepatitis C virus (HCV), hepatitis D virus (HDV), and human immunodeficiency virus (HIV)

TABLE 36-8 Characteristics of Viral Hepatitis

Characteristic	Hepatitis A	Hepatitis B	Hepatitis D	Hepatitis C	Hepatitis E
Virus	27-nm RNA virus	42-nm DNA virus	36-nm RNA virus	30- to 60-nm RNA virus	32-nm RNA virus
Antigens or antibodies	Anti-HAV	HBsAg HBcAg HBeAg	Anti-HDV	Anti-HCV	Anti-HEV
Incubation period	30 days	60–180 days	30–180 days	35–60 days	15–60 days
Route of transmission	Fecal–oral (most common), parenteral, sexual	Parenteral, sexual, across placenta	HBV co-infection Parenteral (?), fecal–oral, sexual	Parenteral, sexual, across placenta	Fecal–oral
Onset	Nonspecific Acute with fever	Insidious	Insidious	Insidious	Acute
Carrier state	Negative	Positive	Positive	Positive	Negative
Severity	Mild	Severe; may be prolonged or chronic	Severe	Unknown	Severe in pregnant women
Chronic hepatitis	No	Yes Increased risk for HCC	Yes	Yes Increased risk for HCC	No
Age group affected	Children and young adults	Any	Any	Any	Children and young adults
Prophylaxis	Hygiene, immune serum globulin, HAV vaccine	Hygiene, HBV vaccine, blood screening	Hygiene, HBV vaccine	Hygiene, blood screening, interferon-alpha	Hygiene, safe water
Pathophysiology	Hepatocyte injury caused by cellular immune responses (T cells, NK cells, and cytokines)	Viral replication, co-infection with viral mutation, inflammation, and cellular necrosis	Co-infection with HBV, severe cell injury, inflammation progressing to cirrhosis	Hepatocyte injury caused by immune response, inflammation, and fibrosis leading to cirrhosis	Viral replication, liver is cytotoxic, immune response causes inflammation and cholestasis
Treatment	Immune globulin within 2 weeks of exposure Symptomatic support	Interferon-alpha, peginterferon-alpha, antivirals (lamivudine [3TC], adefovir [Hepsera], entecavir [Baraclude], telbivudine [Sebivo], tenofovir [Viread])	Interferon-alpha	Interferon-alpha, peginterferon-alpha, antivirals (ribavirin [Virazole], boceprevir [Victrelis], telaprevir [Incivek], simeprevir [Olysio], daclatasvir [DAKLINZA], sofosbuvir [Sovaldi]), combinations of antivirals	Symptomatic support similar to HAV

HAAg, Hepatitis A antigen; *HAV*, hepatitis A virus; *HBcAg*, hepatitis B core antigen; *HBeAg*, hepatitis B e antigen; *HBsAg*, hepatitis B surface antigen; *HBV*, hepatitis B virus; *HCC*, hepatocellular carcinoma; *HCV*, hepatitis C virus; *HDV*, hepatitis D virus; *HEV*, hepatitis E virus; *NK cells*, natural killer cells.

occurs because these viruses share the same route of transmission (contact between infected body fluids and broken skin or mucous membranes, or intravenously). Progression of liver disease is more rapid in these cases.[164]

CLINICAL MANIFESTATIONS The clinical manifestations of the various types of hepatitis are very similar. The spectrum of manifestations ranges from absence of symptoms to fulminating hepatitis, with rapid onset of liver failure and coma. Acute viral hepatitis causes abnormal liver function test results. The serum aminotransferase values, aspartate transaminase (AST) and alanine transaminase (ALT), are elevated but not consistent with the extent of cellular damage. The clinical course of hepatitis usually consists of three phases. The **incubation phase** and manifestations vary depending on the virus (see Table 36-8):

1. **Prodromal (preicteric) phase.** Begins about 2 weeks after exposure and ends with the appearance of jaundice; marked by fatigue, anorexia, malaise, nausea, vomiting, headache, hyperalgia, cough, and low-grade fever; infection is highly transmissible during this phase.
2. **Icteric phase.** Begins 1 to 2 weeks after the prodromal phase and lasts 2 to 6 weeks; jaundice, dark urine, and clay-coloured stools are common; the liver is enlarged, smooth, and tender, and percussion or palpation of the liver causes pain; GI and respiratory symptoms subside, but fatigue and abdominal pain may persist or become more severe. This is the actual phase of illness. Individuals who develop chronic HBV, HDV, or HCV infection do not become jaundiced and may not be diagnosed.
3. **Recovery phase.** Begins with resolution of jaundice, about 6 to 8 weeks after exposure; symptoms diminish, but the liver remains enlarged and tender; liver function returns to normal 2 to 12 weeks after the onset of jaundice.

Chronic active hepatitis is the persistence of clinical manifestations and liver inflammation after acute stages of HBV, HBV/HDV co-infection, and HCV infection. Liver function tests remain abnormal for longer than 6 months, and hepatitis B surface antigen (HBsAg) persists. Chronic active HBV or HCV is a predisposition to cirrhosis and primary hepatocellular carcinoma.[165,166] Chronic active hepatitis constitutes a carrier state, and HBV and HCV can be transmitted from mothers to infants.

EVALUATION AND TREATMENT Diagnosis of hepatitis A virus (HAV) and HCV is based on the presence of anti-HAV and anti-HCV antibodies. The most specific diagnostic test for HBV is serological analysis for specific hepatitis virus antigens (i.e., HBsAg, which is the marker for HBV). Other markers for HBV include antibody to hepatitis B surface antigen (anti-HBs), hepatitis B e antigen (HBeAg), antibody to hepatitis B e antigen (anti-HBe), antibody to hepatitis B core antigen (anti-HBc), immunoglobulin M (IgM), and immunoglobulin G (IgG).[167] The assay for HDV is the measurement of total antibody to hepatitis D antigen (anti-HDV) and serum HDV RNA.[168] HCV RNA quantification is important for evaluation of viral load to evaluate antiviral therapy for chronic HCV. Hepatitis E virus (HEV) is diagnosed from the presence of serum anti-HEV IgG and HEV RNA. HEV is usually a self-limiting disease except in undeveloped countries, where it causes chronic hepatitis, with increased risk in pregnant women. Liver enzyme levels and function tests also can indicate other viral liver diseases, medication toxicity, or alcoholic hepatitis.[169]

Treatments for different types of viral hepatitis are summarized in Table 36-8. Physical activity may be restricted and a low-fat, high-carbohydrate diet is beneficial if bile flow is obstructed. For chronic hepatitis, treatment is directed at suppressing viral replication before irreversible liver cell damage or hepatic carcinoma occurs. Cyclic and combination therapy may prevent medication resistance, and new agents are being developed.[170,171]

After ingestion and GI uptake, HAV replicates in the liver and is secreted into the bile, feces, and sera. To prevent transmission of hepatitis A, proper hand hygiene and the use of gloves for disposing of bedpans and fecal matter are imperative. HAV may be shed in the feces for up to 3 months after onset of symptoms. Molecular procedures are available for direct surveillance of HAV in food.[172] Direct contact with blood or body fluids of individuals with HBV or HBV/HDV co-infection or HCV should be avoided. The administration of immunoglobulin before exposure or early in the incubation period can prevent hepatitis A and hepatitis B. A combined vaccine is available to protect against HAV and HBV infection. There is no vaccine for HCV.[173] A vaccine for HEV exists and is widely used in China, but it is not currently licensed in Canada or other industrialized countries.[174] Pre-exposure vaccination is recommended for health care workers, liver transplant recipients, and others who are at risk for contact with infected body fluids, particularly children.

> **✔ QUICK CHECK 36-7**
> 1. How does hepatitis A virus differ from hepatitis B virus?
> 2. What vaccines are available to prevent viral hepatitis?
> 3. What are the three phases of hepatitis viral infection?
> 4. What complications are associated with chronic active hepatitis?

Disorders of the Gallbladder

Obstruction and inflammation are the most common disorders of the gallbladder. Obstruction is caused by **gallstones**, which are aggregates of substances in the bile. The gallstones may remain in the gallbladder or be ejected, with bile, into the cystic duct. Gallstones that become lodged in the cystic duct obstruct the flow of bile into and out of the gallbladder and cause inflammation. Gallstone formation is termed **cholelithiasis**. Inflammation of the gallbladder or cystic duct is known as **cholecystitis**.

Cholelithiasis (Gallstones)

Cholelithiasis (gallstones) is a prevalent disorder in developed countries. Up to 20% of Canadian women and 10% of men have had cholelithiasis by the age of 60. Moreover, 70 to 80% of the First Nations population is affected by this disorder. Risk factors include obesity, middle age, female gender, use of oral contraceptives, rapid weight loss, First Nations ancestry, genetic predisposition, and gallbladder, pancreatic, or ileal disease.[175,176]

PATHOPHYSIOLOGY Gallstones are formed from impaired metabolism of cholesterol, bilirubin, and bile acids. All gallstones contain cholesterol, unconjugated bilirubin, bilirubin calcium salts, fatty acids, calcium carbonates and phosphates, and mucin glycoproteins. Gallstones are of three types, depending on chemical composition: *cholesterol* (70% cholesterol and the most common [70 to 80%]); *pigmented* (black [hard] and brown [soft] with less than 30% cholesterol); and *mixed*.[177] *Cholesterol gallstones* form in bile that is supersaturated with cholesterol produced by the liver. Supersaturation sets the stage for cholesterol crystal formation, or the formation of "microstones." More crystals then aggregate on the microstones, which grow to form "macrostones." This process usually occurs in the gallbladder, which may have decreased motility. The stones may lie dormant or become lodged in the cystic or common duct, causing pain when the gallbladder contracts and cholecystitis. The stones can accumulate and fill the entire gallbladder (Figure 36-16).

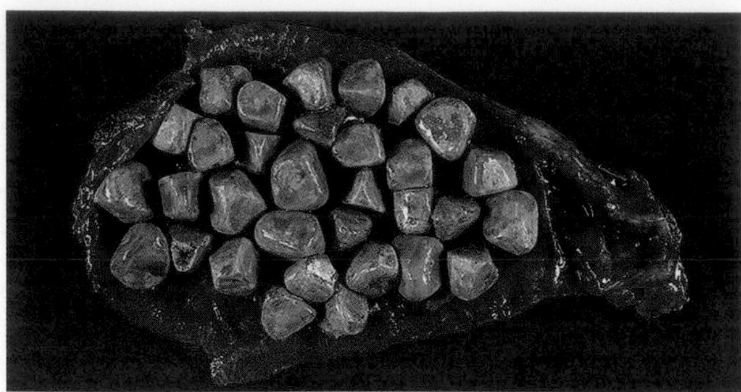

FIGURE 36-16 Resected Gallbladder Containing Mixed Gallstones. (From Kissane, J.M. [Ed.]. [1990]. *Anderson's pathology* [9th ed.]. St. Louis: Mosby.)

Pigmented brown gallstones form from calcium bilirubinate and fatty acid soaps that bind with calcium. They are associated with biliary stasis, bacterial infections, and biliary parasites. They are more common in East Asia. *Pigmented black gallstones* are rare. They are associated with chronic liver disease and hemolytic disease, and are composed of calcium bilirubinate with mucin glycoproteins.[178]

CLINICAL MANIFESTATIONS Cholelithiasis is often asymptomatic. Epigastric and right hypochondrium pain and intolerance to fatty foods are the cardinal manifestations of cholelithiasis. Vague symptoms include heartburn, flatulence, epigastric discomfort, and food intolerances, particularly to fats and cabbage. The pain (biliary colic) occurs 30 minutes to several hours after eating a fatty meal. It is caused by the lodging of one or more gallstones in the cystic or common duct during contraction of the gallbladder. It can be intermittent or steady and usually occurs in the right upper quadrant, radiating to the mid-upper area of the back. Jaundice indicates that the stone is located in the common bile duct.

EVALUATION AND TREATMENT Diagnosis is based on medical history, physical examination, and imaging evaluation. An oral cholecystogram usually outlines the stones. Intravenous cholangiography is used to differentiate cholelithiasis from other causes of extrahepatic biliary obstruction if the cholecystogram is negative. Endoscopic or percutaneous cholangiography and endoscopic or transabdominal ultrasonography are diagnostic options. Oral bile acids (ursodeoxycholic acid or chenodeoxycholic acid) may prevent or dissolve cholesterol stones, but the stones may recur when the medication is discontinued. Dietary factors may prevent the development of gallstones, including reducing the intake of polyunsaturated fat, monounsaturated fat, and caffeine, and increasing the consumption of fibre.[179] Endoscopic removal of gallstones by sphincterotomy or endoscopic papillary balloon dilation is the preferred treatment for uncomplicated gallstones causing obstruction of the bile ducts. Large stones may be managed by lithotripsy.[180]

Cholecystitis

Cholecystitis can be acute or chronic, but both forms are almost always caused by a gallstone lodged in the cystic duct.[181] Obstruction causes the gallbladder to become distended and inflamed. The pain is similar to that caused by gallstones. Pressure against the distended wall of the gallbladder decreases blood flow and may result in ischemia, necrosis, and perforation. Fever, leukocytosis, rebound tenderness, and abdominal muscle guarding are common findings. Serum bilirubin and alkaline phosphatase levels may be elevated. Cholescintigraphy is the most sensitive imaging for cholecystitis. The acute abdominal pain of cholecystitis must be differentiated from that caused by pancreatitis, myocardial infarction, and acute pyelonephritis of the right kidney. Narcotics may be required to control pain, and antibiotics often are prescribed to manage bacterial infection in severe cases. Acute attacks usually require laparoscopic gallbladder resection (cholecystectomy). Obstruction also may lead to reflux of bile into the pancreatic duct, causing acute pancreatitis.[182]

Disorders of the Pancreas

Pancreatitis, or inflammation of the pancreas, is a relatively rare and potentially serious disorder. The incidence is about equal in men and women, is more common between 50 and 60 years of age, and is more likely to occur in Blacks. Risk factors include obstructive biliary tract disease (particularly cholelithiasis), alcoholism, obesity, peptic ulcers, trauma, dyslipidemia, hypercalcemia, smoking, certain medications, and genetic factors (hereditary pancreatitis, cystic fibrosis). The cause is unknown in 15 to 25% of cases. Pancreatitis can be acute or chronic.

According to the Canadian Digestive Health Foundation, acute care inpatient costs for pancreas diseases are ranked as the fifth most expensive digestive disease in Canada; it costs $120 million per year for 13 000 patients. In Canada, pancreatitis affects 1 million people. Acute pancreatitis affects more than 600 000 people, while chronic pancreatitis affects more than 300 000 people. In Canada, similar to other Western countries, obesity is the main risk factor for developing acute pancreatitis.[183]

Acute Pancreatitis

Acute pancreatitis is usually a mild disease and resolves spontaneously, but about 20% of those with the disease develop a severe, acute pancreatitis requiring hospitalization. Pancreatitis develops because of obstruction to the outflow of pancreatic digestive enzymes caused by bile and pancreatic duct obstruction (e.g., gallstones). Acute pancreatitis also results from direct cellular injury from alcohol, medications, or viral infection.[184]

PATHOPHYSIOLOGY In obstructive disease, there is backup of pancreatic secretions and activation and release of enzymes (activated trypsin activates chymotrypsin, lipase, and elastase) within the pancreatic acinar cells. The activated enzymes cause autodigestion of pancreatic cells and tissues, resulting in inflammation. The autodigestion causes vascular damage, coagulation necrosis, fat necrosis (see Chapter 4), and formation of pseudocysts (walled-off collections of pancreatic secretions). Edema within the pancreatic capsule leads to ischemia and can contribute to necrosis. There also may be independent activation of inflammation within acinar cells contributing to the local and systemic responses occurring in acute pancreatitis[185] (Figure 36-17). In cases of alcohol abuse, the pancreatic acinar cell metabolizes ethanol with the generation of toxic metabolites that injure pancreatic acinar cells, causing release of activated enzymes. Chronic alcohol use may also cause formation of protein plugs in pancreatic ducts and spasm of the sphincter of Oddi, resulting in obstruction. The obstruction leads to intrapancreatic release of activated enzymes, autodigestion, inflammation, and pancreatitis.

Systemic effects of acute pancreatitis are related to release of proinflammatory cytokines (e.g., interleukin-6, tumour necrosis factor-alpha, and platelet-activating factor) into the bloodstream. There is activation of leukocytes, injury to vessel walls, and coagulation abnormalities with development of vasodilation, hypotension, and shock. Complications can include acute respiratory distress syndrome (ARDS), heart failure, kidney failure, coagulopathies, intra-abdominal hypertension, and systemic inflammatory response syndrome (SIRS) (see Chapter 24). Paralytic ileus and GI bleeding can occur. Translocation of intestinal bacteria to the bloodstream may cause peritonitis or sepsis.

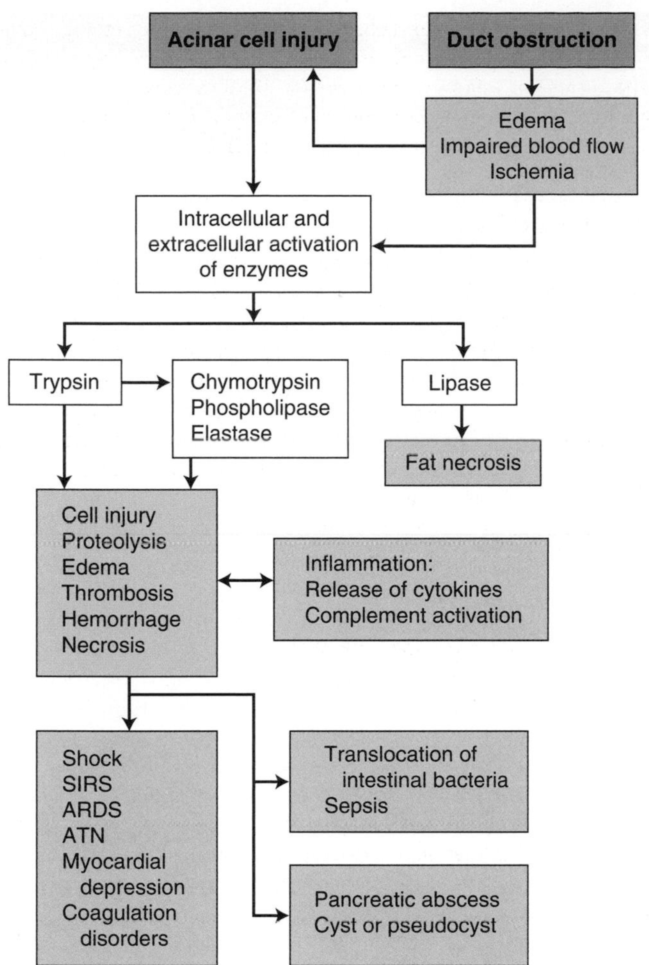

FIGURE 36-17 Pathophysiology of Acute Pancreatitis. *ARDS,* Acute respiratory distress syndrome; *ATN,* acute tubular necrosis; *SIRS,* systemic inflammatory response syndrome.

Recurrent inflammation activates pancreatic stellate cells, causing pancreatic fibrosis, strictures, and duct obstruction that lead to chronic pancreatitis.[186]

CLINICAL MANIFESTATIONS The cardinal manifestation of acute pancreatitis is epigastric or midabdominal constant pain ranging from mild abdominal discomfort to severe, incapacitating pain. The pain may radiate to the back. Pain is caused by (1) edema, which distends the pancreatic ducts and capsule; (2) chemical irritation and inflammation of the peritoneum; (3) irritation or obstruction of the biliary tract; and (4) inflammation of nerves. Fever and leukocytosis accompany the inflammatory response. Nausea and vomiting are caused by paralytic ileus secondary to the pancreatitis or peritonitis. Jaundice can occur from obstruction of the bile duct (e.g., a gallstone) or from pancreatic edema pressing on the duct. Abdominal distension accompanies bowel hypomotility and the accumulation of fluids in the peritoneal cavity. Hypovolemia, hypotension, tachycardia, myocardial insufficiency, and shock occur because plasma volume is lost as inflammatory mediators released into the circulation increase vascular permeability and dilate vessels. Tachypnea and hypoxemia develop secondary to ascites, pulmonary edema, atelectasis, or pleural effusions. Hypovolemia can decrease renal blood flow sufficiently to impair renal function and can cause kidney failure. Tetany may develop as a result of hypocalcemia when calcium is deposited in areas of fat necrosis or as a decreased response to parathormone. Transient hyperglycemia also can occur if glucagon is released from damaged alpha cells in the pancreatic islets. In severe acute pancreatitis, some individuals develop flank or periumbilical ecchymosis, a sign of poor prognosis. Multiple organ failure or SIRS accounts for most deaths of those with severe acute pancreatitis.

EVALUATION AND TREATMENT Diagnosis is based on clinical findings, identification of associated disorders, laboratory studies, and imaging results. Elevated serum amylase concentration is characteristic but is not diagnostic of severity or specificity of disease. Elevated serum lipase level is the primary diagnostic marker for acute pancreatitis.

The goal of treatment for acute pancreatitis is to stop the process of autodigestion and prevent systemic complications. Narcotic medications may be needed to relieve pain. To decrease pancreatic secretions and "rest the gland," oral food and fluids may be withheld initially and continuous gastric suction instituted. Nasogastric suction may not be necessary with mild pancreatitis, but it helps to relieve pain and prevent paralytic ileus in individuals who are nauseated and vomiting. Feeding is usually initiated within 24 to 48 hours if ileus is not present. Parenteral fluids are essential to restore blood volume and prevent hypotension and shock. In severe pancreatitis, enteral nutrition with use of jejunal tube feeding usually is well tolerated, may decrease pancreatic enzyme secretion, prevents gut bacterial overgrowth, and maintains gut barrier function. Medications that decrease gastric acid production (e.g., H2 receptor antagonists) can decrease stimulation of the pancreas by secretin. Antibiotics are used if there is infection. The risk for mortality increases significantly with the development of infection or pulmonary, cardiac, and renal complications.[187]

Chronic Pancreatitis

Chronic pancreatitis is a process of progressive fibrotic destruction of the pancreas. Chronic alcohol abuse is the most common cause. Obstruction from gallstones, smoking, and genetic factors increase the risk for chronic pancreatitis.[188] Toxic metabolites and chronic release of inflammatory cytokines contribute to the destruction of acinar cells and islets of Langerhans. The pancreatic parenchyma is destroyed and replaced by fibrous tissues, strictures, calcification, ductal obstruction, and pancreatic cysts. The cysts are walled off areas or pockets of pancreatic juice, necrotic debris, or blood within or adjacent to the pancreas. New imaging techniques have advanced evaluation of disease severity.[189]

Continuous or intermittent abdominal pain and weight loss are common. The pain is difficult to manage and is associated with increased intraductal pressure, ischemia, neuritis, intra-abdominal hypertension (compartment syndrome), ongoing injury, and both peripheral and central pain sensitization.[190] Manifestations of pancreatic enzyme deficiency, such as steatorrhea or a malabsorption syndrome, are present in late stages of chronic pancreatitis. To correct enzyme deficiencies and prevent malabsorption, oral enzyme replacements are taken before and during meals. Loss of islet cells can cause insulin-dependent diabetes and requires treatment. Cessation of alcohol intake is essential for the management of both acute and chronic pancreatitis. Endoscopic or surgical drainage of cysts or partial resection of the pancreas may be required to relieve pain and to prevent cystic rupture.[191] Chronic pancreatitis is a risk factor for pancreatic cancer.

CANCER OF THE DIGESTIVE SYSTEM

Cancer of the Gastro-Intestinal Tract

Table 36-9 contains information on the various GI cancers by organ, percentage of death compared with all cancer deaths, risk factors, type of cell, and common manifestations. The biology of cancer is presented in Chapter 10.

TABLE 36-9 Cancer of the Gut, Liver, and Pancreas

Organ	Projected Deaths Out of All Cancer Deaths in Canada, 2017 (%)	Risks	Cell Type	Common Manifestations
Esophagus	Males: 3.9% Females: 1.3%	Malnutrition Alcohol Tobacco Chronic reflux	Squamous cell Adenocarcinoma	Chest pain Dysphagia
Stomach	Males: 2.9% Females: 2.1%	Salty food Fried red meat Nitrates–nitrosamines	Adenocarcinoma Squamous cell	Anorexia Malaise Weight loss Upper abdominal pain Vomiting Occult blood
Colorectal	Males: 12.0% Females: 11.3%	Polyps Long-term inflammatory bowel disease Diverticulitis Highly refined carbohydrates; low-fibre, high-fat diets	Adenocarcinoma (left colon grows as ring; right colon grows as mass)	Pain Mass Anemia Bloody stool Obstruction Distension
Liver	Males: 2.2%[a] Females: 0.7%[a]	HBV, HCV, HDV Cirrhosis Intestinal parasite Aflatoxin from mouldy peanuts and corn	Hepatomas Cholangiomas	Pain Anorexia Bloating Weight loss Portal hypertension Ascites Jaundice
Pancreas	Males: 5.6% Females: 6.3%	Chronic pancreatitis Cigarette smoking Alcohol (?) Diabetic women	Adenocarcinoma (exocrine part of gland, ductal epithelium)	Weight loss Weakness Nausea Vomiting Abdominal pain Depression ± jaundice May have insulin-secreting tumours with symptoms of hypoglycemia

[a]Liver deaths are underestimated.

From American Cancer Society. (2015). *Cancer facts & figures 2015.* Retrieved from https://www.cancer.org/research/cancer-facts-statistics/all-cancer-facts-figures/cancer-facts-figures-2015.html; Canadian Cancer Society, & Government of Canada. (2017). *Canadian cancer statistics 2017.* Toronto: Author. Retrieved from http://www.cancer.ca/~/media/cancer.ca/CW/publications/Canadian%20Cancer%20Statistics/Canadian-Cancer-Statistics-2017-EN.pdf.

Cancer of the Esophagus

Carcinoma of the esophagus is a rare type of cancer with an estimated incidence of 1.7% in males and 0.5% in females. The Canadian Cancer Society estimated that over 2 300 Canadians (1 800 men and 530 women) were diagnosed with esophageal cancer in 2017. It also estimated that 2 200 Canadians (1 650 men and 480 women) died of this disease in 2017.[192] Risk factors are summarized in *Risk Factors:* Esophageal Cancer.

PATHOPHYSIOLOGY Carcinoma of the esophagus includes squamous cell carcinoma and adenocarcinoma. The main risk factors for squamous cell carcinoma include chronic alcohol use combined with smoking or chewing tobacco, hot and irritant (alcohol) drinks, food containing nitrosamines, and achalasia.[193] Squamous cell carcinomas are more common in the thoracic and cervical areas of the esophagus.

Adenocarcinomas are more prevalent in males and are associated with cigarette smoking, obesity, and GERD. Adenocarcinoma development is often secondary to infiltration by a gastric carcinoma or to the presence

RISK FACTORS

Esophageal Cancer

- Age greater than 60 years
- Male
- Tobacco use
- Alcoholism
- Dietary factors: deficiencies of trace elements and vitamins
- Malnutrition associated with poor economic conditions or special dietary habits (e.g., very hot drinks, fish preserved in lye; diet deficient in fruits and vegetables)
- Reflux esophagitis with dysplasia
- Sliding hiatal hernia
- Obesity

of Barrett dysplasia, also known as **Barrett esophagus** (columnar rather than squamous epithelium in the lower esophagus), and can progress to metaplasia.[194] Adenocarcinoma is more common at the gastroesophageal junction. The CagA-positive strain of *H. pylori* may be a protection against esophageal carcinoma.[195]

CLINICAL MANIFESTATIONS The two frequent symptoms of esophageal carcinoma are chest pain and dysphagia. The most common type of pain is heartburn. It is initiated by eating spicy or highly seasoned foods and by assuming the recumbent position. Odynophagia (pain on swallowing) may be initiated by the swallowing of cold liquids. Spontaneous chest pain is more difficult to diagnose positively. Some individuals with esophageal cancer complain of a constant retrosternal pain that radiates to the back. Dysphagia (difficulty swallowing) is usually pressurelike and may radiate posteriorly between the scapulae. Dysphagia usually progresses rapidly. Esophageal carcinoma is asymptomatic during the early stages and presents at an advanced stage. Esophageal cancer metastasizes rapidly and, therefore, has a poor prognosis.

EVALUATION AND TREATMENT Individuals with dysphagia undergo endoscopy so that specimens can be obtained and examined for neoplastic change. Endoscopic ultrasound and CT studies of the thorax are used for diagnosis and staging. Prevention of gastroesophageal reflux and removal of high-grade dysplasia are essential to the management of Barrett esophagus.[196] It is impossible to remove all lymph nodes with the tumour, but removal of the primary lesion and the local lymph nodes can benefit the individual with esophageal cancer. If the malignancy has not spread beyond these sites, cure is likely. If metastasis has occurred, however, an incomplete resection is of little survival benefit. Treatment is combined radiation and chemotherapy.[197,198]

Cancer of the Stomach

The Canadian Cancer Society estimated that 3 500 Canadians (2 200 men and 1 300 women) were diagnosed with stomach cancer (also called *gastric cancer*) in 2017. It also estimated that 2 100 Canadians (1 250 men and 780 women) died of this disease in 2017.[199]

In Canada, the incidence rates of stomach cancer continue to decline in both males (2.2% per year) and females (1.3% per year); current rates are about half of what they were in 1985. This decline may be due to long-term improvements in diets and decreases in smoking and heavy alcohol use. The declining incidence rates of stomach cancer may also be related to the more recent recognition and treatment of infection caused by the bacterium *H. pylori*, an important risk factor for stomach cancer.[200]

The case fatality rate for stomach cancer is 75%.[201] Stomach cancer is more prevalent in Asia, particularly China.[202] Loss of tumour-suppressor genes and other genetic alterations may be important in stomach cancer.[203]

PATHOPHYSIOLOGY Gastric adenocarcinomas are associated with atrophic gastritis and *H. pylori* that carry the *CagA* gene product VacA. It also causes gastric B-cell mucosa-associated lymphoid tissue lymphoma. Hereditary diffuse adenocarcinoma is rare and occurs at a younger age.[204] Most adenocarcinomas are sporadic and associated with consumption of heavily salted and preserved foods (e.g., nitrates in pickled foods or in salted foods such as bacon), low intake of fruits and vegetables, and use of tobacco and alcohol. Dietary salt enhances the conversion of nitrates to carcinogenic nitrosamines in the stomach. Salt and nitrates converted to nitrites are caustic to the stomach, delay gastric emptying, and can cause chronic atrophic gastritis. Insufficient acid secretion by the atrophic mucosa creates a relatively alkaline environment that permits bacteria to multiply and act on nitrates. The resulting increase in nitrosamines damages the DNA of mucosal cells, further promoting metaplasia and neoplasia.

Gastric adenocarcinoma usually begins in the glands of the distal stomach mucosa. Duodenal reflux also may contribute to an intestinal-like metaplasia. The reflux contains caustic bile salts that destroy the mucosal barrier that normally protects the stomach.

CLINICAL MANIFESTATIONS The early stages of stomach cancer are generally asymptomatic or produce vague symptoms such as loss of appetite (especially for meat), malaise, and indigestion. Later manifestations of stomach cancer include unexplained weight loss, upper abdominal pain, vomiting, change in bowel habits, and anemia caused by persistent occult bleeding. The prognosis is poor because symptoms do not occur until the tumour has spread and caused distant metastases, particularly to the liver and peritoneal structures. Generally, the first manifestations of carcinoma are caused by distant metastases, and the disease is already in an advanced stage.

EVALUATION AND TREATMENT There are no specific biomarkers for stomach cancer. Micro RNAs are being evaluated as a specific diagnostic and prognostic marker.[205] Most symptoms suggest a problem in the upper GI tract, and a barium X-ray film shows the lesion. Direct endoscopic visualization, lavage, and cellular examination or biopsy establish the diagnosis. Screening and treatment for *H. pylori* infection are the best preventive approaches to stomach cancer. Surgery is the usual treatment for early stages of disease. Staging is determined by pathological findings after resection. Early diagnosis and chemotherapy combined with radiation improves postsurgical outcomes.[206]

QUICK CHECK 36-8
1. How do gallstones form?
2. Compare acute and chronic pancreatitis.
3. What factors are associated with cancer of the esophagus?
4. What dietary factors are associated with stomach cancer?

Cancer of the Colon and Rectum

In Canada, from the mid-1980s to the mid-1990s, overall incidence rates for colorectal cancer declined for both sexes (this decline was more prominent for females). Incidence rates then rose through 2000, only to decline slightly thereafter. This change is most likely due to the increased use of colorectal cancer screening, which can identify and remove precancerous polyps and in turn reduce incidence. The decline in colorectal cancer incidence rates appears mostly in older adults, as rates are increasing among adults under the age of 50 years.[200]

As of 2014, nine provinces had organized colorectal cancer screening programs available, and the remaining province has announced the intention to implement one. Participation rates vary within and between the existing organized programs and do not meet the target of 60%. Colorectal cancer is linked to several modifiable risk factors, including obesity, physical inactivity, consumption of red and processed meat, and smoking.[207] Diabetes may also increase risk for colorectal cancer. (See *Risk Factors:* Cancer of the Colon and Rectum.)

The Canadian Cancer Society estimated that 26 800 Canadians (14 900 men and 11 900 women) were diagnosed with colorectal cancer in 2017. This number represents 13% of all predicted new cancer cases in 2017. The Canadian Cancer Society also estimated that 9 400 Canadians (5 100 men and 4 300 women) died of this disease in 2017. This total represents 12% of all predicted cancer deaths in 2017.[207] Colorectal cancer incidence rates for both males and females are highest in Newfoundland and Labrador. For females, high rates are also seen in Nova Scotia, Prince

RISK FACTORS

Cancer of the Colon and Rectum

- Advanced age
- High-fat (especially egg consumption) diet, red and processed meat, low-fibre diet
- High consumption of alcohol
- Cigarette smoking
- Obesity
- Familial polyposis or family history of colorectal cancer
- Low levels of physical activity
- Inflammatory bowel disease
- Type 2 diabetes mellitus

Edward Island, and Manitoba. The lowest rates for both sexes are in British Columbia.[200] In males, colorectal cancer is now the second most common cancer, and it accounts for approximately 14% of all new male cases. In females, colorectal cancer is the third most common cancer, and it accounts for approximately 12% of all new female cases.[200] Colorectal cancer typically occurs in women 10 years later than in men.

Worldwide, the prevalence and death rate of colorectal cancer are highest in Black populations, possibly because of lack of access to screening and treatment.[208]

PATHOPHYSIOLOGY Most colorectal cancers are sporadic (acquired) or associated with a family history of colorectal cancer. They are caused by multiple gene alterations and environmental interactions (see Chapter 3 for epigenetics and Chapter 10 for mechanisms of oncogenesis). **Familial adenomatous polyposis (FAP)** is a mutation of the *APC* gene (adenomatous polyposis coli, a tumour-suppressor gene) and is the most common hereditary cause of colorectal cancer. **Hereditary nonpolyposis colorectal cancer (HNPCC)**, or **Lynch syndrome**, is associated with several DNA mismatch repair (MMR) gene mutations. Both FAP and HNPCC have a rare, family-linked autosomal dominant inheritance trait that accounts for about 3 to 5% of colorectal cancers.[209,210] Sporadic tumours are also thought to involve the loss of function or mutation of tumour-suppressor genes (i.e., *APC, kRAS, p53* genes). Colorectal cancer begins with the formation of an adenoma and is termed "tumour initiation." The progression to carcinoma is termed *tumour progression* and is a multistep process of genetic mutations that may take 8 to 10 years.

Colorectal polyps are closely associated with the development of cancer. A polyp, or papilloma, is a projection arising from the mucosal epithelium. The most common types of polyps are hyperplastic (a non-neoplastic, or benign, polyp). Adenomatous polyps are neoplastic. They can be pedunculated (have a stalk) or sessile (flat with no stalk). **Neoplastic polyps** are premalignant lesions and are further classified as tubular (the most prevalent), villous (usually sessile), or tubulovillous adenomas (Figure 36-18). Serrated sessile polyps have a sawtooth appearance and can be difficult to detect. Serrated sessile polyps are associated with oncogene mutations and should be removed.[211] The larger the polyp, the greater the risk for colorectal cancer. Although lesions larger than 1.5 cm occur less often, they are more likely to be malignant than those smaller than 1.0 cm. Thus, screening colonoscopy with polypectomy is performed when polyps are found.

Adenocarcinomas of the colon and rectum usually arise from adenomatous polyps and undergo a multistep cascade of genetic events that leads to carcinoma and metastasis[212] (see Figure 10-7). Most colorectal cancers are moderately differentiated adenocarcinomas. These tumours have a long preinvasive phase and when they invade, they tend to grow slowly. Colorectal carcinoma begins from epithelial stem cells

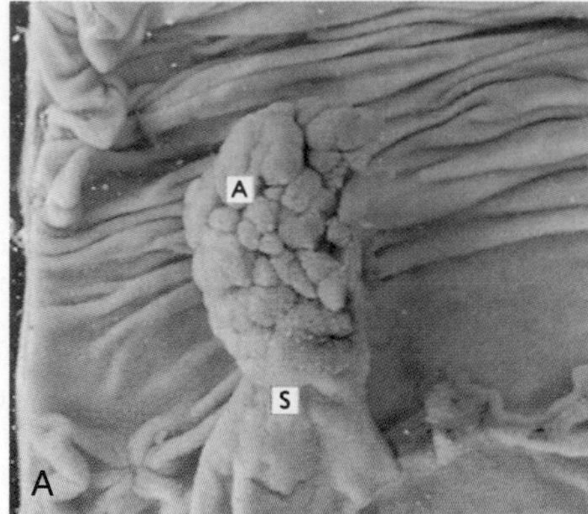

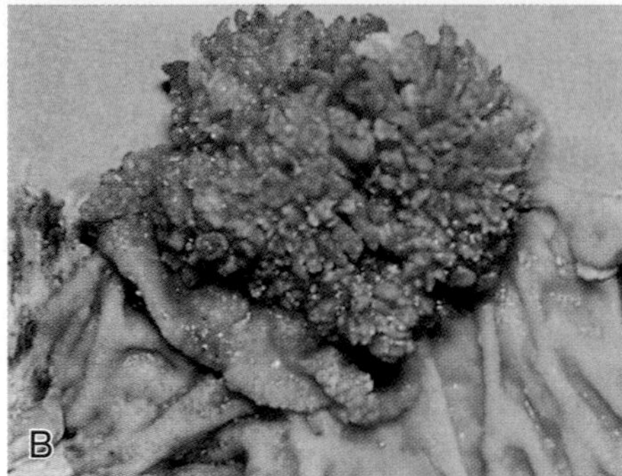

FIGURE 36-18 Neoplastic Polyps. A, Tubular adenomata (*A*) are rounded lesions 0.5 to 2 cm in size that are generally red and sit on a stalk (*S*) of normal mucosa that has been dragged up by traction of the polyp in the bowel lumen. **B,** Villous adenomata are velvety lesions about 0.6 cm thick that occupy a broad area of mucosa generally 1 to 5 cm in diameter. (From Stevens, A., Lowe, J., & Scott, I. [2009]. *Core pathology* [3rd ed.]. London: Mosby.)

located in the glands at the base of the intestinal crypts. Because the lymphatic channels are located under the muscularis mucosae, the lesions must traverse this layer before the multistep process of metastasis can occur. Once the malignant cells of an adenoma traverse the muscularis mucosae, tumour cells enter the bloodstream and lymphatics and become invasive, spreading to other organs. Adenomas can be detected early, however, because the submucosa may not be penetrated for several years.

Small intestinal carcinoma is very rare and is usually located in the duodenum.[213]

CLINICAL MANIFESTATIONS Symptoms of colorectal cancer depend on the location, size, and shape of the lesion and are silent in the early stages (Figure 36-19). Tumours of the right (ascending) colon and left (descending) colon evolve into two distinct tumour types.[214] On the right side (proximal colon), the lesions are polypoid and extend along one wall of the cecum and ascending colon. These tumours may be silent, evolving to pain, palpable mass in the lower-right quadrant, anemia, fatigue, and dark red or mahogany-coloured blood mixed with the stool. These tumours can become large and bulky with necrosis and ulceration, contributing to persistent blood loss and anemia. Obstruction is unusual because the growth does not readily encircle the colon. These tumours are more common in women.

Tumours of the left, or descending, colon (distal colon) start as small, elevated, buttonlike masses. This type grows circumferentially, encircling the entire bowel wall, and eventually ulcerating in the middle as the tumour penetrates the blood supply. Obstruction is common but occurs slowly, and stools become narrow and pencil shaped.

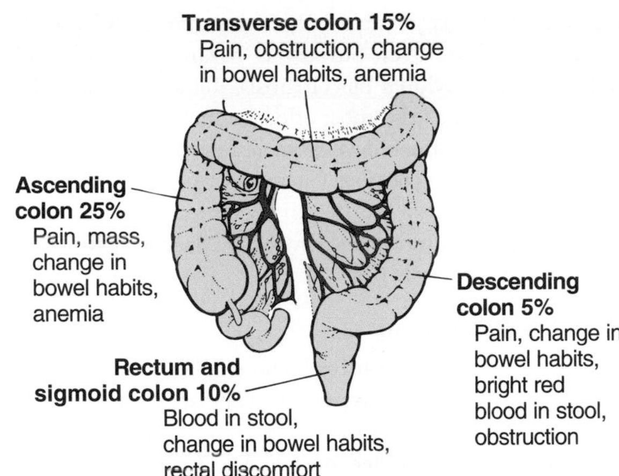

FIGURE 36-19 Signs and Symptoms of Colorectal Cancer by Location of Primary Lesion. Clinical manifestations are listed in order of frequency for each region (lymphatics of colon also shown).

Manifestations include progressive abdominal distension, pain, vomiting, constipation, need for laxatives, cramps, and bright red blood on the surface of the stool. These tumours are more common in men.

Systematic lymphatic distribution occurs along the aorta to the mesenteric and pancreatic lymph nodes. Liver metastasis is common and follows invasion of the mesenteric veins (left colon) or superior veins (right colon), which drain into the portal circulation.

Rectal carcinomas (about 30% of colorectal carcinomas) are defined as tumours occurring up to 15 cm from the anal opening. Tumours of the rectum can spread through the rectal wall to nearby structures: the prostate in men and the vagina in women. Penetration occurs more readily in the lower third of the rectum because it has no serosal covering. Systemic and pulmonary metastases occur through the hemorrhoidal plexus, which drains into the vena cava.

EVALUATION AND TREATMENT Individuals with hereditary polyposis should begin screening at an early age (10 to 12 years) using colonoscopy, with removal of polyps when they are found. Specific, sensitive, and affordable molecular markers are being evaluated to assist with early diagnosis and evaluation of therapy. Carcinoembryonic antigen (CEA) is evaluated during and after cancer treatment. Screening procedures for detection of nonhereditary colorectal cancer are summarized in Box 36-4. Aspirin and celecoxib (Celebrex) may reduce the incidence of colorectal cancer in the general population, but risk for GI bleeding must be considered. Vitamin D, calcium, fibre, folate, dietary modification, weight control, exercise, and other nondietary lifestyle changes can decrease the risk for colorectal cancer.[215]

The staging of colorectal cancer involves imaging and operative exploration.[216] Physical examination of the abdomen detects liver enlargement and ascites; appropriate lymph nodes are palpated. Imaging is useful for pretreatment staging.[216] Operative staging consists of careful exploration during surgery and biopsy of possible metastases. The World Health Organization's TNM classification is widely used for staging of colorectal cancer[217] (see http://www.cancer.ca/en/cancer-information/cancer-type/colorectal/staging/?region=on; see also Figure 10-23).

Treatment for all stages of cancer of the colon is surgical. Chemotherapy and radiation therapy may be given before surgery in the hope that they will shrink the tumour or alter the malignant cells, or both, so that these cells will not survive after surgery. Resection and anastomosis can be performed for cancer of the ascending, transverse, descending, or sigmoid colon and upper rectum. These surgeries are performed through abdominal incisions and assisted with radiofrequency ablation.

BOX 36-4 Screening for Colorectal Cancer

Beginning at age 50, both men and women should follow one of these testing schedules:

Tests That Find Polyps and Cancer

Flexible sigmoidoscopy every 5 years,* *or*
Colonoscopy every 10 years, *or*
Double-contrast barium enema every 5 years,* *or*
CT colonography (virtual colonoscopy) every 5 years*

Tests That Primarily Find Cancer

Every 2 years fecal occult blood test (gFOBT),† *or*
Yearly fecal immunochemical test (FIT),† *or*
Stool DNA or RNA tests (sDNA, sRNA), interval uncertain†

*All positive tests should be followed up with colonoscopy.
†The multiple stool take-home test should be used.
From American Cancer Society. (2015). *Cancer facts & figures 2015*. Retrieved from https://www.cancer.org/research/cancer-facts-statistics/all-cancer-facts-figures/cancer-facts-figures-2015.html; Koga, Y., Yamazaki, N., & Matsumura, Y. (2014). *Expert Rev Mol Diagn, 14*(1), 107–120; Canadian Cancer Society. (2017). *Screening for colorectal cancer*. Retrieved from http://www.cancer.ca/en/prevention-and-screening/early-detection-and-screening/screening/screening-for-colorectal-cancer/?region=bc.

Natural defecation is preserved. Growths in the lower portion of the rectum require removal of the entire rectum with the formation of a permanent colostomy. Chemotherapy, including immunotherapy, is used to treat metastatic disease and cases with a high risk for recurrence. New chemotherapeutic agents are improving personalized, first-line therapy. Immunotherapy, vaccines, and viral vectors for the treatment of colon cancer are under continuing investigation.[218,219] Resection of liver metastases or hepatic intra-arterial chemotherapy may prolong survival.[220,221]

Cancer of the Accessory Organs of Digestion

Cancer of the Liver

Cancer of the liver is a leading cause of cancer death worldwide and is highest in East and Southeast Asia.[222] Liver cancer is one of the fastest rising cancers in Canada. While it is still considered a rare cancer, accounting for an estimated 1% of all new cancer diagnoses and deaths in 2013, the incidence rate of liver cancer has tripled in Canadian men and doubled in women since 1970.[223] Primary liver cancer is rare before the age of 40 years and is most common after 60 years. Cancer in the liver is usually caused by metastatic spread from a primary site elsewhere in the body.[224] Risk factors for primary liver cancer are summarized in *Risk Factors:* Primary Liver Cancer. Risks associated with HBV and HCV are decreasing with antiviral therapy.[225]

RISK FACTORS

Primary Liver Cancer

- Exposure to mycotoxins (aflatoxins), particularly those produced by *Aspergillus flavus*, a mould found on spoiled corn, peanuts, and grain
- Alcohol abuse
- Obesity
- Chronic liver disease, especially cirrhosis
- Infection with hepatitis B virus, hepatitis C virus, and hepatitis D virus, particularly in conjunction with cirrhosis; these infections act either as carcinogens or as co-carcinogens in chronically infected hepatocytes

The Canadian Cancer Society estimated that approximately 2 500 Canadians (1 900 men and 580 women) were diagnosed with liver cancer in 2017. It also estimated that 1 200 Canadians (950 men and 270 women) died of this disease in 2017.[226] As these numbers indicate, men are more affected by liver cancer than women. From 1992 to 2012, the incidence rate of liver cancer rose for males (2.8% per year) and females (1.7% per year). These increases may be at least partially explained by rising immigration from regions of the world where risk factors for liver cancer, such as hepatitis B and C infection and exposure to aflatoxin, are more common.[200]

In Canada, between 2001 and 2010, the mortality rate of liver cancer increased significantly for both males (3.1% per year) and females (2.2% per year). The upward trend in mortality rates is associated with the increase in liver cancer incidence rates.[200]

PATHOPHYSIOLOGY Primary carcinomas of the liver are hepatocellular or cholangiocellular. **Hepatocellular carcinoma (HCC)** develops in the hepatocytes and can be nodular (consisting of multiple, discrete nodules), massive (consisting of a large tumour mass having satellite nodules), or diffuse (consisting of small nodules distributed throughout most of the liver). It is closely associated with chronic hepatitis and cirrhosis. Because carcinoma of the liver invades the hepatic and portal veins, it often spreads to the heart and lungs. Other sites of metastases are the brain, kidney, and spleen.

Cholangiocellular carcinoma (cholangiocarcinoma) is rare (less than 1% of liver cancers), develops in the bile ducts, and occurs less often than hepatocellular carcinoma.[227] It is associated with primary sclerosing cholangitis (a rare autoimmune disease often associated with UC) and is geographically associated with areas where liver fluke infestation is prevalent, such as Southeast Asia. Cholangiocellular carcinoma can occur anywhere along the bile duct and extend directly into the liver, usually as a solitary lesion. A combined form of HCC is known as combined (mixed) hepatocellular–cholangiocellular carcinoma. It is difficult to distinguish an invasion of cholangiocellular carcinoma from a metastatic adenocarcinoma except by neoplastic changes found in nearby ducts.

CLINICAL MANIFESTATIONS HCC is usually asymptomatic. Manifestations can develop slowly or abruptly and include vague abdominal symptoms such as nausea and vomiting, fullness, pressure, and dull ache in the right hypochondrium. In individuals with cirrhosis, deepening jaundice or abrupt lack of appetite is a sign of hepatocellular carcinoma. Obstruction by the tumour can cause sudden worsening of portal hypertension and development of ascites. As the tumour enlarges, it causes pain. Cholangiocellular carcinoma more commonly presents insidiously as pain, loss of appetite, weight loss, and gradual onset of jaundice. Some carcinomas of the liver rupture spontaneously, causing hemorrhage. Others are discovered accidentally during laboratory evaluation, imaging, or surgery for other diseases or trauma.

EVALUATION AND TREATMENT There is no specific test for the diagnosis of liver cancer. Biopsy is not recommended because of the risk for tumour seeding. For high-risk individuals, alpha fetoprotein associated with HBV and abdominal ultrasound are common screening tools. Diagnosis is based on clinical manifestations, laboratory findings, imaging, and exploratory laparotomy. In individuals without cirrhosis, liver scans can document filling defects. CT or ultrasonography is used to detect solid tumours, but neither can distinguish benign from malignant tumours. Primary prevention may be achieved by vaccinating against HBV, preventing and treating HBV and HCV, screening all donated blood for the presence of HBV, and reducing contamination of food with aflatoxins.[228]

Surgical resection is possible only if the tumour is localized to a removable lobe of the liver. Surgery is hazardous and usually not undertaken if the individual has cirrhosis. Radiofrequency (thermal) ablation has emerged as the most effective method for local tumour destruction. Most individuals develop metastases after surgical resection, but long-term survival is possible. Chemotherapeutic agents, immunotherapy, and radiotherapy are treatment options.[229] Liver transplant offers a cure if the waiting time is short. The prognosis for those with symptomatic liver cancer is poor.[230]

Cancer of the Gallbladder

Risk factors for gallbladder cancer include gallstones, advancing age, female gender (2 : 1), anomalous pancreaticobiliary ductal junction, and obesity. Gallbladder cancer occurs rarely before the age of 40 years and is most common between the ages of 50 and 60 years. Primary carcinoma of the gallbladder is rare and associated with larger gallstones. Most gallbladder cancer is caused by metastasis.

The Canadian Cancer Society estimated that 470 Canadians (175 men and 300 women) were diagnosed with gallbladder cancer in 2013. It also estimated that 264 Canadians (97 men and 167 women) died of this disease in 2013.[231]

PATHOPHYSIOLOGY Most primary carcinomas of the gallbladder are adenocarcinomas, and more rarely squamous cell carcinomas. The pathogenesis is not clear. Chronic inflammation may trigger dysplasia and progression to metaplasia. The molecular mechanisms involve mutation of several genes, including tumour-suppressor genes and oncogenes, and alterations in the extracellular matrix.[232] Invasion of the liver and lymph nodes occurs early. Direct invasion of the stomach and the duodenum can cause pyloric obstruction. Infection often accompanies cancer of the gallbladder. Generalized peritonitis, gangrene, perforation, and liver abscesses are potential complications of infection.

CLINICAL MANIFESTATIONS Early stages of gallbladder cancer are asymptomatic, and the disease usually presents at an advanced stage. When symptoms develop, there is usually steady pain in the upper-right quadrant for about 2 months. Other manifestations include diarrhea, belching, weakness, loss of appetite, weight loss, and vomiting. Obstructive jaundice can occur if an enlarging tumour presses on the extrahepatic ducts.

EVALUATION AND TREATMENT Early diagnosis of gallbladder cancer is rare and is often found incidentally. Therefore, older adults with gallstones, particularly women, are evaluated for disease. Inflammatory disorders, such as cholangitis (bile duct inflammation) and peritonitis, often obscure an underlying malignancy. Diagnostic procedures include ultrasonography and further imaging with suspicious findings.[233] Complete surgical resection of the gallbladder is the only effective treatment for early stages of disease, and recurrence is common. Complete removal of tumour tissue and lymph nodes with chemoradiation therapy is performed for more advanced stages. Because advanced malignancies cannot be resected, gallbladders containing stones are removed as a preventive measure. The prognosis of unresectable gallbladder cancer is extremely poor. Molecular therapies are under development.[234]

Cancer of the Pancreas

The Canadian Cancer Society estimated that 5 500 Canadians (2 800 men and 2 700 women) were diagnosed with pancreatic cancer in 2017. It also estimated that 4 800 Canadians (2 400 men and 2 400 women) died of this disease in 2017.[235]

The incidence of pancreatic cancer rises steadily with age. Males are affected slightly more often than females, and Blacks more often than

Whites. Mortality is nearly 100% at 5 years. The cause of pancreatic cancer is not known, but there are modest risks associated with tobacco smoking, certain dietary factors (e.g., high-fat foods and processed meat), obesity, diabetes mellitus, chronic pancreatitis, family history of pancreatic cancer, HNPCC (Lynch syndrome), and *BRCA1* and *BRCA2* mutations.[225]

PATHOPHYSIOLOGY Pancreatic cancer can arise from exocrine or endocrine cells. Most pancreatic tumours arise from metaplastic exocrine cells in the ducts and are called *ductal adenocarcinomas.* Chronic pancreatitis and inflammatory cytokines support tumour growth.[236] There is significant expansion of the extracellular matrix (stroma) from activation of pancreatic stellate cells, a type of fibroblast in the pancreas, that contributes to therapeutic resistance.[237] Tumours arising in small ducts invade nearby glandular tissue, penetrate the covering of the pancreas, and extend into surrounding tissues.[238] Tumours of the head of the pancreas quickly spread to obstruct the common bile duct and portal vein. These tumours can then infiltrate the superior mesenteric artery, the vena cava, and the aorta and form emboli. Tumours of the body and tail of the pancreas infiltrate the posterior abdominal wall. Lymphatic invasion occurs early and rapidly. Venous invasion causes metastases to the liver. Tumour implants on the peritoneal surface can obstruct veins and promote development of ascites.

CLINICAL MANIFESTATIONS Early stages of pancreatic cancer are asymptomatic. When symptoms occur there usually has been a malignant transformation. Typically, vague upper abdominal pain that radiates to the back develops. Jaundice arises in most cases, usually caused by obstruction of the bile duct. Because obstruction impairs enzyme secretion and flow to the duodenum, pancreatic cancer causes fat and protein malabsorption, resulting in weight loss. Distant metastases are found in the cervical lymph nodes, the lungs, and the brain. Most individuals die of hepatic failure, malnutrition, or systemic diseases.

EVALUATION AND TREATMENT There is no specific biomarker for pancreatic cancer and the diagnosis is usually made after the tumour has spread. Several molecular markers are under investigation.[239] Endoscopic ultrasound and CT are used initially for diagnosis.[239] Laparotomy is often used to establish a definitive diagnosis, evaluate the extent of disease, and determine whether palliative bypass surgery (i.e., cholecystojejunostomy and gastrojejunostomy) is needed. Many surgeons recommend a total pancreatectomy because cancer of the pancreas seldom consists of a single lesion. Adjuvant chemotherapy, immunotherapy, radiochemotherapy, and combination therapy may produce favourable controls in locally advanced cancer.[240] Pain management includes opioids and celiac plexus nerve block. Supportive therapy involves an interdisciplinary team.[241] Five-year survival is about 20% with resectable disease (a small subset) and less than 6% for metastatic disease. There is a need for new approaches for earlier diagnosis and more effective treatment.

QUICK CHECK 36-9

1. What are the primary risk factors for colorectal carcinoma?
2. Compare tumours of the right colon with those of the left colon.
3. What is the most common cause of liver cancer?

DID YOU UNDERSTAND?

Disorders of the Gastro-Intestinal Tract

1. Anorexia is lack of a desire to eat despite physiological stimuli that would normally produce hunger.
2. Vomiting is the forceful emptying of the stomach effected by gastro-intestinal (GI) contraction and reverse peristalsis of the esophagus. It is usually preceded by nausea and retching, with the exception of projectile vomiting, which is associated with direct stimulation of the vomiting centre in the brain.
3. Constipation is difficult or infrequent defecation often caused by unhealthy dietary and bowel habits combined with lack of exercise. Constipation can result from a disorder that impairs intestinal motility or obstructs the intestinal lumen.
4. Diarrhea is the presence of frequent loose, watery stools and can be caused by excessive fluid drawn into the intestinal lumen by osmosis (osmotic diarrhea), excessive secretion of fluids by the intestinal mucosa (secretory or infectious diarrhea), or excessive GI motility (motility diarrhea).
5. Abdominal pain is caused by stretching, inflammation, or ischemia (insufficient blood supply). Abdominal pain originates in the organs themselves (visceral pain) or in the peritoneum (parietal pain) and can be acute or chronic. Visceral pain is often referred to the back.
6. Obvious manifestations of GI bleeding are hematemesis (vomiting of blood), melena (dark, tarry stools), and hematochezia (frank bleeding from the rectum). Occult bleeding can be detected only by testing stools or vomitus for the presence of blood.
7. Dysphagia is difficulty swallowing. It can be caused by a mechanical or functional obstruction of the esophagus. Functional obstruction is an impairment of esophageal motility.
8. Achalasia is a form of functional dysphagia caused by loss of esophageal innervation.
9. Gastroesophageal reflux disease is the regurgitation of chyme from the stomach into the esophagus, resulting in an inflammatory response (reflux esophagitis) when the esophageal mucosa is repeatedly exposed to acids and enzymes in the regurgitated chyme.
10. Hiatal hernia is the protrusion of the upper part of the stomach through the hiatus (esophageal opening in the diaphragm) at the gastroesophageal junction. Hiatal hernia can be sliding or paraesophageal or a combination of both.
11. Gastroparesis is delayed gastric emptying in the absence of mechanical gastric outlet obstruction.
12. Pyloric obstruction is the narrowing or blockage of the pylorus, which is the opening between the stomach and the duodenum. It can be caused by a congenital defect, inflammation and scarring secondary to a gastric ulcer, or tumour growth.
13. Intestinal obstruction prevents the normal movement of chyme through the intestinal tract. It can be mechanical (i.e., caused by torsion, herniation, or tumour) or functional as a result of paralytic ileus.
14. The most severe consequences of intestinal obstruction are fluid and electrolyte losses, hypovolemia, shock, intestinal necrosis, and perforation of the intestinal wall.
15. Gastritis is an acute or chronic inflammation of the gastric mucosa.
16. Regurgitation of bile, use of anti-inflammatory drugs or alcohol, *Helicobacter pylori* infection, and some systemic diseases are associated with gastritis.
17. Chronic gastritis of the fundus (immune) and antrum (nonimmune) is the most severe form of gastritis. It can result in gastric atrophy and decreased secretion of hydrochloric acid, pepsinogen, and intrinsic factor.

18. Chronic gastritis of the antrum, the most common type, is not usually associated with impaired secretion or gastric atrophy.
19. A peptic ulcer is a circumscribed area of mucosal inflammation and ulceration caused by excessive secretion of gastric acid, disruption of the protective mucosal barrier, or infection with *H. pylori*.
20. Zollinger-Ellison syndrome is a rare syndrome associated with peptic ulcers caused by a gastrin-secreting neuroendocrine tumour or multiple tumours (gastrinoma) of the pancreas or duodenum.
21. There are three types of peptic ulcers: duodenal, gastric, and stress ulcers.
22. Duodenal ulcers, the most common peptic ulcers, are associated with *H. pylori* infection, chronic use of nonsteroidal anti-inflammatory drugs, increased numbers of parietal (acid-secreting) cells in the stomach, elevated gastrin levels, and rapid gastric emptying. Pain occurs when the stomach is empty, and it is relieved with food or antacids. Duodenal ulcers tend to heal spontaneously and recur frequently.
23. Gastric ulcers develop near parietal cells, generally in the antrum, and tend to become chronic. Gastric secretions may be normal or decreased, and pain may occur after eating.
24. Stress ulcers develop suddenly after severe illness, systemic trauma, or neural injury. Ulceration follows mucosal damage caused by ischemia (decreased blood flow to the gastric mucosa).
25. Cushing ulcer is a stress ulcer caused by head trauma. Ulceration follows hypersecretion of hydrochloric acid caused by overstimulation of the vagal nuclei.
26. Curling ulcer is associated with burn trauma.
27. Postgastrectomy syndromes are long-term complications that follow gastrectomy—the resection of all or part of the stomach. The postgastrectomy syndromes include dumping syndrome, alkaline reflux gastritis, afferent loop obstruction, diarrhea, weight loss, and anemia.
28. Dumping syndrome is the rapid emptying of chyme into the small intestine. It causes an osmotic shift of fluid from the vascular compartment to the intestinal lumen, which decreases plasma volume.
29. Alkaline reflux gastritis is stomach inflammation caused by the reflux of bile and pancreatic secretions from the duodenum into the stomach. These substances disrupt the mucosal barrier and cause inflammation.
30. Afferent loop obstruction is an obstruction of the duodenal stump on the proximal side of a gastrojejunostomy. Biliary and pancreatic secretions accumulate in the stump, causing distension, intermittent pain, and vomiting.
31. Malabsorption syndromes result in impaired digestion or absorption of nutrients and usually cause diarrhea.
32. Pancreatic exocrine insufficiency causes malabsorption associated with impaired digestion. The pancreas does not produce sufficient amounts of the enzymes that digest protein, carbohydrates, and fats into components that can be absorbed by the intestine.
33. Deficient lactase production in the brush border of the small intestine inhibits the breakdown of lactose. It prevents lactose absorption and causes osmotic diarrhea.
34. Bile salt deficiency causes fat malabsorption and steatorrhea (fatty stools). Bile salt deficiency can result from inadequate secretion of bile, excessive bacterial deconjugation of bile, or impaired reabsorption of bile salts caused by ileal disease.
35. Ulcerative colitis (UC) is a chronic inflammatory bowel disease that causes ulceration, abscess formation, and necrosis of the colonic and rectal mucosa. Cramping pain, bleeding, frequent diarrhea, dehydration, and weight loss accompany severe forms of the disease. A course of frequent remissions and exacerbations is common.
36. Crohn's disease (CD) is similar to UC but it affects the GI tract from the mouth to the anus and tends to involve all the layers of the intestinal lumen. "Skip lesion" fissures and granulomata are characteristic of CD. Abdominal tenderness, diarrhea, and weight loss are the usual symptoms.
37. Microscopic colitis is an inflammation that involves either mucosal lymphocytic infiltration or a thickened subepithelial collagen layer with symptoms of watery diarrhea.
38. Irritable bowel syndrome (IBS) is described as a functional disorder with recurring abdominal pain and bloating. IBS can be diarrhea prevalent or constipation prevalent or may alternate between diarrhea and constipation. Alterations in the brain–gut axis, gut microflora, gut immune responses, gut neuroendocrine cell function, genetic susceptibility, and epigenetic factors contribute to intestinal hypersensitivity, intestinal inflammation, increased permeability, and symptoms caused by alterations in motility and secretion.
39. Diverticula are outpouchings of colonic mucosa through the muscle layers of the colon wall. Diverticulosis is the presence of these outpouchings; diverticulitis is inflammation of the diverticula.
40. Appendicitis is the most common surgical emergency of the abdomen. Obstruction of the lumen leads to increased pressure, ischemia, and inflammation of the appendix. Without surgical resection, inflammation may progress to gangrene, perforation, and peritonitis.
41. Mesenteric vascular insufficiency in the intestine is most often associated with occlusion or obstruction of the mesenteric vessels or insufficient intestinal arterial blood flow. The resulting ischemia and necrosis produce abdominal pain, fever, bloody diarrhea, hypovolemia, and shock.
42. Obesity is a metabolic disorder with an increase in body fat mass and a BMI greater than 30.
43. The causes of obesity are complex and involve the interaction of adipokines produced by fat cells and other body weight control signals at the level of the hypothalamus. Metabolic dysregulation includes leptin resistance, insulin resistance, and a proinflammatory state that contribute to the complications of obesity.
44. Visceral obesity and normal weight obesity increase the risk of developing systemic inflammation, dyslipidemia, and insulin resistance with predisposition to atherosclerosis, hypertension, cardiovascular disease, cancer, and type 2 diabetes mellitus. Metabolically healthy obesity delays obesity-related complications until an older age.
45. Malnutrition is lack of nourishment from inadequate amounts of calories, protein, vitamins, or minerals. Starvation is an extreme state of malnutrition. Cachexia is physical wasting associated with chronic disease.
46. Short-term starvation, or lack of dietary intake for 3 or 4 days, stimulates mobilization of stored glucose by two metabolic processes: glycogenolysis (splitting of glycogen into glucose) and gluconeogenesis (formation of glucose from noncarbohydrate molecules).
47. Long-term starvation triggers the breakdown of ketone bodies and fatty acids. Eventually proteolysis (protein breakdown) begins, and death ensues if nutrition is not restored.

Disorders of the Accessory Organs of Digestion

1. Portal hypertension, ascites, hepatic encephalopathy, jaundice, and hepatorenal syndrome are complications of many liver disorders.
2. Portal hypertension is an elevation of portal venous pressure to at least 10 mm Hg. It is caused by increased resistance to venous flow

in the portal vein and its tributaries, including the sinusoids and hepatic vein.

3. Portal hypertension is the most serious complication of liver disease because it can cause potentially fatal complications, such as bleeding varices, ascites, and hepatic encephalopathy.
4. Varices (esophageal, gastric, hemorrhoidal) are distended, tortuous, collateral veins resulting from prolonged elevation of pressure in the portal vein.
5. Splenomegaly is enlargement of the spleen caused by increased pressure in the splenic vein, which branches from the portal vein.
6. Hepatopulmonary syndrome and portopulmonary hypertension are complications of portal hypertension caused by release of nitric oxide and carbon monoxide in the presence of liver injury.
7. Ascites is the accumulation and sequestration of fluid in the peritoneal cavity, often as a result of portal hypertension and decreased concentrations of plasma proteins.
8. Hepatic encephalopathy (portal-systemic encephalopathy) is impaired cerebral function caused by bloodborne toxins (particularly ammonia) not metabolized by the liver. Toxin-bearing blood may bypass the liver in collateral vessels opened as a result of portal hypertension, or diseased hepatocytes may be unable to carry out their metabolic functions.
9. Manifestations of hepatic encephalopathy range from confusion and asterixis (flapping tremor of the hands) to loss of consciousness, coma, and death.
10. Jaundice (icterus) is a yellow or greenish pigmentation of the skin or sclera of the eyes caused by increases in plasma bilirubin concentration (hyperbilirubinemia).
11. Obstructive jaundice is caused by obstructed bile canaliculi (intrahepatic obstructive jaundice) or obstructed bile ducts outside the liver (extrahepatic obstructive jaundice). Bilirubin accumulates proximal to the sites of obstruction, enters the bloodstream, and is carried to the skin and deposited.
12. Hemolytic jaundice is caused by destruction of red blood cells at a rate that exceeds the liver's ability to metabolize unconjugated bilirubin.
13. Hepatorenal syndrome is functional kidney failure caused by advanced liver disease, particularly cirrhosis with portal hypertension. Kidney failure is caused by a sudden decrease in blood flow to the kidneys usually caused by massive GI hemorrhage, liver failure, or inadequate circulating blood volume associated with ascites. The chief clinical manifestation is oliguria.
14. Acute liver failure is severe impairment or necrosis of liver cells with or without pre-existing liver disease or cirrhosis. It is commonly associated with acetaminophen overdose or as a complication of viral hepatitis.
15. Cirrhosis is an inflammatory disease of the liver that causes disorganization of lobular structure, fibrosis, and nodular regeneration. Cirrhosis can result from hepatitis or exposure to toxins, such as acetaldehyde (a product of alcohol metabolism). The disease causes progressive irreversible liver damage, usually over a period of years.
16. Alcoholic liver disease includes fatty liver and alcoholic steatohepatitis from accumulations of fat in the liver and is a precursor to alcoholic cirrhosis.
17. Alcoholic cirrhosis impairs the hepatocytes' ability to oxidize fatty acids, synthesize enzymes and proteins, degrade hormones, and clear portal blood of ammonia and toxins. The inflammatory response includes excessive collagen formation, fibrosis, and scarring, which obstruct bile canaliculi and sinusoids. Bile obstruction causes jaundice. Vascular obstruction causes portal hypertension, shunting, and varices.
18. Nonalcoholic fatty liver disease and nonalcoholic steatohepatitis involve accumulation of fat in the liver not associated with alcohol intake and are commonly associated with obesity.
19. Primary biliary cirrhosis is an autoimmune inflammatory destruction of intrahepatic bile ducts. Its cause is unknown.
20. Secondary biliary cirrhosis develops from prolonged obstruction of bile flow with increased pressure in the hepatic bile ducts that causes pooling of bile and necrosis of tissue. Relief of obstruction allays symptoms of jaundice and pruritus. Continued obstruction causes cirrhosis and liver failure.
21. Viral hepatitis is an infection of the liver caused by a strain of the hepatitis virus (i.e., hepatitis A virus, hepatitis B virus [HBV], hepatitis C virus, and hepatitis E virus). Although they differ with respect to modes of transmission and severity of acute illness, all can cause hepatic cell necrosis, Kupffer cell hyperplasia, and infiltration of liver tissue by mononuclear phagocytes. These changes obstruct bile flow and impair hepatocyte function.
22. The clinical manifestations of viral hepatitis depend on the stage of infection. Fever, malaise, anorexia, and liver enlargement and tenderness characterize the prodromal phase (stage 1). Jaundice and hyperbilirubinemia mark the icteric phase (stage 2). During the recovery phase (stage 3), symptoms resolve. Recovery takes several weeks.
23. Cholelithiasis (the formation of gallstones) is a common disorder of the gallbladder. Gallstones form in the bile as a result of the aggregation of cholesterol crystals (cholesterol stones) or precipitates of unconjugated bilirubin (pigmented stones). Gallstones that fill the gallbladder or obstruct the cystic or common bile duct cause abdominal pain and jaundice.
24. Cholecystitis is an acute or chronic inflammation of the gallbladder usually associated with obstruction of the cystic duct by gallstones.
25. Acute pancreatitis (pancreatic inflammation) is a serious but relatively rare disorder. Pancreatic duct obstruction and injury permits leakage of digestive enzymes into pancreatic tissue, where they become activated and begin the process of autodigestion, inflammation, and destruction of tissues. Release of pancreatic enzymes into the bloodstream or abdominal cavity causes damage to other organs.
26. Chronic pancreatitis results from structural or functional impairment of the pancreas. It causes recurrent abdominal pain and digestive disorders.

Cancer of the Digestive System

1. Cancer of the esophagus is rare and tends to occur in people older than 60 years of age. Alcohol and tobacco use, reflux esophagitis, and nutritional deficiencies are associated with esophageal carcinoma.
2. Dysphagia and chest pain are the primary manifestations of esophageal cancer. Early treatment of tumours that have not spread into the mediastinum or lymph nodes results in a good prognosis.
3. Gastric adenocarcinomas are associated with *H. pylori* that carries the *CagA* gene product cytotoxin-associated vacuolating antigen A, a diet high in salt and food preservatives (nitrates, nitrites), and atrophic gastritis.
4. Approximately 50% of all stomach cancers are located in the prepyloric antrum. Clinical manifestations (weight loss, upper abdominal pain, vomiting, hematemesis, anemia) develop only after the tumour has penetrated the wall of the stomach.
5. Pre-existing polyps are highly associated with adenocarcinoma of the colon. Familial adenomatous polyposis accounts for about 3 to 5% of colorectal cancer cases.

6. Tumours of the right (ascending or proximal) colon are usually large and bulky; tumours of the left (descending, sigmoid or distal) colon develop as small, buttonlike masses. Manifestations of colon tumours include pain, bloody stools, and a change in bowel habits.
7. Rectal carcinomas occur up to 15 cm from the opening of the anus. The tumour spreads transmurally to the vagina in women or the prostate in men.
8. Metastatic invasion of the liver is more common than primary cancer of the liver.
9. Primary liver cancers are associated with chronic liver disease (cirrhosis, hepatitis B). Hepatocellular carcinomas arise from the hepatocytes, whereas cholangiocellular carcinomas arise from the bile ducts. Primary liver cancer spreads to the heart, lungs, brain, kidney, and spleen through the circulation.
10. Cancer of the gallbladder occurs rarely before the age of 40 years and is most common between the ages of 50 and 60 years. Adenocarcinoma is the most common type. Because clinical manifestations occur late in the disease, metastases to lymph channels have usually occurred by the time of diagnosis, and the prognosis is poor.
11. Cancer of the pancreas is the fourth leading cause of cancer deaths in Canada. Most tumours are adenocarcinomas that arise in the exocrine cells of ducts in the head, body, or tail of the pancreas. Symptoms may not be evident until the tumour has spread to surrounding tissues. In Canada, on average, about 8% of people diagnosed with pancreatic cancer will survive for at least 5 years.

KEY TERMS

Achalasia, 925
Acute colonic pseudo-obstruction, 929
Acute gastritis, 930
Acute liver failure (fulminant liver failure), 947
Acute pancreatitis, 952
Adiponectin, 941
Afferent loop obstruction, 934
Alcoholic cirrhosis, 948
Alcoholic fatty liver (steatosis), 948
Alcoholic steatohepatitis (alcoholic hepatitis), 948
Alkaline reflux gastritis, 934
Anemia, 935
Anorexia, 921
Appendicitis, 939
Ascites, 944
Barrett esophagus, 955
Biliary cirrhosis, 949
Bone and mineral disorder, 935
Cachexia, 943
Cholangiocellular carcinoma (cholangiocarcinoma), 958
Cholecystitis, 951
Cholelithiasis, 951
Chronic active hepatitis, 951
Chronic gastritis, 931
Chronic pancreatitis, 953
Cirrhosis, 947
Colorectal polyp, 956
Constipation, 922
Crohn's disease (CD), 937
Curling ulcer, 933
Cushing ulcer, 933
Diarrhea, 935
Diverticula, 938
Diverticulitis, 938
Diverticulosis, 938
Dumping syndrome, 934
Duodenal ulcer, 932
Dysphagia, 925
Eosinophilic esophagitis, 927
Esophageal varices, 943
Familial adenomatous polyposis (FAP), 956
Gallstone, 951
Gastric ulcer, 933
Gastritis, 930
Gastroesophageal reflux disease (GERD), 926
Gastroparesis, 927
Ghrelin, 941
Gluconeogenesis, 943
Glycogenolysis, 942
Hematochezia, 924
Hemolytic jaundice, 946
Hepatic encephalopathy, 945
Hepatocellular carcinoma (HCC), 958
Hepatopulmonary syndrome, 943
Hepatorenal syndrome, 946
Hereditary nonpolyposis colorectal cancer (HNPCC), 956
Hiatal hernia, 927
Hyperbilirubinemia, 945
Icteric phase of hepatitis, 951
Incubation phase, 951
Intestinal obstruction, 928
Irritable bowel syndrome (IBS), 938
Ischemic ulcer, 933
Jaundice (icterus), 945
Lactase deficiency, 935
Large bowel obstruction, 929
Leptin, 941
Leptin resistance, 941
Long-term starvation, 943
Lower gastro-intestinal bleeding, 924
Lynch syndrome, 956
Malabsorption, 935
Maldigestion, 935
Malnutrition, 942
Melena, 924
Microscopic colitis, 938
Mixed hiatal hernia (type 3), 927
Motility diarrhea, 923
Nausea, 921
Neoplastic polyp, 956
Nonalcoholic fatty liver disease (NAFLD), 948
Nonalcoholic steatohepatitis (NASH), 948
Obesity, 940
Obstructive jaundice, 945
Occult bleeding, 924
Osmotic diarrhea, 922
Pancreatic cancer, 959
Pancreatic insufficiency, 935
Pancreatitis, 952
Paraesophageal hiatal hernia (type 2), 927
Paralytic ileus, 928
Parietal pain, 924
Peptic ulcer, 931
Peptide YY, 941
Portal hypertension, 943
Portopulmonary hypertension, 943
Primary biliary cirrhosis, 949
Prodromal (preicteric) phase of hepatitis, 951
Projectile vomiting, 922
Pyloric obstruction (gastric outlet obstruction), 927
Recovery phase of hepatitis, 951
Rectal carcinoma, 957
Refeeding syndrome, 943
Referred pain, 924
Retching, 921
Secondary biliary cirrhosis, 949
Secretory diarrhea, 923
Short-term starvation, 942
Sliding hiatal hernia (type 1), 927
Small bowel obstruction (SBO), 928
Small intestinal carcinoma, 956
Splenomegaly, 943
Starvation, 942
Steatorrhea, 923
Stress-related mucosal disease (stress ulcer), 933
Ulcerative colitis (UC), 937
Upper gastro-intestinal bleeding, 924
Varices, 943
Viral hepatitis, 950
Visceral pain, 924
Vomiting (emesis), 921
Weight loss, 935
Zollinger-Ellison syndrome, 931

REFERENCES

1. Babic, T., & Browning, K. N. (2014). The role of vagal neurocircuits in the regulation of nausea and vomiting. *European Journal of Pharmacology, 722*, 38–47. doi:10.1016/j.ejphar.2013.08.047.
2. Costilla, V. C., & Foxx-Orenstein, A. E. (2014). Constipation: Understanding mechanisms and management. *Clinics in Geriatric Medicine, 30*(1), 107–115. doi:10.1016/j.cger.2013.10.001.
3. Lacy, B. E., Levenick, J. M., & Crowell, M. (2012). Chronic constipation: New diagnostic and treatment approaches. *Therapeutic Advances in Gastroenterology, 5*(4), 233–247. doi:10.1177/1756283X12443093.
4. Costilla, V. C., & Foxx-Orenstein, A. E. (2014). Constipation in adults: Diagnosis and management. *Current Treatment Options in Gastroenterology, 12*(3), 310–321. doi:10.1007/s11938-014-0025-8.
5. Guerrant, R. L., Van Gilder, T., Steiner, T. S., et al. (2001). Practice guidelines for the management of infectious diarrhea. *Clinical Infectious Diseases, 32*(3), 331–351. doi:10.1086/318514.
6. World Gastroenterology Organisation. (2012). *Acute diarrhea in adults and children: A global perspective*. Retrieved from http://www.worldgastroenterology.org/guidelines/global-guidelines/acute-diarrhea/acute-diarrhea-english.
7. Dickinson, B., & Surawicz, C. M. (2014). Infectious diarrhea: An overview. *Current Gastroenterology Reports, 16*(8), 399. doi:10.1007/s11894-014-0399-8.
8. Schiller, L. R. (2012). Definitions, pathophysiology, and evaluation of chronic diarrhea. *Best Practice & Research. Clinical Gastroenterology, 26*(5), 551–562. doi:10.1016/j.bpg.2012.11.011.
9. Juckett, G., & Trivedi, R. (2011). Evaluation of chronic diarrhea. *American Family Physician, 84*(10), 1119–1126.
10. Millham, F. H. (2016). Acute abdominal pain. In M. Feldman, L. S. Friedman, & L. J. Brandt (Eds.), *Sleisenger and Fordtran's gastrointestinal and liver disease: Pathophysiology, diagnosis, management* (10th ed., pp. 161–174). Philadelphia: Saunders.
11. Vermeulen, W., De Man, J. G., Peickmans, P. A., et al. (2014). Neuroanatomy of lower gastrointestinal pain disorders. *World Journal of Gastroenterology, 20*(4), 1005–1020. doi:10.3748/wjg.v20.i4.1005.
12. Feinman, M., & Haut, E. R. (2014). Upper gastrointestinal bleeding. *The Surgical Clinics of North America, 94*(1), 43–53. doi:10.1016/j.suc.2013.10.004.
13. Sánchez-Capilla, A. D., De La Torre-Rubio, P., & Redondo-Cerezo, E. (2014). New insights to occult gastrointestinal bleeding: From pathophysiology to therapeutics. *World Journal of Gastrointestinal Pathophysiology, 5*(3), 271–283. doi:10.4291/wjgp.v5.i3.271.
14. Roden, D. F., & Altman, K. W. (2013). Causes of dysphagia among different age groups: A systematic review of the literature. *Otolaryngologic Clinics of North America, 46*(6), 965–987. doi:10.1016/j.otc.2013.08.008.
15. Kahrilas, P. J., & Boeckxstaens, G. (2013). The spectrum of achalasia: Lessons from studies of pathophysiology and high-resolution manometry. *Gastroenterology, 145*(5), 954–965. doi:10.1053/j.gastro.2013.08.038.
16. Richter, J. E. (2013). Esophageal motility disorder achalasia. *Current Opinion in Otolaryngology and Head and Neck Surgery, 21*(6), 535–542. doi:10.1097/MOO.0b013e3283658f4f.
17. Boeckxstaens, G., El-Serag, H. B., Smout, A. J., et al. (2014). Symptomatic reflux disease: The present, the past and the future. *Gut, 63*(7), 1185–1193. doi:10.1136/gutjnl-2013-306393.
18. Achem, S. R., & DeVault, K. R. (2014). Gastroesophageal reflux disease and the elderly. *Gastroenterology Clinics of North America, 43*(1), 147–160. doi:10.1016/j.gtc.2013.11.004.
19. Zerbib, F., Bruley des Varannes, S., Simon, M., et al. (2012). Functional heartburn: Definition and management strategies. *Current Gastroenterology Reports, 14*(3), 181–188. doi:10.1007/s11894-012-0255-7.
20. Mikami, D. J., & Murayama, K. M. (2015). Physiology and pathogenesis of gastroesophageal reflux disease. *The Surgical Clinics of North America, 95*(3), 515–525. doi:10.1016/j.suc.2015.02.006.
21. Hershcovici, T., & Fass, R. (2013). Step-by-step management of refractory gastroesophageal reflux disease. *Diseases of the Esophagus, 26*(1), 27–36. doi:10.1111/j.1442-2050.2011.01322.x.
22. Roman, S., & Kahrilas, P. J. (2014). The diagnosis and management of hiatus hernia. *BMJ (Clinical Research Ed.), 349*, g6154. doi:10.1136/bmj.g6154.
23. Schweigert, M., Dubecz, A., Ofner, D., et al. (2014). Gangrene of the oesophago-gastric junction caused by strangulated hiatal hernia: Operative challenge or surgical dead end. *Irish Journal of Medical Science, 183*(2), 323–330. doi:10.1007/s11845-013-0981-3.
24. Camilleri, M., Parkman, H. P., Shafi, M. A., et al. (2013). Clinical guideline: Management of gastroparesis. *The American Journal of Gastroenterology, 108*(1), 18–37. doi:10.1038/ajg.2012.373.
25. No, J. H., Kim, S. W., Lim, C. H., et al. (2013). Long-term outcome of palliative therapy for gastric outlet obstruction caused by unresectable gastric cancer in patients with good performance status: Endoscopic stenting versus surgery. *Gastrointestinal Endoscopy, 78*(1), 55–62. doi:10.1016/j.gie.2013.01.041.
26. Hucl, T. (2013). Acute GI obstruction. *Best Practice & Research. Clinical Gastroenterology, 27*(5), 691–707. doi:10.1016/j.bpg.2013.09.001.
27. Taylor, M. R., & Lalani, N. (2013). Adult small bowel obstruction. *Academic Emergency Medicine : Official Journal of the Society for Academic Emergency Medicine, 20*(6), 528–544. doi:10.1111/acem.12150.
28. Brown, C. V. (2014). Small bowel and colon perforation. *The Surgical Clinics of North America, 94*(2), 471–475. doi:10.1016/j.suc.2014.01.010.
29. Sawai, R. S. (2012). Management of colonic obstruction: A review. *Clinics in Colon and Rectal Surgery, 25*(4), 200–203. doi:10.1055/s-0032-1329533.
30. Lahner, E., & Annibale, B. (2009). Pernicious anemia: New insights from a gastroenterological point of view. *World Journal of Gastroenterology, 15*(41), 5121–5128.
31. Smolka, A. J., & Backert, S. (2012). How *Helicobacter pylori* infection controls gastric acid secretion. *Journal of Gastroenterology, 47*(6), 609–618. doi:10.1007/s00535-012-0592-1.
32. Levenstein, S., Rosenstock, S., Jacobsen, R. K., et al. (2014). Psychological stress increases risk for peptic ulcer, regardless of *Helicobacter pylori* infection or use of nonsteroidal anti-inflammatory drugs. *Clinical Gastroenterology and Hepatology, 13*(3), 498–506. doi:10.1016/j.cgh.2014.07.052.
33. Canadian Digestive Health Foundation. (2016). *Statistics (H. pylori)*. Retrieved from http://www.cdhf.ca/en/statistics#11.
34. Epelboym, I., & Mazeh, H. (2014). Zollinger-Ellison syndrome: Classical considerations and current controversies. *The Oncologist, 19*(1), 44–50. doi:10.1634/theoncologist.2013-0369.
35. Cekin, A. H., Taskoparan, M., Duman, A., et al. (2012). The role of *Helicobacter pylori* and NSAIDs in the pathogenesis of uncomplicated duodenal ulcer. *Gastroenterology Research and Practice, 2012*, 189373. doi:10.1155/2012/189373.
36. Gisbert, J. P., & Cakvet, X. (2009). Review article: *Helicobacter pylori*-negative duodenal ulcer disease. *Alimentary Pharmacology and Therapeutics, 30*(8), 791–815. doi:10.1111/j.1365-2036.2009.04105.x.
37. Graham, D. Y. (2014). History of *Helicobacter pylori*, duodenal ulcer, gastric ulcer and gastric cancer. *World Journal of Gastroenterology, 20*(18), 5191–5204. doi:10.3748/wjg.v20.i18.5191.
38. Nirula, R. (2014). Gastroduodenal perforation. *The Surgical Clinics of North America, 94*(1), 31–34. doi:10.1016/j.suc.2013.10.002.
39. Ubukata, H., Nagata, H., Tabuchi, T., et al. (2011). Why is the coexistence of gastric cancer and duodenal ulcer rare? Examination of factors related to both gastric cancer and duodenal ulcer. *Gastric Cancer, 14*(1), 4–12. doi:10.1007/s10120-011-0005-9.
40. Najm, W. I. (2011). Peptic ulcer disease. *Primary Care, 38*(3), 383–394, vii. doi:10.1016/j.pop.2011.05.001.
41. Patel, S. K., Pratap, C. B., Jain, A. K., et al. (2014). Diagnosis of *Helicobacter pylori*: What should be the gold standard? *World Journal of Gastroenterology, 20*(36), 12847–12859. doi:10.3748/wjg.v20.i36.12847.
42. Federico, A., Gravina, A. G., Miranda, A., et al. (2014). Eradication of *Helicobacter pylori* infection: Which regimen first? *World Journal of Gastroenterology, 20*(3), 665–672. doi:10.3748/wjg.v20.i3.665.
43. Bardou, M., Quenot, J. P., & Barkun, A. (2015). Stress-related mucosal disease in the critically ill patient. *Nature Reviews: Gastroenterology & Hepatology, 12*(2), 98–107. doi:10.1038/nrgastro.2014.235.
44. Bolton, J. S., & Conway, W. C., 2nd. (2011). Postgastrectomy syndromes. *The Surgical Clinics of North America, 91*(15), 1105–1122. doi:10.1016/j.suc.2011.07.001.
45. Ersan, Y., Karatas, A., Carkman, S., et al. (2009). Late results of patients undergoing remedial operations for alkaline reflux gastritis syndrome. *Acta Chirurgica Belgica, 109*(3), 364–370.
46. De Martino, C., Calazzo, P., Albano, M., et al. (2012). Acute afferent loop obstruction treated by endoscopic decompression. Case report and review of literature. *Annali Italiani Di Chirurgia, 83*(6), 555–558.
47. Tack, J., & Deloose, E. (2014). Complications of bariatric surgery: Dumping syndrome, reflux and vitamin deficiencies. *Best Practice & Research. Clinical Gastroenterology, 28*(4), 741–749. doi:10.1016/j.bpg.2014.07.010.
48. Lindkvist, B. (2013). Diagnosis and treatment of pancreatic exocrine insufficiency. *World Journal of Gastroenterology, 19*(42), 7258–7266. doi:10.3748/wjg.v19.i42.7258.
49. Levitt, M., Wilt, T., & Shaukat, A. (2013). Clinical implications of lactose malabsorption versus lactose intolerance. *Journal of Clinical Gastroenterology, 47*(6), 471–480. doi:10.1097/MCG.0b013e3182889f0f.
50. Barr, S. I. (2013). Perceived lactose intolerance in adult Canadians: A national survey. *Applied Physiology, Nutrition, and Metabolism, 38*(8), 830–835. doi:10.1139/apnm-2012-0368.
51. Johnston, I., Nolan, J., Pattni, S. S., et al. (2011). New insights into bile acid malabsorption. *Current Gastroenterology Reports, 13*(5), 418–425. doi:10.1007/s11894-011-0219-3.
52. Burisch, J., & Munkholm, P. (2013). Inflammatory bowel disease epidemiology. *Current Opinion in Gastroenterology, 29*(4), 357–362. doi:10.1097/MOG.0b013e32836229fb.
53. Laass, M. W., Roggenbruck, D., & Conrad, K. (2014). Diagnosis and classification of Crohn's disease. *Autoimmunity Reviews, 13*(4–5), 467–471. doi:10.1016/j.autrev.2014.01.029.
54. Zhang, Y. Z., & Li, Y. Y. (2014). Inflammatory bowel disease: Pathogenesis. *World Journal of Gastroenterology, 20*(1), 91–99. doi:10.3748/wjg.v20.i1.91.
55. Pedersen, G. (2015). Development, validation and implementation of an in vitro model for the study of metabolic and immune function in normal and inflamed human colonic epithelium. *Danish Medical Journal, 62*(1), B4973.
56. Beaugerie, L., & Itzkowitz, S. H. (2015). Cancers complicating inflammatory bowel disease. *The New*

England Journal of Medicine, 372(15), 1441–1452. doi:10.1056/NEJMra1403718.
57. Kostic, A. D., Xavier, R. J., & Gevers, D. (2014). The microbiome in inflammatory bowel disease: Current status and the future ahead. *Gastroenterology, 146*(6), 1489–1499. doi:10.1053/j.gastro.2014.02.009.
58. Mantzaris, G. J. (2014). When can we cure Crohn's? *Best Practice & Research: Clinical Gastroenterology, 28*(3), 519–529. doi:10.1016/j.bpg.2014.04.008.
59. Crohns and Colitis Foundation of Canada. (2012). *The impact of inflammatory bowel disease in Canada: 2012 final report and recommendations.* Toronto: Author. Retrieved from http://www.isupportibd.ca/pdf/ccfc-ibd-impact-report-2012.pdf.
60. Lunney, P. C., & Leong, R. W. (2012). Review article: Ulcerative colitis, smoking and nicotine therapy. *Alimentary Pharmacology and Therapeutics, 36*(11–12), 997–1008. doi:10.1111/apt.12086.
61. Feuerstein, J. D., & Cheifetz, A. S. (2014). Ulcerative colitis: Epidemiology, diagnosis, and management. *Mayo Clinic Proceedings, 89*(11), 1553–1563. doi:10.1016/j.mayocp.2014.07.002.
62. Tontini, G. E., Vecchi, M., Pastorelli, L., et al. (2015). Differential diagnosis in inflammatory bowel disease colitis: State of the art and future perspectives. *World Journal of Gastroenterology, 21*(1), 21–46. doi:10.3748/wjg.v21.i1.21.
63. Bressler, B., Marshall, J. K., Bernstein, C. N., et al. (2015). Clinical practice guidelines for the medical management of nonhospitalized ulcerative colitis: The Toronto Consensus. *Gastroenterology, 148*(5), 1035–1058.e3. doi:10.1053/j.gastro.2015.03.001.
64. Papi, C., Fasci-Spurio, F., Rogai, F., et al. (2013). Mucosal healing in inflammatory bowel disease: Treatment efficacy and predictive factors. *Digestive and Liver Disease, 45*(12), 978–985. doi:10.1016/j.dld.2013.07.006.
65. Dayan, B., & Turner, D. (2012). Role of surgery in severe ulcerative colitis in the era of medical rescue therapy. *World Journal of Gastroenterology, 18*(29), 3833–3838. doi:10.3748/wjg.v18.i29.3833.
66. Shen, B. (2012). Acute and chronic pouchitis—Pathogenesis, diagnosis and treatment. *Nature Reviews: Gastroenterology & Hepatology, 9*(6), 323–333. doi:10.1038/nrgastro.2012.58.
67. Cabré, E., & Domènech, E. (2012). Impact of environmental and dietary factors on the course of inflammatory bowel disease. *World Journal of Gastroenterology, 18*(29), 3814–3822. doi:10.3748/wjg.v18.i29.3814.
68. Cheifetz, A. S. (2013). Management of active Crohn disease. *The Journal of the American Medical Association, 309*(20), 2150–2158. doi:10.1001/jama.2013.4466.
69. Kane, J. S., Rotimi, O., Everett, S. M., et al. (2015). Development and validation of a scoring system to identify patients with microscopic colitis. *Clinical Gastroenterology and Hepatology, 13*(6), 1125–1131. doi:10.1016/j.cgh.2014.12.035.
70. Ohlsson, B. (2015). New insights and challenges in microscopic colitis. *Therapeutic Advances in Gastroenterology, 8*(1), 37–47. doi:10.1177/1756283X14550134.
71. Canavan, C., West, J., & Card, T. (2014). The epidemiology of irritable bowel syndrome. *Clin Epidemiology [Electronic Resource], 6*, 71–80. doi:10.2147/CLEP.S40245.
72. Bolino, C. M., & Bercik, P. (2010). Pathogenic factors involved in the development of irritable bowel syndrome: Focus on a microbial role. *Infectious Disease Clinics of North America, 24*(4), 961–975. doi:10.1016/j.idc.2010.07.005.
73. Catanzaro, R., Occhipinti, S., Calabrese, F., et al. (2015). Irritable bowel syndrome: New findings in pathophysiological and therapeutic field. *Minerva Gastroenterologica E Dietologica, 60*(2), 151–163.
74. Vaiopoulou, A., Karamanolis, G., Psaltopoulou, T., et al. (2014). Molecular basis of the irritable bowel syndrome. *World Journal of Gastroenterology, 20*(2), 376–383. doi:10.3748/wjg.v20.i2.376.
75. Mayer, E. A., Savidge, T., & Shulman, R. J. (2014). Brain–gut microbiome interactions and functional bowel disorders. *Gastroenterology, 146*(6), 1500–1512. doi:10.1053/j.gastro.2014.02.037.
76. Coss-Adame, E., & Rao, S. S. (2014). Brain and gut interactions in irritable bowel syndrome: New paradigms and new understandings. *Current Gastroenterology Reports, 16*(4), 379. doi:10.1007/s11894-014-0379-z.
77. Nasser, Y., Boeckxstaens, G. E., Wouters, M. M., et al. (2014). Using human intestinal biopsies to study the pathogenesis of irritable bowel syndrome. *Neurogastroenterology and Motility, 26*(4), 455–469. doi:10.1111/nmo.12316.
78. Beatty, J. K., Bhargava, A., & Buret, A. G. (2014). Post-infectious irritable bowel syndrome: Mechanistic insights into chronic disturbances following enteric infection. *World Journal of Gastroenterology, 20*(14), 3976–3985. doi:10.3748/wjg.v20.i14.3976.
79. Piche, T. (2014). Tight junctions and IBS—The link between epithelial permeability, low-grade inflammation, and symptom generation? *Neurogastroenterology and Motility, 26*(3), 296–302. doi:10.1111/nmo.12315.
80. Quigley, E. M. (2014). Small intestinal bacterial overgrowth: What it is and what it is not. *Current Opinion in Gastroenterology, 30*(2), 141–146. doi:10.1097/MOG.0000000000000040.
81. Ghoshal, U. C., & Srivastava, D. (2014). Irritable bowel syndrome and small intestinal bacterial overgrowth: Meaningful association or unnecessary hype. *World Journal of Gastroenterology, 20*(10), 2482–2491. doi:10.3748/wjg.v20.i10.2482.
82. El-Salhy, M., Gilja, O. H., Gundersen, D., et al. (2014). Interaction between ingested nutrients and gut endocrine cells in patients with irritable bowel syndrome (Review). *International Journal of Molecular Medicine, 34*(2), 363–371. doi:10.3892/ijmm.2014.1811.
83. Fukudo, S. (2013). Stress and visceral pain: Focusing on irritable bowel syndrome. *Pain, 154*(Suppl. 1), S63–S70. doi:10.1016/j.pain.2013.09.008.
84. Lovell, R. M., & Ford, A. C. (2012). Effect of gender on prevalence of irritable bowel syndrome in the community: Systematic review and meta-analysis. *The American Journal of Gastroenterology, 107*(7), 991–1000. doi:10.1038/ajg.2012.131.
85. Chey, W. D., Kurlander, J., & Eswaran, S. (2015). Irritable bowel syndrome: A clinical review. *JAMA: The Journal of the American Medical Association, 313*(9), 949–958. doi:10.1001/jama.2015.0954.
86. Sayuk, G. S., & Gyawali, C. P. (2015). Irritable bowel syndrome: Modern concepts and management options. *The American Journal of Medicine, 128*(8), 817–827. doi:10.1016/j.amjmed.2015.01.036.
87. Ferreira-Aparicio, F. E., Gutiérrez-Vega, R., Gálvez-Molina, Y., et al. (2012). Diverticular disease of the small bowel. *Case Reports in Gastroenterology, 6*(3), 668–676. doi:10.1159/000343598.
88. Tursi, A. (2015). The role of colonoscopy in managing diverticular disease of the colon. *Journal of Gastrointestinal and Liver Diseases, 24*(1), 85–93. doi:10.15403/jgld.2014.1121.tur.
89. Humes, D. J., & Spiller, R. C. (2014). Review article: The pathogenesis and management of acute colonic diverticulitis. *Alimentary Pharmacology and Therapeutics, 39*(4), 359–370. doi:10.1111/apt.12596.
90. Templeton, A. W., & Strate, L. L. (2013). Updates in diverticular disease. *Current Gastroenterology Reports, 15*(8), 339.
91. Tursi, A. (2014). New physiopathological and therapeutic approaches to diverticular disease: An update. *Expert Opinion on Pharmacotherapy, 15*(7), 1005–1017. doi:10.1517/14656566.2014.903922.
92. McDermott, F. D., Collins, D., Heeney, A., et al. (2014). Minimally invasive and surgical management strategies tailored to the severity of acute diverticulitis. *The British Journal of Surgery, 101*(1), e90–e99. doi:10.1002/bjs.9359.
93. Buckius, M. T., McGrath, B., Monk, J., et al. (2012). Changing epidemiology of acute appendicitis in the United States: Study period 1993–2008. *The Journal of Surgical Research, 175*(2), 185–190. doi:10.1016/j.jss.2011.07.017.
94. Vissers, R. J., & Lennarz, W. B. (2010). Pitfalls in appendicitis. *Emergency Medicine Clinics of North America, 28*(1), 103–118. doi:10.1016/j.emc.2009.09.003.
95. Drake, F. T., & Flum, D. R. (2013). Improvement in the diagnosis of appendicitis. *Advances in Surgery, 47*, 299–328.
96. (2015). Correction: Acute appendicitis—Appendectomy or the "antibiotics first" strategy. *The New England Journal of Medicine, 372*(23), 2274. doi:10.1056/NEJMx150021.
97. Bobadilla, J. L. (2013). Mesenteric ischemia. *The Surgical Clinics of North America, 93*(4), 925–940, ix. doi:10.1016/j.suc.2013.04.002.
98. Singal, A. K., Kamath, P. S., & Tefferi, A. (2013). Mesenteric venous thrombosis. *Mayo Clinic Proceedings, 88*(3), 285–294. doi:10.1016/j.mayocp.2013.01.012.
99. Sise, M. J. (2014). Acute mesenteric ischemia. *The Surgical Clinics of North America, 94*(1), 165–181. doi:10.1016/j.suc.2013.10.012.
100. Sundermeyer, A., Zapenki, A., Moysidis, T., et al. (2014). Endovascular treatment of chronic mesenteric ischemia. *Interventional Medicine & Applied Science, 6*(3), 118–124. doi:10.1556/IMAS.6.2014.3.4.
101. Acosta, S., & Björck, M. (2014). Modern treatment of acute mesenteric ischaemia. *The British Journal of Surgery, 101*(1), e100–e108. doi:10.1002/bjs.9330.
102. Flegal, K. M., Carroll, M. D., Kit, B. K., et al. (2012). Prevalence of obesity and trends in the distribution of body mass index among US adults, 1999–2010. *The Journal of the American Medical Association, 307*(5), 491–497. doi:10.1001/jama.2012.39.
103. Flegal, K. M., Kit, B. K., Orpana, H., et al. (2013). Association of all-cause mortality with overweight and obesity using standard body mass index categories: A systematic review and meta-analysis. *The Journal of the American Medical Association, 309*(1), 71–82. doi:10.1001/jama.2012.113905.
104. World Health Organization. (2016). *Obesity and overweight: Fact sheet.* Retrieved from http://www.who.int/mediacentre/factsheets/fs311/en.
105. Wang, Y., Beydoun, M. A., Liang, L., et al. (2008). Will all Americans become overweight or obese? Estimating the progression and cost of the U.S. obesity epidemic. *Obesity, 10*, 2323–2330. doi:10.1038/oby.2008.351.
106. Dixon, J. B. (2010). The effect of obesity on health outcomes. *Molecular and Cellular Endocrinology, 316*(2), 104–108. doi:10.1016/j.mce.2009.07.008.
107. Das, U. N. (2010). Obesity: Genes, brain, gut, and environment. *Nutrition, 26*(5), 459–473. doi:10.1016/j.nut.2009.09.020.
108. Cao, H. (2014). Adipocytokines in obesity and metabolic disease. *The Journal of Endocrinology, 220*(2), T47–T59. doi:10.1530/JOE-13-0339.
109. Ahima, R. S., & Antwi, D. A. (2008). Brain regulation of appetite and satiety. *Endocrinology and Metabolism Clinics of North America, 37*(4), 811–823. doi:10.1016/j.ecl.2008.08.005.
110. Jauch-Chara, K., & Oltmanns, K. M. (2014). Obesity—A neuropsychological disease? Systematic review and neuropsychological model. *Progress in Neurobiology, 114*, 84–101. doi:10.1016/j.pneurobio.2013.12.001.
111. Murray, S., Tulloch, A., Gold, M. S., et al. (2014). Hormonal and neural mechanisms of food reward, eating behaviour and obesity. *Nature Reviews: Endocrinology, 10*(9), 540–552. doi:10.1038/nrendo.2014.91.
112. Sáinz, N., Barrenexte, J., Moreno-Aliaga, M. J., et al. (2015). Leptin resistance and diet-induced obesity: Central and peripheral actions of leptin. *Metabolism: Clinical and Experimental, 64*(1), 35–46. doi:10.1016/j.metabol.2014.10.015.
113. Exley, M. A., Hand, L., O'Shea, D., et al. (2014). Interplay between the immune system and adipose tissue in obesity. *The Journal of Endocrinology, 223*(2), R41–R48. doi:10.1530/JOE-13-0516.
114. Jung, U. J., & Choi, M. S. (2014). Obesity and its metabolic complications: The role of adipokines

and the relationship between obesity, inflammation, insulin resistance, dyslipidemia and nonalcoholic fatty liver disease. *International Journal of Molecular Sciences, 15*(4), 6184–6223. doi:10.3390/ijms15046184.
115. Sam, S., & Mazzone, T. (2014). Adipose tissue changes in obesity and the impact on metabolic function. *Translational Research: The Journal of Laboratory and Clinical Medicine, 164*(4), 284–292. doi:10.1016/j.trsl.2014.05.008.
116. Palmer, B. F., & Clegg, D. J. (2015). The sexual dimorphism of obesity. *Molecular and Cellular Endocrinology, 402*, 113–119. doi:10.1016/j.mce.2014.11.029.
117. Goyal, A., Nimmakayala, K. R., & Zonstein, J. (2014). Is there a paradox in obesity? *Cardiology in Review, 22*(4), 163–170. doi:10.1097/CRD.0000000000000004.
118. Tchernof, A., & Després, J. P. (2013). Pathophysiology of human visceral obesity: An update. *Physiological Reviews, 93*(1), 359–404. doi:10.1152/physrev.00033.2011.
119. Oliveros, E., Somers, V. K., Sochor, O., et al. (2014). The concept of normal weight obesity. *Progress in Cardiovascular Diseases, 56*(4), 426–433. doi:10.1016/j.pcad.2013.10.003.
120. Marques-Vidal, P., Pécoud, A., Hayoz, D., et al. (2008). Prevalence of normal weight obesity in Switzerland: Effect of various definitions. *European Journal of Nutrition, 47*(5), 251–257. doi:10.1007/s00394-008-0719-6.
121. Kramer, C. K., Zinman, B., & Retnakaran, R. (2013). Are metabolically healthy overweight and obesity benign conditions? A systematic review and meta-analysis. *Annals of Internal Medicine, 159*(11), 758–769. doi:10.7326/0003-4819-159-11-201312030-00008.
122. Thibault, R., & Pichard, C. (2012). The evaluation of body composition: A useful tool for clinical practice. *Annals of Nutrition & Metabolism, 60*(1), 6–16. doi:10.1159/000334879.
123. Biro, F. M., & Wien, M. (2010). Childhood obesity and adult morbidities. *The American Journal of Clinical Nutrition, 91*(5), 1499S–1505S. doi:10.3945/ajcn.2010.28701B.
124. Joo, J. K., & Lee, K. S. (2014). Pharmacotherapy for obesity. *Journal of Menopausal Medicine, 20*(3), 90–96. doi:10.6118/jmm.2014.20.3.90.
125. Yanovski, S. Z., & Yanovski, J. A. (2014). Long-term drug treatment for obesity: A systematic and clinical review. *The Journal of the American Medical Association, 311*(1), 74–86. doi:10.1001/jama.2013.281361.
126. Aronne, L. J. (2014). Evolving directions in obesity management. *The Journal of Family Practice, 63*(7, Suppl.), S27–S33.
127. Colquitt, J. L., Pickett, K., Loveman, E., et al. (2014). Surgery for weight loss in adults. *The Cochrane Database of Systematic Reviews*, (8), CD003641, doi:10.1002/14651858.CD003641.pub4.
128. Mason, J. B. (2016). Nutritional principles and assessment of the gastroenterology patient. In M. Feldman, L. S. Friedman, & L. J. Brandt (Eds.), *Sleisenger and Fordtran's gastrointestinal and liver disease: Pathophysiology, diagnosis, management* (10th ed., pp. 57–82). Philadelphia: Saunders.
129. Walmsley, R. S. (2013). Refeeding syndrome: Screening, incidence, and treatment during parenteral nutrition. *Journal of Gastroenterology and Hepatology, 28*(Suppl. 4), 113–117. doi:10.1111/jgh.12345.
130. Suzuki, H., Asakawa, A., Amitani, H., et al. (2013). Cancer cachexia—Pathophysiology and management. *Journal of Gastroenterology, 48*(5), 574–594. doi:10.1007/s00535-013-0787-0.
131. Bloom, S., Kemp, W., & Lubel, J. (2015). Portal hypertension: Pathophysiology, diagnosis and management. *Internal Medicine Journal, 45*(1), 16–26. doi:10.1111/imj.12590.
132. Biecker, E. (2013). Portal hypertension and gastrointestinal bleeding: Diagnosis, prevention and management. *World Journal of Gastroenterology, 19*(31), 5035–5050. doi:10.3748/wjg.v19.i31.5035.
133. Møller, S., Henriksen, J. H., & Bendtsen, F. (2014). Extrahepatic complications to cirrhosis and portal hypertension: Haemodynamic and homeostatic aspects. *World Journal of Gastroenterology, 20*(42), 15499–15517. doi:10.3748/wjg.v20.i42.15499.
134. Tripathi, D., & Hayes, P. C. (2014). Beta-blockers in portal hypertension: New developments and controversies. *Liver International, 34*(5), 655–667. doi:10.1111/liv.12360.
135. Liou, I. W. (2014). Management of end-stage liver disease. *The Medical Clinics of North America, 98*(1), 119–152. doi:10.1016/j.mcna.2013.09.006.
136. Hou, W., & Sanyal, A. J. (2009). Ascites: Diagnosis and management. *The Medical Clinics of North America, 93*(4), 801–817. doi:10.1016/j.mcna.2009.03.007.
137. Pedersen, J. S., Bendtsen, F., & Møller, S. (2015). Management of cirrhotic ascites. *Therapeutic Advances in Chronic Disease, 6*(3), 124–137. doi:10.1177/2040622315580069.
138. Sturgeon, J. P., & Shawcross, D. L. (2014). Recent insights into the pathogenesis of hepatic encephalopathy and treatments. *Expert Review of Gastroenterology & Hepatology, 8*(1), 83–100. doi:10.1586/17474124.2014.858598.
139. Vilstrup, H., Amodio, P., Bajaj, J., et al. (2014). Hepatic encephalopathy in chronic liver disease. 2014 practice guideline by the European Association for the Study of the Liver and the American Association for the Study of Liver Diseases. *Journal of Hepatology, 61*(3), 642–659. doi:10.1016/j.jhep.2014.05.042.
140. Amodio, P., Bemeur, C., Butterworth, R., et al. (2013). The nutritional management of hepatic encephalopathy in patients with cirrhosis: International Society for Hepatic Encephalopathy and Nitrogen Metabolism Consensus. *Hepatology (Baltimore, Md.), 58*(1), 325–336. doi:10.1002/hep.26370.
141. Bañares, R., Catalina, M. V., & Vaquero, J. (2014). Molecular adsorbent recirculating system and bioartificial devices for liver failure. *Clinics in Liver Disease, 18*(4), 945–956. doi:10.1016/j.cld.2014.07.011.
142. Winger, J., & Michelfelder, A. (2011). Diagnostic approach to the patient with jaundice. *Primary Care, 38*(3), 469–482, viii. doi:10.1016/j.pop.2011.05.004.
143. Roche, S. P., & Kobos, R. (2004). Jaundice in the adult patient. *American Family Physician, 69*(2), 299–304.
144. Low, G., Alexander, G. J., & Lomas, D. J. (2015). Hepatorenal syndrome: Aetiology, diagnosis, and treatment. *Gastroenterology Research and Practice, 2015*, 207012. doi:10.1155/2015/207012.
145. Barbano, B., Sardo, L., Gigante, A., et al. (2014). Pathophysiology, diagnosis and clinical management of hepatorenal syndrome: From classic to new drugs. *Current Vascular Pharmacology, 12*(1), 125–135. doi:10.2174/1570161111201140327163930.
146. Stem Cell Network. (2013). *Liver failure*. Ottawa: Author. Retrieved from http://oirm.ca/sites/default/files/disease-liver_failure.pdf.
147. Moreau, R., Jalan, R., & Arroyo, V. (2015). Acute-on-chronic liver failure: Recent concepts. *Journal of Clinical and Experimental Hepatology, 5*(1), 81–85. doi:10.1016/j.jceh.2014.09.003.
148. Shalimar, & Acharya, S. K. (2015). Management in acute liver failure. *Journal of Clinical and Experimental Hepatology, 5*(Suppl. 1), S104–S115. doi:10.1016/j.jceh.2014.11.005.
149. O'Grady, J. (2014). Timing and benefit of liver transplantation in acute liver failure. *Journal of Hepatology, 60*(3), 663–670. doi:10.1016/j.jhep.2013.10.024.
150. Novo, E., Cannito, S., Paternostro, C., et al. (2014). Cellular and molecular mechanisms in liver fibrogenesis. *Archives of Biochemistry and Biophysics, 548*, 20–37. doi:10.1016/j.abb.2014.02.015.
151. Canadian Liver Foundation. (2013). *Liver disease in Canada. A crisis in the making*. Markham, ON: Author. Retrieved from http://www.liver.ca/files/PDF/Liver_Disease_Report_2013/Liver_Disease_in_Canada_-_E.pdf.
152. Huang, Y. W., Yang, S. S., & Kao, J. H. (2011). Pathogenesis and management of alcoholic liver cirrhosis: A review. *Hepatic Medicine, 3*, 1–11. doi:10.2147/HMER.S10265.
153. Eagon, P. K. (2010). Alcoholic liver injury: Influence of gender and hormones. *World Journal of Gastroenterology, 16*(11), 1377–1384. doi:10.3748/wjg.v16.i11.1377.
154. Division of Population Health, National Center for Chronic Disease Prevention and Health Promotion (2012). *Alcohol and public health*. Atlanta, GA: Centers for Disease Control and Prevention.
155. Wiegand, J., & Berg, T. (2013). The etiology, diagnosis and prevention of liver cirrhosis: Part 1 of a series on liver cirrhosis. *Deutsches Ärzteblatt International, 110*(6), 85–91. doi:10.3238/arztebl.2013.0085.
156. Cubero, F. J., Urtasun, R., & Nieto, N. (2009). Alcohol and liver fibrosis. *Seminars in Liver Disease, 29*(2), 211–221. doi:10.1055/s-0029-1214376.
157. Setshedi, M., Wands, J. R., & Monte, S. M. (2010). Acetaldehyde adducts in alcoholic liver disease. *Oxidative Medicine and Cellular Longevity, 3*(3), 178–185. doi:10.4161/oxim.3.3.12288.
158. Orman, E. S., Odena, G., & Bataller, R. (2013). Alcoholic liver disease: Pathogenesis, management, and novel targets for therapy. *Journal of Gastroenterology and Hepatology, 28*(Suppl. 1), 77–84. doi:10.1111/jgh.12030.
159. Struecker, B., Raschzok, N., & Sauer, I. M. (2014). Liver support strategies: Cutting-edge technologies. *Nature Reviews: Gastroenterology & Hepatology, 11*(3), 166–176. doi:10.1038/nrgastro.2013.204.
160. Corrado, R. L., Torres, D. M., & Harrison, S. A. (2014). Review of treatment options for nonalcoholic fatty liver disease. *The Medical Clinics of North America, 98*(1), 55–72. doi:10.1016/j.mcna.2013.09.001.
161. Rinella, M. E. (2015). Nonalcoholic fatty liver disease: A systematic review. *The Journal of the American Medical Association, 313*(22), 2263–2273. doi:10.1001/jama.2015.5370.
162. Purohit, T., & Cappell, M. S. (2015). Primary biliary cirrhosis: Pathophysiology, clinical presentation and therapy. *World Journal of Hepatology, 7*(7), 926–941. doi:10.4254/wjh.v7.i7.926.
163. Jayakumar, S., Chowdhury, R., Ye, C., et al. (2013). Fulminant viral hepatitis. *Critical Care Clinics, 29*(3), 677–697. doi:10.1016/j.ccc.2013.03.013.
164. Price, J. (2014). An update on hepatitis B, D, and E viruses. *Topics in Antiviral Medicine, 21*(5), 157–163.
165. Aydeniz, A., Namiduru, M., Karaoglan, I., et al. (2010). Rheumatic manifestations of hepatitis B and C and their association with viral load and fibrosis of the liver. *Rheumatology International, 30*(4), 515–517. doi:10.1007/s00296-009-1010-8.
166. Chacko, E. C., Surrun, S. K., Mubarack Sani, T. P., et al. (2010). Chronic viral hepatitis and chronic kidney disease. *Postgraduate Medical Journal, 86*(1018), 486–492. doi:10.1136/pgmj.2009.092775.
167. Trépo, C., Chan, H. L., & Lok, A. (2014). Hepatitis B virus infection. *Lancet, 384*(9959), 2053–2063. doi:10.1016/S0140-6736(14)60220-8.
168. Alvarado-Mora, M. V., Locarini, S., Rizzetto, M., et al. (2014). An update on HDV: Virology, pathogenesis and treatment. *Antiviral Therapy, 18*(3 Pt. B), 541–548. doi:10.3851/IMP2598.
169. Pérez-Gracia, M. T., Suay, B., & Mateos-Lindemann, M. L. (2014). Hepatitis E: An emerging disease. *Infection, Genetics and Evolution: Journal of Molecular Epidemiology and Evolutionary Genetics in Infectious Diseases, 22*, 40–59. doi:10.1016/j.meegid.2014.01.002.
170. Halegoua-De Marzio, D., & Hann, H. W. (2014). Then and now: The progress in hepatitis B treatment over the past 20 years. *World Journal of Gastroenterology, 20*(2), 401–413. doi:10.3748/wjg.v20.i2.401.
171. Kohli, A., Shaffer, A., Sherman, A., et al. (2014). Treatment of hepatitis C: A systematic review. *The Journal of the American Medical Association, 312*(6), 631–640. doi:10.1001/jama.2014.7085.
172. Sánchez, G., Bosch, A., & Pintó, R. M. (2007). Hepatitis A virus detection in food: Current and

future prospects. *Letters in Applied Microbiology, 45*(1), 1–5. doi:10.1111/j.1472-765X.2007.02140.x.
173. Honegger, J. R., Zhou, Y., & Walker, C. M. (2014). Will there be a vaccine to prevent HCV infection? *Seminars in Liver Disease, 34*(1), 79–88. doi: 10.1055/s-0034-1371081.
174. Government of Canada. (2015). *Prevention of hepatitis E.* Retrieved from https://www.canada.ca/en/public-health/services/diseases/hepatitis-e/prevention-hepatitis-e.html#s1.
175. Stinton, L. M., & Shaffer, E. A. (2012). Epidemiology of gallbladder disease: Cholelithiasis and cancer. *Gut and Liver, 6*(2), 172–187. doi:10.5009/gnl.2012.6.2.172.
176. Canadian Liver Foundation. (2016). *Gallstones.* Retrieved from http://www.liver.ca/liver-disease/types/gallstones.aspx.
177. Reshetnyak, V. I. (2012). Concept of the pathogenesis and treatment of cholelithiasis. *World Journal of Hepatology, 4*(2), 18–34. doi:10.4254/wjh.v4.i2.18.
178. O'Connell, K., & Brasel, K. (2014). Bile metabolism and lithogenesis. *The Surgical Clinics of North America, 94*(2), 361–375. doi:10.1016/j.suc.2014.01.004.
179. Gaby, A. R. (2009). Nutritional approaches to prevention and treatment of gallstones. *Alternative Medicine Review, 14*(3), 258–267.
180. Itoi, T., & Wang, H. P. (2010). Endoscopic management of bile duct stones. *Digestive Endoscopy, 22*(Suppl. 1), S69–S75. doi:10.1111/j.1443-1661.2010.00953.x.
181. Barie, P. S., & Eachempati, S. R. (2010). Acute acalculous cholecystitis. *Gastroenterology Clinics of North America, 39*(2), 343–357, x. doi:10.1016/j.gtc.2010.02.012.
182. Knab, L. M., Boller, A. M., & Mahvi, D. M. (2014). Cholecystitis. *The Surgical Clinics of North America, 94*(2), 455–470. doi:10.1016/j.suc.2014.01.005.
183. Canadian Digestive Health Foundation. (2016). *Pancreatitis.* Retrieved from http://www.cdhf.ca/en/statistics#22.
184. Lankisch, P. G., Apte, M., & Banks, P. A. (2015). Acute pancreatitis. *Lancet, 386*(9988), 85–96. doi:10.1016/S0140-6736(14)60649-8.
185. Sah, R. P., Dawra, R. K., & Saluja, A. K. (2013). New insights into the pathogenesis of pancreatitis. *Current Opinion in Gastroenterology, 29*(5), 523–530. doi:10.1097/MOG.0b013e328363e399.
186. Muniraj, T., Aslanian, H. R., Farrell, J., et al. (2014). Chronic pancreatitis, a comprehensive review and update. Part I: Epidemiology, etiology, risk factors, genetics, pathophysiology, and clinical features. *Disease-A-Month, 60*(12), 530–550. doi:10.1016/j.disamonth.2014.11.002.
187. Bakker, O. J., Issa, Y., van Santvoort, H. C., et al. (2014). Treatment options for acute pancreatitis. *Nature Reviews: Gastroenterology & Hepatology, 11*(8), 462–469. doi:10.1038/nrgastro.2014.39.
188. Brock, C., Nielsen, L. M., Lelic, D., et al. (2013). Pathophysiology of chronic pancreatitis. *World Journal of Gastroenterology, 19*(42), 7231–7240. doi:10.3748/wjg.v19.i42.7231.
189. Sze, K. C., Pirola, R. C., Apte, M. V., et al. (2014). Current options for the diagnosis of chronic pancreatitis. *Expert Review of Molecular Diagnostics, 14*(2), 199–215. doi:10.1586/14737159.2014.883277.
190. Poulsen, J. L., Olesen, S. S., Malver, L. P., et al. (2013). Pain and chronic pancreatitis: A complex interplay of multiple mechanisms. *World Journal of Gastroenterology, 19*(42), 7282–7291. doi:10.3748/wjg.v19.i42.7282.
191. Johnson, M. D., Walsh, R. M., Henderson, J. M., et al. (2009). Surgical versus nonsurgical management of pancreatic pseudocysts. *Journal of Clinical Gastroenterology, 43*(6), 586–590. doi:10.1097/MCG.0b013e31817440be.
192. Canadian Cancer Society. (2017). *Esophageal cancer statistics.* Retrieved from http://www.cancer.ca/en/cancer-information/cancer-type/esophageal/statistics/?region=bc#ixzz4SASyuSY8.
193. Shimizu, M., Zaninotto, G., Nagata, K., et al. (2013). Esophageal squamous cell carcinoma with special reference to its early stage. *Best Practice & Research: Clinical Gastroenterology, 27*(2), 171–186. doi:10.1016/j.bpg.2013.03.010.
194. Halland, M., Katzka, D., & Iyer, P. G. (2015). Recent developments in pathogenesis, diagnosis and therapy of Barrett's esophagus. *World Journal of Gastroenterology, 21*(21), 6479–6490. doi:10.3748/wjg.v21.i21.6479.
195. Xie, F. J., Zhang, Y. P., Zheng, Q. Q., et al. (2013). *Helicobacter pylori* infection and esophageal cancer risk: An updated meta-analysis. *World Journal of Gastroenterology, 19*(36), 6098–6107. doi:10.3748/wjg.v19.i36.6098.
196. Spechler, S. J. (2013). Barrett esophagus and risk of esophageal cancer: A clinical review. *The Journal of the American Medical Association, 310*(6), 627–636. doi:10.1001/jama.2013.226450.
197. Cowie, A., Noble, F., & Underwood, T. (2014). Strategies to improve outcomes in esophageal adenocarcinoma. *Expert Review of Anticancer Therapy, 14*(6), 677–687. doi:10.1586/14737140.2014.895668.
198. Nakajima, M., & Kato, H. (2013). Treatment options for esophageal squamous cell carcinoma. *Expert Opinion on Pharmacotherapy, 14*(10), 1345–1354. doi:10.1517/14656566.2013.801454.
199. Canadian Cancer Society. (2017). *Stomach cancer statistics.* Retrieved from https://www.cancer.ca/en/cancer-information/cancer-type/stomach/statistics/?region=on.
200. Canadian Cancer Society, & Government of Canada. (2015). *Cancer statistics 2015: Special topic: Predictions of the future burden of cancer in Canada.* Toronto: Author. Retrieved from https://www.cancer.ca/~/media/cancer.ca/CW/cancer%20information/cancer%20101/Canadian%20cancer%20statistics/Canadian-Cancer-Statistics-2015-EN.pdf.
201. Fock, K. M. (2014). Review article: The epidemiology and prevention of gastric cancer. *Alimentary Pharmacology and Therapeutics, 40*(3), 250–260. doi:10.1111/apt.12814.
202. de Martel, C., Forman, D., & Plummer, M. (2013). Gastric cancer: Epidemiology and risk factors. *Gastroenterology Clinics of North America, 42*(2), 219–240. doi:10.1016/j.gtc.2013.01.003.
203. Resende, C., Ristimäki, A., & Machado, J. C. (2010). Genetic and epigenetic alteration in gastric carcinogenesis. *Helicobacter, 15*(Suppl. 1), 3434–3439. doi:10.1111/j.1523-5378.2010.00782.x.
204. Yakirevich, E., & Resnick, M. B. (2013). Pathology of gastric cancer and its precursor lesions. *Gastroenterology Clinics of North America, 42*(2), 261–284. doi:10.1016/j.gtc.2013.01.004.
205. Wu, H. H., Lin, W. C., & Tsai, K. W. (2014). Advances in molecular biomarkers for gastric cancer: miRNAs as emerging novel cancer markers. *Expert Reviews in Molecular Medicine, 16*, e1. doi:10.1017/erm.2013.16.
206. Blakely, A. M., & Miner, T. J. (2013). Surgical considerations in the treatment of gastric cancer. *Gastroenterology Clinics of North America, 42*(2), 337–357. doi:10.1016/j.gtc.2013.01.010.
207. Canadian Cancer Society. (2016). *Colorectal cancer statistics.* Retrieved from http://www.cancer.ca/en/cancer-information/cancer-type/colorectal/statistics/?region=on#ixzz4SAeT4t3q.
208. Tammana, V. S., & Laiyemo, A. O. (2014). Colorectal cancer disparities: Issues, controversies and solutions. *World Journal of Gastroenterology, 20*(4), 869–876. doi:10.3748/wjg.v20.i4.869.
209. Cunningham, D., Atkin, W., Lenz, H. J., et al. (2010). Colorectal cancer. *Lancet, 375*(9719), 1030–1047. doi:10.1016/S0140-6736(10)60353-4.
210. Jasperson, K., Tuohy, T. M., Neklason, D. W., et al. (2010). Hereditary and familial colon cancer. *Gastroenterology, 138*(6), 2044–2058. doi:10.1053/j.gastro.2010.01.054.
211. Kalady, M. F. (2013). Sessile serrated polyps: An important route to colorectal cancer. *Journal of the National Comprehensive Cancer Network, 11*(12), 1585–1594.
212. Zoratto, F., Rossi, L., Verrico, M., et al. (2014). Focus on genetic and epigenetic events of colorectal cancer pathogenesis: Implications for molecular diagnosis. *Tumour Biology, 35*(7), 6195–6206. doi:10.1007/s13277-014-1845-9.
213. Aparicio, T., Zaanan, A., Svrcek, M., et al. (2014). Small bowel adenocarcinoma: Epidemiology, risk factors, diagnosis and treatment. *Digestive and Liver Disease, 46*(2), 97–104. doi:10.1016/j.dld.2013.04.013.
214. Lee, G. H., Malietzis, G., Askari, A., et al. (2014). Is right-sided colon cancer different to left-sided colorectal cancer? A systematic review. *European Journal of Surgical Oncology, 41*(3), 300–308. doi:10.1016/j.ejso.2014.11.001.
215. Song, M., Garrett, W. S., & Chan, A. T. (2015). Nutrients, foods, and colorectal cancer prevention. *Gastroenterology, 148*(6), 1244–1260.e16. doi:10.1053/j.gastro.2014.12.035.
216. Tan, Y. N., Li, X. F., Li, J. J., et al. (2014). The accuracy of computed tomography in the pretreatment staging of colorectal cancer. *Hepato-Gastroenterology, 61*(133), 1207–1212.
217. Canadian Cancer Society. (2017). *Staging colon cancer.* Retrieved from http://www.cancer.ca/en/cancer-information/cancer-type/colorectal/staging/?region=on.
218. Grady, W. M., & Pritchard, C. C. (2014). Molecular alterations and biomarkers in colorectal cancer. *Toxicologic Pathology, 42*(1), 124–139. doi:10.1177/0192623313505155.
219. Linnekamp, J. F., Wang, X., Medema, J. P., et al. (2015). Colorectal cancer heterogeneity and targeted therapy: A case for molecular disease subtypes. *Cancer Research, 75*(2), 245–249. doi:10.1158/0008-5472.CAN-14-2240.
220. Allard, M. A., & Malka, D. (2014). Place of hepatic intra-arterial chemotherapy in the treatment of colorectal liver metastases. *Journal of Vascular Surgery, 151*(Suppl. 1), S21–S24. doi:10.1016/j.jviscsurg.2013.12.003.
221. Sorbye, H. (2014). Recurrence patterns after resection of liver metastases from colorectal cancer. *Recent Results in Cancer Research, 203*, 243–252. doi:10.1007/978-3-319-08060-4_17.
222. Bosetti, C., Turati, F., & La Vecchia, C. (2014). Hepatocellular carcinoma epidemiology. *Best Practice & Research: Clinical Gastroenterology, 28*(5), 753–770. doi:10.1016/j.bpg.2014.08.007.
223. Canadian Cancer Society. (2013). *Liver cancer on the rise.* Retrieved from http://www.cancer.ca/en/about-us/for-media/media-releases/national/2013/liver-cancer-on-the-rise-cancer-statistics/?region=on.
224. Nault, J. C. (2014). Pathogenesis of hepatocellular carcinoma according to aetiology. *Best Practice & Research: Clinical Gastroenterology, 28*(5), 937–947. doi:10.1016/j.bpg.2014.08.006.
225. American Cancer Society (2015). *Cancer facts and figures 2015.* Atlanta: Author.
226. Canadian Cancer Society. (2017). *Liver cancer statistics.* Retrieved from http://www.cancer.ca/en/cancer-information/cancer-type/liver/statistics/?region=on.
227. Razumilava, N., & Gores, G. J. (2014). Cholangiocarcinoma. *Lancet, 383*(9935), 2168–2179. doi:10.1016/S0140-6736(13)61903-0.
228. Colombo, M., & Iavarone, M. (2014). Role of antiviral treatment for HCC prevention. *Best Practice & Research: Clinical Gastroenterology, 28*(5), 771–781. doi:10.1016/j.bpg.2014.07.017.
229. Rasool, M., Rashid, S., Arooj, M., et al. (2014). New possibilities in hepatocellular carcinoma treatment. *Anticancer Research, 34*(4), 1563–1571.
230. Weledji, E. P., Enow Orock, G., Ngowe, M. N., et al. (2014). How grim is hepatocellular carcinoma? *Annals of Medicine and Surgery, 3*(3), 71–76. doi:10.1016/j.amsu.2014.06.006.
231. Canadian Cancer Society. (2017). *Gallbladder cancer statistics.* Retrieved from http://www.cancer.ca/en/cancer-information/cancer-type/gallbladder/statistics/?region=bc.
232. Maurya, S. K., Tewari, M., Mishra, R. R., et al. (2012). Genetic aberrations in gallbladder cancer. *Surgical Oncology, 21*(1), 37–43. doi:10.1016/j.suronc.2010.09.003.

233. Wernberg, J. A., & Lucarelli, D. D. (2014). Gallbladder cancer. *The Surgical Clinics of North America*, *94*(2), 343–360. doi:10.1016/j.suc.2014.01.009.
234. Marino, D., Leone, F., Cavalloni, G., et al. (2013). Biliary tract carcinomas: From chemotherapy to targeted therapy. *Critical Reviews in Oncology/Hematology*, *85*(2), 136–148. doi:10.1016/j.critrevonc.2012.06.006.
235. Canadian Cancer Society. (2017). *Pancreatic cancer statistics.* Retrieved from http://www.cancer.ca/en/cancer-information/cancer-type/pancreatic/statistics/?region=on.
236. Roshani, R., McCarthy, F., & Hagemann, T. (2014). Inflammatory cytokines in human pancreatic cancer. *Cancer Letters*, *345*(2), 157–163. doi:10.1016/j.canlet.2013.07.014.
237. Lunardi, S., Muschel, R. J., & Brunner, T. B. (2014). The stromal compartments in pancreatic cancer: Are there any therapeutic targets? *Cancer Letters*, *343*(2), 147–155. doi:10.1016/j.canlet.2013.09.039.
238. Pinho, A. V., Chantrill, L., & Rooman, I. (2014). Chronic pancreatitis: A path to pancreatic cancer. *Cancer Letters*, *345*(2), 203–209. doi:10.1016/j.canlet.2013.08.015.
239. Poruk, K. E., Firpo, M. A., & Mulvihill, S. J. (2014). Screening for pancreatic cancer. *Advances in Surgery*, *48*, 115–136. doi:10.1016/j.yasu.2014.05.004.
240. Mian, O. Y., Ram, A. N., Tuli, R., et al. (2014). Management options in locally advanced pancreatic cancer. *Current Oncology Reports*, *16*(6), 388. doi:10.1007/s11912-014-0388-y.
241. Erdek, M. A., King, L. M., & Ellsworth, S. G. (2013). Pain management and palliative care in pancreatic cancer. *Current Problems in Cancer*, *37*(5), 266–272. doi:10.1016/j.currproblcancer.2013.10.003.

37

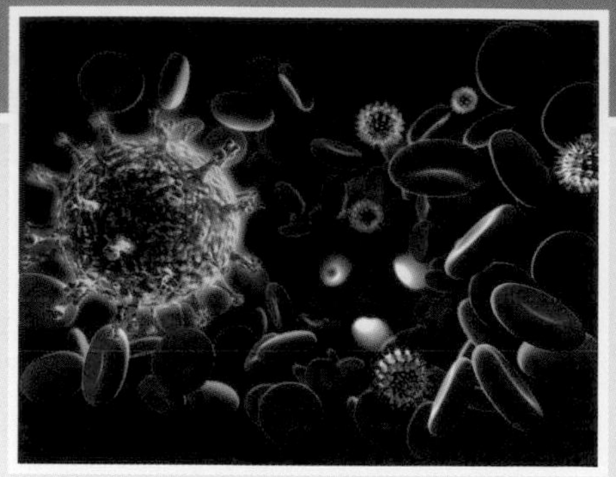

Alterations of Digestive Function in Children

Sharon Sables-Baus, Sara J. Fidanza, and Mohamed El-Hussein

EVOLVE WEBSITE

http://evolve.elsevier.com/Canada/Huether/pathophysiology
Student Review Questions
Key Points
Case Studies
Animations
Quick Check Answers

CHAPTER OUTLINE

Disorders of the Gastro-Intestinal Tract, 968
Congenital Impairment of Motility, 968
Acquired Impairment of Motility, 972
Impairment of Digestion, Absorption, and Nutrition, 974
Diarrhea, 979
Disorders of the Liver, 979
Disorders of Biliary Metabolism and Transport, 979
Inflammatory Disorders, 980
Portal Hypertension, 981
Metabolic Disorders, 982
Gastro-Intestinal Malignancies in Children, 982
Hepatoblastoma, 982
Pancreatic Tumours, 982

Disorders of the Gastro-Intestinal (GI) tract, liver, and pancreas in children include congenital anomalies with structural and functional alterations, enzyme deficiencies, infections, and malignancies. These disorders lead to impairment of motility, digestion, absorption, nutrition, and normal growth and development.

DISORDERS OF THE GASTRO-INTESTINAL TRACT

Congenital Impairment of Motility

Cleft Lip and Cleft Palate

There are numerous types of congenital orofacial anomalies, the most common of which is cleft lip (CL) or cleft palate (CP), or both (CLP). A cleft is a congenital anomaly that features a defect of the lip, alveolus, and/or palate and could be unilateral or bilateral. The incidence of CL, with or without CP, is about 1 in 1 000 live births. In Canada specifically, 1 in 700 children are born with a cleft of the lip, palate, or both.[1] CL and CP can occur in isolation or as part of a broad range of chromosomal, mendelian, or teratogenic syndromes. When CL occurs as part of a chromosomal, mendelian, or teratogenic syndrome, the defect may be referred to as syndromic CLP. If CP occurs alone, the defect may be referred to as nonsyndromic or isolated CP. CP is more common in females, and CL with or without CP is more common in males. Both anomalies can be unilateral or bilateral, or partial or complete.[2] Periconceptional intake of B vitamins, folate, and folic acid and reduced tobacco and alcohol use may prevent orofacial clefts.[3]

PATHOPHYSIOLOGY Cleft lip (CL) and cleft palate (CP) are embryonic developmental anomalies and vary in severity (Figure 37-1). There may be genetic and environmental triggers for syndromic and nonsyndromic CLP. Epigenetic influences include maternal smoking, alcohol steroid or statin use; folate deficiency, or disordered metabolism. CL and CP also may be associated with other malformations (i.e., cardiac, skeletal, or central nervous system). This phenomenon, called *multifactorial inheritance*, is discussed in Chapter 2. Together, the genetic and epigenetic factors reduce the amount of neural crest mesenchyme that migrates into the area that will develop into the face of the embryo.[4]

CL is caused by the incomplete fusion of the nasomedial or intermaxillary process beginning in the fourth week of embryonic development, a period of rapid development. The cleft causes structures of the face and mouth to develop without the normal restraints of encircling lip muscles. The facial cleft may affect not only the lip but also the external nose, nasal cartilages, nasal septum, and alveolar processes. The cleft is usually just beneath the centre of one nostril. The defect may occur bilaterally and may be symmetric or asymmetric. The more complete the CL, the greater the chance that teeth in the line of the cleft will be missing or malformed.

CP is often associated with CL but may occur without it. The fissure may affect only the uvula and soft palate or may extend forward to the nostril and involve the hard palate and the maxillary alveolar ridge. It may be unilateral or bilateral, with the cleft occupying the midline posteriorly and as far forward as the alveolar process, where it deviates to the involved side. Clefts involving the palate only are usually but not necessarily in the midline. In some cases, the vomer and nasal septum are partly or completely undeveloped. When these facial bones are involved, the nasal cavity may freely communicate with the oral cavity. Teeth in the CP area may be missing or deformed. There is increased risk for middle ear infections.

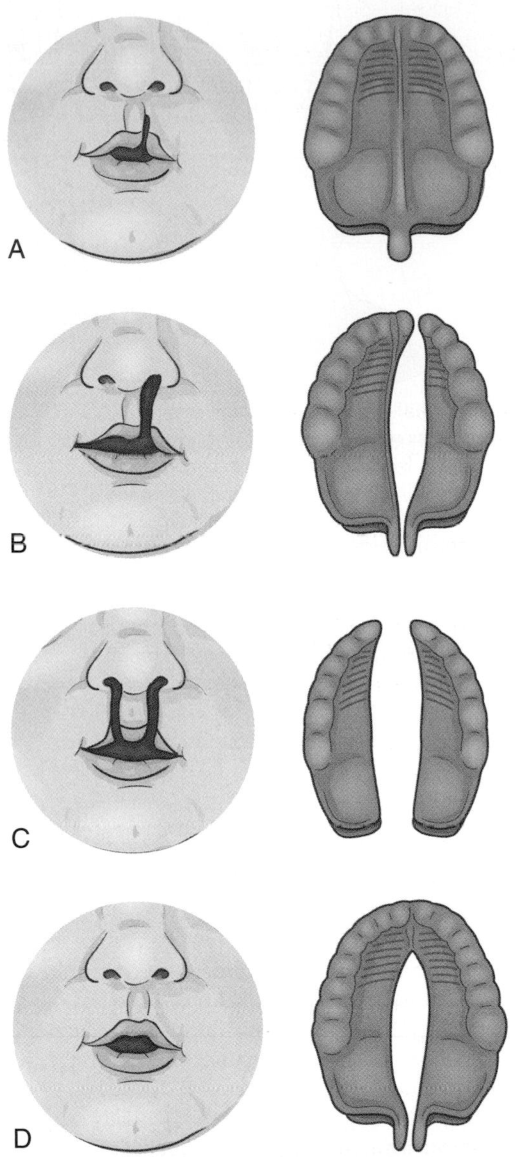

FIGURE 37-1 Variations in Clefts of the Lip and Palate. A, Notch in vermilion border. B, Unilateral cleft lip and palate. C, Bilateral cleft lip and cleft palate. D, Cleft palate.

CLINICAL MANIFESTATIONS Clefts of the lip or palate, or both, are immediately recognizable disruptions of normal facial structure. Feeding difficulty is the most significant clinical manifestation because of the oronasal communication and inability to generate negative pressure needed for normal sucking.[5] There also may be swallowing difficulty.

EVALUATION AND TREATMENT Prenatal diagnosis is made by ultrasound, and postnatal imaging confirms the extent of bone deformity. Soft tissue alterations are evaluated by history and physical examination. The nature and extent of the cleft, the infant's condition, and the method of surgical correction proposed determine the course of treatment. Surgical correction is planned at about the third to sixth month and may be performed in stages.[6,7] There are limited long-term outcome studies.[8]

Feeding the infant with CL usually presents no difficulty if the CL is simple and the palate intact. A baby with a complete CP requires consultation with a feeding and swallowing specialist to ensure adequate and safe nutritional intake. Bottles with nipples specialized for feeding an infant with a CP are required. Breastfeeding may be possible for some infants.[7] An orthodontic prosthesis for the roof of the mouth may facilitate sucking for some infants. Parental education and support is required for the long-term care of children with CP. Longitudinal monitoring requires a cleft/orofacial multidisciplinary team including a plastic surgeon, speech therapist, orthodontist, and nurse.[9]

Esophageal Atresia

Congenital malformations of the esophagus occur in 1 of 3 000 to 4 500 live births. **Esophageal atresia (EA)** is the most common congenital atresia of the esophagus. The esophagus ends in a blind pouch. EA is usually accompanied by a fistula between the esophagus and the trachea (**esophageal atresia/tracheoesophageal fistula [EA/TEF]**).[10] Either defect can occur alone (Figure 37-2). There is a high frequency of anomalies and syndromes associated with EAs.[11]

Environmental risk factors include maternal exposure to methimazole (Tapazole), exogenous sex hormones, infectious diseases, alcohol, or smoking; maternal diabetes; advanced maternal age; and maternal employment in agriculture.[12] Many genes and chromosomal abnormalities have been implicated; 10 to 30% of infants with EA/TEF have associated *v*ertebral, *a*nal, *c*ardiovascular, *t*racheo*e*sophageal, *r*enal, and *l*imb anomalies (VACTERL).[13]

PATHOPHYSIOLOGY The pathogenesis of esophageal abnormalities is unknown. Defective growth of endodermal cells and impaired embryonic foregut development of the trachea and esophagus lead to atresia.[10]

CLINICAL MANIFESTATIONS Antenatal diagnosis of EA/TEF increases with the findings of polyhydramnios (excessive amniotic fluid).[11,12] Swallowed amniotic fluid is usually absorbed into the placental circulation; therefore if the fetus cannot swallow, amniotic fluid accumulates in the uterus. EA will be diagnosed at birth on the basis of drooling, inability to swallow secretions or choking with feeding, and respiratory distress. Confirmation is established by inability to pass a gastric tube into the stomach. If a fistula connects the trachea with the distal esophagus, the abdomen fills with air and becomes distended, possibly interfering with breathing (Figure 37-2, *C–E*). Intermittent cyanosis may result.

Pulmonary complications are compounded by reflux of air and gastric secretions into the tracheobronchial tree through the fistula, causing severe chemical irritation. Infants with EA but no fistulae have scaphoid (boat-shaped), gasless abdomens. In infants with fistulae but without atresia (see Figure 37-2, *E*), the usual symptoms are recurrent aspiration, pneumonia, and atelectasis that remains unexpressed for days or even months.

EVALUATION AND TREATMENT Infants presenting with EA are evaluated with ultrasound, echocardiogram, and vertebral and limb radiographs. Following diagnosis, a tube should be placed into the upper pouch and continuous suction applied to decrease risk for aspiration. The head of the bed should be elevated slightly to assist drainage of the upper pouch. The infant should not be fed orally. Surgical repair is completed in the majority of cases.[14] The overall survival rate for infants with esophageal defects is 95%.[15]

Infantile Hypertrophic Pyloric Stenosis

Infantile hypertrophic pyloric stenosis (IHPS) is an acquired narrowing and distal obstruction of the pylorus and a common cause of postprandial vomiting. The incidence of pyloric stenosis is approximately 2 to 5 in 1 000 live births for males and 1 in 1 000 live births for females.[16] The etiology is unclear but probably multifactorial, involving genetic and environmental factors.

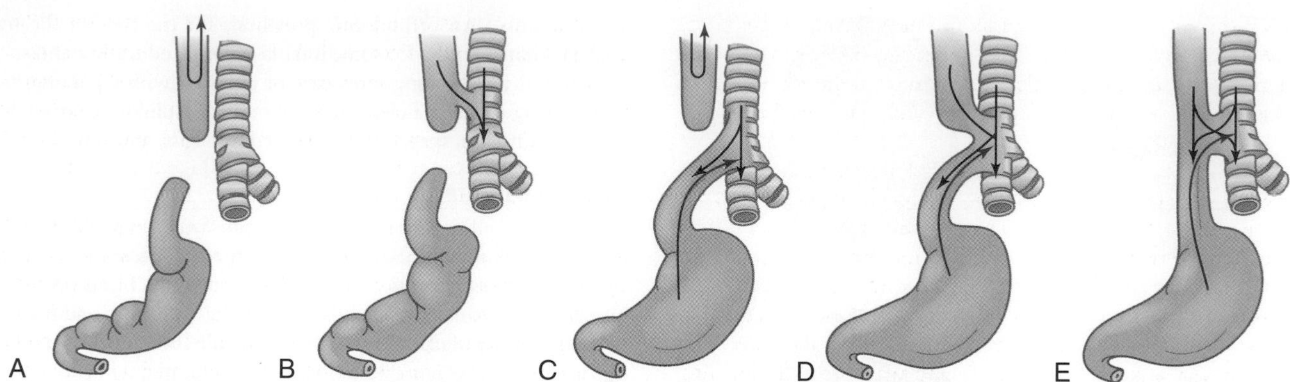

FIGURE 37-2 Five Types of Esophageal Atresia and Tracheoesophageal Fistulae. A, Simple esophageal atresia. Proximal esophagus and distal esophagus end in blind pouches, and there is no tracheal communication. Nothing enters the stomach; regurgitated food and fluid may enter the lungs. **B,** Proximal and distal esophageal segments end in blind pouches, and a fistula connects the proximal esophagus to the trachea. Nothing enters the stomach; food and fluid enter the lungs from the mouth. **C,** Proximal esophagus ends in a blind pouch, and a fistula connects the trachea to the distal esophagus. Air enters the stomach; regurgitated gastric secretions enter the lungs through the fistula. **D,** Fistula connects both proximal and distal esophageal segments to the trachea. Air, food, and fluid enter the stomach and the lungs from the mouth; regurgitated gastric secretions enter the lungs through the fistula. **E,** Simple tracheoesophageal fistula between otherwise normal esophagus and trachea. Air, food, and fluid enter the stomach and the lungs from the mouth through the fistula; and regurgitated gastric secretions enter the lungs through the fistula. Between 85 and 90% of esophageal anomalies are type **C;** 6 to 8% are type **A;** 3 to 5% are type **E;** and fewer than 1% are type **B** or **D.**

PATHOPHYSIOLOGY Individual muscle fibres thicken, so the entire pyloric sphincter becomes enlarged and inflexible. The mucosal lining of the pyloric opening is folded and narrowed by the encroaching muscle. Because of the extra peristaltic effort necessary to force the gastric contents through the narrow pylorus, the muscle layers of the stomach may become hypertrophied as well.

CLINICAL MANIFESTATIONS Between 2 and 8 weeks after birth, an infant who has fed well and gained weight begins forceful, nonbilious vomiting immediately after feeding.[17,18] The infant then demands to be refed. Constipation occurs because little food reaches the intestine.

In severe, untreated cases, increased gastric peristalsis and vomiting lead to severe fluid and electrolyte imbalances, malnutrition, and weight loss that can be fatal within 4 to 6 weeks. Infants with pyloric stenosis are irritable because of hunger, and they may have esophageal discomfort caused by repeated vomiting and esophagitis. The vomitus may be blood-streaked because of rupture of gastric and esophageal vessels.

EVALUATION AND TREATMENT Diagnosis is based on the history, clinical manifestations, and findings on abdominal ultrasound. The force and timing of the vomiting can help distinguish IHPS from gastroesophageal reflux (GER), for which episodes of vomiting are not forceful and occur 10 minutes or more after a feeding. The hypertrophied pylorus is palpable as a firm, small, movable mass, approximately the size of an olive, and is felt in the right upper quadrant in 70 to 90% of infants with pyloric stenosis. The hypertrophied pyloric muscles and narrowed pyloric channel are identified with ultrasound and radiographs.

The standard treatment for hypertrophic pyloric stenosis is a laparoscopic pyloromyotomy, in which the muscles of the pylorus are split and separated. Preoperative and postoperative medical management to correct fluid and electrolyte imbalance has been the key to the high success rate and low complication rates associated with this surgery.[19]

Obstructions of the Duodenum, Jejunum, and Ileum

High intestinal obstruction should be considered whenever persistent vomiting occurs. With duodenal obstruction there will be upper abdominal distension, visible peristaltic waves, a decrease in the size and frequency of meconium stools, progressive weight loss, persistent vomiting, and dehydration. Congenital obstruction of the duodenum can be caused by intrinsic malformations, such as atresia (complete blockage), stenosis (partial obstruction or narrowing), or external pressure, and its incidence is 2.5 to 10 in 100 000 live births.[20] The obstruction may be partial or complete and is usually located at or near the major duodenal papilla. The classic "double bubble" sign is seen on imaging of the abdomen and represents duodenal obstruction. The larger, proximal "bubble" is air in a dilated stomach. The more distal, smaller "bubble" is air in a dilated proximal duodenum. There is usually little or no air in the bowel distal to the obstruction. Double bubble also may be seen on prenatal ultrasounds. An annular pancreas—a defect in which the head of the pancreas surrounds part of the duodenum—can obstruct the duodenum. Congenital obstructions of the jejunum and ileum can be attributable to atresia, stenosis, meconium ileus (MI), megacolon (Hirschsprung's disease), intussusception, Meckel diverticulum, intestinal duplication, or strangulated hernia. In ileal or jejunal atresia, the intestine ends blindly, proximal and distal to an interruption in its continuity, with or without a gap in the mesentery. Stenosis (narrowing of the lumen) causes dilation proximal to the obstruction and luminal collapse distal to it.

Malrotation

Malrotation is the term used to describe the spectrum of abnormalities of embryonic development of the midgut associated with abnormal intestinal rotation or fixation, or both. The incidence is between 1 in 500 and 1 in 600 live births.[20]

PATHOPHYSIOLOGY In malrotation, the small intestine lacks a normal posterior attachment. The mobile loops of intestine can twist upon themselves (volvulus), leading to symptoms of bowel obstruction (see Figure 36-4). The twisting can partly or completely occlude the superior mesenteric artery, causing infarction and necrosis of the entire midgut. Peritoneal (Ladd) bands may press against and obstruct the duodenum.

CLINICAL MANIFESTATIONS Most cases of malrotation-associated volvulus and infarction develop during the neonatal period (90% of infants are younger than 1 year). Some develop during childhood or adulthood. Classic symptoms in infants are intermittent or persistent bile-stained vomiting after feedings and epigastric distension. Dehydration and electrolyte imbalance may occur rapidly. Fever usually ensues with pain and scanty stools. Diarrhea and bloody stools are associated with progressive volvulus, vascular compression, and infarction of the intestine. Intermittent or partial volvulus is more common in older children and adults. It may be asymptomatic or cause minor abdominal discomfort and be discovered during unrelated abdominal surgery.

EVALUATION AND TREATMENT Diagnosis of malrotation with volvulus and infarction is based on clinical manifestations. Radiographic films of the abdomen and barium studies show intestinal gas bubbles and distension proximal to the site of obstruction.

Treatment includes laparoscopic or open surgery to reduce the volvulus.[21] Necrotic bowel may be resected and a primary anastomosis performed. An enterostomy may be created. Most children have a good outcome; however, there is risk for adhesion-related bowel obstruction in about 15% of cases. Resection of large segments of the small intestine results in short bowel syndrome and its long-term sequelae.[22,23]

Meckel Diverticulum

Diverticula are small outpouches, or sacs, that have formed and pushed outward through weak spots of the intestinal wall. **Meckel diverticulum** is a remnant of the embryonic yolk sac and the most prevalent congenital abnormality of the small bowel (usually in the ileum). It is a true diverticulum in that it contains all layers of the intestinal wall. Ectopic gastric mucosal cells are contained in the diverticuli and may cause peptic ulcer and painless bleeding or mimic colonic diverticulitis. Often referred to as "the rule of 2s," a Meckel diverticulum occurs in approximately 2% of the general population, is typically located within 2 feet (61 cm) of the ileocecal valve (on the antimesenteric border of the ileum), is 2 inches (5 cm) in length on average, and its clinical symptomatology often occurs before 2 years of age.[24] Although most Meckel diverticuli are asymptomatic, the most common symptom is painless rectal bleeding. Intestinal obstruction, intussusception, and volvulus can occur, more commonly in adults. Diagnosis is made by symptom presentation and radionucleotide scintigraphy. The scan shows the gastric mucosal cells in the diverticuli. Treatment in those with symptoms is surgical resection.[25-28]

> **QUICK CHECK 37-1**
> 1. What structures are affected in cleft palate and cleft lip?
> 2. What is esophageal atresia?
> 3. What produces pyloric stenosis?

Meconium Syndromes

Meconium is a substance that fills the entire intestine before birth. It is a dark greenish mass of desquamated cells, mucus, and bile that accumulates in the bowel of a fetus and is typically discharged during the first 12 to 48 hours after birth.

Meconium ileus (MI) is an intestinal obstruction in the neonatal period caused by meconium formed in utero that is abnormally thick and sticky, which leads to a partial or complete obstruction at the level of the terminal ileum. There are two forms of MI: simple and complex. Complex MI is a surgical emergency and there is usually an associated GI pathology, such as bowel atresia, necrosis, or perforation. MI occurs in 10 to 15% of infants with cystic fibrosis (CF), and is thought to result from abnormal mucous production in the intestine or impaired pancreatic enzymes, or both[29,30] (see Chapter 28).

Meconium plug syndrome (MPS), also called *functional immaturity of the colon*, is a transient disorder of the newborn colon characterized by delayed passage (greater than 24 to 48 hours) of meconium and intestinal dilatation. **Meconium disease (MD)** is often associated with severe prematurity and low birth weight. It results from a combination of extremely sticky meconium in the colon or terminal ileum and poor intestinal motility, resulting in mechanical bowel obstruction. In both MPS and MD, plugs of meconium are found in the distal ileum and proximal colon, resulting in obstruction of passage of meconium from the rectum.

Distal intestinal obstruction syndrome (DIOS), formerly called *meconium ileus equivalent*, is seen in about 7.4% of children and adults with CF.[31] It is characterized by complete or incomplete intestinal obstruction of viscid fecal accumulation in the terminal ileum and proximal colon.[32]

PATHOPHYSIOLOGY The terminal ileum is plugged with thick, viscous meconium resulting from the formation of an insoluble, calcium–glycoprotein compound in abnormal mucus. The segment of the ileum proximal to the obstruction is distended with liquid contents, and its walls may be hypertrophied. The segment distal to the obstruction is collapsed and filled with small pellets of pale-coloured stool. Meconium in the obstructed segment has the consistency of thick syrup or glue. Peristalsis fails to propel this viscous material through the ileum, and it becomes impacted. Volvulus, atresia, or perforation of the bowel sometimes accompanies MI.

CLINICAL MANIFESTATIONS Abdominal distension usually develops during the first few hours after birth. As air is swallowed, the distension increases and the infant begins to vomit bile-stained material. Infants with CF may have signs of pulmonary involvement, such as tachypnea, intercostal retractions, and grunting respirations. The distended abdomen shows patterns of dilated intestinal loops that feel doughlike when palpated. Some of the loops contain scattered, firm, movable masses. Despite hyperactive peristalsis, the rectal ampulla is empty.

EVALUATION AND TREATMENT Radiological examination confirms the presence of meconium in the ileum or ileocecum. The sweat test measures the amount of chloride in the sweat, is performed to detect or rule out CF, and is accurate in 90% of infants. Defective chloride channels in CF cause increased chloride concentration in sweat. About 50% of cases are complicated with volvulus or perforation. In most cases, the obstruction is relieved by intestinal lavage and administration of oral laxatives.[32,33] If this is not possible, the meconium is removed surgically.[34] Survival of infants with simple MI is improving, with rates approaching 100%. Mortality of infants with complex MI with perforation and subsequent peritonitis or septicemia is about 70%.[29,33] DIOS is treated with hydration and stool softeners.

Idiopathic Intestinal Pseudo-Obstruction

Idiopathic intestinal pseudo-obstruction is a disorder of impaired intestinal motility. The pseudo-obstruction is caused by nerve or peristaltic muscle dysfunction that affects the movement of food, fluid, or air through the intestine. Children present with abdominal swelling or bloating, crampy abdominal pain, nausea, vomiting, constipation, or diarrhea. Idiopathic intestinal pseudo-obstruction is difficult to diagnose and treatment includes intestinal decompression, nutritional support, and symptom management.[35-37]

Hirschsprung's Disease

Hirschsprung's disease, or *aganglionic megacolon*, is a functional obstruction of the colon. It is the most common cause of colon obstruction, accounting for about one-third of all GI obstructions in infants. The incidence is approximately 1 in 5 000 live births and varies among ethnic groups. There is a predominance in males. Hirschsprung's disease is a multifactorial malformation.[38-40]

PATHOPHYSIOLOGY Hirschsprung's disease is characterized by the absence of parasympathetic intrinsic ganglion cells in the submucosal and myenteric plexuses along with the absence of peristaltic movement in the bowels (see Figure 35-13 for normal colon structure). In 80% of cases, the aganglionic segment is limited to the rectal end of the sigmoid colon. In rare cases, the entire colon lacks ganglion cells. The abnormally innervated colon impairs fecal movements, causing the proximal colon to become distended—hence the term *megacolon* (Figure 37-3).

CLINICAL MANIFESTATIONS The infant typically becomes symptomatic during the first 24 to 72 hours after birth with delayed passage of meconium. Mild to severe constipation is the usual manifestation of Hirschsprung's disease, with poor feeding, poor weight gain, and progressive abdominal distension. However, diarrhea may be the first sign because only water can travel around the impacted feces.

The most serious complication in the neonatal period is enterocolitis related to fecal impaction. Bowel dilation stretches and partly occludes the encircling blood and lymphatic vessels, causing edema, ischemia, infarction of the mucosa, and significant outflow of fluid into the bowel lumen. Copious liquid stools result. Infarction and destruction of the mucosa enable enteric microorganisms to penetrate the bowel wall. Frequently, gram-negative sepsis occurs, accompanied by fever and vomiting. Severe and rapid fluid and electrolyte changes may take place, causing hypovolemic or septic shock or death.

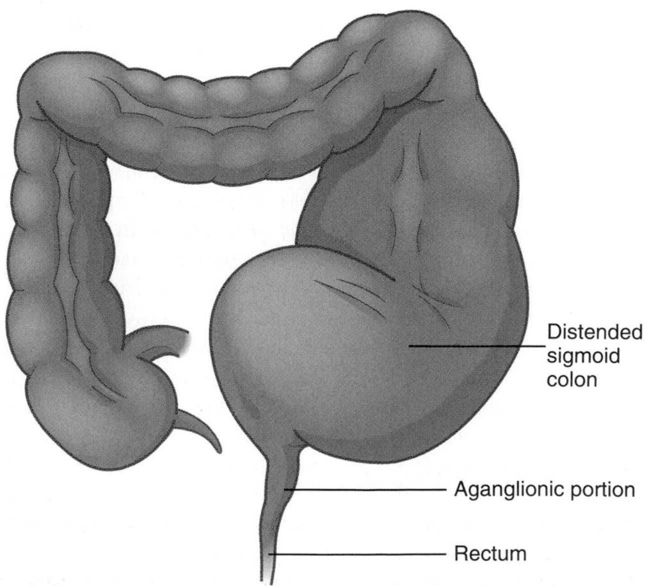

FIGURE 37-3 Hirschsprung's Disease.

EVALUATION AND TREATMENT Radiocontrast enema and anorectal manometry are screening tools for the diagnosis of Hirschsprung's disease. The definitive diagnosis is made by rectal biopsy showing an absence of ganglion cells in the submucosa of the colon.[41] Surgery is the definitive treatment in all cases of Hirschsprung's disease. In general, the prognosis of congenital megacolon is satisfactory for children who undergo surgical treatment. Bowel training may be prolonged; most children achieve bowel continence before puberty but some have long-term constipation or fecal incontinence.[42-46]

Anorectal Malformations

Anorectal malformations (ARMs) represent a spectrum of anomalies of the anus and rectum (Figure 37-4). ARMs include anorectal stenosis, imperforate anus, anorectal atresia, and rectal atresia. Persistent cloaca is the most severe type of ARM and occurs exclusively in girls. The rectum, urethra, and vagina fail to develop separately; instead, they drain through a single, common channel onto the perineum.[47-49] Approximately 40% of infants with anorectal malformations have other developmental anomalies (i.e., Down syndrome, Hirschsprung's disease, and duodenal atresia).[50]

Most ARMs are identified in routine physical examination during the neonatal period. Types of imperforate anus include an anal opening that is narrow or misplaced, a membrane (covering) may be present over the anal opening, the rectum may not connect to the anus, the rectum may connect to part of the urinary tract or to the reproductive system through an opening called a fistula, or the anal opening is not present. Treatment recommendations depend on the type of imperforate anus, the presence and type of associated abnormalities, and the child's overall health status. Anal stenosis can be treated by dilations. Infants with an imperforate anus and other anorectal malformations require surgical correction. Overall mortality is approximately 10%. Lower lesions have better functional outcomes than higher lesions.[49,51]

Acquired Impairment of Motility

Gastroesophageal Reflux

Gastroesophageal reflux (GER) is the passage of gastric contents into the esophagus independent of swallowing. GER is normal and nonpathological in healthy infants and may be asymptomatic or exhibited by regurgitation and vomiting.[52] The frequency of GER is highest in premature infants and occurs in about 70% of healthy infants; however, GER resolves without treatment in 95% of infants by 12 to 14 months of age.[53] Gastroesophageal reflux disease (GERD) is different from GER and occurs when it is the cause of troublesome symptoms or complications, or both, described as esophageal or extraesophageal in nature.[54] Children at greatest risk for complicated GERD are those with prematurity, neurological impairment, EA, obesity, hiatal hernia, achalasia, chronic lung diseases, and certain genetic disorders, including CF.

PATHOPHYSIOLOGY GERD is influenced by genetic, environmental, anatomical, hormonal, and neurogenic factors. Although transient lower esophageal sphincter relaxations (TLESRs) are the most common pathophysiological cause of GER, inadequate adaptation of sphincter tone to changes in abdominal pressure also may be implicated. Factors that maintain lower esophageal sphincter integrity in children include the location of the gastroesophageal junction in a high-pressure zone within the abdomen, mucosal gathering within the sphincter, and the angle at which the esophagus is inserted into the stomach. Reflux persists if any one of these pressure-maintaining factors is altered. Other mediators of GER are esophageal peristalsis or clearance, mucosal resistance that mediates the noxiousness of the refluxate, and delayed

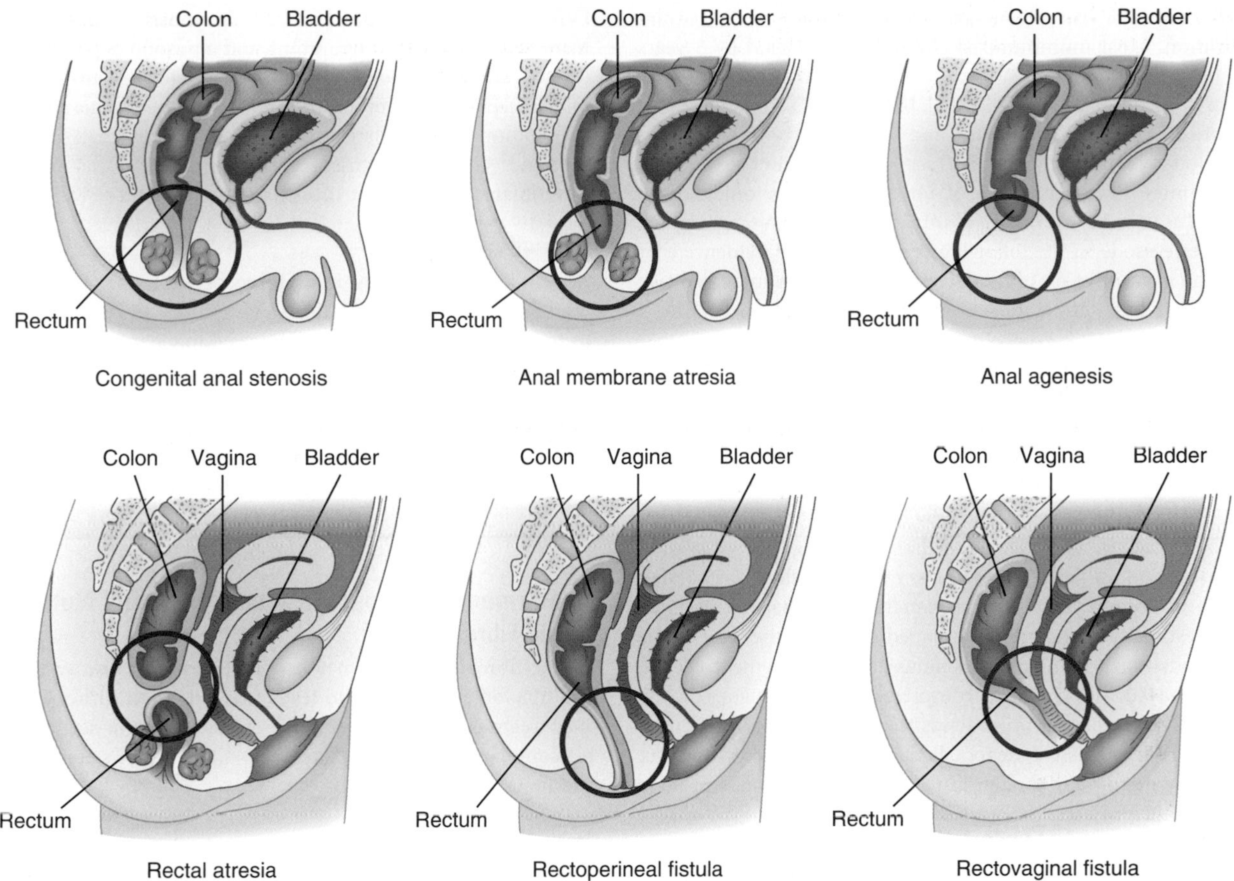

FIGURE 37-4 Anorectal Stenosis and Imperforate Anus. NOTE: With the exception of the rectovaginal fistula, all of the malformations shown occur in both males and females.

gastric emptying. Reflux of acidic gastric contents results in inflammation of the esophageal epithelium (esophagitis) and stimulation of the vomiting reflex.

Esophageal inflammation resulting from GERD is differentiated from eosinophilic esophagitis (EoE), which can occur in children. EoE is thought to be an allergic esophageal disease involving both immediate and delayed hypersensitivity reactions to food ingestion. An eosinophilic infiltrate is associated with inflammation of the entire esophagus that is nonresponsive to acid-suppression therapy. The hallmark symptoms of EoE are dysphagia, food refusal or impaction, and throat and chest pain. Treatment involves food elimination and oral steroids.[55]

CLINICAL MANIFESTATIONS The clinical manifestations of GERD include excessive regurgitation or vomiting; food refusal/anorexia; unexplained crying, choking, or gagging; sleep disturbance; dysphagia; and abdominal or epigastric pain, or both.[54] Esophageal complications of GER can be significant, such as esophagitis, hemorrhage, stricture, Barrett esophagus (metaplasia) (see Chapter 36), and, rarely, adenocarcinoma. Extraesophageal symptoms include cough and wheezing, laryngitis, pharyngitis, dental erosions, sinusitis, recurrent otitis media, and Sandifer syndrome (a neurological disorder).[56] This constellation of symptoms is often indistinguishable from those of cow's milk protein allergy, which may coexist with or overlap GERD.

EVALUATION AND TREATMENT The clinical manifestations are often adequate to confirm a diagnosis of GERD. Esophageal pH monitoring with a probe for 24 hours and endoscopy are routinely used for diagnosis.

Normal physiological GER resolves without treatment. In breastfed babies, maternal elimination of cow's milk protein is recommended, whereas formula-fed infants may require feeding volume and frequency adjustments using extensively hydrolyzed protein or amino acid–based formulas. Using thickened feedings has shown to improve symptoms of GER. Prone positioning is only recommended for infants older than 1 year of age because of the risk for sudden unexpected infant death (SUID). Lifestyle changes for children and adolescents include weight loss, smoking cessation, and avoidance of caffeine, chocolate, alcohol, and spicy foods.

Medications are used to buffer or decrease gastric acid secretion, increase motility, or increase lower esophageal sphincter pressure to treat GER.[57] If no improvement is seen with medical management or the child has life-threatening events with reflux, an antireflux surgical procedure, including gastropexy and fundoplication, is performed. More evidence is needed to evaluate long-term surgical outcomes.[58]

Intussusception

Intussusception is the telescoping of a proximal segment of intestine into a distal segment, causing an obstruction. It is the most common cause of small bowel obstruction in children. Most cases occur between 5 and 7 months of age. Intussusception is more common in males and can occur in children with polyps or tumours (lead points), CF, Meckel diverticulum, intestinal adhesions, or immediately after abdominal surgery.[59] There is a small risk for intussusception associated with rotavirus vaccination but the vaccine is generally safe.[60]

In Canada, rotavirus is a common cause of gastroenteritis in children; approximately 36% of children with rotavirus gastroenteritis see a physician, 15% visit an emergency department, and 7% require hospitalization. Most unimmunized children are infected by 5 years of age.[61]

Rotavirus vaccines are well tolerated, but there is a small increased risk for intussusception in between 1 and 7 cases per 100 000 doses in the 7 days following both the first and second doses.[61] In Canada, as a precaution, infants with a history of intussusception should not be given rotavirus vaccine. About 4% of infants with intussusception will have another episode in the following year; there is no evidence that children who have a history of intussusception are at an increased risk for another intussusception after receiving rotavirus vaccine.[61]

PATHOPHYSIOLOGY In intussusception, the ileum commonly telescopes into the cecum and part of the ascending colon by collapsing through the ileocecal valve, although intussusception can occur anywhere from the duodenum to the rectum. The proximal portion of the intestine (the intussusceptum) collapses into the distal portion (the intussuscipiens) in the direction of peristaltic flow (Figure 37-5). The intussusceptum then drags its mesentery into the enveloping lumen, causing an intussusception. Initially, the mesentery is constricted, obstructing venous return. Compression of the mesenteric vessels between the two layers of intestinal wall and at the U-shaped angle at either end of the intussusceptum leads within hours to venous stasis, engorgement, edema, exudation, and further vascular compression. The tension of the mesentery on the intussusceptum tends to arch the bowel in a curve having its centre at the mesenteric root. Edema and compression obstruct the flow of chyme through the intestine. Unless the intussusception is treated, ischemia and necrosis ensue.

CLINICAL MANIFESTATIONS The classic symptoms of intussusception include colicky abdominal pain, irritability, knees drawn to the chest, abdominal mass, vomiting, and bloody (currant-jelly) stools. Not all of these symptoms may occur, and intussusception has been discovered incidentally by computed tomography (CT) or magnetic resonance imaging (MRI) scan for other indications. Abdominal tenderness and distension develop as intestinal obstruction becomes more acute.

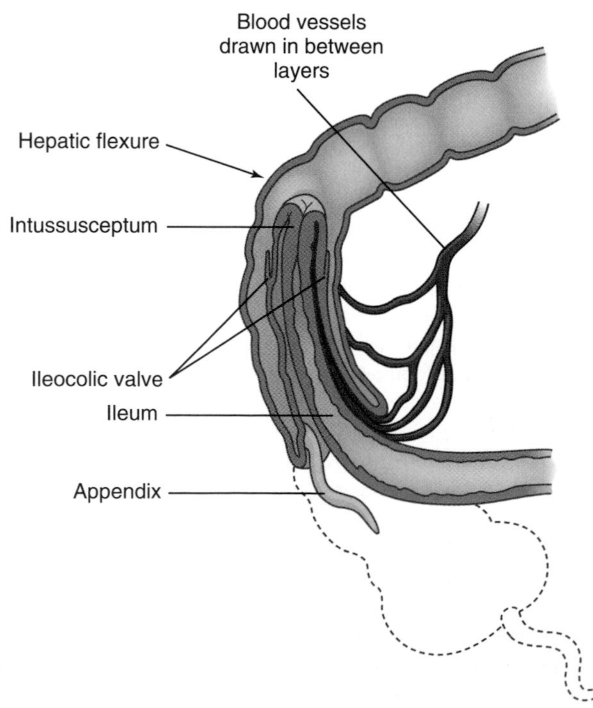

FIGURE 37-5 Ileocolic Intussusception.

EVALUATION AND TREATMENT Diagnosis is based on clinical manifestations, onset of symptoms, and ultrasonographic or radiological imaging studies. An enema reduction is usually effective for large bowel intussusception and prevents the progression to ischemia and perforation. Laparotomy remains the treatment of choice for small bowel intussusception.[62] Untreated intussusception in infants is nearly always fatal. Most infants recover if the intussusception is reduced within 24 hours.[63]

Appendicitis

Appendicitis is common in children between the ages of 10 and 11 years.[64] The mechanisms of disease, symptoms, and treatment are similar to those for adults and can be reviewed in Chapter 36.

> **QUICK CHECK 37-2**
> 1. Describe the pathological defect in meconium ileus.
> 2. Why is there poor bowel motility with Hirschsprung's disease?
> 3. Describe the defect in intussusception.

Impairment of Digestion, Absorption, and Nutrition

Cystic Fibrosis

Cystic fibrosis (CF) is an autosomal recessive disease that involves multiple organ systems and leads to death at an earlier age, although new treatments are extending life expectancy. This section focuses on GI complications of CF; Chapter 28 discusses CF's epidemiology and pulmonary involvement.

PATHOPHYSIOLOGY The GI presentation of CF is caused by a dysfunction of the cystic fibrosis transmembrane regulator (CFTR) protein, which is located on epithelial membranes and regulates chloride and sodium ion channels. It is found throughout the airways, sweat glands, digestive tract, pancreas, hepatobiliary system, and reproductive system (also called *mucoviscidosis* or *fibrocystic disease of the pancreas*). The hallmark pathophysiological triad of CF includes obstruction, infection, and inflammation that are evident throughout the GI tract and within the airways. The full spectrum of involvement is summarized in Table 37-1.

Dysfunction of the CFTR protein results in altered sodium, chloride, and potassium resorption, all of which remain external to the surface of the epithelial membrane, with reduced clearance from tubular structures lined by affected epithelia.[65] Maldigestion of proteins, carbohydrates, fats, and fat-soluble vitamins occurs because mucous obstruction of the pancreatic ducts blocks the flow of pancreatic enzymes, causing intestinal malabsorption and degenerative and fibrotic changes in the pancreas and GI tract. Diabetes mellitus commonly develops from damage to insulin-producing beta cells and insulin resistance.[66]

CLINICAL MANIFESTATIONS Clinical manifestations are summarized in Table 37-1. GI symptoms often precede pulmonary manifestations. Approximately 85% of those with CF present early in life with pancreatic insufficiency (PI). PI is the cause of nutrient malabsorption and failure to thrive in children with CF. Steatorrhea and abdominal distension are common symptoms with potential sequelae that include DIOS, fibrotic colonopathy, or focal biliary cirrhosis. Children who are pancreatic sufficient (PS) are at greater risk of developing pancreatitis.[67] Those with CF are at greater risk for many GI complications, including GI cancers and hepatobiliary abnormalities, which may lead to pancreatic transplant or death.

EVALUATION AND TREATMENT Genetic screening and the sweat test are required for diagnosis. Evaluation of pancreatic sufficiency also is

TABLE 37-1 Pathophysiology, Clinical Manifestations, and Complications of Cystic Fibrosis

Organ Involved	Secretory Dysfunction	Clinical Manifestations	Complications
Sweat glands	Elevated concentration of sodium and chloride in sweat	Hyponatremia; hypochloremia	Heat prostration; shock
Intestine			
Newborn	Viscid meconium	Meconium ileus with intestinal obstruction	Meconium peritonitis; growth failure
Older child and adult	Inspissated (dried out) mucofecal masses (intestinal sludging)	Partial intestinal obstruction with severe cramping pains	Volvulus (obstruction), intussusception (prolapse) Distal intestinal obstruction syndrome Growth failure
Pancreas (enzyme deficiency)	Inspissation and precipitation of pancreatic secretions, causing obstruction of pancreatic ducts Insulin deficiency	Absence of pancreatic enzymes, causing malabsorption of food and fatty, bulky stools Decreased vitamin A, D, E, and K absorption Glucose intolerance	Hypoproteinemia; iron deficiency anemia; malnutrition Vitamins A, D, E, and K deficiency and rectal prolapse Diabetes mellitus (see Chapter 19)
Liver	Inspissation and precipitation of bile and biliary system	Focal biliary cirrhosis; shrunken, "hobnail" liver; fatty liver	Portal hypertension with esophageal varices and hematemesis
Salivary glands	Inspissation and precipitation of secretions in small ducts of submaxillary and sublingual salivary glands	Mild patchy fibrosis of salivary glands	None
Respiratory Tract			
Paranasal structures	Viscid mucus	Retention of mucus; clouding seen on sinus roentgenograms	Mucopyoceles (pus accumulations) with nasal deformity or orbital cavity extension
Nose	Nasal polyps	Obstruction of nasal air flow	Sinusitis
Lungs	Viscid mucus in bronchioles and bronchi	Obstruction of bronchioles causing bronchiolectasis, bronchiectasis, and chronic lung infection	Atelectasis, hemoptysis; pneumothorax; cor pulmonale; respiratory failure
Reproductive Tract			
Male	Viscid genital tract secretions during embryological development, causing failure of formation of normal vas deferens; aspermia	Sterility	None
Female	Distension of endocervical epithelial cells with cytoplasmic mucin	Decreased fertility	Polypoid cervicitis (cervical inflammation) while taking oral contraceptives

Data from Marcdante, K.J., & Kliegman, R.M. (2015). *Nelson essentials of pediatrics* (7th ed.). Philadelphia: Saunders.

essential. The extent of pancreatic function is determined by 72-hour fecal fat measurements, which are not easily obtained. Therefore, the most common measurement of fat malabsorption is fecal elastase. A serum test for trypsinogen also can be used to detect pancreatic insufficiency in children older than 8 years of age.

The goal of treatment for PI is to reduce malabsorption of nutrients and improve growth. Most children with CF take pancreatic enzyme replacement therapy (PERT) for the rest of their lives. PERT is administered before or with every meal, snack, or enteral feeding supplementation. High doses of PERT are associated with DIOS; therefore, minimal effective doses are indicated. High-caloric, high-protein diets with frequent snacks and vitamin supplements are used to treat malnutrition. Nutritional status and growth should be carefully monitored, and growth hormone may be included with nutritional supplements.[68]

Celiac Disease

Celiac disease (CD), formerly called *celiac sprue*, is an autoimmune disease that damages small intestinal villous epithelium when there is ingestion of gluten (gliadin), the protein component of cereal grains. CD is a common multiorgan disease with a strong genetic predisposition associated with human leukocyte antigen DQ2 (HLA-DQ2) and HLA-DQ8.[69] The disease has a prevalence of about 1% worldwide, although evidence suggests only 10 to 15% of the population have been diagnosed and treated.[70] It is estimated that 1 in 133 persons in Canada is affected by CD.[71] **Nonceliac gluten sensitivity (NCGS)**, or wheat allergy, should not be confused with CD; although it presents similarly after the ingestion of gluten, the individual does not have positive autoantibodies or classic intestinal villous atrophy but instead has variable HLA status with similar symptoms as CD.[72]

The pathogenesis of CD is complex and involves genetic and immunological factors. Environmental factors include early infections, gut microbiota in infants, feeding patterns, and timing and amount of gluten. CD presents with greater frequency in children with type 1 diabetes mellitus, autoimmune thyroid or liver disease, Down syndrome, Turner's syndrome, Williams syndrome, selective immunoglobulin A (IgA) deficiency, Addison's disease, and first-degree relatives with CD.[70]

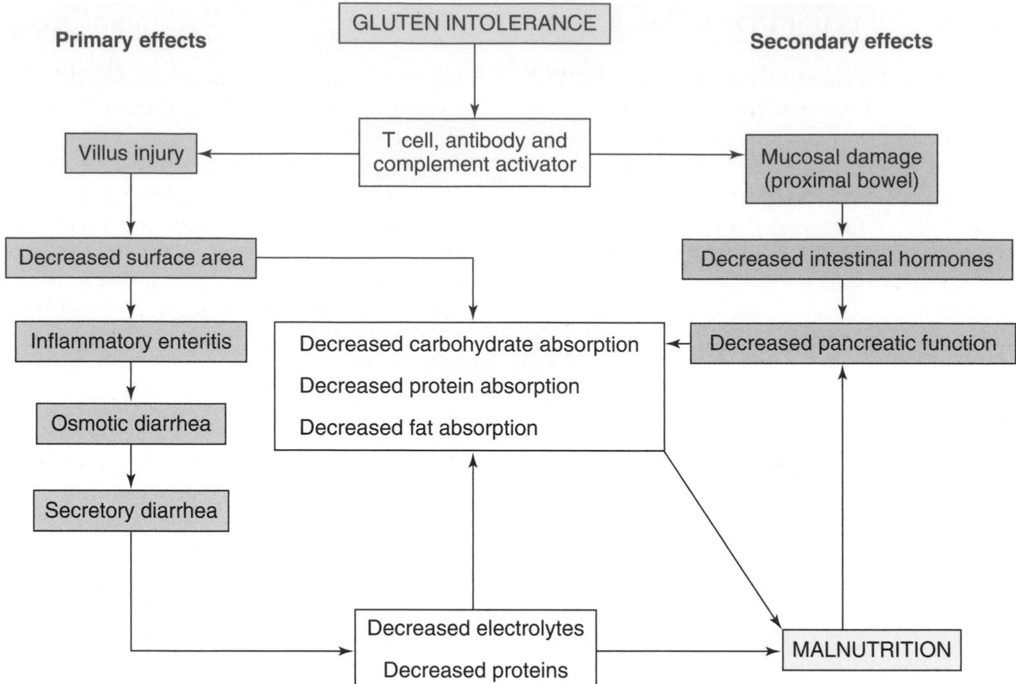

FIGURE 37-6 Pathophysiology of Celiac Disease.

PATHOPHYSIOLOGY The major pathophysiological characteristic of CD is T-cell–mediated autoimmune injury to the small intestinal epithelial cells of genetically susceptible individuals. There is atrophy and flattening of villi, crypt hyperplasia in the upper small intestine, and malabsorption of most nutrients in the presence of cereal gluten, particularly wheat, rye, and barley (Figure 37-6).[73]

Damage to the mucosa of the duodenum and jejunum exacerbates malabsorption. The secretion of intestinal hormones, such as secretin and cholecystokinin–pancreozymin, may be diminished; consequently, secretion of pancreatic enzymes and expulsion of bile from the gallbladder decrease, contributing to malabsorption.

Destruction of mucosal cells causes inflammation, and water and electrolytes are secreted, leading to watery diarrhea. Potassium loss leads to muscle weakness. Magnesium and calcium malabsorption can cause seizures or tetany. Unabsorbed fatty acids combine with calcium, and secondary hyperparathyroidism increases phosphorus excretion, resulting in bone reabsorption. Calcium is no longer able to bind oxalate in the intestine and is absorbed, which causes hyperoxaluria. Gallbladder function may be abnormal, and bile salt conjugation may decrease.

Fat malabsorption in the jejunum is the major cause of steatorrhea (fatty stools). Deficiencies of fat-soluble vitamins are common in children with CD. Vitamin K malabsorption leads to hypoprothrombinemia. In one-third of cases, iron and folic acid malabsorption is manifested as cheilosis, anemia, and a smooth, red tongue. Vitamin B_{12} absorption is impaired in those with extensive ileal disease, and folate and iron deficiencies are common.

CLINICAL MANIFESTATIONS The onset of clinical manifestations of CD depends on the age of the infant when gluten-containing substances are added to the diet. Although in 50% of affected children onset occurs by 18 months of age, it is not uncommon to be diagnosed later in life. Severity of symptoms can vary tremendously, and many children older than 3 years of age present with nongastrointestinal symptoms.[70] GI and extraintestinal symptoms of CD are listed in Box 37-1.

BOX 37-1 Symptoms of Celiac Disease

Gastro-Intestinal Symptoms	Extraintestinal Symptoms
Diarrhea	Fatigue
Abdominal pain and distension	Weight loss, growth failure
Vomiting	Delayed puberty
	Dermatitis herpetiformis
Anorexia	Dental enamel hypoplasia, aphthous stomatitis
Constipation	Arthritis
	Osteoporosis
	Fractures
	Neurological manifestations: ataxia, neuropathy, seizures

Data from Ferraz, E.G., de Jesus Campos, E., Sarmento, V.A., et al. (2012). *Pediatr Dent*, 34(7), 485–488; Guandalini, S., & Assiri, A. (2014). *JAMA Pediatr, 168*(3), 274; Hadjivassiliou, M., Duker, A.P., & Sanders, D.S. (2014). *Handb Clin Neurol, 120*, 607–619.

An unusual complication of CD in infancy is celiac crisis. **Celiac crisis** is characterized by severe diarrhea, dehydration, and hypoproteinemia as a result of malabsorption and protein loss.

EVALUATION AND TREATMENT Diagnosis includes confirmation with serological autoantibody measurement against tissue transglutaminase IgA (tTG IgA) (most sensitive and specific), antiendomysial antibody (anti-EMA) IgA, or deaminated gliadin peptides (DGPs), which are more sensitive in children younger than 2 years of age. A negative genetic screening for HLA haplotypes would rule out CD.[74] Currently, there is controversy regarding treatment for those children who are HLA-positive but asymptomatic. If an autoantibody or genetic screen is positive, a small intestinal biopsy is obtained to detect the classic mucosal changes caused by gluten-induced enteropathy. A wide variety of screening tests for malabsorption also may be useful. Even though there are very useful screening tools to diagnose CD, many children remain undiagnosed.

Treatment consists of lifelong adherence to a gluten-free diet (GFD), which includes elimination of wheat, rye, barley, and malt. Lactose intolerance also may be present from damage to villi; therefore, lactose (milk sugar) also may be excluded from the diet but should be resumed after treatment. Infants are routinely given vitamin D, iron, and folic acid supplements to treat deficiencies. Bone mineral density (BMD) screening is required. For most children, the long-term prognosis is excellent. There is an increased incidence of malignant disease, particularly lymphoma, in individuals who fail to respond or are nonadherent to a GFD.[75]

Malnutrition

Pediatric malnutrition is an imbalance between nutrient requirements and intake that results in energy, protein, and micronutrient deficits that negatively impact growth and development. Malnutrition also involves impaired absorption and altered nutrient utilization. **Kwashiorkor** (deficiency of dietary protein) and **marasmus** (all forms of inadequate nutrient intake) are the two most common types of malnutrition in children. Collectively, they are known as **protein-energy malnutrition (PEM)**. PEM describes the effects of malnutrition but not the etiology or interactions that contribute to nutrient depletion.

Both kwashiorkor and marasmus are states of long-term starvation and are the result of widespread nutritional deficiencies among children in developing countries and economically destitute populations, particularly when associated with human immunodeficiency virus (HIV) infection.[76] Kwashiorkor usually occurs in infants or children from 1 to 4 years of age who have been weaned from breast milk to a high-starch, protein-deficient diet. The death rate of kwashiorkor is higher than that for marasmus.

Marasmus can occur at any age but it is common in children younger than 1 year. In marasmus, starvation is attributable to lack of protein and carbohydrates, and in neglected children it can have a psychogenic basis. In developing countries and impoverished populations, early weaning of breastfed infants to overdiluted commercial formulas is a risk factor for marasmus.

Although PEM is common in developing countries, it is underestimated in hospitalized children. A new paradigm used to define pediatric malnutrition includes etiology (illness or environmental), identification of pathogenesis and chronicity, associations with inflammation, and resulting impact on functional outcomes.[77] PEM is a known complication of chronic diseases, such as chronic fever; infectious diseases like tuberculosis; malignancy; digestive and malabsorptive disorders; cardiac, pulmonary, kidney, and neurological diseases; burns or hypermetabolic states; anorexia and bulimia; and psychogenic illness. Treatments such as radiation therapy and chemotherapy also can contribute to malnutrition. PEM contributes to hospital-acquired conditions (HACs), longer time on mechanical ventilation, increased hospital length of stay, and increased morbidity and mortality rates.[78]

PATHOPHYSIOLOGY The pathogenesis of kwashiorkor is uncertain but includes inadequate dietary protein, leaky gut syndrome (compromised gut barrier), and intestinal inflammation. Recent studies are now implicating alterations in gut microbiota as the central cause of kwashiorkor.[77] There is evidence that children with kwashiorkor show stunting of gut microbiota maturation, which may generate products, such as inhibitors of enzymes in the tricarboxylic acid cycles, that compromise energy metabolism.[79] Support for this theory of causation includes an antibiotic treatment study that demonstrated significant improvement in recovery and mortality rates of malnourished Malawian children.[80]

The lack of sufficient plasma proteins results in generalized edema with a substantial loss of potassium. The liver swells with stored fat because no hepatic proteins are synthesized to form and release lipoproteins. Pancreatic atrophy and fibrosis may be present. Kwashiorkor also causes malabsorption, reduced bone density, and impaired renal function. If the condition is not reversed, the prognosis is very poor.

The metabolic response in marasmus is different, allowing sustained protein and lipid supply during periods of decreased dietary intake. Metabolic processes, including liver function, are preserved, but growth is severely developmentally delayed. Caloric intake is too low to support protein synthesis for growth or the storage of fat. Muscle and fat wasting occur, and anemia is common and can be severe.[81]

CLINICAL MANIFESTATIONS Children with kwashiorkor have appropriate stores of protein and fat that are mobilized inadequately. They have marked generalized edema, dermatoses, hypopigmented hair, distended abdomen, hepatomegaly, and almost normal weight for age (because of edema). Children with marasmus demonstrate greater wasting of protein and fat stores yet have improved survival. Marasmus is characterized by muscle wasting, fatty liver and hepatomegaly, diarrhea, dermatosis, low hemoglobin level, and infection. There is loss of subcutaneous fat and an absence of edema. Both conditions lead to delays in physical, behavioural, and cognitive development and academic performance. Lastly, micronutrient deficiencies, especially with zinc, selenium, iron, and antioxidant vitamins, can lead to immune deficiency and infections. Severe vitamin A deficiency commonly results in blindness.[82]

EVALUATION AND TREATMENT Evaluation of PEM is based on nutritional history and clinical manifestations, including anthropometric measurements. Laboratory monitoring is used to assess for macronutrient and micronutrient deficiencies, aminotransaminase alterations, and response to refeeding. The provision of deficient nutrients will resolve clinical symptoms in 4 to 6 weeks. Use of antibiotics has been shown to improve recovery of PEM and decrease mortality.[83] Developmental sequelae of PEM may be irreversible; therefore early intervention is recommended. Nutritional rehabilitation with appropriate environmental stimulation for infants and young children has been shown to resolve or improve cerebral shrinkage, physical growth, and psychomotor development.

Failure to Thrive or Growth Faltering

Failure to thrive (FTT) or **growth faltering (GF)** is a physical sign demonstrating that a child is receiving inadequate nutrition for optimal growth and development. It is manifested as a deceleration in weight gain, a low weight/height or body-mass-index ratio, or a low weight/height/head circumference ratio. FTT is a common problem and can present at any time in childhood.[84] Approximately 80% of children with FTT present before 18 months of age.[84]

PATHOPHYSIOLOGY Currently, there is a move away from describing FTT as organic versus nonorganic; instead, it is considered a multifactorial condition that includes biological, psychosocial, and environmental contributions that are illness related or nonillness related (Box 37-2). An underlying medical condition is never found in more than 80% of cases of FTT. Categories of FTT include inadequate caloric intake, inadequate caloric absorption, and excessive caloric expenditure. Infants and children are at risk for FTT if their parents or primary caregivers are unable to provide nurturance.

CLINICAL MANIFESTATIONS Clinical manifestations of FTT are delayed growth accompanied by manifestations of malnutrition or an underlying

BOX 37-2 Factors Associated With Failure to Thrive or Growth Faltering

Mechanical feeding difficulties (oromotor dysfunction, congenital anomalies, central nervous system disorders)
Inadequate caloric intake or caloric absorption: infant feeding problems, underlying chronic disease or malabsorption syndromes
Incorrect preparation of formula (too diluted, too concentrated)
Unsuitable feeding habits (food fads, excessive juice)
Behaviour problems affecting eating
Disturbed parent–child relationship; parental stress, parental lack of knowledge; child neglect

Data from Kyle, U.G., Shekerdemian, L.S., & Coss-Bu, J.A. (2015). *Nutr Clin Pract, 30*(2), 227–238; Mehta, N.M., Corkins, M.R., Lyman, B., et al. (2013). *J Parenter Enteral Nutr, 37*(4), 460–481.

disease, or both. Infants who present with FTT frequently have feeding problems. Symptoms include delayed growth; pallid or dry, cracked skin; sparse hair; poorly developed musculature; decreased subcutaneous fat; and swollen abdomen with malabsorption, diarrhea, anorexia, and signs of vitamin deficiencies such as rickets. Social or emotional manifestations include reduced energy level, reduced responsiveness and interaction with the environment, social isolation, spasticity and rigidity when held or touched, inability to make eye contact or smile, refusal to eat, and rejection of foods. There may be long-term side effects on cognitive, behavioural, and academic performance.[85]

EVALUATION AND TREATMENT FTT is suggested if a child falls below the 3rd percentile for weight, or shows stagnation in length or weight.[86] Underlying medical conditions are evaluated. If illness is ruled out, a thorough review of psychosocial, emotional, and environmental components of care is necessary. Screening tools are available to assist with evaluation of nutrition status and to guide therapy, particularly in hospitalized children.[87]

Treatment of FTT includes treating an underlying illness (if found), increasing volume or caloric density of formula, increasing frequency of breastfeeding (if found to be insufficient), structuring meals and snacks, and adding high-calorie foods and additives. Eliminating fruit juice, soda, or excessive milk also will improve appetite and absorption of nutrients. Medications are used to stimulate appetite. Nutrient deficiencies are supplemented. If unable to gain weight, an oral enteral supplement may be added to the diet, or a nasogastric or gastrostomy tube can be used to supplement oral intake.

If the cause is not medical, management then involves the immediate total care of the child and measures to address (1) the psychosocial and emotional problems of the caregivers and (2) parent–child interactions. Counselling, parental modelling, and long-term family support are sometimes required.[88]

Hospital admission and evaluation is recommended if the diagnosis is unclear or the child is in nutritional or emotional jeopardy. Eating patterns, food preferences, caloric intake, and family interactions can be assessed and treatment plans implemented during the hospital stay.

Necrotizing Enterocolitis

Necrotizing enterocolitis (NEC) is an ischemic inflammatory condition that causes bowel necrosis and perforation. NEC is not a specific diagnosis but a constellation of signs and symptoms with several proposed etiologies. It is the most common severe neonatal GI emergency that predominantly affects the smallest and most premature infants.[89,90] Approximately 12% of infants born weighing less than 1 500 g will develop NEC; of those, about 30% will not survive.[91] Isolated or focal intestinal perforation is sometimes confused with NEC and generally is not accompanied by an inflammatory component or by diffuse necrosis.[92]

Despite recent improvements in the survival of extremely preterm infants, the incidence of NEC in Canadian hospitals has not changed significantly over the past 50 years. According to the Canadian Neonatal Network, the prevalence fluctuates around 5% among very-low-birth-weight infants in Canada.[93] These findings align with those of a study by Sankaran and colleagues that examined 16 883 infants admitted to 17 tertiary-level Canadian neonatal intensive care units from January 1996 to October 1997.[94] That study found that the incidence of NEC was 6.6% ($n = 238$) among 3 628 infants with birth weight less than 1 500 grams, and 0.7% ($n = 98$) among 14 606 infants with birth weight greater than 1 500 grams. The study also concluded that NEC was associated with infants with lower gestational age and greater need for assisted ventilation and treatment of patent ductus arteriosus.[94]

PATHOPHYSIOLOGY The exact etiology of NEC is unclear. Factors contributing to the development of NEC include infections, abnormal bacterial colonization, intestinal ischemia, immature immune responses, exaggerated inflammatory responses, immature intestinal motility and barrier function, perinatal stress, effects of medications and feeding practices, and genetic predisposition. The immature mucosal barrier delays digestion and motility is slower, allowing for the accumulation of noxious substances that damage the intestine, increase permeability, and increase the risk for infection. Translocation of intestinal bacteria and other substances contributes to injury, inflammation, and development of systemic inflammatory disease. Immature intestinal innate immunity and an unfavourable balance between normal and pathogenic bacteria promote intestinal inflammation and release of proinflammatory cytokines. Accumulation of gas in the intestine can cause pressure that decreases blood flow, and an imbalance between vasodilator and vasoconstrictor inputs in the immature gut may lead to vasoconstriction, promoting ischemia, injury, and necrosis.[95]

CLINICAL MANIFESTATIONS Manifestations of NEC usually appear suddenly and within weeks of premature birth, and sooner for term neonates. Signs and symptoms of "classic" NEC include feeding intolerance, abdominal distension and bloody stools after 8 to 10 days of age, septicemia with elevated white blood cell count, and falling platelet levels. Unstable temperature, bradycardia, and apnea are nonspecific signs. In late preterm or term infants, NEC is more likely to be associated with other predisposing factors, such as low Apgar scores, chorioamnionitis, exchange transfusions, prolonged rupture of membranes, congenital heart disease, or neural tube defects.

EVALUATION AND TREATMENT Abdominal radiographs show pneumatosis intestinalis or portal venous gas, or both. Symptoms usually progress rapidly, often within hours, from subtle signs to abdominal discoloration, intestinal perforation, and peritonitis or even death. Systemic hypotension requires intensive medical support or bowel resection, or both. A study is in progress to identify predictive biological markers for early diagnosis.[95] Preventive strategies include encouragement of breast milk feeding, judicious fluid management to prevent vascular fluid overload, confirmation of patent ductus arteriosus (see Chapter 25), administration of arginine and glutamine supplements to support intestinal epithelial cell growth, and utilization of enteral probiotics to support normal gut bacteria.[89,96] The rapid onset of symptoms makes primary prevention difficult.

Treatments include cessation of feeding, implementation of gastric suction to decompress the intestines, maintenance of fluid and electrolyte balance, and administration of antibiotics to control sepsis. Surgical resection is the treatment of choice for perforation, and peritoneal drainage may be used as an adjunct to laparotomy.[97] Overall mortality is high, particularly for infants who have surgery.[90]

> **QUICK CHECK 37-3**
> 1. Why do individuals with cystic fibrosis have pancreatic insufficiency?
> 2. Why does loss of villi occur with gluten-sensitive enteropathy?
> 3. Compare kwashiorkor and marasmus.

Diarrhea

Diarrhea is an increase in the water content, volume, or frequency of stools and can be acute or chronic. Diarrhea is usually defined as three or more watery or loose stools in 24 hours.[98] Children with acute gastroenteritis often remain mildly symptomatic for up to 4 weeks; therefore, diarrhea that persists longer than 4 weeks is considered chronic. Diarrhea is a common GI problem during infancy and early childhood and is the leading cause of death in young children, particularly among preterm infants and children in developing countries, with 760 000 deaths per year.[99,100] Severe, acute infectious diarrhea occurs one to three times during the first 3 years of life. Most episodes are self-limiting and resolve within 72 hours.

The pathophysiological mechanisms of diarrhea in children are similar to those described for adults—osmotic, secretory, motility, or inflammatory diarrhea (see Chapter 36). Prolonged diarrhea is more dangerous in infants and children, however, because they have much smaller fluid reserves and more rapid peristalsis and metabolism than adults. Therefore dehydration can develop rapidly if any disturbance increases fluid secretion into the GI lumen (secretory diarrhea), draws fluid into the lumen by osmosis (osmotic diarrhea), reduces intestinal transit time with luminal fluid retention (motility diarrhea), or causes inflammation that results in malabsorption and increased luminal osmotic load from nutrients, fluid, and blood, which may increase gut motility (inflammatory diarrhea).[101]

Diarrhea in Infants and Children

There are numerous causes of diarrhea in infants and young children, including bacterial and systemic infections, malabsorption syndromes, autoimmune disorders, congenital malformations, and genetic disorders.[101] Acute infection is a common cause of childhood diarrhea worldwide.

Acute infectious diarrhea in infants and young children is usually associated with viral or bacterial gastroenteritis. Viruses include rotaviruses, noroviruses, and adenoviruses. Rotavirus is the most common cause in young children and is associated with a higher death rate in low-income countries. Rotavirus vaccine is an effective preventive strategy.[102] Numerous bacteria or parasites can contaminate food or water and cause diarrhea. Specific bacteria can be identified using molecular analysis or stool culture. *Clostridium difficile* is often associated with previous antibiotic therapy.

Infectious diarrhea has a rapid onset, with watery stools sometimes mixed with blood, abdominal cramping, fever, vomiting, and weight loss. Severe dehydration, acidosis, and shock can occur quickly from diarrhea and vomiting.[103] Hemolytic uremic syndrome and kidney failure can develop when diarrhea is associated with *Shigella* toxin and *Escherichia coli* infection (see Chapter 31). Other causes of acute diarrhea in children include antibiotic therapy, appendicitis, chemotherapy, inflammatory bowel disease, parasitic infestation, parenteral infections, and ingestion of toxic substances.

Treatment of diarrhea requires evaluation of cause through history, stool testing for common pathogens, and laboratory analysis. Treatment of underlying illness is warranted when identified. Other treatments include fluid and electrolyte replacement, and antibiotics if a pathogen is found. Antispasmodics may relieve abdominal cramping, and probiotics can reduce duration and improve morbidity and mortality.[104] Intravenous solutions are used only when oral solutions are not tolerated.[105] Prevention includes clean water, environmental sanitation, and good hygiene.

Primary lactose intolerance. **Lactose malabsorption** and **lactose intolerance**, the inability to digest milk sugar, is caused by inadequate production or impaired activity of the enzyme lactase. It is a common cause of diarrhea, particularly in non-White children under the age of 7 years. The malabsorption of lactose results in osmotic diarrhea accompanied by abdominal pain, bloating, and flatulence. Systemic manifestations include skin disease, rheumatological complaints, chronic fatigue, and FTT.[106] Diagnosis includes elimination of dietary lactose or implementation of hydrogen lactose breath testing. Treatment consists of reducing milk consumption or supplementing the diet with oral lactase. Some children can tolerate lactose in fermented forms, such as cheese and yogourt, or by adding soy food. Utilization of a diet low in fermentable oligosaccharides, disaccharides, and monosaccharides and polyols (FODMAPs) or administration of probiotics to alter intestinal flora has been found to be effective in children with lactose-intolerant irritable bowel syndrome and persistent symptoms.[107]

DISORDERS OF THE LIVER

Disorders of Biliary Metabolism and Transport

Neonatal Jaundice

Jaundice (icterus) is a yellow pigmentation of the skin caused by an increased level of bilirubin in the bloodstream (total serum bilirubin [TSB]) that exceeds the 95th percentile for the infant's age in hours or greater than 342 mcmol/L, except in the low-birth-weight population. Jaundice usually becomes clinically apparent when the serum bilirubin concentration is greater than 34 mcmol/L. **Physiological jaundice (hyperbilirubinemia) of the newborn**, or *neonatal bilirubinemia*, is a frequently encountered problem in otherwise healthy newborns caused by lack of maturity of bilirubin uptake and conjugation. Poor caloric intake or dehydration, or both, associated with inadequate breastfeeding also may contribute to the high levels of bilirubin. Although up to 60% of term newborns have clinical jaundice in the first week of life, with a higher percentage in the preterm population, few have significant underlying disease. High bilirubin levels in the newborn period can be associated with hemolytic disease of the newborn, metabolic and endocrine disorders, anatomical abnormalities of the liver, and infections. For older infants and children, the most common causes of unconjugated hyperbilirubinemia are hemolytic processes resulting in bilirubin overproduction. *Pathological jaundice* is a bilirubin concentration greater than 342 mcmol/L in the newborn period associated with a severe illness, or a total serum bilirubin level that rises by more than 85.5 mcmol/L during the newborn period.

Risk factors for development of pathological jaundice include fetal–maternal blood type incompatibility (ABO and Rh incompatibility, hemolytic disease of the newborn), premature birth, exclusive breastfeeding in some infants, maternal age greater than or equal to 25 years, male gender, delayed meconium passage, glucose-6-phosphate dehydrogenase deficiency, and excessive birth trauma such as bruising or cephalohematomas.[107,108]

PATHOPHYSIOLOGY Pathological jaundice results from the complex interaction of factors that cause (1) increased bilirubin production (e.g., hemolysis), (2) impaired hepatic uptake or excretion of unconjugated bilirubin, or (3) delayed maturation of liver bilirubin conjugating mechanisms.[109] The most common cause is hemolytic disease of the newborn (ABO blood incompatibility) (see Chapters 8 and 22), and all pregnant women should be tested for ABO and Rh incompatibility. Unconjugated bilirubin (indirect bilirubin) is lipid soluble and bound to albumin in the blood, and in the free form it readily crosses the blood–brain barrier in infants. Chronic bilirubin encephalopathy (kernicterus) is caused by the deposition of toxic, unconjugated bilirubin in brain cells and usually does not occur in healthy, full-term infants. The mechanism of injury is not clearly known. Elevated conjugated bilirubin level is a sign of underlying disease.

CLINICAL MANIFESTATIONS Physiological jaundice develops during the second or third day after birth and usually subsides in 1 to 2 weeks in full-term infants and in 2 to 4 weeks in premature infants. After this period, increasing bilirubin values and persistent jaundice indicate pathological hyperbilirubinemia. Manifestations include yellowing of skin, dark urine, light-coloured stools, and weight loss. Premature infants with respiratory distress, acidosis, or sepsis are at greater risk for kernicterus (brain damage related to unconjugated hyperbilirubinemia) and the development of athetoid cerebral palsy and speech and hearing impairment.[110]

EVALUATION AND TREATMENT Jaundice is detected by clinical assessment. Both total and direct (conjugated) bilirubin levels are monitored as described previously. Other causes of jaundice must be eliminated to confirm physiological jaundice. Treatment depends on the degree of hyperbilirubinemia. Physiological jaundice is commonly treated by phototherapy and several techniques are available.[111] Pathological jaundice requires an exchange transfusion and treatment of the underlying disorder.

Biliary Atresia

Biliary atresia (BA) is a rare congenital malformation (from 1 in 8000 to 1 in 18000 live births) characterized by the absence or obstruction of intrahepatic or extrahepatic bile ducts; the most common cause of BA is neonatal cholestasis.[112] The etiology of duct injury is not clear but is thought to be related to an embryonic, congenital, or genetic abnormality or an acquired, perinatal, viral-induced progressive inflammation with innate autoimmune destruction. The disease expression is a continuum in which the principal process is one of bile duct destruction.[113] The atresia or obstruction of the bile ducts leads to plugging, inflammation, fibrosis of the bile canaliculi, and cholestasis. Progressive obstruction leads to secondary biliary cirrhosis (see Chapter 36), portal hypertension, or liver failure.

Jaundice is the primary clinical manifestation of BA, along with hepatomegaly and acholic (clay-coloured) stools. Fat absorption is impaired because of the lack of bile salts. Abdominal distension caused by hepatomegaly and ascites may cause anorexia and FTT. Fat-soluble vitamin (A, D, E, K) deficiencies require supplementation. Manifestations of cirrhosis and liver failure include ascites, hypoalbuminemia, hypercoagulation, pruritus, esophageal varices, and GI bleeding that may lead to death.

Early diagnosis of BA is essential, with the best outcome occurring when it is diagnosed and treated in the first 30 to 45 days of life. Late diagnosis of BA does not respond well to current surgical treatment. Diagnosis of BA is based on clinical manifestations, abnormal liver function tests, liver biopsy results, and intraoperative cholangiogram. Serum aminotransaminase and alkaline phosphatase levels are elevated and conjugated (direct) serum bilirubin levels rise progressively. BA can be relieved by hepatoportoenterostomy (HPE; also called the *Kasai procedure*). Even with initial restoration of bile flow, however, obliteration of intrahepatic bile ducts can continue and cirrhosis results. Liver transplantation is a successful long-term therapy for BA.[114] Eighty percent of children with BA die before the age of 3 years if not treated.

Inflammatory Disorders

Hepatitis

Viral hepatitis is discussed in Chapter 36, and the characteristics of the types of viruses that cause hepatitis are presented in Table 36-8.

Hepatitis A virus. Approximately 30 to 50% of reported cases of hepatitis A virus (HAV) occur in children,[115] particularly children of nursery school age. Since the introduction of the hepatitis A vaccine in Canada in 1996, the incidence of HAV has decreased. The number of cases of HAV reported annually in Canada has varied from 2978 (in 1991) to 246 (in 2012). From 2006 to 2012, the incidence in children was highest among 5 to 9 year olds (2.24 per 100000), followed by 1 to 4 year olds.[61]

Outbreaks tend to occur in day care centres with large numbers of children who are not toilet trained and staff members who practice poor handwashing techniques.[116] Vertical transmission from mother to newborn or from a transfusion is rare. HAV in children is usually mild and asymptomatic, but it may involve nausea, vomiting, and diarrhea. Jaundice appears in more than 70% of older children. Almost all children recover from hepatitis A without residual liver damage. Relapse HAV occurs in 3 to 20% of individuals.[117,118]

Given the underdiagnosis and under-reporting of HAV in Canada, and the occurrence of subclinical infections, the actual number of HAV cases is estimated to be seven times higher than reported.[61]

Hepatitis B virus. Risk factors for hepatitis B virus (HBV) include infants of mothers who are chronic hepatitis B surface antigen (HBsAg) carriers; children who immigrated with their families or through adoption from endemic areas; children who live with HBsAg-positive household members; and children who abuse parenteral medications or engage in unprotected sex. Ninety percent of newborns are infected by their mothers (vertical transmission); 25 to 50% of children between the ages of 1 and 5 years of age who are acutely infected will develop chronic infection.[119] Chronic hepatitis may develop because the infant's immune system is immature. Infected infants are at risk for cirrhosis and hepatocellular carcinoma.[120] The most serious consequence of HBV infection is fulminant hepatitis, which occurs in 1% of cases. Hepatitis D virus (HDV) infection depends on active infection with HBV. Exacerbation of HBV is more common in children with superinfected HDV. There is evidence that the risk for fulminant hepatitis is higher in individuals with combined infection of HBV and HDV than in those with HBV infection alone.[121] There also is a higher risk for hepatocellular carcinoma and increased mortality in this group. Aggressive HBV vaccination programs have reduced the incidence of HBV; HDV reduction has mirrored this response.[122] To prevent perinatal transmission of HBV, immunoprophylaxis and HBV vaccination within the first 12 hours of birth are recommended with close follow-up visits.[123] Treatment is conservative and antivirals are used for chronic disease. Children aged 2 to 17 years who are HBsAg seropositive for more than 6 months with elevated serum alanine transaminase (ALT) and HBV DNA levels for more than 3 months may be eligible for treatment with antivirals. Maternal antiviral therapy may be given during the third trimester when there is impending liver decompensation.[124]

In Canada in 2013, rates of reported cases of acute HBV ranged from 0.0 to 0.8 per 100000 across all jurisdictions. Rates of reported cases above the national rate of 0.5 per 100000 were observed in Ontario, Saskatchewan, and Alberta. These HBV rates are likely an underestimation of the true burden of infection in Canada. As acute HBV infection is asymptomatic in over 90% of children and 50 to 70% of adults, the majority of individuals recently infected will not present to a health care provider for testing and therefore will not be reported to the Canadian Notifiable Disease Surveillance System (CNDSS) as an acute case of HBV.[125]

Hepatitis C virus. Hepatitis C virus (HCV) in children is most commonly transmitted vertically and is enhanced with maternal co-infection with HIV. Risk factors for vertical transmission include internal fetal monitoring, prolonged rupture of membranes, and fetal anoxia.[126] HCV transmission also can occur through exposure to infected blood or contaminated materials (as in injection medication use or tattooing and body piercing) and, less commonly, following sexual encounters with HCV-infected partners. Transmission from blood transfusions has become a negligible risk with universal HCV screening of blood. With vertical transmission, spontaneous resolution of HCV is high, up to 40%; otherwise, the disease is usually mild in children and cirrhosis is rare.[126] Because of adverse drug events, only children with persistently elevated serum aminotransferases or those with progressive liver disease are treated with antiviral medications.

In Canada between 2005 and 2013, the rate of reported cases of hepatitis C decreased steadily from 40.3 per 100 000 to 29.6 per 100 000.[125] Advances in blood donation screening and infection control practices in health care settings have almost certainly contributed to the observed reductions in rates of reported HCV cases in Canada.

Chronic hepatitis. HBV and HCV are the main causes of chronic hepatitis in children. Manifestations of chronic hepatitis include malaise, anorexia, fever, GI bleeding, hepatomegaly, edema, and transient joint pain. Often there are no symptoms. Serum alanine aminotransferase and bilirubin levels are elevated. There may be evidence of impairment of synthetic functions of the liver: prolonged prothrombin time, thrombocytopenia, and hypoalbuminemia. Diagnosis is based on the clinical manifestations and liver biopsy results. There is no curative therapy for chronic HBV. Children are treated with antiviral medications and should continue to be monitored.[127] Liver transplant may ultimately be required for chronic hepatitis.

There also is an autoimmune form of chronic hepatitis, known as *autoimmune hepatitis* (AIH) or *primary sclerosing cholangitis* (PSC), with unknown etiology. The pathogenic mechanism is thought to be immunological, environmental, or genetic in nature. These diseases present with elevations in the levels of aminotransferases, autoantibodies, and immunoglobulin G (IgG). AIH is more common in female children, and both are treated with immunosuppressive therapy; about 50 to 80% will achieve remission and long-term survival.[128] A recent pediatric retrospective cross-sectional study of 34 patients with AIH and PSC showed that a greater proportion of females had AIH (74%) than PSC (45%). It also showed that the majority of patients with PSC were Black (55%), while the rest were White (36%) and Latin American (9%), suggesting a possible relation to race. By contrast, no race difference existed for AIH.[129]

Between 2009 and 2013, the rate of reported cases of chronic HBV decreased from 13.6 to 12.0 per 100 000 in Canada. In 2013, chronic HBV rates were higher for males than females overall. However, the rates for females aged 20 to 24 years and 25 to 29 years were higher than the rates for males. Males in the 30-to-39 age group had the highest rates of reported chronic HBV in 2013, followed by females in the 25-to-29 age group (25.9 and 25.7 per 100 000, respectively). In 2013, the following provinces had chronic HBV rates above the national average of 13.0 per 100 000: British Columbia (23.4 per 100 000), Ontario (15.1 per 100 000), and Alberta (14.6 per 100 000).[125]

A number of factors may explain these trends. Canada's universal immunization program targeted at newborns, school-aged children, and, in some jurisdictions, high-risk populations has likely contributed to declining rates of acute HBV. Other public health and infection control interventions aimed at preventing transmission of HBV may also have affected these trends.[125] At the same time, it is important to note that Canadian national HBV rates are heavily influenced by variations in temporal and geographical reporting practices and should be interpreted with caution. HBV reporting across the country is not uniform, and many hepatitis B cases are reported as "unspecified." Moreover, because HBV infection is asymptomatic in most individuals, a number of infected people may not visit their health care provider for HBV testing.[125]

An estimated 0.64 to 0.71% of Canadians (220 000 to 245 000 people) have chronic HCV infection, and approximately 44% of those may be undiagnosed. Not all people with chronic HCV infection will develop cirrhosis or signs or symptoms indicative of liver disease. It is estimated that approximately 84% of people infected with HCV do not develop cirrhosis 20 years after acute infection, and 59% after 30 years. Progression of liver fibrosis is variable and influenced by factors such as alcohol consumption, age at time of infection, male gender, and HIV co-infection.[130]

Treatment and self-care, including reducing alcohol intake, can prevent progressive liver disease and improve quality of life. Treatment of HCV is shifting from older, poorly tolerated interferon-based therapies, which cure approximately 55% of those treated, to new well-tolerated short-course (8 to 12 weeks) interferon-free direct-acting antiviral drugs with cure rates approaching more than 95%. However, treatment can only occur if undiagnosed people get tested and if diagnosed people are engaged in care.[131]

Cirrhosis

Cirrhosis is fibrotic scarring of the liver in response to inflammation and tissue damage resulting in obstruction to the flow of blood and bile. Most forms of chronic liver diseases in children can progress to cirrhosis, but they seldom do so. The complications of cirrhosis in children are the same as those in adults: portal hypertension, the opening of collateral vessels between the portal and systemic veins, and varices. In addition, children with cirrhosis experience growth failure caused by nutritional deficits, as well as developmental delay, particularly in gross motor function because of ascites and weakness. The cause of cirrhosis may influence its severity and course. Some types of cirrhosis can be stabilized if the cause is identified and treated early.[132] The risk for cirrhosis is increasing in obese children who have nonalcoholic fatty liver disease (NAFLD). (See *Health Promotion*: Childhood Obesity and Fatty Liver Disease in Canada.)

Portal Hypertension

Portal hypertension is increased pressure in the portal venous system (see Chapter 36) and a major cause of morbidity and mortality in children with liver disease. There are two basic causes of portal hypertension in children: (1) increased resistance to blood flow within the portal system and (2) increased volume of portal blood flow. The second cause is rare in children and is not discussed here. Increased resistance to flow can occur anywhere in the portal circulatory system. Portal hypertension can accompany cirrhosis, intra-abdominal infections, portal vein thrombosis, congenital anomalies of the portal vein, and congenital hepatic fibrosis.

Types of Portal Hypertension

Extrahepatic portal hypertension. Extrahepatic (prehepatic) portal venous obstruction causes 50 to 70% of the cases of extrahepatic portal hypertension in children. In approximately two-thirds of these children, no specific cause can be found.[133] Obstruction is almost always in the portal vein and is usually caused by thrombosis as a complication of abdominal trauma, pancreatitis, abdominal infections, and some systemic disorders; however, these causes are rare. Life-threatening bleeding and coagulation disorders can occur. Mesoportal bypass (anastomosis of portal vein to mesenteric vein) restores normal physiological portal flow to the liver and corrects portal hypertension.[134]

HEALTH PROMOTION

Childhood Obesity and Fatty Liver Disease in Canada

Canada is in the midst of a childhood obesity epidemic. More than 1 in 4 children and youth in Canada are overweight or obese. A complex and interacting system of factors, complicated by a variety of policy decisions made in a number of different sectors, contributes to increasing rates of overweight and obesity. Key factors that have a direct effect on childhood obesity are the marketing of foods and beverages high in fat and sugar (fructose), greater food availability, and large portion sizes.

Increasingly, obese children are being diagnosed with alterations in health conditions, such as fatty liver disease, that were previously only prevalent among adults. According to the Canadian Liver Foundation, a person is considered to have a fatty liver if the fat builds up to more than 5% of the liver. Nonalcoholic fatty liver disease (NAFLD) affects about 20% of Canadians, making it the most common liver disease in Canada. It is prevalent in people who are overweight or obese. The Canadian Liver Foundation estimates that NAFLD affects almost 3% of children and 25 to 55% of obese children. NAFLD can be found in children as young as 2 years of age. In children, increased waist circumference is an indicator of possible NAFLD, which can range from a simple fatty liver to a liver with inflammation and fibrosis (nonalcoholic steatohepatitis [NASH]) to cirrhosis.

Canadian researchers have strong evidence indicating that reductions in fructose intake, particularly of high-fructose corn syrup (HFCS), can result in significant reductions in metabolic dysregulation and hepatic injury in children with NAFLD. In a recent study, researchers at the University of Alberta examined the impact of dietary intervention (fructose and glycemic index, glycemic load diet [FRAGILE]) on body composition, liver function, and metabolic markers in obese children with NAFLD. The researchers noted that other studies found a direct correlation between higher intakes of simple sugars (fructose, specifically HFCS) and saturated fat with an increased risk for liver damage in childhood NAFLD. Based on their study's findings, they concluded that modest reductions in fructose intake (total fructose, free fructose, and HFCS) result in improvements of plasma markers of liver dysfunction and cardiometabolic risk in childhood NAFLD.

Policymakers across government sectors should coordinate their efforts to reach a consensus to limit and prevent the addition of fructose (particularly in processed foods) to reach a potential therapeutic target for children with NAFLD.

Data from Canadian Liver Foundation. (2016). *Fatty liver disease.* Markham, ON: Author. Retrieved from http://www.liver.ca/files/PDF/New_format_info_sheets_-_2011_-_english/CLF_InfoSheet_FattyLiverDisease_E.pdf; Mager, D.R., Iniguez, I.R., Gilmour, S., et al. (2013). *J Parenter Enteral Nutr, 39*(1), 73–84. doi:10.1177/0148607113501201; Public Health Agency of Canada. (2011). *Curbing childhood obesity: A federal, provincial, and territorial framework for action to promote healthy weights.* Ottawa: Author. Retrieved from http://www.phac-aspc.gc.ca/hp-ps/hl-mvs/framework-cadre/pdf/ccofw-eng.pdf.

Intrahepatic portal hypertension. Liver fibrosis is the primary cause of intrahepatic portal hypertension. The fibrosis can lead to cirrhosis with increased resistance to portal blood flow by constricting and reducing the compliance of hepatic sinusoids. Chronic hepatitis, BA, NAFLD, and congenital hepatic fibrosis are causes of liver fibrosis in children.[135-137]

The clinical manifestations of portal hypertension are (1) splenomegaly, (2) upper GI tract bleeding, (3) ascites, (4) hepatopulmonary syndrome, (5) hepatorenal syndrome, and (6) hepatic encephalopathy (see Chapter 36).

The objectives of the clinical investigation are to (1) locate the site of the venous block and (2) identify the disease responsible for the portal hypertension. The following may be included in the diagnostic evaluation: thorough physical examination; laboratory evaluation of liver function, white blood count, and platelet count; ultrasonographic imaging; endoscopic evaluation; and biopsy. Treatment in children is the same as that in adults (see Chapter 36).

The outcome of portal hypertension depends almost entirely on its cause. Children with extrahepatic disease are expected to recover with little morbidity. For children with intrahepatic disease, the prognosis varies.

Metabolic Disorders

More than 5 000 genetically determined metabolic pathways have been identified in liver tissue. The earliest possible identification of metabolic disorders is essential because (1) early treatment may prevent permanent damage to vital organs, such as the liver or brain; (2) precise genetic counselling may be possible with prenatal diagnosis; and (3) complications can be minimized, even if cure is not possible. Galactosemia, fructosemia, glycogen storage disease (GSD), and Wilson's disease are the most common metabolic disorders. They are treatable and have hepatic clinical manifestations. The mechanisms of disease, clinical manifestations, and evaluation and treatment of these disorders are presented in Table 37-2.

GASTRO-INTESTINAL MALIGNANCIES IN CHILDREN

Globally, cancers in children (0 to 14 years of age) differ from those occurring in adults in terms of their origin and their malignant behaviour. Tumours in children generally have shorter latency periods and are more aggressive and invasive than tumours in adults.

Hepatoblastoma

Hepatoblastoma is the most common pediatric liver cancer, representing more than 90% of malignant liver tumours diagnosed in children under 5 years of age.[138] It usually affects young children within the first 3 years of life, and boys are more affected than girls. Children with hepatoblastoma typically present with an abdominal mass that causes pain and discomfort. Parents often report that their child has lost his or her appetite and is losing weight. Patients also develop weakness and fatigue in addition abdominal swelling and hepatomegaly on physical examination.

Hepatoblastomas are heterogeneous tumours that usually display combinations of epithelial, mesenchymal, undifferentiated, and/or other components. The most common epithelial component is the embryonal pattern, which is characterized by histological patterns recapitulating liver development, and is sometimes associated with genetic disorders.[139]

Hepatoblastoma is often associated with aberrant activation of developmental pathways similar to other embryonal tumours in children. Hepatoblastoma therapy generally includes a combination of surgical resection and chemotherapy. If surgical removal presents a high risk for mortality, due to the size and location of this tumour inside the liver, cure is still possible with liver transplantation. Unfortunately, the prognosis is still poor for children with unresectable or disseminated hepatoblastoma.[140]

Pancreatic Tumours

Malignant pancreatic tumours are a heterogeneous assortment of benign or malignant neoplasms, arising from exocrine cells or endocrine cells that are extremely rare in pediatric age. While pancreatic cancer is one

TABLE 37-2 Galactosemia, Fructosemia, and Wilson's Disease

	Galactosemia	Fructosemia	Wilson's Disease
Mechanism of disease	Deficiency of galactose-1-phosphate uridylyltransferase Autosomal recessive trait Inability to convert galactose to glucose Toxic accumulation of galactose in body tissues, liver, and brain	Deficiency of fructose-1-phosphate aldolase Autosomal recessive trait Inability to metabolize fructose, sucrose, or honey; occurs when breast milk is replaced with cow's milk Toxic accumulation of fructose in body tissues	Autosomal recessive: defect on chromosome 13 (ATP 7B) Defect in copper excretion by liver Impaired transport of copper into bile/blood caused by diminished transport protein (ceruloplasmin) Toxic accumulations of copper in liver, brain, kidney, corneas
Clinical manifestation	High levels of blood galactose Vomiting Hypoglycemia May have failure to thrive Symptoms of cirrhosis at 2–6 months—jaundice Intellectual disabilities if not treated Cataracts if not treated	High levels of blood fructose Vomiting Hypoglycemia May have failure to thrive Hepatomegaly Jaundice Seizures	Intention tremors Indistinct speech Dystonia Greenish yellow rings in cornea Hepatomegaly Jaundice Anorexia Renal tubular defects
Evaluation	Newborn screening Presence of reducing substances in urine when infant is receiving lactose	Detailed dietary history Liver or intestinal mucosa biopsy	Low plasma ceruloplasmin level
Treatment	Galactose-free diet	Fructose, sucrose, honey-free diet Vitamin C supplementation	Chelation therapy to remove copper from body Decreased dietary intake of copper Liver transplant

of the most frequent fatal malignancies in adults, only very small series and a few case reports have been published in the pediatric oncology literature.[141] The main clinical symptom is abdominal pain associated with a palpable mass on examination. Patients also often report a lack of appetite and vomiting.

QUICK CHECK 37-4

1. Why is diarrhea such a serious disorder in infants and children?
2. What is biliary atresia?
3. What are the four most common metabolic disorders that cause liver damage in children?

DID YOU UNDERSTAND?

Overview

1. Alterations of digestive function in children include congenital obstructions of the intestinal tract; disorders of digestion, absorption, or nutrition; or liver disease.

Disorders of the Gastro-Intestinal Tract

1. Cleft lip and cleft palate (failure of the bony palate to fuse in the midline) may occur separately or together. The fissure may affect the uvula, soft palate, hard palate, nostril, and maxillary alveolar ridge, with difficulty sucking and swallowing.
2. Esophageal atresia, a condition in which the esophagus ends in a blind pouch, may occur with or without tracheoesophageal fistula. As the infant swallows oral secretions or ingests milk, the pouch fills, causing either drooling or aspiration into the lungs.
3. Infantile hypertrophic pyloric stenosis is an obstruction of the pyloric outlet caused by hypertrophy of circular muscles in the pyloric sphincter.
4. In intestinal malrotation, the small intestine lacks a normal posterior attachment during fetal development, causing volvulus (twisting of the bowel on itself) that may partly or completely occlude the Gastro-Intestinal (GI) tract and its blood vessels.
5. Meckel diverticulum is a congenital malformation of the GI tract involving all layers of the small intestinal wall; it usually occurs in the ileum.
6. Meconium ileus is a newborn condition in which intestinal secretions and amniotic waste products produce a thick, tarry plug that obstructs the intestine; it occurs in 10 to 15% of newborns with cystic fibrosis (CF).
7. Idiopathic intestinal pseudo-obstruction is a disorder of impaired intestinal motility.
8. Hirschsprung's disease (aganglionic megacolon) is caused by a malformation of the parasympathetic nervous system in a segment of the colon needed for peristalsis, resulting in colon obstruction.
9. Malformations of the anus and rectum range from mild congenital stenosis of the anus to complex deformities, all of which are classified as imperforate anus.
10. Gastroesophageal reflux disease is the presence of symptoms related to the return of stomach contents into the esophagus caused by relaxation or incompetence of the lower esophageal sphincter that results from immaturity of the gastroesophageal sphincter.
11. Intussusception is the telescoping of a proximal segment of intestine into a distal segment, causing an obstruction.
12. CF is an inherited fibrocystic disease that involves mucosal chloride and sodium ion channels in many organs, including the GI tract and pancreas; CF causes pancreatic enzyme deficiency with maldigestion.
13. Celiac disease is caused by hypersensitivity to gluten protein, with autoimmune injury and loss of the villous epithelium. It results in malabsorption and growth failure.

14. Pediatric malnutrition is an imbalance between nutrient requirements and intake that results in energy, protein, and micronutrient deficits, which negatively impact growth and development.
15. Kwashiorkor is a severe protein deficiency. Marasmus is a deficiency of all dietary nutrients, including carbohydrates.
16. Failure to thrive or growth faltering is a multifactorial condition that includes biological, psychosocial, and environmental contributions; it may or may not be illness related; and it results in inadequate physical growth and development of a child.
17. Necrotizing enterocolitis is an ischemic inflammatory disorder in neonates, particularly premature infants, thought to result from immaturity, infection, stress, and anoxia of the bowel wall.
18. Acute diarrhea in infants and children is three or more watery or loose stools in 24 hours; it is commonly caused by viral or bacterial enterocolitis.
19. Chronic diarrhea (diarrhea persisting longer than 4 weeks) can be caused by a wide variety of underlying conditions and often leads to growth failure and slow development.
20. Primary lactose intolerance is the inability to digest milk sugar because of a lack of the enzyme lactase, resulting in osmotic diarrhea.

Disorders of the Liver

1. Physiological jaundice of the newborn is caused by mild hyperbilirubinemia that subsides in 1 or 2 weeks. Pathological jaundice is caused by severe hyperbilirubinemia and can cause brain damage (kernicterus).
2. Biliary atresia is a congenital malformation of the bile ducts that obstructs bile flow and causes jaundice, cirrhosis, and liver failure.
3. Acute hepatitis is usually caused by a virus, and hepatitis A is the most common form of childhood hepatitis. Chronic hepatitis B or C usually occurs by maternal transmission.
4. Cirrhosis results from fibrotic scarring of the liver and is rare in children, but it can develop from most forms of chronic liver disease.
5. Portal hypertension in children usually is caused by extrahepatic obstruction, and the cause is often unknown. Intrahepatic obstruction is related to diseases that cause liver fibrosis.
6. The four most common metabolic disorders that cause liver damage in children are galactosemia, fructosemia, glycogen storage disease, and Wilson's disease. All are inherited as genetic traits and allow toxins to accumulate in the liver.

Gastro-Intestinal Malignancies in Children

1. Children with hepatoblastoma often present with an abdominal mass that causes pain and is associated with loss of appetite and weight loss.
2. The main clinical symptom of a pancreatic tumour is abdominal pain associated with a palpable mass on examination, loss of appetite, and vomiting.

KEY TERMS

Anorectal malformation (ARM), 972
Biliary atresia (BA), 980
Celiac crisis, 976
Celiac disease (CD), 975
Cirrhosis, 981
Cleft lip (CL), 968
Cleft palate (CP), 968
Cystic fibrosis (CF), 974
Diarrhea, 979
Distal intestinal obstruction syndrome (DIOS), 971
Eosinophilic esophagitis (EoE), 973
Esophageal atresia (EA), 969
Esophageal atresia/tracheoesophageal fistula (EA/TEF), 969
Extrahepatic portal hypertension, 981
Failure to thrive (FTT), 977
Fructosemia, 982
Galactosemia, 982
Gastroesophageal reflux (GER), 972
Gastroesophageal reflux disease (GERD), 972
Glycogen storage disease (GSD), 982
Growth faltering (GF), 977
Hepatitis A virus (HAV), 980
Hepatitis B virus (HBV), 980
Hepatitis C virus (HCV), 981
Hepatitis D virus (HDV), 980
Hepatoblastoma, 982
Hirschsprung's disease, 972
Idiopathic intestinal pseudo-obstruction, 971
Infantile hypertrophic pyloric stenosis (IHPS), 969
Intrahepatic portal hypertension, 982
Intussusception, 973
Jaundice (icterus), 979
Kernicterus, 980
Kwashiorkor, 977
Lactose intolerance, 979
Lactose malabsorption, 979
Malrotation, 970
Marasmus, 977
Meckel diverticulum, 971
Meconium, 971
Meconium disease (MD), 971
Meconium ileus (MI), 971
Meconium plug syndrome (MPS), 971
Necrotizing enterocolitis (NEC), 978
Nonceliac gluten sensitivity (NCGS), 975
Nonsyndromic (isolated) CP, 968
Physiological jaundice (hyperbilirubinemia) of the newborn, 979
Protein-energy malnutrition (PEM), 977
Rotavirus, 973
Syndromic CLP, 968
Wilson's disease, 982

REFERENCES

1. University of Toronto, Division of Plastic & Reconstructive Surgery. (2016). *Cleft lip and palate*. Retrieved from https://www.uoftplasticsurgery.ca/programs/cleft-lip-palate/.
2. Leslie, E. J., & Marazita, M. L. (2013). Genetics of cleft lip and cleft palate. *American Journal of Medical Genetics: Part C, Seminars in Medical Genetics, 163C*(4), 246–258. doi:10.1002/ajmg.c.31381.
3. Molina-Solana, R., Yáñez-Vico, R. M., Iglesias-Linares, A., et al. (2013). Current concepts on the effect of environmental factors on cleft lip and palate. *International Journal of Oral and Maxillofacial Surgery, 42*(2), 177–184. doi:10.1016/j.ijom.2012.10.008.
4. Mossey, P. A., Little, J., Munger, R. G., et al. (2009). Cleft lip and palate. *Lancet, 374*(9703), 1773–1785. doi:10.1016/S0140-6736(09)60695-4.
5. Reilly, S., Reid, J., Skeat, J., et al. (2007). ABM Clinical Protocol #17: Guidelines for breastfeeding infants with cleft lip, cleft palate, or cleft lip and palate. *Breastfeeding Medicine, 2*(4), 243–250. doi:10.1089/bfm.2007.9984.
6. Farronato, G., Kairyte, L., Giannini, L., et al. (2014). How various surgical protocols of the unilateral cleft lip and palate influence the facial growth and possible orthodontic problems? Which is the best timing of lip, palate and alveolus repair? Literature review. *Stomatologija, 16*(2), 53–60.
7. Jayaram, R., & Huppa, C. (2012). Surgical correction of cleft lip and palate. *Frontiers of Oral Biology, 16*, 101–110. doi:10.1159/000337664.
8. Shaye, D. (2014). Update on outcomes research for cleft lip and palate. *Current Opinion in Otolaryngology and Head and Neck Surgery, 22*(4), 255–259. doi:10.1097/MOO.0000000000000064.
9. Sitzman, T. J., Allori, A. C., & Thorburn, G. (2014). Measuring outcomes in cleft lip and palate treatment. *Clinics in Plastic Surgery, 41*(2), 311–319. doi:10.1016/j.cps.2013.12.001.
10. El-Gohary, Y., Gittes, G. K., & Tovar, J. A. (2010). Congenital anomalies of the esophagus. *Seminars in Pediatric Surgery, 19*(3), 186–193. doi:10.1053/j.sempedsurg.2010.03.009.
11. Holland, A. J., & Fitzgerald, D. A. (2010). Oesophageal atresia and tracheo-oesophageal fistula: Current management strategies and complications. *Paediatric Respiratory Reviews, 11*(2), 100–106, quiz 106–107. doi:10.1016/j.prrv.2010.01.007.
12. de Jong, E. M., Felix, J. F., de Klein, A., et al. (2010). Etiology of esophageal atresia and tracheoesophageal fistula: "Mind the gap".

Current Gastroenterology Reports, 12(3), 215–222. doi:10.1007/s11894-010-0108-1.
13. Solomon, B. D., Baker, L. A., Bear, K. A., et al. (2014). An approach to the identification of anomalies and etiologies in neonates with identified or suspected VACTERL (vertebral defects, anal atresia, tracheo-esophageal fistula with esophageal atresia, cardiac anomalies, renal anomalies, and limb anomalies). *The Journal of Pediatrics, 164*(3), 451–457. doi:10.1016/j.jpeds.2013.10.086.
14. Pinheiro, P. F., Simões e Silva, E. C., & Pereira, R. M. (2012). Current knowledge on esophageal atresia. *World Journal of Gastroenterology, 18*(28), 3662–3672. doi:10.3748/wjg.v18.i28.3662.
15. Alberti, D., Boroni, G., Corasaniti, L., et al. (2011). Esophageal atresia: Pre and post-operative management. *The Journal of Maternal-Fetal and Neonatal Medicine, 24*(Suppl. 1), 4–6. doi:10.310 9/14767058.2011.607558.
16. Krogh, C., Gørtz, S., Wohlfahrt, J., et al. (2012). Pre- and perinatal risk factors for pyloric stenosis and their influence on the male predominance. *American Journal of Epidemiology, 176*(1), 24–31. doi:10.1093/aje/kwr493.
17. Askew, N. (2010). An overview of infantile hypertrophic pyloric stenosis. *Paediatric Nursing, 22*(8), 27–30.
18. Peters, B., Oomen, M. W., Bakx, R., et al. (2014). Advances in infantile hypertrophic pyloric stenosis. *Expert Review of Gastroenterology & Hepatology, 8*(5), 533–541. doi:10.1586/17474124.2014.903799.
19. Ranells, J. D., Carver, J. D., & Kirby, R. S. (2011). Infantile hypertrophic pyloric stenosis: Epidemiology, genetics, and clinical update. *Advances in Pediatrics, 58*(1), 195–206. doi:10.1016/j.yapd.2011.03.005.
20. Kliegman, R. M., Stanton, B. F., Gemell, J. W., et al. (Eds.), (2011). *Nelson textbook of pediatrics* (19th ed.). Philadelphia: Saunders.
21. Ooms, N., Matthyssens, L. E., Draaisma, J. M., et al. (2016). Laparoscopic treatment of intestinal malrotation in children. *European Journal of Pediatric Surgery, 26*(4), 376–381. doi: 10.1055/s-0035-1554914.
22. Daneman, A. (2009). Malrotation: The balance of evidence. *Pediatric Radiology, 39*(Suppl. 2), S164–S166. doi:10.1007/s00247-009-1152-6.
23. El-Gohary, Y., Alagtal, M., & Gillick, J. (2010). Long-term complications following operative intervention for intestinal malrotation: A 10-year review. *Pediatric Surgery International, 26*(2), 203–206. doi:10.1007/s00383-009-2483-y.
24. Kotecha, M., Bellah, R., Pena, A. H., et al. (2012). Multimodality imaging manifestations of the Meckel diverticulum in children. *Pediatric Radiology, 42*(1), 95–103. doi:10.1007/s00247-011-2252-7.
25. St-Vil, D., Brandt, M. L., Panic, S., et al. (1991). Meckel's diverticulum in children: A 20-year review. *Journal of Pediatric Surgery, 26*(11), 1289–1292.
26. Thurley, P. D., Halliday, K. E., Somers, J. M., et al. (2009). Radiological features of Meckel's diverticulum and its complications. *Clinical Radiology, 64*(2), 109–118. doi:10.1016/j.crad.2008.07.012.
27. Uppal, K., Tubbs, R. S., Matusz, P., et al. (2011). Meckel's diverticulum: A review. *Clinical Anatomy (New York, N.Y.), 24*(4), 416–422. doi:10.1002/ca.21094.
28. Yahchouchy, E. K., Marano, A. F., Etienne, J. C., et al. (2001). Meckel's diverticulum. *Journal of the American College of Surgeons, 192*(5), 658–662.
29. Carlyle, B. E., Borowitz, D. S., & Glick, P. L. (2012). A review of pathophysiology and management of fetuses and neonates with meconium ileus for the pediatric surgeon. *Journal of Pediatric Surgery, 47*(4), 772–781. doi:10.1016/j.jpedsurg.2012.02.019.
30. Karimi, A., Gorter, R. R., Sleeboom, C., et al. (2011). Issues in the management of simple and complex meconium ileus. *Pediatric Surgery International, 27*(9), 963–968. doi:10.1007/s00383-011-2906-4.
31. Lavie, M., Manowitz, T., Vilozni, D., et al. (2015). Long-term follow-up of distal intestinal obstruction syndrome in cystic fibrosis. *World Journal of Gastroenterology, 21*(1), 318–325. doi:10.3748/wjg.v21.i1.318.
32. van der Doef, H. P., Kokke, F. T., van der Ent, C. K., et al. (2011). Intestinal obstruction syndromes in cystic fibrosis: Meconium ileus, distal intestinal obstruction syndrome, and constipation. *Current Gastroenterology Reports, 13*(3), 265–270. doi:10.1007/s11894-011-0185-9.
33. Colombo, C., Ellemunter, H., Houwen, R., et al. (2011). Guidelines for the diagnosis and management of distal intestinal obstruction syndrome in cystic fibrosis patients. *Journal of Cystic Fibrosis, 10*(Suppl. 2), S24–S28. doi:10.1016/S1569-1993(11)60005-2.
34. Copeland, D. R., St. Peter, S. D., Sharp, S. W., et al. (2009). Diminishing role of contrast enema in simple meconium ileus. *Journal of Pediatric Surgery, 44*(11), 2130–2132. doi:10.1016/j.jpedsurg.2009.06.005.
35. Ambartsumyan, L., & Rodriguez, L. (2014). Gastrointestinal motility disorders in children. *Gastroenterology & Hepatology, 10*(1), 16–26.
36. Gariepy, C. E., & Mousa, H. (2009). Clinical management of motility disorders in children. *Seminars in Pediatric Surgery, 18*(4), 224–238. doi:10.1053/j.sempedsurg.2009.07.004.
37. Mallick, S., Prasenjit, D., Prateek, K., et al. (2014). Chronic intestinal pseudo-obstruction: Systematic histopathological approach can clinch vital clues. *Virchows Archiv: An International Journal of Pathology, 464*(5), 529–537. doi:10.1007/s00428-014-1565-y.
38. Amiel, J., & Lyonnet, S. (2001). Hirschsprung disease, associated syndromes, and genetics: A review. *Journal of Medical Genetics, 38*(11), 729–739.
39. McKeown, S. J., Stamp, L., Hao, M. M., et al. (2013). Hirschsprung disease: A developmental disorder of the enteric nervous system. *Wiley Interdisciplinary Reviews: Developmental Biology, 2*(1), 113–129. doi:10.1002/wdev.57.
40. Moore, S. W. (2012). Chromosomal and related Mendelian syndromes associated with Hirschsprung's disease. *Pediatric Surgery International, 28*(11), 1045–1058. doi:10.1007/s00383-012-3175-6.
41. Butler Tjaden, N. E., & Trainor, P. A. (2013). The developmental etiology and pathogenesis of Hirschsprung disease. *Translational Research: The Journal of Laboratory and Clinical Medicine, 162*(1), 1–15. doi:10.1016/j.trsl.2013.03.001.
42. Amiel, J., Sproat-Emison, E., Garcia-Barcelo, M., et al. (2008). Hirschsprung disease, associated syndromes and genetics: A review. *Journal of Medical Genetics, 45*(1), 1–14. doi:10.1136/jmg.2007.053959.
43. Chumpitazi, B. P., & Nurko, S. (2011). Defecation disorders in children after surgery for Hirschsprung disease. *Journal of Pediatric Gastroenterology and Nutrition, 53*(1), 75–79. doi:10.1097/MPG.0b013e318212eb53.
44. Dillon, P. W. (2002). *Congenital pediatric colorectal disorders*. Retrieved from http://www.fascrs.org.
45. Feichter, S., Meier-Ruge, W. A., & Bruder, E. (2009). The histopathology of gastrointestinal motility disorders in children. *Seminars in Pediatric Surgery, 18*(4), 206–211. doi:10.1053/j.sempedsurg.2009.07.002.
46. Gourlay, D. M. (2013). Colorectal considerations in pediatric patients. *The Surgical Clinics of North America, 93*(1), 251–272. doi:10.1016/j.suc.2012.09.017.
47. Bischoff, A., Levitt, M. A., & Peña, A. (2011). Laparoscopy and its use in the repair of anorectal malformations. *Journal of Pediatric Surgery, 46*(8), 1609–1617. doi:10.1016/j.jpedsurg.2011.03.068.
48. Bischoff, A., Levitt, M. A., & Peña, A. (2013). Update on the management of anorectal malformations. *Pediatric Surgery International, 29*(9), 899–904. doi:10.1007/s00383-013-3355-z.
49. Herman, R. S., & Teitelbaum, D. H. (2012). Anorectal malformations. *Clinics in Perinatology, 39*(2), 403–422. doi:10.1016/j.clp.2012.04.001.
50. Levitt, M. A., & Peña, A. (2007). Anorectal malformations. *Orphanet Journal of Rare Diseases, 2*, 33. doi:10.1186/1750-1172-2-33.
51. England, R. J., Warren, S. L., Bezuidenhout, L., et al. (2012). Laparoscopic repair of anorectal malformations at the Red Cross War Memorial Children's Hospital: Taking stock. *Journal of Pediatric Surgery, 47*(3), 565–570. doi:10.1016/j.jpedsurg.2011.08.006.
52. Lightdale, J. R., Gremse, D. A., & Section on Gastroenterology, Hepatology, and Nutrition. (2013). Gastroesophageal reflux: Management guidance for the pediatrician. *Pediatrics, 131*(5), e1684–e1695. doi:10.1542/peds.2013-0421.
53. Wyllie, R., Hyams, J., & Kay, M. (2011). *Pediatric gastrointestinal and liver disease* (4th ed., p. 233). Philadelphia: Saunders.
54. Vandenplas, Y., Rudolph, C. D., Di Lorenzo, C., et al. (2009). Pediatric gastroesophageal reflux clinical practice guidelines: Joint recommendations of the North American Society for Pediatric Gastroenterology, Hepatology, and Nutrition (NASPGHAN) and the European Society for Pediatric Gastroenterology, Hepatology, and Nutrition (ESPGHAN). *Journal of Pediatric Gastroenterology and Nutrition, 49*(4), 498–547. doi:10.1097/MPG.0b013e3181b7f563.
55. Gupta, S. K. (2014). Diagnostic and therapeutic challenges in pediatric eosinophilic esophagitis: Past, present and future. *Digestive Diseases (Basel, Switzerland), 32*(1–2), 107–109. doi:10.1159/000357084.
56. Sherman, P. M., Hassall, E., Fagundes-Neto, U., et al. (2009). A global, evidence-based consensus on the definition of gastroesophageal reflux disease in the pediatric population. *The American Journal of Gastroenterology, 104*(5), 1278–1295. doi:10.1038/ajg.2009.129.
57. Tighe, M., Afzal, N. A., Bevan, A., et al. (2014). Pharmacological treatment of children with gastro-oesophageal reflux. *The Cochrane Database of Systematic Reviews*, (11), CD008550, doi:10.1002/14651858.CD008550.pub2.
58. Martin, K., Deshales, C., & Emil, S. (2014). Outcomes of pediatric laparoscopic fundoplication: A critical review of the literature. *Canadian Journal of Gastroenterology & Hepatology, 28*(2), 97–102.
59. Parikh, M., Samujh, R., Kanojia, R., et al. (2010). Does all small bowel intussusception need exploration? *African Journal of Paediatric Surgery, 7*(1), 30–32. doi:10.4103/0189-6725.59358.
60. Yih, W. K., Lieu, T. A., Kulldorff, M., et al. (2014). Intussusception risk after rotavirus vaccination in U.S. infants. *The New England Journal of Medicine, 370*(6), 503–512. doi:10.1056/NEJMoa1303164.
61. Government of Canada. (2016). *Canadian immunization guide: Part 4*. Retrieved from http://healthycanadians.gc.ca/publications/healthy-living-vie-saine/4-canadian-immunization-guide-canadien-immunisation/index-eng.php?page=19.
62. Apelt, N., Featherstone, N., & Giuliani, S. (2013). Laparoscopic treatment of intussusception in children: A systematic review. *Journal of Pediatric Surgery, 48*(8), 1789–1793. doi:10.1016/j.jpedsurg.2013.05.024.
63. Gray, M. P., Li, S. H., Hoffmann, R. G., et al. (2014). Recurrence rates after intussusception enema reduction: A meta-analysis. *Pediatrics, 134*(1), 110–119. doi:10.1542/peds.2013-3102.
64. Pepper, V. K., Stanfill, A. B., & Pearl, R. H. (2012). Diagnosis and management of pediatric appendicitis, intussusception, and Meckel diverticulum. *The Surgical Clinics of North America, 92*(3), 505–526, vii. doi:10.1016/j.suc.2012.03.011.
65. Gelfond, D., & Borowitz, D. (2013). Gastrointestinal complications of cystic fibrosis. *Clinical Gastroenterology and Hepatology, 11*(4), 333–342. doi:10.1016/j.cgh.2012.11.006.
66. Ode, K. L., & Moran, A. (2013). New insights into cystic fibrosis-related diabetes in children. *The Lancet. Diabetes & Endocrinology, 1*(1), 52–58. doi:10.1016/S2213-8587(13)70015-9.
67. Borowitz, D., & Gelfond, D. (2013). Intestinal complications of cystic fibrosis. *Current Opinion in*

Pulmonary Medicine, 19(6), 676–680. doi:10.1097/MCP.0b013e3283659ef2.
68. Phung, O. J., Coleman, C. I., Baker, E. L., et al. (2010). Recombinant human growth hormone in the treatment of patients with cystic fibrosis. *Pediatrics, 126*(5), e1211–e1226. doi:10.1542/peds.2010-2007.
69. Husby, S., Koletzko, S., Korponay–Szabó, I. R., et al. (2012). European Society for Pediatric Gastroenterology, Hepatology, and Nutrition guidelines for the diagnosis of coeliac disease. *Journal of Pediatric Gastroenterology and Nutrition, 54*(1), 136–160. doi:10.1097/MPG.0b013e31821a23d0.
70. Guandalini, S., & Assiri, A. (2014). Celiac disease: A review. *JAMA Pediatrics, 168*(3), 272–278. doi:10.1001/jamapediatrics.2013.3858.
71. Canadian Celiac Association. (2016). *About celiac disease.* Retrieved from http://www.celiac.ca/?page_id=882.
72. Kabbani, T. A., Vanga, R. R., Leffler, D. A., et al. (2014). Celiac disease or non-celiac gluten sensitivity? An approach to clinical differential diagnosis. *The American Journal of Gastroenterology, 109*(5), 741–746. doi:10.1038/ajg.2014.41.
73. Kaukinen, K., Lindfors, K., Collin, P., et al. (2010). Coeliac disease—A diagnostic and therapeutic challenge. *Clinical Chemistry and Laboratory Medicine, 48*(9), 1205–1216. doi:10.1515/CCLM.2010.241.
74. Liu, E., Lee, H. S., Aronsson, C. A., et al. (2014). Risk of pediatric celiac disease according to HLA haplotype and country. *The New England Journal of Medicine, 371*(1), 42–49. doi:10.1056/NEJMoa1313977.
75. Elli, L., Discepolo, V., Bardella, M. T., et al. (2014). Does gluten intake influence the development of celiac disease-associated complications? *Journal of Clinical Gastroenterology, 48*(1), 13–20. doi:10.1097/MCG.0b013e3182a9f898.
76. Fergusson, P., & Tomkins, A. (2009). HIV prevalence and mortality among children undergoing treatment for severe acute malnutrition in sub-Saharan Africa: A systematic review and meta-analysis. *Transactions of the Royal Society of Tropical Medicine and Hygiene, 103*(6), 541–548. doi:10.1016/j.trstmh.2008.10.029.
77. Garrett, W. S. (2013). Kwashiorkor and the gut microbiota. *The New England Journal of Medicine, 368*(18), 1746–1747. doi:10.1056/NEJMcibr1301297.
78. Prieto, M. B., & Cid, J. L. (2011). Malnutrition in the critically ill child: The importance of enteral nutrition. *International Journal of Environmental Research and Public Health, 8*(11), 4353–4366. doi:10.3390/ijerph8114353.
79. Smith, M. I., Yatsunenko, T., Manary, M. J., et al. (2013). Gut microbiomes of Malawian twin pairs discordant for kwashiorkor. *Science, 339*(6119), 548–554. doi:10.1126/science.1229000.
80. Trehan, I., Goldbach, H. S., LaGrone, L. N., et al. (2013). Antibiotics as part of the management of severe acute malnutrition. *The New England Journal of Medicine, 368*(5), 425–435. doi:10.1056/NEJMoa1202851.
81. Grover, Z., & Ee, L. C. (2009). Protein energy malnutrition. *Pediatric Clinics of North America, 56*(5), 1055–1068. doi:10.1016/j.pcl.2009.07.001.
82. Maida, J. M., Mathers, K., & Alley, C. L. (2008). Pediatric ophthalmology in the developing world. *Current Opinion in Ophthalmology, 19*(5), 403–408. doi:10.1097/ICU.0b013e328309f180.
83. Kismul, H., Van den Broeck, J., & Lunde, T. M. (2014). Diet and kwashiorkor: A prospective study from rural DR Congo. *PeerJ, 2*, e350. doi:10.7717/peerj.350.
84. Cole, S. Z., & Lanham, J. S. (2011). Failure to thrive: An update. *American Family Physician, 83*(7), 829–834.
85. Jaffe, A. C. (2011). Failure to thrive: Current clinical concepts. *Pediatrics in Review, 32*(3), 100–107. doi:10.1542/pir.32-3-100.
86. Nützenadel, W. (2011). Failure to thrive in childhood. *Deutsches Ärzteblatt International, 108*(38), 642–649. doi:10.3238/arztebl.2011.0642.
87. Joosten, K. F., & Hulst, J. M. (2014). Nutritional screening tools for hospitalized children: Methodological considerations. *Clinical Nutrition, 33*(1), 1–5. doi:10.1016/j.clnu.2013.08.002.
88. Black, M. M., Dubowitz, H., Krishnakumar, A., et al. (2007). Early intervention and recovery among children with failure to thrive: Follow-up at age 8. *Pediatrics, 120*(1), 59–69. doi:10.1542/peds.2006-1657.
89. Neu, J., & Mihatsch, W. (2012). Recent developments in necrotizing enterocolitis. *Journal of Parenteral and Enteral Nutrition, 36*(1, Suppl.), 30S–35S. doi:10.1177/0148607111422068.
90. Srinivasan, P. S., Brandler, M. D., & D'Souza, A. (2008). Necrotizing enterocolitis. *Clinics in Perinatology, 35*(1), 251–272. doi:10.1016/j.clp.2007.11.009.
91. Caplan, M. S. (2008). Neonatal necrotizing enterocolitis [introduction]. *Seminars in Perinatology, 32*(2), 69. doi:10.1053/j.semperi.2008.02.001.
92. Gordon, P. V., & Swanson, J. R. (2014). Necrotizing enterocolitis is one disease with many origins and potential means of prevention. *Pathophysiology, 21*(1), 13–19. doi:10.1016/j.pathophys.2013.11.015.
93. Shah, P., Yoon, E. W., Chan, P., & Members of the Annual Report Review Committee. (2013). *Canadian Neonatal Network annual report 2013.* Retrieved from http://www.canadianneonatalnetwork.org/Portal/LinkClick.aspx?fileticket=lreR0871sjA%3D&tabid=39.
94. Sankaran, K., Puckett, B., Lee, D. S. C., et al. (2004). Variations in incidence of necrotizing enterocolitis in Canadian neonatal intensive care units. *Journal of Pediatric Gastroenterology and Nutrition, 39*(4), 366–372. doi:10.1097/00005176-200410000-00012.
95. Kim, J. H. (2014). Necrotizing enterocolitis: The road to zero. *Seminars in Fetal and Neonatal Medicine, 19*(1), 39–44. doi:10.1016/j.siny.2013.10.001.
96. Alfaleh, K., Anabrees, J., Bassler, D., et al. (2011). Probiotics for prevention of necrotizing enterocolitis in preterm infants. *The Cochrane Database of Systematic Reviews*, (3), CD005496, doi:10.1002/14651858.CD005496.pub3.
97. Sola, J. E., Tepas, J. J., 3rd., & Koniaris, L. G. (2010). Peritoneal drainage versus laparotomy for necrotizing enterocolitis and intestinal perforation: A meta-analysis. *The Journal of Surgical Research, 161*(1), 95–100. doi:10.1016/j.jss.2009.05.007.
98. Churgay, C. A., & Aftab, Z. (2012). Gastroenteritis in children: Part 1. Diagnosis. *American Family Physician, 85*(11), 1059–1062.
99. Mehal, J. M., Esposito, D. H., Holman, R. C., et al. (2012). Risk factors for diarrhea-associated infant mortality in the United States, 2005–2007. *The Pediatric Infectious Disease Journal, 31*(7), 717–721. doi:10.1097/INF.0b013e318253a78b.
100. World Health Organization. (2013). *Diarrhoeal disease: Fact sheet No. 330.* Retrieved from http://www.who.int/mediacentre/factsheets/fs330/en/.
101. Zella, G. C., & Israel, E. J. (2012). Chronic diarrhea in children. *Pediatrics in Review, 33*(5), 207–217. doi:10.1542/pir.33-5-207.
102. Kollaritsch, H., Kundi, M., Giaquinto, C., et al. (2015). Rotavirus vaccines: A story of success. *Clinical Microbiology and Infection, 21*(8), 735–743. doi:10.1016/j.cmi.2015.01.027.
103. Pawlowski, S. W., Warren, C. A., & Guerrant, R. (2009). Diagnosis and treatment of acute or persistent diarrhea. *Gastroenterology, 136*(6), 1874–1886. doi:10.1053/j.gastro.2009.02.072.
104. Bernaola Aponte, G., Bada Mancilla, C. A., Carreazo, N. Y., et al. (2013). Probiotics for treating persistent diarrhoea in children. *The Cochrane Database of Systematic Reviews*, (8), CD007401, doi:10.1002/14651858.CD007401.pub3.
105. Grimwood, K., & Forbes, D. A. (2009). Acute and persistent diarrhea. *Pediatric Clinics of North America, 56*(6), 1343–1361. doi:10.1016/j.pcl.2009.09.004.
106. Misselwitz, B., Pohl, D., Frühauf, H., et al. (2013). Lactose malabsorption and intolerance: Pathogenesis, diagnosis and treatment. *United European Gastroenterology Journal, 1*(3), 151–159. doi:10.1177/2050640613484463.
107. Maisels, M. J. (2006). What's in a name? Physiologic and pathologic jaundice: The conundrum of defining normal bilirubin levels in the newborn. *Pediatrics, 118*(2), 805–807. doi:10.1542/peds.2006-0675.
108. Porter, M. L., & Dennis, B. L. (2002). Hyperbilirubinemia in the term newborn. *American Family Physician, 65*(4), 599–606.
109. Colletti, J. E., Kothari, S., Jackson, D. M., et al. (2007). An emergency medicine approach to neonatal hyperbilirubinemia. *Emergency Medicine Clinics of North America, 25*(4), 1117–1135. doi:10.1016/j.emc.2007.07.007.
110. Shapiro, S. M. (2010). Chronic bilirubin encephalopathy: Diagnosis and outcome. *Seminars in Fetal and Neonatal Medicine, 15*(3), 157–163. doi:10.1016/j.siny.2009.12.004.
111. Watson, R. L. (2009). Hyperbilirubinemia. *Critical Care Nursing Clinics of North America, 21*(1), 97–120. doi:10.1016/j.ccell.2008.11.001.
112. Bassett, M. D., & Murray, K. F. (2008). Biliary atresia: Recent progress. *Journal of Clinical Gastroenterology, 42*(6), 720–729. doi:10.1097/MCG.0b013e3181646730.
113. Petersen, C., & Davenport, M. (2013). Aetiology of biliary atresia: What is actually known? *Orphanet Journal of Rare Diseases, 8*, 128. doi:10.1186/1750-1172-8-128.
114. Tessier, M. E., Harpavat, S., Shepherd, R. W., et al. (2014). Beyond the pediatric end-stage liver disease system: Solutions for infants with biliary atresia requiring liver transplant. *World Journal of Gastroenterology, 20*(32), 11062–11068. doi:10.3748/wjg.v20.i32.11062.
115. Degertekin, B., & Lok, A. S. (2009). Update on viral hepatitis: 2008. *Current Opinion in Gastroenterology, 25*(3), 180–185. doi:10.1097/MOG.0b013e328324f478.
116. Klevens, R. M., Miller, J. T., Igbal, K., et al. (2010). The evolving epidemiology of hepatitis A in the United States: Incidence and molecular epidemiology from population-based surveillance, 2005–2007. *Archives of Internal Medicine, 170*(20), 1811–1818. doi:10.1001/archinternmed.2010.401.
117. Suchy, F. J., Sokol, R. J., & Balistreri, W. F. (Eds.), (2014). *Liver disease in children* (4th ed.). Cambridge, UK: Cambridge University Press.
118. Matheny, S. C., & Kingery, J. E. (2012). Hepatitis A. *American Family Physician, 86*(11), 1027–1034.
119. Haber, B. A., Block, J. M., Jonas, M. M., et al. (2009). Recommendations for screening, monitoring, and referral of pediatric chronic hepatitis B. *Pediatrics, 124*(5), e1007–e1013. doi:10.1542/peds.2009-0567.
120. Slowik, M. K., & Jhaveri, R. (2005). Hepatitis B and C viruses in infants and young children. *Seminars in Pediatric Infectious Diseases, 16*(4), 296–305. doi:10.1053/j.spid.2005.06.009.
121. Grabowski, J., & Wedemeyer, H. (2010). Hepatitis delta: Immunopathogenesis and clinical challenges. *Digestive Diseases (Basel, Switzerland), 28*(1), 133–138. doi:10.1159/000282076.
122. Jonas, M. M., Block, J. M., Haber, B. A., et al. (2010). Hepatitis B Foundation. Treatment of children with chronic hepatitis B virus infection in the United States: Patient selection and therapeutic options. *Hepatology (Baltimore, Md.), 52*(6), 2192–2205. doi:10.1002/hep.23934.
123. Sorrell, M. F., Belongia, E. A., Costa, J., et al. (2009). National Institutes of Health consensus development conference statement: Management of hepatitis B. *Hepatology (Baltimore, Md.), 49*(5, Suppl.), S4–S12. doi:10.1002/hep.22946.
124. Pan, C. Q., & Lee, H. M. (2013). Antiviral therapy for chronic hepatitis B in pregnancy. *Seminars in Liver Disease, 33*(2), 138–146. doi:10.1055/s-0033-1345718.
125. Government of Canada. (2016). *Report on hepatitis B and C in Canada: 2013.* Retrieved from https://www.canada.ca/en/public-health/services/publications/diseases-conditions/report-hepatitis-b-c-canada-2013.html.

126. Mack, C. L., Gonzalez-Peralta, R. P., Gupta, N., et al. (2012). NASPGHAN practice guidelines: Diagnosis and management of hepatitis C infection in infants, children, and adolescents. *Journal of Pediatric Gastroenterology and Nutrition, 54*(6), 838–855. doi:10.1097/MPG.0b013e318258328d.
127. El-Shabrawi, M., & Hassanin, F. (2014). Treatment of hepatitis B and C in children. *Minerva Pediatrica, 66*(5), 473–489.
128. Floreani, A., Liberal, R., Vergani, D., et al. (2013). Autoimmune hepatitis: Contrasts and comparisons in children and adults—A comprehensive review. *Journal of Autoimmunity, 46*, 7–16. doi:10.1016/j.jaut.2013.08.004.
129. Rojas, C. P., Bodicharla, R., Campuzano-Zuluaga, G., et al. (2014). Autoimmune hepatitis and primary sclerosing cholangitis in children and adolescents. *Fetal and Pediatric Pathology, 33*(4), 202–209. doi:10.3109/15513815.2014.898721.
130. Canadian Task Force on Preventive Health Care. (2016). *Screen for hepatitis C—Clinician summary*. Retrieved from https://canadiantaskforce.ca/wp-content/uploads/2017/04/Hep-C-Screening_Clinician-Summary 20170421 ENGLISH FINAL.pdf.
131. Janua, N., McGuinness, L., Buller-Taylor, T., et al. (2015). Education and resources for people affected by hepatitis C. *BC Medical Journal, 57*(1), 27.
132. Badizadegan, K., Jonas, M. M., Ott, M. J., et al. (1998). Histopathology of the liver in children with chronic hepatitis C viral infection. *Hepatology (Baltimore, Md.), 28*(5), 1416–1423. doi:10.1002/hep.510280534.
133. Mack, C. L., Zelko, F. A., Lokar, J., et al. (2006). Surgically restoring portal blood flow to the liver in children with primary extrahepatic portal vein thrombosis improves fluid neurocognitive ability. *Pediatrics, 117*(3), e405–e412. doi:10.1542/peds.2005-1177.
134. Sharif, K., McKiernan, P., & de Ville de Goyet, J. (2010). Mesoportal bypass for extrahepatic portal vein obstruction in children: Close to a cure for most! *Journal of Pediatric Surgery, 45*(1), 272–276. doi:10.1016/j.jpedsurg.2009.08.019.
135. Brunt, E. M. (2009). Histopathology of non-alcoholic fatty liver disease. *Clinics in Liver Disease, 13*(4), 533–544. doi:10.1016/j.cld.2009.07.008.
136. Haafiz, A. B. (2010). Liver fibrosis in biliary atresia. *Expert Review of Gastroenterology & Hepatology, 4*(3), 335–343. doi:10.1586/egh.10.29.
137. Peters, L., & Rockstroh, J. K. (2010). Biomarkers of fibrosis and impaired liver function in chronic hepatitis C: How well do they predict clinical outcomes? *Current Opinion in HIV and AIDS, 5*(6), 517–523. doi:10.1097/COH.0b013e32833e3ee6.
138. Lopez-Terrada, D. H. (2014). Hepatoblastoma. *Diagnostic Histopathology, 20*(2), 67. doi:10.1016/j.mpdhp.2014.01.002.
139. Lopez-Terrada, D., & Finegold, M. J. (2012). Tumors of the liver. In F. J. Suchy (Ed.), *Liver disease in children*. New York: Cambridge University Press.
140. Children's Hospital of Pittsburgh. (2017). *Hepatoblastoma (liver cancer) in children: Symptoms and treatment*. Retrieved from http://www.chp.edu/our-services/transplant/liver/education/liver-disease-states/hepatoblastoma-liver-cancer.
141. Dall'Igna, P., Cecchetto, G., Bisogno, G., et al. (2010). Pancreatic tumors in children and adolescents: The Italian TREP project experience. *Pediatric Blood & Cancer, 54*, 675–680. doi:10.1002/pbc.22385.

38

Structure and Function of the Musculo-skeletal System

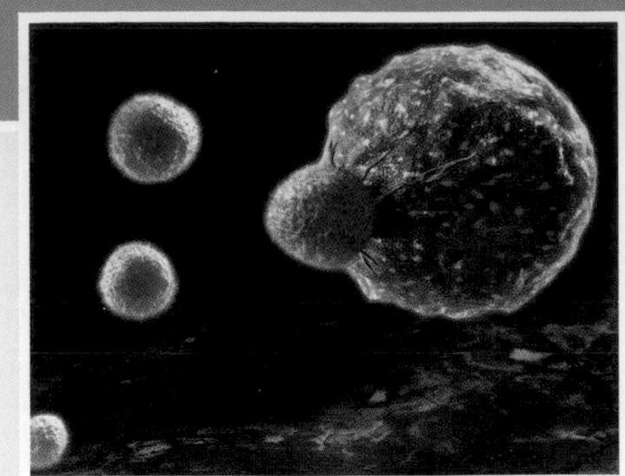

Christy L. Crowther-Radulewicz, Kathryn L. McCance, and Stephanie Zettel

EVOLVE WEBSITE

http://evolve.elsevier.com/Canada/Huether/pathophysiology
Student Review Questions
Key Points
Case Studies
Animations
Quick Check Answers

CHAPTER OUTLINE

Structure and Function of Bones, 988
Elements of Bone Tissue, 988
Types of Bone Tissue, 992
Characteristics of Bone, 994
Maintenance of Bone Integrity, 995
Structure and Function of Joints, 995
Fibrous Joints, 995
Cartilaginous Joints, 995
Synovial Joints, 998
Structure and Function of Skeletal Muscles, 998
Whole Muscle, 999
Components of Muscle Function, 1003
Tendons and Ligaments, 1006
Aging and the Musculo-skeletal System, 1006
Aging of Bones, 1006
Aging of Joints, 1007
Aging of Muscles, 1007

The way an individual functions in daily life, moves about, or manipulates objects physically depends on the integrity of the musculo-skeletal system. The musculo-skeletal system is actually two systems: (1) the skeleton, composed of bones and joints, and (2) soft tissues (skeletal muscles, tendons, and ligaments). Each system contributes to mobility. The skeleton supports the body and provides leverage to the skeletal muscles so that movement of various parts of the body is possible. Contraction of the skeletal muscles and bending or rotation at the joints facilitate movements of the various body parts.

STRUCTURE AND FUNCTION OF BONES

Bones give form to the body, support tissues, and permit movement by providing points of attachment for muscles. Many bones meet in movable joints that determine the type and extent of movement possible. Bones also protect many of the body's vital organs. For example, the bones of the skull, thorax, and pelvis are hard exterior shields that protect the brain, heart and lungs, and reproductive and urinary organs, respectively.

The marrow cavities within certain bones serve as sites of blood cell formation. In adults, blood cells originate exclusively in the marrow cavities of the skull, vertebrae, ribs, sternum, shoulders, and pelvis. The development of blood cells is discussed in Chapter 20. Bones also have a crucial role in mineral homeostasis (storing minerals [i.e., calcium, phosphate, carbonate, magnesium] that are essential for the proper performance of many delicate cellular mechanisms), play a role in hormone homeostasis, and assist in maintaining normal immunological function.

Elements of Bone Tissue

Mature bone is a rigid connective tissue consisting of cells, fibres, a gelatinous material termed **ground substance**, and large amounts of crystallized minerals, mainly calcium, that give bone its rigidity. Ground substance consists of proteoglycans and hyaluronic acid secreted by chondroblasts. The structural elements of bone are summarized in Table 38-1.

Bone cells enable bone to grow, repair itself, change shape, and continuously synthesize new bone tissue and **resorb** (dissolve or digest) old tissue. The fibres in bone are made of collagen, which gives bone its tensile strength (the ability to hold itself together). Ground substance acts as a medium for the diffusion of nutrients, oxygen, metabolic wastes, biochemicals, and minerals between bone tissue and blood vessels.

Bone formation begins during fetal life with the growth of cartilage—the precursor of bone tissue. In mature bone, the formation of new tissue begins with the production of an organic matrix by the bone cells. This **bone matrix** consists of ground substance, collagen, and other proteins (see Table 38-1) that take part in bone formation and maintenance.

The next step in bone formation is **calcification**, in which minerals are deposited and then crystallize. Minerals bind tightly to collagen fibres, producing tensile and compressional strength in bone and allowing it to withstand pressure and weight-bearing.

Bone Cells

Bone contains three types of cells: osteoblasts, osteocytes, and osteoclasts (Figure 38-1). Both osteoblasts and osteocytes originate from

TABLE 38-1 Structural Elements of Bone

Structural Elements	Function
Bone Cells	
Osteoblasts	Synthesize collagen and proteoglycans, mineralize osteoid matrix; produce receptor activator of nuclear factor kappa-B ligand (RANKL), which in turn stimulates osteoclast resorption of bone; also produce osteoprotegerin, which inhibits osteoclast formation by binding to RANKL
Osteoclasts	Resorb bone; major role in bone homeostasis
Osteocytes	Transform osteoblasts trapped in osteoid; signal both osteoblasts and osteoclasts; maintain bone matrix; mechanosensory receptors to reduce or augment bone mass; produce sclerostin, which inhibits bone growth
Bone Matrix	
Bone morphogenic proteins (BMPs)	Induce and regulate bone and cartilage formation; affect all other organ systems; a subfamily of transforming growth factor-beta cytokine growth factors
BMP-1	Plays a key role in extracellular matrix formation; is unrelated to other BMPs (is a metalloprotease)
BMP-2	Promotes chondrogenesis, bone formation; clinically used to enhance bone formation in spine surgery
BMP-3 (osteogenin)	Inhibits bone formation
BMP-4	Is involved in osteoblast differentiation; involved in cartilage repair, endochondral bone formation, enhances chondrogenesis
BMP-6	Found in human plasma; promotes osteoblast differentiation from mesenchymal stem cells (MSCs)
BMP-7	Is involved in osteogenic cell formation from MSCs; enhances bone formation in spine surgery; induces formation of brown fat
BMP-9	Promotes osteoblast formation from MSCs
BMP-13	Inhibits bone formation by reducing calcium mineralization
Collagen fibres	Lend support and tensile strength
Proteoglycans	Control transport of ionized materials through matrix
Glycoproteins	
Albumin	Transports essential elements to matrix; maintains osmotic pressure of bone fluid
α-Glycoproteins	Promote calcification
Laminin	Stabilizes basement membranes in bones
Osteocalcin	Inhibits calcium phosphate precipitation (attracts calcium ions to incorporate into hydroxyapatite crystals); serum osteocalcin is a sensitive marker of bone formation; is a vitamin K–dependent protein present in bone
Osteonectin	Binds calcium in bone; necessary for normal bone formation
Sialoprotein	Promotes calcification, osteoblast formation
Minerals	
Calcium	Crystallizes, providing bone rigidity and compressive strength
Phosphate	Regulates vitamin D, promoting mineralization; a balance of organic and inorganic phosphate required for proper bone mineralization
Alkaline phosphatase	Promotes mineralization
Vitamins	
Vitamin D	Assists with differentiation, mineralization of osteoblasts
Vitamin K	Increases bone calcification; reduces serum osteocalcin

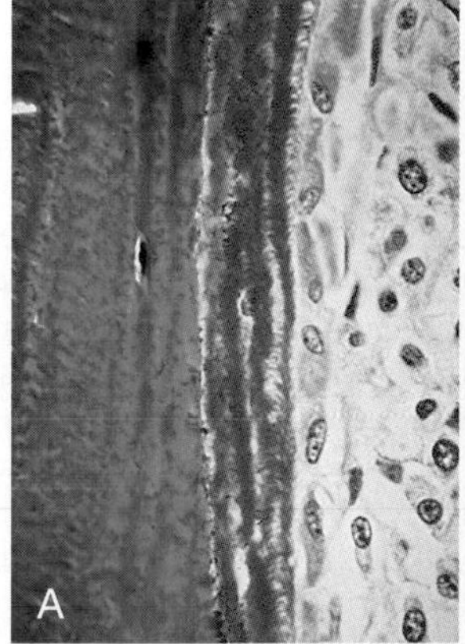

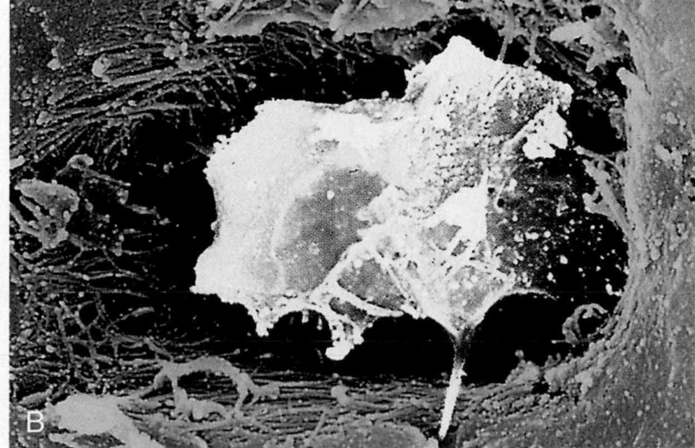

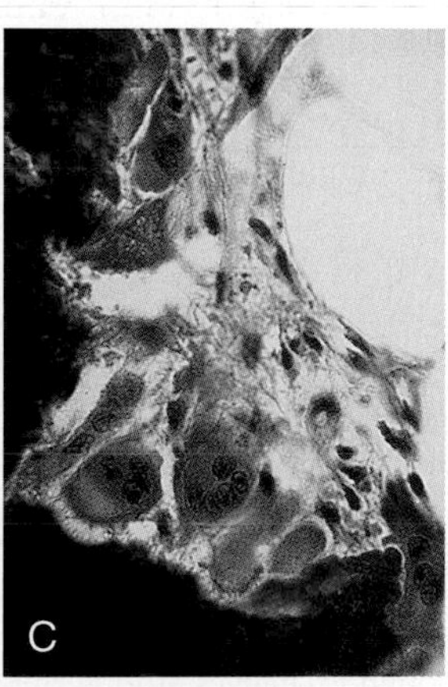

FIGURE 38-1 Bone Cells. A, Osteoblasts are responsible for the production of collagenous and noncollagenous proteins that compose osteoid. Active osteoblasts are aligned on the osteoid. Note the eccentrically located nuclei. **B,** Electron photomicrograph of an osteocyte. Osteocytes reside within the lacunae of compact bone. **C,** Osteoclasts actively resorb mineralized tissue. The scalloped surface in which the multinucleated osteoclasts rest is termed *Howship lacuna.* (**A** and **C,** from Damjanov, I., & Linder, J. [Eds.]. [1996]. *Anderson's pathology* [10th ed.]. St. Louis: Mosby; **B,** from Wikimedia Commons, courtesy Robert M. Hunt.)

osteoprogenitor cells found in the mesenchymal stem cell (MSC) lineage. Unlike osteoblasts and osteocytes, osteoclasts originate from hematopoietic stem cells. Osteoblasts are the bone-forming cells. Once this function is complete, osteoblasts become osteocytes. Osteocytes, the most numerous cells within bone, are osteoblasts that have become imprisoned within the mineralized bone matrix. They have multiple important duties in maintaining bone homeostasis, including synthesizing new bone matrix molecules and initiating osteoclast function. Osteoclasts primarily resorb (remove) bone during processes of growth and repair.

Osteoblasts. Originating from MSCs, osteoblasts are the primary bone-producing cells, and are involved in many functions related to the skeletal system (see Table 38-1). Osteoblasts are responsive to parathyroid hormone (PTH) and produce osteocalcin when stimulated by 1,25-dihydroxy-vitamin D_3.[1] Osteoblasts are active on the outer surfaces of bones, where they form a single layer of cells. Osteoblasts initiate new bone formation by their synthesis of osteoid (nonmineralized bone matrix). Osteoblasts also mineralize newly formed bone matrix. Stimulation of new bone formation and orderly mineralization of bone matrix occur by concentrating some of the plasma proteins (growth factors) found in the bone matrix and by facilitating the deposit and exchange of calcium and other ions at the site. Enzymes, signalling proteins, and growth factors, including bone morphogenic proteins (BMPs) and other members of the transforming growth factor-beta (TGF-β) superfamily, are critical components of bone formation, maintenance, and remodelling (Table 38-2).

Osteoblasts use intercellular calcium signalling to include osteoclastic activity. One of the most important discoveries linking osteoblast and osteoclast function is that of the cytokine receptor activator nuclear factor kappa-B ligand, or RANKL (see "OPG/RANKL/RANK System"). RANKL is expressed by osteoblasts and osteocytes and is necessary for forming osteoclasts[2-4] (see "Osteoclasts"). Thus, the cells of the osteoblastic lineage (osteoblasts, osteocytes) form a network of cells in bone that sense the shape and structure of bone and determine where it is appropriate that bone be formed or resorbed, according to Wolff's law (bone is shaped according to its function).

Osteoblasts synthesize and secrete osteoid when active, and in the resting state they are termed *satellite cells*. If appropriately stimulated, however, the resting osteoblasts are capable of resuming activity.

Osteocytes. Osteocytes, the most abundant cells in bone, are transformed osteoblasts trapped or surrounded in osteoid as it hardens because of minerals that enter during calcification (Figure 38-1, *B*). The osteocyte is within a space in the hardened bone matrix called a lacuna. Each osteocyte contains long, thin cytoplasmic extensions, called *processes*, which run through the canaliculi, providing communication with osteoblasts lying on the bone surface. Another form of extracellular communication used by osteocytes is through transmembrane channels called *gap junctions*, which connect the cytoplasm of adjacent cells.

Osteocytes have numerous functions, including acting as mechanoreceptors and synthesizing certain matrix molecules, playing a major role in controlling osteoblast differentiation and production of growth factors, and maintaining bone homeostasis.[5] As the major source of sclerostin, RANKL, and osteoprotegerin (OPG), osteocytes are thought to be key regulators of both bone formation and bone resorption.[6-8] They also help concentrate nutrients in the matrix. Osteocytes obtain nutrients from capillaries in the canaliculi, which contain nutrient-rich fluids. Through exchanges among these cells, hormone catalysts, and minerals, optimal levels of calcium, phosphorus, and other minerals are maintained in blood plasma.

One of the osteocyte's primary functions is to act as a mechanoreceptor, responding to changes in weight-bearing or other stressors ("loading") on bone. Lying within the lacunae are the osteocyte's primary cilia, which are likely the primary mechanoreceptors in bone.[9,10] Once changes in bone, such as mechanical stress, hormonal imbalance, loading, or unloading, are detected by the osteocyte's mechanoreceptors, multiple molecular signals are produced and the process of bone remodelling begins.[4,11] Remodelling is described on p. 995.

Osteoclasts. Osteoclasts are large (typically 20 to 100 μm in diameter), multinucleated cells that develop from the hematopoietic monocyte/macrophage lineage. Osteoclasts are the major resorptive cells of bone. They migrate over bone surfaces to resorption areas that have been prepared and stripped of osteoid by enzymes, such as collagenases produced by osteoblasts in the presence of PTH, which is necessary for the resorptive process. Osteoclasts travel over the prepared bone surfaces, creating irregular, scalloped cavities known as *Howship lacunae* or *resorption bays*, as they resorb bone areas and then acidify hydroxyapatite (HAP) to dissolve it.

A specific area of the cell membrane forms adjacent to the bone surface and develops multiple infoldings to permit intimate contact with the resorption bay. These infoldings, known as the ruffled border, greatly increase the surface areas of cells under their scalloped or ruffled borders. Osteoclasts resorb bone by secretion of hydrochloric acid, acid proteases (such as cathepsin K), and matrix metalloproteinases (MMPs) that help digest collagen, along with the action of cytokines (see Table 38-2). Osteoclasts also resorb bone through the action of lysosomes (digestive vacuoles) filled with hydrolytic enzymes in their mitochondria.

Osteoclasts bind to the bone surfaces through attachments called podosomes, which are footlike structures that cluster together along a sealing membrane that forms a "belt" containing multiple proteins, enzymes, and integrin receptors.[12,13] Once resorption is complete, the osteoclasts retract and loosen from the bone surface under the ruffled border through the action of calcitonin. Calcitonin binds to receptor areas of the osteoclasts' cell membranes to effectively loosen the osteoclasts from the bone surfaces. Once resorption is completed, osteoclasts disappear by the process of degeneration, either by reverting to the form of their parent cells or by undergoing cell movements away from the site, in which the osteoclast becomes an inactive, or "resting," osteoclast.

In addition to resorption of bone, osteoclasts assist the endocrine and renal systems in maintaining appropriate serum calcium and phosphorus levels. Osteoclasts also appear to have a role in the body's immune response.[12]

OPG/RANKL/RANK System

Osteoprotegerin (OPG) is a glycoprotein belonging to the tumour necrosis factor (TNF) superfamily and inhibits bone remodelling/resorption, inhibiting osteoclast formation. Numerous cells, including osteoblasts and osteocytes, produce it. OPG is key in the interaction between osteoblasts and osteoclasts.[14] Osteoblasts and osteoclasts cooperate (a process called *coupling*) to maintain normal bone homeostasis. RANKL is an essential cytokine needed for the formation and activation of osteoclasts. RANKL, like an automobile's accelerator, increases bone loss. OPG, similar to an automobile's brakes, decreases bone loss because when it is activated it promotes bone formation. When RANKL binds to its receptor, RANK, on osteoclast precursor cells, it triggers their proliferation and increases bone resorption. OPG is secreted by osteoblasts and B lymphocytes[15] and serves as a decoy by binding to RANK, preventing RANKL binding to RANK, and thus preventing bone resorption. Therefore, the overall balance between RANKL and OPG determines the amount of bone loss. The balance between RANKL and OPG is regulated by cytokines and hormones.[16] Alterations of the OPG/RANKL/RANK system can

TABLE 38-2 Selected Factors Affecting Bone Formation, Maintenance, and Remodelling

Factor	Function
Transforming growth factor-beta (TGF-β)	Regulates bone formation, many other cellular processes through signalling; a superfamily of polypeptides
Platelet-derived growth factor (PDGF)	Increases number of osteoblasts
Fibroblast growth factor-2 (FGF-2)	FGF-2 increases osteoblast population, but not function; inhibits alkaline phosphatase activity, osteocalcin, type I collagen, and osteopontin
Insulinlike Growth Factor (IGF)	
IGF-1	Increases peak bone mass during adolescence; decreases osteoblast apoptosis; maintains bone matrix
IGF-2	Increases BMP-9–induced endochondral ossification
Smad proteins	Mediate signalling cascade of TGF-β, especially in embryonic bone development; play role in crosstalk between BMP/TGF-β and Wnt signalling pathways
Bone morphogenic proteins (BMPs)	Have many functions outside skeletal system; stimulate endochondral bone and cartilage formation and function, promote osteoblast maturation; augment bone remodelling by affecting both osteoblasts and osteoclasts; members of TGF-β superfamily of polypeptides
Tumour necrosis factors (TNFs)	Play major role in regulating bone metabolism, especially osteoclast function; superfamily of cytokines
Osteoprotegerin (OPG)	Inhibits bone remodelling/resorption; produced by several cells, including osteoblasts; is a decoy receptor for RANKL (binds to RANKL, inhibiting RANK/RANKL interactions, suppressing osteoclast formation and bone resorption); also may directly interfere with ability of osteoclasts' podosomes to attach to bone matrix
Receptor activator of nuclear factor kappa-B (RANK)	Stimulates differentiation of osteoclast precursors; activates mature osteoclasts
Receptor activator of nuclear factor kappa-B ligand (RANKL)	Promotes osteoclast differentiation/activation; inhibits osteoclast apoptosis
Bone morphogenic protein antagonists	Prevent BMP signalling
Noggin	Binds BMP-2 and -4, reducing osteoblast function
Gremlin	Has multiple effects in and out of skeletal system, but also binds BMP-2, -4, and -7, thus reducing BMP signalling; may play role in development of osteoporosis
Twisted gastrulation	Acts as either a BMP agonist or a BMP antagonist
Activin (a BMP-related protein)	Affects both osteoblasts and osteoclasts; may promote bone formation and fracture healing; expressed by both osteoblasts and chondrocytes; helps regulate bone mass
Annexins	Help mineralize matrix vesicles; may influence bone formation; a class of calcium-binding proteins
Inhibin	Is dominant over activin and BMPs; helps regulate bone mass and strength by affecting formation of osteoblasts and osteoclasts
Leptin	Plays a role in bone formation and resorption
Wnt Antagonists	
Dickkopf (Dkk) family	Disrupt Wnt signalling, leading to reduced bone mass
Sclerostin	Is a protein secreted by osteocytes, osteoblasts, and osteoclasts; binds to BMP-6 and -7; interferes with Wnt signalling pathway, inhibiting bone formation by osteoblasts
Transcription Factors	
β-Catenin pathway	Is a protein with multiple functions; one of most important is activation of genetic transcription factors; balance between Wnt/β-catenin signalling promotes normal bone formation/resorption
Wnt (complex signalling pathway)	Is important in differentiating osteoblasts, bone formation; has overlapping effects with BMPs, helps regulate bone formation and remodelling; crosstalks with other signalling pathways
Nuclear factor of activated B cells (NF-κB)	Affects embryonic osteoclastogenesis; plays role in certain osteoclast, osteoblast, and chondroblast functions
Matrix Metalloproteinases (MMPs)	
Family of endopeptidases (enzymes) that includes collagenases, gelatinases, stromelysins, matrilysins	Help maintain equilibrium of extracellular matrix (ECM); break down almost all components of ECM
A disintegrin and metalloproteinase (ADAM)	Are proteolytic enzymes; also have cell-signalling functions, usually linked to cell membrane
A disintegrin and metalloproteinase with thrombospondin motifs (ADAMTs)	Are similar to ADAMs but are secreted into circulation, are found around cells; various subgroups affect multiple tissues
Cysteine protease	Expressed by osteoclasts as cathepsin K; assists in bone remodelling by cleaving proteins, such as collagen type I, collagen type II, and osteonectin
MMP Inhibitors	
Tetracyclines (especially doxycycline [Teva-Doxycycline]), bisphosphonates	Block enzymatic function of MMPs
Tissue inhibitors of metalloproteinases (TIMPs)	Balance effect of MMPs in maintaining ECM equilibrium

From Boyce, B.F., Yao, Z., & Xing, L. (2010). *Ann N Y Acad Sci, 1192*, 367–375; Genetos, D.C., Wong, A., Weber, T.J., et al. (2014). *PLoS One, 9*(9), e107482; Kim, Y-S., Paik, I.Y., Rhie, Y.J., et al. (2010). *J Korean Med Sci, 25*, 985–991; Norrie, J.L., Lewandowski, J.P., Bouldin, C.M., et al. (2014). *Dev Biol, 393*(2), 270–281; Stewart, A., Guan, H., & Yang, K. (2010). *J Cell Physiol, 223*(3), 658–666; Wang, R.N., Green, J., Wang, Z., et al. (2014). *Genes Dis, 1*(1), 87–105; Zhao, H., Liu, X., Zou, H., et al. (2014). *Cytokine, 71*(2), 199–206.

lead to dysregulation and pathological conditions, including primary osteoporosis, immune-mediated bone diseases, malignant bone disorders, and inherited skeletal diseases (see Figure 38-5).

Bone Matrix

Bone matrix is made of the extracellular elements of bone tissue, specifically collagen fibres, structural proteins (such as proteoglycans and certain glycoproteins), carbohydrate–protein complexes, ground substance, and minerals.

Collagen fibres. Collagen fibres make up the bulk of bone matrix. They are formed as follows:

1. Osteoblasts synthesize and secrete type I collagen and osteocalcin.
2. Collagen molecules assemble into three thin chains (alpha chains) to form fibrils.
3. Fibrils organize into the staggered pattern, with each fibril overlapping its nearest neighbour by about one-fourth of its length. This process creates gaps into which mineral crystals are deposited.
4. After mineral deposition, fibrils interlink and twist to form ropelike fibres.
5. The fibres join to form the framework that gives bone its tensile and supportive strength.

Proteoglycans. Proteoglycans are large complexes of numerous polysaccharides attached to a common protein core. They strengthen bone by forming compression-resistant networks between the collagen fibres. Proteoglycans also control the transport and distribution of electrically charged particles (ions), particularly calcium, through the bone matrix, thereby playing a role in bone calcium deposition and calcification. Proteoglycans are important constituents of ground substance.

Glycoproteins. Glycoproteins are carbohydrate–protein complexes that control the collagen interactions that lead to fibril formation. They also may function in calcification. Four glycoproteins are present in bone: sialoprotein, which binds easily with calcium; osteocalcin, which binds preferentially to crystallized calcium; bone albumin, which is identical to serum albumin and possibly transports essential nutrients to and from bone cells and maintains the osmotic pressure of bone fluid; and α-glycoprotein, which probably plays a significant role in calcification and also may facilitate bone resorption by activating osteoclasts (see Table 38-1).

Bone Minerals

After collagen synthesis and fibre formation, mineralization, the final step, occurs in areas known as matrix vesicles that "bud" from the surfaces of osteoblasts, chondrocytes (cartilage cells), and odontoblasts (cells that form dentin in teeth).[17] Mineralization has two distinct phases: (1) formation of the initial mineral deposit (initiation) and (2) proliferation or accretion of additional mineral crystals on the initial mineral deposits (growth). The majority of the minerals in the body are an analogue of the naturally occurring mineral hydroxyapatite (HAP). The HAP crystals then penetrate the matrix vesicle membrane and enter into the extracellular space.[17]

Table 38-3 lists the sequence in which calcium and phosphate form amorphous (fluid) calcium phosphate compounds that are converted, in stages, to solid hexagonal crystals of HAP. As the calcium and phosphorus concentrations increase in the bone matrix, the first precipitate to form is dicalcium phosphate dihydrate (DCPD). Once DCPD precipitation begins, the remaining phases of bone crystal formation proceed until insoluble HAP is produced, with approximately 80 to 90% of the HAP incorporated into the collagen fibres. Amorphous calcium phosphate is distributed throughout the bone matrix.

TABLE 38-3 Sequence of Calcium and Phosphate Compound Formation and Crystallization[a]

Formula	Name	Abbreviation
$Ca(HPO_4)\bullet 2H_2O$	Dicalcium phosphate dihydrate	DCPD
$Ca_4H(PO_4)_3$	Octacalcium phosphate	OCP
$Ca_9(PO_4)_6$ (var.)	Amorphous calcium phosphate	ACP
$Ca_3(PO_4)_2$	Tricalcium phosphate	TCP
$Ca_5(PO_4)_3OH$	Hydroxyapatite	HAP

[a]Compounds are listed in the order in which precipitation and crystal formation occur.

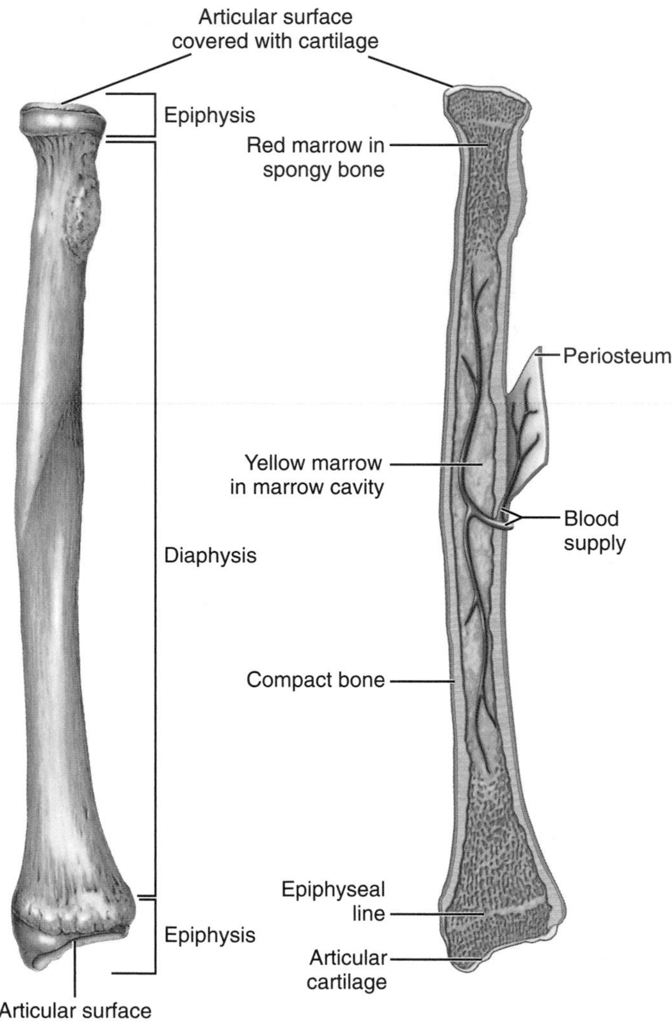

FIGURE 38-2 Anatomy of the Bone. A, External anatomy of a long bone. **B,** Internal structure of a long bone showing spongy (cancellous) and compact bone. (From Solomon, E. [2016]. *Introduction to human anatomy and physiology* [4th ed.]. St. Louis: Saunders.)

Types of Bone Tissue

Bone is composed of two types of bony (osseous) tissue: compact bone (cortical bone) and spongy bone (cancellous bone) (Figure 38-2). Cortical bone is about 85% of the skeleton; cancellous bone makes up the remaining 15%. Both types of bone tissue contain the same structural elements, with a few exceptions. In addition, both compact tissue and spongy tissue are present in every bone. The major difference between the two types of tissue is the organization of the elements.

Compact bone is highly organized, solid, and extremely strong. The basic structural unit in compact bone is the **haversian system** (Figure 38-3). Each haversian system consists of the following:

1. A central canal called the **haversian canal**
2. Concentric layers of bone matrix called **lamellae** (*sing.*, **lamella**)
3. Tiny spaces (lacunae) between the lamellae
4. Bone cells (osteocytes) within the lacunae
5. Small channels or canals called **canaliculi** (*sing.*, **canaliculus**)

Spongy bone is less complex and lacks haversian systems. In spongy bone, the lamellae are not arranged in concentric layers but in plates or bars termed **trabeculae** (*sing.*, **trabecula**) that branch and unite with one another to form an irregular meshwork. The pattern of the meshwork is determined by the direction of stress on the particular bone. The spaces between the trabeculae are filled with red bone marrow. The osteocyte-containing lacunae are distributed between the trabeculae and interconnected by canaliculi. Capillaries pass through the marrow to nourish the osteocytes.

All bones are covered with a double-layered connective tissue called the **periosteum**. The outer layer of the periosteum contains blood vessels and nerves, some of which penetrate to the inner structures of the bone through channels called *Volkmann canals* (see Figure 38-3). The inner layer of the periosteum is anchored to the bone by collagenous fibres (Sharpey fibres) that penetrate the bone. Sharpey fibres also help hold or attach tendons and ligaments to the periosteum of bones.

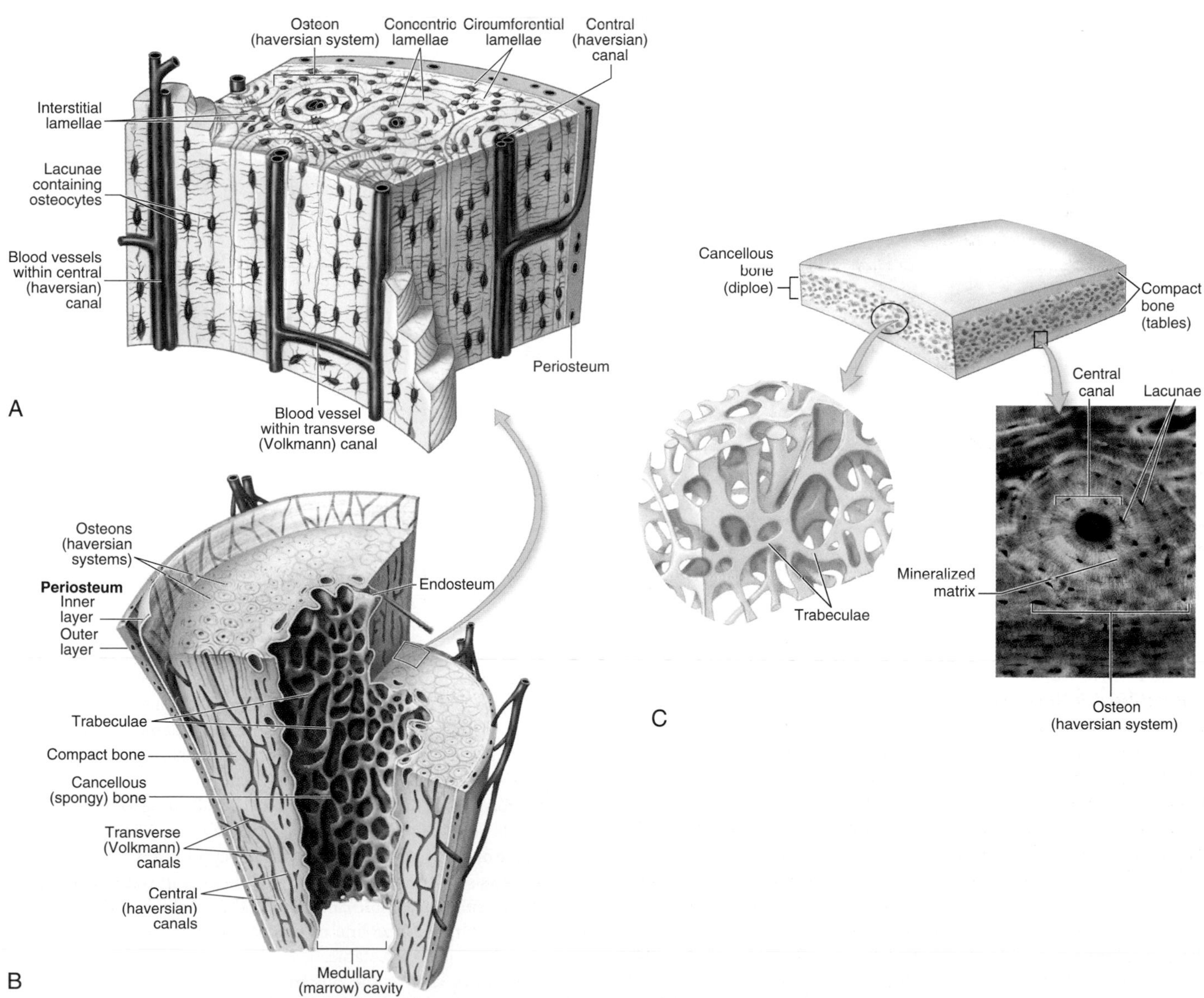

FIGURE 38-3 Structure of Compact and Cancellous Bone. A, Magnified view of compact bone. **B,** Longitudinal section of a long bone showing both cancellous and compact bone. **C,** Section of a flat bone. Outer layers of compact bone surround cancellous bone. Fine structure of compact and cancellous bone is shown in the electron photomicrograph. (From Patton, K.T., & Thibodeau, G.A. [2016]. *Anatomy & physiology* [9th ed.]. St. Louis: Mosby. Photo by Steve Gschmeissner/Science Source.)

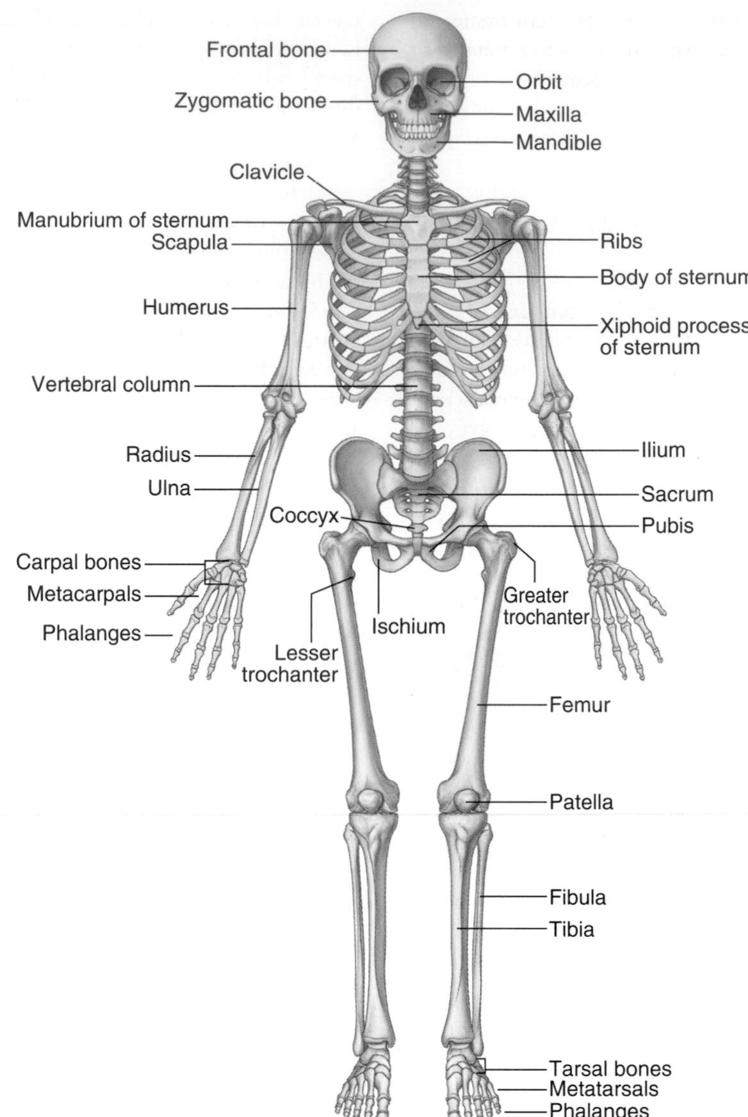

FIGURE 38-4 **Anterior View of the Skeleton.** (From Drake, R., Vogl, A.W., Mitchell, A.W.M., et al. [2015]. *Gray's atlas of anatomy* [2nd ed.]. Philadelphia: Churchill Livingstone.)

Characteristics of Bone

The 206 bones of the human skeleton are distributed between the axial skeleton and the appendicular skeleton. The **axial skeleton**—the skull, vertebral column, and thorax—consists of 80 bones. The other 126 bones of the **appendicular skeleton** comprise the upper and lower extremities, the shoulder girdle (pectoral girdle), and the pelvic girdle (os coxae) (Figure 38-4). The skeleton contributes approximately 14% of an adult's body weight.

Bones can be classified by shape as long, flat, short (cuboidal), or irregular. **Long bones** are longer than they are wide and consist of a narrow tubular midportion (**diaphysis**) that merges into a broader neck (**metaphysis**) and a broad end (**epiphysis**) (see Figure 38-2).

The diaphysis consists of a shaft of thick, rigid compact bone that is able to tolerate bending forces. Contained within the diaphysis is the elongated marrow (medullary) cavity. The marrow cavity of the diaphysis contains primarily fatty tissue, which is referred to as *yellow marrow.* The yellow marrow assists red bone marrow in hematopoiesis only during times of stress. The yellow marrow cavity of the diaphysis is continuous with marrow cavities in the spongy bone of the metaphysis and diaphysis. The marrow contained within the epiphysis is red because it contains primarily blood-forming tissue (see Chapter 20). A layer of connective tissue, the **endosteum**, lines the outer surfaces of both types of marrow cavity.

The broadness of the epiphysis allows weight-bearing to be distributed over a wide area. The epiphysis is made up of spongy bone covered by a thin layer of compact bone. In a child, the epiphysis is separated from the metaphysis by a cartilaginous **growth plate (epiphyseal plate)**. After puberty, the epiphyseal plate calcifies and the epiphysis and metaphysis merge. By adulthood, the line of demarcation between the epiphysis and metaphysis is undetectable.

In **flat bones**, such as the ribs and scapulae, two plates of compact bone are nearly parallel to each other. Between the compact bone plates is a layer of spongy bone. **Short bones**, such as the bones of the wrist or ankle, are often cuboidal. They consist of spongy bone covered by a thin layer of compact bone.

Irregular bones, such as the vertebrae, mandibles, or other facial bones, have various shapes that include thin and thick segments. The thin part of an irregular bone consists of two plates of compact bone surrounding spongy bone. The thick part consists of spongy bone surrounded by a layer of compact bone.

Maintenance of Bone Integrity

Remodelling

The internal structure of bone is maintained by **remodelling**, a three-phase process in which existing bone is resorbed and new bone is laid down to replace it. Clusters of bone cells, termed **basic multicellular units**, carry out remodelling. The basic multicellular units are made up of bone precursor cells that differentiate into osteoclasts and osteoblasts. Precursor cells are located on the free surfaces of bones and along the vascular channels (especially the marrow cavities).

In phase 1 (activation) of the remodelling cycle, a stimulus (e.g., hormone, medication, vitamin, physical stressor) activates the cytokine system, particularly the TNF superfamily, to form osteoclasts.[14] Osteoclasts attach to the bone matrix by actin microfilaments and multiple other proteins that form footlike structures called *podosomes*. Once attached, the osteoclasts' integrin receptors anchor its microfilaments to the extracellular matrix, thus providing receptor pathways between the osteocyte and bone matrix. Lysosomal enzymes produced by osteoclasts "digest" bone; the osteoclasts then release the degraded bone products into the vascular system.[12] After bone is resorbed, the osteoclast leaves behind an elongated cavity termed a *resorption cavity.* The resorption cavity in compact bone follows the longitudinal axis of the haversian system, whereas the resorption cavity in spongy bone parallels the surface of the trabeculae.

New bone formation begins as osteoblasts lining the walls of the resorption cavity express osteoid and alkaline phosphatase, forming sites for calcium and phosphorus deposition. As the osteoid mineralizes, new bone is formed. Successive layers (lamellae) in compact bone are laid down, until the resorption cavity is reduced to a narrow haversian canal around a blood vessel. In this way, old haversian systems are destroyed and new haversian systems are formed. New trabeculae are formed in spongy bone. The entire process of remodelling takes about 3 to 6 months.

Repair

The remodelling process can repair microscopic bone injuries, but gross injuries, such as fractures and surgical wounds (osteotomies), heal by the same stages as soft tissue injuries, except that new bone, instead of scar tissue, is the final result (see Chapter 6). The stages of bone healing are listed here and shown in Figure 38-5:

1. Inflammation or hematoma formation
2. Procallus formation
3. Callus formation
4. Replacement, by basic multicellular units, of the callus with lamellar or trabecular bone
5. Remodelling of the periosteal and endosteal surfaces of the bone to the size and shape of the bone before injury

The speed with which bone heals depends on the severity of the bone disruption; the type and amount of bone tissue that need to be replaced (spongy bone heals faster); the blood and oxygen supply available at the site; the presence of growth and thyroid hormones, insulin, vitamins, and other nutrients; the existence of systemic disease; the effects of aging (see "Osteoporosis" in Chapter 39 on p. 1021); and the availability of effective treatment, including immobilization and the prevention of complications such as infection. In general, however, hematoma formation occurs within hours of fracture or surgery, formation of procallus by osteoblasts within days, callus formation within weeks, and replacement and contour modelling within years—up to 4 years in some cases.

✔ QUICK CHECK 38-1

1. Name the different types of bone cells.
2. What are the major cells involved in bone resorption?
3. Briefly describe the process of remodelling.
4. What are the stages of bone healing?

STRUCTURE AND FUNCTION OF JOINTS

The site where two or more bones are attached is called a **joint**, or **articulation** (Figure 38-6). The primary function of joints is to provide stability and mobility to the skeleton. A joint's function depends on both its location and its structure. Generally, joints that stabilize the skeleton have a simpler structure than those that enable the skeleton to move. Most joints provide both stability and mobility to some degree.

Joints are classified based on the degree of movement they permit or on the connecting tissues that hold them together. Based on movement, a joint is classified as a **synarthrosis (immovable joint)**, an **amphiarthrosis (slightly movable joint)**, or a **diarthrosis (freely movable joint)**. On the basis of connective structures, joints are classified broadly as fibrous, cartilaginous, or synovial. Each of these three structural classifications can be subdivided according to the shape and contour of the articulating surfaces (ends) of the bones and the type of motion the joint permits.

Fibrous Joints

A joint in which bone is united directly to bone by fibrous connective tissue is called a **fibrous joint**. These joints have no joint cavity and allow little, if any, movement.

Fibrous joints are further subdivided into three types: sutures, syndesmoses, and gomphoses. A **suture** has a thin layer of dense fibrous tissue that binds together interlocking flat bones in the skulls of young children. Sutures form an extremely tight union that permits no motion. By adulthood, the fibrous tissue has been replaced by bone. A **syndesmosis** is a joint in which the two bony surfaces are united by a ligament or membrane. The fibres of ligaments are flexible and stretch, permitting a limited amount of movement. The paired bones of the lower arm (radius and ulna) and the lower leg (tibia and fibula) and their ligaments are syndesmotic joints. A **gomphosis** is a special type of fibrous joint in which a conical projection fits into a complementary socket and is held in place by a ligament. The teeth held in the maxilla or mandible are gomphosis joints.

Cartilaginous Joints

There are two types of cartilaginous joints: symphyses and synchondroses. A **symphysis** is a cartilaginous joint in which bones are united by a pad or disc of fibrocartilage. A thin layer of hyaline cartilage usually covers the articulating surfaces of these two bones, and the thick pad of fibrocartilage acts as a shock absorber and stabilizer. Examples of symphyses are the symphysis pubis, which joins the two pubic bones, and the intervertebral discs, which join the bodies of the vertebrae. A **synchondrosis** is a joint in which hyaline cartilage, rather than fibrocartilage, connects the two bones. The joints between the ribs and the sternum are synchondroses. The hyaline cartilage of these joints is called *costal cartilage.* Slight movement at the synchondroses between the ribs and the sternum allows the chest to move outward and upward during breathing.

Joint (Articular) Capsule

The **joint (articular) capsule** is fibrous connective tissue that covers the ends of bones where they meet in a joint; Sharpey fibres firmly attach the proximal and distal capsule to the periosteum, and ligaments

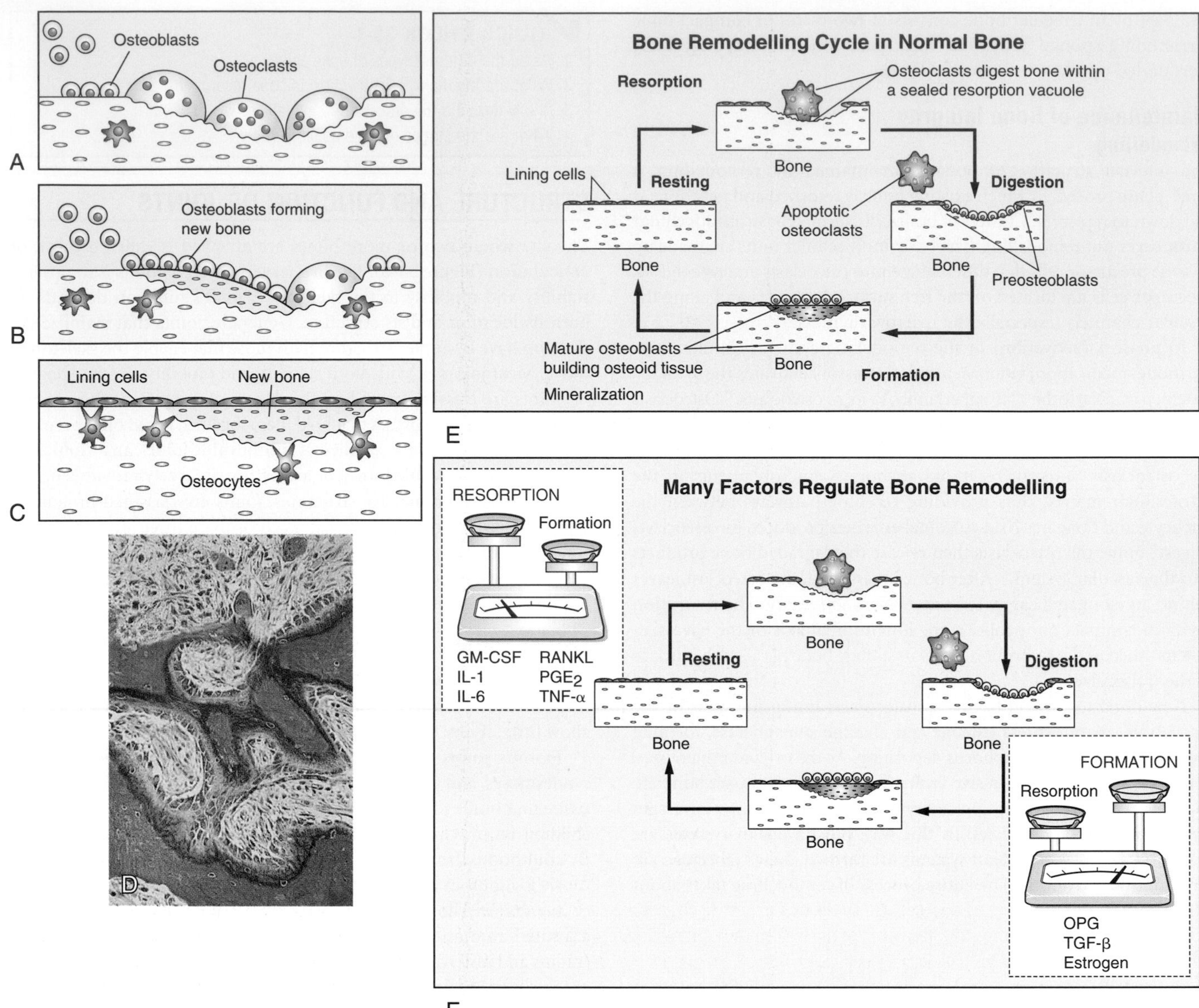

FIGURE 38-5 Bone Remodelling. All bone cells participate in bone remodelling. In the remodelling sequence bone sections are removed by bone-resorbing cells (osteoclasts) and replaced with a new section laid down by bone-forming cells (osteoblasts). Bone remodelling is necessary because it allows the skeleton to respond to mechanical loading, maintains quality control (repair and prevent microdamage), and allows the skeleton to release growth factors and minerals (calcium and phosphate) stored in bone matrix to the circulation. The cells work in response to signals generated in the environment (see **F**). Only the osteoclastic cells mediate the first phase of remodelling. They are activated, scoop out bone **(A)**, and resorb it; then the work of the osteoblasts begins **(B)**. They form new bone that replaces bone removed by the resorption process **(C)**. The sequence takes 4 to 6 months. **D,** Micrograph of active bone remodelling seen in the settings of primary or secondary hyperparathyroidism. Note the active osteoblasts surmounted on red-stained osteoid. Marrow fibrosis is present. **E,** Bone remodelling cycle in normal bone with **(F).** Numerous signalling factors are necessary for remodelling. Factors most important for resorption include granulocyte-macrophage colony-stimulating factor (*GM-CSF*), interleukin-1 (*IL-1*) and *IL-6*, receptor activator of nuclear factor kappa-B ligand (*RANKL*), prostaglandin E_2 (*PGE_2*), and tumour necrosis factor-alpha (*TNF-α*). Important factors for bone formation include osteoprotegerin (*OPG*), transforming growth factor-beta (*TGF-β*), and estrogen. (Adapted from Nucleus Medical Art. **D,** from Damjanov, I., & Linder, J. [Eds.]. *Anderson's pathology* [10th ed.]. St. Louis: Mosby.)

and tendons also may reinforce the capsule. It is composed of parallel, interlacing bundles of dense, white fibrous tissue richly supplied with nerves, blood vessels, and lymphatic vessels. Nerves in and around the joint capsule are sensitive to rate and direction of motion, compression, tension, vibration, and pain.

Synovial Membrane

The **synovial membrane** is a smooth, delicate inner lining of joint capsule found in the nonarticular portion of the synovial joint and any ligaments or tendons that traverse this cavity. It is composed of two

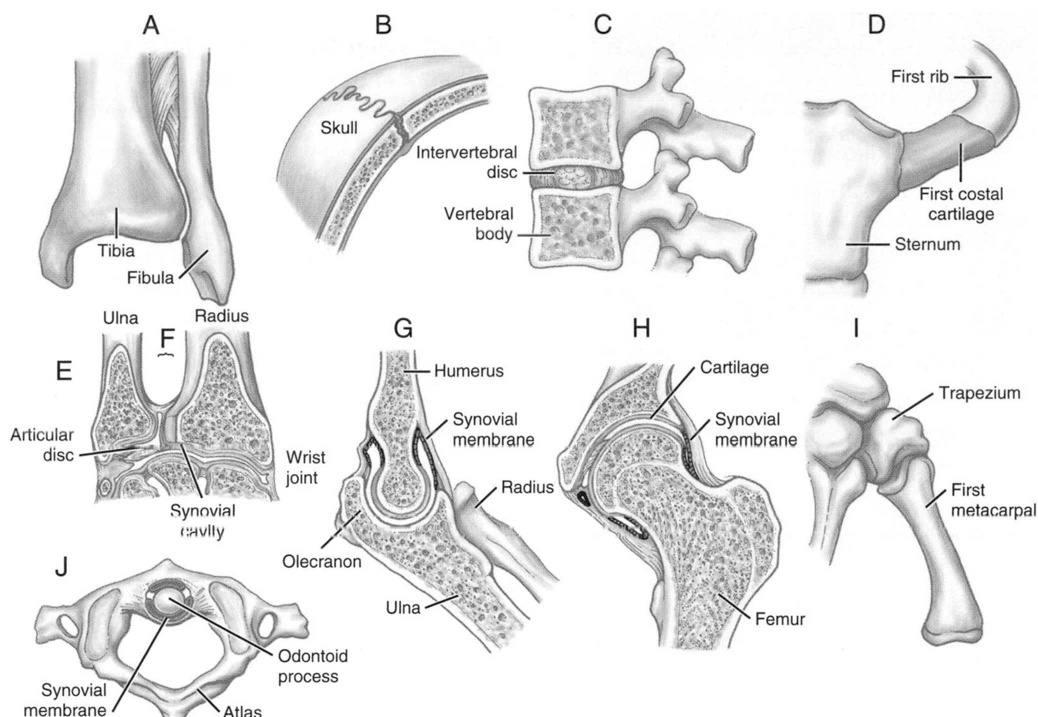

FIGURE 38-6 Various Kinds of Joints. *Fibrous:* **A**, syndesmosis (tibiofibular); **B**, suture (skull). *Cartilaginous:* **C**, symphysis (vertebral bodies); **D**, synchondrosis (first rib and sternum). *Synovial:* **E**, condyloid (wrist); **F**, gliding (radioulnar); **G**, hinge or ginglymus (elbow); **H**, ball and socket (hip); **I**, saddle (carpometacarpal of thumb); **J**, pivot (atlantoaxial). (From Dorland. [2012]. *Dorland's medical illustrated dictionary* [32nd ed.]. St. Louis: Saunders.)

layers: the vascular subintima and the thin cellular intima. The vascular subintima merges with the fibrous joint capsule and is composed of loose fibrous connective tissue, elastin fibres, fat cells, fibroblasts, macrophages, and mast cells; the cellular intima consists of rows of synovial cells embedded in fibre-free intercellular matrix and contains two types of cells—A and B. A cells (macrophages) ingest and remove (phagocytose) bacteria and particles of debris in the joint cavity; B cells (fibroblasts) are the most numerous and secrete hyaluronate, which gives synovial fluid its viscous quality. The synovial membrane is richly supplied with blood and lymphatic vessels and is capable of rapid repair and regeneration.

Joint (Synovial) Cavity

The joint (synovial) cavity is an enclosed, fluid-filled space between articulating surfaces of two bones, also called *joint space.* It enables two bones to move "against" one another and is surrounded by synovial membrane and filled with synovial fluid.

Synovial Fluid

Synovial fluid is superfiltrated plasma from blood vessels that lubricates the joint surfaces, nourishes the pad of the articular cartilage, and covers the ends of the bones. Hyaluronic acid in the synovial fluid gives it important biomechanical properties. It also contains free-floating synovial cells and various leukocytes that phagocytose joint debris and microorganisms.

Articular Cartilage

Articular cartilage is a layer of hyaline cartilage that covers the end of each bone; it may be thick or thin, depending on the size of the joint, the fit of the two bone ends, and the amount of weight and shearing force the joint normally withstands. The function of articular cartilage is to reduce friction in the joint and to distribute the forces of weight-bearing. Articular cartilage is composed of chondrocytes (cartilage cells) (about 2% of the tissue) and an intercellular matrix consisting of type II collagen (about 10 to 30% of weight), proteoglycans (about 5 to 10% of weight), and water. The water content ranges from 60 to almost 80% of the net weight of the cartilage, and individual molecules rapidly enter or exit the articular cartilage to contribute to the resiliency of the tissue.

At the surface of articular cartilage, the collagen fibres run parallel to the joint surface and are closely compacted into a dense, protective mat. (Loss of this dense, compacted configuration at the surface subjects the underlying fibres to splitting and thinning, in which case the cartilage is unable to tolerate weight-bearing.) In the middle layer (the proliferative zone) of the cartilage, the fibres are arranged tangential to the surface, which allows them to deform and absorb some of the weight-bearing (Figure 38-7). In the bottom layer (the hypertrophic zone) of the cartilage, the fibres are perpendicular to the joint surface, allowing them to resist shear forces, and are embedded in a calcified layer of cartilage called the *tidemark.*[18] The tidemark anchors the collagen fibres to the underlying (subchondral) bone. Collagen fibres are important components of the cartilage matrix because they account for approximately 60% of the dry weight and because they (1) anchor the cartilage securely to underlying bone, (2) provide a taut framework for the cartilage, (3) control the loss of fluid from the cartilage, and (4) prevent the escape of protein polysaccharides (proteoglycans) from the cartilage. The proteoglycans give articular cartilage its stiff quality and regulate the movement of synovial fluid through the cartilage. The proteoglycans are macromolecules consisting of proteins, carbohydrates (glycosaminoglycans), and hyaluronic acid.

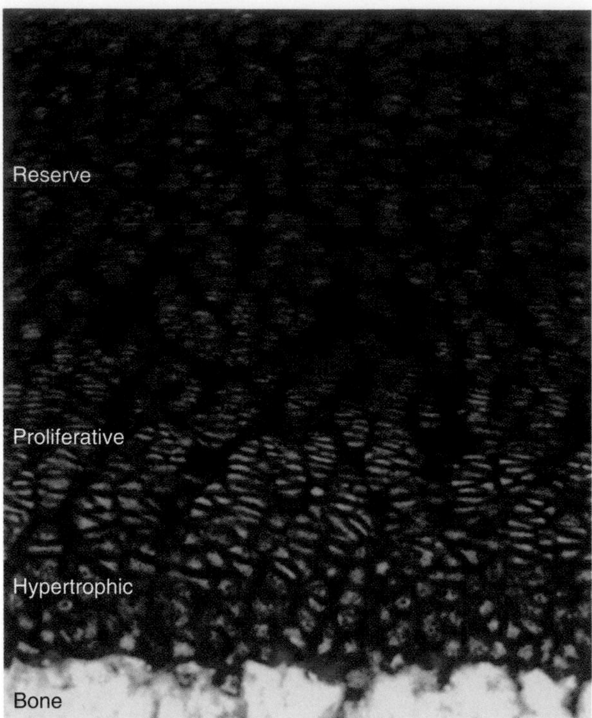

FIGURE 38-7 Collagen Zones. The three collagen zones (reserve, proliferative, and hypertrophic) are distinctly shown in a growth plate. (Reprinted from *Bone,* 41(4), Rebecca Hjorten, Uwe Hansen, et al, "Type XXVII collagen at the transition of cartilage to bone during skeletogenesis," Pages 535–542, Copyright 2007, with permission from Elsevier.)

Synovial Joints

Structure of Synovial Joints

Synovial joints (diarthroses) are the most movable and the most complex joints in the body (Figure 38-8).

Movement of Synovial Joints

Synovial joints are described as uniaxial, biaxial, or multiaxial according to the shapes of the bone ends and the type of movement occurring at the joint (Figure 38-9). Usually, one of the bones is stable and serves as an axis for the motion of the other bone. The body movements made possible by various synovial joints are either circular or angular (Figure 38-10).

> **✔ QUICK CHECK 38-2**
> 1. How do the following joints differ from each other: synarthrosis, amphiarthrosis, and diarthrosis?
> 2. Name at least two characteristics of each of the joints in the previous question that either facilitate or hinder movement.
> 3. Name three functions of articular cartilage.

STRUCTURE AND FUNCTION OF SKELETAL MUSCLES

Skeletal muscles arise from mesodermal precursor cells that then form myoblasts. The millions of individual fibres of skeletal muscle contract and relax to perform the work necessary to move the body (Figure 38-11). Muscle constitutes 40% of an adult's body weight and 50% of a child's weight. Muscle is 75% water, 20% protein, and 5% organic and inorganic compounds. Thirty-two percent of all protein stores for

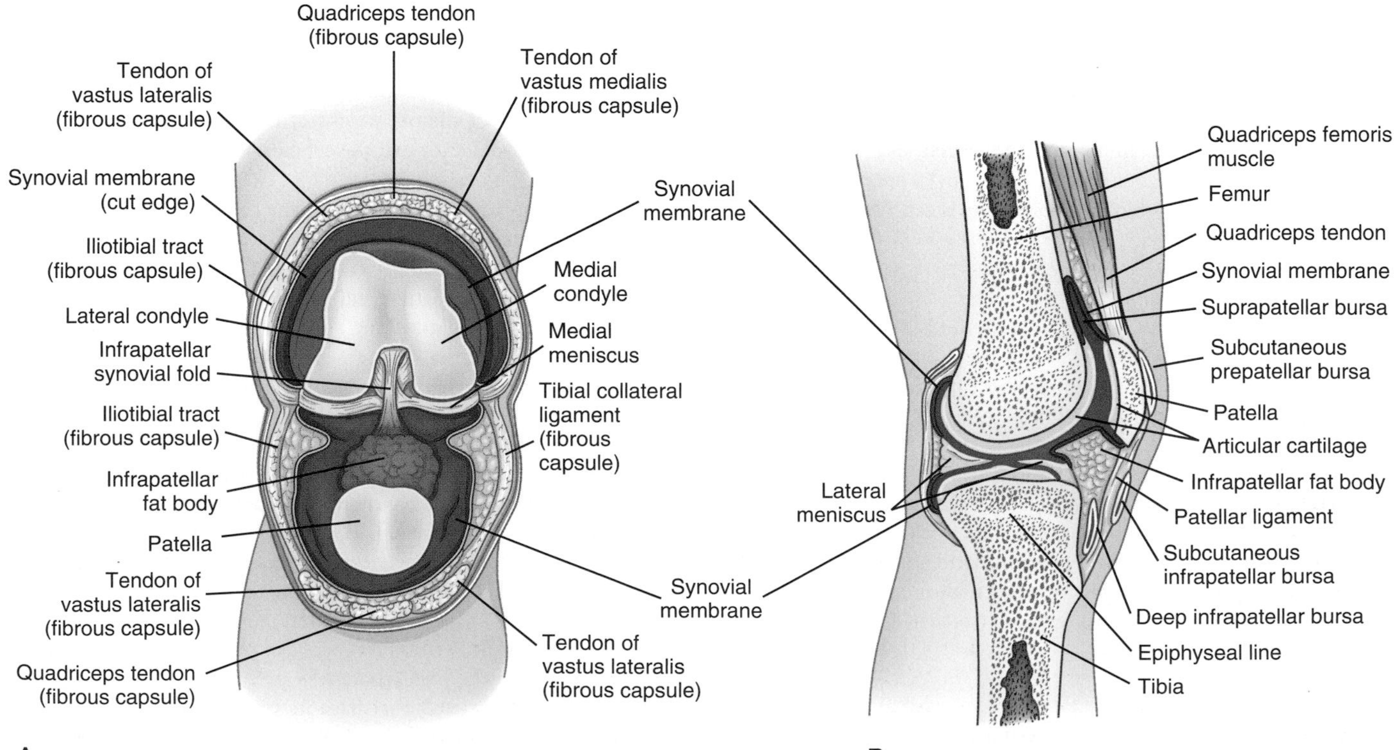

FIGURE 38-8 Knee Joint (Synovial Joint). **A,** Frontal view. **B,** Lateral view.

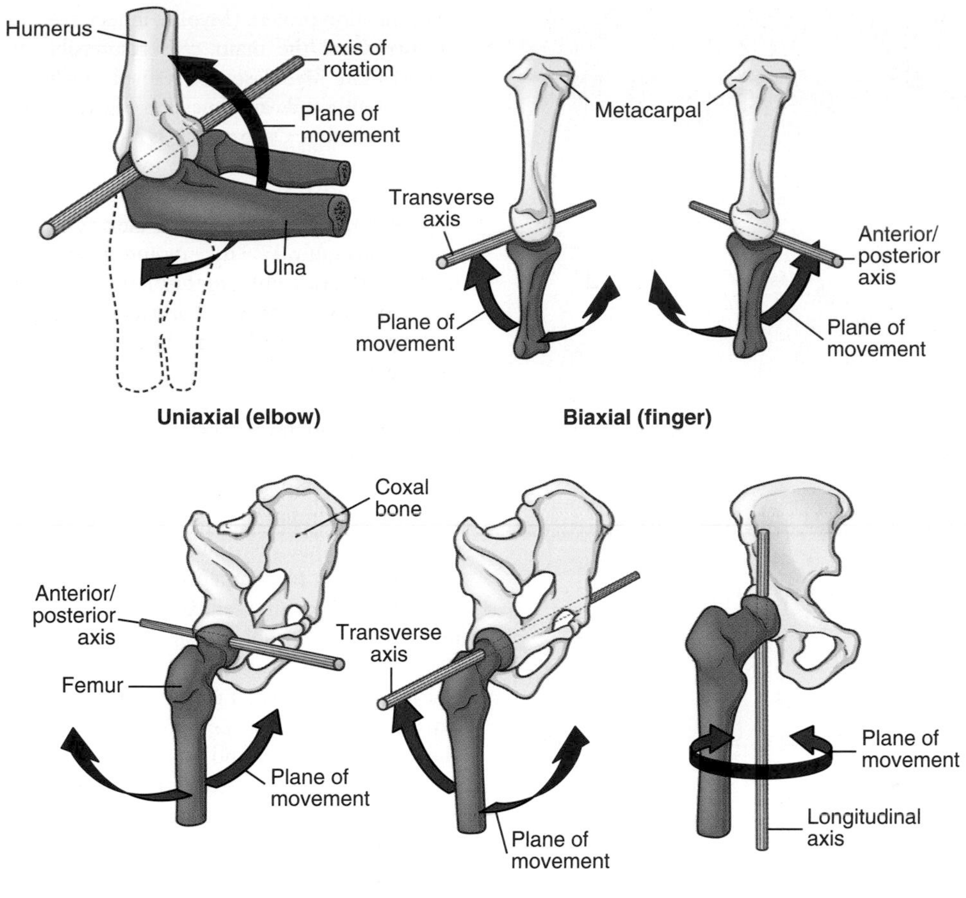

FIGURE 38-9 Movements of Synovial (Diarthrodial) Joints.

energy and metabolism are contained in muscle. Between the ages of 30 and 60, muscle mass decreases by about 225 grams of muscle each year. For each 225 grams of muscle lost, about 450 grams of fat is typically gained.

Whole Muscle

There are more than 600 skeletal muscles in the body. The body's muscles vary dramatically in size and shape. They range from 2 to 60 cm in length and are shaped according to function. **Fusiform muscles** are elongated muscles shaped like straps and can run from one joint to another. The biceps brachii and psoas major are examples of fusiform muscles. **Pennate muscles** are broad, flat, and slightly fan shaped, with fibres running obliquely to the muscle's long axis. The multipennate deltoid muscle, which flexes and extends the arm, is a good example of a muscle shaped according to its function.

Each skeletal muscle is a separate organ, encased in a three-part connective tissue framework called **fascia**. The layers of connective tissue protect the muscle fibres, attach the muscle to bony prominences, and provide a structure for a network of nerve fibres, blood vessels, and lymphatic channels. The layers are as follows:

1. The outermost layer, the **epimysium**, is located on the surface of the muscle and tapers at each end to form the tendon (Figure 38-12, also see p. 1006 for a discussion of tendons). Tendons allow short muscles to exert power on a distant joint, whereas a thick muscle would interfere with the joint's mobility.
2. The **perimysium** further subdivides the muscle fibres into bundles of connective tissue, or **fascicles**.
3. The smallest unit of muscle visible without a microscope is the **endomysium**, which surrounds the muscle.

The ligaments, tendons, and fascia are made up of connective tissue that also buffers the limbs from the effects of sudden strains or changes in speed. The rapid recovery necessary for strenuous exercise is supported by the elastic property of muscle and its connective tissue.

Skeletal muscle has been designated as **voluntary** (controlled directly by the nervous system), **striated** (has a striped pattern when viewed under a light microscope), or **extrafusal** (to distinguish from other contractile fibres in the sensory organ of the muscle). Components that are visible on gross inspection of the whole muscle include the motor and sensory nerve fibres. These function together with the muscle, innervating portions of it and providing the electrical impulses needed for motor function.

Motor Unit

From the anterior horn cell of the spinal cord, the axons of motor nerves branch to innervate a specific group of muscle fibres. Each anterior horn cell, its axon (part of the lower motor neuron; see Chapter 13), and the muscle fibres innervated by it are called a **motor unit** (Figure 38-13). The motor units are composed of lower motor neurons, which extend to skeletal muscles. Often termed the *functional unit* of the neuromuscular system, the motor unit behaves as a single entity and contracts as a whole when it receives an electrical impulse.

The whole muscle may be controlled by several motor nerve axons. These branch to innervate many motor units within the muscle. The whole muscle then may be made up of many motor units. The number

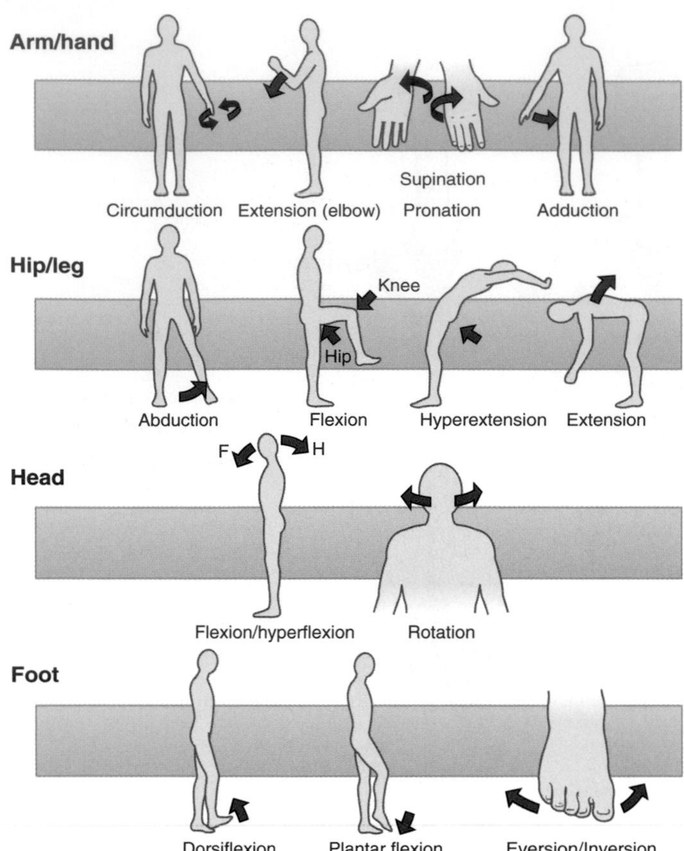

FIGURE 38-10 Body Movements Made Possible by Synovial (Diarthrodial) Joints.

of motor units per individual muscle varies greatly. In the calf, for example, 1 motor axon innervates approximately 2 000 muscle fibres, out of a total of 1 200 000 muscle fibres. This is a high innervation ratio of muscle fibres to axons, and it contrasts markedly with the low innervation ratio found in laryngeal muscles, where two to three muscle fibres constitute each motor unit and the innervation ratio can be of great functional significance. The greater the innervation ratio of a particular organ, the greater its endurance. Higher innervation ratios prevent fatigue, whereas lower innervation ratios allow for precision of movement.

Sensory receptors. Although muscles function as effector organs, they also contain sensory receptors and are involved in sending different signals to the central nervous system. Among these are the muscle spindles and Golgi tendon organs. **Spindles** are mechanoreceptors that lie parallel to muscle fibres and respond to muscle stretching. **Golgi tendon organs** are dendrites that terminate and branch to tendons near the neuromuscular junction. The muscle spindles, Golgi tendon organs, and free nerve endings provide a means of reporting changes in length, tension, velocity, and tone in the muscle. This system of afferent signals is responsible for the muscle stretch response and maintenance of normal muscle tone.

Muscle fibres. Each **muscle fibre** is a single **muscle cell** that is cylindrical in structure and surrounded by a membrane capable of excitation and impulse propagation. The muscle fibre contains bundles of **myofibrils**, the fibre's functional subunits, in a parallel arrangement along the longitudinal axis of the muscle (Figure 38-14). At birth, the muscle fibres have completed development from precursor cells called **myoblasts**. All **voluntary muscles** are derived from the mesodermal layer of the embryo. Genetic transcription factors, most notably myoblast determination protein (MyoD), induce skeletal muscle differentiation. Myoblasts are the main cells responsible for muscle growth and regeneration. Myoblasts are termed *satellite cells* when in a dormant state. **Satellite cells** are crucial in muscle growth, maintenance, repair, and regeneration. Once muscle is injured, satellite cells become activated and increase the number of transcriptional factors necessary to form myoblasts and assist in repair.[19]

The type of peripheral nerve influences the muscle fibre and motor unit considerably. Whether motor nerves are fast or slow determines the type of muscle fibres in the motor unit. White muscle (**type II fibres [white fast-twitch fibres]**) is innervated by relatively large type II alpha motor neurons with fast conduction velocities. These fibres rely on a short-term anaerobic glycolytic system for rapid energy transfer. Red muscle (**type I fibres [red slow-twitch fibres]**) depends on aerobic oxidative metabolism. Table 38-4 describes the specific characteristics of type I and type II fibres.

The overlap of muscle fibres that appears with staining gives a checkerboard appearance to muscle biopsy specimens. This overlap provides an equal distribution of fibre types throughout the muscle and also helps to compensate for muscle fibre loss and fatigue of individual motor units during activity. In spite of this overlap, some muscles contain proportionally more of one fibre type than another. Postural muscles have more type I fibres, allowing them the high resistance to fatigue that is necessary to maintain the same position for extended periods. The ocular muscles have more type II muscle fibres, allowing them to respond rapidly to visual changes.

The number of muscle fibres varies according to location. Large muscles, such as the gastrocnemius, have more fibres (1 200 000) than smaller muscles, such as the lumbrical muscles in the hand (10 000). The diameter of muscle fibres also varies. The closely packed polygons are small (10 to 20 μm) until puberty, when they attain the normal adult diameter of 40 to 80 μm. Women usually have smaller-diameter fibres than men. Small muscles, such as the ocular muscles, are 15 μm in diameter; larger, more proximal muscles are 40 μm in diameter. Fibre size can have functional significance. Studies have shown that larger fibre diameter is associated with generation of greater forces. Fibre diameter can be increased by exercise or occupational overuse, activities that cause hypertrophied muscle.

The major components of the muscle fibre include the muscle membrane, myofibrils, sarcotubular system, sarcoplasm, and mitochondria (see Figure 38-14). The **muscle membrane** is a two-part membrane. It includes the **sarcolemma**, which contains the plasma membrane of the muscle cell, and the cell's **basement membrane**. The sarcolemma is 7.5 μm thick and is capable of propagating electrical impulses to initiate contraction. At the motor nerve end plate, where the nerve impulse is transmitted, the sarcolemma forms the highly convoluted synaptic cleft. The sarcolemma is made up of lipid molecules and protein systems. The protein systems perform special functions, such as transport of nutrients and protein synthesis. They also provide the sodium–potassium pump and include the cell's cholinergic receptor. The basement membrane is 50 μm thick and is composed primarily of proteins and polysaccharides. It also serves as the cell's microskeleton and maintains the shape of the muscle cell. The basement membrane also may function in some way to restrict further diffusion of electrolytes once they have crossed the sarcolemma.

The **sarcoplasm** is the cytoplasm of the muscle cell and contains myoglobin plus the intracellular components that are common to all cells (see Chapter 1). **Myoglobin** is a protein found primarily in skeletal and heart muscle. Related to hemoglobin in the blood, myoglobin stores oxygen and iron in the muscle. The sarcoplasm is an aqueous substance that provides a matrix that surrounds the myofibrils. It contains numerous enzymes and proteins that are responsible for the cell's energy production,

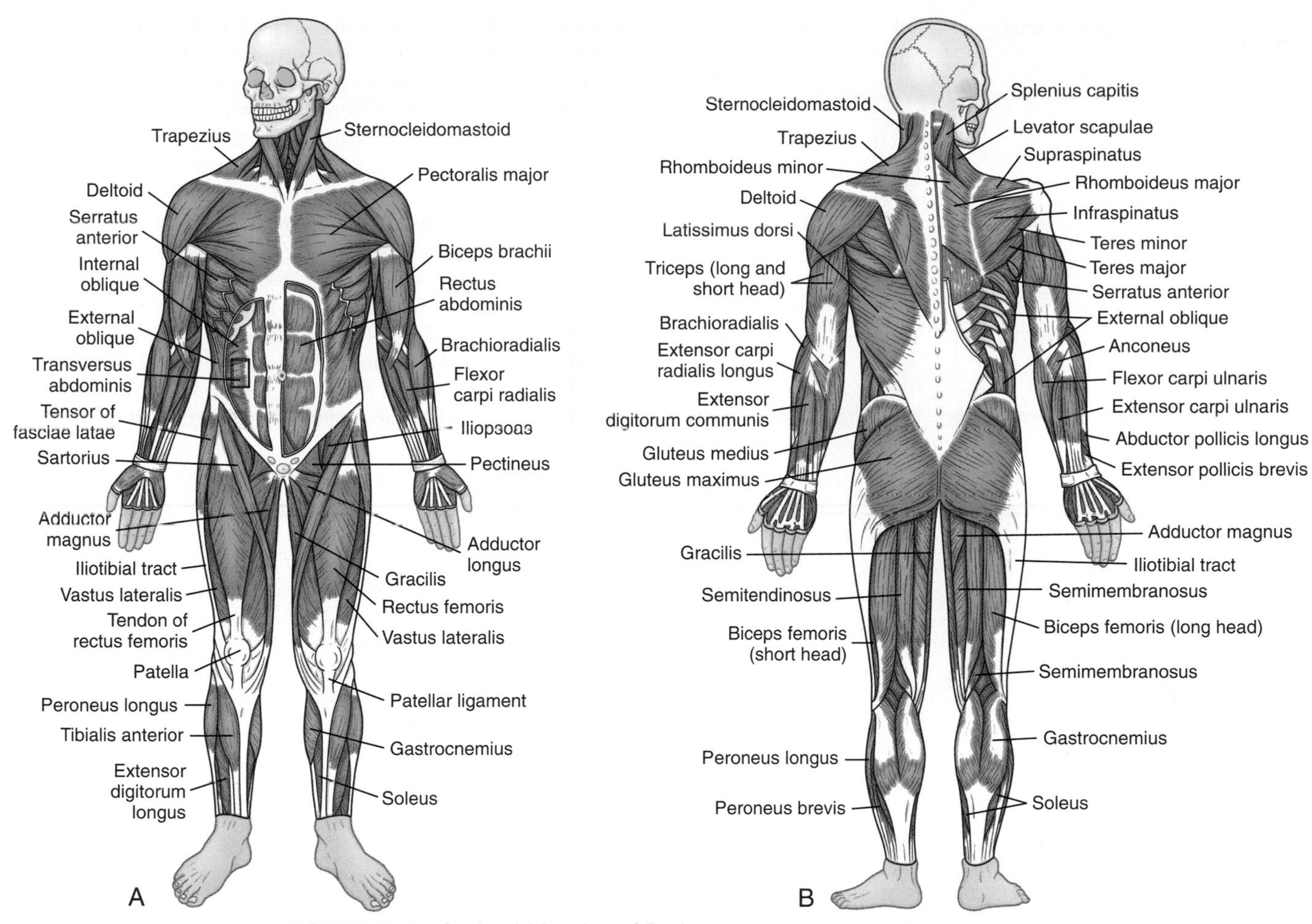

FIGURE 38-11 Skeletal Muscles of Body. **A,** Anterior view. **B,** Posterior view.

TABLE 38-4 Characteristics of Human Skeletal Muscle Fibres

Characteristics	Type I (Red) (Oxidative Fibres [OFs])	Type II (White) Type II-1A (Fast Oxidative Glycolic Fibres [FOGs])
Anatomical location	Deep axial portion of muscle	Surface portion of muscle
Fibre diameter	Small	Large
Motor neuron size	Small	Large
Contraction speed	Slow	Fast
Motor neuron type	Type I, α	Type II-A, II-B, II-X, and II-D II-A: fatigue resistant; II-B: fast fatigable; II-X and II-D: intermediate fatigability
Glycogen content (at rest)	Low	High
Oxidative capacity	High	High (for short periods)
Myosin-ATPase activity	Low	High
Metabolism	Oxidative (also most effective in removing glucose from bloodstream)	Some oxidative pathways, mostly glycolysis
Used for	Maintaining body posture, skeletal support, aerobic activity	Short, intense activity (e.g., sprinting)
Aerobic metabolic capacity	High	Low
Fatigue resistance	High	Intermediate to low
Myoglobin content	High	Low
Capillary supply	Profuse	Intermediate to low
Mitochondria	Many	Few
Intensity of contraction	Low	High
Example (most muscles are mixed)	Soleus muscle	Laryngeal
Satellite cell content	High	Low

ATPase, Adenosinetriphosphatase.
From Schiaffino, S., & Reggiani, C. (2011). *Physiol Rev, 91*, 1447–1531; Verdijk, L.B., Snijders, T., Drost, M., et al. (2014). *Age, 36*(2), 545–547.

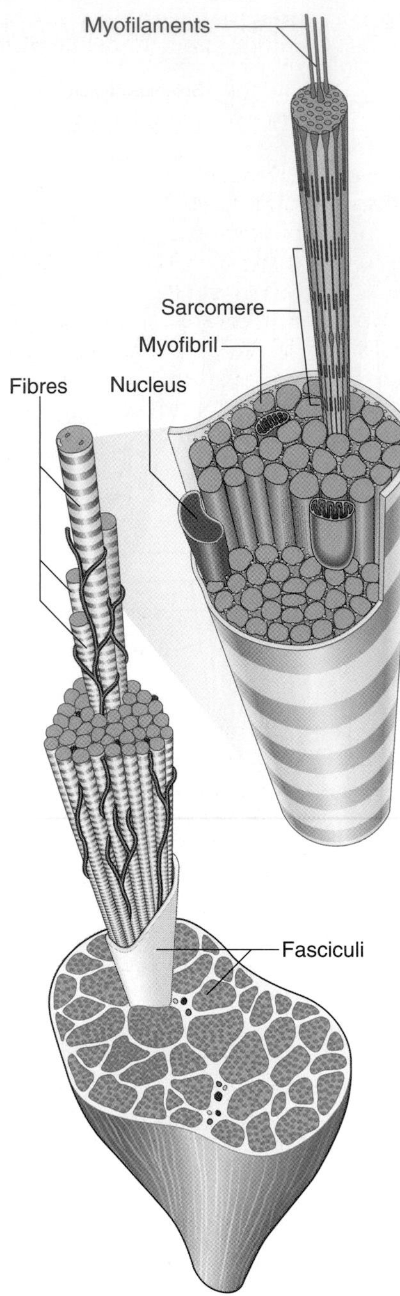

FIGURE 38-12 Levels of Organization Within a Skeletal Muscle Showing Muscle Fibres and Their Coverings. (From Standring, S. [2008]. *Gray's anatomy* [40th ed.]. Edinburgh: Churchill Livingstone.)

protein synthesis, and oxygen storage. The mitochondria house enzyme systems for energy production, particularly those that regulate processes such as the citric acid cycle and adenosine triphosphate (ATP) formation. Many other structures are present in the sarcoplasm. The ribosomes are composed of primarily RNA and participate in the process of protein synthesis. The cell nucleus, satellite cells, glycogen granules, and lipid droplets are suspended in the sarcoplasmic matrix. Blood vessels, nerve endings, muscle spindles, and Golgi tendon organs are also directly located within this structure.

Unique to the muscle is the **sarcotubular system**, a network that includes the transverse tubules and the sarcoplasmic reticulum, which crosses the interior of the cell. The **sarcoplasmic reticulum** is constructed like the endoplasmic reticulum in other cells. The sarcoplasmic reticulum is composed of tubules that run parallel to the myofibrils. The longitudinal tubules are termed **sarcotubules**. In muscle cells, the sarcoplasmic reticulum contains a network of intracellular receptors known as *ryanodine receptors* (RyRs). In response to a nerve impulse, RyR1 (found in skeletal muscle cells) releases intracellular calcium and initiates muscle contraction at the **sarcomere**, a portion of the myofibril. The **transverse tubules**, which also contain calcium release channels and are closely associated with the sarcotubules, run across the sarcoplasm and communicate with the extracellular space. Together, the tubules of this membrane system allow for uptake and regulation of intracellular calcium, release of calcium during muscle contraction, and storage of calcium during muscle relaxation.[20-22]

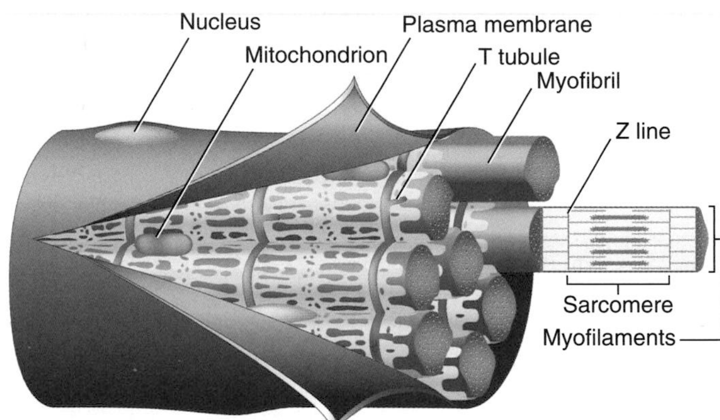

FIGURE 38-14 Muscle Structure. A skeletal muscle consists of fascicles (bundles) of muscle fibres. Each fibre is a cell containing myofibrils that consist of actin and myosin filaments. The filaments are organized into repeating units called sarcomeres. (From Solomon, E. [2016]. *Introduction to human anatomy and physiology* [4th ed.]. St. Louis: Saunders.)

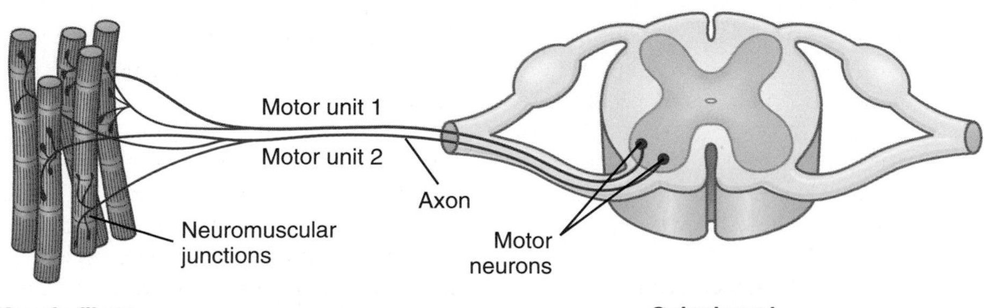

FIGURE 38-13 Motor Units of a Muscle. Each motor unit consists of a motor neuron and all the muscle fibres (cells) supplied by the neuron and its axon branches.

TABLE 38-5 **Contractile Proteins of Skeletal Muscle Sarcomere**

Protein	Location	Function
Actinin	Z disc	Attaches actin to Z discs; helps coordinate sarcomere contraction; cross-links thin filaments in adjacent sarcomeres
Actin	I band (thin filaments)	Is involved in contraction; activates myosin-ATPase; interacts with myosin
α-Actin	Z disc	Is main ligand of titin; links and controls filament length
β-Actin	Z disc	Has regulatory and structural functions; links filaments, controls filament length
Myosin	A band (thick filament)	Is involved in contraction force; two distinct types: myosin heavy chain (MyHC) and myosin light chain (MyLC); hydrolyzes ATP and develops tension
Titin[a] (largest and third most abundant muscle protein)	Half of sarcomere (from Z disc to M band)	Coordinates assembly of proteins that comprise sarcomere; regulates resting length of sarcomere; important for myofibril assembly, stabilization, and maintenance
Nebulin[a]	I band (with α-actin)	Interacts with myosin to produce contraction; binding site for actin, desmin, titin, other proteins; stabilizes and regulates length of actin filaments; plays role in assembly, structure, and maintenance of Z discs
Obscurin[a]	Surrounds sarcomere (mainly at Z disc and M band)	May mediate interaction of sarcoplasmic reticulum and myofibrils; plays role in muscle response to injury; has role in formation and stabilization of M bands and A band

[a]Also may function as molecular scaffolds for myofibril formation.
ATP, Adenosine triphosphate; *ATPase*, adenosinetriphosphatase.
Data from Herzog, J.A., Leonard, T.R., Jinha, A., et al. (2014). *Mol Cell Biomech, 11*(1), 1–17; Luther, P.K. (2009). *J Muscle Res Cell Motil, 30*, 171–185; Pappas, C.T., Krieg, P.A., & Gregorio, C.C. (2010). *J Cell Biol, 189*(5), 859–870; Schiaffino, S., & Reggiani, C. (2011). *Physiol Rev, 91*, 1447–1531.

Myofibrils. The myofibrils are the functional units of muscle contraction. Each myofibril contains sarcomeres, which appear at intervals (see Figure 38-14). The speed with which sarcomeres lengthen and shorten during movement directly influences the strength and function of skeletal muscles. Sprinters tend to have more fast-twitch (FT) fibres than slow-twitch (ST) fibres in their leg muscles, and endurance runners have more ST fibres in their leg muscles. Sarcomeres are composed of several proteins. The two most abundant are actin and myosin, but three other giant, muscle-specific proteins (titin, nebulin, and obscurin) play important roles in myofibril formation and function (Table 38-5).

The myofibrils are the most abundant subcellular muscle component, equalling 85 to 90% of the total volume. On cross-section, they are seen to be irregular polygons with a mean diameter of less than 1 μm. Each myofibril is composed of serially repeating sarcomeres, separated by Z bands (also called *Z discs*), which give the muscle its striped, cross-striated appearance. Each sarcomere has a dark A band and is flanked by two light I bands (Figure 38-15). The A band is 1.5 to 1.6 μm long and contains the thick myosin filaments. Included in the A band is a lighter zone called the *H band*, and in the centre of the H band is the dark *M line*, or *M band*. The I band, which contains actin, is divided at the midpoint of each sarcomere by the Z band. Its length varies with the start of muscle contraction. The Z band marks the boundaries of the sarcomere.[23]

Myofibrils are composed of myofilaments. Each myofilament is structured in a closely packed hexagonal arrangement, with two thin filaments for every thick filament. The thick filament, along with C protein and M line protein, is made up of myosin. Myosin has two subunits—heavy and light meromyosin, which resemble twisted golf club shafts. The thin filaments are twisted double strands consisting of actin, troponin, and tropomyosin (see Chapter 23 and Figure 23-13).

Muscle proteins. A multitude of muscle proteins have been identified and their functions are still being discovered. Table 38-5 summarizes the location and function of some of the important muscle proteins.

Nonprotein constituents of muscle. Substances such as nitrogen, creatine, creatinine, phosphocreatine, purines, uric acid, and amino acids all serve in the complex process of muscle metabolism. Energy is provided by glycogen and its derivatives.

Creatine metabolism and creatinine metabolism have been used to measure muscle mass. Plasma creatine is taken up by muscle and converted into the high-energy phosphate compound phosphocreatine by the enzyme creatine kinase. Creatinine is formed in muscle from creatine at a constant rate of 2% per day. (Measurement of plasma creatinine concentration is discussed in Chapter 29.) Creatine excretion is increased in muscle wasting. This change reflects the reduction in total body creatine stores and the loss of muscle mass.

Inorganic compounds, anions (phosphate, chloride), and cations (calcium, magnesium, sodium, potassium) are important in the regulation of protein synthesis, muscle contraction, and enzyme systems as well as in the stabilization of cell membranes. Total body potassium (TBK) level in adults, measured by the K40 method, has been used to estimate muscle mass, also called *lean body mass.* Total body potassium levels reflect changes in muscle mass seen during growth, malnutrition, and muscle wasting.

Components of Muscle Function

The ultimate function of muscle is to accomplish work. Although variously expressed in such measures as foot-pounds or kilogram-metres, work usually refers to the amount of energy liberated or force exerted over a distance (work = force × distance). Muscles usually contract or tense while doing work. Muscle contraction occurs on the molecular level and leads to the observable phenomenon of muscle movement.

Muscle Contraction at the Molecular Level

The four steps of muscle contraction are (1) excitation, (2) coupling, (3) contraction, and (4) relaxation. The process involves the electrical properties of all cells and the movement of ions across the plasma membrane (see Chapter 1). The muscle fibre is an excitable tissue. At rest, an electrical charge of −90 mV is continually maintained across the sarcolemma. This resting potential, generated by the separation of positive and negative charges on either side of the membrane, creates an electrochemical equilibrium caused by the selective permeability of the sarcolemma to electrolytes in the intracellular and extracellular fluids, particularly potassium and sodium.

Excitation, the first step of muscle contraction, begins with the spread of an action potential from the nerve terminal to the neuromuscular

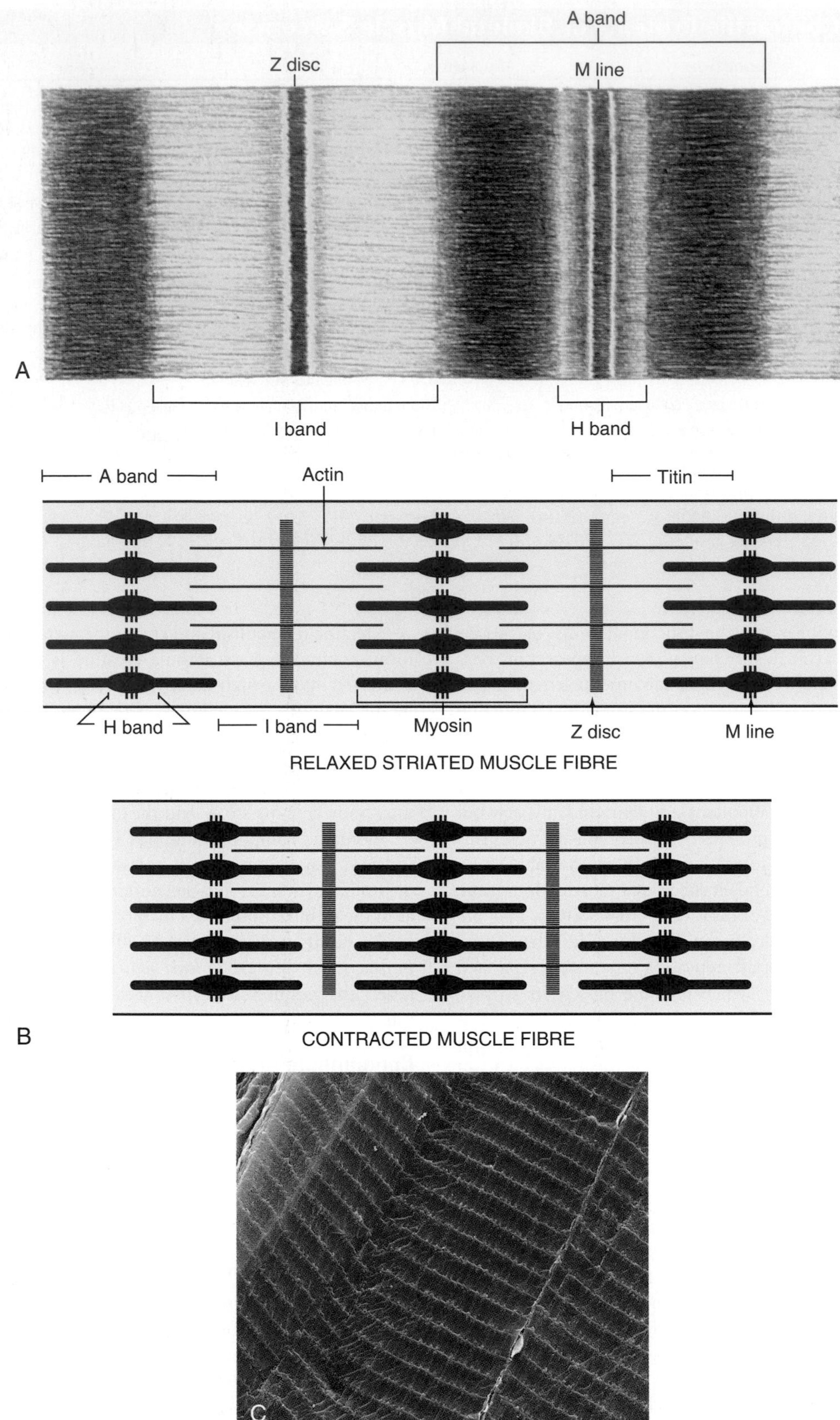

FIGURE 38-15 Muscle Fibres. A, The Z discs define the end of an individual sarcomere. The M line (which lies within the H band) is made of cross-connecting elements of the cytoskeleton. **B,** Actin is the primary protein of the I band (thin filament). Nebulin also extends along the I band and contains binding sites for actin and myosin. Myosin (thick filament) extends through the A band. Titin extends from the Z disc to the M band, binding with myosin; strong titin anchoring within the I band is necessary for proper muscle function. During contraction, the I bands and H bands shorten, moving the Z discs closer together. **C,** Electron photomicrograph of human muscle tissue corresponding to schematics in **A** and **B.** (**A,** modified from Thompson, J.M., McFarland, G.K., Hirsch, J.E., et al. [2002]. *Mosby's clinical nursing* [5th ed.]. St. Louis: Mosby; **C,** SPL/Science Source.)

junction. The rapid depolarization of the membrane initiates an electrical impulse in the muscle fibre membrane called the **muscle fibre action potential**. As the action potential advances along the sarcolemmal membrane, it spreads to the transverse tubules. (The velocity of conduction is much slower in muscle fibres than in myelinated nerve fibres—only 3 to 5 m/sec compared with 54 to 90 m/sec in nerve fibres.) A receptor on the transverse tubule opens, allowing calcium to enter the cell.[24]

The second stage, **coupling**, follows the depolarization of the transverse tubules. This triggers the release of calcium ions from the sarcoplasmic reticulum through RyR1 channels into the sarcoplasm. The calcium then binds to a protein on the actin filament. (Calcium affects troponin and tropomyosin, muscle proteins that bind with actin when the muscle is at rest.) In the presence of calcium, however, both these proteins are attracted to calcium ions, leaving the actin free to bind with myosin. The release of intracellular calcium ions is the critical link between a nerve impulse (electrical excitation) and muscle contraction.[25]

Contraction begins as the calcium ions combine with troponin, a reaction that overcomes the inhibitory function of the troponin–tropomyosin system. Myosin binds to actin, forming cross-bridges. The myosin heads attach to the exposed actin-binding sites, pulling actin (the thin filament) inward. The thin filament, actin, then slides toward the thick filament, myosin. The two ends of the myofibril shorten after contraction when the myosin heads attach to the actin molecules, forming a cross-bridge that constitutes an actin–myosin complex. ATP, located on the actin–myosin complex, is released when the cross-bridges attach. The process of contraction was first described by A.F. Huxley in the 1950s. It is commonly known as the **cross-bridge theory** because the actin and myosin proteins form cross-bridges as they contract. The useful distance of contraction of a skeletal muscle is approximately 25 to 35% of the muscle's length.

The last step, **relaxation**, begins as calcium ions are actively transported back into the sarcoplasmic reticulum, removing ions from interaction with troponin. The cross-bridges detach, and the sarcomere lengthens. (The cross-bridge theory of muscle contraction is discussed in Chapter 23.)

Muscle Metabolism

Skeletal muscle requires a constant supply of ATP and phosphocreatine. These substances are necessary to fuel the complex processes of muscle contraction, driving the cross-bridges of actin and myosin together and transporting calcium from the sarcoplasmic reticulum to the myofibril. Other internal processes of the muscular system that require ATP include protein synthesis, which replenishes muscle constituents and accommodates growth and repair. The rate of protein synthesis is related to hormone levels (particularly insulin), the presence of amino acid substrates, and overall nutritional status. At rest, the rate of ATP formation by oxidation of glucose or acetoacetate is sufficient to maintain internal processes, given normal nutritional status. During activity, the need for ATP increases 100-fold. The metabolic pathways for muscle activity in Table 38-6 show reactions to the immediate need for increased ATP caused by contraction. Activity lasting longer than 5 seconds expends the available stored ATP and phosphocreatine.

Stored glycogen and blood glucose are converted anaerobically to sustain brief activity without increasing the demand for oxygen. Anaerobic glycolysis is much less efficient than aerobic glycolysis, using six to eight times more glycogen to produce the same amount of ATP. With increased activity, such as intense exercise, or with ischemia, an increase in the amount of lactic acid occurs because of the breakdown of glycogen, thus causing a shift in muscle pH (see Table 38-6). This short-term mechanism buys time by allowing ATP formation in spite of inadequate energy stores or oxygen supply. When the anaerobic threshold is reached and more oxygen is required, physiological changes occur, including

TABLE 38-6 Energy Sources for Muscular Activity

Sources	Reactions
Short-term (anaerobic) sources	ATP → ADP + P_i + Energy
	Phosphocreatine + ADP ⇌ Creatine + ATP
	Glycogen/glucose + P_i + ADP → Lactate + ATP
Long-term (aerobic) sources	Glycogen/glucose + ADP + P_i + O_2 → H_2O + CO_2 + ATP
	Free fatty acids + ADP + P_i + O_2 → H_2O + CO_2 + ATP
	Creatine kinase catalyzes reversible reaction of ATP to ADP: Creatine phosphate + ATP $\xrightleftharpoons{\text{Creatine Kinase}}$ Creatine + ATP

ADP, Adenosine diphosphate; *ATP*, adenosine triphosphate; *CO_2*, carbon dioxide; *H_2O*, water; *O_2*, oxygen; *P_i*, inorganic phosphate.
From Spence, A.P., & Mason, E.E. (1992). *Human anatomy and physiology* (4th ed.). St. Paul, MN: West Publishing.

an increase in lactic acid level and increases in oxygen consumption, heart rate, respiratory rate, and muscle blood flow.

Strenuous exercise requires oxygen, which activates the aerobic glycogen pathway for ATP formation. During maximal exercise, free fatty acid mobilization and the aerobic glycogen pathways provide ATP over an extended time. These pathways require oxygen both to maintain maximal activity and to return the muscle to the resting state. Maximal exercise increases oxygen uptake by 15 to 20 times over the resting state. When this system becomes exhausted or inadequate to respond to the need for ATP, fatigue and weakness finally force the muscle to reduce activity with a resultant buildup of lactic acid in muscle fibres. Creatine supplementation may provide some protective effects on muscle in older adult athletes as well as after strenuous physical activity.[26]

Sustaining maximal muscular activity accumulates an **oxygen debt**, which is the amount of oxygen needed to oxidize the residual lactic acid, convert it back to glycogen, and replenish ATP and phosphocreatine stores. For example, after running at maximal speed for 10 seconds, the average person has consumed 1 L of oxygen. At rest, oxygen consumption for the same period is approximately 40 mL. As the person recovers, the measured oxygen debt is 4 L greater than the amount used during activity.

Oxygen consumption is measured to calculate the metabolic cost of activity in normal and diseased muscle. It is an indirect measure of energy expenditure, along with timed tests of activity, heart rate, and respiratory quotient (ratio of carbon dioxide to expired oxygen consumed). Energy expenditure is measured directly by heat production because heat is released whenever work is accomplished.

Another factor that changes energy requirements is muscle fibre type. Type II fibres rely on anaerobic glycolytic metabolism and fatigue readily. Type I fibres can resist fatigue for longer periods because of their capacity for oxidative metabolism.

Muscle Mechanics

Muscle contraction cannot be viewed in isolation. Several factors determine how force is transmitted from the cross-bridges on individual muscle fibres to accomplish whole-muscle contraction. First, when a motor unit responds to a single nerve stimulus, it develops a phasic contraction, also called a *twitch*. Because the motor unit contracts in an all-or-nothing manner, the contraction that is generated will be a maximal contraction. The central nervous system smoothly grades the force generated by recruiting additional motor units and varying the discharge frequency of each active motor unit. This adding of motor units within the muscle is called **repetitive discharge**.

Recruitment and repetitive discharge of motor units allow the muscle to activate the number of motor units needed to generate the desired force. The total force developed is the sum of the force generated by each motor unit. If the motor units are stimulated again, and the muscle unit has not been able to relax between stimulation and the next contraction, the second contraction will fuse with the first, causing **physiological tetanus** (not to be confused with the disease tetanus).

Other variables, such as fibre type, innervation ratio, muscle temperature, and muscle shape, influence the efficiency of muscular contraction. The two muscle fibre types differ in their responses to electrical activity. Tetanus and duration of phasic contractions, which take microseconds to accomplish, are achieved more rapidly in type II (white fast-twitch) than in type I (red slow-twitch) muscle fibres. Low innervation ratios promote control and coordination, whereas high ratios promote strength and endurance. Muscles work best at normal body temperature, 37°C (98.6°F). Finally, muscles with a large cross-sectional area, such as the fan-shaped pennate muscles, develop greater contractile forces than smaller-diameter muscles. The initial length of a muscle and the range of shortening that occurs when the muscle contracts also determine the force it can generate. The long fusiform muscles have a greater range of shortening and can contract up to 57% of their resting length. A certain amount of elongation is necessary to generate sufficient tension and muscular force. The elongation that occurs during the swing of a golf club or tennis racket is an example of how stretch improves contractile force.

Types of Muscle Contraction

During **isometric** (or **static**) **contraction**, the muscle maintains constant length as tension is increased (Figure 38-16). Isometric contraction occurs, for example, when the arm or leg is pushed against an immovable object. The muscle contracts, but the limb does not move. Isometric contraction is also called **static (holding) contraction**.

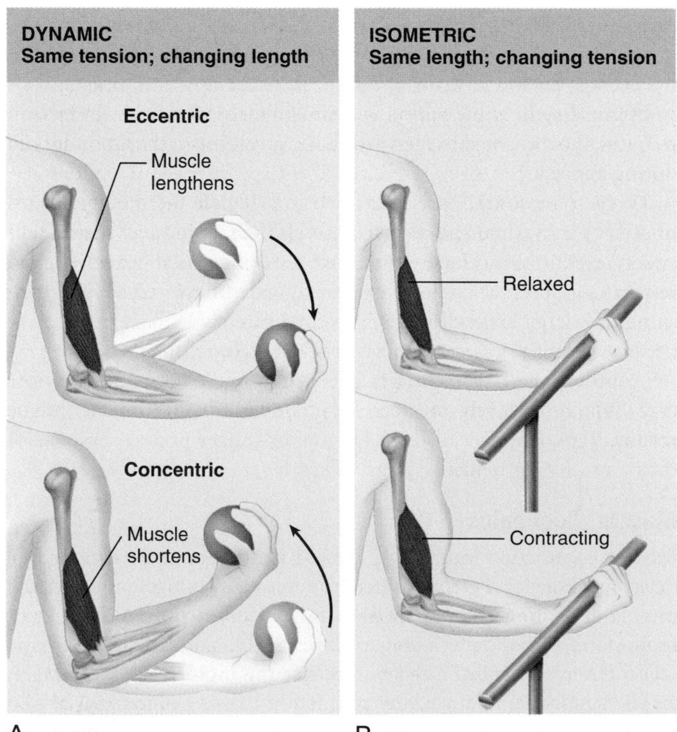

FIGURE 38-16 Dynamic and Isometric Contraction. **A,** In dynamic contraction, the muscle shortens, producing movement. **B,** In isometric contraction, the muscle pulls forcefully against a load but does not shorten. (From Patton, K.T., & Thibodeau, G.A. [2016]. *Structure & function of the body* [15th ed.]. St. Louis: Mosby.)

During **dynamic** (formerly **isotonic**) **contraction**, the muscle maintains a constant tension as it moves. Dynamic contractions can be **eccentric (lengthening)** or **concentric (shortening)**. Positive work is accomplished during concentric contraction, and energy is released to exert force or lift a weight. In contrast, during an eccentric contraction the muscle lengthens and absorbs energy (such as extending the elbow while lowering a weight). Eccentric contraction requires less energy to accomplish and has been said to result in the development of pain and stiffness after unaccustomed exercise.

Movement of Muscle Groups

Muscles do not act alone but in groups, often under automatic control. When a muscle contracts and acts as a prime mover, or **agonist**, its reciprocal muscle, or **antagonist**, relaxes. To illustrate this, hold the right arm in the horizontal position in front of the body and bend the elbow; use the other hand to feel the biceps on the top and the triceps on the bottom of the arm. When the elbow is bent, the biceps are firm, and the triceps are soft. As the arm is extended, the muscles change. When the elbow is completely extended, the biceps are soft and the triceps firm. Completing this movement causes the agonist and antagonist to change automatically; only the movement is commanded, not the alternate contraction and relaxation of the specific muscle groups.

Other associated actions may be seen during walking; as the foot leaves the ground, the paravertebral and gluteal muscles on the opposite sides of the body contract to maintain balance. One notices the loss of the associated muscle's action when paralysis offsets this process and decreases balance. If a person is paralyzed, difficulty in maintaining balance is noticeable.

Tendons and Ligaments

Tendons are important musculo-skeletal structures that attach muscle to bone at a site called an **enthesis**. **Ligaments** attach bone to bone, helping to form joints as well as stabilizing them against excessive movement. Both tendons and ligaments are primarily composed of types III, IV, V, and VI collagen and fibroblasts (termed *tenocytes* in tendons).[27] The fibroblasts in a tendon are arranged in parallel rows; fibroblasts appear less organized in ligaments. Collagen fibres and fibroblasts form fascicles, with multiple fascicles then forming a whole tendon or ligament. In the proteoglycan matrix of tendons, collagen oligomeric matrix protein (COMP) assists in providing gliding and viscoelastic properties. Compared with tendons, ligament fibres typically contain a greater proportion of elastin.

Two main functions of tendons are (1) transferring forces from muscle to bone and (2) acting as a type of biological spring for muscles to allow additional stability during movement. Ligaments stabilize joints by restricting movement. Although both tendons and ligaments can withstand significant distraction (stretching) force, they tend to buckle when compressive force is applied.

Both tendons and ligaments have complex structures at the attachment site of two dissimilar tissues. Figure 38-17 illustrates the transition of tissue between tendon/ligament and bone. These complex structures and differences in mechanical and structural characteristics (either tendon and bone or ligament and bone) make healing and repair of damaged tissue complicated (see *Health Promotion:* Tendon and Ligament Repair).

AGING AND THE MUSCULO-SKELETAL SYSTEM

Aging of Bones

Aging is accompanied by the loss of bone tissue. Bones become less dense, less strong, and more brittle with aging. The bone remodelling cycle takes longer to complete, and the rate of mineralization also slows.

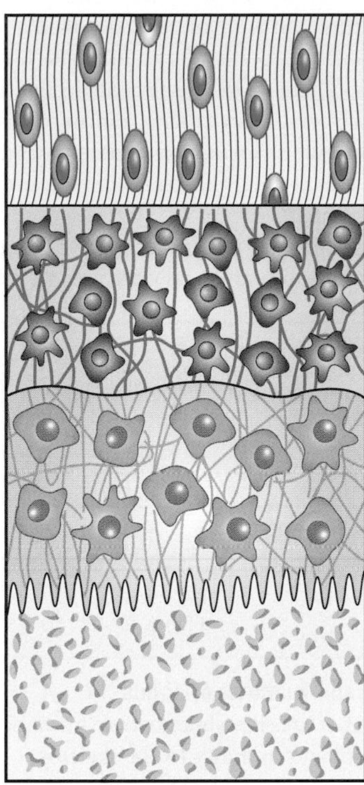
Tendon/ligament
Aligned collagen fibrils (lines)
Fibroblasts embedded throughout (blue oval cells)
Collagen fibrils extend into uncalcified fibrocartilage
Uncalcified fibrocartilage
Larger, less parallel collagen bundles (vertical blue lines)
Collagen types I and II, aggrecan (irregular-shaped cells)
Avascular (yellow background)
Ovoid-shaped, aligned cells (smooth-edged cells)
Wavy tidemark (marks beginning of calcification)
Calcified fibrocartilage
Mineralized tissue
Hypertrophic, more circular chondrocytes
Consists of collagen types I, II, and X
Bone
Interdigitation at surface (zigzag line)
Calcified tissue

FIGURE 38-17 Cartilage–Bone, Tendon/Ligament–Bone, Meniscus–Bone, and Muscle–Tendon Interfaces. This diagram depicts the cartilage–bone, tendon/ligament–bone, meniscus–bone, and muscle–tendon interfaces and their compositions. Gradients of matrix composition, interdigitation of tissue zones, and interconnecting collagen fibres all enable load transfer between disparate tissues. (From Yang, P.J., & Temenoff, J.S. [2009]. *Tissue Eng Part B Rev, 15*[2], 128.)

HEALTH PROMOTION

Tendon and Ligament Repair

Injury of tendons and ligaments constitutes one of the greatest challenges in musculo-skeletal rehabilitation. When these types of structures are damaged, attempts to engineer suitable tissue replacements have proved disappointing. The structures and intricate protein composition of tendons and ligaments are the basis for their complex biomechanical properties. One reason for poor clinical outcome in synthetic tendon structures has been the inability to replicate any material that can bear the high mechanical stresses that occur at the interface between two dissimilar materials (i.e., either tendon and bone or ligament and bone). One promising area of investigation is finding or engineering a biodegradable material, or "scaffold," implanted with specific cells that would regenerate into normal tendon or ligament. The scaffold must be strong enough to withstand the forces at the tissue–bone interface and then gradually break down as it is completely replaced by new cells. Currently, investigators are using synthetic polymers, silk, and collagen as scaffolds, with tendon or ligament fibroblasts and mesenchymal stem cells as the implanted cells. Once these biochemical hurdles are overcome, the repair of damaged tendons and ligaments will be revolutionized.

Data from Jahr, H., Matta, C., & Mobasheri A. (2015). *Curr Rheumatol Rep, 17*(3), 22.

With aging, women experience loss of bone density, accelerated with the rapid bone loss that occurs during early menopause from increased osteoclastic bone resorption, fewer osteocytes, and decreased numbers of osteoblasts.[28] By age 70, susceptible women have, on average, lost 50% of their peripheral cortical bone mass (see Chapter 39). Bone mass losses to such an extent can lead to deformity, pain, stiffness, and high risk for fractures. Men experience bone loss also but at later ages and at a much slower rate than seen in women. Also, initial bone mass in men is approximately 30% higher than in women; therefore bone loss in men causes less risk for disability than it does for women. Men's peak bone mass is related to their race, heredity, hormonal factors, physical activity, and calcium intake during childhood. Bone loss in both genders is related to smoking, calcium deficiency, alcohol intake, and physical inactivity. Bone mass can be gained in healthy young women up to the third decade through participation in physical activity, intake of dietary calcium and other minerals, and use of oral contraceptives. Height is also lost with aging because of intervertebral disc degeneration and, sometimes, osteoporotic spinal fractures.

Stem cells in the bone marrow perform less efficiently with aging, predisposing older adults to acute and chronic illnesses. Such illnesses cause weakness and confusion in older adults and may increase the risk for injury or falling.

Aging of Joints

With aging, cartilage becomes more rigid, fragile, and susceptible to fraying because of increased cross-linking of collagen and elastin, decreased water content in the cartilage ground substance, and reduced concentrations of glycosaminoglycans. Decreased range of motion of the joint is related to the changes in ligaments and muscles. Bones in joints develop evidence of osteoporosis with fewer trabeculae and thinner, less dense bones, making them prone to fractures. Intervertebral disc spaces decrease in height. The rate of loss of height accelerates at age 70 and beyond. Tendons shrink and harden.

Aging of Muscles

The function of skeletal muscle depends on many influences that are affected by cellular factors, such as reduced mitochondrial volume associated with aging.[29] Other influences include the nervous, vascular, and endocrine systems. In the young child, the development of muscle tissue depends greatly on continuing neurodevelopmental maturation. Muscle loss begins at about age 50; however, muscle function remains trainable even into advanced age. Maintaining musculo-skeletal fitness at any age can improve overall health.[30,31]

Age-related loss in skeletal muscle is referred to as **sarcopenia** and is a direct cause of the age-related decrease in muscle strength. As the body ages, muscle mass and strength decline slowly; thus, strength is maintained through the fifth decade, with a slow decline in dynamic and isometric strength evident after age 70. The amount of type II fibres also decreases. There is reduced synthesis of RNA, loss of mitochondrial function,[29,32] and reduction in the size of motor units. The regenerative function of muscle tissue remains normal in older adults. As much as 30 to 40% of skeletal muscle mass and strength may be lost from the third to ninth decade. Muscle fatigue also may contribute to loss of function with aging.[32] Sarcopenia is thought to be secondary to progressive neuromuscular changes and diminishing levels of anabolic hormones. There is an age-related decline in the synthesis of mixed proteins, myosin heavy chains, and mitochondrial protein.[33] Changes in these muscle proteins are related to reduced levels of insulinlike growth factor 1 (IGF-1), testosterone, and dehydroepiandrosterone (DHEA) sulphate.

Maximal oxygen intake declines with age. Basal metabolic rate is reduced and lean body mass decreases in the older adult population.

✔ QUICK CHECK 38-3

1. Name three differences between slow-twitch and fast-twitch muscle fibres.
2. Why is adenosine triphosphate used for muscle contraction?
3. Define the differences between tendons and ligaments.
4. Describe significant changes in the musculo-skeletal system with aging.

DID YOU UNDERSTAND?

Structure and Function of Bones

1. Bones provide support and protection for the body's tissues and organs and are important sources of minerals and blood cells.
2. Bone formation begins with the production of an inorganic matrix by bone cells. Bone minerals crystallize in and around collagen fibres in the matrix, giving bone its characteristic hardness and strength.
3. Bone tissue is continuously being resorbed and synthesized by basic multicellular units of osteoclasts and osteoblasts, respectively.
4. Osteoblasts are multifunctional mononuclear cells derived from osteogenic mesenchymal stromal cells; they are the primary bone-producing cells and are involved in many functions related to the skeletal system.
5. Osteocytes are the most numerous cells in bone and represent the final stage of an osteoblast's life. Though imbedded in the bone matrix, osteocytes have important functions in directing bone remodelling.
6. Osteoclasts are large (typically 20 to 100 μm in diameter), multinucleated cells that develop from the hematopoietic monocyte/macrophage lineage. Osteoclasts are the major resorptive cells of bone.
7. Bones in the body are made up of compact bone tissue and spongy bone tissue. Compact bone is highly organized into haversian systems that consist of concentric layers of crystallized matrix surrounding a central canal that contains blood vessels and nerves. Dispersed throughout the concentric layers of crystallized matrix are small spaces containing osteocytes. Smaller canals, called *canaliculi*, interconnect the osteocyte-containing spaces. The crystallized matrix in spongy bone is arranged in bars or plates. Spaces containing *osteocytes* are dispersed between the bars or plates and interconnected by canaliculi.
8. There are 206 bones in the body divided into the axial skeleton and the appendicular skeleton. Bones are classified by shape as long, short, flat, or irregular. Long bones have a broad end (epiphysis), broad neck (metaphysis), and narrow midportion (diaphysis) that contains the medullary cavity.
9. Bone injuries are repaired in stages. Hematoma formation provides the fibrin framework for formation and organization of granulation tissue. The granulation tissue provides a cartilage model for the formation and crystallization of bone matrix. Remodelling restores the original shape and size to the injured bone.

Structure and Function of Joints

1. A joint is the site where two or more bones attach. Joints provide stability and mobility to the skeleton.
2. Joints are classified as synarthroses, amphiarthroses, or diarthroses, depending on the degree of movement they allow. Joints are also classified by the type of connecting tissue holding them together. Fibrous joints are connected by dense fibrous tissue, ligaments, or membranes. Cartilaginous joints are connected by fibrocartilage or hyaline cartilage. Synovial joints are connected by a fibrous joint capsule. Within the capsule is a small fluid-filled space. The fluid in the space nourishes the articular cartilage that covers the ends of the bones meeting in the synovial joint.
3. Articular cartilage is a highly organized system of collagen fibres and proteoglycans. The fibres firmly anchor the cartilage to the bone, and the proteoglycans control the loss of fluid from the cartilage.
4. Joints help move bones and muscle.

Structure and Function of Skeletal Muscles

1. Skeletal muscle is made up of millions of individual fibres.
2. Between the ages of 30 and 60, muscle mass decreases by about 225 grams of muscle each year. For each 225 grams of muscle lost, about 450 grams of fat is typically gained.
3. Whole muscles vary in size (2 to 60 cm) and shape (fusiform, pennate). They are encased in a three-part connective tissue framework. The fundamental unit of muscle contraction is the motor unit, defined as those muscle fibres innervated by a single motor nerve, its axon, and an anterior horn cell.
4. Satellite cells are dormant myoblasts; however, when activated, they can regenerate muscle.
5. Muscle fibres contain bundles of myofibrils arranged in parallel along the longitudinal axis and include the muscle membrane, myofibrils, sarcotubular system, sarcoplasm, and mitochondria. There are two types of muscle fibres, type I and type II, determined by motor nerve innervation.
6. Myofibrils and myofilaments contain the major muscle proteins actin and myosin, which interact to form cross-bridges during muscle contraction. The nonprotein muscle constituents provide an energy source for contraction and regulate protein synthesis and enzyme systems as well as stabilize cell membranes.

7. Muscle contraction includes excitation, coupling, contraction, and relaxation.
8. Muscle strength is graded by the all-or-nothing phenomenon and recruitment. Speed of contraction is affected by several factors: muscle fibre type, temperature, stretch, and weight of the load.
9. Skeletal muscle requires a constant supply of adenosine triphosphate (ATP) and phosphocreatine to fuel muscle contraction and for growth and repair. ATP and phosphocreatine can be generated aerobically or anaerobically.
10. There are two types of muscle contraction: isometric (static) and dynamic (formerly *isotonic*). Muscle shortening occurs during contraction but can also be seen during pathological and physiological contracture.
11. The site at which tendons attach muscle to bone is called an *enthesis*.
12. Ligaments attach bone to bone, helping to form joints as well as stabilizing them against excessive movement. Both tendons and ligaments are mostly composed of types III, IV, V, and VI collagen and fibroblasts (termed *tenocytes* in tendons).

Aging and the Musculo-skeletal System

1. Sarcopenia, or age-related loss in skeletal muscle, is a direct cause of decrease in muscle strength. A slow decline in dynamic and isometric strength is evident after age 70.
2. The regenerative function of muscle tissue remains normal in older adults.
3. Reduced basal metabolic rate and decreased lean body mass are also noted in the older adult population.

KEY TERMS

Agonist, 1006
α-Glycoprotein, 992
Amphiarthrosis (slightly movable joint), 995
Antagonist, 1006
Appendicular skeleton, 994
Articular cartilage, 997
Axial skeleton, 994
Basement membrane, 1000
Basic multicellular unit, 995
Bone albumin, 992
Bone fluid, 992
Bone matrix, 988
Calcification, 988
Canaliculus (*pl.*, canaliculi), 993
Chondrocyte, 997
Collagen fibre, 992
Compact bone (cortical bone), 992
Concentric (shortening) contraction, 1006
Contraction, 1005
Coupling, 1005
Cross-bridge theory, 1005
Diaphysis, 994
Diarthrosis (freely movable joint), 995
Dynamic (isotonic) contraction, 1006
Eccentric (lengthening) contraction, 1006
Endomysium, 999
Endosteum, 994
Enthesis, 1006
Epimysium, 999
Epiphysis, 994
Excitation, 1003
Fascia, 999
Fascicle, 999
Fibril, 992
Fibrous joint, 995
Flat bone, 994
Fusiform muscle, 999
Glycoprotein, 992
Golgi tendon organ, 1000
Gomphosis, 995
Ground substance, 988
Growth plate (epiphyseal plate), 994
Haversian canal, 993
Haversian system, 993
Hydroxyapatite (HAP), 992
Integrin, 990
Irregular bone, 994
Isometric (static) contraction, 1006
Joint (articular) capsule, 995
Joint (articulation), 995
Joint (synovial) cavity, 997
Lacuna, 990
Lamella (*pl.*, lamellae), 993
Ligament, 1006
Long bone, 994
Metaphysis, 994
Mineralization, 992
Motor unit, 999
Muscle fibre action potential, 1005
Muscle fibre (muscle cell), 1000
Muscle membrane, 1000
Myoblast, 1000
Myofibril, 1000
Myoglobin, 1000
Osteoblast, 990
Osteocalcin, 992
Osteoclast, 990
Osteocyte, 990
Osteoid, 990
Osteoprotegerin (OPG), 990
Oxygen debt, 1005
Pennate muscle, 999
Perimysium, 999
Periosteum, 993
Physiological tetanus, 1006
Podosome, 990
Proteoglycan, 992
Receptor activator of nuclear factor kappa-B ligand (RANKL), 990
Relaxation, 1005
Remodelling, 995
Repetitive discharge, 1005
Resorb, 988
Ruffled border, 990
Sarcolemma, 1000
Sarcomere, 1002
Sarcopenia, 1008
Sarcoplasm, 1000
Sarcoplasmic reticulum, 1002
Sarcotubular system, 1002
Sarcotubule, 1002
Satellite cell, 1000
Short bone, 994
Sialoprotein, 992
Skeletal muscle (voluntary, striated, or extrafusal muscle), 999
Spindle, 1000
Spongy bone (cancellous bone), 992
Static (holding) contraction, 1006
Suture, 995
Symphysis, 995
Synarthrosis (immovable joint), 995
Synchondrosis, 995
Syndesmosis, 995
Synovial fluid, 997
Synovial joint, 998
Synovial membrane, 996
Tendon, 1006
Tidemark, 997
Trabecula (*pl.*, trabeculae), 993
Transverse tubule, 1002
Type I fibre (red slow-twitch fibre), 1000
Type II fibre (white fast-twitch fibre), 1000
Voluntary muscle, 1000

REFERENCES

1. van der Meijden, K., Lips, P., van Driel, M., et al. (2014). Primary human osteoblasts in response to 25-hydroxyvitamin D3, 1,25-dihydroxyvitamin D3, and 24R,25-dihydroxyvitamin D3. *PLoS ONE*, *9*(10), e110283. doi:10.1371/journal.pone.0110283.
2. Boyce, B. F., Yao, Z., & Xing, L. (2010). Functions of NF κB in bone. *Annals of the New York Academy of Sciences*, *1192*, 367–375. doi:10.1111/j.1749-6632.2009.05315.x.
3. Nakashima, T., Hayashi, M., Fukunaga, T., et al. (2011). Evidence for osteocyte regulation of bone homeostasis through RANKL expression. *Nature Medicine*, *17*(10), 1231–1234. doi:10.1038/nm.2452.
4. Xiong, J., & O'Brien, C. A. (2012). Osteocyte RANKL: New insights into control of bone remodeling. *Journal of Bone and Mineral Research*, *27*(3), 499–505. doi:10.1002/jbmr.1547.
5. Hughes, J. M., & Petit, M. A. (2010). Biological underpinnings of Frost's mechanostat thresholds: The important role of osteocytes. *Journal of Musculoskeletal and Neuronal Interactions*, *10*(2), 128–135.
6. Bellido, T. (2014). Osteocyte-driven bone remodeling. *Calcified Tissue International*, *94*(1), 25–34. doi:10.1007/s00223-013-9774-y.

7. Komori, T. (2013). Functions of the osteocyte network in the regulation of bone mass. *Cell and Tissue Research, 352*(2), 191–198. doi:10.1007/s00441-012-1546-x.
8. Sapir-Koren, R., & Livshits, G. (2014). Osteocyte control of bone remodeling: Is sclerostin a key molecular coordinator of the balanced bone resorption–formation cycles? *Osteoporosis International, 25*(12), 2685–2700. doi:10.1007/s00198-014-2808-0.
9. Nguyen, A. M., & Jacobs, C. R. (2013). Emerging role of primary cilia as a mechanoreceptor in osteocytes. *Bone, 54*(2), 196–204. doi:10.1016/j.bone.2012.11.016.
10. Schaffler, M. B., & Kennedy, O. D. (2012). Osteocyte signaling in bone. *Current Osteoporosis Reports, 19*(2), 118–125. doi:10.1007/s11914-012-0105-4.
11. Hambli, R. (2014). Connecting mechanics and bone cell activities in the bone remodeling process: An integrated finite element modeling. *Frontiers in Bioengineering and Biotechnology, 2*, 6. doi:10.3389/fbioe.2014.00006.
12. Cappariello, A., Maurizi, A., Veeriah, V., et al. (2014). The great beauty of the osteoclast. *Archives of Biochemistry and Biophysics, 561*, 13–21. doi:10.1016/j.abb.2014.08.009.
13. Luxenburg, C., Winograd-Katz, S., Addadi, L., et al. (2012). Involvement of actin polymerization in podosomes dynamics. *Journal of Cell Science, 125*(Pt. 7), 1666–1672. doi:10.1242/jcs.075903.
14. Martin, T. J. (2013). Historically significant events in the discovery of RANK/RANKL/OPG. *World Journal of Orthopedics, 4*(4), 186–197. doi:10.5312/wjo.v4.i4.186.
15. Manilay, J. O., & Zouali, M. (2014). Tight relationships between B lymphocytes and the skeletal system. *Trends in Molecular Medicine, 20*(7), 405–412. doi:10.1016/j.molmed.2014.03.003.
16. Weitzman, M. N. (2013). The role of inflammatory cytokines, the RANKL/OPG axis, and the immunoloskeletal interface in physiological bone turnover and osteoporosis. *Scientifica, 2013*, 125705. doi:10.1155/2013/125705.
17. Orimo, H. (2010). The mechanism of mineralization and the role of alkaline phosphatase in health and disease. *Journal of Nippon Medical School, 77*(1), 4–12.
18. Li, X., & Majumdar, S. (2013). Quantitative MRI of articular cartilage and its clinical applications. *Journal of Magnetic Resonance Imaging, 38*(5), 991–1008. doi:10.1002/jmri.24313.
19. Tsivitse, S. (2010). Notch and Wnt signaling, physiological stimuli and postnatal myogenesis. *International Journal of Biological Sciences, 6*(3), 268–281.
20. Catterall, W. A. (2011). Voltage-gated calcium channels. *Cold Spring Harbor Perspectives in Biology, 3*(8), a003947. doi:10.1101/cshperspect.a003947.
21. Lanner, J. T. (2012). Ryanodine receptor physiology and its role in disease. *Advances in Experimental Medicine and Biology, 1*(74), 217–234. doi:10.1007/978-94-007-2888-2_9.
22. Ramachandran, S., Chakraborty, A., Xu, L., et al. (2013). Structural determinants of skeletal muscle ryanodine receptor gating. *The Journal of Biological Chemistry, 288*(9), 6154–6165. doi:10.1074/jbc.M112.433789.
23. Luther, P. K. (2009). The vertebrate muscle Z-disc: Sarcomere anchor for structure and signaling. *Journal of Muscle Research and Cell Motility, 30*(5–6), 171–185. doi:10.1007/s10974-009-9189-6.
24. Rebbeck, R. T., Karunasekara, Y., Board, P. G., et al. (2014). Skeletal muscle excitation–contraction coupling: Who are the dancing partners? *The International Journal of Biochemistry & Cell Biology, 48*, 28–38. doi:10.1016/j.biocel.2013.12.001.
25. Prosser, B. L., Hernandez-Ochoa, E. O., & Schneider, M. F. (2011). S100A1 and calmodulin regulation of ryanodine receptor in striated muscle. *Cell Calcium, 50*(4), 323–331. doi:10.1016/j.ceca.2011.06.001.
26. Bassit, R. A., Pinheiro, C. H., Vitzel, K. F., et al. (2010). Effect of short-term creatine supplementation on markers of skeletal muscle damage after strenuous contractile activity. *European Journal of Applied Physiology, 108*(5), 945–955. doi:10.1007/s00421-009-1305-1.
27. Kuo, C. K., Marturano, J. E., & Tuan, R. S. (2010). Novel strategies in tendon and ligament tissue engineering: Advanced biomaterials and regeneration motifs. *BMC Sports Science, Medicine and Rehabilitation, 2*, 20. doi:10.1186/1758-2555-2-20.
28. Almeida, M., & O'Brien, C. A. (2013). Basic biology of skeletal aging: Role of stress response pathways. *The Journals of Gerontology. Series A, Biological Sciences and Medical Sciences, 68*(10), 1197–1208. doi:10.1093/gerona/glt079.
29. Konopka, A. R., & Streekumaran, N. K. (2013). Mitochondrial and skeletal muscle health with advancing age. *Molecular and Cellular Endocrinology, 397*(1–2), 19–29. doi:10.1016/j.mce.2013.05.008.
30. Pratesi, A., Tarantini, F., & Di Bari, M. (2013). Skeletal muscle: An endocrine organ. *Clinical Cases in Mineral and Bone Metabolism, 10*(1), 11–14. doi:10.11138/ccmbm/2013.10.1.011.
31. Waters, D. L., Baumgartner, R. N., Garry, P. J., et al. (2010). Advantages of dietary, exercise-related, and therapeutic interventions to prevent and treat sarcopenia in adult patients: An update. *Clinical Interventions in Aging, 5*, 259–270.
32. Burton, L. A., & Sumukadas, D. (2010). Optimal management of sarcopenia. *Clinical Interventions in Aging, 5*, 217–228.
33. Lang, T., Streeper, T., Cawthon, P., et al. (2010). Sarcopenia: Etiology, clinical consequences, intervention, and assessment. *Osteoporosis International, 21*(4), 543–559. doi:10.1007/s00198-009-1059-y.

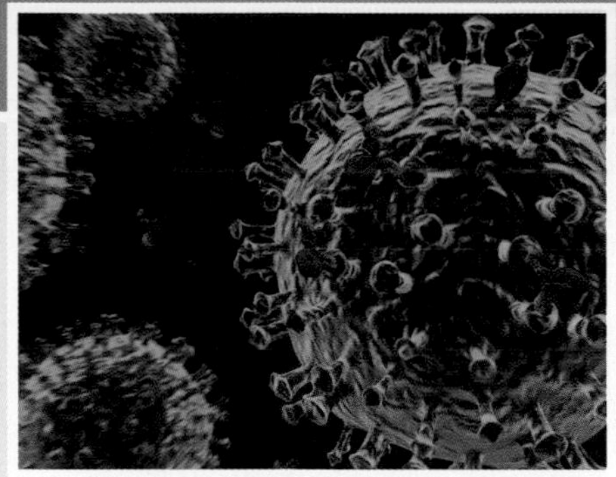

39

Alterations of Musculo-skeletal Function

Christy L. Crowther-Radulewicz, Kathryn L. McCance, and Stephanie Zettel

EVOLVE WEBSITE

http://evolve.elsevier.com/Canada/Huether/pathophysiology
Student Review Questions
Key Points
Case Studies
Animations
Quick Check Answers

CHAPTER OUTLINE

Musculo-skeletal Injuries, 1011
- Skeletal Trauma, 1011
- Support Structures, 1015

Disorders of Bones, 1020
- Metabolic Bone Diseases, 1020
- Infectious Bone Disease: Osteomyelitis, 1028

Disorders of Joints, 1029
- Osteoarthritis, 1029
- Classic Inflammatory Joint Disease, 1032

Disorders of Skeletal Muscle, 1041
- Secondary Muscular Dysfunction, 1041
- Fibromyalgia, 1041
- Chronic Fatigue Syndrome, 1042
- Muscle Membrane Abnormalities, 1043
- Metabolic Muscle Diseases, 1043
- Inflammatory Muscle Diseases: Myositis, 1044
- Toxic Myopathies, 1046

Musculo-skeletal Tumours, 1047
- Bone Tumours, 1047
- Muscle Tumours, 1051

Musculo-skeletal injuries include fractures, dislocations, sprains, and strains. Metabolic disorders, infections, inflammatory or noninflammatory diseases, or tumours may cause alterations in bones, joints, and muscles. The most common disease affecting bone is osteoporosis; much attention and debate has been focused on its risk factors and pathophysiology. Soft tissue disorders—including muscle, tendon, and ligament injuries; tumours; and metabolic derangements—also affect the musculo-skeletal system.

MUSCULO-SKELETAL INJURIES

Trauma is referred to as the "neglected disease." It is the leading cause of death in people ages 1 to 44 years of all ethnicities and socioeconomic levels.[1] In 2010–11, there were 15 190 cases of hospitalization for major injury (with an injury severity score [ISS] of 12 or greater) in Canada. Each increase in the ISS represents an 8% increase in the chance of in-hospital death. Musculo-skeletal injuries were the second most common type of injury (73%) of all of these cases of major injury.[1]

Musculo-skeletal injuries have a major impact on the affected individuals, families, and society in general because of the physical and psychological effects of limitation on mobility and daily activities, pain, and decreased quality of life. In addition, there are direct costs of diagnosis and treatments, and indirect economic costs related to loss of employment and decreased productivity.

Skeletal Trauma

Fractures

A **fracture** is a break in the continuity of a bone. A break occurs when force is applied that exceeds the tensile or compressive strength of the bone. The incidence of fractures varies for individual bones according to age and gender, with the highest incidence of fractures in young males (between the ages of 15 and 24 years) and older adults (65 years of age and older). Fractures of healthy bones, particularly the tibia, clavicle, and lower humerus, tend to occur in young persons as the result of trauma. Fractures of the hands and feet are often caused by accidents in the workplace. The incidence of fractures of the upper femur, upper humerus, vertebrae, and pelvis is highest in older adults and is often associated with osteoporosis (see p. 1021). Hip fractures, the most serious outcome of osteoporosis, have a wide variation in geographical occurrence.[2]

Classification of fractures. There are numerous classification systems for various types of fractures, but the simplest systems describe the basic features of the broken bone. Fractures can be classified as complete or incomplete and as open or closed (Figure 39-1). In a **complete fracture** the bone is broken entirely, whereas in an **incomplete fracture** the bone is damaged but still in one piece. Complete and incomplete fractures also can be called **open** (formerly referred to as **compound**) **fractures** if the skin is open and **closed** (formerly called *simple* or **incomplete**) **fractures** if it is not. A fracture in which a bone breaks into more

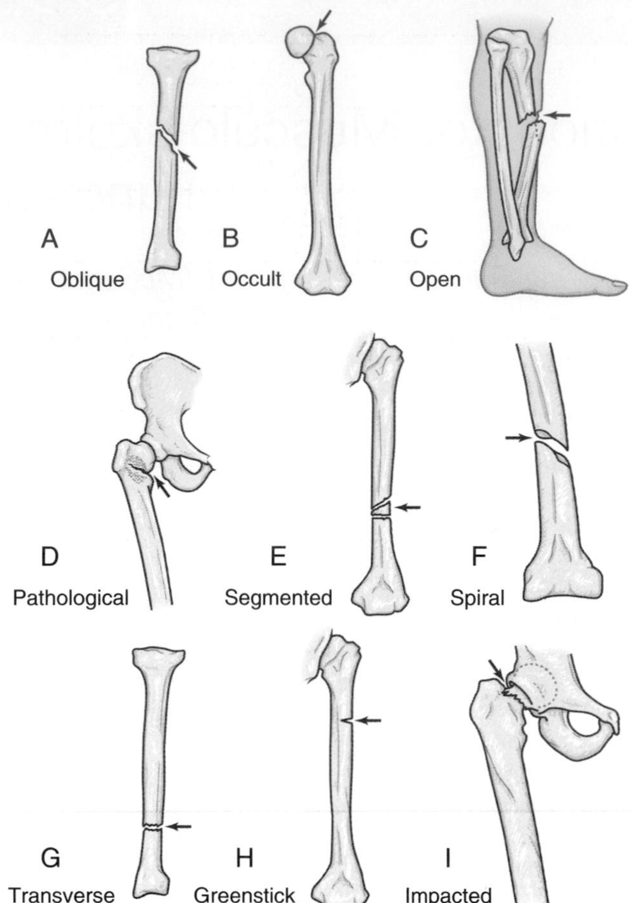

FIGURE 39-1 Examples of Types of Bone Fractures. A, Oblique: fracture at oblique angle across both cortices. *Cause:* Direct or indirect energy, with angulation and some compression. **B,** Occult: fracture that is hidden or not readily discernible. *Cause:* Minor force or energy. **C,** Open: skin broken over fracture; possible soft tissue trauma. *Cause:* Moderate to severe energy that is continuous and exceeds tissue tolerance. **D,** Pathological: transverse, oblique, or spiral fracture of bone weakened by tumour pressure or presence. *Cause:* Minor energy or force, which may be direct or indirect. **E,** Segmented: fracture with two or more pieces or segments. *Cause:* Direct or indirect moderate to severe force. **F,** Spiral: fracture that curves around cortices and may become displaced by twist. *Cause:* Direct or indirect twisting energy or force, with distal part held or unable to move. **G,** Transverse: horizontal break through bone. *Cause:* Direct or indirect energy toward bone. **H,** Greenstick: break in only one cortex of bone. *Cause:* Minor direct or indirect energy. **I,** Impacted: fracture with one end wedged into opposite end of inside fractured fragment. *Cause:* Compressive axial energy or force directly to distal fragment. (Redrawn from Mourad, L. [2002]. Musculoskeletal system. In J.M. Thompson, G.K. McFarland, J.E. Hirsch, et al. [Eds.], *Mosby's clinical nursing* [7th ed.]. St. Louis: Mosby.)

than two fragments is called a **comminuted fracture**. Fractures are also classified according to the direction of the fracture line. A **linear fracture** runs parallel to the long axis of the bone. An **oblique fracture** occurs at a slanted angle to the shaft of the bone. A **spiral fracture** encircles the bone, and a **transverse fracture** occurs straight across the bone.

Incomplete fractures tend to occur in the more flexible, growing bones of children. The three main types of incomplete fractures are greenstick, torus, and bowing fractures. A **greenstick fracture** perforates one cortex and splinters the spongy bone. The name is derived from the damage sustained by a young tree branch (a green stick) when it is bent sharply. The outer surface is disrupted, but the inner surface remains intact. Greenstick fractures typically occur in the metaphysis or diaphysis of the tibia, radius, and ulna. In a **torus fracture**, the cortex buckles but does not break. **Bowing fractures** usually occur when longitudinal force is applied to bone. This type of fracture is common in children and usually involves the paired radius–ulna or the fibula–tibia. A complete diaphyseal fracture occurs in one of the bones of the pair, which disperses the stress sufficiently to prevent a complete fracture of the second bone, which bows rather than breaks. A bowing fracture resists correction (**reduction**) because the force necessary to reduce it must be equal to the force that bowed it. Treatment of bowing fractures is also difficult because the bowed bone interferes with reduction of the fractured bone. Types of fractures are summarized in Table 39-1.

TABLE 39-1 Types of Fractures

Type of Fracture	Definition
Typical Complete Fractures	
Closed	Noncommunicating wound between bone and skin
Open	Communicating wound between bone and skin
Comminuted	Multiple bone fragments
Linear	Fracture line parallel to long axis of bone
Oblique	Fracture line at an angle to long axis of bone
Spiral	Fracture line encircling bone (as a spiral staircase)
Transverse	Fracture line perpendicular to long axis of bone
Impacted	Fracture fragments pushed into each other
Pathological	Fracture at a point where bone has been weakened by disease, for example, by tumours or osteoporosis
Avulsion	Fragment of bone connected to a ligament or tendon detaches from main bone
Compression	Fracture wedged or squeezed together on one side of bone
Displaced	Fracture with one, both, or all fragments out of normal alignment
Extracapsular	Fragment close to joint but remains outside joint capsule
Intracapsular	Fragment within joint capsule
Typical Incomplete Fractures	
Greenstick	Break in one cortex of bone with splintering of inner bone surface; commonly occurs in children and older adults
Torus	Buckling of cortex
Bowing	Bending of bone
Stress	Microfracture
Transchondral	Separation of cartilaginous joint surface (articular cartilage) from main shaft of bone

Fractures may be further classified by cause as pathological, stress, or transchondral fractures. A **pathological** (also known as **insufficiency** or **fragility**) **fracture** is a break at the site of a pre-existing abnormality, resulting from force that would not fracture a normal bone. In any bone that lacks normal ability to deform and recover, these fractures can occur with normal weight-bearing or activity. Rheumatoid arthritis (RA), osteoporosis, Paget's disease, osteomalacia, rickets, hyperparathyroidism, and radiation therapy all cause bone to lose its normal ability to deform and recover. Pathological fractures are generally a result of bone weakness caused by another disease such as cancer, metabolic bone disorders, or infection. Although usually considered insufficiency fractures, breaks in the bone attributable to osteoporosis can also be referred to as pathological fractures. Any disease process that weakens a bone (especially the cortex) predisposes the bone to pathological fracture.

During activities that subject a bone to repeated strain, such as certain athletics, a **stress fracture** can occur in normal or abnormal bone. The forces placed on the bone are cumulative, eventually causing a fracture. A **fatigue fracture** is caused by repetitive, sometimes abnormal stress or torque applied to a bone with normal ability to deform and recover. Fatigue fractures usually occur in individuals who engage in a new or different activity that is both strenuous and repetitive (e.g., joggers, skaters, dancers, military recruits). Because gains in muscle strength occur more rapidly than gains in bone strength, the newly developed muscles place exaggerated stress on the bones that are not yet ready for the additional stress. The imbalance between muscle and bone development causes microfractures to develop in the cortex. If the activity is controlled and increased gradually, new bone formation catches up to the increased demands and microfractures do not occur.

A **transchondral fracture** consists of fragmentation and separation of a portion of the articular cartilage. (Joint structures are defined in Chapter 38.) Single or multiple sites may be fractured, and the fragments may consist of cartilage alone or cartilage and bone. Typical sites of transchondral fracture are the distal femur, the ankle, the patella, the elbow, and the wrist. Transchondral fractures are most prevalent in adolescents.

PATHOPHYSIOLOGY Fracture healing is a complex process that occurs primarily in one of two ways: direct or indirect healing.[3] Both types of healing require integration of cells, signalling pathways, and various molecules. In **direct** (or **primary**) **healing**, intramembranous bone formation occurs when adjacent bone cortices are in contact with one another. Direct bone healing most often occurs when surgical fixation is used to repair a broken bone. No callus formation occurs with this process. **Indirect** (or **secondary**) **healing** involves both intramembranous and endochondral bone formation, development of callus, and eventual remodelling of solid bone.[4] Bone formation that begins with an underlying cartilage scaffold is termed **endochondral bone formation**.

A hallmark of indirect fracture healing is the formation of callus. Indirect fracture healing is most often observed when a fracture is treated with a cast or other nonsurgical method. When a bone is broken, the periosteum and blood vessels in the cortex, marrow, and surrounding soft tissues are disrupted. Bleeding occurs from the damaged ends of the bone and from the neighbouring soft tissue. A clot (hematoma) forms within the medullary canal, between the fractured ends of the bone, and beneath the periosteum (Figure 39-2). Bone tissue immediately adjacent to the fracture dies. This dead tissue (along with any debris in the fracture area) stimulates an intense inflammatory response characterized by vasodilation, exudation of plasma and leukocytes, and infiltration by inflammatory leukocytes, growth factors, and mast cells that simultaneously decalcify the fractured bone ends. Within 48 hours after injury, vascular tissue from surrounding soft tissue and the marrow cavity invades the fracture area, and blood flow to the entire bone increases. Bone-forming cells in the periosteum, endosteum, and marrow are activated to produce subperiosteal procallus along the outer surface of the shaft and over the broken ends of the bone (see Figure 39-2). Osteoblasts within the procallus synthesize collagen and matrix, which becomes mineralized to form callus. As the repair process continues, remodelling occurs, during which unnecessary callus is resorbed and trabeculae are formed along lines of stress as the repair tissues align with the tissue cells of the host (Figure 39-3). Except for the liver, bone is unique among all body tissues in that it will form new bone, not scar tissue, when it heals after a fracture.

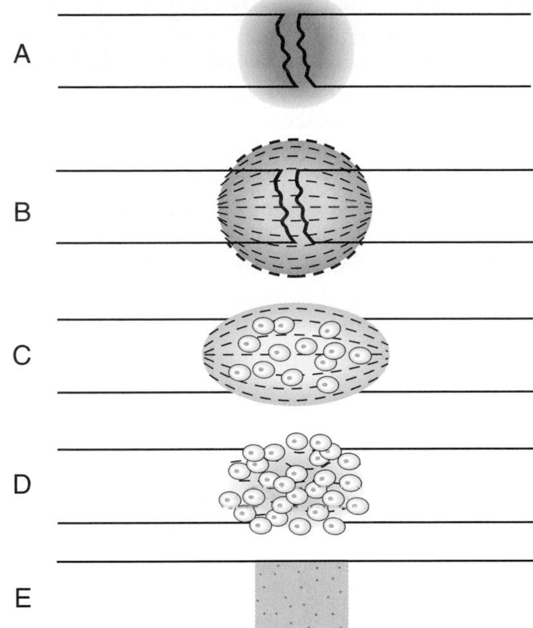

FIGURE 39-2 Bone Healing (Schematic Representation). **A,** Bleeding at broken ends of the bone with subsequent hematoma formation. **B,** Organization of hematoma into fibrous network. **C,** Invasion of osteoblasts, lengthening of collagen strands, and deposition of calcium. **D,** Callus formation; new bone is built while osteoclasts destroy dead bone. **E,** Remodelling is accomplished while excess callus is reabsorbed and trabecular bone is deposited. (From Monahan, F.D., Sands, J., Neighbors, M., et al. [2007]. *Phipps' medical-surgical nursing: Health and illness perspectives* [8th ed.]. St. Louis: Mosby.)

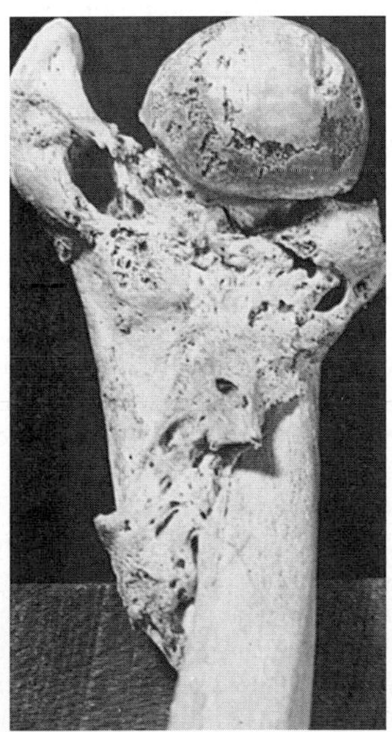

FIGURE 39-3 Exuberant Callus Formation Following Fracture. (From Rosai, J. [1996]. *Ackerman's surgical pathology* [8th ed.]. St. Louis: Mosby.)

CLINICAL MANIFESTATIONS The signs and symptoms of a fracture include unnatural alignment (deformity), swelling, muscle spasm, tenderness, pain and impaired sensation, and decreased mobility. The position of the broken bone segments is determined by the pull of attached muscles, gravity, and the direction and magnitude of the force that caused the fracture.

Immediately after a bone is fractured, there often is numbness at the fracture site because of trauma to the nerve or nerves at the injury site. The numbness may last several minutes, during which time the injured person can continue to use the fractured bone. However, once the numbness dissipates, the subsequent pain is quite severe and may be incapacitating until relieved with medication and treatment of the fracture. Pain can be caused by muscle spasms at the fracture site, overriding of the fracture segments, or damage to adjacent soft tissues.

Pathological fractures can cause angular deformity, painless swelling, or generalized bone pain. Stress fractures are painful because of accelerated remodelling; initially, pain occurs during activity and is usually relieved by rest. Stress fractures also cause local tenderness and soft tissue swelling. Transchondral fractures may be entirely asymptomatic or may be painful during movement. Range of motion in the joint is limited, and movement may evoke audible clicking sounds (crepitus).

EVALUATION AND TREATMENT Adequate immobilization with a splint or cast is often all that is required for healing of fractures that are *not* misaligned. Treatment of a displaced fracture involves realigning the bone fragments (reduction) close to their normal or anatomical position and holding the fragments in place (**immobilization**) so that bone union can occur. Several methods are available to reduce a fracture: *closed manipulation*, *traction*, and *open reduction*. Many displaced fractures can be reduced by closed manipulation and reduction. The bone is moved or manipulated into place without opening the skin. Closed reduction is used when the contour of the bone is in fair anatomical alignment and can be manually placed into normal alignment, and then maintained with immobilization. Splints and casts are used to immobilize and hold a closed reduction in place.

Traction may be used to accomplish or maintain reduction. When bone fragments are displaced (not in their anatomical position), weights may be used to apply firm, steady traction (pull) and countertraction to the long axis of the bone. Traction stretches and fatigues muscles that have pulled the bone fragments out of place, more readily allowing the distal fragment to align with the proximal fragment. Traction can be applied to the skin (skin traction) or directly to the involved bone (skeletal traction). Skin traction is used when only a few kilograms of pulling force are needed to realign the fragments or when the traction will be used only for a brief time, such as before surgery or, for children with femoral fractures, for 3 to 7 days before applying a cast. In skeletal traction, a pin or wire is drilled through the bone distal to the fracture site, and a traction bow, rope, and weights are attached to the pin or wire to apply tension and to provide the pulling force required to overcome the muscle spasm and help realign the fracture fragments. More often, surgical repair (open reduction and internal fixation) or external fixation devices are used to realign displaced fractures.

Open reduction is a surgical procedure that exposes the fracture site; the fragments are then manipulated into alignment under direct visualization. Some form of hardware, such as a screw, plate, nail, or wire, is used to maintain the reduction (**internal fixation**). **External fixation**, a procedure in which pins or rods are surgically placed into uninjured bone near the fracture site and then stabilized with an external frame of bars, is another method used to treat fractures that would not be adequately stabilized with a cast. Bone grafts—using donor bone from the individual (autograft), a cadaver (allograft), or bone substitutes (ceramic composites, bioactive cement)—can fill voids in the bone.

Improper reduction or immobilization of a fractured bone may result in nonunion, delayed union, or malunion. **Nonunion** is failure of the bone ends to grow together. The gap between the broken ends of the bone fills with dense fibrous and fibrocartilaginous tissue instead of new bone. Occasionally, the fibrous tissue contains a fluid-filled space that resembles a joint and is termed a *false joint*, or *pseudoarthrosis*. **Delayed union** is union that does not occur until approximately 8 to 9 months after a fracture. **Malunion** is the healing of a bone in an incorrect anatomical position.

Dislocation and Subluxation

Dislocation and subluxation are usually caused by trauma. **Dislocation** is the displacement of one or more bones in a joint in which the opposing joint surfaces entirely lose contact with one another. If contact between the opposing joint surfaces is only partially lost, the injury is called a **subluxation**.

Dislocation and subluxation are most common in persons younger than 20 years of age and are generally associated with fractures. However, they may be the result of congenital or acquired disorders that cause (1) muscular imbalance, as occurs with congenital dislocation of the hip or neurological disorders; (2) incongruities in the articulating surfaces of the bones, as occur with RA (see p. 1032); or (3) joint instability.

The joints most often dislocated or subluxated are the joints of the shoulder, elbow, wrist, finger, hip, and knee. The shoulder joint most often injured is the glenohumeral joint. Finger dislocations are common injuries in contact sports such as basketball, football, and rugby.

Traumatic dislocation of the elbow joint is common in the immature skeleton. In adults, an elbow dislocation is usually associated with a fracture of the ulna or head of the radius. Traumatic dislocation of the wrist usually involves the distal ulna and carpal bones. Any one of the eight carpal bones can be dislocated after an injury. Dislocation in the hand usually involves the metacarpophalangeal (MCP) and interphalangeal joints.

Considerable trauma is needed to dislocate the hip. Anterior hip dislocation is rare in healthy persons; it is caused by forced abduction—for example, when an individual lands on his or her feet after falling from an elevated height. Posterior dislocation of the hip can occur as a result of an automobile accident in which the flexed knee strikes the dashboard, causing the head of the femur to be pushed posteriorly from the hip joint.

The knee is an unstable weight-bearing joint that depends heavily on the soft tissue structures around it for support. It is exposed to many different types of motion (flexion, extension, rotation) and is one of the most commonly injured joints. A knee dislocation can be anterior, posterior, lateral, medial, or rotary. It is often the result of an injury that occurs during contact sports activities, such as soccer, lacrosse, or football.

PATHOPHYSIOLOGY Dislocations and subluxations are often accompanied by fracture because stress is placed on areas of bone not usually subjected to stress. In addition, as the joint loses its normal congruity, there may be bruising or tearing of adjacent nerves, blood vessels, ligaments, supporting structures, and soft tissue. Dislocations of the shoulder may damage the shoulder capsule and the axillary nerve. Damage to axillary nerves can cause anaesthesia or dysesthesia in the sensory distribution of the nerve and paralysis of the deltoid muscle. Dislocations also may disrupt circulation, leading to ischemia and possibly even permanent disability of the affected extremity tissues.

CLINICAL MANIFESTATIONS Signs and symptoms of dislocations or subluxations include pain, swelling, limitation of motion, and joint deformity. Pain may be caused by effusion of inflammatory exudate into the joint or by associated tendon and ligament injury. Joint deformity is typically caused by muscle contractions that exert pull on the dislocated or subluxated joint. Limitation of motion results from effusion into the joint or the displacement of bones.

EVALUATION AND TREATMENT Evaluation of dislocations and subluxations is based on clinical manifestations and radiographic evaluation. Treatment consists of reduction and immobilization for 2 to 6 weeks to allow healing of damaged structures, followed by exercises to restore normal range of motion in the joint. Depending on the joint and severity of injury, complete healing can take months to sometimes years.

Support Structures

Sprains and Strains of Tendons and Ligaments

Tendon and ligament injuries often accompany fractures and dislocations. A **tendon** is fibrous connective tissue (composed primarily of type I collagen) that attaches skeletal muscle to a bone or other structure; the area of attachment on a bone is called an **enthesis**. The enthesis serves to evenly distribute tension differences between the bone and tendon. The zone where muscle transitions into tendon is known as the *myotendinous junction*. Functionally, muscles and tendons work together as a single, integrated unit allowing motion.[5,6] A **ligament** is a band of fibrous connective tissue that connects bones where they meet in a joint. Ligaments are structurally quite similar to tendons, although ligaments have a higher proportion of small-diameter collagen fibrils. The primary difference between tendons and ligaments is their anatomical location.[7] Tendons and ligaments support the bones and joints and either facilitate or limit motion, respectively. Either structure can be completely separated from bone at their points of attachment, torn, lacerated, or ruptured.

Tearing or stretching of a muscle or tendon is commonly known as a **strain**. Major trauma can tear or rupture a tendon at any site in the body. Most commonly injured are the tendons of the hands and feet, the knee (patellar), the upper arm (biceps and triceps), the thigh (hamstring), the ankle, and the heel (Achilles).

Ligament tears are commonly known as **sprains**. Ligament tears and ruptures can occur at any joint but are most common in the wrist, ankle, elbow, and knee joints. A complete separation of a tendon or ligament from its bony attachment site is known as an **avulsion** and is commonly seen in young athletes, especially sprinters, hurdlers, and distance runners.

Strains and sprains are classified as first degree (mild), second degree (moderate), and third degree (severe). In first-degree injuries, the fibres are stretched but the muscle (strain) or joint (sprain) remains stable. In second-degree strains or sprains, there is more tearing of the tendon or ligament fibres, with muscle weakness (strain) or some joint instability (sprain) but incomplete tearing of fibres. Third-degree strains and sprains result in an inability to contract the muscle normally (strain) and cause significant joint instability (sprain).

PATHOPHYSIOLOGY When a tendon or ligament is torn, an inflammatory exudate develops between the torn ends. Multiple growth factors that direct the repair process are released. Later, granulation tissue containing macrophages, fibroblasts, and capillary buds grows inward from the surrounding soft tissue and cartilage to begin the repair process. Within 4 to 5 days after the injury, collagen formation begins. At first, collagen formation is random and disorganized. As the collagen fibres interweave and connect with pre-existing tendon fibres, they become organized parallel to the lines of the musculotendinous unit. Eventually vascular fibrous tissue fuses the new and surrounding tissues into a single mass. Collagen fibres reconnect the tendon and bone, forming a type of enthesis.[7] Usually a healing tendon or ligament lacks sufficient strength to withstand some stress for 4 to 5 weeks after the injury; it may take more than 3 months to achieve mechanical stability of a joint.[8] If powerful muscle pull does occur during healing, the tendon or ligament ends may separate again, which causes the tendon or ligament to heal in a lengthened shape or with an excessive amount of scar tissue, resulting in poor tendon or ligament function.

CLINICAL MANIFESTATIONS Tendon and ligament injuries are painful and are usually accompanied by soft tissue swelling, changes in tendon or ligament contour, and dislocation or subluxation of bones. Pain is generally sharp and localized, and tenderness persists over the distribution of the tendon or ligament. Movement or weight-bearing increases pain. Even with prompt treatment, depending on the tendon or ligament involved, significant injuries may result in decreased mobility, instability, and weakness of the affected joints.

EVALUATION AND TREATMENT Evaluation is based on mechanism of injury, clinical manifestations, stress radiography, arthroscopy, or arthrography. Initial treatment consists of PRICE (*p*rotection, *r*est, *i*ce, *c*ompression, and *e*levation) for the first 48 to 72 hours. Once swelling and acute pain subside, in most cases, support of the affected tendon or ligament with a compression dressing or brace will provide appropriate reinforcement while the tissues heal. Rehabilitation is crucial to regaining good functional outcome.[9] In severe (third-degree) injuries, treatment may include suturing the tendon or ligament ends in close approximation. If this is not feasible because of the extent of damage, tendon or ligament grafting may be necessary. Prolonged, functional rehabilitation programs help ensure return of near-normal functions, but recovery may be complicated by post-traumatic arthritis.

Tendinopathy, Epicondylopathy, and Bursitis

Trauma also can cause painful inflammation of tendons (tendinopathy [tendonitis]) and bursae (bursitis). Other causes of damage to tendons include reduced tissue perfusion, mechanical irritation, crystal deposits, postural misalignment, and hypermobility of a joint. Thus, *tendinopathy* is a more accurate term than *tendonitis* in most cases. Studies have shown that vascular ingrowth in tendinopathy (neovascularization) is accompanied with nerve ingrowth, facilitating pain transmission in Achilles and patellar tendinopathy.[10]

The histopathology of common conditions, such as lateral epicondylopathy ("tennis elbow") or medial epicondylopathy ("golfer's elbow"), is a degenerative process[11,12] (Figure 39-4). A bony prominence at the end of a bone where tendons or ligaments attach is termed an **epicondyle**. When force is sufficient to cause microscopic tears (microtears) in tissue, the result is known as **tendinopathy** or **epicondylopathy**. Microtears in the tendon, the presence of disorganized collagen fibres, and neovascularization are indicative of incomplete tissue repair. Initial inflammatory changes cause thickening of the tendon sheath, limiting movements and causing pain.[13] Microtears cause bleeding, edema, and pain (because of the presence of substance P) in the involved tendon or tendons. At times, after repeated microtears, calcium may be deposited in the tendon origin area.

Lateral epicondylopathy (tennis elbow) is caused by irritation and overstretching of the extensor carpi radialis brevis (ECRB) tendon and forearm extensor muscles, resulting in tissue degradation, loss of grip strength, and pain.[14] **Medial epicondylopathy (golfer's elbow)** is the result of similar forces affecting the forearm muscles responsible for forearm flexion and pronation (see Figure 39-4). Repetitive load-bearing activities or acute injuries that involve flexion, extension, pronation, or supination of the elbow and forearm can lead to either lateral or medial elbow symptoms.

Clinical manifestations of epicondylopathy are usually localized to one side of the joint. In general, there is local tenderness and more pain with active motion than with passive motion. With tendinopathy or tendonitis, the pain is localized over the involved tendon. Stressing the tendon with simple activities, such as lifting even a few kilograms of

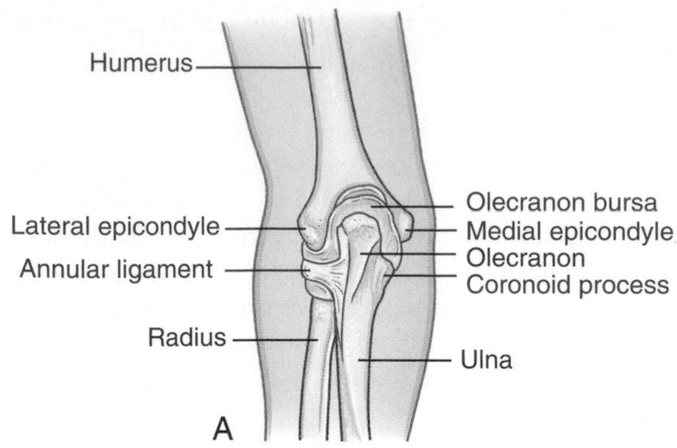

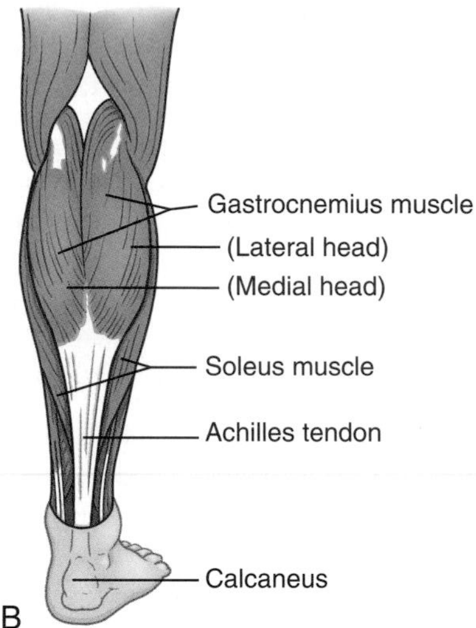

FIGURE 39-4 Epicondylopathy and Tendinopathy. A, Lateral and medial epicondyles of the distal humerus, sites of tennis elbow (lateral) and golfer's elbow (medial). **B,** Achilles tendon, common site of tendinopathy.

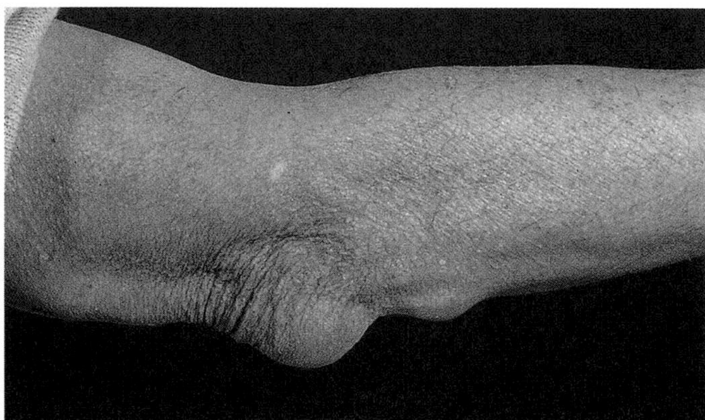

FIGURE 39-5 Olecranon Bursitis. Note swelling at the point of the elbow (olecranon). A smaller, rheumatoid nodule also is present. (From Hochberg, M.C., Silman, A.J., Smolen, J.S., et al. [2015]. *Rheumatology* [6th ed.]. Philadelphia: Elsevier.)

weight, can increase pain. Pain and sometimes weakness limit joint movement.

Bursae are small sacs lined with synovial membrane and filled with synovial fluid that are located between bony prominences and soft tissues such as tendons, muscles, and ligaments (Figure 39-5). Bursae can be either "constant" (those formed during embryological development) or "adventitious" (bursae that develop as a result of chronic friction and degeneration of fibrous tissue between adjacent structures). The primary function of a bursa is to separate, lubricate, and cushion these structures. When irritated or injured, these sacs become inflamed and swell. Because most bursae lie outside joints, joint movement is rarely compromised with bursitis. Acute bursitis occurs primarily in middle age and is caused by trauma. Chronic bursitis can result from repeated trauma. Septic bursitis is caused by wound infection or bacterial infection of the skin overlying the bursae. Bursitis commonly occurs in the shoulder, hip, knee, and elbow but also can affect the spine, wrist, foot, and ankle.

PATHOPHYSIOLOGY Bursitis usually is an inflammation that is reactive to overuse or excessive pressure but also can be caused by infection, autoimmune diseases, crystal deposition, or acute trauma. The inflamed bursal sac becomes engorged, and the inflammation can spread to adjacent tissues. The inflammation may decrease with rest, ice, and aspiration of the fluid. (Inflammation is discussed in Chapter 6.)

CLINICAL MANIFESTATIONS Joint motion is rarely limited in bursitis, except by pain. Shoulder pain may impair arm abduction. Bursitis in the knee produces pain when climbing stairs, and crossing the legs is painful in bursitis of the hip. Lying on the side of the inflamed trochanteric bursa is also very painful. Signs of infectious bursitis may include the presence of pain, a puncture site, warmth and erythema, prior corticosteroid injection, severe inflammation, or an adjacent source of infection, such as from total joint replacement surgery.

EVALUATION AND TREATMENT The diagnosis of tendinopathy, epicondylopathy, and bursitis is primarily based on clinical history and physical examination. Other imaging techniques, such as ultrasound or magnetic resonance imaging (MRI), may be used to evaluate the severity of the problem. Treatment may include temporary immobilization of the joint with a sling, splint, or cast; administration of systemic analgesics; application of ice or heat; or local injection of an anaesthetic, a corticosteroid, platelet-rich plasma (PRP), or a combination local anaesthetic/corticosteroid. Physical therapy to prevent loss of function begins after acute inflammation subsides (see *Health Promotion*: Managing Tendinopathy).

Muscle Strains

Muscle strain is a general term for local muscle damage. Mild injury such as **muscle strain** is usually seen after traumatic or sports injuries. It is often the result of sudden, forced motion causing the muscle to become stretched beyond normal capacity. Strains often involve the tendon as well. Penetrating injuries, such as knife and gunshot wounds, can cause traumatic rupture (see Chapter 4). Muscles are ruptured more often than tendons in young people; the opposite is true in the older population. Muscle strain may be chronic when the muscle is repeatedly stretched beyond its usual capacity. There is evidence of tissue disruption with subsequent signs of muscle regeneration and connective tissue repair when a biopsy is performed. Hemorrhage into the surrounding tissue and signs of inflammation also may be present.

Muscle healing occurs in three phases:

1. *Destruction*, in which the myofibres of the damaged muscle contract and necrose, beginning an inflammatory reaction. The gap between torn fibres is filled by a hematoma.
2. *Repair*, which begins with monocytes phagocytizing the dead tissue and activating satellite cells, which become myoblasts. The myoblasts infiltrate the scar tissue, and new capillary formation begins at the site of injury. The first two phases occur within a week of injury.
3. *Remodelling* occurs as the myofibres mature, form contractile tissue, and attach to the ends of scar tissue.[15] Regeneration may take up to

HEALTH PROMOTION

Managing Tendinopathy

Tennis and golfer's elbow, Achilles tendinopathy, and other tendon problems account for a large percentage of sports-related overuse injuries. Successful treatment of these conditions is challenging because of the mechanisms of tendon healing as well as inconsistent results, with many interventions still not completely understood. Persistent pain is common and may be the result of ingrowth of nerves that accompanies ingrowth of new blood vessels during the healing process. Recent studies suggest that the traditional approach of corticosteroid injections is helpful only for the short term. Other therapies that show promise include the following:

Prolotherapy: An irritant such as glucose or lidocaine (2% Lidocaine Hydrochloride Injection USP) is injected into the affected tendon, inducing an inflammatory response, thereby stimulating growth of new tendon fibres.

Eccentric exercises: The tendon is "prestretched," increasing its resting length and resulting in less strain during movement. The load on the tendon is gradually increased, causing the tendon itself to strengthen.

Extracorporeal shockwave therapy (SWT): External acoustic or sonic waves are focused on the affected area. The shockwaves stimulate soft tissue healing and inhibit pain receptors.

Needling: This treatment involves multiple insertions of a sterile needle into affected tissue. It is thought that the pain sensation is reduced by stimulating A-nerve fibres. This technique is often referred to as "dry needling," since no fluid is introduced.

Platelet-rich plasma (PRP): This autologous source of concentrated platelets is obtained by centrifugation of plasma. The resulting solution contains high concentrations of cytokines and growth factors, such as platelet-derived growth factor (PDGF) and transforming growth factor-beta (TGF-β), which are thought to promote the growth of new, healthy tissue.

Autologous tenocyte injections: Autologous injection of tenocytes at the site of tendinopathy is thought to provide necessary mediators of tissue healing.

From Andarawis-Puri, N., Flatow, E.L., & Soslowsky, L.J. (2015). *J Orthop Res, 33*(6), 780–784; Krey, D., Borchers, J., & McCamey, K. (2015). *Phys Sportsmed, 43*(1), 80–86; Langer, P.R. (2015). *Clin Podiatr Med Surg, 32*(2), 183–193; Mautner, K., & Kneer, L. (2014). *Phys Med Rehabil Clin North Am, 25*(4), 865–880; Wang, A., Mackie, K., Breidahl, W., et al. (2015). *Am J Sports Med, 43*(7), 1775–1783.

TABLE 39-2 Muscle Strain

Type	Manifestations	Treatment
First degree (example: bench press in untrained athlete)	Muscle overstretched, pain but no muscle deformity	Ice should be applied 5 or 6 times in first 24–48 hours; gradual resumption of full weight-bearing after initial rest for up to 2 weeks Exercises individualized to specific injury
Second degree (example: any muscle strain with bruising and pain)	Muscle intact with some tearing of fibres, swelling, pain	Treatment similar to that for first-degree strains
Third degree (example: traumatic injury)	Caused by tearing of fascia, marked weakness, deformity	Surgery to approximate ruptured edges; immobilization and non-weight-bearing status for 6 weeks

6 weeks, and the affected muscle should be protected during that time.

Degrees of acute muscle strain, together with their manifestations and treatment, are summarized in Table 39-2.

A late complication of some muscle injuries is **myositis ossificans**, also known as **heterotopic ossification (HO)**. Its exact pathophysiology remains unknown, but the basic problem seems to be the inability of mesenchymal cells to differentiate into osteoblastic stem cells and inappropriate differentiation of fibroblasts into bone-forming cells. Though uncommon, HO is associated with burns, joint surgery, and trauma to the musculo-skeletal system or central nervous system (CNS). HO may involve the muscle or tendons, ligaments, or bones near the muscle, causing stiffness or deformity of an extremity. Soft tissue calcifications may be seen on plain radiographs.

Rhabdomyolysis

Once used interchangeably with the term *myoglobinuria*, **rhabdomyolysis** is the rapid breakdown of muscle that causes the release of intracellular contents, including the protein pigment myoglobin, into the extracellular space and bloodstream. Physical interruptions in the sarcolemma membrane, called delta lesions, are the route by which muscle constituents are released. (The sarcolemma membrane, the plasma membrane of the muscle cell, is described in Chapter 38.) **Myoglobinuria**, first described in victims of crush injuries in London during World War II, refers to the presence of the muscle protein myoglobin in the urine.

PATHOPHYSIOLOGY Rhabdomyolysis is sometimes incorrectly used interchangeably with *crush injury* (a description of injuries resulting from crushing of a body part), *compartment syndrome* (the consequences of increased intracompartmental pressures of a muscle), or *crush syndrome* (the systemic pathophysiological events caused by rhabdomyolysis, primarily involving the kidneys and coagulation syndrome).[16,17] Although relatively rare, rhabdomyolysis has many causes (Box 39-1) and can result in serious complications, including hyperkalemia (because of the release of intracellular potassium into the circulation) and cardiac dysrhythmias. The most clinically significant complication is acute kidney failure (myoglobin precipitates in the tubules, obstructing flow through the nephron and producing injury).[18] Other complications include metabolic acidosis (from liberation of intracellular phosphorus and sulphate) and even disseminated intravascular coagulation (DIC) (likely caused by activation of the clotting cascade by sarcolemma damage and release of intracellular components from the damaged muscles).

CLINICAL MANIFESTATIONS A *classic triad* of muscle pain, weakness, and dark urine is considered typical of rhabdomyolysis, but those affected may have no complaint of pain or muscle weakness.[16] Abnormally dark urine caused by myoglobinuria may be the first and only symptom; however, the presence of myoglobin in urine is not a reliable test for rhabdomyolysis.[19] The renal threshold for myoglobin is low (approximately 285 nmol/L of urine); therefore, only 200 grams

BOX 39-1 Selected Causes of Rhabdomyolysis

Direct Trauma
Blunt trauma or crush injury (motor vehicle crashes, collapsed buildings)
Burns (thermal)
Electrical injury
Excessive compression (from immobility attributable to stroke, alcohol or medication intoxication)

Medications, Drugs, and Substances
Alcohol
Amphetamines
Anaesthetic and paralytic agents (halothane [Fluothane], propofol [Diprivan], succinylcholine [Anectine]—malignant hyperthermia syndrome)
Antihistamines (diphenhydramine [Benadryl], doxylamine [Unisom])
Antihyperlipidemic agents (statins, clofibrate [Atromid S], bezafibrate [Bezalip SR])
Antipsychotics and antidepressants (amitriptyline [Elavil], doxepin [Apo-Doxepin], fluoxetine [Apo-Fluoxetine], haloperidol [Apo-Haloperidol], lithium [PMS-Lithium Carbonate], protriptyline [Triptil], perphenazine [Perphenazine], promethazine [Histantil], chlorpromazine [Chlorprom], trifluoperazine [Novo-flurazine], venlafaxine [Effexor])
Caffeine
Cocaine
Corticosteroids
Fibrinates (antilipid agents: bezafibrate, ciprofibrate [Modalim], clofibrate, ezetimibe [Ach-exetimibe], gemfibrozil [Dom-gemfibrozil])
Heroin
HIV integrase inhibitor (raltegravir [Isentress])
Hypnotics and sedatives (benzodiazepines, barbiturates)
LSD (lysergic acid diethylamide)
Methadone
Methamphetamine
Methylenedioxymethamphetamine (MDMA; "ecstasy")
Miscellaneous medications (amphotericin B [Abelcet], azathioprine [Imuran], ε-aminocaproic acid [Amicar], quinidine [Quin-G], penicillamine [Cuprimine], salicylates, theophylline [Slo-bid], terbutaline [Bricanyl], thiazides, vasopressin [Pressyn])
Phencyclidine
Protease inhibitors
Statins (atorvastatin [Lipitor], fluvastatin [Lescol], lovastatin [Mevacor], pravastatin [Pravachol], rosuvastatin [Crestor], simvastatin [Zocor])
Miscellaneous medications (amphotericin B, arsenic, azathioprine, halothane, naltrexone [Revia], quinidine, penicillamine, propofol, salicylates, succinylcholine, theophylline, terbutaline, thiazides, vasopressin)

Excessive Muscular Contraction
Status epilepticus
Delirium tremens
Acute psychosis
Severe dystonia
Sporadic strenuous exercise (e.g., marathons, squats)
Tetanus

Infectious Agents
Bacteria (group B streptococci, *Streptococcus pneumoniae, Staphylococcus epidermidis, Borrelia burgdorferi, Escherichia coli, Clostridium perfringens, Clostridium tetani, Streptococcus viridans; Bacillus, Brucella, Legionella, Listeria, Leptospira, Mycoplasma, Plasmodium, Rickettsia, Salmonella,* and *Vibrio* species)
Fungal organisms (*Aspergillus, Candida* species)
Viruses (influenza types A and B, coxsackievirus, dengue, Epstein-Barr, HIV, cytomegalovirus, parainfluenza, varicella-zoster, West Nile)

Toxins
Carbon monoxide
Envenomation (black widow spider, Africanized honey bees, vipers)
Hemlock
Methanol
Toluene

Hereditary Enzyme Disorders (Rare)
McArdle's disease (myophosphorylase deficiency)
Tarui's disease (type VII glycogen storage disease)
Phosphoglycerate mutase deficiency (glycogen storage disease type X)
Carnitine palmitoyltransferase deficiency (CPT1 deficiency)

Miscellaneous Causes
Diabetic ketoacidosis
Endocrinopathy
Heatstroke
Hypothermia
Nonketotic hyperosmolar coma
Polymyositis
Severe electrolyte disorders (near-drowning or water intoxication, severe vomiting or diarrhea)

Data from Cervellin, G., Comelli, I., & Lippi, G. (2010). *Clin Chem Lab Med, 48*(6), 749–756; Croce, F., Vitello, P., Dalla Pria, A., et al. (2010). *Int J STD AIDS, 21*(11), 783–785; Halpern, P., Moskovich, J., Avrahami, B., et al. (2011). *Hum Exp Toxicol, 30*(4), 259–266; Keltz, E., Khan, F.Y., & Mann, G. (2014). *Muscles Ligaments Tendons J, 3*(4), 303–312; Torres, P.A., Helmstetter, J.A., Kaye, A.M., et al. (2015). *Ochsner J, 15*(1), 58–69; Zutt, R., van der Kooi, A.J., Linthorst, G.E., et al. (2014). *Neuromuscul Disord, 24*(8), 651–659.

of muscle needs to be damaged to cause visible changes in the urine. Myoglobin is rapidly cleared, and levels may return to normal within 24 hours of injury. Along with the release of myoglobin, creatine kinase (CK) and other serum enzymes are released in massive quantities (normal CK levels are 5 to 25 units/L for women and 5 to 35 units/L for men). The efflux of intracellular proteins and enzymes includes loss of potassium, phosphate, nucleotides, creatinine, and creatine. Serum hypocalcemia is seen early in the course of myoglobinuria and is followed by late hypercalcemia. The risk for kidney failure increases proportionately to the increase in the levels of serum CK, potassium, and phosphorus.

EVALUATION AND TREATMENT The most important and clinically useful measurement in rhabdomyolysis is serum CK level. A level 5 to 10 times the upper limit of normal (about 1 000 units/L) is used to identify rhabdomyolysis.[18] Once CK levels exceed 15 000 units/L, acute kidney failure is likely. Other laboratory tests may include electrolytes (elevated serum potassium level [hyperkalemia] can cause life-threatening cardiac abnormalities) and blood urea nitrogen (BUN)/creatinine ratio (decreased ratio because of creatine released from damaged muscle being converted to creatinine). Additional laboratory tests—such as measurement of hemoglobin, hematocrit, and platelet levels and determination of activated partial thromboplastin time—may be indicated in the presence of other trauma or suspected bleeding. A recent study evaluated the ultrasonographic appearance of rhabdomyolysis in damaged muscle from earthquake victims and found abnormalities in muscle texture and subcutaneous tissue, as well as liquid areas in the damaged tissue.[20]

Maintaining adequate urinary flow and prevention of kidney failure are goals of treatment. Rapid intravenous hydration maintains adequate kidney flow. Other issues, such as hyperkalemia, may require temporary hemodialysis. Treatments such as using mannitol (Osmitrol) to cause an osmotic diuresis or bicarbonate to alkalinize the urine have not been shown to consistently improve outcomes, though in most instances these types of therapy are unlikely to cause additional complications.[16,17]

Compartment Syndrome

Compartment syndrome is the result of increased pressure within a muscle compartment. Several layers of fibrous fascia (that do not expand) surround skeletal muscles. Increased pressure on the muscle tissue causes diminished capillary blood flow, resulting in local tissue hypoxia and necrosis. Causes of compartment syndrome include conditions that increase the contents of the compartment (such as bleeding after a fracture), decrease the compartment volume (such as a tight bandage or cast), or a combination of both conditions that result in disturbing the muscle's microvasculature (Box 39-2).[21-23] Any condition that disrupts the vascular supply to an extremity (such as severe burns, bleeding disorders, crush injury, snake or insect bites, extremely tight bandages, or casts) can cause increased pressure within the muscle compartments.

PATHOPHYSIOLOGY The weight of a limb extremity can generate enough pressure to produce muscle ischemia (Figures 39-6 and 39-7). Muscle ischemia causes edema, rising compartment pressure, and tamponade, leading to muscle infarction and neural injury and eventually resulting in cell loss.

CLINICAL MANIFESTATIONS Compartments often affected are the anterior and deep posterior tibial compartments in the leg, the forearm, the gluteal compartments in the buttocks, and the abdominal wall. Diagnosis is initiated by clinical examination. The "6 Ps" of compartment syndrome are *P*ain (out of proportion to the injury), *P*ressure (swelling, tenseness of the affected area), *P*allor, *P*aresthesia, *P*aresis (of the involved extremity), and *P*ulselessness. None of these signs is truly dependable, although pain with passive extension of the fingers or toes in the affected extremity and paresthesia tend to be most suggestive of compartment syndrome.[21,24]

A condition known as **Volkmann ischemic contracture** can develop when compartment syndrome is unrecognized or is not adequately treated. Irreversible neurovascular damage can occur. Contracture deformities of the fingers, hand, and wrist can lead to partial or complete disability of the affected limb.

EVALUATION AND TREATMENT Direct measurement of intracompartmental pressure, using a manometer or an electronic transducer, is essential to confirm the diagnosis.[25,26] Laboratory tests, ultrasonography, and imaging studies may help exclude other conditions but generally are not helpful in diagnosing compartment syndrome. Once intracompartmental pressures reach 30 mm Hg, surgical intervention is warranted to relieve pressure within the compartment.

Surgical intervention consists of performing a fasciotomy of the affected area to decompress the compartment and allow return of normal blood supply. Skin grafts are often required to close the resultant opening, but vacuum-assisted wound closure devices also have been used successfully in accelerating wound closure.

BOX 39-2 Factors Affecting Development of Compartment Syndrome

Increased Intracompartmental Pressure

Fracture (open or closed)
Traction
Crush syndrome
Vigorous exercise or nonroutine activity/overuse in nonathletes
High-energy soft tissue injury (blast injuries, blunt force trauma)
Fluid infusion
Arterial puncture
Ruptured abdominal aortic aneurysm
Ruptured ganglion/other cyst
Envenomation (venomous snakes, black widow spiders)
Nephrotic syndrome
Viral myositis
Acute hematogenous osteomyelitis
Orthopedic procedures (e.g., osteotomy, joint replacement)
Seizures
Tetany

Reduced Compartment Volume

Burns
Repair of muscle herniation
Circumferential dressings
Casts that are too tight

Conditions That Disturb Microcirculation

Diabetes
Hypothyroidism
Bleeding disorders (hemophilia, von Willebrand's disease, leukemia, vitamin K deficiency, viral hemorrhagic fevers [dengue])
Excessive anticoagulation
Malignancies

Data from Raza, H., & Mahapatra, A. (2015). *Adv Orthop, 2015,* 543412; Shadgan, B., Menon, M., Sanders, D., et al. (2010). *Can J Surg, 53*(5), 329–334.

Malignant Hyperthermia

Malignant hyperthermia (MH) is an autosomal dominant inherited muscle disorder characterized by a hypermetabolic reaction to certain volatile anaesthetics or certain depolarizing muscle relaxants (such as succinylcholine [Anectine]) that activate a prolonged release of intracellular calcium from the sarcoplasmic reticulum. Recently, advances in molecular genetics have shown that a mutation in the ryanodine receptor of skeletal muscle (RyR1) is responsible for the majority of cases, though other genetic mutations also may be involved.[27,28] The normal excitation-coupling process of muscle contraction is altered in MH. Mutations of RyR1 receptors release uncontrolled amounts of calcium from the sarcoplasmic reticulum into the cytoplasm, causing continuous muscle contraction.[29] This process also causes hypermetabolism with extremely high body temperature, muscle rigidity, rhabdomyolysis, and death if not quickly treated with dantrolene (Dantrium) infusion.[30]

Though reported in all countries, ages, and both genders, young males tend to be more susceptible to MH. Common signs and symptoms are respiratory acidosis (with elevated end tidal carbon dioxide), tachycardia, masseter and skeletal muscle spasm, and elevated body temperature.[29,31]

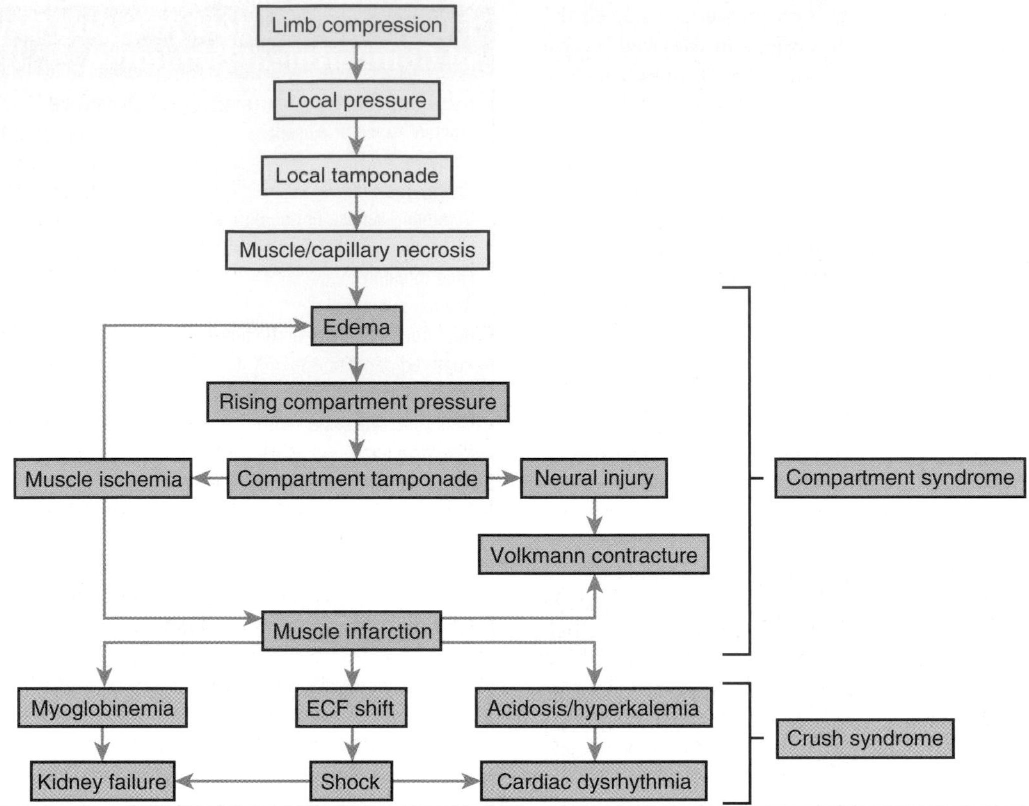

FIGURE 39-6 **Pathogenesis of Compartment Syndrome and Crush Syndrome Caused by Prolonged Muscle Compression.** *ECF*, Extracellular fluid.

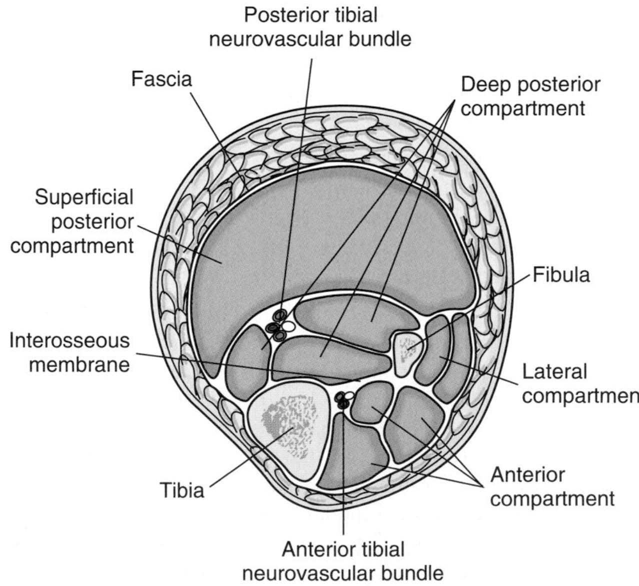

FIGURE 39-7 **Muscle Compartments of the Lower Leg.** (From Mohahan, F.D., Sands, J., Neighbors, M., et al. [2007]. *Phipps' medical-surgical nursing: Health and illness perspectives* [8th ed.]. St. Louis: Mosby.)

EVALUATION AND TREATMENT Careful and thorough preoperative assessment should alert the anaesthesiologist to the possibility of an individual being susceptible to MH. A family history of anaesthetic problems and previous untoward anaesthetic experiences (muscle cramping, unexplained fevers, dark urine) are criteria that require further clarification before administration of a volatile anaesthetic, such as halothane (Fluothane), or of the muscle relaxant succinylcholine. Currently, the muscle contracture test is considered the best predictor of developing MH. A muscle biopsy is obtained from the individual, and the tissue is then separately exposed to standardized amounts of halothane and caffeine. If the muscle bundles exhibit a contracture at specified limits, the individual is considered susceptible to MH.[31] Molecular and DNA testing are promising future means of identifying at-risk individuals.

Priorities in treatment of MH include identifying and treating the underlying disorder and preventing life-threatening kidney failure. MH and myoglobinuria can be treated by infusing dantrolene sodium (Dantrium). Secondary problems include electrolyte imbalance, volume depletion, acidosis, hyperuricemia, hyperkalemia, and calcium imbalance; these need specific treatment. Short-term dialysis also may be necessary.

> **QUICK CHECK 39-1**
> 1. How are fractures classified?
> 2. What is the primary pathology of epicondylopathy?
> 3. What are some causes of compartment syndrome?
> 4. Why is myoglobinuria a dangerous complication of rhabdomyolysis?

DISORDERS OF BONES

Metabolic Bone Diseases

Metabolic bone disease is characterized by abnormal bone structure that is caused by altered or inadequate biochemical reactions, which may be attributable to genetics, diet, or hormones.

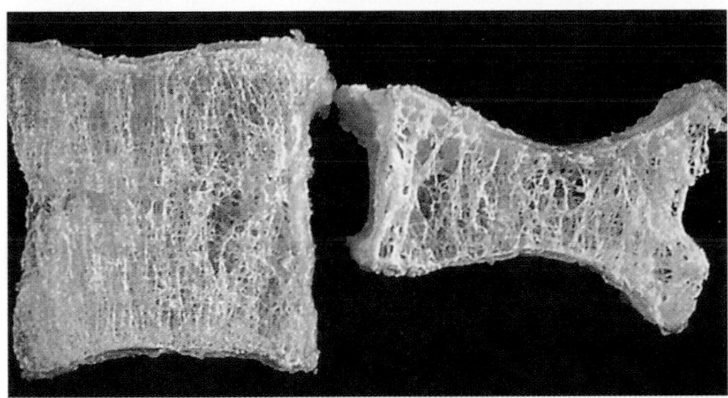

FIGURE 39-8 Vertebral Body. Osteoporotic vertebral body (*right*) shortened by compression fractures compared with a normal vertebral body. Note that the osteoporotic vertebra has a characteristic loss of horizontal trabeculae and thickened vertical trabeculae. (From Kumar, V., Abbas, A.K., & Aster, J.C. [Eds.]. [2015]. *Robbins and Cotran pathologic basis of disease* [9th ed.]. Philadelphia: Saunders.)

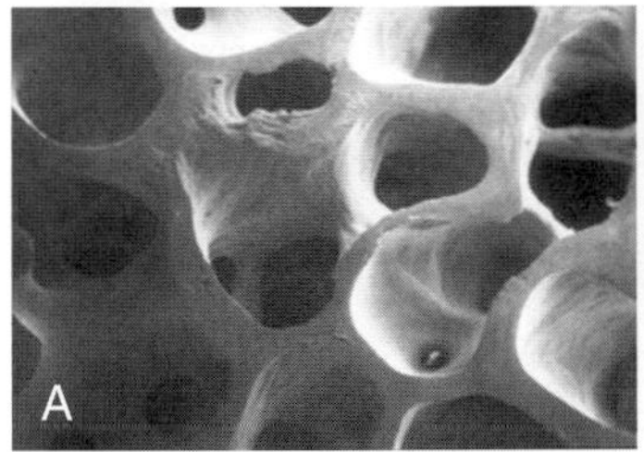

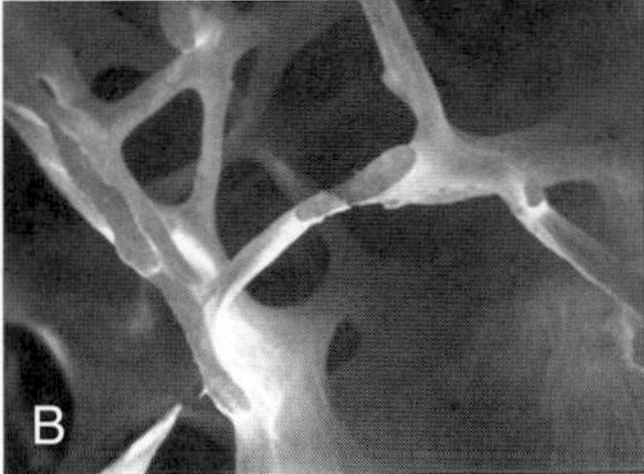

FIGURE 39-9 Electron Microscopic Comparison of Normal and Osteoporotic Bone. A, Normal trabecular structure. **B,** Osteoporotic bone; note the loss of supporting trabeculae. (Reprinted from *Med Clin North Am,* 99[3], Golob, A.L., & Laya, M.B., "Osteoporosis: Screening, prevention, and management," Pages 587–606, Copyright 2015, with permission from Elsevier.)

Osteoporosis

Osteoporosis, or **porous bone**, is generally described as decreased bone mineral density (BMD) and an increased risk for fractures because of alterations in bone microarchitecture. It is a complex, multifactorial, chronic disease that often progresses silently for decades until fractures occur. It is the most common disease that affects bone but is not necessarily a consequence of the aging process because some older adults retain strong, relatively dense bones. In osteoporosis, old bone is being resorbed faster than new bone is being made, causing the bones to lose density, becoming thinner and more porous. A progressive loss of bone mass may continue until the skeleton is no longer strong enough to support itself. Eventually, bones can fracture spontaneously. As bone becomes more fragile, falls or bumps that would not have caused a fracture previously now cause bone to break (a fragility fracture). The most common sites for osteoporosis-related fractures are the spine, femoral neck, and wrist.[32]

Bone tissue can be normally mineralized in osteoporosis, but the mass (density) of bone is decreased and the structural integrity of trabecular bone is impaired. Cortical bone becomes more porous and thinner, making bone weaker and prone to fractures (Figures 39-8 and 39-9). The World Health Organization (WHO) has defined *osteoporosis* as "a systematic skeletal disease characterized by low bone density and microarchitectural deterioration of bone tissue with a consequent increase in bone fragility."[33]

Bone density is based on the number of standard deviations that an adult's bone density differs from the mean BMD of a young-adult reference population (a T-score). Table 39-3 lists these categories. Bone

TABLE 39-3 T-Score and World Health Organization Diagnosis of Bone Density

T-Score	Diagnosis
0 to −0.99 SD	Normal BMD
−1.0 to −2.49 SD	Low bone density (osteopenia)
≤2.5 SD	Osteoporosis
≤2.5 SD with any fracture	Severe osteoporosis

BMD, Bone mineral density; *SD*, standard deviation.

density between 1.5 and 2.5 standard deviations below normal is considered osteopenia. A T-score of 2.5 or more standard deviations below normal bone density is considered osteoporotic. Severe or established osteoporosis is identified when there has been a fragility fracture associated with low bone density. The disease can be (1) generalized, involving major portions of the axial skeleton, or (2) regional, involving one segment of the appendicular skeleton.

Skeletal homeostasis depends on a narrow range of plasma calcium and phosphate concentrations, which are maintained by the endocrine system. Therefore, endocrine dysfunction ultimately can cause metabolic bone disease. In addition to declining levels of sex steroids, the hormones most commonly associated with osteoporosis are parathyroid hormone (PTH), cortisol, thyroid hormone, and growth hormone. (Endocrine function is discussed in Chapters 18 and 19.)

Other factors that can adversely affect normal bone homeostasis include multiple medications (such as glucocorticoids, proton pump inhibitors, thiazolidinediones, antiseizure medications, aromatase inhibitors, selective serotonin reuptake inhibitors [SSRIs], and anticoagulants), vitamin D deficiency, underlying diseases (rheumatoid disease, Paget's disease, cancer, diabetes), low physical activity, and abnormal body mass index.[34-38]

Throughout a lifetime, old bone is removed (resorption) and new bone is added (formation) to the skeleton. During childhood and teenage years, new bone is added faster than old bone is removed. Consequently, bones become larger, heavier, and denser. Bone formation continues at a pace faster than resorption until **peak bone mass** or maximum bone density and strength is reached, around age 30. Up to 90% of peak bone mass is obtained by age 20. After age 30, bone resorption slowly exceeds bone formation. In women, bone loss is most rapid in the first years after menopause but persists throughout the postmenopausal years. The *2010 Clinical Practice Guidelines for the Diagnosis and Management of Osteoporosis in Canada* included a new recommendation that all men and women age 65 and older be routinely screened for osteoporosis.[39] Fractures are the major complication of osteoporosis and it has been estimated that the fracture risk for osteoporosis is a worldwide problem with significant economic and health implications.[40-42] Hip fractures, in particular, can have devastating effects on an individual's life. In addition to direct medical costs, studies have shown decreased quality of life as well as excess loss of life-years for those experiencing hip or osteoporotic fractures.[43-45] The major complications for persons with osteoporosis are fractures (see *Health Promotion:* The Cost of Osteoporosis: Facts and Figures). Bone structure in men allows for improved torque strength, and although men lose bone density with aging, it is at a slower, steadier rate than that of women.[46] Nevertheless, men are more likely to die after a hip fracture than are women.[47,48]

Vertebral fractures tend to occur in the later years of life; however, they are more difficult to ascertain because people may be unaware of the fracture. The degree of compression necessary to define a vertebral fracture is not standardized, although attempts have been made to standardize the definition and diagnosis of vertebral fractures. Thus, the true prevalence is unknown but fractures do increase in frequency

HEALTH PROMOTION

The Cost of Osteoporosis: Facts and Figures

Osteoporosis is the most common bone disease of adults and the foremost cause of fractures in older adults.

- Fewer than 20% of patients with fractures undergo diagnosis and treatment for osteoporosis.
- 80% of fractures in individuals older than 50 years are due to osteoporosis.
- 1 out of every 3 women and 1 out of every 5 men will develop osteoporosis in their lifetime.
- 15–25% of people with hip fractures end up going to a nursing home.
- The cost of fractures to the health care system was $2.3 billion in 2010, with the total cost increasing to $3.9 billion (including costs of long-term care).
- Costs per person directly related to care post-hip fracture are $21 285 in the first year, with a cost of $44 156 if the person is institutionalized.

Data from Papaioannou, A., Morin, S., Cheung, A.M., et al. (2010). *CMAJ, 182*(17), 1864–1873. doi:10.1503/cmaj.100771

TABLE 39-4 Comparison of Fracture Risk Assessment Tools Not Utilizing Bone Mineral Density

Risk Factor	FRAX	SCORE	OSIRIS	ORAI	OST
Age	X	X	X	X	X
Weight	X	X	X	X	X
Previous low-energy fracture	X	X	X		
Estrogen therapy		X	X	X	
Rheumatoid arthritis	X	X			
Height	X				
Parental hip fracture	X				
Smoking	X				
Alcohol	X				
Glucocorticoid therapy	X				
Secondary osteoporosis	X				
Sex	X				
Ethnicity		X			

FRAX, World Health Organization's "Fracture Risk Assessment Tool"; *ORAI,* osteoporosis risk assessment instrument; *OSIRIS,* osteoporosis index of risk; *OST,* osteoporosis self-assessment tool; *SCORE,* simple calculated osteoporosis risk estimation.
Chart from Rubin, K.H., Abrahamsen, B., Friis-Holmberg, T., et al. (2013). *Bone, 56,* 18.

by the sixth and seventh decades. Approximately 1 in 6 women and 1 in 12 men will sustain a vertebral fracture.[49]

Age-related loss of bone density and osteoporosis is most common in White women but affects all races. Asian and Black women have only about half the fracture rate of Whites, but that percentage is expected to increase with improved life expectancy.[50] In spite of lower incidence, mortality in Black women after a hip fracture is higher than among White women. Other factors may include lower calcium intake, a high percentage of lactose intolerance, and increased prevalence of diseases such as sickle cell disease and lupus that increase the risk of developing osteoporosis.[51] Both Black women and Black men have generally been undertreated for osteoporosis.

Fracture prevention is a primary goal of osteoporosis treatment. Measuring BMD by using dual X-ray absorptiometry (DXA) to calculate an individual's T-score continues to be the most common method of evaluating bone health and predicting fracture risk. Unfortunately, the technology to perform DXA scans is not available in all areas of the world. As a result, several tools that do not require BMD testing have been developed and validated to predict future fracture risk. These tools are summarized in Table 39-4. Interestingly, when BMD measurement is not available, there is little difference in fracture prediction between the Internet-based FRAX® and the other tools, including the simplest screening tool—the Osteoporosis Self-assessment Tool, or OST.[52]

Bone quality is not defined by bone mass alone (as measured by BMD) but also by the microarchitecture of the bone. Thus, other variables include crystal size and shape, brittleness, vitality of bone cells, structure of the bone proteins, integrity of the trabecular network, and the ability to repair tiny cracks. Because bone density relates to *quantity* of bone, *quality* of bone is not accurately identified by bone density testing alone. As a result, bone density testing may not accurately identify those who will eventually be susceptible to fractures.

Postmenopausal osteoporosis is bone loss that occurs in middle-aged and older women. It can occur because of estrogen deficiency as well as from estrogen-independent age-related mechanisms (e.g., secondary causes such as hyperparathyroidism and decreased mechanical stimulation). Estrogen deficiency can also increase with stress, excessive exercise, and low body weight. Postmenopausal changes include alterations in the OPG/RANKL/RANK system, resulting in a substantial increase in bone turnover—that is, a remodelling imbalance between the activity of osteoclasts (bone destroyers) and osteoblasts (bone formers). Increased formation and activity of osteoclasts causes removal or resorption of bone and results in a cascade of proinflammatory cytokines. Increased cytokine activation, especially tumour necrosis factor (TNF), can occur with declining estrogen levels.[53] In addition, estrogen helps osteoclast apoptosis (programmed cell death), so a decrease in estrogen levels is associated with *survival* of the bone-removing osteoclasts. Biologically, these processes involve the receptor activator of nuclear factor kappa-B ligand (RANKL), osteoprotegerin (OPG) signalling pathways, and insulinlike growth factor (IGF) (see Chapter 38 and Figures 38-5 and 39-10). Other causes may include a combination of inadequate dietary calcium intake and lack of vitamin D (and possibly decreased magnesium), lack of exercise, low body mass, and family history. IGF is known to help in fracture healing and collagen synthesis and improves conditions for bone mineralization. IGF levels significantly decline by age 60. Excessive phosphorus intake, chiefly through the intake of highly processed foods, hampers the calcium–phosphorus balance by interfering with PTH and fibroblast growth factor-23 (FGF-23).[54,55]

Sex hormones, particularly estradiol (estrogen), are major determinants of bone density in both females and males.[56,57] Androgens (i.e., testosterone and dihydrotestosterone) have long been recognized as stimulants of bone formation. Increasing age in both men and women is associated with declining levels of estradiol and androgen, leading to losses in BMD. Other factors, such as inadequate dietary calcium intake, decreases in weight-bearing exercise, and sarcopenia, also are associated with osteoporosis. Other risk factors are identified in *Risk Factors:* Osteoporosis.

Insufficient intake or malabsorption of dietary minerals is a factor in the development of osteoporosis. Calcium absorption from the intestine decreases with age, and studies of individuals with osteoporosis show that their calcium intake is lower than that of age-matched controls. Other mineral deficiencies, including magnesium, also may be important. Vitamin deficiencies, particularly vitamin D, as well as either deficiencies or excesses of protein also contribute to bone loss. Decreased serum levels of trace elements (zinc, copper, iron, magnesium, and manganese) have been associated not only with lower peak bone mass in developing bone but also with later development of osteoporosis.[58-60] Excessive

RISK FACTORS

Osteoporosis

Genetic
Family history of osteoporosis
White race
Increased age
Female gender

Anthropometric
Small stature
Fair or pale-skinned
Thin build
Low bone mineral density

Hormonal and Metabolic
Early menopause (natural or surgical)
Late menarche
Nulliparity
Obesity
Hypogonadism
Gaucher's disease
Cushing's syndrome
Weight below healthy range
Acidosis

Dietary
Low dietary calcium and vitamin D
Low endogenous magnesium
Excessive protein*
Excessive sodium intake
Anorexia
Malabsorption

Lifestyle
Sedentary
Smoker
Alcohol consumption (excessive)
Low-impact fractures as an adult
Inability to rise from a chair without using one's arms

Concurrent
Hyperparathyroidism

Illness and Trauma
Renal insufficiency, hypocalciuria
Rheumatoid arthritis
Spinal cord injury
Systemic lupus erythematosus

Liver Disease
Marrow disease (myeloma, mastocytosis, thalassemia)

Medications
Corticosteroids
Phenytoin (Dilantin)
Gonadotropin-releasing hormone agonists
Loop diuretics
Methotrexate (Apo-Methotrexate)
Thyroid medications
Heparin
Cyclosporine (Sandimmune)
Medroxyprogesterone acetate (Depo-Provera)
Retinoids

*Low levels of protein intake also have been reported.

intake of caffeine, phosphorus, alcohol, and nicotine along with low body fat (weight less than 57 kg) has been shown to lower BMD.[61-63] Secondary osteoporosis is osteoporosis caused by other conditions, including hormonal imbalances (endocrine disease, diabetes, hyperparathyroidism, hyperthyroidism), medications (e.g., heparin, corticosteroids, phenytoin, barbiturates, lithium), and other substances (e.g., tobacco, ethanol). Other conditions, including rheumatoid disease, human immunodeficiency virus (HIV), malignancies, malabsorption syndrome, and liver or kidney disease, also increase the risk of developing osteoporosis (see *Risk Factors:* Osteoporosis).

Secondary osteoporosis sometimes develops temporarily in individuals receiving large doses of heparin by decreasing osteoblast formation and increasing bone resorption by reducing OPG and, thus, increasing osteoclast formation.[64] Osteoporosis caused by heparin therapy usually resolves when therapy ceases. Other medications increasing risk for osteoporosis include glucocorticoids, proton pump inhibitors, aromatase inhibitors, lithium, methotrexate, anticonvulsants, cyclophosphamide (Procytox), thiazolidinediones, and cyclosporine.

Regional osteoporosis—osteoporosis confined to a segment of the appendicular skeleton—often has no known cause. Classic regional osteoporosis is associated with disuse or immobilization of a limb because of fractures or bone or joint inflammation. A negative calcium balance develops early and continues throughout the period of immobilization. After 8 weeks of immobilization, significant osteoporosis is present. One result of weightlessness has been a uniform distribution of osteoporosis observed in astronauts and in individuals treated with air suspension therapy.

Transient regional osteoporosis has no known etiology and is characterized by bone marrow edema and, sometimes, severe pain. Transient regional osteoporosis is usually self-limiting, and tends to occur in middle-aged men and in women during their late second or third trimester of pregnancy.[65,66] Bone marrow edema can be seen on MRI, and areas of localized bone demineralization are seen in plain radiographs.[67] The lower extremity is most often affected but other areas also can be involved. Treatment is primarily symptomatic and the condition usually resolves spontaneously over 3 to 6 months, with no long-term side effects.

PATHOPHYSIOLOGY Osteoporosis develops when the remodelling cycle (coupling)—bone resorption and bone formation—is disrupted, leading to an imbalance in the coupling process. Osteoclasts are differentiated cells that function to resorb bone. The explosion of new information in the field of bone biology has led to new understandings of osteoclast biology and bone pathophysiology. Of primary importance is the osteoclast differentiation pathway that is dependent on various processes, including proliferation, maturation, fusion, and activation. These processes, in turn, are dependent on the availability of stem cells to allow differentiation to occur and are controlled by hormones, cytokines, and paracrine stromal cell interactions. Thus, proper intracellular communication within bone among its molecular regulators is necessary for normal bone homeostasis. Numerous interleukins, TNF, transforming growth factor-beta (TGF-β), prostaglandin E_2, and hormones interact to control osteoclasts (Figure 39-10). Staggering in its importance to understanding osteoclast biology is the cytokine receptor activator of nuclear factor kappa-B ligand (RANKL); its receptor activator of nuclear factor kappa-B (RANK); and its decoy receptor osteoprotegerin (OPG), a glycoprotein (see Chapter 36 and Figure 36-5).

Glucocorticoid-induced osteoporosis (e.g., prednisone, cortisone) is the most common type of secondary osteoporosis. Glucocorticoids have a direct impact on bone quality by improving osteoclast survival, inhibiting osteoblast formation and function, and increasing osteocyte apoptosis.[68-70] Glucocorticoids increase RANKL expression and inhibit OPG production by osteoblasts. Overall, these alterations result in decreased thickness of the bone cortex and fewer, thinner, and more widely spaced trabeculae in the marrow.[71]

Age-related bone loss begins in the third to fourth decade.[72] The cause remains unclear, but it is known that decreased serum growth hormone and insulinlike growth factor 1 (IGF-1) levels, along with increased binding of RANKL and decreased OPG production, affect osteoblast and osteoclast function.[73] Loss of trabecular bone in men proceeds in a linear fashion with thinning of trabecular bone rather than complete loss, as is noted in women (Figure 39-11).[74] Men have approximately 30% greater bone mass than women, which may be a factor in their later involvement with osteoporosis (Figure 39-12). In addition, men have a more gradual decrease in the levels of testosterone and estradiol (and possibly progesterone), thereby maintaining their bone mass longer than women. Reduced physical activity in older adults is also a likely factor.

CLINICAL MANIFESTATIONS The specific clinical manifestations of osteoporosis depend on the bones involved. The most common

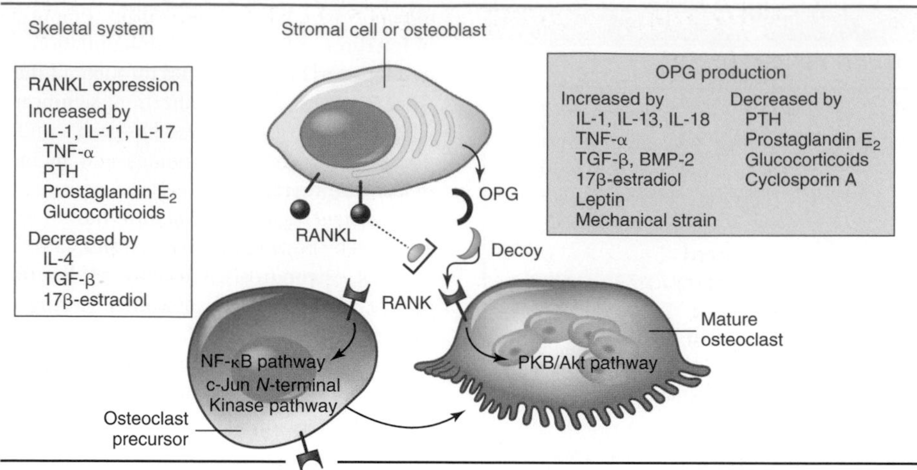

FIGURE 39-10 OPG/RANKL/RANK System. Expression of RANKL, a cytokine and part of the TNF family, and OPG, a glycoprotein receptor antagonist, is modulated by various cytokines, hormones, medications, and mechanical strains (see inserts). In bone, RANKL is expressed by both stromal cells and osteoblasts. RANKL stimulates the receptor RANK on osteoclast precursor cells and mature osteoclasts and activates intracellular signalling pathways to promote osteoclast differentiation and activation as well as cytoskeletal reorganization and survival (PKB/Akt pathway), which increase resorption and bone loss. OPG, secreted by stromal cells and osteoblasts, acts as a "decoy" receptor and blocks RANKL binding to and activation of RANK. *BMP*, Bone morphogenetic protein; *IL*, interleukin; *OPG*, osteoprotegerin; *PKB/Akt pathway*, protein kinase B pathway; *PTH*, parathyroid hormone; *RANK*, receptor activator of nuclear factor kappa-B; *RANKL*, receptor activator of nuclear factor kappa-B ligand; *TGF-β*, transforming growth factor-beta; *TNF-α*, tumour necrosis factor-alpha. (Adapted from Hofbauer, L.C., & Schoppet, M. [2004]. *JAMA, 292*[4], 490–495.)

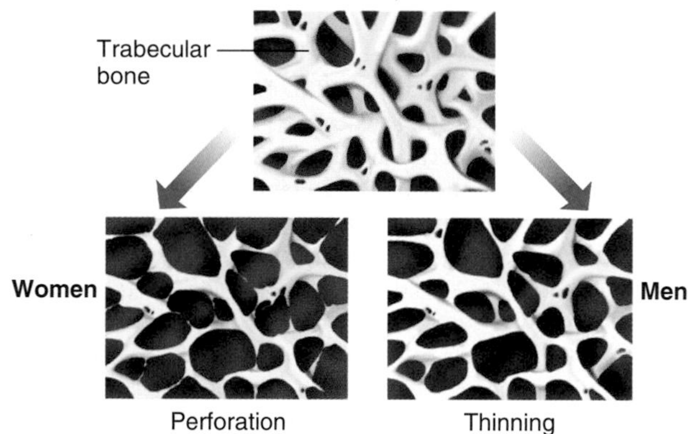

FIGURE 39-11 Mechanism of Loss of Trabecular Bone in Women and Trabecular Thinning in Men. Bone thinning predominates in men because of reduced bone formation. Loss of connectivity and complete trabeculae predominates in women.

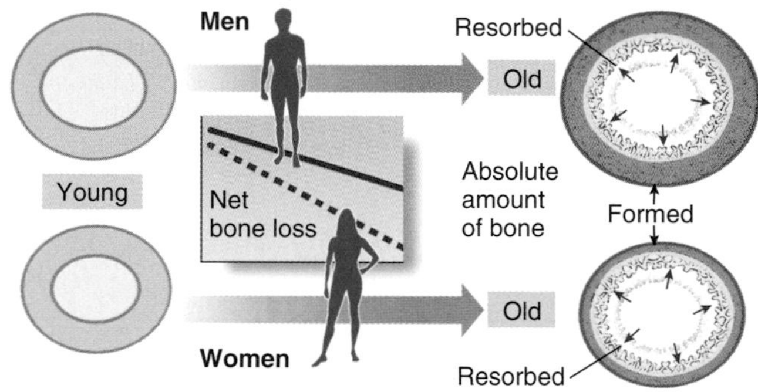

FIGURE 39-12 Bone Loss in Men and Women. Absolute amount of bone resorbed on the inner bone surface and formed on the outer bone surface is more in men than women during aging.

manifestations, however, are pain and bone deformity because of fracture. Unfortunately, these manifestations occur only in an advanced disease state. Fractures are likely to occur because the trabeculae of spongy bone become thin and sparse, and compact bone becomes porous. As the bones lose volume, they become brittle and weak and may collapse or become misshapen. Vertebral collapse causes **kyphosis** (hunchback) and diminishes height (Figure 39-13). Fractures of the long bones (particularly the femur),[75] distal radius, ribs, and vertebrae are most common. Fracture of the neck of the femur—the so-called broken hip—tends to occur in older women with osteoporosis. Fatal complications of fractures include fat or pulmonary embolism, pneumonia, hemorrhage, and shock. Approximately 20% of persons may die as a result of surgical complications. Osteoporosis in men, as in women, also may be related to hypogonadism, with estradiol levels being more clinically important than testosterone levels in both genders. Adequate dietary intake of calcium, vitamin D, magnesium, and other trace minerals (see *Health Promotion:* Calcium, Vitamin D, and Bone Health); adherence to a regular regimen of weight-bearing exercise; and avoidance of alcoholism, tobacco, and glucocorticoids seem to help prevent primary osteoporosis.

EVALUATION AND TREATMENT In general, osteoporosis is detected radiographically as increased radiolucency of bone. By the time abnormalities are detected by radiological examination, up to 25 to 30% of bone tissue may have been lost.

Dual X-ray absorptiometry (DXA) is the current gold standard for detecting and monitoring osteoporosis; however, bone density is not necessarily indicative of bone quality. The utility of DXA in predicting fracture risk has recently been enhanced by development of a trabecular

HEALTH PROMOTION

Calcium, Vitamin D, and Bone Health

Adequate calcium intake is essential for developing and maintaining normal bone structure, but the following question remains a topic of discussion and research: "What is adequate calcium intake?" Calcium is the most abundant mineral in the body and plays a role in maintaining muscle function, hormonal secretion, neurotransmission, and vascular health. Recent conflicting evidence about the effect of calcium on heart disease, for example, has been hotly debated in the medical literature. The conflicting reports about extraskeletal health benefits of vitamin D also were reviewed by the US Institute of Medicine (IOM) and were found to lack enough evidence to be considered reliable.

The role of vitamin D in bone health is unquestioned; the clinical effects of inadequate vitamin D (osteomalacia, rickets) have been well known for many years. Vitamin D is essential for absorbing and maintaining calcium homeostasis in the body. Recently, vitamin D has been postulated to be involved in many extraskeletal functions, such as reducing cancer risk, improving cognitive function in the older adult, preventing autoimmune diseases, improving resistance to infection, providing cardiovascular support, stabilizing posture, and inhibiting metabolic syndrome. Some of these potentially beneficial effects are from data gleaned from the US National Health and Nutrition Examination Survey III (NHANES III), whereas other descriptions are based on observational or small studies. Vitamin D levels are evaluated by measuring serum 1,25-dihydroxy-vitamin D_3 levels. There is still disagreement about what constitutes an "optimal" vitamin D level, but many sources indicate it should be at least 50 nmol/mL. Based on these levels, it has been estimated that nearly 32% of the adult population in Canada has low vitamin D levels (2009–11 data). The average vitamin D level in Canada is 64 nmol/L, with two-thirds of Canadians above the cut-off.

The IOM recently evaluated and summarized clinical evidence and literature reviews regarding the roles of calcium and vitamin D in disease reduction and other health outcomes in North America. Review of these findings resulted in updates of the recommended daily intake of both nutrients. In general, daily calcium intakes of 500 mg for ages 1 through 3, 800 mg for ages 4 through 8, 1 100 to 1 300 mg for ages 9 to 13, and 800 to 1 000 mg for ages 14 through adulthood are adequate for maintaining proper bone health. Recommended dietary allowances for vitamin D vary from 400 to 600 units per day for all ages. Additionally, the IOM found that once calcium intake exceeds more than 2 000 mg a day or vitamin D intake is more than 4 000 units per day, there is increased risk for harm.

Data from Adams, J.S., & Hewison, M. (2010). *J Clin Endocrinol Metab, 95*(2), 471–478; Annweiler, C., Montero-Odasso, M., Schott, A.M., et al. (2010). *J Neuroeng Rehabil, 7,* 50; Binkley, N., Ramamurthy, R., & Krueger, D. (2010). *Endocrinol Metab Clin North Am, 39*(2), 287–301; Bolland, M.J., Avenell, A., Baron, J.A., et al. (2010). *BMJ, 341,* 3691; Dawson-Hughes, B. (2010). *BMJ, 341,* 4993; Grove, M.L., & Book, D. (2010). *BMJ, 342,* 5003; Heiss, G., Hsia, J., Pettinger, M., et al. (2010). *BMJ, 341,* 4995; Janz, T., & Pearson, C. (2013). Health at a glance: Vitamin D levels of Canadians. Retrieved from http://www.statcan.gc.ca/pub/82-624-x/2013001/article/11727-eng.htm; National Institutes of Health Office of Dietary Supplements. (2014). Vitamin D fact sheet for health professionals. Retrieved from https://ods.od.nih.gov/factsheets/VitaminD-HealthProfessional/; Newberry, S.J., Chung, M., Shekelle, P.G., et al. (2014). *Vitamin D and calcium: A systematic review of health outcomes (update).* [AHQR Pub. No. 14-E004-EF]. Rockville, MD: Agency for Healthcare Research and Quality.

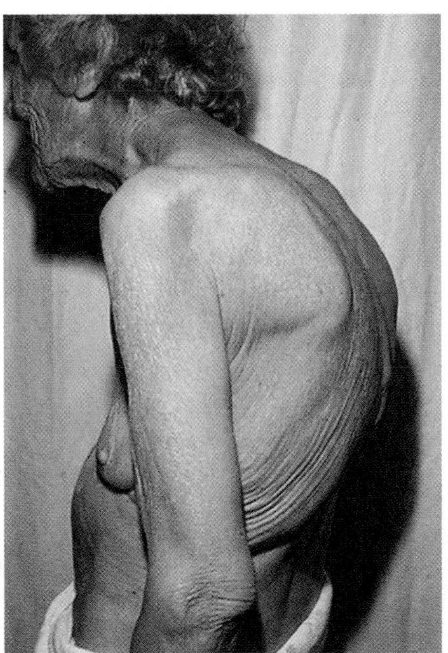

FIGURE 39-13 Kyphosis. This older adult woman's condition was caused by a combination of spinal osteoporotic vertebral collapse and chronic degenerative changes in the vertebral column. (From Kamal, A., & Brocklehurst, J.C. [1992]. *Color atlas of geriatric medicine* [2nd ed.]. St. Louis: Mosby.)

BOX 39-3 Biochemical Markers of Bone Turnover

Biochemical markers of bone turnover are useful in monitoring osteoporosis treatment. Markers of resorption include urinary N-telopeptide (NTx), C-telopeptide (CTx), and deoxypyridinoline. Markers of bone formation include bone-specific alkaline phosphatase (BSAP) and osteocalcin. However, these tests have diurnal variability within the same individual, so there must be significant changes in levels to indicate a difference in bone turnover.

bone score (TBS). TBS evaluates pixel variations in the grey-level areas of lumbar spine images from DXA scans and has been shown to correlate with high-resolution peripheral quantitative computed tomography (HRpQCT) and be a reliable predictor of fractures.[76-79] High-resolution imaging techniques, such as quantitative computed tomography (QCT) scans and HRpQCT imaging, show changes of trabecular and cortical microarchitecture in osteopenic women.[80] Newer MRI techniques also show promise for providing more detailed information about cortical and trabecular bone and have the added safety of no radiation exposure.[80,81] Other evaluation procedures include measurement of serum and urinary biochemical markers to monitor bone turnover (Box 39-3).

The goals of osteoporosis treatment are risk reduction and the prevention of fractures. Bisphosphonates are first-line medications for treating osteoporosis; they primarily work by inhibiting hydroxyapatite breakdown, reducing bone resorption. New medications formulated to prevent or treat osteoporosis are currently being prescribed and evaluated. There are new treatments that help rebuild the skeleton (see *Health Promotion:* New Treatments for Osteoporosis). Selective steroid agents—for example, raloxifene (Evista)—also may be prescribed (see Chapter

33). Regular, moderate weight-bearing exercise can slow the rate of bone loss and, in some cases, reverse demineralization because the mechanical stress of exercise stimulates bone formation. An exercise program to enhance strength and balance has the added benefits of reducing the risk for falls and promoting bone quality.

HEALTH PROMOTION

New Treatments for Osteoporosis

Although bisphosphonates remain the first line of osteoporosis therapy, not all individuals are able to tolerate them, and side effects can include bisphosphonate-related osteonecrosis of the jaw (BRONJ), atrial fibrillation, and fractures. Zoledronic acid (Aclasta), a third-generation bisphosphonate, is given as an annual intravenous infusion and has demonstrated efficacy in treating glucocorticoid-associated osteoporosis, in addition to reducing vertebral and nonvertebral fractures in women and men. However, it can cause an acute phase response in recipients and still carries some risk for BRONJ. Several new treatment options promise progress in treating osteoporosis and may be better tolerated than bisphosphonates.

Denosumab (Prolia) is the first commercially available human monoclonal antibody for treatment of osteoporosis. It binds to the RANKL (see Chapter 38), preventing activation of osteoclasts. By reducing osteoclast activity, bone density is increased and bone resorption is reduced, thus lessening the incidence of fractures. Because denosumab is not cleared by the kidneys (as are bisphosphonates), it has the potential to be useful in those with chronic kidney disease. It is given every 6 months as a 60-mg subcutaneous injection.

Raloxifene, a selective estrogen receptor modulator (SERM), has been in use for several years to treat postmenopausal osteoporosis. It has been effective in reducing vertebral fractures but not hip or other nonspinal fractures. Newer SERMs, including lasofoxifene (which is approved for use in Europe, but not in North America), have been shown to reduce both vertebral and nonvertebral fractures. Bazedoxifene, in combination with estrogen, has been designated as a tissue-selective estrogen complex (TSEC), and is approved for use in Japan and Europe. It has been shown to reduce both vertebral and nonvertebral fractures in postmenopausal women. Neither of these agents, given as daily oral doses, stimulates endometrial or breast tissue.

Other biological agents for treating osteoporosis include odanacatib, a cathepsin K inhibitor. By affecting this enzyme (produced by osteoclasts), bone density is increased. Odanacatib reached phase III trials in the United States, with participants taking it once weekly as an oral agent. However, further development was stopped because of its risk for stroke. Agents directed at signalling pathways of bone formation and homeostasis are another target of osteoporosis intervention. One of the main signalling targets is the Wnt pathway (see Chapter 38). Wnt stimulates osteoblast function and bone formation but is blocked by sclerostin (which is produced by the osteocyte gene *SOST*). Parathyroid hormone (PTH) inhibits sclerostin expression, which may result in increased numbers of osteoblasts. The development of monoclonal antibodies to sclerostin may provide another means to increase bone formation and density.

Data from Bone, H.G., Dempster, D.W., Eisman, J.A., et al. (2015). *Osteoporosis Int, 26*(2), 699–712; Choi, H.J. (2015). *J Menopausal Med, 21*(1), 1–11; Reid, I.R. (2015). *Nat Rev Endocrinol, 11*(7), 418–428; Reyes, C., Hitz, M., Prieto-Alhambra, D., et al. (2016). *J Cell Biochem, 117*(1), 20–28, doi:10.1002/jcb.25266; Suresh, E., & Abrahamsen, B. (2015). *Cleve Clin J Med, 82*(2), 105–114.

The anabolic or bone-building medication PTH has been widely studied and is a major regulator of calcium homeostasis. PTH acts directly on osteocytes, stimulates bone formation, and promotes migration of progenitor bone cells from the marrow into the bloodstream, increasing the production of osteoblasts when intermittently administered.[82,83]

Osteomalacia

Osteomalacia is a metabolic disease characterized by inadequate and delayed mineralization of osteoid in mature compact and spongy bone. In osteomalacia, the remodelling cycle proceeds normally through osteoid formation, but mineral calcification and deposition do not occur. Bone volume remains unchanged, but the replaced bone consists of soft osteoid instead of rigid bone. Rickets is similar to osteomalacia in pathogenesis, but it occurs in the growing bones of children, whereas osteomalacia occurs in adult bone. (Rickets is described in Chapter 40.)

Both osteomalacia and rickets are relatively rare in Canada (rates of incidence are higher in the north—Yukon, Northwest Territories, and Nunavut), but are significant health problems in other parts of the world, such as Great Britain, Ethiopia, Pakistan, Iran, and India. Concomitant diseases, such as HIV, chronic kidney or liver disease, certain cancers, and impaired nutrient absorption from bariatric surgery, can result in vitamin D deficiency and secondary osteomalacia. In Canada, other causes include prematurity with very low birth weight and adhering to a rigid macrobiotic vegetarian diet. Breastfed infants with darker skin who do not receive vitamin D supplementation have been shown to be at risk for developing nutritional rickets.[84]

Many factors contribute to the development of osteomalacia, but the most important is a deficiency of vitamin D. The major risk factors in vitamin D deficiency are diets deficient in vitamin D, decreased endogenous production of vitamin D, intestinal malabsorption of vitamin D, renal tubular diseases, certain types of tumours (particularly of mesenchymal origin), and anticonvulsant therapy. Classic vitamin D deficiency is rare in Canada because of the addition of synthetic vitamin D to dairy products and bread.

Disorders of the small bowel, hepatobiliary system, and pancreas are causes of vitamin D deficiency in Canada. In malabsorptive disease of the small bowel, both vitamin D and calcium absorption are decreased, so vitamin D is lost in feces. Liver disease interferes with the metabolism of vitamin D to its more active form, and diseases of the pancreas and biliary system cause a deficiency of bile salts, which are necessary for normal intestinal absorption of vitamin D.

The mechanism by which anticonvulsant medication therapy results in vitamin D deficiency is not completely understood, but researchers think that the anticonvulsants phenobarbital (PMS-Phenobarbital) and phenytoin interfere with calcium absorption and increase degradation of vitamin D metabolism in the liver. Renal osteodystrophy is another cause of osteomalacia.

PATHOPHYSIOLOGY Crystallization of minerals in osteoid requires adequate concentrations of calcium and phosphate. When the concentrations are too low, crystallization (and hence ossification) does not proceed normally.

Vitamin D deficiency disrupts mineralization because vitamin D normally regulates and enhances the absorption of calcium ions from the intestine. A lack of vitamin D causes the plasma calcium concentrations to fall. Low plasma calcium levels stimulate increased synthesis and secretion of PTH. Although the increase in circulating PTH level raises the plasma calcium concentration, it also stimulates increased renal clearance of phosphate. When the concentration of phosphate in the bone decreases below a critical level, mineralization cannot proceed normally. Newer research has identified a complex interplay of matrix proteins, hormones, metallopeptidases, and certain proteins as also being involved in the development of osteomalacia.

Abnormalities occur in both spongy and compact bone. Trabeculae in spongy bone become thinner and fewer, whereas haversian systems in compact bone develop large channels and become irregular. Because osteoid continues to be produced but not mineralized, abnormal quantities of osteoid accumulate, coating the trabeculae and the linings of the haversian canals. Excessive osteoid also can accumulate in areas beneath the periosteum. The excess of osteoid leads to gross deformities of the long bones, spine, pelvis, and skull.

CLINICAL MANIFESTATIONS Osteomalacia causes varying degrees of diffuse muscular and skeletal pain and tenderness. Pain is noted particularly in the hips, and the individual may be hesitant to walk.[85] Muscular weakness is common and may contribute to a waddling gait. Facial deformities and bowed legs or "knock-knees" may be present. Bone fractures and vertebral collapse occur with minimal trauma. Low back pain may be an early complaint, but pain may also involve ribs, feet, other areas of the vertebral column, and other sites. Fragility fractures may occur. Uremia may be present in renal osteodystrophy.

EVALUATION AND TREATMENT Laboratory data may include elevated BUN and creatinine levels, normal or low serum calcium levels, and a serum inorganic phosphate level that is usually more than 5.5 mg. Alkaline phosphatase and PTH levels are usually elevated. Radiographic findings may show symmetric bowing deformities and fractures with callus formation, particularly in the lower extremities. These types of fractures, known as pseudofractures, along with radiolucent bands perpendicular to the surface of involved bones can help differentiate osteomalacia from fragility fractures that are seen in osteoporosis. A bone biopsy is used to obtain information on bone structure and remodelling and evaluate the presence of subclinical renal osteodystrophy to determine bone architecture, turnover, and even aluminum deposits.[86,87]

Treatment of osteomalacia may vary, depending on its etiology, but the following general principles are included:

1. Adjustment of serum calcium and phosphorus levels to normal
2. Suppression of secondary hyperthyroidism
3. Chelation of bone aluminum if needed
4. Administration of calcium carbonate to decrease hyperphosphatemia
5. Administration of vitamin D supplements (oral or infusion)
6. Administration of bisphosphonate
7. Implementation of renal dialysis, if indicated

Paget's Disease

Paget's disease of bone (PDB, osteitis deformans, or Paget's disease), the second most common bone disease after osteoporosis, is a state of increased metabolic activity in bone characterized by localized abnormal and excessive bone remodelling. Chronic accelerated remodelling eventually enlarges and softens the affected bones, causing bowing deformity, fracture, or neurological problems.

Paget's disease can occur in any bone but most often affects the vertebrae, skull, sacrum, sternum, pelvis, and femur. The disease process may occur in one or more bones without causing significant clinical manifestations.

Paget's disease occurs with equal frequency in men more than 55 years of age and women older than 40 years of age. It is often symptomless and diagnosis is often suspected when an elevated serum alkaline phosphatase level or abnormal X-ray is noted.[88] Radioisotope bone scan, X-rays, and computed tomography (CT) are used to confirm the diagnosis.[89] Serum plasma procollagen-1 N-peptide (PINP) is another serum marker that may provide a more accurate diagnosis.[90] Autopsy data from England and Germany indicate that approximately 3 to 4% of the population older than 40 years of age has Paget's disease. This disease is most prevalent in Australia, Great Britain, New Zealand, and the United States. It affects several members of the same family in 5 to 25% of cases.

The cause of Paget's disease is not yet fully known, but studies have implicated both genetic and environmental factors. Environmental factors that seem to be implicated are primarily viruses, particularly the paramyxovirus family (that includes mumps, parainfluenza, and measles viruses), but no definitive microorganism has yet been identified.[91,92] Of individuals diagnosed with Paget's disease, 10 to 30% have mutations of a specific gene, *sequestosome-1* (*SQSTM1*).[93,94] Interaction between genetic and environmental factors appears to increase osteoclast activity in Paget's disease.

PATHOPHYSIOLOGY Certain chromosomes on *SQSTM1* are known to affect osteoclast differentiation and function, although the exact locus of the genetic abnormality has yet to be identified.[92,95] Paget's disease begins with excessive resorption of spongy bone and deposition of disorganized bone. The trabeculae diminish, and bone marrow is replaced by extremely vascular fibrous tissue.

The resorption phase of Paget's disease is followed by the formation of abnormal new bone at an accelerated rate. The collagen fibres are disorganized, and glycoprotein levels in the matrix decrease. Mineralization may extend into the bone marrow. Bone formation is excessive around partially resorbed trabeculae, causing them to thicken and enlarge. The net result of this accelerated remodelling process is increased bone fragility and an increased risk for bone tumours.[96]

CLINICAL MANIFESTATIONS In the skull, abnormal remodelling is first evident in the frontal or occipital regions; then it encroaches on the outer and inner surfaces of the entire skull. The skull thickens and assumes an asymmetric shape. Thickened segments of the skull may compress areas of the brain, producing altered mentality and dementia. Impingement of new bone on cranial nerves causes sensory abnormalities, impaired motor function, deafness (because of involvement of the middle ear ossicles or compression of the auditory nerve), atrophy of the optic nerve, and obstruction of the lacrimal duct. Headache is commonly noted.

Extensive alterations of the facial bones are rare except in the jaw, where sclerosis and thickening of the maxilla and mandible displace teeth and produce malocclusion. In long bones, resorption begins in the subchondral regions of the epiphysis and extends into the metaphysis and diaphysis. Occasionally, Paget's disease affects both ends of a tubular bone. In the femur, Paget's disease produces an exaggerated lateral curvature. In the tibia, anterior curvature is also exaggerated. Stress fractures are common in the lower extremities.

Clinical manifestations of Paget's disease in the vertebral column depend on the level of involvement and are caused by compression of adjacent structures. In the cervical spine, cord compression can lead to spastic quadriplegia. Approximately 1% of persons with Paget's disease develop osteogenic sarcoma.

EVALUATION AND TREATMENT Evaluation of Paget's disease is made on the basis of radiographic findings of irregular bone trabeculae with a thickened and disorganized pattern. Early disease is detected by bone scanning that shows increased uptake of bone radionuclides. Plasma alkaline phosphatase and urinary hydroxyproline levels are elevated.

Many individuals require no treatment if the disease is localized and does not cause symptoms. Treatment during active disease is for relief of pain and prevention of deformity or fracture. Bisphosphonates are the treatment of choice; a one-time infusion of zoledronic acid can provide long-term reduction of biochemical markers and even remission.[97,100] Newer agents, including monoclonal antibodies (denosumab), interleukin-6 (IL-6) receptor inhibitors (tocilizumab [Actemra]), cathepsin K inhibitors, and Dickkopk-1 inhibitors, are under study for treatment of Paget's disease.[89,96]

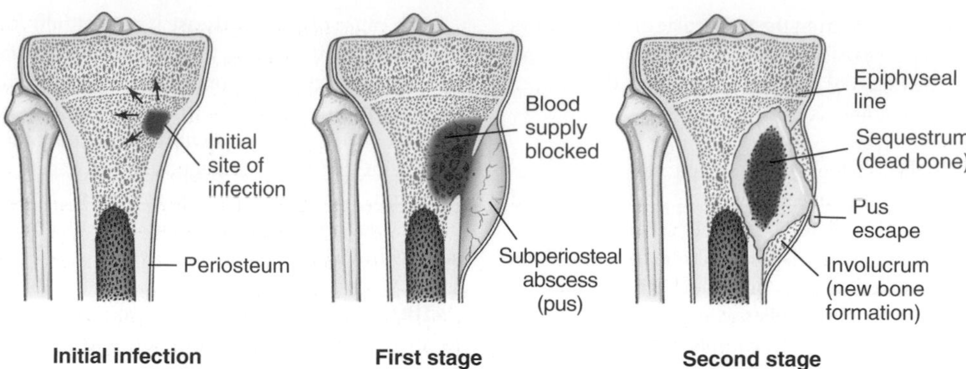

FIGURE 39-14 Osteomyelitis Showing Sequestration and Involucrum.

Infectious Bone Disease: Osteomyelitis

Osteomyelitis is a bone infection most often caused by bacteria; however, fungi, parasites, and viruses also can cause bone infection (Figure 39-14). Multiple classification systems have been used to describe osteomyelitis; the simplest refers to the mode of infection. A bone infection caused by pathogens carried through the bloodstream is termed **hematogenous osteomyelitis**. Acute hematogenous osteomyelitis is more often seen in children and is characterized by fever, pain, and voluntary immobility of the affected limb. (Osteomyelitis in children is discussed in Chapter 40.) **Contiguous osteomyelitis** occurs when infection spreads to an adjacent bone and is often caused by open fractures, penetrating wounds, or surgical procedures. Other causes of osteomyelitis include metabolic and vascular diseases (diabetes, peripheral vascular disease), lifestyle risks (smoking, alcohol or drug abuse), and advanced age.[101] In infants, incidence rates among males and females are approximately equal. In children and older adults, however, males are most commonly affected. A new category of autoimmune, noninfectious osteomyelitis, known as chronic nonbacterial osteomyelitis (CNO), has recently been identified as a cause of chronic bone pain in children.[102]

Staphylococcus aureus remains the primary microorganism responsible for osteomyelitis.[103-105] Other microorganisms include group B streptococcus, *Haemophilus influenzae*, *Salmonella*, and gram-negative bacteria. Group B streptococcus and *H. influenzae* tend to infect young children; *Salmonella* infection is associated with sickle cell anemia; and gram-negative infections are most common in older adults and immunocompromised individuals with impaired immunity. Mycobacterial, viral, and fungal infections occur in immunocompromised individuals.

Cutaneous, sinus, ear, and dental infections are the primary sources of bacteria in hematogenous bone infections. Soft tissue infections, disorders of the gastro-intestinal tract, infections of the genitourinary system, and respiratory tract infections are also sources of bacterial contamination. In addition, infections that occur after total joint replacement procedures are sometimes the cause. The vulnerability of specific bone depends on the anatomy of its vascular supply.

In adults, hematogenous osteomyelitis is more common in the spine, pelvis, and small bones. Microorganisms reach the vertebrae through arteries, veins, or lymphatic vessels. The spread of infection from pelvic organs to the vertebrae is well documented. Vaginal, uterine, ovarian, bladder, and intestinal infections can lead to iliac or sacral osteomyelitis.

Superficial animal or human bites inoculate local soft tissue with bacteria that later spread to underlying bone. Deep bites can introduce microorganisms directly onto bone. The most common infecting organism in human bites is *S. aureus*. In animal bites, the most common infecting organism is *Pasteurella multocida*, which is part of the normal mouth flora of cats and dogs.

Direct contamination of bones with bacteria can also occur in open fractures or dislocations with an overlying skin wound. Intervertebral disc surgery and operative procedures involving implantation of large foreign objects, such as metallic plates or artificial joints, are associated with contiguous osteomyelitis. Osteomyelitis of the arm and hand bones tends to occur in persons who abuse medications. In general, persons who are chronically ill, have diabetes or alcoholism, or are receiving large doses of steroids or immunosuppressive medications are particularly susceptible to chronic osteomyelitis or recurring episodes of this disease.

PATHOPHYSIOLOGY Regardless of the source of the pathogen, the pathological features of bone infection are similar to those in any other body tissue (see Chapter 6). First, the invading pathogen provokes an intense inflammatory response. *S. aureus*, in addition to producing toxins that destroy neutrophils, also forms colonies of microorganisms, called *biofilms*, that adhere to surfaces (such as implants) and increase antibiotic resistance. Biofilms also can reduce the duration of osteoblast activity while enhancing osteoclast activity and promoting inflammation[106-108] (also see Chapter 8). Primarily through activation of the cytokine pathway, the biofilm and inflammation alter the normal balance between osteoblast and osteoclast activity.[105,109] Inflammation in bone is characterized by vascular engorgement, edema, leukocyte activity, and abscess formation. Once inflammation is initiated, the small terminal vessels thrombose and exudate seals the bone's canaliculi. Inflammatory exudate extends into the metaphysis and the marrow cavity and through small metaphyseal openings into the cortex. In children, exudate that reaches the outer surface of the cortex forms abscesses that lift the periosteum of underlying bone. Lifting of the periosteum disrupts blood vessels that enter bone through the periosteum, which deprives underlying bone of its blood supply. This leads to necrosis and death of the area of bone infected, producing **sequestrum**, an area of devitalized bone. Lifting of the periosteum also stimulates an intense osteoblastic response. Osteoblasts lay down new bone that can partially or completely surround the infected bone. This layer of new bone surrounding the infected bone is called an **involucrum** (Figure 39-15). Openings in the involucrum allow the exudate to escape into surrounding soft tissue and ultimately through the skin by way of sinus tracts.

In adults, this complication is rare because the periosteum is firmly attached to the cortex and resists displacement. Instead, infection disrupts and weakens the cortex, which predisposes the bone to pathological fracture.

CLINICAL MANIFESTATIONS Clinical manifestations of osteomyelitis vary with the age of the individual, the site of involvement, the initiating event, the infecting organism, and the type of infection—acute, subacute, or chronic. Osteomyelitis is generally considered acute if diagnosed

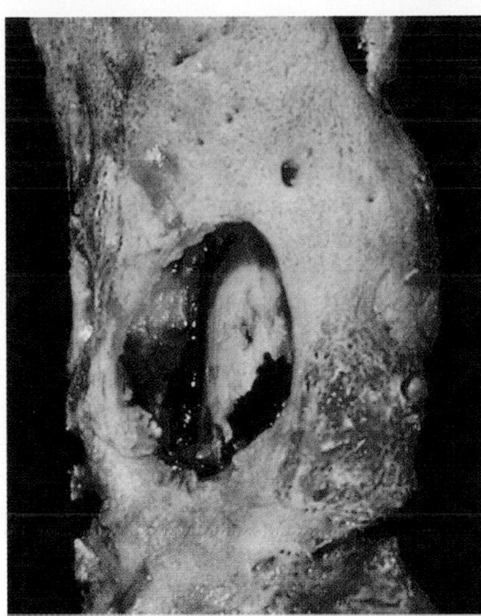

FIGURE 39-15 Resected Femur in a Person With Draining Osteomyelitis. The drainage tract in the subperiosteal shell of viable new bone (involucrum) reveals the inner native necrotic cortex (sequestrum). (From Kumar, V., Abbas, A.K., & Aster, J.C. [Eds.]. [2015]. *Robbins and Cotran pathologic basis of disease* [9th ed.]. Philadelphia: Saunders.)

within 2 weeks after symptom onset and is associated with abrupt onset of inflammation (see Figure 39-15). Subacute osteomyelitis is disease that has been present for 1 to several months, and chronic disease is that which has been present for many months to even years.[101,110]

If an acute infection is not completely eliminated, the disease may become subacute or chronic. In subacute osteomyelitis, signs and symptoms are usually vague. In the chronic stage, infection is indolent or silent between exacerbations. The microorganisms persist in small abscesses or fragments of necrotic bone and produce occasional exacerbations of acute osteomyelitis. The progression from acute to subacute osteomyelitis may be the result of inadequate or inappropriate therapy, or the development of medication-resistant microorganisms.

In the adult, hematogenous osteomyelitis has an insidious onset. The symptoms are usually vague and include fever, malaise, anorexia, weight loss, and pain in and around the infected areas. Edema may or may not be evident. Recent infection (urinary, respiratory, cutaneous) or instrumentation (catheterization, cystoscopy, myelography, discography) usually precedes onset of symptoms.

Single or multiple abscesses (Brodie abscesses) characterize subacute or chronic osteomyelitis. Brodie abscesses are circumscribed lesions 1 to 4 cm in diameter that are found usually in the ends of long bones and surrounded by dense ossified bone matrix. The abscesses are thought to develop when the infectious microorganism has become less virulent or the individual's immune system is resisting the infection somewhat successfully.

In contiguous osteomyelitis, signs and symptoms of soft tissue infection predominate. Inflammatory exudate in the soft tissues disrupts muscles and supporting structures and forms abscesses. Low-grade fever, lymphadenopathy, local pain, and swelling usually occur within days of contamination by a puncture wound.

EVALUATION AND TREATMENT Laboratory data show an elevated white cell count and an elevated level of noncardiac C-reactive protein (CRP). Radiographic studies include radionuclide bone scanning, CT, functional imaging using a combination of radionuclide scanning (using fluorodeoxyglucose [FDG]) and single-photon emission computed tomography (SPECT), positron emission tomography (PET), and MRI. MRI scanning with gadolinium contrast shows both bone and soft tissue, providing more accurate assessment of infection. MRI also shows early changes of bone marrow edema. FDG-SPECT imaging is highly sensitive for evaluating osteomyelitis of the extremities.[111]

Treatment of osteomyelitis includes bone biopsy to identify the causative organism, use of antimicrobial agents, and débridement of infected bone.[104,112] Biodegradable antibiotic-impregnated bioabsorbable beads have also benefited many individuals; newer therapies include the promise of injectable scaffolds impregnated with antibiotics and other antimicrobial substances.[113] Chronic conditions may require surgical removal of the inflammatory exudate followed by continuous wound irrigation with antibiotic solutions in addition to systemic treatment with antibiotics. The ideal antibiotic regimen for treating osteomyelitis has not yet been developed. **Hyperbaric oxygen therapy** with 100% oxygen may stimulate healing by suppressing proinflammatory cytokines and prostaglandins. Implants for total joint replacements may be removed to treat the infected joint more thoroughly.

QUICK CHECK 39-2
1. What are the causes associated with osteoporosis in women and men?
2. How does osteoporosis differ from osteomalacia? Name three differences.
3. What are the risk factors for osteomyelitis?

DISORDERS OF JOINTS

The Canadian Rheumatology Association (https://rheum.ca) recognizes several groups of joint disease (arthropathies). Most of these disorders can be placed into two major categories: noninflammatory joint disease and inflammatory joint disease. With the improvement in detection methods, however, inflammatory pathways are now being identified in conditions previously classified as noninflammatory, such as osteoarthritis.

Osteoarthritis

Osteoarthritis (OA) is the most common age-related disorder of synovial joints. Affecting the entire joint, OA is characterized by local areas of loss and damage of articular cartilage, inflammation, new bone formation of joint margins (osteophytosis), subchondral bone changes, variable degrees of mild synovitis, and thickening of the joint capsule (Figure 39-16). Pathology centres on load-bearing areas. Advancing disease shows narrowing of the joint space attributable to cartilage loss, bone spurs (**osteophytes**), and sometimes changes in the subchondral bone. OA can arise in any synovial joint but is commonly found in the knees, hips, hands, and spine. It is less common in people younger than 40 years of age, and its prevalence increases with age. Although the exact causes of OA are unclear, obesity and trauma are well-known risk factors.[114] Recent research has identified specific microRNAs that affect gene expression in chondrocytes and that may play a role in developing OA.[115,116] OA involves a complex interaction of transcription factors, cytokines, growth factors, matrix molecules, the immune system, mechanical stresses on joints, and enzymes[117-119] (see the following "Pathophysiology" section). Emerging understanding of synovitis and inflammation in OA has led to the recognition of the role played by the body's immune system in OA.[120]

Although incidence rates are quite similar in men and women, after age 50, women typically are more severely affected. OA usually occurs in those persons who put exceptional stress (or joint loading) on joints (e.g., obese persons, gymnasts, long-distance runners or marathoners); persons participating in such sports as basketball, soccer, or football have been shown to develop OA at earlier ages than usual. Obesity itself seems to be an independent risk factor for developing

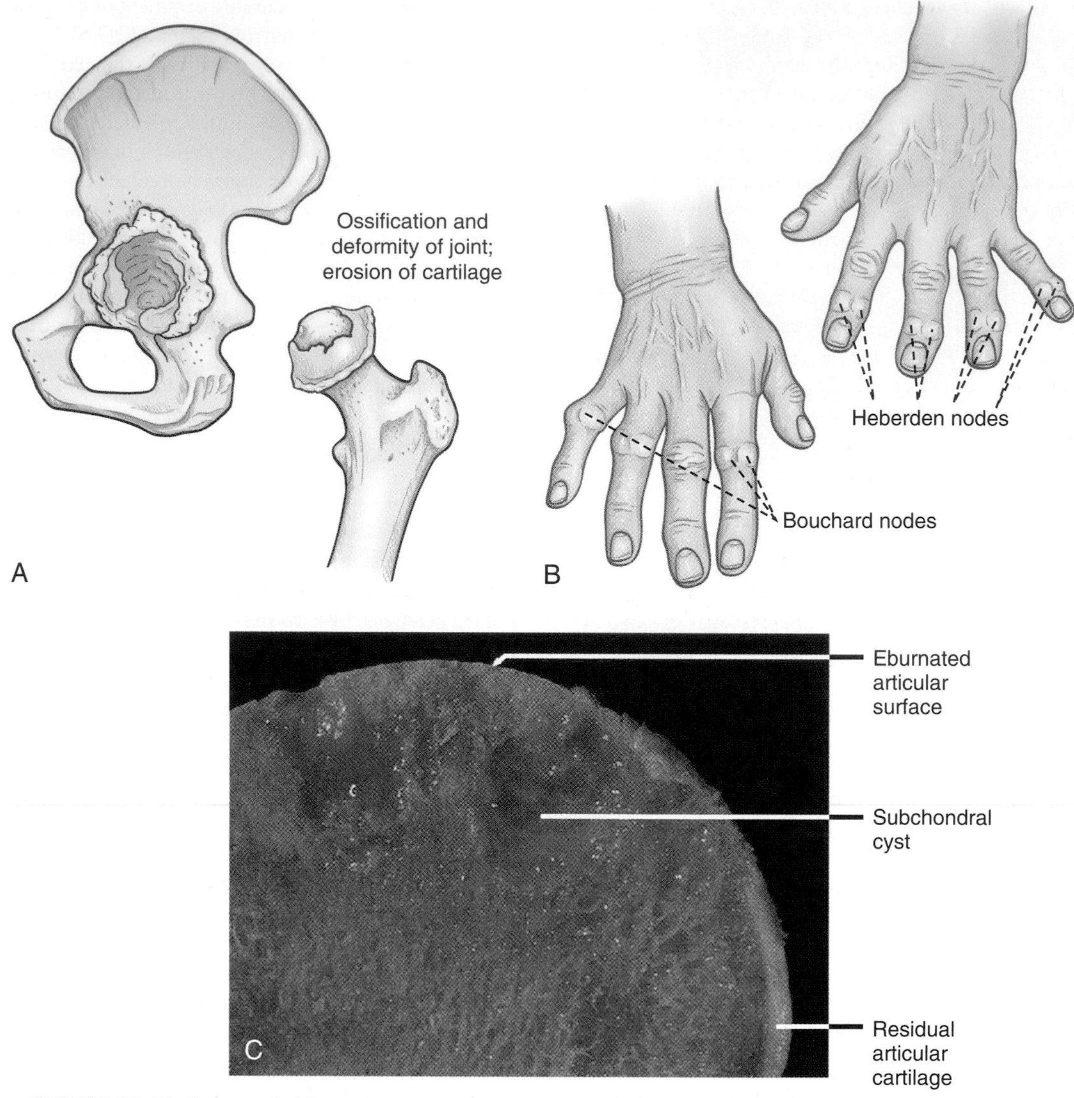

FIGURE 39-16 Osteoarthritis. A, Cartilage and degeneration of the hip joint from osteoarthritis. **B,** Heberden nodes and Bouchard nodes. **C,** Severe osteoarthritis with small islands of residual articular cartilage next to exposed subchondral bone. (**C,** from Kumar, V., Abbas, A.K., & Aster, J.C. [2015]. *Robbins and Cotran pathologic basis of disease* [9th ed.]. Philadelphia: Saunders.)

OA of the knee.[121-124] Chondrocyte death because of mitochondrial release of reactive oxygen species (ROS) is thought to be caused by increased stress on joints.[118] A previously torn anterior cruciate ligament or meniscectomy increases the risk for accelerated OA of the knee.[125,126]

Types of Osteoarthritis

PATHOPHYSIOLOGY The primary defect in OA is loss of articular cartilage.[127] Early in the disease, the articular cartilage loses its glistening appearance, becoming yellow-grey or brownish grey. As the disease progresses, surface areas of the articular cartilage flake off, and deeper layers develop longitudinal fissures (fibrillation). The cartilage becomes thin and may be absent over some areas, leaving the underlying bone (subchondral bone) unprotected. Consequently, the unprotected subchondral bone becomes sclerotic (dense and hard). Cysts sometimes develop within the subchondral bone and communicate with the longitudinal fissures in the cartilage. Pressure builds in the cysts until the cystic contents are forced into the synovial cavity, breaking through the articular cartilage on the way. As the articular cartilage erodes, cartilage-coated osteophytes may grow outward from the underlying bone and alter the bone contours and joint anatomy. These spurlike bony projections enlarge until small pieces, called *joint mice*, break off into the synovial cavity. If osteophyte fragments irritate the synovial membrane, synovitis and joint effusion result. Interestingly, joint pain may be more related to inflammation of the synovium than subsequent cartilage damage or the radiographic extent of arthritis.[128,129] The joint capsule also becomes thickened and at times adheres to the deformed underlying bone, which may contribute to the limited range of motion of the joint (see Figure 39-16).

Articular cartilage is lost through a cascade of signalling, cytokine, and anabolic growth factor pathways.[130,131] Enzymatic processes (including matrix metalloproteinases [MMPs]) assist in breaking the macromolecules of proteoglycans, glycosaminoglycans, and collagen into large, diffusible fragments. Then the fragments are taken up by the cartilage cells (chondrocytes) and digested by the cell's own lysosomal enzymes. (Processes of cellular uptake and lysosomal digestion are described in Chapter 1.) The loss of proteoglycans from articular cartilage is a hallmark of the osteoarthritic process.

Enzymatic destruction of articular cartilage begins in the matrix with destruction of proteoglycans and collagen fibres. Enzymes, particularly stromelysin and acid metalloproteinases, affect proteoglycans by interfering with assembly of the proteoglycan subunit or the proteoglycan aggregate (see Chapter 38); levels of these enzymes are markedly elevated in OA. Changes in the conformation of proteoglycans disrupt the pumping action that regulates movement of water and synovial fluid into and out of the cartilage. Without the regulatory action of the proteoglycan pump, cartilage imbibes too much fluid and becomes less able to withstand the stresses of weight-bearing. With aging, the proteoglycan content is decreased, and water content in cartilage can be increased by as much as 8%, affecting the strength of the cartilage. Persons with OA, even those with fairly extensive cartilage destruction, have elevated levels of proteoglycans or fragments in their synovial fluid, perhaps indicative of the degree of disease activity. MicroRNAs, small nucleic acids that do not code for proteins (but appear to regulate the RNAs that do), may have a direct effect on developing OA by targeting specific genes involved in cartilage development and homeostasis.[116,132,133] Disruptions in cellular signalling pathways, particularly the TGF-β superfamily, play a significant role in developing OA.[134] Other studies indicate that cytokines, such as interleukin-1 (IL-1) and TNF (see Chapter 7 for discussion of cytokines), play a major role in cartilage degradation[130] as a result of release and activation of proteolytic and collagenolytic enzymes associated with an imbalance of cell responses to growth factor activity.[135,136]

Cell-signalling proteins, particularly adipokines such as adiponectin and collagenases (enzymes that degrade collagen), contribute to collagen breakdown in cartilage.[137] Collagen breakdown destroys the fibrils that give articular cartilage its tensile strength and exposes the chondrocytes to mechanical stress and enzyme attack. The osteochondral junction formed by cartilage and its underlying subchondral bone allows alterations in one tissue to affect the adjacent one (biomechanical coupling). When articular cartilage is damaged, abnormal subchondral bone remodelling occurs.[138,139] Thus, a cycle of destruction begins that involves all the components of a joint: cartilage, bone, and the synovium.

CLINICAL MANIFESTATIONS Clinical manifestations of OA typically appear during the fifth or sixth decade of life; although often asymptomatic, articular surface changes are common after the age of 40. Pain in one or more joints—usually with weight-bearing, use of the joint, or load bearing—is the first and most predominant symptom of the disease. Resting the joint often relieves pain. If present, nocturnal pain is usually not relieved by rest and may be accompanied by paresthesias (numbness, tingling, or prickling sensations). Sometimes pain is referred to another part of the body. For example, OA of the lumbosacral spine may mimic sciatica, causing severe pain in the back of the thigh along the course of the sciatic nerve. OA in the lower cervical spine may cause brachial neuralgia (pain in the arm) and is aggravated by movement of the neck. Osteoarthritic conditions in the hip cause pain that may be referred to the lower thigh and knee area. Sleep deprivation adds to the stress of the persistent pain of OA. Physical examination of the person with OA usually shows general involvement of both peripheral and central joints. Peripheral joints most often involved are in the hands, wrists, knees, and feet. Central joints most often afflicted are in the lower cervical spine, lumbosacral spine, shoulders, and hips.

Joint structures are capable of generating a limited number of signs and symptoms. The primary signs and symptoms of osteoarthritic joint disease are pain, stiffness, enlargement or swelling, tenderness, limited range of motion, muscle wasting, partial dislocation, and deformity (see *Risk Factors:* Osteoarthritis).

RISK FACTORS

Osteoarthritis

- Trauma, sprains, strains, joint dislocations, and fractures
- Long-term mechanical stress—athletics, ballet dancing, repetitive physical tasks, and obesity
- Inflammation in joint structures
- Joint instability from damage to supporting structures
- Neurological disorders (e.g., diabetic neuropathy, Charcot neuropathic joint) in which pain and proprioceptive reflexes are diminished or lost
- Congenital or acquired skeletal deformities
- Hematological or endocrine disorders, such as hemophilia, which causes chronic bleeding into the joints, or hyperparathyroidism, which causes bone to lose calcium
- Medications (e.g., colchicine, indomethacin [Indocin], steroids) that stimulate the collagen-digesting enzymes in the synovial membrane

The origin of joint stiffness is unknown. **Joint stiffness** is generally defined as difficulty initiating joint movement, immobility, or a loss of range of motion. The stiffness usually occurs as joint movement begins, and it dissipates rapidly after a few minutes. Stiffness lasting longer than 30 minutes is uncommon in OA. Enlargement and bulging of bone contour, commonly described as swelling, may be caused by bone enlargement or the proliferation of osteophytes around the margins of the joint. In the hands, these areas are called Heberden and Bouchard nodes, where they are typical features of OA (see Figure 39-16). Inflammation of the joint lining, known as synovitis, is thought to be initiated by the release of cartilage extracellular matrix into the joint, which then activates the body's complement system.[140] Swelling also occurs if inflammatory exudate or blood enters the joint cavity, thereby increasing the volume of synovial fluid. This condition, termed **joint effusion**, is caused by (1) the presence of osteophyte fragments in the synovial cavity, (2) drainage of cysts from diseased subchondral bone, or (3) acute trauma to joint structures, resulting in hemorrhage and inflammatory exudation into the synovial cavity (Figure 39-16, *C*).

Range of motion is limited to some degree, depending on the extent of cartilage degeneration. Frequently, joint motion is accompanied by sounds of crepitus, creaking, or grating. Hypermobility and subluxation of joints occur in OA secondary to a neurological disorder. Abnormal knee alignment (either varus or valgus) has been shown to be a risk factor for and can increase progression of the disease.[141,142]

As OA of the lower extremity progresses, the person may begin to noticeably limp (Figure 39-17). Having a limp is distressing because it affects the person's independence and ability to perform the usual activities of daily living. The affected joint is also more symptomatic after use, such as at the end of a period of strenuous activity.

EVALUATION AND TREATMENT Evaluation consists primarily of clinical assessment and radiological studies. More expensive studies, including CT scan, arthroscopy, and MRI, are rarely needed. Newer imaging technologies, such as compositional MRI, are showing promise in identifying structural changes in cartilage; improvements in technology may also allow better monitoring of OA treatment.

Treatment is either conservative or surgical. Conservative treatment includes both pharmacological and nonpharmacological therapies; surgery is a last resort. Both exercise and weight loss have been shown to be two of the most important nonpharmacological treatments in improving knee OA symptoms. Exercise can reduce pain and improve physical function in people with knee OA.[143-147] Exercises to improve muscle tone, range of motion, and balance; stretch the joint capsule;

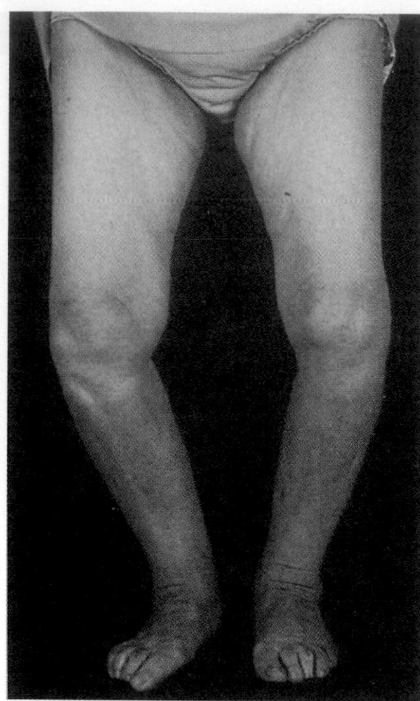

FIGURE 39-17 Typical Varus Deformity of Knee Osteoarthritis. (From Doherty, M. [1994]. *Color atlas and text of osteoarthritis*. London: Wolfe.)

and decrease fear of falling also have shown promise in reducing OA symptoms.[148,149] Braces and foot orthoses may help correct biomechanical abnormalities, thereby reducing pain and improving mobility.[150] Dietary and nutritional supplements can sometimes also improve symptoms. Nutraceuticals, such as chondroitin and glucosamine, have shown success in relieving OA pain in some individuals.[151] Other nonsurgical therapies include analgesic and anti-inflammatory medication therapy to reduce swelling and pain. Acetaminophen (Tylenol) was once considered first-line treatment, but it has been shown to be less effective than nonsteroidal anti-inflammatory drugs (NSAIDs), such as ibuprofen (Advil). However, prolonged use significantly increases the risk for serious associated side effects that are common.[152] Intra-articular injection of corticosteroids and high-molecular-weight viscose supplements, such as hyaluronic acid, also decreases knee pain with OA.[153,154] Recently, because of its high concentration of growth factors, PRP also has been injected into osteoarthritic knee joints with some success in reducing pain and markers of inflammation.[155] Current evidence does not support low-level laser therapy for knee OA.[156] Newer agents, including inhibitors of cytokines, MMPs, and leptin, are under investigation and may prove more effective in treating OA. Surgery is used to improve joint movement, correct deformity or malalignment, or create a new joint with artificial implants. It has been estimated by some researchers that 1 in 4 individuals has a lifetime risk of developing symptomatic OA of the hip.[157] In Canada, 49 503 total hip and 60 136 total knee replacement surgeries were performed in 2013–14, and most were related to OA.[158]

Classic Inflammatory Joint Disease

Inflammatory joint disease is commonly called **arthritis**. Inflammatory joint disease is characterized by inflammatory damage or destruction in the synovial membrane or articular cartilage and by systemic signs of inflammation (fever, leukocytosis, malaise, anorexia, hyperfibrinogenemia).

Inflammatory joint disease can be infectious or noninfectious. Infectious inflammatory joint disease is caused by invasion of the joint by bacteria, mycoplasmas, viruses, fungi, or protozoa. These agents can invade the joint through a traumatic wound, surgical incision, or contaminated needle, or they can be delivered by the bloodstream from sites of infection elsewhere in the body—typically bones, heart valves, or blood vessels. Noninfectious inflammatory joint disease, the most common form, is caused by immune reactions or the deposition of crystals of monosodium urate (MSU) in and around the joint. RA, psoriatic arthritis, and ankylosing spondylitis (AS) are noninfectious inflammatory diseases caused by immune reactions and possibly hypersensitivity reactions; gouty arthritis is a noninfectious inflammatory disease caused by crystal deposition.

Rheumatoid Arthritis

Rheumatoid arthritis (RA) is a chronic, systemic, inflammatory autoimmune disease distinguished by joint swelling and tenderness and destruction of synovial joints, leading to disability and premature death.[159] (Autoimmune disease is described in Chapter 8.) The first joint tissue to be affected is the synovial membrane, which lines the joint cavity (see Chapter 36, Figure 36-9). The two primary types of synovial cells are fibroblastlike synovial cells and macrophagelike synovial cells. Though the initiating mechanism of RA is still unknown, its pathology is fairly well understood. Some factor activates the synovial fibroblasts (SFs) that line the joint cavity.[160-162] The SFs undergo significant changes and develop an exaggerated immune response. Once activated, both types of SF abnormally proliferate and produce proinflammatory cytokines, enzymes, and prostaglandins that perpetuate the inflammatory process,[163] including increasing their lining depth from the normal 1 to 2 cells deep up to 10 to 20 cells thick. This thickened synovial tissue, called "pannus," invades the bone and acts like a localized tumour, where other factors (including increased osteoclast activity) cause bone destruction.[164] Some of the most significant synovial changes involve altered signalling pathways for immune reactions, where SFs attach to articular cartilage and attack it, causing more inflammation; the release of enzymes, such as MMPs, inflammatory chemokines, and cytokines (interleukins and TNF); and ingrowth of blood vessels. Increased blood vessel formation improves the opportunity for activated SFs to enter the bloodstream and affect other joints.[165-167] Eventually, inflammation spreads to the fibrous joint capsule and surrounding ligaments and tendons, causing pain, joint deformity, and loss of function (Figure 39-18). The joints most commonly affected are in the fingers, feet, wrists, elbows, ankles, and knees, but the shoulders, hips, and cervical spine also may be involved, as well as the tissues of the lungs, heart, kidneys, and skin.

The incidence and prevalence of RA have decreased over the past five decades; RA now affects about 1% of the adult population in developed countries.[168] The frequency of RA increases with age. Besides inflammation and destruction of the joints, RA can cause fever, malaise, rash, lymph node or spleen enlargement, and Raynaud phenomenon (transient lack of circulation to the fingertips and toes).

Despite intensive research, the exact cause of RA remains obscure. It is likely a combination of genetic factors interacting with inflammatory mediators. There is a strong genetic predisposition to developing RA. The chronic inflammation characteristics of RA result from an intricate interplay of chemokines that are powerful mediators of inflammation. Ligand/receptor chemokines attract T lymphocytes (T cells) and produce inflammatory changes.[165] A key genetic element has been localized to the human leukocyte antigen (HLA) areas of the major histocompatibility complex in all ethnic groups. Recent research reveals the possibility of specific amino acid malpositions in the HLA molecule as a major factor in developing rheumatic diseases.[169] A surprising new discovery is the presence of T-cell abnormalities in individuals with RA, indicating a defect in telomere repair that may result in faster aging of telomeres

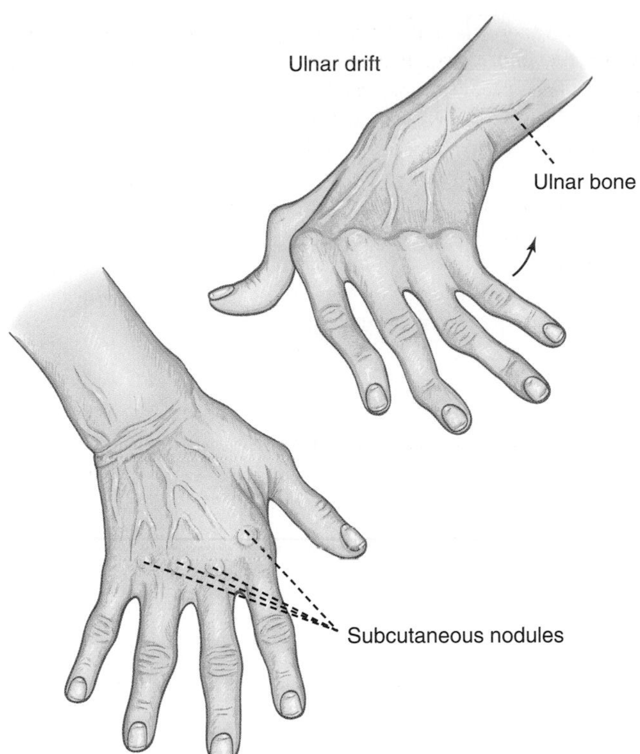

FIGURE 39-18 Rheumatoid Arthritis of the Hand. Note swelling from chronic synovitis of metacarpophalangeal joints, marked ulnar drift, subcutaneous nodules, and subluxation of metacarpophalangeal joints with extension of proximal interphalangeal joints and flexion of distal joints. Note also deformed position of thumb. Hand has wasted appearance. (From Mourad, L.A. [1991]. *Orthopedic disorders.* St. Louis: Mosby.)

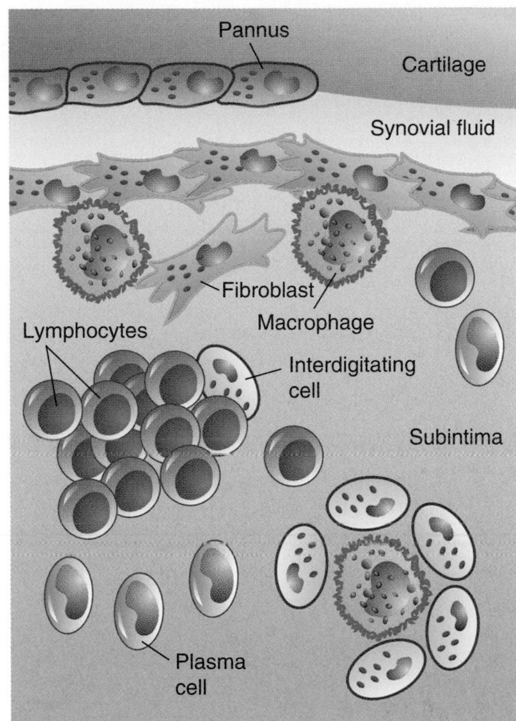

FIGURE 39-19 Synovitis. Inflamed synovium showing typical arrangements of macrophages and fibroblastic cells.

and consequent less efficient immune function. With long-term or intensive exposure to the antigen, normal antibodies (immunoglobulins [Igs]) become autoantibodies—antibodies that attack host tissues (self-antigens). Because they are usually present in individuals with RA, the altered antibodies are termed **rheumatoid factors (RFs)**. The RFs usually consist of two classes of immunoglobulin antibodies (antibodies for IgM and IgG) but occasionally involve antibodies for IgA. Their main antigenic targets are portions of the Ig molecules. RFs bind with their target self-antigens in blood and synovial membrane, forming immune complexes (antigen–antibody complexes). (See Chapter 7 for a discussion about antigen–antibody binding in the immune response.)

Environmental factors, including geographical area of birth, diet, socioeconomic status, and especially smoking, have been identified as risk factors for developing and having higher disease activity of RA.[170,171] RA and other autoimmune diseases have a higher prevalence among women. Additionally, because disease symptoms lessen during pregnancy and are increased again in the postpartal period, researchers are including hormonal involvement in their studies.

PATHOPHYSIOLOGY Although no specific events (such as trauma, illness, or environmental conditions) have been identified that would cause immune abnormalities to develop into localized tissue and joint inflammation, the pathology of RA is fairly well understood. During inflammation, arginine (an α-amino acid) can be enzymatically modified into another α-amino acid, citrulline. This process (citrullination) changes the structure and function of the protein. Other proteins, such as fibrin and vimentin, become citrullinated during cell death and tissue inflammation.[172] In turn, the citrullinated proteins can be seen as antigens by the body's immune system.[173] Thus, both T cells and B cells (B lymphocytes) play a role in the autoimmune response. T cells express RANKL, which promotes osteoclast formation and causes bony erosion.

Basically, cartilage damage in RA is the result of at least three processes: (1) neutrophils and other cells in the synovial fluid become activated, degrading the surface layer of articular cartilage; (2) inflammatory cytokines, particularly tumour necrosis factor-alpha (TNF-α), interleukin-1beta (IL-1β), IL-6, IL-7, and IL-21 induce enzymatic (metalloproteinase) breakdown of cartilage and bone; and (3) T cells also interact with SFs through TNF-α, converting synovium into a thick, abnormal layer of granulation tissue known as **pannus** (see Chapter 7). Macrophages, components of pannus (Figure 39-19), stimulate the release of IL-1, platelet-derived growth factor (PDGF), and fibronectin. The B cells are stimulated to produce more RFs. The newly targeted self-antigens (Igs) are in relatively constant supply and can thus perpetuate inflammation and the formation of immune complexes indefinitely (Figure 39-20).

Inflammatory and immune processes have several damaging effects on the synovial membrane. Along with the swelling caused by leukocyte infiltration, the synovial membrane undergoes hyperplastic thickening as its cells proliferate and abnormally enlarge. As synovial inflammation progresses to involve its blood vessels, small venules become occluded by hypertrophied endothelial cells, fibrin, platelets, and inflammatory cells, which decrease vascular flow to the synovial tissue. Compromised circulation, coupled with increased metabolic needs as a result of hypertrophy and hyperplasia, causes hypoxia and metabolic acidosis. Acidosis stimulates the release of hydrolytic enzymes from synovial cells into the surrounding tissue, initiating erosion of the articular cartilage and inflammation in the supporting ligaments and tendons. Pannus formation does not lead to synovial or articular regeneration but rather to formation of scar tissue that immobilizes the joint.

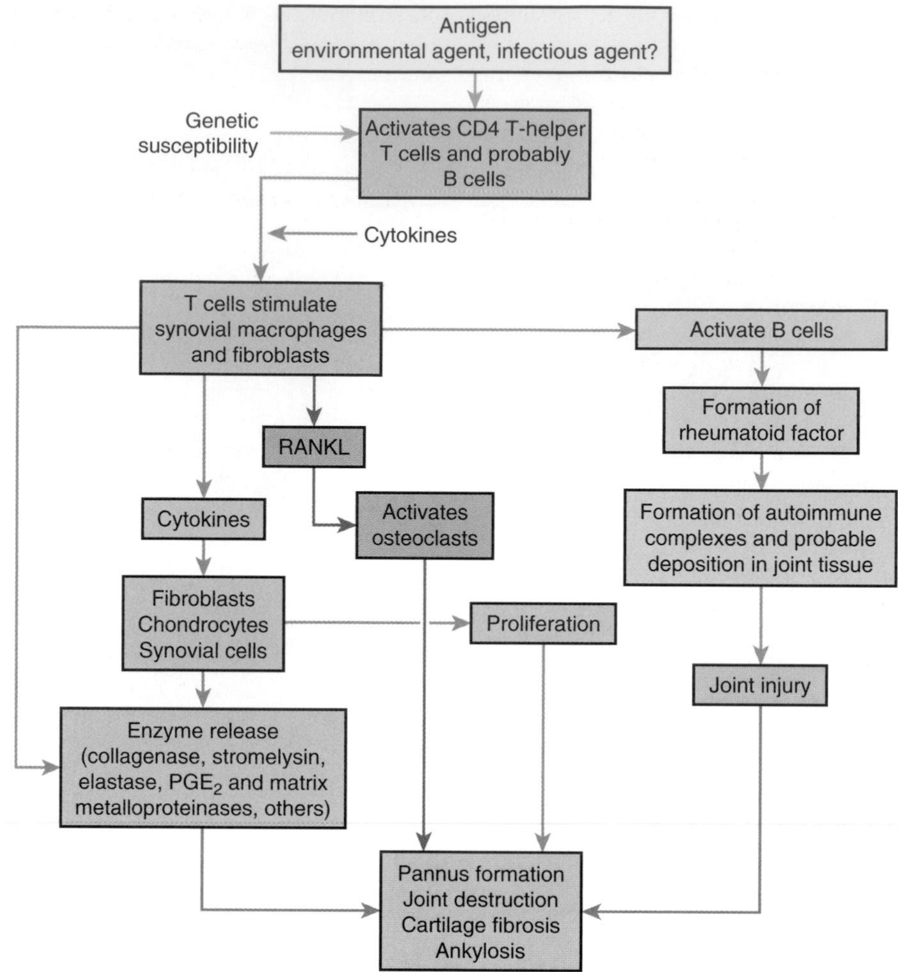

FIGURE 39-20 Emerging Model of Pathogenesis of Rheumatoid Arthritis. Rheumatoid arthritis is an autoimmune disease of a genetically susceptible host triggered by an unknown antigenic agent. Chronic autoimmune reaction with activation of CD4+ T-helper cells and possibly other lymphocytes and the local release of inflammatory cytokines and mediators eventually destroy the joint. T cells stimulate cells in the joint to produce cytokines that are key mediators of synovial damage. Apparently, immune complex deposition also plays a role. Tumour necrosis factor and interleukin-1, as well as some other cytokines, stimulate synovial cells to proliferate and produce other mediators of inflammation, such as prostaglandin E_2 (*PGE_2*), matrix metalloproteinases, and enzymes that all contribute to destruction of cartilage. Activated T cells and synovial fibroblasts also produce receptor activator of nuclear factor kappa-B ligand (*RANKL*), which activates the osteoclasts and promotes bone destruction. Pannus is a mass of synovium and synovial stroma with inflammatory cells, granulation tissue, and fibroblasts that grows over the articular surface and causes its destruction.

CLINICAL MANIFESTATIONS The onset of RA is usually insidious, although as many as 15% of cases have an acute onset. RA begins with general systemic manifestations of inflammation, including fever, fatigue, weakness, anorexia, weight loss, and generalized aching and stiffness. Local manifestations also appear gradually over a period of weeks or months. Typically, the joints become painful, tender, and stiff. Pain early in the disease is caused by pressure from swelling. Later in the disease, pain is caused by sclerosis of subchondral bone and new bone formation. Pain and inability to perform normal functions are the main reasons people seek medical help.[174] Stiffness usually lasts for about 1 hour after rising in the morning and is thought to be related to synovitis. Initially the joints most commonly involved are the MCP joints, proximal interphalangeal (PIP) joints, and wrists, with later involvement of larger weight-bearing joints.

Widespread, symmetric joint swelling is caused by increasing amounts of inflammatory exudate (leukocytes, plasma, plasma proteins) in the synovial membrane, hyperplasia of inflamed tissues, and formation of new bone. On palpation, the swollen joint feels warm and the synovial membrane feels boggy. The skin over the joint may have a ruddy, cyanotic hue and may look thin and shiny.

An inflamed joint may lose some of its mobility. Even mild synovitis can lead to reduced range of motion, which becomes evident after inflammation subsides. Extension becomes limited and is eventually lost if flexion contractures develop. Limited range of motion can progress to permanent deformities of the fingers, toes, and limbs, including ulnar deviation of the hands, boutonnière and swan neck deformities of the finger joints, plantar subluxation of the metatarsal heads of the foot, and hallux valgus (angulation of the great toe toward the other toes). Flexion contractures of the knees and hips are also common.

Joint deformities cause the physical limitations experienced by persons with RA (see Figure 39-18). Loss of joint motion is quickly followed by secondary atrophy of the surrounding muscles. With secondary muscle atrophy, the joint becomes unstable, which further aggravates joint pathology.

Two complications of chronic RA are caused by excessive amounts of inflammatory exudate in the synovial cavity. One complication is the formation of cysts in the articular cartilage or subchondral bone. Occasionally, these cysts communicate with the skin surface (such as in the sole of the foot) and can drain through passages called *fistulae*. The second complication is rupture of a cyst or of the synovial joint itself, usually caused by strenuous physical activity that places excessive pressure on the joint. Rupture releases inflammatory exudate into adjacent tissues, thereby spreading inflammation.

Extrasynovial **rheumatoid nodules**, seen in up to 30% of individuals with RA, are the most common extra-articular manifestations. Each nodule is a collection of inflammatory cells surrounding a central core of fibrinoid and cellular debris. T cells are the predominant leukocytes in the nodule. B cells, plasma cells, and phagocytes are found around the periphery. Nodules are most often found in subcutaneous tissue over the extensor surfaces of elbows and fingers. Less common sites are the scalp, back, feet, hands, buttocks, and knees.

Rheumatoid nodules also may invade the skin, cardiac valves, pericardium, pleura, lung parenchyma, and spleen. These nodules are identical to those encountered in some individuals with rheumatic fever and are characterized by central tissue necrosis surrounded by proliferating connective tissue. Also noted are large numbers of lymphocytes and occasional plasma cells. Acute glaucoma may result with nodules forming on the sclera. Pulmonary involvement may result in diffuse pleuritis or multiple intraparenchymal nodules. Together, the occurrence of pulmonary nodules and pneumoconiosis (chronic inflammation of the lungs from inhalation of dust) creates the syndrome called **Caplan's syndrome**. Diffuse pulmonary fibrosis may occur because of immunologically mediated immune complex deposition.

Rheumatoid nodules within the heart may cause valvular deformities, particularly of the aortic valve leaflets, and pericarditis. Lymphadenopathy of the nodes close to the affected joints may develop. Rheumatoid nodules within the spleen result in splenomegaly. Involvement of blood vessels results in an acute necrotizing vasculitis, characteristic of that noted in other immunological/inflammatory states. Thromboses of such involved vessels may lead to myocardial infarctions, cerebrovascular occlusions, mesenteric infarction, kidney damage, and vascular insufficiency in the hands and fingers (Raynaud phenomenon). Fortunately, the development of vascular changes (particularly systemic vasculitis) is decreasing in frequency as more effective RA treatments are becoming available.[175] Changes in skeletal muscle are often noted in the form of nonspecific atrophy secondary to joint dysfunction.

EVALUATION AND TREATMENT The diagnosis of RA relies on clinical evaluation of joint swelling; however, limitation of movement and control of pain often prevent identification of individuals who would benefit from treatment in early stages of the disease. Early treatment can be effective in preventing the systemic and joint abnormalities of chronic disease. Research has shown that the autoantibodies RF and anti-citrullinated protein antibody (ACPA) can be present for years to decades before synovial or radiographic involvement becomes apparent.[176,177] Compared with RF, ACPA is a much more specific serum marker for RA. The American College of Rheumatology and the European League Against Rheumatism revised their RA classification criteria in 2010 to better identify the early stage of RA.[159] These criteria are shown in Table 39-5. Similarly, the Canadian Rheumatology Association revised its clinical guidelines on the management of RA in 2012 to reflect recent research on effective methods in achieving remission from the condition.[178] Clinical examination and history are the mainstays of RA diagnosis, but new imaging techniques show promise for earlier diagnosis, leading to earlier treatment with a better chance for avoiding disability and joint destruction (see *Health Promotion:* Musculo-skeletal Molecular Imaging).

HEALTH PROMOTION

Musculo-skeletal Molecular Imaging

With improved understanding of the molecular and cellular mechanisms responsible for the effects of rheumatoid arthritis (RA), new imaging techniques promise benefits in earlier and more accurate diagnosis and monitoring of cartilage and bone involvement. Imaging on that same molecular level can provide a "biological read-out" of disease progression and response to treatment. Nuclear medicine imaging, positron emission tomography (PET), and magnetic resonance imaging (MRI) all incorporate some element of molecular imaging.

New modalities of molecular imaging use various probes and contrast agents that have an affinity for specific targets, such as cells, hormones, antigens, and enzymes. Certain monoclonal antibodies have already been successfully labelled with various nuclides and could be used to identify disease progression. Bioluminescent and fluorescent imaging techniques have the advantage of being radiation-free tests and are being used to view in vivo activity, osteoblast activity, osteocalcin expression in bone damage, and osteoclast activity and gene expression during inflammation. A significant area of promise for molecular imaging in RA is recognition of the initial molecular events that occur before cartilage and joint damage becomes apparent. Better monitoring of response to medications also may allow more accurate dosing with the potential for fewer side effects. Because certain bioluminescent and fluorescent agents have specific affinities for particular cells, more efficient bone regeneration may be possible by targeted delivery of appropriate growth factors or stem cells to damaged bone and cartilage.

Data from Malviya, G., Conti, F., Chianelli, M., et al. (2010). *Eur J Med Mol Imaging, 37*(2), 386–398; Reumann, M.K., Weiser, M.C., & Mayer-Kuckuk, P. (2010). *Trends Biotechnol, 28*(2), 93–101.

Early treatment of RA begins with disease-modifying antirheumatic drugs (DMARDs), such as methotrexate, azathioprine (Imuran), sulfasalazine (Salazopyrin), hydroxychloroquine (Plaquenil), leflunomide (Arava), and cyclosporine (Sandimmune). These agents have been shown to slow the progression of RA and may prevent complications such as joint deformities and extra-articular complications. Methotrexate remains the first line of treatment. More recently, targeted treatment for RA has involved use of agents aimed at interrupting the pathogenesis of the disease. Known as biological DMARDs (bDMARDs), these medications affect specific processes in the development of RA and include TNF inhibitors, such as etanercept (Enbrel), adalimumab (Humira), and infliximab (Remicade). They have recently been augmented by the monoclonal antibodies golimumab (Simponi) and certolizumab (Cimzia). Other agents interfere with cytokine function (anakinra [Kineret] inhibits IL-1 function, and tocilizumab targets IL-6), inhibit T-cell activation (abatacept [Orencia]), or deplete B cells (rituximab [Rituxan]).

Education for individuals with RA is fundamental to treatment. Other treatments and therapies include NSAIDs, glucocorticoids, intra-articular steroid injections, physical and occupational therapy with therapeutic exercise, and use of assistive devices. Surgery is used to treat deformities or mechanical deficiencies of joints and can include synovectomy or joint replacement surgery.

Ankylosing Spondylitis

Ankylosing spondylitis (AS) is the most common of a group of inflammatory arthropathies known as *spondyloarthropathies* (SpAs). The Assessment of SpondyloArthritis International Society (ASAS) has

TABLE 39-5 The 2010 American College of Rheumatology/European League Against Rheumatism Classification Criteria for Rheumatoid Arthritis

Target population to be tested:
1. Persons who have at least one joint with definite clinical synovitis (swelling)[a]
2. Persons who have synovitis not better explained by another disease[b]

Classification criteria for RA (score-based algorithm: add scores of categories A to D; a score of ≥6/10 is needed for positive RA diagnosis)[c]

Clinical Finding	Score
A. Joint involvement[d]	
1 large joint[e]	0
2–10 large joints	1
1–3 small joints (with or without involvement of large joints)[f]	2
4–10 small joints (with or without involvement of large joints)	3
>10 joints (at least 1 small joint)[g]	5
B. Serology (at least 1 test result is needed for classification)[h]	
Negative RF *and* negative ACPA	0
Low-positive RF *or* low-positive ACPA	2
High-positive RF *or* high-positive ACPA	3
C. Acute-phase reactants (at least 1 test result is needed for classification)[i]	
Normal CRP *and* normal ESR	0
Abnormal CRP *or* abnormal ESR	1
D. Duration of symptoms[j]	
<6 weeks	0
≥6 weeks	1

[a]The criteria are aimed at classification of newly presenting persons. In addition, persons with erosive disease typical of RA with a history compatible with prior fulfillment of the 2010 criteria should be classified as having RA. Persons with longstanding disease—including those whose disease is inactive (with or without treatment) and who, based on retrospectively available data, have previously fulfilled the 2010 criteria—should be classified as having RA.

[b]Differential diagnoses vary among persons with different presentations, but may include conditions such as systemic lupus erythematosus, psoriatic arthritis, and gout. If it is unclear about the relevant differential diagnoses to consider, an expert rheumatologist should be consulted.

[c]Although persons with a score <6/10 are not classifiable as having RA, their status can be reassessed and the criteria might be fulfilled cumulatively over time.

[d]Joint involvement refers to any *swollen* or *tender* joint on examination, which may be confirmed by imaging evidence of synovitis. Distal interphalangeal joints, first metacarpophalangeal joints, and first metatarsophalangeal joints are *excluded from assessment.* Categories of joint distribution are classified according to the location and number of involved joints, with placement into the highest category possible based on the pattern of joint involvement.

[e]"Large joints" refer to shoulders, elbows, hips, knees, and ankles.

[f]"Small joints" refer to the metacarpophalangeal joints, proximal interphalangeal joints, second through fifth metatarsophalangeal joints, thumb interphalangeal joints, and wrists.

[g]In this category, at least one of the involved joints must be a small joint; the others can include any combination of large and additional small joints, as well as other joints not specifically listed elsewhere (e.g., temporomandibular, acromioclavicular, sternoclavicular).

[h]Negative refers to unit values that are less than or equal to the upper limit of normal (ULN) for the laboratory and assay; low-positive refers to values that are higher than the ULN but ≤3 times the ULN for the laboratory and assay; high-positive refers to unit values that are >3 times the ULN for the laboratory and assay. Where rheumatoid factor (RF) information is only available as positive or negative, a positive result should be scored as low-positive for RF.

[i]Normal/abnormal is determined by local laboratory standards.

[j]Duration of symptoms refers to individual's self-report of the duration of signs and symptoms of synovitis (e.g., pain, swelling, tenderness) of joints that are clinically involved at the time of assessment, regardless of treatment status.

ACPA, Anti-citrullinated protein antibody; *CRP,* C-reactive protein; *ESR,* erythrocyte sedimentation rate; *RA,* rheumatoid arthritis.

Data from Aletaha, D., Neogi, T., Silman, A.J., et al. (2010). *Arthritis Rheum, 62*(9), 2574.

recommended classifying SpAs to include individuals who do not have visible radiographic changes of the skeleton, as well as those who do. There would then be two subgroups: (1) mainly axial disease, including AS, and (2) peripheral SpA.[179] AS is a chronic inflammatory joint disease characterized by stiffening and fusion (ankylosis) of the spine and sacroiliac joints. Like RA, ankylosing spondylitis is a systemic, autoimmune inflammatory disease. Although inflammation is the primary pathological process in both RA and AS, the two diseases differ in the primary site of inflammation and the end result. In RA, the primary site of inflammation is the synovial membrane, resulting in the destruction and instability of synovial joints. In AS, excessive bone formation occurs. The primary pathological site is the enthesis (the point at which ligaments, tendons, and the joint capsule are inserted into bone), and the end result is fibrosis, ossification, and fusion of the joint, primarily the sacroiliac joints and the vertebral column (axial skeleton).

AS occurs worldwide, with the lowest prevalence in South Asian countries and the highest prevalence in North America and Europe; it affects men more often than women.[180] In women, AS may affect the peripheral joints of the appendicular skeleton rather than the axial skeleton, progress less rapidly, and cause less dramatic spinal changes. Primary AS usually develops in late adolescence and young adulthood, with peak incidence at about 20 years of age. Secondary AS affects older age groups and is often associated with other inflammatory diseases (e.g., psoriatic arthropathy, inflammatory bowel disease, Reiter's syndrome).

The exact cause of AS is unknown, but its high association with histocompatibility antigen human leukocyte antigen (HLA-B27) has been known for decades. Misfolding of HLA-B27 in the endoplasmic reticulum may play a key role in developing AS. As misfolded proteins accumulate, they may cause an unfolded protein response (UPR) that disrupts normal cellular functions and causes a stress response of the endoplasmic reticulum (also see Chapter 4). That stress response increases production of interleukin-17 and -23 (IL-17, IL-23), potent cytokines that also may act on T-helper 17 (Th17) cells, promoting their survival.[181,182] Th17 cells are important mediators in human immune diseases. Additional studies have revealed that HLA-B27 itself has many forms; to date more than 100 subtypes have been identified.[183] Certain variations in the endoplasmic reticulum aminopeptidase 1 (ERAP1) protein appear to increase the likelihood of developing AS in people who are HLA-B27 positive.

PATHOPHYSIOLOGY AS begins with inflammation of fibrocartilage in cartilaginous joints. In men, the sacroiliac joint is often affected first, usually before any damage can be radiographically detected.[181] Knee pain may be the initial symptom in women.[184] Inflammatory cells infiltrate the fibrous tissue of the joint capsule, the cartilage that surrounds intervertebral discs, the entheses, and the periosteum. As inflammatory cells (chiefly macrophages) and lymphocytes infiltrate and erode bone and fibrocartilage in joint structures, repair begins. Repair of cartilaginous structures begins with the proliferation of fibroblasts. Fibroblasts synthesize and secrete collagen. The collagen becomes organized into fibrous scar tissue that eventually undergoes calcification and ossification. With time, all the cartilaginous structures of the joint are replaced by ossified scar tissue, causing the joint to fuse, or lose flexibility.

Repair of eroded bone begins with osteoblast activation and proliferation. Osteoblasts lay down new bone (callus), which is remodelled and replaced by compact, lamellar bone. Bone repair changes the contour of the bone's surface because the new bone grows outward (outside the normal border of unaffected bone) to form a new enthesis with the end of the eroded ligament. The new enthesis, which forms on top of the old one, is called a **syndesmophyte**. As calcification of the spinal ligaments progresses, the vertebral bodies lose their concave anterior contour and appear square. The spine assumes the classic bamboo spine appearance of AS.

CLINICAL MANIFESTATIONS The most common signs and symptoms of early AS are low back pain and stiffness. Typically, the individual with primary disease develops low back pain during their early 20s. The pain is at first insidious but progressively becomes persistent. It is often worse after prolonged rest and is alleviated by physical activity. Early morning stiffness usually accompanies the low back pain, and the individual typically has difficulty sitting up or twisting the spine. Forward flexion, rotation, and lateral flexion of the spine are restricted and painful. Early pain and resultant loss of motion are caused by the underlying inflammation and reflex muscle spasm rather than by soft tissue or bony fusion.

As the disease progresses, the normal convex curve of the lower spine (lumbar lordosis) diminishes and concavity of the upper spine (kyphosis) increases. The individual becomes increasingly stooped. The thoracic spine becomes rounded, the head and neck are held forward on the shoulders, and the hips are flexed (Figure 39-21).

Inflammation in the tendon insertions of the many costosternal and costovertebral muscles can cause pleuritic chest pain and restricted chest movement. The pain is usually worse on inspiration. Movement of the diaphragm is normal and full. Pressure on the anterior chest wall over the sternum, ribs, and costal cartilages may cause tenderness. Tenderness over the pelvic brim may cause discomfort at night and interfere with sleep because turning onto the iliac crests causes pain. Tenderness over the ischial tuberosities may make sitting on hard seats unbearable. Tenderness in the heels may contribute to a limp or cautious placement of the feet during walking.

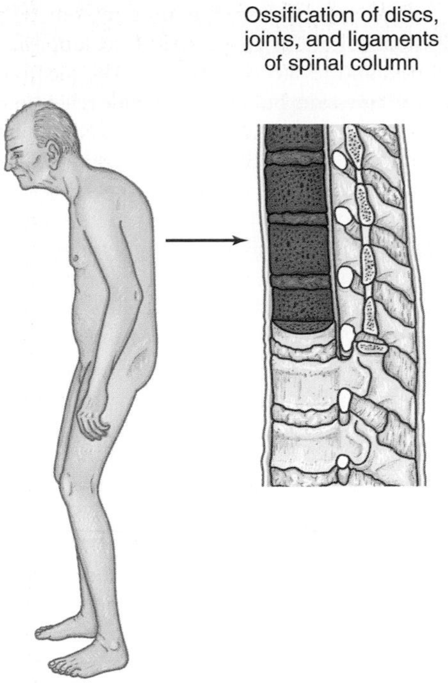

FIGURE 39-21 Ankylosing Spondylitis. Characteristic posture and primary pathological sites of inflammation and resulting damage. (Redrawn from Mourad, L.A. [1991]. *Orthopedic disorders.* St. Louis: Mosby.)

Along with low back pain and sacroiliac pain, inflammation of the bowels, anterior uveitis, aortic regurgitation, fibrosis of the upper lobes of the lung, Achilles tendonitis, and immune-related (IgA) kidney disease frequently accompany AS.[185] Elevated erythrocyte sedimentation rate (ESR) and elevated level of CRP also are common.

EVALUATION AND TREATMENT Diagnosis of AS is based on specific criteria. One of the previous problems with diagnosing AS has been a requirement for radiographic (X-ray) evidence of sacroiliitis; MRI can discover sacroiliitis an average of 7.7 years before there is evidence on X-rays.[186] Both MRI and plain radiographic findings are important in detecting early disease and for evaluating individuals younger than 45 years of age with back pain of at least 3 months' duration.[187]

In addition to sacroiliitis being present on imaging, one or more of the following features allow a diagnosis of spondyloarthritis: inflammatory back pain, arthritis, anterior uveitis, heel pain, dactylitis, psoriasis, Crohn's disease or ulcerative colitis, good response to NSAIDs, family history of spondyloarthritis, positive HLA-B27, or elevated CRP. If the individual has a positive HLA-B27, at least two of the previously mentioned items must be present along with sacroiliitis on MRI or radiographic imaging to make a diagnosis.[188]

Treatment of individuals with AS consists of education about the disease, as well as physical therapy to maintain skeletal mobility and prevent the natural progression of contractures. Prevention of deformity and maintenance of mobility require a continuous program of physical therapy. Supervised group exercises have been shown to reduce pain and to maintain and improve chest expansion and respiratory function, spine mobility, and complete range of motion in the proximal joints.[189]

NSAIDs will often provide temporary symptom relief within 48 hours. Analgesic medications are prescribed to suppress some of the pain and stiffness and to facilitate exercise. The medications do not prevent disease progression, but they do provide relief from symptoms. Biological response modifying agents, such as TNF inhibitors (certolizumab, golimumab) or B-cell depleting agents (rituximab), are increasingly being used to treat AS. Newer agents that target cytokines of Th17 and small nanoparticles that alter certain inflammatory pathways are showing promise in treating AS.[190,191] Surgical procedures, such as osteotomy, total hip replacement, and cervical spinal fusion, and radiation therapy are sometimes used to provide relief for individuals with end-stage disease or intolerable deformity. Individuals should stop smoking to lessen pulmonary problems.

Gout

The prevalence of gout has steadily increased over the past several decades and is now considered the most common inflammatory arthritis worldwide.[192,193] **Gout** is a syndrome caused by either overproduction or underexcretion of uric acid and is characterized by inflammation and pain of the joints. Incomplete purine metabolism results in excess serum uric acid levels (hyperuricemia). Either excessive uric acid production or underexcretion of uric acid by the kidneys will cause hyperuricemia. Underexcretion of uric acid is responsible for about 90% of the cases of elevated uric acid level and appears to have a strong genetic basis.[194,195]

When uric acid reaches a certain concentration in fluids, it crystallizes, forming insoluble precipitates that are deposited in connective tissues throughout the body. Crystallization in synovial fluid triggers the TNF-α inflammatory pathway, causing the release of various chemokines and interleukins, resulting in painful inflammation of the joint, a condition known as **gouty arthritis**. Urate crystal deposits cause oxidative stress reactions in other tissues as well. With time, crystal deposition in subcutaneous tissues causes the formation of small, white nodules, or **tophi**, that are visible through the skin. Tophi are associated with joint damage and an increased death rate, primarily because of cardiovascular events.[196] Hyperuricemia is associated with hypertension, heart disease, type 2 diabetes, kidney disease, and metabolic syndrome.[197]

In classic gouty arthritis, MSU crystals form and are deposited in joints and their surrounding tissues, initiating a powerful inflammatory response.[198] Pseudogout is caused by the formation of calcium pyrophosphate-dihydrate crystals. The effect of either crystal is the same—the onset of an acute inflammatory response (see Chapter 6).

Gout is rare in children and premenopausal women and is uncommon in males younger than 30 years. Male gender, increasing age, and high intake of alcohol, red meat, and fructose are all risk factors for gout.[193] The peak age of onset in males is between 40 and 50 years. The risk of developing gouty arthritis is similar in males and females for a particular urate concentration. Females tend to have onset at a later age and have greater use of diuretics, more coexisting diseases (hypertension, renal insufficiency), more frequent involvement of other joints, and fewer recurrent episodes.[199] Plasma urate concentration is the single most important determinant of the risk of developing gout (Table 39-6).

Uric acid is a weak acid that is ionized at normal body pH and thus occurs in the blood or tissues in the form of urate ion. When ionized, uric acid can form salts with various cations, but 98% of extracellular uric acid is in the form of monosodium urate (uric acid salt). At any time the proportion of uric acid or urate is pH dependent, so the ratio of these two forms varies considerably in urine.

The solubility of urate and uric acid is critical to the development of crystals. Urate is more soluble in plasma, synovial fluid, and urine than in aqueous solutions. The solubility of uric acid in urine rises dramatically as the pH increases. There is little change, however, in the solubility of urate within the normal pH range that exists in the plasma, synovial fluid, and other tissues. The pH can be 5.0 in the collecting tubules of the kidney, thus favouring formation of uric acid. Decreasing temperatures cause both urate and uric acid solubility to fall. The pathways of production of uric acid are shown in Figure 39-22.

TABLE 39-6 Mean Urate Concentrations by Age and Gender

Characteristic	Mean Urate Levels (mcmol/L)
Prepuberty	208.18
Males (at puberty)	Steep rise to 309.3
Females (puberty to after premenopause)	Slow rise to ≈237.9
Females (after menopause)	279.6
Hyperuricemia	
Males	416.4
Females	356.8

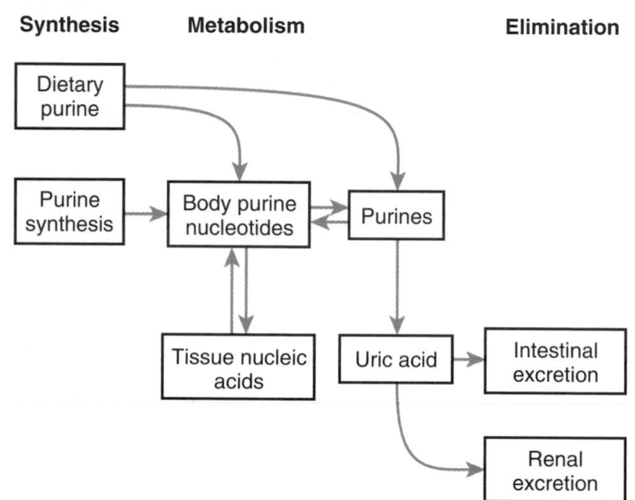

FIGURE 39-22 Uric Acid Synthesis and Elimination. Uric acid is derived from purines ingested or synthesized from ingested foods, as well as being recycled after cell breakdown. Uric acid is then eliminated through the kidneys and gastro-intestinal tract. (Redrawn from Klippel, J.H., & Dieppe, P.A. [Eds.]. [1998]. *Rheumatology* [2nd ed.]. St. Louis: Mosby.)

PATHOPHYSIOLOGY The pathophysiology of gout is closely linked to purine metabolism (or cellular metabolism of purines) and kidney function. Most mammals, except humans, have the enzyme uricase, which catalyzes the conversion of uric acid to allantoin, thus preventing overproduction of uric acid. Environmental and genetic factors also play a role in an individual's urate concentration. At the cellular level, purines are synthesized to purine nucleotides, which are used in the synthesis of nucleic acids, adenosine triphosphate (ATP), cyclic adenosine monophosphate (cAMP), and cyclic guanosine monophosphate (cGMP). Uric acid is a breakdown product of purine nucleotides (urate synthesis and elimination are illustrated in Figure 39-23).

Most uric acid is eliminated from the body through the kidneys. Urate is filtered at the glomerulus and undergoes both reabsorption and excretion within the renal tubules. In primary gout, urate excretion by the kidneys is sluggish. The sluggish excretion may be the result of a decrease in glomerular filtration of urate or acceleration in urate reabsorption. In addition, MSU crystals are deposited in renal interstitial

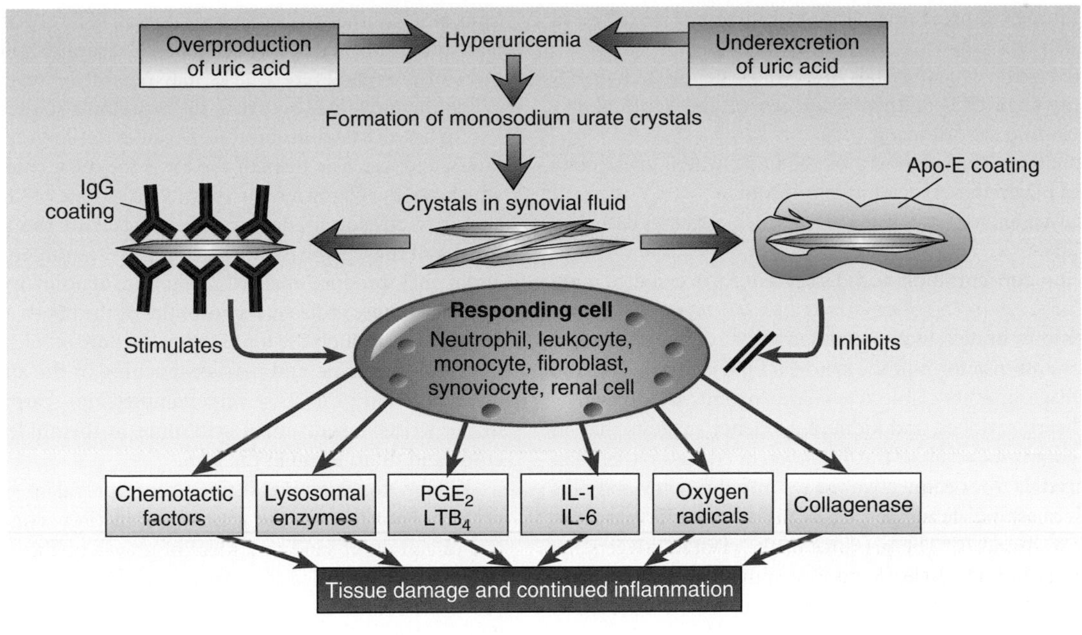

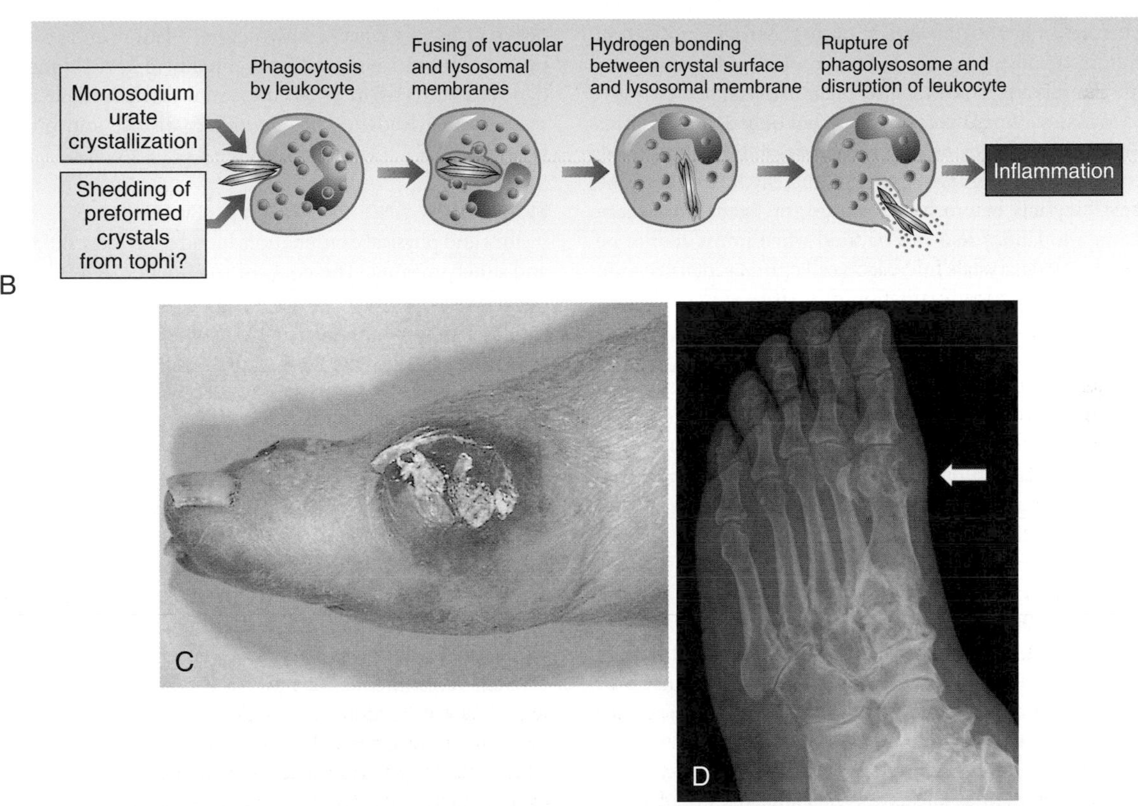

FIGURE 39-23 Pathogenesis of Acute Gouty Arthritis. A, Depending on the urate crystal coating, a variety of cells may be stimulated to produce a wide range of inflammatory mediators. **B,** Sequence of events in the production of the inflammatory response to urate crystals. **C,** Gouty tophus on right foot. **D,** Bone destruction of first metatarsal because of gout. *Apo-E,* Apolipoprotein E; *IgG,* immunoglobulin G; *IL,* interleukin; *LTB_4,* leukotriene B_4; *PGE_2,* prostaglandin E_2. (**C,** from Dieppe, P.A., Kirwan, J., Cooper, C., et al. [1991]. *Arthritis and rheumatism in practice.* London: Gower; **D,** Reprinted from *Rheum Dis Clin North Am,* 40[2], Chhana, A., & Dalbeth, N., "Structural joint damage in gout," Pages 291–309, Copyright 2014, with permission from Elsevier.)

tissues, causing impaired urine flow. (Kidney function is described in Chapter 29.)

The exact process by which crystals of MSU are deposited in joints and induce gouty arthritis is unknown, but several mechanisms may be involved, including the following:

1. MSU precipitates at the periphery of the body, where lower body temperatures may reduce the solubility of MSU.
2. Albumin or glycosaminoglycan levels decrease, which causes decreased urate solubility.
3. Changes in ion concentration and decreases of pH enhance urate deposition.
4. Trauma promotes urate crystal precipitation.

The MSU crystals may form in the synovial fluid or in the synovial membrane, cartilage, or other connective tissues in joints and elsewhere, such as in the heart, earlobes, and kidneys. Evidence suggests that an acute attack of gout is the result of the *formation* of crystals rather than the release of crystals from connective tissues into the synovial fluid.

MSU crystals can stimulate and perpetuate the inflammatory response (see Figure 39-23, *A* and *B*). The presence of the crystals triggers the acute inflammatory response, releasing proinflammatory cytokines and TNFs, during which neutrophils are attracted out of the circulation and begin to phagocytose (ingest) the crystals.

Importantly, deposits of MSU in joints and other tissues can be present years before an acute gout attack occurs. Early identification and intervention in treating gout can reduce morbidity and mortality associated with the disease. Traditionally, plain radiographs (X-rays) have been used to assess joints affected by gout, but only damaged joints can be seen. Newer technologies, including high-resolution ultrasound, dual-energy computed tomography (DECT), and MRI, can assess the presence of MSU crystals before joint, tendon, or ligament damage occurs.[200] Imaging modalities also can be used when joints cannot be aspirated to look for MSU crystals microscopically. Earlier identification allows timely as well as ongoing evaluation of treatment.[201]

CLINICAL MANIFESTATIONS Gout is manifested by (1) an increase in serum urate concentration (hyperuricemia); (2) recurrent attacks of monoarticular arthritis (inflammation of a single joint); (3) deposits of MSU monohydrate (tophi) in and around the joints; (4) kidney disease involving glomerular, tubular, and interstitial tissues and blood vessels; and (5) the formation of kidney stones. These manifestations appear in three clinical stages:

1. **Asymptomatic hyperuricemia**. The serum urate level is elevated but arthritic symptoms, tophi, and kidney stones are not present; this stage may persist throughout life.
2. **Acute gouty arthritis**. Attacks develop with increased serum urate concentrations; tends to occur with sudden or sustained increases of hyperuricemia but also can be triggered by trauma, medications, and alcohol.
3. **Tophaceous gout**. This third and chronic stage of the disease can begin as early as 3 years or as late as 40 years after the initial attack of gouty arthritis. Progressive inability to excrete uric acid expands the urate pool until MSU crystal deposits (tophi) appear in cartilage, synovial membranes, tendons, and soft tissue.

Trauma is the most common aggravating factor of an acute gouty exacerbation. Attacks of gouty arthritis occur abruptly, usually in a peripheral joint (Figure 39-23, *C*). The primary symptom is severe pain. Approximately 50% of the initial attacks occur in the metatarsophalangeal joint of the great toe (a condition known as *podagra*). The other 50% can occur in almost any joint, but most often involve the heel, ankle, instep of the foot, knee, wrist, or elbow. The pain is usually noted at night. Within a few hours the affected joint becomes hot, red, and extremely tender and may be slightly swollen. Lymphangitis and systemic signs of inflammation (leukocytosis, fever, ESR) are occasionally present. Untreated, mild attacks usually subside in several hours but may persist for 1 or 2 days. Severe attacks may persist for several days or weeks. When the individual recovers, the symptoms resolve completely.

Tophaceous deposits produce irregular swellings of the fingers, hands, knees, and feet. The helix of the ear is the most common site of tophi, which are the characteristic diagnostic lesions of chronic gout. Tophi also may develop along the ulnar surface of the forearm, the tibial surface of the leg, the Achilles tendon, olecranon bursa, or other areas. Tophi may produce marked limitation of joint movement and can eventually cause grotesque deformities of the hands and feet (see Figure 39-23, *C*). Although the tophi themselves are painless, they often cause progressive stiffness and persistent aching of the affected joint. Tophi in the extremities can cause nerve compression—carpal tunnel syndrome in the wrists, tarsal tunnel syndrome in the ankles. Tophi also may erode and drain through the skin.

Kidney stones are 1 000 times more prevalent in individuals with primary gout than in the general population. The stones can be the size of a grain of sand or a piece of gravel, or they can accumulate in massive deposits called *staghorn calculi*. They range in colour from pale yellow to brown to reddish black, depending on their composition. Some stones consist of pure MSU; others consist of calcium oxalate or calcium phosphate. Kidney stones can form in the collecting tubules, pelvis, or ureters, causing obstruction, dilation, and atrophy of the more proximal tubules and leading eventually to acute kidney failure. Stones deposited directly in renal interstitial tissue initiate an inflammatory reaction that leads to chronic kidney disease and progressive kidney failure.

EVALUATION AND TREATMENT Evaluation of gout may include history and physical examination, blood tests, joint fluid test, ultrasound, and other imaging. The goals of treatment are to terminate the acute gouty attack as promptly as possible, decrease serum uric acid levels (to dissolve MSU crystals), prevent acute attacks of gout by removing tophi, and, finally, cure gout.[202] Acute gouty arthritis should be treated with anti-inflammatory medications within 24 hours after the attack. The medications of choice are NSAIDs, corticosteroids, and colchicine.[203] Newer medications include interleukin inhibitors.[204] In persons unable to tolerate NSAIDs, colchicine is useful but can be poorly tolerated because of a number of side effects. Once infection has been ruled out, steroids may be injected into the joint to relieve pain. Local application of ice reduces pain during an acute attack.[205] Weight-bearing on the involved joint is avoided until the acute attack subsides. A diet that includes mostly vegetables and fruit with little meat, avoidance of alcohol, and weight loss can help lower serum uric acid concentration.[206] Current recommendations are to decrease serum urate levels to less than 356.9 mcmol/L (or less than 297.4 mcmol/L if the individual has marked MSU crystal deposits on clinical examination or imaging studies).[200] High fluid intake, particularly water, can increase urinary output. Long-term use of antihyperuricemic medications, including newer agents such as pegloticase (Krystexxa), helps reduce serum urate concentrations. Allopurinol (Zyloprim) and febuxostat (Adenuric) are both used to lower serum urate levels by inhibiting the activity of xanthine oxidase.

QUICK CHECK 39-3

1. How does noninflammatory joint disease differ from inflammatory joint disease? Describe two principal features of each.
2. How does rheumatoid arthritis affect the skin, heart, lungs, and kidneys?
3. How do monosodium urate crystals cause gout to develop?

DISORDERS OF SKELETAL MUSCLE

Muscle diseases (myopathies) encompass many entities. Muscle weakness and muscle fatigue are common symptoms. In many cases, neural, traumatic, and psychogenic causes provide an adequate explanation for the failure to generate force (weakness) or sustain force (fatigue) seen in myopathies. The pathophysiological mechanisms in some of the metabolic and inflammatory muscle diseases have been explored, but the cause of many of the myopathies remains obscure. The complex interaction between muscles and nerves affects muscular function as well. Only inherited and acquired disorders of skeletal muscles are discussed here.

Secondary Muscular Dysfunction

Muscular symptoms arise from a variety of causes unrelated to the muscle itself. Secondary muscular phenomena (contracture, stress-related muscle tension, immobility) are common disorders that influence muscular function.

Contractures

Contractures are described as the loss of full passive range of motion secondary to joint, muscle, or other soft tissue limitations[207] and can be pathological or physiological. A physiological muscle contracture occurs in the absence of a muscle action potential in the sarcolemma. Muscle shortening is explained on the basis of failure of the calcium pump in the presence of plentiful ATP. A physiological contracture is seen in McArdle's disease (muscle myophosphorylase deficiency) and MH. The contracture is usually temporary if the underlying pathology is reversed.

A pathological contracture is a permanent muscle shortening caused by muscle spasm or weakness. Heel cord (Achilles tendon) contractures are examples of pathological contractures. They are associated with plentiful ATP and occur in spite of a normal action potential. The most common contractures are seen in stroke, neuromuscular diseases (such as muscular dystrophy), Charcot-Marie-Tooth disease, amyotrophic lateral sclerosis, and CNS injury. Lower-extremity contractures are more common than those in the upper extremity. Prolonged splinting in a single position or an imbalance between agonist–antagonist muscles also can cause joint stiffness and contractures. Contractures also may develop secondary to scar tissue contraction in the flexor tissues of a joint, as in scarring of burned tissues in the antecubital area of the forearm, leading to a flexion contracture.

Stress-Induced Muscle Tension

Abnormally increased muscle tension has been associated with chronic anxiety as well as a variety of stress-related muscular symptoms, including neck stiffness, back pain, and headache.[208] Abnormalities in the CNS, reticular activating system, and autonomic nervous system (ANS) have been implicated. For example, as an individual progressively relaxes, the amplitude of the knee jerk reflex diminishes. Conversely, individuals with absent reflexes increase tension by such manoeuvres as clenching the teeth or strengthening the handgrip. The underlying pathophysiology may be related to the fact that as a muscle contracts, the muscle spindle is activated. This gamma-feedback system produces a series of impulses that are transmitted to the brain by the sensitive 1A afferent fibres. Unconscious tension is thought to increase the activity of the reticular activating system as well, which stimulates firing of the efferent loop of the gamma fibres, produces further muscle contraction, and increases muscle tension. ANS function that regulates increased blood flow to the muscle during sympathetic activity may be related to increased muscle contraction tension.

Various forms of treatment have been used to reduce the muscle tension associated with stress. Progressive relaxation training, yoga, meditation, and biofeedback are examples of stress reduction therapies. Biofeedback uses integrated electromyography (EMG) to make recordings from the skin surface. The goal is to teach the individual to control maladaptive tension. It is particularly useful in individuals who have a connection between skeletal muscle tension and pain. Progressive relaxation training emphasizes the individual's ability to perceive the difference between tension and relaxation. This technique involves sequential tensing and a relaxing environment. The individual is taught to practise this routine daily, often with the use of audio instructions. By teaching the individual to recognize excessive contraction of skeletal muscle, one hopes to enhance the person's ability to relax specific muscle groups to relieve tension and thus reduce CNS arousal as well as ANS arousal.

Disuse Atrophy

The term disuse atrophy describes the pathological reduction in normal size of muscle fibres after prolonged inactivity from bed rest, trauma (casting), or local nerve damage as can be seen with spinal cord trauma or poliomyelitis. Decreased muscle activity reduces muscle mass through both decreased muscle protein synthesis and increased muscle protein breakdown.[209] Reduced protein synthesis is primarily responsible for muscle atrophy. The effects of muscular deconditioning associated with lack of physical activity may be apparent in a matter of days. A normal individual prescribed bed rest loses muscle strength from baseline levels at a rate of 3% per day. Bed rest also is associated with cardiovascular, skeletal, and other organ system changes. Likewise, as people age, their muscles atrophy and become weaker (sarcopenia).

Measures to prevent atrophy include frequent forceful isometric muscle contractions and passive lengthening exercises. Artificial gravity (through the use of a "human centrifuge") has shown benefit in maintaining muscle strength. One of the simplest ways to improve disuse atrophy is to restore a load to the muscle, such as returning to walking, starting active motion to a limb, and adding resistance to movements.[210] If reuse is not restored within 1 year, regeneration of muscle fibres becomes impaired.

Fibromyalgia

Fibromyalgia (FM) is a chronic musculo-skeletal syndrome characterized by diffuse pain, fatigue, increased sensitivity to touch (i.e., tender points), the absence of systemic or localized inflammation, and the presence of fatigue and nonrestorative sleep; anxiety and depression also are frequently present. FM has often been misdiagnosed or completely dismissed by clinicians because there are few objective clinical findings on examination. A common misdiagnosis has been chronic fatigue syndrome (CFS). Of affected individuals, 80 to 90% are women, and the peak age of onset is 30 to 50 years of age. New research supports the possible role of inflammation in FM.[211-213] FM and its symptoms are viewed as the result of CNS dysfunction, where pain transmission and interpretation are amplified, a condition called central sensitization. Although the incidence is unknown, the prevalence is reported to be 2 to 8% and increases with age.[214] Certain autoimmune diseases, especially systemic lupus erythematosus and irritable bowel syndrome, are often seen in association with FM and may coexist if not initially present with FM.

PATHOPHYSIOLOGY Genetic factors are increasingly being suggested as important in developing FM. Relatives of individuals with FM have an increased risk of developing FM. Studies of genetic factors have implicated alterations in genes affecting serotonin, catecholamines, and dopamine—all of these substances are involved in the stress response and sensory processing.[215-217] In spite of these studies, the role of genetic factors has not yet been fully identified in FM. External stressors, such

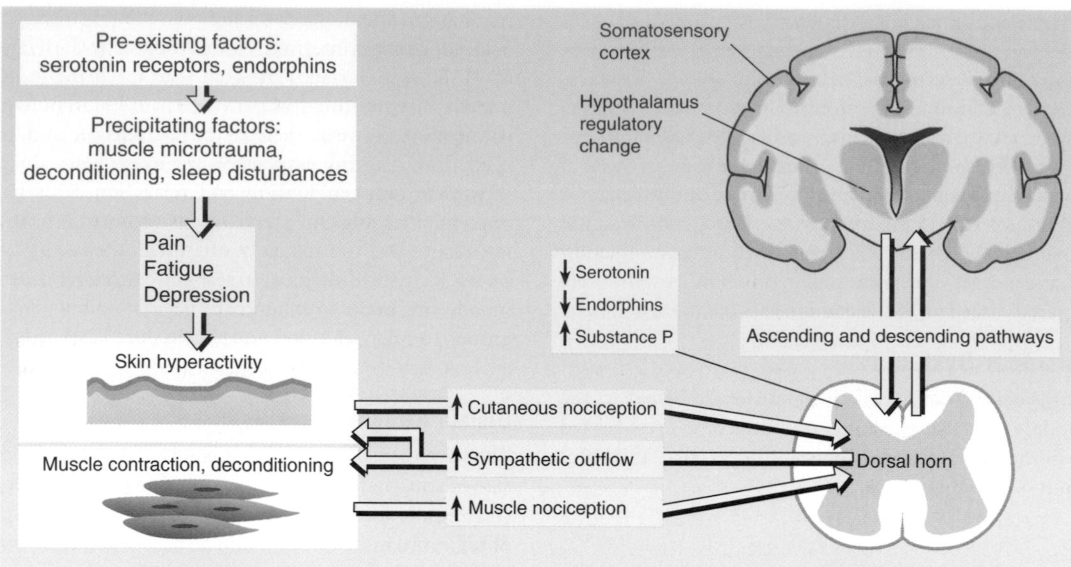

FIGURE 39-24 Theoretical Pathophysiological Model of Fibromyalgia.

as infection, psychosocial stress, and physical or emotional trauma, have been proposed as mechanisms precipitating FM; however, as yet, there is no definitive scientific evidence supporting these theories.[218]

Functional magnetic resonance imaging (fMRI) and PET scans of the brains of individuals with FM have shown activity in different areas of the brain than normally seen in healthy individuals exposed to painful stimuli.[219] These functional abnormalities within the CNS are shown in Figure 39-24. Other pathophysiological evidence includes hypothalamic-pituitary axis alterations that show abnormal response to stress.[220]

CLINICAL MANIFESTATIONS The prominent symptom of FM is diffuse, persistent pain. Persistent pain is defined as pain that is present for more than 3 months. Traditionally, to be classified as FM, tenderness in 11 of 18 specific points was required along with widespread pain. The 2012 classification of FM was simplified and expanded to include other important nonpain symptoms.[221] The pain often begins in one location, especially the neck and shoulders, but then becomes more generalized. People describe the pain as "burning" or "gnawing." Fatigue is profound. The effect on everyday life is considerable. Fatigue is most notable when arising from sleep and in midafternoon. Headaches and memory loss are common complaints. There is a strong association between FM, Raynaud phenomenon, and irritable bowel syndrome. Individuals with FM are light sleepers and awake frequently, which may explain why individuals feel nonrefreshed upon waking.

Almost 25% of individuals seek psychological support for depression. Anxiety, particularly with regard to their diagnosis and future, is almost universal.

EVALUATION AND TREATMENT Because the manifestations of chronic, generalized pain and fatigue are present in many musculo-skeletal (e.g., rheumatic) disorders, these disorders should be considered in the differential diagnosis of FM. In an effort to simplify and more accurately diagnose FM, a panel of experts from across Canada developed the Canadian Guidelines for the Diagnosis and Management of Fibromyalgia Syndrome.[221] According to these guidelines, the symptom complex for FM includes the following:

- Pain that has been present at a similar level for at least 3 months, with insidious onset, usually localized to a particular area (often in muscles and joints); pain might also be neuropathic in nature (i.e., burning); there is no other underlying pathology to explain the pain
- Other associated symptoms: fatigue, nonrestorative sleep, cognitive dysfunction, changes in mood

BOX 39-4 Educating and Providing Reassurance for Individuals With Fibromyalgia

Stress that the illness is real, not imagined.
Explain that fibromyalgia is presumably not caused by infection.
Explain that fibromyalgia is not a deforming or deteriorating condition.
Explain that fibromyalgia is neither life-threatening nor markedly debilitating, although it is an irritating presence.
Discuss the role of sleep disturbances and the relationship of neurohormones to pain, fatigue, abnormal sleep, and mood.
Reassure that although the cause is unknown, some information is known about the physiological changes responsible for the symptoms.
Use muscle "spasms" and, perhaps, "low muscle blood flow" to lay the groundwork for exercise recommendations.
Assist the individual to use aerobic exercise to reduce stress and increase rapid eye movement (REM) sleep.

FM treatment should be highly individualized and can include mind–body interventions (such as biofeedback), movement therapies, and relaxation techniques as well as medication.[222] No one regimen of medication has proved successful for FM. Exercise regimens are beneficial in reducing symptoms. Recommended exercises for individuals with FM include aerobic activities (including kickboxing and weightlifting), stretching, and gentle strengthening programs. Medications such as NSAIDs, opioids, cannabinoids, antidepressants and anticonvulsants with pain-modulating effects, as well as medications that alter the level of neurotransmitters in the brain are also helpful. Two of the most important aspects of treatment are physical activity and patient education (Box 39-4).[223-225]

Chronic Fatigue Syndrome

Chronic fatigue syndrome (CFS) is a chronic debilitating disease that is likely best described as neuroimmunoendocrine disease that is characterized by cognitive impairment, severe postexertional fatigue (including physical, emotional, or cognitive activity), unrefreshing sleep, and decreased physical activity that affects daily functioning.[226,227] Other frequent symptoms include sore throat, tender lymph nodes, pain, and psychiatric complaints. CFS has often been a diagnosis of exclusion because it cannot be objectively identified by any laboratory or specific clinical tests.[228] Because of the difficulty finding objective data to diagnose CFS, the disease also has been termed **myalgic encephalomyelitis (ME)** and has been considered a psychiatric disorder. CFS/ME has remained a controversial diagnosis until recently.

Though there seems to be some psychological involvement in CFS/ME, there is emerging evidence for a physiological basis. New research has revealed a number of physiological abnormalities associated with CFS/ME. Some of these processes include skeletal muscle abnormalities, mitochondrial dysfunction, diminished activity of several types of immune cells, abnormal cytokine regulation, and dysfunction of the hypothalamic-pituitary-adrenal (HPA) axis.[229-232] Because of the continued controversy surrounding CFS/ME and the difficulties diagnosing and treating it, the IOM recommended a new term for the condition in 2015: **systemic exertional intolerance disease (SEID)**.[233] Treatment for SEID remains challenging and must be individualized because there are both physical and psychological components to the disease. Learning how to adapt to stressors and improving physical activity may assist in improving symptoms.[234,235]

Muscle Membrane Abnormalities

Two defects of the muscle membrane (plasma membrane of the muscle fibre) have been linked to clinical syndromes: the hyperexcitable membrane seen in myotonic disorders and the intermittently unresponsive membrane seen in periodic paralyses. Although these are rare disorders, research into their pathological processes has led to an improved understanding of cell membrane channelopathies (ion channels are described in Chapter 13).

Myotonia

Myotonias are genetically inherited diseases caused by alterations in skeletal muscle sodium and calcium ion channels that result in delayed relaxation after voluntary muscle contraction, such as handgrip, eye closure, or muscle percussion.[236,237] Definitive diagnosis is made by genetic testing. Needle EMG is useful in determining likelihood of disease; the distinctive "dive bomber" noise, audible on needle EMG, is caused by the prolonged depolarization of the muscle membrane.

Myotonia comprises various disorders: myotonia congenita, paramyotonia congenita, myotonic muscular dystrophy, and some forms of periodic paralysis. With the exception of myotonic muscular dystrophy, most are mild in symptomatology. Treatment includes sodium channel blocking agents, such as mexiletine (Mexitil Cap). However, in the United States, no pharmacological agents have yet received US Food and Drug Administration approval for treating myotonia.[238,239] In Canada, little information is available on the use of pharmacological agents for treating myotonia. Other treatment modalities include genetic counselling as well as lifestyle and dietary modifications.[240]

Periodic Paralysis

Periodic paralysis encompasses a rare group of muscle diseases characterized by episodes of flaccid weakness. Most are hereditary (autosomal dominant) and caused by calcium or sodium channel abnormalities (pore gating anomalies) because of specific genetic mutations. In normal skeletal muscle, the cellular inflow and outflow of potassium are balanced to maintain the cell's resting potential. Sodium channels, in response to nerve stimulation, create the action potentials that initiate muscle contraction. Calcium channels interact with ryanodine receptors to initiate fast muscle contraction.[241] In susceptible individuals, some instigating factor (such as hyperthyroidism, strenuous exercise, or intake of a high-carbohydrate meal) allows increased muscle uptake of potassium from the plasma. This results in slightly decreased plasma potassium levels but it triggers depolarization of the sarcolemma and allows more potassium to enter the cell, causing hypokalemia.[242] Hypokalemic periodic paralysis also can be triggered by exposure to cold or by rest after strenuous exercise. During an attack of hypokalemic periodic paralysis, the resting muscle membrane potential both is unresponsive to neural stimuli and is reduced from −90 to −45 mV. This condition can last hours to days.

Thyrotoxic periodic paralysis (TPP) is caused by a potassium channelopathy that causes increased flow of potassium into the cell; it does not indicate a potassium deficiency.[243,244] Most common in Asian males, TPP is increasingly being seen in all ethnic groups.[244] The main consequence of increased concentration of intracellular potassium is depolarization of the muscle and resulting weakness. Prevention is aimed at correcting the hyperthyroidism. β-Adrenergic blockers, such as propranolol (Apo-Propranolol), are sometimes given until thyroid function is normal. Oral and intravenous administration of potassium can relieve acute hypokalemic attacks.

Hyperkalemic periodic paralysis is another genetic disorder and is characterized by episodes of flaccid paralysis. It can be activated by several factors, including pregnancy, alcohol, illness, certain medications, eating potassium-rich foods, exposure to cold, and rest after exercising.[245] Although the most striking feature of the condition is flaccid paralysis, many individuals have myotonia present on examination.[245] The sodium channel fails to completely inactivate, causing more sodium to enter the cell and forcing potassium into the extracellular space, thus blocking sodium channels from depolarizing. Though hyperkalemic periodic paralysis episodes are typically shorter in duration than those of hypokalemic periodic paralysis, there is often a lifelong trend to have increasing frequency of attacks. In addition, hyperkalemic periodic paralysis can cause permanent muscle weakness. Respiratory insufficiency can be a life-threatening situation.

Preventive measures include avoiding alcohol and diet soda, potassium-rich foods, or activities that provoke symptoms. Maintaining adequate water intake, eating carbohydrate-rich foods, and keeping warm seem to help some individuals.[246] In acute hyperkalemic periodic paralysis, inhaled albuterol (Ventolin) or glucose/insulin therapy can reduce symptoms. Preventive medications include potassium-lowering agents, such as hydrochlorothiazide (HCTZ, Urozide) or mexiletine.

Metabolic Muscle Diseases

Disorders in muscle metabolism can be caused by endocrine abnormalities or diseases of energy metabolism, such as glycogen storage disease, enzyme deficiencies, and abnormalities in lipid metabolism and mitochondrial function. The term *metabolic myopathies* refers to a group of hereditary muscle disorders caused by defective genes.

Endocrine Disorders

Often the systemic effects of hormonal imbalance overshadow the individual's muscular symptoms. For example, individuals with thyrotoxicosis may have signs of proximal weakness, paresis of the extraocular muscles (exophthalmic ophthalmoplegia), and, rarely, hypokalemic periodic paralysis. Hypothyroidism is often associated with a decrease in muscle mass and strength, with weak, flabby skeletal muscles and sluggish movements.

Thyroid hormone is believed to regulate muscle protein synthesis and electrolyte balance. Alterations in muscle protein synthesis and electrolyte balance may therefore explain the changes in muscle mass and contractility seen in endocrine disorders. The muscular symptoms subside with appropriate treatment of the primary hormonal disorder.

Diseases of Energy Metabolism

Muscles rely on carbohydrates (such as glycogen) and lipids (free fatty acids) for energy. When stored glycogen or lipids cannot be metabolized because of lack of enzymes necessary to generate ATP for muscle contraction, the individual experiences cramps, fatigue, and exercise intolerance. Disorders of muscle metabolism can be self-limiting, such as McArdle's disease and some lipid disorders, or they can cause widespread irreparable muscle destruction, as in acid maltase deficiency.

McArdle's disease. McArdle's disease, or *myophosphorylase deficiency*, is also known as *glycogen storage disease type V*. It was the first myopathy in which a single enzyme defect was identified. It is now one of nine diseases identified to date that have in common an underlying defect in glycogen synthesis, glycogenolysis, or glycolysis. These diseases are often referred to as glycogen storage diseases (GSDs) because each defect results in the abnormal deposition and accumulation of glycogen in skeletal muscle. Individuals with McArdle's disease lack muscle phosphorylase, an enzyme responsible for the breakdown of glycogen in muscle. Normally, after the body uses the short-term ATP and phosphocreatine stores, intramuscular lactic acid accumulated as glycogen is used (see Chapter 18). The individual with McArdle's disease is not able to metabolize glycogen or produce lactic acid.

The altered energy production manifests itself in exercise intolerance, fatigue, and painful muscle cramps. When exercise is carried to an extreme, painful muscle contracture and myoglobinuria can develop. Some individuals describe a "second wind" phenomenon, in which exercise tolerance increases if they slow their pace once the initial sensation of fatigue commences.[247] The muscles of persons with McArdle's disease are able to readily utilize glucose and lactate from the bloodstream. After it is converted to pyruvate, lactate has been shown to be an energy substrate that is oxidized more quickly than either fructose or glucose.[248,249] Higher levels of lactate found in skeletal muscles of those with McArdle's disease may account for this "second wind." As the disease progresses, some individuals have pronounced muscle weakness and wasting. Other organs are not involved, because the absence of phosphorylase is limited to muscle. In general, individuals with McArdle's disease learn to adapt their daily routine to avoid muscle symptoms.

Acid maltase deficiency. Acid maltase deficiency (*glycogen storage disease type II*, or *Pompe's disease*) is an autosomal recessive neuromuscular disease because of mutations of the acid α-glucosidase gene (*GAA*). This deficiency results in an accumulation of glycogen in the lysosomes of muscle cells and other tissues because of the lack of the enzyme acid maltase (also known as acid α-glucosidase).[250,251] The exact mechanism of disease progression is still unknown, but mitochondrial dysfunction and abnormal autophagy of cells appear to play a major role in the disease's clinical manifestations.

The infantile form, which is more severe, is called Pompe's disease (PD) and is recognized shortly after birth by hypotonia, dysreflexia, and an enlarged heart, tongue, and liver. Hypertrophy of these tissues is thought to be the result of glycogen deposition. Muscle biopsy is an important diagnostic tool in identifying PD.[252] In the past, children died of cardiac or respiratory failure within 1 year of diagnosis, but new treatments have improved survival. Late-onset Pompe's disease (LOPD) occurs from childhood into adulthood. Muscular symptoms of LOPD are highly variable and can range from muscle cramping and weakness to varying degrees of respiratory insufficiency.[253] The mainstay of treatment is enzyme replacement therapy with recombinant GAA, but dietary modifications also may improve the course of the disease.[254]

Myoadenylate deaminase deficiency. An enzyme deficiency that produces changes in skeletal muscle and is associated with exercise intolerance is myoadenylate deaminase deficiency (MDD). More often referred to as *adenosine monophosphate deaminase deficiency* (AMDD), this autosomal recessive condition has a wide variation in symptoms.[255] Because individuals with MDD lack myoadenylate deaminase, they have a poor capacity for sustained energy production, yet some with the condition have been able to perform as high-level athletes. The most common symptoms appear to be postexercise muscle cramping or pain, or both, and easy fatigability. Myoadenylate deaminase is the catalytic enzyme that forms phosphocreatine and ATP during exercise through a metabolic pathway that binds the purine and phosphate molecules that constitute ATP. Individuals with MDD differ from those with McArdle's disease in that, during the ischemic exercise test, lactate production is normal in MDD when ATP and phosphocreatine are synthesized. The enzyme defect has been reported to be quite common, but in practice it may be rarely recognized as a cause of exercise intolerance.

Lipid deficiencies. Disorders of lipid metabolism are uncommon but account for severe changes in muscle metabolism. These disorders are caused by abnormalities in the transport and processing of fatty acids for energy. The lipid content of muscle cells consists of free fatty acids, which are oxidized in the mitochondria. These acids require carnitine and the enzyme carnitine palmitoyltransferase (CPT) to transport long-chain fatty acids to the mitochondria. There are two types of CPT: CPT1 is found in liver, muscle, and brain tissue; only deficiencies of the liver type have been found in humans. Children younger than 18 months are most often affected. CPT2 deficiency, most often seen in adolescents or young adults, is an autosomal recessive disorder that invariably causes attacks of severe myalgia and may cause myoglobinuria.[256] Carnitine deficiency causes abnormal lipid deposition in skeletal muscles.

Measuring the CPT and carnitine content in muscle is essential to diagnosis. Cells in the muscle biopsy show vacuoles and lipid deposits. Treatments with riboflavin, medium-chain triglycerides, oral carnitine, prednisone (Deltasone), and propranolol have been beneficial to some individuals. Bezafibrate (Bezalip SR), a medication used to lower lipid levels, also has shown promise in treating CPT2 deficiency.[256]

Inflammatory Muscle Diseases: Myositis

Viral, Bacterial, and Parasitic Myositis

Viral, bacterial, and parasitic infections of varying severity are known to produce inflammatory changes in skeletal muscle, a group of conditions collectively described by the term myositis. In tuberculosis and sarcoidosis, chronic inflammatory changes and granulomata are found in muscle as well as in other affected tissues. In the parasitic infection trichinellosis, *Trichinella* larvae reside in infected meat (primarily pork, but wildlife and even horses can carry the microorganism), migrate to the intestinal mucosa after ingestion, and then travel through the circulatory system to various tissues. The larvae that penetrate into skeletal muscle are able to survive and grow, causing symptoms such as severe pain, rash, and muscle stiffness. Treatment includes the administration of corticosteroids, immunotherapeutic agents, and the antiparasitic agent thiabendazole (Mertect). Toxoplasmosis, a common parasitic infection, is also associated with a generalized polymyositis that responds rapidly to therapy.

In the tropics, more prevalent disorders include bacterial infections with *S. aureus* and parasites such as cysticercus, the larva of the tapeworm *Taenia solium*. Viral infections can be associated with an acute myositis. Muscle pain, tenderness, signs of inflammation, and CK elevation are common manifestations of viral myositis. The self-limiting symptoms of muscle aches and pains during a bout of influenza may actually be a subacute form of viral myopathy.

Polymyositis, Dermatomyositis, and Inclusion Body Myositis

Idiopathic inflammatory myopathies (IIMs) are a group of autoimmune diseases that target skeletal muscle in both children and adults. There are generally four diseases included in this group: dermatomyositis (DM), polymyositis (PM), necrotizing myopathy (NM), and sporadic inclusion body myositis (IBM). The most common form, DM, has been further subclassified into additional subgroups, including the juvenile form—juvenile dermatomyositis (JDM). The exact cause of IIMs is unknown, but recent investigations have uncovered strong links between genetic, environmental, and immunological factors.[257,258] Though still relatively rare, IIMs seem to have a geographical distribution, with greater incidence in northern latitudes, further supporting the hypotheses of genetic and environmental influences in their development.[259,260] The pathophysiology of IIMs remains fully unknown, but it involves interplay between specific autoantibodies, cytokine-mediated inflammation of muscle, and genetic factors.[261,262]

Several characteristics differentiate IBM from the other IIMs in that IBM affects men more often than women and can cause asymmetric weakness. Compared with DM and PM, IBM does not respond as well to anti-inflammatory and immunosuppressive medications.

CLINICAL MANIFESTATIONS IIMs are characterized by progressive, symmetric proximal (shoulder girdle and quadriceps) muscle weakness and myalgia that develops over weeks to months. Because of their progressive nature, these illnesses can be initially confused with other myopathies. A thorough evaluation is required to exclude other disorders. Clinical features common in both PM and DM are joint pain, dysphagia, reduced esophageal motility, vasculitis, Raynaud phenomenon, cardiomyopathy, and interstitial pulmonary fibrosis. Reduced mobility with frequent falls is a common symptom in IBM because both proximal and distal muscles are affected. Some individuals have other coexisting collagen vascular disorders, such as RA, systemic lupus erythematosus, and progressive systemic sclerosis (formerly called *scleroderma*).

Although PM and DM have similar histories of onset, DM includes cutaneous manifestations. The presence of skin involvement is significant in that it can precede muscle involvement by months or even years.[263] The two most classic signs of skin involvement are (1) rashes—a typical heliotrope (reddish purple) rash that generally covers the eyelids and periorbital tissue (Figure 39-25), and (2) erythematous, scaly lesions that cover joints such as the knees and elbows, known as *Gottron lesions*. Other differences between PM and DM include their suspected pathology. PM may be caused by T-cell invasion of the muscle fibres.[264] DM, PM, and NM are associated with an increased risk for malignancy.[265] Both PM and DM seem to respond to prednisone, with or without the addition of immunosuppressives as well as intravenous Ig administration.[266]

IBM is the most common acquired muscle disease affecting individuals older than age 50. IBM differs from both PM and DM in several important ways. Muscle biopsy and histopathological studies of IBM show degenerative changes of muscle, accumulation of multiple proteins within muscle fibres, and evidence of endoplasmic reticular stress with misfolding of proteins.[267,268] Clinical presentation may show earlier onset of asymmetric atrophy and weakness of the quadriceps as well as the wrists and finger flexors. Additionally, IBM generally does not improve with standard immunosuppressants or immune-modifying medications.[269]

EVALUATION AND TREATMENT Muscle biopsy results are striking in DM, with most individuals showing inflammatory cells grouped around blood vessels and atrophy of cells in muscle fascicles. This change, perifascicular atrophy, is absent in PM. CK level is often extremely elevated in both disorders and is a helpful indicator of disease activity. Levels of other muscle enzymes, including aldolase, aspartate aminotransferase (AST), alanine aminotransferase (ALT), and lactate dehydrogenase (LDH), are also found to be elevated in most individuals. The presence of serum antinuclear antibodies (ANAs) also may be helpful in diagnosis. Muscle biopsy is indispensable for a diagnosis of PM or DM as opposed to other myotonic disease.[265] MRI reveals inflammation and edema of the muscles, as well as changes in muscles that may not show clinical evidence of disease. Contrast-enhanced ultrasound can differentiate between IBM and myositis.[270,271] EMG is useful in guiding the site for muscle biopsy.

Treatment primarily includes immunosuppressive medications, although they are not always successful, particularly in the case of IBM. Most clinicians choose corticosteroids initially, usually prednisone on a daily or alternating day schedule, tapering the dosage as the symptoms subside. Successful treatment with azathioprine, methotrexate, creatine (Creatine Systemic), and cyclosporine also has been reported.[265,272] High-dose intravenous Ig administration is sometimes used during active disease. Individuals with muscle weakness require careful physiotherapy to design a regular exercise program that prevents contractures and maximizes functional ability.

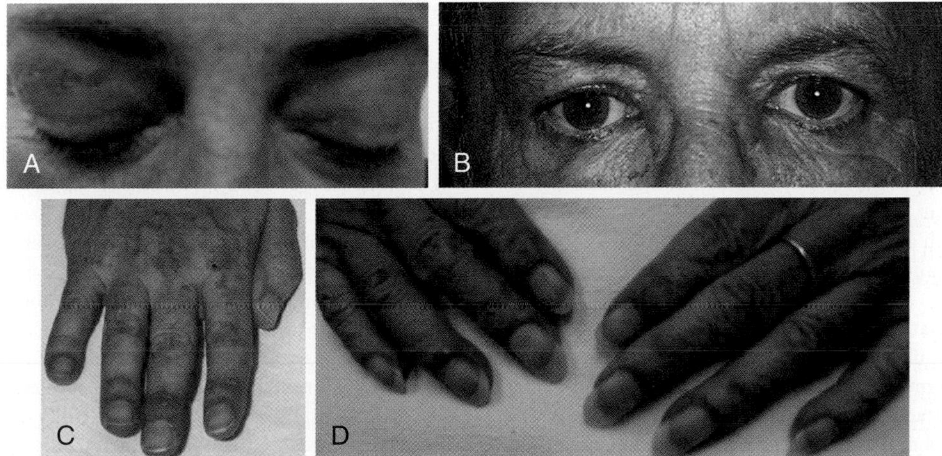

FIGURE 39-25 Clinical Manifestations of Dermatomyositis. **A** and **B**, Heliotrope (violaceous) discoloration around the eyes and periorbital edema. **C**, Gottron lesions. **D**, Increased erythema around nail beds. (**A**, **C**, **D**, from Dimachkie, M.M., Barohn, R.J., & Amato, A.A. [2014]. *Neurol Clin, 32*[3], 595–628; **B**, from Habif, T.P. [1996]. *Clinical dermatology* [3rd ed.]. St. Louis: Mosby.)

BOX 39-5 Agents That Can Cause Toxic Myopathy

Medications, Drugs, and Substances
Alcohol
Amiodarone (Cordarone; and other medications that inhibit CYP3A4 when combined with a statin)
Amphotericin B
Azathioprine
Chloroquine (Teva-Chloroquine)
Clofibrate
Colchicine
Diuretics
Ethanol
Finasteride (CO Finasteride)
Illicit drugs and drugs of abuse (heroin, cocaine, amphetamine, meperidine, pentazocine)
Ipecac (withdrawn from Canadian and US markets)
Isotretinoin (Accutane)
Labetalol (Trandate)
3,4-Methylenedioxymethamphetamine (MDMA, "ecstasy")
Omeprazole (Losec)
Pentachlorophenol (PCP)
Propofol
Retrovirals (AZT [zidovudine])
Statins
Steroids (especially with prolonged high doses; doses >25 mg/day; fluorinated steroids)
Vincristine (Oncovin)

Endocrine Disorders
Adrenal disorders (Addison's disease, Cushing's disease)
Hyperparathyroidism
Hyperthyroidism (creatine kinase may be normal)
Hypothyroidism (creatine kinase may be mildly elevated)

Infectious Agents
Coxsackie A and B viruses
Human immunodeficiency virus (HIV)
Influenza
Lyme disease
Staphylococcus aureus muscle infection (frequent cause of pyomyositis)
Toxoplasmosis
Trichinosis

Miscellaneous
Licorice
Certain edible wild mushrooms
Lead poisoning
Malignant hyperthermia
Organophosphates
Red yeast rice
Snake venom
European migratory quail (quail eat toxic hemlock, hellebore seeds)
Any medication that alters serum concentrations of sodium, potassium, calcium, phosphorus, or magnesium

Data from Pasnoor, M., Barohn, R.J., & Dimachkie, M.M. (2014). *Neurol Clin, 32*, 647–670; Valiyil, V.R., & Christopher-Stine, O. (2010). *Curr Rheumatol Rep, 12*(3), 213–220.

Toxic Myopathies

Muscle damage caused by medications or toxins is also called **toxic myopathy**. Alcohol, lipid-lowering agents (fibrates and statins), antimalarial medications, steroids, thiol derivatives, and narcotics (particularly heroin) can all cause symptoms. Many medications, diseases, and infectious and environmental agents can cause myopathy. The combination of certain medications can also cause muscle injury.[273] Box 39-5 lists some of the causes of toxic myopathy.

Alcohol remains the most common cause of toxic myopathy. Two clinical syndromes are prevalent: (1) an acute attack of muscle weakness, pain, and swelling after a drinking binge or (2) a more chronic, progressive proximal weakness in a long-term drinker.[274] The incidence of acute alcoholic myopathy has been estimated as being up to 20% of individuals admitted with acute alcoholic withdrawal.

The pathological abnormalities include necrosis of individual muscle fibres; whole segments can be found in the same stage of degeneration. The mechanism by which alcohol affects the muscle fibre is uncertain, but a direct toxic effect and nutritional deficiency have both received experimental support.

Acute alcoholic myopathy can range from benign cramps and pain resolving in a matter of hours to severe weakness and markedly increased CK level associated with myoglobinuria and kidney failure. Individuals are prone to repeated attacks following recovery. The only treatment is abstinence from alcohol and improved nutrition. The individual with chronic alcoholic myopathy often has coexisting peripheral neuropathy that complicates the diagnosis.

The most severe complication of toxic myopathy is rhabdomyolysis (acute muscle fibre necrosis with leakage of muscle protein into the bloodstream) that leads to myoglobinuria and acute kidney failure. Most individuals with toxic myopathy present with acute muscle weakness. Pain is an unreliable indicator because many toxic myopathies are painless, but necrotizing toxic myopathies can cause severe pain. Dark-coloured urine may indicate rhabdomyolysis, a serious complication that can lead to death (see p. 1017). Other serious complications can include involvement of respiratory and cardiac muscles.

Measurement of serum creatine levels is helpful in determining muscle damage. Other tests such as EMG may show characteristic changes in function. MRI can demonstrate muscle edema. Features of myopathy can be seen on muscle biopsy.

Repeated intramuscular injections have also been associated with changes in muscle fibres. Local necrosis of muscle fibres and elevated CK level have been reported after intramuscular injections of cephalothin (Averon-1), lidocaine, diazepam (Apo-Diazepam), and digoxin (Toloxin); these effects were not produced with injections of saline. When medications are injected over long periods, a chronic focal myopathy develops. Proliferation of connective tissue in both the muscle fibre and the overlying skin and subcutaneous tissue has been reported. Over time, segments of the muscles, particularly the deltoid and quadriceps, are converted into fibrotic bands. Pathophysiological mechanisms for these changes include repeated needle trauma and infection, along with the nonphysiological acidity or alkalinity of the injected material.

Treatment primarily consists of removing or stopping the offending agent and providing supportive care. Supportive care may include hemodialysis and respiratory or cardiovascular support, depending on severity of symptoms.

✔ QUICK CHECK 39-4

1. What is the main objective clinical finding in fibromyalgia?
2. How do metabolic muscle diseases develop? What causes them?
3. Name one toxic myopathy, and explain why it develops.

MUSCULO-SKELETAL TUMOURS

Bone Tumours

Many different types of tumours involve the skeleton. Although the skeleton is the major site for metastatic spread of multiple myeloma and breast, lung, and prostate cancers, primary bone tumours are relatively rare. **Bone tumours** may originate from bone cells, cartilage, fibrous tissue, marrow, or vascular tissue. Based on the tissue of origin, bone tumours are classified as osteogenic, chondrogenic, collagenic, or myelogenic. Box 39-6 contains the classification of major primary bone tumours. Each type arises from one of the four stem cells that are ultimately derived from the primitive mesoderm (Figure 39-26). In addition, bone tumours may be classified as being of histiocytic, notochordal, lipogenic, or neurogenic origin.

The mesoderm contributes the primitive fibroblast and reticulum cells. The fibroblast is the progenitor of the osteoblast and chondroblast cells. Each cell synthesizes a specific type of intercellular ground substance, and the type of ground substance produced by the cell generally characterizes the tumour derived from that cell. For example, osteogenic tumours usually contain cells that have the appearance of osteoblasts and produce an intercellular substance that can be recognized as osteoid. Chondrogenic tumours contain chondroblasts and produce an intercellular substance similar to chondroid (cartilage). Collagenic tumours contain fibrous tissue cells and produce an intercellular substance similar to the type of collagen found in fibrous connective tissue.

Tumours are also classified as benign or malignant, based on characteristics of the tumour cells (see Chapter 10). The criteria used to identify tumour cells as malignant are (1) an increased nuclear/cytoplasmic ratio, (2) an irregular nuclear border, (3) an excess of chromatin, (4) a prominent nucleolus, and (5) an increase in the number of cells undergoing mitosis. However, many young, rapidly growing normal cells and cells subjected to inflammation and change in their blood supply also exhibit many of these same characteristics. (Tumour characteristics in general are described in Chapter 10.)

Epidemiology

The incidence rate of bone tumours varies with age. In children younger than 15 years, the rate of bone tumours is relatively low, constituting approximately 5% of all malignancies. Adolescents have the highest incidence of bone tumours, and adults between the ages of 30 and 35 have the lowest incidence. After age 35, the incidence rate slowly increases until at age 60 it nearly equals the incidence rate in adolescents, primarily related to secondary metastatic tumours.

The most recent incidence statistics for bone cancer in Canada are from 2013. The Canadian Cancer Society estimated that 405 Canadians (220 men and 150 women) were diagnosed with bone cancer in 2013. It also estimated that 173 Canadians (77 men and 96 women) died of this disease in 2013.[275]

Patterns of Bone Destruction

The general pathological features of bone tumours include bone destruction, erosion or expansion of the cortex, and periosteal response to changes in underlying bone. The least amount of pathological damage occurs with benign bone tumours, which push against neighbouring tissue. Because they usually have a symmetric, controlled growth pattern, benign bone tumours tend to compress and displace neighbouring

BOX 39-6 Classification of Major Primary Tumours Involving Bone

Category and Fraction (%)	Behaviour	Tumour Type	Common Locations	Age (Years)	Morphology
Hematopoietic (20)	Malignant	Myeloma Lymphoma	Vertebrae, pelvis	50–60	Malignant plasma cells or lymphocytes replacing marrow space
Cartilage forming (30)	Benign	Osteochondroma	Metaphysis of long bones	10–30	Bony excrescence with cartilage cap
		Chondroma	Small bones of hands and feet	30–50	Circumscribed hyaline cartilage nodule in medulla
		Chondroblastoma	Epiphysis of long bones	10–20	Circumscribed, pericellular calcification
		Chondromyxoid fibroma	Tibia, pelvis	20–30	Collagenous to myxoid matrix, stellate cells
	Malignant	Chondrosarcoma (conventional)	Pelvis, shoulder	40–60	Extends from medulla through cortex into soft tissue, chondrocytes with increased cellularity and atypia
Bone forming (26)	Benign	Osteoid osteoma	Metaphysis of long bones	10–20	Cortical, interlacing microtrabeculae of woven bone
		Osteoblastoma	Vertebral column	10–20	Posterior elements of vertebrae, histology similar to osteoid osteoma
	Malignant	Osteosarcoma	Metaphysis of distal femur, proximal tibia	10–20	Extends from medulla to lift periosteum, malignant cells producing woven bone
Unknown origin (15)	Benign	Giant cell tumour	Epiphysis of long bones	20–40	Destroys medulla and cortex, sheets of osteoclasts
		Aneurysmal bone cyst	Proximal tibia, distal femur, vertebrae	10–20	Vertebral body, hemorrhagic spaces separated by cellular, fibrous septae
	Malignant	Ewing sarcoma	Diaphysis of long bones	10–20	Sheets of primitive small round cells
		Adamantinoma	Tibia	30–40	Cortical, fibrous, bone matrix with epithelial islands
Notochordal (4)	Malignant	Chordoma	Clivus, sacrum	30–60	Destroys medulla and cortex, foamy cells in myxoid matrix

From Kumar, V., Abbas, A.K., & Aster, J.C. (Eds.). (2015). *Robbins and Cotran pathologic basis of disease* (9th ed.). Philadelphia: Saunders. Adapted from Unni, K.K., & Inwards, C.Y. (2010). *Dahlin's bone tumors* (6th ed.). Philadelphia: Lippincott Williams & Wilkins; by permission of Mayo Foundation.

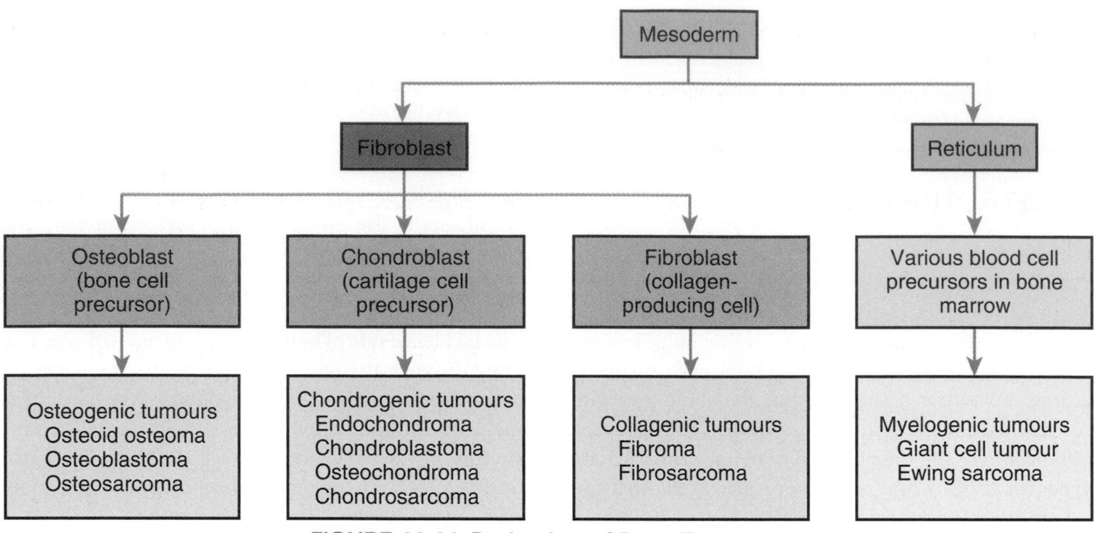

FIGURE 39-26 Derivation of Bone Tumours.

TABLE 39-7 Patterns of Bone Destruction Caused by Bone Tumours

Type	Features
Geographical pattern	Least aggressive type Generally indicative of slow-growing or benign tumour Well-defined margins on tumour, easily separated from surrounding normal bone Uniform and well-defined lytic area in bone Margin smooth or irregular, demarcated by short zone of transition between normal and abnormal bone tissue
Moth-eaten pattern	Characteristic of rapidly growing, malignant bone tumours More aggressive pattern Tumour margin less defined or demarcated; cannot easily be separated from normal bone Areas of partially destroyed bone adjacent to completely lytic areas
Permeative pattern	Caused by aggressive malignant tumour with rapid growth potential Margins of tumour poorly demarcated Abnormal bone merges imperceptibly with normal bone

TABLE 39-8 Surgical Staging System for Bone Tumours of Mesenchymal Origin

Stage	Grade	Site (T)	Metastasis (M)
IA	Low (G_1)	Intracompartmental (T_1)	None (M_0)
IB	Low (G_1)	Extracompartmental (T_2)	None (M_0)
IIA	High (G_2)	Intracompartmental (T_1)	None (M_0)
IIB	High (G_2)	Extracompartmental (T_2)	None (M_0)
IIIA	Low (G_1)	Intracompartmental or extracompartmental (T_1 or T_2)	Regional or distant (M_1)
IIIB	High (G_2)	Intracompartmental or extracompartmental (T_1 or T_2)	Regional or distant (M_1)

Data from Jawad, M.U., & Scully, S.P. (2010). *Clin Orthop Relat Res, 468*(7), 2000–2002; Simon, S.R. (Ed.). (1994). *Orthopaedic basic science.* Chicago: American Academy of Orthopaedic Surgeons.

normal bone tissue, which weakens the bone's structure until it is incapable of withstanding the stress of ordinary use, leading to pathological fracture. Other tumours invade and destroy adjacent normal bone tissue by producing substances that promote resorption by increasing osteoclast activity or by interfering with a bone's blood supply. Three patterns of bone destruction by bone tumours have been identified: (1) the geographical pattern, (2) the moth-eaten pattern, and (3) the permeative pattern (Table 39-7).

Tumours that erode the cortex of the bone usually stimulate a periosteal response—that is, new bone formation at the interface between the surface of the bone and the periosteum. Slow erosion of the cortex usually stimulates a uniform periosteal response. Additional layers of bone are added to the exterior surface of the bone to buttress the cortex. Eventually, the additional layers expand the bone's contour. Aggressive penetration of the cortex, often seen with malignant tumours, usually elevates the periosteum and stimulates erratic patterns of new bone formation. Examples of erratic patterns include concentric layers of new bone; a sunburst pattern, in which delicate rays of new bone radiate toward the periosteum from a single focus on the underlying surface; and rays of new bone that grow perpendicularly, creating a brush or bristle pattern.

EVALUATION A malignant bone tumour must be identified early to allow survival of the individual and preservation of the affected limb. However, individuals often have only vague symptoms that may be attributed to minor trauma, degenerative changes, or inflammatory conditions. In addition, other conditions may obscure the diagnosis.

Thorough diagnostic studies are needed to determine the exact type and extent of bone tumour present, which also helps determine the optimal treatment regimen. Serum alkaline phosphatase levels are elevated in bone lytic tumours and significantly elevated in osteosarcoma. Radiological studies, including plain radiographic films, radionucleotide bone scans, CT scan, MRI, and PET combined with CT (PET/CT), are used to evaluate bone lesions. MRI and PET/CT have become the examination of choice for the local staging of bone tumours, especially the staging of peripheral osteosarcomas (Table 39-8). MRI and PET/

CT are used to monitor the response of osteosarcomas to radiation or chemotherapy and to detect recurrent disease. A PET/CT, particularly when augmented by injection of the radioisotope FDG, provides earlier, more detailed information on tumour location, differentiation, metastases, and response to therapy than other imaging modalities.[276] (Tumour staging is discussed in Chapter 10.)

Additional diagnostic studies done for specific bone tumours include a complete blood count and ESR (to rule out infection or myeloma) and measurement of serum levels of calcium and phosphorus to detect hypercalcemia. Serum glucose levels may be elevated in chondrosarcoma. Bone-specific alkaline phosphatase is elevated when there is bone metastasis.[277] Acid phosphatase level may be moderately elevated in bone metastases, multiple myeloma, and advanced Paget's disease. Serum protein electrophoresis and immunoelectrophoresis are performed to exclude other diseases. To determine the exact tumour type, core needle biopsy is usually done at the time of surgery.[278]

Types

A large number of lesions are classified as bone tumours. Bone tumours are typically classified according to their origin—osteogenic, chondrogenic, collagenic, and myelogenic tumours. They are described in the following sections (Figure 39-27).

Osteogenic tumours: osteosarcoma. **Osteogenic (bone-forming) tumours** are characterized by the formation of bone or osteoid tissue with a sarcomatous tissue. The tissue can have the appearance of callus or compact or spongy bone. The most common malignant bone-forming tumour is the **osteosarcoma**.

The incidence of osteosarcomas, the most commonly diagnosed primary bone tumour, peaks around the second decade, with a slight preference for males.[279,280] Sixty percent of osteosarcomas occur in persons younger than 20 years. A secondary peak incidence for osteosarcoma occurs in the 50- to 60-year age group, primarily in individuals with a history of radiation therapy several years previously for pelvic or other malignancies or for Paget's disease of bone.[281,282] Though considered a bone-forming tumour because of formation of immature osteoid that shows a "lacelike" pattern of bone growth, the radiological appearance of sarcoma is quite variable and often shows a moth-eaten (lytic) pattern of destruction with the tumour extending into the adjacent soft tissue.[283] Occasionally, the tumour may spread to nonadjacent bone or across a joint with normal-appearing areas of bone between tumours (i.e., "skip lesions"). Radionuclide bone scans are used to find skip lesions. MRI and PET/CT are useful in determining bony changes associated with the tumour.

The borders of the tumour are indistinct and merge into adjacent normal bone. Osteosarcomas contain osteoid produced by anaplastic stromal cells, which are atypical, abnormal cells not seen in normal developing bone; they are neither normal nor embryonal. Many tumours are heterogeneous; for example, the osteosarcoma also may contain chondroid (cartilage) and fibrinoid tissue that may form the bulk of the tumour. The osteoid is deposited as thick masses or "streamers," which infiltrate the normal compact bone, destroy it, and replace it with masses of osteoid. Bone tissue produced by osteosarcomas never matures to compact bone.

Ninety percent of osteosarcomas are located in the metaphyses of long bones, especially the distal femoral metaphysis, with 50% around the knee area. The tumour typically impregnates the cortex, lifts the periosteum, and forms a soft tissue mass that is not covered by a smooth shell of new bone. Lifting of the periosteum stimulates bizarre patterns of new bone formation called a *periosteal reaction.* Distinct osteosarcomas occur on the surface of long bones, called parosteal, periosteal, and high-grade surface osteosarcomas; dedifferentiated parosteal and central osteosarcomas also occur.

The most common initial symptoms are pain and an enlarging mass.[284] Initially, the pain is slight and intermittent, but within a short time the pain increases in severity and duration. Pain is usually worse at night and gradually requires medication. Systemic symptoms are uncommon. Often, a coincidental history of trauma is noted. Occasionally, the individual may present with a pathological fracture.

Bone biopsy is critical to diagnosis. Because the most frequent site of metastasis is the lung, a chest CT or MRI of the thorax also should be performed. There are no specific laboratory tests that aid in diagnosing sarcoma but laboratory studies are helpful in assessing overall health before beginning treatment. Once osteosarcoma has been diagnosed, measuring serum alkaline phosphatase and LDH levels can be useful in following response to treatment. The best clinical outcomes occur in those who receive both preoperative and postoperative chemotherapy

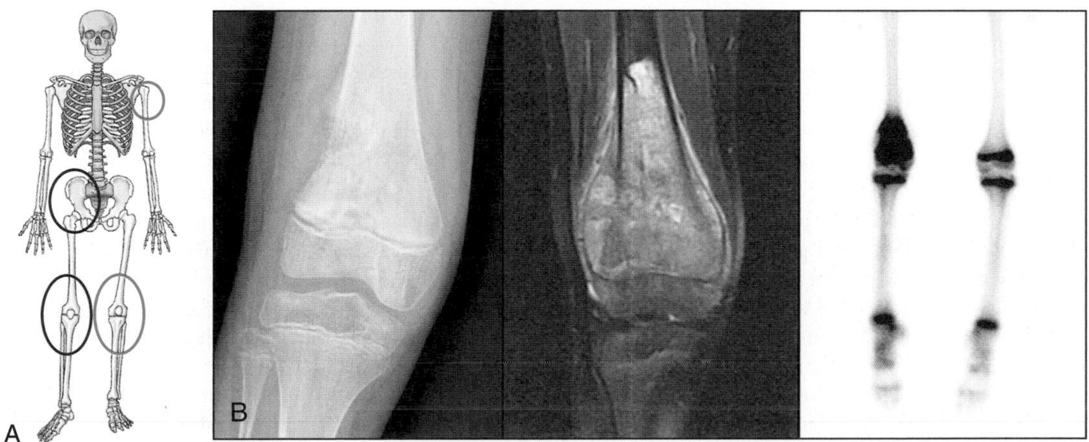

FIGURE 39-27 Osteosarcoma. A, Common locations of Ewing sarcoma and osteosarcoma. *Blue,* osteosarcoma; *red,* Ewing sarcoma. **B,** Comparison of plain radiograph, MRI, and nuclear bone scan appearances of osteosarcoma of the distal femur. Note destruction of the bone cortex and soft tissue component. (**A,** adapted from Bontrager, K.L., & Lampignanno, J.P. [Eds.]. [2013]. *Textbook of radiographic positioning and related anatomy.* St. Louis: Elsevier; **B,** Reprinted from *Pediatr Clin N Am,* 62, HaDuong, J.H., Martin, A.A., Skapek, S.X., & Mascarenhas, L., "Sarcomas," Pages 179–200, Copyright 2015, with permission from Elsevier.)

in addition to surgery.[285,286] Surgery is directed at salvaging the affected limb.[280,284]

Surgery is the major treatment of choice, with the tumour's location and size, the extent of malignancy, and evidence of metastasis dictating the type and extent of surgery (see Table 39-8). Preoperative chemotherapy has greatly increased the number of individuals qualifying for limb salvage surgery. Limb-salvaging procedures have been made possible by advances in reconstructive techniques and endoprosthetics. If an amputation is done, individuals are monitored closely with chest radiographs and CT. Pulmonary metastases are surgically resected, and chemotherapy is now a common therapy given both before and after surgery, using combinations of chemotherapeutic agents. Despite advances in chemotherapy and surgical techniques, overall long-term survival in osteosarcoma with metastases has not significantly improved in the past 30 to 40 years. Osteosarcomas are very difficult to treat with current chemotherapeutic agents.[287,288]

Other sarcomas include Ewing sarcoma (consisting of malignant small round blue cells that originate in the bone and surrounding soft tissue and affect mainly children and adolescents) and synovial sarcoma (originating in the joints), each of which demonstrates specific genetic alterations.[289,290] Others include rhabdomyosarcoma (a soft tissue sarcoma that likely originates in the skeleton but with features more like skeletal muscle) and sarcomas that have no definite morphological pattern, such as leiomyosarcoma (a soft tissue sarcoma) and pleomorphic liposarcoma (a rare and aggressive cancer that affects mainly fat cells in many different sizes and shapes within the same tumour).

Chondrogenic tumours: chondrosarcoma. Chondrogenic (cartilage-forming) tumours produce cartilage or chondroid, a primitive cartilage or cartilagelike substance. The most common chondrogenic tumour is chondrosarcoma.

Chondrosarcoma is the second most common primary malignant bone tumour[291] and is a tumour of middle-aged and older adults. Chondrosarcomas that develop from a pre-existing benign bone lesion (such as an enchondroma) are known as secondary chondrosarcomas. Individuals with certain conditions, such as multiple osteochondromas, may be at greater risk of developing secondary chondrosarcoma. Secondary chondrosarcomas are rare, occurring most often in young adults between 20 and 30 years of age. The tumour is more common in men than in women.

A chondrosarcoma is a large, cartilage-producing, ill-defined malignant tumour that infiltrates trabeculae in spongy bone. It occurs most often in the metaphysis or diaphysis of long bones, especially the femur or proximal humerus, and in the bones of the pelvis.[292] If located near the end of the bone, the tumour will infiltrate into the joint space. The tumour expands and enlarges the contour of the bone, causes extensive erosion of the cortex, and grows into the soft tissues.

Symptoms associated with a chondrosarcoma have an insidious onset. Local swelling and pain are the usual presenting symptoms. At first the pain is dull and intermittent, then gradually intensifies and becomes constant; it may awaken the person at night.

Diagnostic studies include radiographs, which must be reviewed carefully for an accurate diagnosis. MRI is useful in determining the extent of soft tissue involvement.[293,294] Biopsy is done at the time of surgery. (If biopsy is conducted before scheduled surgical incision, seeding of tumour cells could occur.) Sufficient tumour material must be obtained to facilitate an accurate diagnosis.

Surgical excision is generally regarded as the treatment of choice because chemotherapy is generally ineffective.[291] Tumours more centrally located (in the appendicular skeleton) are more likely to metastasize. Consequently, individuals with tumours located in the limbs may have a better prognosis than those with pelvic lesions. Recent advances in understanding the pathophysiology of bone sarcomas has led to development of targeted therapies that show promise for improving outcomes.[295,296]

Collagenic tumours: fibrosarcoma. Collagenic (collagen-forming) tumours originate from mesenchymal cells and produce fibrous connective tissue. Fibrosarcoma is the most common collagenic tumour and can affect bone or soft tissue.

Fibrosarcomas represent 4% of the primary malignant bone tumours, with a broad age distribution. They may occur at any age but are most common in adults between 30 and 50 years of age. The incidence is slightly greater in females. Fibrosarcoma also may be a secondary complication of radiation therapy, Paget's disease, and longstanding osteomyelitis.

Fibrosarcoma is a rare, malignant, solitary tumour that most often affects the metaphyseal region of the femur or tibia. The tumour is composed of a firm, fibrous mass of tissue that contains collagen, malignant fibroblasts, and occasional osteoclastlike giant cells. Secondary fibrosarcoma, which tends to have a worse prognosis, can occur after prior radiation to an area.

The tumour begins in the marrow cavity of the bone and infiltrates the trabeculae. It demonstrates a permeative growth pattern, destroys the cortex, and extends into the soft tissue. Metastasis to the lung is common.

Symptoms associated with the tumour have an insidious onset, which delays diagnosis. Pain and swelling are the usual presenting symptoms and usually indicate that the tumour has infiltrated the cortex. Local tenderness, a palpable mass, and limitation of motion also may be present. A pathological fracture in the affected bone is often the reason for seeking medical help. Diagnostic studies include radiographs and MRI.

Radical surgery and amputation are the treatments of choice for fibrosarcoma. There is a high probability of metastases. Radiation therapy is generally considered ineffective treatment for this tumour. Promising investigations of MMP inhibitors and even injectable compounds may alter future treatment of fibrosarcoma.[297,298]

Giant cell tumour (myelogenic tumours). Giant cell tumour (GCT), along with myeloma (see Chapter 21), are myelogenic tumours, ones that originate from various bone marrow cells. GCT is the sixth most common of the primary bone tumours, accounting for 4 to 5% of bone tumours. It is generally benign but can become malignant after radiation treatment. GCTs have a wide age distribution; however, they are rare in persons younger than 10 years or older than 70 years. Most GCTs are found in persons between 20 and 40 years of age. Unlike most other bone tumours, GCTs affect females more often than males.

The GCT is a solitary, circumscribed tumour that causes extensive bone resorption because of its osteoclastic origin and RANKL overexpression.[299] GCTs are typically located in the epiphyseal regions of the femur, tibia, radius, or humerus.[300] The tumour has a slow, relentless growth rate and is usually contained within the original contour of the affected bone. It may, however, extend into the articular cartilage. When the tumour extends, it is usually covered by periosteum or periosteal bone growth; it may extend into surrounding soft tissue. GCTs have a low rate of metastasis to other organs or tissues, although they have a high rate of recurrence.

The most common symptoms associated with GCT are pain, local swelling, and limitation of movement. Diagnostic studies include radiographs, CT, and MRI. Cryosurgery and resection of the tumour with the use of adjuvant polymethylmethacrylate (PMMA) for bone grafts decrease recurrence and are more successful treatments than curettage and radiation.[299] The monoclonal antibody denosumab has been approved for treating GCTs in cases of recurrence or where surgery is not feasible.[301,302] Depending on the extent of the tumour and its recurrence, amputation may be necessary.

Muscle Tumours

Rhabdomyoma

Rhabdomyoma is an extremely rare benign tumour of muscle that generally occurs in the tongue, neck muscles, larynx, uvula, nasal cavity, axilla, vulva, and heart. These tumours are usually treated by surgical excision and typically do not recur.

Rhabdomyosarcoma

About 3 to 5% of childhood cancers are malignant tumours of striated muscle called *rhabdomyosarcoma.* Infants, children, and teenagers account for more than 85% of cases; there is a slight preference in males. This tumour is highly malignant with rapid metastasis. Rhabdomyosarcomas are located in the muscle tissue of the head, neck, and genitourinary tract in 75% of cases, with the remainder found in the trunk and extremities. Recent animal studies have established a link between chemical, biological, and physical triggers of rhabdomyosarcoma.[303] Recent advances in treatment have improved the 5-year survival for children to greater than 80% in cases of localized tumours.[304] Unfortunately, survival in adults remains poor.

Three types of rhabdomyosarcoma are differentiated on pathological section: anaplastic (formerly known as *pleomorphic*), embryonal, and alveolar. Each type differs from the other molecularly; they are all aggressive tumours and are typically more resistant to therapy. Although rare, the anaplastic, or spindle cell, type is considered to be one of the most highly malignant tumours of the extremities seen in adulthood. Microscopically, embryonal tumours resemble a tadpole or tennis racquet and are most often seen in infancy and childhood. Alveolar-type tumours appear latticelike, similar to lung tissue alveoli, and are more often found in adolescents and adults.

The diagnosis of rhabdomyosarcoma is made by careful incisional biopsy or core needle aspiration and examination of the specimen by a pathologist. CT scan also helps define the tissue borders. PET/CT is useful in identifying involvement of bones, lymph nodes, and bone marrow. Staging is based on the tumour's size, location, presence of metastases, and lymph node involvement. Pathological grading of the tumour is helpful in determining prognosis and treatment.

Treatment consists of a combination of surgical excision, systemic chemotherapy, and radiation therapy. Cure is unlikely when distant metastases are present.

Other Tumours

Metastatic tumours in muscles are rare in spite of the extensive vascular supply of skeletal muscles. It is suggested that local pH or metabolic changes within muscles prevent metastatic involvement from other tumours. When adjacent carcinomas do cause muscle damage, it is usually related to the compression of tissue and resultant muscle atrophy.

QUICK CHECK 39-5

1. From what cells do bone tumours originate?
2. Compare five major characteristics of benign bone tumours with those of malignant bone tumours.
3. How does the presence of metastatic tumours affect treatment options and prognosis of persons with osteosarcoma?

DID YOU UNDERSTAND?

Musculo-skeletal Injuries

1. The most serious musculo-skeletal injury is a fracture. A bone can be completely or incompletely fractured. A closed fracture leaves the skin intact. An open fracture has an overlying skin wound. The direction of the fracture line can be linear, oblique, spiral, or transverse. Greenstick, torus, and bowing fractures are examples of incomplete fractures that occur in children. Stress fractures occur in normal or abnormal bone that is subjected to repeated stress. Fatigue fractures occur in normal bone subjected to abnormal stress. Normal weight-bearing can cause an insufficiency (or fragility) fracture in abnormal bone.
2. Dislocation is complete loss of contact between the articular surfaces of two bones. Subluxation is partial loss of joint contact between two bones. As a bone separates from a joint, it may damage adjacent nerves, blood vessels, ligaments, tendons, and muscle.
3. Tendon tears are called *strains,* and ligament tears are called *sprains.* A complete separation of a tendon or ligament from its attachment is called an *avulsion.*
4. Rhabdomyolysis, often manifested by the presence of myoglobinuria, can be a life-threatening complication of severe muscle trauma, genetic predisposition, or toxic effects of certain medications.

Disorders of Bones

1. Metabolic bone diseases are characterized by abnormal bone structure. In osteoporosis, the density or mass of bone is reduced because the bone remodelling cycle is disrupted. Osteomalacia is a metabolic bone disease characterized by inadequate bone mineralization. Excessive and abnormal bone remodelling occurs in Paget's disease.
2. Osteomyelitis is a bone infection caused *most often* by bacteria. Bacteria can enter bone from outside the body (exogenous osteomyelitis) or from infection sites within the body (hematogenous osteomyelitis).

Disorders of Joints

1. Because of improved imaging technology, inflammation has been identified as an important feature of osteoarthritis (OA).
2. OA is a common age-related disorder of synovial joints. The primary defect in OA is loss of articular cartilage.
3. Rheumatoid arthritis (RA) is an inflammatory joint disease characterized by inflammatory destruction of the synovial membrane, articular cartilage, joint capsule, and surrounding ligaments and tendons. Rheumatoid nodules also may invade the skin, lung, and spleen and involve small and large arteries. RA is a systemic disease that affects the heart, lungs, kidneys, and skin, as well as the joints.
4. Ankylosing spondylitis is a chronic, systemic autoimmune disease characterized by stiffening and fusion of the sacroiliac and spine joints.
5. Gout is a syndrome caused by defects in uric acid metabolism with high levels of uric acid in the blood and body fluids. Uric acid crystallizes in the connective tissue of a joint, where it initiates inflammatory destruction of the joint.

Disorders of Skeletal Muscle

1. A pathological contracture is permanent muscle shortening caused by muscle spasticity, as seen in central nervous system injury or severe muscle weakness.
2. Stress-induced muscle tension is presumably caused by increased activity in the reticular activating system and gamma loop in the muscle fibre. The use of progressive relaxation training and biofeedback has been advocated to reduce muscle tension.

3. Fibromyalgia (FM) is a chronic musculo-skeletal syndrome characterized by diffuse pain and tender points. Theories have proposed that the muscle is the end organ responsible for the pain and fatigue, although they have not been confirmed. Most cases of FM involve women, and the peak age of onset is 30 to 50 years of age. Genetic factors are being increasingly recognized as agents in developing FM.
4. Atrophy of muscle fibres and overall diminished size of the muscle are seen after prolonged inactivity. Isometric contractions and passive lengthening exercises decrease atrophy to some degree in immobilized persons.
5. Because of ion channel disorders, hyperexcitable membranes cause the physical and electrical phenomenon of myotonia. The disorder is treated with medications that reduce muscle fibre excitability. The biochemical defect is related to changes in the muscle membrane and sarcoplasmic reticulum.
6. Metabolic muscle diseases are caused by endocrine disorders, glycogen storage diseases, enzyme deficiencies, and abnormal lipid function. The muscle depends on a complex system of carbohydrates and fats converted by enzymes to produce energy for the muscle cell. Abnormalities in these pathways can inhibit function or cause damage to the muscle fibre. These illnesses are rare, yet they account for significant functional abnormalities.
7. Viral, bacterial, and parasitic infections of muscles produce the characteristic clinical and pathological changes associated with inflammation. These infections are usually treatable and self-limiting.
8. Polymyositis (generalized muscle inflammation) and dermatomyositis (polymyositis accompanied by skin rash) are characterized by inflammation of connective tissue and muscle fibres and muscle fibre necrosis. Cell-mediated and humoral immune factors have been implicated. Treatment with immunosuppressive agents is effective in many cases.
9. The most common cause of toxic myopathy is alcohol abuse. It has been suggested that alcohol use affects muscle fibres both directly (by causing necrosis) and indirectly (by the concomitant nutritional deficiencies typically associated with excessive use of alcohol). Medication administration can also lead to toxic myopathy; a needle used during an injection, secondary infection, and alterations in the acidity and alkalinity of muscle fibres can mechanically damage muscle fibres.

Musculo-skeletal Tumours

1. Bone tumours originate from bone cells, cartilage cells, fibrous tissue cells, or vascular marrow cells. Each cell produces a specific type of ground substance that is used to classify the tumour as osteogenic (bone cell), chondrogenic (cartilage cell), collagenic (fibrous tissue cell), or myelogenic (vascular marrow cell). Malignant bone tumours are usually large, aggressively destroy surrounding bone, invade surrounding tissue, and initiate independent growth outside the site of origin. Benign bone tumours are generally less destructive, limit their growth to the anatomical confines of the bone, and have a well-demarcated border. Certain benign tumours can become malignant.
2. Sarcomas of muscle tissue are rare. Rhabdomyosarcoma has a uniformly poor prognosis, particularly in adults, because of an aggressive invasion and early, widespread dissemination. The usual treatment includes surgical excision, radiation therapy, and systemic chemotherapy.

KEY TERMS

Acid maltase deficiency, 1044
Acute gouty arthritis, 1040
Age-related bone loss, 1023
Ankylosing spondylitis (AS), 1035
Asymptomatic hyperuricemia, 1040
Avulsion, 1015
Biofeedback, 1041
Bone tumour, 1047
Bowing fracture, 1012
Bursa (*pl.*, bursae), 1016
Caplan's syndrome, 1035
Central sensitization, 1041
Chondrogenic (cartilage-forming) tumour, 1050
Chondrosarcoma, 1050
Chronic fatigue syndrome (CFS), 1042
Closed (incomplete) fracture, 1011
Collagenic (collagen-forming) tumour, 1050
Comminuted fracture, 1012
Compartment syndrome, 1019
Complete fracture, 1011
Contiguous osteomyelitis, 1028
Contracture, 1041
Delayed union, 1014
Direct (primary) healing, 1013
Dislocation, 1014
Disuse atrophy, 1041
Dual X-ray absorptiometry (DXA), 1024
Endochondral bone formation, 1013
Enthesis, 1015
Epicondyle, 1015
Epicondylopathy, 1015
Ewing sarcoma, 1050
External fixation, 1014
Fatigue fracture, 1013
Fibromyalgia (FM), 1041
Fibrosarcoma, 1050
Fracture, 1011
Giant cell tumour (GCT), 1050
Glucocorticoid-induced osteoporosis, 1023
Glycogen storage disease (GSD), 1044
Gout, 1038
Gouty arthritis, 1038
Greenstick fracture, 1012
Hematogenous osteomyelitis, 1028
Heterotopic ossification (HO), 1017
Hyperbaric oxygen therapy, 1029
Idiopathic inflammatory myopathy (IIM), 1045
Immobilization (of a fracture), 1014
Incomplete fracture, 1011
Indirect (secondary) healing, 1013
Inflammatory joint disease (arthritis), 1032
Internal fixation, 1014
Involucrum, 1028
Joint effusion, 1031
Joint stiffness, 1031
Kyphosis, 1024
Lateral epicondylopathy (tennis elbow), 1015
Leiomyosarcoma, 1050
Ligament, 1015
Linear fracture, 1012
Malignant hyperthermia (MH), 1019
Malunion, 1014
McArdle's disease, 1044
Medial epicondylopathy (golfer's elbow), 1015
Muscle strain, 1016
Myalgic encephalomyelitis (ME), 1043
Myelogenic tumour, 1050
Myoadenylate deaminase deficiency (MDD), 1044
Myoglobinuria, 1017
Myositis ossificans, 1017
Myositis, 1044
Myotonia, 1043
Nonunion, 1014
Oblique fracture, 1012
Open (compound) fracture, 1011
Osteoarthritis (OA), 1029
Osteogenic (bone-forming) tumour, 1049
Osteomalacia, 1026
Osteomyelitis, 1028
Osteophyte, 1029
Osteoporosis (porous bone), 1021
Osteoprotegerin (OPG), 1023
Osteosarcoma, 1049
Paget's disease of bone (PDB, osteitis deformans, or Paget's disease), 1027
Pannus, 1033
Pathological (insufficiency or fragility) fracture, 1012
Peak bone mass, 1021
Periodic paralysis, 1043
Pleomorphic liposarcoma, 1050

Pompe's disease (PD), 1044
Postmenopausal osteoporosis, 1022
Progressive relaxation training, 1041
Receptor activator of nuclear factor kappa-B (RANK), 1023
Receptor activator of nuclear factor kappa-B ligand (RANKL), 1023
Reduction (of a fracture), 1012
Regional osteoporosis, 1023
Rhabdomyolysis, 1017
Rhabdomyoma, 1051
Rhabdomyosarcoma, 1050
Rheumatoid arthritis (RA), 1032
Rheumatoid factor (RF), 1033
Rheumatoid nodule, 1035
Secondary osteoporosis, 1023
Sequestrum, 1028
Spiral fracture, 1012
Sprain, 1015
Strain, 1015
Stress fracture, 1013
Subluxation, 1014
Syndesmophyte, 1037
Synovial sarcoma, 1050
Systemic exertional intolerance disease (SEID), 1043
Tendinopathy, 1015
Tendon, 1015
Tophaceous gout, 1040
Tophus (*pl.*, tophi), 1038
Torus fracture, 1012
Toxic myopathy, 1046
Transchondral fracture, 1013
Transverse fracture, 1012
Volkmann ischemic contracture, 1019

REFERENCES

1. Canadian Institute for Health Information (2013). *National trauma registry report 2013: Hospitalizations for major injury in Canada, 2010–2011 data*. Ottawa: Author. Retrieved from https://secure.cihi.ca/free_products/NTR_Annual_Report_2013_EN.xls.
2. Kanis, J. A., Oden, A., McCloskey, E. V., et al. (2012). Systematic review of hip fracture incidence and probability of fracture worldwide. *Osteoporosis International*, *23*, 2239–2256. doi:10.1007/s00198-012-1964-3.
3. Marsell, R., & Einhorn, T. A. (2011). The biology of fracture healing. *Injury*, *42*(6), 551–555. doi:10.1016/j.injury.2011.03.031.
4. Secreto, F. J., Hoeppner, L. H., & Westendorf, J. J. (2009). Wnt signaling during fracture repair. *Current Osteoporosis Reports*, *7*(2), 64–69.
5. Bunker, D. L. J., Ilie, V., & Nicklin, S. (2014). Tendon to bone healing and its implications for surgery. *Muscles, Ligaments and Tendons Journal*, *4*(3), 343–350.
6. Charvet, B., Ruggiero, F., & Le Guellec, D. (2012). The development of the myotendinous junction. A review. *Muscles, Ligaments and Tendons Journal*, *2*(2), 53–63.
7. Birch, H. L., Thorpe, C. T., & Rumian, A. P. (2013). Specialisation of extracellular matrix for function in tendons and ligaments. *Muscles, Ligaments and Tendons Journal*, *3*(1), 12–22. doi:10.11138/mltj/2013.3.1.012.
8. Hubbard, T. J., & Hicks-Little, C. A. (2008). Ankle ligament healing after an acute ankle sprain: An evidence-based approach. *Journal of Athletic Training*, *43*(5), 523–529. doi:10.4085/1062-6050-43.5.523.
9. Kaminski, T. W., Hertel, J., Amendola, N., et al. (2013). National Athletic Trainers' Association position statement: Conservative management and prevention of ankle sprains in athletes. *Journal of Athletic Training*, *48*(4), 528–545. doi:10.4085/1062-6050-48.4.02.
10. Knobloch, K. (2008). The role of tendon microcirculation in Achilles and patellar tendinopathy. *Journal of Orthopaedic Surgery and Research*, *3*, 18. doi:10.1186/1749-799X-3-18.
11. Luk, J. K., Tsang, R. C., & Leung, H. B. (2014). Lateral epicondylalgia: Midlife crisis of a tendon. *Hong Kong Medical Journal*, *20*(2), 145–151. doi:10.12809/hkmj134110.
12. Orchard, J., & Kountouris, A. (2011). The management of tennis elbow. *British Medical Journal*, *342*, d2687. doi:10.1136/bmj.d2687.
13. Waseem, M., Nuhmani, S., Ram, C. S., et al. (2012). Lateral epicondylitis: A review of the literature. *Journal of Back and Musculoskeletal Rehabilitation*, *25*(2), 131–142.
14. Chourasia, A. O., Buhr, K. A., Rabago, D. P., et al. (2013). Relationships between biomechanics, tendon pathology, and function in individuals with lateral epicondylosis. *The Journal of Orthopaedic and Sports Physical Therapy*, *43*(6), 368–378. doi:10.2519/jospt.2013.4411.
15. Järvinen, T. A. H., Järvinen, M., & Kalimo, H. (2013). Regeneration of injured skeletal muscle after the injury. *Muscles, Ligaments and Tendons Journal*, *3*(4), 337–345.
16. Cervellin, G., Comelli, I., & Lippi, G. (2010). Rhabdomyolysis: Historical background, clinical, diagnostic, and therapeutic features. *Clinical Chemistry and Laboratory Medicine*, *48*(6), 749–756. doi:10.1515/CCLM.2010.151.
17. Genthon, A., & Wilcox, S. R. (2014). Crush syndrome: A case report and review of the literature. *The Journal of Emergency Medicine*, *46*(2), 313–319. doi:10.1016/j.jemermed.2013.08.052.
18. Zutt, R., van der Kooi, A. J., Linthorst, G. E., et al. (2014). Rhabdomyolysis: Review of the literature. *Neuromuscular Disorders*, *24*(8), 651–659. doi:10.1016/j.nmd.2014.05.005.
19. Young, S. E., Miller, M. A., & Docherty, M. (2009). Urine dipstick testing to rule out rhabdomyolysis in patients with suspected heat injury. *The American Journal of Emergency Medicine*, *27*(7), 875–877. doi:10.1016/j.ajem.2008.06.020.
20. Su, B.-H., Qiu, L., Fu, P., et al. (2009). Ultrasonic appearance of rhabdomyolysis in patients with crush injury in the Wenchuan earthquake. *Chinese Medical Journal*, *122*(16), 1872–1876.
21. Ali, P., Santy-Tomlinson, J., & Watson, R. (2014). Assessment and diagnosis of acute limb compartment syndrome: A literature review. *International Journal of Orthopaedic and Trauma Nursing*, *18*(4), 180–190. doi:10.1016/j.ijotn.2014.01.002.
22. McDonald, S., & Bearcroft, P. (2010). Compartment syndromes. *Seminars in Musculoskeletal Radiology*, *14*(2), 236–244. doi:10.1055/s-0030-1253164.
23. Shadgan, B., Menon, M., Sanders, D., et al. (2010). Current thinking about acute compartment syndrome of the lower extremity. *Canadian Journal of Surgery*, *53*(5), 329–334.
24. Raza, H., & Mahapatra, A. (2015). Acute compartment syndrome in orthopedics: Causes, diagnosis, and management. *Advances in Orthopedics*, *2015*, 543412. doi:10.1155/2015/543412.
25. Collinge, C., & Kuper, M. (2010). Comparison of three methods for measuring intracompartmental pressure in injured limbs of trauma patients. *Journal of Orthopaedic Trauma*, *24*(6), 364–368. doi:10.1097/BOT.0b013e3181cb5866.
26. Hammerberg, E. M., Whitesides, T. E., Jr., & Seller, J. G., 3rd. (2012). The reliability of measurement of tissue pressure in compartment syndrome. *Journal of Orthopaedic Trauma*, *26*(1), 24–31. doi:10.1097/BOT.0b013e31822908cf.
27. Bandschapp, O., & Girard, T. (2012). Malignant hyperthermia. *Swiss Medical Weekly*, *142*, w13652. doi:10.4414/smw.2012.13652.
28. Stowell, K. M. (2014). DNA testing for malignant hyperthermia: The reality and the dream. *Anesthesia and Analgesia*, *118*(2), 397–406. doi:10.1213/ANE.0000000000000063.
29. Schneiderbanger, D., Johannsen, S., Roewer, N., et al. (2014). Management of malignant hyperthermia: Diagnosis and treatment. *Therapeutics and Clinical Risk Management*, *10*, 355–362. doi:10.2147/TCRM.S47632.
30. Correia, A. C., Silva, P. C., & da Silva, B. A. (2012). Malignant hyperthermia: Clinical and molecular aspects. *Revista Brasileira de Anestesiologia*, *62*(6), 820–837. doi:10.1016/S0034-7094(12)70182-4.
31. Kim, D. C. (2012). Malignant hyperthermia. *Korean Journal of Anesthesiology*, *65*(5), 391–401. doi:10.4097/kjae.2012.63.5.391.
32. Chen, H., & Kubo, K. Y. (2014). Bone three-dimensional microstructural features of the common osteoporotic fracture sites. *World Journal of Orthopedics*, *5*(4), 486–495. doi:10.5312/wjo.v5.i4.486.
33. World Health Organization Scientific Group on the Prevention and Management of Osteoporosis (2000). *WHO Technical Report Series, No. 921*. Geneva, Switzerland: Author.
34. Dede, A. D., Lyritis, G. P., & Tournis, S. (2014). Bone disease in anorexia nervosa. *Hormones (Athens, Greece)*, *13*(1), 38–56.
35. Gonnelli, S., Caffarelli, C., & Nuti, R. (2014). Obesity and fracture risk. *Clinical Cases in Mineral and Bone Metabolism*, *11*(1), 9–14.
36. Jackuliak, P., & Payer, J. (2014). Osteoporosis, fractures, and diabetes. *International Journal of Endocrinology*, *2014*, 820615. doi:10.1155/2014/820615.
37. Misra, M., & Klibanski, A. (2014). Anorexia nervosa and bone. *The Journal of Endocrinology*, *221*(3), R163–R176. doi:10.1530/JOE-14-0039.
38. Panday, K., Gona, A., & Humphrey, M. B. (2014). Medication-induced osteoporosis: Screening and treatment strategies. *Therapeutic Advances in Musculoskeletal Disease*, *6*(5), 185–202. doi:10.1177/1759720X14546350.
39. Osteoporosis Canada. (2010). *2010 clinical practice guidelines for the diagnosis and management of osteoporosis in Canada*. Retrieved from http://www.osteoporosis.ca/health-care-professionals/guidelines/.
40. Lange, A., Zeidler, J., & Braun, S. (2014). One-year disease-related health care costs of incident vertebral fractures in osteoporotic patients. *Osteoporosis International*, *25*(10), 2435–2443. doi:10.1007/s00198-014-2776-4.
41. Svedbom, A., Hemlund, E., Ivergård, M., et al. (2013). Osteoporosis in the European Union: A compendium of country-specific reports. *Archives of Osteoporosis*, *8*(1–2), 137. doi:10.1007/s11657-013-0137-0.
42. Viswanathan, H. N., Curtis, J. R., Yu, J., et al. (2012). Direct healthcare costs of osteoporosis-related fractures in managed care patients receiving pharmacological osteoporosis therapy. *Applied Health Economics and Health Policy*, *10*(3), 163–173. doi:10.2165/11598590-000000000-00000.
43. Adachi, J. D., Adami, S., Gehlbach, S., et al. (2010). Impact of prevalent fractures on quality of life: Baseline results from the global longitudinal study of osteoporosis in women. *Mayo Clinic Proceedings*, *5*(9), 806–813. doi:10.4065/mcp.2010.0082.
44. Leslie, W. D., & Morin, S. N. (2014). Osteoporosis epidemiology 2013: Implications for diagnosis, risk assessment, and treatment. *Current Opinion in Rheumatology*, *26*(4), 440–446. doi:10.1097/BOR.0000000000000064.
45. Rao, S. S., Budhwar, N., & Ashfaque, A. (2010). Osteoporosis in men. *American Family Physician*, *82*(5), 503–508.

46. Dy, C. J., Lamont, L. E., Ton, Q. V., et al. (2011). Sex and gender considerations in male patients with osteoporosis. *Clinical Orthopaedics and Related Research, 469*(7), 1906–1912. doi:10.1007/s11999-011-1849-3.
47. Cawthorn, P. M. (2011). Gender differences in osteoporosis and fractures. *Clinical Orthopaedics and Related Research, 469*(7), 1900–1905. doi:10.1007/s11999-011-1780-7.
48. Haentjens, P., Magaziner, J., Colón-Emeric, C. S., et al. (2010). Meta-analysis: Excess mortality after hip fracture among older women and men. *Annals of Internal Medicine, 152*(6), 380–390. doi:10.7326/0003-4819-152-6-201003160-00008.
49. Gerdhem, P. (2013). Osteoporosis and fragility fractures: Vertebral fractures. *Best Practice and Research: Clinical Rheumatology, 27*(6), 743–755. doi:10.1016/j.berh.2014.01.002.
50. Cauley, J. A. (2011). Defining ethnic and racial differences in osteoporosis and fragility fractures. *Clinical Orthopaedics and Related Research, 469*(7), 1891–1899. doi:10.1007/s11999-011-1863-5.
51. NIH Osteoporosis and Related Bone Diseases National Resource Center. (2010). *Osteoporosis and African American women*. Retrieved from http://www.niams.nih.gov/Health_Info/Bone/Osteoporosis/Background/default.asp.
52. Rubin, K. H., Abrahamsen, B., Friis-Holmberg, T., et al. (2013). Comparison of different screening tools (FRAX®, OST, ORAI, OSIRIS, SCORE and age alone) to identify women with increased risk of fracture. A population-based prospective study. *Bone, 56*(1), 16–22. doi:10.1016/j.bone.2013.05.002.
53. Khosla, S. (2013). Pathogenesis of age-related bone loss in humans. *The Journals of Gerontology: Series A, Biological Sciences and Medical Sciences, 68*(10), 1226–1235. doi:10.1093/gerona/gls163.
54. Calvo, M. S., & Tucker, K. L. (2013). Is phosphorus intake that exceeds dietary requirements a risk factor in bone health? *Annals of the New York Academy of Sciences, 1301*, 29–35. doi:10.1111/nyas.12300.
55. Calvo, M. S., & Uribarri, J. (2013). Public health impact of dietary phosphorus excess on bone and cardiovascular health in the general population. *The American Journal of Clinical Nutrition, 98*(1), 6–13. doi:10.3945/ajcn.112.053934.
56. Cauley, J. A. (2015). Estrogen and bone health in men and women. *Steroids, 99*(Pt. A), 11–15. doi:10.1016/j.steroids.2014.12.010.
57. Vandenput, L., Lorentzon, M., Sundh, D., et al. (2014). Serum estradiol levels are inversely associated with cortical porosity in older men. *The Journal of Clinical Endocrinology and Metabolism, 99*(7), E1322–E1326. doi:10.1210/jc.2014-1319.
58. Aaseth, J., Bolvin, G., & Andersen, D. (2012). Osteoporosis and trace elements—An overview. *Journal of Trace Elements in Medicine and Biology, 26*(2–3), 149–152. doi:10.1016/j.jtemb.2012.03.017.
59. Okyay, E., Ertugrul, C., Acar, B., et al. (2013). Comparative evaluation of serum levels of main minerals and postmenopausal osteoporosis. *Maturitas, 76*(4), 320–325. doi:10.1016/j.maturitas.2013.07.015.
60. Zofkova, I., Nemcikova, P., & Matucha, P. (2013). Trace elements and bone health. *Clinical Chemistry and Laboratory Medicine, 51*(8), 1555–1561. doi:10.1515/cclm-2012-0868.
61. Body, J. J., Bergmann, P., Boonen, S., et al. (2011). Non-pharmacological management of osteoporosis: A consensus of the Belgian Bone Club. *Osteoporosis International, 22*(11), 2769–2788. doi:10.1007/s00198-011-1545-x.
62. Celec, P., & Behuliak, M. (2010). Behavioural and endocrine effects of chronic cola intake. *Journal of Psychopharmacology (Oxford, England), 24*(10), 1569–1572. doi:10.1177/0269881109105401.
63. Hallström, H., Byberg, L., Glynn, A., et al. (2013). Long-term coffee consumption in relation to fracture risk and bone mineral density in women. *American Journal of Epidemiology, 178*(8), 898–909. doi:10.1093/aje/kwt062.
64. Panday, K., Gona, A., & Humphrey, M. B. (2014). Medication-induced osteoporosis: Screening and treatment strategies. *Therapeutic Advances in Musculoskeletal Disease, 6*(5), 185–202. doi:10.1177/1759720X14546350.
65. Cano-Marquina, A., Tarin, J. J., Garcia-Perez, M. A., et al. (2014). Transient regional osteoporosis. *Maturitas, 77*(4), 324–329. doi:10.1016/j.maturitas.2014.01.012.
66. Rocchietti March, M., Tovaglia, V., Meo, A., et al. (2010). Transient osteoporosis of the hip. *Hip International, 20*(3), 297–300.
67. Klontzas, M. E., Vassalou, E. E., Zibis, A. H., et al. (2015). MR imaging of transient regional osteoporosis of the hip: An update on 155 hip joints. *European Journal of Radiology, 84*(3), 431–436. doi:10.1016/j.ejrad.2014.11.022.
68. Dore, R. K. (2010). How to prevent glucocorticoid-induced osteoporosis. *Cleveland Clinic Journal of Medicine, 77*(8), 529–536. doi:10.3949/ccjm.77a.10003.
69. Henneicke, H., Gasparini, S. J., Brennan-Speranza, T. C., et al. (2014). Glucocorticoids and bone: Local effects and systemic implications. *Trends in Endocrinology and Metabolism, 25*(4), 197–211. doi:10.1016/j.tem.2013.12.006.
70. Seibel, M. J., Cooper, M. S., & Zhou, H. (2013). Glucocorticoid-induced osteoporosis: Mechanisms, management, and future perspectives. *The Lancet: Diabetes & Endocrinology, 1*(1), 59–70. doi:10.1016/S2213-8587(13)70045-7.
71. Sutter, S., Nishiyama, K. K., Kepley, A., et al. (2014). Abnormalities in cortical bone, trabecular plates, and stiffness in postmenopausal women treated with glucocorticoids. *The Journal of Clinical Endocrinology and Metabolism, 99*(11), 4231–4241. doi:10.1210/jc.2014-2177.
72. Khosla, S. (2012). Pathogenesis of age-related bone loss in humans. *The Journals of Gerontology. Series A, Biological Sciences and Medical Sciences, 68*(10), 1226–1235. doi:10.1093/gerona/gls163.
73. Perrini, S., Laviola, L., Carreira, M. C., et al. (2010). The GH/IGF1 axis and signaling pathways in the muscle and bone: Mechanism underlying age-related skeletal muscle wasting and osteoporosis. *The Journal of Endocrinology, 205*(3), 201–210. doi:10.1677/JOE-09-0431.
74. Giusti, A., & Bianchi, G. (2015). Treatment of primary osteoporosis in men. *Clinical Interventions in Aging, 10*, 105–115. doi:10.2147/CIA.S44057.
75. Warriner, A. H., Patkar, N. M., Curtis, J. R., et al. (2011). Which fractures are most attributable to osteoporosis? *Journal of Clinical Epidemiology, 64*(1), 46–53. doi:10.1016/j.jclinepi.2010.07.007.
76. Hans, D., Goertzen, A. L., Krieg, M. A., et al. (2011). Bone microarchitecture assessed by TBS predicts osteoporotic fractures independent of bone density: The Manitoba study. *Journal of Bone and Mineral Research, 26*(11), 2762–2769. doi:10.1002/jbmr.499.
77. Popp, A. W., Buffat, H., Eberli, U., et al. (2014). Microstructural parameters of bone evaluated using HR-pQCT correlate with the DXA-derived cortical index and the trabecular bone score in a cohort of randomly selected premenopausal women. *PLoS ONE, 9*(2), e88946. doi:10.1371/journal.pone.0088946.
78. Silva, B. C., Leslie, W. D., Resch, H., et al. (2014). Trabecular bone score: A noninvasive analytical method based upon the DXA image. *Journal of Bone and Mineral Research, 29*(3), 518–530. doi:10.1002/jbmr.2176.
79. Ulivieri, F. M., Silva, B. C., Sardanelli, F., et al. (2014). Utility of the trabecular bone score (TBS) in secondary osteoporosis. *Endocrine, 47*(2), 435–438. doi:10.1007/s12020-014-0280-4.
80. Link, Y. M. (2010). The founder's lecture 2009: Advances in imaging of osteoporosis and osteoarthritis. *Skeletal Radiology, 39*(10), 943–955. doi:10.1007/s00256-010-0987-0.
81. Honig, S. (2010). Osteoporosis—New treatments and updates. *Bulletin of the NYU Hospital for Joint Diseases, 68*(3), 166–170.
82. Bellido, T., Saini, V., & Pajevic, P. D. (2013). Effects of PTH on osteocyte function. *Bone, 54*(2), 250–257. doi:10.1016/j.bone.2012.09.016.
83. Huber, B. C., Grabmaier, U., & Brunner, S. (2014). Impact of parathyroid hormone on bone marrow-derived stem cell mobilization and migration. *World Journal of Stem Cells, 6*(5), 637–643. doi:10.4252/wjsc.v6.i5.637.
84. Ward, L. M., Gaboury, I., Ladhani, M., et al. (2007). Vitamin D-deficiency rickets among children in Canada. *Canadian Medical Association Journal, 177*(2), 161–166. doi:10.1503/cmaj.061377.
85. Bhan, A., Rao, A. D., & Rao, D. S. (2010). Osteomalacia as a result of vitamin D deficiency. *Endocrinology and Metabolism Clinics of North America, 39*(2), 321–331. doi:10.1016/j.ecl.2010.02.001.
86. Babayev, R., & Nickolas, T. L. (2014). Can one evaluate bone disease in chronic kidney disease without a biopsy? *Current Opinion in Nephrology and Hypertension, 23*(4), 431–437. doi:10.1097/01.mnh.0000447014.36475.58.
87. Kulak, C. A., & Dempster, D. W. (2010). Bone histomorphometry: A concise review for endocrinologists and clinicians. *Arquivos Brasileiros de Endocrinologia E Metabologia, 54*(2), 87–98.
88. Ferraz-de-Souza, B., & Correa, P. H. (2013). Diagnosis and treatment of Paget's disease of bone: A mini-review. *Arquivos Brasileiros de Endocrinologia E Metabologia, 57*(8), 577–582.
89. Michou, L., & Brown, J. P. (2011). Emerging strategies and therapies for treatment of Paget's disease of bone. *Drug Design, Development and Therapy, 5*, 225–239. doi:10.2147/DDDT.S11306.
90. Cundy, T., & Reid, I. R. (2012). Paget's disease of bone. *Clinical Biochemistry, 45*(1–2), 43–48. doi:10.1016/j.clinbiochem.2011.09.026.
91. Galson, D. L., & Roodman, G. D. (2014). Pathobiology of Paget's disease of bone. *Journal of Bone Metabolism, 21*(2), 85–98. doi:10.11005/jbm.2014.21.2.85.
92. Ralston, S. H., & Layfield, R. (2012). Pathogenesis of Paget disease of bone. *Calcified Tissue International, 91*(2), 97–113. doi:10.1007/s00223-012-9599-0.
93. Roodman, G. D. (2010). Insights into the pathogenesis of Paget's disease. *Annals of the New York Academy of Sciences, 1192*, 176–180. doi:10.1111/j.1749-6632.2009.05214.x.
94. Visconti, M. R., Langston, A. L., Alsonso, N., et al. (2010). Mutations of SQSTM1 are associated with severity and clinical outcome in Paget disease of bone. *Journal of Bone and Mineral Research, 25*(11), 2368–2373. doi:10.1002/jbmr.132.
95. Chung, P. Y., & Van Hul, W. (2012). Paget's disease of bone: Evidence for complex pathogenic interactions. *Seminars in Arthritis and Rheumatism, 41*(5), 619–641. doi:10.1016/j.semarthrit.2011.07.005.
96. Brandi, M. L. (2010). Current treatment approaches for Paget's disease of bone. *Discovery Medicine, 10*(52), 209–212.
97. Baykan, E. K., Saygili, L. F., Erdogan, M., et al. (2014). Efficacy of zoledronic acid treatment in Paget disease of bone. *Osteoporosis International, 25*(9), 2221–2223. doi:10.1007/s00198-014-2752-z.
98. Bolland, M. J., & Cundy, T. (2014). Republished: Paget's disease of bone: Clinical review and update. *Postgraduate Medical Journal, 90*(1064), 328–331. doi:10.1136/postgradmedj-2013-201688rep.
99. Seton, M. (2013). Paget disease of bone: Diagnosis and drug therapy. *Cleveland Clinic Journal of Medicine, 80*(7), 452–462. doi:10.3949/ccjm.80a.12142.
100. Wat, W. Z. (2014). Current perspectives on bisphosphonate treatment in Paget's disease of bone. *Therapeutics and Clinical Risk Management, 10*, 977–983. doi:10.2147/TCRM.S58367.
101. Romanò, C. L., Romanò, D., Logoluso, N., et al. (2011). Bone and joint infections in adults: A comprehensive classification proposal. *European Orthopaedics and Traumatology, 1*(6), 207–217. doi:10.1007/s12570-011-0056-8.
102. Stern, S. M., & Ferguson, P. J. (2013). Autoinflammatory bone diseases. *Rheumatic Disease Clinics of North America, 39*(4), 735–749. doi:10.1016/j.rdc.2013.05.002.

103. Jorge, L. S., Chueire, A. G., & Rossit, A. R. (2010). Osteomyelitis: A current challenge. *The Brazilian Journal of Infectious Diseases, 14*(3), 310–315.
104. Kim, B. N., Kim, E. S., & Oh, M. D. (2014). Oral antibiotic treatment of staphylococcal bone and joint infections in adults. *The Journal of Antimicrobial Chemotherapy, 69*(2), 309–322. doi:10.1093/jac/dkt374.
105. Wright, J. A., & Nair, S. P. (2010). Interaction of staphylococci with bone. *International Journal of Medical Microbiology, 300*(2–3), 193–204. doi:10.1016/j.ijmm.2009.10.003.
106. Aman, A. J., & Adhikari, R. P. (2014). Staphylococcal bicomponent pore-forming toxins: Targets for prophylaxis. *Toxins, 6*(3), 950–972. doi:10.3390/toxins6030950.
107. Chung, P. Y., & Toh, Y. S. (2014). Anti-biofilm agents: Recent breakthrough against multi-drug resistant *Staphylococcus aureus. Pathogens and disease, 79*(3), 231–239. doi:10.1111/2049-632X.12141.
108. Dapunt, U., Maurer, S., Giese, T., et al. (2014). The macrophage inflammatory proteins MIP1α (CCL3) and MIP2α (CXCL2) in implant-associated osteomyelitis: Linking inflammation to bone degradation. *Mediators of Inflammation, 2014*, 728619. doi:10.1155/2014/728619.
109. Sanchez, C. J., Jr., Ward, C. L., Romano, D. R., et al. (2013). *Staphylococcus aureus* biofilms decrease osteoblast viability, inhibits osteogenic differentiation, and increases bone resorption in vitro. *BMC Musculoskeletal Disorders, 14*, 187. doi:10.1186/1471-2474-14-187.
110. Prieto-Pérez, L., Pérez-Tanoira, R., Petkova-Saiz, E., et al. (2014). Osteomyelitis: A descriptive study. *Clinics in Orthopedic Surgery, 6*(1), 20–25. doi:10.4055/cios.2014.6.1.20.
111. Gotthardt, M., Bleeker-Rovers, C. P., Boerman, O. C., et al. (2013). Imaging of inflammation by PET, conventional scintigraphy, and other imaging techniques. *Journal of Nuclear Medicine Technology, 41*(3), 157–169. doi:10.2967/jnumed.110.076232.
112. Conterno, L. O., & Turchi, M. D. (2013). Antibiotics for treating chronic osteomyelitis in adults. *The Cochrane Database of Systematic Reviews*, (9), CD004439, doi:10.1002/14651858.CD004439 .pub3.
113. McLaren, J. S., White, L. J., Cox, H. C., et al. (2014). A biodegradable antibiotic-impregnated scaffold to prevent osteomyelitis in a contaminated in vivo bone defect model. *European Cells and Materials, 27*, 332–349.
114. Losina, E., Weinstein, A. M., Reichmann, W. M., et al. (2013). Lifetime risk and age at diagnosis of symptomatic knee osteoarthritis in the US. *Arthritis Care & Research, 65*(5), 703–711. doi:10.1002/acr.21898.
115. Evangelou, E., Vaides, A. M., Kerkhof, H. J., et al. (2011). Meta-analysis of genome-wide association studies confirms a susceptibility locus for knee osteoarthritis on chromosome 7q22. *Annals of the Rheumatic Diseases, 70*(2), 349–355. doi:10.1136/ard.2010.132787.
116. Tsezou, A. (2014). Osteoarthritis year in review 2014: Genetics and genomics. *Osteoarthritis and Cartilage, 22*(12), 2017–2024. doi:10.1016/j.joca.2014.07.024.
117. Andriacchi, T. P., Favre, J., Erhart-Hiedik, J. C., et al. (2015). A systems view of risk factors for knee osteoarthritis reveals insights into the pathogenesis of the disease. *Annals of Biomedical Engineering, 43*(2), 376–387. doi:10.1007/s10439-014-1117-2.
118. Buckwalter, J. A., Anderson, D. D., Brown, T. D., et al. (2013). The roles of mechanical stresses in the pathogenesis of osteoarthritis: Implications for treatment of joint injuries. *Cartilage, 4*(4), 286–294. doi:10.1177/1947603513495889.
119. Orlowsky, E. W., & Kraus, V. B. (2015). The role of innate immunity in osteoarthritis: When our first line of defense goes on the offensive. *The Journal of Rheumatology, 42*(3), 363–371. doi:10.3899/jrheum.140382.
120. Sokolove, J., & Lepus, C. M. (2013). Role of inflammation in the pathogenesis of osteoarthritis: Latest findings and interpretations. *Therapeutic Advances in Musculoskeletal Disease, 5*(2), 77–94. doi:10.1177/1759720X12467868.
121. Karlsson, M. K., Magnusson, H., Cöster, M., et al. (2015). Patients with knee osteoarthritis have a phenotype with higher bone mass, higher fat mass, and lower lean body mass. *Clinical Orthopaedics and Related Research, 473*(1), 258–264. doi:10.1007/s11999-014-3973-3.
122. Losina, E., Walensky, R. P., Reichmann, W. M., et al. (2011). Impact of obesity and knee osteoarthritis on morbidity and mortality in older Americans. *Annals of Internal Medicine, 154*(4), 217–226. doi:10.7326/0003-4819-154-4-201102150-00001.
123. Silverwood, V., Blagojevic-Bucknall, M., Jinks, C., et al. (2015). Current evidence on factors for knee osteoarthritis in older adults: A systematic review and meta-analysis. *Osteoarthritis and Cartilage, 23*(4), 507–515. doi:10.1016/j.joca.2014.11.019.
124. Wang, X., Hunter, D., Xu, J., et al. (2015). Metabolic triggered inflammation in osteoarthritis. *Osteoarthritis and Cartilage, 23*(1), 22–30. doi:10.1016/j.joca.2014.10.002.
125. Dare, D., & Rodeo, S. (2014). Mechanisms of post-traumatic osteoarthritis after ACL injury. *Current Rheumatology Reports, 16*(10), 448. doi:10.1007/s11926-014-0448-1.
126. Stein, V., Li, L., Lo, G., et al. (2013). Pattern of joint damage in persons with knee osteoarthritis and concomitant ACL tears. *Rheumatology International, 32*(5), 1197–1208. doi:10.1007/s00296-010-1749-y.
127. Amoako, A. O., & Pujalte, G. A. (2014). Osteoarthritis in young, active, and athletic individuals. *Clinical Medicine Insights: Arthritis and Musculoskeletal Disorders, 7*, 27–32. doi:10.4137/CMAMD.S14386.
128. Hall, M., Doherty, S., Courtney, P., et al. (2014). Synovial pathology on ultrasound correlates with the severity of radiographic knee osteoarthritis more than with symptoms. *Osteoarthritis and Cartilage, 22*(10), 1627–1633. doi:10.1016/j.joca.2014.05.025.
129. Haugen, I. K., Slatkowsky Christensen, B., Bøyesen, P., et al. (2016). Increasing synovitis and bone marrow lesions are associated with incident joint tenderness in hand osteoarthritis. *Annals of the Rheumatic Diseases, 75*(4), 702–708. doi:10.1136/annrheumdis-2014-206829.
130. Kapoor, M., Martel-Pelletier, J., Lajeunesse, D., et al. (2011). Role of proinflammatory cytokines in the pathophysiology of osteoarthritis. *Nature Reviews: Rheumatology, 7*, 33–42. doi:10.1038/nrrheum.2010.196.
131. van der Kraan, P. M. (2014). Age-related alterations in TGF beta signaling as a causal factor of cartilage degeneration in osteoarthritis. *Bio-Medical Materials and Engineering, 24*(1, Suppl.), 75–80. doi:10.3233/BME-140976.
132. Clement, T., Salone, V., Charpentier, B., et al. (2014). Identification of new microRNAs targeting genes regulating the Pi/PPi balance in chondrocytes. *Bio-Medical Materials and Engineering, 24*(1, Suppl.), 3–16. doi:10.3233/BME-140969.
133. Trzeciak, T., & Czarny-Ratajczak, M. (2014). MicroRNAs: Important epigenetic regulators in osteoarthritis. *Current Genomics, 15*(6), 481–484. do i:10.2174/138920291566614024212506.
134. van der Kraan, P. M. (2014). Age-related alterations in TGF beta signaling as a causal factor of cartilage degeneration in osteoarthritis. *Bio-Medical Materials and Engineering, 24*(1, Suppl.), 75–80. doi:10.3233/BME-140976.
135. Mrosewski, I., Jork, N., Gorte, K., et al. (2014). Regulation of osteoarthritis-associated key mediators by TNFα and IL-10; effects of IL-10 overexpression in human synovial fibroblasts and a synovial cell line. *Cell and Tissue Research, 357*(1), 207–223. doi:10.1007/s00441-014-1868-y.
136. Sauerschnig, M., Stolberg-Stolberg, J., Schulze, A., et al. (2014). Diverse expression of selected cytokines and proteinases in synovial fluid obtained from osteoarthritic and healthy human knee joints. *European Journal of Medical Research, 19*(1), 65. doi:10.1186/s40001-014-0065-5.
137. Francin, P.-J., Abot, A., Guillaume, C., et al. (2014). Association between adiponectin and cartilage degradation in human osteoarthritis. *Osteoarthritis and Cartilage, 22*(3), 519–526. doi:10.1016/j.joca.2014.01.002.
138. Findlay, D. M., & Atkins, G. J. (2014). Osteoblast–chondrocyte interactions in osteoarthritis. *Current Osteoporosis Reports, 12*(1), 127–134. doi:10.1007/s11914-014-0192-5.
139. Li, G., Gao, J., Cheng, T. S., et al. (2013). Subchondral bone in osteoarthritis: Insight into risk factors and microstructural changes. *Arthritis Research and Therapy, 15*(6), 223. doi:10.1186/ar4405.
140. Liu-Bryan, R. (2013). Synovium and the innate inflammatory network in osteoarthritis progression. *Current Rheumatology Reports, 15*(5), 323. doi:10.1007/s11926-013-0323-5.
141. Felson, D. T., Niu, J., Gross, K. D., et al. (2013). Valgus malalignment is a risk factor for lateral knee osteoarthritis incidence and progression: Findings from the Multicenter Osteoarthritis Study and the Osteoarthritis Initiative. *Arthritis and Rheumatism, 65*(2), 355–362. doi:10.1002/art.37726.
142. Stief, F., Böhm, H., Dussa, C. U., et al. (2014). Effect of lower limb malalignment in the frontal plane on transverse plane mechanics during gait in young individuals with varus knee alignment. *The Knee, 21*(3), 688–693. doi:10.1016/j.knee.2014.03.004.
143. Felson, D. T., Niu, J., Yang, T., et al. (2013). Physical activity, alignment and knee osteoarthritis: Data from MOST and the OAI. *Osteoarthritis and Cartilage, 21*(6), 789–795. doi:10.1016/j.joca.2013.03.001.
144. Fransen, M., McConnell, S., Harmer, A. R., et al. (2015). Exercise for osteoarthritis of the knee. *The Cochrane Database of Systematic Reviews*, (1), CD004376, doi:10.1002/14651858.CD004376 .pub3.
145. Juhl, C., Christensen, R., Roos, E. M., et al. (2014). Impact of exercise type and dose on pain and disability in knee osteoarthritis: A systematic review and meta-regression analysis of randomized controlled trials. *Arthritis & Rheumatology, 66*(3), 622–636. doi:10.1002/art.38290.
146. Koonce, R. C., & Bravman, J. T. (2013). Obesity and osteoarthritis: More than just wear and tear. *The Journal of the American Academy of Orthopaedic Surgeons, 21*(3), 161–169. doi:10.5435/JAAOS-21-03-161.
147. Messier, S. P., Mihalko, S. L., Legault, C., et al. (2013). Effects of intensive diet and exercise on knee joint loads, inflammation, and clinical outcomes among overweight and obese adults with knee osteoarthritis. *The Journal of the American Medical Association, 310*(12), 1263–1273. doi:10.1001/jama.2013.277669.
148. Chyu, M. C., von Bergen, V., Brismée, J. M., et al. (2011). Complementary and alternative exercises for management of osteoarthritis. *Arthritis, 2011*, 364319. doi:10.1155/2011/364319.
149. Yan, J. H., Gu, W. J., Sun, J., et al. (2013). Efficacy of Tai Chi on pain, stiffness and function in patients with osteoarthritis: A meta-analysis. *PLoS ONE, 8*(4), e61671. doi:10.1371/journal.pone.0061672.
150. Raja, K., & Dewan, N. (2011). Efficacy of knee braces and foot orthoses in conservative management of knee osteoarthritis: A systematic review. *American Journal of Physical Medicine and Rehabilitation, 90*(3), 247–262. doi:10.1097/PHM.0b013e318206386b.
151. Fransen, M., Agaliotis, M., Votrubec, M., et al. (2015). Glucosamine and chondroitin for knee osteoarthritis: A double-blind randomized placebo-controlled clinical trial evaluating single and combination regimens. *Annals of the Rheumatic Diseases, 74*(5), 851–858. doi:10.1136/annrheumdis-2013-203954.
152. Fibel, K. H., Hillstrom, H. J., & Halpern, B. C. (2015). State-of-the-art management of knee osteoarthritis. *World Journal of Clinical Cases, 3*(2), 89–101. doi:10.12998/wjcc.v3.i2.89.
153. Ayhan, E., Kesmezacar, H., & Akgun, I. (2014). Intraarticular injections (corticosteroid, hyaluronic acid, platelet rich plasma) for the knee

osteoarthritis. *World Journal of Orthopedics, 5*(3), 351–361. doi:10.5312/wjo.v5.i3.351.

154. Bannuru, R. R., Schmid, C. H., Kent, D. M., et al. (2015). Comparative effectiveness of pharmacologic interventions for knee osteoarthritis: A systematic review and network meta-analysis. *Annals of Internal Medicine, 162*(1), 46–54. doi:10.7326/M14-1231.
155. Sundman, E. A., Cole, B. J., Karas, V., et al. (2014). The anti-inflammatory and matrix restorative mechanisms of platelet-rich plasma in osteoarthritis. *The American Journal of Sports Medicine, 42*(1), 35–41. doi:10.1177/0363546513507766.
156. Huang, Z., Chen, J., Ma, J., et al. (2015). Effectiveness of low-level laser therapy in patients with knee osteoarthritis: A systemic review and meta-analysis. *Osteoarthritis and Cartilage, 23*(9), 1437–1444. doi:10.1016/j.joca.2015.04.005.
157. Murphy, L. B., Helmick, C. G., Schwartz, T. A., et al. (2010). One in four people may develop symptomatic hip osteoarthritis in his or her lifetime. *Osteoarthritis and Cartilage, 18*(11), 1372–1379. doi:10.1016/j.joca.2010.08.005.
158. Canadian Institute for Health Information (2015). *Hip and knee replacements in Canada: Canadian Joint Replacement Registry, 2015 annual report.* Ottawa: Author. Retrieved from https://secure.cihi.ca/free_products/CJRR_2015_Annual_Report_EN.pdf.
159. Aletaha, D., Neogi, T., Silman, A. J., et al. (2010). The 2010 American College of Rheumatology/European League Against Rheumatism classification criteria for rheumatoid arthritis: An American College of Rheumatology/European League Against Rheumatism collaborative initiative. *Arthritis and Rheumatism, 62*(9), 2569–2581. doi:10.1002/art.27584.
160. Klein, K., Ospelt, C., & Gay, S. (2012). Epigenetic contributions in the development of rheumatoid arthritis. *Arthritis Research and Therapy, 14*(6), 227. doi:10.1186/ar4074.
161. Korczowska, I. (2014). Rheumatoid arthritis susceptibility genes: An overview. *World Journal of Orthopedics, 5*(4), 544–549. doi:10.5312/wjo.v5.i4.544.
162. Mohan, V. K., Ganesan, N., & Gopalakirshnan, R. (2014). Association of susceptible genetic markers and autoantibodies in rheumatoid arthritis. *Journal of Genetics, 93*(2), 597–605.
163. You, S., Yoo, S. A., Choi, S., et al. (2015). Identification of key regulators for the migration and invasion of rheumatoid synoviocytes through a systems approach. *Proceedings of the National Academy of Sciences of the United States of America, 111*(1), 550–555. doi:10.1073/pnas.1311239111.
164. Choy, E. (2012). Understanding the dynamics: Pathways involved in the pathogenesis of rheumatoid arthritis. *Rheumatology (Oxford, England), 51*(Suppl. 5), v3–v11. doi:10.1093/rheumatology/kes113.
165. Roeleveld, D. M., & Koenders, M. I. (2014). The role of the Th17 cytokines IL-17 and IL-22 in rheumatoid arthritis pathogenesis and developments in cytokine immunotherapy. *Cytokine, 74*(1), 101–107. doi:10.1016/j.cyto.2014.10.006.
166. Bartok, B., & Firestein, G. S. (2010). Fibroblast-like synoviocytes: Key effector cells in rheumatoid arthritis. *Immunological Reviews, 233*(1), 233–255. doi:10.1111/j.0105-2896.2009.00859.x.
167. Lefevre, S., Meier, F. M., Neumann, E., et al. (2015). Role of synovial fibroblasts in rheumatoid arthritis. *Current Pharmaceutical Design, 21*(2), 130–141.
168. Gibofsky, A. (2012). Overview of epidemiology, pathophysiology, and diagnosis of rheumatoid arthritis. *The American Journal of Managed Care, 18*(13, Suppl.), S295–S302.
169. van Heemst, J., Huizinga, T. J., van der Woude, D., et al. (2015). Fine-mapping the human leukocyte antigen locus in rheumatoid arthritis and other rheumatic diseases: Identifying causal amino acid variants? *Current Opinion in Rheumatology, 27*(3), 256–261. doi:10.1097/BOR.0000000000000165.
170. Klein, K., & Gay, S. (2015). Epigenetics and rheumatoid arthritis. *Current Opinion in Rheumatology, 27*(1), 76–82. doi:10.1097/BOR.0000000000000128.
171. Putrik, P., Ramiro, S., Keszei, A. P., et al. (2016). Lower education and living in countries with lower wealth are associated with higher disease activity in rheumatoid arthritis: Results from the multinational COMORA study. *Annals of the Rheumatic Diseases, 75*(3), 540–546. doi:10.1136/annrheumdis-2014-206737.
172. Song, Y. W., & Kang, E. H. (2010). Autoantibodies in rheumatoid arthritis: Rheumatoid factors and anticitrullinated protein antibodies. *The Quarterly Journal of Medicine, 103*(3), 139–146. doi:10.1093/qjmed/hcp165.
173. Valesini, G., Gerardi, M. C., Iannuccelli, C., et al. (2015). Citrullination and autoimmunity. *Autoimmunity Reviews, 14*(6), 490–497. doi:10.1016/j.autrev.2015.01.013.
174. Gong, G., Li, J., Li, X., et al. (2013). Pain experiences and self-management strategies among middle-aged and older adults with arthritis. *Journal of Clinical Nursing, 22*(13–14), 1857–1869. doi:10.1111/jocn.12134.
175. Ntatsaki, E., Mooney, J., Scott, D. G., et al. (2015). Systemic rheumatoid vasculitis in the era of modern immunosuppressive therapy. *Rheumatology (Oxford, England), 53*(1), 145–152. doi:10.1093/rheumatology/ket326.
176. Goronzy, J. J., & Weyand, C. M. (2009). Developments in the scientific understanding of rheumatoid arthritis. *Arthritis Research and Therapy, 11*(5), 249. doi:10.1186/ar2758.
177. Pruijn, G. J., Wilk, A., & van Venrooij, W. J. (2010). The use of citrullinated peptides and proteins for the diagnosis of rheumatoid arthritis. *Arthritis Research and Therapy, 12*(1), 203. doi:10.1186/ar2903.
178. Karsh, J. (2012). Management of Rheumatoid Arthritis 2012: A Canadian State of the Art. *The Journal of Rheumatology, 39*(8), 1497–1499. doi:10.3899/jrheum.120407.
179. Raychaudhuri, S. P., & Deodhar, A. (2014). The classification and diagnostic criteria of ankylosing spondylitis. *Journal of Autoimmunity, 48–49*, 128–133. doi:10.1016/j.jaut.2014.01.015.
180. Dean, L., Jones, G. T., MacDonald, A. G., et al. (2014). Global prevalence of ankylosing spondylitis. *Rheumatology (Oxford, England), 53*(4), 650–657. doi:10.1093/rheumatology/ket387.
181. Colbert, R. A., DeLay, M. L., Klenk, E. I., et al. (2010). From HLA-B27 to spondyloarthritis: A journey through the ER. *Immunological Reviews, 233*(1), 181–202. doi:10.1111/j.0105-2896.2009.00865.x.
182. Colbert, R. A., Tran, T. M., & Layh-Schmitt, G. (2015). HLA-B27 misfolding and ankylosing spondylitis. *Molecular Immunology, 57*(1), 44–51. doi:10.1016/j.molimm.2013.07.013.
183. Khan, M. A. (2013). Polymorphism of HLA-B27: 105 subtypes currently known. *Current Rheumatology Reports, 15*(10), 362. doi:10.1007/s11926-013-0362-y.
184. Roussou, E., & Sultana, S. (2012). Early spondyloarthritis in multiracial society: Differences between gender, race, and disease subgroups with regard to first symptom at presentation, main problem that the disease is causing to patients, and employment status. *Rheumatology International, 32*(6), 1597–1604. doi:10.1007/s00296-010-1680-2.
185. Rozin, A. P., Hasin, T., Toledano, K., et al. (2010). Seronegative polyarthritis as severe systemic disease. *The Netherlands Journal of Medicine, 68*(6), 236–241.
186. Haroon, N., & Inman, R. D. (2010). Ankylosing spondylitis: New criteria, new treatments. *Bulletin of the NYU Hospital for Joint Diseases, 68*(3), 171–174.
187. Rudwaleit, M., van der Heijde, D., Landewé, R., et al. (2009). The development of assessment of SpondyloArthritis International Society classification criteria for axial spondyloarthritis (part II): Validation and final selection. *Annals of the Rheumatic Diseases, 68*(6), 777–783. doi:10.1136/ard.2009.108233.
188. Golder, V., & Schachna, L. (2013). Ankylosing spondylitis: An update. *Australian Family Physician, 42*(11), 780–784.
189. O'Dwyer, T., O'Shea, F., & Wilson, F. (2014). Exercise therapy for spondyloarthropathies: A systematic review. *Rheumatology International, 34*(7), 887–902.
190. Braun, J., Klitz, U., Heldmann, F., et al. (2015). Emerging drugs for the treatment of axial and peripheral spondyloarthritis. *Expert Opinion on Emerging Drugs, 20*(1), 1–14. doi:10.1517/14728214.2015.993378.
191. Van den Bosch, F., & Dodhar, A. (2014). Treatment of spondyloarthritis beyond TNF-alpha blockade. *Best Practice and Research: Clinical Rheumatology, 28*(5), 819–827. doi:10.1016/j.berh.2014.10.019.
192. Rees, F., Hui, M., & Doherty, M. (2014). Optimizing current treatment of gout. *Nature Reviews: Rheumatology, 10*(5), 271–283. doi:10.1038/nrrheum.2014.32.
193. Roddy, E., & Choi, H. K. (2014). Epidemiology of gout. *Rheumatic Disease Clinics of North America, 40*(2), 155–175. doi:10.1016/j.rdc.2014.01.001.
194. Merriman, T. R., Choi, H. K., & Dalbeth, N. (2014). The genetic basis of gout. *Rheumatic Disease Clinics of North America, 40*(2), 279–290. doi:10.1016/j.rdc.2014.01.009.
195. Richette, P., & Bardin, T. (2010). Gout. *Lancet, 375*(9711), 318–328. doi:10.1016/S0140-6736(09)60883-7.
196. Sriranganathan, M. K., Vinik, O., Bombardieer, C., et al. (2014). Interventions for tophi in gout. *The Cochrane Database of Systematic Reviews*, (10), CD010069, doi:10.1002/14651858.CD010069.pub2.
197. Perez-Ruiz, F., Martinez-Indart, L., Carmona, L., et al. (2014). Tophaceous gout and high level of hyperuricaemia are both associated with increased risk of mortality in patients with gout. *Annals of the Rheumatic Diseases, 73*(1), 177–182. doi:10.1136/annrheumdis-2012-202421.
198. VanItallie, T. B. (2010). Gout: Epitome of painful arthritis. *Metabolism: Clinical and Experimental, 59*(Suppl. 1), S32–S36. doi:10.1016/j.metabol.2010.07.009.
199. Dirken-Heukensfeldt, K. J., Teunissen, T. A., van de Lisdonk, H., et al. (2010). Clinical features of women with gout arthritis: A systemic review. *Clinical Rheumatology, 29*(6), 575–582. doi:10.1007/s10067-009-1362-1.
200. Perez-Ruiz, F., Dalbeth, N., & Bardin, T. (2015). A review of uric acid, crystal deposition disease, and gout. *Advances in Therapy, 32*(1), 31–41. doi:10.1007/s12325-014-0175-z.
201. Chowalloor, P. V., Siew, T. K., & Keen, H. I. (2014). Imaging in gout: A review of recent developments. *Therapeutic Advances in Musculoskeletal Medical, 6*(4), 131–143. doi:10.1177/1759720X14542960.
202. Sivera, F., Andrés, M., Carmona, L., et al. (2014). Multinational evidence-based recommendations for the diagnosis and management of gout: Integrating systematic literature review and expert opinion of a broad panel of rheumatologists in the 3e initiative. *Annals of the Rheumatic Diseases, 73*(2), 328–335. doi:10.1136/annrheumdis-2013-203325.
203. Crittendon, D. B., & Pillinger, M. H. (2013). The year in gout: A walk through the 2012 ACR treatment guidelines. *Bulletin of the Hospital for Joint Diseases, 71*(3), 189–193.
204. Edwards, N. L., & So, A. (2014). Emerging therapies for gout. *Rheumatic Disease Clinics of North America, 40*(2), 375–387. doi:10.1016/j.rdc.2014.01.013.
205. Moi, J. H., Sriranganathan, M. K., Edwards, C. J., et al. (2013). Lifestyle interventions for gout. *The Cochrane Database of Systematic Reviews*, (11), CD010519, doi:10.1002/14651858.CD010519.pub2.
206. Kanbara, A., Hakoda, M., & Seyama, I. (2010). Urine alkalization facilitates uric acid excretion. *Nutrition Journal, 9*, 45. doi:10.1186/1475-2891-9-45.
207. Skalsky, A. J., & McDonald, C. M. (2012). Prevention and management of limb contractures in neuromuscular diseases. *Physical Medicine and*

Rehabilitation Clinics of North America, 23(3), 675–687. doi:10.1016/j.pmr.2012.06.009.
208. Larsman, P., Kadefors, R., & Sandsjö, L. (2013). Psychosocial work conditions, perceived stress, perceived muscular tension, and neck/shoulder symptoms among medical secretaries. *International Archives of Occupational and Environmental Health, 86*(1), 57–63. doi:10.1007/s00420-012-0744-x.
209. Powers, S. K. (2014). Can antioxidants protect against disuse muscle atrophy? *Sports Medicine (Auckland, N.Z.), 44*(Suppl. 2), S155–S165. doi:10.1007/s40279-014-0255-x.
210. Brooks, N. E., & Myburgh, K. H. (2014). Skeletal muscle wasting with disuse atrophy is multi-dimensional: The response and interaction of myonuclei, satellite cells and signaling pathways. *Frontiers in Physiology, 5*, 99. doi:10.3389/fphys.2014.00099.
211. Pernambuco, A. P., Schetino, L. P., Alvim, C. C., et al. (2013). Increased levels of IL-17A in patients with fibromyalgia. *Clinical and Experimental Rheumatology, 31*(6, Suppl. 79), S60–S63.
212. Rodriguez-Pintò, I., Agmon-Levin, N., Howard, A., et al. (2014). Fibromyalgia and cytokines. *Immunology Letters, 161*(2), 200–203. doi:10.1016/j.imlet.2014.01.009.
213. Sturgill, J., McGee, E., & Menzies, V. (2014). Unique cytokine signature in the plasma of patients with fibromyalgia. *Journal of Immunology Research, 2014*, 938576. doi:10.1155/2014/938576.
214. Clauw, D. J. (2014). Fibromyalgia: A clinical review. *The Journal of the American Medical Association, 311*(15), 1547–1555. doi:10.1001/jama.2014.3266.
215. Arnold, L. M., Fan, J., Russell, I. J., et al. (2013). The fibromyalgia family study: A genome-wide linkage scan study. *Arthritis and Rheumatism, 65*(4), 1122–1128. doi:10.1002/art.37842.
216. Diatchenko, L., Fillingim, R. B., Smith, S. B., et al. (2013). The phenotypic and genetic signatures of common musculoskeletal pain conditions. *Nature Reviews: Rheumatology, 9*(6), 340–350. doi:10.1038/nrrheum.2013.43.
217. Docampo, E., Escaramis, G., Gratacòs, M., et al. (2014). Genome-wide analysis of single nucleotide polymorphisms and copy number variants in fibromyalgia suggest a role for the central nervous system. *Pain, 15*(6), 1102–1109. doi:10.1016/j.pain.2014.02.016.
218. Wolfe, F., Häuser, W., Walitt, B. T., et al. (2014). Fibromyalgia and physical trauma: The concepts we invent. *The Journal of Rheumatology, 41*(9), 1737–1745. doi:10.3899/jrheum.140268.
219. Cagnie, B., Coppieters, J., Denecker, S., et al. (2014). Central sensitization in fibromyalgia? A systematic review on structural and functional brain MRI. *Seminars in Arthritis and Rheumatism, 44*(1), 68–75. doi:10.1016/j.semarthrit.2014.01.001.
220. Harbeck, B., Süfke, S., Harten, P., et al. (2013). High prevalence of fibromyalgia-associated symptoms in patients with hypothalamic-pituitary disorders. *Clinical and Experimental Rheumatology, 31*(6, Suppl. 79), S16–S21.
221. Fitzcharles, M. A., Ste-Marie, P. A., Goldenbereg, D. L., et al. (2012). *2012 Canadian guidelines for the diagnosis and management of fibromyalgia syndrome.* Retrieved from http://fmguidelines.ca/?page_id=19.
222. Theadom, A., Cropley, M., Smith, H. E., et al. (2015). Mind and body for fibromyalgia. *The Cochrane Database of Systematic Reviews*, (4), CD001980, doi:10.1002/14651858.CD001980.pub3.
223. Bidone, J. M., Busch, A. J., Webber, S. C., et al. (2014). Aquatic exercise training for fibromyalgia. *The Cochrane Database of Systematic Reviews*, (10), CD011336, doi:10.1002/14651858.CD011336.
224. Bidone, J., Busch, A. J., Bath, B., et al. (2014). Exercise for adults with fibromyalgia: An umbrella systematic review with synthesis of best evidence. *Current Rheumatology Reviews, 10*(1), 45–79.
225. O'Connor, S. R., Tully, M. A., Ryan, B., et al. (2014). Walking exercise for chronic musculoskeletal pain: Systemic review and meta-analysis. *Archives of Physical Medicine and Rehabilitation, 96*(4), 724–734. doi:10.1016/j.apmr.2014.12.003.
226. Aerenhouts, D., Ickmans, K., Clarys, P., et al. (2015). Sleep characteristics, exercise capacity and physical activity in patients with chronic fatigue syndrome. *Disability and Rehabilitation, 37*(22), 2044–2050.
227. Kallestad, H., Jacobsen, H. B., Landro, N. I., et al. (2015). The role of insomnia in the treatment of chronic fatigue. *Journal of Psychosomatic Research, 78*(5), 427–432. doi:10.1016/j.jpsychores.2014.11.022.
228. Rosenblum, H., Shoenfeld, Y., & Amital, H. (2011). The common immunogenic etiology of chronic fatigue syndrome: From infections to vaccines via adjuvants to the ASIA syndrome. *Infectious Disease Clinics of North America, 25*(4), 851–863. doi:10.1016/j.idc.2011.07.012.
229. Brown, A. E., Jones, D. E., Walker, M., et al. (2015). Abnormalities of AMPK activation and glucose uptake in cultured skeletal muscle cells from individuals with chronic fatigue syndrome. *PLoS ONE, 10*(4), e0122982. doi:10.1371/journal.pone.0122982.
230. Gambuzza, M. E., Salmeri, F. M., Soraci, L., et al. (2015). The role of Toll-like receptors in chronic fatigue syndrome/myalgic encephalomyelitis: A new promising therapeutic approach? *CNS and Neurological Disorders Drug Targets, 14*(7), 903–914.
231. Kempke, S., Luyten, P., De Coninck, S., et al. (2015). Effects of early childhood trauma on hypothalamic-pituitary-adrenal axis function in patients with chronic fatigue syndrome. *Psychoneuroendocrinology, 52*, 14–21. doi:10.1016/j.psyneuen.2014.10.027.
232. Romano, G. F., Tomassi, S., Russell, A., et al. (2015). Fibromyalgia and chronic fatigue: The underlying biology and related theoretical issues. *Advances in Psychosomatic Medicine, 34*, 61–77. doi:10.1159/000369085.
233. Committee on the Diagnostic Criteria for Myalgic Encephalomyelitis/Chronic Fatigue Syndrome, Board on the Health of Select Populations, & Institute of Medicine (2015). *Beyond myalgic encephalomyelitis/chronic fatigue syndrome: Redefining and illness.* Washington, DC: National Academies Press.
234. Bourke, J. (2015). Fibromyalgia and chronic fatigue syndrome: Management issues. *Advances in Psychosomatic Medicine, 34*, 78–91. doi:10.1159/000369087.
235. Olson, K., Zimka, O., & Stein, E. (2015). The nature of fatigue in chronic fatigue syndrome. *Qualitative Health Research, 25*(10), 1410–1422. doi:10.1177/1049732315573954.
236. Drost, G., Stunnenberg, B. C., Trip, J., et al. (2015). Myotonic discharges discriminate chloride from sodium muscle channelopathies. *Neuromuscular Disorders, 25*(1), 73–80.
237. Statland, J. M., & Barohn, R. J. (2013). Muscle channelopathies: The nondystrophic myotonias and periodic paralysis. *Continuum, 19*(6), 1598–1614. doi:10.1212/01.CON.0000440661.49298.c8.
238. Novak, K. R., Norman, J., Mitchell, J. R., et al. (2015). Sodium channel slow inactivation as a therapeutic target for myotonia congenital. *Annals of Neurology, 77*(2), 320–322. doi:10.1002/ana.24331.
239. Sharp, L., & Trivedi, J. R. (2014). Treatment and management of neuromuscular channelopathies. *Current Treatment Options in Neurology, 16*(10), 313. doi:10.1007/s11940-014-0313-6.
240. Statland, J., Phillips, L., & Trivedi, J. R. (2014). Muscle channelopathies. *Neurologic Clinics, 32*(3), 601–615.
241. Catterall, W. A. (2011). Voltage-gated calcium channels. *Cold Spring Harbor Perspectives in Biology, 3*(8), a003947. doi:10.1101/cshperspect.a003947.
242. Cheng, C.-J., Kuo, E., & Huang, C. L. (2013). Extracellular potassium homeostasis: Insights from hypokalemic periodic paralysis. *Seminars in Nephrology, 33*(3), 237–247. doi:10.1016/j.semnephrol.2013.04.004.
243. Lin, S. H., & Huang, C.-L. (2012). Mechanism of thyrotoxic periodic paralysis. *Journal of the American Society of Nephrology, 23*(6), 985–988. doi:10.1681/ASN.2012010046.
244. Rolim, A. L., Lindsey, S. C., Kunii, I. S., et al. (2010). Ion channelopathies in endocrinology: Recent genetic findings and pathophysiological insights. *Arquivos Brasileiros de Endocrinologia E Metabologia, 54*(8), 673–681.
245. Jurkat-Rott, K., Holzherr, B., Fauler, M., et al. (2010). Sodium channelopathies of skeletal muscle result from gain or loss of function. *Pflügers Archiv: European Journal of Physiology, 460*(2), 239–248. doi:10.1007/s00424-010-0814-4.
246. Charles, G., Zheng, C., Lehmann-Horn, F., et al. (2013). Characterization of hyperkalemic periodic paralysis: A survey of genetically diagnosed individuals. *Journal of Neurology, 260*(10), 2606–2613. doi:10.1007/s00415-013-7025-9.
247. Das, A. M., Steuerwald, U., & Illsinger, S. (2010). Inborn errors of energy metabolism associated with myopathies. *Journal of Biomedicine and Biotechnology, 2010*, 340849.
248. Kitaoka, Y. (2014). McArdle disease and exercise physiology. *Biology, 3*(1), 157–166. doi:10.3390/biology3010157.
249. Kitaoka, Y., Hoshino, D., & Hatta, H. (2012). Monocarboxylate transporter and lactate metabolism. *Journal of Sports Medicine and Physical Fitness, 1*(2), 247–252.
250. Bhengu, L., Davidson, A., du Toit, P., et al. (2014). Diagnosis and management of Pompe disease. *South African Medical Journal, 104*(4), 273–274.
251. Kishnani, P. S., Beckemeyer, A. A., & Mendelsohn, N. J. (2012). The new era of Pompe disease: Advances in the detection, understanding of the phenotypic spectrum, pathophysiology and management. *American Journal of Medical Genetics: Part C, Seminars in Medical Genetics, 160C*(1), 1–7. doi:10.1002/ajmg.c.31324.
252. Werneck, L. C., Lorenzoni, P. J., Kay, C. S., et al. (2013). Muscle biopsy in Pompe disease. *Arquivos de Neuro-psiquiatria, 71*(5), 284–289.
253. Lachmann, R., & Schoser, B. (2013). The clinical relevance of outcomes used in late-onset Pompe disease: Can we do better? *Orphanet Journal of Rare Diseases, 8*, 160. doi:10.1186/1750-1172-8-160.
254. Pascual, J. M., & Roe, C. R. (2013). Systemic metabolic abnormalities in adult-onset acid maltase deficiency: Beyond muscle glycogen accumulation. *JAMA Neurology, 70*(6), 756–763. doi:10.1001/jamaneurol.2013.1507.
255. Hayes, L. D., Houston, F. E., & Baker, J. S. (2013). Genetic predictors of adenosine monophosphate deaminase deficiency. *Journal of Sports Medicine and Doping Studies, 3*(124), doi:10.4172/2161-0673.1000124.
256. Bonnefont, J. P., Bastin, J., Laforêt, P., et al. (2010). Long-term follow-up of bezafibrate treatment in patients with the myopathic form of carnitine palmitoyltransferase 2 deficiency. *Clinical Pharmacology and Therapeutics, 88*(1), 101–108. doi:10.1038/clpt.2010.55.
257. Lu, X., Peng, Q., & Wang, G. (2015). Discovery of new biomarkers of idiopathic inflammatory myopathy. *Clinica Chimica Acta, 444*, 117–125. doi:10.1016/j.cca.2015.02.007.
258. van der Kooi, A. J., & de Visser, M. (2014). Idiopathic inflammatory myopathies. *Handbook of Clinical Neurology, 119*, 495–512. doi:10.1016/B978-0-7020-4086-3.00032-1.
259. Dobloug, G. C., Antal, E. A., Sveberg, L., et al. (2015). High prevalence of inclusion body myositis in Norway: A population-based clinical epidemiology study. *European Journal of Neurology, 22*(4), 672–e41. doi:10.1111/ene.12627.
260. Meyer, A., Meyer, N., Schaeffer, M., et al. (2015). Incidence and prevalence of inflammatory myopathies: A systematic review. *Rheumatology (Oxford, England), 54*(1), 50–63. doi:10.1093/rheumatology/keu289.
261. Rothwell, S., Cooper, R. G., Lamb, J. A., et al. (2013). Entering a new phase of immunogenetics in the idiopathic inflammatory myopathies. *Current Opinion in Rheumatology, 25*(6), 735–741. doi:10.1097/01.bor.0000434676.70268.66.
262. Tansley, S., & Gunawardena, H. (2014). The evolving spectrum of polymyositis and dermatomyositis—Moving towards clinicoserological syndromes: A critical review.

Clinical Reviews in Allergy and Immunology, 47(3), 264–273. doi:10.1007/s12016-013-8387-6.

263. Auriemma, M., Capo, A., Meogrossi, G., et al. (2014). Cutaneous signs of classical dermatomyositis. *Giornale Italiano Di Dermatologia E Venereologia: Organo Ufficiale, Societa Italiana Di Dermatologia E Sifilografia, 149*(5), 505–517.
264. Dalakas, M. C. (2010). Inflammatory muscle diseases: A critical review on pathogenesis and therapies. *Current Opinion in Pharmacology, 10*(3), 346–352. doi:10.1016/j.coph.2010.03.001.
265. Carstens, P. O., & Schmidt, J. (2014). Diagnosis, pathogenesis and treatment of myositis: Recent advances. *Clinical and Experimental Immunology, 175*(3), 349–358. doi:10.1111/cei.12194.
266. Dalakas, M. C. (2010). Immunotherapy of myositis: Issues, concerns and future prospects. *Nature Reviews: Rheumatology, 6*(3), 129–137. doi:10.1038/nrrheum.2010.2.
267. Dimachkie, M. M., & Barohn, R. J. (2013). Inclusion body myositis. *Current Neurology and Neuroscience Reports, 13*(1), 321. doi:10.1007/s11910-012-0321-4.
268. Schmidt, J., & Dalakas, M. C. (2013). Inclusion body myositis: From immunopathology and degenerative mechanisms to treatment perspectives. *Expert Review of Clinical Immunology, 9*(11), 1125–1133. doi:10.1586/1744666X.2013.842467.
269. Mastaglia, F. L., & Needham, M. (2015). Inclusion body myositis: A review of clinical and genetic aspects, diagnostic criteria and therapeutic approaches. *Journal of Clinical Neuroscience, 22*(1), 6–13. doi:10.1016/j.jocn.2014.09.012.
270. Iaccarino, L., Ghirardello, A., Bettio, S., et al. (2014). The clinical features, diagnosis and classification of dermatomyositis. *Journal of Autoimmunity, 48–49*, 122–127. doi:10.1016/j.jaut.2013.11.005.
271. Schiffenbauer, A. (2014). Imaging: Seeing muscle in new ways. *Current Opinion in Rheumatology, 26*(6), 712–716. doi:10.1097/BOR.0000000000000105.
272. Kley, R. A., Tarnopolsky, M. A., & Vorgerd, M. (2013). Creatine for treating muscle disorders. *The Cochrane Database of Systematic Reviews*, (6), CD0044760, doi:10.1002/14651858.CD004760.pub4.
273. Kuncl, R. W. (2009). Agents and mechanisms of toxic myopathy. *Current Opinion in Neurology, 22*(5), 506–515. doi:10.1097/WCO.0b013e32833045a0.
274. Pasnoor, M., Barohn, R. J., & Dimachkie, M. M. (2014). Toxic myopathies. *Neurologic Clinics, 32*(3), 647–670. doi:10.1016/j.ncl.2014.04.009.
275. Canadian Cancer Society. (2017). *Bone cancer statistics*. Retrieved from http://www.cancer.ca/en/cancer-information/cancer-type/bone/statistics/?region=on.
276. Peller, P. J. (2013). Role of positron emission tomography/computed tomography in bone malignancies. *Radiologic Clinics of North America, 51*(5), 845–864. doi:10.1016/j.rcl.2013.05.005.
277. Du, W. X., Duan, S. F., Chen, J. J., et al. (2014). Serum bone-specific alkaline phosphatase as a biomarker for osseous metastases in patients with malignant carcinomas: A systematic review and meta-analysis. *Journal of Cancer Research and Therapeutics, 10*(Suppl.C), 140–143. doi:10.4103/0973-1482.145842.
278. Traina, F., Errani, C., Toscano, A., et al. (2015). Current concepts in the biopsy of musculoskeletal tumors. *The Journal of Bone and Joint Surgery. American Volume, 97*(1), e7.
279. Berner, K., Johannesen, T. B., Berner, A., et al. (2015). Time-trends on incidence and survival in a nationwide and unselected cohort of patients with skeletal osteosarcoma. *Acta Oncologica (Stockholm, Sweden), 54*(1), 25–33. doi:10.3109/0284186X.2014.923934.
280. HaDuong, J. H., Martin, A. A., Skapek, S. X., et al. (2015). Sarcomas. *Pediatric Clinics of North America, 62*(1), 179–200. doi:10.1016/j.pcl.2014.09.012.
281. Burningham, Z., Hashibe, M., Spector, L., et al. (2012). The epidemiology of sarcoma. *Clinical Sarcoma Research, 2*(1), 14. doi:10.1186/2045-3329-2-14.
282. Moore, D. D., & Luu, H. H. (2014). Osteosarcoma. *Cancer Treatment and Research, 162*, 65–92. doi:10.1007/978-3-319-07323-1_4.
283. Green, J. T., & Mills, A. M. (2014). Osteogenic tumors of bone. *Seminars in Diagnostic Pathology, 31*(1), 21–29. doi:10.1053/j.semdp.2014.01.001.
284. Lietman, S. A., & Joyce, M. J. (2010). Bone sarcomas: Overview of management, with a focus on surgical treatment considerations. *Cleveland Clinic Journal of Medicine, 77*(Suppl. 1), S8–S12. doi:10.3949/ccjm.77.s1.02.
285. Knops, R. R., van Dalen, E. C., Mulder, R. L., et al. (2013). The volume effect in paediatric oncology: A systematic review. *Annals of Oncology, 24*(7), 1749–1753. doi:10.1093/annonc/mds656.
286. Luetke, A., Meyers, P. A., Lewis, I., et al. (2014). Osteosarcoma treatment—Where do we stand? A state of the art review. *Cancer Treatment Reviews, 40*(4), 523–532. doi:10.1016/j.ctrv.2013.11.006.
287. Forscher, C., Mita, M., & Figlin, R. (2014). Targeted therapy for osteosarcomas. *Biologics : Targets and Therapy, 8*, 91–105. doi:10.2147/BTT.S26555.
288. Kansara, M., Teng, M. W., Smyth, M. J., et al. (2014). Translational biology of osteosarcoma. *Nature Reviews: Cancer, 14*(11), 722–735. doi:10.1038/nrc3838.
289. Choi, E. Y., Gardner, J. M., Lucas, D. R., et al. (2014). Ewing sarcoma. *Seminars in Diagnostic Pathology, 31*(1), 39–47. doi:10.1053/j.semdp.2014.01.002.
290. Moore, D. D., & Haydin, R. C. (2014). Ewing's sarcoma of bone. *Cancer Treatment and Research, 162*, 93–115. doi:10.1007/978-3-319-07323-1_5.
291. Leddy, L. R., & Holmes, R. E. (2014). Chondrosarcoma of bone. *Cancer Treatment and Research, 162*, 117–130. doi:10.1007/978-3-319-07323-1_6.
292. Bindiganaville, S., Han, I., Yun, J. Y., & Kim, H. S. (2015). Long-term outcome of chondrosarcoma: A single institutional experience. *Cancer Research and Treatment, 47*(4), 897–903. doi:10.4143/crt.2014.135.
293. Choi, B. B., Jee, W. H., Sunwoo, H. J., et al. (2013). MR differentiation of low-grade chondrosarcoma from enchondroma. *Clinical Imaging, 37*(3), 542–547. doi:10.1016/j.clinimag.2012.08.006.
294. Logie, C. I., Walker, E. A., Forsberg, J. A., et al. (2013). Chondrosarcoma: A diagnostic imager's guide to decision making and patient management. *Seminars in Musculoskeletal Radiology, 17*(2), 101–115. doi:10.1055/s-0033-1342967.
295. Heymann, D., & Rédini, F. (2013). Targeted therapies for bone sarcomas. *BoneKEy Reports, 2*, 378. doi:10.1038/bonekey.2013.112.
296. Radaelli, S., Stacchiotti, S., Casali, P. G., et al. (2014). Emerging therapies for adult soft tissue sarcoma. *Expert Review of Anticancer Therapy, 14*(6), 689–704. doi:10.1586/14737140.2014.885840.
297. Bao, Q., Niess, H., Djafarzadeh, R., et al. (2014). Recombinant TIMP-1-GPI inhibits growth of fibrosarcoma and enhances tumor sensitivity to doxorubicin. *Targeted Oncology, 9*(3), 251–261. doi:10.1007/s11523-013-0294-5.
298. Li, L., Gu, J., Zhang, J., et al. (2015). Injectable and biodegradable pH-responsive hydrogels for localized and sustained treatment of human fibrosarcoma. *ACS Applied Materials and Interfaces, 7*(15), 8033–8040. doi:10.1021/acsami.5b00389.
299. van der Heijden, L., Dijkstra, P. D., van de Sande, M. A., et al. (2014). The clinical approach toward giant cell tumor of bone. *The Oncologist, 19*(5), 550–561. doi:10.1634/theoncologist.2013-0432.
300. Raskin, K. A., Schwab, J. H., Mankin, H. J., et al. (2013). Giant cell tumor of bone. *The Journal of the American Academy of Orthopaedic Surgeons, 21*(2), 118–126. doi:10.5435/JAAOS-21-02-118.
301. Lewin, J., & Thomas, D. (2013). Denosumab: A new treatment option for giant cell tumor of bone. *Drugs of Today (Barcelona, Spain: 1998), 49*(11), 693–700. doi:10.1358/dot.2013.49.11.2064725.
302. Xu, S. F., Adams, B., Yu, X. C., et al. (2013). Denosumab and giant cell tumor of bone—A review and future management considerations. *Current oncology, 20*(5), e442–e447. doi:10.3747/co.20.1497.
303. Zanola, A., Rossi, S., Faggi, F., et al. (2012). Rhabdomyosarcomas: An overview on the experimental animal models. *Journal of Cellular and Molecular Medicine, 16*(7), 1377–1391. doi:10.1111/j.1582-4934.2011.01518.x.
304. Sultan, I., Qaddoumi, I., Yaser, S., et al. (2009). Comparing adult and pediatric rhabdomyosarcomas in the surveillance, epidemiology and end results program, 1973 to 2005: An analysis of 2600 patients. *Journal of Clinical Oncology, 27*(20), 3391–3397. doi:10.1200/JCO.2008.19.7483.

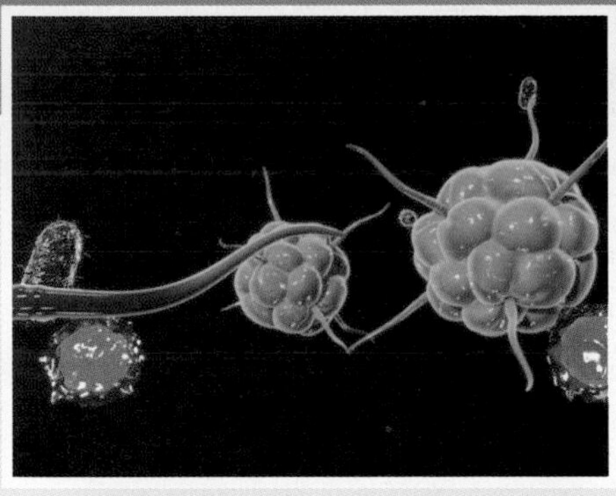

40

Alterations of Musculo-skeletal Function in Children

Kristen Lee Carroll, Lynne M. Kerr, Kathryn L. McCance, and Stephanie Zettel

EVOLVE WEBSITE

http://evolve.elsevier.com/Canada/Huether/pathophysiology

Student Review Questions
Key Points
Case Studies
Animations
Quick Check Answers

CHAPTER OUTLINE

Congenital Defects, 1059
- Clubfoot, 1059
- Developmental Dysplasia of the Hip, 1059
- Osteogenesis Imperfecta, 1060

Bone Infection, 1062
- Osteomyelitis, 1062
- Septic Arthritis, 1063

Juvenile Idiopathic Arthritis, 1064

Osteochondroses, 1065
- Legg-Calvé-Perthes Disease, 1065
- Osgood-Schlatter Disease, 1065

Scoliosis, 1066

Muscular Dystrophy, 1067
- Duchenne Muscular Dystrophy, 1067
- Becker Muscular Dystrophy, 1068
- Facioscapulohumeral Muscular Dystrophy, 1068
- Myotonic Muscular Dystrophy, 1068

Musculo-skeletal Tumours, 1069
- Benign Bone Tumours, 1069
- Malignant Bone Tumours, 1069

Nonaccidental Trauma, 1071
- Fractures in Nonaccidental Trauma, 1071

Musculo-skeletal problems in children can be either congenital or acquired. Both pathology and treatment can cause long-term sequelae because of the growing nature of the immature skeleton. In addition, the emotional trauma of an injured or malformed child is substantial and requires that careful attention be paid to the emotional health of both the child and his or her family.

CONGENITAL DEFECTS

Clubfoot

Clubfoot describes a range of foot deformities in which the foot turns inward and downward. It can affect one or both feet. Technically called **congenital equinovarus** (Table 40-1), the heel is positioned varus (inwardly deviated) and equinus (plantar flexed) (Figures 40-1 and 40-2). The clubfoot deformity can be positional (correctable passively), idiopathic, or teratological (as a result of another syndrome, such as spina bifida). The idiopathic clubfoot occurs in 1 per 1 000 live births, with males twice as likely as females to be affected.

The clubfoot deformity can be corrected by an above-knee casting regimen popularized by Ponseti.[1] In almost 90% of idiopathic and up to 70% of teratological clubfeet, the Ponseti method of serial casting infants' feet is effective (Figure 40-1, *B*). The hindfoot equinus portion of the deformity often requires lengthening of the Achilles tendon, which can be performed in a clinic with the use of a local anaesthetic. Achilles tenotomy (complete transection of the tendon) can be safely performed with local anaesthetic until 8 or 9 months after birth. After this age, a formal lengthening and repair procedure using a general anaesthetic is required. Bracing is required until age 3. Idiopathic feet resistant to these procedures require repeat casting or, in very rare cases, a surgical posteromedial release (PMR). The PMR includes lengthening of the Achilles, posterior tibialis, and flexor tendons, and surgical release of the capsules of the ankle, subtalar, and midfoot joints. Teratological clubfeet require surgical intervention more often than idiopathic clubfeet (see Figure 40-1, *B*) and more prolonged bracing, often through childhood. The Ponseti technique has revolutionized clubfoot treatment around the world. The ability to correct such a crippling deformity without the need for surgery has helped countless children.[2]

Developmental Dysplasia of the Hip

Developmental dysplasia of the hip (DDH) describes imperfect development of the hip joint and can affect the femur, the acetabulum, or both (Figure 40-3). Although most often present congenitally, dysplasia may develop later in the newborn or infant period. Like clubfoot, DDH can be idiopathic or teratological. Teratological hips (i.e., those attributable to another disorder such as cerebral palsy, spina bifida, or arthrogryposis) are more difficult to treat and often need operative intervention. In idiopathic DDH, 70% of cases involve the left side only and 10 to 15% are bilateral. Girls are four times as likely as boys to be affected. Positive family history, breech presentation, and oligohydramnios (low levels of intrauterine fluid) all predispose children to DDH. Children in these groups are considered high risk and must be carefully evaluated with physical examination and, possibly, ultrasound.[3,4] Variants of

TABLE 40-1 Terms Used to Describe Foot Abnormalities

Term	Definition
Position[a]	
Abduction	Lateral deviation away from the midline of the body
Adduction	Lateral deviation toward the midline of the body
Eversion	Twisting of the foot outward along its long axis
Inversion	Twisting of the foot inward on its long axis
Dorsiflexion	Bending of the foot upward and backward
Plantar flexion	Bending of the foot downward and forward
Abnormality	
Talipes	Congenital abnormality of the foot (clubfoot)
Pes	Acquired deformity of the foot
Varus	Inversion and adduction of the heel and forefoot
Valgus	Eversion and abduction of the heel and forefoot
Equinus	Plantar flexion of the foot in which the heel is lower than the toes
Calcaneus	Dorsiflexion of the foot in which the heel is lower than the toes
Planus	Flattening of the medial longitudinal arch of the foot (flatfoot)
Cavus	Elevation of the medial longitudinal arch of the foot (high arch)
Equinovarus	Coexistent equinus and varus deformities
Calcaneovarus	Coexistent calcaneus and varus deformities
Equinovalgus	Coexistent equinus and valgus deformities
Calcaneovalgus	Coexistent calcaneus and valgus deformities

[a]The positions listed can all be achieved by voluntary movement of the normal foot; an abnormality exists if the foot is fixed in one or more of the positions while at rest.

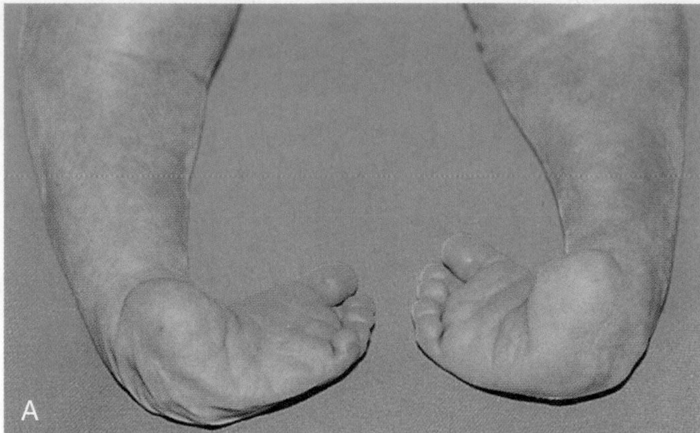

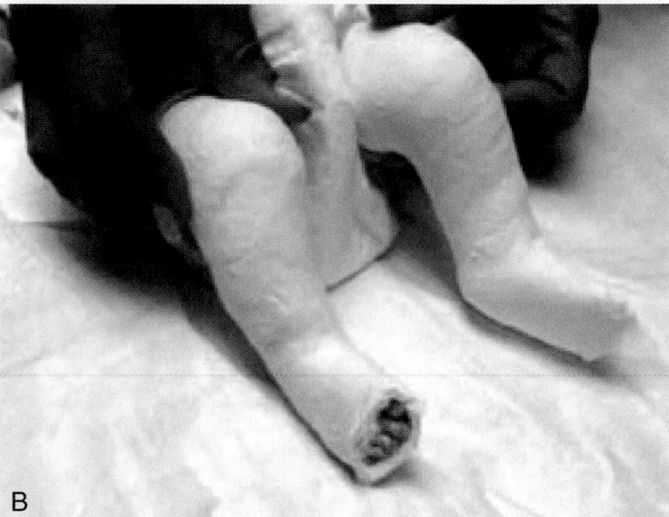

FIGURE 40-1 A, Infant With Bilateral Congenital Talipes Equinovarus. B, Ponseti Casting. (**A,** courtesy Dr. A.E. Chudley, Section of Genetics and Metabolism, Department of Pediatrics and Child Health, Children's Hospital and University of Manitoba, Winnipeg, Manitoba. In Moore, K.L., Persaud, T.V.N., & Torchia, M.G. [Eds.]. [2016]. *The developing human* [10th ed.]. Philadelphia: Saunders. **B,** Reprinted from *Operative Techniques in Orthopaedics,* 15(4), Scher, DM., "The Ponseti method for clubfoot correction," Pages 345–349, Copyright 2005, with permission from Elsevier.)

idiopathic DDH are **dislocated hip** (no contact between the femoral head and acetabulum), **subluxated hip** (partial contact only), and **acetabular dysplasia** (the femoral head is located properly but the acetabulum is shallow). Idiopathic instability of the hip ranges from 3 to 7 per 1 000 live births, but a true dislocation is present in only 1 of 1 000 live births.

Clinical examination is the mainstay of diagnosis. The examination must be performed on a relaxed infant for accuracy. Absolute indications for treatment include a positive Barlow sign (hip reduced, but dislocatable) (Figure 40-4, *A*) or positive Ortolani sign (hip dislocated, but reducible) (Figure 40-4, *B*). Other indicators for further evaluation are limitation of abduction[5] or apparent shortening of the femur (Galeazzi sign). Asymmetric skin folds at the groin also can be a clinical sign of hip pathology.

In children younger than 4 months, bracing with a Pavlik harness is successful in 90% of DDH cases. A Barlow-positive hip (hip reduced, but dislocatable) is easier to treat with a Pavlik harness, and success rates approach 95 to 98% (Figure 40-5). An Ortolani-positive hip (hip dislocated, but reducible) must be followed closely with ultrasound and examination; the success rate with Pavlik harness is 70% in this situation. If a stable reduction is not attained within 2 to 3 weeks of treatment, the Pavlik harness should be abandoned and casting or surgery pursued instead. A partially reduced hip applies pressure on the rim of the acetabulum by the femoral head and can worsen dysplasia and make treatment more difficult. In older children (6 to 12 months), or those who failed bracing with a Pavlik harness, closed reduction of the hip and spica (body) casting performed using a general anaesthetic are required. The spica cast is worn for 3 months. Children older than 12 months require surgery on the joint, the femur, or the acetabulum, or all three (see Figure 40-3). The incidence of good or excellent outcome falls to only 20% by age 4, underscoring the need for early diagnosis and treatment.[6]

Osteogenesis Imperfecta

Osteogenesis imperfecta (OI; brittle bone disease) is a spectrum of disease caused by genetic mutation in the gene that encodes for type I collagen, the main component of bone and blood vessels. The Sillence classification defines six types. Types I and IV are milder forms and are inherited in an autosomal dominant pattern. Types II and III are more severe and are inherited in a recessive pattern. Types V and VI are very rare and are autosomal recessive. Children with type II often die during infancy because of extreme bone fragility.

The classic clinical manifestations of OI are osteopenia (decreased bone mass) and an increased rate of fractures. Children can also have fatigue, pain, hearing loss, and abnormal dentition. With recurrent fractures, bone deformity (bowing) often occurs. In type III OI, the

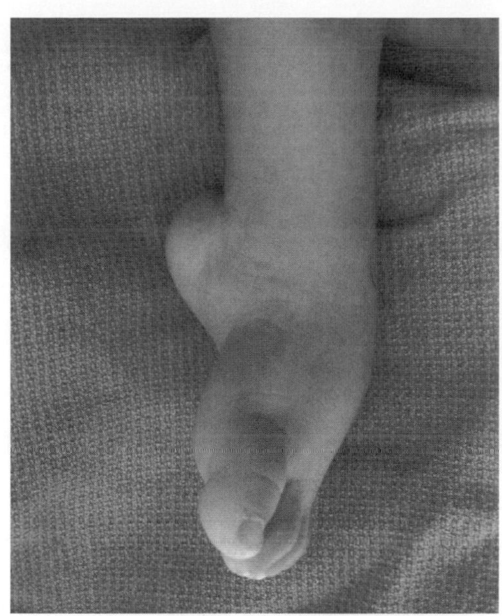

FIGURE 40-2 Idiopathic Clubfoot. Idiopathic clubfoot displaying forefoot adduction (toward midline of body) and supination (upturning) and hindfoot equinus (pointed downward). Note skin creases along arch and back of heel.

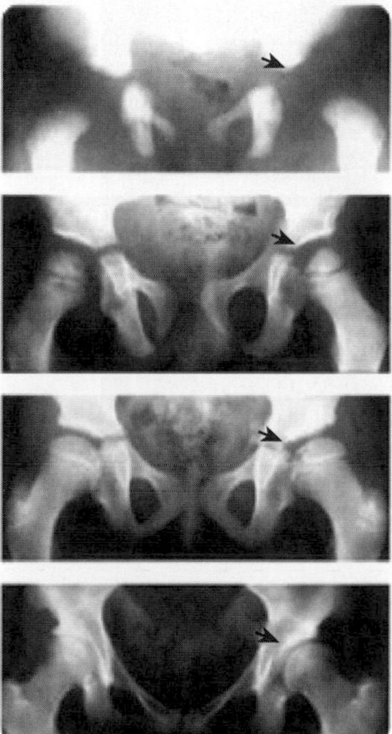

FIGURE 40-3 Hip Dysplasia in Children. Development dysplasia of the hip with residual acetabular dysplasia. Radiographs at birth and 3, 10, and 19 years (top to bottom) show persisting dysplasia.

most severe form compatible with life, children have short stature and triangular faces, possibly blue sclerae, and poor dentition. Because type I collagen also is the main component of blood vessels, vascular deformity, such as aortic aneurysm, can occur. Type IV OI can be subtle, with the child presenting with more normal stature and with fractures often not occurring until the child is older; it can be misdiagnosed as child abuse. Analysis of skin fibroblasts is diagnostic in 85% of children with OI.

Treatment is a combination of medical and surgical approaches (Figure 40-6). For fractures and deformity, intramedullary rodding of

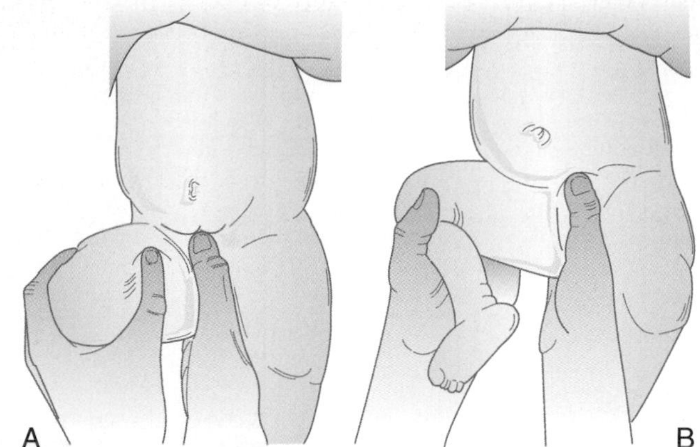

FIGURE 40-4 Congenital Dislocation of the Hip. A, Barlow manoeuvre (*left side*). With one hand pressing the symphysis in front and the sacral spine in back, lateral pressure is applied to the thigh with the thumb of the other hand while pressure is applied with the palm to the knee on the side being examined. The hip that has been flexed to 90° is then adducted. A positive sign is a sensation of abnormal movement, indicating dislocation of the femoral head from the acetabulum. The hands are reversed for examining the other hip. This sign and Ortolani sign may be found only in the first weeks of life. **B,** Ortolani manoeuvre (*right side*). Sign of jerking into correct position. After Barlow manoeuvre **(A),** the hip should be abducted to about 80° while the femur is lifted anteriorly with the fingers along the thigh. A positive sign is a sensation of a jerk or snap with reduction into the joint socket. (Adapted from Specht, E.E. [1974]. *Am Fam Physician, 9,* 88–96.)

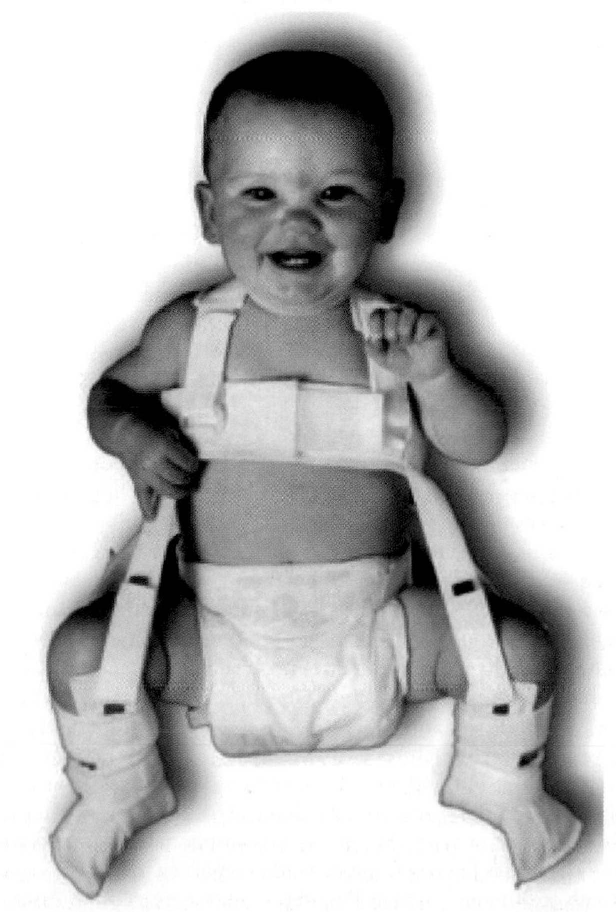

FIGURE 40-5 Pavlik Harness for Bilateral Hip Dislocation. (Wheaton Pavlik Harness. Courtesy of Wheaton Brace Co., Carol Stream, IL.)

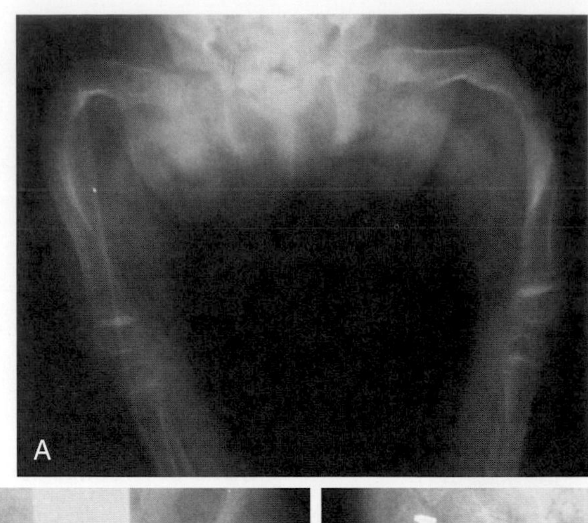

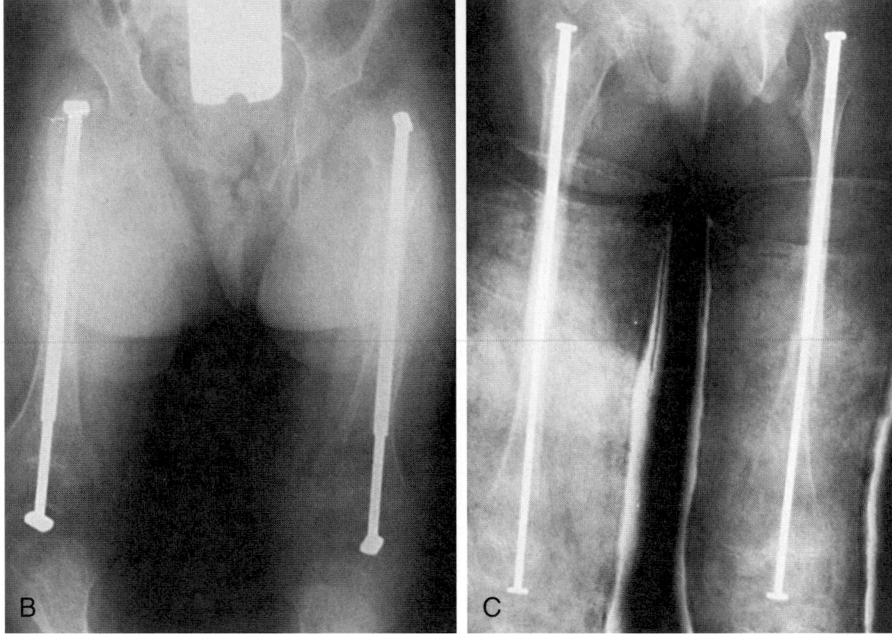

FIGURE 40-6 Osteogenesis Imperfecta Treated With Osteotomies and Telescoping Medullary Rods. A, Severe deformity of both femurs. **B,** Same individual after multiple osteotomies with telescoping medullary rod fixation. **C,** Same individual 4 years later demonstrating growth of femurs, no recurrence of deformity, and elongation of rods. (Plaster casts are in place for immobilization of tibial osteotomies.) (From Crenshaw, A.H. [Ed.]. [1992]. *Campbell's operative orthopaedics* [8th ed., vol. 3]. St. Louis: Mosby.)

the long bones improves position and also splints new fractures. Telescoping rods, which grow with the child, are improving in efficacy. Unfortunately, these children may have to undergo multiple surgeries and re-roddings with growth. The medical treatment, classically involving calcium and vitamin D supplementation, is under intense study. Pamidronate (Aredia) and other bisphosphates, such as alendronate (Fosamax), which decrease bone resorption by inhibiting osteoclasts, are now frequently used. In a multicentre trial,[7] pamidronate was given at 2- to 4-month intervals to children with severe (type III) and mild (type IV) OI. In the 30 children in the study, bone mineral density increased by 41.9%, fractures decreased by 1.7% per year, and mobility increased in 51% of the children. All children claimed their fatigue and chronic bone pain improved.[8] A Cochrane review, however, states it is unclear whether oral or intravenous bisphosphonate treatment consistently decreases fractures, and no studies report an increased fracture rate with treatment.[9] Further long-term studies are needed. Fracture healing remained unchanged. A large multicentre study is now trying to refine these treatments for all children with OI.

BONE INFECTION

Osteomyelitis

Osteomyelitis, or bone infection, is caused by either bacterial or granulomatous (e.g., tuberculosis) infective processes (Box 40-1, Figures 40-7 and 40-8). Antibiotic medications and often surgical interventions are used to treat these infections. Morbidity and mortality resulting from osteomyelitis declined drastically until the 1980s. Unfortunately, with the escalation of methicillin-resistant *Staphylococcus aureus* (MRSA) infections, serious increases in morbidity and mortality have developed.

Acute hematogenous osteomyelitis is the most common form in children. The infection usually begins as an abscess in the metaphysis of a long bone where blood flow is sluggish and bacteria can collect. With increasing pressure, the infection will rupture out of the periosteum and spread along the diaphysis of the bone. A new shell of bone can develop under the elevated periosteum and can become an **involucrum**. The portion of bone that is separated from adequate blood supply by the infection can die, thereby leading to an involucrum. All three of

BOX 40-1 Causative Microorganisms of Osteomyelitis According to Age

Newborns

Staphylococcus aureus (both methicillin-sensitive [MSSA] and methicillin-resistant [MRSA])
Group B streptococcus
Gram-negative enteric rods

Infants

S. aureus (MSSA and MRSA)
Haemophilus influenzae (decreasingly less common secondary to immunization)

Older Children

S. aureus (MSSA and MRSA)
Pseudomonas
Salmonella
Neisseria gonorrhoeae

Adolescents and Adults

Pseudomonas
Mycobacterium tuberculosis

these changes are apparent on radiograph and signify the need for surgical débridement as well as antibiotic treatment.

These radiographic bone changes take 2 to 3 weeks to develop. Initially, osteomyelitis presents as pain, swelling, and warmth. Children often will have fever, decreased appetite, fatigue, elevated white blood cell (WBC) count (50 to 70%), elevated C-reactive protein (CRP) (98%) level, and elevated erythrocyte sedimentation rate (ESR) (90%). Blood culture is positive in only 40 to 60% of cases. Without changes on plain radiograph, magnetic resonance imaging (MRI) can help define the location and extent of the infectious process. In infants, where osteomyelitis can be multifocal in up to 40% of cases, bone scan identifies other locations of infection that may need surgical intervention.

Treatment of osteomyelitis consists of appropriate antibiotic management for 6 weeks. If blood cultures are negative, bone aspirate must be analyzed to determine the bacterial source of the infection. With MRSA or bone changes on MRI, surgical débridement is required. MRSA often leads to more systemic illness, such as endocarditis (infection of the heart valves), organ failure, and infected thrombotic events.[10]

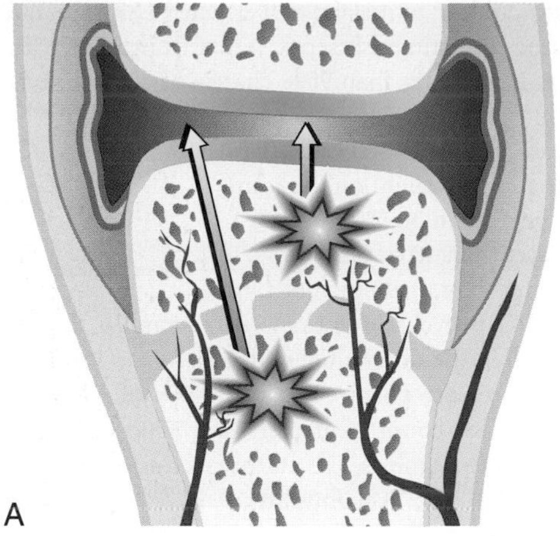

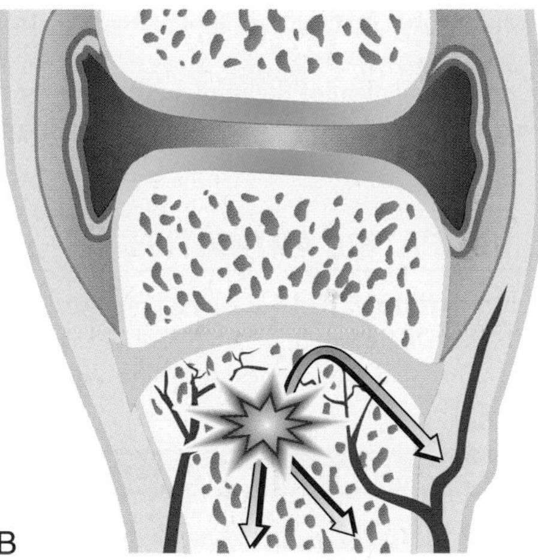

FIGURE 40-7 Pathogenesis of Acute Osteomyelitis Differs With Age. **A,** In infants younger than 1 year the epiphysis is nourished by arteries penetrating through the physis, allowing development of the condition within the epiphysis. **B,** In children up to 15 years of age, the infection is restricted to below the physis because of interruption of the vessels.

Septic Arthritis

Septic arthritis is a bacterial or granulomatous infection of the joint space. This is always a surgical emergency. The bacteria, and the lysosomes created by WBCs fighting the bacteria, can quickly destroy the articular cartilage of the joint and affect the blood supply to the epiphyseal bone nearby. Both of these complications have poor outcomes and can lead to a lifetime of disability.

Septic arthritis can occur primarily or secondary to osteomyelitis that spreads from the metaphysis of the bone into the joint space. The metaphyses of the pediatric hip, shoulder, proximal radius, and distal lateral tibia are all located within the joint capsule, and therefore osteomyelitis in these regions must be carefully monitored for secondary septic arthritis. The most common sites for septic arthritis are knees, hips, ankles, and elbows.

Children with septic arthritis present with severe joint pain, "pseudoparalysis" or marked guarding to motion of the joint, inability to bear weight, and malaise, often with anorexia. Children appear quite ill with this diagnosis. Nonpyogenic arthritis, such as juvenile idiopathic arthritis (JIA), can be difficult to distinguish clinically from septic arthritis

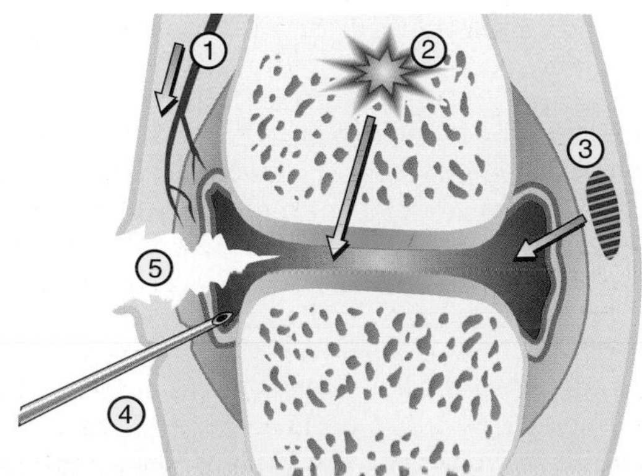

FIGURE 40-8 Routes of Infection to the Joint. **1,** Hematogenous route. **2,** Dissemination from osteomyelitis. **3,** Spread from an adjacent soft tissue infection. **4,** Diagnostic or therapeutic measures. **5,** Penetrating damage by puncture or cutting.

because both can lead to malaise and elevated ESR. The Kocher criteria are often used to distinguish septic joints from joint pain of another cause. There is a greater than 90% chance of a septic joint if three of the five following criteria are met:[11,12]

1. WBC greater than 12 000 cells/μL
2. Inability to bear weight on the joint
3. Fever greater than 38.5°C (101.3°F)
4. ESR greater than 40 mm/hr
5. CRP greater than 0.190 mcmol/L

Fever and CRP level greater than 0.190 mcmol/L appear to have the most influence in the differential diagnosis.

Blood cultures are positive in 30 to 40% of cases. Joint aspirate positive for a WBC count of greater than 7 000 per high-power field (HPF) defines the diagnosis, and culture of this fluid often determines bacterial etiology. As in osteomyelitis, *S. aureus* is the most common bacteria; however, MRSA is now present in up to 30% of affected children.[10,13] Emerging is the understanding that *Kingella kingae* is an important pathogen, occurs in children between 6 months and 4 years of age, and can involve many joints and bone, less frequently the endocardium and other locations.[13]

After surgical débridement of the joint, antibiotics are required for 2 to 3 weeks. Long-term follow-up to assess articular or physeal damage is required.

JUVENILE IDIOPATHIC ARTHRITIS

Juvenile idiopathic arthritis (JIA) is the childhood form of rheumatoid arthritis (see Chapter 39) and accounts for 5% of all cases of rheumatoid arthritis. JIA has three distinct modes of onset: **oligoarthritis** (fewer than three joints), **polyarthritis** (more than three joints), and **Still disease** (severe systemic onset) (Table 40-2). JIA differs from rheumatoid arthritis in several ways:

- Large joints are most commonly affected.
- Chronic uveitis (inflammation of the anterior chamber of the eye) is common if the blood test for antinuclear antibody (ANA) is positive; slit lamp examination by a trained ophthalmologist is required every 6 months to avoid vision loss.
- Serum tests may be negative for rheumatoid factor (RF); RF-positive children have a worse prognosis.
- Subluxation and ankylosis may occur in the cervical spine if disease progresses.
- Rheumatoid arthritis that continues through adolescence can have severe effects on growth and adult morbidity.

Many children with oligoarthritis who are "seronegative" (blood tests negative for RF or ANA) will resolve their symptoms over time. Systemic onset, or "seropositivity," of the disease is more likely consistent with lifelong arthritis. Therefore, treatment is supportive, not curative. Nonsteroidal anti-inflammatory drugs are a mainstay of treatment, and methotrexate (Apo-Methotrexate) is also being used with success. The goals are to minimize inflammation and deformity.

QUICK CHECK 40-1

1. Why is an early diagnosis of developmental dysplasia of the hip imperative?
2. How does osteomyelitis develop?
3. How has MRSA changed musculo-skeletal infections in children?
4. How does juvenile idiopathic arthritis differ from the adult form?

TABLE 40-2 Characteristics of Juvenile Idiopathic Arthritis Related to Mode of Onset

	Systemic Onset	Pauciarticular (Two or Three Subtypes)	Polyarticular (Two Subtypes)
Percentage of patients	30	45	25
Age at onset	Bimodal distribution 1–3 years of age 8–10 years of age	Type I: younger than 10 years Type II: older than 10 years	Throughout childhood and adolescence
Gender ratio (female/male)	1.5:1	Type I: almost all female Type II: 1:9	Mostly female
Joints involved	Any Only 20% have joint involvement at time of diagnosis	Usually confined to lower extremities—knee, ankle, and eventually sacroiliac; sometimes elbow	Any joint; usually symmetric involvement of small joints Hip involvement in 50% Spine involvement in 50%
Extra-articular manifestations	Fever, malaise, myalgia, rash, pleuritis or pericarditis, adenomegaly, splenomegaly, hepatomegaly Systemic signs minimal	Type I: chronic iridocyclitis; mucocutaneous lesions Type II: acute iridocyclitis; sacroiliitis common; eventual ankylosing spondylitis in many	Possible low-grade fever, malaise, weight loss, rheumatoid nodules, or vasculitis
Laboratory test results	Elevated ESR, CRP levels; RF negative; ANA rarely positive; anemia; leukocytosis	Elevated ESR, CRP levels; ANA positive Type I: HLA-DRW5 positive Type II: HLA-B27 positive Type III: HLA-TMo positive	Elevated ESR, CRP levels Type I: RF positive Type II: RF negative
Long-term prognosis	Mortality: 1–2% of all JIA patients Joint destruction in 40%	Continuous disease; eventual remission in 60% Type I: ocular damage; functional blindness in 10% Type II: ankylosing spondylitis Type III: best outlook for recovery	Longer duration; more crippling; remission in 25% Type I: high incidence of crippling arthritis Type II: outlook good

ANA, Antinuclear antibody; *CRP*, C-reactive protein; *ESR*, erythrocyte sedimentation rate; *HLA*, human leukocyte antigen; *JIA*, juvenile idiopathic arthritis; *RF*, rheumatoid factor.

From Hockenberry, M.J., & Wilson, D. (2007). *Wong's nursing care of infants and children* (8th ed.). St. Louis: Mosby.

OSTEOCHONDROSES

The osteochondroses are a series of childhood diseases involving areas of significant tensile or compressive stress (e.g., tibial tubercle, Achilles insertion, hip epiphysis). The pathophysiology is partial loss of blood supply, death of bone (osseous necrosis), progressive bony weakness, and then microfracture. The cause of the decreased blood supply is controversial; trauma, a change in clotting sensitivity, vascular injury, genetic predisposition, or a combination of these factors is presently considered most likely. Additionally, during the years of rapid bone growth, blood supply to the growing ends of bones (epiphyses) may become insufficient, resulting in necrotic bone, usually near joints. Because bone is normally undergoing a continuous rebuilding process, the necrotic areas can self-repair over a period of weeks or months.

Use of anti inflammatory medications, modification of activities, immobilization, and rest are recommended during active stages of the disease. Reparative correction by revascularization is the rule, although years may be required for full healing, and deformity from compression during the period of osseous necrosis can persist.

Legg-Calvé-Perthes Disease

Legg-Calvé-Perthes (LCP) disease is a common osteochondrosis usually occurring in children between the ages of 3 and 10 years, with a peak incidence at 6 years. The disorder is bilateral in 10 to 20% of children, and boys are affected five times more often than girls. Boys have a more poorly developed blood supply to the femoral head than do girls of the same age, and this is thought to be the reason for male predilection. The role of genetics is unclear, but LCP disease is more common in northern European and Japanese children and rare in Black children; family history is positive in 20% of cases. This self-limited disease of the hip, which runs its natural course in 2 to 5 years, is presumably created by recurrent interruption of the blood supply to the femoral head. The ossification centre first becomes necrotic (osteonecrosis) and then is gradually replaced by live bone.

PATHOPHYSIOLOGY Several causative theories have been proposed, including a generalized disorder of epiphyseal cartilage growth, thyroid hormone deficiency, trauma, infection, and blood clotting disorders. However, a Harvard study did not show increases in thrombotic disorders in consecutive children with LCP disease.[14] Boys with a hypercoagulable state are three times more likely to acquire LCP disease than girls with the same disorder.[15] Another study has shown the risk for LCP disease is five times greater in children exposed to passive smoke as opposed to children living in a smoke-free environment.[16] Increased risk has been associated with smoke from indoor use of a wood stove.[17]

In the first stage of LCP disease, the soft tissues of the hip (synovial membrane and joint capsule) are swollen, edematous, and hyperemic, often with fluid present in the joint (Figure 40-9). In the second necrotic stage, the anterior 50% or more of the epiphysis of the femoral head dies because of a lack of blood supply, and the metaphyseal bone at the junction of the femoral neck and capital epiphyseal plate is softened because of increased blood supply and decalcification. Granulation tissue (procallus) and blood vessels then invade the dead bone. The third, or regenerative healing, stage ordinarily lasts 2 to 4 years. The dead bone in the femoral head is replaced by procallus, and new bone is established (see Figure 40-9). In the fourth, or residual, stage, remodelling takes place and the newly formed bone is organized into a live spongy bone.

CLINICAL MANIFESTATIONS Injury or trauma precedes the onset of LCP disease in approximately 30 to 50% of children with LCP disease. For several months the child complains of a limp and pain that can be referred to the knee, inner thigh, and the groin, following the path of the obturator nerve. The pain is usually aggravated by activity and relieved by rest and administration of anti-inflammatory medications.

The typical physical findings include spasm on rotation of the hip, limitation of internal rotation and abduction, and hip flexion–adduction deformity. If the child is walking, an early abnormal gait termed an antalgic (painful) abductor lurch, or a "Trendelenburg gait" (gluteus medius gait pattern), is apparent. If the hip pain or limp has been present for a prolonged period, muscles of the hip and thigh atrophy.

EVALUATION AND TREATMENT The goals of treatment are to preserve normal congruity of the femoral head and acetabulum and maintain spasm-free and pain-free range of motion in the hip joint. Currently, most children can be managed with anti-inflammatory medications and activity modification during periods of synovitis. Serial radiographs are obtained to monitor the progress of the disease and to ensure that the femoral head remains congruent in the acetabulum. Surgery may be necessary if the femoral head becomes subluxated or incongruent with the acetabulum (Figure 40-10).[18-20] Children older than age 6 (by bone age) have a worse prognosis attributable to poorer remodelling potential. Older children require surgery more often to avoid poor congruence of the hip. Poor congruence predisposes to early osteoarthritis, with nearly 50% requiring hip replacement surgery by age 40.

Osgood-Schlatter Disease

Osgood-Schlatter disease consists of osteochondrosis of the tibia tubercle and associated patellar tendonitis. Osgood-Schlatter disease occurs most often in preadolescents and adolescents who participate in sports and is more prevalent in boys than in girls. Osgood-Schlatter disease is one of the most common ailments reported in the 30 million children who are involved in sports.[21]

The severity of the lesion varies from mild tendonitis to a complete separation of the anterior tibial apophysis, a part of the tibial tubercle. The mildest form of Osgood-Schlatter disease causes ischemic (avascular) necrosis in the region of the bony tibial tubercle, with hypertrophic

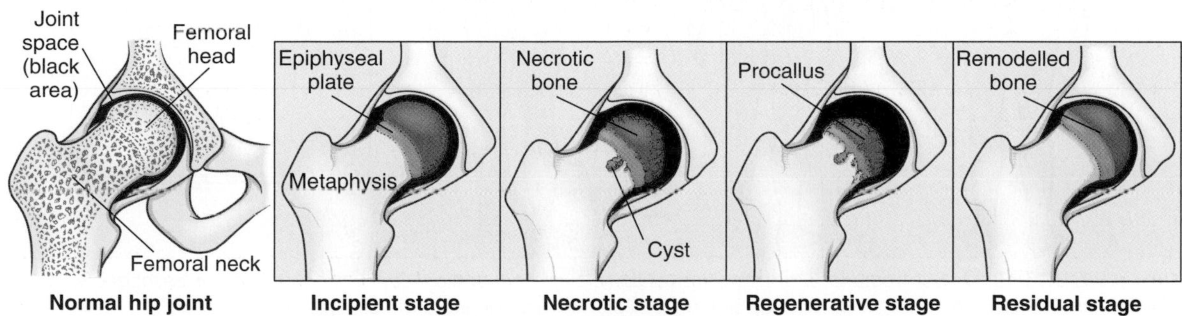

FIGURE 40-9 Stages of Legg-Calvé-Perthes Disease, a Form of Osteochondrosis.

cartilage formation during the stages of repair. In more severe cases, the abnormality involves a true apophyseal separation of the tibial tubercle with avascular necrosis.

The child complains of pain and swelling in the region around the patellar tendon and tibial tubercle, which becomes prominent and is tender to direct pressure. The pain is most severe after physical activity that involves vigorous quadriceps contraction (jumping or running) or direct local trauma to the tibial tubercle area.

The goal of treatment for Osgood-Schlatter disease is to decrease the stress at the tubercle. Often a period of 4 to 8 weeks of restriction from strenuous physical activity, administration of anti-inflammatory medications, and stretching of the quadriceps muscle are sufficient. Bracing with a tubercle band can be very helpful. If the pain is not relieved, a cast or knee immobilizer is required, a situation that is particularly difficult if the condition is bilateral.

Gradual resumption of activity is permitted after 8 weeks, but return to unrestricted athletic participation requires an additional 8 weeks to allow for revascularization, healing, and ossification of the tibial tubercle.[18,22] With skeletal maturity and closure of the apophysis, Osgood-Schlatter disease resolves.

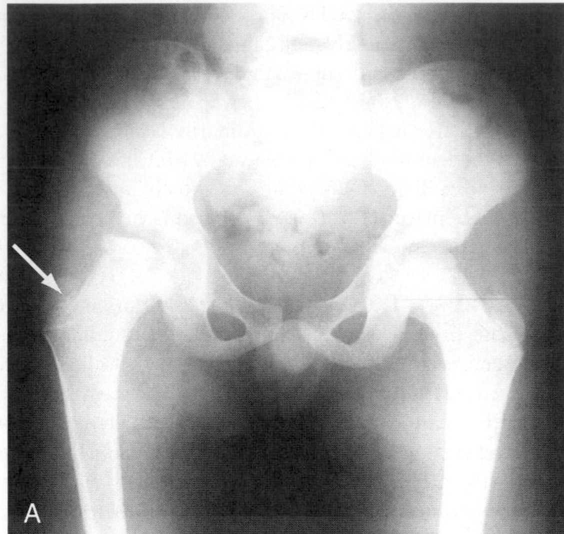

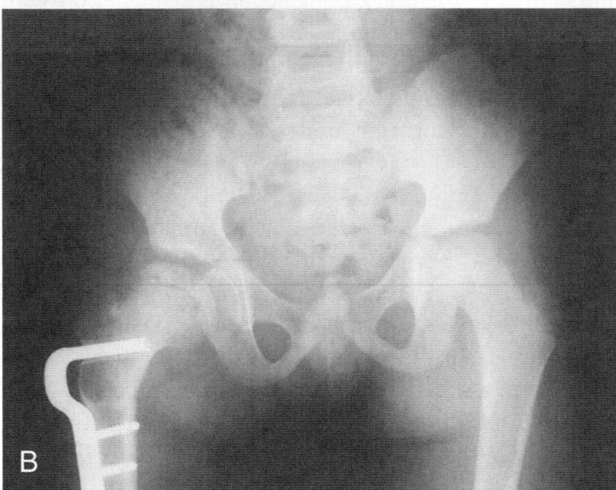

FIGURE 40-10 Pelvis of a 7-Year-Old Boy with Legg-Calvé-Perthes Disease. **A,** The femoral head is flat and extruded from the edge of the joint. This hip is at risk for early arthritis if left to revascularize and heal in this position. **B,** Surgical replacement of the femoral head. As the Perthes heals, the ball has assumed a round shape that matches the socket well.

Sever Disease

Sever disease is the "Osgood-Schlatter" of the calcaneus (heel bone). The insertion of the Achilles pulls on the cartilaginous apophysis of the calcaneus, causing pain. It is more common in athletic children and children who have underlying Achilles tendon tightness, for example, soccer players between the ages of 8 and 12. It is relieved by a heel lift in the shoe, rest, stretching, and anti-inflammatory medications.

SCOLIOSIS

Scoliosis is a rotational curvature of the spine most obvious in the anteroposterior plane (Figure 40-11). It can be classified as nonstructural or structural. **Nonstructural scoliosis** results from a cause other than the spine itself, such as posture, leg length discrepancy, or splinting from pain. **Structural scoliosis** is a curvature of the spine associated with vertebral rotation. Nonstructural scoliosis can become structural if the underlying cause is not found and treated.

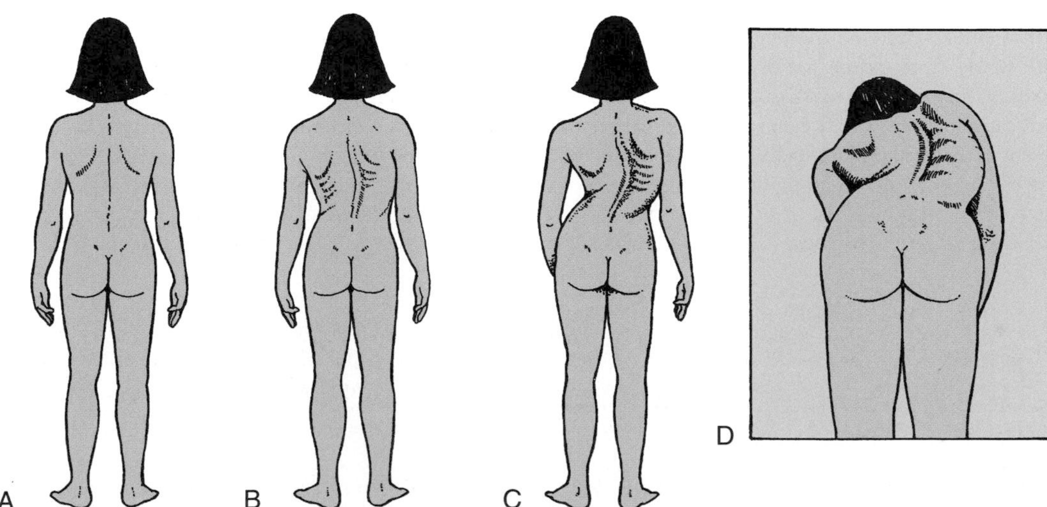

FIGURE 40-11 Scoliosis in Children. Normal spine alignment and abnormal spinal curvatures associated with scoliosis. **A,** Normal. **B,** Mild. **C,** Severe. **D,** Rotation and curvature of scoliosis.

There are three main types of structural scoliosis: idiopathic; congenital (attributable to bony deformity such as hemivertebrae); and teratological (caused by another systemic syndrome such as cerebral palsy). Eighty percent of all scoliosis is idiopathic, which may have a genetic component. Although girls and boys are equally affected, once the curve becomes more than 20 degrees, girls are five times more likely to be affected. Ninety-eight percent of curves are apex right thoracic. If a left thoracic curve appears in the adolescent with idiopathic scoliosis, MRI is performed to rule out a neurological cause. MRI should be performed in scoliotic children with loss of abdominal reflexes and those who have exertional headaches or a congenital curve.[22,23]

Idiopathic curves progress while a child is growing, and progression can be very rapid during growth spurts. When idiopathic curves progress to 25° or greater, and the child is skeletally immature, bracing is required. The total number of hours a brace is worn correlates to efficacy of treatment; 82% of children who wore the brace as prescribed had minimal progression.[24] In braced curves, 72% required no surgery compared with only 48% of those who wore no brace.[25]

Curves of more than 50° will progress after skeletal maturity, so spinal fusion is required to stop progression. Bracing is the only nonoperative measure known to slow scoliotic progression. Chiropractic manipulation, physical therapy, exercise, and diet regimens have not been shown to alter natural history. Bracing is less successful in teratological or congenital curves; therefore, these conditions may require surgical intervention more often.

MUSCULAR DYSTROPHY

The **muscular dystrophies** are a group of inherited disorders that cause progressive muscle fibre loss leading to weakness, mostly of the voluntary muscles. Some dystrophies cause disease in infancy, others in childhood, and others not until adulthood. Muscular dystrophies have different inheritance patterns and different biochemical alterations that cause each specific type. Three are discussed in detail in this chapter. Individuals with Duchenne muscular dystrophy (DMD) have a mutation in a specific gene that leads to alterations in the muscle protein dystrophin. Individuals with myotonic muscular dystrophy (MMD) have a genetic alteration that leads to systemic disease. Although there is no cure for any of the muscular dystrophies, aggressive preventive management has increased the life expectancy and quality of life of children with these disorders. Common forms of muscular dystrophy are described in Table 40-3.

Duchenne Muscular Dystrophy

PATHOPHYSIOLOGY **Duchenne muscular dystrophy (DMD)** is X-linked, generally occurring in boys, and is present in about 1 in 3 500 male births. It is the most common childhood dystrophy. DMD is caused by mutations in the **dystrophin** gene, which lead to alterations or deletions of the muscle protein dystrophin.

The protein dystrophin mediates anchorage of the actin cytoskeleton of skeletal muscle fibres to the basement membrane through a membrane–glycoprotein complex. With lack of dystrophin, the poorly anchored fibres tear themselves apart under the repeated stress of contraction. Free calcium then enters the muscle cells, causing cell death and fibre necrosis (Figure 40-12).

CLINICAL MANIFESTATIONS Boys with DMD will present in the preschool years with muscle weakness, difficulty walking, and large calves (pseudohypertrophy) caused by normal muscle fibre replacement with fat and connective tissue (Figure 40-12, *B* and *C*). Although the calves are large, the muscle is actually weak. Clinical weakness starts in the pelvic girdle, initially causing difficulty rising from the floor (Gower sign) and climbing stairs, and a waddling gait because of weakness in the lumbar and gluteal muscles. Boys with DMD often toe-walk because of weakness of the anterior tibial and peroneal muscles, causing the feet to assume a talipes equinovarus position. The weakness worsens over the subsequent few years, resulting in the loss of ability to ambulate by 8 to 13 years of age. Muscle weakness also leads to contractures of the knees, hips, and other joints, and scoliosis develops in most boys with DMD. Once scoliosis begins, it is relentlessly progressive. Curves of more than 20° are treated surgically to maintain pulmonary function. Muscle weakness and inactivity, particularly once a person is in a wheelchair full time, lead to osteoporosis and pathological fractures. If fracture occurs, bisphosphonates may be used to strengthen bone, although long-term studies on safety have not been performed in this population.

As children age, muscle weakness progresses and respiratory weakness leads to breathing difficulty, particularly when sleeping. Susceptibility to respiratory tract infections and progressive deterioration of pulmonary function generally lead to premature death, usually in the 20s. Cardiomyopathy also may occur and, despite treatment, is generally progressive. Bowel and bladder functions are often mildly affected, with constipation and urinary urgency as frequent symptoms. Mild to moderate cognitive problems are common but not universal.

EVALUATION AND TREATMENT Diagnosis is suggested (a high creatine kinase [CK] level does not confirm the diagnosis because many other alterations can also increase CK) by measuring the blood CK level, which can be 100 times the normal level, with confirmation by genetic testing for mutations in the dystrophin gene.

Management involves maintaining function for as long as possible. Treatment with steroids can prolong the ability to walk by several years and improves life expectancy.[26] Deflazacort (Alnacort) is a corticosteroid that is not easily accessible in Canada and has just been approved for use in treating DMD in the United States.[27,28] It is a steroid that may have fewer side effects than prednisone (Deltasone). Treatment also involves range-of-motion exercises, bracing, and surgical release of contracture deformities and scoliosis when necessary. Children with DMD require a multidisciplinary approach to care, including attention to heart and breathing problems, weight loss/gain, constipation, rehabilitative/developmental problems, psychosocial needs, and neurological and orthopedic problems (Figure 40-13). New guidelines for

TABLE 40-3 Major Muscular Dystrophy Syndromes

Disease	Mode of Inheritance	Age at Clinical Onset	Distribution of Weakness
Duchenne muscular dystrophy/Becker muscular dystrophy (DMD/BMD)	X-linked, sporadic	2–3 years/5–7 years	Proximal with pseudohypertrophy
Facioscapulohumeral muscular dystrophy (FSHD)	Autosomal dominant	Early adolescence	Face, arms, legs
Myotonic muscular dystrophy (MMD)	Autosomal dominant	Variable—birth to adulthood	Distal muscles, face

From Moxley, R.T., 3rd., Ashwal, S., Pandya, S., et al. (2005). *Neurology, 64*(1), 13–20.

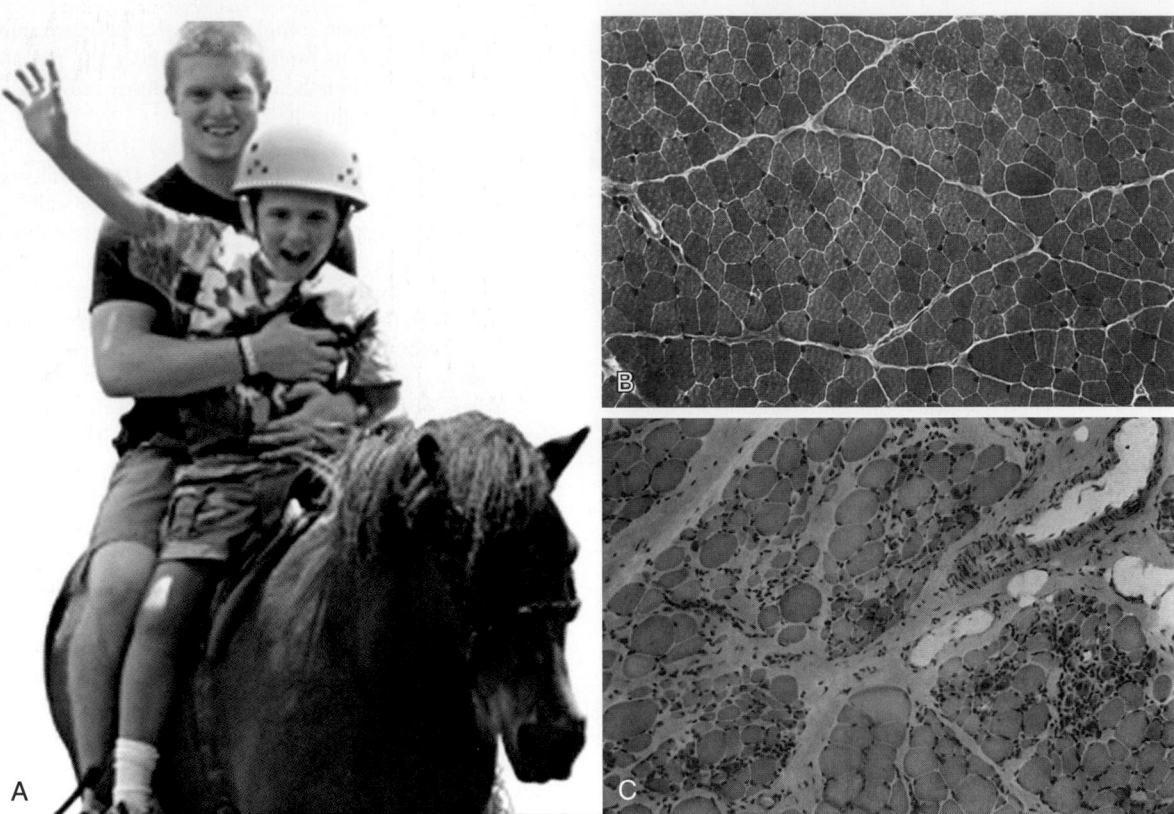

FIGURE 40-12 Duchenne Muscular Dystrophy. A, Young boy with Duchenne muscular dystrophy (DMD) on horseback. B, Transverse section of gastrocnemius muscle from a healthy boy. C, Transverse section of gastrocnemius muscle from a boy with DMD. Normal muscle fibre is replaced with fat and connective tissue. (From Jorde, L.B., Carey, J.C., & Bamshad, M.J. [2010]. *Medical genetics* [4th ed.]. Philadelphia: Mosby.)

the evaluation and treatment of DMD were developed after reviewing thousands of clinical scenarios and are presented as a multisystem, two-part approach. One part is for diagnosis and the other part for management.

The care for individuals with DMD across Canada is delivered in multidisciplinary teams and includes corticosteroid treatment (which tends to prolong ambulation and preserve both cardiac and respiratory function) as well as routine calcium and vitamin D supplementation, and the use of night splints to prevent foot drop.[28] If appropriate, families should receive genetic counselling for recurrence risk and prenatal screening. Family support is necessary throughout the lifespan of the child because needs vary depending on the stage of the disease.

Becker Muscular Dystrophy

Although Becker muscular dystrophy (BMD) has been designated historically as a separate muscular dystrophy, it is actually caused by alterations of the same dystrophin gene (i.e., dystrophinopathies) and protein as seen in DMD. Children with BMD present later and have a longer life expectancy than those with DMD; however, they are part of the same clinical spectrum.

Facioscapulohumeral Muscular Dystrophy

Facioscapulohumeral muscular dystrophy (FSHD), one of the most common muscular dystrophies, is inherited in an autosomal dominant fashion. It is more variable in presentation than DMD. FSHD is usually observed in *late* childhood. Progression is usually slow and lifespan is normal or near normal. FSHD occurs because of a deletion on chromosome 4 that is not associated with any particular gene and causes disease by still unknown mechanisms.

Muscle weakness, which is often asymmetric, usually begins in the face and is then observed in the shoulders and legs. Individuals with FSHD often have weak eye closure, are not able to whistle or inflate a balloon, and have scapular winging.

Diagnosis is by genetic testing, although sometimes biopsies or electrodiagnostic testing may also be performed as part of the diagnostic evaluation. FSHD also may be associated with mild hearing loss, retinal abnormalities, and mild cardiac problems. Unlike DMD or BMD, children with FSHD often have muscle pain, particularly in their arms and shoulders.

Treatment involves administration of nonsteroidal anti-inflammatory drugs to decrease pain and inflammation. Massage and heat treatments also may be helpful. Bracing may be performed for function; for example, dorsiflexion of the feet with ankle-foot orthotics to prevent tripping or to provide support and comfort.

Myotonic Muscular Dystrophy

PATHOPHYSIOLOGY Myotonic muscular dystrophy (MMD) is a multisystem disease that can occur because of mutations in either of two genes resulting in type 1 (*DMPK* gene) and type 2 (*CNBP* gene) MMD. MMD1 may demonstrate a genetic mechanism called *anticipation*, in which children born to a mother with MMD usually have a more severe form of the disease.

CLINICAL MANIFESTATIONS MMD affects the brain, skeletal and smooth muscles, the eyes, the heart, and the endocrine system, manifesting as distal muscle weakness, learning problems or intellectual disability, or both. Additionally, children can have dysphagia, constipation, cardiac dysrhythmias that if untreated may be life-threatening, diabetes,

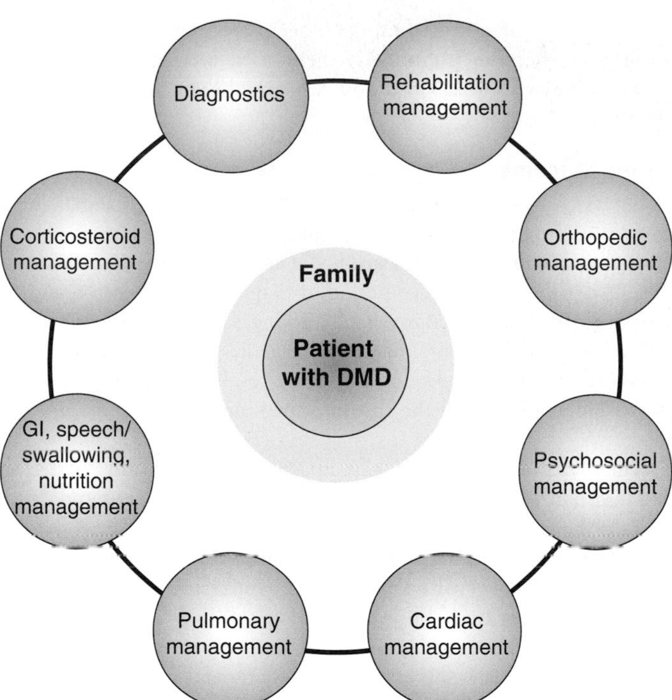

FIGURE 40-13 Multisystem Approach for Evaluation and Treatment of Duchenne Muscular Dystrophy. (Adapted from Bushby, K., Finkel, R., Birnkrant, D.J., et al. [2010]. Diagnosis and management of Duchenne muscular dystrophy part 1: Diagnosis and pharmacological and psychosocial management. *Lancet, 9*(1), 77–93; Bushby, K., Finkel, R., Birnkrant, D.J., et al. [2010]. Diagnosis and management of Duchenne muscular dystrophy part 2: Implementation of multidisciplinary care. *Lancet, 9*(2), 177–189.)

and cataracts. Boys with MMD also may manifest testicular atrophy and early male-pattern baldness. A hallmark of the disease is myotonia—individuals have difficulty relaxing muscles; for example, they may have difficulty relaxing their hand grip after a handshake or opening their eyes after closing them tightly.

Children with mild disease do not develop symptoms until adolescence or older and may display mild muscle weakness (usually more pronounced in the distal muscles), cataracts, and myotonia, but have normal lifespans. Children with a more classic form of the disease also have onset of symptoms in the teenage years but have progressive muscle weakness, cataracts, and cardiac conduction abnormalities; they may have a shortened lifespan and require a wheelchair for mobility. The congenital form, the most severe, may be present at birth or become obvious over the first few years of life.

EVALUATION AND TREATMENT Diagnosis is made by genetic testing for the two genes known to cause MMD. In each case, an abnormal segment of DNA, caused by an abnormally large trinucleotide, repeat expansion of a cytosine–thymine–guanine (CTG) triplet in an untranslated region of a gene, causes abnormal functioning of muscle and other cells. Type 1 is more common and can present in infancy (the congenital form). Infants with MMD may have life-threatening breathing and swallowing problems and developmental delay or intellectual disability, although MMD is not observed until childhood or even adolescence.

Steroids are not useful for the treatment of MMD; however, maintaining muscle function is important, including range-of-motion exercises, bracing, and surgical release of contractures when necessary. Children need to be followed closely by neurologists and primary care providers with treatment for the various aspects of the disease, such as dysphagia, heart dysrhythmias, and constipation, as well as other problems.

QUICK CHECK 40-2

1. What is the pathophysiology of osteochondrosis?
2. What is the cause of Duchenne muscular dystrophy (DMD)?
3. Discuss the clinical manifestations of DMD.
4. Which dystrophy is really a systemic disease?
5. What is the difference between Becker and Duchenne muscular dystrophies?

MUSCULO-SKELETAL TUMOURS

Benign Bone Tumours

The two most common forms of benign bone tumours are osteochondroma and nonossifying fibroma.

Osteochondroma

Osteochondroma (or exostosis) can occur as a solitary lesion or as an inherited syndrome of **hereditary multiple exostoses (HME)**. HME is an autosomal dominant condition with exostoses occurring throughout the skeleton. Osteochondromas appear as bony protuberances because of *EXT1* and *EXT2* genetic anomalies near active growth plates of the proximal humerus, distal femur, or proximal tibia. The most common presentation is a palpable mass that is painful when traumatized. Rarely, the lesion can cause neurological or vascular problems, or tendon rupture from local compression. The lesions can lead to growth disturbance and mildly short stature. Knee valgus (knock-knee), ankle valgus, and hip problems are common. Upper extremity lesions can lead to a pronounced deformity in the forearm with a very short ulna bone. These lesions grow until skeletal maturity; growth or pain after skeletal maturity is a sign of possible malignant transformation, especially in the pelvis or scapular region. Transformation to chondrosarcoma is very rare, occurring in less than 1% of children.

Treatment involves minimizing growth disturbance, local tissue compression, and pain by resection of symptomatic lesions. The regrowth rate is 30% when lesions are removed in early childhood; therefore only symptomatic lesions should be surgically addressed in the growing child.[29]

Nonossifying Fibroma

Of all benign bone tumours, 50% are nonossifying fibromas or fibrous cortical defects. **Nonossifying fibromas** are sharply demarcated, cortically based lesions of fibrocytes that have replaced normal bone. The lesion can occur in any bone, at any age. Nearly 30% of all children have at least one.

Microscopically, these benign nonmetastasizing lesions appear as whorled bundles of fibroblasts and osteoclastlike giant cells. As the tumour grows, lipids make the fibroblasts foamy in appearance, and they are known as *foam cells.*

Treatment is observational only. If these lesions grow too large, however, they will compromise the biomechanical strength of the bone and lead to pathological fractures. Curettage and bone grafting is suggested after pathological fracture or if impending fracture (nonossifying fibroma greater than 50% of the diameter of the bone or greater than 3 or 4 cm) is noted radiographically.

Malignant Bone Tumours

Malignant bone tumours are uncommon tumours in childhood, accounting for fewer than 5% of childhood malignancies and occurring mostly during adolescence. The two main tumours are osteosarcoma and Ewing sarcoma (see Chapter 39).

Osteosarcoma

Osteosarcoma is the most common malignant bone tumour found during childhood and originates in bone-producing mesenchymal cells. Tumours can be broadly classified as those arising within the bone and those arising on the surface of bone. Approximately 75% of these tumours occur in persons between the ages of 10 and 25 years, with most being diagnosed between 15 and 19 years of age during the adolescent growth spurt. Incidence is the same for males and females.

Osteosarcoma may develop as a result of rapid local growth, which increases the likelihood of mutation. It can be induced by ionizing radiation, even with relatively low doses, and can be a tragic consequence of therapeutic radiation for other forms of cancer. The latent period after radiation exposure is 5 to 40 years. There also has been a link to individuals with retinoblastoma (a hereditary eye tumour).

Osteosarcoma has not been linked to chemical carcinogens or viruses. No DNA or RNA virus has been isolated.

Molecular analysis has demonstrated deletion of genetic material on the long arm of chromosome 13, which led to the identification of a tumour-suppressor gene as being part of the mechanism for tumour development. The oncogene *src* also has been associated with osteosarcoma.

PATHOPHYSIOLOGY Osteosarcoma occurs mainly in the metaphyses of long bones near sites of active physeal growth. The tumour most commonly occurs at the distal femur, proximal tibia, or proximal humerus. As a tumour of mesenchymal cells, osteosarcoma demonstrates production of osteoid cells.

Osteosarcoma is a bulky tumour that extends beyond the bone into a soft tissue mass. It may encircle the bone and destroy the trabeculae of the diseased area. Osteosarcoma disseminates through the bloodstream, usually to the lung. As many as 25% of children diagnosed with osteosarcoma exhibit lung metastases at diagnosis. Other sites of metastatic spread include other bones and visceral organs.

CLINICAL MANIFESTATIONS The most common presenting complaint is pain. Night pain, awakening a child from sleep, is a particularly foreboding sign. There may be swelling, warmth, and redness caused by the vascularity of the tumour. Symptoms also may include cough, dyspnea, and chest pain if lung metastasis is present. If a lower extremity is involved, a child may limp or suffer a pathological fracture. Although osteosarcoma is not the result of trauma, trauma may call attention to a pre-existing tumour.

EVALUATION AND TREATMENT The five histological types of osteosarcoma are determined by the predominant cell type. The tumour is graded according to degree of malignancy; the higher the grade, the worse the prognosis.

Surgery and chemotherapy are the primary treatments for osteosarcoma. The tumour is resistant to radiation. Traditionally, surgery includes amputation at the joint above the involved bone; however, more recent limb salvage procedures have gained acceptance, and amputation may be avoided in many children.

Chemotherapy is an important component of treatment. Children routinely receive chemotherapy preoperatively; then the disease is restaged with MRI and surgical biopsy to determine rate of "tumour kill." If more than 90% of tumour cells are killed by chemotherapy, the prognosis is markedly improved. Chemotherapy is then used after surgery for any additional cell spill during surgery. The use of chemotherapy with surgery has increased the 5-year survival rate to 60% or more.[30]

A number of approaches have been used to treat pulmonary metastases. Because pulmonary metastases are generally solitary, thoracotomy with wedge resection has proved to be the most effective treatment.

Ewing Sarcoma

Ewing sarcoma is the second most common and most lethal malignant bone tumour that occurs during childhood. This tumour is named after James Ewing, who first identified it as a separate clinical diagnosis in 1921. The most common period of diagnosis is between 5 and 15 years of age; it is rare after age 30. Ewing sarcoma is slightly more common in males than females. Cytogenic studies have shown a translocation of chromosomes 11 and 22 resulting in a fusion protein (EWS-FLI 1) forming at the chromosomal junction.

PATHOPHYSIOLOGY Ewing sarcoma is most commonly located in the midshaft of long bones or in flat bones. The most common sites include the femur, pelvis, and humerus (Figure 40-14).

Arising from bone marrow, Ewing sarcoma can penetrate the cortex of the bone to form a soft tissue mass. Unlike osteosarcoma, Ewing sarcoma does not make bone and radiographically appears as a permeative, destructive lesion (Figure 40-15). Ewing sarcoma metastasizes to nearly every organ. Metastasis occurs early and is usually apparent at diagnosis or within 1 year. The most common sites are the lung, other bones, lymph nodes, bone marrow, liver, spleen, and central nervous system.

CLINICAL MANIFESTATIONS As with osteosarcoma, the most common complaint is pain that increases in severity. A soft tissue mass is often present. Additional symptoms may include fever, malaise, and anorexia. The radiographic appearance is similar to that of osteomyelitis, and diagnosis is only confirmed with biopsy.

EVALUATION AND TREATMENT Evaluation is determined from genetic testing, elevated sedimentation rate, and lactate dehydrogenase (LDH)

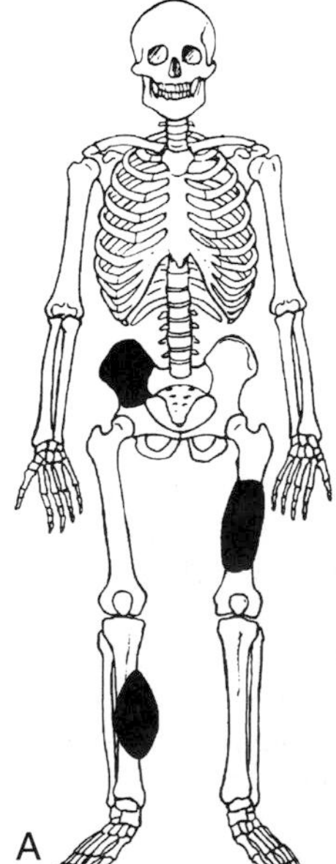

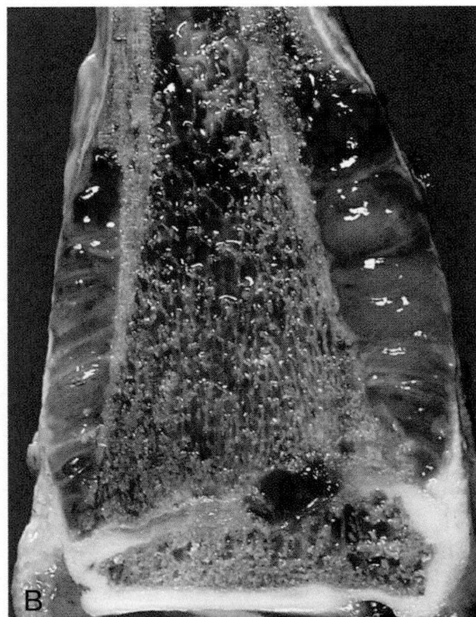

FIGURE 40-14 Ewing Sarcoma. **A,** Most common anatomical sites. **B,** Close-up view of Ewing sarcoma of the distal end of the tibia. Tumour extends into the soft tissue. (From Damjanov, I., & Linder, J. [Eds.]. [1996]. *Anderson's pathology* [10th ed.]. St. Louis: Mosby.)

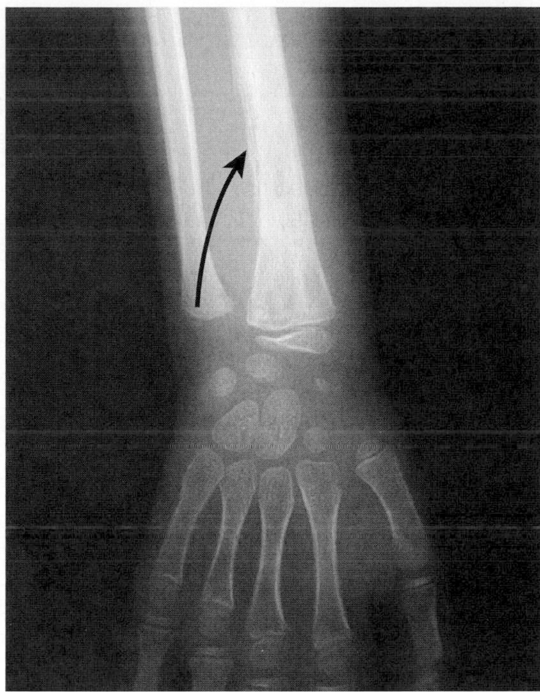

FIGURE 40-15 Ewing Sarcoma of the Distal Radius. Radiograph of an 8-year-old boy showing a permeative lesion of the distal radius. Note the loss of bone cortex on the ulnar border (*arrow*), suggesting an aggressive process. Bone biopsy revealed Ewing sarcoma.

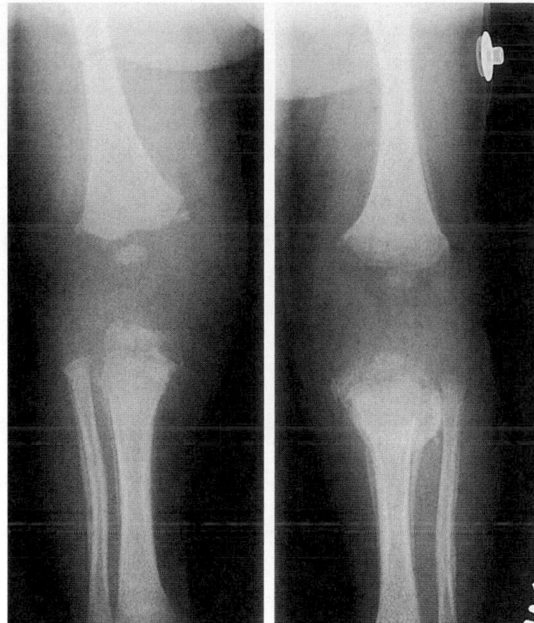

FIGURE 40-16 Corner Fracture. Bilateral knee radiograph showing healing corner fractures of bilateral proximal tibias and distal femurs. Note the varying amount of callus formation signifying fractures at different stages of healing.

levels. Biopsy is used to conclusively establish the diagnosis of a small round cell tumour.

Treatment includes radiation, chemotherapy, and, if possible, surgical débridement. Chemotherapy is continued for 12 to 18 months after resection. Present 5-year survival with this tritherapeutic approach is 60%; however, tumours of the pelvis have a markedly worse prognosis. Metastasis at diagnosis is another poor prognostic indicator, with 5-year survival rate dropping to less than 40%.

QUICK CHECK 40-3

1. What are the most common benign bone tumours of children?
2. What are the two malignant bone tumours found in children?
3. What is the most lethal bone tumour in children?

NONACCIDENTAL TRAUMA

It is estimated that approximately 32% of Canadians have experienced some form of child abuse (physical, emotional, sexual, or neglect).[31] Maltreatment may be psychological, sexual, or physical.[32] Thirty percent of children who have been physically abused are seen by an orthopedist. Accurate and appropriate referrals to child protection agencies are not only legally mandated but also essential for the well-being of the child. An abused child who is returned to the same situation without intervention has a 10 to 15% chance of subsequent mortality.

Fractures in Nonaccidental Trauma

Children who are not yet ambulatory and present with a long bone fracture have more than a 75% chance of that fracture being caused by nonaccidental trauma (NAT).[33] "Corner" metaphyseal fractures are nearly always from abuse but occur only 25% of the time (Figure 40-16). Fractures at multiple stages of healing also suggest abuse; however, OI or other causes of systemic osteomalacia must be ruled out. The most common presentation is a transverse tibia fracture. After walking age, only 2% of long bone fractures are the result of NAT.[34]

EVALUATION NAT necessitates early consultation with child protective services. The child should undergo skeletal survey (especially if less than 2 years of age) and have a complete physical examination to evaluate for pattern bruising, burns, or multiple soft tissue injuries. A thorough history must be obtained for all identified injuries. It is important to remember that social isolation can lead to an increased likelihood of abuse, but no social status is immune. One study reported that racial differences may exist in the evaluation and reporting of NAT. Skeletal trauma is present in a significant number of abused children.[35-37]

When the cause of injury is unclear, bone scan can be helpful in diagnosing subtle injuries, especially rib fractures. Posterior rib fractures are especially likely to be the result of abuse. An MRI and a computed tomography (CT) scan of the brain to check for subdural hematoma and retinal examination to look for hemorrhages are essential.

TREATMENT The treating health care provider must have a nonjudgemental attitude. The child and family involved in NAT are emotionally delicate and require not only physical but also emotional care. Social workers need to be involved early to ensure that the child receives appropriate medical care. Fortunately, fractures tend to heal quickly for those in this age group. Neurological injury and social disease, however, are much more difficult to cure.

QUICK CHECK 40-4

1. Describe the incidence and types of child maltreatment or abuse.
2. What is the most common orthopedic injury in NAT?

DID YOU UNDERSTAND?

Congenital Defects

1. Clubfoot is a common deformity in which the foot is twisted out of its normal shape or position. Clubfoot can be positional, idiopathic, or teratological.
2. Developmental dysplasia of the hip (DDH) is an abnormality in the development of the femoral head, acetabulum, or both. Like clubfoot, DDH can be idiopathic or teratological. It is a serious and disabling condition in children if not diagnosed and treated early, with best outcomes when treated before walking age.
3. Osteogenesis imperfecta (brittle bone disease) is an inherited disorder of collagen that affects primarily bones and results in serious fractures of many bones.

Bone Infection

1. Osteomyelitis is a local or generalized bacterial or granulomatous (e.g., tuberculosis) infection of bone and bone marrow. Bacteria are usually introduced by direct extension from a nearby infection, through the bloodstream, or by trauma.
2. Septic arthritis can occur de novo or secondary to osteomyelitis in very young children in which the metaphysis is still located within the joint capsule of certain joints.

Juvenile Idiopathic Arthritis

1. Juvenile idiopathic arthritis is an inflammatory joint disorder characterized by pain and swelling. Large joints are most commonly affected.

Osteochondroses

1. Avascular diseases of the bone are collectively referred to as osteochondroses and are caused by an insufficient blood supply to growing bones.
2. Legg-Calvé-Perthes disease is one of the most common osteochondroses. This disorder is characterized by epiphyseal necrosis or degeneration of the head of the femur followed by regeneration or recalcification. Children older than 7 years of age at onset have a worse prognosis.
3. Osgood-Schlatter disease is characterized by tendonitis of the anterior patellar tendon and inflammation or partial separation of the tibial tubercle caused by chronic irritation, usually as a result of overuse of the quadriceps muscles. The condition is seen primarily in muscular, athletic adolescent males.

Scoliosis

1. Scoliosis is a rotational curvature of the spine most obvious in the anteroposterior plane, and can be classified as nonstructural or structural. Nonstructural scoliosis results from a cause other than the spine itself, such as posture, leg length discrepancy, or splinting from pain. Structural scoliosis is a curvature of the spine associated with vertebral rotation.

Muscular Dystrophy

1. The muscular dystrophies are a group of genetically transmitted diseases characterized by progressive atrophy of skeletal muscles. There is an insidious loss of strength in all forms of the disorder with increasing disability and deformity. The most common type in childhood is Duchenne muscular dystrophy.

Musculo-skeletal Tumours

1. The two most common forms of benign bone tumours are osteochondroma and nonossifying fibroma.
2. The two main types of malignant childhood bone tumours are osteosarcoma and Ewing sarcoma.
3. Osteosarcoma, the most common malignant childhood bone tumour, originates in bone-producing mesenchymal cells and is most often located near active growth plates, such as the distal femur, proximal tibia, or proximal humerus.
4. Most children with osteosarcoma are diagnosed between 15 and 19 years of age, and osteosarcoma occurs equally in males and females.
5. Ewing sarcoma originates from cells within the bone marrow space and is most often located in the midshaft of long bones or in flat bones. The most common sites include the femur, pelvis, and humerus.
6. Ewing sarcoma is more common in males and is diagnosed most often between the ages of 5 and 15 years.
7. Pain is the usual presenting symptom for either osteosarcoma or Ewing sarcoma.
8. The primary treatments for osteosarcoma are surgery and chemotherapy. The primary treatment for Ewing sarcoma is a combination of chemotherapy, radiation, and surgery.

Nonaccidental Trauma

1. Nonaccidental trauma (NAT) must be considered with any long bone injury in the preambulatory child.
2. The presence of soft tissue injury, corner fractures, and multiple fractures at different stages of healing is extremely helpful for making a diagnosis of NAT.
3. When NAT is suspected, a child must be evaluated radiographically for other fractures, heat trauma, and retinal hemorrhage.
4. All social strata are at risk.
5. The health care provider is legally responsible to report suspected NAT.

KEY TERMS

Acetabular dysplasia, 1060
Acute hematogenous osteomyelitis, 1062
Antalgic (painful) abductor lurch, 1065
Becker muscular dystrophy (BMD), 1068
Clubfoot, 1059
Congenital equinovarus, 1059
Developmental dysplasia of the hip (DDH), 1059
Dislocated hip, 1060
Duchenne muscular dystrophy (DMD), 1067
Dystrophin, 1067
Ewing sarcoma, 1070
Facioscapulohumeral muscular dystrophy (FSHD), 1068
Hereditary multiple exostoses (HME), 1069
Involucrum, 1062
Juvenile idiopathic arthritis (JIA), 1064
Legg-Calvé-Perthes (LCP) disease, 1065
Malignant bone tumour, 1069
Muscular dystrophy, 1067
Myotonic muscular dystrophy (MMD), 1068
Nonossifying fibroma, 1069
Nonstructural scoliosis, 1066
Oligoarthritis, 1064
Osgood-Schlatter disease, 1065
Osteochondroma, 1069
Osteochondrosis, 1065
Osteogenesis imperfecta (OI; brittle bone disease), 1060
Osteomyelitis, 1062
Osteosarcoma, 1070
Polyarthritis, 1064
Scoliosis, 1066
Septic arthritis, 1063
Still disease, 1064
Structural scoliosis, 1066
Subluxated hip, 1060

REFERENCES

1. Morcuende, J. A., Weinstein, S. L., Dietz, F. R., et al. (1994). Plaster cast treatment of clubfoot: The Ponseti method of manipulation and casting. *Journal of Pediatric Orthopedics*, *3*(2), 161–167.
2. Janicki, J. A., Narayanan, U. G., Harvey, B., et al. (2009). Treatment of neuromuscular and syndrome-associated (nonidiopathic) clubfeet using the Ponseti method. *Journal of Pediatric Orthopedics*, *29*(4), 393–397. doi:10.1097/BPO.0b013e3181a6bf77.
3. Woolacott, N. F., Puhan, M. A., Steurer, J., et al. (2005). Ultrasonography in screening for developmental dysplasia of the hip in newborns: Systematic review. *British Medical Journal*, *330*(7505), 1413. doi:10.1136/bmj.38450.646088.E0.
4. Le Ba, T. B., Carmichael, K. D., Patton, A. G., et al. (2015). Ultrasound for infants at risk for developmental dysplasia of the hip. *Orthopedics*, *38*(8), e722–e726. doi:10.3928/01477447-20150804-61.
5. Jari, S., Paton, R. W., & Srinivasan, M. S. (2002). Unilateral limitation of abduction of the hip: A valuable clinical sign for DDH? *The Journal of Bone and Joint Surgery: British Volume*, *84*(1), 104–107.
6. Holman, J., Carroll, K. L., Murray, K. A., et al. (2012). Long term follow-up of open reduction surgery for developmental dysplasia of the hip. *Journal of Pediatric Orthopedics*, *32*(2), 121–124. doi:10.1097/BPO.0b013e3182471aad.
7. Glorieux, F. H., Bishop, N. J., Plotkin, H., et al. (1998). Cyclic administration of pamidronate in children with severe osteogenesis imperfecta. *The New England Journal of Medicine*, *339*(14), 947–952. doi:10.1056/NEJM199810013391402.
8. Poyrazoglu, S., Gunoz, H., Darendeliler, F., et al. (2008). Successful results of pamidronate treatment in children with osteogenesis imperfecta with emphasis on interpretation of bone mineral density for local standards. *Journal of Pediatric Orthopedics*, *28*(4), 483–487. doi:10.1097/BPO.0b013e318173a923.
9. Dwan, K., Phillipi, C. A., Steiner, R. D., et al. (2014). Bisphosphonate therapy for osteogensis imperfecta. *The Cochrane Database of Systematic Reviews*, (7), CD005008, pub 3, doi:10.1002/14651858.CD005088. pub3..
10. Vader Have, K. L., Karmazyn, B., Verma, M., et al. (2009). Community-associated methicillin-resistant *Staphylococcus aureus* in acute musculoskeletal infection in children: A game changer. *Journal of Pediatric Orthopedics*, *29*(8), 927–931. doi:10.1097/BPO.0b013e3181bd1e0c.
11. Caird, M. S., Flynn, J. M., Leung, Y. L., et al. (2006). Factors distinguishing septic arthritis from transient synovitis of the hip in children. A prospective study. *The Journal of Bone and Joint Surgery: American Volume*, *88*(6), 1251–1257. doi:10.2106/JBJS.E.00216.
12. Kocher, M. S., Zurakowski, D., & Kasser, J. R. (1999). Differentiating between septic arthritis and transient synovitis of the hip in children: An evidence-based clinical prediction algorithm. *The Journal of Bone and Joint Surgery: American Volume*, *81*(12), 1662–1670.
13. Principi, N., & Esposito, S. (2015). Kingella kingae infections in children. *BMC Infectious Diseases*, *15*, 260. doi:10.1186/s12879-015-0986-9.
14. Hresko, M. T., McDougall, P. A., Gorlin, J. B., et al. (2002). Prospective reevaluation of the association between thrombotic diathesis and Legg-Perthes disease. *The Journal of Bone and Joint Surgery: American Volume*, *84-A*(9), 1613–1618.
15. Vosmaer, A., Pereira, R. R., Koenderman, J. S., et al. (2010). Coagulation abnormalities in Legg-Calvé-Perthes disease. *The Journal of Bone and Joint Surgery: American Volume*, *92*(1), 121–128. doi:10.2106/JBJS.I.00157.
16. Garcia Mata, S., Ardanaz Aicua, E., Hidalgo Overjero, A., et al. (2000). Legg-Calvé-Perthes disease and passive smoking. *Journal of Pediatric Orthopedics*, *20*(3), 326–330.
17. Daniel, A. B., Shah, H., Kamath, A., et al. (2012). Environmental tobacco and wood smoke increase the risk of Legg-Calvé-Perthes disease. *Clinical Orthopaedics and Related Research*, *470*(9), 2369–2375. doi:10.1007/s11999-011-2180-8.
18. McCullough, L., & Lyman, K. S. (1998). Musculoskeletal considerations across the life span. In S. J. Gates & P. A. Mooar (Eds.), *Musculoskeletal primary care*. Philadelphia: Lippincott.
19. Morrissy, R., & Weinstein, S. (Eds.), (1996). *Lovell and Winter's pediatric orthopaedics* (4th ed.). Philadelphia: Lippincott-Raven.
20. Jorde, L. B., Carey, J. C., Bamshad, M. J., et al. (2006). *Medical genetics* (3rd ed.). St. Louis: Mosby.
21. Cassas, K. J., & Cassettari-Wayhs, A. (2006). Childhood and adolescent sports-related overuse injuries. *American Family Physician*, *73*(6), 1014–1022.
22. Kaeding, C. C., & Whitehead, R. (1998). Musculoskeletal injuries in adolescents. *Primary Care*, *25*(1), 211–223.
23. Davids, J. R., Chamberlin, E., & Blackhurst, D. W. (2004). Indications for magnetic resonance imaging in presumed adolescent idiopathic scoliosis. *The Journal of Bone and Joint Surgery: American Volume*, *86-A*(10), 2187–2195.
24. Katz, D. E., Herring, J. A., Browne, R. H., et al. (2010). Brace wear control of curve progression in adolescent idiopathic scoliosis. *The Journal of Bone and Joint Surgery: American Volume*, *92*(6), 1343–1352. doi:10.2106/JBJS.I.01142.
25. Weinstein, S. L., Dolan, L. A., Wright, J. G., et al. (2013). Effects of bracing in adolescents with idiopathic scoliosis. *The New England Journal of Medicine*, *369*(16), 1512–1521. doi:10.1056/NEJMoa1307337.
26. Moxley, R. T., III, Ashwal, S., Pandya, S., et al. (2005). Practice parameter: Corticosteroid treatment of Duchenne dystrophy: Report of the Quality Standards Subcommittee of the American Academy of Neurology and the Practice Committee of the Child Neurology Society. *Neurology*, *64*(1), 13–20. doi:10.1212/01.WNL.0000148485.00049.B7.
27. Weeks, C. (2017, February 24). Without rare-disease policy, patients in Canada face steep costs for drugs. *The Globe and Mail*. Retrieved from https://beta.theglobeandmail.com/life/health-and-fitness/health/without-rare-disease-policy-patients-in-canada-face-steep-costs-for-drugs-health/article34129051/?ref=http://www.theglobeandmail.com&.
28. McAdam, L. C., Mayo, A. L., Alman, B. A., et al. (2012). The Canadian experience of long term deflazacort treatment in Duchenne muscular dystrophy. *Acta Myologica*, *31*(1), 16–20.
29. Cummings, R. J., Davidson, R. S., Armstrong, P. F., et al. (2002). Congenital clubfoot. *Instructional Course Lectures*, *51*, 385–400.
30. Hayden, J. B., & Hoang, B. H. (2006). Osteosarcoma: Basic science and clinical implications. *The Orthopedic Clinics of North America*, *37*(1), 1–7. doi:10.1016/j.ocl.2005.06.004.
31. Affifi, T. O., McMillan, H. O., Boyle, M., et al. (2014). Child abuse and mental disorders in Canada. *Canadian Medical Association Journal*, *186*(7), E324–E332. doi:10.1503/cmaj.131792.
32. Administration for Children and Families Children's Bureau. (2010). *Child maltreatment 2009*. Washington, DC: U.S. Department of Health and Human Services. Retrieved from http://www.acf.hhs.gov/programs/cb/stats_research/index.htm#can.
33. Rex, C., & Kay, P. R. (2000). Features of femoral fractures in nonaccidental injury. *Journal of Pediatric Orthopedics*, *20*(3), 411–413.
34. Thomas, S. A., Rosenfield, N. S., Leventhal, J. M., et al. (1991). Long-bone fractures in young children: Distinguishing accident injuries from child abuse. *Pediatrics*, *88*(3), 471–476.
35. Lane, W. G., Rubin, D. M., Monteith, R., et al. (2002). Racial differences in the evaluation of pediatric fractures for physical abuse. *The Journal of the American Medical Association*, *288*(13), 1603–1609.
36. Swoboda, S. L., & Feldman, K. W. (2013). Skeletal trauma in child abuse. *Pediatric Annals*, *42*(11), e236–e243. doi:10.3928/00904481-20131022-11.
37. Wood, J. N., French, B., Song, L., et al. (2015). Evaluation for occult fractures in injured children. *Pediatrics*, *136*(2), 232–240. doi:10.1542/peds.2014-3977.

41

Structure, Function, and Disorders of the Integument

Sue Ann McCann, Noreen Heer Nicol, Sue E. Huether, and Stephanie Zettel

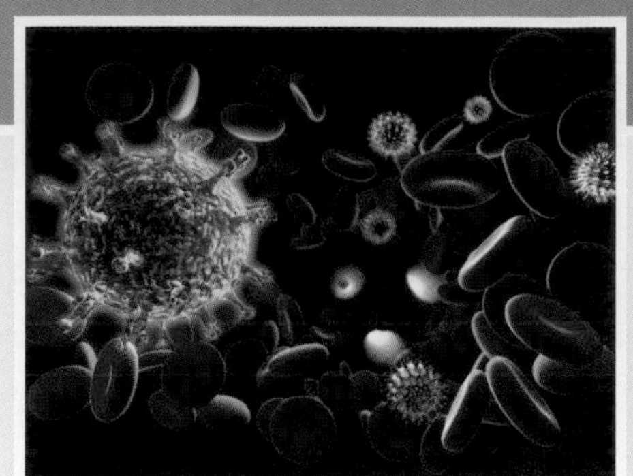

EVOLVE WEBSITE

http://evolve.elsevier.com/Canada/Huether/pathophysiology
Student Review Questions
Key Points
Case Studies
Animations
Quick Check Answers

CHAPTER OUTLINE

Structure and Function of the Skin, 1074
Layers of the Skin, 1074
Clinical Manifestations of Skin Dysfunction, 1076
Disorders of the Skin, 1081
Inflammatory Disorders, 1081
Papulosquamous Disorders, 1083
Vesiculobullous Diseases, 1085
Infections, 1087
Vascular Disorders, 1089
Benign Tumours, 1091
Skin Cancer, 1091
Burns, 1095
Cold Injury, 1099
Disorders of the Hair, 1101
Alopecia, 1101
Hirsutism, 1101
Disorders of the Nail, 1101
Paronychia, 1101
Onychomycosis, 1101
GERIATRIC CONSIDERATIONS: **Aging and Changes in Skin Integrity, 1102**

The skin covers the entire body and is the largest organ of the body, accounting for about 20% of body weight. Combined with the accessory structures of hair, nails, and glands, it forms the integumentary system. The skin's primary function is protection from the environment by serving as a barrier against microorganisms, ultraviolet radiation (UVR), loss of body fluids, and the stress of mechanical forces. The skin regulates body temperature and is involved in immune surveillance and the activation of vitamin D. Touch and pressure receptors provide important protective functions and pleasurable sensations. The commensal (normal) microorganisms of the skin protect against pathological bacteria.

STRUCTURE AND FUNCTION OF THE SKIN

Layers of the Skin

The skin is formed of two major layers: (1) a superficial or outer layer of **epidermis** and (2) a deeper layer of **dermis** (the true skin) (Figure 41-1). The **subcutaneous layer (hypodermis)**, the lowest-lying layer of connective tissue, contains macrophages, fibroblasts, fat cells, nerves, fine muscles, blood vessels, lymphatics, and hair follicle roots. Each skin layer contains cells that represent progressive stages of skin cell differentiation and function as the skin grows. These are summarized in Table 41-1.

Dermal Appendages

The **dermal appendages** include the nails, hair, sebaceous glands, and the eccrine and apocrine sweat glands. The **nails** are protective keratinized plates that appear at the ends of fingers and toes. They have the following structures: (1) the proximal nail fold, (2) the eponychium (cuticle), (3) the matrix from which the nail grows and its nail root, (4) the hyponychium (nail bed), (5) the nail plate, and (6) the paronychium (lateral nail fold) (Figure 41-2). Nail growth continues throughout life at 1 mm or less per day.

Hair colour, density, grain, and pattern of distribution vary considerably among people and depend on age, sex, and ethnicity. Hair follicles arise from the matrix (or bulb) located deep in the dermis. They extend from the dermis at an angle and have an erector pili muscle attached near the mid-dermis that straightens the follicle when contracted, causing the hair to stand up. Hair growth begins in the bulb, with cellular differentiation occurring as the hair progresses up the follicle. Hair is fully hardened, or cornified, by the time it emerges at the skin surface. Hair colour is determined by melanin-secreting follicular melanocytes. Hair growth is cyclic, with periods of growth and rest that vary over different body surfaces.

The **sebaceous glands** open onto the surface of the skin through a canal. They are found in greatest numbers on the face, chest, and back, with modified glands on the eyelids, lips, nipples, glans penis, and prepuce. Sebaceous glands secrete sebum, composed primarily of lipids, which oils the skin and hair and prevents drying. Androgens stimulate the growth of sebaceous glands, and their enlargement is an early sign of puberty.

The **eccrine sweat glands** are distributed over the body, with the greatest numbers in the palms of the hands, soles of the feet, and forehead.

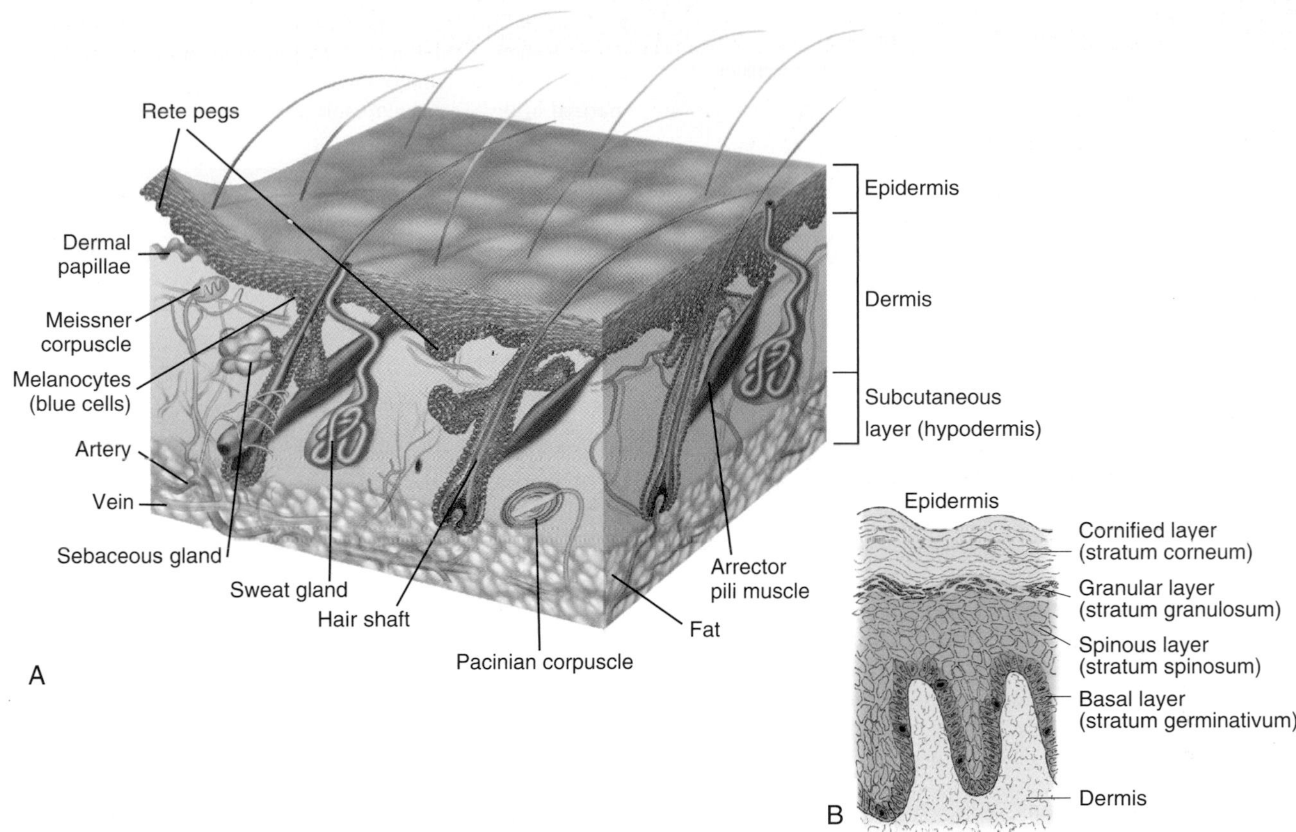

FIGURE 41-1 Structure of the Skin. A, Cross-section showing major skin structures. **B,** Layers of the epidermis. (**A,** from Kumar, V., Abbas, A.K., & Aster, J.C. [Eds.]. [2015]. *Robbins and Cotran pathologic basis of disease* [9th ed.]. Philadelphia: Saunders; **B,** from Baker, S.R. [2007]. *Local flaps in facial reconstruction* [3rd ed.]. Philadelphia: Saunders.)

TABLE 41-1 **Layers of the Skin**

Structure	Cell Types	Characteristics
Epidermis	Keratinocytes	Most important layer of skin; normally very thin (0.12 mm) but can thicken and form corns or calluses with constant pressure or friction; includes rete pegs that extend into papillary layer of dermis
	Langerhans cells	Cells with dendrite process and immune functions
Stratum corneum	Keratinocytes	Tough superficial layer covering body
Stratum lucidum	Keratinocytes	Clear layers of cells containing eleidin, which becomes keratin as cells move up to corneum layer
Stratum granulosum	Keratinocytes Melanocytes	Keratohyalin gives granular appearance to this layer
Stratum spinosum	New keratinocytes	Polygonal shaped with spinous processes projecting between adjacent keratinocytes
Stratum basale (germinativum)	Keratinocytes	Basal layer where keratinocytes divide and move upward to replace cells shed from surface
	Melanocytes	Melanocytes synthesize pigment melanin
	Merkel cells	Function of Merkel cells is not clearly known; they are associated with sensory nerve endings
Dermis Papillary layer (thin)	Macrophages Mast cells	Irregular connective tissue layer with rich blood, lymphatic, and nerve supply; contains sensory receptors and sweat glands (apocrine, eccrine, sebaceous), macrophages (phagocytic and important for wound healing), and mast cells (release histamine and have immune functions) (see Chapter 6)
Reticular layer (thick)	Histiocytes	Histiocytes are wandering macrophages that collect pigments and inflammatory debris
Subcutaneous Layer (Hypodermis)		Subcutaneous tissue or superficial fascia of varying thickness that connects overlying dermis to underlying muscle; contains macrophages, fibroblasts, fat cells, nerves, blood vessels, lymphatics, and hair follicle roots

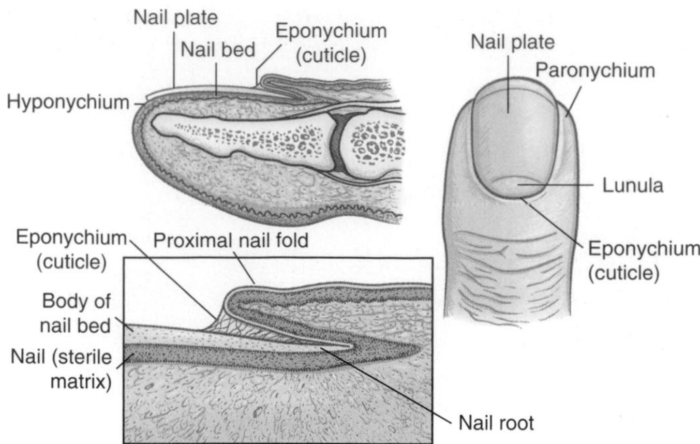

FIGURE 41-2 Structures of the Nail. (Redrawn from Thompson, J.M., McFarland, G.K., Hirsch, J.E., et al. [2002]. *Mosby's clinical nursing* [5th ed.]. St. Louis: Mosby.)

They open onto the surface of the skin and are important in thermoregulation and cooling of the body through evaporation. The **apocrine sweat glands** are fewer in number but produce significantly more sweat than the eccrine glands. They are located near the bulb of hair follicles in the axillae, scalp, face, abdomen, and genital area. Their ducts open into the hair follicle. The interaction of sweat with commensal (normal) flora bacteria contributes to the odour of perspiration.

Blood Supply and Innervation

The blood supply to the skin is limited to the **papillary capillaries**, or plexus, of the dermis. These capillary loops are supplied by a deeper arterial plexus. Branches from the deep plexus also supply hair follicles and sweat glands. A subpapillary network of veins drains the capillary loops. Arteriovenous anastomoses in the dermis facilitate the regulation of body temperature. Heat loss is regulated by (1) variations in skin blood flow through the opening and closing of arteriovenous anastomoses and (2) the evaporative heat loss of sweat. The sympathetic nervous system regulates both vasoconstriction and vasodilation through α-adrenergic receptors in the skin. The lymphatic vessels of the skin arise in the papillary dermis and drain into larger subcutaneous trunks, removing cells, proteins, and immunological mediators.

The structure and function of the skin change with advancing age. A summary of aging changes is included in the box titled *Geriatric Considerations:* Aging and Changes in Skin Integrity (p. 1100).

QUICK CHECK 41-1

1. Describe the two layers of the skin.
2. How do the skin blood vessels and sweat glands regulate body temperature?
3. What are some changes that occur in skin with aging?

Clinical Manifestations of Skin Dysfunction

Lesions

Identification of the morphological structure of the skin, including differentiation between primary and secondary lesions, and assessment of the appearance of the skin in combination with obtaining a health history are essential to identify underlying pathophysiology. Tables 41-2 and 41-3 describe and illustrate the basic lesions of the skin. Clinical manifestations of select skin lesions are described in Table 41-4.

Pressure ulcers. **Pressure ulcers** (sometimes called *pressure sores*) are ischemic ulcers resulting from unrelieved pressure, shearing forces, friction, and moisture. The term *decubitus ulcer* refers to ulcers that develop when unrelieved pressure interrupts normal blood flow to the skin and its underlying tissues. The risks for pressure ulcers are summarized in *Risk Factors:* Pressure Ulcer.[1]

RISK FACTORS

Pressure Ulcer

External Factors

- Prolonged pressure
- Immobilization
- Lying in bed or sitting in chair or wheelchair without changing position or relieving pressure over an extended period
- Lying for hours on hard X-ray, emergency department, and operating room tables
- Prolonged moisture exposure
- Neurological disorders (coma, spinal cord injuries, cognitive impairment, or cerebrovascular disease)
- Fractures or contractures
- Debilitation: older adults in hospitals and nursing homes
- Pain
- Sedation
- Friction and shearing forces
- Coarse bed sheets used for turning by dragging, which produces friction and a shearing force
- Inadequate caretaking staff
- Lack of communication and education regarding pressure ulcer care

Disease and Tissue Factors

- Impaired perfusion; ischemia
- Fecal or urinary incontinence; prolonged exposure to moisture
- Malnutrition, dehydration
- Chronic diseases accompanied by anemia, edema, kidney failure, malnutrition, peripheral vascular disease, or sepsis
- Previous history of pressure ulcers
- Thin skin associated with aging or prolonged use of steroids

Data from Bogie, K., Powell, H.L., & Ho, C. (2012). *Handb Clin Neurol, 109*, 235–246; Coleman, S., Gorecki, C., Nelson, E.A., et al. (2013). *Int J Nurs Stud, 50*(7), 974–1003; García-Fernández, F.P., Agreda, J.J., Verdú, J., et al. (2014). *J Nurs Scholarsh, 46*(1), 28–38; Michel, J.M., Willebois, S., Ribinik, P., et al. (2012). *Ann Phys Rehabil Med, 55*(7), 454–465.

Pressure ulcers usually develop over bony prominences, such as the sacrum, heels, ischia, and greater trochanters. Continuous pressure on tissue between the bony prominence and a resistant outside surface distorts capillaries and occludes the blood supply. Pressure ulcers also can occur in soft tissues from unrelieved pressure, for example, from nasal cannulas or endotracheal tubes. If the pressure is relieved within a few hours, a brief period of reactive hyperemia (redness) occurs and there may be no lasting tissue damage. If the pressure continues unrelieved, the endothelial cells lining the capillaries become disrupted with platelet aggregation, forming microthrombi that block blood flow and cause anoxic necrosis of surrounding tissues (Figure 41-3). Shearing and friction are mechanical forces moving parallel to the skin (dragging) and can extend to the bony skeleton, causing detachment and injury of tissues. Pressure ulcers are staged or graded, and one classification scheme is as follows:[2]

Stage 1—Nonblanchable erythema of intact skin, usually over a bony prominence; darkly pigmented skin may not have visible blanching

Text continued on p. 1081

TABLE 41-2 Primary Skin Lesions

Macule

A flat, circumscribed area that is a change in colour of skin; less than 1 cm in diameter

Examples: Freckles, flat moles (nevi), petechiae, measles, scarlet fever

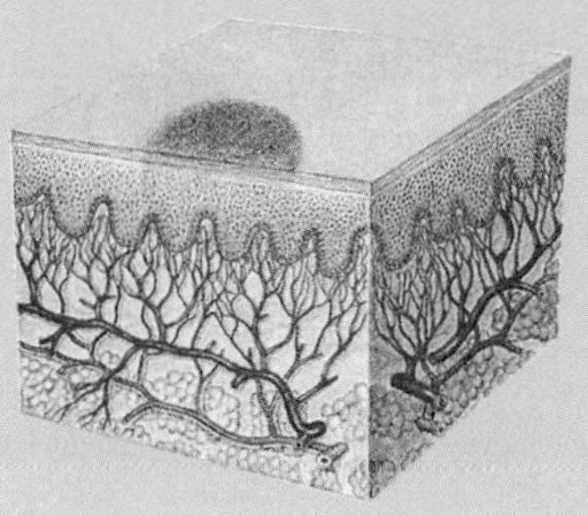

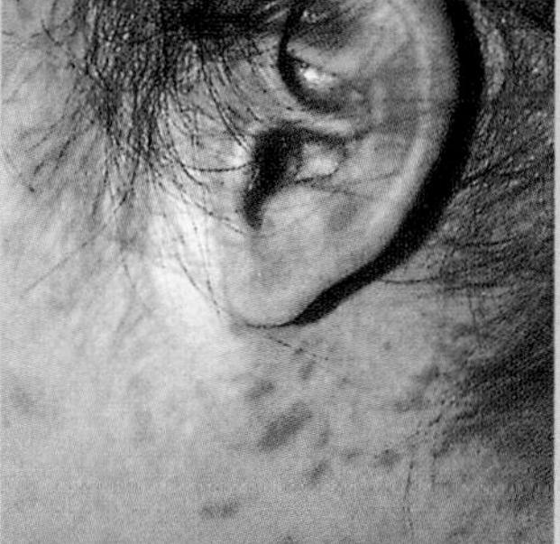

Macules[a]

Papule

An elevated, firm, circumscribed area less than 1 cm in diameter

Examples: Wart (verruca), elevated moles, lichen planus, fibroma, insect bite

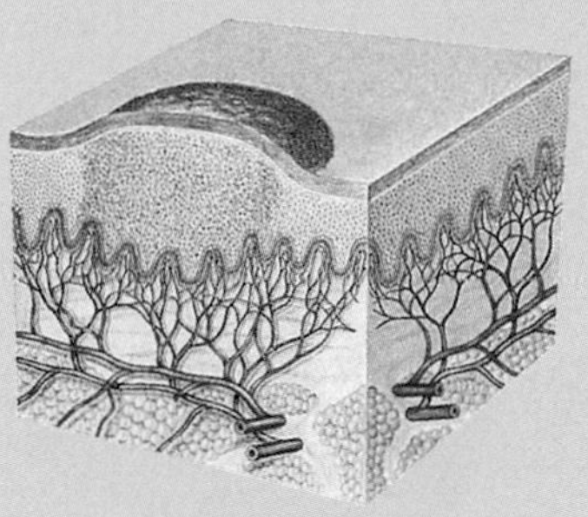

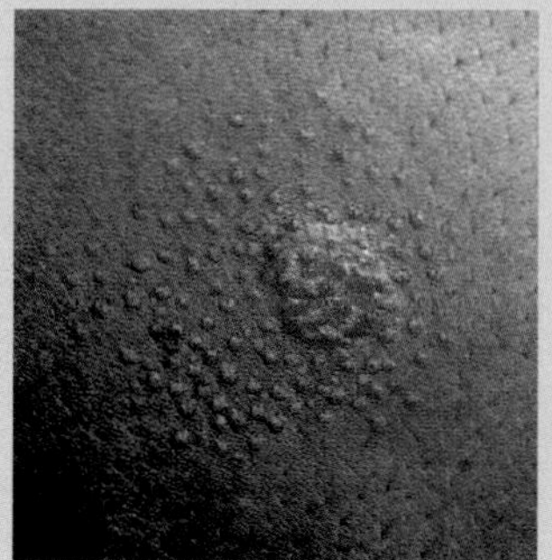

Lichen planus[b]

Patch

A flat, nonpalpable, irregular-shaped macule more than 1 cm in diameter

Examples: Vitiligo, port-wine stains, mongolian spots, café-au-lait spots

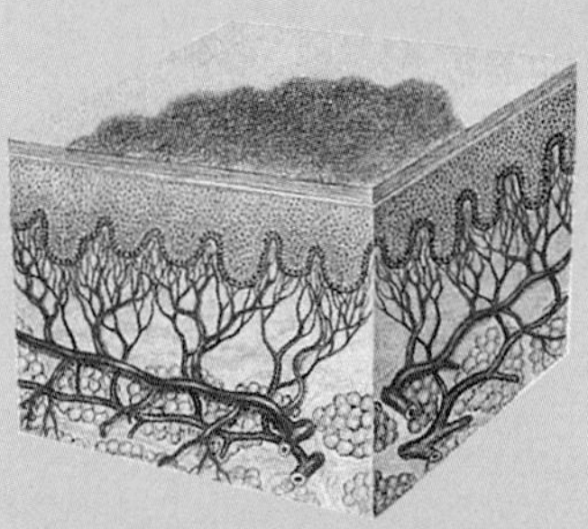

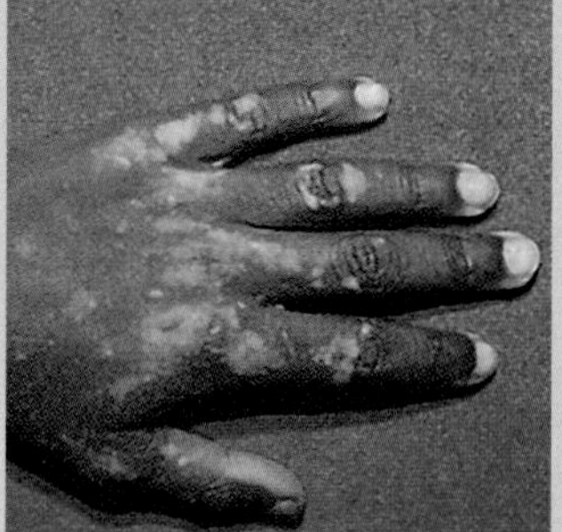

Vitiligo[c]

Plaque

Elevated, firm, and rough lesion with flat top surface greater than 1 cm in diameter

Examples: Psoriasis, seborrheic and actinic keratoses

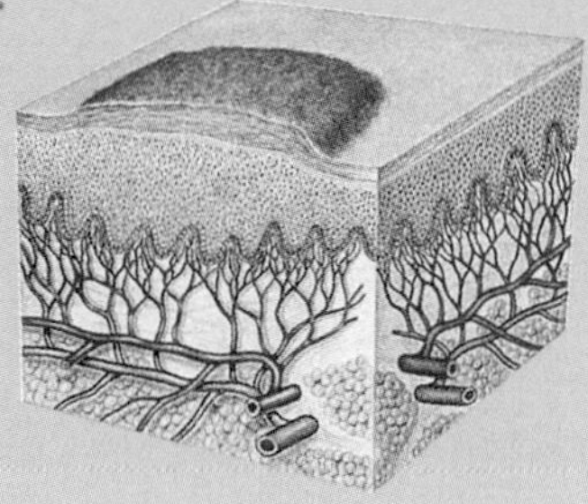

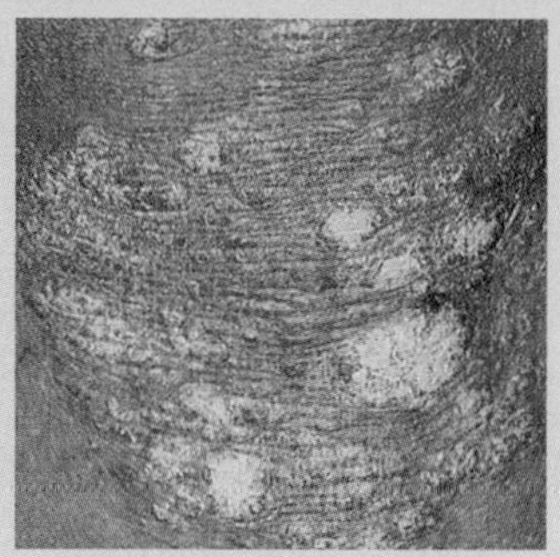

Plaque[d]

Wheal

Elevated, irregular-shaped area of cutaneous edema; solid, transient; variable diameter

Examples: Insect bites, urticaria, allergic reaction

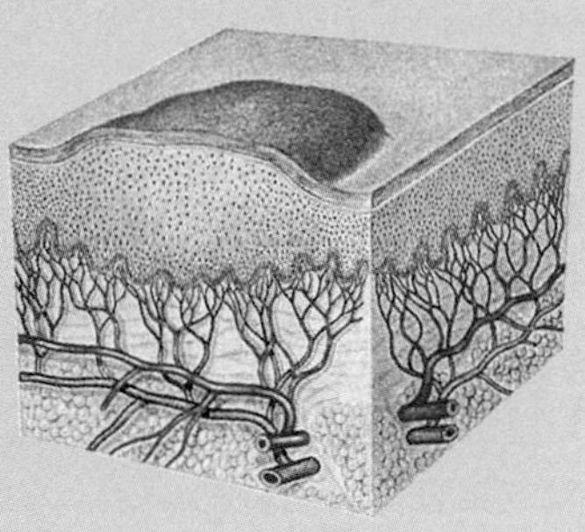

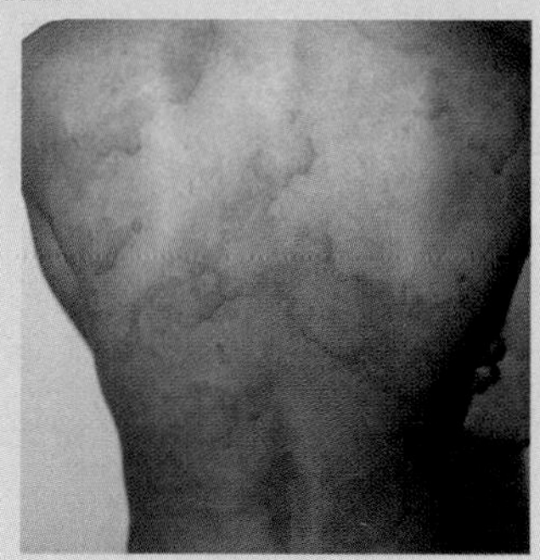

Wheal[e]

Nodule

Elevated, firm, circumscribed lesion; deeper in dermis than a papule; 1–2 cm in diameter

Examples: Erythema nodosum, lipomas

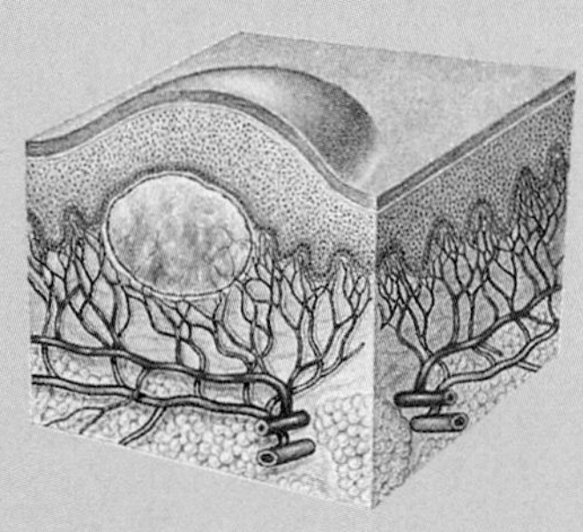

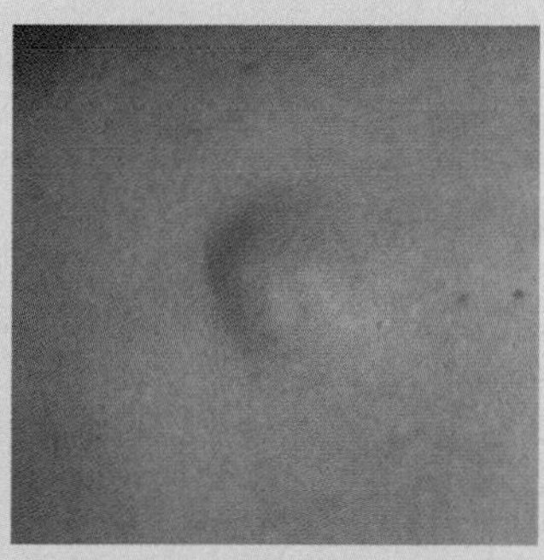

Lipoma[f]

Continued

TABLE 41-2 Primary Skin Lesions—cont'd

Tumour

Elevated, solid lesion; may be clearly demarcated; deeper in dermis; more than 2 cm in diameter

Examples: Neoplasms, benign tumour, lipoma, neurofibroma, hemangioma

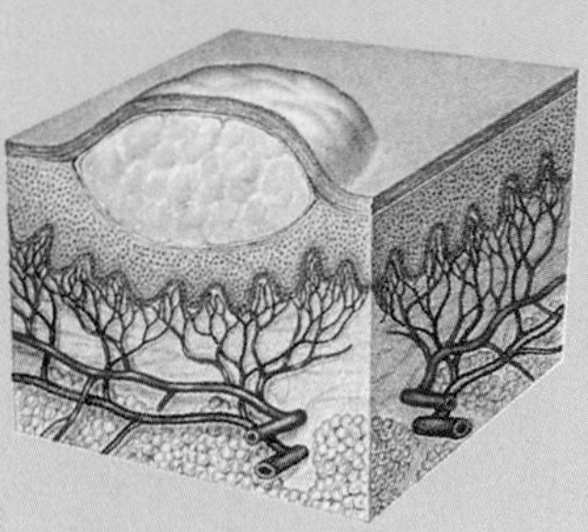

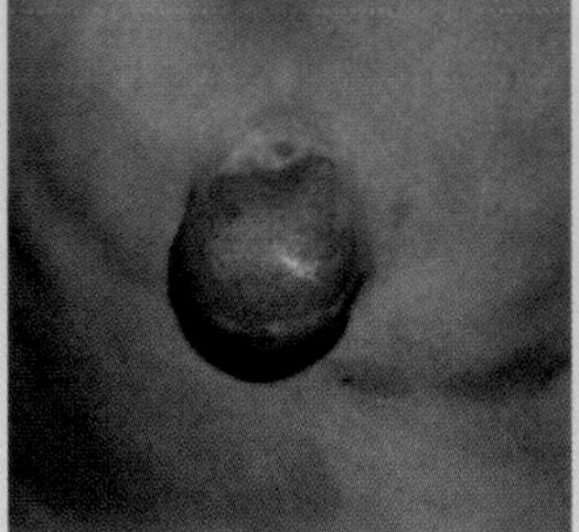

Neurofibroma[f]

Vesicle

Elevated, circumscribed, superficial; does not extend into dermis; filled with serous fluid; less than 1 cm in diameter

Examples: Varicella (chickenpox), herpes zoster (shingles), herpes simplex

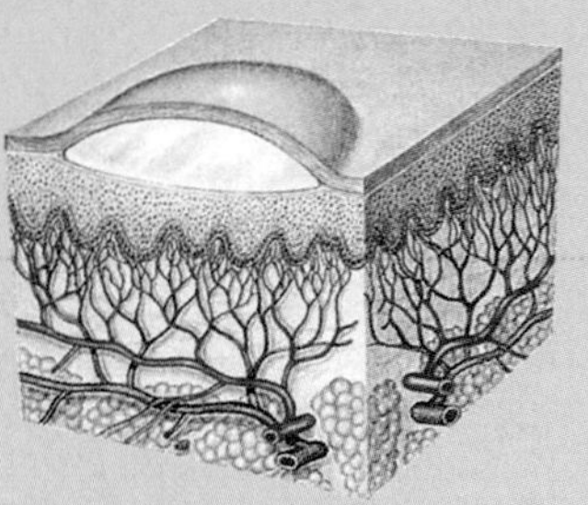

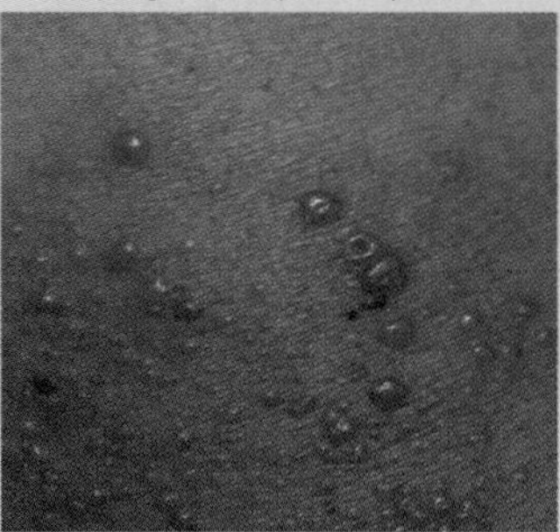

Vesicles[g]

Bulla

Vesicle more than 1 cm in diameter

Examples: Blister, pemphigus vulgaris

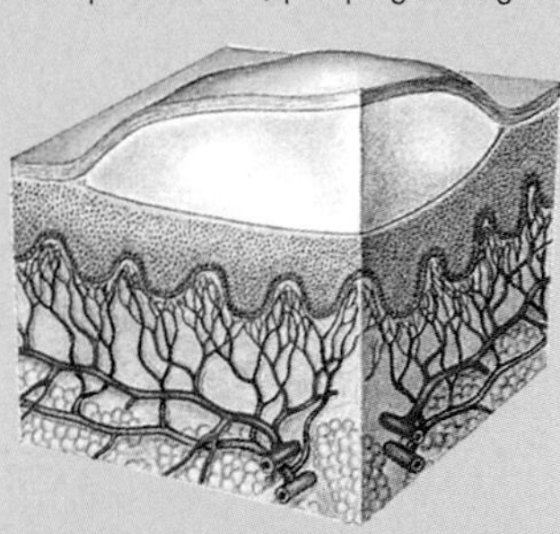

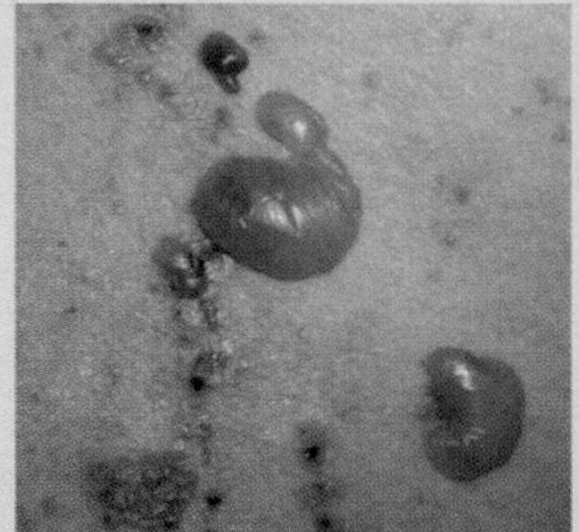

Bulla[h]

Pustule

Elevated, superficial lesion; similar to a vesicle but filled with purulent fluid

Examples: Impetigo, acne

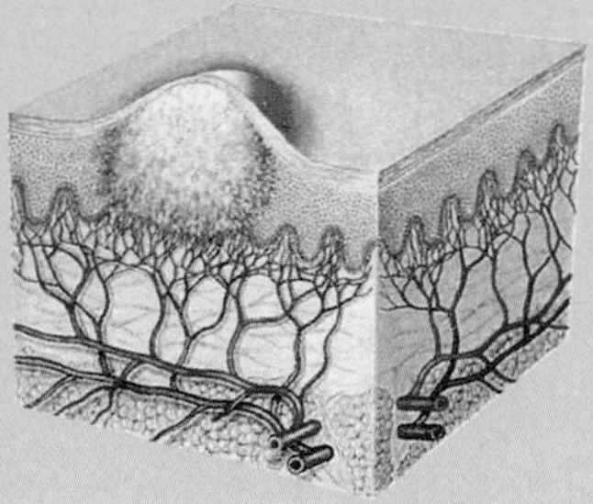

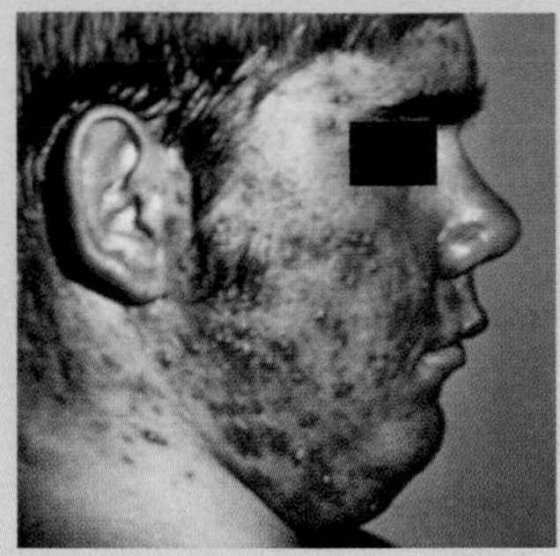

Acne[c]

Cyst

Elevated, circumscribed, encapsulated lesion; in dermis or subcutaneous layer; filled with liquid or semisolid material

Examples: Sebaceous cyst, cystic acne

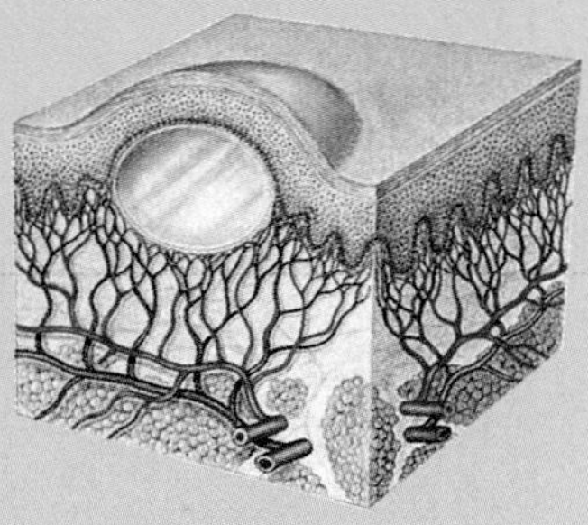

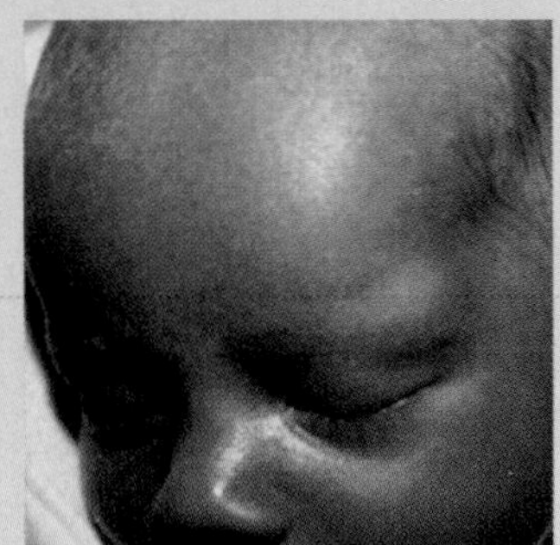

Sebaceous cyst[c]

Telangiectasia

Fine (0.5–1.0 mm), irregular red lines produced by capillary dilation; can be associated with acne rosacea (face), venous hypertension (spider veins in legs), systemic sclerosis, or developmental abnormalities (port-wine birthmarks)

Example: Telangiectasia in rosacea

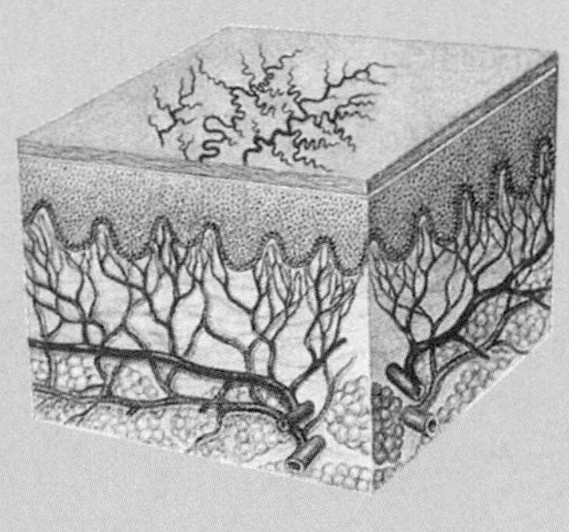

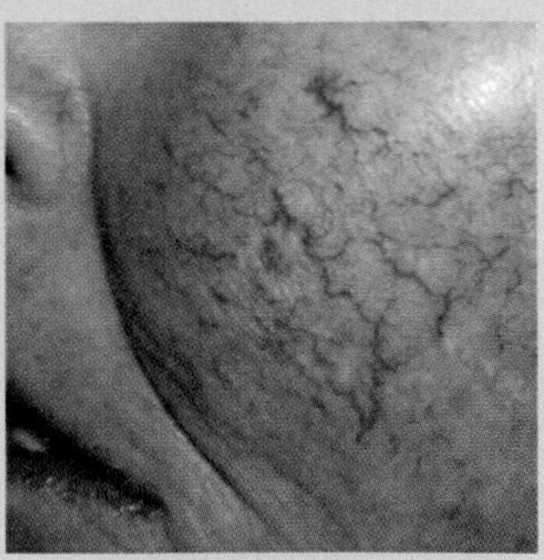

Telangiectasia[e]

[a]Farrar, W.E., Wood, M.J., Innes, J.A., et al. (1992). *Infectious diseases* (2nd ed.). London: Gower.
[b]James, W.D., Berger, T.G., & Elston, D.M. (2011). *Andrews' diseases of the skin* (11th ed.). Philadelphia: Saunders.
[c]Weston, W.L., & Lane, A.T. (2002). *Color textbook of pediatric dermatology* (3rd ed.). Philadelphia: Mosby.
[d]Habif, T.P. (2010). *Clinical dermatology: A color guide to diagnosis and therapy* (5th ed.). Philadelphia: Mosby.
[e]Bolognia, J.L., Jorizzo, J., & Schaffer, J. (2012). *Dermatology* (3rd ed.). Philadelphia: Saunders.
[f]Weston, W.L., Lane, A.T., & Morelli, J.G. (2007). *Color textbook of pediatric dermatology* (4th ed.). St. Louis: Mosby.
[g]Black, M.M., Ambros-Rudolph, C., Edwards, L., et al. (2008). *Obstetric and gynecologic dermatology* (3rd ed.). Philadelphia: Mosby.
[h]Marks, J.G., & Miller, J.J. (2006). *Lookingbill & Marks' principles of dermatology* (4th ed.). London: Saunders.

TABLE 41-3 Secondary Skin Lesions

Scale

Heaped-up, keratinized cells; flaky skin; irregular shape; thick or thin; dry or oily; variation in size

Examples: Flaking of skin with seborrheic dermatitis following scarlet fever, or flaking of skin following a medication reaction; dry skin

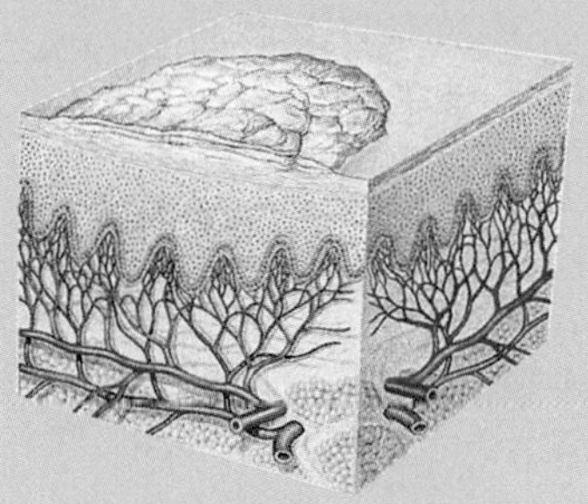
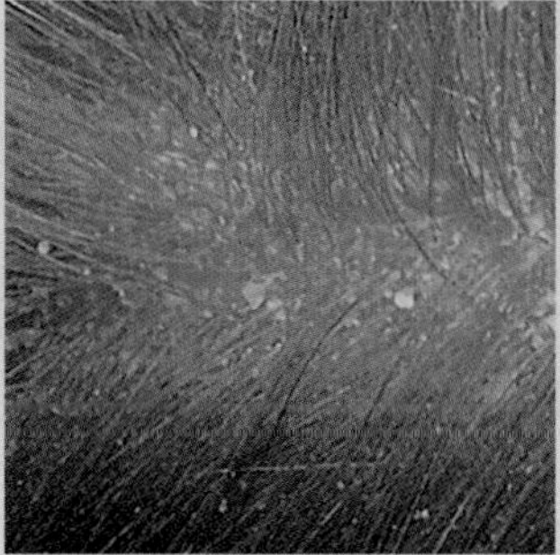

Fine scaling[a]

Lichenification

Rough, thickened epidermis secondary to persistent rubbing, itching, or skin irritation; often involves flexor surface of extremity

Example: Chronic dermatitis

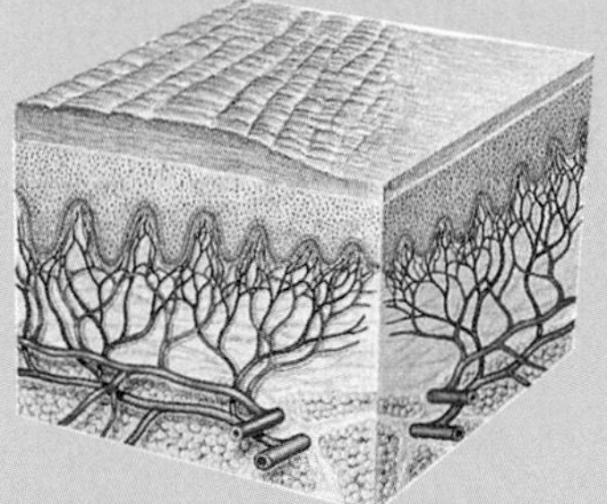
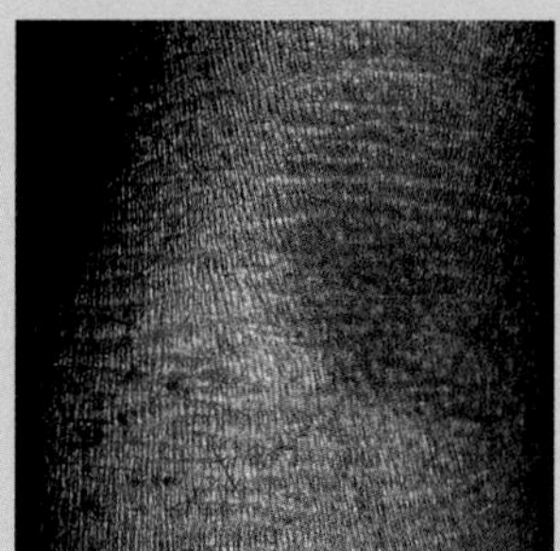

Atopic dermatitis of arm[b]

Keloid

Irregular-shaped, elevated, progressively enlarging scar; grows beyond boundaries of wound; caused by excessive collagen formation during healing

Examples: Keloid formation following surgery

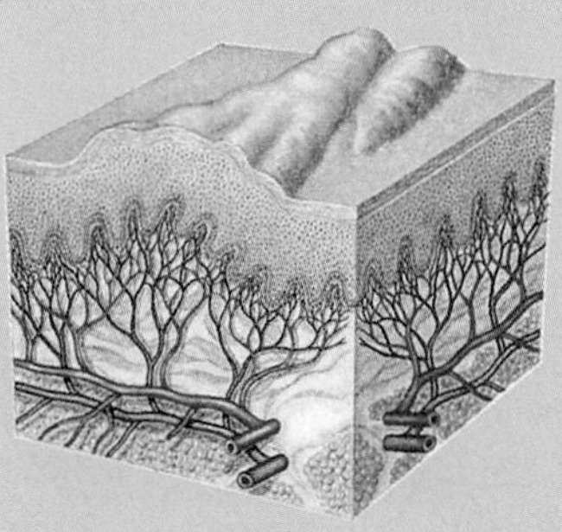
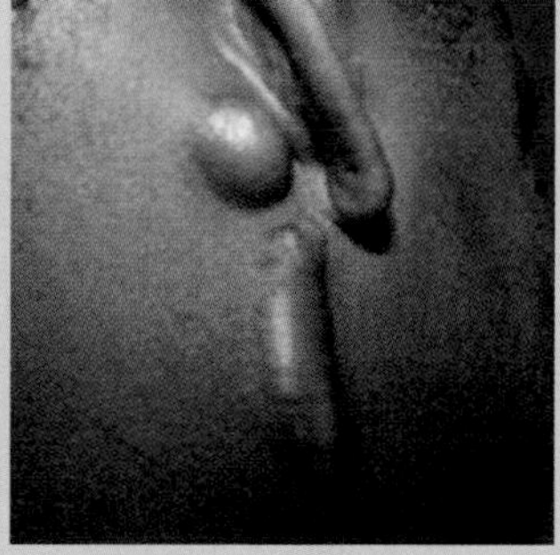

Keloid[c]

Scar

Thin to thick fibrous tissue that replaces normal skin following injury or laceration to the dermis

Examples: Healed wound or surgical incision

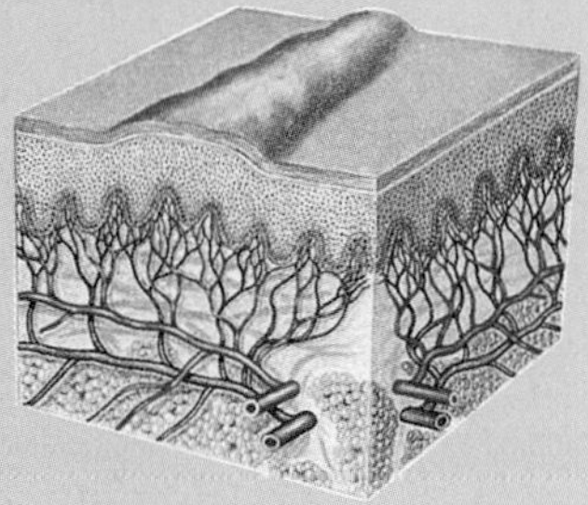
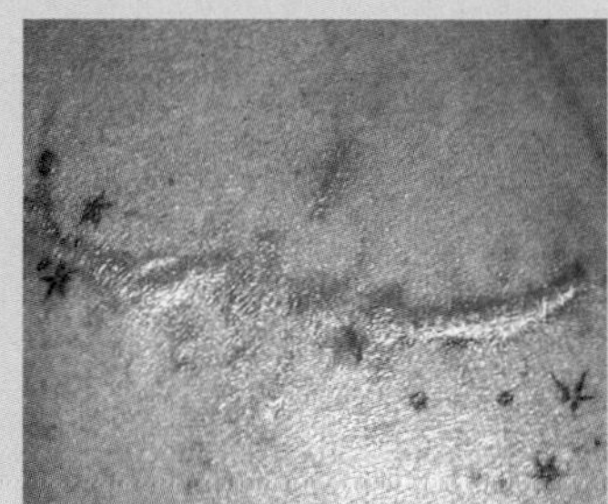

Hypertrophic scar[d]

Excoriation

Loss of epidermis; linear, hollowed-out, crusted area

Examples: Abrasion or scratch, scabies

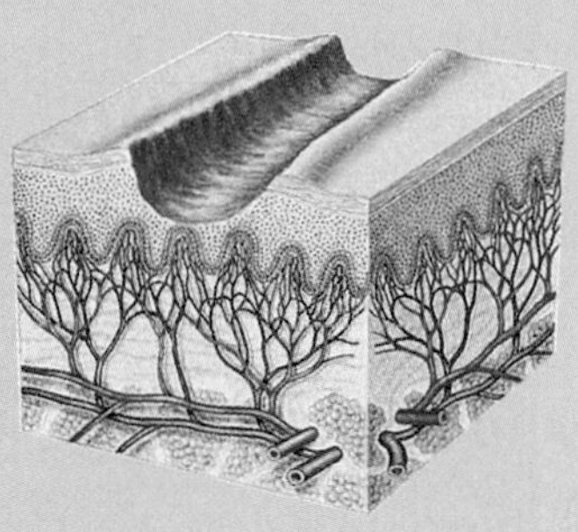
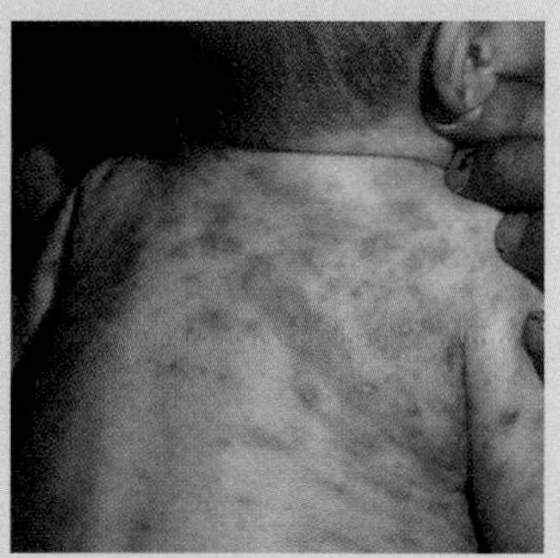

Scabies[c]

Fissure

Linear crack or break from the epidermis to the dermis; may be moist or dry

Examples: Athlete's foot, cracks at the corner of mouth, anal fissure, dermatitis

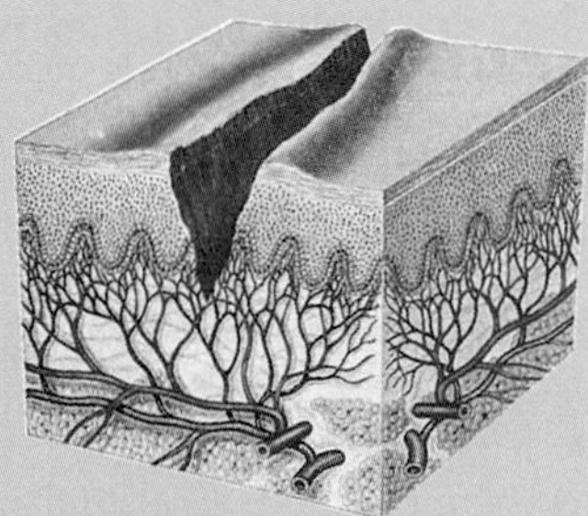
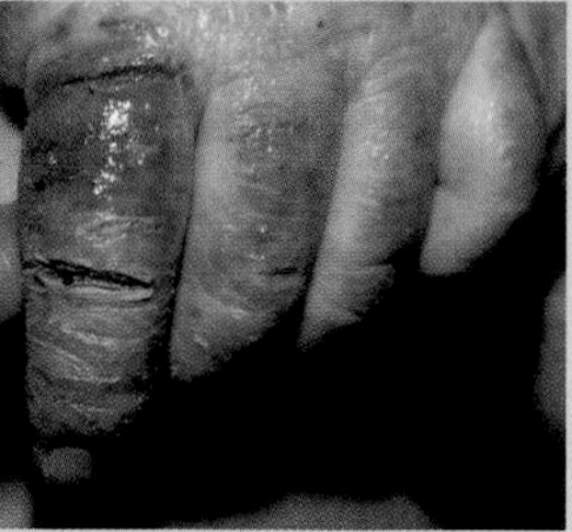

Fissures from infected dermatitis[c]

Continued

TABLE 41-3 Secondary Skin Lesions—cont'd

Erosion

Loss of part of the epidermis; depressed, moist, glistening; follows rupture of a vesicle or bulla or chemical injury

Example: Chemical injury

Erosion on leg[e]

Ulcer

Loss of epidermis and dermis; concave; varies in size

Examples: Pressure ulcer, stasis ulcers

Pressure ulcer on heel[f]

Atrophy

Thinning of skin surface and loss of skin markings; skin appears translucent and paperlike

Examples: Aged skin, striae

Aged skin[g]

[a]Baran, R., Dawber, R.P.R., & Levene, G.M. (1991). *Color atlas of the hair, scalp, and nails.* St. Louis: Mosby.
[b]James, W.D., Berger, T.G., & Elston, D.M. (2011). *Andrews' diseases of the skin* (11th ed.). Philadelphia: Saunders.
[c]Weston, W.L., Lane, A.T., & Morelli, J. (2007). *Color textbook of pediatric dermatology* (4th ed.). St. Louis: Mosby.
[d]Nouri, K., & Leal-Khouri, S. (2003). *Techniques in dermatologic surgery.* Philadelphia: Mosby.
[e]Bolognia, J.L., Jorizzo, J., & Schaffer, J. (2012). *Dermatology* (3rd ed.). Philadelphia: Saunders.
[f]Robinson, J.K., Hanke, C.W., Siegel, D.M., et al. (2015). *Surgery of the skin* (3rd ed.). Philadelphia: Saunders.
[g]Ball, J.W., Dains, J.E., Flynn, J.A., et al. (2015). *Seidel's guide to physical examination* (8th ed.). St. Louis: Mosby.

TABLE 41-4 Clinical Manifestations of Select Skin Lesions

Type	Clinical Manifestation
Comedone	Plug of sebaceous and keratin material lodged in opening of hair follicle; open comedone has dilated orifice (blackhead) and closed comedone has narrow opening (whitehead)
Burrow	Narrow, raised, irregular channel caused by parasite
Petechiae	Circumscribed area of blood less than 0.5 cm in diameter
Purpura	Circumscribed area of blood greater than 0.5 cm in diameter
Telangiectasia	Dilated, superficial blood vessels

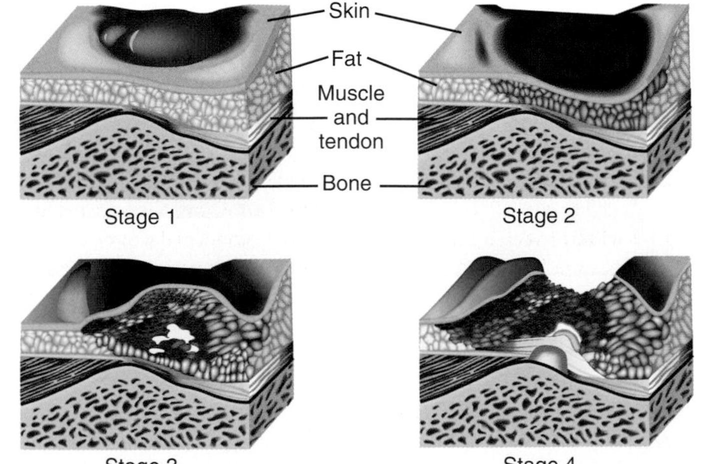

FIGURE 41-3 Progression of Pressure Ulcer. Sustained pressure over a bony prominence compresses the tissue and reduces blood flow, resulting in progressive ischemia and necrosis of tissue.

Stage 2—Partial-thickness skin loss (erosion or blistering) involving epidermis or dermis

Stage 3—Full-thickness skin loss involving damage or necrosis of subcutaneous tissue that may extend to, but not through, underlying fascia

Stage 4—Full-thickness tissue loss with exposure of muscle, bone, or supporting structures (tendons or joint capsules); can include undermining and tunnelling

Suspected deep tissue injury—Localized in an area of purple or maroon discoloured intact skin or blood-filled blister caused by underlying soft tissue damage from pressure, shear, or both

Unstageable—Full-thickness tissue loss with base of ulcer covered by slough or eschar, or both, in the wound bed

Superficial damage results in a layer of dead tissue that forms as an abrasion, blister, erosion, or nonblanchable red or darkened skin or as a reddish blue discoloration when there is deeper tissue damage. Superficial ulcers are more common on the sacrum as a result of shearing or friction forces (forces parallel to the skin). Deep ulcers develop closer to the bone as a result of tissue distortion and vascular occlusion from pressure perpendicular to the tissue (over the heels, trochanter, and ischia). Bacteria colonize the dead tissue, and infection is usually localized and self-limiting. Proteolytic enzymes from bacteria and macrophages dissolve necrotic tissues and cause a foul-smelling discharge that resembles, but is not, pus. The necrotic tissue initiates an inflammatory response with potential pain, fever, and leukocytosis. If the ulceration is large, toxicity and pain lead to a host of possible complications, including loss of appetite, debility, local or systemic infections, and renal insufficiency.

The primary goal for those at risk for pressure ulcers is prevention and early detection. Preventive techniques include frequent assessment of the skin with repositioning and turning of the individual; promotion of movement; implementation of pressure reduction (type of positioning and use of specialty beds), pressure removal (positioning interval), and pressure distribution devices (positioning aids); and elimination of excessive moisture and drainage. Adequate nutrition, oxygenation, and fluid balance must be maintained.[3,4]

Superficial ulcers should be covered with flat, moisture-retaining dressings (e.g., hydrogel dressings) that cannot wrinkle and cause increased pressure or friction. Successful healing requires continued adequate relief of pressure, débridement of necrotic tissue, opening of deep pockets for drainage, and repair of damaged tissue by construction of skin flaps for large, deep ulcers. Infection requires treatment with antibiotics, and pain should be controlled.[5,6]

Keloids and Hypertrophic Scars

Keloids are rounded, firm, elevated scars with irregular clawlike margins that extend beyond the original site of injury. They are most common in darkly pigmented skin types and generally appear weeks to months after a stable scar has formed. **Hypertrophic scars** are elevated erythematous fibrous lesions that do not extend beyond the border of injury. Hypertrophic scars appear within 3 to 4 months and usually regress within 1 year. Both lesions are caused by abnormal wound healing with excessive fibroblast activity and collagen formation, and loss of control of normal tissue repair and regeneration.[7] Genetic susceptibility is likely.[8]

Excessive or poorly aligned tension on a wound, introduction of foreign material into the skin, infection, and certain types of trauma (e.g., burns) are all provocative factors. Those parts of the body at risk include shoulders, back, chin, ears, and lower legs. Individuals 10 to 30 years of age develop lesions much more commonly than do prepubescent children or older adults.

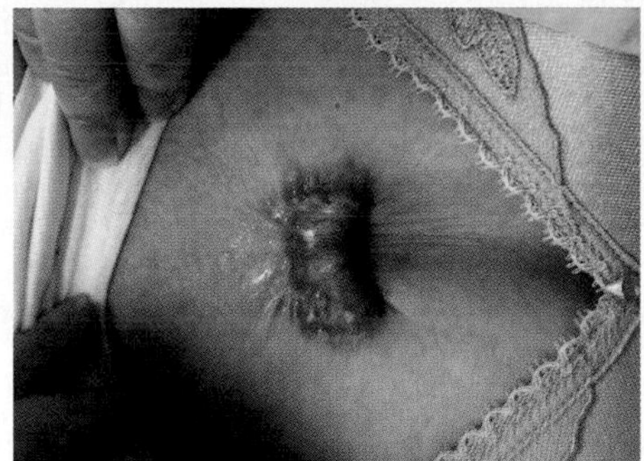

FIGURE 41-4 Keloid. (Courtesy Dr. Jeschke.)

Keloids start as pink or red, firm, well-defined, rubbery plaques that persist for several months after trauma. Later, uncontrolled overgrowth causes extension beyond the site of the original wound, and the overgrowth becomes smoother, irregularly shaped, hyperpigmented, harder, and more symptomatic. The fibrous tissue that accumulates in keloids is associated with increased cellularity and metabolic activity of fibroblasts. The tendency to form **clawlike prolongations** is typical (Figure 41-4).

Various treatments are available for the management of keloids and hypertrophic scars. There also is a need for research to improve treatment outcome.[7]

Pruritus

Pruritus, or itching, is a symptom associated with many primary skin disorders, such as eczema, psoriasis, or insect infestations, or it can be a manifestation of systemic disease (e.g., chronic kidney disease, cholestatic liver disease, thyroid disorders, iron deficiency, neuropathies, or malignancy) or the use of opiate drugs. It may be acute or chronic (neuropathic itch), localized or generalized, and migratory (moves from one location to another).[9] Multiple stimuli can produce itching, and there is interaction between itch and pain sensations. There are many itch mediators, including histamine, serotonin, prostaglandins, bradykinins, neuropeptides, acetylcholine, and interleukin-2 (IL-2) and IL-31. Small unmyelinated type C nerve fibres transmit itch sensations, and specific spinal pathways may carry itch sensations to the brain.[10]

Management of pruritus is challenging and depends on the cause, and the primary condition must be treated. Both topical and systemic therapies are used.[11]

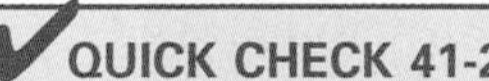

QUICK CHECK 41-2

1. What areas are at greatest risk for pressure ulcers?
2. How does a keloid differ from a normal scar?
3. What stimulates pruritus?

DISORDERS OF THE SKIN

Disorders of the skin may be precipitated by trauma, abnormal cellular function, infection, immune responses and inflammation, and systemic diseases.

Inflammatory Disorders

The most common inflammatory disorders of the skin are eczema and dermatitis. **Eczema** and **dermatitis** are general terms that describe a particular type of inflammatory response in the skin and can be used interchangeably. Eczematous disorders are generally characterized by pruritus, lesions with indistinct borders, and epidermal changes. These lesions can appear as erythema, papules, or scales; they can present in an acute, subacute, or chronic phase. Edema, serous discharge, and crusting occur with continued irritation and scratching. In chronic eczema, the skin becomes thickened, leathery, and hyperpigmented from recurrent irritation and scratching. The location of eczema is related to the underlying cause. Eczematous inflammations need to be differentiated from other rashes and dermatoses, particularly psoriasis.

Allergic Contact Dermatitis

Allergic contact dermatitis is a common form of T-cell–mediated or delayed hypersensitivity. (See Chapter 8 for different types of allergic responses.) The response is an interaction of skin barrier function, reaction to irritants, and neuronal responses, such as pruritus. Genetic susceptibility involves several genes, including loss-of-function mutations in the gene encoding the epidermal protein filaggrin. Various allergens (e.g., microorganisms, chemicals, foreign proteins, latex, medications, metals) can form the sensitizing antigen. Contact with poison ivy is a common example (Figure 41-5). As the allergen contacts the skin, the allergen is bound to a carrier protein, forming a sensitizing antigen. The Langerhans cells (antigen-presenting dendritic cells) process the antigen and present it to T lymphocytes (T cells). T cells then become sensitized to the antigen, inducing the release of inflammatory cytokines and the symptoms of dermatitis.[12] In latex allergy, there is either a type IV hypersensitivity reaction to chemicals used in latex rubber processing or a type I immediate hypersensitivity reaction with immunoglobulin E (IgE) antibodies formed in response to latex rubber protein.[13]

In delayed hypersensitivity (type IV), several hours pass before an immunological response is apparent. The T cells play an important role because they differentiate and secrete lymphokines that affect macrophage (Langerhans cells) movement and aggregation, coagulation, and other inflammatory responses (see Chapter 8). Sensitization usually develops with first exposure to the antigen, and symptoms of dermatitis occur with re-exposure.

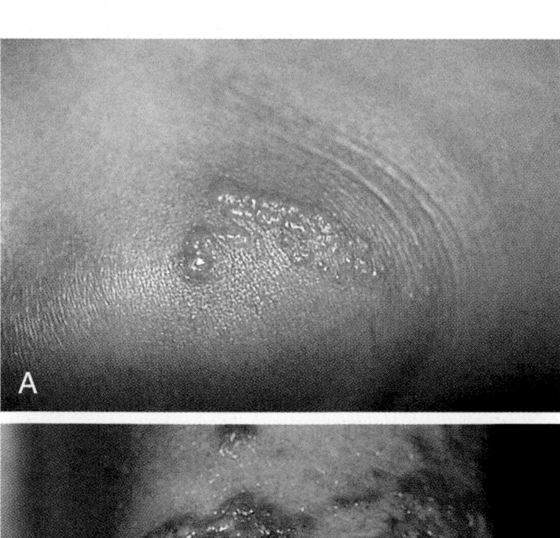

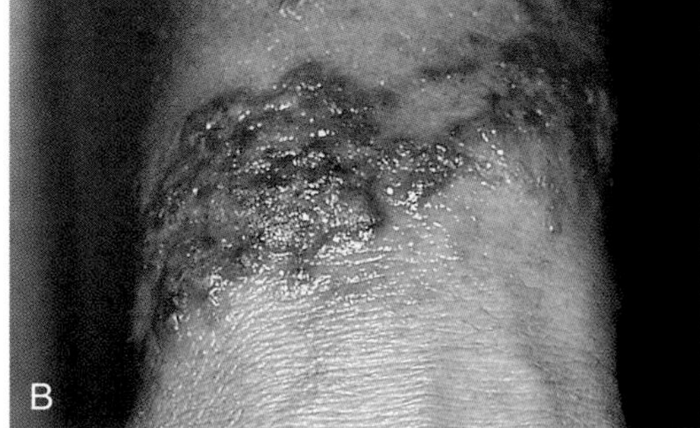

FIGURE 41-5 Poison Ivy. A, Poison ivy on knee. **B,** Poison ivy dermatitis. (Courtesy Department of Dermatology, School of Medicine, University of Utah, Salt Lake City, UT.)

The manifestations of allergic contact dermatitis include erythema and swelling with pruritic (itching) vesicular lesions in the areas of allergen contact. The pattern of distribution provides clues to the source of the antigen (e.g., hands exposed to chemical solutions or boundaries from rings and bracelets). The antigen must be removed for the inflammatory response to resolve and tissue repair to begin. Treatment may require topical or systemic steroids.

Irritant Contact Dermatitis

Irritant contact dermatitis is a nonspecific inflammatory dermatitis caused by activation of the innate immune system by proinflammatory properties of chemicals. The severity of the inflammation is related to the concentration of the irritant, length of exposure, and disruption of the skin barrier.[14] Chemical irritation from acids and prolonged exposure to soaps, detergents, and various agents used in industry can cause inflammatory lesions. The skin lesions resemble allergic contact dermatitis. Removing the source of irritation and using topical agents provide effective treatment.

Atopic Dermatitis

Atopic dermatitis (allergic dermatitis) is common in individuals with a history of hay fever or asthma and is associated with IgE antibodies. It is more common in infancy and childhood; however, some individuals are affected throughout life. Specific details of this disorder are presented in Chapter 42.

Stasis Dermatitis

Stasis dermatitis usually occurs on the lower legs as a result of chronic venous stasis and edema and is associated with varicosities, phlebitis, and vascular trauma (see Chapter 24). Pooling of venous blood traps neutrophils that may release oxidants and proteolytic enzymes. Increased venous pressure widens interendothelial pores with deposition of red blood cells, fibrin, and other macromolecules, making them unavailable for repair while promoting inflammation.[15] First, erythema and pruritus develop followed by scaling, petechiae, and hyperpigmentation. Progressive lesions become ulcerated, particularly around the ankles and pretibial surface (Figure 41-6).

Treatment includes elevating the legs as often as possible, not wearing tight clothes around the legs, and not standing for long periods. Defined infections are treated with antibiotics. Chronic lesions with ulceration are treated with moist dressings, external compression or dressings, and vein ablation surgery.[16]

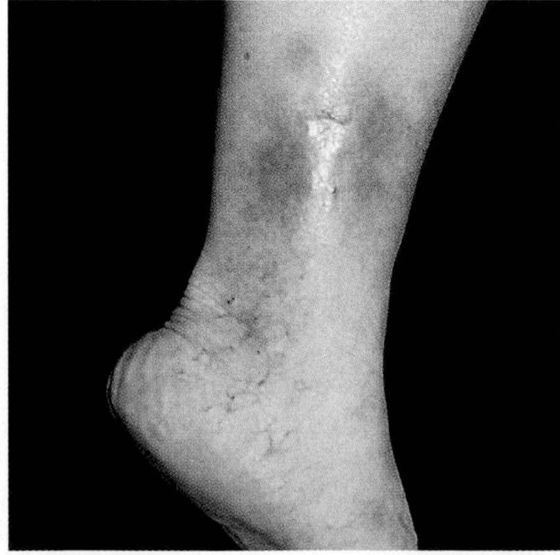

FIGURE 41-6 Stasis Ulcer. (Courtesy Department of Dermatology, School of Medicine, University of Utah, Salt Lake City, UT.)

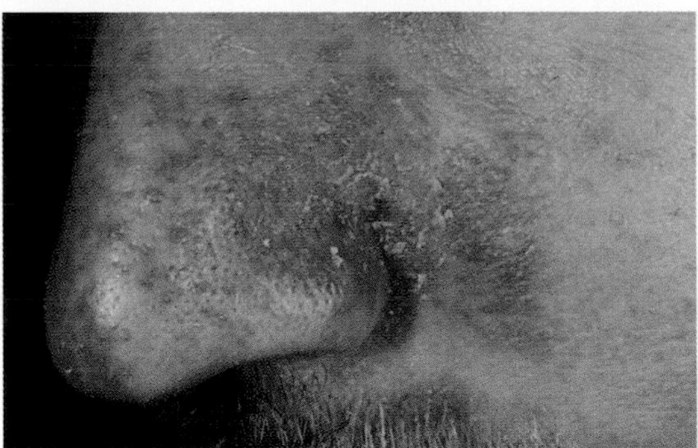

FIGURE 41-7 Seborrheic Dermatitis. (Courtesy Department of Dermatology, School of Medicine, University of Utah, Salt Lake City, UT.)

Seborrheic Dermatitis

Seborrheic dermatitis is a common chronic inflammation of the skin involving the scalp, eyebrows, eyelids, ear canals, nasolabial folds, axillae, chest, and back (Figure 41-7). In infants it is known as *cradle cap*. The cause is unknown. Proposed theories include genetic predisposition, phospholipases from *Malassezia* yeasts, immunosuppression, and epidermal hyperproliferation.[17]

The lesions develop from infancy to old age with periods of remission and exacerbation. The lesions appear as scaly, white or yellowish inflammatory plaques with mild pruritus. Topical therapy includes antifungal shampoos, calcineurin inhibitors, and low-dose steroids for acute flares. Corticosteroids should not be used for maintenance therapy.

Papulosquamous Disorders

Psoriasis, pityriasis rosea, lichen planus, acne vulgaris, acne rosacea, and lupus erythematosus are characterized by papules, scales, plaques, and erythema. Collectively they are described as papulosquamous disorders.

Psoriasis

Psoriasis is a chronic, relapsing, proliferative, inflammatory disorder that involves the skin, scalp, and nails and can occur at any age. Psoriasis affects about 1 to 4% of the population in countries north of the equator. The onset is generally established by 40 years of age. A family history of psoriasis is common and the genetic mechanisms are complex. The onset of psoriasis later in life is less familial and more secondary to comorbidities, such as obesity, smoking, hypertension, and diabetes.[18,19]

The inflammatory cascade of psoriasis involves the complex interactions between macrophages, fibroblasts, dendritic cells, natural killer cells, T helper cells, and T regulatory cells. These immune cells lead to the secretion of numerous inflammatory mediators, such as interferon (IFN), tumour necrosis factor-alpha (TNF-α), and various other cytokines, including IL-12, IL-23, and IL-17. These inflammatory markers are the target for several therapeutic medications known as biologics (biotherapy).[20]

Both the dermis and the epidermis are thickened because of cellular hyperproliferation, altered kerotinocyte differentiation, and expanded dermal vasculature. The turnover time for shedding the epidermis is decreased to 3 to 4 days from the normal of 14 to 20 days, with many more germinative cells and increased transit time through the dermis. Cell maturation and keratinization are bypassed, and the epidermis thickens and plaques form. The loosely cohesive keratin gives the lesion a silvery appearance. Capillary dilation and increased vascularization accommodate the increased cell metabolism but also cause erythema. The disease can be mild, moderate, or severe, depending on the size,

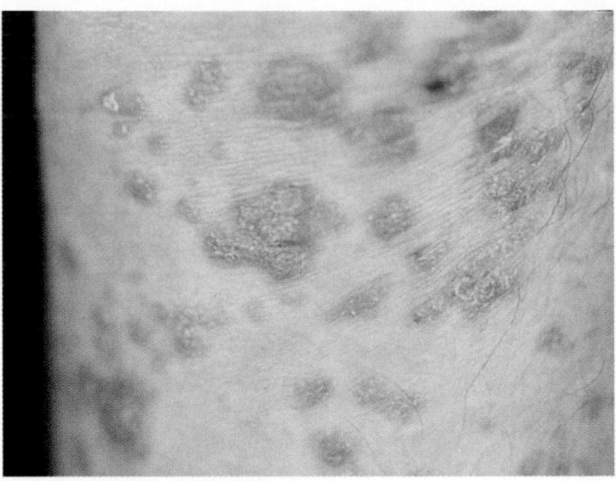

FIGURE 41-8 Psoriasis. Typical oval plaque with well-defined borders and silvery scale. (Courtesy Department of Dermatology, School of Medicine, University of Utah, Salt Lake City, UT.)

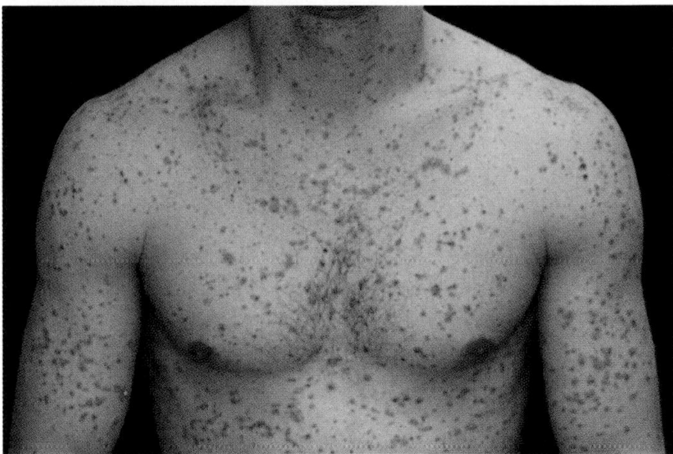

FIGURE 41-9 Guttate Psoriasis Following Streptococcal Infection. Numerous uniformly small lesions may abruptly occur following streptococcal pharyngitis. (Courtesy Department of Dermatology, School of Medicine, University of Utah, Salt Lake City, UT.)

distribution, and inflammation of the lesions. Psoriasis is marked by remissions and exacerbations.

The types of psoriasis include plaque (psoriasis vulgaris), inverse, guttate, pustular, and erythrodermic. Plaque psoriasis is the most common and affects 80 to 90% of individuals with psoriasis. The typical plaque psoriatic lesion is a well-demarcated, thick, silvery, scaly, erythematous plaque surrounded by normal skin (Figure 41-8). Small erythematous papules enlarge and coalesce into larger inflammatory lesions on the face, scalp, elbows, and knees and at sites of trauma (Koebner phenomenon).

Inverse psoriasis is rare and involves lesions that develop in skin folds (i.e., axilla or groin). In guttate psoriasis, small papules appear suddenly on the trunk and extremities (Figure 41-9) a few weeks after a streptococcal respiratory tract infection. Guttate psoriasis may resolve spontaneously in weeks or months. Pustular psoriasis appears as blisters of noninfectious pus (collections of neutrophils), and erythrodermic (exfoliative) psoriasis is often accompanied by pruritus or pain with widespread red, scaling lesions that cover a large area of the body.

Psoriatic arthritis of hands, feet, knees, and ankle joints develops in 5 to 30% of cases. Psoriatic nail disease can occur in all psoriasis subtypes with pitting, onycholysis, subungal hyperkeratosis, and nail plate dystrophy. A number of comorbidities are associated with the inflammatory mechanisms of psoriasis (see *Health Promotion:* Psoriasis and Comorbidities).

HEALTH PROMOTION

Psoriasis and Comorbidities

In addition to skin and joint manifestations, including rheumatoid arthritis, severe psoriasis is associated with inflammatory bowel disease and metabolic syndrome, which includes hypertension, insulin resistance, dyslipidemias, abdominal obesity, nonalcoholic fatty liver disease, and increased risk for atherosclerosis and myocardial infarction that is independent of traditional risk factors for these diseases. The underlying mechanisms are thought to be related to increased levels of systemic proinflammatory mediators, such as tumour necrosis factor-alpha (TNF-α) and chemokines, which are central to the chronic inflammation, oxidative stress, and angiogenesis of psoriasis. The increased prevalence of cancer, particularly lymphoma, may be related to the pathogenesis of psoriasis or could be a consequence of immune modulation therapies. Crohn's disease also is associated with psoriasis, and there may be a genetic overlap between these two diseases. Treatment considerations need to include screening, monitoring, and managing these comorbidities.

Data from Baeta, I.G.R., Bittencourt, F.V., Gontijo, B., et al. (2014). *An Bras Dermatol, 89*(5), 735–744; Boehncke, W.H., & Schön, M.P. (2015). *Lancet, 6736*(14), 61909–61917; Gisondi, P., Galvan, A., Idolazzi, L., et al. (2015). *Front Med (Lausanne), 2*, 1; Ni, C., & Chiu, M.W. (2014). *Clin Cosmet Investig Dermatol, 7*, 119–132.

Treatment is individualized and related to maintaining skin moisture, reducing epidermal cell turnover and pruritus, and promoting immunomodulation. Mild psoriasis is treated with skin-directed therapy, such as medium- to high-strength topical corticosteroids, vitamin D analogues, emollients, and keratolytic agents (such as salicylic acid), and narrow-band ultraviolet (UV) light therapy. Systemic therapy is indicated for moderate to severe disease or in the presence of psoriatic arthritis. Current medications used in Canada to treat this condition include methotrexate (Apo-Methotrexate), oral retinoids, acitretin (Soriatane), and cyclosporine (Sandimmune) (short term). Newer biologics are being used with more frequency as our understanding of the pathophysiology of psoriasis continues to grow. These biologics include the anti-TNF medications infliximab (Remicade), adalimumab (Humira), and etanercept (Enbrel). Ustekinumab (Stelara) is the most recent injectable biological treatment targeting IL-12 and IL-23. The IL-17 inhibitors are currently under investigation for their safety and efficacy.[21,22] A potential complication of biotherapy is the development of antimedication antibodies.[23]

Pityriasis Rosea

Pityriasis rosea is a self-limiting inflammatory disorder that occurs more often in young adults. The cause is thought to be a herpeslike virus (e.g., human herpesvirus 6 [HHV6] and HHV7).[24] Pityriasis rosea begins as a single lesion (**herald patch**) that is circular, demarcated, and salmon-pink, approximately 3 to 10 cm in diameter, and usually located on the trunk. Early lesions are macular and papular. Secondary lesions develop within 14 to 21 days and extend over the trunk and upper part of the extremities (Figure 41-10), although rarely on the face. The small erythematous rose-coloured papules expand into characteristic oval lesions that are bilateral and symmetrically distributed. The pattern of distribution on the back follows the skin lines around the trunk and resembles a drooping pine tree. The scales are sloughed from the margin of the lesions, forming a collarette pattern. Itching is the most common symptom. Occasionally, headache, fatigue, or sore throat precedes the development of the lesions.

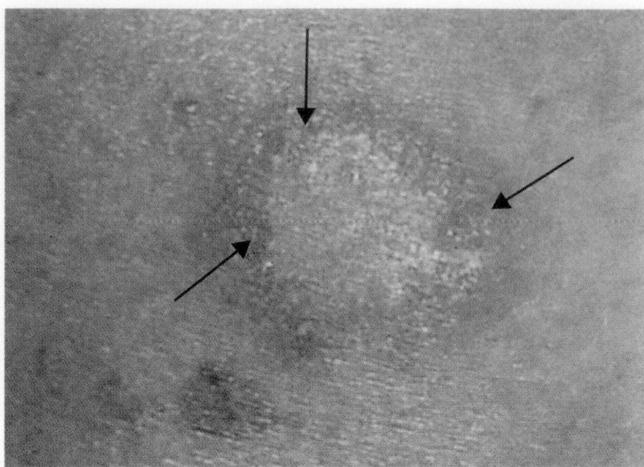

FIGURE 41-10 Pityriasis Rosea Herald Patch. A collarette pattern has formed around the margins (*arrows*). (Courtesy Department of Dermatology, School of Medicine, University of Utah, Salt Lake City, UT.)

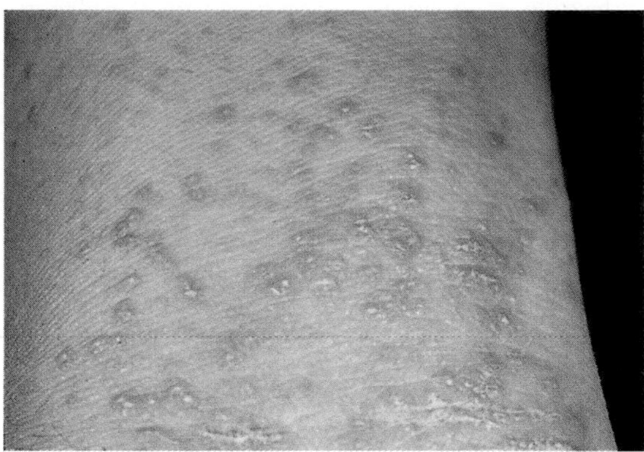

FIGURE 41-11 Hypertrophic Lichen Planus on Arms. (Courtesy Department of Dermatology, School of Medicine, University of Utah, Salt Lake City, UT.)

The diagnosis of pityriasis rosea follows the clinical appearance of the lesion. Secondary syphilis, psoriasis, medication eruption, nummular eczema, and seborrheic dermatitis are among the differential diagnosis considerations. The disorder is usually self-limiting and resolves in a few months with symptomatic treatment for pruritus or cosmetic concerns. UV light (with some risk for hyperpigmentation) or systemic corticosteroids may be used to control pruritus. Acyclovir (Zovirax) and erythromycin (Erythrocin) also may be used for treatment.[25]

Lichen Planus

Lichen planus (LP) is a benign autoimmune inflammatory disorder of the skin and mucous membranes.[26] The age of onset is usually between 30 and 70 years. The cause is unknown, but T cells, adhesion molecules, inflammatory cytokines, perforin, and antigen-presenting cells are involved. LP also is linked to numerous medications and hepatitis C virus.[27] The disorder begins with nonscaling, purple-coloured, flat-topped, polygonal pruritic papules 2 to 4 mm in size, usually located symmetrically on the wrists, ankles, lower legs, and genitalia (Figure 41-11). New lesions are pale pink and evolve into a dark violet colour. Persistent lesions may be thickened and red, forming hypertrophic LP. Oral lesions (oral LP) appear as lacy white rings that must be differentiated from leukoplakia or oral candidiasis.[28] Usually, oral lesions do not ulcerate, but localized or extensive painful ulcerations can occur, and there may be increased risk for oral cancer.[28] Chronic ulcerated lesions become malignant in 1% of individuals with the disease. Thinning and splitting of nails are common, and part or the entire nail may be shed.

Pruritus is the most distressing symptom. The lesions are self-limiting and may last for months or years, with an average duration of 6 to 18 months. Postinflammatory hyperpigmentation is a common consequence of the lesion. Approximately 20% of individuals have a recurrence. Diagnosis is made by the clinical appearance and histopathology of the lesion. Treatment is individualized and includes topical, intralesional, or systemic corticosteroids (second line for resistant LP), and systemic acitretin with or without adjuvant light therapy. Antihistamines are given for itching, and short-term use of topical or systemic corticosteroids may be used to control inflammation. Mucous membrane lesions are treated with topical steroids, topical retinoids or immunomodulators (or both), and systemic glucocorticoids.[29]

QUICK CHECK 41-3

1. Why does inflammation occur with contact dermatitis?
2. What factors are associated with atopic dermatitis?
3. What lesions are associated with papulosquamous disorders?
4. Give three examples of papulosquamous disorders.

Acne Vulgaris

Acne vulgaris is an inflammatory disorder of the pilosebaceous follicle (the sebaceous gland contiguous with a hair follicle) that usually occurs during adolescence. It is discussed in Chapter 42.

Acne Rosacea

Acne rosacea is a chronic inflammation of the skin that develops in middle-aged adults. There are four subtypes of lesions: erythematotelangiectatic, papulopustular, phymatous, and ocular (eyelids and ocular surface). The exact cause is unknown, but factors that trigger an altered innate immune response are involved (i.e., sun exposure and damage, drinking alcohol or hot beverages, hormonal fluctuations, and *Demodex folliculorum* [mites]).[30] The most common lesions are erythema, papules, pustules, and telangiectasia. They occur in the middle third of the face, including the forehead, nose, cheeks, and chin (Figure 41-12). The lesions are associated with chronic, inappropriate vasodilation resulting in flushing and sun sensitivity. Sebaceous hypertrophy, fibrosis, and telangiectasia may be severe enough to produce an irreversible bulbous appearance of the nose (rhinophyma). Disorders of the eye often accompany rosacea, particularly conjunctivitis and keratitis, which can result in visual impairment. Facial application of fluorinated topical steroids may increase the severity of telangiectasias.

Photoprotection, using sunscreens, is essential along with avoidance of other triggers. Both topical (metronidazole [Flagyl], azelaic acid [Finacea]) and oral medications (tetracyclines and doxycline [Teva-Doxycline]) may be effective. Surgical excision of excessive tissue may be required for rhinophyma.[31]

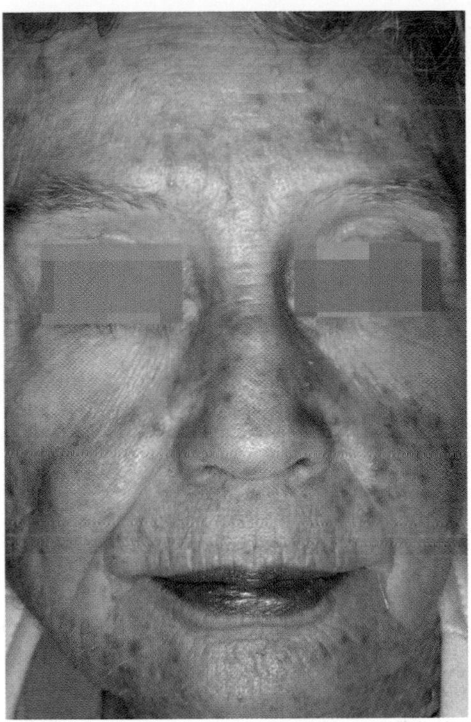

FIGURE 41-12 Granulomatous Rosacea. Pustules and erythema occur on the forehead, cheeks, and nose. (From Habif, T.P. [2016]. *Clinical dermatology* [6th ed.]. Philadelphia: Saunders.)

Lupus Erythematosus

Lupus erythematosus is a systemic, inflammatory autoimmune disease with cutaneous manifestations (see Chapter 8). Discoid (or cutaneous) lupus erythematosus (DLE) is limited to the skin and can progress to systemic lupus erythematosus.[32]

Discoid (cutaneous) lupus erythematosus. Discoid (cutaneous) lupus erythematosus (DLE) usually occurs in genetically susceptible adults, particularly women in their late 30s or early 40s, but people of any age can be affected. The disease can be acute, subacute, intermittent, or chronic. Differentiation of subtypes is by physical examination, laboratory studies, histological analysis, and antibody serology direct immunofluorescence.[33] The lesions may be single or multiple and vary in size. Often the lesions are located on light-exposed areas of the skin, and photosensitivity is common. The face is the most common site of lesion involvement, with a butterfly pattern of distribution found over the nose and cheeks.

The cause is unknown but is related to genetic and environmental factors and an altered immune response to an unknown antigen or to ultraviolet B (UVB) wavelengths. There is development of self-reactive T cells and B cells (B lymphocytes), decreased number of regulatory T cells, and increased levels of proinflammatory cytokines. Autoantibodies and immune complexes cause tissue damage and inflammation[34] (Figure 41-13). On skin biopsy with immunofluorescent observation, there are lumpy deposits of Igs, especially IgM (lupus band test).[35]

The early lesion is asymmetric, with a 1- to 2-cm raised red plaque with a brownish scale. The scale penetrates the hair follicle and leaves a visible follicle opening (carpet-tack appearance) when removed. The lesions persist for months and then resolve spontaneously or atrophy. Healing progresses outward from the centre of the lesion, with residual telangiectasia and hypopigmented scarring. Atrophy of the dermis and epidermis can cause a depressed scar. Treatment options include protection from the sun and use of topical steroids, calcineurin inhibitors, antimalarial medications (e.g., hydroxychloroquine sulphate [Plaquenil sulphate]), and immunosuppressors. These medications must be used with caution to prevent serious side effects.[35]

Vesiculobullous Diseases

Vesiculobullous skin diseases share a common characteristic of vesicle, or blister, formation. Two such diseases are pemphigus and erythema multiforme.

Pemphigus

Pemphigus (meaning "to blister or bubble") is a group of rare autoimmune blistering diseases of the skin and oral mucous membranes caused by circulating autoantibodies directed against the cell surface adhesion molecule desmoglein at the desmosomal cell junction in the

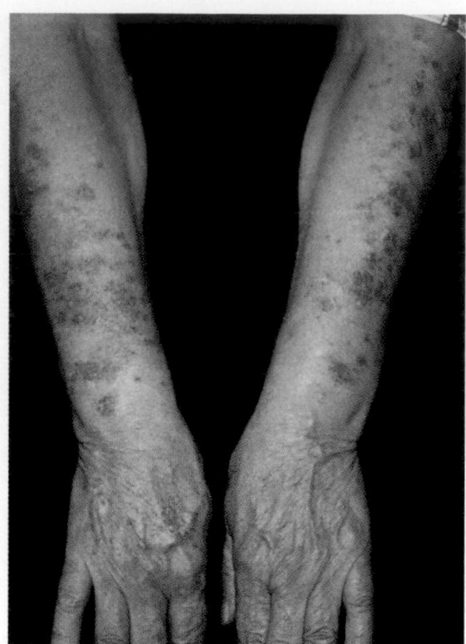

FIGURE 41-13 Subacute Cutaneous Lupus (Discoid Lupus Erythematosus). (Courtesy Department of Dermatology, School of Medicine, University of Utah, Salt Lake City, UT.)

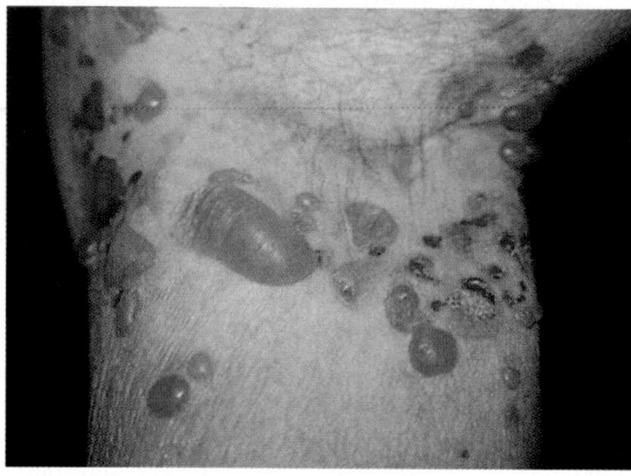

FIGURE 41-14 Bullous Pemphigoid. Generalized eruption with blisters arising from an edematous, erythematous annular base. (Courtesy Department of Dermatology, School of Medicine, University of Utah, Salt Lake City, UT.)

suprabasal layer of the epidermis. IgG autoantibodies and complement component C3 bind to the desmoglein adhesion molecules, resulting in the destruction of cell-to-cell adhesion (acantholysis) in the basal layer of the epidermis (see Table 41-1) with fluid accumulation and the resulting symptom of blister formation (Figure 41-14). Pemphigus can occur in all age groups but is more prevalent in persons between 40 and 50 years of age. There is a genetic predisposition as well as environmental (viral infections, medication-induced, dietary intake, or physical effects such as radiation or surgery) and endogenous (emotional or hormonal stressors) influences. Pemphigus presents in varying forms, often with painful, superficial erosions prone to infection:[36,37]

- **Pemphigus vulgaris** is the most common form. Oral lesions precede the onset of skin blistering, which is more prominent on the face, scalp, and axilla. The blisters rupture easily because of the thin, fragile overlying portion of the epidermis.
- **Pemphigus vegetans** is a variant of pemphigus vulgaris in which large blisters develop in tissue folds of the axilla and groin.
- **Pemphigus foliaceus** is a milder form of the disease and involves acantholysis at the more superficial, subcorneal level of the epidermis (see Table 41-1), with blistering, erosions, scaling, crusting, and erythema usually of the face and chest. Oral mucous membranes are rarely involved.
- **Pemphigus erythematosus** is a subset of pemphigus foliaceus often associated with systemic lupus erythematosus with positive antinuclear antibodies. The lesions are generally less widely distributed.
- **Paraneoplastic pemphigus** is the most severe form of pemphigus and is associated with lymphoproliferative neoplasms.
- **Immunoglobulin A pemphigus** is the most benign form of pemphigus characterized by tissue-bound and circulating IgA antibodies targeting desmosomal or nondesmosomal cell surface components in the basement membrane of the epidermis.
- **Pemphigus herpetiformis** is a very rare form of pemphigus that resembles dermatitis herpetiformis (blistering lesions that have the appearance of herpes lesions) but with immunological and histological findings consistent with pemphigus.

The diagnosis of pemphigus is made from the clinical and histological findings of the skin. Immunofluorescence demonstrates the presence of antibodies at the site of blister formation. The clinical course of the disease may range from rapidly fatal to relatively benign. The primary treatment for pemphigus is systemic corticosteroids in combination with adjuvant immunosuppressants. Newer methods of treatment and a clearer understanding of the pathogenesis have improved the prognosis and decreased mortality.[38]

Erythema Multiforme

Erythema multiforme is a syndrome characterized by inflammation of the skin and mucous membranes, often associated with a T-cell–mediated immunological reaction to a medication or microorganisms (e.g., herpes simplex virus [HSV]) that targets small blood vessels in the skin or mucosa.[39] **Bullous erythema multiforme** involves the mucous membranes. It is relatively rare and occurs more often during the second to fourth decade of life; however, it can occur at any age. Immune complex formation and deposition of C3, IgM, and fibrinogen around the superficial dermal blood vessels, basement membrane, and keratinocytes are common histological findings. Edema develops in the superficial dermis, so vesicles and bullae form. The lesions vary in clinical presentation and may involve the skin or mucous membranes, or both. The characteristic "bull's-eye," or "target," lesions occur on the skin surface with a central erythematous region surrounded by concentric rings of alternating edema and inflammation. The lesions usually occur suddenly in groups over a period of 2 to 3 weeks. Urticarial plaques, 1 to 2 cm in diameter, can develop without the target lesion. A vesiculobullous form is characterized by mucous membrane lesions and erythematous plaques on the extensor surfaces of the extremities. Single or multiple vesicles or bullae may arise on a part of the plaque accompanied by pruritus and burning. The lesions heal within 3 to 4 weeks.

The most common forms of erythema multiforme are usually associated with severe medication reactions and include **Stevens-Johnson syndrome** (severe mucocutaneous bullous form involving 10% of body surface area) and **toxic epidermal necrolysis (TEN)** (severe mucocutaneous bullous form involving 30% of body surface area). T-cytotoxic cells in a human leukocyte antigen–restricted fashion mediate the immune mechanism related to medication reactions[40,41] (see Chapter 42 for pediatric considerations).

Prodromal symptoms of erythema multiforme, including fever, headache, malaise, sore throat, and cough, develop in approximately one-third of the cases. The bullous lesions form erosions and crusts when they rupture. There is necrosis of the epidermis in TEN. The mouth, air passages, esophagus, urethra, and conjunctiva may be involved when mucous membranes are affected. Blindness can result from corneal ulcerations. Difficulty eating, breathing, and urinating may develop with severe consequences. The disease can involve the kidneys and extend from the upper respiratory passages into the lungs. Severe forms of the disease can be fatal.

Recognizing the person's medication history that preceded the target lesion and performing a skin biopsy are required to establish the diagnosis. Mild acute forms of the disease last 10 to 14 days and require no treatment. Any ongoing medication therapy should be withdrawn and reevaluated and underlying infections treated. Fluid and electrolyte balance should be monitored in severe forms of the disease, and mucous membranes should be carefully managed with a bland diet, warm saline eyewashes, topical anaesthetics, or corticosteroids to maintain comfort and prevent infection. Cutaneous blisters can be treated with wet compresses of Burow solution. Ophthalmic, kidney, and lung involvement require special care. Resolution occurs in 8 to 10 days, usually without scarring. Mucosal lesions may take 6 weeks to heal.

QUICK CHECK 41-4

1. Describe the inflammatory lesion associated with lupus erythematosus.
2. Compare the three forms of pemphigus.
3. What is the characteristic lesion of erythema multiforme?

Infections

Cutaneous infections are common forms of skin disease. They generally remain localized, although serious complications can develop with systemic involvement that can be life-threatening. The types of skin infection include bacterial, viral, and fungal. The commensal (normal) flora of the skin consists of aerobes, yeast, and anaerobes and often provides protection against pathogens that cause skin infections, including *Staphylococcus* and *Streptococcus*.

Bacterial Infections

Most bacterial infections of the skin are caused by local invasion of pathogens. Coagulase-positive *Staphylococcus aureus* and, less often, beta-hemolytic streptococci are the common causative microorganisms. Community-acquired methicillin-resistant *Staphylococcus aureus* (CA-MRSA [see Chapter 8]) also is a cause of serious skin infection, particularly skin abscesses.[42]

Folliculitis. Folliculitis is an infection of the hair follicle and can be caused by bacteria, viruses, or fungi, although *S. aureus* is the common culprit. The infection develops from proliferation of the microorganism around the opening and inside the follicle. Inflammation is caused by the release of chemotactic factors and enzymes from the bacteria. The lesions appear as pustules with a surrounding area of erythema. They are most prominent on the scalp and extremities and rarely cause systemic symptoms. Prolonged skin moisture, skin trauma (e.g., shaving facial hair), occlusive clothing, topical agents, and poor hygiene are associated contributing factors. Cleaning with soap and water and topical application of antibiotics are effective treatments.

Furuncles and carbuncles. Furuncles, or "boils," are inflammations of hair follicles (Figure 41-15). They may develop after folliculitis that spreads through the follicular wall into the surrounding dermis. The invading microorganism is usually *S. aureus*, including CA-MRSA (see Chapter 8). The infecting strain may spread to the skin from the anterior nares. Any skin area with hair can be infected, and one or several lesions may be present. The initial lesion is a deep, firm, red, painful nodule 1 to 5 cm in diameter. Within a few days, the erythematous nodules change to a large, fluctuant, and tender cystic nodule accompanied by cellulitis.

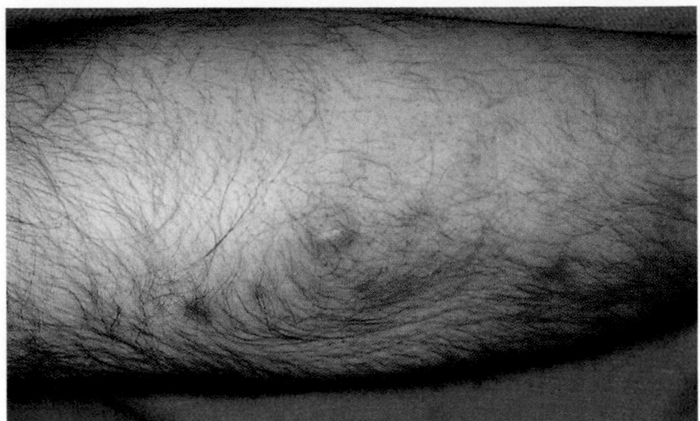

FIGURE 41-15 Furuncle of the Forearm. (Courtesy Department of Dermatology, School of Medicine, University of Utah, Salt Lake City, UT.)

No systemic symptoms are present, and the lesion may drain large amounts of pus and necrotic tissue.

Carbuncles are a collection of infected hair follicles and usually occur on the back of the neck, the upper back, and the lateral thighs. The lesion begins in the subcutaneous tissue and lower dermis as a firm mass that evolves into an erythematous, painful, swollen mass that drains through many openings. Abscesses may develop. Chills, fever, and malaise can occur during the early stages of lesion development.

Furuncles and carbuncles are treated with warm compresses to provide comfort and promote localization and spontaneous drainage. Abscess formation, recurrent infections, extensive lesions, or lesions associated with cellulitis or systemic symptoms require incision and drainage and are treated with systemic antibiotics.

Cellulitis. Cellulitis is an infection of the dermis and subcutaneous tissue usually caused by *S. aureus*, CA-MRSA, or group B streptococci.[43] Cellulitis can occur as an extension of a skin wound, as an ulcer, or from furuncles or carbuncles. The infected area is warm, erythematous, swollen, and painful. The infection is usually in the lower extremities and responds to systemic antibiotics, as well as therapy to relieve pain. Cellulitis also can be associated with other diseases, including chronic venous insufficiency and stasis dermatitis.

Cellulitis must be differentiated from necrotizing fasciitis. Necrotizing fasciitis is a rare, rapidly spreading infection. It is commonly caused by *Streptococcus pyogenes* starting in the fascia, muscles, and subcutaneous fat with subsequent necrosis of the overlying skin. Treatment requires antibiotics and, often, surgical débridement.[44]

Erysipelas. Erysipelas is an acute superficial infection of the upper dermis most often caused by *S. pyogenes*, beta-hemolytic streptococci, and *S. aureus*. The face, ears, and lower legs are involved. Chills, fever, and malaise precede the onset of lesions by 4 hours to 20 days. The initial lesions appear as firm, red spots that enlarge and coalesce to form a clearly circumscribed, advancing, bright red, hot lesion with a raised border. Vesicles may appear over the lesion and at the border. Pruritus, burning, and tenderness are present. Cold compresses provide symptomatic relief, and systemic antibiotics are required to arrest the infection.[45]

Impetigo. Impetigo is a superficial lesion of the skin that is caused by coagulase-positive *Staphylococcus* or beta-hemolytic streptococci. The disease occurs in adults but is more common in children (see Chapter 42).

Lyme disease. Lyme disease is a multisystem inflammatory disease caused by the spirochete *Borrelia burgdorferi* transmitted by *Ixodes* tick bites and is the most frequently reported vectorborne illness. The highest incidence of Lyme disease is among children. The microorganism is difficult to culture, escapes immunodefences, and hides in tissue. It spreads to other tissues by entering capillary beds.[46]

Symptoms of the disease occur in three stages, although 50% of infected individuals are symptom free.[47] *Localized infection* occurs soon after the bite (within 3 to 32 days) with erythema migrans (bull's-eye rash), a T-cell–mediated response usually with fever. Within days to weeks after the onset of the illness, there is *disseminated infection* with secondary erythema migrans, usually with myalgias, arthralgias, and more rarely meningitis, neuritis, or carditis. *Late persistent infection* (more common in Europe) can continue for years with arthritis, encephalopathy, polyneuropathy, or heart failure. The diagnosis of Lyme disease is based on the clinical presentation and history of the tick bite, if known. Serological tests are used to confirm the diagnosis, although there is a delayed antibody response and the test may be negative during the first 3 weeks after infection.[48] Antibiotics (e.g., doxycycline [Teva-Doxycycline], which is not used in children younger than 8 years of age or in pregnant or breastfeeding women, or amoxicillin [Amoxil]) are used for treatment.[49] Re-infection can occur. There is currently no vaccine for Lyme disease.[50]

Viral Infections

Herpes simplex virus. Skin infections with **herpes simplex virus (HSV)** are commonly caused by two types of HSV: HSV-1 and HSV-2. Either type can occur in different parts of the body, including oral and genital locations. Their differences are distinguished by laboratory tests. HSV-1, transmitted by contact with infected saliva, is generally associated with oral infections (cold sore or fever blister) or infection of the cornea (herpes keratitis), mouth (gingivostomatitis), and orolabia (lips/labialis), but it can also cause genital herpes. With initial (primary) infection, the virus is imbedded in sensory nerve endings and it moves by retrograde axonal transport to the dorsal root ganglion, where the virus develops lifelong latency. During the secondary phase, the lesions occur at the same site from reactivation of the virus. The virus travels down the peripheral nerve to the site of the original infection, where it is shed. Exposure to UV light, skin irritation, fever, fatigue, or stress may cause reactivation.[51]

The lesions for HSV-1 appear as a rash or clusters of inflamed and painful vesicles (e.g., within the mouth, over the tongue, on the lips, around the nose) (Figure 41-16). Increased sensitivity, paresthesias, pruritus, and mild burning may occur before onset of the lesions. The vesicles rupture, forming a crust. Lesions may last from 2 to 6 weeks but usually resolve within 2 weeks. Treatment is symptomatic and includes topical or oral antiviral agents.[52]

Genital infections are more commonly caused by HSV-2. The virus is spread by skin-to-skin mucous membrane contact during viral shedding. Risk for infection is high in immunosuppressed persons or in persons who have sexual contact with infected individuals. Vertical transmission from mother to neonate is associated with significant neonatal neurological morbidity and mortality.[53] The initial infection is asymptomatic. With recurrent exposure, the lesions begin as small vesicles that progress to ulceration within 3 to 4 days with pain, itching, and weeping. Treatment is symptomatic and includes topical or oral antiviral agents. A vaccine has been effective in controlling recurrent infection, and progress is being made with prophylactic vaccines.[54]

Herpes zoster and varicella. **Herpes zoster (shingles)** and **varicella (chickenpox**, see Chapter 42) are caused by the same herpesvirus—varicella-zoster virus (VZV). VZV occurs as a primary infection followed years later by activation of the virus to cause herpes zoster (shingles). During this time, the virus remains latent in trigeminal and dorsal root ganglia.

Herpes zoster has initial symptoms of pain and paresthesia localized to the affected dermatome (the cutaneous area innervated by a single spinal nerve; see Chapter 13), followed by vesicular eruptions that follow a facial, cervical, or thoracic lumbar dermatome (Figure 41-17). Local symptoms are alleviated with compresses, calamine lotion, or baking soda. Approximately 15 to 20% of individuals experience postherpetic neuralgia (pain) with reactivation of the virus.[55] Antiviral medications, tricyclic antidepressants, and analgesics are helpful treatments. The varicella vaccine is safe and effective in both children and adults, particularly those older than age 60. In children, the vaccine is given to prevent chickenpox; and in adults, particularly the older adult, the vaccine is given to prevent herpes zoster (shingles).[56]

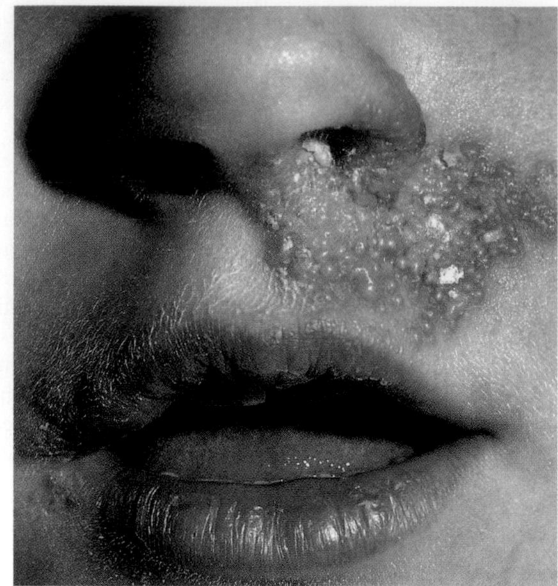

FIGURE 41-16 Herpes Simplex of the Lips (Labialis). Typical presentation with tense vesicles appearing on the lips and extending onto the skin. (From Habif, T.P. [2004]. *Clinical dermatology: A color guide to diagnosis and therapy* [4th ed.]. St. Louis: Mosby.)

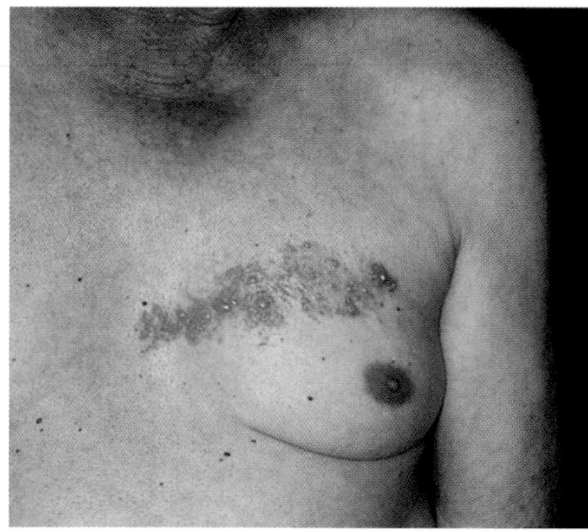

FIGURE 41-17 Herpes Zoster. Diffuse involvement of a dermatome. (Courtesy Department of Dermatology, School of Medicine, University of Utah, Salt Lake City, UT.)

Warts. **Warts** (verrucae) are benign lesions of the skin caused by the many different types of **human papillomavirus (HPV)** that infect the stratified epithelium of skin and mucous membranes. The lesions can occur anywhere and are flat, round, or fusiform and elevated with a rough, greyish surface. Warts are transmitted by touch. Common warts

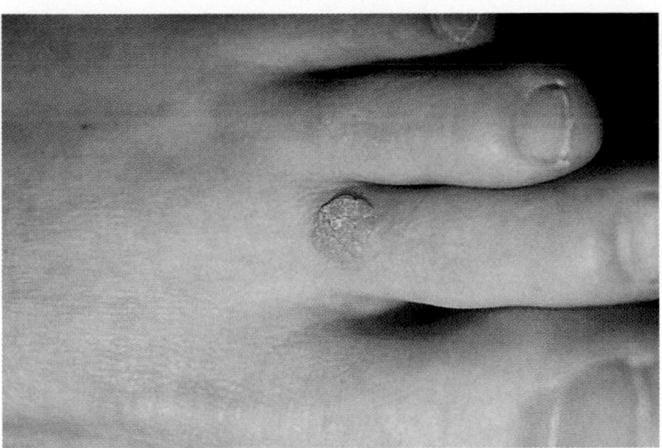

FIGURE 41-18 Verruca Vulgaris (Near Toes). (Courtesy Department of Dermatology, School of Medicine, University of Utah, Salt Lake City, UT.)

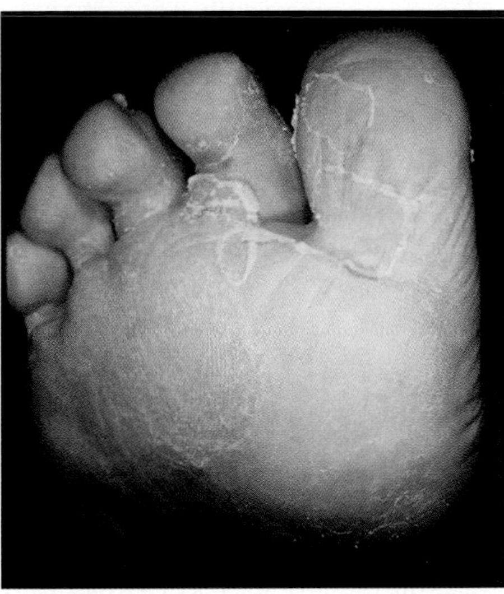

FIGURE 41-19 Tinea Pedis. Inflammation has extended from the web area onto the dorsum of the foot. (Courtesy Department of Dermatology, School of Medicine, University of Utah, Salt Lake City, UT.)

(verruca vulgaris) occur most often in children and are usually on the fingers (Figure 41-18). Plantar warts are usually located at pressure points on the bottom of the feet. Warts are commonly treated with cryotherapy or topical salicylic acid; new agents are being investigated.[57,58]

Condylomata acuminata (venereal warts) are highly contagious and sexually transmitted. The cauliflowerlike lesions occur in moist areas, along the glans of the penis, vulva, and anus. Oncogenic types of HPV are a primary cause of cervical and other types of cancer[59] (see Chapter 33).

Fungal Infections

The fungi causing superficial skin infections are called *dermatophytes*, and they thrive on keratin (stratum corneum, hair, nails). Fungal disorders are known as *mycoses*; when caused by dermatophytes, the mycoses are termed *tinea* (dermatophytosis or ringworm).

Tinea infections. Tinea infections are classified according to their location on the body. The most common sites are summarized in Table 41-5 (Figure 41-19).

Tinea is diagnosed by culture, microscopic examination of skin scrapings prepared with potassium hydroxide (KOH) wet mount, or observation of the skin with a UV light (Wood's lamp). Cultures establish the particular type of fungus; identification is necessary for diagnosis

TABLE 41-5 Common Sites of Tinea Infections

Site	Clinical Manifestations
Tinea capitis (scalp)	Scaly, pruritic scalp with bald areas; hair breaks easily
Tinea corporis (skin areas, excluding scalp, face, hands, feet, groin)	Circular, clearly circumscribed, mildly erythematous scaly patches with slightly elevated ringlike border; some forms are dry and macular, and other forms are moist and vesicular
Tinea cruris (groin, also known as "jock itch")	Small, erythematous, and scaling vesicular patches with well-defined borders that spread over inner and upper surfaces of thighs; occurs with heat and high humidity
Tinea pedis (foot; also known as "athlete's foot")	Lesions between toes, which may spread to soles of feet, nails, and skin or toes; slight scaling; macerated, painful skin, occasionally with fissures and vesiculation
Tinea manus (hand)	Dry, scaly, erythematous lesions, or moist, vesicular lesions that begin with clusters of intensely pruritic, clear vesicles; often associated with fungal infection of feet
Tinea unguium or onychomycosis (nails)	Superficial or deep inflammation of nail that develops yellow-brown accumulations of brittle keratin over all or portions of nail

of hair and nail infections. Fungi have characteristic spores and filaments known as *hyphae* that are more prominent when prepared in KOH. The spores fluoresce blue-green when exposed to UV light. Treatment is related to the type of fungi and includes both topical and systemic antifungal medication.[60]

Candidiasis. Candidiasis is caused by the yeastlike fungus *Candida albicans* and normally can be found on mucous membranes, on the skin, in the gastro-intestinal tract, and in the vagina. *C. albicans* can, under certain circumstances, change from a commensal (normal) microorganism to a pathogen, particularly in the critically ill and those who are immunosuppressed.[61]

Factors that predispose to infection include (1) local environment of moisture, warmth, maceration, or occlusion; (2) systemic administration of antibiotics; (3) pregnancy; (4) diabetes mellitus; (5) Cushing's disease; (6) debilitated states; (7) infants younger than 6 months of age, as a result of decreased immune reactivity; (8) immunosuppressed persons; and (9) certain neoplastic diseases of the blood and monocyte/macrophage system. The commensal (normal) bacteria on the skin, mainly cocci, inhibit proliferation of *C. albicans. C. albicans* can activate the complement system by the alternative pathway and produce small abscesses. Candidiasis affects only the outer layers of mucous membranes and skin and occurs in the mouth, vagina, uncircumcised penis, nail folds, interdigital areas, and large skin folds. Table 41-6 lists the points of differentiation of various sites of candidiasis habitation.

The initial lesion is a thin-walled pustule that extends under the stratum corneum with an inflammatory base that may burn or itch. The accumulation of inflammatory cells and scale produces a whitish yellow curdlike substance over the infected area. The lesion ceases to spread when it reaches dry skin.[62] Topical antifungal agents are commonly used for treatment.

Vascular Disorders

Vascular abnormalities are commonly associated with skin diseases; they may be congenital or may involve vascular responses to local or

TABLE 41-6 Sites of Candidiasis Infection

Site	Risk Factors	Clinical Manifestations	Treatment
Vagina (vulvovaginitis)	Heat, moisture, occlusive clothing Pregnancy Systemic antibiotic therapy Diabetes mellitus Sexual intercourse with infected male	Vaginal itching; white, watery, or creamy discharge Red, swollen vaginal and labial membranes with erosions Lesions, which may spread to anus and groin	Miconazole (Monistat) cream Clotrimazole (Canesten) tablets or cream Nystatin (Nyaderm) tablets Ketoconazole (Nizoral) cream Loose cotton clothing
Penis (balanitis)	Uncircumcised Sexual intercourse with infected female	Pinpoint, red, tender papules and pustules on glans and shaft of penis	Any of the creams listed above Topical steroids for severe inflammation
Mouth	Diabetes mellitus Immunosuppressive therapy Inhaled steroid therapy	Red, swollen, painful tongue and oral mucous membranes Localized erosions and plaques appear with chronic infection	Nystatin (Nyaderm) oral suspension Clotrimazole troches Ketoconazole

systemic vasoactive substances. Blood vessels may increase in number, dilate, constrict, or become obliterated by disease processes.

Cutaneous Vasculitis

Vasculitis (angiitis) is an inflammation of the blood vessel wall that can result in bleeding aneurysm formation, or occlusion with ischemia or infection of surrounding tissue. The extensive vascular bed in the skin results in vasculitic syndromes that may be localized and self-limiting or generalized with multiorgan involvement. The initiating site may be the blood, the vessel wall, or the adjacent tissue. Small vessels are usually affected.

Cutaneous vasculitis develops from the deposit of immune complexes in small blood vessels as a toxic response to medications (phenothiazines, barbiturates, sulfonamides), allergens, or streptococcal or viral infection, or as a component of systemic vasculitic syndromes. The deposits activate complement, which is chemotactic for polymorphonuclear leukocytes, and proinflammatory cytokines.

The disorder is also known as *cutaneous leukocytoclastic angiitis* (from the presence of leukocytes [i.e., neutrophils] in and around vessel walls). A systemic form (cutaneous systemic vasculitis) can involve other organs, including the kidneys, lungs, and gastro-intestinal tract. The pattern of skin involvement includes palpable purpura in the lower legs and feet (from the leakage of blood from damaged vessels) that may progress to hemorrhagic bullae with necrosis and ulceration from occlusion of the vessel. Lesions appear in clusters and persist for 1 to 4 weeks. The disease may be self-limiting and occur as a single episode. Biopsy confirms the diagnosis.

Identifying and removing the antigen (chemical, medication, or source of infection) is the first step of treatment. Corticosteroids and immunosuppressants may be used when symptoms are severe.[63]

Urticaria

Urticaria (hives) is a circumscribed area of raised erythema and edema of the superficial dermis. **Urticarial lesions** are most commonly associated with type I hypersensitivity reactions to medications (penicillin, Aspirin), certain foods (strawberries, shellfish, food dyes), environmental exposure (pollen, animal dander, insect bites), systemic diseases (intestinal parasites, lupus erythematosus), or physical agents (heat or cold) (see Chapter 8). The lesions are mediated by histamine release from sensitized mast cells or basophils, or both, which causes the endothelial cells of skin blood vessels to contract. The leakage of fluid from the vessel appears as wheals, welts, or hives, and there may be few or many that may be distributed over the entire body. Most lesions resolve spontaneously within 24 hours, but new lesions may appear. All possible causes of the reaction should be removed. Antihistamines usually reduce hives and provide relief of itching. Corticosteroids and β-adrenergic agonists may be required for severe attacks. **Chronic urticaria** (recurrent wheals for more than 6 weeks) is either idiopathic or autoimmune in origin and involves inappropriate activation of mast cells.[64] Angioedema (welts or swelling deeper within the skin or mucous membranes) is associated with both groups and more commonly affects the eyes and mouth.

Scleroderma

Localized scleroderma (morphea) means sclerosis of the skin and underlying tissue. The disease is rare and more common in females, and the cause is unknown. Genetic predisposition, autoimmunity, and an immune reaction to a toxic substance are possible initiating mechanisms of the disease. Autoantibodies are often recovered from the skin and serum of individuals with scleroderma. Impaired regulation of collagen gene expression by fibroblasts probably underlies the persistent fibrosis. There are subtypes of localized scleroderma but all involve thickening of the skin. Localized scleroderma is differentiated from the systemic form of the disease by the absence of the following: sclerodactyly, Raynaud phenomenon, abnormalities of the nail bed capillaries, or internal organ involvement.[65]

Systemic scleroderma involves the connective tissues of the skin and many organs, including the kidneys, gastro-intestinal tract, and lungs. There are massive deposits of type I collagen with progressive fibrosis accompanied by inflammatory reactions as well as vascular changes in the capillary network with a decrease in the number of capillary loops, dilation of the remaining capillaries, formation of perivascular infiltrates, and development of occlusion and ischemia.[66]

The clinical features of systemic scleroderma can be summarized using the CREST acronym as a guide:

*C*alcinosis—calcium deposits in the subcutaneous tissue that cause pain
*R*aynaud phenomenon—episodes of arteriolar vasoconstriction or spasm in response to cold or stress
*E*sophageal changes—swallowing difficulty related to acid reflux and increased esophageal fibrosis
*S*clerodactyly—tightening of skin over the fingers and toes leading to tapering of the digits with scarring and tissue atrophy
*T*elangiectasias—dilation of capillaries causing small (0.5 cm), weblike red marks on skin surface

The cutaneous lesions are most often on the face and hands, the neck, and the upper chest, although the entire skin can be involved. The skin is hard, hypopigmented, taut, shiny, and tightly connected to the underlying tissue. The tightness of the facial skin projects an immobile masklike appearance, and the mouth may not open completely. The

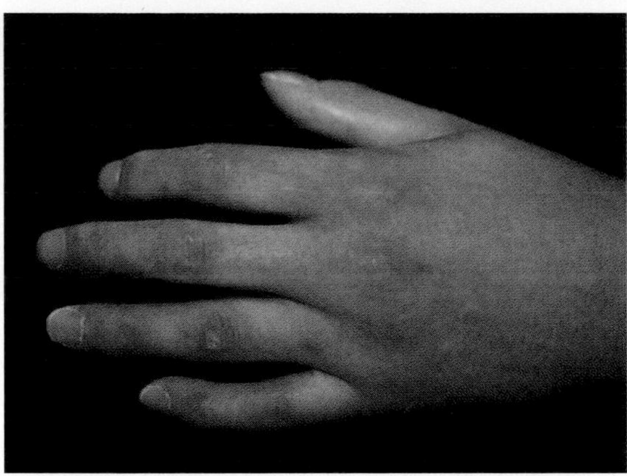

FIGURE 41-20 Scleroderma. Note the inflammation and shiny skin resulting from a combination of Raynaud phenomena and scleroderma affecting the fingers (acrosclerosis). (Courtesy Department of Dermatology, School of Medicine, University of Utah, Salt Lake City, UT.)

nose may assume a beaklike appearance. The hands are shiny and sometimes red and edematous (Figure 41-20). Progression to body organs may occur, and death is caused by subsequent respiratory failure, kidney failure, cardiac dysrhythmias, or esophageal or intestinal obstruction or perforation.[67]

Suitable clothing and a warm environment are essential for protecting the hands. Trauma and smoking should be avoided. Treatment is individualized and based on severity and progression of the disease. Immunosuppression, UV treatment, and other therapies are prescribed.[68]

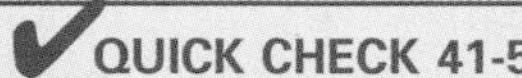

QUICK CHECK 41-5

1. Name two bacterial skin infections, and describe the typical lesions.
2. Compare herpes zoster and varicella.
3. What features distinguish urticarial lesions?

Benign Tumours

Most benign tumours of the skin are associated with aging. Benign tumours include seborrheic keratosis, keratoacanthoma, actinic keratosis, and moles.

Seborrheic Keratosis

Seborrheic keratosis is a benign proliferation of cutaneous basal cells that produces flat or slightly elevated lesions that may be smooth or warty in appearance. The pathogenesis is unknown. These benign tumours are usually seen in older adults and occur as multiple lesions on the chest, back, and face. The colour varies from tan to waxy yellow, flesh coloured, or dark brown-black. Lesion size varies from a few millimetres to several centimetres, and they are often oval and greasy appearing with a hyperkeratotic scale (Figure 41-21). Cryotherapy with liquid nitrogen and laser therapy are effective treatments.

Keratoacanthoma

A **keratoacanthoma** is a benign, self-limiting tumour of squamous cell differentiation arising from hair follicles. It usually occurs on sun-damaged skin of older adults. Incidence is highest among smokers and males. The most commonly affected sites are the face, back of the hands, forearms, neck, and legs. The lesion develops in stages (proliferative, mature, and involution) over a period of 1 to 2 months with a histological pattern resembling squamous cell carcinoma (SCC).

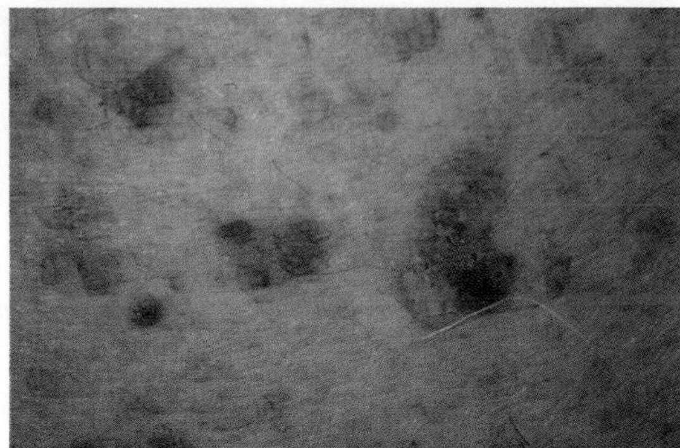

FIGURE 41-21 Seborrheic Keratosis. Typical lesion that is broad, flat, and comparatively smooth surfaced. (Courtesy Department of Dermatology, School of Medicine, University of Utah, Salt Lake City, UT.)

Although the lesions resolve in 3 to 4 months, they can be removed by curettage or excision to improve cosmetic appearance and reduce the risk for evolution to SCC. A biopsy is performed to rule out SCC.

Actinic Keratosis

Actinic keratosis is a premalignant lesion composed of aberrant proliferations of epidermal keratinocytes caused by prolonged exposure to UVR. The prevalence is highest in individuals with unprotected, fair skin and is rare in those with darkly pigmented skin. The lesions appear as rough, poorly defined papules, which may be felt more than seen. Surrounding areas may have telangiectasias. Treatment options include cryoablation, photodynamic therapy, laser surgery, and topical therapies, such as 5-fluorouracil [Adrucil], diclofenac [Voltaren], imiquimod cream [Aldara], and ingenol mebutate [Picato].[69]

Excisions also may be performed, providing tissue for cellular analysis. The lesions should continue to be evaluated for progression to SCC. Protection from the sun with clothing or a sun-blocking agent to prevent lesions from developing elsewhere is advised.

Nevi (Moles)

Nevi (*sing.*, **nevus**) (also known as *moles* or *birthmarks*) are benign pigmented or nonpigmented lesions. Melanocytic nevi, formed from melanocytes, may be congenital or acquired and small (less than 1 cm) or large (greater than 20 cm). Congenital melanocytic nevi may be removed to reduce risk for cutaneous malignant melanoma.[70] During the early stages of development, the cells accumulate at the junction of the dermis and epidermis and are macular lesions. Over time, the cells move deeper into the dermis and the nevi become nodular and symmetric without irregular borders. Nevi may appear on any part of the skin, vary in size, occur singly or in groups, and may undergo transition to malignant melanoma (see p. 1093). Classification of nevi is summarized in Table 41-7. Nevi irritated by clothing or trauma or large lesions may be excised. Multiple and changing moles require regular evaluation.[71]

QUICK CHECK 41-6

1. List two diseases caused by insect bites.
2. Compare keratoacanthoma and actinic keratosis.

Skin Cancer

Basal cell carcinoma (BCC) and SCC (collectively known as *nonmelanoma skin cancers*) are the most prevalent forms of cancer. Malignant melanoma is the most serious and most common cause of death from skin cancer. Important trends related to skin cancer are described in Box 41-1.

BOX 41-1 Important Trends for Skin Cancer

Incidence
- Skin cancer is the seventh most commonly diagnosed cancer in Canada.
- Malignant melanoma is the most serious form of skin cancer; however, it is not as common as the other forms of skin cancer; an estimated 5 800 new cases were predicted in 2012, with 970 deaths.
- One in 3 cancers diagnosed worldwide is skin cancer.
- Skin cancer is the second most common cancer among young adults.

Mortality
- Total estimated deaths from skin cancer in 2015 were 13 340: 9 940 from malignant melanoma and 3 400 from other nonepithelial skin cancers.

Survival
- Basal and squamous cell carcinoma can be cured when detected early.
- Five-year survival for melanoma: it can be cured if diagnosed and removed early.

Risk Factors
- Excessive exposure to ultraviolet radiation from the sun or tanning salons
- Fair complexion
- Darkly pigmented skin: in people with darkly pigmented skin, skin cancer is less common, is diagnosed at a more advanced stage, and has a higher morbidity and mortality than in people with fair skin; it is often found on the palms of hands and soles of feet
- Occupational exposure to coal tar, pitch, creosote, arsenic compounds, and radium
- Immunosuppression

Warning Signs
- Any unusual skin condition, especially a change in the size, borders, or colour of a mole or other darkly pigmented growth or spot

Prevention and Early Detection
- Avoid the sun when ultraviolet light is strongest (e.g., 10 a.m. to 3 p.m.), avoid sun tanning beds, seek shade, use sunscreen preparations, especially those containing ingredients such as PABA (*para*-aminobenzoic acid), and wear protective clothing.
- Basal and squamous cell skin cancers often form a pale, waxlike pearly nodule or a red, scaly, sharply outlined patch.
- Melanomas usually have dark brown or black pigmentation; they start as small molelike growths that increase in size, change colour, become ulcerated, and bleed easily from slight injury.

Treatment
- Options for treatment include surgery, electrodesiccation (tissue destruction by heat), radiation therapy, cryosurgery (tissue destruction by freezing).
- Malignant melanomas require wide and often deep excisions and removal of nearby lymph nodes; selective lymphadenectomy or immunotherapy can be used; vaccines and gene therapy are in development.

Survival
- For basal cell and squamous cell cancers, cure is virtually ensured with early detection and treatment; malignant melanoma, however, metastasizes quickly and accounts for a lower 5-year survival rate.

Data from Canadian Cancer Society, & Statistics Canada. (2016). Canadian cancer statistics 2016. Retrieved from http://www.cancer.ca/~/media/cancer.ca/CW/cancer%20information/cancer%20101/Canadian%20cancer%20statistics/Canadian-Cancer-Statistics-2016-EN.pdf?la=e; Canadian Skin Cancer Foundation. (n.d.). About skin cancer. http://www.canadianskincancerfoundation.com/about-skin-cancer.html.

TABLE 41-7 Classification of Nevi

Type	Common Characteristics
Junctional nevus	Flat, well-circumscribed; vary in size up to 2 cm; dark-coloured hairs may be present; originate in basal layer of epidermis and can eventually reach cutaneous surface; most likely to develop into melanoma
Compound nevus	Most common in adolescents; majority of pigmented lesions in children; rarely does this lesion develop into melanoma; usually 1 cm in size; hairs may be present; surface is elevated and smooth
Intradermal nevus	Small, less than 1 cm, with regular edges and bristlelike hairs; colour ranges from fair skin tone to light brown; has slight likelihood of developing into melanoma

Chronic exposure to UVR causes most skin cancers. Lesions are most common on the face, neck, hands, and other areas with intense sunlight exposure. Protection from the sun and avoidance of tanning beds, particularly during childhood, significantly reduce the risk for skin cancer in later years. Genetic mutations in oncogenes and tumour-suppressor genes (see Chapter 10) are associated with skin cancers. These mutations lead to loss of keratinocyte repair functions and apoptosis resistance of DNA-damaged cells.[72] People with darkly pigmented skin and those who avoid sunlight are significantly less likely to develop these malignant tumours. In people with darkly pigmented skin, basal cells contain more of the pigment melanin, a protective factor against sun exposure. Vitamin D may be an important tumour suppressor for the skin, but more research is needed.[73]

Basal Cell Carcinoma

Basal cell carcinoma (BCC) of the skin is the most common cancer in the world, making it the most common skin cancer by default. BCC is thought to be caused by UVR exposure and also is associated with arsenic in food or water.

BCCs have numerous subtypes, including superficial, nodular, pigmented, morpheaform, and combinations of each; thus, they can have very different clinical presentations—from superficial erythematous papules; to thick, pigmented nodules resembling melanomas; to erosive, necrotic, and ulcerating lesions (Figure 41-22). As the tumour grows it usually has a depressed centre, a rolled border, and small blood vessels on the surface (telangiectasias) (see Figure 41-22). Early tumours are so small they are not clinically apparent. The lesion grows slowly, often ulcerates, develops crusts, and is firm to the touch. If left untreated, basal cell lesions invade surrounding tissues and, over months or years, can destroy a nose, eyelid, or ear (for treatment, see Box 41-1). Metastasis is rare because these tumours do not invade blood or lymph vessels.

Squamous Cell Carcinoma

Squamous cell carcinoma (SCC) of the skin is a tumour of the epidermis and is the second most common human cancer. Two types are characterized: in situ (including Bowen's disease) and invasive. UVR exposure causes SCC and actinic keratosis is a precursor lesion. Other

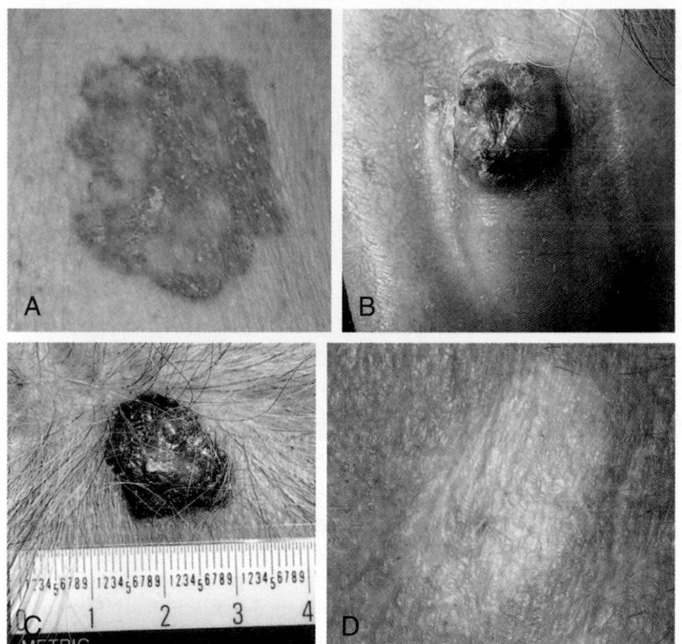

FIGURE 41-22 Types of Basal Cell Carcinoma. A, Superficial. **B,** Nodular. **C,** Pigmented. **D,** Morpheaform—recurrent tumour. (**A** and **D,** from Bolognia, J.L., Jorizzo, J., & Schaffer, J. [2012]. *Dermatology* [3rd ed.]. Philadelphia: Saunders; **B** and **C,** from James, W.D., Berger, T.G., & Elston, D.M. [2009]. *Andrews' diseases of the skin: Clinical dermatology* [11th ed.]. Philadelphia: Saunders.)

risk factors include arsenic at a higher level in drinking water, exposure to X-rays and gamma rays, immunosuppression, and fair skin. *P53* gene mutations are common in SCC and produce tumour cells resistant to apoptosis.[72]

Premalignant lesions include actinic keratosis, leukoplakia (whitish discoloured areas), scars, radiation-induced keratosis, tar and oil keratosis, and chronic ulcers. In situ SCC is usually confined to the epidermis (intraepidermal) but may extend into the dermis. Bowen's disease is a dysplastic epidermal lesion often found on unexposed areas of the body such as the penis and demonstrated by flat, reddish, scaly patches. These lesions rarely invade surrounding tissue and, although they rarely metastasize, they do so more often than BCCs. Other components of the skin (e.g., sweat glands, hair follicles) can develop into skin cancer, but this outcome is relatively uncommon.

SCC is the most common cause of lip cancer, prevalent in older White men, with about 3 000 new cases per year.[74] The lower lip is the most common site. Long-term environmental exposure results in dryness, chapping, hyperkeratosis, and predisposition to malignancy. Immunosuppression, pipe smoking, and chronic alcoholism increase the risk for lip cancer. The most common lesion is termed *exophytic* and usually develops in the outer part of the lip along the vermilion border. The lip becomes thickened and evolves to an ulcerated centre with a raised border (Figure 41-23). These lesions have an irregular surface, follow cracks in the lip, and tend to extend toward the inner surface.

Invasive SCC can arise from premalignant lesions of the skin; it rarely develops from normal-appearing skin and is usually confined to the epidermis (intraepidermal), but may extend into the reticular layer of the dermis (see Table 41-1). Invasive SCCs grow more rapidly than BCCs and can spread to regional lymph nodes. These tumours are firm and increase in both elevation and diameter. The surface may be granular and bleed easily (Figure 41-24). Treatment includes surgical excision

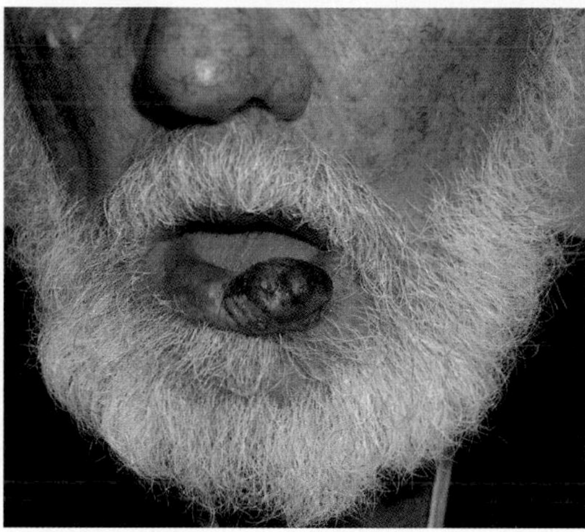

FIGURE 41-23 Lip Cancer. Biopsy confirmed squamous cell carcinoma. Lip vermilion shows diffuse actinic keratosis. (From Bagheri, S.C., Bell, B., & Khan, H.A. [2012]. *Current therapy in oral and maxillofacial surgery.* Philadelphia: Saunders.)

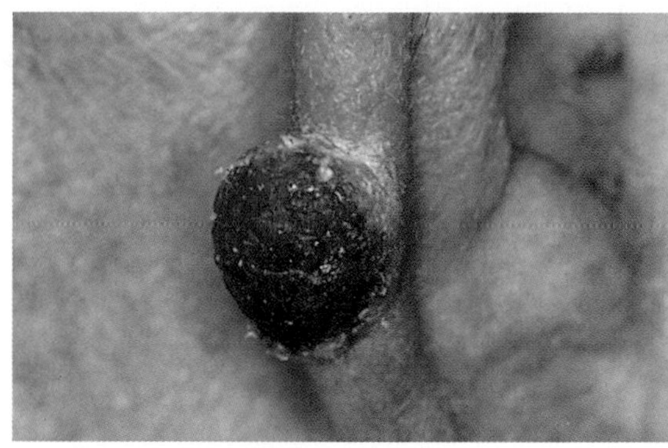

FIGURE 41-24 Squamous Cell Carcinoma. The sun-exposed ear is a common site for squamous cell carcinoma. (Courtesy Department of Dermatology, School of Medicine, University of Utah, Salt Lake City, UT.)

and radiotherapy with consideration of adjuvant chemotherapy or epithelial growth factor receptor inhibitors for advanced disease.[75]

Cutaneous Melanoma

Cutaneous melanoma is a malignant tumour of the skin originating from melanocytes, cells that synthesize the pigment melanin, and arise from the neural crest. Malignant melanoma is the most serious skin cancer. The Canadian Cancer Society estimated that 7 300 Canadians (4 000 men and 3 300 women) were diagnosed with melanoma skin cancer in 2017. It also estimated that about 1 250 Canadians (790 men and 450 women) died of this disease in 2017.[76]

Melanoma also can arise in the uvea of the eye and on mucous membranes.[77] The incidence is increasing worldwide. Risk factors include a personal or family history (or both), UVR exposure (including sunbed use before age 30), immunosuppression, fair hair, fair skin with repeated sunburns, freckles, being a younger female, being an older male, geographical location, past pesticide exposure, and three or more clinically atypical (dysplastic) nevi[78] (see *Health Promotion:* Melanoma in People With Darkly Pigmented Skin). Melanoma is the most common cancer in White women 25 to 29 years old.[79]

Cutaneous melanomas arise as a result of malignant degeneration of melanocytes located either along the basal layer of the epidermis (see Figure 41-1) or in a benign melanocytic nevus. The clinical varieties

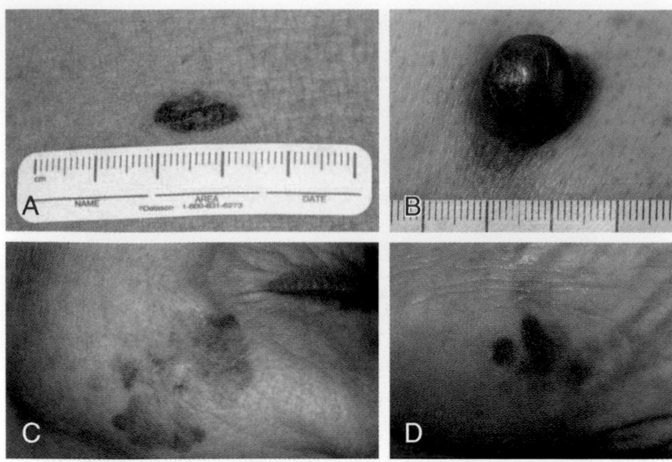

FIGURE 41-25 **Lentigo Malignant Melanoma.** **A,** Superficial spreading melanoma. **B,** Nodular melanoma. **C,** Lentigo malignant melanoma. **D,** Acral lentiginous melanoma on plantar surface of foot. (From Bolognia, J.L., Schaffer, J., Duncan, K., et al. [2014]. *Dermatology essentials.* Philadelphia: Saunders.)

HEALTH PROMOTION

Melanoma in People With Darkly Pigmented Skin

The risk for melanoma is lower in people with darkly pigmented skin. However, they have more advanced disease when diagnosed and a higher death rate. Associated factors include location of the lesion on palms, soles, and subungual sites (e.g., acral lentiginous melanoma) and lower socioeconomic status and education level. These melanomas may represent molecularly distinct cancers that are inherently more aggressive. The location of the lesions may contribute to delayed detection or misdiagnosis. The role of ultraviolet radiation in the risk for melanoma in people with darkly pigmented skin is not clear and research is needed. Genetic mutations may be a contributing factor. Educational programs to increase awareness of risk for melanoma among people with darkly pigmented skin, screening, and self-examination can improve outcomes.

Data from Alexandrescu, D.T., Maslin, B., Kauffman, C.L., et al. (2013). *Dermatol Surg, 39*(9), 1291–1303; Rouhani, P., Hu, S., & Kirsner, R.S. (2008). *Cancer Control, 15*(3), 248–253; Stubblefield, J., & Kelly, B. (2014). *Surg Clin North Am, 94*(5), 1115–1126.

of cutaneous melanoma include superficial spreading melanoma (SSM), the most common; lentigo malignant melanoma (LMM) (Figure 41-25), frequently found in older adults and confused with age spots; primary nodular melanoma (PNM), an aggressive tumour; and acral lentiginous melanoma (ALM), which is rare and aggressive and occurs on non-hair-bearing surfaces (i.e., palms of the hands and soles of the feet) and mucous membranes in people with darker skin.

The pathogenesis of malignant melanoma is complex. Most familial melanomas are associated with cyclin-dependent kinase 4 gene (*CDK4*) and cyclin-dependent kinase inhibitor 2A gene (*p16/CDKN2A*), located on chromosome 9p21. The *CDKN2A* gene encodes two potent tumour-suppressor proteins (p16 and $p14^{ARF}$) that are cell-cycle inhibitors. Both *CDKN2A* and *CDK4* are highly penetrant susceptibility genes and result in melanomas. A number of proto-oncogenes have been identified, including *BRAF* point mutations and genes involved in the regulation of mitogen-activated protein kinase (MAPK), and other signalling pathways. Melanomas have a high mutation rate stimulated by UVR, making gene sequencing difficult.[80]

The relationship between nevi and melanoma makes it important for the clinician to understand the various forms of nevi (see Table 41-7). Most nevi never become suspicious; however, suspicious pigmented nevi need to be evaluated and removed.[71] Indications for biopsy, including sentinel lymph node biopsy, are colour change, size change, irregular notched margin, itching, bleeding or oozing, nodularity, scab formation, and ulceration or an unusual pattern of presentation. The ABCDE rule is used as a guide: *A*symmetry, *B*order irregularity, *C*olour variation, *D*iameter larger than 6 mm, and *E*levation or *E*volving, which includes raised appearance or rapid enlargement. Staging is determined by lesion thickness (presence of *t*umour), lymph *n*ode involvement, and presence of *m*etastasis (TNM staging).[81]

Treatment of melanoma with no evidence of metastatic disease involves a wide surgical excision of the primary lesion site. A lymph node biopsy of the peripherally draining lymph node (sentinel node) is warranted for lesions greater than 1 mm deep. Lesions on the extremities have the best surgical prognosis. Radiation therapy, chemotherapy, and immunotherapy inhibiting the MAPK pathway and *BRAF* mutations are used to treat metastatic disease and have demonstrated long-term improvement in disease outcome.[82] Promising new immunotherapies are used for advanced disease, including checkpoint inhibitors (anti-PD1 antibodies [pembrolizumab (Keytruda), nivolumab (Opdivo)], anti-CTLA4 (cytotoxic T-lymphocyte associated protein 4) antibody [ipilimumab (Yervoy)]), and targeted therapy (*BRAF* or *MEK* inhibition, or both).[83] Vaccines, cell therapy, and biomarkers are under continuing investigation.[84] Early detection is critical to decreasing mortality from metastatic disease.

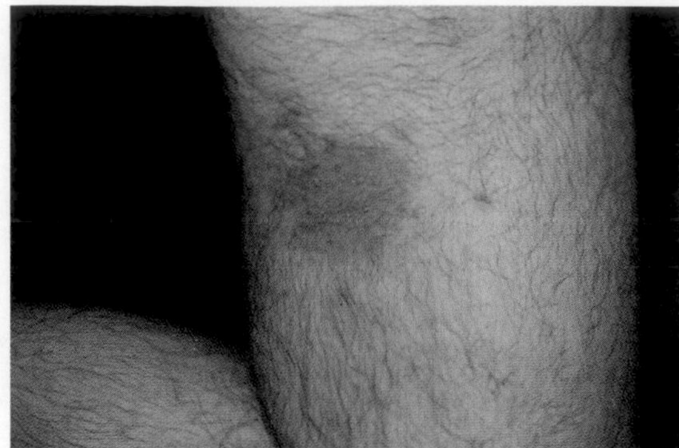

FIGURE 41-26 **Kaposi Sarcoma.** The purple lesion commonly seen on the skin. (Courtesy Department of Dermatology, School of Medicine, University of Utah, Salt Lake City, UT.)

Kaposi Sarcoma

Kaposi sarcoma (KS) is a vascular malignancy associated with immunodeficiency states and occurs among transplant recipients taking immunosuppressive medications. Genetic and environmental cofactors determine disease progression. Human herpesvirus 8 (HHV8) is found in the lesions of KS. Four forms of the disease have been described: classic (more benign), epidemic (rapidly progressive and associated with acquired immune deficiency syndrome [AIDS]), African endemic, and iatrogenic (associated with immunosuppressant treatment, including organ transplant).[85]

The endothelial cell is thought to be the progenitor of KS. The lesions emerge as purplish-brown macules and develop into plaques and nodules with angioproliferation. They tend to be multifocal rather than spreading by metastasis. The lesions initially appear over the lower extremities in the classic form (Figure 41-26). The rapidly progressive form associated with AIDS tends to spread symmetrically over the upper body, particularly the face and oral mucosa. The lesions are often pruritic and painful. About 75% of individuals with epidemic KS have involvement of lymph nodes, particularly in the gastro-intestinal tract and lungs. Organ involvement is much less common in the classic form. The rapidly progressive form has a poor prognosis and shorter survival rates than the classic form. (See Chapter 8 for a further discussion of AIDS.)

Diagnosis is by medical history, physical examination, and skin biopsy, with a high index of suspicion for those with immunodeficiency. Chest X-ray reveals lesions in the lungs. Local lesions can be excised. Multiple disseminated lesions may be treated with a combination of α-interferon, radiotherapy, and cytotoxic medications. Antiangiogenic agents are being tested. Individuals receiving highly active antiretroviral therapy (HAART) have a markedly reduced incidence of KS.[86]

Primary Cutaneous Lymphomas

Primary cutaneous lymphomas are cutaneous T-cell and B-cell lymphomas present in the skin without evidence of extracutaneous disease at the time of diagnosis (see Chapter 21 for classification and general pathophysiology of lymphomas). Cutaneous lymphomas are rare but are the second most common site of extranodal non-Hodgkin lymphoma. The incidence rate is about 1 per 100 000, and the cause of these lesions is unknown.[87] Cutaneous lymphomas are more common in men and generally present after age 50.

Cutaneous lymphomas develop from clonal expansion of B cells, T-helper cells, and rarely T-suppressor cells. The most common is cutaneous T-cell lymphoma (66%), and mycosis fungoides is the most prominent subtype. **Mycosis fungoides** can present as focal or widespread erythematous patches or plaques, follicular papules, comedonelike lesions, and tumours. There may be patches of alopecia. The lesions progress over a period of months or years.

The differential diagnosis of the different types of cutaneous lymphomas is based on clinical manifestations, histological appearance, immunological and cytogenetic features, and response to appropriate treatment. Treatment is based on staging of the disease and includes topical and systemic medications and phototherapy.[88,89]

> **QUICK CHECK 41-7**
> 1. What is the most common skin cancer?
> 2. What malignancy can arise from melanocytes?
> 3. How is Kaposi sarcoma related to AIDS?

Burns

The incidence of burn injuries has declined in the past several years. In 2010, there were 234 deaths due to burns in Canada, with 43 684 hospital visits.[90] Burns may be caused by thermal or nonthermal sources including chemical, electrical, or radioactive sources. Thermal injuries result from thermal contact, scalds, or radiation. Direct contact, inhalation, and ingestion of acids, alkalis, or blistering agents cause chemical burns. Electrical burns occur with the passage of electrical current through the body to the ground or electrical flames or flashes. In addition to cutaneous injury, burns can be associated with smoke inhalation and other traumatic injuries that exacerbate local and systemic responses. Ventilatory support is often needed with inhalation injury.[91]

Burn Wound Depth

The depth of injury identifies the level of tissue destruction; the extent of injury determines clinical management, healing, and mortality. The depth of the burn is divided into four categories and is summarized in Table 41-8.

First-degree burns require no treatment unless the person is an older adult or an infant, in which case severe nausea and vomiting may lead to inadequate fluid intake and dehydration. Fluid therapy may be required in these cases. First-degree burns heal in 3 to 5 days without scarring.

Second-degree burns are either superficial partial-thickness burns or deep partial-thickness burns. Superficial partial-thickness burns are thin-walled, fluid-filled blisters that develop within just a few minutes after injury (Figure 41-27). Tactile and pain sensors remain intact throughout the healing process, and wound care can cause extreme pain. Wounds heal in 3 to 4 weeks with adequate nutrition and no wound complications. Scar formation is unusual and is genetically determined. **Deep partial-thickness burns** (Figure 41-27) look waxy white and take weeks to heal. Necrotic tissue is surgically removed followed by an application of the person's own unburned skin from another body area (autograft). Healing commonly results in hypertrophic scarring with poor functional and cosmetic results (Figure 41-28).

Third-degree burns, or **full-thickness burns**, have a dry, leathery appearance from loss of dermal elasticity (Figure 41-29). In areas of circumferential burns, distal circulation may be compromised from pressure caused by edema. **Escharotomies** (tissue decompression by cutting through burned skin) are performed to release pressure and prevent compartment syndrome (the compression of blood vessels, veins, muscles, or abdominal organs resulting in ischemia, necrosis, and irreversible injury).[92] Full-thickness burns are painless because all nerve endings have been destroyed by the injury.

Fourth-degree burns require skin grafting or reconstructive surgery.

The extent of **total body surface area (TBSA)** burned is estimated using either the "rule of nines" (Figure 41-30) or the modified Lund and Browder chart.[93] The severity of burn injury also considers many factors, including age, medical history, extent and depth of injury, and body area involved. The Ontario Injury Prevention Centre has defined criteria to assist health care providers in identifying who should be referred to a specialized multidisciplinary burn centre in their Burns Centre Consultation Guidelines (see http://www.oninjuryresources.ca/downloads/news/CCSO_BurnsCentreGuidelines_11x14-EN.PDF).

PATHOPHYSIOLOGY AND CLINICAL MANIFESTATIONS Burn injury results in dramatic changes in many physiological functions of the body within the first few minutes after the event. Burns exceeding 20% of TBSA in most adults are considered to be major burn injuries and are associated with massive evaporative water losses and fluctuations of large amounts of fluids, electrolytes, and plasma proteins into the body

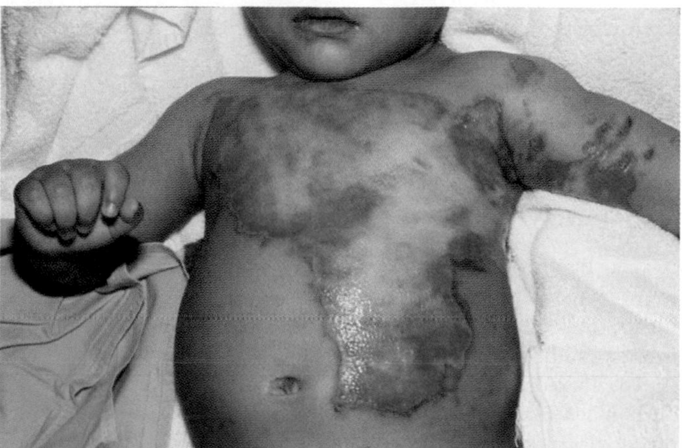

FIGURE 41-27 Superficial Partial-Thickness Burn vs. Deep Partial-Thickness Burn. Superficial partial-thickness burn around edges (after debridement of blister and nonadherent epithelium), with deep partial-thickness burn in centre (note pale appearance and minimal exudates in the centre). (Courtesy Dr. Rogers.)

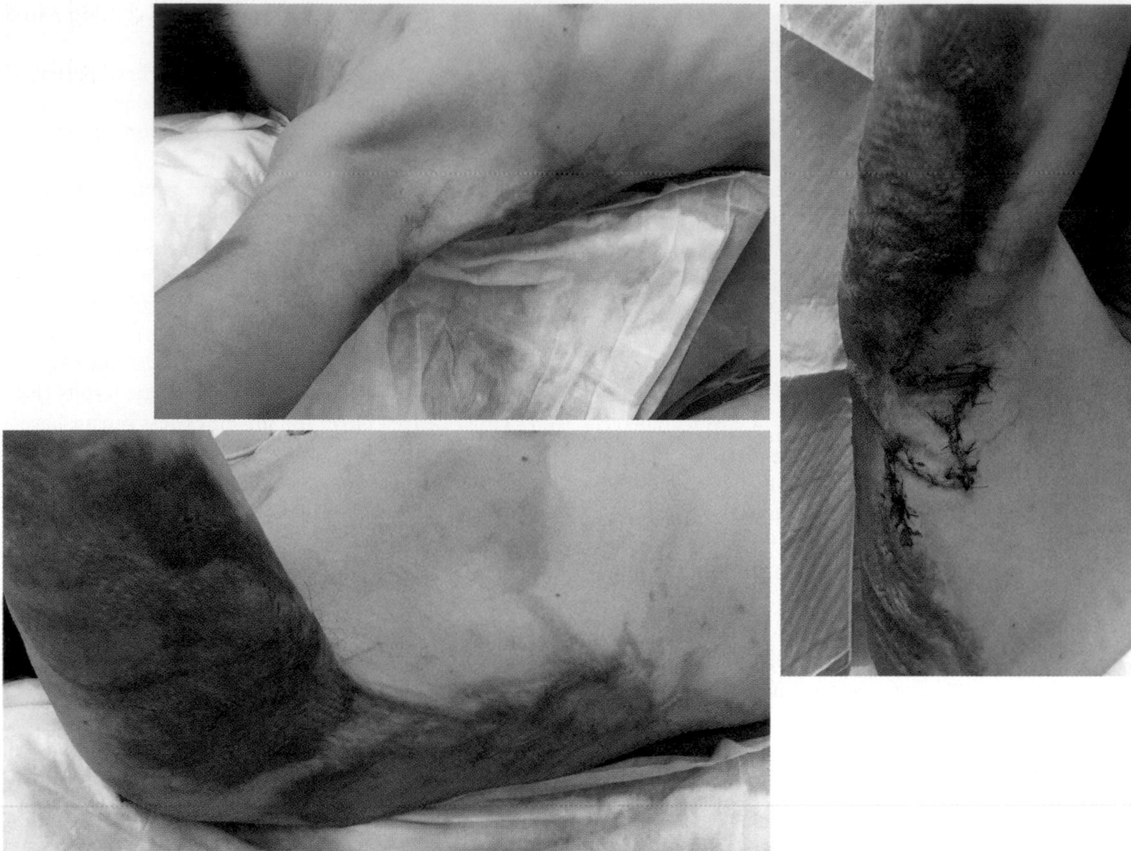

FIGURE 41-28 Axillary Burn Scar Contracture. Note the blanching of the anterior axillary fold and small ulceration from a deep partial-thickness burn, both indicating the diminished range of motion. (Courtesy Dr. Rogers.)

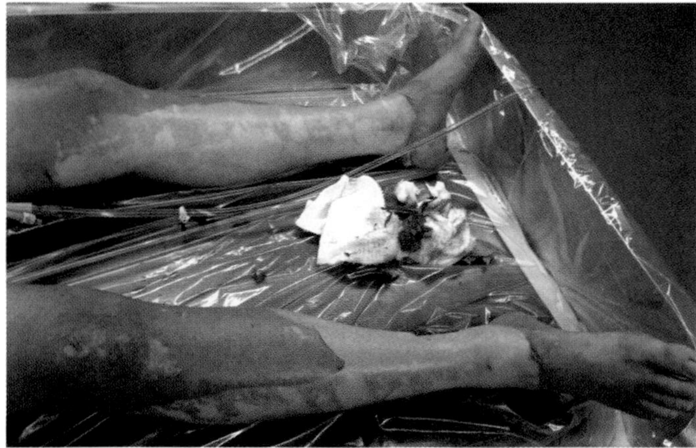

FIGURE 41-29 Full-Thickness Burn. The wound is dry and insensate. (Courtesy Dr. Jeschke.)

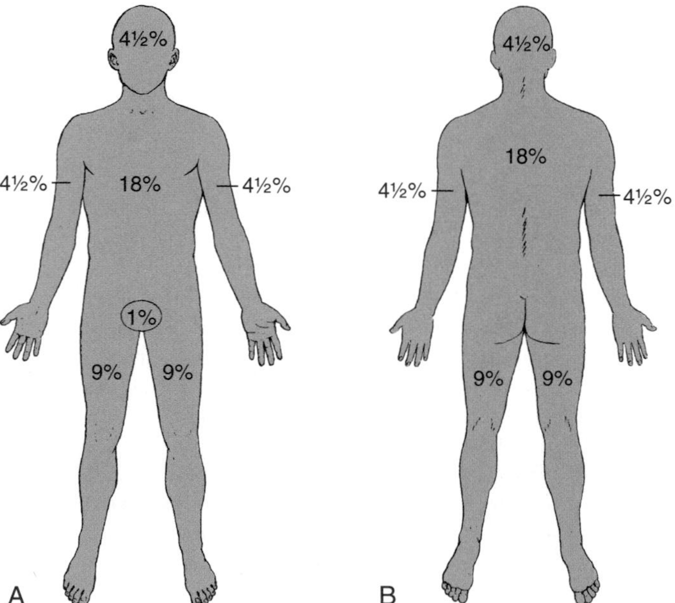

FIGURE 41-30 Estimation of Burn Injury: Rule of Nines. A commonly used assessment tool with estimates of the percentages (in multiples of 9) of the total body surface area burned. **A,** Adults (*anterior view*). **B,** Adults (*posterior view*).

tissues, manifested as generalized edema, circulatory hypovolemia, and hypotension.

The immediate (acute) systemic physiological consequences of major burn injury focus on the profound, life-threatening hypovolemic shock that occurs in conjunction with cellular and immunological disruption within a few minutes of injury (Figure 41-31). **Burn shock** is a condition consisting of a hypovolemic cardiovascular component and a cellular component.

Hypovolemia associated with burn shock results from massive fluid losses and shifts to the interstitial space from the circulating blood volume. The losses are caused by an increase in capillary permeability

TABLE 41-8 Depth of Burn Injury

		SECOND DEGREE		THIRD DEGREE	FOURTH DEGREE
Characteristic	**First Degree**	**Superficial Partial Thickness**	**Deep Partial Thickness**	**Full Thickness**	**Full Thickness and Deeper Tissue**
Morphology	Destruction of epidermis only; local pain and erythema	Destruction of epidermis and some dermis	Destruction of epidermis and dermis, leaving only skin appendages	Destruction of epidermis, dermis, and underlying subcutaneous tissue	Destruction of epidermis, dermis, and underlying subcutaneous tissue, tendons, muscle, and bone
Skin function	Intact	Absent	Absent	Absent	Absent
Tactile and pain sensors	Intact	Intact	Intact but diminished	Absent	Absent
Blisters	Usually none or present after first 24 hr	Present within minutes; thin walled and fluid filled	May or may not appear as fluid-filled blisters; often is layer of flat, dehydrated tissue paper like skin that lifts off in sheets	Blisters rare; usually is layer of flat, dehydrated tissue paper like skin that lifts off easily	None
Appearance of wound after initial débridement	Skin peels at 24–48 hr; normal or slightly red underneath	Red to pale ivory, moist surface	Mottled with areas of waxy, white, dry surface	White, cherry red, or black; may contain visible thrombosed veins; dry, hard, leathery surface	Black and charred-appearing wound
Healing time	3–5 days	21–28 days	30 days to many months	Will not heal; may close from edges as secondary healing if wound is small	Will not heal; requires skin grafting; may require amputation, reconstructive surgery, or both
Scarring	None	May be present; low incidence influenced by genetic predisposition	Highest incidence because of slow healing rate promoting scar tissue development; also influenced by genetic predisposition	Skin graft; scarring minimized by early excision and grafting; influenced by genetic predisposition	Degree of scarring associated with reconstruction and grafting success

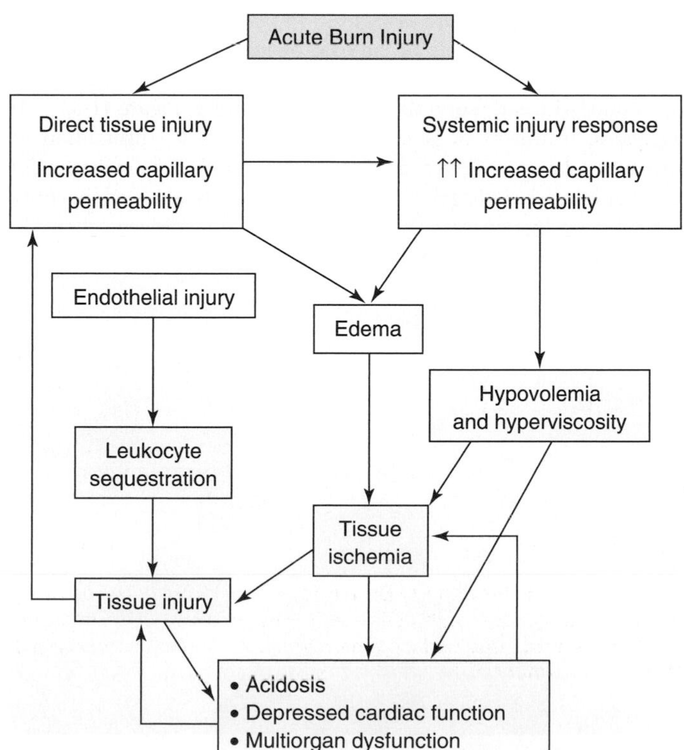

FIGURE 41-31 Immediate Cellular and Immunological Alterations of Burn Shock.

that persists for approximately 24 hours after burn injury. There is decreased cardiac contractility and decreased blood volume. Blood is shunted away from the liver, kidney, and gut—known as the "ebb phase" of the burn response. This phase lasts during the first 24 hours after burn injury and most organ systems are affected. Decreased perfusion of the viscera can decrease gut barrier function and result in translocation of bacteria and endotoxemia with sepsis. Intravenous **fluid resuscitation** is critical to restore the circulating blood volume during this phase, often using lactated Ringer solution. The rate of fluid replacement must be carefully monitored to prevent complications associated with fluid overload. Formulas are available (i.e., Parkland formula or the modified Brooke formula) to guide calculation of fluid volume replacement.[94,95]

Cellular metabolism is disrupted with onset of the burn wound, resulting in altered cell membrane permeability and loss of normal electrolyte homeostasis. Many cytokines and inflammatory mediators in burn serum play a role in these cellular processes. The cardiovascular and systemic responses to burn injury are integrated with the cellular response but are described separately for clarification.

Cardiovascular and Systemic Response to Burn Injury

The clinical manifestations of burn shock are the result of multiple physiological alterations related to burn injury and release of inflammatory cytokines, in addition to the loss of fluid. The hallmark of burn shock is decreased cardiac contractility and decreased cardiac output with inadequate capillary perfusion in most tissues. Decreased cardiac output is related to myocardial depressant factor, as well as decreased intravascular volume.

Fluid and protein movement out of the vascular compartment results in an elevated hematocrit level and white blood cell count, and hypoproteinemia. If not treated immediately, profound hypovolemic shock and inadequate perfusion lead to irreversible shock and death within a few hours. Restoration of capillary integrity and renewal of a functional lymphatic system are required for resolution of the edema. Usually this occurs within 24 hours, but in extensive burns, it may take days or weeks. After the individual has reached the endpoint of burn shock, the term used to describe the person's condition is **capillary seal**.

The liver, with its metabolic, inflammatory, immune, and acute phase functions, plays a pivotal role in burn injury survival and recovery by modulating multiple metabolic pathways. Hepatic changes are common following a major burn, including fatty changes and hepatomegaly, which can influence burn wound recovery.[96] The hepatic response also alters clotting factors, leads to a hypercoagulable state, and can increase the risk for disseminated intravascular coagulation (systemic formation of microthrombi and abnormal bleeding).[97]

Cellular Response to Burn Injury

In addition to capillary endothelial permeability changes resulting in vascular fluid, electrolyte, and protein losses, there are transmembrane potential changes in cells not directly damaged by heat.[98] Cellular dysfunction resulting from burn injury impairs the sodium–potassium pump and results in increased amounts of intracellular sodium and water and decreased potassium level with disruption of the transmembrane potential. Intracellular calcium concentration also may be elevated, thereby influencing myocardial function.[99] Loss of intracellular magnesium and phosphate, hypocalcemia,[100] and elevated serum lactic dehydrogenase (LDH) level occur.[101]

Metabolic Response to Burn Injury

Major burn injury (greater than 40% of TBSA) initiates a systemic hypermetabolic response with an increase in metabolic rate and a hyperdynamic circulation that begins 24 hours after burn injury—known as the "flow phase."[102] This phase can persist for up to 2 years following a burn.[103] Metabolic responses involve the sympathetic nervous system and other homeostatic regulators. Levels of catecholamines, cortisol, glucagon, and insulin (insulin resistance) are elevated with a corresponding increase in energy expenditure and increased gluconeogenesis, glycogenolysis, lipolysis, proteolysis, and lactic acidosis. Myocardial oxygen consumption is elevated and there is catabolic loss of muscle mass.[104] Hyperglycemia and insulin resistance can be prolonged in severe burns and require management with intensive insulin therapy to improve postburn morbidity and mortality.[105,106]

Burn injury initiates an inflammatory response with local activation and recruitment of inflammatory cells, such as leukocytes and monocytes, at the site of injury. These cells release inflammatory cytokines that contribute to the hypermetabolic state.[107] The metabolic rate increases in proportion to burn size and compensates for the profound water and heat loss associated with the burn. The inflammatory response and the release of cytokines at the wound level are magnified into a generalized systemic inflammatory response syndrome that can lead to multiple organ dysfunction.[108] Acute kidney injury is associated with hypovolemia, hypervolemia, and the inflammatory response.[109]

Hypermetabolism also increases the thermal regulatory set point and core and skin temperatures. There is persistent tachycardia, hypercapnia, and body wasting. Wound healing may be impaired, contributing to increased risk for infection and sepsis. Increasing the ambient temperature and early excision and grafting can decrease resting energy expenditure and improve mortality after major burns.[110] Inflammatory mediators circulating to the lung result in pulmonary edema that can be life-threatening.[111]

Immunological Response to Burn Injury

The immunological and inflammatory response to burn injury is immediate, prolonged, and severe. The result in individuals surviving burn shock is *immunosuppression* with increased susceptibility to potentially fatal systemic burn wound sepsis. White blood cells are altered at a time when their need to inhibit sepsis is vital.[112] Phagocytosis is impaired, and cellular and humoral immunity is abnormal. Individuals with altered immunocompetence or chronic disease before burn injury are at additional risk for complications, including wound sepsis.[113]

Macrophages, neutrophils, lymphocytes, and platelets release large amounts of inflammatory cytokines and antibodies, with their levels remaining elevated for weeks after burn injury. When combined with bacterial products, they produce peripheral vasodilation, pulmonary vasoconstriction, increased capillary permeability, and local tissue ischemia in the burn wound. There is distant organ dysfunction and multiple organ failure.[114]

Evaporative Water Loss

With major burn injury, there is loss of the skin's barrier function and ability to regulate evaporative water loss. Normally, the skin is the major source of insensible water loss (75%), and the lungs are minor sources (25%), with a total loss of only approximately 600 to 800 mL/day. This changes dramatically with burns because both the skin and the lungs have increased loss of water as a result of hypermetabolism and hyperventilation, especially in an intubated individual. Total evaporative losses exceed many litres per day in an adult with large burn wounds. Replacement of the loss is mandatory to prevent volume deficit and shock.

EVALUATION AND TREATMENT Burn recovery is complex and prolonged, with complications being the rule rather than the exception. Severity of inhalation injury is also a significant morbidity and mortality factor. The goal of burn management is wound débridement and closure in a manner that promotes survival. Scar formation with contractures is often a consequence of healing in deep partial-thickness and third-degree burns (Figure 41-32).

The essential elements of survival of major burn injury are (1) provision of adequate fluids and nutrition, (2) meticulous management of wounds with early surgical excision and grafting (Figure 41-33), (3) aggressive treatment of infection or sepsis, and (4) promotion of thermoregulation.[114] Several medications are used for the management of severe burns, including β-adrenergic antagonists, β-adrenergic agonists, recombinant human growth hormone, insulin, androgenic steroids, and antibiotics.[102] Burn pain is almost always acute and severe, and

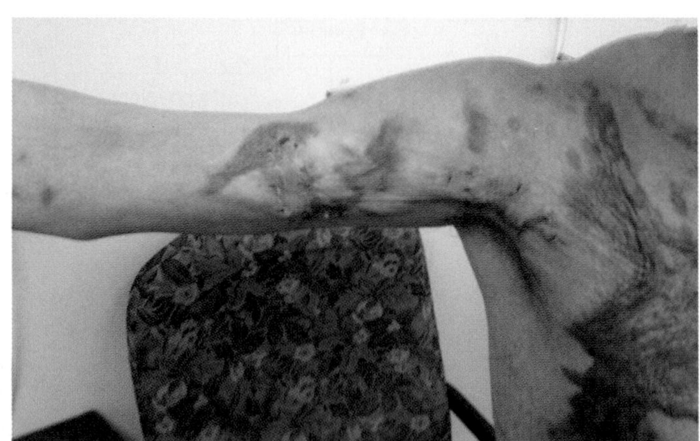

FIGURE 41-32 Hypertrophic Scarring. Deep partial-thickness thermal injury can result in extensive hypertrophic scarring. (Courtesy Dr. Jeschke.)

treatment strategies are aggressive.[115] The risk of developing stress ulcers (Curling ulcers) is reduced with antacids or histamine H2-receptor antagonists.

Nutritional therapy focuses on early enteral therapy to reduce gut-mediated sepsis and to reduce the catabolic state.[116,117] Advancements in skin replacement procedures promote wound closure and healing.[118,119] Reconstructive surgery reduces complications associated with scarring and contractures.[120]

Cold Injury

Exposure to extreme cold includes a spectrum of injuries:[121]

- *Frostnip*—mild and completely reversible injury characterized by skin pallor and numbness
- *Chilblains*—more serious than frostnip; violaceous skin colour with plaques or nodules, pain, and pruritus, but no ice crystal formation; chronic vasculitis can develop and is usually located on the face, anterior lower leg, hands, and feet
- *Frostbite*—tissues freeze and form ice crystals at temperatures less than −2°C (28°F); progresses from distal to proximal and potentially reversible
- *Flash freeze*—rapid cooling with intracellular ice crystals associated with contact with cold metals or volatile liquids

The most common areas affected are fingers, toes, ears, nose, and cheeks. Mild frostbite (frostnip) is cold exposure without tissue freezing. It causes pallor and pain followed by redness and discomfort during rewarming, with no tissue damage. Frostbite occurs when tissues freeze slowly with ice crystal formation. Frozen skin becomes white or yellowish and has a waxy texture. There is numbness and no sensation of pain. Frostbite injury is related to direct cold injury to cells, indirect injury from ice crystal formation, and endothelial cell damage. During

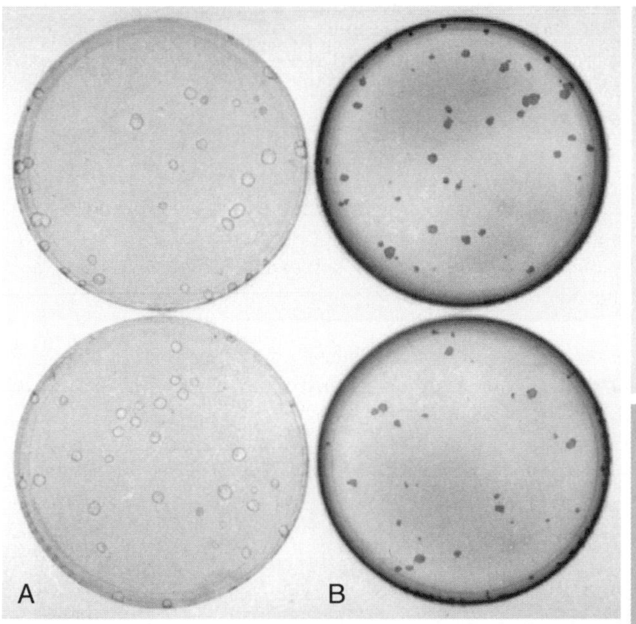

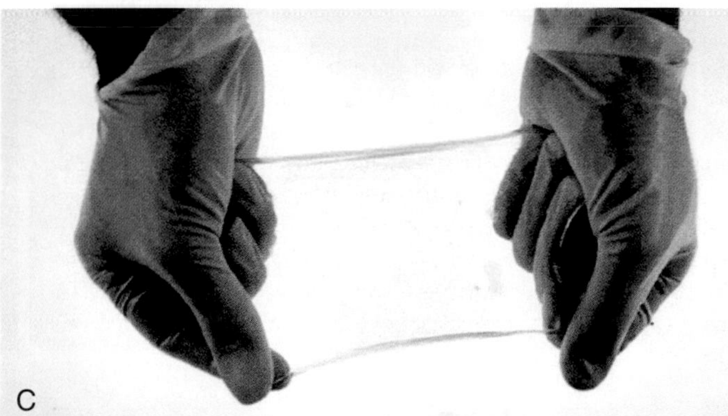

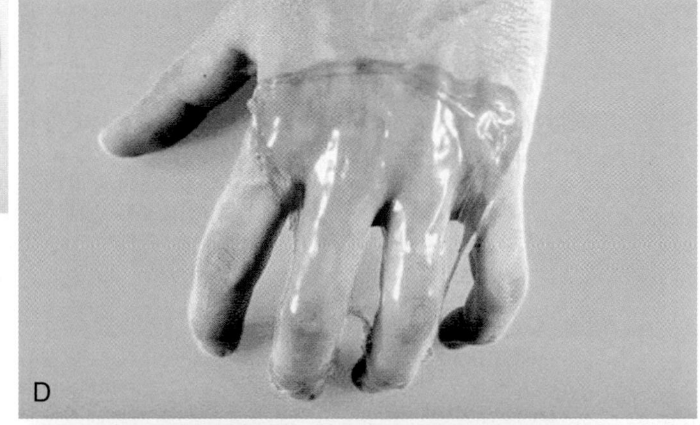

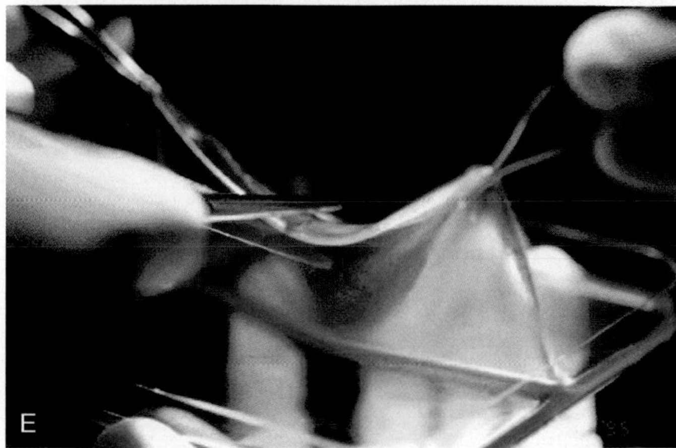

FIGURE 41-33 Cultured Epithelial Autografts. A, B, Keratinocyte culture. Keratinocytes from a severely burnt patient were isolated from a biopsy of unaffected skin and keratinocytes SC colonies, called holoclones, were cultivated in vitro for 2 or 3 weeks to form sheets of epidermal cells. C–E, These epidermal sheets were grafted onto the patient's burnt skin following Barrandon and Green's procedure.

Continued

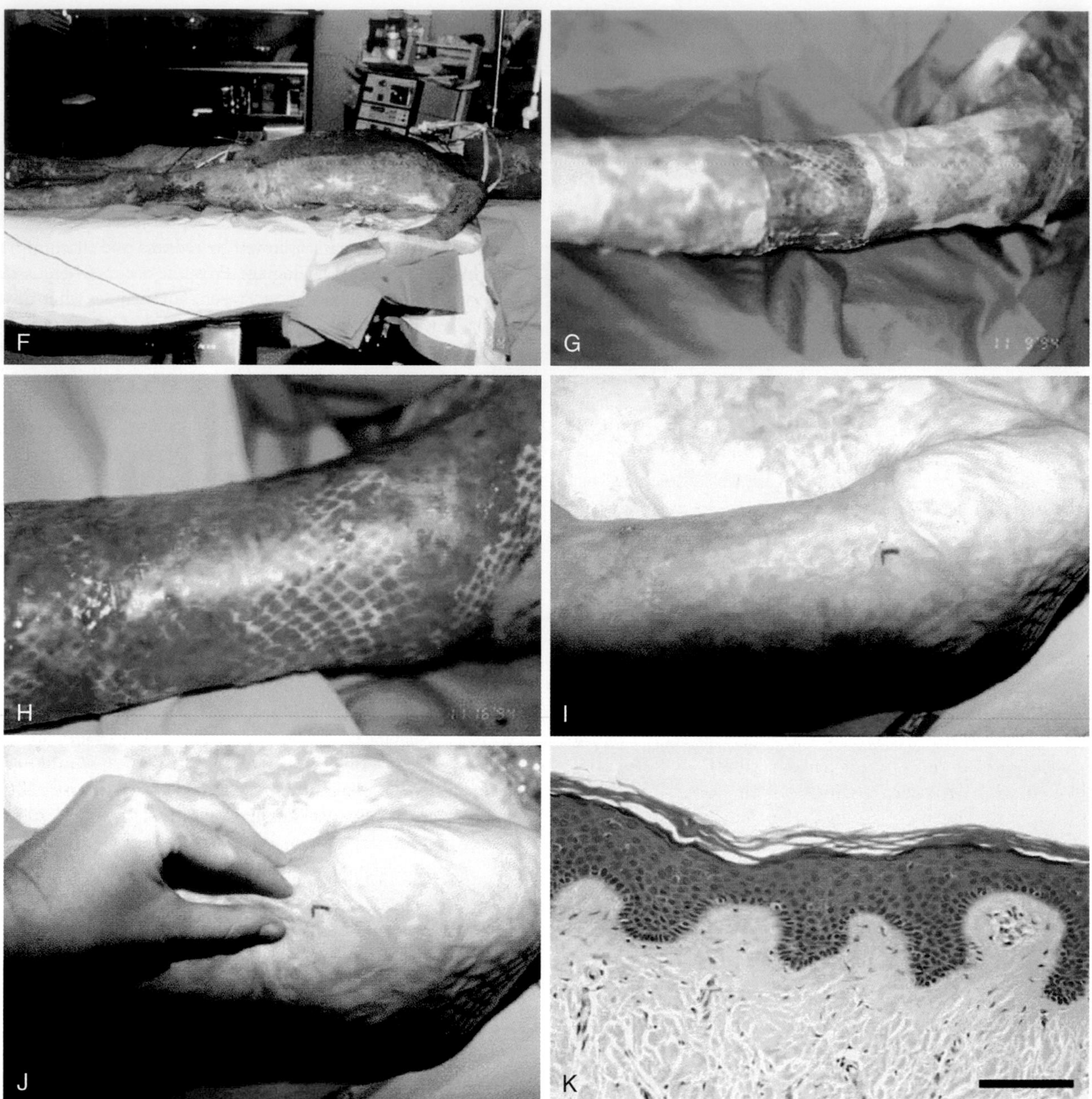

FIGURE 41-33, cont'd F–K, The graft skin is well differentiated and similar to non-grafted skin except the lack of hair follicle and sebaceous gland. (From Ronfard, V. Rives, J.M. Neveux, Y. Carsin, H. Barrandon, Y. (2000). Long-term regeneration of human epidermis on third degree burns transplanted with autologous cultured epithelium grown on a fibrin matrix. Transplantation, 70, 1588–1598. DOI:10.1097/00007890-200012150-00009. Reprinted by permission from Lippincott, Williams and Wilkins.)

rewarming, there is progressive microvascular thrombosis followed by reperfusion injury with release of inflammatory mediators (including thromboxanes, prostaglandins, bradykinins, and histamines) and with impaired circulation and anoxia to the exposed area. Cyanosis and mottling develop followed by redness, edema, and burning pain on rewarming in more severe cases. Edema can cause capillary compression and vascular stasis. Within 24 to 48 hours, vesicles and bullae appear that resolve into crusts that eventually slough, leaving thin, newly formed skin. Frostbite may be classified by depth of injury: superficial includes partial skin freezing (first degree) and full-thickness skin freezing (second degree); deep includes full-thickness and subcutaneous freezing (third degree) and deep tissue freezing (fourth degree). Third-degree and fourth-degree frostbite result in gangrene with loss of tissue.[122]

Immediate treatment of frostbite is to cover affected areas with other body surfaces and warm clothing. The area should not be rubbed or massaged. Rewarming for severe frostbite should occur after emergency transport. Immersion in a warm water bath (40 to 42°C [104 to 107.6°F) until frozen tissue is thawed is the best treatment. Pain is severe and should be treated with potent analgesics. Antibiotics may be given. Vasodilators, thrombolytics, hyperbaric oxygen, and sympathectomy may improve healing responses. Débridement or amputation of necrotic tissue occurs when there is a clear line of demarcation.[123]

DISORDERS OF THE HAIR

Alopecia

Alopecia means loss of hair from the head or body. Hair loss occurs when there is disruption in the growth phase of the hair follicle. Hair loss can be associated with systemic disorders such as hypothyroidism and iron deficiency, chemotherapy for cancer, malnutrition, compulsive hair pulling (trichotillomania), traction on hair from braiding and ponytails, use of hair treatment chemicals, hormonal alterations, and immune reactions.[124]

Androgenic Alopecia

Androgenic alopecia is localized hair loss and occurs in about 80% of men. It is not a disease but a genetically predisposed response to androgens that clusters in families. Within the distribution of hair over the scalp, androgen-sensitive hair follicles are on top and androgen-insensitive follicles are on the sides and back. In genetically predisposed men, the androgen-sensitive follicles are transformed into vellus follicles. Male-pattern baldness begins with frontotemporal recession and progresses to loss of hair over the top of the scalp. Minoxidil (Loniten) may be used to stimulate hair growth and finasteride (Apo-Finasteride) (a 5α-reductase inhibitor) may decrease the effect of androgens on hair follicles.[125]

Female-Pattern Alopecia

Some genetically susceptible women in their 20s and 30s experience progressive thinning and loss of hair over the central part of the scalp, and prevalence increases with advancing age. Contrary to male-pattern baldness, there is usually no loss of hair along the frontal hairline, but the hairs are shorter and thinner (follicular miniaturization). The mechanism of hair loss is unknown but related to genetic and hormonal changes.[126]

Alopecia Areata

Alopecia areata is an autoimmune T-cell–mediated chronic inflammatory disease directed against hair follicles and results in hair loss. There is rapid onset of hair loss in multiple areas of the scalp, usually in round patches. The eyebrows, eyelashes, beard, and other areas of body hair are rarely involved. Stressful events, cell-mediated immune cytokines, genetic susceptibility, and metabolic disorders, such as Addison's disease, thyroid disease, and lupus erythematosus, are associated with alopecia areata.[127]

The affected areas of skin are smooth or may have short shafts of poorly developed hair that breaks at the surface ("exclamation mark" hair). Regrowth occurs within 1 to 3 months, but hair loss may recur at the same site. Permanent regrowth of hair usually occurs. Diagnosis is made by observation of the pattern of hair loss. Biopsy may show a lymphocytic infiltrate around the follicle. There are several treatments for alopecia areata, including corticosteroids and topical immunotherapy, and new treatments are being tested.[128,129]

Hirsutism

Hirsutism occurs in women and is the abnormal growth and distribution of hair on the face, body, and pubic area in a male pattern. There is also frontotemporal hair recession. These areas of hair growth are androgen sensitive. Variations of hair growth in women are great, and a male pattern may be normal. Women who develop hirsutism may be secreting hormones associated with polycystic ovarian syndrome, adrenal hyperplasia, or adrenal tumours, and these disorders require treatment. If no hormonal pathological conditions exist, treatment may include cosmetic removal of hair, suppression of excessive androgen production, or blockage of peripheral androgen receptors.[130]

DISORDERS OF THE NAIL

Paronychia

Paronychia is an acute or chronic infection of the cuticle. One or more fingers or toes may be involved. Individuals whose hands are frequently exposed to moisture are at greatest risk. The most common causative microorganisms are staphylococci and streptococci. Occasionally *Candida* will be present. Acute paronychia is manifested by the rapid onset of painful inflammation of the cuticle, usually after minor trauma. An abscess may develop, requiring incision and drainage for relief of pain. The skin around the nail becomes more edematous and painful with progressive infection. Pus may be expressed from the proximal nail fold and an abscess may develop. The nail plate is usually not affected, although it can become discoloured with ridges. Chronic paronychia develops slowly, with tenderness and swelling around the proximal or lateral nail folds.[131]

Treatment includes prevention by keeping the hands dry. Oral antifungals are not effective because they do not penetrate the affected tissues. Topical application of thymol is usually effective.[132]

Onychomycosis

Onychomycosis (tinea unguium) is a fungal or dermatophyte infection of the nail unit. The most common pattern is a nail plate that turns yellow or white and becomes elevated with the accumulation of hyperkeratotic debris within the plate. Fungal infections of the nail are differentiated from psoriasis, LP, and trauma by culture and microscopy and the absence of pitting on the nail surface, which is characteristic of psoriasis. Treatment is difficult because topical or systemic antifungal agents do not penetrate the nail plate readily. Systemic antifungal medications are more effective. Surgical excision of the nail may be required. Education is essential to preventing recurrence.[133]

QUICK CHECK 41-8

1. Describe the four degrees of burn injury.
2. What dangers accompany frostbite?
3. What is alopecia? Compare the different types.
4. Describe two disorders of the nail.

GERIATRIC CONSIDERATIONS

Aging and Changes in Skin Integrity

- Skin becomes thinner, dryer, and more wrinkled.
- DNA repair of damaged skin decreases.
- Epidermal cells contain less moisture and change shape.
- The dermis thins, producing translucent, paper-thin quality that is more susceptible to tearing.
- The dermis becomes more permeable and less able to clear substances, so those substances accumulate and cause irritation.
- There is a loss of epidermal rete pegs, which weakens the connection to the dermis and gives skin a smooth, shiny, and wrinkled appearance with an increased likelihood to tear from shearing forces.
- There is a loss of elastin, contributing to wrinkling.
- There is a loss of flexibility of collagen fibres, so skin cannot stretch and regain shape as readily.
- The barrier function of the stratum corneum is reduced, increasing risk for injury and infection.
- The significantly decreased number of Langerhans cells reduces the skin's immune response.
- The dermoepidermal border flattens, shortening and decreasing the number of capillary loops.

Other Skin Changes With Aging

- Wound healing decreases as a result of decreased estrogen in both men and women, decreased blood flow, and slower rate of basal cell and fibroblast turnover.
- There are fewer melanocytes; pigmentation becomes irregular, giving decreased protection from ultraviolet radiation and leading to greying of hair.
- Atrophy of eccrine, apocrine, and sebaceous glands causes dry skin.
- Pressure and touch receptors and free nerve endings decrease in number, causing reduced sensory perception.
- With compromised temperature regulation, loss of cutaneous vasomotion, and decreased eccrine sweat production, there is an increased risk for heat stroke and hypothermia.
- The nail plate thins, and nails are more brittle.

Data from Amaro-Ortiz, A., Yan, B., & D'Orazio, J.A. (2014). *Molecules, 19*(5), 6202–6219; Chang, A.L., Wong, J.W., Endo, J.O., et al. (2013). *J Am Med Dir Assoc, 14*(10), 724–730; Emmerson, E., & Hardman, M.J. (2012). *Biogerontol, 13*(1), 3–20; Kottner, J., Lichterfeld, A., & Blume-Peytavi, U. (2013). *Br J Dermatol, 169*(3), 528–542; Ramos-e-Silva, M., Boza, J.C., & Cestari, T.F. (2012). *Clin Dermatol, 30*(3), 274–276.

DID YOU UNDERSTAND?

Overview

1. The skin is the largest organ of the body and equals 20% of body weight. The major functions are to provide a protective barrier and to regulate body temperature.

Structure and Function of the Skin

1. The skin has two layers: the dermis and epidermis. The underlying hypodermis contains connective tissue, fat cells, fibroblasts, and macrophages.
2. The epidermis contains basal and spinous layers with melanocytes, Langerhans cells, and Merkel cells.
3. The dermis is composed of connective tissue elements, hair follicles, sweat glands, sebaceous glands, blood vessels, nerves, and lymphatic vessels.
4. The dermal appendages include nails, hair, sebaceous glands, and eccrine and apocrine sweat glands.
5. The papillary capillaries provide the major blood supply to the skin, arising from deeper arterial plexuses.
6. Heat loss and heat conservation are regulated by arteriovenous anastomoses that lead to the papillary capillaries in the dermis.
7. Pressure ulcers develop from pressure and shearing forces that occlude capillary blood flow with resulting ischemia and necrosis. Areas at greatest risk are pressure points over bony prominences, such as the greater trochanters, sacrum, ischia, and heels.
8. Keloids are sharply elevated scars that extend beyond the border of traumatized skin. Hypertrophic scars do not extend beyond the border of injury.
9. Pruritus is itching and is associated with many skin disorders. Small unmyelinated type C nerve fibres transmit itch sensation.

Disorders of the Skin

1. Allergic contact dermatitis is a form of delayed hypersensitivity that develops with sensitization to allergens, such as metal, chemicals, or poison ivy.
2. Irritant contact dermatitis develops from prolonged exposure to chemicals, such as acids or soaps, with disruption of the skin barrier.
3. Atopic or allergic dermatitis is associated with a family history of allergies, hay fever, elevated immunoglobulin E levels, and increased histamine sensitivity. Pruritus and scratching predispose the skin to infection, scaling, and thickening.
4. Stasis dermatitis occurs on the legs and results from chronic venous stasis and edema.
5. Seborrheic dermatitis involves scaly, yellowish, inflammatory plaques of the scalp, eyebrows, eyelids, ear canals, nasolabial folds, axillae, chest, and back. The cause is unknown, but *Malassezia* yeasts have been implicated.
6. Papulosquamous disorders are characterized by papules, scales, plaques, and erythema.
7. Psoriasis is a chronic inflammatory skin disease associated with a complex inflammatory cascade involving multiple immune cells, resulting in cellular proliferation of both the epidermis and the dermis; it is characterized by scaly, erythematous, pruritic plaques.
8. Pityriasis rosea is a self-limiting inflammatory disease characterized by oval lesions with scales around the edges; it is located along skin lines of the trunk and may be caused by a herpeslike virus.
9. Lichen planus is an autoimmune papular, violet-coloured inflammatory lesion of unknown origin manifested by severe pruritus.
10. Acne vulgaris is an inflammation of the pilosebaceous follicle.
11. Acne rosacea develops on the middle third of the face with hypertrophy and inflammation of the sebaceous glands and is associated with altered innate immune responses.
12. Discoid (cutaneous) lupus erythematosus is an autoimmune disease that can affect only the skin. The systemic form also presents cutaneous lesions. The cutaneous inflammatory lesions usually occur in sun-exposed areas with a butterfly distribution over the nose and cheeks.

13. Pemphigus is a chronic, autoimmune, blistering disease that begins in the mouth or on the scalp and spreads to other parts of the body, often with a fatal outcome.
14. Erythema multiforme is an acute inflammation of the skin and mucous membranes (bullous form) with lesions that appear targetlike with alternating rings of edema and inflammation; it is often associated with T-cell–mediated allergic reactions to medications.
15. Folliculitis is an infection of the hair follicle caused by bacteria, viruses, or fungi, although *Staphylococcus aureus* is the common culprit.
16. A furuncle is an infection of the hair follicle that extends to the surrounding tissue.
17. A carbuncle is a collection of infected hair follicles that forms a draining abscess.
18. Cellulitis is a diffuse infection of the dermis and subcutaneous tissue.
19. Erysipelas is an acute superficial infection of the skin upper dermis most often caused by *Streptococcus pyogenes*, beta-hemolytic streptococci, and *S. aureus*. It commonly affects the face, ears, and lower legs.
20. Impetigo may have a bullous or an ulcerative form and is caused by *Staphylococcus* or beta-hemolytic streptococci.
21. Ticks transmit numerous diseases, including Lyme disease, which is caused by an immune response to the spirochete *Borrelia burgdorferi.*
22. Herpes simplex virus type 1 (HSV-1) causes cold sores but can infect the cornea, mouth, and labia; it can also cause genital herpes. Genital infections are more commonly caused by HSV-2, which is usually spread by sexual contact.
23. Herpes zoster (shingles) and varicella (chickenpox) are both caused by the varicella-zoster virus.
24. Warts are benign, rough, elevated lesions caused by human papillomavirus. Condylomata acuminata, or venereal warts, are spread by sexual contact.
25. Tinea infections (fungal infections) can occur anywhere on the body and are classified by location (i.e., tinea pedis, tinea corporis, tinea capitis).
26. Candidiasis is a yeastlike fungal infection (*Candida albicans*) occurring on skin and mucous membranes, in the gastro-intestinal tract, and in the vagina.
27. Cutaneous vasculitis is an inflammation of skin blood vessels related to immune complex deposition with purpura, ischemia, and necrosis resulting from vessel necrosis.
28. Urticarial lesions are most commonly associated with type I hypersensitivity reactions to medications, certain foods, environmental exposure, systemic diseases, or physical agents. The lesions appear as wheals, welts, or hives.
29. Scleroderma is an autoimmune-mediated sclerosis of the skin that may also affect systemic organs and cause kidney failure, intestinal obstruction, or cardiac dysrhythmias.
30. Seborrheic keratosis is a proliferation of basal cells that produce elevated, smooth, or warty lesions of varying size. They are most common among the older adult population.
31. Keratoacanthoma arises from hair follicles on sun-exposed areas. Three stages of development characterize the lesion, which results in a dome-shaped, crusty lesion filled with keratin that resolves in 3 to 4 months.
32. Actinic keratosis is a pigmented scaly lesion that develops in sun-exposed individuals with fair skin. The lesion may become malignant in the form of squamous cell carcinoma (SCC).
33. Nevi arise from melanocytes and may be pigmented or fleshy pink. They occur singly or in groups and may undergo transition to malignant melanoma.
34. Basal cell carcinoma is the most common skin cancer in the world, and is thought to occur most often as a result of ultraviolet radiation exposure.
35. SCC is a tumour of the epidermis and can be localized (in situ) or invasive.
36. Cutaneous melanoma is a malignant tumour that arises from melanocytes, and if not excised early, metastasis occurs through the lymph nodes.
37. Kaposi sarcoma is a vascular malignancy associated with human herpesvirus 8 and immunodeficiency.
38. Burns are classified according to depth and extent of injury as first-, second-, third-, or fourth-degree burns.
39. Major burn injury causes profound edema and burn shock related to an inflammatory response throughout the cardiovascular system with loss of capillary seal. Fluid resuscitation is critical to prevent shock and death.
40. Major burn injury also causes a hypermetabolic response with increased cortisol, glucagon, and insulin levels and with gluconeogenesis.
41. Immune suppression associated with inflammatory cytokine release from burned tissue increases the risk for infection and can delay wound healing.
42. Cold injury usually occurs on the face and digits, with direct injury to cells and impaired circulation.

Disorders of the Hair

1. Alopecia is loss of hair from the head or body.
2. Male-pattern alopecia is an inherited form of irreversible baldness with hair loss in the central scalp and recession of the frontotemporal hairline.
3. Female-pattern alopecia is a thinning of the central hair of the scalp beginning in women at 20 to 30 years of age.
4. Alopecia areata is an autoimmune-mediated loss of hair and may be associated with stress or metabolic diseases; it is usually reversible.
5. Hirsutism is a male pattern of hair growth in women that may be normal or the result of excessive secretion of androgenic hormones.

Disorders of the Nail

1. Paronychia is an inflammation of the cuticle that can be acute or chronic and is usually caused by staphylococci, streptococci, or fungi.
2. Onychomycosis is a fungal or dermatophyte infection of the nail unit.

KEY TERMS

Acne rosacea, 1085
Acne vulgaris, 1085
Actinic keratosis, 1091
Allergic contact dermatitis, 1082
Alopecia, 1101
Alopecia areata, 1101
Androgenic alopecia, 1101
Apocrine sweat gland, 1076
Atopic dermatitis (allergic dermatitis), 1082
Basal cell carcinoma (BCC), 1092
Bullous erythema multiforme, 1086
Burn shock, 1096
Candidiasis, 1089
Capillary seal, 1098
Carbuncle, 1087
Cellulitis, 1087
Chronic urticaria, 1090
Clawlike prolongation, 1081
Condylomata acuminata (venereal warts), 1089
Cutaneous melanoma, 1093
Cutaneous vasculitis, 1090
Deep partial-thickness burn, 1095
Dermal appendage, 1074
Dermatitis, 1081
Dermis, 1074
Discoid (cutaneous) lupus erythematosus (DLE), 1085
Eccrine sweat gland, 1074
Eczema, 1081
Epidermis, 1074
Erysipelas, 1087
Erythema multiforme, 1086
Erythrodermic (exfoliative) psoriasis, 1083
Escharotomy, 1095
First-degree burn, 1095
Fluid resuscitation, 1097
Folliculitis, 1087
Fourth-degree burn, 1095
Furuncle, 1087
Guttate psoriasis, 1083
Herald patch, 1084
Herpes simplex virus (HSV), 1088
Herpes zoster (shingles), 1088
Hirsutism, 1101
Human papillomavirus (HPV), 1088
Hypertrophic scar, 1081
Immunoglobulin A pemphigus, 1086
Impetigo, 1087
Inverse psoriasis, 1083
Irritant contact dermatitis, 1082
Kaposi sarcoma (KS), 1094
Keloid, 1081
Keratoacanthoma, 1091
Lichen planus (LP), 1084
Lip cancer, 1093
Localized scleroderma (morphea), 1090
Lupus erythematosus, 1085
Lyme disease, 1087
Mycosis fungoides, 1095
Nails, 1074
Necrotizing fasciitis, 1087
Nevus (*pl.*, nevi), 1091
Onychomycosis (tinea unguium), 1101
Papillary capillary, 1076
Papulosquamous disorder, 1083
Paraneoplastic pemphigus, 1086
Paronychia, 1101
Pemphigus, 1085
Pemphigus erythematosus, 1086
Pemphigus foliaceus, 1086
Pemphigus herpetiformis, 1086
Pemphigus vegetans, 1086
Pemphigus vulgaris, 1086
Pityriasis rosea, 1084
Plaque psoriasis, 1083
Pressure ulcer, 1076
Primary cutaneous lymphoma, 1095
Psoriasis, 1083
Psoriatic arthritis, 1083
Psoriatic nail disease, 1083
Pustular psoriasis, 1083
Sebaceous gland, 1074
Seborrheic dermatitis, 1083
Seborrheic keratosis, 1091
Second-degree burn, 1095
Squamous cell carcinoma (SCC), 1092
Stasis dermatitis, 1082
Stevens-Johnson syndrome, 1086
Subcutaneous layer (hypodermis), 1074
Systemic scleroderma, 1090
Third-degree burn (full-thickness burn), 1095
Tinea infection, 1089
Total body surface area (TBSA), 1095
Toxic epidermal necrolysis (TEN), 1086
Urticaria (hives), 1090
Urticarial lesion, 1090
Varicella (chickenpox), 1088
Wart, 1088

REFERENCES

1. de Laat, E. H., Schoonhoven, L., Pickkers, P., et al. (2006). Epidemiology, risk and prevention of pressure ulcers in critically ill patients: A literature review. *Journal of Wound Care, 15*(6), 269–275. doi:10.12968/jowc.2006.15.6.26920.
2. National Pressure Ulcer Advisory Panel. (2007). *Pressure ulcer stages revised by NPUAP, Feb 2007.* Retrieved from http://www.npuap.org/resources/educational-and-clinical-resources/npuap-pressure-ulcer-stagescategories/.
3. Thomas, D. R. (2014). Role of nutrition in the treatment and prevention of pressure ulcers. *Nutrition in Clinical Practice, 29*(4), 466–472. doi:10.1177/0884533614539016.
4. Black, J., Clark, M., Dealey, C., et al. (2014). Dressings as an adjunct to pressure ulcer prevention: Consensus panel recommendations. *International Wound Journal, 12*(4), 484–488. doi:10.1111/iwj.12197.
5. Cushing, C. A., & Phillips, L. G. (2013). Evidence-based medicine: Pressure sores. *Plastic and Reconstructive Surgery, 132*(6), 1720–1732. doi:10.1097/PRS.0b013e3182a808ba.
6. Smith, M. E., Totten, A., Hickam, D. H., et al. (2013). Pressure ulcer treatment strategies: A systematic comparative effectiveness review. *Annals of Internal Medicine, 159*(1), 39–50. doi:10.7326/0003-4819-159-1-201307020-00007.
7. Arno, A. I., Gauglitz, G. G., Barret, J. P., et al. (2014). Up-to-date approach to manage keloids and hypertrophic scars: A useful guide. *Burns, 40*(7), 1255–1266. doi:10.1016/j.burns.2014.02.011.
8. Shih, B., & Bayat, A. (2010). Genetics of keloid scarring. *Archives of Dermatological Research, 302*(5), 319–339. doi:10.1007/s00403-009-1014-y.
9. Ikoma, A. (2013). Updated neurophysiology of itch. *Biological and Pharmaceutical Bulletin, 36*(8), 1235–1240.
10. Hassan, I., & Haji, M. I. (2014). Understanding itch: An update on mediators and mechanisms of pruritus. *Indian Journal of Dermatology, Venereology and Leprology, 80*(2), 106–114. doi:10.4103/0378-6323.129377.
11. Tominaga, M., & Takamori, K. (2013). An update on peripheral mechanisms and treatments of itch. *Biological and Pharmaceutical Bulletin, 36*(8), 1241–1247.
12. Peiser, M. (2013). Role of Th17 cells in skin inflammation of allergic contact dermatitis. *Clinical and Developmental Immunology, 2013*, 261037. doi:10.1155/2013/261037.
13. Cabañes, N., Igea, J. M., de la Hoz, B., et al. (2012). Latex allergy: Position paper. *Journal of Investigational Allergology and Clinical Immunology, 22*(5), 313–330.
14. Lee, H. Y., Stieger, M., Yawalker, N., et al. (2013). Cytokines and chemokines in irritant contact dermatitis. *Mediators of Inflammation, 2013*, 916497. doi:10.1155/2013/916497.
15. McDaniel, J. C., Roy, S., & Wilgus, T. A. (2013). Neutrophil activity in chronic venous leg ulcers—A target for therapy? *Wound Repair and Regeneration, 21*(3), 339–351. doi:10.1111/wrr.12036.
16. White-Chu, E. F., & Conner-Kerr, T. A. (2014). Overview of guidelines for the prevention and treatment of venous leg ulcers: A US perspective. *Journal of Multidisciplinary Healthcare, 7*, 111–117. doi:10.2147/JMDH.S38616.
17. Dessinioti, C., & Katsambas, A. (2013). Seborrheic dermatitis: Etiology, risk factors, and treatments: Facts and controversies. *Clinics in Dermatology, 31*(4), 343–351. doi:10.1016/j.clindermatol.2013.01.001.
18. Boehncke, W. H., & Schön, M. P. (2015). Psoriasis. *Lancet, 386*(9997), 983–994. doi:10.1016/S0140-6736(14)61909-7.
19. Lynde, C. W., Poulin, Y., Vender, R., et al. (2014). Interleukin 17A: Toward a new understanding of psoriasis pathogenesis. *Journal of the American Academy of Dermatology, 71*(1), 141–150. doi:10.1016/j.jaad.2013.12.036.
20. Baliwag, J., Barnes, D. H., & Johnston, A. (2015). Cytokines in psoriasis. *Cytokine, 73*(2), 342–350. doi:10.1016/j.cyto.2014.12.014.
21. Brezinski, E. A., & Armstrong, A. W. (2014). Strategies to maximize treatment success in moderate to severe psoriasis: Establishing treatment goals and tailoring of biologic therapies. *Seminars in Cutaneous Medicine and Surgery, 33*(2), 91–97.
22. Olivieri, I., D'Angelo, S., Palazzi, C., et al. (2014). Advances in the management of psoriatic arthritis. *Nature Reviews: Rheumatology, 10*(9), 531–542. doi:10.1038/nrrheum.2014.106.
23. Jullien, D., Prinz, J. C., & Nestle, F. O. (2015). Immunogenicity of biotherapy used in psoriasis: The science behind the scenes. *The Journal of Investigative Dermatology, 135*(1), 31–38. doi:10.1038/jid.2014.295.
24. Rebora, A., Drago, F., & Broccolo, F. (2010). Pityriasis rosea and herpesviruses: Facts and controversies. *Clinics in Dermatology, 28*(5), 497–501. doi:10.1016/j.clindermatol.2010.03.005.
25. Amatya, A., Rajouria, E. A., & Karn, D. K. (2012). Comparative study of effectiveness of oral acyclovir with oral erythromycin in the treatment of Pityriasis rosea. *Kathmandu University Medical Journal, 10*(37), 57–61.

26. Sharma, A., Bialynicki-Birula, R., Schwartz, R. A., et al. (2012). Lichen planus: An update and review. *Cutis, 90*(1), 17–23.
27. Carrozzo, M., & Scally, K. (2014). Oral manifestations of hepatitis C virus infection. *World Journal of Gastroenterology, 20*(24), 7534–7543. doi:10.3748/wjg.v20.i24.7534.
28. Di Stasio, D., Guida, A., Salerno, C., et al. (2014). Oral lichen planus: A narrative review. *Frontiers in Bioscience, 6*, 370–376.
29. Le Cleach, L., & Chosidow, O. (2012). Clinical practice. Lichen planus. *The New England Journal of Medicine, 366*(8), 723–732. doi:10.1056/NEJMcp1103641.
30. Tüzün, Y., Wolf, R., Kutlubay, Z., et al. (2014). Rosacea and rhinophyma. *Clinics in Dermatology, 32*(1), 35–46. doi:10.1016/j.clindermatol.2013.05.024.
31. Layton, A., & Thiboutot, D. (2013). Emerging therapies in rosacea. *Journal of the American Academy of Dermatology, 69*(6, Suppl. 1), S57 S65. doi:10.1016/j.jaad.2013.04.041.
32. Chong, B. F., Song, J., & Olsen, N. J. (2012). Determining risk factors for developing systemic lupus erythematosus in patients with discoid lupus erythematosus. *The British Journal of Dermatology, 166*(1), 29–35. doi:10.1111/j.1365-2133.2011.1061 0.x.
33. Kuhn, A., & Landmann, A. (2014). The classification and diagnosis of cutaneous lupus erythematosus. *Journal of Autoimmunity, 48–49*, 14–19. doi:10.1016/j.jaut.2014.01.021.
34. Yu, C., Chang, C., & Zhang, J. (2013). Immunologic and genetic considerations of cutaneous lupus erythematosus: A comprehensive review. *Journal of Autoimmunity, 41*, 34–45. doi:10.1016/j.jaut.2013.01.007.
35. Okon, L. G., & Werth, V. P. (2013). Cutaneous lupus erythematosus: Diagnosis and treatment. *Best Practice and Research: Clinical Rheumatology, 27*(3), 391–404. doi:10.1016/j.berh.2013.07.008.
36. Porro, A. M., de Caetano, L. V., de Maehara, L. S., et al. (2014). Non-classical forms of pemphigus: Pemphigus herpetiformis, IgA pemphigus, paraneoplastic pemphigus and IgG/IgA pemphigus. *Anais Brasileiros De Dermatologia, 89*(1), 96–106. doi:10.1590/abd1806-4841.20142459.
37. Ruocco, V., Ruocco, E., Lo Schiavo, A., et al. (2013). Pemphigus: Etiology, pathogenesis, and inducing or triggering factors: Facts and controversies. *Clinics in Dermatology, 31*(4), 374–381. doi:10.1016/j.clindermatol.2013.01.004.
38. Ruocco, E., Wolf, R., Ruocco, V., et al. (2013). Pemphigus: Associations and management guidelines: Facts and controversies. *Clinics in Dermatology, 31*(4), 382–390. doi:10.1016/j.clindermatol.2013.01.005.
39. Samim, F., Auluck, A., Zed, C., et al. (2013). Erythema multiforme: A review of epidemiology, pathogenesis, clinical features, and treatment. *Dental Clinics of North America, 57*(4), 583–596. doi:10.1016/j.cden.2013.07.001.
40. Cheng, C. Y., Su, S. C., Chen, C. H., et al. (2014). HLA associations and clinical implications in T-cell mediated drug hypersensitivity reactions: An updated review. *Journal of Immunology Research, 2014*, 565320. doi:10.1155/2014/565320.
41. Tomasini, C., Derlino, F., Quaglino, P., et al. (2014). From erythema multiforme to toxic epidermal necrolysis. Same spectrum or different diseases? *Giornale Italiano Di Dermatologia E Venereologia: Organo Ufficiale, Societa Italiana Di Dermatologia E Sifilografia, 149*(2), 243–261.
42. Mistry, R. D. (2013). Skin and soft tissue infections. *Pediatric Clinics of North America, 60*(5), 1063–1082. doi:10.1016/j.pcl.2013.06.011.
43. Chira, S., & Miller, L. G. (2010). *Staphylococcus aureus* is the most common identified cause of cellulitis: A systematic review. *Epidemiology and Infection, 138*(3), 313–317. doi:10.1017/S0950268809990483.
44. Al Shukry, S., & Ommen, J. (2013). Necrotizing fasciitis—Report of ten cases and review of recent literature. *Journal of Medicine and Life, 6*(2), 189–194.
45. Gunderson, C. G., & Martinello, R. A. (2012). A systematic review of bacteremias in cellulitis and erysipelas. *The Journal of Infection, 64*(2), 148–155. doi:10.1016/j.jinf.2011.11.004.
46. Radolf, J. D., Caimano, M. J., Stevenson, B., et al. (2012). Of ticks, mice and men: Understanding the dual-host lifestyle of Lyme disease spirochaettes. *Nature Reviews: Microbiology, 10*(2), 98–99. doi:10.1038/nrmicro2714.
47. Bratton, R. L., Whiteside, J. W., Hovan, M. J., et al. (2008). Diagnosis and treatment of Lyme disease. *Mayo Clinic Proceedings, 83*(5), 566–571. doi:10.4065/83.5.566.
48. Eshoo, M. W., Schutzer, S. E., Crowder, C. D., et al. (2013). Achieving molecular diagnostics for Lyme disease. *Expert Review of Molecular Diagnostics, 13*(8), 875–883. doi:10.1586/14737159.2013.850418.
49. Stanek, G., Wormser, G. P., Gray, J., et al. (2012). Lyme borreliosis. *Lancet, 379*(9814), 461–473. doi:10.1016/S0140 6736(11)60103 7.
50. Embers, M. E., & Narasimhan, S. (2013). Vaccination against Lyme disease: Past, present, and future. *Frontiers in Cellular and Infection Microbiology*, 3, 6. doi:10.3389/fcimb.2013.00006.
51. Bloom, D. C., Giordani, N. V., & Kwiatkowski, D. L. (2010). Epigenetic regulation of latent HSV-1 gene expression. *Biochimica et Biophysica Acta, 1799*(3–4), 246–256. doi:10.1016/j.bbagrm.2009.12.001.
52. Vere Hodge, R. A., & Field, H. J. (2013). Antiviral agents for herpes simplex virus. *Advances in Pharmacology, 67*, 1–38. doi:10.1016/B978-0-12-405880-4.00001-9.
53. Pinninti, S. G., & Kimberlin, D. W. (2013). Neonatal herpes simplex virus infections. *Pediatric Clinics of North America, 60*(2), 351–365. doi:10.1016/j.pcl.2012.12.005.
54. Zhu, X. P., Muhammad, Z. S., Wang, J. G., et al. (2014). HSV-2 vaccine: Current status and insight into factors for developing an efficient vaccine. *Viruses, 6*(2), 371–390. doi:10.3390/v6020371.
55. Ruocco, V., Sangiuliano, S., Brunetti, G., et al. (2012). Beyond zoster: Sensory and immune changes in zoster-affected dermatomes: A review. *Acta Dermato-Venereologica, 92*(4), 378–382. doi:10.2340/00015555-1284.
56. Kim, S. R., Khan, F., Ramirez-Fort, M. K., et al. (2014). Varicella zoster: An update on current treatment options and future perspectives. *Expert Opinion on Pharmacotherapy, 15*(1), 61–71. do i:10.1517/14656566.2014.860443.
57. Bruggink, S. C., Gussekloo, J., Egberts, P. F., et al. (2015). Monochloroacetic acid application is an effective alternative to cryotherapy for common and plantar warts in primary care: A randomized controlled trial. *The Journal of Investigative Dermatology, 135*(5), 1261–1267. doi:10.1038/jid.2015.1.
58. On, S. C., Linkner, R. V., Haddican, M., et al. (2014). A single-blinded randomized controlled study to assess the efficacy of twice daily application of sinecatechins 15% ointment when used sequentially with cryotherapy in the treatment of external genital warts. *Journal of Drugs in Dermatology, 13*(11), 1400–1405.
59. Grce, M., & Mravak-Stipetić, M. (2014). Human papillomavirus-associated diseases. *Clinics in Dermatology, 32*(2), 253–258. doi:10.1016/j.clindermatol.2013.10.006.
60. Del Rosso, J. Q., & Kircik, L. H. (2013). Optimizing topical antifungal therapy for superficial cutaneous fungal infections: Focus on topical naftifine for cutaneous dermatophytosis. *Journal of Drugs in Dermatology, 12*(11, Suppl.), s165–s171.
61. Yapar, N. (2014). Epidemiology and risk factors for invasive candidiasis. *Therapeutics and Clinical Risk Management, 10*, 95–105. doi:10.2147/TCRM.S40160.
62. Habif, T. P. (2009). *Clinical dermatology* (5th ed., p. 523). St. Louis: Mosby.
63. Marzano, A. V., Vezzoli, P., & Berti, E. (2013). Skin involvement in cutaneous and systemic vasculitis. *Autoimmunity Reviews, 12*(4), 467–476. doi:10.1016/j.autrev.2012.08.005.
64. Jain, S. (2014). Pathogenesis of chronic urticaria: An overview. *Dermatology Research and Practice, 2014*, 674709. doi:10.1155/2014/674709.
65. Bielsa Marsol, I. (2013). Update on the classification and treatment of localized scleroderma. *Actas Dermo-Sifiliograficas, 104*(8), 654–666. doi:10.1016/j.adengl.2012.10.012.
66. Wigley, F. M. (2009). Vascular disease in scleroderma. *Clinical Reviews in Allergy and Immunology, 36*(2–3), 150–175. doi:10.1007/s12016-008-8106-x.
67. Hudson, M., & Fritzler, M. J. (2014). Diagnostic criteria of systemic sclerosis. *Journal of Autoimmunity, 48–49*, 38–41. doi:10.1016/j.jaut.2013.11.004.
68. Kreuter, A. (2012). Localized scleroderma. *Dermatologic Therapy, 25*(2), 135–147. doi:10.1111/j.1529-8019.2012.01479.x.
69. Chetty, P., Choi, F., & Mitchell, T. (2015). Primary care review of actinic keratosis and its therapeutic options: A global perspective. *Dermatology and Therapy, 5*(1), 19–35. doi:10.1007/s13555-015-0070-9.
70. Ibrahimi, O. A., Alikhan, A., & Eisen, D. B. (2012). Congenital melanocytic nevi: Where are we now? Part II. Treatment options and approach to treatment. *Journal of the American Academy of Dermatology, 67*(4), 515. doi:10.1016/j.jaad.2012.06.022.
71. Puig, S., & Malvehy, J. (2013). Monitoring patients with multiple nevi. *Dermatologic Clinics, 31*(4), 565–577. doi:10.1016/j.det.2013.06.004.
72. Emmert, S., Schön, M. P., & Haenssle, H. A. (2014). Molecular biology of basal and squamous cell carcinomas. *Advances in Experimental Medicine and Biology, 810*, 234–252.
73. Reichrath, J., & Rass, K. (2014). Ultraviolet damage, DNA repair and vitamin D in nonmelanoma skin cancer and in malignant melanoma: An update. *Advances in Experimental Medicine and Biology, 810*, 208–233.
74. American Cancer Society. (2015). *Cancer facts & figures 2015*. Atlanta: Author.
75. Bejar, C., & Maubec, E. (2014). Therapy of advanced squamous cell carcinoma of the skin. *Current Treatment Options in Oncology, 15*(2), 302–320. doi:10.1007/s11864-014-0280-x.
76. Canadian Cancer Society. (2017). *Melanoma skin cancer statistics*. Retrieved from http://www.cancer.ca/en/cancer-information/cancer-type/skin-melanoma/statistics/?region=on.
77. Sondak, V. K., & Messina, J. L. (2014). Unusual presentations of melanoma: Melanoma of unknown primary site, melanoma arising in childhood, and melanoma arising in the eye and on mucosal surfaces. *The Surgical Clinics of North America, 94*(5), 1059–1073. doi:10.1016/j.suc.2014.07.010.
78. Azoury, S. C., & Lange, J. R. (2014). Epidemiology, risk factors, prevention, and early detection of melanoma. *The Surgical Clinics of North America, 94*(5), 945–962. doi:10.1016/j.suc.2014.07.013.
79. Little, E. G., & Eide, M. J. (2012). Update on the current state of melanoma incidence. *Dermatologic Clinics, 30*(3), 355–361. doi:10.1016/j.det.2012.04.001.
80. Lo, J. A., & Fisher, D. E. (2014). The melanoma revolution: From UV carcinogenesis to a new era in therapeutics. *Science, 346*(6212), 945–949. doi:10.1126/science.1253735.
81. Kauffmann, R. M., & Chen, S. L. (2014). Workup and staging of malignant melanoma. *The Surgical Clinics of North America, 94*(5), 963–972. doi:10.1016/j.suc.2014.07.001.
82. Robert, C., Karaszewska, B., Schachter, J., et al. (2015). Improved overall survival in melanoma with combined dabrafenib and trametinib. *The New England Journal of Medicine, 372*(1), 30–39. doi:10.1056/NEJMoa1412690.
83. Hao, M., Song, F., Du, X., et al. (2015). Advances in targeted therapy for unresectable melanoma: New drugs and combinations. *Cancer Letters, 359*(1), 1–8. doi:10.1016/j.canlet.2014.12.050.

84. Ozao-Choy, J., Lee, D. J., & Faries, M. B. (2014). Melanoma vaccines: Mixed past, promising future. *The Surgical Clinics of North America, 94*(5), 1017–1030. doi:10.1016/j.suc.2014.07.005.
85. Ruocco, E., Ruocco, V., Tornesello, M. L., et al. (2013). Kaposi's sarcoma: Etiology and pathogenesis, inducing factors, causal associations, and treatments: Facts and controversies. *Clinics in Dermatology, 31*(4), 413–422. doi:10.1016/j.clindermatol.2013.01.008.
86. Luu, H. N., Amirian, E. S., Chiao, E. Y., et al. (2014). Age patterns of Kaposi's sarcoma incidence in a cohort of HIV-infected men. *Cancer Medicine, 3*(6), 1635–1643. doi:10.1002/cam4.312.
87. Klemke, C. D. (2014). Cutaneous lymphomas. *Journal der Deutschen Dermatologischen Gesellschaft, 12*(1), 7–28. doi:10.1111/ddg.12237.
88. Jawed, S. I., Myskowski, P. L., Horwitz, S., et al. (2014). Primary cutaneous T-cell lymphoma (mycosis fungoides and Sézary syndrome). Part II: Prognosis, management, and future directions. *Journal of the American Academy of Dermatology, 70*(2), 223. doi:10.1016/j.jaad.2013.08.033.
89. Kempf, W., Kazakov, D. V., & Kerl, K. (2014). Cutaneous lymphomas: An update. Part 1: T-cell and natural killer/T-cell lymphomas and related conditions. *The American Journal of Dermatopathology, 36*(2), 105–123. doi:10.1097/DAD.0b013e318289b1db.
90. Parachute Canada. (2015). *The cost of injury in Canada*. Toronto: Author, p. 4, Table 3. Retrieved from http://www.parachutecanada.org/downloads/research/Cost_of_Injury-2015.pdf.
91. Dries, D. J., & Endorf, F. W. (2013). Inhalation injury: Epidemiology, pathology, treatment strategies. *Scandinavian Journal of Trauma, Resuscitation and Emergency Medicine, 21*, 31. doi:10.1186/1757-7241-21-31.
92. Sheridan, R. L., & Chang, P. (2014). Acute burn procedures. *The Surgical Clinics of North America, 94*(4), 755–764. doi:10.1016/j.suc.2014.05.014.
93. Yu, C. Y., Lin, C. H., & Yang, Y. H. (2010). Human body surface area database ad estimation formula. *Burns, 36*(5), 616–629. doi:10.1016/j.burns.2009.05.013.
94. Cancio, L. C. (2014). Initial assessment and fluid resuscitation of burn patients. *The Surgical Clinics of North America, 94*(4), 741–754. doi:10.1016/j.suc.2014.05.003.
95. Pruitt, B. A., Jr. (2014). Reflection: Evolution of the field over seven decades. *The Surgical Clinics of North America, 94*(4), 721–740. doi:10.1016/j.suc.2014.05.001.
96. Jeschke, M. G. (2009). The hepatic response to thermal injury: Is the liver important for postburn outcomes? *Molecular Medicine (Cambridge, Mass.), 15*(9–10), 337–351. doi:10.2119/molmed.2009.00005.
97. Lippi, G., Ippolito, L., & Cervellin, G. (2010). Disseminated intravascular coagulation in burn injury. *Seminars in Thrombosis and Hemostasis, 36*(4), 429–436. doi:10.1055/s-0030-1254051.
98. Kramer, G. C. (2012). Pathophysiology of burn shock and burn edema. In D. N. Herndon (Ed.), *Total burn care* (4th ed.). Philadelphia: Saunders.
99. White, D. J., Maass, D. L., Sanders, B., et al. (2002). Cardiomyocyte intracellular calcium and cardiac dysfunction after burn trauma. *Critical Care Medicine, 30*(1), 14–22.
100. Klein, G. L., Przkora, R., & Herndon, D. N. (2012). Effects of burn injury on bone and mineral metabolism. In D. N. Herndon (Ed.), *Total burn care* (4th ed.). Philadelphia: Saunders.
101. Liu, Z. J., Wang, W., & He, C. S. (2000). Comparison of serum and plasma lactate dehydrogenase in postburn patients. *Burns, 26*(1), 46–48.
102. Pruitt, B. A., Jr., & Wolf, S. E. (2009). An historical perspective on advances in burn care over the past 100 years. *Clinics in Plastic Surgery, 36*(4), 527–545. doi:10.1016/j.cps.2009.05.007.
103. Jeschke, M. G., Gauglitz, G. G., Kulp, G. A., et al. (2011). Long-term persistence of the pathophysiologic response to severe burn injury. *PLoS ONE, 6*(7), e21245. doi:10.1371/journal.pone.0021245.
104. Mecott, G. A., Al-Mousawi, A. M., Gauglitz, G. G., et al. (2010). The role of hyperglycemia in burned patients: Evidence-based studies. *Shock (Augusta, Ga.), 33*(1), 5–13. doi:10.1097/SHK.0b013e3181af0494.
105. Ballian, N., Rabiee, A., Andersen, D. K., et al. (2010). Glucose metabolism in burn patients: The role of insulin and other endocrine hormones. *Burns, 36*(5), 599–605. doi:10.1016/j.burns.2009.11.008.
106. Williams, F. N., Branski, L. K., Jeschke, M. G., et al. (2011). What, how, and how much should patients with burns be fed? *The Surgical Clinics of North America, 1*(3), 609–629. doi:10.1016/j.suc.2011.03.002.
107. Norbury, W. B., & Herndon, D. N. (2012). Modulation of the hypermetabolic response after burn injury. In D. N. Herndon (Ed.), *Total burn care* (4th ed.). Philadelphia: Saunders.
108. Kallinen, O., Maisniemi, K., Böhling, T., et al. (2012). Multiple organ failure as a cause of death in patients with severe burns. *Journal of Burn Care and Research, 33*(2), 206–211. doi:10.1097/BCR.0b013e3182331e73.
109. Fagan, S. P., Bilodeau, M. L., & Goverman, J. (2014). Burn intensive care. *The Surgical Clinics of North America, 94*(4), 765–779. doi:10.1016/j.suc.2014.05.004.
110. Saaiq, M., Ziab, S., & Ahmad, S. (2012). Early excision and grafting versus delayed excision and grafting of deep thermal burns up to 40% total body surface area: A comparison of outcome. *Annals of Burns and Fire Disasters, 25*(3), 143–147.
111. Turnage, R. H., Nwariaku, F., Murphy, J., et al. (2002). Mechanisms of pulmonary microvascular dysfunction during severe burn injury. *World Journal of Surgery, 26*(7), 848–853. doi:10.1007/s00268-002-4063-3.
112. Xiu, F., & Jeschke, M. G. (2013). Perturbed mononuclear phagocyte system in severely burned and septic patients. *Shock (Augusta, Ga.), 40*(2), 81–88. doi:10.1097/SHK.0b013e318299f774.
113. Mann-Salinas, E. A., Baun, M. M., Meininger, J. C., et al. (2013). Novel predictors of sepsis outperform the American Burn Association sepsis criteria in the burn intensive care unit patient. *Journal of Burn Care and Research, 34*(1), 31–43. doi:10.1097/BCR.0b013e31826450b5.
114. Rex, S. (2012). Burn injuries. *Current Opinion in Critical Care, 18*(6), 671–676. doi:10.1097/MCC.0b013e328359fd6e.
115. Gamst-Jensen, H., Vedel, P. N., Lindberg-Larsen, V. O., et al. (2014). Acute pain management in burn patients: Appraisal and thematic analysis of four clinical guidelines. *Burns, 40*(8), 1463–1469. doi:10.1016/j.burns.2014.08.020.
116. Nordlund, M. J., Pham, T. N., & Gibran, N. S. (2014). Micronutrients after burn injury: A review. *Journal of Burn Care and Research, 35*(2), 121–133. doi:10.1097/BCR.0b013e318290110b.
117. Rousseau, A. F., Losser, M. R., Ichai, C., et al. (2013). ESPEN endorsed recommendations: Nutritional therapy in major burns. *Clinical Nutrition, 32*(4), 497–502. doi:10.1016/j.clnu.2013.02.012.
118. Mogoşanu, G. D., & Grumezescu, A. M. (2014). Natural and synthetic polymers for wounds and burns dressing. *International Journal of Pharmaceutics, 463*(2), 127–136. doi:10.1016/j.ijpharm.2013.12.015.
119. Wasiak, J., Cleland, H., Campbell, F., et al. (2013). Dressings for superficial and partial thickness burns. *The Cochrane Database of Systematic Reviews*, (3), CD002106, doi:10.1002/14651858.CD002106.pub4.
120. Orgill, D. P., & Ogawa, R. (2013). Current methods of burn reconstruction. *Plastic and Reconstructive Surgery, 131*(5), 827e–836e. doi:10.1097/PRS.0b013e31828e2138.
121. Mohr, W. J., Jenabzadeh, K., & Ahrenholz, D. H. (2009). Cold injury. *Hand Clinics, 25*(4), 481–496. doi:10.1016/j.hcl.2009.06.004.
122. Petrone, P., Asensio, J. A., & Marini, C. P. (2014). Management of accidental hypothermia and cold injury. *Current Problems in Surgery, 51*(10), 417–431. doi:10.1067/j.cpsurg.2014.07.004.
123. Handford, C., Buxton, P., Russell, K., et al. (2014). Frostbite: A practical approach to hospital management. *Extreme Physiology and Medicine, 3*, 7. doi:10.1186/2046-7648-3-7.
124. Qi, J., & Garza, L. A. (2014). An overview of alopecias. *Cold Spring Harbor Perspectives in Medicine, 4*(3), a013615. doi:10.1101/cshperspect.a013615.
125. Piraccini, B. M., & Alessandrini, A. (2014). Androgenetic alopecia. *Giornale Italiano Di Dermatologia E Venereologia: Organo Ufficiale, Societa Italiana Di Dermatologia E Sifilografia, 149*(1), 15–24.
126. Vujovic, A., & Del Marmol, V. (2014). The female pattern hair loss: Review of etiopathogenesis and diagnosis. *BioMed Research International, 2014*, 767628. doi:10.1155/2014/767628.
127. Alkhalifah, A., Alsantali, A., Wang, E., et al. (2010). Alopecia areata update: Part I. Clinical picture, histopathology, and pathogenesis. *Journal of the American Academy of Dermatology, 62*(2), 177–188. doi:10.1016/j.jaad.2009.10.032.
128. Alkhalifah, A., Alsantali, A., Wang, E., et al. (2010). Alopecia areata update: Part II. Treatment. *Journal of the American Academy of Dermatology, 62*(2), 191–202. doi:10.1016/j.jaad.2009.10.031.
129. Hordinsky, M. K. (2013). Overview of alopecia areata. *The Journal of Investigative Dermatology: Symposium Proceedings, 16*(1), S13–S15. doi:10.1038/jidsymp.2013.4.
130. Blume-Peytavi, U. (2013). How to diagnose and treat medically women with excessive hair. *Dermatologic Clinics, 31*(1), 57–65. doi:10.1016/j.det.2012.08.009.
131. Relhan, V., Goel, K., Bansal, S., et al. (2014). Management of chronic paronychia. *Indian Journal of Dermatology, 59*(1), 15–20. doi:10.4103/0019-5154.123482.
132. Rigopoulos, D., Larios, G., Gregoriou, S., et al. (2008). Acute and chronic paronychia. *American Family Physician, 77*(3), 339–346.
133. Westerberg, D. P., & Voyack, M. J. (2013). Onychomycosis: Current trends in diagnosis and treatment. *American Family Physician, 88*(11), 762–770.

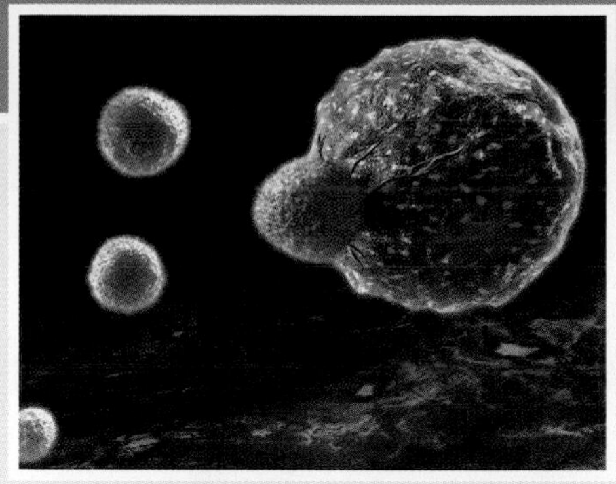

42

Alterations of the Integument in Children

Noreen Heer Nicol, Sue E. Huether, and Stephanie Zettel

EVOLVE WEBSITE

http://evolve.elsevier.com/Canada/Huether/pathophysiology
Student Review Questions
Key Points
Case Studies
Animations
Quick Check Answers

CHAPTER OUTLINE

Acne Vulgaris, 1107
Dermatitis, 1108
Atopic Dermatitis, 1108
Diaper Dermatitis, 1109
Infections of the Skin, 1109
Bacterial Infections, 1109
Fungal Infections, 1110
Viral Infections, 1111
Insect Bites and Parasites, 1113
Scabies, 1114
Pediculosis (Lice Infestation), 1114
Fleas, 1114
Bedbugs, 1114
Cutaneous Hemangiomas and Vascular Malformations, 1115
Cutaneous Hemangiomas, 1115
Cutaneous Vascular Malformations, 1116
Other Skin Disorders, 1116
Miliaria, 1116
Erythema Toxicum Neonatorum, 1116

Children frequently develop alterations of the skin that may be minor or severe and either localized or generalized. Skin diseases in children may have different causative mechanisms and different patterns of distribution than those found in adults, although there may be similarities (e.g., children can also get pressure ulcers). Some skin diseases resolve spontaneously and require no treatment. Diagnosis is commonly made from the history, appearance, and distribution of the lesion or lesions. Common skin diseases of childhood are presented here.

ACNE VULGARIS

Acne vulgaris is the most common skin disease and occurs primarily between the ages of 12 and 25 years. Acne tends to occur in families, and genetic susceptibility may determine the severity of the disease. The incidence of acne is the same in both genders, although severe disease affects males more often.[1] Diets high in simple carbohydrates and dairy products are associated with acne.[2-4]

Acne develops at distinctive pilosebaceous units known as *sebaceous follicles.* Located primarily on the face and upper parts of the chest and back, these follicles have many large sebaceous glands, a small vellus hair (very short, nonpigmented, and very thin hair), and a dilated follicular canal that is visible as a pore on the skin surface. Acne lesions may be noninflammatory or inflammatory (cystic) (Figure 42-1). In **noninflammatory acne**, the comedones are open (blackheads) and closed (whiteheads), with the accumulated material causing distension of the follicle and thinning of follicular canal walls. **Inflammatory (cystic) acne** develops in closed comedones when the follicular wall ruptures, expelling sebum into the surrounding dermis and initiating inflammation. Pustules form when the inflammation is close to the surface; papules and cystic nodules can develop when the inflammation is deeper, causing mild to severe scarring. Both types of lesions may exist in the same individual.

The principal causative factors are (1) hyperkeratinization of the follicular epithelium, (2) excessive sebum production, (3) follicular proliferation of anaerobic *Propionibacterium acnes*, and (4) inflammation and rupture of a follicle from accumulated debris and bacteria (see Figure 42-1). *P. acnes* shifts from being symbiotic to pathogenic and from being noninflammatory to inflammatory. The causal mechanism is unknown.[5] Androgens (dehydroepiandrosterone sulphate and testosterone), synthesized in increasing amounts during puberty, increase the size and productivity of the sebaceous glands, which promotes *P. acnes. P. acnes* produces extracellular porphyrins and proinflammatory molecules, including chemotactic factors and lipolytic and proteolytic enzymes. The hydrolytic action of the enzymes converts triglycerides into free fatty acids (FFAs). FFAs activate Toll-like receptors, T-cell–associated and T-helper 17 (Th17)–associated inflammation, and edema that results in pus formation and breakdown of the follicle wall.[6]

The treatment of acne should be individualized according to severity. Combinations of a topical retinoid [Retin-A], benzoyl peroxide, and antimicrobial agents are preferred. Retinoids are anticomedogenic and comedolytic and have some anti-inflammatory effects. Benzoyl peroxide is antimicrobial with some keratolytic effects. Antibiotics have anti-inflammatory and antimicrobial effects. Use of systemic therapies, including oral antibiotics, sex hormones, corticosteroids, and isotretinoin

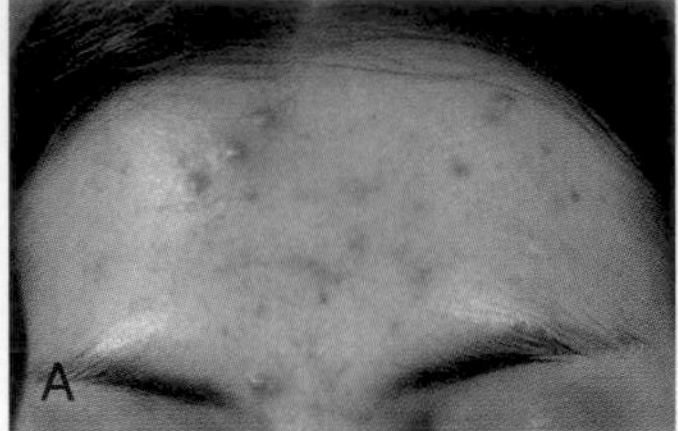

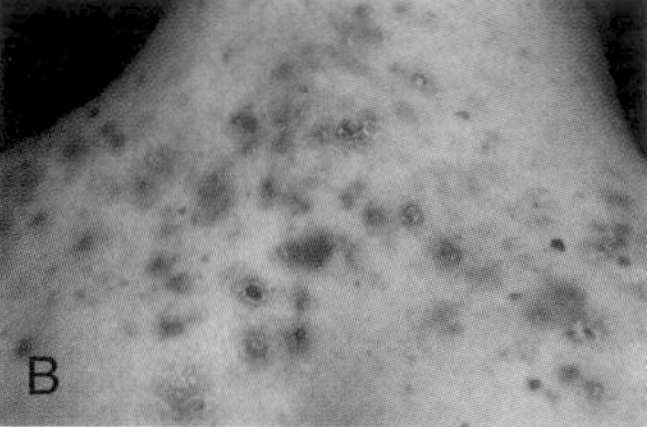

FIGURE 42-1 Acne. A, Inflammatory papules and pustules. **B,** Severe nodular cystic acne. (From Kliegman, R.M., Stanton, B.F., Gemell, J.W., et al. [Eds.]. [2011]. *Nelson textbook of pediatrics* [19th ed.]. Philadelphia: Saunders.)

(Accutane; this medication requires pregnancy prevention), may be limited by side effects.[7] Acne surgery, including comedo extraction, intralesional steroids, and cryosurgery, is useful in selected individuals. Severe scarring may be treated with dermabrasion, lasers, and resurfacing techniques. Diets should avoid high glycemic index foods. Psychological support is important because acne negatively affects quality of life, self-esteem, and mood in adolescents and is associated with an increased risk for anxiety, depression, and suicidal ideation.[8] Special consideration must be given to treatment for those with darker skin because they have greater risk for hyperpigmentation and keloidal scarring.[9] Research is continuing on the development of vaccines to prevent acne.[10]

Acne conglobata is a highly inflammatory form of acne with communicating cysts and abscesses beneath the skin that can cause scarring. Remissions tend to occur during the summer, perhaps from more exposure to sunlight. This type of acne requires the use of systemic and combination therapies to prevent medication resistance.

Hydradinitis suppurativa (inverse acne) is a chronic inflammatory disease characterized by recurrent abscesses, sinus tract formation, and scarring. There is hyperkeratosis and occlusion of the pilosebaceous follicular ducts involving areas of skin where there are folds, hair follicles, and apocrine (sweat) glands (i.e., axillary, inguinal, inframammary, genital, buttocks, and perineal areas of the body). The cause is unknown, but the incidence is estimated at 1 to 4% of the population and is more common in females. Aggravating factors include obesity, stress, and smoking. The lesions present as deep, firm, painful subcutaneous nodules that track and rupture horizontally under the skin. Treatment can include incision and drainage of nodules, culture of exudate, and administration of antibiotics (with concern about the presence of methicillin-resistant *Staphylococcus aureus* [MRSA]), topical or intralesional corticosteroids, and retinoids. The disease can recur for years, with negative effects on quality of life.[11]

DERMATITIS

Atopic Dermatitis

Atopic dermatitis (AD), also known as *atopic eczema*, is the most common cause of eczema in children. Approximately 17% of Canadians experience this at least one point in their lives.[12] More than half of these individuals develop asthma and allergies later in life.[13] Onset is usually from 2 to 6 months of age, and 85% of cases develop within the first 5 years of life.

The cause of this chronic relapsing form of pruritic eczema involves an interplay of genetic predisposition; altered skin barrier function associated with filaggrin gene mutations and filaggrin deficiency (proteins that bind keratin in the epidermis); reduced ceramide (a stratum corneum lipid) levels; decreased antimicrobial peptides; altered innate immunity; and altered immune responses to allergens, irritants, and microbes.[14] Filaggrin gene mutations also are associated with increased risk for asthma in AD and ichthyosis vulgaris (dry, scaly skin)[15] (Figure 42-2).

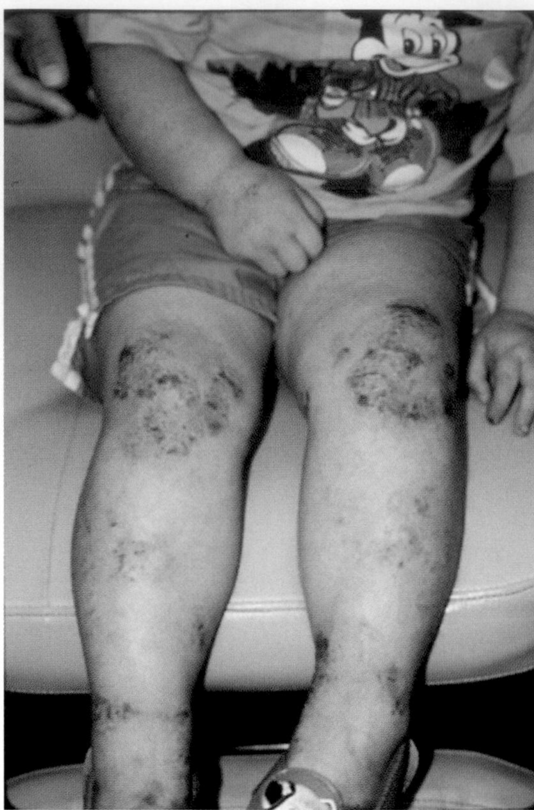

FIGURE 42-2 Atopic Dermatitis. Characteristic lesions with crusting from irritation and scratching over knees and around ankles. (Courtesy Department of Dermatology, School of Medicine, University of Utah, Salt Lake City, UT.)

There is an altered skin microbiome with formation of biofilm by *S. aureus* that may act as superantigens causing exacerbations of eczema.[16]

AD has a constellation of clinical features that include severe pruritus and a characteristic eczematoid appearance with redness, edema, and scaling. The skin becomes increasingly dry, itchy, sensitive, and easily irritated because the barrier function of the skin is impaired. Itching is the hallmark of AD, and rubbing and scratching to relieve the itch are responsible for many of the clinical skin changes of AD. In young children, a rash appears primarily on the face, scalp, trunk, and extensor surfaces of the arms and legs (see Figure 42-2). In older children and adults, the rash tends to be found on the neck, antecubital and popliteal fossae, and hands and feet. Individuals with AD also tend to develop viral, bacterial, and fungal skin infections in the eczematous areas. There are no specific laboratory features of AD that can be used for diagnostic and treatment purposes.[17] Most affected individuals show increased serum levels of immunoglobulin E (IgE), interleukin-4, and eosinophils (eosinophilia) and positive skin tests to a variety of common food and inhalant allergens.

Management of individuals with AD includes accurate diagnosis and comprehensive evaluation of triggers and response to treatment; management of confounding factors, including sleep disruption; and education of individuals and caregivers. Avoidance of triggers and promotion of skin hydration, including soaking baths and emollients, are key to good therapy.[18] Anti-inflammatory agents, such as topical corticosteroids and calcineurin inhibitors, are necessary during active flare-ups of eczema. Immunomodulator therapy and wet wrap therapy[19] are used for severe eczema. Systemic therapy includes the use of sedating antihistamines and antibiotics. Research is in progress to develop molecule-specific targets to produce long-term disease remission.[20]

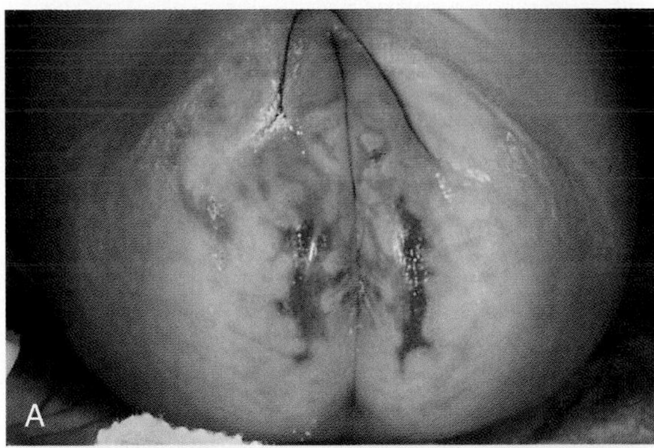

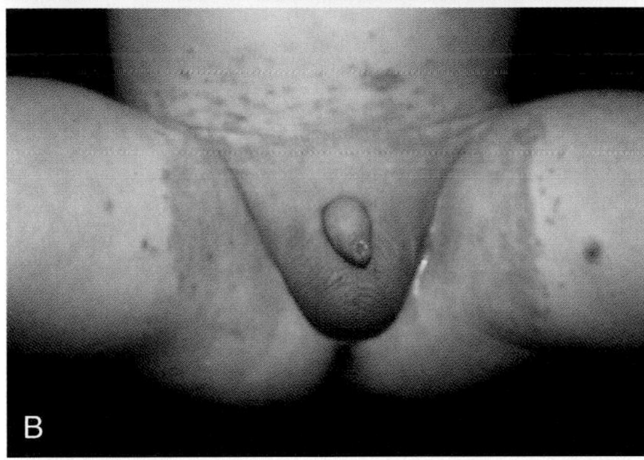

FIGURE 42-3 Diaper Dermatitis. A, Diaper dermatitis with erosions. **B,** Diaper dermatitis with *Candida albicans* secondary infection. (Courtesy Department of Dermatology, School of Medicine, University of Utah, Salt Lake City, UT.)

BOX 42-1 Impetigo

Vesicular Impetigo

- Contagious, acute, superficial, vesiculopustular are the most common forms
- Caused by group A *Streptococcus pyogenes* (alone or with *Staphylococcus aureus*)
- Spread by direct physical contact with other infected individuals or through insect bites
- Presents as small vesicles with a honey-coloured serum; yellow to white-brown crusts form as vesicles rupture and extend radially
- Untreated lesions last for weeks and cover large area
- Regional lymphadenitis common
- Most significant complication is acute glomerulonephritis
- Treatment is aggressive in light of this complication

Bullous Impetigo

- Caused by *S. aureus*
- Bacterial toxin (exfoliative toxin) produced causes disruption in cellular adhesion with blister formation
- Occurs in neonates
- Highly contagious
- Source is family member with pustule or asymptomatic carrier with pathogen in anterior nares, perineal region, or fingernails
- Transmitted by contact with individual or contaminated equipment
- Presents with vesicles that enlarge or coalesce to form superficial bullae, few localized lesions, or many lesions scattered over the skin surface; as bullae rupture, thin, flat, honey-coloured crust appears (hallmark of impetigo)
- Lesions found on face around the nose and mouth; hands and other exposed areas also susceptible

Diaper Dermatitis

Diaper dermatitis (diaper rash) is a form of irritant contact dermatitis initiated by a combination of factors, including prolonged exposure to and irritation by urine and feces as well as maceration by wet diapers or airtight plastic diaper covers. Disposable diaper designs have decreased the incidence of diaper dermatitis in infants. Often, diaper dermatitis is secondarily infected with *Candida albicans*. The resulting inflammation affects the lower aspect of the abdomen, genitalia, buttock, and upper portion of the thigh.

The lesions vary from mild erythema to erythematous papular lesions. Candidal (monilial) diaper dermatitis is usually very erythematous, with sharp margination and pustulovesicular satellite lesions (Figure 42-3).

Treatment involves frequent diaper changes to keep the affected area clean and dry or regular exposure of the perineal area to air, use of superabsorbent diapers, and topical protection with a product containing petrolatum or zinc oxide, or both. Topical antifungal medication is used to treat *C. albicans*, when present.[21]

QUICK CHECK 42-1

1. What causes the inflammation of acne vulgaris?
2. What lesions are typical of atopic dermatitis in children?
3. What causes diaper dermatitis?

INFECTIONS OF THE SKIN

Infectious diseases caused by bacteria, viruses, and fungi constitute the major forms of skin disease. Breaks in skin integrity, particularly those that inoculate pathogens into the dermis and epidermis, may cause or exacerbate infections. Most infections tend to occur superficially; however, systemic signs and symptoms develop occasionally and can be life-threatening in immunosuppressed children.

Bacterial Infections

Impetigo Contagiosum

Impetigo is the most common bacterial skin infection in children 2 to 5 years of age. *S. aureus* and, less commonly, *Streptococcus pyogenes* cause impetigo. The mode of transmission is by both direct and indirect contact. The disease is more common in midsummer to late summer, with a higher incidence in hot, humid climates. Impetigo is particularly infectious among people living in crowded conditions with poor sanitary facilities or in settings such as day care facilities. It affects children in good health, but conditions such as anemia and malnutrition are predisposing factors.

Bacterial invasion occurs through minor breaks in the cutaneous surface or as a secondary infection of a pre-existing dermatosis or infestation. The staphylococci produce bacterial toxins called *exfoliative toxins* (ETs) that cause a disruption in desmosomal adhesion molecules with blister formation. There are two types of impetigo: nonbullous and, more rarely, bullous (caused only by *S. aureus*), where blisters enlarge or coalesce to form bullae (Box 42-1). Both forms of impetigo begin as vesicles with a thin vesicular roof composed of stratum corneum that ruptures to form a honey-coloured crust (Figure 42-4). The lesions are often located on the face, around the nose and mouth, but the hands and other exposed areas also are involved. Impetigo is clinically characterized by crusted erosions or ulcers that may arise as a primary infection or as a secondary infection of a pre-existing dermatosis or infestation.

The treatment of choice for both types of impetigo is topical mupirocin (Bactroban) or fusidic acid (Fucidin) for uncomplicated

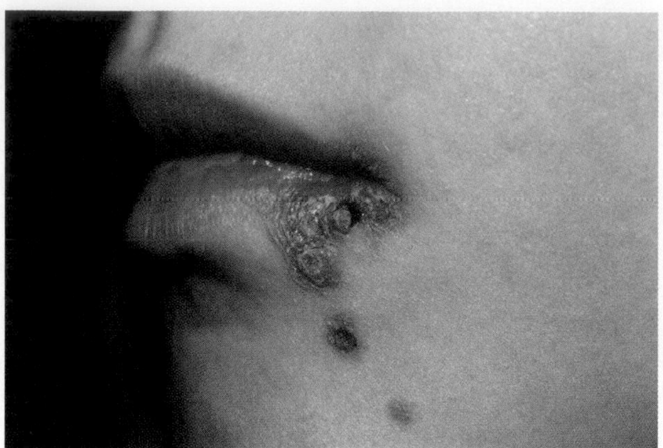

FIGURE 42-4 Impetigo. Multiple crusted and oozing lesions of impetigo. (From Kliegman, R.M., Stanton, B.F., Gemell, J.W., et al. [Eds.]. [2011]. *Nelson textbook of pediatrics* [19th ed.]. Philadelphia: Saunders.)

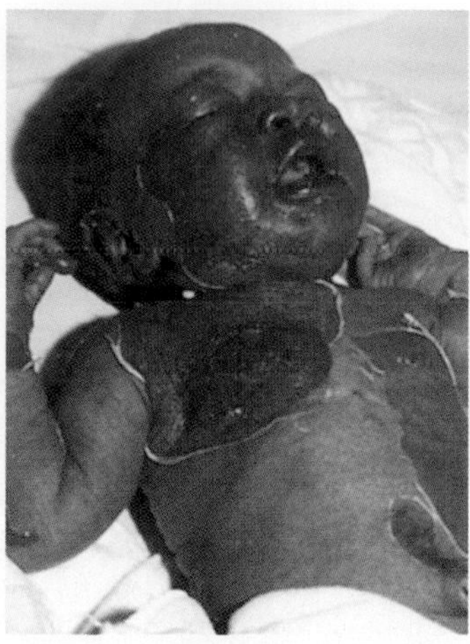

FIGURE 42-5 Staphylococcal Scalded-Skin Syndrome. The skin lesions, showing desquamation and wrinkling of the skin margins, appeared 1 day after drainage of a staphylococcal abscess. (From Kliegman, R.M., Stanton, B.F., Gemell, J.W., et al. [Eds.]. [2011]. *Nelson textbook of pediatrics* [19th ed.]. Philadelphia: Saunders.)

lesions. For extensive or complicated impetigo, systemic antibiotics may be warranted, but β-lactam antibiotics should be avoided if MRSA is suspected.[22] Prompt treatment prevents complications, such as glomerulonephritis, necrotizing fasciitis, and septic shock syndrome. Lesions usually resolve in 2 to 3 weeks without scarring. Using good handwashing techniques and isolating the infected child's washcloth, towels, drinking glass, and linen are important for prevention.[23]

Staphylococcal Scalded-Skin Syndrome

Staphylococcal scalded-skin syndrome (SSSS) is the most serious staphylococcal infection that affects the skin and is usually seen in infants and children younger than 5 years of age. SSSS is caused by virulent group II strains of staphylococci that produce an exfoliative toxin. The toxin attacks desmoglein and adhesion molecules and causes a separation of the skin just below the granular layer of the epidermis (see Figure 41-1).[24] The toxin is usually produced at body sites other than the skin and arrives at the epidermis through the circulatory system. Staphylococci typically are not found in the skin lesions themselves. Adults have circulating antistaphylococcal antibodies and are better able to metabolize and excrete the toxin. Neonates are at the highest risk because of their lack of immunity with no prior exposure to the toxin.[25] A source of the infection in neonates may be from health care workers who are nasal carriers of the microorganism. This reinforces the need for good infection control practices with all neonates.[26]

The clinical symptoms begin with fever, malaise, rhinorrhea, and irritability followed by generalized erythema with exquisite tenderness of the skin. There may be associated impetigo, but the infection often begins in the throat or chest. The erythema spreads from the face and trunk to cover the entire body except for the palms, soles, and mucous membranes. Within 48 hours, blisters and bullae may form, giving the child the appearance of being scalded. The pain is severe (Figure 42-5). Fluid loss from ruptured blisters and water evaporation from denuded areas may cause dehydration. Perioral and nasolabial crusting and fissures develop. In severe cases, the skin of the entire body may slough. When secondary infection can be prevented, healing of the involved skin occurs in 10 to 14 days, usually without scarring.

Before medical intervention is initiated, culture and histological or exfoliative cytological studies must be performed to differentiate SSSS from erythema multiforme (EM) and toxic epidermal necrolysis (TEN), both of which are usually caused by an immune reaction to medications.[27] When SSSS infection is confirmed, treatment with oral or intravenous antibiotics begins. The skin should be treated in the same manner as a severe burn, with meticulous aseptic technique. Skin substitutes may be used for adjuvant therapy.[28] Special care is required when there is involvement of the lips and eyelids.

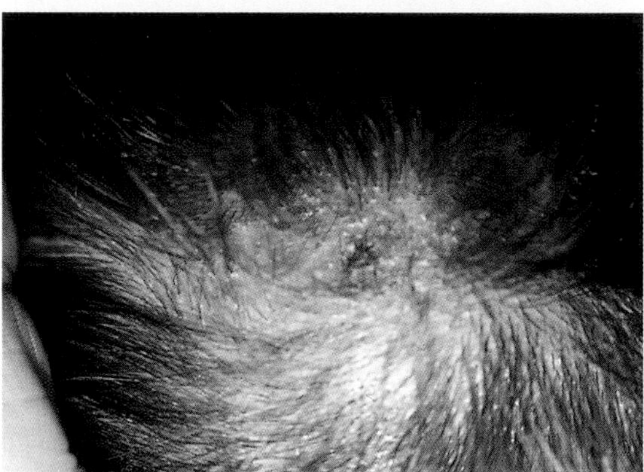

FIGURE 42-6 Tinea Capitis. (Courtesy Department of Dermatology, School of Medicine, University of Utah, Salt Lake City, UT.)

Fungal Infections

Tinea Capitis

Tinea capitis, a fungal infection of the scalp (scalp ringworm), is the most common fungal infection of childhood. It rarely affects infants and is seen in children between 2 and 10 years of age. The primary microorganism responsible for this disease is *Trichophyton tonsurans*.[29] *Microsporum canis* also continues to be a pathogenic microorganism in this disease and is found on cats, dogs, and certain rodents. Humans appear to be a terminal host for *M. canis.* Children who handle such animals are possible hosts. Direct transmission between humans does not occur. However, there is direct human transmission of *T. tonsurans* in crowded areas, the most prevalent environment of the fungus.[30]

The lesions are often circular and manifested by broken hairs 1 to 3 mm above the scalp, leaving a partial area of alopecia from 1 to 5 cm in diameter (Figure 42-6). A slight erythema and scaling with raised borders can be observed.

Diagnosis is best confirmed by potassium hydroxide (KOH) examination and fungal culture. Tinea capitis always requires systemic treatment because topical antifungal agents do not penetrate the hair follicle. Several oral antifungal agents, particularly griseofulvin (Fulvicin), are available for treatment.[31] Use of Wood's light examination has become less popular because there are a number of dermatophytes that fluoresce under an ultraviolet light.

Tinea Corporis

Tinea corporis (ringworm) is a common superficial dermatophyte infection in children. The organisms most commonly responsible for this disease are *M. canis* and *Trichophyton mentagrophytes.* As in tinea capitis, contact with young kittens and puppies is a common source of the disorder. Tinea corporis preferentially affects the nonhairy parts of the face, trunk, and limbs. Lesions are often erythematous, round or oval scaling patches that spread peripherally with clearing in the centre, creating the ring appearance, which is why this disease is commonly referred to as *ringworm.* The lesions are distributed asymmetrically, and multiple lesions, when present, overlap. Transmission occurs by direct contact with an infected lesion and through indirect contact with personal items used by the infected person. KOH examination of the scale from the border of the lesions confirms the diagnosis. Most lesions respond well to applications of appropriate topical antifungal medications.[32]

Thrush

Thrush is the term used to describe the presence of *C. albicans* in the mucous membranes of the mouths of infants. It occurs less commonly in adults, and infected adults are usually immunocompromised. *C. albicans* penetrates the epidermal barrier more easily than other microorganisms because of its keratolytic proteases and other enzymes. Thrush is characterized by the formation of white plaques or spots in the mouth that lead to shallow ulcers caused by keratolytic proteases from the microorganism. The tongue may have a dense, white covering. The underlying mucous membrane is red and tender and may bleed when the plaques are removed. The disease is often accompanied by fever and gastro-intestinal irritation. The infection commonly spreads to the groin, buttocks, and other parts of the body. Treatment may be difficult and includes oral antifungal washes, such as nystatin (Nyaderm) oral suspension. Simultaneous treatment of a *Candida* nipple infection or vaginitis in the mother is helpful in reducing the *C. albicans* surface colonization of the infant. Feeding bottles and nipples should be sterilized to prevent reinfection. The diaper area should be kept clean and dry.

Viral Infections

Viral infections of the skin in children are caused by poxvirus, papovavirus, and herpesvirus.

Molluscum Contagiosum

Molluscum contagiosum is a common, highly contagious viral infection of the skin and, occasionally, conjunctiva that affects school-aged children, sexually active young adults, and immunocompromised individuals. The incidence is higher among children who swim or have eczema; however, the mechanism of disease is not clear.[33] The disease is transmitted by skin-to-skin contact or from autoinoculation.[34]

The poxvirus proliferates within the follicular epithelium and induces epidermal cell proliferation. The epidermis grows down into the dermis to form saccules containing clusters of virus. The characteristic molluscum body is composed of mature, immature, and incomplete viruses and cellular debris.[35]

The lesions of molluscum are discrete, slightly umbilicated, dome-shaped papules 1 to 5 mm in diameter that appear anywhere on the skin or conjunctiva. The lesions are mainly on the trunk, face, and extremities in children (Figure 42-7). There is usually no inflammation surrounding molluscum lesions unless they are traumatized or secondary infection occurs. Scarring may occur with healing.

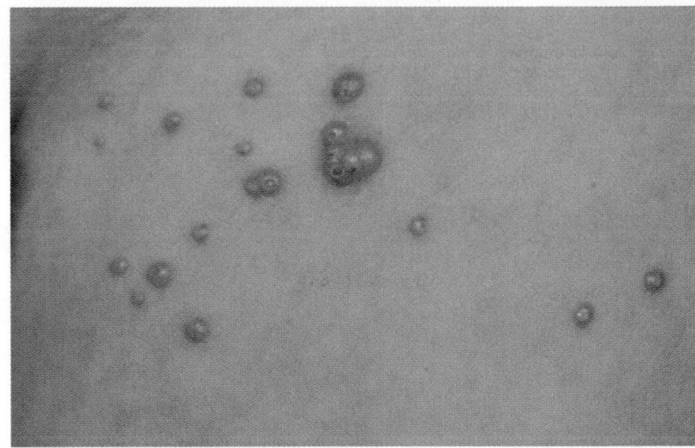

FIGURE 42-7 Molluscum Contagiosum. Waxy pink globules with umbilicated centres. (From Habif, T.P. [2004]. *Clinical dermatology: A color guide to diagnosis and therapy* [4th ed.]. St. Louis: Mosby.)

The three best diagnostic procedures are (1) staining smears of the expressed molluscum body, (2) examining a biopsy specimen, or (3) inoculating a molluscum suspension into cell cultures to demonstrate the cytotoxic reactions. Most lesions are self-limiting and clear in 6 to 9 months if not manipulated.

Treatment options include immunomodulatory and antiviral therapy and destructive procedures (cryotherapy, curettage, or laser ablation); however, no treatment is universally effective. KOH solution applications can be safe, effective, and inexpensive.[36] Treatment is recommended for genital molluscum to prevent sexual transmission and autoinoculation.[37] Measures to prevent spread of infection must be taken. Recurrences are common.

Rubella (German or 3-Day Measles)

Rubella is a common communicable disease of children and young adults caused by an RNA virus that enters the bloodstream through the respiratory route. This disease is mild in most children. The incubation period ranges from 14 to 21 days. Prodromal symptoms include enlarged cervical and postauricular lymph nodes, low-grade fever, headache, sore throat, rhinorrhea, and cough. A faint-pink to red coalescing maculopapular rash develops on the face with spread to the trunk and extremities 1 to 4 days after the onset of initial symptoms (Figure 42-8). The rash is thought to be the result of virus dissemination to the skin. The rash subsides after 2 to 3 days, usually without complication. Children are usually not contagious after development of the rash (Table 42-1).

Vaccination for rubella is usually combined with vaccines for measles, mumps, and rubella (MMR). Measles is known to occur in previously immunized children. The *Canadian Immunization Guide* includes vaccine recommendations and is available at https://www.canada.ca/en/public-health/services/canadian-immunization-guide.html (and for measles, specifically, see https://www.canada.ca/en/public-health/services/publications/healthy-living/canadian-immunization-guide-part-4-active-vaccines/page-12-measles-vaccine.html). Rubella has almost been eliminated in North America because of vaccination campaigns. However, challenges to maintaining elimination include large outbreaks of measles in highly travelled developed countries, frequent international travel, and clusters of both Americans and Canadians who remain unvaccinated because of personal belief exemptions.[38] Although MMR vaccine may rarely be associated with adverse neurological events, studies conclude that MMR immunization does not cause autism.[39] Lack of vaccination, however, leads to significant morbidity and mortality, with pneumonia, croup, and encephalitis being causes of death worldwide.

Women of childbearing age are immunized if their rubella hemagglutination-inhibition titre is low. Pregnancy should be avoided for 3 months after vaccination because the attenuated virus in the vaccine may remain viable for this period. Pregnant women who have rubella early in the first trimester may have a fetus who develops congenital defects.

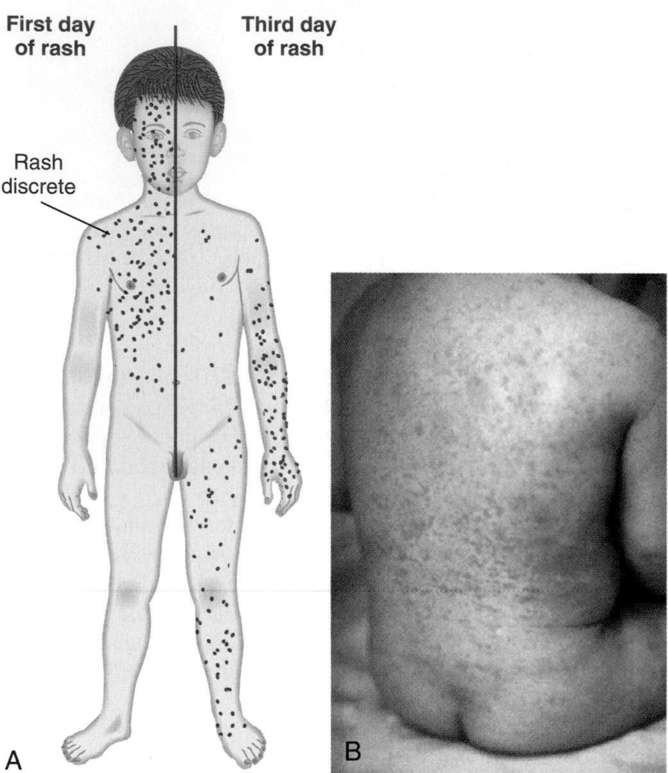

FIGURE 42-8 Rubella (3-Day Measles). **A,** Typical distribution of full-blown maculopapular rash with tendency to coalesce. **B,** Rash of rubella. (From Centers for Disease Control and Prevention Image Bank, Figure #712. Retrieved from http://phil.cdc.gov/phil/.)

There is no specific treatment for rubella. Recovery is spontaneous, although lymph nodes may remain enlarged for weeks. Supportive therapy includes rest, fluids, and use of a vaporizer. In rare cases, a mild encephalitis or peripheral neuritis may follow rubella.

Rubeola (Red Measles)

Rubeola is a highly contagious, acute viral disease of childhood. Transmitted by direct contact with droplets from infected persons, rubeola is caused by an RNA-containing paramyxovirus with an incubation period of 7 to 12 days, during which there are no symptoms. The virus enters the respiratory tract and attaches to dendritic cells and alveolar macrophages, amplifies in local lymphatic tissue, and progresses to systemic disease.[40] Prodromal symptoms include high fever (up to 40.5°C [104.9°F]), malaise, enlarged lymph nodes, rhinorrhea, conjunctivitis, and barking cough. Within 3 to 4 days, an erythematous maculopapular rash develops over the head and spreads distally over the trunk, extremities, hands, and feet. Early lesions blanch with pressure, followed by a brownish hue that does not blanch as the rash fades. Characteristic pinpoint white spots surrounded by an erythematous ring develop over the buccal mucosa and are known as *Koplik spots.* These spots precede the rash by 1 to 2 days. The rash then subsides within 3 to 5 days.

Complications associated with measles may be caused by the primary infection or by a secondary bacterial infection. Measles encephalitis occurs in about 1 of 800 cases, and most children recover completely. Only a small minority of children develop permanent brain damage or die. Bacterial complications include otitis media and pneumonia, usually caused by group A hemolytic streptococcus, *Haemophilus influenzae*, or *S. aureus* infection.

Measles is prevented by vaccination. As discussed in the "Rubella" section (p. 1111), immunization is key to prevention. There is no specific treatment for measles, and supportive therapy is the same as that recommended for rubella. Antibiotic therapy is initiated if secondary bacterial infections develop.

Roseola (Exanthema Subitum)

Roseola is a presumed viral infection of children between 6 months and 2 years of age and can be seen in children up to 4 years of age. The

TABLE 42-1 Differential Presentation of Viral Diseases Producing Rashes

Viral Disease	Incubation Period	Prodromal Symptoms	Duration/Characteristics	Clinical Symptoms
Rubella (German measles)	14–21 days	1–2 days Mild fever Malaise Respiratory symptoms	1–3 days Pink-red maculopapular rash Face and trunk	Enlarged and tender occipital and periauricular lymph nodes
Rubeola (red measles)	7–12 days	2–5 days Fever Cough Respiratory symptoms	3–5 days Purple-red to brown maculopapular rash Face, trunk, extremities	Koplik spots 1–3 days before rash
Roseola (exanthema subitum)	5–15 days	2–5 days High fever	1–3 days Red macular rash Neck and trunk	Rash develops when fever subsides
Varicella (chickenpox)	11–20 days	1–2 days Low-grade fever Cough May be asymptomatic	7–14 days Red papules, vesicles, pustules in clusters	Eruption of new lesions for 4–5 days Occasional ulcerative lesion in mouth
Fifth disease (human parvovirus B19, erythrovirus)	4–28 days	May be asymptomatic Low-grade fever, malaise before rash	7–10 days "Slapped-cheek" rash on face; lacy red rash on trunk and limbs; may itch	Rash develops when fever subsides

incubation period is 5 to 15 days, followed by the sudden onset of fever (38.9° to 40.5°C [101.3° to 104.9°F]) that lasts 3 to 5 days. Following the fever, an erythematous macular rash that lasts about 24 hours develops primarily over the trunk and neck. Children usually feel well, eat normally, and have few other symptoms. There is usually no treatment.

Smallpox

Smallpox (variola) was a highly contagious and deadly, but also preventable, disease caused by poxvirus variolae. Smallpox was eradicated worldwide in 1977. Routine immunization programs for infants were discontinued in 1972, in 1977 for health care workers, and in 1988 for Canadian Forces.[41]

Chickenpox and Herpes Zoster

Chickenpox (varicella) and herpes zoster (shingles) are both produced by the varicella-zoster virus (VZV). VZV is a complex deoxyribonucleic acid (DNA) virus of the herpes group. The incubation period is 10 to 27 days, averaging 14 days. Vesicular lesions occur in the epidermis, as infection occurs within keratinocytes. An inflammatory infiltrate is often present. Vesicles eventually rupture, followed by crust formation or the development of transient ulcers on mucous membranes. Varicella occurs in people not previously exposed to VZV, whereas herpes zoster (shingles) occurs in individuals who had varicella in the past. The virus enters the dorsal root ganglia and remains latent. Since the introduction of live attenuated VZV vaccine in 1995, there has been a significant reduction in varicella incidence and its associated complications.[42]

Chickenpox. Chickenpox (varicella) is a disease of early childhood, with 90% of children contracting the disease during the first decade of life. Being a highly contagious virus, chickenpox is spread by close person-to-person contact and by airborne droplets. Introduction of an infected person into a household results in a 90% possibility of susceptible persons developing the disease within the incubation period, usually 14 days. Children are contagious for at least 1 day before development of the rash. Transmission of the virus may occur until approximately 5 to 6 days after the onset of the first skin lesions in healthy children. In immunocompromised children, the virus is recoverable for a longer period, but infected children must be considered contagious for at least 7 to 10 days. Transmission occurs more readily in temperate climates than in tropical climates.

Normally, children who develop chickenpox have no prodromal symptoms. The first sign of illness may be pruritus or the appearance of vesicles, usually on the trunk, scalp, or face. The rash later spreads to the extremities. Characteristically, lesions can be seen in various stages of maturation, with macules, papules, and vesicles present in a particular area at the same time (Figure 42-9). The vesicular lesions are superficial and rupture easily. New lesions will erupt for 4 to 5 days, until there are approximately 100 to 300 in different stages of development. The vesicles become crusted, and over time only the crust remains, although there may be an occasional vesicle on the palm later in the disease. Although uncommon, ulcerative lesions are sometimes seen in the mouth and, less commonly, on the conjunctiva and pharynx. Fever usually lasts 2 to 3 days, with body temperature ranging from 38.5 to 40°C (101.3 to 104°F).

Complications are rare in children but more common in adults. They can include transient hematuria (from rupture of vesicles in the bladder), epistaxis, laryngeal edema, and varicella pneumonia. One case of chickenpox produces almost complete immunity against a second attack. Rarely, the fetus may be malformed (congenital varicella syndrome) if chickenpox develops in the first half of pregnancy. Infants whose mothers have chickenpox at any stage of pregnancy have a higher risk of developing herpes zoster during the first few years of life.[43] Varicella-zoster immunoglobulin should be administered to neonates

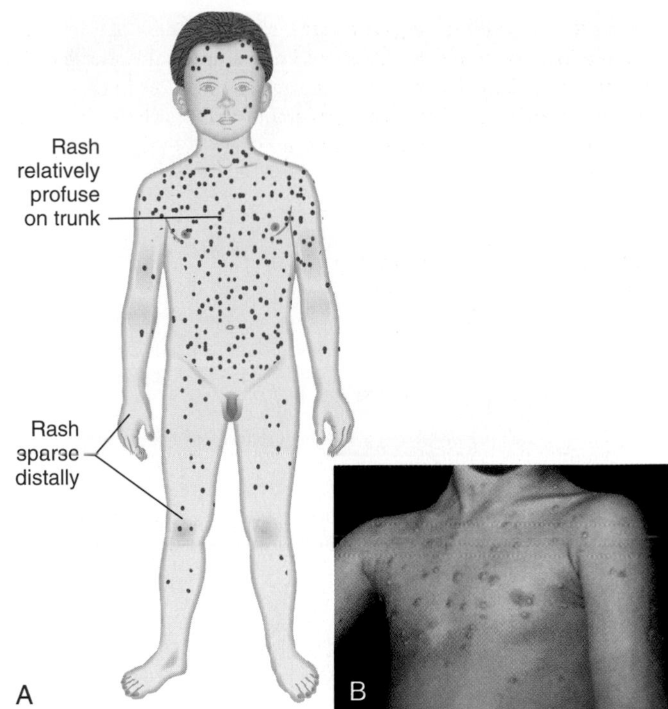

FIGURE 42-9 Chickenpox. A, Pattern of generalized, polymorphous eruption. **B,** Chickenpox lesions on fifth day of illness. (From Centers for Disease Control and Prevention Image Bank, Figure #2882. Retrieved from http://phil.cdc.gov/phil/).

whenever the onset of maternal disease is between 5 days before and 2 days after delivery.[44]

Uncomplicated chickenpox requires no specific therapy. Baths, wet dressings, and oral antihistamines occasionally help to relieve pruritus and to prevent secondary infection from developing as a result of scratching. Oral antistaphylococcal medications should be given if secondary bacterial infection is present. Zoster immune globulin may be administered to immunodeficient individuals if given within 72 hours after exposure to chickenpox. Oral acyclovir (Zovirax) may be valuable in immunosuppressed or other select groups of children. The varicella vaccine protects against both varicella and herpes zoster. However, wild-type (vaccine-resistant) viruses are a continuing threat.[45]

Herpes zoster. Although herpes zoster (shingles) occurs mainly in adults, approximately 5% of cases are in children younger than 15 years. The pathophysiology and treatment are reviewed in Chapter 41.

QUICK CHECK 42-2

1. Compare the cause and presentation of impetigo and staphylococcal scalded-skin syndrome.
2. Describe rubella and rubeola.
3. How are chickenpox and herpes zoster related?

INSECT BITES AND PARASITES

Insect bites and infestations are common causes of skin disorders in children and adults. Skin damage occurs by various mechanisms, including trauma of bites and stings, allergic reactions, transmission of disease, injection of substances that cause local or systemic reactions, and inflammatory reactions resulting from embedded and retained insect mouth parts and scratching of the skin.

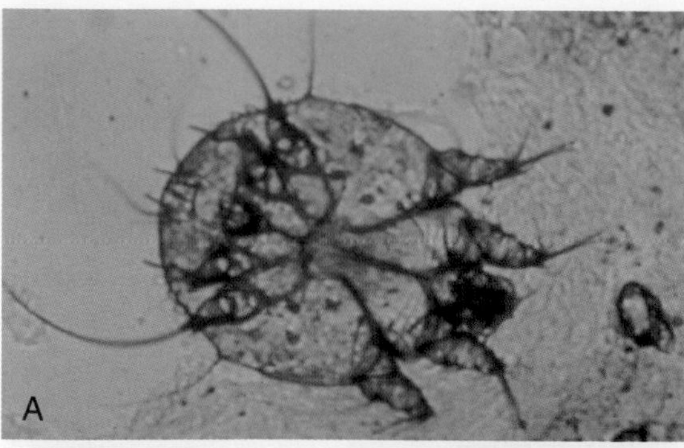

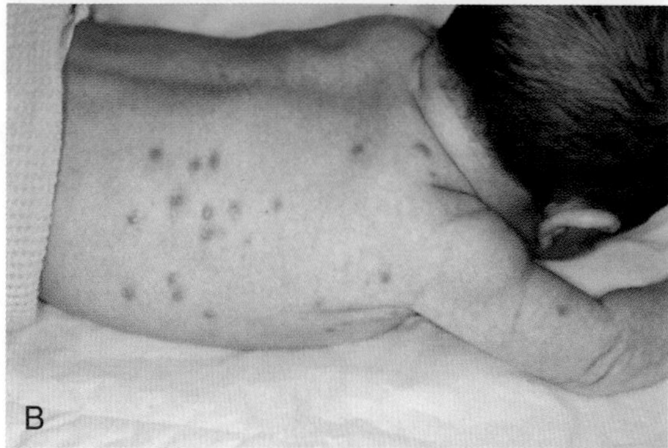

FIGURE 42-10 **Scabies. A,** Scabies mite, as seen clinically when removed from its burrow. **B,** Characteristic scabies bites. (Courtesy Department of Dermatology, School of Medicine, University of Utah, Salt Lake City, UT.)

Scabies

Scabies is a contagious disease caused by the itch mite *Sarcoptes scabiei* (Figure 42-10, *A*), which can colonize the human epidermis. Scabies is a common skin infection in tropical settings, affecting large numbers of people, particularly children. It is transmitted by close personal contact and by infected clothing and bedding. Scabies is often epidemic in areas of overcrowded housing and poor sanitation. Immunocompromised individuals are at greater risk. Scabies can facilitate *S. pyogenes* and *S. aureus* skin coinfections with systemic complications. The scabies mite has adapted mechanisms to overcome host defences, including complement inhibitors.[46] Infestation is initiated by a female mite that tunnels into the stratum corneum, depositing eggs and creating a burrow several millimetres to 1 cm long. Over a 3-week period, the eggs mature into adult mites, which sometimes are recognized as tiny dots at the ends of intact burrows.

Symptoms appear 3 to 5 weeks after infestation. The primary lesions are burrows, papules, and vesicular lesions, with severe pruritus that worsens at night. Pruritus is thought to be related to sensitization to the larval stages of the parasite. In older children and adults, the lesions occur in the webs of fingers; in the axillae; in the creases of the arms and wrists; along the belt line; and around the nipples, genitalia, and lower buttocks. Infants and young children have a different pattern of distribution, with involvement of the palms, soles, head, neck, and face (Figure 42-10, *B*). Secondary infections and crusting develop as a result of scratching and eczematous changes.

Diagnosis of scabies is made by observation of the tunnels and burrows and by microscopic examination of scrapings of the skin to identify the mite or its eggs or feces. Treatment involves the application of a scabicide, which is curative. All clothing and linens should be washed and dried in hot cycles or dry-cleaned.[47]

Pediculosis (Lice Infestation)

The three known types of human lice are (1) the head louse (*Pediculus capitis*), (2) the body louse (*Pediculus corporis*), and (3) the crab or pubic louse (*Phthirus pubis*). They are parasites and survive by sucking blood. The female louse reproduces every 2 weeks, producing hundreds of nits as newly hatched lice mate with older lice. The mouthparts are shaped for piercing and sucking and are attached to the skin of the host while the louse is feeding. When piercing the skin, the louse secretes toxic saliva, and the mechanical trauma and toxin produce a pruritic dermatitis. Head and body lice are acquired directly by personal contact or indirectly by sharing of combs, brushes, or towels or contact with infested clothes, toys, furniture, carpets, or bedding. Crab lice are spread by close body contact, usually with an infected adult. Other common sources of transmission include sharing clothing or headphones.

Pruritus is the major symptom of lice infestation. With head lice, the ova attach to hairs above the ears and in the occipital region. The primary lesion caused by the body louse is a pinpoint red macule, papule, or wheal with a hemorrhagic puncture site. The primary lesion often is not seen, because it is masked by excoriations, wheals, and crusts. The crab louse is found on pubic hairs but also may be found in other body hair, such as eyelashes, mustache, beard, and underarm hair. Young children in particular may become infected with crab lice on their eyebrows or eyelashes.

The live louse, 2 to 3 mm long, is rarely observed. The ova, or nits, can be observed as oval, yellowish, pinpoint specks fastened to a hair shaft. The ova fluoresce under an ultraviolet light (Wood's lamp) and are observed best with a microscope. Nits are removed with a nit comb, and pediculicides, such as lindane shampoo or lotion, are the most effective treatment. Success or failure of therapy for ectoparasitic infestation depends much more on proper use of the topical preparation than on the type of scabicide or pediculicide used.[48]

All clothes, towels, bedding, combs, and brushes should be washed and dried in hot air or instead washed in boiling water, or clothes can be ironed to rid them of lice. Individuals who have close personal contact with the infected person should also be treated.

Fleas

Young children are very susceptible to fleabites. Bites occur in clusters along the arms and legs or where clothing is tight fitting, such as near elastic bands that circle the thigh or waist. The bite produces a urticarial wheal with a central hemorrhagic puncture (Figure 42-11). Itching can be controlled with antihistamines.[49] Treatment includes spraying carpets, crevices, and furniture with malathion or lindane powder. Infected animals should be treated, and clothes and bedding should be washed in hot water.

Bedbugs

Bedbugs (*Cimex lectularius*) are blood-sucking parasites that live in the crevices and cracks of floors, walls, and furniture and in bedding or furniture stuffing. They are 3 to 5 mm long and reddish brown. Bedbugs are nocturnal, emerging to feed in darkness by attaching to the skin to suck blood, and are attracted by warmth and carbon dioxide. Feeding occurs for 5 to 15 minutes, and the bedbug then leaves. It will move long distances to search for food and can travel from house to house.

Immunological reactions to bedbug saliva vary, but bites typically yield erythematous and pruritic papules. The face and distal extremities, areas uncovered by sleeping clothes or blankets, are preferentially involved. If the host has not been previously sensitized, the only symptom is a red macule that develops into a nodule, lasting up to 14 days. In sensitized children and adults, pruritic wheals, papules, and vesicles may form.

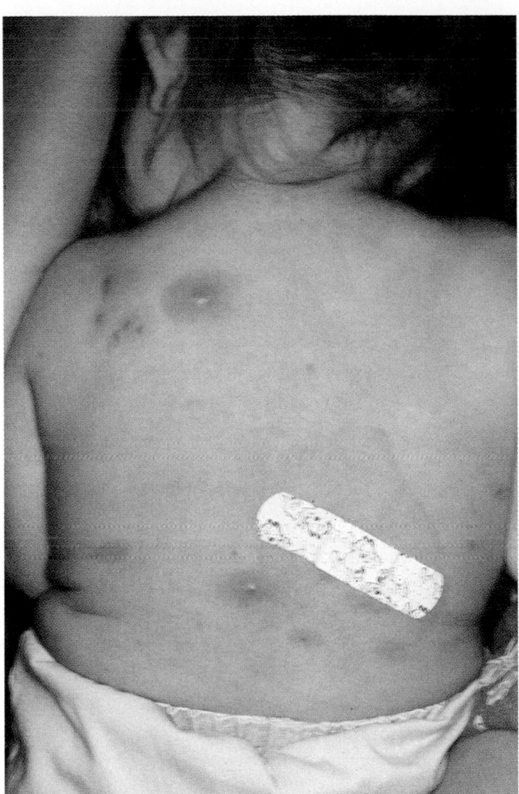

FIGURE 42-11 Fleabites. Fleabite producing a urticarial wheal with central puncture.

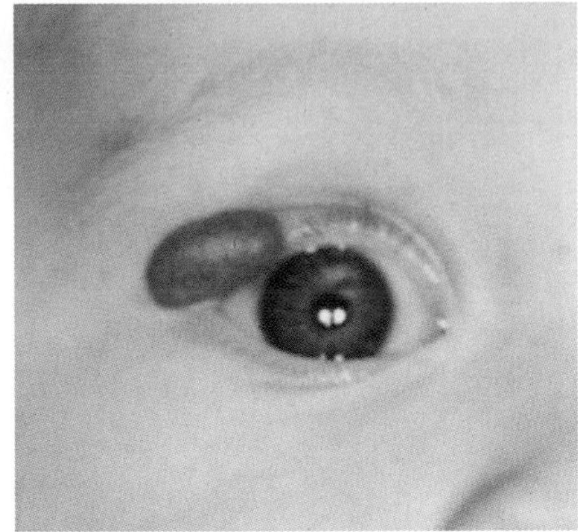

FIGURE 42-12 Superficial (Capillary) Hemangioma. (Courtesy Department of Dermatology, School of Medicine, University of Utah, Salt Lake City, UT.)

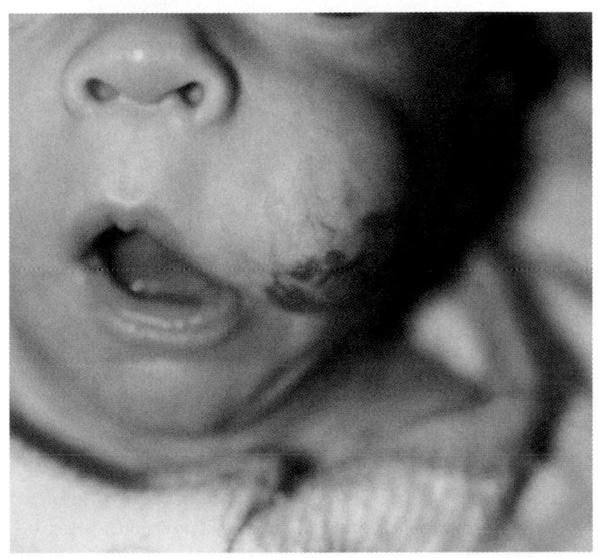

FIGURE 42-13 Cavernous Hemangioma. (Courtesy Department of Dermatology, School of Medicine, University of Utah, Salt Lake City, UT.)

Most lesions respond to oral antihistamines or topical corticosteroids, or both. Secondary infections require antibiotic treatment. Bedbugs are eliminated by inspecting and cleaning or disposing of bedding, mattresses, furniture, and other contaminated items and by using applications of approved insecticides, usually by a professional.[50]

CUTANEOUS HEMANGIOMAS AND VASCULAR MALFORMATIONS

Cutaneous vascular anomalies are frequent tumours of early infancy and are categorized as either hemangiomas or vascular malformations.

Cutaneous Hemangiomas

Cutaneous hemangiomas are benign tumours that form from the rapid growth of vascular endothelial cells, which results in formation of extra blood vessels. Hemangiomas can be superficial or deep.[51] *Superficial hemangiomas* are known as infantile (capillary) or **strawberry hemangiomas**. Deep lesions are known as *cavernous or congenital hemangiomas*. The etiology may be related to embolization of fetal placental endothelial cells with placental trauma or loss of placental angiogenic inhibitor of placental and maternal origin. Superficial hemangiomas are associated with endothelial glucose transporter 1 (GLUT1). There is proliferation of mast cells, which are thought to promote the angiogenesis. Infiltration of fat cells, fibrosis, and the rich vascular network give the lesions a firm, rubbery feel. Females are affected more often than males.

About 30% of infantile hemangiomas are apparent at birth, but they usually emerge 3 to 5 weeks after birth. They grow rapidly during the first few years of life and become bright red and elevated with minute capillary projections that give them a strawberry appearance. Only one lesion is usually present and is located on the head and neck area or trunk (Figure 42-12). After the initial growth, the lesion grows at the same rate as the child and then starts to involute at 12 to 16 months of age. Approximately 90% of strawberry hemangiomas involute by 5 to 9 years of age, usually without scarring. Most superficial hemangiomas require no treatment.

Hemangiomas located over the eye, ear, nose, mouth, urethra, or anus may require treatment because they interfere with function and have a higher risk for infection or injury.

Cavernous hemangiomas are a rare variant of superficial hemangiomas and are GLUT1-negative (Figure 42-13). They are present and fully grown at birth and are usually solitary lesions on the head or limbs that appear as a spongy purplish mass of tissue. They have larger and more mature vessels within the lesion. There are two groups of cavernous hemangiomas: rapidly involuting and noninvoluting. Rapidly involuting cavernous hemangiomas disappear by 12 to 14 months of age, leaving an area of thin skin. Noninvoluting cavernous hemangiomas do not undergo involution.

Rapidly progressing hemangiomas are treated with a beta-blocker (e.g., propranolol [Apo-Propranolol]), with regression occurring within

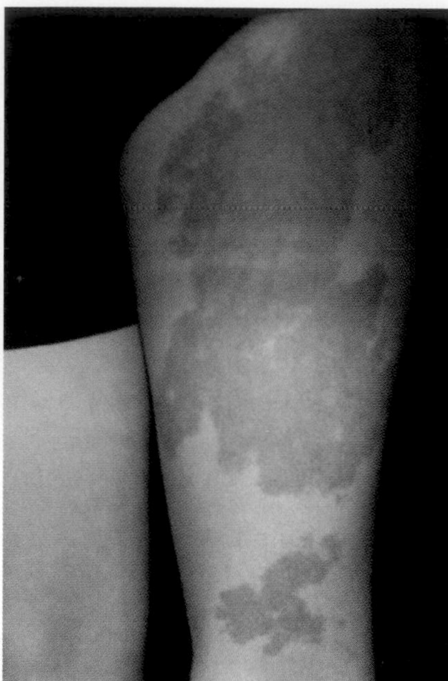

FIGURE 42-14 Port-Wine Hemangioma. Port-wine hemangioma in a child. (Courtesy Department of Dermatology, School of Medicine, University of Utah, Salt Lake City, UT.)

2 weeks and should be considered a first-line agent.[52] Other therapies include systemic or intralesional steroids. Cryosurgery, laser surgery, sclerotherapy, and embolization are alternative treatment options. Interferons, vincristine (Oncovin), cyclophosphamide (Procytox), and radiotherapy can suppress angiogenesis.[53]

Cutaneous Vascular Malformations

Cutaneous vascular malformations are rare congenital anomalies of blood vessels present at birth but may not be apparent for several years.[54] They grow proportionately with the child and never regress. The malformations occur equally among males and females. Occasionally they expand rapidly, particularly during the hormonal changes of puberty or pregnancy and in association with trauma. Vascular malformations are classified as low flow or high flow. *Low-flow malformations* involve capillaries, veins, and lymphatics. *High-flow malformations* involve arteries. In addition to locations within the skin, they may involve the gastro-intestinal tract, bone (Maffucci's syndrome or Sturge-Weber syndrome),[55] facial capillary malformation, skin, eye, or brain (leptomeningeal hemangioma). *Overgrowth syndromes* can occur with either high-flow or low-flow malformations, with overgrowth of the underlying structures (i.e., legs, arms, facial bones). The most common vascular malformations are nevus flammeus (port-wine stains) and salmon patches (stork bite, angel kiss).

Port-wine (nevus flammeus) stains are congenital malformations of the dermal capillaries. The lesions are flat, and their colour ranges from pink to dark reddish purple. They are present at birth or within a few days after birth and do not fade with age. Involvement of the face and other body surfaces is common, and the lesions may be large (Figure 42-14). Treatments using cryosurgery or tattooing are not satisfactory. The pulsed dye laser is the treatment of choice to successfully lighten the colour and flatten the more nodular and cavernous lesions. Waterproof cosmetics may be used to cover the lesions.

Salmon patches are macular pink lesions present at birth and located on the nape of the neck, forehead, upper eyelids, or nasolabial fold region. They are a variant of nevus flammeus, more superficial, and one of the most common congenital malformations in the skin. The pink colour results from distended dermal capillaries, and 95% of patches fade by 1 year of age. Those located at the nape of the neck may persist for a lifetime. They generally do not present a cosmetic problem.

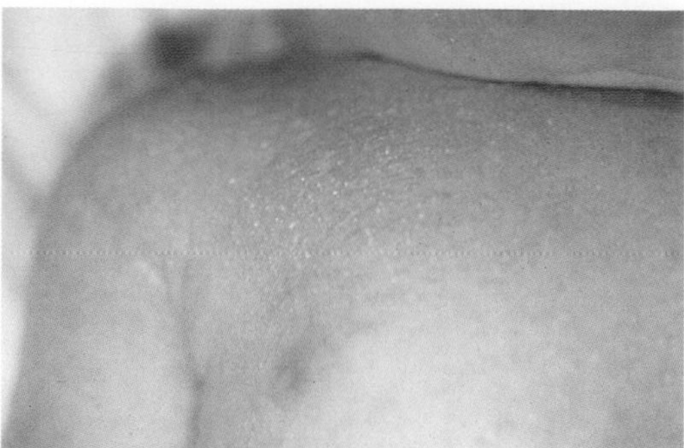

FIGURE 42-15 Miliaria Rubra. Note discrete erythematous papules or papulovesicles. (Courtesy Department of Dermatology, School of Medicine, University of Utah, Salt Lake City, UT.)

OTHER SKIN DISORDERS

Miliaria

Miliaria is a dermatosis commonly seen in infants that is characterized by a vesicular eruption after prolonged exposure to perspiration with subsequent obstruction of the eccrine ducts. There are two forms of miliaria: miliaria crystallina and miliaria rubra. In miliaria crystallina, ductal rupture occurs within the stratum corneum and appears as 1- to 2-mm clear vesicles without erythema. They rupture within 24 to 48 hours and leave a white scale. In miliaria rubra, the ductal rupture occurs in the lower epidermis, with inflammatory cells attracted to the site of the rupture. Miliaria rubra (prickly heat) is characterized by 2- to 4-mm discrete erythematous papules or papulovesicles (Figure 42-15). Both forms may become secondarily infected, requiring systemic antibiotics. The key to management is avoidance of excessive heat and humidity, which cause sweating. Light clothing, cool baths, and air conditioning assist in keeping the skin surface dry and cool.

Erythema Toxicum Neonatorum

Erythema toxicum neonatorum (toxic erythema of the newborn) is a benign erythematous accumulation of macules, papules, or pustules that appears at birth or 3 to 4 days after birth. The lesions first appear as a blotchy, macular erythematous rash. The macules vary from 1 mm to 1 cm in diameter. When papules or pustules develop, they are light yellow or white and 1 to 3 mm in diameter. There may be a few or several hundred lesions, and any body surface can be affected, with the exception of the palms and soles, where there are no pilosebaceous follicles. The cause of the lesion is unknown but may be related to an innate immune response to the first commensal microflora with release of mast cell mediators. It is self-limiting and resolves spontaneously within a few weeks after birth. No treatment is required.

QUICK CHECK 42-3

1. Give two examples of insect bites or parasites that affect children. What features are observed in each?
2. Compare a strawberry hemangioma with a cavernous hemangioma.

DID YOU UNDERSTAND?

Acne Vulgaris

1. Acne vulgaris is the most common skin disease and is related to obstruction of pilosebaceous follicles and proliferation of *Propionibacterium acnes*, primarily of the face, neck, and upper trunk. It is characterized by both noninflammatory and inflammatory lesions.
2. Hydradinitis suppurativa is a chronic inflammatory disease with occlusion of the pilosebaceous follicles, primarily where there are folds of skin. The lesions include inflammatory nodules, sinus tracts, fistulae, and scarring.

Dermatitis

1. Atopic dermatitis is an alteration in the skin barrier; occurs as red, scaly lesions on the face, cheeks, and flexor surfaces of the extremities in infants and young children; and is associated with inflammatory cytokines, elevated IgE levels, and a family history of asthma and hay fever.
2. Diaper dermatitis is a type of irritant contact dermatitis that develops from prolonged exposure to urine and feces and often becomes secondarily infected with *Candida albicans.*

Infections of the Skin

1. Impetigo is a contagious bacterial disease occurring in two forms: bullous and vesicular. The toxins from the bacteria produce a weeping lesion with a honey-coloured crust.
2. Staphylococcal scalded-skin syndrome (SSSS) is a staphylococcal skin infection that produces an exfoliative toxin with painful blisters and bullae formation over large areas of the skin, requiring systemic antibiotic treatment.
3. Tinea capitis and tinea corporis are fungal infections of the scalp and body caused by dermatophytes.
4. Thrush is a fungal infection of the mouth caused by *C. albicans.*
5. Molluscum contagiosum is a poxvirus of the skin that produces pale papular lesions filled with viral and cellular debris.
6. Rubella (German or 3-day measles) is a communicable viral disease characterized by fever, sore throat, enlarged cervical and postauricular lymph nodes, and a generalized maculopapular rash that lasts 1 to 4 days.
7. Rubeola is a viral contagious disease with symptoms of high fever, enlarged lymph nodes, conjunctivitis, and a red rash that begins on the head and spreads to the trunk and extremities. The rash subsides within 3 to 5 days. Both bacterial and viral complications may accompany rubeola.
8. Roseola is a benign disease of infants with a sudden onset of fever that lasts 3 to 5 days, followed by a rash that lasts 24 hours.
9. Smallpox (variola) was a highly contagious and deadly viral disease that has been eradicated worldwide by vaccination.
10. Chickenpox (varicella) is a highly contagious disease caused by the varicella-zoster virus. Vesicular lesions occur on the skin and mucous membranes. Individuals are contagious from 1 day before the development of the rash until about 5 to 6 days after the rash develops.
11. Herpes zoster (shingles) is a viral eruption of vesicles on the skin along the distribution of a sensory nerve caused by chickenpox virus that persists in sensory nerve ganglia.

Insect Bites and Parasites

1. Scabies is a pruritic lesion caused by the itch mite, which burrows into the skin and forms papules and vesicles. The mite is very contagious and is transmitted by direct contact.
2. Pediculosis (lice infestation) is caused by blood-sucking parasites that secrete toxic saliva and damage the skin to produce pruritic dermatitis. Lice are spread by direct contact and are recognized by the ova or nits that attach to the shafts of body hairs.
3. Fleabites produce a pruritic wheal with a central puncture site and occur as clusters in areas of tight-fitting clothing.
4. Bedbugs are blood-sucking parasites that live in cracks of floors, furniture, or bedding and feed at night. They produce pruritic wheals and nodules.

Cutaneous Hemangiomas and Vascular Malformations

1. Cutaneous hemangiomas are benign tumours that form from the rapid growth of vascular endothelial cells and result in formation of extra blood vessels.
2. Cutaneous vascular malformations are rare congenital anomalies of blood vessels present at birth.
3. A strawberry hemangioma is a vascular lesion present at birth that proliferates in size and then grows at the same rate as the child. Most lesions resolve spontaneously by 5 years of age.
4. A cavernous hemangioma is present at birth, with larger vessels than a strawberry hemangioma, and is bluish red. Cavernous hemangiomas usually involute by 9 years of age and may require surgical removal if located near the eyes, nares, or genitalia.
5. Port-wine stains are congenital malformations of dermal capillaries that do not fade with age.
6. Salmon patches are macular pink lesions with dilated capillaries that usually resolve by 1 year of age.

Other Skin Disorders

1. Miliaria are small pruritic papules or vesicles that result from obstruction of the sweat duct opening in infants.
2. Erythema toxicum neonatorum is a benign accumulation of macules, papules, and pustules that spontaneously resolves within a few weeks after birth.

KEY TERMS

Acne conglobata, 1108
Acne vulgaris, 1107
Atopic dermatitis (AD), 1108
Bedbug, 1114
Chickenpox (varicella), 1113
Cutaneous hemangioma, 1115
Cutaneous vascular malformations, 1116
Diaper dermatitis (diaper rash), 1109
Erythema toxicum neonatorum, 1116
Fleabite, 1114
Herpes zoster (shingles), 1113
Hydradinitis suppurativa (inverse acne), 1108
Impetigo, 1109
Inflammatory (cystic) acne, 1107
Miliaria, 1116
Miliaria crystallina, 1116
Miliaria rubra (prickly heat), 1116
Molluscum contagiosum, 1111
Noninflammatory acne, 1107
Roseola, 1112
Rubella, 1111
Rubeola, 1112
Scabies, 1114
Smallpox (variola), 1113
Staphylococcal scalded-skin syndrome (SSSS), 1110
Strawberry (capillary) hemangioma, 1115
Thrush, 1111
Tinea capitis, 1110
Tinea corporis (ringworm), 1111

REFERENCES

1. Bate, K., & Williams, H. C. (2013). Epidemiology of acne vulgaris. *The British Journal of Dermatology, 168*(3), 474–485. doi:10.1111/bjd.12149.
2. Grossi, E., Cazzaniga, S., Crotti, S., et al. (2016). The constellation of dietary factors in adolescent acne: A semantic connectivity map approach. *Journal of the European Academy of Dermatology and Venereology, 30*(1), 96–100. doi:10.1111/jdv.12878.
3. Mahmood, S. N., & Bowe, W. P. (2010). Diet and acne update: Carbohydrates emerge as the main culprit. *Journal of Drugs in Dermatology, 13*(4), 428–435.
4. Melnik, B. C., John, S. M., & Plewig, G. (2013). Acne: Risk indicator for increased body mass index and insulin resistance. *Acta Dermato-Venereologica, 93*(6), 644–649. doi:10.2340/00015555-1677.
5. Harvey, A., & Huynh, T. T. (2014). Inflammation and acne: Putting the pieces together. *Journal of Drugs in Dermatology, 13*(4), 459–463.
6. Lwin, S. M., Kimber, I., & McFadden, J. P. (2014). Acne, quorum sensing and danger. *Clinical and Experimental Dermatology, 39*(2), 162–167. doi:10.1111/ced.12252.
7. Eichenfield, L. F., Krakowski, A. C., Piggott, C., et al. (2013). Evidence-based recommendations for the diagnosis and treatment of pediatric acne. *Pediatrics, 131*(Suppl. 3), S163–S186. doi:10.1542/peds.2013-0490B.
8. Bhate, K., & Williams, H. C. (2014). What's new in acne? An analysis of systematic reviews published in 2011–2012. *Clinical and Experimental Dermatology, 39*(3), 273–277. doi:10.1111/ced.12270.
9. Yin, N. C., & McMichael, A. J. (2014). Acne in patients with skin of color: Practical management. *American Journal of Clinical Dermatology, 15*(1), 7–16. doi:10.1007/s40257-013-0049-1.
10. Simonart, T. (2013). Immunotherapy for acne vulgaris: Current status and future directions. *American Journal of Clinical Dermatology, 14*(6), 429–435. doi:10.1007/s40257-013-0042-8.
11. Gill, L., Williams, M., & Hamzvi, I. (2014). Update on hidradenitis suppurativa: Connecting the tracts. *F1000prime Reports, 6*, 112. doi:10.12703/P6-112.
12. Asiniwasis, R., Sajic, D., & Skotnicki, S. (2016). Atopic dermatitis: The skin barrier and the role of ceramides. *Skin Therapy Letter©: A physician's guide to dermatology treatment information*. Retrieved from http://www.skintherapyletter.ca/ped/2012/3.1/1.html.
13. Darlenski, R., Kazandjieva, J., Hristakieva, E., et al. (2014). Atopic dermatitis as a systemic disease. *Clinics in Dermatology, 32*(3), 409–413. doi:10.1016/j.clindermatol.2013.11.007.
14. Lyons, J. J., Milner, J. D., & Stone, K. D. (2015). Atopic dermatitis in children: Clinical features, pathophysiology, and treatment. *Immunology and Allergy Clinics of North America, 35*(1), 161–183. doi:10.1016/j.iac.2014.09.008.
15. McAleer, M. A., & Irvine, A. D. (2013). The multifunctional role of filaggrin in allergic skin disease. *The Journal of Allergy and Clinical Immunology, 131*(2), 280–291. doi:10.1016/j.jaci.2012.12.668.
16. Oranje, A. P., & de Waard-van der Spek, F. B. (2015). Recent developments in the management of common childhood skin infections. *The Journal of Infection, 71*(Suppl. 1), S76–S79. doi:10.1016/j.jinf.2015.04.030.
17. Eichenfield, L. F., Tom, W. L., Chamlin, S. L., et al. (2014). Guidelines of care for the management of atopic dermatitis: Section 1. Diagnosis and assessment of atopic dermatitis. *Journal of the American Academy of Dermatology, 70*(2), 338–351. doi:10.1016/j.jaad.2013.10.010.
18. Kanchongkittiphon, W., Gaffin, J. M., & Phipatanakul, W. (2015). Child with atopic dermatitis. *Annals of Allergy, Asthma and Immunology, 114*(1), 6–11. doi:10.1016/j.anai.2014.08.016.
19. Nicol, N. H., Boguniewicz, M., Strand, M., et al. (2014). Wet wrap therapy in children with moderate to severe atopic dermatitis in a multidisciplinary treatment program. *The Journal of Allergy and Clinical Immunology: In Practice, 2*(4), 400–407. doi:10.1016/j.jaip.2014.04.009.
20. Schäkel, K., Döbel, T., & Bosselmann, I. (2014). Future treatment options for atopic dermatitis—small molecules and beyond. *Journal of Dermatological Science, 73*(2), 91–100. doi:10.1016/j.jdermsci.2013.11.009.
21. Shin, H. T. (2014). Diagnosis and management of diaper dermatitis. *Pediatric Clinics of North America, 61*(2), 367–382. doi:10.1016/j.pcl.2013.11.009.
22. Hartman-Adams, H., Banvard, C., & Juckett, G. (2014). Impetigo: Diagnosis and treatment. *American Family Physician, 90*(4), 229–235.
23. Pereira, L. B. (2014). Impetigo—Review. *Anais Brasileiros de Dermatologia, 89*(2), 293–299.
24. Aalfs, A. S., Oktarina, D. A., Diercks, G. F., et al. (2010). Staphylococcal scalded skin syndrome: Loss of desmoglein 1 in patient skin. *European Journal of Dermatology, 20*(4), 451–456. doi:10.1684/ejd.2010.1007.
25. Neylon, O., O'Connell, N. H., Slevin, B., et al. (2010). Neonatal staphylococcal scalded skin syndrome: Clinical and outbreak containment review. *European Journal of Pediatrics, 169*(12), 1503–1509. doi:10.1007/s00431-010-1252-1.
26. Paranthaman, K., Bentley, A., Milne, L. M., et al. (2014). Nosocomial outbreak of staphylococcal scalded skin syndrome in neonates in England, December 2012 to March 2013. *Euro Surveillance, 19*(33), pii–20880.
27. Williams, P. M., & Conklin, R. J. (2005). Erythema multiforme: A review and contrast from Stevens-Johnson syndrome/toxic epidermal necrolysis. *Dental Clinics of North America, 49*(1), 67–76, viii. doi:10.1016/j.cden.2004.08.003.
28. Baartmans, M. G., Dokter, J., den Hollander, J. C., et al. (2011). Use of skin substitute dressings in the treatment of staphylococcal scalded skin syndrome in neonates and young infants. *Neonatology, 100*(1), 9–13. doi:10.1159/000317997.
29. Mirmirani, P., & Tucker, L. Y. (2013). Epidemiologic trends in pediatric tinea capitis: A population-based study from Kaiser Permanente Northern California. *Journal of the American Academy of Dermatology, 69*(6), 916–921. doi:10.1016/j.jaad.2013.08.031.
30. Abdel-Rahman, S. M., Schuenemann, E., Stering, T. K., et al. (2010). The prevalence of infections with *Trichophyton tonsurans* in schoolchildren: The CAPITIS study. *Pediatrics, 125*(5), 966–973.
31. Kakourou, T., & Uksal, U. (2010). European Society for Pediatric Dermatology. Guidelines for the management of tinea capitis in children. *Pediatric Dermatology, 27*(3), 226–228. doi:10.1111/j.1525-1470.2010.01137.x.
32. Andrews, M. D., & Burns, M. (2008). Common tinea infections in children. *American Family Physician, 77*(10), 1415–1420.
33. Olsen, J. R., Gallacher, J., Piguet, V., et al. (2014). Epidemiology of molluscum contagiosum in children: A systematic review. *Family Practice, 31*(2), 130–136. doi:10.1093/fampra/cmt075.
34. Butala, N., Siegfried, E., & Weissler, A. (2013). Molluscum BOTE sign: A predictor of imminent resolution. *Pediatrics, 131*(5), e1650–e1653. doi:10.1542/peds.2012-2933.
35. Smith, K. J., & Skelton, H. (2002). Molluscum contagiosum: Recent advances in pathogenic mechanisms, and new therapies. *American Journal of Clinical Dermatology, 3*(8), 535–545.
36. Can, B., Topaloglu, F., Kavala, M., et al. (2014). Treatment of pediatric molluscum contagiosum with 10% potassium hydroxide solution. *The Journal of Dermatological Treatment, 25*(3), 246–248. doi:10.3109/09546634.2012.697988.
37. Zichichi, L., & Maniscalco, M. (2012). The challenges of a neglected STI: *Molluscum contagiosum. Giornale Italiano Di Dermatologia E Venereologia: Organo Ufficiale, Societa Italiana Di Dermatologia E Sifilografia, 147*(5), 447–453.
38. Parker Fiebelkorn, A., Redd, S. B., Gallagher, K., et al. (2010). Measles in the United States during the postelimination era. *The Journal of Infectious Diseases, 202*(10), 1520–1528. doi:10.1086/656914.
39. Maglione, M. A., Das, L., Raaen, L., et al. (2014). Safety of vaccines used for routine immunization of U.S. children: A systematic review. *Pediatrics, 134*(2), 325–337. doi:10.1542/peds.2014-1079.
40. de Vries, R. D., Mesman, A. W., Geijtenbeek, T. B., et al. (2012). The pathogenesis of measles. *Current Opinion in Virology, 2*(3), 248–255. doi:10.1016/j.coviro.2012.03.005.
41. Ontario Ministry of Health and Long-Term Care. (2012). *Diseases: Smallpox*. Retrieved from http://www.health.gov.on.ca/english/providers/pub/disease/smallpox.html.
42. Gershon, A. A., & Gershon, M. D. (2013). Pathogenesis and current approaches to control of varicella-zoster virus infections. *Clinical Microbiology Reviews, 26*(4), 728–743. doi:10.1128/CMR.00052-13.
43. Smith, C. K., & Arvin, A. M. (2009). Varicella in the fetus and newborn. *Seminars in Fetal and Neonatal Medicine, 14*(4), 209–217. doi:10.1016/j.siny.2008.11.008.
44. Shrim, A., Koren, G., Yudin, M. H., et al. (2012). Management of varicella infection (chickenpox) in pregnancy. *Journal of Obstetrics and Gynaecology Canada, 34*(3), 287–292.
45. Quinlivan, M., & Breuer, J. (2014). Clinical and molecular aspects of the live attenuated Oka varicella vaccine. *Reviews in Medical Virology, 24*(4), 254–273. doi:10.1002/rmv.1789.
46. Swe, P. M., Reynolds, S. L., & Fischer, K. (2014). Parasitic scabies mites and associated bacteria joining forces against host complement defence. *Parasite Immunology, 36*(11), 585–593. doi:10.1111/pim.12133.
47. Mounsey, K. E., & McCarthy, J. S. (2013). Treatment and control of scabies. *Current Opinion in Infectious Diseases, 26*(2), 133–139. doi:10.1097/QCO.0b013e32835e1d57.
48. Wolf, R., & Davidovici, B. (2010). Treatment of scabies and pediculosis: Facts and controversies. *Clinics in Dermatology, 28*(5), 511–518. doi:10.1016/j.clindermatol.2010.03.008.
49. Juckett, G. (2013). Arthropod bites. *American Family Physician, 88*(12), 841–847.
50. Studdiford, J. S., Conniff, K. M., Trayes, K. P., et al. (2012). Bedbug infestation. *American Family Physician, 86*(7), 653–658.
51. Elluru, R. G. (2013). Cutaneous vascular lesions. *Facial Plastic Surgery Clinics of North America, 21*(1), 111–126. doi:10.1016/j.fsc.2012.11.001.
52. Gunturi, N., Ramgopal, S., Balagopal, S., et al. (2013). Propranolol therapy for infantile hemangioma. *Indian Pediatrics, 50*(3), 307–313.
53. Greene, A. K. (2011). Management of hemangiomas and other vascular tumors. *Clinics in Plastic Surgery, 38*(1), 45–63. doi:10.1016/j.cps.2010.08.001.
54. Huang, J. T., & Liang, M. G. (2010). Vascular malformations. *Pediatric Clinics of North America, 57*(5), 1091–1110. doi:10.1016/j.pcl.2010.08.003.
55. Chen, J. K., Ghasri, P., Aguilar, G., et al. (2012). An overview of clinical and experimental treatment modalities for port wine stains. *Journal of the American Academy of Dermatology, 67*(2), 289–304. doi:10.1016/j.jaad.2011.11.938.

INDEX

A

A band, 585, 585*f*
A beta (Aβ) fibres, 339
A delta (Aδ) fibres, 339
Abbreviations, pulmonary, 689*t*
Abdominal pain, 924
Abducens nerve, 330*t*
Aberrant conduction, 645*t*–646*t*
ABGs. *See* Arterial blood gases
Abnormal uterine bleeding, 820–821, 821*t*
ABO blood group, 210, 210*f*
Abscesses, 150
  brain, 413
  cavitation of, 715
  peritonsillar, 727
  respiratory tract, 715
  spinal cord, 413
  tonsillar, 727
Abscopal effects, 288*b*
Absence seizure, 436*t*
Absolute polycythemia, 526
Absolute refractory period, 24
Absorption atelectasis, 701
Acanthosis nigricans, 257*t*
Accelerated junctional rhythm, 644*t*–645*t*
Accelerated ventricular rhythm, 644*t*–645*t*
Accessory organs of digestion, 899. *See also* Exocrine pancreas; Gallbladder; Gastro-intestinal tract; Liver
  anatomy of, 910, 911*f*
  cancer of, 957–959
  disorders of, 943–953
Accidental hyperthermia, 346–347
Accommodation, 349–350, 352
Acetabular dysplasia, 1059–1060
Acetaminophen (Tylenol), 86, 88*f*
  acute liver failure and, 915*b*
  for osteoarthritis, 1031–1032
Acetazolamide, 753*t*
Acetylcholine, 314*t*, 331, 903*t*
Acetylcholine receptors (AChRs), 417
Achalasia, 925–926, 926*f*
Achilles tenotomy, 1059
AChRs. *See* Acetylcholine receptors
Acid maltase deficiency, 1044
Acid-base balance
  buffer systems in, 126–128, 128*t*
  CKD progression and, 777–778, 777*t*
  compensatory changes for, 131*f*
  hydrogen ion in, 126
  pH and, 126, 128*t*
Acid-base imbalances
  ABGs, 131–132
  compensatory changes for, 131*f*
  description of, 128, 131*f*
  metabolic acidosis, 128, 130*t*
  metabolic alkalosis, 128–129, 131*f*
  respiratory acidosis, 129–130, 131*f*
  respiratory alkalosis, 130–131, 131*f*
Acidemia, 128, 683
Acidosis
  definition of, 128
  ECF hydrogen ions in, 125
  metabolic (*See* Metabolic acidosis)
  oxyhemoglobin dissociation curve affected by, 691–692
  respiratory, 129–130, 131*f*
Acids
  bile, 912
  carbonic, 126
  nonvolatile, 126
  renal excretion of, 130*f*
  strong, 126
  titratable, 130*f*
  volatile, 126
  weak, 126
Acinus, 680, 805
Aclasta, 1026*b*
Acne conglobata, 1108
Acne rosacea, 1085, 1085*f*
Acne vulgaris, 1085, 1107–1108, 1108*f*
Acoustic nerve, 330*t*
ACPA. *See* Anti-citrullinated protein antibody
Acquired heart disease, 673–677
Acquired hypercoagulability, 554
Acquired immune deficiency. *See* Secondary immune deficiency
Acquired immunity. *See* Adaptive immunity
Acquired immunodeficiency syndrome (AIDS)
  cardiac complications in, 638
  in children, 198–199, 307
  clinical manifestations of, 195–196, 200*f*
  CNS involvement in, 198–199
  definition of, 195
  epidemiology of, 195
  HIV progression to, 199*f*
  lymphocytopenia and, 531
  neurologic complications of, 414–415
  opportunistic infections associated with, 196*b*
  pathogenesis of, 196, 197*f*
  pediatric, 198–199
  prevalence of, 195
  sexual transmission of, 196*b*
  treatment and prevention of, 196–198, 198*f*
Acquired sideroblastic anemia, 525
Acral lentiginous melanoma, 1093–1094
Acrocephaly, 431*f*
Acromegaly, 469, 470*f*
ACTH. *See* Adrenocorticotropic hormone
ACTH-independent hypercortisolism, 487
Actin, 585–586, 585*f*, 1003*t*
Actinic keratosis, 1091
Actinin, 1003*t*
Action potentials
  cardiac, 580, 582–583, 582*t*, 583*f*
  definition of, 24
  propagation of, 24*f*
Activated partial thromboplastin time, 916*t*
Activated platelets, 146
Activator protein-1, 290
Active immunity, 160
Active immunization, 189–190
Active transport, 18, 18*f*
  of potassium and sodium, 21, 21*f*, 22*t*
Activin, 794*t*, 804, 991*t*
Acute alcoholism, 91–92
Acute bacterial conjunctivitis, 353
Acute bacterial meningitis, 435
Acute bacterial prostatitis, 878–879, 878*b*
Acute bleeding, 924, 924*t*
Acute bronchitis, 711
Acute colonic pseudo-obstruction, 929
Acute confusional states, 369*b*, 371–374, 374*t*
Acute coronary syndromes, 617, 623–628
  myocardial infarction (*See* Myocardial infarction)
  pathophysiology of, 623, 623*f*
  unstable angina, 623–624, 624*b*, 625*f*
  unstable plaque, 623–624, 623*f*–624*f*
Acute cough, 696
Acute cystitis, 765–766
Acute encephalopathies, 434–435
Acute epiglottitis, 727, 730*t*
Acute gastritis, 930
Acute gouty arthritis, 1040
Acute hematogenous osteomyelitis, 1062–1063, 1063*f*
Acute hydrocephalus, 380
Acute idiopathic TTP, 548
Acute infectious diarrhea, 979
Acute inflammation, 150, 150*t*
Acute inflammatory response, 139, 139*f*, 149–150
Acute kidney injury (AKI)
  classification of, 772–775, 773*t*
  clinical manifestations of, 774–775
  definition of, 772
  evaluation of, 775, 775*t*
  intrarenal, 773–774, 773*t*
  oliguria in, 125, 773*f*, 774
  pathophysiology of, 772–775, 773*f*, 773*t*
  postrenal, 773*t*, 774
  prerenal, 773, 773*t*
  RIFLE criteria for, 772, 773*t*
  treatment of, 775
Acute laryngotracheitis, 725, 726*t*
Acute liver failure, 915*b*, 947
Acute lung injury (ALI), 704
  in children, 735
Acute lymphocytic leukemia, 305, 533–536, 534*t*
  in children, 570
Acute myeloid leukemia, 533–536, 534*t*
  in children, 570
Acute organic brain syndromes, 371
Acute otitis media, 356
Acute pain, 342–343, 344*t*
Acute pancreatitis, 952–953, 953*f*
Acute pericarditis, 629, 629*f*
Acute poststreptococcal glomerulonephritis, 786–787
Acute pyelonephritis, 767, 767*t*, 788
Acute rejection, 211
Acute respiratory distress syndrome (ARDS), 704, 705*f*
  in children, 735
Acute rheumatic fever, 634–637, 636*f*, 636*t*
Acute toxic inhalation, 702–703
Acute tubular necrosis (ATN), 772
Acute-phase reactants, 150, 150*t*
Acyanotic heart defects, 662–663
ADA deficiency. *See* Adenosine deaminase deficiency
Adaptation
  cellular (*See* Cellular adaptation)
  definition of, 74
  diseases of, 216–217
  potassium, 123
Adaptation stage, of general adaptation syndrome, 216–217
Adaptive immunity
  cells of, 142
  description of, 135, 136*t*
  inflammation compared to, 159
  innate immunity interaction with, 159
Adaptive resizing, 281
ADCC. *See* Antibody-dependent cellular cytotoxicity
Addison's disease, 125, 490
Adenocarcinomas
  characteristics of, 718*t*, 719, 719*f*
  definition of, 236
  ductal, 959
  mammary, 236
Adenoid cystic carcinoma, 856*t*
Adenomas
  pituitary, 469
  renal, 763–764
  toxic, 472–473
Adenomyosis, 831–832
Adenosine deaminase deficiency (ADA deficiency), 191, 195
Adenosine diphosphate (ADP), 16
Adenosine monophosphate deaminase deficiency, 1044
Adenosine triphosphate (ATP), 345, 585
  in cellular metabolism, 16, 16*b*, 643–647
  sodium-potassium pump affected by, 81–82
Adenotonsillar hypertrophy, 348
Adenotonsillectomy, 348
ADH. *See* Antidiuretic hormone
ADHD. *See* Attention-deficit/hyperactivity disorder
Adipocytes
  cancer-associated, 283
  interlobular, 104*f*
Adipocytokines, 940–941, 941*b*
Adipokines, 481
  CAD and, 620
Adiponectin, 854, 941, 941*b*
Adipose tissue, 31*t*–33*t*, 32*f*, 854
Adjuvant chemotherapy, 263
Adolescents, TBW in, 132*b*. *See also* Children
Adoptive cell therapy, 263
ADP. *See* Adenosine diphosphate
Adrenal cortex
  aldosterone secretion by, 459, 459*f*
  anatomy of, 457, 457*f*
  androgens secretion by, 459
  cortisol secretion by, 458–459, 459*f*
  disorders of, 487–490
    Addison's disease, 125, 490
    adrenocortical hypofunction, 489–490
    congenital adrenal hyperplasia, 489
    Cushing's syndrome and Cushing's disease, 487–489, 488*f*
    hyperaldosteronism, 489
    hypocortisolism, 489–490
  estrogen secretion by, 459
  glucocorticoids produced by, 457–459
Adrenal glands
  aging and, 461*b*
  alterations of, 487–491
  anatomy of, 457, 457*f*
  hormones produced by, 457–460
Adrenal medulla
  catecholamine secretion by, 459–460, 461*f*
  tumours of, 260–261, 490–491
Adrenarche, 795–796
Adrenergic receptors
  α, 224, 331, 333*t*
  β, 224, 331, 333*t*
Adrenergic transmission, 331
Adrenocortical hypofunction, 489–490
Adrenocorticotropic hormone (ACTH), 220, 227, 448–451, 449*f*, 451*t*
  Cushing's syndrome caused by excessive secretion of, 487–489, 488*f*
  deficiency of, 468
Adrenomedullin, 597
ADT. *See* Androgen-deprivation therapy
Advil (ibuprofen), 619
Aerobic glycolysis, 249
Affective-motivational system, 340
Afferent arteriole, 745
Afferent loop obstruction, 934
Afferent neuron, 321–322
Afferent pathways, 309, 339
Afterload, 588, 588*f*, 639, 641*f*
Agammaglobulinemia, 192
Aganglionic megacolon, 972, 972*f*
Age-related bone loss, 1023, 1024*f*
Age-related macular degeneration, 352, 352*f*
Ageusia, 356
Agglutination, 163
Aging
  adrenal gland changes and, 461*b*
  of bone, 1006–1007
  breast changes secondary to, 849–850
  cellular, 107–109, 109*f*
  chest wall and, 692
  chronological, 107–108
  definition of, 107
  ECM changes with, 108
  endocrine glands and, 461*b*
  erythrocytes affected by, 516*b*
  esophagus by, 918

Page numbers followed by "*f*" indicate figures; "*t*" indicate tables; "*b*" indicate boxes. Syndromes and Disorders appear in boldface.

Aging (*Continued*)
female reproductive system and, 811–812, 811*f*
frailty and, 109
gallbladder affected by, 917*t*
gas exchange and, 692
gastro-intestinal tract and, 918
GH changes and, 451*b*, 461*b*
gonads changes and, 461*b*
hearing changes with, 357
hematological system affected by, 516*b*, 517*t*
hemoglobin affected by, 516*b*
IGF changes and, 451*b*, 461*b*
immune response and, 174*b*
innate immunity and, 155*b*
of joints, 1007
libido and, 812
liver affected by, 917*t*
lungs and, 692
male reproductive system and, 812
menstrual cycle and, 802
of muscles, 1007–1008
nervous system changes with, 335
normal, 108
olfaction changes with, 357*b*
pancreas changes and, 461*b*, 917*t*
pituitary gland changes and, 461*b*
presbyopia and, 352
prostate cancer risk with, 887
pulmonary system and, 692
renal function affected by, 756
replicative, 108
reproductive system and, 811–812
of skeletal muscles, 1007–1008
skin changes in, 1102
small intestine affected by, 918
stomach affected by, 918
stress-age syndrome and, 230
systemic, 109
taste changes with, 357*b*
testes and, 812
thyroid gland changes and, 461*b*
tissue, 109
vision changes with, 357*b*
Agitated delirium, 371–373
Agnosia, 371
Agonal rhythm, 644*t*–645*t*
Agonist, of muscles, 1006
Agranulocytes, 499, 507
Agranulocytosis, 531
AIDS. *See* Acquired immunodeficiency syndrome
Air embolism, 613*t*
Air pollution
CAD and, 620
cancer and, 293–294, 294*f*
diseases caused by, 86*b*
lung health and, 709*b*
Air trapping, 711, 711*f*
Airway obstruction, 706–707, 725, 726*f*
Airway remodelling, 706
Airway resistance, 688
Airways. *See also* Pulmonary system
conducting, 679–680, 681*f*–682*f*
gas-exchange, 680–681, 682*f*–683*f*
lower, 682*f*
disorders of, 728–737
upper, 679, 681*f*
Akathisia, 383*t*
AKI. *See* Acute kidney injury
Akinesia, 384
Alanine aminotransferase, 916*t*
Alarm stage, of general adaptation syndrome, 216–217, 217*f*
Albinism, 99
Albumin, 100, 117, 496, 771, 916*t*, 945, 989*t*
Alcohol
cancer and, 283, 285*f*, 285*t*
cellular injury caused by, 90–93
daily intake of, recommended, 91
deaths caused by, 90
epigenetics and gestation exposure to, 67
immune defects caused by, 92
low-risk guidelines for, 92*b*
metabolism of, 91, 91*f*, 285*f*
nutritional status affected by, 90–91
prenatal exposure to, 92–93, 93*f*
toxic myopathies and, 1046, 1046*b*
Alcohol dehydrogenase, 91
Alcoholic cirrhosis, 948
Alcoholic fatty liver, 948
Alcoholic hepatitis, 948
Alcoholic liver disease, 92, 92*f*
cirrhosis and, 948
Alcoholic steatohepatitis, 948
Alcoholism, 91–92, 92*f*
Aldactone, 753*t*
Aldosterone
blood pressure affected by, 580*f*, 597
blood volume regulation and, 747, 748*f*
hypertension and, 607–608
nephron function affected by, 752
potassium regulation by, 123
secretion of, 459, 459*f*
sodium balance affected by, 118
urine regulation and, 747, 748*f*
Alendronate, 1061–1062
Algor mortis, 110
ALI. *See* Acute lung injury
Alkalemia, 128
Alkaline phosphatase, 916*t*, 989*t*
Alkaline reflux gastritis, 934
Alkalosis
contraction, 129
definition of, 128
metabolic, 128–129, 131*f*
hypochloremic, 128
respiratory, 130–131, 131*f*
Alkylphenols, 855
Alleles
autosomal dominant, 50
description of, 49
recombination of, 57
Allergens, 208
Allergic alveolitis, 205
Allergic conjunctivitis, 353–354
Allergic contact dermatitis, 208*f*, 1082, 1082*f*
Allergy
bee sting, 208–209
description of, 199–201
gastro-intestinal, 202
Alloantigens, 210
Allodynia, 343
Alloimmune diseases
description of, 201
transfusion reactions as, 210–211
transplant rejection as, 211
Alloimmunity
alloantigens and, 210
description of, 201
Allopurinol (Zyloprim), 536
All-or-none response, 313
Allostasis, 219
Allostatic overload, 219
Alnacort, 1067–1068
Alopecia, 260, 1101
Alopecia areata, 1101
Alpha cells, 455, 455*f*
Alpha globulins, 496–497
Alpha rigidity, 381, 381*t*
α-Thalassemias, 567–568
ALS. *See* Amyotrophic lateral sclerosis
Alternative pathway, of complement system, 141
Alveolar dead space, 698, 698*f*
Alveolar ducts, 680, 682*f*
Alveolar hypoventilation, 129
Alveolar hypoxia, chronic, 683
Alveolar macrophages, 681, 682*f*
Alveolar pressure, 690, 690*f*
Alveolar sac, 680*f*
Alveolar septum, 682
Alveolar surface tension, 686–687
Alveolar ventilation, 684
Alveoli, 680, 682*f*–683*f*
Alveolocapillary membrane
anatomy of, 682, 683*f*
oxygen diffusion across, 690, 691*f*, 698
oxygen toxicity damage to, 703
Alzheimer's disease, 374–376, 375*f*, 375*t*–376*t*, 376*b*
Amalgams, dental, 93
Amblyopia, 350, 351*t*
Ambulatory blood pressure monitoring, 676
Amenorrhea, 819–820, 841*f*
Amiloride, 753*t*
Amino acid metabolism defects, 433–434
Amino acids, 39
as neurotransmitters, 314*t*
Ammonia, 643–648
Ammonium, 130*f*
Amnesia, 369, 370*t*
Amniotic fluid embolism, 613*t*
Amphiarthrosis, 995
Amphipathic lipids, 3–5
Ampulla, of fallopian tube, 800, 800*f*
Ampulla of Vater, 911, 915
α-Amylase, 899–901
Amylin, 456, 477, 481
Amyloidosis, 543–544
Amyotrophic lateral sclerosis (ALS), 388–389
Anabolism, 14
Anaerobic glycolysis, 17
Anal cancer, 270*t*–273*t*
Anaphase, 25
Anaphylactic shock, 650, 650*f*
Anaphylatoxins, 141
Anaphylaxis, 202, 650
Anaplasia, 236
Androgen insensitivity syndrome, 816
Androgen receptors
in prostate cancer, 851
signalling, 882, 882*f*, 885
Androgen-deprivation therapy (ADT), 884
Androgenic alopecia, 1101
Androgens, 459, 795–796, 810
in female reproductive system, 801
hypersecretion of, 489, 490*f*
in prostate cancer, 882, 882*f*
testosterone as source of, 882, 885
Andropause, 812
Anemia
aplastic, 521*t*, 527*t*
cancer and, 257*t*, 258
in children, 560–563, 561*b*, 561*t*
of chronic disease, 521*t*, 527*t*
classification of, 520–522, 521*t*
clinical manifestations of, 520–522, 527*t*
Cooley's, 567
Fanconi, 305
folate deficiency, 521*t*, 523–524
hemolytic, 527*t*, 560, 562–563
hypoplastic, 526
hypoxemia associated with, 522
iron deficiency, 521*t*, 524–525, 524*f*–525*f*
in children, 560–562, 561*b*
clinical manifestations of, 562
evaluation and treatment of, 562
pathophysiology of, 561–562
leukemia and, 536*t*
macrocytic-normochromic, 521*t*, 522–524
mechanisms of, 258
megaloblastic, 258, 522–524
microcytic-hypochromic, 521*t*, 524–526
normocytic-normochromic, 521*t*, 526, 527*t*
pernicious, 521*t*, 522–523, 522*f*
postgastrectomy, 935
posthemorrhagic, 521*t*, 527*t*
progression of, 527*t*
sickle cell, 521*t*, 564–565
sideroblastic, 521*t*, 525–526
Anencephaly, 429
Aneuploid cell, 43
Aneuploidy, 43–46, 45*f*
autosomal, 46, 46*f*, 47*t*
sex chromosome, 46, 48*f*
Aneurysms
arterial, 611
berry, 408, 409*f*
cerebral, 611–612
clinical manifestations of, 611–612
definition of, 611
false, 611, 612*f*
fusiform, 408, 611
giant, 408
intracranial, 408–409, 409*f*
saccular, 408, 611
thoracic aortic, 611–612
Aneurysms (*Continued*)
true, 611, 612*f*
types of, 612*f*
Angelman syndrome, 52, 64–65, 65*f*
Angina pectoris
microvascular, 621*b*
Prinzmetal, 621
stable, 620–621
unstable, 623–624, 624*b*, 625*f*
Angioedema, hereditary, 141–142
Angiogenesis, 153, 578–579
cancer cell inducement of, 247–248, 248*f*
tumour-induced, 248*f*
Angiogenesis factors, 153
Angiogenic factors, 247–248
Angiogenic inhibitors, 247–248
Angiomas, 419*t*
Angiotensin I, 118
Angiotensin II, 118
arteriolar remodelling mediated by, 608
endothelial dysfunction and, 607–608
Angiotensin receptor blockers (ARBs), 608
Angular stomatitis, 524–525
ANH. *See* Atrial natriuretic hormone
Anhidrotic ectodermal dysplasia, 62–63
Anion gap, 128, 130*t*
Anions, 18–19
Anisotropic band, 585, 585*f*
Ankylosing spondylitis, 209, 1035–1038, 1037*f*
Anoikis, 255
Anomic aphasia, 371, 372*t*–373*t*
Anorectal malformations, 972, 973*f*
Anorexia, 535, 921
Anorgasmia, 842
Anosmia, 356
ANP. *See* Atrial natriuretic peptide
ANS. *See* Autonomic nervous system
Antagonist, of muscles, 1006
Antalgic abductor lurch, 1065
Anterior columns, 320–321, 321*f*
Anterior fontanelle, 426, 427*f*
Anterior fossa, 323
Anterior horn, 320–321
Anterior pituitary gland
anatomy of, 448–452
chromophils of, 448
chromophobes of, 448
diseases of, 468–471
acromegaly, 469, 470*f*
hyperpituitarism, 469
hypopituitarism, 468, 469*f*
prolactinomas, 470–471
hormones produced by, 448–452, 451*t*
regions of, 448
Anterior spinal artery, 327, 329*f*
Anterior spinothalamic tracts, 323
Anterograde amnesia, 369, 370*t*
Anthropogenic emissions, 93
Antibiotic resistance, 183, 189
UTI and, 766*b*
Antibiotics
bactericidal, 188–189
bacteriostatic, 188–189
broad-spectrum, 138
micro-organisms destroying, 188–189, 188*t*
Antibodies, 159
antigen binding to, 163
clinical use of, 160*t*
colostral, 165
functions of, 163–165, 164*f*
heterophilic, 532
immunoglobulins compared to, 161–162
molecular structure of, 162–163
monoclonal, 165*b*, 264
in newborns, 174*b*
plasma cells production of, 496
predominantly antibody deficiencies, 192–193, 192*t*
in umbilical cord blood, 174*b*
Antibody screen test, 514*t*–516*t*
Antibody-dependent cellular cytotoxicity (ADCC), 173, 204, 206*f*
Antibody-mediated hemorrhagic disease, 569–570

Anticipatory stress responses, 217
Anti-citrullinated protein antibody (ACPA), 1035
Anticoagulants, 514*t*–516*t*
Anticodon, 42
Antidiuretic hormone (ADH)
  blood volume regulation and, 747, 748*f*
  diabetes insipidus and, 467–468, 467*t*
  homeostatic function of, 452
  nephron function affected by, 752
  secretion of, 452
  syndrome of inappropriate, 122, 257*t*, 466–467, 467*t*
  synthesis of, 447–448
  urine regulation and, 747, 748*f*
  water balance regulated by, 117–119, 119*f*
Antiemetics, 260
Antigen processing, 168–169, 169*f*–170*f*
Antigen receptors, 9
  B cell, 167, 167*f*
  cell surface, 159–160
  T cell, 167*f*, 168
Antigen-binding fragments, 162, 164*f*
Antigen-binding site, 163
Antigenic determinant, 163
Antigenic drift, 185
Antigenic shifts, 185, 185*f*
Antigenic variation, 185
Antigen-presenting cells (APCs), 168, 221–222
Antigens
  antibodies binding to, 163
  blood group, 210
  clinical use of, 160*t*
  definition of, 159–160
  description of, 141
  endogenous, 168–169
  exogenous, 168–169
  human leukocyte, 169, 195, 211, 211*f*–212*f*
  immunogens compared to, 161
  processing and presentation of, 168–169, 169*f*–170*f*
  self, 167–168
  superantigens, 169–170, 172*f*
  T-cell-independent, 171, 172*f*
Antigravity posture, 389
Antimetabolites, 262
Antimicrobial peptides, 137
Antimicrobials, 188–189, 188*t*
Antiphospholipid syndrome (APS), 554
Antiport, 18, 19*f*
Antiretroviral therapy, 196–197
Antithrombin III (AT-III), 513
Antitoxins, 163–164, 182–183
α1-Antitrypsin, 149
Antivascular endothelial growth factor (anti-VEGF), 352
Antrum, 902, 902*f*
Anuria, 774
Anus, 909, 909*f*
Aorta, 577
  coarctation of, 664, 665*f*
  semilunar valves, 577, 577*f*–578*f*
Aortic regurgitation, 634
Aortic stenosis, 633, 633*f*, 664–666, 665*f*
APCs. *See* Antigen-presenting cells
Aphasia, 371, 372*t*–373*t*
Aplastic anemia, 521*t*, 527*t*
Aplastic crisis, 566
Apneusis, 366*t*
Apocrine sweat glands, 1074–1076
Apoferritin, 508
Apoptosis
  cancer cell resistance to, 249–250, 250*f*
  definition of, 14, 74, 101, 105
  dysregulated, 105
  extrinsic pathway of, 249, 250*f*
  features of, 102*t*
  intrinsic pathway of, 249, 250*f*
  mechanisms of, 106*f*
  morphological changes associated with, 103*f*
  muscle wasting and, 257–258
Apoptotic bodies, 101
Apotransferrin, 508–509
Appendicitis, 939
  in children, 974
Appendicular skeleton, 994, 994*f*
Apraxia, 390
Aprosody, 389–390
APS. *See* Antiphospholipid syndrome
Aquaporins, 116
Aquaretics, 753*t*
Aqueduct of Sylvius, 319
Aqueous humour, 349–350
Arachnoid, 323
Arachnoid villi, 323–324
ARBs. *See* Angiotensin receptor blockers
Arcuate arteries, 745
Arcus senilis, of eye, 621–622
ARDS. *See* Acute respiratory distress syndrome
Aredia, 1061–1062
Areflexia, 387
Areola, 806
Arnold-Chiari malformation, 429–430
Aromatase, 882, 882*f*
Arousal
  alterations in, 363–369
    brain death secondary to, 368, 368*b*
    breathing patterns and, 364, 365*f*, 366*t*
    cerebral death secondary to, 368–369
    clinical manifestations of, 364–367, 364*t*
    infratentorial disorders as cause of, 364, 365*t*
    level of consciousness and, 364, 365*t*
    metabolic disorders as cause of, 364, 365*t*
    motor responses and, 367, 367*f*–368*f*, 368*t*
    oculomotor responses and, 364–367, 367*f*
    outcomes of, 368–369
    pathophysiology of, 363–364
    pupillary changes and, 364, 366*f*
    structural, 363
    supratentorial disorders as cause of, 363–364, 365*t*
  mediation of, 363
Arrested state, 26–27
Arrhythmias, 643
Arsenic, inorganic, 295
Arterial aneurysms, 611
Arterial blood gases (ABGs), 131–132
Arterial blood pressure, 595, 595*f*
Arterial chemoreceptors, 596, 596*f*
Arterial oxygenation, 690–691, 691*f*
Arterial pressure
  of carbon dioxide, 685–686, 689*t*
  of oxygen, 685–686, 689*t*
Arterial thrombi, 553
Arterial thromboembolism, 613*t*
Arterial thrombosis, 612–613
Arterial vessels, 589–590, 592*f*
Arteries
  arcuate, 745
  collateral, 578–579
  coronary
    anatomy of, 578, 579*b*, 581*f*
    calcification of, 100
    obstruction of, 80–81
  disorders involving, 606–628
  elastic, 589
  functions of, 575
  hypertension (*See* Hypertension)
  interlobar, 745
  muscular, 589
  renal, 744–745
  structure of, 589–590, 592*f*
  systemic circulation, 589, 590*f*–591*f*
Arteriogenesis, 578–579
Arteriolar remodelling, angiotensin II mediating, 608
Arterioles, 589, 590*f*–591*f*
  afferent, 745
  efferent, 745
Arteriosclerosis, 614
Arthritis
  gouty, 1038, 1039*f*, 1040
  juvenile idiopathic, 1064, 1064*t*
  oligoarthritis, 1064
  osteoarthritis, 1029–1032, 1030*f*, 1031*b*, 1032*f*
Arthritis *(Continued)*
  polyarthritis, 1064
  psoriatic, 1083–1084
  rheumatoid (*See* Rheumatoid arthritis)
  septic, 1063–1064
Arthus reactions, 205
Articular capsule, 995–996
Articular cartilage, 997
  loss of, osteoarthritis and, 1030–1031
Asbestos-silicate mineral, 295, 703
Ascending colon, 909, 909*f*
Ascending pathways, 309
Ascites, 117, 944–945, 944*f*–945*f*
Aseptic meningitis, 412, 435
Ask-Upmark kidney, 786
Aspartate, 314*t*
Aspartate aminotransferase, 916*t*
Asphyxial Injuries, 93–96
Aspiration
  foreign body, 727
  pulmonary, 701
Aspiration pneumonitis, 733
Assessment of SpondyloArthritis International Society, 1035–1036
Association fibres, 316–317
Associational neurons, 310
Asterixis, 383*t*
Asthma
  acute responses in, 708*f*
  bronchial, 706, 706*f*
  in children, 733–735, 734*b*
  clinical manifestations of, 707
  definition of, 705–706
  evaluation of, 707–708
  hygiene hypothesis of, 706
  incidence of, 706*b*
  indigenous people in Canada and, 706*b*
  pathophysiology of, 706–707, 706*f*–708*f*
  risk factors for, 706
  status asthmaticus and, 707
  treatment of, 707–708
Astigmatism, 352, 352*f*
Astrocytes, 310–311, 312*t*
  swelling of, 398
Astrocytomas, 418–420, 419*t*–420*t*, 437–438, 437*t*
Asymptomatic hyperuricemia, 1040
Asystole, 644*t*–645*t*
Ataxia telangiectasia, 534
Ataxic breathing, 366*t*
Ataxic cerebral palsy, 433
Ataxic gait, 389
Atelectasis, 701, 702*f*
Atherogenesis, 608, 614
Atherogenic diet, 619
Atherosclerosis, 80–81, 614–617
  arterial aneurysms and, 611
  CAD from, 616*f*, 617
  clinical manifestations of, 614–617
  diabetes mellitus and, 485, 487*f*
  evaluation and treatment of, 617
  pathophysiology of, 614, 615*f*–616*f*
Athetosis, 383*t*
AT-III. *See* Antithrombin III
Atmospheric pressure, 688–689
ATN. *See* Acute tubular necrosis
Atonic seizure, 436*t*
Atopic dermatitis, 892*t*–894*t*, 1082
  in children, 1108, 1108*f*
Atopic individuals, 203
ATP. *See* Adenosine triphosphate
Atria, of heart, 577, 577*f*
Atrial fibrillation, 644*t*–645*t*
Atrial flutter, 644*t*–645*t*
Atrial natriuretic hormone (ANH), 118, 119*f*
Atrial natriuretic peptide (ANP), 752
Atrial receptors, heart rate and, 589
Atrial septal defect, 667–668
Atrial tachycardia, 644*t*–645*t*
Atrioventricular bundle (AV bundle), 582, 582*f*
Atrioventricular canal defect, 668, 668*f*
Atrioventricular dissociation, 645*t*–646*t*
Atrioventricular node (AV node), 581–583, 582*f*
Atrioventricular septal defect, 668
Atrioventricular valves (AV valves), 577, 578*f*
Atrophy, 75–76, 75*f*, 1079*t*–1080*t*
Attention-deficit/hyperactivity disorder (ADHD), 369, 369*b*
Attenuated virus, 189
Atypical ductal hyperplasia, 845, 846*f*
Atypical hyperplasia, 77, 845, 846*f*
Atypical lobular hyperplasia, 845, 846*f*
Atypical pneumonia, 733
Auerbach plexus, 902, 906
Auricle, 354, 354*f*
Autoantibodies, 201
Autocrine signalling, 12–13, 14*f*
Autocrine stimulation, 242
Autografts, 1098–1099, 1099*f*–1100*f*
Autoimmune diseases
  definition of, 201
  examples of, 201*t*
  systemic lupus erythematosus, 209–210
Autoimmune gastritis, 523
Autoimmune thyroiditis, 473
Autoimmune type 1 diabetes mellitus, 476–477
Autoimmunity, 201, 209–210
Autolysis, 101–102
Automatic cells, 583
Automaticity, of heart, 583
Autonomic dysfunction, 411
Autonomic hyper-reflexia, 402, 403*f*–404*f*
Autonomic nervous system (ANS)
  components of, 309, 328–334
  functions of, 331–334, 334*f*
  lung innervation by, 685
  neuroreceptors and neurotransmitters of, 331, 333*t*
  parasympathetic nervous system, 224, 331, 332*f*
  preganglionic and postganglionic neurons of, 328, 331*f*
  salivation in, 901
  sympathetic nervous system, 222–224, 328–331, 332*f*
Autonomic regulation, 599
Autophagic vacuoles, 75–76
Autophagolysosome, 106–107
Autophagosome, 106–107
Autophagy, 74, 106–107, 106*b*, 107*f*
Autoreactive T cells, 201
Autoregulation, 378
  coronary circulation and, 598–599
Autosomal aneuploidy, 46, 46*f*, 47*t*
Autosomal dominant inheritance
  delayed age of onset, 51
  epigenetics and, 52, 53*f*
  expressivity and, 51–52, 52*f*
  genomic imprinting and, 52
  pedigrees and, 50, 51*f*
  penetrance and, 51–52, 51*f*
  recurrence risks of, 50–51
Autosomal recessive inheritance
  consanguinity and, 54
  pedigrees in, 52–53, 53*f*
  recurrence risks and, 53–54, 54*f*
Autosomes, 42
AV bundle. *See* Atrioventricular bundle
AV node. *See* Atrioventricular node
AV valves. *See* Atrioventricular valves
Avanafil, 888
Avastin (bevacizumab), 263*t*
Avulsions, 1015
Awareness
  alterations in, 369–371
    clinical manifestations of, 370*t*, 371
    evaluation and treatment of, 371
    pathophysiology of, 369–371
  definition of, 369
  mediation of, 363
Axial skeleton, 994, 994*f*
Axon hillock, 310
Axons, 310, 310*f*
5-Azacytidine, 70, 70*f*
Azidothymidine, 189
Azotemia, 772

B

B cell antigen receptor, 167, 167*f*
B cells (B lymphocytes)
  bone marrow as origin of, 165–167
  class switch in maturation of, 170–171
  clonal diversity generation and, 165–168, 167*t*
  clonal selection of, 170–171, 172*f*
  description of, 159–160
  development of, 167–168
  differentiation sites of, 162*f*, 168
  in immune response, 165–171
B lymphocytes. *See* B cells
B vitamins, 280
B_{12} vitamin, 522–523
Bacille Calmette-Guérin (BCG), 714
Bacilli, 178
Bacteremia, 183
Bacteria
  antibiotic resistance of, 183, 189
  definition of, 178
  growth of, 178–183
  pyrogenic, 183
  self-protein coating on, 182
  structure of, 177*f*
  survival of, 178–183
  toxins secreted by, 163–164
Bacterial embolism, 613*t*
Bacterial infections
  in children, 1109–1110, 1109*b*, 1110*f*
  examples of, 180*t*–181*t*
  of skin, 1087–1088, 1087*f*
Bacterial meningitis, 412–413, 435
Bacterial pneumonia, 732, 732*t*
Bacterial tracheitis, 727, 730*t*
Bactericidal antibiotics, 188–189
Bacteriostatic antibiotics, 188–189
Bactrim, 766*b*
Bainbridge reflex, 589
Balanitis, 871, 871*f*
Ballism, 383*t*
Balloon angioplasty, 665
Bare lymphocyte syndrome, 191, 192*t*
Bariatric surgery, 942
Barometric pressure, 688–689
Baroreceptor reflexes, 589
Baroreceptors, 119–120, 596, 596*f*
Barr bodies, 54, 54*f*
Barrett esophagus, 69, 954–955
Bartholinitis, 827, 827*f*
Basal cell carcinoma, 290, 1092, 1093*f*
Basal ganglia, 315–317, 316*f*, 319*f*
Basal ganglia motor syndromes, 390
Basal ganglion gait, 389
Basal ganglion posture, 389
Basal lamina, 11
Basal nuclei, 317
Base pair substitutions, 39, 41*f*
Basement membrane, 10–11, 1000
Bases, 38–39
Basic fibroblast growth factor, 247–248
Basic multicellular units, 995
Basilar skull fractures, 397
Basis pedunculi, 319
Basopenia, 530*t*, 531
Basophil count, 514*t*–516*t*
Basophilia, 530*t*, 531
Basophils, 142*f*, 145–147, 499, 499*t*, 530*t*
Bazedoxifene, 1026*b*
BBB. *See* Blood-brain barrier
B-cell receptors, 142
BCG. *See* Bacille Calmette-Guérin
Bcl-2, 250
BCR-ABL gene, 305, 536–537
BCR-ABL protein, 242–243
Becker muscular dystrophy, 1067*t*, 1068
Beckwith-Weidemann syndrome, 52, 65–66
Bedbugs, 1114–1115
Bee sting allergy, 208–209
Behavioral stress, 217*f*
Bell's palsy, 388*b*
Bence Jones protein, 543, 545
Benign breast disease, 844–845
Benign prostatic hyperplasia, 77, 876–878, 877*f*
Benign rolandic epilepsy, 436*t*
Benign tumours
  of adrenal medulla, 260–261
  description of, 235–236
  malignant tumours compared to, 236*f*
  of skin, 1091, 1091*f*, 1092*t*
Bent nail syndrome, 870–871, 871*f*
Benuryl (probenecid), 826*b*
Benzol, 295
Beriberi, 643
Berry aneurysms, 408, 409*f*
Beta cells, 455, 455*f*
Beta globulins, 496–497
Beta-cell dysfunction, 481
β-Thalassemias, 567–568, 568*f*
Bevacizumab (Avastin), 263*t*
Biallelic expression, 64
Bicarbonate, 118, 130*f*
Bicornuate uterus, 817*f*
Bicuspid valve, 577, 577*f*–578*f*
Bidi smoking, 276–277
Bile
  acids, 912
  components of, 912
  definition of, 912
  liver secretion of, 913*f*, 914
Bile acid pool, 912
Bile acid-dependent fraction, 912
Bile acid-independent fraction, 912
Bile canaliculi, 911, 912*f*
Bile duct cancer, 270*t*–273*t*
Bile salt deficiency, 935
Bile salts, 912, 935
Biliary atresia, 980
Biliary cirrhosis, 949
Bilirubin, 99–100, 507–508, 508*f*
  conjugated, 913, 946
  definition of, 913
  liver and metabolism of, 913, 913*f*, 916*t*
  unconjugated, 913
Binding proteins, hormones and, 444, 445*t*
Binding site, 9
Binge drinking, 92
Bioassays, 446*b*
Biofeedback, 1041
Biofilms, 179–182
Biotransformation, 84–85
Biphasic effects, of hormones, 446
Bipolar neurons, 310
Birthmarks, 1091, 1092*t*, 1094
Bisphenol A, 855
Bisphosphonate therapy, 545, 1061–1062
Bisphosphonate-related osteonecrosis of jaw, 1026*b*
Bladder
  anatomy of, 746, 746*f*
  cancer of, 270*t*–273*t*, 295, 764–765
  exstrophy of, 785, 785*f*
  innervation of, 746
  low bladder wall compliance, 763
  neurogenic, 762, 762*t*, 767*t*
  outflow obstruction of, 878
  overactive bladder syndrome, 762–763
  tumours of, 764–765
  underactive bladder syndrome, 762
Bladder function tests, 754, 755*t*
Bladder outlet obstruction, 763
  in children, 785
Blalock-Taussig shunt, 669–670
Blast cells, 571, 571*f*
Blastocysts, 505, 800
Blebs, 711
Bleeding. *See also* Hemorrhage
  abnormal uterine, 820–821, 821*t*
  acute, 924, 924*t*
  gastric, 931
  gastro-intestinal, 924, 924*t*, 925*f*
  leukemia and, 536*t*
  in menstrual cycle, 803
  occult, 924, 924*t*
  types of, 510*t*
Bleeding time, 514*t*–516*t*
Blepharitis, 353
Blindness, 484–485, 484*t*, 485*f*
Blood
  composition of, 496–500, 497*f*
    erythrocytes, 505–506
    leukocytes (*See* Leukocytes)
    plasma, 496–497, 498*t*
    plasma proteins, 496–497
Blood *(Continued)*
  functions of, 496
  oxygen transport in, 690–692
Blood cells, 499*t*, 504–505. *See also* Erythrocytes; Hematopoiesis; Leukocytes; Platelets
  components of, 142, 142*f*
  development of, 503–510
Blood clots
  definition of, 141, 512
  dissolution of, 512*f*
  laboratory tests for, 514*t*–516*t*
  lysis of, 513–514, 514*f*
  mechanism of, 513*f*
  retraction of, 513–514
Blood flow
  in cardiac cycle, 578, 579*f*–580*f*
  definition of, 593
  to exocrine pancreas, 915
  factors affecting, 593–595
  through heart, 576–578, 577*f*
  intrarenal, autoregulation of, 746–747, 747*f*
  laminar, 594, 594*f*
  pressure effects on, 593–594
  pulmonary
    congenital heart disease and decreased, 668–670
    congenital heart disease and increased, 667–668
  renal, 746–747, 747*f*, 753
  resistance effects on, 593–594
  splanchnic, 910
  turbulent, 594, 594*f*
  in vasa recta, 751
  velocity of, 594, 594*f*
Blood group antigens, 210
Blood lead levels, 88–89
Blood pressure
  aldosterone effects on, 580*f*, 597
  ambulatory monitoring of, 676
  arterial, 595, 595*f*
  baroreceptors effect on, 596, 596*f*
  cardiac output effects on, 595
  checking, 606
  chemoreceptor reflex control of, 596, 596*f*
  in children, 674*t*
  classification of, 606*t*
  diastolic, 595
  hormone effects on, 597
  pericardial sac causing reflex changes in, 576
  postmortem changes in, 110
  regulation of, 595–598
  systolic, 595
  total peripheral resistance effects on, 595–596
  vasopressin effects on, 580*f*, 597
  venous, 598
Blood supply
  to brain, 325–326, 326*f*–327*f*, 327*t*
  to CNS, 325–327
  to liver, 911, 912*f*
  to skin, 1076
  to spinal cord, 327, 329*f*
Blood urea nitrogen (BUN), 754, 775
Blood velocity, 594, 594*f*
Blood vessel tumours, 419*t*
Blood vessels. *See also* Arteries; Capillaries
  arterioles, 589, 590*f*–591*f*
  damage to, 512*f*
  endothelium of, 575, 590–591, 592*f*–593*f*, 593*t*
  function of, in hemostasis, 510–511
  of kidney, 744–745
  lumen of, 589, 593–594
  metarterioles, 591–593, 592*f*
  of nephron, 744*f*
  stiffness of, 595
  of stomach, 902, 902*f*
  structure of, 589–593, 592*f*
  vascular compliance of, 595
Blood volume, 496
  ADH and aldosterone regulating, 747, 748*f*
  aging effects on, 516*b*, 517*t*
Blood-brain barrier (BBB), 326, 328*f*
Bloom's syndrome, 244–246, 305, 534
Blowout hemorrhage, 510*t*
Blue spells, 669
Blunt-force injuries, 94*t*–95*t*
BMI. *See* Body mass index
BNP. *See* B-type natriuretic peptide
Body fluids. *See also* Total body water (TBW)
  distribution of, 115–116, 132*b*
  hydrogen ions in, 126
  pH of, 126, 128*t*
Body heat, production and loss of, 345, 345*t*
Body mass index (BMI), 283, 283*t*
Body of stomach, 902, 902*f*
Body temperature
  death-related decreases in, 110
  menstrual cycle and, 805
  normal range of, 344
  regulation of (*See* Thermoregulation)
Body weight, 115, 116*t*
Bone. *See also* Joints
  age-related loss of, 1023, 1024*f*
  aging of, 1006–1007
  anatomy of, 988–995, 989*f*, 989*t*, 992*f*, 994*f*
  calcification of, 988
  calcium and, 778, 989*t*, 1025*b*
  cancellous, 992–993, 992*f*
  cells of, 988–990, 989*f*, 989*t*
  characteristics of, 31*t*–33*t*, 33*f*
  compact, 992–993, 992*f*–993*f*
  cortical, 992–993, 992*f*–993*f*
  density, 1021–1022, 1021*t*
  destruction, bone tumours and, 1047–1049, 1048*t*
  flat, 994
  formation of, 991*t*
    endochondral, 1013, 1013*f*
  function of, 988–995
  healing, 1013, 1013*f*
  irregular, 994–995
  long, 994
  maintenance of, 991*t*, 995
  marrow cavities in, 988
  metastases to, 256
  mineralized, 1021
  minerals of, 992
  osteoblasts of, 988–990, 989*f*, 989*t*
  osteoclasts of, 988–990, 989*f*, 989*t*
  osteocytes of, 988–990, 989*f*, 989*t*
  pain, leukemia and, 536*t*
  phosphate and, 778, 989*t*
  remodeling of, 991*t*, 995, 996*f*
  repair of, 995, 1037
  short, 994
  spongy, 992–993, 992*f*
  tissue, elements of, 988–992
  turnover, biochemical markers of, 1025*b*
  types of, 992–993
  vitamins D and, 1025*b*
Bone cancer, 270*t*–273*t*
Bone disorders
  metabolic bone diseases, 1020–1027
  osteomalacia, 1026–1027
  osteomyelitis, 1028–1029, 1028*f*–1029*f*
  osteoporosis (*See* Osteoporosis)
  Paget's disease, 856*t*, 1027
  postgastrectomy, 935
Bone fluid, 992
Bone infections
  osteomyelitis, 1028–1029, 1028*f*–1029*f*, 1062–1063, 1063*b*, 1063*f*
  septic arthritis, 1063–1064
Bone marrow
  B cells from, 165–167
  hematopoiesis in, 504–505, 504*f*
  multiple myeloma and, 542–543, 543*f*
  niches in, 504–505, 504*f*
  transplants
    childhood cancer patients and, 307*b*
    for SCID, 195
Bone matrix, 988, 992
Bone mineral density, 1021, 1021*t*
Bone morphogenetic proteins, 989*t*, 991*t*
Bone tumours
  bone destruction patterns of, 1047–1049, 1048*t*
  in children, 1069–1071, 1070*f*–1071*f*
  chondrosarcoma, 1050
  classification of, 1047, 1047*b*

Bone tumours *(Continued)*
collagenic, 1050
derivation of, 1048*f*
epidemiology of, 1047
evaluation of, 1048–1049, 1048*t*
giant cell tumour, 1050
malignant, in children, 1069–1071
osteosarcoma, 1049–1050, 1049*f*
pathological features of, 1047–1049
staging for, 1048*t*
types of, 1049–1050
BOOP. *See* Bronchiolitis obliterans organizing pneumonia
Botulinum toxin (Botox), 763
Bowing fractures, 1012, 1012*t*
Bowman capsule, 742*f*, 743
Bowman space, 743
BPD. *See* Bronchopulmonary dysplasia
Brachial plexus, 328
Brachycephaly, 431*f*
Brachytherapy, 262
Bradykinesia, 384
Bradykinin, 141
Brain. *See also* Hypothalamus
blood supply to, 325–326, 326*f*–327*f*, 327*t*
cerebellum in, 313–314, 319
cerebral hemispheres of, 314–318, 316*f*
in children, 426
CSF flow to, 324*f*
development of, 426
diencephalon of, 317–318
divisions of, 313–314, 315*f*, 315*t*
edema of, 379–380, 379*f*
forebrain, 313–318, 315*t*
hindbrain, 313–314, 315*t*, 319–320
intracerebral hematomas and, 395*t*, 397, 397*f*
malformations of, 431–432, 431*f*–432*f*, 434*t*
metencephalon of, 319
midbrain, 313–314, 315*t*, 319
myelencephalon of, 319–320
overview of, 313–320
pons of, 313–314, 319
postnatal growth of, 426
telencephalon of, 314–318, 316*f*
Brain abscesses, 413
Brain cancer, 270*t*–273*t*
Brain death, 368, 368*b*
Brain herniation syndromes, 378–379, 379*b*, 379*f*
Brain injuries. *See also* Traumatic brain injury
classification of, 395*t*
closed, 394–395, 395*t*
diffuse, 395*t*, 397–398
focal, 394–397, 395*t*, 396*f*
open, 395*t*, 397
secondary, 395*t*, 398
Brain networks, 314, 315*b*
Brain tumours, 304
astrocytomas, 418–420, 419*t*–420*t*
in children, 436–438, 437*f*, 437*t*, 438*b*
of CNS, 417–421, 418*f*, 419*t*–420*t*
ependymomas, 419*t*, 420
glioblastoma multiforme, 419–420, 419*t*
gliomas, 418–420, 419*t*
meningiomas, 419*t*, 420
metastatic, 421
neurofibromas, 419*t*, 420–421
oligodendroglioma, 419*t*, 420
primary intracerebral, 418–420, 419*t*
Brainstem
anatomy of, 313–314, 315*f*
gliomas of, 437*t*, 438
respiratory centre in, 684, 685*f*
reticular formation and, 313–314, 315*f*
BRCA1, 247, 855, 883–884, 891
BRCA2, 247, 855, 883–884, 891
Breast cancer
clinical manifestations of, 860, 860*f*
description of, 270*t*–273*t*
diet and, 853–854
ductal carcinoma in situ, 237–238, 847*b*, 856*t*, 857–860, 859*f*
EMT and, 855
environmental causes of, 853–855
environmental chemicals and, 854–855
Breast cancer *(Continued)*
estrogen and risk of, 851–852
evaluation of, 860
genes involved in, 57, 247
genetic heterogeneity and, 855
GH and, 852
hormonal factors in, 850–852, 850*f*–851*f*
hormone replacement therapy and risk of, 852
IGF and, 819
incidence of, 845, 848*f*
inherited syndromes, 855–857
lobular carcinoma in situ, 856*t*, 859–860
lobular involution and, 849–850, 850*f*
male, 891
mammography for, 847*b*, 852–853, 852*f*
melatonin and, 852
menopausal hormone therapy and, 850, 852
metastasis of, 255
obesity and, 854
oral contraceptives and, 852
pathogenesis of, 855–857, 857*f*–859*f*
physical activity and, 283–285, 855
postlactational involution and, 849–850, 850*f*
pregnancy and, 845–849
progesterone and risk of, 851
prolactin and, 852
radiation exposure causing, 853
reproductive factors in, 845–849
risk factors in, 845, 849*t*
screening for, 847*b*, 857–858
treatment of, 860
tumour dormancy and, 856–857
types of, 856*t*
vascular mimicry and, 857
Breast disorders
atypical ductal hyperplasia, 845, 846*f*
benign breast disease, 844–845
galactorrhea, 843–844
male, 890–891
Breast lesions
nonproliferative, 844
proliferative, with atypia, 845
proliferative, without atypia, 844–845
Breasts
aging effects on, 849–850
anatomy of, 805–807, 805*f*
areola, 806
cysts of, 844
definition of, 805
development of, 806, 818
estrogen effects on, 806
functions of, 806–807
lobular involution and, 849–850, 850*f*
lymphatic drainage of, 806, 806*f*
male, 807
nipple, 806
postlactational involution and, 849–850, 850*f*
sarcoma of, 856*t*
sex hormones and development of, 850
terminal duct lobular units of, 849
Breathing
abnormal patterns of, 696
airway resistance in, 688
alveolar surface tension and, 686–687
elastic properties in, 687–688, 687*f*
laboured, 696
mechanics of, 686–688
muscles of, 686, 686*f*
restricted, 696
work of, 688, 688*f*
Breathing patterns, 364, 365*f*, 366*t*
Brittle bone disease, 1060–1062, 1062*f*
Broad-spectrum antibiotics, 138
Broca area, 316, 318*f*
Broca dysphasia, 371, 372*t*–373*t*
Brodmann area, 315–316, 316*f*
Brodmann area 4, 316, 317*f*
Brodmann areas 44, 45, 316, 318*f*
Bromosulfophthalein excretion, 916*t*
Bronchi, 680, 682*f*
Bronchial asthma, 706, 706*f*
Bronchial circulation, 681–683
Bronchial metaplasia, 78, 79*f*
Bronchiectasis, 701–702
Bronchioles, 680, 682*f*–683*f*
Bronchiolitis, 702
in children, 730–732
Bronchiolitis obliterans, 702
in children, 733
Bronchiolitis obliterans organizing pneumonia (BOOP), 702
Bronchitis
acute, 711
chronic, 709–710, 709*f*–710*f*, 709*t*
Bronchoconstriction, 688
Bronchodilation, 688
Bronchopulmonary dysplasia (BPD), 730, 730*b*, 730*t*, 731*f*
Brudzinski sign, 409–410
Brush border, 906
Bruton agammaglobulinemia, 192–193, 192*t*
B-type natriuretic peptide (BNP), 118, 119*f*
heart failure and, 598*b*, 673
Budesonide, 726
Buerger's disease, 613
Buffering
acid-base balance and, 126–128, 128*t*
carbonic acid-bicarbonate, 126
definition of, 126
protein, 126, 130*f*
renal, 126–128, 130*f*
Buffers, 126
Bulbar palsy, 388
Bulbourethral glands, 809, 809*f*
Bulla, 1077*t*–1078*t*
Bullets, wounding potential of, 94*t*–95*t*
Bullous erythema multiforme, 1086
Bumetanide, 753*t*
BUN. *See* Blood urea nitrogen
Bundle of His, 582, 582*f*
Burinex, 753*t*
Burkitt lymphoma, 242, 541–542, 542*f*
in children, 571–572
Burn shock, 1096, 1097*f*
Burning mouth syndrome, 524
Burns
cardiovascular response to, 1097–1098
cellular response to, 1098
clinical manifestations of, 1095–1097, 1097*f*
deep partial-thickness, 1095, 1097*t*
evaluation of, 1098–1099
evaporative water loss in, 1098–1099
first-degree, 1095, 1097*t*
fourth-degree, 1095, 1097*t*
full-thickness, 1095, 1096*f*, 1097*t*
healing, 1095, 1096*f*, 1098–1099, 1098*f*–1100*f*
immunological response to, 1098
incidence, 1095
metabolic response to, 1098
pathophysiology of, 1095–1097, 1097*f*
rule of nines in, 1095, 1096*f*
second-degree, 1095, 1095*f*, 1097*t*
superficial partial-thickness, 1095, 1095*f*, 1097*t*
third-degree, 1095, 1096*f*, 1097*t*
total body surface area in, 1095, 1096*f*
treatment of, 1098–1099, 1098*f*–1100*f*
wound depth, 1095–1097, 1097*t*
Bursae, 1016, 1016*f*
Bursitis, 1015–1016, 1016*f*
Butyrate, 280
Bystander effects, 288, 288*f*

C

C cells, of thyroid gland, 453, 453*f*
C fibres, 339
C1, 141
C1 esterase inhibitor, 141–142
C1 INH deficiency, 141–142
C3, 141
deficiency of, 192*t*, 193
C5, 141
Cachexia, 256–258, 258*f*–259*f*, 943
CAD. *See* Coronary artery disease
Caenorhabditis elegans, 108
Calcaneovalgus, 1060*t*
Calcaneovarus, 1060*t*
Calcification, of bone, 988
Calcitonin, 453, 454*t*
Calcitonin gene-related peptide, 225*t*–226*t*, 411
Calcium
balance, alterations in, 126, 127*t*
bone and, 778, 989*t*, 1025*b*
as cellular accumulations, 100, 101*f*–102*f*
CKD and phosphate balance with, 777*t*, 778
cytosolic, 83
formation of, 992*t*
intracellular concentrations of, 82
Calcium hydroxide, 100
Calcium salts, 100
Calcium stones, 761
Calcium-calmodulin complex, 447
Calcium-troponin complex, 586
Calculi, urinary, 760–761
Caloric ice water test, 367*f*
Calyces, 741, 742*f*
cAMP. *See* Cyclic adenosine monophosphate
CAMs. *See* Cell adhesion molecules
Canadian Cystic Fibrosis Registry, 737
Canadian Diabetes Association, 476, 482
Canadian Nuclear Safety Commission, 286
Canaliculi, 993, 993*f*
Cancellous bone, 992–993, 992*f*
Cancer
of accessory organs of digestion, 957–959
adenocarcinomas (*See* Adenocarcinomas)
bladder, 270*t*–273*t*, 295, 764–765
bone, 270*t*–273*t*
brain, 270*t*–273*t*
breast cancer (*See* Breast cancer)
in Canada, 274
carcinomas (*See* Carcinomas)
causes of, 269*f*
cell surface antigens expressed by, 252
cellular differentiation during, 237*f*
cervical (*See* Cervical cancer)
characteristics of, 235–238, 260–264
chemotherapy for, 262–263
childhood (*See* Childhood cancers)
classification of, 270*t*–273*t*
clinical manifestations of, 256–260
anemia and, 257*t*, 258
cachexia and, 256–258, 258*f*–259*f*
fatigue associated with, 256
GI tract and, 260
hair and, 260
infection and, 259, 259*t*
leukopenia and, 259
pain and, 256
paraneoplastic syndromes and, 256, 257*t*
skin and, 260
thrombocytopenia and, 259
colorectal, 270*t*–273*t*, 837, 954*t*, 955–957, 956*b*–957*b*, 956*f*–957*f*
definition of, 235
development of, 268
diagnosis of, 260–264
of digestive system, 953–959
DNA methylation and, 68–69, 69*f*, 246, 274–275
early life conditions, 274–276
endometrial, 836–838, 837*f*–838*f*, 838*t*
environmental-lifestyle factors and, 268, 269*f*
air pollution and, 293–294, 294*f*
alcohol and, 283, 285*f*, 285*t*
chemicals and, 294–295
diet, 277, 279*f*
electromagnetic radiation and, 291–292, 292*f*
infection and, 292–293, 293*t*
ionizing radiation and, 285–289, 286*t*, 287*f*
nutrition, 277–282, 279*f*–282*f*
obesity and, 283, 283*t*, 284*f*
occupational hazards and, 294–295
physical activity and, 283–285
sexually transmitted infections and, 292–293, 293*t*
tobacco smoking, 276–277, 277*f*
ultraviolet radiation and, 289–291

Cancer *(Continued)*
epigenetic screening for, 69
epigenetics and, 68–70, 69*f*, 268, 269*f*, 282*f*
of esophagus, 270*t*–273*t*, 954–955, 954*b*, 954*t*
familial, 244, 244*t*
of gallbladder, 270*t*–273*t*, 958
genes, 243, 243*t*
genetic lesions in, 262*b*
genetics of, 238–240, 268, 269*f*
of GI tract, 953–957, 954*t*
global burden of, 274, 274*b*
glucose requirement in, 250*f*
growth factor signaling pathways in, 242*f*
hallmarks of, 238, 239*f*
hereditary nonpolyposis colorectal, 837
heterogeneity of, 240
HPV and, rising incidence of, 293*b*
immunotherapy for, 263
incidence of, 268, 274
laryngeal, 270*t*–273*t*, 717–718, 717*f*
lip, 270*t*–273*t*, 1093, 1093*f*
of liver, 954*t*, 957–958, 957*b*
lung (*See* Lung cancer)
metabolism in, 249*f*
microenvironments of, 241*f*
miRNAs and, 69
mortality trends with, 274, 274*b*
nasopharyngeal, 270*t*–273*t*
neovascularization of, 255
ocular, 270*t*–273*t*
oral cavity, 270*t*–273*t*
ovarian (*See* Ovarian cancer)
pain, 256, 344*t*
pancreatic, 270*t*–273*t*, 954*t*, 958–959
penis, 270*t*–273*t*, 871–872, 872*b*
prevention of, 277
process of, 236*f*
progression of, 284*f*
prostate (*See* Prostate cancer)
radiation therapy for, 262
sites of, 270*t*–273*t*
skin (*See* Skin cancer)
staging of, 260–261, 260*t*, 261*f*
stomach, 954*t*, 955
surgery for, 262
targeted disruption of, 263–264, 263*t*
terminology of, 235–238
testicular, 270*t*–273*t*, 875–876, 875*b*, 875*f*
tissue differentiation during, 237*f*
TNM staging of, 260, 261*f*, 720
treatment of, 260–264
tumour markers for, 260–261, 261*t*
tumours (*See* Tumours)
in utero conditions, 274–276
vaginal, 270*t*–273*t*, 835–836
viruses associated with, 252
vulvar, 270*t*–273*t*, 836
World Health Organization prevention strategy for, 275*b*
wound healing and, 240
Cancer cells
anaplasia of, 236
angiogenesis inducement by, 247–248, 248*f*
apoptosis resistance by, 249–250, 250*f*
biology of, 238–255
dormancy of, 255
EMT and, 253, 254*f*, 255
energy metabolism reprogramming by, 248–249, 249*f*
genomic instability of, 244–247
growth suppressor evasion by, 243–244
heterogeneity of, 247
immune system destruction evasion by, 252–253, 253*f*
invasion activation by, 253–255
metastasis of, 253–255, 254*f*
proliferative signaling by, 240–243, 242*f*
in prostate cancer, 886
replication immortality of, 247
transformation of, 238–240
tumour-promoting inflammation and, 250–252, 251*t*
Cancer cells *(Continued)*
tumour-specific antigens expressed by, 241*f*
Cancer-associated adipocytes, 283
Cancer-associated fibroblasts, 249, 885–886
Candida albicans, 138, 186, 826
Candidiasis, 187, 1089, 1090*t*
Cannabinoids, 86*t*, 342
Cannabis. *See* Marihuana
Cannon, Walter B., 216
Capillaries
anatomy of, 590
coronary, 579
fenestrations in, 590
functions of, 575
glomerular, 745
lymphatic, 906
papillary, 1076
peritubular, 745
permeability of, inflammation effects on, 117
systemic circulation, 589, 590*f*–591*f*
Capillary hydrostatic pressure, 116–117
Capillary oncotic pressure, 116
Capillary pressures, glomerular filtration and, 741*f*, 747–748, 750*f*
Capillary seal, 1098
Caplan's syndrome, 1035
CAR cells. *See* CXCL12-abundant reticular cells
Carbohydrate metabolism, in CKD, 778
Carbohydrates
as cellular accumulations, 97–98
collectin reaction with, 137
liver metabolism of, 914
in plasma membrane, 2–3, 6*f*, 9
small intestine absorption of, 908*b*
Carbon, 99
Carbon dioxide
arterial pressure of, 685–686, 689*t*
from cellular metabolism, 684
diffusion of, 692
partial pressure of, 689*t*, 691*f*
Carbon monoxide poisoning, 90
Carbon tetrachloride, 83, 88*f*
Carbonic acid, 126, 130*f*
Carbonic acid–bicarbonate buffering, 126
Carbonic anhydrase, 126–128
Carbonic anhydrase inhibitors, 753*t*
Carboxyhemoglobin, 90
Carboxypeptidase, 141
Carbuncles, 1087
Carcinogenesis, 294–295
Carcinogens
chemicals as, 294–295
definition of, 268
dietary sources of, 277
occupational hazards as, 294–295
Carcinoid syndrome, 257*t*
Carcinoma in situ, 237–238, 855
Carcinomas. *See also* Cancer
adenocarcinomas, 236, 718*t*, 719, 719*f*
adenoid, 856*t*
basal cell, 290, 1092, 1093*f*
cholangiocellular, 958
definition of, 236
ductal carcinoma in situ, 237–238, 847*b*, 856*t*, 857–860, 859*f*
hepatocellular, 958
infiltrating lobular, 856*t*
inflammatory, 856*t*
intraductal, 856*t*
large cell, 718*t*, 719
lobular carcinoma in situ, 856*t*, 859–860
medullary, 856*t*
metaplastic, 856*t*
mucinous, 856*t*
nipple retraction and, 860*f*, 860*t*
non-small cell, 718*t*, 719, 719*f*
oat cell, 719–720
papillary, 856*t*
rectal, 957
renal cell, 763–764, 764*f*
renal transitional cell, 763–764
small cell, 718*t*, 719–720
small intestinal, 956
squamous cell, 290, 718*t*, 719, 719*f*, 856*t*, 1092–1093, 1093*f*
Carcinomas *(Continued)*
thyroid, 474
transitional cell, 764–765
tubular, 856*t*
Carcinomatous meningitis, 421
Cardiac action potentials, 580, 582–583, 582*t*, 583*f*
Cardiac cycle, 578, 579*f*–580*f*
Cardiac muscle
cells of, 584–586
hypertrophy of, 76–77, 76*f*
skeletal muscle compared to, 584–585
structure of, 33*f*, 33*t*–34*t*
Cardiac orifice, 902
Cardiac output
afterload, 588, 588*f*
blood pressure affected by, 595
in elderly, 587*t*
factors affecting, 587–589
heart rate effects on, 588–589
myocardial contractility and, 588, 588*f*
preload, 587–588, 587*f*
Cardiac sphincter, 901
Cardiogenic shock, 648, 649*f*
Cardiomyocytes, 576, 584
Cardiomyopathies, 630–632, 631*f*
Cardiopulmonary resuscitation (CPR), 737
Cardiovascular disorders
acute coronary syndromes (*See* Acute coronary syndromes)
in AIDS patients, 638
aneurysms (*See* Aneurysms)
arterial thrombosis, 612–613
atherosclerosis, 80–81, 485, 487*f*, 611, 614–617, 615*f*–616*f*
cardiomyopathies, 630–632, 631*f*
in children
acquired heart disease, 673–677
congenital heart disease (*See* Congenital heart disease)
hypertension, 674–677, 674*t*, 675*b*, 676*t*
Kawasaki disease, 673–674, 674*b*
obesity and, 676*b*
chronic venous insufficiency, 604–605
congenital heart disease (*See* Congenital heart disease)
coronary artery disease (*See* Coronary artery disease)
deep venous thrombosis, 605
diabetes mellitus complications with, 484*t*, 485
embolism, 613, 613*t*
heart failure (*See* Heart failure)
hypertension (*See* Hypertension)
MI (*See* Myocardial ischemia)
MODS (*See* Multiple organ dysfunction syndrome)
Orthostatic hypotension, 611
peripheral artery disease, 617
PVD, 484*t*, 486, 613–614
Raynaud phenomenon, 205, 613–614
thromboangiitis obliterans, 613
renin-angiotensin-aldosterone system and, 607–609
shock (*See* Shock)
superior vena cava syndrome, 605–606
varicose veins, 604–605, 605*f*
Cardiovascular vasomotor control centre, 588–589
Caretaker genes, 243*t*, 244
Carina, 680, 680*f*
Carnitine palmitoyltransferase, 1044
Carpopedal spasm, 131
Carrier detection tests, 53–54
Carriers
definition, 49–50
heterozygous, 53
obligate, 51
Cartilage
articular, 997
types of, 31*t*–33*t*, 32*f*
Cartilage intermediate layer protein, 403–404
Cartilaginous joints, 995–997, 997*f*
Cascade, 140
Caseous necrosis, 103, 104*f*
Caspases, 105–106, 250
Catabolism
definition of, 14
phases of, 16, 16*f*
protein, 75, 220
Cataracts, 350, 351*t*
Catecholamines
adrenal medulla secretion of, 459–460, 461*f*
description of, 221
neuroreceptors and, 331
physiological effects of, 224, 224*t*
proinflammatory cytokine production affected by, 224
Cathelicidins, 137
Cations, 18–19
Cat's eye reflex, 440
Cauda equina, 320
Cauda equina syndrome, 403, 762, 762*t*
Caudate nucleus, 317, 319*f*
Caveolae, 3, 4*t*, 23–24
Cavernous hemangiomas, 1115, 1115*f*
Cavernous sinus, 325
Cavitation, of abscesses, 715
CCR5 antagonist, 196–197
CD. *See* Crohn's disease
CD3, 168
CD4, 168
CD4+ T cells, 195
CD8, 168
CD59, 142
Cecum, 909, 909*f*
Cefizox (ceftizoxime), 826*b*
Cefoxitin (Mefoxin Pws), 826*b*
Ceftizoxime (Cefizox), 826*b*
Ceftriaxone (Rocephin), 826*b*
Celiac crisis, 976
Celiac disease, 975–977, 976*b*, 976*f*
Cells, 27*f*. *See also* Blood cells
of adaptive immunity, 142
aging of, 107–109, 109*f*
bone, 988–990, 989*f*, 989*t*
burn response of, 1098
dendritic, 147
differentiation, 2
ECM of, 10–12, 11*f*
eukaryotes, 1
functions of, 2
of inflammation, 142–149, 142*f*
of innate immunity, 142
membrane transport in
active, 18, 18*f*, 21, 21*f*, 22*t*
description of, 17–24
mediated, 17–18, 19*f*
membrane potentials and, 24, 24*f*
passive, 17–20, 18*f*–21*f*
systems of, 22*t*
by vesicle formation, 21–24
memory, 160, 171
of nervous system, 309–311
plasma, 160
prokaryotes, 1
protein regulation in, 8–9, 9*f*
reproduction of, 25–27
signaling of, 12–14, 14*f*–15*f*
structure and functions of components in
cytoplasmic organelles, 2, 4*t*
illustration of, 3*f*
nucleus, 2, 3*f*–4*f*
plasma membrane (*See* Plasma membrane)
Cell adhesion molecules (CAMs), 7–8
Cell cortex, 8
Cell cycle
cell division rates in, 26
cytokinesis in, 25–26
description of, 25–27
growth factors and, 26–27, 26*f*, 26*t*
interphase in, 25
meiosis, 25, 42, 44*f*
mitosis in, 25–26, 25*f*, 42, 44*f*
phases of, 25, 25*f*
regulation of, 281*f*
Cell junctions, 12, 13*f*
Cell polarity, 2, 5*f*
Cell surface antigen receptors, 159–160
Cell-mediated hypersensitivity reactions, 202*t*, 205–207, 207*f*
Cell-mediated immunity, 171–173

Cell-to-cell adhesions
- cell junctions and, 12, 13f
- description of, 10–12
- ECM of, 10–12, 11f

Cellular accumulations
- calcium and, 100, 101f–102f
- carbohydrates and, 97–98
- definition of, 96
- glycogen and, 98–99
- hemoproteins and, 99–100, 100f
- lipids and, 97–98, 98f
- mechanisms of, 96, 96f
- melanin and, 99
- pigments and, 99–100
- proteins and, 99
- urate and, 100–101
- water and, 97, 98f

Cellular adaptation
- atrophy and, 75–76, 75f
- definition of, 74
- description of, 75
- dysplasia and, 77, 78f
- hyperplasia and, 77, 78f
- hypertrophy and, 76–77, 76f
- metaplasia and, 78, 79f
- stages of, 79f

Cellular communication, 12–14, 14f

Cellular death. *See also* Apoptosis
- autophagy and, 74, 106–107, 106b, 107f
- classification of, 101
- necrosis (*See* Necrosis)
- pathologic calcification caused by, 74
- programmed, 14, 105
- stages of, 79f

Cellular immunity, 160

Cellular injury, 78–96
- alcohol causing, 90–93
- carbon monoxide as cause of, 90
- causes of, 74
- chemical agents causing, 83–93, 85f
- definition of, 75
- to ECM, 78
- free radicals causing, 82–83
- hypoxia and, 80–82
- irreversible, 78, 78t, 79f
- lead as cause of, 88–90
- mechanisms of, 79, 79t, 97t
- mercury exposure as cause of, 93
- mitochondria in, 83, 84b
- reversible, 78, 78t, 79f
- ROS causing, 82–83, 84f
- stages of, 79f
- systemic manifestations of, 101
- types of, 78t

Cellular metabolism
- ATP in, 16, 16b, 643–647
- carbon dioxide from, 684
- definition of, 14
- food of, 16, 16f
- impairment of, in shock, 643–648, 647f
- oxidative phosphorylation in, 16–17, 17f
- production of, 16, 16f
- thiamine deficiency effects on, 643

Cellular receptors, 10–12, 15t

Cellular swelling, 97

Cellulitis, 1087

Central canal, 320–321

Central chemoreceptors, 685–686

Central diabetes insipidus, 467

Central fever, 347

Central herniation, 379b, 379f

Central line-associated bloodstream infections, 651b

Central nervous system (CNS). *See also* Brain; Spinal cord; Vertebral column
- AIDS involvement of, 198–199
- BBB of, 326, 328f
- blood supply to, 325–327
- components of, 309, 313–327
- cranium of, 323
- CSF and ventricular system in, 323–324
- deafferentation pain and, 344t
- divisions of, 315t
- infections of, 435
- inherited metabolic disorders of, 433–434, 433t, 434f

Central nervous system (CNS) *(Continued)*
- intoxications of, 434–435, 434t
- malformations of, 427–432
  - craniostenosis, 430, 431f
  - neural tube defects and, 427–430, 428f–430f, 430t
- meninges of, 323, 324f
- motor pathways of, 318f, 322
- neoplasms of, HIV and, 415
- protective structures of, 323–325
- sensory pathways of, 322–323
- tumours of, 417–421
  - brain, 417–421, 418f, 419t–420t

Central nervous system disorders, 394–416. *See also* Spinal cord injuries; Stroke; Traumatic brain injury
- AIDS-related neurologic complications, 414–415
- brain abscesses, 413
- cerebrovascular accidents, 406–410
- cerebrovascular disease, 406
- degenerative disorders of spine, 402–406
  - low back pain, 402–403
- degenerative joint disease, 403–405
- encephalitis, 413–414, 413t, 414b, 435
- Guillain-Barré syndrome, 310, 388, 416, 416t
- headaches, 410–411, 410t
- herniated intervertebral disc, 405–406, 405f
- infections and, 411–415, 412f
- inflammation and, 411–415
- intracranial aneurysms, 408–409, 409f
- meningitis, 412–413
- multiple sclerosis, 415–416, 415f
- spinal cord abscesses, 413
- subarachnoid hemorrhage, 408–410, 410t
- vascular malformations, 399–402
- vertebral injuries, 399, 400f, 400t

Central neurogenic hyperventilation, 366t

Central neuropathic pain, 343

Central pontine myelinolysis, 467

Central sensitization, 343, 1041

Central sulcus, 315–316, 316f

Central thyroid disorders, 471

Central tolerance, 167–168

Centromere, 25

Cerebellar astrocytomas, 437–438

Cerebellar gait, 389

Cerebellar motor syndromes, 390

Cerebellar tremor, 383t

Cerebellum, 313–314, 319

Cerebral aneurysms, 611–612

Cerebral aqueduct, 319

Cerebral artery vasospasm, 409

Cerebral blood flow, 377–380, 378b

Cerebral blood oxygenation, 378b

Cerebral blood volume, 378b

Cerebral cortex, 314, 316f

Cerebral death, 368–369

Cerebral edema, 379–380, 379f

Cerebral hemispheres (telencephalon), 314–318, 316f

Cerebral hemodynamics. *See also* Hydrocephalus
- alterations in, 377–380
  - increased intracranial pressure and, 378–379, 378f
- terminology associated with, 378b

Cerebral hypoxia, 93, 704

Cerebral infarction, 407

Cerebral nuclei, 317

Cerebral palsy, 433
- female sexual dysfunction and, 843t

Cerebral peduncles, 319

Cerebral perfusion pressure, 377–378, 378b

Cerebral thromboses, 407

Cerebral vasoconstriction, 131

Cerebrospinal fluid (CSF)
- brain flow of, 324f
- composition of, 323t
- pH of, 685
- ventricular system and, 323–324

Cerebrovascular accidents, 406–410. *See also* Stroke
- female sexual dysfunction and, 843t

Cerebrovascular disease, 406
- in children, 435–436

Cerebrum, 317

Ceruloplasmin, 497

Cervical cancer, 252
- classification for precursor lesions to, 836t
- clinical manifestations of, 834
- description of, 270t–273t
- evaluation of, 835
- HPV and development of, 833–834, 836b, 892t–894t
- incidence of, 833
- pathogenesis of, 833–834, 834f–835f
- precursor lesions for, 892t–894t
- prevention of, 836b
- screening for, 834b
- staging of, 836t
- treatment of, 835

Cervical carcinoma in situ, 833, 836t

Cervical intraepithelial neoplasia, 833, 835f, 836t

Cervicitis, 826–827

Cervix
- anatomy of, 799–800, 800f
- dysplasia of, 78f
- inflammation of, 826–827
- neoplasm progression in, 238f

CFTR proteins. *See* Cystic fibrosis transmembrane conductance regulator proteins

CG (cytosine-guanine) dinucleotide repeats, 67–68

cGMP. *See* Cyclic guanosine monophosphate

Chalazion, 353

Channels, 17, 18f

Chemical asphyxiants, 95

Chemical carcinogenesis, 294–295

Chemical epididymitis, 876

Chemical synapses, 12–13

Chemical-induced cellular injury, 83–93, 85f

Chemicals Management Plan, 854

Chemokines, 143, 251

Chemoreceptor trigger zone, 921

Chemoreceptors
- central, 685–686
- peripheral, 684, 686

Chemotactic factors, 141

Chemotaxis, 145

Chemotherapy
- adjuvant, 263
- alopecia caused by, 260
- cancer treatment with, 262–263
- induction, 263
- for leukemia, 536
- multiple myeloma treated with, 545
- neoadjuvant, 263

Chest muscle retraction, 725, 727f

Chest physiotherapy, 710

Chest radiography, 714

Chest wall
- aging and, 692
- anatomy of, 683, 684f
- disorders of, 699–700
- elastic properties of, 687–688, 687f
- restriction, 699, 699f

Cheyne-Stokes respiration, 364, 366t, 696

Chiari II malformation, 429–430

Chickenpox, 1088, 1112t, 1113, 1113f

Chief cells, 905

Childhood cancers
- bone marrow transplants and, 307b
- brain tumours and, 304
- chromosomal abnormalities with, 305
- congenital factors associated with, 304t
- death rates for, 303
- embryonic tumours and, 303
- environmental factors with, 305–307, 306b
- Epstein-Barr virus and, 307
- etiology of, 303–307, 304t
- genetic and genomic factors in, 305, 305t

Childhood cancers *(Continued)*
- incidence of, 303–307
- magnetic fields and, 306b
- mesodermal germ layer as source of, 303, 304f
- multiple causation theory of, 305
- oncogenes associated with, 305, 305t
- prenatal drug exposures as cause of, 305–306, 306t
- prognosis for, 307
- survival rates for, 307
- **tumor-suppressor genes associated with**, 305, 305t
- types of, 303–307

Children
- AIDS in, 198–199, 307
- blood pressure in, 674t
- bone tumours in, 1069–1071, 1070f–1071f
- brain growth and development in, 426
- cardiovascular disorders in
  - acquired heart disease, 673–677
  - congenital heart disease (*See* Congenital heart disease)
  - hypertension, 674–677, 674t, 675b, 676t
  - Kawasaki disease, 673–674, 674b
  - obesity and, 676b
- coagulation disorders in, 569–570
  - hemophilias, 569, 569t
  - ITP, 569–570
- congenital heart disease (*See* Congenital heart disease)
- CT scans risks for, 306b
- diarrhea in, 979
- erythrocyte disorders in, 560–568
  - anemia, 560–563, 561b, 561t
  - hemolytic anemia, 560, 562–563
  - iron deficiency anemia, 560–562, 561b
  - sickle cell disease, 564–567, 564f–567f, 565t
  - thalassemias, 567–568
- fever in, 346b
- G6PD deficiency in, 560
- gastro-intestinal tract disorders in
  - anorectal malformations, 972, 973f
  - appendicitis, 974
  - celiac disease, 975–977, 976b, 976f
  - cleft lip, 968–969
  - cleft palate, 968–969
  - cystic fibrosis, 974–975, 975t
  - diarrhea, 979
  - duodenum obstruction, 970
  - esophageal atresia, 969, 970f
  - failure to thrive, 977–978, 978b
  - GER, 972–973
  - growth faltering, 977–978, 978b
  - hepatoblastoma, 982
  - Hirschsprung's disease, 972, 972f
  - idiopathic intestinal pseudo-obstruction, 971–972
  - ileum obstruction, 970
  - infantile hypertrophic pyloric stenosis, 969–970
  - intussusception, 973–974, 974f
  - jejunum obstruction, 970
  - lactose intolerance, 979
  - malignancies, 982–983
  - malnutrition, 977
  - malrotation, 970–971
  - Meckel diverticulum, 971
  - meconium syndromes, 971
  - necrotizing enterocolitis, 978–979
  - pancreatic tumours, 982–983
  - tracheoesophageal fistula, 969, 970f
- GH deficiency in, 468, 469f
- hydrocephalus in, 426
- lead exposure and, 88b, 89, 90f
- leukemia in, 303, 570–571, 571f
  - clinical manifestations of, 570–571
  - evaluation and treatment of, 571
  - pathophysiology of, 570
- liver disorders in
  - biliary atresia, 980
  - cirrhosis, 981
  - hepatitis, 980–981
  - metabolic disorders, 982, 983t
  - neonatal jaundice, 563, 979–980
  - portal hypertension, 981–982

Children *(Continued)*
lymphomas in, 303, 571–572
Burkitt, 571–572
Hodgkin's, 572, 572*f*
non-Hodgkin's, 571–572
medication-related poisoning of, 85*b*
metabolic syndrome in, 479, 480*b*
musculo-skeletal disorders in
bone tumours, 1069–1071, 1070*f*–1071*f*
clubfoot, 1059, 1060*f*–1061*f*, 1060*t*
developmental dysplasia of hip, 1059–1060, 1061*f*
Ewing sarcomas, 1070–1071, 1070*f*–1071*f*
juvenile idiopathic arthritis, 1064, 1064*t*
Legg-Calvé-Perthes disease, 1065, 1065*f*–1066*f*
malignant bone tumours, 1069–1071
muscular dystrophies, 1067–1069, 1067*t*, 1068*f*–1069*f*
nonaccidental trauma, 1071, 1071*f*
nonossifying fibromas, 1069
Osgood-Schlatter disease, 1065
osteochondromas, 1069
osteochondroses, 1065–1066, 1065*f*–1066*f*
osteogenesis imperfecta, 1060–1062, 1062*f*
osteomyelitis, 1062–1063, 1063*b*, 1063*f*
osteosarcomas, 1070
scoliosis, 1066–1067, 1066*f*
septic arthritis, 1063–1064
Sever disease, 1066
nervous system development in, 426–427
neurologic disorders in
amino acid metabolism defects, 433–434
anencephaly, 429
brain malformations, 431–432, 431*f*–432*f*, 434*t*
brain tumours, 436–438, 437*f*, 437*t*, 438*b*
cerebral palsy, 433
cerebrovascular disease, 435–436
Chiari II malformation, 429–430
CNS malformations, 427–432
congenital hydrocephalus, 432, 432*f*
cortical dysplasias, 431–432
craniostenosis, 430, 431*f*
cyclopia, 427
Dandy-Walker malformation, 432
encephalocele, 429
encephalopathies, 433–435
epilepsy, 436, 436*t*
inherited metabolic disorders of CNS, 433–434, 433*t*, 434*f*
meningitis, 435
meningocele, 429, 429*f*
microcephaly, 431, 431*f*, 434*t*
myelomeningocele, 429–430, 429*f*
neural tube defects, 427–430, 428*f*–430*f*, 430*t*
neuroblastomas, 438–439
perinatal stroke, 435
phenylketonuria, 433–434, 434*f*
retinoblastoma, 439–440, 439*f*
seizure disorders, 436, 436*t*
spina bifida, 427, 429*f*
spina bifida occulta, 430
storage diseases, 434
stroke, 435–436
pain perception in, 341*t*
poisoning of, 85*b*, 434, 434*t*
pulmonary diseases and disorders in
acute epiglottitis, 727, 730*t*
ALI, 735
ARDS, 735
aspiration pneumonitis, 733
asthma, 733–735, 734*b*
bacterial tracheitis, 727, 730*t*
BPD, 730, 730*b*, 730*t*, 731*f*
bronchiolitis, 730–732
bronchiolitis obliterans, 733
croup, 725–727, 726*f*–727*f*
cystic fibrosis, 735, 736*b*, 736*f*
foreign body aspiration, 727

Children *(Continued)*
OSAS, 727–728
pneumonia, 732–733, 732*t*
RDS, 728–730, 728*b*, 729*f*
respiratory tract infections, 730–733
SUID, 737, 737*b*
tonsillar infections, 727
upper airways infections, 725–727, 726*t*
renal disorders in
acute poststreptococcal glomerulonephritis, 786–787
glomerular disorders, 786–788
hemolytic uremic syndrome, 787–788
hypoplastic kidneys, 786
immunoglobulin A nephropathy, 787
incidence of, 784
nephroblastoma, 788, 788*t*
nephrotic syndrome, 787
polycystic kidney disease, 786
renal agenesis, 786
skin disorders in
acne vulgaris, 1107–1108, 1108*f*
atopic dermatitis, 1108, 1108*f*
bacterial infections, 1109–1110, 1109*b*, 1110*f*
bedbugs, 1114–1115
chickenpox, 1088, 1112*t*, 1113, 1113*f*
cutaneous hemangiomas, 1115–1116, 1115*f*
cutaneous vascular malformations, 1116, 1116*f*
dermatitis, 1108–1109
diaper dermatitis, 1109, 1109*f*
erythema toxicum neonatorum, 1116
fleabites, 1114, 1115*f*
fungal infections, 1110–1111, 1110*f*
herpes zoster, 1112*t*, 1113
impetigo, 1109–1110, 1109*b*, 1110*f*
infections, 1109–1113
insect bites, 1113–1115, 1114*f*–1115*f*
lice infections, 1114
miliaria, 1116, 1116*f*
molluscum contagiosum, 1111, 1111*f*
parasites, 1113–1115, 1114*f*–1115*f*
roseola, 1112–1113, 1112*t*
rubella, 1111–1112, 1112*f*, 1112*t*
rubeola, 1112, 1112*t*
scabies, 1114, 1114*f*
smallpox, 1113
staphylococcal scalded-skin syndrome, 1110, 1110*f*
thrush, 1111
tinea capitis, 1110–1111, 1110*f*
tinea corporis, 1111
viral infections, 1111–1113, 1111*f*–1113*f*, 1112*t*
strabismus in, 350
TBW in, 132*b*
urinary system disorders in
bladder exstrophy, 785, 785*f*
bladder outlet obstruction, 785
epispadias, 785
hypospadias, 784–785, 785*f*
incidence of, 784
ureteropelvic junction obstruction, 785–786
urinary incontinence, 790, 790*t*
UTI, 788–789, 789*b*
vesicoureteral reflux, 789–790, 789*f*–790*f*
Chimeric, 536–537
Chlamydia, 891–894
Chlamydia trachomatis, 892*t*
Chlamydial conjunctivitis, 353–354
Chlamydial ophthalmia, 892*t*–894*t*
Chlamydophila pneumonia, 732*t*, 733
Chloride
balance, 117–120
alterations in, 120–122, 120*f*, 120*t*
hypertonic alterations to, 120*f*, 121
hypotonic alterations to, 120*f*, 121–122
isotonic alterations to, 120*f*, 121

Chloride *(Continued)*
bicarbonate and, 118
transport of, 118
Chloride reabsorption inhibitors, 753*t*
Choking asphyxiation, 93
Cholangiocellular carcinoma, 958
Cholecystitis, 952
Cholecystokinin, 903, 903*t*
Cholelithiasis, 951–952, 952*f*
Choleresis, 912–913
Choleretic agent, 912–913
Cholesterol, 618, 619*b*
Choline deficiency, in pregnancy, 280
Cholinergic crisis, 417
Cholinergic transmission, 331
Chondrocytes, 997
Chondrogenic tumours, 1050
Chondrosarcoma, 1050
Chopping wound, 94*t*–95*t*
Chordae tendineae, 577, 577*f*
Chordee, 784
Chorea, 383*t*
Choroid plexuses, 323, 324*f*
Chromaffin cell tumours, 490–491
Chromatids, 25
Chromatin, 25, 63
Chromophils, 448
Chromophobes, 448
Chromosomes, 38
childhood cancers and abnormalities of, 305
fragile sites on, 49
homologous, 42, 44*f*
instability of, 247
karyotype of, 42, 44*f*
sex
aneuploidy of, 46
description of, 42
structure of
abnormalities of, 46–49, 48*f*–49*f*
description of, 42–49, 45*f*
translocations
description of, 47–49, 49*f*
oncogene activation by, 242, 243*f*
Chromosomal mosaics, 46
Chromosome 5p deletion syndrome, 663*t*
Chromosome aberrations
aneuploidy, 43–46, 45*f*–46*f*, 48*f*
deletions, 46–47, 48*f*
Down syndrome (*See* Down syndrome)
duplications, 47
Fragile X syndrome, 49
incidence of, 42
inversions, 47
Klinefelter's syndrome, 46, 47*t*, 48*f*, 54
polyploidy, 42–43
tetraploidy, 42–43
translocations, 47–49, 49*f*
triploidy, 42–43
Turner's syndrome, 46, 47*t*, 48*f*, 54
Chromosome bands, 42, 44*f*
Chromosome breakage, 46
Chromosome theory of inheritance, 50
Chromosome translocations, 238–240
Chronic alcoholism, 92, 92*f*
Chronic alveolar hypoxia, 683
Chronic bacterial prostatitis, 878*b*, 879
Chronic bronchitis, 709–710, 709*f*–710*f*, 709*t*
Chronic cluster headaches, 411
Chronic conjunctivitis, 353–354
Chronic cough, 696
Chronic cyanosis, 669
Chronic fatigue syndrome, 1041–1043
Chronic gastritis, 931
Chronic granulomatous disease, 192*t*, 193
Chronic hepatitis, in children, 981
Chronic immune gastritis, 931
Chronic inflammation, 150–152, 151*f*, 251, 251*t*
Chronic kidney disease (CKD)
acid-base balance and, 777–778, 777*t*
carbohydrate metabolism in, 778
cardiovascular system and, 776*t*, 778–779
clinical manifestations of, 777
creatinine and urea clearance in, 777, 777*t*

Chronic kidney disease (CKD) *(Continued)*
definition of, 775
dyslipidemia and, 777*t*, 778
endocrine system and, 776*t*, 779
evaluation of, 779
female sexual dysfunction and, 843*t*
gastro-intestinal system and, 776*t*, 779
hematological system and, 776*t*, 779
immune system and, 776*t*, 779
neurological system and, 776*t*, 779
pathophysiology of, 775–777, 777*f*, 777*t*
phosphate and calcium balance and, 777*t*, 778
progression of, 777, 777*t*
protein metabolism in, 778
pulmonary system and, 776*t*, 779
reproductive system and, 776*t*, 779
skin and, 776*t*, 779
stages of, 775*t*
systemic effects of, 776*t*
treatment of, 779
Chronic Kidney Disease Epidemiology Collaboration, 754
Chronic lymphocytic leukemia, 533, 534*t*, 536–538
Chronic lymphocytic thyroiditis, 473
Chronic migraines, 411
Chronic mucocutaneous candidiasis, 192*t*, 193
Chronic myeloid leukemia, 242–243, 533, 534*t*, 536–538, 537*f*
in children, 571
Chronic nonbacterial osteomyelitis, 1028
Chronic nonimmune gastritis, 931
Chronic obstructive pulmonary disease (COPD), 708–709, 711*f*
Chronic orthostatic hypotension, 611
Chronic pancreatitis, 953
Chronic pelvic pain syndrome, 878*b*, 879
Chronic postoperative pain, 344*t*
Chronic prostatitis, 878*b*, 879
Chronic pyelonephritis, 767, 767*t*, 788
Chronic rejection, 211
Chronic relapsing TTP, 548
Chronic tension-type headache, 411
Chronic traumatic encephalopathy, 399
Chronic urticaria, 1090
Chronic venous insufficiency, 604–605
Chronological aging, 107–108
Chronotropic effect, 224
Chylomicrons, 617–618
Chylothorax, 700, 700*t*
Chyme, 902, 910–911
Cialis, 888
Cigar smoking. *See* Smoking, tobacco
Cigarette smoking. *See* Smoking, tobacco
Ciliated simple columnar epithelium, 29*t*–30*t*, 30*f*
Cingulate gyrus herniation, 379*b*, 379*f*
Circadian rhythm sleep disorders, 349
Circle of Willis, 325–326, 326*f*
Circulating anticoagulants, 514*t*–516*t*
Circulation
bronchial, 681–683
collateral, 578–580
coronary, 578–580, 579*b*, 581*f*
autonomic regulation and, 599
autoregulation and, 598–599
regulation of, 598–599
pulmonary
anatomy of, 681–683, 683*f*
control of, 683
perfusion distribution in, 689–690
systemic (*See* Systemic circulation)
Circulatory system. *See also* Blood; Heart
anatomy of, 576*f*
functions of, 575
Cirrhosis
alcoholic, 948
alcoholic liver disease and, 948
ascites caused by, 944, 944*f*
biliary, 949
causes of, 948*b*
in children, 981
clinical manifestations of, 944*f*
definition of, 947–948

Cirrhosis *(Continued)*
 nonalcoholic fatty liver disease and, 948–949
 nonalcoholic steatohepatitis and, 948–949
Citrate (Clomid), 822
Citric acid cycle, 16
CKD. *See* Chronic kidney disease
Clara cell, 682*f*
Class switch, 170–171
Classic cerebral concussions, 398
Classical pathway, of complement system, 141
Clastogens, 46
Clathrin, 21–23, 23*f*
Clawlike prolongations, 1081, 1081*f*
Clear cell tumours, 764
Cleft lip, 968–969
Cleft palate, 968–969
Clinical breast examination, 857–858
Clitoris, 797, 797*f*
Cloacal exstrophy, 785
Clomid (citrate), 822
Clonal diversity
 definition of, 165–167
 description of, 159–160
 generation of, 165–168, 167*t*
 illustration of, 161*f*
Clonal expansion, 238–240, 240*f*
Clonal selection
 B cell, 170–171, 172*f*
 description of, 160, 168–171
 generation of, 165–168, 167*t*
 illustration of, 161*f*
Clonic phase, 376–377
Closed brain injuries, 394–395, 395*t*
Closed fractures, 1011–1012, 1012*f*, 1012*t*
Clostridium botulinum, 182–183
Clostridium difficile, 138
 diarrhea and, 923*b*
Clot retraction test, 514*t*–516*t*
Clotting cascade, 140
Clotting factors
 function of, 497, 512–513, 513*f*
 laboratory tests for, 514*t*–516*t*
Clotting system, 140*f*, 141, 512
Clubbing, 697, 697*f*
Clubfoot, 1059, 1060*f*–1061*f*, 1060*t*
Cluster breathing, 366*t*
Cluster headache, 410*t*, 411
Clustered regularly interspaced short palindromic repeats (CRISPR), 52
CNS. *See* Central nervous system
COA. *See* Coarctation of the aorta
Coagulation disorders. *See also* Disseminated intravascular coagulation
 in children, 569–570
  hemophilias, 569, 569*t*
  ITP, 569–570
 consumptive thrombohemorrhagic disorders, 550–553
 impaired hemostasis, 550
 liver disease, 550
 pathologic conditions that cause, 550
 thromboembolic disorders, 553–554, 553*f*
 vitamin K deficiency, 550
Coagulation system. *See* Clotting system
Coagulative necrosis, 103, 104*f*
Coal, 703
Coarctation of the aorta (COA), 664, 665*f*
Coated vesicles, 21–23, 23*f*
Cocaine, 89*t*
Cocci, 178
Cochlea, 354, 354*f*–355*f*
Cockcroft–Gault formula, 754
Codominance, 49
Codons, 39
Cognitive function. *See also* Arousal; Awareness; Data-processing deficits; Seizure/seizure disorders
 alterations in, 363–377
 neural systems in, 363
Cognitive-evaluative system, 340
Cogwheel rigidity, 381, 381*t*
Cold injury, 1099–1101
Collagen, 10, 153–154, 510–511
 dysfunctional synthesis of, 154
Collagen fibres, 992
Collagen zones, 997, 998*f*
Collagenic tumours, 1050
Collateral arteries, 578–579
Collateral circulation, 578–580
Collateral ganglia, 328–331
Collecting duct, 744, 744*f*
Collectins, 137, 686
Colloid osmotic pressure, 20
Colon, 909, 909*f*
 cancer of, 270*t*–273*t*, 837, 954*t*, 955–957, 956*b*–957*b*, 956*f*–957*f*
 diverticular disease of, 938–939, 939*f*
Colony-stimulating factor-1, 251
Colony-stimulating factors, 505
Colorado tick fever, 413*t*
Colorectal cancer, 270*t*–273*t*, 837, 954*t*, 955–957, 956*b*–957*b*, 956*f*–957*f*
Colorectal polyps, 956
Colostral antibodies, 165
Colour blindness, 352
Colour vision alterations, 352
Coma
 irreversible, 368–369
 myxedema, 474
Combined immune deficiency, 191–192, 192*t*, 193*f*
Combined oral contraceptive pills, 833
Commensal relationship, 137
Comminuted fractures, 1011–1012, 1012*t*
Commissural fibres, 317
Common bile duct, 911, 912*f*
Communicating hydrocephalus, 380, 380*t*
Communicating pneumothorax, 700
Community-acquired pneumonia, 712, 712*b*
Compact bone, 992–993, 992*f*–993*f*
Compartment I disorders, 819–820
Compartment II disorders, 819–820
Compartment III disorders, 819–820
Compartment syndrome, 1019, 1019*b*, 1020*f*
Compensatory hyperplasia, 77, 152–153
Compensatory hypertrophy, 760
Complement
 activation of, 82
 deficiencies of, 192*t*, 193
 functions of, 96
 in septic shock, 652*b*
Complement cascade, 140
Complement receptors, 143
Complement system, 140–141, 140*f*
Complementarity determining regions, 162–163
Complementary base pairing, 39
Complete fractures, 1011–1012, 1012*t*
Complete precocious puberty, 818, 819*b*, 868–869, 869*b*
Complex motor performance alterations, 389–390
Compliance
 lung, 687
 vascular, 595
Complicated hypertension, 609–611, 609*t*
Complicated plaque, 614
Compound fractures, 1011–1012, 1012*f*, 1012*t*
Compound skull fractures, 397
Compression atelectasis, 701
Compressive syndrome, 421
Computed tomography (CT) scans
 children risks with, 306*b*
 high-resolution peripheral quantitative, 1025
 ionizing radiation risks with, 287*b*
Concentration gradient, 19, 19*f*
Concentric muscle contraction, 1006
Concussions, 398
Conducting airways, 679–680, 681*f*–682*f*
Conduction system, of heart, 580–583, 582*f*
Conductive dysphasia, 371, 372*t*–373*t*
Conductive hearing loss, 355
Condylomata acuminata, 892*t*–894*t*, 1089
Cones, 349
Congenital adrenal hyperplasia, 489
 maternal conditions associated with, 663*t*
Congenital equinovarus, 1059, 1060*f*, 1060*t*
Congenital heart disease
 acyanotic heart defects, 662–663
 aortic stenosis, 664–666, 665*f*
 atrial septal defect, 667–668
 atrioventricular canal defect, 668, 668*f*
 categorization of, 662–663, 663*f*
 COA, 664, 665*f*
 cyanotic heart defects, 662–663
 endocarditis risks and, 666*b*
 environmental factors associated with, 662, 663*t*
 genetic factors associated with, 662, 663*t*
 heart failure caused by, 672–673, 673*b*, 673*t*
 hypoplastic left heart syndrome, 672, 672*f*
 incidence of, 662
 naming of, 663
 patent ductus arteriosus, 667, 667*f*
 pulmonary blood flow and, 667–670
 pulmonary stenosis, 666–667, 666*f*
 shunt, 662–663, 664*f*
 TAPVC, 670–671, 671*f*
 tetralogy of Fallot, 662–663, 664*f*, 668–669, 669*f*
 TGA, 670
 TGV, 670, 671*f*
 tricuspid atresia, 669–670, 670*f*
 truncus arteriosus, 671–672, 672*f*
 ventricular septal defect, 668
Congenital hydrocephalus, 432, 432*f*
Congenital hypothyroidism, 473–474
Congenital immune deficiency. *See* Primary immune deficiency
Congenital nephrotic syndrome, 787
Congenital sideroblastic anemia, 525
Congestive splenomegaly, 545–546
Conivaptan, 753*t*
Conjugated bilirubin, 913, 946
Conjugated vaccine, 190
Conjunctivitis, 353
Connective tissue
 fibroblasts in, 11–12, 11*f*
 types of, 31*t*–33*t*
Connexons, 12, 13*f*
Conn's syndrome, 489
Consanguinity, 54
Consciousness
 definition of, 363 (*See also* Arousal; Awareness)
 level of, 364, 365*t*
Constipation, 922
Constrictive pericarditis, 630, 630*f*
Consumptive thrombohemorrhagic disorders, 550–553
Contact activation pathway, of clotting system, 141
Contact dermatitis, 207, 208*f*
Contact range entrance wound, 94*t*–95*t*
Contact-dependent signalling, 12–13, 14*f*
Contaminated food, 855
Contiguous osteomyelitis, 1028
Contractile proteins, of skeletal muscles, 1003, 1003*t*
Contraction alkalosis, 129
Contractures, 1041
Contralateral control, 316, 318*f*, 320
Contrecoup injury, 394–395, 395*t*, 396*f*
Contusions, 94*t*–95*t*
 description of, 394–395, 395*t*
Conus medullaris, 320
Convergence, 310, 313
Convulsion, 376
Cooley's anemia, 567
Cooper ligaments, 805
COPD. *See* Chronic obstructive pulmonary disease
Coping, with stress, 228–229, 230*f*
Cor pulmonale, 698, 717
Cornea, 349, 349*f*
Cornification, 805
Coronary arteries
 anatomy of, 578, 579*b*, 581*f*
 calcification of, 100
 obstruction of, 80–81
 oxygen delivery by, 586, 588
Coronary artery disease (CAD), 609
 adipokines and, 620
 air pollution and, 620
 atherogenic diet and, 619
 atherosclerosis as cause of, 616*f*, 617
 development of, 617–620
 diabetes mellitus, 618
 dyslipidemia and, 617–618, 618*t*
 HDL and, 618
 hypertension and, 618
 infections and, 620
 inflammation markers and, 619
 insulin resistance and, 618
 LDL and, 618
 MI caused by, 617
 nontraditional risk factors in, 619–620
 obesity and, 618–619
 sedentary lifestyle and, 618–619
 tobacco smoking and, 618
 troponin I and, 619–620
Coronary capillaries, 579
Coronary circulation, 578–580, 579*b*, 581*f*
 autonomic regulation and, 599
 autoregulation and, 598–599
 regulation of, 598–599
Coronary heart disease, 223*b*
Coronary ligament, 911
Coronary ostia, 578, 581*f*
Coronary perfusion pressure, 598
Coronary sinus, 578, 581*f*
Coronary veins, 578, 580, 581*f*
Coronary vessels, 578–580
Corpora cavernosa, 808–809, 809*f*
Corpora quadrigemina, 319
Corpora spongiosum, 808–809, 809*f*
Corpus callosum, 316*f*, 317
Corpus luteum, 800–801, 801*f*
 cysts, 830
Cortex, of kidney, 741, 742*f*
Cortical bone, 992–993, 992*f*–993*f*
Cortical dysplasias, 431–432
Cortical nephrons, 743
Corticobulbar tract, 316
 axons of, 322
Corticospinal tracts, 316, 318*f*
Corticotropin-releasing hormone (CRH), 220, 224, 449*t*, 458, 459*f*
Cortisol, 220–221, 221*t*
 hypercortisolism and, 487–489
 secretion of, 458–459, 459*f*
Cough, 695–696
Cough reflex, 684
Coup injury, 394–395, 395*t*, 396*f*
Cowper glands, 809, 809*f*
Cow's milk allergy, 561
COX. *See* Cyclo-oxygenase
COX-1, 146
CpG dinucleotides, 62
CpG islands, 52
CPK-MB. *See* Creatine phosphokinase-myocardial bound
CPR. *See* Cardiopulmonary resuscitation
Crack, 89*t*
"Cracked pot" sign, 432
Cranial nerve palsy, 388
Cranial nerves, 309
 list of, 330*t*
 structure of, 328, 329*f*
Craniopharyngioma, 437*t*, 438
Craniosacral division, 331
Craniostenosis, 430, 431*f*
Cranium, 323
C-reactive protein, 1029
Creatine kinase, 1017–1018, 1067
Creatine phosphokinase-myocardial bound (CPK-MB), 625
Creatinine, CKD progression and clearance of, 777, 777*t*
Creutzfeldt-Jakob disease, 373–374, 375*t*
CRH. *See* Corticotropin-releasing hormone
Cri du chat syndrome, 46–47, 663*t*
CRISPR. *See* Clustered regularly interspaced short palindromic repeats

Crista ampullaris, 354
Critical micelle concentration, 935
Critical region, 65
Crohn's disease (CD), 936–938, 936*t*
Cross-bridge theory of muscle contraction, 586, 1005
Cross-bridges, 585
Crossover, 56–57, 56*f*
Croup, 725–727, 726*f*–727*f*
Crush injury, 1017
Crush syndrome, 1017, 1020*f*
Crying, pathological, 389–390
Cryoglobulins, 205
Cryptorchidism, 873–874
Crypts of Lieberkühn, 905*f*, 906
Crystallizable fragment, 162
CSF. *See* Cerebrospinal fluid
CT scans. *See* Computed tomography scans
Cul-de-sac, 798, 798*f*
Curcumin, 280, 880*b*–881*b*
Curling ulcers, 933
Cushing ulcer, 933
Cushing's disease, 487–489, 488*f*
Cushing's syndrome, 222*b*, 257*t*, 487–489, 488*f*
Cushing's-like syndrome, 487
Cutaneous hemangiomas, 1115–1116, 1115*f*
Cutaneous lupus erythematosus, 1085, 1086*f*
Cutaneous melanoma, 1093–1094, 1094*b*, 1094*f*
Cutaneous vascular malformations, 1116, 1116*f*
Cutaneous vasculitis, 1090
CXCL12-abundant reticular (CAR) cells, 504–505
Cyanide, 95
Cyanosis, 662–663, 669, 696–697
Cyanotic heart defects, 662–663
Cyclic adenosine monophosphate (cAMP), 446–447, 447*f*, 447*t*
Cyclic guanosine monophosphate (cGMP), 446–447, 447*t*
Cyclin-dependent kinase inhibitor 2A, 291
Cyclomen (danazol), 833
Cyclo-oxygenase (COX), 146
Cyclopia, 427
Cystatin C, 753–754, 775
Cystic duct, 914
Cystic fibrosis, 52, 53*f*
  in children, 735, 736*b*, 736*f*, 974–975, 975*t*
Cystic fibrosis transmembrane conductance regulator (CFTR) proteins, 735
Cystinuric stones, 761
Cystitis, 765–767, 788
Cystocele, 828, 829*f*
Cystometric test, 763
Cystometrogram, 755*t*
Cystometry, 755*t*
Cystosarcoma phyllodes, 856*t*
Cysts, 150
  breast, 844
  corpus luteum, 830
  dermoid, 830
  epididymal, 873
  follicular, 829–830
  functional, 829
  ovarian, benign, 829–830, 829*f*
  skin, 1077*t*–1078*t*
Cytochrome P-450, 91
Cytochromes, 16–17, 99
Cytokines, 26, 143, 222, 224. *See also* Growth factors
  adipocytokines and, 940–941, 941*b*
  inflammatory, 481
  proinflammatory, 941*b*
Cytokinesis, 25–26, 42
Cytoplasm, 2, 4*t*
Cytoplasmic matrix, 2
Cytosine-guanine (CG) dinucleotide repeats, 67–68
Cytosines, 38
  methylated, 62
Cytoskeleton, 4*t*
Cytosol, 2
Cytotoxic edema, 380
Cytotoxic T cells, 160, 170, 172*f*–173*f*, 173, 221–222

D

D vitamins, 454, 454*b*, 989*t*
  bone and, 1025*b*
  deficiency, 771
  kidneys and, 752
  supplementation of, 752*b*, 778
DAF. *See* Decay accelerating factor
Damage-associated molecular patterns (DAMPs), 142, 608
Danazol (Cyclomen), 833
Dandy-Walker malformation, 432
Dark adaptation, 351*t*
Data-processing deficits
  acute confusional states, 369*b*, 371–374, 374*t*
  agnosia, 371
  Alzheimer's disease, 374–376, 375*f*, 375*t*–376*t*, 376*b*
  delirium, 369*b*, 371–374, 374*t*
  dementia, 373–374, 374*t*–375*t*
  dysphasia, 371, 371*f*, 372*t*–373*t*
  frontotemporal dementia, 375*t*, 376
Daughter cells, 25–26
Dawn phenomenon, 482
Daytime incontinence, 790
D-dimer, 514
D-dimer test, 553
de Quervain's thyroiditis, 473
Deafferentation pain, 344*t*
Deamination, 914
Death, somatic, 109–110
Decay accelerating factor (DAF), 142
Decerebrate posture/response, 368*f*
Decerebrate posture/response, 389
Decornification, 805
Decorticate posture/response, 368*f*
Decorticate posture/response, 389
Decubitus ulcer, 152
Deep partial-thickness burns, 1095, 1097*t*
Deep venous thrombosis, 605
  in thrombocythemia, 549
Defecation reflex, 910
Defence mechanisms, 135–149, 136*t*. *See also* Immunity
Defensins, 137
Deflazacort, 1067–1068
Degenerative disc disease, 403–404
Degenerative joint disease, 403–405
Degranulation, 145, 145*f*–146*f*
Dehiscence, wound, 154
Dehydration
  definition of, 119–121
  isotonic fluid loss as cause of, 121
  signs and symptoms of, 121*b*
Dehydroepiandrosterone, 794*t*
Delayed age of onset, 51
Delayed hypersensitivity reactions, 202
Delayed hypersensitivity skin test, 207
Delayed puberty, 818, 818*b*, 818*t*, 868, 869*b*
Delayed repolarization, 124
Deletions, 46–47, 48*f*
Delipidation, 284*f*
Delirium, 369*b*, 371–374, 374*t*
Delta cells, 455
Demadex, 753*t*
Demeclocycline, 467
Dementia, 373–374, 374*t*–375*t*
Dementia of Alzheimer's type, 374
Dementia with Lewy body, 375*t*, 384
Dendrites, 310, 310*f*
Dendritic cells, 147
Dengue, 413*t*
Denosumab, 1026*b*
Dense irregular connective tissue, 31*f*, 31*t*–33*t*
Dense regular (white fibrous) connective tissue, 31*f*, 31*t*–33*t*
Dental amalgams, 93
Deoxyhemoglobin, 507
Deoxyribonucleic acid (DNA), 1, 38
  composition of, 38–39
  demethylating agents, 70, 70*f*
  double-helix model of, 38–39, 40*f*
  as genetic code, 39
  mitochondrial, 108
Deoxyribonucleic acid (DNA) *(Continued)*
  mutations, 39, 41*f*
  replication of, 39, 40*f*
  structure of, 38–39
Depolarization, 24, 582, 644*t*–645*t*
Depot medroxyprogesterone acetate, 833
Dermal appendages, 1074–1076, 1076*f*
Dermatitis, 1081–1082
  allergic contact, 208*f*, 1082, 1082*f*
  atopic, 892*t*–894*t*, 1082, 1108, 1108*f*
  in children, 1108–1109
  diaper, 1109, 1109*f*
  irritant contact, 1082
  seborrheic, 1083, 1083*f*
  stasis, 1082, 1082*f*
Dermatomes, 328, 329*f*
Dermatomyositis, 257*t*, 1045, 1045*f*
Dermatophytes, 186
Dermis, 1074, 1075*f*, 1075*t*
Dermoid cysts, 830
Descending colon, 909, 909*f*
Descending facilitatory pathways, 342
Descending inhibitory pathways, 342
Descending pathways, 309
Desensitization, to allergens, 209
Desire disorders, 842
Desmosomes, 12, 13*f*
Detrusor areflexia, 762, 762*t*
Detrusor hyper-reflexia, 762, 762*t*
Detrusor muscle, 746
Developmental basis of health and disease, 274–275
Developmental dysplasia of hip, 1059–1060, 1061*f*
Developmental plasticity, 274–275
Diabetes insipidus, 467–468, 467*t*
Diabetes mellitus
  CAD and, 618
  categories of, 476
  complications of
    acute, 482–483, 482*f*, 483*t*
    atherosclerosis, 485, 487*f*
    cardiovascular disease, 484*t*, 485
    chronic, 483–487, 484*t*
    diabetic nephropathy, 484*t*, 485
    diabetic neuropathies, 484*t*, 485, 486*f*
    diabetic retinopathy, 484–485, 484*t*, 485*f*
    DKA, 246*f*, 482–483, 483*t*
    HHS, 482–483, 482*f*, 483*t*
    hypoglycemia, 257*t*, 482, 483*t*
    infection, 484*t*, 486
    macrovascular disease, 484*t*, 485–486
    microvascular disease, 484–485, 484*t*, 485*f*
    PVD, 484*t*, 486
    stroke, 484*t*, 486
  diagnostic criteria for, 476, 476*b*
  epidemiology of, 477*t*
  etiology of, 477*t*
  female sexual dysfunction and, 843*t*
  gestational, 482
  insulin resistance and, 852
  maturity-onset diabetes of youth, 482
  type 1, 476–479, 478*f*, 478*t*, 479*b*
  type 2, 222*b*, 479–482, 479*f*–480*f*, 481*b*, 837
  wound healing and, 154
Diabetic glomerulopathy, 771*f*
Diabetic ketoacidosis (DKA), 246*f*, 478, 482–483, 483*t*
Diabetic nephropathies, 484*t*, 485, 770
Diabetic neuropathies, 484*t*, 485, 486*f*
Diabetic retinopathy, 484–485, 484*t*, 485*f*
Diamox, 753*t*
Diapedesis, 147
Diaper dermatitis, 1109, 1109*f*
Diaphragm, 686, 686*f*
Diaphysis, 994
Diarrhea
  acute infectious, 979
  in children, 979
  clinical manifestations of, 923
  Clostridium difficile and, 923*b*
  definition of, 922, 979
  evaluation of, 923–924
  hypokalemia as cause of, 124
Diarrhea *(Continued)*
  in infants, 979
  motility, 923
  osmotic, 922–923
  pathophysiology of, 922–923
  postgastrectomy, 935
  secretory, 923
  stool volume in, 922
  treatment of, 923–924
Diarthrosis, 995
Diastole, 578
Diastolic blood pressure, 595
Diastolic depolarization, 583
Diastolic dysfunction, 642
Diastolic heart failure, 641
DIC. *See* Disseminated intravascular coagulation
Dichlorodiphenyltrichloroethane, 855
Diencephalon, 317–318
Diet. *See also* Nutrition
  breast cancer and, 853–854
  cancer and, 277, 279*f*
  prostate cancer and, 880, 880*b*–881*b*
Dietary acculturation, 607
Dietary fat, small intestine and, 906*b*
Diethylstilbestrol, 275, 305–306
Differentiated cells, 28*f*
Differentiation, cellular, 2
Diffuse axonal injuries, 394, 395*t*, 397–398
Diffuse brain injury, 395*t*, 397–398
Diffuse noxious inhibitory control, 342
Diffuse papillomatosis, 844
Diffusion, in passive transport, 19–20, 19*f*
DiGeorge syndrome, 191–192, 192*t*, 193*f*, 475
Digestion, extracellular, 16, 16*f*
Digestive system. *See also* Accessory organs of digestion; Gastro-intestinal tract
  anatomy of, 899, 900*f*
  cancer of, 953–959
  mouth, 899–902
Digestive tract cancer, 270*t*–273*t*
Digital rectal examination, 886–887
Digoxin (Toloxin), 641
Dihydrotestosterone, 876–877
1,25-Dihydroxy-vitamin D_3, 454
Dilantin (phenytoin), 398–399
Dilated cardiomyopathy, 630–631, 631*f*
Dilutional hyponatremia, 122
Dimorphic fungi, 186
Dioxins, 855
Diplegia, 386*b*
Diploid cells, 42
Diplopia, 350
Dipsogenic polydipsia, 467
Direct antiglobulin test, 514*t*–516*t*
Direct effects, of hormones, 446
Discoid lupus erythematosus, 1085, 1086*f*
Disease-modifying antirheumatic drugs (DMARDs), 1035
Diseases of adaptation, 216–217
Dislocation, 1014–1015
Disse space, 911–912
Disseminated intravascular coagulation (DIC), 550–553
  clinical course of, 550–551
  clinical manifestations of, 552–553, 552*b*
  conditions associated with, 551, 551*b*
  D-dimer test for, 553
  definition of, 550
  diagnosis of, 551
  evaluation of, 553
  hemorrhage and, 552
  pathophysiology of, 551–552, 551*f*
  treatment of, 553
Distal convoluted tubule, 744, 744*f*, 750–752
Distal intestinal obstruction syndrome, 971
Disuse atrophy, 75, 1041
Diuresis, postoperative, 760
Diuretics, urine flow and, 752, 753*t*
Divergence, 310, 313
Diverticula, 938–939
Diverticular disease, 938–939, 939*f*
Diverticulitis, 938–939

Diverticulosis, 928*t*, 938–939
DKA. *See* Diabetic ketoacidosis
DMARDs. *See* Disease-modifying antirheumatic drugs
DMD. *See* Duchenne muscular dystrophy
DNA. *See* Deoxyribonucleic acid
DNA methylation
Alzheimer's disease and, 374–375
cancer and, 68–69, 69*f*, 246, 274–275
description of, 52, 53*f*, 62–63, 63*f*, 67
gene expression alteration by, 238–240
DNA methyltransferase, 280
DNA polymerase, 39
DNA sequencing, 57
DNA-binding proteins, 2
Dolichocephaly, 431*f*
Doll's eyes phenomenon, 367*f*
Dominance, 49–50
Dominant effects, 49
Dopamine
muscle movement alterations and, 381–382
properties of, 314*t*
substantia nigra synthesis of, 319
Dormancy, of cancer cells, 255
Dorsal horn, 320–321
Dorsal respiratory group, 684
Dorsal root ganglion, 320–321
Dosage compensation, 54
Double uterus, 817*f*
Double vagina, 817*f*
Double-helix model, of DNA, 38–39, 40*f*
Double-strand break, 287*f*
Down syndrome, 534, 663*t*
features of, 46*f*, 47*t*
leukemia risks with, 305
maternal age and, 46, 46*f*
prevalence of, 46
Downregulation, 444–446, 446*f*
Doxycycline (Teva-Doxycycline), 826*b*
Driver mutations, 238–240
Drosophila melanogaster, 108
Drowning, 95–96
Droxia, 528
Drugs. *See also specific drugs*
abuse of, 85–86, 86*t*
child poisoning caused by, 85*b*
childhood cancers and prenatal exposure to, 305–306, 306*t*
pupils and, 364
social or street, 89*t*
wound healing affected by, 154
Dry-lung drowning, 95
Dual X-ray absorptiometry, 1024–1025
Duchenne muscular dystrophy (DMD), 55, 1067–1068, 1067*t*, 1068*f*–1069*f*
Ductal adenocarcinomas, 959
Ductal carcinoma in situ, 237–238, 847*b*, 856*t*, 857–860, 859*f*
Ductal intraepithelial neoplasia, 857–858
Duke criteria, 638
Dumping syndrome, 934
Duodenum
anatomy of, 905–906, 905*f*
obstruction of, 970
ulcers of, 932–933, 932*f*, 933*t*
Duplications, 47
Dura matter, 323
Dusts, 703
Dutch Famine Birth Cohort, 274–275
Dwarfism, hypopituitary, 468, 469*f*
Dynamic muscle contraction, 1006, 1006*f*
Dynorphins, 341–342
Dysfunctional uterine bleeding, 820–821
Dysgeusia, 356
Dyskinesia, 382
Dyslipidemia, 617–618, 618*t*
CKD progression and, 777*t*, 778
Dysmenorrhea, 819
Dyspareunia, 842
Dysphagia, 611–612, 925–926, 926*f*
Dysphasia, 371, 371*f*, 372*t*–373*t*
Dysplasias
acetabular, 1059–1060
anhidrotic ectodermal, 62–63
bronchopulmonary, 730, 730*b*, 730*t*, 731*f*
Dysplasias *(Continued)*
cellular adaptation and, 77, 78*f*
of cervix, 78*f*
cortical, 431–432
of hip, developmental, 1059–1060, 1061*f*
Dyspnea, 611–612, 695
Dyspraxia, 375, 390
Dysreflexia, 402
Dysregulated apoptosis, 105
Dysrhythmias, 643, 644*t*–646*t*
Dyssomnias, 348–349
Dyssynergia, 762
Dystonia, 381*t*, 389
Dystonic cerebral palsy, 433
Dystonic movements, 389
Dystonic postures, 389
Dystrophic calcification, 100, 102*f*
Dystrophin, 55, 1067

E

E vitamins, 880*b*–881*b*
Ear
dysfunctions of, 342
external, 354, 354*f*
infections of, 342
inner, 354–355, 354*f*–355*f*
normal, anatomy of, 354–355
Eastern equine encephalitis, 413*t*
EBV. *See* Epstein-Barr virus
Eccentric muscle contraction, 1006
Ecchymosis, 510*t*
Eccrine sweat glands, 1074–1076
ECF. *See* Extracellular fluid
ECF-A. *See* Eosinophil chemotactic factor of anaphylaxis
ECG. *See* Electrocardiogram
ECM. *See* Extracellular matrix
Ectopic kidneys, 784
Ectopic testes, 873–874
Eczema, 1081–1082
Edecrin, 753*t*, 945
Edema
brain, 379–380, 379*f*
cerebral, 379–380, 379*f*
clinical manifestations of, 117
cytotoxic, 380
evaluation of, 117
formation mechanisms of, 116–117, 118*f*
generalized, 117
interstitial, 380
localized, 117
macular, 484–485
metabolic, 380
pathophysiology of, 116–117
pitting, 117, 118*f*
pulmonary, 703–704, 703*f*
treatment of, 117
vasogenic, 379
Effective osmolality, 20
Effective renal blood flow, 753
Effective renal plasma flow, 753
Effector organs, 309
Efferent arteriole, 745
Efferent lymphatic vessels, 599, 600*f*
Efferent neuron, 321–322
Efferent pathways, 309, 339
Efferent tubules, 807, 808*f*
EGF. *See* Epidermal growth factor
Eisenmenger's syndrome, 668
Ejaculation, of penis, 809
Ejaculatory duct, 809
Ejection fraction, 587
heart failure with preserved, 641–642, 642*t*
heart failure with reduced, 632, 639–641, 641*f*, 642*t*
Elastic arteries, 589
Elastic cartilage, 31*t*–33*t*, 32*f*
Elastic connective tissue, 31*f*, 31*t*–33*t*
Elastic recoil, 687
Elastin, 10
Elderly. *See also* Aging
age-related macular degeneration and, 352, 352*f*
cardiac output in, 587*t*
cardiovascular function in, 587*t*
fever in, 346*b*
hearing changes in, 357
Elderly *(Continued)*
hematological system in, 517*b*
hyponatremia in, 122*b*
immune response and, 174*b*
innate immunity and, 155*b*
MODS and, 653
olfaction changes in, 357*b*
pain perception in, 341*t*
presbyopia and, 352
renal function and, 756
sleep characteristics of, 348*b*
taste changes in, 357*b*
TBW in, 132*b*
thermoregulation in, 345–346
vision changes in, 357*b*
Electrocardiogram (ECG)
for complicated hypertension, 610
description of, 582–583, 583*f*
hyperkalemia findings with, 124*f*
hypokalemia findings with, 124*f*
MI and, 622, 622*f*
myocardial infarction diagnosis using, 626, 628*f*
Electrolytes, 7–8
distribution of, 115–116, 116*t*
small intestine absorption of, 908*b*
as solutes, 18–21
Electromagnetic radiation, 291–292, 292*f*
Electromechanical dissociation, 644*t*–645*t*
Electromyography, 755*t*
Electron-transport chain, 16–17
Electrophiles, 84–85
ELISA. *See* Enzyme-linked immunosorbent assay
Embolic stroke, 407
Embolism
cardiovascular, 613, 613*t*
pulmonary, 715–716, 715*f*
Embolus, 553, 613, 613*t*
Embryonal tumours, 438–440
Embryonic stem cells, 64
Embryonic tumours, 303
Emesis, 921
Emission, 809
Emphysema, 709*t*, 710–711, 710*f*–711*f*
Empirical risks, 58
Empyema, 700, 700*t*
EMT. *See* Epithelial-mesenchymal transition
Encephalitis, 413–414, 413*t*, 414*b*, 435
Encephalocele, 429
Encephalopathies, 433–435
hepatic, 945
Endocannabinoids, 342
Endocardial cushion defect, 668
Endocardial disorders
acute rheumatic fever, 634–637, 636*f*, 636*t*
aortic regurgitation, 634
aortic stenosis, 633, 633*f*
infective endocarditis, 637–638, 637*b*, 637*f*–638*f*
mitral regurgitation, 634
mitral stenosis, 633–634, 633*f*
MVPS, 634, 635*f*
rheumatic heart disease, 634–637, 636*f*
tricuspid regurgitation, 634
valvular dysfunction, 632–634, 632*t*, 633*f*
Endocarditis, 666*b*
Endocardium, 576, 576*f*
Endocervical canal, 799, 800*f*
Endocervical gonorrhea, 892*t*–894*t*
Endochondral bone formation, 1013, 1013*f*
Endocrine disorders, 1043–1044
Endocrine glands. *See also* Adrenal glands; Pancreas; Parathyroid glands; Pituitary gland; Thyroid gland
aging effects on, 461*b*
anatomy of, 443, 444*f*
dysfunction of, 465
pineal gland, 452
structure and function of, 447–460
Endocrine pancreas, 455–457. *See also* Diabetes mellitus
dysfunction of, 467
Endocrine system
anatomy of, 443, 444*f*
CKD and, 776*t*, 779
female, 850*f*
functions of, 443
Endocrine-disrupting chemicals, 854–855
Endocytic matrix, 23*b*
Endocytosis, 21–23, 22*f*–23*f*, 23*b*
Endogenous antigens, 168–169
Endogenous opioids, 341–342, 341*f*
Endogenous pyrogens, 150, 346
Endolarynx, 679
Endometrial cancer, 270*t*–273*t*, 836–838, 837*f*–838*f*, 838*t*
Endometrial polyps, 830, 830*f*
Endometriosis, 832–833, 832*f*
Endometrium
anatomy of, 799, 800*f*
hyperplasia of, 77
Endomitosis, 509–510
Endomorphins, 341–342
Endomysium, 999
Endoplasmic reticulum
characteristics of, 4*t*
dilation of, 81–82
protein folding in, 8*b*, 8*f*
stress, 8*b*, 105
Endorphins
as endogenous opioids, 341–342, 341*f*
properties of, 314*t*
β, in stress response, 225*t*–226*t*
Endosome, 21–23, 23*f*
Endosteum, 994
Endothelial cells, 146, 590–591
inflammation of injured, 614
Endothelial dysfunction, 607–608
Endothelial injury, 554, 614
Endothelium
description of, 146
inflammation of, 146, 612–613
vascular, 575, 590–591, 592*f*–593*f*, 593*t*
Endothelium-derived relaxing factor, 597
Endotoxic shock, 183
Endotoxins, 183
End-stage kidney disease, 772
Energy metabolism diseases, 1044
Engulfment, 148*f*–149*f*, 149
Enkephalins
as endogenous opioids, 341–342
properties of, 314*t*
Enteric plexus, 899, 900*f*
Enterocele, 828
Enterocytes, 906
Enteroglucagon, 903*t*
Enterohepatic circulation, 912, 913*f*
Enthesis, 1006, 1015
Entrance wound, 94*t*–95*t*
Entropion, 353
Enuresis, 790, 790*t*
Environmental chemicals, 854–855
Environmental tobacco smoke, 276
Enzyme-linked immunosorbent assay (ELISA), 292, 446*b*
Eosinopenia, 530*t*, 531
Eosinophil chemotactic factor of anaphylaxis (ECF-A), 145, 165*f*
Eosinophil count, 514*t*–516*t*, 516*b*
Eosinophilia, 530*t*, 531
Eosinophilic esophagitis, 927, 973
Eosinophils, 142*f*, 147, 499, 499*t*, 530*t*, 706
Ependymal cells, 310–311, 312*t*
Ependymomas, 419*t*, 420, 437–438, 437*t*
Epicardium, 576, 576*f*
Epicondylopathy, 1015–1016, 1016*f*
Epicritic information, 322–323
Epidermal growth factor (EGF), 26*t*, 240–242
Epidermis, 1074, 1075*f*, 1075*t*
Epididymal cysts, 873
Epididymis, 808–809, 808*f*
inflammation of, 876, 876*f*
Epididymitis, 876, 876*f*, 892*t*–894*t*
Epidural hematomas, 94*t*–95*t*, 395–396, 395*t*
Epigallocatechin gallate, 880*b*–881*b*
Epigenetic diseases
in genetic abnormality context, 67–68, 67*f*

Epigenetic diseases *(Continued)*
molecular approaches to, 68
treatment of, 69–70
Epigenetics
alcohol exposure during gestation and, 67
alcohol metabolism and, 285*f*
autosomal dominant inheritance and, 52, 53*f*
cancer and, 68–70, 69*f*, 268, 269*f*, 282*f*
definition of, 62
genomic imprinting, 64–66, 65*f*–66*f*
in human development, 64
inheritance of states of, 66–68
maternal care and, 66–67
mechanisms of, 62–64
DNA methylation, 52, 53*f*, 62–63, 63*f*
histone modification, 63–64, 63*f*
RNA-based, 64
mental illness and, 67
nutrition and, 66
twin studies on, 68, 68*f*
Epiglottitis, 727, 730*t*
Epilepsy, 376–377
in children, 436, 436*t*
Epileptogenic focus, 376–377
Epimysium, 999
Epinephrine, 224, 459, 588
nebulized, 726
Epiphyseal plate, 994
Epiphysis, 994
Epispadias, 785
Epithalamus, 317–318
Epithelial cells, 137
of lungs, 681
Epithelial tissues, 29*t*–30*t*
Epithelialization, 152–153
Epithelial-mesenchymal transition (EMT), 253, 254*f*, 255
breast cancer and, 855
prostate cancer and, 886
Epithelioid cells, 151
Epitopes, 163
EPSPs. *See* Excitatory postsynaptic potentials
Epstein-Barr virus (EBV), 252, 531
Burkitt lymphoma and, 541–542
childhood cancers and, 307
description of, 183
infectious mononucleosis and, 531–532
Equatorial plate, 25
Equilibrium receptors, 354
Equinovalgus, 1060*t*
Equinovarus, 1060*t*
Erectile dysfunction treatments, 888
Erectile reflex, of penis, 809, 812
Erlotinib (Tarceva), 263*t*
Erosion, 1079*t*–1080*t*
Eryptosis, 522
Erysipelas, 1087
Erythema, 207
Erythema multiforme, 1086–1087
Erythema toxicum neonatorum, 1116
Erythroblasts, 506
Erythrocyte osmotic fragility test, 514*t*–516*t*
Erythrocytes, 505–506
aging effects on, 516*b*
childhood disorders of, 560–568
anemia, 560–563, 561*b*, 561*t*
hemolytic anemia, 560, 562–563
iron deficiency anemia, 560–562, 561*b*
sickle cell disease, 564–567, 564*f*–567*f*, 565*t*
thalassemias, 567–568
description of, 142, 142*f*
development of, 506–509
erythropoiesis, 506–507, 506*f*, 508*t*
hemoglobin synthesis and, 506–507, 507*f*
iron cycle and, 508–509, 509*f*
disorders involving, 520–526
absolute polycythemia, 526
anemia (*See* Anemia)
familial polycythemia, 528*t*
hereditary hemochromatosis, 529
iron overload, 529
myeloproliferative, 526–529
Erythrocytes *(Continued)*
polycythemia vera, 526–528, 528*t*
relative polycythemia, 526
secondary polycythemia, 526, 528*t*
functions of, 497, 499*t*
laboratory tests for, 514*t*–516*t*
senescent, normal destruction of, 507–509
sickled, 565, 565*f*–566*f*
size and shape of, 497
in spleen, 501*f*
Erythrodermic psoriasis, 1083
Erythromelalgia, 549
Erythropoiesis, 506, 506*f*
nutritional requirements for, 507, 508*t*
Erythropoietin, 258, 506, 506*f*
kidneys and, 753
Escharotomies, 1095
Escherichia coli, 435, 700, 765–766
Esophageal atresia, 969, 970*f*
Esophageal phase of swallowing, 901
Esophageal varices, 943
Esophagitis, 926, 973
Esophagus
aging effects on, 918
anatomy of, 899–902, 899*f*
Barrett, 69, 954–955
cancer of, 270*t*–273*t*, 954–955, 954*b*, 954*t*
eosinophilic esophagitis and, 927
GER, 972–973
GERD, 925–926, 972–973
GERD and inflammation of, 973
Essential thrombocythemia, 549
Essential tremor, 383*t*
Estradiol, 444, 801, 838*f*, 851–852
Estriol, 801
Estrogen
adrenal cortex secretion of, 459
biological effects of, 801, 802*t*
biosynthesis of, 851*f*
breast cancer risk and, 851–852
breast development and, 806
carcinogenicity of, 852
endometrial cancer and, 837
functions of, 794*t*, 801
hypersecretion of, 489
nonreproductive effects of, 802*b*
in sexual differentiation, 794
in stress response, 225*t*–226*t*
tumours secreting, 489
Estrogen receptors, 837–838
signalling, 882, 882*f*
Estrogen receptor-α, 885
Estrogen receptor-β, 885
Estrone, 801
Ethacrynic acid, 753*t*, 945
Ethanol. *See* Alcohol
Ethylenediaminetetraacetic acid, 547
Euchromatin, 63
Eugonadism, 818*b*
Eukaryotes, 1
Euploid cells, 42–43
Eustachian tube, 354, 354*f*
Evista, 1025–1026, 1026*b*
Ewing sarcoma, 236, 304, 1050, 1070–1071, 1070*f*–1071*f*
Exanthema subitum, 1112–1113, 1112*t*
Excess relative risks, with ionizing radiation, 286
Excitatory neurotransmitters, 340
Excitatory postsynaptic potentials (EPSPs), 313
Excited delirium syndrome, 371–373
Excoriation, 1079*t*–1080*t*
Excretion, 747, 750*f*
Executive attention deficits, 369, 370*t*
Exhaustion stage, of general adaptation syndrome, 216–217
Exit wound, 94*t*–95*t*
Exocrine pancreas
anatomy of, 911*f*, 915, 917*f*
blood flow to, 915
enzymatic secretion in, 916–918
innervation of, 915
laboratory tests for, 917*t*
Exocytosis, 21–23, 22*f*
Exogenous antigens, 168–169
Exogenous pyrogens, 346
Exons, 41
Exotoxins, 182–183
Expectancy-related cortical activation, 342
Expiration
forces during, 687*f*
muscles of, 686
Expression disorders, 389–390
Expressive aprosody, 389–390
Expressive dysphasia, 371, 372*t*–373*t*
Expressivity, 51–52, 52*f*
Exstrophy of bladder, 785, 785*f*
External anal sphincter, 909, 909*f*
External auditory canal, 354, 354*f*
External ear, 354, 354*f*
External fixation, of fractures, 1014
External intercostal muscles, 686, 686*f*
External urethral sphincter, 746, 746*f*
Extinction, 369–371
Extracellular fluid (ECF)
in acidosis, 125
definition of, 115
description of, 18–19
hypokalemia in, 123
potassium concentration in, 123, 125
sodium in, 117–118
water movement between ICF and, 116
Extracellular matrix (ECM), 5, 849, 850*f*
aging changes to, 108
cellular injury to, 78
description of, 10–12, 11*f*
fibroblasts excretion of, 11–12, 11*f*
Extradural hematomas, 395–396, 395*t*
Extradural space, 323, 324*f*
Extrafusal muscles, 999
Extrahepatic portal hypertension, 981
Extramedullary hematopoiesis, 504
Extrapyramidal cerebral palsy, 433
Extrapyramidal motor syndromes, 390, 390*t*
Extrapyramidal symptoms, 382
Extrapyramidal system, 315–317, 316*f*
Extrinsic allergic alveolitis, 703
Extrinsic tissue factor, 141
Exudate, 150
Exudative pleural effusion, 700, 700*t*
Eye
anatomy of, 349–350, 349*f*
arcus senilis of, 621–622
external, structure and disorders of, 353–354, 353*f*
extrinsic muscles of, 350, 350*f*
infections of, 180*t*–181*t*, 353–354
movement-related disorders of, 350
Eyelids, 353, 353*f*

F

F cells, 455
Facial nerve, 330*t*
Facilitation, 313
Facioscapulohumeral muscular dystrophy (FSHD), 67*f*, 68, 1067*t*, 1068
Factor XII. *See* Hageman factor
FAD. *See* Flavin adenine dinucleotide
Failure to thrive, 977–978, 978*b*
Fallopian tubes, 800, 800*f*
salpingitis and, 825–826, 825*f*
False vocal cords, 679, 681*f*
Falx cerebri, 323
Familial adenomatous polyposis, 262, 956
Familial polycythemia, 528*t*
Familial tremor, 383*t*
Fanconi anemia, 305
Fas-associated death domain signaling complex, 250
Fas/CD95, 250
Fascia, 999
Fascicles, 327, 329*f*, 999
Fasciculations, 387
Fasciculus cuneatus, 322–323
Fasciculus gracilis, 322–323
Fast-twitch fibres, 1000
Fat embolism, 613*t*
Fat-free mass, 109
Fatigue, cancer and, 256
Fatigue fractures, 1013
Fats
liver metabolism of, 914
small intestine absorption of, 908*b*
Fatty change, 98, 98*f*
Fatty liver, 98, 98*f*
alcoholic, 948
nonalcoholic, 948–949
Fatty necrosis, 103, 104*f*
Fatty streak, 614, 615*f*
Fc receptors, 148–149, 203
FDPs. *See* Fibrin degradation products
Febrile seizure, 436*t*
Fecal mass, 910
Fecal mass, 928*t*
Feedback systems, 443–444, 445*f*
Female reproductive system
aging and, 811–812, 811*f*
androgens in, 801
breasts (*See* Breasts)
clitoris, 797, 797*f*
development of, 793–796
external genitalia of, 796*f*
fallopian tubes, 800, 800*f*
function of, 796
internal genitalia of, 795*f*, 798–801, 798*f*
labia majora, 797, 797*f*
labia minora, 797, 797*f*
menopause, 811–812, 811*f*
menstrual cycle (*See* Menstrual cycle)
mons pubis, 797, 797*f*
ovaries, 800–801, 801*f*
perineum in, 797*f*, 798
sex hormones of, 794*t*, 801–802, 802*b*, 802*t*
uterus (*See* Uterus)
vagina (*See* Vagina)
vestibule in, 797–798, 797*f*
vulva, 796–798, 797*f*
Female reproductive system disorders
abnormal uterine bleeding, 820–821, 821*t*
adenomyosis, 831–832
amenorrhea, 819–820, 841*f*
bartholinitis, 827, 827*f*
breast cancer (*See* Breast cancer)
cervical cancer (*See* Cervical cancer)
cervicitis, 826–827
delayed puberty, 818, 818*b*, 818*t*
dysmenorrhea, 819
endometrial cancer, 836–838, 837*f*–838*f*, 838*t*
endometrial polyps, 830, 830*f*
endometriosis, 832–833, 832*f*
infections, 823–827
infertility, 843
inflammations, 823–827
leiomyomas, 235–236, 236*f*, 831, 831*f*
ovarian cancer (*See* Ovarian cancer)
ovarian cysts, 829–830, 829*f*
PCOS, 822, 822*f*, 823*b*
pelvic organ prolapse, 763, 827–828, 828*b*, 828*f*–829*f*, 830*b*
PID, 824–825, 824*f*, 825*b*–826*b*
PMDD, 822–823
PMS, 822–823, 824*b*
precocious puberty, 818, 819*b*
reproductive tract abnormalities, 816–817, 817*f*
salpingitis, 825–826, 825*f*
sexual dysfunction, 842–843, 843*t*
sexual maturation alterations, 817–818, 818*b*–819*b*, 818*t*
vaginal cancer, 835–836
vaginitis, 826
vaginosis, 826
vulvar cancer, 270*t*–273*t*, 836
vulvodynia vestibulitis, 827
Female reproductive tract abnormalities, 816–817, 817*f*
Female sexual trauma, 767*t*
Female-pattern alopecia, 1101
Fenestrations, 590
FEP. *See* Free erythrocyte protoporphyrin
Ferritin, 508
serum, determination, 514*t*–516*t*
Fetal alcohol spectrum disorder, 92–93, 93*f*
prevention of, 427*b*
Fetus
drug exposure and, 305–306, 306*t*
vulnerability of, to environments, 275*f*

Fever, 338
acute rheumatic, 634–637, 636*f*, 636*t*
benefits of, 346
central, 347
in children, 346*b*
Colorado tick, 413*t*
in elderly, 346*b*
inflammation-related, 150
pathogenesis of, 346, 346*f*
of unknown origin, 346
FGF. *See* Fibroblast growth factor
Fibrillation, 387
Fibrils, 992
Fibrin, 154
Fibrin degradation products (FDPs), 514, 551–552
Fibrin split products (FSPs), 551–552
Fibrin-fibrinogen degradation products, 514*t*–516*t*
Fibrinogen, 496–497
Fibrinogen assay, 514*t*–516*t*
Fibrinolysis, 514
Fibrinolytic system, 141, 513–514, 514*f*
Fibrinopeptides, 141
Fibrinous exudate, 150
Fibroadenomas, 236
simple, 845
Fibroblast growth factor (FGF), 26*t*, 153, 991*t*
Fibroblast growth factor receptor, 837–838
Fibroblasts
cancer-associated, 249, 885–886
in connective tissue, 11–12, 11*f*
ECM excretion by, 11–12, 11*f*
in prostate cancer, 885–886
in wound healing, 153–154
Fibrocystic changes, 844
Fibrocystic disease of pancreas, 974
Fibromyalgia, 1041–1042, 1042*b*, 1042*f*
Fibronectin, 10–11
Fibrosarcoma, 856*t*, 1050
Fibrous adhesions, 928*t*
Fibrous cartilage, 31*t*–33*t*, 32*f*
Fibrous joints, 995, 997*f*
Fibrous plaque, 614, 616*f*
Fight-or-flight response, 216, 328–331
Filtration, in passive transport, 20, 20*f*
Filtration fraction, 746
Filtration slits, 743
Filum terminale, 320, 320*f*
Fimbriae, 800, 800*f*
First messengers, 446–447, 447*f*
First-degree block, 645*t*–646*t*
First-degree burns, 1095, 1097*t*
Fissure, 1079*t*–1080*t*
Fissure of Rolando, 315–316
Flaccid paresis/paralysis, 387
Flaccidity, 381*t*
Flagyl (metronidazole), 826*b*
Flail chest, 699, 699*f*
Flat bones, 994
Flavin adenine dinucleotide (FAD), 16–17
Fleabites, 1114, 1115*f*
Fluid resuscitation, 1096–1097
FMR1, 67–68
Foam cells, 614
Focal brain injury, 394–397, 395*t*, 396*f*
Focal segmental glomerulosclerosis, 787
Focal seizure, 436*t*
Folate, 523–524
Folate deficiency anemia, 521*t*, 523–524
Folic acid, 523–524
Folic acid deficiency, 90–91
Follicle cells, of thyroid gland, 452, 453*f*
Follicle-stimulating hormone (FSH), 448–451, 449*f*, 451*t*
deficiency of, 468
functions of, 794*t*
in menstrual cycle, 804
production of, 794
Follicular cysts, 829–830
Folliculitis, 1087
Follistatin, 804
Fontan procedure, 672
Fontanelles, 426, 427*f*
Food additives, 855
Food allergy, 938
Food poisoning, 180*t*–181*t*
Foramen of Luschka, 323–324
Foramen of Magendie, 323–324
Foramen of Monro, 323–324
Foramen ovale, 667
Forebrain, 313–318, 315*t*
Foreign body aspiration, 727
Foreign matter, 613*t*
Foreskin, 808
Fornix, of vagina, 798
Fosamax, 1061–1062
Fossae, 323
Fourth-degree burns, 1095, 1097*t*
Fovea centralis, 349, 349*f*
Fractures, 94*t*–95*t*
basilar skull, 397
bowing, 1012, 1012*t*
classification of, 1011–1014, 1012*f*, 1012*t*
clinical manifestations of, 1013–1014
closed, 1011–1012, 1012*f*, 1012*t*
comminuted, 1011–1012, 1012*t*
complete, 1011–1012, 1012*t*
compound, 1011–1012, 1012*f*, 1012*t*
compound skull, 397
definition of, 1011
delayed union of, 1014
evaluation of, 1014
external fixation of, 1014
fatigue, 1013
greenstick, 1012, 1012*f*, 1012*t*
healing, 1013, 1013*f*
impacted, 1012*f*, 1012*t*
incomplete, 1011–1012, 1012*t*
insufficiency, 1012–1013
internal fixation of, 1014
linear, 1011–1012, 1012*t*
malunion of, 1014
of nonaccidental trauma, 1071, 1071*f*
nonunion of, 1014
oblique, 1011–1012, 1012*f*, 1012*t*
occult, 1012*f*
open, 1011–1012, 1012*f*, 1012*t*
open reduction of, 1014
osteoporosis causing, 1021–1022, 1022*t*
pathological, 1012–1013, 1012*f*, 1012*t*
pathophysiology of, 1013, 1013*f*
segmented, 1012*f*
spiral, 1011–1012, 1012*f*, 1012*t*
stress, 1012–1013, 1012*t*
torus, 1012, 1012*t*
traction of, 1014
transchondral, 1012*t*, 1013
transverse, 1011–1012, 1012*f*, 1012*t*
treatment of, 1014
vertebral, 399–400, 400*t*
Fragile sites, on chromosomes, 49
Fragile X syndrome, 49, 67–68, 67*f*
Fragile X tremor ataxia syndrome (FXTAS), 67–68
Fragile X-associated primary ovarian insufficiency, 67–68
Frailty, aging and, 109
Frameshift mutations, 39, 41*f*
Framework regions, 162–163
Free erythrocyte protoporphyrin (FEP), 525
Free fatty acids, 481
Free radicals, 286–287, 287*f*
cellular injury caused by, 82–83
definition of, 82–83
diseases and disorders linked to, 83*b*
generation of, 83
inactivation of, 84*t*
oxidative stress from, 82–83, 83*t*, 108
termination of, 84*t*
types of, 83*t*
Freely movable joints, 995
Frontal lobe, 315–316, 316*f*
Frontal lobe ataxic gait, 389
Frontotemporal dementia, 375*t*, 376
Fructosemia, 982, 983*t*
FSH. *See* Follicle-stimulating hormone
FSHD. *See* Facioscapulohumeral muscular dystrophy
FSPs. *See* Fibrin split products
Full-thickness burns, 1095, 1096*f*, 1097*t*
Functional constipation, 922
Functional cysts, 829
Functional dysphagia, 925
Functional hearing loss, 355
Functional incontinence, 762*t*
Functional residual capacity, 687
Fungal diseases
description of, 186–187
examples of, 187*t*
morphology of, 186*f*
opportunistic, 196*b*
Fungal infections, 1089, 1089*f*, 1089*t*–1090*t*
in children, 1110–1111, 1110*f*
Fungal meningitis, 412
Fungi, 186–187, 186*f*, 187*t*
Furosemide, 753*t*, 945
Furuncles, 1087, 1087*f*
Fusiform aneurysms, 408, 611
Fusiform muscles, 999
FXTAS. *See* Fragile X tremor ataxia syndrome

G

G_0 phase, in cell cycle, 25, 25*f*
G_1 phase, in cell cycle, 25, 25*f*
G_2 phase, in cell cycle, 25, 25*f*
G6PD deficiency. *See* Glucose-6-phosphate dehydrogenase deficiency
GABA. *See* Gamma-aminobutyric acid
Gait, 1065
Gait disorders, 389
Galactorrhea, 843–844
Galactosemia, 982, 983*t*
Galea aponeurotica, 323
Gallbladder
aging effects on, 917*t*
anatomy of, 911*f*, 914, 917*f*
cancer of, 270*t*–273*t*, 958
disorders of, 951–952, 952*f*
hormonal regulation of, 914–915
Gallstones, 951–952, 952*f*
Gametes, 42
Gamma globulins, 496–497
Gamma rigidity, 381, 381*t*
Gamma-aminobutyric acid (GABA), properties of, 314*t*
Gamma-glutamyltranspeptidase, 916*t*
Ganglia, 310
basal, 315–317, 316*f*, 319*f*
collateral, 328–331
paravertebral, 328–331
sympathetic, 328–331
Gangrenous cystitis, 765
Gangrenous necrosis, 103–105, 104*f*
Gap junctions, 12, 13*f*, 288
Gas exchange, 692
Gas gangrene, 105
Gas pressure, 688–689, 689*f*
Gas transport, 688–692
Gas-exchange airways, 680–681, 682*f*–683*f*
Gasping breathing pattern, 366*t*
Gastric acid, 904–905, 905*f*
Gastric bleeding, 931
Gastric emptying, 903–904
delayed, 928
Gastric glands, 904, 904*f*
Gastric inflammation, 251
Gastric inhibitory peptide, 903*t*
Gastric motility, 903–904, 903*t*
Gastric secretion, 904–905, 904*f*
Gastric ulcers, 933, 933*t*
Gastrin, 457, 903, 903*t*
Gastrin-releasing peptide, 903*t*
Gastritis, 930–931
Gastrocolic reflex, 910
Gastroduodenal junction, 902, 902*f*
Gastroesophageal reflux (GER), 972–973
Gastroesophageal reflux disease (GERD), 925–926, 972–973
Gastroileal reflex, 909
Gastro-intestinal allergy, 202
Gastro-intestinal bleeding, 924, 924*t*, 925*f*
Gastro-intestinal infections, 180*t*–181*t*
Gastro-intestinal system. *See also specific organs*
CKD and, 776*t*, 779
MODS in, 654–655
Gastro-intestinal (GI) tract. *See also* Accessory organs of digestion
aging and, 918
cancer manifestations of, 260
cancer of, 953–957, 954*t*
esophagus (*See* Esophagus)
immunity and, 910
large intestine, 909–910, 909*f*, 917*t*
microbiome of, 910
mouth, 899–902
stomach (*See* Stomach)
wall of, 899, 900*f*
Gastro-intestinal tract disorders
abdominal pain, 924
anorexia, 535, 921
appendicitis, 939
bile salt deficiency, 935
CD, 936–938, 936*t*
in children (*See* Children, gastro-intestinal tract disorders in)
clinical manifestations of, 921–924
constipation, 922
diarrhea (*See* Diarrhea)
diverticular disease, 938–939, 939*f*
dysphagia, 611–612, 925–926, 926*f*
gastritis, 930–931
gastro-intestinal bleeding, 924, 924*t*, 925*f*
GERD, 925–926, 972–973
hiatal hernia, 927, 927*f*
IBD, 935–938, 936*b*, 936*t*
IBS, 938, 938*b*
intestinal obstruction (*See* Intestinal obstruction)
lactase deficiency, 935
malabsorption syndromes, 935
mesenteric vascular insufficiency, 939–940
microscopic colitis, 938
motility disorders, 925–929
nutrition disorders, 940–943
pancreatic exocrine insufficiency, 935
peptic ulcer disease (*See* Peptic ulcer disease)
pyloric obstruction, 927–928
UC, 936–937, 936*t*
vomiting, 367, 921–922
Gastroparesis, 928
Gate control theory, 339
Gating, 12
GCT. *See* Glucose change test
Gegenhalten. *See* Paratonia
Gene amplification, 238–240, 243, 244*f*
Gene expression, 238–240
Gene mapping, 57, 57*f*
Gene splicing, 41
General adaptation syndrome, 216–217, 217*f*
Generalized clonic-tonic seizure, 377, 436*t*
Generalized edema, 117
Generalized lymphadenopathy, 538
Generic conflict hypothesis, 64
Genes, 38
cancer, 243, 243*t*
Genetic diseases
autosomal dominant inheritance
delayed age of onset, 51
epigenetics and, 52, 53*f*
expressivity and, 51–52, 52*f*
genomic imprinting and, 52
pedigrees and, 50, 51*f*
penetrance and, 51–52, 51*f*
recurrence risks of, 50–51
autosomal recessive inheritance
consanguinity and, 54
pedigrees in, 52–53, 53*f*
recurrence risks and, 53–54, 54*f*
multifactorial inheritance, 58–59, 58*f*, 59*b*
transmission of, 50–56
X-linked inheritance
pedigrees and, 55
recurrence risks in, 55–56, 56*f*
sex determination and, 54–55, 55*f*
sex-limited and sex-influenced traits in, 56
X inactivation and, 54, 54*f*
Genetic heterogeneity, 855

Genetics
  definition of, 38
  DNA as code for, 39
  dominance, 49–50
  elements of, 49–50
  genotype, 49
  phenotype, 49
  recessiveness, 49–50
Genital herpes, 892*t*–894*t*
Genomic imprinting, 52, 64–66, 65*f*–66*f*
Genomic instability
  of cancer cells, 244–247
  ionizing radiation causing, 288
Genotype, 49
GER. *See* Gastroesophageal reflux
GERD. *See* Gastroesophageal reflux disease
Germ cell inheritance, 276*t*
Germ cell mutation, 244
Germ cell tumours, 419*t*
German measles, 1111–1112, 1112*f*, 1112*t*
Germline mosaicism, 51
Gestational diabetes mellitus, 482
GH. *See* Growth hormone
Ghrelin, 457, 481, 903*t*, 941, 941*b*
GHRH. *See* Growth hormone-releasing hormone
GI tract. *See* Gastro-intestinal tract
Giant aneurysms, 408
Giant cell tumour, 1050
Giant cells, 151
Giantism, pituitary, 469, 469*f*
Gibbs-Donnan equilibrium, 20
Glands of Montgomery, 806
Glans, 808, 809*f*
Glasgow Coma Scale, 394, 395*t*
Glaucoma, 350, 351*t*, 352*f*
Gleason score, 880*b*–881*b*
Gleevec (imatinib), 242–243, 263*t*, 538
Glenn shunt, 670
Glioblastoma multiforme, 419–420, 419*t*
Gliomas, 418–420, 419*t*
  brainstem, 437*t*, 438
  optic, 437*t*, 438
Glisson capsule, 911
Global dysphasia, 371, 372*t*
Globins, 506–507
Globulins, 496–497, 916*t*
Globus pallidus, 317, 319*f*
Glomerular capillaries, 745
Glomerular disorders
  in children, 786–788
  glomerulonephritis (*See* Glomerulonephritis)
Glomerular filtration
  capillary pressures and, 741*f*, 747–748, 750*f*
  definition of, 747
  in distal convoluted tubule, 750–752
  Loop of Henle and, 750–752
  in proximal convoluted tubule, 749–750
  substances transported in, 750*b*
  urine formation and, 747, 750*f*
Glomerular filtration membrane, 742*f*, 743
Glomerular filtration rate, 746, 748–749
  renal clearance and, 753–754
Glomerular injury
  mechanisms of, 768*f*
  primary, 767–768
  secondary, 767–768
Glomerular lesions, 769*t*
Glomerulonephritis
  acute, 767–768
  acute poststreptococcal, 786–787
  chronic, 770–771, 771*f*
  clinical manifestations of, 769
  evaluation of, 769
  immunological pathogenesis of, 769*t*
  nephritic syndrome associated with, 770*t*
  nephrotic syndrome associated with, 770*t*
  pathophysiology of, 768–769, 768*f*
  soluble immune-complex, 769*t*
  treatment of, 769
  types of, 769–770, 770*t*
Glomerulotubular balance, 750
Glomerulus, 743, 745*f*
Glossitis, 525*f*
Glossopharyngeal nerve, 330*t*
Glucagon, 456–457, 477, 481
Glucocorticoid-induced osteoporosis, 1023
Glucocorticoids, 726. *See also* Cortisol
  adrenal cortex producing, 457–459
  exogenous, stress affected by, 221–222
  functions of, 457–458, 458*f*
  secretion of, 217*f*, 227
Gluconeogenesis, 942–943
Glucophage (metformin), 481–482, 822
Glucose
  impaired, in shock, 647–648, 647*f*
  insulin promoting uptake of, 455–456
Glucose change test (GCT), 482
Glucose transporters (GLUTs), 455
Glucose-6-phosphate dehydrogenase (G6PD) deficiency
  in children, 560
  test, 514*t*–516*t*
Glutamate, 314*t*
Glutathione-S-transferases, 281–282, 883–884
GLUTs. *See* Glucose transporters
Glycerol, 753*t*
Glycine, 314*t*
Glycocalyx, 9
Glycogen, 98–99
Glycogen storage diseases, 98–99, 982, 1044
Glycogenolysis, 942–943
Glycolipids, 2–3, 6*f*, 9
Glycolysis
  aerobic, 249
  anaerobic, 17
  process of, 16, 17*f*
  pyruvate from, 17, 17*f*
Glycoprotein hormones, 448–451, 451*t*
Glycoprotein PIIb/IIIa (GPIIb/IIIa), 510
Glycoproteins, 2–3, 6*f*, 9, 989*t*, 992
Glycosylated hemoglobin, 476
α-Glycoprotein, 992
GM_2 gangliosidosis, 434
GnRH. *See* Gonadotropin-releasing hormone
Goblet cells, 680
Golfer's elbow, 1015
Golgi complex, 4*t*
Golgi tendon organs, 1000
Gomphosis, 995
Gonadarche, 795–796
Gonadostat, 794–795
Gonadotropin-releasing hormone (GnRH), 449*t*
  functions of, 794*t*
  in menstrual cycle, 804
  production of, 794
Gonadotropin-releasing hormone pulse generator, 794–795
Gonads, 793, 795*f*
  aging and, 461*b*
  hormonal stimulation of, 797*f*
Gonococcal infections, 892*t*–894*t*
Gonorrhea, 891–894, 892*t*–894*t*
Gorlin syndrome, 290
Gout, 1038–1040, 1038*f*–1039*f*, 1038*t*
Gouty arthritis, 1038, 1039*f*, 1040
GPIIb/IIIa. *See* Glycoprotein PIIb/IIIa
Graft-*versus*-host disease, 195, 307
Granulation tissue, 153
Granulocytes, 142, 142*f*, 498–499, 507, 509, 529–531, 530*t*
Granulocytopenia, 531
Granulocytosis, 530, 530*t*
Granuloma, 151–152, 151*f*
Granulosa cells, 801
Grasp reflex, 367*f*
Graves' dermopathy, 472
Graves' disease, 471–473, 472*f*
Great cardiac vein, 580, 581*f*
Great vessels, of heart, 577, 577*f*
Green tea, 880*b*–881*b*
Greenstick fractures, 1012, 1012*f*, 1012*t*
Gremlin, 991*t*
Grey matter, 314, 317
Ground substance, 988
Growth factor-regulated kinases, 243
Growth factors
  cell proliferation stimulated by, 26*f*
  definition of, 26–27
  signaling pathways, in cancer, 242*f*
  types of, 26*t*
Growth faltering, 977–978, 978*b*
Growth hormone (GH)
  aging and, 451*b*, 461*b*
  breast cancer and, 852
  deficiency of, 468, 469*f*
  function of, 448–451, 449*f*, 451*t*
  hypersecretion of, 469, 470*f*
  in stress response, 225*t*–226*t*
Growth hormone-releasing hormone (GHRH), 448–451, 449*t*
Growth plate, 994
Guanine, 38
Guillain-Barré syndrome, 310, 388, 416, 416*t*
Gunshot wounds, 94*t*–95*t*
Guttate psoriasis, 1083, 1083*f*
Gynecomastia, 890–891
Gyri, 314, 316*f*

H

H1 receptors, 145
H1N1 (swine influenza virus), 185
H2 receptors, 145
H5N1 avian influenza virus, 185
Haemophilus influenzae, 435, 1028
Hageman factor (factor XII), 141, 512
Hair
  cancer manifestations of, 260
  colour of, 1074
  disorders of, 1101
  structures of, 1074
Hair cells, 354
Haldane effect, 692
Hallucinogens, 86*t*
Hand, rheumatoid arthritis of, 1033*f*
Hand sanitizer, 709*b*
Hanging strangulations, 93–95
Haploid cells, 42
Haplotypes, 211
Haptens, 161
Hashimoto's disease, 473
Haustra, 909, 909*f*
Haustral segmentation, 908
Haversian canal, 993, 993*f*
Haversian system, 993, 993*f*
Hayflick limit, 247
HDL. *See* High-density lipoprotein
Headaches, 410–411, 410*t*
Health care-associated pneumonia, 712, 712*b*
Healthy immigrant effect, 607
Hearing, 354–357, 354*f*–355*f*. *See also* Ear
Hearing loss, 355
Heart
  action potentials of, 580, 582–583, 582*t*, 583*f*
  ATP for, 585
  automaticity of, 583
  blood flow through, 576–578, 577*f*
  capillaries of, 579
  cardiac cycle of, 578, 579*f*–580*f*
  chambers of, 577, 577*f*
  conduction system of, 580–583, 582*f*
  coronary vessels of, 578–580
  emotional stress effects on, 228*b*
  energy synthesis for, 585
  fibrous skeleton of, 577, 578*f*
  functions of, 575–576
  great vessels of, 577, 577*f*
  hypertrophy of, 584
  innervation of, 583–584, 584*f*
  intracardiac pressures in, 578, 578*t*
  left, 575, 576*f*
  parasympathetic nerves of, 583–584, 584*f*
  rhythmicity of, 583
  right, 575, 576*f*
  Starling's law of, 587, 587*f*
  structures of, 576–578
  sudden cardiac death, 626, 627*f*
  sympathetic nerves of, 583–584, 584*f*
  valves of, 577, 577*f*–578*f*
  veins of, 578, 580, 581*f*
  weight of, 575–576
Heart disease
  acquired, in children, 673–677
  congenital (*See* Congenital heart disease)
  dysrhythmias, 643, 644*t*–646*t*
  manifestations of, 638–643
  rheumatic, 634–637, 636*f*
Heart failure, 485
  afterload in, 639, 641*f*
  BNP and, 598*b*, 673
  Canadian statistics on, 639*b*
  congenital heart disease causing, 672–673, 673*b*, 673*t*
  definition of, 638–639
  diastolic, 641
  high-output, 642–643, 643*f*
  left
    clinical manifestations of, 641
    description of, 639–642
    in HIV, 638
    in infants, 672–673
    management of, 641
  with preserved ejection fraction, 641–642, 642*t*
  with reduced ejection fraction, 632, 639–641, 641*f*, 642*t*
  right, 642, 642*f*
  risk factors of, 638–639
  systolic, 639
Heart rate
  atrial receptors and, 589
  cardiac output and, 588–589
  cardiovascular vasomotor control centre and, 588–589
  hormone effects on, 589
  neural reflexes and, 589
  pericardial sac causing reflex changes in, 576
Heart rate variability, 224
Heart wall
  anatomy of, 576, 576*f*
  disorders of, 629–638
    acute pericarditis, 629, 629*f*
    constrictive pericarditis, 630, 630*f*
    pericardial effusion, 629–630, 630*f*
Heat cramps, 346
Heat exhaustion, 346
Heat stroke, 346–347
HeLa cells, 247
Helicobacter pylori, 251, 523
  peptic ulcer disease caused by, 931–933
Heliox, 726
Helminths, 187*t*
Helper T cells, 160, 169, 171*f*, 221–222
Hemagglutinin protein, 183
Hemangioblastomas, 419*t*
Hematemesis, 924*t*
Hematochezia, 924, 924*t*
Hematocrit, 777*t*
Hematocrit determination, 514*t*–516*t*
Hematogenous osteomyelitis, 1028
Hematological system. *See also* Blood
  aging effects on, 516*b*, 517*t*
  blood tests for, 514*t*–516*t*
  CKD and, 776*t*, 779
  components of, 496–503
  in elderly, 517*b*
  lymphoid organs
    description of, 500–503
    lymph nodes, 502–503, 503*f*
    mononuclear phagocyte system, 503, 503*t*
    primary, 165–167, 500
    secondary, 160, 162*f*, 500
    spleen, 500–502, 502*f*
Hematomas
  epidural, 94*t*–95*t*, 395–396, 395*t*
  extradural, 395–396, 395*t*
  intracerebral, 395*t*, 397, 397*f*
  subdural, 94*t*–95*t*, 395*t*, 396–397
Hematopoiesis
  in bone marrow, 504–505, 504*f*
  cellular differentiation and, 505–506, 505*f*
  definition of, 503–504
  extramedullary, 504
Hematopoietic cell growth factors, 26*t*, 505
Hematopoietic stem cell transplantation, 545, 568

Hematopoietic stem cells (HSCs), 504, 504*f*
Hematuria, 771
Heme, 507–508, 508*f*
Hemiagnosia, 344*t*
Hemidesmosome, 12, 13*f*
Hemiparesis, 386*b*
Hemiplegia, 386*b*
Hemiplegic posture, 389
Hemizygous individuals, 54
Hemochromatosis, 57, 529
Hemodynamic stroke, 407
Hemoglobin, 126
  aging effects on, 516*b*
  glycosylated, 476
  laboratory tests for, 514*t*–516*t*
  NO binding to, 507, 507*f*
  oxygen transport by, 690–692
  sickle cell, 564, 564*f*, 565*t*
  structure of, 506–507, 507*f*
  synthesis of, 506–507, 507*f*
Hemoglobin desaturation, 691
Hemoglobin determination, 514*t*–516*t*
Hemoglobin electrophoresis, 514*t*–516*t*
Hemoglobin H disease, 567
Hemoglobin S, 564, 564*f*
Hemolysis, 522
Hemolytic anemia, 527*t*
  in children, 560, 562–563
Hemolytic disease of newborn, 211
  clinical manifestations of, 562–563
  evaluation and treatment of, 563
  incidence of, 562
  pathophysiology of, 562, 563*f*
Hemolytic jaundice, 99–100, 946, 947*t*
Hemolytic uremic syndrome, 787–788
Hemophilias, 569, 569*t*
Hemoproteins, as cellular accumulations, 99–100, 100*f*
Hemoptysis, 696
Hemorrhage
  blowout, 510*t*
  DIC and, 552
  intracranial, 408, 435
  petechial, 510*t*
  subarachnoid, 408–410, 410*t*
Hemorrhagic cystitis, 765
Hemorrhagic disorders
  antibody-mediated, 569–570
  classification of, 546*t*
  inherited, 569
Hemorrhagic exudate, 150
Hemorrhagic infarcts, 407
Hemorrhagic stroke, 408, 435
Hemosiderin, 99, 100*f*, 508
Hemosiderosis, 99
Hemostasis
  blood vessels function in, 510–511
  definition of, 510
  function of, 520
  platelet function in, 510–511, 546
Hemothorax, 700, 700*t*
Henoch-Schönlein purpura nephritis, 787
Heparin-induced thrombocytopenia (HIT), 547
Hepatic artery, 911, 911*f*–912*f*
Hepatic encephalopathy, 945
Hepatic porta vein, 911, 912*f*
Hepatic vein, 899, 911, 912*f*
Hepatitis, in children, 980–981
Hepatitis A virus, 950–951, 950*t*
  in children, 980
Hepatitis B virus, 252, 292, 950–951, 950*t*
  in children, 980
Hepatitis C virus, 252, 292, 950–951, 950*t*
  in children, 981
Hepatitis D virus, 950–951, 950*t*
  in children, 980
Hepatitis E virus, 950–951, 950*t*
Hepatoblastoma, 982
Hepatocellular carcinoma, 958
Hepatocytes, 64, 911, 912*f*
Hepatopulmonary syndrome, 943
Hepatorenal syndrome, 946–947
Hepcidin, 258, 509
Herceptin (trastuzumab), 263*t*
Herd immunity, 190
Hereditary angioedema, 141–142
Hereditary hemochromatosis, 529
Hereditary multiple exostoses, 1069
Hereditary nonpolyposis colorectal cancer (HNPCC), 52, 69, 244–246, 837, 956
Hereditary sideroblastic anemia, 525
Hereditary thrombophilias, 554
Hering-Breuer reflex, 684
Hernia, 928*t*
  hiatal, 927, 927*f*
Herniated intervertebral disc, 405–406, 405*f*
Heroin, 89*t*
Herpes simplex virus, 892*t*–894*t*, 1088, 1088*f*
Herpes zoster, 1088, 1088*f*
  in children, 1112*t*, 1113
Herpesviruses, 184, 252
Hesitation marks, 94*t*–95*t*
Heterochromatin, 63
Heterochronic parabiosis, 108
Heterochronic transplantations, 108
Heterophilic antibodies, 532
Heteroplasmy, 109
Heterosegmental pain inhibition, 342
Heterotopic ossification, 1017
Heterozygotes, 49
Heterozygous carriers, 53
Heterozygous individuals, 49
Hexose-monophosphate shunt, 149, 193
HHS. *See* Hyperosmolar hyperglycemic syndrome
Hiatal hernia, 927, 927*f*
Hibernating myocardium, 625
Hiccups, 367
Hidradenitis suppurativa, 1108
HIF. *See* Hypoxia-inducible transcription factor
High-density lipoprotein (HDL), 618
Highly active antiretroviral therapy, 414
High-output failure, 642–643, 643*f*
High-resolution peripheral quantitative computed tomography (HRpQCT), 1025
High-sensitivity C-reactive protein, 614
Hila, 680
Hilum, 741, 742*f*
Hindbrain, 313–314, 315*t*, 319–320
Hip
  developmental dysplasia of, 1059–1060, 1061*f*
  dislocated, 1059–1060
  subluxated, 1059–1060
Hirschsprung's disease, 972, 972*f*
Hirsutism, 1101
Histaminase, 141
Histamine, 145, 146*f*, 202, 224–227, 225*f*, 903*t*
  properties of, 314*t*
Histone acetyl transferase, 280
Histone acetylation, 63
Histone deacetylase inhibitors, 70
Histone modification, 63–64, 63*f*
Histones, 1, 63
HIT. *See* Heparin-induced thrombocytopenia
HIV. *See* Human immunodeficiency virus
HIV distal symmetric polyneuropathy, 414
HIV fusion inhibitors, 196–197
HIV integrase, 195
HIV integrase inhibitors, 196–197
HIV protease, 195
HIV protease inhibitors, 196–197
HIV transcriptase inhibitors, 196–197
HIV-associated neurocognitive disorder, 414
HIV-associated peripheral neuropathy, 414
Hives. *See* Urticaria
HLA-B27, 209, 1037
HLAs. *See* Human leukocyte antigens
HLHS. *See* Hypoplastic left heart syndrome
HNPCC. *See* Hereditary nonpolyposis colorectal cancer
Hodgkin's disease, 236, 263
Hodgkin's lymphoma, 303–304
  in children, 572, 572*f*
  clinical manifestations of, 539, 539*f*, 542*f*
  pathophysiology of, 539, 539*f*
  stages of, 540, 540*t*
  treatment of, 540
Homeostasis, 12, 216
  protein, 8–9, 9*f*
Homologous chromosomes, 42, 44*f*
Homozygotes, 49
Homozygous individuals, 49
Homunculus, 315*f*, 316
Hordeolum, 353
Hormonal hyperplasia, 77
Hormonal signalling, 12–13, 14*f*
Hormone receptors, 444–447, 446*f*
Hormone replacement therapy, breast cancer risk and, 852
Hormones
  adrenal gland, 457–460
  alterations of, 465–466, 467*t*
  binding proteins and, 444, 445*t*
  biphasic effects of, 446
  blood pressure affected by, 597
  breast cancer and, 850–852, 850*f*–851*f*
  characteristics of, 443
  direct effects of, 446
  ectopic sources of, 465
  feedback systems of, 443–444, 445*f*
  first messengers and, 446–447, 447*f*
  gallbladder regulation by, 914–915
  heart rate affected by, 589
  of HPA system, 227, 447–452, 449*f*
  hypothalamic, 449*t*, 466*f*
  lipid-soluble, 444, 444*t*, 447, 448*f*
  mechanisms of action of, 444–447, 446*f*
  in menstrual cycle, 804, 804*t*
  nephron functions and, 752
  neuroendocrine, 227
  pancreatic, 455–457
  parathyroid, 454–455, 474–476
  permissive effects of, 446
  pineal gland, 452
  pituitary
    anterior, 448–452, 451*t*
    posterior, 452
  in prostate cancer, 882, 882*f*, 884–885
  protein, 444
  regulation of, 443–444
  release of, 443–444
  second messengers and, 446–447, 447*f*, 465
  secretion of, 443
  steroid, 443, 497
  stress response affected by, 224–227, 225*t*–226*t*
  structural categories of, 443, 444*t*
  target cells for, 14, 444–447, 446*f*, 465
  thyroid gland, 453–454, 454*t*
  transport of, 444
  vasoconstrictor, 597
  vasodilator, 597
  water-soluble, 444, 444*t*
Horseshoe kidney, 784
Hospital-acquired pneumonia, 712, 712*b*
HPA system. *See* Hypothalamic-pituitary-adrenal system
HPV. *See* Human papillomavirus
HPV DNA test, 834*b*
HRpQCT. *See* High-resolution peripheral quantitative computed tomography
HSCs. *See* Hematopoietic stem cells
HTLV-1. *See* Human T-cell lymphotropic virus type 1
Human chorionic gonadotropin, 794*t*
Human development, epigenetics in, 64
Human epidermal growth factor receptor, 242
Human Genome Project, 57, 57*f*
Human immunodeficiency virus (HIV)
  AIDS progression from, 199*f*
  antiretroviral therapy for, 196–197
  CD4+ T cells and, 195
  CNS neoplasms and, 415
  description of, 195
  genetic map of, 197*f*
  in infants, 199
Human immunodeficiency virus (HIV) *(Continued)*
  left ventricular failure in, 638
  life cycle and possible sites of, 198*f*
  myelopathy, 414
  neurocognitive disorder associated with, 414
  opportunistic infections and, 414–415
  peripheral neuropathy associated with, 414
  prevalence of, 195
  structure of, 197*f*
  transmission of, in pregnancy, 198–199
  vaccinations in, 198
  viral meningitis and, 414
Human leukocyte antigens (HLAs), 169, 195, 211, 211*f*, 476–477, 1032–1033
  inheritance of, 212*f*
Human papillomavirus (HPV), 252, 292–293
  cervical cancer development and, 833–834, 836*b*, 892*t*–894*t*
  rising incidence of cancer and, 293*b*
  warts caused by, 1088–1089, 1089*f*
Human papillomavirus DNA test, 834*b*
Human T-cell lymphotropic virus type 1 (HTLV-1), 252
Humoral immunity, 160
Hunt and Hess subarachnoid hemorrhage grading system, 410, 410*t*
Huntington's disease, 51, 373
Huxley, A. F., 1005
Hyaline cartilage, 31*t*–33*t*, 32*f*
Hyaline membrane disease. *See* Respiratory distress syndrome of newborn
Hydrea, 549
Hydrocele, 873, 873*f*
Hydrocephalus, 319
  in children, 426
  clinical manifestations of, 380
  congenital, 432, 432*f*
  definition of, 380
  evaluation and treatment of, 380
  pathophysiology of, 380
  types of, 380*t*
Hydrochlorothiazide, 753*t*
Hydrogen, 752
Hydrogen ions, 126
Hydrogen peroxide, 83*t*
Hydrogen sulfide, 95
Hydronephrosis, 759–760, 760*f*
Hydrostatic pressure, 20, 20*f*
  capillary, 116–117
  interstitial, 116
Hydroureter, 759–760
Hydroxyapatite, 992
Hydroxyl radicals, 83*t*
11β-Hydroxysteroid dehydrogenase type 1, 222*b*
5-Hydroxytryptamine, 903*t*
Hydroxyurea, 528, 549
  for sickle cell disease, 567
Hygiene, 709*b*
Hyperactive confusional state. *See* Delirium
Hyperactivity, 383*t*
Hyperacute rejection, 211
Hyperaldosteronism, 128, 489
  primary, 124
Hyperalgesia, 344*t*
Hyperbaric oxygen therapy, 1029
Hyperbilirubinemia, 99–100, 563, 945
Hypercalcemia, 100, 127*t*, 257*t*, 475, 543–545
Hypercapnia, 129
  oxyhemoglobin dissociation curve affected by, 691–692
  pulmonary diseases causing, 697
Hyperchloremia, 121
Hypercoagulability, 554
Hypercortisolism, 487–489
Hypercyanotic spells, 669
Hyperemesis, 389–390
Hyperfunction, 760
Hyperglycemia, 470, 476–477, 479–481, 480*f*
Hypergonadotropic hypogonadism, 818*b*, 818*t*, 869*b*
Hyperhemolytic crisis, 566

Hyperkalemia
  clinical manifestations of, 125, 125t
  ECG findings with, 124f
  evaluation of, 125–126
  hypoxia as cause of, 125
  neuromuscular effects of, 125
  pathophysiology of, 125
  treatment of, 125–126
Hyperkinesia, 382, 383t
Hypermagnesemia, 127t
Hypermenorrhea, 821t
Hypermetabolism, MODS and, 654
Hypermethylation, 68–69
Hypernatremia, 121
Hyperopia, 352, 352f
Hyperosmolar hyperglycemic syndrome (HHS), 482–483, 482f, 483t
Hyperparathyroidism, 474–475
Hyperphosphatemia, 127t
Hyperpituitarism, 469
Hyperplasia
  atypical, 77, 845, 846f
  atypical ductal, 845, 846f
  atypical lobular, 845, 846f
  benign prostatic, 77, 876–878, 877f
  cellular adaptation and, 77, 78f
  compensatory, 152–153
  congenital adrenal, 489
  of endometrium, 77
  hormonal, 77
  mild, 844
  pathological, 77
  prostatic, 883
  usual ductal, 844
Hyperpolarization, 582
Hyperpolarized state, 24
Hypersecretion of GH, 469, 470f
Hypersensitivity
  definition of, 199–201
  examples of, 200t
  incidence of, 200t
  mechanisms of, 202–207, 202t
Hypersensitivity pneumonitis, 703
Hypersensitivity reactions
  antigenic targets of, 208–211
  characteristics of, 202, 202t
  definition of, 199–201
  delayed, 202
  immediate, 202
  type 1 (IgE-mediated)
    clinical manifestations of, 202–203, 204f, 205t
    evaluation and treatment of, 203
    mechanisms of, 202, 202t, 203f
  type II (tissue-specific), 202t, 203, 206f
  type III (immune complex-mediated), 202t, 205, 207f
  type IV (cell-mediated), 202t, 205–207, 207f
  types of, 86–88
Hypersomnia, 348
Hypersplenism, 545
Hypertension
  acromegaly-associated, 470
  aldosterone and, 607–608
  CAD and, 618
  Canadian prevention efforts for, 608b
  in children, 674–677, 674t, 675b, 676t
  classification of, 606, 606t
  complicated, 609–611, 609t
  coronary heart disease and, 223b
  diagnostic algorithm for, 606, 606f
  dietary potassium and lower risk of, 123b
  incidence of, 606
  intracranial, 378–379, 378f
  malignant, 609–610
  portal, 943–944, 944f, 981–982
  portopulmonary, 943
  primary, 674–675, 675b
    Indigenous people of Canada and, 607
    inflammation and, 608
    insulin resistance and, 608–609
    new immigrants and, 607
    obesity and, 608, 609b
    pathophysiology of, 607–609, 610f
    pressure-natriuresis relationship and, 607, 607f
    renin-angiotensin-aldosterone system in, 607–609
Hypertension *(Continued)*
    risk factors associated with, 606–607, 607b
    sympathetic nervous system and, 606–607, 634
  pulmonary artery, 698, 716–717, 716f
  secondary, 606, 674–675, 675b
    pathophysiology of, 609
Hypertensive crisis, 609–610
Hypertensive hypertrophic cardiomyopathy, 631
Hyperthermia, 346–347
  malignant, 347, 1014–1015
Hyperthyroidism, 471–473, 471f–472f, 643
Hypertonia, 381, 381f–382f, 381t
Hypertonic fluid alterations, 120f, 121
Hypertrophic cardiomyopathy, 631, 631f
Hypertrophic obstructive cardiomyopathy, 631, 631f
Hypertrophic osteoarthropathy, 257t
Hypertrophic scars, 154, 155f, 1081, 1081f, 1098f
Hypertrophy, 76–77, 76f
  compensatory, 760
  of heart, 584
  myocardial, 609
Hyperuricemia, 100–101
  asymptomatic, 1040
Hyperventilation, 696
Hypervolemic hypernatremia, 121
Hypervolemic hyponatremia, 122
Hypoactive confusional state, 371–373
Hypoactive delirium, 371–373
Hypoactive sexual desire, 842
Hypoalbuminemia, 771
Hypocalcemia, 127t, 475
Hypocapnia, 130–131, 696
Hypochloremia, 122
Hypochloremic metabolic alkalosis, 128
Hypocortisolism, 489–490
Hypodermis, 1074, 1075f, 1075t
Hypogammaglobulinemia, 192
Hypogeusia, 356
Hypoglossal nerve, 330t
Hypoglycemia, 257t, 482, 483t
Hypogonadotropic hypogonadism, 818b, 818t, 869b
Hypokalemia
  cardiac effects of, 124
  clinical manifestations of, 124, 125t
  diarrhea caused by, 124
  in ECF, 123
  ECG findings of, 124f
  evaluation of, 124–125
  insulin and, 124
  pathophysiology of, 123–124
  predisposing factors, 123
  treatment of, 124–125
Hypokinesia, 384
Hypomagnesemia, 127t, 475
Hypomethylation, 68–69
Hypomimesis, 389–390
Hyponatremia, 122, 122b
Hypoparathyroidism, 475–476
Hypoperfusion, 407
Hypophosphatemia, 127t, 475
Hypophysial portal system, 447–448, 450f
Hypopituitarism, 468, 469f
Hypopituitary dwarfism, 468, 469f
Hypoplastic anemia, 526
Hypoplastic kidneys, 786
Hypoplastic left heart syndrome (HLHS), 672, 672f
Hypopolarized state, 24
Hypoprothrombinemia, 976
Hyporeflexia, 387
Hyposmia, 356
Hypospadias, 784–785, 785f
Hypotension, orthostatic, 611
Hypothalamic-pituitary-adrenal (HPA) system
  alterations of, 466–471
  feedback mechanisms of, 221
  hormones of, 227, 447–452, 449f
  regulation of, 220–222
  schematic diagram of, 220f
  stress effects on, 223b
Hypothalamohypophysial tract, 447–448, 450f
Hypothalamus
  anatomy of, 447–448
  body heat conservation and, 345
  description of, 317–318
  functions of, 319b
  hormones produced by, 449t, 466f
  neurosecretory cells of, 447–448
  sleep and, 348
Hypothermia, 347, 347b
Hypothyroidism, 472f–474f, 473–474, 844
Hypotonia, 380–381, 381t
Hypotonic fluid alterations, 120f, 121–122
Hypoventilation, 696
Hypovolemia, 1096–1097
Hypovolemic hypernatremia, 121
Hypovolemic hyponatremia, 122
Hypovolemic shock, 648, 649f
Hypoxemia, 522
  clubbing from, 697, 697f
  pulmonary diseases causing, 697–698, 698f
Hypoxia, 487, 697
  cellular injury caused by, 80–82
  cellular responses to, 81–82
  cerebral, 93, 696
  chronic alveolar, 683
  hyperkalemia caused by, 125
  inflammation and, 80, 81f
  ischemia causing, 80–81, 80f
  progressive, 80–81
  tissue, 522
Hypoxia-inducible factor-1α, 247–248
Hypoxia-inducible transcription factor (HIF), 80
Hypoxic pulmonary vasoconstriction, 683

I

I bands, 585, 585f
IARC. *See* International Agency for Research on Cancer
IBD. *See* Inflammatory bowel disease
IBS. *See* irritable bowel syndrome
Ibuprofen (Advil), 619
ICF. *See* Intracellular fluid
Icterus gravis neonatorum, 563, 945
Icterus neonatorum, 563
Ictus, 377
Idiojunctional rhythm, 644t–645t
Idiopathic Addison's disease, 490
Idiopathic calcium urolithiasis, 761
Idiopathic inflammatory myopathies, 1045, 1045f
Idiopathic intestinal pseudo-obstruction, 971–972
Idiopathic pulmonary arterial hypertension, 716
Idiopathic pulmonary fibrosis (IPF), 702
Idioventricular rhythm, 644t–645t
IFNs. *See* Interferons
IgA deficiency, 192
IgE-mediated hypersensitivity reactions. *See* Immunoglobulin E-mediated hypersensitivity reactions
IGF-1. *See* Insulinlike growth factor 1
IGF-2. *See* Insulinlike growth factor 2
IGFs. *See* Insulinlike growth factors
IL-1. *See* Interleukin-1
IL-1β. *See* Interleukin-1β
IL-2. *See* Interleukin-2
IL-4. *See* Interleukin-4
IL-6. *See* Interleukin-6
IL-7. *See* Interleukin-7
IL-10. *See* Interleukin-10
IL-13. *See* Interleukin-13
Ileocecal valve, 905–906, 905f, 909
Ileogastric reflex, 909
Ileum, 905–906, 905f
  obstruction of, 970
IM. *See* infectious mononucleosis
Image processing, 369, 370t
Imatinib (Gleevec), 242–243, 263t, 538
Immediate hypersensitivity reactions, 202
Immigrants, primary hypertension and new, 607
Immovable joints, 995
Immune complex-mediated hypersensitivity reactions, 202t, 205, 207f
Immune (peripheral) CRH, 224
Immune deficiency. *See also* Acquired immunodeficiency syndrome
  care for, 193
  clinical presentation of, 190–191
  combined, 191–193, 192t, 193f
  definition of, 190
  evaluation for, 193, 194t
  primary (congenital), 190–193, 192t
  replacement therapies for, 193–195
  secondary (acquired), 190, 193, 194b
Immune response
  aging and, 174b
  B cells in, 165–171
  cellular interactions in, 169–171
  clonal diversity and clonal selection generation in, 165–168, 167t
  elderly and, 174b
  overview of, 161f
  primary, 168
  secondary, 168
  T cells in, 165–171
  from vaccination, 189
Immune system
  burn response of, 1098
  cancer cell evasion from, 252–253, 253f
  CKD and, 776t, 779
  micro-organisms defenses against, 180t
  neuropeptides effect on, 227
  secretory, 165, 166f
  in stress, 227, 227f
  systemic, 165
Immune thrombocytopenic purpura (ITP), 549
  in children, 569–570
Immunity. *See also* Adaptive immunity; Innate immunity
  active, 160
  cell-mediated, 171–173
  cellular, 160
  description of, 135, 136t
  GI tract and, 910
  herd, 190
  humoral, 160
  lymphocytes and, 149
  NK cells and, 149, 173
  passive, 160
Immunization, active, 189–190
Immunocompetent cells, 160
Immunocytes, 507
Immunogenicity, 190
Immunogens, antigens compared to, 161
Immunoglobulin A nephropathy, 787
Immunoglobulin A pemphigus, 1086
Immunoglobulin E-mediated (IgE-mediated) hypersensitivity reactions
  clinical manifestations of, 202–203, 204f, 205t
  evaluation and treatment of, 203
  mechanisms of, 202, 202t, 203f
Immunoglobulins
  A, 162
  antibodies compared to, 161–162
  classes of, 162–163, 163f, 163t
  D, 162
  E, 162, 164–165, 165f
  G, 162
  M, 162
  molecular structure of, 162–163, 163f
  polypeptide chains of, 162–163
  secretory, 165
Immunological injury, 96
Immunoreactive trypsinogen, 737
Immunotherapy
  cancer treatment with, 263
  passive, 190
Impacted fractures, 1012f, 1012t
Impaired hemostasis, 550
Impetigo, 1087, 1109–1110, 1109b, 1110f
Imprinting, genomic. *See* Genomic imprinting
Inbreeding, 54

Incised wound, 94*t*–95*t*
Inclusion body myositis, 1045
Incomplete fractures, 1011–1012, 1012*t*
Incomplete penetrance, 51
Incontinence, 762*t*, 790, 790*t*
Increased intracranial pressure, 378–379, 378*f*
Incretins, 481
Incus, 354, 354*f*
Indeterminate range entrance wound, 94*t*–95*t*
Indigenous people in Canada
  asthma and, 706*b*
  primary hypertension and, 607
  tuberculosis and, 194*b*
Indirect Coombs test, 514*t*–516*t*
Indomethacin, 667
Induced pluripotent stem cells, 108
Induction chemotherapy, 263
Induration, 207
Infantile hypertrophic pyloric stenosis, 969–970
Infantile spasms, 436*t*
Infants
  diarrhea in, 979
  HIV in, 199
  hypothyroidism in, 473–474
  innate immunity and, 155*b*
  left ventricular failure in, 672–673
  oxygen toxicity in, 703
  pain perception in, 341*t*
  reflexes in, 426–427, 427*t*
  renal function and, 756
  skull of, 426
  sleep characteristics of, 348*b*
  SUID and, 737, 737*b*
  TBW in, 132*b*
  thermoregulation in, 345–346
Infarct, 103
Infarction, 617
Infections. *See also* specific infections
  active immunization against, 189–190
  antimicrobials treating, 188–189, 188*t*
  bacterial, 180*t*–181*t*, 1087–1088, 1087*f*, 1109–1110, 1109*b*, 1110*f*
  bone
    osteomyelitis, 1028–1029, 1028*f*–1029*f*, 1062–1063, 1063*b*, 1063*f*
    septic, 1063–1064
  CAD and, 620
  cancer and, 259, 259*t*, 292–293, 293*t*
  central nervous system disorders and, 411–415, 412*f*
  of CNS, 435
  control measures for, 188
  countermeasures against, 188, 188*t*
  diabetes mellitus complications with, 484*t*, 486
  of ear, 355
  eye, 180*t*–181*t*, 353–354
  female reproductive system disorders with, 823–827
  fungal, 1089, 1089*f*, 1089*t*–1090*t*, 1110–1111, 1110*f*
  gastro-intestinal, 180*t*–181*t*
  global prevalence of, 177
  leukemia and, 536*t*
  opportunistic, 177–178
    AIDS and, 196*b*
    HIV and, 414–415
  otitis media, 180*t*–181*t*, 356
  passive immunotherapy for, 190
  pleural effusion, 700
  respiratory tract (*See* Respiratory tract infections)
  sexually transmitted, 180*t*–181*t*
  skin, 180*t*–181*t*, 1087–1089, 1087*f*–1089*f*, 1089*t*
    in children, 1109–1113
  tonsillar, 727
  upper airway, in children, 725–727, 726*t*
  urinary tract (*See* Urinary tract infection)
  viral, 1088–1089, 1088*f*–1089*f*, 1111–1113, 1111*f*–1113*f*, 1112*t*
  wound, 180*t*–181*t*
  zoonotic, 180*t*–181*t*, 183
Infectious diseases, 177
Infectious injuries, 96
Infectious mononucleosis (IM), 531–532
Infectious viral encephalitides, 413, 413*t*
Infective endocarditis, 637–638, 637*b*, 637*f*–638*f*
Inferior colliculi, 319
Inferior vena cava, 577, 577*f*
Infertility, 843
Infiltrating lobular carcinoma, 856*t*
Infiltrations. *See* Cellular accumulations
Infiltrative splenomegaly, 546
Inflammasomes, 143
Inflammation
  activation of, 138–139
  acute, 150, 150*t*
  acute-phase reactants during, 150, 150*t*
  adaptive immunity compared to, 159
  benefits of, 139
  biologic mediators during, 145*f*
  in cachexia, 256
  CAD and markers of, 619
  capillary permeability affected by, 117
  cellular components of, 142–149, 142*f*
  cellular products of, 143–145
  central nervous system disorders and, 411–415
  of cervix, 826–827
  chronic, 150–152, 151*f*, 251, 251*t*
  of endothelium, 146, 612–613
  of epididymis, 876, 876*f*
  exudate of, 150
  female reproductive system disorders with, 823–827
  fever and, 150
  gastric, 251
  hypoxia and, 80, 81*f*
  of injured endothelial cells, 614
  ischemic injury as cause of, 82
  leukocytosis in, 150
  local changes in, 138*f*
  mediators of, 144*f*, 146
  in MODS, 653, 654*t*
  phagocytes in, 146–149
  plasma protein synthesis and, 150
  plasma protein systems in, 140–142, 140*f*
  platelets in, 146
  primary hypertension and, 608
  prostate cancer and chronic, 883, 883*f*–884*f*
  resolution phase of, 152
  signs of, 138–139
  tumour-promoting, 250–252, 251*t*
  type 2 diabetes mellitus and, 222*b*
  wound healing and, 153, 153*f*
Inflammatory acne, 1107
Inflammatory bowel disease (IBD), 935–938, 936*b*, 936*t*
Inflammatory carcinoma, 856*t*
Inflammatory cytokines, 481
Inflammatory injury, 96
Inflammatory joint disease, 1031–1032. *See also* Arthritis
  ankylosing spondylitis, 209, 1035–1038, 1037*f*
  gout, 1038–1040, 1038*f*–1039*f*, 1038*t*
  infectious, 1032
  noninfectious, 1032
  rheumatoid arthritis (*See* Rheumatoid arthritis)
Inflammatory response
  acute, 139, 139*f*, 149–150
  definition of, 135, 138
Influenza
  antigenic shifts in, 185, 185*f*
  description of, 185
Infratentorial disorders, 364, 365*t*
Infratentorial herniation, 379*b*, 379*f*
Infundibulum, 800, 800*f*
Inguinal canals, 807, 807*f*
Inhalation disorders, 702–703
Inheritance
  autosomal dominant
    delayed age of onset, 51
    epigenetics and, 52, 53*f*
    expressivity and, 51–52, 52*f*
    genomic imprinting and, 52
Inheritance (*Continued*)
    pedigrees and, 50, 51*f*
    penetrance and, 51–52, 51*f*
    recurrence risks of, 50–51
  autosomal recessive
    consanguinity and, 54
    pedigrees in, 52–53, 53*f*
    recurrence risks and, 53–54, 54*f*
  chromosome theory of, 50
  of epigenetic states, 66–68
  mode of, 50
  multifactorial, 58–59, 58*f*, 59*b*
  sex linked, 54
  X-linked
    pedigrees and, 55
    recurrence risks in, 55–56, 56*f*
    sex determination and, 54–55, 55*f*
    sex-limited and sex-influenced traits in, 56
    X inactivation and, 54, 54*f*
Inherited hemorrhagic disease, 569
Inherited metabolic disorders of CNS, 433–434, 433*t*, 434*f*
Inhibin, 794*t*, 804
Inhibitory neurotransmitters, 341
Inhibitory postsynaptic potentials (IPSPs), 313
Injuries
  asphyxial, 93–96
  immunological, 96
  infectious, 96
  inflammatory, 96
  intentional, 93–96, 94*t*–95*t*
  unintentional, 93–96, 94*t*–95*t*
Innate immunity. *See also* Inflammation
  adaptive immunity interaction with, 159
  aging and, 155*b*
  cells of, 142
  defects in, 191, 192*t*, 193
  definition of, 135
  description of, 136*t*
  elderly and, 155*b*
  infants and, 155*b*
  microbiome and, 137–138, 137*t*
  natural barriers in, 135
  physical barriers and, 135, 135*f*
Inner dura, 323
Inner ear, 354–355, 354*f*–355*f*
Inorganic ions, in plasma, 497
Inositol triphosphate, 447, 447*t*
Inotropic agents, 588
Inotropic effect, 224
Insect bites, 1113–1115, 1114*f*–1115*f*
Insomnia, 348
Inspiration
  forces during, 687*f*
  muscles of, 686, 686*f*
Institute of Medicine, US, 853
Insufficiency fractures, 1012–1013
Insula, 317
Insular lobe, 317
Insulin, 222*b*, 914
  actions of, 456*f*, 456*t*
  glucose uptake affected by, 455–456
  hypokalemia caused by, 124
  potassium regulation by, 123
  secretion of, 443, 455
  synthesis of, 455
Insulin resistance
  CAD and, 618
  definition of, 479–481
  diabetes mellitus and, 852
  obesity contributing to, 481
  in PCOS, 822
  primary hypertension and, 608–609
Insulinlike growth factor 1 (IGF-1), 26*t*
Insulinlike growth factor 2 (IGF-2), 26*t*, 65–66
Insulinlike growth factors (IGFs)
  aging and, 451*b*, 461*b*
  in bone formation, 991*t*
  breast cancer and, 819
  functions of, 448–451
Integral membrane proteins, 7
Integrin, 990
Integrin αIIbβ3, 510
Integumentary system. *See* Skin
Intensity of pain, 338–339
Intentional injuries, 93–96, 94*t*–95*t*
Intentional tremor, 383*t*
Intercalated cells, 744
Intercalated discs, 584–585, 584*f*
Intercostal muscles, 686, 686*f*
Intercourse pain, 842
Interferon regulatory factors (IRFs), 142–143
Interferons (IFNs), 145
Interleukin-1 (IL-1), 144, 169, 183
Interleukin-1β (IL-1β), 652*b*
Interleukin-2 (IL-2), 26*t*, 169
Interleukin-4 (IL-4), 170–171
Interleukin-6 (IL-6), 144, 183, 652*b*
Interleukin-7 (IL-7), 168
Interleukin-10 (IL-10), 145
Interleukin-13 (IL-13), 170–171
Interleukins, 143
Interlobar arteries, 745
Interlobular adipocytes, 104*f*
Intermediate range entrance wound, 94*t*–95*t*
Intermittent claudication, 617
Internal anal sphincter, 909
Internal capsule, 317, 319*f*
Internal carotid arteries, 325, 326*f*
Internal fixation, of fractures, 1014
Internal hydrocephalus, 380, 380*t*
Internal urethral sphincter, 746, 746*f*
International Agency for Research on Cancer (IARC), 268, 276–277, 293–294
International Myeloma Working Group, 544–545
Interneurons, 310
Interphase, 25
INTERPHONE study, 291
Interpretive centres, 339
Interstitial cystitis, 766–767
Interstitial edema, 380
Interstitial fluid
  definition of, 115
  lymphatic system absorption of, 117
  water movement between plasma and, 115–116, 117*f*
Interstitial hydrostatic pressure, 116
Interstitial oncotic pressure, 116
Interventricular foramen, 323–324
Intervertebral disc, 324–325, 325*f*
Intestinal obstruction
  causes of, 928, 928*t*
  classification of, 929*t*
  clinical manifestations of, 929
  evaluation of, 929
  pathophysiology of, 928–929, 930*f*
  treatment of, 929
Intestinointestinal reflex, 909
Intoxications, of CNS, 434–435, 434*t*
Intracardiac pressures, 578, 578*t*
Intracellular fluid (ICF)
  definition of, 115
  description of, 18–19
  potassium concentration in, 123, 125
  water movement between ECF and, 116
Intracellular overhydration, 121–122
Intracerebral hematomas, 395*t*, 397, 397*f*
Intracranial aneurysm, 408–409, 409*f*
Intracranial hemorrhage, 408, 435
Intracranial hypertension, 378–379, 378*f*
Intracranial pressure, 377–379, 378*b*, 378*f*
Intractable pain, 343
Intraductal carcinoma, 856*t*
Intraductal papillomas, 844
Intrahepatic jaundice, 945–946, 947*t*
Intrahepatic portal hypertension, 982
Intramural plexus, 899, 900*f*
Intraparenchymal hemorrhagic stroke, 408
Intraprostatic conversion, 882, 882*f*
Intrarenal acute kidney injury, 773–774, 773*t*
Intrarenal blood flow, autoregulation of, 746–747, 747*f*
Intravascular fluid, 115
Intraventricular hydrocephalus, 380, 380*t*
Intrinsic tissue factor, 141, 523, 904
Introns, 41, 64
Intussusception, 973–974, 974*f*

Inverse acne, 1108
Inverse psoriasis, 1083
Inversions, 47
Involucrum, 1028, 1029*f*, 1062–1063
Iodine deficiency, 854
Ionizing radiation
  acute effects of, 288–289
  breast cancer caused by, 853
  bystander effects of, 288, 288*f*
  cancer and, 285–289, 286*t*, 287*f*
  CT scans and, 287*b*
  definition of, 286–287
  excess relative risks with, 286
  exposure to, 286, 286*t*
  genomic instability caused by, 288
  latent effects of, 288–289
  low-dose, 289, 289*b*
  microenvironmental effects of, 288–289
  nontargeted effects of, 288, 288*f*
  responses to, 288*b*
Ions, 7–8, 18–19
IPF. *See* Idiopathic pulmonary fibrosis
IPSPs. *See* Inhibitory postsynaptic potentials
IRFs. *See* Interferon regulatory factors
Iron
  dietary sources of, 560–561
  tissue cell storage of, 99
Iron cycle, 508–509, 509*f*
Iron deficiency anemia, 521*t*, 524–525, 524*f*–525*f*
  in children, 560–562, 561*b*
    clinical manifestations of, 562
    evaluation and treatment of, 562
    pathophysiology of, 561–562
Iron overload, 529
Iron replacement therapy, 525
Irregular bones, 994–995
Irreversible coma, 368–369
Irritable bowel syndrome (IBS), 938, 938*b*
Irritant contact dermatitis, 1082
Irritant receptors, 684
Irritative syndrome, 421
Ischemia, 154, 611–612, 697. *See also* Myocardial ischemia
  hypoxia caused by, 80–81, 80*f*
  inflammation caused by, 82
  mental stress-induced, 621, 621*f*–622*f*
  peripheral artery disease and, 617
  silent, 621, 621*f*–622*f*
Ischemia-reperfusion injury, 82, 82*f*
Ischemic infarcts, 407
Ischemic penumbra, 407
Ischemic phase, 803, 803*f*
Ischemic stroke, 407–408, 435
Ischemic ulcers, 933
Islets of Langerhans, 455, 455*f*
Isoflavones, 854
Isohemagglutinins, 210
Isolated cleft palate, 968
Isometric muscle contraction, 1006, 1006*f*
Isothiocyanates, 281–282
Isotonic fluid alterations, 120*f*, 121
Isotonic fluid excess, 121
Isotonic fluid loss, 121
Isotropic bands, 585, 585*f*
Isovolemic hypernatremia, 121
Isovolemic hyponatremia, 122
Isthmus, 452
ITP. *See* Immune thrombocytopenic purpura

J

JAK2 gene (Janus kinase gene), 526–528
Jamestown encephalitis, 413*t*
Janus family of tyrosine kinases, 447
Janus kinase gene (*JAK2 gene*), 526–528
Jaundice, 99–100
  hemolytic, 946, 947*t*
  intrahepatic, 945–946, 947*t*
  liver disorders and, 945–946, 946*f*
  neonatal, 563, 979–980
  in newborns, 945
  obstructive, 945–946, 947*t*
  types of, 947*t*
Jaw, bisphosphonate-related osteonecrosis of, 1026*b*
Jejunum, 905–906, 905*f*
  obstruction of, 970
Jerk nystagmus, 350
Joint capsule, 995–996
Joint cavity, 997
Joint disorders, 1029–1032, 1030*f*, 1031*b*, 1032*f*
Joint effusion, 1031
Joint stiffness, 1031
Joints. *See also* Bone
  aging of, 1007
  cartilaginous, 995–997, 997*f*
  definition of, 995
  fibrous, 995, 997*f*
  freely movable, 995
  immovable, 995
  slightly movable, 995
  synovial, 997*f*–1000*f*, 998
  types of, 995, 997*f*
Jones criteria, 636, 636*t*
J-receptors, 684
Junctional bradycardia, 644*t*–645*t*
Junctional complex, 12, 13*f*
Junctional tachycardia, 644*t*–645*t*
Juvenile dermatomyositis, 1045
Juvenile idiopathic arthritis, 1064, 1064*t*
Juvenile myoclonic epilepsy, 436*t*
Juxtaglomerular apparatus, 742*f*, 743
Juxtamedullary nephrons, 743, 744*f*

K

K vitamins, 989*t*
  deficiency, 550
Kaposi sarcoma, 252, 270*t*–273*t*, 307, 1094–1095, 1094*f*
Karyogram, 42
Karyolysis, 101–102
Karyorrhexis, 101–102
Karyotype, 42, 44*f*
Kawasaki disease, 673–674, 674*b*
Kegel exercises, 828
Keloids, 154, 155*f*, 1079*t*–1080*t*, 1081, 1081*f*
Keratitis, 354
Keratoacanthoma, 1091
Kernicterus, 563, 979–980
Kernig sign, 409–410
Kidney disorders
  acute kidney injury (*See* Acute kidney injury)
  Ask-Upmark, 786
  in children (*See* Children, renal disorders in)
  chronic kidney disease (*See* Chronic kidney disease)
  hypoplastic, 786
  kidney dysfunction, 772
  polycystic kidney disease, 786
  renal agenesis, 786
Kidney failure, 754*b*, 772
Kidney stones, 760–761, 767*t*
Kidneys
  acid excretion by, 130*f*
  acid-base buffering by, 126–128, 130*f*
  anatomy of, 741–745, 742*f*–745*f*
  Ask-Upmark, 786
  blood vessels of, 744–745
  cancer of, 270*t*–273*t*
  damage to, 775
  definition of, 741
  dysfunction of, 772
  ectopic, 784
  erythropoietin and, 753
  function of, 741, 747–753
  glomerulus (*See* Glomerulus)
  horseshoe, 784
  hydronephrosis of, 759–760, 760*f*
  hypoplastic, 786
  lobes of, 741, 742*f*
  nephron (*See* Nephron)
  structures of, 741–745, 742*f*–745*f*
  substances transported in tubules of, 750*b*
  vitamin D and, 752
  Wilms tumour and, 305
Kinin cascade, 140
Kinin system, 140*f*, 141
Kissing disease, 532
Klebsiella pneumoniae, 700
Klinefelter's syndrome, 46, 47*t*, 48*f*, 54
Klinefelter's variant, 663*t*
Knee joints. *See* Synovial joints
Koilonychia, 524, 525*f*
Konno procedure, 665
Krebs cycle, 16
Kupffer cells, 507–508, 911–913
Kussmaul respirations, 128, 696
Kwashiorkor, 977
Kyphosis, 1023–1024, 1025*f*, 1037

L

La Crosse encephalitis, 413*t*
Labia majora, 797, 797*f*
Labia minora, 797, 797*f*
Lacerations, 94*t*–95*t*
Lacrimal apparatus, 353, 353*f*
β-Lactamase, 183
Lactase deficiency, 935
Lactate dehydrogenase (LDH), 548, 916*t*
Lactation, inappropriate, 843–844
Lacteal, 906
Lactic acid, 17
Lactobacillus sp., 138, 186
Lactose intolerance, 979
Lactose malabsorption, 979
Lacuna, 990
Lacunar infarcts, 407
Lacunar strokes, 407
Lamellae, 993, 993*f*
Lamina propria, 905*f*, 906
Laminar blood flow, 594, 594*f*
Laminin, 989*t*
Laplace's law, 587, 686
Large bowel obstruction, 928*t*, 929
Large cell carcinoma, 718*t*, 719
Large intestine, 909–910, 909*f*, 918
  obstruction of, 929
Laryngeal box, 679
Laryngotracheitis, 725, 726*t*
Larynx
  anatomy of, 679, 680*f*–681*f*
  cancer of, 270*t*–273*t*, 717–718, 717*f*
Lasix, 753*t*, 945
Latent tuberculosis infection (LTBI), 714
Late-onset Pompe's disease, 1044
Lateral apertures, 323–324
Lateral columns, 320–321, 321*f*
Lateral corticospinal tract, 322
Lateral epicondylopathy, 1015
Lateral fissure, 315–316
Lateral horn, 320–321
Lateral spinothalamic tracts, 323
Lateral sulcus, 315–316, 316*f*
Laughter, pathological, 389–390
LBB. *See* Left bundle branch
LDH. *See* Lactate dehydrogenase
LDL. *See* Low-density lipoprotein
Lead
  blood levels of, 88–89
  cellular injury caused by, 88–90
  children exposed to, 88*b*, 89, 90*f*
  exposure sources of, 90*t*
Lead poisoning, 435
Lead-pipe rigidity, 381, 381*t*
Leak point pressure measurement, 755*t*
Lectin pathway, of complement system, 141
Lee-White coagulation time, 514*t*–516*t*
Left atrioventricular valve, 577, 577*f*–578*f*
Left atrium, 577, 577*f*
Left bundle branch (LBB), 582
Left coronary artery, 578, 579*b*, 581*f*
Left ventricle, 577, 577*f*
Left ventricular failure
  clinical manifestations of, 641
  description of, 639–642
  in HIV, 638
  in infants, 672–673
  management of, 641
Left ventricular hypertrophy (LVH), 76–77
Left-to-right shunting, 662–663, 664*f*
Legg-Calvé-Perthes disease, 1065, 1065*f*–1066*f*
Leiomyomas, 235–236, 236*f*, 831, 831*f*
Leiomyosarcoma, 1050
Lennox-Gastaut syndrome, 436*t*
Lens, 349–350
Lentiform nucleus, 317, 319*f*
Lentigo malignant melanoma, 1093–1094, 1094*f*
Leptin, 854, 941, 941*b*
Leukemia, 270*t*–273*t*
  acute lymphocytic, 305, 533–536, 534*t*
    in children, 570
  acute myeloid, 533–536, 534*t*
    in children, 570
  anemia and, 536*t*
  bleeding and, 536*t*
  bone pain and, 536*t*
  chemotherapy for, 536
  in children, 303, 570–571, 571*f*
    clinical manifestations of, 570–571
    evaluation and treatment of, 571
    pathophysiology of, 570
  chronic lymphocytic, 533, 534*t*, 536–538
  chronic myeloid, 242–243, 533, 534*t*, 536–538, 537*f*
    in children, 571
  classification of, 533
  clinical manifestations in, 535, 536*t*, 537
  definition of, 236, 532, 570
  Down syndrome risks with, 305
  genetic factors with, 305
  infections and, 536*t*
  new cases and deaths from, in Canada, 534*t*
  origin of, 533*f*
  pathophysiology of, 533–537
  Philadelphia chromosome in, 533–534, 534*f*
  related pathophysiology in, 535, 536*t*
  risk factors for, 534
  stem-like cancer cells progressing to, 535, 535*f*
  treatment of, 535–538
  weight loss and, 536*t*
Leukemic cells, 570
Leukemoid reaction, 530–531
Leukocoria, 440
Leukocytes. *See also* Lymphocytes; Phagocytes
  agranulocytes, 499, 507
  basophils, 142*f*, 145–147, 499, 499*t*, 530*t*
  description of, 142, 142*f*
  development of, 509
  disorders involving, 529–538
    agranulocytosis, 531
    basopenia, 530*t*, 531
    basophilia, 530*t*, 531
    eosinopenia, 530*t*, 531
    eosinophilia, 530*t*, 531
    granulocytopenia, 531
    granulocytosis, 530, 530*t*
    infectious mononucleosis, 531–532
    leukemia (*See* Leukemia)
    lymphocytosis, 530*t*, 531
    monocytopenia, 530*t*, 531
    monocytosis, 530*t*, 531
    neutropenia, 530*t*, 531
    neutrophilia, 530, 530*t*
    quantitative alterations, 529–538
  eosinophils, 142*f*, 147, 499, 499*t*, 530*t*, 706
  function of, 501*f*, 507
  granulocytes, 142, 142*f*, 498–499, 507, 509, 529–531, 530*t*
  immunocytes, 507
  laboratory tests for, 514*t*–516*t*
  lymphocytopenia, 530*t*, 531
  monocytes, 142, 142*f*, 147, 499, 499*t*, 509, 529–531, 530*t*
  neutrophils, 142*f*, 147, 498–499, 530*t*
  NK cells, 149, 173, 221–222, 499, 499*t*
Leukocytosis, 150, 529
Leukopenia, 259, 529
Leukotrienes, 146
Level of consciousness, 364, 365*t*
Levitra, 888
Leydig cells, 807
LH. *See* Luteinizing hormone
Libido
  aging and, 812
  decreased, 842
  testosterone and, 810

Lice infections, 1114
Lichenification, 1079*t*–1080*t*
Lieberkühn crypts, 909, 909*f*
Life expectancy, 108
Lifespan
  definition of, 107
  normal, 108
Li-Fraumeni syndrome, 244, 305
Ligaments, 1006, 1007*f*
  sprains and strains of, 1015
Ligands, 9
Ligature strangulations, 95
Limbic system, 317, 319*f*
Linear fracture, 1011–1012, 1012*t*
Linkage analysis, 56–57, 56*f*
Linoleic acid, 880*b*–881*b*
Lipid bilayer, of plasma membrane
  description of, 2–3, 5*f*
  proteins associated with, 7, 8*f*
Lipid deficiency, 1044
Lipid peroxidation, 83, 86
Lipid rafts, 5, 6*f*–7*f*
Lipids
  amphipathic, 3–5
  as cellular accumulations, 97–98, 98*f*
  liver cell accumulation of, 98, 98*f*
  metabolism of, 617–618
  of plasma membrane, 3–5, 7*f*
Lipid-soluble hormones, 444, 444*t*, 447, 448*f*
Lipofuscin, 75–76
Lipoid nephrosis, 787
Lipomas, 235–236
Lipopolysaccharide, 183
Lipoprotein(a), 618
Lipoproteins, 497
  definition of, 617
  high-density, 618
  low-density, 548
    CAD and, 618
    oxidation of, 614, 616*f*
  very-low-density, 617–618
Lips
  cancer of, 270*t*–273*t*, 1093, 1093*f*
  cleft, 968–969
Liquefactive necrosis, 103, 104*f*
Liver
  aging effects on, 917*t*
  anatomy of, 911, 911*f*
  bile secretion of, 913*f*, 914
  bilirubin metabolism and, 913, 913*f*, 916*t*
  blood supply to, 911, 912*f*
  cancer of, 954*t*, 957–958, 957*b*
  function, tests of, 916*t*
  hematological functions of, 913–914
  injury to, chemicals causing, 85, 87*f*–88*f*
  lobules, 911, 912*f*
  metabolic detoxification of, 914
  metabolic functions of, 911, 912*f*
  mineral storage in, 914
  nutrient metabolism of, 914, 914*t*
  vascular functions of, 913–914
  vitamin storage in, 914
Liver cells, 98, 98*f*
Liver disease, 550, 948
Liver disorders
  acute liver failure, 915*b*, 947
  in children
    biliary atresia, 980
    cirrhosis, 981
    hepatitis, 980–981
    metabolic disorders, 982, 983*t*
    neonatal jaundice, 563, 979–980
    portal hypertension, 981–982
  cirrhosis (*See* Cirrhosis)
  complications of
    ascites, 117, 944–945, 944*f*–945*f*
    hepatic encephalopathy, 945
    hepatorenal syndrome, 946–947
    jaundice, 945–946, 946*f*
    portal hypertension, 943–944, 944*f*
  viral hepatitis, 950–951, 950*t*
Lobes, of kidney, 741, 742*f*
Lobular carcinoma in situ, 856*t*, 859–860
Lobular involution, 849–850, 850*f*
Localized edema, 117
Localized lymphadenopathy, 538
Localized scleroderma, 1090
Locked-in syndrome, 369
Locus, 49
Long bones, 994
Longitudinal fissure, 315–316
Long-term starvation, 943
Loop of Henle, 743–744, 743*f*, 750–752
Loose areolar connective tissue, 31*f*, 31*t*–33*t*
Low back pain, 402–403
Low bladder wall compliance, 763
Low-density lipoprotein (LDL), 548
  CAD and, 618
  oxidation of, 614, 616*f*
Low-dose ionizing radiation, 289, 289*b*
Lower airways, 682*f*
  disorders of, 728–737
Lower esophageal sphincter, 901–902
Lower gastro-intestinal bleeding, 924
Lower motor neuron syndromes, 385*t*, 386–387, 387*f*
Lower motor neurons, 322
Lower respiratory tract infections, 180*t*–181*t*
Lown-Ganong-Levine syndrome, 645*t*–646*t*
LTBI. *See* Latent tuberculosis infection
Lumbar lordosis, 1037
Lumbar plexus, 328
Lumen, 589, 593–594
Lung cancer
  clinical manifestations of, 720
  definition of, 718
  description of, 270*t*–273*t*
  evaluation of, 720
  genetic risks of, 718–719
  incidence of, 720*b*
  pathophysiology of, 720
  TNM staging of, 720
  tobacco smoking causing, 718–719
  treatment of, 720
  types of, 718*t*, 719–720, 719*f*
Lung receptors, 684–685
Lungs
  acinus of, 680
  aging and, 692
  air pollution and health of, 709*b*
  alveolar pressure in, 690, 690*f*
  alveoli of, 680, 682*f*–683*f*
  ANS innervation of, 685
  bronchi of, 680, 682*f*
  capacity of, 688*f*
  compliance of, 687
  defense mechanisms of, 679, 680*t*
  elastic properties of, 687–688, 687*f*
  epithelial cells of, 681
  gravity effects on, 689–690, 690*f*
  health guidelines for, 709*b*
  hila of, 680
  lobes of, 679
  oxygen transport in, 690–692
  restrictive diseases of, 701–704
  tobacco smoking and, 709*b*
  vasculature of, 683
Lupus erythematosus, 1085, 1086*f*
  systemic, 209–210
Lupus nephritis, 770
Luteal phase, 803, 803*f*
Luteinizing hormone (LH), 448–451, 449*f*, 451*t*
  deficiency of, 468
  functions of, 794*t*
  in menstrual cycle, 804
  production of, 794
LVH. *See* Left ventricular hypertrophy
Lyme disease, 1087–1088
Lymph, 502–503, 575
  composition of, 599
Lymph nodes, 502–503, 503*f*, 599, 600*f*
  enlargement of, 538, 538*f*–539*f*
  RS cells and, 539, 539*f*
Lymphadenopathy, 538, 538*f*
Lymphatic capillary, 906
Lymphatic system
  anatomy of, 599, 600*f*
  of breasts, 806, 806*f*
  definition of, 599
  disorders involving, 538–545
    lymphadenopathy, 538, 538*f*
    lymphomas (*See* Lymphomas)
  functions of, 599
  interstitial fluid absorption by, 117
Lymphatic veins, 599, 600*f*
Lymphatic venules, 599
Lymphatic vessels, 580, 581*f*
  efferent, 599, 600*f*
Lymphedema, 117
Lymphoblastic lymphoma, 542
Lymphoblasts, 570
Lymphocyte count, 514*t*–516*t*, 516*b*
Lymphocytes
  alterations to, 530*t*, 531
  description of, 142, 142*f*, 159–160, 160*f*, 499, 499*t*
  immunity and, 149
  tumour-infiltrating, 253
Lymphocytopenia, 530*t*, 531
Lymphocytosis, 530*t*, 531
Lymphogranuloma venereum, 892*t*–894*t*
Lymphoid organs
  description of, 500–503
  lymph nodes, 502–503, 503*f*
  mononuclear phagocyte system, 503, 503*t*
  primary, 165–167, 500
  secondary, 160, 162*f*, 500
  spleen, 500–502, 502*f*
Lymphoid stem cells, 165–167
Lymphoid tissues, of secretory immune system, 165
Lymphokines, 143
  T cells secreting, 173
Lymphomas, 270*t*–273*t*
  Burkitt, 242, 541–542, 542*f*
    in children, 571–572
  in children, 303, 571–572
    Burkitt, 571–572
    Hodgkin's, 572, 572*f*
    non-Hodgkin's, 571–572
  definition of, 236, 571
  Hodgkin's, 303–304
    in children, 572, 572*f*
    clinical manifestations of, 539, 539*f*, 542*f*
    pathophysiology of, 539, 539*f*
    stages of, 540, 540*t*
    treatment of, 540
  incidence rates of, in Canada, 538
  lymphoblastic, 542
  malignant, 538–545
  mucosa-associated lymphoid tissue, 251
  multiple myeloma, 542–545, 543*f*–544*f*
  non-Hodgkin's, 304
    in children, 571–572
    clinical manifestations of, 541, 541*t*
    definition of, 540
    incidence of, 540
    pathophysiology of, 540–541
    treatment of, 541
  primary cutaneous, 1095
Lynch syndrome, 956
Lysosomal storage diseases, 434
Lysosomes, 21–23, 23*f*
  characteristics of, 4*t*
Lysozyme, 137
Lytic lesions, 543–544

M

M line, 585, 585*f*
M phase, in cell cycle, 25, 25*f*
M protein, 543, 544*f*
MAC. *See* Membrane attack complex
Macewen sign, 432
Macrocytic-normochromic anemia, 521*t*, 522–524
Macromolecules, 10–11
Macrophages, 31*t*–33*t*, 96–97, 499
  alveolar, 681, 682*f*
  in atherogenesis, 614
  steroids effects on, 154
  tissue, 911–912
  tumour-associated, 251–252, 255
  in wound healing, 147, 153
Macrovascular disease, 484*t*, 485–486
Macula densa, 743, 745*f*
Macula lutea, 349, 349*f*
Maculae, 354–355
Macular edema, 484–485
Macule, 1077*t*–1078*t*
Magnesium balance, alterations in, 126, 127*t*
Magnetic fields, childhood cancers and, 306*b*
Magnetic resonance imaging (MRI), 1029
Major duodenal papilla, 910–911
Major histocompatibility complex (MHC), 169, 191, 211
Malabsorption, 935
Malabsorption syndromes, 935
Maladaptive coping, 229
Malaria, 187–188
Maldigestion, 935
Male breast, 807
Male breast cancer, 891
Male breast disorders, 890–891
Male reproductive system
  aging and, 812
  andropause and, 812
  bulbourethral glands, 809, 809*f*
  development of, 793–796
  ejaculatory duct, 809
  epididymis, 808–809, 808*f*
  external genitalia of, 796*f*, 807–809, 807*f*–809*f*
  internal genitalia of, 795*f*, 809
  penis (*See* Penis)
  prostate gland, 763, 809, 809*f*
  scrotum, 808, 808*f*
  seminal vesicles, 809, 809*f*
  sex hormones of, 794*t*, 810
  spermatogenesis, 810, 810*f*
  testes (*See* Testes)
  vas deferens, 809*f*
Male reproductive system disorders
  benign prostatic hyperplasia, 876–878, 877*f*
  cryptorchidism, 873–874
  delayed puberty, 868, 869*b*
  ectopic testes, 873–874
  epididymitis, 876, 876*f*
  gynecomastia, 890–891
  hydrocele, 873, 873*f*
  male breast cancer, 891
  male breast disorders, 890–891
  orchitis, 874–875, 875*f*
  penis disorders (*See* Penis disorders)
  precocious puberty, 868–869, 869*b*
  prostate cancer (*See* Prostate cancer)
  prostate gland disorders, 876–887
  prostatitis, 878–879, 878*b*
  scrotal disorders, 872–876, 873*f*
  sexual dysfunction, 888–890
  sexual maturation alterations, 868–869
  sexually transmitted infections, 891–894, 892*t*–894*t*
  sperm production impairment, 888–890
  spermatocele, 873, 873*f*
  testicular appendages, 874
  testicular cancer, 875–876, 875*b*, 875*f*
  testicular torsion, 874, 874*f*
  urethral strictures, 763, 869
  urethritis, 869
  variocele, 872–873, 873*f*
Male-pattern baldness, 56
Malignant bone tumours, in children, 1069–1071
Malignant hypertension, 609–610
Malignant hyperthermia, 347, 1014–1015
Malignant melanoma, 1093–1094, 1094*f*
Malignant pleural mesothelioma, 718*t*
Malignant tumours, 235–236, 236*f*
Malleus, 354, 354*f*
Malnutrition, 75–76, 942–943
  in children, 977
Malrotation, 970–971
Mammary adenocarcinoma, 236
Mammary stem cells, 851
Mammographic density, 852–853, 852*f*
Mammography, 847*b*, 852–853, 852*f*
Mannitol, 753*t*
Mannose-binding lectin (MBL), 137, 141
  deficiency of, 192*t*, 193
Manual strangulation, 95
Marasmus, 977
Marfan's syndrome, 634
Marginating storage pool, 505–506

Margination, 147
Marihuana, 89*t*, 342
MASP-1, 141
MASP-2, 141
Mast cells, 145–146, 145*f*–146*f*, 165, 224, 225*f*
Mastoid air cells, 354
Mastoid process, 354
Maternal care, epigenetics and, 66–67
Matrix metalloproteinases (MMPs), 153, 248, 291
Maturity-onset diabetes of youth (MODY), 482
MBL. *See* Mannose-binding lectin
McArdle's disease, 1044
Mean arterial pressure, 595
Mean corpuscular hemoglobin, 514*t*–516*t*
Mean corpuscular hemoglobin concentration, 514*t*–516*t*
Mean corpuscular volume, 514*t*–516*t*
Meckel diverticulum, 971
Meconium disease, 971
Meconium ileus, 971
Meconium plug syndrome, 971
Meconium syndromes, 971
Medial epicondylopathy, 1015
Median aperture, 323–324
Median eminence, 452
Mediastinal shift, 700
Mediastinum, 575–576, 679
Mediated transport, 17–18, 19*f*
Mediterranean diet, 853–854
Medroxyprogesterone (Provera), 821
Medroxyprogesterone acetate, 837
Medulla, 313–314
Medulla, of kidney, 741, 742*f*
Medulla oblongata, 319–320
Medullary carcinoma, 856*t*
Medulloblastomas, 419*t*, 437–438, 437*t*
Mefoxin Pws (cefoxitin), 826*b*
Megakaryocytes, 146, 499–500
Megaloblastic anemia, 258, 522–524
Meiosis, 25, 42, 44*f*
Meissner corpuscles, 356
Meissner plexus, 902, 906
Melanin, as cellular accumulations, 99
Melanocortin-1, 291
Melanocytes, 99
Melanocyte-stimulating hormone (MSH), 448
Melanoma, 290–291, 1093–1094, 1094*b*, 1094*f*
Melanosomes, 99
Melatonin, 225*t*–226*t*, 452
  breast cancer and, 852
Melena, 924, 924*t*
Membrane attack complex (MAC), 141
Membrane lipid rafts (MLRs), 5, 6*f*–7*f*
Membrane potentials, 24, 24*f*, 582
Membrane transport proteins, 17
Membrane-associated IgM, 167
Memory, 369, 370*t*
Memory cells, 160, 171
Memory disorders, 369, 370*t*
Mendel, Gregor, 49–50
Mendelian traits, 49
Ménière's disease, 355
Meninges, 323, 324*f*
Meningiomas, 419*t*, 420
Meningitis, 412–413, 435
Meningocele, 429, 429*f*
Menometrorrhagia, 821*t*
Menopausal hormone therapy, 850, 852
Menopause, 811–812, 811*f*
Menorrhagia, 524, 821*t*
Menorrhea, 821*t*
Menses, 803, 803*f*
Menstrual cycle
  aging and, 802
  bleeding in, 803
  body temperature and, 805
  duration of, 802, 803*f*
  hormonal control of, 804, 804*t*
  ovarian cycle of, 804
  phases of, 802–803
  vaginal response in, 805
Menstrual disorders
  abnormal uterine bleeding, 820–821, 821*t*
Menstrual disorders *(Continued)*
  amenorrhea, 819–820, 841*f*
  dysmenorrhea, 819
  PCOS, 822, 822*f*, 823*b*
Menstrual phase, 803, 803*f*
Menstruation, 803, 803*f*
  retrograde, 832
Mental illness, epigenetics and, 67
Mental stress-induced ischemia, 621, 621*f*–622*f*
Mercury
  anthropogenic emissions and, 93
  cellular injury caused by exposure to, 93
  thimerosal, 190
Merkel discs, 356
Mesangial cells, 743, 745*f*
Mesangial matrix, 743, 745*f*
Mesencephalon. *See* Midbrain
Mesenchymal stem cells (MSCs), 195, 504, 504*f*
Mesenchymal tissue, 78
Mesenchymal-epithelial transition (MET), 886
Mesenteric vascular insufficiency, 939–940
Mesentery, 905*f*, 906
Mesodermal germ layer, 303, 304*f*
Mesonephric ducts, 793, 795*f*
Mesothelium, 270*t*–273*t*
Messenger RNA (mRNA), 41, 247
MET. *See* Mesenchymal-epithelial transition
Metabolic acidosis, 643
  acid-base imbalances and, 128, 130*t*
  causes of, 130*t*
  clinical manifestations of, 128
  sodium bicarbonate for, 125–126
Metabolic alkalosis, 128–129, 131*f*
  hypochloremic, 128
Metabolic disorders, 364, 365*t*
  in children, 982, 983*t*
Metabolic edema, 380
Metabolic pathway, 16
Metabolic syndrome, 479, 480*b*, 618–619
Metabolic tremor, 383*t*
Metabolically healthy obesity, 943
Metabolism
  of alcohol, 91, 91*f*, 285*f*
  amino acid metabolism defects, 433–434
  of bilirubin, liver and, 913, 913*f*, 916*t*
  burn response of, 1098
  of carbohydrates, liver and, 914
  cellular
    ATP in, 16, 16*b*, 643–647
    carbon dioxide from, 684
    definition of, 14
    food of, 16, 16*f*
    impairment of, in shock, 643–648, 647*f*
    oxidative phosphorylation in, 16–17, 17*f*
    production of, 16, 16*f*
    thiamine deficiency effects on, 643
  fat, liver and, 914
  of lipids, 617–618
  muscle, 1005
    disorders of, 1043–1044
  of myocardium, 586–587
  nutrient, liver and, 914, 914*t*
  protein
    cortisol effects on, 220
    liver and, 914, 914*t*
Metals, 855
Metaphase, 25
Metaphase plate, 25
Metaphase spread, 42
Metaphysis, 994
Metaplasia, 78, 79*f*
Metaplastic carcinoma, 856*t*
Metarterioles, 591–593, 592*f*
Metastases
  to bone, 256
  of breast cancer, 255
  cancer cell, 253–255, 254*f*
  definition of, 236, 253
  of ovarian cancer, 841, 842*f*
  in prostate cancer, 886, 887*f*
Metastatic brain tumours, 421
Metastatic calcification, 100
Metastatic disease, 764
Metencephalon, 319
Metformin (Glucophage), 481–482, 822
Methamphetamine, 89*t*
Methemoglobin, 507
Methicillin-resistant *Staphylococcus aureus* (MRSA), 183, 712
Methylated cytosines, 62
Methylenetetrahydrofolate reductase (MTHFR), 554
Methylome, 275–276
Metronidazole (Flagyl), 826*b*
Metrorrhagia, 821*t*
Mexiletine, 1043
Mexitil Cap, 1043
MGUS. *See* Monoclonal gammopathy of undetermined significance
MHC. *See* Major histocompatibility complex
MI. *See* Myocardial ischemia
Microalbuminuria, 485, 609
Microbiome, 137–138, 137*t*
  GI tract and, 910
Microcephaly, 426, 431, 431*f*, 434*t*
Microcytic-hypochromic anemia, 521*t*, 524–526
Microdomains, 2–3
Microenvironmental niches, 28*f*
Microfilaments, 310
Microglia, 310–311, 312*t*
β2-Microglobulin, 545
β_2-Microglobulin, 169
Micro-organisms
  antibiotic resistant, 189
  antibiotics destroying, 188–189, 188*t*
  classes of, 178*t*
  countermeasures against infectious, 188, 188*t*
  description of, 177–188
  immune system defenses of, 180*t*
  opportunistic, 138
  of osteomyelitis by age, 1063*b*
  parasitic, 187
  pathogenic, 178, 179*t*
  PID and, 824
  pneumonia caused by, 712, 712*b*
  tissue damage caused by, 178, 179*t*
MicroRNA (miRNA), 64, 247
  cancer and, 69
  coding, 70
Microscopic colitis, 938
Microsomal ethanol-oxidizing system, 91, 91*f*
Microtubules, 310
Microvascular angina, 621*b*
Microvascular disease, 484–485, 484*t*, 485*f*
Microvasculature thrombosis, 549
Microvilli, 906
Micturition (urination), 745–746
Micturition reflex, 746
Midamor, 753*t*
Midbrain, 313–314, 315*t*, 319
Midcortical nephrons, 743
Middle ear, 354, 354*f*–355*f*
Middle fossa, 323
Migraines, 410–411, 410*t*
Migratory testis, 874
Mild concussions, 398
Mild diffuse axonal injury, 398
Miliaria, 1116, 1116*f*
Miliaria crystallina, 1116
Miliaria rubra, 1116, 1116*f*
Mineral disorders, postgastrectomy, 935
Mineralization, 992
Mineralocorticoids, 459, 459*f*
Minerals
  of bone, 992
  liver storage of, 914
  small intestine absorption of, 908*b*
Minimal change nephropathy, 787
Minimally conscious state, 369
Minute volume, 684
Mirror focus, 377
Missense mutations, 39, 41*f*
Mitochondria
  in cellular injury, 83, 84*b*
  characteristics of, 4*t*
  ROS damaging, 83
Mitochondrial DNA (mtDNA), 108
Mitofusin-2, 256–257
Mitogen-activated protein kinase, 291
Mitosis, 25–26, 25*f*, 42, 44*f*
Mitotic cells, 235–236
Mitral and tricuspid complex, 577
Mitral regurgitation, 634
Mitral stenosis, 633–634, 633*f*
Mitral valve, 577, 577*f*–578*f*
  infective endocarditis of, 638, 638*f*
Mitral valve prolapse syndrome (MVPS), 634, 635*f*
Mixed hearing loss, 355
Mixed hiatal hernia, 927, 927*f*
Mixed incontinence, 762*t*
Mixed nerves, 327–328
Mixed precocious puberty, 819*b*, 869*b*
MLH1, 69
MLRs. *See* Membrane lipid rafts
MMPs. *See* Matrix metalloproteinases
Mobitz I block, 645*t*–646*t*
Mobitz II block, 645*t*–646*t*
Moderate diffuse axonal injury, 398
Modification of Diet in Renal Disease, 754
MODS. *See* Multiple organ dysfunction syndrome
MODY. *See* Maturity-onset diabetes of youth
Moles, 1091, 1092*t*, 1094
Molluscum contagiosum, 1111, 1111*f*
Monoallelic expression, 64
Monoamines, 314*t*
Monoclonal antibodies, 165*b*, 264
Monoclonal gammopathy of undetermined significance (MGUS), 544
Monocyte chemotactic protein-1, 251
Monocyte count, 514*t*–516*t*
Monocytes, 142, 142*f*, 147, 499, 499*t*, 509, 529–531, 530*t*
Monocytopenia, 530*t*, 531
Monocytosis, 530*t*, 531
Monokines, 143
Mononuclear phagocyte system, 503, 503*t*
Monosaturated fatty acids, 906*b*
Monosodium urate crystals, 1032, 1038–1040
Mons pubis, 797, 797*f*
Motilin, 903, 903*t*
Motility diarrhea, 923
Motility disorders, 925–929
  acquired, 972–974
  congenital, 968–972
Motor dysphasia, 371, 372*t*–373*t*
Motor neuron diseases, 387–388, 388*b*
Motor neurons, 310, 321–322
  lower, 322
  upper, 322
Motor pathways, 318*f*, 322
Motor responses, in arousal alterations, 367, 367*f*–368*f*, 368*t*
Motor units, 322
Motor units, of skeletal muscles, 999–1003, 1002*f*
Mouth
  anatomy of, 899–902
  salivation in, 899–901, 901*f*
Moyamoya disease, 436
MPNs. *See* Myeloproliferative neoplasms
MRI. *See* Magnetic resonance imaging
mRNA. *See* Messenger RNA
MRSA. *See* Methicillin-resistant *Staphylococcus aureus*
MSCs. *See* Mesenchymal stem cells
MSH. *See* Melanocyte-stimulating hormone
mtDNA. *See* Mitochondrial DNA
MTHFR. *See* Methylenetetrahydrofolate reductase
Mucinous carcinoma, 856*t*
Mucopolysaccharidoses, 97–98
Mucopurulent cervicitis, 826–827
Mucosa, of small intestine, 903*t*
Mucosa, of stomach, 903*t*
Mucosa-associated lymphoid tissue lymphoma, 251
Mucosal barrier, 905
Mucoviscidosis, 974
Mucus, 905

Müllerian ducts, 793, 795*f*
Müllerian inhibitory hormone, 793–794
Multichannel urodynamic testing, 763
Multifactorial diseases, 74
Multifactorial inheritance, 58–59, 58*f*, 59*b*, 968
Multigenerational phenotypes, 276*t*
Multiple causation theory, of childhood cancers, 305
Multiple myeloma, 542–545, 543*f*–544*f*
Multiple organ dysfunction syndrome (MODS)
clinical manifestations of, 654–655
definition of, 643
elderly and, 653
evaluation of, 655
gastro-intestinal system in, 654–655
hypermetabolism and, 654
inflammatory processes in, 653, 654*t*
myocardial depression in, 654
oxygen delivery in, 654
pathogenesis of, 653, 653*f*
pathophysiology of, 653–654
supply-dependent oxygen consumption and, 654
treatment of, 655
triggers of, 654*b*
Multiple sclerosis, 415–416, 415*f*
female sexual dysfunction and, 843*t*
Multiple-antibiotic resistance, 189
Multipolar neurons, 310
Multipotent cells, 27, 28*f*
Muscle cells, 1000
Muscle contraction
calcium-troponin complex in, 586
concentric, 1006
cross-bridge theory of, 586, 1005
dynamic, 1006, 1006*f*
eccentric, 1006
excitation-contraction coupling in, 586
isometric, 1006, 1006*f*
molecular basis for, 585*f*, 1003–1005
static, 1006
steps in, 1003–1005
types of, 1006, 1006*f*
Muscle fibre action potential, 1003–1005
Muscle fibres, 1000–1002, 1001*t*, 1002*f*
Muscle membrane, 1000
abnormalities of, 1014–1015
Muscle movement alterations
akinesia, 384
bradykinesia, 384
description of, 381–385
dopamine and, 381–382
Huntington's disease, 373
hyperkinesia, 382, 383*t*
hypokinesia, 384
Parkinson's disease, 384–385, 384*f*–385*f*
paroxysmal dyskinesia, 382
tardive dyskinesia, 382
Tourette syndrome, 382, 382*b*
Muscle pumps, 587, 593*f*
Muscle strain, 1016–1017, 1017*t*
Muscle tissues, 33*t*–34*t*
Muscle tone alterations, 380–381, 381*t*
Muscle tumours, 1051
Muscle wasting
in cachexia, 257–258, 259*f*
in Cushing's syndrome, 488
protein depletion causing, 648
Muscles
aging of, 1007–1008
agonist of, 1006
antagonist of, 1006
cardiac (*See* Cardiac muscle)
fibres, 1004*f*
functions of, 1003–1006
healing phases of, 1016–1017
mechanics of, 1005–1006
metabolism of, 1005
disorders of, 1043–1044
movement of, 1006
skeletal (*See* Skeletal muscles)
strains of, 1016–1017, 1017*t*
Muscular arteries, 589
Muscular dystrophies, 1067–1069, 1067*t*, 1068*f*–1069*f*
Muscular ventricular septal defects, 668
Musculo-skeletal disorders
bone tumours (*See* Bone tumours)
bursitis, 1015–1016, 1016*f*
in children (*See* Children, musculo-skeletal disorders in)
compartment syndrome, 1019, 1019*b*, 1020*f*
dislocation, 1014–1015
epicondylopathy, 1015–1016, 1016*f*
fractures (*See* Fractures)
incidence of, 1011
joints disorders (*See* Joint disorders)
ligament sprains and strains, 1015
malignant hyperthermia, 347, 1014–1015
muscle strain, 1016–1017, 1017*t*
muscle tumours, 1051
rhabdomyolysis, 1017–1019, 1018*b*
skeletal trauma, 1011–1015
subluxation, 1014–1015
tendinopathy, 1015–1016, 1016*f*, 1017*b*
tendon sprains and strains, 1015
Mutagens, 39
Mutational hot spots, 39, 39*b*
Mutations, 39, 41*f*, 238–240, 244, 248
Mutualistic relationship, 137
MVPS. *See* Mitral valve prolapse syndrome
Myalgic encephalomyelitis, 1042–1043
Myasthenia gravis, 257*t*
clinical manifestations of, 417
definition of, 417
evaluation and treatment of, 417
pathophysiology of, 417
Myasthenic crisis, 417
MYC proto-oncogene, 242
Mycobacterium tuberculosis, 103
Mycoplasmal pneumonia, 732*t*, 733
Mycoses, 186
Mycosis fungoides, 1095
Myelencephalon, 319–320
Myelin, 310
Myelin sheath, 310
Myelodysplasia, 430*t*
Myelodysplastic syndrome, 525
Myelogenic tumours, 1050
Myeloid tissue, 504
Myeloma cells, 542–543
Myelomeningocele, 429–430, 429*f*
Myeloperoxidase–hydrogen peroxide system, 193
Myeloproliferative disorders, 536
Myeloproliferative erythrocyte disorders, 526–529
Myeloproliferative neoplasms (MPNs), 526–527, 549
Myenteric plexus, 902, 906
Myoadenylate deaminase deficiency, 1044
Myoblasts, 1000
Myocardial depression, 654
Myocardial hypertrophy, 609
Myocardial infarction, 80–81, 624*f*
clinical manifestations of, 626
complications with, 628*t*
CPK-MB release after, 625
definition of, 627*b*
ECG for diagnosis of, 626, 628*f*
evaluation of, 626–628, 628*f*
female sexual dysfunction and, 843*t*
functional changes caused by, 625, 626*f*
functional impairment caused by, 626
non-ST elevation, 623, 625*f*
oxygen deprivation in, 625
pathophysiology of, 624–626, 626*f*
ST elevation, 623, 625*f*
structural changes caused by, 625, 626*f*
sudden cardiac death and, 626, 627*f*
transmural, 624, 625*f*
treatment for, 626–628
VEDV affected by, 626
Myocardial ischemia (MI)
CAD causing, 617
clinical manifestations of, 620–621
ECG and, 622, 622*f*
evaluation and treatment of, 621–623
pathophysiology of, 620, 620*f*
PCI and, 623
Prinzmetal angina and, 621
Myocardial ischemia (MI) *(Continued)*
silent, 621, 621*f*–622*f*
SPECT and, 622–623
stable angina pectoris and, 620–621
stress echocardiography and, 622–623
Myocardial oxygen consumption, 586, 588
Myocardial remodeling, 625
Myocardial stunning, 625
Myocardium, 576, 576*f*, 580
cardiomyopathies of, 630–632, 631*f*
cells of, 584–586, 584*f*
contractility of, 586–588, 588*f*
hibernating, 625
metabolism of, 586–587
oxygen delivery to, 586, 588
relaxation of, 586–587
sympathetic nervous system effecting, 583–584
Myoclonic seizure, 436*t*
Myoclonus tremor, 383*t*
Myofascial pain, 344*t*
Myofibrils, 584, 1000, 1002*f*, 1003
Myofibroblasts, 154
Myoglobin, 508, 598, 1000–1002
in urine, 1017–1018
Myoglobinuria, 1017
Myomas, 831, 831*f*
Myometrium, 799, 800*f*
Myoneural junction. *See* Neuromuscular junction
Myophosphorylase deficiency, 1044
Myopia, 352, 352*f*
Myosin, 585–586, 585*f*, 1003*t*
Myositis, 1044–1045, 1045*f*
Myositis ossificans, 1017
Myotonia, 1043
Myotonic muscular dystrophy, 1067*t*, 1068–1069
Myxedema, 474, 474*f*
Myxedema coma, 474

N

NAD. *See* Nicotinamide adenine dinucleotide
Nails
disorders of, 1101
psoriatic nail disease, 1083–1084
structures of, 1074, 1076*f*
Naloxone (Narcon), 342
Narcolepsy, 348–349
Narcon (naloxone), 342
Nasal cavity cancer, 270*t*–273*t*
Nasopharynx
anatomy of, 679, 680*f*–681*f*
cancer of, 270*t*–273*t*
National Cancer Institute, 307
National Council on Radiation Protection and Measurements, 286
National Kidney Foundation, 754
Natriuretic peptides, 597
nephron function affected by, 752
Natural immunity. *See* Innate immunity
Natural killer (NK) cells, 149, 173, 221–222, 499, 499*t*, 911–912
Nausea, 921
NAUTICA. *See* North American Urinary Tract Infection Collaborative Alliance
NCF. *See* Neutrophil chemotactic factor
ncRNA. *See* Noncoding RNA
Nebulin, 1003*t*
Nebulized epinephrine, 726
Necroptosis, 101
Necrosis, 74
caseous, 103, 104*f*
coagulative, 103, 104*f*
definition of, 101–102
description of, 101–105
fatty, 103, 104*f*
features of, 102*t*
gangrenous, 103–105, 104*f*
liquefactive, 103, 104*f*
morphological changes associated with, 103*f*
programmed, 101
Necrotizing enterocolitis, 978–979
Necrotizing fasciitis, 1087
Necrotizing myositis, 1045
Negative feedback, 443–444
Neglect syndrome, 369–371
Neisseria gonorrhoeae, 163, 188–189
Neisseria meningitidis, 435
Neoadjuvant chemotherapy, 263
Neonatal jaundice, 563, 979–980
Neoplasms
clonal proliferation model of, 238–240, 240*f*
HIV and CNS, 415
infectious agents associated with, 251*t*
inflammatory conditions associated with, 251*t*
myeloproliferative, 526–527, 549
opportunistic, 196*b*
progression of, in cervix, 238*f*
Neoplastic polyps, 956, 956*f*
Neovascularization, 247, 255
Nephritic syndrome
clinical manifestations of, 771
definition of, 771
evaluation of, 772
glomerulonephritis associated with, 770*t*
pathophysiology of, 771
treatment of, 772
Nephroblastoma, 788, 788*t*
Nephrogenic diabetes insipidus, 467
Nephron
blood vessels of, 744*f*
components of, 741, 742*f*
cortical, 743
definition of, 741
distal convoluted tubule, 750–752
distal convoluted tubule of, 744, 744*f*
functions of, 747–752, 749*f*
ADH effects on, 752
aldosterone effects on, 752
hormones and, 752
natriuretic peptides effects on, 752
juxtamedullary, 743, 744*f*
loop of Henle of, 743–744, 743*f*
midcortical, 743
proximal convoluted tubule of, 742*f*, 743–744, 749–750
Nephropathy
diabetic, 484*t*, 485
minimal change, 787
Nephrotic syndrome, 257*t*
in children, 787
clinical manifestations of, 771, 772*t*
definition of, 771
evaluation of, 772
glomerulonephritis associated with, 770*t*
pathophysiology of, 771
primary, 787
secondary, 787
treatment of, 772
Nerve growth factor (NGF), 26*t*
Nerve impulse, 313, 314*t*
Nerve sheath tumours, 420–421
Nerves
injury to, 311
regeneration of, 311, 312*f*
Nervous system. *See also* Autonomic nervous system; Central nervous system; Peripheral nervous system; Somatic nervous system
aging changes to, 335
cells of, 309–311
children and development of, 426–427
CKD effects on, 776*t*
components of, 309
Nestin-expressing cells, 504–505
Net filtration, 116, 117*f*
Net filtration pressure, 747–748
Neural lobe, 452
Neural reflexes, heart rate and, 589
Neural tube defects, 427–430, 428*f*–430*f*, 430*t*
Neuraminidase, 183
Neurilemma cells. *See* Schwann cells
Neurilemmoma, 419*t*
Neuritic plaques, 374–375
Neuroblastomas, 438–439
Neuroendocrine hormones, 227
Neuroendocrine tumours, 718*t*, 719–720
Neurofibrillary tangles, 99, 374–375, 375*f*
Neurofibrils, 310
Neurofibromas, 419*t*, 420–421
Neurofibromatosis, 51–52, 52*f*

Neurofibromatosis type 1, 420
Neurofibromatosis type 2, 420–421
Neurogenic bladder, 762, 762*t*, 767*t*
Neurogenic diabetes insipidus, 467
Neurogenic shock, 402, 648–650, 650*f*
Neuroglia, 310–311, 312*f*
Neuroglial cells, 309–311, 312*f*
Neurohormonal signalling, 12–13, 14*f*
Neurological determination of death, 368
Neurological system, CKD and, 776*t*, 779
Neuromatrix theory, 339
Neuromotor function alterations
  ALS, 388–389
  hypertonia, 381, 381*f*–382*f*, 381*t*
  hypotonia, 380–381, 381*t*
  lower motor neuron syndromes, 385*t*, 386–387, 387*f*
  motor neuron diseases, 387–388, 388*b*
  muscle movement
    akinesia, 384
    bradykinesia, 384
    description of, 381–385
    Huntington's disease, 373
    hyperkinesia, 382, 383*t*
    hypokinesia, 384
    Parkinson's disease, 384–385, 384*f*–385*f*
    paroxysmal dyskinesia, 382
    tardive dyskinesia, 382
    Tourette syndrome, 382, 382*b*
  muscle tone, 380–381, 381*t*
  upper motor neuron syndromes, 385–386, 385*t*, 386*b*, 386*f*–387*f*
Neuromuscular junction, 310, 322, 322*f*
Neuromuscular junction disorders, 417
Neurons, 27
  afferent, 321–322
  associational, 310
  bipolar, 310
  components of, 310, 310*f*
  definition of, 309
  description of, 310
  efferent, 321–322
  interneurons, 310
  motor, 310, 321–322
    lower, 322
    upper, 322
  multipolar, 310
  postganglionic, 328, 331*f*
  postsynaptic, 313
  preganglionic, 328, 331*f*
  presynaptic, 313
  pseudounipolar, 310
  sensory, 310
  synapse between, 311*f*
  third order, 322–323
  transmission by, 311*f*
  unipolar, 310
Neuropathic pain, 343
Neuropathies, 416*t*
  diabetic, 484*t*, 485, 486*f*
Neuropeptides
  properties of, 314*t*
  Y, 224, 225*t*–226*t*
Neuroplasticity, 313, 313*b*
Neuroreceptors, 331, 333*t*
Neurotransmitters
  of ANS, 331, 333*t*
  chemical signaling through, 12–13, 14*f*
  description of, 313
  excitatory, 340
  inhibitory, 341
  of pain modulation, 340–342, 341*f*
  types of, 314*t*
Neutralization, 163
Neutropenia, 530*t*, 531
Neutrophil chemotactic factor (NCF), 145
Neutrophil count, 514*t*–516*t*, 516*b*
Neutrophilia, 530, 530*t*
Neutrophils, 142*f*, 147, 498–499, 499*t*, 530*t*
Nevi, 99, 1091, 1092*t*, 1094
Newborns
  antibodies in, 174*b*
  hemolytic disease of, 211
    clinical manifestations of, 562–563
    evaluation and treatment of, 563
    incidence of, 562
    pathophysiology of, 562, 563*f*
Newborns *(Continued)*
  jaundice in, 945
  RDS, 728–730, 728*b*, 729*f*
NGF. *See* Nerve growth factor
Niches, in bone marrow, 504–505, 504*f*
Nicotinamide adenine dinucleotide (NAD), 16–17
Nicotinamide adenine dinucleotide phosphate oxidase, 193
Night terrors, 349
Nipple, 806
  carcinoma and retraction of, 860*f*, 860*t*
NIPPV. *See* Noninvasive positive-pressure ventilation
Nissl substances, 310
Nitric oxide (NO), 83, 83*t*, 510
  hemoglobin binding to, 507, 507*f*
  in septic shock, 652*b*
  vascular function of, 597
NK cells. *See* Natural killer cells
NLRs. *See* NOD-like receptors
N-*MYC* oncogene, 243, 244*f*
NO. *See* Nitric oxide
Nociceptin/orphanin FQ, 341–342
Nociception, 339
Nociceptive pain, 339
Nociceptive transmission, 339
Nociceptors, 339, 339*t*
Nodes of Ranvier, 310, 311*f*
NOD-like receptors (NLRs), 143
Nodular thyroid disease, 472–473
Nodule, 1077*t*–1078*t*
Noggin, 991*t*
Nonaccidental trauma, 1071, 1071*f*
Nonalcoholic fatty liver disease, 948–949
Nonalcoholic steatohepatitis, 948–949
Nonbacterial infectious cystitis, 766
Nonbacterial prostatitis, 879
Nonbacterial thrombotic endocarditis, 637–638
Nonceliac gluten sensitivity, 975
Noncoding RNA (ncRNA), 64, 247
  gene expression alteration by, 238–240
Noncommunicating hydrocephalus, 380, 380*t*
Nondisjunction, 45–46, 45*f*
Nondividing support cells, 810, 810*f*
Nonerosive reflux disease, 926
Nonfluent dysphasia, 371, 372*t*–373*t*
Non-Hodgkin's lymphoma, 304
  in children, 571–572
  definition of, 540
Non-Hodgkin's lymphomas
  clinical manifestations of, 541, 541*t*
  incidence of, 540
  pathophysiology of, 540–541
  treatment of, 541
Nonhomologous end joining pathway, 286–287
Nonimmunologic urticaria, 202–203
Noninfectious cystitis, 766
Noninflammatory acne, 1107
Noninvasive positive-pressure ventilation (NIPPV), 701
Nonmyelinating Schwann cells, 310–311, 312*t*
Non-nociceptive stimulation, 339
Nonoliguric renal failure, 774
Nonossifying fibromas, 1069
Nonpuerperal hyperprolactinemia, 843
Nonpurulent meningitis, 412, 435
Non-REM (NREM) sleep, 347–348
Nonsense mutations, 39, 41*f*
Non-small cell carcinoma, 718*t*, 719, 719*f*
Nonspastic cerebral palsy, 433
Non-ST elevation myocardial infarction, 623, 625*f*
Nonsteroidal anti-inflammatory drugs (NSAIDs)
  gastritis caused by, 930
  for osteoarthritis, 1031–1032
  peptic ulcer disease caused by, 931–932
Nonstructural scoliosis, 1066
Nonsyndromic cleft palate, 968
Nontargeted effects, 288, 288*f*
Nonunion, 1014
Nonvolatile acid, 126
Norepinephrine, 331, 459, 588
  properties of, 314*t*
Norethisterone acetate, 837
Normal flora, 137
Normal microbiome, 137–138, 137*t*
Normal transit constipation, 922
Normal weight obesity, 943
Normal-pressure hydrocephalus, 380
Normoblasts, 506
Normocytic-normochromic anemia, 521*t*, 526, 527*t*
North American Urinary Tract Infection Collaborative Alliance (NAUTICA), 766*b*
Norwood procedure, 672
NREM. *See* Non-REM sleep
NS1 protein, 185–186
NSAIDs. *See* Nonsteroidal anti-inflammatory drugs
Nuclear envelope, 2, 4*f*
Nuclear factor of activated B cells, 991*t*
Nuclear pores, 2, 4*f*
Nucleic acid amplification tests, 733
Nucleolus, 2, 4*f*
Nucleophiles, 84–85
Nucleosomal remodeling, 245*f*
5′-Nucleotidase, 916*t*
Nucleus, 2, 3*f*–4*f*
Nucleus accumbens, 317, 319*f*
Nucleus pulposus, 324–325, 325*f*
Nutrient metabolism, liver and, 914, 914*t*
Nutrigenomics, 277, 279*f*
Nutrition
  alcohol intake effects on, 90–91
  cancer and, 277–282, 279*f*–282*f*
  epigenetics and, 66
  erythropoiesis requirements with, 507, 508*t*
  wound healing and, 154
Nutrition disorders, 940–943
  malnutrition, 75–76, 942–943, 977
  obesity (*See* Obesity)
  starvation, 942–943
Nystagmus, 350

O

Oat cell carcinoma, 719–720
O'Beirne sphincter, 909
Obesity
  adipocytokines and, 940–941, 941*b*
  breast cancer and, 854
  CAD and, 618–619
  cancer and, 283, 283*t*, 284*f*
  in children with cardiovascular disorders, 676*b*
  clinical manifestations of, 941
  definition of, 940
  evaluation of, 941–942
  incidence of, 940
  insulin resistance from, 481
  metabolic changes of, 284*f*
  metabolically healthy, 943
  normal weight, 943
  overweight compared to, 941–942
  pathophysiology of, 940–941, 942*f*
  primary hypertension and, 608, 609*b*
  treatment of, 941–942
  type 2 diabetes mellitus and, 222*b*
  wound healing delayed by, 154
Obesity hypoventilation syndrome, 348
Obligate carriers, 51
Oblique fractures, 1011–1012, 1012*f*, 1012*t*
Obscurin, 1003*t*
Obstructive jaundice, 945–946, 947*t*
Obstructive lung diseases, 705–711
  asthma (*See* Asthma)
  chronic bronchitis, 709–710, 709*f*–710*f*, 709*t*
  COPD, 708–709, 711*f*
  emphysema, 709*t*, 710–711, 710*f*–711*f*
Obstructive sleep apnea syndrome (OSAS), 348
  in children, 727–728
Obstructive uropathy, 759
Occipital lobe, 316*f*, 317
Occlusive stroke, 435
Occult bleeding, 924, 924*t*
Occult fractures, 1012*f*
Occupational hazards, as carcinogens, 294–295
Ocular cancer, 270*t*–273*t*
Ocular movement alterations, 350
Oculocephalic reflex response, 367*f*
Oculomotor nerve, 330*t*
Oculomotor responses, in arousal alterations, 364–367, 367*f*
Oculovestibular reflex, 367*f*
Ogilvie syndrome, 929
Olfaction, 356, 356*f*, 357*b*
Olfactory hallucinations, 356
Olfactory nerve, 330*t*
Oligoarthritis, 1064
Oligodendrocytes, 310–311, 312*t*
Oligodendroglia, 310–311, 312*t*
Oligodendroglioma, 419*t*, 420
Oligomenorrhea, 821*t*
Oliguria, 125, 773*f*, 774
Omalizumab (Xolair), 708
Oncogenes
  activation mechanisms of, 239*f*
  childhood cancers associated with, 305, 305*t*
  definition of, 242
  dominant, 243, 243*t*
  gene amplification of, 243, 244*f*
  genetic events that activate, 242
  mutations in, 248
  N-*MYC*, 243, 244*f*
  signal cascade activation by, 242
  translocations effect on, 242, 243*f*
Oncomirs, 247
Oncosis vacuolar degeneration, 97, 98*f*
Oncotic pressure, 20, 20*f*
  capillary, 116
  interstitial, 116
Onychomycosis, 1101
Open brain injury, 395*t*, 397
Open fractures, 1011–1012, 1012*f*, 1012*t*
Open pneumothorax, 700
Open reduction, of fractures, 1014
Open trauma, 394
Open wounds, 152
OPG. *See* Osteoprotegerin
Opioids
  abuse of, 86*t*
  endogenous, 341–342, 341*f*
Opportunistic infections, 177–178
  AIDS and, 196*b*
  HIV and, 414–415
Opportunistic micro-organisms, 138
Opsonins, 141
Opsonization, 148–149
Optic chiasm, 349–350
Optic disc, 349, 349*f*
Optic glioma, 437*t*, 438
Optic nerves, 330*t*, 349–350, 349*f*, 353*f*
Optic neuritis, 415
Oral cavity, cancer of, 270*t*–273*t*
Oral contraceptives, breast cancer and, 852
Orchitis, 874–875, 875*f*
Organ of Corti, 354, 355*f*
Organelles, 1
  cytoplasmic, 2, 4*t*
Organs, 27*f*
Organ-specific autoimmune adrenalitis, 490
Orgasmic dysfunction, 842
Oropharyngeal phase of swallowing, 901
Oropharynx, 679, 680*f*–681*f*
Orthopnea, 695
Orthostatic hypotension, 611
OSAS. *See* Obstructive sleep apnea syndrome
Osgood-Schlatter disease, 1065
Osmitrol, 753*t*
Osmolality, 20
  plasma, 118–119
Osmolarity, 20
Osmoreceptors, 118–119
Osmosis, in passive transport, 20, 21*f*
Osmotic diarrhea, 922–923
Osmotic diuretics, 753*t*
Osmotic pressure, 20
Osseous labyrinths, 354
Osteitis deformans, 841
Osteoarthritis, 1029–1032, 1030*f*, 1031*b*, 1032*f*
Osteoblastic niche, 504–505, 504*f*

Osteoblasts, 988–990, 989*f*, 989*t*, 1037
Osteocalcin, 989*t*, 992
Osteochondromas, 1069
Osteochondroses, 1065–1066, 1065*f*–1066*f*
Osteoclasts, 988–990, 989*f*, 989*t*
Osteocytes, 988–990, 989*f*, 989*t*
Osteogenesis imperfecta, 1060–1062, 1062*f*
Osteogenic tumours, 1049–1050
Osteoid, 990
Osteomalacia, 1026–1027
Osteomyelitis, 1028–1029, 1028*f*–1029*f*
  in children, 1062–1063, 1063*b*, 1063*f*
Osteophytes, 1029
Osteoporosis
  clinical manifestations of, 1023–1024, 1024*f*
  definition of, 1021
  electron microscopic image of, 1021*f*
  evaluation of, 1024–1026, 1025*b*
  facts and figures on, 1022*b*
  fractures caused by, 1021–1022, 1022*t*
  glucocorticoid-induced, 1023
  pathophysiology of, 1023, 1024*f*
  postmenopausal, 1022
  regional, 1023
  risk factors of, 1023*b*
  secondary, 1022–1023
  transient regional, 1023
  treatment of, 1024–1026, 1026*b*
  in vertebral body, 1021*f*
Osteoprotegerin (OPG), 990–992, 991*t*, 1022–1023, 1024*f*
Osteosarcoma, 1049–1050, 1049*f*, 1070
Ostium primum atrial septal defect, 667
Ostium secundum atrial septal defect, 667
Otitis externa, 355–356
Otitis media infections, 180*t*–181*t*, 356
Otitis media with effusion, 356
Otoliths, 354–355
Outlet dysfunction, 922
Oval window, 354, 354*f*–355*f*
Ovarian cancer, 270*t*–273*t*
  clinical manifestations of, 841, 842*f*
  evaluation of, 842
  global incidence of, 838, 839*f*
  metastasis of, 841, 842*f*
  pathogenesis of, 838–841, 841*f*
  risk factors of, 838, 840*t*
  staging of, 842*t*
  treatment of, 842
Ovarian cycle, 800–801, 804
Ovarian cysts, 829–830, 829*f*
Ovarian follicles, 800, 801*f*
Ovarian tumours, 841*f*
Ovaries
  anatomy of, 800–801, 801*f*
  PCOS, 822, 822*f*, 823*b*
  torsion of, 830
Overactive bladder syndrome, 762–763
Overflow incontinence, 762*t*
Over-the-counter drugs, 85*b*
Overweight, obesity compared to, 941–942
Oviducts, 800
Ovulation, 803, 803*f*
Ovum, 793
Oxidation, 16, 17*f*
Oxidative phosphorylation, 16–17, 17*f*, 248–249
Oxidative stress
  in chronic alcoholism, 92
  definition of, 82–83
  free radicals and, 82–83, 83*t*, 108
  intracellular signaling pathways activated by, 83
  reperfusion injury caused by, 82
  ROS and, 82–83
Oximeter, 691
Oxycephaly, 431*f*
Oxygen
  arterial pressure of, 685–686, 689*t*
  coronary artery delivery of, to myocardium, 586, 588
  diffusion of, across alveolocapillary membrane, 690, 691*f*, 698
  impairment of, in shock, 643–647
  MODS and delivery of, 654
Oxygen *(Continued)*
  myocardial infarction and deprivation of, 625
  partial pressure of, 688–689, 691*f*, 729
  supply-dependent consumption of, 654
  transport of, 690–692
Oxygen debt, 1005
Oxygen saturation, 691
Oxygen toxicity, 703
Oxygenation, arterial, 690–691, 691*f*
Oxygen-dependent killing mechanisms, 149
Oxyhemoglobin, 507, 691
Oxyhemoglobin dissociation curve, 691–692, 691*f*
Oxytocin, 806
  function of, 452
  in stress response, 225*t*–226*t*
  synthesis of, 447–448

P

P wave, 582–583, 583*f*
Pacinian corpuscles, 356
PAF. *See* Platelet-activating factor
Paget's disease, 856*t*, 1027
PAH. *See Para*-aminohippuric acid
Pain
  abdominal, 924
  acute, 342–343, 344*t*
  bone, leukemia and, 536*t*
  cancer and, 256, 344*t*
  categories of, 342*b*
  central neuropathic, 343
  chronic postoperative, 344*t*
  clinical descriptions of, 342–343
  deafferentation, 344*t*
  definition of, 338
  heterosegmental inhibition of, 342
  intensity of, 338–339
  intercourse, 842
  intractable, 343
  low back, 402–403
  modulation of, 340–342
    neurotransmitters of, 340–342, 341*f*
    pathways of, 342
  myofascial, 344*t*
  neuroanatomy of, 339–340
  neuropathic, 343
  nociceptive, 339
  parietal, 924
  perception of, 340, 341*t*
  peripheral neuropathic, 343
  persistent, 343, 344*t*
  phantom limb, 344*t*
  pulmonary disease signs with, 697
  radicular, 403
  referred, 342–343, 343*f*, 924
  segmental inhibition of, 342
  somatic, 342–343
  theories of, 338–339
  threshold for, 340, 341*t*
  tolerance for, 340, 341*t*
  transduction of, 339
  transmission of, 339–340, 340*f*
  visceral, 342–343, 924
Painful bladder syndrome/interstitial cystitis (PBS/IC), 766–767
Painless thyroiditis, 473
Palate, cleft, 968–969
Palmomental reflex, 367*f*
Pamidronate, 1061–1062
PAMPs. *See* Pathogen-associated molecular patterns
Pancreas. *See also* Diabetes mellitus
  aging and, 461*b*, 917*t*
  anatomy of, 455, 455*f*
  cancer of, 270*t*–273*t*, 954*t*, 958–959
  disorders of, 952–953
  endocrine, 455–457
    dysfunction of, 467
  exocrine
    anatomy of, 911*f*, 915, 917*f*
    blood flow to, 915
    enzymatic secretion in, 916–918
    innervation of, 915
    laboratory tests for, 917*t*
  fibrocystic disease of, 974
  hormones secreted by, 455–457
  tumours of, in children, 982–983
Pancreatic duct, 915
Pancreatic exocrine insufficiency, 935
Pancreatic polypeptide, 457, 903*t*
Pancreatitis
  acute, 952–953, 953*f*
  chronic, 953
Paneth cells, 910
Panhypopituitarism, 468
Pannus, 1033
Papanicolaou (Pap) test, 834*b*
Papillary apocrine change, 844
Papillary capillaries, 1076
Papillary carcinoma, 856*t*
Papillary muscles, 577, 577*f*
Papilledema, 351*t*
Papillomas, 419*t*
  intraductal, 844
Papule, 1077*t*–1078*t*
Papulosquamous disorders, 1083–1085, 1083*f*–1085*f*, 1084*b*
Para-aminohippuric acid (PAH), 753
Parabens, 855
Paracentesis, 945
Paracetamol. *See* Acetaminophen
Paracrine signalling, 12–13, 14*f*
Paraesophageal hiatal hernia, 927, 927*f*
Parafollicular cells, 453
Paralysis, 385–386
  periodic, 1043
  thyrotoxic periodic, 1043
Paralysis agitans, 384
Paralytic ileus, 928, 928*t*
Paramesonephric ducts, 793, 795*f*
Paranasal sinus cancer, 270*t*–273*t*
Paraneoplastic pemphigus, 1086
Paraneoplastic syndromes, 256, 257*t*
Paraparesis, 386*b*
Paraphimosis, 869–870, 870*f*
Paraplegia, 386*b*
Paraprotein, 543–544
Parasites, 1113–1115, 1114*f*–1115*f*
Parasitic diseases, 187–188, 187*t*
Parasitic micro-organisms, 187
Parasomnias, 349
Parasympathetic nervous system
  anatomy of, 331, 332*f*
  in stress response, 224
Parathyroid glands
  anatomy of, 453*f*, 454
  disorders of, 474–476
    hyperparathyroidism, 474–475
    hypoparathyroidism, 475–476
  hormones of, 454–455, 474–476
Paratonia, 367, 367*f*, 381, 381*t*, 382*f*
Paratopes, 163
Paravertebral ganglia, 328–331
Parenting, 66–67
Paresthesias, 478*t*
Parietal cells, 904
Parietal lobe, 316–317, 316*f*
Parietal lobe disease, 369–371
Parietal pain, 924
Parietal peritoneum, 799
Parietooccipital sulcus, 316*f*, 317
Parkinsonian syndrome, 384
Parkinsonian tremor, 383*t*
Parkinsonism, 384, 384*f*
Parkinson's disease, 384–385, 384*f*–385*f*
Parkinson's syndrome, 384
Paronychia, 1101
Parosmia, 356
Paroxysmal dyskinesia, 382
Paroxysmal nocturnal dyspnea, 695
Pars distalis, 448, 449*f*
Pars intermedia, 448, 449*f*
Pars nervosa, 450*f*, 452
Pars tuberalis, 448, 449*f*
Partial pleura, 683, 684*f*
Partial precocious puberty, 819*b*, 869*b*
Partial pressure of carbon dioxide, 689*t*, 691*f*
Partial pressure of oxygen, 688–689, 691*f*, 729
Partial seizure, 436*t*
Partial thromboplastin time, 514*t*–516*t*
Partial trisomy, 46
Particulate matter, 293–294
Passenger mutations, 238–240
Passive immunity, 160
Passive immunotherapy, 190
Passive transport, 17–18, 18*f*
  diffusion in, 19–20, 19*f*
  filtration in, 20, 20*f*
  osmosis in, 20, 21*f*
Pasteurella multocida, 1028
Patch (skin lesion), 1077*t*–1078*t*
Patched 1 tumor-suppressor gene, 290
Patent ductus arteriosus, 667, 667*f*
Patent foramen ovale, 667
Pathogen-associated molecular patterns (PAMPs), 142
Pathogenic micro-organisms, 178, 179*t*
Pathologic calcification, 74
Pathological atrophy, 75
Pathological crying, 389–390
Pathological fractures, 1012–1013, 1012*f*, 1012*t*
Pathological fungi, 186
Pathological hyperplasia, 77
Pathological laughter, 389–390
Pattern recognition receptors (PRRs), 142, 183
Pattern theory, 339
Pavementing, 147
Pavlik harness, 1060, 1061*f*
PBS/IC. *See* Painful bladder syndrome/interstitial cystitis
PCI. *See* Percutaneous coronary intervention
PCOS. *See* Polycystic ovary syndrome
PDE5i. *See* Phosphodiesterase type 5 inhibitors
PDGF. *See* Platelet-derived growth factor
Peak bone mss, 1021
Pediculosis, 892*t*–894*t*, 1114
Pedigrees
  analysis of, 56–57, 56*f*
  autosomal dominant inheritance and, 50, 51*f*
  autosomal recessive inheritance and, 52–53, 53*f*
  cystic fibrosis and, 52, 53*f*
  Prader-Willi syndrome and, 66*f*
  symbols used in, 50, 50*f*
  X-linked inheritance and, 55
Pelvic floor dysfunction, 922
Pelvic inflammatory disease (PID), 824–825, 824*f*, 825*b*–826*b*, 891
Pelvic nerve, 331
Pelvic organ prolapse, 763, 827–828, 828*b*, 828*f*–829*f*, 830*b*
Pemphigus, 1085–1086, 1086*f*
Pemphigus erythematosus, 1086
Pemphigus foliaceus, 1086
Pemphigus herpetiformis, 1086
Pemphigus vegetans, 1086
Pemphigus vulgaris, 1086
Pendular nystagmus, 350
Penetrance, 51–52, 51*f*
Penetrating trauma, 394
Penis
  anatomy of, 808–809, 808*f*–809*f*
  cancer of, 270*t*–273*t*, 871–872, 872*b*
  ejaculation of, 809
  erectile reflex of, 809, 812
  functions of, 808
  hypospadias and, 784–785, 785*f*
  sexual excitement of, 809
  torsion of, 784
  tumours of, 871
Penis disorders
  balanitis, 871, 871*f*
  cancer, 270*t*–273*t*, 871–872, 872*b*
  paraphimosis, 869–870, 870*f*
  Peyronie disease, 870–871, 871*f*
  phimosis, 869–870, 870*f*
  priapism, 871, 871*f*
  tumours, 871
Pennate muscles, 999
Pepsin, 905
Peptic ulcer disease
  definition of, 931
  duodenal ulcers, 932–933, 932*f*, 933*t*
  gastric ulcers, 933, 933*t*
  Helicobacter pylori causing, 931–933
  lesions caused by, 931*f*
  NSAIDs causing, 931–932
  postgastrectomy syndromes, 934–935
  risk factors of, 931*b*

Peptic ulcer disease *(Continued)*
stress ulcers, 933
surgical treatment of, 934
Zollinger-Ellison syndrome and, 931
Peptide YY, 903*t*, 941, 941*b*
Percutaneous coronary intervention (PCI), 623
Perfusion, 595, 689–690
Pericardial cavity, 576
Pericardial effusion, 117, 629–630, 630*f*
Pericardial fluid, 576
Pericardial sac, 576
Pericarditis
acute, 629, 629*f*
constrictive, 630, 630*f*
Pericardium, 576, 576*f*
disorders of, 629–630
Perilymph, 354
Perimembranous ventricular septal defects, 668
Perimenopause, 811, 811*f*
Perimetrium, 799, 800*f*
Perimysium, 999
Perinatal stroke, 435
Perineum, 797*f*, 798
Periodic paralysis, 1043
Periosteal reaction, 1049
Periosteum, 323, 993, 993*f*
Peripheral artery disease, 617
Peripheral chemoreceptors, 684, 686
Peripheral (immune) CRH, 224
Peripheral cyanosis, 696
Peripheral membrane proteins, 7
Peripheral nervous system (PNS)
components of, 309, 327–328, 329*f*
disorders of, 416–417, 416*t*
spinal nerves and, 320*f*, 327–328
Peripheral neuropathic pain, 343
Peripheral tolerance, 173
Peripheral vascular disease (PVD), 484*t*, 486, 613–614
Raynaud phenomenon, 205, 613–614
thromboangiitis obliterans, 613
Peripheral vascular resistance-mediated ischemic cellular injury, 608
Peripheral vascular system, 589, 590*f*–591*f*
Peristalsis, 901, 908
Peritoneal cavity, 906
Peritoneum, 906
Peritonsillar abscesses, 727
Peritubular capillaries, 745
Permissive effects, of hormones, 446
Pernicious anemia, 521*t*, 522–523, 522*f*
Peroxisome-proliferator-activated receptor-γ coactivator-1 alpha, 256–257
Peroxisomes, characteristics of, 4*t*
Persistent pain, 343, 344*t*
Persistent vegetative state, 369
Personalized medicine, 262
Pertussis vaccine, 190
Pessary, 828
Pesticides, 855
Petechial hemorrhage, 510*t*
Peyer patches, 910
Peyronie disease, 870–871, 871*f*
PGI_2. *See* Prostacyclin
pH
of body fluids, 126, 128*t*
of CSF, 685
maintenance of, 130*f*
of vagina, 798–799, 826
Phagocytes, 139, 507. *See also* Macrophages
basophils, 142*f*, 145–147
defects of, 192*t*, 193
dendritic cells, 147
eosinophils, 142*f*, 147
in inflammation, 146–149
monocytes, 142, 142*f*, 147
neutrophils, 142*f*, 147
Phagocytosis, 21–23, 147–149, 148*f*
Phagolysosomes, 148*f*–149*f*, 149
Phagophore, 106–107
Phagosomes, 148*f*–149*f*, 149
Phantom limb pain, 344*t*
Pharyngeal cancer, 270*t*–273*t*
Pharyngotympanic tube, 354, 354*f*
Phase I activation enzymes, 281
Phase II detoxification enzymes, 281
PHDs. *See* Prolyl hydroxylases
Phencyclidine, 86*t*
Phenotype, 49
Phenylalanine hydroxylase, 434
Phenylketonuria (PKU), 49, 433–434, 434*f*
Phenytoin (Dilantin), 398–399
Pheochromocytomas, 490–491
Philadelphia chromosome, 242–243, 533–534, 534*f*
Phimosis, 869–870, 870*f*
Phlebotomy, 526
Phosphate
balance, alterations in, 126, 127*t*
bone and, 778, 989*t*
CKD and calcium balance with, 777*t*, 778
formation of, 992*t*
Phosphatidylserine, 143
Phosphodiesterase type 5 inhibitors (PDE5i), 888
Phospholipids, 5
Phthalates, 855
Phthirus pubis, 892*t*
Physical activity
breast cancer and, 855
Canadian schools promoting, 940*b*
cancer and, 283–285
Physical barriers, 135, 135*f*
Physiological atrophy, 75
Physiological jaundice of newborn, 979
Physiological stress, 216, 217*f*
Physiological tetanus, 1005–1006
Pia mater, 323, 324*f*
Pica, 435
Pick disease, 376
PID. *See* Pelvic inflammatory disease
PIF. *See* Prolactin-inhibiting factor
Pigments, as cellular accumulations, 99–100
PIN. *See* Prostatic intraepithelial neoplasia
Pineal gland, 452
Pinkeye, 353
Pinna, 354, 354*f*
Pinocytosis, 21–23
Pipe smoking. *See* Smoking, tobacco
Pit cells, 911–912
Pitting edema, 117, 118*f*
Pituitary adenomas, 469
Pituitary giantism, 469, 469*f*
Pituitary gland
aging and, 461*b*
anatomy of, 448, 449*f*–450*f*
anterior
acromegaly and, 469, 470*f*
anatomy of, 448–452
chromophils of, 448
chromophobes of, 448
diseases of, 468–471
hormones produced by, 448–452, 451*t*
hyperpituitarism and, 469
hypopituitarism and, 468, 469*f*
prolactinomas and, 470–471
regions of, 448
posterior
anatomy of, 452
diabetes insipidus and, 467–468, 467*t*
diseases of, 466–468
hormones of, 452
SIADH and, 122, 257*t*, 466–467, 467*t*
tumours of, 470–471
Pituitary stalk, 450*f*, 452
Pituitary tumours, 419*t*
PKU. *See* Phenylketonuria
Plagiocephaly, 431*f*
Plaque, 614
complicated, 614
fibrous, 614, 616*f*
rupture of, 614
unstable, 623–624, 623*f*–624*f*
Plaque (skin lesion), 1077*t*–1078*t*
Plaque psoriasis, 1083, 1083*f*
Plasma
composition of, 496–497, 498*t*
hydrostatic pressure in, 20, 20*f*
inorganic ions in, 497
oncotic pressure in, 20, 20*f*
Plasma *(Continued)*
osmolality, 118–119
serum compared to, 496
water movement between interstitial fluid and, 115–116, 117*f*
Plasma albumin, 117
Plasma cell count, 514*t*–516*t*
Plasma cells, 160
antibody production by, 496
in asthma, 706
Plasma creatinine concentration, 754
Plasma membrane
carbohydrates in, 2–3, 6*f*, 9
composition of, 2–9, 5*f*
functions of, 2–9, 5*f*, 5*t*
lipid bilayer of
description of, 2–3, 5*f*
proteins associated with, 7, 8*f*
lipids of, 3–5, 7*f*
proteins of, 5–8, 8*f*
receptors, 9, 10*f*
classes of, 14, 15*t*
signaling molecules and, 14, 15*f*
Plasma protein systems
clotting system and, 140*f*, 141
complement system and, 140–141, 140*f*
control of, 141–142
in inflammation, 140–142, 140*f*
interaction of, 141–142
kinin system and, 140*f*, 141
Plasma proteins
albumin, 100, 117, 496
classification of, 497
composition of, 496–497
globulins, 496–497
regulatory, 497
synthesis of, 150
transport, 497
Plasmin, 141, 513–514
Plasminogen, 141
Plasmodium, 187–188
Plastic rigidity, 381, 381*t*
Plasticity, developmental, 274–275
Platelet count, 514*t*–516*t*
Platelet-activating factor (PAF), 146, 652*b*
Platelet-derived growth factor (PDGF), 26–27, 26*t*, 991*t*
Platelets
activated, 146
activation of, 510, 511*f*
adhesion studies, 514*t*–516*t*
aggregation tests, 514*t*–516*t*
altered functions of, 549–550
characteristics of, 499–500, 499*t*, 501*f*
development of, 509–510
disorders of, 546–549
thrombocythemia, 548–549
thrombocytopenia, 547–548
hemostasis function of, 510–511, 546
in inflammation, 146
laboratory tests for, 514*t*–516*t*
micrograph of, 501*f*
normal concentration of, 500
sticky, 511*b*
Pleomorphic liposarcoma, 1050
Pleura
abnormalities of, 699–700, 699*f*, 700*t*
anatomy of, 683, 684*f*
Pleural cavity, 683, 684*f*
Pleural effusion, 117, 700, 700*t*
Pleural space, 683, 684*f*
Plexus injuries, 416, 416*t*
Plexuses, 310, 327–328
brachial, 328
lumbar, 328
sacral, 328
PMDD. *See* Premenstrual dysphoric disorder
PMS. *See* Premenstrual syndrome
Pneumococcal pneumonia, 190, 713, 713*f*, 732, 732*t*
Pneumococcus, 713
Pneumoconiosis, 703
Pneumonia
atypical, 733
bacterial, 732, 732*t*
in children, 732–733, 732*t*
chlamydophila, 732*t*, 733
clinical manifestations of, 713–714
Pneumonia *(Continued)*
community-acquired, 712, 712*b*
definition of, 711–712
evaluation of, 714
health care-associated, 712, 712*b*
hospital-acquired, 712, 712*b*
micro-organisms causing, 712, 712*b*
mycoplasmal, 732*t*, 733
pathophysiology of, 712–713, 713*f*
pneumococcal, 190, 713, 713*f*, 732, 732*t*
staphylococcal, 732, 732*t*
streptococcal, 732, 732*t*
treatment of, 714
urine antigen testing of, 714
ventilator-associated, 712, 712*b*
viral, 713, 732, 732*t*
Pneumothorax, 699–700, 699*f*
PNS. *See* Peripheral nervous system
Podocytes, 743
Podosomes, 990
Point mutations, 238–240
Poiseuille's law, 593
Poison ivy, 207, 208*f*, 1082, 1082*f*
Poisoning
carbon monoxide, 90
in children, 85*b*, 434, 434*t*
lead, 435
Polarity, 18–19
Poliovirus, 189–190
Pollution, air
CAD and, 620
cancer and, 293–294, 294*f*
diseases caused by, 86*b*
Polyarthritis, 1064
Polychlorinated biphenyls, 855
Polycystic kidney disease, 786
Polycystic ovary syndrome (PCOS), 822, 822*f*, 823*b*
Polycythemia, 257*t*
absolute, 526
familial, 528*t*
relative, 526
secondary, 526, 528*t*
Polycythemia vera, 526–528, 528*t*
Polydipsia, 467
in type 1 diabetes mellitus, 478*t*
Polygenic traits, 58
Polymenorrhea, 821*t*
Polymerase chain reaction, 733
Polymorphism, 49
Polymorphonuclear neutrophil, 147. *See also* Neutrophils
Polymyositis, 1045
Polypeptides, 5–7, 39
Polyphagia, 478*t*
Polyphenols, 280
Polyploid cells, 42–43
Polyploidy, 42–43
Polyps
colorectal, 956
endometrial, 830, 830*f*
neoplastic, 956, 956*f*
Polysomnography, 348
Polyunsaturated fatty acids, 906*b*
Polyuria, 478*t*
Pompe's disease, 1044
Pons, 313–314, 319
Pores of Kohn, 680–681, 702*f*
Porphyrin analysis, 514*t*–516*t*
Portal hypertension, 943–944, 944*f*, 981–982
Portopulmonary hypertension, 943
Port-wine stains, 1116, 1116*f*
Position effect, 47
Positive feedback, 443–444
Postcentral gyrus, 316–317, 316*f*
Postconcussion syndrome, 398
Posterior columns, 320–323, 321*f*
Posterior fontanelle, 426, 427*f*
Posterior fossa, 323
Posterior horn, 320–321
Posterior pituitary gland
anatomy of, 452
diseases of, 466–468
diabetes insipidus and, 467–468, 467*t*
SIADH, 122, 257*t*, 466–467, 467*t*
hormones of, 452
Posterior spinal artery, 327, 329*f*
Postganglionic neurons, 328, 331*f*

Postgastrectomy syndromes, 934–935
Posthemorrhagic anemia, 521*t*, 527*t*
Posthyperventilation apnea, 364, 366*t*
Postictal phase, 377
Postinflammatory IBS, 938
Postlactational involution, 849–850, 850*f*
Postmenopausal osteoporosis, 1022
Postmortem autolysis, 110
Postmortem changes, 109–110
Postoperative diuresis, 760
Postpartum thyroiditis, 473
Postrenal acute kidney injury, 773*t*, 774
Postsynaptic neurons, 313
Post-translational modifications (PTMs), 5–7
Post-traumatic seizures, 398–399
Post-traumatic stress disorder (PTSD), 217
Postural abnormalities, 385, 385*f*
Posture disorders, 389
Postvoid residual urine, 755*t*
Postvoid urine, 763
Potassium, 123*b*, 777*t*. *See also* Hyperkalemia; Hypokalemia
  active transport of, 21, 21*f*, 22*t*
  adaptation, 123
  aldosterone regulation of, 123
  alterations in, 122–126
    clinical manifestations of, 125*t*
  dietary, hypertension and stroke lower risk with, 123*b*
  in ECF, 123, 125
  in ICF, 123, 125
  insulin regulation of, 123
  renal losses of, 124
  total body, 123–124
  urinary excretion of, 125
Potassium-sparing diuretics, 753*t*
Pouchitis, 937
Powassan encephalitis, 413*t*
PP cells, 455
PR interval, 582–583, 583*f*
Prader-Willi syndrome, 52, 64–65, 65*f*–66*f*
Precapillary sphincter, 591–593, 592*f*
Precentral gyrus, 316, 317*f*
Precipitation, 163
Preclinical diastolic dysfunction, 642
Precocious puberty, 818, 819*b*, 868–869, 869*b*
Precursor cells, 28*f*
Predominantly antibody deficiencies, 192–193, 192*t*
Pre-excitation syndromes, 645*t*–646*t*
Preganglionic neurons, 328, 331*f*
Pregnancy
  breast cancer and, 845–849
  choline deficiency in, 280
  pyelonephritis and, 767*t*
  sickle cell test and, 566, 567*f*
Preictal phase, 377
Prekallikrein, 141
Preload, 587–588, 587*f*
Premature atrial contractions, 644*t*–645*t*
Premature junctional contractions, 644*t*–645*t*
Premature ventricular contractions, 644*t*–645*t*
Premenstrual dysphoric disorder (PMDD), 822–823
Premenstrual syndrome (PMS), 822–823, 824*b*
Premotor area, 315–316, 316*f*
Prepuce, 808
Prerenal acute kidney injury, 773, 773*t*
Presbycusis, 355
Presbyopia, 352
Pressure, blood flow affected by, 593–594
Pressure flow study, 755*t*
Pressure ulcers, 1076–1081, 1076*b*, 1080*f*
Pressure-natriuresis relationship, 607, 607*f*
Presynaptic neurons, 313
Pretibial myxedema, 472
PRF. *See* Prolactin-releasing factor
Priapism, 871, 871*f*
Primary adrenal insufficiency, 490
Primary aldosteronism, 489
Primary amenorrhea, 819–820
Primary bile acids, 912
Primary biliary cirrhosis, 949
Primary cutaneous lymphomas, 1095
Primary dysmenorrhea, 819
Primary emphysema, 710
Primary glomerular injury, 767–768
Primary hyperaldosteronism, 124, 489
Primary hyperparathyroidism, 474–475
Primary hypertension, 674–675, 675*b*
  Indigenous people of Canada and, 607
  inflammation and, 608
  insulin resistance and, 608–609
  new immigrants and, 607
  obesity and, 608, 609*b*
  pathophysiology of, 607–609, 610*f*
  pressure-natriuresis relationship and, 607, 607*f*
  renin-angiotensin-aldosterone system in, 607–609
  risk factors associated with, 606–607, 607*b*
  sympathetic nervous system and, 606–607, 634
Primary hypothyroidism, 473–474, 473*f*
Primary (congenital) immune deficiency, 190–193, 192*t*
Primary immune response, 168
Primary incontinence, 790
Primary intention wound healing, 152, 152*f*
Primary intracerebral tumours, 418–420, 419*t*
Primary lymphoid organs, 165–167, 500
Primary motor area, 316, 317*f*
Primary nodular melanoma, 1093–1094
Primary particles, 294
Primary peristalsis, 901
Primary pneumothorax, 699–700
Primary polycythemia. *See* Polycythemia vera
Primary polydipsia, 467
Primary spermatocytes, 810, 810*f*
Primary spinal cord injury, 399
Primary thrombocythemia, 549
Primary thyroid disorders, 471
Primary voluntary motor area, 316, 317*f*
Primary-progressive multiple sclerosis, 415–416
Principal cells, 744
Principle of independent assortment, 50
Principle of segregation, 50
Prinzmetal angina, 621
Proband, 50
Probenecid (Benuryl), 826*b*
Prodroma, 377
Proerythroblasts, 506
Progesterone, 794*t*, 838*f*
  biological effects of, 801–802, 802*t*
  breast cancer risk and, 851
  secretion of, 801–802
Progesterone receptor, 837–838
Programmed necrosis, 101
Progressive bulbar palsy, 388
Progressive hypoxia, 80–81
Progressive relaxation training, 1041
Progressive spinal muscular atrophy, 388
Progressive-relapsing multiple sclerosis, 415–416
Proinflammatory cytokines, 941*b*
Projectile vomiting, 922
Prokaryotes, 1, 178
Prolactin
  breast cancer and, 852
  secretion of, 470–471
  in stress response, 225*t*–226*t*
Prolactin-inhibiting factor (PIF), 449*t*, 843
Prolactinomas, 470–471
Prolactin-releasing factor (PRF), 449*t*
Prolia, 1026*b*
Proliferative inflammatory atrophy, 883
Proliferative phase, of wound healing, 153–154
Prolyl hydroxylases (PHDs), 80
Promotor sites, 41
Propionibacterium acnes, 1107
Proprioception, 356–357
Prostacyclin, 598
Prostacyclin (PGI_2), 146, 510
Prostaglandins, 146
Prostate cancer
  aging and risk of, 887
  androgen receptor in, 851
  cancer cells in, 886
  chronic inflammation and, 883, 883*f*–884*f*
  clinical manifestations of, 886
  description of, 270*t*–273*t*
  diet and, 880, 880*b*–881*b*
  EMT and, 886
  epigenetic factors in, 883–884
  evaluation of, 886–887
  fibroblasts in, 885–886
  genetic factors in, 883–884
  Gleason score for, 880*b*–881*b*
  hormones involved in, 882, 882*f*, 884–885
  incidence of, 879–880, 879*f*
  metastasis sites in, 886, 887*f*
  pathogenesis of, 884, 884*f*
  prostate epithelial neoplasia and, 885, 886*f*
  race and, 887
  screening for, 887, 888*f*
  staging for, 889*b*–890*b*
  stromal environment in, 885–887, 887*f*
  treatment of, 886–887
  vasectomy and risk of, 882–883
Prostate epithelial neoplasia, 885, 886*f*
Prostate gland
  anatomy of, 809, 809*f*
  disorders of, 876–887
  enlargement of, 763
Prostate-specific antigen (PSA), 261, 886–887
Prostatic hyperplasia, 883
Prostatic intraepithelial neoplasia (PIN), 885, 886*f*
Prostatitis, 878–879, 878*b*
Protamines, 64
Proteases, 224
Proteasomes, 75
Protein adducts, 84–85
Protein C, 513
Protein folding, in endoplasmic reticulum, 8*b*, 8*f*
Protein kinases, 447
Protein S, 513
Protein wasting, 488
Protein-energy malnutrition, 977
Protein-free fluid, 749
Proteins
  BCR-ABL, 242–243
  buffering, 126, 130*f*
  cartilage intermediate layer, 403–404
  catabolism of, 75, 220
  as cellular accumulations, 99
  CFTR, 735
  contractile, of skeletal muscles, 1003, 1003*t*
  depletion of, 647–648
  formation of, 39–42
  function of, 914*t*
  homeostasis of, 8–9, 9*f*
  hormones, 444
  importance of, 914*t*
  integral membrane, 7
  liver metabolism of, 914, 914*t*
  metabolism
    in CKD, 778
    cortisol effects on, 220
  peripheral membrane, 7
  plasma membrane, 5–8, 8*f*
  receptor, 14
  regulation of, in cells, 8–9, 9*f*
  serum, 916*t*
  small intestine absorption of, 908*b*
  synthesis, 42, 43*f*, 99
  transmembrane, 7, 8*f*
Proteinuria
  CKD progression and, 777*t*
  in multiple myeloma, 544
Proteoglycans, 9, 992
Proteolytic systems, 8–9
Proteomes, 5–7
Proteomics, 5–7
Prothrombin time, 514*t*–516*t*, 916*t*
Prothrombinase complex, 513
Prothrombotic state, 547
Proton pump inhibitors, 926
Proto-oncogenes, 242
Protopathic modalities, 323
Protoporphyrin, 507
Protoporphyrin analysis, 514*t*–516*t*
Protozoan parasites, 187–188, 187*t*, 196*b*
Provera (medroxyprogesterone), 821
Proximal convoluted tubule, 742*f*, 743–744, 749–750
PRRs. *See* Pattern recognition receptors
Pruritus, 1081, 1085, 1114
PSA. *See* Prostate-specific antigen
Psammoma bodies, 100
Pseudohypoparathyroidism, 475
Pseudomonas aeruginosa, 138
Pseudostratified ciliated columnar epithelium, 29*t*–30*t*, 30*f*
Pseudounipolar neurons, 310
Psoriasis, 1083–1084, 1083*f*, 1084*b*
Psoriatic arthritis, 1083–1084
Psoriatic nail disease, 1083–1084
Psychological stressors, 217
Psychomotor stimulants, 86*t*
Psychoneuroimmunology, 217–219
Psychosocial distress, 227–228
Psychosocial stress, 223*b*
PTMs. *See* Post-translational modifications
PTSD. *See* Post-traumatic stress disorder
Puberty
  age of onset, 817–818
  definition of, 795
  delayed, 818, 818*b*, 818*t*, 868, 869*b*
  precocious, 818, 819*b*, 868–869, 869*b*
  reproductive system and, 795–796
Puerperal infections, 824
Pulmicort, 726
Pulmonary artery, 577, 577*f*
  anatomy of, 682
  constriction of, 683
  pressure, 683
Pulmonary artery hypertension, 698, 716–717, 716*f*
Pulmonary atresia, 666
Pulmonary blood flow
  congenital heart defects with decreased, 668–670
  congenital heart defects with increased, 667–668
  gravity effects on, 690*f*
Pulmonary circulation. *See also* Heart
  anatomy of, 576*f*, 681–683, 683*f*
  control of, 683
  functions of, 575
  perfusion distribution in, 689–690
Pulmonary diseases and disorders
  acute bronchitis, 711
  ALI, 704
  ARDS, 704, 705*f*
  aspiration, 701
  asthma (*See* Asthma)
  atelectasis, 701, 702*f*
  bronchiectasis, 701–702
  bronchiolitis, 702, 730–732
  in children (*See* Children, pulmonary diseases and disorders in)
  chronic bronchitis, 709–710, 709*f*–710*f*, 709*t*
  conditions caused by
    hypercapnia, 697
    hypoxemia, 697–698, 698*f*
    respiratory failure, 698–699
  COPD, 708–709, 711*f*
  cor pulmonale, 698, 717
  emphysema, 709*t*, 710–711, 710*f*–711*f*
  inhalation disorders, 702–703
  obstructive lung diseases, 705–711
  pneumonia (*See* Pneumonia)
  pulmonary artery hypertension, 698, 716–717, 716*f*
  pulmonary edema, 703–704, 703*f*
  pulmonary embolism, 715–716, 715*f*
  pulmonary fibrosis, 702
  respiratory tract infections (*See* Respiratory tract infections)
  restrictive lung diseases, 701–704
  signs and symptoms of
    breathing pattern abnormalities, 696
    clubbing, 697, 697*f*
    cough, 695–696

Pulmonary diseases and disorders *(Continued)*
cyanosis, 696–697
dyspnea, 695
hemoptysis, 696
hyperventilation, 696
hypoventilation, 696
pain, 697
sputum abnormalities, 696
tuberculosis (*See* Tuberculosis)
Pulmonary edema, 703–704, 703*f*
Pulmonary embolism, 715–716, 715*f*
Pulmonary fibrosis, 702
Pulmonary function tests, 688
Pulmonary stenosis, 666–667, 666*f*
Pulmonary system
abbreviations for, 689*t*
aging and, 692
anatomy of, 679–683, 680*f*–684*f*
bronchial circulation in, 681–683
chest wall in, 683, 684*f*
CKD and, 776*t*, 779
conducting airways of, 679–680, 681*f*–682*f*
defense mechanisms of, 679, 680*t*
functions of, 679
breathing mechanics, 686–688
gas transport, 688–692
overview of, 684, 684*f*
ventilation (*See* Ventilation)
gas-exchange airways of, 680–681, 682*f*–683*f*
larynx (*See* Larynx)
lower airway, 682*f*
lungs (*See* Lungs)
pleura in, 683, 684*f*
trachea (*See* Trachea)
upper airway, 679, 681*f*
Pulmonary vascular resistance (PVR), 668
Pulmonary veins, 577, 682
Pulmonic semilunar valves, 577, 577*f*–578*f*
Pulse pressure, 595
Pulsus paradoxus, 630, 707
Puncture wound, 94*t*–95*t*
Punnett square, 50, 51*f*, 54*f*
Pupil, 364, 366*f*
Purified protein derivative, 714
Purines, 38
Purkinje fibres, 582, 582*f*
Purpura fulminans, 412
Purulent exudate, 150
Pustular psoriasis, 1083
Pustule, 1077*t*–1078*t*
Putamen, 317, 319*f*
PVD. *See* Peripheral vascular disease
PVR. *See* Pulmonary vascular resistance
Pyelonephritis, 767, 767*t*, 788
Pyknosis, 101–102
Pyloric obstruction, 927–928
Pyloric sphincter, 902, 902*f*
Pyloric stenosis, threshold of liability for, 58, 58*f*
Pylorus, 902, 902*f*
Pyramidal cerebral palsy, 433
Pyramidal motor syndrome, 385, 387*f*, 390*t*
Pyramidal system, 316, 318*f*
Pyramids, of kidney, 741, 742*f*
Pyrogenic bacteria, 183
Pyrogens, 150
Pyruvate, 17, 17*f*

Q

QRS complex, 582–583, 583*f*
QT interval, 582–583, 583*f*
Quadriparesis, 386*b*
Quadriplegia, 386*b*
Quality-adjusted life year, 108

R

RAAS. *See* Renin-angiotensin-aldosterone system
Rabies vaccine, 198
Radial scar, 844–845
Radiation therapy
for cancer, 262
secondary malignancies caused by, 853
Radicular pain, 403
Radicular syndrome, 421
Radiculopathy, 405, 416*t*
Radiofrequency electromagnetic radiation, 291
Radioimmunoassay (RIA), 446*b*
Radiolysis, 286–287
Radon, 294
Raloxifene, 1025–1026, 1026*b*
RANK. *See* Receptor activator nuclear factor kappa-B
RANKL. *See* Receptor activator nuclear factor kappa-B ligand
Rapamycin, 108
Rapid eye movement (REM) sleep, 347–348
RAS (rat sarcoma), 240–242
Raynaud phenomenon, 205, 613–614
RBB. *See* Right bundle branch
RDS. *See* Respiratory distress syndrome of newborn
Reactive oxygen species (ROS), 80
cellular injury caused by, 82–83, 84*f*
mitochondria damaged by, 83
oxidative stress and, 82–83
sun exposure as cause of, 290
Reactive stress response, 217
Rebound headaches, 411
Receptive aprosody, 389–390
Receptive dysphasia, 371, 372*t*–373*t*
Receptor activator nuclear factor kappa-B (RANK), 990–992, 991*t*, 1022–1023, 1024*f*
Receptor activator nuclear factor kappa-B ligand (RANKL), 990–992, 991*t*, 1022–1023, 1024*f*
Receptor protein, 14
Receptor-mediated endocytosis, 23, 23*f*
Recessive effects, 49
Recessiveness, 49–50
Reciprocal translocation, 47
Recombinant human erythropoietin (r-HuEPO), 506
Recombinant human granulocyte colony-stimulating factor, 259
Recombination, of alleles, 57
Recombination activating genes, 167
Rectal carcinomas, 957
Rectocele, 828, 829*f*
Rectosigmoid sphincter, 909
Rectosphincteric reflex, 910
Rectum, 910
cancer of, 270*t*–273*t*, 837, 954*t*, 955–957, 956*b*–957*b*, 956*f*–957*f*
Recurrence risks
in autosomal dominant inheritance, 50–51
in autosomal recessive inheritance, 53–54, 54*f*
in X-linked inheritance, 55–56, 56*f*
Red cell count, 514*t*–516*t*
Red measles, 1112, 1112*t*
Red muscle, 1000, 1001*t*
Red nucleus, 319
Reed-Sternberg (RS) cells, 539, 539*f*, 572, 572*f*
Refeeding syndrome, 943
Referred pain, 342–343, 343*f*, 924
Reflex arcs, 321–322, 322*f*
Reflexes, in infants, 426–427, 427*t*
Refraction alterations, 352, 352*f*
Refractory period, 582
Regeneration, tissue, 152
Regional osteoporosis, 1023
Regulatory T cells, 160, 173
Regurgitation
aortic, 634
mitral, 634
tricuspid, 634
valvular, 632, 632*t*, 633*f*, 634
Relative polycythemia, 526
Relative refractory period, 24
Relaxin, 794*t*
REM. *See* Rapid eye movement sleep
Remitting-relapsing multiple sclerosis, 415–416
Renal adenomas, 763–764
Renal agenesis, 786
Renal aplasia, 786
Renal arteries, 744–745
Renal autoregulation, 746–747, 747*f*
Renal blood flow, 746–747, 747*f*, 753
Renal cancer, 270*t*–273*t*
Renal capsule, 741, 742*f*
Renal cell carcinoma, 763–764, 764*f*
Renal clearance
BUN and, 754
glomerular filtration rate and, 753–754
plasma creatinine concentration and, 754
renal blood flow and, 753
Renal colic, 761
Renal columns, 741, 742*f*
Renal corpuscle, 742*f*, 743
Renal disorders. *See* Children, renal disorders in
Renal fascia, 741
Renal function
aging effects on, 756
elderly and, 756
infants and, 756
tests of, 753–754, 755*t*
Renal insufficiency, 772
Renal papillae, 745–746
Renal plasma flow, 746, 753
Renal system, 741–746. *See also* Kidneys
Renal transitional cell carcinoma, 763–764
Renal tumours, 763–764, 764*f*
Renal veins, 745
Renalase, 747
Renin, 118
Renin-angiotensin-aldosterone system (RAAS), 118, 119*f*, 607–609
renal blood flow regulation by, 747
Repair, of scar tissue, 152
Reperfusion injury, 82, 82*f*
Repetitive discharge, 1005–1006
Replicative aging, 108
Repolarization, 24, 582
delayed, 124
Reproductive system
aging and, 811–812
CKD effects on, 776*t*, 779
development of, 793–796
female (*See* Female reproductive system)
male (*See* Male reproductive system)
maturation and, 795–796
puberty and, 795–796
sexual differentiation in utero, 793–795
Resistance, blood flow affected by, 593–594
Resistance stage, of general adaptation syndrome, 216–217
Resistin, 941*b*
Resolution, of inflammation, 152
Respiration. *See also* Breathing; Ventilation
brainstem control of, 684, 685*f*
Cheyne-Stokes, 364, 366*t*, 696
Kussmaul, 128, 696
neurochemical control of, 684–686, 685*f*
physiology of, 699*f*
Respiratory acidosis, 129–130, 131*f*
Respiratory alkalosis, 130–131, 131*f*
Respiratory bronchioles, 680, 682*f*–683*f*
Respiratory burst, 149
Respiratory distress syndrome of newborn (RDS), 728–730, 728*b*, 729*f*
Respiratory failure, 698–699
Respiratory rate, 684
Respiratory tract
laryngeal cancer of, 270*t*–273*t*, 717–718, 717*f*
lung cancer (*See* Lung cancer)
malignancies of, 270*t*–273*t*, 717–720
Respiratory tract infections, 180*t*–181*t*
abscesses, 715
acute bronchitis, 711
in children, 730–733
pneumonia (*See* Pneumonia)
tuberculosis (*See* Tuberculosis)
Rest legs syndrome, 349
Resting membrane potential, 24
Restricted breathing, 696
Restrictive cardiomyopathy, 631–632, 631*f*
Restrictive lung diseases, 701–704
ALI, 704
ARDS, 704, 705*f*
aspiration, 701
atelectasis, 701, 702*f*
bronchiectasis, 701–702
bronchiolitis, 702, 730–732
inhalation disorders, 702–703
pulmonary edema, 703–704, 703*f*
pulmonary fibrosis, 702
Resveratrol, 280
Retching, 921
Rete testis, 807, 808*f*
Reticular activating system, 313–314, 315*f*
Reticular formation, 313–314, 315*f*
Reticulocyte, 506
Reticulocyte count, 514*t*–516*t*
Reticuloendothelial system, 913
Retina, 349, 349*f*
Retinal detachment, 351*t*
Retinoblastoma, 26, 305
in children, 439–440, 439*f*
familial, 243
gene for, 51, 243
Retinoids, 1107–1108
Retractile testis, 874
Retrograde amnesia, 369, 370*t*
Retrograde menstruation, 832
Retropulsion, 903
Reverse transcriptase, 195
Reverse transcriptase inhibitors, 196–197
Reverse Warburg effect, 249
Reversible sideroblastic anemia, 525
Rh blood group, 211
Rh incompatibility, 562–563
Rhabdomyolysis, 774, 1017–1019, 1018*b*
Rhabdomyomas, 1051
Rhabdomyosarcomas, 236, 304, 1050–1051
Rheumatic heart disease, 634–637, 636*f*
Rheumatoid arthritis
ankylosing spondylitis compared to, 1035–1036
cause of, 1032–1033
classification criteria for, 1036*t*
clinical manifestations of, 1034–1035
evaluation of, 1035
female sexual dysfunction and, 843*t*
of hand, 1033*f*
HLAs and, 1032–1033
incidence of, 1032
mechanisms of, 1032
molecular imaging of, 1035*b*
pathophysiology of, 1033, 1033*f*–1034*f*
treatment of, 1035
Rheumatoid factors, 1032–1033
Rheumatoid nodules, 1035
Rhinovirus, 183
r-HuEPO. *See* Recombinant human erythropoietin
Rhythmicity, of heart, 583
RIA. *See* Radioimmunoassay
Ribonucleic acid (RNA), 1
messenger, 41, 247
micro, 64, 247
cancer and, 69
coding, 70
noncoding, 64, 238–240, 247
ribosomal, 42
transcription, 41, 42*f*–43*f*
transfer, 42
translation, 42, 43*f*
Ribosomal RNA (rRNA), 42
Ribosomes
biogenesis of, 75
characteristics of, 4*t*
protein synthesis and, 42, 99
Rickets, 1026
RIFLE criteria, 772, 773*t*
Right atrium, 577, 577*f*
Right bundle branch (RBB), 582
Right coronary artery, 578, 579*b*, 581*f*
Right lymphatic duct, 599, 600*f*
Right ventricle, 577, 577*f*
Right ventricular failure, 642, 642*f*
Right-to-left shunting, 662–663, 664*f*
Rigidity, 381, 381*t*
Rigor mortis, 110
Rilutek (riluzole), 389
Riluzole (Rilutek), 389

Ringed sideroblasts, 525
Rituximab (Rituxan), 263*t*, 548
RNA. *See* Ribonucleic acid
RNA polymerase, 41
Robertsonian translocation, 47
Rocephin (ceftriaxone), 826*b*
Rods, 349
ROS. *See* Reactive oxygen species
Roseola, 1112–1113, 1112*t*
Ross procedure, 665
Rotavirus, 973–974
rRNA. *See* Ribosomal RNA
RS cells. *See* Reed-Sternberg cells
Rubella, 1111–1112, 1112*f*, 1112*t*
Rubeola, 1112, 1112*t*
Rubral tremor, 383*t*
Rubrospinal tract, 322
Ruffini endings, 356
Ruffled border, 990
Rugae, 798
Rule of nines, in burns, 1095, 1096*f*
Russell-Silver Syndrome, 66

S

S phase, in cell cycle, 25, 25*f*
SA node. *See* Sinoatrial node
Sabin vaccine, 165, 189–190
Saccular aneurysms, 408, 611
Sacral plexus, 328
SAGs. *See* Superantigens
Saliva, 899–901, 901*f*
Salivary glands, cancer of, 270*t*–273*t*
Salivary α-amylase, 899–901
Salivation, 899–901, 901*f*
Salivatory glands, 899–901, 901*f*
Salk vaccine, 165, 189–190
Salmonella, 1028
Salpingitis, 825–826, 825*f*
Saltatory conduction, 310
Saphenous veins, 604
Sarcolemma, 1000
Sarcomas, 236
of breast, 856*t*
Ewing, 236, 304, 1050, 1070–1071, 1070*f*–1071*f*
fibrosarcoma, 1050
Kaposi, 252, 270*t*–273*t*, 307, 1094–1095, 1094*f*
leiomyosarcoma, 1050
osteosarcomas, 1049–1050, 1049*f*, 1070
pleomorphic liposarcoma, 1050
rhabdomyosarcomas, 236, 304, 1050–1051
synovial, 1050
Sarcomeres, 584, 584*f*, 1002
Sarcopenia, 109, 1008
Sarcoplasm, 1000–1002
Sarcoplasmic reticulum, 1002
Sarcotubular system, 1002
Sarcotubules, 1002
Satellite cells, 309, 1000
Saturated fatty acids, 906*b*
Scabies, 892*t*–894*t*, 1114, 1114*f*
Scale (skin lesion), 1079*t*–1080*t*
Scaphocephaly, 431*f*
Scar tissue
contracture of, 154–155
definition of, 152
repair of, 152
Scars
hypertrophic, 154, 155*f*, 1081, 1081*f*, 1098*f*
keloids, 154, 155*f*, 1079*t*–1080*t*, 1081, 1081*f*
radial, 844–845
Scavenger receptors, 143
Schilling test, 523
Schwann cells, 309–311, 312*f*
Sciatica, 403
SCIDs. *See* Severe combined immunodeficiencies
Sclera, 349, 349*f*
Scleroderma, 1090–1091, 1091*f*
Sclerosing adenosis, 844
Scoliosis, 1066–1067, 1066*f*
Scotoma, 351*t*
Scrotum, 808, 808*f*
disorders of, 872–876, 873*f*
Sebaceous glands, 1074
Seborrheic dermatitis, 1083, 1083*f*
Seborrheic keratosis, 1091, 1091*f*
Second messengers, 446–447, 447*f*, 465
Secondary amenorrhea, 819–820, 841*f*
Secondary bile acids, 912
Secondary biliary cirrhosis, 949
Secondary brain injury, 395*t*, 398
Secondary dysmenorrhea, 819
Secondary glomerular injury, 767–768
Secondary hyperaldosteronism, 489
Secondary hyperparathyroidism, 475
Secondary hypertension, 606, 609, 674–675, 675*b*
Secondary hypocortisolism, 490
Secondary hypothyroidism, 473–474, 473*f*
Secondary (acquired) immune deficiency, 190, 193, 194*b*
Secondary immune response, 168
Secondary incontinence, 790
Secondary intention wound healing, 152–153, 152*f*
Secondary lymphoid organs, 160, 162*f*, 500
Secondary osteoporosis, 1022–1023
Secondary Parkinsonism, 384
Secondary particles, 294
Secondary peristalsis, 901
Secondary pneumothorax, 699–700
Secondary polycythemia, 526, 528*t*
Secondary spermatocytes, 810, 810*f*
Secondary spinal cord injury, 399
Secondary thrombocythemia, 549
Secondary thyroid disorders, 471
Secondary ureteropelvic junction obstruction, 785–786
Secondary-progressive multiple sclerosis, 415–416
Second-degree block, 645*t*–646*t*
Second-degree burns, 1095, 1095*f*, 1097*t*
Secondhand smoke, 276, 709*b*
Secretin, 903, 903*t*
Secretory diarrhea, 923
Secretory IgA, 192
Secretory immune system, 165, 166*f*
Secretory immunoglobulin, 165
Secretory phase, 803, 803*f*
Sedative-hypnotics, 86*t*
Sedentary lifestyle, 618–619
Segmental pain inhibition, 342
Segmented fractures, 1012*f*
Seizure/seizure disorders
absence, 436*t*
atonic, 436*t*
in children, 436, 436*t*
clinical manifestations of, 377
conditions associated with, 376, 377*t*
definition of, 376
evaluation and treatment of, 377
febrile, 436*t*
focal, 436*t*
generalized clonic-tonic, 377, 436*t*
myoclonic, 436*t*
partial, 436*t*
post-traumatic, 398–399
types of, 376–377, 377*t*
Selective attention, 369, 370*t*
Selective attention deficits, 369
Selective auditory attention, 369
Selective estrogen receptor modulator, 1026*b*
Selective IgA deficiency, 192, 192*t*
Selective visual attention, 369
Selenium, 880*b*–881*b*
Self-antigens, 167–168
Self-renewal cells, 27, 28*f*
Selye, Hans, 216
Semen, 809
Semicircular canals, 354, 354*f*–355*f*
Semilunar valves, 577, 577*f*–578*f*
Seminal vesicles, 809, 809*f*
Seminiferous tubules, 807, 808*f*
Senescence, 108
Senile disease complex, 374
Sensorimotor syndrome, 421
Sensorineural hearing loss, 355
Sensory dysphasia, 371, 372*t*–373*t*
Sensory inattentiveness, 369–371
Sensory neurons, 310
Sensory pathways, 322–323
Sensory speech area, 316*f*, 317
Sensory-discriminative system, 340
Sepsis
central line-associated bloodstream infections as cause of, 651*b*
deaths involving, 650–651
description of, 183
guidelines for surviving, 652, 652*b*
Septic arthritis, 1063–1064
Septic shock, 650–652, 651*t*, 652*b*, 652*f*
Septicemia, 183, 643
Sequestosome-1, 1027
Sequestration crisis, 566
Sequestrum, 1028
Serotonin, 903*t*
properties of, 314*t*
Serous cell, 682*f*
Serous exudate, 150
Sertoli cells, 810, 810*f*
Serum, 496
Serum electrolytes, 945
Serum electrophoresis, 496–497
Serum enzymes, 916*t*
Serum ferritin determination, 514*t*–516*t*
Serum proteins, 916*t*
Serum sickness, 205
Sever disease, 1066
Severe combined immunodeficiencies (SCIDs), 191, 192*t*, 195
Severe congenital neutropenia, 192*t*, 193
Severe diffuse axonal injury, 398
Sex chromosomes
aneuploidy of, 46
description of, 42
Sex hormones
breast development and, 850
definition of, 793
female, 794*t*, 801–802, 802*b*, 802*t*
male, 794*t*, 810
Sex linked inheritance, 54
Sex-influenced traits, 56
Sex-limited traits, 56
Sexual differentiation, 793–795
Sexual dysfunction
female, 842–843, 843*t*
male, 888–890
Sexual maturation alterations, 817–818, 818*b*–819*b*, 818*t*, 868–869
Sexual trauma, female, 767*t*
Sexually transmitted infections/ diseases, 180*t*–181*t*, 891–894, 892*t*–894*t*
cancer and, 292–293, 293*t*
SGLT2. *See* Sodium-glucose cotransporter 2
Shaken baby syndrome, 94*t*–95*t*
Sharp-force injuries, 94*t*–95*t*
Shear stress, 578–579
Sheehan's syndrome, 468
Shift to the left, 530–531
Shift to the right, 530–531
Shift work sleep disorder, 349
Shingles, 1088, 1113
Shock, 696
anaphylactic, 650, 650*f*
cardiogenic, 648, 649*f*
cellular metabolism impairment in, 643–648, 647*f*
clinical manifestations of, 648
compensatory mechanisms for, 643
description of, 643
glucose impairment in, 647–648, 647*f*
hypovolemic, 648, 649*f*
neurogenic, 648–650, 650*f*
oxygen use impairment in, 643–647
septic, 650–652, 651*t*, 652*b*, 652*f*
treatment for, 648
types of, 648–652
vasogenic, 648–650
Short bones, 994
Short-term starvation, 942–943
Shunt, 662–663, 664*f*, 669–670
Shunting
left-to-right, 662–663, 664*f*
right-to-left, 662–663, 664*f*
ventilation-perfusion mismatch caused by, 698, 698*f*
Shwachman syndrome, 534
SIADH. *See* Syndrome of inappropriate antidiuretic hormone
Sialoprotein, 989*t*, 992
Sickle cell anemia, 521*t*, 564–565
Sickle cell disease, 564–567, 564*f*–567*f*, 565*t*
Sickle cell test, 514*t*–516*t*, 566, 567*f*
Sickle cell trait, 564–565
Sickle cell-hemoglobin C disease, 564–566
Sickle cell-thalassemia disease, 564–566
Sickled erythrocytes, 565, 565*f*–566*f*
Sideroblastic anemia, 521*t*, 525–526
Sigmoid colon, 909, 909*f*
Signal transduction pathways, 14, 15*f*
Signalling cell, 14
Sildenafil, 888
Silent ischemia, 621, 621*f*–622*f*
Silent mutations, 39
Silent thyroiditis, 473
Simple columnar epithelium, 29*t*–30*t*, 30*f*
Simple cuboidal epithelium, 29*f*, 29*t*–30*t*
Simple fibroadenomas, 845
Simple sinus tachycardia, 644*t*–645*t*
Simple squamous epithelium, 29*f*, 29*t*–30*t*
Single gene defects, 191
Single nucleotide polymorphisms, 277
Single-photon emission computed tomography (SPECT), 622–623
Sinoatrial node (SA node), 581, 582*f*, 583
Sinus block, 645*t*–646*t*
Sinus bradycardia, 644*t*–645*t*
Sinus dysrhythmias, 644*t*–645*t*
Sinus venosus atrial septal defect, 667
Sinusoids, 911, 912*f*
SIRS. *See* Systemic inflammatory response syndrome
Sister chromatids, 25
Skeletal muscle disorders
acid maltase deficiency, 1044
chronic fatigue syndrome, 1041–1043
contractures, 1041
dermatomyositis, 1045, 1045*f*
disuse atrophy, 75, 1041
endocrine disorders, 1043–1044
energy metabolism diseases, 1044
fibromyalgia, 1041–1042, 1042*b*, 1042*f*
idiopathic inflammatory myopathies, 1045, 1045*f*
inclusion body myositis, 1045
lipid deficiency, 1044
McArdle's disease, 1044
myoadenylate deaminase deficiency, 1044
myositis, 1044–1045, 1045*f*
myotonia, 1043
periodic paralysis, 1043
polymyositis, 1045
stress-induced muscle tension, 1041
toxic myopathies, 1046, 1046*b*
Skeletal muscles
cardiac muscle compared to, 584–585
contractile proteins of, 1003, 1003*t*
extrafusal, 999
fast-twitch, 1000
fibres, 1000–1002, 1001*t*, 1002*f*
function of, 998–999
fusiform, 999
motor units of, 999–1003, 1002*f*
myofibrils of, 1002*f*, 1003
nonprotein constituents of, 1003
pennate, 999
sensory receptors of, 1000
slow-twitch, 1000
striated, 999
structure of, 33*f*, 33*t*–34*t*, 998–1006, 1001*f*–1002*f*
voluntary, 999–1000
skeletal muscles, aging of, 1007–1008
Skeletal system, CKD and, 776*t*
Skeletal trauma, 1011–1015
Skeleton, 994, 994*f*
Skin
aging changes to, 1102
anatomy of, 1074–1081, 1075*f*, 1075*t*
apocrine sweat glands of, 1074–1076
blood supply to, 1076
cancer manifestations of, 260
CKD effects on, 776*t*, 779
cysts, 1077*t*–1078*t*
dermal appendages, 1074–1076, 1076*f*

Skin *(Continued)*
dermis, 1074, 1075*f*, 1075*t*
eccrine sweat glands of, 1074–1076
epidermis, 1074, 1075*f*, 1075*t*
layers of, 1074–1076, 1075*f*, 1075*t*
sebaceous glands of, 1074
subcutaneous layer of, 1074, 1075*f*, 1075*t*
tumours of, 1077*t*–1078*t*
ulcers, 1079*t*–1080*t*
Skin cancer, 260
basal cell carcinoma, 290, 1092, 1093*f*
cutaneous melanoma, 1093–1094, 1094*b*, 1094*f*
description of, 270*t*–273*t*
Kaposi sarcoma, 252, 270*t*–273*t*, 307, 1094–1095, 1094*f*
melanoma, 290–291
multistep, theoretical scheme of, 290
primary cutaneous lymphomas, 1095
squamous cell carcinoma, 290, 1092–1093, 1093*f*
sun exposure and, 290
trends for, 1092*b*
types of, 290
ultraviolet radiation as cause of, 1092
Skin disorders
acne rosacea, 1085, 1085*f*
acne vulgaris, 1085
actinic keratosis, 1091
allergic contact dermatitis, 208*f*, 1082, 1082*f*
atopic dermatitis, 892*t*–894*t*, 1082
bacterial infections, 1087–1088, 1087*f*
benign tumours, 1091, 1091*f*, 1092*t*
burns (*See* Burns)
candidiasis, 1089, 1090*t*
carbuncles, 1087
cellulitis, 1087
chickenpox, 1088
in children (*See* Children, skin disorders in)
cold injury, 1099–1101
cutaneous vasculitis, 1090
eczema, 1081–1082
erysipelas, 1087
erythema multiforme, 1086–1087
folliculitis, 1087
fungal infections, 1089, 1089*f*, 1089*t*–1090*t*
furuncles, 1087, 1087*f*
herpes simplex virus, 892*t*–894*t*, 1088, 1088*f*
herpes zoster, 1088, 1088*f*
hypertrophic scars, 154, 155*f*, 1081, 1081*f*
impetigo, 1087
infections, 180*t*–181*t*, 1087–1089, 1087*f*–1089*f*, 1089*t*
inflammatory, 1081–1083
irritant contact dermatitis, 1082
keloids, 154, 155*f*, 1079*t*–1080*t*, 1081, 1081*f*
keratoacanthoma, 1091
lesions, 1076–1081, 1077*t*–1080*t*
lupus erythematosus, 1085, 1086*f*
Lyme disease, 1087–1088
necrotizing fasciitis, 1087
papulosquamous, 1083–1085, 1083*f*–1085*f*, 1084*b*
pemphigus, 1085–1086, 1086*f*
pressure ulcers, 1076–1081, 1076*b*, 1080*f*
pruritus, 1081, 1085
psoriasis, 1083–1084, 1083*f*, 1084*b*
scleroderma, 1090–1091, 1091*f*
seborrheic dermatitis, 1083, 1083*f*
shingles, 1088
stasis dermatitis, 1082, 1082*f*
tinea infections, 1089, 1089*f*, 1089*t*
urticaria, 202–203, 204*f*, 1090
varicella, 1088
vascular, 1089–1091
vesiculobullous diseases, 1085–1087, 1086*f*
viral infections, 1088–1089, 1088*f*–1089*f*
warts, 1088–1089, 1089*f*
Skin lesions, 1076–1081, 1077*t*–1080*t*
Skull
fontanelles of, 426, 427*f*
of infants, 426
malformations of, 430, 431*f*
periosteum of, 323
sutures of, 426, 427*f*
Sleep
definition of, 347
deprivation, 219, 338
disorders of, 348–349
elderly characteristics of, 348*b*
hypothalamus and, 348
infant characteristics of, 348*b*
non-REM, 347–348
REM, 347–348
Sleepwalking, 349
Sliding hiatal hernia, 927, 927*f*
Slightly movable joints, 995
Slit membranes, 743
Slow-reacting substances of anaphylaxis (SRS-A), 146
Slow-transit constipation, 922
Slow-twitch fibres, 1000
Small bowel obstruction, 928–929, 928*t*
Small cell carcinoma, 718*t*, 719–720
Small intestinal carcinoma, 956
Small intestine
aging effects on, 918
anatomy of, 905–906, 905*f*
dietary fat and, 906*b*
digestion and absorption in, 906–907, 907*f*–908*f*, 908*b*
duodenum, 905–906, 905*f*
ileum, 905–906, 905*f*
jejunum, 905–906, 905*f*
motility in, 908–909
mucosa of, 903*t*
nutrients absorbed in, 908*b*
obstruction of, 929
villi, 905*f*, 906
Small lymphocytic lymphoma, 536
Small vessel disease, 407
Smallpox, 1113
Smoking, tobacco, 855
CAD and, 618
cancer and, 276–277, 277*f*
environmental tobacco smoke, 276
facts on, 718*b*
health consequences of, 278*f*
lung cancer and, 718–719
lung health and, 709*b*
prevalence of, in Canada, 277*f*
secondhand, 276
Smooth muscle, 33*t*–34*t*, 34*f*
Snout reflex, 367*f*
Social drugs, 89*t*
Social support, 229
Society of Obstetricians and Gynaecologists of Canada (SOGC), 293
Sodium
active transport of, 21, 21*f*, 22*t*
balance
aldosterone effects on, 118
alterations in, 120–122, 120*f*, 120*t*
hypertonic alterations to, 120*f*, 121
hypotonic alterations to, 120*f*, 121–122
isotonic alterations to, 120*f*, 121
maintenance of, 117–120
CKD progression and water balance with, 777*t*
in ECF, 117–118
functions of, 117–118
Sodium bicarbonate, 125–126
Sodium reabsorption inhibitors, 753*t*
Sodium-glucose cotransporter 2 (SGLT2), 481
Sodium-potassium pump, ATP levels effect on, 81–82
SOGC. *See* Society of Obstetricians and Gynaecologists of Canada
Soluble immune-complex glomerulonephritis, 769*t*
Solute, 17
Solutes, electrolytes as, 18–21
Somatic cell inheritance, 276*t*
Somatic cell mutation, 244
Somatic cell nuclear transfer, 108
Somatic cells, 42, 43*f*
Somatic death, 109–110
Somatic nervous system, components of, 309
Somatic pain, 342–343
Somatic recombination, 167
Somatosensory function, 356–357
Somatostatin, 225*t*–226*t*, 449*t*, 457, 903*t*
Somatotropic hormones, 448–451, 451*t*
Somnambulism (sleepwalking), 349
Somogyi effect, 482
Spasmodic croup, 725–727
Spastic cerebral palsy, 433
Spasticity, 381, 381*f*–382*f*, 381*t*, 386
Spatial summation, 313
Specific immunity. *See* Adaptive immunity
Specificity theory, 338–339
SPECT. *See* Single-photon emission computed tomography
Sperm cells, 793, 807, 809, 810*f*
production impairment, 888–890
Sperm motility, 890
Spermatids, 810
Spermatocele, 873, 873*f*
Spermatocytes, 810, 810*f*
Spermatogenesis, 810, 810*f*, 888–890
Spermatogonia, 810
Spermatozoon, 793
Sphincter of Oddi, 910–911, 914–915
Spina bifida, 427, 429*f*
Spina bifida occulta, 430
Spinal accessory nerve, 330*t*
Spinal cord
anatomy of, 320–322, 320*f*–322*f*
blood supply to, 327, 329*f*
central canal of, 320–321
coverings of, 320, 321*f*
cross section of, 321–322, 322*f*
description of, 315*t*
reflex arcs of, 321–322, 322*f*
tracts of, 321*f*
tumours of, 421
in vertebral column, 320, 320*f*
Spinal cord abscesses, 413
Spinal cord injuries
clinical manifestations of, 400–402, 401*t*–402*t*
evaluation and treatment of, 402
female sexual dysfunction and, 843*t*
pathophysiology of, 399–400
primary, 399
secondary, 399
types of, 399*t*
Spinal multiple sclerosis, 415
Spinal nerves, 320*f*, 327–328
Spinal shock, 386, 401*t*–402*t*
Spinal stenosis, 405
Spinal tracts, 321–322
Spindle fibres, 25
Spindles, 1000
Spine
axial compression injuries of, 400*f*, 400*t*
degenerative disorders of, 402–406
low back pain, 402–403
flexion injuries of, 400*f*, 400*t*
flexion-rotation injuries of, 400*f*, 400*t*
hyperextension injuries of, 400*f*, 400*t*
Spinnbarkeit mucus, 799–800
Spinothalamic tract, 320–321, 321*f*
anterior, 323
lateral, 323
Spiral fractures, 1011–1012, 1012*f*, 1012*t*
Spirochetes, 178
Spironolactone, 753*t*
Splanchnic blood flow, 910
Splanchnic nerves, 328–331
Spleen
absence of, 502
anatomy of, 500–502, 502*f*
disorders involving, 545–546, 545*b*
erythrocytes in, 501*f*
functions of, 500
Splenectomy, 546
Splenic pulp, 501
Splenomegaly, 532, 537, 943
congestive, 545–546
diseases related to, 545, 545*b*
infiltrative, 546
Spondyloarthropathies, 1035–1036
Spondylolisthesis, 404
Spondylolysis, 404
Spongy bone, 992–993, 992*f*
Spontaneous mutations, 39
Spousal death, 228*b*
Sprains, 1015
Sputum abnormalities, 696
Squamocolumnar junction, 799
Squamous cell carcinoma, 290, 718*t*, 719, 719*f*, 856*t*, 1092–1093, 1093*f*
SRS-A. *See* Slow-reacting substances of anaphylaxis
SRY gene, 55, 793
ST elevation myocardial infarction, 623, 625*f*
ST interval, 582–583, 583*f*
St. Louis encephalitis, 413*t*
Stab wound, 94*t*–95*t*
Stable angina pectoris, 620–621
Staghorn calculus, 761
Stance disorders, 389
Stapes, 354, 354*f*
Staphylococcal pneumonia, 732, 732*t*
Staphylococcal scalded-skin syndrome, 1110, 1110*f*
Staphylococcus aureus, 169–170, 178–179, 182*f*, 700
methicillin-resistant, 183
osteomyelitis and, 1028
Starling forces, 116
Starling's law of the heart, 587, 587*f*
Starvation, 942–943
Stasis dermatitis, 1082, 1082*f*
Static encephalopathies, 433
Static muscle contraction, 1006
Status asthmaticus, 707
Status epilepticus, 377, 436*t*
Steatorrhea, 923
Steatosis, 96, 98, 98*f*
Stellate cells, 911–912
Stem cells, 281
definition of, 27
embryonic, 64
hematopoietic, 504, 504*f*
induced pluripotent, 108
mammary, 851
mesenchymal, 195, 504, 504*f*
properties of, 28*f*
Stem-like cancer cells, 535, 535*f*
Stendra, 888
Stenosis, 578–579
aortic, 633, 633*f*, 664–666, 665*f*
mitral, 633–634, 633*f*
pulmonary, 666–667, 666*f*
valvular, 632, 632*t*, 633*f*
Steroid hormones, 443, 497
Stevens-Johnson syndrome, 1086
Sticky platelets, 511*b*
Still disease, 1064
Stomach
aging effects on, 918
anatomy of, 902, 902*f*
blood vessels of, 902, 902*f*
cancer of, 270*t*–273*t*, 954*t*, 955
gastric motility in, 903–904, 903*t*
gastric secretion in, 904–905, 904*f*
mucosa of, 903*t*
Storage diseases, 96–97
in children, 434
Strabismus, 350
Strains
ligament, 1015
muscle, 1016–1017, 1017*t*
stress and, 216
tendon, 1015
Strangulation, 93–95
Stratified squamous epithelium, 29*f*, 29*t*–30*t*
Stratified squamous transitional epithelium, 29*f*, 29*t*–30*t*
Strawberry hemangiomas, 1115
Street drugs, 89*t*
Streptococcal pneumonia, 732, 732*t*
Streptococcus pneumoniae, 190, 435
Streptococcus pyogenes, 169–170
Stress
acute, 216
adverse heart effects of, 228*b*
anti-inflammatory effects of, 224–227
behavioral, 217*f*
chronic, 227
coping with, 228–229, 230*f*
coronary heart disease and, 223*b*

Stress *(Continued)*
cortisol secretion during, 220–221, 221*t*
cytokine secretion affected by, 224
definition of, 216
diseases and conditions associated with, 219*t*
exogenous glucocorticoids effect on, 221–222
good types of, 230*f*
health outcome determination in, 228, 229*f*
historical background on, 216–219
HPA system and, 223*b*
immune system in, 227, 227*f*
nonlinear and complex interactions of, 223*f*
overview of, 219
physiological, 216, 217*f*
proinflammatory effects of, 224–227
psychosocial, 223*b*
shear, 578–579
sleep deprivation caused by, 219
strain and, 216
type 2 diabetes mellitus and, 222*b*
Stress echocardiography, 622–623
Stress fractures, 1012*t*, 1013
Stress incontinence, 762*t*
Stress response
anticipatory, 217
definition of, 216
hormones influencing, 224–227, 225*t*–226*t*
HPA system regulation and, 220–222
mechanisms of, 220–227
neuroendocrine regulation of, 222–224
parasympathetic nervous system in, 224
reactive, 217
schematic diagram of, 218*f*
sympathetic nervous system in, 222–224
Stress ulcers, 933
Stress-age syndrome, 230
Stress-induced muscle tension, 1041
Stressors
definition of, 216
personality characteristics and, 228
psychological, 217
repetitive exposure to, 227
Stress-related mucosal disease, 933
Stretch receptors, 684
Striated muscles, 999. *See also* Skeletal muscle
Striatum, 317, 319*f*
Stroke, 80–81
childhood, 435–436
diabetes mellitus complications with, 484*t*, 486
dietary potassium and lower risk of, 123*b*
embolic, 407
heat, 346–347
hemodynamic, 407
hemorrhagic, 408, 435
ischemic, 407–408, 435
lacunar, 407
occlusive, 435
perinatal, 435
prevention of, in women, 406*b*
signs of, 399–402
thrombotic, 407
Stroke volume, 587–588
Stroma, 26, 235–236, 236*f*, 885–886
Stromal cells, 240, 504
Strong acid, 126
Structural scoliosis, 1066
Struvite stones, 761
Stye, 353
Subacute thyroiditis, 473
Subarachnoid hemorrhage, 408–410, 410*t*
Subarachnoid space, 323, 324*f*
Subclinical hypothyroidism, 473–474
Subclinical thyroid disease, 471
Subcutaneous layer of skin, 1074, 1075*f*, 1075*t*
Subdural hematomas, 94*t*–95*t*, 395*t*, 396–397
Subdural space, 323, 324*f*
Subluxation, 1014–1015
Submucosal plexus, 902, 906
Substance P, 449*t*
properties of, 314*t*
in stress response, 225*t*–226*t*
Substantia gelatinosa, 320–321
Substantia nigra, 317, 319, 319*f*
Substrate, 16
Substrate phosphorylation, 17
Subthalamic nucleus, 317, 319*f*
Subthalamus, 317–318
Subvalvular aortic stenosis, 664–665
Succussion splash, 927
Suck reflex, 367*f*
Sudden cardiac death, 626, 627*f*
Sudden unexpected infant death (SUID), 737, 737*b*
Suffocation, 93
SUID. *See* Sudden unexpected infant death
Sulci, 314, 316*f*
Summation, 313
Sun burn, 290
Sun exposure, 290
Superantigens (SAGs), 169–170, 172*f*
Superficial hemangiomas, 1115, 1115*f*
Superficial mycoses, 186
Superficial partial-thickness burns, 1095, 1095*f*, 1097*t*
Superficial spreading melanoma, 1093–1094
Superior colliculi, 319
Superior vena cava, 577, 577*f*
Superior vena cava syndrome, 605–606
Superoxide, 83*t*
Supply-dependent oxygen consumption, 654
Suppurative cystitis, 765
Suppurative exudate, 150
Suprachiasmatic nucleus, 349–350
Supratentorial disorders, 363–364, 365*t*
Supratentorial herniation, 379*b*, 379*f*
Supravalvular aortic stenosis, 664–666
Surface tension, 686–687
Surfactant, 681, 682*f*, 686–687
deficiency, RDS from, 728
impairment of, 701
Surgery, for cancer, 262–264
Sustained attention deficits, 369
Sutures, 995
cranial, 426, 427*f*
Swallowing, 901–902
dysphagia and, 611–612, 925–926, 926*f*
Sweat glands, 1074–1076
Swine influenza virus (H1N1), 185
Sylvian fissure, 315–316, 316*f*
Sympathetic ganglia, 328–331
Sympathetic nervous system
anatomy of, 328–331, 332*f*
myocardial performance affected by, 583–584
primary hypertension and, 606–607, 634
in stress response, 222–224
Symphysis, 995
Symport, 18, 19*f*
Synapses, 27, 311*f*, 313
Synaptic bouton, 313
Synaptic cleft, 311*f*, 313
Synarthrosis, 995
Synchondrosis, 995
Syndesmophyte, 1037
Syndesmosis, 995
Syndrome of inappropriate antidiuretic hormone (SIADH), 122, 257*t*, 466–467, 467*t*
Syndromic cleft palate, 968
Synovial cavity, 997
Synovial fluid, 997
Synovial joints, 997*f*–1000*f*, 998
Synovial membrane, 996–997
Synovial sarcoma, 1050
Synovitis, 1033*f*
Syphilis, 892*t*–894*t*
Systemic aging, 109
Systemic circulation
anatomy of, 576*f*, 589, 590*f*–591*f*
arterioles of, 589, 590*f*–591*f*
blood vessel structure in, 589–593, 592*f*
Systemic circulation *(Continued)*
bronchial circulation, 682–683
capillaries, 589, 590*f*–591*f*
function of, 575
Systemic exertional intolerance disease, 1043
Systemic immune system, 165
Systemic inflammatory response syndrome (SIRS), 650
Systemic lupus erythematosus, 209–210
Systemic scleroderma, 1090
Systemic vascular resistance, 588
Systole, 578
Systolic blood pressure, 595
Systolic compressive effect, 598
Systolic heart failure, 639

T

T cell antigen receptor, 167*f*, 168
T cells (T lymphocytes), 147
autoreactive, 201
CD4+, 195
clonal diversity generation and, 165–168, 167*t*
cytotoxic, 160, 170, 172*f*–173*f*, 173, 221–222
description of, 159–160
development of, 168
differentiation sites of, 162*f*
functions of, 171–173
helper, 160, 169, 171*f*, 221–222
in immune response, 165–171
lymphokine-secreting, 173
regulatory, 160, 173
subsets of, 169, 171*f*
thymus as origin of, 165–167
T lymphocytes. *See* T cells
T wave, 582–583, 583*f*
Tadalafil, 888
Talipes, 1060*t*
Tamm-Horsfall protein, 751
Tamponade, 629
TAPVC. *See* Total anomalous pulmonary venous connection
Tarceva (erlotinib), 263*t*
Tardive dyskinesia, 382
Target cells, for hormones, 14, 444–447, 446*f*, 465
Taste, 356, 356*f*, 357*b*
Tay-Sachs disease, 434
TBI. *See* Traumatic brain injury
TBW. *See* Total body water
T-cell receptors, 142
T-cell-independent antigens, 171, 172*f*
Tears, 353, 353*f*
Tegmentum, 319
TEL-AML1 gene, 305
Telangiectasia, 1077*t*–1078*t*
Telencephalon (cerebral hemispheres), 314–318, 316*f*
Telomerase, 247, 247*f*
Telomeres, 108, 247, 247*f*
Telophase, 25–26
Templates, 39
Temporal fossa, 323
Temporal lobe, 316*f*, 317
Temporal summation, 313
Tenase complex, 513
Tendinopathy, 1015–1016, 1016*f*, 1017*b*
Tendons, 1006, 1007*f*
sprains and strains of, 1015
Teniae coli, 909, 909*f*
Tennis elbow, 1015
Tension pneumothorax, 700
Tension-type headache, 410*t*, 411
Tentorium cerebelli, 323
Terminal duct lobular units, 849
Termination sequence, 41
Tertiary hyperparathyroidism, 475
Testes
aging and, 812
anatomy of, 807–808, 807*f*–808*f*
cancer of, 270*t*–273*t*, 875–876, 875*b*, 875*f*
development of, 818
ectopic, 873–874
function of, 807
torsion of, 874, 874*f*
tumours of, 875, 875*f*
Testes-determining factor, 793–794
Testicular appendages, 874
Testosterone
androgens and, 882, 885
functions of, 794*t*, 810
libido and, 810
in sexual differentiation, 794
in stress response, 225*t*–226*t*
Tet spells, 669
Tethered cord syndrome, 430
Tetralogy of Fallot, 662–663, 664*f*, 668–669, 669*f*
Tetraploidy, 42–43
Teva-Doxycycline (doxycycline), 826*b*
TF. *See* Tissue factor
TFPI. *See* Tissue factor pathway inhibitor
TGA. *See* Transposition of great arteries
TGF-β. *See* Transforming growth factor-beta
TGV. *See* Transposition of great vessels
Th1 cells, 169, 221–222
Th1 to Th2 shift, 222
Th2 cells, 169, 221–222
Th17 cells, 169
Thalamus, 317–318
Thalassemias, 521*t*, 526
in children, 567–568
discovery of, 567
sickle cell, 564–566
α-, 567–568
β-, 567–568, 568*f*
Thalidomide, 85–86, 545
Theca cells, 801
Thelarche, 795, 818
T-helper cells, 706
Therapeutic hyperthermia, 346
Thermoregulation. *See also* Fever
disorders of, 346–347
in elderly, 345–346
in infants, 345–346
mechanisms of, 344–345, 345*t*
trauma and, 347
Thiamine deficiency, 643
Thiazides, 753*t*
Thimerosal, 190
Third order neurons, 322–323
Third-degree block, 645*t*–646*t*
Third-degree burns, 1095, 1096*f*, 1097*t*
Thoracic aortic aneurysms, 611–612
Thoracic cavity, 683, 684*f*
Thoracic duct, 599, 600*f*
Thoracolumbar division, 328–331
3-Day Measles, 1111–1112, 1112*f*, 1112*t*
Threshold of liability, 58, 58*f*
Threshold potential, 24
Thrombin time, 514*t*–516*t*
Thromboangiitis obliterans, 613
Thrombocytes. *See* Platelets
Thrombocythemia, 548–549
Thrombocytopenia, 259
Thrombocytopenia, 547–548
Thrombocytopenia-absent radius syndrome, 547
Thrombocytosis, 548–549
Thromboembolic disease, 546
Thromboembolic disorders, 553–554, 553*f*
Thromboembolus, 605
Thrombolysis, 407–408
Thrombomodulin, 513
Thrombophilia, 554
Thrombopoietin, 510
Thrombosis, 546. *See also* Deep venous thrombosis
arterial, 612–613
microvasculature, 549
Thrombospondin-1, 248
Thrombotic crisis, 565–566
Thrombotic strokes, 407
Thrombotic thrombocytopenic purpura (TTP), 548
Thromboxane A_2 (TXA_2), 146
Thrombus, 553–554, 553*f*
venous, 605
Thrush, 1111
Thymine, 38
Thymus, T cells from, 165–167
Thyroid carcinoma, 474
Thyroid gland
aging and, 461*b*
anatomy of, 452, 453*f*
C cells of, 453, 453*f*

Thyroid gland *(Continued)*
disorders of, 471–474
carcinoma, 474
central, 471
Graves' disease, 471–473, 472*f*
hyperthyroidism, 471–474, 471*f*–472*f*
hypothyroidism, 472*f*–474*f*, 473–474
nodular thyroid disease, 472–473
primary, 471
secondary, 471
subclinical thyroid disease, 471
thyrotoxic crisis, 473
thyrotoxicosis, 471–473, 471*f*–472*f*
follicle cells of, 452, 453*f*
hormones of
actions of, 453–454, 454*t*
regulation of, 453, 454*t*
synthesis of, 453
Thyroid storm, 473
Thyroid-stimulating hormone (TSH), 345, 443–444, 448–451, 449*f*, 451*t*
deficiency of, 468
regulation of, 453, 454*t*
Thyrotoxic crisis, 473
Thyrotoxic periodic paralysis, 1043
Thyrotoxicosis, 471–473, 471*f*–472*f*
Thyrotropin-releasing hormone (TRH), 443–444, 449*t*
regulation of, 453, 454*t*
Thyrotropin-stimulating hormone-releasing hormone, 345
Thyroxine, 443–444, 454*t*
Thyroxine-binding globulin, 453
Tidemark, 997
Tight junctions, 12, 13*f*, 584–585
Tinea capitis, 1110–1111, 1110*f*
Tinea corporis, 1111
Tinea unguium, 1101
Tinnitus, 355
TIPS. *See* Transjugular intrahepatic portosystemic shunts
Tissue factor (TF), 141
Tissue factor pathway, of clotting system, 141
Tissue factor pathway inhibitor (TFPI), 513
Tissue hypoxia, 522
Tissue inhibitors of metalloproteinases, 991*t*
Tissue macrophages, 911–912
Tissue plasminogen activator, 513–514
Tissue thromboplastin, 512
Tissues, 27*f*
aging of, 109
connective, 11–12, 11*f*, 31*t*–33*t*
description of, 27
epithelial, 29*t*–30*t*
formation of, 27
granulation, 153
micro-organisms causing damage to, 178, 179*t*
muscle, 33*t*–34*t*
regeneration of, 152
types of, 27
wound healing formation of, 153–154
Tissue-specific antigens, 203–204
Tissue-specific hypersensitivity reactions, 202*t*, 203, 206*f*
Titin, 585–586, 1003*t*
Titratable acid, 130*f*
TLRs. *See* Toll-like receptors
TNF-α. *See* Tumour necrosis factor-alpha
TNM staging, 260, 261*f*, 720
Tobacco. *See* Smoking, tobacco
Tolerance, 209
Toll-like receptors (TLRs), 142–143, 143*t*
Toloxin (digoxin), 641
Tongue, glossitis and, 525*f*
Tonić phase, 376–377
Tonicity, 20, 21*f*
Tonsil cancer, 270*t*–273*t*
Tonsillar abscesses, 727
Tonsillar infections, 727
Tophaceous gout, 1040
Tophi, 1038
Torsemide, 753*t*
Torsion
intestinal obstruction from, 928*t*
of ovaries, 830
of penis, 784
of testes, 874, 874*f*
Torus fractures, 1012, 1012*t*
Total anomalous pulmonary venous connection (TAPVC), 670–671, 671*f*
Total body surface area, in burns, 1095, 1096*f*
Total body water (TBW)
in adolescents, 132*b*
age-related changes in, 115
body weight in relation to, 115, 116*t*
in children, 132*b*
distribution of, 115–116, 116*t*
in elderly, 132*b*
in infants, 132*b*
Total iron-binding capacity, 514*t*–516*t*
Total peripheral resistance, 588, 595–596
Total resistance, 594
Touch, 356
Tourette syndrome, 382, 382*b*
Toxic adenoma, 472–473
Toxic epidermal necrolysis, 1086
Toxic gas exposure, 702–703
Toxic multinodular goitre, 472–473
Toxic myopathies, 1046, 1046*b*
Toxicophores, 84–85
Toxins, bacteria secreting, 163–164
Toxoids, 190
TP53 (tumour protein p53), 243–244, 246*f*, 250
Trabeculae, 993, 993*f*
Trabecular bone score, 1025
Trachea, anatomy of, 680, 680*f*–681*f*
Tracheitis, 727, 730*t*
Tracheoesophageal fistula, 969, 970*f*
Trachoma, 353–354
Traction, of fractures, 1014
Trafficking, 7
Trait anger, 223*b*
Transcalvarial herniation, 379*b*, 379*f*
Transchondral fractures, 1012*t*, 1013
Transcortical dysphasia, 371, 372*t*
Transcription, 41, 42*f*–43*f*
Transfer RNA (tRNA), 42
Transferrin, 99, 497, 508–509, 916*t*
Transferrin saturation, 514*t*–516*t*
Transformation, of cancer cells, 238–240
Transformation zone, 799
Transforming growth factor-beta (TGF-β), 26*t*, 145, 153, 991*t*
Transforming growth factors, 145
Transfusion reactions, 210–211
Transgenerational phenotypes, 276*t*
Transient ischemic attacks, 407
Transient regional osteoporosis, 1023
Transitional cell carcinoma, 764–765
Transjugular intrahepatic portosystemic shunts (TIPS), 943–945
Translation, 42, 43*f*
Translocations, chromosome
description of, 47–49, 49*f*
oncogene activation by, 242, 243*f*
Transmembrane proteins, 7, 8*f*
Transmural myocardial infarction, 624, 625*f*
Transplant rejection, 211
Transport maximum, 749
Transporter pumps, 18, 18*f*
Transporters, 17, 18*f*
Transposition of great arteries (TGA), 670
Transposition of great vessels (TGV), 670, 671*f*
Transthoracic echocardiography (TTE), 632–633
Transudative pleural effusion, 700, 700*t*
Transverse colon, 909, 909*f*
Transverse fibres, 317
Transverse fractures, 1011–1012, 1012*f*, 1012*t*
Transverse tubules, 1002
Trastuzumab (Herceptin), 263*t*
Trauma
skeletal, 1011–1015
thermoregulation and, 347
Traumatic brain injury (TBI)
closed, 394–395, 395*t*
complications of, 398–399
definition of, 394
diffuse axonal injuries and, 395*t*, 397–398
focal brain injury, 394–397, 395*t*, 396*f*
open, 395*t*, 397
primary, 394–398
secondary, 395*t*, 398
Treitz ligament, 905–906, 905*f*
Tremors, 383*t*
Trendelenburg gait, 1065
TRH. *See* Thyrotropin-releasing hormone
Triamterene, 753*t*
Tricarboxylic acid cycle, 16
Trichinella larvae, 1044
Trichomoniasis, 892*t*–894*t*
Tricuspid regurgitation, 634
Tricuspid valve, 577, 577*f*–578*f*
atresia of, 669–670, 670*f*
Trigeminal autonomic cephalalgias, 411
Trigeminal nerve, 330*t*
Trigone, 746, 746*f*
Triiodothyronine, 443–444, 454*t*
Trimethoprim-sulfamethoxazole, 766*b*
Triploidy, 42–43
Trisomy, 43
partial, 46
Trisomy 13 syndrome, 663*t*
Trisomy 18 syndrome, 663*t*
Trisomy 21. *See* Down syndrome
Trisomy 21 syndrome, 663*t*
Trochlear nerve, 330*t*
Tropism, 183
Tropomyosin, 585–586, 585*f*
Troponin C, 585–586
Troponin I, 585–586, 626–627
CAD and, 619–620
Troponin T, 585–586
Troponin-tropomyosin complex, 585–586, 585*f*–586*f*
Trousseau phenomenon, 257*t*
True aneurysms, 611, 612*f*
True vocal cords, 679
Truncus arteriosus, 671–672, 672*f*
Trypanosoma brucei, 188
Trypanosoma cruzi, 188
TSH. *See* Thyroid-stimulating hormone
TTE. *See* Transthoracic echocardiography
TTP. *See* Thrombotic thrombocytopenic purpura
Tuberculin skin test, 714
Tuberculosis
clinical manifestations of, 714
definition of, 714
evaluation of, 714–715
granuloma with, 151–152, 151*f*
Indigenous people in Canada and, 194*b*
latent infection of, 714
pathophysiology of, 714
risk factors of, 714
treatment of, 714–715
Tubular carcinoma, 856*t*
Tubular reabsorption, 747, 750*f*
Tubular secretion, 747, 750*f*
Tubuloglomerular feedback, 746–747
Tubulointerstitial fibrosis, 759–760
Tubulus rectus, 807, 808*f*
Tumour markers, 260–261, 261*t*
Tumour necrosis factor-alpha (TNF-α), 143–144, 222*b*, 652*b*
Tumour protein p53 (TP53), 243–244, 246*f*, 250
Tumour-associated macrophage, 251–252, 255
Tumour-infiltrating lymphocytes, 253
Tumours
of adrenal medulla, 260–261, 490–491
angiogenesis induced by, 248*f*
benign (*See* Benign tumours)
bladder, 764–765
bone tumours (*See* Bone tumours)
chondrogenic, 1050
chromaffin cell, 490–491
classification of, 235–238, 261–262
Tumours *(Continued)*
clear cell, 764
of CNS, 417–421
brain, 417–421, 418*f*, 419*t*–420*t*
collagenic, 1050
dormancy of, 856–857
embryonal, 438–440
estrogen-secreting, 489
giant cell, 1050
inflammation promotion by, 250–252, 251*t*
initiation of, 238
intestinal obstruction from, 928*t*
malignant, 235–236, 236*f*
muscle, 1051
myelogenic, 1050
neuroendocrine, 718*t*, 719–720
nomenclature for, 235–238
osteogenic, 1049–1050
ovarian, 841*f*
pancreatic, in children, 982–983
of penis, 871
of pituitary gland, 470–471
progression of, 238
promotion of, 238
renal, 763–764, 764*f*
skin, 1077*t*–1078*t*
spinal cord, 421
testicular, 875, 875*f*
Wilms, 305, 788, 788*t*
Tumour-suppressor genes
childhood cancers associated with, 305, 305*t*
deactivation of, 245*f*
description of, 51, 63
familial cancer caused by function loss of, 244*t*
functions of, 243, 243*t*
retinoblastoma gene and, 243
silencing, 245*f*
TP53, 243–244, 246*f*
Tunica albuginea, 807, 808*f*
Tunica externa, 589, 592*f*
Tunica intima, 589, 592*f*
Tunica media, 589, 592*f*
Tunica vaginalis, 807, 807*f*
Turbulent blood flow, 594, 594*f*
Turner's syndrome, 46, 47*t*, 48*f*, 54, 663*t*
TXA_2. *See* Thromboxane A_2
Tylenol. *See* Acetaminophen
Tympanic cavity, 354
Tympanic membrane, 354, 354*f*
Tyrosine, 99
Tyrosine kinase inhibitors, 242
Tyrosine kinases, 446–447, 447*t*

U

Ubiquitin, 75
Ubiquitin–proteasome pathway, 75
Ubiquitin–proteasome system (UPS), 8–9
Ulcerative colitis (UC), 936–937, 936*t*
Ulcerative cystitis, 765
Ulcers
curling, 933
Cushing, 933
duodenal, 932–933, 932*f*, 933*t*
gastric, 933, 933*t*
ischemic, 933
peptic (*See* Peptic ulcer disease)
pressure, 1076–1081, 1076*b*, 1080*f*
skin, 1079*t*–1080*t*
stress, 933
surgical treatment of, 934
venous stasis, 604, 605*f*
Ultraviolet radiation, 289–291, 1092
Umbilical cord blood, antibodies in, 174*b*
Uncal herniation, 379*b*, 379*f*
Unconjugated bilirubin, 913
Underactive bladder syndrome, 762
Unfolded-protein response (UPR), 8*b*
Unicornuate uterus, 817*f*
Unilateral neglect syndrome, 369–371
Unintentional injuries, 93–96, 94*t*–95*t*
Uniparental disomy, 65–66
Unipolar neurons, 310
Uniport, 18, 19*f*
Universal donors, 210–211
Unsaturated fatty acids, 906*b*

Unstable angina, 623–624, 624*b*, 625*f*
Upper airway
  anatomy of, 679, 681*f*
  infections of, in children, 725–727, 726*t*
Upper esophageal sphincter, 901
Upper gastro-intestinal bleeding, 924
Upper motor neuron gate, 389
Upper motor neuron paresis/paralysis, 385, 386*b*
Upper motor neuron syndromes, 385–386, 385*t*, 386*b*, 386*f*–387*f*
Upper motor neurons, 322
Upper respiratory tract infections, 180*t*–181*t*
UPR. *See* Unfolded-protein response
Upregulation, 444–446, 446*f*
UPS. *See* Ubiquitin–proteasome system
Urate, 100–101, 1038, 1038*t*
Urea, 751, 753*t*
  CKD progression and clearance of, 777, 777*t*
Ureaphil, 753*t*
Uremia, 772
Uremic syndrome, 772
Ureterocele, 785–786
Ureterohydronephrosis, 759–760, 760*f*
Ureteropelvic junction obstruction, 785–786
Ureterovesical junction obstruction, 785–786
Ureters, anatomy of, 745–746
Urethra
  anatomy of, 746, 746*f*
  partial obstruction of, 763
Urethral strictures, 763, 869
Urethritis, 869
Urge incontinence, 762*t*
Uric acid, 1038–1040, 1038*f*
Uric acid stones, 761
Urinalysis, 754, 755*t*
Urinary bladder. *See* Bladder
Urinary calculi, 760–761
Urinary incontinence, 762*t*, 790, 790*t*
Urinary system
  disorders, in children (*See* Children, urinary system disorders in)
  structures, 745–746
Urinary tract infection (UTI)
  acute cystitis, 765–766
  antibiotic resistance and, 766*b*
  causes of, 765
  in children, 788–789, 789*b*
  complicated, 765
  mechanisms of, 771*f*
  uncomplicated, 765
Urinary tract obstruction
  anatomical obstructions in, 763
  definition of, 759
  kidney stones, 760–761, 767*t*
  lower, 761–763, 762*t*
  major sites of, 760*f*
  neurogenic bladder, 762, 762*t*, 767*t*
  overactive bladder syndrome, 762–763
  upper, 759–761, 760*f*
Urination (micturition), 745–746
Urine
  ADH and aldosterone regulating, 747, 748*f*
  composition of, 752
  concentration of
    countercurrent exchange system and, 750, 751*f*
    in Loop of Henle, 750–751
  diuretics and flow of, 752, 753*t*
  flow, anatomical obstructions to, 763
  glomerular filtration and, 747, 750*f*
  myoglobin in, 1017–1018
  postvoid, 763
  properties of, 755*t*
  tubular reabsorption and, 747, 750*f*
  tubular secretion and, 747, 750*f*
Urine antigen testing, 714
Urobilinogen, 913
Urodilatin, 118, 747
Urodynamic tests, 755*t*
Uroflowmetry, 755*t*, 763
Urokinaselike plasminogen activator, 513–514
Uromodulin, 751
Urticaria (hives), 202–203, 204*f*, 1090
Urticarial lesions, 1090
Urushiol, 161
Usual ductal hyperplasia, 844
Uterine cancer, 270*t*–273*t*
Uterine fibroids, 831, 831*f*
Uterine phases, of menstrual cycle, 804–805
Uterine tubes, 800
Uterus
  abnormal bleeding of, 820–821, 821*t*
  abnormalities of, 816–817, 817*f*
  anatomy of, 799–800, 799*f*–800*f*
  bicornuate, 817*f*
  corpus of, 799, 800*f*
  double, 817*f*
  fundus of, 799
  isthmus of, 799, 800*f*
  positions of, 799, 799*f*
  prolapse of, 828, 828*f*
  unicornuate, 817*f*
  wall of, 799, 800*f*
UTI. *See* Urinary tract infection

V

Vaccinations
  fears with, 190
  in HIV, 198
  immune response from, 189
  mass, 189
  purpose of, 189
  rabies, 198
Vaccines, 189–190
Vagina
  anatomy of, 796–798, 798*f*
  cancer of, 270*t*–273*t*, 835–836
  double, 817*f*
  fornix of, 798
  menstrual cycle response by, 805
  pH of, 798–799, 826
  prolapse of, 828*b*
  self-cleansing action of, 798–799
  wall of, 798
Vaginismus, 842
Vaginitis, 826
Vaginosis, 826, 892*t*–894*t*
Vagus nerve, 330*t*
Valence, 19
Valsalva manoeuvre, 910
Valvular aortic stenosis, 664
Valvular dysfunction, 632–634, 632*t*, 633*f*
Valvular hypertrophic cardiomyopathy, 631
Valvular regurgitation, 632, 632*t*, 633*f*, 634
Valvular stenosis, 632, 632*t*, 633*f*
Vaprisol, 753*t*
Vaptans, 467
Vardenafil, 888
Varicella, 1088, 1112*t*, 1113, 1113*f*
Varices, 943, 944*f*
Varicose veins, 604–605, 605*f*
Variocele, 872–873, 873*f*
Variola, 1113
Vas deferens, 809*f*
Vasa recta, 745, 751
Vasa vasorum, 589
Vascular compliance, of blood vessels, 595
Vascular dementia, 375*t*
Vascular endothelial growth factor (VEGF), 26*t*, 153, 247–248
Vascular endothelium, 575, 590–591, 592*f*–593*f*, 593*t*
Vascular malformations, 399–402
Vascular mimicry, 857
Vascular niche, 504–505, 504*f*
Vascular permeability, 138–139
Vasectomy, prostate cancer risk and, 882–883
Vasoactive intestinal peptide, 225*t*–226*t*, 903*t*
Vasoactive intestinal polypeptide, 439
Vasoconstriction, 589
  hypoxic pulmonary, 683
Vasoconstrictor hormones, 597
Vasodilation, 138, 589
Vasodilator hormones, 597
Vasogenic edema, 379
Vasogenic shock, 402, 648–650
Vasomotor flushes, 811
Vaso-occlusive crisis, 565–566
Vasopressin, 467
  blood pressure affected by, 580*f*, 597
Vasopressin blockers, 753*t*
Vaults, 4*t*
VDLs. *See* Very-low-density lipoproteins
VEDP. *See* Ventricular end-diastolic pressure
VEDV. *See* Ventricular end-diastolic volume
Vegetables, 880*b*–881*b*
Vegetative state, 369
VEGF. *See* Vascular endothelial growth factor
Veins
  anatomy of, 591–593, 592*f*
  blood pressure in, 598
  chronic venous insufficiency of, 604–605
  coronary, 578, 580, 581*f*
  distension of, 604
  lymphatic, 599
  renal, 745
  saphenous, 604
  valves in, 587, 593*f*
  varicose, 604–605, 605*f*
Venereal warts, 1089
Venezuelan encephalitis, 413*t*
Venous sinuses, 501
Venous stasis ulcers, 604, 605*f*
Venous thrombi, 553
Venous thromboembolism, 613*t*
Venous thrombosis, 257*t*
Ventilation. *See also* Breathing
  alveolar, 684
  alveolar surface tension and, 686–687
  chemoreceptors in, 684–686
  definition of, 684
  distribution of, 689–690, 690*f*
  lung receptors in, 684–685
  maintaining adequate, 688, 688*f*
  muscles of, 686, 686*f*
  neurochemical control of, 684–686, 685*f*
  noninvasive positive-pressure, 701
Ventilation-perfusion mismatch, 698, 698*f*
Ventilation-perfusion ratio, 690, 698, 698*f*
Ventilator-associated pneumonia, 712, 712*b*
Ventral horn, 320–321
Ventral respiratory group, 684
Ventricles, 323
  of heart, 577, 577*f*
Ventricular block, 645*t*–646*t*
Ventricular bradycardia, 644*t*–645*t*
Ventricular end-diastolic pressure (VEDP), 587–588
Ventricular end-diastolic volume (VEDV), 587–588, 587*f*
  myocardial infarction effects on, 626
Ventricular fibrillation, 644*t*–645*t*
Ventricular remodelling, 639
Ventricular septal defect, 668
Ventricular standstill, 644*t*–645*t*
Ventricular system, 323–324
Ventricular tachycardia, 644*t*–645*t*
Venules
  functions of, 575
  lymphatic, 599
  systemic circulation, 589, 590*f*–591*f*
Vermiform appendix, 909, 909*f*
Vermis, 319
Vertebral arteries, 325, 326*f*
Vertebral body osteoporosis, 1021*f*
Vertebral column
  anatomy of, 324–325, 325*f*
  spinal cord in, 320, 320*f*
Vertebral fractures, 399–400, 400*t*
Vertebral injuries, 399, 400*f*, 400*t*
Vertigo, 357
Very-low-density lipoproteins (VLDLs), 617–618
Vesicle, 1077*t*–1078*t*
Vesicosphincter dyssynergia, 762
Vesicoureteral reflux, 767*t*
  in children, 789–790, 789*f*–790*f*
Vesiculobullous diseases, 1085–1087, 1086*f*
Vestibular nystagmus, 357
Vestibule, 354–355, 354*f*–355*f*
  in female reproductive system, 797–798, 797*f*
Vestibulitis, 827
Vestibulocochlear nerve, 330*t*
Vestibulospinal tract, 322
Viagra, 888
Video urodynamics, 755*t*, 763
Villi, 905*f*, 906
Viral conjunctivitis, 353–354
Viral diseases
  description of, 183–186
  examples of, 184*t*
  opportunistic, 196*b*
  stages of, 183*f*
Viral encephalitis, 435
Viral hepatitis, 950–951, 950*t*
Viral infections, 1088–1089, 1088*f*–1089*f*
  in children, 1111–1113, 1111*f*–1113*f*, 1112*t*
Viral meningitis, 412, 435
  HIV and, 414
Viral pneumonia, 713, 732, 732*t*
Virchow triad, 554, 605
Virilization, 489, 490*f*
Viruses
  attenuated, 189
  cancer associated with, 252
  cellular effects of, 184
  life cycle of, 183, 183*f*
  pathogenicity of, 183
  poliovirus, 189–190
Visceral pain, 342–343, 924
Visceral pleura, 683, 684*f*
Visfatin, 941*b*
Vision. *See also* Eye
  aging changes in, 357*b*
  colour, alterations in, 352
  diabetic retinopathy impact on, 484–485, 484*t*, 485*f*
  dysfunctions of, 350–353
    neurological disorders causing, 352–353, 353*f*
  elderly changes in, 357*b*
  overview of, 349–354
Visual acuity alterations, 350–352, 351*f*, 351*t*
Vitamins
  B, 280
  B_{12}
    deficiency of, 522–523
    oral replacement of, 523
  D, 454, 454*b*, 989*t*
    bone and, 1025*b*
    deficiency, 771
    kidneys and, 752
    supplementation of, 752*b*, 778
  E, 880*b*–881*b*
  K, 989*t*
    deficiency, 550
  liver storage of, 914
  small intestine absorption of, 908*b*
Vitreous humour, 349–350
Vocal cords
  false, 679, 681*f*
  true, 679
Volatile acid, 126
Volkmann canals, 993, 993*f*
Volkmann ischemic contracture, 1019
Volume-sensitive receptors, 119–120
Voluntary muscles, 999–1000
Voluntary phase of swallowing, 901
Vomiting, 367, 921–922, 927
von Recklinghausen disease, 51–52
von Willebrand factor (vWF), 510–511
Vulva, 796–798, 797*f*
Vulvar cancer, 270*t*–273*t*, 836
Vulvitis, 827
Vulvodynia vestibulitis, 827
Vulvovestibulitisdynia, 827
vWF. *See* von Willebrand factor

W

Waist-hip ratio, 854
Wallerian degeneration, 311
Wandering, 383*t*
Warts, 1088–1089, 1089*f*

Water. *See also* Total body water
balance
ADH regulating, 117–119, 119*f*
alterations in, 120–122, 120*f*, 120*t*
hypertonic alterations to, 120*f*, 121
hypotonic alterations to, 120*f*, 121–122
isotonic alterations to, 120*f*, 121
maintenance of, 117–120
burns and evaporative loss of, 1098–1099
cellular accumulations and, 97, 98*f*
CKD progression and sodium balance with, 777*t*
gaining of, 116*t*
intoxication with, 122
loss of, 116*t*
movement of
alterations in, 116–117
between ECF and ICF, 116
between plasma and interstitial fluid, 115–116, 117*f*
small intestine absorption of, 908*b*
Water-soluble hormones, 444, 444*t*
Weak acid, 126
Weight gain, in Cushing's syndrome, 487, 488*f*
Weight loss
in cachexia, 256
leukemia and, 536*t*
postgastrectomy, 935
Weight loss surgery, 942
Wenckebach block, 645*t*–646*t*
Wernicke area, 316*f*, 317
Wernicke dysphasia, 371, 372*t*–373*t*
West Nile virus, 413, 413*t*, 414*b*
Western equine encephalitis, 413*t*
West's syndrome, 436*t*
Wheal, 1077*t*–1078*t*
Wheal and flare reaction, 202–203
White adipose tissue, 257–258
White fibrous connective tissue, 31*f*, 31*t*–33*t*
White graft, 211
White matter, 314
White muscle, 1000, 1001*t*
White reflex, 440
Whole blood clotting time, 514*t*–516*t*
Wilms tumour, 305, 788, 788*t*
Wilson's disease, 982, 983*t*
Wirsung duct, 915
Wiskott-Aldrich syndrome, 191, 192*t*, 547
Wnt signals, 27
Wolffian ducts, 793, 795*f*
Wolff-Parkinson-White syndrome, 645*t*–646*t*
Women. *See also* Female reproductive system
microvascular angina and, 621*b*
stroke prevention in, 406*b*
Work of breathing, 688, 688*f*
World Health Organization, cancer prevention strategy of, 275*b*
Wound healing
cancer and, 240
diabetes mellitus and, 154
drug effects on, 154
dysfunctional, 154–155, 155*f*
fibrin deposition in, 154
fibroblasts in, 153–154
inflammation phase of, 153, 153*f*
macrophages in, 147, 153
maturation phase of, 154
new tissue formation phase of, 153–154
nutrition and, 154
obesity delaying, 154
open, 152
primary intention, 152, 152*f*
proliferative phase of, 153–154
remodeling phase of, 154
secondary intention, 152–153, 152*f*
Wounds. *See also specific wounds*
contraction of, 154–155
dehiscence and, 154
disruption of, 154
infections of, 180*t*–181*t*

X

X chromosomes, 62–63
X inactivation, 54, 54*f*
Xanthelasmas, 621–622
Xanthine stones, 761
Xenobiotics, 83–84, 87*f*, 281
Xenoestrogen, 855
Xeroderma pigmentosum, 244–246
X-linked inheritance
pedigrees and, 55
recurrence risks in, 55–56, 56*f*
sex determination and, 54–55, 55*f*
sex-limited and sex-influenced traits in, 56
X inactivation and, 54, 54*f*
X-linked SCID, 191, 192*t*
Xolair (omalizumab), 708
X-ray absorptiometry, 1022

Y

Yawning, 367

Z

Z line, 585, 585*f*
Zeranol, 855
Zoledronic acid, 1026*b*
Zollinger-Ellison syndrome, 931
Zona fasciculata, 457, 457*f*
Zona glomerulosa, 457, 457*f*
Zona reticularis, 457, 457*f*
Zoonotic infections, 180*t*–181*t*, 183
Zyloprim (allopurinol), 536

PREFIXES AND SUFFIXES USED IN MEDICAL TERMINOLOGY

Prefix	Meaning
a-	Without, not
acantho-	Spiny, thorny
af-	Toward
an-	Without, not
ante-	Before
anti-	Against; resisting
auto-	Self
bi-	Two; double
blast-	Immature cell, embryonic
circum-	Around
co-, con-	With; together
contra-	Against
crine-	Secrete, separate
de-	Down from, undoing
dia-	Across; through
dipl-	Twofold, double
dys-	Bad; disordered; difficult
ecto-	Displaced, outside
ef-	Away from
em-, en-	In, into
endo-	Within
epi-	Upon, above
eu-	Good
ex-, exo-	Out of, out from
extra-	Outside of
hapl-	Single
hem-, hemat-	Blood
hemi-	Half
hom(e)o-	Same; equal
hyper-	Over; above
hypo-	Under; below
infra-	Below, beneath
inter-	Between
intra-	Within
iso-	Same, equal
juxta-	Near
macro-	Large
mega-	Large; million(th)
mes-	Middle
meta-	Beyond, change, after
micro-	Small; millionth
milli-	Thousandth
mono-	One (single)
necro-	Death
neo-	New
non-	Not
oligo-	Few, scanty
ortho-	Straight; correct, normal
para-	By the side of; near
per-	Through
peri-	Around; surrounding
poly-	Many
post-	After
pre-	Before
pro-	First; promoting
quadri-	Four
re-	Back again
retro-	Behind
semi-	Half
sub-	Under
super-, supra-	Over, above, excessive
trans-	Across; through
tri-	Three; triple

Suffix	Meaning
-al, -ac	Pertaining to
-algia	Pain
-aps, -apt	Fit; fasten
-arche	Beginning; origin
-ase	Signifies an enzyme
-blast	Sprout; make
-centesis	A piercing
-cide	To kill
-clast	Break; destroy
-crine	Release; secrete
-cytosis	Increase in number
-ectomy	A cutting out
-emesis	Vomiting
-emia	Refers to blood condition
-flux	Flow
-gen	Creates; forms
-genesis	Creation, production
-gram	Something written
-graph(y)	To write, draw
-hydrate	Containing H_2O (water)
-ia, -sia	Condition; process
-iasis	Abnormal condition
-ic, -ac	Pertaining to
-in	Signifies a protein
-ism	Signifies "condition of"
-itis	Signifies "inflammation of"
-lemma	Sheath, covering
-lepsy	Seizure
-lith	Stone; rock
-logy	Study of
-lunar	Moon; moonlike
-malacia	Softening
-megaly	Enlargement
-metric, -metry	Measurement, length
-oid	Like; in the shape of
-oma	Tumour
-opia	Vision, vision condition
-oscopy	Viewing
-ose	Pertaining to, sugar
-osis	Condition, process
-ostomy	Formation of an opening
-otomy	Cut
-penia	Lack
-philic	Loving
-phobic	Fearing
-phragm	Partition
-plasia	Growth, formation
-plasm	Substance, matter
-plasty	Shape; make
-plegia	Paralysis
-pnea	Breath, breathing
-(r)rhage, -(r)rhagia	Breaking out, discharge
-(r)rhaphy	Sew, suture
-(r)rhea	Flow
-some	Body
-tensin, -tension	Pressure
-tonic	Pressure, tension
-tripsy	Crushing
-ule	Small, little
-uria	Refers to urine condition